Procedures

Fundamentals of Nursing

CONCEPTS, PROCESS, AND PRACTICE

PATRICIA A. POTTER, RN, BSN, MSN
Director of Nursing Practice
Barnes-Jewish Hospital
St. Louis, Missouri

ANNE GRIFFIN PERRY, RN, BSN, MSN, EdD
Professor
Saint Louis University School of Nursing
Coordinator, Cardiopulmonary Specialty
Saint Louis University Health Sciences Center
St. Louis, Missouri

FOURTH EDITION

with over 977 color illustrations

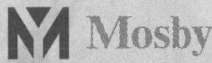

St. Louis Baltimore Boston
Carlsbad Chicago Naples New York Philadelphia Portland
London Madrid Mexico City Singapore Sydney Tokyo Toronto Wiesbaden

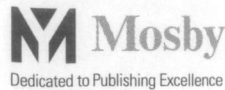
Mosby
Dedicated to Publishing Excellence

A Times Mirror
Company

Vice President and Publisher: Nancy L. Coon
Senior Editor: Susan R. Epstein
Senior Developmental Editor: Beverly J. Copland
Project Manager: John Rogers
Senior Production Editor: Lavon Wirch Peters
Layout Artist: Jeanne Genz
Designer: Amy Buxton
Manufacturing Manager: Theresa Fuchs

FOURTH EDITION

Printed in the United States of America
Composition by Graphic World, Inc.
Lithography/color film by Color Associates
Printing/binding by Von Hoffmann Press

Mosby–Year Book, Inc.
11830 Westline Industrial Drive
St. Louis, Missouri 63146

Library of Congress Cataloging-in-Publication Data

Potter, Patricia Ann.
    Fundamentals of nursing : concepts, process, and practice /
Patricia A. Potter, Anne Griffin Perry. — 4th ed.
        p.   cm.
    Includes bibliographical references and index.
    ISBN 0-8151-6909-4
    1. Nursing.   I.   Perry, Anne Griffin.   II.   Title.
    [DNLM: 1. Nursing Care. 2. Nursing Process. 3. Nurse-Patient
    Relations.   WY 100 P868f 1997]
RT41.P844   1997
610.73—dc20
DNLM/DLC   96-19177
for Library of Congress   CIP

96 97 98 99 00 / 9 8 7 6 5 4 3 2 1

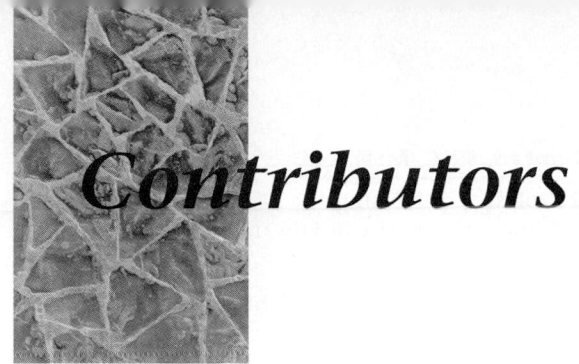

Contributors

Elizabeth A. Ayello, RN, BSN, MS, PhD, CS, CETN

Clinical Assistant, Professor of Nursing
New York University School of Education—Nursing
New York, New York

Penny S. Brooke, RN, BSN, MS, JD

Assistant Dean, Student Affairs—Associate Professor
University of Utah College of Nursing
Salt Lake City, Utah

Judith A. Chaney, RN, BSN, MS, PhD, AAMFT

Private Practice
Highland, Illinois

Sharon H. Cox, RN, MSN, CNAA

Principal Consultant, Founder
Cox and Associates
Brentwood, Tennessee

Rick Daniels, RN, BSN, MSN, PhD

Associate Professor of Nursing
Oregon Health Sciences University at Southern
Ashland, Oregon

Lynne Dearing, RN, BSN, MSN, MA

Instructor in Nursing
Grays Harbor College
Aberdeen, Washington

Jana L. Weindel Dees, RN, BSN, MSN

Staff Nurse/Unit Based Educator
Barnes-Jewish Hospital
St. Louis, Missouri

Carole Edelman, RN, MS, CS

Director of Nursing, Waverly Care Center
New Canaan, Connecticut
Adjunct Faculty, Columbia University
New York, New York

Sally M. Featherstone, RN, BA, BSN, MN, CS, CGC, CDE

Director of Psychiatry
Dartmouth Hitchcock Medical Center
Lebanon, New Hampshire

Susan Jane Fetzer, RN, BA, BSN, MSN, MBA, PhD(c), CCRN

Assistant Professor of Nursing
University of New Hampshire
Durham, New Hampshire

Joyce J. Hamlin, RNC, BSN, MSN, CNS

Learning Resources Nurse Educator
Helene Fuld School of Nursing
Trenton, New Jersey

Susan A. Hauser Jeffers, RN, BA, BSN, MS

Instructor, School of Nursing
Mansfield General Hospital
Mansfield, Ohio

Martina K. Jones, RN, BSN, MSN(R)

Instructor in Nursing
Southern Illinois University at Edwardsville
Edwardsville, Illinois

Judith Ann Kilpatrick, RNC, BSN, MSN

Lecturer in Nursing
Widener University
Chester, Pennsylvania

Carl A. Kirton, RN, BSN, MA, CCRN

Clinical Assistant Professor of Nursing
New York University
New York, New York

Mary Ann Lavin, RN, BSN, MS, MSN, DSc, FAAN, ANP

Assistant Professor of Nursing
Saint Louis University
St. Louis, Missouri

Annette Giesler Lueckenotte, RN, BSN, MS, CS

Gerontologic Nurse Practitioner
Alexian Brothers Senior Health Center
St. Louis, Missouri

Mary Kay Knight Macheca, RN, BSN, MSN(R), CDE

Diabetes Clinical Nurse Specialist
Barnes-Jewish Hospital
St. Louis, Missouri

Jeffrey C. McManemy, RN, BSN, MSN, CS

Coordinator, Nursing Education, Clinical Instructor
Saint Louis University Health Sciences Center
St. Louis, Missouri

Sharon L. Merritt, RN, BSN, MSN, EdD

Associate Professor/Director, Center for
Narcolepsy Research
University of Illinois at Chicago
Chicago, Illinois

Mary Dee Miller, RN, BSN, MS, CIC

Nurse Epidemiologist
Mercy Hospitals, Hamilton/Fairfield
Hamilton, Ohio

Kathleen Mulryan, RN, BSN, MSN

Professor of Nursing
LaGuardia Community College
New York, New York

Marsha Evans Orr, RN, MS, CS

Regional Clinical Manager
Apria Healthcare
Phoenix, Arizona

Veronica (Ronnie) Peterson, RN, BA, BSN, MS

Nursing Supervisor
University of Wisconsin Hospital and Clinics
Madison, Wisconsin

Judith Roos, RN, BSN, MSN

Associate Professor of Nursing
Jewish Hospital College
St. Louis, Missouri

Patsy Ruchala, RN, BSN, MSN, DNSc

Associate Professor of Nursing
Coordinator, Perinatal Nursing Master's Specialty
Saint Louis University School of Nursing
St. Louis, Missouri

Janice Rumfelt, RNC, MSN, EdD

Assistant Professor of Nursing
Southern Illinois University at Edwardsville
Edwardsville, Illinois

Thomas J. Smith, RN, BSN, MN, PhD

Associate Professor of Nursing
Nicholls State University
Thibodaux, Louisiana

Rachel E. Spector, RN, BS, MS, PhD, CTN, FAAN

Associate Professor of Nursing
Boston College School of Nursing
Chestnut Hill, Massachusetts

Ann Bernadette Tritak, RN, BSN, MA, EdD

Associate Professor of Nursing
Fairleigh Dickinson University
Teaneck, New Jersey

JoEtta A. Vernon, RN, MS, PhD

Research Consultant
Omaha, Nebraska

Mary E. Walker, RN, BSN, MA

Psychiatric Clinical Nurse Specialist
Veterans Administration Medical Center
Knoxville, Iowa

Pamela Becker Weilitz, RN, MSN(R), CS

Manager, Nursing Practice
Barnes-Jewish Hospital
St. Louis, Missouri

Valerie J. Yancey, RN, BA, BSN, MSN, CCRN

Staff Nurse, MICU
Barnes-Jewish Hospital
St. Louis, Missouri

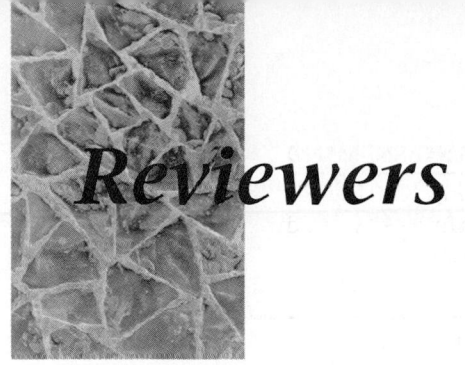

Reviewers

Cheryl Anema, RN, BSN, MSN
Assistant Professor of Nursing
Trinity Christian College
Palos Heights, Illinois

Sue A. Beeson, RN, BSN, MSN, PhD
Assistant Professor of Nursing
University of North Carolina, Greensboro
Greensboro, North Carolina

Margaret Bellak, RN, MN
Associate Professor of Nursing
Indiana University of Pennsylvania
Indiana, Pennsylvania

Julie Beshore Bliss, RN, BS, MA, MEd, DEd
Assistant Professor of Nursing
William Paterson College of New Jersey
Wayne, New Jersey

Joy H. Boarini, RN, BSN, MSN, ET
Education Manager
Hollister Incorporated
Libertyville, Illinois

Karen Bowers, RN, BA, BSN, MEd
Professor of Nursing
Columbus State Community College
Columbus, Ohio

Jean Brannon, RN, BSN, MA
Associate Professor of Nursing
San Antonio College
San Antonio, Texas

Peggy Breckinridge, BSN, MSN, FNP
Associate Professor of Nursing
College of Health Sciences
Roanoke, Virginia

Sister Mary Rosita Brennan, CSSF, RN, BSN, MSN, DNSc
Chair, Department of Associate Nursing
Felician College
Lodi, New Jersey

Margie E. Brown, RNC, BSN, MSN, ANP
Professor of Nursing, ADN Program
Long Beach City College
Long Beach, California

Jerri Bryant, RN, BSN, MPH, CIC
Director, Quality Assessment/Improvement
Emerald Health Network, Inc.
Cleveland, Ohio

M. Petrine Churchill, RN, BN
Staff Nurse, OPD/Emergency Department
Western Regional Health Complex
Yarmouth, Nova Scotia, Canada

Sheila Cunningham, RN, BSN, MSN
Assistant Professor of Nursing
Neumann College
Aston, Pennsylvania

Rick Daniels, RN, BSN, MSN, PhD
Associate Professor of Nursing
Oregon Health Sciences University at Southern
Ashland, Oregon

Sharon Davis, RN, BSN, MN
Freshman Coordinator, Associate Degree Nursing
HINDS Community College
Jackson, Mississippi

Ingeborg Haug Digiacomo, RN, BS, MA, EdD
Associate Professor of Nursing
County College of Morris
Randolph, New Jersey

Heyward Michael Dreher, RN, BSN, MN
Assistant Professor of Nursing
LaSalle University School of Nursing
Philadelphia, Pennsylvania

Helen Edwards, RN, BA, MS
Queensland University of Technology
Brisbane, Queensland, Australia

Dorothy Thomas, RN, MSN
Associate Professor of Nursing
St. Louis Community College at Florissant Valley
St. Louis, Missouri

Carole J. Petrosky Vozel, RNC, BSN, MSN, PhD
Senior Nurse Instructor
Western Pennsylvania Hospital School of Nursing
Pittsburgh, Pennsylvania

Debra Walden, RNP, BA, BSN, MNSc
Assistant Professor of Nursing
Arkansas State University
Jonesboro, Arkansas

Geoff Wilson, RN, B app Sc, DNE, MN
Senior Lecturer, Department of Nursing
Director, Cardiovascular Health Centre
University of Southern Queensland
Toowoomba, Queensland, Australia

Leah Wichmann Wilson, RN, MS, CIC
Infection Control Consultant
Infection Control Consultants
Phoenix, Arizona

Emily Yale, RN, MSN
Instructor
St. Louis Community College, Meramec
St. Louis, Missouri

MaryLou Yam, RN, BSN, MA, PhD, CS
Assistant Professor of Nursing
Saint Peter's College
Jersey City, New Jersey

*This book is dedicated to **Virginia Henderson***
and the professional nurses of today. The nursing profession
lost a passionate leader who envisioned a rewarding and
promising future for nursing. The professional nurses of today
embrace that vision and challenge us all to achieve even more.

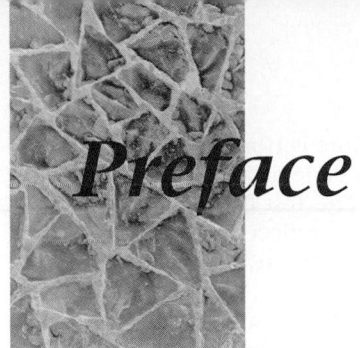

Preface

The future of nursing promises dynamic change and continual challenges. Nurses of tomorrow need a broad knowledge base from which to provide care. The role of the nurse includes assuming the lead in preserving nursing practice and demonstrating its contribution to the health care of our nation. Nurses of tomorrow, therefore, need to become critical thinkers, client advocates, clinical decision makers, and client educators within a broad spectrum of care services.

The fourth edition of *Fundamentals of Nursing: Concepts, Process, and Practice* has been revised to prepare today's students to meet the challenges of tomorrow. This textbook is designed for beginning students in all types of professional nursing programs. The comprehensive coverage provides fundamental nursing concepts, skills, and techniques of nursing practice and a firm foundation for more advanced areas of study.

As nursing education addresses changes in practice, so must nursing textbooks. This fourth edition has been thoroughly updated with a contemporary approach to nursing education that focuses on primary, acute, and restorative care. The increased focus on primary care includes health promotion for clients in the home and community-based settings, addressing the commonalities and uniqueness of various settings. The important themes of managed health care, cultural diversity, client education, nursing research, care of the older adult, and critical thinking are integrated throughout to prepare students for practice. We are indebted to the many educators and students who have shared their thoughts, visions, and ideas with us, and we credit each of them as valuable collaborators for this revision.

▍FEATURES

We have carefully developed this fourth edition with the student in mind. We have designed this text to welcome the new student to nursing, communicate our own love for the profession, and promote learning and understanding. Key features of the text include the following:

- Students will appreciate the **clear, engaging writing style**. Even complex technical and theoretical concepts are presented in language that is readily understandable.
- The book's **visual appeal** has been carefully planned as an integral and functional part of the text. Nearly 1000 large, clear, full-color drawings and photographs illustrate the text, reinforcing and clarifying key concepts and techniques. The clear, readable type and bold headings make the book easy to read and follow. Far more than merely adding bright and attractive colors to the page, each accented special element is consistently color-keyed so that students can immediately identify important information that supports the narrative.
- A new **critical thinking chapter** has been created to emphasize the broad scope of expertise needed to become a professional nurse. A nurse's knowledge base, experience, intuition, and ethical standards all merge to assist the nurse in making clinical judgments.
- The **five-step nursing process** serves as the organizing framework for all discussions of clinical content. The process is introduced and clearly explained in Unit 2. Students learn how the nursing process is an important part of critical thinking. In each clinical chapter, nursing process is discussed in narrative and enhanced by a series of boxes that illustrate the application of the nursing process to client care. These boxes provide pertinent examples of NANDA diagnoses, samples of the diagnostic process, sample care plans, and sample evaluations of interventions against expected outcomes. A distinct logo alerts students to nursing process content. This logo precedes each step in the narrative and is repeated in each box, visually linking the narrative discussion to the boxed displays. As the discussion guides students through the process, the boxes demonstrate how to apply it.
- Essential **nursing procedures** are presented in a clear, step-by-step, 2-column format with research-based rationales. Large, full-color photos and drawings clarify important or difficult steps to ensure understanding and mastery.
- A three-tiered approach on **primary, acute, and restorative care** provides a contemporary, logical framework for discussing today's broad spectrum of health care services and clinical care issues in diverse settings.
- A **health promotion focus** reflects the emphasis of today's practice on maintaining wellness and preventing illness, deemphasizing the importance of the hospital as the center for health care. Activities and interventions that promote health are provided throughout the text to assist the student in identifying appropriate strategies.
- Throughout the text, providing nursing care in both **acute** and **community-based settings** reflects the diverse settings of current health care delivery.
- **Client education** is one of the nurse's most vital responsibilities in today's practice. Special boxes highlight what to teach clients and families to ensure that they become knowledgeable, active participants in their health care.

- **Research Highlight boxes** with implications for nursing practice can be found in clinical chapters to emphasize the relevance of research to everyday client care.
- Both nurses and clients may be greatly influenced by their ethnic or cultural heritage. A separate chapter on cultural diversity emphasizes the importance of ascertaining each client's cultural beliefs and practices as they pertain to health care. New **Cultural Aspects of Care boxes** stress the importance of adapting a client's cultural/ethnic preferences into the health care plan.
- **Learning aids** to help students identify, review, and apply important content in each chapter include Learning Objectives, Key Concepts, Key Terms, Critical Thinking Exercises, References, and Additional Readings. To assist students to learn important terminology, **key terms** are boldfaced and defined in each chapter.

NEW AND EXPANDED CONTENT

As the scope of nursing practice broadens, so must the knowledge base for even beginning students. To truly prepare students for today's practice, this knowledge must reflect the most current guidelines and techniques. We have therefore totally updated all content and added and expanded coverage in key areas. Incorporated throughout are the latest standards and guidelines from the CDC, JCAHO, OSHA, AHCPR, ACS, and NANDA.

- New **Clinical Pathways** and **CareMaps®** from progressive hospitals across the country provide examples of this collaborative approach to planning, implementing, and documenting care.
- Caring for the older adult client presents a unique challenge. New **Gerontological Nursing boxes** alert students to special concerns and provide guidelines to help them meet the needs of these clients.
- **Delegation** of care to unlicensed assistive personnel is a new element of the RN's role in today's practice. Thorough discussion of this issue helps students understand the importance of delegation and when it is appropriate.
- **New chapters** on Critical Thinking and Nursing Judgment, Health Promotion and Primary Health Care, Acute Care, and Restorative and Home Health Care address new nursing roles and changes in practice.
- **Completely revised chapters** on Spiritual Health, Documentation and Reporting, Infection Control, Sleep, and Comfort reflect current clinical practice.
- New **1996 CDC Isolation and Standard Precaution Guidelines** replace universal precautions and body substance isolation.
- New **mental status** and **substance abuse assessment** and health promotion coverage in the physical examination chapter.

TEACHING AND LEARNING PACKAGE

In recognition of the challenges faced by both faculty and students, we have developed an unsurpassed array of teaching/learning materials:

- The **_Instructor's Resource Manual with Test Bank_** has been totally revised and includes the following features for all chapters: objectives, topical outline with page source, key concepts, a wide variety of classroom/clinical experiences, and answers to the critical thinking exercises from the text. Procedure Performance Checklists are also included and are available as a separate booklet for student purchase as well. The Test Bank includes all new, higher-level questions that reflect the NCLEX format. The Test Bank is also available in computerized format for IBM or Macintosh.
- More than 100 full-color **Transparency Acetates** have been selected for effective use in class discussions and for instructional value.
- **Mosby's Nursing Skills Video Series** is an ideal complement to the text, providing visual reinforcement to enhance learning. The _Instructor's Resource Manual_ provides a section that details how to maximize the benefit of the videos, including questions for each video to assist in evaluating student learning.
- The popular **_Study Guide_** to accompany this text has been completely revised to provide a comprehensive, self-paced resource for students. Each chapter includes numerous short-answer questions designed to test knowledge of the chapter's content. This approach teaches students how to "pull out" key information from the chapters and reinforces learning by requiring them to actively write in answers in the outline. This written outline can later serve as a review tool for tests. The final section of each chapter includes review questions in NCLEX format that also requires the student to provide the rationale for the selected answer. Answers are keyed back to the page in the text where relevant content is presented.
- A new series of **interactive videodiscs** on **Applying Critical Thinking to Nursing Skills** has been developed to help students learn to incorporate critical thinking in the performance of basic skills, even in the earliest stages of their nursing education.

* * * * * * * * * *

We are pleased to note the growing number of men currently involved in the practice of nursing, and we acknowledge their dedication, skill, and professionalism. We have therefore made every effort to eliminate any gender-specific pronouns. In a very few instances, we have used "she" to refer to the nurse and "he" to refer to the client in order to clearly communicate to the reader.

ACKNOWLEDGMENTS

The development of this textbook resulted from the combined efforts of many talented professionals committed to excellence. We appreciate their dedication and enthusiasm. Throughout the text we have attempted to acknowledge the contributions of our professional nurse colleagues who make a difference in the lives of their clients and the communities they serve. We are very proud to be associated with such fine individuals.

We wish to give special recognition to the editorial and production teams who have helped to make this textbook a reality. We especially wish to thank:

- Suzi Epstein, Senior Editor, and Beverly Copland, Senior Developmental Editor, for their guidance and support. This text is truly a team effort. Their leadership has ensured a quality textbook with innovative design and informative content. Both Suzi and Bev have committed long hours to keep us on schedule and on target with regard to the objectives for this project. Bev continues to be a first-class tracker of contributors, manuscript, and authors!

- Lavon Peters, for her detailed and methodical approach to the very important production process. She is a critical part of the *Fundamentals* team.
- Amy Buxton, Book Designer, whose innovative design gives the book its exciting and attractive visual appeal.
- Michael Clement, MD, Mesa, Arizona, for his photographic contributions that bring visual life to each page.
- Jack Reuter, for his computer expertise, which provides clear, detailed illustrations to enhance and complement the text.
- Angelica Uniforms of St. Louis, for contributing uniforms worn in many of the photographs.
- Our contributors and reviewers, whose painstaking critique of content and design ensures a high-quality textbook. Their work often goes unnoticed; however, they have helped to set the standard for a comprehensive and accurate text.

- To the professional managers and nursing staff at Barnes-Jewish Hospital, the faculty and students of Jewish College of Nursing and Allied Health, the nursing faculty of Saint Louis University School of Nursing, and the nursing staff of Saint Louis University Hospital. We hope to capture and reveal the accomplishments they achieve daily through the case studies, clinical examples, and photographic images within the text. Their example of clinical excellence motivates us to develop an instructive textbook.

The creation of a nursing textbook is no small feat. We continue to be very grateful to the faculty and students who use our text. The partnership that we have forged during the last two decades has been a very rewarding one. We hope to continue to meet the standard of excellence you, our readers, expect.

Patricia A. Potter

Anne Griffin Perry

Contents

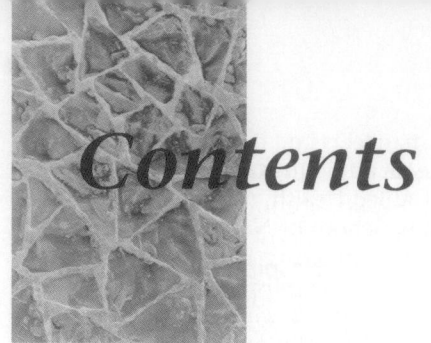

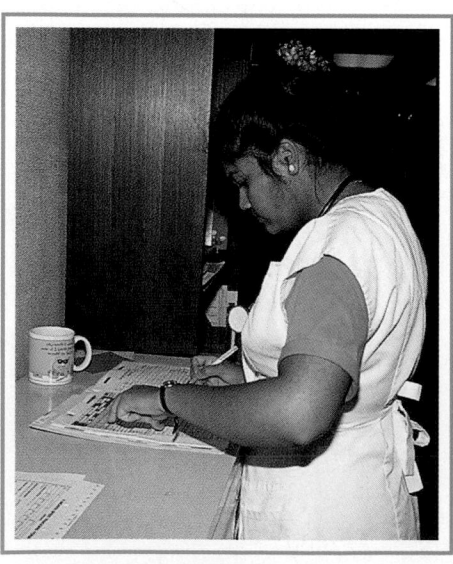

3 Health Promotion and Primary Health Care, 47

Mary Ann Lavin

4 Acute Care, 61

Anne Griffin Perry

5 Restorative and Home Health Care, 79

Thomas J. Smith

UNIT 2

The Nursing Process and Critical Thinking, 96

6 Critical Thinking and Nursing Judgment, 97

Patricia A. Potter

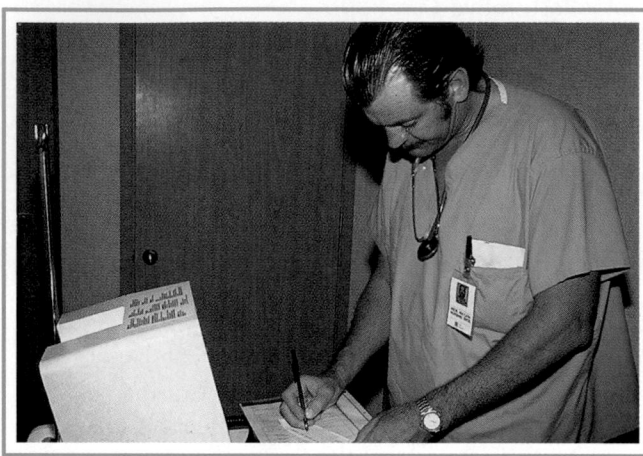

7 Assessment, 107
Patricia A. Potter

8 Nursing Diagnosis, 124
Anne Griffin Perry

9 Planning, 136
Anne Griffin Perry

10   Implementation, 155
Anne Griffin Perry

11   Evaluation, 165
Patricia A. Potter

12   Documentation and Reporting, 179
Rick Daniels

UNIT 3

*Professional Nursing Concepts
and Practices, 206*

13   Profession of Nursing, 207
Anne Griffin Perry

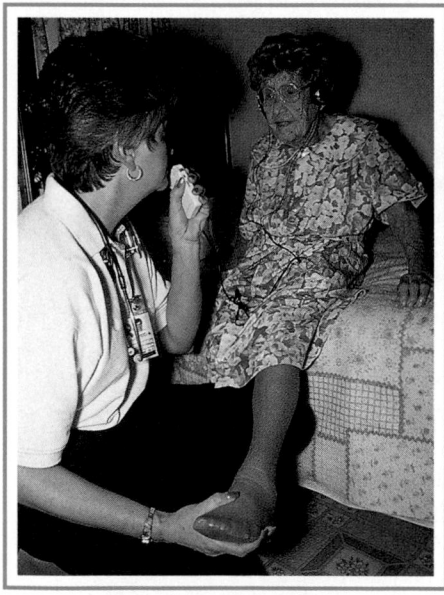

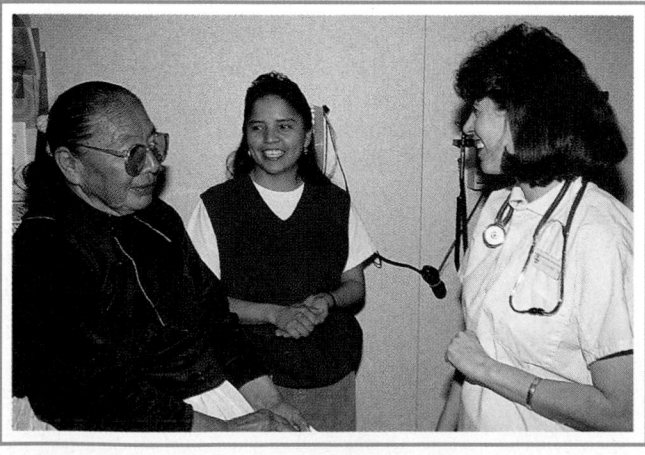

UNIT 5

Promoting Wellness Throughout the Lifespan, 477

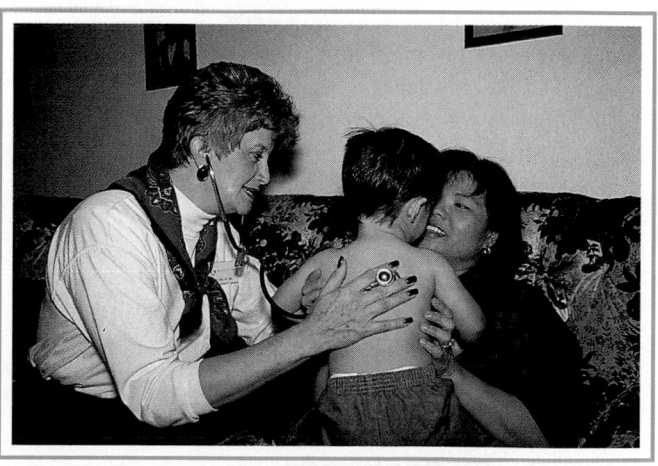

UNIT 6

Professional Nursing Skills, 593

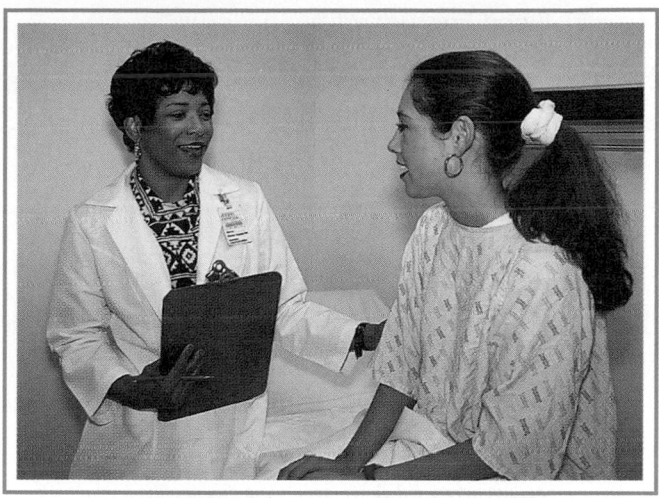

34 Infection Control, 741

Mary Dee Miller

35 Administration of Medications, 789

Carl A. Kirton

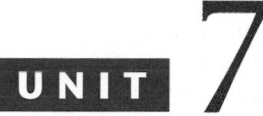

UNIT 7

Providing a Safe Environment, 869

36   Safety, *870*
Kathleen Mulryan

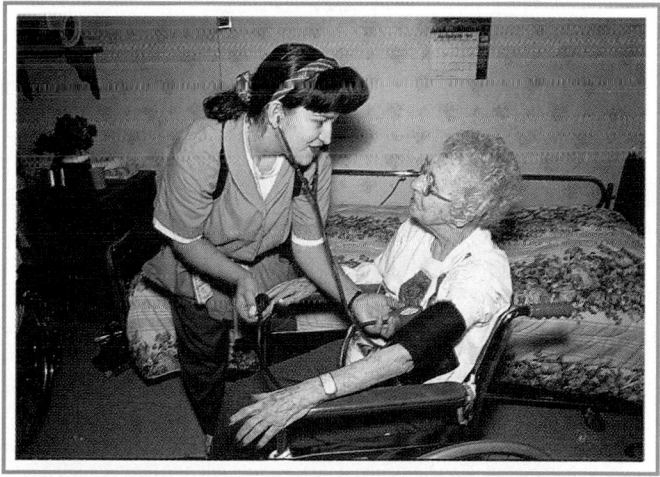

37   Mobility and Immobility, *893*
Jana L. Weindel Dees

UNIT 8

Basic Physiological Needs, 1015

42 Sleep, *1128*
Sharon L. Merritt

43 Comfort, *1153*
Patricia A. Potter

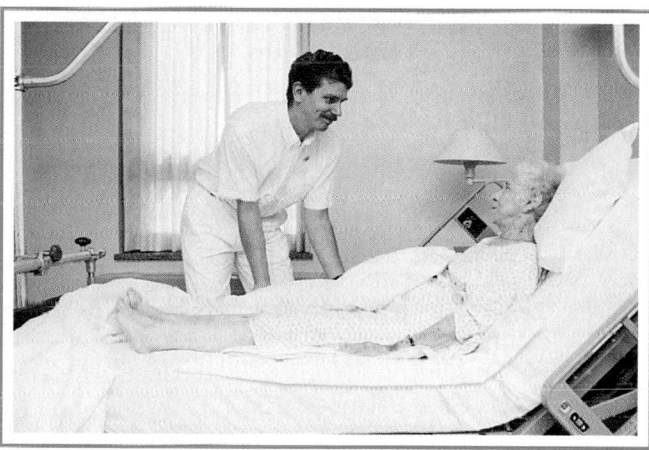

44 Oxygenation, *1191*
Pamela Becker Weilitz

UNIT 9

Caring for the Perioperative Client, 1379

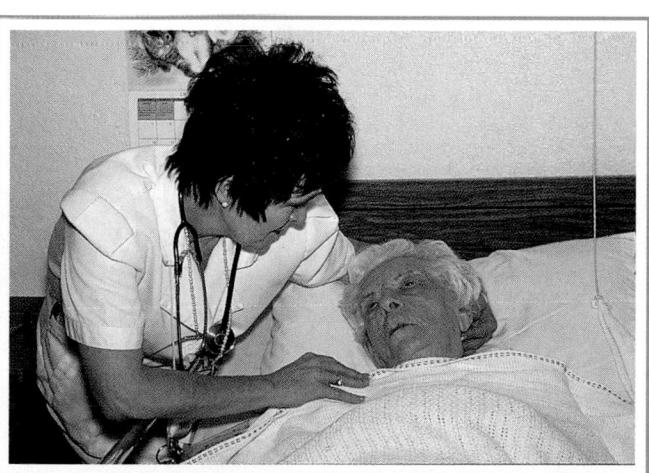

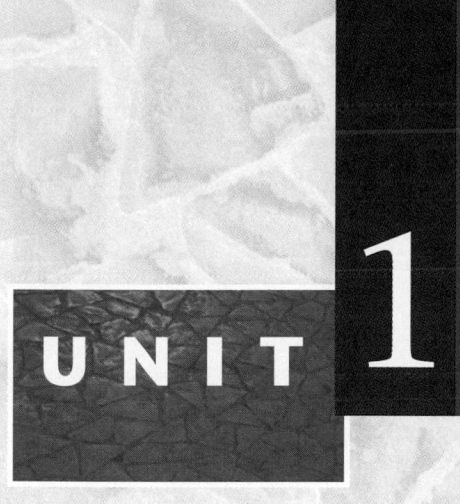

Coordinating
Health Care Delivery

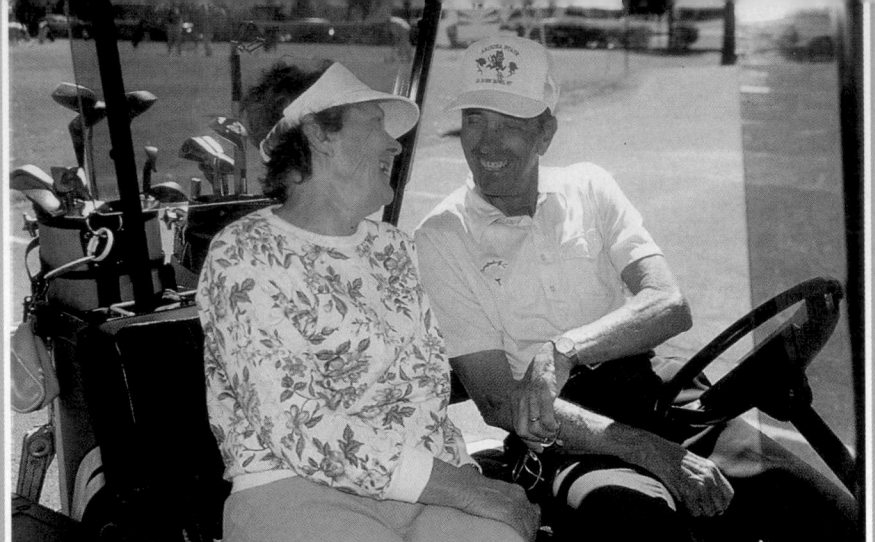

## Chapter 1

Health-Illness Continuum

Objectives

Mastery of content in this chapter will enable the student to:

▶ Define the key terms listed.

▶ List Healthy People 2000 goals.

▶ Discuss the definition of health and related concepts.

▶ Discuss the health-illness continuum, high-level wellness, agent-host-environment, health-belief, and health-promotion models.

▶ Describe health-promotion and illness-prevention activities.

▶ List and discuss the three levels of preventive care and four types of risk factors.

▶ Describe variables influencing health beliefs and practices.

▶ Describe variables influencing illness behavior.

▶ List and discuss the stages of illness behavior.

▶ Describe the impact of illness on the client and family.

▶ Discuss the nurse's role in health and illness.

▶ Utilize the Wellness Checkup Tool.

In the past, most individuals and societies viewed good health or wellness as the opposite or absence of disease. This simple "either/or" attitude can be easily applied; a person is considered healthy or ill, with no range in between. Viewing health as an either/or situation ignores the health-illness continuum. In the approaching twenty-first century, health will be viewed from a broader perspective. The broader aspect of health may include such elements as a feeling of empowerment, loving relationship, zest for living, a strong social support network, a sense of meaning in life, or a certain level of independence (Haber, 1994). Psychosocial and functional dimensions (Duffy and MacDonald, 1990) become increasingly integral components of good health in this new view. Nurses and other health care professionals will encourage a clearer definition of health promotion and disease prevention. When they become primary care specialists, nurses are more involved in identifying health patterns. Research will enable them to identify methods to decrease health risks. When risk reduction and health promotion can be demonstrated and related to cost and quality of life, the government may be persuaded to finance preventive care (Gordon, 1994).

Health care (defined by the narrower domain of medical care) in the United States has maintained its status as a very high priority. The United States spends a far higher percentage of its gross national product (GNP) on health care than does any other country (Haber, 1994). Ironically health itself has not been a high priority. At present only 3% of the nation's health care costs are spent on health promotion and disease prevention, and of this 3% less than 1% is spent on changing unhealthy behavior (Haber, 1994). Although there has been little attention at the federal level to unhealthy lifestyles or risk factors among Americans, the recent document *Healthy People 2000* promotes a new federal focus on health promotion and disease prevention.

This document serves as the framework for the 1990s as the United States begins to focus more on health promotion and disease prevention instead of illness care.

HEALTHY PEOPLE 2000

In 1980 an influential document, *Healthy People: The Surgeon General's Report on Health Promotion and Disease Prevention* was published. This report has been widely cited by the popular media as well as in professional journals and at health conferences. This document was pivotal in fostering health-promoting initiatives throughout the nation (McTernan and Rice, 1986; Willis, 1986).

A decade later in 1990 a national follow-up effort, *Healthy People 2000,* was initiated by the U.S. Public Health Service (PHS) in an effort to reduce preventable death and disability for Americans by the year 2000 (PHS, 1992). The strategy announced by the Secretary of Health and Human Services requires a cooperative effort by government, voluntary and professional organizations, businesses, and individuals.

During the 1990s the *Healthy People 2000* initiative focuses on three broad public health goals for Americans: (1) to increase the span of healthy life, (2) to reduce health disparities, and (3) to achieve access to preventive services (see the box below). Three hundred specific objectives designed to help achieve these goals were set in 22 priority areas (see the box on p. 4).

Setting health care priorities is no longer a simple matter of tabulating the number of deaths from a few diseases and then organizing a campaign against the most prevalent ones, like heart disease and cancer. The *Healthy People 2000* initiative is health oriented, not disease oriented, and as such recognizes the complexity of socioeconomic, lifestyle, and other nonmedical influences that affect attainment and maintenance of health.

Nation's Year 2000 Goals

1. *Increase the span of healthy life for Americans.* Data indicate that Americans had a life expectancy of 73.7 years in 1980 (it was actually 75 in 1987). However, on average, only 62 of those years were spent in a healthy state; 11.7 years included dysfunctions such as acute and chronic illnesses, impairments, and handicaps. One goal of the Year 2000 National Health Objectives is to decrease the number of dysfunctional years.
2. *Reduce health disparities among Americans.* Even as average life expectancy increased, lifespan for African Americans has actually declined since 1986. The average life expectancy for whites in 1988 was 75.6. For blacks it was 69.4. Futhermore, whites experience fewer years of dysfunction than do blacks or Native Americans, although more years of dysfunction than experienced by Hispanics. One goal of the Year 2000 National Health Objectives is to reduce this disparity.
3. *Achieve access to preventive health services for all Americans.* One of the reasons for the disparity in life expectancy is the inequitable use of preventive health services. For example, whereas 79% of white pregnant women received first-trimester prenatal care, only 61% of black pregnant women did. The result is that the infant mortality rate for black infants is 17.9 deaths per 1000 live births, but the rate for whites is only 8.6. Another result of the inequitable use of preventive health services can be found in the death rate statistics for people age 74 and younger. In 1987, the death rate for whites was 367 per 100,000 population, whereas for blacks it was 628 per 100,000 population. One goal of the Year 2000 National Health Objectives is to assure access to preventive services for all Americans so as to improve health and ensure years of healthy life.

Modified from Public Health Service, US Department of Health and Human Services, vol 40, no 8, suppl 2, Washington, DC, 1992, US Goverment Printing Office.

Healthy People 2000: Priority Areas and Lead PHS Agencies

1. Physical Activity and Fitness	President's Council on Physical Fitness and Sports
2. Nutrition	National Institutes of Health
	Food and Drug Administration
3. Tobacco	Centers for Disease Control and Prevention
4. Alcohol and Other Drugs	Alcohol, Drug Abuse, and Mental Health Administration
5. Family Planning	Office of Population Affairs
6. Mental Health and Mental Disorders	Alcohol, Drug Abuse, and Mental Health Administration
7. Violent and Abusive Behavior	Centers for Disease Control and Prevention
8. Educational and Community-Based Programs	Centers for Disease Control and Prevention
	Health Resources and Services Administration
9. Unintentional Injuries	Centers for Disease Control and Prevention
10. Occupational Safety and Health	Centers for Disease Control and Prevention
11. Environmental Health	National Institutes of Health
	Centers for Disease Control and Prevention
12. Food and Drug Safety	Food and Drug Administration
13. Oral Health	National Institutes of Health
	Centers for Disease Control and Prevention
14. Maternal and Infant Health	Health Resources and Services Administration
15. Heart Disease and Stroke	National Institutes of Health
16. Cancer	National Institutes of Health
17. Diabetes and Chronic Disabling Conditions	National Institutes of Health
	Centers for Disease Control and Prevention
18. HIV Infection	National AIDS Program Office
19. Sexually Transmitted Diseases	Centers for Disease Control and Prevention
20. Immunization and Infectious Disease	Centers for Disease Control and Prevention
21. Clinical Preventive Services	Health Resources and Services Administration
	Centers for Disease Control and Prevention
22. Surveillance and Data Systems	Centers for Disease Control and Prevention

From US Department of Health and Human Services, PHS: *Healthy people 2000: national health promotion and disease prevention objectives*, Washington, DC, 1990, US Government Printing Office.

■ DEFINITION OF HEALTH

Good **health** or wellness is not merely the absence of illness. Defining good health is difficult because each person has a personal concept of health. Health is not acquired scientific knowledge; nor is it a thing, a part of the body, or a function of the body such as hearing, seeing, or breathing. Health is a state of being that people define in relation to their own values.

The shift in focus from illness to health is significant. The World Health Organization (WHO) formulated a campaign for health for all by the year 2000. The campaign implies a collective responsibility by WHO to provide access to health care to everyone worldwide, starting with each country's own national area of need. During a survey of the WHO health conference in 1991, experts attending the conference stated that health promotion in America was misdirected. In addition, the gap widened between health promotion as practiced in the United States and the world view of health promotion pursued in other countries (WHO, 1992). The differences are particularly strong in three areas: equity, power, and scope (see the box on p. 5).

The WHO definition of health has the following characteristics that promote a positive concept of health (Edelman and Mandle, 1994):
1. A concern for the individual as a total system

2. A view of health that identifies internal and external environments
3. An acknowledgment of the importance of an individual's role in life

Nurses can differ on their definitions of health. They plan care based on a definition of health and accepted standards of health care. Neuman's system model (1989, 1990) focuses on health as the totality of life processes and includes disease as a process.

Health in its broadest sense is a dynamic state in which the individual adapts to changes in internal and external environments to maintain a state of well-being. The internal environment includes many factors that influence health, including genetic and psychological variables, intellectual and spiritual dimensions, and disease processes. The external environment includes factors outside the person that may influence health, including the physical environment, social relationships, and economic variables. Because both environments continuously change, the person must adapt to maintain a state of well-being.

Health and *illness* therefore must be defined in terms of the individual. Health can include conditions that the client or nurse may have previously considered to be illness. For example, a person with epilepsy who has learned to control seizures with medication and who functions at home and at work may now not consider himself ill. Health

---

Health Promotion: United States Versus World Health Organization

Equity. In the world view of health promotion, the goal of equal access to health carries more importance than optimizing each person's individual health. The WHO emphasizes providing basic health services to all people before moving on to the more sophisticated needs of subgroups.

Power. In other countries, power and control are central issues in health promotion. "Health Promotion in Developing Countries: A Call to Action," a 1990 WHO strategy document, declares: "Focus of health promotion is social action for health." The goal is to give people a voice in changing unhealthy environments. Showing people how to adapt to or make the most of their situations through behavioral changes has less value. "Knowledge alone, without adequate supportive systems and facilities, is not enough to lead people to action." In the United States, most health promotion efforts steer clear of political involvement for social action.

Scope. In the world community, the scope of health promotion includes broad social aspects of quality of life. Good housing, safe transportation, basic education, good food supplies, and strong social relationships are within the domain of health promotion. American health promotion rarely addresses these broader determinants of health.

Modified from World Health Organization: Health promotion in developing countries: a call for action, *Am J Health Promotion* 6(3):174, 1992.

---

is also closely related to an individual's work place and home life, and stressors can be the result of those environments.

CASE STUDY Although Mary held an important management position, she recently experienced numerous stressors that taxed her ability to adapt. Her personal stressors, which included her husband's job loss, her son's recent hospitalization, and her car being stolen; in conjunction with her job responsibilities to listen to her staff's problems caused her to feel overwhelmed. As these feelings escalated, Mary thought more about running away from it all. She decided to seek out the nurse in the medical department of her company.

Distress can be shared with a professional when health is negatively affected and the distressed person wants to change the causes of distress. In this case study Mary was able to express her feelings to the company nurse. Once the nurse accepted Mary's reaction to the stressors in her life and they formed a trusting relationship, the nurse could begin assisting Mary to learn how to better manage the stressors of home and work. ■

■ MODELS OF HEALTH AND ILLNESS

A model is a theoretical way of understanding a concept or idea. Because health and illness are complex concepts, models are used to understand the relationships between these concepts and the client's attitudes toward health and health practices.

Health beliefs are a person's ideas, convictions, and attitudes about health and illness. Health beliefs may be based on factual information or misinformation, common sense or myths, or reality or false expectations. Because health beliefs usually cause **health behavior**, they can positively or negatively affect a client's level of health. Positive health behaviors are activities related to maintaining, attaining, or regaining good health and preventing illness. Common positive health behaviors include immunizations, proper sleep patterns, adequate exercise, and nutrition. Negative health behaviors include practices actually or potentially harmful to health, such as smoking, drug or alcohol abuse, poor diet, and refusal to take necessary medication.

Nursing models help define health and assist in understanding clients' health behavior and beliefs so that effective health care can be provided. These models allow nurses to understand and predict clients' health behavior, including how they use health services and adhere to recommended therapy.

A client's health beliefs depend on many factors, including perception of the level of health, modifying factors such as demographics (such as the type and site of housing), personality, and perception of benefits resulting from positive health behavior. Health models usually incorporate these components.

The health-illness continuum, high-level wellness, and agent-host-environment models describe the relationships between health and illness. The health-belief model explains and predicts a client's health behavior; the evolutionary-based and health-promotion models were developed by nurses and focus on health promotion. These models represent different ways of approaching complex issues and understanding a client's attitudes and values about health and illness.

Health-Illness Continuum

According to Neuman (1990), "health on a continuum is the degree of client wellness that exists at any point in time, ranging from an optimal wellness condition, with available energy at its maximum, to death, which represents total energy depletion." According to this **health-illness continuum model**, health is a dynamic state that continuously alters as a person adapts to changes in the internal and external environments to maintain a state of physical, emotional, intellectual, social, developmental, and spiritual well-being. Illness is a process in which the functioning of a person is diminished or impaired in one or more dimensions when compared with the person's previous condition. Because health and illness are relative qualities, existing in varying degrees, it is more accurate to consider health and illness in terms of a point on a scale or continuum rather than an either/or, absolute state (Fig. 1-1).

Literature supports the view that health and the attain-

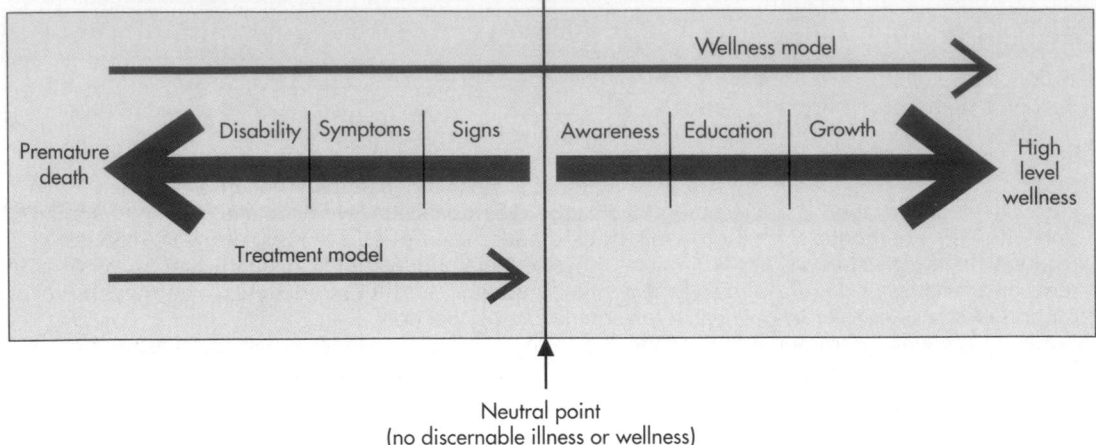

Fig. 1-1 Wellness-illness continuum. *(Redrawn from Ryan RS, Travis JW:* Wellness workbook, *Berkeley, Calif, 1981, Ten Speed Press; used with permission of John W Travis, MD, Yukiah, Calif. © 1975, 1988.)*

ment of it is a central concept and a goal of nursing practice (Pender, 1975, 1987, 1990; Parse, 1981, 1990; Pender and Pender, 1986; Neuman, 1989, 1990; Meleis, 1990). A nurse can determine a client's level of health at any point on the health-illness continuum. High-level wellness and severe illness are the opposite ends of the continuum, with a full range of states in between. A client's risk factors (variables that make illness more likely in any dimension) are important in identifying level of health. Risk factors include genetic and physiological variables such as age, family history, lifestyle, and environment. As a person progresses through human developmental stages, certain risk factors are more common than others. For example, an adolescent is more likely than an adult to experience stressors related to body image and self-concept, and an older adult is more likely than a child to develop cardiac disease.

Clients' views of their level of health depend on attitudes toward health and values, beliefs, and perceptions of their physical, emotional, intellectual, social, developmental, and spiritual well-being. The nurse and client mutually set goals to reach the client's optimal level of health (Meleis, 1990).

The drawback of the health-illness continuum is that it is not always easy to describe a client's level of health in terms of one point between two extremes. For example, is a man who has a broken leg, but who has adapted to limited mobility more or less healthy than a physically healthy man experiencing severe depression after the death of his spouse? This model is effective when it is used to compare a client's present level of health with previous levels of health. Subsequently it is useful as the nurse helps the client set goals to attain a future level of health.

High-Level Wellness Model

First developed in the late 1950s and revised by Dunn (1977), the high-level wellness model is oriented toward maximizing the health potential of an individual. This model requires the individual to maintain a continuum of balance and purposeful direction within the environment. It involves progress toward a higher level of functioning, an open-ended and ever-expanding challenge to live at the

fullest potential. Last, there is continued integration of health practices by the individual at increasingly higher levels throughout life (Dunn, 1959, 1977; Pender, 1993).

Nursing models of wellness are directed at behavioral change and have been successful in nurse-managed centers for older adults (Gilpatrick, 1989; Smith and Sorrell, 1989). In this approach to wellness, nurses implement nursing interventions that help clients modify selected high-risk behaviors. These interventions are in broad categories and are based on principles of adult learning (Gilpatrick, 1989). High-level wellness is a dynamic process, not a passive, static state. The high-level wellness model can also be applied to family and community health. Families and communities have many functions, and high-level wellness involves successful functioning in an integrated manner.

NURSE-CLIENT PARTNERSHIP

The nurse who practices within a holistic health model attempts to create conditions that promote optimal health. The client's current belief system is the beginning framework from which the nurse helps the client find healthy ways to meet individual needs (Rawlins, Williams, and Beck, 1993). In this model, nurses utilizing the nursing process consider clients the ultimate experts regarding their own health and respect clients' subjective experience as relevant in maintaining health or assisting in healing. Clients in the holistic model are coparticipants in health promotion, working closely with the nurse to determine necessary and appropriate interventions (Rawlins, Williams, and Beck, 1993).

Holistic nurses' most powerful healing and teaching capacities come from who they are and how they relate to others. Holistic nurses who pursue their own personal growth and strive toward optimal health for themselves are better able to facilitate healing and optimal health in others.

Agent-Host-Environment Model

The agent-host-environment model of health and illness originated in the community health work of Leavell et al. (1965) and has since been expanded as a model for describing the cause of illness in other health areas. According to this approach the level of health or illness of an individual or group depends on the dynamic relationship of the agent, host, and environment.

The **agent** is any internal or external factor that by its presence or absence can lead to disease or illness. Agents can be biological, chemical, physical, mechanical, or psychosocial. The presence of these agents does not mean a person will become ill, but an agent must be present (or absent, as in a lack of adequate nutrition) for a particular illness to occur.

The **host** is the person or persons who may be susceptible to a particular illness or disease. Host factors are physical or psychosocial situations or conditions that put an individual or group at risk for becoming ill. Examples of such factors are the host's family history, age, or lifestyle.

The **environment** consists of all factors outside of the host. Physical environment includes economic level, climate, living conditions, and elements such as light and sound levels. Social environment consists of factors involving a person's or group's interaction with others, including stress, conflicts with others, economic hardships, and life crises such as the death of a spouse.

The agent-host-environment model emphasizes that health and illness depend on the dynamic interaction of all three variables. Community health nursing has further developed the interaction between agent-host-environment into a causal model for addressing the health needs for homeless families (Fig. 1-2). This model, first developed by Pesznecker (1984) and recently reported by Berne et al. (1990), proposes that health-promoting or health-damaging responses are shaped by interaction between the individual or group and the environment and that the responses are further mediated by public policy. For example, homeless persons may be faced with a variety of stressors or agents that affect their levels of health. These stressors (e.g., inadequate shelter, exposure to crime, and exposure to nature's elements) increase the homeless client's risk for illness (Fig. 1-3).

The agent-host-environment model was expanded into a general theory of the multiple causes of disease. Until recent decades, it was commonly believed that single causes of a disease could be identified. Infectious diseases in particular were thought to have single causes; the agents (e.g., the bacteria or viruses) were considered solely responsible. It is now recognized that most diseases have multiple

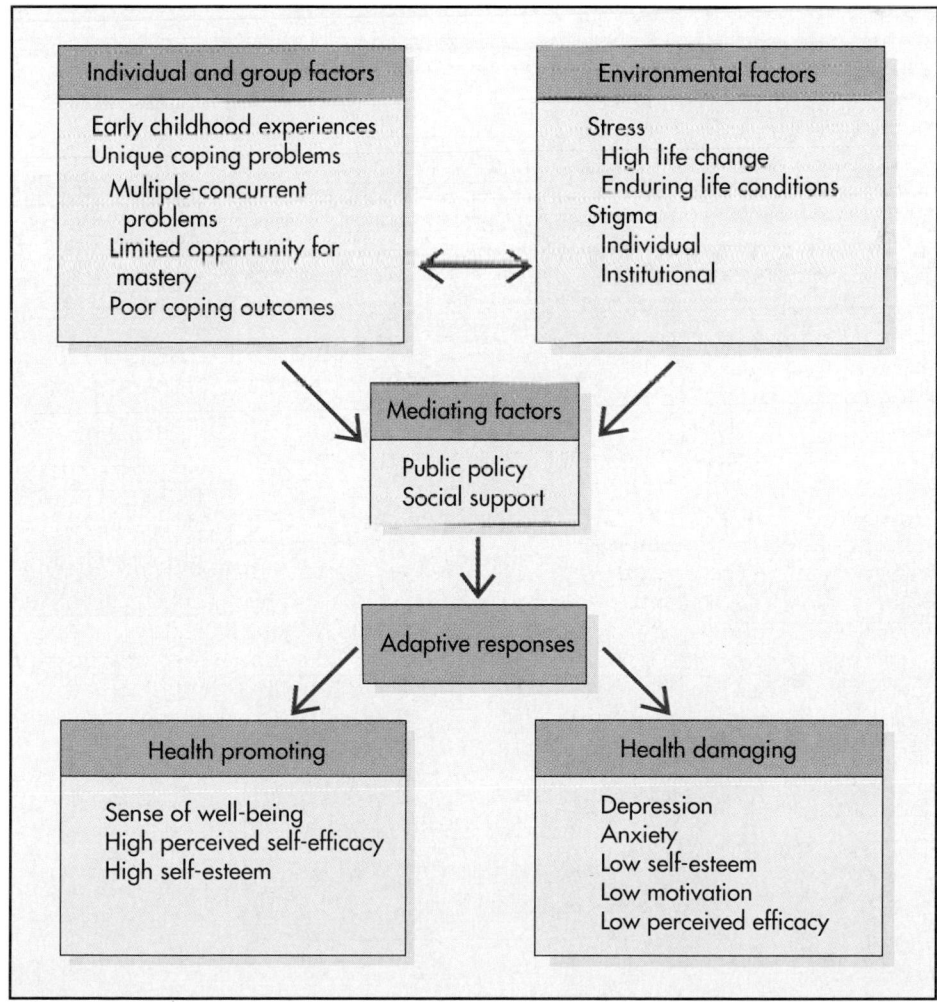

Fig. 1-2 Adaptational model of poverty. *(Redrawn from Pesznecker E: The poor: a population at risk,* Public Health Nurs *1(4):237, 1984.)*

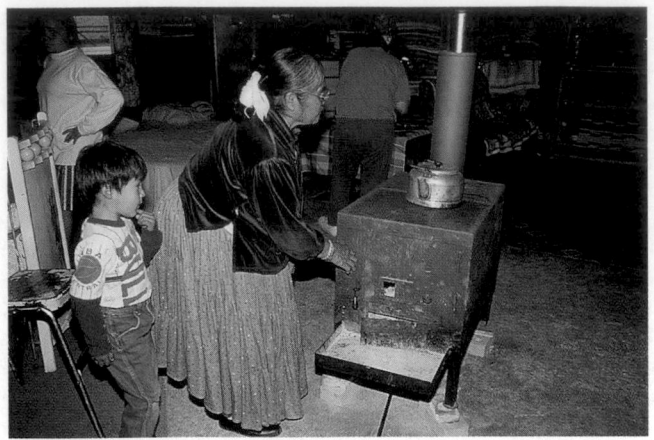

Fig. 1-3 Homeless shelter offers food, sleeping accommodations, and support for child care.

causes, as the agent-host-environment model demonstrates. The theory of the multiple causes of disease is important from nursing's holistic perspective. Care of the client is based on knowledge of environmental, psychosocial, and lifestyle factors.

Health-Belief Model

Rosenstoch's (1974) and Becker and Maiman's (1975) **health-belief model** (Fig. 1-4) addresses the relationship between a person's belief and behavior. It provides a way of understanding and predicting how clients will behave in relation to their health and how they will comply with health care therapies.

> **CASE STUDY**   Tom has several health problems. His poor diet, increased weight, lack of exercise, and smoking clogged his coronary vessels. His stressful lifestyle and job responsibilities aggravated this condition. The sources of Tom's illness are found not only in the many interrelationships that make up his life, but his family's predisposition. His problems have their roots in the health habits of his family and in his family history of coronary disease. ■

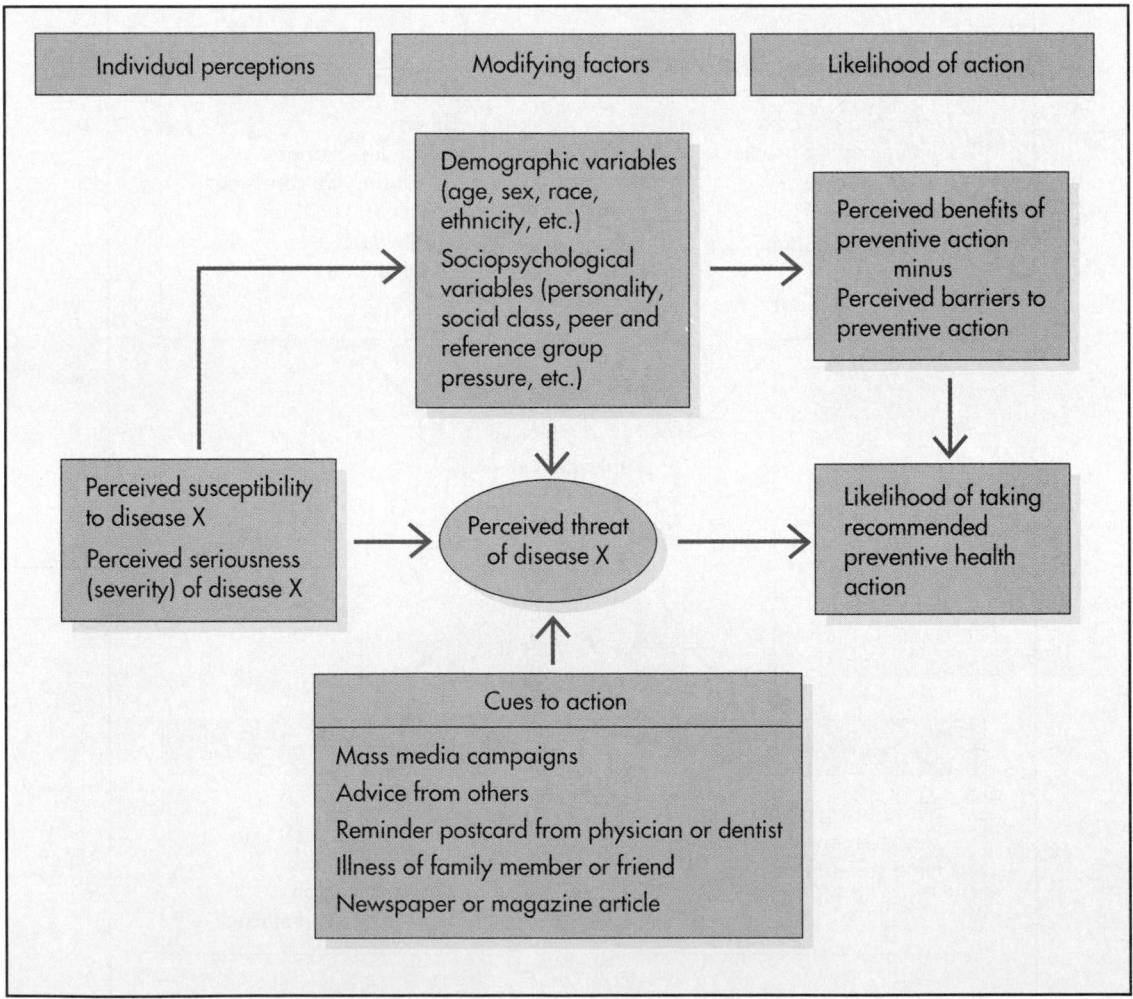

Fig. 1-4 Health-belief model. *(Redrawn from Becker MH, Maiman LA: Sociobehavioral determinants of compliance with health and medical care recommendations,* Med Care *33(1):1021, 1975.)*

The first component in this model involves the individual's perception of susceptibility to an illness. For example, a client needs to recognize the familial link for coronary artery disease.

After this link is recognized, particularly when one parent and two siblings have died in their fourth decade from myocardial infarction, the client may perceive the personal risk of heart disease. The second component is the individual's perception of the seriousness of the illness. This perception is influenced and modified by demographic and sociopsychological variables, perceived threats of the illness, and cues to action (e.g., mass media campaigns and advice from family, friends, and medical professionals).

The third component—the likelihood that a person will take preventive action—is the person's perception of the benefits of taking action. Preventive action may include lifestyle changes, increased adherence to medical therapies, or a search for medical advice or treatment.

The health-belief model helps nurses understand factors influencing clients' perceptions, beliefs, and behavior, and plan care that will most effectively assist clients in maintaining or regaining health and preventing illness.

Health-Promotion Model

The health-promotion model proposed by Pender (1982, 1993a, 1996) was designed to be a "complementary counterpart to models of health protection." Health promotion is directed at increasing a client's level of well-being (Pender, 1993a, 1996). The model focuses on three functions (Fig. 1-5). It identifies factors (e.g., demographic and social) that enhance or decrease participation in health promotion. The model also organizes cues into a pattern to explain the likelihood of a client's participation in health-promotion behavior (Pender, 1993, 1996). The focus of this model is to explain the reasons that individuals engage in health activities. It is not designed for use with families or communities.

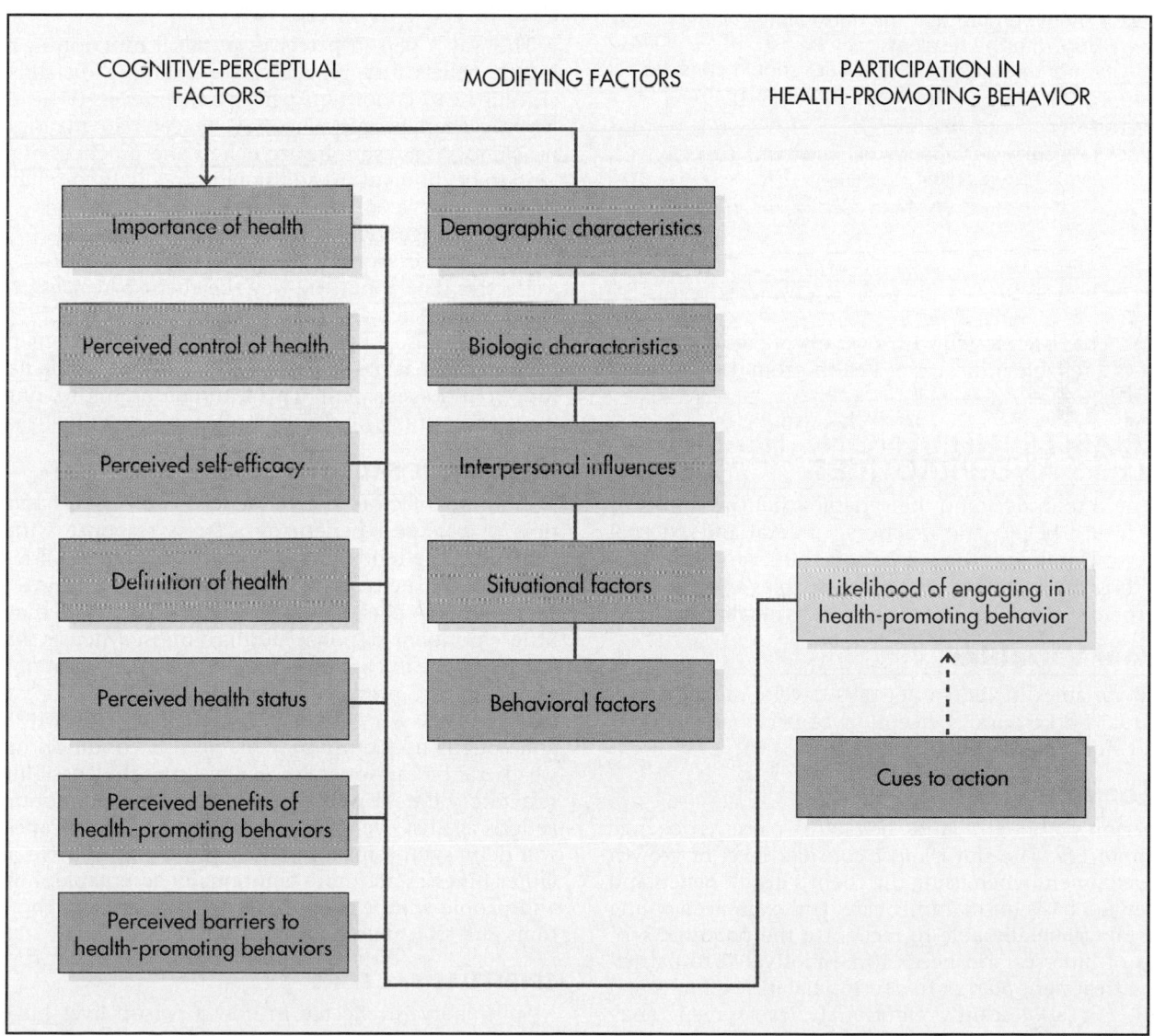

Fig. 1-5 Health-promotion model. *(Redrawn from Pender NJ:* Health promotion in nursing practice, *ed 3, Norwalk, Conn, 1996, Appleton & Lange.)*

RESEARCH HIGHLIGHT

RESEARCH ABSTRACT

Older adults who live in nursing facilities often become fixtures in their chairs. They have little to no active exercise except to go between their rooms and the common room for meals. A study conducted by Gueldner and Spradley (1988) looked at 64 residents in nursing homes. They divided the group into two groups using a quasi-experimental design. One group routinely went for a walk outside each day as weather permitted and the others had no walk. The study concluded that regular outdoor walking should be instituted for all residents of nursing facilities because there was a positive correlation to self-esteem and increased activity in the residents who had the walks.

IMPLICATION FOR PRACTICE
▶ Older adults enjoy exercise.
▶ Routine exercise enables positive feelings of self.
▶ Outside walks need to be offered more frequently to residents of nursing homes.
▶ Nurses should ensure that the nurse aide includes more walking with the residents they help.
▶ Activity programs in nursing facilities should consider walking an important component of their program.

REFERENCE
Gueldner S, Spradley J: Outdoor walking lowers fatigue, *J Gerontol Nurs* 14(10):6, 1988.

This model has been tested with a variety of populations because it is a reliable indicator of health promotion (see the box above).

■ VARIABLES INFLUENCING HEALTH BELIEFS AND PRACTICES

Nurses need to understand the variables that can influence clients' health beliefs and practices. Internal and external variables can influence how a person thinks and acts. Understanding the way in which these variables affect a client allows the nurse to plan and deliver individualized care.

Internal Variables

Internal variables include a person's developmental stage, intellectual background, perception of personal functioning, and emotional and spiritual factors.

DEVELOPMENTAL STAGE

A person's thought and behavior patterns change throughout life. The nurse must consider level of growth and development when using the client's health beliefs and practices as a basis for planning care. For example, a young child is not generally able to recognize the potential seriousness of illnesses and needs to be motivated to participate in a treatment plan or to develop habits for illness prevention. An adolescent's emotional development may influence personal beliefs about health-related matters such as the use of contraception, and the nurse thus uses different techniques of teaching than would be used for an adult.

Knowledge of the stages of growth and development helps the nurse predict the client's response to the present illness or the threat of future illness. The planning of nursing care is then adapted to these expectations, as well as to the client's abilities to participate in self-care.

INTELLECTUAL BACKGROUND

A person's beliefs about health are shaped in part by intellectual variables, including knowledge (or misinformation) about body functions and illnesses, educational background, and past experiences. These variables influence a person's thoughts. In addition, cognitive abilities shape the *way* a person thinks, including the ability to understand factors involved in illness and to apply knowledge of health and illness to personal health practices. Cognitive abilities also relate to a person's developmental stage. A nurse considers intellectual background when trying to understand a client's beliefs about health and health practices so that these variables can be incorporated into nursing care (Edelman and Mandle, 1994).

PERCEPTION OF FUNCTIONING

The way a person perceives physical functioning affects health beliefs and practices. For example, persons with chronic heart conditions perceive their levels of health differently than people who have never had major health problems. As a result, health beliefs and practices of people tend to be different. In addition, individuals who have successfully recovered from severe acute illnesses may subsequently change their health beliefs and practices.

When nurses assess a client's level of health, they gather subjective data about the way the client perceives physical functioning, such as level of fatigue, shortness of breath, or pain. They also obtain objective data about actual functioning, such as blood pressure, height measurements, and lung sound assessment. This information allows nurses to more successfully plan and implement individualized care.

EMOTIONAL FACTORS

Emotional factors also influence health beliefs and practices. A person experiencing a stress response with each change in life tends to respond to any sign of illness (see Chapter 22), perhaps by worrying that the illness is life threatening. A person who generally is very calm may have little emotional response during illness, whereas an individual unable to cope emotionally with the threat of illness may deny the presence of symptoms and not take therapeutic action. For example, a man who is short of breath and coughs frequently may blame this condition on cold weather if he cannot emotionally accept the possibility of a respiratory illness. Many people have strong emotional reactions against even thinking about the risk of cancer and will deny symptoms and refuse to take preventive action. Other illnesses are more emotionally acceptable, however, and people will be more likely to acknowledge the symptoms and seek appropriate care.

SPIRITUAL FACTORS

Spirituality is reflected in how a person lives his or her life, including the value and beliefs exercised, the relationships established with family and friends, and the ability to find hope and meaning in life. Spirituality serves as an integrating theme in peoples' lives (see Chapter 25). A person's spirituality influences the views held about health from a broad perspective. Fryback (1992) has found health to be associated with belief in a higher power that gives individuals faith and the ability to love. Health is viewed by many as the ability to live one's life fully. Religious practices are one way people exercise spirituality. There are some religions that restrict the use of certain forms of medical treatment. Nurses must understand client's spiritual dimensions to involve them effectively in nursing care.

External Variables

External variables influencing a person's health beliefs and practices include family practices, socioeconomic factors, and cultural variables.

FAMILY PRACTICES

The way that clients' families use health care services generally affects their health practices. Healthy families generally seek ways to help all members achieve their highest potential. Flexibility in healthy families encourages members to change role responsibilities, because members are able to temporarily perform each other's tasks (deChesnay and Magnuson, 1988).

If a child's parents treated every virus and illness as a potentially severe disease and immediately sought health care, the child generally does the same in adulthood. A person with this type of family background would be more likely to stay home from school or work with a cold, whereas others would attempt to carry on as usual. Likewise, clients are more likely to practice prevention if their families did so. For example, people whose parents took them for annual checkups as children are more likely to take their own children for regular checkups.

SOCIOECONOMIC FACTORS

Social and psychosocial factors can increase the risk for illness and influence the way that a person defines and reacts to illness. Psychosocial variables include the stability of the person's marital or intimate relationship, lifestyle habits, and occupational environment.

Neighbors, peers, and co-workers are usually aware of a person's level of health, and if the person is unexpectedly absent from work or a planned activity or is experiencing a symptom of illness, a member of the social network may encourage medical attention. A person generally seeks approval and support from social groups, and this desire for approval and support affects health beliefs and practices. For example, if it is socially acceptable in a particular peer group for teenage girls to smoke, the pressure to conform may be stronger than the concern about smoking being harmful to health.

Social variables partly determine how the health care system provides medical care. Because the health care system is organized in certain ways, it determines how clients can obtain care. The system provides care for clients with health problems that society considers "legitimate" and "acceptable." In addition, the system defines the treatment method, the economic cost to the client, and potential reimbursement to the health care agency or client. The health care system is a complex structure on which clients depend for care.

Like social variables, economic variables may affect a client's level of health by increasing the risk for disease and influencing how or at what point the client enters the health care system.

A worker who has health insurance is more likely to seek care and treatment for a chronic cough than an individual who is out of work and has no insurance. A person's compliance with the treatment that is designed to maintain or improve health is also affected by economic status. A person who has high utility bills, a large family, and a low income tends to give a higher priority to food and shelter than to costly drugs or treatment or expensive foods for special diets.

CULTURAL BACKGROUND

Cultural background influences individual beliefs, values, and customs. It influences entry into the health care system and personal health practices. For example, a study of health education practices for African Americans showed that most individuals did not have access to health education as a means for primary prevention (Airhihenbuwa, 1989).

If nurses are not aware of their own and other cultural patterns of behavior and language, they may not be able to recognize and understand a client's behavior and beliefs and may have difficulty interacting with the client. For example, a client from a culture that strongly values and expects close, warm, and supportive family relationships may experience cultural conflict with a nurse who does not value or has not experienced close kinship ties (Leininger, 1977). The nurse must identify and incorporate cultural factors into a client's care plan to avoid conflict between goals and methods of care and the client's cultural background (see Chapter 21).

HEALTH PROMOTION AND DISEASE PREVENTION

Nurses emphasize health-promotion and illness-prevention activities as important forms of health care. Nurses assist clients in maintaining good health and improving their levels of health instead of merely providing care after illness occurs. Health promotion and illness prevention are closely related concepts and, in practice, overlap to some extent. Activities involving **health promotion** help clients maintain or enhance their present levels of health. Activities for **illness prevention** protect clients from actual or potential threats to health. Both types of activities are future oriented. The difference between them involves motivations and goals. Health-promotion activities motivate people to act positively to reach the goal of more stable levels of health. Illness-prevention activities motivate people to avoid declines in health or functional levels.

Health-promotion activities can be passive or active. With **passive strategies of health promotion**, individuals gain from the activities of others without doing anything themselves. The fluoridation of municipal drinking water and the fortification of homogenized milk with vitamin D are two examples of passive health-promotion strategies.

With **active strategies of health promotion**, individuals are motivated to adopt specific health programs. Weight reduction and smoking cessation programs require clients to be actively involved in measures to improve their present and future levels of wellness while decreasing the risk of disease.

Health-promotion and illness-prevention activities have become an important focus of health care. Although scientific and medical advances since the 1940s have resulted in cures for many infectious diseases, there are still no cures for many chronic diseases. Thus there is greater motivation for preventing the occurrence of these diseases. In addition, the rapid rise of health care costs has motivated consumers to seek ways of decreasing the incidence and minimizing the results of illness or disability. Last, society as a whole has become increasingly conscious of health and the value of maintaining or increasing the level of health.

Pender (1993) has developed the Lifestyle and Health Habits Assessment (LHHA), which is divided into 10 sections. The assessment tool uses *yes* and *no* responses. The rating in each section, as well as the total score, provides the information necessary to design an individualized health-protection and health-promotion program for the client. In primary care settings, the use of the model may increase the client's awareness of living patterns and assist in motivating behavior changes (Pender, 1993) (see Chapter 3).

The goal of a total health program is to improve a client's level of well-being in all dimensions, not just physical health. Total programs are based on the belief that many factors can affect health. Health can be influenced by individual practices such as poor eating habits and little or no exercise. It can also be affected by physical stressors, a poor living environment, exposure to air pollutants, and an unsafe environment. Psychological stressors and hereditary factors can also influence level of health. Total health-promotion programs are directed at changing lifestyle by developing habits that can improve level of health. The fol-lowing categories are identified as important determinants of health status (Edelman and Mandle, 1994):

1. Smoking
2. Nutrition
3. Alcohol use
4. Habituating drug use
5. Driving
6. Exercise
7. Sexuality and contraceptive or barrier use
8. Family relationships
9. Risk-factor modification
10. Coping and adaptation

Other programs are aimed at specific health care problems. For example, support groups exist to help people with acquired immunodeficiency syndrome (AIDS). Exercise programs encourage participants to exercise regularly to reduce their risk of cardiac disease. Stress-reduction programs teach participants to cope with stressors and reduce their risks for multiple illnesses, such as infections, gastrointestinal disease, and cardiac disease.

Some health-promotion and illness-prevention programs are operated by health care agencies. Others are independently operated. Many corporations have developed on-site health-promotion activities for employees. Likewise, colleges and community centers offer health-promotion and illness-prevention programs. Nurses may be actively involved in these programs or may serve as consultants or give referrals. The goal of these activities is to improve health through preventive health services, environmental protection, and health education.

Health-promotion and illness-prevention activities are important to the consumer and the health care provider. Whether an activity uses the active or passive strategy, the goal is to maintain or improve the level of physical, emo-

Table 1-1	**The Three Levels of Prevention**				
PRIMARY PREVENTION		**SECONDARY PREVENTION**		**TERTIARY PREVENTION**	
HEALTH PROMOTION	**SPECIFIC PROTECTION**	**EARLY DIAGNOSIS AND PROMPT TREATMENT**	**DISABILITY LIMITATIONS**	**RESTORATION AND REHABILITATION**	
Health education	Use of specific immunizations	Case-finding measures: individual and mass	Adequate treatment to arrest disease process and prevent further complications	Provision of hospital and community facilities for retraining and education to maximize use of remaining capacities	
Good standard of nutrition adjusted to developmental phases of life	Attention to personal hygiene	Screening surveys	Provision of facilities to limit disability and prevent death	Education of the public and industries to use rehabilitated persons to the fullest possible extent	
Attention to personality development	Use of environmental sanitation	Selective examinations			
Provision of adequate housing and recreation and agreeable working conditions	Protection against occupational hazards	Cure and prevention of disease process to prevent spread of communicable disease, prevent complications, and shorten period of disability		Selective placement	
Marriage counseling and sex education	Protection from accidents			Work therapy in hospitals	
Genetic screening	Use of specific nutrients			Use of sheltered colony	
Periodic selective examinations	Protection from carcinogens				
	Avoidance of allergens				

Modified from Leavell HR et al: *Preventive medicine for doctors in the community,* ed 3, New York, 1965, McGraw-Hill.

tional, intellectual, social, developmental, and spiritual well-being. Although activities are often organized in specific programs, nurses in all areas of practice often have opportunities to assist clients in adopting activities to promote health and decrease risks of illness.

Levels of Preventive Care

Nursing care oriented to health promotion and illness prevention can be understood in terms of health activities on the primary, secondary, and tertiary levels (Table 1-1).

PRIMARY PREVENTION

Primary prevention is true prevention; it precedes disease or dysfunction and is applied to clients considered physically and emotionally healthy. It is not therapeutic, does not use therapeutic treatments, and does not involve symptom identification (Edelman and Mandle, 1994). Healthy activities are directed at decreasing the probability of specific illnesses or dysfunctions. In addition, primary prevention includes health education programs, immunization, and physical and nutritional fitness activities. Primary prevention can be provided to an individual or to a general population, or it can focus on individuals at risk for developing specific diseases.

SECONDARY PREVENTION

Secondary prevention focuses on individuals who are experiencing health problems or illnesses and who are at risk for developing complications or worsening conditions. Activities are directed at diagnosis and prompt intervention, thereby reducing severity and enabling the client to return to normal health as early as possible (Pender, 1993; Edelman and Mandle, 1994). A large portion of secondary level nursing care is delivered in the home, hospital, or skilled nursing facility, to prevent complications. Secondary prevention includes screening techniques and treatment of early stages of disease to limit disability by averting or delaying the consequences of advanced disease.

TERTIARY PREVENTION

Tertiary prevention occurs when a defect or disability is permanent and irreversible. It involves minimizing the effects of the disease or disability by interventions directed at preventing complication and deterioration (Edelman and Mandle, 1994). Activities are directed at rehabilitation rather than diagnosis and treatment (Pender, 1993). Care at this level aims to help clients achieve as high a level of functioning as possible, despite the limitations caused by illness or impairment. This level of care is called *preventive care* because it involves prevention of further disability or reduced functioning. A nurse who provides tertiary care to a recently blinded client, for example, not only assists the client in adapting to the disability through activities such as teaching techniques to perform personal hygiene, but also directs attention to the goal of preventing future problems such as accidents in the home or potential problems with child rearing (see Table 1-1).

■ RISK FACTORS

A **risk factor** is any situation, habit, environmental condition, physiological condition, or other variable that increases the vulnerability of an individual or group to an illness or accident. For example, a person whose father and paternal grandfather died of acute myocardial infarctions in their forties is at risk for coronary disease. Likewise, members of a community exposed to industrial air pollution are at risk for developing pulmonary disease. Risk factors include variables other than physical conditions. For example, a person who has experienced emotional stressors over a long period risks developing many kinds of illness.

The presence of risk factors does not mean that a disease will develop, but risk factors increase the chances that the individual will experience a particular disease. Risk factors can occur in different aspects of a person's internal or external environment. Nurses and other health care professionals are concerned with them for several reasons. Risk factors play a major role in how a nurse identifies a client's health status. They can also influence health beliefs and practices if a person is aware of their presence. Identifying risk factors is also important for health-promotion and illness-prevention activities; such identification allows modification or elimination of the risk factors.

Risk factors can be placed in the following interrelated categories: genetic and physiological factors, age, physical environment, and lifestyle.

Genetic and Physiological Factors

Physiological risk factors involve the physical functioning of the body. Certain physical conditions, such as being overweight, place increased stress on a person's physiological systems (e.g., the circulatory system), increasing susceptibility to illness in these areas. Heredity, or genetic predisposition to specific illness, is a major physical risk factor. For example, a person with a family history of diabetes mellitus is at risk for developing the disease later in life. Other documented genetic risk factors include family histories of cancer, coronary disease, and renal disease.

Age

Age increases susceptibility to certain illnesses. For example, the risk of cardiovascular disease increases with age for both sexes. The risks of birth defects and complications of pregnancy increase in women bearing children after age 35. Many kinds of cancer pose a greater risk for persons over age 45 than for younger persons. Age risk factors are often closely associated with other risk factors such as family history and personal habits. For example, a man at age 60 who has smoked 40 years is at a greater risk for developing lung cancer than a man at age 30 who has smoked 10 years. Nurses need to educate their clients about the importance of regularly scheduled checkups for their age group (Fig. 1-6).

Environment

The physical environment in which a person works or lives can increase the likelihood that certain illnesses will occur. For example, some kinds of cancer and other diseases are more likely to develop when industrial workers are exposed to certain chemicals or when people live near toxic waste disposal sites. Screening for these environmentally based risk factors is directed at the short-term effects of the exposure and the potential for long-term effects (Edelman and Mandle, 1994).

Air, water, and noise pollution increase the risk of illness.

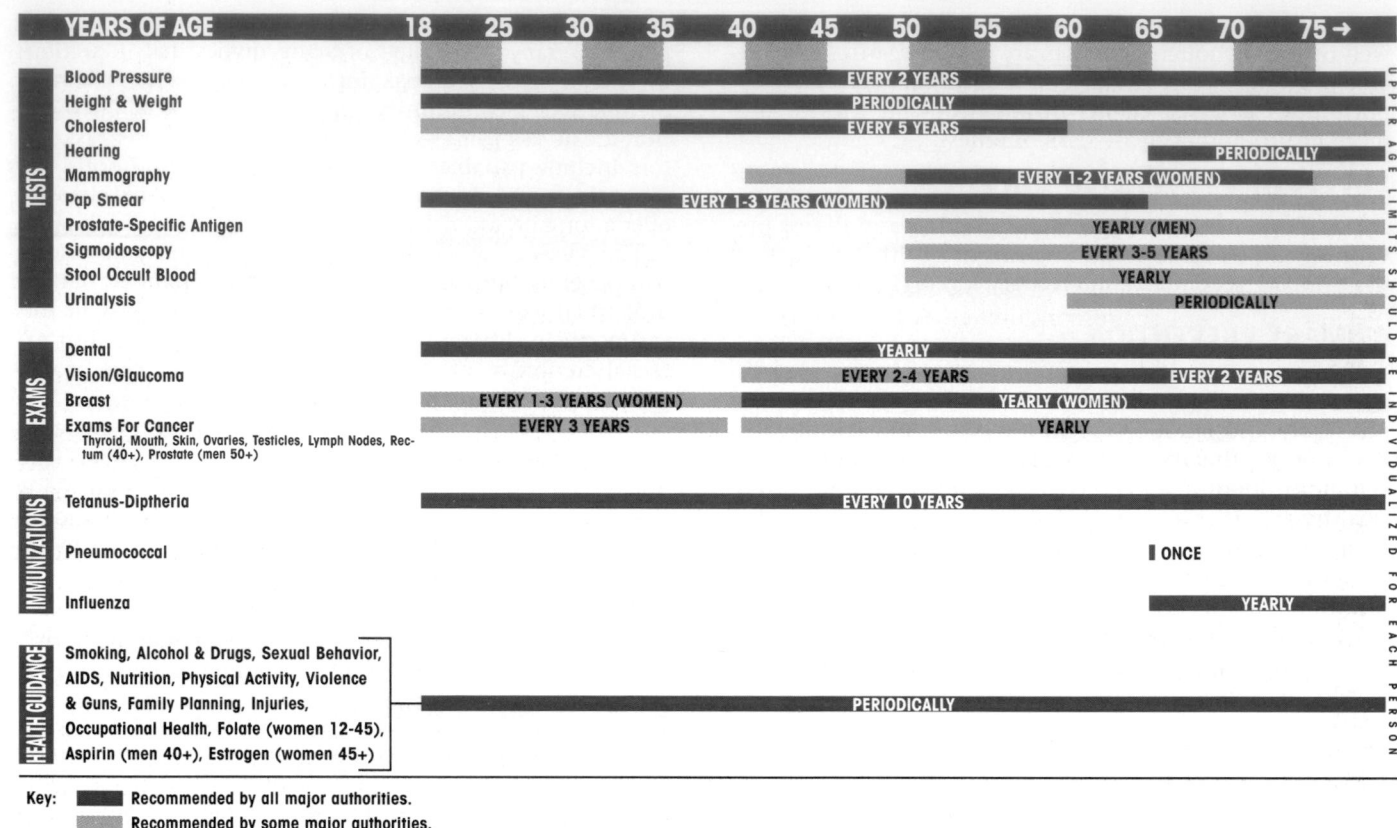

Fig. 1-6 Adult preventive care timetable: recommendation of major authorities. *(Redrawn from ANA: Clinician's handbook of preventive services:* Put prevention into practice, *1994, ANA; modified from* Healthy People 2000.)

High crime rates or overcrowding can also lead to stresses that make individuals more susceptible to disease.

In the home the physical environment may include conditions that pose risks to an individual or family. Unclean, poorly heated or cooled, or overcrowded dwellings increase the likelihood that diseases will be contracted and spread. Within the family, conflicts or other problems may create stressors that put individual members or the family as a whole at increased risk of illness.

Lifestyle

Many activities, habits, and practices involve risk factors; the stresses of life crises and frequent lifestyle changes also are risk factors. Health practices and behaviors can have positive or negative effects on health. Practices with potential negative effects are risk factors; these include overeating or poor nutrition, insufficient rest and sleep, and poor personal hygiene. Other habits that put a person at risk for illness include smoking, alcohol or drug abuse, and activities involving a threat of injury such as skydiving or mountain climbing. Some habits are risk factors for specific diseases. For example, excessive sunbathing increases the risk of skin cancer, and being overweight increases the risk of cardiovascular disease.

Any emotional stress can be a risk factor if it is severe or prolonged or the person is unable to cope adequately. In such a case, emotional stress may increase the chance of illness. Emotional stressors may occur with events such as divorce, pregnancy, and arguments. Any area of life that leads to long-term emotional stress can be a risk factor. Job-related stresses, for example, may overtax a person's cognitive skills and decision-making ability, leading to "mental overload" or "burnout" (see Chapter 22).

ILLNESS AND ILLNESS BEHAVIOR

Illness is not merely the presence of a disease process. **Illness** is a state in which a person's physical, emotional, intellectual, social, developmental, or spiritual functioning is diminished or impaired compared with that person's previous experience. Cancer is a disease process, but one client with leukemia who is responding to treatment may continue to function as usual, whereas another client with breast cancer who is preparing for surgery may be affected in dimensions other than the physical.

Illness, therefore, is not synonymous with disease. Although nurses must be familiar with different kinds of diseases and their treatments, they are concerned more with illness, which may include disease but also the effects on functioning and well-being in all dimensions.

People who are ill generally act in a way that medical sociologists call **illness behavior.** Illness behavior involves the ways persons monitor their bodies, define and interpret their symptoms, take remedial actions, and use the health care system (Mechanic, 1982). If individuals perceive themselves to be ill, illness behavior can serve as coping mechanisms. For example, illness behavior may be a means of obtaining reassurance. A person who has been off work for a week because of illness may need to be reassured that his employer missed his contribution and that others care about him (Lambert and Lambert, 1987). The health team can also be a source of support and reassurance for clients. This support is particularly important for clients with chronic diseases. Clients with severe cardiac impairments who are unable to care for themselves look to the health team for support. Clients may need reassurance that the inability to care for themselves is due to the physical disease and not to a lack of motivation or desire. In addition, illness behavior can result in clients being released from roles, social expectations, or responsibilities. For a homemaker, for example, the "flu" may be a temporary release from child care and household responsibilities.

Variables Influencing Illness Behavior

Just as health behavior is affected by internal and external variables, so is illness behavior. To understand the client's behavior and plan individualized care, the nurse needs to understand the influences of these variables. They are complex in their origins and effects.

INTERNAL VARIABLES

Important internal variables influencing the way clients behave when they are ill are their perceptions of symptoms and the nature of the illness. If clients believe that the symptoms of their illnesses disrupt their normal routine, they are more likely to seek health care assistance than if they do not perceive the symptoms to be disruptive. An example might be a carpenter with back pain. If clients believe that the symptoms are serious or perhaps life threatening, they are also more likely to seek assistance. Persons awakened by crushing chest pains in the middle of the night generally view this event as a symptom of a potentially serious and life-threatening illness and will probably be motivated to seek assistance. However, such a perception can also have the opposite effect. Individuals may fear serious illness, react by denying it, and not seek medical assistance.

A client's illness behavior can also be affected by the nature of the illness. **Acute illnesses** involve symptoms of relatively short duration that are usually severe and may affect functioning in any dimension. **Chronic illnesses** persist, usually longer than 6 months, and can affect functioning in any dimension. Several variables influence the illness behavior of a client with a chronic illness. The client may fluctuate between maximal functioning and serious recurrences that may be life threatening. If a chronic illness cannot be cured and the symptoms are only partially relieved by therapy, the client may not be motivated to comply with the therapy plan. In addition, in the present system health care professionals are sometimes not highly motivated to remain involved in a client's care, and the client's own motivation may also lessen.

Clients with acute illnesses are more likely to seek health care and comply readily with therapy. Chronically ill clients may become less actively involved in their care, may experience greater frustration, and may comply less readily with care. Because nurses generally spend more time than other health care professionals with chronically ill clients, they are in the unique position of being able to assist these clients in overcoming problems related to illness behavior.

EXTERNAL VARIABLES

External variables influencing a client's illness behavior include the visibility of symptoms, social group, cultural background, economic variables, accessibility of the health care system, and social support.

The visibility of the symptoms of an illness can affect body image and illness behavior. For example, a person who has a draining sore on the lip may seek assistance sooner than a person with a sore throat because people may comment on the sore, the sore changes the person's appearance, and the drainage requires continual care.

Clients' social groups may assist them in recognizing the threat of illness or support the denial of potential illness. For example, two 35-year-old women in two different social groups have identified breast masses while performing breast self-examination; both discuss the finding with their friends. The first woman's friends might encourage her to seek medical attention to determine whether a biopsy is necessary, whereas the second woman's friends might tell her that the lump probably represents only fibrocystic disease and that she does not need to rush to a doctor. These examples show the influence that friends may have on a client. The client's interaction with family members, peers, and others may have similar results.

Illness behavior can be interpreted and explained in terms of personal experiences and expectations. Cultural and ethnic background teaches an individual how to be healthy, recognize illness, and be ill. Meanings attached to health and illness are related to the basic culture-bound values by which a person defines a given experience and perception (Spector, 1991).

Therefore to develop individualized therapy, a nurse needs to understand a client's cultural background. Western culture has emphasized a specific, systematic, causal explanation for trying to understand disease. The effects of disease and its interpretation also vary according to cultural circumstances. For example, there is a higher mortality rate from measles in underdeveloped countries than in western cultures (Moore et al, 1980).

Clients' access to the health care system is closely related to the influence of economic factors. The health care system is a socioeconomic system that clients must enter, interact within, and exit. For many clients, entry into the system is complex or confusing, and some clients may seek nonemergency medical care in an emergency room because they do not know how otherwise to obtain health services. The physical proximity of clients to a hospital, clinic, or health care agency often influences how soon they enter the system after deciding to seek care. In addition, some clients are reluctant to seek care from a large, complex medical center and will more readily visit a community agency. Clients frequently feel that a large medical center is impersonal, that care is provided in a mechanized, assembly line approach, and that health care personnel are always looking for the worst. Some clients, however, may seek care only from a large medical center because they believe diagnosis and treatment procedures are more current.

There are options now available in the health care system that are more pro-health promotion. One of them is the Health Maintenance Organization (HMO). HMOs have taken a leadership role in health promotion activities. In addition to routine checkups and screenings, seminars and classes are offered on such topics as diet and weight control, smoking, stress management, and physical fitness. Health maintenance members consider health education to be an important component of their membership services at the HMO. Another option for individuals to keep healthy is to join a health club. Increasingly health clubs are offering aerobic exercises and physical and nutritional programs. Facilities include swimming pools, tennis, basketball, weight rooms, saunas, massage therapy areas, and others. More and more individuals who can afford the cost of club memberships are becoming active members.

Stages of Illness Behavior

Although the behavior of ill individuals is influenced by internal and external variables, people generally pass through five stages of illness behavior (Fig. 1-7). This pattern involves how a person seeks, finds, and completes health care.

A nurse encounters clients in various stages of illness behavior. Knowledge of these stages enables the nurse to assess client behavior, determine the stage of illness behavior, and develop interventions to promote optimal physical, emotional, intellectual, social, and spiritual functioning throughout the illness.

STAGE 1: SYMPTOM EXPERIENCE

During the initial stage, a person is aware that "something is wrong." A person usually recognizes a physical sensation or a limitation in functioning but does not suspect a specific diagnosis.

The person's perception of a symptom includes awareness of a physical change such as pain, a rash, or a lump; evaluation of this change and a decision that it is a symptom of an illness; and an emotional response.

For example, a 38-year-old woman detects a lump during monthly breast self-examination. She knows the lump is not related to hormonal changes because she recently completed her menstrual period. She decides that the lump means that something is wrong and that it may be a symptom of cancer. She becomes anxious and fearful about this diagnosis.

If she regards the symptoms as severe or life threatening, immediate care may be sought or the symptoms' presence or implications may be denied. If she denies the symptoms or their meaning for future wellness, advice or treatment may be delayed. Before progressing to the next stage of illness behavior, the person must acknowledge the presence of a health problem.

STAGE 2: ASSUMPTION OF THE SICK ROLE

If symptoms persist and become severe, clients assume the sick role. At this point the illness becomes a social phenomenon, and sick people seek confirmation from their families and social groups that they are indeed ill and that they should be excused from normal duties and role expectations (Coe, 1978). The social group recognizes the illness and may also support continued self-medication.

The assumption of the sick role results in emotional changes, such as withdrawal or depression, and physical changes. Emotional changes may be simple or complex, depending on the severity of the illness, the degree of disability, and the anticipated length of the illness.

In the case of an illness requiring intervention from health professionals, the person may deny that such intervention is necessary and thus delay contact with the health care system. After accepting the persistent nature of the symptoms or the potential threat to present and future levels of wellness, the person seeks contact with the health care system and becomes a client.

STAGE 3: MEDICAL CARE CONTACT

If symptoms persist despite home remedies, become severe, or require emergency care, the person is motivated to seek professional health services. In this stage the client seeks expert acknowledgment of the illness, as well as treatment. In addition, the client seeks an explanation of the symptoms, the cause of the symptoms, the course of the illness, and the implications of the illness for future health.

Clients' illnesses can be validated at any point on the health-illness continuum. A health professional may determine that they do not have an illness or that illnesses are present and may be life threatening. Clients then accept or deny this diagnosis, depending on several factors. The variables that affect illness behavior influence client reaction. If clients accept the diagnosis, they usually follow with the prescribed treatment plan. If they deny the diagnosis, they may begin "shopping" within the health care system. In such a case, clients consult several health care providers until they find one who makes the desired diagnosis or until they accept the initial diagnosis. Clients who consider themselves ill, even if health professionals regard them as healthy, may "shop" with a variety of doctors and therapists to obtain the desired diagnosis of illness. Conversely, clients initially diagnosed as ill, particularly with life-threatening illnesses, may seek another expert to tell them that their health or lives are not threatened. Clients with diagnosed cancer may seek opinions from several physicians in an attempt to avoid facing the diagnosis.

STAGE 4: DEPENDENT CLIENT ROLE

After accepting the illness and seeking treatment, the client enters the fourth stage of illness behavior. In this stage, the client depends on health care professionals for the relief of symptoms. The client accepts care, sympathy, and protection from the demands and stresses of life. A client can adopt the dependent role in a health care institution, at home, or in a community setting.

It is socially permissible for clients in the dependent role to be relieved of normal obligations and tasks. The more ill the clients, the more they are excused from responsibilities.

After entering the dependent stage, the client must also adjust to the disruption of a daily schedule. This disruption affects the client's role in occupation, family, and community and may lead to stress in the emotional, intellectual, social, developmental, and spiritual dimensions.

STAGE 5: RECOVERY AND REHABILITATION

The final stage of illness behavior—recovery and rehabilitation—can arrive suddenly, such as when a fever subsides. If recovery is not prompt, long-term care may be required before the client is able to resume an optimal level of functioning (e.g., the case of a fractured leg). In the case of chronic illness, the final stage may involve an adjustment to a prolonged reduction in health and functioning.

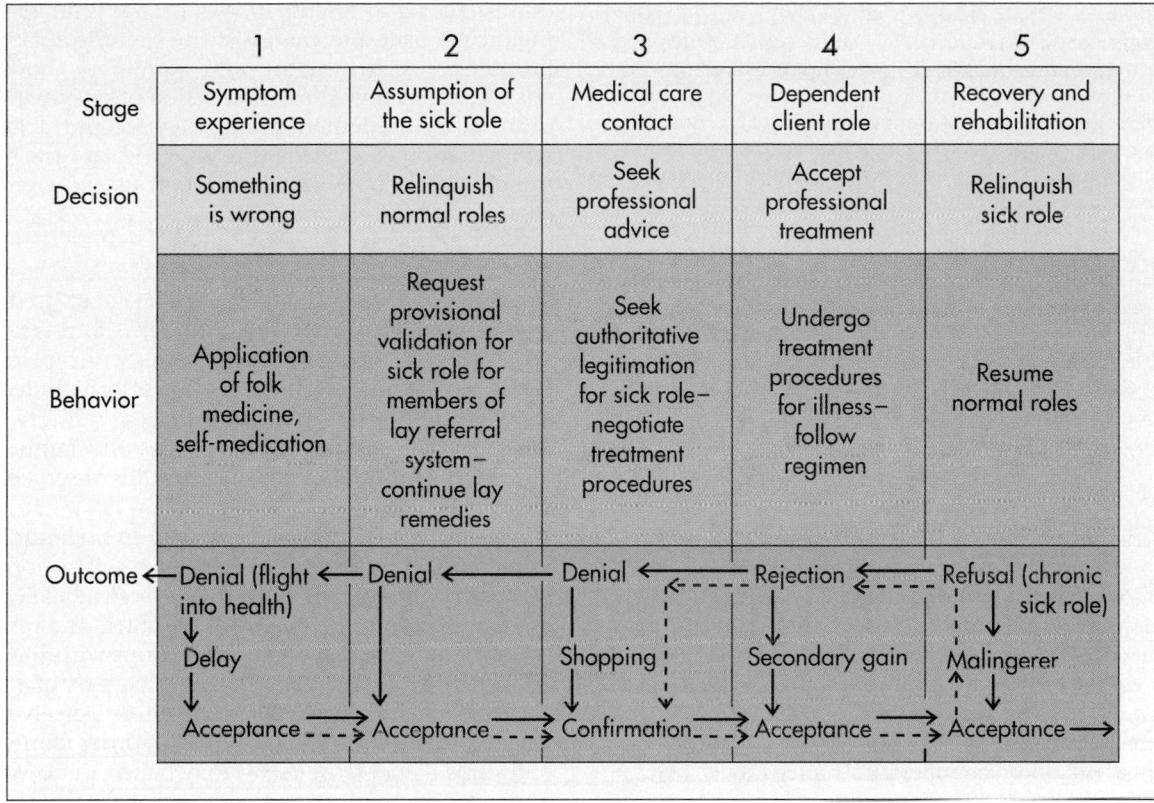

	1	2	3	4	5
Stage	Symptom experience	Assumption of the sick role	Medical care contact	Dependent client role	Recovery and rehabilitation
Decision	Something is wrong	Relinquish normal roles	Seek professional advice	Accept professional treatment	Relinquish sick role
Behavior	Application of folk medicine, self-medication	Request provisional validation for sick role for members of lay referral system— continue lay remedies	Seek authoritative legitimation for sick role— negotiate treatment procedures	Undergo treatment procedures for illness— follow regimen	Resume normal roles
Outcome	← Denial (flight into health) ↓ Delay ↓ Acceptance	← Denial ↓ Acceptance	← Denial ↓ Shopping ↓ Confirmation	← Rejection ↓ Secondary gain ↓ Acceptance	← Refusal (chronic sick role) ↓ Malingerer ↓ Acceptance →

Fig. 1 7 Stages of illness behavior. *(Redrawn from Suchman EA: Stages of illness and medical care, J Health Hum Behav 6:114, 1965.)*

Not all clients go through each stage, nor do they all move through them at the same rate or in the same manner. People who have been in good health but suddenly suffer heart attacks and are taken to the emergency room, for example, are put immediately into the dependent client role, even though they have not progressed emotionally through the earlier stages. Nonetheless, the described pattern of illness behavior occurs in many cases, and an understanding of these stages helps a nurse identify clients' changing illness behavior and plan effective nursing care with clients.

IMPACT OF ILLNESS ON CLIENT AND FAMILY

Illness is never an isolated life event. The client and family must deal with changes resulting from illness and treatment. Each client responds uniquely to illness, and therefore nursing interventions must be individualized. The client and family commonly experience behavioral and emotional changes, as well as changes in roles, body image, self-concept, and family dynamics.

Behavioral and Emotional Changes

People react differently to illness or the threat of illness. Individual behavioral and emotional reactions depend on the nature of the illness, the client's attitude toward it, the reaction of others to it, and the variables of illness behavior.

Short-term, non–life-threatening illnesses evoke few behavioral changes in the functioning of the client or family.

A husband and father who has a cold, for example, may lack the energy and patience to spend time in family activities and may be irritable and prefer not to interact with his family. This is a behavioral change, but the change is subtle and does not last long. Some may even consider such a change a normal response to illness.

Severe illness, particularly one that is life threatening, can lead to more extensive emotional and behavioral changes, such as anxiety, shock, denial, anger, and withdrawal. These are common responses to the stress of illness. The nurse develops interventions to assist the client and family in coping with this stress because the stressor itself cannot usually be changed.

Impact on Family Roles

People have many roles in life, such as wage earner, decision maker, professional, and parent. When an illness occurs, the roles of client and family may change. Such a change may be subtle and short term or drastic and long term. An individual and family generally adjust more easily to subtle, short-term changes. In most cases they know that the role change is only temporary. For example, the mother of two preschool children has a viral infection, and her illness continues for a week; during this time, she gives up her roles of homemaker and child-care provider. Initially she may welcome giving up these roles to be able to care for herself. As she gets better, however, she begins to look forward to resuming her roles.

With short-term role changes, a client does not go

CASE STUDY Mr. Lampe is a married 40-year-old construction worker with three sons. The family is very active in outdoor activities and goes hiking and camping every 2 weeks during the summer and fall. Mr. Lampe is injured while hiking, and his injury requires the amputation of one leg. Because of the injury, Mr. Lampe has to change jobs and as a result receives a lower salary. The family activities change from active outdoor ones to passive indoor ones. Mrs. Lampe becomes angry because the reduction in income makes it difficult for the family to maintain its previous standard of living. The three sons become angry because their dad no longer takes them camping and hiking. Mr. Lampe becomes angry because he feels that his wife and children should be grateful that he is alive and should not worry about material things. The anger in the family gradually increases to the point that Mr. Lampe becomes unable to function at his highest level. The visiting nurse notices these changes in the family and observes angry outbursts. She refers the family for counseling sessions with a family therapist to help them cope with the anger resulting from the changes in Mr. Lampe's roles. ■

through prolonged adjustment phases. Long-term changes, however, require an adjustment process similar to the grief process. The client and family often require specific counseling and guidance to assist them in coping with the role changes. The preceding case study illustrates the way that such changes can occur.

In some cases family members may mistakenly assume that the ill person needs to be free of decisions and responsibilities. Family members take over all the roles of the client, including wage earner and decision maker. For instance, although Mr. Lampe needs to recover physically from his illness, he does not have to relinquish all of his roles in the family. If the family attempts to relieve him of all responsibility, he may feel isolated and withdraw from them. Because changes in a client's role affect family, nurses must incorporate the family into the plan of care (deChesnay and Magnuson, 1988).

Impact on Body Image

Body image is the subjective concept of physical appearance. Some illnesses result in changes in physical appearance, and clients and families react differently to these changes. The reactions of clients and families to changes in body image depend on the following:

1. The types of changes (e.g., loss of a limb, a special sense, or an organ)
2. Their adaptive capacity
3. The rate at which changes take place
4. Supportive services available

When a change in body image occurs, such as results from a leg amputation, the client generally adjusts in the following phases: shock, withdrawal, acknowledgment, acceptance, and rehabilitation. Initially the client may be shocked by the change or impending change and may depersonalize it and talk about it as though it were happening to someone else. As the client and family recognize the reality of the change, they become anxious and may with-

draw, refusing to discuss it. Withdrawal is an adaptive coping mechanism that can assist the client in making the adjustment. As the client and family acknowledge the change, they move through a period of grieving. At the end of the acknowledgment phase, they accept the loss. During rehabilitation, the client is ready to learn how to adapt to the change in body image through use of a prosthesis or changes in lifestyle and goals.

Impact on Self-Concept

Self-concept is individuals' mental image of themselves, including how they view their strengths and weaknesses in all aspects of their personalities. Self-concept depends in part on body image and roles but also includes other aspects of the psychological and spiritual self. The impact of illness on the self-concept of clients and family members may be more complex and less readily observed than role changes.

Self-concept is important in a person's relationships with other family members. A client whose self-concept changes because of illness may no longer meet the expectations of the family, leading to tension or conflict. As a result, family members may change their interactions with the client. For example, the client may no longer be part of the family's decision-making process or may not be perceived as being able to provide emotional support to other family members or friends. Finally, the client may be left out of social functions. In the course of providing care, a nurse is able to observe changes in the client's self-concept—or in the self-concepts of family members—and develop a care plan to help them adjust to the impact of illness (see Chapter 23).

Impact on Family Dynamics

Because of the effects of illness on the client and family, family dynamics often change. Nursing interventions need to be directed toward the family and client (Reeder, 1991). Family dynamics is the process by which the family functions, makes decisions, gives support to individual members, and copes with everyday changes and challenges. If a parent in a family becomes ill, family activities and decision making often come to a halt as the other family members wait for the illness to pass, or they delay action because they are reluctant to assume the ill person's roles or responsibilities. In some cases of prolonged illness, the family often has to shift to a new pattern of functioning, a change that can lead to emotional stress. Young children, for example, may experience a strong sense of loss if either parent is hospitalized or is unable to provide affection and a sense of security. Emotional difficulty may continue even when the other parent or family members are successful in assuming the roles and responsibilities of the hospitalized parent. If a parent of an adult becomes ill and cannot carry out usual activities, the adult child often assumes many of the parent's responsibilities and in essence becomes a parent to the parent. Such a reversal of the usual situation can lead to stress, conflicting responsibilities for the adult child, or direct conflict over decision making (see Chapter 27).

■ KEY CONCEPTS ■

► A healthy individual adapts to changes in internal and external environments and thus maintains a state of well-being in all dimensions.

► An illness may be a disease, but it also includes reduced functioning in any human dimension.

► A person's state of health or illness should be considered in relation to individual values, personality, and lifestyle rather than be measured by any absolute standard.

► According to the health-illness continuum model, health and illness are in a dynamic, relative relationship. This model allows a nurse to compare a client's state of health with past states.

► The high level wellness model describes health as an integrated method of functioning oriented at maximizing an individual's potential.

► The agent-host-environment model describes disease or illness as the result of the dynamic interaction of factors related to the agent, host, and environment. No one factor is the cause of disease or illness.

► The health-belief model helps nurses understand and predict the behavior of clients in seeking or complying with health care.

► The health-promotion model is directed at increasing an individual's level of well-being and self-actualization.

► Health beliefs and practices are influenced by internal variables, including developmental stage, intellectual background, perception of functioning, and emotional and spiritual factors, and by external variables, including family practices and socioeconomic and cultural factors.

► Nursing incorporates health-promotion and disease-prevention activities rather than simply treating illness after it occurs.

► Primary preventive care helps healthy people maintain and increase their levels of health.

► Secondary preventive care helps ill persons avoid complications or further health problems.

► Tertiary preventive care helps clients adapt to or overcome disability or reduced functioning caused by illness.

► Risk factors threaten a person's health, influence health practices, and are important considerations in illness-prevention activities.

► Illness behavior, like health practices, is influenced by many variables and must be considered by the nurse when planning care.

► Although no two ill individuals behave in exactly the same way, most pass through the following stages of illness behavior: symptom experience, assumption of the sick role, medical care contact, the dependent role, and recovery and rehabilitation.

► Illness can have many effects on the client and family, including behavioral and emotional changes and changes in roles, body image, self-concept, and family dynamics.

► To plan and implement holistic nursing care that assists in attaining states of maximal functioning and well-being, a nurse must consider all of the effects of an illness on a client and family.

■ KEY TERMS ■

Active strategies of health promotion, p. 11

Acute illness, p. 15

Agent, p. 7

Chronic illness, p. 15

Environment, p. 7

Health, p. 4

Health behavior, p. 5

Health-belief model, p. 8

Health promotion, p. 11

Health-illness continuum, p. 5

Host, p. 7

Illness, p. 14

Illness behavior, p. 14

Illness prevention, p. 11

Passive strategies of health promotion, p. 11

Primary prevention, p. 13

Risk factor, p. 13

Secondary prevention, p. 13

Tertiary prevention, p. 13

■ CRITICAL THINKING EXERCISES ■

1. You are working in a day-care setting. You're asked to design an early education health promotion program for the 4-year-old group. You initially focus on diet and exercise. How do you begin to design the program? What resources do you need?

2. One of the students in your school seeks your advice for smoking cessation programs. How do you identify appropriate resources? Which programs would be suitable for this person? What information does the client need about the potential programs?

3. Assess your own lifestyle. Identify three areas for change. Select one area, determine what needs to change, how to identify resources to promote change, how to select and implement the resources, and how to evaluate the effectiveness of the change.

REFERENCES

Airhihenbuwa CO: Health education for African Americans: a neglected task, *Health Educ* 20:9, 1989.

ANA: *Clinician's handbook of preventive services: put prevention into practice*, Washington, DC, 1994, ANA.

Becker MH, Maiman LA: Sociobehavioral determinants of compliance with health and medical care recommendations, *Med Care* 33(1):1021, 1975.

Berne AS et al: A nursing model for addressing the health needs of homeless families, *Image J Nurs Sch* 22:8, 1990.

Coe R: *Sociology of medicine,* ed 2, New York, 1978, McGraw-Hill.

deChesnay M, Magnuson N: How healthy families cope with stress, *AAOHN J* 36:361, 1988.

Duffy M, MacDonald E: Determinants of functional health of older persons, *Gerontologist* 30(4):503, 1990.

Dunn HL: High-level wellness for man and society, *Am J Public Health* 49:789, 1959.

Dunn H: What high level wellness means, *Health Values* 1:9, 1977.

Edelman CL, Mandle CL: *Health promotion throughout the life span,* ed 2, St Louis, 1994, Mosby.

Fryback PB: Health for people with a terminal diagnosis, *Nurs Sci Q* 6(3):147, 1992.

Gilpatrick DM: Moving clients toward wellness: behavioral change, *Clin Nurse Spec* 3(1):25, 1989.

Gordon M: *Nursing diagnosis process and application,* ed 3, St Louis, 1994, Mosby.

Gueldner S, Spradley J: Outdoor walking lowers fatigue, *J Gerontol Nurs* 14(10):6, 1988.

Haber D: *Health promotion and aging,* New York, 1994, Springer.

Lambert CE, Lambert VA: Psychosocial impacts created by chronic illness, *Nurs Clin North Am* 22:527, 1987.

Leavell HR et al: *Preventive medicine for doctors in the community,* ed 3, New York, 1965, McGraw-Hill.

Leininger M: Cultural diversities of health and nursing care, *Nurs Clin North Am* 12(1):5, 1977.

McTernan EJ, Rice NC: An overview of the role of allied health professionals in the health promotion and disease prevention movement, *J Allied Health* 15(4):289, 1986.

Mechanic D: The epidemiology of illness behavior and its relationship to physical and psychological distress. In Mechanic D, editor: *Symptoms, illness behavior, and help seeking,* New York, 1982, Prodist.

Meleis AI: Being and becoming healthy: the core of nursing knowledge, *Nurs Sci Q* 3:107, 1990.

Moore LG et al: *The biocultural basis of health: expanding views of medicine anthropology,* Prospect Heights, Ill, 1980, Waveland.

Neuman B: *The Neuman systems model,* ed 2, Norwalk, Conn, 1989, Appleton & Lange.

Neuman B: Health as a continuum based on the Neuman systems model, *Nurs Sci Q* 3:129, 1990.

Parse RR: *Man-living-health: a theory of nursing,* New York, 1981, Wiley.

Parse RR: Health: a personal commitment, *Nurs Sci Q* 3:136, 1990.

Pender NJ: A conceptual model for preventive health behavior, *Nurs Outlook* 23:385, 1975.

Pender NJ: Expressing health through lifestyle patterns, *Nurs Sci Q* 3:115, 1990.

Pender NJ: Health promotion and illness prevention. In Werley HH, Fitzpatrick JJ, editors: *Annual review of nursing research,* New York, 1993a, Springer.

Pender NJ: *Health promotion and nursing practice,* Norwalk, Conn, 1982, Appleton-Century-Crofts.

Pender NJ: *Health promotion and nursing practice,* ed 3, Norwalk, Conn, 1996, Appleton & Lange.

Pender NJ, Pender AR: Attitudes, subjective norms, and intentions to engage in health behaviors, *Nurs Res* 35(1):15, 1986.

Pesznecker E: The poor: a population at risk, *Public Health Nurs* 1(4):237, 1984.

Public Health Service, US Department of Health and Human Services, vol 40, no 8, suppl 2, Washington, DC, 1992, US Government Printing Office.

Rawlins R, Williams S, Beck C: *Mental health-psychiatric nursing: a holistic life cycle approach,* St Louis, 1993, Mosby.

Reeder JM: Family perception: a key to intervention. In American Association of Critical-Care Nurses: *AACN clinical issues in critical care nurse,* Mission Viejo, Calif, 1991, The Association.

Rosenstoch I: Historical origin of the health belief model, *Health Educ Monogr* 2:334, 1974.

Ryan RS, Travis JW: *Wellness workbook,* Berkeley, Calif, 1981, Ten Speed Press.

Smith JM, Sorrell V: Developing wellness programs: a nurse-managed stay-well center for senior citizens, *Clin Nurse Spec* 3(1):198, 1989.

Spector RE: *Cultural diversity in health and illness,* ed 3, Norwalk, Conn, 1991, Appleton & Lange.

Suchman EA: Stages of illness and medical care, *J Health Hum Behav* 6:114, 1965.

US Department of Health and Human Services, PHS: *Healthy people 2000: national health promotion and disease prevention objectives,* Washington, DC, 1990, US Government Printing Office.

Willis CR: The future of allied health in the health promotion and disease prevention movement, *J Allied Health* 15(4):349, 1986.

World Health Organization: Health promotion in developing countries: a call for action, *Am J Health Promotion* 6(3):174, 1992.

ADDITIONAL READINGS

Advisory Committee on Immunization Practices (ACIP): Prevention and control of influenza: part 1, vaccines, *MMWR* 42(RR-6):1. 1993.

Broome CV, Breiman RF: Neumococcal vaccine: past, present and future, *N Engl J Med* 325:1506, 1991.

Brown RL: Identification and office management of alcohol and drug disorders. In Fleming MF, Barry KL, editors: *Addictive disorders,* St Louis, 1992, Mosby.

Centers for Disease Control and Prevention: Prevention and control of tuberculosis in US communities with at-risk minority populations and prevention and control of tuberculosis among homeless persons: recommendations of Advisory Council for Elimination of Tuberculosis, *MMWR* 41(RR-5):1, 1992.

Centers for Disease Control and Prevention: Recommendations for HIV testing services for inpatients and outpatients in acute-care hospital settings and technical guidance on HIV counseling, *MMWR* 42:1, 1993.

Collier JAH: Developmental and systems perspectives on chronic illness, *Holistic Nurs Pract* 5(1):1, 1990.

Frank E et al: Predictors of physicians' smoking cessation advice, *JAMA* 266:3139, 1991.

Friedan TR, Sterling T, Pablos-Mendez A: The emergence of drug-resistance tuberculosis: we can't afford not to try it, *N Engl J Med* 328:576, 1993.

Lewis BS, Lynch WD: The effect of physician advice on exercise behavior, *Prev Med* 22:110, 1993.

Simons-Morton DG et al: Characteristics of controlled studies of patient education and counseling for preventive health behaviors, *Pat Educ Couns* 19:175, 1992.

Turner RC, Wauvers LE, O'Brien KO. The effect of patient-carried reminder cards on the performance of health maintenance measures, *Arch Intern Med* 150:645, 1990.

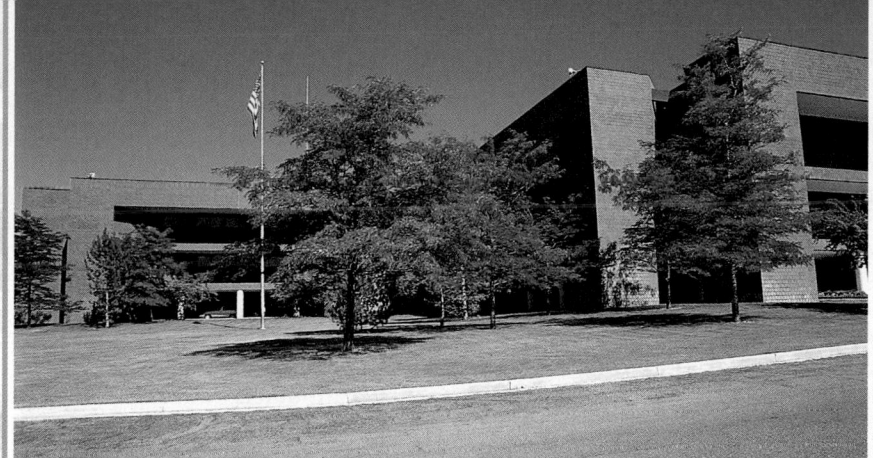

 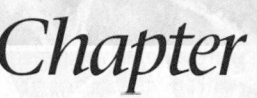 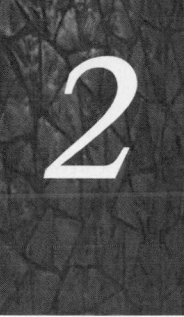
The Health Care Delivery System

Objectives

Mastery of content in this chapter will enable the student to:

▶ Define the key terms listed.

▶ Discuss major events in the evolution of the health care system.

▶ Discuss the principal factors influencing health care reform.

▶ Describe the type of quality measures that will be used to measure health system performance.

▶ Discuss factors influencing access to the health care system.

▶ Differentiate between primary, secondary, and tertiary levels of health care.

▶ Describe the types of health care agencies.

▶ Discuss the client's right to health care and describe client rights within the health care delivery system.

▶ Compare the various methods for financing health care.

▶ Explain the advantages and disadvantages of a capitated reimbursement system.

▶ Discuss nursing's role within delivery of care and work redesign methodologies.

The United States health care system is changing. Many health care institutions are no longer thriving economically, even though health care spending is climbing (Solovy, 1994). Experts estimate that by the year 2000 health care spending will be approximately 16% to 18% of the gross domestic product. Because business, industry, and the government are paying the majority of health care bills, they are demanding greater controls over use of resources and evidence that quality health care is being received by clients (Sovie, 1990). Health care institutions are scrambling to find better ways to provide health care at a lower cost. At the same time, they are being evaluated very closely by regulatory agencies such as the Joint Commission on Accreditation of Health Care Organizations (JCAHO), professional review organizations (PROs), and state health departments. The reviews focus on the outcomes of health care and whether clients leave health care institutions in an improved state of health with the capacity to manage their continued health care needs.

The consumers of health care are also changing. There are greater demands placed upon care providers due to an increase in the older adult and the chronically ill populations. The social environment for many clients is very difficult and demanding because of diminishing support from family and friends and changes in the economic environment (Bower, 1993). Clients are leaving acute care settings earlier at earlier stages of recovery, yet there are fewer resources at home for support.

Consumers of health care are concerned about accessing appropriate, cost-effective, quality health care. Access refers to consumers being able to easily use a broad range of health care providers including advanced practice nurses, primary care physicians, and medical specialists, at a variety of community health care sites (AONE, 1994). Furthermore, access should not be limited to those individuals who are healthy or those who have insurance coverage. Today, many consumers are penalized because of preexisting conditions, making insurance unobtainable. It is important for clients to be able to acquire needed health services easily, in cost-effective settings. Consumers also want health care institutions to be accountable for quality and to be able to show the influence interaction with health care systems has on clients' overall lives and their functional health status.

Nursing is a major component of the health care delivery system, and nurses make up the largest employment group within the system. Nursing services are necessary for virtually every client seeking care of any type, including primary, secondary, tertiary, and restorative. Because nursing is such an important part of the health care delivery system, the nurse needs to understand the system to effectively deliver quality care within it. Every nurse practicing today needs to appreciate that health care is a business. The success of any health care business depends on nursing's participation in creating the systems needed for delivering cost-effective care and creating strategies to ensure that clients receive quality care.

EVOLUTION OF THE HEALTH CARE DELIVERY SYSTEM

It is important to understand the developments leading to the creation of the current American health care delivery system. At the turn of the century, only a few urban hospitals existed in the United States. These institutions served the poor, whereas the affluent and middle-class members of the population were treated at home (McMahon, 1987). The early hospitals were primarily financed by voluntary donations and supported by groups such as churches. By the late 1920s, because of the very high losses faced by hospitals (many clients were unable to pay), a new system of payment was introduced—third-party payment (Smith, 1990). Hospital insurance plans quickly developed, and the cost of health care has grown ever since.

From the mid-1920s to mid-1930s there was much discussion at the government level regarding costs of medical care. No public assistance was available until 1935 brought the passage of the Social Security Act, which facilitated public assistance to blind persons, older adults, and dependent children. A major national health care conference in 1938 resulted in the first national discussion of a national health care program in the United States. A general consensus emerged from the conference about principles for improving the nation's health, but there was no agreement about how the costs of health care would be divided between federal and state governments (Smith, 1990). That problem still exists.

The end of World War II came in 1945. Prior to that time the U.S. government was not involved in the health care industry. The Hill-Burton Act of 1945 was passed, providing money for hospital construction, expansion, or improvement. As a result, new hospitals were built in suburban and rural settings. Large urban medical centers were expanded for scientific research and technological advances. The focus of teaching and research in larger academic settings resulted in higher costs in delivering care. For example, a client hospitalized in a teaching hospital would undergo a greater variety of diagnostic tests and procedures than one hospitalized in a smaller, private, community hospital. Academic medical centers continue to have higher costs in managing client care, making it difficult for these centers to compete with lower cost hospitals.

With the passage of the Medicare and Medicaid amendments to the Social Security Act in 1965, the U.S. government established national and state health insurance programs for certain segments of the population. The Medicare program provides health insurance for persons who are over 65 years of age or disabled. The Medicaid program provides a joint federal and state health insurance program for low-income persons in specific groups, including families with dependent children, older adults, blind or disabled persons, and persons who cannot afford medical care. Medicaid and Medicare are regulated through different eligibility requirements and benefits across states. The Medicaid program is voluntary. In Canada, similar but more inclusive medical services are provided by provincial medical care plans. The Social Security Amendments Act of 1972 changed the Medicare and Medicaid program, largely to control costs. From 1974 to 1981, succeeding amendments were made to control costs and improve cost-effectiveness strategies. In 1977 a new federal Health Care Financing Administration (HCFA) was created to administer the Medicare and Medicaid programs.

The National Health Planning and Resources Development Act of 1974 (PL 93-641) introduced a comprehensive system of health care planning. The law intended to bring together the work of new health systems agencies (HSAs) with that of state planning agencies. Previously fragmented federal programs for health planning were combined into one system. Consumers would shape local health plans and cut medical costs. A purpose of the Act was to improve planning and health care accessibility. For example, the construction of any new facility or the addition of beds to a hospital would be reviewed by planning groups. Local governments, private health care providers, and community groups failed to support the local and state planning agencies. Thus an abundance of hospital beds and expensive technology became available in most larger cities.

Although legislation was designed to provide for the expansion of hospitals and payment of services and to develop a system of health care planning, some legislation did affect certain professionals. The Rural Health Clinics Act of 1978 represented the U.S. government's willingness to allow nurse practitioners to deliver primary health care. This act provided for the development of rural health clinics in medically underserved areas, for the use of nurse practitioners as clinic staff, and for direct reimbursement to clinics for services provided by nurse practitioners to Medicare and Medicaid recipients. This law began the trend toward involving nurses in primary health care delivery.

During the 1970s, research was underway to identify similarities and differences between hospitals. Much attention was paid to the resources used by hospitals. Resource use depended on the types of clients for whom a hospital cared and the severity of their conditions, as well as usual treatments and procedures used. Yale University collaborated with the federal Social Security Administration and the State of New Jersey to determine whether the concept of defining groups of similar clients for resource **utilization review** could be used as a system for payment (Smith, 1990). In other words, if research showed that clients with similar diagnoses could be cared for at similar costs and with favorable results, diagnostic categories could be used for establishing payment of hospital costs nationally. The outcome of the research was the 1983 Medicare prospective pricing plan approved by Congress for most inpatient services as part of the Social Security Amendments of 1983. Hospitals were no longer reimbursed for all costs incurred in the care of a client. Instead payment for hospital services to Medicare clients was based on flat rates per admission based on **diagnosis-related groups (DRGs)**. The **prospective payment** system has been one of the most significant factors affecting the health care industry. Health care institutions no longer had unlimited resources. Fewer dollars were available for health care service provision and capital expenses, for example, addition and renovation to hospital facilities, acquisition of computer systems, and purchase of diagnostic equipment.

As Yale was conducting its research, there was considerable public attention to finding ways to control health care costs. By the end of 1969 the federal government supported the formation of comprehensive, prepaid, group practice corporations to stimulate competition, improve health system efficiency, raise quality of care, and increase access to health services (Drew, 1989). The **Health Maintenance Organization (HMO)** Act of 1973 established HMOs to provide comprehensive preventive and treatment services to a specific group of voluntarily enrolled persons under a fixed, prepaid plan. Members of an HMO made periodic payments in advance for expected costs of benefits for a population group. The HMOs promised to deliver specifically defined services within a fixed, prepaid system, offering an incentive to contain costs and unnecessary use of services. Thus began the concept of **managed care.**

Health care is a business whose central issues are rising costs and the availability of quality health care services. Financial pressures have forced hospitals and other health care institutions to shift organizational priorities. Less visionary institutions have attempted to control costs through reduction in the work force and support services needed to provide direct client care. There is a concern that institutions have made financial incentives a priority over quality humane care. Nursing professionals are in a position to help restructure care delivery systems while assuming responsibility for maintaining a level of excellence in health care. More than ever, the role of nursing in client advocacy will be critical to ensure that the health care needs of all populations are served.

■ HEALTH CARE REFORM

Health care reform has been discussed at every level in American life. The United States health care system has been scrutinized and compared with other systems in Canada, England, and Australia. Few people would disagree that change is needed within the United States system, even though it is seen by many as the best health care system in the world.

People usually have little or no interaction with the health care delivery system while experiencing good health. However, if they become ill, feel ill, or are motivated for other reasons to seek health care, they must enter the health care delivery system. Some clients enter the system easily by walking into a clinic or hospital emergency room or by making an appointment with a physician in private practice. Other clients experience difficulties in entering the system because of confusion or unfamiliarity with the agencies or because of inadequate health insurance. There are too many rural areas that lack accessible health care services. Populations in large cities may have better access but serious health problems, such as infant mortality, exist. Problems in urban areas are often due to a lack of primary care services. Urban areas have an excess of secondary and tertiary health care settings.

Too many people cannot afford health care. Health care costs continue to rise for three reasons. First, rising poverty levels reduce the percentage of mothers receiving prenatal care. Hence, premature births, low–birth-weight infants, and infant mortality and morbidity rates increase in the indigent population. The cost for the care of these clients is considerable. Second, the increase in the number of clients with chronic disease and AIDS or AIDS-related illness is costly to the health care system, as well as to public and private insurance carriers. Third, modern technology provides physicians and nurses with skills and treatments to care for victims of trauma and disease who, 10 years ago, would have died from the same problems. The costs of care within intensive care units are the highest in the health care system.

The care that is received may be unnecessary and is often fragmented, with resources used for the acute episode of illness rather than prevention. This results in more hospital days and higher costs. The challenge for America is to create a health care system that offers universal access to all members of the population, provides comprehensive care, is portable, accessible, and appropriate.

Legislative Initiatives

Health care reform is occurring in spite of the difficulties the U.S. government has had in selecting the best legislative package for change. It is important, however, to understand the issues in health care reform at the legislative level (Table 2-1). Because of the problems of universal access and rising costs there is growing public interest in a national health care plan. The goal of such a plan would be to provide all Americans with health insurance coverage. Options that have been considered include:

- Incremental expansion of public programs (Medicare and Medicaid).
- Mandatory requirements for employers to offer private health insurance to employees.
- A comprehensive national health plan (acute, long term, rehabilitation, dental, and occupational health) financed through progressive taxes.

The expansion of existing public programs would greatly benefit the poor. Long-term care proposals are particularly popular among older adults and the disabled. As of 1990 only 52% of nursing home services were covered by public or private insurance (Harrington, 1990). A problem with Medicare expansion proposals is that new voluntary programs could still not be paid for by persons of low income, who need the services the most. A single, integrated program is needed to ensure fair distribution to all.

The employer-based financing programs combine public and private financing mechanisms. Employers offer private insurance plans or pay taxes for public insurance coverage (Harrington, 1990). In addition, employers can buy insurance directly through public sponsors, and individuals would be encouraged to join managed care plans such as HMOs. Medicaid and Medicare would continue with most of these plans; however, there could be some restructuring to shift resources from acute to chronic and long-term care.

The problem with this category of plan is that many people might not be covered because small businesses, the self-employed, and part-time workers may be exempt.

The comprehensive national health plan may be modeled like the Canadian health plan. The plan would be mandatory and cover all individuals for comprehensive health services. Private-sector providers would provide services. Costly copayments and deductibles common with traditional insurance would be eliminated. It is believed that a single well-administered health plan would save millions of dollars in paper work alone. The concerns over the national health plan come from the proposed progressive tax system needed to fund the plan and a mistrust of the government bureaucracy needed to administer the plan.

Restructuring

The health care system in the next century will ensure access to more Americans. Hospitals, clinics, and physician practice groups have already begun to merge into large health care networks or systems. The larger networks will have greater resources through a variety of services than single hospitals. A network will have the bargaining power of buying larger volumes of supplies or equipment at a lower cost. The integrated networks will be designed to deliver a seamless continuum of comprehensive health care. This means any client who accesses the health care system will be able to do so at a single point and receive primary, preventive, acute, and rehabilitative care in a well-coordinated manner.

Providers will be paid based on **capitation**, with health care systems assuming responsibility for covered lives at a fixed cost per client, regardless of the amount of care given (hospitalization and outpatient). Capitated payments will be made on a periodic basis for each covered life within a health plan. Primary care providers will act as the gatekeepers to the system, controlling access. The focus will shift from acute, episodic care to a continuum of care provided for a large population. Primary care and prevention will achieve greater importance. Capitation will place financial risk on the providers who deliver services, thus offering an incentive to keep clients healthy and out of hos-

Table 2-1	**Health Care Reform Issues**	
ISSUE	**DEFINITION**	**IMPLICATIONS**
Universal access	A provision that would ensure all Americans receive insurance coverage through government support with employer subsidies.	Will require all employers (including small businesses) to offer or provide coverage.
Coverage	Pertains to who is to be included in a health care plan, and the components of the plan (e.g., HMO, standard benefit plan, or fee-for-service plan).	Federal government will pay for individuals below poverty level.
Restructured delivery	Allows community health service organizations (CHSO) to be formed. These are same as HMOs, providing comprehensive care on a capitated basis or annual budget basis. Network formation (merging of hospitals, clinics, MD practice groups) is encouraged to provide a seamless continuum of care.	Places more emphasis on primary care. Ultimately will reduce number of hospital beds.
Uniform benefits	The services offered in a universal health plan might include doctor's bills, hospital bills, prescription drugs, mental health, preventive care for children, and substance abuse treatment.	Limited coverage for long-term care. Congress will likely determine benefit package.

pitals. Hospitals will no longer become the primary center for health care, and thus the number of hospital beds within communities will decline. Community clinics, home health services, and outpatient centers will grow in importance. Use of a capitated payment system will encourage health care providers to promote the health of clients and prevent future, more costly illnesses; collaborate with other providers to avoid duplication of services; and conserve health care resources by providing appropriate and necessary care (Fraser et al, 1993).

Work Redesign

A trend that has appeared as a result of health care reform is **work redesign.** This refers to changing the actual structure and ultimately the responsibilities of the jobs people perform (Hackman and Oldham, 1980). Specifically, many health care institutions have looked at how care is delivered to clients. Are there ways to make work more efficient, help care providers become more productive, and improve clients' satisfaction with the level of care delivered?

Most hospitals can point to inefficiencies in services as a source of increasing costs. The work of client care often involves a variety of care providers, each often duplicating the work of others. In work redesign, an analysis is made of the work process being performed, for example, the admission of clients. Each task or activity (e.g., nursing history, delivering supplies, gathering specimens) associated with the process is reviewed to determine if it is necessary or appropriate. Then the analysis asks who is performing the task and should that person be doing it? In many work redesign studies it becomes apparent that indirect or nonnursing activities (e.g., gathering supplies, delivering meals, changing beds) occupy a high proportion of nurses' time (Tonges, 1992). Work redesign of nursing delivery systems ultimately involves identifying the aspects of traditional nursing care that can be safely and appropriately assigned to nonlicensed staff. This may mean the creation of multipurpose roles that combine elements such as housekeeping, dietary, supply clerk, and nurse's aide, to better facilitate work on a nursing unit (Tonges, 1992). Services formerly centralized in hospital departments (e.g., pharmacy or physical therapy) are distributed to client care units. The professional nurse's roles become focused on clinical decision making, coordination of care in collaboration with physicians, and client education and discharge planning. Ultimately when work redesign is well organized, staff are better satisfied and clients gain more efficient care.

Quality Measures of Performance

Quality health care has often been difficult to define. Unless health care providers can define quality, the purchasers of health care (employers, insurers, HMOs, etc.) will buy based upon price alone. For many years hospitals gathered information on mortality rates, length of stay, and patient satisfaction. Although these measures can be useful, health care providers are defining quality in terms of outcomes. Examples of outcomes are the readmission rates for sickle cell clients, functional health status of clients following discharge (e.g., ability and time frame for returning to work), and the rate of postoperative infection. Not all providers agree on what outcomes are most important, there are few measures that are comparable across institutions, and not

all health care systems have the same data available for measurement.

Governmental and regulatory agencies such as the Joint Commission on Accreditation of Health Care Organizations (JCAHO, 1996) are beginning to define the outcome indicators used to determine a health system's performance. These same indicators can be used to compare a given system with others in the same community. The JCAHO has already developed the Indicator Measurement System (IMS). Participation is currently voluntary, but it will likely become a mandatory part of health care institutions' accreditation process. The IMS, unlike many state or local initiatives, is well designed, tested, and **risk adjusted.** Clients of both low and high acuity are measured by the IMS so that outcomes are a fair reflection of the specific institutions' client population.

Systems like the IMS will provide consumers with a quality "report card" of various health agencies to help in deciding what system provides the best care (Fig. 2-1). The Health Care Advisory Board (1994) predicts that health systems will be asked to report on indicators that reflect treatment of disease as well as managing clients' health (see the box on p. 26). All of the measures can help an institution manage cost and quality. The indicators that will have the greatest impact on payers and consumers selecting a health system are yet unknown, however, the Health Care Advisory Board rates access, appropriateness, service quality, encounter outcomes, and disease management as having the greatest potential influence. It is clear that by the turn of the century health systems will be required to not only manage costs so as to remain competitive but also to demonstrate measurably how quality of care is achieved.

■ LEVELS OF HEALTH CARE

Health care is provided at three levels: primary care, secondary or acute care, and tertiary care. Each provides a structure for how health care services are organized and de-

	Star Health plan	Winner Health plan	Quality Health plan
Wait time for referrals	0	+	0
Time waiting in emergency	#	0	+
Unplanned readmissions	0	#	@
C-section rate	+	#	0
Childhood flu immunization rates	0	@	@
Pneumonia mortality	+	#	0
Hospital satisfaction	0	#	+
Overall ranking	85.0	76.2	80.4

Fig. 2-1 Example of a health system report card.

Health System Quality Measures

Access:	Information tells consumers how easy it is to gain access to medical services (e.g., timeliness of care, availability of physicians, and geographical convenience).
Appropriateness:	Indicators that show discrepancies between actual care given and level of care considered "necessary", thereby representing a system's ability to provide cost effective care. Examples: length of stay, frequency of procedure versus ideal rate.
Service quality:	Indicators of whether consumers believe that a health plan or system is responsive, pleasant, and "user friendly." Examples: overall satisfaction with care, time spent waiting in ER, speed of billing.
Screening measures:	Rate-based indicators of the effectiveness of a plan's efforts to screen a targeted population for early detection of a disease. Examples: pap smear or cholesterol screening rate.
Encounter outcomes:	Measures of the results of specific clinical encounters. Examples: mortality rates, unplanned return to emergency, disease specific complications (postoperative shock, wound infection, respiratory arrest).
Disease management:	Indicators of the health plan's or system's success in treating an entire disease across a continuum of care. Examples: heart disease, diabetes, primary care (utilization rates of preventive services), specialty care (diagnosis specific health status scores).
Prevention measures:	Indicators of the frequency and effectiveness of the preventive care provided to consumers of a health plan. Examples: annual number of prevention visits, percentage of women receiving prenatal care during first trimester.
Consumer health status:	Indicators of a health plan's ability to maintain the health of its enrolled population. Examples: incidence and prevalence of cancer or heart disease, general health index.

Modified from Health Care Advisory Board: *Next generation of outcomes tracking: implications for health plans and systems,* vol 2, *Quality measures,* Washington, DC, 1994, The Advisory Board Co.

livered. For example, primary care tends to be delivered in physician's offices and community clinics and tertiary care is more commonly provided in hospitals and rehabilitation facilities.

In addition there are three levels of prevention that help to explain clients' health behavior at different stages of illness. A client may be receiving one level of health care while participating in different levels of prevention, depending on the complexity of health care needs. The nurse assumes significant responsibility for delivering care to clients at all levels and in initiating preventive measures. Levels of health care and the levels of prevention are defined as follows:

- Primary Care—Primary care involves the first contact a client makes in a given episode of illness that leads to a decision regarding a course of action to resolve any real or potential health problem. The providers of primary health care are often internists, pediatricians, obstetricians, and nurse practitioners. Settings for primary care include physician's offices, nurse-managed clinics, schools, and occupational health settings.
- Primary Prevention—Aimed toward health promotion and protection against illness. Primary preventive measures are applied before a disease manifests itself through signs and symptoms. Health promotion includes good measures of nutrition and attention to personality development.
- Secondary Care—Secondary care involves provision of a specialized medical service by a physician specialist or a hospital on referral by a primary care physician. A client has developed recognizable signs and symptoms that are either definitively diagnosed or require further diagnostic review. Secondary care settings include hospitals and ambulatory care clinics.

- Secondary Prevention—Directed toward health maintenance for clients experiencing health problems, complications, or disabilities. Secondary prevention occurs during the period of pathogenesis after a disease has manifested signs and symptoms. Two levels of secondary prevention include early diagnosis and prompt treatment (e.g., hypertension screening) and acute care.
- Tertiary Care—A level of care that is specialized and highly technical in diagnosing and treating complicated or unusual health problems. Clients who require teritary care present with an extensive and often complicated pathological condition.
- Tertiary Prevention—Deals with the rehabilitation and return of clients to a status of maximal function within the limits posed by disease or disability. This level of prevention occurs after a disease has caused extensive damage, as in the case of a stroke.

With health care reform, greater emphasis is being placed on primary care and prevention. Nursing has the chance to provide leadership to communities and health care systems who are aligning resources to better serve their populations. Critical to the success of improving primary care delivery is the ability to find strategies that successfully change client behavior and link clients to resources so that healthier lifestyles can be pursued.

█ HEALTH CARE SERVICES

A broad variety of health care services (see the box on p. 27) are available to clients and families, depending on the nature and extent of a health problem and level of care required. The types of services offered also often depend on the site in which clients seek health care (e.g., a hospital or mental health clinic).

Examples of Health Care Services

HEALTH PROMOTION
- Prenatal classes
- Classes on care of elderly parents
- Nutrition counseling
- Exercise classes
- Stress management
- Smoking cessation classes
- Family planning

ILLNESS PREVENTION
- Screening programs (e.g., hypertension, high cholesterol levels, breast cancer [mammography])
- Mental health counseling and crisis prevention
- Immunizations
- Occupational health and safety measures (e.g., work place ventilation, protective eye wear, noise control)
- Public legislation (e.g., seat belts, air bags, helmets, school bus codes)
- Poison control information

PRIMARY CARE
- School and college health units
- Routine checkups or physical examinations
- Follow-up for chronic illness
- Community mental health centers

DIAGNOSIS
- Radiological procedures (e.g., MRI and CT scans, x-ray studies)
- Physical examinations (system focused)
- Blood testing

TREATMENT
- Client education for specific disease management
- Surgical intervention
- Laser therapies
- Pharmacological therapies

REHABILITATION
- Cardiovascular programs
- Pulmonary programs
- Sports medicine
- Alcohol- and drug-dependence programs
- Mental illness programs
- Stroke and spinal-cord–injury programs
- Home health care

CONTINUING CARE
- Geriatric day care
- Hospice
- Domiciliary homes
- Psychiatric day care

Health Promotion and Prevention

Health-promotion services are a key to quality health care. By keeping people healthy, the overall costs of health care decline. Preventive care also involves health-promotion activities, including specific health education programs designed to help clients reduce the risk of illness, maintain maximal function, and promote habits related to good health. Health-promotion activities take place in many settings. For example, community clinics offer programs such as prenatal nutrition classes in which the essentials of good nutrition during pregnancy, after childbirth, and for the infant are taught. These classes promote the general health of the woman, fetus, and infant.

Illness prevention is an important component of health care. It is a service that assists clients and families in reducing risk factors for disease. Immunization programs are one example of a service that improves the health not only of individuals but also a community as a whole (see Chapter 3).

Primary Care

Primary care services involve the client directly and usually involve the first contact with a primary care provider, for example, physician or nurse practitioner. The focus is on early detection as well as routine care (Fig. 2-2). For example, primary care services include annual physical examinations as well as routine follow-up for clients with known health problems such as high blood pressure. Primary care services should be easily accessible to clients either in their community or place of work. Critical to the success of primary care is understanding a client's health belief values and using strategies that respect the client's cultural and socioeconomic resources. This is important in assisting clients

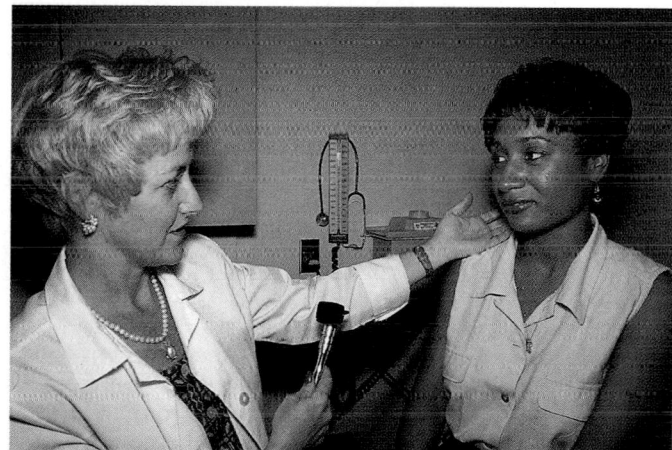

Fig. 2-2 Advance practice nurses play an important role in primary care delivery.

to accept whatever health care practices are necessary to prevent or reverse episodes of illness.

Diagnosis and Treatment

The diagnosis and treatment of illness are traditionally the most commonly used services of the health care system. These services can be delivered in primary care settings. However, once a client develops a more complicated problem and the primary care provider is not able to care for a particular condition, a medical specialist is often needed (see Chapter 4). Typically, secondary care delivered in acute care setting is quite costly, particularly if clients wait to have health care after symptoms have developed.

Clients with serious complications or who suffer from chronic disease require ongoing care and frequently are readmitted to hospitals. Acute episodes of illness that require hospitalization often result in use of sophisticated diagnostic procedures and complex therapeutic procedures, all of which are costly. With health care reform there has been greater attention paid to determining whether highly technological diagnostic procedures are needed in all cases. These procedures can be expensive and their use may not contribute to better quality care or outcomes.

On the positive side, advances in technology and computers have resulted in diagnostic procedures that improve the chance of early diagnosis. Many new diagnostic tests are noninvasive and painless. Furthermore, diagnostic services can now be brought to a client; hospitals have equipped motorized vans with diagnostic x-ray equipment and offer services at sites such as shopping malls and public libraries.

Treatment methods have also expanded because of advances in technology and knowledge. Clients are receiving newer, more innovative health care treatments based on the most recent research. Treatment of illnesses has also expanded outside hospitals and other institutions into the home. When treatment is initiated within a health care institution, nurses teach the client and family to complete the treatment plan at home and in the outpatient setting.

Rehabilitation

Rehabilitation is the restoration of a person to normal or near-normal function after a physical or mental illness, injury, or chemical addiction. Rehabilitation was once available primarily for clients with illnesses or injury to the nervous system, but the health care delivery system has expanded its scope of such services. Today, specialized rehabilitation services, such as cardiovascular and pulmonary rehabilitation programs, help clients and families adjust to necessary changes in lifestyle and learn to function with limitations of their disease (see Chapter 5).

Rehabilitation services begin the moment a client enters the health care system. Initially, rehabilitation may focus on the prevention of complications related to the illness or injury. As the condition stabilizes, rehabilitation is directed at maximizing the client's functioning and level of independence.

Continuing Care

Continuing care services offer clients ongoing supportive care for chronic, long-term health problems. This includes services for clients with physical disabilities as well as mental illness. Continuous medical care is not necessary to keep these clients functional and active. Clients and families are given alternatives that allow clients to remain within the home setting. A psychiatric day hospital offers therapeutic programs for individuals as well as groups of clients during daytime hours. Clients receive ongoing therapy but return to their homes in the evenings. Many continuing care services, such as hospice and geriatric day-care centers, relieve the burden of families having to provide all of the support to loved ones.

■ TYPES OF HEALTH CARE AGENCIES

Health care is provided in a variety of settings. With health care reform, fewer clients are cared for in hospitals. Alternatives include outpatient, institutional, community-based, volunteer, hospice, and government health care agencies.

Outpatient Agencies

Clients who do not require hospitalization can receive health care in an alternative site such as a clinic or other ambulatory care facility. **Outpatient services** are generally directed at primary and secondary care. An outpatient setting is designed to be convenient and easily accessible to clients.

PRIMARY PROVIDER OFFICES

Primary provider offices offer primary care for a large segment of the population. Physicians in office practice tend to focus on the diagnosis and treatment of specific illnesses rather than on health promotion and other services. However, this trend is slowly changing. More health care plans require enrollees to have regular physical examinations or "checkups" with their primary physician. During these visits physicians screen for possible health problems and make recommendations to minimize or control risk factors. With more competition in health care, physicians' offices now offer a wider range of diagnostic and therapeutic services. Some offices have complete laboratory facilities for analyzing specimens and obtaining electrocardiograms and radiographs (x-ray films). Diagnostic procedures such as sigmoidoscopy and ultrasound can also be performed. Simple surgical procedures such as biopsies and removal of skin lesions are offered.

Nurses employed in physicians' offices can assume many roles. Some nurses have the traditional role of registering clients, taking vital signs, preparing the client for examination or laboratory studies, and providing basic information. Other nurses work collaboratively with physicians in advanced practice roles, conducting physical examinations and histories, offering health education, and recommending therapies for clients in stable health states. Advanced practice nurses can directly manage caseloads of stable, healthy client populations with great success. These nurses provide follow-up care to their clients during repeat visits.

CLINICS

Clinics traditionally involve a department in a hospital where clients not requiring hospitalization receive medical care (Fig. 2-3). They may also exist in the form of a group practice of physicians, a nurse-run ambulatory clinic, or a community agency that delivers a particular type of health service such as immunizations. Frequently clients who use clinics are from a lower socioeconomic level or are older adults with fixed incomes. Clients who suffer chronic disease are frequent visitors to clinics. Costs for clinic services are generally lower than for other health services. However, the services are often fragmented. Clients may not see the same health care provider consistently and there may be poor communication of the client's health status when care transfers to the acute setting.

Nurse-managed clinics or nursing centers have developed over the past 20 years to provide high-quality nursing

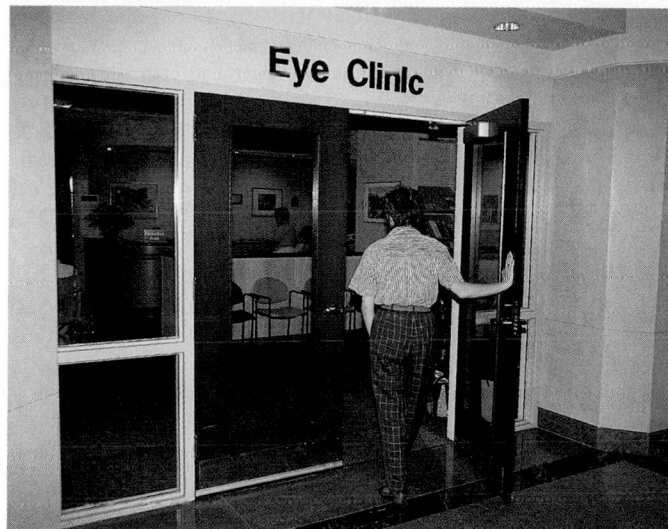

Fig. 2-3 Health care clinics offer early detection and education to clients seeking preventive care.

Nurse-Managed Clinic Services

- Physical and developmental assessment
- Health risk appraisal
- Wellness counseling
- Health education
- Psychosocial counseling
- Care and prevention of common diseases
- Acute and chronic care management
- Home care services
- Imaging, visualization, and therapeutic touch

services with a focus on health promotion and health education, disease prevention, chronic disease management, and support for self-care and care givers (Aydelotte and Gregory, 1989; Riesch, 1992). The clinics are typically managed by nurses in advanced practice roles such as nurse practitioners and clinical nurse specialists. However, registered nurses in traditional roles also are actively involved in the clinics. Many of the clinics operate in association with academic centers to combine teaching and research in a nurse-controlled environment (Phillips and Steel, 1994). The clinics maintain a collaborative and consultative relationship with physicians. This is necessary in most states to guarantee reimbursement for services. The services offered in a nurse-managed clinic are varied (see the box above). It is how the services are delivered that makes a nurse-managed clinic unique.

Primary care services delivered by nurses are different than those delivered by physicians in primary care settings. The nurse in an advanced practice role combines nursing and medical knowledge within a perspective of client-centered care (Phillips and Steel, 1994). This means that nursing stresses education and self-care. Clients who suffer chronic illness must partner with families in order to do the work of managing their illness. A nurse-managed clinic designs services to help people assume more responsibility for their health and to acquire necessary coping skills. Over the long term, advanced practice nurses are very effective in improving client outcomes by enabling clients to remain functional within their home and community.

AMBULATORY CARE CENTERS

Ambulatory care centers, like clinics, provide health services on an outpatient basis. The centers may be affiliated with hospitals or function independently under a corporation or a single physician or group of physicians. An ambulatory care center may be located within an inpatient facility; however, most are stand-alone centers located away from a major inpatient institution. A "Surgi-Center" is one

example of an ambulatory care center where clients come for minor surgical procedures such as cataract extraction, plastic surgery, and endoscopic procedures. An "urgent-care center" provides 24-hour service to clients for minor injuries or illnesses such as lacerations and influenza. The urgent-care center offers an alternative to a hospital emergency room.

Institutions

Institutional agencies include hospitals, extended care facilities, psychiatric facilities, and rehabilitation centers. All offer health care services to **inpatients** (clients admitted to a stay within an institution for diagnosis, treatment, or rehabilitative services). Most also offer services to outpatients (clients visiting the institution for an episode of diagnosis or treatment lasting only a few hours).

HOSPITALS

Hospitals traditionally have been the major agency of the health care system. Typically a client came to a hospital for diagnosis and treatment and remained hospitalized until almost fully recovered. However, prospective reimbursement has changed how clients are cared for in hospitals. A client within a certain diagnostic-related group (DRG) is expected to be cared for and discharged within a projected period. For example, a woman who delivers a baby without complications is expected to be discharged home within 24 to 48 hours in most hospitals.

Today, clients who enter hospitals are acutely ill and need comprehensive and specialized tertiary health care. The services provided by hospitals vary considerably. Small rural hospitals with only 40 beds may offer only limited emergency and diagnostic services, as well as general inpatient services. In comparison, large urban medical centers offer comprehensive, state-of-the-art diagnostic services, emergency care, surgical intervention, intensive care units, inpatient services, and rehabilitation facilities. Larger hospitals also offer professional staff from a variety of specialties such as social service, respiratory therapy, physical and occupational therapy, and speech therapy. The focus in hospitals is to provide the highest quality of care possible so that clients can be discharged early but safely to the home or a facility that can adequately manage remaining health care needs. If clients are not fully recovered, alternative care sites are found, including extended care facilities, nursing homes, and home care. Many insurers even deny hospitalization for clients with "minor" conditions.

Hospitals are classified as *public* or *private*. Public and private hospitals exist throughout Canada and the United States. A public hospital is financed and operated by a government agency at the local, state, provincial, or national level. Many clients in public hospitals cannot afford to pay for care. The hospitals provide services at a not-for-profit rate. Private hospitals are owned and operated by groups such as churches, corporations, businesses, and charitable organizations. The majority of clients who enter private hospitals have some type of insurance or medical assistance to pay for care. Private hospitals are operated on a for-profit or not-for-profit basis. The profit status influences how revenue can be used for services and taxation purposes. Many large corporations such as Humana and the Hospital Corporation of America (HCA) operate groups of for-profit hospitals across the United States.

Another type of hospital is the military hospital. Military hospitals are located throughout the United States and in countries around the world to provide medical care for members of the armed forces and their families.

A nurse who works within a hospital has the opportunity to work in a variety of roles and different departments. The care of clients on an inpatient nursing unit or within an intensive care unit requires the nurse to have the knowledge and skills for applying the nursing process (see Unit II) using critical thinking, providing client education, coordinating health care services and discharge planning, and delivering a variety of therapies. As the depth of nursing knowledge increases, many nurses specialize their practice. This allows them to become expert in the care of select client populations. Many hospitals have, for example, specialized units for the care of clients with oncological, orthopedic, pulmonary, or cardiac problems. Other opportunities within a hospital setting may include the role of client educator, nurse manager, clinical nurse specialist, and infection control coordinator.

SUBACUTE CARE

There has been a recent growth in **subacute care** units, designated sites that provide medical specialty care for clients who need a greater intensity of care than generally provided in a skilled nursing facility but who no longer require acute care (Stahl, 1994). Generally clients who have suffered an acute illness, injury, or worsening of a disease and require continued hospitalization are candidates for subacute care. Clients receive goal-oriented treatment given immediately after or instead of acute hospitalization to treat one or more specific, active complex medical conditions or to administer technically complex treatments (Stahl, 1994). Many of the clients who require subacute care are outliers (those who have exhausted their inpatient DRG days). Thus a hospital can transfer a client to a subacute unit and reduce its financial risk since the stay on the unit meets different reimbursement guidelines. In addition, physicians have less concern over releasing clients to an outside setting when a hospital-based subacute unit is available. Subacute units are located in hospitals, as well as skilled nursing and rehabilitation facilities.

EXTENDED CARE FACILITIES

An **extended care facility** is an institution providing intermediate and long-term medical, nursing, or custodial care for clients recovering from acute illness or clients with chronic illnesses or disabilities. Extended care facilities include intermediate care and skilled nursing facilities, long-term care and nursing homes, and some retirement community institutions. At one point, extended care facilities primarily cared for older adults. However, as hospitals manage clients toward early discharge, there is a greater need for intermediate care settings for clients of all ages. For example, a young client who has experienced a stroke or traumatic accident may be transferred to an extended care facility for rehabilitative or supportive care until discharge to the home becomes a safe option. The growth of extended care facilities will increase as the number of older adults grows. With a "graying" population on the rise, more extended care facilities are needed.

Intermediate Care. An intermediate care or **skilled nursing facility** offers skilled care from a licensed nursing staff. This may include administration of intravenous fluids, wound care, long-term ventilator management, and physical rehabilitation. Extensive supportive care is provided until clients can move back into the community or into residential care. Third-party payers cover skilled nursing care. Extended care facilities provide around-the-clock nursing coverage. Nurses employed in such a setting have expertise similar to that of nurses working in acute-care inpatient settings. In addition, the nurse should have a background in gerontological nursing principles.

Long-Term Care. A long-term care facility or nursing home provides 24-hour intermediate and custodial care such as bathing, dressing, feeding, and exercise therapy for clients of any age with chronic or debilitating illnesses. The majority of clients in long-term care facilities are older adults. Custodial care is not reimbursed by most insurers. Long-term care has been under attack for years because of claims regarding inadequate care and abuses. Many of the claims have been justified. However, much of the negative public opinion about nursing homes is based on misconceptions about the level of care provided. The box on p. 31 compares nursing functions in long-term and acute care institutions. It is important for a nurse working in a long-term care facility to accept the philosophy that long-term care is not the end for the older adult, that life continues with meaning and value, and that the nurse is an important person in the older adult's life. The nurse can assist the individual to move in a more positive direction to attain or retain that meaning and value.

Residential Community. A third type of extended care facility is a residential or retirement community. Clients live in separate apartments or condominiums that compose a residential center. The clients remain relatively independent within a partially protective setting. Usually people keep all personal possessions in their residences. Services available within retirement communities include 24-hour nursing care, emergency medical care, housekeeping, laundry, transportation, social activities, and food service. The residential community bridges the gap between independent living and placement in a nursing home.

PSYCHIATRIC FACILITIES

Clients who suffer emotional and behavioral problems such as depression, violent behavior, and eating disorders often require special counseling and treatment in psychi-

---

Nursing Functions in Caring for Older Adults in Institutions

LONG-TERM CARE

- Provide a milieu for living rather than illness and dying.
- Teach clients and families.
- Counsel clients and family.
- Learn about and use community resources, advise family and client of same.
- Establish short-term and long-term goals; evaluate progress toward both periodically.
- Secure and maintain health, recreation, and social history.
- Plan and coordinate care.
- Teach ancillary personnel.
- Communicate clients' needs in written and verbal form.
- Give treatments, medications, and rehabilitative exercises.
- Observe and evaluate client response to treatment, medications, and care plan.
- Teach health care maintenance to staff and clients.
- Keep physician aware of changes in clients' condition.
- Institute life-saving measures in the absence of a physician.
- Perform physical assessment of clients.
- Ensure adequate medical, dental, and podiatric care for clients.
- Maintain hydration, nutrition, aeration, and comfort.

ACUTE CARE

- Support client in achieving highest level of autonomy possible in situation.
- Provide appropriate information to client and family about treatment plan, medications, and diagnosis in collaboration with physician.
- Collaborate with multiprofessionals, client, and family to develop a comprehensive care plan.
- Supervise ancillary personnel.
- Recognize implications of syndromes for client care (e.g., renal failure, coronary disease, emphysema).
- Protect clients from injury or iatrogenic disease.
- Perform physical and psychosocial assessments and integrate in nursing care plan.
- Initiate action as outlined in nursing protocols regarding various conditions.
- Provide emergency treatment as needed (e.g., cardiopulmonary resuscitation, amelioration of shock, hemorrhage, convulsions, poisoning).
- Alert physician to changes in client status and abnormal findings of tests.
- Maintain hydration, nutrition, aeration, and comfort.

From Ebersole P, Hess P: *Toward healthy aging: human needs and nursing response*, ed 4, St Louis, 1994, Mosby.

---

atric facilities. Located in hospitals, independent outpatient clinics, or private mental health hospitals, psychiatric facilities offer inpatient and outpatient services, depending on the seriousness of the problem. Clients may enter these facilities voluntarily or involuntarily.

Voluntary hospitalization involves relatively short stays with the purpose of stabilizing the client. A comprehensive multidisciplinary treatment plan involving clients and families is established for clients with psychiatric illness. Medicine, nursing, social work, and activity therapy collaborate to develop a plan of care that will enable clients to return to functional states within the community. At discharge from inpatient facilities, clients are usually referred for follow-up care at clinics or with counselors.

REHABILITATION CENTER

A **rehabilitation center** is a residential institution providing therapy and training to restore clients to optimal levels of functioning and independence. Rehabilitation centers actively involve clients and families in providing health care. The goal of rehabilitation is to decrease the clients' dependence on the care provided so that they assume responsibility for personal care.

Rehabilitation centers employ persons from nursing, medicine, and the allied health fields such as physical therapy. Many rehabilitation centers focus on physical rehabilitation programs to teach the client and family to achieve maximal physical function after a stroke, head or spinal cord injury, or other physical impairment. **Drug rehabilitation centers** help the client become free from drug dependence and return to the community. Nurses employed

in rehabilitation centers are committed to long-term continuity of nursing services and must be knowledgeable in their specialized area.

Community-Based Agencies

Community-based health care agencies focus on providing health care to clients within their neighborhoods. Examples of such agencies are adult day-care centers, home health care agencies, rural primary care hospitals, crisis intervention centers, and specialized support groups such as Alcoholics Anonymous. Nurses may have a variety of roles within these agencies.

ADULT DAY-CARE CENTERS

Adult day-care centers provide health care to specific client populations during the day. They may be associated with a hospital or nursing home or exist as independent centers. Frequently the clients of such centers do not require hospitalization but need continuous health care services while their families or support persons work. These clients include older adults needing daily physical rehabilitation, individuals with emotional illnesses needing daily counseling, and individuals with chemical dependence problems who are involved in rehabilitation programs. Adult day-care centers reduce the cost of health care and allow clients to retain more independence by living at home.

Nurses working in day-care centers provide continuity between care delivered in the home and in the center. For instance, nurses can ensure that the client continues to take prescribed medication, and can administer specific treatments; the nurse can also assist the client through counseling sessions. Knowledge of community needs and resources is essential in providing adequate support of clients who often spend only a few hours a week in the day-care setting (Ebersole and Hess, 1994).

HOME HEALTH CARE AGENCIES

A **home health care agency** is an organization providing professional and nonprofessional health care services in the home (see Chapter 5). Home health care has been one of the fastest growing areas of health care due to the emphasis on early discharge by hospitals. Many hospitals now operate home health care agencies. Other corporations, such as the Visiting Nurses Association and community health centers, provide home care.

RURAL HOSPITALS

In 1989 the Omnibus Budget Reconciliation Act (OBRA) directed the Department of Health and Human Services to create a new health care entity, rural primary care hospitals (RPCH). An RPCH provides 24-hour emergency care, with no more than six inpatient beds for providing temporary care for 72 hours or less to clients needing stabilization before transfer to a larger hospital. Physicians, nurse practitioners, or physician assistants staff the RPCH (Sharp, 1991). Access to health care in rural areas has been a serious problem. Most rural hospitals have had a severe shortage of primary care providers. Many have been forced to close because of economic failure. The RPCH can provide inpatient care to acutely ill or injured persons before they are transferred to better-equipped facilities. Basic radiological and laboratory services are also available.

With health care reform, more big-city health care systems are branching out and establishing affiliations or mergers with rural hospitals. The rural hospitals provide a referral base to the larger tertiary care medical centers. Recently, federal laws have granted higher cost-based rates of payment from Medicare and Medicaid to certified rural health clinics (Montague, 1994). The number of these clinics has grown significantly in the last few years. Better partnerships and reimbursement should ensure survival of rural health care and improve access for millions of citizens.

Nurses who work in rural hospitals or clinics often function independently in the absence of a physician. Competence in physical assessment, clinical decision making, and emergency care is essential. Nurse practitioners use medical protocols or work under collaborative agreements with staff physicians.

CRISIS INTERVENTION CENTERS

Crisis intervention centers provide emergency psychiatric care and counseling to clients experiencing extreme stress or conflict, often involving suicide attempts or drug or alcohol abuse. These centers, which are usually self-contained units within a hospital or community health care center, provide services 24 hours a day. The services may be delivered directly on the premises, or counseling may be provided over the telephone. The primary objectives of crisis intervention centers are to help the person cope with the immediate problem and to offer guidance and support for long-term therapy (see Chapter 22).

Support Groups

Support groups provide self-help services for clients with select health problems, for example, loss of spouse, drug addiction, or cancer. Participants receive emotional support and information on ways to adjust to personal and health problems. For example, Alcoholics Anonymous is an international nonprofit organization of recovering alcoholic persons whose purpose is to help alcoholics stop drinking and remain sober through group support, shared experiences, and faith in a higher power. Meetings are held in a central community location such as a church, school, or hospital. Al-Anon assists families in helping alcoholic family members, and Alateen helps teenagers cope with alcoholism in their families.

Support groups are usually organized by groups of clients who have experienced common health problems. Reach to Recovery is an example of a support group comprising clients who have undergone mastectomy or breast reconstruction surgery. Through support groups, clients can discuss problems and learn that other people share those problems. Participants also learn to problem solve and offer each other the emotional support needed to deal with crises.

Volunteer Agencies

Volunteer agencies are not-for-profit health care agencies established nationally or within a community to meet a specific need. Examples are the American Lung Association and the American Cancer Society and, in Canada, the Canadian Lung Association and the Canadian Heart Foundation. Most volunteer agencies do not provide treatment but have programs for the prevention and detection of specific illnesses; public education is a major focus. In addition, some volunteer agencies provide financial support for training of physicians and nurses, as well as for biomedical research directed at the prevention, detection, or treatment of certain diseases.

Volunteer agencies depend heavily on professional and lay volunteers to perform many of their activities. Financial support is generally derived from fund-raising activities, federal grants, and donations from individuals. Many health professionals donate time and resources to agencies within their specialty.

Hospices

A **hospice** is a system of family-centered care designed to allow clients to live and remain at home with comfort, independence, and dignity while alleviating the strains caused by terminal illness. The focus of hospice care is palliative care, not curative treatments (see Chapter 26). Hospices can benefit a client in the terminal phases of any disease, such as cardiomyopathy, multiple sclerosis, acquired immunodeficiency syndrome (AIDS), cancer, emphysema, or renal disease.

A client entering a hospice has reached the terminal phase of illness (generally final 6 weeks), and the client, family, and physician have agreed that no further treatment can reverse the disease process. An attempt is made to provide care that ensures death with dignity in the client's home. The client and family must accept the fact that the hospice will not use emergency measures such as cardiopulmonary resuscitation to prolong life. Instead, the hospice provides pain control and comfort measures to maintain the quality of life. A multidisciplinary approach involving physician, nurses, social workers, pharmacists, and pastoral care staff is critical to the hospice program.

Hospice care is focused within the home, but occasionally clients require readmission to a hospital or care unit because the physical care becomes too burdensome for the family. Hospices are operated by independent agencies that are not affiliated with a hospital, by home care agencies, and by hospitals where special units are established in a separate area of the institution.

Nurses who work in hospices are employed in institutional and community settings. Hospice nurses are committed to the philosophy and objectives of the facilities for which they work. They provide care and support for the client and family during the terminal phase, at the time of death, and continue to offer bereavement counseling and follow-up to the family following the client's death.

Most hospice programs rely on community volunteers to make ongoing visits to clients' homes and to offer **respite care.** Caring for a terminally ill spouse or relative can be emotionally and physically draining. Respite care provides a primary care provider such as a spouse or family member the opportunity to have some time alone. A nurse or specially trained volunteer comes to the home so that the primary care provider can run errands or have a break from the responsibility of direct care. The respite care service is important in maintaining the health of the care giver and family.

Government Agencies

Government agencies are clinics, hospitals, and other health services supported by local, state, provincial, or national taxes. Local government agencies include city hospitals and public health clinics. Agencies at the state or provincial level include state psychiatric hospitals and hospitals for clients with pulmonary disease. National agencies include primary research institutions such as the National Institutes of Health (NIH) and agencies administering health and welfare programs for a country, such as the Canadian Department of National Health and Welfare.

The types of local and state or provincial agencies and the allocation of resources for these agencies vary from one city, state, or province to another. Usually, agency funds originate in the tax base and are controlled by elected or appointed officials.

Health departments at the city or county level are generally concerned with specific health needs of the community (e.g., immunization and prenatal care) and may receive additional support from the state or provincial health organization. Federal agencies provide specific kinds of health services on a national level. Of the many health-related national agencies in the United States and Canada, two are described in the following paragraphs: VA hospitals and the Canadian health care system.

VETERANS ADMINISTRATION HOSPITALS

VA hospitals were established after World War II to provide care for injured and disabled veterans. They are generally near medical schools and major medical centers with teaching and training functions. Many of the medical staff members in a VA hospital are supplied by the medical school. Nursing services in VA hospitals are provided around the clock. Nursing services and nursing roles in these hospitals are similar to those in nongovernment hospitals.

CANADIAN HEALTH CARE SYSTEM

The Canadian health care system includes a Department of National Health and Welfare, which is responsible for enforcing federal laws about harmful foods and drugs, providing health care services for certain categories of people, promoting fitness and amateur sports, administrating social welfare programs, and overseeing financial and technical programs (Stewart, 1985). Universal health care is available in Canada, supported by tax dollars. Most general and specialized hospital costs are financed by provincial hospital insurance plans.

▌ HEALTH CARE DELIVERY ISSUES

Health care delivery, the methods used to provide health care services, is changing in response to the critical issues of health care reform. A shift is occurring, with more health care delivered in outpatient settings. Hospitals are seeking new ways to deliver care to gain efficiency and shorten length of stay. Greater attention is being paid to the importance of preventive health care, with institutions offering services that help individuals and families maintain health or detect illness in an early phase. Health care providers are also learning that the health of a community and its citizens are closely interrelated. Greater accountability is required of health care providers by the consumers of their services.

In the midst of so much change, nursing emerges as a leader in developing new care delivery strategies. It is important, however, to understand the factors in society influencing health care delivery so that appropriate changes can be made to create better ways of providing nursing care, and to develop new nursing roles.

Competency of Health Care Providers

As the health care system changes, so must the competencies of its professionals. A consumer of health care should be able to expect that the standards of nursing care and practice in any health care setting are appropriate, safe, and efficacious. There are two principal mechanisms designed to ensure competent professional nursing practice. An established nursing education program must set professional standards for its students and meet educational outcomes based upon national accreditation guidelines. Graduates of these programs should be able to assume entry level positions within health care settings and perform competently within their defined responsibilities. Health care organizations, such as hospitals or home care agencies, ensure quality by establishing policies, procedures, and protocols that meet national accrediting standards. An additional assurance that high quality standards are met by professionals is certification of individuals in general and specialty practices.

The Pew Health Professions Commission (Shugars,

O'Neil, and Bader, 1991) investigated the trends in health care, the preparation of professionals, and identified six critical competencies needed for health professions by the year 2005:

- Care for the community's health
- Practice primary care and prevention
- Promote healthy lifestyles
- Involve clients and families in health care decision making
- Assess and use technology appropriately
- Accommodate expanded accountability

Clearly, changes will be necessary in professional education curriculums. Students will receive more clinical opportunities in "nontraditional" settings such as clinics, neighborhood health centers, HMOs, and day-care facilities, rather than traditional hospitals. It will be important for students to learn to understand the variables influencing a person's willingness and ability to remain healthy. Colleges and schools of nursing have already begun to deemphasize a focus on illness and have stressed the importance of understanding health and illness along a continuum. Nurses will play a key role in primary care and health promotion. Thus graduates of professional nursing programs must acquire the knowledge and skills needed to build strong relationships with clients and family members so that they may actively participate in the plan of care.

Health care organizations are spending more resources on the education and training of staff members. The Joint Commission on Accreditation of Health Care Organizations (1994) requires regular competency assessment of all direct care providers. With changing technology and innovations in medical treatment, staff who work in acute care settings are particularly challenged to remain current and competent. The move toward specialization adds to the burden of a professional to pursue necessary education.

Society and the Consumer's Movement

Consumers of health care have increased their knowledge and awareness of health promotion, illness prevention, and treatment practices. As a result, consumers are exerting influence on health care and its delivery. No longer do consumers simply accept a health care professional's recommendations. Consumers are curious. They eagerly seek out information about their health. They expect that information will be provided so that they may collaborate with care providers in making the right decisions about their health problems and the implications on their lifestyles. As consumers have become more knowledgeable about health in general, they have become more aware of the impact of lifestyle on health. As a result, consumers have expressed a greater need for knowledge and services related to illness prevention and health promotion (see Chapter 3). Similarly, businesses and corporations have started programs to promote wellness and fitness. A business can reduce its overall costs if employees enjoy better health. Increased sick time and disability of employees cause significant financial loss. The interest society holds for more information about health care is growing. More people wish to learn about self-care so that they may remain as independent as possible.

Another major influence on societal trends has been the "baby boomers," people born during the decade after World War II. That segment of the population is now middle-aged and is beginning to express concerns about the availability and quality of health care. As this group approaches old age, significant changes will probably occur in health care delivery systems. For example, health maintenance services, which allow persons with chronic disease to achieve a high level of wellness and functioning, will become more important.

The health care beliefs and practices of society are complex, depending on citizens' values, ethics, concepts of health, and other factors. In general, however, consumers' desire for health promotion, health maintenance, and new cures and treatments has led to changes in the health care delivery system. Many institutions and community-based agencies provide a wide range of outpatient health-promotion and health-maintenance programs regularly. Volunteer agencies have arisen to meet specific needs in health maintenance and promotion, and consumers have become more active in fund raising to support research in these areas.

New Knowledge and Technology

Scientific knowledge continues to rapidly increase. Research has led to new treatments and cures for life-threatening conditions such as cancer and cardiovascular disease. Clients have the opportunity to receive the most advanced treatment in the form of organ transplantation, laser surgery, and gene-alteration therapies.

The disadvantages of this knowledge explosion are threefold. First, it is increasingly difficult for health care professionals to remain well-informed about advances in their field. With the volume of knowledge available, it is difficult to stay a generalist. For example, a practicing nurse has trouble staying competent in all areas of general nursing practice. Many care givers have become specialized so that they can focus on exclusive areas of knowledge and skills. Nurses may choose oncology or critical care as a specialty. However, the demands for more primary care will require competent generalists in the future.

A second disadvantage is the costs related to technology. New third-generation antibiotics, diagnostic imaging equipment, and specialized beds or support surfaces are just a few examples of technologies that are introduced daily into health care settings. Consumers must ask whether these new technologies improve the quality of care and are cost effective. Statistics have shown an overuse of existing technologies, accounting for up to 50% of the rise in overall health care costs (Institute of Medicine, 1985). Nurses play a key role in evaluating new products and determining whether they help improve nursing practice. The costs of technologies are eventually transferred to clients. The ultimate factors in the use of technologies may be the economic resources available and the wants and needs of society as a whole.

The third disadvantage of advanced technology relates to its impact on health care delivery. Because technology causes greater specialization in health care, there is a risk of more fragmentation in care. It is important to have a single care giver who coordinates a client's health management. For example, one physician directs the course of therapy, using advice from radiologists, surgeons, and perhaps rehabilitation experts. However, diverse specialization usually introduces multiple care givers who do not always communicate clearly to ensure well-coordinated client care. Increased fragmentation of care adds to health care costs and the risk of an adverse event.

Legal Issues and Ethics

As people become more aware of their rights to health care and humane treatment, legal and ethical issues arise when care becomes compromised (see Chapters 19 and 20). Health care providers are under increased scrutiny as consumers gain a better understanding of their health problems. Safe, efficacious, and humane health care is an expectation of society. When this expectation is unmet, legal actions can be taken against care givers, and the ethical dilemmas that arise are enormous.

A legal right is that to which a person is entitled by law. A client has a legal right to competent and safe care. Ethics are the principles or standards governing proper conduct. A person's ethical right, such as a desire to refuse lifesaving therapy, has no legal guarantee. The legal and ethical concerns raised by consumers have changed the health care system. Standards have been implemented by various regulatory agencies to ensure that health care staff are competently educated. Policies within an institution dictate proper procedures for obtaining client consent to treatment. Institutions have created ethics committees to review professional practices and offer guidance when client rights are threatened. More attention is being given to client advocacy. Health care institutions are more intent on keeping clients and families informed and ensuring that staff members are responsible for their practice.

■ THE CLIENT AND THE HEALTH CARE DELIVERY SYSTEM

Clients entering the health care system have rights. Society generally believes that all people have a right to health care. After persons enter the health care delivery system, they become clients and thus have certain rights *within* the system. Health care consumers have a general right to determine *what* kind of health care should be available for present and future needs. Each of these rights affects how health care is delivered, but practices ensured by these rights are also influenced by society's attitudes and the system itself.

Right to Health Care

Society has generally come to believe that all people have a right to health care, regardless of cultural, economic, or other factors. In the 1960s, this belief led to the development of the federal Medicare and Medicaid programs. However, the Medicare and Medicaid programs do not cover all health care costs. Therefore rising overall costs require clients to assume more and more of the cost.

Quality of care should be an inherent right of all clients. In the face of budget tightening and fewer resources, the quality of nursing care cannot be compromised. In acute care settings, considerable emphasis is placed on getting clients home as quickly as possible. The clients who are found in hospitals are acutely ill to begin with. With a shortened length of stay, the time during which nurses care for clients is very intense. In some institutions, a high ratio of nurses to clients is viewed as too expensive, so there has

been an analysis of the appropriate methods for delivering care with fewer nurses. In addition, in an attempt to further reduce nursing costs, lower-salaried, unlicensed health care workers have been hired. Proactive nursing departments, who recognize that quality professional nursing care is imperative to good health care outcomes, are finding ways to restructure care delivery without compromising quality.

Rights Within the System

In 1973 the American Hospital Association developed a Patient's Bill of Rights (see Chapter 4), which was revised in 1992 and lists 12 specific rights of hospitalized clients. The bill offers some guidance and protection to clients by stating the responsibilities of the hospital and staff to clients and families. However, it is not a legally binding document. The Patient's Bill of Rights supports consumer activities for clients in the health care system. Clients have the right to information pertaining to diagnosis and treatment, fees for services, and continuity of care. Clients have the right to refuse any diagnostic or treatment procedures. Above all, the Patient's Bill of Rights reaffirms clients' rights to information and privacy while receiving health care.

One of the client's specific legal rights in any health care facility is **informed consent.** This is a person's agreement to allow something to happen, such as surgery or a diagnostic procedure. Informed consent is based on a full disclosure of the potential significant risks, benefits, and alternatives available to a client. Chapter 20 describes in detail the criteria for informed consent.

Clients' rights and informed consent affect the way the health care system delivers care. Most agencies now have committees to evaluate client suggestions and complaints about the delivery of health care. In many institutions, this committee is called a *patient care committee.* Another committee, an institutional review board, ensures that elements of informed consent are consistent with federal guidelines. Although the need to protect clients' rights sometimes results in increased work and paper work, this protection is necessary to ensure that all clients maintain their rights within the health care delivery system.

Entry Into the System

The three most common ways that clients enter the health care system are entry by referral from a health team member, entry when the client has a specific health need, and entry related to financial resources. Other methods of entry are self-referral, employer referral, and social referral.

A client may enter the system by referral from a health team member in the case of an acute, potentially life-threatening problem, such as severe chest pain, or in the case of a less threatening problem such as a rash of unknown cause. In an emergent situation a client typically calls a physician who refers the client directly to emergency services. In less acute situations the nurse is frequently the professional in a position to refer the client to the system. Such referrals may be given to a neighbor seeking advice, a child and family at a school where the nurse practices or does volunteer work, and the family of a client to whom the nurse has previously provided care.

Clients also enter the system on their own because of a specific need. For example, a college student may seek health care for treatment of a sore throat or gastrointestinal upset and thus may enter the health care system at the primary care level through the student health center. Another student may be involved in a severe automobile accident and enter the health care system through a hospital emergency room.

Finally, entry into the health care system may be influenced by financial situations. People who are employed and have insurance may readily enter hospitals for elective surgical or diagnostic procedures because they have the financial resources to seek and pay for primary health care. However, employers may only offer certain health care plans, thus restricting employees' choices of physicians and agencies. Unemployed persons with limited resources may seek care only if the illness becomes acute and may then go to hospital emergency rooms. Frequently the only type of care some clients can obtain is that supported by local, state, provincial, or federal programs.

Clients meet nurses whenever they enter the health care system. The first impression that the client has of the care delivered by a nurse may form a significant and lasting impression about nursing and health care in general. Nurses therefore have the opportunity to increase client awareness of health care services and the types of quality care they can and should expect.

■ FINANCING HEALTH CARE SERVICES

Health care spending in the United States as of 1994 climbed to nearly 14% of the gross domestic product (Solovy, 1994). In 1990, only 8.6% of Canada's GNP was spent on health care (Harrington, 1990). Despite the differences in spending between the two countries, studies have failed to show significant differences in the outcomes. It has become increasingly difficult, if not impossible, for people to meet health care costs with their own resources.

In fact, many Americans have no means to pay for health care. Approximately 60% of insured Americans are underinsured, and 33 million Americans have no insurance at all. Government agencies and private companies have developed a variety of prepaid health care, insurance, and social service programs to subsidize the cost of health care.

Private Insurance Plans

Traditionally, health care systems operated on a fee-for-service basis, receiving payment for each episode of care. Even though this trend is rapidly changing, there are still "private-pay" insurance options that support fee-for-service activities. Such an insurance policy can be obtained by an individual or through a group plan offered by employers. This type of plan is a retrospective fee-for-service option. Health insurance programs pay for some, most, or all of the expenses of health care for the client. Such payments are called **third-party reimbursements** because the costs of health care services are met, not by the health care agency or the client, but by the third party, the insurer. Ultimately, of course, consumers bear the costs through insurance premiums. In the United States the current trend includes for-profit commercial health insurers and Blue Cross and Blue Shield plans.

Managed Care Plans

Today there are a variety of health maintenance organizations that receive capitated payment to cover a variety of services for enrollees or members: preventive care, acute care, emergent care, and psychiatric care, for example. In 1992 a survey of employee health benefits in the United States for workers in settings with more than 200 employees showed only 4% still had traditional "private insurance" plans that involved no precertification or other form

Table 2-2 **Types of Managed Care Programs**		
TYPE	**DEFINITION**	**CHARACTERISTICS**
Preferred Provider Organization (PPO)	One that limits an enrollee's choice to a list of "preferred" hospitals, MDs, and providers. An enrollee pays more out-of-pocket for using a provider not on the list.	Contractual agreement exists between a set of providers and one or more purchasers (self-insured employers or insurance plans). Comprehensive health services at a discount to companies under contract. Focus on health maintenance.
Exclusive Provider (EPO)	One that limits an enrollee's choice to providers belonging to one organization. May or may not be able to use outside providers at additional expense.	Limited contractual agreement. Less access to select specialists.
Health Maintenance	Provide comprehensive, preventive, and treatment services to a specific group of voluntarily enrolled persons. Structures include a variety of models: Staff Model—MDs are salaried employees of the HMO. Group Model—HMO contracts with single group practice. Network Model—The HMO contracts with multiple group practices and/or integrated organizations. Independent Practice Association (IPA)—The HMO contracts with MDs who usually are not members of groups and whose practices include fee-for-service and capitated clients.	Focus on health maintenance, primary care. All care provided by a primary care physician.

of managed care (Friedman, 1993). Another 43% had traditional plans that did use precertification and other utilization controls. The remainder of employers provided benefits through HMOs and other managed care programs.

Any managed care program limits an enrollee's ability to choose any provider and to self-refer through the health care system. The primary care provider becomes a gatekeeper. Specific guidelines are established for levels of health care service, length of hospitalization, and medical specialist access. For example, if a client develops an acute muscle sprain and perhaps wishes to see an orthopedic physician, it will be necessary to first see the primary care provider (such as a medical internist). The aim is to reduce unnecessary utilization of health care resources (e.g., specialized medical care), and to manage the client so that hospitalization is not required. If the client has a problem requiring treatment, **precertification** authorization is conducted to determine whether the treatment is covered by the managed care plan and what is the most appropriate setting for the treatment to be delivered. There are select procedures and diagnoses that must be treated on an outpatient basis only.

There are several reasons why managed care plans have been growing. One is the belief that it is better to merge different services into an organized system. Second, capitation through managed care plans serves as an incentive to the provider to manage a client's care more efficiently. Third, managed care programs tend to reduce hospital utilization rates and total costs. Managed care programs rely on the process of utilization management. There are many employment opportunities becoming available to nurses in this specialty.

There are several types of managed care programs (Table 2-2). Many mixed models are also emerging. The models for hospital/HMO relationships should match local market conditions and consumer needs. For example, one managed care model might include several integrated hospitals, nursing homes, outpatient services, and a staff model HMO. Another model might be designed for psychiatric hospitals, clinics, and day-care services with an Independent Practice Association (IPA) model HMO.

Long-Term Insurance

About 75% of the elderly in the United States are covered by some type of private health insurance; however, most plans cover the same as Medicare (Ebersole and Hess, 1994). As a result, there is little if any coverage for long-term care. Most persons who are 50 years or older will need some form of long-term care for themselves or their parents. Nursing home care for a spouse or parent can cost $22,000 to $50,000 per year (Ebersole and Hess, 1994). The unavailability of long-term care insurance is a national concern.

Private insurance companies have begun to add long-term care policies. The policies provide an insured person $24 to $100 daily for an unlimited period of time or for as little as 2 years (Ebersole and Hess, 1994). There is also discussion to expand Medicare long-term care benefits. Perhaps the most promising plan is to offer long-term care benefits through a national health care plan. Several legislative proposals have been submitted to the U.S. Congress in the past for consideration (Harrington, 1990; Curtin, 1991).

U.S. Government Insurance Plans

The Social Security Act of 1965 provided two plans for a national health insurance program. Beneficiaries include older adults and impoverished or disabled persons. Medicare and Medicaid were designed to improve access to health care for those most in financial need.

MEDICARE

Persons entitled to **Medicare** coverage include adults who are 65 years of age or older, persons of any age with permanent kidney failure, and select individuals with disabling illnesses. The program is administered by the Health Care Financing Administration (HCFA) and is funded in part through Social Security (FICA) taxes. The original Medicare program (Title XVIII) has undergone numerous changes since its inception. There are still two parts to the program, however. Part A is basically acute-care hospital insurance; Part B covers physician and certain outpatient services (see the box below). Most persons do not pay monthly premiums directly for Medicare because of deductions of premiums from monthly social security checks.

Medicare does not pay for the full cost of certain services. For example, a diagnostic test such as a mammogram is reimbursed only for a flat amount of $50. If a radiological center charges more than the flat rate, the client must pay the remainder. Hospitals and physicians voluntarily choose to

---

Examples of Health Care Services Covered and Not Covered by Medicare

EXAMPLES OF COVERED SERVICES
- Acute hospital care
- Selected skilled nursing care
- Home health care within defined limits
- Diagnostic laboratory testing
- Diagnostic radiological testing
- Physical therapy
- Speech pathology services
- Ambulance (when health is at risk)
- Kidney dialysis or transplant
- Medications given in the hospital or skilled nursing facility
- Selected outpatient medications
- Physician care for medical and surgical services, treatments, tests, and procedures
- Outpatient and emergency care for illness or accidents
- Prosthetic devices
- Durable medical equipment (e.g., oxygen, wheelchairs, home dialysis)
- Medical supplies (e.g., syringes, dressings)
- Hospice benefits
- Respite care under specific conditions
- Mental health services (only 180 days paid for a lifetime)
- Selected immunizations (influenza)

EXAMPLES OF SERVICES NOT COVERED
- Long-term care
- Preventive health services (e.g., physical examinations)
- Hearing examinations and hearing aids
- Dental care (nonserious)
- Eye examinations and eyeglasses

participate in Medicare, although many states are considering making it mandatory for licensure. If a physician accepts assignment (i.e., the Medicare payment), there is a percentage of the fee (e.g., 20%) paid by the client. Participants in the program are encouraged to purchase supplemental insurance plans through private insurers. Coverage by Medicare can be confusing to a client. The Social Security Administration offers pamphlets explaining all benefits.

Payment by the government for services offered under Medicare is based on the DRG classification system. This classification system is based on 23 major diagnostic categories (e.g., diseases of the respiratory system or diseases of the circulatory system). Most of the categories contain a medical and surgical division. Each division is then further broken down into DRGs, totaling 494. The specific DRG assigned depends primarily on a client's principal medical diagnosis. However, secondary diagnoses, operating room procedures, age, discharge status, complications, and comorbidities (preexisting conditions) are also considered. A hospital receives one payment for each Medicare discharge based on the DRG classification, regardless of actual cost for caring for a client. The formula for determining payment is weighted, depending on the intensity and changes in resource consumption. Each DRG is assigned an average length of stay.

Because Medicare reimburses the hospital a fixed amount, regardless of actual costs, the hospital is at risk for operating at a loss. The hospital is given the incentive to find other methods of providing quality care to recover costs and make a profit. The hospital is also motivated not to keep the client hospitalized longer than necessary because the reimbursement is the same regardless of the client's actual length of stay.

In theory, prospective payments should help contain costs and even be an incentive for improved quality. Hospitals know the projected length of stay for each DRG and the anticipated payment. Opportunities to reduce system delays and inefficiencies, find better diagnostic measures,

coordinate care more efficiently, and reduce unnecessary procedures should improve quality care. The longer clients are hospitalized, the greater risk for complications. On the other hand, there is public concern that prospective payments might reduce the quality of care in certain cases. Regulatory mechanisms within the Medicare system protect clients from premature discharge and reduced standards of care. Protection of clients is ensured by audits of records by federal authorities. If these audits identify a trend to prematurely discharge clients, resulting in readmission to the hospital within 7 days, the hospital risks losing reimbursement funds.

MEDICAID

Medicaid is the government insurance program for persons of very low income. Coverage is regulated by states. Nationally, the average income eligibility requirement for Medicaid is less than half of the 1990 federal poverty level (nationally defined income level below which a family is considered "poor") (Rooks, 1990). Specifically, a family of three with an income of more than $5000 per year is too well off to qualify for Medicaid.

Medicaid has financed a large portion of maternal and child care for the poor. Since 1963 the Medicaid program has helped improve child health and reduce infant mortality rates through prenatal care. However, in 1981, major cuts in Medicaid programs were instituted by the Reagan administration. A financial crisis threatened most government-funded social and health programs.

With demands exceeding resources, many states toughened Medicaid eligibility rules. A study in 1988 showed that the United States had the nineteenth lowest infant mortality rate among industrialized nations. This embarrassing statistic prompted Congress to take steps to restore Medicaid funding. As of 1989, all states must provide Medicaid coverage for pregnant women and for children up to the age of 6 if family income is less than 133% of the federal poverty level.

An increased number of impoverished people who fail to qualify for Medicaid do not have access to health care. With the growing number of poor, the funds for Medicaid are dwindling. Many hospitals and other agencies are taking measures to minimize treatment of Medicaid clients because they are not reimbursed for their costs. Obvious reforms to the Medicaid system are needed, such as requiring Medicaid-eligible citizens to enter HMO plans for better managed medical care.

CATASTROPHIC HEALTH INSURANCE

The advanced technology of medical care in the United States has created challenging problems. More people are surviving illness and are living longer. Conditions that in the past would have proved fatal can now be treated successfully. The high costs associated with major and chronic illness are not covered by most insurance programs. In July 1988 the Medicare Catastrophic Coverage Act was passed to provide protection against the overwhelming out-of-pocket costs of major lengthy illnesses. Medicare recipients must pay flat premiums for the coverage. In addition, Medicare recipients who file income tax returns pay an additional fee based on taxable income.

The catastrophic coverage includes benefits for clients

CASE STUDY   *Case description:* Mr. Truman was admitted to the hospital on November 1 after experiencing chest pain and shortness of breath. He had undergone cardiac surgery almost 10 years before but was beginning to have symptoms again. He was scheduled for a cardiac catheterization, but it was delayed until November 3. The physician also referred Mr. Truman for diet counseling for a low-cholesterol diet. The cardiac catheterization proceeded without complications, and surgery was unnecessary. Mr. Truman remained hospitalized overnight to ensure that no problems developed. He was discharged on November 4.

Principal diagnosis: Ischemia, heart

Secondary diagnosis: Disturbances heart, functional, long-term effect of cardiac surgery

DRG assigned: DRG 125: circulatory disorders except acute myocardial infarction with cardiac catheterization without complex diagnosis

Assigned or allowed length of stay: 2.2 days

Actual length of stay: 3.1 days *Payment calculation (based on 2.2 days):* Payment per discharge × DRG weight = $3400 × 0.7015 = $2385

Actual hospital costs for Mr. Truman: $2960

Loss for hospital: $575 ■

hospitalized over 60 days. There is also a limit on the amount that clients will be required to pay for physician fees. Expanded coverage for medications has also been added. Despite the revisions, it is estimated that only 17% of Medicare enrollees will benefit from the change (Ebersole and Hess, 1994).

Canadian Government Health Insurance

The Canadian government has an integrated health care system with national health insurance. All citizens of Canada are covered by the mandatory program financed with tax dollars. Benefits are comprehensive, including short- and long-term care, and involve use of private-sector providers of services. The plan bypasses middlemen. Thus the government negotiates directly with providers to establish reasonable health care rates. Canada has substantially lower health care costs than the United States. The Canadian health care plan is more cost effective in that it has fewer expenditures on insurance, prepayment, and administration costs, and the costs to hospitals and physicians are also lower. However, unlike the United States, clients may experience long waiting periods for elective procedures.

■ INNOVATIONS IN HEALTH CARE DELIVERY

It seems that nursing has had an opportunity to make significant contributions to health care throughout history. The twenty-first century will be no different. Health care re-

form is giving nurses the opportunity to expand their roles, develop better quality of care services, and thus ensure healthier outcomes for clients and families. Nursing's Agenda for Health Care Reform (ANA, 1991) presented nursing's recommendations for steps to achieve immediate health care reform (see the box below). Many of these recommendations have begun. Successful achievement of the agenda will shift the focus of health care from illness and cure to wellness and care (ANA, 1991).

Care Management and Critical Pathways

In the past, care givers from all disciplines such as nursing, medicine, and social work managed a client's care within a hospital by contributing their own plans of care. There has always been an objective to coordinate the work of all care givers so that a single plan was followed with favorable outcomes. This was not always easy to accomplish, depending on the nursing delivery-of-care model or the collaboration of all care givers. For example, team nursing was so focused on the tasks of nursing care that little effort was given to ensure continuity of discharge planning and participation by all care givers. Frequently, members of the team were unaware of each discipline's plan.

An innovative approach that has met with success is **care management;** structuring accountability for client outcomes at the care delivery level within a unit or area of care (Zander, 1994). With care management, typically one care giver coordinates care from admission through discharge within an acute-care setting. A single, multidisciplinary

---

Nursing's Agenda for Health Care Reform

The basic components of nursing's "core of care" include:
- A restructured health care system that:

Enhances consumer access to services by delivering primary health care in community settings

Fosters consumer responsibility for personal health, self-care, and informed decision making in selecting health care services

Facilitates the use of the most cost-effective providers and therapeutic options

- A federally defined standard package of essential health care services available to all citizens and residents of the United States, provided and financed through an integration of public and private plans and sources

- A phase-in of essential services, so that the health care delivery system can be fiscally responsible in the:

Coverage of pregnant women and children, which is critical

Design of services that specifically assist vulnerable populations who have had limited access to the health care delivery system (A "Healthstart Plan" is proposed to improve the health status of these individuals.)

- Planned change to anticipate health care service needs that correlate with changing national demographics
- Steps to reduce health care costs, including:

Required use of managed care in a public health plan and encouraged in private plans

Incentives for consumers and providers to use managed-care arrangements

Controlled growth of the health care delivery system through planning and prudent resource allocation

Incentives for consumers and providers to be more cost efficient in exercising health care options

Development of health care policies based on effectiveness and outcomes research

Ensurance of direct access to a full range of qualified providers

Elimination of unnecessary bureaucratic controls and administrative procedures

- Case management required for clients with continuing health care needs
- Provisions for long-term care, including:

Public and private funding for services of short duration to prevent personal impoverishment

Public funding for extended care

Emphasis on the consumer's responsibility to financially plan for long-term care needs

- Insurance reforms to ensure improved access to coverage
- Access to services ensured by no payment at the point of service and elimination of balance billing in public and private plans
- Establishment of public or private-sector review—operating under federal guidelines and including payers, providers, and consumers—to determine resource allocation, cost reduction approaches, allowable insurance premiums, and fair and consistent reimbursement levels (This review would progress in a climate sensitive to ethical issues.)

Modified from ANA: *Nursing's agenda for health care reform,* Washington, DC, 1991, The Association.

BARNES

CARE PATH	1
100 CHEMOTHERAPY	

SERVICE	PHYSICIAN
PRIMARY NURSE	PRIMARY NURSE

DC DATE	ADM DATE	DATE OF SURGERY	A-8

PROBLEM NUMBER	*IF APPLICABLE PATIENT PROBLEMS / NURSING DIAGNOSES
#1	LACK OF KNOWLEDGE
#2	ALTERATION IN NUTRITION R/T DECREASED INTAKE, NAUSEA, VOMITING, ANOREXIA, INCREASED CALORIC REQUIREMENT
#3	POTENTIAL FOR INFECTION R/T MYELOSUPPRESSION, IMMUNO-SUPPRESSION
#4	POTENTIAL ALTERATION IN MUCOUS MEMBRANES R/T STOMATITIS, ESOPHAGITIS, VAGINITIS
#5	ALTERATION IN URINARY ELIMINATION R/T NEPHROTOXIC EFFECTS OF CHEMOTHERAPY, POTENTIAL FOR HEMORRHAGIC CYSTITIS
#6	POTENTIAL FOR INJURY R/T THROMBOCYTOPENIA, SEDATION

PROBLEM NUMBER		PRE-ADMIT	DAY 1	DAY 2
#2 #3 #4 #5 #6 #7 #8	ASSESSMENT / MONITORING	Evaluate IV access Evaluate response to previous treatment **Patient tolerated previous treatment without complications** Patient has adequate IV access (peripheral or VAD)	Nutritional status Nausea, vomiting Weight Bowel Function I & O Pain / comfort Skin / mucous membrane integrity Fall prevention Understanding of therapy / knowledge deficits Emotional response / coping mechanisms IV / vascular access site condition / type Results of CBC, SMA6 Vital signs **Pt will have stable vital signs** **Pt will have adequate urinary output without evidence of hematuria**	Nausea, vomiting Effectiveness of antiemetics Bowel Function I & O Pain / comfort Skin / mucous membrane integrity Patient response to treatment Emotional response / coping mechanisms IV / vascular access site condition Vital signs **Pt will have stable vital signs** **Pt will have adequate urinary output without evidence of hematuria**
#2 #7	CONSULTS	*Surgery for access placement	*SW - Emotional support, community resources, financial resources *Dietary - If patient has lost 5% of TBW within one month BHH / *BHIV - IF portion of tx to be done at home. If nursing required at home. *CNS *Pastoral Care *Psychological Resource Nurse (Gyn / Onc only)	*SW-consult completed *Dietary consult completed *CNS consult completed
	PROC. TEST	CBC *SMA 6 *Cr Cl	**CBC / SMA6 results adequate for chemotherapy administration**	*SMA 6 *Mg
#4 #5 #8	TREATMENT		Initiate and monitor IV fluid Administer antiemitic therapy Initiate Chemotherapy Regimen Initiate oral hygiene	Monitor IV fluid Administer antiemitic Rx Continue Chemotherapy Regimen Continue oral hygiene Determine accuracy of IV rate - determine if rate needs to be increased with MD approval to facilitate DC

Fig. 2-4 Example of sections of a care path. *(Courtesy Barnes-Jewish Hospital, St Louis.)*

③

100

			DAY 1	DAY 2
	ACTIVITY		Up with assistance Institute fall prevention protocol	Up with assistance Continue fall prevention protocol
	MEDS / IV		Initiate IV access within 2 hours of admission **IV site / VAD without redness, swelling, tenderness and with adequate blood return**	**IV site / VAD without redness, swelling, tenderness and with adequate blood return**
#2	NUTRITION		Diet as tolerated **Pt will have 2 or less episodes of nausea / vomiting.** **Pt will have 2 or less episodes of diarrhea**	Diet as tolerated **Pt will have 2 or less episodes of nausea / vomiting.** **Pt will have 2 or less episodes of diarrhea**

#1
 	
#7
	PATIENT / FAMILY EDUCATION		**Develop and Initiate Teaching Plan**
			1. Reason for and implication of chemotherapy
			2. Method of administration
			3. Anticipated length of therapy
			4. Names of drugs
			5. Review of each drug
			6. Side effects / management
			  A. Nausea / Vomiting
			  B. Anorexia
			  C. Diarrhea
			  D. Constipation
			  E. Alopecia
			  F. Stomatitis
			  G. Skin Changes
			  H. Fatigue
			  I. Myelosuppression
			  J. Sexuality implications
			  *K. Renal Toxicity
			  *L. Hemorrhagic Cystitis
			  *M. Cardiotoxicity
			  *N. Neurotoxicity
			  *O. Ototoxity
			7. Resources:
			  Cancer Information Center (CIC)
			  American Cancer Society
			  Support Groups (refer to CIC)
			*Care of VAD
			Informed consent signed (If chemotherapy is investigational)
			Give drug information and symptom management sheets to pt
			Pt will have written information outlining chemotherapy drug names, method of administration, common side effects and their management.
			Pt will have information regarding support groups, community resources and Cancer Information Center
				Reassess Comprehension
				Reinforce teaching.
				Teach signs and symptoms to report to MD after discharge
				1. Severe nausea, vomiting, diarrhea, constipation
				2. Temperature greater than 38.5C
				3. Sore which will not heal
				4. Spontaneous bleeding / bruising
				5. Cough which does not resolve
				6. Frequent, painful urination or blood in urine
				7. Rash of any kind
				8. Sudden weight gain or loss
				9. Pain of unusual intensity or distribution.
				
				Medications to **AVOID** without MD order.
				Aspirin
				Antibiotics
				Anticonvulsants
				Anticoagulants
				Barbiturates
				Antihypertensives
				Cough Medications
				Darvon
				Hypoglycemics
				Diuretics
				Hormones
				Tranquilizers
				Nasal Spray
				Vitamins

	DISCHARGE PLANNING	Evaluate for appropriateness of home infusional therapy	**Pt / Family verbalizes understanding of Care Path. Plan of care mutually set with pt / family.**	
#1 #7	PSYCHOSOCIAL / EMOTIONAL NEEDS		Provide opportunity to discuss implications / issues relating to disease / treatment **Patient / family exhibits positive coping skills related to disease / treatment**	Provide opportunity to discuss implications / issues relating to disease / treatment **Patient / family exhibits positive coping skills related to disease / treatment**
	SIGNATURES			

3100-22 REV. 9/92

Fig. 2-4, cont'd Example of sections of a care path.

plan is implemented so that all care givers work with one plan to achieve the same client outcomes. A popular tool used in care management is critical pathways. A **critical pathway** is a multidisciplinary treatment plan that sequences clinical interventions over a projected length of stay or a projected time frame (e.g., home health visits) for specific case types (Fig. 2-4), such as normal vaginal delivery, total hip replacement, or congestive heart failure. A pathway is developed by members of all disciplines that normally care for the particular client type. One model for a pathway is the **CareMap®**. Initially developed at the New England Medical Center in Boston, a CareMap® describes the clinical work of each professional discipline and department as it relates to clients' and families' measurable outcomes of care (Zander, 1992). A CareMap® is unique in that it incorporates day to day expected outcomes as well as those outcomes anticipated at discharge or at the end of a treatment phase.

Each day the CareMap® outlines clinical assessments, treatments and procedures, dietary interventions, activity and exercise therapies, patient education, and other discharge planning activities necessary to ensure a smooth, uneventful course of recovery. The CareMap® tells care givers what care needs to be given and when, so that a client is discharged on time and in as healthy a condition as possible. Outcomes incorporated into a CareMap® give nurses, physicians, and other care providers important signs for determining if care is appropriate and if the client is responding as desired. If a client does not proceed as predicted and if interventions or outcomes do not occur as planned, the team analyzes these variances (see Chapter 11) to decide how to revise the CareMap®. When a CareMap® is used 24 hours a day by each professional caring for a client, care management toward outcomes is tightly structured (Zander, 1992). In many hospitals a primary nurse coordinates a client's progress through a CareMap®. The nurse is responsible for communicating with other care givers so that a client's progress is uninterrupted. Proactive organizations are developing CareMaps® for home health, outpatient procedures, and clinic visits.

Case Management

As the health care environment continues to change, case management is an approach that coordinates and links health care services to clients and their families. The concept is not new. Various models have been used to arrange and connect health and social services for clients who have ongoing health problems. Case management is defined by Zander (1994) as the coordination of client care across care areas, between agencies, and (where possible) extending into wellness. What is unique about case management is that clinicians, either as individuals or part of collaborative groups, are overseeing the management of case-type–based care (e.g., clients with specific diagnoses) and are usually held accountable to some standard of cost management and quality of care. Case management involves managing a client's care across a continuum. For example, in one model a client with a chronic disease such as congestive heart failure may be assigned a nurse as a case manager in a medicine outpatient clinic. Whenever the client is hospitalized, the same case manager coordinates care so that all providers understand the client's unique needs. When the client is discharged, the case manager determines if home care or other services are necessary to sustain and support the client's health status. The case manager may choose to visit the client in the home to ensure that health promotion behavior is maintained. All institutions have different models based on their services and needs of clients.

All clients need their health care managed but not all require case management. Typically, formal case management is needed for approximately 20% of clients who enter acute health care settings (Zander, 1994). Clients requiring case management are high risk, usually experiencing complicated medical problems, and have limited resources for ongoing health care.

In many institutions, case managers are clinical nurse specialists or primary nurses who have demonstrated an expert level of nursing practice. The case manager, once assigned a client, becomes accountable for short- and long-range clinical outcomes as well as overall financial outcomes. In other words, the case manager partners with the physician and other care providers to ensure diagnostic and treatment approaches are appropriate and delivered promptly. Duplication of services and use of unnecessary resources are effectively managed by a case manager. In addition the case manager establishes a plan of care with the client, coordinates any consults, updates the client and family on progress in care, and facilitates discharge to an appropriate health care facility or the home. In many cases the case manager is accountable for placing clients on CareMaps® and utilizing the clinical guidelines for effective management of client care. A nurse who assumes the role of a case manager must have skills and knowledge in negotiating, obtaining and coordinating services and resources, intervening at key points for clients, and analyzing the trends in care that create negative clinical outcomes. Case managers are an extremely important part of managed care.

One system that has moved case management beyond hospital walls is Carondelet St. Mary's Hospital and Health Center. The hospital, located in Tucson, Arizona, identified the high-risk elderly population most in need of case management. This population is often chronically ill and likely to become acutely ill without intervention. The Carondelet system has developed a nursing health maintenance organization (HMO) that allows nurses to manage clients across the spectrum of health care, such as in ambulatory care, community health centers, acute care, home care, and extended care and hospice settings (Michaels, 1992). The case managers assume responsibility for client care outside of the hospital setting by assessing and monitoring health, providing education, directing clients at lower levels of illness to physician and hospital services, and interacting with home care agencies (Hyde, 1993). The program at Carondelet has had positive outcomes. Their clients have experienced fewer hospital admissions, fewer readmissions, and shorter hospital length of stays than the U.S. Medicare HMO (Ethridge, 1991).

Patient-Focused Care

Many hospitals have begun to look at redesigning the work of care providers so that staff work smarter rather than harder. The process of caring for clients is a complex one. Many different types of professionals and nonprofessionals are involved. Too often in the past, attention has focused

---

**Components of a
Patient-Focused Care Model**

- Cross training of staff to provide up to 90% of required client services
- Flattening management structure to empower staff with decision making on the unit level
- Moving services closer to the client
- Grouping similar client populations together
- Organizing staff into work teams
- Assigning ancillary personnel directly to the units
- Designing streamlined documentation systems
- Designing methods to provide client care items at the bedside

Modified from Clouten K, Weber R: Patient-focused care . . . playing to win, *Nurs Manag* 25(2):34, 1994.

---

on the tasks, functions, and structures involved in caring for clients. However, this has created numerous inefficiencies in care delivery. The focus instead should be on client need.

The concept of patient-focused care was first implemented in 1989 (Clouten and Weber, 1994). It involves bringing all care providers and services to the client. Cross-trained care givers from multidisciplinary backgrounds form self-governed teams, responsible for the "whole" work process that delivers care to clients (Clouten and Weber, 1994). The assumption is that if the tasks that are normally provided by ancillary personnel, for example, phlebotomy, ECG testing, physical therapy, or respiratory therapy, are moved closer to clients, the number of staff involved and number of steps to get the work done are reduced. Thus hospitals realize cost savings and clients perceive better overall care and service. A typical patient-focused care unit has its own admitting, pharmacy, lab, and radiology areas. Variations exist within different hospitals.

In a patient-focused care model the nurse is still a key player in coordinating client care. Nurses are more likely performing professional nursing activities, for example, education or clinical assessment, than ancillary functions such as bed making or specimen collection. Cross-trained care providers can deliver multiple services and reduce the number of personnel a client must see. This can significantly add to client satisfaction and staff satisfaction.

To develop a patient-focused care model, all staff members must be able to participate in the redesign of their work. In addition, staff must be ready and willing to change. The process involves several components (see the box above). Nursing's challenge is to take the care production process apart and to recombine its elements into a new, more adaptable delivery system that achieves favorable outcomes (Tonges, 1992).

Assistive Personnel

There are many hospitals and other health care institutions that have responded to health care reform by placing more unlicensed assistive personnel such as certified nurse assistants, nurse technicians, and orderlies in acute-care settings and lowering the number of registered nurses. This change creates the fear among RNs that nursing will return to a task-based focus and quality of care will suffer. At the heart of the issue is the concern RNs have in being able to trust less-trained individuals to manage delegated care activities. Traditionally, nurses have assumed responsibility for all aspects of client care, but it is not necessary for registered nurses to participate in repetitive, low-risk client care tasks that can be reassigned to others.

If the number of assistive personnel is changed haphazardly, without attention to the work processes that occur on a nursing unit, the outcomes can be negative. Unplanned change may add to the burden of an RN and negate the intent of redistributing routine, repetitive tasks to less-skilled personnel. If assistive personnel are improperly trained, nurses find themselves frequently supervising staff instead of attending to client education, clinical assessment, and discharge planning. The American Nurses Association (ANA) issued a position statement on unlicensed assistive personnel (1992). The association clarified the importance of nurses being in the position to direct patient care activities and to know what activities can be safely delegated or assigned (see Chapter 4).

The addition of alternate care providers can be done in an innovative way that successfully reduces RN workload, delegates appropriate tasks to unlicensed personnel, and improves client and staff satisfaction. The organizations that have successfully added assistive personnel without compromising quality of care have recognized the importance of having RNs and assistive personnel doing the right work and engaging in team building. An initial step to changing the "mix" of staff on a nursing unit is to spend time gaining staff support and willingness to change. Staff must recognize that the way work is performed will be different. A formal work analysis, involving all levels of staff on a unit, helps to identify the type of activities that take place and who is in the best position to perform them. Typically, a work analysis shows RNs that there are many activities that can be safely delegated to less-skilled staff. For example, activities that can be delegated include those of a repetitive nature and that do not require nursing judgment (e.g., bathing, assisting clients with feeding, specimen collection, and measuring height and weight). The assistive personnel must be involved in the change process so that they feel a sense of belonging, recognition, self-worth, and control (Hayes, 1994). Assistive personnel spend a significant amount of time with clients and can be valuable sources of information to RNs as they work together. Both RNs and assistive personnel must learn to value one another's contribution to client care. The formation of trust helps the RN learn to delegate tasks appropriately and to focus time on professional nursing responsibilities.

Advance Practice Nursing

An advance practice nurse (APN) is not an innovation. However, the roles that advance practice nurses are beginning to assume with health care reform are innovative and challenging. Advance practice nurses consist of clinical nurse specialists (CNS), nurse practitioners (NP), nurse midwives, and nurse anesthetists. They are considered APNs because of their advanced education and experience. In most states, certification for these roles is a requirement.

An APN, particularly a CNS, NP, or nurse midwife, has the opportunity to be a leader in providing primary care.

Working collaboratively with physicians, APNs can provide primary care less expensively and often more effectively than physicians alone. This is due in part to the nurse's holistic approach to clients' health care needs. The nurse is able to assess a client's health in the context of the family and social setting and make recommendations that ultimately improve a client's health habits. One area of practice that APNs can especially influence is that of gerontological care. The number of older adults within our population is increasing. APNs with gerontological certification are able to apply specialized knowledge about the aged to create approaches that help older adults increase health-conducive behavior, minimize health losses and disability, and facilitate the diagnosis, palliation, and treatment of disease. Keeping the older adult population healthy and functional not only is a significant contribution to quality care but also reduces health care costs created by frequent hospitalization.

An APN in a primary care setting usually partners with a physician or group of physicians under a collaborative agreement. This agreement allows the nurse to prescribe medications (narcotics are a usual exception) and treat presenting health problems within the scope of the nurse's practice. The APN assumes a case load of clients, manages their ongoing health care problems, and refers to the partnering physician when more complicated problems arise. In addition, APNs can receive reimbursement for their services. With a shortage of primary care physicians in the United States, nurses in advance practice roles have an opportunity to establish the systems needed to create effective health-promotion programs (see Chapter 13).

Quality Improvement

Efforts in ensuring and improving the quality of health care have never been as important as they are today. The health care agencies that survive in the twenty-first century will be able to guarantee a superior level of quality of care. Third-party payers will likely contract with successful organizations. For example, if a hospital uses managed care to successfully lower complications and improve clients' functional states after treatment for cancer, the hospital will receive payer support.

Health care is behind industry in regards to quality management. The terms most frequently discussed in the health care literature have been *quality assurance* and *quality improvement* (see Chapter 11). Quality assurance (QA) is the ongoing systematic monitoring or evaluation of nursing prac-

---

JCAHO's Standards for Improving Organizational Performance

The organization has a planned, systematic, organizationwide approach to design, measure, assess, and improve its performance.

New processes are designed well, based on the organization's mission, client expectations, up-to-date sources of information about processes, and the performance of the processes and their outcomes.

Organization systematically measures performance of processes that affect a large percentage of clients, place clients at risk, or have been shown to be problem prone.

Organization identifies areas for possible improvement of existing processes and determine if changes improved the processes.

Modified from JCAHO: *Accreditation manual for hospitals*, Oakbook Terrance, Ill, 1996, The Joint Commission.

---

tice, medical practice, or practice of other disciplines. Traditionally, QA has focused on clinical practice, providing information on the appropriateness of nursing care processes and activities. QA programs directed staff to inspect existing processes and repair rather than prevent problems and create innovative processes (Schroeder, 1988).

Quality improvement (QI) has become the new focus in health care. Other terminology for the quality improvement effort includes total quality management (TQM), performance improvement, and continuous quality improvement (CQI). It is a more integrated, coordinated approach to find ways to continually improve practices (e.g., fall prevention or client instruction on self-medication) and services (e.g., client admission process and radiology turnaround). A focus is the elimination of barriers that impede clients' use of the health care system at a nursing unit or agency. The JCAHO (1996) has established standards (see the box above) that require members of all health care disciplines to collaborate in identifying the best possible clinical practice that can guarantee repeated favorable outcomes for clients. The skills and knowledge needed to participate in a successful QI program are many (see Chapter 11). Health care institutions must commit resources for staff development and more importantly, staff involvement in ongoing QI activities.

∎ KEY CONCEPTS ∎

▶ Health care reform is being driven by escalating costs, forcing health care institutions to deliver care more efficiently without sacrificing quality.

▶ A national health care plan will likely address expansion of existing public programs, provision of private health insurance to all employed individuals, and a comprehensive health plan.

▶ Restructuring is resulting in hospitals and physician practices merging into systems that have greater resources to provide a continuum of care.

▶ Capitation forces providers to assume the risk to keep clients healthy.

▶ Work redesign involves identifying aspects of traditional nursing care that can be safely and appropriately assigned to nonlicensed staff.

▶ Health care services are provided in a large number of settings, across all age groups, and for the chronically and acutely ill.

▶ Chronically ill and disabled clients seek knowledge and skills to maximize their levels of wellness and independence.

▶ Health systems in the future will be evaluated on the basis of outcomes, such as access, service quality, prevention of illness, encounter outcomes, consumer health status, and success in treating disease.

▶ The Medicare prospective reimbursement system is based on payment calculated on the basis of DRG assignment.

▶ Health-promotion activities are designed to help clients reduce the risk of illness, maintain maximal function, and promote lifestyle habits related to good health.

▶ Illness-prevention activities are directed at helping the client and family reduce risk factors.

▶ Once a client develops signs and symptoms of a disease, secondary prevention is needed to maintain a desired level of health and minimize complications.

▶ Rehabilitation allows an individual to return to a level of normal or near-normal function after a physical or mental illness, injury, or chemical dependency.

▶ Community-based agencies focus on providing health care to clients within their neighborhoods.

▶ Nurse-managed clinics offer primary care delivered by advanced practice nurses with a focus on client-centered care.

▶ Alternative health care settings that manage clients with disabilities or complicated illnesses include subacute care, skilled nursing facilities, and rehabilitation centers.

▶ Managed care plans establish specific guidelines for covered medical benefits available to enrollees as well as length of hospitalization for which the plan will pay and access to medical specialists.

▶ Consumers of health care should be guaranteed that all practitioners are competent.

▶ CareMaps® are an example of a multidisciplinary plan of care for each day of a client's expected length of stay or episode of treatment.

∎ KEY TERMS ∎

Adult day-care centers, p. 31

Capitation, p. 24

Care management, p. 39

CareMap®, p. 42

Crisis intervention centers, p. 32

Critical pathway, p. 42

Diagnosis-related group (DRG), p. 23

Drug rehabilitation centers, p. 31

Extended-care facility, p. 30

Health Maintenance Organization (HMO), p. 23

Home health care agency, p. 32

Hospice, p. 32

Informed consent, p. 35

Inpatients, p. 29

Managed care, p. 23

Medicaid, p. 38

Medicare, p. 37

Outpatient services, p. 28

Precertification, p. 37

Prospective payment, p. 23

Rehabilitation, p. 28

Rehabilitation center, p. 31

Respite care, p. 33

Risk-adjusted, p. 25

Skilled nursing facility, p. 30

Subacute care, p. 30

Third-party reimbursements, p. 36

Utilization review, p. 23

Volunteer agencies, p. 32

Work redesign, p. 25

■ CRITICAL THINKING EXERCISES ■

1. Trinity hospital is a 300-bed acute-care hospital that provides outpatient and inpatient services. Recently the percentage of clients cared for under Medicare has risen from 35% to 42%. In addition, another 36% of the clients belong to PPOs. Approximately 10% have Medicaid and the remainder have private insurance. The director of nursing reports that the costs for providing care to clients are increasing. The average length of stay in the hospital is 6.5 days. What can be done to improve the hospital's ability to be profitable? What would the role of the nurse be in those improvements?

2. Consider Mr. Wilson, a 68-year-old client who will have major surgery to replace the joint in his hip. Afterward, extensive therapy will be needed for him to again walk normally. Describe the type of health care agencies that might become involved in the care of Mr. Wilson.

3. Mrs. Ramirez is a 42-year-old client who is employed as an advertising agent for a large corporation. She travels 65% of the time. Her business requires her to have a physical exam every 2 years. During a recent checkup Mrs. Ramirez was found to have an elevated cholesterol and triglyceride level. Her blood pressure is 134/84, up from 2 years ago. The nurse who conducted a health history learned that Mrs. Ramirez eats "on the go" and only exercises when at home. She also smokes 2 packs of cigarettes a day. What level of health care did Mrs. Ramirez pursue? What level of prevention should the nurse initiate and why?

4. Ms. Yim is a 65-year-old client who experienced a stroke 8 days ago. She has lost movement on her left side and is unable to speak clearly. Mr. Rogers is a 60-year-old client who is in the hospital 2 days following a total knee replacement operation. Which client would benefit from case management and why?

REFERENCES

American Nurses Association: *Nursing's agenda for health care reform,* Washington, DC, 1991, The Association.

American Nurses Association: *Progress report on unlicensed assistive personnel: informational report,* Report CNP-CNE-B, Washington, DC, 1992, The Association.

AONE: The consumer healthcare reform agenda, *Nurs Manag* 25(5):17, 1994.

Aydelotte MK, Gregory MS: Nursing practice: innovative models. In *Nursing centers: meeting the demand for quality health care,* NLN Pub 21-2311, New York, 1989, National League for Nursing.

Bower KA: Case management: work redesign with patient outcomes in mind. In McDonagh KJ, editor: *Patient-centered hospital care: reform from within,* Ann Arbor, 1993, Health Administration Press.

Clouten K, Weber R: Patient-focused care . . . playing to win, *Nurse Manag* 25(2):34, 1994.

Curtin L: Rube Goldberg and the great American healthcare system, *Nurs Manag* 22(5):9, 1991 (editorial).

Donabedian A: Evaluating the quality of medical care, *Milbank Memorial Fund Quarterly* 44:166, 1966.

Drew JC: Health maintenance organizations: history, evolution and survival, *Nurs Health Care* 11(3):145, 1989.

Ebersole P, Hess P: *Toward healthy aging: human needs and nursing response,* ed 4, St Louis, 1994, Mosby.

Ethridge P: A nursing HMO: Carondelet St. Mary's experience, *Nurs Manag* 22(7):24, 1991.

Fraser I et al: Capitation and reform: challenges and choices for hospital leadership, *Hospitals* 67(7):23, 1993.

Friedman E: Managed care, where will your hospital fit in? *Hospitals* 67(7):18, 1993.

Hackman J, Oldham G: *Work Redesign,* Menlo Park, Calif, 1980, Addison-Wesley.

Harrington C: Policy options for a national health care plan, *Nurs Outlook* 38(5):223, 1990.

Hayes PM: Team building: bringing RNs and NAs together, *Nurs Manag* 25(5):52, 1994.

Health Care Advisory Board: *Next generation of outcomes tracking: implications for health plans and systems,* vol 2, *Quality measures,* Washington, DC, 1994, The Advisory Board Co.

Hyde J: *Case Study: Carondelet St. Mary's Hospital and Health Center, Nursing Issue Tracking,* Washington, DC, 1993, Health Care Advisory Board.

Institute of Medicine: *Assessing medical technologies,* Washington, DC, 1985, National Academy Press.

Joint Commission on Accreditation of Health Care Organizations: *Accreditation manual for hospitals,* Oakbrook Terrace, Il, 1996, The Joint Commission.

McMahon LF: The development of diagnosis-related groups. In Burdsley M, Coles J, Jenkins L, editors: *DRGs and health care,* London, 1987, King Edward Hospital Fund for London.

Michaels C: Carondelet St. Mary's nursing enterprise, *Nurs Clin North Am* 27(1):77, 1992.

Montague J: Rural and primary care across the nation, *Hospitals and Health Networks* 68(8):60, 1994.

Phillips DL, Steel JE: Factors influencing scope of practice in nursing centers, *J Professional Nsng* 10(2):84, 1994.

Riesch SK: Nursing centers: state of the art survey results. In *Nursing centers: meeting the demand for quality health care,* NLN Pub 21-2311, New York, 1992, National League for Nursing.

Rooks JP: Let's admit we ration health care—then set priorities, *Am J Nurs* 90:39, 1990.

Schroeder P: Directions and dilemmas in nursing quality assurance, *Nurs Clin North Am* 23(3):657, 1988.

Sharp N: Rural healthcare: new opportunities for nurses, *Nurs Manag* 22(3):22, 1991.

Shugars D, O'Neil E, Bader J, editors: *Health America: Practitioners for 2005,* Durham, NC, 1991, The Pew Health Professions Commission.

Smith JP: The politics of American healthcare, *J Adv Nurs* 15:487, 1990.

Solovy A: Taming the tiger: the economics of health care reform, *Hospitals and Health Networks* 68(5):26, 1994.

Sovie M: Redesigning our future: whose responsibility is it? *Nurs Econ* 8(1):21, 1990.

Stahl D: Subacute care: the future of health care, *Nurs Manag* 25(10):34, 1994.

Stewart M et al: *Community health nursing in Canada,* Toronto, 1985, Gage.

Tonges MC: Work designs: sociotechnical systems for patient care delivery, *Nurs Manag* 23(1):27 1992.

Zander K: Quantifying, managing and improving quality, *The New Definition* 7(2):1, 1992.

Zander K: Responsive restructuring. IV. Care management and case management, *The New Definition* 9(2):1, 1994.

ADDITIONAL READINGS

Bargar SE: The delivery of early and periodic screening, diagnosis, and treatment program services by NPs in a nursing center, *Nurse Practitioner* 18(6):65, 1993.

Borkowski V: Implementation of a managed care model in an acute care setting, *JHQ* 16(2): 25, 1994.

Bostrom J, Zimmerman J: Restructuring nursing for a competitive health care environment, *Nursing Economics* 11(1):35, 1993.

Cerne F: Shaping up for capitation, *Hospitals and Health Networks* 68(7):28, 1994.

Deming WE: *Out of the crisis,* Cambridge, Mass, 1986, MIT Center for Advanced Engineering.

Huber DG et al: Use of nursing assistants: staff nurse opinions, *Nurs Manag* 25(5):64, 1994.

Hudson Institute: *Workforce 2000: work and workers for the 21st century,* Indianapolis, 1987, The Institute.

Lorenz E: *DRG working guidebook,* Alexandria, Va, 1992, St. Anthony's.

Ponte PR et al: Development needs of advance practice nurses in a managed care environment, *JONA* 23(11) 13, 1993.

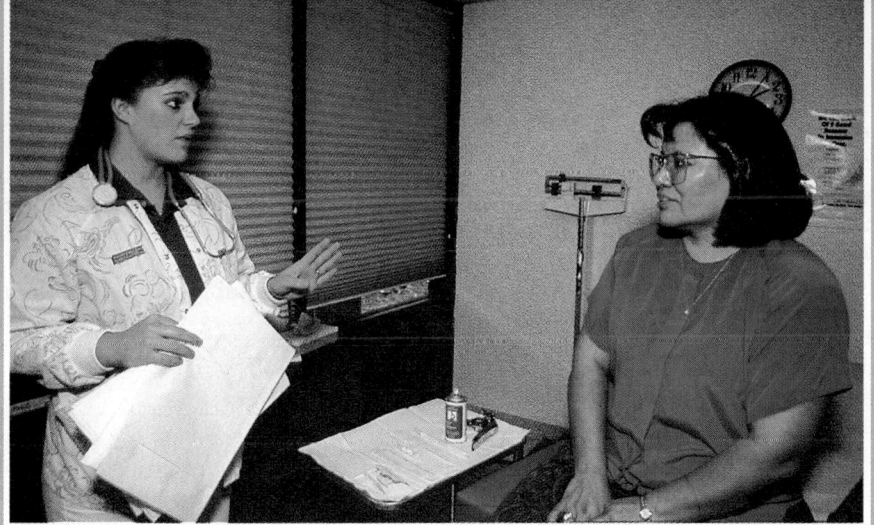

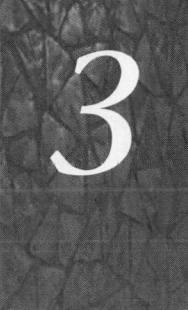

## Chapter 3

Health Promotion and Primary Health Care

Objectives

Mastery of content in this chapter will enable the student to:

▶ Define the key terms listed.

▶ Describe basic guidelines for developing a primary health care program.

▶ Identify various primary care settings.

▶ Recognize that health-promotion activities are appropriate in every health care setting.

▶ Discuss how technology may be used and creatively applied for health-promotion purposes in primary care settings.

▶ Describe the role of nurses in primary care settings.

▶ Distinguish between primary, secondary, and tertiary prevention.

▶ Discuss four types of core competencies in nursing especially needed for promoting health in primary care.

▶ Discuss issues related to the delivery of primary nursing care.

Health promotion involves behaviors that help prevent disease and protect health. Promoting health and providing primary health care are vital nursing functions. Clients pursue information and assistance from a variety of health care providers in order to maintain wellness. This may include selecting a physician, learning about infant care, or starting an exercise program. The nurse has perhaps the best perspective of a client's total health needs. The primary care environment is an ideal site for therapeutic nurse-client interactions and interventions that can influence the quality of health promotion.

Primary care is a personal health care system that provides for first-contact, continuous, comprehensive, and coordinated care. It is designed to meet the common health care needs of clients within a community. Preventive, curative, and restorative services are provided to maximize the health and well-being of clients (Stanhope and Lancaster, 1996). Primary care is the major component of an overall primary health care system. A **primary health care system** is one in which essential health care services are universally accessible to individuals and families within a specific community, are made available to them through their full participation, and are provided at a cost that the community and county can afford (World Health Organization [WHO], 1978).

The focus of primary care is wellness. The focus of the United States health care system has primarily been the treatment of illness. Health care resources have been aimed at curing rather than caring. As a result of managed care initiatives, the current development of primary health care organizations and networks offers some hope that health promotion and disease prevention will be increasingly emphasized. Achievement of a primary care–based health care delivery model will require the transfer of financial as well as professional resources from our current acute care–based system.

To date, the model for the delivery of care in the United States does not consistently emphasize efficient, available, cost-effective primary care to all individuals.

■ HEALTH PROMOTION AND DISEASE PREVENTION

Nursing's role in health promotion within primary care settings has three main components. First, health is a human right and needs to be promoted for its own sake. A healthy lifestyle has the potential to increase or maintain a client's level of wellness and functioning. Second, impairment and disability take their toll on clients, their families, and society. These can be prevented or minimized through early screening and detection of illness or risk factors known to cause illness or trauma. Third, health care includes not only the diagnosis and treatment of illness, but also the return of an acutely or chronically impaired client, family, or community to a level of optimal health. Health care is also directed at preventing further decline. These three components correspond to the public health definitions of primary, secondary, and tertiary prevention.

Primary Prevention

Primary prevention involves health promotion and disease prevention. Eating a well-balanced diet, engaging in a reg-

ular program of exercise, maintaining a healthy weight, and not smoking are examples of primary prevention. Primary prevention activities can extend beyond the health care environment. For example, in grade schools children are now better informed about healthy eating habits, abstinence from smoking and substance abuse, and the importance of routine exercise. These measures promote optimal health and may help prevent coronary artery disease in later years (Fig. 3-1).

Secondary Prevention

Secondary prevention involves early detection of illness and its complications. Increasing women's awareness of breast cancer and encouraging breast self-examination and mammography are examples of secondary prevention (Fig. 3-2). These activities help to detect illness in its earliest stages and to prevent or minimize its complications.

Once illnesses are diagnosed in their earliest stages, clients are usually able to return to their daily activities and jobs. As a result, they may feel that they have more control over their life, and the social and financial costs of the illness are reduced.

Tertiary Prevention

Tertiary prevention involves maintaining optimal health once a disease or disability has developed. It also involves

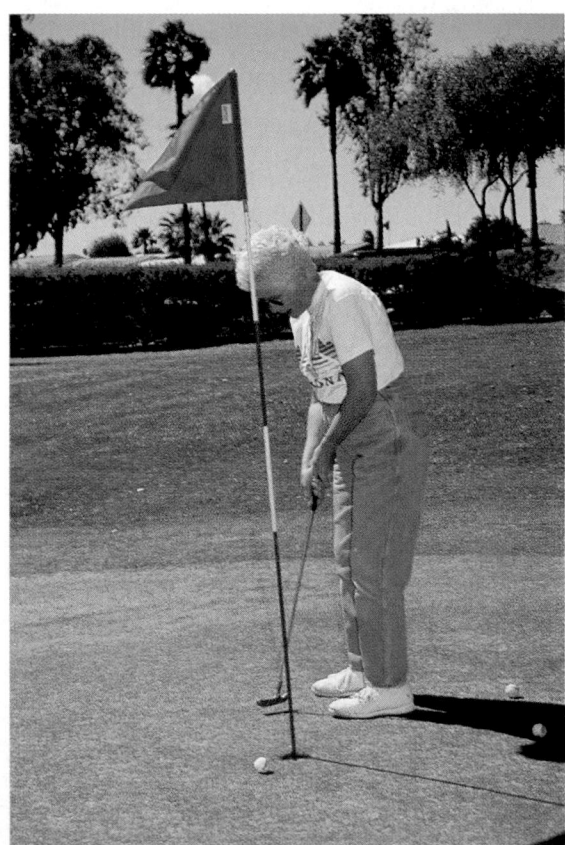

Fig. 3-1 Regular exercise as a health-promotion activity.

preventing further decline in health. For example, recovery from alcoholism is a continuous process, even after years of sobriety. For members of Alcoholics Anonymous, it is a way of life, based on a 12-step program, that provides a way of thinking not only about alcohol but about one's self, others, and the world. Following the program helps to prevent further decline and to maintain optimal health.

We can thus see that health-promotion and disease-prevention activities include encouraging behavioral changes along with communicating health-related information. Clients need this information and knowledge to make decisions about behavioral changes. Nurses can also make unique contributions by diagnosing or identifying health needs and referring clients to appropriate resources. Use of education teaching guides (see the box on p. 50) and applying new research (see the box below) are ways to help clients achieve optimal health.

PRIMARY HEALTH CARE

Primary health care is based on practical, scientifically sound and socially acceptable methods and technology. Such care is delivered in multiple settings, such as community nursing centers, health maintenance organizations, and community-based clinics. It must be an integral part of the nation's health care system and of the social and economic development of the community. Essential services are provided at this primary level of contact (see the box on p. 51, top).

Primary health care should ideally include universal access. **Universal access** ensures that health care is provided to all citizens, regardless of their employment or insurance status. The Health Security Act introduced in 1993 offered universal access to a basic benefit package of hospital, preventive, physician, and long-term care services (Stanhope and Lancaster, 1996). All employed workers would have received insurance through their employers. The unemployed would have received benefits through a government-paid system (Richardson, 1995). However, our current health care systems and settings have not achieved this goal. Health professionals do their best with the resources available to deliver primary care to as many people as possible. Today the poor and uninsured are still underserved by our primary health care system.

Primary Care Environment

To deliver care in a primary care environment, the nurse must be knowledgeable of the needs of society, the primary care delivery system, the expectations of the client and family, and the available technological resources. In addition, trends in demographics, economic resources, and the workforce all affect the primary care environment.

Demographic trends point to several factors. In the United States and Canada decreased mortality and increased longevity are going to result in an increase in the older adult population. Thus, there is a greater need for primary health care and health promotion in community-based settings for this population.

Economic trends demostrate that a larger base of the population remains at the low income level (Johnson, 1992). As a result, there continues to be an increased demand for government-based health care services. To date, little of this health care dollar is directed toward primary health care.

Trends in the workforce are threefold. First, as the "baby boomer" generation ages, the demands on Medicare are expected to increase. Second, the corporate job sector has had

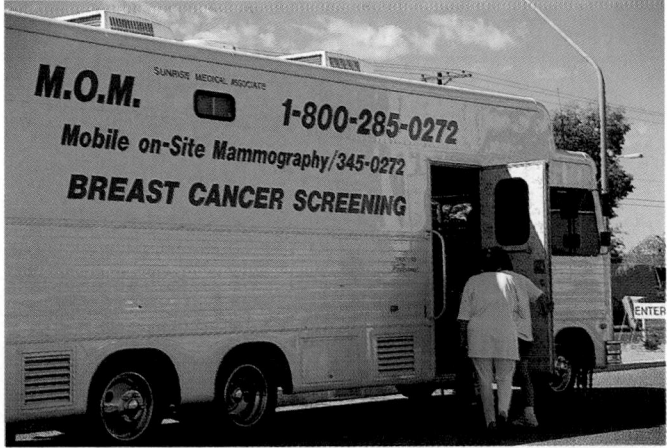

Fig. 3-2 Mammography vans bring service to client's community setting.

► **RESEARCH HIGHLIGHT**

RESEARCH ABSTRACT

Most studies of the problems and information needs of cardiac patients in early recovery describe these only for the period of hospitalization. In this study, however, the authors focused on the first 6 months after discharge. Eighty two cardiac patients, admitted to a university hospital with a myocardial infarction (MI) or for coronary artery bypass surgery (CABS), were interviewed 6 months after discharge. Questions required them to describe problems they experienced in early recovery and what information they needed. All but one of the 82 patients stated they had problems during the first 6 months after discharge. Most problems described concerned emotional reactions (59%), their change in physical condition (59%), deleterious effects of treatment (56%) and convalescence (54%). Topics on which most patients needed additional or different information were deleterious effects of the treatment (26%), physical condition (24%), risk factors (24%), convalescence (24%), and knowledge of the disease (24%).

IMPLICATIONS FOR PRACTICE

► Give patients an opportunity to express their postdischarge concerns and problems they may be encountering.

► Develop postdischarge health education programs for cardiac patients.

► Develop cardiac patient support groups whereby patients can learn from the experience of others.

REFERENCE

Jaarsma T et al: Problems of cardiac patients in early recovery, *J Adv Nurs* 21:21 1995.

Smoking and Your Lungs

Chances are, you started smoking because it was cool, sophisticated, and glamorous. Or your friends smoked and you were curious about what smoking was like.

Now you know smoking is anything but cool. It makes you cough, cuts your "wind," gives you bad breath, and stains your teeth. It's also expensive; in 1 year, a heavy smoker may spend $1000 or more on cigarettes.

More important, smoking causes emphysema, chronic bronchitis, lung cancer, heart disease, and gum disease. It increases your chances of having a stroke, diseases of the blood vessels, and stomach ulcers. Women who smoke during pregnancy may have premature babies. Smoking increases the risk of osteoporosis in women. And smoke in the air harms nonsmokers.

YOU AND YOUR DEFENSE SYSTEM

The insides of your lungs are exposed to the environment every time you breathe. To protect them from foreign particles that could enter the body through this route, the lungs have several defense mechanisms.

Tiny hairlike cilia line your bronchial tubes. Normally they are in constant movement, sweeping germs, dirt, and mucus out of your lungs. But tobacco smoke slows down and actually paralyzes the cilia. Dirt particles and germs that enter the lungs are not removed. And the mucus that collects in the lungs provides a fertile environment for germs to multiply. This is the reason smokers suffer more respiratory infections.

Mucus lining the airways serves two purposes: it helps remove dirt and germs and it moistens the air you breathe. Smoking dries out the mucus, further hampering the defensive action of removing foreign matter. Smokers often experience dry, scratchy throat because the normal moisture is absent.

THE CHEMICALS IN TOBACCO

Tar is a cancer-causing substance that clings to the inside of your lungs, forming a brown, sticky coat. All tobacco contains tar. Many people switched to low-tar cigarettes in the belief that these brands were less damaging. But the fact is, even small amounts of tar can still cause cancer. In addition, many smokers who switch to low-tar brands take deeper draws and smoke more cigarettes.

Nicotine causes the blood vessels to constrict, raising your blood pressure and forcing your heart to work harder than it should. Smokers suffer from cold hands and feet caused by poor circulation. In time, this can cause vascular diseases.

Burning tobacco produces carbon monoxide. Each time you inhale the hot smoke, you are taking carbon monoxide into your lungs. The tiny blood vessels in your lungs pick up this carbon monoxide instead of oxygen. Tests on smokers have found that carbon monoxide levels in their blood are 15 times higher than in the blood of nonsmokers. As a smoker, your entire body is chronically oxygen-deficient.

IT'S NOT TOO LATE TO QUIT

Even if you have been smoking for years—even if you already have a lung disease—quitting smoking now will greatly improve your health. The cilia will begin working again and help keep your lungs swept clean. Your blood vessels will relax, allowing the blood to flow normally, so your heart will no longer work so hard. Your lung tissue will become healthier and you will breathe easier.

This guide may be copied for distribution to patients and families. All rights reserved.

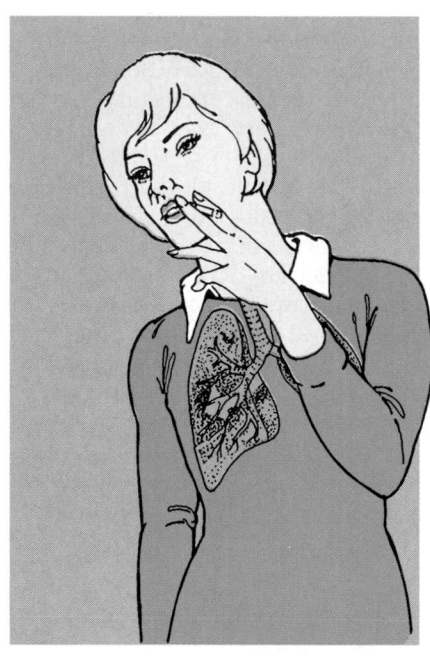

From *Mosby's patient teaching guides,* St Louis, 1995, Mosby.

---

a period of downsizing, and more employers no longer carry health insurance as an employment benefit. Last, there are factors in the health care workforce that affect the delivery of primary care. The health care delivery system is currently overspecialized, which adds to the cost of care as well as to the poor availability of primary care services.

SOCIETY

The impact of society on health promotion and primary care revolves around the client's fundamental right to a standard of living that is adequate for optimal health and well-being. The Declaration of Alma Alta (WHO, 1978) specifies the basic components to be included in primary health care programs. This declaration reaffirmed that "health, which is a state of complete physical, mental and social well-being, and not merely the absence of disease or infirmity, is a fundamental human right . . ."

In addition, the current emphasis on health care reform has provided a stimulus to emphasize healthy lifestyles. The box on p. 51, bottom, is an example of a national strategy to promote health that involves a selected series of objectives developed by the United States Department of Health and Human Services (USDHHS, 1991). Called *Healthy People 2000,* it includes health status, risk reduction, service and

Essential Services at Primary Level of Contact

- Obtaining health histories and performing complete health exams
- Assessing and evaluating symptoms of common and acute illnesses (e.g., colds, infections)
- Prescribing and managing medication regimens for common or acute conditions
- Managing long-term health problems (e.g., diabetes, hypertension, depression)
- Promoting healthy lifestyles (e.g., nutrition and exercise counseling, stress management planning)
- Providing screening and preventive services (e.g., immunizations, blood pressure screening, smoking cessation programs)
- Networking with health protection and support programs (e.g., safe houses for domestic abuse victims)
- Managing prenatal care, delivery of normal pregnancies, family planning needs
- Identifying health needs that require referral for more specialized care

protection objectives, and research needs. Each objective has a measurable outcome and frequently specifies concrete health promotion behaviors. For example, all primary health care providers need to promote healthy behaviors in clients to combat coronary disease or adolescent weight problems. These behaviors would include changing dietary and physical activity habits that lead to heart disease and weight problems (USDHHS, 1994a). Specific intervention strategies are outlined in the box below.

PRIMARY CARE DELIVERY SYSTEM

Primary care services must be the major component of the primary care delivery system. The primary care delivery system is composed of accessible community based settings, such as physicians' offices, health maintenance organizations (HMOs), community nursing centers, and community health centers. The emphasis of these facilities is to deliver cost-effective primary health care. These services are often provided through a managed-care type of model (see Chapter 2). In a managed-care model, health care, which includes primary care services as well as emergency, preventive, and hospital treatment, is provided at a fixed fee. Clients in this model agree to receive all their health care from the designated health care providers, such as an HMO (Chapter 2). Specialty care is received and reimbursed only after referral from the primary care provider (Stanhope and Lancaster, 1996). Primary health care providers include physicians, nurses, nurse practitioners, and advanced practice nurses.

A Look at Selected National Health Promotion and Disease Prevention Objectives and Research Needs of *Healthy People 2000*

1.0 PHYSICAL ACTIVITY AND FITNESS

Health Status Objectives

1.1 Reduce coronary heart disease deaths to no more than 100 per 100,000 people (age-adjusted baseline: 135 per 100,000 in 1987).

1.2 Reduce overweight to a prevalence of no more than 20% among people aged 20 and older and no more than 15% among adolescents aged 12 through 19. (Baseline: 26% for people aged 20 through 74 in 1976-1980, 24% for men and 27% for women; 15% for adolescents aged 12 through 19 in 1976-1980.)

Risk Reduction Objectives

1.3 Increase to at least 30% the proportion of people age 6 and older who engage regularly, preferably daily, in light to moderate physical activity for at least 30 minutes per day. (Baseline: 22% of people aged 18 and older were active for at least 30 minutes five or more times per week, and 12% were active seven or more times per week in 1985.)

Services and Protection Objectives

1.12 Increase to at least 50% the proportion of primary care providers who routinely assess and counsel their patients regarding the frequency, duration, type, and intensity of physical activity practices. (Baseline: Physicians provided exercise counseling for about 30% of sedentary patients in 1988.)

Research Needs

Research is needed, especially for population subgroups, to further define the relationships between physical activity, physical fitness, and:
- the incidence of cardiovascular disease;
- the incidence of colon cancer;
- the incidence of osteoporosis and osteoporosis-related hip fractures;
- the incidence of and disability from osteoarthritis;
- the incidence of low back pain, injury, and disability;
- the incidence of injuries;
- the incidence of obesity and selected types of body fat patterns;
- nutritional patterns;
- the adoption of healthy behavior patterns;
- the prevention and cessation of cigarette smoking;
- the treatment of alcohol and drug abuse;
- the incidence of depressive episodes among depressed people;
- improved mental well-being;
- the cognitive and functional ability of older adults; and
- quality of life.

Research on the determinants of regular physical activity is also needed to identify the knowledge, attitudes, and behavioral and social skills associated with a high probability of adopting and maintaining a regular exercise program.

Modified from US Department of Health and Human Services, Public Health Service: *Healthy people 2000: national health promotion and disease prevention objectives—full report, with commentary,* Pub No 91–50212, Washington, DC, 1991.

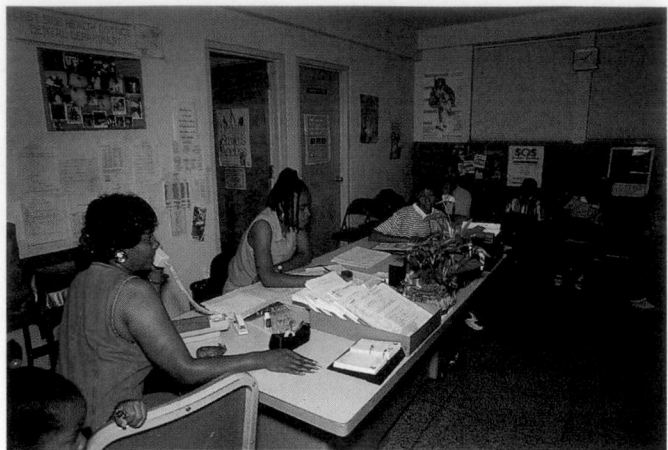

Fig. 3-3 Community-based primary care clinic.

In some settings the nurse engages in health-promotion activities on an individual or family basis. In other settings these activities are directed to specific groups or to general health education programs. In still other settings health-promotion activities are directed to the general community, its people, and its services (Fig. 3-3).

Some settings are for-profit, whereas others are non-profit. Some are clinical sites only, whereas others are learning and research sites. Some are rural, some are urban, some are well financed, and some are poor.

Health care delivery settings have changed over time. Historically the focus has been on hospital-based or private medical care settings. With the emphasis now on controlling overall health care costs, the focus is shifting to community-based and primary care settings.

PRIMARY HEALTH CARE PROVIDERS

Providers of primary health care services are **primary care generalists,** and they must have competencies in health promotion and disease prevention, assessment and evaluation of symptoms and physical signs, management of common acute and chronic medical conditions, and identification and appropriate referral for other needed health care services (USDHHS, 1992). Primary health care generalists include family physicians, general internists, pediatricians, and advanced practice nurses. Advanced practice nurses (APNs) in primary care settings include nurse practitioners (NPs) in specialties such as family, pediatric, adult, and gerontologic nursing, as well as certified nurse midwives (CNMs) (Chapter 13). NPs and CNMs collaborate with physicians within the primary care setting, managing a caseload of clients and families. These nurses are certified for practice by nursing credentialing bodies. Some nurses also have postgraduate-level training and become certified practitioners in specialties that complement general primary care nursing (see Chapter 13).

To provide competent primary care the nurse must demonstrate professional, interpersonal, intraprofessional and interprofessional, and multicultural competencies.

Professional Competence. Professional nursing competence involves being well informed and optimally educated. Because the depth and breadth of nursing practice is always increasing, nurses have a professional obligation to remain current with ongoing research, continuing education, and certification and recertification programs.

Interpersonal Competence. Interpersonal competence involves the ability to relate well with others, whether they are clients, coworkers, peers, or those in positions of authority.

Intraprofessional and Interprofessional Competence. Intraprofessional and interprofessional competence involves a demonstrated ability to relate well with one's nursing peers and with other professionals. It is based on a proactive stance of cordiality, flexibility, trust, and an ability to articulate and uphold one's professional goals, standards, and responsibilities in a manner that fosters respect and cooperation.

Multicultural Competence. Multicultural competence involves a sensitivity to diverse groups, an awareness that we are all members of a global village closely united as a result of a global community, and an ability to act appropriately based on this sensitivity and awareness. Multicultural competence also involves being aware of one's own cultural influences and behaviors and the difficulties these may pose for others. Nurses must be willing and able to provide client education and supportive care that fits a client's cultural needs and definition of health (see Chapter 21).

Client and Family

In the primary setting, as in other health care settings, the "client" can include the person seeking health care and that person's family or significant other. References to the client encompass all these options. Nurse-client interactions take place in a variety of settings that provide access to care across the lifespan (see the box on p. 53, top). Some of these interactions are general and some are specialized: for example, concentrating on the care of children, workers, or older adults. Health promotion, disease prevention, and primary care are focused on the needs of the client.

HEALTH PROMOTION

Health-promotion behaviors are those in which the client views health as a goal in itself and attends health care programs or performs activities designed to achieve or maintain optimal health (Walker, Sechrist, and Pender, 1987). Health-promotion activities in primary care settings include well-baby classes, diet counseling, development of routine exercise programs, and stress management techniques.

DISEASE PREVENTION

Disease-prevention behaviors are those in which the client performs activities designed to decrease the risk of illness. Health-promotion and disease-prevention behaviors necessarily complement one another in their desired outcome of the client's optimal health. Thus, health-promoting and disease-preventing behaviors are subcategories of health-behavior.

We can illustrate health promoting behaviors in primary care settings by referring to Pender's (1987) Health-promotion Model as an example (see Chapter 1). The Health-Promoting Lifestyle Profile in the box on p. 53, bottom, highlights the criteria for assessing specific client behaviors consistent with Pender's model. The results obtained from its application in a worker setting have

Nurse-Client Interaction Settings

NURSE-MANAGED CENTERS (NMCs)

Nurse-managed centers "are organizations that provide direct access to professional nurses who offer client-centered health services for reimbursement. With the use of nursing models of health, professional NMCs diagnose and treat human responses to potential and actual health problems. Examples of professional nursing services include health education, health promotion, and health-related research. Services are frequently targeted to underserved individuals and groups. An effective referral system and collaboration with other health care professionals are an integral part of NMCs. As models of professional nursing practice and research, NMCs are ideal sites for faculty and student practice. They are administered by a professional nurse" (Fehring, Schulte, and Riesch, 1986).

COLLABORATIVE PRACTICE SETTINGS

Collaborative practice settings involve nurses and physicians, in partnership or in groups, together delivering health care outlined in written agreements and jointly agreed-on guidelines or standing orders.

HEALTH CARE NETWORK CENTERS

Health care network centers are settings in which nurses assess clients, provide support, and, when necessary, link them to health care providers or human service agencies. Clients include those with increased vulnerability related to prehospitalization and posthospitalization, grieving, or unemployment or those with few if any health care resources (see Archbishop's Commission on Community Health, 1991).

PUBLIC HEALTH DEPARTMENT SETTINGS

Public health department settings are those in which nurses provide immunization services, home visit follow-up of women during prenatal and postnatal periods,

well-baby and well-child assessments, and infectious disease case-finding and control. Nurses also conduct home visits, make community assessments, and report actual or potential health problems.

NEIGHBORHOOD HEALTH CENTERS

Neighborhood health centers are sites established by city, regional, state, or federal funds, or are financed by local churches, parishes, or volunteer groups. A multidisciplinary team approach, for example, involving nurses, physicians, social workers, and dietitians, is used to deliver primary health care. Community members are often invited to become members of the center's advisory body or governing board.

HEALTH MAINTENANCE ORGANIZATIONS (HMOs)

Health maintenance organizations are settings in which comprehensive health maintenance and treatment services are provided for a group of enrolled persons who pay a prenegotiated fee and are charged fixed payments for health care services (Edelman and Gavan, 1994).

SCHOOLS

Schools are settings in which nurses provide health promotion, immunization, health education, and screening services. They also provide assessments needed for the early detection of acute illnesses (especially infectious diseases), administer first aid, and offer counseling.

OCCUPATIONAL HEALTH SETTINGS

Occupational health settings are settings in business or industry in which nurses promote health, report environmental hazard, conduct screening for high risks, treat common health problems using guidelines developed jointly with the physicians responsible for medical care, administer first aid, and issue referrals.

Health-Promoting Lifestyle Profile

SELF-ACTUALIZATION

Is enthusiastic and optimistic, likes self, grows and changes, has long-term goals, feels happy and content, is aware of strengths and weaknesses, looks forward to future, sets realistic goals, knows what is important, respects own accomplishments, finds days challenging, finds life has purpose, finds satisfying environment.

HEALTH RESPONSIBILITY

Checks cholesterol level, reports symptoms to physician, reads books about health, questions physician, obtains second opinions, discusses health concerns, checks blood pressure, seeks information, attends environmental programs, observes body for changes, attends health care programs.

EXERCISE

Participates in stretching exercise, vigorously exercises three times a week, enrolls in supervised programs, engages in recreational activities, checks pulse rate.

NUTRITION

Eats breakfast, eats three meals daily, uses no preservatives, reads labels, takes in essential nutrients, selects from basic food groups.

INTERPERSONAL SUPPORT

Discusses concerns or problems, praises others easily, enjoys touching, maintains meaningful interpersonal relationships, spends time with close friends, expresses concern and love, touches, is touched.

STRESS MANAGEMENT

Has daily relaxation time, is aware of stress sources, uses meditation and relaxation exercises, relaxes muscles before sleep, uses pleasant bedtime thoughts, expresses feelings, uses stress control methods.

Modified from Walker SN, Sechrist KR, Pender NJ: The health-promoting lifestyle profile: development and psychometric characteristics, *Nurs Res* 36:76, 1987.

RESEARCH HIGHLIGHT

RESEARCH ABSTRACT

The health-promoting lifestyles of blue-collar, skilled trade, and white-collar workers are examined. Specific purposes included determining differences in health-promoting behaviors, especially according to worker category, as well as ethnic identification, age, gender, education, and marital status. A convenience sample of 638 workers in a Midwestern automotive components plant completed the Health-Promoting Lifestyle Profile (HPLP) and demographics questionnaire. Significant main effects on lifestyle were noted on the basis of category of worker, age, gender, and education.

White-collar workers were significantly higher than the other two groups on self-actualization, exercise, and interpersonal support scales. Blue-collar workers were significantly lower than the other groups on nutrition and health-promoting lifestyle.

Younger workers had significantly higher scores than the other groups on self-actualization, exercise, and interpersonal support. Older workers had signifcantly higher scores on health responsibility and nutrition.

Women scored higher on total health-promoting lifestyle scale and on the health responsibility, exercise, and interpersonal support subscales.

Higher education consistently predicted higher scores. When education was controlled, ethnicity, including race, had no main effects on the subscales (except African Americans exercised more). More specifically, the results of this study did not support an assumption of disadvantage in terms of health awareness and practices by African Americans.

IMPLICATIONS FOR PRACTICE

▶ Do not offer the same program or set of health promotion interventions to all clients.

▶ Do not assume disadvantage on the basis of race.

▶ Systematically assess and diagnose health-promoting behaviors and lifestyle. May use the HPLP for this purpose.

▶ Tailor interventions and strategies specific to the health-promotion needs of the individuals or groups with whom you are working.

▶ Recognize that education and age are important variables to consider in tailoring a health-promotion program.

REFERENCE

Lusk SL, Kerr MJ, Ronis DL: Health-promoting lifestyles of blue-collar, skilled trade, and white-collar workers, *Nurs Res* 44(1):20, 1995.

Preventive Service Recommendations for Adults and Older Adults

SCREENING
- Anemia and hemoglobinopathies
- Blood pressure
- Body measurement
- Cancer detection by physical examination
  - Breast
  - Oral cavity
  - Pelvic organs
  - Rectum and prostate
  - Skin
  - Testes
  - Thyroid
- Cholesterol
- Cognitive and functional impairment
- Depression
- Fecal occult blood
- Hearing
- Mammography
- Papanicolaou smear
- Plasma glucose
- Prostate-specific antigen
- Sexually transmitted diseases and HIV infection
- Sigmoidoscopy
- Thyroid function
- Tuberculosis
- Urinalysis
- Vision

IMMUNIZATION/PROPHYLAXIS
- Aspirin
- Estrogen and progestin
- Hepatitis B
- Influenza
- Pneumococcus
- Rubella
- Tetanus and diphtheria

COUNSELING
- Alcohol and other drug abuse
- Dental and oral health
- Injury and violence prevention
- Nutrition
- Physical activity
- Polypharmacy
- Sexually transmitted diseases and HIV infection
- Smoking cessation
- Unintended pregnancy

From US Department of Health and Human Services, Public Health Service: *Clinician's handbook of preventive services*, Washington, DC, 1994, USDHHS.

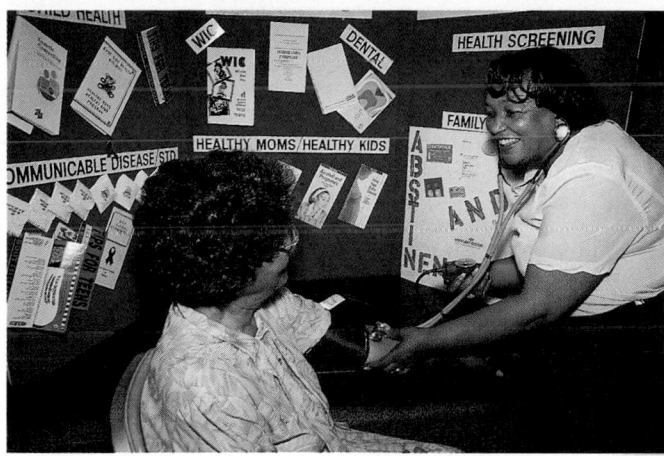

Fig. 3-4 Blood pressure screening.

important implications for occupational health nursing (see the box on p. 54, top).

The box on p. 54, bottom, illustrates selected preventive services for adults and older adults. These include screenings, immunization/prophylaxis, and counseling (Fig. 3-4). Their systematic assessment is important in all primary health care settings.

HEALTH PROTECTION

Health-protecting behaviors are sometimes listed separately and may be considered a third subcategory of health behavior. Thorough assessment may reveal the need for vehicular safety, home safety, domestic-violence recognition, recreational safety, and occupational safety and health education (see the box below). The nurse may choose to use many of the assessment guides currently available for assistance in assessing the client's behavior within these categories (e.g., USDHHS, 1994b; Stanhope and Knollmueller, 1992).

Using proper health-protection strategies or interventions is as important as correct assessment and diagnosis of clients at risk. When a nursing intervention involves client education and client advocacy, the education for the client should be explicit and thorough. For example, to reduce lead toxicity among children, parents need to be thoroughly informed about how they can eliminate lead hazards in the home (see the box on p. 56).

But client education may not be sufficient to solve the problem. Making a home nonhazardous for lead may also require lead-based paint testing, repair, and renovation; the cost may be too expensive for the client to pay alone. However, partnerships among government, community, charitable, and corporate institutions may be forged to help individuals and families help cover the expense (USDHHS, 1991). The nurse as a client advocate can assist in establishing these partnerships.

Although client advocacy is usually directed solely at the client, it may also involve nurses reflecting on their own risk-taking behaviors. Self-reflection provides valuable insights concerning nurse and client vulnerability. Nurse self-reflection also has a professional purpose: it is an essential part of nursing leadership (Gebbie, 1994).

Technological Resources

Technological developments are becoming increasingly important for nurses striving to provide the best possible primary health care. Technology has the potential to increase accessibility to health care services. As these technological applications further develop, nurses and clients may soon be computer networking and routinely interacting with each other through voice-activated computers and video conferences (American Nurses Association [ANA] Task Force, 1994). As more computer programs are developed, the more they are used and the more cost per use is decreased. For example, the Sisters of Saint Mary (SSM) Rehabilitation Institute (1994) has established a computerized bulletin board designed especially for disabled clients. It helps clients communicate with each other and provides

---

Health-Protection Assessment Categories for Age-Appropriate Counseling

VEHICULAR SAFETY
- Safety belts, adult and child
- Motorcycle and bicycle helmets
- Inflatable safety restraints
- Designated driver usage

HOME SAFETY
- Kitchen safety
- Food safety
- Fall prevention practices
- Fire prevention safety, including electrical safety
- Smoke detector usage
- Carbon monoxide poisoning precautions
- Lead poisoning precautions
- Prescribed and over-the-counter (OTC) drug precautions
- Accidental poisoning precautions
- Rat and pest control
- Firearms safety

DOMESTIC VIOLENCE RECOGNITION
- Child abuse
- Partner abuse
- Elder abuse

RECREATIONAL SAFETY
- Swimming
- Boating
- Skiing, water and snow
- Contact sports
- Jogging
- Horseback riding

OCCUPATIONAL SAFETY AND HEALTH
- Lung pollutants
- Skin irritants
- Injury risk
- Noise exposure
- Lead or other heavy metal exposure
- Hepatitis, tuberculosis, or HIV exposure

Lead Poisoning Protection Strategies

- Be alert for chipping and flaking paint.
- Make sure child puts only safe, clean items in mouth.
- Feed well-balanced meals that are low in fat and high in iron, calcium, and zinc.
- Do not allow child to eat snow or icicles.
- Use safe interior paints on toys, walls, and furniture.
- Use pottery only for display if unsure about the glaze.
- Store food in glass, plastic, or stainless steel containers, not in opened cans.
- Have your water tested, and draw drinking water only from the cold tap after allowing water to run for a few minutes (if you suspect lead danger).
- Have children wash hands before eating.
- Ask your local public health or housing official about an evaluation of lead hazards in your residence.
- *If you work with lead,* shower and change before coming home.
- Wash clothes separately from those of other family members.

TESTING
Every child between the ages of 6 months and 6 years should be tested for lead at least once a year with a simple blood test. This may be done with a finger stick or by venipuncture. If anyone in the household is diagnosed with lead poisoning, all other household members should be tested.

From Stanhope M, Knollmueller RN: *Handbook of community and home health nursing,* ed 2, St Louis, 1996, Mosby.

online library options, updated listings of community activities, and descriptions of available services and resources.

Human service organizations benefit from computer networks. For example, through HandsNet,* a nonprofit information and communications network, service organizations can access information about AIDS/HIV; alcohol and substance abuse prevention; children, youth, and family issues; welfare and health care reform; housing and community development; and hunger and nutrition policies (HandsNet, 1995).

The general public may also have access to health information networks (e.g., NUS-NCI CancerNet and the Dana Farber Cancer Center) and electronic discussion groups that focus on health-related issues (e.g., gerinet [listserve@uvbm.cc.buffalo.edu], which is a geriatric health care discussion group, and minhlth [listserve@dawn.hampshire.edu], which addresses minority health issues).

Technology has also enhanced health care providers' ability to extend life and prolong death. A large proportion of health care dollars are spent during a person's last few weeks of life. Critical care, for example, is the most expensive health care option. These technological advances are expensive and have the potential to divert health care dollars away from primary care and health-promotion and illness-prevention activities.

■ NURSES' ROLE IN THE DELIVERY OF PRIMARY CARE

The professional nurse is in a position to deliver cost-effective, resource-efficient, and competent primary care and health-promotion and disease-prevention activities. Primary care nurses financed by, linked to, or subcontracted by a primary care organization could assume the major responsibility for community health-promotion and disease-prevention services. Some of these services might include following up on clients who fail to keep immunization appointments, providing growth and development assessments of high-risk infants and toddlers in their homes, diabetic education classes, infectious disease control and follow-up services, domestic abuse prevention and follow-up services, healthy lifestyles, stress management programs, and compliance evaluations. The focus would then be on maintaining or maximizing health *before* a new problem or a complication of an old problem occurs.

Community-Based Practice

Clients may be members of groups or aggregates, such as the workers in a factory, students in a school district, or the older adults in a retirement home. Clients may also be perceived as communities. Thus the nurse must assess a community's strengths, potential or actual health problems, and health-promotion needs. The nurse then uses the nursing process to derive relevant diagnoses, to develop a plan, and to implement and evaluate the outcomes (see Unit 2).

One contemporary example of a primary care nurse in this situation is the parish nurse. The parish nurse works in a specific neighborhood, has links to a broadly defined health care network, and works with community health care providers. This parish nurse model may be useful for any health care organization or network interested in maximizing the health of the population served and minimizing the expenses associated with preventable illnesses or complications.

Another example of community-based practice is the home health care nurse, who focuses on acute and restorative care in the home. Although the nurse interacts with the client and family after an acute illness, the care is directed toward restoring the client's level of health and function to the preillness status. Availability of home health nurses maintains clients' continuity of care from the hospital into the community (see Chapter 5).

---

*For information, contact HandsNet, 20195 Stevens Creek Blvd, Suite 120, Cupertino, Calif; e-mail: HN3187@handsnet.org or HN00X0@handsnet.org; Calif; phone: 408/257-4500; fax: 408/257-4500.

Community-based practice can assist in resolving the dilemma of access to care. Some clients may belong to a primary care organization but are unable to reach it. Lack of transportation thus becomes a barrier to access. Accessibility may also be a problem for the uninsured. Many people who are self-employed, work only part-time, or are unemployed may not be able to afford insurance coverage for themselves or their families. Their access to most primary care facilities is thus extremely limited. Nurses must be aware of accessibility concerns and must work with community health care providers and primary health care organizations to provide adequate care for all community members.

COMMUNITY-ORIENTED PRIMARY CARE

Community-oriented primary care is a community-responsive model of health care delivery that integrates both primary care and public health (Stanhope and Lancaster, 1996). This model is designed to combine the care of individuals, families, and groups into cost-effective, easily access-

---

CASE STUDY

BACKGROUND

Eliciting a chief complaint or health concern, asking the correct branching questions, performing the correct examinations, and arriving at a diagnosis are important parts of the health assessment of an individual. Battered women, however, frequently cover up or mask the fact that they are battered. Even after eliciting several health concerns, it is wise to ask if there are any other questions or issues she would like to discuss.

ASSESSMENT

Twenty-four-year-old Jan was accompanied to the clinic by 28-year-old Robert. They had been living together for the past 2 years. She came to the clinic because she was tired. Her embarrassed, mostly toothless smile was warm and pleasant. They recently moved into the city from another Midwestern state. Jan had a history of emotional problems and was receiving disability. Robert had back problems and no job or income. Both were in need of health care and employment.

Robert controlled most of the conversation. His eye contact was usually good. He had to think about how to use words and answer questions, however. His speech, therefore, had a halting, unsure quality about it. Nevertheless, he seemed knowledgeable about his own health history and Jan's. Whenever Jan spoke he became angry and told her to "shut up."

The social and emotional contexts in which this assessment took place are important. Robert answered all questions regarding himself and Jan. He was sitting in a chair and Jan was curled up on the end of a second chair. Only when Robert stalled did she contribute facts.

Becoming increasingly concerned about her demeanor and Robert's anger, the nurse directed the assessment and conversation to Jan. The nurse asked Jan directly if she had any health concerns. Only then did she bring up the possibility that she might be pregnant, since her last menstrual period was 3 months ago. At this point she smiled and said both she and Robert were looking forward to the baby.

NURSING DIAGNOSIS

The diagnosis of risk for violence directed at others is defined as a state in which an individual exhibits behaviors that are or can be physically harmful to others (Kim, McFarland, and McLane, 1995). Robert's high need for control of the situation, his anger, and his contempt for Jan (manifested in the words "shut-up") lead the nurse to suspect that Robert is at risk of violence, directed at Jan. Jan's submissiveness, unwillingness to control the situation, toothlessness, and pregnancy lead the nurse to suspect that Jan may be a victim of domestic abuse.

PLANNING AND IMPLEMENTATION

First, it was necessary to get Jan away from Robert, and he was asked go to the waiting area. When pursuing information regarding abuse or providing interventions, the victim needs to be away from the abuser. If the issue of abuse is brought up in front of the abuser, the victim's safety is further threatened. One plan was quickly made: Jan needed an alternative place to go should she decide her safety would warrant it. While in the clinic setting

Jan was given the name, address, and phone number of a shelter for abused women and the domestic abuse hotline with the local police department. During the clinic visit, she requested assistance from the police department and was given transportation to the women's shelter.

EVALUATION

Jan remained in the shelter and sought prenatal care through the women's health clinic. During her pregnancy she finished her GED, took parenting classes, and volunteered with domestic violence community groups. At her postpartum examination, Jan was planning to return to her parents, who promised to help her with her baby daughter, which allowed Jan to enter a job training program. Jan's long-term plans are to remain in the city where her parents live, but to eventually be self-supporting. She is undergoing therapy to improve her self-image and to avoid being a repeat victim of abuse.

REVIEW

This case study demonstrates health-protecting behavior on the part of a woman at risk of being physically abused. In terms of assessment, the nurse picked up on three sets of cues. One set concerned Jan (i.e., her toothlessness, lack of eye contact, and withdrawn body language). A second set revolved around the possible pregnancy. The nurse knew that the probability of abuse increases during pregnancy as the mother's interest naturally turns somewhat away from her partner and increasingly to herself and the child she is bearing. The third set was provided by Robert's angry responses whenever Jan spoke. Putting these three sets of cues together, the nurse arrived at the diagnosis that there was an immediate and high risk for domestic violence in the situation in which Jan and Robert were living.

Once the diagnosis was made, the nurse began to implement a plan consisting of short- and long-term goals and interventions. Because the risk for violence was immediate, the nurse needed to intervene immediately. Long-term interventions centered on giving Jan the information and support she needed to decide her future's course freely.

The initial contact of a health professional with a woman who is being abused is often in the provider's office or in an emergency department. Because of the reticence of women to speak about being battered, special interviewing techniques are needed. Still, many victims of abuse go undetected. The knowledgeable, observant, and sensitive nurse working in any primary care setting is capable of making an important contribution to the prevention, recognition, and treatment of abused women.

Primary care settings offer the nurse opportunities to assist clients to develop health-promotion and disease-prevention behaviors. In addition, the nurse is involved in primary, secondary, and tertiary prevention strategies. Nurses have the potential to affect the health care of their clients while participating in collaborative practice settings. ■

ible health care programs. To succeed in delivering this kind of primary health care, nurses cannot depend only on themselves. They must also work with community health care workers, who can then extend the capabilities of the nurse. Drawn from the local community, these health care workers may relate well to community members and may carry out many health-promotion and disease-prevention tasks.

The Community as a Partner in Primary Care

At the same time, there is another challenge, which is to see the community not as a client but as a partner (Anderson, Gottschalk, and Martin, 1993). This type of model is more amenable to a community development approach to health promotion, which works with the community in the assessment of its own health-promotion needs, priorities, strategies, and evaluation mechanisms.

SAMPLE FLOW SHEET FOR ADULT PREVENTATIVE CARE

Vaccine Administration Record

Vaccine	Date Given	Vaccine Manufacturer	Vaccine Lot Number	Site Given	Initials of Vaccine Administrator	Signature of Patient

*Signature of vaccine administrator / *Signature of vaccine administrator

REPETITIVE HEALTH SCREENING MEASURES* — Hearing, Glaucoma/Vision, Breast Exam, Mammogram, Rectal, Stool Guaiac, Flex Sig, Pap/Testicular Exam, Pelvic/Prostate, Cholesterol, Other (Specify)

SELECTIVE SCREENING* — RPR, HIV, PPD, FBS, Other (Specify)

PT. EDUCATION* — ETOH, Smoking, Self Exam, Nutritional Counseling, Exercise, Other (Specify)

*date in box - ADD TO PROBLEM LIST WHEN INDICATED

Fig. 3-5 Sample flow sheet for adult preventive care. *(Modified from St Louis University Medical Center: Master Problem List/Preventive Profile, St Louis University Medical Center, Form MR.3 1992.)*

The key component in developing a health care partnership with a community is involvement of the community leaders. These leaders have an accurate understanding of the health, housing, economic, and development needs of the community. Such a partnership provides the power, information, financial support, and resources to the community-oriented primary care program. Together community leaders and health care professionals are a powerful force in meeting the primary care and health-promotion and illness-prevention needs of a community.

THE NURSING PROCESS AND THE DELIVERY OF PRIMARY CARE SERVICES

This section uses a case study method to demonstrate how the nursing process is used in a primary care setting. In such settings, the standard written nursing care plans are not generated. Rather, a nurse does a complete history and physical, diagnoses health care needs, intervenes, and evaluates outcomes appropriately. The client's medical record is maintained in a narrative format and uses flow sheets (Fig. 3-5) to track health-promotion and illness-prevention strategies.

■ KEY CONCEPTS ■

▶ Primary health care includes universal access.

▶ Whereas health professionals attempt to deliver primary care to all, the end result today is often a fragmented care system for the poor and the uninsured.

▶ Primary care settings are the first level of contact for clients and their families with the health care system.

▶ Health promotion activities are appropriate in every health care setting and at every level of care.

▶ The nurse is interested in client behaviors that affect health, whether they be health promoting, health protecting, or disease preventing.

▶ Self-reflection is essential if nurses are to become leaders.

▶ Technology may be put to creative use in health promotion and in primary care.

▶ Role of nursing refers to the professional responsibilities nurses assume and to how nurses view and define themselves and their goals.

▶ Health-promotion activities may be used at the primary, secondary, and tertiary levels of prevention.

▶ The delivery of primary nursing care involves striving to achieve universal access and to work with other health care professionals.

■ KEY TERMS ■

Community-oriented primary care, p. 57

Health-protecting behaviors, p. 55

Interpersonal competence, p. 52

Intraprofessional and interprofessional competence, p. 52

Multicultural competence, p. 52

Primary care, p. 48

Primary care generalists, p. 52

Primary health care system, p. 48

Professional nursing competence, p. 52

Universal access, p. 49

■ CRITICAL THINKING EXERCISES ■

1. A nurse and social worker want to develop a health promotion program. They are specifically interested in offering a community an opportunity to form women's groups, a major purpose of which is to decrease infant mortality through education regarding, and promotion of, adequate infant nutrition and care. How would you decide which program to begin first?

2. A self-reflection exercise: What are the thought processes you employ to justify continuing an activity that presents a risk to your health?

3. Using the major categories listed in the sample plan for the delivery of primary health care provided in the box on p. 51, bottom, develop a health-promotion program of your own choice.

REFERENCES

American Nurses Association Task Force: *Scope of practice for nursing informatics*, Washington, DC, 1994, American Nurses Association.

Anderson ET, Gottschalk J, Martin DA: Contemporary issues in the community. In Mason DJ, Talbot SW, Leavitt JK, eds: *Policy and politics for nurses: action and change in the workplace, government, organizations and community,* Philadelphia, 1993, WB Saunders.

Archbishop's Commission on Community Health, *Elements to consider when planning a health ministry program*, St Louis, 1994, Catholic Community Services.

Edelman CL, Gavan CS: Health policy and the delivery system. In Edelman CL, Mandle CL, eds: *Health promotion throughout the lifespan,* St Louis, 1994, Mosby.

Fehring RJ, Schulte J, Riesch SK: Toward a definition of nurse-managed centers, *J Comm Health Nurs* 3(2):59, 1986.

Gebbie K: What would Florence have done? *Acad Nurs* Summer:28, 1994.

HandsNet, HandsNet at a Glance, Cupertino, Calif, 1995.

Jaarsma T, Kastermans M, Dassen T, et al: Problems of cardiac patients in early recovery, *J Adv Nurs* (21):21, 1995.

Johnson T: Changing demographics in minority populations of the United States. In *Caring for the emerging majority: creating a new diversity in nurse leadership*, Rockville, MD, 1992, Division of Nursing in the Office of Minority Health.

Kim MJ, McFarland GK, McLane AM: *Pocket guide to nursing diagnoses,* ed 6, St Louis, 1995 Mosby.

Lusk SL, Kerr MJ, Ronis DL: Health-promoting lifestyles of blue-collar, skilled trade, and white-collar workers, *Nurs Res*, 44:20, 1995.

Mosby's patient teaching guides, St Louis, 1995, Mosby.

Pender NJ: *Health promotion in nursing practice,* ed 2, Norwalk, Conn, 1987, Appleton & Lange.

Richardson H: Longterm care. In Kovner A, ed: *Health care delivery in the United States.* New York, 1995, Springer.

St. Louis University Medical Center: *Master problem list/preventive profile,* Form MR3, 1992.

Sisters of Saint Mary: Insights, St Louis: SSM Rehabilitation Institute, 6:1, 1994.

Stanhope M, Knollmueller RN: *Handbook of community and home health nursing,* ed 2, St Louis, 1996, Mosby.

Stanhope M, Lancaster J: *Community health nursing: promoting health of aggregates, families, and individuals,* St Louis, 1996, Mosby.

U.S. Department of Health and Human Services, Public Health Service: *Healthy people 2000: national health promotion and disease prevention objectives—full report, with commentary,* Pub. No. 91-50212, Washington, D.C., 1991, US Government Printing Office.

U.S. Department of Health and Human Services, Public Health Service: *Health personnel in the United States: eighth report to congress,* Pub. No. HRS-P-OD-92-1, Washington, D.C., 1992, US Government Printing Office.

U.S. Department of Health and Human Services, Public Health Service, Centers for Disease Control and Prevention (CDC): Prevalence of overweight among adolescents. In *MMWR Morb Mortal Wkly Rep* 43(44):818, 1994a.

U.S. Department of Health and Human Services, Public Health Service: *Clinician handbook of preventive services,* ISBN 0-16-043115-8, Washington, D.C., 1994b.

Walker SN, Sechrist KR, Pender NJ: The health-promoting lifestyle profile: development and psychometric characteristics, *Nurs Res* 36:76, 1987.

World Health Organization, *Primary health care,* Geneva, 1978.

World Health Organization, *Alma-ata 1978: primary health care, health for all,* Series No.1, Geneva, 1978

ADDITIONAL READINGS

Babcock DE, Miller MA: *Client education: theory and practice,* St Louis, 1994, Mosby.

Bullough B, Bullough V: *Nursing in the community,* St Louis 1990, Mosby.

Clark MJ: *Nursing in the community,* Norwalk, CT, 1992, Appleton & Lange.

Cox HC, et al: *Clinical applications of nursing diagnosis: adult, child, women's, psychiatric, gerontic and home health considerations,* ed 2, Philadelphia, 1993, FA Davis.

Family Care Health Centers: *Abuse protocols,* St Louis, 1995, 6827 S Broadway, St Louis, Mo, 63111.

Werner D, Bower B: *Helping health workers learn: a book of methods, aids, and ideas for instructors at the village level* (9th printing), Palo Alto, CA, 1991, The Hesperian Foundation.

Werner D, Thuman C, and Maxwell J: *Where there is no doctor: a village health care handbook* (revised edition), Palo Alto, CA, 1992, The Hesperian Foundation.

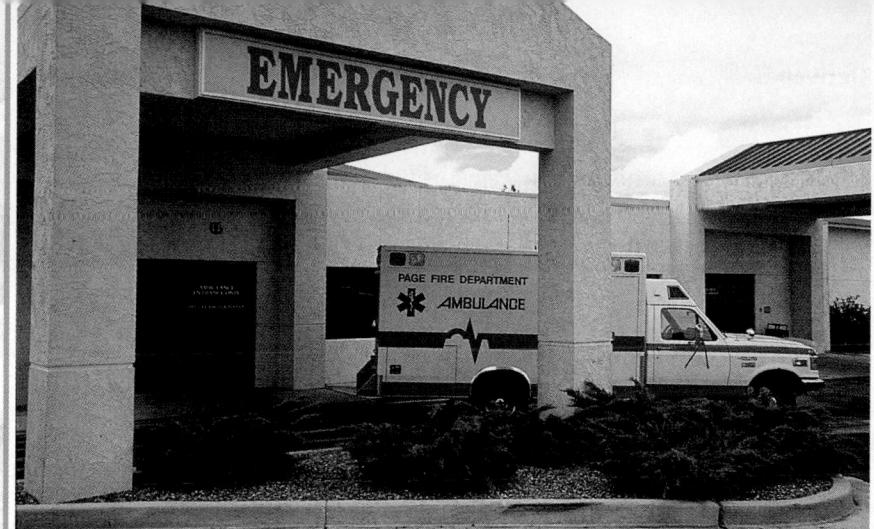

## Chapter 4

Acute Care

Objectives

Mastery of content in this chapter will enable the student to:

▶ Define the key terms listed.

▶ Identify the influence reimbursement has had on acute care agencies.

▶ Explain the relationship registered nurses should have with unlicensed assistive personnel.

▶ Describe the Five Rights of Delegation.

▶ Discuss the dimensions of client satisfaction.

▶ Describe nursing's roles and responsibilities in an acute care facility.

▶ Identify purposes of health care referrals.

▶ Identify clients in need of comprehensive discharge planning.

▶ Identify future trends in health care and the way they affect clinical practice in acute care settings.

When clients experience an abrupt or severe episode of illness, major surgery, or the physical injuries of trauma, **acute health care** becomes necessary. Acute care is typically provided in the emergency rooms, medical-surgical units, and intensive care units of hospitals. Specialized personnel use complex and sophisticated technology to diagnose and treat clients' medical problems. The time during which a client remains in an acute care setting is typically short, but the impact it has on a client physically, emotionally, and economically is significant.

When clients enter the health care system for their acute care needs, nursing becomes the most essential health care service (Joel, 1994). Clients come to hospitals for nursing because of the need for monitoring and surveillance on a continuous basis and because of self-care deficits and compromised functional states. In addition, clients require symptom management, education, coordination of services, counseling, and referral to community support systems. The nurse is the one health care professional available 24 hours a day to coordinate the complex care a client requires.

The health care system is changing (see Chapter 2). Under the economic constraints created by the Medicare prospective pricing system, managed care, and capitation, fewer dollars are available for health care. The acute care setting has been most dramatically affected. To remain profitable, hospitals have pushed to reduce a client's length of stay, reduce use of ancillary services such as respiratory therapy, and minimize the use of diagnostic testing. As a result, physicians have tried to treat clients in the community and choose hospitalization as a last resort (Joel, 1994). The hospitalized client today, compared with the client of 10 years ago, is more severely ill, stays in the hospital a shorter time, and undergoes an aggressive treatment program. Nursing requirements have grown as clients continue to require critical and rapid assessments, comprehensive nursing care plans, well-coordinated services from other health care disciplines, and effective and timely discharge planning. The professional nurse must be highly competent to skillfully manage a client's clinical needs while minimizing the unnecessary use of costly medical resources.

▌ THE ACUTE CARE ENVIRONMENT

The acute care hospital is in the middle of health care reform. Every hospital in the United States is undergoing changes that are influencing how hospitals are staffed, who makes up the staff, and how care is delivered. Chapter 2 summarizes types of acute care settings and issues pertaining to hospital restructuring; work redesign; and the use of unlicensed, assistive personnel. The changes are influencing nursing staff, clients, physicians, and the services they provide.

Staff

The nurse who works in an acute care setting is the most critical health care provider. It is the professional nurse who is found at the heart of client care delivery. Many hospitals have reduced the percentage of registered nurses who staff acute care units. As a result, the nurse's responsibilities become less involved with basic direct care activities (e.g., hygienic care and ambulation) and more involved with client assessment, delivery of complex treatments requiring problem solving and individualization, and coordination of other health care provider services. Registered nurses are being asked to assume greater accountability for the efficient and timely clinical management of clients. Active collaboration with the whole health care team is critical to the nurse's success in coordinating client care.

More unlicensed assistive personnel have been added to provide a supportive work force at a lower cost. Unlicensed, assistive personnel include any unlicensed staff member, regardless of title, to whom nursing tasks are delegated (National Council, 1995), for example, nurse assistant, patient care technician, or nurse technician. With proper training, unlicensed, assistive personnel can become valuable partners with the nurse in providing basic care measures safely and effectively. Curtin (1994) stresses the importance of assistive personnel being at the "nurse's side" rather than "at the bedside." The assistive personnel must work closely with the nurse in performing those tasks that help make the nurse more productive and available for complex nursing care measures.

In a typical situation an acute care nurse assigned to the care of five clients cannot be in each client's room at the same time. Each client has a different set of needs. The nurse must be the one to make the decision as to which clients require direct intervention and which ones need care that can be delegated to an assistive personnel. For example, a client recovering 2 days after major surgery will need to be ambulated more frequently and involved more in self-care activities. Another client, admitted from the emergency room with gastrointestinal bleeding, will require frequent monitoring and administration of pharmacological and intravenous therapies. Which client will the nurse delegate to the care of assistive personnel? The answer is both. **Delegation** is not based upon which client requires care but rather what tasks can best be delivered by unlicensed, assistive personnel. The nurse can delegate the

---

The Five Rights of Delegation

RIGHT TASK
Tasks that are repetitively performed, require minimal problem solving or innovation. One that is delegable for a specific client

RIGHT CIRCUMSTANCES
Appropriate client setting with available resources and right timing

RIGHT PERSON
Right person is delegating the right task to the right person to be performed on the right client

RIGHT DIRECTION
Clear, concise description of the task, including its purpose, limits and expectations. Right information about a client must also be communicated if any variation is needed in how the task is to be performed

RIGHT SUPERVISION
Appropriate monitoring, evaluation, intervention, and feedback

Modified from National Council: Delegation, concepts and decision-making process, National Council of State Boards of Nursing, Inc., Chicago, Illinois, 1995.

bath of the 2-day postoperative client but may decide that if the client continues to have an irregular heart rhythm, it might be wise to accompany the client during ambulation. In the case of the client admitted from the emergency room, assistive personnel can help by obtaining lab specimens and helping to turn and reposition the client in bed.

The box on p. 62 lists the five rights of delegation. Appropriate delegation requires critical thinking on the part of the nurse in deciding the needs of each client and making sure appropriate supervision is available as needed.

The role of the nurse is changing as hospitals reengineer the processes of care and redesign who performs the work. This provides opportunities for the nurse to take the lead in how to design care delivery models. The focus must always be on the client and how to ensure that high quality care can always be delivered.

Clients

Consumers of health care are becoming more knowledgeable about health care issues and pay greater attention to what they hear about hospitals, physicians, and the perceived quality of nursing. No matter how advanced a hospital might be in the technology it uses, a client's experience with illness and medical care is a truer measure of quality. What clients experience and what they think of that experience, will influence how they choose to use a health care system in the future (Gerteis et al, 1993). With the competition that now exists between hospitals and health care systems, it is time for all health care providers to pay very close attention to clients' expectations of care.

The Joint Commission on Accreditation of Health Care Organizations (1996) requires hospitals to monitor client satisfaction with their health care. As a result, most hospitals conduct regular surveys throughout the year to measure client satisfaction. In many metropolitan areas, the client satisfaction scores of competing hospitals are being published so that consumers (clients, businesses, and insurers) can make decisions about the quality of care at each hospital. In response to client satisfaction issues, many hospitals are developing customer service programs. Customer service includes primary services (e.g., hospital lodging, nursing care, and medical treatment) and secondary services (e.g., referral to areas of comfort and convenience) (Leming, 1991). In delivering primary services, staff learn to become customer focused first. This means always holding the highest respect for the client as a discriminating and knowledgeable individual. This sounds like common sense, particularly for nurses who learn to develop the therapeutic nurse-client relationship, but *customer service* is a modern term for what nurses value most (Brickhill, 1995). It is becoming more of an important principle to apply during any client interactions.

The Picker/Commonwealth Program for Patient-Centered Care was established in 1987 to explore clients' needs and concerns, as clients define them, and to promote models of care that make the experience of illness and hospitalization more humane (Gerteis et al, 1993). The researchers from this organization conducted focus sessions with clients and their family members. As a result of their work, seven dimensions of patient-centered care were defined (see the box on p. 64). The seven dimensions encompass much of the scope of what is nursing practice. The Picker/Commonwealth program has developed a tool that measures client satisfaction along the seven dimensions. The survey looks globally at client perceptions of the care they received in a hospital in an attempt to understand how all hospital departments contribute to or influence client satisfaction. Nonetheless, nursing plays a key role in client satisfaction because nursing is one of the professions that is most likely to influence each of the seven dimensions.

Client satisfaction is becoming the basis for many quality improvement efforts within hospitals (see Chapter 11). Satisfaction instruments like the Picker/Commonwealth tool can begin to identify potential areas for improvement. However, the unique needs of individual client populations require health care professionals to look at client satisfaction in more detail to truly understand client expectations. For example, nurses working on an oncology unit will have different client satisfaction issues around physical comfort than nurses caring for new mothers in a postpartum hospital suite. Making client satisfaction a priority will help nurses and other health care providers develop the types of therapies and approaches that not only improve a client's state of health but also make them interested, participative partners in care.

Physicians

Physicians find themselves in a difficult situation in today's health care system. Their image with clients has been changing. The medical profession is not held in the same high regard as it was 10 or more years ago. The causes for the profession's fall from grace can be attributed to greater public consciousness of the fallibility of medical science, doctors' incomes, publicized stories about medical malpractice and fraud, and current debate over access to care (Gerteis et al, 1993). Coupled with this change in consumer perception is the change in reimbursed medical services. Just as hospitals are receiving less revenue for services, so are physicians.

As doctors worry about attracting and retaining clients, hospitals have placed more demands on physicians to work more efficiently and to maintain or improve clinical outcomes. In other words, physicians are expected to treat their clients at a lower cost, while achieving positive results. For example, in academic medical centers, where the cost for providing health care is higher than in community hospitals, physicians are being asked to use fewer resources, for example, laboratory or radiology tests, antibiotics, or specialists. Physicians worry that the focus on cost reduction will endanger the quality of care delivered to their clients. However, there are many physicians who acknowledge that unnecessary resources have been used excessively in the past.

Clearly hospitals are seeing the need to partner more closely with physicians and vice versa. Physicians want to believe that hospitals are focused on the client's needs and welfare. Doctors will join in efforts to improve quality of care within hospitals if staff invite them to collaborate (Gerteis et al, 1993). One example is the development of critical pathways (see Chapters 9 and 12). A multidisciplinary team is successful in developing sound clinical guidelines only when a physician plays an active role in pathway development. The pathway is designed on the basis of best clinical practice as well as the judicious use of resources,

The Dimensions of Patient-Centered Care

I. Respect for clients' values, preferences, and expressed needs
    ■ Clients expect to be treated with dignity and respect.
    ■ Clients want to be informed and involved in decisions about their care.
    ■ A client's perception of needs should not be completely different from those identified by a health care provider.

II. Coordination and integration of care
    ■ Clients' feelings of powerlessness can be minimized by a competent and caring staff.
    ■ The client looks for someone to be in charge of his or her care and to communicate clearly with other health team members.
    ■ Clients look to have services and procedures well coordinated.
    ■ Clients need to know at all times who to call for help.

III. Information, communication, and education
    ■ Clients expect to receive accurate and timely information about their clinical status, progress, or prognosis.
    ■ Clients and families need to be informed of major changes in therapies or status.
    ■ Tests and procedures must be explained in language a client can understand.
    ■ Clients and family members want to know how to manage care on their own to the extent they desire or are able.

IV. Physical comfort
    ■ Physical care that comforts clients is one of the most elemental services care givers can provide.
    ■ Nurses should respond in a timely and effective way to any request for pain medication, explain the extent of pain the client can expect, and offer alternatives for pain management.
    ■ Clients expect to have privacy and to have their cultural values respected.
    ■ The hospital environment should be kept clean and comfortable.

V. Emotional support and alleviation of fear and anxiety
    ■ Clients look to care providers to share their fears and concerns.
    ■ Clients need to understand the impact illness will have on their ability to care for themselves and their family.
    ■ Clients worry about their ability to pay for their medical care and hospitalization. Are there staff who can help with those worries?

VI. Involvement of family and friends
    ■ Care providers must recognize and respect the family and friends on whom clients rely for support.
    ■ Clients have the right to determine if family members are to be involved in decisions about their care.
    ■ Clients expect those family or friends who will provide physical support and care after discharge to be properly informed.

VII. Transition and continuity
    ■ Clients want information about medications to take, dietary or treatment regimens to follow, and danger signals to look for after hospitalization.
    ■ Clients expect to have their continuing health care needs met after discharge with well-coordinated services.
    ■ Clients and family members expect access to any necessary health care resources after discharge.

Modified from Gerteis M et al: *Through the patient's eyes*, San Francisco, 1993, Jossey-Bass.

giving all staff members a clearer road map for managing a client's clinical care more successfully.

More hospitals are conducting surveys to measure physician satisfaction. Physicians appreciate the interest generated when hospitals ask about their satisfaction with delivery of services, staff competency, staff communication, and client perceptions. Hospitals then must take action to improve services or respond to those problems physicians identify. For example, automated client records, staff development programs, client information and education services, and partnerships with advanced practice nurses are just some of the approaches being used to improve physician satisfaction, while also improving health care services.

Services

The changes in health care bring new services into the acute care setting. Since managed care now limits the type of procedures or conditions that require hospitalization, more hospitals have added special procedure and recovery units to manage clients on an outpatient basis. These units may provide services such as endoscopy, pheresis, cardiac catheterization, special wound care, and intravenous access placement. Outpatient surgical units are also quite common in hospital settings. Both procedure and surgical units require nurses to be highly competent in client assessment, intravenous sedation, and client education. Clients enter the units, undergo a procedure, and are discharged all in the same day. Nurses must know how to act quickly and make the right judgments to ensure clients receive safe and appropriate care. Family members and friends become important resources when clients undergo outpatient procedures. The nurse ensures that clients reach a condition to be safely discharged and that family members know how to assume care for the client until the client can resume normal activities at home.

Medical-surgical and intensive care units have become busier since client acuity has risen. Clients do not come to hospitals unless it is absolutely necessary. Perhaps one of the greatest challenges for nurses within acute care settings is remaining knowledgeable about new technology. Intravenous fluid delivery pumps, support surface mattresses, medications, monitoring devices, and dressing materials are just some of the technologies that are constantly changing. The nurse must understand how to use the technology as well as what information is needed about a client to apply the technology safely.

■ THE ACUTE CARE CONTINUUM

Admission to a hospital is an extremely stressful event. Once hospitalized, a client may move to various locations within an institution, depending on the nature of the health care problem being treated. Nurses play a key role in coordinating care from admission through discharge by maintaining a holistic approach necessary to recognize and anticipate the client's total health care needs.

Continuum of Care

The concept of a continuum of care has become more important with the arrival of prospective reimbursement for hospitals (see Chapter 2). When a client enters the acute care hospital, the cost for hospitalization in most cases is predetermined, regardless of the resources used by care givers. As a result, for hospitals to survive financially, there is pressure to discharge clients as soon as possible. Given a client's usual limited length of stay in a hospital, the timely and accurate determination of health care needs and their prioritization are critical. To ensure a continuum of care, all care givers must know the client's prioritized needs so that a thoroughly integrated plan of care can be administered. Fragmentation of care occurs when a client receives a variety of services that may be repetitious, unrelated, or inappropriate. This fragmentation is expensive and unacceptable. A well-coordinated, multidisciplinary approach ensures a continuum of care from admission to discharge.

Examples of JCAHO Standards for Admission and Discharge

NURSING AND HEALTH TEAM RESPONSIBILITIES

Before hospital admission

Identifies and uses available information sources about the client's needs.

Communicates with other care settings and organizations.

During admission

The hospital:

Provides services consistent with its mission, population served, and settings.

Makes arrangements with other organizations and settings to facilitate the client's admission.

Clients are referred and transferred to meet their needs based on intensity, risk, and staffing level.

When appropriate, clinical consultants and contractual arrangements are used for referrals and transfers.

In the hospital

Services flow continuously from assessment through treatment and reassessment.

The client's care is coordinated among practitioners.

Before discharge

The need for discharge planning assessment is determined. The hospital has a way of identifying those clients for whom discharge planning is critical.

Education prepares the client for discharge.

At discharge

The client is directly referred to practitioners, settings, and organizations to meet his or her continuing needs.

The use and value of continuing care to meet the client's needs are reassessed.

The hospital provides information or data to help others meet the client's continuing care needs.

Modified from Joint Commission on Accreditation of Healthcare Organizations: Manual of hospital accreditation: 1996 standards, Chicago, 1996, The Commission.

Regulatory Requirements

The purpose of regulatory agency standards for the acute care setting is to ensure the quality and appropriateness of the care delivered. At present, it is believed that a client receives the best quality care within a shorter time frame if the health care is well coordinated immediately upon admission to the acute care facility. The U.S. government, through Medicare and the health departments of all 50 states, has created specific standards addressing the importance of **discharge planning** and a continuum of care from hospital to home. The Joint Commission on Accreditation of Healthcare Organizations (JCAHO) conducts regular accreditation visits of hospitals throughout the United States. The JCAHO seeks to improve the quality of health care provided to the public and stimulate health care organizations to meet or exceed standards of practice (JCAHO, 1996). Specific standards pertaining to the continuum of care, emphasizing the importance of a well-coordinated admission and discharge process, can be found in the box below, left.

■ ADMISSION TO AN ACUTE CARE AGENCY

A client can access the health care system in a variety of ways (e.g., hospital, emergent care center, clinic, or physician's office) (see Chapter 2). This section focuses primarily on admission into a hospital system. Commonalities exist for all settings (see the box below).

Initial Admission Procedures

Each institution follows a different set of policies and procedures for admitting a client. A client's condition determines the extent of the admitting procedure. For example, a client entering through the emergency department may not be in a condition to undergo the same interview process that takes place in a hospital admission office. In the case of an emergency admission, friends or family members provide pertinent information for the hospital's records while the client is transported directly to a nursing unit. In contrast, an elderly client who can no longer attend to daily chores but who is still independent enough to perform some self-care activities will undergo extensive screening before being accepted as a nursing home resident.

Admission officers and technicians are the personnel primarily involved with the preliminary procedures for admitting clients into an agency. Some hospitals have a small

---

Common Procedures for Admission to a Health Care Agency

- Placement of client in appropriate receiving area
- Assessment of client's health care problems and needs
- Determination of client's payment source for health care
- Explanation of client's rights
- Orientation to the health care agency's policies and procedures
- Preliminary testing and screening (specific for each agency)
- Development of an individualized plan of care
- Initiation of discharge plan

A PATIENT'S BILL OF RIGHTS

INTRODUCTION

Effective health care requires collaboration between patients and physicians and other health care professionals. Open and honest communication, respect for personal and professional values, and sensitivity to differences are integral to optimal patient care. As the setting for the provision of health services, hospitals must provide a foundation for understanding and respecting the rights and responsibilities of patients, their families, physicians, and other caregivers. Hospitals must ensure a health care ethic that respects the role of patients in decision making about treatment choices and other aspects of their care. Hospitals must be sensitive to cultural, racial, linguistic, religious, age, gender, and other differences, as well as the needs of persons with disabilities.

The American Hospital Association presents *A Patient's Bill of Rights* with the expectation that it will contribute to more effective patient care and be supported by the hospital on behalf of the institution, its medical staff, employees, and patients. The American Hospital Association encourages health care institutions to tailor this bill of rights to their patient community by translating and/or simplifying the language of this bill of rights as may be necessary to ensure that patients and their families understand their rights and responsibilities.

BILL OF RIGHTS*

1. The patient has the right to considerate and respectful care.

2. The patient has the right to and is encouraged to obtain from physicians and other direct caregivers relevant, current, and understandable information concerning diagnosis, treatment and prognosis.
   Except in emergencies when the patient lacks decision-making capacity and the need for treatment is urgent, the patient is entitled to the opportunity to discuss and request information related to the specific procedures and/or treatments, the risks involved, the possible length of recuperation, and the medically reasonable alternatives and their accompanying risks and benefits. Patients have the right to know the identity of physicians, nurses, and others involved in their care, as well as when those involved are students, residents, or other trainees. The patient also has the right to know the immediate and long-term financial implications of treatment choices, insofar as they are known.

3. The patient has the right to make decisions about the plan of care prior to and during the course of treatment and to refuse a recommended treatment or plan of care to the extent permitted by law and hospital policy and to be informed of the medical consequences of this action. In case of such refusal, the patient is entitled to other appropriate care and services that the hospital provides or transfer to another hospital. The hospital should notify patients of any policy that might affect patient choice within the institution.

4. The patient has the right to have an advance directive (such as living will, health care proxy, or durable power of attorney for health care) concerning treatment or designating a surrogate decision maker with the expec-

tation that the hospital will honor the intent of that directive to the extent permitted by law and hospital policy.
Health care institutions must advise patients of their rights under state law and hospital policy to make informed medical choices, ask if the patient has an advance directive, and include that information in patient records. The patient has the right to timely information about hospital policy that may limit its ability to implement fully a legally valid advance directive.

5. The patient has the right to every consideration of privacy. Case discussion, consultation, examination, and treatment should be conducted so as to protect each patient's privacy.

6. The patient has the right to expect that all communications and records pertaining to his/her care will be treated as confidential by the hospital, except in cases such as suspected abuse and public health hazards when reporting is permitted or required by law. The patient has the right to expect that the hospital will emphasize the confidentiality of this information when it releases it to any other parties entitled to review information in these records.

7. The patient has the right to review the records pertaining to his/her medical care and to have the information explained or interpreted as necessary, except when restricted by law.

8. The patient has the right to expect that, within its capacity and policies, a hospital will make reasonable response to the request of a patient for appropriate and medically indicated care and services. The hospital must provide evaluation, services, and/or referral as indicated by the urgency of the case. When medically appropriate and legally permissible, or when a patient has so requested, a patient may be transferred to another facility. The institution to which the patient is to be transferred must first have accepted the patient for transfer. The patient must also have the benefit of complete information and explanation concerning the need for, risk, benefits, and alternatives to such a transfer.

9. The patient has the right to ask and be informed of the existence of business relationships among the hospital, educational institutions, other health care providers, or payers that may influence the patient's treatment and care.

10. The patient has the right to consent to or decline to participate in proposed research studies or human experimentation affecting care and treatment or requiring direct patient involvement, and to have those studies fully explained prior to consent. A patient who declines to participate in research or experimentation is entitled to the most effective care that the hospital can otherwise provide.

11. The patient has the right to expect reasonable continuity of care when appropriate and to be informed by physicians and other caregivers of available and realistic patient care options when hospital care is no longer appropriate.

12. The patient has the right to be informed of hospital policies and practices that relate to patient care, treat-

From American Hospital Association, Chicago, Ill., 60611. Catalog No. 157759, 1992.
*These rights can be exercised on the patient's behalf by a designated surrogate or proxy decision maker if the patient lacks decision-making capacity, is legally incompetent, or is a minor.

A PATIENT'S BILL OF RIGHTS—cont'd

ment, and responsibilities. The patient has the right to be informed of available resources for resolving disputes, grievances, and conflicts, such as ethics committees, patient representatives, or other mechanisms available in the institution. The patient has the right to be informed of the hospital's charges for services and available payment methods.

The collaborative nature of health care requires that patients, or their families/surrogates, participate in their care. The effectiveness of care and patient satisfaction with the course of treatment depend, in part, on the patient fulfilling certain responsibilities. Patients are responsible for providing information about past illnesses, hospitalizations, medications, and other matters related to health status. To participate effectively in decision making, patients must be encouraged to take responsibility for requesting additional information or clarification about their health status or treatment when they do not fully understand information and instructions. Patients are also responsible for ensuring that the health care institution has a copy of their written advance directive if they have one. Patients are responsible for informing their physicians and other caregivers if they anticipate problems in following prescribed treatment.

Patients should also be aware of the hospital's obligation to be reasonably efficient and equitable in providing care to other patients and the community. The hospital's rules and regulations are designed to help the hospital meet this obligation. Patients and their families are responsible for making reasonable accommodations to the needs of the hospital, other patients, medical staff, and hospital employees. Patients are responsible for providing necessary information for insurance claims and for working with the hospital to make payment arrangements, when necessary.

A person's health depends on much more than health care services. Patients are responsible for recognizing the impact of their life-style on their personal health.

CONCLUSION

Hospitals have many functions to perform, including the enhancement of health status, health promotion, and the prevention and treatment of injury and disease; the immediate and ongoing care and rehabilitation of patients; the education of health professionals, patients, and the community; and research. All these activities must be conducted with an overriding concern for the values and dignity of patients.

satellite admission office within the emergency department. Clients usually experience considerable anxiety about the admission process, so all personnel should treat them courteously and professionally. This is where customer service begins. If one person shows an uncaring attitude, clients may assume that all the personnel are unprofessional. By making clients and families feel welcome, nurses and other staff members begin to establish a therapeutic relationship with the client.

The first step in admitting a client is to acquire identifying information, including full legal name, age, birth date, address, next of kin, admitting physician, religion, occupation, social security number, and type of insurance. This information ensures correct legal identification of the client. Data may be entered into a computer that provides a printout of an admission sheet that is placed within the client's permanent medical record. Each client receives a permanent identification number for the hospital record.

After this identifying information is gathered, the client receives an identification bracelet used when therapies or procedures such as medication administration or x-ray examinations are performed. The bracelet should be secure so that it remains in place throughout hospitalization. It is especially important for children or confused or comatose clients to have identification bracelets.

The hospital is responsible for ensuring the clients' legal rights at admission. The admission officer will instruct clients or legal guardians about the general consent form for treatment. The signature on the consent form gives the hospital permission to perform routine procedures and selected therapies. In addition, the hospital must give clients written information about their rights under state law to make decisions about medical care, including the right to accept or refuse medical or surgical treatment. Clients must

receive information about their rights to formulate advance directives such as durable power of attorney for health care. The Patient Self-Determination Act became effective in December 1991. Each state determines how the law concerning advance directives is to be stated. Finally, it is important for the client to receive information regarding the "Patient's Bill of Rights" from the American Hospital Association (AHA, 1992). This document must be posted within an admission office for all clients to see. In addition, most institutions give clients copies of the "Patient's Bill of Rights" in their admission booklets. The information must be understandable and easy to read. The bill describes clients' rights to be well informed and receive respectful, competent, continuous, and confidential health care (see the box on pp. 66 to 67).

Each hospital has policies and procedures of which the client should be informed. Usually the client or family receives a brochure explaining available services (e.g., pastoral care and social work), visiting hours, meal schedules, smoking policies, and any other policies or rules that affect the person's conduct as a client. At admission, a client is usually quite anxious and unable to remember a great deal of information. A booklet gives the client a resource to be used at any time.

In some cases, clients may undergo laboratory and x-ray testing in the admission office. However, the majority of testing is now done on an outpatient, preadmission basis to control the costs of inpatient care. Such tests can be performed safely and more economically before the client is hospitalized.

After all necessary information has been collected and the client is thoroughly informed, the next step is transportation of the client to the nursing unit. To begin ensuring continuity of care, the admission office notifies the nursing unit of the client's admission, current status, and room assignment. This allows nursing staff to prepare a room and obtain necessary equipment for the arrival. In some hospitals the nursing department determines room assignments. This ensures that the client who requires frequent observation and therapy is placed in a room accessible to the nursing staff.

Admission to a Nursing Unit
(Procedure 4-1)

Members of the admission office, transport service, or emergency department transport the client to the nursing unit. The client's condition determines whether ambulation or the use of a wheelchair or stretcher is most appropriate. Upon arrival at the unit the client and family are introduced to the nurse responsible for the client's care. The initial moments spent with a client begin the orientation phase of the nurse-client relationship (see Chapter 14).

The nurse completes a number of procedures during the admission process, including orientation of the client and family to the room and unit procedures, collection of a nursing history (see Chapter 7) and physical assessment (see Chapter 33), collection of specimens, and a clarification of client questions and expectations. The nurse must always be conscious of the client's level of fatigue and comfort. The admission process can be exhausting, especially if there is a delay in the admission office for a room assignment. When the client is experiencing physical or psychological symptoms, the nurse determines whether any portion of the admission process can be completed later.

■ MULTIDISCIPLINARY DISCHARGE PLANNING

As soon as a client is admitted to a hospital, all members of the health care team begin preparations for discharge (Fig. 4-1). Successful **discharge planning** is a centralized, coordinated, multidisciplinary process that ensures that the client has a plan for continuing care after leaving the hospital (AHA, 1983). Discharge planning facilitates the transition of the client from one environment to another (see the box below). The following outcomes must be ensured for a client's successful discharge plan:

1. Client and family understand the diagnosis, anticipated level of functioning, discharge medications and treatments, anticipated medical follow-up care, and response to take in an emergency.
2. Specialized education is provided to the client and family to ensure proper care after discharge.
3. Community support systems are coordinated to enable the client to return home and to assist the client and family in coping with changes in health status.
4. Relocation of the client and coordination of support systems or transfer to another health care facility are performed.

Every client in a hospital requires discharge planning. There are conditions, however, that place a client at greater risk for being unable to meet continuing health care needs after discharge, such as the terminally ill or clients with permanent disabilities (see the box below). When clients have one of these conditions, it is especially important to assess their desire and ability to manage health care needs at home (Rice, 1992).

Clients who should be considered for home care include those needing assistance while recovering from acute illness, or to prevent or manage exacerbations of chronic illness, and families needing assistance in the care of the terminally ill (Cookfair, 1991).

All care givers who care for a client with a specific health problem must participate in discharge planning. Development of a plan with mutually accepted outcomes and ongoing communication about its progress is essential. For example, a client admitted to the hospital for a major surgical procedure involving the lung will probably require the collaboration of the physician, nurses, respiratory therapists, physical therapists, social workers, and home health care staff. The client will need pain management, early physical ambulation, aggressive pulmonary therapy, and education for improved exercise tolerance. The client's smooth transition from hospital to home may not be accomplished if, for example, the nurse's pain management measures are not used before physical therapy; the physician chooses to prescribe bed rest for an extra day; or the social worker is not informed of the lack of family support. All care givers must work together for a discharge plan to be successful.

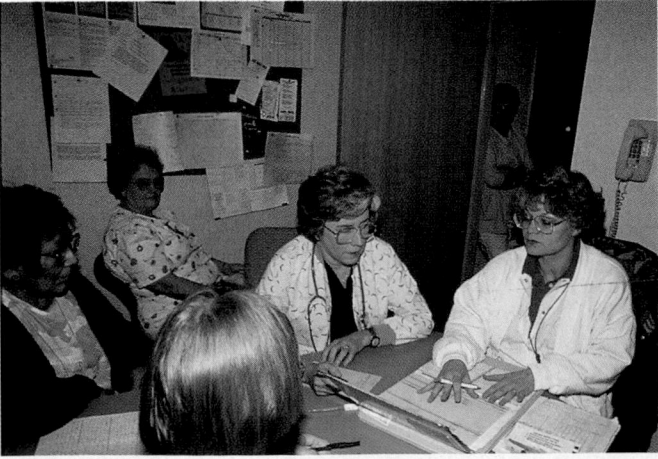

Fig. 4-1 Staff participating in discharge planning conference.

Client Risk Factors for Discharge Planning
■ Lack of knowledge of treatment plan
■ Newly diagnosed chronic disease
■ Major surgery
■ Radical surgery
■ Prolonged recuperation from major surgery or illness
■ Social isolation
■ Emotional or mental instability
■ Complex home care regimen
■ Lack of financial resources
■ Lack of available or appropriate referral sources
■ Terminal illness

PROCEDURE 4-1

Admitting a Client to a Nursing Division

STEPS	RATIONALE

ROOM PREPARATION

1. Wash hands.

Reduces spread of microorganisms.

2. Prepare assigned room with necessary equipment and personal care items:
  a. Bedpan and urinal
  b. Wash basin
  c. Bath towel and washcloth
  d. Toiletry items (e.g., soap, toothpaste, hand lotion)
  e. Tissue paper
  f. Water pitcher and drinking glass
  g. Kidney or emesis basin
  h. Thermometer
  i. Sphygmomanometer

Promotes comfort by preventing unnecessary delays during care. (Clients often prefer to bring personal care items from home into health care agency.)

3. Prepare bed by adjusting it to the lowest horizontal position. Turn down top sheet and bedspread.

Makes getting into bed easier and safer. If client is to be transferred to bed from stretcher, place bed in high position.

4. Arrange room furniture for easy access to the bed.

5. Assemble special equipment such as suction equipment, oxygen supplies, and pole for intravenous line. Be sure that it is in working order.

Prevents delays in case immediate treatment is necessary.

ADMISSION PROCESS

6. Greet client and family cordially. Introduce self by name and job title; state that you are responsible for client's care. (Primary nurse may be assigned at this time.)

Reduces anxiety about admission and expedites client requests.

7. Escort client and family to assigned room. Introduce them to roommate If semiprivate room is assigned.

Orientation begins with introduction to roommate.

8. Assess client's general appearance, noting signs or symptoms of physical distress.

Provides baseline assessment. (If client is having acute physical problems, postpone routine admission procedures until client's immediate needs are met.)

9. Assess client's and family's psychological status by noting nonverbal behaviors and verbal responses to greetings and explanations.

Anxiety influences ability to adapt to health care environment and amount of instructions that will be retained.

10. Check physician's orders for treatment measures that should be initiated immediately.

Delay can cause worsening of condition.

11. Orient client to nursing division.
  a. Introduce staff members who enter room. Always introduce client by last name.

Promotes ability to recognize care givers.

  b. Tell client name of head nurse or charge nurse of division and role in solving problems.

Provides means for client to communicate problems.

  c. Explain visiting hours and their purpose.
  d. Discuss smoking policy.

Willingness to observe visiting-hour policy ensures that client will receive adequate rest.

  e. Demonstrate equipment use (e.g., bed, overbed table, lighting).

Client's safety depends on understanding correct use of equipment.

  f. Show client how to use nurse call light and position it in a convenient place. Have client demonstrate use of light (see the illustration).

Ensures that client knows how to call for assistance.

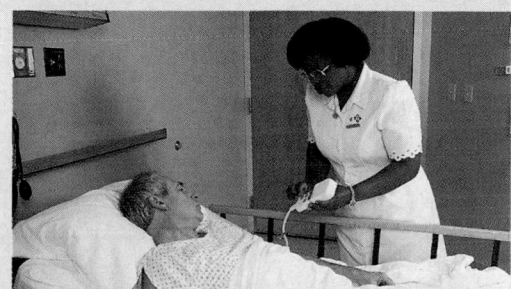

Step 11f

Continued.

Admitting a Client to a Nursing Division—cont'd

STEPS	RATIONALE
g. Escort client to bathroom (if able to ambulate).	
h. Explain hours for mealtime and nourishments.	
i. Describe services available (e.g., chaplain visitation, gift shop, activity therapy).	Offers client options for making decisions.
12. Have family leave room unless they choose to assist client with undressing. Close door and curtains. Help client undress and assist into comfortable position.	Provides for privacy; prepares client for care.
13. Assess vital signs (see Chapter 32).	Provides baseline measurement to compare future findings; determines alterations from normal expected range.
14. Obtain nursing history to include the following assessment categories (see Chapter 33):	Provides data necessary to develop individualized plan of care based on client's identified health problems.
a. Client's perceptions of illness.	
b. Past medical history.	
c. Presenting signs and symptoms.	
d. Risk factors for illness.	
e. History of allergies. (Provide client with allergy band, similar to size of identification band, listing allergies of foods, drugs, or substances.)	Alerts nurses to substances to which client is allergic.
f. Medication history. If medications are brought to agency, have client or family take drugs home; otherwise, medications are stored on unit for safekeeping. (Follow individual hospital policy.)	Therapeutic drug administration depends on correct dosages, proper timing of dosages, and avoidance of drug incompatibilities.
g. Alterations in activities of daily living.	Helps identify client and family needs on discharge to the home.
h. Family resources and support.	
i. Client's knowledge of health problems and implications for long-term care.	Allows nurse to plan necessary instruction to prepare client for discharge.
15. Conduct physical assessment of appropriate body systems (see Chapter 33).	Provides objective data and baseline data for identifying health problems.
16. If urine specimen was not obtained prior to admission, instruct client on acquiring urine specimen. Inform client about technicians who will obtain blood specimens and perform tests.	Urinalysis, complete blood cell count, electrocardiogram, and chest x-ray study are basic screening tests.
17. Inform client about procedures or treatments scheduled for the next shift or day (e.g., visits by physician or dietitian).	Client has right to be informed of any scheduled procedures or treatments; being able to anticipate planned therapies minimizes anxiety.
18. Give client chance to ask questions about procedures or therapies.	Provides opportunity to clarify expectations and misconceptions.
19. Collect valuables client chooses to keep. Complete listing sheet (see agency policy) and have client or family member sign it. Place valuables in safe.	Accounts for placement of valuables and prevents loss.
20. Allow client and family time together to spend alone, if desired.	Admission procedure can be stressful and fatiguing; allows time for decision making.
21. Be sure that call light is within easy reach, bed is in low position, and side rails are raised.	Provides for client's safety.
22. Wash hands.	Reduces spread of microorganisms.
23. Record history and assessment findings on appropriate forms.	Prompt, thorough documentation prevents deletion of data.
24. Notify physician of client's arrival; report any unusual findings.	Client's condition may require immediate attention.
25. Begin to develop nursing plan of care. Confer again with client as needed.	Provides for continuity of care.

NURSING ROLES AND RESPONSIBILITIES

Clinical Practice

Clinical nursing practice must change with the health care delivery system. Competent nursing is critical to the financial integrity of the hospital. Skillful clinical practice in caring for the acutely ill can minimize the client's functional deficits, reduce the costs of care, return the client to the home environment in a timely manner, and assist the family in home care activities (Collier, Schirm, 1992).

The nursing process (see Unit 2) is a systematic, purposeful method of helping clients regain, maintain, or promote health. The nurse is often the first health care provider to encounter a client and must ensure that an organized approach to care begins immediately. Application of the nursing process ensures effective discharge planning. Assessment of a client's health care problems and responses to those problems, identification of specific problems requiring intervention, development of a plan to eliminate or modify problems, provision of appropriate interventions, and evaluation of interventions is the nursing process. If any step is incorrectly performed, discharge will not go smoothly (Fig. 4-2).

Nurses in different hospitals conduct the discharge planning process differently. When the delivery-of-care system is primary nursing, a single nurse is responsible for coordinating care from admission to discharge for a select group of clients. Even though the primary nurse is unable to be with the client every day, it is that nurse's responsibility to identify the client's discharge planning needs and then to be sure that all members of the health care team are aware of these needs. The primary nurse may team up with unlicensed, assistive personnel to ensure that care is well coordinated on a day-to-day basis. However, the primary nurse retains accountability for the client's nursing care outcomes. Clear communication of discharge planning information in the client's medical record is essential. Many hospitals also have discharge planning rounds on nursing units. During rounds, various members of the health care team discuss the status of each client with respect to potential discharge. Rounds allow members of all disciplines to interact and discuss the best treatment options for each client.

In some hospitals, nurses assume the role of case manager. The role builds on the accountability practiced in primary nursing (Zander, 1988, 1994). The case manager is responsible for specific client outcomes during the course of the client's stay in the hospital. Care expected to be delivered by various disciplines throughout a hospital may be planned and managed through formal **case management** plans, sometimes called *critical paths* (Zander, 1988). The critical paths are multidisciplinary treatment plans that predict certain interventions and clinical outcomes over a projected length of stay. The plan of care from each discipline, such as nursing, medicine, pharmacy, social work, and dietary, is integrated into a single plan, the critical path. The case manager uses the critical path as a blueprint for a client's treatment and management. All members of the team have one common plan from which to anticipate how to manage a client's care. Discharge planning is integral to the critical path. The case manager can always individualize a plan of care, but the critical pathway provides a useful standard of practice for a particular health problem (see Chapter 9).

Not all clients follow a clinical course that can be standardized on a clinical path. Many will experience complications or have conditions that cannot easily be predicted. In this case, case managers play a key role in identifying the unique problems of these clients and collaborating aggressively with physicians and other care providers to ensure responsive and appropriate care.

Referrals for Health Care Services

Often a client requires the services of various disciplines within a hospital, such as dietary, social work, and/or physical therapy. The nurse is often the first to recognize the client's needs. For example, a client may have had a poor appetite for several days and may reveal to the nurse a dislike for many of the food choices on the menu. A referral to a dietitian could result in identifying food preferences that are appropriate to the client's diet. It is important to remember that other health professionals specialize in skills and knowledge that give a client services that the nurse cannot offer. Referrals should be made as soon as possible after the client's need is identified.

In many agencies a physician's order is needed for a referral, especially when specific therapies are planned (e.g., physical therapy). It is ideal to have clients participate in referral processes so that they are involved in decision making. If clients fail to understand the purpose of referrals, they may refuse proposed treatment measures. The roles that various disciplines can play in a treatment plan are identified in the box on p. 72.

When multiple referrals are made for a client's plan of care, the staff nurse or case manager coordinates referral activities. Often it is necessary to have different therapists col-

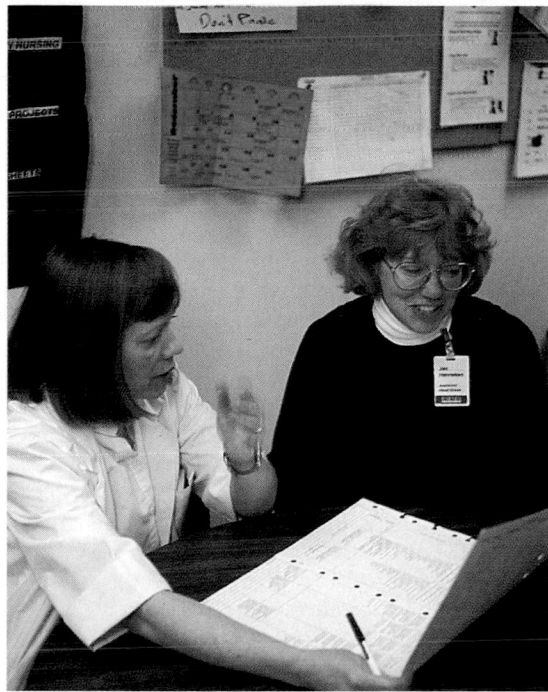

Fig. 4-2 Planning care based on client individual care needs.

Health Disciplines Used in Referrals

DIETITIAN
- Provides proper nutrient and food source requirements in clients' diets
- Instructs clients on meal planning and diet restrictions

SOCIAL WORKER
- Provides counseling for major life crises such as terminal illness and family problems
- Assists in finding community resources such as equipment for home health care or an agency that will accept clients after discharge from a hospital
- Assists in finding financial resources to cover medical costs

PHARMACIST
- Receives orders for medications ordered for home use
- Prepares medication for administration by home health care nurse
- Checks laboratory results for therapeutic drug levels
- Reviews risk for drug interactions

PHYSICAL THERAPIST
- Assists in the examination and treatment of physically disabled or handicapped persons
- Assists in rehabilitating clients and restoring normal musculoskeletal function

OCCUPATIONAL THERAPIST
- Trains clients to adapt to physical handicaps by learning new vocational skills or activities of daily living

SPEECH THERAPIST
- Assists clients with disorders affecting normal oral communication

CLINICAL NURSE SPECIALIST
- Consults with nursing staff on appropriate interventions for complex nursing diagnoses
- Provides instruction to clients and family members who will assume self-care

HOME HEALTH CARE NURSE
- Provides follow-up discharge visits to a client's home for the delivery of nursing services

---

laborate so that a client's care is uninterrupted. For example, there may be certain times in the day when a client can better tolerate physical therapy or is most receptive to instruction. The nurse attempts to plan referral activities at these times.

Transfers Within an Agency

Discharge planning can become more complicated when a client transfers from one nursing unit to another. This often occurs when the client requires a different type of medical service. For example, a client may be admitted to a medical nursing unit for diagnosis of chest pain but is eventually transferred to a surgical nursing unit for an open-heart procedure. Transfers to different units require considerable preparation. Nurses on the sending unit coordinate activities with nurses on the receiving unit. These activities include assessing the client's stability for transfer, preparing the client's medical record, transporting medications and personal supplies, orienting the client and family to the transfer procedure, and transporting the client to the new unit. Before a transfer is initiated, it is critical to determine a client's physical condition. A client who is not stable may require special equipment such as oxygen, a cardiac monitor, or intravenous fluids during transfer to a new unit. Regardless of where a client is transferred, the discharge care plan must remain current and appropriate for all team members to follow. Nurses on a receiving unit must acquire complete information about the client's medical needs and nursing care so that continuity of care is not sacrificed. Frequently this is a role of the case manager. Nurses from the sending unit provide a complete report (see the box on p. 73) to nurses on the receiving unit. The client's discharge plan may stay the same regardless of a transfer to a new area, but it is important for the client, family, nurses, and other health care providers to validate it. Nurses must have a clear understanding of the client's progress and the interventions planned.

After a client arrives on a new unit, the nursing staff is responsible for assessing the client's condition and determining whether revisions to the plan of care are needed. Throughout the transfer process, the client and family are kept informed, to minimize their anxiety and fear.

Teaching as Part of the Discharge Plan

Teaching the client, family, and other care givers is an important responsibility for all members of the health care team. The nurse has the primary responsibility for instructing the client on the nature of any health problems, anticipated restrictions, discharge medication use, types of complications to inform a physician about, and resources available for assistance. However, other health care providers, such as pharmacists, dietitians, social workers and physical or occupational therapists, can also contribute to the client's education. What is most important is to have an agreed upon plan so that all care givers are giving the same information. Conflicting explanations between two different care providers can be very confusing to a client and can ultimately lead to improper self-care decisions. Nurses need to be alert for possible learning barriers that affect all clients, and, in particular, the older adult client (see the box on p. 73). Ultimately the goal of education is to provide clients and care givers with essential knowledge and skills to meet continuing health care needs. When planning discharge, it is important to identify support persons who will be assisting the client at home. Because of the advancing age of our population, it is common for clients over the age of 80 to be cared for by persons over 65 years of age (Knapp, 1994).

Nurses are challenged to provide effective client education while having limited contact with clients. Clients admitted to hospitals for short 23-hour stays should receive education before coming to the hospital or should be instructed on priority issues just before discharge.

The JCAHO (1996) has set minimum standards for infor-

Elements of Reporting a Client Transfer

- Reason for hospitalization (i.e., diagnosis)
- Health history
- Allergies
- Review of client's current condition
- Review of current nursing diagnoses
- Review of nursing plan of care
- Review of client's medications and medical therapies, clarification of treatments ordered for the day
- Acquisition of special equipment for client care

GERONTOLOGICAL PRINCIPLES for Barriers to Learning

- Sensory changes (e.g., decreased vision and hearing)
- Pain
- Bladder frequency or urgency
- Limited endurance
- Decreased attention span
- Physical inability to perform motor tasks
- Environmental noise, which is distracting and disruptive
- Environmental temperature, especially drafts or chilling
- Depression with low energy levels

Data from Lueckenotte AG: *Gerontologic Nursing*, St Louis, 1996, Mosby.

---

mation to be provided to clients and their families (see Chapter 15). Nurses and all members of the health care team must document any instruction provided and evaluate the client's understanding.

Discharge From the Hospital

If discharge planning is successful, the discharge of a client from a hospital should be uneventful. The nurse monitors the client's progress on an ongoing basis. As a client successfully meets the expected outcomes of care, the goals of care are met, and the client achieves an improved level of health or maintenance of a preexisting health state. At the same time the nurse assists in coordinating the care of other disciplines. Procedure 4-2 outlines the steps taken in the successful discharge of a client.

At discharge, clients must have the necessary knowledge, skill, and resources to meet self-care needs. Most clients are able to return home. The nurse and health care team determine whether resources are available to assist clients at home or whether home health care services are required. Clients who require more extensive care may enter skilled nursing facilities or rehabilitation programs, or they may become residents of nursing homes. When health care continues after discharge, health care providers must receive a thorough review of the client's needs. The hospital nurse may talk directly with care givers in other agencies or provide a detailed summary of the care plan on a discharge document. Care should continue in the new setting with little interruption.

DISCHARGE AGAINST MEDICAL ADVICE

Occasionally a client chooses to leave a hospital against medical advice (AMA). In this situation, there is a risk that the client will suffer complications from leaving the hospital prematurely. The client must sign a form that releases the physicians and hospital from any legal liability for the client's health. Before an AMA form is completed, the nurse and/or physician discusses with the client the possible outcomes of the decision. The client must clearly understand all the risks. The AMA form is signed by the client and is witnessed by the physician or nurse (depending on agency policy). Usually the staff informs the risk-management department of any AMAs.

Home Health Care Planning

Discharge planning is a major function of most home health care agencies, especially those affiliated with hospitals (see Procedure 4-2). Agencies hire experienced nurses to function as home health coordinators or discharge planners. Nurses attend discharge planning rounds and consult with medical, nursing, and social work staffs in hospitals and clinics. They facilitate access to all home health equipment and services during a client's discharge from the hospital or clinic. The coordinator screens all referrals to see whether the client is eligible for home health services in terms of insurance coverage, health care needs, and family and home situation (see Chapter 5). After determining that a client is eligible for home health care services, the coordinator completes a referral form based on information obtained from the following:

1. Client and family interviews
2. Consultation with physicians, other nurses, and staff members
3. The client's medical records

Thorough assessment and data collection by the coordinator before hospital discharge facilitates continuity of care and, in many cases, can speed the discharge process. To promote independence, initial teaching begins before the client leaves the acute care facility. A complete discharge assessment allows home health care nurses to better understand the client's medical problems. It provides more information for making decisions about home health care planning.

Another aspect of discharge planning occurs when the client is discharged from home health care. The home health nurse (case manager) usually collaborates with the client, family, and other home health care staff (such as nurses, therapists, and social workers) to plan the discharge. All necessary referrals are made to community resources for follow-up care. For example, a client with chronic lung disease may be referred to breathing clubs, support groups, or outpatient rehabilitation programs. The home health care staff follows up on these referrals to assess client satisfaction.

∎ DELIVERY OF ACUTE NURSING CARE

Delivery of care in an acute setting is unique by the nature of the acuity of clients, the urgency often times in providing treatments, and the challenges faced in coordinating the contributions of multiple health care providers. This section attempts to emphasize the important principles for applying the nursing process in an acute care setting.

Discharging a Client

STEPS	RATIONALE

DISCHARGE PLANNING

1. From time of admission, assess client's health care needs for discharge, using nursing history, care plan, and ongoing assessments of physical abilities and cognitive function (see Unit 2).

Plan for discharge begins at admission and continues throughout client's stay in agency.

2. Assess client's and family's need for health teaching related to home therapies, restrictions resulting from health alterations, and possible complications.

Will improve understanding of health care needs and ability to achieve self-care at home; inclusion of family member in teaching sessions provides client with available resource.

3. Assess with client and family environmental factors within home that might interfere with self-care (e.g., size of rooms, doorway clearances, steps, bathroom facilities). (A home health care nurse may be available on referral to assist with assessment.)

May pose risks to safety as a result of limitation created by illness or need for certain therapies.

4. Collaborate with physician and other disciplines (e.g., physical therapy) in assessing need for referral for skilled home health care services or an extended care facility.

Clients eligible for home health care are confined to home as result of illness, are under physician's care, and require skilled nursing care on intermittent basis; a multidisciplinary assessment ensures a comprehensive discharge plan.

5. Assess acceptance of health problems and related restrictions.

Acceptance of health status can affect willingness to adhere to therapies and restrictions after discharge.

6. Consult other health team members about needs after discharge (e.g., dietitian, social worker, home health care nurse). Make appropriate referrals.

Members of all health care disciplines should collaborate to determine client's needs and functional abilities.

7. Develop appropriate nursing diagnoses (see Chapter 7) and care plan (see Chapter 8). Implement plan of care (see Chapter 9). Evaluate progress on an ongoing basis (see Chapter 10). Develop relevant goals for discharge, as follows:

Well-coordinated plan of care ensures that client will meet desired clinical outcomes by discharge.

   a. Client will understand health care problems and related implications.

Client and family teaching will better prepare client to care for individual needs.

   b. Client will be able to care for individual needs.

Planned discussion periods will give client opportunity to ask questions and clarify information.

   c. Home environment will be safe.

Family members can make changes before client's arrival to make home safer. A home health care nurse may be able to assess home.

   d. Health care resources in the home will be available.

Early referral to home health care services will allow nurses to assess client's needs more thoroughly.

PREPARATION BEFORE DAY OF DISCHARGE

8. Suggest ways to change physical arrangement of home to meet client's needs.

Client's level of independence and ability to retain function can be maintained within safe environment.

9. Provide client and family with information about community health care resources.

Community resources often offer services client or family cannot provide.

10. Conduct teaching sessions with client and family as soon as possible during hospitalization (e.g., signs and symptoms of complications; information regarding medications, use of medical equipment follow-up care, diet, exercise, restrictions imposed by illness or surgery). Pamphlets or books may be given to client.

Gives opportunities to practice new skills, ask questions, and obtain necessary feedback to ensure learning.

Discharging a Client—cont'd

STEPS	RATIONALE

DAY OF DISCHARGE

11. Let client and family ask questions or discuss issues related to home health care (optional).

Allows for final clarification of information previously discussed; helps relieve anxiety.

12. Check physician's discharge orders for prescriptions, change in treatments, or need for special appliances. (Orders should be written as early as possible.)

Discharge is authorized only by physician; early check of orders permits you to attend to any last-minute treatments or procedures well before discharge.

13. Determine whether client or family has arranged for transport home.

Client's condition at discharge will determine method for transport.

14. Offer assistance as client dresses and packs all personal belongings. Provide privacy as needed.

Promotes comfort.

15. Check all closets and drawers for belongings. Obtain copy of valuables list signed by client and have security or appropriate administrator deliver valuables to client. Account for all valuables.

Prevents loss of personal items; client's signature will verify receipt of items; relieves nursing department of liability for losses.

16. Provide client with prescriptions or medications ordered by physician. Review previous instruction.

Review of drug information provides feedback to determine success in learning about medications.

17. Contact agency's business office to determine whether client needs to finalize arrangements for payment of bill. Arrange for client or family to visit office.

Source of concern for many clients is whether agency has accepted insurance or other payment forms.

18. Acquire utility cart to move client's belongings. Obtain wheelchair for clients unable to ambulate. Clients leaving by ambulance will be transported on ambulance stretchers.

Provides for safe transport of client.

19. Assist client to wheelchair or stretcher using proper body mechanics and transfer techniques. Escort client to entrance of agency where source of transportation is waiting (see agency policy).

Prevents injury to you and client; agency policy requires escort to ensure client's safe exit.

20. Lock wheelchair wheels. Assist client in transferring into automobile or transport vehicle. Help family place personal belongings in vehicle.

Agency's liability ends once client is safely in vehicle.

21. Return to unit and notify admitting or appropriate department of time of discharge.

Allows agency to prepare for admission of next client.

22. Document discharge on discharge summary form (see Chapter 12). In many institutions, client receives signed copy of form (see Step 10).

Discharge summary is essential for documenting client's status when leaving health care agency; signed copy demonstrates plan was communicated to and agreed to by client.

23. Document status of health problems at discharge.

Allows final evaluation of plan of care.

Assessment

Client and family assessment is always the first responsibility the nurse assumes when a client enters a health care setting. In the acute care setting, assessment becomes more important because decisions about the data must often be made very quickly. In the emergency room and intensive care unit, clients can deteriorate very quickly. Nurses therefore must be able to detect changes in a client's condition immediately.

During admission (Procedure 4-1), the nurse follows agency procedure and collects a variety of data from the client, including nursing history, demographic data, previous medical conditions and surgeries, past medications and treatments, client goals, and functional limitations and activities. The condition of the client will influence the amount and type of data the nurse collects. In an emergent setting the nurse may focus on the ABCs of assessment (*Ai*rway, *B*reathing, *C*irculation), while admission to a general nursing unit will likely have the nurse collect more extensive information. A comprehensive assessment will include the following information:

1. Nursing history and physical assessment of all body systems, with emphasis on the present illness (see Chapters 7 and 33)
2. Psychosocial assessment (education, ethnicity, and social relations)
3. Family dynamics (decision making and rituals)
4. Community resources (need for financial assistance and follow-up care)
5. Environmental factors (housing, transportation, and neighborhood)
6. Functional limitations (inabilities related to activities of daily living)
7. Client and family knowledge and attitudes toward illness and health behaviors, the impact on their lifestyle, and the need for follow-up care in the client's home
8. Significance illness has on client's values, beliefs, and spiritual health

Discharge planning begins during the assessment phase. Any special discharge needs and concerns should be communicated to social workers, home health care staff, or case managers, depending on the staff available to assist. Time may be required to plan for a client's placement into home care or extended care facilities once discharge occurs. In complicated specialty cases (e.g., IV therapy, mechanical ventilation, and hospice care), home health nurses may visit the client in the hospital before discharge to identify needs, initiate discharge teaching, and prepare the client and family for care (see Chapter 5).

Nursing Diagnosis

The diagnostic function is central to a nurse's role, especially in acute care where a client's condition can change quickly. After collecting data about the client, priority nursing diagnoses are developed. The client will likely have numerous nursing diagnoses, otherwise hospitalization would be unnecessary. However, nurses in the acute care setting must be able to intervene for those problems that create the most risk for the client. Those diagnoses that are less of a

priority still need to be communicated in home health or other settings where the client's care may be continued.

Nursing diagnoses are individualized to client needs; the clinical chapters in later sections of this text provide specific examples of nursing diagnoses for a variety of health care problems. If the nurse has assessed an insufficient number of defining characteristics for a diagnosis, additional information from family or friends may help confirm a nursing diagnosis (see Chapter 8). The diagnostic process requires the correct use of assessment skills in revealing defining characteristics for client problems.

Planning

The plan of care identifies nursing diagnoses and establishes goals and outcomes. In the acute care setting, short-term goals are more realistic than long-term goals. Any long-term goals are likely to be met after a client is discharged. Short- and long-term goals must be measurable and must include the involvement of the client and family. Overall, goals and outcomes are established to help the client achieve an improved level of health by the time of discharge. Goals and outcomes for the terminally ill or clients with serious disabilities are often directed at maintaining existing function and ensuring the client's comfort.

The acute care setting often offers more resources to the client and family than any other setting. Clients can benefit from a diverse group of health care providers and therapies. This is especially true for large acute care teaching hospitals. The challenge is to have clients receive the right resources in the most timely manner possible. Planning must involve the client and family. Clients now expect this level of involvment. Client, family, or significant other involvement in planning leads to better long-term compliance with care. The client is urged to take an active, responsible role. There are multiple factors that the nurse must then consider if the client's care is extended into the home (see Chapter 5).

Implementation

In an acute care setting, there is one domain of nursing practice that has particular importance. Benner (1984) describes this as "effective management of rapidly changing situations." The nurse must be able to respond skillfully in life-threatening emergencies, match client demands to resources in emergencies, and deal with medical crises until a physician arrives. This requires a competent individual who knows the scope of safe nursing practice but who also can begin to anticipate the life support measures a client will need. For example, if a client begins to show a rapid fall in blood pressure and pulse and shows changes in level of consciousness, the nurse will ready necessary equipment and resources to begin more aggressive intravenous and pharmacological therapy. The client's priorities are always reordered during emergent situations to ensure that appropriate therapies are being used.

The demands created within an acute care setting also require a nurse to competently coordinate daily care activities. Each client has a unique set of needs and nursing interventions selected for his or her care. When the nurse is responsible for multiple clients, application of good management skills is a priority (see Chapter 17). The nurse must work effectively will all levels of care providers to be sure the most important interventions are carried out. Even though the acute care setting is hectic, the nurse must not lose sight of the importance of keeping the client and family well informed and showing a caring and compassionate attitude.

 ## Evaluation

Evaluation of the outcomes of care is an ongoing process. Because there is the push to discharge clients from hospitals as quickly as possible, evaluation has never been more important. Nurses must critically review and determine whether a client is improving and how the client is responding to therapies. Are nursing and medical interventions effective? If not, are appropriate changes in therapy being made? A critical pathway has been shown to be an excellent tool for guiding the care of clients. However, if a client does not progress on a pathway as predicted, the nurse is frequently the one who must bring the health care team together to decide on a new course of action.

Another important aspect of evaluation is determining the client's continuing needs at the time of discharge. The remaining nursing diagnoses may require the client and family to assume more self-care responsibilites. The client's care may continue to be at a level of complexity such that home care or admission to an extended care facility will be needed. The nurse evaluates the extent to which teaching, counseling, and referral are needed to ensure the successful transfer of the client's care to other care givers.

Outcomes of care must be documented for continuity of care, reimbursement, accreditation, and research. The ability or inability to meet outcomes for various client populations is becoming the focus of quality improvement efforts (see Chapter 11).

The acute care setting is changing as a result of societal trends, reimbursement challenges, and the demands of health care consumers. The nurse who works in an acute care setting must be highly competent and able to work with various staff members in coordinating and delivering care. Client satisfaction is becoming an important theme for nurses working in acute care to understand. Nurses must know their clients' expectations and anticipate how to make the hospitalization experience less threatening.

The challenge in health care today is to provide clients with appropriate services as quickly as possible. The nurse plays a key role in helping a client adjust and know what to expect from various health care providers. From admission through discharge, the nurse coordinates client care so that a smooth transition from hospital to the home or alternative health care facility occurs. A multidisciplinary approach is needed to ensure that clients receive all available resources. Discharge planning ensures a continuum of care after the client leaves the hospital.

▪ KEY CONCEPTS ▪

▶ Health care providers need to know that what clients think, feel, and experience is important.

▶ Clients expect to be involved in decisions about their care.

▶ In the acute care setting, registered nurses are working with unlicensed, assistive personnel who partner with the nurse to improve delivery of basic care measures.

▶ The Five Rights of Delegation are the right task, right circumstances, right person, right direction and communication, and right supervision.

▶ Admission into a hospital begins with ensuring that a client knows what to expect during the hospital stay.

▶ Prospective reimbursement has created pressure to discharge clients as soon as possible.

▶ Discharge planning begins when a client is admitted to a hospital.

▶ During admission, clients are given information about their rights in making decisions about medical care, including the right to refuse treatment.

▶ A medical condition may place a client at risk for needing thorough discharge planning.

▶ A nurse should refer clients to other health care providers when it becomes apparent that the expertise of other disciplines is needed.

▶ The ultimate outcome of discharge planning is to give clients the knowledge, skills, and resources needed to assume self-care after discharge.

▶ In the acute care setting the nurse must be able to make quick and timely assessments, prioritize nursing diagnoses, set appropriate short-term goals, deliver safe and effective interventions, and evaluate the outcomes of the client's care.

▪ KEY TERMS ▪

Case management, p. 71
Delegation, p. 62
Discharge planning, p. 68

▪ CRITICAL THINKING EXERCISES ▪

1. Ms. Johnson is assigned the care of five clients. A nurse technician, Mr. Sanchez, is teaming up with Ms. Johnson to assist in client care. At the beginning of the shift, Ms. Johnson learns that two of the clients are being discharged that morning. One client is going to surgery within the hour. The other two clients are recovering from surgery (1 and 2 days postoperatively, respectively). What are some of the factors that the nurse will consider in delegating care to Mr. Sanchez? Consider examples of some of the tasks Ms. Johnson may choose to delegate.

2. Mr. Simon is a 60-year-old client, newly diagnosed with cancer, who enters the hospital for removal of a portion of his colon. Until this time, he has been very healthy. He lives alone in a small rural community, with family residing in a town about 300 miles away. He belongs to the local Catholic church. As the nurse assigned to Mr. Simon, consider his risks for needing comprehensive discharge planning. Develop a discharge plan.

3. Mr. Oaks is a 70-year-old man with a neurogenic bladder requiring self-catheterization. His vision is poor. He lives alone and is very independent. He has received some instruction in the technique of self-catheterization. Describe your approach to teaching this client.

REFERENCES

American Hospital Association: *Patients' bill of rights,* Catalog No 157759, 1992.

American Hospital Association: *Introduction to discharge planning for hospitals,* Chicago, 1983, American Hospital Publishing.

Benner P: *From novice to expert,* Menlo Park, Calif, 1984, Addison Wesley.

Brickhill C: ICU for the '90s: The "Intensive Customer Unit," *Nurs Manage* 26(1):44, 1995.

Collier JAH, Schirm V: Family-focused nursing care of hospitalized elderly in acute care settings, *Int J Nurs Stud,* 29(1):49, 1992.

Cookfair JM: *Nursing process and practice in the community,* St Louis, 1991, Mosby.

Curtin, LL: The heart of patient care, *Nurs Manage* 25(5):7, 1994.

Gerteis M et al: *Through the patient's eyes,* San Francisco, 1993, Jossey-Bass.

Griffith E: Homecare prophecies and predictions. I. *Home Healthc Nurs* 5(6):10, 1987.

Joel LA: Changes in the hospital as a place of practice. In McCloskey JC, Grace HK: *Current issues in nursing,* St Louis, 1994, Mosby.

Joint Commission on Accreditation of Healthcare Organizations: *Manual of hospital accreditation: 1996 standards,* Chicago, 1996, The Commission.

Knapp M: Acute care gerontological nursing: its time has come, *J Gerontol Nurs* 20(5):9, 1994.

Leming, T: Quality customer service: nursing's new challenge, *Nurs Admin Q* 15(4):5, 1991.

Lueckenotte AG: *Gerontologic nursing,* St Louis, 1996, Mosby.

McCloskey JC, Grace HK: *Current issues in nursing,* St Louis, 1994, Mosby.

National Council: *Delegation, concepts and decision making process,* Chicago, Ill, 1995, National Council of State Boards of Nursing, Inc.

National League for Nursing and American Nurses Association: *Nursing's agenda for health care reform,* New York, 1991, National League for Nursing.

Nolan M: Helping "new careers" of the frail elderly patients: the challenge for nurses in acute care settings, *J Clin Nurs* 1(6):303, 1992.

Rice R: *Homehealth nursing practice, concepts, and applications,* St Louis, 1992, Mosby.

Zander K: Managed care within acute care settings: design and implementation via nursing care management, *Health Care Superv* 6(2):27, 1988.

Zander K: Nurses and case management. In McCloskey JC, Grace HK: *Current issues in nursing,* St Louis, 1994, Mosby.

ADDITIONAL READINGS

American Nurses Association: *Standards of nursing care for home health care practice,* Kansas City, Mo, 1986, The Association.

Benefield LE, editor: *Home health care management,* Englewood Cliffs, NJ, 1988, Prentice-Hall.

Cronin SN, Owsley VB: Identifying nursing research priorities in an acute care hospital, *J Nurs Admin* 23(11):58, 1993.

Farren E: Discharge planning: quality care—financial savings. *Nurs Health Care: The Supplement,* New York, 1990, National League for Nursing, Pub. No. 41-2365.

Handy CM: Home care of patients with technically complex nursing needs, *Nurs Clin North Am* 23(2):315, 1988.

Holly CM: The ethical quandaries of acute care nursing practice, *J Prof Nurs* 9(2):110, 1993.

Mitchell MK, Storfield JL, editors: *Standards of excellence for home care organizations: Community Health Accreditation Program (CHAP),* New York, 1989, National League for Nursing.

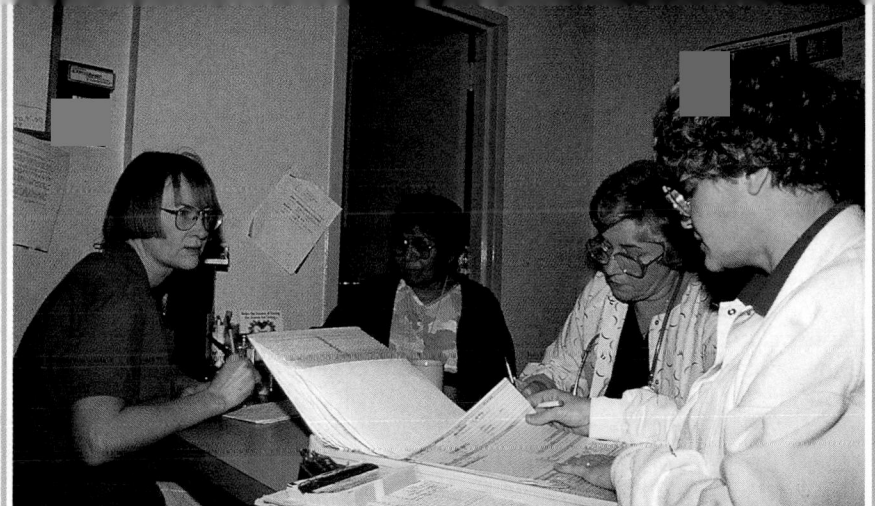

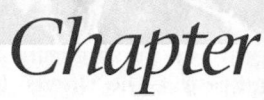 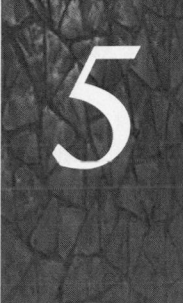
Restorative and Home Health Care

Objectives

Mastery of content in this chapter will enable the student to:

▶ Define key terms listed.

▶ Discuss historical, current, and future trends in restorative care.

▶ Describe the team approach to restorative care.

▶ Discuss the roles of the nurse in restorative care.

▶ Describe the use of the nursing process in restorative care.

▶ Discuss quality improvement issues related to restorative care.

▶ Identify types of home health care agencies and reimbursement mechanisms.

▶ Describe how regulatory standards and quality assurance guidelines affect the clinical practice of home health nursing.

▶ Identify future trends in home health care and the way they affect clinical practice in both acute care and home health care settings.

The overall goals of nursing care are to promote, maintain, and restore the clients' health. Although many definitions of health exist, the definition of health advanced by the World Health Organization (WHO) is applicable for clients in all health care settings, including the restorative care areas (see Chapter 1). Nurses assist clients to achieve their maximum level of health and function by intervening at the primary level to promote health, at the secondary level to maintain health, or at the tertiary level to restore health (Edelman and Mandle, 1994).

■ RESTORATIVE CARE

Restorative care settings are numerous. They include but are not necessarily limited to inpatient and outpatient rehabilitation facilities, subacute care facilities, clinics, and home health care agencies. The services provided in the restorative care settings are those designed to bring the client to the maximal level of health and function. In some instances restorative services are used to assist the family in providing for a terminally ill family member in the home setting.

Historical Perspective

Since the opening of the first rehabilitation facility in 1893, restorative care has become an increasingly vital component of the health care delivery system. Initially, restorative services were primarily needed for younger persons who were the victims of traumatic injuries or accidents or for certain debilitating diseases such as polio (Raymond, 1986). However, twentieth-century advances in the control of infectious diseases, treatment of life-threatening conditions, nutrition, technology, and other aspects of health care have

widened the expanse of restorative care and will continue to do so at an ever-increasing pace into the twenty-first century (McCourt, 1993). At present in the United States, with the demand for cost-effective, quality care across all health care settings, the need for and the extent of restorative services in health care is predicted to rapidly expand.

In general, the need for restorative care services is directly proportional to longevity. However, the longer a person lives, the greater the person's chance of experiencing health problems, which create functional problems and require restorative services to maximize the residual functional capacity (see the box below, left). Simply put, as mortality decreases, morbidity increases. Restorative care minimizes the impact of morbidity, so as morbidity increases, so does the need for restorative services (Avillon and Mirgon, 1989).

Before the end of World War II, restorative services were increasing as a segment of the health care delivery system. These services were primarily available in association with military service. The Social Security Act of 1935 was the first attempt to extend restorative services to the American public (McCourt, 1993). Also, during that era restoration was viewed solely as a medical specialty, and physicians were virtually the only restorative care professionals (McKeown, 1979).

Initially the inclusion of the nurse on these restorative care teams was limited. Not until 1965 did it become necessary for the American Nurses Association to publish its *Guidelines for the Practice of Nursing on the Rehabilitation Team: An Answer to a Growing Need* as standards of care for the nurse on the restorative care team.

A most important event in the development of restorative care in the United States occurred with the passage of the Rehabilitation Act of 1973 (Avillon and Mirgon, 1989), which was designed to increase awareness of the need for restorative services and to extend these resources throughout the community. The goals of restorative care were to return clients to the community and to increase their control of and participation in their care. Subsequent addenda to the act, such as the Americans with Disabilities Act of 1990, have made physical barriers and discrimination bias against the "disabled" illegal. These changes have further advanced the importance and prevalence of restorative care in the

---

Common Health Problems That Limit Functioning and Require Restorative Care

DISEASE CONDITIONS
- Heart diseases like coronary artery disease and congestive heart failure
- Pulmonary diseases like chronic obstructive pulmonary disease and restrictive lung disorders (e.g., black lung)
- Neurological and vascular diseases like parkinsonism, cerebrovascular accidents, and peripheral vascular diseases

CONGENITAL CONDITIONS
- Cystic fibrosis
- Club feet
- Heart defects (e.g., arteriovenous malformations)

TRAUMATIC CONDITIONS
- Motor vehicular accidents, falls, or other injuries, particularly involving the spinal cord (e.g., spinal cord injury) or the brain (e.g., closed head injury)

MENTAL AND COGNITIVE CONDITIONS
- Drug-induced psychoses
- Mood disorders (e.g., depression)
- Memory loss
- Dementia (e.g., Alzheimer's disease)

Modified from Hoeman S: *Rehabilitation nursing: process and application*, St Louis, 1996, Mosby.

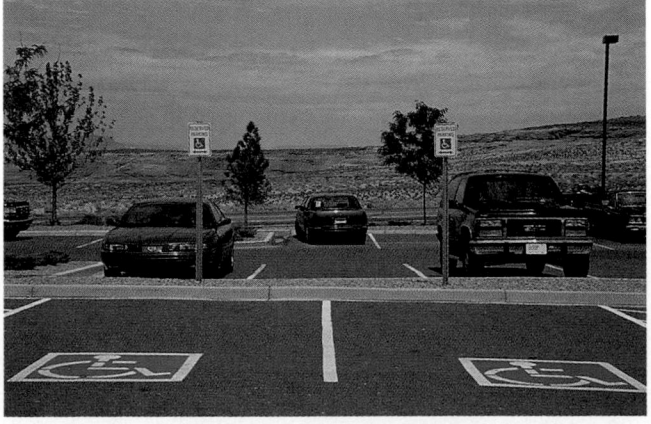

Fig. 5-1 "Handicap" parking.

community settings (Thompson-Hoffman and Storck, 1991). The current widespread availability of structural modifications such as wheelchair access ramps, raised toilet seats in enlarged stalls in public restrooms, and widened "handicap" parking places are notable examples of such physical enhancements (Fig. 5-1).

With the Rehabilitation Act of 1973 the role of nursing in restorative care rapidly expanded. Increasingly, nurses assisted the clients as restorative care managers, care givers, and advocates. The nurse became a dominant member and, with the client, a co-leader of the restorative care team. In 1974 the Association of Rehabilitations Nurses was formed (McCourt, 1993). Ten years later, that association began to grant credentials to specialists in rehabilitation nursing.

■ FUNCTIONAL STATUS AND RESTORATIVE CARE

Clients have a baseline level of functioning, which is referred to as their **functional capacity**. Many health problems afflict clients and result in one or more problems that limit this capacity. Classifications of common health problems that limit functioning and necessitate restorative care are multiple (see the box on p. 80).

The reduced functional capacity created by one or more health problems is referred to as the **residual functional capacity**, which is the level of functioning remaining after the health problem occurred. The difference in functioning between the original functional capacity (before the health problem occurred) and the residual functional capacity is referred to as the **residual functional deficit** (Fig. 5-2).

Restorative care or restorative nursing is synonymous with the more traditional terms "rehabilitation care" or "rehabilitation nursing." In nursing literature the word *restoration* represents the positive focus of the nurse to assist the client in the acute and restorative aspects of care, and it gradually replaces the word **rehabilitation** in an effort to gain distance from the sometimes negative connotation associated with the latter. Likewise, the terms "residual functional deficit" and "residual functional capacity" are being used instead of "**handicap**" or "**disability**," and the term "restorative client" is being used in place of the terms "the disabled" and "the handicapped" (Thompson-Hoffman and Storck, 1991).

Restorative care is an effort by a health care team, including the nurse, to assist the client to return to the maximal functional status (Fraley, 1992). In other words, restorative care is devoted to minimizing the residual functional deficit and maximizing the residual functional capacity (Figs. 5-3 and 5-4).

The **restorative health care team** supports the client's efforts to maximize independence within the constraints of the residual functional capacity and, as soon as possible, to reintegrate the client into the community in the previous or modified role and setting (Gallagher and Kreider, 1987).

Ideally the nurse desires to eliminate the residual functional deficit, thereby restoring the client to the original functional capacity. In reality, however, that may not be possible. There will usually be some residual functional deficit after a function-compromising health problem such as a cerebro-vascular accident. The nurse's realistic role is to minimize the effects of the deficit, which includes preventing complications and further deterioration, in order to re-

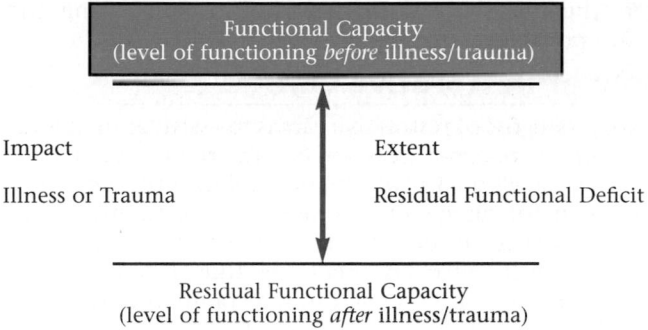

Fig. 5-2 The relationship of functional capacity, residual functional capacity, and residual functional deficit *before* restoration.

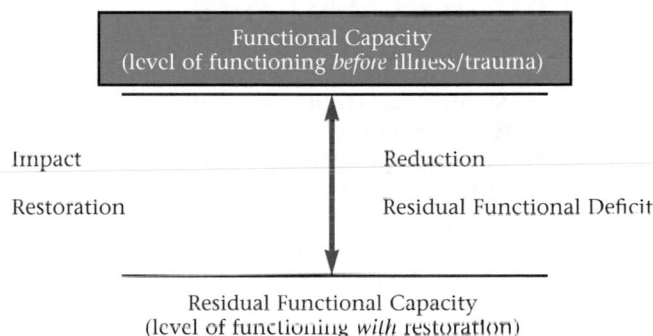

Fig. 5-3 The relationship of functional capacity, residual functional capacity, and residual functional deficit *with* restoration.

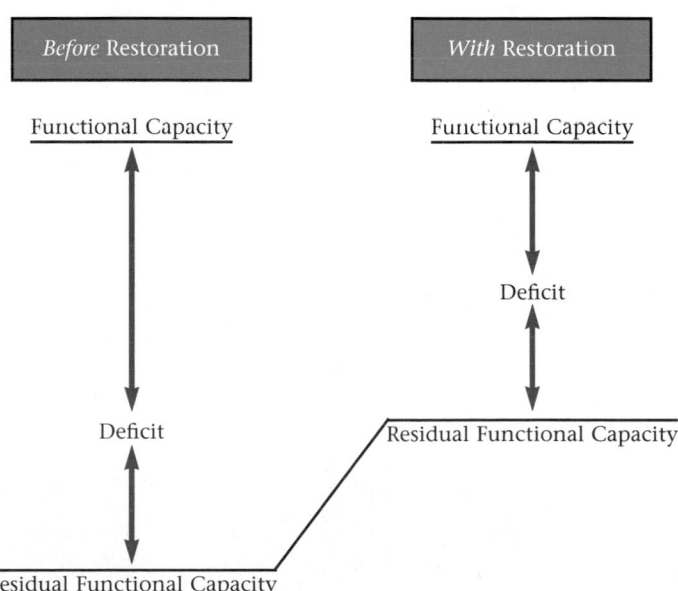

Fig. 5-4 Comparison of functional capacity and residual functional capacity *before* and *with* restoration.

store the client to the highest level of functioning and health possible (Edelman and Mandle, 1994).

Goal of Restorative Care

The overall goal of restorative care is to assist an individual to regain the maximal functional status, thereby enhancing the individual's quality of life. Although health care professionals, including the nurse, and various health institutions are involved in restorative care, the intent is to promote client independence and self-care, thus facilitating the client's resumption of a place in the community (Kemp et al, 1990).

Central to restorative care are the client's adaptation to the problems necessitating restorative care and fulfillment of all needs in Maslow's hierarchy (see Chapter 27). The restorative health care team supports the client's adaptation to or adjustment of the loss of function, maximization of the residual functional capacity, and return of the client to the community (Hoeman, 1990).

Restorative Health Care Team

Restorative health care requires an interdisciplinary team approach to ensure the delivery of comprehensive, cost-effective, nonfragmented, quality care. This team is composed of a variety of health care professionals, the client, and the client's family and significant others (Fig. 5-5).

The core members of the restorative health care team are the client, the client's family and significant others, the nurse, and the physician. Besides the nurse and the physician, other health care professionals may be on the team on an as-needed basis. In addition, other persons may be included in the restorative team less frequently and for a shorter duration (see the box on p. 83).

The restorative care team functions as a unit to assist the client to achieve the maximal possible level of functioning and to reintegrate into the community. As a whole, the team engages in clinical decision making involving assessment, diagnosis, planning, implementation, and evaluation (American Congress of Rehabilitation Medicine, 1992).

Although the health care professionals work together as a team, members participate and contribute from the specific focus of their respective disciplines (McCourt, 1993). For example, if the team is concerned with a functional problem related to mobility, the physical therapist focuses on the physical adjustments to enhance mobility while the nutritionist focuses on foods and feeding schedules to increase activity tolerance during mobility; or for a client with a bathing self-care deficit, the nurse assists with the bathing while supervising and reinforcing the client's use of transfer techniques taught by the physical therapist and assistive devices provided by the occupational therapist (McCourt, 1993).

For the restorative care team to function efficiently, the following must occur:

1. Leadership must be determined. Ultimately the client is the leader of the team. Because of nursing's constant interaction with the client, the nurse assumes responsibility for coordinating the activities of the restorative care team and managing the client's case and care, and is in fact the team leader (Campbell, 1992) (Fig. 5-6). The nurse also ensures proper use of resources and facilitates timely discharge of clients (McCourt, 1993).
2. Communication has to be effective, frequent, and documented. Case conferences involving as many members of the team as possible, especially the client and family or significant others, and shared written reports are central to this communication (Commission on Accreditation of Rehabilitation Facilities, 1991).
3. Collaboration among team members must be complete and genuine. All areas of expertise of the team are used in the plan of care (Howard, 1991).
4. Conflict resolution among disciplines must be quick. Boundaries and roles for specific disciplines must be well defined and respected but must not become the predominant concern (Cohen et al, 1992). Conflicts are best resolved by maintenance of mutual respect

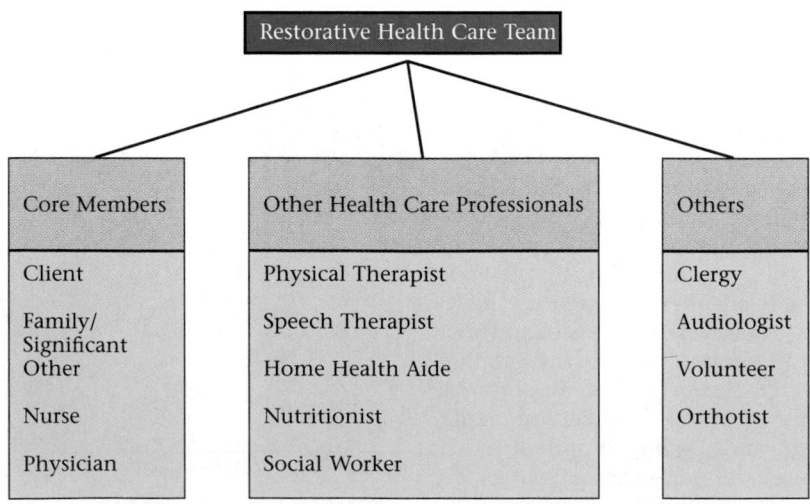

Restorative Health Care Team		
Core Members	**Other Health Care Professionals**	**Others**
Client	Physical Therapist	Clergy
Family/ Significant Other	Speech Therapist	Audiologist
	Home Health Aide	Volunteer
Nurse	Nutritionist	Orthotist
Physician	Social Worker	

Fig. 5-5 The restorative health care team. *(Data from JCAHO, 1995.)*

among team members, unfailing focus on the team's purpose, effective communication—especially involving attentive listening and clarification—acceptance of necessary trade-offs, and common sense and logic (Frank and Elliot, 1992).

Research studies have documented that when the previously mentioned behaviors occur, the effectiveness of the interdisciplinary team approach to restorative care is evident (O'Toole, 1992).

Restorative Care: Functional Problems and Considerations

Various illnesses or injuries create the need for restorative care to maximize the client's functional abilities. Most commonly, functional limitation or impairment exists that decreases the client's ability to perform tasks. Trauma, illness, and the client's functional limitations are the important considerations in restorative care. However, if the interdisciplinary team is to assist a client to effectively adapt to limitations, the overall focus of care is directed to all of the client's needs (Falvo, 1991).

In some instances the client's functional deficit will remain. However, the client and family are taught how to adapt so that the client's maximal level of health and independence is achieved. When working in a restorative care setting, the following must be taken into account: the client's willingness to participate in care, family structure and relationships, environmental situation and living arrangements, and resource availability. As the emphasis for early discharge continues, there are more clients receiving their restorative care in the home setting.

Possible Other Members of the Restorative Team and Their Functions

VOLUNTEER
- Visit or call clients
- Run errands

CLERGY
- Meeting spiritual needs
- Support and counsel clients and their significant others

PSYCHOLOGIST
- Meeting mental health needs
- Support and counsel clients and their significant others

RESPIRATORY THERAPIST
- Meeting oxygenation needs
- Technical support for oxygen therapies (e.g., ventilator set-up)

AUDIOLOGIST
- Meeting auditory and balance needs
- Diagnose and counsel concerning hearing aids and other assist devices

BIOMEDICAL ENGINEER
- Design and manufacture various prosthetic and adaptive devices to meet particular client needs (e.g., design special fork for self-feeding)

OSTHETIST AND ORTHOTIST
- Design and manufacture various prosthetic and adaptive devices to meet particular client needs (e.g., design artificial limb)

HOME HEALTH IN THE CONTINUUM OF CARE

Home health care is the provision of medically related professional and paraprofessional services and equipment to clients and families in their places of residence for health maintenance, education, illness prevention, diagnosis and treatment of disease, palliation, and rehabilitation. The most common services include nursing; medical and social work; physical, occupational, speech, and respiratory therapy; nutritional therapy; and physician care. Of these services, nursing is used most often as a result of client needs.

Paraprofessional services include home health care aides, housekeepers, and companions. Many of these care givers provide personal care and household support services that prevent the need for costly hospitalization or care in a skilled nursing facility.

Home health care equipment is any medically related product adapted for home use, including highly technical items such as mechanical ventilators, intravenous (IV) infusion pumps, and nontechnical items such as hospital beds and walkers.

Home health care agencies have extended almost every type of health care service into the client's residence. Health promotion and education are traditionally the primary objectives of home care. The focus is encouragement of client and family independence through teaching of self-care. Recovery and stabilization of illness must be addressed in the home, where problems related to lifestyle, safety, environment, family dynamics, and health care practices can be readily identified.

Clients who need home health care have a variety of physical, socioeconomic, and psychological problems. Some of these clients are in medically unstable conditions and may have an acute problem such as wound infection or an exacerbation of a chronic condition such as lung disease. They usually require home treatment, professional assessment, education, and frequent changes in therapy. Some clients may be in medically stable condition (e.g., persons with chronic insulin-dependent diabetes), but they require long-term care to prevent exacerbations and hospitalization. Insurance reimbursement for medically unstable

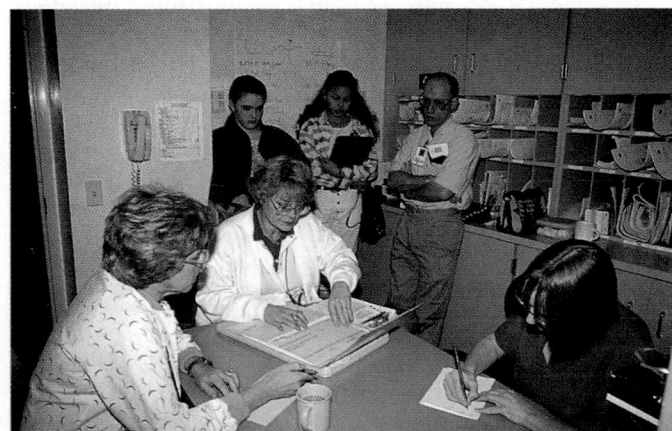

Fig. 5-6 Nurse conducting meeting of restorative health care team.

clients has improved, but most policies and government funds do not reimburse clients for long-term care.

■ TYPES OF HOME HEALTH CARE SERVICES AND REIMBURSEMENT

To meet client needs for home health care services and equipment and to ensure adequate reimbursement, nurses must understand the services available and the way clients are reimbursed. Home health care services are reimbursed by three mechanisms: government funds, private insurance, and private pay.

Home Health Care Agencies

Home health care agencies provide skilled, intermittent professional and home health care aide services, usually once or twice a day for up to 7 days a week. Visits usually last 1 hour. Professional services include the implementation of a plan of treatment and skilled assessment and instruction. Home health care aides provide personal care such as bathing, feeding, and bed making. Use of these services allows clients to live independently, usually with the help of family members.

Approved agencies that provide these services usually receive reimbursement from the government (such as Medicare and Medicaid in the United States), private insurance, and private pay. The Medicare and Medicaid programs have strict, elaborate regulations governing reimbursement for home health care services. An agency cannot simply charge for a service and expect to receive full reimbursement. Most professional services provided through a Medicare-licensed agency are reimbursed at the costs for providing the service by government programs. Commercial payers, such as Blue Cross, often negotiate contract rates or provide reimbursement for billed charges. Because of the increasing costs of health care, all reimbursement mechanisms are closely evaluated.

Private Duty Agencies

Private duty agencies provide professional and paraprofessional home health care services on a more continuous basis, usually by registered nurses, licensed practical nurses, housekeepers, companions, or home health care aides. These agencies provide nursing coverage for 4 to 24 hours a day.

The cost of 24-hour, private-duty nursing care ranges from $7000 to $12,000 (U.S.) a month, depending on the level of the professional providing the care (Association of Rehabilitation Nurses, 1991). Government funds will not pay for private-duty nursing care, so reimbursement is provided primarily by private insurance and private pay. Some government programs are available for homemaker services. As expected, these services are generally affordable only to people for whom commercial insurance provides reimbursement or to those who can afford to pay privately.

Durable Medical Equipment Companies

Most **durable medical equipment (DME)** companies provide medical equipment such as hospital beds, wheelchairs, commodes, and ventilators, as well as disposable supplies. Home oxygen is also available from most DME companies. Reimbursement is through government and private insurance. Fairly stringent guidelines exist for determining reimbursement for equipment. Many DME companies are now encouraged to seek accreditation from the Joint Commission on Accreditation of Healthcare Organizations to ensure quality of equipment and services (JCAHO, 1995).

The DME industry is one of the most rapidly growing areas in the health care field. Nurses and therapists are frequently employed by these companies to provide client education and assist with sales and marketing activities. Referrals can be made to DME companies by any health care professional. The physician must certify medical necessity by signing a prescription for the equipment.

■ INCREASED DEMAND FOR HOME HEALTH CARE

Home health care has evolved into a challenging, rapidly growing field. Because of recent economic, social, governmental, and technological developments, home health care professionals are caring for clients who are more ill, who go home from the hospital sooner, and who have more needs for highly technical care and complex equipment than ever before.

Other forces causing more demand for restorative and home health care services include increases in the number of older adults and chronically ill persons, advances in home health care technology, and the breakdown of the extended family (see the box below). Most households require two incomes, which leaves fewer family members at home to care for the older adults and disabled persons. Clients are more acutely ill when discharged from the hospital and require more intensive services.

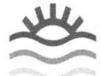 **GERONTOLOGICAL PRINCIPLES for *Restoration***

As persons get older, the process of meeting their restorative needs involves a longer, more involved intervention because, in comparison with younger persons, older persons:

■ Are more prone to injuries (such as hip fracture) and illnesses (such as cardiovascular accident) requiring prolonged, complex restorations.

■ Have more chronic conditions (diabetes mellitus, parkinsonism, etc.) with unknown origins, extensive therapeutic regimens, and multiple complications of their own, which complicate and slow any recovery or restoration.

■ "Heal" or recover more slowly because of functional decrements in perfusion, oxygenation, nutrition, skin integrity, and tissue integrity. The quantity and efficiency of delivery of oxygen, glucose, and other nutrients to affected areas is decreased.

■ Respond less quickly because of sensory deficits (decreased vision, hearing, etc.) and slower transmission of both sensory and motor neurological impulses. Client's perception, comprehension, and mobility are limited, and safety and self-care are at risk. Client learning and active participation in the restoration may be impaired.

■ Have less resources available (social, financial, etc.) to support or aid restoration.

The U.S. government's health care payment system has resulted in major cutbacks that have made an impact on the home health care industry. Funding for hospital care has been drastically cut, especially for older adults, resulting in a tremendous increase in the need for home health care services by clients who would have previously been hospitalized. As a result, many of these clients require more highly skilled and technical services.

Many agencies are able to provide many highly technical services in the home; these include IV therapy, mechanical ventilation, infant apnea monitoring, and preterm labor monitoring. Because of the nature of these services, the agency is required to provide 24-hour staff availability and services 7 days a week. Although the cost for providing many of these services at home is much less than in an institutional setting, less government funding of the health care system has forced home health care agencies to operate efficiently or fail.

▌ NURSING ROLES AND THE RESTORATIVE CARE TEAM

Nurses assume many roles, from nurse to agency owner and director. Home health care provides a great deal of autonomy and flexibility and offers opportunities for independent clinical practice, management, marketing, teaching, clinical specialization, and research. The nurse continuously assists the client in restoration and coordinates the restorative care team (American Nurses Association and Association of Rehabilitation Nurses, 1988).

Clinical Practice

Home health care nurses provide creative, adaptive care to clients in the home (Fig. 5-7). A holistic, nonjudgmental,

and family-centered philosophy is essential for the nurse in the home. The nurse must understand another person's value systems and beliefs. The nurse helps clients grow and develop independence and usually has an interest in health promotion and maintenance. Most of all, home health care nurses must take the initiative to assess and diagnose client problems, implement appropriate therapies, and evaluate outcomes (see the box below). Some agencies use the nurse as a case manager, who is the person responsible for initiating the plan of care and ensuring continuous follow-up with progress toward discharge.

Home health care nurses provide individualized care and have one-on-one contact with clients and families. They are independent and have their own caseloads, and they help clients adapt to the plan of care and disease processes. For example, a terminally ill client receiving daily heparin injections is helped by the nurse to establish a medication schedule that complements daily home routines. Nurses also help clients adjust to the influences of cultural and en-

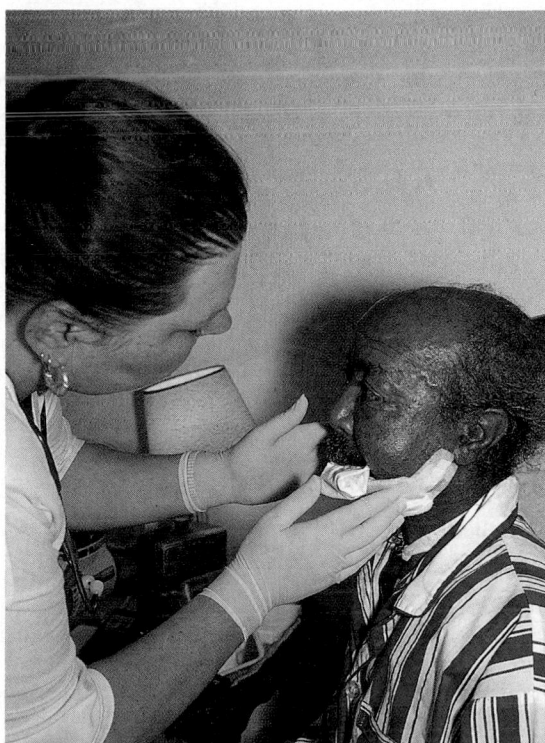

Fig. 5-7 Care provided in client's home.

Home Health Care Nursing Skills

WOUND CARE
Sterile dressings, debridement and irrigation of wounds, packing, assessment of drainage, assessment and culture of wounds, and instructing clients and families in wound care.

RESPIRATORY CARE
Management of oxygen therapy, mechnical ventilation, and suctioning and care of tracheotomies.

VITAL SIGNS
Monitoring blood pressure, cardiopulmonary status, and instructing clients and families in pulse taking (when appropriate).

ELIMINATION
Clients with new ostomy appliances often need assistance with irrigation and skin care procedures, as well as with learning to use specialized equipment. Assessment and teaching, insertion of urinary catheters, irrigation, observation for infection, and instruction of family in intermittent catheterization are also provided.

NUTRITION
Assessment of nutrition and hydration status, instruction on prescribed diet, administration of tube feedings, and instructing families in tube feedings.

REHABILITATION
Instructing clients and families in the use of assistive devices, range of motion exercises, ambulation, and transfer techniques.

MEDICATIONS
Instructing clients and families on medication actions, administration, and side effects; monitoring compliance and effectiveness of prescribed medications.

INTRAVENOUS THERAPY
Assessment and management of dehydration; giving antibiotic medications, parenteral nutrition, blood products, and analgesic and chemotherapeutic agents.

SELECTED LABORATORY STUDIES
Drawing blood for studies related to disease processes or medications.

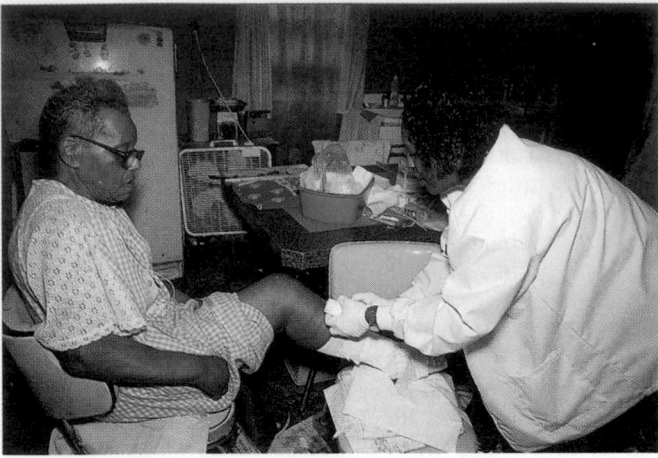

Fig. 5-8 Educating client in home setting.

vironmental factors and have the opportunity to develop the nurse-client relationship more fully than do nurses in hospitals.

Home health care nursing requires clinical assessment and judgment, teaching skills, and the ability to coordinate and document care provided. A home health care nurse needs a broad knowledge of community resources, cultural and socioeconomic factors, family dynamics, and psychology (Fig. 5-8). Writing skills that include demonstrated knowledge and application of regulatory and reimbursement guidelines are essential abilities. In most settings the home health care nurse is a generalist, one who applies nursing care skills and knowledge for clients of all ages and a wide range of health problems.

Home Health Care Management

Most home health care agency directors, managers, and field supervisors are nurses who possess advanced training in administration and experience in home health care practice. They provide a vital link among care givers, clients, physicians, community resources, advisory board members, and regulatory and reimbursement agencies. In addition to clinical and personnel management, they are responsible for financial management, quality assurance, and program development. Home health care nursing management requires a strong ability to promote staff excellence while containing costs and complying with reimbursement and regulatory guidelines.

Teaching and Research Activities

Most nurses in home health care agencies are involved in many educational activities. In fact, the primary focus of home health care nursing is client and family education to establish self-care and independence. Nurses determine client and family learning abilities and needs, develop and implement individualized teaching plans, and evaluate the success of the client in meeting learning objectives. Frequent visits to homes allow the nurse to evaluate whether clients are successfully applying new knowledge to health care practices.

Most home health care agencies coordinate staff educa-

tional activities, including orientation, case conferences, monthly in-service workshops, and physical assessment courses. Workshops about specialty services are also important as home care becomes more technical and intensive.

The home health care nurse must also know how to solve problems. Frequently the nurse enters a client's home to find an absence of resources. Managers and field staff must refine problem-solving skills and further develop them into more formalized research activities. Many agencies are engaged in formalized studies to document the following:

1. Cost effectiveness of clinical problems
2. Staffing needs
3. Consumer satisfaction
4. Quality assurance and improvement activities

The preceding research activities will become important as competition and regulations increase and funding sources decrease.

Legal and Ethical Responsibilities

Nurses are legally able to perform independent nursing activities based on educational preparation and experience. Nurses can evaluate clients for home health care services without a medical order but must provide care under the direction of a written plan of treatment signed by a physician. Home health care nurses often establish the plan of care and then collaborate with the physician for medical treatment plans. The most controversial legal issues in home health clinical practice include the following:

1. Risks associated with providing highly technical procedures, such as administration of IV medication and blood products, in the home
2. Legal aspects of client teaching such as liability for errors made by family care givers based on misuse of information provided by the nurse
3. Compliance with Medicare or other government home health care regulations

Because of limited, highly fragmented funding for home health care, home health care nurses must determine whether to continue providing services when there is risk of inadequate reimbursement. Often, Medicare coverage expires and clients need ongoing care but are unwilling or unable to pay for it. Many nurses face ethical dilemmas when torn between complying with regulations and caring for the needs of older adults and indigent and chronically ill clients. The nurse must be very knowledgeable about home health care policies to provide clinical documentation that will result in optimal reimbursement for the client. Nursing managers must also be very knowledgeable about regulations and follow the legal steps necessary to overturn coverage denials when appropriate.

Discharge Planning

Discharge planning is a major function of most home health care agencies, especially those affiliated with hospitals. Nurses attend discharge planning rounds and consult with medical, nursing, and social work staffs in hospitals and clinics. Nurses facilitate access to all home health care equipment and services during a client's discharge from the hospital or clinic. Thorough assessment and data collection by the coordinator before hospital discharge facilitates continuity of care and in many cases can speed the discharge process (see Chapter 4).

Sample Functional Aspects for Holistic Assessment in Restorative Care

PHYSICAL FUNCTIONAL ASPECTS
Review of body systems
- System by system
- Basic senses
- Swallowing
- Continence

Endurance/tolerance of activity
Mobility
- Active range of motion (ROM)
- Passive ROM
- Body movement and locomotion
- Assistive devices required
- Travel needs and arrangements
- Activities of daily living
- Activities of independent living: Meal preparation, shopping, cleaning, laundry, telephoning

MENTAL FUNCTIONAL ASPECTS
Level of cognitive functioning
- Alertness
- Attention span
- Orientation
- Memory: short-term, long-term
- Language
- Learning
- Communication: Ability to speak and express, ability to receive and understand
- Understanding and comprehension
- Reasoning and judgment

EMOTIONAL FUNCTIONAL ASPECTS*
Determination of coping style(s)
- Negative: Denial, regression and so forth
- Positive: Compensation and the like

Acceptance of residual function deficits
- Motivation for restoration
- Mood and affect
- Depression
- Fear and anxiety
- Anger and guilt
- Cooperation with restoration care and team

SOCIAL FUNCTIONAL ASPECTS
Study of social supports and contacts
- Significant others and family
- Community: Place of residence, social interaction, social support

VOCATIONAL FUNCTIONAL ASPECTS
Level of education and training
- Past employment
- Transferable skills
- Current job analysis

RESOURCES FOR RESTORATIVE CARE
Availability and means of transportation
- Access to public transportation

*Modified from Favlo D: *Medical and psychosocial aspects of chronic illness and disability,* Gaithersburg, Md, 1991, Aspen.

▌ RESTORATIVE CARE AND THE NURSING PROCESS

The nurse uses the nursing process to individualize care so that the client is assisted to regain the maximal possible level of function and independence. Effective use of the nursing process requires that the nurse use critical thinking and clinical decision making to focus on the client's needs.

 ### Assessment

The assessment must focus on the total functional needs of the client (see the box above). Gordon's eleven Functional Health Patterns (FHPs) provide one type of assessment framework to provide a data base that focuses on the client's total needs and functional status (Edelman and Mandle, 1994; Carpenito, 1993, 1995). Client and family assessment begins at referral. The coordinator submits written referral forms to the home health nurses. These forms usually include demographic data, physician's orders, medications, treatments, nursing and medical diagnoses, goals and prognoses, and functional limitations and activities.

Special problems and concerns at discharge should be communicated to the home health care staff. In complicated specialty cases (e.g., IV therapy, mechanical ventilation, and hospice care) home health nurses may also visit the client in the hospital before discharge to identify needs, initiate discharge teaching, and prepare the client and family for care.

Before the nurse can thoroughly assess the client and family, a preassessment phase must take place. This phase involves incorporating information about the client's environment and gradually establishing a nurse-client relationship. The nurse combines information from the referral with an assessment of the client and family in the home; the nurse uses interviews, physical assessments, and histories to do this. For this reason, the assessment is complex and time consuming. An assessment usually includes data about the following areas:

1. Physical assessment and history of all body systems, with emphasis on the present illness
2. Psychosocial assessment (education, ethnicity, and social relations)
3. Family dynamics (decision making and rituals)
4. Spiritual health (life values, hope, and a sense of community with others)
5. Community resources (need for financial assistance and follow-up care)
6. Environmental factors (housing, transportation, and neighborhood)
7. Functional limitations (problems resulting in inabilities related to activities of daily living)
8. Client and family knowledge and attitudes toward illness and health behaviors and the impact on their lifestyle

Examples of NANDA Nursing Diagnoses Routinely Identified for Clients Requiring Home Health Care

Impaired skin integrity *related to:*
- Physical immobility
- Radiation
- Pressure

Altered nutrition *related to:*
- Inability to ingest or digest food
- Inability to absorb nutrients

Bathing/hygiene self-care deficit *related to:*
- Pain
- Musculoskeletal impairment
- Decreased endurance

Pain *related to:*
- Decreased joint mobility

Knowledge deficit *related to:*
- Lack of experience
- Cognitive limitation

Risk for infection *related to:*
- Inadequate primary or secondary defenses
- Inadequate acquired immunity
- Malnutrition

Nursing Diagnosis

After collecting data about the client and the home, the home health care nurse selects nursing diagnoses. Any nursing diagnosis may apply to a client in the home; however, some health problems are seen routinely (see the nursing diagnoses box at left). If the nurse has assessed an insufficient number of defining characteristics for a diagnosis, additional information from family or friends may help confirm a diagnosis. The diagnostic process (see the diagnostic process box on p. 89) requires the correct use of assessment skills in revealing the defining characteristics for client problems. Gordon's FHPs are listed in the box on p. 89 along with a sampling of specific restorative concerns.

Planning

The plan of care identifies nursing diagnoses and establishes long- and short-term goals (see the care plan below). The nursing diagnoses and goals should be related to the primary disease processes, treatment plan, functional limitations, and psychosocial, financial, and environmental problems.

Sample Nursing Care Plan for Knowledge Deficit

NURSING DIAGNOSIS: **knowledge deficit** regarding home intravenous (IV) antibiotic administration related to lack of previous experience.
DEFINITION: Knowledge deficit is the state in which specific information is lacking.*

GOAL	EXPECTED OUTCOMES	INTERVENTIONS	RATIONALE
Client will acquire knowledge and skill of basic IV therapy by 7/16.	Client demonstrates correct handwashing and aseptic technique by second visit.	While in the client's home, demonstrate and watch client return demonstration of proper handwashing and aseptic technique.	Learning that is applied immediately is retained longer and is more subject to immediate use than that which is not.
	Client demonstrates correct preparation and administration of IV fluids and medication by third visit.	Demonstrate and watch client return demonstration of inspection of bag label for date and name, inspection of solution, priming of tubing with fluid, and insertion of needle into cap.	
	Client explains knowledge of effects of medication by second visit.	Instruct client on three side effects of medication. Praise client for correct answer.	Learning is facilitated when learner receives feedback.
	Client safely disposes of used equipment by third visit.	Demonstrate proper disposal of IV equipment and explain safety issues. Place needles in an empty plastic milk carton. Dispose of used intravenous bags and tubing in garbage.	Relating skill to home improves retention of information.

*Data from Kim MJ, McFarland GK, McLane AM: *Pocket guide to nursing diagnoses*, ed 6, St Louis, 1995, Mosby.

Sample Nursing Diagnostic Process for Home Health Care

ASSESSMENT ACTIVITIES	DEFINING CHARACTERISTICS	NURSING DIAGNOSIS
Ask if client has had experience with self-administering IV medications.	Client communicates never having given IV medications in past and requests information.	**Knowledge deficit** regarding home IV antibiotic administration related to lack of previous experience
Instruct client to read written instructions, and note level of reading comprehension.	Client reads written words but demonstrates poor retention (e.g., why catheter is flushed).	
Observe client's behavior when receiving instruction on how to flush catheter.	Client hesitates to hold syringe and defers all teaching to significant other.	

Gordon's FHPs With Sampling of Specific Restorative Concerns

PATTERN
- Health perception/management

Restorative concerns
- Self-care capability
- Maintenance of safety
- Adherence to prescribed therapy

PATTERN
- Nutrition-metabolic

Restorative concerns
- Suitability of diet
- Integrity of skin
- Energy for daily activities

PATTERN
- Elimination

Restorative concerns
- Bowel control
- Bladder control
- Interaction in public/community

PATTERN
- Activity-exercise

Restorative concerns
- Endurance for/in activities
- Impairments in mobility
- Home maintenance management

PATTERN
- Sleep-rest

Restorative concerns
- Decreased daytime alertness
- Interference with/interrupted sleep
- Sleep/activity asynchrony

PATTERN
- Cognitive-perceptual

Restorative concerns
- Capacity to learn
- Acute pain and chronic pain
- Sensory impairments

PATTERN
- Self-perception/self-concept

Restorative concerns
- Body image disturbances
- Feelings of self-worth
- Feelings of powerlessness

PATTERN
- Role-relationship

Restorative concerns
- Altered family/living arrangements
- Capability for vocation/employment
- Social contact and involvement

PATTERN
- Sexuality-reproductive

Restorative concerns
- Methods of contraception
- Facilitation of conception
- Alternate means of sexual activity

PATTERN
- Coping-stress tolerance

Restorative concerns
- Perception of intense stressors
- Dealing with change and loss
- Exhaustion of adaptive abilities

PATTERN
- Value-belief

Restorative concerns
- Maintenance of the human spirit
- Holistic well-being
- Worth of life and health

CLIENT TEACHING
for Home IV Therapy

OBJECTIVE
■ Client demonstrates, with assistance of care giver, the correct technique for administering home intravenous (IV) antibiotic therapy.

TEACHING STRATEGIES
■ Teach correct handwashing technique.
■ Discuss the importance of infection control and safe IV administration.
■ Demonstrate and have client demonstrate mixture, administration, and discontinuance of IV solution.
■ Have family member or significant other observe administration procedure.

EVALUATION
■ Client correctly washes hands.
■ Client gathers all necessary equipment.
■ Client correctly administers first dose of medication.

The planning process in home health care requires involvement of the client, family, and significant others. All care is given in the home. The client and family are accustomed to having control, and the nurse must not lose sight of this fact. Home health care professionals have minimal control over the environment, unlike hospital nurses who work in a very controlled environment. Client involvement in planning and teaching can lead to better compliance with care. The client is urged to take an active role by assuming responsibility for care. The following factors must be considered when planning home care:
1. Socioeconomic, cultural, and environmental factors
2. Family and community resources
3. Client teaching (see the box at left)
4. Interdisciplinary collaboration between home health care and hospital professionals
5. The client's physician and other health care providers, who must be consulted and informed on a regular basis

Short- and long-term goals must be realistic, measurable, and based on expected outcomes. Home health care staff must foster independence to prepare the client for discharge from home health care services. The plan for

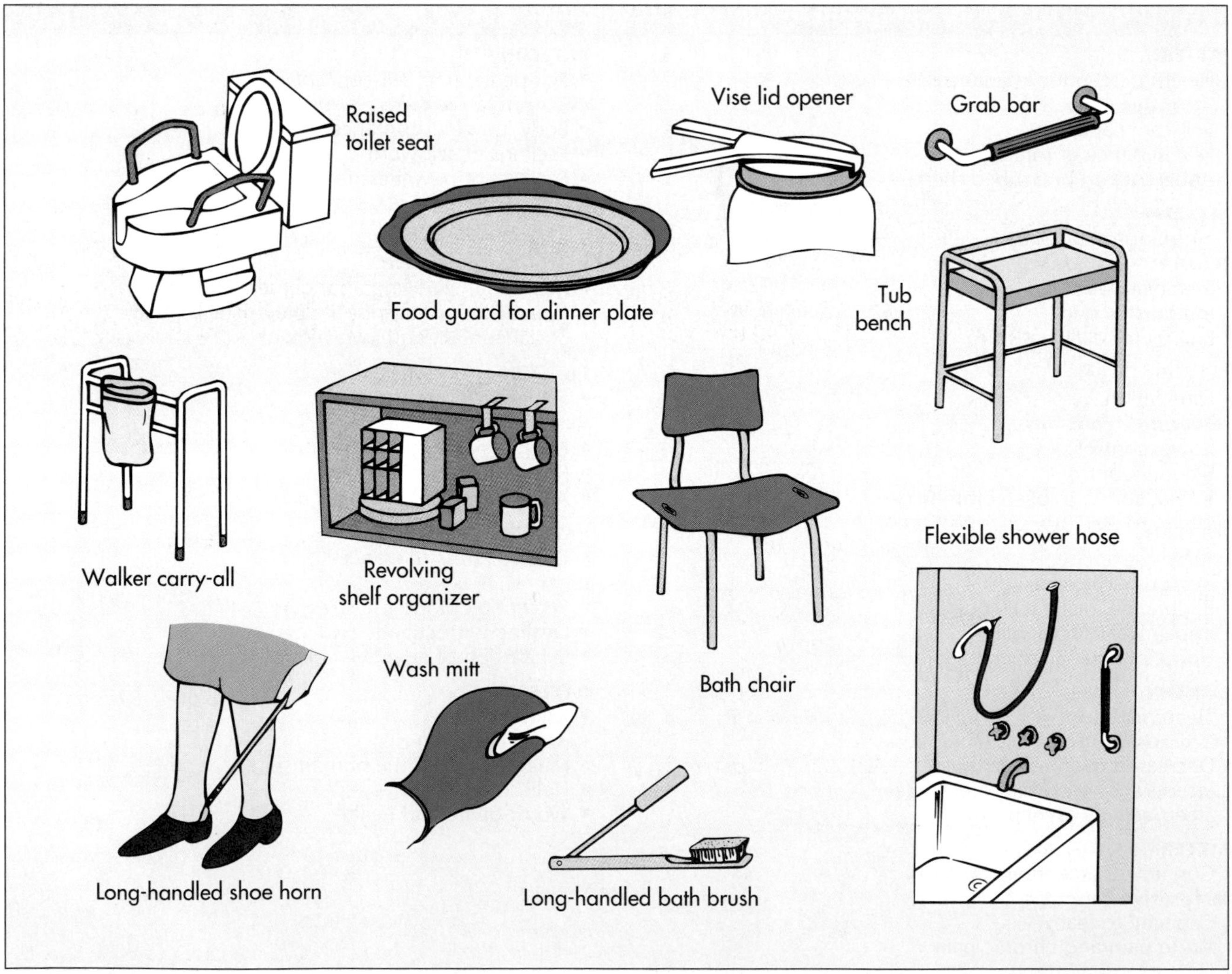

Raised toilet seat

Vise lid opener

Grab bar

Food guard for dinner plate

Tub bench

Walker carry-all

Revolving shelf organizer

Bath chair

Flexible shower hose

Wash mitt

Long-handled shoe horn

Long-handled bath brush

Fig. 5-9 Special equipment commonly used in the home setting for clients recovering from a stroke.

restorative care may include some of the following client-centered goals:

- Client's activity tolerance is maintained or increased
- Client/family performs a specific nursing skill independently.
- Client's ability to perform self-care activities is maintained or increased.
- Client continues to participate in care decisions.

Implementation

Implementation of the plan of care requires close collaboration among clients, family members, restorative health care personnel, and physicians (see the box below). Skilled interventions include assessments, teaching, consultation with physicians about changes in therapy, and initiation of complex procedures such as dialysis, IV therapy, phototherapy, and mechanical ventilation. Clients are taught how to use special equipment and adaptive aids to improve mobility, coordination, and independence when performing activities of daily living (Fig. 5-9). Most procedures can be taught to the client and family. Government and private insurers pay for visits only until the client and family have had time to learn procedures. Interventions such as prenatal assessments and the administration of blood products require the skill of a registered nurse. These interventions are not taught to the family. Thorough documentation of the visit supports reimbursement resulting from the necessity of skilled care.

Planned interventions are not always easily achieved in many homes (see the box below). Nurses in home health care must adapt interventions to all types of environmental, social, financial, and cultural constraints. Family and community resources must be used to assist with implementation.

Evaluation

Evaluation of outcomes of care is an ongoing process, which is the key to the success of home health care (see the evaluation box on p. 92). Outcomes of care must be documented for continuity of care, reimbursement, accreditation, and research. Evaluation of client response to teaching, treatments, and medications results in identification of changes needed in therapy. It also helps identify obstacles that may interfere with the effectiveness of the care plan. Effective, ongoing evaluation of outcomes and thorough follow-up for necessary changes are the most important functions of home health care personnel.

■ CLINICAL ASPECTS OF QUALITY IMPROVEMENT

Many government and private regulatory agencies have established standards and guidelines for the operation and reimbursement of restorative health care agencies. All regulations directly or indirectly have an impact on the clinical and administrative practice of home health care nurses.

The U.S. and Canadian governments have established specific reimbursement guidelines for coverage of home health care services. Government agencies, specifically the

---

Nursing Implementation for the Restorative Client

ROLES OF THE NURSE IN IMPLEMENTATION
- Care provider implementing nursing interventions
- Supervisor of ancillary nursing care personnel: orienting them to the nursing plan of care, instructing them concerning the nursing orders, evaluating their implementation of the nursing orders
- Case manager of the client's case
- Coordinator of the restorative care team

CONCERNS OF THE NURSE IN IMPLEMENTATION
- Ensurance of delivery of quality care to the client by meeting and exceeding all standards for care published by either the American Nurses Association or the Association of Rehabilitation Nurses* and all criteria for accreditation enforced by either the Commission on Accreditation of Rehabilitation Facilities† or the Joint Commission on Accreditation of Healthcare Organizations‡
- Accountability for the conduct of the nursing plan of care and the collaboration of the restorative care team
- Documentation of the nursing plan of care and its implementation, to facilitate reimbursement
- Ultimately, facilitation of client's discharge to independence in care (self-care)

---

*American Nurses Association and Association of Rehabilitation Nurses: *Rehabilitation nursing: scope of practice, process, and outcome criteria,* Washington DC, 1988, The Associations.
†Commission on Accreditation of Rehabilitation Facilities: *1991 standards manual for organizations serving people with disabilities,* Tucson, Ariz, 1991, The Commission.
‡Joint Commission on Accreditation of Healthcare Organizations: *Accreditation manual for hospitals,* Oakbrook Terrace, Ill, 1995, Joint Commission on Accreditation of Healthcare Organizations.

Nursing Implementation for the Restorative Client: Logistics for Implementation

ENVIRONMENT OF THE CARE SETTING: CLIENT'S HOME OR WORKPLACE
- What is its layout and structure?
- Does it have adequate means for meeting hygienic and sanitation needs?
- Will the client be safe there, especially if alone or isolated?
- Can it be modified to accommodate the client's needs?

TRANSPORTATION TO, FROM, AND WITHIN THE CARE SETTING
- How will the client get to, in, and out of the home?
- Can the client get to the workplace?
- How will the client get to the employee cafeteria on the second floor of the workplace?

RESOURCES FOR THE HEALTH CARE SETTING
- What is the *willingness* of the client's employer and co-workers to accommodate the client's needs?
- Are necessary supports *available* in the workplace?
- Does the homebound client have *access* to emergency health services (i.e., "911" service)?
- What is the *suitability* of the nurse providing restorative services for the client in the client's workplace?
- Can the nurse be *reimbursed* for care provided to the client in the workplace?

Sample Evaluation of Interventions for Knowledge Deficit

GOAL	EVALUATIVE MEASURES	EXPECTED OUTCOMES
Client will acquire knowledge and skill of basic intravenous (IV) therapy by 7/16.	Client demonstrates appropriate use of aseptic technique.	Client will demonstrate correct handwashing and aseptic technique by second visit.
	Observe IV sites routinely.	Signs/symptoms of infection and infiltration will be absent from catheter site. There will be no evidence of unresolved infection or lack of healing.
	Have client demonstrate preparation and administration of IV fluids.	Client will demonstrate correct preparation and administration of IV fluids and medication by third visit. Correct number of doses will be administered. No unused, expired medication will be found in home.
	Have client describe side effects of medication.	There will be no side effects of medication from improper administration. Client will list three side effects of medication by second visit.
	Observe client disposing of equipment; check disposal containers.	Needle container will be filled with appropriate waste. Client will have no incidence of needle sticks or exposures in home. There will be no improperly disposed of needles, bags, or tubing in home by third visit.

Health Care Financing Administration, distribute funds for all claims and monitor for compliance with guidelines.

Two independent organizations have established comprehensive standards for home health care. They are the JCAHO and the Community Health Accreditation Program (CHAP). To receive accreditation, all hospital-based home health care agencies must meet the standards of the JCAHO. Other organizations elect to achieve JCAHO or CHAP accreditation for quality improvement and reimbursement purposes (JCAHO, 1995). Most states also require licensure of home health care agencies. State guidelines follow those of Medicare but may also include additional regulations. Accreditation standards focus on documentation and case management because they affect the day-to-day practice of home health care nurses.

The client's clinical record must contain comprehensive, updated care plans and detailed nursing notes from each visit. Visit reports must contain evidence that a visit was necessary and that skilled care was given (e.g., assessments, which reflect medical instability, and client teaching and consultation with physicians). Homebound status, safety measures, progress toward discharge, client comprehension of instruction, and functional limitations must also be well documented.

Each client must be assigned a case manager, who coordinates all aspects of care, including planning and collaboration with all home health care disciplines, community resources, and physicians. The case manager plans the client's discharge from a home health care program and imple-

ments follow-up as needed. A monthly case conference must be held on each client and followed by written documentation.

The goal of case management is to ensure the quality of interdisciplinary planning and coordination of care. The purpose of quality improvement is to ensure delivery and documentation of quality care and agency compliance with regulatory and reimbursement guidelines. Although direct client care must be the primary consideration of the home health care nurse, these regulatory procedures must also be performed. Failure to comply with these guidelines can result in considerable damage to clients and possibly the lifetime loss of their home health care benefits.

❚ SPECIALTY NURSING AREAS

Home health care clients increasingly need more specialized and technically advanced services. Most agencies realize that general home health care nurses are not trained to provide this level of care. As a result, agencies have developed specialty nursing teams in areas such as hospice care, IV and pulmonary therapy, obstetrics, psychiatry, pediatrics, oncology, and diabetes care. Many larger agencies employ clinical nurse specialists to develop and manage specialty nursing programs.

Hospice

Hospice is a philosophy of care. It exists to provide support and care for persons in the last months of an incurable illness so that life can be lived as fully and comfortably as possible.

Hospice care has evolved into a specialization. Nurses working in this area need highly technical skills related to pain control and other palliative therapies. They also need to know the psychology of dealing with dying clients and their families (see Chapter 26). This specialized philosophy of care is applied to clients and families in the comfort of their own homes. In the United States about 80% of certified hospice care is provided in the home. Most programs are managed by home health care agencies. Home hospice care is preferred over inpatient hospice care for clients whose family members provide home care.

Home Intravenous Therapy

Clients are now receiving **home IV therapies**, including hydration, antibiotic medications, parenteral nutrition, blood products, and analgesic and chemotherapeutic agents (see the box at right).

In the United States many agencies require national IV therapy certification offered through the Intravenous Nurses Society for nurses who administer home IV therapy. These nurses are usually certified in chemotherapy as well. Intravenous therapy nurses must have good teaching and assessment skills (see the box on p. 90). A multidisciplinary approach is often used to offer the client a complete range of IV therapy services. A pharmacist, dietitian, nurse, and physician are part of the infusion therapy team of many home health care agencies. Comprehensive discharge planning is needed to ensure safe and effective home care.

Home Respiratory Care

Clients with chronic lung and other debilitating diseases are discharged sooner, are more ill, and need more complicated and technical care and equipment. They may require oxygen, mechanical ventilation, and tracheotomies (see Chapter 44).

Respiratory care technology has responded to the needs of these clients. Small, portable ventilators are now as efficient and effective as most hospital ventilators. Nurses caring for these clients not only need to know procedures for operating this equipment but also must have advanced knowledge and skills in respiratory nursing care and client and family teaching.

▌ ISSUES AND CONSIDERATIONS IN RESTORATIVE CARE

Currently access to health care is a major political and legislative issue (McCourt, 1993). Historically the majority of health care services were in acute care settings (Chapter 4). By the year 2000 there will be a 100% increase in the need for restorative care services in the United States (Avillon and Mirgon, 1989). This increase is due to increased longevity, early discharge from acute care settings, and legislation that prevents discrimination against impaired clients in the community or workplace settings. Restorative

▶ **RESEARCH HIGHLIGHT**

RESEARCH ABSTRACT
This article presents a case-study analysis of home infusion therapy. The study identifies how the responsibilities for the education and care of the client and family, the maintenance of the infusion equipment, and the ordering and administration of the intravenous medications are shared between nursing and pharmacy. The case study highlights the strengths of a preplanned model for implementing home infusion therapy. In this model, the plan is designed to meet the usual needs for these clients and families. Once it is determined that home infusion therapy is required, the nurse, in collaboration with the pharmacist, modifies the existing plan to include the individual needs of the client and family. A list of potential problems with specific interventions is developed in case problems should arise.

A review of clients who received home infusion therapy with this model noted a decreased rate of complications, received their therapy in a timely manner, and were comfortable with receiving such care in the home.

IMPLICATIONS FOR PRACTICE
▶ Early education of the client and family increases the likelihood of successful implementation of this therapy in the client's home.
▶ Good communication between the nurse and the pharmacy must be established before initiating home infusion therapy.
▶ Although the nurse and pharmacist are primary members of the team, the client's and family's needs, schedules, and responsibilities all must be coordinated with both the nurse and pharmacist.

REFERENCE
Haddad MA, Keefer KR, Stein JE: Teamwork in home infusion therapy: the relationship between nursing and pharmacy, *Home HealthCare Nurse* 11(1):40, 1993.

care has a legislative mandate, in addition to a professional obligation, to provide services (Pope and Tarlov, 1991).

Major considerations for restorative care are the reimbursement mechanisms. Federal, state, and private groups are including restorative care services within their payment criteria. This trend continues. Cost-benefit analyses reveal lower cost and greater benefit to clients and families who use these services (Thompson-Hoffman and Storck, 1991).

As technology becomes more pervasive in a health care system, the providers can use this same technology in multiple settings (e.g., in the home as well as in acute care settings). Nurses are in the forefront of restorative care. Nurses are bringing the knowledge, technology, and caring of the discipline into the community settings and assisting clients and their families in achieving the highest level of independence.

■ KEY CONCEPTS ■

▶ The services provided in restorative settings are those designed to bring the client to the maximal level of health and function.

▶ Clients have a baseline level of functioning, which is referred to as their *functional capacity.*

▶ The restorative health care team supports the client's efforts to maximize independence within the constraints of the residual functional capacity and, as soon as possible, to reintegrate the client into the community in the previous or modified role and setting.

▶ Restorative care requires an interdisciplinary team approach to ensure the delivery of comprehensive, cost-effective, nonfragmented, quality care.

▶ Home health care is the provision of medically related professional and paraprofessional services and equipment to clients and families in their places of residence for health maintenance, education, illness prevention, diagnosis and treatment of disease, palliation, and rehabilitation.

▶ To meet client needs for home health care services, adequate reimbursement, which includes three payment mechanisms (government funds, private insurance, and private pay) must be obtained.

▶ Home health care professionals now care for clients who are more ill, who go home from the hospital sooner, and who have more needs for highly technical care and complex equipment than ever before.

▶ Home health nursing requires clinical assessment and judgment, teaching skills, and the ability to coordinate and document care provided.

▶ Discharge planning is a major function of most home health care agencies, especially those affiliated with hospitals.

▶ Many government and private regulatory agencies have established standards and guidelines for the operation and reimbursement of restorative health care agencies.

▶ Two independent organizations have established comprehensive standards for home health care. They are the JCAHO and the Community Health Accreditation Program (CHAP).

▶ Home health care clients increasingly need more specialized and technically advanced services such as hospice care, IV and pulmonary therapy, obstetrics, psychiatry, pediatrics, oncology, and diabetes care.

▶ Nurses bring the knowledge, technology, and caring of the discipline into the community and assist clients and their families in achieving the highest level of independence.

■ KEY TERMS ■

Disability, p. 81
Durable medical equipment (DME), p. 84
Functional capacity, p. 81
Handicap, p. 81
Home health care, p. 83
Home health care agencies, p. 84
Home intravenous (IV) therapies, p. 93
Hospice care, p. 93
Private-duty agencies, p. 84
Rehabilitation, p. 81
Residual functional capacity, p. 81
Residual functional deficit, p. 81
Restorative care, p. 81
Restorative health care team, p. 81

■ CRITICAL THINKING EXERCISES ■

1. You are the restorative nurse for a young adult woman client with a spinal cord injury who refuses to leave her home because she may urinate and "not even know it." How will you approach this client and this health care situation? What interventions will you perform or suggest to assist this client?

2. A middle-aged woman neighbor has a daughter who was involved in a motor vehicle accident (MVA) 2 years ago and who has just finished her restoration. Several days ago, this woman's elderly mother was involved in a similar MVA; this neighbor now tells you that she knows that "this" (her mother's restoration) will be a lot "rougher" than was her daughter's restoration. What is the basis for this woman's statement? As a nurse, how can you be of assistance to this neighbor?

3. You are the restorative nurse and case manager for a client who is a successful professional man and who insists on returning to work full-time as soon as possible. What are your concerns as you interact with this client?

4. A restorative care client has just returned to live with his large, extended family in their home. Among the family members there are several who are able to provide care for the client but are unwilling to do so. How will you approach this health care situation? Which nursing diagnoses are applicable to this health care situation? What interventions will you perform or suggest to assist this client?

REFERENCES

American Congress of Rehabilitation Medicine: *Guide to interdisciplinary practice in rehabilitation settings*, Skokie, Ill, 1992, American Congress of Rehabilitation Medicine.

American Nurses Association and Association of Rehabilitation Nurses: *Rehabilitation nursing: scope of practice, process, and outcome Criteria*, Washington DC, 1988, The Association.

Association of Rehabilitation Nurses: *The rehabilitation clinical nurse specialist*, Skokie Ill, 1991, The Association.

Avillon A, Mirgon B: *Quality assurance in rehabilitation nursing: A practical guide*, Rockville, Md, 1989, Aspen.

Campbell L: Team maintenance and enhancement. In *American Congress of Rehabilitation Medicine guide to interdisciplinary practice in rehabilitation settings*, Skokie, Ill, 1992, American Congress of Rehabilitation Medicine.

Carpenito LJ: *Nursing diagnoses: application to clinical practice*, ed 5, Philadelphia, 1993, Lippincott.

Carpenito LJ: *Nursing diagnoses: application to clinical practice*, ed 6, Philadelphia, 1995, Lippincott.

Cohen H, Rubin A, Gombash L: The team approach to treatment of a dizzy patient, *Arch Phys Med Rehabil* 73:703, 1992.

Commission on Accreditation of Rehabilitation Facilities: *1991 standards manual for organizations serving people with disabilities*, Tucson, Ariz, 1991, The Commission.

Edelman C, Mandle C: *Health promotion throughout the lifespan*, St Louis, 1994, Mosby.

Falvo D: *Medical and psychosocial aspects of chronic illness and disability*, Gaithersburg, Md, 1991, Aspen.

Fraley A: *Nursing and the disabled across the lifespan*, Boston, 1992, Jones & Bartlett.

Frank R, Elliot T: Conflict resolution and feedback. In *American Congress of Rehabilitation Medicine's guide to interdisciplinary practice in rehabilitation settings*, Skokie, Ill, 1992, American Congress of Rehabilitation Medicine.

Gallagher L, Kreider M: *Nursing and Health*, Norwalk, Conn, 1987, Appleton & Lange.

Haddad MA, Keefer KR, Stein JE: Teamwork in home infusion therapy: the relationship between nursing and pharmacy, *Home HealthCare Nurse* 11(1):10, 1993.

Hoeman S: Interdisciplinary team treatment in acute care. In Deutsch P, Fralish K, editors: *Innovations in head injury rehabilitation*, New York, 1990, Matthew Bender.

Hoeman S: *Rehabilitation nursing: process and application*, St Louis, 1996, Mosby.

Howard M: Interdisciplinary team treatment in acute care. In Deutsch P, Fralish K, editors: *Innovations in head injury rehabilitation*, New York, 1991, Matthew Bender.

Joint Commission on Accreditation of Healthcare Organizations: *Accreditation manual for hospitals*, Oakbrook Terrace, Ill, 1995, Joint Commission on Accreditation of Healthcare Organizations.

Kemp B, Brummel-Smith K, Ramsdell J: *Geriatric rehabilitation*, Austin, Tx, 1990, Pro-Ed.

Kim MJ, McFarland GK, McLane AM: *Pocket guide to nursing diagnoses*, ed 6, St Louis, 1995, Mosby.

McCourt A: *The specialty practice of rehabilitation nursing: a core curriculum*, ed 3, Skokie, Ill, 1993, The Rehabilitation Nursing Foundation of The Association of Rehabilitation Nurses.

O'Toole J: The interdisciplinary team: research and education, *Holist Nurs Pract* 6(2):76, 1992.

Pope A, Tarlov A: *Disability in America: toward a national agenda for prevention*, Washington, DC, 1991, National Academy.

Raymond C: Polio survivors spurred rehabilitation advances, *J Am Med Assoc*, 255:1404, 1986.

Thompson-Hoffman S, Storck I, editors: *Disability in the United States: a review of the state of knowledge*, New York, 1991, Springer.

ADDITIONAL READINGS

American Nurses Association: *Guidelines for the practice of nursing on the rehabilitation team: an answer to a growing need*, Washington, DC, 1965, The Association.

Bronstein K, Popovich J, Stewart-Amidei C: *Promoting stroke recovery*, St Louis, 1991, Mosby.

Butler M: Geriatric rehabilitation nursing, *Rehabil Nurs* 16:318, 1991.

Catanzaro M: Rehabilitation nursing, *J Adv Nurs* 2(1):32, 1993.

Flaherty B: The nurse legal consultant and disabling injuries, *Rehabil Nurs* 16:30, 1991.

Fanning R, Judge J, Weihe F et al: Housing needs of individuals with severe mobility impairments: a case study, *J Rehabil* 57(2):7, 1991.

Greenwood R, Schriner K, Johnson V: Employer concerns regarding workers with disabilities and the business-rehabilitation partnership, *J Rehabil* 57(1):21, 1991.

Groch S: Public services available to persons with disabilities in major U.S. cities, *J Rehabil* 57(3):23, 1991.

Heffner R: *The rehabilitation survival guide*, St Louis, 1994, Mosby.

Hoeman S: Community-based rehabilitation, *Holist Nurs Pract* 6(2):32, 1992.

Hoeman S: *Rehabilitation nursing: process and application*, St Louis, 1995, Mosby.

Leath C: Team managed care for older adults: a clinical demonstration of a community model, *J Gerontol Nurs* 17(7):25, 1991.

Mullahy C: Making case management count, *Case Manager* 2(3):40, 1991.

North M, Meeusen M, Hollnsworth P: Discharge planing: increasing client and nurse satisfaction, *Rehabil Nurs* 16:327, 1991.

Nosek M, Roth P, Zhu Y: Independent living programs: the impact of program age, consumer control, and budget on program operation, *J Rehabil* 57(4):28, 1991.

Resources for Rehabilitation, Inc: *Resources for people with disabilities and chronic conditions*, Lexington, Mass, 1991, Resources for Rehabilitation.

US Architectural and Transportation Barriers Compliance Board: Accessibility guidelines for buildings and facilities, *Fed Reg* 56(144):35, 408, 1991.

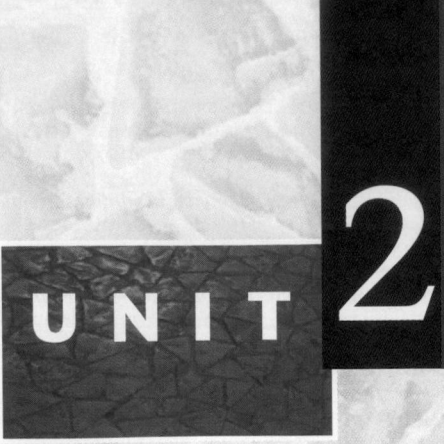

UNIT 2

The Nursing Process and Critical Thinking

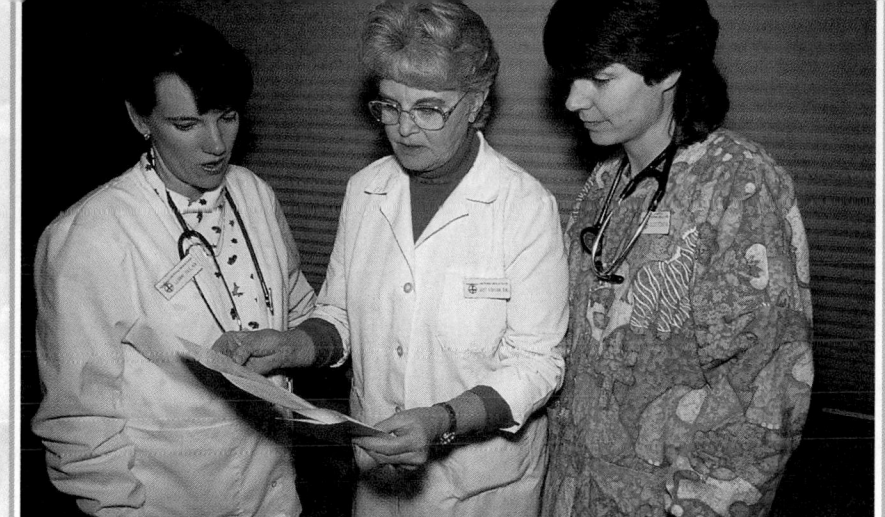

## Chapter 6

Critical Thinking and Nursing Judgment

Objectives

Mastery of content in this chapter will enable the student to:

► Define the key terms listed.

► Describe components of a critical thinking model for nursing judgment.

► Explain the difference between problem solving and decision making.

► Explain the importance of clinical experience in critical thinking.

► Discuss the relationship of the nursing process to a model for critical thinking.

► Describe how attitudes influence the ability to make critical judgments.

► Summarize the standards to be applied in critical thinking in nursing.

► Explain the relationship between the scientific method and the nursing process.

► Describe the five steps of the nursing process.

A nurse's role is to assist individuals, sick or well, in the performance of activities contributing to health and its recovery, or to a peaceful death (International Council of Nurses, 1973). This definition captures the complexity of nursing. When given the responsibility to assist a person in regaining or improving health, a nurse must be able to think critically in order to problem solve and find the best solution to a client's needs. Critical thinking is a process that challenges an individual to interpret and evaluate information to derive judgments. Over time, a nurse's expertise develops as he or she cares for many clients, testing and refining nursing approaches, learning from successes and failures, and always applying new knowledge that is appropriate to a client's needs. The ability to think critically, apply knowledge and experience, problem solve, and make decisions is central to nursing practice.

Clients present a wide variation of experiences, symptoms, known medical diseases, behaviors, values, and social perspectives when they make contact with a health care provider. To add to the complexity of what a nurse does, these same variables can change. In the presence of such variation it is a nurse's responsibility to make relevant observations about a client; examine ideas, **inferences**, assumptions, and principles; recognize health problems; and develop an approach to care that eliminates or minimizes the client's problems. Within any health care setting a nurse must be able to use knowledge from nursing and other disciplines, think quickly and creatively, and make sound decisions to ensure a client's well-being, for, as Renee Fox (1980) noted, "however familiar and routine it may be, or seemingly unthreatening and nontragic, no nursing action or interaction that involves a patient is trivial or completely ordinary."

CRITICAL THINKING

Consider a situation in which a nurse enters a client's hospital room and observes a client's "scared" facial expression. Making the observation that the client is "scared" may result from the nurse's experience with other clients or from having worked with the same client the previous day and knowing that a change has occurred. The nurse pursues the situation further. When the client provides further information on "not feeling well," the nurse begins to consider the client's reason for seeking health care, observes for subtle signs of how the client lies in bed, and begins to ask the client questions. The questions may be direct, such as "Tell me what you are feeling" or "Are you having pain?" Measurement of the client's pulse, blood pressure, and respiratory rate may provide further information about the client's status. How the nurse uses information to reason, make inferences, and form a mental picture of what is happening to this client is **critical thinking**.

Thinking is making use of the mind and involves forming conclusions, making decisions, drawing inferences, and reflecting (Gordon, 1995). It is an active and organized process (Chaffee, 1994). When a nurse directs thinking toward understanding and finding solutions to a client's health problems, the process becomes purposeful and goal oriented. In relationship to nursing, the critical thinking process is reflective, reasonable thinking about nursing problems without a single solution and is focused on de-

---

Critical Thinking Abilities

- Thinking actively by using one's intelligence, knowledge, and skills to answer questions
- Carefully exploring situations by asking and trying to answer relevant questions
- Thinking for ourselves by carefully examining various ideas and arriving at thoughtful conclusions
- Viewing situations from different perspectives to develop an in-depth, comprehensive understanding
- Discussing ideas in an organized way to exchange and explore ideas with others

Modified from Miller MA, Babcock DE: *Critical thinking applied to nursing,* St Louis, 1996, Mosby.

---

ciding what to believe and do (Kataoka-Yahiro and Saylor, 1994). Learning to think creatively and deeply enables a nurse to care for clients as their advocate and to become more astute in the choices made about their care. Critically thinking challenges a person to examine assumptions about current information and to interpret and evaluate arguments with the intent of reaching a conclusion from a new perspective (Strader, 1992). To think critically involves an integrated set of thinking abilities and attitudes (see the box above). One must be able to take in information, use recent and past memory, apply reason and logic, review data in a disciplined manner, and make decisions fairly and creatively.

Consider the nurse who cares for a dying client. The nurse knows that during grieving a client may show certain behaviors. The nurse recalls the theory of grieving, which predicts certain behaviors the client may display. If the client speaks of death at one time but later expresses a feeling of improvement, the nurse incorporates this experience into the concept of grief work. The nurse intervenes on the basis of the client's specific response and needs rather than just on the basis of the "textbook picture" of the grief response. Therapeutic decisions are based on the unique factors that affect the client so that innovative approaches can be used to provide the client comfort. Then, when the nurse cares for another dying client, the previous experience enables the nurse to critically reflect on and consider the right decisions for the new client. When a nurse makes decisions about another person's health, bias, prejudice, and application of "traditional" thinking are inappropriate. Critical thinking frees individuals to think for themselves and to take action after a problem or situation is clearly understood.

Thinking and Learning

Learning is a lifelong process. To grow, each of us acquires new knowledge and refines the ability to think, problem solve, and make judgments. Learning and thinking are inseparable. Over time, as we engage in new experiences and apply the knowledge we have, we become better able to form assumptions, present ideas, and make valid conclusions.

As a professional nurse, one must always look and think ahead. One cannot allow thinking to become routine or standardized. Nursing practice must always change. That is to say, as new knowledge becomes available, professional nurses must always challenge traditional ways of doing things and look to what is most effective, has scientifically supported evidence, and results in better client outcomes. To think critically gives a nurse the ability to learn and to positively influence nursing practice. A nurse's maturity is measured by the ability to use new knowledge and engage in a process of discovery that benefits clients as well as the profession.

A CRITICAL THINKING MODEL

Kataoka-Yahiro and Saylor (1994) have developed a model of critical thinking for nursing judgment (Fig. 6-1). The model defines the outcome of critical thinking as nursing judgment that is relevant to nursing problems in a variety of settings. The model is designed to address nursing judgment in clinical, managerial, leadership, and educational roles. For the purpose of this chapter, the discussion focuses on clinical nursing judgment. When a nurse enters into any clinical experience, the model proposes, there are five components of critical thinking, which ultimately leads the nurse to make the clinical judgments that are necessary for safe, effective nursing care (see the box below).

Specific Knowledge Base

The first component of critical thinking is the nurse's specific knowledge base in nursing. This varies according to the basic nursing education program from which the nurse graduated, additional continuing education, and any ad-

vanced degrees that the nurse may pursue. A nurse's knowledge base includes information and theory from the sciences, humanities, and nursing that are needed to think about nursing problems. Such information provides the data that are used in the various critical thinking processes. It is important that this knowledge base include approaches that reinforce the nurse's ability to think critically about nursing problems (Fig. 6-2).

Experience

The second component of the critical thinking model is experience in nursing. Unless a nurse has the opportunity to practice in a clinical setting and make decisions about client care, critical thinking will not develop. When a nurse has an encounter with a client, a wealth of information can be learned from observing, sensing, talking with the client, and then reflecting actively on the experience. Clinical experience provides the laboratory for testing nursing knowledge. The nurse will learn that "textbook" approaches lay an important groundwork for practice but that adaptations must be made to accommodate the setting, the unique qualities a client presents, and the experiences the nurse has gained from previous clients. Benner (1984) notes that the expert nurse understands the context of a clinical situation, recognizes cues, and interprets them as relevant or irrelevant. This level of competency comes only from experience. Perhaps the best lesson to be learned by a new nursing student is to value all client experiences. Use each

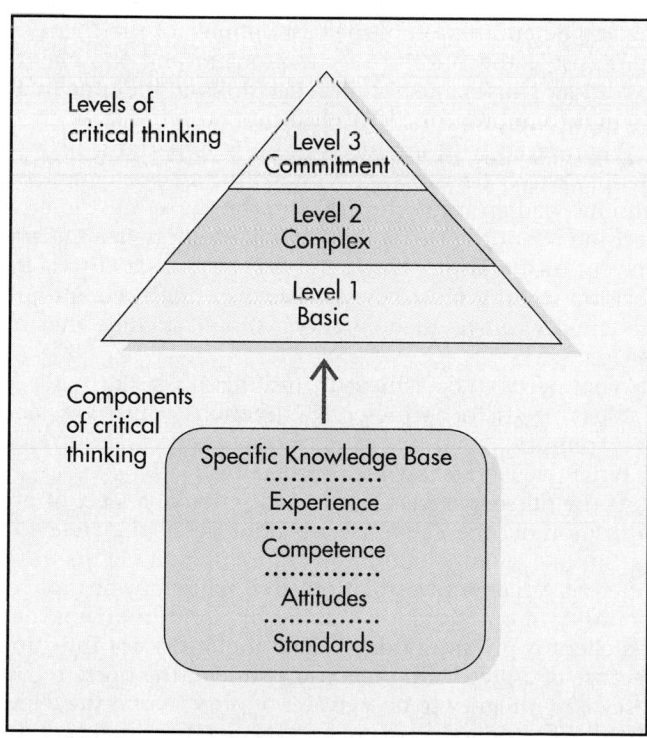

Fig. 6-1 Critical thinking model for nursing judgment. *(Redrawn from Kataoka-Yahiro M, Saylor C: A critical thinking model for nursing judgment, J Nurs Educ, 33(8):351, 1994. Modified from Glaser, 1941; Miller and Malcolm, 1990; Paul, 1993; and Perry, 1970.)*

Components of Critical Thinking in Nursing

SPECIFIC KNOWLEDGE BASE IN NURSING

EXPERIENCE IN NURSING

CRITICAL THINKING COMPETENCIES
- General competencies
- Specific competencies in clinical situations
- Specific competency in nursing

ATTITUDES FOR CRITICAL THINKING
- Confidence
- Independence
- Fairness
- Accountability
- Risk Taking
- Discipline
- Perseverance
- Creativity
- Curiosity
- Integrity
- Humility

STANDARDS FOR CRITICAL THINKING
Intellectual standards
- Clear
- Precise
- Specific
- Accurate
- Relevant
- Plausible
- Consistent
- Logical
- Deep
- Broad
- Complete
- Significant
- Adequate
- Fair

Professional standards
- Ethical criteria for nursing judgment
- Criteria for evaluation
- Professional responsibility

Modified from Kataoka-Yahiro M, Saylor C: A critical thinking model for nursing judgment, *J Nurs Educ*, 33(8):351, 1994.

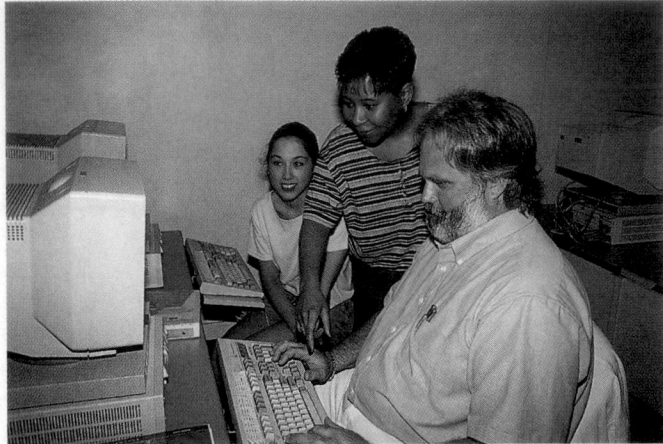

Fig. 6-2 In the computer laboratory, students begin to learn clinical scenarios that stimulate critical thinking.

one as a stepping-stone to build and acquire new knowledge, make comparisons and contrasts, and stimulate innovative thinking.

Competencies

Critical thinking competencies are the cognitive processes a nurse uses to make nursing judgments. There are three types of these competencies; general critical thinking, specific critical thinking in clinical situations, and specific critical thinking in nursing. General critical thinking processes include the scientific method (see p. 104), problem solving, and decision making. They are also used in other disciplines (e.g., social work and medicine) and in nonclinical situations. Problem solving involves obtaining information when there is a gap between what is occurring and what should be occurring. When a person begins to water the lawn and finds that the water is not flowing from the nozzle, a quick problem-solving approach involves locating the spot along the hose where it is kinked. Problem solving in a clinical situation might involve a nurse entering a client's room and finding the client in pain. An assessment of the client's position in bed finds the client lying in a twisted manner. A catheter tube is pinching the client's skin. The nurse repositions the client and realigns the tube away from the client's body; as a result, the client expresses relief of discomfort. The nurse obtained information that clarified the client's source of discomfort and tested a solution that was successful. Effective problem solving also involves the nurse evaluating the solution over time to ensure that it is still effective. The nurse returns to the client's room to evaluate whether the discomfort has returned. It may become necessary to try different options if the problem recurs. Having solved a problem in one situation allows the nurse to apply that knowledge to future client situations.

In decision making a person selects actions to meet a goal. For example, decision making occurs when a person decides how to use his or her time or what food to cook for a dinner meal. To make a decision, one must assess all options, weigh each against a set of criteria, and then make a final choice. For example, when a nurse makes a decision about a place of employment, several criteria are usually considered: location, reputation of institution, level of staffing, opportunity for professional advancement, and compensation. A decision should be made freely on the basis of a person's values and preferences. Once a decision is made, the individual should believe that it was the best possible choice.

Specific critical thinking competencies in clinical situations include diagnostic reasoning, clinical inferences, and clinical decision making. Physicians, social workers, and other health care professionals use these same competencies. An example of diagnostic reasoning involves the nurse who makes ongoing assessments on the basis of a client's medical problems (Carnevali and Thomas, 1993). Although the nurse does not make medical diagnoses, he or she looks for anticipated signs and symptoms that are common to a diagnosis to assist in making the clinical inferences about a client's progress. For example, a client who has had a history of a myocardial infarction ("heart attack") must be monitored for recurrent chest pain or irregularity of vital signs. The nurse is the eyes and ears of a physician and must be able to critically analyze changing clinical situations so that a client's immediate needs can be anticipated. This is the important collaborative role that the nurse assumes. Any diagnostic conclusions made by the nurse help the physician pinpoint the nature of a problem more quickly and select proper medical therapies.

Whenever a nurse approaches a clinical problem, such as a client who is in pain, is anxious about an impending diagnostic procedure, or has an injury to the skin, a decision must be made in choosing the best approach to reach a desired goal. The goal is generally the relief or resolution of the client's problem. The clinical decision-making process for selecting the best approach requires thoughtful reasoning and determination of the best options for the client on the basis of the priority of the problem and the client's condition. Nurses make clinical decisions all the time in an attempt to improve a client's health.

When faced with any decision, it is important, first, to identify why a decision is necessary. In the case of a client who has had an injury to the skin, the nurse must make a decision about the therapies that will promote healing and prevent further injury. Strader (1992) notes that criteria for decision making must be established so that the appropriate choices can be made. Criteria should include the following:

What needs to be achieved? (healing of the skin)
What needs to be preserved? (mobility, nutrition, and comfort)
What needs to be avoided? (infection)

As the nurse considers each of the criteria, a level of prioritization occurs. The nurse sets priorities as they relate to the specific client situation. Because different clients bring different variables to a situation, an activity may be more of a priority in one situation and less of a priority in another. If a client is physically dependent and at risk for infection because of a preexisting medical problem, the nurse recognizes skin integrity to be a greater priority than if the client was mobile and able to eat a normal diet, in which case the priority of skin integrity might have less urgency.

Once the nurse prioritizes the decision to be made, nursing therapies are selected for relieving the problem. A wide range of choices may be available, from nursing therapies to client strategies. The nurse selects, tests, and evaluates each approach. Strader (1992) notes that troubleshooting is also a part of decision making. The nurse tries to anticipate what might go wrong and considers alternative approaches to minimize or prevent problems. For example, the nurse assesses the client's elimination status to ensure that urinary or fecal incontinence is not an underlying problem that might interfere with skin healing. The nurse takes steps to control elimination problems so that the area of the skin is not exposed to irritating or infectious drainage.

Nurses make decisions about individual clients, but they also make decisions about groups of clients. A nurse who works during the busy day shift on a hospital unit is likely to care for several clients. The nurse uses criteria for determining which clients have the greatest priorities. Criteria might include factors such as the acuity of the client, the risk involved in delaying treatment, and the client's expectations of the nurse's care. For example, a client who has just returned from surgery is likely to have a greater priority than a client who is recovering as expected and is awaiting discharge the next day. Similarly, a client who is having a sudden drop in blood pressure along with a change in consciousness warrants the nurse's attention over a client who needs to be assisted for a walk down the hallway. The nurse visits the client who has had no visitors and has recently been given a diagnosis of cancer before checking on the surgical client whose family has just arrived. In order for nurses to be able to manage the wide variety of problems groups of clients present (see the box at right), ongoing decision making is critical. In addition, time management is a part of decision making and ensures that the nurse's time is well spent and that the nurse is responsive to client needs.

One category of critical thinking competencies is specific to nursing. The nursing process is a systematic approach that is used to critically assess and review a client's condition, identify the client's response to a health problem, take appropriate action, and then evaluate whether the action is effective. The format for the nursing process is unique to the discipline of nursing and provides a common language and process for nurses to "think through" clients' clinical problems (Kataoka-Yahiro and Saylor, 1994). The nursing process is a systematic, comprehensive approach for nursing care.

Attitudes for Critical Thinking

The fourth component of the critical thinking model is attitudes for critical thinking. Paul (1993) has summarized attitudes that are central aspects of a critical thinker. These attitudes are the values that a critical thinker must exhibit to be successful. A person must exhibit cognitive skills to think critically, but it is also important to ensure that these skills are used fairly and responsibly. The following are examples of attitudes for critical thinking.

ACCOUNTABILITY

When a person approaches a situation that calls for critical thinking, it is the individual's duty to be answerable for whatever decision is made. As a professional nurse, one must make decisions in response to a client's rights, needs, and interests. The nurse must assume accountability for whatever judgment is made on the client's behalf.

Clinical Decision Making for Groups of Clients

- Identify the problems of each client.
- Compare clients and determine which problems are most urgent on the basis of basic needs, the client's changing or unstable status, and problem complexity.
- Anticipate the time it will take to attend to priority problems.
- Decide how to combine activities to resolve more than one problem at a time.
- Consider how to involve the client as a decision maker and participant in care.

THINKING INDEPENDENTLY

As persons mature and acquire new knowledge, they learn to consider a wide range of ideas and concepts and then make their own judgments. This does not mean they discount other people's ideas. All perspectives of a given situation should be considered. However, a critical thinker does not accept another person's ideas without question. To think independently, one challenges traditional ways of thinking, and looks for rational and logical answers to problems. Independent thinking is at the heart of nursing research (Chapter 16). For many years nurses routinely massaged areas of clients' skin exposed to pressure, thinking the circulation to the affected area would improve. An independent thinker asked the following question: What did massage do to the integrity of underlying tissues? As a result, nursing practice has changed, and massage of pressure areas is now avoided.

RISK TAKING

A person must be willing to have his or her ideas examined and be receptive to new thinking. The beliefs we hold can often be challenged by more logical and rational alternatives. It is easy to make quick, impulsive decisions. It takes courage and a willingness to take risk to recognize what beliefs are false and to then take action based on beliefs that are supported by solid reasoning and facts. Unless one is able to take a risk, one can have difficulty accepting change. There is much discussion going on now about the use of unlicensed assistive personnel to replace registered nurses. Many nurses have resisted, arguing that only registered nurses are equipped to care for clients. However, data show that a good percentage of the routine work performed within hospital settings is repetitive and can be safely delegated to an unlicensed staff member. Having the courage to look at alternative ways to deliver nursing care without compromising quality is critical for nurse managers in dealing with the rapid changes that are occurring in health care.

HUMILITY

It is important to admit one's own limitations. Critical thinkers admit what they do not know and try to acquire the knowledge needed to make a proper decision. A client's safety and welfare may be at risk if a nurse is unable to acknowledge his or her inability to deal with a practice problem. The nurse must rethink a situation, pursue additional knowledge, and then use the information to form a conclusion. Whenever a nurse is pulled to a different nursing unit within a hospital to work, there may be clients with conditions for which the nurse has not provided care. The nurse may be reluctant to admit his or her inexperience. A willingness to confer with a more experienced nurse and to acquire the information needed to properly manage a client's problems enables the nurse to mature professionally.

INTEGRITY

Critical thinkers question and test personal knowledge and beliefs as rigorously as they test the knowledge and beliefs of others. Personal integrity builds trust from peers and subordinates. A person of integrity is quickly willing to admit and evaluate any inconsistencies in his or her own ideas and beliefs. Nursing executives who are strong leaders learn to readily admit when their ideas no longer serve to provide direction to a nursing service. They entertain new information and encourage subordinates to provide solutions to difficult management problems (Fig. 6-3).

PERSEVERANCE

A critical thinker is determined to find effective solutions to client care problems. Quick solutions are not acceptable. The nurse learns as much as possible about a problem, tries various approaches to care, and continues to seek additional resources until the right approach is discovered. For example, the nurse may use a variety of wound care therapies for a diabetic client. This particular type of client can have complicated wounds because the normal healing process is impaired. To find a therapy that works, the nurse may consult with a nurse specialist or dietitian or even refer to a research article on wound care.

CREATIVITY

Creativity involves original thinking. This means finding solutions outside what is traditionally done. Frequently clients pose problems that require unique approaches. For example, an arthritic client might have serious limitation of movement in the hips and knees. One creative approach to helping the client remain mobile is to elevate all chairs

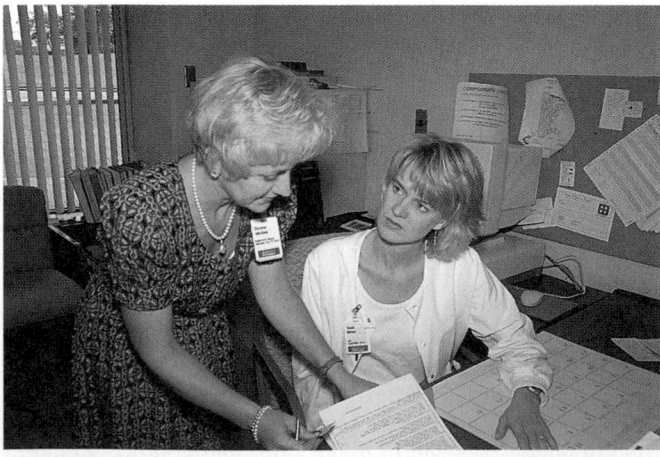

Fig. 6-3 Nursing managers face complex decisions involving clients and staff.

in the home on small blocks nailed to the chair legs, so that it becomes unnecessary for the client to bend at an extreme angle while sitting.

Standards for Critical Thinking

The fifth component of critical thinking includes intellectual and professional standards. Paul (1993) identified intellectual standards to be universal for critical thinking. When a nurse considers a client problem, it is important to use these standards to ensure that the right decisions are made. For example, when attempting to understand the extent of a client's pain, the nurse seeks clear information from the client and clarifies any confusing statements. Any measurements, such as the degree of swelling around the painful area, are precisely made. The nurse examines the client and ensures that findings are specifically located and accurately interpreted. As the nurse collects all the information about the client's pain, additional questions may be asked to ensure that information is in depth and complete.

Professional standards for critical thinking refer to ethical criteria for nursing judgments and criteria for professional responsibility and accountability (see Chapter 19). These standards express the goals and values of the nursing profession. Application of these standards requires that nurses use critical thinking for the good of individuals or groups (Kataoka-Yahiro and Saylor, 1994).

Levels of Critical Thinking in Nursing

A critical thinking model helps show the complexity of the clinical decision-making process in nursing. As a nurse gains new knowledge and matures into a competent professional, the ability to critically think expands. Kataoka-Yahiro and Saylor's model (1994) identifies three levels of critical thinking in nursing: basic, complex, and commitment levels. The levels tend to parallel the five levels of proficiency as described by Benner (1984): novice, advanced beginner, competent, proficient, and expert.

In the basic level the learner assumes that authorities have the right answers for every problem. Thinking tends to be concrete and based on a set of rules or principles. This is an early step in development of reasoning ability (Kataoka-Yahiro and Saylor, 1994). The individual has had limited experience in applying critical thinking. Despite the tendency to be governed by others, a person learns to accept the diverse opinions and values among authorities. In the case of a novice nurse, critical thinking while performing a nursing procedure is limited. The step-by-step approach is used to provide care and may not be adapted to the client's unique or unusual needs.

In the complex level of critical thinking a person continues to recognize the diversity of individual outlook and perception. What changes is the person's abilities and initiative. Experience helps the individual gain the ability to detach from authorities and analyze and examine alternatives more independently and systematically. In the case of nursing, a practitioner begins to see how nursing actions have long-term benefits for clients. The nurse begins to anticipate better and explore a broader range of alternatives. There is a willingness to consider deviations from standard protocols or rules when complex client situations develop. There is often more than one solution to a problem. Nurses learn a variety of different approaches for the same therapy.

The third level of critical thinking is commitment. At this level the nurse chooses actions or beliefs based on the alternatives identified at the complex level of thinking. The nurse is able to anticipate the need to make critical choices after analyzing the merits of other alternatives. The nurse's maturity is reflected in the routine pursuit of the best, most innovative, and most appropriate options for a client's care.

NURSING PROCESS OVERVIEW

The nursing process is one approach to problem solving that enables a nurse to organize and deliver nursing care. It is an element of critical thinking that allows nurses to make judgments and take actions based on reason. A process is a series of steps or components leading to achievement of a goal. The three characteristics of a process are purpose, organization, and creativity (Bevis, 1978). Purpose is the goal or specific aim of the process. The nursing process is used to diagnose and treat human responses to health and illness (American Nurses Association, 1980). Organization is the series of steps or components needed to achieve the goal. The nursing process includes five steps: assessment, nursing diagnosis, planning, implementation, and evaluation (Fig. 6-4). Creativity is the continual development of the process itself. The nursing process is dynamic and continuous. It provides a blueprint for critical thinking so that a nurse can individualize care and respond to client needs in a timely and reasonable manner to improve or maintain the client's level of health.

The nursing process is a creative, organizational structure and framework for providing nursing care, yet it is flexible

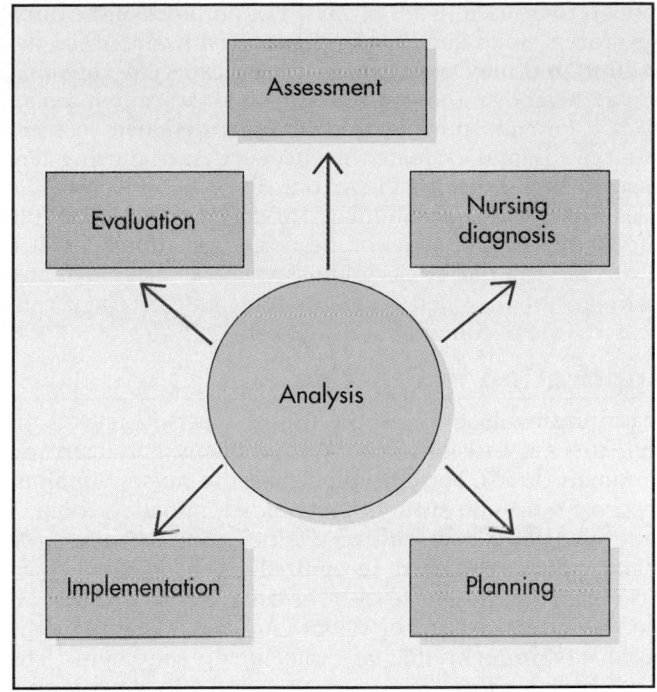

Fig. 6-4 Five-step nursing process model.

Table 6-1	Summary of Nursing Process	
COMPONENT	PURPOSE	STEPS
Assessment	To gather, verify, and communicate data about client so that database is established	1. Collecting nursing health history 2. Performing physical examination 3. Collecting laboratory data 4. Validating data 5. Clustering data 6. Documenting data
Nursing diagnosis	To identify health care needs of client, to formulate nursing diagnoses	1. Analyzing and interpreting data 2. Identifying client problems 3. Formulating nursing diagnoses 4. Documenting nursing diagnosis
Planning	To identify client's goals; to determine priorities of care, to determine expected outcomes, to design nursing strategies to achieve goals of care	1. Identifying client goals 2. Establishing expected outcomes 3. Selecting nursing actions 4. Delegating actions 5. Writing nursing care plan 6. Consulting
Implementation	To complete nursing actions necessary for accomplishing plan	1. Reassessing client 2. Reviewing and modifying existing care plan 3. Performing nursing actions
Evaluation	To determine extent to which goals of care have been achieved	1. Comparing client response to criteria 2. Analyzing reasons for results and conclusions 3. Modifying care plan

enough to be used in all settings. The purposes of the nursing process are to identify the client's health care needs, determine priorities, establish goals and expected outcomes of care, establish and communicate a client-centered plan of care, provide nursing interventions designed to meet client needs, and evaluate the effectiveness of nursing care in achieving expected client outcomes and goals (Table 6-1). Bandman and Bandman (1995) describe the whole nursing process as a series of means-ends relationships. The means are the nurse's accurate assessment, diagnosis, and treatment of the client, and the ends are the client's increased level of function and well-being.

Application in Practice

Reasoning is one way people think. A person reflects on and arrives at decisions and solves problems (Bandman and Bandman, 1995). For example, when the nurse, Ms. Sims, observes Mr. Sierra sitting in a clinic examination room, a variety of thoughts begin to cross her mind. What are the client behaviors that are recognized? What do the behaviors mean? Has the nurse seen the behaviors before? How is the nurse reacting to the client? Are there factors in the clinic environment that are influencing the client? The nurse begins to use reasoning to succeed in determining the client's health care interests and needs. For example, reasoning helps the nurse decide what to say to Mr. Sierra after the client asks, "Am I going to have to go to the hospital?" One response might be, "Only your doctor knows." A deceptive answer might be, "Don't worry, you are going to feel better." Another response might be, "Tell me what led you to think you need to go to the hospital." The latter approach neither denies nor avoids the client's concerns. Instead, the nurse facilitates the client's own reasoning so that the client may state facts or inferences about his own condition. Depending on what the client says, the nurse may ask further questions, choose to examine the client, or perhaps step outside the examination room to review the client's medical chart.

The scientific method is one approach to reasoning that moves from observable facts of experience to reasonable explanations of these facts (Bandman and Bandman, 1995). It is an approach that allows for identification and resolution of problems. The client in the clinic may tell the nurse that pain in his lower back has developed after a fall from a ladder. With closer observation the nurse notices the client's bent posture, grimacing, and slow movement from chair to examination table. The client's behaviors might imply the presence of pain, but the nurse will ask, "Are you having pain? If so, tell me exactly where it is located. Does the pain increase when you try to sit down?" The nurse may have the client slowly bend forward or to the side. Intuitions about the client's problem are not as trustworthy as actual or measurable observations. The nurse continues to use a problem-solving approach to learn more about the client, to determine the nature of the problem, and ultimately to offer approaches to relieve his discomfort.

The nursing process involves scientific reasoning (Table 6-2). The nurse makes inferences about the meaning of a client's response to a health problem or generalizes about the client's functional state of health. A pattern will begin to form; for example, the client is having acute pain and his mobility is limited. The nurse continues to gather more information until an accurate classification of the client's problem is determined, such as the following nursing diagnosis: impaired physical mobility related to acute back pain. The clear definition of the client's problem then provides the basis for nursing interventions and evaluation of outcomes. The nurse's interventions are designed to relieve the pain so as to improve the client's mobility.

The nursing process is simply one variation of scientific reasoning that allows nurses to organize, systematize, and conceptualize nursing practice (Bandman and Bandman, 1995). It is a general approach to client systems of individuals, families, groups, or communities. It is an approach that allows nurses to differentiate their practice from that of physicians and other health care professionals. When nurses think critically, the client becomes an active participant and the ultimate outcome is a comprehensive, individualized approach to care.

To succeed in using the nursing process, a nurse must op-

	Table 6-2 Comparison of Steps in Problem Solving, the Scientific Method, and the Nursing Process	
PROBLEM SOLVING	**COPI AND COHEN'S SEVEN-STEP SCIENTIFIC METHOD***	**NURSING PROCESS**
Encountering problem	The Problem Preliminary **hypothesis**	Assessing
Collecting data	Collecting additional facts	
Identifying exact nature of problem	Formulating hypotheses	Forming a nursing diagnosis
Determing plan of action	Deducing further consequences	Planning (outcome identification)
Carrying out plan	Testing consequences	Implementing
Evaluating plan in new situation	Application	Evaluating
Plan of action		

*Copi IM, Cohen C: *Introduction to logic,* ed 9, New York, 1994, Macmillan.

erate within a set of assumptions or concepts as a frame of reference (Bandman and Bandman, 1995). To be useful, data collection must be made in reference to the intended purpose of nursing, for example, pain relief or client learning. These concepts (pain management or adult learning) are the basis for nursing judgments in the form of diagnosis, nursing plans, implementation, and evaluation. Conceptual frameworks such as pain management or theoretical models such as Orem's self-care deficit theory give the nurse a basis for determining the information to be collected, diagnostic areas to be considered, and nursing goals and therapies.

The Five-Step Nursing Process

The framework of the nursing process includes the following steps: assessment, nursing diagnosis, planning (including expected outcome identification), implementation, and evaluation. Each step of the nursing process is essential for accurate problem solving and is closely interrelated with the other steps. Gordon (1995) describes the first two steps of assessment and diagnosis as problem identification components and the remaining three steps as problem-solving components. During assessment the nurse collects data about the client from a variety of sources (Fig. 6-5). The nature and amount of data are always changing, requiring the nurse to take the data and form meaningful patterns. The

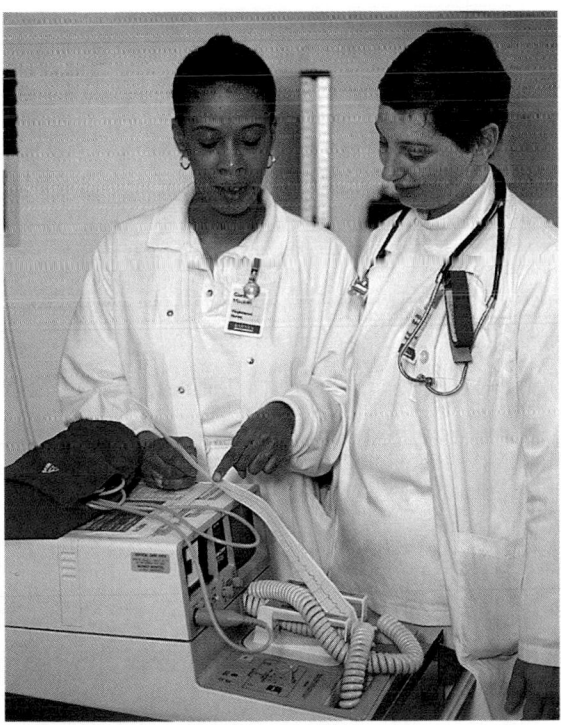

Fig. 6-5 Nurses may collaborate when collecting and interpreting data from selected diagnostic tests, such as with an electrocardiogram.

nurse's clinical problem solving is sometimes linear, sometimes branching when data from new problems are recognized, and at other times cyclical when the nurse must reassess and validate information (Yura and Walsh, 1988). Accuracy is essential so that the nurse makes the proper conclusions that will direct a plan of care.

The nursing diagnosis step involves taking assessment data and formulating diagnostic statements that identify the client's health-related problems. The accuracy of these statements depends on the thoroughness of data collection, sorting, clustering, and validation. The identified nursing diagnoses form the framework for the client's plan of care. Thus the nursing diagnoses provide the nurse with an individualized, client-centered focus.

During the planning step of the process a care plan is formulated. It is individualized based on the assessment database and the client's nursing diagnoses. A component of planning is outcome identification. It is important for the nurse to identify the expected outcomes (responses or behaviors) that the client will achieve if the plan of care is successful. Outcomes are stated in behavioral terms such as "the client will correctly prepare prescribed medications." Nursing interventions that are selected for the plan of care, such as supervised demonstration for medication preparation, focus on meeting expected outcomes. The nursing care plan contains expected client outcomes and goals, appropriate nursing interventions, and criteria for evaluation.

Implementation is the action step of the nursing process. The nurse uses a variety of approaches to resolve the client's health problems. Interventions are problem oriented and individualized according to the client's care plan. Interventions are continually modified based on an ongoing evaluation of the client's response and the nurse's diagnostic analysis. The success of this step is examined during evaluation.

The fifth step of the nursing process is evaluation. The nurse determines the client's progress toward meeting expected outcomes and achieving goals and the success of nursing interventions. If interventions are successful, the client's nursing diagnoses are resolved. If the client's health problems remain, the process of evaluation guides the nurse to revise, eliminate, or add therapies. Evaluation is the completion of a cycle of activities in which the results have a continuing effect on the other steps of the process. Evaluation is the stage of clinical problem solving that helps foster a client's desired outcomes by checking and adjusting other stages of the nursing process. This step provides for the revision of the nursing care plan as necessary to resolve health problems.

The entire process is sequential and interrelated. Each step depends on the previous one. The sequence is logical because client information is gathered before health care needs are determined. The plan is based on client needs, and nursing care is provided according to that plan. Nursing care is evaluated in terms of achievement of expected outcomes.

■ KEY CONCEPTS ■

► Critical thinking involves thinking beyond a single solution for a problem and focusing on deciding what the best alternatives are.

► The nursing process is a critical thinking competency that guides the nurse to make judgments about client care.

► Critical thinking is based on knowledge, experience, critical thinking competencies, attitudes, and standards.

► Clinical decision making requires the nurse to establish and weigh criteria in deciding on the best choice of therapy for a client.

► Practical experience in the daily care of clients gives a nurse the opportunity to make decisions and to develop greater expertise in making nursing judgments.

► Having the proper attitudes when engaging in critical thinking ensures a fair, responsible, and innovative approach to reasoning.

► The purpose of the nursing process is to identify the client's health care needs, establish a nursing care plan, and complete nursing interventions designed to meet these needs.

► The nursing process includes five steps—assessment, nursing diagnosis, planning, implementation, and evaluation—with outcome identification as a part of planning.

► The nursing process is a standard for professional nursing practice.

■ KEY TERMS ■

Critical thinking, p. 98

Decision making, p. 100

Diagnostic reasoning, p. 100

Hypothesis, p. 104

Inference, p. 98

Nursing process, p. 103

Problem solving, p. 100

Scientific method , p. 100

■ CRITICAL THINKING EXERCISES ■

1. You are instructed to go to a client's room and administer a subcutaneous injection of heparin. The procedure manual outlines the steps to take in selecting an injection site in the abdomen. When you enter the room, the client says, "My stomach is killing me, I feel nauseated." What would you do?

2. Mr. Javier is 66 years old and lives alone. He has a neighbor, Ms. Pena, who lives next door. He comes to the community clinic 1 month after having been diagnosed with diabetes. His eyesight is poor, and while talking with him you learn that he has forgotten instructions given during the last clinic visit regarding his diet and medication schedule. It will be necessary for Mr. Lopez to follow his diet and medication regimen to control his blood suger properly. How might you apply creativity and responsibility in your critical thinking approach to Mr. Javier's care?

3. Mr. Stein is to have regular range-of-motion exercises performed following knee surgery. How might the nurse adapt the approach to assist the client if all the following variables are known: the client reports pain in the knee; the client has never before had surgery; the client is a professional athlete.

REFERENCES

American Nurses Association: Nursing and social policy statement, Kansas City, Mo, 1980, The Association.

Bandman EL, Bandman B: Critical thinking in nursing, ed 2, Norwalk, Conn, 1995, Appleton & Lange.

Benner P: From novice to expert, Menlo Park, Calif, 1984, Addison Wesley.

Bevis EM: Curriculum building in nursing: a process, St Louis, 1978, Mosby.

Carnevali DL, and Thomas MD: Diagnostic reasoning and treatment decision making in nursing, Philadelphia, 1993, JB Lippincott.

Chaffee J: Thinking critically, ed 3, Boston, 1994, Houghton Mifflin.

Copi IM, Cohen C: Introduction to logic, ed 9, New York, 1994, Macmillan.

Fox RC: The evolution of medical uncertainty, Milbank Memorial Fund Quarterly/Health and Society 58(1):1, 1980.

Glaser E: An experiment in the development of critical thinking, New York, 1941, Bureau of Publications, Teacher's College, Columbia University.

Gordon M: Nursing diagnosis: process and application, ed 3, St Louis, 1995, Mosby.

International Council of Nurses: Code for nurses, Geneva, 1973, The Council.

Kataoka-Yahiro M, Saylor C: A critical thinking model for nursing judgment, J Nurs Educ 33(8):351, 1994.

Miller M, Malcolm N: Critical thinking in the nursing curriculum, Nurs Health Care 11:67, 1990.

Miller MA, Babcock DE: Critical thinking applied to nursing, St Louis, 1996, Mosby.

Paul R: The art of redesigning instruction. In J Willsen, and AJA Binker, editors: Critical thinking: how to prepare students for a rapidly changing world, Santa Rosa, Calif, 1993, Foundation for Critical Thinking.

Perry W: Forms of intellectual and ethical development in the college years: a scheme, New York, 1970, Holt, Rinehart, and Winston.

Strader M: Critical thinking. In Sullivan EJ, Decker PJ: Effective management in nursing, ed 3, Redwood City, Calif, 1992, Addison Wesley Nursing.

Yura H, Walsh M: The nursing process: assessing, planning, implementing, and evaluating, ed 5, Nowalk, Conn, 1988, Appleton & Lange.

ADDITIONAL READINGS

Brooks K, Shepherd J: The relationship between clinical decision-making skills in nursing and general critical thinking abilities of senior nursing students in four types of nursing programs, J Nurs Educ 29:391, 1990.

Hughes K, Young W: Decision making: stability of clinical decisions, Nurse Educator 17(3):12, 1992.

Tanner C et al: The phenomenology of knowing the patient, Image J Nurs Sch 25:273, 1993.

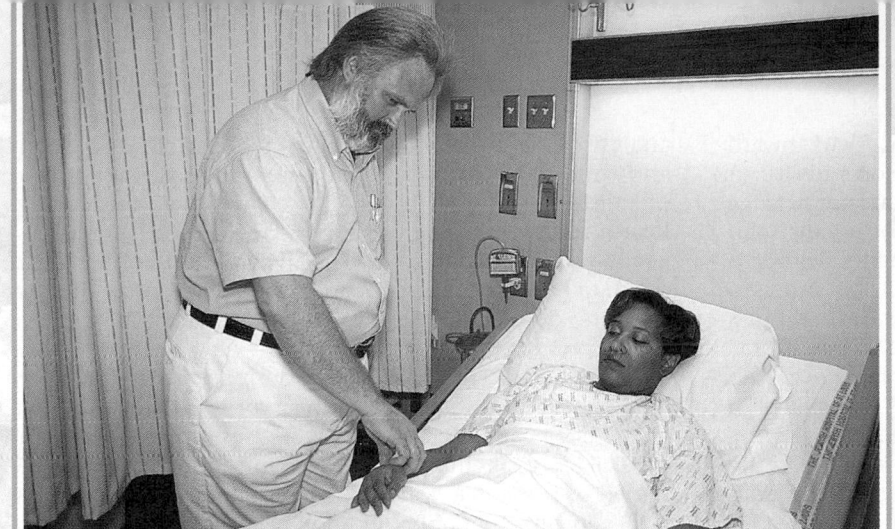
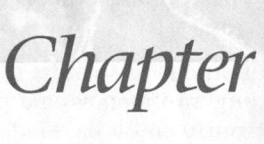
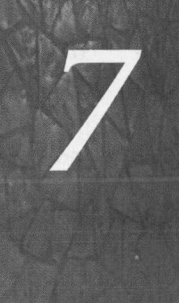

Chapter 7

Assessment

Objectives

Mastery of content in this chapter will enable the student to:

▶ Define the key terms listed.

▶ Explain the relationship of data collection and data analysis in critical thinking.

▶ Discuss the purpose of nursing assessment.

▶ Explain the difference between a comprehensive and problem-oriented assessment.

▶ Explain why client expectations are important to include in assessment.

▶ Describe how assessment is a flexible approach to problem solving.

▶ Differentiate between objective and subjective data.

▶ State the sources of data for a nursing assessment.

▶ Describe the four interviewing techniques.

▶ State the purpose of a nursing history.

▶ State the purpose of a physical examination.

▶ Conduct and record a nursing assessment.

Nursing is unique because of its broad focus toward understanding and managing a person's health. A competent nurse must have adequate knowledge in physiology, pathophysiology, psychopathology, and medical treatment to safely perform treatments delegated by physicians. For example, when a physician orders a medication such as insulin, the nurse must know the drug's effect, the symptoms the client might have if side effects develop, and the actions to take when problems occur. In this same example the nurse must also have knowledge in therapeutic communication, dimensions of daily living that affect a person's health situation, and adult learning principles, to instruct and support the client in daily self-administration of insulin injections. The nurse has two focuses in clinical practice: as a collaborator with other disciplines and as a primary provider of nursing care (Carpenito, 1993).

A diagnosis of diabetes mellitus (for which insulin is prescribed) is a lifetime medical diagnosis. However, a client's response to this health problem, defined as a *nursing diagnosis,* changes many times throughout the person's life. Over time the client may have trouble following a diabetic diet, managing resources to purchase syringes, or facing any of a number of factors that affect the ability to cope with the disease. A nurse must always think critically about clients and their responses to their health problems to provide the most effective and appropriate level of care. Whenever there is a change in a client, medical treatment, daily living functions, the environment, or external resources, the nurse must think critically to make the right judgments. A hallmark of expert nursing practice is the ability to remain open to changes in a clinical situation (Carnevali and Thomas, 1993).

The first step of the nursing process, assessment, begins with the nurse applying knowledge and experience to collect data about a client. Just as an astronomer uses knowledge of the galaxies to explore through a telescope, the nurse applies knowledge of science and the discipline of nursing to explore and discover clients' unique and personal health care problems.

Assessment is used in the nurse's collaborative role. The nurse makes clinical observations of a client, reports the client's situation relative to a medical problem, and then follows delegated medical activities prescribed by the physician. In the independent role of a health care provider, the nurse assesses a client's health care needs and institutes nursing interventions to maintain or improve the client's health. Accurate assessment is crucial to ensure needs are properly identified and the right course of action is implemented by the nurse.

■ A CRITICAL THINKING APPROACH TO ASSESSMENT

In today's complex health care environment, nurses must be able to solve problems accurately, thoroughly, and quickly. This means that the nurse must be able to review a tremendous amount of information to make critical judgments. Nursing **assessment** is the systematic process of gathering, verifying, and communicating data about a client. This phase of the nursing process includes two steps: collection of data from a primary source (the client) and secondary sources (family, health professionals), and the analysis of data as a basis for nursing diagnoses (Bandman and Bandman, 1995). The purpose of the assessment is to establish a data base about the client's perceived needs, health problems, related experiences, health practices, goals, values, and lifestyle. The information contained in the **data base** is the basis for an individualized plan of nursing care, developed and refined throughout the time the nurse cares for the client.

To be most useful, data collection must pertain to a particular health problem. In other words, assessment data must be relevant. Nurses often work in settings where standardized assessment forms are available. These forms are designed to provide a minimal accountability of the nursing profession to the public (Gordon, 1994). Use of the forms ensures a comprehensive level of assessment. However, the nurse cannot become a slave to an assessment form. It is not meant to restrict the nurse's approach. These forms cover a broad array of questions that may lead to volumes of data that prove interesting but not necessarily relevant to a specific client's health problem. For example, a client who comes to a clinic because of an upper respiratory viral infection may not require a comprehensive review of sexual patterns and neurological status. Such issues may not be relevant to identifying the client's current problems and treatment. In addition, the nurse-client interaction period is brief; thus a focused assessment must review the client's respiratory condition, energy level, nutrition, and the ability to follow medical treatments prescribed.

It is important for a nurse to learn to critically think about what to assess. The independent judgement of when a question or measurement is appropriate is influenced by the nurse's clinical knowledge and experience (Gordon, 1994). When a nurse first encounters a client, there is a chance for a quick overview. This overview is usually based on the nurse's specialty of practice or the treatment situation: an emergency room nurse uses the A-B-C (airway-breathing-circulation) approach; a psychiatric nurse may focus on the client's reality, anxiety level, and violence potential (Carnevali and Thomas, 1993). It is possible that other important cues may be missed with such an intense focused assessment. However, the nurse interprets cues from the client to know how in-depth an assessment should be. Assessment is dynamic; it should allow the nurse to freely explore relevant problems as they appear.

Typology of 11 Functional Health Patterns

- Health perception–health management pattern
- Nutritional-metabolic pattern
- Elimination pattern
- Activity-exercise pattern
- Cognitive-perceptual pattern
- Sleep-rest pattern
- Self-perception–self-concept pattern
- Role-relationship pattern
- Sexuality-reproductive pattern
- Coping-stress-tolerance pattern
- Value-belief pattern

From Gordon M: *Nursing diagnosis: process and application,* ed 3, St Louis, 1994, Mosby.

An initial scanning of a client's situation allows the nurse to use key assessment data to respond to priorities. If a client in the emergency room enters in respiratory distress, the nurse must recognize the client's signs and symptoms and respond quickly. After a client's situation stabilizes there may be a need to collect more data. A comprehensive client data base includes a nursing health history, physical examination, results of laboratory and diagnostic tests, and information from health care team members and the client's family. It is important for the nurse to recognize that situations can change at any time during assessment. The data collected must be relevant and appropriate.

Carnevali and Thomas (1993) suggest two approaches to collecting comprehensive data. One is a structured comprehensive data base format, such as Gordon's 11 functional health patterns (see the box on p. 108), and the other is a problem-oriented approach focusing on the client's presenting situation. The comprehensive approach moves from general to specific. For example, a nurse may use a history tool organized by Gordon's functional patterns. Data are collected in all 11 categories and then reviewed to see if patterns of problems are revealed. For each of the 11

patterns the nurse assesses clients by organizing patterns of behavior and physiological responses that pertain to a functional health category. The nurse then compares assessment data with the client's base line (e.g., usual blood pressure, weight, and nutritional intake); established norms based on age, gender, height, and weight; and cultural, social, or other norms, such as religious practices, ethnic dietary guidelines, and health care practices (Gordon, 1987). The assessment of each of the 11 patterns represents the interaction of the client and the environment, which Gordon calls *biopsychosocial integration*. No one health pattern can be understood without knowledge of the other patterns (Gordon, 1991). Description and evaluation of health patterns assist the nurse in identifying functional patterns (client strengths) and dysfunctional patterns (nursing diagnoses), which assist in developing the nursing care plan (Gordon, 1987, 1991).

The problem approach to assessment begins with problematic areas such as pain and spreads out to relevant areas of the client's life. A comprehensive pain assessment begins with a review of the nature of the pain itself and then broadens to categories such as the influence of pain on

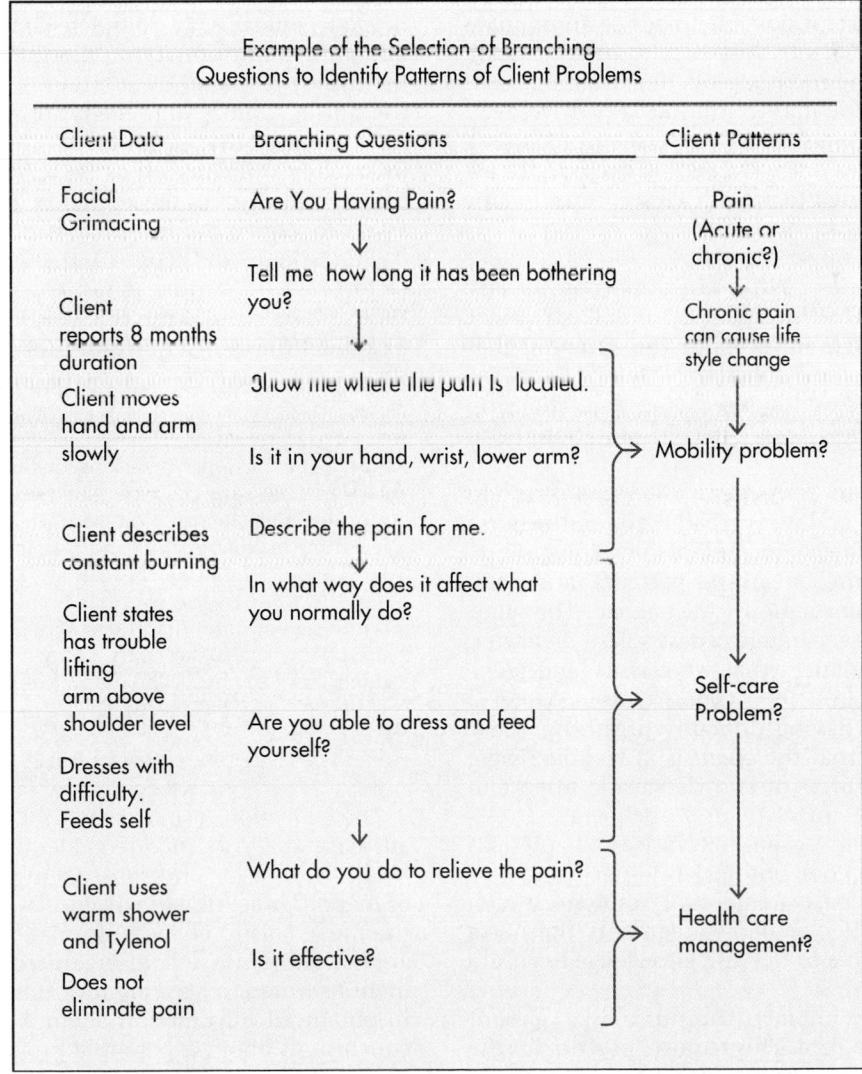

Fig. 7-1 Example of branching logic for selecting assessment questions.

lifestyle, family relationships, and work habits. Once completed, the problem of pain will be thoroughly analyzed so that a comprehensive approach can be used to provide pain relief.

Whatever approach is used, the nurse must cluster cues of information and begin to identify emerging patterns and potential problems. To do this well, a nurse critically anticipates. In other words, the nurse always tries to stay a step ahead of the assessment. Once a question has been asked of a client or an observation has been made, the information often branches to an additional series of questions or observations (Fig. 7-1). The risk the nurse takes in not anticipating assessment questions is to fail to recognize problems or to dismiss relevant problems (Hurst et al, 1991). Knowing how to frame questions is a basic skill, refined over time. The nurse decides which questions are relevant to the situation while at the same time being sure the assessment is complete. The nurse's thoughts about the client proceed from something given, a cue or data, to a conclusion. The extent of a nurse's ability to grasp the meaning of all the data being collected and analyzed is related to the nurse's knowledge and experience.

Organization of Data Gathering

Accurate assessment makes it possible to devise appropriate goals and strategies for clients. The faculty of Ohio State University developed one methodology for teaching nursing students problem-solving techniques (Ryan-Wenger, 1990). The approach emphasizes how assessment requires a level of detail to ensure accuracy (Table 7-1). Steps in the assessment phase are outlined to provide clearer direction for how nurses make client care decisions.

It is important for the nurse's assessment to first consider the nurse-client interaction. What is the purpose of any nurse-client interaction? Who will be involved? What knowledge does the nurse have about the situation that brings the nurse and client together? These factors influence the nurse's success in developing a relationship with the client that leads to a directed and purposeful assessment.

As a nurse conducts an assessment, there are considerable interactions (verbal and nonverbal) between the nurse and client. In addition the client presents physiological responses such as posturing, breathing patterns, and body movement that relay information to the nurse. The nurse must use all senses to accurately assess client behavior. Our senses collect experiences that we classify and judge (Bandman and Bandman, 1995). For example, when a nurse observes a client having difficulty breathing, sense impressions are formed that the client is in trouble. These sense impressions are sources of knowledge and often reliable clues that lead the nurse to more deliberate assessment. The skills of physical examination (see Chapter 33) enable the nurse to explore physical findings accurately and in detail, such as measurement of respiratory rate, rhythm, and depth. When making judgments the nurse connects sense experiences to nursing knowledge to ensure accurate reasoning.

As a client and nurse interact, the nurse asks relevant questions to gather more data. This requires practice for the beginning nurse to become proficient. If the nurse stops prematurely in asking questions, the data base can be incomplete and the resultant conclusions, made in the form of nursing diagnoses, can be inaccurate. Any inferences about the client or about the nurse's own behavior toward the client are separated from actual data.

Data Collection

The nurse collects data that are descriptive, concise, and complete. Assessment does not include **inferences** or interpretative statements that are unsupported with data. Descriptive data originate in the client's perception of a symptom, the perceptions and observations of the family, the nurse's observations, or reports from other members of the health care team. For example, a client may describe pain as a "sharp, throbbing pain in the abdomen." The nurse's observation may be, "The client lies on the right side holding the abdomen. Facial grimacing present." The nurse conducts a focused examination and records only observations and avoids interpreting behavior (e.g., "The client tolerates pain poorly."). Concise data briefly describe the information obtained. The information is summarized in a short format using correct medical terms (e.g., "Client describes a constant, sharp, throbbing pain in the upper right quadrant of the abdomen. Pain began 48 hours before hospitalization, 2 hours after a high-fat meal. Pain was not relieved by antacids."). Complete data collection results from obtaining all information relevant to the actual or potential health problem, in addition to the client's reaction to the nurse. A nurse and client are each affected by the behavior of the other. Assessment must consider whether this interaction influences how the client behaves. To confirm that complete data have been collected, the nurse might ask, "Do I have the information to answer the questions: 'When, where, and what are the duration and influencing factors?' " For example, a nurse in an outpatient clinic uses these questions to write the assessment of a client seeking treatment for recurrent headaches.

CASE STUDY   Mrs. Cooper is seeking treatment for recurrent headaches. She describes the headaches as occurring every morning after she rises from bed. The pain is localized over the left front maxillary sinus and is described by Mrs. Cooper as "pulsating." The headaches last anywhere from 1 hour to "all day." In the past the pain has been relieved with ibuprofen, but the client states that the medication has not been effective during the past 10 days. Mrs. Cooper notices an increase in the intensity of the headache during cold, damp weather. ▪

The collection of inaccurate, incomplete, or inappropriate data leads to incorrect identification of the client's health care needs and subsequent inaccurate, incomplete, or inappropriate nursing diagnoses. Inaccurate data result if the nurse fails to collect information relevant to a specific area or if the nurse is disorganized or unskilled in assessment techniques. Data are incomplete if the nurse neglects to obtain all information about a specific area, jumps to conclusions about a potential problem, or makes assumptions without validation. Inappropriate data are unrelated to the area being assessed.

Table 7-1	A Methodology for Nursing Assessment
ELEMENT	**NURSING ACTIVITY**
Nurse-Client Interaction	Identify purpose of the nurse-client interaction (e.g., to provide hygiene care, administer a tube feeding, interact with an anxious client). Identify the system of study along with important subsystems (e.g., the client, nurse-client, group of clients, community). Recognize relationships between client and the environment that influence client's behavior and/or nurse-client interaction. Know the purpose of each nursing experience and type of client to prepare for the interaction. For example, practice hygiene skills before giving hygiene care.
Recording Nurse and Client Behavior	Nurse and client are affected by each other's behavior and characteristics. Observe own verbal and nonverbal behavior to assess effect on client. Use all senses to accurately observe and record client's verbal/nonverbal behavior. Use tools and instruments (stethoscope, thermometer, height/weight chart) to accurately measure behavior and physiological signs.
Questions and Inferences	Ask relevant questions to gather more data. *Do not be satisfied with simple answers.* For example: *Nurse:* Are you feeling nauseated? *Client:* Yes. *Nurse:* Tell me when it began; are you having other symptoms? Be aware of inferences about your own behavior: "My nervousness is showing;" "The client and I are not communicating well." *Keep inferences separate from data.* Use appropriate follow-up questions to clarify. The client responds to questions asked and other data are collected to support or refute inferences.
Identifying Patterns	Based on knowledge and data, identify patterns of nurse and client behavior. A pattern is similar to a nursing diagnosis and is defined as a particular behavior occurring over time (e.g., client walks 4 miles a day—has a pattern of regular exercise), or a pattern may be a cluster of behavior (e.g., client has shortness of breath, increased heart rate, rapid respirations following routine exercise—indicating poor activity tolerance). Identify positive and negative patterns. A positive pattern might be a client's spiritual strengths; a negative pattern might be poor eating habits. It is important to recognize and maintain positive health patterns as well as decrease effects of negative health patterns. Identify interaction patterns based on observation of nurse-client interaction. For example, nurse asks questions and client responds in one-word phrases with no eye contact.
Apply Theories and Concepts	Concepts and theories help to support, refute, or give meaning to observed patterns. For example, while administering medication a student identifies a pattern of grief over a client's loss of a spouse and supports the finding by documentation that expression of guilt, crying, and poor eating habits are signs of dysfunctional grieving. Previously identified patterns are assessed for their potential or real effect on a client. Patterns with a negative effect on health (e.g., poor compliance in taking medication) are noted. Patterns that positively affect health (e.g., getting regular sufficient sleep) are reviewed. Also consider patterns of nurse behavior or client-nurse interaction that have positive or negative effects.
Validation	Document interpretation of patterns of data with reliable sources (e.g., literature, other nurses, family, health care professionals).

Ryan-Wenger NM: A nursing process methodology, *Nurs Outlook* 38(4):190, 1990.

∎ TYPES OF DATA

During assessment, the nurse obtains two types of data, subjective and objective. **Subjective data** are clients' perceptions about their health problems. Only clients can provide this kind of information. For example, the presence of pain is a subjective finding. Only clients can provide information about its frequency, duration, location, and intensity. Subjective data usually include feelings of anxiety, physical discomfort, or mental stress. Although only clients can provide subjective data relevant to these feelings, the nurse must be aware that these problems can result in physiological changes, which are identified through objective data collection.

Objective data are observations or measurements made by the data collector (Fig. 7-2). Assessment of a client's blood pressure and identification of the size of a localized body rash are examples of observed objective data. The measurement of objective data is based on an accepted standard, such as the Fahrenheit or celsius measure on a thermometer, or centimeters on a measuring tape. Body temperature and head circumference are examples of measured objective data.

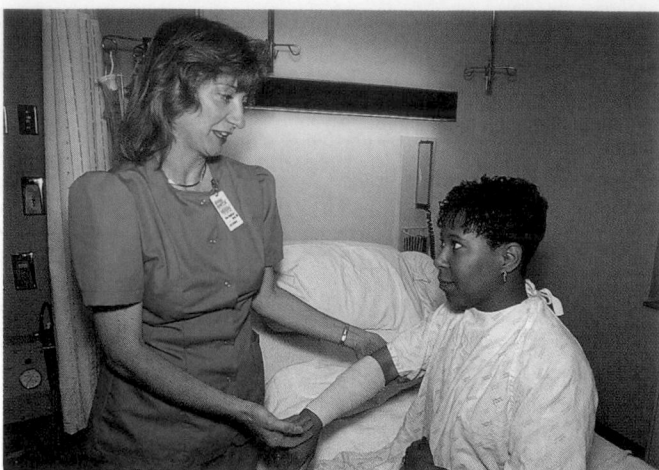

Fig. 7-2 Nurse palpates temperature of skin to assess circulation.

CASE STUDY Ms. Johnson is taking care of Mr. Woods 1 day after an appendectomy. Ms. Johnson asks Mr. Woods about any pain or discomfort. He replies, "I have an occasional twinge in my right side, but I'm fine." Ms. Johnson observes that Mr. Woods is diaphoretic and has tachycardia, and that his blood pressure is elevated. ■

Mr. Woods' description of his pain is subjective, but the physiological changes of elevated blood pressure, tachycardia, and diaphoresis are the objective findings the nurse assesses.

■ SOURCES OF DATA

Data are obtained from the client, family, significant others, health care team members, health records, physical examination, results of diagnostic and laboratory tests, and pertinent nursing and medical literature. The nurse's own experience with similar types of clients is an additional source of data. Each source provides information about the client's level of wellness, anticipated prognosis, risk factors, health practices and goals, and patterns of health and illness, as well as information relevant to the client's health care needs.

Client

In most situations the client is the best source of information. The client who is oriented and answers questions appropriately can provide the most accurate information about health care needs, lifestyle patterns, present and past illnesses, perception of symptoms, and changes in activities of daily living. It is important, however, to consider the setting where the nurse interacts with a client. A client experiencing acute symptoms in an emergency room will not be able to offer the same depth of information as one who comes to a primary care clinic for a routine checkup.

Family and Significant Others

Families and significant others can be interviewed as primary sources of information about infants or children and critically ill, mentally handicapped, disoriented, or unconscious clients. In cases of severe illness or emergency situations, families may be the only available sources of data about clients' health-illness patterns, current medications, allergies, onset of illness, and other information needed by nurses and physicians.

The family and significant others are also important secondary sources of information. It is important to include them in assessment of the client when appropriate. Often spouses or close friends will sit in during an assessment and provide their view of the client's health problems or needs. They can not only supply data about the client's current health status but also often they are able to indicate when changes in the client's status occurred and how the client's functioning was affected. Finally, family and friends can make pertinent observations about the client's needs that can affect the way care is delivered.

Health Care Team Members

The health care team consists of physicians, nurses, allied health professionals, and nonprofessional employees working in a health care setting (see Chapter 13). Because assessment is an ongoing process, the nurse must communicate with other health care team members, including physical therapists, social workers, community health workers, and spiritual advisers, whenever possible. Health care team members can provide data about the way the client interacts within the health care environment, reacts to information about diagnostic tests, and responds to visitors. Every member of the health care team is a potential source of information, and the team can identify and communicate data and verify information from other sources.

Medical Records

The present and past medical records of the client can verify information about past health patterns and treatments or can provide new information. By reviewing medical records, the nurse can identify patterns of illness, previous responses to treatment, and past methods of coping.

Other Records

Other records such as educational, military, and employment records may contain pertinent health care information. If the client received services at a community health center or day-care clinic, the nurse should obtain data from these records but must first obtain written permission from the client or guardian to see them. Any information obtained is confidential and is treated as part of the client's legal medical record (see Chapter 20).

Literature Review

Reviewing nursing, medical, and pharmacological literature about an illness helps the nurse complete the data base. The review increases the nurse's knowledge about the symptoms, treatment, and prognosis of specific illnesses, and established standards of therapeutic practice. The knowledgeable nurse is able to obtain pertinent, accurate, and complete information for the assessment data base.

Nurse's Experience

Benner (1984) notes that a nurse's expertise develops after testing and refining propositions, questions, and principle-based expectations. For example, after a nurse has cared for a client with abdominal pain there are lessons learned. The nurse will recognize more quickly the behavior the client showed while in acute pain. The nurse will have noted the extent to which positioning techniques helped the client to relax and have less discomfort. The principle of administering a pain medication regularly rather than when the client requests it, to achieve better pain control, will have been tested. Critical thinking is strengthened by practical experience and the opportunity to make decisions. A nurse's ability to make an assessment will improve from using past experience, applying relevant knowledge, and focusing on data collection that avoids wasteful consideration of unnecessary information.

METHODS OF DATA COLLECTION

The nurse uses the interview, the nursing health history, the physical examination, and results of laboratory and diagnostic tests to establish the data base. Each method allows the nurse to collect complete information about the client's past and present level of wellness.

Interview

The first step in establishing the data base is to interview the client. The **interview** is a pattern of communication initiated for a specific purpose and focused on a specific content area. In nursing, the major purposes of the interview are to obtain a nursing health history, identify health needs and risk factors, and determine specific changes in level of wellness and pattern of living. Perhaps most important, the interview should help clients relate their own interpretation and understanding of their condition. This means the nurse and client must be partners during the interview rather than the nurse controlling the interview. Unless an interview allows a client to express needs, the interaction may be unsuccessful.

An interview may be focused, as in the case of a client admitted to the emergency room, or it can be comprehensive. The interviewer obtains information about the client's health, lifestyle, support systems, patterns of illness, patterns of adaptation, strengths and limitations, and resources. As the nurse listens and considers the information shared, the client may be directed to give more detail or discuss a topic that seems to reveal a possible problem. Since the client's report will include subjective information, the nurse uses data from the interview for later validation with objective information. For example, if the client reports difficulty in walking, the nurse will later assess the client's gait and muscle strength.

When conducting the interview, the nurse uses specific communication skills to focus attention on the client's level of wellness. The nurse also helps the client understand the changes that are occurring or will occur once health care begins. This chapter describes communication skills and the interview, whereas Chapter 14 discusses the total communication process and details the various communication techniques necessary for nursing practice.

The nursing interview achieves several objectives (see the

Objectives of the Nursing Interview
■ Establish a therapeutic relationship with the client.
■ Establish the nurse's sense of caring for the client as an individual.
■ Introduce the client to the facility in a manner that is not threatening.
■ Gain insight about the client's concerns.
■ Determine the client's expectations of health care providers and the health care delivery system.
■ Obtain cues about parts of the data collection phase that require in-depth investigation (branching).

---

box above). First, the nurse-client relationship is initiated. A **nurse-client relationship** is the association between the nurse and the client that has a mutual concern, the client's well-being. This relationship builds a professional interpersonal closeness that develops and aids in the investigation and discussion of the client's responses to health and illness. This relationship encourages the sharing of information, ideas, and emotions, and enables the nurse to express a level of caring for the client.

During the interview the nurse obtains information about a client's physical, developmental, emotional, intellectual, social, and spiritual dimensions. Physical and developmental information reflects normal functioning and the pathological changes in a person's pattern of living induced by illness, trauma, or developmental crisis. Emotional information includes the behavioral responses to changes in health and pattern of living. Relevant emotional information includes mood, perceptions, body image, self-concept, and attitudes about sexuality. Intellectual information includes intellectual performance, problem-solving ability, educational level, communication patterns, and attention span. Social information involves environmental, cultural, ethnic, or social patterns that can affect the present or future level of wellness. The nurse also collects information about values, beliefs, and religious practices, which are part of the spiritual dimension.

The interview also provides the nurse with the opportunity to observe the client. The nurse observes interactions between the client and family and between the client and the health care environment; the nurse also observes the use of eye contact, nonverbal communication, and other body language. While observing this behavior, appearance, and interaction with the environment, the nurse determines whether the data obtained by observation are consistent with those obtained by verbal communication. For example, if the client states no concern about an upcoming diagnostic test but appears anxious and irritable, the data conflict. Observations during an interview lead the nurse to gather additional objective information to form accurate conclusions.

The interview is a mechanism by which the client can obtain information as well. If a positive nurse-client relationship has been established, the client will feel comfortable asking the nurse questions about the health care environment, treatments, diagnostic testing, and available resources. The client needs this information to participate in decision making regarding goals and the plan of care. It is important for the nurse to ask the client about his or her expectations of health care providers. In addition, the interview is a first step toward establishing a therapeutic relationship between the nurse and client so that health interventions such as education or counseling can occur. To interview a client successfully and achieve the purpose and objectives of the interview, the nurse needs skills in initiating the nurse-client relationship, using the various types of interview techniques, and moving from one phase of the interview to the next.

TYPES OF INTERVIEW TECHNIQUES

The client's personality and health care needs, the health care setting, and the nurse's skill and experience affect the interview process. An emergency situation may require a type of interview technique in which the nurse asks focused questions pertaining to the client's physical status. A client entering an extended care facility with a chronic illness requires an interview approach that includes more elaboration and desciption of data. The interview in an emergency room usually centers on the present illness or trauma, precipitating factors, medications, and allergies. By contrast, an interview with a client undergoing extensive rehabilitation may focus on past and present illnesses and coping strategies, family and community resources, and present limitations and goals for rehabilitation. The nurse can use many interview techniques to elicit the necessary information from the client or another source.

A comprehensive approach or a problem-solving approach to assessment also influences techniques the nurse will use. For example, when the interview focuses on a problem presented by the client, more direct questions are used. If the interview is more comprehensive, open-ended questions are very useful.

Problem-Seeking Technique. The **problem-seeking interview** identifies the client's potential problems, and subsequent data collection focuses on those problems. For example, the nurse may ask the client about changes in digestion, such as lack of appetite, nausea, vomiting, or diarrhea. If the client says that some of these symptoms have occurred, the nurse proceeds with problem-solving questions that focus on the specific change in digestion.

Problem-Solving Technique. The **problem-solving interview** technique focuses on gathering in-depth data on specific problems identified by the client or nurse (Ivey, 1988). For example, if the client reports vomiting has been present for 2 days, the nurse asks what precipitated the first event, whether the client has other symptoms, whether it occurs each time the client eats or drinks, and what characterizes the vomitus. Information about the onset, aggravating factors, associated symptoms, relief measures that the client has tried, and the effectiveness of these measures ultimately guide the nurse's selection of nursing interventions.

Direct-Question Technique. The **direct-question interview** is a structured format requiring one- or two-word answers and is frequently used to clarify previous information or provide additional information (Ivey, 1988). For example, "Are you having pain when you vomit?" is a direct question. With this technique, the questions do not en-

courage the client to volunteer more information than is directly requested. This type of questioning is useful in obtaining biographical data and specific information about health problems, such as symptoms, precipitating factors, and relief measures.

Open-Ended Question Technique. The **open-ended question interview** is aimed at obtaining a response of more than one or two words. This technique leads to a discussion in which clients actively describe their health status. This method strengthens the nurse-client relationship because it demonstrates that the nurse wants to invest time in hearing clients' thoughts. Examples of open-ended questions follow:

1. "What are your health care needs?"
2. "How have you been feeling?"
3. "Tell me what coming to the hospital means to you."

PHASES OF THE INTERVIEW

The interview involves orientation, working, and termination phases. Before interviewing the client, the nurse prepares by considering the purpose of the interview, reading the client's past medical record, obtaining information about the present illness, reviewing literature on the health problem, and creating an environment conducive to an interview. If it is likely the interview will lead the nurse to perform any skills, a review of those skills is useful for a beginning nurse. An interview with a hospitalized client should be scheduled for a time when interruptions by other health care professionals or family will be minimal and the client will not be receiving visitors. An environment in which the client is comfortable and relaxed is also conducive to a good interview. A client interviewed at home may prefer that the interview take place in a bedroom away from other family members, or in the living room with a spouse present. Remember to let the client decide when to involve family. Finally, the nurse selects a place private enough to allow the client to be comfortable when providing personal information (Hickey, 1990).

Orientation Phase. Before beginning, the nurse reviews the purpose for the interview, the types of data to be obtained, and the methods most appropriate for conducting the interview. The interview helps establish the nurse-client

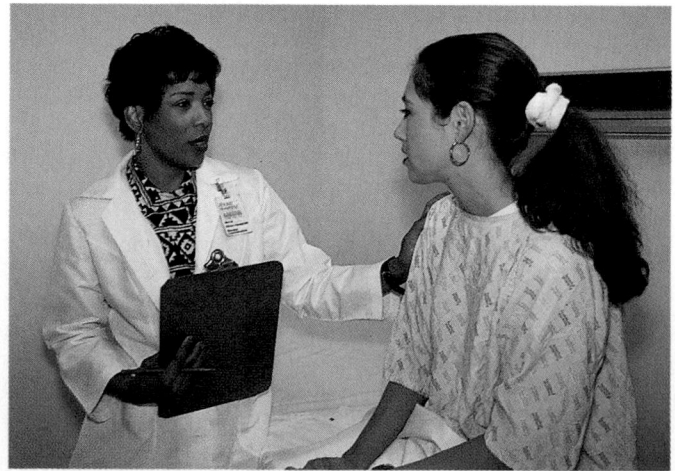

Fig. 7-3 Nurse explains purpose of interview.

relationship, which influences the ability of the nurse to establish trust with the client. While conducting the interview, the nurse remains aware that the client is forming an impression about nursing.

The nurse opens the interview by explaining the purposes of the interview (Fig. 7-3). The nurse also discusses the types of questions that will be asked and the client's role in the process. Then the nurse spends a few minutes becoming acquainted with the client.

CASE STUDY   Mr. Coffey is preparing an admission history on Mr. Rose, a 21-year-old man hospitalized for the first time.

Mr. Coffey: Good afternoon, Mr. Rose. I'm Bill Coffey, and I'm the nurse who will be managing your care during your hospital stay and through discharge to your home.

Mr. Rose: Hi, Bill. Please call me Jim. What do you mean by managing my care?

Mr. Coffey: That means I'm responsible for coordinating your nursing care with the rest of the nurses while you're hospitalized. I will work with them to plan for your discharge back to your home. Although other nurses will sometimes take care of you when I'm off, I'm the nurse who plans your care. Once you're discharged, I'll call you at home to see how you are doing and if you have any questions.

Mr. Rose: I guess that's a lot like being a coach. You may not play the game, but you're responsible for winning or losing.

Mr. Coffey: I suppose that's one way of looking at it. To better plan your care I will be asking some questions about your health. We call this a *health interview*. Any information you give me is confidential. The total interview should take about 20 to 30 minutes. Is it okay if I begin the interview in a few minutes?

Mr. Rose: How about giving me a half hour? My wife is about to leave. She needs to go pick up the kids at day care. That way we can have some time together. I'll be ready after that.

Mr. Coffey: That's fine. Since you're in a private room, I will do the health interview here. (Mr. Rose nods.)

Thirty minutes later, Mr. Coffey returns to the room.

Mr. Coffey: Okay. Before I get started, do you have any questions for me?

Mr. Rose: Yes. Why is there an outlet for oxygen on the wall above my bed? Does that mean that I'm really sick—did they put me in a special room?

Mr. Coffey: No, that's not it. Every bed in this hospital has an oxygen outlet located on the wall above the head of the bed. The reason is that this hospital has a central oxygen delivery system, and when a patient needs oxygen, we're able to supply it quickly, easily, and safely.

Mr. Rose: Okay. I wasn't actually worried. I was basically just curious. That was the only piece of equipment I couldn't explain.

Mr. Coffey: (pause) Jim, you mentioned that you and your wife have children in day care. Tell me a bit about your family. ■

In this example, Mr. Coffey introduced his role to the client. He reviewed the interview process and its objectives, confidentiality, and length. The nurse and client agreed mutually on an interview time. Before beginning the interview, Mr. Coffey asked his client if he had any questions. Mr. Coffey's answer about the oxygen allowed Mr. Rose to

---

Strategies for Effective Communication

- *Silence* is helpful for making observations and provides the client with time to organize thoughts and present complete information to the interviewer.
- *Attentive listening* demonstrates interest in the client's needs, concerns, and problems. Listening can be facilitated by maintaining eye contact, remaining relaxed, and using appropriate touch techniques.
- *Conveying acceptance* demonstrates the interviewer's willingness to listen to the client's beliefs, values, and practices without being judgmental.
- *Related questions* are planned. When asking these questions, the nurse uses words and word patterns in the client's normal sociocultural context.
- *Paraphrasing* provides an opportunity for the interviewer to validate information from the client without changing the meaning of the statement. Paraphrasing is the interviewer's formulation of what the client has said in more specific words.
- *Clarifying* facilitates correct communication of information. It is achieved by asking the client to restate the information or by providing an example.
- *Focusing* eliminates vagueness in communication, limits the area of discussion, and helps the interviewer direct attention to the pertinent aspects of a client's message.
- *Stating observations* provides the client with feedback about how the interviewer observes behavior, action, facial expression, or activities.
- *Offering information* allows the interviewer to clarify treatments, initiate health teaching, and identify and correct misconceptions.
- *Summarizing* condenses the data into an organized review. It validates data because the client has the opportunity to confirm that they are correct. Summarizing indicates the end to a particular part of the interview.

---

clarify his concern so that he would not be distracted during the interview. Mr. Coffey asked an open-ended question about Mr. Rose's family to encourage Mr. Rose to talk.

Working Phase. As the interview progresses, the nurse asks questions to form a data base from which the nursing care plan will be developed. The four techniques of interviewing are implemented as needed. In addition, the nurse uses 10 communication strategies (see the box above) to facilitate communication and ensure that nurse and client clearly understand each other (see Chapter 14).

Termination Phase. As in the other phases of the interview, termination requires skill on the part of the interviewer. Ideally the client should be given a clue that the interview is coming to an end. For example, the nurse may say, "There are just two more questions," or "We'll be finished in 5 to 6 minutes." With this method the client can maintain attention without being distracted by wondering how much longer the interview will last. Also, the client may ask any final questions before the interview ends.

The nurse should be as organized during this phase as during the opening. The interview is terminated in a friendly manner, with the nurse indicating specifically when there will be additional contact. For example, an appropriate way to end an interview would be, "Thank you for your help. The information you have shared will be

BARNES HOSPITAL
ST. LOUIS, MISSOURI

Person to Contact: | Emergency Phone:

Why you came to the hospital?

Allergies (food, drugs, latex, environment)?

Items brought in from home?
☐ Medications ☐ Dentures
☐ Contacts ☐ Glasses
☐ Hearing Aid

Did you bring:
☐ Money ☐ Jewelry ☐ Credit Cards ☐ Checkbook/Checks ☐ Other _____
(These need to be locked up with security or sent home. Hospital will not be responsible for valuables left in room)

MEDICINE NAMES	Dose & How Often Taken	Reason You Take Medicine	Time of Last Dose
Prescribed by a Doctor			
Non-Prescription			

Do you have any problems with your medicines?

Do you smoke? ☐ Yes ☐ No   Do you use "street" drugs? ☐ Yes ☐ No   How much caffeine do you drink or eat?
Do you chew tobacco? ☐ Yes ☐ No   How much alcohol do you drink?_____   _____

Medical History: ☐ Epilepsy ☐ Cancer ☐ Chicken Pox/Shingles ☐ Menstrual Disease
☐ Heart Disease ☐ Stroke ☐ Hepatitis ☐ Fainting/Dizzy Spells ☐ Circulation Problems
☐ Lung Disease ☐ Diabetes ☐ High Blood Pressure ☐ Stomach Problems ☐ Swelling
☐ Liver Disease ☐ TB ☐ Rheumatic Disease ☐ Bladder Problems ☐ Bleeding
☐ Immune Disorders   ☐ Sexually Transmitted Disease: _____
☐ Other _____

HISTORY COMMENTS:

Could you be pregnant? ☐ Yes ☐ No   When was your last Period?_____

What surgeries or procedures have you had? (Date)

Family Health History: ☐ Hypertension ☐ Diabetes ☐ Heart Disease ☐ Stroke ☐ Cancer ☐ Other _____

Which of the following have you had in the past 12 months?
☐ Self Breast Exam ☐ Prostate Check ☐ Glaucoma Check ☐ Rectal Check (over 40) ☐ Dental Exam
☐ Mammogram (over 40) ☐ Testicular Check ☐ Pelvic Exam ☐ Hearing Check ☐ Vision Check

Are your immunizations current? ☐ Yes ☐ No ☐ Unknown
(Call ID Specialist)

Fig. 7-4 Nursing health history. *(Courtesy Barnes-Jewish Hospital, St Louis.)*

Are you on a special diet?	How is your appetite?
Any foods you can't eat, and why?	Any difficulty eating or swallow-
Nutritional supplements/or diet substitutions (e.g., vitamins, artificial sweeteners, salt, substitutes)	Weight loss/gain (amount) in the last 12 months?

How often do you have a BM?
Do you have any difficulty having a bowel movement?
☐ use laxatives   ☐ hemorrhoids
☐ use stool softeners   ☐ black/tarry stools

Do you have any difficulty urinating?

☐ burning   ☐ blood   ☐ leaking   ☐ frequency

Do you tire easily?   ☐ Yes   ☐ No

Do you get regular exercise?   ☐ Yes   ☐ No
What kind?_____   How often?_____

Have you fallen recently?   ☐ Yes   ☐ No

What activities do you need help with?
☐ Feeding/eating   ☐ Meal preparation   ☐ Walking on level surfaces
☐ Dressing   ☐ Transportation   ☐ Walking on stairs
☐ Grooming/bathing   ☐ Housework   ☐ Paying for Medicines
☐ Taking medications   ☐ Handling finances
☐ Toileting   ☐ Grocery shopping
☐ Moving/positioning   **(RN consider appropriate consults)**

Aides used at home:
☐ Eye glasses   ☐ Contact lenses
☐ Hearing aid   ☐ Cane
☐ Walker   ☐ Wheelchair
☐ Prosthesis:_____
DENTURES: ☐ Upper ☐ Lower
PARTIALS: ☐ Upper ☐ Lower

Is it difficult for you to carry out prescribed health care regimens (Diet, Activity, Medications)?   ☐ Yes   ☐ No
If **YES**, explain:

How much sleep do you normally get?

What helps you fall asleep?

Who do you live with?   ☐ Alone   ☐ Spouse only   ☐ Family   ☐ Friends   ☐ Nursing Home

Who helps you at home?   ☐ Spouse   ☐ Family   ☐ Friends   ☐ Home Health   ☐ Visiting Nurse

Do you have concerns about your family while you are in the hospital?

What major changes have you had in your life in the past 12 months?

Do you feel you deal successfully with stress?   ☐ Yes   ☐ No

Would you like additional resources?   ☐ Yes   ☐ No

Do you have concerns that your illness/hospitalization will affect:
☐ appearance   ☐ job   ☐ male/female roles   ☐ how you feel about yourself

Is religion important in your life?   ☐ Yes   ☐ No

Will this illness/hospitalization interfere with any religious beliefs/practices?   ☐ Yes   ☐ No

What do you expect from us while in the hospital?

Do you have a Living Will?   ☐ Yes   ☐ No   Do you have a Power of Attorney?   ☐ Yes   ☐ No
Do you have a copy with you?   ☐ Yes   ☐ No

Patient/Significant Other Signature: Relationship:	Date	Staff Signature Title:	Date

☐ REVIEWED BY REGISTERED NURSE   SIGNATURE: DATE:

TO BE COMPLETED BY STAFF ONLY

Patient provided: ☐ Admit kit   ☐ ID band   ☐ Sensitivity/Allergy band on patient   ☐ Allergy sticker on chart
Patient instructed: ☐ Valuables policy   ☐ Waiver signed   ☐ Smoking   ☐ Visitation
☐ Nursing call/Emergency   ☐ TV/phone   ☐ Fall precautions/band on wrist
☐ Patient's Rights/responsibilities   ☐ Received copy of Personal Directions for My Healthcare

Time patient arrived on Division:_____   SIGNATURE:_____

Fig. 7-4, cont'd Nursing health history.

helpful in planning your care. Another nurse will be caring for you this evening, but I'll be back on duty tomorrow morning. Do you have any other questions? Is there anything I can do for you now?"

The nurse's interviewing skills and techniques are essential in developing a good data base. The skillful interviewer is able to adapt interview strategies based on the client's responses. Pertinent health data are obtained when the nurse is prepared for the interview and is able to carry out each interview phase with minimal interruption.

ESTABLISHING THE NURSE-CLIENT RELATIONSHIP

Perhaps the most difficult client interview for a nurse to conduct is the first. It is an important time for the nurse to establish a relationship that fosters trust and confidence with a client. For some clients, being interviewed by a nurse is a new experience. An important goal for the initial interview is to lay the groundwork for the nurse to understand the client's needs and to begin a relationship that allows the client to become an active partner in decisions about care.

After the orientation phase of an interview, a client should begin to feel more comfortable speaking with the nurse. This is important, because the working phase requires the nurse to gather information of a more personal and focused nature. The nurse consciously communicates a sense of trust and confidentiality to clients. Illnesses that cause people to seek help are often accompanied by anxiety, helplessness, disruption of family relationships, and changes in self-image. Frequently, clients are asked to provide very personal information about themselves and their families. Generally, people share such information only with close friends, and there is a certain amount of trust that this information will not be shared with others. The nurse assures clients that interviews are confidential before asking them to share personal information.

Finally, the nurse-client relationship is enhanced by the professionalism and competence conveyed by the nurse. The nurse's attitude, professional manner, and appearance encourage a supportive therapeutic relationship with the client. Their free communication allows for ongoing identification of health care needs and objectives. The nurse is involved with the client and family and becomes an advocate for the client. The nurse acts for the client and encourages others to put the client's needs high on their list of priorities.

Nursing Health History

The **nursing health history** is data collected about the client's level of wellness (present and past), family history, changes in life patterns, sociocultural history, spiritual health, and mental and emotional reactions to illness. The nursing history is obtained during an interview, and it is the first step in performing assessment. The objective is to identify patterns of health and illness, risk factors for physical and behavioral health problems, deviations from normal, and available resources for adaptation. Although many health history forms are structured, the nurse learns to use the questions as starting points (Fig. 7-4). A good assessor learns to refine and broaden questions as needed so that the client's unique needs are correctly assessed.

Patterns of a client's health and illness are identified by collecting data about the physical and developmental, intellectual, emotional, social, and spiritual dimensions (Fig. 7-5). Incorporating data from all dimensions enables the nurse to develop a complete plan of care. Although many formats for the nursing health history have been given in the literature, all contain similar basic components.

BIOGRAPHICAL INFORMATION

Biographical information is factual demographic data about the client. The client's age, address, occupation and working status, marital status, and types of insurance coverage should be included.

REASON FOR SEEKING HEALTH CARE

The nurse asks why the client sought health care, because the information contained on the initial admission form may differ greatly from the client's subjective reason for seeking health care. For example:

CASE STUDY   Mr. Brown has been seen in the outpatient clinic for chronic diarrhea and is scheduled for a series of gastrointestinal diagnostic tests. During the nursing health history the nurse asks Mr. Brown his reason for seeking health care. "To find out why I have this pain in my stomach," the client replies. The information can make the nurse aware of any discomfort that may be related to chronic diarrhea. In addition, an unknown source of pain may be causing the client much anxiety. ■

The client's statement is not diagnostic; instead, it is the client's perception of reasons for seeking health care. Clarification of the client's perception identifies potential areas for education, counseling, or community resources required throughout all phases of diagnosis and recovery. When recorded, the statement is enclosed in quotation marks to indicate the client's words.

CLIENT EXPECTATIONS

The assessment of client expectations is not the same as the reason for seeking medical care, although they are often related. It is becoming more important for nurses to acknowledge what is important to the client who is seeking health care. Failure to identify a client's expectations of health care providers and a health care institution can result in poor client satisfaction. Client satisfaction is becoming a standard measure of quality for all hospitals throughout the country.

Clients typically have expectations in the following areas:

- Information needed to care for their health problems independently
- Caring and compassion expressed by care providers
- Timeliness of care givers' response to client requests
- Relief of pain and symptoms
- Involvement in decision making
- Cleanliness of the care environment

The initial interview can establish the client's expectations when entering the health care setting. Later, as the client has had interactions with health care providers, it is valuable to reassess expectations.

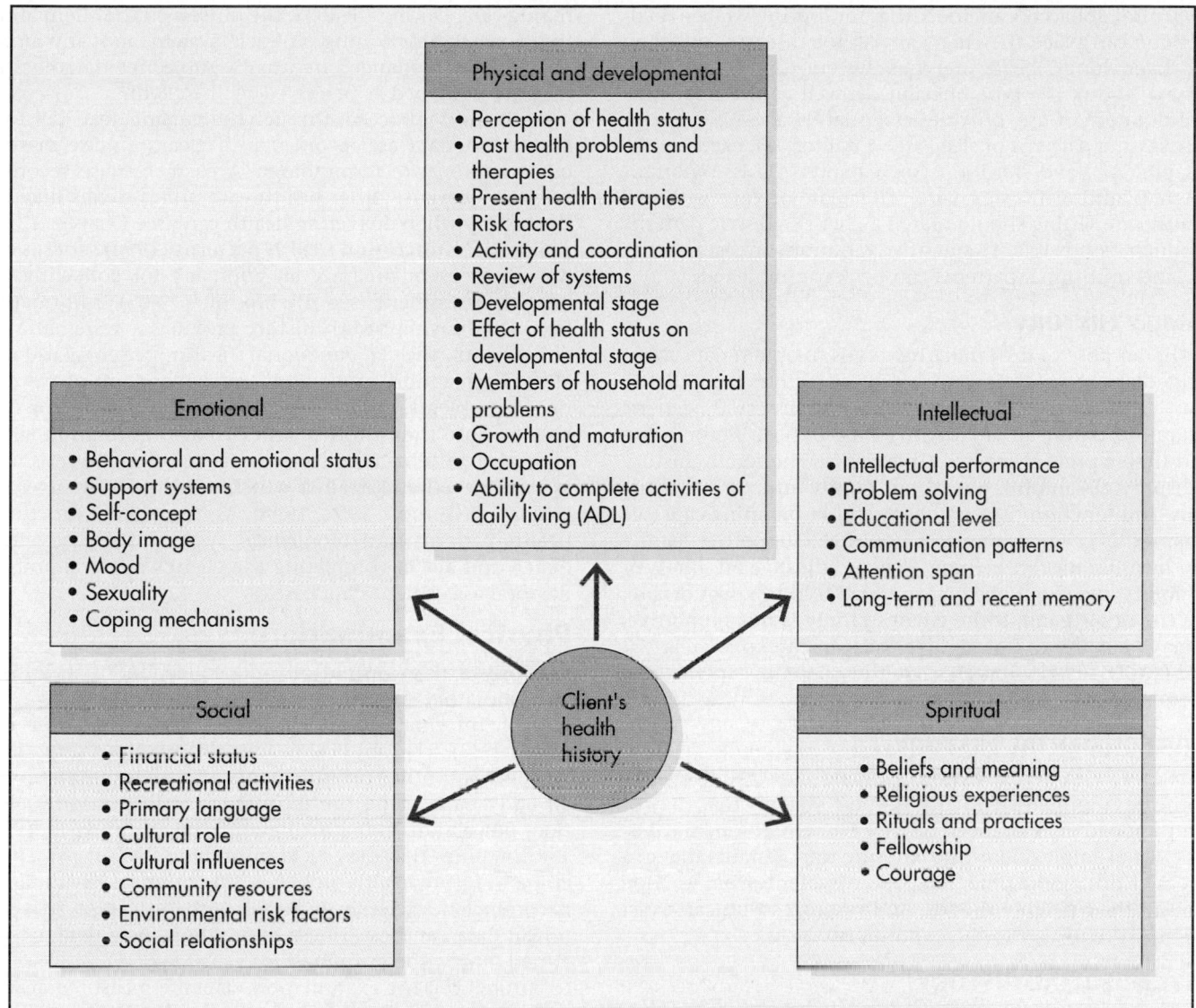

Physical and developmental

- Perception of health status
- Past health problems and therapies
- Present health therapies
- Risk factors
- Activity and coordination
- Review of systems
- Developmental stage
- Effect of health status on developmental stage
- Members of household marital problems
- Growth and maturation
- Occupation
- Ability to complete activities of daily living (ADL)

Emotional

- Behavioral and emotional status
- Support systems
- Self-concept
- Body image
- Mood
- Sexuality
- Coping mechanisms

Intellectual

- Intellectual performance
- Problem solving
- Educational level
- Communication patterns
- Attention span
- Long-term and recent memory

Social

- Financial status
- Recreational activities
- Primary language
- Cultural role
- Cultural influences
- Community resources
- Environmental risk factors
- Social relationships

Spiritual

- Beliefs and meaning
- Religious experiences
- Rituals and practices
- Fellowship
- Courage

Client's health history

Fig. 7-5 Dimensions for gathering data for a health history.

PRESENT ILLNESS

If an illness is present, nurses gather essential and relevant data about the onset of symptoms. The nurse determines when the symptoms began, whether they began suddenly or gradually, and whether they are always present or come and go. The nurse also asks about the duration of symptoms. In the section of the history on present illness, the nurse records specific information such as location, intensity, and quality of a symptom. For example, when the client indicates the symptom of pain, the nurse asks the client to point to or outline the area of the body affected, asks the client to rate the intensity on a scale of 1 to 10, and has the client describe what the pain feels like (see Chapter 43). The nurse needs to know whether any action precipitates the symptoms, makes them worse, or provides relief.

It is also appropriate to learn clients' expectations of the health care providers. The nurse determines whether clients expect to be "cured," "free of pain," or "able to care for themselves." This information assists in establishing the goals of nursing care, as well as in determining whether clients' expectations of themselves and the health care providers are realistic. In addition, such expectations provide the nurse with information on client perceptions about patterns of illness or changes in lifestyle.

PAST HEALTH HISTORY

The information collected about past history provides data on the client's health care experiences. The nurse assesses whether the client has ever been hospitalized or has undergone surgery. Also essential in planning nursing care are descriptions of allergies, including allergic reactions to food, drugs, or pollutants. If an allergy is present, the specific reaction and treatment are noted on the assessment form.

The nurse also identifies habits and lifestyle patterns. Use of alcohol, tobacco, caffeine, drugs, or routinely taken medications can place the client at risk for diseases involving the liver, lungs, heart, nervous system, or thought processes. Noting the type of habit, as well as the frequency and duration of use, provides essential data.

Assessing patterns of sleep (see Chapter 42), exercise (see Chapter 37), and nutrition (see Chapter 41) is important when planning nursing care. The plan of care within a health care setting should match a client's lifestyle patterns as much as possible. Frequently, variations in sleep, activity, and nutritional patterns can be accommodated.

FAMILY HISTORY

The purpose of the family history is to obtain data about immediate and blood relatives. The objectives are to determine whether the client is at risk for illnesses of a genetic or familial nature and to identify areas of health promotion and illness prevention (see Chapter 1). The family history also provides information about family structure, interaction, and function that may be useful in planning care (see Chapter 27). For example, a cohesive, supportive family can be a resource in helping a client adjust to an illness or disability and should be incorporated into the plan of care. On the other hand, if the client's family is not supportive, it may be better to not involve them in care, particularly if the family history reveals that the client is experiencing stress related to familial relationships.

ENVIRONMENTAL HISTORY

The environmental history provide data about clients' home environments and any support systems that they or family members may need to use. The environmental history, for example, identifies exposure to pollutants that can affect health, high crime that prevents clients from walking around their neighborhoods, and resources that can assist clients in returning to the community.

PSYCHOSOCIAL HISTORY

A complete psychosocial history reveals who the support systems are for the client, including spouse, children, other family members, or close friends. The psychosocial history includes information about ways that the client and family typically cope with stress (see Chapter 22). The same behavior, such as taking a walk, reading, or talking with a friend, can be used as a nursing intervention if the client experiences stress while receiving health care. The nurse also learns if the client has experienced any recent losses that create a sense of grief (see Chapter 26).

SPIRITUAL HEALTH

Life experiences and events are shaped by one's spirituality. The spiritual dimension repesents the totality of one's being and is difficult to assess quickly. A nurse reviews with clients their beliefs about life, their source for guidance in acting on beliefs, and the relationship they have with family in exercising their faith. Rituals and religious practices as a way to express spirituality are also assessed.

REVIEW OF SYSTEMS

The **review of systems (ROS)** is a systematic method for collecting data on all body systems. The systems that are assessed depend on the client's condition and urgency in initiating care. During the ROS, the nurse asks the client about the normal functioning of each system and any noted changes. Such changes are usually subjective data because they are described as perceived by the client.

As the nurse proceeds through the nursing health history, assessment data are recorded in a clear, concise manner using appropriate terminology. A clear, concise record is necessary because other health care professionals may use the history when delivering health care (see Chapter 12).

Gordon's **functional health patterns** (1994) serve as one way to focus or organize an approach for collecting the nursing assessment (see the box on p. 108). Information from the nursing health history provides a systematic description of the 11 functional health patterns and the client's perception, evaluation, and explanation of any particular problems. The 11 patterns establish the nursing data base because the historical and current information about all health patterns is collected and the information is used as baseline criteria against which any future changes are evaluated (Gordon, 1991, 1994). Assessments of functional health patterns and biomedical systems are easily integrated and aid in completing the client's physical and behavioral assessment data base.

Physical Examination

The **physical examination** and collection of diagnostic and laboratory data involve the gathering of objective, observable information undistorted by client perceptions (see Chapter 33). The physical examination is the taking of vital signs and other measurements and the examination of all body parts using the techniques of inspection, palpation, percussion, and auscultation. The examiner looks for abnormalities that may yield information about past, present, and future health problems. The physical examination is conducted after the nursing health history so that historical data can be verified. In addition, new data are obtained during the examination.

Throughout the examination, data are measured against a **standard**, which is an established rule or basis of comparison in measuring or judging capacity, quantity, content, and value of objects in the same category. The term *norm* is frequently used interchangeably with the term *standard* in the literature. Selected standards are reliable and relevant for the category being compared. For example, established standards for ideal height and weight are used to determine whether an individual is taller or shorter than the standard or is overweight or underweight. There are standards for blood pressure ranges for clients of select age groups. The nurse conducts the physical examination to verify information and collect further data, which are compared with the standards to determine whether the findings are normal or abnormal. Chapter 33 discusses these skills in more detail.

Before conducting the physical examination, the nurse prepares the client, environment, and necessary equipment. The nurse informs the client about the process of the physical examination, specifically its purposes, the nurse's role, the client's role, and the approximate duration.

ORDER OF EXAMINATION

The physical examination is carried out in a systematic manner similar to the ROS in the health history. This component of assessment usually begins with data on the client's height, weight, and vital signs (see Chapter 32).

Next the examiner writes a general statement about perceptions of the client and the client's level of health. This statement, called the *general survey,* includes information about mental status, body development, nutritional status, sex and race, chronological versus apparent age, behavior, appearance, and speech. Last is a head-to-toe examination of the body systems. The examiner records objective data obtained, using clear, concise, and appropriate language in describing each system examined.

PHYSICAL EXAMINATION TECHNIQUES

The nurse uses **inspection, palpation, percussion,** and **auscultation** to thoroughly examine a client. Each technique requires that certain principles be followed to ensure accurate data collection. Throughout an examination the nurse works closely with a client to minimize any anxiety or discomfort. Chapter 33 describes each of the examination techniques in detail.

Diagnostic and Laboratory Data

The final source of assessment data is the results of diagnostic and laboratory tests. The tests are ordered by physicians or advanced practice nurses. It is important for the nurse to review the results to verify alterations identified in the nursing health history and physical examination. They include base line information about the response to illness and information about the effects of later treatment measures. Laboratory data can help to identify actual or potential health care problems not previously noted by the client or examiner.

Laboratory data are compared with the established norms for a particular test, age group, and sex. The nurse identifies variations from normal and interprets findings according to the disease process and treatments. In addition, laboratory data can be used to evaluate the success or failure of nursing and medical interventions.

Laboratory tests are selected according to the symptoms or disease. However, common tests may be used for a large number of clients. Specific laboratory tests and the nursing responsibilities associated with them are detailed in Units 8 and 9.

■ FORMULATING NURSING JUDGMENTS

To be useful, assessment data must refer to the intended purpose of nursing and relate to the client's health problems (Bandman and Bandman, 1995). These interrelated concepts are the basis for nursing judgments. The nurse critically chooses the type of information to collect about a client, interprets the information to determine abnormalities, conducts further observations to clarify information, and then names the client's problem(s) in the form of nursing diagnoses (see Chapter 8).

Data Interpretation

The nurse may collect extensive information about a client. Through a process of inferential reasoning and judgment the nurse decides what information has meaning in relation to the client's health status (Gordon, 1994). Inferential reasoning involves the process of attaching new meaning

to known clinical data. For example, consider the following situation: When entering the client's room at 6 AM the nurse notices the client's bed linen is pulled down to the end of the bed and twisted in a lump, with the blanket on the floor. (Inference: the bed linen is in disarray.) Closer inspection finds the client sitting up in the chair next to the bed, holding his incision firmly, breathing slowly, and stating, "I didn't get much sleep last night." (Inference: the client received inadequate sleep.)

In this example of inference in practice, one nurse will infer inadequate sleep and then assess further the nature of the problem. In this case, assessment of the client's comfort level may reveal important additional cues. Another nurse may not make the second inference, and simply tidy up the bed and leave the room. Interpretation of data summarizes the data and provides a focus for attention (Gordon, 1994).

Problem assessment means collecting, estimating, and judging the value and significance of data (Lauri, 1982). This means the nurse is always thinking, analyzing data about a client to make accurate and meaningful interpretations of the client's problems. Assessment enables the nurse to understand problems further, to judge the extent of the problem, and to trace relationships between problems (Vitale et al, 1978). This is the heart of critical thinking and clinical problem solving. To prevent errors, the nurse validates and verifies any inferences or assumptions. Validation is obtained by comparing data with another source. For example, while summarizing an interview the nurse asks the client about accuracy of the most pertinent information. Findings gained in a physical exam can be validated with another nurse or with the medical record summary.

Data Clustering

After collecting and validating subjective and objective data and interpreting the data, the nurse organizes the information into meaningful clusters. This is dependent on recognizing significant cues. There are times when assessment data point clearly to a certain nursing diagnosis. For example, a client who has recently been diagnosed with diabetes, has had no opportunity to talk with a physician, and is asking questions about insulin obviously has a problem related to inadequate knowledge. As the nurse clusters cues, such as, the client asking questions and reporting no previous experience with insulin use, a pattern of meaning forms. Clustering of data helps to focus on identification of the correct problem. In the case of the diabetic client, data interpretation is relatively simple and routine; the nurse recognizes similarity to past situations.

During data clustering certain cues alert the nurse's thinking processes more than others (Gordon, 1994). These cues help to generate nursing diagnoses. The nurse becomes experienced in recognizing features of health problems, such as pain, anxiety, or immobility. Over time the nurse stores knowledge from previous experiences so that more complicated clustering becomes recognizable. This explains the difference in the skill of a beginning nurse versus a more expert nurse.

During data clustering, the nurse organizes data and focuses attention on client functions needing support and assistance for recovery. The next step is to form nursing diagnoses from the clusters of data to develop specific nursing interventions for the client's care. The

Focused Data Clustering

SYSTEM-ORIENTED FORMAT
Integumentary System
- Intact, flushed skin that is hot and dry to touch
- Dry oral mucosa, coated tongue, and cracked lips

Gastrointestinal System
- Distended, firm abdomen that is tender to palpation in lower quadrants
- Hyperactive bowel sounds in all quadrants
- History of anorexia, nausea, vomiting, and diarrhea for 2 days

Medical Record
- Laboratory tests indicating elevated white blood cell (WBC) count and hematocrit level: hypernatremia
- Abdominal x-ray examination showing gas-filled loops of bowel
- Admitting diagnosis of gastroenteritis

FUNCTIONAL HEALTH PATTERN FORMAT
Activity and Exercise Pattern
- Statement of increased fatigue when walking
- Demonstration of ability to perform activities of daily living (ADLs)
- Fatigued, dyspneic, and diaphoretic appearance when performing ADLs
- Increased pulse from 90 to 126 beats per minute during ADLs

Sleep and Rest Pattern
- Report of difficulty in falling and remaining asleep
- Denial of use of sleeping aids

Medical Record
- Previous history of decreased activity tolerance and poor sleeping 2 weeks before hospital admission for congestive heart failure
- Chest x-ray film showing pulmonary congestion

box at left demonstrates focused data clustering using system-oriented assessment and functional health pattern assessment.

■ DATA DOCUMENTATION

Data documentation is the last part of a complete assessment. Thoroughness and accuracy are necessary when recording data. If an item is not recorded, it is lost and unavailable to the data base.

Thoroughness in data documentation is essential for two reasons. First, all data pertinent to client status are included. Even information that does not seem to indicate an abnormality should be recorded. It may become pertinent later, serving as a base line for a change in status. A general rule of thumb is that if it is assessed it should be recorded. Second, observation and recording of client status is a legal and professional responsibility. The nurse practice acts in all states and the ANA *Policy Statement* (1980) and *Standards of Clinical Practice* (1991) mandate accurate data collection and recording as independent functions essential to the role of the professional nurse (see Chapter 13).

Being factual is easy after it becomes a habit. The basic rule is to record all observations. When recording data, a nurse should pay attention to facts and should make an effort to be as descriptive as possible. Anything heard, seen, felt, or smelled should be reported exactly. Conclusions about such data become nursing diagnoses. Because assessment includes the collection and documentation of subjective and objective data, the nurse should make certain that the data base is complete and factual before data clustering. Premature clustering can lead to inaccurate nursing diagnoses. In situations in which the client has just been admitted or when the client's status is changing rapidly, it is better to continually collect and document the new data and delay clustering.

■ KEY CONCEPTS ■

► Good assessment requires the nurse to apply knowledge and experience in making the necessary observations and measurements to gather data about clients.

► Written data statements should be descriptive, concise, and complete and should not include inferences or interpretative statements.

► Collection of inaccurate, incomplete, or inappropriate data may result in incorrect identification of the client's health care needs.

► The nature and amount of data in assessment are always changing, requiring a nurse to anticipate and ask questions to be sure assessment is accurate and complete.

► Gordon's 11 functional health patterns are a framework for a comprehensive assessment that moves inquiry from the general to the specific so that patterns of problems can be identified.

► Subjective findings can be related to physiological changes identified through objective data gathering.

► Subjective data are the client's perceptions.

► Good assessment requires communicating with all health care team members.

► Families can be an important source of information about the client's health status.

► The interview enables a nurse to establish a nurse-client relationship through caring, which fosters the sharing of ideas for a thorough assessment.

► The problem-solving interview technique explores in-depth data about specific problems.

► An interview includes an orientation, working, and termination phase.

► An interview with a client seeking health care should include assessment of the client's expectations.

▶ Learning a client's expectations of health care providers assists in establishing goals of care.

▶ To form a nursing judgment, the nurse critically assesses a client, interprets the information gathered, conducts further assessment for clarification, and names the client's problems.

▶ During the interview, information is obtained about the physical, developmental, intellectual, emotional, social, and spiritual dimensions of the client.

▶ The nursing health history involves data about level of wellness, past medical history, family history, environmental history, psychosocial and cultural history, and a review of the body systems.

▶ Laboratory and diagnostic tests add to the data base and verify data gathered through the nursing health history and physical examination.

▪ KEY TERMS ▪

Assessment, p. 108

Auscultation, p. 121

Data base, p. 108

Direct-question interview, p. 114

Functional health patterns, p. 120

Inspection, p. 121

Inference, p. 110

Interview, p. 113

Norm, p. 120

Nurse-client relationship, p. 113

Nursing health history, p. 118

Objective data, p. 111

Open-ended question interview, p. 114

Palpation, p. 121

Percussion, p. 121

Physical examination, p. 120

Problem-seeking interview, p. 114

Problem-solving interview, p. 114

Review of systems (ROS), p. 120

Standard, p. 120

Subjective data, p. 111

▪ CRITICAL THINKING EXERCISES ▪

1. Mrs. Kinsey is a 61-year-old woman who is being seen at home following hospitalization for her arthritis. She greets you at the door and you enter the home. The two of you sit down at the kitchen table. You notice many unwashed dishes in the sink, and the counter is covered with stacks of mail. On the kitchen table are six bottles of medication. What inferences might you make from your observations? How might you assess the client to gather more objective information about her health status?

2. Miss Fong has been assigned to your care for the first time. The nurse from the previous shift tells you she had surgery on her left lower leg and has a very large bandage. During the night she required an analgesic to help her sleep. She is able to drink liquids without nausea. You know that one of your responsibilities is to do an assessment of the client's condition. What are three priorities you would focus assessment on?

3. Mr. Rossi comes to the clinic with the following history: for the last 3 days he has had ringing in his ears and dizziness. Within the last 24 hours he has experienced nausea and headache as well. Identify three different open-ended questions that will prompt Mr. Rossi to discuss his condition.

REFERENCES

American Nurses Association: *Nursing: a social policy statement,* Kansas City, Mo, 1980, The Association.

American Nurses Association: *Standards of clinical nursing practice,* Washington, DC, 1991, The Association.

Bandman EL, Bandman B: *Critical thinking in nursing,* ed 2, Norwalk, Conn, 1995, Appleton & Lange.

Benner P: *From novice to expert: excellence and power in clinical practice,* Menlo Park, Calif, 1984, Addison-Wesley.

Carnevali DL, Thomas MD: *Diagnostic reasoning and treatment decision making in nursing,* Philadelphia, 1993, JB Lippincott.

Carpenito LJ: *Nursing diagnosis,* ed 5, Philadelphia, 1993, JB Lippincott.

Gordon M: *Manual of nursing diagnoses: 1991-1992,* St Louis, 1991, Mosby.

Gordon M: *Nursing diagnosis: process and application,* ed 2, St Louis, 1987, Mosby.

Gordon M: *Nursing diagnosis: process and application,* ed 3, St Louis, 1994, Mosby.

Hickey PW: *Nursing process handbook,* St Louis, 1990, Mosby.

Hurst K et al: The recognition and non-recognition of problem-solving stages in nursing practice, *J Adv Nurs* 16:1444, 1991.

Ivey AE: *Intentional interviewing and counseling: facilitating client development,* ed 2, Pacific Grove, Calif, 1988, Brooks/Cole.

Lauri S: Development of the nursing process through action research, *J Adv Nurs* 7:301, 1982.

Ryan-Wenger NM: A nursing process methodology, *Nurs Outlook* 38(4):190, 1990.

Vitale B et al: *A problem-solving approach to nursing care plans,* St Louis, 1978, Mosby.

ADDITIONAL READINGS

Bryn DD et al: Evaluation of nursing process documentation, *J Adv Nurs* 19:960, 1994.

Edelman C, Mandle CC: *Health promotion throughout the lifespan,* ed 2, St Louis, 1990, Mosby.

Kaplan SM: The nurse as change agent, *Ped Nurs* 16(6): 603, 1990.

Luekenotte AG: *Pocket guide to gerontologic assessment,* St Louis, 1990, Mosby.

McCain RF: Nursing by assessment, not intuition, *Am J Nurs* 65:82, 1965.

Miller MA, Babcock DE: *Critical thinking applied to nursing,* St Louis, 1996, Mosby.

Moss AR: Determinants of patient care: nursing process or nursing attitudes? *J Adv Nurs* 13:615, 1988.

Roberts JD et al: Problem solving in nursing practice: application, process, skill acquisition, and measurement, *J Adv Nurs* 18:886, 1993.

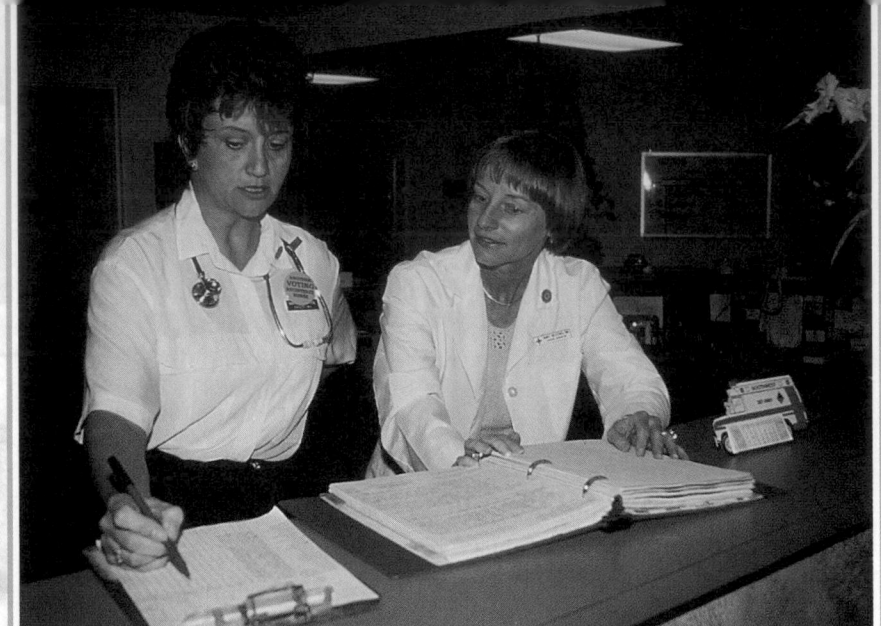

## Chapter 8

Nursing Diagnosis

Objectives

Mastery of content in this chapter will enable the student to:

▶ Define the key terms listed.

▶ Describe the way defining characteristics and the etiological process individualize a nursing diagnosis.

▶ List and discuss the steps of the nursing diagnostic process.

▶ Demonstrate the nursing diagnostic process.

▶ Differentiate between a nursing diagnosis and a medical diagnosis.

▶ Explain what makes a nursing diagnosis correct.

▶ Discuss the advantages of nursing diagnoses for the client and the nursing profession.

▶ Discuss the limitations of nursing diagnoses.

▶ Formulate nursing diagnoses from a nursing assessment.

After completing the nursing assessment, the nurse proceeds to the nursing diagnosis, which is a clinical judgment about individual, family, or community responses to actual or potential health problems or life processes. A nursing diagnosis is a statement that describes the client's actual or potential response to a health problem that the nurse is licensed and competent to treat. Impaired skin integrity related to decreased mobility and potential for infection related to poor nutritional intake are examples of nursing diagnoses. Nursing diagnoses provide the basis for selection of interventions to achieve outcomes for which the nurse is accountable (NANDA, 1990; Carpenito, 1993). Outcomes and interventions are selected in relationship to particular nursing diagnoses (McCloskey and Bulechek, 1992). The reasons for formulating a nursing diagnosis after analyzing assessment data are to identify health problems involving the client and family and to provide direction for the nursing care. The statement of a nursing diagnosis is the result of a diagnostic process during which the nurse uses critical thinking. Nursing diagnoses are developed for a client, family, or community; and take into account the physical, developmental, intellectual, emotional, social, and spiritual data obtained during assessment.

EVOLUTION OF NURSING DIAGNOSIS

Nursing has attempted to define itself professionally and functionally since the writings of Nightingale, who stated that the purpose of nursing care was "to put the patient in the best condition for nature to act upon him" (Nightingale, 1860).

Initially, nursing curricula were organized around disease entities or medical models. However, in the mid-1950s and early 1960s, nursing leaders and educators started to revise curricula around **client-centered problems** (Carpenito, 1995). According to McFarland and McFarlane (1989), nursing diagnosis was first introduced in the nursing literature in 1950. Fry (1953) proposed that nursing could be more creative by the formulation of nursing diagnoses and an individualized nursing care plan. This was not supported by professional nursing, and in 1955 the Model Nurse Practice Act of the American Nurses Association (ANA) excluded diagnosis or prescriptive therapies (ANA, 1955). As a result, nurses were hesitant to use nursing diagnostic labels.

However, the works of Henderson, Abdellah, and other theorists encouraged defining nursing in terms of client problems. These early theorists, by defining nursing action in terms of client-centered problems, were partly responsible for the interest and eventual use of nursing diagnosis in contemporary nursing education, practice, administration, and research (see Chapter 13).

In 1973, the first national conference for the classification of nursing diagnosis was held to identify nursing functions and establish a classification system. Participants of conferences have developed the nursing diagnostic categories (see the box on p. 126). In 1982 a professional association, the **North American Nursing Diagnosis Association (NANDA)** was established. The purpose of NANDA was "to develop, refine, and promote a taxonomy of nursing diagnostic terminology of general use for professional nurses" (Kim, McFarland, and McLane, 1984). In other words, NANDA's work provides a common language for the health problems nurses deal with. Just as the medical diagnosis diabetes mellitus informs physicians about the nature and treatment of a specific disease, the nursing diagnosis impaired skin integrity informs nurses about the nature of and care activities required for this specific health problem. The ANA has officially sanctioned NANDA as the organization to govern the development of a classification system of nursing diagnoses (Carpenito, 1995).

Nursing diagnosis was first incorporated into the ANA's *Standards of Nursing Practice* in 1971 (ANA, 1973), and it remains in the current standards (ANA, 1991). In 1980 and 1994, the ANA supported nursing diagnosis in *Nursing: A Social Policy Statement,* which defined nursing as "the diagnosis and treatment of human responses to actual or potential health problems" (ANA, 1980, 1994). In 1987 the definition of nursing diagnosis was strengthened in the refined definition of nursing in ANA's paper *Scope of Nursing Practice,* which defines nursing as the diagnosis and treatment of human responses to health and illness (ANA, 1987).

As nursing curricula continue to incorporate nursing diagnosis into the educational preparation of nurses, the research in this field will continue to grow. As a result, new diagnostic labels are continually developed, researched, and added to the NANDA listing, which is by no means complete. The continued evolution of nursing diagnosis draws from the collective wealth of nursing knowledge. Through the ongoing collaboration of nursing educators, administrators, researchers, and practitioners, the further development of nursing diagnoses has the potential to enrich the nursing profession.

DEFINITION

Nursing literature contains many definitions for *nursing diagnosis.* These definitions evolved as the profession's acceptance of nursing diagnosis strengthened. Table 8-1 lists some definitions and their sources. However, some common components of these definitions include nursing, client, and health problems. In addition, each definition implies that the nurse uses critical thinking skills to analyze the client's assessment data to form nursing diagnoses.

The definition of a nursing diagnosis presented in this text is to assist the student in using diagnoses as a framework for delivering nursing care. This component, like all components of the nursing process, enables the student to critically plan individualized nursing care.

A **nursing diagnosis** is a statement that describes the client's actual or potential response to a health problem that the nurse is licensed and competent to treat. The client's actual and potential responses are obtained from the assessment data base, a review of pertinent literature, the client's past medical records, and consultation with other professionals, all of which are collected during assessment. Last, the client's actual or potential responses require interventions from the domain of nursing practice (Carlson et al, 1991; Carpenito, 1995).

CRITICAL THINKING AND THE NURSING DIAGNOSTIC PROCESS

Critical thinking is a complex process (see Chapter 6). **Critical thinking** is the examination of data, the gathering of

North American Nursing Diagnosis Association (NANDA) Accepted Nursing Diagnoses

Activity Intolerance
Activity Intolerance, Risk for
Adaptive Capacity, Decreased: Intracranial*
Adjustment, Impaired
Airway Clearance, Ineffective
Anxiety
Aspiration, Risk for
Body Image Disturbance
Body Temperature, Altered, Risk for
Bowel Incontinence
Breastfeeding, Effective
Breastfeeding, Ineffective
Breathing Pattern, Ineffective
Cardiac Output, Decreased
Caregiver Role Strain
Caregiver Role Strain, Risk for
Communication, Impaired Verbal
Community Coping, Potential for Enhanced*
Community Coping, Ineffective*
Confusion, Acute*
Confusion, Chronic*
Constipation
Constipation, Colonic
Constipation, Perceived
Coping, Defensive
Coping, Family: Potential for Growth
Coping, Ineffective Family: Compromised
Coping, Ineffective Family: Disabling
Coping, Ineffective Individual
Decisional Conflict (Specify)
Denial, Ineffective
Diarrhea
Disuse Syndrome, Risk for
Diversional Activity Deficit
Dysreflexia
Energy Field Disturbance*
Environmental Interpretation Syndrome: Impaired*
Family Processes, Altered: Alcoholism*
Family Processes, Altered
Fatigue
Fear
Fluid Volume Deficit (1)
Fluid Volume Deficit (2)
Fluid Volume Deficit, Risk for
Fluid Volume Excess
Gas Exchange, Impaired
Grieving, Anticipatory
Grieving, Dysfunctional
Growth and Development, Altered
Health Maintenance, Altered
Health-Seeking Behaviors (Specify)
Home Maintenance Management, Impaired
Hopelessness
Hyperthermia
Hypothermia
Incontinence, Functional
Incontinence, Reflex
Incontinence, Stress
Incontinence, Total
Incontinence, Urge
Infant Behavior, Disorganized*
Infant Behavior, Disorganized: Risk for*
Infant Behavior Organized: Potential for Enhanced*
Infant Feeding Pattern, Ineffective
Infection, Risk for
Injury, Perioperative Positioning: Risk for*

Injury, Risk for
Knowledge Deficit (Specify)
Loneliness, Risk for*
Management of Therapeutic Regimen,
  Community: Ineffective*
Management of Therapeutic Regimen, Families: Ineffective*
Management of Therapeutic Regimen,
  Individuals: Effective*
Management of Therapeutic Regimen, Individuals: Ineffective
Memory, Impaired*
Mobility, Impaired Physical
Noncompliance (Specify)
Nutrition, Altered: Less Than Body Requirements
Nutrition, Altered: More Than Body Requirements
Nutrition, Altered: Risk for More Than Body Requirements
Oral Mucous Membrane, Altered
Pain
Pain, Chronic
Parent/Infant/Child Attachment Altered, Risk for*
Parental Role Conflict
Parenting, Altered
Parenting, Altered, Risk for
Peripheral Neurovascular Dysfunction, Risk for
Personal Identity Disturbance
Poisoning, Risk for
Post-Trauma Response
Powerlessness
Protection, Altered
Rape-Trauma Syndrome
Rape-Trauma Syndrome: Compound Reaction
Rape-Trauma Syndrome: Silent Reaction
Relocation Stress Syndrome
Role Performance, Altered
Self-Care Deficit, Bathing/Hygiene
Self-Care Deficit, Dressing/Grooming
Self-Care Deficit, Feeding
Self-Care Deficit, Toileting
Self-Esteem Disturbance
Self-Esteem, Chronic Low
Self-Esteem, Situational Low
Self-Mutilation, Risk for
Sensory/Perceptual Alterations (Specify) (visual, auditory,
  kinesthetic, gustatory, tactile, olfactory)
Sexual Dysfunction
Sexuality Patterns, Altered
Skin Integrity, Impaired
Skin Integrity, Impaired Risk for
Sleep Pattern Disturbance
Social Interaction, Impaired
Social Isolation
Spiritual Distress (Distress of the Human Spirit)
Spiritual Well-Being, Potential for Enhanced*
Suffocation, Risk for
Swallowing, Impaired
Thermoregulation, Ineffective
Thought Processes, Altered
Tissue Integrity, Impaired
Tissue Perfusion, Altered (Specify Type) (renal, cerebral,
  cardiopulmonary, gastrointestinal, peripheral)
Trauma, Risk for
Unilateral Neglect
Urinary Elimination, Altered
Urinary Retention
Ventilation, Inability to Sustain Spontaneous
Ventilatory Weaning Process, Dysfunctional
Violence, Risk for: Self-Directed or Directed at Others

*1994 additions.

Table 8-1	Definitions of Nursing Diagnosis
AUTHOR	**DEFINITION**
Abdellah (1957)	"The determination of the nature and extent of nursing problems presented by the individual patients or families receiving nursing care."
Durand, Prince (1966)	"A statement of a conclusion resulting from a recognition of a pattern derived from a nursing investigation of the patient."
Gebbie, Lavin (1975)	"The judgment or conclusion that occurs as a result of nursing assessment."
Bircher (1975)	"An independent nursing function. . . . An evaluation of a client's personal responses to his or her human experience throughout the life cycle, be they developmental or accidental crises, illness, hardship, or other stresses."
Aspinall (1976)	"A process of clinical inference from observed changes in patient's physical or psychological condition; if it is arrived at accurately and intelligently, it will lead to identification of the possible causes of symptomatology."
Gordon (1976)	"Actual or potential health problems which nurses, by virtue of their education and experience, are capable and licensed to treat."
Roy (1982)	"Nursing diagnosis is a concise phrase or term summarizing a cluster of empirical indicators representing patterns of unitary man."
Shoemaker (1984)	"A nursing diagnosis is a clinical judgment about an individual, family, or community that is derived through a deliberate, systematic process of data collection and analysis. It provides the basis for prescriptions for definitive therapy for which the nurse is accountable. It is expressed concisely and includes the etiology of the condition when known."
Carpenito (1987)	"A nursing diagnosis is a statement that describes the human response (health state or actual/ potential altered interaction pattern) of an individual or group which the nurse can legally identify and for which the nurse can order the definitive interventions to maintain the health state or to reduce, eliminate, or prevent alteration."
NANDA (1990)	"A nursing diagnosis is a clinical judgment about individual, family, or community responses to actual and potential health problems and life processes. Nursing diagnoses provide the basis for selection of nursing interventions to achieve outcomes for which the nurse is accountable."
Carlson et al. (1991)*	"Nursing diagnosis is a summary statement about the health status of a client(s) derived through the assessment process and requiring intervention from the domain of nursing."

*Modified from Carlson JH et al: *Nursing diagnosis: a case-study approach,* Philadelphia, 1991, Saunders.

information from the literature, the organization of observations, and drawing upon past experiences (Bandman and Bandman, 1995). Its use in formulating a nursing diagnosis is essential. As nursing care expands into a variety of health care settings, more aspects of critical thinking are required in diagnostic reasoning and judgment (Gordon, 1994).

The **diagnostic process** incorporates the skills of critical thinking in the decision-making steps the nurse uses to develop a diagnostic statement (Carnevali et al, 1984; Carnevali and Thomas, 1993). This process includes analysis and interpretation of assessment data, identification of problems, and formulation of nursing diagnoses (Fig. 8-1).

Analysis and Interpretation of Data

During assessment, data are collected from a variety of sources, validated, and sorted into clusters that form patterns. The data base is continually revised as changes in the client's physical and emotional status occur. This includes the results of laboratory and diagnostic tests. During this step, the nurse uses knowledge and experience, analyzes and interprets, and draws conclusions about the data clusters and patterns (Benner, 1984; Carnevali et al, 1984; Carlson et al, 1991; Bandman and Bandman, 1995).

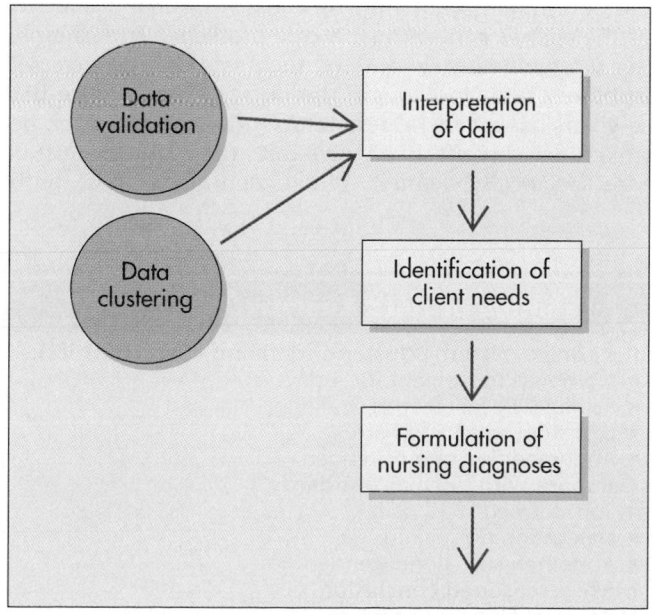

Fig. 8-1 Nursing diagnostic process.

CLUSTERING DATA

The analysis of data involves recognizing patterns or trends, comparing these patterns with normal health patterns, and drawing conclusions about the client's response (see the box below). The nurse looks for patterns or trends while examining clusters of data. When a relationship among these patterns is identified, a list of client-centered problems or needs begins to emerge.

The clusters of data consist of defining characteristics. **Defining characteristics** are the clinical criteria that support (validate) the presence of the diagnostic category. Clinical criteria are objective or subjective signs and symptoms or risk factors (Carpenito, 1995). Multiple defining characteristics resulting from assessment data support the nursing diagnosis (Carpenito, 1995). The presence of one sign or symptom is not sufficient to support the nursing diagnostic label. Absence of defining characteristics suggests that the diagnosis should be rejected. Diagnostic categories and their defining characteristics provide structure for the cognitive process in the identification of client needs and actual formulation of nursing diagnoses (Hurley, 1986; Carpenito, 1995).

Critically organizing and identifying patterns is demonstrated through the following example. Gray hair alone does not necessarily indicate that a person is an older adult. However, gray hair, wrinkled skin, age spots, and a slower gait are clusters of data that characterize a pattern known as an older adult.

The identified pattern is compared with normal standards. The nurse uses widely accepted norms, such as normal laboratory and diagnostic test values, and professional knowledge as the basis for comparison and judgment. When comparing the patterns, the nurse decides whether the grouped signs and symptoms are within normal standards (Gordon, 1994). Defining characteristics that are beyond healthful norms form the basis for problem identification.

Identification of Client Problems

Before formulating the nursing diagnosis, the nurse identifies the client's general health care problems. For example, after receiving clusters of data, such as dyspnea, increased respiratory rate, and cough, the nurse may recognize that the client has a general respiratory problem. However, before a nurse can effectively give care, the problem must be more specifically defined. When identifying these problems, the nurse considers all assessment data and focuses on pertinent and abnormal data (Gordon, 1994). It may help the inexperienced nurse to think of this identification phase as the general health care problem and the formulation of the nursing diagnosis as the specific health care problem. The nurse moves from general to specific.

To identify the client's needs, the nurse first determines what the client's health problems are and whether they are actual or potential problems. An **actual health problem** is one that is perceived or experienced by the client, such as a sleep pattern disturbance related to a noisy environment. An **at risk health problem** alerts the nurse to the need for preventive interventions (Gordon, 1994). The risk factors for risk and at risk nursing diagnoses represent those situations that increase the vulnerability of a client or group to an illness or accident (Carpenito, 1995). For example, during the postoperative course, an overweight smoker is at risk for ineffective airway clearance related to incisional pain.

The problem-identification step brings the nurse closer to forming a nursing diagnosis. Making general analyses from the clustered data assists the nurse in recognizing specific problems and then making a nursing diagnosis.

■ NURSING DIAGNOSIS STATEMENT
Nursing Diagnosis Format

The nursing diagnosis format (that is, how the actual diagnosis is stated) flows from the diagnostic process. This format provides the beginning nurse with familiarity and rationale for the structure of a nursing diagnostic statement.

Throughout this text, nursing diagnoses are stated in a two-part format accepted by NANDA (McLane, 1987; NANDA, 1990): the diagnostic label followed by a statement of related factors (Table 8-2). The diagnostic labels are categories approved by NANDA (see the box on p. 126). The related factor is a condition or etiology that affects the client's actual or potential response, which can be changed by nursing interventions.

This two-part format is accepted by the majority of nursing leaders (Soares O'Hearn, 1990; Carlson et al, 1991; Gordon, 1994; Carpenito, 1995). It assists the nurse in individualizing a client's nursing diagnoses and provides

---

Example of Data Analysis

Recognize pattern (cluster of defining characteristics).
- No bowel movement for 4 days
- Painful defecation with straining
- Last stool small and hard
- Abdomen firm and distended

Compare with normal standards.
- Soft, formed stool daily
- Defecation not painful
- Abdomen soft, nondistended

Make a reasoned conclusion.
- Bowel elimination problem

Table 8-2	NANDA Nursing Diagnosis Format
DIAGNOSTIC STATEMENT	**RELATED FACTORS**
Constipation	Inadequate dietary fiber
	Effects of medications
	Inadequate fluid intake
	Decreased activity
Fatigue	Discomfort
	Excessive role demands
	Increased energy requirement
Impaired skin integrity	Fluid retention
	Excessive secretions
	Immobilization
	Altered circulation

direction for the selection of appropriate interventions. The nursing interventions are directed toward altering or resolving the etiological or related factors (McCloskey and Bulechek, 1992). This format supports the delivery of individualized nursing care for one client or a group of clients.

Formulation of the Nursing Diagnosis

Formulation of the nursing diagnosis is based on identification of client needs. Once assessment data begin to reveal problems, the nurse is directed toward selection of appropriate nursing diagnoses. The diagnostic label is supported by defining characteristics present in the client's assessment data base. The label is the problem (for example, risk for injury) and its related factor (for example, related to confusion). The problem is an actual or potential client response to health or illness. The related factors are etiological or other contributing conditions that influence the client's response (Carpenito, 1995).

The "related to" phrase identifies the etiology or cause of the problem. This is not a cause-and-effect statement, but rather it indicates that the etiology can contribute to or be associated with the problem (Fig. 8-2). Including the phrase requires the nurse to use critical thinking skills to individualize the nursing diagnosis and subsequent interventions (Table 8-3).

The **etiology** or cause of the nursing diagnosis must be within the domain of nursing practice and a condition that

responds to nursing interventions. In some settings, medical diagnoses are recorded as the etiology of the nursing diagnosis. This is incorrect. Nursing interventions cannot change the medical diagnosis. However, nursing interventions can be directed at etiological factors and the diagnostic label. For example, the nursing diagnosis, pain related to breast cancer, is incorrect. Nursing actions cannot affect the medical diagnosis of breast cancer. Rewording the diagnosis to read, pain related to impaired skin integrity secondary to mastectomy incision results in nursing interventions directed at improving comfort through and pain control and incision care.

As the client's health status changes, nursing diagnoses are modified. For example, a client's pertinent assessment data may include the following: decreased dietary fiber and limited fluid intake, no bowel movement for 3 days, decreased bowel sounds, distention of the lower abdomen, hard fecal material extracted during digital rectal examination, and a guaiac-negative stool specimen. The most appropriate nursing diagnosis is, constipation related to limited dietary fiber intake. However, once a high-fiber diet is initiated and the client's constipation is resolved, a risk for constipation remains based on the client's past history.

If a health problem has been resolved, the nursing diagnosis no longer exists. When the client's physiological and emotional status changes, the health problem may remain relevant, but the etiology may change. Therefore the nurse must modify the nursing diagnoses by changing the etiology (Fig. 8-3). If a new problem arises, the nurse develops new nursing diagnoses reflecting changes in the client's needs and status.

The modification of nursing diagnoses is ongoing. As the level of nursing care and level of wellness change, these changes are reflected in the statement of nursing diagnoses. Outdated nursing diagnoses do not accurately reflect the client's current needs.

Assessment Data and the Diagnostic Statement

Nursing assessment data must support the diagnostic label and the related factors must support the etiology. In order to collect correct data it may help to identify assessment ac-

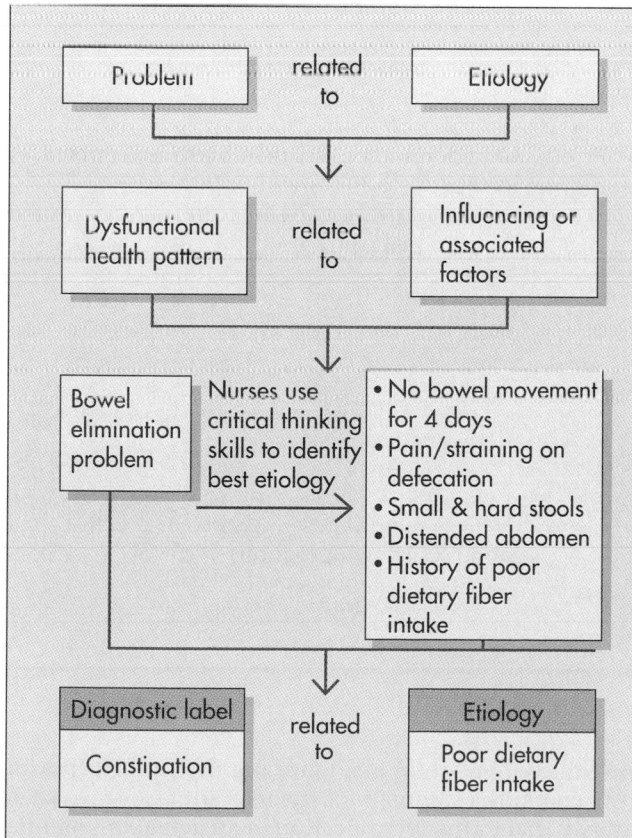

Fig. 8-2 Relationship between diagnostic statement and format. *(Redrawn from Hickey P: Nursing process handbook, St Louis, 1990, Mosby.)*

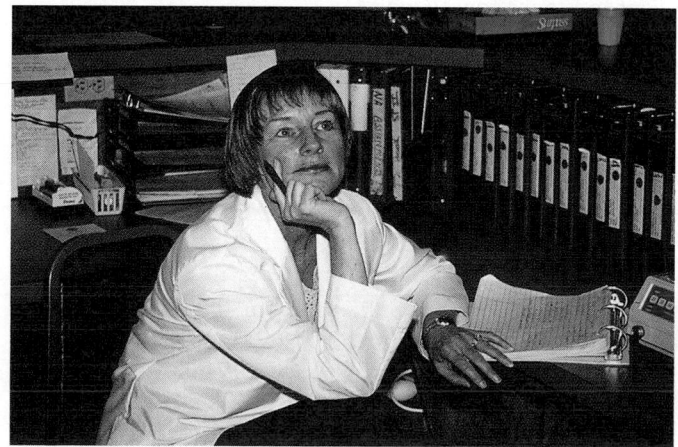

Fig. 8-3 Nurse uses critical thinking to modify nursing care plan.

Table 8-3	Comparison of Interventions for Nursing Diagnoses With Different Etiologies

NURSING DIAGNOSES	INTERVENTIONS
CLIENT A	
Ineffective airway clearance related to obesity	Place client in high Fowler's position. Have client cough and deep breathe every 2 hours while awake. Start weight-reduction diet (1200 calories) to decrease obesity.
Feeding self-care deficit related to inability to bend arms secondary to bilateral arm casts	Encourage family to visit during meals. Be certain staff or family members are available to feed client. Provide high-calorie milkshakes with straw at 3 and 8 PM.
Anxiety related to social isolation secondary to protective isolation	Plan staffing patterns to include visits to client's room four times a day. Provide diversional activities.
CLIENT B	
Ineffective airway clearance related to poor coughing technique	Teach client deep breathing and coughing. Splint client's abdominal incision during coughing.
Feeding self-care deficit related to inability to grasp feeding utensils	Provide large-handled eating utensils. Offer finger foods cut in large pieces for between-meal snacks: 10-2-8.
Social isolation related to effects of neighborhood	Provide client with phone numbers and location of local senior citizens' center. Draw client a map of neighborhood stores, restaurants, and libraries.

Table 8-4	Formulation of Nursing Diagnoses

CLUSTERING DATA	IDENTIFICATION OF CLIENT NEED	NURSING DIAGNOSIS FORMULATION
Diarrhea for 3 weeks Distended abdomen Family history of stomach cancer	Alteration elimination patterns	Diarrhea related to unknown cause
Weight loss: 15 pounds	Excessive weight loss	Altered nutrition: less than body requirements related to chronic diarrhea for 3 weeks
Anemia, hemoglobin level of 10 g 40 pack-year history of smoking Slight change of emphysema shown on chest x-ray film Crackles auscultated in lung fields Productive cough on rising each morning	Risk for postoperative respiratory complications	Ineffective airway clearance after surgery related to incisional pain
Temporary colostomy Abdominal incision Client resistance to viewing of abdomen	Change in body image	Self-esteem disturbance related to change in body image
Client verbalization of fear of stomach cancer Client withdrawal after biopsy report Anxiety	Changes in interpersonal interactions	Ineffective individual coping related to fear about unknown prognosis

tivities that produce specific kinds of data. For example, asking the client about the quality and perception of pain results in subjective data. However, palpating an area, which may elicit a painful grimace, provides objective information. Likewise, asking a client to describe the perception of an irregular heartbeat elicits subjective information, and using auscultation to obtain a pulse produces an ob-

jective measurement for heart rate and rhythm. The box on p. 131 contains a summary of the relevant assessment data that may lead to the identification of an actual or potential health care problem. Table 8-4 demonstrates data clustering, identification of client need, and formulation of nursing diagnoses from the pertinent assessment data presented in the box on p. 131.

Table 8-5 uses the two nursing diagnoses, ineffective airway clearance, and self-esteem disturbance, to demonstrate how defining characteristics and probable related factors assist in the development of the total diagnostic label. The defining characteristics and relevant etiologies are from the text *Pocket Guide to Nursing Diagnoses,* by Kim, McFarland, and McLane (1995) and are derived from the NANDA classification.

Nursing Diagnosis and Medical Diagnosis

Nursing diagnosis focuses on and defines the nursing needs of the client (Gordon, 1994). It reflects the client's level of health or response to a disease or pathological process, an emotional state, a sociocultural phenomenon, or a developmental stage. A **medical diagnosis** predominately identifies a specific disease state. The medical focus is on the diagnosis and treatment of the disease.

Medical and nursing diagnoses are developed using assessment data bases. In both professions the diagnostic label directs the direction of care. However, the nursing data base is global, and includes an in-depth assessment of the physiological, psychological, sociocultural, developmental, and spiritual dimensions of the client. Medicine's data base includes the physiological systems and the personal and social systems. The personal and social systems may be lim-

---

Summary of Relevant Assessment Data

PHYSICAL AND DEVELOPMENTAL DATA
- Diarrhea for 3 weeks
- Productive cough on rising each morning
- 15-pound weight loss 2 weeks before hospitalization
- Hemoglobin level of 10 g
- Slight change of emphysema shown on chest x-ray film
- Crackles in bilateral lung bases
- Distended abdomen
- Squamous cell cancer
- 20-year history of smoking, 2 packs a day (10 pack-years)
- Family history of stomach cancer
- Family history of heart attacks
- 40-year marriage
- 20-year self-employment
- One adult son, 35 years old
- Two sisters, 50 and 48, with no major health problems
- Temporary colostomy
- Abdominal incision

INTELLECTUAL DATA
- Talkative
- Frequent questions about whether he has cancer
- Good attention span
- Fearful of stomach cancer

EMOTIONAL DATA
- Anxiety
- Withdrawal after biopsy report of squamous cell cancer
- Avoidance of viewing abdomen incision

SOCIAL DATA
- Tennis three times a week
- Active role in his neighborhood

SPIRITUAL DATA
- Methodist
- Weekly church attendance
- Daily Bible reading

Table 8-5	**Defining Characteristics and Etiologies to Support Nursing Diagnoses**		
ASSESSMENT ACTIVITIES	**DEFINING CHARACTERISTICS**	**NURSING DIAGNOSES**	**ETIOLOGIES ("RELATED TO")**
Auscultate lungs.	Abnormal breath sounds	Ineffective airway clearance	Decreased energy or fatigue
Observe respiration.	Changes in rate or depth of respiration		Tracheobronchial infection, obstruction, or secretion
Observe cough.	Cough		Pain
Inspect skin color.	Cyanosis		
Ask client about shortness of breath and observe for it.	Dyspnea		
Ask client about smoking.	Smoking history		
Observe client's grooming.	Verbal or nonverbal response to actual or perceived change in structure or function	Self-esteem disturbance	Biophysical factors (e.g., amputation or loss of function of extremity)
Observe client's willingness to participate in rehabilitation.	Missing or impaired body part, not looking or touching body or body part		Cognitive or perceptual factors (e.g., expressions of worthlessness and sorrow)
Review history of trauma injury.	Trauma to body		Psychosocial factors (e.g., withdrawal behavior or excessive crying)
	Refusal to acknowledge change		

ited to a family medical history and the economic and insurance history of the client (Gordon, 1994).

The goals and objectives of a nursing diagnosis differ from those of a medical diagnosis. The goal of a nursing diagnosis is to direct a plan of care to assist clients and their families to adapt to their illness and to resolve health care problems. The goals of a medical diagnosis are to identify and to design a treatment plan for curing the disease or the pathological process.

The objective of a nursing diagnosis is development of an individualized plan of care so that the client and family are able to cope with changes and to meet the challenges resulting from health problems. The objective of the medical diagnosis is to prescribe treatment. For example, a 20-year-old college student is admitted with right lower quadrant abdominal pain. The physician makes a medical diagnosis of appendicitis, and the client undergoes an emergency appendectomy to remove the infected appendix. After the appendectomy the nurse develops several nursing diagnoses, one of which is impaired physical mobility related to pain secondary to an abdominal incision. The nursing care will be directed at gradually increasing the client's mobility to preoperative levels.

■ SOURCES OF DIAGNOSTIC ERROR

The diagnostic process is not error free. In the diagnostic process the nurse relies on four areas. First, there must be an assessment data base present. Second, the nurse analyzes and interprets these data. Third, the data are clustered into meaningful groups. Last, the nurse identifies client problems that result in the identification of the diagnostic label. Each of these four areas is a potential source of diagnostic error, which can alter the health outcomes of the client.

Errors in Data Collection

This type of error occurs during the assessment process. If data are incompletely collected, omitted, or misinterpreted, diagnoses are missed. If data collection is disorganized, the diagnostic process is scattered.

The following practices are essential during assessment to avoid data collection errors. First, prior to assessment, the nurse critically reviews his or her level of comfort and competence with interview and physical assessment skills. The beginner should approach assessment in steps. For example, the first experience may be completing an interview on a family member or collecting physical assessment data on one system. The learner then moves on to more complex assessments.

Second, the nurse must determine the accuracy of data collected. For example, the nurse who auscultates abnormal lung sounds for the first time may be unsure of what is being heard through the stethoscope. To minimize the risk of inaccuracy, the nurse must have a more experienced colleague validate findings or explain why they are incorrect.

Third, when developing assessment skills, the nurse needs to check completeness of assessment data. Reviewing client assessments in clinical or classroom settings provides the nurse with a constructive learning opportunity to determine when assessments are complete or when further revisions are needed.

Last, errors in data collection are reduced when an organized approach is used for the assessment. Prior to assess-

ment the nurse should have the appropriate forms and examination equipment. The nurse can achieve an organized assessment if the environment is private, quiet, and comfortable for the client.

Errors in Interpretation and Analysis of Data

Following assessment the nurse reviews the data base. During this review the nurse determines if data are accurate and complete. The nurse reviews the data to validate that subjective data are supported by measurable objective physical findings when necessary. The nurse may also review supportive literature to ensure an adequate knowledge base to form a correct nursing diagnosis. Last, the nurse begins to identify and organize relevant assessment patterns to support the presence of client problems.

Errors in Data Clustering

After data are interpreted and analyzed, data clustering occurs. Errors in data clustering occur when data are clustered prematurely, incorrectly, or not at all (Gordon, 1982, 1994). Premature closure of clustering occurs when the nurse makes the nursing diagnosis before all data have been grouped. Incorrect clustering occurs when the nurse tries to make the nursing diagnosis fit the signs and symptoms obtained. The nursing diagnosis should be derived from the data, not the reverse. An incorrect nursing diagnosis affects quality of care.

Errors in the Diagnostic Statement

The last type of error that can occur is the manner in which the nursing diagnosis is stated. There are some common guidelines to reduce errors in the diagnostic statement itself. The statement should be worded in appropriate, concise, and precise language, which involves using correct terminology reflecting the client's response to the illness or condition. A diagnostic statement such as "unhappy and worried about health" can lead to errors. The language needs to be more precise and appropriate, such as, ineffective individual coping related to fear of medical diagnosis. Also, the problem and etiology portions must be within the scope of *nursing* to diagnose and treat. Concise wording ensures that the nursing need can be easily communicated to other nurses and health care professionals. The box below lists suggestions in writing nursing diagnoses.

Avoiding Diagnostic Errors

Identify client's response to illness.
State a NANDA diagnostic statement.
Identify an etiology treatable by nursing.
Identify a client need associated with a treatment or test.
Identify client's response to equipment.
Identify client's, not nurse's, problem.
Identify client's problem, not interventions.
Identify client's problem, not goals.
Avoid prejudicial statements.
State the etiology legally.
Identify a problem and an etiology.
Identify only one client problem in a diagnostic statement.

Table 8-6	Examples of Errors in Formulating the Nursing Diagnostic Statement		
CORRECT STATEMENT	**STATED AS MEDICAL DIAGNOSIS**	**STATED IN MEDICAL TERMINOLOGY**	**STATED AS A NURSING INTERVENTION**
Diarrhea related to unknown cause	Diarrhea	Alteration in bowel elimination related to lesion in descending colon	Offer bedpan frequently because of diarrhea.
Altered nutrition: less than body requirements related to chronic diarrhea for 3 weeks	Potential malnutrition	Alteration in nutrition: less than body requirements owing to malnutrition	Provide high-protein diet due to high risk for altered nutrition.
Ineffective airway clearance after surgery related to discomfort secondary to incisional pain	Potential postoperative pneumonia	Ineffective airway clearance owing to emphysema	Have client cough frequently because of ineffective airway clearance.
Self-esteem disturbance related to change in body image	Avoidance reaction to colostomy	Disturbance in self-concept owing to colostomy	Encourage client to interact with others.

In addition, there are three incorrect ways to state the diagnostic label, including nursing diagnoses stated as medical diagnoses, use of medical terminology to describe the cause, and statement of the nursing diagnosis as an intervention. These are errors because they shift the focus of the statement from nursing to medicine or shift the focus from the cause to the intervention. Table 8-6 states the correct nursing diagnoses and compares them with the three errors of medical diagnosis, medical terminology, and nursing intervention. As expertise with the diagnostic process is gained, the likelihood of errors is reduced, and the nurse is able to develop nursing diagnoses based on the actual or potential nursing needs of the client. Errors in the diagnostic process result in the development of an incomplete or inappropriate nursing care plan.

▌ NURSING DIAGNOSES: APPLICATION TO CARE PLANNING

The use of nursing diagnoses is a mechanism for identifying the domain of nursing. The formulated nursing diagnoses provide direction for the planning process and the selection of nursing interventions to achieve the desired outcomes. The care plan (see Chapter 9) is a mechanism for demonstrating accountability (Carlson et al, 1991; Carpenito, 1993). In addition, the nursing diagnoses and subsequent care plan assist in communicating to other professionals the client-centered problems through the nursing care plan, consultations, discharge planning, and client care conferences (Fig. 8-4).

Advantages of Nursing Diagnoses

Nursing diagnoses are advantageous for both nurses and clients. They facilitate communication among nurses about a client's level of wellness and assist in discharge planning. The health care delivery system today requires greater numbers of health care professionals. As more people become responsible for the care of a client, it is essential that these professionals are able to clearly communicate about the client's problems. Nursing diagnoses facilitate communication in several ways. The initial list of nursing diagnoses is an easily obtainable reference to the client's current health care needs. Nursing diagnoses also help prioritize the client's needs. As the nurse communicates with other professionals, the use of nursing diagnoses encourages organized communication relevant to the client's goals and priorities.

Nursing diagnoses are also used for charting in the progress notes, writing referrals, and providing effective transition of care from one unit to another, from one clinic to another, or from the hospital to the community. Discharge planning is the set of decisions and activities designed to give continuity and coordination to nursing care. Discharge planning is necessary when a client is discharged from one hospital to another or from the hospital to a community-based agency. In discharge planning, nursing diagnoses are the mechanism for communicating and delineating care the client still requires (Carpenito, 1995; Gordon, 1994).

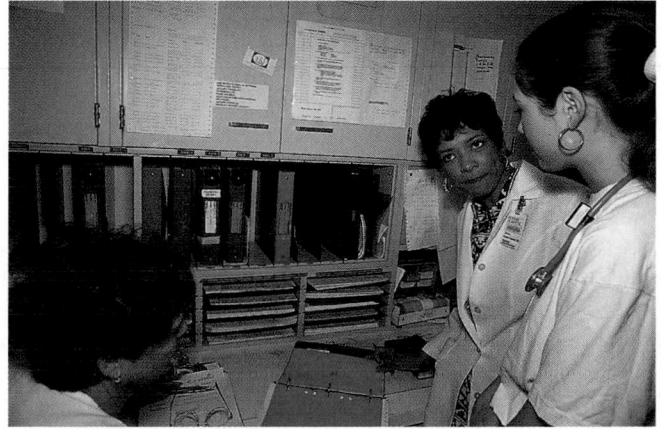

Fig. 8-4 Nurses discuss client's health care needs.

Nursing diagnoses can also serve as a focus for quality improvement (Gordon, 1994). Quality improvement is the monitoring and evaluation of process and outcomes in health care or any other business to identify opportunities for improvement. The nursing diagnosis is a method of identifying the focus of nursing activity. When focusing on the nursing diagnosis, the reviewer can determine whether nursing care was correct and delivered according to standards of practice.

The benefits of nursing diagnoses for the profession are also important for the client and family. Better communication among health care professionals helps eliminate potential problems in giving care and maintains a focus on meeting the client's health care goals. Similarly, the ultimate reason for improvement and peer review is to ensure that high-quality care is given to clients and families. Furthermore, the client benefits from the individualization of nursing care resulting from appropriate goal setting, correct selection of priorities, selection of appropriate interventions, and establishment of outcome criteria.

Limitations of Nursing Diagnoses

Nursing diagnoses have limitations, and the beginning practitioner should be aware of their existence. Because of the continuous evolution of the terms and use of nursing diagnoses, the language can occasionally be verbose and contain jargon. This may limit the use of nursing diagnoses to only nursing professionals and result in confusion among other members of the health care team (Seahill, 1991; Carpenito, 1995).

Imprecise language of the diagnosis may incorrectly "label" a client. One such diagnostic label is *noncompliance*. The term is value laden and incomplete (Stantis and Ryan, 1982; Edel, 1985).

In addition, the evolution of a standardized terminology in the form of a taxonomy has resulted in confusion about the language of the diagnostic label (Lunney, 1986; Porter, 1986). The 1986 National Conference for the Classification of Nursing Diagnosis first proposed a taxonomic structure for an organizational framework of current and future diagnostic labels (McLane, 1987). To date, the revised taxonomic structure serves as a classification system for nursing diagnosis (Carpenito, 1995).

The evolving taxonomy can limit nursing practice. Nursing diagnoses, developed by the Task Force of the National Group for the Classification of Nursing Diagnoses, are only the beginning of a total classification system. Through formulation and use of other nursing diagnoses, the taxonomy will grow and expand the focus of professional nursing.

■ KEY CONCEPTS ■

▶ The diagnostic process includes critical analysis and interpretation of data, identification of client problems, and formulation of nursing diagnoses.

▶ The interpretation of data requires the nurse to validate and cluster data.

▶ Nursing diagnoses state the actual or potential problems of the client's health status.

▶ Nursing diagnoses are written for the physical, developmental, intellectual, emotional, social, and spiritual dimensions of the client.

▶ Nursing diagnoses are necessary to develop a plan of care that will help the client and family adapt to changes resulting from an illness or change in lifestyle.

▶ Nursing diagnostic errors can occur by errors in data collection, interpretation and analysis of data, clustering of data, or in the diagnostic statement.

▶ Nursing diagnoses improve communication between nurses and other health professionals.

▶ Nursing diagnoses can serve as a focus for quality assurance and improvement and peer review.

■ KEY TERMS ■

Actual health problem, p. 128

At risk health problem, p. 128

Client-centered problems, p. 125

Critical thinking, p. 125

Defining characteristics, p. 128

Diagnostic process, p. 127

Etiology, p. 129

Medical diagnosis, p. 131

North American Nursing Diagnosis Association (NANDA), p. 125

Nursing diagnosis, p. 125

■ CRITICAL THINKING EXERCISES ■

1. Your client's nursing Kardex contains a care plan for bathing/hygiene and toileting self-care deficit related to decreased mobility of right arm. What data do you need from the assessment data base to determine whether the nursing diagnosis is relevant?

2. Using a client's assessment cluster data from the history and physical examination components, identify which trends are fully supported by data and which trends need more data. (Using multicolored highlighters can assist with this exercise.)

3. How do you organize assessment data to derive nursing diagnoses that reflect client response to illness, hospitalization, and lifestyle changes?

REFERENCES

American Nurses Association: *Model nurse practice act,* Washington, DC, 1955, The Association.

American Nurses Association: *Standards of nursing practice,* Washington, DC, 1973, The Association.

American Nurses Association: *Nursing: a social policy statement,* Washington, DC, 1980, The Association.

American Nurses Association: *Scope of nursing practice,* Washington, DC, 1987, The Association.

American Nurses Association: *Standards of clinical nursing practice,* Washington, DC, 1991, The Association.

American Nurses Association: *Nursing: a social policy statement, 1994 Revision,* Washington, DC, 1994, The Association.

Bandman EL, Bandman B: *Critical thinking in nursing,* ed 2, Norwalk, Conn, 1995, Appleton and Lange.

Benner P: *From novice to expert,* Menlo Park, Calif, 1984, Addison-Wesley.

Carlson JH et al: *Nursing diagnosis: a case-study approach,* Philadelphia, 1991, WB Saunders.

Carnevali DL et al: *Diagnostic reasoning in nursing,* Philadelphia, 1984, JB Lippincott.

Carnevali DL, Thomas MD: *Diagnostic reasoning and treatment decision making in nursing,* Philadelphia, 1993, JB Lippincott.

Carpenito LJ: *Nursing diagnoses: application to clinical practice,* ed 5, Philadelphia, 1993, JB Lippincott.

Carpenito LJ: *Nursing diagnoses: application to clinical practice,* ed 6, Philadelphia, 1995, JB Lippincott.

Edel MK: Noncompliance: an appropriate nursing diagnosis? *Nurs Outlook* 33:183, 1985.

Fry VS: The creative approach to nursing, *Am J Nurs* 53:301, 1953.

Gordon M: *Nursing diagnoses: process and practice,* New York, 1982, McGraw-Hill.

Gordon M: *Nursing diagnosis: process and application,* ed 3, St Louis, 1994, Mosby.

Hickey P: *Nursing process handbook,* St Louis, 1990, Mosby.

Hurley ME: *Classification of nursing diagnoses,* St Louis, 1986, Mosby.

Iowa Intervention Project, 1992.

Nursing interventions classification (NIC), ed 2, St Louis, 1996, Mosby.

Kim MJ, McFarland GK, McLane AM, editors: *Classification of nursing diagnoses: proceedings of the Fifth Conference (NANDA),* St Louis, 1984, Mosby.

Kim MJ, McFarland GK, McLane AM: *Pocket guide to nursing diagnoses,* ed 6, St Louis, 1995, Mosby.

Lunney M: Nursing diagnoses: refining the system, *Am J Nurs* 82:456, 1986.

McCloskey JC, Bulechek GM: *Nursing interventions classification (NIC),* ed 2, St Louis, 1996, Mosby.

McFarland GK, McFarlane EA: *Nursing diagnosis and intervention: planning for patient care,* St Louis, 1989, Mosby.

McLane AM, editor: *Classification of nursing diagnoses: proceedings from the Seventh Conference (NANDA),* St Louis, 1987, Mosby.

Nightingale F: *Notes on nursing: what it is and is not,* London, 1860, Harrison & Sons.

North American Nursing Diagnosis Association: *Proceedings of the ninth national conference,* Orlando, Fla, March 17-21, 1990.

Porter EJ: Critical analysis of NANDA nursing diagnoses taxonomy. I, *Image J Nurs Sch* 18:137, 1986.

Seahill L: Nursing diagnosis vs. goal-oriented treatment planning in child psychiatry, *Image J Nurs Sch* 23:95, 1991.

Soares O'Hearn CA: Nursing diagnosis: a phenomenological structural description and multidimensional taxonomy or typological redefinition. In Chaska N: *The nursing profession: turning points,* St Louis, 1990, Mosby.

Stantis MA, Ryan J: Noncompliance, an unacceptable diagnosis, *Am J Nurs* 82:941, 1982.

ADDITIONAL READINGS

Benner P, Tanner C: How expert nurses use intuition, *Am J Nurs* 87:23, 1987.

Carpenito LJ: *Nursing diagnoses: application to clinical practice,* ed 2, Philadelphia, 1987, JB Lippincott.

Dalton J: A descriptive study: defining characteristics of the nursing diagnosis: cardiac output, alterations in, decreased, *Image J Nurs Sch* 17:113, 1985.

Fehring RJ: Validating diagnostic labels: standardized methodology. In Hurley M, editor: *Classification of nursing diagnoses: proceedings of the Sixth Conference (NANDA),* St Louis, 1986, Mosby.

Gebbie KM, Lavin MA: Classifying nursing diagnoses, *Am J Nurs* 74:250, 1974.

Gleit CJ, Tatro S: Nursing diagnoses for healthy individuals, *Nurs Health Care* 8:456, 1981.

Gordon M: Nursing diagnoses and the diagnostic process, *Am J Nurs* 76:1298, 1976.

Gordon M: The concept of nursing diagnoses, *Nurs Clin North Am* 14:487, 1979.

Jacoby MK: The dilemma of physiological problems: eliminating the double standard, *Am J Nurs* 85:281, 1985.

Kim MJ: Nursing diagnoses in critical care, *Dimens Crit Care Nurs* 2:5, 1983.

Kim MJ: Without collaboration, what's left? *Am J Nurs* 85:281, 1985.

Martens K: Let's diagnose strengths, not just problems, *Am J Nurs* 86:192, 1986.

Miller K: *Critical thinking and nursing process,* 1996, St Louis, Mosby.

Nettle C et al: Community nursing diagnosis, *J Community Health* 6(3):135, 1989.

Popkess SA: Diagnosing your patient's strengths, *Nurs 81* 11:34, 1981.

Shamansky SL, Yanni CR: In opposition to nursing diagnosis: a minority opinion, *Image J Nurs Sch* 17:47, 1985.

Shoemaker JK: Essential features of a nursing diagnosis. In Kim MJ et al, editors: *Classification of nursing diagnoses: proceedings of the Fifth Conference (NANDA),* St Louis, 1984, Mosby.

Walker L: Nursing diagnoses and interventions: new tools to define nursing's unique role, *Nurs Health Care* 7(6):323, 1986.

## Chapter 9

Planning

Objectives

Mastery of content in this chapter will enable the student to:

▶ Define the key terms listed.

▶ Discuss the process of priority setting.

▶ Describe goal setting.

▶ List the seven guidelines of a written outcome statement.

▶ Discuss the difference between a goal and an expected outcome.

▶ Discuss the process of selecting nursing interventions.

▶ Define the three types of interventions.

▶ Discuss the differences between nurse-initiated, physician-initiated, and collaborative interventions.

▶ List the purposes of critical pathways.

▶ Describe the differences between care plans used in hospital and community health settings.

▶ Describe the similarities and differences between nursing care plans and critical pathways.

▶ Develop a care plan from a nursing assessment.

▶ List the six steps involved in consultation.

▶ Discuss the consultation process.

Nursing assessment and the formulation of nursing diagnoses initiate the planning step of the nursing process. **Planning** is a category of nursing behavior in which client-centered goals and expected outcomes are established and nursing interventions are selected to achieve the goals. During planning, priorities are set. In addition to collaborating with the client and family, the nurse consults with other members of the health care team, reviews pertinent literature, modifies care, and records relevant information about the client's health care needs and clinical management.

ESTABLISHING PRIORITIES

After formulating specific nursing diagnoses, the nurse uses critical thinking skills to establish priorities for the diagnoses by ranking them in order of importance. Priorities are established to identify the sequencing of nursing interventions when a client has multiple problems or alterations (Carpenito, 1995).

Establishing priorities is not merely a matter of numbering the nursing diagnoses on the basis of severity or physiological importance. Rather, priority selection is the method the nurse and client use to mutually rank the diagnoses in order of importance based on the client's desires, needs, and safety.

Maslow's (1970) hierarchy of needs can be one useful method for designating priorities. The hierarchy of human needs arranges the basic needs in five levels of priority (Fig. 9-1). The most basic, or first, level includes physiological needs such as air, water, and food. The second level includes safety and security needs, which involve physical and psychological security. The third level contains love and belonging needs, including friendship, social relationships, and sexual love. The fourth level encompasses esteem and self-esteem needs, which involve self-confidence, usefulness, achievement, and self-worth. The final level is the need for self-actualization, the state of fully achieving potential and having the ability to solve problems and cope realistically with life's situations. Basic physiological and safety needs are usually first priority. The nurse may encounter situations in which there are no emergent physical or safety needs, but in which high priority must be given to the psychological, sociocultural, developmental, or spiritual needs of the client (see Chapter 27).

Clients entering the health care system generally have unmet needs. For example, a person brought to an emergency room experiencing acute pneumonia has an unmet need for oxygen, the most basic physiological need. An older woman in a high-crime area may be concerned about physical safety; and, while hospitalized, may have a need for psychological security from fear that her home will be burglarized. A widowed homemaker whose children have moved away may feel that she does not belong or is not loved. Nurses in all practice settings encounter clients whose needs might be unmet. Nursing care includes helping clients, and often the family, meet these needs.

The hierarchy of needs is a useful way for nurses to plan for the needs of a client. One need may take priority over another (such as restoration of an adequate airway before education that will help the client adjust to an emotional conflict). The nurse uses priorities to organize interventions to achieve goals and expected outcomes to meet the client's needs.

Priorities are classified as high, intermediate, or low. Priorities depend on the urgency of the problem, the nature of the treatment indicated, and the interactions among the nursing diagnoses. Nursing diagnoses that, if untreated, could result in harm to the client or others have the highest priorities (Gordon, 1987, 1994). For example, risk for vi-

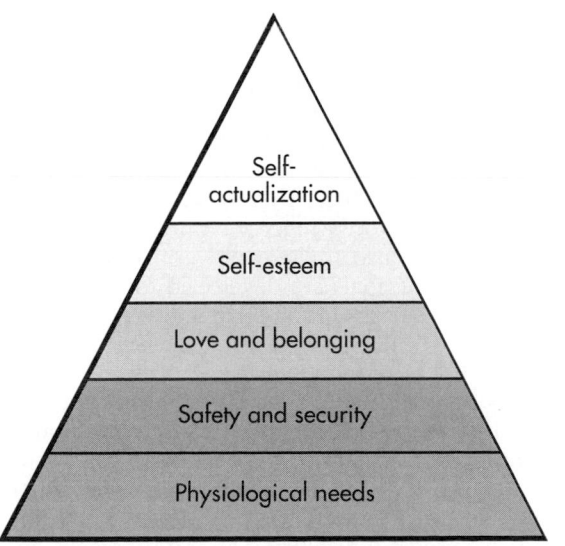

Fig. 9-1 Maslow's hierarchy of needs.

Table 9-1	Priority Setting	
Nursing Diagnoses	**Rationale**
HIGH PRIORITY	
Diarrhea related to unknown cause	Prompt resolution of diarrhea and cause prevents further decline in physiological and emotional status.
Ineffective individual coping related to anxiety of unknown diagnosis	Prompt intervention for ineffective coping will help client prepare for a diagnostic test, treatment, or diagnosis.
Ineffective airway clearance after surgery related to abdominal incisional pain	Because of the risk of postoperative pulmonary complictions, nurse will institute preventive client education early in nursing care.
INTERMEDIATE PRIORITY	
Altered nutrition: less than body requirements related to chronic diarrhea for 3 weeks	This nursing diagnosis does not affect client's immediate physiological or emotional status. Possible surgery will also assist in resolving diagnosis.
LOW PRIORITY	
Risk for infection related to history of smoking for 20 years	This nursing diagnosis reflects client's long-term needs.

olence, impaired gas exchange, and decreased cardiac output are high-priority nursing diagnoses. High priorities can occur in both the psychological and physiological dimensions, and the nurse should avoid classifying only physiological nursing diagnoses as high priority.

Intermediate priority nursing diagnoses involve the nonemergency, non–life-threatening needs of the client. Low priority nursing diagnoses are client needs that may not be directly related to a specific illness or prognosis.

Whenever possible, the client should be involved in priority setting. In some situations the client and nurse assign different priority rankings to the nursing diagnoses. If both place different values on health care needs and treatments, these differences can be resolved through open communication. However, when the client's physiological and emotional needs are at stake, the nurse needs to assume primary responsibility for setting priorities.

When the nurse uses clinical judgment and diagnostic reasoning to assign priorities to nursing diagnoses, the needs of the client, resources of the health care system, and limitations of time are considered (Kataoka-Yahiro and Saylor, 1994; Gordon et al, 1994). Table 9-1 displays priority settings and rationales. These priorities involve client needs and resources and limitations of the health care system.

■ CRITICAL THINKING AND ESTABLISHING GOALS AND EXPECTED OUTCOMES

Establishing goals and expected outcomes requires that the nurse critically evaluate the preestablished priority diagnoses, the urgency of the problems, and the resources of the client and the health care delivery system (Bandman and Bandman, 1995). Goals and expected outcomes are specific statements of client behavior or responses that the nurse anticipates from nursing care. After assessing, diagnosing, and establishing priorities about the client's health care needs, the nurse formulates goals and expected outcomes with the client for each nursing diagnosis (Gordon, 1994).

The purposes for writing goals and expected outcomes are twofold. First, goals and expected outcomes provide direction for individualized nursing interventions. Second, the goals and outcomes are used to determine the effectiveness of the interventions.

In this text, the terms *goals* and *expected outcomes* are used to indicate anticipated client responses. Fig. 9-2 illustrates the relationships among nursing diagnoses, goals, expected outcomes, and nursing interventions.

Each goal and expected outcome statement must have a time frame for evaluation. The time element depends on the nature of the problem, etiology, overall condition of the client, and treatment setting.

Goals of Care

Nursing care is planned according to nursing diagnoses and the priority set for each diagnosis. Whenever possible, the nurse and client work together in developing the goals of care. The nursing diagnoses formulated are based on the client's response and perception of changes in level of wellness, activities of daily living, lifestyle patterns, and role performance. Because each person responds uniquely to a situation, the nursing diagnoses and client goals of health care are also unique.

Individual nursing diagnoses and priority setting helps determine the goals of care. Bulechek and McCloskey (1985), define **goals** as "guideposts to the selection of nursing interventions and criteria in the evaluation of nursing interventions." Mutual goal setting is an activity that includes the client and family to prioritize the goals of care, then develop a plan of action to achieve those goals (McCloskey and Bulechek, 1994).

ROLE OF THE CLIENT IN GOAL SETTING

A **client-centered goal** is a specific, measurable objective designed to reflect the client's highest level of wellness and independence in function. Client-centered goals require active involvement by the client. Goals should be realistic and based on client needs and resources.

For clients to participate in goal setting, they should be alert and have some degree of independence in completing activities of daily living, problem solving, and decision making. When developing goals, the nurse can act as an advocate for the client to prevent further deterioration in the level of wellness or cognitive and physical functioning.

When clients' cognitive and physical impairments are so severe that they are unable to actively participate in goal setting, the nursing team acts in their behalf to develop client-centered goals. These clients may include comatose individuals, totally disoriented individuals, individuals unable to participate in decision making, and children.

Goals should not only meet the immediate needs of the client but should also include prevention and rehabilitation. Two types of goals are developed for the client; they are short-term goals and long-term goals.

SHORT-TERM GOALS

A short-term goal is an objective that is expected to be achieved in a short period of time, usually less than a week (Carpenito, 1995). With the present health care system and shorter hospital stays, short-term goals are the direction for the immediate care plan. (Long-term goals may be more appropriate for problem resolution after discharge [Carpenito, 1989]). A short-term goal for a client with ineffective air-

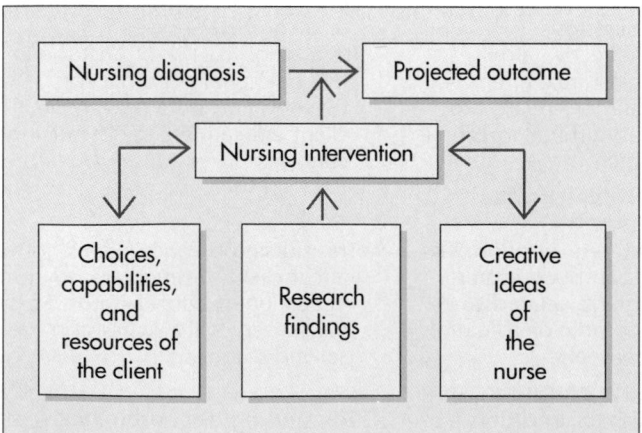

Fig. 9-2 From diagnosis to outcome. *(Redrawn from Gordon M:* Nursing diagnosis: process and application, *ed 3, St Louis, 1994, Mosby.)*

Table 9-2	Examples of Goal Setting with Expected Outcomes

NURSING DIAGNOSES	GOALS	EXPECTED OUTCOMES
Ineffective individual coping related to fear of negative prognosis	Client will openly discuss diagnosis.	Client will ask pertinent questions about diagnosis by 6/1. Client will express fears by 6/2. Client will identify at least two strategies for dealing with fears by 6/4.
Ineffective airway clearance related to incisional pain	Client's lungs will remain clear throughout postoperative period.	Client will turn, cough, and deep breathe every hour. Client achieves incentive spirometer goal of 90% every 2 hours. Client pain level remains ≤4 on a scale of 0-10.
Knowledge deficit regarding postoperative care at home related to inexperience	Client will state four postoperative risks before discharge.	Client drinks 2 to 3 L of fluid every day by 6/2. Client will name three signs of wound infection by 6/3. Client will demonstrate aseptic wound care by 6/3. Client will state home activity restrictions by 6/5.
Altered peripheral tissue perfusion related to postoperative venous status and risk for thrombophlebitis	Client will maintain adequate tissue perfusion by discharge.	Client performs active range of motion exercises every 2 hours while restricted to bed. Client's toes remain warm, dry with capillary refill of ≤2 seconds. Client increases ambulation by 50 feet every day.

way clearance, for example, may be "absence of abnormal lung sounds within 2 days."

LONG-TERM GOALS

A long-term goal is an objective that is expected to be achieved over a longer period of time, usually over weeks or months (Carpenito, 1995). Long-term goals may be carried over into discharge to skilled nursing facilities, rehabilitation settings, or return to the home. For example, a long-term goal for a client with an ineffective airway clearance may be to "remain free of upper respiratory infection for 6 months." These goals often focus on prevention, rehabilitation, discharge, and health education. Failure to set long-term goals may prevent the client from receiving continuity of care.

Goal setting establishes the framework for the nursing care plan. Table 9-2 shows the progression from nursing diagnoses to goals, which are individualized to meet client needs. Through goals, the nurse is able to provide continuity of care and promote optimal use of time and resources. Ultimately the goal leads to the development of expected outcomes.

Expected Outcomes

An **expected outcome** is the specific, step-by-step objective that leads to attainment of the goal and the resolution of the etiology for the nursing diagnosis (see Table 9-2). An outcome is a measurable change of the client's status in response to nursing care (Gordon, 1994; Carpenito, 1995).

Outcomes are the desired responses of a client's condition in the physiological, social, emotional, developmental, or spiritual dimensions. This change in condition is documented through observable or measurable client responses. The expected outcomes determine when a specific, client-centered goal has been met and later assist in evaluating the response to nursing care and resolution of the nursing diagnosis.

Expected outcomes have several functions. Projected before nursing actions are selected, expected outcomes provide a direction for nursing activities (Gordon, 1987, 1994). Outcomes include observable client behavior and measurable criteria for each goal. They also provide a projected time span for goal attainment and an opportunity to state any additional resources that may be required to achieve the goal, including additional equipment, personnel, or knowledge. Finally, the nurse uses expected outcomes as criteria to evaluate the effectiveness of nursing activities.

Expected outcomes are derived from short- and long-term client-centered goals and are based on nursing diagnoses developed (see Table 9-2). When writing expected outcomes, the nurse should ensure that the outcome statement is written in measurable behavioral terms. This allows the nurse to note specifically the behavior expected for resolution of the problem. The expected outcome statements should be written sequentially, with time frames. This provides the nurse with an order for the interventions, as well as a time reference for resolution of the problem.

Several expected outcomes are usually developed for

each goal and nursing diagnosis. The rationale for the multiple expected outcomes is that few client problems can be resolved by one nursing action. In addition, the listing of the step-by-step expected outcomes gives the nurse practical guidance in planning interventions.

Guidelines for Writing Goals and Expected Outcomes

There are seven guidelines for writing goals and expected outcomes. These seven guidelines involve client-centered, singular, observable, measurable, time-limited, mutual, and realistic factors.

CLIENT-CENTERED FACTORS

Because nursing care is directed from nursing diagnoses, the goals and expected outcomes focus on the client. These statements reflect expected client behavior and responses as a result of nursing interventions.

A common error in writing goals and expected outcomes is to write the statement as an intervention. The correct statement is, "client will ambulate in the hall three times a day." A common error is to write, "nursing assistant will ambulate client in the hall three times a day."

SINGULAR FACTORS

Each goal or expected outcome statement should address only *one* behavioral response. This singularity provides a more precise method to evaluate client response to the nursing action. An incorrect statement may read, "client's lungs will be clear to auscultation and respiratory rate will be 20/min by 8/22" and the lungs are clear but the respiratory rate is 28/min after nursing actions, it is difficult to determine whether the expected outcome has been achieved. By splitting the statement into two parts, "lungs will be clear to auscultation by 8/22" and "respiratory rate will be 20/min by 8/22," the nurse can determine specifically the outcome that has been achieved. In addition, singularity assists the nurse in modification of the care plan.

OBSERVABLE FACTORS

The desired outcome of nursing care must be observable. Through observation the nurse notes that the change has taken place. Observable changes can occur in physiological findings, the client's level of knowledge, and behavior. The results can be obtained by directly asking the client about the condition or can be observed using assessment skills. Examples of outcomes involving assessment skills are, "lungs will be clear on auscultation by 8/22" and "nonpurulent wound drainage will occur by 9/12."

MEASURABLE FACTORS

Goals and expected outcomes are written to give the nurse a standard against which to measure the client's response to nursing care. Examples are "body temperature will remain 98.6" and "apical pulse will remain between 60 and 100 beats/min." A goal or an outcome that is stated in measurable terms allows the nurse to objectively quantify changes in the client's status.

Common mistakes are made when the nurse uses vague qualifiers such as *normal, stable, acceptable,* or *sufficient* in the expected outcome statement. Vague qualifiers have different meanings to different people. Using such terms results in guesswork in determining the client's response to care. Terms specifically describing quality, quantity, frequency, and weight allow the nurse to evaluate whether the expected outcome was achieved.

TIME-LIMITED FACTORS

The time frame for each goal and expected outcome indicates when the expected response should occur. Time frames assist the nurse and client in determining that progress is being made at a reasonable rate. When the date of evaluation arrives, the nurse assesses the client to determine whether that particular expected outcome has been reached. If the outcome is unmet, but it is still appropriate for the client's care, another future evaluation date is set.

MUTUAL FACTORS

Mutual setting of goals and expected outcomes ensures that the client and nurse agree on the direction and time limits of care. Mutual goal setting can increase the client's motivation and cooperation.

During this mutual setting of goals and outcomes, the nurse does not impose personal values on the client. However, the nurse must also be aware of client safety and basic human needs. Using experience and acquired knowledge, the nurse may need to direct some of the goals and expected outcomes to keep the client physically and emotionally stable and safe.

REALISTIC FACTORS

Short, realistic goals and expected outcomes can quickly provide the client and nurse with a sense of accomplishment. In turn, this sense of accomplishment can increase the client's motivation and cooperation. When establishing realistic goals, the nurse, through assessment, must know the resources of the health care facility, family, and client; the client's physiological, emotional, cognitive, and sociocultural potential; and the economic cost and resources available to reach expected outcomes in a timely manner. Establishing goals and expected outcomes without a thorough assessment of client, environment, or resources can be frustrating to the client and nurse because the plan then contains unrealistic goals.

■ CRITICAL THINKING AND DESIGNING NURSING INTERVENTIONS

Nursing interventions, strategies, or actions are selected after goals and expected outcomes are established (see Fig. 9-2). Nursing interventions are those actions designed to assist the client in moving from the present level of health to that described in the expected outcome (Gordon, 1994). However, implementation of these interventions occurs during the implementation phase of the nursing process (see Chapter 10).

Choosing suitable nursing interventions is a decision-making process (Bulechek and McCloskey, 1990). A nursing intervention is any direct care treatment that the nurse performs on behalf of a client. These treatments include nurse-initiated, physician-initiated, and collaborative interventions for the client (McCloskey and Bulechek, 1994). The nurse critically evaluates assessment data, priorities, knowledge, and experience to select actions that will successfully meet the established goals and expected outcomes (Gordon, 1994; Gordon et al, 1994).

The nurse chooses interventions to achieve each outcome. The method of intervention selection is always the same, but the types of interventions are individualized to the client's needs. Fig. 9-2 illustrates the relationship of interventions to goals and expected outcomes.

Types of Interventions

There are three categories of nursing interventions: nurse-initiated, physician-initiated, and collaborative interventions. Category selection is based on client needs. One client may require all three categories, whereas another client may need only nurse- and physician-initiated interventions.

NURSE-INITIATED INTERVENTIONS

Nurse-initiated interventions are the response of the nurse to the client's health care needs and nursing diagnoses. This type of intervention is "an autonomous action based on scientific rationale that is executed to benefit the client in a predicted way related to the nursing diagnosis and client centered goals" (Bulechek and McCloskey, 1994). Nurse-initiated interventions involve aspects of professional nursing practice encompassed by licensure and law. These interventions require no supervision or direction from others. For example, interventions for increasing a client's knowledge about adequate nutrition or activities of daily living related to hygiene are independent nursing actions.

In delineating the scope of nursing practice, the ANA (1980) listed 10 areas in nursing's domain (see the box below). This list, with the continuing work of NANDA, Nursing Intervention Classification (NIC) project at the University of Iowa, and nurse researchers, clarifies and elaborates the realm of independent nursing practice.

Nurse-initiated interventions do not require a physician's order or an order from another professional. Physicians frequently include in their written orders the specifics of independent nursing interventions. However, according to the nurse practice acts in a majority of states, nursing actions pertaining to activities of daily living, health education, health promotion, and counseling are in the domain of nursing practice. These acts delineate the legal scope of the practice of nursing within the geographical boundaries of the jurisdiction (see Chapter 20).

PHYSICIAN-INITIATED INTERVENTIONS

Physician-initiated interventions are based on the physician's response to a medical diagnosis, and the nurse completes the physician's written orders (Bulechek and McCloskey, 1994). Administering a medication, implementing an invasive procedure, changing a dressing, and preparing a client for diagnostic tests are examples of such interventions. It is not always within the legal practice of nursing for the nurse to prescribe and order these treatments, but it is within the practice of nursing for the nurse to complete such orders and to individualize aproaches to their administration. For example, a physician may order a dressing change twice a day, an intravenous (IV) medication every 6 hours, and a bone scan for Mr. Diaz. The nurse incorporates each of these orders into Mr. Diaz's plan of care so that they are safely and efficiently completed.

Each physician-initiated intervention requires specific nursing responsibilities and technical nursing knowledge. When administering medications, the nurse is responsible for knowing the classification of the drug, its physiological action, normal dosage, side effects, and nursing interventions related to its action or side effects (see Chapter 35). Nursing interventions associated with administering medication depend on the physician's written order.

Delineation of Nursing Practice

- Self-care limitations
- Impaired functioning in areas such as rest, sleep, ventilation, circulation, activity, nutrition, elimination, skin, or sexuality
- Pain and discomfort
- Emotional problems related to illness and treatment, life-threatening events, or daily experiences such as anxiety, loss, loneliness, or grief
- Distortion of symbolic function, reflected in interpersonal and intellectual processes such as hallucinations
- Deficiencies in decision making and the ability to make personal choices
- Self-image changes required by health status
- Dysfunctional perceptual orientations to health
- Strains related to life processes such as birth, growth and development, and death
- Problematic affiliative relationships

From American Nurses Association: *Nursing: a social policy statement,* Kansas City, Mo, 1980, The Association.

CASE STUDY Ms. Kline, RN, is caring for a preoperative client, Mrs. Wells, who has the following medication order: "Atropine sulfate, 0.4 mg intramuscular at 8 AM today." Ms. Kline recalls that atropine is an anticholinergic medication and that the desired preoperative effect is to control salivation, bronchial secretions, and rhinorrhea during surgical anesthesia. She consults a resource to determine that 0.4 mg is an appropriate preoperative dose. Ms. Kline prepares Mrs. Wells for the injection and tells Mrs. Wells to expect an increase in thirst caused by medication. After administration of the drug, she observes the client for side effects such as flushing, tachycardia, restlessness, or disorientation, and she records in the client's medication administration record (MAR) that the drug has been administered. ■

With an invasive procedure or dressing change, the nurse is responsible for knowing when the procedure is necessary, the clinical skills necessary to complete it, and its expected outcome and possible side effects; the nurse is also responsible for adequate preparation of the client and proper communication of the results.

When a specific diagnostic or laboratory test is ordered by a physician, the nurse is responsible for scheduling the test, preparing the client, and knowing the normal findings and nursing implications associated with it.

COLLABORATIVE INTERVENTIONS

Collaborative interventions are therapies that require the knowledge, skill, and expertise of multiple health care professionals. For example, Mr. Joseph is a 78-year-old man who is a hemiplegic from a recent cerebrovascular accident and also has a long-term history of dementia. His cognitive functions are limited, he is at risk for problems related to impaired sensation and mobility, and he is unable to independently complete activities of daily living. In order for Mr. Joseph to maintain his present level of health, he requires specific nursing interventions to prevent pressure ulcers; physical therapy interventions to prevent musculoskeletal changes from immobility; and occupational therapy interventions for eating and hygiene needs, etc. The care for this client requires the coordination of collaborative interventions from multiple health care professionals all directed toward the long-term goal of maintaining Mr. Joseph's present level of health.

Nurse-initiated, physician-initiated, and collaborative interventions require critical nursing judgment and decision making. When encountering physician-initiated or collaborative interventions, the nurse does not automatically implement the therapy, but must determine whether it is appropriate for the client. Every nurse encounters an inappropriate or incorrect order at some time. The nurse with a strong knowledge base recognizes the error and seeks to correct it. The ability to recognize incorrect therapies is particularly important when administering medications or implementing procedures. An error can occur in writing the order or transcribing it to the Kardex or medication card. Clarifying an order is competent nursing practice, and it protects the client and members of the health care delivery system. The nurse carrying out an incorrect or inappropriate intervention is as much in error as the person who wrote or transcribed the original order, and is liable for any complications resulting from the error. Chapter 20 explains legal issues affecting nursing practice.

Selection of Interventions

When selecting interventions, the nurse, using clinical decision-making skills, deliberates about six factors to select nursing interventions for a specific client. These factors, elaborated in the box at right, include (1) characteristics of the nursing diagnosis, (2) expected outcomes, (3) research base (nursing knowledge) for the interventions, (4) feasibility of the intervention, (5) acceptability to the client, and (6) competency of the nurse (Bulechek and McCloskey, 1987, 1994). To achieve this the nurse also reviews standardized care plans, policy or procedure manuals, textbooks, and nursing and related health care literature; and collaborates with other health care professionals. During deliberation, the nurse reviews client needs, priorities, and previous experiences to select nursing interventions that have the best potential for achieving the expected outcomes. As the nurse gains experience, this deliberation process becomes more efficient and experience based (Benner, 1984).

Research of standardized care plans, policy and procedure manuals, textbooks, and nursing and related literature addresses usual problems and nursing actions for given conditions. Although they are written in general terms, the nurse may use these resources to acquire new knowledge.

Choosing Nursing Interventions

1. **Characteristics of the Nursing Diagnosis**
   - Interventions must be directed toward altering the etiological factors or signs and symptoms associated with the diagnostic label.
   - Interventions may be directed toward altering or eliminating risk factors, which are associated with **"risk for"** nursing diagnoses.
2. **Expected Outcomes**
   - Outcomes are stated in measurable terms and used to evaluate the effectiveness of the interventions.
3. **Research Base**
   - Review clinical nursing research related to diagnostic label and client problem.
   - Review articles that describe the utilization of research findings in similar clinical situations and settings.
4. **Feasibility**
   - Interaction of nursing interventions with treatments being provided by other health professionals.
   - Cost: Is intervention both clinically effective and cost efficient?
   - Time: Are time and personnel resources well managed?
5. **Acceptability to the client**
   - Treatment plan must be congruent with client's goals and health care values.
   - Mutually decided nursing goals.
   - Client must have required self-care abilities or have a person who can assist with health care.
6. **Competencies of the nurse**
   - Knowledgeable of scientific rationale for the intervention.
   - Possession of necessary psychosocial and psychomotor skill to complete interventions.
   - Ability to function within setting and effectively and efficiently use health care resources.

Modified from Bulechek GM, McCloskey JC: Nursing interventions: what they are and how to choose them, *Holistic Nurs Pract* 1(3):36, 1987.

This knowledge assists in the individualization of the intervention.

Collaboration completes the selection of interventions. Through collaboration the nurse is able to tap the best resources to individualize the nursing actions to meet the expected outcomes. During collaboration the nurse includes the client to select suitable interventions. The collaboration process is discussed in a later section of this chapter.

The Nursing Interventions Classification (NIC) project, developed at the University of Iowa, is a system to classify 336 direct care treatments that nurses perform (McCloskey and Bulechek, 1994). The purpose of the NIC is to provide standardization of language for nursing treatments, which will facilitate communication and documentation of care (Carter et al, 1995). The classification is designed to be comprehensive, including independent and collaborative interventions that cover all specialty areas (Carter et al, 1995).

Interventions are subdivided into six domains, which comprise the Taxonomy of Nursing Interventions (Table 9-3). The advantages of the taxonomy are five. First, the domains and classes help clinicians locate and select inter-

Table 9-3 | NIC TAXONOMY

DOMAIN 1	DOMAIN 2	DOMAIN 3	DOMAIN 4	DOMAIN 5	DOMAIN 6

LEVEL 1 DOMAINS

DOMAIN 1	DOMAIN 2	DOMAIN 3	DOMAIN 4	DOMAIN 5	DOMAIN 6
1. Physiological: Basic Care that supports physical functioning	**2. Physiological: Complex** Care that supports homeostatic regulation	**3. Behavioral** Care that supports psychosocial functioning and facilitates life-style changes	**4. Safety** Care that supports protection against harm	**5. Family** Care that supports the family unit	**6. Health System** Care that supports effective use of the health care delivery system

LEVEL 2 CLASSES

DOMAIN 1	DOMAIN 2	DOMAIN 3	DOMAIN 4	DOMAIN 5	DOMAIN 6
A *Activity and Exercise Management:* Interventions to organize or assist with physical activity and energy conservation and expenditure	G *Electrolyte and Acid-Base Management:* Interventions to regulate electrolyte/acid base balance and prevent complications	O *Behavior Therapy:* Interventions to reinforce or promote desirable behaviors or alter undesirable behaviors	U *Crisis Management:* Interventions to provide immediate short-term help in both psychological and physiological crises	W *Childbearing Care:* Interventions to assist in understanding and coping with the psychological and physiological changes during the childbearing period	Y *Health System Mediation:* Interventions to facilitate the interface between patient/family and the health care system
B *Elimination Management:* Interventions to establish and maintain regular bowel and urinary elimination patterns and manage complications due to altered patterns	H *Drug Management:* Interventions to facilitate desired effects of pharmacological agents	P *Cognitive Therapy:* Interventions to reinforce or promote desirable cognitive functioning or alter undesirable cognitive functioning	V *Risk Management:* Interventions to initiate risk-reduction activities and continue monitoring risks over time	X *Lifespan Care:* Interventions to facilitate family unit functioning and promote the health and welfare of family members throughout the lifespan	a *Health System Management:* Interventions to provide and enhance support services for the delivery of care
C *Immobility Management:* Interventions to manage restricted body movement and the sequelae	I *Neurologic Management:* Interventions to optimize neurologic functions	Q *Communication Enhancement:* Interventions to facilitate delivering and receiving verbal and nonverbal messages			b *Information Management:* Interventions to facilitate communication among health care providers
D *Nutrition Support:* Interventions to modify or maintain nutritional status	J *Perioperative Care:* Interventions to provide care before, during, and immediately after surgery	R *Coping Assistance:* Interventions to assist another to build on own strengths, to adapt to a change in function, or to achieve a higher level of function			
E *Physical Comfort Promotion:* Interventions to promote comfort using physical techniques	K *Respiratory Management:* Interventions to promote airway patency and gas exchange	S *Patient Education:* Interventions to facilitate learning			
F *Self-Care Facilitation:* Interventions to provide or assist with routine activities of daily living	L *Skin/Wound Management:* Interventions to maintain or restore tissue integrity	T *Psychological Comfort Promotion:* Interventions to promote comfort using psychological techniques			
	M *Thermoregulation:* Interventions to maintain body temperature within a normal range				
	N *Tissue Perfusion Management:* Interventions to optimize circulation of blood and fluids to the tissue				

© Iowa Intervention Project, 1992. In McCloskey JC, Bulechek GM: *Nursing interventions classification (NIC),* ed 2, St Louis, 1996, Mosby.

ventions appropriate to their clients. Second, it helps in the design and revision of curricula for beginning and advanced nurses. Third, the structure of the taxonomy permits numerical coding, which can facilitate computer use and ease in analysis of data (Iowa Intervention Project [IIP], 1993). This feature assists in furthering nursing knowledge through nursing research. Fourth, the taxonomy can easily be expanded to include more interventions. Last, the taxonomy provides a mechanism to effectively determine the cost of nursing care (IIP, 1993; Carter et al, 1995).

Usually the nurse will have more interventions than are necessary to meet the desired outcome. Some are discarded as inappropriate, others are adapted to the client's needs and abilities. As a result the list of possible interventions is narrowed down to those suitable to the client (Redman, 1993). These interventions are then written on the nursing care plan.

■ PLANNING NURSING CARE

There are multiple methods to communicate a client's nursing care. One is the nursing care plan, which is based on assessment data and includes the nursing diagnoses, goals, expected outcomes, and specific nursing activities and strategies. In many settings nursing care plans are being integrated into multidisciplinary plans of care. The nursing component of the plan is easily recognizable.

A second method is **critical pathways.** Critical pathways are multidisciplinary treatment plans that prescribe interventions and the time frame for achieving expected outcomes for select clients over a projected length of stay (London, 1993).

Purpose of Care Plans

The **nursing care plan** is a written guideline for client care. Written care plans document the client's health care needs, which are determined by assessment and the nursing diagnoses, goals, and expected outcomes formulated during planning. In addition, the written care plan communicates to other nurses and health care professionals the client's pertinent assessment data, a list of problems, and therapies. A written care plan decreases the risk of incomplete, incorrect, or inaccurate care.

The care plan is organized so that any nurse can quickly identify the nursing actions to be delivered. In hospitals and outpatient and community-based settings, the client often receives care from more than one nurse, physician, or allied health professional. The written nursing care plan makes possible the coordination of nursing care, subspecialty consultations, and scheduling of diagnostic tests.

The care plan can also identify and coordinate resources used to deliver nursing care. The listing of specific equipment and supplies necessary for nursing actions is an economically efficient mechanism for selecting equipment. If all equipment and supplies are included in the care plan, the nurse's time is used more effectively in providing care.

The nursing care plan enhances the continuity of nursing care by listing specific nursing actions necessary to achieve the goals of care. These nursing activities can be carried out daily. A correctly formulated nursing care plan facilitates the continuity of care from one nurse to another. As a result, all nurses have the opportunity to deliver high-quality, consistent care.

Written nursing care plans organize information exchanged by nurses in change-of-shift reports. Nurses focus these reports on nursing care and treatments delineated in care plans. At the end of shifts, nurses discuss care plans with the next care givers. Thus all nurses are able to discuss current and pertinent information about the client's care plan.

The written care plan also includes the long-term needs of the client. Incorporating the goals of the care plan into discharge planning is particularly important for a client who will be undergoing long-term rehabilitation in the community. A complete care plan enhances the continuity of nursing care between nurses in the hospital and community.

Same-day surgeries and earlier discharges from hospitals require the nurse to plan discharge needs on the care plan the moment the client enters a health care agency. Mortensen and McMullin (1986) note that incomplete assessments and the absence of measurable outcome criteria extend client stays in short-term, 1-day surgical centers. Client stays were lengthened because there were no documented, measurable criteria for discharge readiness on the postoperative nursing care plans. As a result, there was confusion among the health care team as to when the client could safely be discharged from the setting.

When developing an individualized care plan, the nurse involves the family and client. The family is a resource that can be used to help the client meet health goals. In addition, meeting some of the family's needs can improve the client's level of wellness.

The last item documented on the nursing care plan is the expected outcome criteria used in evaluation of care. Proper listing of the criteria provides the nurse with objective statements that help determine whether the goals of care have been achieved.

The complete care plan is the blueprint for nursing action. It provides direction for implementation of the plan and a framework for evaluation of the client's response to nursing actions.

Care Plans in Various Settings

The structure of the nursing care plan varies from one health care setting to another. For example, the care plan used in a hospital is different from one used in a community health setting. The nursing care plan developed for the client returning home is usually based solely on long-term health needs. In addition, the client, family, and significant others are more involved and assume more responsibility for care because the client is receiving nursing care in the home. Although the structure of the care plan varies depending on the setting, its overall purpose is to provide a written guideline for care so that the health care needs of the client and subsequent therapies are communicated among the health care team.

INSTITUTIONAL CARE PLANS

Institutional (staff) care plans are concise documents that become part of the client's medical record. Many hospitals use the Kardex nursing care plan. **Kardex** is a trade name for a card-filing system that allows quick reference to the particular needs of the client for certain aspects of nursing care. Information about medications, activity levels, level of self-care, diet, treatments, and procedures is usually included on the outside of the card. The nursing care plan is commonly placed on the inside (Fig. 9-3). Each institution has its own format for the Kardex, but the basic information contained on it is universal. The care plan section of the Kardex also has institutional variations. One institution might use a three-column nursing care plan, which includes the problem, goal, and nursing action. Another institution may incorporate a four-column nursing care plan, which includes the nursing diagnosis, goal, nursing action, and evaluation.

Computerized Care Plans. The use of computers and the need to efficiently organize the nurse's time have resulted in standardized care plans, which are forms created for a specific nursing diagnosis or clinical area (for example, coronary care, abdominal surgery, postpartum, and same-day surgery units). For example, the nurse selects a nursing diagnosis and then individualizes a care plan by making selections from menus. Each care plan lists generalized nursing diagnoses, goals, outcome criteria, and interventions for specific clients (Fig. 9-4).

After completing a nursing assessment, the nurse determines whether a standardized form should be used for that particular client. Even if the care plan is generally appropriate for a client, the nurse must add or delete information on the standardized form to individualize it for the client's needs. Failure to do so can result in incomplete and inaccurate care.

Computerized/standardized nursing care plans are a method to streamline and augment care planning, and provide documentation for third party reimbursement (Hirtzel-Trexler, 1994). They are designed to incorporate current practice guidelines to achieve the desired client outcomes for a specific group of clients. In addition these plans encourage the nurse to incorporate individual client care needs into the plan of care (Hirtzel-Trexler, 1994).

STUDENT CARE PLANS

Nursing students learn to write and use a nursing care plan as part of their education. The student care plan is essential for learning the problem-solving technique, the

Medical Diagnosis and other pertinent medical information:						1083 13160 23-4
10/25 LBP c̄ RLE Sciatica						Smith, Phil
10/26 Laminectomy L4-L5 c̄ Bone Graft						

Condition	Satis			PMH:
Allergies (Drugs, food, other)	PCN, ASA, Codeine			DM

Adm. Date 10/23	Age 64	Religion Cath.	Mode of Travel
Service Ortho	Doctor Ford	Resident Kowalski	Intern

FREQUENTLY ORDERED ITEMS		Date	Specimens/Daily Lab	Date	Treatments
Temp. Pulse & Resp.	> q4°	10/25	Adm. Blood work	10/24	BR and Logroll q2°
BP		10/25	UA c̄ Micro		
		10/25	BS		
I & O	q8°				
Weights					
Spot Checks					
Chest P.T.					
Incentive Spirometer					
P.T.					

ACTIVITIES		NUTRITION		Date	Diagnostic Procedures		
Ad lib		Diet Regular					
Ambulate	X2						
Chair							
BRP				10/25	Myelogram		
Bedrest					CT Scan		
Bath	Feedings			10/25	CXR		
Self				10/25	ECG		
Tub	Assist c̄ meals						
Shower	FLUID BALANCE						
Bed ✓	Force						
Assist.	D E N						
	Restrict						
	D E N						

Orderlies Needed	
Family:	

NURSING CARE PLAN

Date	Nursing Diagnosis	Expected Outcomes	Nursing Plan/Orders
10/26	Pain related to incisional Swelling	1. Client requests for pain med. decreases by 10/28. 2. Client respiratory expansion ↑ by 10/27.	1. Encourage client to Log Roll when turning. 2. Instruct client in relaxation exercizes.
10/27	Impaired physical mobility related to pain	1. Client increases ambulation from BID to QID or greater by 10/28. 2. Client assumes ADL by 10/29.	1. Ambulate in Hall c̄ client 20 min. after administration of analgesic. 2. Encourage family to walk client. 1. Allow client extra time to do self-care for hygiene needs.

Discharge Planning:	Destination:	Transportation:	Probable Date:	Referral Agencies:	Appointment:
				Supplies:	

Patient Name	

Fig. 9-3 Nursing care plan on a nursing Kardex.

NURSING STANDARD CARE PLAN

Nursing Diagnosis: INEFFECTIVE BREATHING PATTERN

Related to: _____
(respiratory muscle fatigue, anxiety, pain, impaired respiratory
mechanics such as chest tubes, incisions, anatomy)

Date Initiated/ Initials	Expected Outcomes	Date to be Met/Initials	Date Met/ Initials
_____	Patient will verbalize understanding of _____ .	_____	_____
_____	Patient will demonstrate ability to perform _____ .	_____	_____
_____	Patient will pace and schedule activities.	_____	_____
_____	Patient will use relaxation techniques for breating control.	_____	_____
_____	Patient will maintain respiratory rate of _____ with PaC02 of _____ .	_____	_____
_____	Other: _____	_____	_____

Relevant baseline data: _____
_____

Referrals: (date contacted)

☐ Nurse Specialist: _____   ☐ Home Care: _____   ☐ Social Work: _____
☐ Other: _____   ☐ Other: _____

Date Initiated/ Initials	Nursing Interventions	Date Inactivated/ Initials
	1. Assess respiratory function for rapid, shallow, irregular, or slow breathing, dyspnea, use of accessory muscles, breath sounds, restlessness, confusion, and cyanosis every _____ .	
	2. Monitor patient's mental status/LOC every _____ .	
_____ _____ _____	3. Maintain adequate airway by: ☐ a. cough/splinting every _____ ☐ b. suction every _____ ☐ c. incentive spirometry every _____	_____ _____ _____
	4. Pace and schedule activity to avoid dyspnea resulting from fatigue. Schedule is _____ _____	
	5. Provide physical and emotional support during episodes of respiratory distress by: _____	
_____ _____ _____ _____ _____	6. Provide teaching specific to patient or support person's needs. Initiate individual plan: ☐ a. pursed lip breathing ☐ b. coughing/splinting techniques (specify) _____ _____ ☐ c. relaxation techniques (specify) _____ _____ ☐ d. diaphragmatic breathing _____ _____ ☐ e. other: _____ _____	_____ _____ _____ _____ _____
_____ _____ _____ _____	7. Other interventionsl specific to patient: a. _____ b. _____ c. _____ d. _____	_____ _____ _____ _____
	Signature/Initials: _____	

☐ **PLAN OF CARE MUTUALLY SET WITH PATIENT AND/OR FAMILY.**

Fig. 9-4 Standardized nursing care plan. *(Courtesy Barnes-Jewish Hospital, St Louis, Mo.)*

Table 9-4	Scientific Rationale for the Student Care Plan

NURSING DIAGNOSIS: **Risk for impaired skin integrity** related to immobility resulting from coma
DEFINITION: Risk for impaired skin integrity is the state in which an individual's skin is at risk of being adversely altered.*

ASSESSMENT	GOALS	IMPLEMENTATION	RATIONALE	EXPECTED OUTCOMES
Fever: higher than 102° F for 72 hours Diaphoresis Incontinence of urine	Skin remains intact Absence of decreased muscle mass over bony prominences	Turn client every 2 hours in following sequence: 8 AM—supine 10 AM—left side Noon—prone Repeat, beginning with supine position.	Critical time for skin tissue breakdown is between 1 and 2 hours of constant pressure.†	No skin breakdown is noted. Skin color, temperature, and capillary return are normal. Client is afebrile.
Decreased skin turgor No skin breakdown noted		Keep client's skin dry at all times.	Moisture increases maceration of skin and promotes bacterial growth.‡	Skin remains dry and intact. Skin turgor is improved.

*Data from Kim MJ, McFarland GK, McLane AM: *Pocket guide to nursing diagnoses*, ed 5, St Louis, 1995, Mosby.
†Data from Bereck KH: *Nurs Clin North Am* 10(1):160, 1975
‡Data from Kavchack-Keys MA: *Nurs 77* 7:60, 1977.

nursing process, skills of written communication, and organizational skills needed for nursing care. Most important, by using the nursing care plan students can apply the knowledge gained from nursing and medical literature and the classroom to a practice situation.

The student care plan is more elaborate than a care plan in a hospital or community health care agency because its purpose is to teach the process of planning care. To learn the care planning process, the student must progress in a step-by-step manner, beginning with assessment and ending with evaluation. Student care plans vary from one educational program to another and between beginning and more advanced students. Some educational institutions model the student care plan on the care plan used in the affiliated health care agency. The only modification may be that the instructor requires the beginning student to include the scientific rationale for the nursing interventions selected (Table 9-4). A **scientific rationale** is the reason that, based on supporting literature, a specific nursing action was chosen.

CARE PLANS FOR COMMUNITY-BASED SETTINGS

Planning care for clients in community-based settings, for example, clinics, community centers, or clients' homes, involves using the same principles of nursing practice. However, in these settings the nurse must complete a more comprehensive community, home, and family assessment. In this setting, the client/family unit is in equal partnership with health care professionals (Bond, Phillips, and Rollins, 1994). Ultimately the client/family must be able to independently provide the majority of health care. The nurse designs a plan to (1) educate client/family about the necessary care techniques, (2) teach client/family how to integrate care within family activities, and (3) allow client/family to assume a greater percentage of care in graduated increments (Bond, Phillips, and Rollins, 1994; Lund, 1994). Last, the plan is designed to include nurses' and the client's/family's evaluation of expected outcomes.

Critical Pathways

Critical pathways allow staff from all disciplines, such as medicine, nursing, and pharmacy, to develop integrated care plans for a projected length of stay for clients with a specific case type (Fig. 9-5). The pathways clearly communicate the standard of care for a client. For example, the pathway here is for a lung transplant evaluation, which recommends on a day-by-day basis the client's activities, consults, procedures, discharge planning, and educational topics expected for the client's progression through the transplantation process. The nurse and other health team members use the pathway to monitor a client's progress and as a documentation tool. The pathway can be individualized. The pathway also helps staff make decisions on an ongoing basis to ensure the client's progress. Due to the arrival of managed care (see Chapter 2), documentation tools that integrate the standards of care for multiple disciplines are necessary. Critical pathways meet this need, and charting by exception is frequently the method of choice (see Chapter 12). When using critical pathways to plan care, many other forms, for example, nursing care plans, nurses notes, and teaching forms, are eliminated because all the pertinent components are included on the pathway format.

▍WRITING THE NURSING CARE PLAN

As an initial step in planning, the nurse assigns a priority to each nursing diagnosis; priority can be based on Maslow's hierarchy of needs, urgent client physiological and safety needs, and important needs perceived by the client. The nursing diagnosis with the highest priority is the beginning point for the nursing care plan and is followed by other nursing diagnoses in order of assigned priority.

When using the five-column plan, in the assessment column (column 1), the nurse includes all data relevant to the corresponding nursing diagnosis. The nurse includes the previously developed goals in the next column (column 2). At this point, the nurse begins to translate the short- and

Text continued on p. 152.

1

BARNES

CARE PATH®
501
LUNG TRANSPLANT EVALUATION

SERVICE		PHYSICIAN		
PRIMARY NURSE		PRIMARY NURSE		
DC DATE	ADM DATE	DATE OF SURGERY	**A-8**	

Problem Number	PATIENT PROBLEMS / NURSING DIAGNOSES
#1	LACK OF KNOWLEDGE R/T LUNG TRANSPLANT EVALUATION EXPERIENCE
#2	DECREASE IN EXERCISE CAPACITY R/T IMPAIRED OXYGENATION/VENTILATION/DECONDITIONING
#3	POTENTIAL FOR ALTERATION IN COPING R/T SITUATIONAL CRISIS/TRANSITION
#4	POTENTIAL FOR ALTERATION IN FAMILY PROCESSES R/T SITUATIONAL CRISIS/TRANSITION
#5	POTENTIAL FOR ALTERATION IN NUTRITION R/T INAPPROPRIATE INTAKE/DYSPNEA
#6	IMPAIRED GAS EXCHANGE R/T ALVEOLAR-CAPILLARY MEMBRANE CHANGE/ALTERED BLOOD FLOW *IF APPROPRIATE

#	1 - 12	1 - 12	1 - 2, 6 - 8, 12	2, 10, 12	1
	ASSESSMENT / MONITORING	CONSULTS	PROCEDURES / TEST	TREATMENT	ACTIVITY
PRE ADMIT		Transplant office to preschedule following as needed for pt.: 2-D Echo, Quant. V-Q, Resting RVG, PFTs, MRI, Cardiac Cath, Chest CT, Transesophageal echocardiogram			
DAY 1	Braden scale Respiratory status Fall prevention Assess/individualize pt. problem list	Notify consults as per orders. Check with transplant P.A. for additional tests which may be needed. SMA 6 and 12, CBC, CMV, HSV, EBV, Vz titers, HbsAq, HbsAb, HIV, Hep. A, Hep. C titers, T & S, PT, PTT HLA (A,B,C,DR) Typing, incl. cytotoxic screen, u/a - routine & micro, CXR-AP & lat	Apply skin tests 07 ⎫ 08 ⎬ Nursing, Pulm. Rehab., & H.O. 09 ⎭ 10 11 ⎫ 12 ⎬ Psychologist 13 ⎭ 14 ⎫ CDL 15 ⎬ 16 ⎫ PFTs 17 ⎬ ⎫ Chaplain 18 ⎭ 19 Cardiology Consult 20	Appropriate bed surface for Braden scale O₂ • At rest • Activity _____ CPT x1 x2 x3 x4 by Nursing, Physical Therapy, family Aerosols x1 x2 x3 x4 (Self)	Continue activity as done at home
	SIGNATURE	INIT.	SIGNATURE	INIT.	SIGNATURE	INIT.

Fig. 9-5 Critical pathway. *(Courtesy Barnes-Jewish Hospital, St Louis.)*

			2

BARNES

CARE PATH®
501
LUNG TRANSPLANT EVALUATION

CNS	DIETARY	RT	
HOME HEALTH	OT	OTHER	
PT	SW	OTHER	**A-8**

Problem Number	PATIENT PROBLEMS / NURSING DIAGNOSES
#7	POTENTIAL FOR INEFFECTIVE AIRWAY CLEARANCE R/T EXCESSIVE SECRETIONS/FATIGUE
#8	INEFFECTIVE BREATHING PATTERN R/T INCREASED WORK OF BREATHING
#9	POTENTIAL FOR INFECTION R/T ALTERED NUTRITION/CHRONIC DISEASE
#10	POTENTIAL FOR INJURY R/T PHYSICAL DECONDITIONING
#11	SPIRITUAL DISTRESS R/T CHALLENGED BELIEF AND VALUE SYSTEM
#12	POTENTIAL FOR ALTERED SKIN INTEGRITY R/T POOR NUTRITION/DECREASED MOBILITY

1	1, 5, 9, 12	1 - 12	1 - 12	1, 2, 4, 11	INITIALS (SEE KEY AT BOTTOM)		
MEDS / IVS	**NUTRITION**	**PATIENT / FAMILY EDUCATION**	**DISCHARGE PLANNING**	**PSYCHOSOCIAL/ EMOTIONAL/ SPIRITUAL NEEDS**			
		Give LTE manual, 6200 pt. letter.					
Pt. to do self meds.; Initiate IV access within 2 hrs. of admission	Continue home diet	Lung transplant evaluation Review tests for day 1 & 2 Personalize instruction to pts. individual learning needs. **Pt./family able to verbalize purpose and any special preparation for follow-up care for tests.**	Plan of care has been mutually set with pt./ family. Educational and DC planning needs will be assessed. **Pt./family verbalizes understanding of care path.**	Allow pt./ family to verbalize concerns and questions and relate problems back to appropriate discipline.			

SIGNATURE	INIT.	SIGNATURE	INIT.	SIGNATURE	INIT.

Fig. 9-5, cont'd Critical pathway.

Continued

#	1 - 12	1 - 12		1 - 2, 6 - 8, 12	2, 10, 12
	ASSESSMENT / MONITORING	CONSULTS	PROCEDURES / TESTS	TREATMENT	ACTIVITY
DAY 2		Start 24 hr. urine	07 08 09 } Psychol-ogist 10 11 } V-Q } Tread mill 12 13 14 15 } PTFs 16 } Dr. 17 Trulock 18 19 20	Appropriate bed surface for Braden scale O_2 • At rest _____ • Activity _____ CPT x1 x2 x3 x4 by Nursing, Physical Therapy, family Aerosols x1 x2 x3 x4 (Self)	
DAY 3		Complete 24 hr. urine - creatinine, cr. cl. Labs: HDL chol. battery, fasting glu-cose Serum Creatinine	07 08 09 10 } PT 11 } nutrition 12 13 } Tread mill 14 15 } RVG 16 17 18 } Cath. 19 } consult 20	Appropriate bed surface for Braden scale O_2 • At rest _____ • Activity _____ CPT x1 x2 x3 x4 by Nursing, Physical Therapy, family Aerosols x1 x2 x3 x4 (Self)	
DAY 4		**Social Work, Physical Therapy, Pulm. Rehab. follow-up; Cardiac Cath**	07 08 09 10 } Cardiac cath.; 11 } follow-up by 12 } Social Worker, 13 } PT, 14 } Rehab. 15 } Nutrition, 16 } Transplant 17 } Coordinator 18 19 20	Appropriate bed surface for Braden scale O_2 • At rest _____ • Activity _____ CPT x1 x2 x3 x4 by Nursing, Physical Therapy, family Aerosols x1 x2 x3 x4 (Self)	
DAY 5 DISCHARGE		**Home Care/DC follow-up instruction from consults: Physical Therapy, Pulm. Rehab. Social Work** **Pt. is to see Dr. Patterson or designee prior to DC**		Appropriate bed surface for Braden scale O_2 • At rest _____ • Activity _____ CPT x1 x2 x3 x4 by Nursing, Physical Therapy, family Aerosols x1 x2 x3 x4 (Self) **Pt./family able to perform home treatment plan.**	**Pt./family able to verbalize plans to implement out-pt./home exercise program**
	SIGNATURE	INIT.	SIGNATURE	INIT.	SIGNATURE	INIT.

Fig. 9-5, cont'd Critical pathway.

1	1, 5, 9, 12	1 - 12	1 - 12	1, 3, 4, 11	INITIALS (SEE KEY AT BOTTOM)		
MEDS / IVS	NUTRITION	PATIENT / FAMILY EDUCATION	DISCHARGE PLANNING	PSYCHOSOCIAL/ EMOTIONAL/ SPIRITUAL NEEDS			
		Review tests for days 2 & 3					
		Review tests for days 3 & 4					
		Review tests for days 4 & 5	Social Work to begin planning for home O$_2$ and other resources.	Pt. identifies caregivers and/or emotional support systems. Pt./family anticipate possible lifestyle change. Pt. develops with chaplain faith/values component of ongoing recovery plan.			
d/c IV **IV site free of phlebitis** **Verbalize understanding of home medications.**	**Tolerating PO intake**	**Verbalizes understanding of home care instructions from physiotherapy, nutrition, Social Work and Pulm. Rehab.**	Social Work to finalize plans for transportation/ equipment. Pt./family is ready for DC and has necessary information/ oxygen and equipment for care.	Pt. able to express feelings r/t Transplant program and disease process.			
SIGNATURE	INIT.	SIGNATURE	INIT.	SIGNATURE			INIT.

Fig. 9-5, cont'd Critical pathway.

long-term goals into action plans that anticipate the needs of the client, coordinate nursing care, and select appropriate nursing measures.

The nurse writes the action plan in the implementation column (column 3) of the care plan. Each nursing action is written to include information necessary to implement nursing care. It may help the beginning nurse to ask whether the stated interventions answer the following questions:

1. *What* is the intervention?
2. *When* should each intervention be implemented?
3. *How* should the intervention be performed?
4. *Who* should be involved in each aspect of intervention?

In addition, the nurse should understand the rationale (column 4) for a specific intervention. Nonspecific nursing interventions result in incomplete or inaccurate nursing care, lack of continuity among care givers, and poor use of resources.

Common omissions in writing nursing interventions include action, frequency, quantity, method, or person to perform them. These errors can occur if the nurse is unfamiliar with the planning process. Table 9-5 illustrates these types of errors by showing incorrect and correct statements of nursing interventions.

Column 5 of the nursing care plan contains the projected outcome criteria previously identified. Listing the criteria on the care plan gives a written estimation of when the goal of care has been achieved, thus indicating when a particular nursing diagnosis is no longer relevant to the client's plan of care.

■ WRITING CRITICAL PATHWAYS

The writing of a critical pathway is a lengthy process, involving all members of a multidisciplinary health care team. Staff who are most familiar with a select client group develop the comprehensive clinical guidelines for managing the client's care. Consideration is given to best clinical practices, appropriate use of resources (such as lab tests), and expected outcomes. The resultant pathway reflects each discipline's clinical standards. Critical pathways are a case management tool, which delineates client outcomes within specific time frames (Windle, 1994). To write and use a critical pathway the nurse must understand each component of the nursing process (Zander and McGill, 1994).

Critical pathways delineate specific care, but also provide a mechanism for timely revision of the plan of care (Zander, 1988). This method of care delivery reframes the work of nursing so that it is clear to the health care team as well as to the client and family (Zander, 1988; Zander and McGill, 1994). When writing a critical pathway the nurse must be familiar with other pathways developed in the agency, and the literature as it is related to a specific disease or surgical procedure. The pathway delineates related nursing diagnoses and interventions. Expected outcomes are developed during the planning phase, and a specific time interval for achieving the outcome is included. In addition, the critical pathway is written so that all members of the health care team can document delivery of care or changes in status (see Chapter 12).

■ CONSULTING OTHER HEALTH CARE PROFESSIONALS

Planning nursing care involves consultation with other members of the health care team (Fig. 9-6). Consultation may occur at any step in the nursing process, but it is needed most often in the planning and intervention steps when the nurse is more likely to identify a problem requiring additional knowledge, skills, or resources (Lund, 1994).

Table 9-5	Frequent Errors in Writing Nursing Interventions	
TYPE OF ERROR	**INCORRECTLY STATED NURSING INTERVENTION**	**CORRECTLY STATED NURSING INTERVENTION**
Failure to precisely or completely indicate nursing actions	Nurse assistant will turn client every 2 hours.	Nurse assistant will turn client every 2 hours, using the following schedule: 8 AM—supine, 10 AM—left side, Noon—prone, 2 PM—right side. Repeat at 4 PM and 2 AM
Failure to indicate frequency	Nurse assistant will observe client cough and deep breathe.	Nurse assistant will observe client cough and deep breathe at 10 AM—2 PM—6 PM—10 PM.
Failure to indicate quantity	Primary nurse will provide hydrogen peroxide (H_2O_2) mouthwash to client every 2 hours while awake: 8-10-12-2-4-6-8-10.	Primary nurse will provide 50 ml of H_2O_2 mouthwash to client every 2 hours while awake: 8-10-12-2-4-6-8-10.
Failure to indicate method	Primary nurse will change client's dressing once a shift: 6 AM—2 PM—10 PM.	Primary nurse will replace client's dressing, with Neosporin ointment to wound and two dry 4 × 4 dressings secured with hypoallergenic tape, once a shift: 2 PM—10 PM—6 AM.
Failure to indicate person to perform the action	Irrigate nasogastric (NG) tube every 2 hours (even) round the clock with 30 ml of normal saline (NS).	Primary nurse will irrigate NG tube every 2 hours (even) around the clock with 30 ml NS.

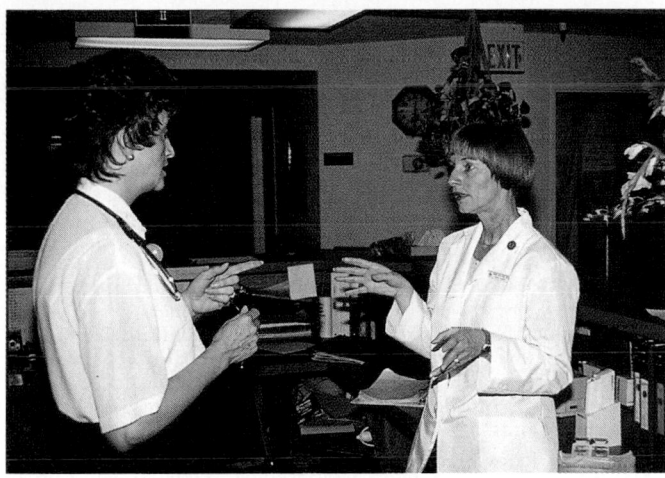

Fig. 9-6 Consultation and planning care.

Consultation is a process in which the expertise of a specialist is sought to identify ways to handle problems in client management or the planning and implementation of programs. Consultation is based on the problem-solving approach, and the consultant is the stimulus for change.

In clinical nursing, consultation is used to solve problems in the delivery of nursing care or the use of resources. Nurse consultants are most frequently approached for advice about difficult clinical problems. Nurses are consulted for their clinical expertise, client education skills, or staff education skills.

Nurses also consult with other members of the health care team, such as physical therapists, nutritionists, and social workers. Again, the consultant focuses on problems in nursing.

When to Consult

The need for consultation in nursing occurs when the nurse has identified a problem that cannot be solved using personal knowledge, skills, and resources. Consultation increases the nurse's knowledge about the problem and helps in learning skills and obtaining the resources needed to solve the problem. After the consultation, the nurse may be able to resolve similar problems in the future. For example, a nurse encountering a client with a recent colostomy might request a consultation from an enterostomal therapist to determine the materials needed to clean the colostomy site and the specific techniques to use during the procedure.

Consultation is also used when the exact problem remains unclear. A consultant objectively entering a situation can more clearly assess and identify the exact nature of the problem, whether it is client, personnel, or equipment oriented. An unbiased consultant can often objectively identify the problem and outline a method for resolving it.

How to Consult

The first step in the consultation process is identification of the general problem area, which will give the consultant a starting point for identifying the problem. Second, the consultation should be directed to the appropriate professional, who may be another nurse or another member of the health care team.

Third, the nurse provides the consultant with pertinent information and resources about the problem area. Pertinent information includes a brief summary of the problem, methods used to resolve the problem, and the outcome of those methods. Other resources can include the client's medical record, nurses and other members of the health team, and the client's family.

Fourth, the nurse should not provide biased information to the consultant. Consultants are in the clinical setting to identify and resolve a nursing problem, and biasing them can hinder problem resolution. Bias can be avoided by not overloading consultants with subjective and emotional conclusions about the client and problem.

Fifth, the nurse requesting consultation should be available to discuss the findings and recommendations. When a consultation is requested, the nurse provides a private, comfortable atmosphere in which the consultant and client can meet. However, this does not mean that the nurse leaves the environment. A common mistake is turning the whole problem over to the consultant. The consultant is not there to take over the problem, but is there to assist the nurse in resolving it. The nurse requesting assistance should request the consultation for a day when both are scheduled to work and a time when distractions are minimal.

Finally, the nurse incorporates the consultant's recommendations into the care plan. The success of the advice depends on the implementation of the problem-solving techniques suggested.

Consultants are a valuable adjunct to nursing care. In clinical nursing practice, competent and experienced nurses encounter problems beyond their knowledge or experience. Professional and competent nurses recognize their limitations, seek appropriate consultation, and learn from the findings and recommendations.

■ KEY CONCEPTS ■

▶ During the planning component, client goals are determined and prioritized, expected outcomes of nursing care are developed, and a nursing care plan is written.

▶ Nursing care is planned and organized around specific nursing diagnoses, resulting in individualized care plans.

▶ Goals include prevention, rehabilitation, and addressing the crisis or urgent needs of the client.

▶ Goal setting establishes a framework for the care plan.

▶ Using expected outcomes, the nurse evaluates the effectiveness of the care plan.

▶ The care plan is a written guideline for client care so

that the care given can be quickly understood by all members of the health care team.

▶ Critical pathways are multidisciplinary treatment plans that predict the interventions and outcomes to be met for selected clients over a projected length of stay.

▶ Care plans and critical pathways increase communication among nurses and facilitate the continuity of care from one nurse to another and from one health care setting to another.

▶ The planning of individualized care requires involvement of the client and family.

▶ The care plan is a method for teaching students to transfer knowledge gained from nursing and medical literature and the classroom into practical experience.

▶ Poorly written plans for care result in incomplete or inaccurate nursing care, lack of continuity among care givers, and poor use of resources.

▶ Correctly written nursing interventions include actions, frequency, quantity, method, and the person to perform them.

▶ Nurse-initiated or independent nursing interventions can solve the client's problems without consultation or collaboration with physicians or other health care professionals.

▶ Physician-initiated or dependent nursing interventions are completed with a physician's order, but require nursing judgment or decision making.

▶ Planning nursing care often involves consultation with other members of the health care team.

■ KEY TERMS ■

Client-centered goal, p. 138

Collaboration, p. 142

Collaborative interventions, p. 142

Consultation, p. 153

Critical pathway, p. 144

Expected outcome, p. 139

Goals, p. 138

Kardex, p. 144

Nurse-initiated interventions, p. 141

Nursing care plan, p. 144

Physician-initiated interventions, p. 141

Planning, p. 137

Scientific rationale, p. 147

■ CRITICAL THINKING EXERCISES ■

1. How do you link goals and expected outcomes of nursing care from nursing diagnoses?

2. What criteria do you use to determine expected outcomes for a given set of client-centered goals?

3. What information do you need to plan nursing interventions for your clients? If you had nursing assistants, how would you plan those nursing strategies that could be delegated to these persons?

REFERENCES

American Nurses Association: *Nursing: a social policy statement,* Kansas City, Mo, 1980, The Association.

Bandman EL, Bandman B: *Critical thinking in nursing,* ed 2, Norwalk, Conn, 1995, Appleton & Lange.

Benner P: *From novice to expert: excellence and power in clinical nursing practice,* Menlo Park, Calif, 1984, Addison-Wesley.

Bereck KH: *Nurs Clin North Am* 10(1):160, 1975.

Bond N, Phillips P, Rollins JA: Family-centered care at home for families with children who are technology dependent, *Pediatric Nursing* 20:123, 1994.

Bulechek GM, McCloskey JC: *Nursing interventions: treatments for nursing diagnoses,* Philadelphia, 1985, WB Saunders.

Bulechek GM, McCloskey JC: Nursing interventions: what they are and how to choose them, *Holistic Nurs Pract* 1(3):36, 1987.

Bulechek GM, McCloskey JC: Nursing intervention taxonomy development. In McCloskey JC, Grace H, eds, *Current issues in nursing,* ed 3, St Louis, 1990, Mosby.

Bulechek GM, McCloskey JC: Nursing interventions classification: defining nursing care. In McCloskey JC, Grace H, eds: *Current issues in nursing,* ed 4, St Louis, 1994, Mosby.

Carpenito LJ: *Nursing diagnosis application to clinical practice,* ed 3, Philadelphia, 1989, JB Lippincott.

Carpenito LJ: *Nursing diagnosis application to clinical practice,* ed 6, Philadelphia, 1995, JB Lippincott.

Carter et al: Using the nursing interventions classification to implement Agency for Health Care Policy and Research guidelines, *J Nurs Care Qual* 9(2):76, 1995.

Gordon M: *Nursing diagnosis: process and application,* ed 2, New York, 1987, McGraw-Hill.

Gordon M: *Nursing diagnosis: process and application,* ed 3, St Louis, 1994, Mosby.

Gordon M et al: Clinical judgement: an integrated model, *Adv Nurs Sci* 16:55, 1994.

Hirtzel-Trexler BJ: Commentary on practice guidelines: a standard whose time has come, *AONE's Leadership Perspectives* 2(2):22, 1994.

Iowa Intervention Project, 1992.

Iowa Intervention Project (IIP): The NIC taxonomy structure, *Image: Journal of Nursing Scholarship, 25:*187, 1993.

Kataoka-Yahiro M, Saylor C: A critical thinking model for nursing judgment, *J Nurs Educ* 33(8):351, 1994.

Kavchack-Keys MA: *Nurs 77* 7:60, 1997.

Kim MJ, McFarland GK, McLane AM: *Pocket guide to nursing diagnosis,* ed 5, St Louis, 1995, Mosby.

London J: On the right path: collaborative case management makes nurses partners in the care-planning process, *Health Progress* 74(5):36, 1993.

Lund SM: Family-centered nurse coordinator-early childhood intervention: development and implementation of the CNS role, *Clinical Nurse Specialist* 8:109, 1994.

Maslow AH: *Motivation and personality,* ed 2, New York, 1970, Harper & Row.

McClosky JC, Bulechek GM: Standardizing the language for nursing treatments: an overview of the issues, *Nurs Outlook* 42:56, 1994.

Mortensen M, McMullin C: Discharge score for surgical outpatients, *Am J Nurs* 86:1347, 1986.

Redman BK: *The Process of Patient Education,* ed 7, St Louis, 1993, Mosby.

Windle PE: Critical pathways: an integrated documentation tool, *Nurs Management* 25(9):80F, 1994.

Zander K: Nursing case management-resolving the DRG paradox, *Nurs Clin North Am* 23:503, 1988.

Zander K, McGill R: Critical and anticipated recovery paths: only the beginning, *Nurs Management* 25(8):34, 1994.

ADDITIONAL READINGS

Hendrix MJ, LaGodna GE: Consultation: a political process aimed at change. In Lancaster J, Lancaster W, eds: *Concepts for advanced clinical nursing practice,* St Louis, 1982, Mosby–Year Book.

Pilcher MW: Post-discharge care: how to follow-up, *Nurs 86* 16:50, 1986.

Sanborn CW, Blount M: Standard plans for care and discharge, *Am J Nurs* 84:1394, 1984.

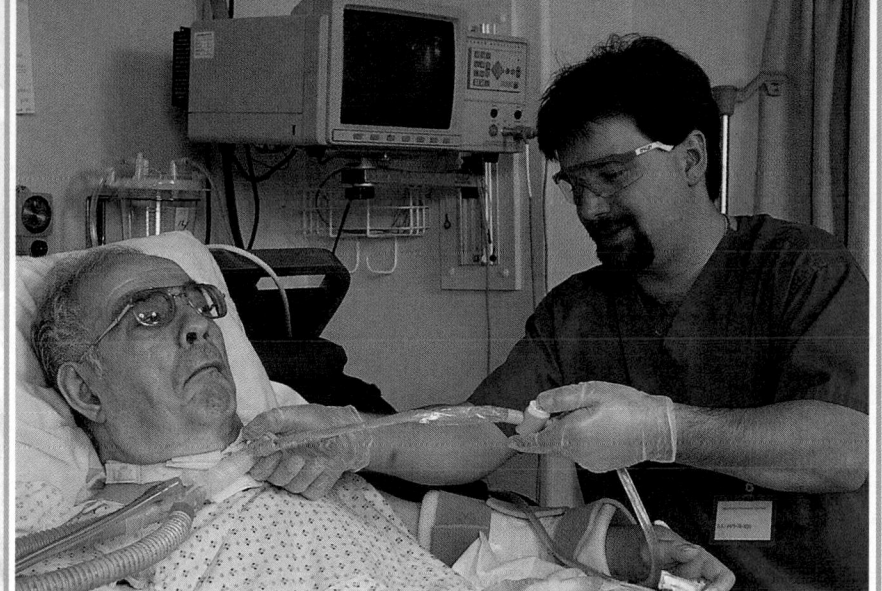

 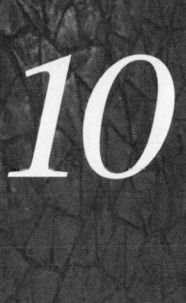
Implementation

Objectives

Mastery of content in this chapter will enable the student to:

▶ Define the key terms listed.

▶ Discuss the differences between protocols and standing orders.

▶ Describe the information-processing model for selecting nursing interventions.

▶ List and discuss the five steps of the implementation process.

▶ Describe the five different implementation methods.

▶ Select appropriate implementation methods for an assigned client.

Implementation, a component of the nursing process, is a category of nursing behavior in which the actions necessary for achieving the goals and expected outcomes of nursing care are initiated and completed. In theory, implementation of the nursing care plan follows the planning component of the nursing process. However, in many health care settings implementation may begin directly after assessment. For example, immediate implementation is necessary when the nurse identifies urgent needs of the client, in situations such as cardiac arrest, sudden death of a loved one, or loss of a home in a fire.

Implementation includes performing, assisting, or directing the performance of activities of daily living, counseling and teaching the client or family, giving direct care to achieve client-centered goals, supervising and evaluating the work of staff members, and recording and exchanging information relevant to the client's continued health care.

In noncrisis situations, implementation begins after the care plan has been developed and focuses on the initiation of nursing interventions to achieve the goals and expected outcomes of care. A **nursing intervention** is any action taken by the nurse to help the client move from a present health state to the health state described in the expected outcomes (Gordon, 1994). The client may require intervention in the form of support, medication, treatment for the current condition, client-family education, or treatment to prevent future health problems.

Implementation is continuous and interactive with the other components of the nursing process. During implementation, the nurse reassesses the client, modifies the care plan, and rewrites expected outcomes as necessary. For effective implementation, the nurse must be knowledgeable about types of interventions, the implementation process, and specific implementation methods.

TYPES OF NURSING INTERVENTIONS

Implementation puts the care plan into action. After the plan has been developed, according to client needs and priorities, the nurse performs specific nursing interventions, which include nurse-initiated and physician-initiated treatments (Bulechek and McCloskey, 1995) (see Chapter 9). Nursing interventions may be entirely based on protocols or standing orders. A clear description of protocols and standing orders is necessary for safe nursing practice.

Protocols and Standing Orders

A **protocol** is a written plan specifying the procedures to be followed during care of a client with a select clinical condition or situation, such as care of a postoperative client. Nurses providing primary care for clients in an outpatient setting follow treatment and diagnostic protocol. In such a setting, nurses assess the client and identify abnormalities. The protocol delineates the conditions that nurses are permitted to treat, such as controlled hypertension, and the types of treatment they are permitted to administer, such as well baby immunizations.

A protocol can also be strictly within the framework of nursing, such as a protocol for admission and discharge, pain management, or initiating cardiopulmonary resuscitation (CPR). Protocols are also used in interdisciplinary settings for diagnostic testing and physical, occupational, and speech therapies.

A **standing order** is a document containing orders for the conduct of routine therapies, monitoring guidelines, and/or diagnostic procedures for specific clients with identified clinical problems. The orders direct the conduct of client care in various clinical settings. Standing orders are approved and signed by the physician in charge of care before their implementation. They are commonly found in critical care settings, where clients' needs can change rapidly and require immediate attention. Such a standing order might specify a certain drug, such as lidocaine or propanol, for an irregular heart rhythm. After assessing the client and identifying the irregular rhythm, the critical care nurse gives the specified medication without first notifying the physician. Standing orders are also common in the community health setting, in which the nurse encounters situations that do not permit immediate contact with a physician. Thus standing orders and protocols give the nurse legal protection to intervene appropriately in the client's best interest.

Nursing interventions implemented during the nursing process include nurse- and physician-initiated interventions. Before implementing any therapy, including any included in protocols and standing orders, the nurse must use sound judgment in determining whether the intervention is correct and appropriate. Second, the nurse implementing any intervention has the responsibility to obtain correct theoretical knowledge and develop the clinical competency necessary to perform the intervention. Nursing responsibility is equally great for all types of interventions.

CRITICAL THINKING SKILLS AND IMPLEMENTING NURSING INTERVENTIONS

Nurses make two major types of decisions in the nursing process. The diagnostic process defines the client's strengths and problems at the conclusion of the assessment and throughout the diagnostic stage (Bandman and Bandman, 1994; McFarland and McFarlane, 1989). The nurse then uses a methodical, systematic, research-based approach to plan and select appropriate interventions (Bulechek and McCloskey, 1995; Gordon, 1987, 1994).

The student must carefully select interventions designed to achieve expected outcomes and know how nurse-initiated and physician-initiated interventions differ. Several factors make decision making more difficult when choosing among nurse-initiated (independent) interventions (Gordon, 1994; Snyder, 1985). One factor is the absence of objective data concerning the probable consequences of the interventions. Another factor is that nurse-initiated interventions are often not mutually exclusive from medical therapies. For example, the nurse may need to augment relaxation, massage, and guided imagery techniques with prescribed analgesics for pain management (see Chapter 43).

Snyder (1985) proposes an information-processing model of decision making (Table 10-1). The objective of this model is to characterize the sequence of the thought process used by problem solvers. In addition, Snyder incorporates a behavioral decision model for decision making; this model focuses on decisions that will be made rather than the ways in which they are made. Therefore, the information-processing model identifies how decisions are made, and the behavioral decision model denotes the type

Table 10-1	Information-Processing Model for Impaired Physical Mobility Related to Pain Secondary to Abdominal Incision		
POSSIBLE ACTIONS	**POSSIBLE CONSEQUENCES ASSOCIATED WITH ACTION**	**PROBABILITY OF CONSEQUENCE**	**VALUE OF CONSEQUENCE TO CLIENT**
Teach relaxation exercises.	Client is able to control perception of pain.	Moderate	Ability to control perception and response to pain
	Pain is unrelieved.	Moderate	
	Pain increases.	Low	
Teach client use of controlled analgesia.	Client is able to control administration of analgesia within preset limits.	High	Ability of client to use analgesia to continuously relieve pain
	Pain is relieved.	High	
	Pain is unrelieved.	Moderate	
	Pain increases.	Low	
Administer narcotic analgesia every 4 hours.	Client is unable to control administration of analgesia.	High	Inability to control administration of analgesia
	Pain increases in intensity before nurse administers narcotic analgesia.	Moderate to high	Increase or decrease of pain perception based on blood levels of narcotic analgesia
	Pain is relieved.	Moderate to high	
	Client is confused after administration of narcotic analgesia.	Low to moderate	

of decisions made. With the information-processing model, the nurse uses the following components of decision making when determining nursing interventions (Snyder, 1985):

1. The set of all possible nursing actions. For example, pain-control measures including analgesia, relaxation, and positioning.
2. A listing of all possible consequences associated with each possible nursing action, such as relief of pain, no relief of pain, and adverse reaction to analgesia.
3. The determination of the probability that each of the consequences will occur. For example, the client's pain decreased with previous analgesia and positioning, therefore adverse reactions are unlikely.
4. A judgment based on the value of that consequence to the client. For example, the client's pain will most likely be decreased with analgesia and positioning.

This model is effective in teaching the student clinical decision making. However, the beginning student or practitioner still needs supervision from an instructor or experienced nurse to guide the decision-making process.

There will be cases when the nurse may delegate care to another care provider such as an unlicensed nurse assistant. The nurse recognizes that priorities for one client may require delegation of another client's care to competent staff.

IMPLEMENTATION PROCESS

The implementation component of the nursing process has five steps: reassessing the client, reviewing and modifying the existing nursing care plan, identifying areas of assistance, implementing nursing interventions, and communicating interventions.

Reassessing the Client

Assessment is a continuous process, which may focus on only one dimension or system. Each time a nurse interacts with a client, additional data are gathered to reflect physical, developmental, intellectual, emotional, social, and spiritual needs. When new data are obtained and a new need is identified, the nurse modifies nursing care.

CASE STUDY A nursing care plan has been developed for Mrs. Coyle (Table 10-2). The nursing diagnosis, altered urinary elimination related to perineal swelling after vaginal delivery, provided the focus for the plan. Before inserting the straight catheter the nurse reassesses Mrs. Coyle to determine that she has not voided spontaneously, because if she has, the catheterization procedure is no longer appropriate. ■

The reassessment phase of the implementation component thus provides a mechanism for the nurse to determine whether the proposed nursing action is appropriate.

Reviewing and Modifying the Existing Nursing Care Plan

Although the nursing care plan was developed according to the nursing diagnoses identified during assessment, changes in the client's status can necessitate modification of planned nursing care. Before beginning care, the nurse reviews the care plan and compares it with assessment data to validate the stated nursing diagnoses and determine whether the nursing interventions are the most appropriate for the clinical situation. If the client's status has changed and the nursing diagnosis and related nursing interventions are no longer appropriate, the nursing care plan needs to be modified (see Chapter 9).

Modification of the existing care plan includes several steps. First, data in the assessment column are revised to reflect the client's current status. New data entered in the care plan should be dated to inform other members of the health care team of the time that the change occurred.

Table 10-2	Sample Nursing Care Plan			

NURSING DIAGNOSIS: Altered urinary elimination related to perineal swelling after vaginal delivery.
DEFINITION: Altered urinary elimination is the state in which an individual experiences a disturbance in urine elimination.*

ASSESSMENT	GOAL	IMPLEMENTATION	EVALUATION
Client has not voided in 8 hr. Fluid intake for last 8 hr is 2400 ml. Client states that she "feels the urge to void" and experiences bladder discomfort. Bladder is palpable to 2 cm below umbilicus.	Acheive emptying of bladder (8/17).	Insert straight catheter, using sterile technique, if client has not voided in 8 hr and bladder is palpable.	1000 ml of clear yellow urine is returned via straight catheter (8/16). Bladder is not palpable (8/16). Client no longer has sensation to void (8/17). Client no longer complains of bladder discomfort (8/17).

*Data from Kim MJ, McFarland GK, McLane AM: *Pocket guide to nursing diagnoses,* ed 6, St Louis, 1995, Mosby.

Second, nursing diagnoses are revised. Nursing diagnoses that are no longer relevant are deleted, and new nursing diagnoses are added and dated. Because the client's status and health care needs have changed, the priorities, goals, and expected outcomes also must be revised. The revisions are also dated on the care plan.

Third, specific implementation methods are revised to correspond to the new nursing diagnoses and client goals. This revision reflects the client's present status. In addition, revised implementation can include the client's specific needs for health care resources.

Finally, the nurse evaluates client response to the nursing actions. If client response is not consistent with the expected outcomes, further revisions to the plan of care are needed. For example, a preoperative care plan was developed for Mr. Diaz. As he progressed through the postoperative period, his nursing needs changed. The nurse made modifications in the care plan for one nursing diagnosis: ineffective breathing pattern after surgery related to abdominal incisional pain (Table 10-3). On the second postoperative day, the nurse assessed the client and noted decreased chest wall movements, crackles that were auscultated in the right lower lobes, and an elevated temperature (39° C). Mr. Diaz had a standing order for a chest x-ray examination, which was taken immediately and revealed the collapse of alveoli in the right lower lobe. The nursing diagnosis was revised to read ineffective airway clearance related to abdominal incisional pain. The nursing diagnostic label was revised due to the presence of right lower lobe crackles and decreased chest wall movement. The goal of maintaining a patent airway was still appropriate. Specific nursing interventions were developed to assist in achieving a patent airway. Finally, the projected outcomes were rewritten to reflect the desired level of wellness and indicate when the need had been resolved.

The astute nurse is sensitive to changes in the client's status and readily incorporates these changes into the care plan. The health status of the client changes continuously. Therefore the care plan needs to be flexible to incorporate necessary changes. An out-of-date or incorrect care plan compromises the quality of nursing care, whereas review and modification enable the nurse to provide nursing care that best meets the client's needs.

Identifying Areas of Assistance

Some nursing situations require the nurse to seek assistance. The assistance can be additional personnel, knowledge, or nursing skills. Before implementing care, the nurse evaluates the plan to determine the need for assistance and the type required.

Situations requiring additional personnel vary. For example, a nurse assigned to care for an immobilized client may need additional personnel to help turn, transfer, and position the client because of the physical work involved. The nurse also needs to determine when the personnel are needed. If the client needs to be turned and repositioned every 2 hours, additional personnel will be needed every 2 hours. The nurse then must determine the number of persons needed and must discuss the need for assistance with potential resources. Finally, the nurse needs to take time to plan care so that the other team members do not become overburdened. Additional personnel are also required when a client's health status declines or when the number of clients increases. In both situations the required level of nursing care is too much for one nurse to deliver safely.

CASE STUDY   Mr. Douglas, RN, is assigned to care for two postoperative clients, Mr. Huan and Mrs. Jade. Two hours into the shift, Mr. Huan begins to hemorrhage and goes into shock. Mr. Douglas spends the next hour stabilizing Mr. Huan's condition. At this point he reviews the care plan for Mrs. Jade and the new care plan for Mr. Huan. The nurse's assessment of the situation is that for the next 2 hours he will need to spend all of his time with Mr. Huan. He approaches his supervisor with this assessment and requests additional help for the next 2 hours. ■

Some nursing situations require additional knowledge and skills. A nurse needs additional knowledge when administering a new medication or implementing a new procedure. Such information can be obtained from a hospital's formulary or procedure book. If the nurse still is uncertain about the new medication or procedure, other members of the health care team can be consulted.

Because of the continual growth of health care professions and related technology, a nurse may lack the skills needed to carry out a procedure. When this occurs, infor-

Table 10-3	**Modified Nursing Care Plan for Mr. Diaz**

NURSING DIAGNOSIS: Ineffective airway clearance related to abdominal incisional pain
DEFINITION: Ineffective airway clearance is the state in which an individual is unable to clear secretions or obstructions from the respiratory tract to maintain airway patency.*

ASSESSMENT	GOALS	IMPLEMENTATION	EVALUATION
Smoked two packs/day 20 years; chest x-ray film showing slight change of emphysema; crackles auscultated in lung field; scheduled for abdominal surgery	Maintain a patent airway (11/8).	Demonstrate turn, cough, and deep breathing to client. Have client perform exercises every 2 hours while awake.	Productive cough produced. Airway clear to auscultation.
MODIFIED 24 HOURS AFTER SURGERY			
Decreased chest wall movements; crackles in base that do not clear with coughing	Promote airway clearance (11/8).	Administer chest physiotherapy to all lobes of the lung: 8-12-4-8-12-4. Ensure that Mr. Diaz coughs and deep breathes every 2 hours around the clock. Suction nasotracheal area every 2 hours if client is unable to cough productively. Teach client to splint incision with pillow before and during coughing.	Lung fields are clear on auscultation. Client becomes afebrile. Chest x-ray film demonstrates atelectasis resolving. Client does not report increased pain during coughing.

*Data from Kim MJ, McFarland GK, McLane AM: *Pocket guide to nursing diagnoses,* ed 6, St Louis, 1995, Mosby.

mation about the procedure is obtained from the literature and the agency's procedure book. Next, all equipment necessary for the procedure is collected. Finally, another nurse who has correctly and safely completed the procedure provides assistance. The assistance can come from another staff nurse, a supervisor, an educator, or a nurse specialist. Requesting assistance occurs frequently in all types of nursing practices and is a learning process that continues throughout educational experiences and into professional development.

Implementing Nursing Interventions

The nurse selects from the following nursing intervention methods to achieve the goals of nursing care:
1. Assisting in the performance of activities of daily living
2. Counseling and educating the client and family
3. Providing direct nursing care
4. Supervising and evaluating the work of other staff members

Nursing practice is composed of cognitive, interpersonal, and psychomotor (technical) skills. Each type of skill is needed to implement interventions. The nurse is responsible for knowing when one of these methods is preferred over another and for having the necessary theoretical knowledge and psychomotor skills to implement each. A later section introduces the general theoretical information for each method and refers to subsequent chapters that detail the necessary theoretical and psychomotor skills.

COGNITIVE SKILLS

Cognitive skills involve nursing knowledge. The nurse must know the rationale for each therapeutic intervention,

understand normal and abnormal physiological and psychological responses, be able to identify client learning and discharge needs, and recognize the client's health promotion and illness prevention needs.

INTERPERSONAL SKILLS

Interpersonal skills are essential to effective nursing action. The nurse must communicate clearly with the client, family, and other members of the health care team. Caring and trust are conveyed when nurses communicate openly and honestly. Client teaching and counseling must be done to the level of the client's understanding and expectations. The nurse must also be sensitive to the client's emotional response to the illness and treatment. Proper use of interpersonal skills enables the nurse to be perceptive to the client's verbal and nonverbal communication (see Chapter 14).

PSYCHOMOTOR SKILLS

Psychomotor skills involve the direct care needs of clients, such as changing a dressing, giving an injection, or suctioning a tracheostomy. The nurse has a professional responsibility to acquire these skills. In the case of a new skill, nurses assess their level of competency and obtain the necessary resources to ensure that the client receives the treatment safely.

Communicating Nursing Interventions

Nursing interventions are written or communicated orally. When written, nursing interventions are incorporated into the nursing care plan and client's medical record. The care plan usually reflects proposed nursing interventions. After the interventions are implemented, the client's response to the treatment is recorded on the appropriate record (see Chapter 12). This information usually includes a brief description of the nursing assessment, the specific procedure, and the client's response.

A brief description of pertinent assessment findings and client response in the client's medical record validates the need for a specific nursing intervention. Writing the time and the details of the intervention documents that the procedure was completed.

Nursing interventions are also communicated orally from one nurse to another or to other health care professionals. Nurses commonly communicate orally when changing shifts, transferring a client to another unit, or discharging a client to another health care agency. Whether the nursing intervention is written or communicated orally, the language should be clear, concise, and to the point.

■ IMPLEMENTATION METHODS

The nurse carries out the nursing care plan by using several implementation methods. For example, a client with the nursing diagnosis, impaired physical mobility related to bilateral arm casts, may require assistance in performing activities of daily living. The client with ineffective individual coping related to fear of medical diagnosis may require counseling as a method of nursing intervention. The client with a knowledge deficit needs client health education focused on the area of need. The totally immobilized or disoriented client requires nursing interventions providing total client care. Another method of implementation involves the supervision and evaluation of other members of the health care team.

For each nursing diagnosis the nurse identifies appropriate interventions, each of which requires specific theoretical knowledge and clinical skills.

Assisting With Activities of Daily Living

Activities of daily living (ADLs) are activities usually performed in the course of a normal day; they include ambulating, eating, dressing, bathing, brushing the teeth, and grooming. Conditions resulting in the need for assistance with ADLs can be acute, chronic, temporary, permanent, or rehabilitative. An acute disease is characterized by symptoms that are usually severe and are present for a relatively short time, usually less than 6 months. An episode of acute disease results in recovery to a state of health and activity comparable to the state before the disease, passage into a chronic phase of the disease, or death. For example, the postoperative client who is unable to independently complete all ADLs. While progressing through the postoperative period, the client gradually depends less on nurses for completing ADLs.

A chronic disease persists longer. Although the symptoms are usually less severe than those of the acute phase of the same disease, chronic disease may result in complete or partial disability. A client with partial paralysis after a cerebrovascular accident may have a chronic impairment requiring long-term assistance with ADLs.

The client's need for assistance with ADLs may be temporary, permanent, or rehabilitative. In the case of temporary assistance with ADLs, the client needs assistance during a specific period. A client with impaired mobility

because of bilateral arm casts has a temporary need for assistance. After the casts are removed, the client will gradually assume responsibility for ADLs. However, a client with a total self-care deficit related to an irreversible injury high in the cervical spinal cord has a permanent need for assistance. It is unrealistic for the nurse to plan a rehabilitation program with the goal that this client will be able to independently complete all ADLs. However, through restorative care, the client will learn new ways to perform ADLs, thus becoming more independent and better able to perform some self-care (see Chapter 5).

Through assessment, the nurse collects data that verify the need for assistance with ADLs. As the nurse analyzes this data, nursing diagnoses are formed in relation to such assistance.

Counseling

Counseling is an implementation method that helps the client use a problem-solving process to recognize and manage stress and that facilitates interpersonal relationships among the client, family, and health care team. Nurses provide counseling to help the client accept actual or impending changes resulting from stress. Counseling is emotional, intellectual, spiritual, and psychological support. A client and family who need nursing counseling have normal adjustment difficulties and are upset or frustrated, but are not necessarily psychologically disabled. Clients with psychiatric diagnoses require therapy by nurses specializing in psychiatric nursing or by social workers, psychiatrists, or psychologists.

Many counseling techniques are used to foster cognitive, behavioral, developmental, experiential, and emotional growth in clients (see the box below). Counseling encourages individuals to examine available alternatives and to decide which choices are useful and appropriate. When clients are able to examine alternatives, they can develop a sense of control and are able to better manage stress. To assist clients in need of counseling techniques, the nurse must be able to identify the need for counseling and possess communication skills to develop a therapeutic relationship (Sundeen et al, 1995).

Clients or families needing counseling include persons who must adjust lifestyle patterns, as in smoking cessation, weight reduction, or increasing activity. Clients coping with chronic or disabling diseases require counseling to help them adapt to changes in lifestyle or body image as the disease progresses. During life-threatening illnesses, clients and families need counseling to cope with the possibility of death.

Teaching

Counseling is closely aligned to teaching. Both involve using communication skills to effect a change in the client.

Examples of Counseling Strategies Used by Nurses	
■ Behavior modification	■ Reality orientation
■ Bereavement counseling	■ Crisis intervention
■ Biofeedback	■ Guided imagery
■ Relaxation training	■ Play therapy

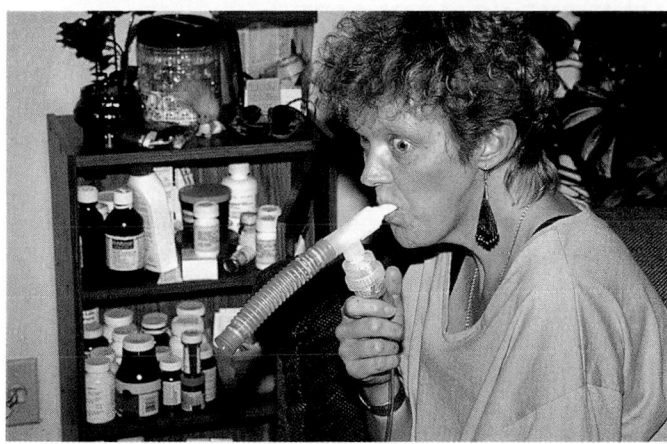

Fig. 10-1 Teaching client in home setting to use an aerosol medication delivery device.

However, with counseling the change results in the development of new attitudes and feelings, whereas in teaching the focus of change is intellectual growth or the acquisition of new knowledge or psychomotor skills (Redman, 1993).

Teaching is an implementation method used to present correct principles, procedures, and techniques of health care to clients and to inform clients about their health status (see Chapter 17). As a nursing responsibility, teaching is implemented in all health care settings, such as in acute care, home care, and community based settings (Fig. 10-1). The nurse is responsible for assessing the learning needs of clients and is accountable for the quality of education delivered.

The teaching-learning process is an interaction between the teacher and learner in which specific learning objectives are presented (Redman, 1993). This process provides the organizational structure and framework for client education. The teaching-learning process is much like the basic nursing process.

During assessment, the nurse determines the client's learning needs and readiness to learn. The nurse then interprets the data to formulate nursing diagnoses reflecting the identified needs. During planning, the nurse and client establish goals for learning. Implementation is the initiation of the teaching strategies designed to achieve the learning goal. Finally, evaluation measures the learning that has occurred. The purpose of the teaching-learning process is to develop and implement a teaching plan individualized for the client's needs, level of knowledge, and learning resources.

Providing Direct Nursing Care

To achieve the therapeutic goals for the client, the nurse initiates interventions to compensate for adverse reactions, uses precautionary and preventive measures in providing care, applies correct techniques in administering care and preparing the client for special procedures, and initiates lifesaving measures in emergency situations. The following sections briefly discuss the nursing interventions in these areas. The specific knowledge and skills needed to carry out these nursing procedures are detailed in subsequent chapters.

COMPENSATION FOR ADVERSE REACTIONS

An **adverse reaction** is a harmful or unintended effect of a medication, diagnostic test, or therapeutic intervention. Adverse reactions can follow independent, dependent, or interdependent nursing interventions. Nursing actions that compensate for adverse reactions reduce or counteract the reaction. To intervene, the nurse must have knowledge of the potential undesired effects. For example, when administering a medication, the nurse understands the known and potential side effects of the drug. After administration of the medication the nurse assesses the client for any adverse effects. The nurse should be aware of drugs that can counteract the side effects. For example, a client may have an unknown hypersensitivity to penicillin and may develop hives after three doses. The nurse records the reaction and stops further administration of the drug. The nurse also consults the physician's standing orders and administers Benadryl, an antipruritic medication to relieve the itching and an antihistamine to reduce the allergic response.

When caring for a client who is undergoing or has undergone a particular diagnostic test, the nurse must understand the test and any potential adverse effects. For example, a client has not had a bowel movement in 24 hours after a barium enema. Because a bowel impaction is a potential side effect of a barium enema, the nurse increases fluid intake and instructs the client to let the nursing personnel know when a bowel movement occurs.

Therapeutic interventions may also have potential adverse effects.

CASE STUDY Ms. Rice, RN, assesses a stage I pressure ulcer on Mr. Blaskowitz's sacrum. She develops interventions designed to prevent further skin breakdown and promote wound healing. She obtains an order for an alternating air mattress and film dressing (Tegaderm). Ms. Rice also changes Mr. Blaskowitz's turning schedule from every 2 hours to every hour while awake and every 2 hours while asleep (2200 to 0700 hours). After the second day of treatment, Ms. Rice reassesses Mr. Blaskowitz's skin and notes stage I pressure ulcers on both heels; the sacral ulcer has also progressed to a stage III ulcer. To counteract the continued skin breakdown, the nurse discontinues the air mattress and obtains an order for the Clinitron bed, Tegaderm for the heel ulcers, and a hydrogel dressing for the sacral ulcer (see Chapter 38). ∎

Although adverse effects are not common, they do occur. The nurse learns potential side effects, recognizes the presence of an adverse reaction, and intervenes accordingly.

PREVENTIVE MEASURES

Preventive nursing actions are directed at promoting health and preventing illness to avoid the need for acute or rehabilitative health care. Prevention includes assessment and promotion of the client's health potential, application of prescribed measures such as immunizations, health teaching, and early diagnosis and treatment.

In the case of a client who has a hypersensitivity to penicillin, the nurse can implement several preventive measures. The nurse indicates the penicillin allergy in the client's medical record, informs the client and family of the need for a Medic-Alert bracelet, and teaches them actions they should take if the client is given penicillin again. The nurse also teaches the client and family that this is a potentially life-threatening allergy and which specific drugs to avoid.

Preventive nursing actions are used to meet the therapeutic goals of the client. Through preventive actions the nurse is able to help the client attain the highest level of wellness.

CORRECT TECHNIQUES IN ADMINISTERING CARE AND PREPARING A CLIENT FOR PROCEDURES

The administration of nursing care requires the nurse to be experienced in many **techniques**, which are methods followed in performing specific procedures such as administering medications, changing clients' dressings, or inserting Foley catheters. Client care, particularly in the home and hospital, involves many techniques. Every procedure the nurse does for the client is carried out by a specific method.

To carry out a procedure, the nurse must be knowledgeable about the procedure itself, the frequency, the steps, and the expected outcomes. In a hospital the nurse completes many procedures each day. Some of these procedures might be new, so before conducting a new procedure the nurse assesses personal competencies and determines the need for assistance, new knowledge, or new skills.

LIFESAVING MEASURES

A **lifesaving measure** is implemented when a client's physiological or psychological state is threatened. The purpose of the lifesaving measure is to restore physiological or psychological equilibrium. Such measures include administering emergency medications, instituting cardiopulmonary resuscitation (Fig. 10-2), restraining a confused or violent client, and obtaining immediate counseling from a crisis center for a severely anxious client.

The initiation of lifesaving measures is an essential component of nursing practice. As with any procedure, the nurse must be knowledgeable about the lifesaving procedure itself, steps, and expected outcomes. If an inexperienced nurse encounters a situation requiring emergency measures, the proper nursing action may be to get an experienced professional.

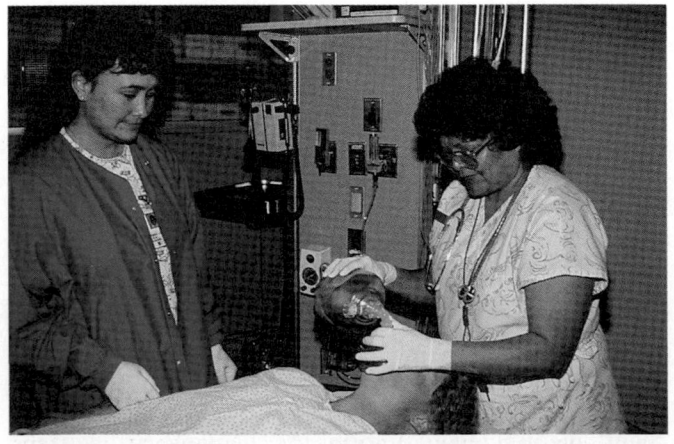

Fig. 10-2 Initiating artificial respirations.

ACHIEVING GOALS OF CARE

The client's health care goals can be achieved by providing an environment conducive to meeting such goals; adjusting care in accordance with clients' expressed or implied needs; stimulating and motivating clients, thereby enabling them to achieve self-care and independence; and encouraging clients to accept care or adhere to the treatment regimen. For each nursing intervention, the nurse and client work together to meet the mutually developed goals. The nurse assumes a more active or more passive role depending on the intervention.

Nurses can help create a health care environment conducive to achieving clients' goals. Ideally the nurse creates an environment that provides clients with adequate privacy for meeting basic needs and allows them to feel safe and free to interact with the health care team. An early step in establishing an appropriate environment is to orient clients and families to the health care agency. If it is a hospital, clients need to be oriented to their rooms, the health care team, and other clients. Clients in clinics should be oriented to clinic policies and procedures, the location of restrooms and cafeterias, and the health care team. When clients receive care in the home, the nurse should take time to acquaint clients and their families with the purposes and expectations of the home visits.

Whether clients are in the hospital, outpatient clinic, or a community setting, the nurse takes measures to provide privacy. Obviously, clients need privacy to carry out activities of hygiene, grooming, and elimination. In addition, they need privacy to talk with family, friends, or members of the health care team. In an environment of privacy, clients may feel free to share concerns, ask questions about diagnosis and treatment, and resolve personal problems.

Nursing care and other therapeutic measures are designed to meet the client's needs. As a further aid in the attainment of health care goals, the nursing care plan should be flexible so the client is not placed into a fixed routine. Obviously the degree of flexibility depends on the nature of the need, the severity of the client's disability or illness, and the client's dependence on nursing care. However, even the smallest degree of flexibility, giving the client an opportunity to have some choice about the type or timing of nursing care, is valuable.

Clients with severe and chronic diseases should be encouraged to increase their levels of self-care and indepen-

CASE STUDY Mr. Porter is a 50-year-old executive, husband, and father of three teenagers. He is recovering from a severe myocardial infarction (heart attack) and cardiac arrest. For the past 3 days, all of Mr. Porter's hygiene and grooming needs have been met by the nursing staff. One day, Mr. Porter expresses doubts of ever getting his energy back and being able to care for himself. That evening Mr. Martin, a student nurse, assesses Mr. Porter and develops a nursing care plan. One of the goals is complete self-care by Mr. Porter within 1 week. With the help of his instructor, Mr. Martin implements the following plan, which is designed to achieve the overall goal of independence in various phases:
Day 1 Wash face, shave, and comb hair
Day 2 Feed himself meals, wash face, shave, and comb hair
Day 4 Perform grooming activities and feed himself
Day 6 Shower ■

dence. To avoid discouraging clients, it is best to attempt to achieve this nursing goal gradually. The care plan is implemented so that clients successfully achieve one level of independence before attempting the next.

Each day includes achievable tasks for Mr. Porter. Placing the tasks in sequential order serves the following purposes: (1) each task was developed with the knowledge that Mr. Porter could indeed successfully complete the activity, (2) a sequence of successes will motivate Mr. Porter to continue with the plan, and (3) the sequence was designed to gradually increase Mr. Porter's activity tolerance.

Clients with chronic diseases may need to adhere to many treatment modalities. **Client adherence** means that clients and families must invest time in carrying out the required home treatments. For example, a client with chronic obstructive pulmonary disease (COPD) may need to spend several hours a day performing respiratory therapies designed to keep the airway open and maintain an acceptable level of wellness.

Some treatment plans include the need for the client and family to adjust to functional changes as a result of medications. For example, a client with high blood pressure being treated with atenolol (Tenormin) occasionally feels increasingly fatigued during the early stages of treatment. Another client with cancer who is undergoing chemotherapy may have changes in energy level and body image as a result of the medication.

Finally, adherence to treatment plans can require an increased financial investment by the client and family. For example, for a client who has cardiac disease, a two-story house may no longer be suitable because the client is unable to climb stairs without feeling short of breath. Thus the client and family may need to invest in a new house or have their present home modified.

Investments of time, money, and personal resources for a long period can be discouraging. The discouraged client may neglect the treatment regimen. After the client begins to reduce adherence to treatment, levels of wellness may decline.

Nurses are able to intervene and assist the client in adhering to a treatment plan. Adequate discharge planning and education of the client and family help promote a smooth transition from one health care setting to another or to the home. They also help increase the client's level of knowledge about the treatment plan. Counseling helps the client and family adapt to change resulting from the disease process or treatment. Continuity of care also provides a supportive professional who is familiar with the client's pattern of living, pattern of wellness, and treatment. In addition, reinforcing successes with the treatment plan encourages the client to adhere to the regimen.

Supervising and Evaluating the Work of Other Staff Members

The nurse who develops the care plan frequently does not perform all of the nursing interventions. Some interventions may be delegated to other members of the health care team. For example, noninvasive interventions such as skin care, range of joint motion exercises, ambulation, grooming, and hygiene measures can be assigned to a nursing assistant. In the case of a licensed practical nurse, medication administration and vital sign assessment may be delegated. The nurse assigning tasks is responsible for ensuring that each task is appropriately assigned and is completed according to the standard of care.

■ KEY CONCEPTS ■

▶ Implementation requires the nurse to reassess the client, review and modify the existing care plan, identify areas in which assistance is needed, implement nursing interventions, and communicate nursing interventions.

▶ The care plan is modified as a client's level of wellness and health care needs change.

▶ The implementation of nursing care may require additional knowledge, nursing skills, and personnel.

▶ After implementation, the nurse writes in the client's record a brief description of the nursing assessment, specific procedures, and client's response to nursing care.

▶ Counseling helps the client use problem solving to recognize and manage stress and facilitates interpersonal relationships among the client, family, and health care team.

▶ Teaching is used to present correct principles, procedures, and techniques of health care to clients; inform

clients about their health status; and refer clients and families to appropriate resources.

▶ Nursing actions to achieve therapeutic goals include compensation for adverse reactions, preventive measures, correct techniques for administering care and preparing the client for procedures, and lifesaving measures.

▶ Nursing actions that achieve the attainment of health care goals include providing a conducive environment, adjusting care to fit the client's needs, and stimulating and motivating the client.

▶ Delegating care to other personnel involves ensuring that the individuals are skilled in the tasks and complete them according to the standard of care.

▶ To complete any nursing procedure, the nurse must be knowledgeable about the procedure, frequency, the steps, and the expected outcomes.

■ KEY TERMS ■

Activities of daily living (ADLs), p. 160

Adverse reaction, p. 161

Client adherence, p. 163

Counseling, p. 160

Implementation, p. 156

Lifesaving measure, p. 162

Nursing intervention, p. 156

Preventive nursing actions, p. 161

Protocol, p. 156

Standing order, p. 156

Techniques, p. 162

■ CRITICAL THINKING EXERCISES ■

1. Your client is voiding infrequently and producing small amounts of urine. A physician writes an order for insertion of a straight catheter to relieve bladder distension. What additional data must you obtain from the client to determine whether this is an appropriate intervention?

2. You are assigned to ambulate Mr. Clay, who had abdominal surgery 24 hours ago. Mr. Clay weighs 270 lbs and is 6 feet tall. What questions do you need to answer before you attempt to ambulate this client?

3. Your client needs a complicated wound irrigation and dressing change. What measures will you take to reduce the risk of an adverse reaction to this intervention?

REFERENCES

Bandman EL, Bandman B: *Critical thinking in nursing,* ed 2, Norwalk, Conn, 1995, Appleton & Lange.

Bulechek GM, McCloskey JC: *Nursing interventions classification (NIC),* ed 2, St Louis, 1995, Mosby.

Gordon M: *Nursing diagnosis: process and application,* ed 2, New York, 1987, McGraw-Hill.

Gordon M: *Nursing diagnosis: process and application,* ed 3, St Louis, 1994, Mosby.

Kim MJ, McFarland GK, McLane AM: *Pocket guide to nursing diagnoses,* ed 6, St Louis, 1995, Mosby.

McFarland GK, McFarlane EA: *Nursing diagnosis and intervention: planning for patient care,* St Louis, 1989, Mosby–Year Book.

Redman BK: *The process of patient education,* ed 7, St Louis, 1993, Mosby.

Snyder M: *Independent nursing interventions,* New York, 1985, Wiley.

Sundeen SJ et al: *Nurse-client interaction: implementing the nursing process,* ed 5, St Louis, 1995, Mosby.

ADDITIONAL READINGS

American Nurses Association: *Nursing: a social policy statement,* Kansas City, Mo, 1980, The Association.

Carpenito LJ: *Nursing diagnosis application to clinical practice,* ed 4, Philadelphia, 1993, Lippincott.

Kim MJ: Degree of independence of nursing interventions for nursing diagnoses. In Hurley MA, editor: *Classification of nursing diagnoses: proceedings of the Sixth Conference (NANDA),* St Louis, 1986, Mosby–Year Book.

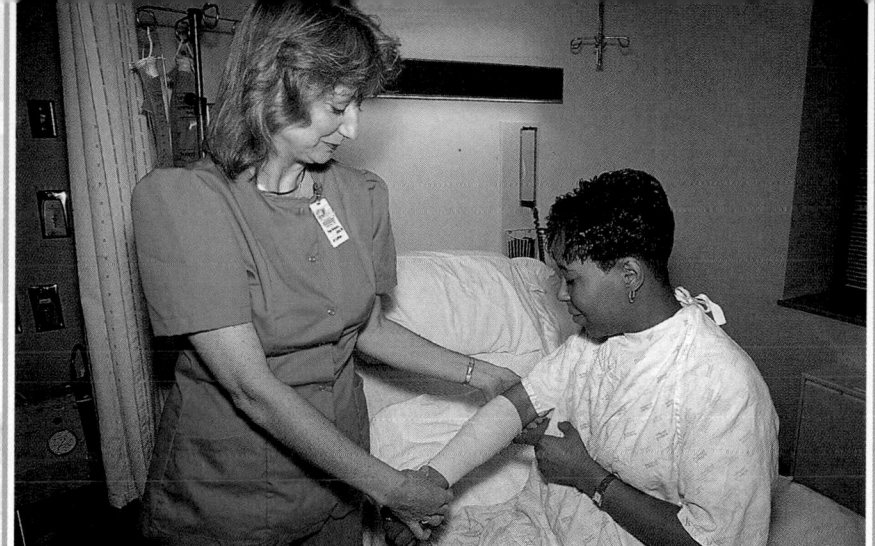

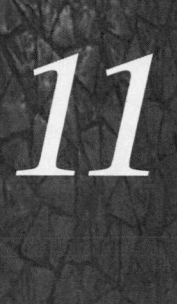

## Chapter 11

Evaluation

Objectives

Mastery of content in this chapter will enable the student to:

▶ Define the key terms listed.

▶ Explain the relationship between expected outcomes and goals of care.

▶ Explain how the step of evaluation involves critical thinking.

▶ Give examples of evaluation measures used to determine a client's progress toward outcomes.

▶ Evaluate nursing actions selected for a client.

▶ Describe how evaluation can lead to revision or modification of a plan of care.

▶ Explain the purpose of quality improvement (QI).

▶ Discuss the dimensions of performance that should be incorporated into an organization's QI program.

▶ Describe the common features in models used for QI.

▶ Describe the steps of a process improvement for QI.

Whenever a nurse delivers care and provides therapy, certain questions must be asked: Was the therapy effective in improving the client's function? Did the client benefit? It is important to evaluate each client according to the level of wellness or recovery the health care team and client have established in the goals of care. The **evaluation** step of the nursing process measures the client's response to nursing actions and the client's progress toward achieving goals. Data are collected on an ongoing basis to measure changes in functioning, in daily living, and in availability or use of external resources (Carnevali and Thomas, 1993). Evaluation occurs whenever the nurse has contact with a client. The emphasis is on client outcomes. The nurse evaluates whether the client's behaviors or responses reflect a reversal or improvement in a nursing diagnosis or maintenance of a healthy state. During evaluation, the nurse decides if the previous steps of the nursing process were effective by examining the client's responses and comparing them with the behaviors stated in the expected outcomes.

Another aspect of evaluation involves measurement of the quality of nursing care provided in a health care setting. Nurses evaluate each client's progress and recovery, but this is not enough. A health care organization must be accountable and responsible for evaluating and improving the quality of nursing and other client care services being provided to all clients. The quality of health care is a focus of the Joint Commission on Accreditation of Healthcare Organizations (JCAHO) and **professional standards review organizations (PSROs)**. The JCAHO (1995) defines quality of care as the "degree to which health services for individuals and populations increase the likelihood of desired health outcomes and are consistent with current professional knowledge." Each health care professional must be competent, but to achieve high-quality care, an organization must have the right systems and processes to provide care that is appropriate and efficacious. There are always opportunities to improve because client care is complex, involving numerous variables. The larger the organization, the greater the variables influencing how care is delivered. Nursing plays a key role in helping an organization find ways to improve the quality of client care. The emphasis is on client outcomes, professional practice, and the systems in which professionals practice.

■ DYNAMICS OF EVALUATING THE NURSING PROCESS

While caring for clients, the nurse compares subjective and objective data gathered from the client, other nurses or care givers, and the family to determine the degree of success in meeting expected outcomes established during planning. If outcomes are met, the overall goals for the client are also met. The nurse compares client behaviors and responses assessed before nursing interventions are delivered with the behaviors and responses that occur following nursing care. The nurse applies knowledge about the client's condition, considers previous experience with similar clients, and reviews data from the assessed baseline to critically analyze if the client's condition is changing. Critical thinking directs the nurse to analyze the findings from evaluation. Is the client's condition improved? Can the client improve, or are there physical factors preventing recovery? Does the

client's motivation or willingness to pursue healthier behavior influence response to therapies?

During evaluation the nurse continually redirects nursing care to best meet client needs. For example, when evaluating a client for a change in vital signs, the nurse applies knowledge of disease processes and physiological responses to interpret whether a change has indeed occurred and whether the change is desirable. A client with acute pain may have an increased heart rate and increased muscular tension. The nurse knows this is a sympathetic nervous system response to painful stimuli. After administering a pain medication and repositioning the client, the nurse will return to evaluate if vital signs have returned either to the client's baseline (prior to experiencing pain) or to a more acceptable level. Positive evaluations occur when desired results are met, leading the nurse to conclude that the dosage of medication and the nursing intervention effectively met the client's goal of improved comfort. Negative evaluations or undesired results indicate that the problem was not resolved or that potential problems were not avoided. As a result, the nurse must change the care plan and try different therapies or a different approach in administering existing therapies.

This sequence of critically evaluating and revising therapies continues until problems are appropriately resolved. Outcomes must be realistic and adjusted on the basis of the client's prognosis and condition. The nurse must realize that evaluation is dynamic and ever changing, depending on the client's nursing diagnoses and condition. A client whose health status continuously changes requires more frequent evaluation. In addition, priority diagnoses are often evaluated first. For example, a nurse evaluates a client's acute pain before evaluating the status of knowledge deficit.

Goals

A goal specifies the behavior or response that indicates resolution of a nursing diagnosis or maintenance of a healthy state. It is a summary statement of what is to be accomplished when all expected outcomes have been met. Each nursing diagnosis in the client's care plan has a goal, and every goal has a time frame for evaluation. The nurse evaluates goals after comparing evaluative findings with all expected outcomes. When a goal has been accomplished, the nurse knows that interventions have been successful and that the client is progressing.

As hospital stays become shorter, many clients are discharged before all goals are met and all nursing diagnoses are resolved. When preparing a client for discharge, the nurse evaluates the status of each nursing diagnosis and writes an evaluative statement identifying the client's progress toward goal achievement and problem resolution. Appropriate revisions to the care plan are made for home or follow-up care (for example, an extended-care facility). The nurse must clearly distinguish between goals that have been met and goals that require continued intervention. A home health nurse will probably revise interventions to adapt them to the client's home.

Expected Outcomes

Expected outcomes are the expected results of a goal-oriented process (see Chapter 9). They are statements of progressive, step-by-step responses or behaviors that the client needs to accomplish to achieve the goals of care provided. When outcomes are achieved, the related factors for a nursing diagnosis no longer exist. For example, for a nursing diagnosis of impaired skin integrity related to pressure of physical immobilization, the client must achieve the goal of attaining intact skin in the area of injury. This will be accomplished by meeting the outcomes of "the skin lesion will be clean without drainage in 3 days" and showing evidence of healing through "reduction in size by 1 cm and inflammation in 1 week." If the outcomes are met the nurse has successfully eliminated pressure over the skin and used therapies that have healed the skin lesion. Expected outcomes have short time frames (depending on the health care setting) and include as few as one or two intervention sessions (Hickey, 1991). To provide truly objective measurements the outcomes are measurable, stated in behavioral terms, and have time frames for evaluation (see Chapter 9).

After a specified interval or when all interventions in the plan of care have been completed, the nurse evaluates the client's ability to demonstrate the behavior or response stated in the outcomes. Evaluation of each expected outcome and its place in the sequence of care is essential. Failure to evaluate each expected outcome results in an inability to determine the place in which the sequence faltered. In other words, the nurse is not able to revise and redirect the plan of care at the most appropriate time.

If the client achieves the expected outcome, the nurse either continues the care plan or discontinues interventions because the goal of care is met. If evaluation determines that the expected outcome was not met or only partially met, the nurse begins reassessment and revision of the care plan.

■ EVALUATION OF GOAL ACHIEVEMENT

The purpose of nursing care is to assist the client with resolving actual health problems, preventing the occurrence of potential problems, and maintaining a healthy state. Evaluation of the goals of care determines whether this purpose was accomplished. The nurse matches the client's behavior (e.g., self-administration of insulin or anxiety-free behavior) or physiological response (e.g., decrease in size of pressure ulcer or fall in body temperature) with the behavior or response specified in the goal. For example, during an initial assessment, a client may report acute abdominal pain, rate the pain as 8 on a scale of 0 to 10 (see Chapter 43), and grimace or hold the abdomen during attempts to move in bed. This baseline is used by the nurse to identify the nursing diagnosis of pain and establish the goal of "client will perceive a reduction in pain within 48 hours." The nurse's evaluation determines if the outcomes that reflect goal accomplishment were met. Did the interventions of positioning, proper and timely administration of analgesics, and use of relaxation successfully reduce the client's pain? Outcomes may include "client will verbalize pain at 3 on a scale of 0 to 10 in 24 hours" and "client will position self without nonverbal signs of discomfort." After providing appropriate comfort measures, the nurse reassesses the client by measuring the subjective report of pain, observing facial expressions, and noting if the client initiates turning and repositioning. The new data or client responses are compared with outcome criteria to determine whether predicted changes have occurred (Table 11-1). To objectively evaluate the degree of success in achieving a goal, the nurse should use the following steps:

1. Examine the goal statement to identify the exact desired client behavior or response.
2. Assess the client for the presence of that behavior or response.
3. Compare the established outcome criteria with the behavior or response.
4. Judge the degree of agreement between outcome criteria and the behavior or response.
5. If there is no agreement (or only partial agreement) between the outcome criteria and the behavior or response, what is/are the barriers? Why did they not agree?

There are different degrees of goal attainment. If the client's response matches or exceeds the outcome criteria, the goal is met. If the client's behavior begins to show changes but does not yet meet criteria set, the goal is partially met. If there is no progress, the goal is not met (Table 11-2). A clearly defined goal with specific outcomes is easily measured (see Chapter 9).

Table 11-1	Evaluation Measures to Determine the Success of Goals and Expected Outcomes	
GOALS	**EVALUATIVE MEASURES**	**EXPECTED OUTCOMES**
Client's pressure ulcer will heal within 7 days.	Inspect color, condition, and location of pressure ulcer. Measure diameter of ulcer daily. Note odor and color of drainage from ulcer.	Erythema will be reduced in 2 days. Diameter of ulcer will decrease in 5 days. Ulcer will have no drainage in 2 days. Skin overlying ulcer will be closed in 7 days.
Client will tolerate ambulation to end of hall by 11/20.	Palpate client's radial pulse before exercise. Palpate client's radial pulse 10 minutes after exercise. Assess respiratory rate during exercise. Observe client for dyspnea or breathlessness during exercise.	Pulse will remain below 110 beats per minute during exercise. Pulse rate will return to resting baseline within 10 minutes after exercise. Respiratory rate will remain within two breaths of client's baseline rate. Client will deny feeling of breathlessness.

Table 11-2	Examples of Objective Evaluation of Goal Achievement		
GOALS	**OUTCOME CRITERIA**	**CLIENT RESPONSES**	**EVALUATION FINDINGS**
Client will self-administer insulin by 12/18.	Client prepares insulin dosage in syringe by 12/17. Client demonstrates self-injection by 12/18.	Client prepared accurate dosage in syringe on 12/17. Client administered morning insulin dosage; self-injection was correctly performed on 12/18.	Client has progressed and achieved desired behavior.
Client's lungs will be free of secretions by 11/30.	Coughing will be nonproductive by 11/29. Lungs will be clear to auscultation by 11/30. Respirations will be 20 per minute by 11/30.	Client coughed frequently and productively on 11/29. Lungs were clear to auscultation on 11/30. Respirations were 18 per minute on 11/29.	Client will require continued threapy. Condition is improving.
Client will be able to perform self-care measures without discomfort in 2 days.	Client will verbalize pain at 3 on a scale of 10 within 2 days. Client will initiate bathing within 2 days.	Client reports severe right-sided abdominal pain at 5 on a scale of 10 while attempting bathing on day 2.	Client's condition still indicates a problem. Continued therapy with possibly new care measures is required.

Evaluative Measures and Sources

Evaluative measures are simply the assessment skills and techniques used to collect data for evaluation. For example, auscultation of lung sounds, observation of a client's skill performance, inspection of the skin, and inquiry regarding the severity of pain are all evaluative measures (Fig. 11-1). In fact, they are the same as assessment measures but are performed at the point of care when decisions are made about the client's status and progress. The intent of assessment is to identify what if any problems exist. The intent of evaluation is to determine if the known problems have improved, worsened, or otherwise changed.

The new data collected from evaluation measures are critically analyzed and compared with expected outcomes to determine whether changes occurred (see Table 11-1). After caring for a client over a long period, the nurse is able to make subtle comparisons of responses and behaviors. Previous experience coupled with a scientific knowledge base are key to critical thinking. The accuracy of any evaluation improves when the nurse is familiar with the client's behavior and physiological status. Evaluation is also more exact after the nurse has seen more than one client with a similar type of problem.

The primary source of data for evaluation is the client. However, the nurse also uses the family and other care givers. Documentation and reporting in the evaluation process is of critical importance. Written nursing progress notes, assessment flow sheets, and information shared among nurses during change-of-shift reports (see Chapter 12) should communicate a client's progress toward meeting expected outcomes and goals for the nursing plan of care. If a client is cared for using a critical pathway or CareMap® (see Chapter 12), the nurse and team members clearly know what outcomes are to be met for a given day (Fig. 11-2). The CareMap® as a documentation tool includes expected outcomes that the care team predicts will be met during the client's projected length of stay. The nurse and other team members refer to the outcomes on the

CareMap® on an ongoing basis. If there is variance (unexpected outcomes or outcomes occurring at a different time than expected), the nurse reports these responses and revises the plan of care as needed. By having outcomes clearly documented on either a CareMap® or other documentation form, the nurse and other health care providers clearly know what to evaluate. All members of the health care team should have a sense of the client's progress. Each nurse summarizes data on an ongoing basis to ensure that the client is progressing to a better level of health.

■ CARE PLAN REVISION AND CRITICAL THINKING

As goals are evaluated, adjustments to the care plan are made as indicated. If a goal was successfully met, that portion of the care plan is discontinued. Unmet and partially met goals require the nurse to reactivate the nursing process sequence. After a nurse reassesses a client, nursing diagnoses may be modified or added with appropriate goals, expected outcomes, and interventions established. The nurse also redefines priorities. This is an important step in critical thinking—knowing how the client is progressing and how problems either resolve or worsen. The nurse's careful monitoring and early detection of problems are a client's first line of defense (Benner, 1984). Benner describes the importance of nurses learning how to anticipate the client's future course. It is based on the nurse's observations of what is occurring with a specific client and not merely what may happen to clients in general. Frequently changes are very subtle. Evaluation must be client specific, based on a close familiarity with each client's behavior, physical status, and reaction to care givers. Accurate evaluation leads to the appropriate revision of ineffective care plans and discontinuation of therapy that has been successful.

Discontinuing a Care Plan

After determining that expected outcomes and goals have been achieved, the nurse confirms this evaluation with the client. If the nurse and client agree that the expected outcomes have been met, the nurse discontinues that care plan. For example, a client has the nursing diagnosis, knowledge deficit regarding insulin therapy related to inexperience. To achieve the ultimate goal of accurate client administration of insulin, the nurse establishes outcomes, including "client will describe the purpose of insulin by 9/20," "client will correctly prepare insulin in syringe by 9/20," and "client will administer insulin injection independently by 9/22." The nurse discusses the information with the client and learns whether the client understands explanations and is comfortable with the information provided. In addition, the nurse will observe the client's preparation of the medication and actual self-injection. Once outcomes are met successfully it is unnecessary to teach additional information about insulin administration. The care plan can be documented as discontinued. This ensures that other nurses will not unnecessarily continue a care plan. Continuity of care assumes that care provided is relevant to client needs. Significant time is wasted when achieved goals are not communicated.

Modifying a Care Plan

When goals are not met, the nurse identifies the variables or factors that interfered with goal achievement. Usually a change in the client's condition, needs, or abilities makes alteration of the care plan necessary. For example, when teaching self-administration of insulin, the nurse discovers that the client has a literacy problem or a visual impairment that prevents the reading of insulin dosages on the syringe. As a result, original outcomes cannot be met. Thus the nurse uses new interventions and revises outcomes to meet the goal of care.

Lack of goal achievement may also result from an error in nursing judgment or failure to follow each step of the nursing process. Clients frequently have very complex problems. The nurse should always remember the possibility of overlooking or misjudging something. When there is failure to achieve a goal, no matter what the reason, the entire nursing process sequence is repeated to discover changes that need to be made to promote, maintain, or restore the client's health.

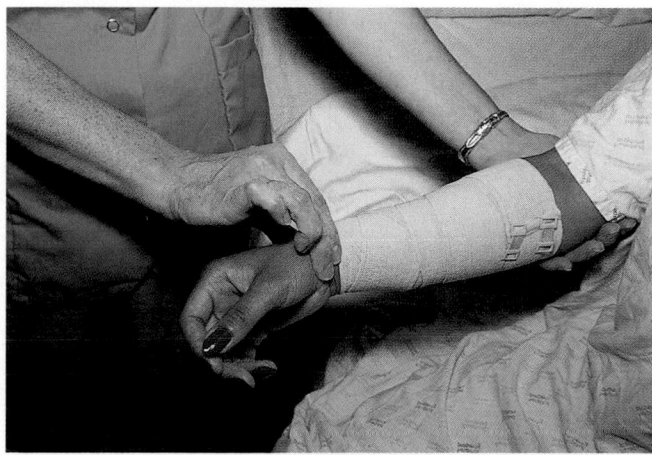

Fig. 11-1 Nurse evaluates circulation following bandage application.

REASSESSMENT

A complete reassessment of all client factors relating to the nursing diagnosis and etiology is the first step in reactivating the nursing process. Reassessment requires critical thinking when the nurse compares new data about the client's condition with previously assessed information. Often a nurse applies intuitive knowledge from experiences with other clients to direct the reassessment process. Encounters over time with clients and families who have similar health problems give nurses a strong background of knowledge to use for anticipating client needs and planning care. For example, consider Mr. Landis, who has the nursing diagnosis of pain related to trauma of a surgical incision. Two days following surgery the client continues to have a poor appetite, despite the fact that there are no obvious surgical complications. If the client continues to have pain the nurse may automatically associate loss of appetite with discomfort. However, the experienced nurse may recall a previous client who became almost depressed following surgery. After exploring the problem further, the nurse learns that Mr. Landis' family has not been visiting, the client is fearful of losing his job, and in addition to experiencing loss of appetite the client is not sleeping well. Although the client continues to have pain, a new priority diagnosis may be anticipatory grieving related to losses associated with illness. Refocus on this diagnosis may improve the client's appetite. As in the original assessment, data are collected from all available sources. Depending on the nurse's findings, it often becomes necessary to assess variables that were not covered on the initial assessment.

Reassessment ensures that the data base is accurate and current. It may also reveal the missing link, that is, a critical piece of new information that was overlooked and thus interfered with goal achievement. All new data are sorted, validated, and clustered to analyze and interpret differences from the original data base. The nurse documents reassessment data to alert other nursing staff to the client's status.

NURSING DIAGNOSES

After reassessment, the nurse reevaluates all nursing diagnoses and determines whether the diagnostic statement was accurately formulated for the situation. The nurse asks whether the correct diagnosis was selected and whether it and the etiological factor are current. The problem list should then be revised to reflect the client's changed status. A new diagnosis may be made. If a previous diagnosis no longer accurately reflects the problem, it should be discontinued and a modified statement should be entered. For example, if the nurse finds that a client with diabetes has a serious visual impairment, it may be unlikely that the client will be able to self-administer insulin. The nurse's assessment reveals that a family member is available as a resource. To develop a plan designed to educate an alternate care giver about the administration of insulin, the nurse then establishes a new diagnosis, altered health maintenance related to visual impairment.

A nurse's care is based on an accurate list of nursing diagnoses. Accuracy is more important than the number of diagnoses selected. As the client's condition changes, the diagnoses do too.

SERVICE ORTHO_____ PHYSICIAN _____ CARE PATH 804
PRIMARY NURSE_____ ADM DATE _____
DC DATE _____

PATIENT PROBLEMS/NURSING DIAGNOSIS	
#1	Pain
#2	Impaired physical mobility
#3	Lack of knowledge
#4	High risk for injury

PROBLEM NUMBER		ED ADM DATE	MED CLEARANCE	DAY DOS	DAY POD 1
	ASSESSMENT MONITORING	Total Nursing Admission/Assessment Assess for hip or leg deformity Assess skin condition q shift NV status check	Assess NV status q 4o	Dressing D/I HMV patent to SS NV assessment q 1o x4 then q 2o to hip/LE Assess bowel sounds Assess lung sounds Assess abdominal distention Skin assessment q shift	Dressing D/I HMV patent to SS NV assessment q 2o Assess bowel sounds Assess lung sounds Assess abdominal distention Skin assessment q shift
	CONSULTS	Pre-Screening		Consults… P.T. O.T. S.W.	Initiate… P.T. O.T.
	PROCEDURE/ TEST	Admit labs CBC, 6, PT/PTT SMA 12, T & S UA with micro EKG CXR Hip x-ray Overhead frame Trapeze Advance 2000 bed	Medical clearance tests	X-ray post op m PAR/OU CBC, 6 post op in PAR	CBC, 6 Hgh/Hct > than transfuse
	TREATMENT	Traction (skeletal or Buck's 5lb) Foley cath Ice to hip prn I/O I.S. every 2o WA TCDB every 2o	Bucks tx I.S. every 2o Foley cath care	HMV I/O I.S. every 1o TCDB every 2o Foley cath care Check hip dressing	DC Foley cath I/O I.S. every 1o TCDB every 2o Check hip dressing
	ACTIVITY	Bedrest Turn 45o every 2o	Bedrest Turn 45o every 2o	Bedrest Turn every 2o	Chair BID MD to determine weight bearing status Stand with walker and P.T. Assist with ADL's
	MEDS/IVS	Heplock 20 gauge of > Prn analgesic LOC AAOC	PRN analgesics Flush HL every 8o IVF's stated after MN day before surgery	IVF's PCA Ancef x6 doses #1/#2	IVF to KVO PCA Ancef #3/4/5
	NUTRITION	Req. NPO after MN	Req. NPO after MN	Clear/full liquids	Advance to regular
	PATIENT/ FAMILY EDUCATION	Nursing Pre-op teaching Use of I.S. Traction Post-op routine Potential need for 730cu	Nursing Continue — pre-op post-op teaching	Reinforce pre-op Post-op teaching i.e., activity, I/O, I.S., PCA, diet	P.T./Nursing Wt bearing status Transfers OOB to chair
	DISCHARGE PLANNING	Nursing Assess condition at home Determine need for: Social Services P.T. O.T. Home Health **Pt./Family verbalizes understanding of Care Path. Plan of care has been mutually set with pt/family**	**High risk screening** Social Worker		Initiate P.T.
	PSYCHO-SOCIAL/ EMOTIONAL	Provide emotional support		Provide emotional support	Give positive feedback on activity
	VARIANCE				
	SIGNATURES				

Fig. 11-2 Portion of total hip care path. *(Courtesy Barnes-Jewish Hospital, St Louis.)*

BARNES - JEWISH HOSPITAL

DAY POD 2	DAY POD 3	DAY POD 4	DAY POD 5	DC OUTCOMES
Dressing D/I DC HMV per HO dressing over old HMV site NV assessment q shift	Incision line clean, dry, well approximated 4 x 4 over old HMV site D/I Minimal HMV site drainage Afebrile	Incision line clean, dry, well approximated No drainage from old HMV site	Staples/sutures removed per H.O. if not on Prednisone (If on Prednisone — remove 14 days in office/clinic) Check walker/crutches to go home with patient for safety	No signs or symptoms infection No evidence of dislocation
		Potential evaluation Home Health		
		Hip x-ray taken CBC		Wound clean and dry Hgh/Hct stable
I.S. every 2o WA	I.S. every 2o WA	I.S. every 4o WA		Lungs clear or WNL
Check hip dressing				
Chair BID P.T. BID Assist with ADL's	Chair		Chair TID P.T.–bid Transfers OOB indep. Amb. indep. with walker and steady gait Indep. with ADL's	Ind. ambulate with steady gait/walker Uses O.T. equipment correctly to perform self care activity
IVF's chd to HL DC PCA DC Ancef after #6 Initiate p.o. pain medications	DC H.L. if Hct > 28 p.o. pain medications	p.o. pain medications	p.o. pain meds	Pain controlled with p.o. analgesics
Regular	Regular	Regular	Regular	
P.T./Nursing	P.T./Nursing OT–instructions	P.T./Nursing	P.T./Nursing	Able to verbalize and demonstrate correct precautions/weight bearing status. Able to verbalize understanding of home care exercises.
ADL Equipment form OT– reacher, etc.	Follow-up with P.T. concerning DC plans ADL training with O.T. Initial eval. of DC by S.W.		DC pt with discharge instructions, prescriptions, home equipment	DC to appropriate level of care with MD/clinic follow-up
Verbal praise for accomplishment	Accepting D/O plan and motivated to	DC plan accepted	DC plan accepted with positive attitude	Demonstrated appropriate coping and emotional response

Fig. 11-2, cont'd Portion of total hip care path.

GOALS AND EXPECTED OUTCOMES

When care plans are revised, the nurse reviews goals and expected outcomes for needed changes. Even the goals for unchanged nursing diagnoses should be examined for appropriateness. Determining that each goal and expected outcome is realistic for the problem, etiology, and time frame is particularly important. Unrealistic expected outcomes and time frames make goal achievement difficult.

The nurse clearly documents goals and expected outcomes for new or revised nursing diagnoses so that all team members are aware of the revised care plan. When the goal is still appropriate but has not yet been met, the nurse may change the evaluation date to allow more time. All goals and expected outcomes should be client centered, with realistic expectations for client achievement.

INTERVENTIONS

The evaluation of interventions examines two factors: the appropriateness of the interventions selected and the correct application of the implementation process. The appropriateness of an intervention may be based on the **standard of care** for a client's health problem. If the client who is postoperative for abdominal surgery has a specific nursing diagnosis, such as ineffective airway clearance, the standard of care established by a nursing department for this problem may include pain control measures with coughing or deep breathing exercises to help a client breathe more easily with a clear airway. The nurse reviews the standard of care to determine whether the right interventions have been chosen or if additional ones are required.

It may only be necessary to increase or decrease the frequency of interventions. The nurse uses judgment based on previous experience, as well as the client's actual response to therapy. For example, if a client continues to have congested lung sounds, the nurse increases the frequency of coughing exercises to remove secretions.

During evaluation, the nurse may determine that some planned interventions are designed for an inappropriate level of nursing care. If the level of care needs to be changed, a different action verb, such as *assist* in place of *provide,* may be substituted. Sometimes the level of care is appropriate, but the interventions are unsuitable because of a change in the expected outcome. In this case, the interventions should be discontinued and new ones should be planned.

During implementation, the nurse evaluates the client's response during and immediately after intervention. This is the beginning of the evaluation process. Evaluation must be integrated with ongoing nursing care activity. If the response is favorable, implementation continues. Reevaluation occurs when the intervention proves unsuccessful. The nurse then examines the other components of implementation such as client and environment preparation, anticipated complications, or use of personal or technical skills during care delivery (Hickey, 1991).

Changes in implementation should be guided by the nature of the client's unfavorable response. Consulting with other nurses may yield suggestions for improving the approach to care delivery. Senior nurses are often excellent resources because of their experience. Simply changing the care plan is not enough. The nurse must implement the new plan and reevaluate the client's response to the nursing actions. Evaluation is continuous.

Occasionally an error during care planning and delivery is discovered during evaluation. This should be anticipated. The nursing process is designed to be a systematic, problem-solving approach to individualized client care, but there is a wide array of variables for each client with a health care problem. Clients with the same health care problem are not treated the same way. As a result the nurse sometimes makes errors in judgment. The systematic use of evaluation provides a way for nurses to catch these errors in judgment. The nurse consistently incorporates evaluation into practice to minimize errors and ensure that the most appropriate interventions are used.

Evaluation is the final step of the nursing process, a systematic method for organizing and delivering nursing care. The exclusion of evaluation from the nursing process prevents the nurse from evaluating nursing practice and determining whether the outcomes of client care are beneficial. The regular application of evaluation ensures that a client's care plan is current and appropriate.

■ QUALITY IMPROVEMENT

The evaluation of health care is a process used to determine the quality of care and service provided to clients. Each professional nurse is expected to evaluate his or her success in delivering effective nursing care. However, good client outcomes are a product of all individual actions and interactions that relate directly or indirectly to the care received by a client (Scoble and Hembrough, 1993). The outcomes of care are a measure of the performance of the entire health care team. For example, following surgery for a total hip repair, does the client regain functional mobility without severe pain and without complications such as wound infection? To achieve such results requires collaboration by nurses, physical therapists, physicians, dietitians, and perhaps even infection control specialists. More and more, emphasis is being placed on monitoring and evaluating the systems and processes that influence client care. This process is receiving more attention than ever before because of the increasing costs of health care.

Today consumers are more informed and thus more interested in the quality of health care because of rising costs. Accrediting and regulatory agencies are attempting to set a uniform set of standards so that quality comparisons can be made across health care institutions (Health Care Advisory Board, 1994). There are wide variations in the quality of health care within and among institutions. High costs of care do not necessarily ensure high quality and therefore there is significant room for improvement within all health care organizations. The focus of quality improvement at one point was only on hospitals. Now even health care plans (see Chapter 2) are being asked to demonstrate quality since their coverage often restricts employers and consumers from choosing their provider of health care.

As health care institutions look for ways to differentiate themselves from other organizations, quality of care is the answer. Nursing has participated in the monitoring of quality for many years and, for this reason, nurses are leading the efforts within organizations to better understand how to measure quality of care. The JCAHO (1995) defines **quality improvement** (QI) as an approach to the continuous

---

Dimensions of Performance

DOING THE RIGHT THING

- **Efficacy** of a procedure or treatment (e.g., pain management, skin care) in relation to a client's condition. Does the procedure or treatment produce the desired result?
- **Appropriateness** of a test, procedure, or service to meet the client's needs. Is the level of care given the level of care considered necessary (e.g., use of pulse oximetry instead of arterial blood gases)?

DOING THE RIGHT THING WELL

- **Availability** of a needed test, procedure, treatment, or service to the client who needs it (e.g., appointment scheduling in clinics, access to emergency care)
- **Timeliness** with which a needed test, procedure, treatment, or service is provided to the client (e.g., response time for stat x-ray, delays in operating room cases)
- **Effectiveness** with which tests, procedures, treatments, and services are provided (e.g., success with established

standard of care on a CareMap® in meeting client outcomes)
- **Continuity** of the services provided to the client with respect to other services, practitioners, and providers over time (e.g., prompt and appropriate referrals to home health; use of a teaching plan preadmission, during a hospital stay, and postadmission)
- **Safety** of the client (and others) to whom the services are provided (e.g., use of physical restraints, use of Standard Precautions)
- **Efficiency** with which services are provided, showing the relationship between outcomes and the resources used to deliver care (e.g., readmission rate to hospital, comparing client's functional status with the cost of providing care)
- **Respect and caring** with which services are provided (e.g., client satisfaction ratings, informing clients about advance directives)

---

study and improvement of the processes of providing health care services to meet the needs of clients and others. Staff within an organization work together in teams to identify what opportunities exist for improving care and what actions are necessary to achieve success. The purpose of QI is not to identify problems retrospectively, but to identify opportunities prospectively to improve the quality of care or service (Patton and Stanley, 1993). There are several dimensions of performance that a health care institution should include to have a comprehensive QI program (see the box above). Assessment of whether an organization is doing the right thing or doing the right thing well should be the focus of QI activities.

Multidisciplinary Approach

Historically, most QI efforts have been conducted by individual departments within health care organizations. For example, nursing would have an individual QI plan, as would social service, pharmacy, and respiratory therapy. Clearly, all health care providers contribute to the outcomes of client care. Therefore, it makes more sense for staff who are most familiar with client care activities to collaborate on QI efforts. For example, if a team of staff identifies an opportunity to improve the timeliness and efficiency of the admission process to its unit, it makes sense to include nursing, admitting, transporters, pharmacy, and all other departments that make early contact with the client. A nursing plan alone would not improve the admission process as successfully as a multidisciplinary plan. To be successful the members of the team must share respect for one another's contributions to client care and be open to new ideas and change.

Unit-Based QI Teams

In many health care organizations the units that provide client care have unit-based QI teams. In a unit-based program, members identify clinical priorities for a unit, monitor quality indicators, evaluate monitoring results, and recommend changes in service or practice. Unit-based teams are participative, decentralizing decision making and ac-

countability for practice and placing it on the level of the staff. Ultimately an effective QI program will lead to improved clinical practice, better participation by professional staff members, and increased sophistication of evaluation. It will also achieve better outcomes for clients.

Components of a QI Program

A well-organized QI program uses a systematic approach to improve processes throughout an organization. This ensures that everyone speaks the same language in regard to QI projects. The JCAHO's 10 steps to QI (see the box below) are incorporated within many health care organization's programs. The 10 steps ensure a systematic approach for identifying opportunities to improve quality of care and to take appropriate action to resolve any problems. In addition to the JCAHO's 10 steps, there are numerous process-improvement models to be found across the country (Table 11-3). All of the models have similar elements, such as identification of a process or problem. Although they appear in Table 11-3 to be linear, the processes are cyclical (Keill and Johnson, 1994). The models use a scientific ap-

---

JCAHO's 10 Steps for Quality Improvement

1. Establish responsibility and accountability for a QI program.
2. Define the scope of service for a clinical area.
3. Define the key aspects of service for the clinical area.
4. Develop quality indicators to monitor the outcomes and appropriateness of care delivered.
5. Establish thresholds for evaluation of indicators.
6. Collect and analyze data from monitoring activities.
7. Evaluate results of monitoring activities to determine the need for change in practice.
8. Resolve problems through development of action plans.
9. Reevaluate to determine if plan was successful.
10. Communicate QI results to the organization.

Table 11-3	Models for Process Improvement	
PRIDE	**FOCUS-PDCA**	**FADE**
Process—select one to improve	Find process to improve Organize team that knows process	Focus on a problem

Relevant dimensions of
  performance measurement
	Clarify current knowledge
	  of process
		Analyze the problem

Interpret data and evaluate
  variance
	Understand causes of
	  process variation	

Design or redesign the process	Select process improve- ment	Develop a plan

Execute the plan	PDCA: Plan
	        Do
	        Check
	        Act
		Execute the plan

Improve—validate by remeasuring		

Modified from Keill P, Johnson T: Optimizing performance through process improvement, *J Nurs Care Qual* 9(1):1, 1994.

proach to problem solving, similar to the nursing process, that often requires returning to various steps in the model to evaluate and then reassess work that needs to be done. An organization may use the JCAHO's 10-step program to organize its QI program but use a QI model such as FOCUS-PDCA to structure problem analysis and resolution.

RESPONSIBILITY FOR PROGRAM

A director of QI can be found within each organization to assume responsibility for a QI program. Often the department of nursing has a director or assistant director whose responsibilities include ensuring that nursing plays a key role in the organization's QI program. In nursing care areas, clinics, or within home health sections, a nurse manager is often responsible for supporting a unit-based program. That manager assists in bringing together the multidisciplinary team that will conduct QI projects. Individual staff members are responsible for monitoring quality, making decisions about practice, and ensuring that high-quality care is administered.

SCOPE OF SERVICE

Each nursing unit or practice area involved in the care of a select group of clients provides a well-defined set of services. An analysis of a unit's scope of service reveals the types of clients who receive nursing care and the types of processes involved in delivering care. An example might be a general medicine unit in an acute care hospital that cares for middle and older adult clients who have diabetes, heart failure, and gastrointestinal disorders. The unit is involved in processes including medication administration, diabetes education, referrals for cardiac diagnostic testing, and endoscopy. An understanding of the scope of service allows staff to focus on quality issues related to typical client groups.

KEY ASPECTS OF SERVICE

The unit-based committee reviews activities or services considered most important to providing high-quality service to clients. Examples of key aspects of service on the medicine unit might include client education, postdiagnostic monitoring, and administration of IV therapy.

To identify the greatest opportunity for measuring quality, nurses categorize the key aspects of service by high-volume, high-risk, and problem areas. Aspects of care are high volume if more than 50% of the unit's clients receive that service. An aspect of care is high risk if performing or omitting the activity could result in trauma or death for the client or litigation or loss of license. Finally, problem-prone aspects of care are those that have the potential to produce problems for the client, staff, or institution (Patton and Stanley, 1993). This method for prioritizing helps staff to focus on the most important care activities. In the example of the medicine unit, if a high volume of clients are diabetic and if the unit has seen a problem of readmissions resulting from poor glucose control, an opportunity may exist to improve client education and support.

DEVELOPING QUALITY INDICATORS

A **quality indicator** is a quantitative measure of an important aspect of care that determines whether quality of service conforms to requirements. Examples include the percentage of clients who successfully self-administer insulin, the incidence of wound infection, and the percentage of serious medication errors. It is a standard of performance. The quality indicator is the focus for a QI project with staff monitoring criteria that will show if an indicator is being met. There are three types of indicators: structure, process, and outcome.

Structure indicators evaluate the structure or systems for delivering care (e.g., the percentage of staff on nights, compliance in checking emergency cart contents, and nurse's attendance at required courses). **Process indicators** evaluate the manner in which care is delivered (e.g., the use of a pain assessment, recovery of clients from sedation, and client education methods). **Outcome indicators** evaluate the end result of care delivered (Patton and Stanley, 1993). They represent measurable changes in a client's status after receiving care (e.g., the client's ability to administer insulin after instruction or the condition of the client's skin following use of a skin care protocol).

Processes of care are obviously closely related to outcomes, and the structure in which a process of care occurs enhances or hinders the effectiveness of care (Donabedian, 1988). When a unit-based team selects an indicator for QI monitoring, it is important that the indicator be relevant. It is often appropriate to measure both a process and the anticipated outcome to know if standards of care are being met. For example, the staff on the medicine unit may choose to measure its success in implementing diabetes instruction early while measuring whether clients learn to administer insulin correctly. When a unit-based team sits together to select quality indicators for a QI project, it helps to ask which processes and related outcomes need improvement (Keill and Johnson, 1994). Processes to improve may include:

- A weak process that is causing problems (e.g., poor pain management for sickle cell clients)
- A stable process that is adequate but can benefit from improvement (e.g., waiting time for ambulatory surgery can be improved to heighten client satisfaction)
- A process linked to negative outcomes (e.g., education of newly diagnosed diabetes with an incidence of readmission to the hospital for poor glucose control)

When staff then analyze the processes that are high volume, high risk, and problem prone, the team will select indicators that are most relevant to improve.

ESTABLISHING THRESHOLDS FOR EVALUATION

After selecting a quality indicator, staff must determine ways to quantitatively measure the indicator. The occurrence of an indicator, or the percentage of times the indicator is observed (e.g., the number of clients who can successfully explain self-care instructions compared with the number instructed), is one common measure. The **threshold** is a standard for determining whether a problem with quality exists. A measurement that falls below a threshold indicates a problem. For example, staff may set a threshold that states 90% of clients who receive instruction will correctly self-administer insulin. If after monitoring the results show only 88% of clients correctly self-administer insulin, the threshold is not met. Staff will then thoroughly review the factors interfering with successful client education. When QI is an ongoing process, staff continuously work to improve outcomes or performances by raising thresholds.

It is important to understand that almost all processes have variation. For example, consider the process of diabetic instruction and the associated outcome of clients administering insulin. Possible variations in this process and outcome might include time when teaching begins, the materials available for instruction, the number of staff who teach, and learner motivation. Setting a specific threshold (e.g., clients score 90% on a diabetes skills test and staff complete instruction 100% of the time) may not be routinely achievable. The intent of any QI program is to seek ways to improve continuously. This means to define the acceptable level of performance and allow for normal variability.

DATA COLLECTION AND ANALYSIS

On unit-based committees, nurses and staff colleagues monitor criteria for each quality indicator for a predetermined number of clients or cases. Staff must collect meaningful information on a sufficient number of clients to allow for accurate analysis of the appropriateness of care. In the example of diabetic instruction and insulin administration, staff might monitor criteria including use of recommended teaching materials, staff's compliance with teaching standards (e.g., topics and content), and each client's score on a return demonstration test. Additional criteria might include time when teaching begins, age of clients, and client's experience with previous instruction. Collection of relevant data allows accurate analysis of potential problems with quality and their possible causes. For example, if diabetic clients perform poorly on their demonstration test, staff can analyze if standards are inconsistently met or if teaching is unnecessarily delayed. Learning ability may also differ between older adults and younger clients.

EVALUATION OF CARE

Monitoring of quality indicators evaluates if specifically defined processes reach desired outcomes. If results exceed or meet a threshold or if performance is within the controls set for a process, no problem has been identified and the process is performing well. When thresholds for satisfactory care have not been met or when performance is below the control limits set, staff must attempt to determine the cause of problems. For example, if clients who receive diabetic instruction are able to score only an average of 70% on a return demonstration test, staff must determine the reasons for this. This step requires nurses and colleagues to honestly review practice activities and look for opportunities to reinforce nursing care standards or improve practice.

This is a time when the team may choose to use one of the models for QI. The **FOCUS-PDCA** model allows staff to find the aspect of the process to improve, to organize an expert team who knows the process, to clarify knowledge about the process, to understand any sources of variation, and to select an improvement or solution. A key requirement is to be sure the right experts are involved in reviewing the process. In the case of diabetic instruction, it will be important to have dietitians, nursing staff, diabetes nurse specialists, educators, and pharmacists involved as part of the team. Many of these staff might have been on the original QI committee. However, once a problem is identified, additional team members may be needed. The group will use the steps of FOCUS-PDCA to clarify the process used for client instruction, to understand what sources of variation may be occurring, and to recommend an approach to improve client learning through demonstration of injections.

RESOLUTION OF PROBLEMS

After evaluating factors contributing to quality problems, staff develop action plans to improve the process and expected outcomes. It is important to establish actions that will result in success. For example, the action of merely notifying staff that a problem exists is unlikely to change practice or improve outcomes. An action plan should be more direct. In FOCUS-PDCA the staff will *p*lan the action or improvement to make, *d*o or implement the change, *c*heck or analyze results of the change, and then *a*ct on the findings. For example, the team may identify that clients are not performing well with insulin administration because teaching is not being started as soon as the client learns that insulin will be a form of therapy. In addition, the staff is having difficulty acquiring teaching materials needed for instruction. In this case, the team recommends having the pharmacy send instructional materials when insulin is sent to the unit. A clinical pharmacist will assist with instruction on insulin. The staff nurses and nurse specialist develop a protocol that outlines specific content to teach daily until the client learns to administer injections. Collectively the team develops an innovative approach to teaching that is designed to get appropriate information more quickly and efficiently to the client so learning can take place.

EVALUATION OF IMPROVEMENT

After implementing an action plan to improve quality of care, staff must reevaluate the success of the plan. In the example, staff will repeat monitoring of the teaching process and the results of client testing to see if improvement has been made. The change may be positive or negative. For example, if client test scores improve, the team has successfully improved outcomes. Similarly, if test scores show no improvement or even worsen, a new plan of action will be needed. The QI process is similar to the nursing process. When desired outcomes (QI criteria) are not met, staff reinstitute the QI process.

COMMUNICATION OF RESULTS

The results of QI activities must be communicated to staff in all appropriate organizational departments. If findings and results are not communicated, practice changes are not likely to occur. Regular discussion of QI activities in staff meetings, distribution of QI newsletters or memos, and a mechanism for QI committee members to personally report to other colleagues are examples of communication strategies. Often a QI study reveals information that applies to other units or departments. In this case the organization must be responsible for responding to the problem with resources needed to make changes. Revision of policies and procedures, modification of standards of care, or implementation of system changes are examples of the ways that an organization may respond to quality issues.

The incorporation of a QI program within a health care setting benefits the client, professional staff, and institution. With a focus on client outcomes, QI activities will lead to a selection of interventions that result in improved client care. Professional staff members learn from their own practice, identify opportunities to change practices, and gain greater satisfaction from improved client outcomes. An institution will benefit from an improved level of care delivery that reduces excessive use of resources and improved client satisfaction with services.

■ KEY CONCEPTS ■

▶ Evaluation determines a client's response to nursing actions and the extent to which goals of care have been met.

▶ The nurse compares the client's response to nursing actions with expected outcomes established during planning.

▶ Evaluation measures are assessment skills used to collect data for evaluation.

▶ The nursing care plan is modified based on data obtained during evaluation.

▶ As a result of evaluation, client priorities may change.

▶ Expected outcomes are stated in behavioral terms to describe the desired effect of nursing actions.

▶ Evaluation enables the nurse to determine the reason that the care plan was successful or unsuccessful.

▶ For nurses to be accountable for their practice, they must know the outcomes of care.

▶ Evaluation involves critical thinking because the nurse determines the optimal way to deliver nursing care.

▶ Quality improvement is a disciplined approach to find ways to improve the processes and outcomes of health care.

▶ The three types of quality indicators are structure, process, and outcome.

▶ To successfully improve a process, all staff familiar with the process need to be involved.

▶ Establishing thresholds or statistical controls allows staff to determine if changes to a process are successful.

■ KEY TERMS ■

Evaluation, p. 166

FOCUS-PDCA, p. 175

Outcome indicators, p. 175

Process indicators, p. 175

Professional standards review organizations (PSROs), p. 166

Quality improvement (QI), p. 172

Quality indicator, p. 174

Standard of care, p. 172

Structure indicators, p. 174

Threshold, p. 175

■ CRITICAL THINKING EXERCISES ■

1. Mr. Vacaro has been visiting the clinic for more than a month. He visits weekly for follow-up care for a chronic venous stasis ulcer of the left leg. The nurse's note at the time of his first visit contained the following information: "Ulcer with irregular margins, 4 cm wide by 5 cm long, approximately .5 cm deep, draining foul-smelling purulent yellowish drainage. Only subcutaneous tissue visible. Skin around ulcer, brownish rust in color. Zinc oxide and calamine gauze applied to ulcer; Ace bandage applied to gauze. Client instructed to return in 2 weeks." As the nurse who is caring for the client on the follow-up visit, what expected outcomes would you anticipate for the goal of "wound will demonstrate healing within 4 weeks"? What evaluative measures would you use to determine if the wound was healing?

2. Ms. Ikado is a 55-year-old woman who experienced a heart attack and is now recovering on a medical cardiology unit. Her primary nurse has identified the need to teach Ms. Ikado about activity restriction, diet, stress management, and medications. Ms Ikado will likely be in the hospital for 3 more days. Explain why evaluation is important in this case. How will the nurse's evaluation of Ms. Ikado's learning influence the plan of care at discharge?

3. Write a response to the following: "It is more important for nurses to have expert assessment skills than to know how to evaluate care."

4. As a nurse on a neurological unit you care for a number of clients with parkinsonism, a disorder that causes an unsteady gait, muscle weakness, and muscular rigidity. Over the last month five clients with parkinsonism have fallen. Develop a quality indicator and monitoring criteria to measure this practice problem.

REFERENCES

Benner P: *From novice to expert: excellence and power in clinical nursing practice,* Menlo Park, Calif, 1984, Addison-Wesley.

Carnevali DL, Thomas MD: *Diagnostic reasoning and treatment decision making in nursing,* Philadelphia, 1993, JB Lippincott.

Donabedian A: The quality of care: how can it be assessed? *JAMA* 260:1743, 1988.

Health Care Advisory Board: *Next generation of outcomes tracking: implications for health plans and systems, vol 2: quality measures,* Washington, DC, 1994, The Advisory Board.

Hickey PW: *Nursing process handbook,* St Louis, 1991, Mosby.

Joint Commission on Accreditation of Healthcare Organizations: *1995 Accreditation manual for hospitals, vol 1, standards,* Chicago, 1995, The Commission.

Keill P, Johnson T: Optimizing performance through process improvement, *J Nurs Care Qual* 9(1):1, 1994.

Patton S, Stanley J: Bridging quality assurance and continuous quality improvement, *J Nurs Care Qual* 7(2):15, 1993.

Scoble KB, Hembrough B: Nursing clinical pertinence review: a step toward quality improvement, *J Nurs Care Qual* 7(2):52, 1993.

ADDITIONAL READINGS

Davies AR et al: Outcomes assessment in clinical settings: a consensus statement on principles and best practices in project management, *J Qual Improve* 20(1):6, 1994.

Green E, Katz JK: Practice guidelines: a standard whose time has come, *J Nurs Care Qual* 8(1):23, 1993.

Hegyvary ST: Issues in outcomes research, *J Nurs Qual Assur* 5(2):1, 1991.

Marek KD: Outcome measurement in nursing, *J Nurs Qual Assur* 4(1):1, 1989.

Potter PA: An assessment tool for developing quality indicators, *J Nurs Care Qual* 6(1):30, 1991.

Recker D, Oie M: Application of total quality management to unit-based quality assessment and improvement, *J Nurs Care Qual* 8(4):25, 1994.

Visalli HN: Blending the clinical nurse specialist functions and quality improvement leadership: a partnership in care, *J Nurs Care Qual* 8(3):75, 1994.

Williams AD: Development and application of clinical indicators for nursing, *J Nurs Care Qual* 6(1):1, 1991.

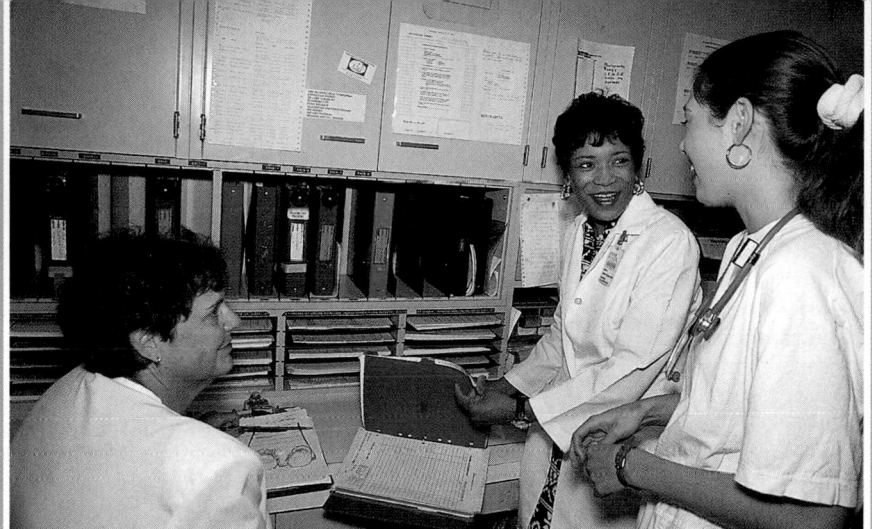

## Chapter 12

Documentation and Reporting

Objectives

Mastery of content in this chapter will enable the student to:

▶ Define the key terms listed.

▶ Discuss the relationship between documentation and health care financial reimbursement.

▶ Identify purposes of a health care record.

▶ Describe guidelines for effective documentation and reporting.

▶ Discuss legal guidelines for recording.

▶ Describe the different methods used in record keeping.

▶ Discuss the advantages and disadvantages of standardized documentation forms.

▶ Identify elements to include when documenting a client's discharge plan.

▶ Describe the role of critical pathways in multidisciplinary documentation.

▶ Describe the influences of home care documentation.

▶ Identify the important aspects of long-term care documentation.

▶ Discuss the role of computerization in documentation.

▶ Identify ways to maintain confidentiality of records and reports.

▶ Describe the purpose of a change-of-shift report.

▶ Explain how to verify telephone orders.

Documentation is a vital aspect of nursing practice. Over time, the format and quality of documentation have evolved, but the focus continues to be a positive impact on client care. Today one of the most challenging issues in nursing is how to document quality client care within the constraints imposed by regulations, resources, and finances. The ideal documentation system should provide comprehensive client information, address client outcomes and standards, facilitate reimbursement from government and insurance company payors, and serve as a legal document (Twardon and Gartner, 1993).

Nursing documentation has become increasingly important because of its fiscal connection in determining the cost of client care. Regulations require health care institutions to monitor and evaluate the quality and appropriateness of client care. Such monitoring requires a thorough review of the documentation in a client's medical record. **Accreditation** agencies such as the Joint Commission on Accreditation of Healthcare Organizations (JCAHO) specify guidelines for information to be documented. Under the prospective payment system, hospitals are reimbursed a set dollar amount by Medicare for each **diagnosis-related group (DRG)** (see the box below). Everything that is done for a client should be documented in the medical record. If the documentation is incomplete, a health care institution will not recover its costs.

As members of the health care team, nurses must communicate information about clients accurately and in a timely, effective manner. The quality of client care depends on care givers' ability to communicate with one another. All health care providers require the same information about clients so that they can plan an organized, comprehensive care plan. Unless the client's care plan is communicated to all members of the health care team, care becomes fragmented, repetition of tasks occurs, and therapies are often delayed or even deleted. The result of poor communication is often poor client outcomes such as delayed recovery and complications that could have been avoided. Nurses are accountable for their actions; as a result, information in the record must be clear and logical, describing exactly all care delivered.

The health care environment creates many challenges for accurately documenting and reporting the care delivered to clients. The quality of care deserved by clients, the standards of regulatory agencies, the reimbursement structure in the health care system, and the legal guidelines for nursing practice make documentation and reporting two of the most important functions of a nurse. Any information about a client's care should be communicated with careful thought. All members of the health care team depend on recorded and reported information. Accurate information ensures continuity and quality of care.

■ MULTIDISCIPLINARY COMMUNICATION WITHIN THE HEALTH CARE TEAM

Client care requires proficient communication among members of the health care team. As a result, care givers use a variety of ways to exchange information about clients. **Reports** are oral or written exchanges of information shared between care givers in a number of ways (Fig. 12-1). After completing a work shift, nurses give a verbal report to nurses on the next shift. A physician may call a nursing unit to receive a verbal report on a client's progress for the day. The laboratory submits a written report describing the results of diagnostic tests for inclusion in the permanent medical record.

A **record** is a permanent written communication that documents information relevant to a client's health care management, for example, a clinic record or chart. After each clinic visit, information about the client's health care is recorded. With each successive visit the record is available to the physician and other members of the health care team. It is a continuing account of the client's health care status and needs.

Another way that information is communicated is through discussions among team members. Discussions may be informal or formal. They allow a review of information so that problems are identified and solutions are recommended. A formal discussion, for example, is a discharge planning conference in a restorative care unit. The members of all disciplines (e.g., nursing, social work, medicine, and physical therapy) meet to discuss the client's progress toward established discharge goals. **Consultations** are another form of discussion whereby one professional care giver gives formal advice about the care of a client to another. For example, a family nurse practitioner confers

---

■ Diagnosis-Related Groups

■ A diagnosis-related group (DRG) is a series of decision trees designed to cluster groups of clients together by diagnosis, surgical procedures, complications, comorbidities (preexisting illness), and age.
■ The statistical weight of a DRG is multiplied by a hospital's specific rate of reimbursement.
■ The hospital is reimbursed a fixed amount for every client grouped into the DRG regardless of length of stay or cost of treatment.
■ An assigned DRG may change on the basis of documentation.

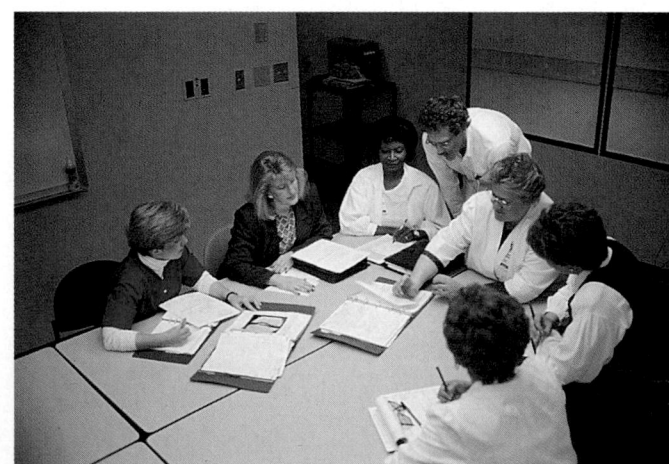

Fig. 12-1 Staff communicate information about their clients during an end-of-shift report.

with a staff nurse about the best choice of nonmedicinal therapies for controlling chronic back pain, or an acute care nurse consults with a dietitian in the selection of the best diet therapy for a client with a diagnosis of diabetes. Both consultations and conferences should be documented in a client's permanent record so that all care givers can benefit from the information and plan care accordingly.

∎ DOCUMENTATION

Documentation is important in health care today. **Documentation** is defined as anything written or printed that is relied on as a record of proof for authorized persons. A medical record should be a comprehensive description of the client's health status and needs, as well as the services provided for the client's care. Good documentation reflects not only quality of care but also evidence of each health care team member's accountability in giving care.

Several types of records are used to communicate information about clients. Although each agency uses a different record format, all records contain basically the following information:

1. Client identification and demographic data
2. Informed consent for treatment and procedures
3. Admission nursing history
4. Nursing diagnoses or problems
5. Nursing or multidisciplinary care plan
6. Record of nursing care treatment and evaluation
7. Medical history
8. Medical diagnosis
9. Therapeutic orders
10. Medical and health discipline's progress notes
11. Reports of physical examinations
12. Reports of diagnostic studies
13. Summary of operative procedures
14. Discharge plan and summary

Purposes of Records

A record is a valuable source of data that is used by all members of the health care team. Its purposes include communication, financial billing, education, assessment, research, auditing, and legal documentation.

COMMUNICATION

The record is a means by which health care team members communicate contributions to the client's care, including individual therapies, client education, and use of referrals for discharge planning. The plan of care should be clear to anyone reading the chart. When a staff member is caring for a client, the record should explain the measures needed to maintain continuity and consistency of care.

FINANCIAL BILLING

The client care record is a document that shows the extent to which health care agencies should be reimbursed for services; it is a client's bill. Diagnosis-related groups have become the basis for establishing reimbursement for client care (see the box on p. 180). Nursing documentation can make a difference to ensure high standards of quality care and maximum reimbursement to health care agencies. Detailed recording helps in establishing codable diagnoses that are used to determine a DRG. The nurse's contribution to documentation can help interpret the type of treatment

a client receives. When client charges exceed the length of stay allowed for a particular DRG, documentation can potentially justify the additional time.

EDUCATION

A client's record contains a variety of information, including medical and nursing diagnoses, signs and symptoms of disease, successful and unsuccessful therapies, diagnostic findings, and client behaviors. Students of nursing, medicine, and other health-related disciplines use these records as educational resources. An effective way to learn the nature of an illness and the response to it is to read the client care record. Although no two clients have identical records, patterns of information can be identified in records of clients who have similar health problems. With this information students learn the patterns to look for in various health problems and become better able to anticipate the type of care required for a client.

ASSESSMENT

The record provides data that nurses use to identify and support nursing diagnoses and plan proper interventions for care. Information from the record adds to the nurse's observations and assessment. The surgical history, for example, is in the record. Thus it is unnecessary for the nurse to collect information that is already available unless there is reason to believe that the information is inaccurate. The medical progress notes detail the physician's findings at the time of assessment. Before caring for any client, the nurse refers to the medical record for new, relevant assessment findings. The nurse is able to enter a client's room, anticipate the status of the client, and then conduct an individualized assessment of the client.

The record provides a total picture of the client's health status. Assessment data entered by each health care team member do not simply describe isolated happenings. Each observation is part of a larger puzzle that, when solved, reveals the client's health status. The record contains data to explain and confirm observations or refute interpretations. For example, after inspection of a wound the nurse may conclude that it is healing poorly; the nurse checks the record, which may give additional information, including the client's appetite, other descriptions of the wound's appearance, laboratory results indicating the onset of infection, and the physician's observation of the wound in the last 24 hours. Any observations or interpretations made by the nurse are compared with data from the record. The record helps explain the reasons for and implications of any findings the nurse gathers.

RESEARCH

Statistical data relating to the frequency of clinical disorders, complications, use of specific medical and nursing therapies, deaths, and recovery from illness can be gathered from client records. Records are a valuable resource for describing characteristics of the client populations in a health care agency.

A nurse may use clients' records during a research study to collect information on certain factors. For example, if a nurse uses a new method of pain control in a group of clients, the records could provide data on the success of therapy. Recording entries that describe the number of analgesic medications that are used or clients' subjective reports of pain relief could be used to evaluate new pain-control measures. Nurses may also research records of previously discharged clients to identify nursing care problems. For example, a study to determine the incidence of infection in clients with specific types of intravenous catheters might be performed by means of a chart review.

AUDITING AND MONITORING

A regular review of information in client records gives a basis for evaluation of the quality and appropriateness of care provided in an institution. The JCAHO requires hospitals to establish quality-improvement programs for conducting objective, ongoing reviews of client care. The JCAHO has standards for types of information to be found in the client's record, such as indications that a plan of care is developed with the client as a participant and that discharge planning and client education have occurred. The JCAHO asks institutions to establish standards for quality care. Nurses monitor or review records throughout the year to determine the degree to which quality-improvement standards are met (see Chapter 11). Deficiencies identified during monitoring are shared with all members of the nursing staff so that corrections in policy or practice can be made. Quality-improvement programs keep nurses informed of standards of nursing practice to maintain excellence in nursing care.

Medical records are also audited to review charges for the client's care. Private insurance carriers and auditors from the federal government review records to determine the reimbursement that a client or a health care agency receives. Thorough documentation of supplies and equipment that have been used ensures that costs are recovered and that clients receive the care they require.

Table 12-1	Examples of Criteria for Reporting and Recording
TOPIC	**ITEMS TO REPORT OR RECORD**
Symptom (e.g., pain, nausea, headache, dizziness)	Description of episode Location of symptom Severity Onset Precipitating factors Frequency and duration Aggravating and relieving factors Associated symptoms
Sign (e.g., rash, tenderness on palpation of body part, decreased breath sounds)	Location of sign Description or quality of findings Aggravating or relieving factors Onset
Nursing care measures (e.g., enema, bath, dressing change)	Time administered Equipment used if appropriate Client's response (positive[+]or negative[−]) Nurse's observations
Client behavior (e.g., anxiety, confusion, hostility)	Onset Behaviors exhibited Precipitating factors Nursing response or action Client's response
Medication administration	Time administered Any required preliminary observations (e.g., pulse rate, blood pressure) Client's response or effect of medication (positive [++] or negative [−−]) Nursing measures taken for negative response
Client teaching	Information or topic presented Method of instruction (e.g., discussion, role playing, demonstration) Resources used (e.g., videotape, booklet) Evidence that client understands instruction (e.g., return demonstration, change in behavior)
Discharge planning	Client goals or expected outcomes Progress toward goals Need for referrals or resources Client's involvement in care plan

+, For example, client denied pain during dressing change.
−, For example, client experienced severe abdominal cramping during enema.
++, For example, client reports that pain is reduced after analgesic.
−−, For example, rash is noted over lower abdomen.

LEGAL DOCUMENTATION

A medical record must be accurate because it is a legal document (see Chapter 20). In the case of a lawsuit the medical record, not the nursing care, is on trial. Consequently, thorough, accurate documentation is one of the best defenses for legal claims associated with nursing care. The record serves as a description of exactly what happened to a client. Nursing care may have been excellent; however, "care not documented is care not done" in a court of law. In addition, even consultations with other health care providers may be worthy of documentation. To protect themselves from a client ignoring nursing instructions, nurses must indicate any instructions or referrals in the medical record (Mandell, 1994). Clients frequently request copies of their medical records, and they have the right to read those records. Each institution has policies for controlling the manner in which records are shared.

Recording should not become merely routine or superficial, nor should nurses wait until the end of a shift of care to record the client's care. Good documentation should be done in a timely manner with careful thought. Four common communication problem areas in malpractice caused by inadequate documentation are (1) not charting the correct time when events occurred, (2) failing to record verbal orders or failing to have them signed, (3) charting actions in advance to save time, and (4) documenting incorrect data (Martin, 1994). Table 12-1 provides guidelines for legally sound documentation.

∎ GUIDELINES FOR QUALITY DOCUMENTATION AND REPORTING

Quality documentation and reporting are necessary to enhance efficient, individualized client care. Six important guidelines must be followed for quality documentation and reporting: factual basis, accuracy, completeness, currentness, organization, and confidentiality.

Factual Basis

Information about clients and their care must be factual. A record should contain descriptive, objective information about what a nurse sees, hears, feels, and smells (Eggland, 1993). An objective description is the result of direct observation and measurement. Factual information is less likely to be misleading or to cause misinterpretation. The use of words such as *appears, seems,* or *apparently* is not acceptable because they lead to conclusions that cannot be supported by objective information. If a nurse documents inferences or conclusions without factual information, errors in care can occur.

The nurse should also document subjective information but only when it is supported by facts. For example, the description, "the client seems anxious" does not accurately communicate information. The description does not inform another care giver of the details regarding the behaviors exhibited by the client that led to the use of the word *anxious*. The phrase *seems anxious* is a conclusion without supported facts. Documentation should clearly explain the nurse's observations of the client's behaviors and not interpret those observations. If a client reports subjective information to the nurse, it should be written with quotations as a subjective entry in the client's own words. For example, "Client states, 'I feel very nervous, and out of control.'"

The nurse can then add any objective findings that more clearly describe the client's anxiety, such as an increased blood pressure and pulse rate.

Accuracy

A client's record must be accurate so that precise documentation is sustained. The use of exact measurements ensures that a record is accurate. The nurse makes descriptions such as "Intake, 360 ml of water" rather than "Client drank an adequate amount of fluid." Measurements are later used as a means to determine whether a client's condition has improved or worsened. Charting that an abdominal wound is "5 cm in length" is more accurate than "large and gaping." Use of an institution's accepted abbreviations, symbols, and system of measures (e.g., metric) ensures that all staff members will use the same language in their reports and records. It is also important to use abbreviations that will not be misinterpreted. For example, *o.d.* (once daily) can be interpreted to mean *OD* (right eye). To avoid any chance of error, abbreviations are spelled in their entirety when terminology is confusing.

Correct spelling is important for accurate documentation and reporting. Terms can easily be confused or misinterpreted (e.g., *dysphagia* or *dysphasia* and *dram* or *gram*). Simple spelling mistakes can also cause serious treatment errors. Medications such as digitoxin and digoxin or morphine and Numorphan must be spelled carefully. If a mistake is made on a medication record, a client may receive the wrong medication.

An accurate entry in a record must reflect what nurses do during the time frame of the entry. Nurses never chart for anyone else or let anyone chart for them. (An exception is when nurses call their units to report a medication or therapy that they had not charted while on duty.) In a court of law it would be easy for a lawyer to create doubt about care when a recorded note did not truly reflect what was done by the nurses. It is acceptable for nurses to later call and ask colleagues to chart information after they leave work. However, the entry must clearly show what was done and by whom (e.g., "At 11 AM Sam Turner, RN, called and reported that at 8 AM Demerol 100 mg IM was administered to client for abdominal pain" [Kopf, 1993]).

Another way to ensure accuracy of records is to correctly countersign entries. Agency policies explain how and when to countersign. For example, registered nurses may be required to countersign a note entered into the record by a nursing student. When a nurse countersigns another nurse's entry, it means that the entry was reviewed and the care given was approved. When a nurse countersigns an entry, it is important that the person administering care is clearly identified. If the record is inaccurate, both nurses can share liability for any client injury that might result.

JCAHO standards (1995) require that "all entries in medical records are dated and authenticated, and a method is established to identify the authors of entries." Therefore any descriptive entry in a client's record ends with the care giver's full name and status, such as "Julie Smith, RN" Nicknames are not used. A nursing student enters the full name and educational institution, such as "David Jones, SN (student nurse), OHSU (Oregon Health Sciences University)." The signature holds a nurse accountable for information recorded.

Completeness

The information within a recorded entry or a report should be complete, containing concise, thorough information about a client's care. Concise data are easy to understand. Lengthy notes are difficult to read. Sketchy or abbreviated notes may leave an impression that nursing care was hurried or incomplete. A long report wastes time and is often boring. Clear, succinct recording and reporting gives only essential information and avoids the use of unnecessary words or irrelevant detail.

A good report or record is thorough and contains complete information about a client. Criteria for thorough communication exist for certain health problems or nursing activities (Table 12-2). The nurse makes written entries in the client's medical record, describing nursing care that is administered and the client's response. An example of a thorough nurses' note follows:

7:15 PM Client verbalizes sharp, throbbing pain localized along radial side of right wrist, beginning approximately 15 minutes ago. Pain increased with movement of wrist, slightly relieved with elevation of hand on pillow. Radial pulses equal bilaterally. Right wrist circumference 1 cm larger than left wrist. Dr. Kent notified at 7:10. Percocet 2 tabs given for pain. Lee Turno, RN.

Currentness

Timely entries are essential in the client's concurrent care (JCAHO, 1995). Delays in recording or reporting can result in serious omissions and untimely delays for needed care. For example, failure to report a drop in blood pressure can delay the administration of a critically needed medication. Legally a late entry in a chart may be interpreted as negligence (see Chapter 20). Ongoing decisions about care must be based on currently reported information. Activities or findings to communicate at the time of occurrence include the following:

1. Vital signs
2. Administration of medications and treatments
3. Preparation for diagnostic tests or surgery
4. Change in status
5. Admission, transfer, discharge, or death of a client
6. Treatment for a sudden change in status

Routine activities such as bathing or giving oral hygiene do not need to be charted immediately. This information is often included in flow sheets. When describing an aspect of care, a nurse should refer to the client's problem, the nursing intervention, and the client's response. A revision or update of a care plan should occur when the client's con-

Table 12-2	Legal Guidelines for Recording	
GUIDELINES	**RATIONALE**	**CORRECT ACTION**
Do not erase, apply correction fluid, or scratch out errors made while recording.	Charting becomes illegible; it may appear as if you were attempting to hide information or deface record.	Draw single line through error, write word error above it; then record note correctly.
Do not write retaliatory or critical comments about client or care by other health care professionals.	Statements can be used as evidence for nonprofessional behavior or poor quality of care.	Enter only objective descriptions of client's behavior; client comments should be quoted.
Correct all errors promptly.	Errors in recording can lead to errors in treatment.	Avoid rushing to complete charting; be sure information is accurate.
Record all facts.	Record must be accurate and reliable.	Be certain entry is factual; do not speculate or guess.
Do not leave blank spaces in nurse's notes.	Another person can add incorrect information in space.	Chart consecutively, line by line; if space is left, draw line horizontally through it and sign your name at end.
Record all entries legibly and in ink.	Illegible entries can be misinterpreted, causing errors and lawsuits; ink cannot by erased; records are photocopied and stored on microfilm.	Never erase entries or use correction fluid, and never use pencil.
If order is questioned, record that clarification was sought.	If you perform order known to be incorrect, you are just as liable for prosecution as the physician is.	Do not record "physician made error." Instead, chart that "Dr. Smith was called to clarify order for_____."
Chart only for yourself.	You are accountable for information you enter into chart.	Never chart for someone else (exception: if care giver has left unit for day and calls with information).
Avoid using generalized, empty phrases such as "status unchanged" or "had good day."	Specific information about client's condition or case can be accidently deleted if information is too generalized.	Use complete, concise descriptions of care.
Begin each entry with time, and end with your signature and title.	This guideline ensures that correct sequence of events is recorded; signature documents who is accountable for care delivered.	Do not wait until end of shift to record important changes that occurred several hours earlier; be sure to sign each entry.

dition changes. It is impossible and unnecessary for a nurse to document every aspect of care in the record when it happens. Therefore it may help to keep a work sheet or notepad close at hand when caring for several clients. Writing notes shortly after the care occurs ensures that an entry recorded later in the record will be accurate.

Each institution uses a system to report the time of day. Military time, a 24-hour system, avoids misinterpretation of AM and PM times that occur with the 12-hour system. In the 24-hour system four-digit number indicates the hours and minutes (Table 12-3).

Organization

The nurse communicates information in a logical format or order. Health care team members understand information better when it is given in the order in which it occurred. For example, an organized note describes the client's pain, nurse's assessment and interventions, and the physician's order in a logical order of occurrence. The disorganized note is fragmented and does not clearly explain what happened first. Poorly organized notes can lead to confusion about whether proper care was given.

Confidentiality

A confidential communication is information given by one person to another with trust and confidence that such information will not be disclosed. The law protects information about clients that is gathered by examination, observation, conversation, or treatment. Nurses should not discuss clients' status with other clients or staff uninvolved in the client's care. Nurses are legally and ethically obligated to keep information about clients' illnesses and treatments confidential. A legal suit can be brought against nurses who disclose information about clients without their consent (see Chapter 20). Only staff members directly involved in care have legitimate access to the records. Nurses and other health care professionals may have reason to use records for data gathering, research, or continuing education. These uses are not breaks in confidentiality, as long as the records are used as specified and permission is granted from hospital internal review boards.

A client's record is accessible to many personnel. Nurses are responsible for protecting records from unauthorized readers such as visitors. The nurse should know the location of the record at all times. If it is misplaced, every effort should be made to find it. The record is stored by the health care agency after treatment ends.

Methods of Recording

The quality of documentation is constantly under review by nursing managers as they attempt to find ways to help nurses improve recording of information. Documentation must follow standards dictated by the JCAHO to maintain institutional accreditation, to lessen liability, and to justify the need for nursing services. For example, the JCAHO (1995) requires that all clients who are admitted to a health care institution have an assessment of physical, psychosocial, environmental, self-care, client education, and discharge-planning needs. In addition, the JCAHO stresses the importance of evaluating client outcomes, including the client's response to treatments, teaching, or preventive

Table 12-3	Comparison of Military and Civilian Time Systems	
MILITARY	**CIVILIAN**	
0100	1:00 AM	
0200	2:00 AM	
0215	2:15 AM	
1200	Noon	
1420	2:20 PM	
1800	6:00 PM	
2400	Midnight	
0001	12:01 AM	

care. Such standards can make documentation time-consuming.

Nurses involved in the direct care of clients often have difficulty in fully documenting their client's care. Lack of time, the feeling that no one reads notes, excess duplication, and a concern about the meaningfulness of information in charts are just some of the concerns nurses have about documentation. These problems have led to more bedside charting and the creation of flow sheets (see Fig. 12-2). Bedside graphics offer nurses the convenience of entering information immediately after it is collected from a client. There is no need to leave the bedside, jot information down on a reminder sheet, and then enter the data in the record at the nurse's station.

In addition, the value of nursing care plans is controversial (Twardon and Gartner, 1993). Some nursing authors propose eliminating care plans; others argue for their continued use. The JCAHO (1996) recommends a multidisciplinary plan of care. Overall, careful scrutiny of the use and value of care plans must be critiqued by nurse clinicians. The outcome of the scrutiny will be a care plan format that is available as a positive tool in documentation of client care.

The nursing service department of each health care agency selects the method that is used to document client care. The method should reflect the philosophy of the nursing service and incorporate the standards of care and practice for the department. For example, if a nursing department's standards of practice use nursing diagnosis or a framework such as Gordon's functional health patterns (Gordon, 1995), the documentation system uses nursing diagnoses and health patterns in care plans and other forms.

Professional care is reflected by professional charting, which proves what the nurse has done and effectively communicates the client's status and progress. Because the nursing process shapes a nurse's approach and direction of care, good documentation reflects the nursing process. Assessment data are recorded to offer to all health care team members a database from which to draw conclusions about the client's problems. Information describing the client's problems or diagnoses then directs care givers to choose an appropriate care plan with nursing therapies. Evaluation of care communicates the client's status, degree of progress, and success in meeting expected outcomes of care.

Many record-keeping methods are found within health care institutions. The difference among them is the manner in which information is organized. A challenge exists to find a record-keeping method that ensures optimal communication, yet simplifies the charting process. The JCAHO requires documentation of nursing diagnoses or problems within the context of the nursing process, as well as evidence of client and family teaching and discharge planning. If more than one discipline regularly cares for a client, the JCAHO also expects a multidisciplinary care plan.

NARRATIVE DOCUMENTATION

Narrative documentation is the traditional method for recording nursing care. It is simply the use of a storylike format to document information specific to client conditions and nursing care. There is no single, "correct" order in which to chart client events. Consequently, nurses chart in varying formats in their use of narrative documentation.

Currently, narrative charting is seldom the primary method of documentation and is being replaced by other formats (e.g., SOAP, PIE, and Focus [described later in this chapter]). Narrative charting is easy to use in emergency situations in which a simple, chronological order is needed, and it is familiar to many nurses. However, narrative documentation is considered the least desirable form of charting in most nursing settings. Among the disadvantages of the narrative style are its likelihood of being subjective, the lack of organized structure, and the lack of analysis and critical decision making on the part of the nurse.

PROBLEM-ORIENTED MEDICAL RECORDS

The **problem-oriented medical record (POMR)** is a method of documentation that places emphasis on the client's problems. The method corresponds to the nursing process and facilitates communication of client needs (Gawlinski and Rasmussen, 1984). Data are organized by problem or diagnosis. Narrative notes are used to incorporate assessment, planning, intervention, and evaluative information specific to the client's health status. Ideally each member of the health care team contributes to a single list of identified client problems. This assists in coordinating a common plan of care. However, in some institutions a modified POMR method of charting is used only by nurses in a nursing notes record section. The POMR has the following major sections: database, problem list, care plan, and progress notes.

Database. The database section contains all available assessment information pertaining to the client (e.g., the physician's physical examination and medical history, the nurse's admission history and ongoing assessment, the dietitian's assessment, laboratory reports, and radiological test results). The database is the foundation for identifying client problems and planning care. The database should remain active and current, and revisions should be made as new data become available. The database accompanies clients through successive hospitalizations or clinic visits. An active database ensures continuity of care.

Problem List. After data are analyzed, problems are identified and a single list is made. The problems are listed in chronological order and filed in the front of the client's

record to serve as an organizing guide for the client's care. New problems are added as they are identified. After a problem has been resolved, the date is recorded and a line is drawn through the problem and its number.

A problem may be well defined, such as a specific medical or nursing diagnosis. The problems include the client's physiological, psychological, social, cultural, spiritual, developmental, and environmental needs. It is important to avoid listing problems that are vague or not supported by data. The nurse lists a diagnosis, if one can be established, rather than a less specific term. For example, the nursing diagnosis of *ineffective airway clearance* is characterized by a cough, dyspnea, and abnormal breath sounds. *Impaired breathing* or *coughing* would be an unacceptable nursing diagnosis.

Care Plan. A care plan is developed for each problem by the disciplines involved in the client's care (see Chapter 9). Nurses document the plan of care in a variety of formats. Generally, these plans of care include nursing diagnoses, expected outcomes, and interventions.

Progress Notes. Health care team members monitor and record the progress of a client's problems. Narrative notes, flow sheets, and discharge summaries are forms used to document the client's progress. **SOAP** is an acronym for the problem-oriented method of documentation as follows:

S—Subjective data (verbalizations of the client)
O—Objective data (that which is measured and observed)
A—Assessment (diagnosis based on the data)
P—Plan (what the care giver plans to do)

An *I* and *E* are sometimes added (as in *SOAPIE*) in various institutions. The *I* stands for intervention, and the *E* represents evaluation. The logic for SOAP (IE) notes is similar to that of the nursing process. Data are collected about each of the client's problems, a conclusion is made, and a care plan

---

Examples of Progress Notes Written in the SOAP and PIE Formats

1/19/95 Knowledge deficit related to inexperience regarding surgery
4:30 PM
S—"I'm worried about what it will be like after surgery."
0—Client asking frequent questions about surgery. Has had no previous experience with surgery. Wife present, acts as a support person.
A—Knowledge deficit regarding surgery related to inexperience. Client also expressing anxiety.
P—Explain routine preoperative preparation. Demonstrate and explain rationale for TCDB exercises. Provide explanation and teaching booklet on postoperative nursing care. S. Lazarus, RN

P—Knowledge deficit regarding surgery related to inexperience.
I—Explained to client normal preoperative preparations for surgery. Demonstrated TCDB exercises. Provided booklet to client on postoperative nursing care.
E—Client demonstrates TCDB exercises correctly. Needs review of postoperative nursing care.
S. Lazarus, RN

is developed. Each SOAP (IE) note is numbered and titled according to the problem on the list it addresses.

PIE documentation is similar to SOAP charting in its problem orientation. However, it differs from the SOAP method in that PIE charting has a nursing origin, whereas SOAP originated from the medical model. PIE is an acronym for problem, intervention, evaluation, as follows:

P—Problem or nursing diagnosis applicable to client
I—Interventions or actions taken
E—Evaluation of the outcomes of nursing interventions and the client's response to nursing therapies

This format simplifies documentation by unifying the care plan and progress notes into a complete record. In the PIE format, unlike the SOAP format, the narrative note does not include assessment information (see the box on p. 186). Daily assessment data appear instead on special flow sheets, thus preventing duplication of information. The PIE notes can be numbered or labeled according to the client's problems. Resolved problems are dropped from daily documentation after the nurse's review. Continuing problems are documented daily.

SOURCE RECORDS

In a **source record** the client's chart is organized so that each discipline (e.g., nursing, medicine, social work, or respiratory therapy) has a separate section in which to record data. Unlike the POMR, the information is not organized by client problems. However, an advantage of a source record is that care givers can easily locate the proper section of the record in which to make entries. Table 12-4 lists the components of a source record.

A disadvantage of the source record is that information is fragmented. Because information is not organized by client problems, details about a specific problem may be distrib-

---

Sample Nurse's Note

8/6 1100 Client states, "I'm having a hard time catching my breath." Respirations, labored at 28/min; P, 96; BP, 112/70. Client using intercostal muscles during inhalation. Breath sounds auscultated, crackles over both lower lobes. Chest excursion equal bilaterally. Elevated head of bed to Fowler's position. Obtained arterial blood gas analysis at 1045 order. Results are pH, 7.34, Pco_2, 44 mm Hg; Po_2, 80 mm Hg. Dr. Stein called. Applied O_2 at 4 L/min per mask as ordered. Remained at bedside to calm client. P. Haske, RN

---

uted throughout the record. It may become necessary to locate data from several different sections before identifying the client's problems and the care plan. For example, the nurse describes the character of abdominal pain and use of relaxation therapy and analgesic medication in the nurses' notes. The physician's notes describe the progress of the client's bowel obstruction and the plan for surgery in a separate section of the record. The results of x-ray examinations that show the location of the bowel obstruction are in the test results section of the record. The method by which source records are organized does not show how information from the disciplines is related or how care is coordinated to meet all of the client's needs.

The nurses' notes section is where nurses enter a narrative description of nursing care and the client's response (see the box above). It is also a section for documenting care that is provided by the physician in the nurse's pres-

---

Table 12-4	Organization of Traditional Source Record	
SECTIONS	**CONTENTS**
Admission sheet	Specific demographic data about client: legal name, identification number, sex, age, birth date, marital status, occupation and employer, health insurance, nearest relative to notify in an emergency, religious preference, name of attending physician, date and time of admission
Physician's order sheet	Record of physician's orders for treatment and medications, with date, time, and physician's signature
Nurse's admission assessment	Summary of nursing history and physical examination
Graphic sheet and flow sheet	Record of repeated observations and measurements such as vital signs, daily weights, and intake and output
Medical history and examination	Results of initial examination performed by physician, including findings, family history, confirmed diagnoses, and medical plan of care
Nurses' notes	Narrative record of nursing process: assessment, nursing diagnosis, planning, implementation, and evaluation of care
Medication records	Accurate documentation of all medications administered to client: date, time, dose, route, and nurse's signature
Physician's progress notes	Ongoing record of client's progress and response to medical therapy and review of disease process
Health care discipline's records	Entries made into record by all health-related disciplines: radiology, social work, and laboratories
Discharge summary	Summary of client's condition, progress, prognosis, rehabilitation, and teaching needs at time of dismissal from hospital or health care agency

ASHLAND COMMUNITY HOSPITAL

GRAPHIC/INTAKE-OUTPUT RECORD
DAILY CARE/ACTIVITY RECORD

DATE																									
Hosp Day / Post OP Day																										
Bath:	PB	BB	Sh	Tub		PB	BB	Sh	Tub		PB	BB	Sh	Tub		PB	BB	Sh	Tub		PB	BB	Sh	Tub	
Daily Care:	AM		PM		HS	AM		PM		HS	AM		PM		HS	AM		PM		HS	AM		PM		HS
Hygiene Oral/Skin																										
Foley Care/PeriCare																										
Stool/GUIAC + –																										
Turn (L.B.R.) Position																										

	24	04	08	12	16	20	24	04	08	12	16	20	24	04	08	12	16	20	24	04	08	12	16	20	24	04	08	12	16	20
Temperature:																														
Pulse:																														
Respiration:																														
Blood Pressure																														
Daily Weight/Time																														

Diet/%					
Snack/%					

INTAKE		11-7	7-3	3-11	24 hr	11-7	7-3	3-11	24 hr	11-7	7-3	3-11	24 hr	11-7	7-3	3-11	24 hr	11-7	7-3	3-11	24 hr
	ORAL																				
	IV																				
	TPN																				
	PC = 250cc																				
	8 Hr. Total																				

OUTPUT																					
	URINE-Vd																				
	URINE-Cath																				
	NG																				
	Emesis																				
	8 Hr. Total																				

EQUIPMENT																					

Diagnostic Studies																					

ACH FORM 118

Fig. 12-2 Nursing care record. *(Courtesy Ashland Community Hospital, Portland, Ore.)*

ence. The nurse may record key diagnostic test results from other sections of the record in the nurses' notes if they are of major importance in the care of the client.

CHARTING BY EXCEPTION

Charting by exception is an innovative approach that is used to streamline documentation. Charting by exception reduces repetition and time spent in charting. It is a shorthand method for documenting normal findings and routine care based on clearly defined standards of practice and predetermined criteria for nursing assessments and interventions. Clearly defined standards of practice that specify nurses' responsibilities to clients provide the framework for routine care of all clients. With standards integrated into documentation forms, such as predefined normal assessment findings or predetermined interventions, a nurse need only document significant findings or exceptions to the predefined norms. In other words, the nurse writes a longhand note only when the standardized statement on the form is not met. Assessments are standardized on forms so that all care givers evaluate and document findings consistently (Fig. 12-2).

Because the standard assessments are located in the chart, client data are already present on the permanent record, so nurses do not have to keep temporary notes for later transcription and care givers have easy access to current data. The assumption with charting by exception is that **all standards are met with a normal or expected response unless otherwise documented.** When nurses see entries in the chart, they know that something out of the ordinary has been observed or has occurred. For that reason when changes in a client's condition have developed, it is easy to track them.

FOCUS CHARTING

Another format for documentation is **focus charting** (Table 12-5). This charting format allows the documentation of any client situation. Each entry includes Data, Actions, and client Response **(DAR)** (see Table 12-5 for the particular client situation). It is not necessary to have each component of the DAR in each charting entry. However, according to Lampe (1994), the use of all three (DAR) helps promote the best documentation.

One distinction of focus charting is its movement away from charting only problems. Focus charting identifies client concerns and does not label them "problems" (which often has a negative connotation). Focus charting structures progress notes according to the focus of the note: a sign or symptom, a condition, a nursing diagnosis, a behavior, a significant event, or an acute change in a client's condition. In addition, focus charting does not require that concerns be worded in the language of nursing diagnoses. This allows for greater flexibility in client documentation.

The advantages of focus charting are that structure is provided for the progress notes, that documentation is written in accordance with the nursing process, that nurses are encouraged to broaden their thinking to include any client concerns, not just problem areas, and that critical thinking is encouraged. Focus charting is easily understood by care givers and adaptable to most health care settings.

CASE MANAGEMENT AND CRITICAL PATHWAYS

The **case management** model of delivering care (see Chapter 2) incorporates a multidisciplinary approach to documenting client care (Crummer and Carter, 1993). The standardized plan of care is summarized into **critical pathways** (Fig. 12-3), which are multidisciplinary integrated care plans for the problems, key interventions, and expected outcomes of the client with a specific disease or condition. The nurse and other team members such as physical or respiratory therapists use the critical pathway to monitor the client's progress during each shift. All care givers use one critical pathway as a monitoring and documentation tool (see Chapter 2). Critical pathways that are incorporated into documentation tools can be developed to eliminate other nursing forms and thus reduce duplication and the amount of charting (Woodyard and Sheetz, 1993). For example, a checklist format could be used while documenting the critical pathway, instead of the more narrative format that is used when charting by exception. In general the checklist tends to eliminate unnecessary written charting and focuses the nurse's attention on the information that is documented.

The critical pathways are used on each shift of care to direct and monitor the flow of client care. The current trends for critical pathways are for agencies to define client-focused outcomes and to specify those interventions necessary for a given day of care. Because of the nature of human response, there are **variances** in the client outcomes as the client deviates from the critical pathway plan. These variances refer to either the positive or the negative changes depending on the clinical situation (Acord-Szczesny, 1994). A

Table 12-5	**Examples of Focus Charting**		
DATE	**TIME**	**FOCUS**	**DATA, ACTIONS, CLIENT RESPONSE (DAR)**
6/20	8:20 AM	Hypotension	D—BP in left arm 90/60, client's skin diaphoretic, client responds to name. A—Placed client in Trendelenburg position, increased IV fluid rate to 100 ml/hr per protocol, called Dr. Arkin. R—Client remains responsive, BP in left arm 94/68 3 min after increasing fluids. S. Wilson, RN
6/30	4:20 PM	Pain	D—Twisting in bed, grimacing with movement, states has sharp lower back pain. A—Administered morphine sulfate 10 mg IM. R—Verbalized relief within 15 minutes, lying quietly. T. Newson, RN

1

BARNES

**CARE PATH® 405
MULTIPLE SCLEROSIS
EXACERBATION**

SERVICE **NEUROLOGY**	PHYSICIAN	
PRIMARY NURSE	PRIMARY NURSE	
DC DATE	ADM DATE	DATE OF SURGERY **A-8**

Problem Number	PATIENT PROBLEMS / NURSING DIAGNOSES
#1	SELF CARE DEFICIT R/T MUSCLE WEAKNESS, PAIN, COORDINATION OR PARALYSIS
#2	IMPAIRED PHYSICAL MOBILITY R/T MUSCLE WEAKNESS
#3	ALTERATION IN ELIMINATION R/T NEUROMUSCULAR IMPAIRMENT
#4	LACK OF KNOWLEDGE R/T UNFAMILIARITY WITH TREATMENT AND DISEASE PROCESS

* IF APPROPRIATE

DATE	#	1, 2 ASSESSMENT / MONITORING	1, 2 CONSULTS	3 PROCEDURES / TEST	1, 2, 3 TREATMENT	1 ACTIVITY
DAY 1		Assess for fall prevention Assess for skin breakdown Assess neuro status and information processing Assess urinary elimination Assess bowel function VS q shift with NC Notify House Officer for Temp ≥ 37.9 Malaise, change in bladder habits, weakness Monitor VS q 30 min. during 1st dose of Solumedrol infusion. House Officer to remain with pt. for 1st 15 min. of infusion.	Physical Therapy evaluation *Occupational Therapy *Social Work *Pastoral Care *Speech-communication and swallow	EKG prior to 1st dose of Solumedrol and after 1st dose completed *MRI *LP Straight cath for PVR *Straight cath q 6 hrs. Guaiac all stools Notify House Officer if + on guaiac Monitor blood glucose 2 hrs. after Solumedrol Notify House Officer if ≥ 250 I & O	Urinalysis	Up with assist Out of bed in chair at least TID for ½ hr. periods
DAY 2		Assess for fall prevention Assess for skin breakdown Assess neuro status and information processing Assess urinary elimination Assess bowel function Notify House Officer if no BM after 48 hrs. VS routine with NC Notify House Officer for Temp ≥ 37.9 Malaise, change in bladder habits, weakness **Skin remains intact Pt. maintains bowel function** **Pt. remains free of injury**	Evaluation completed Frequency of tx and pain established Social Work-Consult Occupational Therapy to address functional performance *Foot care nurse if indicated	Speech-Functional communication established Bedside swallow evaluation completed within 24 hrs. **Stool remains guaiac negative**		

SIGNATURE	INIT.	SIGNATURE	INIT.	SIGNATURE	INIT.

405

Fig. 12-3 Critical path for multiple sclerosis exacerbation. *(Courtesy Barnes-Jewish Hospital, St Louis.)*

BARNES	CARE PATH® 405 MULTIPLE SCLEROSIS EXACERBATION					2

CNS	DIETARY	RT
HOME HEALTH	OT	OTHER
PT	SW	OTHER **A-8**

Problem Number	PATIENT PROBLEMS / NURSING DIAGNOSES

1, 2, 3	2	4	1, 2, 3, 4	1, 2, 4	INITIALS (SEE KEY AT BOTTOM)		
MEDS / IVS	NUTRITION	PATIENT / FAMILY EDUCATION	DISCHARGE PLANNING	PSYCHOSOCIAL/ EMOTIONAL/ SPIRITUAL NEEDS			
IV-Hep lock flush q shift with NS Solumedrol 250mg/100cc NS q 6 hrs.-given over 1/2-1 hr. times 12-30 doses Zantac 150 mg PO BID Oscal 500 mg with Vit. D 1 tab BID Docusate Sodium 100 mg q hs Mylanta 30cc PO pc and hs Dalmane 15-30 mg or Restoril 15-30 mg q hs	*Low sodium Advance diet as tolerated Maintain hydration	Orient to unit Provide information on Solumedrol therapy **Pt. verbalizes understanding of Solumedrol Protocol and IV Therapy**	**Pt./family understands goal of therapy. Pt./family verbalizes understanding of disease process. Pt./family understands safety needs. Pt./family verbalizes understanding of care path. Plan of care has been mutually set with pt./family.**	*Social Work for crises intervention *Pastoral Care- emotional and spiritual			
Evaluate time schedule for Solumedrol to minimize sleep interruption	**Pt. caloric needs met body weight maintained. Pt. adequate fluid intake of 3,000/day.**		Social Work- consult with nursing, MD, and therapists to assess pt. needs. Social Work assessment completed.	Pastoral Care- Pt./family support needs assessed. **Social Work- high risk screening form completed.**			
SIGNATURE	INIT.	SIGNATURE	INIT.	SIGNATURE	INIT.		

Fig. 12-3, cont'd Critical path for multiple sclerosis exacerbation.

Table 12-6	Example of Variance Documentation in Open Text Format

A 56-year-old client is on a surgical unit 1 day after cholycystectomy. He is beginning to have an elevated temperature, his breath sounds are decreased bilaterally in the bases of both lobes of the lungs, and he is slightly confused. The following is an example of the variance documentation for this client.

DATE/TIME	VARIANCE	REASON	COMMENTS/PLAN
9/23/95, 10:00 AM	Decreased breath sounds; Elevated temperature	Decreased ambulation Bilateral consolidation of secretions in bases of both lung lobes	Administer oxygen 2 L per physician's protocol Place continuous pulse oximetry on client; monitor vital signs every hour
	Mental confusion	Decreased oxygenation	Frequently assess client's cerebellar function

positive variance occurs when a client progresses more rapidly than expected (e.g., use of a Foley catheter may be discontinued a day early). A negative variance occurs when the activities on the clinical pathway are not completed as predicted or the client does not meet the expected outcomes. An example of a negative variance is the addition of oxygen therapy and oximetry for a postoperative client with pulmonary problems. A variance analysis is necessary to review the data for trends and for developing and implementing an action plan to respond to the identified client problems (Table 12-6). In addition, variances may result from one-time causes or may result from changes in the client's health, or may occur as a result of other health complications not associated with the primary reason for which the client requires care (Hospital Case Management, 1993). The nurse's responsibility is to "correct" the client change (variance) or to justify the actions taken to manage the critical pathway deviation (Iyer and Camp, 1995).

As the use of critical pathways is refined, the ultimate beneficiary is the client. More accuracy of predicted outcomes will evolve, and variations in client progress will be more easily determined. This will potentiate the proactive nature of client care. In addition, the advantages of multidisciplinary involvement in the plans and interventions for the client are many and varied (see the box below).

Benefits of Case Management and Critical Pathways

The following are the benefits of using critical pathways in client care:
- Continuity of care is more easily communicated.
- Novice health care providers are given a structure within which to provide care.
- Clients are integral to the planning process.
- The entire health care team is involved in all phases of client care.
- Discharge planning and teaching begins very early in the client care process.
- A more creative critical decision-making process is encouraged, which leads to better client outcomes.

Common Record-Keeping Forms

A client's medical record may use a variety of forms to make documentation easy, quick, and comprehensive. Many forms eliminate the need to duplicate repeated data in the nursing notes. The forms present special types of information in a format that is more accessible than long, detailed progress notes.

NURSING HISTORY FORMS

A nursing history form is a special form that is completed at the time a client is admitted to a nursing care unit (see Fig. 7-4, pp. 116 to 117). The form usually contains basic biographical data (e.g., age, method of admission, and physician), the admitting medical diagnosis or chief complaint, a brief medical-surgical history (e.g., previous surgeries or illnesses, allergies, and medication history), the client's perceptions about illness or hospitalization, and a review of health risk factors. A physical assessment of all body systems is either incorporated into the nursing history or included on a separate form. The history form allows the admitting nurse to make a thorough assessment to identify relevant nursing diagnoses or problems for the client's care plan. Data on history forms provide baseline data that can be compared with changes in the client's condition. Each institution designs a nursing history form differently, depending on the standards of practice and philosophy of nursing care.

GRAPHIC SHEETS AND FLOW SHEETS

Client care **flow sheets** are forms that allow nurses to assess the client and document the findings. The checklist facilitates a thorough assessment by providing a framework instead of using open-ended narrative categories (O'Brien and Landstrom, 1994). It is unnecessary to chart a narrative progress note each time the vital signs are checked, a bath is given, or a drug is administered. The flow sheet is a quicker, more efficient way to record information.

The only time that the nurse may wish to duplicate information from a flow sheet into a narrative or progress note is when a significant change occurs that results in specific therapies. For example, if a client's blood pressure becomes dangerously high, the nurse may record the pressure and the medication administered in the narrative progress note.

Benefits of Using a Client Care Flow Sheet

- Information is accessible to all members of the health care team.
- Time spent on documentation is decreased.
- Information is current.
- Errors resulting from transfer of information are decreased.

A flow sheet provides a quick, easy reference to the health care team members in assessing a client's status. It becomes unnecessary to locate data from several different sources. Critical care and acute care units commonly use flow sheets for all types of physiological data. Benefits of using a flow sheet are listed in the box above.

NURSING KARDEX

Nursing information that is needed for the daily care of clients is readily accessible in the nursing **Kardex** (see Chapter 9). The Kardex is a flip-over card that is usually kept in a portable index file or notebook at the nurses' station. Most Kardex forms have two parts, an activity and treatment section and a nursing care plan section. Nurses refer to the Kardex throughout the day. It organizes information in a useful manner as nurses give change-of-shift reports or make walking rounds. The Kardex contains pertinent information about clients and their ongoing care plans. An updated Kardex eliminates the need for continual referral to the chart for routine information. Information commonly found in the Kardex includes the following:

1. Basic demographic data (e.g., age and religion)
2. Primary medical diagnosis
3. Current physician's orders to be carried out by the nurse
4. A written nursing care plan (based on the nursing process and used when a formal plan is not found in the client's record)
5. Nursing orders
6. Scheduled tests and procedures
7. Safety precautions to be used in the client's care
8. Factors related to activities of daily living

In many institutions nurses make Kardex entries in pencil because it is usually necessary to make frequent revisions as the client's needs change. However, entries should be made in ink if the Kardex is a permanent part of the client's record. The Kardex provides the nurse an opportunity to communicate useful information to the nursing team about the client's unique needs. Within the care plan or the "order-entries" sections the nurse can communicate information such as client preferences and diet, specific methods to perform a treatment, methods to incorporate client participation in care, or preferred times to perform a nursing order.

Information within the Kardex should not simply be a reflection of routine nursing responsibilities or standardized care. For example, a client with the nursing diagnosis of altered urinary elimination has a urinary tract infection and is required to drink large amounts of fluids. A Kardex entry of "increase fluid intake" is relevant but not particularly individualized. If, however, the nurse's assessment has revealed that the client prefers iced tea and cranberry juice, a Kardex entry of "offer cranberry juice and iced tea, 1000 ml per shift" addresses the client's preferences and tailors the care plan to the client's needs.

The Kardex care plan has disadvantages. Access is usually limited to nurses. Also, the Kardex does not offer space for writing an extensive plan for the client with multiple problems.

TWENTY-FOUR-HOUR CLIENT CARE RECORDS AND ACUITY CHARTING SYSTEMS

Consolidation of the nursing records into a system that accommodates a 24-hour period is often used. According to Addy-Keller and McElwaney (1993), a 24-hour record-keeping system is essential in the elimination of unnecessary record-keeping forms (Fig. 12-4). Accurate assessment information and documentation of activities of daily living are more easily obtained with 24-hour notations. In addition, 24-hour client care records often use flow sheets and checklists to further enhance efficiency. To illustrate, two hospitals in the Pacific Northwest have used 24-hour client care records for more than 5 years. Staff agree that the 24-hour method is a much better charting system than the shift-by-shift formats that were previously used.

Twenty-four-hour client care records are also foundational for an **acuity charting** system. Acuity charting requires that staff document their interventions, thereby obtaining an overall level of acuity for each client. The acuity level determined by the nursing care allows clients to be rated in comparison to one another. For example, an acuity system might rate clients from 1 to 5 (1 is high, 5 is low). A client returning from surgery with multisystem problems has an acuity level of 1. On the same continuum another client awaiting discharge after a successful recovery from surgery has an acuity level of 5. Staffing patterns can then be determined by examining the acuity levels of the clients on a particular nursing unit. The client-to-staff ratios depend on a composite gathering of data in regard to the 24-hour interventions that are necessary for implementing care.

STANDARDIZED CARE PLANS

Although every professional nurse is responsible for developing an individualized care plan for a client, the process of writing the plan is time-consuming. Nurses caring for several clients may need to write extensive care plans. Many institutions have attempted to make documentation easier for nurses with **standardized care plans.** The plans, based on the institution's standards of nursing practice, are preprinted, established guidelines that are used to care for clients who have similar health problems. After a nursing assessment is completed, the staff nurse identifies the standard care plans that are appropriate for the client. The care plans are placed in the client's medical record. Modifications can be made in ink to the standardized plans to individualize the therapies. Most standardized care plans also allow the nurse to write in specific goals or desired outcomes of care, as well as the dates by which these outcomes should be achieved.

There are several advantages and disadvantages of standardized care plans. One advantage is the establishment of clinically sound standards of care for similar groups of

Oregon Health Sciences University
Hospitals and Clinics

ACUTE CARE
24 HOUR FLOW SHEET
4 YEARS TO ADULT

ACCOUNT NO.
MED. REC. NO.
NAME
BIRTHDATE

YESTERDAY'S

DATE _____ WEIGHT_____ WEIGHT_____

ISOLATION _____

TIME					
F	C				F	C

	F	C
	103.1	39.5
	102.2	39.0
	101.3	38.5
	100.4	38.0
	99.5	37.5
	98.6	37.0
	97.7	36.5
	96.8	36.0
	95.9	35.6
	95.0	35.0

103.1	39.5
102.2	39.0
101.3	38.5
100.4	38.0
99.5	37.5
98.6	37.0
97.7	36.5
96.8	36.0
95.9	35.6
95.0	35.0

PULSE RADIAL
APICAL
RESP.
B/P
PAIN
SA O₂
O₂

PAIN LEVEL
0-NONE
10-SEVERE

DAYS / INITIALS: RN: CNA:

HYGIENE
☐ BED BATH   ☐ SHOWER   ☐ ORAL CARE
☐ CATHETER CARE   COMMENTS:_____
_____

ACTIVITY
☐ BED REST   CHAIR:_____
AMBULATE:_____SLEEP:_____HRS
COMMENTS:_____
_____

SAFETY
☐ SAFETY POLICY
☐ RESTRAINTS   TYPE:_____
☐ SITTER   COMMENTS:_____
_____

EVENINGS / INITIALS: RN: CNA:

HYGIENE
☐ BED BATH   ☐ SHOWER   ☐ ORAL CARE
☐ CATHETER CARE   COMMENTS:_____
_____

ACTIVITY
☐ BED REST   CHAIR:_____
AMBULATE:_____SLEEP:_____HRS
COMMENTS:_____
_____

SAFETY
☐ SAFETY POLICY
☐ RESTRAINTS   TYPE:_____
☐ SITTER   COMMENTS:_____
_____

NIGHTS / INITIALS: RN: CNA:

HYGIENE
☐ BED BATH   ☐ SHOWER   ☐ ORAL CARE
☐ CATHETER CARE   COMMENTS:_____
_____

ACTIVITY
☐ BED REST   CHAIR:_____
AMBULATE:_____SLEEP:_____HRS
COMMENTS:_____
_____

SAFETY
☐ SAFETY POLICY
☐ RESTRAINTS   TYPE:_____
☐ SITTER   COMMENTS:_____
_____

	BREAKFAST	LUNCH	DINNER
DIET			
% TAKEN			
% SNACKS			

ASSIST
S - SELF
P - PARTIAL
F - FEED

RESOURCES/EQUIPMENT USED TO PROVIDE PATIENT CARE:
SCD ☐   K PAD ☐   TRAPEZE ☐ _____ ☐
NUMBER OF IV PUMPS   SINGLE_____DOUBLE_____
NUMBER OF SUCTION UNIITS _____
SPECIAL BED _____
OTHER_____

8.1-4A (1)

Fig. 12-4 Twenty-four-hour client care record. *(Courtesy Oregon Health Sciences University Hospitals and Clinics, Portland, Ore.)*

DATE:															

| START DATE/TIME | STANDARDS AND INTERVENTIONS | ✔ — | ASSESSMENT STANDARD OR PROTOCOL MET. INTERVENTION CARRIED OUT | | ✳ — | VARIANCE FROM STANDARDS OR ORDERED INTERVENTIONS. SEE NARRATIVE ENTRY. | | | → — | VARIANCES REMAIN. NO CHANGES FROM LAST NARRATIVE ENTRY. | | | | | |

RN INITIALS

(Left margin vertical labels: ASSESSMENT STANDARDS; PROTOCOLS / INTERVENTIONS)

TEACHING

ASSESSMENT STANDARDS: ADULTS AND PEDIATRIC PATIENTS ABOVE 4 YEARS. All normal assessments include patient without subjective

NORMAL NEUROLOGICAL ASSESSMENT:
- alert and oriented X3 (person place, time)
- behavior appropriate to situation
- PERL
- full range of motion with symmetry of strength
- no paresthesia
- verbalization clear and coherent
- swallows without coughing or choking on liquids or solids
- gait steady if patient ambulatory
- clear vision (corrective lenses allowable)

PEDIATRIC:
- alert and oriented appropriately for developmental age
- verbalization/vocalization appropriate for developmental age
- tracks and recognizes objects appropriately for developmental age (if unable to assess clear vision)

NORMAL RESPIRATORY ASSESSMENT:
- rate appropriate for age while at rest
- respirations quiet, regular and unlabored
- equal and clear breath sounds over both lung fields
- nail beds and mucous membranes pink
- sputum and nasal drainage clear if present

NORMAL CARDIOVASCULAR ASSESSMENT:
- regular apical or radial pulse
- capillary refill less than 3 seconds
- no edema
- peripheral pulse palpable and of equal quality
- pink nail beds and mucous membranes

NORMAL GASTROINTESTINAL ASSESSMENT:
- abdomen soft and non-distended
- no pain with palpation
- bowel tones present
- tolerates prescribed diet without problem
- bowel movements appropriate in color, volume, and consistency for intake
- if NG present, drainage clear to light green in color, heme negative

NORMAL GENITOURINARY ASSESSMENT:
- able to empty bladder q shift without urgency, frequency, pain, or post-void feeling of fullness or distention
- urine clear yellow to amber without foul odor.
- absence of vaginal or penile drainage
- continent
- if catheter present, patent and draining freely.
PEDIATRIC: urine output 1-3 cc/kg/hour

NORMAL NEUROVASCULAR (CMS) ASSESSMENT:
- pink nail beds
- warm
- full range of motion
- capillary refill less than 3 seconds
- palpable peripheral pulses
- no edema
- no paresthesia

NORMAL MUSCULOSKELETAL ASSESSMENT:
- absence of joint tenderness, swelling, redness, or increased temperature
- full range of motion all joints
- no muscle weakness

NORMAL INTEGUMENTARY ASSESSMENT:
- skin color consistent with race
- skin warm, dry, and intact
- mucous membranes moist and without lesions
- no rashes, petechiae, or purpura
- no signs of infestation

Fig. 12-4, cont'd Twenty-four-hour client care record.

Barnes Hospital

PATIENT DISCHARGE SUMMARY

C-16

Date _10/17/--_ Time _____1030_____

Addressograph Plate

MEANS: ☐ Ambulatory ☒ Wheelchair ☐ Stretcher

METHODS: ☒ M.D. order ☐ AMA with release ☐ AMA with release

Afebrile 24 hours? ☒ Yes ☐ No TPR _36^8-72-16_____ B/P _124/72_____

☐ Physician notified of irregularities

DISCHARGED TO: ☐ Home ☐ Nursing Home ☒ Home with Home Health Care ☐ Other

If discharged to Nursing Home or other facility/service:

Name _____ Address/Phone _____

☐ Release of information form signed ☐ Chart copied ☐ Transfer form completed ☐ Transportation Arranged

DISCHARGE CONSIDERATIONS:

☐ Valuables from cashier ☐ PTA meds returned ☐ Scripts given
☒ NA ☒ NA ☒ NA

DISCHARGE INSTRUCTIONS

FOR PROBLEMS OR FOLLOW-UP:

Physician _Dr. Stan Jones_____ Phone _362-5000___ Appt. _10/24/91_____

Other: _____

_____

Activity: _To remain in bed with Ⓛ foot elevated on two pillows. May be up only_
to go to the bathroom.

Diet: _To follow 1800 calorie ADA diet as instructed by the dietitian. For questions_
about diet, call the dietitian (Sue Marlin) 362-3184.

Medications: _To take usual dosage of 30 units NPH insulin and 8 units of regular_
insulin every morning before breakfast.

Wound Care: _Change dressings to Ⓛ foot daily using moistened fine mesh gauze_
with dry 4x4 gauze and wrap dressings with 4 kling gauze.

Teaching Materials Given: _Copy of "Controlling Your Diabetes" and "Diabetic Menu_
Planning."

Special Instructions: _Call doctor for increased pain, redness, swelling or drainage from_
Ⓛ foot wound. Barnes Home Health nurses will be visiting daily to change
dressing to Ⓛ foot.

My discharge instructions have been explained and a copy has been given to me.

Patient/Significant Other _John Owens_____ Relation _HUSBAND_____

Nurse _B. Rand, RN_____

Fig. 12-5 Discharge summary form. *(Courtesy Barnes-Jewish Hospital, St Louis.)*

clients. These standards can be useful when quality-improvement audits are conducted. Standardized care plans are easy to locate in a client's record; thus all staff can quickly refer to them. Another advantage is education. Nurses learn to recognize the accepted requirements of care for clients. The standardized care plans can also improve continuity of care among professional nurses. In addition, although the plans must be modified for each client, documentation takes less time.

The use of standardized care plans is controversial. The major disadvantage is the risk that the standardized plans inhibit nurses' identification of unique, individualized therapies for clients. Another disadvantage is the need to formally update the plans on a routine basis to ensure that content is current and appropriate. Staff members often develop many standardized care plans for clients who receive care in their institutions. Large numbers of plans take up space for storage and are more costly to print than one common care plan form. There is the trend among many hospitals to computerize care plans. With such a system, daily computer-generated care plans are printed and incorporate several nursing diagnoses or problems in a single care plan. Such a streamlined system improves the daily revision and updating of plans.

When standardized care plans are used in a health care facility, the nurse remains responsible for an individualized approach to care. Therefore if a standardized plan has an intervention that is not specifically tailored to the client's need, there should be a method for the nurse to revise or alter the intervention to individualize it. Standardized care plans are not meant to replace the nurse's professional judgment and decision making.

DISCHARGE SUMMARY FORMS

Much emphasis is placed on preparing a client for an efficient, timely discharge from a health care institution. A prospective payment system based on DRGs encourages health care institutions to be more efficient and to discharge the client as soon as possible. However, it is important to ensure that a client's discharge results in desirable outcomes. The earlier a client is discharged, the more likely it is that a hospital will be fully reimbursed. The Healthcare Financing Administration requires multidisciplinary involvement in discharge planning to ensure that a client leaves the hospital in a timely manner with the necessary resources.

Ideally discharge planning begins at admission. Nurses revise the plan as the client's condition changes. There should be evidence of the involvement of the client and family members in the discharge-planning process. There should be no surprises at the time of the client's discharge. The client should have the necessary information and resources to return home. The box above includes tips on completing discharge summary forms.

When a client is discharged from inpatient care, a clinical resume is prepared by the nurse, the social worker, and other members of the health care team. The reason for hospitalization, significant findings, client's status, and the specific teaching plan are given to the client or family (JCAHO, 1995). Discharge summary forms (Fig. 12-5) make the summary concise and instructive. Many forms include a copy that is given to a client, family member, or home

---

Tips on Writing Discharge Summary Forms

INFORMATION FOR HOME HEALTH CARE NURSES
- Describe nursing interventions (e.g., dressing changes, step-by-step wound care).
- Describe information that is presented to client.
- Describe client's ability to perform health care skills (e.g., administering medications, use of crutches).
- Explain family members' involvement in care.
- Describe resources that are needed in home (e.g., Meals on Wheels, self-help devices).

INFORMATION FOR CLIENTS
- Use clear, concise descriptions in client's own language.
- Provide step-by-step description of how to perform a procedure (e.g., home drug administration); reinforce explanation with printed instructions.
- Identify precautions for the client to follow when performing self-care or administering medications.
- Review signs and symptoms of complications that should be reported to physician.
- List names and phone numbers of health care providers whom client can contact.

---

health care nurse. This transfer of information ensures better continuity of self-care in the home. A summary form emphasizes previous learning by the client and family. The form may be attached to pamphlets or teaching brochures.

Home Health Care Documentation

The home health care business continues to grow as growing proportions of older adults require an ever-increasing use of home health care services. Medicare has specific guidelines for establishing eligibility for home health care reimbursement. In the fulfillment of these Medicare guidelines, documentation by home health care nurses has become the largest problem area: 50% of the nursing time is spent in documentation (Braunstein, 1993).

Documentation in the home health care system has different implications than in other areas of nursing. The primary difference is the nature of the home setting, which dictates that the majority of care is witnessed by a narrower scope of persons (i.e., client, family, direct health care provider). This situation demands that the documented care have accuracy and completeness so that the entire health care team has a valid means of identifying what care is rendered in the home. Home health care requires that the entire health care team work closely together (see the box on p. 198). In addition, the documentation is both the quality control and the justification for reimbursement from Medicare, Medicaid, or private insurance companies. Nurses must document all their services for payment (e.g., direct skilled care, client instructions, skilled observation, and evaluation visits) (JCAHO, 1995). The chart forms are similar to those used in other settings but are somewhat more detailed and greater in number (see the box on p. 198). The nurse is the pivotal person in the documentation of the delivery of home health care.

Home health care documentation has unique problems

Multidisciplinary Example of Health Care Team Working Together

A home health care agency in a five-county region addressed the need to provide quality documentation in its services. A task force of clinical nurse specialists, clinicians, and an education director analyzed the nursing care plan system and identified seven specific goals to guide the new system: (1) improve quality of care, (2) maintain and expand concept of nursing diagnosis, (3) integrate physician's plan of treatment and nursing plan, (4) measure patient outcomes, (5) interface data entry functions, (6) reduce documentation time, and (7) develop outcome standards for the program. The task force elected to use the NANDA taxonomy and developed a concise, operational, and visually appealing nursing plan that integrated the physician's plan with the nursing plan. The revised system exhibits positive benefits of relevance of the nursing plan to client care needs, decreased duplication of documentation, comprehensive record keeping (e.g., physicians, nurses, and others), an enhanced continuity of care, and a severe reduction in care plan development. The increased ease of use and a broader inclusion of members of the health care team make this revised documentation system a positive new method of record keeping.

Twardon C, Gartner M: *Nurse Manage* 24(11):81, 1993.

Home Health Care Forms for Documentation

The usual forms used to document home care include:

- Client assessment
- Referral source information/intake form
- Discipline-specific care plans
- Physician's plan of treatment
- Medication sheet
- Clinical progress notes
- Miscellaneous (conference notes, verbal order forms, telephone calls)
- Discharge summary
- Reports to third-party payors

Modified from Iyer PW, Camp NH: *Nursing documentation: a nursing process approach*, St Louis, 1995, Mosby.

because of the need for different health care providers to access the medical record. Some parts of the record are needed in the home with the client; other chart forms are needed in an office setting. Thus duplication of documentation is necessary, or agency policies are needed regarding what forms nurses should leave at their office versus what forms should be taken into the homes. Computerized client records are evolving as one means of addressing these different needs (Lancaster, 1993). With the use of modems and laptop computers it is possible for the records to be available in multiple locations, which allows greater access to the multidisciplinary needs that are often present in home health care.

Long-Term Health Care Documentation

An ever-increasing number of elderly persons require care in long-term health care facilities. The acuity of conditions in these persons continues to escalate as geriatric clients develop more disabilities commensurate with their age. Nursing personnel often face challenges much different from those in the acute care setting. These differences require a significantly different basis for nursing documentation (Iyer and Camp, 1995).

Outside agencies are instrumental in determining the standards and policies for documentation in long-term health care. For example, the Omnibus Budget Reconciliation Act of 1987 was an extremely significant Medicare and Medicaid legislation for long-term care documentation. Regulated standards for **resident** assessments, individualized care plans, and qualifications for health care providers (e.g., registered nurses, licensed practical nurses, nurse's aides) were requirements of OBRA 1987. In addition, the department of health in each state governs the frequency

of written nursing records of the residents in long-term care facilities.

Long-term care documentation supports a multidisciplinary approach in the assessment (referred to as a minimum data set) and planning process (referred to as resident assessment protocols) of the clients. Communication among such health care providers as nurses, social workers, recreational therapists, and dietitians is essential in the regulated documentation process. The fiscal support for long-term care residents hinges on the justification of nursing care as demonstrated in sound documentation of the services rendered (Eliopoulos, 1992).

Computerized Documentation

Computers are used in health care facilities in a variety of ways. The technology that exists is virtually unlimited, and the future holds incredible potential for the continuing impact of computerization in the health care delivery system. Nurses have traditionally been the primary users of the computerized systems. For example, supplies, equipment, stock medications, and diagnostic testing are services linking nurses to computers. However, the recent trend is that nurses must be encouraged and allowed to use computerized documentation to enhance their professional performance.

There are many benefits to computerized documentation. The new documentation systems that are now available can relieve nurses of repetitive clerical and monitoring tasks and increase the time that is available for direct client care. Software programs allow nurses to quickly enter specific assessment data one time, and the information is automatically transferred to different reports. Computers also help reduce errors, standardize nursing care plans, increase nursing satisfaction and productivity, and document all facets of client care (Town, 1993). Instead of writing lengthy nurses' notes, nurses can select choices on a screen that automatically build a comprehensive record of an event. Another benefit of computerized documentation is improving quality-improvement efforts. According to Town (1993), meeting JCAHO outcome standards is enhanced with computerized documentation because care planning is standardized on the computer.

Computerized documentation can be used in a variety of

Benefits of Automated Speech-Recognition (ASR) Technology

The following are benefits of ASR in the nursing division of an East Coast medical center:
- Comprehensive nursing documentation with minimal nursing effort
- Decreased charting errors and omissions
- Consistent documentation patterns
- Increased interdisciplinary communication
- Considerable time savings for the nurse
- Clear, concise, legible documentation
- Increased compliance with Joint Commission on Accreditation of Healthcare Organization standards (written into the software)

Modified from Trofino J: *Nurs Manage* 24:7, 1993.

client care settings. Computer systems obviously are used in large hospitals, but their use is not limited to facilities with major expenditure budgets. Rural health care organizations have shown that, despite fiscal constraints, commercially available software is affordable. A 53-bed hospital in Jefferson, Iowa, was able to implement a sophisticated, computerized, client-centered documentation system (Gleason, 1993). This system was successful, and the nurses expect continued changes as the computerized documentation system is revised. A community AIDS clinic in Santa Clara, Calif. implemented computerized documentation in its telephone triage system (Henry et al, 1994): the high volume of client contacts made computerized documentation a viable alternative for the triage nurses.

Computerized documentation could change drastically with the increased use of new technological **nursing interfaces** (Chu, 1993). Typical **user interfaces** (e.g., keyboard and monitor) require typing skills and result in data entry errors. The increasingly prevalent **graphic user interfaces** (e.g., trackball, touch pads, mouse, and icons) are not well suited for the large volumes of data that are necessary in nursing documentation. Therefore in the future nursing could use either pen-based or voice-recognition computers in documentation. A notebook-sized computer with handwriting recognition capabilities would allow nurses to document with an ease and a flexibility not possible in the current systems. In addition, **automated speech-recognition** (ASR) or voice-recognition technology allows nursing documentation to expand to a new horizon of capabilities. The benefits of ASR in nursing documentation are multivaried as demonstrated in an ASR project in a large medical center in New Jersey (Trofino, 1993) (see the box at left).

The development of a complete **computer-based patient care record** (CPCR) is envisioned as a futuristic trend

---

Recommendations of the Institute of Medicine for Computer-Based Patient Care Recording

- The computer-based patient record (CPCR) contains a problem list that defines all the client's clinical problems and the status of each. All health care practitioners, including nurses, dentists, social workers, and doctors, would update the list.
- The CPCR supports systematic measurement and recording of the client's health status and functional abilities in order to promote more precise, routine evaluations of client care outcomes.
- The logical basis for all diagnoses or conclusions are contained in the CPCR, serving to document the clinical rationale for decisions about the client.
- The CPCR will contain a lifelong record of events that may have influenced a person's health by incorporating records from various settings and time periods. This shifts the focus to wellness and client outcomes as measures of successful health care.
- Confidentiality of health care information must be ensured in whatever system is developed.
- Authorized health care providers involved in direct client care will have simultaneous and remote access to the CPCR. This would permit an emergency department, for example, to access the client's records from the last inpatient admission, or for the nurses at a tertiary hospital to access the client's records at the home health care agency.
- The CPCR allows users to retrieve information selectively and to choose various formats for examining and interpreting it. By using artificial intelligence technology, the CPCR will help health care providers focus on the most pertinent information needed at a particular moment by creating custom-tailored views of the same information. For example, the nurse could review a number of hospitalizations to determine whether the client had pressure ulcers in the past.
- Local and remote knowledge, literature, administrative databases, and systems can be linked with the CPCR. This will permit ready access to publications, clinical practice guidelines, and clinical decision support systems. For example, the nurse could do a literature search on some aspect of nursing care from the client's bedside.
- The CPCR can assist in the process of clinical problem solving by offering the nurse decision analysis tools, clinical reminders, prognostic risk assessment, and other clinical aids. For example, the computer can help identify clients who are at risk for falls or remind the nurse to evaluate the response to the injection of morphine given an hour ago.
- The CPCR supports structured data collection in a manner that adequately supports practitioners' direct entries and stores that information according to a defined vocabulary. Programs will use standardized vocabulary, such as nursing diagnoses of the North American Nursing Diagnosis Association.
- The quality and costs of care can be evaluated through the use of the CPCR. Better data access, faster data retrieval, more versatility in data display, and clinical reminders should improve health care delivery.
- The CPCR is sufficiently flexible and expandable to support not only today's basic information needs but also the evolving needs of each clinical specialty and subspecialty. As knowledge bases and sophisticated uses of information grow, computer systems must also grow.*

*Simpson R: *Nurs Manage* 22(10):24, and 22(11):26, 1991.

for client records (Simpson, 1991a, 1991b). The CPCR will be a comprehensive system that uses many components of data collection and makes use of a broad scope of computerization capabilities. The idea for this system of record keeping stemmed from the Computer-based Patient Record Institute, which was formed in 1992. This group comprised vendors, health care providers, and professional organizations. Their recommendations for the CPCR were extensive and numerous (see the box on p. 199). The new CPCR would have a much broader scope than the current charting systems, and would have a greater role in the utility of client care and in clinical decision making. The CPCR lends itself to allowing the nurse to have an instrumental role in this new form of documentation.

Nurses must know the risks of computerized documentation. There are legal risks associated with computerized documentation. Computers increase access to information by almost everyone. The password that is used to enter and sign off computer files should not be shared with another care giver. A good system requires frequent changes in personal passwords to prevent unauthorized persons from tampering with records. Nurses must know how to correct charting errors on a computer. Any data that have been permanently saved as part of the record should not be deleted. However, any incorrect entries or misspelled words that have not been stored can be deleted or corrected. If information is accidentally deleted, a brief explanation can be entered into the computer. Some institutions may request an incident report. Printouts of computerized records should be protected. Shredding of printouts or the logging of the number of copies generated by each care giver are ways to minimize duplicate records and protect the confidentiality of clients.

The transition to computerized documentation presents a unique challenge to nurses and nurse managers. However, the obstacles to surmount are minor in comparison to the tremendous benefits of the new computerized systems (Fig. 12-6). The successful implementation of a computerized documentation system requires preparation, involvement, and commitment of the entire nursing staff (Mathews and Zadak, 1993). The results of better standardization of care

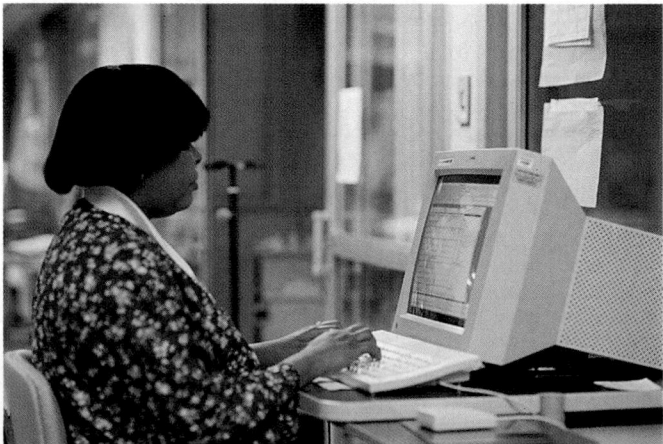

Fig. 12-6 Computerized documentation systems allow nurses to be more productive and ensure comprehensive recording of client information.

plans, more efficient use of the nurse's time, and ultimately, improved quality of client care are inherent in the use of computerized documentation.

▌ REPORTING

Information about clients is exchanged among health care team members, clients, and family members. Nurses communicate information about clients so that all team members can make the best decisions about them and their care. Reports offer a summary of activities or observations seen, performed, or heard. Four types of reports made by nurses include the change-of-shift report, telephone reports, transfer reports, and incident reports.

Change-of-Shift Reports

The **change-of-shift report** occurs two or three times a day on every type of nursing unit in all types of health care settings. At the end of each shift nurses report information about their assigned clients to the nurses working on the next shift. The report is a system of communication aimed at transferring essential information that is necessary for safe, holistic client care. The purpose of the report is to provide better continuity of care among nurses who are caring for a client. If one nurse finds a certain pain-relief measure more effective for a client, it is important that the information be relayed to the next nurse caring for the client so that pain-control interventions can be optimized. A complete report establishes the nurses' accountability in being sure that client care is uninterrupted.

A change-of-shift report may be given orally in person, by audiotape recording, or during rounds at the client's bedside. Oral reports are given in conference rooms, and staff members from both shifts participate. An audiotape report is given by the nurse who has completed care for the client and is left for the nurse on the next shift to review. Taped reports can improve efficiency by allowing staff to report when time is available. A disadvantage of a taped report is that it does not allow staff members to ask questions or clarify explanations. Reports given in person or during rounds permit nurses to obtain immediate feedback when questions are raised about a client's care. When nurses make rounds, the client and family members also have the opportunity to participate in any decisions. Likewise, the nurses can see the client together to perform needed assessments, evaluate progress, and determine the interventions best suited to the client's needs. A disadvantage of rounds is that it takes a long time to complete a report on all clients.

Because of the many responsibilities nurses have to assume, it is important that a change-of-shift report be conducted quickly and efficiently (Table 12-7). Time taken during the report keeps the nurse away from clients. A good report describes clients' health status and lets staff on the next shift know exactly what kind of care the clients will require. Significant facts about clients are reviewed (e.g., the condition of wounds or episodes of chest pain) to provide a baseline for comparison during the next shift. Data about clients should be objective and concise. Interpretation, the result of selecting, comparing, and summarizing, is important because the nurse can report the clinical significance of the shift's events.

An organized report follows a logical sequence. To pre-

Table 12-7	**Comparison of Do's and Dont's of Change-of-Shift Report**

Do's	**Dont's**
Provide only essential background information about client (i.e., name, sex, age, physician's diagnosis, and medical history).	Don't review all routine care procedures or tasks (e.g., bathing, scheduled changes).
Identify client's nursing diagnosis or health care problems and their related causes.	Don't review all biographical information already available on Kardex.
Describe objective measurements or observations about client's condition and response to health problem: emphasize recent changes.	Don't use critical comments about client's behavior, such as "Mrs. Wills is so demanding."
Share significant information about family members as it relates to client's problems.	Don't make assumptions about relationships between family members.
Continuously review ongoing discharge plan (e.g., need for resources, client's level of preparation to go home).	Don't engage in idle gossip.
Relay to staff significant changes in the way therapies are given (e.g., different position for pain relief, new medication).	Don't describe basic steps of a procedure.
Describe instructions given in teaching plan and client's response.	Don't explain detailed content unless staff members ask for clarification.
Evaluate results of nursing or medical care measures (e.g., effect of back rub or analgesic administration).	Don't simply describe results as "good" or "poor." Be specific.
Be clear about priorities to which oncoming staff must attend.	Don't force oncoming staff to guess what to do first.

pare for the report, the nurse gathers information from work sheets, the client's Kardex, and the client's care plan. A systematic approach such as using the nursing process can provide staff with critical information that is needed to continue care. The following is an example of a change-of-shift report:

1. *Background information:* Cy Tolan in bed 4, a 32-year-old client of Dr. Lang, is scheduled for a colon resection this morning. He has had ulcerative colitis for 2 years. He was admitted last night with slight abdominal discomfort. This is his first experience with surgery. He knows he may require a colostomy.
2. *Assessment:* Mr. Tolan expressed difficulty falling asleep last night. He had several questions about surgery. Early in the night he called for assistance several times.
3. *Nursing diagnosis:* His chief nursing care problems are *knowledge deficit* related to inexperience with surgery and *anxiety* related to potential body change.
4. *Teaching plan:* He asks appropriate questions about surgery. We have explained to him that a colostomy may be needed. Staff on evenings explained postoperative routines. I reinforced information with him early in the night. He stated that he felt less anxious.
5. *Treatments:* A cleansing enema was administered until clear at 9 PM; no blood was noted in the return. He complained of some abdominal cramping immediately afterward, but that disappeared. He received a Dalmane 15 mg PO at 11:30 PM and I gave him a back rub. He fell asleep after midnight.
6. *Family information:* His wife remained with him last evening until the end of visiting hours. She has returned and is in the room this morning.
7. *Discharge plan:* Mr. Tolan is a very active person at home. He plays tennis and basketball and swims. Mrs. Tolan is concerned about how he might react to a

colostomy. I suggest making a referral to the enterostomal therapist early, if the colostomy is performed.
8. *Priority needs:* Right now, Mr. Tolan is relaxing in his room. The operative permit has been signed. All preoperative procedures have been completed except for his preop medications, due on call to the operating room.

When giving a report, the nurse discusses clients or family members in a professional manner. It is often necessary to describe the interactions among clients, nurse, and family members in behavioral terms. The nurse avoids using labels such as *uncooperative, difficult,* or *bad* when describing such behaviors. A good report is objective and nonjudgmental. Value-laden terms do not establish working relationships between staff members and clients.

Telephone Reports

Health care team members frequently talk to one another by telephone. For example, a nurse informs a physician of changes in a client's condition, a nurse from one unit communicates information to a nurse on another unit about a client transfer, or the laboratory staff or a radiologist reports results of diagnostic tests. Information in a telephone report should be permanently documented in written form if significant events or changes in a client's condition have occurred. Thus the persons involved with a telephone report should ensure that the information is clear, accurate, and concise.

To document a phone call, the nurse includes when the call was made, who made it (if other than the writer of the information), who was called, to whom information was given, what information was given, and what information was received, for example, "At 10:22 AM called laboratory; S. Thomas, technician, reported Mr. Rush's potassium at 3.2. C. Towns, RN"

Telephone Order Guidelines

- If the physician sounds hurried over the phone, use clarification questions to avoid misunderstandings.
- Clearly determine the client's name, room number, and diagnosis.
- Repeat any prescribed orders back to the physician.
- Write a telephone order to include date and time given; name of client, nurse, and physician; and the complete order.
- Follow agency policies; some institutions require telephone (and verbal) orders to be reviewed and signed by two nurses.
- Have the physician cosign the order within the time frame required by the institution (usually 24 hours).

Telephone Orders

Telephone orders (TOs) involve a physician stating a prescribed therapy over the phone to a registered nurse. Clarifying messages is important when a nurse accepts physician's orders over the telephone. The order must be verified by repeating it clearly and precisely. Then the nurse writes the order on the physician's order sheet in the client's permanent record and signs it. An example follows: "1/16/95: 7:20 PM Darvocet-N PO 1 tab now and q4h prn. T.O. Dr. Reiss/Carol Towns, RN" The physician later verifies the telephone order legally by signing it within a set time period (e.g., 24 hours). Telephone orders are frequently given at night or during an emergency. Telephone orders should be used only when absolutely necessary, not for the sake of convenience. The box above provides guidelines that the nurse can use to prevent errors in receiving telephone orders.

Transfer Reports

Clients frequently transfer from one unit to another to receive different levels of care. For example, clients transfer from intensive care units to general nursing units after the level of care no longer requires intense monitoring. A **transfer report** involves communication of information about clients from the nurse on the sending unit to the nurse on the receiving unit.

Transfer reports may be given by phone or in person. When giving a transfer report, nurses include the following information:

1. Client's name, age, primary physician, and medical diagnosis
2. Summary of medical progress up to the time of transfer
3. Current health status (physical and psychosocial)
4. Current nursing diagnoses or problems and care plan
5. Any critical assessments or interventions to be completed shortly after transfer (helps receiving nurse to establish priorities of care)
6. Any special considerations, such as isolation status or resuscitation status
7. Need for any special equipment

After the sending nurse completes the transfer report, the receiving nurse should have time to ask questions about the client's status.

Incident Reports

An incident is any event that is not consistent with the routine operation of a health care unit or routine care of a client. The client, visitor, or employee may be at risk when anything unusual occurs in a health care area. Examples of incidents include client falls, accidental needle-stick injuries, a visitor having symptoms of illness, medication administration errors, accidental deletion of ordered therapies, and carelessness in performance of a procedure that led to injury or a risk for client injury. Reporting of incidents helps the identification of high-risk trends in nursing care or daily unit operations that warrant correction. Changes in policies and procedures, in-service seminars about nursing care practice, and changes in the operation of a nursing unit are ways in which repeated incidents can be corrected. Incident reports are an important part of a unit's quality-improvement program (see Chapter 11).

When an incident occurs, the nurse involved in the incident or the nurse who witnesses an injury completes an **incident report**. The report is completed even though an injury does not occur or is not apparent. Most institutions have specific incident report forms (Fig. 12-7). The report typically goes to the institution's risk-management office for review. Further review may occur, depending on the nature of the incident. For example, the employee health department might review all incidents involving employee needle-stick injuries. The hospital's legal department may review incidents when possible lawsuits against the hospital are expected.

When a client or visitor is involved in an incident, the nurse observing the incident takes steps to remove the individual from risk and then begins a report describing details of the incident. A physician examines the individual to determine whether any injury has been suffered. If a client is affected, the physician documents the examination and findings in the client's medical record. The nurse documents only an objective description of what happened and follow-up care that occurred. The nurse reports what was actually observed. Examples of an accurate and an inaccurate note follow:

Accurate note: Client found on floor, complained of pain in left hip. Noted external rotation and shortening of left leg. Lifted back into bed with assistance from orderlies. VS: BP, 142/88; P, 90; R, 22. Side rails up, call light within reach, instructed to remain in bed. Dr. Smith notified, portable x-ray ordered STAT.

Inaccurate note: Client fell out of bed, complained of pain in left hip. Noted external rotation and shortening of left leg. Dr. Smith notified.

An incident report should be concise and accurate, reporting exactly what the nurse observes and administers in the way of care. Parisi (1994) states that an incident report for a medication error should include the following: (1) an accurate, concise description of the medication error, (2) addition of relevant information and no making of excuses for the error, and (3) record of any adverse reactions the client has had.

The nurse does not specify in the medical record that an incident report was prepared. When the nurse is a victim of an incident, that nurse reports details of the incident and then seeks medical attention according to institutional policy.

DO NOT COPY
OREGON HEALTH SCIENCES UNIVERSITY
UNIVERSITY HOSPITAL & CLINICS

QA&I CONFIDENTIAL INCIDENT REPORT

Unit No.

Name

Birthdate

Complete immediately for every incident and send to the Quality Management Medical Director/Medical Services Director, MBS.

INCIDENT INVOLVES: (Check all involved)

Patient ☐   **Visitor** ☐   **Other** ☐   **Medical Device** ☐

Address (if
pertinent) _____

Diagnosis (if
patient) _____

Location of Incident
(unit, rm)_____ Date _____ Hour _____

Involved Medical Device:
    Device description _____

    Identifier   (Manufacturers' Model #, Serial # or Clinical Engineering #.

                    _____ / _____ / _____

Involved Medical or _____
Nursing Personnel Names

Were Witnesses Present _____
(List names if pertinent)

Description of Incident incl. immediate action taken _____
(Use back if necessary)

Bed High	☐
Bed Low	☐
Rails Up	☐
Rails Down	☐
Restraints	☐
Activity Orders:	
Bed Rest	☐
Limited	☐
BRP	☐

To Whom was Incident Reported _____

Signature of Person Reporting _____

Physical Findings and Diagnosis

Supervisor's Report and Final Action Taken

_____
Supervisor or Physician's Signature

H:\shared\qm\risksafe\formats\irform\fmt

Fig. 12-7 Incident report. *(Courtesy Oregon Health Sciences University Hospitals and Clinics, Portland, Ore.)*

Nurses usually become involved in client-related incidents at some point in their careers. They must understand the purpose of incident reports and the correct way to report information. The following list provides guidelines for correctly completing an incident report:

1. The nurse who witnessed the incident or who found the client at the time of the incident should file the report.
2. The nurse describes specifically what happened in concise, objective terms.
3. The nurse does not interpret or attempt to explain the cause of the incident.
4. The nurse describes objectively the client's condition when the incident was discovered.
5. Any measures taken by the nurse, other nurses, or physicians at the time of the incident are reported.
6. No nurse is blamed in an incident report.
7. The report is submitted as soon as possible to the appropriate administrator.
8. The nurse should never make a photocopy of the incident report for a personal file because the copy could be subpoenaed in court.

■ KEY CONCEPTS ■

▶ Multidisciplinary communication is essential within the health care team.

▶ A client's health care record is written documentation of the care received.

▶ Accurate record keeping requires an objective interpretation of data with precise measurements, correct spelling, and proper use of abbreviations.

▶ The medical record is a legal document and requires information describing exactly the care that is delivered to a client.

▶ A nurse's signature on an entry in a record designates accountability for the contents of that entry.

▶ Any change in a client's condition warrants immediate documentation, to keep a record accurate.

▶ All information pertaining to a client's health care management that is gathered by examination, observation, conversation, or treatment is confidential.

▶ The medical record is a client's bill or financial record that serves as the basis for reimbursement.

▶ Problem-oriented medical records are organized by the client's health care problems.

▶ The logic of SOAP, SOAPIE, or PIE charting is to organize entries in the progress notes by the nursing process.

▶ Critical pathways are instrumental in documenting methods that will produce a better quality of client outcomes.

▶ Medicare guidelines for establishing a client's home health care cost reimbursement is the basis for documentation by home health care nurses.

▶ Long-term care documentation is multidisciplinary and closely linked with fiscal requirements of outside agencies.

▶ Computerized information systems provide information about clients in an organized and easily accessible fashion.

▶ The major purpose of the change-of-shift report is to maintain continuity of care.

▶ Rounds allow nurses to perform needed assessments, evaluate clients' progress, and determine the best interventions for a client's needs.

▶ When information pertinent to care is communicated by telephone, the information must be verified.

▶ Incident reports objectively describe any event that is not consistent with the routine care of a client.

■ KEY TERMS ■

Accreditation, p. 180

Acuity charting, p. 193

Automated speech recognition, p. 199

Case management, p. 189

Change-of-shift report, p. 200

Charting by exception, p. 189

Computer-based patient care records, p. 199

Consultations, p. 180

Critical pathways, p. 189

DAR, p. 189

Diagnosis-related group (DRG), p. 180

Documentation, p. 181

Flow sheets, p. 192

Focus charting, p. 189

Graphic user interface, p. 199

Incident report, p. 202

Kardex, p. 193

Nursing interface, p. 199

PIE, p. 187

Problem-oriented medical record (POMR), p. 186

Record, p. 180

Reports, p. 180

Resident, p. 198

SOAP, p. 186

Source record, p. 187

■ CRITICAL THINKING EXERCISES ■

1. Mr. J. Reeves is a 63-year-old client who was recently admitted to an oncology unit in an acute care facility. Upon questioning him, the nurse finds that he is most concerned about his difficulty in breathing and the thick secretions that are causing a frequent cough. Hypothesize the documentation for Mr. Reeves's problem of ineffective airway clearance using different charting formats (e.g., SOAP, PIE, and Focus charting).

2. Mrs. Ellis fell (while ambulating alone) while attempting to walk from her bed to the bathroom early in the morning in your acute care facility. She stated that she "simply sat down" and that she "doesn't hurt anywhere." Document the necessary components for an incident report, and give the rationale for the chosen information.

3. A home health care agency has been using POMR for its documentation. Several members of the health care team are interested in changing to a case management system. Describe the argument in favor of supporting such a change. The same agency receives a federal grant to purchase a computerized documentation system. A number of the staff nurses voice their concerns for changing to a computerized system. What advantages could be given for the positive changes that could be predicted in this new system?

4. A client is admitted to your medical unit for alteration in nutrition, less than body requirements. As she is being assessed, she states that she has not been eating well for the past month. She also adds that she is somewhat weak and feels a little dizzy if she is up too much. As you further examine her, you find that her mucous membranes are dry, that her skin turgor is somewhat "rubbery," and that her temperature is 38.2° C. In addition, the client's pulse is fast (heart rate, 94 beats per minute), and she is breathing a little fast (20 respirations per minute). Briefly chart those aspects of the examination that are subjective and those that are objective.

REFERENCES

Acord-Szczesny J: Computer tracking of critical path variations, *Inside Case Management* 1(2):1, 1994.

Addy-Keller J, McElwaney E: A new documentation tool, *Nurs Manage* 24(11):46, 1993.

Braunstein ML: The electronic patient records solution, *Caring* 12(7):30, 1993.

Chu S: Clinical information systems: the nursing interface, *Nurs Manage*, 24(11):58, 1993.

Crummer M, Carter V: Critical pathways, the pivotal tool, *J Cardiovasc Nurs* 7(4):30, 1993.

Eggland ET: *Nursing documentation resource guide*, Gaithersburg, Md, 1993, Aspen.

Eliopoulos C: *Nursing administration manual for long-term care facilities*, Glen Arm, Md, 1992, Health Education Network.

Gawlinski A, Rasmussen S: Improving documentation through change theory, *Focus Crit Care* 11(6):12, 1984.

Gleason B: Rural hospitals set the pace for computerized documentation? *Nurs Manage*, 24(7):49, 1993.

Gordon M: *Manual of nursing diagnosis: 1995-1996*, St Louis, 1995, Mosby.

Henry SB et al: A computer-based approach to quality improvement for telephone triage in a community AIDS clinic, *Nurs Adm Q* 18(2):65, 1994.

Hospital Case Management: Keep focus on the big picture when tackling variance analysis 1(8):1, 1993.

Iyer PW, Camp NH: *Nursing documentation: a nursing process approach*, St Louis, 1995, Mosby.

Joint Commission on Accreditation of Healthcare Organizations: *Standards for the accreditation of home care*, Chicago, 1995, Joint Commission on Accreditation of Healthcare Organizations.

Joint Commission on Accreditation of Healthcare Organizations: *Standards for the accreditation of hospitals*, Chicago, 1996, JCAHO.

Kopf R: Are your medical records a legal asset or liability? Legal documentation guidelines, *J Nurs Law* 1(1):5, 1993.

Lampe S: *Focus charting: documentation for patient-centered care*, Minneapolis, 1994, Creative Nursing Management.

Lancaster L: Nursing information systems in the year 2000: another perspective, *Comput Nurs* 11(1):3, 1993.

Mandell M: Not documented: not done, *Nursing 94* 24(8):62, 1994.

Martin F: Documentation tips: to help you stay out of court, *Nursing 94* 24(6):63, 1994.

Mathews J, Zadak K: Managerial decisions for computerized patient care planning, *Nurs Manage*, 24(7):54, 1993.

O'Brien K, Landstrom G: Using system integration to revise documentation, *Nurs Manage*, 25(2):56, 1994.

Parisi S: What to do after a med error, *Nursing 94* 24(6):59, 1994.

Simpson R: Computer-based patient records: the Institute of Medicine's vision, part I, *Nurs Manage*, 22(10):24, 1991a.

Simpson R: Computer-based patient records: the Institute of Medicine's 12 requisites, part 2, *Nurs Manage*, 22(11):26, 1991b.

Town J: Changing to computerized documentation-plus! *Nurs Manage*, 24(7):44, 1993.

Trofino J: Voice-activated nursing documentation: on the cutting edge, *Nurs Manage*, 24(7):40, 1993.

Twardon C, Gartner M: The nursing plan: innovative home health documentation, *Nurs Manage*, 24(11):81, 1993.

Woodyard LW, Sheetz J: Critical pathway patient outcomes: the missing standard, *J Nurs Care Qual* 8(1):51, 1993.

ADDITIONAL READINGS

Bialorucki T, Blaine M: Protecting patient confidentiality in the pursuit of the ultimate computerized information system, *J Nurs Care Qual* 7(1):53, 1992.

Kerr SD: A comparison of four nursing documentation systems, *J Nurs Staff Dev* 8:27, 1992.

Matz L, Gary G: Patient outcomes measure home health care accomplishments, *Nurs Manage* 24(5):96Y, 1992.

Nadler G: The challenge of a paperless system, *J Nurs Adm*, 23(4):37, 1993.

Pulliam L, Valentine J, Raymond J et al: Implementation of a computerized information system in a long term care facility, *Comput Nurs* 10(5):201, 1992.

Strom CA: Combining patient classification and nursing documentation, *Nurs Manage*, 24(2):79, 1993.

Vlasses FR: Computerized documentation system: blessings or curse? *Orthop Nurs* 12(1):51, 1993.

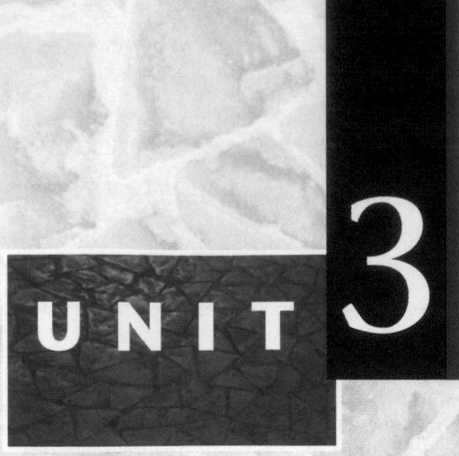

UNIT 3

Professional Nursing Concepts and Practices

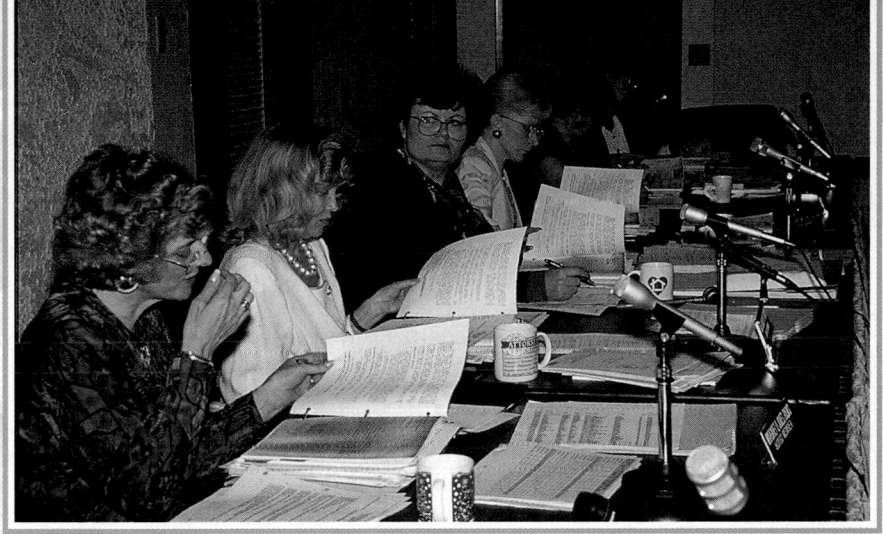

## Chapter 13

Profession of Nursing

Objectives

Mastery of content in this chapter will enable the student to:

▶ Define the key terms listed.

▶ Discuss the historical development of professional nursing.

▶ Discuss the modern definitions, philosophies, and theories of nursing practice.

▶ Describe educational programs for becoming a registered nurse.

▶ Describe practice settings for nurses.

▶ Describe the roles and functions of a nurse.

▶ List the five characteristics of a profession and discuss how nursing demonstrates these characteristics.

▶ Discuss the influence of social and economic changes on nursing practice.

▶ Discuss the influence of nursing on political issues and health care policy.

Modern nursing is an art and a science involving many activities, concepts, and skills related to basic social sciences, physical sciences, ethics sciences, contemporary issues, and other areas. Nursing as a profession is unique because it addresses the many responses of individuals and families to health problems. Nurses have many roles, such as care givers, primary care providers, clinical decision makers, advocates, researchers, and teachers; and they must often assume several roles at the same time. Because of nursing's diversity, nurses need a philosophy of nursing and theories of practice to shape the future growth of the profession. Over the years, nurses have developed many philosophies and definitions of nursing. The following definition, written by Virginia Henderson and adopted by the **International Council of Nurses (ICN)** (1973), is a concise statement with which current nurse theorists agree:

> The unique function of the nurse is to assist the individual, sick or well, in the performance of those activities contributing to health, its recovery, or to a peaceful death that the client would perform unaided if he had the necessary strength, will, or knowledge. And to do this in such a way as to help the client gain independence as rapidly as possible.

The profession of nursing is complex and multifaceted. Nurses practice in many settings that emphasize different aspects of nursing care and nursing roles. In addition, individuals can become registered nurses through a variety of educational programs, and a variety of career opportunities become available as nurses advance their education and increase clinical competencies.

Expertise in nursing is the result of knowledge and clinical experience. The expertise required to interpret clinical situations and make complex decisions is the essence of nursing care, and is the basis for the advancement of nursing practice and the development of nursing science (Benner, 1984; Benner and Tanner, 1987; Carnevali and Thomas, 1993).

Critical thinking skills are essential to nursing (see Chapter 6). Critical thinking is a rational, reasoning process used to deliver nursing care. In critical thinking the nurse must be able to make relevant observations, recognize health problems, develop appropriate solutions, and evaluate the results of those solutions (Tanner et al, 1987; Alfaro-LeFevre, 1995; Bandman and Bandman, 1995). When providing care based on critical thinking skills, the nurse makes clinical judgements about the care needed for clients based on fact, experience, and standards of care (Alfaro-LeFevre, 1995). Knowledge, expertise, and life-long learning is gained through the continual process of critical thinking.

The profession of nursing evolves as society and health care needs and policies change. Nursing responds and adapts to changes, meeting new challenges as they arise.

■ HISTORICAL PERSPECTIVE

Why do this and other introductory nursing texts devote limited and precious space to the profession's history? Knowing the historical roots of nursing enables both students and practicing professionals to prepare for the health care needs of the twenty-first century. Our discipline is a melding of knowledge from the physical sciences, humanities, social sciences, and clinical competencies to meet the individual needs of clients. Knowing the profession's history widens the knowledge base of nurses and promotes an understanding of the social and intellectual origins of the discipline (Keeling and Ramos, 1995).

Nursing was distinguished in its early history as a form of community service and was originally related to a strong instinct to preserve and protect the family (Donahue, 1995). Nursing began as the desire to keep people healthy and provide comfort, care, and assurance to the sick. Although the general goals of nursing have remained relatively the same over the centuries, the practice of nursing has been influenced by society's changing needs, and thus nursing has gradually evolved.

Nursing is as old as medicine. Throughout history, nursing and medicine have been interdependent. During the era of Hippocrates, medicine was practiced without nursing, and during the Middle Ages, nursing was practiced without medicine (Donahue, 1995; Deloughery, 1995).

Christianity greatly influenced the profession. One of the earliest records of Christian nursing detailed the formation of the Order of the Deaconesses, a group somewhat like today's public health or visiting nurses. The Deaconesses of the early church were lay women appointed by bishops. Their role was to visit the sick. Deaconess appointments were highly valued, and given only to women of high social standing (Deloughery, 1995).

Nightingale's views on nursing were derived from a spiritual philosophy, developed in her adolescence and adulthood (Macrae, 1995). Her religious roots were also seen in the statistical analyses that connected poor sanitation with cholera and dysentery. She viewed nursing as a search for truth in finding answers to health care questions or discovering and using God's laws of healing in nursing practice (Macrae, 1995).

Historically, men and women have held the role of nurse. The entry of women into nursing can be traced to approximately AD 300 (Shryock, 1959; Donahue, 1995). Women entered nursing because the social position of Roman women improved (Shryock, 1959), Christians taught that men and women are equal before God (Shryock, 1959; Dolan et al, 1983), and Christians appealed to women "to carry on His work in behalf of all who were in distress" (Shryock, 1959).

The Benedictine order, founded in the sixth century, increased the number of men entering nursing. Although the Benedictines were scholars, librarians, teachers, and agriculturalists, nursing the sick eventually became the chief function and duty of their community life (Donahue, 1995).

During the Middle Ages, charitable institutions were started (AD 1100 to 1200) to care for the aged, sick, and poor (Deloughery, 1995). Nurses delivered custodial care and depended on physicians or priests for direction (Kelly, 1981). One consistent role of the nurse from early civilization is that of the midwife. Throughout medical and nursing histories the midwife has been accepted in the role of assisting women during childbirth.

The Crusades became a stimulus for expanded nursing and health care. Military nursing orders for men were formed, and hospitals were established. After the Crusades, large cities began to develop and grow with the decline of feudalism. The extensive population growth in cities led to

Problems Associated with Illnesses During the Growth of Cities

- Overcrowding
- Poor ventilation
- Poor heating and cooling
- Poor sanitation, garbage collection, and plumbing
- Poor water supply
- Inadequate methods of preserving foods
- Ignorance of elementary hygiene practices

certain health problems (see the box above) and an increased need for health care. Some of these problems still exist in urban areas today, although the mortality rates associated with them have greatly declined.

Secular groups were also formed to meet specific health care needs during the Middle Ages. The Hospital Brothers of St. Anthony cared for victims of the disease called *St. Anthony's fire,* the Brothers of Misericordia in Italy provided transportation services for the ill, and the Alexian Brothers (a group still active today) cared for victims of bubonic plague.

The lack of hygiene and sanitation and the increasing poverty in urban centers resulted in serious health problems in the fifteenth to seventeenth centuries. Societal factors, such as laws punishing the poor and the Window Tax, which led to decreased ventilation because landlords bricked in windows to avoid paying the tax, created conditions and health needs to which nursing responded.

The Sisters of Charity was founded in 1633 by St. Vincent de Paul. The sisters cared for people in hospitals, asylums, and poorhouses. In addition, the sisters became widely known as visiting nurses because they cared for sick people in their homes. The first supervisor of the Sisters of Charity was Louise de Gras, a widow of high social standing. de Gras, who entered the order and was later known as St. Louise de Marillac, established perhaps the first educational program to be associated with a nursing order. She recruited intelligent, refined, and compassionate women (Donahue, 1995). The program included experience in the care of the sick in the hospital, as well as home visits. The Sisters of Charity was introduced in America by Mother Elizabeth Seton in 1809, and later their name was changed to the Daughters of Charity (Donahue, 1995).

In the eighteenth century, the further growth of cities brought an increase in the number of hospitals and a larger role for nurses. Smallpox epidemics in the French colonies and during the Revolutionary War in the English colonies increased the need for nursing services. Nursing skills and knowledge were generally passed on by experienced nurses because there was still little formal education for them.

During the nineteenth century the Deaconess order was revived by Protestant churches. The Deaconess Institute at Kaiserswerth, Germany, was established in 1836 by Pastor Theodore Fliedner (Woodham-Smith, 1983; Donahue, 1995). The regeneration of this nursing order was stimulated by the recognition of the need for the services of nurses.

In October 1846, Florence Nightingale received the *Year-book of the Institution of Deaconesses at Kaiserswerth* (Woodham-Smith, 1983). In 1847, she went to Kaiserswerth to work with the Deaconesses (Woodham-Smith, 1983; Donahue, 1995).

In 1853, Nightingale went to Paris to study with the Sisters of Charity and was later appointed superintendent of the English General Hospitals in Turkey. During this period she brought about major reforms in hygiene, sanitation, and nursing practice, and reduced the mortality rate at the Barracks Hospital in Scutari, Turkey, from 42.7% to 2.2% in 6 months (Woodham-Smith, 1983; Cohen, 1984; Donahue, 1995).

In 1860, Nightingale wrote *Notes on Nursing: What It Is and What It Is Not* for the lay person. Her philosophy of nursing practice reflected the changing needs of society. She saw the role of nursing as having "charge of somebody's health" based on the knowledge of "how to put the body in such a state to be free of disease or to recover from disease" (Nightingale, 1860; Schuyler, 1992). During the same year, she developed the first organized program of training for nurses, the Nightingale Training School for Nurses at St. Thomas' Hospital in London.

The Civil War (1860 to 1865) stimulated the growth of nursing in the United States. Clara Barton, founder of the American Red Cross, tended soldiers on the battlefields, cleansing their wounds, meeting their basic needs, and comforting them in death. The American Red Cross was ratified by the U.S. Congress in 1882 after 10 years of lobbying by Barton. Dorothea Lynde Dix, Mary Ann Ball (Mother Bickerdyke), and Harriet Tubman also influenced nursing during the Civil War (Donahue, 1995). As superintendent of the female nurses of the Union Army, Dix organized hospitals, appointed nurses, and oversaw and regulated supplies to the troops. Mother Bickerdyke organized ambulance services, supervised nurses, and walked abandoned battlefields at night looking for wounded soldiers. Harriet Tubman was active in the Underground Railroad movement and assisted in leading over 300 slaves to freedom (Donahue, 1995).

After the Civil War, nursing schools in the United States and Canada began to pattern their curricula after the Nightingale School. In Canada the first training school, St. Catherine's in Ontario, was founded in 1874 (Donahue, 1995; Raab, 1985). In 1884, Mary Agnes Snively took over the directorship of the Toronto General Hospital. She helped form the Canadian National Association of Trained Nurses in 1908 (Donahue, 1995; Raab, 1985). The name was later changed to the **Canadian Nurses Association (CNA)** in 1924 (Donahue, 1995).

Isabel Hampton (later Isabel Hampton Robb), a graduate of St. Catherine's in Ontario, was the first superintendent of the Johns Hopkins Training School in Baltimore, Maryland. She authored the following textbooks: *Nursing: Its Principles and Practice for Hospital and Private Use* (1894), *Nursing Ethics* (1900), and *Educational Standards for Nurses* (1907) (Donahue, 1995). She helped found the Nurses' Associated Alumnae of the United States and Canada in 1896. The Canadian affiliation was removed in 1899, and the organization became the **American Nurses Association (ANA)** in 1911. Hampton was also one of the original founders of the *American Journal of Nursing* (Donahue, 1995; Wheeler, 1985).

Nursing in hospitals expanded in the late nineteenth

century, but nursing in the community did not increase significantly until 1893 when Lillian Wald and Mary Brewster opened the Henry Street Settlement, which focused on the health needs of poor people who lived in tenements in New York City (Donahue, 1995; Silverstein, 1985). Nurses working in this settlement had greater responsibility for their clients than nurses working in hospitals because they frequently encountered situations requiring action independent of a physician's orders. In addition to the treatment of illness, poor people needed nursing therapies aimed at restoring nutrition, providing shelter, and maintaining hygiene. Wald authored the following books describing her activities with the Henry Street Settlement: *The House on Henry Street* (1915) and *Windows on Henry Street* (1934).

Advances were made in hospital care, public health, and nursing education in the early twentieth century. Mary Adelaide Nutting, a member of the first graduating class at Johns Hopkins Hospital and successor to Isabel Hampton Robb as superintendent of the Johns Hopkins Training School, was instrumental in the affiliation of nursing education with universities. She became the first professor of nursing at Columbia University Teachers College in 1907 (Donahue, 1995).

In 1923 the Rockefeller Foundation funded a survey of nursing education, the Goldmark Report. The report concluded that nursing education needed increased financial support and suggested that the money be given to university schools of nursing. As a result the Rockefeller Foundation funded the expansion of several nursing programs, including Yale and Vanderbilt Universities and the University of Toronto.

As nursing education developed, nursing practice also expanded. In 1901 the Army Nurse Corps was established, followed in 1908 by the Navy Nurse Corps. Nursing specialization was also developing. In the 1920s, graduate nurse-midwifery programs were initiated, and beginning in the 1950s, specialty nursing organizations such as the Association of Operating Room Nurses (1949), American Association of Critical-Care Nurses (1969), and Oncology Nursing Society (1975) were formed.

In 1965 the National Commission on Nursing and Nursing Education explored issues that included the supply of and demand for nurses, clarification of nursing roles and functions, education of nurses, and career opportunities available to nurses. Their report, often called the *Lysaught report* after Jerome P. Lysaught, the director of the study, called for clarification of nursing roles and responsibilities in relation to those of other health care professionals. It also advocated greater financial support for nurses and more career opportunities to attract nurses and retain them in the profession (Lysaught, 1970).

As nursing practice and education evolved to meet the needs of society, nursing's code of ethics, which was initially discussed in 1897, also evolved (Viens, 1989). The first written ANA Code of Ethics was proposed in 1926 at the organization's annual convention. The purpose of this code was to "create a sensitiveness to ethical situations and to formulate general principles which result in the formation of conscious and critical judgment resulting in action in specific situations" (ANA, 1926). Again as technology and the needs of society changed, the Code underwent multiple revisions, the most recent being the 1985 Code for

Nurses with Interpretive Statements (Sward, 1978; ANA, 1985) (see Chapter 19).

Today the profession is faced with greater challenges. Nurses and nurse educators are revising nursing practice and curricula to meet the ever-changing needs of society. Advances in technology, rising acuity of clients, and early discharge of clients from health care institutions require nurses to have a strong and current knowledge base from which to practice. Nursing practice is moving toward more community-based settings, and the challenge is to prepare professional nurses to deliver complex, multifaceted care in the client's home.

■ CONCEPTUAL AND THEORETICAL MODELS OF NURSING PRACTICE

The development of nursing science, conceptual models, and theory is a scholarly activity. A **conceptual model** refers to global ideas about the individuals, groups, situations, or events of interest to a specific discipline. Theories, which are composed of concepts and propositions, focus more specifically on the events and phenomena of the discipline (Fawcett, 1992). Theory contributes to a sound basis of nursing practice (Chinn and Jacobs, 1995). Developing this science involves generating knowledge. Although this knowledge can be used with knowledge from other disciplines, it is designed to advance and support nursing practice and health care (Hinshaw, 1989; Chinn and Jacobs, 1995). One method for creating nursing's scientific knowledge base is through the development and use of **nursing theory.**

The variety of nursing theories contained in this chapter provide the student with insights into client care, open nursing options, and stimulates innovative nursing interventions. Levine (1995) supports the need for a variety of nursing theories, because there is no global theory of nursing that fits every situation. The strength of nursing practice lies in the diversity of its nurses: their experiences, their commitment, their professionalism (Levine , 1995).

Historically, nursing theories were studied in an isolated academic environment independent of nursing practice. There is, however, a contemporary move toward nursing science-based practice (Donaldson, 1995). Nurses now and in the future need to have models of care from which their practice is based (Parse, 1990; Dean, 1995).

As nursing continues to evolve, nurses theorize about the nature of nursing practice, the principles on which practice is based, and the proper goals and functions of nursing in society. Conceptual and theoretical nursing models are used to provide knowledge to improve practice, guide research and curricula, and identify the domain and goals of nursing practice. Nursing theories provide the nurse with goals for assessment, nursing diagnoses, and interventions; common ground for communication; and professional autonomy and accountability. They also guide future directions for nursing research, practice, education, and administration (Meleis, 1985; Torres, 1986; Parse, 1987; Fawcett, 1989; Marriner-Tomey, 1994; Chinn and Jacobs, 1995) (see the box on p. 211).

An historical review demonstrates that nursing has developed a growing body of knowledge. Nursing concepts and theories have evolved since Nightingale, who, in establishing the discipline of nursing, spoke with firm con-

---

Goals of Theoretical Nursing Models

- Guide research to establish empirical knowledge base for nursing
- Identify area to be studied
- Identify research techniques and tools that will be used to validate nursing interventions
- Identify nature of contribution that research will make to advancement of knowledge
- Formulate legislation governing nursing practice, research, and education
- Formulate regulations interpreting nurse practice acts so that nurses and others better understand laws
- Develop curriculum plans for nursing education
- Establish criteria for measuring quality of nursing care, education, and research
- Prepare job descriptions used by employers of nurses
- Guide development of nursing care delivery systems
- Provide knowledge to improve nursing administration, practice, education, and research
- Provide systematic structure and rationale for nursing activities
- Identify domain and goals of nursing

---

viction about the "nature of nursing as a profession that required knowledge distinct from medical knowledge" (Nightingale, 1860; Schuyler, 1992). The overall goal of this knowledge has been to explain the practice of nursing as different and distinct from the practice of medicine, psychology, and social work (Torres, 1986; Fawcett, 1989; Chinn and Jacobs, 1995).

A significant milestone influencing the development of nursing concepts and theory was the establishment of the journal, *Nursing Research,* in 1952. This journal reports on the scientific investigations being conducted by nurses and other professionals. The journal has encouraged scientific productivity and has helped to provide the framework for a questioning attitude that has set the stage for further inquiries into theoretical nursing (Meleis, 1985).

In the mid-1950s, nursing leaders began to formulate theoretical views of nursing and concerns about subjects to include or exclude from nursing curricula. Columbia University Teachers College offered master's and doctoral programs in nursing education and administration (Meleis, 1985). Several prominent nurse theorists graduated from this institution; these include Peplau, Henderson, Hall, Abdellah, King, Wiedenbach, and Rogers.

During the 1960s, Yale University School of Nursing defined nursing even further. "Nursing was considered a process rather than an end, an interaction rather than content, and a relationship between two human beings rather than an interaction between unrelated nurse and patient" (Meleis, 1985). In addition, the ANA's 1965 position paper defined nursing and concluded that one of the most significant goals for nursing was theory development. The ANA supported and lobbied for the need for continuing efforts to develop the body of nursing knowledge (ANA, 1965; Meleis, 1985). As a result, federal support was also provided to nurses pursuing masters and doctoral degrees.

Theory development was emphasized from the mid-1960s to 1970. A series of symposia, sponsored by Case Western Reserve University, was held to assist in the development of nursing theory. During the mid-1970s the **National League for Nursing (NLN)**, the accrediting institution for nursing education programs, made theory-based curriculum a requirement for accreditation. Thus schools of nursing were expected to use a conceptual framework in the development and implementation of their curricula (Meleis, 1985).

Definitions and theories of nursing can help the nursing student understand how the roles and actions of nurses fit together in nursing. The following sections describe, in chronological order, concepts basic to selected nursing theories (Table 13-1).

Nightingale's Theory

Contemporary authors are beginning to explore Florence Nightingale's work as a potential theoretical and conceptual model for nursing (Meleis, 1985; Torres, 1986; Marriner-Tomey, 1994; Chinn and Jacobs, 1995). Meleis (1985) notes that Nightingale's concept of environment as the focus of nursing care and her admonition that nurses need not know all about the disease process are early attempts to differentiate between nursing and medicine.

Nightingale did not view nursing as limited merely to the administration of medications and treatments but rather as oriented toward providing fresh air, light, warmth, cleanliness, quiet, and adequate nutrition (Nightingale, 1860; Torres, 1986). Through observation and data collection, she linked the client's health status with environmental factors and, as a result, initiated improved hygiene and sanitary conditions during the Crimean war.

Torres (1986) notes that Nightingale provided basic concepts and propositions that could be validated and used for practice in nursing. Nightingale's "descriptive theory" provides nurses with a way to think about nursing or a frame of reference that focuses on clients and the environment (Torres, 1986). Nightingale's letters and writings direct the nurse to act on behalf of the client. Her principles encompass the areas of practice, research, and education. Most important, her concepts and principles shaped and delineated nursing practice (Marriner-Tomey, 1994). Nightingale taught and used the nursing process, noting that "vital observation [assessment] . . . is not for the sake of piling up miscellaneous information or curious facts, but for the sake of saving life and increasing health and comfort."

Peplau's Theory

Hildegard Peplau's theory (1952) focuses on the individual, nurse, and interactive process (Peplau, 1952); the result is the nurse-client relationship (Torres, 1986; Marriner-Tomey, 1994). According to this theory the client is an individual with a felt need, and nursing is an interpersonal and therapeutic process. Nursing's goal is to educate the client and family and to help the client reach mature personality development (Chinn and Jacobs, 1995). Therefore the nurse strives to develop a nurse-client relationship in which the nurse serves as a resource person, counselor, and surrogate.

When the client seeks help, the nurse first discusses the nature of the problem and explains the services available. As the nurse-client relationship develops, the nurse and

Table 13-1	Summary of Nursing Theories	
THEORIST	**GOAL OF NURSING**	**FRAMEWORK FOR PRACTICE**
Nightingale (1860)	To facilitate "the body's reparative processes" by manipulating client's environment (Torres, 1986)	Client's environment is manipulated to include appropriate noise, nutrition, hygiene, light, comfort, socialization, and hope.
Peplau (1952)	To develop interaction between nurse and client (Peplau, 1952)	Nursing is a significant, therapeutic, interpersonal process (Peplau, 1952). Nurses participate in structuring health care systems to facilitate natural ongoing tendency of humans to develop interpersonal relationships (Marriner-Tomey, 1994).
Henderson (1955)	To work interdependently with other health care workers (Marriner-Tomey, 1994), assisting client to gain independence as quickly as possible (Henderson, 1964). To help client gain lacking strength (Torres, 1986)	Nurses help client to perform Henderson's 14 basic needs (Henderson, 1966) (see p. 213).
Abdellah (1960)	To provide service to individuals, families, and society. To be kind and caring but also intelligent, competent, and technically well prepared to provide this service (Marriner-Tomey, 1994)	This theory involves Abdellah's 21 nursing problems (Abdellah et al 1960) (see p. 213).
Orlando (1961)	To respond to client's behavior in terms of immediate needs. To interact with client to meet immediate needs by identifying client behavior, reaction of nurse, and nursing action to be taken (Torres, 1986; Chinn and Jacobs, 1995)	Three elements, including client behavior, nurse reaction, and nurse action, compose nursing situation (Orlando, 1961).
Hall (1962)	To provide care and comfort to client during disease process (Torres, 1986)	The client is composed of the following overlapping parts: person (core), pathological state and treatment (cure), and body (care). Nurse is care giver (Marriner-Tomey, 1994; Chinn and Jacobs, 1995).
Wiedenbach (1964)	To assist individuals in overcoming obstacles that interfere with the ability to meet demands or needs brought about by condition, environment, situation, or time (Torres, 1986)	Nursing practice is related to individuals who need help because of behavioral stimulus. Clinical nursing has the following components: philosophy, purpose, practice, and art (Chinn and Jacobs, 1995).
Levine (1966)	To use conservation activities aimed at optimal use of client's resources	This adaptation model of human as integral whole is based on "four conservation principles of nursing" (Levine, 1973).
Johnson (1968)	To reduce stress so that client can move more easily through recovery process	This basic needs framework focuses on seven categories of behavior (see p. 214). Individual's goal is to achieve behavioral balance and steady state by adjustment and adaptation to certain forces (Johnson, 1980; Torres, 1986).
Rogers (1970)	To maintain and promote health, prevent illness, and care for and rehabilitate ill and disabled client through "humanistic science of nursing" (Rogers, 1979)	"Unitary man" evolves along life process. Client continuously changes and coexists with environment.
Orem (1971)	To care for and help client attain total self-care	This is self-care deficit theory. Nursing care becomes necessary when client is unable to fulfill biological, psychological, developmental, or social needs (Orem, 1985).
King (1971)	To use communication to help client reestablish positive adaptation to environment	Nursing process is defined as dynamic interpersonal process between nurse, client, and health care system.
Travelbee (1971)	To assist individual or family to prevent or cope with illness, regain health, find meaning in illness, or maintain maximal degree of health (Marriner-Tomey, 1994)	Interpersonal process is viewed as human-to-human relationship formed during illness and "experience of suffering."
Neuman (1972)	To assist individuals, families, and groups to attain and maintain maximal level of total wellness by purposeful interventions	Stress reduction is goal of systems model of nursing practice (Torres, 1986). Nursing actions are in primary, secondary, or tertiary level of prevention.
Patterson and Zderad (1976)	To respond to human needs and build humanistic nursing science (Patterson and Zderad, 1976; Chinn and Jacobs, 1995)	Humanistic nursing requires participants to be aware of their "uniqueness" and "commonality" with others (Chinn and Jacobs, 1995).

Table 13-1	Summary of Nursing Theories—cont'd	
THEORIST	**GOAL OF NURSING**	**FRAMEWORK FOR PRACTICE**
Leininger (1978)	To provide care consistent with nursing's emerging science and knowledge with caring as central focus (Chinn and Jacobs, 1995)	With this transcultural care theory, caring is the central and unifying domain for nursing knowledge and practice (Leininger, 1980).
Roy (1979)	To identify types of demands placed on client, assess adaptation to demands, and help client adapt	This adaptation model is based on the physiological, psychological, sociological, and dependence-independence adaptive modes (Roy, 1980).
Watson (1979)	To promote health, restore client to health, and prevent illness (Marriner-Tomey, 1994)	This theory involves philosophy and science of caring; caring is interpersonal process comprising interventions that result in meeting human needs (Torres, 1986).
Parse (1981)	To focus on man as living unity and man's qualitative participation with health experience (Parse, 1990) (Nursing as science and art [Marriner-Tomey, 1994])	Man continually interacts with environment and participates in maintenance of health (Marriner-Tomey, 1994). Health is continual, open process rather than state of well-being or absence of disease (Parse 1990; Marriner-Tomey, 1994; Chinn and Jacobs, 1995).

client mutually define the problem and potential solutions. The client gains from this relationship by using available services to meet needs, and nurses assist the client in reducing anxiety related to the health care problem. Peplau's theory is unique in that the collaborative nurse-client relationship creates a "maturing force" through which interpersonal effectiveness assists in meeting the client's needs (Beeber, Anderson, and Sills, 1990). When the original needs have been resolved, new needs may emerge. The nurse-client interpersonal relationship is characterized by the following overlapping phases: orientation, identification, explanation, and resolution (Chinn and Jacobs, 1995).

Peplau's theory and ideas were developed to provide a design for the practice of psychiatric nursing. Nursing research on anxiety, empathy, behavioral tools, and tools to evaluate verbal responses resulted from Peplau's conceptual model (Marriner-Tomey, 1994).

Henderson's Theory

Virginia Henderson's nursing theory (Harmer and Henderson, 1955) involves basic needs of the whole person. Henderson (1964) defines nursing as

assisting the individual sick or well in the performance of those activities contributing to health or its recovery . . . that he would perform unaided if he had the necessary strength, will, or knowledge. And to do this in such a way as to help him gain independence as rapidly as possible.

The following needs, often called *Henderson's 14 basic needs*, provide a framework for nursing care (Henderson, 1966):

1. Breathe normally.
2. Eat and drink adequately.
3. Eliminate by all avenues of elimination.
4. Move and maintain a desirable position.
5. Sleep and rest.
6. Select suitable clothing; dress and undress.
7. Maintain body temperature within normal range.

8. Keep the body clean and well groomed.
9. Avoid dangers in the environment.
10. Communicate with others.
11. Worship according to faith.
12. Work at something that provides a sense of accomplishment.
13. Play or participate in various forms of recreation.
14. Learn, discover, or satisfy the curiosity that leads to normal development and health.

Abdellah's Theory

The nursing theory developed by Faye Abdellah et al. (1960) emphasizes delivering nursing care for the whole person to meet the physical, emotional, intellectual, social, and spiritual needs of the client and family. When using this approach, the nurse needs knowledge and skills in interpersonal relations, psychology, growth and development, communication, and sociology, as well as a knowledge of the basic sciences and specific nursing skills. The nurse is a problem solver and decision maker. The nurse formulates an individualized view of the client's needs, which may occur in the following areas:

1. Comfort, hygiene, and safety
2. Physiological balance
3. Psychological and social factors
4. Sociological and community factors

In these four areas, Abdellah et al. (1960) identified the following specific client needs, which are often referred to as *Abdellah's 21 nursing problems:*

1. To maintain good hygiene and physical comfort
2. To achieve optimal activity, exercise, rest, and sleep
3. To prevent accident, injury, or other trauma and prevent the spread of infection
4. To maintain good body mechanics and prevent and correct deformities
5. To facilitate the supply of oxygen to all body cells
6. To facilitate the maintenance of nutrition to all body cells

7. To facilitate the maintenance of elimination
8. To facilitate the maintenance of fluid and electrolyte balance
9. To recognize the physiological responses of the body to disease conditions—pathological, physiological, and compensatory
10. To facilitate the maintenance of regulatory mechanisms and functions
11. To facilitate the maintenance of sensory function
12. To identify and accept positive and negative expressions, feelings, and reactions
13. To identify and accept the interrelatedness of emotions and organic illness
14. To facilitate the maintenance of effective verbal and nonverbal communication
15. To facilitate the development of productive interpersonal relationships
16. To facilitate progress toward achievement of personal spiritual goals
17. To create and/or maintain a therapeutic environment
18. To facilitate awareness of the self as an individual with varying physical, emotional, and developmental needs
19. To accept the optimum possible goals in light of limitations—physical and emotional
20. To use community resources as an aid in resolving problems arising from illness
21. To understand the role of social problems as influencing factors in the cause of illness

Orlando's Theory

To Ida Orlando (1961), the client is an individual with a need that, when met, diminishes distress, increases adequacy, or enhances well-being (Chinn and Jacobs, 1995). Orlando's theory radically shifted the nurse's focus from the client's medical diagnosis and automatic activities to the client's behavior in terms of the client's immediate need and determining if the needs were achieved with nursing action (Schmieding, 1995). Orlando's theory contains a conceptual framework for professional nursing. Three elements—client behavior, nurse reaction, and nurse actions—compose the nursing situation (Marriner-Tomey, 1994). After nurses thoroughly assess the client's needs, they recognize the impact of that need on the client's level of health and then act automatically or deliberately to meet the need, ultimately reducing the client's distress (Chinn and Jacobs, 1995).

Levine's Theory

Myra Levine's nursing theory, formulated in 1966 and published in 1973, views the client as an integrated being who interacts with and adapts to the environment. Levine believes that nursing intervention is a conservation activity, with conservation of energy as a primary concern (Fawcett, 1989). Health is viewed in terms of the conservation of energy in the following areas, which Levine calls the *four conservation principles of nursing:*

1. Conservation of client energy
2. Conservation of structural integrity
3. Conservation of personal integrity
4. Conservation of social integrity

With this approach, nursing care involves conservation activities aimed at the optimal use of the client's resources.

Johnson's Theory

Dorothy Johnson's theory of nursing (1968) focuses on how the client adapts to illness and how actual or potential stress can affect the ability to adapt. The goal of nursing is to reduce stress so that the client can move more easily through recovery (Johnson, 1968). Johnson's theory focuses on basic needs in terms of the following categories of behavior:

1. Security-seeking behavior
2. Nurturance-seeking behavior
3. Master of oneself and one's environment according to internalized standards of excellence
4. Taking in nourishment in socially and culturally acceptable ways
5. Ridding the body of waste in socially and culturally acceptable ways
6. Sexual and role-identity behavior
7. Self-protective behavior

According to Johnson, the nurse assesses the client's needs in these categories of behavior, called *behavioral subsystems.* Under normal conditions the client functions effectively in the environment. When stress disrupts normal adaptation, however, behavior becomes erratic and less purposeful. The nurse identifies this inability to adapt and provides nursing care to resolve problems in meeting the client's needs.

Rogers' Theory

In her theory, Martha Rogers (1970) considers man (unitary human being) as an energy field coexisting within the universe. Man is in continuous interaction with the environment (Lutjens, 1995). In addition, man is a unified whole, possessing personal integrity and manifesting characteristics that are more than the sum of the parts (Rogers, 1970). Unitary man is a "four dimensional energy field identified by pattern and manifesting characteristics that are specific to the whole and which cannot be predicted from the knowledge of parts" (Marriner-Tomey, 1994). The four dimensions used in Rogers' theory—energy fields, openness, pattern and organization, and four dimensionality—are used to derive principles about how human beings develop.

Rogers views nursing primarily as a science and is committed to nursing research. Nursing therefore incorporates knowledge of the basic sciences and physiology, as well as nursing knowledge:

> The science of nursing aims to provide a body of abstract knowledge growing out of scientific research and logical analysis and capable of being translated into nursing practice. Nursing's body of scientific knowledge is a new product specific to nursing. . . . Nursing is a humanistic science.

Orem's Theory

Dorothea Orem (1971) developed a definition of nursing that emphasizes the client's self-care needs. Orem describes her philosophy of nursing in this way:

> Nursing has as a special concern man's needs for self-care action and the provision and management of it on a continuous basis in order to sustain life and health, recover from disease or injury, and cope with their effects. Self-care is a requirement of every person— man, woman, and child. When self-care is not maintained, illness,

disease, or death will occur. Nurses sometimes manage and maintain required self-care continually for persons who are totally incapacitated. In other instances, nurses help persons to maintain required self-care by performing some but not all care measures, by supervising others who assist patients, and by instructing and guiding individuals as they gradually move toward self-care.

Thus the goal of Orem's theory is helping the client perform self-care. According to Orem, nursing care is necessary when the client is unable to fulfill biological, psychological, developmental, or social needs. The nurse determines why a client is unable to meet these needs, what must be done to enable the client to meet them, and how much self-care the client is able to perform. The goal of nursing is to increase the client's ability to independently meet these needs (Hartweg, 1995).

King's Theory

Imogene King's goal attainment theory (1971, 1981, 1987) focuses on three interacting systems: personal systems, interpersonal systems, and social systems. There forms a personal relationship between client and nurse. The nurse-client relationship is the vehicle for the delivery of nursing care, which is a dynamic interpersonal process in which the nurse and client are affected by each other's behavior, as well as by the health care system (King, 1971, 1981). The nurse's goal is to use communication to assist the client in reestablishing or maintaining a positive adaptation to the environment.

Neuman's Theory

Betty Neuman (1972) defines a total-person model incorporating the holistic concept and an open-systems approach (Marriner-Tomey, 1994). To Neuman, the person is a dynamic composite of physiological, sociocultural, and developmental variables that function as an open system. As an open system, the person interacts with, adjusts to, and is adjusted by the environment, which is viewed as a stressor (Chinn and Jacobs, 1995). The internal environment consists of those influences (intrapersonal) within the client. The external environment is influences (interpersonal) outside the client. The created environment is the client's attempt to create a safe setting, which may be made up of conscious or unconscious mechanisms (Reed, 1995). Each environment has potential threats from stressors, which disrupt the system. Neuman's model includes intrapersonal, interpersonal, and extrapersonal stressors (Neuman, 1982, 1995; Marriner-Tomey, 1994).

Neuman believes that nursing is concerned with the whole person. The goal of nursing is to assist individuals, families, and groups in attaining and maintaining a maximal level of total wellness (Neuman and Young, 1972). The nurse assesses, manages, and evaluates client systems. Nursing focuses on the variables affecting the client's response to the stressor (Chinn and Jacobs, 1995). Nursing actions are in the primary, secondary, and tertiary levels of prevention. Primary prevention focuses on strengthening a line of defense through the identification of actual or potential risk factors associated with stressors. Secondary prevention strengthens internal defenses and resources by establishing priorities and treatment plans for identified symptoms, and tertiary prevention focuses on readaptation. The principal goal in tertiary prevention is to strengthen resistance to stressors through client education and to assist in preventing a recurrence of the stress response (Neuman, 1982; Torres, 1986; Marriner-Tomey, 1994; Chinn and Jacobs, 1995).

Roy's Theory

Sister Callista Roy's adaptation theory (Roy and Obloy, 1979; Roy, 1980, 1984, 1989) views the client as an adaptive system. According to Roy's model, the goal of nursing is to help the person adapt to changes in physiological needs, self-concept, role function, and interdependent relations during health and illness (Marriner-Tomey, 1994). The need for nursing care arises when the client cannot adapt to internal and external environmental demands. All individuals must adapt to the following demands:

1. Meeting basic physiological needs
2. Developing a positive self-concept
3. Performing social roles
4. Achieving a balance between dependence and independence

The nurse determines what demands are causing problems for a client and assesses how well the client is adapting to them. Nursing care is then directed at helping the client adapt.

Watson's Theory

Watson's philosophy of caring (1979, 1985, 1988) attempts to define the outcome of nursing activity in regard to the humanistic aspects of life (Watson, 1979; Marriner-Tomey, 1994). The action of nursing is directed at understanding the interrelationship of health, illness, and human behavior. Nursing is concerned with promoting and restoring health and preventing illness.

Watson's model is designed around the caring process, assisting clients to attain or maintain health or to die peacefully. Interventions are related to the human care process. Human care requires that the nurse be knowledgeable about human behavior and human responses to actual or potential health problems, individual needs, how to respond to others, and strengths and limitations of the client and family, as well as those of the nurse. In addition, the nurse comforts and offers compassion and empathy to clients and their families. Caring represents all of the factors the nurse uses to deliver health care to the client (Watson, 1987).

■ AMERICAN NURSES ASSOCIATION (ANA) DEFINITION OF NURSING PRACTICE

In 1955 the ANA published the following official definition of nursing practice*:

The practice of professional nursing means the performance for compensation of any act in the observation, care, and counsel of the ill, injured, or infirm or in the maintenance of health or prevention of illness of others, or in the supervision and teaching of other personnel, or in the administration of medications and treatments as prescribed by licensed physician or dentist, requiring substantial specialized judgment and skill and based on knowledge and application of the principles of biological, physical, and social sciences. The foregoing shall not be deemed to include acts of diagnosis or prescription of therapeutic or corrective measures.

*From ANA: *Am J Nurs* 55:1474, 1955.

This early definition by the ANA is significant in its attempt to define nursing practice in a fairly specific manner. Nonetheless, it tends to stress nursing's dependent role, an emphasis no longer accepted. In 1965 the ANA Committee on Education issued a position paper that presents a fuller definition of nursing and emphasizes nursing as an independent profession[†]:

Nursing is a helping profession and, as such, provides services which contribute to the health and well-being of people.

Nursing is a vital consequence to the individual receiving services; it fills needs that cannot be met by the person, family, or other persons in the community.

Three essential components of professional nursing are care, cure, and coordination. The care aspect is more than "to take care of"; it is also "caring for" and "caring about." It is dealing with human beings under stress, frequently over long periods of time. It is providing comfort and support in times of anxiety, loneliness, and helplessness. It is listening, evaluating, and intervening appropriately.

The promotion of health and healing is the cure aspect of professional nursing. It is assisting clients to understand their health problems and helping them cope. It is the administration of medications and treatments. It is also the use of clinical nursing judgment in determining, on the basis of patient outcomes, whether the plan of care needs to be maintained or changed. It is knowing when and how to use existing and potential resources to help patients toward recovery and adjustment by mobilizing their own resources.

[†]From ANA: *Am J Nurs* 65:106, 1965.

Professional nursing practice is this and more. It is sharing responsibility for the health and welfare of all people in the community, and it is participating in programs designed to prevent illness and maintain health. It is coordinating and synchronizing medical and other professional and technical services that affect patient care. It is supervising, teaching, and directing all those involved in nursing care.

In 1979 the Committee of Chairpersons of the ANA determined that the **Congress for Nursing Practice** should define the nature and scope of nursing practice. The Congress is the part of the ANA concerned with legal aspects of nursing practice, public recognition of the significance of nursing practice to health care, and implications for nursing practice of trends in health care.

In 1980 the Congress defined nursing as the diagnosis and treatment of human responses to actual or potential health problems (ANA, 1980). This definition involves the following characteristics of nursing: phenomena, theory application, nursing action, and evaluation of the effects of action (Fig. 13-1). *Phenomena* are the human responses to actual or potential health problems. The nurse identifies the client's responses by assessing health status and obtaining data. The nurse applies nursing *theory* to understand these responses. The nurse takes *actions* to resolve actual or potential health care problems. The nurse then evaluates the *effects* of the actions on the client's responses. These four characteristics are related to the nursing process, which is described in Unit 2.

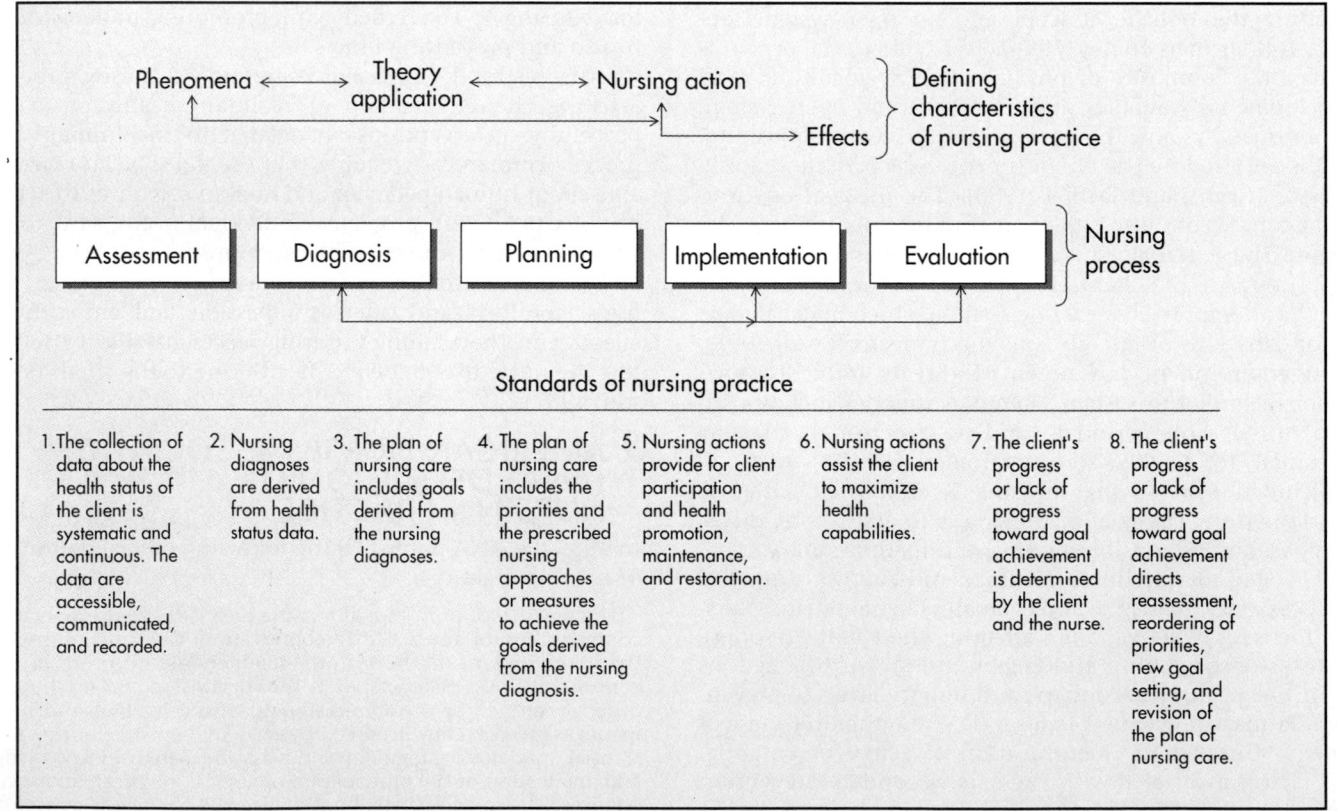

Fig. 13-1 Defining characteristics of nursing practice: relationship to the nursing process and the standards of nursing practice. *(Redrawn from the American Nurses Association:* Nursing and social policy statement, *Kansas City, Mo, 1980, The Association.)*

CANADIAN NURSES ASSOCIATION (CNA) DEFINITION OF NURSING PRACTICE

The CNA in the 1986 *Definition of Nursing and Standards for Nursing Practice* defined nursing. Nursing practice can be generally defined as a dynamic, caring, helping relationship in which the nurse assists the client to achieve and maintain optimal health. The nurse fulfills this purpose by applying knowledge and skills from nursing and related fields using the nursing process, the substance of which is determined by a conceptual model(s) for nursing. Founded in 1908, the CNA provides leadership to practicing nurses in the Canadian provinces. Through the actions and activities of the CNA, nurses can meet the health care demands of the changing Canadian society (Meilicke and Larsen, 1988).

EDUCATIONAL PREPARATION

Registered Nurse Education

As the profession of nursing grew, various educational routes for becoming a **registered nurse (RN)** were developed. Initially, hospital schools of nursing were developed to educate nurses who would work within those institutions.

As nursing increasingly defined its own body of knowledge, formalized educational processes developed to ensure a consistent level of education in institutions. Such consistency was also necessary for RN licensure.

Currently in the United States an individual can become an RN through an associate degree, diploma, or baccalaureate degree program. In Canada there are diploma and baccalaureate degree programs.

ASSOCIATE DEGREE EDUCATION

The associate degree program in the United States is a 2-year program usually offered by a college or junior college. This program focuses on the basic sciences and on theoretical and clinical courses related to the practice of nursing. Graduates of this type of program take the state board examination for RN licensure.

DIPLOMA EDUCATION

The diploma program in the United States is a 2- or 3-year program usually associated with a hospital. Diploma programs also focus on the basic sciences and on theoretical and clinical courses related to nursing practice. Some diploma programs are affiliated with colleges or universities, which grant college credit for nonnursing courses. Graduates of a diploma program receive a diploma from the hospital and take the state board examination for RN licensure. In the United States, diploma programs are declining in numbers. In Canada, diploma programs are offered in community colleges or hospitals and are 2-year programs (or 3 years in some hospital-based programs) compared with associate degree programs in the United States.

BACCALAUREATE EDUCATION

The baccalaureate degree program usually encompasses 4 years of study in a college or university. The program focuses on the basic sciences and on theoretical and clinical courses, as well as courses in the social sciences, arts, and humanities to support nursing theory. In Canada, a Bachelor of Science in Nursing (BScN) or a Bachelor in Nursing (BN) is the equivalent to the Bachelor of Science in Nursing (BSN) in the United States.

The American Association of Colleges of Nursing (AACN) published the *Essentials of College and University Education for Professional Nursing* (1986). This document delineated essential knowledge, practice and values, attitudes, personal qualities, and professional behavior for the baccalaureate-prepared nurse. The goal of this document was to provide standards by which "faculty can measure the content of the curriculum and the performance of the graduate" (AACN, 1986).

Accreditation and Licensure

To be accredited, nursing programs must meet certain criteria established by the National League for Nursing (NLN). This voluntary accreditation is available for basic nursing education programs and master's degree programs in nursing (National Commission on Nursing, 1983).

RN licensure for practice in most states and provinces requires that the student complete a prescribed course of study from an approved program. In the United States the program must be approved by the State Board of Nursing in the state in which the student is seeking licensure. In Canada the program must be approved by a Provincial Board of Nursing in the province in which the student is seeking licensure.

In the United States, RN candidates must pass the National Council Licensure Examination for Registered Nurses (NCLEX-RN), which is administered by each state's board of nursing. In Canada the CNA Testing Service (CNATS) administers the test to qualified candidates in each province.

Characteristics of Graduate Education in Nursing Leading to the Master's Degree

The master's program in nursing is offered by an educational institution of higher learning and is built on a baccalaureate curriculum, including an upper-division major in nursing. It provides students with an opportunity to:
- Acquire advanced knowledge from the sciences and the humanities to support advanced nursing practice and role development
- Expand knowledge of nursing theory as a basis for advanced nursing practice
- Develop expertise in a specialized area of clinical nursing practice
- Acquire the knowledge and skills related to a specific functional role in nursing
- Acquire initial competence in conducting research
- Plan and initiate change in the health care system and in the practice and delivery of health care
- Further develop and implement leadership strategies for the betterment of health care
- Actively engage in collaborative relationships with others to improve health care
- Acquire a foundation for doctoral study

Modified from National League for Nursing: *Characteristics of graduate education in nursing leading to the master's degree,* New York, 1978, The League.

Whether nurses can practice in a state or province other than their own depends on the agreement between the states or provinces involved.

Graduate Nursing Education

As expressed by the ANA (1969), the purpose of a graduate program in nursing is to prepare nurse clinicians capable of improving nursing care through the advancement of nursing theory and sciences. A person completing a graduate program can receive the degree of Master of Arts in Nursing (MA), Master in Nursing (MN), or Master of Science in Nursing (MSN). The NLN has described the characteristics of and standards for accredited master's degree nursing programs (see the box on p. 217).

A master's degree in nursing can be valuable for nurses seeking roles of nurse educator, clinical nurse specialist, nurse administrator, or nurse practitioner. These roles are described later in this chapter.

The first nursing doctorate program opened in 1953 at the University of Pittsburgh. The need for nurses with doctorate degrees is rising (Institute of Medicine, 1983). Professional doctoral programs in nursing (DSN or DNSc) emphasize the application of research findings to clinical nursing. Other programs emphasize more basic research and theory and award the Doctor of Philosophy (PhD) in nursing (Holzemer, 1987).

Continuing Education

Because nursing is a dynamic profession, **continuing education** programs help nurses remain current in nursing skills, knowledge, and theory. Continuing education involves formal, organized, and educational programs offered by State Nurses' Associations (Fig. 13-2) and educational and health care institutions. As expressed by the ANA (1991), the goals of continuing education in nursing are to improve and maintain nursing practice, promote and exercise leadership in effecting change in health care delivery systems, and fulfill professional learning needs. Other goals include helping nurses become specialized in a particular area of practice and teaching nurses new skills and techniques.

In general, continuing education programs are short term and are designed for all nurses. The ANA or the state

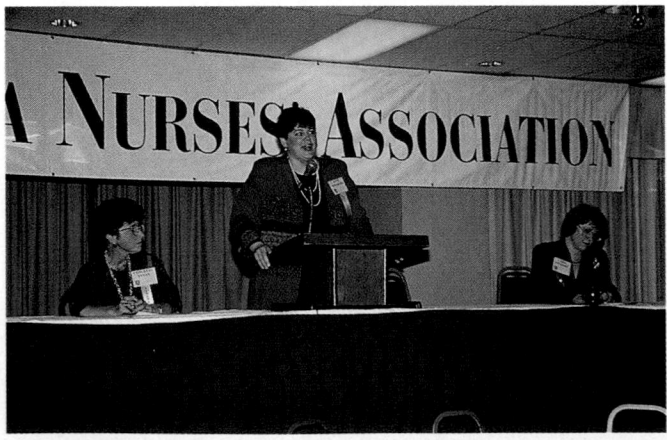

Fig. 13-2 Participating at State Nurses' Association provides continuing education and networking opportunities.

board of nursing is the accrediting agency for these programs. The ANA awards continuing education units on completion of specific courses. Some states require nurses to take continuing education courses for license renewal.

In-Service Education

An **in-service education** program is instruction or training provided by a health care agency or institution. An in-service program is held in the institution and is designed to increase the knowledge, skills, and competencies of nurses and other health care professionals employed by the institution. For example, a hospital might offer an in-service program to inform nurses about primary nursing before it is implemented at the hospital.

All nurses have access to continuing education and in-service programs organized and conducted by a university, private hospital, private continuing education service, or the employing institution or agency. Such programs assist the practicing nurse in acquiring new knowledge and skills necessary for today's highly technical and fast-changing health care delivery system.

Licensed Practical Nurse Education

A licensed practical or vocational nurse is trained in basic nursing techniques and direct client care. The **licensed practical nurse (LPN)** or **licensed vocational nurse (LVN)** practices under the supervision of a registered nurse in a hospital or community health practice setting. A licensed practical nurse, or in Canada a registered nurse's assistant (RNA), generally receives 1 year of education and training in a hospital, community college, or other agency. The LPN or LVN is licensed by a board after completing the educational program and passing the licensure examination.

Career Mobility and Clinical Ladder

Education continues to be important after the nurse begins practice, whether the practice setting focuses on the adult or child, the chronically or acutely ill, or the home or hospital. Nursing encompasses an ever-widening range of roles. Multiple career paths and goals are open to new and experienced practitioners (Hefferin and Kleinknecht, 1986).

Opportunities for career mobility are increasing. The clinical ladder unifies clinical practice and nursing administration, fosters collaboration between nursing education and service, and is a professional advancement system.

A clinical ladder contains structure, criteria for clinical competencies, promotional procedures, and incentives for advancement within a health care organization (Huey, 1982). The structure is individualized for a specific institution and may include multiple levels on the clinical, administration, research, and education pathways (ANA, 1984). There are specific objective, measurable criteria for each level within the structure. Within a clinical ladder system, nurses are no longer promoted strictly on the basis of education and seniority within the institution. Promotional procedures within the clinical ladder are clearly delineated, thereby promoting self-appraisal and peer appraisal for career mobility within the system. The incentive for advancement may include increased autonomy of practice, raise in salary or promotion within the organizational structure itself, increased expertise, and personal self-fulfillment.

The clinical ladder is a method for career mobility by which one program can encourage and motivate nurses to remain in the health care setting. Career counseling is another method for retention and promoting within the settings.

Hefferin and Kleinknecht (1986) developed the Nursing Career Preference Inventory to assist nurses in determining which of the four primary nursing practice areas—clinical, administration, research, or education—reflects their personal work activity interests or preferences. Career inventories are valuable in retaining bright, talented nurses within an institution and decreasing the risk of experienced nurses leaving the profession.

∎ NURSING PRACTICE

Nurses practice in a variety of settings, in many roles within those settings, and with other care givers in the allied health professions. The practice of nursing is guided only in part by administrators in hospitals and other health care agencies and institutions. State and provincial nurse practice acts establish specific legal regulations for practice, and professional organizations establish standards of practice as criteria for nursing care.

Standards of Nursing Practice

As nursing has gained independence as a profession, it has increasingly set its own standards for practice. Standards for practice are important as objective guidelines for nurses to provide care and as criteria for evaluating care. When standards are clearly defined, clients can be assured they are receiving high-quality care, nurses know exactly what is necessary to give nursing care, and administrators can determine that care meets acceptable standards. Moreover, standards of practice are important if a legal dispute arises over whether a nurse practiced appropriately in a particular case (see Chapter 20). The ANA and the CNA have published standards of nursing practice (Table 13-2; see the box below). In addition, the ANA has published standards of professional performance (see the box at right).

Nurse Practice Acts

In all states in the United States and all provinces in Canada, nurse practice acts regulate the licensure and practice of nursing. Each state or province defines for itself the scope of nursing practice, but most have similar practice acts. The definition of nursing practice published by the ANA in 1955 (see p. 215) is in some ways representative of the scope of nursing practice as defined in most states and provinces. In the last decade, however, many states have revised their nurse practice acts to reflect nursing's growing autonomy and the expanded roles of nurses in practice. The 1955 ANA prohibition against diagnosis and treatment, for example, has been removed from nurse practice acts in many states or rephrased to differentiate between nursing diagnosis and treatment and medical diagnosis and treatment. Nurse practice acts are discussed in more detail in Chapter 20.

Practice Settings

Nursing practice settings are expanding due to the changes in the health care delivery system. Nurses need an educational basis to prepare them to address the ever-changing health care needs of their clients, develop research skills to monitor client outcomes, and increase their psychomotor skills and cognitive knowledge as technology increases (NLN, 1992; AACN, 1993). There is a greater emphasis on community-based practice and the knowledge base for this practice developed from traditional and nontraditional methods. Table 13-3 gives statistics on the numbers of nurses in practice settings.

HOSPITALS, SKILLED NURSING, AND RESTORATIVE SETTINGS

The largest group of practicing nurses is those working in hospitals. Current reimbursement practices of private and federal or state insurance groups have resulted in shorter hospital stays (see Chapter 2). Thus clients are being discharged from hospitals sooner, frequently requiring continued nursing care in the home. Today's hospital-based professional nurse is not only adept in providing nursing care but is also able, through early discharge planning and collaborative practice, to meet the home care needs of clients (McEwen, 1994).

Nursing practice in hospital and skilled nursing facilities is becoming more complex due in part to the increased older adult population, rising acuity of clients, and new

Canadian Nurses Association Standards for Nursing Practice

Nursing practice requires that a conceptual model(s) for nursing be the basis of practice.
Nursing practice requires the effective use of the nursing process.
Nursing practice requires that the helping relationship be the nature of the client-nurse interaction.
Nursing practice requires nurses to fulfill professional responsibilities.

Modified from Canadian Nurses Association: *A definition of nursing practice. Standards for nursing practice*, Ottawa, 1986, The Association.

Standards of Professional Performance

∎ The nurse systematically evaluates the quality and effectiveness of nursing practice.
∎ The nurse evaluates his/her own nursing practice in relation to professional practice standards and relevant statutes and regulations.
∎ The nurse acquires and maintains current knowledge in nursing practice.
∎ The nurse contributes to the professional development of peers, colleagues, and others.
∎ The nurse's decisions and actions on behalf of clients are determined in an ethical manner.
∎ The nurse collaborates with the client, significant others, and health care providers in providing client care.
∎ The nurse uses research findings in practice.
∎ The nurse considers factors related to safety, effectiveness, and cost in planning and delivering client care.

Modified from American Nurses Association: *Standards of clinical practice*, Washington, DC, 1991, The Association.

Table 13-2	ANA Standards of Nursing Practice	
STANDARD	**ELEMENT**

ASSESSMENT

The nurse collects client health data.

The priority of data collection is determined by the client's immediate condition of needs.

Pertinent data are collected using appropriate assessment techniques.

Data collection involves the client, significant others, and health care providers when appropriate.

The data collection process is systematic and ongoing.

Relevant data are documented in a retrievable form.

NURSING DIAGNOSIS

The nurse analyzes the assessment data in determining diagnoses.

Diagnoses are derived from the assessment data.

Diagnoses are validated with the client, significant others, and health care providers, when possible.

Diagnoses are documented in a manner that facilitates the determination of expected outcomes and plan of care.

The nurse identifies expected outcomes individualized to the client.

Outcomes are derived from the diagnoses.

Outcomes are documented as measurable goals.

Outcomes are mutually formulated with the client and health care providers, when possible.

Outcomes are realistic in relation to client's present and potential capabilities.

Outcomes are attainable in relation to resources available to the client.

Outcomes include a time estimate for attainment.

Outcomes provide direction for continuity of care.

PLANNING

The nurse develops a plan of care that prescribes interventions to attain expected outcomes.

The plan is individualized to the client's condition or needs.

The plan is developed with the client, significant others, and health care providers, when appropriate.

The plan reflects current nursing practice.

The plan is documented.

The plan provides for continuity of care.

IMPLEMENTATION

The nurse implements the interventions identified in the plan of care.

Interventions are consistent with the established plan of care.

Interventions are implemented in a safe and appropriate manner.

Interventions are documented.

EVALUATION

The nurse evaluates the client's progress toward attainment of outcomes.

Evaluation is systematic and ongoing.

The client's responses to interventions are documented.

The effectiveness of interventions is evaluated in relation to outcomes.

Revisions in diagnoses, outcomes, and the plan of care are documented.

The client, significant others, and health care providers are involved in the evaluation process, when appropriate.

Modified from American Nurses Association: *Standards of clinical practice*, Washington, DC, 1991, The Association.

forms of supportive therapy. Infections associated with acquired immunodeficiency syndrome (AIDS), organ transplantation, and technological equipment used in the critical care setting are a few factors contributing to a higher percentage of critically ill clients in hospitals (Pruitt and Campbell, 1994).

In addition to the rising acuity rate, there has been a sharp upward spiraling of health care costs. To adjust for this increase, some hospitals are reducing the number of people on staff without decreasing the workload. Professional nurses are caught in this dilemma (McClure, 1991). Today's professional nurses are challenged to meet the multiple health care needs of clients with reduced resources.

In hospitals, nursing services operate 24 hours a day.

Hospitals use different staffing patterns to meet the need for nursing care. Some hospitals have three 8-hour shifts, whereas other hospitals use two 12-hour shifts or three 10-hour shifts that overlap during the early morning, late afternoon, and night. The roles and responsibilities of nurses employed in hospitals vary because hospitals differ widely in size and organizational structure (see Chapter 2).

Clients in hospitals generally require 24-hour nursing care. Hospitals may be acute, long-term, or rehabilitation care facilities. Nurses employed in an acute-care setting care for clients with severe illnesses and complex problems. Today these clients are usually more dependent and more seriously ill than clients in the past because of shorter periods of hospitalization. As a result, nursing practice in acute-care

Table 13-3	Employment Settings of Registered Nurses		
SETTING		**UNITED STATES***	**CANADA†**
Hospital		67%	73%‡
Nursing homes		7%	—
Community health		10%	12%
Physician and dentist offices		8%	3%
Schools		2%	—
Nursing education		4%	3%
Occupational health		1%	—
Other		4%	3%
Unknown		2%	6%

Moses EB: *The registered nurse population, findings from the National Sample Survey of Registered Nurses,* March 1992, US Department of Health and Human Services; Public Health Service, Division of Nursing, Health Resources, and Services Administration.
†From Kerr JR, MacPhail J: *Canadian nursing issues and perspectives, ed 3,* St Louis, 1994, Mosby.
‡Includes nurses working in hospitals, skilled nursing facilities, and restorative care hospitals.

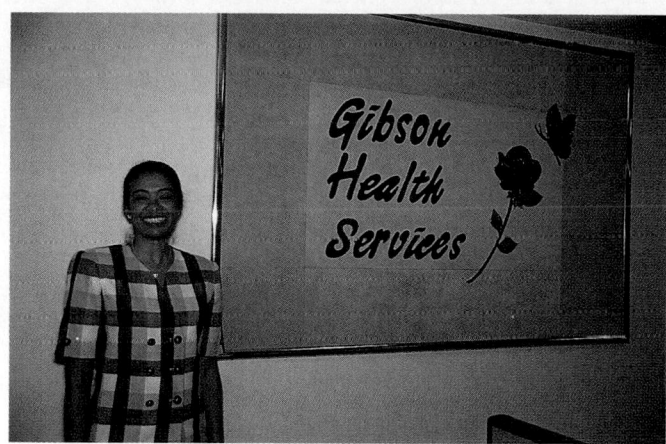

Fig. 13-3 Nursing provides opportunities to create local health care centers.

settings has become more specialized and complex. The skills and knowledge needed to practice in this setting are determined by the clinical area of practice.

The rapid rise in the number of older adults, clients with chronic illnesses, and clients with functional impairments has resulted in the growth of long-term care facilities. Long term care is provided in institutions such as chronic disease hospitals, psychiatric hospitals, and nursing homes. Nursing homes are the most common agencies providing in-house, long-term care.

Restorative care facilities generally employ many types of health care professionals. The goal of these institutions is to teach disabled clients to achieve a maximal level of function and to teach families to help them reach that level (see Chapter 5).

COMMUNITY-BASED PRACTICE SETTINGS

The number of nurses employed in community-based practice settings is increasing substantially. The rising costs of institutional care create the need for community-based nursing services aimed at health promotion, disease prevention, and restorative care.

Nursing in community-based settings is focused on health promotion and maintenance, education and management, and coordination and continuity of restorative care within the client's community. Community-based nurses assess the health needs of individuals, families, and communities and help clients cope with threats to health and problems of illness. Whereas institutional health care focuses on the individual and family, community-based nursing is also directed toward the health of the community and the interaction of individuals within that community. A community can be a particular location such as an urban or rural area or a group of people related by occupation, school, or another common interest or characteristic. Thus community-based nurses are employed in a variety of practice settings, including community and occupational health centers, schools, home health care agencies, health clinics, and private practices.

Community Health Centers. Community health centers offer comprehensive programs for health maintenance and promotion, education and management, and coordination of care within the community. Community health centers provide ambulatory care (care sought by clients able to come to the centers), as well as care within the home.

Nurses employed in these centers often work more independently than nurses in institutional settings. Community health centers also employ other health professionals, but nurses generally provide most of the care, and may in fact own and operate the facility (Fig. 13-3). In some settings, physicians are called in only when specific needs arise. Examples of community health centers are planned parenthood clinics and family care and mental health centers.

Schools. Community-based health services are common in schools and on college campuses. Nursing services include health education in disease prevention, health promotion, and sex education. In addition, nurses working in schools may provide care for students with nonemergency acute illnesses such as upper respiratory tract infections, influenza, and viruses. School nurses also make referrals for students and their families when additional, more specialized health care is needed.

Occupational Health Settings. Many large companies provide health services to employees in occupational health centers located on the premises. Nursing care in these settings involves five areas. The nurse may develop programs aimed at increasing health and safety in the workplace by reducing the number of occupational accidents, the risk of occupational disease, or the transmission of a contagious disease among the workers. The nurse may provide programs for health promotion, disease prevention, and health education. The nurse also treats nonemergency acute illnesses and provides first aid. In emergency situations such as heart attacks or trauma, the nurse gives emergency care and arranges transportation to a hospital. The nurse also refers employees to additional health resources when necessary.

Home Health Care Agencies. A client often needs specific nursing care that can be given efficiently in the home (see Chapter 5). Nurses in these agencies provide home-based nursing care to clients discharged from that particular institution. Other agencies providing home health care include visiting nurse associations, public health nursing agencies, hospices, and private home care agencies.

The nurse who functions in the home must also be skilled at teaching. Rising health care costs have limited the duration and frequency of visits. As a result the home health care nurse often teaches the client or family to competently perform nursing activities and self-care. Caring for the client in the home environment requires the nurse to be flexible, resourceful, creative, and self-confident, as well as clinically competent (see Chapter 5).

OTHER SETTINGS

There are a number of other settings in which nurses practice and where their roles and responsibilities vary widely. A nurse may be employed in a physician's office, a legal office, or a health care consultation service. A nurse may practice in solo or joint practice with other nurses and other health care professionals who provide care independently to well or stable client groups. Nurses are also employed in educational and research positions.

Regardless of the practice environment, nurses are challenged to deliver quality care. Nursing research linking quality client outcome studies with cost effectiveness provides documentation that nurses are meeting the challenge. Nurses are active in speaking out about health care issues at all levels of government (Holzemer, 1990).

■ ROLES AND FUNCTIONS OF THE NURSE

Contemporary nursing requires that the nurse possess knowledge and skills in a variety of areas. In the past the principal role of nurses was to provide care and comfort as they carried out specific nursing functions, but changes in nursing have expanded the role to include increased emphasis on health promotion and illness prevention, as well as concern for the client as a whole. The contemporary nurse functions in the interrelated roles of care giver, clinical and ethical decision maker, protector and client advocate, case manager, rehabilitator, comforter, communicator, and teacher.

Care Giver

As care giver, the nurse helps the client regain health through the healing process. Healing is more than just curing a specific disease, although treatment skills that promote physical healing are important to care givers. The nurse addresses the holistic health care needs of the client, including measures to restore emotional, spiritual, and social well-being. The care giver helps the client and family set goals and meet those goals with a minimal cost of time and energy.

Clinical Decision Maker

To provide effective care, the nurse uses critical thinking skills throughout the nursing process (Fig. 13-4). Before undertaking any nursing action, whether it is assessing the client's condition, giving care, or evaluating the results of care, the nurse plans the action by deciding the best approach for each client. The nurse makes these decisions

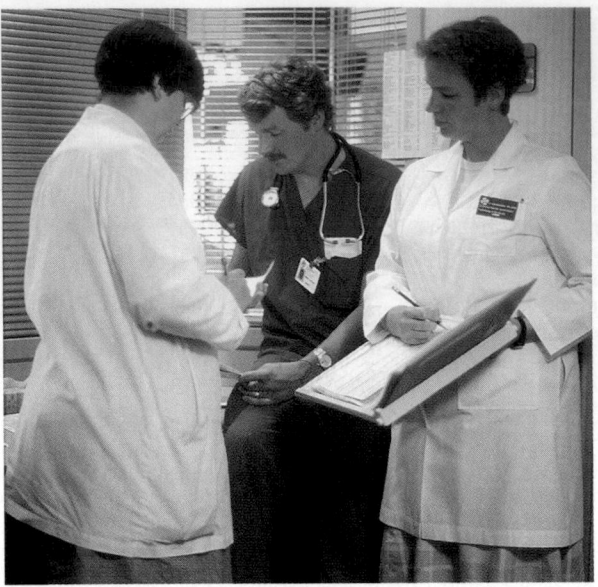

Fig. 13-4 Decision making is at the core of nursing practice.

alone or in collaboration with the client and family. In each of these situations, the nurse collaborates and consults with other health care professionals (Keeling and Ramos, 1995).

Protector and Client Advocate

As protector the nurse helps maintain a safe environment for the client and takes steps to prevent injury and protect the client from possible adverse effects of diagnostic or treatment measures. Confirming that a client does not have an allergy to a medication and providing immunization against disease in a community-based practice are examples of the nurse's protective role.

In the role of client advocate, the nurse protects the client's human and legal rights and provides assistance in asserting those rights if the need arises. For example, the nurse may provide additional information for a client who is trying to decide whether to accept treatment. The nurse may also defend clients' rights in a general way by speaking out against policies or actions that might endanger clients' well-being or conflict with their rights.

Case Manager

As case manager, the nurse coordinates the activities of other members of the health care team, such as nutritionists and physical therapists, when managing a group of clients' care. In addition, nurses must also manage their own time and the resources of the practice settings. Differentiated practice models offer nurses opportunities to make decisions about their career paths. In a differentiated practice setting, nurses can choose between roles as managers of client care or as associate nurses who carry out the case manager's decisions (Manthey, 1990). As managers, nurses coordinate and delegate care responsibilities and supervise other health care workers.

Rehabilitator

Rehabilitation is the process by which individuals return to maximal levels of functioning after illness, accidents, or other disabling events. Frequently clients experience physical or emotional impairments that change their lives, and the nurse helps them adapt as fully as possible. Rehabilitative and restorative care activities range from teaching clients to walk with crutches to helping clients cope with lifestyle changes often associated with chronic illness (see Chapter 5).

Comforter

The role of comforter, caring for the client as a person, is a traditional and historical one in nursing and has continued to be important as nurses have assumed new roles. Because nursing care must be directed to the whole person rather than simply the body, comfort and emotional support often help give the client strength to recover. While carrying out nursing activities, nurses can provide comfort by demonstrating care for the client as an individual with unique feelings and needs. As comforter, nurses should help the client reach therapeutic goals rather than encourage emotional or physical dependence.

Communicator

The role of communicator is central to all other nursing roles. Nursing involves communication with clients and families, other nurses and health care professionals, resource persons, and the community. Without clear communication it is impossible to give care effectively, make decisions with clients and families, protect clients from threats to well being, coordinate and manage client care, assist the client in rehabilitation, offer comfort, or teach. The quality of communication is a critical factor in meeting the needs of individuals, families, and communities (see Chapter 14).

Teacher

As teacher, the nurse explains to clients concepts and facts about health, demonstrates procedures such as self-care activities, determines that the client fully understands, reinforces learning or client behavior, and evaluates progress in learning. Some teaching can be unplanned and informal, such as when a nurse responds to a question about a health issue in casual conversation. Other teaching activities may be planned and more formal, such as when the nurse teaches a client with diabetes to self administer insulin injections. The nurse uses teaching methods that match the client's capabilities and needs and incorporates other resources, such as the family, in teaching plans (see Chapter 15).

Career Roles

The preceding roles and functions apply to all nurses in most practice settings. Career roles, on the other hand, are specific employment positions. Because of increasing educational opportunities for nurses, the growth of nursing as a profession, and a greater concern for job enrichment, the nursing profession offers expanded roles and different kinds of career opportunities. Examples of career roles include nurse educators and advanced practice nurses, such as clinical nurse specialists, nurse practitioners, certified nurse-midwives, anesthetists, administrators, and researchers. Additional nonclinical roles include risk managers, quality improvement nurses, and product consultants.

NURSE EDUCATOR

A **nurse educator** works primarily in schools of nursing, staff development departments of health care agencies, and client education departments. Nursing educators generally have a background in clinical nursing, which provides them with practical skills and theoretical knowledge. A faculty member in a school of nursing prepares students to function as nurses. Nursing faculty members are responsible for teaching current nursing practice theory and necessary skills in laboratories or clinical settings. Nurse educators in nursing schools are usually required to have graduate degrees in nursing education. In addition, they generally have a specific clinical specialty and advanced clinical experience.

Nurse educators in staff development departments of health care institutions provide educational programs for nurses within their institution. These programs include orientation of new personnel, critical care nursing courses, and instruction about new equipment or procedures.

The primary focus of the nurse educator in an agency's department of client education is to teach ill or disabled clients and families to provide care in the home. In most health care agencies, however, the budget does not permit a separate client education department. Therefore staff nurses usually incorporate education into a client's plan of care.

ADVANCED PRACTICE NURSE

The **advanced practice nurse (APN)** has a master's degree in nursing, advanced education in pharmacology and physical assessment, and certification and expertise in a specialized area of practice (ANA, 1995). An APN usually works in primary, acute, restorative, or community health care agency. In addition, an APN may specialize in the management of a disease such as cancer, diabetes, or cardiovascular or pulmonary disease or in a specific field such as pediatrics or gerontology. The APN functions as a clinician, educator, case manager, consultant, and researcher within the area of practice to plan or improve the quality of nursing care for the client and family.

Clinical Nurse Specialist. The **clinical nurse specialist (CNS)** has a masters's degree in nursing and expertise in a specialized area of practice. A CNS may work in primary care, acute care, restorative care, and community-based settings. In addition, the CNS may specialize in specific diseases such as diabetes mellitus, cancer, or congestive heart failure or in a specific field such as pediatrics or gerontology. The CNS functions as an expert clinician, educator, case manager, consultant, and researcher to plan or improve the quality of care provided to the client and family.

Nurse Practitioner. The **nurse practitioner** provides health care to clients, usually in an outpatient, ambulatory care, or community-based setting (Roy and Obloy, 1979; Molde and Diers, 1986). Molde and Diers noted that nurse practitioners care for clients with complex problems and attend more to symptoms of nonpathological conditions, comfort, and comprehensiveness of care.

A significant percentage of primary care encounters extend beyond the boundaries of medicine and demand the expertise of the nurse. The nurse practitioner is able to establish a collaborative provider-client relationship.

A nurse practitioner may work with a specific group of

clients or clients of all ages and health care needs. The major nurse practitioner categories are adult, family, pediatric, obstetrics-gynecology, and geriatric nurse practitioner. A nurse practitioner has the knowledge and skills necessary to detect and manage limited acute and chronic stable conditions. The nurse practitioner's educational preparation includes a practitioner program or a master's degree in nursing.

An adult nurse practitioner (ANP) provides primary, ambulatory care to adults with a nonemergency acute or chronic illness, and in some settings tertiary care. ANPs are usually employed in ambulatory care centers or outpatient clinics and work in collaboration with a primary physician.

A family nurse practitioner (FNP) provides primary ambulatory care for families, usually in collaboration with a family care physician. The FNP meets the family's general health care needs, manages some illnesses by providing direct care, and guides or counsels the family as needed.

A pediatric nurse practitioner (PNP) provides health care to infants and children. An obstetrics-gynecology nurse practitioner (OB-GYN) provides primary ambulatory care to women seeking obstetrical or gynecological health care. The nurse practitioner who is also a certified nurse-midwife may independently deliver infants. A geriatric nurse practitioner (GNP) provides ambulatory or inpatient care to older adults. The GNP's activities include interventions for health maintenance, illness prevention, or health restoration.

Certified Nurse-Midwife. A **certified nurse-midwife (CNM)** is an RN who is also educated in midwifery and is certified by the American College of Nurse-Midwives. The practice of nurse-midwifery involves providing independent care for women during normal pregnancy, labor, and delivery, as well as care for the newborn. It may include some gynecological services such as routine Papanicolaou (Pap) smears, family planning, and treatment for minor vaginal infections. A CNM practices with a health care agency that provides medical consultation, collaborative management, and referral.

Nurse Anesthetist. A **nurse anesthetist** is an RN who has received advanced training in an accredited program in anesthesiology. Nurse anesthetists provide surgical anesthesia under the guidance and supervision of an anesthesiologist, who is a physician with advanced knowledge of surgical anesthesia.

Nurse Administrator. A **nurse administrator** manages client care and the delivery of specific nursing services within a health care agency. This administrator may hold a middle-management position, such as head nurse or supervisor, or an upper-level management position, such as assistant or associate director or director of nursing services. Functions of administrators include budgeting, staffing, strategic planning of programs and services, employee evaluation, and employee development. Middle-management positions usually require at least a baccalaureate degree in nursing, and upper-level positions generally require a master's degree.

Nurse Researcher. The **nurse researcher** investigates problems to improve nursing care and to further define and expand the scope of nursing practice (see Chapter 16). The nurse researcher may be employed in an academic setting, hospital, or independent professional or community-service agency. The minimum educational requirement is now a doctoral degree, with at least a master's degree in nursing.

Health Care Team

In most practice settings the nurse works with other health care professionals to provide total care for clients. The health care team comprises four general types of professionals, including nurses, physicians, allied health professionals such as therapists and technicians, and other specialists such as social workers and chaplains. The involvement of many different persons in the client's health care, however, may cause a fragmenting of care. Because nurses have the greatest opportunity to interact with all of the other professionals in the health care team, they often have the role of coordinating and integrating services within a managed care system.

PHYSICIAN

A **physician** is a professional who has earned a degree of Doctor of Medicine (MD) or Doctor of Osteopathy (DO). The physician has completed a required curriculum, has had a specific period of postgraduate training, and has passed a licensing examination. A physician is licensed for the medical diagnosis and treatment of clients.

Most physicians specialize in diseases involving one body system (e.g., a cardiologist specializes in heart diseases) or in one specific disease (e.g., an oncologist specializes in cancer). Physicians may also specialize in surgery or in treating a certain age group.

Nurses work with physicians in many capacities. One nurse may work in a setting in which most nursing care depends on the physician's orders. An intensive care nurse may follow written standing orders that permit more independent nursing actions. A clinical nurse specialist or nurse practitioner may function in a collaborative capacity with a physician; for example, when preparing a client with newly diagnosed diabetes for discharge, the nurse and physician work together to teach the client and family about home care.

PHYSICIAN ASSISTANT

A **physician assistant (PA)** is trained in certain aspects of the practice of medicine to provide support to physicians, including conducting physical examinations, performing diagnostic procedures, and completing treatments such as cast application and suturing. PAs practice in the United States but not in Canada and must work under the direction and supervision of a physician. In some states PAs may prescribe medications. PAs practice in hospitals, clinics, or private physicians' offices.

ALLIED AND OTHER HEALTH CARE PROFESSIONALS

Therapist. A **physical therapist (PT)** is licensed to assist in the examination, testing, and treatment of physically disabled or handicapped people through the use of special exercises, the application of heat and cold, the use of sonar waves, and other techniques. A PT usually receives training in a 6-year college program leading to a master's of science degree in physical therapy. A PT practices in hospitals, clinics, rehabilitation centers, and community-based agencies.

An **occupational therapist (OT)** is licensed or certified to develop and use adaptive devices that help chronically ill or handicapped clients carry out activities of daily living. OTs usually receive education and training in 4-year college programs, and like a PT, work in a variety of settings.

A **respiratory therapist (RT)** is licensed to deliver treatment designed to improve clients' ventilatory function or oxygenation. Educational and training programs vary. They range from 6-month training programs to educational programs in 4-year colleges. An RT is usually employed in an institutional health care setting.

Nurses work with therapists in a collaborative capacity. Care initiated by therapists is frequently continued and evaluated by nurses. Nurses and therapists together consider the client's progress and develop goals and discharge plans that include the client and family. In addition, nurses refer clients to therapists for further care. For example, a nurse caring for a person with severe pulmonary disease may refer the client to a PT to learn exercises for strengthening the upper arm muscles, to an OT to learn energy-saving techniques for activities of daily living, and to an RT for techniques to promote airway clearance.

Pharmacist. A pharmacist is a licensed professional who formulates and dispenses medications. The pharmacist may practice only within a pharmacy or may be involved in client care conferences or in the development of medication administration systems (see Chapter 35). The pharmacist's education ranges from a bachelor of science degree to a doctorate in pharmacology. A pharmacist practices in an institutional or outpatient setting.

The pharmacist is a valuable resource for nurses. For example, the nurse can request information about new drugs from the pharmacist. The nurse must always know the action, desired effect, correct dosage, and side effects of all drugs administered. If this information is unavailable in standard reference books such as textbooks or hospital formularies, the nurse should consult the pharmacist.

Pharmacists also provide information about which drugs are compatible and which can be mixed or administered together. In addition, pharmacists can tell the nurse which over-the-counter drugs may interact adversely with prescribed drugs so that this information can be incorporated into the discharge teaching plan.

Social Worker. A social worker is trained to counsel clients and families. Counseling services may include providing emotional support for clients and families during severe or terminal illnesses, arranging placement in extended care facilities, and locating financial resources. The social worker generally has a baccalaureate or master's degree in social work and is employed in every type of agency in the health care system. A nurse frequently refers clients to a social worker, and they work together to identify resources for meeting clients' present and future health care needs.

Spiritual Advisors. Spiritual advisors offer spiritual support and guidance to clients and families and may be employed by an agency or institution or be provided by a religious affiliation within the community. Spiritual advisors are ministers, priests, nuns, rabbis, or lay members of religious congregations. A client may request to see a chaplain or spiritual advisor, or the nurse may initiate a referral.

■ NURSING AS A PROFESSION

Professionalism

Nursing is not simply a collection of specific skills, and the nurse is not simply a person trained to perform specific tasks. Nursing is a profession.

No one factor absolutely differentiates a job from a profession, but the difference is important in terms of how nurses practice. When we say a person acts "professionally," for example, we imply that the person is conscientious in actions, knowledgeable in the subject, and responsible to self and others. Professions possess the following primary characteristics:

1. A profession requires an extended education of its members, as well as a basic liberal foundation.
2. A profession has a theoretical body of knowledge leading to defined skills, abilities, and norms.
3. A profession provides a specific service.
4. Members of a profession have autonomy in decision making and practice.
5. The profession as a whole has a code of ethics for practice.

Nursing clearly shares, to some extent, each of these characteristics. Nursing is still evolving as a profession, however, and faces controversial issues as nurses strive for greater professionalism.

EDUCATION

As a profession, nursing requires that its members possess a significant amount of education. The issue of standardization of nursing education is a major controversy today. Most nurses agree that nursing education is important to practice and that it must respond to changes in health care created by scientific and technological advances. The ANA's 1965 position paper on nursing education empha-

---

> **Premises for ANA's First Position Paper on Education for Nursing**
>
> ■ Nursing is a helping profession and, as such, provides services which contribute to the health and well-being of people.
> ■ Nursing is of vital consequence to the individual receiving services; it fills needs which cannot be met by the person, by the family, or by other persons in the community.
> ■ The demand for services of nurses will continue to increase.
> ■ The professional practitioner is responsible for the nature and quality of all nursing care that clients receive.
> ■ The services of professional practitioners of nursing will continue to be supplemented and complemented by the services of nurse practitioners who will be licensed.
> ■ Education for those in the health professions must increase in depth and breadth as scientific knowledge expands.
> ■ In addition to those licensed as nurses, the health care of the public, in the amount and to the extent needed and demanded, requires the services of large numbers of health occupation workers to function as assistants to nurses. These workers are presently designated: nurses' aids, orderlies, assistants, attendants, etc.
> ■ The professional association must concern itself with the nature of nursing practice, the means for improving nursing practice, the education necessary for practice, and the standards for membership in the professional association.

From American Nurses Association: *A position paper: educational preparation for nurse practitioners and assistants to nurses,* Kansas City, Mo, 1965, The Association.

sizes the role of education in the profession (see the box on p. 225).

In 1984 the ANA described two levels of practice, the associate nurse and the professional nurse, which require the bachelor of science in nursing. The NLN also supports a proposal that associate and diploma graduates take one licensing examination. North Dakota was the first state to implement such a policy. In January 1987, North Dakota's Supreme Court ruled that the state board "has the authority . . . to direct that only associate and baccalaureate degree graduates may sit for practical and registered nursing license examinations respectively" (News, 1987).

THEORY

As nursing has emerged as a profession, nursing knowledge has been developed through nursing theories. Theoretical models serve as frameworks for nursing curricula and clinical practice. Nursing theories also lead to further research that increases the scientific basis of nursing practice.

A theory is a way of understanding a reality, and in this general sense, all practicing nurses use the theories they have learned. Several of the approaches described in the section on definitions and philosophies are parts of fully developed nursing theories.

SERVICE

Nursing has always been a service profession, although in the past the service was usually viewed as a charitable one. Today, nursing is a vital and indispensable component of the health care delivery system.

AUTONOMY

Autonomy is an essential element to professional nursing (Schutzenhofer, 1987, 1988). Autonomy means that a person is reasonably independent and self-governing in decision making and practice. Nurses must be prepared to shape health policy, not just respond to change (Schutzenhofer and Musser, 1994). In the past, physicians, hospital administrators, and others in the health care delivery system have found nursing autonomy difficult to understand and support. Research demonstrates that as nurses attain higher levels of educational preparation, professional autonomy rises (Schutzenhofer, 1987; Schutzenhofer and Musser, 1994). Through clinical competence and diverse practice settings, nurses are increasingly taking on independent roles in nurse-run clinics, collaborative practice, and advanced nurse practice settings.

With increased autonomy come greater responsibility and accountability. *Accountability* means that the nurse is responsible, professionally and legally, for the type and quality of nursing care provided. The nurse is accountable for keeping abreast of technical skills and knowledge needed to perform nursing care. The nursing profession itself regulates accountability through nursing audits and standards of practice.

CODE OF ETHICS

Nursing has a code of ethics that defines the principles by which nurses function. In addition, nurses incorporate their own values and ethics into practice. Chapter 19 gives several examples of specific statements of nursing's code of ethics.

Professional Organizations

A **professional organization** is created to deal with issues of concern to those practicing in the profession. In North America the major professional nursing organizations are the ANA, CNA, and NLN. The CNA and the ANA were formed in the late nineteenth century to improve standards of health and availability of health care, to foster high standards for nursing, and to promote the professional development and general and economic welfare of nurses. The ANA and CNA are part of the ICN. The objectives of the ICN parallel those of the CNA and ANA; the ICN promotes national associations of nurses, improves standards of nursing practice, seeks a higher status for nurses, and provides an international power base for nurses.

The NLN is concerned with the improvement of nursing education, nursing service, and health care delivery in the United States. In Canada the Canadian Association of University Schools of Nursing and the Canadian Association of Practical and Nursing Assistants perform similar functions.

Nursing students also take part in organizations such as the National Student Nurses Association (NSNA) in the United States and the Canadian Student Nurses Association (CSNA) in Canada. These organizations consider issues of importance to nursing students and often cooperate in activities and programs with the professional organizations.

Some professional organizations are special-interest groups focusing on specific areas such as critical care, nursing administration or research, or nurse-midwifery. These organizations seek to improve the standards of practice, expand nursing roles, and foster the welfare of nurses within the specialty areas. In addition, professional organizations present education programs and publish journals. Some representative specialty organizations are discussed in the following paragraphs.

The Association of Operating Room Nurses (AORN) in the United States and the National Conference of Operating Room Nurses in Canada are concerned with continuing education for operating room nurses, higher standards for operating room care, and increased research activities.

The Association of Women's Health, Obstetrical, and Neonatal Nurses (AWHONN) includes Canadian and American nurses and promotes standards of practice in obstetrical and gynecological nursing, encourages professional growth for its members, and is an accrediting body for advanced programs in obstetrical and gynecological nursing.

The National Association of Pediatric Nurse Associates/Practitioners (NAPNAP) is a national organization for nurses prepared by training or experience to give primary care to children. NAPNAP works in conjunction with the American Academy of Pediatrics.

The American Association of Critical-Care Nurses (AACN) is a national organization of nurses working in critical care areas. It is concerned with nursing education, practice, and research as they involve critical care nursing.

■ SOCIETY'S INFLUENCE ON NURSING

Throughout history, nursing has responded to society's needs. Contemporary nursing education, practice, and research are an outgrowth of economic, technological, demographic, sociological, and political issues.

Technological Advances

In recent years, scientific and technological advances have affected almost every aspect of life. Health care has changed in many ways, including the use of new equipment, new diagnostic tests and treatment measures, and new drugs. Nursing has adapted and will continue to respond to these changes with continuing education, in-service programs, and other educational approaches. Nursing is also uniquely concerned with the *human* side of technological advances. Society as a whole seems to accept technological advances in health care, but clients often experience problems related to them. For example, dialysis machines have been used for many years to treat clients with kidney problems, but that fact does not lessen the emotional conflict a client may experience after learning that dialysis is needed. As health care technology becomes increasingly complex and sophisticated, nurses must help clients adjust to the use of technology in care.

Demographic Changes

Demographic changes affect the population as a whole. Changes that have influenced health care in recent decades include the population shift from rural areas to urban centers; increasing life span; the higher incidence of chronic, long-term illness; and the increased incidence of diseases such as alcoholism and lung cancer. Nursing as a profession responds to such changes by exploring new methods for providing care, by changing educational emphases, and by establishing practice standards in new areas. To better meet the changing health care needs of clients, the nurse also responds to demographic changes in the population served by the practice setting.

Consumer's Movement

The consumer's movement is a heightened awareness of the value and costs of products and services; in short, consumers want their money's worth. Health care in general has been influenced by the consumer's movement in ways as diverse as new kinds of health care agencies such as health maintenance organizations, new forms of health insurance, and concern about the rising costs of health care (see Chapter 2). Also, consumers are more knowledgeable about health and illness and are becoming more vocal in their desire for high-quality care. Because nurses generally interact with clients more than other health care professionals, they must often answer questions about the quality and costs of health care. Health care consumers are also more aware of their rights as clients, and the nurse supports these rights in the role of client advocate.

Health Promotion

Related to the consumer's movement is a greater emphasis in society on health promotion and illness prevention. Exercise and nutrition are subjects that interest many people. Nursing has responded to this greater concern for health promotion in many ways, from programs in the community to specific health promotion and teaching activities for clients in hospitals and other health care settings. Health promotion activities are a part of many of the roles of a nurse, including care giver, client advocate, rehabilitator, communicator, and teacher (see Chapter 3).

Women's Movement

The women's movement has brought about many changes in society as women have increasingly sought economic, political, occupational, and educational equality. Nursing is responding in two ways. Because most nurses are women, they are increasingly asserting their equal rights as human beings, employees, and health care professionals. The women's movement has encouraged nurses to seek greater autonomy and responsibility in providing care in an environment that has been and continues to be patrician (Bunning and Campbell, 1990). The women's movement has caused female clients to seek more responsibility for and control over their bodies, health, and lives in general. As women become more aware of their own needs and unique qualities, they seek health care that can help them meet those needs.

Human Rights Movement

Like the women's movement, the human rights movement is changing the way society views the rights of *all* of its members, including minorities, clients with terminal illness, pregnant women, and older adults. Many groups have special health care needs, and nursing has responded by respecting all clients as individuals with a right to good care and with basic human rights. Nurses advocate the rights of all clients, but they have also recognized the special needs of some groups and thus have created bills of rights for dying, hospitalized, and pregnant clients, as well as other groups, to ensure that quality care is provided without sacrificing these rights.

▌ TRENDS IN NURSING

This chapter has emphasized that nursing is not a static, unchanging profession but is continuously growing and evolving as society changes, as health care emphases and methods change, as lifestyles change—and as nurses themselves change. To speak of nursing at all is to speak of nursing as it is at a given time, and in this sense, this chapter is about trends in nursing.

The current philosophies and definitions of nursing demonstrate the holistic trend in nursing—to address the whole person in all dimensions, in health and illness, and in interaction with the family and community. Nursing continues to draw on the social sciences and other fields as the focus of nursing care expands.

One trend in nursing education is the growing number of students receiving basic nursing education in community colleges and universities. Professional nursing organizations continue to stress the importance of education for nurses seeking new and expanded roles.

Nursing practice trends include a growing variety of employment settings in which nurses have greater independence. Nurses continue to gain autonomy and respect as members of the health care team. Nursing roles continue to expand with the broadening focus of nursing care.

Trends in nursing as a profession include the growing emphasis on the aspects of nursing that characterize it as a profession, including education, theory, service, autonomy, and ethical codes. The activities of nursing's professional organizations reflect all the trends in nursing education and practice. Finally, all the influences of society on nursing also reflect trends in contemporary nursing.

Two other trends need to be discussed: the increasing political influence of nursing and nursing's influence on health care policy and practice.

Political Influence of Professional Nursing

Historically, nurses' involvement in politics has been limited. Although individual nurses such as Florence Nightingale, Lillian Wald, Margaret Sanger, and Lavinia Dock have influenced decision making in areas such as sanitation, nutrition, and birth control, nurses have accomplished less as a group (Hall-Long, 1995). The women's movement, however, has inspired nurses to address health care issues. In addition, as more college-educated people enter the profession, they bring to nursing the activism and involvement of the university campus.

In 1974, the ANA formed the Nurses Coalition in Politics (N-CAP), which was the first political action committee (PAC) for nurses. This organization, which was later renamed ANA-PAC, is a major PAC that is sought for support for candidates seeking federal offices (Mason, 1990).

Political power is the ability to influence or persuade an individual holding a government office to exert the power of that office to affect a desired outcome (Rogge, 1987). Traditionally, nurses have been uncomfortable with politics because the majority of nurses are women and politics has been male dominated. Nurses are also unaware of historical precedents established by nurses in the political arena, and because they are not politically astute, nurses lack the political education to successfully compete in politics (Mason and Talbott, 1985; Mason, 1990).

Nurses' involvement in politics is receiving greater emphasis in nursing curricula, professional organizations, and health care settings (Stanhope and Belcher, 1993). Professional nursing organizations have employed lobbyists to urge state legislatures and the U.S. Congress to improve the quality of health care. Kalisch and Kalisch (1982) note that the ANA

> works for the improvement of health standards and the availability of health care services for all people; fosters high standards of nursing, stimulates and promotes the professional development of nurses, and advances their economic and general welfare. The purposes are unrestricted by considerations of nationality, race, creed, lifestyle, color, sex, or age.

The ANA employs RNs as lobbyists at the federal level, and state nursing organizations also hire lobbyists and legislative specialists to work on state nursing issues and assist with federal efforts. Finally, lobbyists working on behalf of nursing are employed in Washington, D.C., by professional interest groups such as the American Federation of Teachers, NLN, American College of Nurse-Midwives, American Public Health Association, and AACN. These groups aim to remove financial barriers to health care, increase the quality of nursing care available, increase economic rewards to nurses, and expand professional nursing roles (Aiken, 1982).

In addition, individual nurses can influence policy decisions at all governmental levels, and organized nursing's unified efforts such as with Nursing's Agenda for Health Care Reform (Tri-Council, 1991) will be critical to exert nurses' influence early in the political process (Hall-Long, 1995). Specific strategies include integration of public policy into nursing curricula, early socialization and participation in professional organizations, diverse settings for clinical practice, and running for public office (Hall-Long, 1995). If nurses become serious students of social needs, activists in influencing policy to meet those needs, and generous contributors of time and money to nursing and their organizations and to candidates working for universal good health care, then the future is bright indeed.

Nursing's Influence on Health Care Policy and Practice

Nurses are becoming more involved in health care reform. *Nursing's Agenda for Health Care Reform* supports the creation of a health care system that ensures access, quality, and services at affordable costs (Tri-Council, 1991). The plan for reform focuses on primary health care services and the promotion, restoration, and maintenance of health (Tri-Council, 1991).

Political activism and commitment are a part of professionalism, however, and politics are an important aspect of the delivery of health care. Therefore nurses should not view politics as "dirty business" but as a reality that includes the arts of influence, compromise, and social interaction.

Nurses have been involved in a different sort of politics in schools of nursing and in health care settings when seeking additional resources, more self-direction, and accountability with authority. The skills gained in such experiences can be transferred to the politics of health care policy-making.

As long as nurses maintain involvement in health care policy and practice, misinformed outsiders cannot attempt to impose their will on nursing and nursing practice. Non-nursing groups, often led by other health care providers, have made attempts to impose institutional licensure, mandatory continuing education, curtailment of advanced nursing practice, and other constraints on a profession that should have its own voice in decisions made in these and numerous other areas affecting the quality of nursing care. Although nurses have often successfully prevented infringement on the profession's self-governance, the future of nursing requires that nurses individually and collectively seek a greater influence on health care policies affecting nursing practice.

∎ KEY CONCEPTS ∎

▶ Nursing is an essential part of society; it has grown out of society and has evolved with it.

▶ Nursing has responded to the health care needs of society, which were influenced by economic, social, and cultural variables of a specific era.

▶ Formalized education programs for professional nursing were established in the nineteenth century by Florence Nightingale.

▶ The growth of nursing and nursing education in the United States was stimulated by the Civil War.

▶ The Canadian Nurses Association and the American Nurses Association were established in the late nineteenth century.

▶ Nursing education became affiliated with universities early in the twentieth century.

▶ Expansion of nursing into the military occurred in the early twentieth century, and the development of specialty nursing organizations began in the 1950s and has continued to the present.

▶ The Lysaught report (1970) emphasized the need for clarification of nursing roles and responsibilities, greater financial support for nurses, and more career opportunities.

▶ Nursing definitions reflect changes in the practice of nursing and help bring about changes by identifying the domain of nursing practice and guiding research, practice, and education.

▶ Conceptual and theoretical nursing models provide knowledge to improve practice, guide research and nursing curricula, and identify the domain and goals of nursing practice.

▶ Educational preparation of the registered nurse can be through one of three programs in the United States or two programs in Canada.

▶ Nursing standards provide the guidelines for implementing and evaluating nursing care.

▶ The rapid rise in the number of older adults and rate of chronic illnesses and functional impairments has resulted in an increased number of long-term care facilities.

▶ Community-based agencies focus primarily on health promotion, maintenance, education, and management, as well as coordination and continuity of restorative care within the community.

▶ The multiple roles and functions of the nurse include care giver, decision maker, protector, client advocate, case manager, rehabilitator, comforter, communicator, and teacher.

▶ Specific employment positions include nurse educator, advanced practice nurse, nurse practitioner, certified nurse-midwife, nurse anesthetist, administrator, and researcher.

▶ The health care team is multidisciplinary and includes a nurse, physician, physician assistant, physical therapist, occupational therapist, respiratory therapist, pharmacist, social worker, and spiritual advisor.

▶ Nursing is a profession encompassing educational preparation for the nurse, nursing theory, a provided service, autonomy, and a code of ethics.

▶ Professional nursing organizations deal with issues of concern to specialist groups within the nursing profession.

▶ Changes in society, such as increased technology, new demographic patterns, consumerism, health promotion, and the women's and human rights movements, have led to changes in nursing.

▶ Nurses are becoming more politically sophisticated and, as a result, are able to increase nursing's influence on health care policy and practice.

∎ KEY TERMS ∎

Advanced practice nurse (APN), p. 223

American Nurses Association (ANA), p. 209

Canadian Nurses Association (CNA), p. 209

Certified nurse-midwife (CNM), p. 224

Clinical nurse specialist (CNS), p. 223

Congress for Nursing Practice, p. 216

Conceptual model, p. 210

Continuing education, p. 218

In-service education, p. 218

International Council of Nurses (ICN), p. 208

Licensed practical nurse (LPN), p. 218

Licensed vocational nurse (LVN), p. 218

National League for Nursing (NLN), p. 211

Nurse administrator, p. 224

Nurse anesthetist, p. 224

Nurse educator, p. 223

Nurse practitioner, p. 223

Nurse researcher, p. 224

Nursing theory, p. 210

Occupational therapist (OT), p. 224

Pharmacist, p. 225

Physical therapist (PT), p. 224

Physician, p. 224

Physician assistant (PA), p. 224

Professional organization, p. 226

Registered nurse (RN), p. 217

Respiratory therapist (RT), p. 225

Social worker, p. 225

Spiritual advisors, p. 225

∎ CRITICAL THINKING EXERCISES ∎

1. You are assigned to care for a client who needs to learn how to manage cardiac medication. Describe the criteria you would use to select a nursing theory for a basis for clinical practice.

2. You are assigned to interview a clinical nurse specialist and a nurse practitioner. What information would you need about the roles before conducting your interview?

3. Part of your education includes experiences in different types of health care settings. What differences would you expect between nurses who practice in hospitals, skilled care facilities, and community-based facilities? Would you expect any commonalities?

REFERENCES

Abdellah FG et al: *Patient-centered approaches to nursing,* New York, 1960, Macmillan.

Aiken LH: The impact of federal health policy on nursing. In Aiken LH, editor: *Nursing in the 80's: crises, opportunities, challenges,* Philadelphia, 1982, Lippincott.

Alfaro-LeFevre R: *Critical thinking in nursing: a practical approach,* Philadelphia, 1995, Saunders.

American Association of Colleges of Nursing: *Essentials of college and university education for professional nursing: a final report,* Washington, DC, 1986, The Association.

American Association of Colleges of Nursing: *Nursing education's agenda for the 21st century,* Washington, DC, 1993, The Association.

American Nurses Association: A code of ethics, *Am J Nurs* 26:621, 1926.

American Nurses Association: ANA news, *Am J Nurs* 55:1474, 1955.

American Nurses Association: *A position paper: educational preparation for nurse practitioners and assistants to nurses,* Kansas City, Mo, 1965, The Association.

American Nurses Association: Educational preparation for nurse practitioners, *Am J Nurs* 65(12):106, 1965.

American Nurses Association: *Statement on graduate education in nursing,* New York, 1969, The Association.

American Nurses Association: *Nursing and social policy statement,* Kansas City, Mo, 1980, The Association.

American Nurses Association: *Nursing and social policy statement,* Washington, DC, 1995, The Association.

American Nurses Association: *Career ladders: an approach to professional productivity and job satisfaction,* ANA Pub No N5-27, Kansas City, Mo, 1984, The Association.

American Nurses Association: *Code for nurses with interpretive statements,* ANA Publ No G-56, Kansas City, Mo, 1985, The Association.

American Nurses Association: *Standards for continuing education in nursing,* Washington, DC, 1991, The Association.

American Nurses Association: *Standards of clinical practice,* Washington, DC, 1991, The Association.

American Nurses Association Committee on Education: *A position paper,* New York, 1965, The Association.

Bandman EL, Bandman B: *Critical thinking in nursing,* ed 2, Norwalk, Conn, 1995, Appleton and Lange.

Beeber L, Anderson CA, Sills GM: Peplau's theory in practice, *Nurs Sci Q* 3(1):6, 1990.

Benner P: *From novice to expert: excellence and power in clinical nursing practice,* Menlo Park, Calif, 1984, Addison-Wesley.

Benner P, Tanner C: How expert nurses use intuition, *Am J Nurs* 87(1):23, 1987.

Bunning S, Campbell JC: Feminism and nursing: historical perspectives, *ANS Adv Nurs Sci* 12(4):11, 1990.

Canadian Nurses Association: *A definition of nursing practice. Standards for nursing practice,* Ottawa, 1986, The Association.

Carnevali DL, Thomas MD: *Diagnostic reasoning and treatment decision making in nursing,* Philadelphia, 1993, Lippincott.

Chinn PL, Jacobs MK: *Theory and nursing: a systematic approach,* ed 4, St Louis, 1995, Mosby.

Cohen IB: Florence Nightingale, *Sci Am* 250(128):137, 1984.

Dean H: Science and practice: the nature of knowledge. In Omery A, Kasper CE, Page GG, editors: *In search of nursing science,* Thousand Oaks, Calif,1995, Sage.

Deloughery C: *Issues and trends in nursing,* ed 2, St Louis, 1995, Mosby.

Dolan JA et al: *Nursing in society: a historical perspective,* ed 15, Philadelphia, 1983, Saunders.

Donahue MP: *Nursing: the finest art, an illustrated history,* St Louis, 1995, Mosby.

Donaldson SK: Nursing science for nursing practice. In Omery A, Kasper CE, Page GG, editors: *In search of nursing science,* Thousand Oaks, Calif, 1995, Sage.

Fawcett J: *Analysis and evaluation of conceptual models of nursing,* ed 2, Philadelphia, 1989, Davis.

Fawcett J: Contemporary conceptualization of nursing: philosophy or science? In Kikuchi J, Simmons H: *Philosophic inquiry in nursing,* Newbury Park, Calif, 1992, Sage.

Hall-Long BA: Nursing's past, present, and future political experiences, *Nurs Health Care: Perspectives on Community* 16:24, 1995.

Harmer D, Henderson V: *Textbook of the principles and practice of nursing,* ed 5, Riverside, NJ, 1955, Macmillan.

Hartweg DL: Dorothea Orem: self-care deficit theory. In McQuiston CM, Webb AA: *Foundations of nursing theory,* Thousand Oaks, Calif, 1995, Sage.

Hefferin EA, Kleinknecht MK: Development of the nursing career preference inventory, *Nurs Res* 35(1):44, 1986.

Henderson V: The nature of nursing, *Am J Nurs* 64:62, 1964.

Henderson V: *The nature of nursing,* New York, 1966, Macmillan.

Hinshaw AS: Nursing science: the challenge to develop knowledge, *Nurs Sci Q* 2(4):162, 1989.

Holzemer W: Doctoral education in nursing: an assessment of quality: 1979-1984, *Nurs Res* 36(2):110, 1987.

Holzemer WL: Quality and cost of nursing care: is anybody out there listening, *Nurs Health Care* 11(8):412, 1990.

Huey FL: Looking at ladders, *Am J Nurs* 82:1520, 1982.

Institute of Medicine, Division of Health Care Services: *Nursing and nursing education: public policies and private actions,* Washington, DC, 1983, National Academy Press.

Johnson DE: Theory in nursing: borrowed and unique, *Nurs Res* 11:206, 1968.

Johnson DE: The behavioral system for nursing. In Riehl JP, Roy C, editors: *Conceptual models for nursing practice,* ed 2, New York, 1980, Appleton-Century-Crofts.

Kalisch BJ, Kalisch PA: *Politics of nursing,* Philadelphia, 1982, Lippincott.

Keeling AW, Ramos MC: The role of nursing history in preparing nursing for the future. *Nurs Health Care: Perspectives on Community* 16:30, 1995.

Kelly LY: *Dimensions of professional nursing,* New York, 1981, Macmillan.

Kerr JR, McPhail J: *Canadian nursing issues and perspectives,* ed 3, St Louis, 1994, Mosby.

King IM: *Toward a theory for nursing,* New York, 1971, Wiley.

King IM: *Toward a theory for nursing: systems, concepts, process,* New York, 1981, Wiley.

King IM: King's theory of goal attainment. In Parse RR, editor: *Nursing science: major paradigms, theories, critiques,* Philadelphia, 1987, Saunders.

Leininger MM: Caring: a central focus of nursing and health care services, *Nurs Health Care* 1(3):135, 1980.

Levine MC: *An introduction to clinical nursing,* ed 2, Philadelphia, 1973, Davis.

Levine, ME: The rhetoric of nursing theory, *Image: Journal of Nursing Scholarship* 27:11, 1995.

Lutjens LRJ: Martha Rodgers: the science of unitary human beings. In McQuiston CM, Webb AA: *Foundations of nursing theory,* Thousand Oaks, Calif, 1995, Sage.

Lysaught JP: *An abstract for action,* New York, 1970, McGraw-Hill.

Macrae J: Nightingale's spiritual philosophy and its significance for modern nursing, *Image J Nurs Sch* 27:8, 1995.

Manthey M: 1990 nursing: a profession of choice, *Nurs Manage* 21(9):17, 1990.

Marriner-Tomey A: *Nursing theorists and their work,* ed 3, St Louis, 1994, Mosby.

Mason DJ: Nursing and politics: a profession comes of age, *Orthop Nurs* 9(5):11, 1990.

Mason DJ, Talbott SW: *The political action handbook for nurses,* Menlo Park, Calif, 1985, Addison-Wesley.

McClure ML: Nursing and hospital cost containment, *J Prof Nurs* 7(1):4, 1991.

McEwen M: Promoting interdisciplinary collaboration, *Nurs Health Care* 15(6):304, 1994.

Meilicke D, Larsen, J: Leadership and the leadership of the Canadian Nurses Association. In Baumgart AJ, Larsen J, editors: *Canadian nursing faces the future: development and change,* St Louis, 1988, Mosby.

Meleis AI: *Theoretical nursing: development and progress,* Philadelphia, 1985, Lippincott.

Molde S, Diers D: Nurse practitioner research: selected literature review and research agenda, *Nurs Res* 34(6):362, 1986.

Moses EB: *The registered nurse population, findings from the National Sample Survey of Registered Nurses,* March 1992, US Department of Health and Human Services; Public Health Service; Division of Nursing, Health Resources, and Services Administration.

National Commission on Nursing: *Source book: National Commission on Nursing,* Chicago, 1983, American Hospital Association.

National League for Nursing: *An agenda for nursing education reform. In support of nursing's agenda for health care reform,* New York, 1992, National League for Nursing Press.

National League for Nursing: *Characteristics of graduate education in nursing leading to the master's degree,* New York, 1978, The League.

Neuman B: *The Neuman systems model: application to nursing education and practice,* New York, 1982, Appleton Century-Crofts.

Neuman B: *The Neuman systems model,* ed 3, Norwalk, Conn, 1995, Appleton & Lange.

Neuman BM, Young RJ: A model for teaching total person approach to patient problems, *Nurs Res* 21:264, 1972.

News: North Dakota's High Court frees nursing board to enforce its BSN requirement for RN licensure, *Am J Nurs* 87(3):372, 1987.

Nightingale F: *Notes on nursing: what it is and what it is not,* London, 1860, Harrison & Sons.

Orem DE: *Nursing: concepts of practice,* New York, 1971, McGraw-Hill.

Orem DE: *Nursing: concepts of practice,* ed 3, New York, 1985, McGraw-Hill.

Orlando IJ: *The dynamic nurse-patient relationship: function, process, and principles,* New York, 1961, Putnam.

Parse RR: *Nursing science: major paradigms, theories, and critiques,* Philadelphia, 1987, Saunders.

Parse RR: Nursing theory-based practice: a challenge for the 90s, *Nurs Sci Q* 3(2):53, 1990.

Patterson JG, Zderad LT: *Humanistic nursing,* New York, 1976, Wiley.

Peplau HE: *Interpersonal relations in nursing,* New York, 1952, Putnam.

Pruitt RH, Campbell BF: Educating for health care reform and the community, *Nurs Health Care* 15(6):308, 1994.

Raab DM: Nursing in Canada: perseverance in practice, *Health Care* Sept 1985, p 27.

Reed KS: Betty Neuman: the Neuman systems model. In McQuiston CM, Webb AA: *Foundations of nursing theory,* Thousand Oaks, Calif, 1995, Sage.

Rogers ME: *An introduction to the theoretical basis of nursing,* Philadelphia, 1970, Davis.

Rogge MM: Nursing and politics: a forgotten legacy, *Nurs Res* 36(1):26, 1987.

Roy C: The Roy adaptation model. In Riehl JP, Roy C, editors: *Conceptual models for nursing practice,* New York, 1980, Appleton-Century-Crofts.

Roy C: *Introduction to nursing: adaptation model,* ed 2, Englewood Cliffs, NJ, 1984, Prentice Hall.

Roy C: The Roy adaptation model. In Riehl JP, Roy C, editors: *Conceptual models for nursing practice,* ed 3, New York, 1989, Appleton-Century-Crofts.

Roy C, Obloy SM: The practitioner movement: toward a science of nursing, *Am J Nurs* 79:1698, 1979.

Schmieding NJ: Ida Jean Orlando: a nursing process theory. In McQuiston CM, Webb AA: *Foundations of nursing theory,* Thousand Oaks, Calif, 1995, Sage.

Schutzenhofer KK: The measurement of professional autonomy, *J Prof Nurs* 3:278, 1987.

Schutzenhofer KK: The problem of professional autonomy, *Healthcare Women Int* 9:93, 1988.

Schutzenhofer KK, Musser DB: Nurse characteristics and professional autonomy, *Image J Nurs Sch* 26:201, 1994.

Schuyler CB: Florence Nightingale. In Nightingale F: *Notes on nursing: what it is and what it is not,* commemorative ed, Philadelphia, 1992, Lippincott.

Shryock RH: *The history of nursing: an interpretation of the social and medical factors involved,* Philadelphia, 1959, Saunders.

Silverstein NG: Lillian Wald at Henry Street 1893-1895, *ANS Adv Nurs Sci* 7(2).1, 1985.

Stanhope M, Belcher AE: Political imperatives for nursing practice. In Lancaster J, Lancaster W, editors: *Concepts for advanced nursing practice,* St Louis, 1993, Mosby.

Sward, K: The code for nurses: an historical perspective. In American Nurses Association: *Perspectives on the code for nurses,* Pub No G-132, Kansas City, Mo, 1978, The Association.

Tanner CA et al: Diagnostic reasoning strategies of nursing and nursing students, *Nurs Res* 36(6):358, 1987.

Torres G: *Theoretical foundations of nursing,* Norwalk, Conn, 1986, Appleton-Century-Crofts.

Tri-Council: *Nursing's agenda for health care reform,* Washington, DC, 1991, The Association.

Viens DC: A history of nursing's code of ethics, *Nurs Outlook* 37(1):45, 1989.

Watson J: *Nursing: human science and human care,* Norwalk, Conn, 1985, Appleton-Century-Crofts.

Watson J: *Nursing: the philosophy and science of caring,* Boston, 1979, Little, Brown.

Watson J: Nursing on the caring edge: metaphorical vignettes, *ANS Adv Nurs Sci* 10(1):10, 1987.

Watson J: *Nursing: human science human care: a theory of nursing,* Pub No 15-2236, New York, 1988, National League for Nursing.

Wheeler CE: *The American Journal of Nursing* and the socialization of a profession: 1900-1920, *ANS Adv Nurs Sci* 7(2):20, 1985.

Woodham-Smith C: *Florence Nightingale,* New York, 1983, McGraw-Hill.

ADDITIONAL READINGS

Canadian Nurses Association: *Nursing in Canada: 1985,* Ontario, Canada, 1986, The Association.

Dennis KE, Prescott PA: Florence Nightingale: yesterday, today, and tomorrow, *ANS Adv Nurs Sci* 7(2):66, 1985.

Dickoff J, James P: A theory of theories: a position paper, *Nurs Res* 17(3):197, 1968.

Diers D, Hamman A, Molde S: Complexity of ambulatory care: nurse practitioner and physician caseloads, *Nurs Res* 35(5):310, 1986.

Fairman JA: Sources and references for research in nursing history, *Nurs Res* 36(1):56, 1987.

Kasch CR: Establishing a collaborative nurse-patient relationship: a distinct focus of nursing action of primary care, *Image J Nurs Sch* 18:44, 1986.

Leininger MM: *Transcultural nursing: concepts, theories and practices,* New York, 1978, Wiley.

Leininger MM: *Transcultural care, diversity and universality: a theory of nursing,* Thorofore, NJ, 1985, Slack.

Parse RR: *Man-living-health: theory of nursing,* New York, 1981, Wiley.

Parse RR, Cogne AB, Smith MJ: *Nursing research: qualitative methods,* Bowie, Md, 1985, Brady.

Roy C: Adaptation: a conceptual framework for nursing, *Nurs Outlook* 18(3):42, 1970.

Roy C: *Introduction to nursing: an adaptation model,* ed 2, Englewood Cliffs, NJ, 1984, Prentice Hall.

Roy C, Roberts S: *Theory construction in nursing: an adaptation model,* Englewood Cliffs, NJ, 1981, Prentice Hall.

Shamansky SL, Schilling LS, Holbrook TL: Determining the market for nurse practitioner services: the New Haven experience, *Nurs Res* 34(4):242, 1985.

Taylor MS, Covaleski MA: Predicting nurse's turnover and internal transfer behavior, *Nurs Res* 34(4):237, 1985.

Travelbee J: *Interpersonal agents of nursing,* ed 2, Philadelphia, 1971, Davis.

Walker LO: Toward a clearer understanding of the concept of nursing theory, *Nurs Res* 20(5):428, 1971.

Watson J et al: *A model of caring: an alternative health care model for nursing practice and research,* ANA Pub No NP-59-3M 8179 190, Kansas City, Mo, 1979, American Nurses Association.

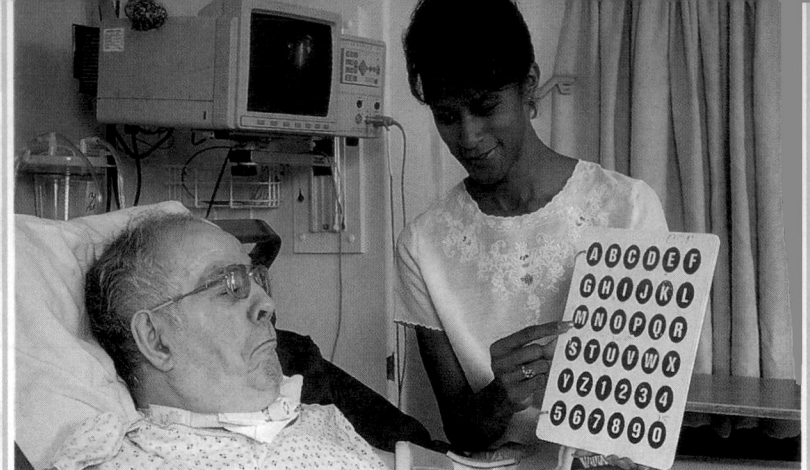

## Chapter 14

Communication

Objectives

Mastery of content in this chapter will enable the student to:

▶ Define the key terms listed.

▶ Describe differences between the three levels of communication.

▶ Identify characteristics of verbal and nonverbal communication.

▶ Discuss the functions of communication in the nurse-client relationship.

▶ Explain the role of communication in the nursing process.

▶ Describe each element of the communication process.

▶ Identify factors that promote and inhibit communication.

▶ Give examples of techniques that promote therapeutic communication.

▶ List and discuss the phases of a therapeutic helping relationship.

▶ Explain the dimensions of a helping relationship.

▶ Discuss nursing care measures for clients with communication alterations.

ommunication is the basic element of human interactions that allows people to establish, maintain, and improve contacts with others. Because communicating is something persons do every day, they often mistakenly think it is simple. However, communication is a complex process that involves behaviors and relationships and allows individuals to associate with others and the world around them. It is an ongoing, dynamic series of events in which meaning is generated and transmitted.

Communication is an interpersonal process that involves verbal and nonverbal exchanges of information and ideas. Communication refers not only to content but also to feelings and emotions that people may convey in a relationship. Silence is also a means of communication; for example a nurse listening to an anguished husband whose wife has died. Communication conveys information, and it is an act of sharing. Communication is one of the most important factors used to establish a therapeutic nurse client relationship.

Nursing is based on establishing a caring and helping relationship. This relationship is the foundation to the interaction that allows the client and health care team to strive for a mutual understanding of the client's needs. In this collaborative manner the client, nurse, and other members of the health care team identify mutually agreed upon goals. Communication generates a means for bringing about change. The nurse listens, speaks, and acts to negotiate change to promote the client's well-being and return to a level of wellness.

LEVELS OF COMMUNICATION

Communication occurs at the intrapersonal, interpersonal, and public levels. **Intrapersonal communication** occurs within an individual. It is self-talk or an internal dialogue that occurs constantly and consciously. The goal of intrapersonal communication is self-awareness, which is influenced by self-concept and feelings of self-worth. Positive self-concept and self-awareness that come through internal dialogue can help nurses express themselves appropriately to others. For example, when a nurse walks into the client's room and thinks, "He looks uncomfortable. I'd better turn him on his side," the communication is intrapersonal. Another situation involving intrapersonal communication is when a nurse notes a grimaced facial expression on the face of a client and thinks, "Is this client in pain? What do I need to do for the client? When was the last dose of pain medication administered?"

Interpersonal communication is the interaction between two people or in a small group. It is often face-to-face and is the type most frequently used in nursing situations. Individuals communicating are continuously aware of one another. Healthy interpersonal communication allows problem solving, sharing of ideas, decision making, and personal growth. In nursing, there are many situations that challenge interpersonal communication skills. Each encounter with a client, such as collecting a blood specimen or taking a health history, requires exchange of information. Meetings with staff members, physicians, social workers, and therapists test the nurse's communication skills with people who may have different opinions and experiences. Being a member of a nursing committee challenges the nurse's ability to express ideas clearly and decisively. Interpersonal communication is the heart of nursing practice. A nurse can help a client by communicating at a meaningful interpersonal level.

Public communication is interaction with large groups of people. Giving a lecture to a roomful of students and speaking to a consumer group on health promotion are examples of public communication. Being a competent communicator with an audience requires the ability to envision oneself speaking to a group. Special platform skills such as use of posture, body movements, and tone of voice help the speaker to express ideas.

ELEMENTS OF THE COMMUNICATION PROCESS

Examination of the components of the communication process helps a person understand communication. A model can simply and graphically demonstrate complex processes, but it can also oversimplify. A model provides the nursing student with a framework for observing, understanding, and predicting what occurs as two people communicate.

A communication model must incorporate several principles. Communication is complex, involving verbal and nonverbal symbols and messages exchanged between persons. Communication is a process. This process allows persons to send messages both intentionally and unintentionally. Often a person can send or convey a message about personality or attitude without being aware of it. Communication is a response between two or more persons as they send and receive stimuli and messages.

Communication occurs on a social level, with participants engaged in intrapersonal and interpersonal contact. The process is dynamic, with the meaning of messages negotiated by participants. During communication, the person may or may not be aware of each element of communication (Fig. 14-1). During casual conversation participants do not bother to analyze the meaning of every gesture or word. For example, a person may become quite animated, using hands to express an idea without consciously thinking, "I'll wave my hand to stress this point." The nurse, however, learns to be conscious of each element of the communication process. In this way, the nurse can interact effectively with clients and remain aware of communication's effect on them. Because of the interaction between sender and receiver involved in communication, the model tends to oversimplify a complex process. However, each element is crucial. Information and meaning can be gained or lost if any element is altered.

Referent

The **referent** or stimulus motivates a person to communicate with another. It may be an object, experience, emotion, idea, or act. Individuals who consciously consider the referent during interpersonal interaction can carefully develop and organize messages.

Sender

The **sender**, also called the *encoder*, is the person who initiates the interpersonal communication or message. The sender puts the referent into a form that can be transmitted and assumes responsibility for the accuracy of the content and the emotional tone of the message. The role of sender

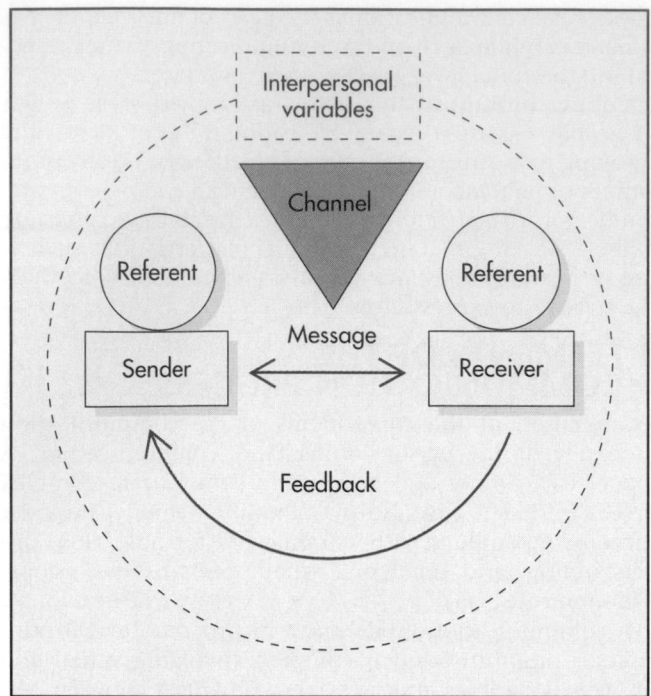

Fig. 14-1 Communication as an active process between sender and receiver.

may switch back and forth between participants at any time when information is transmitted.

Message

The **message** is the information that is sent or expressed by the sender. The most effective message is clear and organized and is expressed in a manner familiar to the person receiving it. An appropriate amount of information must be given, and the receiver must be ready to hear the message. For example, professional jargon (technical terminology used by health care providers) needs to be reserved for interactions between professionals and not between nurses and clients. Likewise, teaching is inappropriate if nurses try to teach the client everything in one sitting or teach the client to manage a colostomy when the client is not willing to look at the stoma. The message may comprise verbal and nonverbal language symbols (e.g., spoken words, facial expressions, or gestures). Unfortunately, not all symbols have universal meaning; therefore difficulties in communication may occur with the message if the sender is not aware of this factor and does not seek clarification.

Channels

The message is sent along a channel of communication. **Channels** are means of conveying messages, such as through visual, auditory, and tactile senses. The sender's facial expression visually conveys a message. The spoken word travels via auditory channels. Placing a hand on an individual while communicating uses the channel of touch. Generally, the more channels the nurse uses to send a message, the better the client will understand it. For example, when attempting to relieve pain, the nurse verbal-

izes concern, expresses compassion, and repositions the client gently to lessen the pain.

Receiver

The **receiver**, also called the *decoder*, is the person to whom the message is sent. For communication to be effective, the receiver must perceive or become aware of the message. The message from the sender then acts as one of the receiver's referents. It prompts the receiver to decode and respond to the sender's message. The nurse learns to engage in intrapersonal communication to analyze and interpret the client's comments. Ideally, the sender's intention is perceived by the receiver. There is no guarantee that this will occur because words and symbols have multiple meanings. However, the more that the sender and receiver have in common, the more likely that the sender's meaning will be communicated.

Feedback

Communication is an ongoing process. The receiver returns a message to the sender. This **feedback** helps to reveal whether the meaning of the message is received. Mere intent to communicate is insufficient to ensure that a message is accurately received. The receiver's verbal and nonverbal response sends feedback to the sender to reveal the receiver's understanding of the message. To be effective, the two must be sensitive and open to each other's message, clarify the message, and modify behavior accordingly. In a social relationship both persons involved assume equal responsibility for seeking openness and clarification, whereas the nurse assumes major responsibility in the nurse-client relationship.

▌ MODES OF COMMUNICATION

People send messages in the verbal and nonverbal modes, which are closely bound together during interpersonal interaction. As we speak, we express ourselves through movements, tone of voice, facial expressions, and general appearance. These modes can convey the same or different messages. The nurse who learns skills of communication masters techniques of each mode.

Verbal Communication

Verbal communication involves spoken or written word. Words are tools or symbols used to express ideas or feelings, arouse emotional responses, or describe objects, observations, memories, or inferences. Words may also be used to convey hidden meanings, test the other's interest or degree of concern, or express hostility, or fear. Language is a code that conveys meaning. A single word can change the meaning of a phrase or sentence. Language is effective only when each person communicating understands the message clearly.

A nurse encounters clients of various cultures who speak different languages. Also, some clients speak the same language as the nurse but use subcultural variations of certain words. For example, the word *dinner* may mean a midday meal to one person and the last meal of the day to another. These dialects and subdialects confuse meaning. Consequently, a nurse often works with clients who speak the same language but interpret messages differently from the way the nurse intended. To make a message clear, the nurse uses effective verbal communication techniques; clear and effective words and phrases at the level of understanding for the client. The nurse frequently incorporates gestures to strengthen the verbal message. For example, in caring for the hearing impaired client, the nurse utilizes an interpreter to facilitate the sending of the verbal message.

CLARITY AND BREVITY

Effective communication is simple, short, and direct. Fewer words spoken result in less confusion. Because of the intrapersonal variables involved, human communication is imprecise in many ways. Vague phrases such as *you know* add little clarity to a message. Clarity is achieved by speaking slowly and enunciating clearly. Using examples can make an explanation easier to understand. For instance, instructing a client with arthritis about self-care measures at home is more meaningful when the nurse provides specific examples, including demonstrations to reinforce the verbal message.

Repeating important parts of a message also makes communication clearer. The receiver should know the what, why, how, when, who, and where of ideas communicated.

Brevity is best achieved by using words that express an idea simply. "Tell me where your pain is" is better than "I would like you to describe for me the location of your discomfort." A simple, clear phrase communicates more effectively.

VOCABULARY

Communication is unsuccessful if the receiver is unable to translate the sender's words and phrases. In nursing and medicine there are many technical terms and jargon. If the nurse uses these terms, the client may become confused and unable to follow instructions or learn important information. Rather than telling the client, "Sit up while your lungs are auscultated," it might be better to say, "Sit up while I listen to your lungs." The first statement might make the client feel anxious. A message spoken in terms the client understands makes communication more effective.

DENOTATIVE AND CONNOTATIVE MEANING

A single word can have several meanings. A **denotative** meaning is one shared by individuals who use a common language. For example, the word *baseball* has the same meaning for all individuals who speak English, and the word *code* denotes cardiac arrest to nurses. The denotative meaning is used to define a word so that it means the same to everyone.

The **connotative** meaning of a word reflects the shade or interpretation of a word's meaning rather than the definition. For example, using the word *serious* to describe a client's condition may suggest to families that the client may be close to death, but nurses may not consider a client to be near death unless the words *critical* or *guarded* are used. Nurses must carefully select words that cannot be easily misinterpreted. This is important throughout the communication process. For example, when charting how a client tolerated endotracheal suctioning, the nurse should avoid using words such as "tolerated well." Instead, the nurse should describe clear objective assessment findings such as respiratory rate, depth, regularity of respirations, and lung sounds.

PACING

Verbal communication is more successful when expressed at an appropriate speed or pace. Talking rapidly, using awkward pauses, or speaking too slowly and deliberately can convey an unintended message. In the following example, the nurse uses awkward pauses during an explanation to a client:

Client: Do you know if the doctor found anything wrong?

Nurse: No (pause), but I'm sure if he did (longer pause) he would have come to explain things to you. (then very rapidly) Now let's get back to where we were.

Long pauses and rapid shifts to another subject may give the client the impression that the truth is being hidden. Also, speed and pace of speech varies, depending on geographical location.

The speed with which a message is verbalized, in addition to the presence, absence, and length of pauses, can determine the degree to which communication satisfies the listener. The nurse should not talk so quickly that words are unclear. Pauses should be used to accentuate or stress a particular point, giving the listener time to hear and comprehend the meaning of words. Proper pacing is achieved by thinking about what to say before saying it. Looking for nonverbal cues from the listener that might suggest confusion or misunderstanding is also useful. A person can also ask a listener if the pace is too fast or too slow or if the message needs repeating.

TIMING AND RELEVANCE

Timing is critical to reception of a message. If the boss is in a bad mood, the time is wrong to ask for a raise. If a client is in pain, the time is wrong to explain the risks of surgery. Even though a message is clearly and concisely stated, poor timing can prevent it from being accurately received. Therefore the nurse must be sensitive to the appropriate time for discussions. Often the best time for interaction is when a client expresses an interest in communicating. By asking a simple question such as, "Would you like to talk about your surgery?" the nurse can avoid wasting time and energy if the client does not.

A person is more likely to communicate when a message is important. For example, when a client is facing open-heart surgery the next day, a discussion of the risks of cigarette smoking has less relevance than a review of preoperative procedures. An explanation of the side effects of birth control pills is relevant to the young woman who has received her first prescription for the medication. Verbal communication is more likely to have an impact when messages pertain to an individual's interests and needs.

HUMOR

Humor can be a powerful tool in promoting well-being. The phrase, "laughter is the best medicine," applies when nurses use humor to help clients adjust to stress imposed by illness. Wootsen (1993) notes that laughter helps relieve stress-related tension and pain, increases the nurse's effectiveness in providing emotional support to clients, and humanizes the experience of illness. Laughter serves as a psychological and physical release. Humor can enhance feelings of well-being, reduce anxiety, and increase pain tolerance (Beare and Myers, 1994).

Nurses can appropriately use humor with clients and colleagues by telling jokes, sharing humorous incidents or situations, and using puns. Wootsen's (1993) discussion of the use of humor reveals that clients and peers relax more readily and feel more at ease when humor is employed in conversation. This also opens the interaction process, facilitating the ease of message sending and receiving. Also, the release of emotional tension with humor improves comfort levels of clients and peers.

Humor is not always appropriate, however, (e.g., after the death of a loved one). Nurses need to be cautious in using humor to mask their own fears and discomforts or their inability to communicate with clients. Humor therefore should not become the only means of communication, but it can be an effective approach in helping clients to interact more openly and honestly.

Nonverbal Communication

Actions often speak louder than words. **Nonverbal communication** is transmission of messages without the use of words. It is one of the most powerful ways people convey messages to others. We continuously communicate nonverbally in every face-to-face encounter. Gestures impart meanings that are more significant than words. In a classic text, Ekman (1965) describes the ways in which nonverbal communication and verbal communication are interrelated. Nonverbal cues add meaning to the verbal message (Table 14-1).

Nonverbal communication is more powerful than verbal communication. The nurse needs to be alert to nonverbal messages accompanying verbal messages sent to clients. Clients may sense a lack of trust, or anxiety, when a mismatch exists between a nurse's verbal and nonverbal messages. The phrase, "Good morning, how are you?" can convey a number of meanings to the client if the nurse's tone of voice and facial expression do not match the words spoken. A verbal message should be reinforced or complemented by appropriate nonverbal cues. For example, when a nurse initially greets a client, maintaining eye contact and speaking in a calm voice can relay a sense of security to the client.

During assessment, the nurse observes clients' verbal and nonverbal messages. Clients who say that they feel fine but grimace during movement are communicating two different messages. Becoming a good observer of nonverbal behavior requires time and practice. The nurse who perceives nonverbal messages is better able to understand clients, detect changes in conditions, and determine nursing care needs.

METACOMMUNICATION

Metacommunication is a message within a message that conveys a sender's attitude toward the self and the message and the attitudes, feelings, and intentions toward the listener. It can be an explicit statement (verbal) or an implicit demonstration of feelings (nonverbal). For example, the client states to the nurse "I know things are getting better." The nurse notes that the client is teary-eyed and has a facial grimace. In this situation, the nurse needs to further explore the true meaning of the client's statement as the message has more meaning than that of the spoken words.

PERSONAL APPEARANCE

The general impression formed of another person influences the response to that person. A person's appearance is one of the first things noticed during an interpersonal encounter. People form an impression about another person within 20 seconds to 4 minutes. This impression is based mostly on appearance. Physical characteristics, dress, grooming, and the presence of jewelry and adornment provide clues to the person's physical well-being, personality, social status, occupation, religion, culture, and self-concept. Paying attention to one's appearance can contribute to positive self-image and professional image.

Nurses can help clients maintain a sense of worth by allowing them to wear their own clothes if possible or if not contraindicated by treatments. Hospital gowns are drab and ill fitting. In restorative care settings, as well as in the home setting, clients are strongly encouraged to wear comfortable, washable, casual clothes. Personal clothes and grooming (make-up, combing hair) give a sense of physical recovery and mental alertness.

Physical characteristics, such as the condition of hair, color of skin, weight, energy level, and presence of a physical deformity, also communicate information about the level of health. There are no established standards for physical characteristics that demonstrate good health. Each individual displays combinations of physical characteristics. The nurse remains alert for changes in physical appearance because they can be significant signs of disease. For example, the nurse analyzes the health history findings and notes that the client has expressed recent weight loss and expresses loss of interest in personal appearance and grooming. The nurse may interpret from the findings early

Table 14-1	Relationships Between Verbal and Nonverbal Communication
RELATIONSHIP	**EXAMPLE**
Repeating—verbal and nonverbal cues saying the same thing but in different ways	When a mother describes how tall her son is, she also holds her hands at a distance above the floor equal to the child's height.
Contradicting—verbal and nonverbal cues conveying different messages	The nurse tells the client that obtaining a blood specimen "won't hurt a bit," but her sarcastic grin delivers a different message.
Complementing—nonverbal messages adding to verbal messages	A client says she is afraid to be admitted to the hospital, and her anxious expression and trembling hands leave little doubt of her fear.
Accenting—nonverbal cues emphasizing verbal messages	A wave of the hand while saying hello accentuates the word spoken.
Relating and regulating—nonverbal cues indicating when to begin or stop talking	A client who continually opens and closes her mouth briefly as her physician is talking is seeking an opportunity to speak.
Substituting—a nonverbal cue being used instead of words	A person nods vigorously to show approval of another's decision.

signs of depression and recommend further evaluation of the potential identified health alteration.

Physical appearance often leads to impressions about personality and self-concept. Unfortunately, stereotyped views regarding the "perfect body" also influence the image of a person's body. Nurses should assess the importance of physical appearance to a client threatened with loss of body parts or function. They also need to consider their own views and values about body image.

The nurse's physical appearance influences the client's perception of care received. Each client has a preconceived image of a nurse. The traditional white uniform can be a symbol of cleanliness and competence. Although the uniform is not a reflection of abilities, it may become more difficult to establish a sense of trust and reliability if the nurse does not meet the client's image. A professional nurse today may wear uniforms, scrubsuits, and laboratory coats, as well as street clothes, to perform duties. A neat, well-tailored look conveys the message of a competent professional. Conversely, a nurse who has bad breath or cigarette breath, "messy" hair, poorly manicured nails, dirty shoes, or excessively strong perfume, for example, may be considered unprofessional and may be taken less seriously than a nurse who has paid attention to these details of personal appearance.

INTONATION

The tone of a speaker's voice can have a significant effect on a message's meaning. Depending on intonation, a message can express enthusiasm, concern, hostility or indifference. The intonation of the message is affected by the person's emotions. It is important for nurses to be aware of how they are sending a message. A simple question such as "How are you doing?" can express genuine interest to indifference depending on the tone of voice used in the message. Voice tone can be a cue to a client's emotional state and energy level.

FACIAL EXPRESSION

The face has rich communication potential. A mutual glance or meeting of eyes between two people can set the tone for an interpersonal encounter. The face and eyes send overt and subtle cues that assist in interpretation of messages. Facial expressions often become the basis for important interpersonal judgments. Because of diversity in facial expressions, their meanings may be difficult to judge. The face may reveal genuine emotions or contradict true emotions, or facial expressions may be suppressed. Often people are unaware of the messages that their expressions convey. Providing clear feedback helps lessen confusion created by conflicting messages and expressions. When facial expressions fail to reveal clear messages, the receiver should seek verbal feedback to be sure of the speaker's intent.

For example, nurses are frequently watched by clients. Consider the impact of a nurse's facial expression on a client who asks, "Am I going to die?" The slightest change of expression can reveal the nurse's true feelings. It is difficult to control all facial expressions, but the nurse learns to be aware of what they can reveal. For example, when caring for a debilitated or deformed client, the nurse should avoid expressions of disgust.

Eye contact is an important facial expression. Wide eyes are associated with frankness, terror, and naiveté; downward glances reflect modesty or shyness. Raised upper eyelids reveal displeasure, and a stare is often associated with anger and coldness. When two people confront each other, eye contact often prefaces a message. Initiating eye contact shows a willingness to communicate. Persons who maintain eye contact during a conversation are perceived as believable. Maintaining eye contact allows a person to become a good observer. It has been suggested that the level at which eye contact occurs significantly influences communication. The nurse should avoid looking down at a client during a discussion. One way this can be avoided is for the nurse to sit down. The nurse appears less dominant and threatening sitting near the client at the same eye level.

POSTURE AND GAIT

The way that people stand and move is a visible form of self-expression. Posture and gait reflect attitudes, emotions, self-concept, and physical wellness. Leaning forward or toward a person conveys attention to that person. Leaning backward in a more relaxed manner shows less interest and caution.

An erect posture and a quick, purposeful gait communicate a sense of well-being and assuredness. A slumped posture and a slow, shuffling gait may indicate depression or discomfort. A bent-over posture may be a protective response to physical disease and injury. Nurses can collect useful information by observing clients' posture and gait. Specific illnesses cause identifiable gaits such as the shuffle of parkinsonism, a neuromuscular disorder. Gait may be altered by many physical factors such as pain, drugs, or fractures.

GESTURES

Gestures are used to illustrate an idea that is difficult or inconvenient to describe in words. A wave of a hand, a salute, and shifting of feet are gestures. They are visual enhancers that emphasize, punctuate, and clarify the spoken word. Pointing to an area of pain may be more accurate than describing the pain's location. Gestures may reveal specific meanings, or with other communication cues, they may send messages.

TOUCH

Touch is a personal form of nonverbal communication. Persons engaged in communication must be close to each other when touch is used. Because touch is more spontaneous than verbal communication, it generally seems more authentic. Various messages, such as affection, emotional support, encouragement, tenderness, and personal attention, are conveyed through touch (Fig. 14-2). Touch is an important part of the nurse-client relationship, but it must be used with discrimination because strong social norms govern its use. Who, when, why, and where people touch are determined by unwritten sociocultural guidelines. Many persons mistakenly perceive touch as having only sexual implications. The nurse must *always* be aware of the appropriate use of touch in varied situations and settings. The nurse should especially exercise discretion with the use of touch in the paranoid individual as the interpretation could be misconstrued by the client as a different meaning than intended by the nurse.

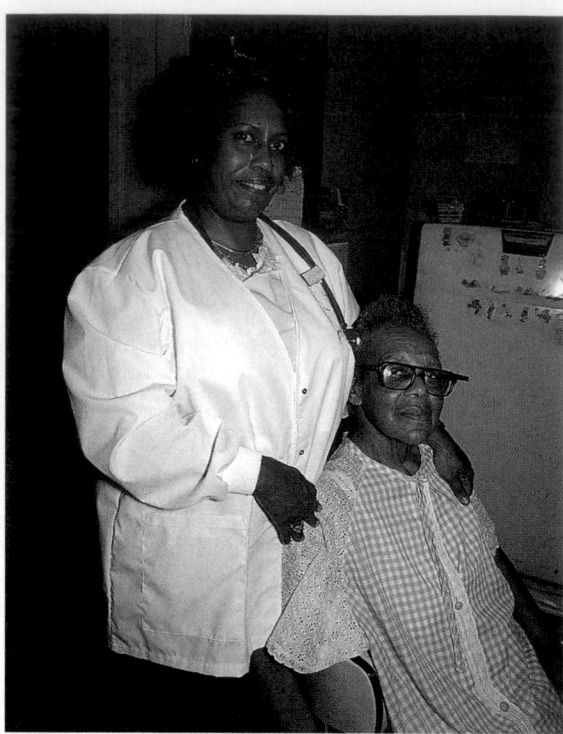

Fig. 14-2 Touching a client conveys acceptance, caring, and empathy.

Nurses rely on touch when carrying out interventions. Nurses can touch clients while performing physical assessments, giving baths, providing backrubs, and assisting with dressing. The nurse who is unaccustomed to touching or being touched may feel uncomfortable when performing interventions.

Similarly, persons who are ill must permit closer physical contact than they normally tolerate. Illness places people in dependent roles that call for the nurse to initiate and maintain closer interpersonal contact. It is important to remain sensitive to clients' dispositions toward touching. If clients shy away from the nurse's touch or refuse to hold the nurse's hand during pain, they are probably uncomfortable with being touched. Finally, touch can be a useful therapeutic tool. Holding the hand of distraught or grieving clients can often convey understanding better than words or other gestures. A nurse must be sure to use touch purposefully during interactions. Although touch can be helpful to clients, its use must be clearly understood and accepted.

FACTORS INFLUENCING COMMUNICATION

Perceptions, values, cultural background, knowledge, roles, and the setting of interaction influence the content of a message and the manner in which it is shared. Interpersonal communication is made more complex because each person is influenced differently by these intrapersonal variables. Intrapersonal variables make each interpersonal communication unique. Each person makes different associations and interprets messages differently. An understanding

of these factors helps a nurse know the reasons that a client may have difficulty communicating and the strategies needed to help.

Development

Most children are born with the physical mechanisms and capacity to develop speech and language skills. Children with developmental disorders such as cerebral palsy, autism, and Down's syndrome may have varied capacity levels for the development of speech and language. The rate of speech development varies and is directly related to neurological and intellectual development (Whaley and Wong, 1995). A child's environment must also offer stimulation for normal development. The environment provided by parents affects the ability to communicate. The nurse uses special techniques to communicate with children of different developmental stages.

To communicate effectively with children, the nurse must understand the influence of development on language and thought processes. Both affect the way children communicate and the manner in which the nurse can successfully interact with them.

Perceptions

Each person senses, interprets, and understands events differently. **Perception** is the personal view of events. A nurse might state, "I've noticed you have been quiet since your family left. Would you like to talk about it?" The client's perception of the nurse's intent will affect the willingness to talk. Perceptions are formed by expectations and experiences. Differences in perceptions between people who are interacting can be a barrier to communication.

Values

Values are standards that influence behavior (see Chapter 18). They are what a person considers important in life and thus influence expression of thoughts and ideas. Values also affect interpretation of messages. Because values are a general guide to behavior, it is important for a nurse to develop awareness of them. Some values may be identified easily and without conflict (e.g., confidentiality or good skin care for an immobile client); others may lead to a high level of conflict and be difficult to articulate (e.g., values about death or the right to die). Knowing and clarifying values are important to clinical decision making and interaction. A nurse does not allow personal values to interfere with professional relationships. Judgmental attitudes destroy trust and can be detrimental to effective communication.

Emotions

Emotions are a person's subjective feelings about events. The way a person relates or communicates with others is influenced by emotions. A client who is angry may react to nurses' instructions differently than one who is frightened. Emotions influence the ability to receive a message successfully. Emotions can also cause a person to misinterpret or not hear a message. Nurses should not take it personally if clients ventilate their emotions on them. Nurses can assess clients' emotions by observing their interactions with family, physicians, or other nurses.

When nurses care for clients they must be aware of their own emotions. It is difficult to hide emotions. Clients are perceptive and can sense anger, frustration, or sadness. It is usually inappropriate to discuss personal emotions with clients. A social support system of colleagues allows nurses to express emotions. Utilization of employee assistance programs, peer group meetings, and the use of interdisciplinary teams such as social work and pastoral care allow the nurse to express feelings and emotions at an appropriate time and place. These interventions should be outcome focused to identify solutions to perceived or identified problems and concerns of the nurse.

Sociocultural Background

Culture is the sum total of learned ways of doing, feeling, and thinking; it is a form of conditioning that shows itself through behavior. Language, gestures, values, and attitudes reflect cultural origin. Culture influences the manner in which the client and nurse relate to each other in varied situations. The nurse learns to be cognizant of cultural meanings in the communication process. The influence of culture sets limits for the way people act and communicate.

Culture also influences methods of communicating symptoms or feelings of distress to others. Differences exist in self-disclosure or the willingness to convey emotions and psychological information to others. For example, European Americans are more open and willing to discuss private family matters, whereas Latin, African, and Asian Americans are reluctant to reveal personal or family information to strangers, such as nurses or physicians. Some groups (e.g., Latin and Asian Americans) value a quiet demeanor and self-restraint; to be open or argumentative is thought to reflect negatively on family honor. In other groups, talking about oneself is considered bragging; Native Americans, for example, value silence and are comfortable with it. For a number of ethnic or racial groups, an inhibited silence occurs only in the presence of strangers or professionals of the dominant culture; sometimes this is due to historical distrust based on discrimination. At other times it can be attributed to family loyalties and an agreement not to share problems outside of the family (see Chapter 21).

Language differences can also hamper communication and relationships. When a nurse cares for a client who speaks another language, an interpreter may be necessary. Except on a social basis or for care activities, a hospital interpreter is preferable to a family member. Hospital interpreters generally understand medical terminology and can convey hospital policies and procedures. If a family member serves as an interpreter, it may be easier for the nurse to devise ways to communicate with the client. The nurse can learn key words such as *water*, *pain*, or *bathroom* to ensure that the client's basic needs are assessed and understood.

Gender

Sex differences affect the communication process. Men and women have different communication styles and each influences the communication process uniquely. Tannen (1990) discusses different communication styles of men and women. From age 3, girls play with a best friend or in a small group and use language to seek confirmation, minimize differences, and establish or reinforce intimacy. Boys, on the other hand, use language to establish independence and negotiate status activities in large groups; even when they want to make friends, they are likely to do it by play-

fully butting heads. In adulthood, women and men have completely different impressions of the same conversation. Tannen (1990) claims that the frictions between the sexes arise because girls and boys grow up in essentially different cultures, so conversation between them is, in effect, cross-cultural. This approach differs from the deference-dominance theories and focuses instead on a predominate female pattern of seeking relationships and connection with others and a predominate male pattern of accomplishing tasks and seeking independence and status. Although such an approach does not explain all problems that arise in relationships between women and men, it makes it possible to explain dissatisfactions without blame and without discarding the relationship.

Certainly nurses need to be aware of these differences when working with clients or other health team members of the opposite sex. Active listening and seeking clarification will help prevent misperceptions and misunderstandings (Ebersole and Hess, 1994).

Knowledge

Communication can be difficult when the persons communicating have different levels of knowledge. A message will not be clear if the words or phrases are not part of the listener's vocabulary. "The incision is well approximated without drainage" means the same as "The incision is clean and healing fine," but the latter is more easily understood by a client.

Nurses communicate with clients and professionals who have different levels of knowledge. A common language is essential when communicating across different knowledge levels. Nurses assess clients' knowledge by noting their responses to questions, abilities to discuss health problems, and questions that they ask. After assessment, nurses use terms and phrases that clients understand to promote attention and interest.

Roles and Relationships

People communicate in a style appropriate to their roles and relationships. Students talk differently with friends than they do with instructors, physicians, or clergy. Words, facial expressions, tone of voice, and gestures depend on the person receiving the communication.

Nurses may feel comfortable communicating with colleagues, joking about daily events, and sharing amusing stories. However, communicating with a client who is entering a clinic for the first time requires a different role. Anticipating apprehension, nurses convey respect by using the client's last name and avoid humor until they can determine the client's reaction to them. The client is probably looking for support rather than funny stories. Later, when the relationship between nurse and client is stronger, casual conversation and addressing the client on a first-name basis may be appropriate, but only with the client's permission (Wootsen, 1993).

People feel more comfortable when expressing ideas to individuals with whom they have developed positive, satisfying relationships. As a nurse-client relationship develops, the nurse and client gain confidence in relating ideas and feelings. Communication is more effective when the participants remain aware of their roles in a relationship. The nurse must avoid using terms of endearment such as "honey" or "sweetie" when addressing any client. Terms such as these may be interpreted as inappropriate and offensive by the client.

Environment

People tend to communicate better in a comfortable environment. A warm room, free of noise and distractions, is best. Noise and lack of privacy or space may create confusion, tension, or discomfort. For example, a client fearful of the diagnosis of cancer would hesitate to discuss the illness in a busy, crowded waiting room. Environmental distractions can distort the messages sent between two people.

The nurse has some control when selecting the setting for communicating with clients. A quiet office or lounge is ideal. When the client is visited at home, a bedroom or den may be best.

In today's health care environment, there is often less time to spend with clients. In the acute care setting a nurse must learn how to use time with clients wisely because of shortened length of hospital stay.

The nurse's efforts to convey information must not be blocked by environmental distractions. Communication must be concise and relevant based on the client's plan of care. This communication process continues as the client enters the posthospitalization phase of care. Clients frequently are transferred to various settings. Communication may require getting information for clients and families about various health care settings. Communication continues in these varied settings, such as the skilled nursing unit or home. Creative methods such as phone interaction or computer faxed reference are commonly employed in facilitating the communication process in today's changing health care environment.

Space and Territoriality

Territoriality defines the meaning of a person's right to an area of space and surroundings. Territory is important because it provides people with a sense of identity, security, and control. In other words, individuals feel threatened when others invade their territory because it disrupts psychological homeostasis, creates anxiety, and produces feelings of loss of control. In a classic text, Hall (1969) coined the term **proxemics**, which means the use of space in interpersonal relationships or the distance between communicators. During social interaction, people consciously maintain a distance between themselves. Personal space is an invisible "bubble," and it is mobile—it goes with a person. Territory can be separated and made visible to others, such as a fenced-in yard, towel on the beach, or hospital bed. When personal space is threatened by intrusion, a defensive response occurs, preventing effective communication. Nurses often work with clients in situations in which space and territory are important. As with touch, the distance separating nurses from clients must be judged by the situation and culture. Physically restraining clients in danger of self-injury, giving mouth-to-mouth resuscitation, holding crying infants, and facilitating the excretory functions of incontinent clients require invasion of intimate space.

Intimate distance or space includes an area of 18 inches in which people are able to touch one another or make physical contact. Clients are sensitive about how nurses use distance.

As the distance becomes greater, the client and nurse feel more at ease. Greater flexibility is afforded when intimate contact is not required. Sitting with a client to conduct an interview, discuss personal feelings or thoughts, or teach are examples of personal distance (18 inches to 4 feet). Increasing the physical distance makes it easier for the client and nurse to communicate because the nurse becomes less imposing. Social distance (4 to 12 feet) is needed when dealing with groups. Making rounds with physicians is an example of group interaction. Communication at a social distance is less threatening than communication in an intimate or personal space because intimate sharing of thoughts and feelings is less likely to occur. Public distance (greater than 4 feet) is the distance maintained for formal speaking. A community health nurse presenting a seminar on hypertension to older adults, or a professor lecturing to a class are examples.

■ THERAPEUTIC COMMUNICATION

Therapeutic communication is the process in which the nurse, utilizing a planned approach, learns about the client. This process focuses on the client but is planned and directed by the professional (Keltner, Schwecke, and Bostrom 1991). Therapeutic communication develops an interpersonal relationship between the client and nurse. This process involves significant skill, since the nurse must pay attention to multiple interacting and nonverbal behaviors. Therapeutic communication conveys confidentiality. Since the client knows all information shared with the nurse remains part of the medical record and is not shared as gossip, the client feels comfortable disclosing pertinent health data, concerns, fears, or family issues. In ideal situations the nurse is alert to the need to share information obtained from the client during disclosure. The nurse purposefully shares the information to benefit the client and maximize the plan of care. *Only* health care team members directly involved with the client's plan of care are privileged to the information. Confidentiality must be secured at all times in dealing with disclosure statements.

Therapeutic communication ultimately enables the nurse to establish a working relationship with the client and family. The nurse must be aware of cultural differences in which some client populations may be reluctant to share information openly with professionals. The process of therapeutic communication involves skill and genuine commitment on the part of the nurse to assist the client in the attainment of mutual care goals (Fig. 14-3).

Social Interaction

The first attempt at communicating with a client usually consists of a brief social interaction. The messages conveyed are superficial in that neither the nurse nor client discusses deeply personal matters of concern. Interpersonal exchange tends to be based on intuitive, unthinking, and automatic responses. Superficial interaction makes participants feel safe because the discussion has no hidden intent for personal disclosures.

A nurse often uses superficial social interaction at the beginning of a conversation with a client to lay a foundation for a closer relationship. For example, the nurse might greet a client by saying, "Good morning, Mrs. Sears, it's nice to see you today," or "Hi, Mr. Simpson, how do you like the great weather we're having?"

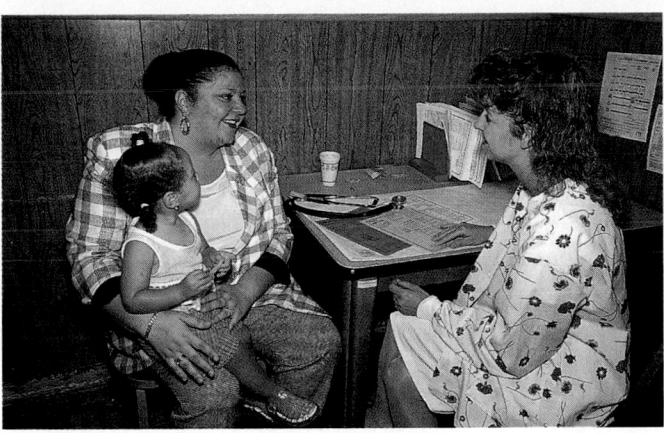

Fig. 14-3 A relaxed atmosphere helps establish a therapeutic relationship.

The skillful nurse does not allow social interaction to dominate a conversation but does maintain a congenial and warm style to build the client's trust. The goal is to help the client feel comfortable in sharing attitudes and feelings.

Caring and Methods of Effective Communication

The nurse uses communication skills while establishing a therapeutic relationship. There is no formula for forming a relationship with a client. Each person communicates uniquely, and each client requires different communication techniques. The nurse should be flexible in techniques used to foster communication with each client.

LISTENING ATTENTIVELY

Listening is one of the most effective therapeutic communication techniques. It is a nonverbal method to convey interest in the client's needs, concerns, and problems. It requires the nurse's complete attention and involves an attempt to understand the entire verbal and nonverbal message that a person is communicating. Listening is an active, learned process, while hearing is a passive, neurological process of receiving information.

Listening effectively may at first seem awkward and time consuming, but like any skill, it requires practice. An effective listener, however, gains satisfaction from working with people and understanding their deeper health concerns. To be an attentive listener, the nurse uses the following skills:

1. Face clients while they speak.
2. Maintain natural eye contact to show willingness to listen.
3. Assume an attentive posture. Avoid crossing the legs and arms because this conveys a defensive posture.
4. Avoid distracting body movements, such as wringing hands, tapping feet, or fidgeting with an object in the hands.
5. Nod in acknowledgment when clients talk about important points or look for feedback.
6. Lean toward speakers to communicate involvement.

The nurse must appear natural while listening to clients. Nonverbal cues, such as leaning toward the speaker, should not become overbearing or threaten intimate space. Listening skillfully during a nursing procedure is beneficial and is

an efficient use of time. For example, much can be learned and conveyed by the nurse who listens while giving clients baths. Clients, not the bath procedures, become the center of attention.

CONVEYING ACCEPTANCE

Showing acceptance means not judging another person and demonstrates the interviewer's willingness to listen to the client's beliefs, values, and practices. This is difficult at times because a nurse meets clients of diverse backgrounds. Acceptance is not the same as agreement. Acceptance is a willingness to hear the person without conveying doubt or disagreement.

Certainly a nurse does not accept all aspects of a client's behavior or illness. The nurse works to bring about change that improves a client's level of health. Acceptance is tolerance toward others that fosters a relationship between nurse and client.

To show acceptance the nurse remains aware of personal nonverbal expressions. The nurse avoids facial expressions and gestures that suggest disapproval, such as frowning, rolling the eyes upward, or shaking the head in disbelief. The following show that the nurse accepts what a client has to say:

1. Listening without interrupting
2. Providing verbal feedback that demonstrates understanding
3. Being sure that nonverbal cues match verbal communication
4. Avoiding arguing, expressing doubts, or attempting to change the client's mind

ASKING RELATED QUESTIONS

Questioning is a direct method of communicating. The nurse's aim is to gain specific information about the client. Questions used during a conversation set the tone of the verbal interaction and control its direction. Questions are most effective when they relate to the topic or subject being discussed and use words and word patterns in the client's normal sociocultural context. During assessment of the client's health status, questions follow a logical sequence. The following example demonstrates this technique:

Nurse: Mr. James, can you tell me where you are having pain?
Client: Well, it seems to be in my back.
Nurse: What part of your back?
Client: Here, in the lower part.
Nurse: How would you describe the pain?
Client: It feels like a knife went through me.

The nurse's line of questioning helps the client tell a story. Each question focuses on a specific aspect of the story. The nurse is careful not to ask more than one question at a time or move on to another subject until the current topic is adequately explored. The nurse selects a question on the basis of the client's previous response so that information flows logically.

If the nurse wants the client to elaborate, open-ended questions are most effective. They give a client a chance to talk more completely about problems or concerns. Such questions cannot be answered with *yes* or *no*. Examples of open-ended questions are:

1. "Would you describe the pain you have been feeling?"
2. "What seems to be the problem?"
3. "Explain to me how your family feels about your illness."

Asking the client open-ended questions allows the nurse to assess a number of factors. The client's verbal and nonverbal responses can reveal emotions. The nurse may be able to judge the level of the client's vocabulary and understanding of health by the response. Often the nurse seeks details of physical signs and symptoms, and the open-ended question elicits more accurate and detailed descriptions. Because an open-ended question prompts a lengthy response, the nurse can assess gaps or discrepancies.

PARAPHRASING

Paraphrasing is restating clients' messages in the nurse's own words. Usually a paraphrased statement uses fewer words than the original statement. Through paraphrasing, the nurse sends feedback that lets clients know whether their messages were understood and prompts further communication. The following example illustrates this point:

Client: I've had it. My doctor won't tell me what's going on. He doesn't seem to care what I think.

Nurse: You're frustrated because you and your doctor haven't talked about your diagnosis?

Client: Yes, he obviously doesn't know what it's like to be sick.

Practice is required to paraphrase accurately. If the meaning of a message is changed or distorted through paraphrasing, communication may become ineffective. For example, a client may say, "I've been overweight all my life and never had any problems. I can't understand why I need to be on a diet." Paraphrasing this statement by saying, "You mean you don't care if you're overweight or not?" is incorrect. "It seems that you're not convinced you need a diet because you've remained healthy," is a more accurate way of paraphrasing the statement.

CLARIFYING

Despite efforts at paraphrasing, the nurse may not understand the client's message. When a misunderstanding occurs, the nurse momentarily stops the discussion to clarify meaning. **Clarification** may be defined as the act of restating what has been stated or sent to the receiver of the message. Without clarification, valuable information can be lost. Information critical to the client's care plan can be incomplete unless confusing or conflicting data are clarified. The nurse can attempt to repeat the message or admit confusion and ask the client to restate the message. In the following example, a client has come to the clinic for a checkup:

Client: I knew I might have a problem. It seems to be in my family. The last time I was here, though, it wasn't bad, so I didn't mention it.

Nurse: Excuse me, Mr. Brewer, can you tell me what type of problem you're having?

The nurse must also clarify messages. Examples can be used to clarify a vague, abstract idea. When using examples, the nurse describes ideas or situations to which the client can easily relate. In the following dialog, a nurse is explaining activity restrictions to a client who has had eye surgery:

Nurse: Now, Mr. Lee, once you go home you are not supposed to place stress on your eye.

Client: I'm not sure I know what you mean.

Nurse: Well, you're not allowed to stoop or bend over with your head down. For example, if you want to pick up your slippers off the floor or pick up a basket of laundry, don't bend over. Instead, bend your knees and keep your head up.

Client: I have a dog at home. I guess I can't bend over to pick him up?

Nurse: That's right. Bend your knees to lower yourself down if you want to pick up your dog.

The more specific a clarifying message, the more likely it will be understood. Clients who are easily confused by the complex terms and jargon of medicine appreciate a simple, down-to-earth explanation that uses familiar examples.

FOCUSING

Focusing may be defined as centering information on the key elements or concepts of the message that has been sent. Focusing eliminates vagueness in communication by limiting the area of discussion. As clients discuss topics related to health, their messages often become vague. For example, a client may say to the nurse, "Well, I've just been feeling funny lately. It doesn't really bother me that much. It's just this feeling I'm having in my head." This description tells little except that the client does not feel well. If the nurse does not help focus specifically on the physical complaint, the client will likely continue to use vague descriptions.

To focus the discussion, the nurse might respond to the client by saying, "You said you've been feeling funny lately. Tell me when this feeling first started," or "Describe the feeling in your head." As in clarifying, the nurse seeks meaning in the client's message. In the case of focusing, however, the nurse understands the client's message but realizes that it is nonspecific or vague.

The nurse does not use focusing if it interrupts clients while discussing an important issue. If conversations continue without new information or clients begin to repeat themselves, focusing is useful.

STATING OBSERVATIONS

When communicating, people are often unaware of the way that their messages are received. Feedback from others tells them whether they communicated the intended message. One way the nurse can provide feedback is by sharing with clients observations of their behavior during communication. The nurse describes the impressions created by the nonverbal cues. The following example illustrates this point:

CASE STUDY   Miss Tucker is sitting in the waiting room of her physician's office. She is slumped in the chair, her body movements are slow, and she yawns while speaking with the nurse. The nurse says, "Miss Tucker, you appear to be quite tired." ∎

If the client's verbal message conflicts with nonverbal cues, the nurse's observation may help convey a clearer message. Stating observations often leads the client to communicate more clearly without the need for extensive questioning, focusing, or clarification.

The nurse does not state observations that might embarrass or anger the client. The nurse in the preceding example would not say, "Miss Tucker, you look a mess." Even if such an observation is made with humor, the client can become resentful.

OFFERING INFORMATION

When two people communicate, the process is rarely one sided. In an interaction with a client, the nurse frequently offers information that gives the client additional data or insight. The client in the following dialog is scheduled to have surgery the next day for an abdominal tumor removal:

Client: My doctor has told me I'm first on the schedule for surgery tomorrow.
Nurse: Yes, we'll be awakening you about 6 AM.
Client: My family would like to be here then.
Nurse: That's no problem. They are free to come at 6, and we'll show them where to wait for you once you've left for the operating room.

Providing the client with additional information encourages further response. Offering information on an ongoing, timely basis not only facilitates communication but also promotes health teaching.

It is usually not helpful to withhold information from clients, particularly when they seek it. If the nurse avoids sharing information or gives only partial information, clients may lose trust in the nurse. If physicians choose to withhold information, the nurse needs to clarify the reasons with them. However, there is a wide range of information the nurse can share. The nurse must avoid advising a client when giving information so as not to influence the client's decision-making process. The nurse provides information that enables clients to reach the decision they feel optimize their sense or state of well-being.

MAINTAINING SILENCE

Silence allows the nurse and client to organize thoughts. The use of silence can be effective but is difficult because pauses in conversation that last several seconds or minutes can cause unease. Beginning nurses may need to practice this technique before feeling comfortable.

The use of silence requires skill and timing. Silence allows the client an opportunity to communicate intrapersonally, organize thoughts, and process information. It gives clients time to search for words or feelings. Silence is particularly useful when clients are confronted with difficult decisions that they are not sure how to share with the nurse. For example, silence may help clients gain the confidence needed to share the decision to refuse medical treatment.

Silence also allows the nurse to observe clients. The nurse pays particular attention to nonverbal messages, such as worried expressions or loss of eye contact. Remaining silent demonstrates the nurse's willingness to wait for a response. Often the nurse has many questions, but some people, especially older adults, are unable to reply quickly. Impatience expressed by the nurse frustrates clients' efforts at communication. Silence shows that the nurse is interested and will accept any response clients can express.

When clients become emotionally upset, silence helps them gather thoughts. A quiet period may diffuse an emotionally tense situation. A nurse's silence acknowledges clients' needs for a few moments of privacy. After clients are ready to talk again, they will more likely express feelings clearly.

USING ASSERTIVENESS

Assertiveness is standing up for one's rights without violating those of others (Stanhope and Lancaster, 1996). Through assertive techniques people express feelings and emotions confidently, spontaneously, and honestly. Assertive persons make choices and decisions and are able to control their lives more effectively than nonassertive individuals. Nurses can teach clients assertiveness skills and how to use them to promote their own health.

Examples of assertiveness skills include speaking clearly, dealing with manipulation, and protecting against criticism. A clear message is complete and specific and includes all information a client needs to understand. The following example illustrates the incorrect technique for communicating a message:

Nurse: Your recovery depends on your ability to exercise right.
Client: Does that mean I can begin running?

The nurse should have been more specific when transmitting the message and should have given the client more information, as shown in the following example:

Nurse: Your recovery will include walking daily, beginning by walking two to three blocks and progressing to one mile per day within a month. Your physician and physical therapist should be consulted before you begin to run.

To avoid being manipulated, nurses acquire skills to protect themselves from others who consciously or unconsciously use them. Learning to say *no* and resisting guilt imposed intentionally by others are two helpful techniques. Learning to say *no* is illustrated in the following case study:

Staff member: Listen, I'm really in a rush. Can you help me get this report completed?
Nurse: I've planned a home visit this morning. Perhaps my schedule will permit it tomorrow. I'll let you know.

Constructive criticism can promote growth, but manipulative criticism makes people vulnerable (Stanhope and Lancaster, 1992). The following example illustrates a method of protecting against criticism:

Supervisor: Nancy, I've been concerned about your performance lately.
Nurse: What have your concerns been?
Supervisor: I see you've been involved in two separate incidents with medication errors.
Nurse: Can you suggest ways I might avoid errors next time?

Negative inquiry is a skill that involves asking for more information when a criticism has been made. The person remains unemotional and low-key when asking for information and avoids sounding angry or sarcastic. Using criticism for growth helps nurses feel good about themselves.

Supervisor: Your nurse's notes need to be more objective in describing the situation.
Nurse: Can you give me some specific examples?

SUMMARIZING

Summarization is a concise review of main ideas that have been discussed. It sets the tone for further interactions between the nurse and client. Beginning a new interaction by summarizing a previous one helps the client recall topics discussed and shows the client that the nurse has analyzed their communication. In the following example, the nurse, Ms. Spier, has been working for several days to help the client, Mrs. Ramos, learn about diabetes:

> **CASE STUDY**   Ms. Spier enters the client's room and says, "Good morning, Mrs. Ramos. I've come to talk with you more about your diabetes. If you recall, yesterday we discussed the purpose of insulin, its side effects, and how to give an injection." ■

Summarizing helps the nurse review key aspects of an interaction. Further communication can then focus on relevant issues. Clients will be able to sense whether the nurse understood their part of the message. With a summary the client is able to review information and make additions or corrections.

Barriers to Effective Communication

Some communication techniques or styles result in interpersonal interactions that are not therapeutic. These barriers can be damaging when a nurse is building a client relationship. Many techniques that normally promote effective communication can be harmful if used improperly.

GIVING AN OPINION

Giving an opinion takes decision making away from the client. It inhibits spontaneity, stalls problem solving, and creates doubt. The following example demonstrates how giving an opinion can be harmful:

Nurse: Mr. Jones, you look like you're deep in thought.
Client: Oh, no, not really. I was just thinking about whether my daughter is coming to see me.
Nurse: Well, if you ask me, she should have been here before now. It would mean so much to you.

Often the client simply needs an opportunity to express feelings. Giving an opinion prevents the client from developing solutions to problems.

At times, clients may require suggestions. For example, when a client is selecting a special diet, the nurse's help may be needed to choose the right food. Suggestions are presented to clients as options because the final decision rests with the client.

OFFERING FALSE REASSURANCE

When a client is seriously ill, the nurse is tempted to offer hope to the client with statements such as "You'll be fine" or "There's nothing to worry about." When a client is

reaching out for understanding, false reassurance from the nurse may discourage open communication. The following example illustrates this point:

Client: I'm so afraid of becoming dependent on my wife. I feel I'm never going to get any better.
Nurse: There's no reason to be so afraid. Things will get better.

Genuine, truthful reassurance, however, is important and helps validate a client's self-worth and sense of hope. Bradley and Edinberg (1990) have identified six basic conditions in which verbal reassurance can be given; a client can be reassured:

1. That there is hope
2. That the nurse is listening
3. That care is available
4. That certain undesirable changes can be expected (e.g., loss of hair from chemotherapy)
5. That the client will be treated like a person
6. That the client's problem is understood

The following dialog shows how the nurse conveys a willingness to understand a client's concerns without falsely reassuring her that the illness or symptoms are minor:

> **CASE STUDY**   Mrs. Stevens is a 58-year-old woman with terminal cancer. Her home health nurse, Mr. Fry, is sitting by her side.
>
> *Mrs. Stevens:* I sometimes think this isn't happening to me. It seems so unfair. . . . Oh, I'm sorry. You don't want to hear my problems.
> *Mr. Fry:* No, please, Mrs. Stevens, I do want to hear how you feel. ■

BEING DEFENSIVE

Defensiveness in response to criticism suggests that the client has no right to an opinion. When a nurse becomes defensive the client's concerns are often ignored. The following example illustrates the point:

> **CASE STUDY**   Mr. Locke has been a regular visitor to the health clinic for several years. The last time he visited the clinic, he had symptoms that resulted in his hospitalization. He now is returning to the clinic for a checkup 1 week after discharge from the hospital.
>
> *Mr. Locke:* Well, I hope I don't have to see Dr. Warren today.
> *Nurse:* I don't understand, Mr. Locke, is something wrong? Dr. Warren has been your doctor here for some time.
> *Mr. Locke:* I don't care. He was the one who put me in the hospital, and that was a waste of time.
> *Nurse:* That's silly. Dr. Warren is an excellent physician.
> *Mr. Locke:* You think so, huh? He hasn't put you in the hospital for no reason.
> *Nurse:* You were very ill, Mr. Locke. I know Dr. Warren made the right decision. ■

The nurse has threatened the relationship with Mr. Locke. He will probably not trust the nurse to keep his concerns confidential. The nurse is ignoring the client's feelings and will probably not take any action to remedy the problem. After this conversation, the nurse will have difficulty continuing a rapport that will prompt the client to discuss additional problems.

When clients express criticism, the nurse should listen to what they have to say. Listening does not imply agreement. To learn the reasons behind the client's criticism, the nurse avoids becoming defensive. There are two sides to any story, and the nurse attempts to learn why clients have become angry or dissatisfied. The following dialog demonstrates this technique:

Mr. Locke: Well, I hope I don't have to see Dr. Warren today.
Nurse: You seem upset, would you like to talk about it?
Mr. Locke: I just don't think he should have put me in the hospital.
Nurse: You believe hospitalization was unnecessary?
Mr. Locke: Yes, they really didn't do much of anything. They took a few tests and did some x-rays.
Nurse: Mr. Locke, did your doctors tell you what the tests showed?
Mr. Locke: No, not really. That's why I'm so angry.

The nurse's patience led to an identification of the client's real concern, not knowing the results of his diagnostic tests. By avoiding defensiveness the nurse defused Mr. Locke's anger so that he could describe his concerns.

SHOWING APPROVAL OR DISAPPROVAL

Expressing excessive approval can be as harmful to a nurse-client relationship as stating disapproval. Offering excessive praise implies that the behavior being praised is the only acceptable one. Often the client shares a decision with the nurse, not in an effort to seek approval but to provide a means to discuss feelings. The following example illustrates this point:

Client: I've decided that when I leave the hospital I'll stay with my son. He doesn't want me to go home and be alone.
Nurse: Oh, I'm so glad to hear that. I think you definitely made the right decision. It's best for you to be with your son.

This nurse's comment will likely end further discussion of the topic. The client may perceive that the nurse agrees with the son. Perhaps the client would be better off with the son. On the other hand, the client may have a strong desire to remain independent, and now that has been discouraged. The nurse's excessive approval did not allow the client to think or act freely and inhibited the potential for decision making. A better response by the nurse might be, "You seem concerned about losing your independence."

On the other hand, disapproval implies that the client must meet the nurse's expectations or standards. In the following example, the nurse's response may hinder the client's positive attitude and recovery:

Client: Oh, I feel good, I was able to get up in the chair once today.
Nurse: Only once? You're going to have to get up more often than that!

It would have been better for the nurse to say, "You're making fine progress. Your doctor would like you to try to be up at least three times today. Do you think you'd like to sit up just before going to bed?" A disapproving statement causes the client to feel rejected. The client may avoid further interaction with the nurse, thus potentially slowing recovery.

STEREOTYPING

Everyone is unique. However, stereotyped responses inhibit uniqueness and oversimplify the situation. **Stereotypes** are generalized beliefs held about people. The use of stereotypes inhibits communication and can threaten a nurse-client relationship. Stereotyping statements, such as "Older adults are always confused" or "Clients with back problems cannot tolerate pain" seriously impair interpersonal communication.

Another nontherapeutic communication is the use of meaningless, stereotyped responses. Their use minimizes the importance of a person's message. The following example illustrates this point:

Client: I slept poorly last night. My incision seemed to be pulling.
Nurse: You can't win them all. At least the incision is healing well.

ASKING WHY

When people disagree with or fail to understand others, they are tempted to ask why the others believe or have acted in such a way. Clients frequently interpret "why" questions as accusations. They may also think that the nurse knows the reasons and is simply testing them. Regardless of clients' perceptions of the nurse's motivation, "why" questions can cause resentment, insecurity, and mistrust.

If the nurse wants additional information, there are more effective ways of phrasing questions. For example, rather than asking, "Why didn't you do your exercises?" the nurse could say, "You didn't do your exercises. Is something wrong?" Rather than asking, "Why are you anxious?" the nurse could say, "You appear upset. Would you like to talk?"

CHANGING THE SUBJECT INAPPROPRIATELY

A nurse might inadvertently stop a client from discussing a subject of importance by changing the subject. Abruptly interrupting conversation is rude and shows a lack of empathy, as the following example shows:

Nurse: Good morning, Mr. Jones. How are you feeling?
Mr. Jones: (facial expression shows discomfort) Oh, not so good. My incision is rather sore.
Nurse: Well, let's get you up in a chair. We need to discuss your exercises.

The nurse's comment shows an unwillingness to discuss Mr. Jones' discomfort. The chance for a therapeutic assessment of his discomfort is lost. In this example, changing the subject was not therapeutic because the nurse ignored a potentially serious problem.

Changing the subject stalls progress of a therapeutic communication. The client's thoughts and spontaneity are interrupted, ideas become tangled, and as a result, the information provided may be inadequate. It is particularly important to avoid changing the subject during assessment. If the client has the opportunity to complete a message, the information shared will be more thorough and useful.

■ HELPING RELATIONSHIPS

The nurse-client relationship is more than a mutual partnership. It is a process in which the helper is asked to intervene in the life of the client to help the client engage in more effective behavior. The nurse-client relationship is a dynamic process involving a collaborative effort of nurse and client to resolve a problem and to promote the client's health and adaptation abilities. The nurse uses skills of interpersonal communication to develop a relationship with clients that allows understanding of them as total persons. This helping relationship is therapeutic, promoting a psychological climate that brings positive client change and growth. The relationship also focuses on meeting clients' needs. Although the nurse may gain much satisfaction from the relationship, clients should be the primary recipients and determiners of benefits.

Creation of a therapeutic environment rests on the nurse's ability to provide physical and psychosocial comfort to the client (see the box below). The nurse ensures that the client's physiological needs are satisfied. For exam-

ple, the nurse positions the client so that breathing is normal for comfortable sleep. The nurse's actions consider the client's preferences. The nurse and client mutually determine how needs are met. The following case study shows how the nurse involves the client in care:

> **CASE STUDY**   Mrs. Greer is a 63-year-old widow who is hospitalized for lung cancer. She makes frequent requests for pain medication before a dose is due. When a nurse delivers the medication, Mrs. Greer criticizes her for being late. Nothing the nurses do seems to satisfy Mrs. Greer.
>
> Ms. Edwards, RN, has cared for Mrs. Greer for the past 2 days and requests to care for her. Ms. Edwards enters her client's room and begins to straighten out the bed linen. Ms. Edwards asks, "Are you comfortable in that position, Mrs. Greer? Would you like a pain shot now?" Mrs. Greer accepts the offer and begins to relax in Ms. Edwards' presence. The nurse helps Mrs. Greer assume a more comfortable position on her side.
>
> Once the client's pain has diminished, Ms. Edwards sits by her bed and says, "I know you've been experiencing much discomfort. Over the past few days we have not always been able to help you feel better. Can you help me to know the best way to make you feel comfortable?" ■

Efforts at improving Mrs. Greer's comfort make her more willing to discuss problems. The nurse soon learns of Mrs. Greer's great fear of death. The client has made frequent requests of the nurses to avoid feeling lonely. By discussing Mrs. Greer's fears, the nurse and client are able to find ways to minimize loneliness. The nurse's concern leads to solutions to the client's problems.

A helping relationship between the nurse and client does not just happen. It is built with care as the nurse uses therapeutic communication techniques.

Dimensions of Helping Relationships

Common features of a helping relationship are trust, empathy, caring, autonomy, and mutuality. They are essential if the nurse wants to establish positive and supportive relationships with clients.

TRUST

Trust may be defined as the belief that other people will provide help in times of need and distress. Unless clients believe that a nurse wishes to care for their needs, a trusting relationship cannot develop. Trust fosters open, therapeutic communication. Previous experiences may affect clients' willingness to trust a nurse. Lack of previous health care experience or traumatic experiences cause clients to hesitate in trusting care givers. To foster trust, the nurse acts consistently, reliably, and competently. Honesty in sharing information with clients also builds trust. Without trust, a nurse-client relationship does not progress beyond social interaction and tending only to superficial needs.

EMPATHY AND SYMPATHY

Empathy is widely accepted as a clinical component of the helping relationship, and within nursing it is considered an essential part of the nurse-client relationship. Definitions of empathy reflect the influence of psychotherapist Carl Rogers, who is well known for his work in identifying

---

![research highlight icon] ## RESEARCH HIGHLIGHT

RESEARCH ABSTRACT

This study describes intensive care unit nurses' experiences and reactions concerning limitations in communicating with mechanically ventilated clients. The methodology included a demographic questionnaire and voluntary participation in an interview that focused on three areas:

1. The nurses' perception of limitations and facilitating factors in communicating with clients on mechanical ventilators.
2. Discussion of past experiences concerning the communication process with clients on mechanical ventilators.
3. The effect of nurse-client perceived relationships influenced by the communication process.

Factors identified as obstacles in establishing a relationship with a client included initial contact with the client, workload of the nurse, and the nurses' personal feelings for the client.

IMPLICATIONS FOR PRACTICE

▶ Collaborative communication processes with the health care team are essential during the course of client care.

▶ Creative communication strategies, such as sign language or touch, reduce communication barriers.

▶ It is essential for nurses to establish a helping relationship with clients who have impaired communication despite stress evoking factors in an ICU environment.

REFERENCE

Bergbom-Engberg I, Haljamäe H: The communication process with ventilator patients in the ICU as perceived by the nursing staff, *Intens Crit Care Nurs* 9:40, 1993.

and describing the characteristics of a helping relationship. Empathy is the ability to try to understand and enter the client's frame of reference (Haber et al, 1994). Empathy is sensing, comprehending, and sharing the client's frame of reference, beginning with the problem the client recognizes. It is a fair, sensitive, and objective look at what another person experiences.

Empathy helps clients explain and explore their feelings so that problem solving might occur. It takes time for empathy to develop in a relationship. A nurse cannot automatically understand a client's feelings or experiences. In the following case study, being open and receptive helps the nurse learn to be empathetic:

> **CASE STUDY** Mr. Vincent has been caring for Mr. Pierce since his admission to the hospital yesterday. Mr. Pierce is scheduled to have open-heart surgery. Mr. Vincent enters the client's room, makes eye contact with him, and sits in the chair beside his bed. The following conversation occurs:
>
> *Mr. Vincent:* Hello, Mr. Pierce. You look as though you're rather deep in thought.
> *Mr. Pierce:* Oh, I suppose I do. It's just that I can't help but think about what tomorrow will bring.
> *Mr. Vincent:* Would you like to talk about your surgery? I imagine you have a lot of questions.
> *Mr. Pierce:* Yes, I would like to know more. ▪

The nurse could easily have avoided Mr. Pierce's true concerns and even attempted to change the subject. An unhelpful remark would have been, "Don't worry, Mr. Pierce. Would you like me to get you something to read?" Such a comment would ignore Mr. Pierce's fears about surgery and prevent development of a meaningful relationship between the nurse and client. The skillful nurse moves the conversation forward to learn more about the client.

In contrast to empathy, sympathy is the expression of one's own feelings about another's predicament. It is the concern, sorrow, or pity shown by the nurse for the client in which the needs of the client are seen as the nurse's needs. This may pose a difficulty by preventing the development of an effective helping relationship. For example, the nurse uses communication skills when expressing condolences to the family of a lost loved one. "I'm sorry that your father died so suddenly. My father also died this way. If there is anything I can do please do not hesitate to find me." By this message, the nurse utilizes both concepts of sympathy and empathy by offering assistance and sharing the client's frame of reference.

CARING

Caring is having a positive regard for another person. It is basic to a helping relationship. Most clients directly or indirectly express a need to be cared for at some time. Nurses show caring by accepting clients for who they are and respecting them as individuals. When clients feel cared for, they feel secure in threatening or anxiety-producing situations. Caring also promotes trust and decreases anxiety. Diminished anxiety and stress increase the body's defenses and help promote healing.

AUTONOMY AND MUTUALITY

Autonomy is the ability to be self-directed. **Mutuality** involves sharing with another. These are important in any helping relationship. The nurse and client work as a team, participating in care. The nurse offers opportunities to make decisions, even if it is as simple as choosing a bath time. As a client becomes more independent, the nurse offers more opportunities for decision making. The nurse also acts as an advocate to keep the client informed of health care alternatives and give support in decision making.

Phases of a Helping Relationship

The helping relationship is established and maintained by the professional nurse and consists of the preinteraction, orientation, working, and termination phases. The relationship is reciprocal; nurse and client relate to each other as they progress to therapeutic rapport. A helping relationship progresses over time as the nurse and client interact, but the helping relationship is not the same as the nursing process. The nursing process is a series of steps taken to manage a client's health problems. A helping relationship is a bond that allows the nurse to be more effective in carrying out the nursing process. The nurse is responsible for directing the client through the helping relationship to ensure that the client's needs are met. The challenge for the nurse is to establish a helping relationship with minimal time by incorporating effective communication patterns with the client, family, and health care team.

Chapter 7 discusses the interview as a method for obtaining a nursing health history and identifying changes in the client's level of wellness and living patterns. Although the phases of an interview and of a helping relationship are the same, communication patterns are different. The interview can initiate a nurse-client relationship because it may be the first encounter. However, the interview is not the mechanism for maintaining a long-term therapeutic relationship that extends past hospitalization. A helping relationship goes beyond the scope of an interview to establish rapport that is the basis for an ongoing resolution of the client's health problems.

PREINTERACTION PHASE

Before a first meeting with a client, the nurse ideally reviews information pertaining to the client. Such information may include the medical or nursing history, an entry in the nurse's notes of the medical record, or a discussion with another nurse who cared for the client. During this review, the nurse thinks about concerns that may develop. For example, before entering a relationship with a young cancer client, the nurse considers how the client is adjusting and whether death may be discussed. The preinteraction phase is a time when the nurse plans an approach. This process helps avoid stereotyping clients and allows the nurse to think about personal values or feelings. Although the nurse may feel anxious about a client, this sharpens mental processes and helps planning. The beginning nursing student should seek assistance from instructors if anxiety becomes intense.

A final step of the preinteraction phase is to choose a location and setting for the first meeting with a client. A comfortable, private, and attractive setting fosters interpersonal interaction. The nurse also allows for sufficient time for discussion.

ORIENTATION

The orientation phase begins when the nurse and the client first meet. It sets the tone for the rest of the nurse-client relationship. The orientation phase is superficial and is often marked by uncertainty and exploration.

During any initial encounter, both participants closely observe each other. The nurse and client make inferences and form judgments about each other's behavior. Therapeutic communication will be more effective if the nurse is genuine, empathetic, and caring.

The nurse and client meet and identify each other by name. It is wise to address the client formally by using last names; for example, the nurse might say, "Good morning, Mr. Spencer. I am Ms. Tucker. I am a student nurse assigned to take care of you today." As the therapeutic relationship develops, a client may ask the nurse to be more informal. Failure to identify oneself can create uncertainty because the client often encounters many personnel when seeking health care.

At the beginning of the relationship neither individual is able to perceive the other's uniqueness. The nurse perceives a person who has a health-related problem. The client perceives the nurse as one of many health care professionals whose job is to help. Engaging in a social interaction initially helps the nurse and client become relaxed. The following dialog demonstrates communication to place a client at ease:

Nurse: It certainly is a lovely day, Mrs. Spier.
Client: Yes, isn't it? If I were home and feeling better, I'd be planting my garden.
Nurse: You're a gardener? What types of plants do you enjoy growing?
Client: Oh, a little of everything. I like some tomatoes, lettuce, radishes, and maybe some squash.

The nurse directs the conversation so that she and Mrs. Spier feel at ease. Rushing into a therapeutically oriented discussion when the client feels uncomfortable serves no purpose. The nurse and Mrs. Spier can come to know each other better and begin to develop a meaningful relationship if the social interaction is properly directed.

Testing. The client often tests the nurse during the orientation phase. This is caused by the client's difficulty in acknowledging a need for help, fear of expressing true feelings, and anxiety over the need to change. The nurse who is aware of the client's concerns attempts to display confidence and competence. The nurse should not be defensive during testing but should be open and interested in the client's concerns. The client may use silence to avoid communicating. The nurse can show a desire to help by explaining the actions taken and performing care smoothly. The following case study shows communication involving testing:

CASE STUDY   Mr. Miles is a 52-year-old businessman who has been hospitalized for treatment of a bleeding stomach ulcer. He is very independent, and he is accustomed to making decisions for himself. Ms. Rains, the nurse, enters the client's room.

Ms. Rains: Good morning, Mr. Miles. I am Ms. Rains, and I will be caring for you today.
Mr. Miles: You will, huh? Tell me, how long have you been a nurse?
Ms. Rains: About 2 years. I have worked in this hospital since graduation.
Mr. Miles: Well, you won't have to worry about me. I can take care of myself.
Ms. Rains: I can imagine it's frustrating to be very independent one minute and then suddenly become ill and feel as though everyone is telling you what to do.
Mr. Miles: You can say that again. I'm just not used to needing help.
Ms. Rains: Mr. Miles, I'm not here to take away your independence. There are a number of things I need to do for you, but there are also many things I want you to be able to do for yourself. Let me explain some of the procedures I will be doing.
Mr. Miles: OK, I appreciate that. ■

Ms. Rains recognizes Mr. Miles' attempt to test her competence. Mr. Miles is fearful of losing his independence. If Ms. Rains had minimal experience in developing relationships with clients, she may have felt the need to remain superficial and nondirective. The client will sense the nurse's superficiality during testing and avoid meaningful discussion. In this case, Ms. Rains acknowledges concerns and acts to eliminate Mr. Miles' fears.

Building Trust. Trust is relying on someone without doubt or question. Confidence, dependability, confidentiality, and credibility result in a trusting relationship. It is not easy for a client to perceive the need for help or to ask for it. Often a client trusts the nurse but is incapable of asking for assistance. Trust provides the foundation for effective communication as an individual becomes more open in expressing feelings and thoughts.

Trusting another person involves risk. As clients begin to share feelings and attitudes with the nurse, they become vulnerable. Clients must become comfortable in revealing personal information. The nurse who is insecure with clients may choose superficial methods to build trust: sharing secrets, telling private jokes, or encouraging clients to establish the relationship on a first-name basis. Some clients accept such behaviors, but others may resent being treated differently. Instead of enjoying the nurse's extra attention, they become distrustful.

Genuine caring is a powerful method for acquiring trust. The nurse shows sensitivity and understanding of the client's needs. Expressing concern is one way to establish trust. By showing concern, the nurse encourages the client's growth and progress. The following case study demonstrates communication to build trust:

CASE STUDY   *Mr. Squires:* I've been home now for 4 days, and I just don't know what to do.
Ms. Ramsey: You're obviously upset. Tell me what the problem is. I'd like to help.
Mr. Squires: The doctor put me on that new diet. It seemed easy in the hospital, but I'm afraid I'm not eating right.
Ms. Ramsey: You've improved so much since your hospitalization. Let's sit down together and see what kinds of foods you should eat. Then we'll look at the types of foods you like that are allowed in your new diet.

Mr. Squires begins to trust Ms. Ramsey, who shows a willingness to help, not out of duty but out of a desire to meet his needs.

Mr. Squires: You shouldn't have to go to so much trouble for me.
Ms. Ramsey: You're not causing me trouble at all. An important part of my job is to help you stay healthy. Helping you to understand your diet better is part of my job.
Mr. Squires: Well, if I can learn to fix and eat the right foods, my doctor says I may stay out of the hospital longer this time.
Ms. Ramsey: Your doctor is right. Now let's go over what you know so far.

Another element that aids establishment of trust is recognizing Mr. Squires' individuality. He realizes that Ms. Ramsey respects him as a unique person.

Mr. Squires: The doctor said I should eat more vegetables and fruits. I really don't like many vegetables.
Ms. Ramsey: Well, let's make a list of what you do like. You know there are different ways to prepare the same kinds of foods. If you're able to eat the things you like, you'll be able to follow the diet more easily.
Mr. Squires: That sounds good. Before I left the hospital I didn't think I would have much choice in what I ate.
Ms. Ramsey: Sure you do. I'll show you that you can have a lot of variety in your diet and even enjoy it. It's important that the diet be planned for you and not someone else.

Trust develops on a foundation of caring. Ms. Ramsey's time, patience, and conscientiousness show her concern for Mr. Squires' welfare. ∎

Identifying Problems and Goals. During the initial encounter, the nurse begins to assess the client's health status. Through observations and interaction the nurse begins to make diagnostic conclusions. The client's health problems may be simple, such as moving without discomfort, choosing foods that will be easily tolerated, or getting out of bed safely. The relationship with the client is strengthened if the nurse identifies important client problems. Also, the client may not be able to recognize problems. During the orientation phase, the nurse uses communication techniques to direct the client to an awareness of problems, focus on the nature of the problems, and explore potential solutions. As problems are identified, the nurse and client mutually set goals. When the client is able to participate in goal setting and see the desired benefits, nursing interventions are more effective.

Sometimes the aim of the interaction is a mutual sharing of information, thoughts, and feelings rather than identification or addressing of problems. The nurse may find that the client is recovering without difficulty or coping well with the situation.

Identification of problems uses attentive listening, open-ended questioning, paraphrasing, and clarifying. Initially the nurse avoids identifying a large number of actual or potential problems. Bombarding the client with too many questions can result in emotional and physical fatigue. Also, it makes the client less trusting and more suspicious of the nurse's intentions. Limiting problem identification facilitates the client's understanding of the client's and nurse's roles. The following case study demonstrates communication to identify problems and goals:

CASE STUDY Mr. Sachs is a 58-year-old man who has suffered a partial paralysis of his right side and is newly admitted to a rehabilitation facility. Mr. Sachs needs to regain function in his right hand to retain his job as a telephone repairman. He is also fearful of damage to his self-image. He feels deformed and unable to live normally again.

Mr. Sachs: So much has happened to me. I know I may never again be able to do the things I once enjoyed.
Nurse: I know it's a difficult time for you now, but there are many things we can do to help you regain normal function.
Mr. Sachs: But there are so many things wrong with me.
Nurse: Let's take one at a time. What is most important to you?
Mr. Sachs: If only I could use my hand.
Nurse: Your doctor has ordered some exercises to increase the strength in your hand. The physical therapist will teach you how to do each one. Are you willing to try them?
Mr. Sachs: You bet I am. If only I could use my hand again to work.
Nurse: Let's start with some simple goals. First we'll help you gain strength in your fingers so you can grasp eating utensils, a comb, or a razor. After that we'll try some more strenuous exercises.
Mr. Sachs: OK, that sounds reasonable. Show me what I need to do. ∎

Clarifying Roles. After a helping relationship is initiated, roles must be clarified. This occurs through a sharing of information, including the client's immediate needs, the client's perception of those needs, nursing care measures to be instituted, and steps for ensuring client participation in care. The helping relationship requires participation from both parties, but the nurse assumes the leadership role. Leadership does not mean control in the manipulative sense. Instead, the nurse takes the initiative in determining the client's point of view. The client assumes a role as receiver of care but also assumes an ongoing role as a participant in care.

Forming Contracts. After goals and roles are clearly defined, the nurse may establish a contract with the client. Generally, this involves a brief verbal interchange. Elements of the contract include location, frequency, and length of contacts with the client and duration of the relationship. The nurse should not present the contract in an overly formal way, but should outline an agreement in a way that clarifies expectations and summarizes steps for facilitating progress toward health. The following example demonstrates communication to form a contract:

Nurse: Mr. Reed, I'll be seeing you at home each morning for the next 4 days. After we practice your exercises together, I'd like you to do them on your own. Practice the exercises as often as you can without feeling pain or fatigue. On Friday, I'll introduce you to Mr. Ikeda, the nurse who will work with you next week. I'll be sure he knows the types of exercises you're doing.

Ideally, it is important to let the client know when the relationship will be terminated. This may not always be possible due to unplanned discharges or transfers within the hospital and the various nurses caring for the client during hospitalization. If the relationship is successful, the nurse and client frequently share respect and concern. The closer the nurse and client become in working together, the more difficult it is to end the relationship. If the client can anticipate the length of the relationship, termination will be less stressful. A student nurse often spends time with only one or two clients, often resulting in close relationships. Clients must be prepared for the end of the student's clinical experience; otherwise the client may become angered or disappointed.

WORKING PHASE

During the working phase of a helping relationship, the nurse strives to meet goals set during the orientation phase. The nurse and client work together. The relationship broadens and becomes more flexible as the nurse and client are more willing to share feelings and discuss problems.

The nurse encourages the client's open expression of feelings. This may best be achieved by listening. If a client is unaccustomed to sharing feelings, the nurse must be patient and understanding. The nurse's empathy and respect help explore the client's true thoughts and feelings.

As the relationship progresses, clients participate in more self-exploration and are better able to discuss relevant issues. The nurse helps clients understand their feelings so that change can occur when necessary. Communication skills that encourage clients to communicate in a manner that facilitates their growth include confrontation, immediacy, and self-disclosure (Haber et al, 1994). If the working phase is successful, clients are able to act on ideas and feelings. This often requires risk, and the nurse must remain supportive. Clients must deal with success and failure as they make decisions and resolve problems. Any attempt at change should be within clients' abilities. Change becomes less of a threat when clients express feelings about change and accept temporary setbacks. The nurse should encourage even the slightest progress.

Confrontation. The nurse makes clients aware of inconsistencies in behavior or thoughts that interfere with self-understanding. The technique helps clients recognize growth or deal with important issues. The following case study demonstrates confrontation:

> **CASE STUDY**   Mrs. Perkins is a 60-year-old client with a history of obesity and high blood pressure. She has been returning to the clinic monthly for checkups.
>
> *Mrs. Perkins:* I feel frustrated, and I'm tired of being fat.
> *Nurse:* When I saw you last month you told me you had lost 10 pounds and your clothes fit better. I can tell the difference.
> *Mrs. Perkins:* You're right, but it takes so much time to lose weight. I just get down on myself. ■

Immediacy. The nurse focuses interaction on the present situation between nurse and client. Clients learn to understand how they interact with others. This involves drawing attention to clients' behavior or statements. The following example demonstrates immediacy.

> *Nurse:* As we've talked, you've seemed distant.
> *Client:* Um-hm.
> *Nurse:* Perhaps you are upset since I was not able to come talk with you as soon as I had promised.
> *Client:* Well, I had been looking forward to talking with you yesterday.

Self-Disclosure. The nurse reveals personal experiences, thoughts, ideas, values, or feelings in context of the relationship. This is not therapy for the nurse. It shows clients that their experiences can be understood. The following dialog illustrates self-disclosure:

> **CASE STUDY**   Ms. Wells' mother died just a month before. Since then, she has had difficulty with following her diet.
>
> *Nurse:* This has been a difficult time for you.
> *Ms. Wells:* It seems as though my world's collapsed.
> *Nurse:* Three years ago I lost my mother. It was a very difficult time. I often struggled, but I had to get on with my life. ■

Integrating Communication With Nursing Actions. Nursing actions can generally be divided into four groups: physiological, psychological, spiritual, and socioeconomic. Physiological actions that attend to a client's physical needs, such as nutrition, elimination, and comfort, have high visibility. Most physiological actions are nonverbal and routinely performed. Traditionally, emphasis has been placed on a nurse's ability to perform physiological actions. Their high visibility allows the client to recognize the nurse as a good practitioner.

In contrast, psychological, socioeconomic, and spiritual nursing actions have low visibility. Psychological actions serve emotional needs. Socioeconomic actions, such as referring clients to community health agencies, assist clients in adapting to an environment. Spiritual actions help clients gain support for their belief systems. Low-visibility tasks are not readily observed or measured by others. Psychological, socioeconomic, and spiritual actions require cognitive and affective skills that are not routine and have traditionally led to less reward for the nurse.

Communication is important in performing both high- and low-visibility tasks (Fig. 14-4). Giving emotional support or educating the client's family obviously requires effective communication, but basic nursing care procedures do too. The following case study shows how the nurse can integrate communication with nursing actions.

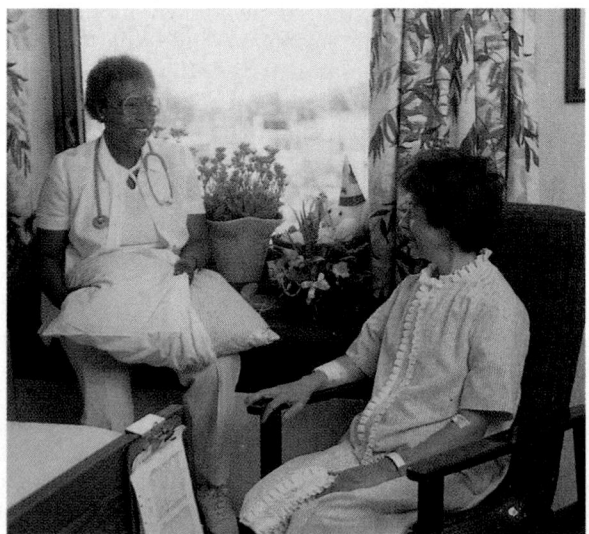

Fig. 14-4 The nurse integrates therapeutic communication skills into all aspects of care.

The nurse silently enters Mr. Richards' room and tells him, "It's time for your pain shot." He is mildly startled and grimaces as he turns. As Mr. Richards starts to ask a question, the nurse quickly reaches for his arm and prepares to inject the needle.

In contrast, a second nurse, Mr. Ives, enters Mr. Richards' room and says, "I have that pain medication you requested. Are you still feeling uncomfortable?" He turns and replies, "Yes, my back feels like a knife went through it. Will the pain ever go away?" Mr. Ives lays the syringe on the table, sits down next to Mr. Richards, and says, "It's normal to have pain the first day or two after surgery. Let me give you that shot, and then I can show you how to move more carefully in bed to avoid worsening the pain." ∎

Through communication, a nurse can convey the confidence, credibility, and knowledge that clients expect. In this example a few words of concern and reassurance (low-visibility communication skills) make receiving an injection more acceptable and encourage Mr. Richards to express his feelings.

Communication facilitates all nursing care measures. Integrating high- and low-visibility tasks allows Mr. Ives to accomplish several goals simultaneously. He quickly and efficiently assesses Mr. Richards' pain, provides a reassuring explanation, and demonstrates an alternative way of relieving pain. Therapeutic communication during high-visibility tasks increases the client's acceptance and understanding of procedures, lessens anxiety, and improves the client's satisfaction and willingness to cooperate.

TERMINATION

During the orientation phase, the nurse tells the client when to expect the relationship to end. When termination occurs, the client should not be surprised. By remaining aware of goals of the relationship, the client should be prepared to function effectively without the nurse's support. Termination can nonetheless be difficult and painful for the client. The primary objective at the end of any helping relationship is termination in a planned and satisfying manner. Summarizing accomplishments and reviewing any unmet needs or follow-up care are helpful.

Evaluation of Goal Achievement. Vital to termination is evaluation of goals. The nurse encourages assessment of the appropriateness and outcome of goals established. The following case study shows communication to evaluate goals.

Mrs. Mercado has worked with the client, Mr. Adams, during his stay in the hospital. Mr. Adams had surgery for repair of a fractured leg. Together, Mrs. Mercado and Mr. Adams set goals for his physical rehabilitation and return home.

Mrs. Mercado: Well, Mr. Adams, your doctor has discharged you for tomorrow morning. How do you feel about going home?
Mr. Adams: Oh, I'll be glad to get out of here. My leg feels pretty good.
Mrs. Mercado: Do you feel comfortable walking with the crutches?
Mr. Adams: Yes, I do. As you suggested, I practiced climbing stairs quite a bit in physical therapy. As you know, I have five stairs to climb up to my front door. I can climb them now without losing my balance.
Mrs. Mercado: You've also worked hard on learning to transfer from the bed and chair to a standing position with the crutches.
Mr. Adams: It's a lot easier now. All the practice you suggested helped. Since you've explained all of the right ways to hold the crutches, they feel like a natural part of me. I do hope I can get rid of them soon though.
Mrs. Mercado: Well, it sounds like you're ready to leave. Continue your leg exercises as you've done them here, and soon you won't need those crutches.
Mr. Adams: Thanks again for your help. I didn't think I'd ever be able to walk with these things, but now the crutches are no problem. ∎

Both Mrs. Mercado and Mr. Adams experience satisfaction in meeting goals, particularly because the goals are mutually set. If goals are left unaccomplished, the reasons are examined, and plans are made for attainment in the future. Mr. Adams has not achieved the ability to walk without his crutches. Mrs. Mercado encourages him to continue his exercise regimen so that he will become strong enough to walk independently.

Separation. Depending on the relationship between nurse and client, the client may have feelings of anxiety or ambivalence as termination nears. Ideally the client expresses feelings regarding termination. The nurse plans time to allow the client to share concerns or fears.

If the client remains in the health care setting and the nurse is the one leaving as a result of a scheduled day off or vacation, the client may feel abandoned. The nurse makes sure the client's care is uninterrupted by introducing the new nurse or communicating the client's needs with a written care plan. The nurse shares information that might foster the development of a helping relationship between other nurses and the client.

∎ COMMUNICATION AND THE NURSING PROCESS

Communication is important to the nursing process. A nurse uses communication skills during each step of the process (see the box on p. 252). Assessment, nursing diagnosis, planning, implementation, and evaluation of a client's care depend on effective communication between the nurse, client, family, and health care team. Through communication a nurse and client come to an agreement about how to meet the goals of care successfully. These functions are part of the ongoing nursing process.

Communication is also important when caring for clients with communication problems. If clients are unable to interact with people because of illness, developmental delays, physical limitations imposed by therapy, or emotional reasons, the nurse encourages communication. The nurse uses the nursing process to ensure that clients communicate in a meaningful and effective way.

 Assessment

Assessment can begin with a review of factors that influence communication. The client's developmental level,

Communication Through the Nursing Process

ASSESSMENT
- Interviewing and history taking
- Physical examination (use of visual, auditory, and tactile channels)
- Observation of nonverbal behavior
- Review of medical records, literature, diagnostic tests

NURSING DIAGNOSIS
- Written analysis of assessment findings
- Discussion of health care needs and priorities with client and family

PLANNING
- Written care plans
- Health team planning sessions
- Discussions with client and family to determine methods of implementation
- Making referrals

IMPLEMENTATION
- Discussion with other health professionals
- Health teaching
- Provision of therapeutic support
- Contact with other health resources
- Record of client's progress in care plan and nurse's notes

EVALUATION
- Acquisition of verbal and nonverbal feedback
- Written results of expected outcomes
- Update of written care plan
- Explanation of revisions to client

Table 14-2	Assessment of Physical Communication Barriers	
SPEECH AND LANGUAGE MECHANISMS	**ALTERATIONS AFFECTING SPEECH**
Respiratory system	Extreme dyspnea (shortness of breath)
	Artificial airways: endotracheal tube or tracheostomy
	Laryngectomy (surgical removal of larynx)
Oral and nasal cavities	Cleft palate
	Loose-fitting dentures
	Neurological disease affecting articulation (e.g., parkinsonism)
Speech center	Aphasia related to cerebrovascular accident (stroke) or brain tumor
Auditory system	Conduction or nerve deafness

Examples of NANDA Nursing Diagnoses Related to Communication Alterations

Impaired verbal communication *related to:*
- Physical barrier or artificial airway
- Neurological deficit
- Cultural language difference
- Developmental deficit

Ineffective individual coping *related to:*
- Situation crises
- Maturational crises

Impaired social interaction *related to:*
- Communication barriers

---

perceptions, emotions, cultural orientation, and knowledge are just a few items that the nurse must understand before planning ways to promote communication. It may be difficult to assess all of these factors if a client has physical barriers to communication. Family or friends then may become important for the nurse's assessment.

PHYSICAL AND PSYCHOLOGICAL BARRIERS TO COMMUNICATION

A client may suffer physical or psychological alterations that impair communication. To speak spontaneously and clearly, a person must have an intact respiratory system, normal oral and nasal cavities, and a functioning speech center in the cerebral cortex. Normal reception of language requires an intact auditory system. In the case of a child, the nurse assesses a child's ability to communicate, including the observation of sounds, gestures, and vocabulary expressed. When an adult develops hearing problems later in life, the ability to receive and understand messages is impaired. Review of medical history and physical assessment provide clues to the client's physical ability to communicate (Table 14-2). Physical barriers cause loss of speech, impaired articulation, or inability to find or name words. Neurological impairments such as cerebral palsy or autism may prevent the development of normal speech or receptive language skills. Such disabilities require the use of alternative communication forms such as wordboards, computers, and signed speech.

The nurse should also consider whether clients are taking medication that impairs speech. Some medications, such as antidepressants, neuroleptics, or sedatives, may cause a client to slur words or use incomplete sentences. The nurse should be familiar with common side effects of such medications.

Some psychological illnesses such as psychosis or depression influence the ability to communicate. The client may demonstrate flight of ideas, constant verbalization of the same words or phrases, or a loose association of ideas. The nurse must isolate psychological causes of speech problems from possible neurological causes.

 ## Nursing Diagnosis

The inability to communicate effectively influences a client's ability to express needs or react to the environment. After collecting assessment data the nurse clusters pertinent defining characteristics for patterns of problems. The nurse's success in identifying the client's communication problem will ensure the formulation of an accurate nursing diagnosis (see the nursing diagnoses box on p. 252). The related diagnostic factor should focus on the cause of the communication disorder so that appropriate interventions are chosen (see the diagnostic process box below). For example, an elderly client who has had a stroke and has aphasia would lead the nurse to develop a diagnosis such as impaired verbal communication related to altered expression, comprehension, or a combination of the two. An accurate related factor must be defined. Different interventions would be used if the nature of the problem were expression rather than comprehension.

The nurse may also diagnose problems in clients who have difficulty with interacting with other persons. In these situations the client's difficulty of expression or a change in communication patterns leads the nurse to make a diagnosis.

Planning

Effective communication takes practice and concentration. The nurse makes a conscious effort at considering ways to help clients and families communicate thoughts and feelings more effectively. Planning an appropriate place and organizing care to allow sufficient time are essential. Consideration must also be given to interventions and communication techniques appropriate for the client's age and culture. Communication aids, such as a writing board for a client with a tracheostomy or a special call light for a client who is paralyzed, may be useful. The nurse also needs to identify family members and other members of the health care team to whom communication problems can be referred or from whom the nurse can seek assistance in designing appropriate communication strategies. Some referrals might include the speech therapist for the client experiencing **aphasia** (neurological condition in which language function is defective or absent), an interpreter for a client who speaks a foreign language, or a psychiatric liaison nurse for the angry or highly anxious client.

It is especially important to have the client make decisions about the care plan. A person must feel comfortable and willing to communicate if effective interaction is to occur.

Success in promoting a client's ability to communicate depends not only on the client's participation in goal setting but also on the nurse's style of communication and the ability to establish a helping relationship. The use of therapeutic communication skills allows the nurse to perceive, react to, and respect the client's uniqueness. Successful interpersonal communication meets the following goals of care for a client:

1. It transmits clear, concise, and understandable messages.
2. The client gains a sense of trust in the nurse as a care giver.
3. The nurse and client send and receive feedback.

After goals are mutually determined, expected outcomes are designated, and specific interventions are planned (see the care plan on p. 254).

Implementation

With all clients the nurse tries to develop a helping therapeutic relationship. Clients will then feel more comfortable in interaction despite communication alterations.

DEVELOPING SOCIAL SKILLS

If ineffective coping or impaired social interaction is present, the nurse's interventions focus on helping clients do the following:

1. Express feelings and needs
2. Develop conversational skills
3. Communicate thoughts and feelings clearly (verbally and nonverbally)
4. Demonstrate assertiveness
5. Solve problems
6. Facilitate conversation with peers and staff

A nurse who has more experience with communication skills and interpersonal dynamics may assist clients through role playing. This allows clients to practice situations in which they have difficulty communicating. The following simple interventions can also be used to reinforce attempts at interaction:

1. Encourage participation in normal social activities
2. Discuss neutral topics or subjects in which clients have interests
3. Give positive reinforcement for acceptable social interactions
4. Help clients identify persons with whom they feel comfortable and encourage activities with them
5. Change bed or room assignments (in hospital) to encourage friendships or associates with same interests
6. Minimize clients' idle time

Sample Nursing Diagnostic Process for Communication Alterations

ASSESSMENT ACTIVITIES	DEFINING CHARACTERISTICS	NURSING DIAGNOSIS
Observe whether client speaks spontaneously	Unable to speak English	**Impaired verbal communication** related to cultural differences (inability to speak English)
Ask client to read menu and describe the items preferred	Inability to recognize/understand words	
Review with family to determine client's primary language	Cultural differences	

Sample Nursing Care Plan for Impaired Verbal Communication

NURSING DIAGNOSIS: **Impaired verbal communication** related to cultural differences, English as a second language.
DEFINITION: Impaired verbal communication is the state in which an individual experiences a decreased or absent ability to attend and respond to messages others send (Haber et al, 1994).

GOAL	EXPECTED OUTCOMES	INTERVENTIONS	RATIONALE
Client will express basic needs with minimal anxiety and frustration.	Client will utilize alternative methods to communicate. Client will use English phrases.	Talk clearly and slowly, using simple, short sentences.	This allows the client to stay focused on one idea when client's vocabulary is limited to yes/no, using short simple questions aids in accurate responses.
		Use attentive listening.	Listening enables the nurse to understand the message that the client is sending and also facilitates the nurse/client relationship.
		Use alternative method of communication, including communication board with English and corresponding Spanish words, and use of interpreter.	Mutual understanding of communication can be enhanced by both verbal and written messages. Important information should be written down for review and use by other health care members. (Gulanick et al, 1994).
		Encourage client and family to teach staff some Spanish words that can be used in basic care or in greetings.	Communication that is familiar to the client diminishes misunderstandings between nurse and client (Barkauskas et al, 1994).
		Utilize nonverbal cues with verbal message.	Nonverbal communication is much stronger in relaying a message to a client. Facial movements, eye contact, and body position add feelings to the verbal message (Davies P, 1994).

Techniques and Tools to Enhance Communication

Communication boards with words, letters, or pictures denoting basic needs (toilet, water)
Paper and pencil, pen, magic marker to allow expression of needs or thoughts
Use of interpreter for sign language or for clients with English as a second language
Involve family and friends in care delivery as appropriate
Keep call bell or light system within reach
Use of nonverbal gestures such as eye blinks or finger movements for yes/no responses
Use words that the client can understand, avoid medical terminology
Keep environment quiet and free from distractions
Always be an attentive listener

CONTROLLING THE ENVIRONMENT

If an environment is uncomfortable or distracting, a client will have difficulty with communicating, regardless of the problem. The nurse can control the environment so that it is conducive to interpersonal interactions. Methods of environmental control include the following:

1. Regulating room temperature to a comfortable level
2. Eliminating or reducing loud noises in the room (e.g., radio or equipment alarm)
3. Making the client comfortable
4. Asking other staff members or family (if appropriate) not to enter room during interaction
5. Reducing bright or glaring light

COMMUNICATING WITH CLIENTS WITH SPECIAL NEEDS

At times, it is necessary for nurses to use special communication techniques for successful nurse-client interactions. Clients with sensory and motor impairments, as well as children and older adults, require individualized approaches to communication.

Providing Alternate Communication Methods. Clients with physical communication barriers (e.g., a client with a laryngectomy or endotracheal tube) may be unable to speak, or clarity of speech is so poor that alternate methods of communication are needed (see the box on p. 254). For these clients the nurse provides methods that are simple to use. Anything complicated can be frustrating and make communication more difficult. The nurse is patient as the client tries to communicate. The client must be physically able to use the method that the nurse provides. Clients must have the communication board or pencil and pad nearby. A client who is unable to speak can be at risk for injury unless personal needs can be quickly communicated.

Communicating With a Child. Communication with a child requires special considerations so that the nurse can develop a working relationship with both the child and family. The nurse receives much information from parents. Because contact between parent and child is usually close, information communicated by parents can be assumed to be reliable. However, some parents may exaggerate. If the client is a young child, it helps to offer toys or materials for play so that the parent can give full attention to the nurse. The nurse gives periodic attention to infants and younger children as they play to make them participants. An older child can be actively involved in communication (see the box below).

Children, particularly the very young, are especially responsive to nonverbal messages. Sudden movements or threatening gestures can frighten them. The nurse walking into an examination room with a broad grin and animated hand movements might inhibit formation of a relationship. The nurse should remain calm and gentle. It helps to let children make the first moves in interpersonal contacts. A quiet, friendly, confident tone of voice is best.

Children dislike being stared at. Adults looking down on them make them feel vulnerable. While communicating with young children, the nurse should meet them at eye level. Children often feel helpless in most situations involving interaction with health care personnel (Whaley and Wong, 1995).

When it is necessary to give explanations or directions, the nurse uses simple, direct language. The nurse must be honest with children. Deceiving children into thinking painful procedures are painless will only make them angry. To minimize fear and anxiety, the nurse should always tell children what to expect immediately before a procedure.

Drawing and play are two effective ways to communicate with young children. Drawing provides an opportunity for them to communicate nonverbally (by making drawings) and verbally (by explaining pictures). The nurse can use children's drawings as bases for initiating conversation. Techniques for communicating with children also vary with age.

Communicating With Older Adults. Communication processes with older adults require special attention. The nurse must be aware of the physical, psychological, emotional, and social changes of aging that influence communication patterns. Age-related changes in the auditory system can result in impaired hearing. Changes in the middle and inner ear predispose the elderly to be intolerant of loud

---

Focuses for Communicating With Children

INFANT (0-1 YEAR)
- The infant communicates primarily nonverbally (e.g., coos, cries) because the infant is unable to use words.
- Infants respond to care giver's nonverbal behavior. They become quiet with close physical contact.
- Infants attain comfort from the sound of a soft voice though words are not understood.
- Loud, harsh sounds and sudden firm handling frighten the infant.
- Older infants (6 months) experience separation anxiety; therefore the parents should be in view while infant is being held by stranger.

TODDLER (1-3 YEARS)
OR PRESCHOOLER (3-5 YEARS)
- The child communicates verbally and nonverbally.
- The child is egocentric and understands things only related to self.
- The child is unable to distinguish fact from fantasy.
- The child understands analogies only in a literal sense (e.g., "coughing your head off").
- The child should be allowed to explore the environment (e.g., handle a stethoscope).
- The child understands simple, short sentences, familiar words and concrete explanations.

SCHOOL-AGE CHILD (5-12 YEARS)
- The child seeks reasons and explanations for everything but requires no validation.
- The child is interested in functional aspects of objects and events. (What is going to occur, why it is being performed.)
- The child is concerned with body integrity.
- The child should be allowed to manipulate equipment (e.g., hold a percussion hammer).
- The child understands simple explanations and demonstrations.
- The child should be allowed to express fears and questions.

ADOLESCENT (13-18 YEARS)
- Adolescents think more abstractly, fluctuating between childlike and adult thinking behavior.
- The nurse should avoid imposing values or judgments.
- Adolescents should be allowed to talk about their feelings.
- Adolescents avoid answering (the nurse should avoid embarrassing questions).
- Adolescents are willing to discuss concerns with adults outside of family.
- Adolescents use a language of their own; unfamiliar terms should be clarified with the adolescent.
- Clarification of adolescent's and parents' point of view essential.

Modified from Wong DL: *Whaley and Wong's nursing care of infants and children*, ed 5, St Louis, 1995, Mosby.

GERONTOLOGICAL PRINCIPLES
for Communication

Keep noise levels to a minimum.
Be an attentive listener! Allow time for conversation.
Ensure proper functioning hearing aid devices (check battery and fit).
Make sure glasses are clean and well-fitting.
Do not speak loudly or shout, direct conversation to the better hearing ear. Stand in front of the client.
Keep sentences short and simple.
Allow the opportunity for the client to reminisce.
Encourage involvement in social activities such as senior centers, church functions.
Make referrals to speech therapy and social services as appropriate.
Talk at the client's level of understanding.
Always ask for feedback, especially when teaching a task or skill.

Modified from Ebersole P, Hess P: *Toward healthy aging*, ed 4, St Louis, 1994, Mosby.

noise and cause problems associated with high and low frequency sound discrimination (Ebersole and Hess, 1994). Impairment of the otic nerve often causes a conditon known as *tinnitus*, which produces a constant ringing sound in the ear. Motor disturbance such as dysarthria interfere with the clarity of pronunciation. Visual acuity and accommodation change as a normal part of aging. This process interferes with nonverbal communication as the older adult experiences difficulty in differentiating fine writing or similar objects. Glaucoma, cataracts, macular degeneration, and other disease-related conditions may affect the vision of the older adult.

Social barriers such as loss of spouse or significant others impair communication pathways. Ebersole and Hess (1994) discuss social concerns of compromised finances, travel expenses, and social activities as barriers to communication

for the elder. The nurse must also take into consideration that dentures are proper fitting, glasses are clean and secure, and hearing aid devices are properly functioning to facilitate communication (see Chapter 39). When obvious deficits exist, the nurse maximizes existing motor and sensory function so that the client can communicate more effectively (see the box at left).

Communicating With the Unconscious Client. Even when persons are unconscious or nonresponsive, they may be able to receive stimuli. Hearing is thought to be the last sensation lost with unconsciousness and the first to be regained with consciousness. Therefore nurses need to be careful not to say anything to unconscious clients or within their hearing range that they would not say to fully conscious clients. Other important nursing interventions include talking with the client while providing care; explaining procedures; providing orientation information, such as the nurse's name, place, date, and time of day; and avoiding bedside conversations with others about the client.

Evaluation

Evaluating whether communication has been therapeutic aids a client in improving communication, and it improves the nurse-client relationship. The nurse evaluates nursing interventions based on the previously established client goals to determine whether strategies or interventions were effective and what client changes resulted because of the interventions.

Successful communication is evaluated by the nurse's observations of client interactions. The nurse not only determines that communication exists, but also that the client appears satisfied that the message was received. For example, the nurse might ask the following questions:

1. Does the client appear more physically comfortable?
2. Does the client talk about feelings, reactions, and thoughts, or was conversation superficial?
3. Were the appropriate team members consulted?

Nurses compare actual outcomes with expected outcomes when determining the success or effect of interven-

Sample Evaluation of Interventions for Impaired Verbal Communication

GOALS	EVALUATIVE MEASURES	EXPECTED OUTCOMES
Client will express basic needs clearly by 10/1.	Observe client use communication board. Ask family to question client about whether needs have been met.	Client will use alternate method of communication by 9/29.
Client sends clear, concise, and understandable messages by discharge from intensive care unit.	Observe client's interactions with nurse and family. Confirm meaning of client's message by paraphrasing it.	Client will use English phrases by second day after surgery. Client voluntarily discusses thoughts or feelings with the nurse by second visit.
Client gains a sense of trust in the nurse as care giver by third home visit.	Observe client's openness and willingness to discuss personal thoughts or feelings.	Client expresses accomplishment of goals of relationship by third visit. Client shares feelings about termination of helping relationship by third visit.

tions (see the evaluation box on p. 256). It is also useful for nurses to evaluate the effectiveness of their own unique communication styles and techniques frequently and to make periodic written "process recordings" of the verbal and nonverbal interactions with clients. Interactions and responses can then be examined by the nurse or the communication specialist. Some questions that could be asked during such examinations follow:

1. Did nurses encourage openness and allow the client to express thoughts and tell the story?

2. Did responses block the client's efforts? If so, how?
3. Were responses supportive or critical, opinionated, or trite?
4. Were open-ended or closed-ended questions used? Were they used appropriately?
5. How could communication be more effective?

If expected outcomes are not met or progress is not satisfactory according to the client, the nurse needs to reassess and modify the plan of care.

■ KEY CONCEPTS ■

▶ Effective communication is the process that allows nurses to establish working relationships with clients.

▶ Successful communication requires the message intended by the speaker to be similar or identical to the meaning acquired by the receiver.

▶ Words that have different connotative meanings can be easily misinterpreted by the person receiving the message.

▶ Effective verbal communication requires clear and concise phrasing of words, a proper pacing of statements, and an understandable vocabulary.

▶ Communication is the means by which the nurse helps clients adjust to changes imposed by illness.

▶ A nurse uses selective communication skills when interacting with clients and all members of the health care team.

▶ Trust, empathy, caring, autonomy, and mutuality are basic dimensions of a helping nurse-client relationship.

▶ The working phase of a helping relationship involves the nurse and client working together so that the client can express thoughts and feelings freely and constructively.

▶ Clients with physical communication barriers may be able to express themselves more effectively with communication aids.

▶ Clients with ineffective social skills may benefit from positive reinforcement and encouragement to participate in interactions.

■ KEY TERMS ■

Aphasia, p. 253
Assertiveness, p. 243
Autonomy, p. 247
Caring, p. 247
Channels, p. 234
Clarification, p. 242
Communication, p. 233
Connotative, p. 235

Denotative, p. 235
Empathy, p. 246
Feedback, p. 234
Focusing, p. 242
Interpersonal communication, p. 233
Intrapersonal communication, p. 233
Listening, p. 241
Message, p. 234
Metacommunication, p. 236
Mutuality, p. 247
Nonverbal communication, p. 236
Paraphrasing, p. 242
Perception, p. 238
Proxemics, p. 240
Public communication, p. 233
Receiver, p. 234
Referent, p. 233
Sender, p. 233
Stereotypes, p. 245
Summarization, p. 244
Verbal communication, p. 234

■ CRITICAL THINKING EXERCISES ■

Juan Acaro, a refugee of Cuba, is admitted to the cardiology unit for severe chest pain. Juan speaks only minimal English and his wife speaks only Spanish. While obtaining the nursing admission data, the nurse recognizes Juan is very anxious. He does not maintain eye contact and is reluctant to participate with physical contact during his examination.

1. Discuss different modes of communication and how they would relate to a client with a cultural variation.

2. What are four types of physical communication barriers?

3. Identify communication aids that may be used for a client with a communication barrier.

4. Discuss communication skills used by the nurse with Juan during the nursing process.

REFERENCES

Barkauskas V et al: *Health and physical assessment*, St Louis, 1994, Mosby.

Beare P, Myers J: *Principles and practices of adult health nursing*, ed 2, St Louis, 1994, Mosby.

Bergbom-Engberg I, Haljamäe H: The communication process with ventilator patients in the ICU as perceived by the nursing staff, *Intens Crit Care Nurs* 9:40, 1993.

Bradley J, Edinberg MA: *Communication in the nursing context*, ed 3, Norwalk, 1990, Appleton and Lange.

Davies P: Non-verbal communication with patients, *Br J Nurs* 3(5):220, 1994.

Ebersole P, Hess P: *Toward healthy aging,* ed 4, St Louis, 1994, Mosby.

Ekman P: Communication through nonverbal behavior: a source of information about an interpersonal relationship. In Tomkins SS, Izard CE, editors: *Affect, cognition, and personality*, New York, 1965, Springer.

Gulanick M et al: *Nursing care plans: nursing diagnosis and intervention*, ed 3, St Louis, 1994, Mosby.

Haber et al: *Comprehensive psychiatric nursing*, ed 4, St Louis, 1994, Mosby.

Hall ET: *The hidden dimension*, New York, 1969, Doubleday.

Keltner N, Schwecke L, Bostrom C: *Psychiatric nursing: a psychiatric management approach*, St Louis, 1991, Mosby.

Stanhope M, Lancaster J: *Community health nursing: process and practice for promoting health*, ed 4, St Louis, 1996, Mosby.

Tannen D: *You just don't understand: women and men in conversation*, New York, 1990, Morrow.

Whaley L, Wong D: *Nursing care of infants and children*, ed 5, St Louis, 1995, Mosby.

Wootsen P: For the health of it, *J Nurs Jocularity* 4(3):41, 1993.

ADDITIONAL READINGS

Armstrong M, Kelly A: Enhancing staff nurses' interpersonal skills: theory to practice, *Clin Nurs Spec* 7(6):313, 1993.

Case B: Walking around the elephant: a critical-thinking strategy for decision making, *J Cont Educ Nurs* 25(3):101, 1994.

Davidhizar R, Shearer R: Soft-spoken managers: a blend of communication styles, *Nurs Manage* 24(7):112L, 1993.

Dellasega C et al: Nursing process: teaching elderly clients, *J Gerontological Nurs* 20(1):31, 1994.

Fiesta J: Duty to communicate—"doctor notified", *Nurs Manage* 25(1):24, 1994.

Johnson L, Mattson S: Communication: the key to crisis prevention in pediatric death, *Crit Care Nurs* 12(8):23, 1992.

Karshmer J: Nine rules of thumb to make communications work, *Nurs Manage* 23(11):80I, 1992.

Manzano J et al: Verbal communication of ventilator-dependent patients, *Crit Care Med* 21(4):512, 1993.

Price MM: Nursing potpourri: one unit's way of sharing needed information, *Crit Care Nurs* 13(5):95, 1993.

Prim R: Communication: coping with the unspoken dance, *Nurs Manage* 24(3):33, 1993.

Sharp N: Nurses link up to high-speed communication network, *Nurs Manage* 24(5):16, 1993.

Moore LN, Proffitt C: Communicating effectively with elderly surgical patients, *AORN J* 58(2):345, 1993.

## Chapter 15

Teaching-Learning Process

Objectives

Mastery of content in this chapter will enable the student to:

- ► Define the key terms listed.
- ► Identify a client's health promotion and restoration needs.
- ► Describe the similarities and differences between teaching and learning.
- ► Identify the purposes of client education.
- ► Describe how to incorporate communication principles into the teaching-learning process.
- ► Describe the domains of learning.
- ► Differentiate factors that determine the readiness to learn from those that determine the ability to learn.

- ► Compare the nursing and teaching processes.
- ► Write learning objectives for a teaching plan.
- ► Describe characteristics of a good learning environment.
- ► Identify principles of effective teaching.
- ► Describe ways to adapt teaching for clients with different learning needs.
- ► Describe ways to incorporate teaching with routine nursing care.
- ► Identify methods for evaluating learning.

Client education has become one of the most important roles for nurses working in any health care setting. Teaching prenatal care to healthy mothers in a physician's office, instructing clients visiting a clinic about immunization of children, and teaching heart attack victims about newly prescribed medications are all examples of client education. Clients and family members have the right to health education so that they are able to make intelligent, informed decisions about their health and lifestyle. Many clients now receive many treatments in their homes or in an outpatient setting or, if they are hospitalized, they are discharged earlier (Kruger, 1991). Effective health education is essential to care for increasing numbers of clients in the community and to minimize the effects of preventable disease (Noble, 1991).

Shorter hospital stays, increased demands on nurses' time, and the need to give seriously ill clients concise, meaningful information as soon as possible emphasize the importance of quality client education (Bull, 1992). As nurses try to find the best way to educate clients, the general public has become more assertive in seeking knowledge and understanding of their health and the resources available within the health care system (Kruger, 1991). Providing clients with needed information about health care is necessary to ensure continuity of care from the hospital to the home (Bull, 1992). A well-designed, comprehensive teaching plan, which fits a client's learning needs, can reduce health care costs, improve the quality of care, and help clients gain optimum wellness and increased independence.

The significance of client education is enhanced because of the client's right to know and to be informed about diagnosis, prognosis, treatments, and risks. Educational materials provided should be readily understandable. It is negligent to assume that clients will learn on their own. Accurate, timely teaching is needed for clients to make decisions about their health and improve their overall health status. More attention is being paid in courts of law as to whether clients are adequately informed about ways to manage their health. Competent professional nursing practice includes client education. The nurse can provide adequate education only by identifying clients' learning needs and by using the most appropriate teaching strategies.

■ STANDARDS FOR CLIENT EDUCATION

Client education has long been a standard for professional nursing practice. According to Virginia Henderson (1966), part of a nurse's role is to "improve the patient's level of understanding and therefore promote health." Accrediting agencies in the United States and Canada set guidelines for providing client education in health care institutions (Barnes, 1993; American Association of Diabetes Educators, 1992). The guidelines ensure that the client and family receive information necessary to maintain the client's opti-

---

Client Education Standards

STRUCTURE
Standards in regard to structure relate to human and material resources, including administration and management of the health care agency. Nurses in both staff and administrative roles should contribute to their development and implementation.

STANDARD 1
The health care agency has a philosophy, goals, and objectives that reflect its mandate and provide direction for client education.

STANDARD 2
Client education is integrated into all areas of nursing practice in the health care system.

STANDARD 3
The nursing department of the health care agency is active in developing a comprehensive plan for client education.

STANDARD 4
An individual/department is responsible for facilitating and coordinating matters of client education.

PROCESS
Process standards outline criteria by which client education is delivered. The educational process includes the same steps as the nursing process.

STANDARD 1
The primary focus of the educational process is the client.

STANDARD 2
An educational assessment is done by the nurse in collaboration with the client.

STANDARD 3
The nurse demonstrates planning in the educational process.

STANDARD 4
The nurse applies principles of the educational process in implementation of client education.

STANDARD 5
A written outline of the educational process is available as a communication tool, a resource to health professionals, and as a record.

OUTCOME
Outcome standards are the criteria to measure results of the educational process.

STANDARD 1
The nurse evaluates the educational process.

STANDARD 2
The client participates in evaluating the educational process.

From the Alberta Association of Registered Nurses: *Client education: position statement and guidelines,* 1985, Edmonton, Alberta, Canada, 1986, The Association.

mal level of health. In the United States the Joint Commission on Accreditation of Healthcare Organizations (JCAHO) (1995) describes the following standards for client/family education:

1. The client/family are provided with education that can enhance knowledge, skills, and behaviors that are necessary to benefit fully from the health care interventions provided by the organization.
2. The organization plans and supports the provision and coordination of client/family education activities and resources.
3. Clients/families have their learning needs, capabilities, and readiness to learn assessed.
4. The client/family educational process is interdisciplinary, as appropriate to the plan of care.
5. The client/family receive education specific to the client's assessed needs, capabilities, and readiness. Such education includes medication administration, use of medical equipment, knowledge about food/drug interactions and diet modification, rehabilitation, and how to obtain further treatment.
6. Information about any discharge instructions given to the client/family is provided to the organization or individual responsible for the continuing care of the client.

The successful accomplishment of these standards depends on participation of all health care professionals. Evidence of successful client education must be noted in the client's medical record.

In 1986, the Alberta Association of Registered Nurses developed a set of client education standards (see the box on p. 260) that address the educational process related to adult clients. The standards help to direct nurses in client education.

■ PURPOSES FOR CLIENT EDUCATION

Nursing's Agenda for Health Care Reform by the American Nurses Association (ANA) (1991) recommends a restructuring of the health care system, focusing on wellness and care rather than illness and cure. The emphasis is on maintaining health. Clients now know more about health and want to be involved in health maintenance. Nursing needs to provide education so that clients receive information about care in more convenient and familiar places (ANA, 1991). Comprehensive client education includes three important purposes, each involving a separate phase of health care (see the box below).

Maintenance and Promotion of Health and Illness Prevention

The public has recently become more health conscious. Participation in fitness clubs, diet programs, regular exercise activities, and health screening programs are examples of ways people pay more attention to their health.

The nurse is a visible, competent resource for clients intent on improving physical and psychological well-being. In the school, home, clinic, or workplace, the nurse provides information and skills that will allow clients to assume healthier behaviors (see the box below). For example, in childbearing classes, nurses teach expectant parents about physical and psychological changes in the woman and about fetal development. After learning about normal childbearing, the mother is more likely to eat healthy foods, engage in physical exercise, and avoid substances that might harm the fetus. Promoting healthy behavior through education increases self-esteem by allowing clients to assume more responsibility for their health. Greater knowledge can result in better health maintenance habits. When clients become more health conscious, they are

---

Topics for Health Education

HEALTH MAINTENANCE AND PROMOTION AND ILLNESS PREVENTION
- First aid
- Avoidance of risk factors (e.g., smoking, alcohol)
- Stress management
- Growth and development
- Hygiene
- Immunizations
- Prenatal care and normal childbearing
- Nutrition
- Exercise
- Safety (in home and hospital)
- Screening (e.g., blood pressure, vision, cholesterol level)

RESTORATION OF HEALTH
- Client's disease or condition
  - Anatomy and physiology of body system affected
  - Cause of disease
  - Origin of symptoms
  - Expected effects on other body systems
  - Prognosis
  - Limitations on function
  - Rationale for treatment
  - Medications
  - Tests and therapies

- Nursing measures
- Surgical intervention
- Expected duration of care
- Hospital or clinic environment
- Hospital or clinic staff
- Long-term care
- Methods for client participation in care
- Limitations posed by disease or surgery

COPING WITH IMPAIRED FUNCTIONS
- Home care
  - Medications
  - Intravenous therapy
  - Diet
  - Activity
  - Self-help devices
- Rehabilitation of remaining function
  - Physical therapy
  - Occupational therapy
  - Speech therapy
- Prevention of complications
  - Knowledge of risk factors
  - Implications of noncompliance with therapy
  - Environmental alterations

more likely to seek early diagnosis of health problems (Redman, 1993).

> **CASE STUDY** Mr. Sim's father died of complications of a malignant melanoma. Mr. Sims routinely wears sunblock and performs regular skin assessments. Noticing the growth of a mole on his thigh, Mr. Sims immediately sought medical attention, the mole was surgically removed, and Mr. Sims enjoyed a favorable health outcome. ■

Restoration of Health

Injured or ill clients need information and skills that will help them regain or maintain their levels of health (see the box on p. 261). Clients who are recovering from illness or injury and are adapting to the resultant changes often seek information about their conditions. However, clients who find it difficult to adapt to illness may become passive and uninterested in learning. The nurse learns to identify clients' willingness to learn and helps to motivate interest.

The family is a vital part of a client's return to health and may need to know as much as the client. If the nurse excludes the family from a teaching plan, conflicts may arise. For example, if the family does not understand a client's need to regain independent function, their efforts may cause the client to become unnecessarily dependent and slow the client's recovery. The nurse should not assume that the family should be involved and must first assess the client-family relationship.

Coping With Impaired Functioning

Not all clients fully recover from illness or injury. Many must learn to cope with permanent health alterations. New knowledge and skills are often necessary for clients to continue activities of daily living (see the box on p. 261). For example, the client whose ability to speak is lost after surgery of the larynx learns new ways of communicating, and the client with severe heart disease learns to modify risk factors that might cause further heart damage.

In the case of serious disability, the client's family role may change; as a result, the client's family needs to understand and accept these changes. The family's ability to provide support can result from education, which begins as soon as the client's needs are identified and the family displays a willingness to help. The nurse teaches family members to assist the client with health care management, for example, giving medications and baths and applying dressings. Families of clients with alterations such as alcoholism, mental retardation, or drug dependence also learn to adapt to the emotional effects of these chronic conditions.

A nurse learns to recognize the information to teach to clients at different levels of wellness by assessing clients' needs and abilities. Learning occurs when information is practical and useful to the learner. Comparing the desired level of health with the actual state enables the nurse to plan effective teaching programs.

■ TEACHING AND LEARNING

It is impossible to separate teaching from learning. **Teaching** is an interactive process that promotes learning. It consists of a conscious, deliberate set of actions that help individuals gain new knowledge or perform new skills (Red-

man, 1993). A teacher provides information that prompts the learner to engage in activities that lead to a desired change.

Learning is the acquisition of new knowledge, attitudes, and skills through reinforced practice and experience. A client with diabetes demonstrates the technique for preparing insulin in a syringe. Preoperatively, a surgical client discusses ways to relieve postoperative pain. Generally, teaching and learning begin when a person identifies a need for knowing or acquiring an ability to do something. According to Knowles (1970), adult learning is an internal process, and there are superior conditions of learning and principles of teaching. Teaching is most effective when it responds to a learner's needs. The teacher assesses these needs by asking questions and determining the learner's interests. Interpersonal communication is essential for successful teaching.

Role of the Nurse in Teaching and Learning

Clients and their families often ask nurses for health information. A client may request information about what will happen during a procedure. Family members may question the reason for their father's pain. A school may ask for information about childhood immunization. Identification of the need for teaching is easy when clients request information. Often, however, a client's need for teaching may be less obvious.

The nurse should try to anticipate clients' needs for information based on their physical conditions or treatment plans. The nurse's responsibility is to teach the information that clients and their families need. The nurse clarifies information provided by physicians and may become the primary source of information for adjusting to health problems.

To be an effective educator, the nurse must do more than just pass on facts. The nurse must carefully determine what clients need to know and find the time when they are ready to learn. Kruger (1991) noted three areas for nurse responsibility in patient education: (1) preparation of clients receiving care (e.g., preoperative teaching, self-injection of insulin); (2) preparation of clients being discharged from a health care facility (e.g., discharge medications and procedures, potential complications that require the client to return to the physician or hospital); and (3) documentation of client education activities (e.g., noting the specific education within the client's health record, educational flow sheet, or discharge summary).

When nurses value client education and are able to implement it, clients are better prepared to assume health care responsibilities. The relationship between client education and favorable client outcomes is an important nursing research issue.

Teaching as Communication

The teaching process closely parallels the communication process (see Chapter 14). Effective teaching depends in part on effective interpersonal communication. A teacher applies each element of the communication process while imparting information to learners. Thus the teacher and student become involved in a teaching process that increases the student's knowledge and skills.

The steps of the teaching process can be compared with

Table 15-1	Comparison of Terms Used in Teaching and Communication

COMMUNICATION	TEACHING
REFERENT Idea that initiates reason for communication	Perceived need to provide person with information, establishment of relevant learning objectives by teacher
SENDER Person who conveys message to another	Teacher who performs activities aimed at assisting other person to learn
INTRAPERSONAL VARIABLES (SENDER) Knowledge, values, emotions, and sociocultural influences that affect sender's thoughts	Teacher's philosophy of education (based on learning theory); knowledge of teaching content; teaching approach; experiences in teaching; teacher's emotions and values
MESSAGE Information expressed or transmitted by sender	Content or information taught
CHANNELS Methods used to transmit message (e.g., visual, auditory, touch)	Methods used to present content (e.g., visual and auditory materials, touch, taste, smell)
RECEIVER Person to whom message is transmitted	Learner
INTRAPERSONAL VARIABLES (RECEIVER) Knowledge, values, emotions, and sociocultural influences that affect receiver's thoughts	Willingness and ability to learn (e.g., physical and emotional health, education, experience, developmental level)
FEEDBACK Information revealing that true meaning of message was received	Determination of whether learning objectives were achieved

those of the communication process (Table 15-1). In teaching, the referent is the need to provide the client with information. The client may request information, or the nurse may perceive a need for information. The nurse then identifies specific learning objectives. A **learning objective** describes what the learner will be able to do after successful instruction.

The nurse is the sender who wants to convey a message to the client. The nurse promotes learning by communicating in a language recognizable to the learner. Many intrapersonal variables influence the nurse's style and approach. The nurse's attitudes, values, emotions, and knowledge influence the way the nurse sends messages. Past experiences with teaching help the nurse choose the best way to present information.

The message or content to be taught is delivered clearly and precisely. The nurse organizes information to be taught in a logical sequence so that the client will more easily understand skills or ideas. Each lesson progresses from the simple to the more complex skills or ideas (Haire-Joshu and Houston, 1992).

The nurse may use a variety of ways to present teaching content. All the senses are channels for presenting information. The auditory channel is the simplest, as in a lecture or discussion. The learning process becomes more active and stimulating, however, when several sensory channels are used together. For example, a client with newly diagnosed heart disease will learn how to measure a pulse best by actually feeling the pulsation of an artery.

The receiver in the teaching-learning process is the learner. A number of intrapersonal variables affect motivation and ability to learn. Clients are ready to learn when they express a desire to do so and are more likely to receive the message when they understand the content. Attitudes, anxiety, and values influence the ability to understand a message. The ability to learn depends on factors such as emotional and physical health, education, stage of development, and previous knowledge.

An effective teacher provides a mechanism for evaluating the success of a teaching plan and providing feedback. Having a client demonstrate a newly learned skill and asking the client to describe the correct dosage schedule for a medication are ways to gather feedback. Feedback must show the success of the learner in achieving objectives; that is, the learner restates information or provides a return demonstration of skills learned.

DOMAINS OF LEARNING

Learning occurs in cognitive (understanding), affective (attitudes), and psychomotor (motor skills) domains. Any topic to be learned may involve all domains or only one. The nurse often works with clients who need to learn in each domain. For example, clients learn to understand about diabetes, the way that it affects the body, and ways to control blood sugar levels for healthier lifestyles (cognitive domain). In addition, clients learn to accept the long-term nature of the disease (affective domain). Many diabetic clients must also learn to administer insulin injections on a daily basis (psychomotor domain). The characteristics of learning within each domain affect the teaching and evaluation methods used. Understanding each learning domain prepares the nurse to select proper teaching techniques. However, the nurse needs to also be able to apply the basic principles of learning to any teaching method (see later section).

Cognitive Learning

Cognitive learning includes all intellectual behaviors. Bloom (1956) classifies cognitive behaviors in an ordered hierarchy. The simplest behavior is acquiring knowledge, whereas the most complex is evaluation.

KNOWLEDGE

Using knowledge is acquiring new facts or information and being able to recall them. For example, a client learns about a prescribed medication and is able to describe its purpose and potential side effects.

COMPREHENSION

Comprehension is the ability to understand the meaning of learned material. For example, the client is able to explain specifically how the new medication will improve physical condition.

APPLICATION

Application involves using abstract, newly learned ideas in concrete situations. For example, the client learns to self-administer the medication according to a meal schedule to minimize side effects.

ANALYSIS

Analysis involves relating ideas in an organized way. It allows a person to distinguish important from unimportant information. For example, the client is able to distinguish which side effects are more likely to be experienced from the medication and to compare them with the effects experienced by another person.

SYNTHESIS

Synthesis is the ability to recognize parts of information as a whole. For example, the client experiences side effects from a medication and is able to take preventive steps.

EVALUATION

Evaluation is a judgment of the worth of a body of information for a given purpose. For example, a client is able to recognize the need for more information about insulin in order to plan an exercise program.

Affective Learning

Affective learning deals with expression of feelings and acceptance of attitudes, opinions, or values. Values clarification (see Chapter 18) is an example of affective learning. The simplest behavior in the hierarchy is receiving, and the most complex is characterizing (Krathwohl et al, 1964).

RECEIVING

Receiving is being willing to attend to another person's words. For example, a woman shows a willingness to listen to a nurse explain the surgical procedure for removal of a breast.

RESPONDING

Responding involves active participation through listening and reacting verbally and nonverbally. The person feels satisfied from the response. For example, the client asks the nurse about the appearance of the incision that she will have.

VALUING

Valuing means attaching worth to an object or behavior. This is shown through the learner's behavior. The person is motivated to act out the behavior. For example, the client expresses a concern about the effect of surgery on her appearance. After surgery, the client refuses to look at the incision and wears a gown with a high neck.

ORGANIZING

Organizing is developing a value system by identifying and organizing values and resolving conflicts. For example, the client learns to accept changes created by surgery and is willing to participate in social activities.

CHARACTERIZING

Characterizing involves acting and responding with a consistent value system. The person behaves consistently when values are tested or challenged. For example, the client assumes a normal lifestyle after having breast surgery. She is able to discuss with others her positive feelings about herself.

Psychomotor Learning

Psychomotor learning involves acquiring skills that require the integration of mental and muscular activity such as the ability to walk or to use an eating utensil. The simplest behavior in the hierarchy is perception, whereas the most complex is origination (Simpson, 1972).

PERCEPTION

Perception is being aware of objects or qualities through the use of sense organs. A person associates a sensory cue with the task to perform. For example, after hearing the siren of an ambulance a person considers driving to the curb to avoid a collision.

SET

A set is a readiness to take a particular action. There are three sets: mental, physical, and emotional. For example, a person uses judgment to determine the best way to perform a motor act (mental readiness). Before performing the act, such as rising from a wheelchair, the person aligns and postures properly (physical readiness). A client might make the commitment (emotional set) to regularly perform exercises.

GUIDED RESPONSE

A guided response is the performance of an act under the guidance of an instructor. This involves imitation of a demonstrated act. For example, a client prepares an insulin injection after watching a nurse's demonstration. The nurse provides immediate reinforcement after the client correctly performs the act.

MECHANISM

A mechanism is a higher level of behavior whereby a person has gained confidence and skill in performing the behavior. Usually the skill is more complex or involves several more steps than a guided response. For example, a client is able to fill the insulin syringe for different insulin doses.

COMPLEX OVERT RESPONSE

A complex overt response involves performing a motor skill involving a complex movement pattern. The person performs the skill smoothly and accurately without hesitation. For example, a client is able to self-administer an insulin injection using several sites.

ADAPTATION

Adaptation occurs when a person is able to change a motor response when unexpected problems arise. For example, as a nurse administers an injection, the appearance of blood during aspiration results in changing the way that the syringe is handled.

ORIGINATION

Origination is a highly complex motor act that involves creating new movement patterns. A person acts on the basis of existing psychomotor skills and abilities. For example, a nurse uses a different method of venipuncture on a client whose arm is swollen.

■ BASIC LEARNING PRINCIPLES

To teach effectively and efficiently, the nurse must first understand how people learn. Learning depends on the motivation to learn, the ability to learn, and the learning environment. Motivation addresses a person's desire to learn (Redman, 1993). The client's willingness to become involved in learning influences a nurse's teaching approach. Previous knowledge, attitudes, and sociocultural factors influence motivation.

The ability to learn depends on physical and cognitive attributes, developmental level, physical wellness, and intellectual thought processes. If a learning ability is impaired, such as with a client in pain, a teacher postpones teaching activities or modifies strategies to better meet the learner's needs.

The environment also impacts the ability to learn. One of the nurse's major tasks is to manipulate environmental conditions to facilitate learning. For example, when the environment is noisy, the nurse should modify conditions to enhance learning. This can be particularly challenging for a nurse in a busy health care setting.

Motivation to Learn

ATTENTIONAL SET

An attentional set is the mental state that allows the learner to focus and comprehend the material. People often use mental pictures to visualize ideas. While a nurse explains how to give support to a dying client, students might envision grasping the fragile hand of a dying person. Before learning anything, students must give attention to, or concentrate on, the information to be learned.

Physical discomfort, anxiety, and environmental distractions can influence the ability to attend. Any physical condition that impairs the ability to concentrate (e.g., pain, fatigue, or hunger) interferes with learning. Therefore, the nurse determines the client's level of comfort and energy before beginning a teaching plan and ensures that the client is comfortable enough for discussion. Nonverbal cues can also reveal that a client is not ready to learn.

Anxiety may increase or decrease the ability of a person to pay attention. Anxiety is uneasiness or uncertainty resulting from anticipating a threat or danger. When faced with change or the need to act differently, a person feels anxious. Learning requires a change in behavior and thus produces anxiety. A mild level of anxiety may motivate learning. However, a high level of anxiety prevents learning from occurring. It incapacitates a person, creating an inability to attend to anything other than to relieve the anxiety.

Environmental distractions (discussed in a later section) interfere with the ability to attend to a teacher and learning activities. Unplanned interruptions or an uncomfortable environment are not conducive to learning.

MOTIVATION

Motivation is an internal impulse (e.g., an idea, an emotion, or a physical need) that causes a person to take action. If a person does not want to learn, it is unlikely that learning will occur. Motivation may result from a social, task, or physical motive.

Social task mastery and physical motives stimulate a person to learn. Social motives are a need for connection, social approval, or self-esteem. People normally seek out others with whom to compare opinions, abilities, and emotions. For example, a student often works hard to win praise from a teacher or the admiration of peers.

Task mastery motives are based on needs such as achievement and competence. A nursing student repeatedly works in a laboratory to learn the technique for giving an injection because of the motivation to master the task or skill. After a person succeeds at a task the person is usually motivated to achieve more.

Often client motives are physical. A client with a physical change in function may be motivated to learn. According to Tanner (1989), knowledge that is necessary for survival creates a stronger stimulus for learning than knowledge that merely promotes health. Teaching strategies reflect the relative importance of each kind of physical motive.

Not all persons are interested in maintaining health. A client with lung disease may continue to smoke. An obese client may worsen a heart condition by refusing to follow a low-fat diet. No therapy will have an effect unless a person is motivated by the belief that health is important. The trend in health care is to treat clients in their homes after they recover from the acute phase of illness. Such treatment is successful only if clients follow the recommendations of the care givers. **Compliance** is a client's adherence to the prescribed course of therapy. The nurse must assess the client's motivation to learn and what the client needs to know in order to adhere to the prescribed therapy.

A client's health beliefs can be powerful motivators, and they are influenced by a number of variables (see Chapter 1). The Health-Belief Model cites the following health beliefs as critical for motivation (Rosenstock, 1974):

1. The clients are susceptible to the disease in question.
2. The disease would have serious effects on their lives if they contracted it.
3. Actions can be taken to reduce the likelihood of contracting the disease or lessen its severity.

4. The threat of taking these actions is not as great as the threat of the disease itself.

The **Health-Belief Model** (see Chapter 1) was originally designed to explain the reasons that persons attempt health actions. Later the model was used to predict compliance with therapies. Motivation now appears to play a role in the application of the Health-Belief Model. Motivation is a cue for preventive health action. Further research is still needed on the usefulness of the model in predicting changes in client behavior. However, proven examples of motivational triggers are interpersonal crisis, interference of symptoms with valued social activity, and the nature and quality of symptoms (Redman, 1993).

Nurses can use the Health-Belief Model in health education. If a nurse can modify a client's perception of disease susceptibility or severity, the client may be more receptive to learning. When the perceived threat of a disease and the benefit of professional intervention are recognized, educational measures can lead to predictable changes in health behavior. The model does not prescribe strategies for changing health behavior. There is no standard method for motivating a person with a given health belief. However, the model can be useful in the assessment of a client's educational needs and willingness to learn.

Health education often involves changing attitudes and values that are not altered by simple teaching of facts. Therefore the nurse gives attention to ideas or beliefs that motivate a person to learn and applies the motivating factor to the teaching plan. For example, when a client is a busy executive with high blood pressure, the nurse can use the following factors to motivate a client to learn new health habits: the client's desire to succeed and the concern that illness will impair work.

PSYCHOSOCIAL ADAPTATION TO ILLNESS

A temporary or permanent loss of health is difficult for clients to accept. The process of grieving gives clients time to adapt psychologically to the emotional and physical implications of illness. The stages of grieving (see Chapter 26) encompass a series of responses that clients experience during illness. People experience these stages at different rates and sequences, depending on their self-concepts before illness, the severity of illness, and the changes in lifestyle that the illness creates. Effective, supportive care guides clients through the grieving process.

Readiness to learn is significantly related to the stage of grieving (Table 15-2). When unwilling or unable to accept the reality of illness, clients cannot learn. However, properly timed teaching can facilitate adjustment to illness or disability.

The nurse identifies the client's stage of grieving on the basis of typically displayed behaviors. When the client enters the stage of acceptance that is compatible with learning, the nurse introduces a teaching plan. Continuous assessment of the client's behaviors determines the stages of grieving. Teaching continues as long as the client remains in a stage conducive to learning.

Table 15-2	Relationship Between Psychosocial Adaptation to Illness and Learning		
STAGE	**CLIENT'S BEHAVIOR**	**LEARNING IMPLICATIONS**	**RATIONALE**
Denial or disbelief	Client avoids discussion of illness ("There's nothing wrong with me"), withdraws from others, and disregards physical restrictions. Client suppresses and distorts information that has not been presented clearly.	Provide support, empathy, and careful explanations of all procedures while they are being done. Let client know you are available for discussion. Explain situation to family. Teach in present tense (e.g., explain current therapy).	Client is not prepared to deal with problem. Any attempt to convince or tell client about illness will result in further anger or withdrawal. Provide only information client pursues or absolutely requires.
Anger	Client blames and complains and often directs anger toward nurse.	Do not argue with client, but listen to concerns. Teach in present tense. Reassure family of client's normality.	Client needs opportunity to express feelings and anger; client is still not prepared to face future.
Bargaining	Client offers to live better life in exchange for promise of better health ("if God lets me live, I promise to be more careful").	Continue to introduce only reality. Teach only in present tense.	Client is still unwilling to accept limitations.
Resolution	Client begins to express emotions openly, realizes that illness has created changes, and begins to ask questions.	Encourage expression of feelings. Begin to share information needed for future, and set aside formal times for discussion.	Client begins to perceive need for assistance and is ready to accept responsibility for learning.
Acceptance	Client recognizes reality of condition, actively pursues information, and strives for independence.	Focus teaching on future skills and knowledge required. Continue to teach about present occurrences. Involve family in teaching information for discharge.	Client is more easily motivated to learn. Acceptance of illness reflects willingness to deal with its implications.

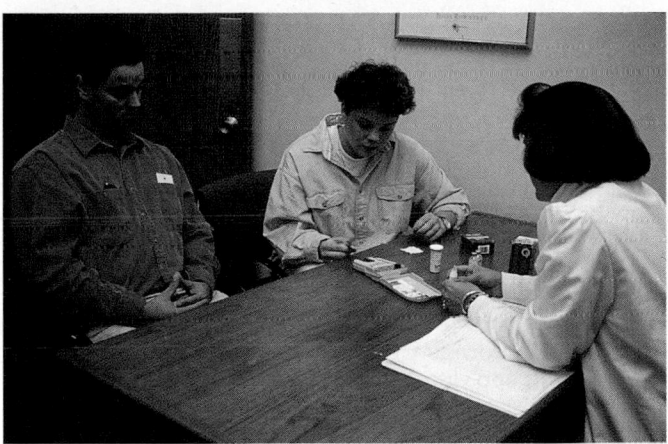

Fig. 15-1 Nurse instructing a client with a glucose meter. *(Courtesy Steve Frazier, Barnes Hospital, St Louis.)*

ACTIVE PARTICIPATION

A client's involvement in learning implies an eagerness to acquire knowledge or skills. It also improves the opportunity for the client to make decisions during teaching sessions. For example, a client with a diagnosis of diabetes learns to monitor blood glucose levels to gain control of the disease. The nurse assists the client in choosing a blood glucose meter and adapting a monitoring system and schedule to personal lifestyle patterns (Fig. 15-1).

Funnell et al. (1991) describe an Empowerment Model for health education in which the client has the knowledge, skills, and responsibility to effect change. The client is not seen as a passive recipient or consumer of health care and education, but as an active partner in the provision of care. Empowering the client will promote overall health and maximize the use of available resources.

Ability to Learn

DEVELOPMENTAL CAPABILITY

Cognitive development influences the client's ability to learn. A nurse can be a competent teacher, but if the client's intellectual abilities are not considered, teaching is unsuccessful. Sometimes a nurse has shared teaching booklets and brochures and then discovered that the client cannot read. Learning, like developmental growth, is an evolving process. The nurse must know the client's level of knowledge and intellectual skills before beginning a teaching plan. For example, reading a thermometer or measuring liquid or solid food portions requires the ability to perform math calculations. Reading a medication label or instructions in a teaching booklet requires reading and comprehension skills, and learning to regulate insulin dosages requires problem-solving skills. Following directions when performing self-care in accordance with limitations requires comprehension and application skills.

A requisite level of maturation and cognitive development must exist before an individual is capable of learning new information. It is wrong to assume that a client has a certain level of knowledge; instead, the nurse should assess the client's level of knowledge. Learning occurs more readily when new information complements existing knowledge.

Age-Group. Age reflects the developmental capability for learning and the type of learning behaviors that can be acquired (Table 15-3). Without proper biological, motor, language, and personal-social development, many types of learning cannot take place. Learning occurs when behavior changes as a result of experience or growth (Wong, 1995).

PHYSICAL CAPABILITY

The ability to learn often depends on the level of physical development and overall physical health. To learn psychomotor skills, a client must possess the necessary level of strength, coordination, and sensory acuity. For example, it is useless to teach a client to transfer from a bed to a wheelchair if the client has insufficient upper body strength. An older client cannot learn to apply an elastic bandage with poor eyesight or the inability to grasp the bandage tightly. Therefore the nurse should not overestimate the client's physical development or status. The following physical attributes are required to learn psychomotor skills:

1. Size (height and weight match the task to perform or the equipment to use [e.g., crutch walking])
2. Strength (ability of client to follow a strenuous exercise program)
3. Coordination (dexterity needed for complicated motor skills such as using utensils or changing a bandage)
4. Sensory acuity (visual, auditory, tactile, gustatory, and olfactory: sensory resources needed to receive and respond to messages taught)

Any condition (e.g., pain) that depletes a person's energy will also impair the ability to learn. A client who spends a morning undergoing rigorous diagnostic studies is unlikely to be capable of the effort needed for any learning discussion. When an illness becomes aggravated by complications, such as a high fever or respiratory difficulty, teaching should be postponed. After working with a client, the nurse assesses energy level by noting a client's willingness to communicate, amount of activity initiated, and responsiveness toward questions. The nurse may halt teaching temporarily if a client needs rest. The nurse achieves greater teaching success when the client is an active participant in learning.

Learning Environment

Factors in the physical environment where teaching takes place make learning a pleasant or difficult experience. The nurse chooses a setting that helps the client focus on the learning task. The number of persons being taught, need for privacy, room temperature, room lighting, noise, room ventilation, and room furniture are important when choosing the setting.

The ideal environment for learning is a room that is well lit and has good ventilation, appropriate furniture, and a comfortable temperature (Fig. 15-2). A darkened room interferes with the client's ability to watch the nurse's actions, especially when demonstrating a skill or using visual aids such as posters or pamphlets. A room that is cold, hot, or stuffy will make the client too uncomfortable to attend to the nurse's activities. Comfortable furniture helps eliminate distractions, such as the need to change position or shift body weight.

Table 15-3	Developmental Capacities for Learning
LEARNING CAPACITY	**TEACHING METHODS**
INFANT Infant relies on parents for basic needs. Infant learns to trust adults when they convey love and compassion. Infant explores environment through senses.	Keep routines (e.g., feeding, bathing) consistent. Hold infant firmly while smiling and speaking softly to convey sense of trust. Have infant touch different textures (e.g., soft fabric, hard plastic).
TODDLER Toddler learns to understand words and express feelings verbally. Toddler learns by associating words with objects. Toddler likes to explore environment through play.	Use play to teach procedure or activity (e.g., handling examination equipment, applying bandage to doll). Offer picture books that describe story of children in hospital or clinic. Use simple words such as *cut* instead of *laceration* to promote understanding.
PRESCHOOLER Vocabulary grows. Preschooler uses language without comprehending meaning of words, especially concepts (e.g., right or left, time). During play, child expresses feelings more through actions than words. Preschooler asks questions and imitates adults.	Use role playing, imitation, and play to make it fun for preschoolers to learn. Encourage questions and offer explanations. Use simple explanations and demonstrations. Encourage children to learn together through pictures and short stories of how to perform hygiene.
SCHOOL-AGE CHILD Child interacts with adults and peers outside family. Child begins to acquire ability to relate series of events and actions to mental representations that can be expressed verbally and symbolically. Child is able to make judgments. Child matures physically. Play becomes more formal and imaginative. Child is inquisitive and asks many questions about health.	Teach psychomotor skills needed to maintain health. (Complicated skills, such as learning to use a syringe, may take considerable practice.) Offer opportunities to discuss health problems and answer questions.
ADOLESCENT Adolescent struggles between childlike feelings of dependence and independence of adults. Teenager wants to be in control but, during illness, fears loss of self-concept or body image. Adolescent is able to solve abstract problems. Teenager learns best when immediate benefit is gained.	Help adolescent learn about feelings and need for self-expression. Allow adolescents to make decisions about health and health promotion (e.g., safety, sex education, substance abuse). Use problem solving to help adolescents make choices.
YOUNG OR MIDDLE ADULT Adult complies with health teaching because client fears the results. Learning occurs when adult values information being taught.	Encourage participation by setting mutual goals. Encourage independent learning. Offer information so that adult can understand effects of health problem.
OLDER ADULT Often, there is decline in visual and auditory acuity, which impairs perception of stimuli. Sensory alterations, mobility limitations, and physical coordination problems affect capacity to learn. Sleep-wake cycles are more fragmented. Older adult takes pride in being independent. There is no decline in intelligence with age.	Teach when client is alert and rested. Involve adult in discussion or activity. Focus on wellness and the person's strength. Use approaches that enhance sensorially impaired client's reception of stimuli (see Chapter 38). Keep teaching sessions short.

It is also important to choose a quiet setting. A quiet setting offers privacy; infrequent interruptions are best. The nurse can provide privacy even in a busy hospital by closing cubicle curtains or taking the client to a quiet spot. In a home a bedroom might separate the client from household activities. If the client desires, family members might share in discussions. However, a client may be reluctant to discuss the nature of the illness when others, even close family members, are in the room.

Teaching a group of clients requires a room that allows everyone to be seated comfortably and within hearing distance of the teacher. The size of the room should not overwhelm the group, tempting participants to sit outside the group along the room's perimeter. Arranging the group to

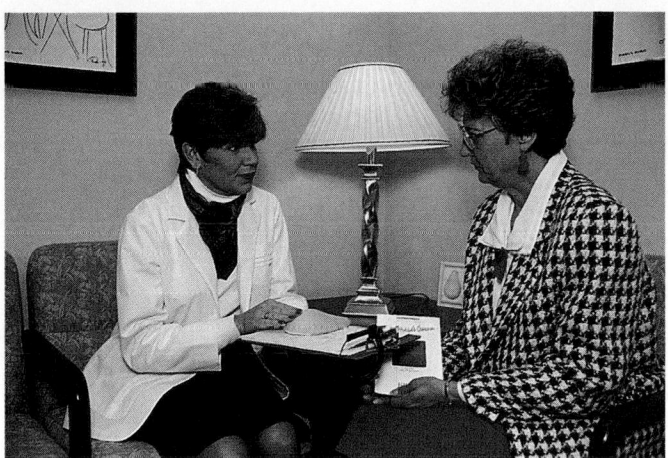

Fig. 15-2 Choosing comfortable, pleasant environments enhances the learning experience. This nurse is explaining the breast self-examination procedure to the client.

allow participants to observe one another further enhances learning. More effective communication occurs as learners observe others' verbal and nonverbal interactions.

INTEGRATING THE NURSING AND TEACHING PROCESSES

A relationship exists between the nursing and teaching processes. With the nursing process a thorough assessment reveals the client's health care needs. The nursing diagnoses that are identified are unique to the client's situation. A care plan is individualized, prescribing nursing therapies designed to improve or maintain the client's level of health. Evaluation determines the level of success in meeting goals of care.

While diagnosing a client's health care problems, the nurse may also identify the need for education. When education becomes a part of the care plan, the teaching process begins. Like the nursing process, the teaching process requires assessment, in this case analyzing the client's need, motivation, and ability to learn (Table 15-4). A diagnostic statement specifies the information or skills the client requires. The nurse sets specific learning objectives and implements the teaching plan using teaching and learning principles to ensure that the client acquires knowledge and skills. Finally, the teaching process requires an evaluation of learning based on learning objectives.

The nursing and teaching processes are not the same. The nursing process requires assessment of all sources of data to determine a client's total health care needs. The teaching process focuses on the client's learning needs and willingness and capability to learn. Table 15-4 compares the teaching and nursing processes.

 Assessment

Success in teaching a client requires the nurse to assess all factors influencing relevant content, the client's ability to learn, and the resources for instruction. The client's learning needs determine the choice of teaching content.

LEARNING NEEDS

The nurse determines the information that is critical for the client to learn, which determines the choice of teaching content. Learning needs change depending on where the client is in the recovery process. Assessment is thus an ongoing activity. An effective assessment is the basis by which instruction can be individualized to each client (Redman, 1993). The nurse assesses the following:

1. Questions raised by the client or family about health issues. When a client feels a need to know something, the nurse recognizes that the client will likely be receptive to learn.
2. Client's level of understanding of current health status, implications of illness, types of therapy, and prognosis. This information helps to determine a client's perception of the threat of illness and its effect on lifestyle.
3. Information or skills needed by the client to perform self-care and to understand the implications of a health problem. Health care team members anticipate learning needs related to specific health problems. For example, a newly diagnosed diabetic client obviously needs to learn about dietary control. A client who has had major surgery must learn the physical restrictions imposed by the procedure.
4. Client's experiences that influence the need to learn. For example, a client who has had previous surgery is more likely to be familiar with preoperative procedures.
5. Information that family members require to support the client's needs. The extent of information depends on the extent of the family's role in helping the client.

MOTIVATION TO LEARN

Nurses use several tools to assess the client's motivation to learn. In the absence of such tools the nurse can ask questions that define the client's motivation. These questions help to determine whether the client is prepared and willing to learn. Although a client may have a variety of learning needs, a lack of motivation seriously threatens the success of the teaching plan. The nurse assesses the following motivational factors:

1. Client behavior (e.g., attention span, tendency to ask questions, memory, and ability to concentrate during questioning).
2. Client's health beliefs and perception of the severity of a health problem, efficacy of current treatment, and extent of possible bodily harm.
3. Client's attitudes about health care providers (e.g., role of client and nurse in making decisions). Mutually set goals are more likely to be valued by the client.
4. Client's knowledge of information to be learned. The client must play an active role in seeking health-based information.
5. Pain, fatigue, anxiety, or other physical symptoms that can interfere with the ability to attend and participate. In acute care settings, a client's physical condition can easily detract from learning.
6. Client's sociocultural background. A client's beliefs and values about health and various therapies may be influenced by sociocultural norms or tradition (see Chapter 21).

Table 15-4	Comparision of the Nursing and Teaching Processes	
BASIC STEPS	**NURSING PROCESS**	**TEACHING PROCESS**
Assessment	Collect data about client's physical, psychological, social, cultural, developmental, and spiritual needs from client, family, diagnostic tests, medical record, nursing history, and literature.	Gather data about client's learning needs, motivation, ability to learn, and teaching resources from client, family, learning environment, medical record, nursing history, and literature.
Nursing diagnosis	Identify appropriate nursing diagnoses.	Identify client's learning needs on basis of three domains of learning.
Planning	Develop individualized care plan. Set diagnosis priorities based on client's immediate needs. Collaborate with client on care plan.	Establish learning objectives, stated in behavioral terms. Identify priorities regarding learning needs. Collaborate with client on teaching plan. Identify type of teaching method to use.
Implementation	Perform nursing care therapies. Include client as active participant in care. Involve family in care as appropriate.	Implement teaching methods. Actively involve client in learning activities. Include family participation as appropriate.
Evaluation	Identify success in meeting desired outcomes and goals of nursing care.	Determine outcomes of teaching-learning process. Measure client's ability to achieve learning objectives. Reteach as needed.

7. Client's learning-style preference. When various options are available for learning (e.g., brochures, videotape, and discussion), a client may perceive one approach as being more interesting. Merritt (1991) studied learning-style preferences of clients who underwent cardiac surgery and found that they preferred organized, detailed instruction using oral and pictorial-graphic modes of presentation over independent instruction modes.

ABILITY TO LEARN

The nurse determines the client's physical and cognitive levels. Health care providers often underestimate the client's cognitive deficits. Many factors can impair the ability to learn, including body temperature, electrolyte levels, oxygenation status, and blood glucose level. In an acute care setting, several of these factors may influence a client at one time. The nurse assesses the following factors related to the ability to learn:

1. Physical strength, movement, and coordination. The nurse determines the extent to which the client can perform skills.
2. Sensory deficits (see Chapter 39) that may affect the client's ability to understand or follow instruction. The following example illustrates this point.

CASE STUDY Mrs. Lyon is a 68-year-old woman who received a prescription from her physician for a heart medication that slows the heart's rate. Mrs. Lyon must learn to check her pulse to be sure that her heart does not beat too slowly. Assessment reveals that Mrs. Lyon is unable to feel an arterial pulse because her fingers are stiff and callused. No one who lives nearby is consistently available to check her pulse. However, Mrs. Lyon's hearing is still good. The nurse chooses instead to teach Mrs. Lyon to listen to her heart beat with a stethoscope. ■

3. Client's reading level. This can be difficult to assess because a functionally illiterate client is often able to conceal it by using excuses such as not having the time or having left his eyeglasses at home. The nurse asks a client to read instructions from a teaching brochure and then explain its meaning.
4. Client's developmental level. This influences the approaches chosen by the nurse during teaching (see Table 15-3).
5. Client's cognitive function, including memory, knowledge, association, and judgment.

TEACHING ENVIRONMENT

The environment for a teaching session must be conducive to learning. The nurse assesses the following factors when seeking a place to teach clients:

1. Distractions or persistent noise. A quiet area should be set aside for teaching.
2. Comfort of the room, including ventilation, temperature, lighting, and furniture.
3. Room facilities and available equipment.

RESOURCES FOR LEARNING

A client may require the support of family members or significant others. In this case the nurse assesses the readiness and ability of family and friends to learn the information necessary for the care of the client. The nurse also needs to understand the home environment. Assessment of resources also includes a review of any teaching tools available. The nurse assesses the following resources for learning:

1. Family members' perceptions and understanding of the client's illness and its implications. Family perceptions should match those of the client; otherwise, conflicts may arise in the teaching plan.
2. Client's willingness to have family members involved in the teaching plan and to provide health care. In-

formation about the client's health care is confidential unless the client chooses to share it. Sometimes it is difficult for the client to accept the help of family members, especially when bodily functions are involved.

3. Family's willingness to participate in care. If the client chooses to share information regarding health status with family members, the family members must be assessed for their abilities and willingness to participate in care of the client. Not all family members may be responsible, willing, or able to assist in care.

4. Resources within the home. These include persons willing to assist the client with procedures such as bathing or taking medications, financial or material resources such as obtaining health care equipment, and architectural resources such as arrangement of rooms or stairways.

5. Teaching tools, including brochures, audiovisual materials, or posters. Printed material should match the client's reading level and present subject material clearly and logically. Brochures or booklets must be current.

 ## Nursing Diagnosis

After assessing information related to the client's ability and need to learn, the nurse interprets data to form diagnoses that reflect the client's specific learning needs (see the nursing diagnoses box at right). This ensures that teaching will be goal directed and individualized. If a client has several learning needs, nursing diagnoses allow for priority setting (see the diagnostic process box below).

Several nursing diagnoses apply to learning needs. Each diagnostic statement describes the specific type of learning need and its cause. Classifying diagnoses by the three learning domains helps the nurse to focus specifically on subject matter and teaching methods.

 Examples of NANDA Nursing Diagnoses for Learning Needs

Altered health maintenance *related to:*
- Lack of knowledge about health practices
- Lack of fine motor skills

Knowledge deficit (affective) *related to:*
- Misunderstanding of prognosis

Knowledge deficit (cognitive) *related to:*
- Newly diagnosed disease
- Newly prescribed therapy

Knowledge deficit (psychomotor) *related to:*
- Inexperience with skill
- Lack of interest in learning

Noncompliance with medications *related to:*
- Poor understanding of therapies
- Disbelief of health risk

Bathing/hygiene self-care deficit *related to:*
- Neuromuscular impairment
- Unfamiliarity with preventive care measures

Impaired social interaction *related to:*
- Poor communication skills

Some health care problems can be managed or eliminated through education. In these situations the related factor of the diagnostic statement is knowledge deficit. For example, a client may have difficulty interacting socially because of a lack of effective communication skills, or a self-care deficit may exist because of an inadequate knowledge base.

Some nursing diagnoses also indicate that teaching may be inappropriate. The nurse may identify conditions that

 ## Sample Nursing Diagnostic Process for Learning Needs

ASSESSMENT ACTIVITIES	DEFINING CHARACTERISTICS	NURSING DIAGNOSES
Ask client to describe understanding of planned surgery. Observe response to discussion about surgery.	States that physician has not yet provided explanation. Unable to describe purpose of surgery. Asks numerous questions and requests further information.	Knowledge deficit (cognitive) regarding impending surgery related to inexperience
Review medical record for history.	No previous surgical experience. Surgery is elective.	
Observe client attempt exercise program. Ask client to describe steps to follow in exercises. Assess body temperature. Ask client to perform simple memory tests.	Unable to follow through with all exercise steps. Cannot describe proper steps in sequence. Fever of 38.8° C (102° F). Unable to repeat sequence of numbers backward. Short-term memory of events is reduced.	Knowledge deficit (psychomotor) regarding ambulation training related to impaired cognition

Sample Nursing Care Plan for Knowledge Deficit

NURSING DIAGNOSIS: Knowledge deficit (cognitive) regarding impending surgery related to inexperience
DEFINITION: Knowledge deficit is the state in which specific information is lacking (Kim, McFarland, and McLane, 1995).

GOALS	EXPECTED OUTCOMES*	INTERVENTIONS	RATIONALE
Client will describe preoperative surgical care experience by 7/8.	Client will describe preoperative routines planned on morning before surgery (7/8), including monitoring and treatments, visit by anesthesiologist, and surgery time.	Five days before surgery, send client brochure on preoperative care. Make follow-up phone call 48 hours before surgery to discuss information.	Early timing and reinforcement of preoperative teaching may improve knowledge of surgery routines (Cupples, 1989). Discussion helps client understand implications of surgery (Merritt, 1991).
Client will participate in preoperative and postoperative surgical care procedures (7/8 and 7/9).	Client will demonstrate breathing and range of motion exercises by 7/8.	Demonstrate and have client return demonstration of breathing and exercise routines, including coughing, deep breathing, turning, and leg exercises.	Return demonstration effectively reveals success in learning motor skill (Redman, 1993). Cognitive learning is needed to give learners understanding of importance of motor skills.
	Client will describe postoperative routines and related rationale for recovery by 7/9.	Discuss benefits exercises have in preventing complications. Discuss procedures to anticipate after surgery. Have client view videotape of postoperative surgical experience.	Discussion is appropriate teaching method for cognitive learning (Redman, 1993). Videotape can be stimulus for follow-up discussion on points of interest.

*Teaching objectives.

cause barriers to effective learning (e.g., pain or activity intolerance). In these cases the nurse delays teaching until the nursing diagnosis is resolved or the health problem is controlled.

Planning

After determining the nursing diagnoses that identify a client's learning needs, the nurse develops a teaching plan, determines goals and expected outcomes, and involves the client in selecting learning experiences (see the care plan above). Expected outcomes guide the choice of teaching strategies and approaches with a client. Client participation ensures a more relevant, meaningful plan.

DEVELOPING LEARNING OBJECTIVES

The first step in forming a teaching plan is developing learning objectives. A learning objective identifies the expected outcome of a planned learning experience and helps establish priorities for learning. Despite all planning, a particular instructional session often leads to unanticipated learning. It may be difficult to anticipate all objectives for a teaching session. However, objectives cause a teacher to plan teaching sessions so that time is maximized and the best resources are available for learning.

Objectives are either short- or long-term. Short-term objectives relate to the client's immediate learning needs,

such as knowing the nature of gallbladder disease to understand an upcoming test. Long-term objectives relate to acquisition of the knowledge and skills that are needed to permanently adapt to a health problem (e.g., learning to plan a diet within restrictions caused by gallbladder disease). Like a goal of care, a long-term objective is usually all-encompassing. Short-term objectives can be compared with the steps taken to achieve long-term goals.

The objectives established by the nurse and client guide the teaching plan. Poorly determined objectives can create confusion throughout the teaching-learning process. Thus a learning objective includes the same criteria as goals or outcomes in a nursing care plan (see Chapter 9), including the following:

1. Singular behaviors
2. Observable or measurable content
3. Timing or conditions under which the objective is measured
4. Goals mutually set between the nurse and client

Each objective is a statement of a singular behavior that identifies the learner's ability to do something after a learning experience. A behavioral objective contains an active verb describing what the learner will do after the objective is met, such as *to perform* a crutch gait, *to administer* an injection, or *to identify* drug dosages. The verb should have few interpretations (e.g., to identify, to describe, to label, to classify, to demonstrate, or to select) and be stated in terms of how the client is to demonstrate learning, rather than what or how the teacher is to teach (Redman, 1993). Singular behaviors are easier to evaluate at the end of instruction.

Behavioral objectives are measurable and observable, indicating how learning is evidenced (e.g., "to perform *the three-point crutch gait*" or "to prepare *foods without using salt*"). The objective describes precise behaviors and content. An example of a vague or nonspecific objective might be "to be familiar with knowledge about diabetes." This example does not explain what the learner is to do, and it raises questions about how the behavior can be measured. If content is missing, the objective cannot guide teaching and learning. The precise behaviors and content set the standard for feedback that reflects learning and forms the basis for evaluation of the teaching plan.

An objective is more precise when it describes the conditions or timing under which the behavior occurs. Conditions or time frames should be realistic and designed for the learner's needs (e.g., "to identify the side effects of Ritalin by discharge"). It also helps to consider conditions under which the client or family will typically perform the learning behavior (e.g., "to walk from bedroom to bath using crutches"). The criteria for acceptable performance set a standard by which achievement of objectives is measured. A teacher sets criteria on the basis of a desired level of accuracy, success, or satisfaction. For example, a client undergoing therapy for a fractured leg will walk on crutches *to the end of the hall within 3 days*. Criteria are more acceptable when established by the teacher and learner. However, the nurse serves as a resource in setting the minimal criteria for success. Criteria on which the client and nurse agree help to define the expected behaviors and the quality of performance. The client also uses these criteria for self-evaluation, which is a powerful motivator of behavior.

After formulating objectives, the nurse and client work to establish a teaching plan. During planning the nurse integrates basic teaching principles and develops a well-timed, organized teaching plan.

INTEGRATING BASIC TEACHING PRINCIPLES

Teaching priorities should reflect the priorities of the nursing diagnoses. Teaching is the process of leading someone to learn. When developing a teaching plan, the nurse considers the principles that improve its effectiveness. The realm of teaching deals with teachers' behavior, the reason teachers behave the way they do, and effects of their behavior on learners. There is no single correct way to teach, since each learning situation determines the best way to teach. The principles of teaching are, in effect, techniques that incorporate the principles of learning.

Setting Priorities. Priorities for teaching are based on nursing diagnoses and the learning objectives established for the client. A client's learning needs must be set in order of priority to conserve the time and energy of the client and nurse. For example, a client with a permanent leg injury has a knowledge deficit regarding the nature of the injury and its implications, as well as the types of skills needed to resume a normal life at home. The client will benefit most from first learning about the injury and the resultant physical changes before learning how to cope with the disability.

Timing. When is the right time to teach? When a client first enters a clinic or hospital? At discharge? At home? Each may be appropriate because clients continue to have learning needs and opportunities as long as they stay in the health care system. The nurse determines the client's readiness to learn. Timing can be difficult because emphasis is placed on a client's early discharge from a hospital. For example, it may take several days after surgery for a client to become free of discomfort so that attention can be given to learning. By the time the client feels ready to learn, discharge may already be scheduled. The nurse should plan teaching activities for a time when the client is most attentive, receptive, and alert. Many hospitals provide information to clients before admission. The client's activities should be organized to provide time for rest and teaching-learning interactions.

The duration of teaching sessions also influences learning ability. Prolonged sessions cause concentration and attentiveness to decrease. Frequent sessions lasting 20 minutes are more easily tolerated and retain the client's interest in the material. However, shorter hospital stays and lack of insurance reimbursement for outpatient education sessions may necessitate longer teaching sessions. The nurse can assess a client's loss of concentration by observing for nonverbal cues, such as poor eye contact or slumped posture. After loss of concentration is noted, the session should be stopped. However, teaching sessions should not be too brief. The client needs time to comprehend the information and to give feedback.

Teaching sessions should be held frequently enough to document the client's learning. The frequency of sessions depends on the learner's abilities and the complexity of the material. For example, a newly diagnosed diabetic will require more visits to an outpatient education center than the client whose insulin dosage was changed after 5 years. Intervals between teaching sessions should not be so long that the client might forget information. For a client discharged from a hospital, home health care nurses must reinforce learning.

Organizing Teaching Material. A good teacher gives careful consideration to the order of information presented. An outline of content helps organize information into a logical sequence. Material should progress from simple to complex ideas because a person must learn the simple facts and concepts before learning how to make associations or complex interpretations of ideas. For example, to teach a client with diabetes to calculate a 1200-calorie diet, the nurse first teaches the client about calories, proteins, fats, and carbohydrates and then uses simple mathematical problems to help the client learn to calculate amounts.

The nurse begins any instruction with essential content. Clients are more likely to remember information that is taught during the first third of a teaching session (Miller, 1985). For example, after surgical removal of a cancerous lung tumor, the client's predisposition to cancer recurrence makes learning the warning signs of cancer crucial. The nurse starts with essential information and then completes a teaching session with informative but less critical content. It helps to summarize important points. Repetition reinforces learning. A concise summary of key topics helps the learner know the most important information.

Maintaining Learning Attention and Participation.
Active participation is key to learning. Persons learn better
when more than one of the body's senses are stimulated.
Audiovisual aids and role playing are good teaching strategies. By actively experiencing a learning event, the person
will be more likely to retain the knowledge gained.

A teacher's actions can also increase learner attention and
interest. When conducting a discussion with a learner, the
teacher should stay active by changing tone and intensity of
voice, making eye contact, and using gestures that accentuate key points of discussion. An effective teacher often uses
as much energy as the learner, talking and moving among a
group rather than remaining stationary behind a lectern or
table. A learner remains interested in a teacher who is actively enthusiastic about the subject under discussion.

Building on Existing Knowledge. A client learns best
on the basis of preexisting cognitive abilities and knowledge. Thus a teacher is more effective by presenting information that builds on a learner's existing knowledge.
The key is assessing the learner's level of knowledge by
discovering how much is known about the topic. Then a
teaching plan must be individualized based on the client's
learning needs. A client quickly loses interest if a nurse begins with familiar information.

Selection of Teaching Methods. During planning the
nurse chooses appropriate teaching methods and encourages the client to offer suggestions. A teaching method is
the way that the teacher delivers information and is based
on the client's learning needs (see the box below). For
example, a client with a psychomotor deficit learns best
through demonstrations and supervised practice. The
client masters skills by manipulating equipment and prac-

ticing manual skills. Discussions, question-and-answer sessions, and formal lectures are effective methods for promoting cognitive learning. Clients with intellectual deficits
are given the opportunity to explore new ideas, recognize
new relationships, and apply knowledge to their unique
needs. A highly effective method for stimulating affective
learning is group discussion. More than one method may
be used for instruction.

WRITING TEACHING PLANS

In all health care settings, nurses develop written teaching plans for use by colleagues. When one nurse, such as a
primary nurse, is responsible for developing the initial
teaching plan, all information about the client is incorporated appropriately.

The teaching plan includes topics for instruction, optional resources (e.g., equipment or teaching booklets),
recommendations for involving family, and objectives of
the teaching plan. A plan may be lengthy or in outline
form.

The setting influences the complexity of any teaching
plan. In an acute care setting, plans are concise and focused
on the primary learning needs of the client because there is
limited time for teaching. A home health care teaching
plan may be more extensive in scope because nurses often
have more time to instruct clients and clients are often less
anxious in the home setting.

A plan should provide continuity of instruction, particularly when several nurses are involved in caring for the
client. The more specific the plan, the easier it is for nurses
to follow through. To avoid duplication, the nurse should
know the point at which the last teaching session ended.

Teaching Methods

COGNITIVE
Discussion (one-on-one or group)
- May involve nurse and client or nurse with several clients
- Promotes active participation and focuses on topics of in-
terest to client
- Allows peer support
- Enhances application and analysis of new information

Lecture
- Is more formal method of instruction because it is controlled by teacher
- Helps learner acquire new knowledge and gain comprehension

Question-and-answer session
- Is designed specifically to address client's concerns
- Assists client in applying knowledge

Role play, discovery
- Allows client to actively apply knowledge in controlled
situation
- Promotes synthesis of information and problem solving

**Independent project (computer-assisted instruction),
field experience**
- Allows client to assume responsibility for completing
learning activities at own pace
- Promotes analysis, synthesis, and evaluation of new information and skills

AFFECTIVE
Role play
- Allows expression of values, feelings, and attitudes

Discussion (group)
- Allows client to acquire support from others in group
- Permits client to learn from other experiences
- Promotes responding, valuing, and organization

Discussion (one-on-one)
- Allows discussion of personal, sensitive topics of interest
or concern

PSYCHOMOTOR
Demonstration
- Provides presentation of procedures or skills by nurse
- Permits client to incorporate modeling of nurse's behavior
- Allows nurse to control questioning during demonstration

Practice
- Gives client opportunity to perform skills using equipment
- Provides repetition

Return demonstration
- Permits client to perform skill as nurse observes
- Is excellent source of feedback and reinforcement

Independent projects, games
- Require teaching method that promotes adaptation and
origination of psychomotor learning
- Permit learner to use new skills

Implementation

Implementation of a teaching plan (see the case study below) involves application of all teaching and learning principles, including the following:

1. Knowing the client's learning needs
2. Selecting a time that coincides with the client's readiness and ability to learn
3. Knowing the client's ability to comprehend (Miller and Bodie, 1994) (see the box on p. 276)
4. Selecting a teaching method that fits the learning domain for the client's learning need
5. Selecting and establishing priorities for content
6. Involving the client and family in the teaching plan
7. Awareness of personal teaching abilities (know content, be interested in the learner, and be aware of personal motives)

CASE STUDY Mrs. Menendez is a 58-year-old woman seen in the clinic for the treatment of type II (non–insulin-dependent) diabetes. She has had diabetes for 2 years and repeatedly returns to the clinic as a result of poor compliance with the prescribed therapy. The nurse, Ms. Sommers, decides that Mrs. Menendez might benefit from a teaching program directed toward improving her ability to cope with diabetes and increasing her self-management skills.

ASSESSMENT

The nurse's assessment reveals that Mrs. Menendez is 5 feet, 1 inch tall and weighs 164 pounds. Her blood sugar levels in the clinic are repeatedly elevated, indicating poor glucose control. Mrs. Menendez is to take an oral hypoglycemic medication every morning, monitor her blood glucose levels twice a day, follow a 1500-calorie diabetic diet, and walk for 20 minutes three to four times per week.

When discussing Mrs. Menendez's condition, Ms. Sommers learns that her client knows only that diabetes is "a touch of bad sugar." The client does not understand the cellular action of insulin or the interplay of diet, exercise, medication, and blood glucose monitoring in blood glucose control. Mrs. Menendez has never seen a nutritionist and is unaware of how her obesity impacts her diabetes. She admits to not adhering to her meal plan, refuses to exercise, and does not monitor her own blood glucose levels. Mrs. Menendez does take her diabetes medication as prescribed but is unaware of its mechanism of action or side effects **(knowledge deficit)**.

Ms. Sommers is concerned that if Mrs. Menendez has a history of poor compliance, she may not benefit from a teaching plan. However, she learns that Mrs. Menendez has an interest in learning more because she asks the nurse several questions (readiness to learn).

The client is unfamiliar with many of the terms Ms. Sommers uses to describe diabetes (cognitive capability).

Mrs. Menendez is married to an employed laborer and has four children, one of whom is 18 years of age and still lives at home. Mrs. Menendez does all of the cooking for her family and has never seen a nutritionist for dietary counseling. When asked if Mr. Menendez could be present at a teaching session, Mrs. Menendez says "Yes, he will come if I ask him to" (family support).

Ms. Sommers reserves a conference room for the first teaching session. She arranges to use a short videotape on general facts of diabetes. She then locates Spanish-translated pamphlets on diabetes medications (teaching resources).

NURSING DIAGNOSIS

Assessment reveals a number of diagnoses:

Knowledge deficit: cognitive regarding illness related to:
- Poor understanding of pathophysiology of diabetes
- Poor understanding of components of diabetes therapy

Knowledge deficit: psychomotor regarding blood glucose monitoring related to:
- Inexperience with blood glucose self–monitoring skills

PLANNING

On the basis of the diagnoses, Ms. Sommers and Mrs. Menendez set mutually agreed on learning objectives. After proper instruction Mrs. Menendez will be able to:

1. Develop a 1500-calorie diabetic meal plan for 1 week.
2. Monitor blood glucose levels independently, two times per day.
3. Describe the action and side effects of her diabetes medication.
4. Lose 2 pounds in 1 month.

The nurse does not plan to cover all topics in one teaching session. Mrs. Menendez agrees to have her husband attend to learn about diabetes and the treatment program. Mrs. Menendez agrees to follow up after the initial session with a nutritionist. The nurse and client agree to hold the initial session on Thursday morning when Mr. Menendez does not work.

IMPLEMENTATION

Ms. Sommers begins the session by getting to know Mr. Menendez and observing how he and his wife interact. She recognizes that Mr. Menendez is interested in helping his wife. The client and her husband are attentive and responsive to Ms. Sommers' questions.

The nurse shows the film to give Mr. and Mrs. Menendez a thorough introduction to diabetes. After the film the nurse and her clients discuss aspects of the film relevant to Mrs. Menendez's condition, and the nurse answers the couple's questions. Ms. Sommers discusses the diabetes medication and its side effects. She also explains how obesity affects diabetes control and Mrs. Menendez's need to see a nutritionist. The nurse asks questions designed to help Mr. Menendez gain an understanding of the long-term impact of his wife's disease. Throughout the discussion Ms. Sommers uses simple terms to explain key concepts. When the Menendezes show confusion, Ms. Sommers clarifies information with illustrations on the blackboard.

Ms. Sommers uses the remaining class time to demonstrate blood glucose self-monitoring with a glucose meter. This type of teaching gets Mr. and Mrs. Menendez actively involved. The nurse demonstrates the cleaning and operation of the meter. She has Mr. and Mrs. Menendez each perform a return demonstration of these procedures. She then explains the proper procedure for recording blood glucose levels and appropriate target ranges.

EVALUATION

The nurse asks the Menendezes to briefly explain the nature of diabetes. After viewing the film they are able to give a simple but complete description of the action of insulin and the treatment components of diabetes. Ms. Sommers understands that it is easy to forget information that is not reinforced. She gives Mr. and Mrs. Menendez a pamphlet to review before the next class and asks them to write down any questions they might have.

It is too early to evaluate Mrs. Menendez's adherence with the diabetic diet or her weight loss. However, Mrs. Menendez is to see the nutritionist within the week.

Mrs. Menendez is to bring her blood glucose meter and record book to the next visit so that Ms. Sommers can evaluate her adherence with her glucose monitoring schedule. Mrs. Menendez is to perform the glucose monitoring herself, relying on Mr. Menendez for assistance and support only if needed. Thus the nurse has begun a constructive teaching plan that will enable Mrs. Menendez and her husband to cope more effectively with her disease. As the teaching process continues, Ms. Sommers will work with Mr. and Mrs. Menendez to reach all the objectives based on the nursing diagnoses. ∎

RESEARCH HIGHLIGHT

RESEARCH ABSTRACT

Functional illiteracy is a growing problem in the United States. Nurses often rely on educational pamphlets or brochures as teaching aids for clients. However, many are written at well above the eighth-grade level. A reading level below fifth grade is considered functional illiteracy.

Miller and Bodie chose a convenience sample of 100 subjects from inpatient and ambulatory care areas of a veterans' affairs center, determined their reading levels, and correlated the reading levels of the subjects with their highest grade completed in school.

Approximately 60% of the sample held a high school diploma, a general education diploma, or a college degree, and the average grade completed was calculated as 11.6. However, 80% of the veterans included in the sample were considered partially illiterate, with the average veteran in the facility reading at a 5.6 grade level.

IMPLICATIONS FOR PRACTICE

▶ The assumption that the last grade level completed equals reading ability is unwarranted.

▶ Health education materials for the veterans in this medical center should be written at a fifth-grade level.

▶ Replication of this study to other populations to increase the generality of the findings should be completed.

REFERENCE

Miller B, Bodie M: Determination of reading comprehension level for effective patient health—education materials, *Nurs Res* 43(2):118, 1994.

---

8. Using appropriate teaching aids and resources
9. Controlling the environment so that it is conducive to learning
10. Using repetition and reinforcement appropriately
11. Giving the client feedback

Implementation involves believing that each interaction with a client is an opportunity to teach. The nurse maximizes opportunities for effective learning and uses a diversified approach to create an active learning environment.

TEACHING APPROACHES

A nurse's approach in teaching is different from teaching methods. Some situations require a teacher to be directive. Others may require a nondirective approach. An effective teacher concentrates on the task and uses teaching approachs according to the learner's needs. A learner's needs and motives can change over time. Thus the teacher must always be aware of the need to modify teaching approaches.

Telling. The telling approach is useful when limited information must be taught (e.g., preparing a client for an emergent diagnostic procedure). If a client is highly anxious but it is vital for information to be given, telling can be effective. When using telling, the nurse outlines the task to be done by the client and gives explicit instructions. There is no opportunity for feedback with this method.

Selling. The selling approach uses two-way communication. The nurse paces instruction based on the client's response. Specific feedback is given to the client who shows success at learning. For example, the client learns a step-by-step procedure for changing a dressing. The nurse uses information from the client to adapt the teaching approach.

Participating. The participating approach involves the nurse and client setting objectives and participating in the learning process together. The client helps decide content, and the nurse guides and counsels the client with pertinent information. For example, a client with diabetes must learn about diet, exercise, and possible complications of the disease. Learning activities must be adapted to incorporate elements of the home environment. In this method there is opportunity for discussion, feedback, and revision of the teaching plan.

Entrusting. The entrusting approach provides the client the opportunity to manage self-care. Responsibilities are accepted, and tasks are performed well by the client. The nurse observes the client's progress and remains available to assist without introducing more new information. For example, a diabetic client has been self-administering insulin for more than 3 months. Injections are performed correctly, and the client can explain signs and symptoms of low blood glucose levels. The nurse instructs the client about a new prescribed dose of insulin and allows the client to perform the self-injection.

Reinforcing. The principle of reinforcement applies to the process of learning; however, the teacher must often be the source of reinforcement. **Reinforcement** is using a stimulus that increases the probability of a response. A learner who receives reinforcement before or after a desired learning behavior is likely to repeat the behavior. Feedback is a common form of reinforcement.

Reinforcers are positive or negative. Positive reinforcement, such as a smile or approval, produces desired responses. Negative reinforcement such as frowning, complaining, or criticizing produces the desired behavior when the reinforcers are removed. People usually respond better to positive reinforcement. The effects of negative reinforcement are less predictable and often undesirable.

Three types of reinforcers are social, material, and activity. When a nurse works with a client most reinforcers are social (e.g., smiles, compliments, words of encouragement, or physical contact), which are used to acknowledge a learned behavior. Examples of material reinforcers are food, toys, and music. These work best with young children. Activity reinforcers rely on the principal that a person is motivated to engage in an activity if promised that, after its completion, the opportunity to engage in more desirable activity will be available. For example, a client will more likely perform a painful exercise if given the chance to take a nap afterward.

Choosing an appropriate reinforcer involves careful thought and attention to individual preferences. Observing behavior often helps reveal the best reinforcer to use. Reinforcers should never be used as threats, and reinforcement is not always effective with every client. A young child responds more to social reinforcers than do older children or adults. An adult with whom the nurse has a good relationship is more effectively reinforced than an adult with whom the nurse has a poor relationship.

INCORPORATING TEACHING WITH NURSING CARE

Many nurses find that they can teach more effectively while delivering nursing care. For example, while bathing a diabetic client the nurse discusses foot care, or while administering drugs the nurse may explain a medication's side effects. An informal, unstructured style relies on the positive therapeutic relationship between nurse and client, which fosters a spontaneity in the teaching-learning process. This does not suggest that teaching should occur without a formal plan. When the nurse follows a teaching plan informally, the client feels less pressure to perform and learning becomes more of a shared activity. Teaching during routine care is efficient and cost-effective (Fig. 15-3).

INSTRUCTIONAL METHODS

Instructional methods that are chosen depend on the client's learning needs, the time available for teaching, the setting, the resources available, and the nurse's own comfort level with teaching. Skilled teachers are flexible in altering teaching methods according to the learner's responses. An experienced teacher uses a variety of techniques and teaching aids. A nurse cannot expect to be an expert educator when first entering nursing practice. Learning to become an effective educator takes time and practice.

When first starting to teach clients, it helps to remember that clients perceive the nurse as an expert. However, this does not mean that the nurse must have all of the answers. It simply means that clients expect that the nurse will keep them appropriately informed. The nurse can provide an effective teaching plan, keeping it simple and focused on clients' needs. A variety of teaching methods can be used, and a variety of teaching aids is usually available.

One-on-One Discussion. Perhaps the most common method of instruction used by a nurse is one-on-one discussion. When teaching a client at the bedside, in a physician's office, or in the home, the nurse directly shares information. Various teaching aids can be used during the discussion, depending on the client's learning needs. Information is usually given in an informal manner, allowing the client to ask questions or share concerns. The nurse

uses unstructured and informal discussion when helping the client understand the implications of illness and ways to cope with health stressors.

Group Instruction. A nurse uses group instruction with clients or families for one of the following reasons (Redman, 1993):

1. Groups are an economical way to teach a number of clients at one time.
2. The experience of being part of a group may be the most likely way for clients to meet learning objectives.

Group instruction often involves both lecture and discussion. Lectures are highly structured and are efficient in helping groups of clients learn standard content about a subject. For example, a nurse might teach groups of clients about the warning signs of breast cancer, the health risks of smoking, or the normal development of a fetus. A lecture does not ensure that learners are actively thinking about the material presented; thus discussion and practice sessions are essential (Redman, 1993).

After hearing information from a lecture, learners need the opportunity to share ideas and seek clarification. Group discussions allow clients and families to learn from each other as they review common experiences. A productive group discussion helps participants solve problems and arrive at solutions toward improving each member's health. To be an effective group leader, the nurse must be able to guide participation. Acknowledging a look of interest, asking questions, and summarizing key issues foster group involvement. However, not all clients benefit from group discussions, and sometimes the physical or emotional level of wellness may prohibit participation.

Preparatory Instruction. Clients frequently face unfamiliar tests or procedures that create significant anxiety. Providing information about procedures helps clients form realistic images of what to anticipate. This is a common expectation of clients in acute care settings because information helps to give them a sense of control. When the experience matches expectations, the client is more likely to attend to the nurse's future explanations. A nurse gains respect when preparatory explanations prove useful. The nurse uses the following guidelines for giving preparatory explanations:

1. Physical sensations during the procedure are described but not evaluated. For example, when drawing a blood specimen, the nurse explains that the client will feel a sticking sensation as the needle punctures the skin.
2. The cause of the sensation is described, preventing misinterpretation of the experience. For example, the nurse explains that a needle insertion burns because alcohol used to cleanse the skin enters the puncture site.
3. Clients are prepared only for aspects of the experience that have commonly been noticed by other clients. For example, the nurse explains that it is normal for a tight tourniquet to cause a person's hand to tingle and feel numb.

The client finds comfort in knowing what to expect. When the nurse's descriptions accurately portray the actual experience, the client is able to cope more effectively with stress from procedures and therapies. The known is less threatening than the unknown.

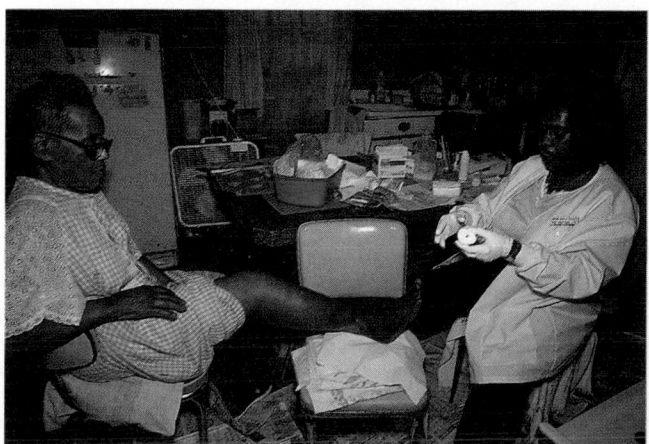

Fig. 15-3 Nurse teaching client about care in the home setting.

Demonstrations. Demonstrations are useful methods for teaching psychomotor skills. Skills such as preparation of a syringe, bathing an infant, crutch walking, measuring a pulse, changing a dressing, and conflict resolution techniques can be taught by demonstration. The client is able to observe a skill before practicing it. Demonstrations are most effective when learners first observe the teacher and then practice the skill in mock or real situations (**return demonstrations**). Nurses commonly use demonstrations for teaching motor skills; however, motor skills are not learned separately from attitudes and factual knowledge (Redman, 1993). A demonstration should be combined with discussion to clarify concepts and feelings. An effective demonstration requires advanced planning, including the following:

1. Be sure that the learner can easily see the demonstration. Position the learner to provide a clear view of the skill being performed.
2. Review the rationale and steps of the procedure.
3. Assemble and organize equipment. Be sure that all equipment works.
4. Perform each step in sequence while analyzing knowledge and skills involved.
5. Determine when explanations are to be given, considering the client's learning needs.
6. Judge proper speed and timing of the demonstration, based on the client's cognitive abilities and anxiety level.

The nurse demonstrates a skill in the same order in which the client will perform it. The demonstration involves the following:

1. Performing each step slowly and accurately
2. Encouraging the client to ask questions so that each step is understood
3. Explaining the rationale for each step
4. Allowing the client to observe each step
5. Avoiding a hurried approach
6. Allowing the client to handle equipment and practice the skill under supervision

The client demonstrates the procedure to ensure that learning has occurred. The independent demonstration should occur under the same conditions found at home or place where the skill is to be performed. For example, if a client is learning to walk with crutches, the nurse simulates the home environment. If short, narrow steps lead to the client's bedroom, the client should learn to climb similar stairs in the hospital.

Analogies. Learning occurs when a teacher translates complex language or ideas into words or concepts that the client understands. In addition, the client benefits by integrating new information into daily routines. **Analogies** supplement verbal instruction with familiar images that make complex information more real and understandable (Redman, 1993). For example, when explaining intestinal peristalsis to a client, an analogy would be the movement of an earthworm as the wave moves down the length of the worm. Another analogy is comparing arterial blood pressure to the flow of water through a hose. To use analogies the nurse follows the following general principles:

1. Be familiar with the concept.
2. Know the client's background, experience, and culture.
3. Keep the analogy simple and clear.

Role Playing. A nurse uses role play for teaching ideas and attitudes. For example, a nurse may teach parents to respond to a child's behavior, help spouses to react to one another's anger, and assist families in communicating with dying relatives. During role play people are asked to play themselves or someone else. The technique involves rehearsing a desired behavior. As a result of role play, clients are taught the skills required and feel more confident in being able to perform independently.

Discovery. Discovery is a useful technique for teaching clients problem solving, application, and independent thinking. During individual or group discussion a nurse may pose a problem or situation for clients to solve. The problem pertains to the clients' learning needs. For example, clients with heart disease may be asked to plan a meal low in cholesterol. The clients in the group work together to decide which foods would be appropriate in the diet. The nurse asks the group members to present their diet, providing an opportunity to identify mistakes and reinforce correct information.

SPEAKING THE CLIENT'S LANGUAGE

It is important to use words a client can understand. The nurse defines unfamiliar medical or nursing terms and uses them consistently throughout a teaching session. Medical jargon can be confusing.

Byrne and Edeani (1984) found that clients understand fewer medical words than health professionals predict. The problem of **functional illiteracy** is also real. Approximately 25 million Americans are functionally illiterate (unable to read above a fifth-grade level), and another 45 million are considered marginally illiterate (unable to use printed or written information to get their everyday needs met). Although illiteracy exists among all races, African Americans, Native Americans, and Hispanics have the highest rates (Fain, 1994). Years of schooling are not accurate indicators of reading ability (Miller and Bodie, 1994).

To compound the problem, the readability of health education material has been researched extensively and has been shown to range from elementary school level to college level (Owen et al, 1993). For example, four American Heart Association and National Heart, Lung, and Blood Institute pamphlets were found to have a mean reading grade level of 14.7 (Merritt et al, 1993). Studies have also shown that clients are more apt to understand information prepared at a grade 5 level than at a grade 9 level (Estey et al, 1994). Thus it appears that the written health information available to a client often exceeds a client's reading ability.

Implications of illiteracy and resulting poor communication skills for client education include the client's inability to analyze instructions or synthesize information and incorporate it into a behavior task. Also, illiterate adults have not acquired the problem-solving skills of drawing conclusions and inferences from experience, and they will not ask questions to obtain or clarify information that has been presented.

The nurse needs to address literacy problems by using simple terminology to enhance the client's understanding. Frequently asking clients for feedback determines whether clients comprehend, and asking for return demonstrations will help clarify instruction and provide a time for repeated review of procedures. Teaching materials should be written

CULTURAL ASPECTS OF CARE

The community health nurse assessed the need to provide acquired immunodeficiency syndrome (AIDS) education to the three teenage sons in a Mexican-American family in her caseload. Substance abuse (alcohol and drug addiction) is higher among Hispanics than among other groups, largely because of *machismo*, a cultural view that drinking and drug use demonstrate strength and masculinity. In addition, some Hispanics share needles and syringes to administer vitamins, medications, or contraceptives purchased in Mexico.

In providing health education to this family, the nurse relied on the interpretation of true cultural *machismo* in which Hispanic men take responsibility for their families and protect them from harm. Using this cultural value, the nurse encouraged these young Hispanic men to protect their loved ones from the threat of diseases such as AIDS. The nurse also discussed appropriate methods of contraception, and proper medication and vitamin administration.

Caudle P: Providing culturally sensitive health care to Hispanic clients, *Nurse Practitioner* 18(12):40, 1993.

on a fifth-grade reading level with attention given to short words and sentences, large type, and simple format.

The nurse must also know of the client's cultural background and beliefs and ability to understand instructions developed outside of the native language (see the box above). Cultural diversity is increasing and poses a great challenge to the nurse trying to provide culturally sensitive care. When educating clients of different ethnic groups the nurse must:

1. Become aware of the distinctive aspects of each culture.
2. Collaborate with other nurses and educators to assist in dealing with cultural diversity.
3. Enlist the help of people in the cultural group to share values and beliefs.
4. Utilize input and experiences of ethnic nurses in providing care to members of their own community (Bernal, 1993).

USING TEACHING TOOLS

Many teaching tools are available for nurses to use when instructing a client. Selection of the right tool depends on the instructional method chosen, the client's learning needs, and the client's ability to learn (Table 15-5). For example, a printed pamphlet may not be the best tool to use for a client with poor reading comprehension, and an audiotape may be the best choice for a client with visual impairment.

SPECIAL NEEDS OF CHILDREN AND OLDER ADULTS

A nurse's choice of instructional methods and application of teaching-learning principles may be based on a client's age. Children, adults, and older adults learn differently. The nurse adapts teaching strategies to each learner.

Children pass through several developmental stages (see

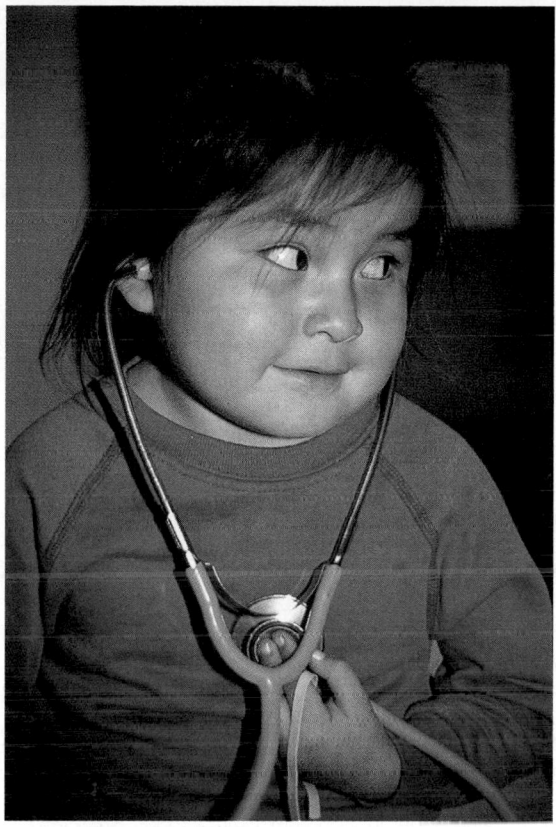

Fig. 15-4 The preschool child learns not to be afraid of medical equipment by being allowed to handle the stethoscope and imitating its use.

Unit 5). In each developmental stage children acquire new cognitive and psychomotor abilities that respond to different types of learning (Fig. 15-4). For example, a nurse can teach school-age children about health as they acquire the ability to see things through the point of view of others. Dental hygiene, nutrition, safety measures, and sex education are examples of topics that may be presented to school children of varying ages. Parental input is incorporated in planning health education for children.

Older adults experience numerous physical and psychological changes as they age (see Chapter 31). These changes can create barriers to learning unless adjustments are made in nursing interventions.

Sensory changes such as visual and hearing deficits require teaching methods that enhance older clients' functioning. For example, the nurse sits to face clients with hearing problems and speaks in a low tone of voice during discussions. Clients with visual problems can benefit from the use of printed materials containing large print. Research demonstrates that older adults learn and remember effectively if the learning is paced properly and the material is relevant to the learner's needs and abilities (Deakins, 1994; Dellasega et al, 1994). Although older adults have slower cognitive function and reduced short-term memory, nurses can facilitate learning in several ways in order to support behaviors that maximize the individual's capacity for self-care (see the box on p. 280). When teacing older

Table 15-5	Teaching Tools for Instruction	
DESCRIPTION	**LEARNING IMPLICATIONS**
PRINTED MATERIAL Written teaching tools available as pamphlets, booklets, brochures	Material must be easily readable for learner. Information must be accurate and current. Method is ideal for understanding complex concepts and relationships.
PROGRAMMED INSTRUCTION Written sequential presentation of learning steps requiring that learners answer questions and that teachers tell them whether they are right or wrong	Instruction is primarily verbal, but teacher may use pictures or diagrams. Method requires active learning, giving immediate feedback, correcting wrong answers, and reinforcing right answers. Learner works at own pace.
COMPUTER INSTRUCTION Use of programmed instruction format in which computers store response patterns for learners and select further lessons on basis of these patterns (programs can be individualized)	Method requires reading comprehension, psychomotor skills, and familiarity with computer.
NONPRINT MATERIALS **Diagrams** Illustrations that show interrelationships by means of lines and symbols	Method demonstrates key ideas, summarizes, and clarifies key concept.
Graphs (bar, circle, or line) Visual presentations of numerical data	Graphs help learner to grasp information quickly about single concept.
Charts Highly condensed visual summary of ideas and facts that may highlight series of ideas, steps, or events	Charts demonstrate relationship of several ideas or concepts. Method helps learners know what to do.
Pictures Photographs or drawings used to teach concepts in which the third dimension of shape and space is not important	Photographs are more desirable than diagrams because they more accurately portray the details of the real item. Drawings are pertinent for removing the superfluous detail present in real objects.
Physical objects Use of actual equipment, objects, or models to teach concepts or skills	Models are useful when real objects are too small, large, or complicated or are unavailable. Learners can manipulate objects that are to be used later in skill.
Other audiovisual materials Slides, audiotapes, television, and videotapes used with printed material or discussion	Materials are useful for clients with reading comprehension problems and visual deficits.

GERONTOLOGICAL PRINCIPLES for Teaching

- Use a slow pace of presentation.
- Give information in short, frequent sessions.
- Repeat information frequently.
- Reinforce teaching with audiovisual material, written exercises, and practice.
- Use analogies and concrete examples.
- Reduce interruptions.
- Allow more time for learners to express themselves, demonstrate learning, and ask questions.
- Establish reachable short-term goals.
- Apply teaching to present situations.
- Base new information on the client's previous level of learning.

Modified from Deakins DA: *Am J Nurs* 94(4):38, 1994.

clients, the nurse should include family members who may be assuming partial care for the client. However, the nurse must be sensitive to the client's desire for assistance, since offering unwanted support may result in negative outcomes and may be perceived as nagging and interference (Connell, 1991).

Evaluation

Client education is not complete until the nurse evaluates outcomes of the teaching-learning process (see the evaluation box on p. 281). The nurse determines whether clients have learned the material. Evaluation reinforces learners' correct behavior, helps learners realize how they should change incorrect behavior, and helps the teacher determine adequacy of teaching (Cronbach, 1977). The nurse evaluates success by observing the client's performance of each

Sample Evaluation of Interventions for Knowledge Deficit

GOALS	EVALUATIVE MEASURES	EXPECTED OUTCOMES
Client will describe preoperative surgical care experience by 7/8.	Ask client to identify procedures anticipated before surgery.	Client will describe preoperative routines planned on morning before surgery.
Client will participate in preoperative and postoperative surgical care procedures by 7/8.	Have client demonstrate breathing exercises. Ask client to explain benefits of breathing exercises.	Client will demonstrate deep breathing exercises by 7/8. Client will describe how exercises help prevent pneumonia by 7/8.

expected behavior (see the evaluation box above). Success depends on the client's ability to meet the established performance criteria.

Direct observation of client behaviors is useful when determining how a person will act in the future. Watching a client demonstrate a skill helps the nurse to know whether the correct technique is being used. However, a client may choose to behave differently later. Observation works best in a situation when a client is unaware of being watched.

Oral and written questioning are other useful evaluation methods. A client's success in cognitive learning can be measured verbally by the client answering questions about a specific topic that was taught. Questions measure behaviors that are not easily observed. The nurse should carefully phrase questions to ensure that the learner understands them and that objectives are truly measured.

Another form of evaluation includes self-reports (oral and written) and self-monitoring (written). This involves the client or family member providing information independently. An example might include a client's report of the foods eaten during a specific week, matched against a newly prescribed diet. The nurse relies on the client's honesty and memory in self-reporting.

Because of the increasing importance of client satisfaction (see Chapter 4), nurses should evaluate whether clients have the information they want. Have their expectations been met? A client may want specific information that he or she knows will be necessary to continue a normal lifestyle at home. Nurses must include client expectations as a part of their evaluation.

During evaluation the nurse also has the client demonstrate the behaviors described in the learning objectives. If the evaluation process indicates a knowledge or skill deficit, the nurse repeats or modifies the teaching plan. Evaluation may reveal new learning needs or the existence of new factors that may interfere with the client's ability to learn. Alternative teaching methods often help clarify information or skills that the client was unable to comprehend or per-

form originally. When a client has difficulty in an acute care setting, the nurse may make a referral to resources such as home health care for further education and evaluation. Like the nursing process, the teaching-learning process is continuous and ever changing.

DOCUMENTATION OF CLIENT TEACHING

Because client teaching often occurs informally between nurse and client (e.g., during medication administration or physical examination), it is difficult to document it consistently. Nurses often fail to take the time to write down material that is taught. However, because a nurse is legally responsible for providing accurate, timely information to clients, it is essential to document the outcomes of teaching. Barron (1987) suggests the following for documenting client education:

1. Specific content. Specifically describe subject matter so that other nurses can follow up and reinforce teaching (e.g., "Insulin injection demonstrated" or "Explained side effects of Inderal"). Avoid generalizations, such as "medications taught," that leave staff uninformed about what content has been taught.
2. Evaluation of learning. Document evidence of learning (e.g., a return demonstration or the ability to describe a medication). This informs staff about the client's progress and determines information that still must be taught.
3. Method of teaching. Describe teaching methods that are used. Knowing the methods used in instruction (e.g., demonstrations or discussion) helps staff follow up more efficiently or offer alternative teaching methods if learning does not occur. When resources such as pamphlets or audiovisual materials are used, the nurse documents this in the client's record. Many institutions have special forms that allow easy documentation. For instance, teaching flow sheets (Fig. 15-5) are excellent records that document the plan, implementation, and evaluation of client teaching.

BARNES

C-33

DIABETIC INSTRUCTION RECORD

TI = TEACHING INITIATED
D/V = DEMONSTRATES/VERBALIZES UNDERSTANDING
FI = FAMILY INCLUDED

ADDRESSOGRAPH PLATE

ASSESSMENT

1. HIGHEST LEVEL OF FORMALIZED
   EDUCATION ATTAINED *High School*
2. VISION *Glasses required for reading*
3. LITERACY *Able to read and explain information in teaching booklet*
4. IDENTIFIED BARRIERS TO
   LEARNING

	DATE & INITIAL			COMMENTS
	TI	D/V	FI	
A) DISEASE OVERVIEW	P.L.	R.K.	P.L.	Wife included in teaching
1. DEFINITION OF DIABETES	3/28	3/29	3/28	session
2. LONGTERM COMPLICATIONS (MICROVASCULAR/MACROVAS-CULAR/NEUROPATHY)	P.L. 3/28	R.K. 3/29	P.L. 3/28	
3. 3 FACTORS OF CONTROL (DIET, EXERCISE, MEDICATION)	P.L. 3/28	R.K. 3/29	P.L. 3/28	
B) DIET	R.K.			
1. TYPE *1800 Cal. ADA*	3/29			
SNACK TIMES *8:00 PM*	3/29 R.K.			
2. MEAL TIMING *8am 12N 6PM*	3/29 R.K.			
3. FOOD TYPES TO AVOID (FRIED FATTY FOODS, SIMPLE SUGARS)				
4. IMPORTANCE OF WEIGHT CONTROL				
C) EXERCISE				
1. TYPE				
2. FREQUENCY				
3. DURATION				
4. EFFECTS ON BLOOD SUGAR CONTROL & INSULIN UTILIZATION				
D) MEDICATION				
1. NAME/DOSAGE				
2. ORAL AGENT				
a. WHEN TO TAKE				
b. ACTION OF MEDICATION				
3. INSULIN				
a. ACTION, KINDS, STORAGE				
b. PREPARATION, ADMINISTRATION				
c. SITE SELECTION/ROTATION				

Fig. 15-5 Documentation tool for client teaching. *(Courtesy Barnes-Jewish Hospital, St Louis.)*

▪ KEY CONCEPTS ▪

► In the health care system today, there is greater emphasis in providing quality health education.

► The nurse must ensure that clients, families, and communities receive information needed to maintain optimal health.

► Health education is aimed at the promotion, restoration, and maintenance of health.

► Teaching is most effective when it is responsive to the learner's needs.

► Teaching is a form of interpersonal communication, with teacher and student actively involved in a process that increases the student's knowledge and skills.

► The ability to learn depends on a person's physical and cognitive attributes.

► The ability to attend to the learning process depends on physical comfort and anxiety levels and the presence of environmental distraction.

► A person's health beliefs influence the willingness to gain knowledge and skills necessary to maintain health.

► Teaching must be timed to coincide with the client's readiness to learn.

► Clients of different age-groups require different teaching strategies as a result of developmental capabilities.

► The client should be an active participant in a teaching plan, agreeing to the plan, helping choose instructional methods, and recommending times for instruction.

► Learning objectives describe what a person is to learn in behavioral terms.

► A combination of teaching methods improves the learner's attentiveness and involvement.

► A teacher is more effective when presenting information that builds on a learner's existing knowledge.

► A teacher who uses reinforcers such as praise or encouragement for a behavior is trying to increase the probability of the behavior recurring.

► The older adult learns most effectively when information is slowly paced and presented in small amounts.

► A nurse evaluates a client's learning by observing performance of expected learning behaviors under desired conditions.

▪ KEY TERMS ▪

Affective learning, p. 264

Analogies, p. 278

Cognitive learning, p. 264

Compliance, p. 265

Functional illiteracy, p. 278

Health-belief model, p. 266

Learning, p. 262

Learning objective, p. 263

Motivation, p. 265

Psychomotor learning, p. 264

Reinforcement, p. 276

Return demonstrations, p. 278

Teaching, p. 262

▪ CRITICAL THINKING EXERCISES ▪

1. Tommy Carter is a 7-year-old who was recently hospitalized with newly diagnosed insulin-dependent diabetes. He has no family history of diabetes. He is being discharged on a regimen that includes a diabetic diet, two insulin injections per day, and blood glucose self-monitoring. He is to return to the clinic in 1 week. Design teaching plans for both Tommy and his parents.

2. Mrs. Jones, who is 38 years old, is scheduled for a breast biopsy. Her mother and sister have a history of breast cancer. They are both currently in remission and are in their sixth and seventh year after initial diagnoses. Mrs. Jones has never had surgery. She is nervous and "scared of the diagnosis." List your teaching priorities for this client.

3. Mr. Taylor, who is 53 years old, has a cast on his right leg after repair of a fractured ankle. He is to begin crutch walking tomorrow and must learn about cast care. You ask Mr. Taylor to read the cast care pamphlet and discuss its content with you. You discover that he is unable to read and comprehend the information in the brochure. Describe the interventions you would employ in developing a teaching plan for this client.

4. Mrs. Johnson is a 62-year-old woman with a long-standing history of non–insulin-dependent diabetes. She is in the clinic for a routine examination, and a blood test reveals that she is "in poor glucose control." You as the nurse approach Mrs. Johnson to do some diabetic instruction, and she says to you, "I really don't want to talk about my diabetes. I know all I want to know about it!" Describe how you would approach teaching with Mrs. Johnson.

REFERENCES

Alberta Association of Registered Nurses: *Client education: position statement and guidelines, 1985*, Edmonton, Alberta, Canada, 1986, The Association.

American Association of Diabetes Educators: The scope of practice for diabetes educators and the standards of practice for diabetes educators, *Diabetes Educator* 18(1):52, 1992.

American Nurses Association: *Nursing's agenda for health care reform*, Kansas City, Mo, 1991, The Association.

Barnes LA: Patient education standards, *MCN: Am J Maternal Child Nurs* 18(1):45, 1993.

Barron S: Documentation of patient education, *Patient Educ Counsel* 9:81, 1987.

Bernal H: A model for delivering culture-relevant care in the community, *Public Health Nurs* 10(4):228, 1993.

Bloom BS, editor: Taxonomy of educational objectives, *Cognitive domain*, vol 1, New York, 1956, Longman.

Bull MJ: Managing the transition from hospital to home, *Qual Health Res* 2(1):27, 1992.

Byrne TJ, Edeani D: Knowledge of medical terminology among hospitalized patients, *Nurs Res* 33(3):178, 1984.

Caudle P: Providing culturally sensitive health care to Hispanic clients, *Nurse Practitioner* 18(12):40, 1993.

Connell CM: Psychosocial contexts of diabetes and older adulthood: reciprocal effects, *Diabetes Educator* 17(5):364, 1991.

Cronbach LJ: *Educational psychology*, ed 3, New York, 1977, Harcourt Brace Jovanovich.

Cupples SA: *Effects of timing and reinforcement of preoperative education on knowledge and recovery of coronary artery bypass graft patients*, doctoral dissertation, Washington, DC, 1989, Catholic University of America.

Deakins DA: Teaching elderly patients about diabetes, *Am J Nurs* 94(4):38, 1994.

Dellasega C et al: Nursing process: teaching elderly clients, *J Gerontol Nurs* 20(1):31, 1994.

Estey A et al: Patient's understanding of health information: a multihospital comparison, *Patient Educ Counsel* 24:73, 1994.

Fain JA: When your patient can't read, *Am J Nurs* 94(5):16B, 1994.

Funnell MM et al: Empowerment: an idea whose time has come in diabetes education, *Diabetes Educator* 17(1):37, 1991.

Haire-Joshu D, Houston C: Promoting behavior change: teaching/learning strategies. In *Management of diabetes mellitus: perspectives of care across the lifespan*, St Louis, 1992, Mosby.

Henderson V: *The nature of nursing: a definition and its implication for practice, research, and education*, New York, 1966, McMillan.

Joint Commission on Accreditation of Healthcare Organizations: *Accreditation manual of hospitals*, Chicago, 1995, The Commission.

Kim MJ, McFarland GK, McLane AM: *Pocket guide for nursing diagnoses*, ed 6, St Louis, 1995, Mosby.

Krathwohl DR et al: *Taxonomy of educational objectives: the classification of educational goals. Handbook II. Affective domain*, New York, 1964, David McKay.

Kruger S: The patient educator role in nursing, *Appl Nurs Res* 4(1):19, 1991.

Merritt S: Learning style preferences of coronary artery disease patients, *Cardiovasc Nurs* 27(2):7, 1991.

Merritt SL et al: Readability levels of selected hypercholesterolemia patient education literature, *Heart Lung* 22(5):415, 1993.

Miller A: When is the time ripe for teaching? *Am J Nurs* 85(7):801, 1985.

Miller B, Bodie M: Determination of reading comprehension level for effective patient health-education materials, *Nurs Res* 43(2):118, 1994.

Noble C: Are nurses good patient educators? *J Adv Nurs* 16:1185a, 1991.

Owen PM et al: Reading, readability and patient education materials, *Cardiovasc Nurs* 29(2):9, 1993.

Redman BK: *The process of patient education*, ed 7, St Louis, 1993, Mosby.

Rosenstock IM: Historical origins of the health belief model, *Health Educ Monogr* 2:354, 1974.

Simpson EJ: The classification of educational objectives in the psychomotor domain. In *Contributions of behavioral science to instructional technology: the psychomotor domain*, Mt Ranier, Md, 1972, Gryphon.

Tanner G: A need to know, *Nurs Times* 85(31):54, 1989.

Wong DL: *Whaley and Wong's nursing care of infants and children*, ed 5, St Louis, 1995, Mosby.

ADDITIONAL READINGS

Blackburn JA: Achieving a multicultural service orientation: adaptive models in service delivery and race and culture training, *Caring Magazine* 11(4):22, 1992.

Byrne DM et al: Evaluation of the efficacy of an instructional programme in the self-management of patients with asthma, *J Adv Nurs* 18(4):637, 1993.

Close A: Strategic planning in patient education, *Nurs Stand* 6(43):32, 1992.

Lorig K: *Patient education: a practical approach*, ed 1, St Louis, 1992, Mosby.

Redman BK: Patient education at 25 years: where we have been and where we are going, *J Adv Nurs* 18(5):725, 1993.

Riley-Clark A et al: How do you evaluate the effectiveness of your patient teacing? *Oncol Nurs Forum* 20(5):825, 1993.

Ross MET: Hardiness and complaince in elderly patients with diabetes, *Diabetes Educator* 17(5):372, 1991.

Saivastava R, Wong K: Promoting cultural sensitivity in the work place, *ANNA J* 19(4):419, 1992.

Wasson D, Anderson MA: Hospital-patient education: current status and future trends, *J Nurs Staff Dev* 10(3):147, 1994.

Wong M: Self-care instructions: do patients understand educational materials? *Focus Crit Care* 19(1):47, 1992.

## Chapter 16

Research

Objectives

Mastery of content in this chapter will enable the student to:

► Define the key terms listed.

► Compare the various ways to acquire knowledge.

► List the characteristics of scientific investigation.

► Compare methods for developing new nursing knowledge.

► Define scientific and nursing research.

► Compare the research process with the nursing process.

► List the American Nurses Association's priorities for nursing research.

► Explain how the rights of human research subjects are protected.

► Explain the rights of others who assist in human research studies.

► Describe a typical research report.

► Discuss methods of locating research reports in nursing and related areas.

► Explain how to organize information from a research report.

► List the characteristics of a clinical nursing problem that can be researched.

► List the criteria for using research findings in nursing practice.

Throughout the history of the profession, nursing leaders and organizations have made considerable efforts to increase nurses' awareness of the importance of nursing research as a foundation for practice. In 1974 the American Nurses Association (ANA) House of Delegates passed a resolution calling for more nursing research to focus on clinical problems that nurses face in professional practice.

■ HISTORICAL PERSPECTIVE

A brief historical perspective enables nurses to understand how past issues influence health and, in turn, their influence on nursing practice (see the box below). It is agreed that Florence Nightingale's detailed observation about the effects of nursing actions during the Crimean War was the initial nursing research study (Polit and Hungler, 1995; Talbot, 1995). After Nightingale, nursing research activities focused primarily on educational issues, specifically resulting in the Goldmark Report, which identified gaps in the educational background in nursing education. Following the Goldmark report the method for educating nurses changed, and more university-based nursing curricula resulted. During the 1940s research activities focused on educational issues. In the 1950s, however, there was an increase in the number of nurses with advanced degrees and the journal *Nursing Research* was initiated. The Walter Reed Army Institute of Research was established. The University of Pittsburgh offered the first doctorial program in nursing in 1954. There were increases in the availability of private and government monies, and the American Nurses Foundation was established (Polit and Hungler, 1995). In the 1960s several professional nursing organizations initiated development of nursing research priorities. The *Lysaught Report* recommended increases in research toward nursing practice and nursing education. Terms such as *conceptual framework, conceptual model, nursing process,* and *theoretical base of nursing practice* began to appear in the nursing literature. In the 1970s nursing studies tended to focus on the roles and characteristics of nurses rather than on problems in delivering professional care to clients (Gortner, 1980). During this time more nurses were receiving doctoral preparation and initiating their own research, and more nursing research journals were published (see the box on p. 287). In 1981 the ANA published specific recommendations for studying research at the different nursing education levels (ANA, Commission on Nursing Research, 1981). A study of nursing by the Institute of Medicine (1983) recommended that the federal government increase funds for

---

Historical Evolution of Nursing Research

1820	Florence Nightingale, the first nurse researcher, is born.	1952	*Nursing Research,* the official research journal of the American Nurses Association (ANA), is published.
1854	Nightingale at military hospital in Scutari during the Crimean War.	1952	Mildred Montag publishes *Community College Education for Nursing.*
1858	Nightingale's *Notes on Matters Affecting the Health, Efficiency and Hospital Administration of the British Army* and *Notes on Hospitals* published in London by Harrison and Sons.	1953	Institute of Research and Service in Nursing Education at Teachers College in Columbia University.
1858	Nightingale made a fellow of the Royal Statistical Society.	1955	The American Nurses Foundation is formed.
1859	*Notes on Nursing* published.	1956	Committee on Research and Studies formed by the ANA.
1860	Nightingale Training School opens at St. Thomas's Hospital, London.	1957	Western Interstate Commission on Higher Education (WICHE), Southern Regional Educational Board (SREB).
1896	Nurses' Associated Alumnae of the United States and Canada organized.	1963	Surgeon General's Consultant Group on Nursing *(Toward Quality in Nursing).*
1900	*American Journal of Nursing* first published.	1964	*International Journal of Nursing Studies* is published.
1903	North Carolina first state to pass permissive licensure law.	1966	*International Nursing Index* published.
1907	Nutting's "The Education and Professional Position of Nurses," Nutting and Dock's *A History of Nursing.*	1970	Lysaught report: *An Abstract for Action.*
1923	Goldmark Report sponsored by the Committee for the Study of Nursing Education.	1976	ANA Commission on Nursing Research publishes *Preparation of Nurses, for Participation in Research.*
1924	Yale University offers first degree in nursing.	1981	ANA Commission on Nursing Research publishes *Research Priorities for the 1980s* and *Guidelines for the Investigative Function of Nurses.*
1924	Teachers College, Columbia University, offers first doctoral program for nurses, granting and EdD.		
1932	The Association of Collegiate Schools of Nursing is organized.	1985	ANA Cabinet on Nursing Research publishes *Directions for Nursing Research: Toward the Twenty-first Century.*
1934	New York University offers first PhD in nursing.	1986	Establishment of the National Center for Nursing Research at the National Institutes of Health.
1936	Sigma Theta Tau awards first grant for research in the United States.	1988	*Nursing Scan in Research* published.
1948	Ginzberg Report published.	1989	Clinical Practice Guidelines published by the Agency for Health Care Policy and Research.
1948	Brown Report prepared for the National Nursing Council.	1992	*Healthy People 2000* published by Department of Health and Human Services.
1949	Murdock Report published.	1993	National Center for Nursing Research renamed the National Institute of Nursing Research.

Modified from Talbot LA: *Principles and practice of nursing research,* St Louis, 1995, Mosby.

Journals Focusing on Nursing Research	
1952	*Nursing Research*
1967	*IMAGE*
1978	*Research in Nursing and Health*
	Advances in Nursing Science
1979	*Western Journal of Nursing Research*
1980s	*Applied Nursing Research*
1990s	*Clinical Nursing Research*
	Qualitative Health Research

scientific research in nursing and that steps be taken to establish a national organization to place nursing research "in the mainstream of scientific investigation." Acting on this recommendation in 1985, the U.S. Congress overrode two presidential vetoes to establish the National Center for Nursing Research (NCNR) under the National Institutes of Health (NIH). In 1993 the NCNR was promoted to the National Institute of Nursing Research (NINR), giving it equal status and accountability with the other institutes of the NIH.

In 1991 the ANA revised the *Standards of Clinical Nursing Practice*. Within this document are the *Standards of Professional Performance* (see Chapter 13, Table 13-2). Standard 7 recommends that the professional nurse use research findings in practice (ANA, 1991). Thus the ANA recommends that nurses incorporate research findings in clinical practice to restore health, prevent illness, and minimize the effects of acute and chronic disease and disability.

SCIENTIFIC RESEARCH IN NURSING
Knowledge Acquisition

Knowledge is information, and discovery is the creative process of obtaining new knowledge (Talbot, 1995). Knowledge is acquired in many ways. A person continuously takes in and processes numerous pieces of information to understand experiences. The scientific researcher also seeks to explain or understand reality, but the scientist's process of acquiring knowledge is systematic and logical. This process, or scientific method, is the foundation of research. Scientific research is the most reliable and objective of all methods of gaining knowledge.

One way of learning is by tradition. One generation passes knowledge to the next. For example, children often learn about traditional holidays such as Christmas and Passover through traditional or customary family practices. In nursing, certain traditional methods of practice such as the change-of-shift report and other daily hospital work practices are passed from one practitioner to the next. Tradition is an efficient way of learning, although it can also limit the ability to seek new ways of doing things. If tradition becomes so ingrained that a person does not question the custom, other, more appropriate or efficient ways may be overlooked.

Knowledge is also acquired by seeking information from experts in a particular field. Experts are often asked to solve problems or answer questions. For example, at income tax time an accountant's help is sought to fill out tax forms. Similarly, nursing students often seek the advice of instructors and practicing nurses when assessing and caring for clients. Authority, like tradition, is not infallible, although it is commonly treated as absolute truth.

A person also learns through experience. Without this process a person would have to relearn a procedure every time it was performed. Practice leads to the development of routines that help build skills. For example, a student nurse taking a blood pressure measurement for the first time may feel awkward and unsure of hearing the sounds, but with practice the student's technique and confidence improve. Although experience is an important way of learning, it has limitations. A person may continue to do something simply because it was learned that way and may overlook improved or other ways of doing the same thing. If experience causes a person to learn something incorrectly, the person uses knowledge inappropriately.

Knowledge is also acquired by investigating ideas from another discipline within the nursing perspective, for example, by using Selye's model of general adaptation and applying it to clinical nursing situations.

Learning by problem solving is yet another way of gaining knowledge. Trying various ways of resolving client's health care needs, developing new staffing patterns, or evaluating health care products will eventually result in problem solving. This method of learning is practical, but it is unsystematic and often a haphazard way of learning. In nursing, because clients' health status depends on nursing actions, the problem-solving method may lead toward specific research questions.

The nurse can use the skills of logical reasoning and critical thinking to analyze information acquired through traditional learning, information seeking, experiential learning, investigating ideas from other disciplines, and problem solving to determine a course of nursing action. In addition, the nurse can use the skills of scientific inquiry to identify and investigate a clinical, professional, or educational issue. The skills of scientific inquiry require the use of the scientific method.

The scientific method is the most advanced, objective means of acquiring knowledge. By use of this method the researcher attempts to understand, explain, predict, or control a nursing phenomenon (Polit and Hungler, 1995). The method is characterized by systematic, orderly procedures that, although not without fault, seek to limit the possibility for error and minimize the likelihood that any bias or opinion by the researcher might influence the results of research and thus the knowledge gained. Polit and Hungler (1995) describe the characteristics of scientific investigation as follows:

1. The steps of planning and conducting an investigation are undertaken in a systematic, orderly fashion.
2. Nurse/scientists attempt to control external factors that are not under direct investigation but that can influence a relationship between phenomena they are studying. For example, if a nurse were studying the relationship between diet and heart disease, other characteristics such as stress would have to be controlled for contributing factors to this disease.
3. Evidence that is part of experience (**empirical data**) is gathered directly or indirectly through use of the observations and assessments and is the basis for discovering new knowledge.

4. The goal is to understand phenomena in such a way that the knowledge gained can be applied generally, not just to isolated cases or circumstances.

5. Scientists strive to conduct investigations that contribute to testing or developing theories, thereby advancing the knowledge that can be applied toward increasing understanding of people, places, or life events.

Nursing and the Scientific Approach

The purpose of the scientific approach is to serve as a method of problem solving, as a system for acquiring knowledge, or to predict nursing phenomena (Polit and Hungler, 1995; Table 16-1).

Compared with other ways of acquiring knowledge, the scientific method is more orderly and objective in its approach. Nurses use this approach to develop knowledge. In the past, much of the information used in nursing practice was borrowed from other disciplines such as biology, physiology, psychology, and sociology. Often, this information was applied to nursing without testing or comparing ways for caring for clients. For example, nurses use several methods to help clients sleep. Interventions such as giving a client a back rub, making sure that the bed is clean and comfortable, preparing the environment by dimming the lights, and talking to a worried or anxious client are frequently used nursing measures and, in general, are logical, common-sense approaches. However, when these measures are considered in greater depth, questions may arise about their applications for different clients in different situations.

Research provides a way for nursing questions and problems to be studied in greater depth within the context of nursing. Frequently nurses rely on personal experience or the statements of nursing experts. If an intervention works for most clients, the nurse may be satisfied with this success without questioning whether there might be a better way. If the intervention is not successful, the nurse might use an

approach practiced by a colleague or try a different sequence of accepted measures. Even if an intervention discovered with this approach is effective for one or more clients, it may not be appropriate for other clients in other settings. Approaches must be tested to determine the measures that work best with specific clients.

Definitions of Scientific and Nursing Research

The **scientific method** is a systematic method of questioning and challenging the validity of scientific assumptions (Polit and Hungler, 1995). Within the scientific method is the **scientific approach**, which is a logical, orderly, and objective means of generating research questions and testable hypotheses. Several factors affect scientific research. When scientists use systematic, controlled methods for studying events or problems, they have more confidence that the results are accurate and are not influenced by opinion or belief. These studies are well organized and follow a specific procedure. For a study to be empirical, the evidence collected must come from objective findings. In addition, other researchers should be able to examine the evidence and see the same **phenomena** (results). To guide the design of a research study, scientists create a hypothetical proposition (**hypothesis**) about what they expect to see before conducting the study. Scientists generally study the way that characteristics or events are different or the way that one event causes another.

When reading research studies, nurses should avoid interpreting results in terms of cause and effect because there is a difference between cause-and-effect and other kinds of relationships. For example, as people get older, they tend to lose their hair, and their skin becomes wrinkled. These factors are related to each other as part of the aging process, but neither causes the other. Researchers often study such relationships without being able to determine why or how these changes take place.

Biomedical research is concerned mainly with discover-

Table 16-1	Purpose of the Scientific Method, Research Question, and Nursing Research	
PURPOSE	**TYPES OF QUESTIONS**	**NURSING RESEARCH EXAMPLE**
Description	How prevalent is the phenomenon? What are the characteristics of the phenomenon? What is the process by which the phenomenon is experienced?	What categories of activities are involved in the at-home care of people with AIDS, and what is the market value of the unpaid care giving? (Ward and Brown, 1994)
Exploration	What is the full nature of the phenomenon? What is going on? What factors are related to the phenomenon?	What information is used by expert critical care nurses, and how do they structure the information when reasoning and making clinical decisions? (Fonteyn and Grobe, 1994)
Explanation	What is the underlying cause? What does the occurrence of the phenomenon mean? Why does the phenomenon exist?	What are the factors that determine perimenstrual symptom patterns in women? (Mitchell et al, 1994).
Prediction and control	If phenomenon *X* occurs, will phenomenon *Y* follow? Can the occurrence of the phenomenon be controlled? Does an intervention result in the intended effect?	What combination of factors best predicts health-promoting behaviors among adults with disabilities? (Stuifbergen and Becker, 1994)

Modified from Polit DF, Hungler BP: *Nursing research: principles and methods,* ed 5, Philadelphia, 1995, Lippincott.

ing the causes and treatments of disease. In contrast, **nursing research** focuses on the full range of human responses and is directed toward helping well people improve their health status and stay healthy, as well as assisting clients who are sick or disabled by an illness to maintain or improve their health.

The Commission on Nursing Research of the ANA (1981a) has defined nursing research as follows:

Nursing research develops knowledge about health and the promotion of health over the full life span, care of persons with health problems and disabilities, and nursing actions to enhance the ability of individuals to respond effectively to actual or potential health problems.

The International Council of Nurses (1986) supports the need for nursing research as a means for improving the health and welfare of people. Nursing research is a way to identify new knowledge, improve professional education and practice, and use resources effectively. The material that follows provides one of the clinical research studies that have changed the practice of nursing.

The effect of preoperative teaching on postoperative recovery is an area that has been studied extensively. Some studies have examined the effect of preoperative teaching on positive postoperative outcomes (Meeker, 1994; Planchock and Wiggins, 1994). Timmons and Bower (1993) examined the effect of preoperative teaching on clients' understanding of patient-controlled analgesia and their management of postoperative pain. The group receiving preoperative education managed their pain significantly better. Teaching clients what they can expect on the day of surgery and in the immediate postoperative period is now a widely accepted and implemented nursing measure. For example, such teaching often includes information about when vital signs will be monitored after surgery and the deep breathing and coughing techniques they will be asked to perform. This information is provided to relieve fear and anxiety and to help clients recover from surgery.

Because nurses are interested in acquiring knowledge about a wide range of human needs and responses to health problems, nursing research uses many methods to study clinical problems (see the box above). The hallmark of scientific research is the **experiment**. In a true experimental study the conditions under which a measure is investigated are tightly controlled. Experimental approaches to studying a problem require that the information about human subjects be collected and quantified in a prescribed manner. **Quantitative research** is rigorous, systematic, objective examination of specific concepts and their relationships to test theory by focusing on numerical data, statistical analysis, and controls to eliminate bias (Polit and Hungler, 1995). The study usually includes a control or **comparison group**, which does not receive the nursing measure being investigated. The results for this group are compared with those of a study or an **experimental group**, the group that receives some form of treatment or intervention. The **subjects**, persons selected for the comparison and experimental groups, are chosen at random from among those eligible for the study. Designing an experiment to study physical causes of disease is less difficult than designing an experiment that also includes psychological or social aspects of health. For example, to study the relationship between postoperative anxiety and preoperative

---

Types of Research

HISTORICAL RESEARCH
Systematic collection and critical evaluation of data relating to past events (Polit and Hungler, 1995)

EXPLORATORY RESEARCH
Initial study designed to develop or refine research questions or to test and refine data-collection methods (Polit and Hungler, 1995)

EVALUATION RESEARCH
Study that tests how well a program, practice, or policy is working

DESCRIPTIVE RESEARCH
Study in which the objective is to accurately identify characteristics of persons, situations, or groups and the frequency with which certain events or characteristics occur

EXPERIMENTAL RESEARCH
Study in which the investigator controls the independent variable and randomly assigns subjects to different conditions

QUASI-EXPERIMENTAL RESEARCH
Study in which subjects cannot be randomly assigned to treatment conditions, although the researcher controls the independent variables

CORRELATIONAL RESEARCH
Study that explores the interrelationships among variables of interest without any active intervention by the researcher

---

teaching, the researcher can control one psychological factor by using only subjects having surgery for the first time. However, the researcher cannot control other experiences that the clients may have had, such as hearing a friend's "horror" stories about surgery or reading about surgical experiences in the newspapers. These psychological factors that cannot be controlled may influence the subject's level of anxiety.

Nursing studies use many methods for investigating clinical problems; some may be similar to the experimental approach. Other research methods may be similar to those used in the social sciences such as anthropology and sociology. The amount of knowledge known about the problem and the type of problem being investigated are factors that determine the methods used. Nursing is a practice discipline that deals with unique physical, emotional, and social problems that people experience in regaining, maintaining, and promoting health.

Qualitative research is the exploration of little-known phenomena that are not easily quantified or categorized in which inductive reasoning is used to develop generalizations or theories from specific observations or interviews (Polit and Hungler, 1995). Qualitative research involves the discovery of important characteristics and the ways they might be related. For example, a qualitative research study might involve a survey measuring clients' perceptions of mechanical ventilation (Knebel et al, 1994). When qualitative methods are used, the investigator uses strategies such as open-ended interviews and case histories to study the area of interest.

Table 16-2	**Comparison of the Nursing Process and the Research Process**

NURSING PROCESS	RESEARCH PROCESS
Assessment	Identify phenomena
Diagnosis	Research problem
	Hypotheses
Planning	Study design
Goals	Review of literature
Patient outcomes	Theoretical or conceptual framework
Implementation	Data collection
Evaluation	Analysis of results
	Recommendations and implications for further research

Modified from Talbot LA: *Principles and practice of nursing research*, St Louis, 1995, Mosby.

Nursing Research and the Nursing Process

The research process consists of phases or steps that can be compared and contrasted with those of the nursing process. Both are problem-solving processes used by nurses in practice (Table 16-2), but they are very different. The nursing process is used to determine health needs and plan nursing care for clients. It is used as a basis for gaining and using information about clients to help them restore, maintain, or promote health. Depending on the nursing diagnosis, knowledge from a number of disciplines may be used in the nursing process to help clients solve particular health problems.

In contrast, the **research process** is used to gain knowledge that can be used in other, similar situations. Nurses may want to gain knowledge about the reason a particular event happens or the best way to provide care for clients with a certain health problem. The research process is used to gain knowledge that can be applied to a whole group or class of clients.

During the assessment phase of the nursing process the nurse caring for a client with sleeping difficulties determines factors that might interfere with the ability to sleep. These may include the client's concern about health status, pain, a noisy environment, or a messy or uncomfortable bed. After assessing these aspects, the nurse formulates a nursing diagnosis, plans interventions, implements these interventions, and evaluates the subjective and objective evidence that indicates whether the client is able to sleep.

In contrast, a researcher studying sleeping difficulties seeks new information that can be applied to more than one client. For example, a nurse notices that many clients seem to have a difficult time sleeping the night before a particular diagnostic procedure. Based on work with these clients, the nurse determines that most of them express concerns about the results of the test. In this situation the nurse might design a research study in which some of the clients receive the usual nursing care and others receive care based on relieving anxiety. After collecting information about the effects of the usual care for one group and the new approach for the other, the nurse researcher com-

	ANA Nursing Research Priorities

Generation of knowledge enabling nurses to:
- Promote health, well-being, and the ability to care for oneself among all age, social, and cultural groups.
- Minimize and prevent behaviorally and environmentally induced health problems that compromise the quality of life and reduce productivity.
- Minimize the negative effects of new health technologies on the adaptive abilities of individuals and families experiencing acute or chronic health problems.
- Ensure that the care needs of particularly vulnerable groups, such as the elderly, children with congenital health problems, individuals from diverse cultures, the mentally ill, and the poor, are met in effective and acceptable ways.
- Classify nursing practice phenomena.
- Ensure that principles of ethics guide nursing research.
- Develop instruments to measure nursing outcomes.
- Develop integrative methodologies for the holistic study of human beings as they relate to their families and lifestyles.
- Design and evaluate alternative models for delivering health care and for administering health care systems so that nurses will be able to balance high quality and cost-effectiveness in meeting the nursing needs of identified populations.
- Evaluate the effectiveness of alternative approaches to nursing education for the kind of practice that requires broad knowledge and a wide repertoire of skills, and for the kind of practice that requires specialized knowledge and a focused set of skills.
- Identify and analyze historical and contemporary factors that influence the shaping of nursing professionals' involvement in national health care policy development.

From American Nurses Association Cabinet on Nursing Research: *Directions for nursing research: toward the twenty-first century*, Washington, DC, 1985, The Association.

pares the results to determine whether clients who received the new care had less difficulty sleeping than those who received the normal care. If the clients receiving the new care slept better, the nurse has acquired new knowledge about how generally to help clients.

Nurse Researchers

In 1981 the ANA's Commission on Nursing Research published guidelines for the academic preparation of nurses conducting research. In this document the Association noted that all levels of nursing preparation have an active role in the process of developing nursing knowledge and implementing this knowledge into practice.

In 1985 the ANA's Cabinet on Nursing Research outlined predictions about consumers of nursing services, health care systems, and nursing for the year 2000. On the basis of these predictions, directions for nursing research were further specified (see the box above). With these priorities the profession demonstrates to nurses, other health care professionals, and the general public the areas in which nurses need further knowledge to improve their services. Nurses can use these priorities to guide policy makers and decisions about participation in a research project.

Nurses conduct research in a variety of settings. Student nurses and practitioners may be asked to participate in studies that investigate client outcomes and the effectiveness of nursing care. These types of research projects are commonly called *quality assurance* or *improvement studies* (see Chapter 11). Data are collected to determine the impact nurses have on achievement of client care objectives in a particular clinical setting. Because the results of such research are usually applicable only in one institution, this is not scientific research as discussed earlier. However, such research is important to the institution because the nursing department can use it to demonstrate the contributions made by nurses to client care.

Clinical nursing research should be undertaken by nurses educated to conduct scientific investigations (Fig. 16-1). Generally, nurse researchers hold master's and doctoral degrees. Any subject who is asked to participate in a nursing study is entitled to receive information about the qualifications of the researcher. The researcher's educational background and biographical sketch give information about the person's qualifications. An experienced researcher is usually more qualified than a beginning researcher to undertake a complex, long-term project. Nurses new to research may, however, make important contributions by assisting with data collection, conducting replicated studies (studies previously performed elsewhere), or conducting less complex studies.

Doctorally prepared nurses are prepared to initiate, design, and conduct all phases of research. Nurses with a master's degree in nursing are prepared to collaborate in the design and conduct of research and provide expertise for reviewing studies and integrating studies into practice (ANA, 1989). At the baccalaureate level nurses are prepared to read research critically and determine the readiness of research for use in practice, promote understanding of ethical research principles, identify clinical problems needing research, and assist experienced investigators in conducting research studies. Nurses with associate's degrees are expected to use research findings in practice, sometimes under the guidance of nurses prepared at higher levels of education; identify clinical problems needing study; and assist in the conduct of nursing studies.

Now and into the next century nursing research has the potential to evaluate practice and determine those practices that should be changed. In addition, the emphasis for health care is toward a health promotion, disease prevention, and primary care model (see Chapter 3). The box below lists health promotional, disease prevention, and nursing care research priorities from the NCNR.

ETHICAL ISSUES IN RESEARCH
Rights of Human Subjects

To refine existing knowledge and develop new knowledge, clinical research is sometimes directed at trying new procedures whose outcome is doubtful or unknown (ANA, 1985a). This kind of research may conflict with the purpose of nursing practice, which is to meet specific clients' needs. In such cases the researcher is responsible for structuring the investigation to avoid or minimize harm to the subjects. Although it is not always possible to anticipate all potential undesirable effects, researchers are obligated to inform everyone involved about the known potential risks. Other basic human rights must also be observed. These principles are set forth by both the Canadian Nurses Association (CNA, 1983, 1991) and the ANA (1985, 1985a).

Informed consent means that research subjects (1) are given full and complete information about the purpose of the study, procedures, data collection, potential harm and benefits, and alternative methods of treatment; (2) are capable of fully understanding the research and the implica-

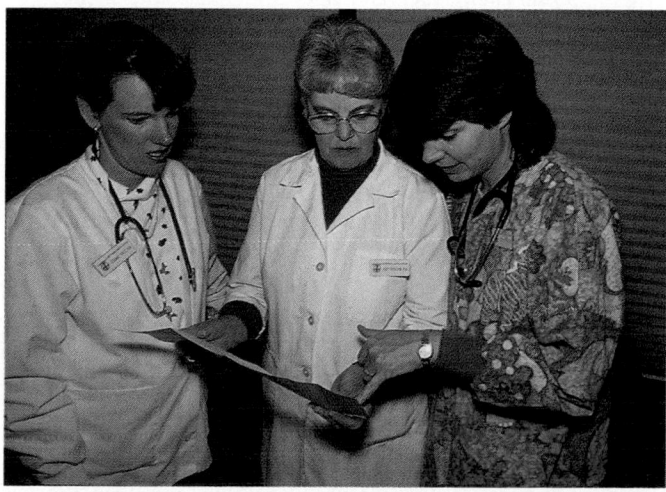

Fig. 16-1 Nurses collaborating on research.

Research Priorities From the National Center for Nursing Research

LOW BIRTH WEIGHT: MOTHERS AND INFANTS
Includes prevention of premature delivery and care of low-birth-weight infants.

HIV INFECTION: PREVENTION AND CARE
Includes ethical issues, and physiological, psychosocial, and systems factors relating to care of persons with HIV infection.

LONG-TERM CARE FOR OLDER ADULTS
Includes such issues as quality of care, continuity of care, and family caregiving.

SYMPTOM MANAGEMENT
Includes biopsychosocial parameters of pain and other symptoms, and measures for symptom assessment and management.

INFORMATION SYSTEMS
Includes development of standardized data sets to document nursing care across settings and a taxonomy to classify nursing phenomena.

HEALTH PROMOTION FOR CHILDREN AND ADOLESCENTS
Includes psychosocial mechanisms underlying health promotion behaviors.

TECHNOLOGY DEPENDENCY ACROSS THE LIFE SPAN
Includes individual and family responses to technology dependency and prevention of complications.

Modified from NCNR: National Center for Nursing Research, Bethesda, Md, 1992, The Center (basic brochure).

tions of participation; and (3) understand how confidentiality or anonymity are maintained. **Confidentiality** guarantees that any information provided by the subject will not be reported in any manner that identifies the subject and will not be made accessible to people outside the research team (Polit and Hungler, 1995). **Anonymity** occurs when even the researcher cannot link the subject to the data (Polit and Hungler, 1995). The subject is assured of free choice in giving consent, including the right to withdraw from the study at any time (Polit and Hungler, 1995; Talbot, 1995). Procedures for obtaining informed consent must be outlined in the study protocol.

In addition, the researcher planning to conduct a study must possess the knowledge and skills necessary to undertake the research. Generally a nurse planning to conduct a study involving psychiatric clients should be familiar with psychiatric nursing principles and theory. Current ANA (1985a) and CNA (1983, 1991) guidelines state that qualified nurse researchers have a right to engage in research and have a right of access to resources needed to conduct studies.

Federal regulations (Federal Register, 1994) require that institutions receiving any federal funding or conducting drug or medical device research regulated by the Food and Drug Administration establish institutional review boards (IRBs). Such a group reviews all studies conducted in the institution to ensure that ethical principles (see Chapter 19) are observed. A major responsibility of the IRB is to determine the risk status of all research projects. The nurse's responsibility is to protect clients' rights at all times.

Rights of Other Research Participants

Student nurses and practicing nurses may be asked to participate in research as data collectors or may be involved in the care of clients participating in a study. All participants, including health care professionals caring for clients, have the right to be fully informed about the study, its procedures (including informed consent and risk factors), and any physical or emotional injury that clients could experience as a result of participation. Often the physical risks are more obvious than the emotional risks. Depending on the problem being studied, clients may be asked to give highly personal, intrusive information. Because this type of research can lead to anxiety or stress for some clients, the researcher should prepare all participants, including nurses delivering care, for this possibility and assist them in coping with the effects. Participants also have the right to see review forms from the IRB that certify approval of the study. Any student, nurse, or other participant has the right to refuse to carry out any research procedures if concerned about their ethical aspects.

Besides dealing with the harmful effects of a research project, nurses may be faced with other ethical dilemmas (Talbot, 1995). For example, some clients may feel they have to participate in an investigation to please the health care professionals on whom they depend for care. They may feel that they will receive inferior care if they refuse to participate. Research ethics require that clients are not made to feel that they are obliged to participate in a study. The ultimate decision rests with the client. Withholding proper care or in any way implying that care will be withheld from clients who refuse to participate is unethical (see Chapter 18).

Another ethical dilemma in research involves withholding a new intervention from clients who might benefit from its use. For example, in an experiment investigating a new intervention the experimental group may receive the new intervention while the comparison group receives the usual care. In such cases clients in the comparison group are deprived of a new treatment that could be beneficial to them. One way of managing this dilemma is to offer the new nursing care to the comparison group after data necessary to the experimental study have been collected.

NURSING RESEARCH IN NURSING PRACTICE

Identifying Research Studies

When reading nursing literature, the registered nurse or nursing student must be able to distinguish a research report or article from other types of writing. This may not be as simple as it seems. Even if the title has the word *research* in it, the article does not necessarily report the results of a research study. The nurse can determine whether an article reports a research study only by examining its contents. Sometimes, however, an article's title can give a clue to its contents. Phrases such as *a study of* or *comparison of* suggest

RESEARCH HIGHLIGHT

RESEARCH ABSTRACT

Engaging older adults in a discussion regarding life-sustaining interventions (cardiopulmonary resuscitation [CPR], tube feeding, and mechanical ventilation) is recommended but remains an uncommon practice among health care providers. This study was conducted to determine the short-term impact of a discussion by a physician with homebound older clients, age 60 to 93 years, concerning areas of urgent, life-sustaining interventions. Data were collected using the Zung Depression Scale, Life Satisfaction Index A and B, Locus of Desired Controls, and an interview with the physician. Clients' knowledge of specific urgent care modalities were assessed during the discussion with the physician. Most clients voiced no specific fears of the future. However, some clients lacked a clear understanding of the concepts and terminology regarding CPR, intubation, and tube feeding.

IMPLICATIONS FOR PRACTICE

▶ Discussing life-sustaining interventions with older adults is not widely used; therefore teaching is an effective nursing strategy, using terminology that the client understands.

▶ Involving older clients in the decision-making process regarding life-sustaining choices may increase their internal locus of control. Nurses should be supportive and encouraging.

▶ Many older adults have not discussed life-sustaining interventions with significant others.

▶ Open communication patterns involve a conscious effort by the health care team to clearly present the client's regimen of care and decision-making process.

REFERENCE

Kellogg F et al: Life-sustaining interventions in frail elderly persons, *Arch Intern Med* 152:2317, 1994.

a research report. The abstract and the introductory paragraphs of an article can also indicate whether the article is based on research.

An **abstract** is a short summary of the purpose of a study, the subjects included in the research, the way the study was conducted, and the results obtained in the investigation (see the box on p. 292). An abstract is often quite brief and does not contain all essential information from the article. The first few paragraphs of the article should provide further clues about whether it describes a research study. Phrases such as *the purpose of this study was* and *this research was carried out to determine* are indications that the article is a research report. If the article describes only the author's experience with a particular aspect of nursing care, it probably is not a research article. In addition to the abstract, a typical research report has the following parts:

1. *Introduction* section: An introductory section presenting the purpose, a summary of literature used to formulate the study, and the hypotheses tested
2. *Methods* section: Description of the methods used to conduct the study, including the sample (what or who was studied), and to collect data, including the device or instrument used to measure empirical information
3. *Results* section: Description of the results obtained in the study, including statistical tests used to analyze data
4. *Discussion* section: Presentation of the author's interpretation of the results, including conclusions and implications that can be drawn from the study
5. *Reference* list (articles used to support the study)

If the report is written by one of the researchers in the study, it is a **primary source.** Any other article about the study is considered a **secondary source** (for example, an article in which the author was not directly involved in conducting the study but collected the information from a primary or another secondary source). Most nursing textbooks are secondary sources of information. Authors of these texts incorporate knowledge and information gathered from nursing and related literature, including research written by original investigators.

The fact that a report is a primary source does not guarantee its accuracy, which depends on the ability of researchers to be scientific, impersonal, and impartial in conducting studies. However, a primary source does report firsthand knowledge, whereas a secondary source may include another person's interpretation of the original work.

Locating Research Studies

Students and practicing nurses often need to find research articles on subjects that interest them (Fig. 16-2). In the health care field a number of resources are useful when searching the literature for research articles.

To locate primary research sources related to a particular subject, the first source is the journals where original research reports are usually published. The most efficient way to locate research articles is to consult an index of journal articles. The *Cumulative Index to Nursing and Allied Health Literature (CINAHL),* published bimonthly, contains listings from over 300 English-language nursing and allied health journals, as well as publications of the ANA and National League for Nursing. The *International Nursing Index,* published four times a year, contains listings from more than 200 nursing journals from around the world. *Index Medicus,*

an international index published monthly, includes listings from approximately 2900 biomedical journals, including about 60 nursing journals. The *Hospital Literature Index,* published quarterly, contains listings from journals dealing with planning and providing health care programs and services. These indexes are generally found in reference sections of medical and nursing libraries. In addition, individual subscribers can purchase CD-ROM formats for these databases.

The indexes just mentioned can save time in locating articles. Each index uses a list of key words that form subject headings and subheadings; article listings are grouped or organized under these headings. For example, a person might find subject headings such as *pain* or *primary nursing,* whereas subheadings might include *physiology* or *history,* respectively. An author listing is also available, making it possible to find articles published during a certain time period by a particular person. Articles on a particular subject are found by first checking the subject headings to see whether the key term listed in the index matches the subject. The key term listing may also lead to other subject groupings that contain articles similar in content. Using an index may at first seem time consuming, but it saves time because the alternative is looking through many journals trying to find articles pertinent to the subject. Many nursing and medical libraries provide computerized searches for articles. A list of articles and abstracts is transmitted over telephone lines within hours of being requested. Nurses having access to microcomputers and modems may access bibliographical services available through the Internet or a database vendor.

Major nursing journals publish research studies or research reports. Some journals, such as *Nursing Research,* are devoted solely to research; other nursing journals, such as the *American Journal of Critical Care,* also publish original reports of research studies. Specialty practice journals publish research articles devoted to the particular specialty.

Secondary literature sources such as books can be helpful in finding primary research sources. Nursing students seeking research articles should use reference lists or bibliographies at the end of textbook chapters. To document the scientific basis for their writing, authors frequently cite

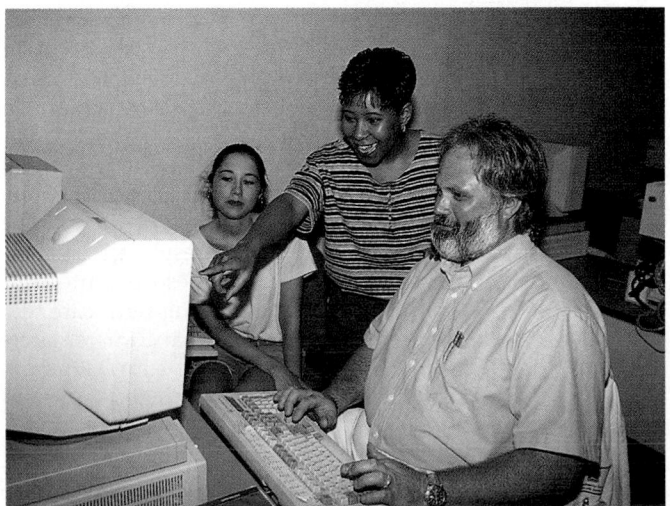

Fig. 16-2 Nursing students using the computer to find research articles.

primary sources as references, and these references are a valuable resource for nursing students who want more information.

Other secondary resources helpful in finding primary nursing research articles are research reviews such as the *Annual Review of Nursing Research* and the *Review of Research in Nursing Education*. Each volume is devoted to a certain topic. A review can help determine the status of research on a topic and can direct the reader toward other primary research sources. Research reviews are relatively new in nursing.

Organizing Information From a Research Study

Articles listed in a bibliography or reference section are called **citations**. A citation provides the author's name and information about where "ideas" or "quotations" were originally published. Writers are ethically obligated to give credit to others whose thoughts are used, even if the original author's exact words are not quoted.

There are many ways to list a citation. The style recommended by the American Psychological Association (1994) is widely used. This format avoids the use of footnotes. All citations are arranged alphabetically at the end of the report. Schools of nursing use many formats, however, and nursing students should ask about the citation format used at their own schools. Listing citations according to the recommended guidelines prevents students from listing incomplete citations.

The date of publication gives the approximate time the study was conducted. Sometimes researchers define the exact time period in the article, because a considerable time (as long as 2 years) may pass between the time a study was completed and the time the article was published. Noting when a study was conducted allows the reader to track the development of knowledge in a particular area.

In nursing, many kinds of clinical problems are studied. The subject of the study provides information about the topics being investigated by nurse researchers. Studies undertaken in a particular problem area can then be collected and evaluated. There are often many ways to investigate a particular research problem. Knowing the way in which researchers studied a question helps students evaluate the thoroughness of the investigation.

A major purpose of scientific research is to increase knowledge about general classes of people or events. Knowledge about the subjects in a research study gives the nurse information about clients to whom the conclusions may be applied. When similar results are obtained with different groups of clients, nurses can be more confident when using the new methods with other clients.

The clinical setting can influence the results of a study. For example, findings from research studies on acute care needs are not necessarily applicable in a long-term care setting. This information is particularly relevant for research involving psychological aspects of nursing care. Different regions of the country have unique traditions and customs. Nursing interventions appropriate for people with certain attitudes and beliefs may not be relevant in regions or settings where attitudes and beliefs differ substantially.

The results summarize the findings about the area of study. When the findings and conclusions are replicated in a number of research studies, the conclusions are more generalizable than in the case of an isolated research project. The effects of preoperative teaching on the postoperative recovery of clients, for example, is a problem area in which collective evidence provides a reasonable scientific foundation for nursing practice.

Learning to find and read nursing research studies is not a simple task. Many books and journal articles in nursing and related disciplines provide more detailed information about reading and evaluating research studies. Nursing research is based on principles of logic, and with a thoughtful approach the nursing student can learn to understand and evaluate nursing research studies.

Identifying Clinical Nursing Problems

Diers (1979) defined a **clinical nursing problem** as "a difference between two states of affairs, a discrepancy between the way things are and the way they ought to be, or between what one knows and what one needs to know to eliminate the problem." The following questions are raised by this definition:

1. Given the nursing interventions recommended for clients with a particular health care problem, how might the suggested care be improved so that the results or outcomes of care are better?
2. Given the knowledge about how to provide nursing care, what additional information would be needed to plan new interventions for clients with a particular health care problem?

Unanswered questions and the desire to improve nursing practice can provide the stimulus for conducting a research study.

Experience can make it possible to identify a researchable clinical nursing problem, but a nurse does not need to have years of clinical practice to identify a nursing problem. Sometimes a person who is relatively new in a situation can more easily see how things could be improved than those who have more experience and who take present conditions for granted. The nurse also considers whether the problem frequently occurs in a particular client group, whether it can be consistently and accurately measured, and whether a possible nursing solution might change the way care is delivered (Fuller, 1982).

Sometimes nursing students or practicing nurses think their ideas about nursing problems for study are not worthwhile unless they are certain that the proposed clinical study would make a radical change in client care. However, research efforts also may have to refine ideas about a clinical problem before the investigator can test alternative nursing interventions. In fact, some nurse researchers think that more investigative work needs to be conducted to describe the client response before research is designed to test an alternative intervention. In addition, the researcher may have to devise correct ways for measuring results before the study can proceed. All these factors may discourage a nurse from undertaking a nursing research project. On the other hand, such projects can be viewed as stimulating challenges because much information has yet to be scientifically tested for its relevance to nursing practice.

Using Findings in Nursing Practice

Nurses should read journals that contain research reports, as well as textbooks and other sources, in nursing and related fields. For example, this text uses *Research Highlight*

boxes to illustrate how research can progress from the phase of clinical problem refinement to the testing of new nursing measures (see the boxes below). To use findings in clinical practice, the nurse must be aware of the problems already studied.

RESEARCH HIGHLIGHT

RESEARCH ABSTRACT
In Virginia, drowning is the second leading cause of "accidental" death after motor vehicle accidents in the age-group 0 to 19 years.
Objective: To determine the epidemiology of drowning in children and adolescents age 0 to 19 in Virginia so that drowning prevention strategies specific to this state may be developed.
Methods: A retrospective review was completed on all medical examiner records of children and adolescents age 0 to 19 who drowned in Virginia from January 1, 1989, to December 31, 1993. Drowning rates were calculated for Virginia residents only, using 1990 population census data.
Results: There were 131 drownings in the age-group 0 to 19 years. Blacks, males (age 15 to 19), and children younger than 5 years of age had the highest drowning rates. Almost 40% of children under 5 years of age drowned in swimming pools, all of which were residential. More than 80% of these children were in the care of a parent, relative, or another adult at the time of the incident. Almost 50% of adolescents age 15 to 19 drowned while engaged in a sport or recreational activity in rivers, lakes, or other natural bodies of water. There was a detectable blood alcohol or drug level, or both, in more than 40% of the 15- to 19-year-olds. Of the seven children or adolescents who drowned in a bathtub, four were less than 2 years old and two had a history of seizure disorder. In each of four cases in which the child was 2 years of age or younger, a parent, relative, or another adult was responsible for the child at the time but left the room momentarily to perform a brief task.

IMPLICATIONS FOR PRACTICE
▶ Teach parents how to safely bathe infants and small children.
▶ Provide ongoing education about the danger of leaving small children unattended around any body of water.
▶ Encourage parents to obtain safe water and swimming instructions for their children.
▶ Reinforce the hazards associated with alcohol use during recreational activities.
▶ At a community level, participate in or lead cardiopulmonary resuscitation classes for parents and youth 14 years of age and older.
▶ At the local and state government levels, promote increased awareness of the dangers involved and support protective public health legislation such as mandatory fences around residential pools.

REFERENCE
Sanders JK, Gaenzle MB, Zanga JR et al: Child and adolescent drownings in Virginia: a population-based study. Presented at the 122nd Annual Meeting and Exhibition of the American Public Health Association, Washington, DC, November 1994 (abstract No. 178).

Not all research related to clinical nursing problems can or should be applied in practice. The nurse must judge the scientific worth of a study before considering its use in practice. This chapter can provide only a foundation for judging the worth of a research study. Other aspects that should be considered follow (Stetler, 1985, 1994; Stetler and DiMaggio, 1985):

1. The amount of supportive evidence provided by other scientific studies that have obtained similar results
2. Determination of whether the subjects and environment in the study are similar to the clients for whom the nurse provides care in the particular practice setting
3. The theoretical basis for present nursing care and the effectiveness of current theory in solving clinical nursing problems
4. The feasibility of applying findings, including ethical and legal limitations, institutional policy, changes in the organization of nursing services that might be required, and potential costs in time, money, and equipment

The nurse must make judgments that involve validating the scientific soundness of a study, comparatively evaluating whether any use can be made of the findings, and deciding the type of application that would be appropriate (Stetler, 1985).

Haller et al. (1979) note that **research utilization** (using research findings in day-to-day practice) begins with the identification of a clinical nursing problem that has been investigated through conceptually related studies; the results of these studies can be used in clinical practice. The

RESEARCH HIGHLIGHT

RESEARCH ABSTRACT
A phenomenological method was used to study 76 South Florida Haitian immigrants who were interviewed regarding their definition of health and methods of promoting health. Health was perceived as life itself. The majority defined health as a combination of characteristics from the social-behavioral dimension and physical examination. Presence of signs or symptoms of illness did not define ill health unless incapacitating. Multiple social and behavioral definers of health contrasted with those of health care providers, who use physical characteristics and laboratory results as the dominant criteria. Such differences may pose problems related to formulating culturally sensitive, effective, and acceptable health education programs.

IMPLICATIONS FOR PRACTICE
▶ Assess client's concept of health.
▶ Acknowledge and respect the client's concept.
▶ Identify and articulate areas of diversity between your concept and the client's.
▶ Identify mutually agreed upon health goals.
▶ Collaborate in developing a health promotion or preventive health plan, or both.
▶ Together, implement and evaluate a plan over time and adjust as needed.

REFERENCE
DeSantis L: *Health Values,* 17(6):3, 1993.

problem area chosen must have an established research base, be relevant to practice, and be reliably evaluated by nurses in clinical settings. When selecting the problem area, the nurse is concerned with whether a solid research base exists for changing practice, the scientific merit of the studies that constitute the research base, and the potential risk to the client in implementing the practice change. The final phases include developing a clinical protocol that can be used to implement the change and clinically evaluating the outcomes of the new nursing care to determine its effectiveness.

Nurses often participate in quality assurance or quality improvement studies that evaluate the processes and outcomes (results) of nursing care (see Chapter 11). These studies measure how well nursing interventions are being implemented with specific clients by examining expected outcomes related to the nursing process protocols and procedures of a specific setting. By examining the quality of care provided for clients in their own setting and changing care as needed, nurses can use research to improve the quality of care.

Nurses should not change from accepted to unproven ways of providing client care without careful deliberation and consultation with colleagues. Experimenting with new nursing measures is inappropriate, especially if an increased risk to clients' health is possible.

■ KEY CONCEPTS ■

▶ People acquire knowledge through tradition, from authorities in a field, through experience, by trial and error, and through application of the scientific method.

▶ A scientific investigation is an orderly, planned, and controlled way of studying reality that can be applied to general situations and contributes to the testing of theories about people, places, or life events.

▶ Nursing research is conducted to study the physical or psychosocial responses of people of all ages in health and illness.

▶ An experimental research study controls factors that could influence the results, includes comparison and experimental treatment groups of subjects, and uses random means for selecting study subjects.

▶ A qualitative research study organizes information in narrative format so that phenomena can be described and patterns of relationships can be discovered.

▶ Participation of human subjects in research studies requires the researcher to obtain informed consent of study subjects, maintain the confidentiality of subjects, and protect subjects from undue risk or injury.

▶ When summarizing data reported in a research study, the nurse should note when, how, where, and by whom the investigation was conducted and who and what was studied.

▶ A researchable clinical nursing problem is one that is not satisfactorily resolved by present nursing interventions, occurs frequently in a particular group, can be consistently and accurately measured, and has a possible solution within the realm of nursing practice.

▶ To determine whether research findings can be used as a basis for nursing practice, the nurse should consider the scientific worth of the study, the substantiating evidence provided in other studies, the similarity of the research setting to the nurse's own clinical practice setting, the status of current nursing theory, and factors affecting the feasibility of application.

■ KEY TERMS ■

Abstract, p. 293
Anonymity, p. 292
Biomedical research, p. 288
Citations, p. 294
Clinical nursing problem, p. 294
Comparison group, p. 289
Confidentiality, p. 292
Empirical data, p. 287
Experiment, p. 289
Experimental group, p. 289
Hypothesis, p. 288
Informed consent, p. 291
Nursing research, p. 289
Phenomena, p. 288
Primary source, p. 293
Qualitative research, p. 289
Quantitative research, p. 289
Research process, p. 290
Research utilization, p. 295
Scientific approach, p. 288
Scientific method, p. 288
Secondary source, p. 293
Subjects, p. 289

■ CRITICAL THINKING EXERCISES ■

1. The nurse is concerned about learning to properly clean a pressure ulcer. Explain the benefits to the client if the nurse learns how to clean the sore by the scientific method versus trial and error.

2. If you wished to determine the best method for cleaning a pressure ulcer, what type of research method would you use for study?

3. The nurses working on an orthopedic unit decided to study the factors that commonly result in client falls on their unit. Explain why this quality improvement study is not scientific research. How could it be made into a scientific research study?

REFERENCES

American Nurses Association: *Directions for nursing research: toward the twenty-first century,* Kansas City, Mo, 1985, The Association.

American Nurses Association: *Education for participating in nursing research,* Kansas City, Mo, 1989, The Association.

American Nurses Association: *Human rights guidelines for nurses in clinical and other research,* Kansas City, Mo, 1985a, The Association.

American Nurses Association: *Human rights guidelines for nurses in clinical and other research,* Washington, DC, 1985b, The Association.

American Nurses Association: *Standards of clinical nursing practice,* Washington, DC, 1991, The Association.

American Nurses Association Cabinet on Nursing Research: *Directions for nursing research: toward the twenty-first century,* Washington, DC, 1985, The Association.

American Nurses Association Commission on Nursing Research: *Guidelines for the investigative function of nurses,* Kansas City, Mo, 1981, The Association.

American Nurses Association Commission on Nursing Research: *Research priorities for the 1980s: generating a scientific basis for nursing practice,* Kansas City, Mo, 1981a, The Association.

American Psychological Association: *Publication manual of the American Psychological Association,* ed 4, Washington, DC, 1994, The Association.

Canadian Nurses Association: *Code of ethics for nurses,* Ottawa, 1991, The Association.

Canadian Nurses Association: *Ethical guidelines for nursing research involving human subjects,* Ottawa, 1983, The Association.

Code of Federal Regulations, *Federal Register,* May 1994.

DeSantis L: Haitian immigrant concepts of health, *Health Values* 17(6):3, 1993.

Diers D: *Research in nursing practice,* Philadelphia, 1979, Lippincott.

Fuller ED: Selecting a clinical nursing problem, *Image* 14:60, 1982.

Gortner SR: Nursing research: out of the past and into the future, *Nurs Res* 29:204, 1980.

Haller KB, Reynolds MA, Horsley JA: Developing research-based innovation protocols: process, criteria, and issues, *Res Nurs Health* 2:45, 1979.

Institute of Medicine Division of Health Care Services: *Nursing and nursing education: public policies and private actions,* Washington DC, 1983, National Academy.

International Council of Nurses: *Nursing research: ICN position statement,* Geneva, 1986, The Council.

Kellogg F, Crain M, Cowrin J et al: Life-sustaining interventions in frail elderly persons, *Arch Intern Med* 152:2317, 1994.

Knebel A, Shekleton ME, Burns S et al: Weaning from mechanical ventilation: concept development, *Am J Crit Care,* 3(6):416, 1994.

Meeker BJ: Preoperative education: evaluating postoperative patient outcomes, *Patient Educ Counsel* 23(1):41, 1994

NCNR: National Center for Nursing Research, Bethesda, Md, 1992, The Center (basic brochure).

Planchock NY, Wiggins MV: Preoperative assessment and teaching: physiological and psychological preparation, *Semin Periop Nurs* 3(2):61, 1994.

Polit DF, Hungler BP: *Nursing research: principles and methods,* ed 5, Philadelphia, 1995, Lippincott.

Sanders JK, Gaenzle MB, Zanga JR et al: Child and adolescent drownings in Virginia: a population-based study. Presented at the 122nd Annual Meeting and Exhibition of the American Public Health Association, Washington, DC, November 1994 (abstract No. 178).

Stetler C: Research utilization: defining the concept, *Image* 17:40, 1985.

Stetler CB: Refinement of the Stetler/Marram model for application of research findings to practice, *Nurs Outlook* 42(1):15, 1994.

Stetler CB, DiMaggio G: Research utilization among clinical nurse specialists, *Clin Nurs Specialist* 5(3):151, 1991.

Talbot LA: *Principles and practice of nursing research,* St Louis, 1995, Mosby.

Timmons ME, Bower FL: The effect of structured preoperative teaching on patients' use of patient-controlled analgesia (PCA) and their management of pain, *Orthop Nurs* 12 (1):23, 1993.

ADDITIONAL READINGS

American Nurses Association Cabinet on Nursing Research: *Establishment of a National Institute of Nursing: a statement of rationale,* Kansas City, Mo, 1983, The Association (mimeographed).

Bergstrom N et al: Collaborative nursing research: anatomy of a successful consortium, *Nurs Res* 33:20, 1984.

Fitzpatrick JJ, Tauton RL, Benoliel JQ: *Annual review of nursing research,* vol 8, New York, 1990, Springer.

Mallison MB: The shortage that destroys, *Am J Nurs* 87:899, 1987.

Merritt DH: The National Center for Nursing Research, *Image* 18:84, 1986.

Sarter B: *Paths to knowledge: innovative research methods for nursing,* New York, 1988, National League for Nursing.

Stetler CB, Marram G: Evaluating research findings for applicability in practice, *Nurs Outlook* 25:559, 1976.

Trussell P, Brandt A, Knapp S: *Using nursing research: discovery, analysis, and interpretation,* Wakefield, Mass, 1981, Nursing Resources.

Werley HH, Fitzpatrick J: *Annual review of nursing research,* vol 4, New York, 1986, Springer.

Woods NF, Catanzaro M: *Nursing research: theory and practice,* St Louis, 1987, Mosby–Year Book.

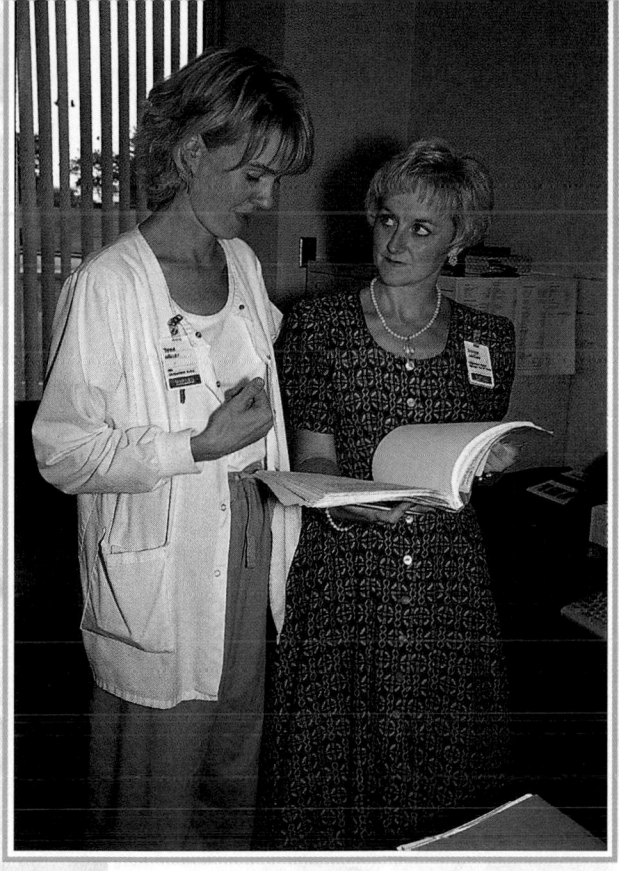

## Chapter 17

Leadership and Management

Objectives

Mastery of content in this chapter will enable the student to:

▶ Define the key terms listed.

▶ Differentiate between leadership and management.

▶ Compare and contrast management theories in respect to their perspectives for improving productivity.

▶ Describe and give examples of the four classic leadership styles: autocratic, democratic, laissez-faire, and situational.

▶ List and give examples of three primary types of management skills that student nurses can begin to develop.

Given the complexity of illness and the variety of settings in which health care is delivered, the need for effective leadership and management in nursing has never been more compelling. For years, staff nurses relied on those above them in the organizational hierarchy to provide leadership and management of their unit. In today's health care environment all professional nurses must rely on their *own* leadership and management skills if they are to be successful. Whether it is in facilitating a client's progression through a critical pathway in a cost effective manner (management of resources at the bedside) or serving on a task force to improve quality of care (leadership at the organizational level) these two skills, leading and managing, are prerequisites for the *professional* practice of nursing.

◼ DEFINITIONS OF LEADERSHIP AND MANAGEMENT

Leadership is the art of getting others to want to do something you are convinced should be done (Kouzes and Posner, 1990). The origin of the word *lead* is a word meaning "to go." **Leaders** typically have a vision of where "to go"—a direction in which others are influenced to follow. Leaders are the ones who show the way and have a grasp of the "big picture."

Management is closely related. The word *management* comes from a word meaning "hand." **Managers** "handle the day-to-day operations" to achieve a desired outcome. Successful organizations require both leadership and management. One author has conceptualized these two functions by saying "management promotes efficiency in climbing the ladder of success; leadership determines whether the ladder is leaning against the right wall" (Covey, 1989).

Nursing has focused more on management—details of day-to-day operations—and less on leadership in the past (Marriner-Tomey, 1992). Today's health care environment requires that nurses manage clinical outcomes for clients while also taking a leadership role in meeting organizational objectives. For example, nurses play a pivotal role in finding ways to manage clinical care at reduced cost. The movement toward staff empowerment in the last several years has enabled nurses in a variety of settings to take on responsibilities that were formerly designated to the manager. Staff nurses are setting standards of care, deciding scheduling and staffing issues, and monitoring quality of care outcomes. Health care settings in the future are likely to continue this trend with fewer managers, more self-directed work teams across department lines, and case managers with responsibility and accountability for resource utilization. This makes the development of leadership and management skills of equal importance to developing clinical skills; these skills are developed in much the same way as clinical skills: through theory, application, and practice.

◼ LEADERSHIP AND MANAGEMENT THEORIES

The industrial revolution and mass production in the early twentieth century marked the origins of leadership theory and the study of management. The development of leadership theory has proceeded along two lines—research on leadership traits and the development of management thought.

The early studies of leadership traits were simplistic in that they focused on personal characteristics of leaders in an attempt to isolate those traits indicative of effective leaders. The list of desirable traits grew to over 100 essential characteristics, many of which were overlapping and inconsistent and none of which could be conclusively proven as a prerequisite for leadership.

One positive contribution of "trait theory," however, was the work of Douglas McGregor in the mid-1960s, in which he described managers by their basic belief system (Hersey and Blanchard, 1988). McGregor described leadership traits from two different views "theory X" and "theory Y." Managers who believe in **theory X** assume that people inherently dislike work and will avoid it when possible. The manager must force employees to work by directing and controlling them and threatening them with punishment. Theory X holds that employees prefer to be controlled and directed, have little ambition, reject personal responsibility, and are motivated only by job security. The manager's emphasis is on organizational goals and meeting these goals with close supervision, coercion, and threats, if necessary. Since organizational goals take precedence over developing personal potential, employees may be frustrated and less productive.

Theory Y managers believe that work is as natural to their employees as play. Theory Y holds that employees are self directed and will engage in goal-directed activity by choice, as long as they agree with the goals. Employees are capable of success and will seek responsibility for problem solving. The theory Y manager delegates responsibility, offers minimal direction, and uses praise and recognition as motivators. Theory Y managers believe in developing human potential and thereby meeting organizational goals.

McGregor suggested that these basic belief systems should not be viewed as opposites, or one bad and the other good. Rather, he stressed the need to structure the work situation so that both personal and organizational goals could be met. He proposed a collaboration between the manager and the employee for the integration of goals as a means of increasing productivity and providing job satisfaction (Table 17-1).

The development of management thinking over the last century has likewise moved from a simplistic to a more comprehensive approach. A familiarity with the development of management thought can be helpful to the student in creating personal ideas about effective management.

Scientific Management Theory

Beginning with Frederick Taylor in the late 1800s, management theory focused on ways to improve productivity of employees through various management approaches. Taylor's theory of **scientific management** emphasized technology as the basis for increasing productivity. Taylor used the principles of observation, measurement, and scientific comparison to develop work standards. He introduced time and motion studies to analyze tasks, based on the belief that improving the performance of tasks would improve the efficiency of the organization. Taylor disregarded rule-of-thumb judgments and replaced them with systematic methods to improve efficiency. Taylor's ideas resulted in reduced waste, performance standards, and selection of qual-

Table 17-1	List of Assumptions of Theory X and Theory Y	
THEORY X		**THEORY Y**
Work is inherently distasteful to most people.		Work is as natural as play if the conditions are favorable.
Most people are not ambitious, have little desire for responsibility, and prefer to be directed.		Self-control is often indispensable in achieving organizational goals.
Most people have little capacity for creativity in solving organizational problems.		The capacity for creativity in solving organizational problems is widely distributed in the population.
Motivation occurs only at the physiological and security levels.		Motivation occurs at the social, esteem, and self-actualization levels, as well as at the physiological and security levels.
Most people must be controlled and often corrected to achieve organizational objectives.		People can be self-directed and creative at work if properly motivated.

From Hersey P, Blanchard K: *Management of organizational behavior: utilizing human resources,* ed 5, Englewood Cliffs, 1988, Prentice-Hall.

ified employees who were offered incentives for meeting production goals. Taylor's scientific approach was the basis for the work analysis done in many hospitals in the mid-1970s, which resulted in client classification systems in nursing. These systems classify clients according to severity of illness and project the number and type of care givers needed for that workload.

Management Process

In the 1920s Henri Fayol, a French industrialist, recognized the universality of management. All managers, regardless of the type of organization, have essentially the same tasks: planning, organizing, staffing, directing, coordinating, reporting, and budgeting. He called this the **management process** and the tasks associated with it became identified with the acronym *POSDCORB*. He also was the first to propose that management could and should be taught in colleges.

Human Relations Movement

In the 1940s and 50s, the humanistic movement came into vogue in response to poor working conditions and a general lack of concern for employee welfare. At the core of **human relations management** is the belief that the social environment is as important as the physical environment in determining productivity. A key development in this line of thinking was the research project commonly known as "Hawthorne Studies," which highlighted the "human side" of the productivity equation. Researchers from Harvard University conducted studies involving workers at the Hawthorne plant of the Western Electric Company in Chicago to determine the effects of changes in the work environment (e.g., lighting, breaks, salary incentives) on productivity. To the surprise of researchers, their studies indicated that work relationships and morale were more influential than physical conditions or money on workers' productivity. These studies were the genesis of the humanistic movement and research quickly turned to group dynamics, motivation, and the informal organization as factors in promoting productivity (Morrison, 1993).

Systems Theory

In the early 1960s attempts were made to integrate research from various disciplines (e.g., sociology, economics, engi-neering, and mathematics) into a single unifying theory—systems theory. This approach views organizations as open systems with each of the parts interdependent on the other and contributing to the success or failure of the whole system. Since all parts of the organization are interrelated, a change in one area often has a ripple effect on the whole organization. Emphasis is on the need for communication and cooperation among all members of the organization, functioning as interdependent groups forming a whole (Bernhard and Walsh, 1990).

■ LEADERSHIP AND MANAGEMENT STYLE

Leadership style is an important factor in determining effectiveness. Style refers to the approach or manner a leader uses to influence the behavior of others in various situations. It is important to observe various leadership styles and begin to develop a sense of the most appropriate style for a particular situation. Leadership styles relate to the amount of control or freedom allowed the group by the manager. Styles range from total control by the manager to extreme permissiveness. The most common styles are autocratic, democratic, and laissez-faire.

Autocratic Style

The **autocratic leader** retains all authority and responsibility and is concerned primarily with tasks and goal accomplishment. This type of leader assigns clearly defined tasks and establishes one-way communication with the group. The autocratic leader is firm, insistent, and dominating. Such a leader stresses prompt, orderly performance and uses power to intimidate or pressure those who fail to adhere to expectations. This leader displays little trust or confidence in employees and, therefore, makes all the decisions. Since employees generally fear this type of manager, individual initiative and creativity may be stifled.

A common variation of the autocratic style is "maternalism," where the group views the leader with a "mother knows best" attitude. Maternalistic leaders have a greater consideration for the welfare of the group than those who are strictly autocratic. They still make all the decisions, but because of their personal relationship with employees, they are viewed as "benevolent" autocrats (Morrison, 1993).

The autocratic style of leadership can be appropriate in

some situations. Neophyte nursing staff members function more productively under the direction of autocratic leaders since this style meets their needs for guidance and structure during the orientation phase. In situations in which immediate action is required and there is no time for group decisions, the autocratic leader is able to take quick action. Autocratic leaders excel in times of crisis (e.g., cardiac arrest) and in situations of disorder (e.g., natural disaster); they often have the reputation for being able to get difficult assignments completed.

Democratic Style

The **democratic style** is a people-centered approach that allows employees more control and individual participation in the decision-making process. The emphasis is on team building and a spirit of collaboration through the joint effort of all team members. Democratic leaders function to facilitate goal accomplishment while stressing the self-worth of each individual. These leaders treat each staff member as an adult and expect the same in return. Criticism focuses on behaviors, not on personality, and is offered in an attempt to promote growth and development of the staff.

The democratic style works best with mature employees who work well together as groups. This style sometimes does not work as well with ancillary staff who may need more direction. The group decision making process may be slow and frustrating to those who expect prompt action on an issue. Disagreements are more likely, which may require more time to resolve. While this style may demand more of the leader, it is often valued for contributing to the growth and development of the staff. Examples of this approach in health care settings include scheduling and assignments made by the staff, shared governance, group problem-solving through task forces composed of staff nurses, or staff involvement in quality improvement efforts.

Laissez-Faire Style

This leadership style is often referred to as the "free run style" or permissive leadership. This type of leader relinquishes control completely and chooses to avoid responsibility by delegating all decision making to the group. **Laissez-faire** leaders want everyone to feel free to do "their own thing" and, as a result, there is no sense of direction unless provided by the group or an informal leader. This style may work well with highly motivated professional groups (e.g., a research staff), however, it seldom works well in health care settings given the complexity of the work environment.

Situational Leadership

Situational leadership theory takes into account the style of the leader, the maturity of the group, and the situation at hand to form a comprehensive approach to the issue of management style. Situational leadership theory contends that there is no single best leadership style but rather that the style used by the manager should be contingent upon the maturity level of the employees or group and the situation at hand. This model for determining the most appropriate management style grew out of a comprehensive study of leadership conducted in the mid 1960s at Ohio State University. Hersey and Blanchard proposed this approach as a means for the manager to facilitate the growth and development of staff. The more managers adapt their leadership styles to meet particular situations and the needs of staff, the more effective they will tend to be in reaching personal and organizational goals (Hersey and Blanchard, 1988).

Situational leadership theory identifies four typical styles for leaders and proposes that leaders use these styles in accommodating the needs of their employees and the situation. The four styles are:

1. Directing. The leader provides specific instructions and supervises the accomplishment of tasks.
2. Coaching. The leader monitors the accomplishment of tasks while also explaining decisions, asking for feedback or suggestions, and recognizing good performance.
3. Supporting. The leader supports the efforts of others, facilitates their goal accomplishment, and shares responsibility for decision making.
4. Delegating. The leader gives the responsibility for decision making and problem solving to mature staff who have demonstrated their competence (Hersey and Blanchard, 1988).

This approach of gradually relinquishing control and giving increasing decision-making authority to staff is in keeping with modern management theory regarding staff empowerment. While there is no one best leadership style, the overall approach of a leader needs to be to foster the growth of others and facilitate their development so that they are less and less dependent on the leader. The cornerstone of situational leadership theory is the flexibility of the manager in adapting to the needs of the individual or group. In a typical work setting the manager may be "directive" in dealing with staff who are in orientation while acting as a "coach" for those on another shift who are more experienced but still need some guidance. The "supporting" style may be apparent as the manager works with a "staff action committee" and assists members in solving a problem with another department. A manager who relies on seasoned staff nurses to monitor quality of care issues and regularly report audit results in a staff meeting is using the "delegating" style to promote the growth and development of staff. Obviously it is important to carefully assess developmental level or job maturity in matching styles to group or individual needs. This approach also demands flexibility of leaders to accommodate to difficult styles rather than those with which they are most comfortable. This approach to developing leadership styles is growth producing both for the manager and the staff. Managers who know the capabilities of their staff and adjust their styles accordingly improve the likelihood of retaining capable, competent, satisfied nurses on staff. In this sense, the understanding of this situational approach to managing is key to success as a manager.

■ LEADING AND MANAGING IN A TYPICAL WORK SETTING

The application of management concepts is often apparent in the day-to-day operations of any health care setting. The nursing staff involved in providing care to clients or families uses leadership and management skills at a clinical level while those in management positions use these same skills at a group or unit-wide level to accomplish the goals of the unit. These leadership/management behaviors are reflected in the work flow on any given day.

Typical Work Flow

The day begins in hospitals, skilled nursing facilities, and long-term care facilities with a "change of shift report" in which nurses from the preceding shift review with those coming on duty the condition and needs of their clients. This allows the nurse coming on duty to plan or organize the day, establish priorities, and take note of some tasks that can be delegated to others (planning, organizing). Beginning with those tasks deemed highest priority, the nurse begins the shift assessing the clients to be cared for and determining their priorities for the day, often involving family members in this process. Throughout the day, the nurse may coordinate care activities with the needs of other departments (e.g., x-ray or laboratory) and report to the physician or social worker perceptions of the client's progress (coordinating, reporting). The nurse may delegate some tasks to unlicensed assistive personnel (e.g., bathing a client or ambulating a client down the hall) in order to make the best use of time with the client and family. At the end of the shift the nurse reflects on the day's activities and reports the highlights, critical events, or teaching activities to those coming on duty to ensure continuity of care (Fig. 17-1). More experienced staff nurses may have also participated in a committee meeting to discuss goals for the unit, reviewed chart audits to monitor quality of care, or perhaps represented their unit in the education council in shared governance. Balancing all these competing needs obviously requires leadership and management skills.

Those on the evening and night shifts experience their own version of these same behaviors. In contrast to the day shift, in which many diagnostic procedures occur, the evening shift is often more involved with families, client teaching, and discharge planning. Nurses who especially enjoy these activities often prefer this shift as there is more contact with families during these hours. The night shift is obviously the quietest of the three shifts in terms of procedures, contact with other departments, and so on, and, therefore, has the fewest staff. This calls for even greater use of management skills, however, in that with fewer resources more care must be taken to prioritize needs, delegate tasks appropriately, and carefully evaluate situations that might escalate into critical events.

A typical day for the manager involves many of these same behaviors but with a different focus. The primary focus for a staff nurse is the client and family; the primary focus for the manager is meeting the needs of the staff. Just as a staff nurse may assist a family in planning for discharge, the manager assists the staff in planning to meet unit goals or organizational objectives. A staff nurse might teach a family member ways to cope with the demands of being a care giver while a manager may provide an in-service for the staff in enhancing self-care or dealing with demanding clients. Although a staff nurse represents the unit on a shared governance council, the manager represents the unit in a community-wide meeting as a means to improve marketing of health care services. Just as a typical day for staff nurses involves a variety of activities (e.g., change of shift report, client teaching, coordination with other departments, etc.), the manager's day is equally varied with activities ranging from interviewing prospective staff, coaching a new staff member to better coordinate activities with another department, or meeting with physicians and administrators to prepare a new service for the department. The leadership and management skills needed are similar—the application of those skills is at a different level. Table 17-2 summarizes the contrasting ways in which these behaviors are applied at the clinical and managerial levels.

In developing an awareness of leadership and management skills, it is important to observe those in leadership roles who can serve as mentors for less experienced nurses. An understanding of the role of the manager can assist the student nurse in identifying role models to assist them in developing leadership skills.

Role of the Nurse Manager

The role of the manager in today's health care setting is undergoing significant changes. Many of these changes began in the mid-1970s and early 1980s when health care organizations decentralized management functions and organized each unit with a manager who had ultimate responsibility for quality of care on the unit. Nurse managers were given responsibility for hiring, developing, and evaluating their staff. They were given responsibility for developing an

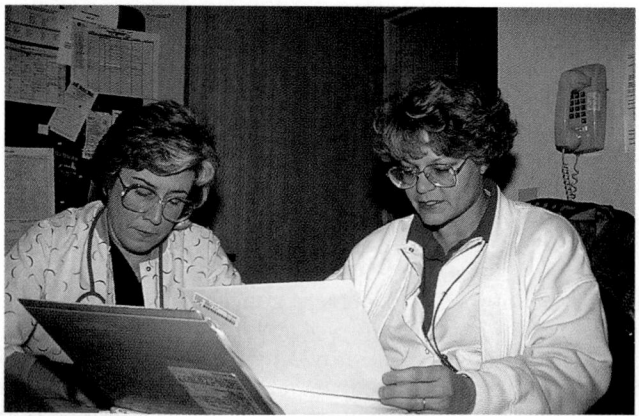

Fig. 17-1 Staff engaged in change of shift report plan for priorities of care.

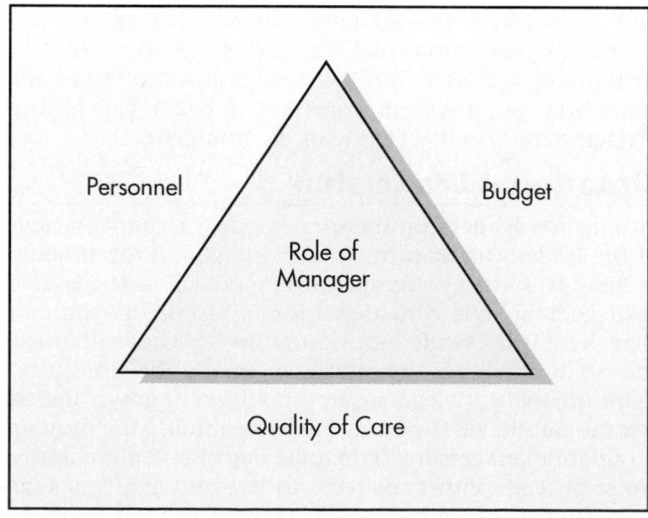

Fig. 17-2 Conceptual model for role of nurse manager.

	Table 17-2	Leading/Managing Behaviors at the Clinical and Managerial Levels	

BEHAVIORS	CLINICAL APPLICATION	MANAGERIAL APPLICATION
Planning/goal setting	Assisting clients and families in formulating their vision of future well-being after hospitalization	Assisting staff in formulating annual goals for the unit and systems needed to accomplish goals
Teaching/coaching	Teaching, interpreting information to promote client/family functioning and well-being	Teaching, interpreting information to promote unit functioning and enhanced services
Coordination with other services/departments	Assisting the family with their use of support services (e.g., social work, chaplain, home health) and/or scheduling client care in concert with needs of other departments (e.g., x-ray, lab)	Developing a staff committee to focus on problem solving and delegating the authority to the group to implement their action plans to improve daily unit operations
Promoting development of others through support and delegation	Encouraging clients and families to assume greater responsibility for maintenance of health	Developing assertive personnel to assume responsibilities within their job description through effective delegation
Representing the work group or profession	Active participation in unit task forces, shared governance councils, etc., or participating in community blood drive	Involvement in organizational initiatives (e.g., marketing new services to physicians) or participating on committees for nursing organizations (ANA, AACN)

Modified from Yoder-Wise P: *Leadership and management in nursing,* St Louis, 1995, Mosby.

annual budget for the unit and held accountable for managing the unit within the budget. Nurse managers have been responsible for monitoring the quality of care, dealing with personnel issues, and doing this in a cost effective manner. In a general sense this role can be conceptualized in three dimensions (Fig. 17-2).

The "ultimate accountability for the quality of care" is a typical one-sentence definition of the role of the nurse manager. To fulfill this responsibility managers develop ways to continually monitor key quality indicators and often enlist staff nurses in this effort. Managers also monitor feedback from clients and families in written client satisfaction surveys or conversations in making client rounds. A similar process of obtaining feedback routinely occurs with physicians, other department directors, and members of the community. Effective listening and follow-up to resolve problems is a key role for the manager.

Personnel issues also cover a wide range of efforts including recruitment of staff, interviewing and hiring staff, developing staff (with the assistance of preceptors), and overseeing regular staff evaluations. Nurse managers rely on their more experienced staff to serve as role models for new employees. However, managers play a key role in "setting the tone" for expectations of staff, fostering customer service attitudes, and professional practice in keeping with standards of care. In the event that the staff nurse fails to meet expected standards for practice, the manager has the responsibility to address the underlying issues. Dealing with personnel issues can be time consuming and complex. However, the on-going growth and development of the staff can be a most rewarding part of the management role.

The third dimension of the management role is intertwined with the others in that the manager must manage the available resources (personnel) to meet the needs of clients (quality of care) in a cost effective manner (budget).

The financial aspects of the management role also cover a wide range of responsibilities. Developing a unit budget each year with the approval of administration, monitoring the use of supplies and personnel on a regular basis, and accounting for underutilization and overutilization of funds requires special skills of the manager. In addition, the manager also participates in decision making about the purchase of new equipment and the development of new services for additional revenue. Staff nurses are increasingly involved in the day-to-day financial operations of the unit in their efforts to reduce overtime, minimize waste, and offer ideas to make work more efficient.

As health care organizations continue to adjust to continuous change, many aspects of the "management role" are gradually being assumed by staff nurses. In many settings, staff are making their own schedules, chairing committees, participating in peer evaluations, and monitoring the quality of care. The next several years will likely bring more decision making to the staff level as the number of managers declines and nurses function more in multidisciplinary teams with other health care professionals. Health care organizations, like their counterparts in business and industry, are downsizing, reducing layers of management, becoming more customer focused, and relying on multiskilled staff to coordinate their activities and function in self-directed teams (Pinchot and Pinchot, 1994). Therefore, it is important that nursing students begin developing leadership and management skills early in their preparation.

LEADERSHIP SKILLS FOR NURSING STUDENTS

Given the multitude of changes in health care affecting nurses at the staff level, it is of increasing importance that nursing students prepare themselves for leadership roles. There are several leadership skills that can be developed that prepare the new graduate for the demands of professional practice.

First among these are organizational skills, including data collection, priority setting, action plan development, and techniques for coordinating activities with others involved in client care. Observing experienced nurses in the clinical setting who have good organizational skills and who practice different ways to "get the job done" are part of this skill development process.

The art of effective delegation is another skill nursing students need to observe and practice to improve their management skills. Delegation is the process of assigning part of one person's responsibility to another person with their consent (Bernhard and Walsh, 1990). The purpose of delegating is to improve efficiency and provide job enrichment for the delegatee. For example, a manager might ask a staff nurse to do a client survey in a new service being proposed within the facility. The information from clients is gathered in the course of a typical work day and gives the nurse an opportunity to elicit and interpret client responses. This feedback is helpful in marketing strategies and provides job enrichment for the staff nurse in the process. It should be remembered that even though the delegation of a task transfers the responsibility and authority to another person, the delegator retains accountability for the delegated tasks. It is important to follow some basic principles for effective delegation. These are listed in the box at right.

By including all the components of proper delegation, the student nurse or staff nurse functions as a partner with the co-worker. The delegator shares liability for the actions or nonactions of the co-worker. These legal parameters apply to both the delegator and the delegatee. When delegation is appropriately done, everyone benefits (Wywialowski, 1993).

Given the workplace changes expected in the twenty-first century, another skill of utmost importance is the ability to be a team player and function as a part of a team. Most models proposed for health care reform speak of "networks" of professionals, "clustered" work groups made up of different disciplines or "cross functional teams" for

Requirements for Delegating Duties and Tasks

- Determine the complexity of client needs or the nature of the work to be delegated.
- Identify the employee to whom tasks are to be delegated.
- Determine that the work is consistent with the employee's job description and normal duties.
- Clearly communicate expectations and desired results using concrete measurable terms; convey both trust and sufficient authority.
- Obtain the employee's voluntary acceptance of the work request.
- Keep communication lines open while providing needed direction, instruction, and supervision.
- Compare actual results with expectations, give constructive feedback, and praise to reward the employee's efforts.

Modified from Wywialowski E: *Managing client care,* St Louis, 1993, Mosby.

client focused care. Clearly the predominant work style for the workplace in the year 2000 will be "teams" in one form or another (Katzenbach and Smith, 1993).

It is important for student nurses to be aware of this trend and use every opportunity to practice interpersonal skills, problem solving skills, and especially a team attitude. Specifically this means fostering a common commitment to quality client care, valuing the diversity of different team members, recognizing the achievement of others, and providing support to each other. Openly discussing conflicts so as to resolve them rather than working around them should become the norm. Finding common ground when working with other departments or with physicians with the client as the primary focus will be essential. Building effective teams and creating a collegial working environment is a process that is beneficial to clients, growth producing for the staff, and fundamental to the success of the organization.

■ KEY CONCEPTS ■

► Leadership involves influencing others toward the accomplishment of a goal.

► The leader moves a group forward with a sense of vision or direction, whereas the manager improves productivity and makes things run smoothly.

► All managers are leaders to some extent in that their actions influence others, preferably in a positive way.

► The human relations approach suggests that morale and attention to growth and development of employees are key to improving productivity of staff.

► A manager plans, organizes, directs, and controls activities so that the plan is actually accomplished.

► Theory X and theory Y deal with the manager's attitudes about employees, which are often reflected in management style.

► Rather than focusing on one "best" leadership style, situational leadership stresses that the leadership style is determined by the needs and maturity of the group being led.

► Management skills that the nurse can begin to develop while still a student include organizational skills, effective delegation, and developing a team player attitude.

■ KEY TERMS ■

Autocratic leader, p. 300

Democratic style, p. 301

Human relations management, p. 300

Laissez-faire, p. 301

Leaders, p. 299

Managers, p. 299

Management process, p. 300

Scientific management, p. 299

Situational leadership, p. 301

Theory X, p. 299

Theory Y, p. 299

■ CRITICAL THINKING EXERCISES ■

1. The nursing staff have voiced displeasure regarding their schedule. They feel that they are working too many weekends and that days off are inconsistent. The nurse manager realizes that it is important to be sure all shifts have an adequate complement of staff. To resolve the problem of a suitable schedule, how might this manager act?

2. Consider the following situations and determine the style of situational leadership that the nurse manager should use in each situation.

    a. Joan is a new staff nurse who is completing her orientation. She is about to perform a tracheostomy dressing change for the first time.

    b. Ken is a staff nurse with 10 years experience. He is an expert clinician and enjoys teaching. He is interested in chairing a staff committee to revise the orientation program.

    c. Sue has been on staff for 3 years. She has chaired the unit practice council for 3 months. She is having trouble setting an agenda for the committee's next meeting.

3. A staff nurse asks an LPN to check the dressing on a client who had surgery several hours earlier. Who has the ultimate accountability in this situation for the judgment used in completing this request?

REFERENCES

Bernhard L, Walsh M: *Leadership-the key to professionalization in nursing*, ed 2, St Louis, 1990, Mosby.

Covey S: *The seven habits of highly effective people*, New York, 1989, Simon & Schuster.

Hersey P, Blanchard K: *Management of organizational behavior: utilizing human resources*, ed 5, Englewood Cliffs, 1988, Prentice-Hall.

Katzenbach J, Smith D: *The wisdom of teams: creating the high performance organization*, Boston, 1993, Harper Business.

Kouzes J, Posner B: *The leadership challenge: how to get extraordinary things done in organizations*, San Francisco, 1990, Jossey-Bass.

Marriner-Tomey A: *A guide to nursing management*, ed 4, St Louis, 1992, Mosby.

Morrison M: *Professional skills for leadership: foundations of a successful career*, St Louis, 1993, Mosby.

Pinchot G, Pinchot E: *The end of bureaucracy and the rise of the intelligent organization*, San Francisco, 1994, Barrett-Koehler.

Wywialowski E: *Managing client care*, St Louis, 1993, Mosby.

Yoder-Wise P: *Leading and managment in nursing*, St Louis, 1995, Mosby.

ADDITIONAL READINGS

Barter M: Unlicensed assistive personnel: issues relating to delegation and supervision, *J Nurs Administration* 94:36, 1994.

Carr JT: Learning to walk the leadership talk, *Healthcare Executive* 9(2):16, 1994.

Chase L: Nurse manager competencies, *J Nurs Administration* 94:56, 1994.

Editors: The new nurse manager: a linchpin in quality care and cost control, *Hospitals* 66:22, 1992.

Kouzes J, Posner B: Transformational leadership: the credibility factor, *Health care forum* 36(4):16, 1993.

Mark B: The emerging role of the nurse manger: implications for educational preparation, *J Nurs Administration* 94:48, 1994.

Sovie M: Nurse manager: a key role in clinical outcomes, *Nursing Management* 25:30, 1994.

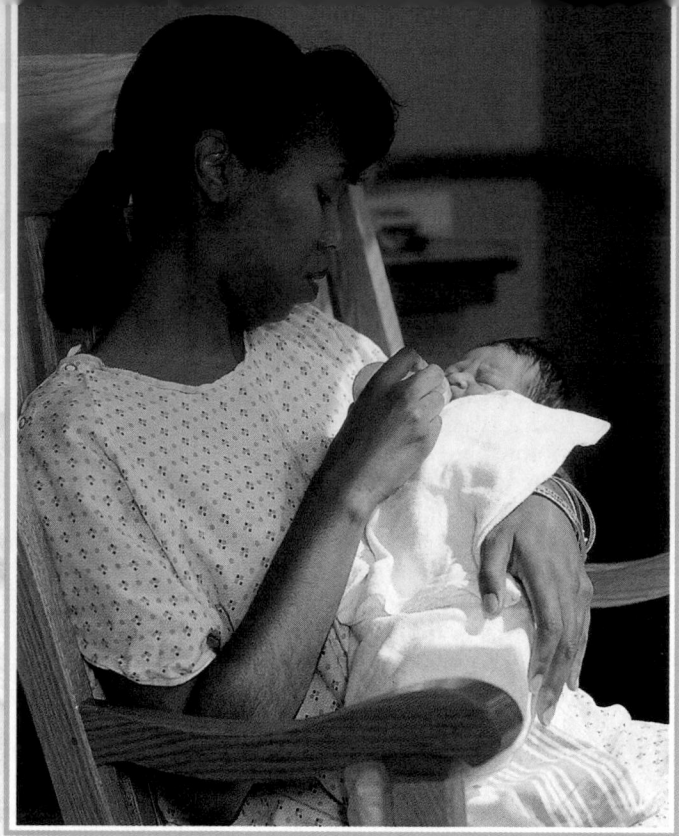

## Chapter 18

Values

Objectives

Mastery of content in this chapter will enable the student to:

▶ Define the key terms listed.

▶ Describe the ways values influence behavior.

▶ Discuss the ways values are learned.

▶ Contrast and compare modes of value transmission.

▶ Discuss the influence of caring on professional nursing practice.

▶ Identify the seven values defined by the American Association of Colleges of Nursing as essential for professional nursing.

▶ Describe the role of the nurse advocate.

▶ Describe how a nurse's values can influence client care.

▶ Describe the process and techniques of values clarification.

▶ Discuss the advantages of values clarification in nursing.

▶ Use a values clarification strategy to examine personal values.

▶ Describe how a nurse might respond to a personal values challenge.

▶ Discuss the values challenges that face the nursing profession.

Values give life and identity to individuals, professions, and societies. Nurses are challenged daily with relationships and decisions influenced by values. Expert practitioners seek to face those challenges with a clear perspective and purposeful action. An understanding of nurse, client, and professional values helps in that process.

CASE STUDY   Michael, who is 15 years old, was wounded by a gunshot to the neck in a street gang incident. The injury has left him paralyzed. You, as his primary nurse, have had a hard time caring for him because he often treats you in a hostile, demanding way. He maintains a tough exterior and brags about "taking a bullet" to his gang friends. You have begun to see through much of his behavior and know that although Michael has long been involved in "adult" situations, he is still a child. Hostility covers up his fear. You notice that often he is on the verge of tears. Michael's physical nursing care, although complex, is nothing compared to the relationship challenges you face with him as you try to help him rehabilitate his life. You have deep empathy for him, but you also feel angry when he continues to glorify gang life and communicates with his old friends. Sometimes his hostility toward you and your teaching efforts makes you dread entering his room. You hope he can now see how "stupid" his choices were and cannot understand why he continues to show loyalty to a way of life that has been so destructive for him. You wonder what he gets out of it. You feel inwardly angry that Michael does not seem to value the possibilities you outline for him. As a nurse you value holistic care but see no way to affect his social situation. As a citizen you are outraged at the social chaos caused by people like Michael. All of these reactions impact your professional relationship with Michael and the care you give him. ∎

Values are formed and maintained by individuals and also by groups of people. In the example above, the nurse witnesses the power of belonging and loyalty values for Michael's gang. In addition to her own personal values, the nurse also feels compelled by a set of values held by the nursing profession. New nurses are "socialized" into the profession. This means that students entering nursing as novices gradually take on the values of nurses, leading to a display of behaviors accepted by the profession and society as unique to nursing.

Good nursing is more than tending to clients' physical and psychological needs. The situation with Michael demonstrates that many challenging aspects of nursing have to do with human values, the subject of this chapter. One cannot have human interactions without engaging the values of others. People take seriously those ideas, events, and practices that are meaningful to them. Because values are so important to us all, they are a source of great satisfaction and a source of conflict. A skillful nurse learns to recognize and work with the power of values while caring for clients.

▌ VALUES DEFINED

A concept as complicated as values can not be simply defined. Three classic writers on values (Kluckhohn, 1951; Maslow, 1959; Rokeach, 1973) state that a **value** is a personal belief about the worth of a given idea, attitude, custom, or object that sets standards that influence behavior. Values are the beliefs that a person acts on and thus become the standards for guiding actions, developing and maintaining attitudes toward relevant objects, morally judging self and others, and comparing self and others. If a person holds a particular value, then he or she has personally chosen, interpreted, justified, and preferred that value over others.

Uustal (1992) summarizes the common elements in values definitions. Valuing has cognitive, selective, affective, and action components. A person thinks about, chooses, feels for, and acts on important personal values. Consider your own choice to pursue a professional nursing education. Certainly you thought carefully about that choice. You carefully chose to further your education over other life alternatives. Perhaps you delayed marriage plans. Maybe you waited until your children were in school to begin your studies or quit a stable job to accomplish an educational goal. Making those difficult choices among competing values and interests required that you feel strongly about the value of professional education. Had you not valued education highly, you would have not acted to begin nursing school. Although people may value many things, actions are often the most clear indicator of what value has highest priority.

The values an individual holds reflect personal needs, cultural and societal influences, and relationships with significant others. Values relate to one another to form a **value system.** For example, a person's religious beliefs and family ties contribute to the formation of health values. Consider a person who has learned through religious teaching that people have obligations to others and that they should consider others' as well as their own interests. This same person lives in a family that shares work responsibilities and decision making. Shaped by experiences and education that give weight to communal needs, this person might be likely to make his or her health care decisions based on the wants and needs of others. For example, a person may not elect further treatment for a progressive illness because of the financial strain it would put on others. The interactive dynamic of the multiple values of concern for others, interdependence, self-sacrifice, and loyalty implied in this example describes a value system. In health care interactions, each client functions from a value system of unique personal needs and preferences.

Nurses have sets of values, too, and should develop an awareness of how their own value system may influence client care. For example, a nurse may value the importance of family involvement with care. If a client fails to hold the same value, a nurse's automatic inclusion of the family in the plan of care may cause conflict. An understanding of value systems helps nurses act in professional and knowledgeable ways.

Health practices are intimately tied to values. The frequency and consistency with which people follow health-promoting behaviors depends on what they value (Fig. 18-1). Illness often causes people to reassess their values. The nurse helps clients clarify or reprioritize personal values, minimize conflict, and achieve consistency among values and behaviors related to health.

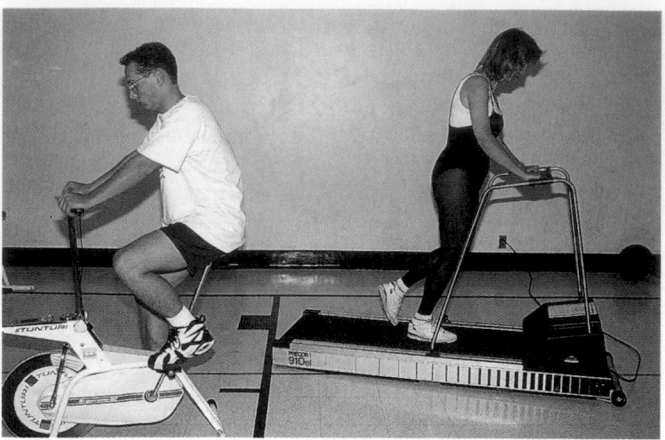

Fig. 18-1 Regular exercise demonstrates a person's value for good health.

■ NATURE AND FUNCTION OF VALUES

The values that influence behavior may be conscious or unconscious. An individual may express values openly or demonstrate them through verbal and nonverbal behaviors. Most persons are consciously aware of only a few prominent values that they acknowledge as significant in their lives. Other values may be operative and influence behavior but are not at a level of the person's awareness. No two individuals give equal importance to the same values. The values that hold the greatest importance in shaping thoughts and actions help create a person's unique identity.

A person's values about health determine the choices made about health promotion and the use of health care resources during a time of illness. Ideally, health behaviors should be realistic. Having realistic goals allows the person to be flexible and attain greater satisfaction from the attitudes, behaviors, and feelings influenced by personal values.

Perceptions of other individuals and our responses toward them are influenced by values. For example, when meeting someone for the first time, a person notes the other person's appearance and behavior. One nurse may be favorably impressed by a male client with a relaxed and friendly manner, wearing tattered blue jeans, long hair, a beard, and an earring. Another nurse, perhaps a person who values a tidy appearance and a more formal, professional manner, may have an initial negative reaction to the same person. Values, then, function as a filter for the many incoming experiences and relationships people encounter in a day. We simply cannot live without values. The filtering function of values helps people make many necessary judgments and gives people a sense of themselves in relationship to others. But it is important to remember that values do not determine the worth of any person nor should one's assessment of others' values determine how they are treated in a professional relationship.

■ FORMATION OF VALUES

Values can be learned through observation, reasoning, and experience (Hamilton, 1992). An individual observes behaviors in certain settings and notes the response it evokes.

Successful or productive behaviors can then be adopted as guides to conduct. For example, when children first enter school, they may observe the positive responses teachers give to students who complete their assignments neatly and correctly. They see parents and teachers reinforcing the behaviors of "good students" with verbal praise, high grades, or special privileges. Many children respond by assimilating the traditional values associated with successful academic performance that they have observed: following directions, being neat and punctual, and giving correct answers to questions.

An illustration of how educational values are formed through a process of reasoning would be those educators who have reconsidered traditional educational values and now work to reinforce different or complementary values. In an effort to enhance creativity, self-expression, and academic questioning in younger children, these educators may place less emphasis on conformity to directions, "right" answers, or proper spelling and penmanship. Children in these educational environments may learn different academic values.

To continue the example of acquiring educational values, some individuals shape their values through experience. Sometimes younger people do not take education seriously until they have had life experiences that cause them to revalue learning and personal growth. When they return to school with this new set of values, they most often are very successful.

Likewise, a client may form health values through the processes of observation, reasoning, and experience. For example, beginning a successful exercise program might follow as a result of education about the benefits of exercise (reasoning), observing the positive results of regular exercise in a family member, or as the result of an experience of illness, such as a heart attack.

The values held by a professional group can also be formed through reasoning, observation, and experience. Nursing students can learn empathy, a nursing value, by using reasoning to consider the meaning behind human behavior. For example, when one understands that young people often join gangs because of the human need for family, belonging, and support, empathy for a young gang member's needs might develop. Students can also observe the powerful effects of empathic care giving. Watching a skilled, compassionate nurse calm a confused person can assist the student in learning to value empathic listening and behavior. The student's own experience of feeling uninformed or confused around more experienced nurses and doctors often gives the student empathy for clients who are also less informed and often afraid to ask questions. Students, knowing what that feels like from their own experience, can generate empathic responses and make useful suggestions to clients.

People form values by interacting with others. Most often, people transmit values to others unconsciously, in the simple sharing of daily life. Other times, values are formed through deliberate transmission, as people attempt to influence others' attitudes and behaviors.

Modes of Value Transmission

Values are learned and evolve over a lifetime. Many values are not consciously chosen as the values people wish to have. Values become a part of an individual during socialization in the family, school, work, church, and other social groups. When children observe parents, family, and friends, they internalize behaviors that form the foundation of their value system.

Using the formation of honesty as an example, people who influence a child are generally unaware of all the ways they transmit values. For example, if a parent consistently demonstrates honesty in dealings with others, especially with the child, most likely the value of truth telling will be transmitted to the child. The child becomes honest without the parent's insistence or threat. Conversely, if the child frequently overhears the parent lie to others, that child may also begin to "use" the truth only for his or her own advantage.

The process of transmitting values can also be deliberate, as when a parent says to a child who has lied, "You should be ashamed of yourself. Good girls don't lie." Five traditional modes of value transmission are described in Table 18-1. These modes can lead to widely varying effects. Some modes are more effective than others, and some may not be effective at all. Careful evaluation of values transmission modes may help parents, teachers, and health care profes-

sionals in their efforts to develop an understanding of values formation and use the most effective methods.

Value formation, modification, and reaffirmation occur throughout a person's life. Cognitive and emotional levels of development influence the way values are learned.

Sociocultural Influences

Values are formed in social settings where the educational, socioeconomic, spiritual, and cultural backgrounds of people may vary (see Chapters 19 and 21). Within the larger culture there may be smaller groups of people, subcultures, with values distinct enough to set them apart from the dominant group.

People take on many values of the dominant culture in which they live. Because people learn to value that which is familiar, the customs, behaviors, rituals, and attitudes of unfamiliar others can seem foolish, ineffective, or even dangerous to an onlooker. This is particularly true with health care practices.

To give effective care, a nurse strives to understand the influence of culture on caring behaviors, value of health promotion, use of health care services, and adjustment to illness. Professional care givers' value systems may differ

Table 18-1	Modes of Value Transmission	
DESCRIPTIONS	**IMPLICATIONS**
MODELING Persons act in way to show others preferred way to behave. People acquire values from variety of role models.	Children initially wish to be like their parents; thus parents can model values they perceive as significant. Modeling may not lead to socially acceptable behavior (e.g., viewing another's aggressive behavior). Unless parents point out the most desirable values, children can follow any role model.
MORALIZING Parents and teachers hold standards for right and wrong and rigidly force children to conform to their sets of values.	This approach can be very authoritarian. Moralizing parents may be unwilling to consider alternative values for children. With this approach, one way is often the only way. Young persons reared by moralizing adults often have difficulty with making independent choices.
LAISSEZ-FAIRE At times, people acquire values by behaving informally without restrictions or limitations. No one value system is right for everyone, and children form values without parents' rigid guidelines.	Parents want children to be free to explore a variety of life experiences. Children are encouraged to be inquisitive and learn from experiences. Parents may refrain from discipline. Limitation is that no one assumes responsibility for children's behavior. Conflict and confusion may arise if children have no direction.
RESPONSIBLE CHOICE Balance of freedom and restriction allows children to select values that lead to personal satisfaction and parental support. Children's choices are more limited as compared with laissez-faire approach.	Values are not strictly imposed by parents. As children choose values, parents, other family members, and teachers allow them to explore within boundaries new behaviors and their consequences. Children who can freely discuss their behavior and its effects will learn to understand their own values.
REWARD AND PUNISHMENT Offering rewards for certain valued behaviors serves to control behavior. When children fail to assume certain behaviors, parents administer punishment.	Parents may choose to use either form of value transmission more frequently. Using rewards can be positive approach to strengthen preferred values. Punishment may teach that violence is acceptable.

from those of clients. However, a nurse realizes that cultural practices are not "right" or "wrong," but rather expressions of meaning. While better alternatives might be available for some health problems, a nurse can show respect for a clients' cultural orientation by attempting to understand the meaning and value behind culture-specific health practices before attempting modifications (Johnson and Rogers, 1994).

VALUES IN PROFESSIONAL NURSING

Because values give identity, influence actions, and sustain what is meaningful, professions are as strong as the values on which they are based. All professions exist in relationship to society and are needed only as long as the underlying values of the profession are shared by the persons they serve. For purposes of identity and education, professions state what they believe to be their organizing and sustaining values. As with people, basic, fundamental values of a profession rarely change significantly. However, professions periodically reassess their values and behaviors and reprioritize or expand them to accommodate new demands. Nursing's most fundamental value is care (caring). Client advocacy has also developed as a primary nursing value. The American Association of Colleges of Nursing (AACN) specifies seven other essential nursing values.

The Value of Caring

Care, like love, is a primal concept known all over the world. Most people can give their own definition of care, but it is difficult, if not impossible to offer one universal definition for this important term. A consensus has emerged within nursing that **caring** serves as nursing's central value, providing an organizing framework for professional research, education, and theory development (Swanson, 1991).

Morse et al. (1990) identified 35 authors who offer definitions of care and give perspectives on its main characteristics. Five perspectives on the nature of caring can be identified in an analysis of the authors' works. Those perspectives include care as a human trait, a moral ideal, an affect, an interpersonal relationship, and therapeutic interventions. Any of these perspectives offer a valid starting point for developing a conceptual understanding of care that is useful for nursing practice.

Those who describe care as a human trait note that it is an innate human characteristic and that all people have the capacity to care. Nurtured in people by their own experiences of being cared for, care exists as a learned behavior. This universal aspect of care as a human trait helps nurses recognize that each culture has developed specific caring gestures and expectations that should be incorporated into professional practice. As a moral ideal, care inspires in humans the desire to dedicate themselves to the well-being of others. Because care makes survival of all living things possible, it takes on a moral character. Caring persons strive to preserve and enhance the dignity and integrity of others. Care's moral dimension has been developed as an "ethic of care" to nurture, repair, and tend to the world and all things in it (see Chapter 19).

To feel care for someone or something is to experience it as an affect. When one expresses an internal experience and acknowledges that "I care about you," he or she has experienced care as an affect. Care extends from an emotional involvement with others and gets its life from the concern and interest this involvement creates. Authors who stress care as an interpersonal relationship assert that care is defined by the interaction between the nurse and the client. Care happens interpersonally and takes on the unique characteristics of each human relationship. Care can refer to the "work" nurses do, the therapeutic interventions performed by nurses for others. Nurses talk about "care plans," personalized care, and client care conferences. All of these terms give reference to the specific activities chosen and undertaken by the nurse to assist individuals, families, and groups to higher levels of wellness.

As the body of caring research and concept development continues, nursing knowledge of its central value will become even more enriched. Leininger (1984), Noddings (1984), Watson (1985), Gadow (1985), and Benner and Wrubel (1989), to name only a few authors, have written foundational works for nursing's caring theory development.

It is important to remember that clients and families also have ideas about what is caring practice. Care always happens within a context, implying that it is not simply an abstract or theoretical value but rather takes its shape and definition by what is needed in each situation (Benner and Wrubel, 1989). For example, when caring for an adolescent with a behavior disorder, firmness, limit setting, and imposing discipline may be the most caring interventions. In a different situation with a disturbed adolescent, offering flexibility and more options may show caring.

Von Essen and Sjoden (1991) studied nurse and client perceptions of the most and least important caring behaviors and found that nurses and clients did not always agree. Clients ranked honesty, giving clear information, and competent clinical practice as the most important caring gestures; nurses ranked affective behaviors such as empathic listening as most valuable. When planning care for a client, engaging his or her participation and paying attention to the caring relationship enhances the quality of care.

Because caring is so important to the profession, nurses must remain diligent in maintaining care as a central value of their practice in all health care settings. Care is easily eroded, needing constant attention and resources to survive. When, because of constraints on their practice, nurses are not able to deliver the nurturing activities designed to assist people, they may feel dissatisfied with nursing. Certain changes within the health care delivery system (see Chapter 2) also threaten nurses' ability to exercise the caring they value. Specialization in health care has divided care givers' responsibilities, which can lead to depersonalization and fragmentation of care. Health care institutions and society expect nurses to do more with fewer resources; yet nurses often lack the autonomy and authority to decide how care will be provided (Kurtz and Warry, 1991).

Advanced technology can endanger the humane approach to nursing care when the nurse's attention turns toward monitoring sophisticated equipment rather than to sustaining the nurse-client relationship. While competence in managing today's technology can be a most valuable expression of caring in many contexts, nurses' diligent attention to the person receiving the care becomes vitally important in sustaining holistic caring (Cooper, 1993). As nursing's primary value, caring influences standards of performance in all professional activities.

American Association of Colleges of Nursing Values

In a document entitled "Essentials of College and University Education for Professional Nursing," the American Association of Colleges of Nursing (AACN) published the results of a project designed to identify the essential knowledge, skilled practice, and values necessary for nursing. The project resulted in a consensus among nursing professionals across the United States that recommended seven values essential for the professional nurse (Table 18-2). They include altruism, equality, esthetics, freedom, human dignity, justice, and truth.

In addition to listing the values, examples of professional

Table 18-2	Essential Nursing Values and Behaviors*	
ESSENTIAL VALUES	**ATTITUDES AND PERSONAL QUALITIES**	**PROFESSIONAL BEHAVIORS**
ALTRUISM Concern for the welfare of others	Caring Commitment Compassion Generosity Perseverance	Gives full attention to the client when giving care. Assists other personnel in providing care when they are unable to do so. Expresses concern about social trends and issues that have implications for health care.
EQUALITY Having the same rights, privileges, or status	Acceptance Assertiveness Fairness Self-esteem Tolerance	Provides nursing care based on the individual's needs irrespective of personal characteristics. Interacts with other providers in a nondiscriminatory manner. Expresses ideas about the improvement of access to nursing and health care.
ESTHETICS Qualities of objects, events, and persons that provide satisfaction	Appreciation Creativity Imagination Sensitivity	Adapts the environment so that it is pleasing to the client. Creates a pleasant work environment for self and others. Presents self in a manner that promotes a positive image of nursing.
FREEDOM Capacity to exercise choice	Confidence Hope Independence Openness Self-direction Self-discipline	Honors individual's right to refuse treatment. Supports the rights of other providers to suggest alternatives to the plan of care. Encourages open discussion of controversial issues in the profession.
HUMAN DIGNITY Inherent worth and uniqueness of an individual	Consideration Empathy Humaneness Kindness Respectfulness Trust	Safeguards the individual's right to privacy. Addresses individuals as they prefer to be addressed. Maintains confidentiality of clients and staff. Treats others with respect regardless of background.
JUSTICE Upholding moral and legal principles	Courage Integrity Morality Objectivity	Acts as a health care advocate. Allocates resources fairly. Reports incompetent, unethical, and illegal practice objectively and factually.
TRUTH Faithfulness to fact or reality	Accountability Authenticity Honesty Inquisitiveness Rationality Reflectiveness	Documents nursing care accurately and honestly. Obtains sufficient data to make sound judgments before reporting infractions of organizational policies. Participates in professional efforts to protect the public from misinformation about nursing.

From American Association of Colleges of Nursing: *Essentials of college and university education for professional nursing,* Washington, DC, 1986, The Association; reprinted from American Nurses Association: *Code for nurses,* Kansas City, Mo, 1976, The Association.
*The values are listed in alphabetical rather than priority order.

behavior demonstrating each of the seven values were added to the document. Professions establish standards of behavior reflective of their set of values. Because professional values are most vividly "lived out" by individual practitioners, the document also includes examples of ideal personal qualities and attitudes of professionals.

In practice, the nurse prioritizes values when making decisions. Incorporation of the AACN values into one's personal and professional value system enables the nurse to uphold the profession's standards and deliver compassionate, competent care. Periodic evaluation and discussion by the nursing profession of its values should occur. Research of nurse and client perceptions of these values would help show whether professional and societal values match (Tompkins, 1993). Because professions flourish only when they meet the felt needs of the individuals and communities they serve, values agreement between a profession and society remains essential.

The Value of Advocacy

As the nursing profession has matured and taken on its primary obligation to protect and enhance the autonomy of clients, the value of client **advocacy** has grown. Nursing's professional code of ethics asserts that the social contract between nurses and clients is based on the fundamental understanding that clients' values are to be supported and upheld. To support, uphold, and speak up for the values of others is advocacy. Health is not an end in itself, but rather a means by which persons live a life that is meaningful to them (American Nurses Association [ANA] Code of Ethics, 1985).

The strong stand for client advocacy within nursing has been influenced by many factors (Pence, 1994). As health care choices become more complex, as the knowledge gap between professionals and clients widens, as costs rise, when the choices for medical treatment become highly risky or burdensome, people become vulnerable. Clients and families need professionals who take the clients' values and interests seriously and who will be there to guide them through confusing decisions and systems. Nurses are ideally positioned for advocacy roles because they are dedicated to holistic care; understand health care systems, wellness and disease processes; and are frequently with clients for extended periods.

Clients' vulnerability increases when they become less able to promote their own interests and values. When clients cannot effectively speak for themselves, the nurse's advocacy role must become more active. Loss of consciousness, debilitating pain, diminished cognitive abilities, and emotional stress impair a person's ability to advocate for himself or herself. Client advocacy, in the most general sense, commits nurses to take those actions necessary for decreasing the client's specific vulnerability. The nurse advocate's frame of reference should always be the client's values and interests, not the nurse's or the profession's.

Although one can recite with ease the obvious reasons why clients may need help, the model of advocacy should not lead nurses to assume that all clients need or want strong forms of advocacy. As with any other specific intervention, an assessment of client needs, values, and preference should be part of the nursing process. The best form of advocacy with all clients comes in the form of appropri-ate teaching, explanation of procedures, updates on test results, involvement in planning, identification of client strengths, and careful listening. These caring interventions are forms of advocacy because they strengthen clients' abilities to pursue their own values and goals.

■ VALUES AND HEALTH PROMOTION

Nursing's goal is to help clients establish health-protecting or health-promoting behaviors, thereby modifying habits to achieve optimal levels of wellness (Edelman and Mandel, 1994). Frequently clients are taught facts and concepts about their conditions, but their health behaviors remain unchanged. The nurse who learns about clients' values devises a more successful teaching program (Fig. 18-2). Giving clients meaningful, practical information increases the likelihood that they will assume behaviors that promote well-being. Keller (1993) states that although research has demonstrated that the value an individual places on health influences health behaviors, the connection between values and behavior remains inconsistently explored. How people come to value health also needs further investigation (see the box on p. 313).

Helping persons identify, prize, and act on their values provides a foundation for nursing interventions that promote health and prevent illness. Values serve an integrating function for spiritual, cultural, psychological, and physiological dimensions of human life and, as such, impact each dimension and the person's overall well-being in many ways. A person's value system can be challenged by any alteration in health status, especially those that require life changes. Changes brought on by injury and illness can result in values fragmentation, ambivalence, apathy, overconforming, inconsistency, and uncertainty, all of which can have a negative impact on a person's health status (Potter and Perry, 1995).

Values Clarification

Nursing interventions can promote health in the human dimension of valuing. Because individuals are not always consciously aware of their values, they can have difficulty when making choices or when they feel forced to change their values. People do not suddenly become aware of their values, and many people are unable to name their values

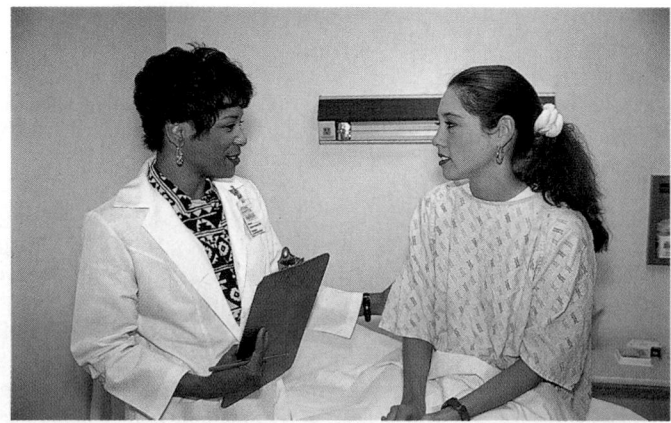

Fig. 18-2 Nurse educating young adult in primary care clinic.

► **RESEARCH HIGHLIGHT**

RESEARCH ABSTRACT

This study examined the health values of a group of African-American women who reported practicing coronary heart disease risk-reduction behaviors. The factors that contribute to the development of the group's valued health behaviors were examined. The investigator interviewed 22 young African-American women between the ages of 18 and 40 and who had a variety of occupations and income levels. Health values information was gathered through extensive interviews with the participants. Four themes emerged from the interviews: (1) becoming aware of values through role models and religion, (2) deciding to undertake behavior change, (3) sustaining the selected changes, and (4) getting "off track." The study found that the participants were strongly influenced in their health value development by seeing observable consequences of risky behaviors. Kinship systems played a critical role in health knowledge transmission and in selecting, practicing, and sustaining chosen health related behaviors. **Kinship systems** are those close people or groups of people, usually related by blood or marriage, who form meaningful family ties with one another. This finding supports the belief that many people change behavior based on how they believe family members will be affected by their choices.

IMPLICATIONS FOR PRACTICE

► Kinship systems provide motivation and support for persons undertaking positive health changes. Families should be included in client teaching sessions.

► Role modeling of positive health behaviors is important for health values formation. Help clients identify role models and incorporate what they value in their models into teaching plans.

► Changing health behaviors is complex. Develop an appreciation of the client's life situation and unique family system considerations.

► Lapses in sustaining positive health behaviors happen to everyone. Offer support, not judgment, during lapses, and help the client identify strengths and sources of support.

► People develop "rules" for themselves for sustaining behaviors. Help clients set attainable goals and reasonable guidelines through client teaching.

REFERENCE

Keller C: Developing and sustaining valued health behaviors in young African-American women, *Health Values* 17(3):49, 1993.

Three Steps of Values Clarification

CHOOSING ONE'S BELIEFS AND BEHAVIORS
- Choosing from alternatives
- Choosing freely
- Considering all consequences

PRIZING ONE'S BELIEFS AND BEHAVIORS
- Prizing and cherishing the choice
- Publicly affirming the choice

ACTING ON ONE'S BELIEFS
- Making the choice part of one's behavior
- Acting with a pattern of consistency and repetition

Modified from Raths LS, Harmin M, Simon SB: *Values and teaching*, ed 2, Columbus, Ohio, 1979, Merrill.

communication with clients becomes more effective because the nurse is able to focus attention on clients' comments and the reasons for them. In the process clients often show a willingness to discuss problems and true feelings, helping the nurse establish an individualized care plan.

Values clarification does not imply that there is a specific set of values that should be accepted by all persons. It is not a form of religious, moral, or cultural indoctrination. Rather, values clarification, or valuing, is a process of self-discovery that helps people gain insights into their own values. By using values clarification, people can more meaningfully make choices when alternatives are presented and determine whether the choices seem consistent with their beliefs. The nurse's role is to shape responses to the client's questions or statements to motivate a client to examine personal thoughts and actions.

Raths, Harmin, and Simon (1979) pioneered values clarification as an approach to appraisal of values, describing a method involving three steps: choosing, prizing, and acting (see the box above). *Choosing* begins values clarification as the person selects, then ranks, personal values. The life values scale (see the box on p. 314) provides an example of how a person may begin the process. It consists of 10 values that clients ranks in an order that accurately reflects their personal value hierarchy. Another way to complete this exercise is by having clients freely name 10 values and then prioritize them. When persons freely choose personal values, they will more likely cherish the final choice. Individuals must also be able to see their alternatives and the values each choice represents. For example, an older woman may experience the sudden loss of her husband. As she shares her concerns with a home health care nurse, it is clear that she has several choices. She can continue to live alone and grieve for her husband, move in with her daughter and away from friends, or live at home and begin to regularly socialize with male and female companions. The nurse helps the woman examine her choices without passing judgment or offering advice. A clear understanding of options and their consequences will ensure that the woman's final choice is the right one for her.

The nurse helps clients clarify alternatives so that they can act on the best possible choices. When the nurse makes a clarifying response, it should be brief, selective, nonjudg-

clearly. To promote a healthy awareness of personal values and behaviors in the change process, individuals can use the cognitive processes of values clarification.

Values clarification can be a useful tool in assisting clients and families to select and act on health-promoting behaviors, adapt to the stress of acute illness or injury, and find the personal resources necessary for maximal return of function in a rehabilitative process. Values clarification helps clients gain awareness of personal priorities, identify unclear values, and resolve major conflicts between values and behavior. While using values clarification strategies,

Life Values Scale

The 10 values listed in alphabetical order below are often important life values. Study the list carefully, and choose the one value that is most important to you by writing the number 1 in the space to the left of that value. Write the number 2 for the value that ranks second in importance. Continue in the same manner for the remaining values until you have included all ranks from 1 to 10. Each value will have a different rank.

_____ Family harmony
_____ Independence
_____ Job satisfaction
_____ Keeping up hobbies (reading, gardening, sports, music)
_____ Maintaining a home
_____ Mobility (being able to get around, travel)
_____ Physical attractiveness
_____ Privacy
_____ Spending time with others
_____ Spiritual growth

mental, thought provoking, and spontaneous. A good clarifying exchange between nurse and client lasts only a short time. To the older woman contemplating living arrangement changes after her husband's death, the nurse might say, "It sounds like you've said that both privacy and relationships are very important to you. Can you keep some privacy if you lived with your daughter?" The nurse's response makes the client think about values after the exchange. The nurse often has little warning when the client seeks solutions to a values dilemma. With experience, a nurse can learn to make clarifying responses without advanced planning. Clarifying responses are best used when a values conflict is the issue. For example, when the home health care nurse explains to the widow changes in her medications, values clarification is not needed. A nurse makes a clarifying response only for situations in which no right or wrong answer exists. Situations lacking answers are those involving beliefs, aspirations, feelings, and attitudes. For example, the woman may say to the nurse, "My daughter is afraid to have me live alone. What should I do?" The nurse responds, "You have a difficult decision to make. Do you have fears about living alone?" Although the response is consciously and deliberately designed to stimulate thought, it should not appear contrived.

Prizing is showing private and public satisfaction with the value chosen. A person holds a value in esteem by feeling good about a choice. A nurse helps a client use values clarification so that the person is able to affirm personal values in the presence of significant others. In the example of the widow, she would prize the decision to begin socializing after her husband's death by being able to share those plans with her daughter. By announcing personal values, individuals reaffirm their importance or relevance.

Acting on a chosen value strengthens its acceptance. Acting requires a translation of values into behavior. The widow begins to attend church socials and volunteers at a local hospital. Raths, Harmin, and Simon (1979) suggest that persons should act consistently and regularly on chosen values. It would be important for the widow to consciously and routinely seek opportunities to spend time with friends and acquaintances. It may, however, be difficult to act consistently on a chosen value. Even though the recently widowed woman wants a more active social life, she may find activities difficult without her husband's company. She may bypass some social invitations not because she does not value company, but because she does not feel emotionally safe yet.

Values clarification goes a step beyond the nursing intervention of allowing clients to express feelings. Naming feelings will not provide adequate information if the real problem is a conflict in values. The nurse who is familiar with values clarification can help the client define values, clarify goals, and seek solutions. The client becomes more aware of the way values influence actions. Awareness is an essential component of health promotion and problem solving.

When several different values are expressed by more than one person in a situation, values clarification alone may not be adequate for resolving conflicts between competing values. The most values clarification can do is help people understand one another's meanings and values. The persons involved may still not agree on what should be done. Because some values are "better" than others, resolution of some value conflicts requires skilled ethical analysis (see Chapter 19).

Values Clarification in Various Settings

Exploring clients' values with them can occur in any setting. The bedside, a clinic office, and the home are all suitable places for clients to enter into values conversations with the nurse. Values clarification is often more successful when the nurse has repeated contacts with clients. It is difficult for the nurse to help clients meaningfully achieve each step of the valuing process when interactions are minimal.

Clients and families in acute care settings may experience an upheaval in their value systems as a result of the crisis of illness or injury. Many times, fundamental issues of life and death surround the acute phases of illness. The nurse in these settings should develop an ability to raise, at the appropriate time, clarifying questions regarding the use of technology, dignified death, and the meaning of life and health itself. Price and Murphy (1994) underscore the nurse's duty to educate clients and families about treatment decisions, particularly those at the end of life, because of the nurse's privileged status of being in meaningful, close relationships with them.

Health care professionals, too, undergo value strain in acute care settings. In the research of Solomon et al. (1993) almost half of the 759 nurses and 687 physicians surveyed reported that they had gone against their own conscience in providing care to the terminally ill. Professionals in acute care settings may value technological interventions very highly because they often witness miraculous recoveries and the saving of lives. An overvaluing of technology and curing can, however, desensitize practitioners to other human values such as comfort and dignity and widen the gap between client and care giver values.

Values questions and the promotion of optimal health in rehabilitative or restorative settings may have unique qualities. In a process of recovering health or pursuing a peaceful death, a reprioritization of values may happen gradually and require significant changes in lifestyle. For example, a young woman in rehabilitation for paralysis sustained after an automobile accident may begin to learn that relationships and needing to gain knowledge are now more important to her than hobbies she previously enjoyed. These shifts in values occur over time. An attentive nurse looks for signals that the client is doing values work and assists in that process. An example of values clarification used in an extended care facility is shown below.

As is demonstrated in this case study, it takes time, interest in others, teaching skills, self-awareness, and nonjudgmental listening for nurses to develop values clarification as an important health promotion exercise in client care. Values clarification is a valuable means for helping persons sort out true feelings and beliefs and gain a better awareness of life's possibilities.

▊ VALUES CHALLENGES IN NURSING

Because values give people meaning and are held very deeply, it is easy to see how conflict arises internally or between people when values are challenged. One has only to look at the American abortion debate to see how intensely people justify their own prioritization of values. Nurses, as part of their job, come into intimate contact with diverse groups of people and may experience values challenges daily.

As nursing matures, critical shifts in professional values have occurred, sparking controversies and creating new

---

CASE STUDY Ms. Cody was an 85-year-old woman who managed her own business for 43 years and raised four children by herself. In her advancing years she had been able to maintain her own apartment, aided by the daily visits of a son who lived close to her. Ms. Cody enjoyed daily walks around the neighborhood, to the store, and to her nearby church. Because of her activity, she remained quite physically fit but began to suffer serious short-term memory loss and diminished cognition, making even simple conversations and daily judgments difficult for her. On one hot summer day, while her son was at work, she set off on one of her walks, wandering about aimlessly until she came, exhausted by the heat, to a neighbor's door looking for her apartment. They offered help and called her son. Neighbors had been questioning her ability to stay in her apartment and threatened to call the abuse hot line if the son did not take action to change his mother's living situation. Reluctantly the son placed his mother in an elder care facility. Her condition deteriorated rapidly; she became withdrawn, refused to eat, and while struggling to get out of a chair, fell and broke her hip. On one of his daily visits with his mother, now bedridden, the son says to Mr. Allen, his mother's primary nurse, "I just don't think I've done the best thing. She has given so much to me. Something's not right." Mr. Allen, who has been developing a relationship with the family, believes that values clarification might help. The son is experiencing a conflict because he values his duty to both keep his mother safe and at the same time, protect her independence and dignity.

CHOOSING FROM ALTERNATIVES

The son, Mr. Cody, has been involved in giving care to his mother for 16 years. He had always tried to make decisions that protected his mother's independence because she valued it highly. When confronted by the neighbors' strong difference of opinion and possible legal action, he acted quickly to remedy the situation. Now, 1 month later, Mr. Cody is looking for more options.

EXAMINING ALL CONSEQUENCES

Although it is never possible to predict all consequences of a decision, creating options by weighing the potential benefits and burdens of a choice offers insight into personal values. Mr. Cody had little reason to believe that his mother's quality of life would improve if she stayed in the elder facility. While the care was good, it "just wasn't home." That concerns him greatly. To bring her home would require increased sacrifices of time, energy, and personal resources. He does not have a background in skilled care interventions but believes he can learn. Through teaching, Mr. Allen is able to increase Mr. Cody's understanding of the complexities involved and direct him toward appropriate resources. Mr. Cody believes that sending his mother to live with one of her other children would still feel like "not being home to die."

CHOOSING FREELY

Mr. Allen understands how important it is for Mr. Cody to own his decision. Mr. Cody had stated that he felt "pressured" before and had not come to terms with his decision. Now he has the chance to weigh the options in accordance with his most cherished values. "I've talked to the home health people and to close friends from church. I can also arrange to do more of my work at home. I want to bring Mother home with me." To which Mr. Allen replies, "You sound determined. How do you feel now that you've made this decision?"

PRIZING THE CHOICE

Mr. Cody acknowledges that he is intimidated by all of the details he has to work out, but that he trusts "it will all happen." He states that he feels determined to see whether bringing his mother home will help her appetite and mood, benefiting her healing process. Mr. Cody is able to conclude, "Inwardly, I feel more peaceful now." Mr. Allen realizes that with a decision of this magnitude, expressing realistic concerns does not necessarily resolve his uncertainty.

AFFIRMING THE CHOICE

Having made the decision, it is now important for Mr. Cody to communicate his choice to others. Mr. Allen helps Mr. Cody explore how he can prize his choice, even when there may be differences of opinion. He asks, "Did your brother and sister seem supportive of your plan?" Mr. Cody and Mr. Allen go on to discuss how best Mr. Cody can inform others and follow through with his value-based choice.

ACTING WITH A PATTERN

Mr. Allen was able to get reports from the home health care nurse who began to see Ms. Cody in her son's home. Mr. Cody worked out a schedule of care giving and gained satisfaction from the fact that his mother began to eat more heartily and offered frequent smiles to her care givers. She died at home of a stroke 2 months later. Had the period of home care extended well past the 2 months Mr. Cody stayed at home with his mother, had his mother shown no signs of improvement, or had the volunteer care givers begun to suffer disproportionate burdens, occasions for reassessing with Mr. Cody his goals and values may have arisen again. As life circumstances change, goals and the prioritization of values may shift accordingly. It may be difficult for a nurse, particularly when she does not agree with a client or family member's initial decision, to be open to reclarifying values nonjudgmentally. Had Mr. Allen thought it impossible for Mr. Cody's plan to work, or had he dismissed Mr. Cody's action as "guilt-driven" instead of value based, the nurse's ability to aid Mr. Cody in values clarification would have been significantly compromised. ▪

ideals. The first nursing code of ethics named obedience to physicians as a primary professional value (Freitas, 1990). Since then, nurses have placed loyalty to clients and their families as a paramount value (Pence, 1994). Nurses individually and collectively face the challenge of renewing and reshaping professional values within rapidly changing health care systems and professional relationships.

Values also affect health at a social level, posing challenges to the nursing profession. Health care reform in the United States has been difficult not because legislators and health care professionals disagree on whether something should be done, but rather because each proposal gives preference to certain values over others. For example, some plans consider basic medical coverage for all citizens (universal health care) a primary value. Others consider personal choice of health care practitioners and medical insurance as most important. Some groups highly value free competition and unlimited growth of medical research and technology. Where does nursing stand on these issues? Have nurses collectively named, prized, and acted on the profession's set of values for health care reform? Skill in negotiating conflict and responding to values challenges emerges as critical for personal and professional growth.

Personal Challenges

Nurses care for clients who possess unique values about life and the human experience. Therefore nurses should be aware of their own values, understanding how they interact with the values of clients. To make intelligent and thoughtful decisions about care, nurses must be aware of the influence personal values have in care giving.

Nurses are people, too, with deeply held sets of convictions and value systems. It is a mistake to presume, as is often done, that because nursing is a caring profession dedicated to the service of others, nurses no longer experience personal disappointment, frustration, sadness, and anger in certain situations. There may even be some embarrassment, personal and professional, in acknowledging that nurses struggle with negative feelings and behavior when their values are challenged.

Sometimes the challenges are easy to identify. A nurse may feel contempt for a family member who has abused a child. Or another nurse can feel very angry at an intoxicated client who has taken a life in a car accident he caused or at a young woman who is giving birth to her third crack-addicted baby. At other times the challenges are more subtle. Perhaps a nurse working in a women's health clinic has strong values concerning human sexuality, believing that sex outside of marriage is wrong. The nurse may be less attentive to an unmarried teenager in a clinic who has a sexually transmitted disease. Situations like these may challenge the values a nurse holds about life and personal responsibility. How can a nurse, as a person, negotiate the conflict he or she feels inside?

First, to meet the challenge, a nurse must have self-knowledge. The nurse will have difficulty assuming the role of a professional when personal values are poorly conceived and unclear. Values clarification, as described above, done alone or with the help of another person, helps nurses explore their values. A nurse can use a source of discomfort, such as frustration or anger in a client situation, as a trigger for recognizing a values challenge. Recognizing and acknowledging conflict is a necessary first step to shaping an appropriate response.

Second, the nurse should attend to the challenge. A number of possibilities exist. Attempting to understand the life situation and experience of the other person often helps. If the client is seen as a person instead of being placed in a behavior category, the possibility for a relationship exists. Values do not determine the worth of a person's life, nor do they make any one person more or less human or valuable. It is important to point out that understanding and respecting inherent human dignity is not the same as excusing a person's behavior. To understand that a person who abuses a child has probably learned that behavior as a result of his or her own abuse may help the nurse see the complexity of value development. It does not excuse or condone abuse of children. Persons who seek help for repeated illness episodes caused by lifestyle choices (e.g., lung disease from smoking) are making poor health choices, as most of us do at some point. If a nurse assesses his or her own life for lapses in health-promoting behaviors, it is likely that he or she will find them. Understanding requires good listening skills, use of therapeutic communication, and a humble willingness to accept the complexities of life stories.

The nurse should try not to judge the client's behavior or assume the underlying value. A client will be unable to reconcile personal values issues if the nurse moralizes or gives unsolicited advice. Nurses should think of themselves as persons who gather data about the health needs of another person. Competent nurses help clients make their own decisions about health care values. It is important to remember that meaningful changes, especially in complicated cases like substance abuse, rarely occur in the context of punishing, judgmental relationships.

There are times, however, when acknowledging feelings, putting aside judgment, and trying to understand do not change a nurse's internal response to a situation, nor do they change client behavior. During times of conflict the nursing profession is clear about what constitutes responsible nursing behavior. Even though a nurse may not approve of the behaviors exhibited or like a client, it remains the nurse's obligation to give care that demonstrates respect for the human dignity of the other person (ANA Code of Ethics, 1985). Sometimes it may be all a nurse can do to render safe, competent, physiological care. For nursing to remain a socially valued profession, in the realm of professional behavior and action the individual nurse's values and attitudes must not interfere with the obligation to give competent, respectful care to everyone in need.

Professional Challenges

As noted above, for a profession to exist and flourish in a society, a need must exist for its services. The people a profession serves must see its function as valuable. In addition to the nursing profession's challenge to uphold its caring ideals through education, research, and expert practice, the nursing profession faces an increasing responsibility to respond collectively to societal health issues.

Nursing has historically been concerned with meeting the health care needs of individuals and families. The value of advocacy in this model has been most commonly interpreted as protecting and enhancing the autonomy of individuals. Muyskens (1993) argues that nurses have a collective responsibility to become more involved in social issues surrounding access to health care for whole populations. In short, nursing's model of individual client advocacy should be expanded to include health advocacy for whole populations. For health advocacy to become more established as a nursing value, the profession must rise to the challenge with political, educational, and research efforts. This does not imply that nurses should abandon the value of individual client advocacy, but rather that advocacy be seen as more encompassing.

Assuming an even greater role as health advocates would challenge nursing to examine societal health care values carefully. It would then support and advocate those values that were most consistent with professional ideals. Priester (1992) names six values (identified in a research project) underlying the United States health care system. They include professional autonomy, client autonomy, client advocacy, consumer sovereignty, high-quality care, and universal access to care. Aroskar (1993) calls for a reconfiguration of those values and challenges nursing to play a key role in that process. A new framework would reorder or redefine current values and add values that place a greater emphasis on community. Nursing could then reevaluate its own set of values and its professional position on health care reform in light of the new values framework. The everescalating issues of health care reform are value driven. The nursing profession and society have much to gain in taking up the challenge.

■ KEY CONCEPTS ■

▶ When nurses are aware of their personal values and professional values, they are better able to be effective practitioners.

▶ Values provide a standard of behavior for the person or group that holds them.

▶ A person acquires values through reasoning, observation, and experience.

▶ A child acquires values from parents, other family members, school, church, and other social institutions.

▶ A person's cultural background influences health values.

▶ A nurse's values influence client care.

▶ The values of caring and advocacy are foundational nursing values.

▶ When making clinical decisions, the nurse acts in ways that reflect the values inherent in the profession.

▶ The nurse who learns about a client's values is better prepared to help the client assume health-protecting or health-promoting behaviors.

▶ Values clarification is a health-promoting process that encourages an understanding of personal values.

▶ A person must be able to choose values freely from available alternatives and understand the consequences of choosing.

▶ Nurses who use values clarification with clients offer clarifying responses that stimulate introspection about values and behavior.

▶ Values clarification promotes effective reasoning and decision making.

▶ A nurse who assists a client in clarifying values and making decisions does so nonjudgmentally.

▶ Nurses experience challenges in practice related to personal and professional values.

▶ Social values are important in determining effective health care reform.

▶ The nursing profession should become more involved with health advocacy, which includes individual client advocacy.

■ KEY TERMS ■

Advocacy, p. 312

Caring, p. 310

Kinship system, p. 313

Value, p. 307

Value system, p. 307

Values clarification, p. 313

■ CRITICAL THINKING EXERCISES ■

1. You have been taking care of a child who has been abused by her parent. The child has become attached to you, and your caring efforts to build trust with the child seem to be working. The child is less withdrawn and does not flinch when people come near her. The abusing parent has begun to visit and the child seems to regress during the visits, appearing frightened. It is very difficult for you to interact naturally or pleasantly with the parent. In report you express your frustration to the next nurse, "People like that shouldn't be allowed to have any more children." Identify the personal and professional values challenges you face, and think through all of your responses, gathering data about your own values and attitudes.

2. As a clinic nurse in an urban area, you are seeing an unmarried teenager who has had several episodes of sexually transmitted disease. The 16-year-old client tells you she wants to have a baby and expresses her desire to show love to a child. Discuss how you might use values clarification with this young woman.

3. As a home health care nurse you have been taking care of an elderly man who has chronic heart disease. He has become increasingly symptomatic and may need hospitalization for management of his illness. He tells you that he does not want to continue "doctoring" and that he is ready to die. He does not feel that people—family or health professionals—are listening to him. Reread the section on the value of advocacy and think of some ways you could be this client's advocate.

REFERENCES

American Association of Colleges of Nursing: *Essentials of college and university education for professional nursing,* Washington, DC, 1986, The Association.

American Nurses Association: *Code for nurses with interpretive statements,* Kansas City, Mo, 1985, The Association.

Aroskar M: A plea for revisiting values in nursing and health care, *J Prof Nurs* 9(5):253, 1993.

Benner P, Wrubel J: *The primacy of caring: stress and coping in health and illness,* Menlo Park, Calif, 1989, Addison Wesley.

Cooper M: The intersection of technology and care in the ICU, *ANS* 15(3):23, 1993.

Edelman C, Mandel C: *Health promotion through the lifespan,* St Louis, 1994, Mosby.

Freitas L: Historical roots and future perspectives related to nursing ethics, *J Prof Nurs* 6(4):197, 1990.

Gadow S: Nurse and patient: the caring relationship. In Bishop A, Scudder J, editors: *Caring, curing, coping,* Birmingham, 1985, University of Alabama Press.

Hamilton PM: *Realities in contemporary nursing,* 1992, Addison Wesley Nursing.

Johnson K, Rogers S: When cultural practices are health risks: the dilemma of female circumcision, *Holistic Nurs Pract* 8(2):70, 1994.

Keller C: Developing and sustaining valued health behaviors in young African-American women, *Health Values* 17(3):49, 1993.

Kluckhohn C: Values and value-orientation in the theory of action: an exploration in definition and classification. In Parsons T, Shils E, editors: *Toward a general theory of action,* New York, 1951, Harper & Row.

Kurtz R, Warry J: Caring ethic: more human kindness, the care of nursing science, *Nurs Forum* 26(1):4, 1991.

Leininger M, editor: *Care: the essence of nursing and health,* Thorofare, NJ, 1984, Slack.

Maslow A: *New knowledge in human values,* New York, 1959, Harper & Row.

Morse J, Solberg S, Neander W et al: Concepts of caring and caring as a concept, *ANS* 13(1):1, 1990.

Muyskens J: Nursing and access to health care, *Bioethics Forum* 9(4):11, 1993.

Noddings N: *Caring: a feminist approach to ethics and moral education,* Berkeley, Calif, 1984, University of California.

Pence T: Nursing's most pressing moral issue, *Bioethics Forum* 10(1):3, 1994.

Potter P, Perry A: *Basic nursing,* ed 3, St Louis, 1995, Mosby.

Preister R: A values framework for health system reform, *Health Affairs* 11(2):84, 1992.

Price D, Murphy D: DNR: still crazy after all these years, *J Nurs Law* 1(3):53, 1994.

Raths L, Harmin M, Simon S: *Values and teaching,* ed 2, Columbus, Ohio, 1979, Merrill.

Rokeach M: *The nature of human values,* New York, 1973, Free Press.

Solomon M, O'Donnell L, Jennings B et al: Decisions near the end of life: professional views on life-sustaining treatments, *Am J Public Health* 83(1):14, 1993.

Swanson K: Empirical development of a middle range theory of caring, *Nurs Res* 40(3):161, 1991.

Tompkins E: Nurse and client perceptions of the AACN nursing values, *West J Nurs Res* 15(3):363, 1993.

Von Essen L, Sjoden PO: Patient and staff perceptions of caring: review and replication, *J Adv Nurs* 16(1):1363, 1991.

Watson J: *Nursing: human science and human care a theory of nursing,* New York, 1985, National League for Nursing.

ADDITIONAL READINGS

Abood D, Conway T: Health value and self-esteem as predictors of wellness behavior, *Health Values* 16(3):20, 1992.

Ashworth P, Longmate M, Morrison P: Patient participation: its meaning and significance in the context of caring, *J Adv Nurs* 17(12):1430, 1992.

Caffrey R, Caffrey P: Nursing: caring or codependent? *Nurs Forum* 29(1),12, 1994.

Eddy D, Elfrink V, Weis D et al: Importance of professional nursing values, *J Nurs Educ* 33(6):257, 1994.

Fetsch S, Mintun M: Strengthening the nurse's role as patient advocate, *Bioethics Forum* 10(1):15, 1994.

Hunstock D: Values and the for-profit healthcare industry: a manageable issue, *JONA* 24(3) 13,16, 1994.

Mohr W: Values and the for-profit healthcare industry: an uneasy fit, *JONA* 24(3): 12,14, 1994.

Muyskens J: Equality vs individuality: American values in conflict, *Sch Inq Nurs Prac: Int J* 6(3):235, 1992.

Northrup D: Self-care myth reconsidered, *ANS* 15(3):59, 1993.

Saarmann L, Freitas L, Rapps J, Riegel B: The relationship of education to critical thinking ability and values among nurses: socialization into professional nursing, *J Prof Nurs* 8(1):26, 1992.

Sullivan J, Deane D: Caring: reappropriating our tradition, *Nurs Forum* 29(2):5, 1994.

Uustal D: *Values and ethics in nursing: from theory to practice,* ed 4, Greenwich RI, 1992, Educational Resources in Nursing and Wholistic Health.

Weis D, Shank M. Eddy D et al: Professional values in baccalaureate nursing education, *J Prof Nurs* 9(6):336, 1993.

Wolf Z, Giardino E, Osborne P et al: Dimensions of nurse caring, *Image J Nurs Sch* 26(2):107, 1994.

## Chapter 19

Ethics

Mastery of content in this chapter will enable the student to:

▶ Define the key terms listed.

▶ Discuss the influence of ethics on nursing practice.

▶ Describe nursing's ethic of care.

▶ Compare responsibility and accountability in nursing practice.

▶ Discuss the content of nurses' professional codes of ethics.

▶ Identify the factors that influence moral reasoning.

▶ Describe the primary and secondary ethical principles.

▶ Discuss the moral basis of informed consent and advance directives.

▶ Apply a method of ethical analysis to a clinical situation.

▶ Identify the major functions of institutional ethics committees.

▶ Discuss how nurses can engage in preventive ethics.

The study of ethics has become increasingly important for nurses. Technological advances have pushed questions about the beginning and end of human life, the quality of life, and professional ethics and virtue to new limits. The most pressing moral questions of our era are being asked in health care settings, for it is there that people come face to face with real-life choices about health, life, and death. As the complex issues of abortion, assisted suicide, organ transplantation, and allocation of scarce medical resources are debated in the media, nurses are finding themselves on the "front lines" of those same questions. Nurses need the necessary skills and insights to make effective contributions in ethically sensitive situations.

Clients are becoming more aware of their rights within the health care system and are concerned about ethical issues. They look to health care professionals to help them with their concerns. Nurses take very seriously their accountability and responsibility for autonomous ethical practice, no longer yielding their responsibility for a full scope of practice to other professionals or institutions. The nursing profession functions under its own code of ethics and is increasingly aware of how this affects nursing practice.

Because ethical issues are often hard to explain and settle, the participation of nurses in this dimension of practice can lead to frustration. Nurses often say that ethical issues leave them feeling trapped, or "in the middle." Although nurses have a primary commitment to clients, they are also accountable to families, physicians, peers, institutions, and society. At times the nurse's duty to one person or group is at odds with other loyalties. Murphy (1993a) encourages nurses to find ways to get out of the middle when it is viewed in the negative sense of feeling powerless. This can be accomplished through expanding one's knowledge base in ethics, seeking professional support, and developing a strong, positive sense of the nurse's moral position. Nurses can learn to see the "in-the-middle" position as a privileged place. From this vantage point the nurse is able to participate as a client advocate, sensitive to differing viewpoints and interests.

■ DEFINITION OF ETHICS

Ethics is a term with many meanings. Simply stated, ethics is concerned with how people ought to act and how they ought to be in relationship with others. Ethics does not just describe how things are, but rather is concerned with establishing norms or standards for how human life and conduct should be (Mandle, Boyle, and O'Donohoe, 1994). It is concerned with questions of good and bad, right and wrong conduct, character or motives. Defined broadly, the terms **morals** and **ethics** are used interchangeably, although subtle differences in meaning exist in ethics literature. Authors who define ethics as a term different from morals reserve the term ethics for the philosophical investigation or study of a particular issue or dilemma, whereas morals describe the actual behaviors, customs, and beliefs of people and groups. Morals have a social character (Davis and Aroskar, 1991). Health care ethics, of which nursing ethics is a part, concerns itself with what is good or right for human health and life.

Many times nurses realize that it is not clear what the right action should be. In such situations the involved persons experience moral uncertainty or distress, or describe their situation as a moral dilemma. The study of ethics in health care has centered on resolving ethical dilemmas. Because so many morally confusing situations arise in health care settings, this emphasis has been appropriate. Ethics, however, should not be reduced to only a consideration of difficult problems. Questions of personal character (virtue) and right relationships should not be overlooked. Ethics can also be used to describe a pattern or way of life. As such, ethics reflects the personal virtues, principles, and standards that govern professional behaviors. Nursing's moral way of life has been described by many as an "ethic of care" (Bevis, 1988; Leininger, 1988; Watson, 1988). Care is a moral word that guides the way a nurse should act and be with others.

Values and ethics are related. Values (see Chapter 18), the building blocks for personal and professional morality, influence one's ethical decision making, relationships, and conduct. Values are based on experience, religion, education, and culture. Additional sources of values for nurses are the nursing profession and employing institutions. A person's ethic flows from his or her values.

The study of ethics is not, however, concerned only with values and what each individual wants, feels, or cherishes. Since all people want, feel, and value different things, ethics would then be the study of competing personal values. Just because a person values something, however sincerely, does not necessarily make it right or good.

Ethics is a study of good conduct, character, and motives and is concerned with determining what is good or valuable for all people. Ethical investigation goes beyond personal preferences to establish norms and standards upon which individuals, professions, and societies agree. Within nursing, specific values and moral requirements are necessary to maintain the integrity of the profession. An ethical nurse will act and treat others in specific ways that are consistent with nursing norms and will be guided by more than personal preferences or values.

■ ETHICS IN NURSING

To become mature professionals who are able to participate effectively in the ethical dimensions of their practice, nurses must continue to develop a strong sense of their moral identity, seek support from available professional resources (Fig. 19-1), and expand their knowledge and skill in the area of ethics. The moral position or identity of nursing, an "ethic of care," is described below. Professional codes of ethics, mandates for nursing accountability and responsibility, and institutional ethics committees offer support and guidance for ethical practice. Familiarity with moral reasoning, moral theory, and ethical principles helps the nurse effectively consider ethical situations.

An Ethic of Care

Care can be described as an action, a virtue, an affect, an ethical principle, or a way of being in the world. Care as an ethic for nursing is concerned not only with the resolution of ethical dilemmas, but also with the ways people behave toward one another. An **ethic of care** is concerned with relationships between people and with a nurse's character and attitude toward others. Caring knowledge is gained through personal and emotional involvement with others

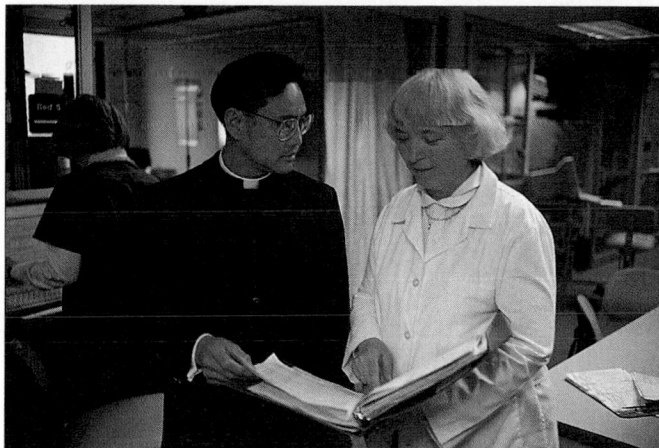

Fig. 19-1 Nurses collaborate with other professionals in making ethical decisions.

and by joining them in their moral struggles (Cooper, 1991).

To be able to care is part of human survival. Being cared for early in life gives a child a moral knowledge about what it is to care and be cared for. People who do not experience care in their lives often find it difficult to act in caring ways. Someone who experiences caring can apply this is his or her profession. Nurses become experts in caring by learning how to attend to the specific needs of the persons with whom they are in relationship. A professional caring nurse is able to have empathy for another person. The nurse should try to understand the situation of the other person and take into account as much of the other's life and experience as possible. The professional care giver is able to go from a self-centered to an other-centered position and is willing to take action on behalf of other persons (Brown, Kitson, and McKnight, 1992).

Practitioners who function from an ethic of care are sensitive to unequal relationships that can lead to an abuse of one person's power over another, intentional or otherwise. In health care settings clients and families are often on unequal footing with professionals because of the client's illness, lack of technical information, regression caused by pain and suffering, and unfamiliar circumstances. The nurse advocacy role is critical in an ethic of care (see Chapter 18).

Caring activities cannot always be determined in advance, since they depend on the situation. A client who has attempted suicide will need different caring behaviors than those appropriate for an older adult with cognitive impairment. An ethic of care leads a nurse to be sensitive to each situation and to respond with technical and moral knowledge, compassion, competence, and personal integrity.

Care can be easily eroded in environments that emphasize technical cure and do not view people in the context of their lives and values. Nurses can use their caring knowledge in situations where client interests are threatened. Senior nursing students report that they recognize how difficult it can be to maintain ideal nursing behavior in certain circumstances (see the box above).

▶ **RESEARCH HIGHLIGHT**

RESEARCH ABSTRACT
Through clinical experience and education nursing students develop expectations about the ethical dimensions of nursing practice. Having role expectations met often contributes to a future nurse's sense of contentment with a profession. If expectations are considerably different from what is experienced in practice, disillusionment may be experienced by new practitioners. Twenty-three senior baccalaureate nursing students were interviewed. A summary of interviews found patterns that centered around the themes of control, power, and respect. The study concludes that senior nursing students (1) were realistic about nursing practice, (2) perceived themselves as quite powerless, (3) verbalized a commitment to the ethical principle of respect for client values and self-determination, (4) felt guilty when they did not speak up when they believed they should have, and (5) were disappointed when practicing nurses did not "stand up" for clients. The study gives information on how the students perceived their future ability to practice nursing as it ought to be done.

IMPLICATIONS FOR PRACTICE
▶ Nursing students would benefit by educational methods that help them process the ethical questions that come up in their experiences.
▶ Students, encouraged by good role modeling, should be exposed to effective methods of nurse advocacy in classrooms and practice settings.
▶ Discussions that allow the expression of positive and negative feelings regarding personal and professional expectations should be encouraged.
▶ Students and faculty should develop teaching and learning strategies that build self-confidence, self-evaluation, and self-reliance.

REFERENCE
Kelly B: The "real world" of hospital nursing practice as perceived by nursing undergraduates, *J Prof Nurs* 9(1):27, 1993.

Nurses' Codes of Ethics

Nursing has developed codes of ethics that describe ideals for professional conduct. Codes reflect ethical principles widely accepted by members of the profession. Because codes are written in general, universal terms, they are not designed to tell nurses what to do in specific ethical situations; rather, they give guidelines to assist nurses in their own moral reasoning. There are several codes for professional nurses (see the boxes on pp. 322 to 323). Note that the codes differ slightly but that all reflect a commitment to the primary principles of respect for autonomy (client self-determination), beneficence (doing good), nonmaleficence (avoiding harm), justice (treating people fairly), and the secondary principles of veracity (truth-telling), fidelity (keeping promises), and confidentiality (respecting privileged information).

American Nurses Association Code of Ethics

- The nurse provides services with respect for human dignity and the uniqueness of the client unrestricted by considerations of social or economic status, personal attributes, or the nature of health problems.
- The nurse safeguards the client's right to privacy by judiciously protecting information of a confidential nature.
- The nurse acts to safeguard the client and the public when health care and safety are affected by the incompetent, unethical, or illegal practice of any person.
- The nurse assumes responsibility and accountability for individual nursing judgments and actions.
- The nurse maintains competence in nursing.
- The nurse exercises informed judgment and uses individual competence and qualifications as criteria in seeking consultation, accepting responsibilities, and delegating nursing activities to others.

- The nurse participates in activities that contribute to the ongoing development of the profession's body of knowledge.
- The nurse participates in the profession's efforts to implement and improve standards of nursing.
- The nurse participates in the profession's efforts to establish and maintain conditions of employment conducive to high-quality nursing care.
- The nurse participates in the profession's effort to protect the public from misinformation and misrepresentation and to maintain the integrity of nursing.
- The nurse collaborates with members of the health professions and other citizens in promoting community and national efforts to meet the health needs of the public.

From American Nurses Association: *Code for nurses with interpretive statements*, Kansas City, Mo, 1985, The Association.

International Council of Nurses Code for Nurses

- The fundamental responsibility of the nurse is fourfold: to promote health, to prevent illness, to restore health, and to alleviate suffering.
- The need for nursing is universal. Inherent in nursing is respect for life, dignity, and rights of man. It is unrestricted by considerations of nationality, race, creed, color, age, sex, politics, or social status.
- Nurses render health services to the individual, the family, and the community and coordinate their services with those of related groups.

NURSES AND PEOPLE
- The nurse's primary responsibility is to those people who require nursing care.
- The nurse, in providing care, promotes an environment in which the values, customs, and spiritual beliefs of the individual are respected.
- The nurse holds in confidence personal information and uses judgment in sharing this information.

NURSES AND PRACTICE
- The nurse carries personal responsibility for nursing practice and for maintaining competence by continual learning. The nurse maintains the highest standards of nursing care possible within the reality of a specific situation.

- The nurse uses judgment in relation to individual competence when accepting and delegating responsibilities.
- The nurse when acting in a professional capacity should at all times maintain standards of personal conduct which reflect credit upon the profession.

NURSES AND SOCIETY
- The nurse shares with other citizens the responsibility for initiating and supporting action to meet the health and social needs of the public.

NURSES AND CO-WORKERS
- The nurse sustains a cooperative relationship with co-workers in nursing and other fields. The nurse takes appropriate action to safeguard the individual when his care is endangered by a co-worker or any other person.

NURSES AND THE PROFESSION
- The nurse plays the major role in determining and implementing desirable standards of nursing practice and nursing education.
- The nurse is active in developing a core of professional knowledge.
- The nurse, acting through the professional organization, participates in establishing and maintaining equitable social and economic working conditions in nursing.

From International Council of Nurses: *ICN code for nurses: ethical concepts applied to nursing*, Geneva, 1973, Imprimeries Populaires.

Accountability and Responsibility

A nurse assumes responsibility and accountability for nursing care provided. **Responsibility** refers to the execution of duties associated with the nurse's particular role (American Nurses Association [ANA], 1985). When administering medications, the nurse is responsible for assessing clients' need for the drugs, giving them safely and correctly, and evaluating the responses. A nurse who acts in a responsible manner gains the trust of clients and other professionals. A responsible nurse remains competent in knowledge and skills and demonstrates a willingness to perform within the ethical guidelines of the profession.

Accountability means being answerable for one's own actions. A nurse is accountable to self, the client, the profession, the employer, and society. If a wrong dose of medication is given, the nurse is accountable to the client who received it, the physician who ordered it, the nursing service that set standards of expected performance, and society, which demands professional excellence. To be accountable, the nurse acts according to the professional code

Canadian Nurses Association Code of Ethics

CLIENTS

Value I
Respect for Needs and Values of Clients
A nurse treats clients with respect for their individual needs and values.

Value II
Respect for Client Choice
Based upon respect for clients and regard for their right to control their own care, nursing care reflects respect for the right of choice held by clients.

Value III
Confidentiality
The nurse holds confidential all information about a client learned in the health care setting.

Value IV
Dignity of Clients
The nurse is guided by consideration for the dignity of clients.

Value V
Competent Nursing Care
The nurse provides competent care to clients.

NURSING ROLES AND RELATIONSHIPS

Value VI
Nursing Practice, Education, Research and Administration
The nurse maintains trust in nurses and nursing.

Value VII
Cooperation in Health Care
The nurse recognizes the contribution and expertise of colleagues from nursing and other disciplines as essential to excellent health care.

Value VIII
Protecting Clients from Incompetence
The nurse takes steps to ensure that the client receives competent and ethical care.

Value IX
Conditions of Employment
Conditions of employment should contribute in a positive way to client care and the professional satisfaction of nurses.

Value X
Job Action
Job action by nurses is directed toward securing conditions of employment that enable safe and appropriate care for clients and contribute to the professional satisfaction of nurses.

NURSING ETHICS AND SOCIETY

Value XI
Advocacy of the Interests of Clients, the Community and Society
The nurse advocates the interests of clients.

Value XII
Representing Nursing Values and Ethics
The nurse represents the values and ethics of nursing before colleagues and others.

THE NURSING PROFESSION

Value XIII
Responsibilities of Professional Nurses' Associations
Professional nurses' organizations are responsible for clarifying, securing and sustaining ethical nursing conduct. The fulfillment of these tasks requires that professional nurses' organizations remain responsive to the rights, needs and legitimate interests of clients and nurses.

From Canadian Nurses Association: *Code of ethics for nursing*, Ottawa, November 1991, The Association.

---

of ethics. Thus when an error is made, the nurse reports it and initiates care to prevent further injury. Accountability calls for an evaluation of a nurse's effectiveness in practice. Professional accountability serves the following purposes:

1. To evaluate new professional practices and reassess existing ones
2. To maintain standards of health care
3. To facilitate personal reflection, ethical thought, and personal growth on the part of health care professionals
4. To provide a basis for ethical decision making

To be accountable, the nurse practices within the codes of the profession. Accountability requires an evaluation of the nurse's performance in providing nursing care. The Joint Commission on Accreditation of Healthcare Organizations (JCAHO) has recommended the establishment of standards for the delivery of nursing care. These standards, developed by nursing clinical experts, provide a basic structure against which nursing care is objectively measured. These standards do not eliminate the need for individualized care plans. Instead, the nurse incorporates the standards into the care plans designed for each client. Accountability can be better ensured and measured when "quality care" has been defined. Most institutions rely on the guidance offered through JCAHO and ANA standards.

FOUNDATIONS FOR ETHICAL DELIBERATIONS

"Doing ethics" involves participating in a critical thought process about right and wrong, good and bad, or most often, thinking about situations in which one has more than one "right" possible course of action. It is a process that occurs in many client-nurse interactions. For example, managing a dying client's pain requires the nurse to decide whether to administer the next ordered dose of morphine or be concerned as to whether the drug might depress the client's respiratory rate. The most difficult cases are those in which there is no clear right or wrong. Developing an understanding of the complex thought process (**moral reasoning**) involved in processing ethical situations helps nurses participate more fully in the discussions. As nurses develop skills in assessing and using good moral reasoning, they can help and support clients in that same process. Most moral reasoning happens after an ethical situation has been recognized and before one acts on the situation. People begin to think though the situation, hoping to determine the best thing to do. Whether they can identify it or not, people also use moral theory in their moral reasoning process. Familiarity with basic moral theories helps the nurse better understand the other person's position. Ethical principles guide one's moral reasoning. Principles offer "universal" norms or standards for guidance in reasoning. A brief discussion of moral reasoning, ethical theory, and ethical principles follows.

Moral Reasoning

Because ethical problems occur in situations involving people who have different approaches to moral reasoning, it is helpful if the nurse can sort through the various factors that influence a persons' thinking. The influences on reasoning that will be discussed are emotions, the law, religious faith, and culture. It is important to remember that in health care, ethics discussions are done in pluralistic settings, involving clients, families, and professional groups who have different ideas about the "good" and what ought to be done.

Emotions play an important role in ethical reasoning. Human emotions can spark awareness of ethical issues and injustices. People often feel very strongly about ethical situations, which can lead to positive or negative outcomes if agreement and resolution are sought in an ethical dilemma. People's feelings or emotions are different and change in the same person from day to day or hour to hour. For example, to decide to start unwanted treatment on a person after he or she becomes unconscious primarily because a family member feels guilt or sadness may not be the best thing to do. Of course, one would need to know more about the situation to be sure of that. Feelings should be honored, acknowledged, and used as a consideration in moral reasoning without making ethics simply a discussion about the validity and sincerity of individuals' feelings. Ethics is concerned with developing a system of shared values in a pluralistic society.

Legal considerations can also affect moral reasoning. Obviously it is important to consider the law of the land, the policies of an institution, or the guidelines of policy and procedure in one's moral thinking. Many people base their reasoning on religious commands or laws. Ethics and the law are often in harmony, but not always. Just because an act is legal does not automatically make it right or good, nor are all illegal actions necessarily morally wrong. An obvious example would be the claims of people who protest against legalized abortion on moral grounds. Sometimes, too, illegal actions can be morally justified, especially when people claim that a higher good is being protected by the action. Relying on the law as the primary consideration of moral standards is a form of **legalism.** For example, to refuse to act on the request of a terminally ill, competent client who wishes to stop treatment because practitioners are afraid of being sued could be an example of legalism. Certainly the practitioners in the situation should consider the legal implications, but that consideration should not be the only basis for ethical reasoning. To fully consider the ethics of a situation, one must account for more than the legal dimensions.

Humans grow up in groups and learn their most cherished values and moral standards from their various cultures, both large and small. People in any culture learn to accept social mores and conventions. Families, professional groups, health care systems, and nations all provide individuals with reasons for ethical action. All of the "cultures" just named establish what is considered right and wrong for the people of those cultures, many times on the basis of what has always been done. Often people do not even notice their inherited cultural standards because the influences are so ingrained and natural. Behaviors are not necessarily ethical, however, just because "everybody does it." One might question the health care cultural practice of performing "slow codes." In a "slow code" professionals with the responsibility to initiate life-prolonging resuscitation (often nurses) do so "slowly" because it is generally agreed that a vigorous attempt would in no way help the person. Nurses question the ethics of violating policy that obligates them to properly initiate cardiopulmonary resuscitation on all persons who do not have a "do not resuscitate" order written by the physician. On the other hand, they may agree that a "code" would be hopeless and unnecessarily invasive. Answering the question of whether slow codes are "right" should involve reasoning that goes beyond the claim that they are commonly done in hospital cultures.

Personally held religious or spiritual convictions, as well as many church teachings, have long guided people in their moral reasoning. Health care institutions that have specific religious affiliations set forth ethical guidelines consistent with their sets of beliefs. Practitioners in those settings should know what those standards are. In many situations, however, because religious talk and convictions are so particular to the group holding them, difficulties arise when religious views are held up as the only answer to morally complicated situations. All the listener has to say is, "I don't believe that set of teachings," and the conversation ends or leads to argument. Moral reasoning that seeks some kind of agreement or resolution tries to get to a common ground in which all people can join in the discussion of right and wrong.

The influences on the moral reasoning just discussed cannot be avoided. They should be acknowledged as important to the people holding them; at the same time, attempts are made to expand the ethical conversation to include a broader range of considerations.

Moral Theories

Ethical theory provides a framework for people to use to determine and distinguish appropriate actions (Mandle, Boyle, and O'Donohoe, 1994). Moral theory covers a complicated, expansive body of knowledge that is beyond the scope of this introduction to health care ethics. However, there are two basic moral theories that play important roles in the reasoning process. Their basic positions are illustrated by an example below. Remember that ethical theories are very complex and that one explanation is only a small part of what any one theory is about.

The first theory, frequently referred to as deontology, focuses more on the act or duty to be performed than on the outcome or consequences of the act. This kind of thinking leads one to consider the inherent rightness or wrongness of an act or duty itself. It follows, then, that if an act is wrong it should not be done and if the act is good or right, one is morally obligated to do it. In the "assisted suicide" debate persons who hold that it should never be done, regardless of the consequences, argue from a deontological theory. It is seen as an act of killing an innocent person and always wrong. It is argued that a person has a duty to one's self and others to protect and preserve human life, even in very difficult times.

Teleological theory considers primarily the consequences of an action. This kind of moral theory "invents" the good by looking at situations to determine what should be done, guided by the consequences the action will have on the involved persons. A person using teleological reasoning might argue that in certain circumstances assisting someone's death would be allowable if the outcome would be more favorable, such as in a case where a competent person asks for help because his or her death is certain and is causing unbearable suffering. It is easy to see how these two positions can oppose one another. Reasoning from a rigid position using either theory can make it difficult to advance or resolve moral discussions.

Ethical Principles

When making clinical judgments, nurses often justify their reasoning using both consequences and universal moral principles and duties. The principles discussed below form the basis of Western ethical and philosophical traditions. The most fundamental of these principles is respect for persons. Four other primary principles stem from this basic principle. They are respect for autonomy, beneficence, nonmaleficence, and justice. Three secondary principles are veracity, confidentiality, and fidelity. They are derived from the primary principles but are discussed here because they are very important in describing the moral responsibilities of professionals. These principles are defined in the preamble to the *Code for Nurses with Interpretive Statements* (ANA, 1985)

RESPECT FOR PERSONS

The principle of **respect for persons** underlies all of health care ethics and implies that humans should revere their own lives and the lives of others and accept death

 CULTURAL ASPECTS OF CARE

A Latina woman was receiving treatment for advanced cancer at a large urban medical center. Her condition deteriorated and meaningful recovery from her illness was highly unlikely. She was taken to an intensive care unit for impending respiratory failure. She was competent and indicated that she did not want any further aggressive medical therapies but believed she needed the approval of the male members of her family, two brothers, who lived in Mexico. Efforts were made to contact them, and they indicated that they would come. Because they had 2 days of travel time, she had to be placed on a regimen of ventilator therapy and blood pressure medication to prolong her life until they could arrive and decide what to do. The client's primary nurse felt moral distress because he believed the client should have been able to make the decision about her own life and death by herself. It seemed wrong that she should have to defer to the decision of her brothers.

(Thiroux, 1990). This principle holds that life is the most basic possession humans have. Without it there can be no ethical questions. Because life is so valuable, humans are morally obligated to preserve and protect it. Nurses must take all reasonable means to protect and sustain human life where there is hope of recovery or when clients can benefit from life-prolonging treatment (ANA, 1985). This principle explains why terminating treatment on a person is never taken lightly.

The principle of respect for persons prompts questions about the quality of life. Although people differ widely on quality of life evaluations, for most people being alive is more than having functioning vital organs. Respect for persons should also include the fact that humans die. To exclude that reality from ethical deliberations can lead to situations where respect for the person is violated.

Respecting persons is directly related to the principle of respect for autonomy. Because people all differ in their values and life plans, respecting them should include an appreciation of their individual differences and personal meanings.

RESPECT FOR AUTONOMY

Autonomy means that individuals should have the freedom to choose their own life plan and ways of being moral. Part of the shared human destiny includes respecting the uniqueness of each person. Because no two people or situations are exactly alike, the principle of autonomy directs nurses' moral concerns toward carefully determining the client's values.

It is important to remember that no one is ever fully autonomous. Critics claim that models of autonomy that are ruggedly individualistic have led to unrealistic health care expectations and inadequate views of the person (Childress and Fletcher, 1994). Others note that the intense interest in individual clients should be modified by expanding our attention to include families and other intimates (Nelson, 1992). Autonomy and individualism are also somewhat culturally relative. Many cultures have a more communal view of the person and find liberal, Western emphasis on the individual very limiting (see the box at left).

The principle of respect for autonomy has received such exaggerated emphasis today, in part, because of health care's traditional emphasis on the principle of beneficence. When the principle of beneficence (the duty to do good for someone) overrides the client's autonomy, the result is paternalism. **Paternalism** is doing what the health professional believes is in the client's best interests, at times regardless of the client's own determinations. Paternalistic behavior has often been justified because professionals have more knowledge and experience in the technical management of health problems. In most cases clients will readily accept the professional's medical expertise and judgment, but as the decisions become more complex, the limits of paternalism become apparent. Although professionals believe they know what is best, they are not the ones who have to live through the illness experience or live with the consequences of the choice. Most health care choices have an ethical as well as a technical component. Increasingly, clients wish to take responsibility for their health decisions and be active partners in both the technical and moral dimensions of their care. Two important methods for respecting autonomy and encouraging client and family participation in decision making are worth noting here. The first, informed consent, has long provided the moral basis for health care communications. The second, advance directives, is a more recent development. The moral basis of these two methods is discussed later in this chapter (see also Chapter 20).

NONMALEFICENCE AND BENEFICENCE

The principles of nonmaleficence and beneficence are viewed on a continuum ranging from not inflicting harm (**nonmaleficence**) to benefiting others by doing good (**beneficence**). The continuum ranges from not inflicting harm through three beneficent actions: removing harm, preventing harm, and taking positive steps to do good for the benefit of others.

Nonmaleficence provides a minimum standard to which practitioners are always held. In clinical situations, however, it is often difficult to draw the line between not inflicting harm and doing good. For example, the nurse at the well-baby clinic who immunizes children against diphtheria, whooping cough, and tetanus inflicts some degree of harm or pain. The action is beneficial, however, because it prevents the serious harm of childhood illness.

In determining the good in health care situations one must calculate the risks and benefits in each case. Few choices in health care are risk free. Benefits promote the client's welfare and health, whereas risks detract from the client's health or welfare. For example, the client with cancer must weigh all the benefits and risks of experimental cancer drugs before choosing to receive the treatments. The weighing of benefits and risks should include all relevant factors, both technical and moral.

The principle of beneficence requires the nurse to provide health benefits to clients, balance the benefits against the risk in situations in which a choice must be made, and determine the best way to assist the client. Most often the concept of weighing risks and benefits is thought of in terms of choosing medical therapies or surgery. In many settings the nurse plays an important role in reinforcing and discussing risks and benefits with the client as determined by the treatment team. The nurse's conversation may help clients identify for themselves the morally relevant benefits and risks, such as quality of life issues. In the daily care of clients nurses encounter seemingly small but very important choices that involve a risk-benefit calculation. For example, a hospital nurse may decide to defer some scheduled activity because a sleep-deprived client is finally resting comfortably. The principle of nonmaleficence requires that the nurse avoid harming clients during delivery of nursing care. For example, the nurse would not ever knowingly use a contaminated needle to draw blood from a client under the principle of nonmaleficence.

JUSTICE

The principle of **justice** requires treating others fairly and giving persons their due. When there are resources to distribute in health care, nurses can allocate them in such a way that equal shares go to all recipients (noncomparative justice) or so that those in the greatest need get what they need for survival (comparative justice).

Distributing health care in a just way is difficult. Not everyone is equal in every way. Sometimes there are situations in which it seems that one person should receive a greater or lesser share than another. Because resources are limited, each person may not be able to receive an equal share.

The distribution of nursing care is determined by the needs of clients and by nurses who establish priorities based on those needs. Certain clients require more attention and more nursing care than others. To live and avoid permanent disability, they require immediate intervention. For example, the client who is admitted to the neurological unit after suffering head trauma usually requires immediate assessment and attention to prevent brain damage associated with edema or hemorrhage. Other clients in the same unit who are in more physically stable condition are cared for on a different time line and at a different intensity level. Some clients die despite any help that the nurse can provide. The criteria of need, added with the client's prognosis, is basic to the practice of **triage**, which is used by nurses and other health care professionals when resources are in short supply or time demands are great.

Unequal treatment of clients always requires justification. For example, should a client who does everything possible to improve his health be cared for differently than a client who refuses to follow medical recommendations? The principle of justice supports the argument that there should be at least equal initial access to health care for assessment of the client's needs. This view has limitations, but it supports a more critical evaluation of distribution of scarce health care resources. Continued support to a client who repeatedly refuses health care advice may not seem to be the best way to use resources. However, the principle of justice requires the nurse to ensure fair allocation of resources to all clients.

VERACITY, CONFIDENTIALITY, AND FIDELITY

The secondary principles of ethical conduct outlined in the ANA Code of Nurses include **veracity**, the duty to tell the truth, **confidentiality**, the duty to protect privileged information, and **fidelity**, the duty to keep promises.

The principle of truth-telling (veracity) directs the practitioner to avoid directly lying to clients or deceiving them. The ethical question of giving a placebo (a medication substituted for one the client thinks he or she is getting, usually with no chemical properties) can be raised under the principle of veracity. Placebos are given with the hope that a desired outcome can be achieved, for example, decreased dependence on an addictive drug. Giving a placebo medication fools the client into accepting a non-addictive substance. Although the nurse does not lie to the person by saying "I'm giving your morphine now," the nurse's actions of silently giving saline after the client's request for a pain medication violate the principle of veracity because of the deception involved. Although arguments are made supporting the benefits of placebos in some cases, desired outcomes are rarely achieved by dishonest means. Clients need to be involved in their own care, no matter how difficult that may be.

Further, veracity does not just imply that nurses should not lie, but also requires that they are positive and forthcoming in offering information relative to the client's situation. At times this requirement can cause problems for nurses and underscores the importance of honoring the team approach to health care. For example, a young man asks the nurse for information about the drugs he would be required to take after a heart transplant. The nurse reviews the side effects of the medications and the life changes associated with chronic drug regimens and answers the client's questions honestly, offering all relevant information even though the client may choose to remove himself from the transplant list. The nurse would also discuss the benefits of the transplant. Some physicians may view a nursing action like this one as interference with the physician-client relationship. Under the principle of veracity, teaching and client advocacy in this situation should be done using a team approach. Issues that the nurse identifies should be brought forward for discussion by the client and health care team.

Confidentiality is a basic ethical principle that ensures a client's privacy. Nurses avoid discussing a client's condition with anyone not directly involved in the client's care. Conflicting obligations may arise when a client chooses to keep confidential information that places the client or others at risk. For example, a client with acquired immunodeficiency syndrome (AIDS) may choose not to tell his or her family members. If family members will be assuming care for the client, the nurse may believe that they have the right to be informed. The principle of veracity guides the nurse in encouraging clients to share information about their illness. The principle of confidentiality helps the nurse understand the serious implications of sharing privileged information against the wishes of a competent person.

The principle of fidelity (faithfulness) requires that nurses keep promises made to clients. When one is faithful and keeps promises that are made, the trust so vital to the nurse-client relationship can be formed. When clients and families cannot depend on the nurse to follow through on agreements, they are put at risk.

INFORMED CONSENT AND ADVANCE DIRECTIVES

Informed consent promotes and respects autonomy by expanding the client's knowledge of his or her options. **Advance directives** are forms of communication in which persons can give direction on how they would like to be treated when they cannot speak for themselves. Both informed consent and advance directives have become part of the legal structure of health care. Before surgery, for example, the physician is legally bound to give the client certain information (see Chapter 48).

Advance directives have legal dimensions, too. In 1990 the Patient Self Determination Act (PSDA) became law and was implemented in all health care institutions effective December 1, 1991. The law requires that all persons receiving medical care in an institution recognized by Medicare and Medicaid be given written information about their legal rights to make decisions about medical care, including the right to accept or refuse medical or surgical treatment. Although the informed consent doctrine and advance directive legislation are most often seen as legal agreements, both have deeply rooted ethical dimensions based on the moral relationships between professionals and clients.

To make autonomous decisions and actions, clients must be offered enough information and be free of internal or

GERONTOLOGICAL PRINCIPLES for Promoting Ethical Care of Older Adults

Discussing life values with clients helps them make meaningful choices in ethical situations. Many older adults have special needs—hearing deficits, cognitive or memory impairments, multiple chronic illnesses, and isolation—that may impact the communication process. The nurse should be prepared to devote the time necessary to communicate with older adults. Listening to older adult clients tell their life stories may give the nurse important moral information about client values.

- Older adult clients may not as readily accept offered medical interventions. Although refusals of treatment may be contrary to the professional's value system, care should be taken to develop a relationship of trust and support with the client to determine his or her values.
- Because of decreasing physical capabilities and cultural bias, older adults are often thought of as mentally incompetent for many decisions. The nurse should support a client's autonomy by directing choices and questions to the client, not a younger relative or caretaker.
- Many older persons have not been as influenced by ideas of client autonomy as younger generations. The nurse should understand that some older adults are uncomfortable questioning or disagreeing with medical authorities. They may view assertiveness as a violation of trust.
- Older persons living in nursing homes should have assistance in preparing advance directives. In collaboration with the client, family, and medical team the nurse can encourage discussions to determine how nursing home residents want their medical care to proceed if they become unable to speak for themselves.

external influences so that they can act. Informed consent helps clients understand their options so that they can make a decision that best reflects their own values. Clients depend on professionals to give them honest, accurate information at a level they can understand to aid them in making medical and moral health care decisions. Professionals guided by an ethic of care recognize that they are in a privileged position of partnership and trust with clients who rely on the professional's integrity, competence, and guidance. The respect for autonomy that is at the heart of informed consent is honored, whether the client agrees or disagrees with professional advice. In supporting clients with informed choice, there are individuals and groups of people to whom professionals must pay particular attention. An example of a group that may have particular needs in the area of informed consent and advance directives would be older adults (see the box above).

The informed consent process occurs when competent clients can be in dialog with their loved ones and the persons providing care. When clients are unable to participate, informed consent can be extended to them through advance directives (Fig. 19-2). Respect for autonomy requires that members of the health care team follow these directives.

Under the PSDA, clients must be provided with information about their rights to formulate advance directives such as a living will or to appoint someone to speak for them a

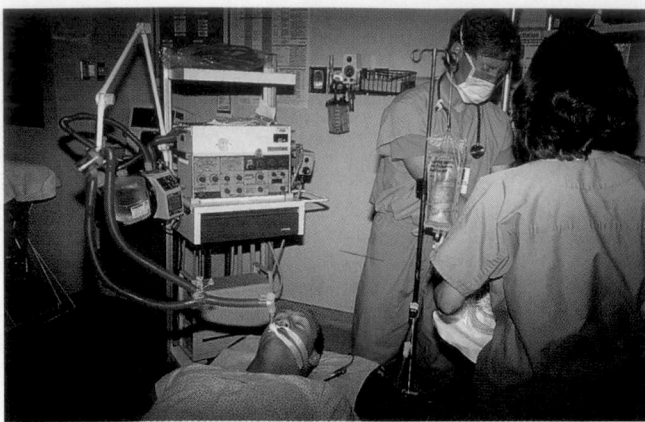

Fig. 19-2 Advance directives convey a client's choices about the level of care to be given in times of critical illness.

> ## Assessment Parameters for Ethical Deliberations
>
> ### CLIENT PREFERENCES
> - Consider client values and preferences.
> - Rely on surrogates or advance directives if client is not competent.
>
> ### FAMILY SYSTEMS
> - Evaluate the burdens and benefits of the decision on family.
> - Assess the capacity of the family to fulfill obligations.
>
> ### SOCIAL CONSIDERATIONS
> - Incorporate employment and financial considerations.
> - Evaluate emotional impact of a decision on client's social situation.
>
> ### MEDICAL DIAGNOSIS AND PROGNOSIS
> - Seek accurate, thorough, and unbiased medical data.
> - Consider health state with and without medical interventions.
>
> ### COMMUNITY SUPPORT
> - Evaluate community resources for increasing care options.
> - Determine sources of physical and emotional community support.
>
> ### STAFF INPUT
> - Validate with staff the extent of care needed.
> - Consider staff assessment of client and family coping mechanisms.
>
> ### IDEAL PICTURE
> - Work toward helping client and family identify their most important goals.
> - Devise strategies that can help achieve the ideal picture.

through a durable power of attorney for health care (Flarey, 1991). A **living will** lists the medical treatment a person chooses to omit or refuse if the person is unable to make decisions and is terminally ill. In a **durable power of attorney for health care** persons appoint a relative or trusted friend to make medical decisions on their behalf in situations when they are not able. The wishes of clients must be documented in medical records.

When a client cannot give informed consent and does not have an advance directive (e.g., an unconscious person in an emergency room) professionals assume that the injured or ill client would want treatment to preserve life. Health care providers have a social contract based on trust requiring that clients be treated and not abandoned if they cannot speak for themselves.

The nurse has an ethical obligation to assist, promote, and support client decision making, to support clients' rights to informed consent, to provide information about advance directives, and to follow the directives clients provide.

METHODOLOGY FOR ETHICAL DECISION MAKING

Ethical deliberations that involve challenging ethical problems and dilemmas can be guided by a method similar to the nursing process. A nurse can best discuss and help resolve ethical dilemmas by considering all relevant information. Each ethical situation or dilemma will be different, but the nurse in any setting can use the following guidelines for ethical processing and decision making.

1. *Presume good will.* It is essential that nurses and all involved persons enter ethical discussions presuming that everyone wants to find the "good." If discussions begin with distrust and hostility, they do not proceed very far. While people may hold very different ideas on what they think is best, that does not make them "bad" people, nor should they be excluded from the reasoning process.

2. *Identify all important persons.* Take time to consider all of the people who are involved in the moral decision-making process. This list may include professional care givers—physicians and nurses—as well as institu-

tional and societal interests. How much weight each person's values and views should be given is another matter. Obviously some people have more at stake than others, and their voices should be clearly heard. To omit the interests of any key person can lead to a decision that is regrettable.

3. *Gather the relevant information.* Relevant information includes data about the client preferences, family systems, medical diagnosis and prognosis, social considerations, and community support. One also should gather information from care givers. It is important that the goal or "ideal picture" be clearly stated, since the goal usually determines how the good should be achieved (see the box above). Data gathering is an extremely important step in the ethical reasoning process. One cannot come to good conclusions on the basis of weak or absent information. Nurses are able to gather most relevant information as they listen while clients reveal their stories and values. Moral information is often buried in stories instead of being measurable and factual.

4. *Identify important ethical principles.* Although the identification of general, universal ethical principles cannot tell nurses what to do in any situation, the principles can help reasoners explore more fully the values

inherent in the dilemma. Once the values are named, it can become easier to seek solutions that protect cherished norms and values.

5. *Propose alternative courses of action.* Many times, ethical problems seem overwhelming because the participants can see only one possible course of action. Creating reasonable options that protect important human values can be freeing to the persons involved.

6. *Take action.* Once the options are openly discussed, the participants can move toward implementing an agreed upon course of action.

No two ethical dilemmas are the same. Using a systematic model for ethical decision making increases the probability that all ethical principles and values involved are reviewed. The nurse acts after evaluating all alternative courses of action. It is also essential that the nurse does not act alone. Communication of the plan for resolving ethical dilemmas must be shared with all health care team members. A systematic approach to ethical decision making allows nurses to practice in a professional manner and to increase their ability to deal with complex, ethical situations.

■ INSTITUTIONAL ETHICS COMMITTEES

Health care workers recognize that scientific and technological advances and increased public awareness and participation in health care issues have raised ethical, legal, and social questions about clients and the care they receive. Ethical issues are rarely best resolved in a "top down" manner in which the persons involved defer to an expert or authority. "Doing" ethics in institutional settings is a community activity, involving input from clients, families, professionals, and administrators. To help facilitate ethical dialog and provide the educational and policy resources necessary to create a climate sensitive to ethical challenges, health care institutions have developed ethics committees. Ethics committees have typically served several purposes including education, policy recommendation, and case consultation or review (see the box below). The case review function of ethics committees should be accessible to any involved person.

The functions of institutional ethics committees are undergoing revision and expansion as health care systems change (Smith, 1994). For example, the shifting of health care delivery from hospital to community settings calls for innovative strategies to engage a broader range of social and ethical issues that are relevant to the clients and professionals outside acute care facilities. The JCAHO, an accreditation organization for health care institutions, has issued revised and new standards on clients rights (JCAHO, 1992). JCAHO standards have pushed forward the development of institutional ethics committees. Committees can serve as the forum for drafting meaningful policies to meet client rights standards within institutions (Heitman, 1993).

Nurses' Relationship to Ethics Committees

Historically nurses have not been fully included on ethics committees. The absence of nurses has not been intentional, but rather may stem from nursing's perceived status in health care environments and the view that decision making, even on ethical matters, is a physician function (Rushton, 1994). Nurses are, however, becoming increasingly involved in the development and function of institutional ethics committees. The composition of an ethics committee should be multidisciplinary and may include nurses from many functional roles, physicians, administrators, educators, social workers, clergy, medical or nursing students, and lay representatives. Having representation from various disciplines helps ensure that the moral interests of all relevant parties are heard. Typically there are not many positions on a committee for any one group. Nurses who care daily for clients should have a direct voice on ethics committees, since they hold valuable moral information on client and family values, health status, and coping. Direct care providers are ideally suited to assume a client advocate role (see Chapter 18). Nurses not on a committee have the responsibility to be knowledgeable about their representatives and how to access committee expertise for clinical ethical situations. Murphy (1993b) describes a model of ethics consultation that successfully uses a nurse-ethicist. Expanded roles for nurses in ethics are on the horizon.

Ethics committees should not be seen as a "quick fix" for the many ethical dilemmas nurses encounter in health care settings. Ethical situations are usually best handled by means of competent, sensitive intervention by the professionals involved. Nurses can be very effective when they assume a proactive teaching and facilitating role with clients and families. Many problems begin because people feel misled or are not aware of their options and do not know when to speak up about their concerns. Formal help from an ethics committee may certainly be sought after all other avenues of communication have been pursued. Although it is not the committee's function to solve problems for people, input from persons who have had experience in similar cases often helps bring about agreement and clarity. Ethics committees do not replace important physician/nurse-client relationships, but rather offer a valuable resource for strengthening them.

■ ETHICAL HEALTH PROMOTION

Nurses are concerned with promoting good health in all dimensions of life. Because of the concern for wellness promotion, nurses not only attend to the crisis of an acute heart attack but also undertake the task of teaching nutritional and exercise behaviors essential to heart disease prevention. So it is with ethics. As discussed in this chapter, nurses need the expertise to attend to multiple ethical

---

Primary Functions of Ethics Committees

- To offer education in ethics to diverse populations: clients, families, professionals, institutional staff, and community members
- To assist institutions in the development and review of policies related to ethical responsibilities
- To ensure that policies are implemented and understood by ever-changing groups of practitioners
- To serve as resource persons or consultants for specific client situations with ethical dimensions

dilemmas and situations of conflict in their practice. Just as important is the preventive role nurses can play in clinical ethics.

Many ethical situations that end in crisis or dilemma happen because good prevention has not been practiced (Forrow, Arnold, and Parker, 1993). For example, end of life treatment decisions are not most ideally discussed when the client is getting worse. Expert nurses are skilled in understanding predictable patterns. Nurses can use their "in-the-middle" position to identify the need for early communication. The nurse not only understands the position of the medical team but also has important information about client and family coping. Facilitating early dialog can prevent misunderstanding later in the process.

One of the best ways to prevent ethical crisis is to work at establishing relationships of trust and understanding with clients and families. Under these conditions, clients can better exercise their autonomy by feeling free to share their values and questions with their care givers. By using an ethic of care, nurses can create the climate of support and encouragement necessary for helping people make meaningful but difficult choices.

■ KEY CONCEPTS ■

▶ Technological advances, increasing public awareness of ethical issues, and enhanced professionalism have encouraged nurses to confront the ethical dimensions of practice.

▶ Professional nurses have an ethical obligation to clients, the profession, employing institutions, and society to provide high-quality care.

▶ The nurse's role in ethical situations provides a unique vantage point from "in the middle."

▶ The relationship between nurse and client is the foundation for nursing's ethic of care.

▶ An ethic of care directs the nurse's attention toward client advocacy, the context of each ethical situation, virtue, and attending to power relationships.

▶ Professional nursing codes of ethics provide guidelines for competent, ethical, client-centered nursing practice.

▶ An ethical nurse maintains skill competency and assumes responsibility for nursing care.

▶ Responsibility refers to the scope of function and duties a nurse is required to perform.

▶ A nurse is accountable when demonstrating a willingness to assume responsibility for nursing care.

▶ Emotions, religious faith, the law, and culture all influence a person's moral reasoning.

▶ Ethical principles provide a basis for common understanding of how people might determine the "good" in a complex situation.

▶ The process of informed consent helps support and ensure client autonomy in health care decisions.

▶ Advance directives provide a source of information about client values when the client is unable to express his or her wishes.

▶ An ethical dilemma results from conflicts in values, causing uncertainty in decision making.

▶ Nurses can benefit by using a systematic approach to thinking through ethical issues.

▶ The nurse considers all relevant information in an ethical dilemma before acting.

▶ The ethics committee provides an excellent resource for nurses and clients needing consultation on a morally perplexing situation.

▶ Nurses' ethical interventions should be focused on preventing acute ethical dilemmas by building appropriate professional-client relationships and by recognizing early ethical "symptoms."

■ KEY TERMS ■

Accountability, p. 322

Advance directives, p. 327

Autonomy, p. 325

Beneficence, p. 326

Confidentiality, p. 326

Durable power of attorney for health care, p. 328

Ethic of care, p. 320

Ethics, p. 320

Fidelity, p. 326

Informed consent, p. 327

Justice, p. 326

Legalism, p. 324

Living will, p. 328

Morals, p. 320

Moral reasoning, p. 323

Nonmaleficence, p. 326

Paternalism, p. 325

Respect for persons, p. 325

Responsibility, p. 322

Triage, p. 326

Veracity, p. 326

■ CRITICAL THINKING EXERCISES ■

1. A home health care nurse has become very frustrated with a client who does not follow through with recommended wound care. The wound is not healing well. Describe how professional accountability and responsibility might guide the nurse's actions.

2. You are caring for a hospitalized client who is preparing for discharge. As she is packing, resident physicians enter her room and tell her that a new pneumothorax was detected on her morning x-ray. They abruptly tell her she won't be going home and that they will be inserting a chest tube as soon as they gather the supplies. The client states her refusal and begins to cry. The physicians, concerned mostly about her need for a chest tube, silently begin to get supplies out of the cabinet in the room. Describe how an understanding of an ethic of care would guide your actions. Write down a plan for how you would proceed in this situation.

3. A client in the clinic where you work wants to prepare an advance directive. Construct a teaching plan for this client that would cover all the relevant information for this process.

4. As a nurse clinician you have worked with a chronically ill person for 3 years. The client has end-stage renal disease from diabetes, is blind, and has had bilateral amputations. He has now developed a seizure disorder and has had trouble regulating his new medications. One afternoon, as you are leaving his home after a visit, he asks you to give him advice on how to end his life. Using the method for ethical decision making, deliberate this nursing dilemma.

5. In caring for an elderly woman who is hospitalized for gastrointestinal tract bleeding and weight loss, she tells you that she does not want aggressive treatment if she has cancer. You notice that the family encourages her vigorously to cooperate with all of the tests. Discuss how you might begin some "preventive ethics" in this situation.

REFERENCES

American Nurses Association: *Code for nurses with interpretive statements*, Kansas City, Mo, 1985, The Association.

Bevis E: Caring: a life force. In Leininger M, editor: *Caring: an essential human need*, Detroit, 1988, Wayne State University.

Brown J, Kitson A, McKnight T: *Challenges in caring: explorations in nursing and ethics*, London, 1992, Chapman & Hall.

Childress J, Fletcher J: Respect for autonomy, *Hast Cent Rep* 24(3):34, 1994.

Cooper M: Principle-oriented ethics and the ethic of care: a creative tension, *ANS* 14(2):22-31, 1991.

Davis A, Aroskar M: *Ethical dilemmas and nursing practice*, Norwalk, Conn, 1991, Appleton & Lange.

Forrow L, Arnold R, Parker L: Preventive ethics: expanding the horizons of clinical ethics, *J Clin Ethics* 4(4):287, 1993.

Flarey D: Advanced directives: in search of self-determination, *JONA* 21(11):16, 1991.

Heitman E: A proactive role for the ethics committee or ethics consultant: meeting the JCAHO standards on patient rights, *Trends Healthcare Law Ethics* 8(4):11, 1993.

Joint Commission on the Accreditation of Healthcare Organizations: *Accreditation manual for hospitals*, Oakbrook Terrace, Ill: JCAHO, 1992.

Kelly B: The "real world" of hospital nursing practice as perceived by nursing undergraduates, *J Prof Nurse* 9(1):27, 1993.

Leininger M: *Caring: an essential human need*, Detroit, 1988, Wayne Sate University.

Mandel C, Boyle P, O'Donohoe J: Ethical issues relevant to health promotion. In Edelman C, Mandel C, editors: *Health promotion through the lifespan*, St Louis, 1994, Mosby.

Murphy P: Clinical ethics: must nurses be forever in the middle? *Bioethics Forum* 9(4):3, 1993a.

Murphy P: A nurse-ethicist model of ethics consultation, *Trends Healthcare Law Ethics* 8(4):23, 1993b.

Nelson J: Taking families seriously, *Hast Cent Rep* 22(4):6, 1992.

Rushton C: The voice of nurses on ethics committees, *Bioethics Forum* 10(4):30, 1994.

Smith M: The future of healthcare ethics committees, *Trends Healthcare Law Ethics* 9(2):7, 1994.

Thiroux J: *Ethics: theory and practice*, New York, 1990, Macmillan.

Watson J: *Nursing: human science and human care: a theory of nursing*, New York, 1988, National League of Nursing.

ADDITIONAL READINGS

Aroskar M: Ethical foundations in nursing for broad health care access, *Sch Inq Nurse Prac: Int J* 6(3):201, 1992.

Barta K, Neighbors M: Nurses knowledge and role in patients' end-of-life decision making, *Trends Healthcare Law Ethics* 8(4):50, 1993.

Basto P: Ethical decision making in the neonatal intensive care unit, *Bioethics Forum* 9(4):22, 1993.

Beauchamp T, Childress J: *Principles of biomedical ethics*, ed 4, New York, 1994, Oxford University.

Chally P: Moral decision making in neonatal intensive care, *JOGNN* 21(6):475, 1992.

Condon E: Nursing and the caring metaphor: gender and political influences on an ethics of care, *Nurs Outlook* 40(1):14, 1992.

Crowley M: The relevance of Noddings' ethic of care to the moral education of nurses, *J Nurse Educ* 33(2):74, 1994.

Davis A: The sources of a practice code of ethics for nurses, *J Adv Nurse* 16(11):1358, 1991.

Husted G, Husted J: *Ethical decision making in nursing*, St Louis, 1995, Mosby.

Miller B, Beck L, Adams D: Nurses' knowledge of the code for nurses, *J Cont Educ Nurs* 22(5):198, 1991.

Moin L, Strumpf N: Use of physical restraints in the hospital setting: implications for the nurse, *Geriatr Nurs* 15(3):127, 1994.

Murphy P: When "there is nothing more to do": ACT, *Trends Healthcare Law Ethics* 9(3):31, 1994.

Olsen D: Controversies in nursing ethics: a historical review, *J Adv Nurse* 17(9):1020, 1992.

Olsen D: Populations vulnerable to the ethics of caring, *J Adv Nurse* 18(11):1696, 1993.

Price D, Murphy P: Nurses are always responsible, *J Nurse Law* 1(2):63, 1993.

Raines D: Moral agency in nursing, *Nurse Forum* 29(1):5, 1994.

Salsberry P: Caring, virtue theory, and a foundation for nursing ethics, *Sch Inq Nurse Prac: Int J* 6(2):155, 1992.

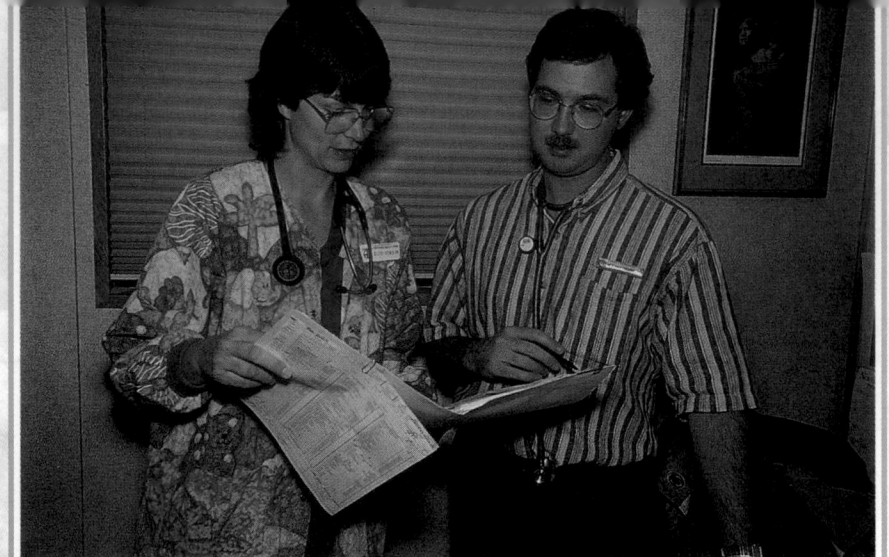

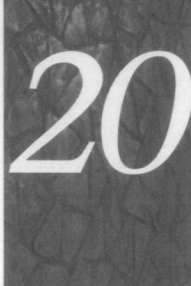

Chapter 20

Legal Issues

Objectives

Mastery of content in this chapter will enable the student to:

► Define the key terms listed.

► Explain legal concepts that apply to nurses.

► Describe the legal responsibilities and obligations of nurses.

► List sources for standards of care for nurses.

► Define legal aspects of nurse-client, nurse-physician, nurse-nurse, and nurse-employer relationships.

► Give examples of legal issues that arise in nursing practice.

Safe nursing practice includes an understanding of the legal boundaries within which nurses must function. As with all aspects of nursing today, an understanding of the implications of the law supports critical thinking on the nurse's part. Nurses must understand the law to protect themselves from liability and to protect their clients' rights. Nurses need not fear the law, but rather should view the information that will follow as the foundation for understanding what is expected by our society from professional nursing care providers. The laws in our society are fluid and constantly changing to meet the needs of the persons the laws are intended to protect. As technology has expanded the role of the nurse, the ethical dilemmas associated with client care have increased and often become legal issues as well. While federal laws apply to all of the states, nurses must also be aware that laws vary widely across the country. It is important for nurses to know the laws in their state that affect their practice.

The public is better informed than in the past about their rights to health care. Nurses' familiarity with the laws enhances their ability to be client advocates.

LEGAL LIMITS OF NURSING

Professional nurses must understand the legal limits influencing their daily practice. This coupled with good judgment and sound decision making ensures safe and appropriate nursing care.

Sources of Law

The legal guidelines that nurses must follow are derived from statutory law, regulatory law, and common law. **Statutory law** is created by elective legislative bodies such as state legislatures and the U.S. Congress. An example of state statutes are the **nurse practice acts** found in all 50 states. These statutory nurse practice acts describe and define the legal boundaries of nursing practice within each state. For example, a nurse practice act defines the responsibilities nurses have for the administration and prescription of medication. An example of a federal statute enacted by the U.S. Congress is the Americans with Disabilities Act. This legislation has become very prominent as the rights of handicapped individuals are being protected in the work place, in educational institutions, and throughout our society. Legislation enacted by the U.S. Congress sets guidelines by which all persons within the various states and jurisdictions must abide. There are few exceptions wherein private institutions choose not to accept federal funding to avoid some federal mandates. When state legislatures enact laws, they cannot conflict with federal guidelines.

Statutory law falls into two separate categories. Laws are designated as either civil or criminal statutes. **Civil laws** are concerned with relationships between individuals. These laws protect the rights of persons within our society and encourage fair and equitable treatment among people. Although violations of civil laws might cause harm to an individual or property, usually no great threat to society as a whole exists. For example, civil laws of torts include malpractice, which protects the client's right to safe and appropriate care. Society is not at risk unless the defendant health care provider (e.g., doctor or hospital) is intentionally causing harm to clients. If the intention was malicious or bad on the health care provider's part, then this action

would fall under the criminal law. Another example of civil law is **defamation**, wherein statements made about a person, for example, their competence as a nurse, that are untrue may lead to personal problems, but they do not threaten society in general. **Slander** is the term used for spoken words that defame another, while written defamation is referred to as **libel**. Penalties for civil violations usually include fines or placing the plaintiff in a position similar to that enjoyed prior to the injury. For example, if someone destroys another person's property, they will be required to replace the item or give the money it would cost to repair the damage they caused.

Criminal penalties are more severe. They include restricting peoples' activities by placing them in jail where their personal freedom is restricted. **Criminal law** is concerned with relationships between individuals and society as a whole when actions threaten the peace and safety of members in society. When a lawsuit is brought under a criminal statute, it is actually the government who steps into the position of the plaintiff to challenge the behavior of the defendant. An example of a criminal law violation is the misuse of controlled substances by nurses.

A **crime** is an offense against society that violates criminal law. There are two classifications of crimes. A **felony** is a crime of a serious nature. It carries a penalty of imprisonment for greater than 1 year or even possibly death. A **misdemeanor** is a less serious crime. The penalty is usually a fine or imprisonment for less than 1 year. There are few crimes nurses can commit if they practice within accepted standards of care, for example, institutional policy, medical protocols, and critical pathways. For the purpose of this chapter, flagrant crimes such as murder and illegally dispensing controlled substances will not be discussed. Laws relating to such offenses apply to nurses and all individuals.

Regulatory law or **administrative law** greatly affects nursing practice. State Boards of Nursing are the legal regulators of the nursing profession. For example, many state boards create rules and regulations that impose a duty upon all nurses in the state to report incompetent or unethical nursing behavior to the state board. Administrative law bodies, such as State Boards of Nursing, have power through the delegation of authority from legislatures to the experts in the various fields. The law recognizes that the practice of nursing is complicated and better understood by professionals in the field. Therefore, the legislature authorizes the State Board of Nursing to establish rules and regulations that define and explain the Nurse Practice Act. Again, each state delegates this authority differently. In some jurisdictions the State Boards of Nursing are the ultimate authority while in other jurisdictions the State Board of Nursing serves in an advisory capacity only.

Administrative laws are often overseen by specific administrative bodies. State Boards of Nursing serve as panels of "judges" when nurses violate the licensure statute or rules created by the nursing board. Administrative law judges are identified to hear cases when a problem arises related to a rule or regulation and the nurse disagrees with the state board's earlier decision. Administrative procedure allows the nurse to appeal to the state or federal court system after the nurse has given the state board or other administrative agency the opportunity to settle the dispute. Administrative procedures are intended to alleviate some of the overcrowding of the court systems in our society.

As previously stated, administrative bodies such as the State Board of Nursing are made up of the experts in the fields they oversee and it is hoped they have a greater understanding of the factors involved in the dispute. The penalties associated with administrative law actions include disciplinary actions and suspension or revocation of the nurse's professional license. Administrative actions may later lead to a civil or criminal action. If a nurse loses his or her professional license and the case involves either civil or criminal wrongs, then further legal charges may follow.

Common law is a source of law that has developed through general customs of accepted behavior in our society as discussed in previous court cases. When either a civil or a criminal case goes to court, previous case rulings are used to argue that the current court decision should be decided based on the similarities and differences of previously decided cases. How courts rule on the circumstances and facts surrounding an incident is called a *precedent*. For example, if a nurse is allowed by a court to take a client off life support systems this action would set a precedent for nurses in future cases. Case law can be overruled if a more recent decision disagrees with the earlier case law. Common law is very fluid. Cases regarding a client's right to refuse treatment, for example, are not found in every state. Therefore, other jurisdictions or states are looked to for guidance. The results of their cases can influence what happens in the nurse's own state. If a jurisdiction does not have current case decisions on a client's right to refuse treatment, nurses cannot be absolutely sure of how the court in their state will view the nurse's actions in either supporting or refusing to support the client's decision to refuse treatment. Nurses must rely upon the statutory laws in their state to give them guidance on how the court will view the nurses' actions.

Although institutional policy is not a literal source of law, when an agency writes policies and procedures for the nursing staff, these guidelines are looked upon as the internal laws of the agency. If nurses do not practice within the stated policies and procedures of their employer, their actions may be viewed as outside of or below the acceptable standard of care as identified by their employer. It is important for nurses to serve on the decision-making committees charged with updating policies and procedures. These guidelines should be reviewed annually. Policies and procedures should be written in such a way that the standard of care identified is in the best interest of the client and can realistically be met by the nursing staff. When policies and procedures are written setting a standard that does not allow staffing patterns to be met, the nurses are set up for falling below the standard of care that their institution has set. It is also important not to allow common practice and self-set standards to fall below what is acceptable and safe nursing care. Most agencies' policies and procedures are written to meet the guidelines and standards of accrediting agencies such as the Joint Commission on Accreditation of Health Care Organizations (JCAHO). Standards of care will be discussed further.

Licensure

All registered nurses are licensed by the Board of Nursing of the state in which they practice. The requirements for li-

censure vary among states, but most nursing licensing acts require minimal education requirements and a licensure examination. All states use the National Council Licensure Examinations (NCLEX) for registered nurse and licensed vocational/practical nurse examinations. Licensure permits persons to offer special skills to the public, but it also provides legal guidelines for protection of the public.

A license can be suspended or revoked by the Board of Nursing if a nurse's conduct violates provisions in the licensing statute. For example, nurses who perform illegal acts such as selling or taking controlled substances jeopardize their license status. Because a license is viewed as a property right, due process must be followed before a license can be suspended or revoked. Due process includes the timely notification of the charges brought against the nurse and the opportunity for the nurse to defend against these charges in a hearing. Hearings do not occur in courts, but are usually conducted by the State Board of Nursing. Some states provide administrative and judicial review of such cases if nurses have used all other forms of appeal.

STUDENT NURSES

Student nurses must also practice nursing in a reasonable and safe manner. If a client is harmed as a direct result of a nursing student's actions or lack of action, the liability for the incorrect action is generally shared by the student, instructor, hospital or health care facility, and university or educational institution. Student nurses should never be assigned to tasks for which they are unprepared and should be carefully supervised by instructors as they learn new procedures. Although student nurses are not considered employees of the hospital, the institution has a responsibility to monitor the acts of student nurses. Student nurses are expected to perform as professional nurses would in providing safe client care. Faculty members are usually responsible for instructing and observing students, but in some situations, staff nurses serving as preceptors may share these responsibilities. Every nursing school should provide clear definitions of preceptor and faculty responsibility. Because students are not considered employees, they are not protected by the worker's compensation laws if they are injured. It is important for student nurses to carry health and disability insurance to protect themselves financially while they are in school.

Sometimes students are employed as nursing assistants or nurses' aides when not attending classes. If student nurses are employed in this capacity, they should not perform tasks that do not appear in a job description for a nurses' aide or assistant. For example, even if a student has learned to administer intramuscular medications in class, this task may not be performed as a nurses' aide.

Supervisory liability occurs when the staff nurse overseeing the assistant or aide knowingly assigns work without regard for the person's ability to safely conduct the task defined in the job description. If you, as a student employed as a nurse's aide are requested to perform a responsibility that you are unprepared to safely complete, bring this information to your supervisor's attention and get the help you need. Continuing education should be available to enable you to perform your role as an employee safely. Nurses, including student nurses, must advocate for the client's right to safe care.

LEGAL LIABILITY IN NURSING

Torts

A **tort** is a civil wrong made against a person or property. Torts may be classified as unintentional or intentional. An example of an unintentional tort is **negligence** or **malpractice**. Malpractice is negligence committed by a professional such as a nurse or physician. Intentional torts are willful acts that violate another's rights. Examples are assault, battery, defamation, and invasion of privacy.

NEGLIGENCE AND MALPRACTICE

The New York Supreme Court discussed the difference between ordinary negligence and malpractice involving health care professionals in the case of *Borrillo v. Beekman Downtown Hospital* (1989). The distinction depends upon whether the acts or omissions involved a matter of "medical science or art requiring special skill not ordinarily possessed by lay persons," or instead can be understood by the everyday experience of lay persons on a jury. If the professional opinion of an expert with special skill and knowledge is required, the theory of malpractice applies rather than ordinary negligence.

Negligence is conduct that falls below a standard of care. Malpractice results when nursing care is below that required for safe nursing practice. No intent is needed for negligence to occur. It is established by law for the protection of others against unreasonable risk of harm. It is characterized chiefly by inadvertence, thoughtlessness, or inattention. Negligence or malpractice may involve carelessness, such as not checking an arm band resulting in administration of the wrong medication. However, carelessness is not always the cause. If nurses perform a procedure for which they have not been trained and do it carefully, but still harm the client, a claim of negligence or malpractice could be made. If nurses give care that does not meet appropriate standards, they may be held negligent. Because these actions are performed by a professional, the negligence of the nurse is termed *malpractice*.

Nurses have been involved in several common negligent acts or professional malpractice. Examples follow:

1. Intravenous therapy errors resulting in infiltration or phlebitis
2. Burns to clients from improperly monitored heat therapy
3. Falls resulting in injuries to clients
4. Failure to use aseptic technique where required
5. Errors in sponge, instrument, or needle counts in surgical cases

Nurses must perform all procedures correctly. They must also use professional judgment as they carry out physicians' orders as well as independent nursing therapies for which they have authority. Any nurse who does not meet accepted standards of practice or care or who performs duties in a careless fashion runs a risk of being found negligent.

Because malpractice is negligence related to a professional's practice, the following criteria must be established in a malpractice law suit against a nurse:

1. The nurse (defendant) owed a duty to the client (plaintiff)
2. The nurse did not carry out that duty or breached the duty of care

3. The client was injured
4. Both the actual and proximate causes of the client's injury were a result of the nurse's failure to carry out the duty

The ability to predict harm is evaluated in malpractice cases. The situation surrounding the injury is evaluated to determine if it was likely that the injury or harm to the client could have been expected from the care that was or was not provided. The cause of the injury is also investigated through the evaluation of the actual and the nearest causes of the injury. Had it not been for what the nurse did or did not do, could an injury have been prevented? The question is also asked if there were any breaks in the chain of events leading to the injury, possibly related to other persons who provided care, that could have led to the client's harm. The *Berdyck v. Shinde* case stated that the negligence of one practitioner does not relieve the negligence of another if both cooperated in causing an injury to a client and no break occurred in the chain of events and the resulting injury. To break the chain, the negligent intervention of the second nurse must be disconnected from the negligence of the first nurse and must be the independent cause of the client's injury.

A nurse's duty of care to a client is defined by the standards of care for safe nursing practice. Duty is the legal obligation on one person to act for the benefit of another person due to the relationship between them (*Berdyck v. Shinde*, 1993). The duty of care to the client can be breached through either omission or commission. Whether a duty of care exists (*Shepherd v. Mielke*, 1994) is a legal question that is answered by foreseeability and policy considerations. In the *Shepherd* case a nursing home client was sexually assaulted by a visitor to her room. The court said that the nursing home had a duty to protect the client by providing a safe environment. A jury had to determine if sexual assault was likely to happen. The resulting harm need not be expected, but must be reasonably within the general field of dangers covered by the nurse's duties to protect the client. The court in *Shepherd* identified the duty of ordinary care as the duty of taking reasonable precautions to protect those who are unable to protect themselves. The client in this case could not lock her door, screen visitors, or generally provide for her own safety. She was in the nursing care facility because she was unable to perform these tasks for herself. When a nursing home or other institution offers services to the public for a fee, it is expected that a duty to protect and safeguard the residents from foreseeable risk of harm is created. If the nurse fails to provide care, then the breach of duty is one of omission. If care is provided in a manner below the expected standard of care, then the nurse has committed negligence or professional malpractice. For example, in the case of *Jackson v. Pleasant Grove Health Care Center* (1993), staff of a nursing home was guilty of malpractice due to failure to protect a confused client from wandering off outside the home in January. The client died from exposure.

The duty of a psychotherapist to warn third parties of threats of violence communicated by a client was first recognized by the California Supreme Court in *Tarasoff v. Regents of the University of California* (1976). The court believed that because a psychotherapist stands in a special relationship with the client, the therapist has a duty to predict whether the client poses a danger to others. Secondly, the therapist must take precautions to protect the foreseeable victim from that danger. If the court could find that the nurse also shares in this "special relationship," then the duty to warn may also exist with nursing. A careful balancing of the need for privacy and confidentiality of privileged communication would need to be weighed. The nurse would be advised to talk with a supervisor before warning the third party. In predicting whether a client's threat is serious enough to justify breaching the confidentiality of the therapist-client relationship, a therapist must exercise reasonable professional judgment. A reasonable effort must be made to warn of the threat of danger to a third party (*Hutchinson v. Patel*, 1994). The duty to warn is not a diagnostic or professional judgment only, but an act based on reasonable care under the circumstances. This distinction removes worrisome threats a client may disclose to a nurse from the privileged communications protected by therapeutic relationships.

Although related to other professional duties, similar reasoning was seen in the case of *Grant v. Touro Infirmary* (1969). The court felt that the surgical nurses' failure to properly count sponges during surgery was not services of a professional nature. The court stated that in determining whether a duty exists depends upon the act being performed rather than the fact that a nurse was performing the act. Counting sponges does not require a degree in nursing.

Minimizing Liability Through Effective Documentation and Client Relationships

Nurses can reduce their chances of being named in lawsuits by following standards of care, giving competent health care, and developing an empathetic rapport with clients. In addition, careful, complete, and objective documentation serves as evidence of the standard of nursing care provided (see Chapter 12). Timely and truthful documentation is important to provide the communication necessary between the health care team members. Documentation is used in many ways that benefit the client and demonstrate that the nurse is an effective care provider. Good documentation also keeps other health care providers up to date on the most recent treatments received by the client so ongoing care can be safely provided.

A number of courts have stated that when a health care provider negligently alters or loses medical records relevant to a malpractice claim the health care provider must demonstrate why these events occurred. An institution has a duty to maintain nursing records. These duties are established by statutes and accreditation regulations. Nursing notes contain substantial evidence needed to understand the care received by a client. If records are lost or incomplete the court will presume that the care that cannot be reviewed was negligent and therefore the cause of the client's injuries. The hospital can, however, provide evidence that it was not negligent and that the injury was not the result of care (Reagan, 1994).

It is very important for documentation to be done in a timely manner. The common practice of carrying the nursing care notes in the nurse's pocket in a notebook and transferring the documentation to the chart at the end of the shift can be dangerous. Other care providers may provide care to the client without up-to-date information if this practice is followed. Harm may come to a client whose record is not accurate and up-to-date. Truthful documentation is also essential. If an error is made in the documentation, it is important to follow the policies and procedures of the institution to correct it. Obliterating or erasing errors may appear to be a coverup and lead to charges of fraud. The credibility of a nurse who goes to court will be negatively affected if it appears that the nurse's initial charting has been changed after an injury has occurred to a client.

Nurse-client relationships are very important, not only in ensuring quality care but also in minimizing legal risks. Trust develops between a nurse and client. Clients who believe that the nurses performed their duties correctly and were concerned with their welfare are less likely to initiate a lawsuit against the nurse. Sincere caring for clients is an essential role of the nurse and is an effective risk management tool. However, caring will not totally protect the nurse if malpractice occurs. When a client is injured the investigation into the incident may implicate the nurses even if the client feels kindly toward them.

Malpractice Insurance

All nurses should consider purchasing personal professional liability insurance, even if the employing institution has coverage. Personal liability insurance protects nurses in all aspects of professional practice. The employer's insurance covers nurses only while working within the scope of their employment. If a nurse does not practice according to the policies and procedures of the institution, negligence or malpractice may be determined as falling outside the scope of the employment and therefore the employer's insurance may not cover the nurse's actions.

Because nurses are professionals, it is often difficult to separate their private lives from their professional skills. Often nurses are called upon by neighbors and friends to provide nursing care on a volunteer basis. This type of professional activity is not covered by the employer's insurance policy because the care given was not the responsibility of the employer. Nurses may act as good Samaritans by providing emergency assistance at an accident scene for example. The good Samaritan laws protect persons who help others while acting reasonably without gross negligence. Because nurses have professional knowledge, the nurse would be held to a higher standard than an ordinary untrained good Samaritan. The definition of gross negligence would be defined by the individual circumstances surrounding the emergency care given and the reasonableness of the nurse's good Samaritan intervention. Gross negligence involves unreasonable recklessness on the part of the good Samaritan whether that person is a professional or a lay person.

Standards of Care

Standards of care are guidelines for nursing practice. Standards establish an expectation for nurses to provide safe and appropriate client care. If nurses do not perform duties within accepted standards of care, they may place themselves in jeopardy of legal action and, more importantly, place their clients at risk for harm and injury. In a malpractice lawsuit, these standards are used to determine whether the nurse has acted as any reasonably prudent nurse in a similar setting with the same credentials would act. If nurses are named as defendants in a malpractice lawsuit and it is shown that neither the accepted standards of care outlined by the state nurse practice act nor the policies of the employing institution were followed, the nurse's legal liability is clear. The guidelines offered by professional organizations do not hold the same weight as law, but will be used to determine whether the expected standard of care has been met.

The law defines the standards of care that nurses must provide. All state legislatures have passed nurse practice acts that define the scope of nursing practice or the framework within which nurses must practice. Nurse practice acts set educational requirements for nurses, distinguish between nursing and medical practice, and generally define nursing practice. The rules and regulations enacted by the state board of nursing or administrative law bodies help to define the practice of nursing more specifically. For example, a state board may develop a rule describing intravenous therapy practice. All nurses are responsible for knowing the provisions of the act for the state in which they work as well as the rules and regulations enacted by the state board of nursing and other regulatory administrative bodies.

Professional organizations are another source for defining standards of care. The American Nurses Association (ANA) has developed standards for nursing practice, policy statements, and similar resolutions (see Chapter 13).

Nursing specialty organizations also have standards of practice defined for certification of nurses who work in specific specialty areas such as the operating room (OR) or critical care. These standards also serve as guidelines to determine whether nurses perform their duties appropriately.

The written policies and procedures of the employing institution detail how nurses are to perform their duties. These internal standards of care are usually quite specific and are found in procedural manuals on most nursing units. For example, a procedure/policy outlining the steps that should be taken when changing a dressing or administering medication gives specific information about how nurses are to perform these tasks. These policies provide another definition of standards of care. Institutional policies and procedures must conform to laws and cannot conflict with legal guidelines that define acceptable standards of care.

The fact that your institution may require you to perform a procedure will not protect you as an individual if this practice is found to be outside the scope of nursing as defined by your state's nurse practice act. The law as written will overrule any agency policy or procedure. In a Texas case a nurse testified to merely following the agency's policy. The court ruled that the state nurse practice act was the rule of law the nurse should have been following. The fact that the nurse was relying upon what the employer recommended was not a good defense.

Standards of care concern nurses' accountability or obligations to account for their actions. General duty nurses are legally responsible for meeting the same standards as other general duty nurses in similar settings. However, specialized nurses such as nurse anesthetists, intensive care nurses, certified nurse-midwives, or operating room nurses are held to standards of care and skill exercised by those in the same specialty as defined by applicable standards. All nurses should know the standards of care they are expected to meet within their specific specialty and work setting. Ignorance of the law or of standards of care is not a defense to malpractice.

One of the first and most important cases to discuss a nurse's liability was *Darling v. Charleston Community Memorial Hospital*. This 1966 Illinois Supreme Court case has been adopted in almost every state. It involved an 18-year-old man with a fractured leg. The man's toes became swollen and discolored, and he developed decreased sensation. He complained to the nursing staff many times. Although the nurses recognized the symptoms as signs of impaired circulation, they failed to tell their supervisor that the physician did not respond to their calls or the client's needs. Gangrene developed and the man's leg had to be amputated. Although the physician was held liable for incorrectly applying the cast, the nursing staff was also liable because they had not adhered to the standards of care for monitoring and reporting the client's symptoms.

Standards of care of the reasonably prudent nurse may also be influenced by the location of the nurse's practice setting. In the past, the standard of care was determined by the locality rule, which looks at the specific geographical area where the nurse practices and the common practices in that area. As we have become a much more mobile nation with the ease of rapid transportation, a national standard of care has developed. This national standard of care also has received wider recognition due to the necessity of having an expert witness testify as to the appropriate standard of care in a nursing malpractice case. It became difficult to find local experts to testify against persons with whom they might work. Therefore the locality rule was extended to include nursing experts from locations outside of, but in practices similar to, the site where the injury occurred.

Today, an expert may be called to define and explain to the court what a reasonably prudent nurse would have been expected to do under the facts of the case from any similar setting around the country. It is recognized and understood that nursing practice differs based on the rural or urban nature of the institutional setting. Additionally, home health care, occupational health nursing, and other community-based clinical settings require that the expert be familiar with the standards of care in these settings versus the traditional hospital or institutional setting. The expert witness, often a clinical nurse specialist or educator, is called upon to explain to the jury and the court what is considered to be "beyond the ken" of the common person. The expert must be certified by the court as having the credentials, experience, and indeed an understanding of what the standard of care should have been in the case at hand. In *Thurman v. Pruitt Corp.* (1994) an RN who worked as a visiting nurse was qualified to serve as an expert witness regarding the standard of care expected for nursing home residents. The expert witness is distinguished from the fact witness. Staff nurses may testify in a court proceeding as a fact witness if they have first hand personal experience with the facts of the case. The expert witness evaluates the nurses' professional judgments and behavior under the circumstances being reviewed by the court.

Confidentiality

Nursing standards for what is confidential information are based upon professional ethics (see Chapter 19). The ideals of privacy and sensitivity to the needs and rights of clients who may not choose to have nurses intrude upon their lives, but who depend upon nurses for their care, guide the nurse's judgment. The nurse's sense of fairness and professionalism demand that confidential information not be shared with others.

In the case of *Wyatt v. St. Paul Fire and Marine Insurance Company* (1994) a client brought an action against a licensed practical nurse employed by a hospital. The LPN gave information to a third party that indicated that the client either had AIDS or was being tested for it. In the *Wyatt* case the court defined an injury involving disclosure of confidential information as any adverse consequences that result.

The American Nurses Association Code for Nurses states, "when individuals become nurses, they make a moral commitment to uphold the values and special obligations expressed in their code" (American Nurses Association, 1976). The code further states, "the client trusts the nurse to hold all information in confidence. This trust could be destroyed and the client's welfare jeopardized by injudicious disclosure of information provided in confidence" (American Nurses Association, 1985).

Confidential information gained while caring for a client may be privileged and therefore immune from disclosure under the law. In other words, if a client shares information confidentially with the nurse, the information does not have to be revealed in any legal proceeding. However, a legal privilege protecting the nurse's communication with the client may or may not exist in the jurisdiction within which the nurse is practicing. If the client believes or knows that what he tells the nurse is not protected from disclosure, it is likely that the client will be guarded in what information is shared. Nurses can be most effective by having complete and accurate information regarding clients' most intimate problems. In a 1985 Utah case, *Hoffman v. Conder*, the nurse caring for the client overheard some very confidential and sensitive information discussed between the client and his attorney. The local police sought to gain this information from the nurse. When the client's attorney objected, the decision as to whether the nurse had to disclose the information to the police was given to the courts. Initially the nurse was ordered to disclose the statement overheard between the client and the attorney. An appeal to the Utah Supreme Court resulted in an order preventing the disclosure of the confidential communication overheard by the nurse. The nurse's knowledge of confidential information was protected in this case not by virtue of the nurse-client relationship, but rather by the attorney-client privilege. Because the nurse's presence was necessary to care for the client, the information overheard between the client and the attorney was privileged, and therefore confidential.

Informed Consent

Clients sign general consent forms when they are admitted to institutions. Separate, special consent forms may need to be signed by the client or representative before specialized procedures are performed. Laws may vary in states as to what form of consent is necessary. The following factors must be verified for a consent to be valid:

1. The person must be mentally and physically competent and be legally an adult (capacity to consent).
2. The consent must be given voluntarily. No forceful measures may be used to obtain it.
3. The person giving consent must thoroughly understand the options available.
4. Persons giving consent must have the opportunity to have all questions answered satisfactorily and to confirm their understanding of the treatment to be given.

Fig. 20-1 is an example of a consent form for admission to a hospital.

Informed consent is a person's agreement to allow something to happen (e.g., surgery, blood transfusion, or invasive procedures). It is based on a full disclosure of the potential significant risks, benefits, and alternatives available to the client. Informed consent allows the client to make an informed decision based on full disclosure of the facts. A person is able to give consent if they are of legal age, competent, or if they have been legally identified as the surrogate decision maker. Parents are the legal guardians of their children and must give their consent for treatment of a child. If the parents are divorced, the parent who has legal custody of the child is the parent to approach to obtain consent for treatment. Other surrogate decision makers may have legally been delegated this authority through special powers of attorney documents or through court guardianship procedures. It is also important that informed consent is received without threat. For example, if consent for surgery is being sought, it is not appropriate to seek such consent as the client is being taken into surgery, unless an emergency situation exists.

Consent must be received from a person who can understand explanations in order for them to truly understand the decision they are making. For example, a client under the effects of a sedative will not be able to understand clearly the implications of an invasive procedure. Will there be pain? What are possible complications? Will the client's activity be limited following the procedure? If the client speaks a language different from the health care provider or is deaf, it is important to involve an interpreter. It is always important to clarify clients' understanding of the information they have been told to ensure that the consent being given is truly informed.

In order to be denied the right to give consent due to incompetence, a legal proceeding must be held to determine that the client is indeed incompetent. The court will then assign a surrogate decision maker to act on behalf of the client. It cannot be assumed that older adults are not competent and thus not able to refuse treatment. Family members must obtain the legal right to give consent on behalf of an elderly family member if they are in disagreement with the client's desires. Psychiatric clients also are not automatically considered incompetent to consent by the courts. Psychiatric clients maintain and retain the right to refuse treatment until a court has legally determined that they are incompetent to decide for themselves.

A client refusing surgery or other medical treatment must be informed about any harmful consequences. If the client continues to refuse, the rejection should be written, signed, and witnessed. Parents are usually the legal

THE CHILDREN'S MERCY HOSPITAL
Kansas City, Missouri

TERMS AND CONDITIONS OF ADMISSION

NECESSARY MEDICAL TREATMENT:
Recognizing the need for hospital care for the child whose name appears herein, consent is hereby given to The Children's Mercy Hospital for hospital services rendered under the general and specific instructions of the attending physician and treatment to be necessary for the safety, welfare and health of the child.

PROFESSIONAL CARE:
The patient is under the professional care of an attending physician who arranges for services for the care and treatment of the patient. The attending physician is usually selected by the patient's parent or guardian, but may when not designated or under emergency circumstances be otherwise selected.

RELEASE OF INFORMATION:
The Hospital is authorized to furnish information from the patient's medical record to any insurer, compensation carrier or welfare agency who may be providing financial assistance for hospital care.

PHOTOGRAPHS:
Photographs of the patient may be taken under the supervision of The Children's Mercy Hospital by members of the Staff or other persons for teaching, medical research purposes or for publicity as deemed proper by the Hospital and the taking of pictures, unless specifically denied in writing, shall not be deemed an invasion of privacy.

PERSONAL VALUABLES:
The Hospital shall not be liable for loss or damage to any personal property of the patient brought into The Children's Mercy Hospital.

PAYMENT FOR HOSPITAL CARE:
I/We do hereby assume financial responsibility for and agree to make payment in full to The Children's Mercy Hospital for all charges for services or medical supplies furnished the above patient. Payment is to be made within 30 days as bills are presented with settlement in full, or arrangements for same to be made in the Financial Counseling Department before departure of the patient.

I/We do certify that the financial information given is true, accurate and complete to the best of my/our knowledge, and further authorize The Children's Mercy Hospital to investigate any and all financial information given on this admission under their normal investigative procedures.

I/We do hereby assign and authorize payment directly to the above named Hospital and physician(s) of all hospitalization or insurance benefits and physician fee benefits and guarantee to pay any balance, with the understanding that the account is not settled or closed until after the insurance benefits are received by the Hospital and if there is a remaining balance I/we agree to pay the same. I/We are aware of the above contents.

I/We hereby certify that I/we have read all parts of this Admission Form and agree and accept all terms and conditions hereon and state that all representations made by me are true.

I am aware of the above contents.

A photocopy of the agreement shall be considered as valid and effective as the original.

SIGNED	ADDRESS	PHONE
RELATION TO PATIENT	DATE	
WITNESS	DATE	
SECOND WITNESS (TELEPHONE CONSENTS)	DATE	

Fig. 20-1 Sample consent form for admission to the hospital. *(Courtesy The Children's Mercy Hospital, Kansas City, Mo.)*

guardians of pediatric clients and therefore are the persons who must sign consent forms. Occasionally a parent or guardian refuses treatment for a child. In these cases, the court may intervene on the child's behalf. The practice of making a child a ward of the court and administering necessary treatment is relatively common in such cases. A nurse involved in such a case should inform the nursing supervisor for assistance.

The law has long recognized that individuals have the right to be free from bodily intrusion. The more intrusive and the more serious the potential outcomes of a procedure, the wiser it is to receive written informed consent. Even with written informed consent, there are still questions as to whether the client was fully informed of the potential consequences of the treatment being suggested. Many procedures that nurses perform (e.g., insertion of IVs or nasogastric tubes) do not require a formal written consent, yet clients still deserve the protection of their right to give or refuse consent to treatment. Implied consent to treatment is very often involved in nursing procedures. For example, when the nurse approaches the client with a syringe in hand and the client rolls to expose the injection site, implied consent has been given. If the client resists the injection either verbally or through actions, the nurse must not proceed with the procedure.

To force treatment upon a client could result in a charge of assault and battery. **Assault** is any willful attempt or threat to harm another, coupled with the ability to actually harm the other person. The victim believes harm will come as a result of the threat. Assault may be subtle; for example, the nurse might try to force the client into taking a drug. Consent must be given voluntarily. A more obvious example might involve a nurse's handling of an uncooperative client in the emergency room. If the exasperated nurse yells, "If you don't take off these filthy clothes, I'm going to rip them off you!" and moves towards the client, the claim of assault could be made. **Battery** is any intentional touching of another without consent. Injury is not a requirement.

More recently, cases involving the client's desire to refuse life-prolonging treatment, including food and nutrition, have recognized the continuing rights of persons to refuse treatment they do not wish to receive.

In some instances, obtaining informed consent is difficult. If the client is unconscious, for example, consent must be obtained from a person legally authorized to give consent on the client's behalf. If an injured person has been declared legally incompetent, consent must be obtained from the person's legal guardian. In emergency situations, if it is impossible to obtain consent from the client or an authorized person, the procedure required to benefit the client (or perhaps save a life) may be undertaken without liability for failure to obtain consent. In those instances, the law presumes the client would wish to be treated.

A signed consent form is required for a client to participate in a research treatment such as a new dressing. It is often difficult to describe the potential risks and benefits of treatment in research projects. If a client participates in an

---

INFORMED CONSENT FOR AMNIOCENTESIS

I. I hereby request and authorize Doctor _____ to perform a diagnostic amniocentesis (pass a needle through the abdominal wall and withdraw some of the amniotic fluid). I further request that an attempt be made to perform the following test(s) on my unborn child:

    A.   Chromosome analysis _____ (Initial)

    B.   Alpha-fetoprotein _____ (Initial)

    C.   Acetylcholinesterase _____ (Initial)
        (If indicated)

    D.   _____ _____ (Initial)

II. I consent to the performance of an ultrasound examination for the purpose of dating the pregnancy, locating the placenta and selecting a site for placement of the needle.

III. I understand that:

    A.   the procedure of amniocentesis involves a small risk to both mother and fetus and that these risks include; discomfort at the site where the needle was inserted, cramping, bloody spotting, leakage of amniotic fluid, intrauterine infection and miscarriage.

    B.   there is a possibility that growing the fetal cells may not be successful and that repeat amniocentesis would then be required.

    C.   although the likelihood of an error is considered to be extremely small, a complete and correct diagnosis of the condition of the fetus based on the test(s) performed cannot be guaranteed.

    D.   the results provided of normal chromosomes or normal biochemical status of the fetus does not eliminate the possibility that the child may have birth defects and/or mental retardation because of other disorders.

    E.   in the case of twins, the results may apply to only one of the pair.

    F.   in some Rh negative mothers Rh sensitization has occurred following amniocentesis.

IV. I have had my questions answered and understand and accept the risks and limitations of this test.

Signed: _____ (Patient)

       _____ (Spouse)

       _____ (Witness)

    Date: _____

Fig. 20-2 Sample consent form for a special procedure. *(Courtesy The Children's Mercy Hospital, Kansas City, Mo.)*

experimental treatment program or submits to the use of experimental drugs or treatments, an even more detailed and stringently regulated informed consent is used. The federal Food and Drug Administration and the institutional review board will review the information in the consent form for research involving human subjects. The client is always given the option of withdrawing from the experiment at any time.

Institutional review boards (IRBs) have been established in most institutions that conduct research involving clients. These review boards review the protocol of the intended research to determine if the client has been protected and is in fact well informed as to the potential risks of being involved in the research project.

Because nurses do not receive a medical education nor do they perform surgery or direct medical procedures, obtaining client consent for medical procedures is not appropriate. Even if the nurse was in the room when the physician provided the necessary information, the nurse does not have the medical training to know if thorough informed consent information was presented to the client. The nurse, however, can serve as a witness to the client's signature on the consent form. When the nurse is asked to witness the signing of a medical consent form, it is advisable to put beside the nurse's signature "witnessed signature only." Nurses are not prepared to know all of the medical risks, benefits, and alternatives of medical treatment. If the nurse suspects or has concern that clients do not understand the procedure for which they have signed an informed consent or a client denies understanding, the nurse is obligated to notify the physician or nursing supervisor to make sure that the client is informed before the treatment occurs. Clients' rights to self-determination give them the right to clear information with which to make decisions. Fig. 20-2 is a sample consent form for a special procedure that is similar to some consent forms for surgery. Note that possible complications are listed to make certain the client understands them. Many advanced practice nurses are now autonomously treating clients. It is therefore likely that formal written consent for nursing procedures will also be expected for the treatment received from advanced practice nurse specialists.

The health care provider giving information to receive informed consent must be culturally sensitive. There are many barriers to effective communication, including cultural, educational, and emotional barriers. The nurse must understand the way in which clients and their family members make important decisions. It is essential for nurses to understand the various cultures with which they interact. The cultural beliefs and values of the client may be very different from those of the nurse. It is important for nurses not to impose their own cultural values upon the client. Insensitivity and stereotyping of different ethnic groups is equally of concern. A conscious awareness of the different values and beliefs held by various cultures is essential for sensitive nursing care.

Physician Interactions

Nurses may share liability for errors made by physicians and other health care personnel or for inadequate care provided by the employing institution. The physician is responsible for directing medical treatment. Nurses are obligated to follow physician's orders unless they believe the orders are in error or would harm clients. Therefore all orders must be assessed, and if one is found to be erroneous or harmful, further clarification from the physician is necessary. If the physician confirms the order and the nurse still believes it is inappropriate, the supervising nurse should be informed. A nurse should not proceed to perform a physician's order if it is foreseeable that harm will come to the client. The nursing supervisor should be informed and written memoranda detailing the events in chronological order and the reasons for refusing to carry out the order should be written to protect the nurse from disciplinary action. The supervising nurse should help resolve the questionable order. A medical consult may be called in to help clarify the appropriate or inappropriateness of the order. A nurse carrying out an inaccurate or inappropriate order may be legally responsible for any harm suffered by the client.

The court in *Berdyck v. Shinde* (1993) identified that although a nurse cannot practice medicine, a nurse employed by a hospital to which a client is admitted by an attending physician is under a duty to keep the attending physician informed of the client's condition. This permits the physician to make a proper diagnosis and devise a plan of treatment. In order to inform a physician properly, nurses must perform a competent nursing assessment of the client to determine the signs and symptoms that are significant in relation to the attending physician's tasks of diagnosis and treatment. Nurses were held by this court to be persons of superior knowledge and skill who must employ that degree of care and skill that an ordinary practitioner utilizing diligence would employ in like circumstances. The standard of care utilized in this case was for nurse practitioners (*Albain v. Flower Hospital*, 1990).

The physician should write all orders, and the nurse must make sure that they are transcribed correctly. Verbal orders are not recommended because they increase the possibilities for error. If a verbal order is necessary (e.g., during an emergency), it should be written and signed by the physician as soon as possible, usually within 24 hours. The nurse should be familiar with the institution's policy and procedures on verbal orders.

A difficult area regarding physician orders involves an order of "no code" or "do not resuscitate" (DNR) for a terminally ill client. Many physicians are reluctant to write such orders because they fear legal repercussions for "abandoning" a client. A "no code" order should be written, not given verbally. The physician should regularly review DNR orders in case the client's condition warrants a change. Partial code or "slow code" verbal instructions have been suggested as a way for a physician to avoid writing a "no code" order. However, "slow codes" may be defined differently by various institutions and may be interpreted as not performing resuscitative procedures as a competent person would. If resuscitative procedures are performed more slowly than recommended by the American Heart Association, they may be interpreted as below the standard of care and therefore be the basis for a lawsuit.

Clients often request medical advice over the telephone. Telephone diagnosis can be risky as the client may not know to describe significant symptoms. Nurses should be cautious in diagnosing or giving advice over the telephone.

Telephone triage should be avoided. Again, the nurse must be familiar with institutional policies and avoid the risks related to miscommunication.

Short Staffing

During nursing shortages or staff downsizing periods, the issue of inadequate staffing may arise. The Joint Commission on Accreditation of Health Care Organizations (JCAHO) requires institutions to have guidelines for determining the number (staffing ratios) of nurses required to give care to a specific number of clients. Legal problems may arise if there are not enough nurses to provide competent care. If assigned to care for more clients than is reasonable, nurses should bring this information to the attention of the nursing supervisor. If nurses are required to accept assignments, they should make written protest to nursing administrators. Although these protests may not relieve nurses of responsibility if a client suffers an injury because of inattention, it would show that they were attempting to act reasonably. Whenever a written protest is made, nurses should keep a copy of this document in their own personal file. Most administrators recognize that knowledge of a potential problem shifts some of the responsibility to the institution. Nurses should not walk out when staffing is inadequate because charges of abandonment could be made. A nurse who refuses to accept an assignment may be considered insubordinate, and clients will not benefit from having even less staff available. It is important to know the institution's policies and procedures on how to handle such reports before the situation arises. If a policy or a procedure does not exist, nurses need to become involved in the policy-making committee that would be responsible for such a guideline.

Floating

Nurses are sometimes required to "float" from the area in which they normally practice to other nursing units. In one case, a nurse in obstetrics was assigned to an emergency room. A client entered the emergency room and complained of chest pain. The client was given an increased dosage of lidocaine by the obstetrical nurse and died after suffering irreversible brain damage and cardiac arrest. The nurse lost the malpractice lawsuit. Nurses who float should inform the supervisor of any lack of experience in caring for the type of clients on the nursing unit. They should also request and be given orientation to the unit. A supervisor can be held liable if a staff nurse is given an assignment he or she cannot safely care for. In the case of *Winkelman v. Beloit Memorial Hospital* (1992) the court remarked that if an employer wishes to rotate nurses to areas outside of their usual area of expertise, the employer should provide the training and education to prepare nurses to work in an area outside of their normal assignment.

Contracts and Employment Agreements

Many nurses are hired without a formal written contract. A contract is a written or oral agreement between two people in which goods or services are exchanged. An oral contract is as legally binding as a written one but may be more difficult to prove. A breach of contract occurs if either party fails to carry out agreed obligations. Even though nurses' employment agreements generally are not in the form of a written contract, employee handbooks and manuals that describe the nurse's responsibilities may be interpreted as the written form of the agreement between the hiring institution and the nurse. Without a written contract, it becomes difficult to prove the terms of the agreement between the employer and the employee nurse, but the court will look to any evidence of what was reasonably agreed upon between the nurse and the employer. Nurses should become aware of the state law related to firing for cause or no cause dismissal in the state in which they work. There are also states that are referred to as "right to work" states. Union activities affecting nursing labor relations differ in these states. It is important for nurses to understand the employment laws in the state where they work.

By accepting a job, a nurse enters into an agreement with an employer. The nurse will perform professional duties competently, adhering to the policies and procedures of the institution. In return, the employer not only pays for the nursing services but also furnishes facilities and equipment in proper working order to enable the nurse to provide efficient and competent care. If nurses sign a contract without reading the agreement, they will be held to the terms of this agreement. Not reading a legally binding contract before signing is no excuse. Institutional policies, procedures, and employee handbooks may be interpreted as the written terms of a nurse's employment contract.

Nurses also enter into contractual arrangements with clients. Nurses agree to give competent care, and clients agree to pay for the services. When clients sign admission forms upon entering a health care agency or agree to nursing care in any health care setting, they initiate the contract. Many private duty nurses have specific written contracts with their clients. It is from such contracts that the client and the nurse identify the specific expectations of both parties.

It is difficult to promise definite outcomes to clients. It is, therefore, unwise to make promises that could be interpreted as a contract. It is possible that a nurse may be sued for breach of contract if a client's condition worsens after the nurse has "promised" the client this would not happen. For example, if the nurse promises the client that pain medication will be given to keep the client comfortable and the physician discontinues the medication order, the nurse cannot keep the promise to the client. If clients do not believe they received the results they were promised a breach of contract suit may result.

■ LEGAL ISSUES IN NURSING PRACTICE

Legal issues in nursing practice reflect changing trends in the lifestyles of people in our society. The following topics are examples of recent developments in the law.

Surrogate Pregnancy Contracts and Adoption

Several states have statutes that prevent enforcement of surrogate parenting agreements. In such agreements couples agree to pay the pregnancy and birth expenses to a woman who is artificially impregnated and gives birth to the couple's baby. Other states have "baby selling" statutes that prohibit the exchange of money for adoption and thus make most surrogacy contracts unenforceable. Legal and public policy considerations determine whether or not surrogacy statutes are enforceable. All states have statutes regulating adoption and prohibit a mother from giving final consent to the adoption of her child prior to birth or prior to the passage of a waiting period after birth. Thus most states' adoption statutes would find surrogacy agreements unenforceable.

Abortion Issues

Abortion is one of this country's more hotly debated issues. Nursing finds itself in the middle. A nurse may work with a client seeking an abortion or one who has had an abortion. Nurses must understand the legal rights of women relative to abortion.

In *Roe v. Wade* (1973), the United States Supreme Court upheld the fundamental right to privacy, including a woman's decision to have an abortion. The *Roe* court concluded that the woman, in consultation with her doctor, is free to end a pregnancy without any state regulations throughout the first trimester, during which the risk of maternal mortality from abortion is less than with normal childbirth. By the second trimester, however, the state has an interest in protecting maternal health. At that time the state may enforce regulations regarding the qualifications of the person performing the abortion, and the features of the abortion facility. The state's interest in protecting potential human life becomes compelling at the point of infant viability, roughly at the beginning of the third trimester (*Roe v. Wade*, 1973). During the third trimester the state prohibits abortion, except when necessary to protect maternal health. In a 1986 case, *Thorneburg v. American College of Obstetrics and Gynecology* (1986), a number of procedural requirements regarding informed consent such as provisions for printed material, detailed reporting, procedures for determining fetal viability, and the presence of a second physician were found to unconstitutionally chill the right to abortion or deter women from seeking an abortion. A spousal consent requirement was invalidated in *Planned Parenthood of Missouri v. Danforth* (1976). The court also struck a requirement that an unmarried woman under 18 get parental consent before receiving an abortion. Requirements that parental notice be given prior to their child having an abortion, however, have been upheld in other cases such as *H.L. v. Mathison*, 1981). Parental consent requirements are illegal and unconstitutional only if they "unduly burden" the right to an abortion or make it too difficult to receive an abortion.

The laws relating to a woman's right to have an abortion have continued to be challenged and limited. The *Webster v. Reproductive Health Services* case in 1989 substantially narrowed the *Roe v. Wade* trimester system. Missouri may require physicians to conduct viability tests prior to conducting abortions if there is reason to believe that the fetus is over 28 weeks' gestational age. The Department of Health and Human Services regulations interpreted the Hyde Amendment and refused federal funding to family planning projects that provide abortion counseling or referrals. In January of 1993 this "gag rule" was overruled by President Clinton's Executive Order.

The case of *Planned Parenthood of Southeastern Pennsylvania v. Casey* (1992) upheld the requirements of informed consent in that the physician must present the woman a description of the nature of the abortion procedure, the health risk related to abortion and childbirth, the probable gestational age of the fetus, the availability of state-published material about medical assistance for childbirth, adoption agencies, and child support from the father. The court decision also upheld a mandatory 24-hour waiting period between when the materials are provided to the client and the abortion. *Casey* upheld the requirement that an emancipated minor get informed consent of one parent or guardian or a judicial determination that the minor woman is mature and has given her informed consent.

Controlled Substances

Another legal issue that might arise for nurses involves the use of controlled substances. In 1970 the Comprehensive Drug Abuse Prevention and Control Act was passed in the United States. It covers substances such as narcotics, depressants, stimulants, and hallucinogens. The Act regulates hospital distribution systems, rehabilitation programs for drug abuse, and research into the medical treatment of addiction. Nurses may administer controlled substances only under the directions of a licensed physician or advanced practice nurse who has prescriptive authority. Many states do not allow advanced practice nurses to prescribe controlled substances.

Controlled substances should be kept securely locked, and only authorized personnel should have access to them (see Chapter 35). Precise records must be maintained regarding the dispensing and storage of controlled substances. There are criminal penalties for misuse of controlled substances. There have been cases in which physicians illegally prescribe and dispense controlled substances, and if nurses employed by such physicians fail to report these activities they are legally accountable for aiding and abetting the physician. Advanced practice nurses are gaining prescriptive authority to varying degrees in the United States. The same precautions relate to any health provider who is prescribing controlled substances.

Acquired Immunodeficiency Syndrome (AIDS)

The care of AIDS and HIV-positive clients has legal implications for nurses. In 1983 the Centers for Disease Control and Prevention (CDC) issued national guidelines regarding blood and body fluid precautions. In 1985 the CDC recognized standard precautions as a necessary protection for both clients and health care personnel. In 1995, the health care workers must protect themselves through following standard precaution procedures with all clients (see Chapter 34). The administrative agency for occupational safety and health (OSHA) has also issued regulations mandating the use of standard precautions.

Health care workers are at risk of being exposed to AIDS. In New York a nurse brought a case against the state because the guards who were assigned to a prisoner the nurse was treating did not help control the client despite the nurse's repeated requests. The nurse received a needle stick and the court awarded her $5.4 million in damages (Letters, 1992). Of the small percentage of documented cases of health care providers who have acquired the HIV virus as a result of their occupation, one third of those persons are nurses. However, only 4.7% of the documented AIDS cases reported to the CDC are known to be health care workers.

Only laboratory workers have contracted AIDS from their jobs in higher numbers than nurses. The majority of health care workers infected on the job receive puncture or cut injuries (Legislative Network for Nurses, 1994).

By 1991 the CDC recommended that health care workers who perform exposure and invasive procedures voluntarily submit to testing. The CDC now urges infected practitioners to receive written permission from clients as well as clearance from a panel of experts prior to performing invasive procedures that pose a danger of exposing a client to their blood. It is important that nurses not only protect their clients through standard precautions, but also protect themselves. The American Nurses Association is opposed to mandatory testing of nurses. It has supported policies to encourage the safety of both the client and the nurse.

The Americans with Disabilities Act (ADA) discusses the rights of disabled people and is the most extensive law on how employers must treat HIV-infected clients and health care workers. The 1987 Supreme Court case of *School Board of Nassau County Florida v. Arline* established that persons with infectious diseases are protected under the handicapped and disabilities laws. In 1990 the ADA codified the *Arline* ruling, stating that an infected person cannot be discriminated against based on the fear of contagiousness. Co-workers who refuse to work with HIV-positive people can leave companies open to indirect charges of discrimination if the employer does not monitor the work environment.

The ADA requires "reasonable accommodation" for disabled employees, including those persons with HIV or AIDS. Reasonable accommodations include altering work schedules or the physical environment itself as well as transferring an employee to a position where the risk of exposure is eliminated. Even if persons are asymptomatic they have the same rights and protections afforded under the ADA. Employees must disclose their needs for special accommodation, but if employers should have known of an obvious disability and discriminate against the employee, they will still be liable for discrimination.

The CDC guidelines for invasive procedures supported a nurse in a Department of Health and Human Services case wherein it was ruled that ICU nurses do not practice "exposure prone" procedures under the CDC definition. Therefore an HIV-positive ICU nurse who was reassigned to a nurse liaison position was inappropriately transferred from a role as an ICU nurse (Headline News, 1992). Nurses must be careful not to discriminate against clients or other health care workers who are HIV infected. Institutional policies and procedures should stress the federal guidelines to discourage discrimination.

Issues of disclosure, privacy, and confidentiality are an important concern when working with HIV- or AIDS-infected clients or peers. The ADA addresses the privacy and confidentiality necessary. Whether health care workers are required to disclose information about their own HIV status to clients is being dealt with mainly on a state-by-state basis. The ADA regulations, however, protect the privacy of infected persons by giving individuals the opportunity to decide whether to disclose their disability. In the 1991 case of *New York Society of Surgeons v. Axelrod*, the court rejected the idea that AIDS be classified as a sexually transmitted disease in order to allow physicians to have this information without consent from the client. This case upheld the privacy protections for AIDS patients. Several cases (*Faya v. Almarza*, 1993; *Kerins v. Hartley*, 1993) have held that health care providers may be obligated to disclose the fact that they are HIV positive. Both of these cases involved a physician/client relationship. A third case, *Carroll v. Sisters of St. Francis Health Services* (1992), allowed damages for a client's visitor who obtained a needle stick, based on the reasonableness of his fear of contracting AIDS.

Most states require the reporting of contagious diseases, including AIDS, to the national Centers for Disease Control and Prevention. Many states also require reporting to the local department of health. If disclosure is allowed to anyone but these reporting agencies, the state regulations generally require that such persons must have a "need to know," for example, spouses, medical or emergency personnel, or other persons who are at risk of acquiring the disease.

In all of the privacy, confidentiality, and disclosure cases, there is a balancing between the rights of the HIV/AIDS-infected persons and those of the public or health care workers. Both civil and criminal liability can result if private information is disclosed without authorization. Nurses must understand the reporting laws in the state in which they practice. Courts can order disclosure of AIDS clients' records in situations that may not be addressed by a statute even without the client's consent. Whenever information is requested on a client by any third parties, including insurance companies or employers, nurses must obtain a signed release by the client prior to releasing confidential information. Every health care worker who comes in contact with a client does not have a need to know of the client's HIV/AIDS status. Confidential information must be protected.

The courts have upheld the employer's right to fire a nurse who refused to care for an AIDS client. The nurse, a home health care nurse in her first trimester of pregnancy, feared that she would contract opportunistic infections from an AIDS client. Her employer had a policy that provided no exceptions for refusing client care assignments. The court did not agree that the nurse had been discriminated against based on gender due to her pregnancy. Nurses who refuse to care for HIV-infected clients may be reprimanded or fired for insubordination.

In summary, nurses must be concerned with balancing the rights of protecting themselves with protecting the client's rights. Both are afforded protection against discrimination and protection of privacy by federal and state laws. Most legal cases involving nurses and AIDS currently relate to the protections needed for nurses as employees. Strict compliance with the standard precautions is the nurse's wisest strategy.

Death and Dying

Many legal issues surround the event of death, including a basic definition of the actual point at which a person is considered dead. The law identifies that death occurs when there is greatly diminished brain function, despite function of other body organs. One reason for the development of this definition is to facilitate recovery of organs for transplantation. Even though the client may be legally "brain dead" the client's organs may be healthy for donation to other clients. This definition is also used when there is question whether to continue life support. Nurses must be aware of legal definitions of death because they must document all events that occur when the client is in their care. Nurses may be assigned the responsibility of discussing the possibility of organ donation with a dying client's family.

Ethical and legal questions are raised by the issue of **euthanasia**. Active euthanasia involves an intentional action to promote the death of a client, for example, administering a lethal dose of morphine. Assisted suicide has been widely debated in recent years. In the 1994 *People v. Kevorkian* case the Michigan Supreme Court dealt with four assisted suicide cases in one opinion. This case challenged the newly enacted Michigan assisted suicide statute and the court found that the statute does not violate the Michigan or U.S. Constitutions. This case had nothing to do with the merits of assisted suicide or nursing procedure. The court described assisted suicide as involving active misconduct or intentionally and artificially curtailing life. Suicide involves an affirmative act to end life, whereas refusing medical treatment simply permits life to run its course. The majority of states treat assisted suicide as a crime separate from murder, with less severe penalties.

The less well defined area of passive euthanasia involves the lack of action that ultimately results in the death of the client. For example, by withholding food and nutrition at the request of a client, the nurse is potentially participating in passive euthanasia. However, the doctrine of informed consent ensures the client the right to refuse treatment. Withholding of food and nutrition has been upheld in court cases that support the client's right to refuse treatment.

When clients will not allow health care providers to attempt to save their lives, the nurse's focus must be upon the goal of caring versus curing. Laws that exist to protect the client's right to give informed consent are further supported by cases that allow a client to die a premature death due to illness or injury. The 1976 case involving Karen Ann Quinlan recognized that means that sustain life artificially may be considered extraordinary. The court allowed the comatose client to be disconnected from the ventilator. Where death is inevitable, the courts have generally honored the client's refusal of treatment. In the 1978 case of *Satz v. Perlmutter*, a 73-year-old man with a terminal disease was also granted the right to have his respirator removed. The court found that since the client would have the right to refuse treatment as a competent adult, he also had the right to discontinue treatment. The court concluded that by allowing the client to have the respirator removed, it was not condoning suicide. The client was not inducing his own condition but just wished to live on his own power.

Withholding of nutrition and fluids has been authorized for a nonterminal comatose client, (*Brophy v. New England Sinai Hospital*, 1986) and the right of a nonterminal competent client to refuse force feeding was upheld in the *Bouvia v. Superior Court* case in 1986. A nursing home client was also granted the right to stop feedings and to be allowed to die in the 1986 New Jersey case of *In Re Requena*. In the *Cruzan v. Missouri Dept. of Health* (1990) case, the U.S. Supreme Court recognized the right of Missouri to require "clear and convincing evidence" of the client's prior wishes. Artificial feeding was recognized as medical treatment that could be withheld; however, other jurisdictions retain the right to set conditions for withdrawing or withholding life-sustaining treatment.

In other situations involving death, nurses have specific legal duties. For example, nurses have the legal obligation to treat the deceased person's remains with dignity (see Chapter 26). Wrongful handling of a deceased person's remains could cause emotional harm to the survivors. In one case, for example, survivors sued when a mislabeling of bodies led to an Orthodox Jew's body being prepared for a Roman Catholic funeral and a Roman Catholic's body being prepared for Jewish burial.

Autopsy consent must be given by the decedent before death or by a close family member after death. Laws in many states give an order of priority for family members who may give consent for an autopsy. For an adult male, for example, his wife, then his adult children, and then other family members may give consent. Sometimes an autopsy consent has exclusions (such as no studies involving the brain). As with any consent, the physician should not use coercion to obtain consent. Autopsies are required in circumstances such as death resulting from an accident or suspected abuse or other criminal activity.

Living Wills and Health Care Surrogates

In light of the attention being given to the rights of the terminally ill and people in a persistently vegetative (permanently comatose) state, the nurse may find that many clients have living wills, special medical directives, or medical powers of attorney identifying health care surrogates. The Patient's Self-determination Act requires health care institutions to inquire whether an advanced directive such as a living will has been created. If the client does not have such a document, the nurse may be asked to provide information about these documents. The nurse should be familiar with the institution's policies complying with the Act.

Living wills are documents instructing physicians to withhold or withdraw life-sustaining procedures when death is imminent. These procedures are considered as prolonging the dying process rather than promoting life. Each state providing for living wills has its own requirements for executing them. Generally, two witnesses, neither of whom can be a relative or doctor, are needed when the client signs the document.

Medical special directives also must be legally prepared with the appropriate witnessing of the client's signature. They give directions to health care providers on the client's desires in specific critical situations. Health care surrogate statutes are sometimes also referred to as *durable powers of attorney*. Clients execute these documents to appoint someone to make health care decisions if and when they are no longer able to make decisions on their own behalf.

Organ Donations

Legally competent persons are free to donate their bodies or organs for medical use. Consent forms are available for this purpose. In many states adults may sign the back of their driver's license indicating consent. State laws define if a nurse may serve as a witness when individuals wish to give consent for the donation of organs or the body. The nurse must be aware of the policies and procedures of the institution and the laws in the state when they are asked to serve as a witness for a person who wishes to give consent for a donation.

In most states Required Request laws stipulate that at the

time of a person's death the qualified health care giver must ask family members to consider organ or tissue donation. In the past, this option has not been regularly offered to the family. Required Request laws came about because of the shortage of suitable organs for transplantation. The Uniform Anatomical Gift Act addresses many problems of organ donation. The physician who certifies death shall not be involved in the removal or transplantation of organs (see Chapter 26).

The National Organ Transplant Act of 1984 prohibits the purchase or sale of organs. Public Law 99-509, Sec. 93-18 established written protocols for identification of potential organ donors. This law increases the awareness of the options to donate or decline donation. The Social Security Act requires hospitals to implement this policy in order to receive Medicare or Medicaid reimbursement (Transplantation Proceedings, 1990).

▌ NURSING ROLES RELATED TO LEGAL PRACTICE

Nurses work in various sites outside of institutionalized nursing settings. Included in community settings are occupational or industrial work sites wherein nurses provide preventative and ongoing primary care to workers; public or community health, where preventative services such as immunizations and well child care are provided in schools, homes and clinics; and home health care, which provides follow-through services following a person's hospitalization. Clients may also be cared for in long-term care facilities. Nurses are professionals who are accountable for the autonomous judgments they make while working in a community setting. The community health nurse must work collaboratively with other health care team members to verify that the care provided and information shared is timely and accurate.

It is important that nurses, especially those employed in community health settings, understand the public health laws. State legislatures enact statutes under the Health Code, which describes the reporting laws for communicable diseases, school immunizations, and laws intended to promote health and reduce health risks in communities. The Centers for Disease Control and Prevention (CDC) and the Occupational Health and Safety Act (OHSA) also provide guidelines on a national level for safe and healthy communities and work environments. The purposes of public health laws are protection of the public's health; advocating for the rights of people, regulating health care and health care financing, and to ensure professional accountability for the care provided. Community health nurses have the legal responsibility to enforce the laws enacted to protect the public health. These laws may include reporting suspected abuse and neglect, reporting communicable diseases, ensuring that required immunizations have been received by clients in the community, and reporting of other health-related issues enacted to protect the public's health.

The Social Security Act, and the Omnibus Budget Reconciliation Act indicate standards of care for nursing facilities. The standards require an initial and periodic comprehensive assessment of each nursing home resident's functional capacity as well as a comprehensive care plan for each resident. The plan must include medical, nursing, and psychosocial needs stated in measurable objectives with a timetable to meet those needs. In the case of *In the Matter of Involuntary Discharge or Transfer of J.S.* (1994), a client who was a nursing home resident refused treatment and was involuntarily discharged. The court held that the nursing care facility had not demonstrated that the presence of the resident who refused treatment for a mental condition endangered other residents, and thus they had no grounds for the involuntary discharge of the resident.

The Nurse as An Advocate

Nurses serve as client advocates by protecting the rights of clients to be informed and to participate in the decisions regarding the care they will receive. The nurse may also become an advocate when a health risk is identified for which there is no legal guidance. The nurse may become actively involved as a lobbyist through the legislative and administrative processes. Nurses serve as client advocates when they become involved to improve health care. A lobbyist is a person who informs decision makers and educates them regarding the needs of clients and the safe practice of nursing. Nurses must serve as experts in educating lawmakers and policy makers on the needs of clients and the community.

The Nurse as A Risk Manager

The nurse is also a risk manager. Through minimizing the risk in providing care for clients, the nurse reduces the possibility that clients will be financially and emotionally devastated through being injured by inappropriate care. The nurse also assists the employer in avoiding lawsuits through risk management efforts that ensure a safe environment for clients. **Risk management** is a system of ensuring appropriate nursing care. Steps involved in risk management include identifying possible risks (e.g., those that predispose clients to falls), analyzing them, acting to reduce them, and evaluating steps taken.

Incident reports are tools used by risk managers. When a client is harmed or placed in danger by incorrect care, such as a drug error, an incident report is completed by the nurse. The report is completed in an objective and thorough manner, stating only the facts involved (see Chapter 12). These reports are analysed by the risk manager to de-

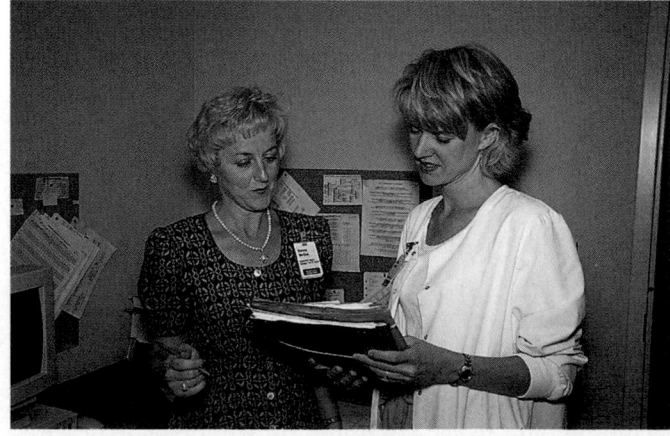

Fig. 20-3 Nurses discussing an incident report.

termine how future problems can be avoided. For example, if incident reports show that drug errors commonly involve a new IV pump, the risk manager will look to see if staff have been properly trained on use of the pump. In-service education may be all that is necessary to reduce future errors. Nurses are advised to check the status of the protection of incident reports (see Fig. 12-7) in the state in which they are practicing as these risk management tools reveal potentially damaging information if used as evidence in a lawsuit (Fig. 20-3).

The underlying rationale for quality assurance in risk management programs is the highest possible quality of care. Some insurance companies, medical and nursing organizations, and the JCAHO require the use of quality assurance and risk management procedures. Quality care is the responsibility of both the employer and the individual provider.

Risk management also entails good documentation. The nurse's documentation can be the nurse's memory of what actually was done for a client and can serve as proof that the nurse acted reasonably and safely. Documentation should be thorough, accurate, and performed in a timely manner (see Chapter 12). These communications to other members of the health care team regarding the client's status and care must be made in a timely manner so that the client's further care will be based on accurate information. When a lawsuit is being evaluated, the nurse's notes are very often the first record to be reviewed by the plaintiff's counsel. If the nurse's credibility becomes questionable as a result of these documents, the risk of greater liability exists for the nurse. The nurse's notes are a risk management and quality assurance tool not only for the employer but also for the individual nurse.

Professional Involvement

Nurses must be involved in their professional organizations and on committees that define the standards of care for nursing practice. If current laws, rules and regulations, or policies under which nurses must practice do not reflect reality, nurses must become involved in lobbying to see that the scope of nursing practice is accurately defined. Nurses must be willing to represent nursing and the client's perspective on community boards as well. The viewpoint of nurses becomes more powerful and nurses become more effective as a profession when organized and cohesive.

■ KEY CONCEPTS ■

► With increased emphasis on client rights, nurses in practice today must understand their legal obligations and responsibilities to clients.

► The civil law system is concerned with the protection of a person's private rights, and the criminal law system deals with the rights of individuals and society as defined by legislative statutes.

► Under the law, practicing nurses must follow standards of care, which originate in nurse practice acts, the guidelines of professional organizations, and the written policies and procedures of employing institutions.

► Registered nurses and licensed practical nurses are licensed by the state in which they practice; licensing is based on educational requirements, the passing of an examination, and other criteria.

► Student nurses are expected to perform as professional nurses, should be assigned only to tasks for which they are prepared, and should be carefully supervised.

► Nurses are responsible for performing all procedures correctly and exercising professional judgment as they carry out physician orders.

► All clients are entitled to confidential health care and freedom from unauthorized release of information.

► Nurses should act and speak carefully to avoid frightening, coercing, or physically intimidating clients (assault).

► Informed consent allows physical procedures to be carried out in a lawful manner, without fear of battery.

► A nurse can be found liable for malpractice if the following criteria are established: the nurse (defendant) owed a duty to the client (plaintiff), the nurse did not carry out that duty, the client was injured, and the nurse's failure to carry out the duty caused the client's injury.

► Nurses are responsible for confirming that informed consent has been given for any surgery or other medical procedure before the procedure is performed.

► Legal issues involving death include documenting all events surrounding the death, treating a deceased person with dignity, and obtaining consent for an autopsy from the decedent (before death) or a close family member (after death).

► Nurses are client advocates and ensure quality of care through risk management and lobbying for safe nursing practice standards.

► A competent adult can legally give consent to donate specific organs, and nurses may serve as witnesses to this decision.

► Nurses are obligated to follow physicians' orders unless they believe the orders are in error or could be detrimental to clients.

► Staffing standards determine the ratio of nurses to clients, and if the nurse is required to care for more clients than is reasonable, a formal protest should be made to the nursing administration.

► Nurses must file incident reports in all situations when someone could or did get hurt.

► Depending on state laws, nurses are required to report

possible criminal activities such as child abuse, and certain communicable diseases.

► All nurses should know the laws that apply to their area of practice.

■ KEY TERMS ■

Administrative law, p. 333

Assault, p. 339

Battery, p. 340

Civil law, p. 333

Common law, p. 334

Crime, p. 333

Criminal law, p. 333

Defamation, p. 333

Euthanasia, p. 345

Felony, p. 333

Incident report, p. 346

Informed consent, p. 338

Libel, p. 333

Living wills, p. 345

Malpractice, p. 335

Misdemeanor, p. 333

Negligence, p. 335

Nurse practice acts, p. 333

Regulatory law, p. 333

Risk management, p. 346

Slander, p. 333

Standards of care, p. 336

Statutory law, p. 333

Tort, p. 335

■ CRITICAL THINKING EXERCISES ■

1. Nurse Smith was en route to the hospital to begin his shift. On the way, he was flagged down by his next-door neighbor. The woman stated that she left her 2-year-old son in the bathtub while she ran down the street to get a carton of cigarettes. When she returned from the store, he was floating face down in the tub. She pulled him out, but he did not begin breathing. She asked Nurse Smith to help her. Nurse Smith told her to call the ambulance, and he began CPR, when he realized he did not carry private malpractice insurance. He continued CPR until the ambulance arrived. The ambulance transported the child to the nearest emergency department, where he was pronounced dead on arrival. The child's mother sued Nurse Smith for malpractice after child welfare workers cited her for neglect, due to Nurse Smith's "hotline" call to the State Department of Children and Family Services.

   a. Was Nurse Smith obligated to stop and render assistance?

   b. Did Nurse Smith have a legal obligation to report the woman to the State Department of Children and Family Services? What was that legal obligation?

   c. Does Nurse Smith have any legal protection from the lawsuit, since he carried no private malpractice insurance? Explain.

2. Mrs. Lee has leukemia and has been hospitalized for acute and extreme anemia. She is married and has two young daughters. The physician has ordered blood transfusions to assist Mrs. Lee over her crisis. Unfortunately, Mrs. Lee's religion prohibits her from receiving blood transfusions. The husband has stated that, although he does not share her religion, he will concur with her wishes. Without the transfusion, Mrs. Lee will die. The physician has told you that he will declare a medical emergency and order you to initiate the transfusions as soon as Mrs. Lee slips into a coma from lack of oxygen. He has told you that if you do not comply, he will report you to the nursing supervisor and make sure that you are fired.

   a. What risks do you face if you administer the transfusion?

   b. What should you do?

   c. Would your answer change if this woman was admitted in a coma and there was no information regarding her wishes concerning blood transfusions?

3. Mr. Andrews is an 80-year-old man admitted for gallbladder surgery. He is recuperating. On the day that the physician allows him to walk down the hall with assistance, he asks you to help him do so. Mr. Andrews has on antiembolism hose, and he has slippers in the closet in his room. You get Mr. Andrews out of bed and assist him in walking down the hall, which has newly-buffed linoleum floor. You forget to put on his slippers, although you know about them. While walking down the hall, you turn to look at a very good-looking resident who has just begun to make rounds for the morning. As you are looking around, Mr. Andrew's foot slips out from under him and he falls to the floor, breaking his hip. Identify the elements of negligence and use this scenario to apply those elements.

REFERENCES

   Albain v Flower Hospital, 553 N.E. 2d 1038, 1990.

   American Nurses Association: *Code for nurses*, Kansas City, 1976, The Association.

   American Nurses Association: *Code for nurses with interpretive statements*, Kansas City, 1985, The Association.

   Americans with Disabilities Act, 42 U.S.C. s 12101 (1990) et. seq. Public Law No. 101-336, 140 Stat. 327.

   Berdyck v Shinde, 613 N.E. 2d 1014, 1993.

   Borrillo v Beekman Downtown Hospital, 537 N.Y.S. 2d 219, 1989.

   Bouvia v Superior Court, 225 Cal. Rptr. 297, 1986.

   Brophy v New England Sinai Hospital, 497 N.E. 2d 626, 1986.

   Carroll v Sisters of St. Francis Health Services, W.L. 276 717, Tenn. App. Ct, 1992.

   Civil Rights Act, 42 U.S.C. s 1975 (1994) et. seq. Public Law No. 103-419 P.L. (Oct. 25, 1994)

   Cruzan v Missouri Dept. of Health, 497 U.S. 261, 269, 1990.

   Darling v Charleston Community Memorial Hospital, 33 Ill2d 326, 1966.

   Faya v Almarza, 620 A.2d 327, 1993.

   Grant v Touro Infirmary, 223 So.2d 148, 1969.

   Headline News: An HIV infected pharmacist, *Am J Nurs* 92(7):9, 1992.

   H.L. v Mathison, 450 U.S. 398, 1981.

   Hoffman v Conder, 712 P.2nd 216, 1985.

   Hutchinson v Patel, 637 So. 2d 415, 1994.

   In the Matter of Involuntary Discharge or Transfer of J.S., 512 N.W. 2d 604, 1994.

   In Re Joseph G., 667 P. 2d 176, 1983.

   In Re Requena, 517 A.2d 869, 1986.

   Jackson v Pleasant Grove Health Care Center, 980 S. 2d 692, 1993.

Kerins v Hartley, 93 Daily Journal D.A. 9850, July 30, 1993.

Legislative Network for Nurses, Silver Spring, Md, Feb. 9, 1994, Business Publishers Inc.

Letters: New York shouldn't contest a court's decision, *RN Magazine* 92(11):8, 1992.

National Organ Transplant Act, Public Law 98-507, Oct 19, 1984.

New York Society of Surgeons v Axelrod, 569 N.Y.S. 2d 922, 1991.

People v Kevorkian, W.L. 700448, Mich. 12, 13, 1994.

Planned Parenthood of Missouri v Danforth, 428 U.S. 52, 1976.

Planned Parenthood of Southeastern Pennsylvania v Casey, 112 S.Ct. 2791, 1992.

Reagan Report on Nursing Law 35 R.R.N.L. 7 Dec. 1994

Roe v Wade, 410 U.S. 113, 1973.

Satz v Perlmutter, 362 So.2d 160, 163, 1978.

School Board of Nassau County Florida v Arline, 480 U.S. 273, 1987.

Shepherd v Mielke, 887 P. 2d 220, 1994.

State v Sexton, 869 P 2d 301, 1994.

Tarasoff v Regents, of the University of California, 551 P. 2d 334, 1976.

Thor v Superior, 21 Cal. Rptr. 2d 3576, 1993.

Thorneburg v American College of Obstetrics and Gynecology, 476 U.S. 747, 1986.

Thurman v Pruitt Corp., 442 S.E. 2d 849, 1994.

Transplantation Proceedings, 22(3):902, 1990.

Webster v Reproductive Health Services, 492 U.S. 490, 1989.

Winkelman v Beloit Memorial Hospital, 483 N.W. 2nd 211, WI. 1992.

Wyatt v St. Paul Fire and Marine Insurance Company, 868 S.W. 2d 505, 1994.

ADDITIONAL READINGS

Aiken TD: *Legal, ethical and political issues in nursing*, Philadelphia, 1994, Davis.

American Hospital Association: *Required request legislation: a guide for hospitals in organ and tissue donation*, Chicago, 1988, The Association.

The basis for the right of committed patients to refuse psychotropic medication, *J Health Hosp Law* 22(6):176, 1989.

Bernzweig EP: *The nurse's liability for malpractice*, ed 4, St Louis, 1990, Mosby.

Cushing M: The right to fire v. public interest, *Am J Nurs* 92(12):18, 1992.

Davis AJ, Aroskar MA: *Ethical dilemmas and nursing practice*, ed 3, Norwalk, Conn, 1991, Appleton & Lange.

Flaskerud JH, Ungvarski PJ: *HIV/AIDS a guide to nursing care*, ed 3, Philadelphia, 1995, Saunders.

Scott DJ: Withholding consent for medical care of a child: the ultimate parental decision, *J Health Hosp Law* 23:3, 1990.

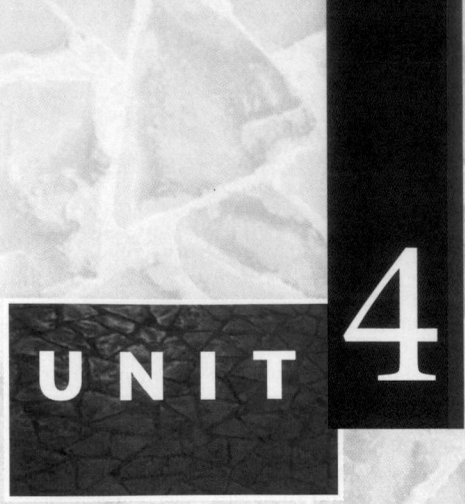

UNIT 4

Basic Psychosocial Needs

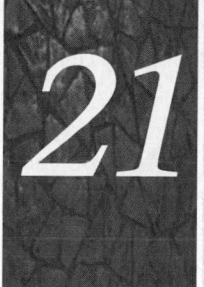

## Chapter 21

Cultural Diversity

Objectives

Mastery of content in this chapter will enable the student to:

▶ Define the key terms listed.

▶ Explain the need for a nurse's self-evaluation when providing care to clients from other sociocultural backgrounds.

▶ Describe heritage-consistent and heritage-inconsistent attributes.

▶ Describe the relationship of sociocultural background to health and illness beliefs and practices.

▶ Describe cultural phenomena—environmental control, biological variations, social organization, communication, space, and time—that apply to culturally sensitive nursing practice.

▶ Compare concepts of traditional and modern health and illness beliefs and practices.

▶ List general health and illness beliefs and practices of Asian, black or African origin, Native, Hispanic origin, and white Americans.

▶ Perform a cultural assessment using the heritage-consistency assessment tool.

▶ Discuss several ways in which planning and implementation of nursing interventions can be adapted to a client's ethnicity.

Nurses often come from different ethnic, cultural, and religious backgrounds than their clients. It is imperative that nurses understand that clients have differing world views and interpretations about health and illness, based on sociocultural and religious beliefs. When awareness of and sensitivity to clients' unique health and illness beliefs and practices are conveyed by the nurse, good rapport is established. This rapport promotes the delivery of safe and culturally effective nursing care.

A broad range of health and illness beliefs exists in the United States. Many of these beliefs have roots in the cultural, ethnic, religious, and/or social background of a person, family, or community. When anticipating or experiencing an illness or crisis, a person may use a **modern** or **traditional** approach to prevention and healing, or both approaches may be used. The following questions must be asked with respect to the nurse's and client's cultural backgrounds.

1. Who is the nurse from a cultural perspective? *Who is the client from a cultural perspective?*
2. What is the nurse's heritage? *What is the client's heritage?*
3. What are the health traditions of the nurse's heritage? *What are the health traditions of the client's heritage?*
4. What cultural phenomena interact with the nurse's health care needs? *What cultural phenomena interact with the client's health care needs?*

The answers to these questions will help the nurse successfully provide care for a client of a different cultural or ethnic background. It will also allow effective transcultural rapport and communication. **Transcultural rapport and communication** occurs when each person attempts to understand the other's point of view from that person's cultural frame of reference. Effective transcultural communication is facilitated by identification of areas of commonalities. After reaching a cultural understanding, the nurse must consider the client's cultural factors throughout the nursing process. In the last decade, major nursing organizations have emphasized the importance of considering cultural factors when delivering nursing care. The subspecialty of **transcultural nursing** represents an effort by nurses from all cultural backgrounds and clinical areas to come together and define concepts that enable them to develop the knowledge and skills needed to provide culturally sensitive care.

■ IMMIGRATION AND DEMOGRAPHY

The population of the United States consists largely of the descendants of immigrants. The only truly Native Americans are the American Indians, Aleuts, and Eskimos because they settled here thousands of years before the Europeans, Asians, and Africans. People came from every nation of the world and they continue to immigrate. The passage of Public Law 99-603, The Immigration Reform and Control Act of 1986, made it possible for several million people to become legal aliens in this country if they have lived here since 1982 and have proof of employment. Many communities now face a critical situation in the delivery of health care services to new immigrants.

The **demographics** of the United States population are changing. The European majority has been shrinking (Fig. 21-1); the black or African origin, Hispanic origin, Asian, and American Indian, Eskimo, or Aleut populations are growing. If current immigration and birth trends continue, it is predicted that by the year 2000 the Hispanic origin population will increase by 21%, the Asian by 22%, black or African origin by 12%, and European by 2% from current levels (Henry, 1990). It is also predicted that by the year 2065 the "average" American resident will be of black or African origin, Asian, Hispanic origin, Arabian, or Pacific Islands descent—not European (Fuller, 1989). Social upheavals in the world, in South America, Cuba, Haiti, the former Yugoslavia, the former Soviet Union; and famines and civil wars in African nations, have caused people to seek refuge in the United States. For example, in 1992, 810,635 immigrants arrived in the United States, representing the second largest flow of immigrants in 70 years. The largest numbers were from Mexico (91,332), Vietnam (77,728), the Philippines (59,179), the Republics of the former Soviet Union (43,590), and the Dominican Republic (40,840). The Immigration and Naturalization Service is expecting between 800,000 and 900,000 immigrants each year under the immigration laws that were passed in 1990. Legal immigrants are now seeking citizenship in record numbers, given the welfare reform measures of 1995 (Verhovek, 1995).

The terms *black or African origin; Asian or Pacific Islander; European; American Indian, Eskimo, or Aleut;* and *Hispanic origin* will be used to address the major cultural groups because they indicate each group's region or country of origin, and these are the categories selected by the United States Bureau of the Census (US Bureau of Census, 1992).

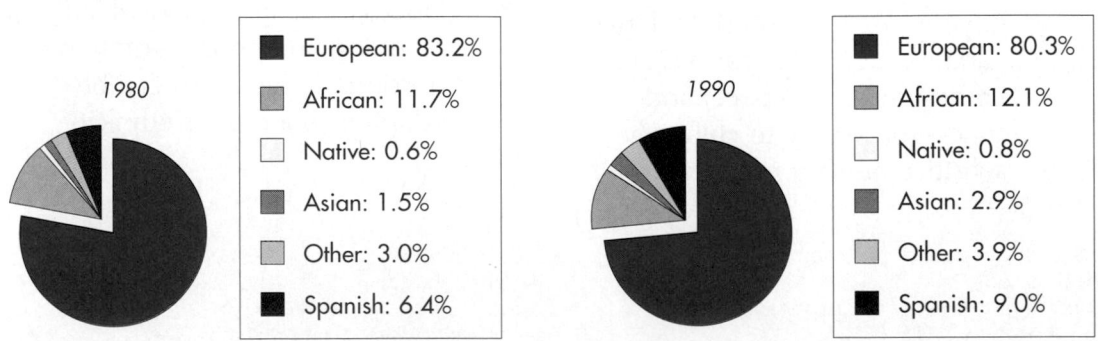

Fig. 21-1 United States population comparison: 1980-1990 census. *(From New York Times, March 11, 1991, p 1.)*

The social explosion in the United States in the mid-1960s resulted in a surge of group consciousness. Blacks, Asian, European, Native, and Hispanic origin Americans asserted their cultural group identities. The rebirth of ethnic identity eroded both the **melting pot** myth and the belief that an American culture would decrease group awareness (Giordano and Giordano, 1977).

Each immigrant group has its own cultural attitudes, beliefs, and practices about health and illness. Health and illness can be interpreted in terms of personal experience and expectations. There are countless ways to explain health and illness, and people base their responses on cultural, religious, and ethnic backgrounds. The responses are culture specific, based on clients' experiences and perceptions.

As the twenty-first century approaches, nurses are affected by enormous demographic, social, and cultural changes, which play a profound role in both the observed health care beliefs and practices and the use of health care services by a given individual, family, or community. The complexity of delivering culturally competent and congruent care has been dramatically increased by attempts to reform both the health care and welfare systems. Nurses must assess, evaluate, and care for people from all cultural backgrounds, including those who are recent immigrants. The provision of nursing care can be challenging when the nurse is from one ethnocultural background and the client is from another. The nurse who is not familiar with the client's cultural background and frame of reference may incorrectly assess and evaluate the client's health care needs.

■ HERITAGE CONSISTENCY

One way of analyzing belief systems is through the melting-pot theory, in which people assume the characteristics of the dominant culture (acculturation) via schools, television, radio, and motion pictures. Another theory is **heritage consistency**, which looks at **acculturation** on a continuum (Table 21-1). Using this theory, the degree to which people identify with dominant and traditional cultures is assessed. It is possible to assess health beliefs by determining people's ties to traditional beliefs and their stage of acculturation. A relationship exists between strong personal identities and heritage or level of acculturation and health beliefs.

Heritage consistency was originally developed by Estes and Zitzow (1980) to assess and counsel alcoholic American Indian, Eskimo, or Aleuts within a cultural context. It describes the degree to which lifestyle reflects tribal culture. The theory has been expanded in an attempt to study the degree to which lifestyle reflects the traditional culture, whether it is black or African origin, Asian, European, Native, or Hispanic origin.

Culture

Culture represents nonphysical traits, such as values, beliefs, attitudes, and customs shared by a group of people and passed from one generation to the next. There is not a single definition of culture. All too often definitions tend to omit salient aspects or to be too general to have any real meaning. There are, however, countless ideas as to the

Table 21-1	Heritage Continuum	
HERITAGE CONSISTENCY FACTORS	**HERITAGE INCONSISTENCY FACTORS**
Childhood development occurred in the individual's country of origin or in a U.S. neighborhood of like ethnic group.	Childhood development did not occur in the individual's country of origin or in an immigrant neighborhood of like ethnic group.
Extended family members encouraged participation in traditional religious or cultural activities.	Extended family members did not encourage participation in traditional religious or cultural activities.
Individual engaged in frequent visits to the country of origin or to the "old neighborhood" in the United States.	Individual does not engage in visits to the country of origin or the "old neighborhood" in the United States.
Family homes are within the ethnic community.	Family home was not in the ethnic community.
Individual participates in ethnic cultural events such as religious festivals, "national holidays," singing, dancing, and costumes.	Individual does not participate in ethnic cultural events.
Individual was raised in an extended family setting.	Individual was not raised in an extended family setting.
Individual maintains regular contact with the extended family.	Individual does not maintain contact with the extended family.
Individual's name has not been Americanized.	Individual's name has been Americanized.
Individual was educated in a parochial (nonpublic) school with a religious or ethnic philosophy similar to personal background.	Individual was educated in public schools.
Individual engages primarily in social activities with others of the same ethnic background.	Individual does not engage primarily in social activities with others of the same ethnic background.
Individual has knowledge about the ethnic culture and language.	Individual does not have knowledge about ethnic culture and language.
Individual possesses elements of personal pride about the national and ethnic origin.	Individual does not possess elements of personal pride about the national and ethnic origin.
Individual incorporates elements of historical beliefs and practices into personal philosphies.	Individual does not incorporate elements of historical beliefs and practices into personal philosophies.

Modified from Spector RE: *Cultural diversity in health and illness*, ed 3, Norwalk, Conn, 1991, Appleton & Lange.

meaning of this term. Culture is also the sum of beliefs, practices, habits, likes, dislikes, norms, customs, and rituals learned from the family during the years of socialization. Many persons' beliefs, thoughts, and actions, both conscious and unconscious, are determined by cultural background (Spector, 1991). Lastly, culture is a "metacommunication system" wherein not only spoken words have meaning, but everything else as well (Matsumoto, 1988). One example of this is the manner in which one person reacts nonverbally to another person's conversation, the way he or she may make eye contact, hold the body, and hold the hands.

Ethnicity

Ethnicity is a sense of identification associated with a cultural group's common social and cultural heritage. Ethnicity is complex, elusive, and not always clearly defined. A person is born into an ethnic group but may also adopt characteristics of another ethnic group. The characteristics of an ethnic group include common language and dialect, migratory status, race, and religious faith and practices. People share traditions, values, symbols, literature, folklore, music, and food preferences. Settlement and employment patterns and special political interests are often similar. People from the same ethnic group often have a sense of uniqueness. These characteristics extend from family to neighborhood to communities. There are at least 106 different ethnic groups in North America and more than 170 American Indian tribes (Thernstrom, 1980).

Religion

Religion is a belief in a divine or superhuman power (or powers) to be obeyed and worshipped as the creator and ruler of the universe (Abramson, 1980). Ethical values and religious beliefs and practices serve to further clarify ethnicity. Religious teachings help formulate a philosophy and system of practices through a system of beliefs, practices, and social controls having specific values, norms, and ethics that vary between religious groups. Some religious practices are health related. For example, some religions teach that adherence to a code or mandate is conducive to harmony and health and that breaking it may cause disharmony or illness (Thernstrom, 1980).

The degree of heritage consistency is evaluated by determining the importance of culture, ethnicity, and religion to a person, although it is difficult to isolate the specific aspects of culture, ethnicity, and religion that shape a person's world view. Fig. 21-2 illustrates the way that culture, ethnicity, and religion relate to the socialization of a person. When religion is discussed, culture and ethnicity must also be included.

The client comes from a distinct heritage involving eth-

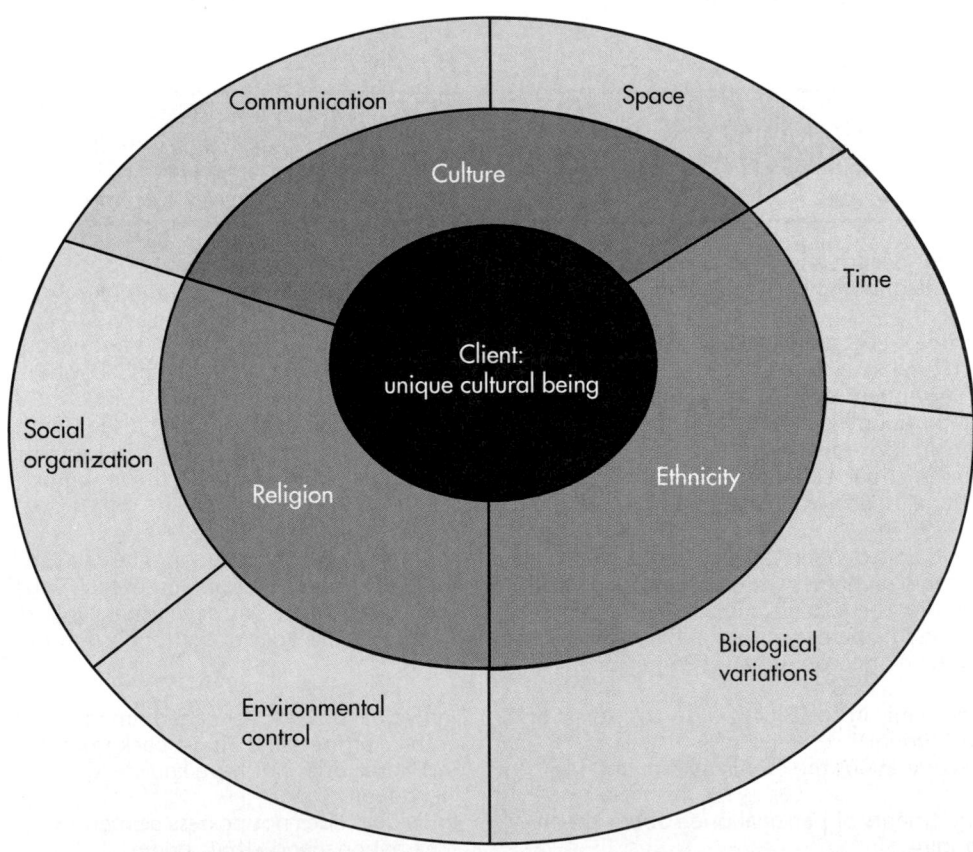

Fig. 21-2 Model of the client within a culturally unique heritage and the cultural phenomena that have an impact on nursing care. *(From Spector RE:* Cultural diversity in health and illness, *ed 3, Norwalk, Conn, 1991, Appleton & Lange; and Giger JN, Davidhizar RE:* Trans-cultural nursing assessment and intervention, *ed 2, St Louis, 1995, Mosby.)*

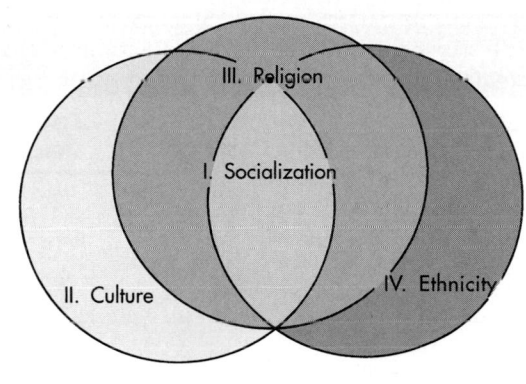

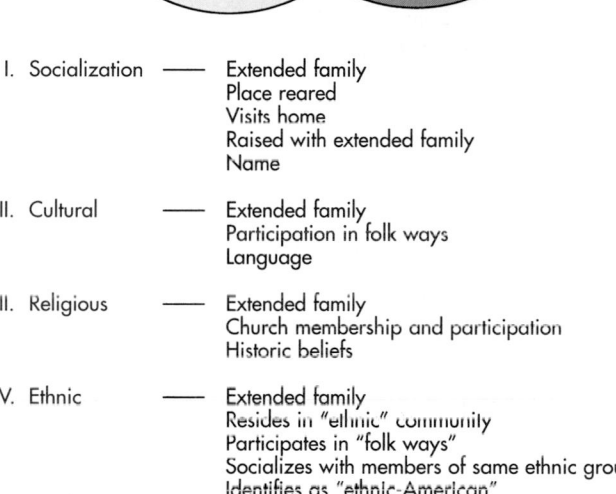

I. Socialization —— Extended family
                    Place reared
                    Visits home
                    Raised with extended family
                    Name

II. Cultural —— Extended family
                Participation in folk ways
                Language

III. Religious —— Extended family
                  Church membership and participation
                  Historic beliefs

IV. Ethnic —— Extended family
              Resides in "ethnic" community
              Participates in "folk ways"
              Socializes with members of same ethnic group
              Identifies as "ethnic-American"

Fig. 21-3 Model of heritage consistency. *(From Spector RE:* Cultural diversity in health and illness, *ed 3, Norwalk, Conn, 1991, Appleton & Lange.)*

nic, cultural, and religious background. Heritage consistency is ever-changing. It is not designed to **stereotype** or diagnose. Rather, it is a way of understanding whether a person interprets a health or illness event in a modern or traditional way. The factors constituting heritage consistency are presented in Fig. 21-3.

■ CULTURAL PHENOMENA

In addition to heritage consistency, there are six cultural phenomena that Giger and Davidhizar (1995) have identified as varying between cultural groups. These are environmental control, biological variations, social organization, communication, space, and time. Fig. 21-2 illustrates how ethnicity, religion, and culture are affected by cultural phenomena, thus further defining heritage consistency.

Environmental Control

Environmental control refers to the ability of members of a particular cultural group to plan activities that control nature or direct environmental factors (Giger and Davidhizar, 1995). Included are the complex systems of traditional health and illness beliefs, the practice of folk medicine, and the use of traditional healers. This particular cultural phenomenon plays an extremely important role in the way clients respond to health-related experiences, including the ways in which they define health and illness and seek and use health and nursing care resources and social supports. Table 21-2 presents a summary of data related to environ-

mental control and other cultural phenomena that affect nursing care.

Biological Variations

There are several ways in which people from one cultural group differ biologically (i.e., physically and genetically) from members of other cultural groups. The following are a few of the significant examples to consider:

1. Body build and structure. There are specific bone and structural differences between groups, such as the smaller stature of Asians.
2. Skin color. There are variations in tone, texture, healing abilities, and hair follicles.
3. Enzymatic and genetic variations. These variations include the way a client may respond to drug and dietary therapies.
4. Susceptibility to disease. Many diseases have higher morbidity rates within certain groups. These include tuberculosis, which is higher in American Indians; diabetes mellitus, which is higher in Hispanic origin and American Indians; and hypertension, which is higher in black or African origin Americans. Other illnesses are listed in Table 21-2.
5. Nutritional variations. There are many examples of nutritional preferences, ranging from the hot and cold preferences found among Hispanic origin Americans, the *yin* and *yang* preferences found among Asian Americans, and the rules of the kosher diet found among Jewish and Islamic Americans. A common nutritional disorder is that of lactose intolerance, found among Mexican, black or African origin, Asian, and Eastern European Jewish Americans (Giger and Davidhizar, 1995).

The high incidence of AIDS in the black or African origin and Hispanic origin communities is an emerging public health concern. As of August 1994, there were a total of 349,971 AIDS cases reported in the United States; 32% of these cases were among black or African origin Americans, who compose 12.1% of the population. About 17% of the AIDS cases were among Hispanic origin Americans, who are 9% of the population (Massachusetts Department of Public Health, 1994). There is an overall disproportionate number of AIDS cases in these two communities.

Social Organization

The social environment in which people grow up and live plays an essential role in their cultural development and identification. Children learn responses to life events from the family and its ethnoreligious group (see Table 21-2). This **socialization** process is an inherent part of heritage—cultural, religious, and ethnic background. *Social organization* refers to the family unit (nuclear, single-parent, or extended family) and the social group organizations (religious or ethnic) with which clients and families may identify.

SOCIAL BARRIERS TO HEALTH CARE

Several social barriers, such as unemployment, underemployment, homelessness, lack of health insurance, and poverty prevent people from entering the health care system. Poverty is by far the most critical factor. *Poverty* is a relative term and changes from time and place. In the United States, poverty is pervasive and found extensively among

Table 21-2	Cross-Cultural Examples of Cultural Phenomena Affecting Nursing Care					
NATIONS OF ORIGIN	**ENVIRONMENTAL CONTROL**	**BIOLOGICAL VARIATIONS***	**SOCIAL ORGANIZATION**	**COMMUNICATION**	**SPACE**	**TIME ORIENTATION**
ASIA China Hawaii Philippines Korea Japan Southeast Asia (Laos, Cambodia, Vietnam)	Traditional health and illness beliefs Use of traditional medicines Traditional practitioners: Chinese doctors and herbalists	Liver cancer Stomach cancer Coccidioidomycosis Hypertension Lactose intolerance	Family: hierarchial structure, loyalty Devotion to tradition Many religions, including Taoism, Shintoism, Buddhism, Islam, and Christianity Community social organizations	National language preference Dialects, written characters Use of silence Nonverbal and contextual cuing	Noncontact people	Present
AFRICA West Coast (as slaves) Many African countries West Indian Islands Dominican Republic Haiti Jamaica	Traditional health and illness beliefs Folk medicine tradition Traditional healer: root-worker	Sickle cell disease Hypertension Cancer of the esophagus Stomach cancer Coccidioidomycosis Lactose intolerance	Family: many female, single parent Large, extended family networks Strong church affiliation within community Community social organizations	National languages Dialect: Pidgen, Creole, Spanish, and French	Close personal space	Present over future
EUROPE Germany England Italy Ireland Other European countries	Primary reliance on modern health care system Traditional health and illness beliefs Some remaining folk medicine tradition	Breast cancer Heart disease Diabetes mellitus Thalassemia	Nuclear families Extended families Judeo-Christian religions Community social organizations	National languages Many learn English immediately	Noncontact people Aloof Distant Southern countries: closer contact and touch	Future over present
NATIVE AMERICAN 170 Native American tribes Aleuts Eskimos	Traditional health and illness beliefs Folk medicine tradition Traditional healer: medicine man	Accidents Heart disease Cirrhosis of the liver Diabetes mellitus	Extremely family oriented Biological and extended families Children taught to respect traditions Community social organizations	Tribal languages Use of silence and body language	Space very important and has no boundaries	Present
HISPANIC COUNTRIES Spain Cuba Mexico Central and South America	Traditional health and illness beliefs Folk medicine tradition Traditional healers: Curandero, Espiritista, Partera, Senora	Diabetes mellitus Parasites Coccidioidomycosis Lactose intolerance	Nuclear family Extended families Compadrazzo: godparents Community social organizations	Spanish or Portuguese primary language	Tactile relationships Touch Handshakes Embracing Value physical presence	Present

Modified from Giger JN, Davidhizar RE: *Transcultural nursing assessment and intervention*, ed 2, St Louis, 1995, Mosby.
*Indicates a high morbidity incidence.

people in certain geographical areas (e.g., Appalachia, other rural areas, and urban areas) and certain groups (e.g., black or African origin, Hispanic origin, and American Indian, Eskimo, or Aleuts; older adults; migrant workers; and illegal aliens). Poor health, crippling diseases, drug and alcohol abuse, and inferior education are contributing social causes of poverty. Much was learned about fighting poverty since 1964, but today there is an emerging new "War on Poverty" wherein the poor are seen as the cause of poverty and not the victims (Shoor, 1995).

Government and private programs aid people with short- and long-term problems. The nurse must be aware of clients' needs and financial resources and the aid programs that are best suited for a given client and/or family in need. This includes staying informed about potential legislative acts such as the Personal Responsibility Act (proposed in 1994), which discouraged illegitimacy and teen pregnancy by prohibiting welfare to minor mothers and denying increased Aid to Families with Dependent Children for additional children (Gingrich, Armey, and The House Republicans, 1994). Nurses must stay abreast of the rapidly changing poverty programs in order to aid clients in this complex political situation.

Communication

Communication differences are presented in many ways, including language differences, verbal and nonverbal behaviors, and silence (see Table 21-2). Language differences are possibly the most important factor in providing transcultural nursing care because these differences impact all stages of the nursing process. Clear and effective communication is important when dealing with any client, especially if language differences create a cultural barrier between the nurse and client (see Chapter 14). If the client does not speak the nurse's language, a translator is necessary. More often, however, the client speaks the nurse's language with limited ability or uses language with denotative or connotative meanings different from the nurse's meanings. For example, a client with limited language ability might know customary greetings such as "How are you?" or "Hello" but not understand health terms such as "pain" or "temperature" that are usually understood by lay persons in the nurse's cultural group.

Failure to communicate effectively with the client not only causes delays in diagnosis and treatment but may also lead to tragic results. In one in-cident, for example, an English-speaking nurse failed to determine that the client truly understood preoperative instructions about washing the surgical site with povidone-iodine (Betadine). The non–English-speaking Asian client, throughout the instruction period, nodded and smiled when the nurse asked her, "Do you understand what I told you?" The nurse judged that the client understood the instructions. Much to the nurse's dismay, the client drank the whole bottle of povidone-iodine solution instead of washing with it.

The nurse should not have assumed that the client understood what was being said. A more appropriate nursing intervention would have been to demonstrate *how* to wash the area with povidone-iodine, then have the client repeat the demonstration. No words have to be spoken; yet by doing this procedure or any other procedure in pantomime, the client grasps what the nurse is teaching and is then able to follow directions.

When deprived of the most common medium of interaction with clients, the spoken word, nurses often become frustrated and ineffective. Nurses need to communicate with clients limited in the use of their language. Some nurses tend to avoid clients with whom they cannot communicate. This creates a vicious circle of cultural misunderstandings. According to Muecke (1970), the nurse might behave toward clients in the following ways that could be misconstrued:

1. The nurse shouts the same words louder. Raising the voice does not make the words more understandable, and such actions could also suggest hostility to clients.
2. The nurse focuses on tasks rather than on clients. This suggests that the nurse is more interested in the tasks than in the clients.
3. The nurse stops talking with clients and starts doing things for them instead of with them, possibly implying clients' inferiority.

The effect of such actions is the painful isolation of clients who do not speak the nurse's language and who are in an unfamiliar environment. Consequently, clients experience cultural shock and may react by withdrawing, becoming hostile or belligerent, or being uncooperative.

Language differences can be bridged. The nurse can ask family members who speak the nurse's language to interpret. The family can also provide information about the client's background that could be valuable in holistic care. The health care institution can also facilitate the search for an interpreter. For example, a list of bilingual or multilingual staff members and volunteers in a hospital might be kept in a central place, such as the information desk.

Medical terms must be clearly explained to all clients, especially those with limited skills in the nurse's language. Jargon presents problems even for alert, oriented, adult clients who speak the nurse's language. For example, there may be many clients who think that *force fluids* means "force urination" or "force elimination of fluids."

Differences in denotative meanings may exist between members of two cultures, causing miscommunication. For instance, when black or African origin American youths say "That's bad" and mean "That's good," European adults might be confused. The youths are speaking in an *argot,* or a special linguistic code of their cultural group. Another linguistic block to communication between ethnic groups comes from differences in connotative meanings for certain words, even when the denotative meanings are the same. For example, to a European American, *hospital* may mean a facility where modern health care is provided. Navajos, however, associate hospitals with death, because they believe the ground and the building where any person dies become contaminated for an indeterminate period with evil spirits that will infect anyone who steps on this ground. Thus they avoid hospitals.

By giving special attention to the communication process, nurses can work to overcome language differences with clients who do not speak their language. Observing nonverbal behaviors, for example, can help clarify communication, although nonverbal communication is also influenced by culture. Nurses can also learn to phrase questions and statements to elicit information from clients whose ethnic background shapes their responses. For example, when a Mexican American man is asked if he feels pain, he may simply say "no" if he believes that admitting pain is a sign he is not manly. The nurse might ask instead whether he feels pain with a change in position, while coughing, or at night.

Finally, the nurse who practices in an area where many members of an ethnic group live should attempt to learn the clients' language. No nurse can learn all the languages that may be encountered in practice, but it is possible for a nurse to learn one other language. With more difficult languages, such as Vietnamese, the nurse can learn some basic terms. Many community health nurses and nurses practicing in community-based settings have learned the languages of their clients.

Space

Personal space involves people's behaviors and attitudes toward the space around them. **Territoriality** is an attitude toward an area people have claimed and defend or react emotionally about when others encroach on it. Both are influenced by culture, and thus different ethnic groups have varying norms related to the use of space (see Table 21-2).

Staff members and other clients frequently encroach on clients' territory in hospitals, including their rooms, beds, closets, and belongings. The nurse should try to respect client's territory as much as possible, especially when performing nursing procedures. The nurse should also welcome visiting members of the family and extended family. This can remind clients of home, lessening the effects of isolation and shock from hospitalization.

Personal space is involved in many nursing activities, and the nurse should be sensitive about the client's attitudes toward personal space (see Chapter 14). For example, providing nursing care often involves touching the client, an action that has different meanings in different cultures and for different individuals. Actions comforting to one client may be threatening to another. Standards of behavior vary also in terms of who, male or female, can touch the client, and where.

The generalizations about the use of personal space are based on studies of the behavior of European North Americans. Use of personal space varies between individuals and ethnic groups. The extreme modesty practiced by members of some cultural groups, such as Hispanic Americans, may prevent members from seeking preventive health care. Much more research must be done on other cultural groups to enable full understanding of the nature of personal space from a multicultural perspective.

Time

Many cultures in the United States and Canada tend to be future oriented. The members of these cultures are concerned with long-range goals and with health care measures in the present to prevent the occurrence of illness in the future. They prefer to plan ahead in making schedules, setting appointments, and organizing activities. **Time orientation** varies among different cultural groups, however, and a nurse who has one attitude toward time may find it difficult to understand and plan care for clients with a different time orientation. Some black or African origin, Hispanic origin, and Southern European Americans are oriented more to the present than the future. These clients may not share a future-oriented nurse's attitude toward matters related to time. Clients may be late for appointments, not because of reluctance or lack of respect for the nurse but because they are less concerned about planning ahead to be on time than with the activity in which they are currently engaged. This time orientation difference may become important in health care measures such as long-term planning and explanations of medication schedules. For example, if a client has not been regularly taking medications prescribed to lower blood pressure, teaching about the potential effects of hypertension should emphasize short-term problems rather than only long-term problems, which may be less important to the client. Table 21-2 further illustrates the time orientation of cultural groups.

▌ TRADITIONAL HEALTH AND ILLNESS BELIEFS

When health beliefs and practices are discussed as they relate to culture, ethnicity, and religion, the word *may* should be used to prevent stereotyping. The range of health and illness definitions, beliefs, and practices is infinite, and there are differences within and between groups. However, some discernible commonalities exist. The nurse must remember that it is important to constantly assess and communicate with clients to clarify their beliefs about health and illness.

Traditional Beliefs

Culturally based folk beliefs often determine the definitions of health and illness for people who have traditional belief systems. The prevention and treatment of an illness depend on understanding its cause. Traditional health beliefs about the cause of illness may differ vastly from the Western model of epidemiology. It is, therefore, important to understand traditional epidemiology, or the causes of illness within a belief system. Cultural, ethnic, and religious backgrounds often reflect the beliefs held about this phenomenon. In the Western epidemiological model, the causes of an illness may be stress and maladaption, viruses, bacteria, or carcinogens. In the traditional epidemiological model, there are vastly different causative agents, including soul loss, spirit possession, spells, evil eyes, and hexes. Illness may be due to people who have the ability to make others ill (e.g., witches). People who believe in these forces must exercise great care to protect themselves. Envy, hate, and jealousy are also forces to be avoided. A person may practice prevention by avoiding situations that could provoke the envy, hate, or jealousy of another. If health is viewed as the reward for good behavior, every effort is made to avoid situations in which social or religious behavior is compromised (Spector, 1991).

Traditional Practices

Many traditional practices are used to prevent and treat illness; these include the use of objects, substances, and religious practices, also known as *folk medicine*. Indeed, folk medicine is related to other types of medicine practiced in society. One example of this is the present popularity of alternative medicine and the use of homeopathic remedies. Folk medicine has coexisted, with increasing tensions, with modern medicine and was derived from academic medicine of earlier generations. Folk practices of ancient times have only in part been abandoned by modern health care belief systems. Many of these beliefs and practices continue to be observed today. Today's "popular medicine" is in a sense commercial folk medicine. The following are varieties of traditional folk medicine (Yoder, 1972):

1. **Natural folk medicine** is one of humankind's earliest uses of the natural environment and is the use of herbs, plants, minerals, and animal substances to prevent and treat illnesses.
2. **Magicoreligious folk medicine** uses charms, holy words, and holy actions to prevent and cure illnesses.

NATURAL FOLK MEDICINE

Natural folk medicine is widely practiced in the United States and the world. In general, this form of prevention and treatment is found in old-fashioned remedies and household medicines. These remedies have been passed down for generations, and many are in common use today. Many of these remedies are herbal, and the customs and rituals related to the use of herbs vary among ethnic groups. The common aspect of the use of herbs is the knowledge that they are present in nature to be used as a source of therapy. The way that these medicines are gathered and the specific uses may vary by group and region. In general, folk-medicine traditions prescribe the time of year in which the herb is picked; the way it is dried and prepared; and the method, amount, and frequency for consumption.

The following are some examples of natural folk medicines:

A person whose heritage is from Jamaica may use cerasee tea to keep his "system" clean.

A person whose heritage is from Italy may use garlic to prevent the evil eye.

A person whose heritage is from Germany may use a potato to treat a wart.

A person whose heritage is from Greece may use chamomile tea to treat stomach disorders.

A person whose heritage is from China may use burned-rice tea to treat diarrhea.

MAGICORELIGIOUS FOLK MEDICINE

Magicoreligious folk medicine, too, has existed for as long as humans have sought to cure their ailments. It is now labeled by some as "superstition"; yet for believers, it may take the form of religious practices related to healing. One example of this is a form of unofficial religious healing known as *powwowing, charming,* or *conjuring.* In these practices charms, amulets, holy water, such as water from Lourdes, and physical manipulations are used in the attempt to heal illness.

USE OF PROTECTIVE OBJECTS

Protective objects can be worn, carried, or hung in the home. Amulets are objects with magical powers (e.g., charms worn on a string or chain around the neck, wrist, or waist to protect the wearer from the evil eye or evil spirits). Amulets exist in societies all over the world and are associated with protection from trouble (Budge, 1978). People may also use talismans or "consecrated religious objects" (Budge, 1978). Talismans are believed to possess extraordi-

nary powers and may be worn on a rope around the waist or carried in a pocket or purse. People who wear amulets or carry a talisman should be allowed to do so in health care agencies. A palm from Palm Sunday in the Catholic home or a mezuzah on the door of a Jewish home are other examples of protective objects that are used to protect the home and family.

USE OF FOOD

Foods are ingested in certain ways or amounts. This practice uses diet and consists of many different observances. In many belief systems the body is kept in balance or harmony by the type of food eaten, so many food taboos and combinations exist. For example, it is believed that some food substances can be ingested to prevent illness. People from many ethnic backgrounds eat raw garlic or onion, wear them on the body, or hang them in the home for this purpose. The rules of kosher practiced among Jewish people mandate the elimination of pork and shellfish from the diet. They allow fish with scales and fins and only certain cuts of beef from animals with cloven hooves that chew cud (cattle and lambs). Jews also believe that milk and meat must never be placed on the same dishes or eaten at the same meal. Moslems also adhere to many dietary practices that are similar to the kosher diet. For example, Moslems do not eat pork. Religious teaching can lead to clients not accepting health care products, such as pork-based insulin for the treatment of diabetes.

RELIGIOUS PRACTICES

Another traditional approach to illness prevention centers around religion and includes practices such as the burning of candles, rituals of redemption, and prayer. Religion strongly affects the way people attempt to prevent illness, and it plays a strong role in rituals associated with health protection. Religion dictates social, moral, and dietary practices designed to keep a people healthy and in balance. Religion also plays a vital role in those persons' perceptions of illness prevention. Many persons believe illness can be prevented by strictly following religious codes, morals, and practices, and view illness as punishment for violating a religious code. Religious practices such as the Catholic custom of blessing of the throats on St. Blaise Day to prevent sore throats and choking are performed for protection from illness.

Traditional Remedies

The use of folk or traditional medicine is increasing, and its practice is seen among people from all cultural and ethnic backgrounds. When people use the medicines that are from within their ethnocultural heritage, it is viewed as "traditional health care" (Fig. 21-4). When people use non-Western medicine that is not of their ethnocultural tradition, it is "alternative medicine." Use of folk medicine is not a new practice among heritage-consistent people, so many of the remedies have been used and passed on for generations. The pharmaceutical properties of vegetation—plants, roots, stems, flowers, seeds, and herbs—have been studied, tested, cataloged, and used for countless centuries. Many of these plants are used by specific communities. Others cross ethnic and community lines and are used in certain geographical areas. These remedies are purchased in special stores or

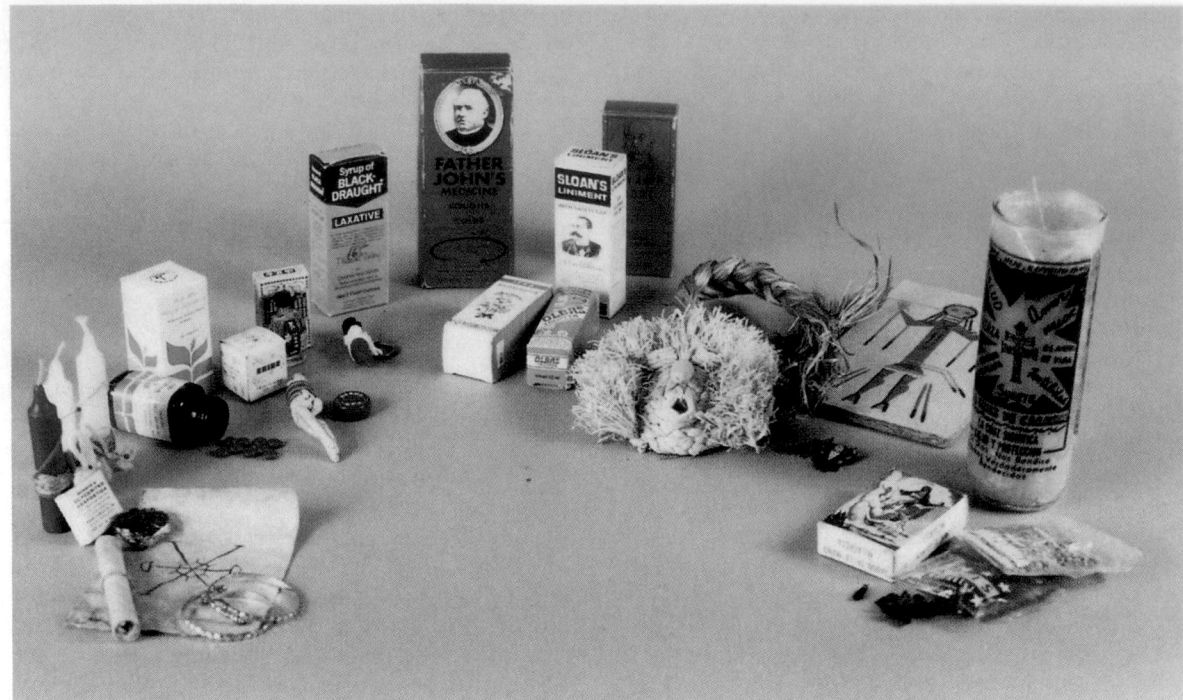

Fig. 21-4 Asian American remedies include *Huo Li Jian Mei Su, Jen Shen Lu Jung Wan,* Ginseng root, White flower, and Tiger balm. *(Courtesy Lucy Rozier, Boston College Audio Visual Services, Boston College, Chestnut Hill, Mass.)*

market places in ethnocultural communities within the United States and may also be purchased in the country of origin.

Nurses must determine whether clients are taking traditional or alternative remedies. This is very important when clients do not take the medications that have been prescribed. Frequently, the active ingredients of folk remedies are unknown. If clients are taking them, the nurse must determine the remedy and its active ingredients. Often these ingredients can be antagonistic or synergistic to prescribed medications. If this is the situation, the medication may have no effect, or a severe overdose may occur. The richness of this pharmacopoeia far exceeds the limits of this chapter; thus only a limited sample of the remedies of each population will be highlighted.

Healers

In the traditional context, healing is the restoration of the person to a state of harmony between the body, mind, and spirit, or the restoration of holistic health. Within a given community, specific people are known to have the power to heal. The healer is thought to have received the gift of healing from a divine source.

In many instances a heritage-consistent person may consult a traditional healer before, instead of, or along with a modern health care provider. Many differences exist between the Western physician and the traditional healer (Kaptchuk and Croucher, 1987) (Table 21-3). The relationship between the person and the healer, for example, is often much closer than that between the person and the health care professional. The person sees the healer as one who understands the problem within the cultural context,

speaks the same language, and shares a similar world view. Examples of traditional healers follow:

1. *Medicine man:* the traditional healer of the American Indian
2. *Senora:* a Puerto Rican woman knowledgeable in the treatment of illness
3. *Espiritista:* a person possessing more sophisticated skills than the *Senora*
4. *Curandero:* a person of Mexican heritage with the God-given ability to heal using a religious-psychiatric approach
5. *Partera:* a Mexican-American midwife
6. *Root-worker:* a black or African origin person able to determine the cause of an illness and the treatment
7. *Chinese doctor:* a doctor often educated in both the traditional Chinese herbal medicines and modern medicine

Traditional healers have always been a part of cultures. The methods used by these healers were developed over generations by trial and error and are often based on religious beliefs and social circumstances. Effective methods have been preserved and adapted to meet the needs of the present time. The traditional healer is aware of the cultural and personal needs of the client and is able to understand the problem in today's world.

■ CULTURAL ASPECTS OF HEALTH AND ILLNESS

Many cultures exist in the United States today (see Table 21-2 and Fig. 21-1). Nurses must be aware of these groups and be familiar with the basic characteristics of each. The following "culture capsules" provide a general overview of

Table 21-3	Comparisons: Traditional Healer Versus Physician

HEALER	PHYSICIAN
Maintains an informal, friendly, affective relationship with the entire family	Is business-like and formal, dealing primarily with the client
Comes to the house day or night	Stays in a physician's office or *clinic* where the client must go for services. Rarely, if ever, makes home visits
For diagnosis, consults with head of house, creates a mood of awe, talks to all family members, is not authoritarian, has social rapport, builds expectation of cure	Deals primarily with the ill person, may address only that person's illness (authoritarian manner can create fear)
Is generally less expensive than the physician	Is generally more expensive than the healer
Has ties to the "world of the sacred," has rapport with the symbolic, spiritual, creative, or holy force	Is primarily secular, pays little attention to the religious beliefs of a client or meanings of an illness
Shares the world view of the client (i.e., speaks the same language, lives in the same neighborhood or in the same similar socioeconomic conditions, may know the same people, understands the lifestyle of the client)	Generally does not share the world view of the client (i.e., may not speak the same language, live in the same neighborhood or in the same socioeconomic conditions, may not understand the lifestyle of the client)

Modified from Spector RE: *Cultural diversity in health and illness,* ed 3, Norwalk, Conn, 1991, Appleton & Lange.

Asian, black or African origin, American Indian, Hispanic origin, and European American cultures. Each capsule includes a synopsis of the culture's background, traditional definitions of health and illness, and traditional beliefs about the causes of illness, methods of prevention, and remedies.

These capsules illustrate the dynamic similarities and differences between groups of people. However, clients must be assessed as individuals. Characteristic beliefs of a cultural group are not necessarily shared by each individual in that group. However, this background may be used as a framework for providing culturally sensitive nursing care.

Asian Americans

Asian Americans originated in China, Hawaii, the Philippines, Korea, Japan, Laos, Cambodia, and Vietnam. Many Asian Americans have lived in the United States for several generations. Others arrived more recently, and others are still entering the country, especially in California (Fig. 21-5). Asians comprise the second largest ethnic group in the American population. The following is a brief demographic sketch of the population:

- The median age of this population in 1990 was 29.8 years (U.S. Bureau of the Census, 1992, p. 23).
- 73.6% of the members over age 25 have completed a high school education (U.S. Bureau of the Census, 1994, p. 9).
- Personal earnings for people working full time in 1989 averaged $31,979 (U.S. Bureau of the Census, 1994, p. 475).
- 11% of people over age 25 in this group were below the poverty level in 1991 (Go, 1994).

The family is composed of a hierarchical structure, and loyalty among members is valued. There is a devotion to tradition and many religions, including Taoism, Buddhism, Islam, and Christianity, are practiced.

Within the Asian community, Chinese medicine provides an overall framework for Asian cultures and teaches that health is a state of spiritual and physical harmony be-

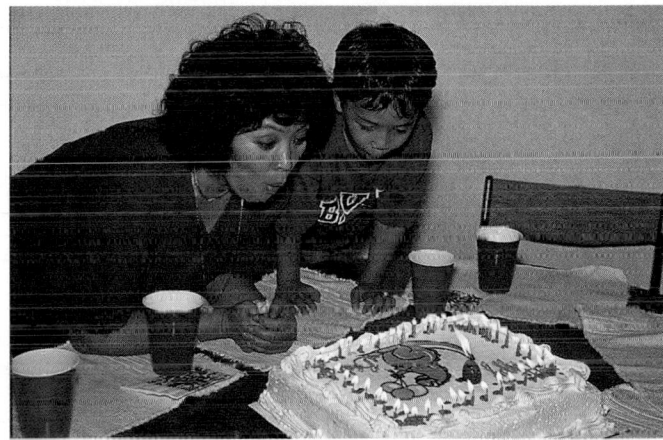

Fig. 21-5 Blending of Asian culture and American practices at a child's birthday party.

tween a body, mind, and spirit in harmony with nature. In addition, the forces of *yin* (female, negative energy) and *yang* (male, positive energy) must be in balance. Illness is the result of imbalance between *yin* and *yang*. The body is viewed as a gift from parents and ancestors. It is not the person's personal property and must be cared for and maintained. The primary role of the physician in ancient China was to help safeguard the body and to prevent illness. If a person became ill despite preventive measures, it was not necessary to pay the physician for treatment.

ILLNESS CAUSE AND PREVENTION

Illness may be caused by an upset in the balance of *yin* and *yang*. The weather, overexertion, and prolonged sitting may also cause illness, which may be prevented by adhering to a proper diet to maintain the body's balance, exercising, avoiding temperature changes, and taking certain remedies.

REMEDIES

The following examples are a few traditional remedies used to prevent and treat ailments among Asian Americans.

Huo Li Jian Mei Su are small, brown, coated pills taken twice a day to counteract senility, for the relief of fatigue, and for the maintenance of youth, health, and beauty. They can also be used to treat insomnia, gastritis, constipation, and abnormal liver function. *Jen Shen Lu Jung Wan* is a brown, gummy substance encased in white wax. It is indicated in the treatment of general debility, anemia, lack of well-being, mental overstrain, loss of appetite, and it may be taken before elective surgery. Ginseng root is the most famous Chinese medicine. It has universal medicinal usage in "building the blood," especially after childbirth. Ginseng is native to the United States and is used in this country as a restorative tonic. White flower is an oily liquid used to treat aches, pains, and sprains and is also effective in treating colds, influenza, headaches, and coughs. Tiger balm is a salve used for temporary relief of minor aches and pains. Other methods of treatment include the use of acupuncture, a method of treating disease by puncturing the skin at certain points of the body with metal needles, and moxibustion, the application of heat to these same points (Spector, 1991).

Black or African Origin Americans

Most black or African origin Americans were brought to the United States as slaves between 1619 and 1860 from the west coast of Africa. Today, many have also immigrated to the United States from black or African origin countries, the West Indies, the Dominican Republic, Haiti, and Jamaica. The 1990 black or African origin population was 29,986,000, or 11.7% of the total population of the United States. The following is a brief demographic sketch of the population:

- The median age of this population in 1990 was 28.1 years (U.S. Bureau of the Census, 1992, p. 23).
- 59.8% of the members over 25 have completed a high school education (U.S. Bureau of the Census, 1994, p. 5).
- Personal earnings for people working full time in 1989 averaged $22,525 (U.S. Bureau of the Census, 1994, p. 475).
- 25% of people over 25 in this group were below the poverty level in 1991 (U.S. Bureau of the Census, 1992, p. 70).

The family is often composed of a matriarchal structure and there are many single parent households headed by females; there are strong and large extended family networks. There is a continuation of tradition and a strong religious affiliation within the community. Many black or African origin Americans tend to use traditional medicines and healers when the people are knowledgeable of and have access to this resource.

The traditional definition of health stems from the black or African origin belief about life and the nature of being. Life is a process rather than a state, and the nature of a person is viewed in terms of an energy force rather than matter. When healthy, a person is in harmony with nature. Illness is seen as a disharmony of the mind, body, and spirit or as a disharmony between man and nature. Researchers and epidemiologists have noted chronic illnesses and illness patterns that are associated with cultural and ethnic groups. Berg and Berg (1989) describe the correlation between psychological stress and hypertension found in black or African origin Americans.

ILLNESS CAUSE AND PREVENTION

Illness (disharmony) is often attributed to demons and evil spirits. Several methods are used as protection from these forces, including the ancient belief and practice of voodoo. Voodoo is believed to cause, as well as prevent, the action of malevolent forces. "White" magic protects against these forces, and "black" magic directs their energy to a specific person or body area. The extent of the belief in this magic is unknown. Traditional beliefs about prevention of illness focus on avoiding people believed to carry evil spirits. Prayer and a well-balanced diet are considered helpful.

REMEDIES

The following examples are a few traditional remedies used to prevent or treat ailments among black or African origin Americans.

Bangles are silver bracelets worn by people originating from the West Indies. They overlap but are open to let out evil and closed to prevent evil from entering the body. They are worn from infancy and are replaced as the person grows. These bracelets tarnish and leave a black ring on the skin when a person is becoming ill. The black ring serves as a signal to rest, improve the diet, and take any other needed precautions. Some people wear many bangles, believing that their sound frightens away evil spirits. Many people believe that they are extremely vulnerable to evil, even to death, when the bangles are removed, so removal of these bracelets can cause a great deal of anxiety. Talismans protect the wearer from all sickness and are worn on a string around the waist or carried in a pocket or in a purse. Asafoetida is a foul-smelling, gummy substance worn to ward off colds and evil. It is known as the *incense of the devil*. Voodoo candles have a peculiar spiritualistic character and are used for sacred rituals and rites. Colors also have significance. For example, pink means love; white means peace, and blue means success and protection from harm (Spector, 1991).

American Indians

There are approximately 170 American Indian tribes in the United States, predominantly in the Western states. Each tribe, or nation, has its own unique cultural heritage and traditional health and illness beliefs and practices (Fig. 21-6). Although many American Indians remain on reservations, many also live off of them. Members of the American Indian nations immigrated to this land long before the Europeans and other immigrants. With a 1990 population of 1.9 million or 0.7% of the total population of the United States, they comprise the smallest group in the American population. The following is a brief demographic sketch of this population:

- The median age of this population in 1990 was 26.2 years (U.S. Bureau of the Census, 1992, p. 23).
- 60.5% of the members over 25 have completed a high school education (U.S. Bureau of the Census, 1994, p. 7).

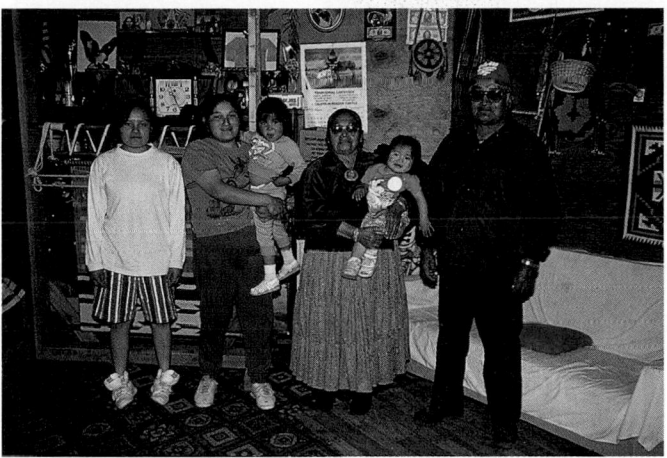

Fig. 21-6 American Indian family in front of a display at a local festival.

- Personal earnings for people working full time in 1989 averaged $23,121; (U.S. Bureau of the Census, 1994, p. 475).
- 23.7% of people over 25 in this group were below the poverty level in 1991 (Go, 1994).

The family is often composed of a nuclear family with strong biological and large extended family networks. Children are taught to respect traditions. There are community organizations that provide social and cultural services that are growing in strength and numbers. Many American Indians tend to use traditional medicines and healers and are knowledgeable of these resources. The people may frequently be treated by a traditional medicine man, and the sweat lodge and herbs are frequently used to treat mental symptoms. Several diagnostic techniques include the use of divination, conjuring, and star-gazing.

Health reflects the ability to live in total harmony with nature and the ability to survive under extremely difficult circumstances. People are believed to have an intimate spiritual relationship with nature. The earth is considered a living organism, the body of a higher individual, with a will and a desire to be well and experience health and illness. The body and earth must be treated with respect. Because the earth provides food, shelter, and medicine to humans, it must be protected. According to Basque (1975), "The land belongs to life, life belongs to the land, and the land belongs to itself." Thus to stay healthy a person must maintain a positive, balanced relationship with nature.

Another explanation of the American Indian view of health is that the body is divided into two halves, plus and minus. There are also, in every whole, two energy poles, positive and negative. People have the power to control themselves, and with this potency, spiritual power (control of the body's energy) is derived. Health is described as the harmony or balance between the two halves or the two energy poles. Illness is the disharmony of the body, mind, and spirit.

ILLNESS CAUSE AND PREVENTION

Sources causing illness vary from nation to nation or tribe to tribe. Hopi Indians associate illness with evil spirits

> ## RESEARCH HIGHLIGHT
>
> **RESEARCH ABSTRACT**
> The purpose of this study was to advance transcultural nursing knowledge predicated on lived experiences of Native Americans with non–insulin-dependent diabetes. Data were collected in rural Oklahoma and consisted of nonstructured interviews and clinical observations. The informants' lived experiences were categorized and described. The reactions included choices made to adapt to recommended health maintenance regimes, fear of amputation, fear of impending death, and grieving related to changes in health. These findings serve to further illustrate in a specific way the need for the nurse to carefully assess the client and to listen to what clients tell regarding their understanding of the given problem.
>
> **IMPLICATIONS FOR PRACTICE**
> ▶ Cultural assessment helps to identify clients' understanding of disease process.
> ▶ Client teaching can be adapted to incorporate cultural beliefs, values, and preferences within the plan of care.
> ▶ Cultural resources can be indentified to assist clients in adjusting to illness.
>
> **REFERENCE**
> Parker JG: The lived experience of Native Americans with diabetes within a transcultural nursing perspective, *J Transcult Nurs* 6(1):5, 1994.

and therefore strive to avoid or ward off these spirits. Navahos see illness as the result of displeasing the holy people, annoying the elements, disturbing animal and plant life, neglecting the celestial bodies, misusing a sacred Indian ceremony, or tampering with witches or witchcraft. Hawk Littlejohn (1979), an Eastern Band Cherokee medicine man, describes illness as the imbalance of the body, mind, or spirit caused by an excess in one domain and the neglect of the other two. For example, a student who spends too much time studying—developing the mind—may neglect the body and spirit and will therefore be vulnerable to disharmony and illness. The main principle for the prevention of illness is the maintenance of harmony with the body, mind, and spirit and the avoidance of factors that cause disharmony (see the box above).

REMEDIES

The following examples are remedies used by American Indians to prevent or treat illness. A mask is worn to hide the self from the devil or evil spirits. Sweet grass is burned as a rite of purification by the medicine man. A sand painting is created by the Navaho medicine man while diagnosing an ailment. The painting is created in an elaborate diagnostic ceremony of motion of the hand. When the hand moves in a certain way, the medicine man knows that it is indicative of a specific illness and is able to prescribe the correct treatment. A thunderbird is an amulet worn for good luck and protection (Spector, 1991).

Hispanic Origin Americans

Members of the Hispanic origin community originate in Spain, Cuba, Mexico, Puerto Rico, and other Spanish- or Portuguese-speaking countries of Central and South America. With a 1990 population of 22,354,059 or 9%, they comprise the most rapidly growing ethnic group in the American population. The following is a brief demographic sketch of this population:

- The median age of this population in 1990 was 25.5 years (U.S. Bureau of the Census, 1992, p. 23).
- 47.1% of the members over 25 have completed a high school education (U.S. Bureau of the Census, 1994, p. 11).
- Personal earnings for people working full time in 1989 averaged $22,383 (U.S. Bureau of the Census, 1994, p. 475).
- 21.3% people over 25 in this group were below the poverty level in 1991 (U.S. Bureau of the Census, 1992, p. 70).

The family is often composed of a nuclear family with strong and large extended family networks and *compadrazzo*-godparents. There is a continuation of tradition and a strong church affiliation within the community. Many, but not all, Hispanics are Catholic.

The people may frequently be treated by a traditional healer such as a *Curandero, Santero,* or *Senora,* and herbs are frequently used to treat mental symptoms. Several diagnostic techniques include the use of divination, observation, and/or exorcism. Health is often believed to be the result of good luck or a reward from God for good behavior. Health represents a state of equilibrium within the universe where the forces of hot, cold, wet, and dry are balanced. Blood is hot and wet, and yellow bile is hot and dry; phlegm is cold and wet, and black bile is cold and dry. The concept originated with the early Hippocratic theory of health and the four humors. Health exists when the four humors are in a balanced state. Health is maintained by the diet and other practices that keep the humors balanced. Illness is viewed as misfortune or bad luck, punishment from God for evil thoughts or actions, or the imbalance of hot and cold.

ILLNESS CAUSE AND PREVENTION

Several factors cause illness. A hot-cold imbalance, for example, is primarily caused by improper diet. Food substances are classified as hot or cold without regard to their actual temperature. This classification can vary from person to person, but essentially, certain foods are known to be hot, and others are known to be cold. Examples of cold food are chicken, honey, avocados, bananas, and lima beans. Examples of hot foods are chocolate, coffee, corn meal, garlic, kidney beans, onions, and peas. Illness can occur if these foods are eaten in improper combinations or amounts. For example, *friadad del estomago* (cold stomach) is caused by eating too many cold foods. There are several conditions in which a person maintains health by adhering to this hot-cold system. A pregnant woman avoids hot foods. During menstruation and after childbirth, she avoids cold foods. An infant who requires formula that contains a hot food such as evaporated milk may also be fed a cold food.

Other factors believed to cause illness are the "dislocation of body parts"(i.e., fallen fontanel) and magic or supernatural causes outside the body such as *mal ojo* (bad eye). *Envidia* (envy) is also a cause of illness and bad luck, and many means are used to prevent it. Many people of Hispanic origin believe that to succeed is to fail (i.e., when a person's success provokes the envy of friends and neighbors, misfortune or illness may follow). Illness may be prevented by proper diet, avoidance of "harmful" people, the wearing of amulets for protection, the use of candles, and prayer.

REMEDIES

The following remedies are used among people of Hispanic origin for the prevention or treatment of illness. The *Mano Negro* (blackhand) amulet of Puerto Rico may be placed on a baby at birth and is believed to protect it from the evil eye. *Jabon de la Mano Milagrosa* (soap of the miraculous hand) is used to cleanse and protect a person. All kinds of novena candles may be burned to ward off evil. One example is *La Cruz De Caravaca* (the Cross of Caravaca) candle, and it is burned for health, courage, strength, fertility, and luck. This "wishing cross" is for good luck, health, and protection against evil. The yellow color symbolizes the power of the mind. Manzanilla is an herb made into tea and used to treat stomach and intestinal pain, uterine cramps, anxiety, and insomnia. Anis are star-shaped seeds used to treat painful gases, upset stomach, colic, and anorexia, and to increase breast milk (Spector, 1991).

European Americans

Members of most European American communities originated in Europe and have been migrating to this country since 1620. This population is a diverse mixture of people from many countries, speaking numerous languages, and observing a wide variety of health beliefs and practices. The 1980 census was the first to attempt to break down the population by country of origin. The largest groups were from Germany, England, Ireland, and France. The following is a brief demographic sketch of the population:

- The median age of this population in 1990 was 34.4 years (U.S. Bureau of the Census, 1992, p. 23).
- 74.6% of the members over 25 have completed a high school education (U.S. Bureau of the Census, 1994, p. 3).
- Personal earnings for people working full time in 1989 averaged $31,419 (U.S. Bureau of the Census, 1994, p. 474).
- 8.8% of people over 25 in this group were below the poverty level in 1991 (U.S. Bureau of the Census, 1992, p. 70).

Health and illness are defined in many ways. Health includes the ability to perform activities of daily living, a state of physical and emotional well-being, and a state free of illness. Illness is described as the inability to perform activities of daily living, the presence of disease symptoms and pain, and the malformation of body organs.

ILLNESS CAUSE AND PREVENTION

To European Americans, traditional beliefs about the causes of illness are many and varied. Examples of these causes include breaking of religious rules, exposure to causative factors such as punishment from God, drafts, climatic changes, and the abuse of the body. A wide variety of

Heritage Assessment Tool

1. Where was your mother born? _____
2. Where was your father born?_____
3. Where were your grandparents born?:
   a. Your mother's mother?_____
   b. Your mother's father? _____
   c. Your father's mother? _____
   d. Your father's father? _____
4. How many brothers _____ and sisters _____ do you have?
5. What setting did you grow up in? Urban _____ Rural _____ Suburban _____
6. What country did your parents grow up in?
   Father _____ Mother _____
7. How old were you when you came to the United States? _____
8. How old were your parents when they came to the United States?
   Mother _____ Father _____
9. When you were growing up, who lived with you?
   Nuclear _____ or Extended _____ Family
10. Have you maintained contact with:
    a. Aunts, uncles, cousins? (1) Yes _____ (2) No _____
    b. Brothers and sisters?   (1) Yes _____ (2) No _____
    c. Parents?   (1) Yes _____ (2) No _____
    d. Your own children?   (1) Yes _____ (2) No _____
11. Did most of your aunts, uncles, cousins live near to your home?
    (1) Yes _____ (2) No _____
12. Approximately how often did you visit your family members who lived outside of your home?
    (1) Daily _____ (2) Weekly _____ (3) Monthly _____ (4) Once a year or less _____ (5) Never _____
13. Was your original family name changed?
    (1) Yes _____ (2) No _____
14. What is your religious preference?
    (1) Catholic _____ (2) Jewish _____
    (3) Protestant _____ Denomination _____ (4) Other _____ (5) None _____
15. Is your spouse the same religion as you?
    (1) Yes _____ (2) No _____
16. Is your spouse the same ethnic background as you?
    (1) Yes _____ (2) No _____
17. What kind of school did you go to?
    (1) Public _____ (2) Private _____ (3) Parochial _____
18. As an adult, do you live in a neighborhood where the neighbors are the same religion and ethnic background as yourself?
    (1) Yes _____ (2) No _____
19. Do you belong to a religious institution?
    (1) Yes _____ (2) No _____
20. Would you describe yourself as an active member?
    (1) Yes _____ (2) No _____
21. How often do you attend your religious institution?
    (1) More than once a week _____ (2) Weekly _____ (3) Monthly _____
    (4) Special holidays only _____ (5) Never _____
22. Do you practice your religion in your home?
    (1) Yes _____ (2) No _____ (if yes, please specify)
    (3) Praying _____ (4) Bible reading _____ (5) Diet _____ (6) Celebrating religious holidays _____
23. Do you prepare foods of your ethnic background?
    (1) Yes _____ (2) No _____
24. Do you participate in ethnic activities?
    (1) Yes _____ (2) No _____ (if yes, please specify)
    (3) Singing _____ (4) Holiday celebrations _____ (5) Dancing _____
    (6) Festivals _____ (7) Costumes _____ (8) Other _____
25. Are your friends from the same religious background as you?
    (1) Yes _____ (2) No _____
26. Are your friends from the same ethnic background as you?
    (1) Yes _____ (2) No _____
27. What is your native language? _____
28. Do you speak this language?
    (1) Prefer _____ (2) Occasionally _____ (3) Rarely _____
29. Do you read your native language?
    (1) Yes _____ (2) No _____

The greater the number of *yes* answers, the more likely the client is to strongly identify with a traditional heritage. (The one *no* answer that indicates heritage identity is "Was your name changed?")

From Spector RE: *Cultural diversity in health and illness,* ed 3, Norwalk, Conn, 1991, Appleton & Lange.

methods for preventing illness may be found among European Americans, including diet, exercise, religious rituals, and the wearing of shawls and/or amulets.

REMEDIES

The following are a few examples of remedies reported among European Americans. *Malocchio* is an Italian horn worn to prevent the evil eye. The hunchbacked man Gobo worn on a horn offers extra protection; he holds a horseshoe for luck in his left hand and points the index and little finger of his right hand to ward off the evil spirit. Syrup of Black Draught is used as an over-the-counter laxative. Father John's Medicine is a family medicine that has been used for colds and coughs since 1855. Swamp root is an over-the-counter liquid used as a diuretic. Sloan's Liniment aids in the temporary relief of minor pains resulting from arthritis and other ailments. *Olbas* and *magentropfen* are medicines sold in Germany to treat sore throats and lack of appetite (Spector, 1991).

■ CULTURAL FACTORS AND THE NURSING PROCESS

When nurses provide care to clients from other backgrounds, they must be aware of and sensitive to their own unique heritage and health traditions and then to the client's sociocultural background. They must assess and listen carefully to health and illness beliefs and practices (see the box on p. 365). The nursing process enables the nurse to provide individualized care and can be adapted to provide culturally sensitive care (Table 21-4).

Assessment

The nurse should begin assessment by determining the client's cultural heritage, social organization background (see Table 21-4), and language skills. The client should be asked about the cause of the illness or problem. The nurse should then determine whether the person is taking any home remedies to treat the symptoms and whether social support services are available.

Community Assessment

When clients receive care in primary care, restorative care, or community-based settings, the assessment process of transcultural nursing comes alive the moment the client leaves the confines of the institutional setting. The nurse must provide culturally competent and sensitive care to the client in the community. One way that sensitivity and appreciation for a given community are developed is when the nurse goes out and witnesses the daily life of that community. The box on p. 367 lists various social organizational factors that the nurse may want to explore as a way of acquiring this awareness. The "answers" to the various areas raised are generally found in libraries or through interviews with people from the community. A second approach to this activity is to walk through the community and view the churches, social organizations, and health-related services available. If possible, the nurse can visit a community health care provider or clinic, a church or community center that serves the target group, or grocery stores

Table 21-4	Cultural Adaptation of the Nursing Process	
PROCESS	**ACTION**	
ASSESSMENT		
Heritage consistency	Perform heritage-consistency assessment (see the box on p. 365) on self and client.	
Environmental control	Ask about the client's beliefs of the nature of the health problem and actions being taken at home or in the community to treat and resolve it.	
	Ask about other health care resources being used.	
Biological variations	Ask about nutritional preferences.	
	Observe body structure, skin tone, and color.	
	Be aware of health problems that may be more common in client's background.	
Social organizations	Conduct community activities.	
Communication skills	Determine the needs of the client who does not speak the nurse's language and provide competent interpreters.	
Space	Be aware of territoriality; seek permission before intruding in the client's territory.	
	Be aware of touch and eye-contact expectations.	
Time	Understand the differences in time orientation.	
NURSING DIAGNOSIS		
Development of problem list	Ask about the client's interpretation of the problem and possible effective interventions.	
PLANNING	Include client, family, and community in plans as needed.	
IMPLEMENTATION	Alter usual ways of interacting to adjust to client's social interaction and etiquette.	
	Incorporate interventions agreeing with client's cultural heritage, educational level, and language skills.	
EVALUATION	With client, determine whether nursing care has met expectations and needs.	

Ethnocultural Social Organization Assessment Tool

- Demographic data that include:
  - Total population size of city or town
  - Breakdown by areas: residential concentrations of target group
  - Breakdown by ages
  - Education
  - Occupations
  - Income
- Traditional health and illness beliefs found within target group
- Traditional health and illness practices within target group
- Use and sources of home remedies
- Identity of traditional healers

and pharmacies to observe differences in foods and over-the-counter remedies. If possible, the nurse should eat a meal in a neighborhood restaurant.

Nursing Diagnosis

Assessment enables the nurse to cluster relevant data and develop actual or potential nursing diagnoses related to the cultural or ethnic needs of the client. In addition, the nursing diagnosis should state the probable cause. The identification of the cause of the problem further individualizes the nursing care plan and encourages selection of appropriate interventions (see Chapter 8).

Planning

When establishing the goals and expected outcomes of care and planning specific interventions, the nurse again considers cultural variables as they relate to the client. The extended family should be involved in care, for example, if the family is the client's strongest support group. Cultural beliefs and practices, such as the use of special prayers and amulets, can be implemented into therapy (Berg and Berg, 1989). The client's cultural heritage, educational level, and language skills should be considered when planning teaching activities. To avoid confusion, misunderstanding, or cultural conflict, explanations of aspects of care usually not questioned by acculturated clients may be required for clients who do not speak the nurse's language or who are not acculturated (DeSantis, Thomas, 1990). The nurse may have to alter usual ways of interacting to avoid offending or alienating a client with different attitudes toward social interaction and etiquette. For example, a client who is modest and self-conscious about the body may need psychological preparation before some procedures and tests that are

usually viewed as routine (e.g., obtaining a chest x-ray film or electrocardiogram [ECG]).

Implementation

The nurse can find out what care clients consider appropriate by involving them and families in planning it and by asking about their expectations. This should be done in every case, even if the nursing care cannot be modified. Because the nurse and clients are likely to take many aspects of their cultures for granted, questions should be clear, and explanations should be explicit. Discussing cultural variables with clients and families during planning helps the nurse implement clients' personal health beliefs and practices so that interventions can be individualized.

Evaluation

The nurse evaluates the results of nursing care by determining the extent to which the individualized goals and expected outcomes of care have been met. Evaluation continues throughout the nursing process and should include feedback from the client and family. Self-evaluation of both a personal and professional nature is crucial as the nurse increases skills for interaction with clients from diverse cultural backgrounds. In order to assist meeting the client's needs and health care goals, the nurse should consider the following questions:

1. Are nurses open to understanding ways in which the client's values differ from theirs?
2. Have nurses given sufficient attention to communicating with the client with limited skills in the nurse's language?
3. Are the client's family and community involved in the nursing process?
4. Are the client's beliefs and practices integrated into nursing therapies?
5. Are nurses' therapeutic relationships with the client grounded on respect for the client, regardless of cultural differences?

Nurses should evaluate their attitudes toward providing transcultural nursing care. Some nurses may believe they should treat all clients the same and simply "act naturally." However, this attitude fails to acknowledge that cultural differences exist and that there is no one natural human behavior. The nurse cannot act the same with all clients and still hope to deliver effective, individualized, holistic care. Sometimes, inexperienced nurses are so self-conscious about cultural differences and so afraid of making a mistake that they impede the nursing process by not asking questions about areas of difference or by asking so many questions that they seem to pry into the client's personal life. The process of self-evaluation can help the nurse become more comfortable when providing care to clients from diverse backgrounds.

▪ KEY CONCEPTS ▪

▶ Cultural heritage affects all dimensions of health; it is vital that the nurse consider cultural background when planning care.

▶ The way that culture influences behaviors, attitudes, and values depends on many factors and thus may not be the same for individual members of a cultural group.

▶ Although basic human needs are the same for all people, the way a person seeks to meet those needs is influenced by culture.

▶ The nurse should have an understanding of the prevalent characteristics of the five major groups in North America—Asian; black or African origin; American Indian, Eskimo, and Aleut; Hispanic origin; and European Americans—but should always individualize care rather than generalize about all clients in these groups.

▶ Before assessing the cultural background of a client, nurses should assess the influence of their own cultures.

▶ Nursing diagnoses for clients should include potential problems in interaction with the health care system and problems involving the effects of culture.

▶ The planning and implementation of nursing interventions should be adapted as much as possible to the client's cultural background.

▶ Evaluation should include the nurse's self-evaluation of attitudes and emotions toward providing nursing care to clients from diverse sociocultural backgrounds.

▪ KEY TERMS ▪

Acculturation, p. 353

Culture, p. 353

Demographics, p. 352

Environmental control, p. 355

Ethnicity, p. 354

Heritage consistency, p. 353

Magicoreligious folk medicine, p. 359

Melting pot, p. 353

Modern, p. 352

Natural folk medicine, p. 359

Personal space, p. 358

Religion, p. 354

Socialization, p. 355

Stereotype, p. 355

Territoriality, p. 358

Time orientation, p. 358

Traditional, p. 352

Transcultural rapport and communication, p. 352

Transcultural nursing, p. 352

▪ CRITICAL THINKING EXERCISES ▪

1. Ms. Sanchez, a recent immigrant from South America, has been admitted to the hospital for the first time in her life. She appears apprehensive. What are two activities that you may undertake to help her adjust to this strange environment?

2. Mr. Jabar is a practicing Muslim and is on a clear liquid diet. He refuses to eat the gelatin dessert that he is served. What intervention would be helpful in respect to his diet?

3. When a client is often late for a clinic appointment, what interventions may prevent this from becoming a problem?

4. Mrs. Chan, a 57-year-old Asian immigrant, is going home and is refusing to accept follow-up nursing care. What assessment questions may be helpful in determining who and what will be helpful for her?

REFERENCES

Abramson HJ: Religion. In Thermstrom S, editor: *The Harvard encyclopedia of American ethnic groups*, Cambridge, Mass, 1980, Harvard University Press.

Basque W: Lecture notes, Boston, 1975, Boston College.

Berg J, Berg BL: Compliance, diet, and cultural factors among black Americans with end-stage renal disease, *J Nat Black Nurses Assoc* 3(2):18, 1989.

Boyle JS: The practice of transcultural nursing, *Transcultural Nursing Society Newsletter* 7:2, 1987.

Budge EAW: *Amulets and superstitions*, New York, 1978, Dover Publications. (Originally published in London, 1930, by Oxford University Press).

DeSantis L, Thomas J: The immigrant Haitian mother: transcultural nursing perspective on preventive health care for children, *J Transcult Nurs* 2:2, 1990.

Estes G, Zitzow D: Heritage consistency as a consideration in counseling American Indian, Eskimo, or Aleuts. Paper presented at the convention of the National Indian Education Association, Dallas, 1980.

Fuller WP: Recent trends in U.S. refugee policy, *America* 161:238, 1989.

Giger JN, Davidhizar RE: *Transcultural nursing assessment and intervention*, ed 2, St Louis, 1995, Mosby.

Gingrich N, Armey D, and The House Republicans: *Contract with America: the bold plan*, New York, 1994, Random House.

Giordano J, Giordano GP: *The ethno-cultural factor in mental health*, New York, 1977, Institute of Pluralism and Group Identity.

Go GV: Changing populations and health. In Edelman CL, Mandle C: *Health promotion through the life-span*, ed 3, St Louis, 1994, Mosby.

Henry WA III: Beyond the melting pot, *Time* 135:28, April 9, 1990.

Kaptchuk T, Croucher M: *The healing arts*, New York, 1987, Summit Books.

Littlejohn H: Personal interview, Boston, 1979.

Massachusetts Department of Public Health, AIDS Surveillance Summary *HIV/AIDS Quarterly Review*, p 3, July/Aug 1994.

Matsumoto M: *The unspoken way*, Tokyo, 1988, Kodansha International.

Muecke MA: Overcoming the language barrier, *Nurs Outlook* 18:53, 1970.

Parker G: The lived experience of Native Americans with diabetes within a transcultural nursing perspective, *J Transcult Nurs* 6(1):5, 1994.

Shoor D: In Lavelle R, editor: *America's new war on poverty-a reader for action*, San Francisco, 1995, KQED Books.

Spector RE: *Cultural diversity in health and illness,* ed 3, Norwalk, Conn, 1991, Appleton & Lange.

Thernstrom S, editor: *The Harvard encyclopedia of American ethnic groups,* Cambridge, Mass, 1980, Harvard University Press.

U.S. Bureau of the Census: *1990 Census of the Population General Population Characteristics United States,* Washington, DC, 1992, U.S. Government Printing Office.

U.S. Bureau of the Census: *1990 Census of the Population, Education in the United States,* Washington, DC, 1994, U.S. Government Printing Office.

Verhovek SH: Legal immigrants seek citizenship in record numbers, *The New York Times* vol 544, No 50,019, April 2, 1995, pp 1, 28.

Yoder D: Folk medicine. In Dorson HR, editor: *Folklore and folklife,* Chicago, 1972, University of Chicago Press.

ADDITIONAL READINGS

Airhihenbuwa CO: Health education for black or African origin Americans: a neglected task, *Health Educ* 20:9, 1989.

Braithwaite RL et al: Community organization and development for health promotion within an urban black community: a conceptual model, *Health Educ* 20:56, 1989.

Carnegie ME: *The path we tread: blacks in nursing: 1854-1984,* Philadelphia, 1987, Lippincott.

Conway FJ, Carmona PE: Cultural complexity: the hidden stressors, *J Adv Med Surg Nurs* 1(4):65, 1989.

DeSantis L: A profile of cultural diversity in nursing practice, *Fla Nurse* 37:15, 1989.

Dresser N, *Our own stories,* White Plains, NY, 1993, Longman.

Flaskerud JH, Rush CE: AIDS and traditional health beliefs and practices of black women, *Nurs Res* 38(4):210, 1989.

Hammerschlag CA: *The dancing healers: a doctor's journey of healing with American Indian, Eskimo, or Aleuts,* San Francisco, 1988, Harper & Row.

Huttlinger K, Wiebe P: Transcultural nursing care: achieving understanding in a practice setting, *J Transcult Nurs* 1:17, 1989.

Leininger M: The transcultural nurse specialist: imperative in today's world, *Nurs Health Care* 10(5):250, 1989.

Leininger M: Transcultural nurse specialists and generalists: new practitioners in nursing, *J Transcult Nurs* 1:4, 1989.

Leininger M: Issues, questions, and concerns related to the nursing diagnosis cultural movement from a transcultural nursing perspective, *J Transcult Nurs* 2:23, 1990.

McNall MCC, Benner P: Healing we cannot explain, *Am J Nurs* 89(9):1162, 1989.

Morrison T: *Beloved,* New York, 1987, Knopf.

Murray P: *Song in a weary throat: an American pilgrimage,* New York, 1987, Harper & Row.

Sullivan LW: Guest editorial: issues on health care, *J Nat Black Nurse Assoc* 3.3, 1989.

Takaki R, *A different mirror,* Boston, 1993, Little, Brown.

Tripp-Reimer T: Cross-cultural perspectives on patient teaching, *Nurs Clin North Am* 24(3):613, 1989.

Walker A: *The temple of my familiar,* New York, 1989, Harcourt, Brace, Jovanovich.

Zahler D, Zahler KA: *Test your cultural literacy,* New York, 1988, Arco.

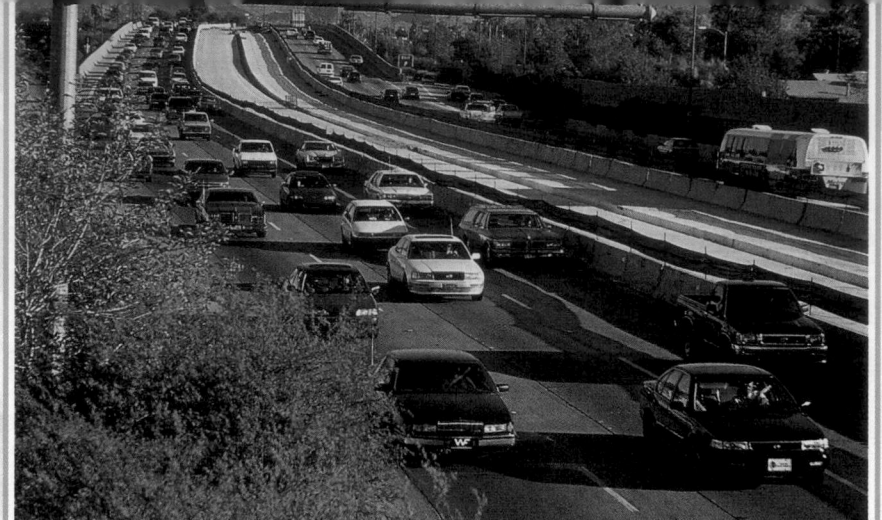

## Chapter 22

Stress and Adaptation

Objectives

Mastery of content in this chapter will enable the student to:

▶ Define the key terms listed.

▶ Discuss the limitations of homeostatic control.

▶ Compare four models of stress as they relate to nursing practice.

▶ Describe how adaptation occurs in each of the five dimensions.

▶ Describe two forms of local physiological adaptation.

▶ Describe the three phases of the general adaptation syndrome.

▶ List and discuss behaviors that are responses to stress.

▶ List and discuss the most common ego-defense mechanisms that are responses to stress.

▶ Discuss the effects of prolonged stress on each of the five dimensions of a person's functioning.

▶ Describe stress-management techniques that nurses can help clients use and use themselves.

▶ Discuss techniques of crisis intervention.

very person experiences forms of stress throughout life. Stress can provide the stimulus for change and growth, and in this respect, some stress is positive and even necessary. However, too much stress can result in poor judgment, physical illness, and inability to cope. A number of studies have proposed a relationship between stressful life events and a wide variety of physical and psychiatric disorders (Yatkin and Labban, 1992). Stress is a phenomenon affecting all dimensions within a person's life.

Claude Bernard, in 1867, was one of the first physiologists to recognize the consequences of stress. He proposed that changes in the internal and external environments disrupted the functioning of an organism and that it was essential for an organism to adapt to a stressor to survive. In 1920, Walter Cannon studied physiological responses to emotional arousal and emphasized the adaptive functions of the "fight-or-flight" reaction. Cannon also noted that these responses were the result of the influence of the emotional state on the body and that the subsequent responses were adaptive and physiological (Robinson, 1990).

Hans Selye developed a biochemical model of stress known as the general adaptation syndrome (GAS), which described physiological events during a stress response. Selye also introduced the concept of stressors, which are internal or external stimuli that cause stress (Selye, 1976). Selye's classic research into stress and stressors has been important for health care professionals. Current research in many disciplines is focused on a variety of stress and stress-related concepts.

∎ CONCEPTS OF STRESS

Stress and Stressors

Everyone experiences stress from time to time, and normally a person is able to adapt to long-term stress or cope with short-term stress until it passes. Stress can place heavy demands on a person, and if the person is unable to adapt, illness can result. **Stress** is any situation in which a nonspecific demand requires an individual to respond or take action (Selye, 1976). It involves physiological and psychological responses. Stress can lead to negative or counterproductive feelings or threaten emotional well-being. It can threaten the way a person normally perceives reality, solves problems, thinks in general; and a person's relationships and sense of belonging. In addition, stress can threaten a person's general outlook on life, attitude toward loved ones, and health status (Kline-Leidy, 1990; Oberst et al, 1991; Kosciulek, McCubbin, and McCubbin, 1993).

An individual's perception or experience of a major change initiates the stress response. The stimuli preceding or precipitating the change are called **stressors.** Stressors represent an unmet need and may be physiological, psychological, social, environmental, developmental, spiritual, or cultural. Stressors can generally be classified as internal or external. **Internal stressors** originate inside a person (e.g., a fever, a condition such as pregnancy or menopause, or an emotion such as guilt). **External stressors** originate outside a person (e.g., a marked change in environmental temperature, a change in family or social role, or peer pressure).

Physiological Adaptation

Physiological adaptation to stress is the body's ability to maintain a state of relative balance. This adaptive ability is a dynamic form of equilibrium in the body's internal environment. The internal environment constantly changes, and the body's adaptive mechanisms continually function to adjust to these changes and thus to maintain equilibrium, or **homeostasis.**

Homeostasis is maintained by physiological mechanisms that control body functions and monitor body organs. For the most part these mechanisms are controlled by the nervous and endocrine systems and do not involve conscious behavior. The body makes adjustments in heart rate, respiratory rate, blood pressure, temperature, fluid and electrolyte balances, hormone secretions, and level of consciousness—all directed at maintaining adaptation.

MECHANISMS OF PHYSIOLOGICAL ADAPTATION

When a person becomes aware of an unmet physiological need, such as food or warmth, deliberate actions can meet the need. For the most part, however, adaptation involves adjustments that the body makes automatically to maintain equilibrium. These homeostatic mechanisms are self-regulatory; in other words, they are automatic. In a person with an illness or injury, however, the mechanisms may not be able to maintain and sustain homeostasis.

Physiological mechanisms of adaptation function through negative feedback, a process by which the controlling mechanism senses an abnormal state, such as lowered body temperature, and makes an adaptive response, such as initiating shivering to generate body heat. Three of the major mechanisms used in adapting to a stressor are controlled by the medulla oblongata, the reticular formation, and the pituitary gland.

Medulla Oblongata. The medulla oblongata controls vital functions necessary to survival. These include heart rate, blood pressure, and respiration. Impulses traveling to and from the medulla oblongata can increase or decrease these vital functions. For example, regulation of the heart beat is the result of sympathetic or parasympathetic nervous system impulses traveling from the medulla oblongata to the heart. The heart rate increases in response to pulses from sympathetic fibers and decreases with impulses from parasympathetic fibers.

Reticular Formation. The reticular formation is a small cluster of neurons in the brainstem and spinal cord. It also controls vital functions and continuously monitors the physiological status of the body through connections with sensory and motor tracts. For example, certain cells within the reticular formation can cause a sleeping person to regain consciousness or increase the level of consciousness when a need arises.

Pituitary Gland. The pituitary gland, a small gland attached to the hypothalamus, supplies hormones that control vital functions. The pituitary gland produces hormones necessary for adaptation to stress. In addition, the pituitary gland regulates the secretion of thyroid, gonadal, and parathyroid hormones. Hormone secretion, like other homeostatic mechanisms, is normally regulated by a feedback mechanism that continuously monitors hormone levels in the blood. When hormone levels drop, the pituitary gland receives a message to increase hormone secretion. When hormone levels rise, the pituitary gland decreases hormone production.

LIMITATIONS OF PHYSIOLOGICAL MECHANISMS OF ADAPTATION

Physiological mechanisms of adaptation work together through complex relationships in the nervous and endocrine systems and other body systems to maintain a relative constancy within the body. In a healthy person these mechanisms affect physiological balance and the body's needs are met. However, physiological mechanisms of adaptation can provide only short-term control over the body's equilibrium. They cannot adapt to long-term changes in hormone secretion or vital functions. Thus illness, injury, or prolonged stress can decrease the adaptive capacity. Decreased functioning can result in continued but inadequate homeostatic control or breakdown of the feedback mechanism that allows control. Either form of decreased function can result in further illness or death.

In severe stress situations, for example, the pituitary gland supplies the body with the necessary hormones. However, these hormones may be insufficient in quantity to provide the physiological energy necessary for coping. In this case the person's condition deteriorates and functioning declines. The feedback mechanism of homeostatic control may break down because of organ abnormality.

Models of Stress

The origins and effects of stress can be examined in terms of medical and behavioral theoretical models. Stress models are used to identify the stressors for a particular individual and predict that person's responses to them. Each model emphasizes a different aspect of stress.

The nurse uses stress models to help a client cope with unhealthy, nonproductive responses to stressors. With modifications, these models can help the nurse respond in a caring, individualized way.

RESPONSE-BASED MODEL OF STRESS

The response-based model is concerned with specifying the particular response or pattern of responses that may indicate a stressor. Selye's model of stress (1976) is a response-based model that defines stress as a nonspecific response of the body to any demand made on it. Stress is demonstrated by a specific physiological reaction, the GAS. Thus the response of a person to stress is purely physiological and is never modified to allow cognitive influences (McNett, 1989).

The response-based model does not allow individual differences in response patterns. This lack of flexibility may produce some difficulties for nurses because individual differences must be identified in the assessment phase. However, it may be most useful when determining physiological responses.

ADAPTATION MODEL

The adaptation model proposes that four factors determine whether a situation is stressful (Mechanic, 1962). The ability to cope with stress, the first factor, usually depends on the person's experience with similar stressors, support systems, and overall perception of the stressor.

The second factor deals with the practices and norms of the person's peer group. If the peer group considers it normal to talk about a particular stressor, the client may respond by complaining about it or discussing it. This response may help adaptation to the stress, or the client may respond in this way simply to conform to peer group behavior.

The third factor is the impact of the social environment in assisting an individual to adapt to a stressor. For example, a homeless woman with schizophrenia may seek assistance from a clinic nurse practitioner about an acute pelvic infection. The nurse may then assess and make a referral to a local community hospital for IV antibiotic therapy. The nurse and the hospital in this example are resources for the client to reduce the severity of a stressor.

The last factor involves the resources that can be used to deal with the stressor. In the example just given, the client needs transportation to the hospital and Medicaid coverage or financial arrangements that will provide for her care. Both of these factors will influence how she can access the resource to help her cope with the physiological stressor.

The adaptation model is based on the understanding that people experience anxiety and increased stress when they are unprepared to cope with stressful situations. Using this model and appropriate interventions, nurses can help clients and families to promote health in all human dimensions.

STIMULUS-BASED MODEL

The stimulus-based model focuses on disturbing or disruptive characteristics within the environment. The classic research that identified stress as a stimulus has resulted in the development of the social readjustment scale, which measures the effects of major life events on illness (Holmes and Rahe, 1976). The stimulus-based model focuses on the following assumptions (McNett, 1989):

1. Life change events are normal, and they require the same type and duration of adjustment.
2. People are passive recipients of stress, and their perceptions of the event are irrelevant.
3. All people have a common threshold of stimulus, and illness results at any point after the threshold.

As with the response-based model, the stimulus-based model does not allow for individual differences in perception and response to stressors. Nurses may experience difficulty when attempting to use this model in stress management because of the lack of flexibility for individual adaptation.

TRANSACTION-BASED MODEL

The transaction-based model views the person and environment in a dynamic, reciprocal, interactive, relationship (Lazarus and Folkman, 1984). This model, developed by Lazarus and Folkman, views the stressor as an individual perceptual response rooted in psychological and cognitive processes. Stress originates from the relationship between the person and the environment. This model focuses on stress-related processes such as cognitive appraisal and coping (Monsen, Floyd, and Brookman, 1992).

Factors Influencing Response to Stressors

The response to any stressor depends on physiological functioning, personality, and behavioral characteristics, as well as the nature of the stressor. The nature of the stressor involves the following factors:

1. Intensity
2. Scope
3. Duration
4. Number and nature of other stressors

Each factor influences the response to a stressor. A person may perceive the intensity or magnitude of a stressor as minimal, moderate, or severe. The greater the magnitude of the stressor, the greater the stress response. Likewise, the scope of a stressor can be described as limited, medium, or extensive. The greater the scope of a stressor, the greater the response of the client to it (Lazarus and Folkman, 1984).

∎ ADAPTATION TO STRESSORS

Adaptation is the process by which the physiological or psychosocial dimensions change in response to stress. Because many stressors cannot be avoided, health promotion often focuses on a person's, family's, or community's adaptation to stress.

There are many forms of adaptation. Physiological adaptations make possible a physiological homeostasis. A similar process of adaptation, however, may occur in the psychosocial and other dimensions.

An adaptive response occurs when a stimulus from the internal or external environment causes a departure from the balanced state of the organism. Adaptation thus is an attempt to maintain optimal functioning. Adaptation involves reflexes, automatic body mechanisms for protection, coping mechanisms, and ideally can lead to adjustment or mastery of a situation (Selye, 1976; Monsen, Floyd, and Brookman, 1992). A stressor that stimulates adaptation may be short term, such as a fever, or long term, such as paralysis of a limb. To function optimally, a person must be able to respond to such stressors and adapt to the required demands or changes. Adaptation requires an active response from the whole person.

Like an individual, a family or group may need to adapt to a stressor. Family adaptation is the process by which a family maintains a balance so that it can fulfill its purposes and tasks, deal with stress, and promote the growth of individual members. For a family to adapt successfully, good communication skills, mutual respect for all family members, adequate resources for adaptation, and previous experience with stressors must exist (Haber, 1990; Fox, 1991).

Dimensions of Adaptation

Stress can affect the physical, developmental, emotional, intellectual, social, and spiritual dimensions. Adaptive resources exist in each of these dimensions. Therefore, when assessing a client's adaptation to a stress a nurse must consider the total person. Table 22-1 highlights adaptive re-

Table 22-1	**Dimensions of Adaptation**				

DIMENSION	ADAPTIVE RESOURCES	EXAMPLE OF STRESSOR	EXAMPLE OF UNSUCCESSFUL OUTCOME	EXAMPLE OF SUCCESSFUL OUTCOME
Physical	Local adaptation syndrome General adaptation syndrome	Fever	Death	Infection resolved
Developmental	Successful coping in past development task/stages Successful adaptation to past stressors	Retirement	Depression	Role functions altered to other meaningful activities
Emotional	Psychological defense mechanisms Individual personality strengths	Rape	Irrational fear of men	Integration of traumatic memory Serves as advocate for others at rape crisis center
Intellectual	Formal education Ability to problem solve Communication skills Realistic perception of stressor Conscious mobilization of past positive coping strategies	Diagnosis of cancer	Denies presence of cancer and foregoes any treatment	Uses an active problem-solving approach to make decisions about care
Social	Social network provides support Others may direct person to needed resources	Alcoholism in a family member	Person with alcoholism withdraws from family and other social contacts	Active participation of all family members in Alcoholics Anonymous support groups
Spiritual	Prayer groups; support from priest, rabbi, or minister	Ill family member feels that God has abandoned him or her	Withdraws from attending church, won't talk with church members or minister	Begins to seek out friends in the church, volunteers for church-related activities

sources found in each dimension and gives examples of positive and negative outcomes of stressors.

■ RESPONSE TO STRESS

The total person is involved in responding and adapting to stresses. Most research into stress responses, however, focuses on psychological or emotional and physiological responses, even though these dimensions overlap and interact with the other dimensions.

When stress occurs, a person uses physiological and psychological energy to respond and adapt. The amount of energy required and the effectiveness of the attempt to adapt depend on the intensity, scope, and duration of the stressor and the number of other stressors. The stress response is adaptive and protective, and the characteristics of this response are the result of integrated neuroendocrine response (see the box below).

Physiological Response

The classic research by Selye (1946, 1976) has identified the two physiological responses to stress: the **local adaptation syndrome (LAS)** and the **general adaptation syndrome (GAS)**. The LAS is a response of a body tissue, organ, or part to the stress of trauma, illness, or other physiological change. The GAS is a defense response of the whole body to stress.

LAS

The body produces many localized responses to stress. These include blood clotting, wound healing (see Chapter 49), accommodation of the eye to light, and response to pressure (see Chapter 38). All forms of the LAS share the following characteristics:

1. The response is localized; it does not involve entire body systems.
2. The response is adaptive, meaning that a stressor is necessary to stimulate it.

Characteristics of the Stress Response

- Stress response is natural, protective, and adaptive.
- There are normal responses to stressors; stressors encountered in everyday circumstances increase catecholamine excretion, which causes an increase in heart rate and blood pressure.
- Physical and emotional stressors trigger similar responses (specificity versus nonspecificity). Magnitude and patterns may differ.
- There are limits in ability to compensate.
- Magnitude and duration of stressors may be so great that homeostatic mechanisms for adjustment fail, leading to death.
- Repeated exposure to stimuli results in adaptive changes; that is, tissue levels of the enzyme tyrosine hydrolase increase, which increases capacity for the body to produce norepinephrine and epinephrine.
- There are individual differences in response to same stressors.

Modified from Lindsay AM, Carrieri VK, Page GG: Stress response. In Lindsay AM, Carrieri VK, editors: *Pathological phenomenon in nursing: human response to illness,* ed 2, Philadelphia, 1993, Saunders.

---

3. The response is short term. It does not persist indefinitely.
4. The response is restorative, meaning that the LAS assists in restoring homeostasis to the body region or part.

Two localized responses, the reflex pain response and the inflammatory response, are described here as examples of the LAS. Nurses encounter these responses in many health care settings.

Reflex Pain Response. The reflex pain response is a localized response of the central nervous system to pain (see Chapter 43). It is an adaptive response and protects tissue from further damage. The response involves a sensory receptor, a sensory nerve to the spinal cord, a connector neuron within the spinal cord, a motor nerve from the spinal cord, and an effector muscle. An example would be the unconscious, reflex removal of the hand from a hot surface. Another example would be a muscle cramp.

Inflammatory Response. The inflammatory response is stimulated by trauma or infection. This response localizes the inflammation, thus preventing its spread, and promotes healing. The inflammatory response may produce localized pain, swelling, heat, redness, and changes in functioning. It occurs in three phases. The first phase involves changes in cells and the circulatory system. Initially, narrowing of blood vessels occurs at the injury to control bleeding. Then histamine is released at the injury, increasing blood flow to the area and increasing the number of white blood cells to combat infection. Almost simultaneously kinins are released to increase capillary permeability to permit the flow of proteins, fluid, and leukocytes to the injury. At this point the localized blood flow decreases, keeping leukocytes in the area to fight infection.

The second phase is characterized by release of exudate from the wound. Exudate is a combination of fluid, cells, and other substances produced in the area of injury. The type and amount of exudate vary from injury to injury and from person to person. Exudate is usually released at the injury, which may be a cut, laceration, or surgical incision. The last phase is repair of tissue by regeneration or scar formation. Regeneration replaces damaged cells with identical or similar cells. Scar formation replaces original tissue that is not functional. The inflammatory response alerts the nurse that the body is adapting to a local injury. During adaptation the inflammatory response protects the body from infection and promotes healing.

GAS

The GAS is a physiological response of the whole body to stress. It involves several body systems, primarily the autonomic nervous system and the endocrine system. Some textbooks refer to the GAS as the neuroendocrine response. The GAS consists of the alarm reaction, the resistance stage, and the exhaustion stage (Fig. 22-1).

Alarm Reaction. The alarm reaction involves the mobilization of the defense mechanisms of the body and mind to cope with the stressor. Hormone levels rise to increase blood volume and thereby prepare the person to act. Other hormones are released to increase blood glucose levels to make energy available for adaptation. Increased levels of other hormones—epinephrine and norepinephrine—result in an increased heart rate, increased blood flow to muscles, increased oxygen intake, and greater mental alertness.

This extensive hormonal activity prepares the person for the **fight-or-flight response.** Cardiac output, oxygen intake, and respiratory rate are increased; the pupils of the eyes are dilated to produce a greater visual field; and the heart rate is increased for more energy. Other changes occur to prepare the person to act (Fig. 22-2). With this increased mental energy and alertness, the person is prepared to flight or flee the stressor.

During the alarm reaction the person is faced with a specific stressor. The person's physiological response is exten-sive, involving major systems of the body, and it may last from a minute to many hours. If the stressor is extreme or remains for a long time, there may be a threat to life. If the stressor is still present after the initial alarm reaction, the person progresses to the second phase of the GAS, resistance.

Resistance Stage. In the resistance stage the body stabilizes, and hormone levels, heart rate, blood pressure, and cardiac output return to normal. The person is attempting to adapt to the stressor. If the stress can be resolved, the body repairs damage that may have occurred. However, if the stressor remains present, as in continued blood loss, de-

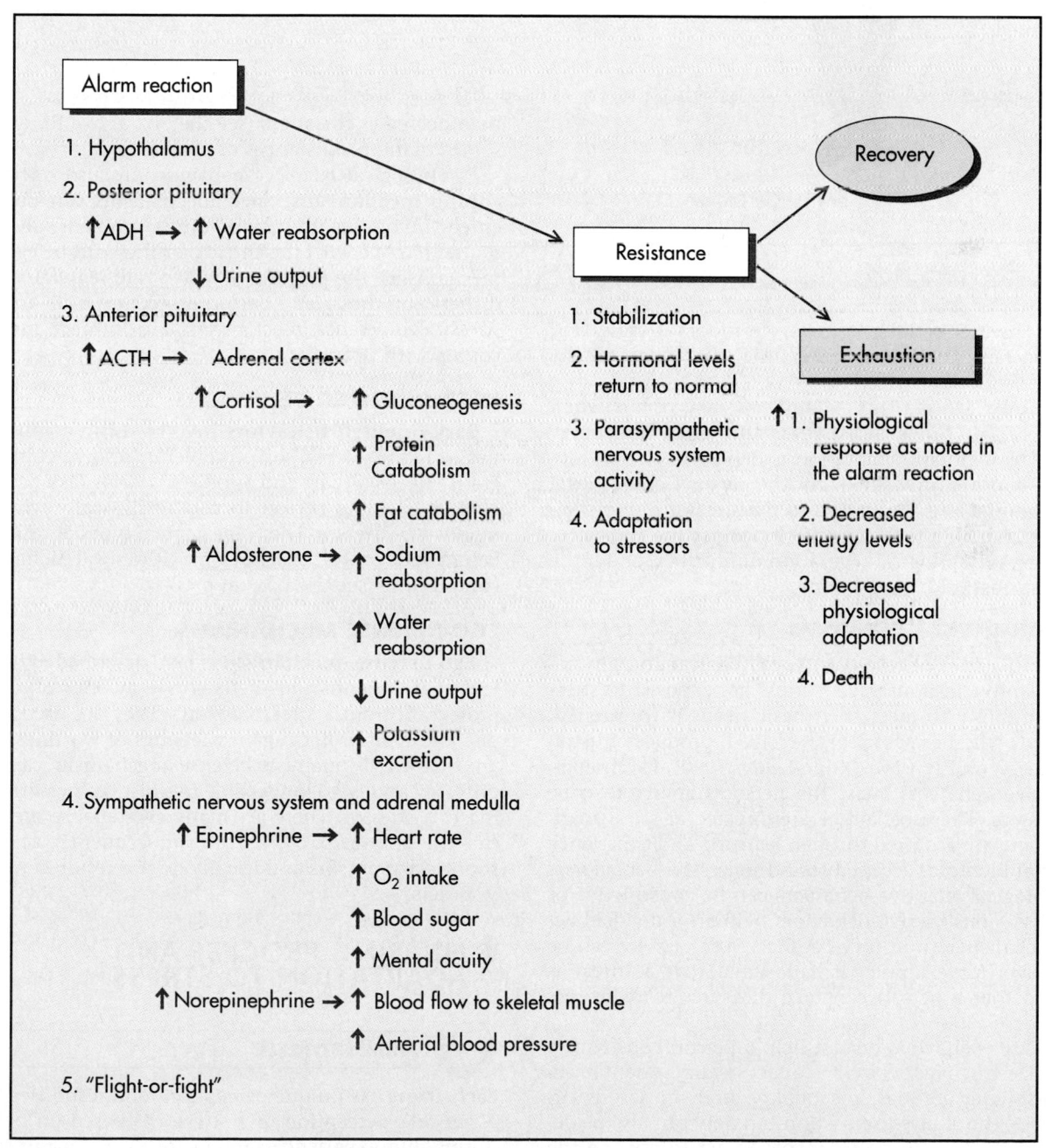

Fig. 22-1 General adaptation syndrome (GAS).

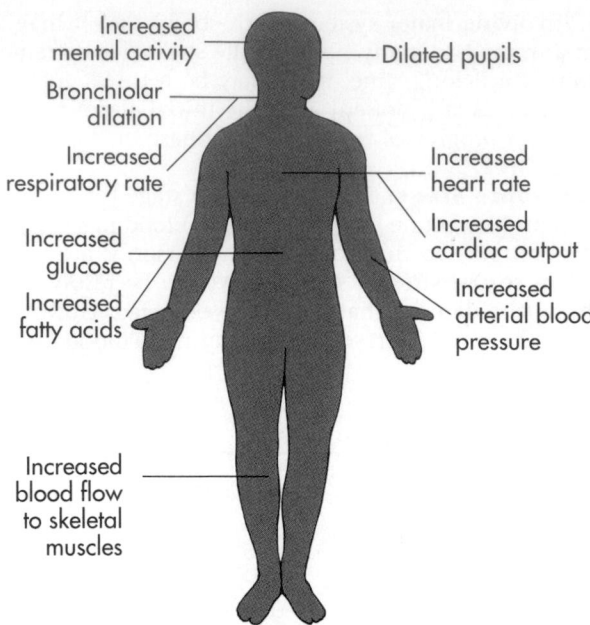

Fig. 22-2 Fight-or-flight response.

Common Drugs of Abuse	
Alcohol	(beer, wine, "hard" liquor)
Amphetamine	(crank)
Caffeine	(coffee, tea, colas)
Cannabis	(marijuana)
Cocaine	(crack)
Hallucinogens	(LSD, peyote)
Inhalants	(glue, gasoline)
Nicotine	(cigarettes)
Opioids	(morphine, heroin)
Sedative, hypnotic,	(diazepam, barbiturates)
anxiolytic	
Anabolic steroids	
PCP	

bilitating disease, or long-term severe mental illness, and adaptation fails, the person enters the third phase of the GAS, exhaustion.

Exhaustion Stage. The exhaustion stage occurs when the body can no longer resist stress and when the energy necessary to maintain adaptation is depleted. The physiological response is intensified, but the person's energy level is compromised and adaptation to the stressor diminishes. The body is unable to defend itself against the impact of the stressor, physiological regulation diminishes, and if the stress continues, death may result.

Psychological Response

Exposure to a stressor results in psychological and physiological adaptive responses. As people are exposed to stressors, their ability to meet their basic needs is threatened. This threat, whether actual or perceived, produces frustration, anxiety, and tension (Kline-Leidy, 1990). Psychological adaptive behaviors assist the person's ability to cope with stressors. These behaviors are directed at stress management and are acquired through learning and experience as a person identifies acceptable and successful behaviors.

Psychological adaptive behaviors can be constructive or destructive. Constructive behaviors help an individual accept the challenge to resolve conflict. Even anxiety can be constructive; for example, it can signal that a threat is present so that a person can take measures to reduce its severity.

Destructive behaviors do not help a person cope with a stressor. Destructive behaviors affect reality orientation, problem-solving abilities, personality, and, in severe circumstances, the ability to function. Anxiety can also be destructive (e.g., if a person is unable to act to remove the stressor). To some, the abuse of alcohol or drugs may seem to be an adaptive behavior; in reality, it increases rather than decreases the stress (see the box above for a listing of some common substances of abuse).

Psychological adaptive behaviors are also referred to as **coping mechanisms.** Such mechanisms can be task oriented, involving the use of direct problem-solving techniques to cope with the threats, or they can be ego-defense mechanisms, the purpose of which is to regulate emotional distress and thus give a person protection from anxiety and stress. Ego-defense mechanisms are indirect methods of coping with stress.

TASK-ORIENTED BEHAVIORS

Task-oriented behaviors involve using cognitive abilities to reduce stress, solve problems, resolve conflicts, and gratify needs (Stuart and Sundeen, 1991). Task-oriented behaviors enable a person to cope realistically with the demands of a stressor. The three general types of task-oriented behavior are attack behavior, withdrawal behavior, and compromise (see the box on p. 377).

EGO-DEFENSE MECHANISMS

Ego-defense mechanisms, first described by Sigmund Freud, are unconscious behaviors that offer psychological protection from a stressful event. They are used by everyone and help protect against feelings of worthlessness and anxiety. Occasionally a defense mechanism can become distorted and is no longer able to assist the person in adapting to a stressor. There are many ego-defense mechanisms (see the box on p. 377). They are frequently activated by short-term stressors and usually do not result in psychiatric disorders.

■ NURSING PROCESS AND ADAPTATION TO STRESS

 Assessment

Each client has unique perceptions and responses to stress. A person's perception of a stressor is based on beliefs and norms, life experiences and patterns, environmental factors, family structure and function, developmental stage, past experiences with stress, and coping mechanisms.

Psychological Adaptive Behaviors

TASK-ORIENTED BEHAVIORS
- Attack behavior is acting to remove or overcome a stressor or to satisfy a need.
- Withdrawal behavior is removing the self physically or emotionally from the stressor.
- Compromise behavior is changing the usual method of operating, substituting goals, or omitting the satisfaction of needs to meet other needs or to avoid stress.

EXAMPLES OF EGO-DEFENSE MECHANISMS
- Compensation is making up for a deficiency in one aspect of self-image by strongly emphasizing a feature considered an asset.
- Conversion is unconsciously repressing an anxiety-producing emotional conflict and transforming it into nonorganic symptoms.
- Denial is avoiding emotional conflicts by refusing to consciously acknowledge anything that might cause intolerable emotional pain.
- Displacement is transferring emotions, ideas, or wishes from a stressful situation to a less anxiety-producing substitute.
- Identification is patterning behavior after that of another person and assuming that person's qualities, characteristics, and actions.
- Regression is coping with a stressor through actions and behaviors associated with an earlier developmental period.

Physiological Indicators of Stress

- Elevated blood pressure
- Increased muscle tension in neck, shoulders, back
- Elevated pulse and increased respiration
- Sweaty palms
- Cold hands and feet
- Slumped posture
- Fatigue
- Tension headache
- Upset stomach
- Higher-pitched voice
- Nausea, vomiting, and diarrhea
- Change in appetite
- Change in weight
- Change in urinary frequency
- Abnormal laboratory findings: elevated adrenocorticotropic hormone, cortisol, and catecholamine levels and hyperglycemia
- Restlessness: difficulty falling asleep or frequent awakening
- Dilated pupils

Because nurses spend a great deal of time with clients and their families or friends, they are in an optimal position to critically analyze coping responses. Nurses also provide care for clients in various settings, and thus they are often able to assess reactions to stress. The nurse assesses for indicators of stress and coping in all dimensions of adaptation.

PHYSIOLOGICAL INDICATORS

Physiological indicators of stress are objective, more readily identified and can be commonly observed or measured (see the box above, right). However, they are not always observed all the time in all clients experiencing stress, and they vary with individuals. Vital signs are usually elevated, and the client may appear restless and be unable to rest or concentrate. These indicators can appear at any stage of stress.

The duration and intensity of the symptoms are directly related to the perceived duration and intensity of the stressor. Physiological indicators arise from a variety of systems. Therefore the assessment of stress involves collecting data from all systems.

The link between psychological stress and disease is frequently called the *mind-body interaction*. Research has shown that stress can affect illness and disease patterns. At the turn of the century, infectious diseases were the leading causes of death, but since then antibiotics, improved living conditions, increased knowledge of nutrition, and better sanitation methods have lowered the death rate. Now the leading causes of death are diseases involving lifestyle stressors.

During any stage there may be physical complaints such as nausea, vomiting, diarrhea, or headache. Physical appearance is changed; posture may be slumped, hygiene and grooming are poor, and style of dress differs. Prolonged stress has been linked with cardiovascular and gastrointestinal diseases. Some cancers and immunological disorders, as well as migraine headaches, burnout, and irritability, are associated with prolonged, unresolved stressors (Peddicord, 1991; Hufft, 1992; Cooper and Faragher, 1993; Schedlowski, 1993).

Mild stress situations do not usually produce chronic physiological damage, but moderate and severe stress can create a risk of medical illness or a worsening of a chronic illness (Kline-Leidy, 1990). **Mild stress situations** are stressors that everyone encounters regularly, such as oversleeping, traffic jams, a flat tire, or criticism from a superior. Such situations usually last a few minutes to a few hours. By themselves, these stressors are not significant risks for symptom development. However, multiple mild stressors over a short time can increase risk of illness (Holmes and Rahe, 1976).

Moderate stress situations last longer, from several hours to days. For example, an unresolved disagreement with a co-worker, a sick child, or the prolonged absence of a family member are moderate stress situations.

Severe stress situations are chronic situations that may last several weeks to several years, such as continual marital disagreements, prolonged financial difficulties, and long-term physical illness. The more frequent and longer the stress situation, the higher the health risk (Wiebe and Williams, 1992). The development of stress-related disease can be examined in terms of the health-illness continuum (Fig. 22-3). As a person's stress increases, stress behaviors increase gradually, which decreases energy and adaptive responses.

Identifying the mind-body interaction is crucial for predicting the risk of stress-related illness. A nurse also criti-

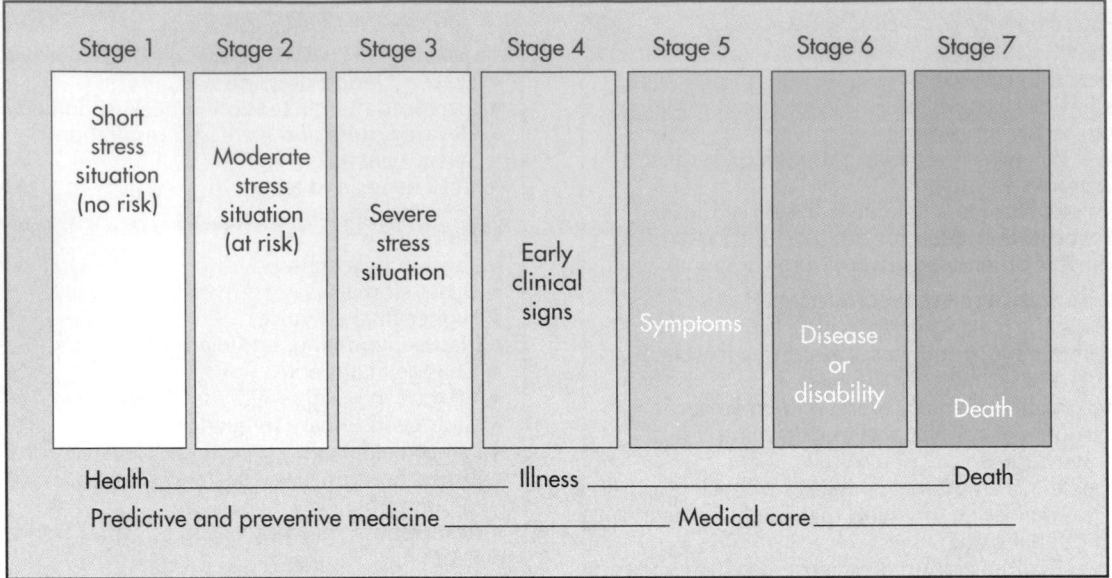

Fig. 22-3 Stages of illness development in stress-related diseases.

cally assesses the client's perception of stressors, for what may seem a mild stress situation to the nurse may be extremely disturbing to the client.

DEVELOPMENTAL INDICATORS

Prolonged stress can affect the ability to complete developmental tasks. In any developmental stage a person normally encounters tasks and engages in behaviors characteristic of the stage. Prolonged stress can interrupt or impede passage through the stage. In extreme forms, prolonged stress can lead to maturational crises.

Infants or young children generally encounter stressors at home. When nurtured in responsive, empathetic environments, they are able to develop healthy self-esteem and ultimately learn healthy adaptive coping responses (Haber et al, 1992). However, the absence of parental figures or their failure to provide the security needed to develop a sense of trust can be stressors. In later life there may be chronic distrust, resulting in withdrawal and disturbed interpersonal relationships. If parents or the environment prevent children from developing a sense of autonomy, the children may experience stress, which is indicated by excessive dependence on others or passive inactive behavior.

School-age children normally develop a sense of adequacy. They begin to realize that accumulation of knowledge and mastery of skills can help them accomplish goals, and self-esteem develops through friendships and sharing with peers. At this stage stress is indicated by the inability or unwillingness to develop friendships.

Adolescents normally develop a strong sense of identity but at the same time need to be accepted by peers. Adolescents with strong social support systems report an increased ability to adjust to stressors, but adolescents without social support systems frequently report increased psychosocial problems (DuBois et al, 1992). There are many stressors in this age group, including conflicts involving sexual drive and expected standards of behavior. Prolonged

conflict may present as indecision and confusion, rebellion, depression, or anxiety.

Young adults are in transition from youthful experiences to adult responsibilities. They must prepare for careers, for living alone, and perhaps for starting families. Conflicts may develop between work and family responsibilities. Stressors include conflicts between expectations and reality. Kolotylo, Parker, and Chapman (1990) studied the stress experience of 15 mothers whose newborns were admitted into neonatal intensive care units or intermediate-care units. The mothers reported frustrations over the expectation of healthy newborns and the reality of having very ill infants. Because of the conflict between expectation and reality, the mothers experienced feelings of helplessness, fear of the unknown, and alienation from other mothers (see the box on p. 379).

Middle-age adults are usually involved in family building, creating stable careers, and perhaps caring for older parents. They are generally able to control desires and in some cases substitute the needs of spouses, children, or parents for their needs. Stress can result, however, if they feel that too many responsibilities have been placed on them. A recent trend is looking at the impact of stressors of the family care giver's role. The middle years have been called the *sandwich generation* in which middle adults are frequently responsible for chronically ill parents while raising their own families. Because of the stressors involved, care givers have reported increases in fatigue, minor illnesses (e.g., colds and influenza), depression, and dissatisfaction with family interaction (Musolf, 1991).

Older adults are commonly faced with adapting to changes in family and perhaps to the deaths of spouses or longtime friends. Older adults must also adjust to changes in physical appearance and physiological functioning. Major life changes such as retirement also are stressful. Some older adults must cope with relocation to some form of institutionalized living. Moving to a nursing home may be

▶ RESEARCH HIGHLIGHT

RESEARCH ABSTRACT

A caring nursing approach involves sensitivity to cultural differences in coping with stress. This study looked at family processes among low income, female headed inner city families that were primarily African American. The researcher found increased family stress and lower levels of social support when compared to white Anglo-Saxon Protestant families. Nursing interventions that targeted family stress and increased coping were recommended.

IMPLICATIONS FOR PRACTICE

▶ Recognize female headed, low income families may be experiencing high stress and have minimal social supports.

▶ If present, the nurse should intervene to assist with stress reduction and augment social support.

REFERENCE

Murata J: Family stress, social support, violence, and son's behavior, *West J Nurs Res* 16(2), 154, 1994.

Behavioral and Emotional Indicators of Stress

- Anxiety
- Depression
- Burnout
- Increased use of chemical substances
- Change in eating habits, sleep, and activity pattern
- Mental exhaustion
- Feelings of inadequacy
- Loss of self-esteem
- Increased irritability
- Loss of motivation
- Emotional outbursts and crying
- Decreased productivity and quality of job performance
- Tendency to make mistakes (i.e., poor judgment)
- Forgetfulness and blocking
- Diminished attention to detail
- Preoccupation (i.e., daydreaming or "spacing out")
- Inability to concentrate on tasks
- Increased absenteeism and illness
- Lethargy
- Loss of interest
- Proneness to accidents

particularly stressful for an older person and can aggravate existing health and emotional problems (Mikhail, 1992; Porter and Clinton, 1992).

EMOTIONAL BEHAVIORAL INDICATORS

Emotions are sometimes assessed directly or indirectly by observing a client's behavior. Stress affects emotional well-being in many ways (see the box above, right). Because an individual personality involves a complex relationship among factors, the reaction to prolonged stress is determined by examining the client's current lifestyle and stressors, prior experiences with stressors, past successful coping mechanisms, role functions, self concept and **hardiness**, which is a combination of three personality characteristics thought to mediate against stress. These three characteristics are sense of control over life events, commitment to meaningful activities, and anticipation of challenge as an opportunity for growth (Wiebe and Williams, 1992; Tartasky, 1993).

INTELLECTUAL INDICATORS

Prolonged stress can manifest itself in the intellectual dimension and have observable indicators. A person's ability to acquire new knowledge or skills is impaired. A person's cognitive appraisal of a situation may also be inaccurate. Stress can impede communication between the client and others. The family may be unable to resolve conflicts. In addition, the client's ability to effectively solve problems is reduced. As a result, increased dependence on others occurs.

SOCIAL INDICATORS

Assessing stressors and coping resources in the social dimension involves exploring with the client the amount, type, and quality of social interactions present. Stressors on the family may create dysfunction that affects the client or the family as a whole (Reis and Heppner, 1993).

The nurse must also be aware of cultural differences in stress responses or coping mechanisms. For example, an

CULTURAL ASPECTS OF CARE

A caring nursing approach involves sensitivity to cultural differences in coping with stress. Nurse researchers, along with a translator, interviewed 120 Cambodian refugee women in two sites in the United States. They found that these women tended to cope by the use of nonconfrontation and withdrawal, two culturally approved strategies. These two themes were seen as ways women control and harmonize stressful situations. Nurses must recognize that coping styles of nonconfrontation and withdrawal may not represent maladaptive responses in the Cambodian cultural group. In addition, communication may not be as direct as in the dominant American culture, underlying problems such as depression may be overlooked, so the nurse may need to gently explore situations that may be mentioned obliquely (Frye and D'Avanzo, 1994).

African American client may prefer obtaining social support from family members rather than professional assistance (Murata, 1994) (see the box above).

SPIRITUAL INDICATORS

People use spiritual resources to adapt to stress in many ways, but stress can also manifest itself in the spiritual dimension. Severe stress may result in anger at the supreme being, or the person may view the stressor as punishment. Stressors such as acute illness or the death of a loved one may threaten a person's meaning of life and can lead to depression. When providing care to a client who is affected spiritually, a nurse should not judge the appropriateness of religious feelings or practices but should examine how beliefs and values have changed (see Chapter 25).

Nursing Diagnosis

A review of assessment data leads the nurse to cluster data that may indicate a potential or actual stressor and the client's response. Clustering of data, along with the application of the nurse's knowledge and experience with clients in stress, leads to a nursing diagnosis. For example, changes in appetite and sleeping patterns and increased frequency of headaches are defining characteristics for ineffective individual coping, which is a frequent nursing diagnosis for clients experiencing stress (see the nursing diagnoses box at right). Identification of a nursing diagnostic label requires the presence of appropriate defining characteristics (see the diagnostic process box on p. 381). The diagnostic label must be supported by the defining characteristics in the data base.

The nursing diagnosis should identify the probable etiology for the problem. Incorrect identification of the cause of a nursing diagnosis can result in an inappropriate care plan and selected interventions. For example, ineffective individual coping related to inadequate support system results in interventions designed to increase the client's support resources (e.g., friends, family, support groups). If the nurse incorrectly identified unmet expectations as the related factor, then the plan of care is not directed toward the resolution of the nursing diagnosis. Stress can result in multiple diagnostic statements. Examples selected here do not represent the entire list. Unit 4 contains additional nursing diagnoses that occur when an individual has unmet needs resulting from stress. Chapters 21, 23 and 25 include nursing diagnoses associated with unmet sociocultural, self-concept, and spiritual needs. This process of nursing diagnosis corresponds with the diagnostic monitoring function domain of nursing practice.

Planning

The formulation of nursing diagnoses initiates the formation of a care plan (see the care plan on p. 381). The care plan is individualized to the client's perception of the stressor and response to stress. The nurse and client mutually develop realistic goals, expected outcomes, and interventions designed to assist the client with coping with the stressor. Whenever appropriate, a friend or family member should be involved in planning. Sensitivity to specific cultural stressors and expressions of adaptation also will promote a sense of being cared about when the plan is made.

In most situations, stress-management plans are long term and are conducted in the client's home or on an outpatient basis. Therefore the nurse must also know about the availability and cost of resources in the community.

Stress-management techniques are designed to match the client's actual and potential stressors. The general goals for clients who require stress management include the following:

1. Reduction in frequency of stress-inducing situations
2. Decreased physiological response to stress
3. Improved behavioral and emotional responses to stress

Examples of NANDA Nursing Diagnoses for Stress

Anxiety *related to:*
- Change in health status
- Maturational or situational crisis

Altered growth and development *related to:*
- Separation from significant others
- Situational crisis (e.g., unplanned pregnancy)

Caregiver role strain *related to:*
- Adjustment to medical diagnosis
- Adjustment to decreased level of physical function

Fatigue *related to:*
- Overwhelming psychological demands
- Excessive role demands

Hopelessness *related to:*
- Long-term stress
- Lost belief in values

Ineffective family coping: compromised or **disabling** or **ineffective individual coping** *related to:*
- Inadequate coping methods
- Prolonged stress (e.g., physiological, maturational, situational)

Risk for injury *related to:*
- Impaired problem-solving abilities

Sleep pattern disturbance *related to:*
- Maturational or situational crisis

Implementation

Stress management may be seen as a health promotion activity or an intervention that modifies a response to illness. The focus depends on the purpose of the nursing interventions based on the client's needs. The nurse is responsible for implementing thoughtful interventions that are carried out in several nursing domains.

Health Promotion

Before specific stress management techniques are taught to the client, the nurse must establish a helping role. Creation of a trusting, caring environment serves as a foundation for any behavior change. "Presencing" or just "being there" for the client fosters a sense of support that facilitates personal growth (Monsen, Floyd, and Brookman, 1992; Campbell-Heider and Hart). When helping the client reduce stress, the nurse reduces stressful situations, decreases the physiological response to stress, and improves the behavioral and emotional responses to stress.

REDUCING STRESSFUL SITUATIONS

It is unrealistic to try to eliminate all stressors. However, the nurse can reduce some stressors and thereby provide the client with a greater sense of control. There are several methods that assist in stress reduction.

Structure. Each client has unique habits and routines that help accomplish day-to-day activities. This life structure serves to decrease a need for energy developed to responding to changing conditions. Illness, crises, or changes

Sample Nursing Diagnostic Process for Care Giver Role Strain

ASSESSMENT ACTIVITIES	DEFINING CHARACTERISTICS	NURSING DIAGNOSIS
Ask client what a typical day is like caring for his wife at home	Client describes 9 months of maintaining constant care and vigilance over activities of spouse	**Care giver role strain** related to adjustment to recent diagnosis of wife's Alzheimers dementia
Determine to what extent the care giving role interferes with other roles or social functions such as a job	Client is awakened frequently during the night to find wife wandering in the house Client reports he regrets not being able to perform duties of church deacon since taking over care of wife Client states he has no outside activities	
Explore the care giver's perception and acceptance of social support and knowledge of community resources Observe client's behavior and mannerisms during assessment	Client states that he hasn't asked anyone to assist him but several close friends live nearby Client has no knowledge of community resources Care giver appears fatigued, sighs occasionally	

Sample Nursing Care Plan for Care Giver Role Strain

NURSING DIAGNOSIS: **Care giver role strain**
DEFINITION: A care giver's felt difficulty in performing the family care giver role (Kim, McFarland, and McLane, 1995).

GOAL	EXPECTED OUTCOME	INTERVENTIONS	RATIONALE
Client appears rested, states he has resumed one outside activity	Client commits to a plan of a balanced daily routine that incorporates time for own rest or relaxation (3/30)	Discuss ways to simplify care routine (e.g., do all meal preparations during one time period; set aside a specific time to read or sew) Assist client in establishing a consistent care routine Explore pros and cons of outside activities client could incorporate into daily/weekly routine	Simplifying routine provides for more manageable functioning (Ugarriza and Gray, 1993) Brings comfort and assists in developing free time (Langer, 1993) Physical and emotional health is an important component of coping (Kosciulek, McCubbin, and McCubbin, 1993)

in living arrangements disturb a client's routine, thereby disturbing the pattern of living and resulting in greater energy expenditure. A plan that assists a client to renew a familiar life structure or develop a new routine consistent with a changed life situation can reduce stress (White, Richter, and Fry, 1992).

Time Management. Persons who use time efficiently generally experience less stress because they feel more in control of their lives. A nurse acting in the teaching-coaching domain may assist clients to prioritize tasks if they are feeling overwhelmed or immobilized. Realistic structuring of time is needed if clients are not allowing enough time for each activity. A client's role functions should be analyzed conjointly to determine if modifications could be made

that would reduce time demands (Peddicord, 1991).

Controlling the demands of others is essential for effective time management. Few people are able to meet all requests made by others. It is important to learn to recognize which requests can be realistically met, which need to be negotiated, and which ones could be assertively declined. Blocking out a period of time to address specific goals also reduces a sense of urgency and increases feelings of control.

Environmental Modification. Tension created by multiple life changes increases the response to stress. Although all stress cannot be avoided, those life changes that are under the client's control can be deliberately postponed so more energy is available for coping with unavoidable stressors.

Avoiding other stressors is also helpful. For example, it

may be possible to minimize contact with people or situations that elicit tension. If minimal and moderate stressors are mediated, the client is better able to resolve severe stressors (White, Richter, and Fry, 1992).

DECREASING PHYSIOLOGICAL RESPONSE TO STRESS

In general, stress-management techniques involve health-promoting habits that can reduce the impact of stress on physical and mental health. These are often common sense approaches that provide a basis for low-stress living. General prerequisites for stress management include regular exercise, humor, good nutrition and diet, adequate rest, and relaxation techniques.

Regular Exercise. A regular exercise program improves muscle tone and posture, controls weight, reduces tension, and promotes relaxation. In addition, exercise reduces the risk of cardiovascular disease and improves cardiopulmonary functioning. A client who has a history of chronic illness, who is at risk for developing an illness, or who is over the age of 35 should begin a physical exercise program only after discussing it with a physician. In general, for a fitness program to have positive physical effects, a person should exercise at least three times a week for 30 to 40 minutes.

Everyone should use warm-up exercises before vigorous exercise such as jogging, aerobic dancing, or tennis. Warm-up exercises stimulate blood flow to the muscles and increase flexibility. They reduce the risk of damage to the musculoskeletal system during exercise. Similarly, after vigorous exercise a person should do cool-down exercises rather than stop abruptly. For example, after jogging or aerobic dancing a person should walk around at a moderate pace, gradually slowing down and stopping. Cool-down exercises allow the cardiovascular, pulmonary, musculoskeletal, and metabolic systems to gradually return to their resting states.

Exercise programs are effective in decreasing the severity of stress-related conditions such as hypertension, obesity, tension headaches, fatigue, mental exhaustion, irritability, and depression. Exercise promotes release of endogenous opioids that create a feeling of well-being (McCubbin, 1993).

Humor. Humor as therapy has been popularized in the lay literature by Norman Cousins (1979). The ability to perceive fun and laugh alleviates stress (Robinson, 1990; Dahl and O'Neal, 1993). The physiological hypothesis is that laughter releases endorphins into the circulation and feelings of stress are relieved. Simon (1990) notes that humor can influence an older adult's perception of health and morale; in turn the ability to observe situational humor is related to successful aging (Fig. 22-4). Through the helping role, nurses can initiate therapeutic activities such as encouraging clients to relate past humorous anecdotes or develop a "humor" scrapbook. The nurse will critically examine the client's receptivity to humor first, though, to ensure it is never demeaning or ill-timed (Hulse, 1994).

Nutrition and Diet. Nutrition and exercise are closely related. Food provides the fuel for activity and increased exercise, which improves circulation and the delivery of nutrients to body tissues.

Everyone is encouraged to maintain weight according to

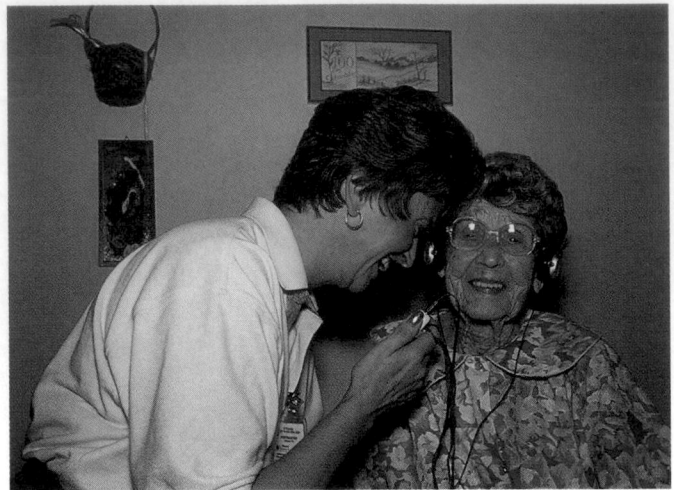

Fig. 22-4 Sharing a joke or laughing with clients can assist in reducing stress and supporting a therapeutic relationship.

standard ranges for sex, age, and body build. In addition to avoiding overeating or undereating, a person should be aware of the nutritional quality of foods. Too much fat, caffeine, salt, or sugar can upset the body's metabolic functioning; deficiencies in vitamins, minerals, and nutrients can also cause metabolic problems. Poor dietary habits can worsen a stress response and make a person irritable, hyperactive, and anxious. This impairs the ability to meet personal, family, and role responsibilities. Nursing measures for helping a client meet nutritional needs are detailed in Chapter 41.

Rest. An established, habitual pattern of sufficient rest and sleep is also important for managing stress. A person experiencing stress should be encouraged to allow time for rest and sleep. Sleep not only refreshes the body but also helps a person become mentally relaxed. A client may need specific help in learning to relax to fall asleep.

Relaxation Techniques. Progressive relaxation with and without muscle tension and imagery techniques reduces the physiological and emotional components of stress (see the box on p. 383). Relaxation techniques are learned behaviors and require training and practice sessions. After the client becomes skilled at these techniques, tension is reduced and physiological parameters are changed (see the box on p. 383).

Spirituality. Spiritual activities can also have a positive effect in decreasing stress (Dahl and O'Neal, 1993). Practices such as prayer, meditation, or reading religious material may be meaningful resources for a client. In one study (Young, 1993) spiritual practices of older clients promoted feelings of productivity and adaptability that assisted coping in chronically ill individuals.

IMPROVED BEHAVIORAL AND EMOTIONAL RESPONSES TO STRESS

Behavioral and emotional responses to stress can be mediated by the use of support systems, crisis intervention, and enhancement of self-esteem.

Support Systems. The saying, "No man is an island," is of particular importance for stress management. A support

Changes Resulting from Relaxation Techniques

- Lowered blood pressure (baseline)
- Lowered heart rate (baseline)
- Decreased cardiac dysrhythmias
- Decreased oxygen demands and oxygen consumption
- Decreased muscle tension
- Lowered metabolic rate
- Increased alpha brain waves, which occur when the client is awake, nonattentive, and relaxed
- Increased restfulness
- Improved concentration
- Improved ability to cope with stressors

CLIENT TEACHING on Deep Abdominal Breathing for a Client With Anxiety

OBJECTIVES
- Clients will exhibit decreased pulse rate.
- Client will report less muscle tension and a heightened sense of relaxation.

TEACHING STRATEGIES
- Discuss with client the importance of incorporating deep breathing into daily routine.
- Reinforce that optimal benefits require practice of the techniques at least 3 to 4 times daily.
- Provide a quiet comfortable environment with low lighting.
- Instruct client to take and record pulse and rate tension on a scale from 1 to 10 (10 being the highest anxiety ever felt and 1 being near sleep).
- Encourage client to assume a comfortable relaxed position with legs and feet uncrossed and arms relaxed and eyes closed.
- Teach client to breathe in slowly through the nostrils, filling the abdomen before filling the lungs.
- Explain to client the need to exhale slowly though the mouth till the abdomen feels flat.
- Tell client to focus thoughts on this slow rhythmic breathing for several minutes.
- Encourage client to give head, neck, and shoulder "permission" to relax during each exhalation.

EVALUATION
- Have client take and report pulse or note difference from prerelaxation rate.
- Ask client to rate self-tension on the scale and report the difference between pre- and postrelaxation.

system of family, friends, and colleagues who will listen and offer advice and emotional support is beneficial to a person experiencing stress. Support systems can reduce stress reactions and promote physical and mental well-being (Revenson and Majerovitz, 1991). Nursing research has documented the correlation of positive social supports and the reduction of symptoms in chronic diseases (White, Richter, and Fry, 1992)

Ulbrich and Bradsher (1993) noted that support moderated the effect of stressors or emotional distress in both white and African American older women especially when the support was viewed as a close confidant. Nurses can use various methods to help clients build support systems such as encouraging family to visit, making support groups available, encouraging involvement in church groups, and encouraging recreational activities. Nurses can use therapeutic communication to teach clients socialization skills if clients do not know how to interact appropriately. All of these methods help clients build stronger support systems. If stress is the result of social isolation, nursing strategies are aimed at helping clients develop new social networks.

Crisis Intervention. Crisis intervention is a therapeutic technique for helping a client resolve a particular, immediate stress problem. Crisis intervention does not involve an in-depth analysis of a situation but addresses the immediate, urgent need for stress reduction. The goal is to restore the person as quickly as possible to the precrisis level of functioning in all dimensions.

Crises occur when people encounter problems or stress situations with which they are unable to cope in usual ways. A crisis can also occur as a reaction to a perceived or threatened loss (Atkins and Amenta, 1991). A crisis does not necessarily denote occurrence of a traumatic event. But even if this happens, it can be an opportunity for personal growth if the crisis is successfully mastered (Younger, 1991).

Clients and nurses are at risk for two types of crises, situational and developmental. A **situational crisis** arises suddenly in response to an external event or conflict involving a specific circumstance. Symptoms associated with situational crises are transient, and the episode is brief. Situational crises include giving birth, major role changes, acute physical illness, physical assault or rape, family changes such as remarriage or the death of a family member, and unexpected unemployment.

A **developmental crisis** occurs when a person is unable to complete the developmental tasks of a psychosocial stage and is therefore unable to continue developing. A developmental crisis can occur at any point in life if circumstances prevent a person from meeting the challenge of a particular stage.

After determining that a client is experiencing a crisis, the nurse plans and implements specific measures to help resolve it. Aguilera (1994) has developed an approach to intervention that can be used for both types of crises (Fig. 22-5).

This approach enables the nurse to understand how a stressful event has led to a state of crisis. Resolution of the crisis depends on the person's realistic perception of the stressful event and use of adequate coping mechanisms. If the crisis has arisen because perception of the event is distorted, the nurse helps the client perceive the stressful event realistically. If the crisis has arisen because of a lack of situational support or coping mechanisms, the nurse initiates measures to assist the client in these areas by maximizing available coping mechanisms, such as incorporating regular diet and exercise into lifestyle, and developing additional supports, such as joining an appropriate support group. The nurse then evaluates the extent to which the client is able to resolve the crisis with these means.

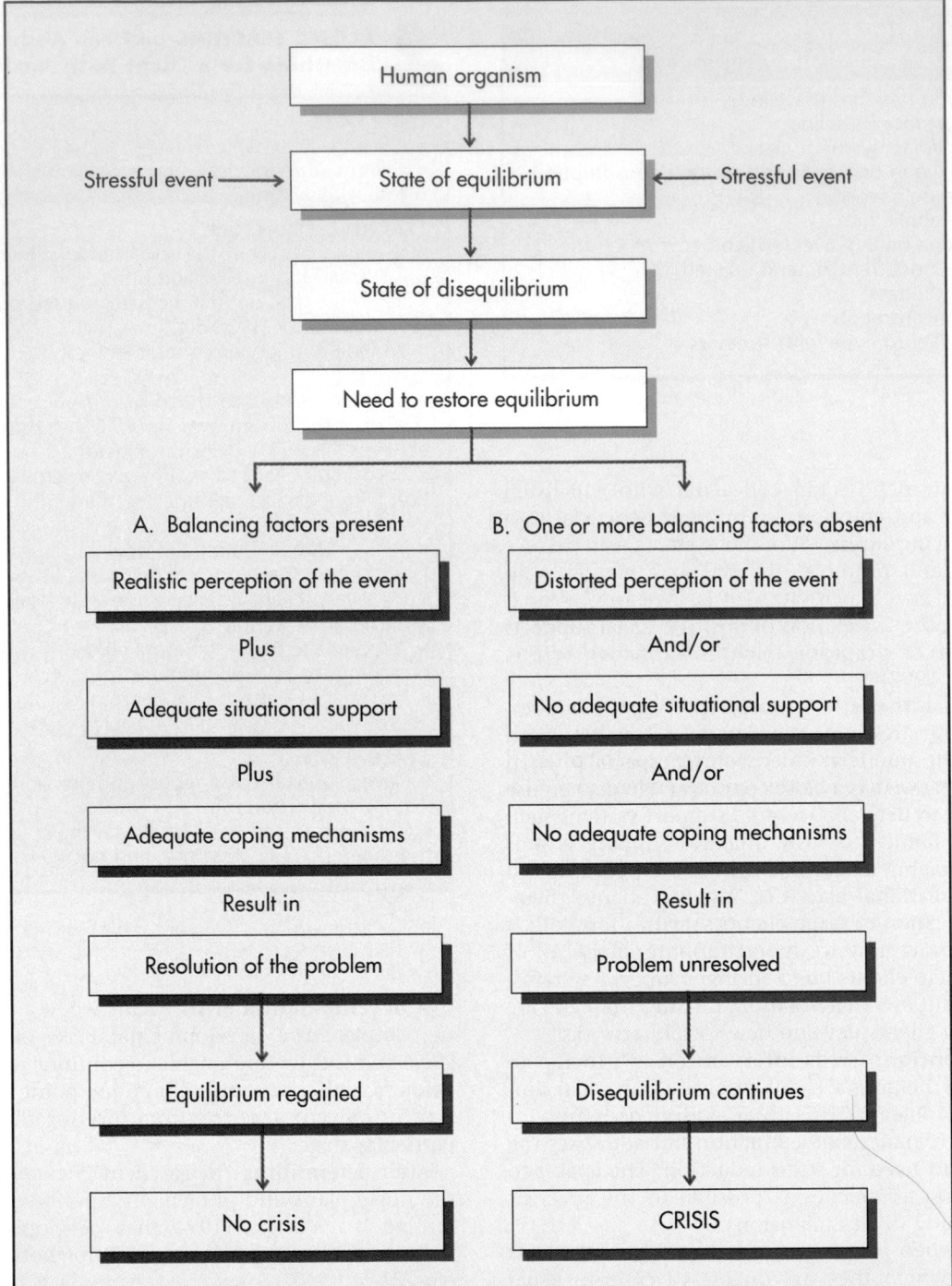

Fig. 22-5 Crisis intervention model. *(Redrawn from Aguilera DC: Crisis intervention: theory and methodology, ed 7, St Louis, 1994, Mosby.)*

Enhancing Self-esteem. Improvement in a client's self-esteem can assist in positive stress-reduction strategies. When clients identify their positive characteristics, it helps them see resources that can be drawn upon to cope with the stressor.

Cognitive restructuring is another intervention that can modify stress responses. This is a technique where the nurse and client analyze the client's appraisals of a stressor. If these are unrealistic or focused only on negative outcomes, the client is assisted to restructure the thinking to more realistic, positive patterns, such as encouraging the client to do something for himself or herself (e.g., getting a haircut or taking 30 minutes each day to read a book). This can serve to modulate the emotional reaction and response (Peddicord, 1991; Badger, 1992).

PROMOTING STRESS MANAGEMENT FOR NURSES

Most nurses experience stress in their work environments. Stressors can consist of workload, institutional policies, conflict with co-workers, or client characteristics

Sample Evaluation of Interventions for Care Giver Role Strain

GOAL	EVALUATIVE MEASURES	EXPECTED OUTCOME
Client appears rested; states he has resumed one outside activity	Note signs of fatigue or energy Review new care routine developed. Ask client what other modifications may need to be made Explore with client how the outside activity is helping him relieve stress Ask client to compare present and previous energy levels. Use visual analog where number 1 represents client's previous energy level	Client commits to a plan of a balanced daily routine that incorporates time for own rest and relaxation (3/30)

(Foxall, Zimmermen, and Bene, 1990; Skipper, Jung, and Coffey, 1990). Reaction to a job-related stressor depends on the nurse's personality, health status, previous experiences with stress, and coping mechanisms.

Job stress frequently results in a condition called **burnout**, which is characterized by a decreased concern for the people with whom one is working. During burnout the client experiences physical and emotional exhaustion (Melamed, Kushnir, and Shirom, 1992). The job or profession no longer has positive rewards and the client may experience anger or apathy.

Nurses are at risk for job stress burnout and benefit from using the same stress management techniques they teach clients. In the organizational and work role competency domain of practice, nurses should identify specific stressors at work and strive to eliminate them. It is also helpful to gain social support from other nurses in order to maintain a caring attitude toward clients.

Evaluation

Because clients' perceptions of stress differ, their perceptions of stress reduction do, too. Therefore evaluation of nursing interventions directed at stress management must consider whether the client's perception of the stress has declined, whether the client is able to control factors that contribute to the stress, and whether the client is able to independently develop stress-reduction strategies.

To evaluate interventions directed at stress management the nurse must obtain objective measures of reduced frequency of stressful situations, decreased physiological response to stress, and improved behavioral and emotional responses to stress.

Achievement of care goals can indicate the degree of stress reduction. The nurse evaluates the effectiveness of stress-management techniques through expected outcome measures (see the evaluation box above).

∎ KEY CONCEPTS ∎

▶ Physiological adaptive mechanisms are controlled by the medulla oblongata, reticular formation, and pituitary gland.

▶ Prolonged stress decreases the adaptive capacity of the body.

▶ Stress is physiological or psychological tension that can affect a person in any or all human dimensions.

▶ An individual may encounter stressors in the internal or external environment.

▶ Stressors necessitate change or adaptation so that a state of equilibrium can be maintained.

▶ A person's response to stress is influenced by the intensity, duration, and scope of the stressor and by the number of stressors present at one time.

▶ A person adapts to stress by using resources in the physical and developmental, emotional, intellectual, social, and spiritual dimensions.

▶ The two forms of physiological response to stress are the local adaptation syndrome and the general adaptation syndrome.

▶ The local adaptation syndrome involves several specific responses to stress, including the reflex pain response and the inflammatory response.

▶ The general adaptation syndrome involves a multisystem physiological response to stress.

▶ The three stages of the general adaption syndrome are the alarm reaction, the resistance stage, and the exhaustion stage.

▶ Psychological responses to stress include task-oriented behaviors and ego-defense mechanisms.

▶ Task-oriented behaviors include attack behavior, withdrawal, and compromise.

▶ Ego-defense mechanisms are unconscious behaviors that offer a person psychological protection from stressful feelings or events.

▶ Stress has an impact on the onset, course, and outcome of illness.

▶ Prolonged stress decreases the ability to adapt to the stress and affects the person in all five dimensions.

▶ People generally learn to use short- and long-term strategies to cope with stress.

▶ Stress-management techniques include health-enhancing habits, crisis intervention, and methods of reducing job stress.

■ KEY TERMS ■

Adaptation, p. 373

Burnout, p. 385

Coping mechanisms, p. 376

Crises, p. 383

Crisis intervention, p. 383

Developmental crisis, p. 383

Ego-defense mechanisms, p. 376

External stressors, p. 371

Fight-or-flight response, p. 375

General adaptation syndrome (GAS), p. 374

Hardiness, p. 379

Homeostasis, p. 371

Internal stressors, p. 371

Job stress, p. 385

Local adaptation syndrome (LAS), p. 374

Medulla oblongata, p. 371

Mild stress situations, p. 377

Moderate stress situations, p. 377

Physiological adaptation, p. 371

Pituitary gland, p. 371

Reticular formation, p. 371

Severe stress situations, p. 377

Situational crisis, p. 383

Stress, p. 371

Stressors, p. 371

Task-oriented behaviors, p. 376

■ CRITICAL THINKING EXERCISES ■

1. During a home visit you note that your older client is apathetic, has vague somatic complaints, and talks about how difficult her life is to manage since the death of her husband 6 months ago. What additional areas would you assess? What social supports would be available in your community for her?

2. Calvin Kleiger had a myocardial infarction yesterday. What are the important physiological responses to stress that can increase the risk for further cardiac damage? What nursing measures can reduce these stress responses?

3. You work in an intensive care unit with a co-worker who has been an outstanding nurse for the past 10 years. Recently, however, she has been irritable with clients and calls in sick frequently. How would you explore the possibility of burnout with her? What stress management techniques could you discuss with her?

REFERENCES

Aguilera DC: *Crisis intervention: theory and methodology,* ed 7, St Louis, 1994, Mosby.

Atkins R, Amenta M: Family adaptation to AIDS: a comparative study, *Hospice Journal* 7:71, 1991.

Badger T: Coping, lifestyle changes, health, perception, and marital adjustment in middle aged women and men with cardiovascular disease and their spouses, *Health Care for Women Int* 13:43, 1992.

Campbell-Heider N, Hart C: Updating the nurse's bedside manner, *Image* 5(2):133, 1993.

Cooper C, Faragher E: Psychosocial stress and breast cancer: the interrelationship between stress events, coping strategies and personality, *Psychol Med* 23:653, 1993.

Cousins N: *Anatomy of an illness,* New York, 1979, Bantam.

Dahl J, O'Neal J: Stress and coping behavior of nurses in desert storm, *J Psychosocial Nurs* 31(12):17, 1993.

DuBois D et al: A prospective study of life stress, social support and adaptation in early adolescence, *Child Dev* 63:542, 1992.

Fox P: Stress related to family change among Vietnamese refugees, *J Community Health Nurs* 8(1):45, 1991.

Foxall MJ, Zimmermen L, Bene B: A comparison of frequency and sources of nursing job stress perceived by intensive care, hospice, and medical-surgical nurses, *J Adv Nurs* 15:77, 1990.

Frye B, D'Avanzo C: Cultural themes in family stress and violence among Cambodian refugee women in the inner city, *Advances in Nursing Science* 16(3):64,1994.

Haber J: A family systems model for divorce and the loss of self, *Arch Psychiatr Nurs* 6(4):228, 1990.

Haber J et al: *Comprehensive psychiatric nursing,* ed 4, St Louis, 1992, Mosby.

Holmes T, Rahe R: The social readjustment scale, *J Psychosom Res* 12:213, 1976.

Hufft A: Psychosocial adaptation to pregnancy in prison, *J Psychosocial Nurs* 30(4):19, 1992.

Hulse J: Humor: a nursing intervention for the elderly, *Geriatr Nurse* 15:88, 1994.

Kim MJ, McFarland GK, McLane AM: *Pocket guide to nursing diagnoses,* ed 6, St Louis, 1995, Mosby.

Kline-Leidy N: A structural model of stress, psychosocial resources, and symptomatic experience in chronic physical illness, *Nurs Res* 39:30, 1990.

Kolotylo CJ, Parker NI, Chapman JS: Mother's perception of their neonates' in-hospital transfers from a neonatal intensive care unit, *JOGN* 20(2):146, 1990.

Kosciulek J, McCubbin M, McCubbin H: A theoretical framework for family adaptation to head injury, *J Rehab* 59(3):40, 1993.

Langer S: Ways of managing the experience of caregiving to elderly relatives, *West J Nurs Res* 15:582, 1993.

Lazarus RS, Folkman S: *Stress appraisal and coping,* New York, 1984, Springer.

Lindsay AM, Carrieri VK, Page GG: Stress response. In Lindsay AM, Carrieri VK, editors: *Pathological phenomenon in nursing: human response to illness,* ed 2, Philadelphia, 1993, Saunders.

McCubbin J: Stress and endogenous opioids: behavioral and circulatory interactions, *Biological Psychology* 35:91, 1993.

McNett SC: Lazarus' theory of stress and coping. In Riegel B, Ehrenreich D, editors: *Psychological aspects of critical care nursing,* Rockville, Md, 1989, Aspen.

Mechanic D: *Students under stress,* Glencoe, Ill, 1962, Free Press.

Melamed S, Kushnir T, Shirom A: Burnout and risk factors for cardiovascular disease, *Behavioral Med* 18(2):55, 1992.

Mikhail M: Psychological responses to relocation to nursing home, *J Gerontology Nurs* 18(3):35, 1992.

Monsen R, Floyd L, Brookman J: Stress-coping-adaptation: concepts for nursing, *Nursing Forum* 27(4):27, 1992.

Murata J: Family stress, social support, violence, and son's behavior, *West J Nurs Res* 16(2):154, 1994.

Musolf JM: Easing the impact of the family caregiver's role, *Rehabil Nurs* 16(2):82, 1991.

Oberst MT et al: Self-care burden, stress appraisal, and mood among persons receiving radiotherapy, *Cancer Nurs* 14(2):71, 1991.

Peddicord K: Strategies for promoting stress reduction and relaxation, *Nurs Clin N Am* 26(4):867, 1991.

Porter E, Clinton J: Adjusting to the nursing home, *West J Nurs Res* 14(4):464, 1992.

Reis S, Heppner P: Examination of coping resources and family adaptation in mothers and daughters of incestuous versus nonclinical families, *J Counseling Psych* 40(1):100, 1993.

Revenson T, Majerovitz D: The effects of chronic illness on the spouse, *Arthritis Care and Research* 4(2):63, 1991

Robinson L: Stress and anxiety, *Nurs Clin North Am* 25(4):935, 1990.

Schedlowski M et al: Psychophysiological, neuroendocrine and cellular immune reactions under psychological stress, *Neuropsychobiology* 28:87, 1993.

Selye H: The general adaptation syndrome and the diseases of adaptation, *Clin Endocrinol* 6:117, 1946.

Selye H: *The stress of life*, ed 2, New York, 1976, McGraw-Hill.

Simon JM: Humor and its relationship to perceived health, life satisfaction, and morale in older adults, *Issues Ment Health Nurs* 11:17, 1990.

Skipper JK, Jung JD, Coffey LC: Nurses and shiftwork: effects on physical health and mental depression, *J Adv Nurs* 15:835, 1990.

Stuart GW, Sundeen SJ: *Principles and practice of psychiatric nursing*, ed 4, St Louis, 1991, Mosby.

Tartasky D: Hardiness: conceptual and methodological issues, *Image* 25(3):225, 1993.

Ugarriza D, Gray T: Alzheimer's disease: nursing interventions for clients and caretakers, *J Psychosocial Nurs M H Ser* 21(10):7, 1993.

Ulbrich P, Bradsher J: Perceived support, help-seeking and adaptation to stress among older black and white women living alone, *J of Aging and Health* 5(3):365, 1993.

White N, Richter J, Fry C: Coping, social support, and adaptation to chronic illness, *West J of Nurs Res* 14(2):211, 1992.

Wiebe D, Williams P: Hardiness and health: a social psychophysiological perspective on stress and adaptation, *J Soc and Clin Psych* 11(3):238, 1992.

Yatkin V, Labban S: Stress and schizophrenia, *J Psychosocial Nurs and M H Ser* 30(6):29, 1992.

Young C: Spirituality and the chronically ill Christian elderly, *Geriatric Nurs* 14: 298, 1993.

Younger J: A theory of mastery, *Advances in Nursing Science* 14(1):76, 1991.

ADDITIONAL READINGS

Cataldo J: Hardiness and death attitudes: predictors of depression in the institutionalized elderly, *Arch of Psych Nurs* 8(5):326, 1994.

Dobratz M: Causal influences of psychological adaptation in dying, *West J Nurs Res* 15(6):708, 1993.

Levy L, Derby J, Martinkowski K: Effects of membership in bereavement support groups on adaptation to conjugal bereavement, *Am J of Comm Psychology* 21(3):361, 1993.

Palinkas L: Going to extremes: the cultural context of stress, illness and coping in Antarctica, *Soc, Sc Med* 35(5):651, 1992.

Selye H: The general adaptation syndrome and the diseases of adaptation, *Clin Endocrinol (Oxf)* 6:117, 1946.

## Chapter 23

Self-Concept

Objectives

Mastery of content in this chapter will enable the student to:

▶ Distinguish the four components of self-concept: identity, body image, self-esteem, and roles.

▶ Describe stressors that can affect self-concept.

▶ Relate factors that can lead to role conflict, role ambiguity, and role strain.

▶ Identify the components of identity confusion.

▶ Define the components of a healthy self-concept, as related to psychosocial and cognitive stages.

▶ Identify and discuss ways in which the nurse's self-concept and nursing activities can affect the client's self-concept.

▶ Describe behaviors that may indicate identity confusion, disturbed body image, low self-esteem, and role conflict.

▶ Identify important aspects of culture that affect nursing care in support of clients' self-concept.

▶ Distinguish factors that promote a healthy self-concept.

▶ Plan the care of a client with a specific self-concept disturbance.

The self is our most intimate relationship, clearly one of the most important aspects of our life experience, yet it is one of the most difficult to define. What we think and feel about ourselves affects the care we give ourselves physically and emotionally and the care we give to others. People with low self-concepts do not feel worthy of care and often will not seek care for physical or emotional health.

The diabetic who does not assume self-care, the adult who repeatedly neglects diet and sleep during infection, and the child who does not keep his or her body bathed all have behaviors that are indicative of a poor self-concept. The young child who is sexually abused or the child who is neglected will be at an increased risk for developing poor self-concept.

Self-concept is an individual's knowledge about the self (e.g., "I am good at math") (Wigfield and Karpathian, 1991). It is a subjective image of the self and a complex mixture of unconscious and conscious feelings, attitudes, and perceptions. Self-concept provides us with a frame of reference that affects our management of situations and our relationships with others. We begin forming our self-concept at a young age. Adolescence is a critical time when many things continually affect the self-concept (Fig. 23-1). If a child has had a stable and secure childhood, the self-concept of an adolescent can be surprisingly stable (Marsh, 1990). Discrepancies between certain aspects of personality and self-concept may become sources of stress or conflict.

Self concept and perception of health are closely associated to each other. A client's belief in good health can enhance self-concept. Statements such as "I'm strong as an ox" or "I've never been sick a day in my life" indicate that a person's thoughts about health are positive. These thoughts are important to one's self-perception. Negative self-perception is reflected in such statements as "It's not worth it anymore" or "I'll never get any better."

Hospitalization, illness, surgery, separation from family, and other factors can also affect self-concept. For example, amputation of an extremity or a breast results in altered body image. Adaptation includes integrating the bodily change into the physical concept of self, the body image. Chronic illness may affect the ability to provide financial support, thereby affecting self-worth and roles within the family. These changes may alter self-concept.

OVERVIEW OF SELF-CONCEPT

Self-concept is developed through a very complex process that involves many variables. The four components of self-concept are identity, body image, self-esteem, and roles. Self-concept is the psychic representation of an individual, the central core of "I" around which all perceptions and experiences are organized. Self-concept is a dynamic combination formulated over years and based on the following:

1. Reactions of others to one's body
2. Ongoing perceptions of the reactions of others to the self
3. Relationships with self and others
4. Personality structure
5. Perceptions of stimuli that have an impact on the self
6. Prior and new experiences
7. Present feelings about the physical, emotional, and social self
8. Expectations about the self

Self-concept gives a sense of continuity, wholeness, and consistency to a person. A healthy self-concept has a high degree of stability and generates positive or negative feelings toward the self (see the box on p. 390).

Our **identity** forms one of the four integrating principals of self concept. People are aware if they are being who they really are versus behaving in a particular way because it is expected of them. Being "oneself" is the crux of identity. Identity is often gained from one's self-observations and from what we are told about ourselves (Stuart and Sundeen, 1991). Important and influential adults often give the child much of its identity until the child is able to self-observe. This is why it is so damaging to tell a child "You are dumb" or "You are ugly." It may be difficult or impossible for the child to make a judgment that this is untrue, so he or she incorporates these negative statements into his or her identity.

When we think of ourselves physically, our mental picture is our **body image**. These mental images are not necessarily consistent with the actual body structure or appearance. Body image is the part of the self-concept that involves attitudes and experiences pertaining to the body, including notions about masculinity and femininity, physical prowess, endurance, and capabilities (Drench 1994). Body image develops gradually over several years as children learn about their bodies and their structures, functions, abilities, and limitations. Body image may change within a few hours, days, weeks, or months, depending on external stimuli on the body and actual changes in appearance, structure, or function. The way others view our body is also influential. For example, a controlling, violent husband might tell his wife she is ugly and that no one else would want her. Over the years of marriage, she believes this image of herself and incorporates it into her self-concept.

In the case of a physical change, if a nurse shows acceptance of a mastectomy scar, the woman will incorporate a more positive, whole view of herself, simply because this is what is being reflected to her by the nurse. If a family member reacts with disgust to an amputated limb, the individual may develop a negative body image. Clients closely watch the reactions of others to their wounds and scars. It

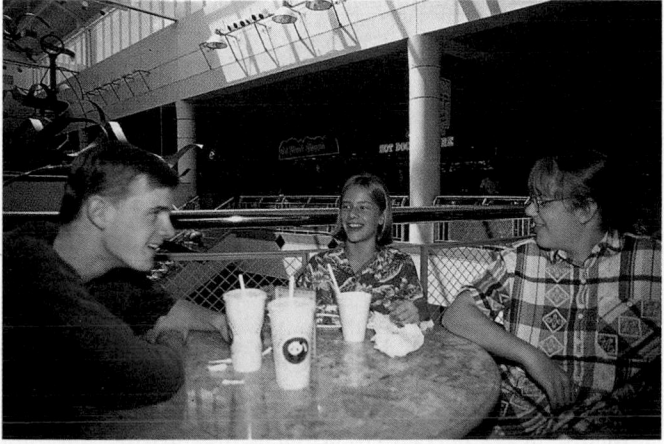

Fig. 23-1 Adolescents can gain self-confidence through group activities.

RESEARCH HIGHLIGHT

RESEARCH ABSTRACT

The "self" is one of the most studied subjects in psychology. Banaji has reviewed studies of the "self" from 1987 to 1994. New research studies how the self is the focus of our behavior with an emphasis on specific social situations. Research also examines self-knowledge and self-improvement (the desire to bring oneself closer to what one should or would like to be).

Long-term changes in self-concept are quite difficult to achieve, but there have been many studies demonstrating temporary changes in self-concept. Often changes in self-concept have occurred during life-transition changes. When people pursue self-knowledge, self-enhancement, or self-improvement, they are motivated to do so. We seem to want to be like the ideal images of ourselves and pursue those things that will bring us closer to our ideal selves.

Also of interest has been the topic of self-presentation. Some studies have shown that when exposed to an evaluative threat, people with high self-esteem will be more assertive and people with low self-esteem will be more self-protective in their actions. Also, those with high self-esteem have been shown to take greater risks. Another exciting expectation of "self" research is the influence of culture and society on the formation and maintenance of the self.

IMPLICATIONS FOR PRACTICE

▶ Often changes in the self will be temporary; long-term changes require continuing support from the nurse to the individual to make those changes. Continuing support to the client's significant others is also needed.

▶ Transition periods such as from health to illness can be periods for great changes within the self. It is important for the nurse to recognize these periods, in addition to normal stages of development.

▶ People with high self-esteem are usually more assertive and will take greater risks. These clients tell nurses about their needs.

▶ Clients with low self-esteem may be less likely to express their needs.

REFERENCE

Banaji M, Prentice D: *Ann Rev Psychol* 45:297, 1994.

is very important for the nurse to monitor responses toward the client. Statements such as "This wound is healing nicely" or "This scar looks good" can be very affirming for the body image of the client.

Self-esteem is derived from two sources, the self and others. It depends on love and approval. Self-esteem involves the acceptance of self because of basic worth, despite weaknesses and limitations. A person who values himself and feels valued by others usually has high self-esteem. A person who feels worthless and receives little respect from others usually has low self-esteem.

People have self-perceptions based on perceived health status, gender, age, background, family roles, occupational and social roles, and use of leisure time. Normally these different aspects of the self are common to all of us. Feelings about ourselves for the most part tend to be fairly constant,

even with good and bad days. Consistency remains, even though a person may be perceived in different ways by others.

The ability to work is an important part of self-concept. Often people who are sick feel a great sense of worthlessness. The nurse must accept ill people with worth and dignity. The nurse's acceptance of a client as an individual with worth and dignity can be crucial in helping to improve self-esteem.

■ COMPONENTS OF SELF-CONCEPT

Self-concept can be described in terms of a continuum from strong to weak or positive to negative, depending on the individual strengths of the four components.

Identity

Identity involves the internal sense of individuality, wholeness, and consistency of a person over time and in various circumstances. The concept of identity thus includes constancy and continuity. Identity implies being distinct and separate from others, yet being a whole and unique self.

The child learns culturally accepted values, behaviors, and roles. A child identifies first with parenting figures and later with teachers, peers, and heroes. To form an identity, the child must be able to bring together learned behaviors into a coherent, consistent, and unique whole (Erikson, 1963). This sense of identity continuously evolves and is influenced by circumstances throughout life.

During adolescence a person's chief emotional task is the development of a sense of self, or identity. Many physical, emotional, cognitive, and social changes occur. If adolescents are unable to meet the self-imposed personal and social expectations that help them define the self, the teenagers may experience identity confusion. A person with a solid sense of identity will feel integrated rather than fragmented (Erikson, 1963).

The achievement of identity is necessary for intimate relationships because one's identity is expressed in relationships with others. Sexuality is a part of one's identity. Sexual identity is a person's image of the self as a man or a woman and the meaning of this image. This image and its meaning depend on culturally determined values that are learned through socialization (see Chapter 24).

Body Image

Body image is made up of a person's perceptions of the body, both internally and externally. It includes feelings and attitudes toward the body. Body image is influenced by personal views of physical characteristics and abilities and by perceptions of others' views.

Body image is affected by cognitive growth and physical development. Normal developmental changes such as growth and aging have a more apparent effect on body image than on other aspects of self-concept. A school-age child's body image is different from an infant's. One of the glaring differences is the ability to walk. This change depends on physical maturation. Hormonal changes occur during adolescence and in later stages of life to influence body image (e.g., menopause during middle adulthood). Aging involves a decrease in visual acuity, hearing, and mobility; these changes may affect body image.

Cultural and societal attitudes and values also influence

body image (see the box below). Youth, beauty, and wholeness are emphasized in American society, a fact apparent in television programs, movies, and advertisements. In Eastern cultures aging is viewed very positively, since the older adult is respected. Western cultures (particularly in the United States) have been socialized to fear and dread the normal aging process. For instance, menopause in other cultures is viewed as a time in which women gain power and wisdom. Until recently in Western culture menopause was the time when women were less desirable sexually. However, this is no longer the prevailing belief, and menopausal and postmenopausal women are maintaining an even stronger sense of themselves and their own attractiveness.

Body image depends only partly on the reality of the body. A person generally does not adapt quickly to changes in the physical body. Physical changes may not be incorporated into a person's ideal body image. Often, for example, people who have experienced significant weight loss do not perceive themselves as thin. Older adults often report that they do not feel different but when they look in the mirror, they are surprised by wrinkled skin or gray hair. Often people who were once thin and have gained a great deal of weight feel that they are still their former body weight until reminded by tight clothes or a mirror.

Self-Esteem

Self-esteem is based on internal and external factors. Self-esteem is our sense of self-worth; it is an evaluation that an individual makes and maintains about the self. According to Erikson (1963), young children begin to develop a sense of usefulness or industry by learning to act on their own initiative. Self-esteem is related to the individual's evaluation of his or her effectiveness at school or work, within the family, and in social settings. Self-efficacy is closely related to this idea (i.e., self-appraisal of one's competence in performing various tasks) (Bandura, 1982).

Self-esteem can be understood by thinking of the relationship between a person's self-concept and the ideal self. The ideal self consists of the aspirations, goals, values, and standards of behavior that a person considers ideal and strives to attain. The **ideal self** originates in the preschool years and develops throughout life; it is influenced by societal norms and the expectations and demands of parents and significant others. In general, a person whose self-concept almost matches the ideal self has high self-esteem, whereas a person whose self-concept varies widely from the ideal self has low self-esteem.

A person's family and society in general set the standards by which individuals evaluate themselves. A child who excels in science is comfortable among peers in a classroom, and self-esteem is high. However, if the same child is placed in a more difficult science class with new classmates, self-esteem may decrease until the child gains confidence within the new environment.

Self-evaluation is an ongoing mental process. Self-worth, or self-esteem, is a basic human need, according to Maslow's hierarchy. People need to feel worthy of living. Self-esteem is important in the maintenance of self-concept.

Self-esteem also is influenced by the amount of control that people believe they have over life goals and successes. A person with high self-esteem tends to attribute success to personal qualities and efforts. When successful, an individual with low self-esteem tends to attribute this to luck or others' help rather than personal ability (Marsh, 1990).

Roles

Roles involve expectations or standards of behavior that have been accepted by the family, community, and culture. Behavior is based on patterns established through socialization. Socialization begins just after birth, when an infant responds to adults and adults respond to the infant's behaviors. The patterns are stable and change only minimally during adulthood. A child learns behaviors that are approved by society through the following processes:

1. **Reinforcement-extinction:** Certain behaviors become common or are avoided, depending on whether they are approved and reinforced or discouraged and punished.
2. **Inhibition:** A child learns to refrain from behaviors, even when tempted to engage in them.
3. **Substitution:** A child replaces one behavior by another, which provides the same personal gratification.
4. **Imitation:** A child acquires knowledge, skills, or behaviors from members of the social or cultural group.
5. **Identification:** A child internalizes the beliefs, behavior, and values of role models into a personal, unique expression of self.

During **socialization**, a child generally develops the skills necessary for functioning in many different roles. Unsuc-

CULTURAL ASPECTS OF CARE

SELF-CONCEPT

Recent issues in the study of the self attempt to explain cultural differences between individuals by looking at the differences cultures have in viewing independence versus collectivism. In this case independence refers to an individualism where one is not dependent on or subject to the control or opinion of others. Collectivism, by contrast, refers to persons considered as members of a group or whole with similarity among members.

Often the concepts of individualism and collectivism are viewed in Eastern versus Western cultural terms. In cultures emphasizing collectivism (e.g., Japan and China) the collective self is more complex and intricate in structure and the individualistic self is more simplistic, whereas in cultures where individualism is emphasized (United States, Canada, and Australia) the individual, private self is the most complex. These cultures have different values in regard to the group. People socialize according to their culture. Culture influences what we tend to value in our lives. How we think about ourselves, what motivates us, and how we behave are all related to the culture within which we are socialized.

The preceding concept applies to dress and body adornment. In Western cultures people value individual expression through clothing and hairstyles. In Eastern cultures there is a more restrictive code of clothing and hairstyles that is acceptable (although this is changing as our society becomes more international). The effect of individualism versus collectivism can be seen in newspapers, movies, and other media from both cultures.

cessful socialization is an inability to function acceptably according to society's values.

An adult is more concerned with the actual behavior that is appropriate to roles than with learning the basic values implicit in roles. An adult is expected to distinguish between ideal role expectations and realistic possibilities. In addition, adults experience many roles, usually with an increased role specificity. Adults are concerned about relationships with other people. The success of various roles and relationships contributes to a sense of well-being or self-esteem. In contrast to adults, a child learns about the personal, physical self and the immediate environment. Only after becoming comfortable with the physical self and establishing trust in parents can a child begin to socialize with other children.

To function effectively in roles, people must know the expected behavior and values, must desire to conform to them, and must be able to meet the role requirements. Most individuals have more than one role. Common roles include mother or father, wife or husband, daughter or son, employee or employer, sister or brother, and friend. Each role involves meeting certain expectations of others. Fulfillment of these expectations leads to rewards. Failure to comply with them leads to disapproval.

■ STRESSORS AFFECTING SELF-CONCEPT

Stressors challenge a person's adaptive capacities. Selye (1956) states that stress is the normal wear and tear of life, not the specific result of any one action or typical response to any one thing. The normal process of maturation and development itself is a stressor. Changes that occur in physical, spiritual, emotional, sexual, familial, and sociocultural health are stressful. A self-concept stressor is any real or perceived change that threatens identity, body image, self-esteem, or role behavior (Fig. 23-2).

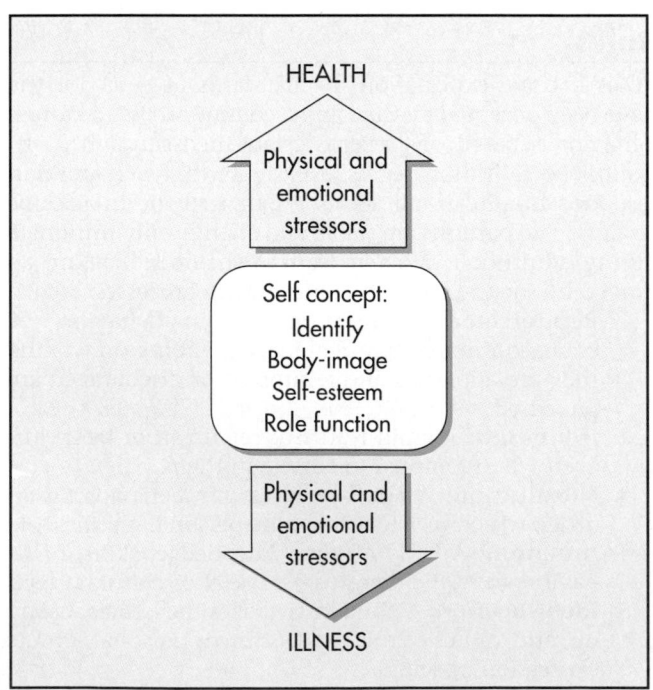

Fig. 23-2 How stressors affect self-concept.

Different individuals react to the same situation with varying degrees of stress. Perception of a stressor is an important factor that influences the response to it. All people learn patterns of behavior that usually provide the means for coping with or adapting to stressors, thus providing methods for coping with future stressors. However, some people are immobilized by perceived threats and require help from other people. Prolonged stress or perceived stress can deplete adaptive ability.

Any change in health can be a stressor that affects self-concept. A physical change in the body leads to an altered body image, in which identity and self-esteem can also be affected. Chronic illnesses often alter roles, which may alter one's identity and self-esteem (Fig. 23-3). The following case study illustrates the interrelationship of the four components of self-concept.

CASE STUDY   A 48-year-old man suffers a stroke. The stroke is unexpected and sudden. He was not even aware that he had hypertension, since he had not been getting yearly checkups. Paul awakens in the hospital bed to find that he cannot move even his hand. He cannot care for himself. Paul cannot even turn himself for days. Finally he is able to pull himself out of bed and into a chair with the nurse's help. He wonders what lies in store for him. Paul's body image has dramatically changed from a man of strength and endurance to that of a helpless individual. Paul worries about his family and what will happen. His daughter, the oldest child, is away at college, and his son is still in high school. Paul and his wife, Meredith, are terrified. Although Meredith works, they have not saved enough money to be able to educate their children without his wages. Paul's role as chief financial provider for the family may be drastically changed if his condition does not change.

Paul's self-esteem wanes as his recovery and rehabilitation move slowly. His self-concept changes from that of a strong laborer, one who did his own plumbing and car repairs, to a man who has to tell his son what to do because he does not have the strength to do these tasks. Although he is now at home in the rehabilitation process, Paul is not able to perform tasks for the family and must wait until his wife and son get home to help him with things that require strength. Paul's adaptation capabilities are stretched to the maximum, although his physician tells him he is very fortunate to be alive. His life is now changed—for how long he does not know. Paul's identity is not clear to him any more, he has no clear role within the family, his body image has been drastically altered, and his self-esteem is spiraling lower and lower.

Paul continues in outpatient physical therapy. It takes much time and hard work even on simple tasks, but he begins to gain some strength. Paul continues to make gains. He is able to return to work. He has some diminished mental quickness and some muscle weakening, but he is able to perform his job. His self-esteem recovers, and his body image is enhanced. Although he still feels somewhat altered, his capabilities closely resemble his capabilities before the stroke. ■

A crisis occurs when a person cannot overcome obstacles with usual methods of problem solving and adapting. Any crisis requires change and thus threatens self-concept. Some crises, such as the case study above, directly affect all four components of self-concept. During self-concept crises, as with other kinds of crises, supportive resources are necessary to help a person learn new ways of coping with and responding to the event or situation to maintain a positive self-concept.

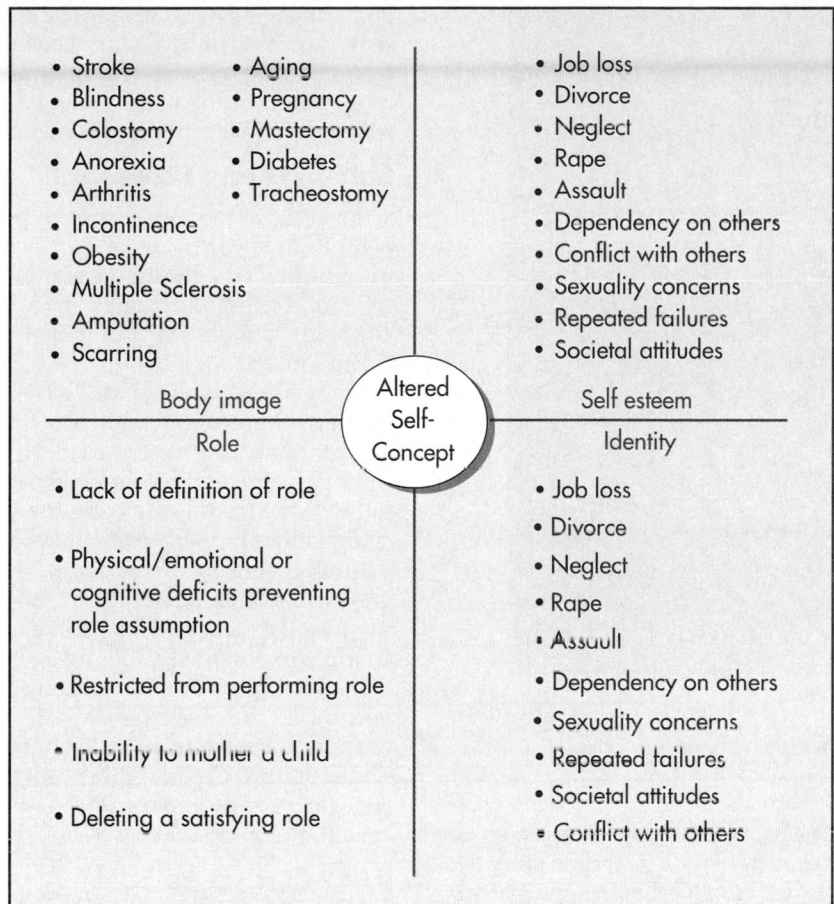

Fig. 23-3 Examples of changes that alter a client's self-concept.

Identity Stressors

The identity is defined as the "organizing principle of the personality system that accounts for the unity, continuity, uniqueness, and consistency of the personality"(Stuart and Sundeen, 1991). Identity is affected by stressors throughout life. Adolescence is a time of great change, causing insecurity and anxiety. Adolescents are trying to adjust to the physical, emotional, and mental changes of increasing maturity. Stressors may arise in any of these areas or as a result of conflicts among them.

An adult generally has a more stable identity and thus a more firmly developed self-concept. Cultural and social stressors rather than personal stressors may have more impact on an adult's identity. For example, an adult may have to decide between career and marriage, cooperation and competition, or dependence and independence in a relationship (Stuart and Sundeen, 1991).

Other developmental markers such as the initiation of menses, puberty, menopause, retirement, decreasing physical abilities, and other factors associated with aging also affect identity. Identity, like body image, is closely related to appearance and abilities (Fig. 23-4). Retirement may mean the loss of an important means of achievement and continued success. People at retirement may begin to question their identities and accomplishments. Physical and emotional isolation may add stress when significant others die.

In fact, depression is common in the retired population. Depression is a diagnosis often missed by health care professionals, since it is often associated with symptoms of physical illness (Reed, 1991).

Identity confusion results when people do not maintain a clear, consistent, and continuous consciousness of personal identity. It may occur at any stage of life if a person is unable to adapt to identity stressors. Under extreme stress an individual may experience depersonalization, a state in which internal and external realities or the differences between the self and others cannot be determined.

Body Image Stressors

Changes in the appearance, structure, or function of a body part will require change in body image. Changes in the appearance of the body, such as an amputation or facial disfigurement, are obvious stressors affecting body image. Mastectomy, colostomy, and ileostomy alter the appearance and function of the body, although the changes are not apparent when people are clothed. Even though not apparent to others, these bodily changes have a significant effect on the individual. Chronic illnesses such as heart and renal disease involve a change in function, in which the body no longer functions at an optimal level. Even "normal" body changes resulting from the normal developmental progress of aging can affect body image. In addi-

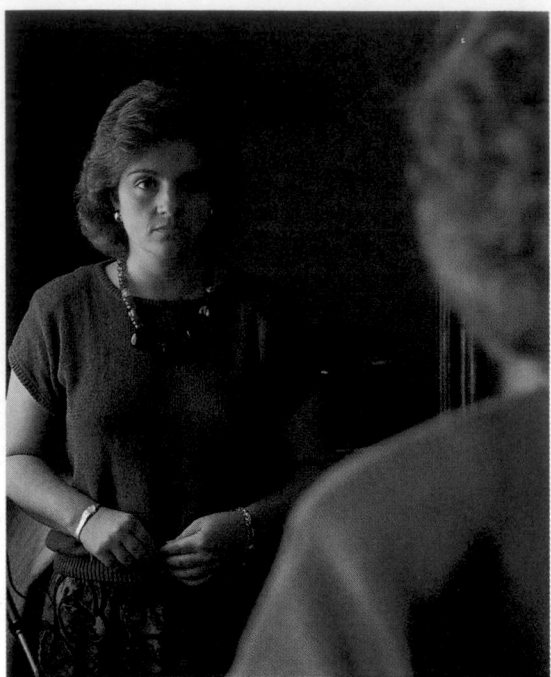

Fig. 23-4 A person's appearance influences his or her identity.

tion, pregnancy and significant weight gain or loss change body image, as well as chemotherapy or radiation therapy.

An individual's perception of body changes may be affected by how the changes came about. Paralysis caused by war injuries may be considered acceptable; veterans may be treated as heroes and praised for bravery; governmental resources will be available for rehabilitation. However, people who have automobile accidents while drunk and suffer paralysis may receive a different response from society.

The significance of a loss of function or a change in appearance is affected by the individual's perception of the alteration. Body image consists of ideal and real elements. For example, if a woman's body image incorporates breasts as the ideal, the loss of a breast by mastectomy may be a very significant alteration. The greater the importance of the body or a specific body part, the greater the threat felt from a change in body image.

Many people associate success with a specific body part or function. For example, athletes may consider their bodies and physical activities to be the focus of personal success. However, if they can never again participate in physical activities because of an accident, their adaptation and rehabilitation may be affected. They must revise long-accepted assumptions about themselves and alter their lifestyles. To regain positive self-concepts and self-esteem and to maintain good health, they must adapt to their body image stressors.

People with altered body images, such as those with facial alterations, often feel rejected and isolated. Feelings of helplessness are also common. This feeling of social isolation is often based in reality; people are afraid of embarrassing or offending individuals who are deformed and thus avoid contact with them.

Positive social changes with regard to illness and altered body image have occurred. The media now frequently present positive stories about persons who have had major body-altering surgery. These stories provide positive role models for individuals undergoing unusual stressors, as well as for their families, friends, and society as a whole.

Self-Esteem Stressors

Self-esteem is the sense of being respected, accepted, competent, and worthy. A person with low self-esteem tends to feel unloved and often experiences depression and anxiety. Self-esteem fluctuates with surrounding conditions, although a basic core of positive or negative feeling is maintained.

Many stressors affect the self-esteem of the infant, toddler, preschooler, and adolescent. Inability to meet parental expectations, harsh criticism, inconsistent punishment, sibling rivalry, and repeated defeats may reduce the level of self-worth. Stressors affecting the self-esteem of an adult include failure in work and failures in relationships.

Illness, surgery, or accidents that change life patterns may also decrease feelings of self-worth. Chronic illnesses such as diabetes, arthritis, and cardiac dysfunction require changes in accepted and long-assumed behavioral patterns. When changes are slow and progressive, people have opportunities for anticipatory grieving. However, a sudden change in health is more likely to create a crisis situation. The more the chronic illness interferes with the ability to engage in activities contributing to feelings of worth or success, the more it affects self-esteem.

Role Stressors

Roles set up socially expected behavior patterns associated with one individual's function in various social groups (Stuart and Sundeen, 1991). Throughout life people undergo numerous role changes. Normal changes associated with growth and maturation result in developmental transitions. Situational transitions occur when parents, spouses, or close friends die or people move, marry, divorce, or change jobs. A health-illness transition is a movement from a state of health or well-being to one of illness or vice versa. Any of these transitions may threaten self-concept, resulting in role conflict, role ambiguity, or role strain. It is important to recognize that a shift along the continuum from illness to wellness is as stressful as a shift from wellness to illness.

ROLE CONFLICTS

Role conflict is a lack of compatible role expectations (Broadwell, 1983). When a person is required to simultaneously assume two or more roles that are inconsistent, contradictory, or mutually exclusive, role conflict may occur. For example, a middle-aged woman with teenage children has to care for her older parents in her home. Conflicts may occur as she interacts with them simultaneously as care giver and as child. Negotiating a balance of time and energy between her children and parents may also create role conflict. The importance of each conflicting role influences the degree of conflict experienced.

There are three basic kinds of role conflict: interpersonal, interrole, and personal role. **Interpersonal conflict** occurs when one or more persons have opposing or incompatible expectations for an individual in a particular role. For example, a woman's friends and her mother may have very different expectations of how she should care for her children.

Interrole conflict occurs when pressures or expectations associated with one role oppose pressures or expectations associated with another. A man who works 10 to 12 hours a day may have problems if his wife expects him to be at home with the family.

Personal role conflict occurs when role requirements violate an individual's personal values. For example, a nurse who values the preservation of life experiences conflict when faced with caring for a client who chooses to refuse life-support therapies.

ROLE AMBIGUITY

Role ambiguity involves unclear role expectations. When there are unclear expectations, people are unsure of what to do, how to do it, or both. Such a situation is often stressful and confusing. Role ambiguity is common in the adolescent years. Adolescents are pressured by parents, peers, and the media to assume adultlike roles, yet remain in the role of a dependent child. Role ambiguity is also common in employment situations. In complex, rapidly changing, or highly specialized organizations employees often become unsure of what is expected of them.

ROLE STRAIN

Role strain blends role conflict and role ambiguity. Role strain may be expressed as a feeling of frustration when a person feels inadequate or feels unsuited to a role. Role strain is often associated with gender role stereotypes (Stuart and Sundeen, 1991). Women in positions typically held by men may be perceived by others as less competent, less objective, or less knowledgeable than their male counterparts. Thus they may feel that they must work harder and be better to compete. Men in typically female roles also encounter gender bias, which frequently questions their masculinity.

The sick role involves the expectations of others and society. Role conflict may occur when general societal expectations (take care of yourself and you'll get better) and the expectations of co-workers (need to get work done) collide. The conflict of taking care of oneself while getting everything done can be a major challenge.

The sick role may also involve role ambiguity. People are expected to be dependent and simultaneously participate actively so that they can get well and leave the sick role quickly. However, chronically ill people cannot do this. The sick role is supposed to be temporary, yet the chronically ill must comply with therapy that may be necessary for the remainder of life.

Role overload occurs when an individual cannot decide with which pressures to comply because of an excessive number of demands and a conflict of priorities. The expectations of the various roles become overwhelming, and the person does not have the physical, intellectual, economic, emotional, and other resources to adapt to or perform the expected roles.

Self-concept can be altered by stressors affecting identity, body image, self-esteem, or roles. These stressors can also affect health. If people are unable to adapt to such stressors, their health may be at risk. If the resulting identity confusion, disturbed body image, low self-esteem, role conflict, strain, or ambiguity is not relieved, illness may result.

Development of Self-Concept

Development of self-concept is a lifelong process. Each stage of development has specific activities that assist the client in developing a positive self-concept (see the box below).

INFANT

What an infant needs initially is a primary caretaker and a relationship with that caretaker. This nurturing role can be fulfilled by a mother, father, or someone responsible for the caretaking of the infant. When the infant has pleasant, nurturing interactions with its caretakers, these are remembered and internalized into the infant's psyche. If the interactions are unsatisfying, painful, or frustrating, these are split from the psyche and repressed from consciousness. These split and repressed feelings will be projected onto others in later life (Scharff and Scharff, 1991). It is very important that the infant's physical and emotional needs be consistently met. This consistency enables trust to form.

Self-Concept: Developmental Tasks

0 TO 1 YEAR
- Begins to trust
- Distinguishes self from environment

1 TO 3 YEARS
- Has control of some language
- Begins to be autonomous in thoughts and actions
- Likes body
- Likes self

3 TO 6 YEARS
- Takes initiative
- Identifies with a gender
- Increases self-awareness
- Language skills increase

6 TO 12 YEARS
- Is industrious
- Interacts with peers
- Self-esteem increases with new skill mastery
- Aware of strengths and limits

12 TO 20 YEARS
- Accepts changed body
- Explores goals for future
- Feels positive about self
- Interacts with those to whom he or she finds sexually attractive

MID-20S TO MID-40S
- Has intimate relationships with family and significant others
- Has stable, positive feelings about self

MID-40S TO MID-60S
- Can accept changes in appearance and endurance
- Reassesses life goals
- Shows contentment with aging

LATE 60S ON
- Feels positive about one's life and its meaning
- Interested in providing a legacy for the next generation

At first, newborns can barely tell the difference between their own pleasurable sensations and the objects from which the sensations are derived. Newborns do not have a clear sense of body boundaries. The external world is an extension of themselves. Only as their perceptive and sensory functions mature do infants gradually learn about their bodies. Infants completely depend on adults to take care of their basic needs. When needs such as feeding and nurturance are met promptly and consistently, infants begin to develop trust in the world. Because infants view themselves as part of the primary care giver, positive experiences help them gain confidence in themselves.

Weaning, contact with others, and exploration of the environment heighten self-awareness. As children approach their first birthdays, coordination of sensory experiences is internalized into their body images.

Without adequate stimulation of the motor abilities and the senses, body image and self-concept development are impaired, as shown by studies of infants in premature incubators who lacked rocking, stroking, and cuddling (Kramer et al, 1975). Infants' initial experiences with their bodies, which are determined largely by care and attitudes of the mother, are the basis for developing body images. Later acceptance and management of the body and the reactions of others to it are the ways we continue to formulate our body image (Murray and Huelskoetter, 1991).

TODDLER

Toddlers (1 to 3 years of age) are more mobile and able to interact with others. Their major psychosocial task is the development of autonomy (see Chapter 28). Children move from total dependence to a greater sense of independence and separateness of themselves from others. They also tend to view others and themselves in terms of "all good" or "all bad". They gain skills by feeding themselves and performing basic hygiene tasks. Toddlers learn to coordinate movements and imitate others. They learn control of their bodies through locomotion, toilet training, speech, and socialization skills.

Parts of themselves may be viewed as "permanent," so getting a haircut or flushing waste products down the toilet may cause stress because they were a part of the self. Toddlers do not always know when they are ill, fatigued, too cold, or thirsty or have wet pants. Toddlers are full of impulse and personify the Sesame Street Cookie Monster: "Want cookie . . . take cookie!" It is the parent's task and society's job to gently put limits on behaviors that are expected.

PRESCHOOLER

Body boundaries, sense of self, and gender of preschoolers become more definite to them because of a developing sexual curiosity and awareness of differences from others of the same and opposite gender. Learning about the body, where it begins and ends, what it looks like, and what it can do, are basic to self-concept and body image formation. Growing self-awareness includes discovery of feelings; for example, preschoolers learn names for their feelings. They begin to learn how they affect others and how others respond to them. They also learn the rudiments of control over feelings and behavior. The concept of body is reflected in the way children talk, move, draw pictures, and play.

Children begin to test roles and imitate people as they identify with the same-sex parent or a family member (see Chapter 28).

Children feel small in relation to adults. They establish positive or negative views of themselves. They hear and experience emotions and pronouncements of others, especially parents, about themselves as people. They also hear about things and events around them. When these expressions are repeated many times, they begin to form a predictable pattern. Children internalize the views of others and begin to see the views of others as part of themselves. They then behave to match these views. This view of the self begins as a judgment made by another. For example, Johnny's parents consider him to be mechanically inclined. As he develops, this perception becomes a part of him and he acts accordingly by putting together or repairing things. Children learn to value what their parents value. Appraisal by a family member becomes self-appraisal. Family is critical to the child's budding self-concept, and negative input at this time creates a decreased self-esteem, which the person as an adult will have to work very hard to overcome.

SCHOOL-AGE CHILD

Until children attend school, self-concept and body image are based primarily on parental attitudes (see Chapter 29). At school others contribute to self-concept and body image. This can have a counterbalancing effect for children whose families have been extremely critical, or it can be negative if the child experiences a negative educational environment.

As the child enters the school years, growth is steady, and more motor, social, and intellectual skills are acquired. The child's body changes, and sexual identity strengthens. Attention span increases, and reading allows expansion of self-concept through imagination into other roles, behaviors, and places. Through games children interact with peers, develop additional motor and intellectual skills, and thereby expand self-concept and body image (Fig. 23-5). Children express feelings through games, literature, drawing, and music. The nurse can use these to gain clues to children's self-concepts. With increased problem-solving abilities, a greater self-awareness of personal strengths and

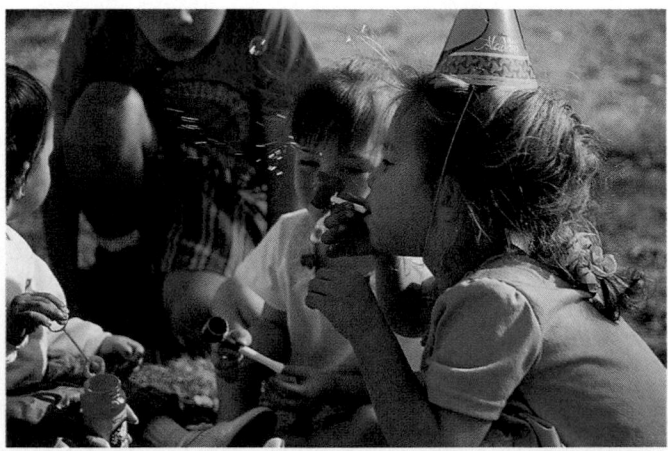

Fig. 23-5 Interaction with peers builds a child's self-concept.

limitations develops. Self-concept and body image can change at this time because the child is changing physically, emotionally, mentally, and socially.

ADOLESCENT

Adolescence brings physical, emotional, and social upheaval. Throughout sexual maturation, new feelings, roles, and values must be integrated into the self. Rapid growth, noticed by the adolescent and others, is an important factor in body image acceptance and revision (see Chapter 29).

Adolescents are forced to alter their mental pictures of themselves. Physical changes in size and appearance cause changes in self-perception and use of the body. Adolescents spend a great deal of time in front of the mirror for hygiene, grooming, and dressing in which they seek to improve their appearance as much as possible. Great distress is felt about perceived body imperfections.

Development of self-concept and body image is closely related to identity formation (Erikson, 1963). Early experiences have important effects. Positive experiences as a child enable adolescents to feel good about themselves. Negative experiences as a child may result in a poor self-concept. Children who enter adolescence with negative feelings find this difficult period even more distressing.

Adolescents may overemphasize appearance; a pointed nose, large ears, short stature, or large body frame may consequently cause adolescents to underevaluate themselves. If adolescents do not feel accepted for themselves or their bodies, they may try to compensate through sports, vocational or academic success, religious commitment, use of alcohol or drugs, or a group of friends to enhance prestige. Compensations may be quite positive or negative, depending on the acceptance of society of that particular activity.

Adolescents also begin to relate to the opposite sex in new ways and with increasing interest. They sample various behavioral roles as they establish a sense of identity, including who they are, what life means, and where they are going.

YOUNG ADULT

Although physical growth has stopped, cognitive, social, and behavioral changes continue for the rest of life. Young adulthood (early 20s to mid-40s) is a period of choice; it is a period of settling into responsibility, gaining stability in the establishment of employment, and beginning intimate relationships. Self-concept and body image become relatively stable at this time.

Self-concept and body image are social creations, and approval and acceptance are given for normal appearance and proper behavior according to societal standards. Self-concept constantly evolves and can be identified in values, attitudes, and feelings about the self.

MIDDLE ADULT

Physical changes such as additional fat deposits, baldness, gray hair, wrinkles, and varicosities confront the middle adult. This developmental stage, resulting from changes in hormone production and, often, a decrease in activity, affects body image, which may in turn alter self-concept. People realize that they look older, and they may feel older as well. Work may be stressful if middle-age people feel that they have less stamina, endurance, and vigor to cope with the task at hand. This reduced energy level is often the result of lower basal metabolism and reduced muscle tone.

Illness or death of loved ones can create concerns about personal health. The person can feel inferior to youth as the previous self-image of a strong and healthy body with boundless energy is replaced with a self-image reflecting the changes of aging. Difficulties in accepting the loss of youth are also caused by fear of the effects of menopause, folklore about sexuality, and social and advertising pressures describing the virtues of youth.

The middle adult years are often the time for a reassessment of life experiences and a redefinition of the self in life roles and values (see Chapter 30). This is called the midlife crisis. This reevaluation might include career or marriage choices. Successful resolution involves the integration of new qualities into self-concept. Most people gradually adjust to their slowly changing bodies and accept the changes as part of maturing. Emotionally mature people realize that they cannot return to youth and acknowledge that their own pasts and experiences are valid and valuable. Middle-age people who are content with their age and have no desire to relive the youthful years exhibit a healthy self-concept.

OLDER ADULT

Physical changes in older adults can be seen as gradual reductions of structure and function (see Chapter 31). Loss of muscle strength and tone occurs. Osteoporosis, which is a loss of bone density and mass, may increase the risk of fractures or create a "dowager's" hump.

Loss of sensory acuity is a factor that influences older adults in interacting with the environment. The normal process of aging causes decreased visual acuity. Hearing loss can cause negative personality changes as older people realize that they are no longer aware of all that is happening or said. Suspiciousness, irritability, impatience, or withdrawal may develop because of impaired hearing. Often, older adults view a hearing aid as another threat to body image. To many older adults, eyeglasses are more socially acceptable because they are worn by all age-groups, but a hearing aid is perceived as direct evidence of age. Adjustment to the use of a hearing aid may be difficult; if motivation is low, hearing aids may be rejected.

Loss of skin tone with accompanying wrinkles and appearance may affect self-esteem and cause older persons to feel ugly in a society that values youth and beauty. Western culture does not discriminate with age and appearance toward men as severely as it does toward women.

Sexual activity may diminish with age, even though the ability to perform remains. Often, many older people do not engage in sexual activity because they lack partners. Changes in body image may deter sexual activity because of anticipated or perceived rejection by a partner or because of feared inability to perform, even though most research indicates that no physical barriers exist.

Self-concept during older adulthood is influenced by experiences throughout life. It is a time when many people reflect on their lives, reviewing successes and disappointments and thereby creating a unified sense of meaning about themselves and the world (see the box on p. 398). Helping the younger generation in a positive way often helps an older adult to develop a feeling of leaving a legacy.

GERONTOLOGICAL PRINCIPLES
for Supporting Self-Concept

- As persons age, it is useful to individuals to focus on memories they have in which they were helpful to another person. These events may have happened a long time ago or very recently.
- As a culture, we often do not provide older adults with opportunities to tell about themselves. It may even be discouraged. Having clients experience this exercise can be ego strengthening.
- Try the following exercise to produce the feeling of a client's positive self-worth:

Find a quiet and comfortable location for a conversation. Ask the client, "As you look back on events that have occurred, tell me about an event in your life of which you are especially proud." Spend about 30 minutes of uninterrupted time listening. Give the client complete attention and good eye contact. An interested person gives self-validation to the client in a way that is very satisfying.

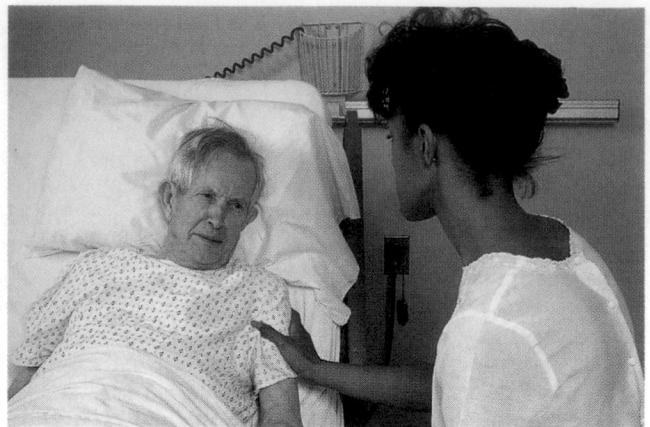

Fig. 23-6 Nurses can use touch and direct eye contact to increase a client's self-concept.

Self-concept is also influenced by people's present perceived health status.

Family Effect on Self-Concept Development

Family plays a key role in creating and maintaining its members' self-concepts. Children learn from parents and siblings a basic sense of who they are and how they are expected to live. Negative self-concepts may be created in children, even by well-meaning parents. Parents who are harsh, inconsistent, or have low self-esteem may have learned these patterns from their parents, thereby creating a cycle that may be difficult to break. To reverse a client's low self-esteem, the nurse may need to first assess the family's style of relating. Self-concept change demands hard work and consistency, supported by the entire nursing staff and physicians as well.

■ NURSE'S EFFECT ON CLIENT'S SELF-CONCEPT

A nurse's acceptance of a client with an altered self-concept helps stimulate positive rehabilitation. With a client whose physical appearance has changed and who must adapt to a new body image, it is likely that both client and family may look to nurses and observe their responses and reactions to the new situation. Nurses have a significant impact on clients in this respect. Nursing plans formulated to help a client with an altered self-concept can be enhanced or defeated by the nurse's unconscious values and feelings. It is critical for nurses to assess and clarify the following about themselves:

1. The nurse's own feelings about health and illness
2. How the nurse reacts to stress
3. The power of nonverbal communication with client and family and how it is being displayed
4. What personal values and expectations are conveyed and affect clients
5. How a nonjudgmental approach can benefit the client

Nurses need to assess themselves honestly before they can begin to understand how they affect their clients with both words and actions. Nurses should pay attention to "triggers," which are heightened feelings that occur in response to a given situation. Nurses cannot deny that they have feelings, ideas, values, and expectations or deny that they make judgments. Self-awareness is critical in initially understanding and accepting others. All people make decisions about themselves, the environment, and other people on the basis of personal frames of reference. As professionals, nurses must be prepared to work with people who have different frames of reference from the nurse. Nurses who are secure in their own identities more readily accept and thus reinforce clients' identities. However, nurses who are unsure of their own identities may be unable to accept clients and may react as if clients should be something or someone else, thus creating a nonaccepting environment for the client.

Nurses also have a significant impact on body image. Clients who must adapt to a changed body image caused by illness or surgery need support, as do their families. For example, if nurses feel that ostomies or mastectomies are horribly disfiguring, they should not express that opinion to clients either verbally or nonverbally. Nurses should talk with people who have had experience in the care and rehabilitation of such clients. Meeting people who have had such surgery and who have recuperated can increase knowledge. Nurses who feel insecure about their own body images will probably react more strongly to changes in clients' physical appearances and functioning.

Inadvertently frowning or grimacing when performing procedures can have profound effects on the client. A nurse who avoids a client should recognize that something is wrong. The nurse's nonverbal behaviors help to convey the level of caring that exists for a client (Fig. 23-6). For example, the self-concept of incontinent clients can be threatened by the perception that the caretakers find the situation unpleasant. Nurses should anticipate these reactions, acknowledge them, and focus on the client instead of the unpleasant task or situation. Otherwise, clients may perceive nurses' behaviors as rejection. If nurses can put themselves in the client's position, they can envision measures to ease embarrassment, frustration, anger, and denial. It is rewarding to display caring for those clients undergoing dramatic changes to the body.

SELF-CONCEPT AND THE NURSING PROCESS

 ## Assessment

In assessing self-concept, the nurse obtains objective and subjective data that focus on actual and potential self-concept stressors and on behaviors associated with an altered self-concept. Examples of stressors that the nurse may identify while collecting the nursing history include loss of job, onset of chronic disease, or homelessness (see Fig. 23-3). Further objective data include behaviors demonstrated by the client, such as preoccupation with a change in body image, hesitancy to try new things, and verbal and nonverbal interactions between the client and others (e.g., expressions of shame or failure to look at a body part). Subjective data are gathered to determine the client's view of the self and the environment. Significant others' perceptions are a vital source of data. How do family and significant others perceive the client's response to threats to self-esteem? Table 23-1 presents assessment questions that may help in the assessment of self-concept.

The nursing assessment should include consideration of previous coping behaviors; the nature, number, and intensity of the stressors; and the client's internal and external resources. Many times the nurse forgets to assess how the client has dealt with prior stressors. Coping may be through avoidance of the problem, information gathering, deferring decisions about themselves to the significant other to make, denial, and so on. Not all issues are addressed in the same way by clients, but many times one uses a significant coping pattern. Client medical records are

another objective source of data that may reveal a history of negative coping through the use of alcohol or other substances.

It is also important to assess the client's health promotion activities. For example, does the client attend a bereavement group or a divorced-singles group to gain support during stressful life events? A review of resources within the client's community (see the box above) and the client's willingness or interest in using them also helps in eventually establishing a plan of care. Hospital and community nurses need to be aware of resources for client referral because the care does not end with the end of hospitalization. Home and community care of the client are rapidly becoming the major source of health care.

> ### Resources in the Community for Self-Concept Support
>
> - ACOA: Adult Children of Alcoholics
> - AA: Alcoholics Anonymous
> - Compassionate Friends: Parents whose children have died
> - NAMI: National Alliance for the Mentally Ill
> - Make Today Count: Women recuperating from mastectomy
> - Overeaters Anonymous: Support for eating disorder of overeating
> - Grief support groups: Often offered by counseling services and churches
> - Women's crisis centers: Support for victims of abuse and assault

Table 23-1	Examples of Self-Concept Assessment Questions	
QUESTIONS FROM THE NURSE	**TYPICAL RESPONSES THAT INDICATE LOW SELF-ESTEEM**	
IDENTITY "If I did not know you, how would you describe yourself to me?"	Answers that are derogatory about oneself (e.g., "I'm not much good," "I don't matter," or "I'm too skinny, fat, ugly")	
BODY IMAGE "Is there something about your body you'd change? If so, what is it?"	It is normal for people to make comments about specific attributes, such as "My nose is too long" or "My thighs are too fat." If the answer focuses on many items, this is not healthy. Answers that indicate marked divergence from what the person is are also cause for concern, such as "I would weigh 150 pounds less" or "I would not be Hispanic," indicate great discomfort.	
SELF-ESTEEM "How do you feel about yourself?" "Are you accomplishing what you want in your life so far?"	Statements of not liking oneself or not achieving what one had hoped are cause for concern. Verbalizing hopelessness or helplessness indicates distress of the self.	
ROLES "Do you feel you've been able to be a (mother, daughter, wife, husband, father, son) in your family, in the way you wanted to be?"	Feelings of dissatisfaction in the role are distressing to the self-concept.	

Examples of NANDA Nursing Diagnoses for Disturbance in Self-Concept

Altered parenting *related to:*
Identity confusion subsequent to earlier conflicts with own parents
Lack of preparation for role
Altered role performance *related to:*
Demands on time as result of entry into college
Perceptions about ageist attitudes encountered in workplace
Anxiety about abilities after myocardial infarction
Anxiety *related to:*
Perception of midlife aging changes and implication for job security
Marital role conflicts
Concerns about sexuality
Body image disturbance *related to:*
Negative perception of self after hysterectomy
Visual impairment
Fear *related to:*
Feelings of powerlessness from recent home burglary
Unresolved crisis of being assaulted
Impaired adjustment *related to:*
Anxiety about body image (amputation)
Fear of terminal illness (AIDS)
Impaired social interaction *related to:*
Role ambiguity (widowhood)
Depression resulting from recent admission to extended care facility
Ineffective individual coping *related to:*
Low self-esteem
Dysfunctional parent-child relationship
Unclear role expectations

Parental role conflict *related to:*
Feeling loss of control as a result of birth of child with congenital defect
Anxiety about upcoming remarriage
Personal identity disturbance *related to:*
Rapid loss of weight
Value conflicts aroused by peer group
Confusion about sexuality
Risk for violence: self-directed *related to:*
Identity confusion in adolescence
Inability to cope with multiple role expectations
Low self-esteem after abuse from spouse
Powerlessness *related to:*
Incompatible role expectations at home and work
Feelings of low self-worth
Rape-trauma syndrome *related to:*
Unresolved crisis of being assaulted sexually
Self-esteem disturbance *related to:*
Job interview anxiety
Perception of sexuality after infertility problems
Situational low self-esteem *related to:*
Unresolved grief
Lack of meaningful support system
Role conflict with colleagues
Spiritual distress (distress of the human spirit) *related to:*
Identity confusion in midlife
Altered body image from accidental paralysis
Alcohol and drug abuse

Sample Nursing Diagnostic Process for Self-Concept Disturbances

ASSESSMENT ACTIVITIES	DEFINING CHARACTERISTICS	NURSING DIAGNOSES
Review presenting clinic history	45-year-old man with amputation of right leg following auto accident	**Body image disturbance** related to negative perception of self following amputation
Ask client to describe how the amputation has affected his life routines	Client states that employment as a construction worker will no longer be possible	
Ask client how he feels about himself	Client states, "I see myself as less of a man. How can I be a husband and father?"	
Ask client what the diagnosis of acquired immunodeficiency syndrome (AIDS) means to her	Client states that she believes blood tests were mixed up and she simply has bad case of "flu"	**Impaired adjustment** related to fear of terminal illness
	Relates how a close friend died a painful AIDS death alone	
Question family regarding perception of client	Family states that client has said she would "rather kill myself than die like my friend"	

Nursing Diagnosis

Assessment data need careful interpretation by the nurse. Clients with defining characteristics for self-concept disturbances may suggest nursing diagnoses pertinent to deficiencies in identity, body image, self-esteem, or role performance. Events that have an impact on the "self" exert stressors on the self-concept. If the stressor is great enough, or if it is exerted on the client for a long enough period, the client will become symptomatic.

The assessment should reveal the presence of defining characteristics and client behaviors that lead to a nursing diagnosis (see the nursing diagnoses box and the diagnostic process box on p. 400). The nurse must be careful to make an accurate diagnosis on the basis of assessment data. For example, consider a client with diagnosed chronic lung disease. The nurse may quickly assume that the client has a poor body image as a result of a loss in body function. However, this information alone will not form a conclusive nursing diagnosis. *Altered role performance* might be an appropriate nursing diagnosis as well, because of the client's change in the physical capacity to assume a role as an employee. More data are needed for the nurse to make an insightful judgment about the client's health problems. The client's verbalization of hopelessness, avoidance in social activities, and negative statements about his body, are signs of *body image disturbance.*

 ## Planning

After determining the nursing diagnoses, the nurse, client, and family need to plan care directed at helping the client regain or maintain a healthy self-concept. The care plan is based on goals and expected outcomes (see the care plan below). The outcomes will provide the measures for determining whether the eventual plan of care is successful. The nurse must determine whether the outcomes established are realistic, given the client's current physical and psychosocial state. For a client beginning to receive chemotherapy and having body image stressors (hair loss, weight loss, decrease in strength) expected outcomes might include describing the physical effects of the medication and expressing feelings about the illness and the treatment taking place. Also, a later goal might be: The client will adapt successfully to the new body (with its strengths and weaknesses) that emerges after the chemotherapy is finished. Other health care team members also have goals and interventions. Physical therapy may have a goal of full muscular strength again, while occupational therapy's goal may be for the client to do most of his activites of daily living, even though there has been some sensory destruction by the chemotherapy. It is important to establish with the client the priority of the goals.

If the client's stay in a health care facility will be short, there may not be enough time to restructure body image,

 ## Sample Nursing Care Plan for Self-Concept Disturbance

NURSING DIAGNOSIS: **Body image disturbance** related to negative perception of self after hysterectomy
DEFINITION: Body image disturbance is a disruption in the way one perceives one's body image (Kim MJ, McFarland GK, and McLane AM, 1995).

GOAL	EXPECTED OUTCOMES	INTERVENTIONS	RATIONALE
Client will verbalize positive, realistic aspects of body image by discharge (projected 3/24).	Client will state one positive effect of surgery by 3/22.	Teach about physical and physiological effects of abdominal hysterectomy (3/19).	Providing clear information about aftereffects of hysterectomy dispels misunderstandings and myths on results of surgery. It also reinforces positive aspects of procedure. Including family members helps ensure reinforcement of information and support for client.
	Client will redefine and share values and beliefs regarding femininity by 3/23.	Encourage client to explore beliefs, perceptions, and values related to sexuality, femininity, and female roles. Begin twice a day on 3/20 (7-3, 3-11).	This gives client opportunity to redefine rigid concepts of gender and roles and reintegrate more positive self-image.
	Client will voice statements indicating some acceptance of physical self by 3/24.		
	Client will be able to look at incision by 3/24.	Encourage client to view and touch abdominal area during bathing.	Personalizes loss of body part.

and if the client has not resolved the problem by discharge, referral to a community resource should be recommended. A psychiatric community health clinic, support groups, and family group counseling services are options to consider. If the client is experiencing an extended period of depression or grief, the family physician, a psychiatric clinical nurse specialist, or a psychiatrist may need to evaluate the individual for necessary therapy.

After establishing goals the nurse plans strategies aimed at resolving the nursing diagnoses. Specifically, the nursing interventions are directed at the related factor for the diagnosis. For example, in the case of *body image disturbance* related to negative perception of self after hysterectomy, the nurse's interventions will aim to help the client regain her femininity and accept the physical changes associated with the abdominal incision. If the related factor were negative perception of self after diagnosis of diabetes, the interventions would be very different. The client in this case would need support to understand the nature of a chronic disease and recognize that a normal, fulfilling life can be maintained.

The care plan presents the goals, expected outcomes, and interventions for a client with a self-concept disorder. Interventions focus on helping the client adapt to the stressors that led to the self-concept disturbance and on supporting and reinforcing the development of coping methods. Often a client perceives a situation as overwhelming and may feel hopeless about returning to the level of previous functioning. The client may need time to adapt to physical changes. The nurse should look for strengths in both the individual and the family and provide resources and education to turn limitations into strengths. Client teaching creates understanding of why certain events have happened (e.g., nature of chronic disease, change in relationships, the effect of loss), and many times, once understood, the sense of hopelessness and helplessness can be lessened.

 ## Implementation

Establishing a therapeutic environment and relationship and supporting self-exploration are critical to intervening with clients who have self-concept problems. The many variables influencing a client's views of the self are personal and private. The nurse must clearly and genuinely convey care for the client. Then and only then will trust develop to enable the nurse to partner with the client in establishing purposeful interventions.

Creating a Therapeutic Environment

The human experience in illness and its treatment affect an individual's self-concept in various ways. The client needs a safe, nonjudgmental, and supportive environment. Some suggestions to create that support are:

1. Accept the client, keeping in mind that most people regress to earlier developmental stages when ill.
2. Understand that anger with one's self or with things not under one's control is often projected onto the nearest person. Usually it is the nurse or a family member. Reacting with anger may be the thing one wants to do, but it is not productive for the nurse or the client. Exploring with the client the true feelings

CLIENT TEACHING
on Approaches for Reducing Anger

OBJECTIVE
- Client will be able to express anger regarding self in a constructive manner.

TEACHING STRATEGIES
- Encourage client to talk about angry situations, write down negative thoughts, and discuss them objectively.
- When anger-producing situations arise, encourage client to try instead a form of physical exercise.
- When anger is directed at another person, learn to stop the thinking with a signal (e.g., rubberband on the wrist, biting the tongue softly, telling self to stop unproductive thinking).
- Plan a discussion of an anger-producing event that will allow the client to explore feelings underneath the anger.

EVALUATION
- Ask client to discuss reasons for being angry with himself or herself.
- Observe interactions with family and friends.

underneath the angry reaction is much more productive (see the box above).

Normal, everyday health care activities are capable of lowering a client's self-concept. For example, a hospitalized client almost always experiences role changes and lowered self-esteem as a result of dependence on those providing care. A physical examination performed in a clinic along with drawing of blood samples threatens the client's body and privacy. Because such nursing activities are anxiety producing for most clients, the client often feels alienated and vulnerable and may react in ways that demonstrate regression.

By encouraging visits from friends and family members the client is assisted to maintain his or her usual role within the family. Discussing procedures with the client and encouraging participation in the care plan itself are examples of ways a nurse can respect client identity. In general, the nurse should assist the client in carrying on as much as possible of the usual activities and relationships that support self-concept. If self-concept depends on activities in which the client is no longer able to participate, the nurse is challenged to encourage adaptation to change through other kinds of activities that rebuild self-concept and a sense of normalcy.

Keep other nurses and other health care professionals up to date on the client's progress because they can be involved in offering support and reinforcement. If a health alteration is particularly severe, staff conferences are useful in helping the nurse handle personal feelings and emotions, as well as a time for receiving input and planning a unified plan of care for the health care team.

The nurse's primary role, perhaps, is as a caring person who is a role model for the client and family. Acceptance of the client as a human being who has ideas, feelings, and values and who is worthy and whole, despite illness or physical alterations, is an essential component of nursing care. Feelings of insecurity, fears of rejection, or loss of self-worth can be lessened through sensitive, knowledgeable nursing care.

Establishing a Therapeutic Relationship

Chapter 14 outlines in detail the techniques used in establishing therapeutic relationships with clients. In the case of clients with self-esteem disturbances, it is important to establish a feeling of acceptance of the individual, creating a sense of harmony by a warm, friendly manner, appropriate smile, and eye contact. The following behaviors are involved in establishing acceptance and trust:

1. Be nonjudgmental, and convey acceptance of the client.
2. Build rapport based on common interests or experiences during conversation.
3. Give the client your full attention, listen carefully, and indicate that there is time to listen.
4. Adopt the client's terminology as much as possible.

In any helping relationship trust is essential. Trust is gained by displaying reliability and following through with what you say. Empathy, or feeling for clients, understanding behavior, and being motivated to act on a client's behalf are other essential characteristics for establishing a helping relationship. The following interventions may be used to help clients who have undergone body image alterations and those clients who have poor self-concepts:

1. Determine client's present abilities and coping.
2. Use effective interviewing techniques.
3. Determine the family's ability to positively reinforce client's perception of self.
4. Convey acceptance and empathy.
5. Encourage appropriate expression of anger.
6. Use interventions to help clients work through hopelessness, sadness, and grief (see Chapter 26).
7. Give positive reinforcement to desired behavior and accomplishments, as appropriate.
8. Promote exploration of understanding of behavior and feelings.
9. Present alternative courses of action and ways to change behavior to be more adaptive.
10. Build on previous client knowledge when teaching and finding "teachable moments" when clients are ready to learn.
11. Assist clients (and families) in identifying resources or support systems.
12. Validate strengths, appropriate ideas, and behaviors.
13. Introduce changes gradually, one at a time if possible, to allow adequate time for adjustment and avoid further threats to self-concept.
14. Encourage clients to express self-affirmations (e.g., "I can" or "I'm still capable of . . .").
15. Reinforce progress in behavior or self-care activities.
16. Encourage evaluation of progress between the nurse and the client.
17. Terminate the nurse-client relationship after working through feelings of separation and termination.

When providing care to clients experiencing stress that affects self-esteem and identity, the nurse should include activities in which clients will achieve success. Tasks should not be so difficult that the client cannot succeed. Ensuring a small success is better than risking a defeat at a larger task.

CASE STUDY Cindy is a 24-year-old factory worker. She lives at home with her disabled mother. Cindy's father was alcoholic for most of her life and recently has become sober, although her mother and father divorced some years ago. Cindy is the second youngest of six children. She has one older sister. As her brothers grew and matured, one by one they were kicked out of the family by Dad. He beat all the boys severely, and one by one they joined the armed services. Cindy's sister was forced to take the younger children with her on dates and the like. The sister married early and left the family also.

Cindy came to her family physician's office saying she was so angry she "didn't know what to do." She had injured her hand by pounding it on her car, after having an argument with her mother. After she has her hand splinted, she begins to tell Marcia, Dr. Stephens' nurse, how she feels. Cindy tells Marcia that two of her brothers have moved in with her mother and her. Neither of them works, and they do not contribute anything toward the family's living expenses. Both have girlfriends, and they invite their girlfriends over in the evenings. Cindy is so angry that she spends her evenings in her own room watching television. She says she gets upset when she sees her brothers lounging around the house when she leaves for work in the mornings. One of her brothers has children that he does not support financially and seldom sees.

Cindy says that her mother has the expectation that she should help support her brothers by continuing to help pay for the rent, for the food, and for some of the utilities. Cindy tells Marcia she is so angry over this that she is starting to be upset over small things and that she is afraid she will lose control. She asks Marcia if she would put up with such a situation. Marcia replies that it is a situation that has evolved in the family and that it is difficult to know what all the dynamics were that allowed this situation to come about. She tells Cindy that perhaps she should seek some counseling from the local community mental health agency. Marcia points out that they have sliding scale fees based on income and they are convenient to Cindy's work location. Cindy responds that she has insurance that would pay for counseling, but she does not want to be seen at the community agency. Marcia gets a list of counselors to whom Dr. Stephens refers clients. She also tells Cindy she can look in the telephone book under "counseling" for more names. Cindy seems greatly relieved and takes the list.

Marcia tells Cindy she will follow up in a week with a phone call to see how things are going and to see whether Cindy was able to select a counselor. Marcia was very conscious of the ethical issue of not referring Cindy to just one counselor or therapist, but of giving her at least three names plus suggesting she check the telephone pages if she wanted to go further. During the 1-week phone call Cindy tells Marcia that she has had her first appointment with a counselor and found it very helpful. She states that she is looking for an apartment but has not found one as yet. Her mother continues to allow the sons to live with her, free of responsibilities. Cindy thanks Marcia for helping her with her anger, and Cindy agrees to update Marcia at her doctor's appointment the next week.

Marcia was insightful in recognizing Cindy's anger and distress about a situation that at first glance may appear harmless. However, seeing the escalating potential in the situation, Marcia wisely intervened. ■

Table 23-2	Levels of Nursing Interventions for Self-Concept Disturbance	
PRINCIPLE	**RATIONALE**	**NURSING ACTIONS**

GOAL: EXPAND CLIENT'S SELF-AWARENESS

PRINCIPLE	RATIONALE	NURSING ACTIONS
Work with resources client possesses.	Some resources, such as self-control and self-perception, are needed as foundations for later nursing care.	Confirm identity. Provide support measures to reduce anxiety. Approach client in undemanding way. Accept and attempt to clarify any verbal or nonverbal communication. Prevent client isolation. Help establish simple routine. Help set limits on inappropriate behavior. Orient client to reality. Reinforce appropriate behavior. Gradually increase activities and tasks that provide positive experiences. Assist in personal hygiene and grooming. Encourage client to care for self.
Maximize client's participation in therapeutic relationship.	Mutuality is necessary for client to assume ultimate responsibility for behavior and coping responses.	Gradually increase client's participation in decisions that affect care. Convey that client is responsible individual.

GOAL: ENCOURAGE CLIENT'S SELF-EXPLORATION

PRINCIPLE	RATIONALE	NURSING ACTIONS
Show interest in and accept client's feelings and thoughts.	When nurse shows interest in and accepts client's feelings and thoughts, the nurse helps client to do so also.	Attend to and encourage client's expression of emotions, beliefs, behavior, and thoughts—verbally, nonverbally, symbolically, or directly. Use therapeutic communication skills and empathic responses. Note use of logical and illogical thinking and reported and observed emotional responses.
Help client clarify self-concept and relationships to others through self-disclosure.	Self-disclosure and understanding self-perceptions are prerequisites to bringing about future change; this may, in itself, reduce anxiety.	Elicit client's perceptions of strengths and weaknesses. Help describe ideal self. Identify self-criticisms. Help describe how client perceives relationships to other people and events.
Be aware and have control of your own feelings.	Self-awareness allows nurse to model authentic behavior.	Be open to your own feelings. Accept your positive and negative feelings. Practice therapeutic use of self: share your feelings with client, describe how another might have felt, and mirror your perception of client's feelings.
Respond empathically, not sympathetically, emphasizing that power to change lies with client.	Sympathy can reinforce client's self-pity; rather, nurse should communicate that client's life situation is subject to one's own control.	Use empathic responses and monitor yourself for feelings of sympathy or pity. Reaffirm that client is not helpless or powerless when dealing with problems. Convey verbally and behaviorally that client is responsible for behavior, including choice of maladaptive or adaptive coping responses. Discuss with client scope of choices, areas of strength, and coping resources available.

GOAL: ASSIST CLIENT IN SELF-EVALUATION

PRINCIPLE	RATIONALE	NURSING ACTIONS
Help client to clearly define problem.	Only after problem is accurately defined can alternative choices be proposed.	Identify relevant stressors with client and ask for appraisal of them. Clarify that client's beliefs influence feelings and behaviors. Mutually identify faulty beliefs, misperceptions, distortions, illusions, and unrealistic goals. Mutually identify areas of strength. Place concepts of success and failure in proper perspective. Explore use of coping resources.
Explore client's adaptive and maladaptive coping responses to problem.	Examination of client's choices made during coping will help define successful and unsuccessful responses.	Describe how coping responses are chosen and have positive and negative consequences. Contrast adaptive and maladaptive responses. Mutually identify disadvantages of client's maladaptive coping responses. Mutually identify advantages or "payoffs" of client's maladaptive coping responses.

Table 23-2	Levels of Nursing Interventions for Self-Concept Disturbance—cont'd	
PRINCIPLE	**RATIONALE**	**NURSING ACTIONS**

GOAL: ASSIST CLIENT IN FORMING REALISTIC GOALS

Help client identify alternative solutions.	Only when all possible alternatives have been evaluated can change be effected.	Help client understand that one can only change oneself, not others.
		If client holds inconsistent perceptions, show that the following can change: beliefs or ideals to bring them closer to reality, and environment to make it consistent with beliefs. If self-concept is not consistent with behavior, client can change the following: behavior to conform to self-concept, beliefs underlying self-concept to include behavior, and self-ideal.
		Mutually review use of coping resources.
Help client conceptualize realistic goals.	Goal setting that includes clear definition of expected change is necessary.	Encourage client to form personal (not nurse's) goals.
		Mutually discuss emotional and practical consequences of each goal.
		Help client define concrete change to be made.
		Encourage client to enter new experiences for growth potential.
		Use role modeling and role playing when appropriate.

GOAL: ASSIST CLIENT IN BECOMING COMMITTED TO DECISION AND IN ACHIEVING GOALS

Help client take necessary action to change maladaptive coping responses and maintain adaptive ones.	Ultimate objective in promoting client's insight is to replace maladaptive coping responses with more adaptive ones.	Provide opportunity for success.
		Reinforce strengths, skills, and healthy aspects of client's personality.
		Assist client in gaining assistance (e.g., vocational, financial, and social services).
		Use family and groups to enhance client's self-esteem.
		Allow client sufficient time to change.
		Provide support and positive reinforcement to maintain progress.

GOAL: ASSIST CLIENT IN ACKNOWLEDGING GOALS ACHIEVED AND EVALUATING THOSE NOT ACHIEVED

Help client to purposefully review achievements and explore reasons for any problems or setbacks.	Reinforcement of gains made in strengthening self-concept will motivate continued change.	Mutually review progress made.
		Affirm achievements with client and family or significant others.
		Evaluate what contributed most to success.
		Help client discuss feelings regarding goals not achieved.

GOAL: ASSIST CLIENT TO RE-FORM PLAN FOR ACHIEVING GOALS

Support client in reviewing goals.	Insight gained from attempts to change will support further progress.	Review with client need for further self-evaluation.
		Encourage client to continue those experiences that were successful.
Identify alternatives not tried previously.	Different approaches may be necessary to achieve desired outcomes.	Explore how new coping resources can be applied to continued change.
		Redefine changes in adaptive behaviors to be made.
		Continue to reinforce strengths and successes.

Modified from Stuart GW, Sundeen SJ: *Principles and practice of psychiatric nursing*, ed 5, St Louis, 1995, Mosby.

Sequential tasks enable the client to build on each success, continuously reinforcing achievement.

Supporting Self-Exploration

Encouraging the client's self-exploration is achieved by accepting the client's feelings and thoughts, by helping the client to clarify interactions with others, and by being empathetic. This encouragement reinforces the client's self-concept, reduces anxiety, and shows that the client has self-control. The nurse encourages self-expression and stresses the client's self-responsibility.

Assisting the client in self-evaluation involves helping the client to define problems clearly and identifying positive and negative coping mechanisms. The nurse works closely with the client to help to analyze adaptive and maladaptive responses, contrast different alternatives, and discuss outcomes. Self-evaluation in a geriatric client often involves a form of life review.

Assisting the client to establish realistic goals involves helping the client to identify alternative solutions and develop realistic goals based on them. The long-term goals of adapting to changes in self-concept or attaining a positive self-concept are based on the premise that the client first develops insight and self-awareness concerning problems and stressors and then acts to solve the problems and cope with the stressors. Stuart and Sundeen (1991) summarize nursing interventions that are appropriate for the client engaging in self-exploration:

1. Increased self-awareness
2. Self-exploration
3. Self-evaluation
4. Formulation of realistic goals
5. Commitment to goals and achievement through action
6. Acknowledgment of goals achieved and evaluation of those not achieved
7. Re-formation of the plan to achieve the goals

Each level of intervention includes specific client goals and actions (Table 23-2). The nurse helps the client proceed step by step through these levels with an individualized approach to the client's needs. If the alteration in self-concept is severe, the nurse should seek assistance from other professionals such as mental health nurses or should refer the client to specialized care. Sometimes self-help groups can provide a forum for clients to learn self-exploration. People in self-help groups are those who have had body-altering experiences (e.g., mastectomy [Reach for Recovery] or laryngectomy [Laryngectomy Club]). Self-help groups are available in most communities. The groups provide a special kind of support. People who have experienced self-concept stressors and who have adapted to them can be very instrumental in helping clients adapt to body image changes. The following case study serves to summarize nursing interventions geared at supporting clients with altered self-esteem.

The following points are essential in addressing a client whose self-concept appears to be in distress:

1. Any extreme emotion that seems stronger than it needs to be in the situation at hand should be carefully assessed.

2. Developmental stifling or thrusting ahead usually creates symptoms.
3. Follow-up of emotional symptoms is always necessary because frequently people do not follow through, once they are out of their immediate distress.
4. Nurses frequently have opportunities for self-concept assessment, whereas physicians may not.
5. Most symptoms are initially discovered by simply listening to the client.

 ## Evaluation

Success in meeting each client goal requires use of objective evaluation criteria (see the evaluation box below). Frequent evaluation of client progress is recommended so that changes can be quickly instituted if necessary. The goals may be unrealistic or inappropriate as the client's condition changes or new information is learned.

Desired outcomes for a client with a self-concept disturbance may include statements of self-acceptance and acceptance of change in appearance or function. Social interaction, adequate self-care, acceptance of use of prosthetic devices, and statements indicating understanding of teaching all indicate progress. A positive attitude toward rehabilitation and increased movement toward independence facilitates a return to preexisting roles at work or at home.

The client's adaptation to major changes may take a year or longer, but the fact that this period is long does not signify maladaptation. The nurse should look for signs that the client has reduced some stressors. Reorganization of self-concept takes time. It takes years for this reorganization to develop, and additional change and development also require time. Although change may be slow, care of the client with a self-concept disturbance can be rewarding.

 ## Sample Evaluation of Interventions for Self-Concept Disturbance

GOAL	EVALUATIVE MEASURES	EXPECTED OUTCOME
Client will verbalize positive, realistic aspects of body image by discharge.	Monitor client's communication with staff and family for gradual movement toward positive view of female body: "Being a woman doesn't just mean being able to have babies" or "I still am an attractive person." Observe nonverbal communication such as neutral-positive facial expressions when focused on abdominal incision. Note whether client verbalizes positive factual information presented in teaching session.	Client will redefine and share values and beliefs regarding femininity.

∎ KEY CONCEPTS ∎

► Self-concept is physiologically, emotionally, and socially formed based on the reactions of others to the client and then by the person's interpretations of those reactions to the self.

► Self-concept is influenced by health, family experiences, social and occupational roles, and intellectual and leisure activities.

► The components of self-concept are identity, body image, self-esteem, and roles.

► Each developmental stage involves factors that are important to the development of a healthy, positive self-concept.

► Identity is the consistent sense of self as a person distinct from others.

► Identity is particularly vulnerable during adolescence.

► Identity stressors during adolescence include the expectations of others to prepare for a career and independence, to cope with one's sexuality, and to make choices about relationships and roles; such stressors may lead to identity confusion.

► Body image is the mental picture of one's body and is not necessarily consistent with actual structure or appearance.

► Body image also includes attitudes, emotions, and personality reactions of the person toward the body.

► Body image is influenced by growth and development, cultural and societal values and attitudes, and individual perceptions of the body.

► Body image stressors include changes in physical appearance, structure, or functioning caused by normal developmental changes or illness.

► Self-esteem depends on a person's perception of the ideal self as it compares with the real self.

► Self-esteem stressors include developmental and relationship changes, illness (particularly chronic illness involving changes in what were normal activities), surgery, and accidents and the responses of other individuals to changes resulting from these events.

► Roles are learned through socialization, from one's family and one's culture.

► Role stressors, including role conflict, role ambiguity, and role strain, may originate in unclear or conflicting role expectations and be aggravated by the effects of illness.

► The nurse's self-concept and nursing actions can have a profound effect on a client's self-concept.

► Planning and implementing nursing interventions for self-concept disturbance involve expanding the client's self-awareness, encouraging self-exploration, aiding in self-evaluation, helping formulate goals in regard to adaptation, and assisting the client in achieving those goals.

∎ KEY TERMS ∎

Body image, p. 389
Ideal self, p. 391
Identification, p. 391
Identity, p. 389
Identity confusion, p. 393
Imitation, p. 391
Inhibition, p. 391
Interpersonal conflict, p. 394
Interrole conflict, p. 395
Reinforcement-extinction, p. 391
Role, p. 391
Role ambiguity, p. 395
Role conflict, p. 394
Role strain, p. 395
Self-concept, p. 389
Self-esteem, p. 390
Socialization, p. 391
Substitution, p. 391

∎ CRITICAL THINKING EXERCISES ∎

1. Your 35-year-old male diabetic client has a history of being noncompliant with his diabetic regimen. His sister tells you he was sexually abused by his older brother. How would this relate to his noncompliance?

2. A 27-year-old woman is admitted to your unit after a severe drug reaction that has left her with only 50% vision in both eyes. She is a systems analyst with the U.S. government and works on computers much of the time. She is very concerned about maintaining her job. What types of changes and solutions would you plan together?

3. A newly divorced male client is hospitalized for a long list of symptoms. His test results have been normal. His physician is impatient with the client's continuous bodily focus and mentions to you that his symptoms do not now seem to have any physical cause. The physician is exasperated with his client. How might you approach this client to begin to assess what the real problem is?

REFERENCES

Bandura A: Self-efficacy mechanism in human aging, *Am Psychol* 37(2):122, 1982.

Banaji M, Prentice D: *Ann Rev Psychol* 45:297, 1994.

Drench M: Changes in body image secondary to disease and injury, *Rehabil Nurs* 19(1):31, 1994.

Erikson EH: *Childhood and society,* ed 2, New York, 1963, Norton.

Kim MJ, McFarland GK, McLane AM: *Pocket guide to nursing diagnoses,* ed 4, St Louis, 1995, Mosby.

Kramer M et al: Extra tactile stimulation of the premature infant, *Nurs Res* 24(5):324, 1975.

Marsh H: A multidimensional, hierarchical model of self-concept: theoretical and empirical justification, *Educ Psychol Rev* 2(2):77, 1990.

Murray RB, Huelskoetter MMW: *Psychiatric-mental health nursing: giving emotional care,* ed 3, Norwalk, Conn, 1991, Appleton & Lange.

Reed P: Self-transcendence and mental health in oldest-old adults, *Nurs Res* 40(1):5, 1991.

Scharff J, Scharff D: *A primer of object relations therapy,* Northvale, NJ, 1992, Jason Aronson.

Stuart GW, Sundeen SJ: *Principles and practice of psychiatric nursing,* ed 5, St Louis, 1995, Mosby.

Wigfield A, Karpathian M: Who am I and what can I do? Children's self-concepts and motivation in achievement situations, *Educ Psychol* 26(3,4):233, 1991.

ADDITIONAL READINGS

Boyd C: Testing a model of mother-daughter identification, *West J Nurs Res* 12(4):448, 1990.

Broadwell DC: Validation of a role conflict, role ambiguity, and role predictability instrument. Doctoral dissertation, Atlanta, 1983, Georgia State University.

Brundage DJ, Broadwell DC: Altered body image. In Phipps WJ et al, editors: *Medical-surgical nursing: concepts and clinical practice,* ed 4, St Louis, 1991, Mosby.

Davenport D, Yurich J: Multicultural gender issues, *J Counsel Dev* 70(9):64, 1991.

Haber J et al: Self awareness. In Haber J et al, editors: *Comprehensive psychiatric nursing,* ed 4, St Louis, 1992, Mosby.

Kaplan H, Sadock B: *Clinical psychiatry,* Baltimore, 1990, Williams & Wilkins.

Murray R, Zentner J: *Nursing assessment and health promotion through the life span,* ed 3, Englewood Cliffs, NJ, 1985, Prentice Hall.

Selye H: *The stress of life,* New York, 1956, McGraw Hill.

Tarolli-Jager K: Personal hardiness: your buffer against burnout, *Am J Nurs* 94(2):71, 1994.

## Chapter 24

Sexuality

Mastery of content in this chapter will enable the student to:

▶ Define the key terms listed.

▶ Identify personal attitudes, beliefs, and biases related to sexuality.

▶ Discuss the nurse's role in maintaining or enhancing a client's sexual health.

▶ Define *sexuality* and describe its dimensions.

▶ Describe key concepts of sexual development during infancy, childhood, adolescence, and adulthood.

▶ Identify male and female genitalia and describe functions related to sexual stimulation and response and reproduction.

▶ Describe the sexual response cycle (Masters and Johnson model).

▶ Describe physical, therapeutic, and psychological issues affecting sexuality.

▶ Identify potential causes of sexual dysfunction.

▶ Assess a client's sexuality.

▶ Define appropriate nursing diagnoses on sexuality.

▶ Identify and describe nursing interventions to promote sexual health.

▶ Evaluate a client's sexual health.

▶ Identify potential referral resources for clients' sexual concerns outside the nurse's level of expertise.

Sex is a topic that was long considered taboo for proper adult conversation. Gradually, over the last 30 to 50 years, knowledge about sex and discussion of issues of sexuality have come to be recognized as important and necessary for human development. Since the mid-1960s, health care professionals have recognized the relevance of sexual health as a component of well-being. Even so, many adult clients lack knowledge regarding sexuality or are reluctant to raise questions related to sexuality. For example, concerns may include postpartum resumption of sexual intercourse, normalcy of development, and anxiety over the effects of antihypertensive medication on sexual function.

Initiating discussion of relevant sexual topics within clients' current developmental and health status is part of the nurse's helping role and teaching-coaching function. Such initiation may help clients feel more comfortable and relate concerns. However, many care givers lack knowledge, comfort, and confidence in addressing sexual matters. To discuss issues of sexuality in practice, the care giver must possess the necessary knowledge base, skills in assessment and communication, and a caring sensitive attitude.

It is also critical that care givers recognize that sexual issues are value laden. Religious teachings, culturally prescribed gender roles, beliefs about sexual orientation, and past and present social and environmental influences affect both the client's and the provider's value system. Acknowledging values and biases and gaining knowledge about sexual issues may broaden understanding of the vast range of normal sexual behavior and enable health care providers to be more effective and caring in working with clients.

■ CONCEPTS OF SEXUALITY

Sexuality is difficult to define because it encompasses so many aspects of our lives and is expressed through a variety of behaviors. It is not only intrinsic to a person's very being but also extends into relationships with others. Intimacy and physical sharing are lifelong biological and social needs. **Sexual health** has been defined as "the integration of the somatic, emotional, intellectual, and social aspects of sexual being, in ways that are positively enriching and that enhance personality, communication, and love" (World Health Organization, 1975).

Many people erroneously think of sexuality only in terms of sex. Sexuality and sex, however, are two different things. The word **sex** is often used in two ways. Most commonly it is used to refer to the physical part of a relationship, genital sexual activity. It is also used to label gender, whether one is female or male (Zawid, 1994). **Sexuality**, on the other hand, is a much broader term. It is expressed through interactions and relationships with people of the opposite sex and/or same sex and includes a person's thoughts, experiences, learnings, ideals, values, fantasies, and emotions. It is related to how persons feel about themselves and how they communicate those feelings to others through their overt actions, such as touching, kissing, hugging, and sexual intercourse, and through more subtle behavior, such as gestures, mannerisms, dress, and vocabulary (Denney and Quadagno, 1992; Zawid, 1994). Sexuality influences and is influenced by life experiences. These influences and experiences are often different for women than for men.

The process by which people come to know themselves as females or males is not clearly understood. Being born with female or male genitalia and subsequently learning female or male social roles seem to be key ingredients; yet this does not explain all variations of sexuality and sexual behavior. This diversity is more understandable when nurses remember that sexuality is intertwined with all aspects of self. Consideration of sexuality and sexual health, therefore, requires a holistic perspective. It has sociocultural, ethical, psychological, and biological dimensions.

Dimensions of Sexuality

SOCIOCULTURAL DIMENSIONS

Sexuality is influenced by cultural rules and norms that determine what is acceptable behavior within the culture. Global cultural diversity creates considerable variability in sexual norms and represents a wide spectrum of beliefs and values. Examples include meaning and behavior allowed during dating, what is considered arousing, types of sexual activity, sanctions and prohibitions on sexual behavior, who one marries, and who is allowed to marry.

Circumcision is an example of cultural sexual tradition. Male circumcision is the removal of the prepuce or foreskin over the glans penis. Although a controversial issue, approximately 80% of newborn boys in the United States are circumcised for "hygienic reasons" or as a symbol of religious or ethnic identity (Denney and Quadagno, 1992). Female circumcision is an ancient tradition that is deeply embedded in some countries (see the box below). It is often referred to as *female genital mutilation* and involves either a removal of the clitoris or infibulation. Infibulation includes the excision of the clitoris, the labia minora, and incision of the labia majora to create raw surfaces. These raw surfaces are stitched together to cover the urethra and the vaginal opening with a hood of skin, leaving only a small posterior opening for flow of urine and menstrual blood. Female circumcision is much more damaging than male circumcision. Often the procedure is performed by nonmedical personnel with unsterile equipment, such as scissors. Complications are significant.

The definitive and comprehensive survey of sexual practices and beliefs in America conducted by University of Chicago researchers confirmed that people are influenced by their social networks and tend to act out social scripts (Michael et al, 1994). Sexual behavior is very similar to any

CULTURAL ASPECTS OF CARE

Female circumcision is now generally limited to some countries in Africa and to a lesser extent other regions of the world. It is primarily practiced by Muslims although it is not required by the Koran (Kopelman, 1994). Immigrants to the United States from these countries may seek a practitioner to perform circumcision on their daughters. In practicing communities, female circumcision is the physical marking of the marriageability of women; it symbolizes social control of their sexual pleasure and their reproduction. Cultural and family values, group identity, and marriage goals rather than individual identity and goals are deeply embedded (Kopelman, 1994; Toubia, 1994).

other social behavior, that is, people behave the way they are rewarded for behaving. They tend to "play by the rules" when choosing someone to have sex with and when choosing someone to marry. How persons understand sexual aspects of their world depends on who they are socially and what society they live in. Specific neighborhoods or societies and specific religions encourage or discourage certain patterns of sexuality. Sexual lives are embedded in social lives that offer opportunities and constraints. For example, partners are approved or disapproved of by important others. As a result, people tend to marry those who resemble them in age, education, race, religion, and social status. Apparently, the freedom to find whomever a person wishes is a myth; in reality, the vast majority of people "see" only a preselected group—their own sociocultural group (Michael et al, 1994).

In summary, every society plays a powerful role in shaping sexual values and attitudes and in structuring or constraining sexual development and expression in its members. Each social group has its own set of rules and norms that guide the behavior of its members. These rules become an integral part of an individual's thinking and underlie sexual behavior, including, for example, how people find partners, who they find as partners, how they relate to one another, how often they have sex, and what they do when they have sex.

RELIGIOUS AND ETHICAL DIMENSIONS

Sexuality is also linked to religious and ethical standards of conduct. Ideas about ethical sexual conduct and emotions related to sexuality form the basis for sexual decision making. The spectrum of attitudes toward sexuality ranges from a traditional view of sex only within marriage to an attitude that allows individuals to determine what is right. Sexual decisions that transgress a person's ethical code may result in internal conflict.

Several general approaches to ethical sexual decision making are suggested by Masters, Johnson, and Kolodny (1982). In one approach, sexual decisions are based primarily on religion. What people consider to be right or wrong sexually is strongly linked to religious attitudes and beliefs. Contemporary religious faiths view sexual values and acceptable behavior and expression differently (Zawid, 1994). Some major church bodies in the United States have developed working papers or statements on sexuality to reflect their positions or beliefs (Catholic Church, 1991; Evangelical Lutheran Church in America, 1993; Episcopal Church, 1994). Even though there are official church positions, individual members hold diverse opinions (Denney and Quadagno, 1992). People may also publicly say they believe in a particular sexual value system but behave quite differently in private. A second approach views any sexual act between consenting adults in private as moral. Some people believe that moral sexuality enhances personal growth and interpersonal relationships. Others believe that the morality of a sexual act must be decided on the basis of the situation in which it occurs.

Consequently, people differ in their sexual beliefs and values. Michael et al. (1994) divided respondents into three categories on the basis of attitudes and beliefs. People in the "traditional" category said that their religious beliefs always guided their sexual behavior, and that homosexuality, abortion, and premarital and extramarital sex were always wrong. The "relational" category believed sex should be a part of a loving relationship but did not necessarily have to be reserved for marriage. The "recreational" category said that sex need not have anything to do with love.

A more individualistic morality became widespread in the 1960s and 1970s. Many people reevaluated their moral codes and began to see sexuality as a mode of self-expression. Women asserted their right to control reproduction and the expression of their sexual feelings. This new morality emphasized ownership of one's own body and feelings, free choice, and self-actualization. The struggle of the 1990s appears to be how to combine this individualistic morality (without losing the gains) with a more monogamous expression of sexuality. The increasing rate of diseases such as gonorrhea, chlamydia, human papilloma virus (HPV), and human immunodeficiency virus (HIV) has influenced the reemphasis on monogamous relationships.

PSYCHOLOGICAL DIMENSIONS

Many of our beliefs and attitudes regarding female and male psychological, moral, and psychosexual development are based on the theories of Freud, Erikson, and Kohlberg (see Chapter 28). Contemporary feminist psychologists, such as Carol Gilligan (1982) and Nancy Chodorow (1974), have challenged these assumptions. They contend that the female self is defined by relation to others while the male self is defined by separation and individuation.

Sexuality does, however, encompass learned behavior. What is appropriate and valued is learned early in life by observing parental behavior. Parents usually have the first significant influence on children. They frequently teach sexuality through subtle or nonverbal communication. Often how people view and feel about themselves as sexual beings is related to what parents have conveyed to them about their bodies and their actions. Messages often differ with gender. Research has shown that parents tend to treat girls and boys differently beginning at birth: they dress them differently, decorate their rooms differently, and even respond to them differently. They encourage and reward boys for exploring and being independent; girls are more often encouraged to be helpers and ask for assistance (Denney and Quadagno, 1992). Both mothers and fathers also tend to reinforce sex-typed play in their preschool children.

In summary, parents treat their children differently based on gender. Such variations are responsible for some of the gender differences in observed behavior. However, it is also possible that some gender differences are biologically determined.

Sexual Identity

BIOLOGICAL IDENTITY

Biological differences between men and women are determined at conception. The genetic material in a fertilized egg is organized in the chromosomes that give rise to sexual differentiation. Under normal conditions, female fetuses receive two X chromosomes, one from each parent, and male fetuses receive an X chromosome from the mother and a Y chromosome from the father. Initially the genitalia of the fetus are undifferentiated. When the sex hormones begin to cue fetal tissues, the genitalia assume male or female characteristics. Hormones influence the individual again at puberty, during which girls develop cyclical menstrual cycles and female secondary sex characteristics and boys develop a relatively constant production of spermatozoa (sperm) and male secondary sex characteristics.

GENDER IDENTITY

Gender identity is the sense of being feminine or masculine. As soon as an infant is born (and perhaps sooner with use of amniocentesis or other antenatal testing) the parents and community label the child as *girl* or *boy*. As discussed earlier, after a label is attached to an infant, adults adjust their behavior to relate to a female or male baby. Different patterns of interaction influence the infant's developing sense of gender identity.

As children begin to explore and understand their own bodies, they combine this information with the way that society treats them to create images of themselves as girls or boys. By age 3, children are aware that they will remain girls and boys and that changes in outward appearance will not alter their gender. This recognition is part of the development of self-concept.

GENDER ROLE

Much research and writing in the last decade has been produced on the origin of the **gender role**—the way that a person acts as female or male. Social learning theorists believe that society influences female and male behavior and is thus the primary source of femaleness or maleness. Because gender-role behavior is encouraged by parents, peers, and the media, differences among individuals' sexual behavior develop.

Environmental factors alone do not satisfactorily explain the differences and similarities between female and male sexual behavior. Some researchers believe that sex hormones influence the development of fetal brain tissue, contributing to the differences in female and male sexual behavior. Most likely, as with other human behavior, sexual behavior is a combination of many interacting biological and environmental factors.

Cultural factors can be key elements in defining sex roles. Culture may tightly prescribe roles as feminine or masculine (e.g., the role of breadwinner and home finance coordinator as masculine roles and child care provider and cook as feminine roles). Other cultural groups may be more flexible in role definition and encourage women or men to explore a variety of roles or behavior without labeling the behavior as sex-linked. The women's movement of the 1970s did much to expand the North American cultural definition of appropriate feminine behavior (e.g., primary breadwinner and mother). Ripple effects of this movement have also offered men a broader range of socially acceptable behavior, allowing them to openly express emotion and increase involvement in child care. These expanded options have created dilemmas. Conflicts may arise in juggling careers with child-rearing responsibilities. Biological reproductive time frames and family attitudes may also cause conflict.

Sexual Orientation

Sexual orientation is the clear, persistent, erotic preference of a person for one sex or the other. Studies of human sex-

uality in the 1940s and 1950s developed a continuum between heterosexuality and homosexuality. Few, if any, individuals are totally confined to one end of the continuum throughout life. Most people cluster near the **heterosexual** end of the continuum, with a smaller percentage at the **homosexual** or **gay**, **lesbian** end; however, some people are **bisexual** and feel comfortable having sexual relations with either sex. Such a continuum provides a conceptual model for understanding the variance of sexual orientation in society and the complexity of human behavior. It is not unusual for an individual to have occasional erotic feelings toward someone of the same sex without acting on these feelings. Likewise, it is not uncommon to have a same-sex encounter during adolescence without settling at the homosexual end of the continuum.

Many misconceptions exist about gay and lesbian lifestyles. The extent to which gays and lesbians decide to be secretive or open about their sexual orientation affects their lifestyle. Some remain "in the closet" while others go through incremental steps in "coming out." This process includes self-acknowledgement, self-acceptance, and self-disclosure (Alexander and LaRosa, 1994). "Coming out" is particularly difficult, however, because of **homophobia**, or irrational fears of homosexuality, displayed by some members of society. Homophobia may result in such activities as acts of aggression, violence, and verbal assault.

Society sometimes thinks of gay men as somehow feminized and wishing to be women and of lesbians as desiring to be like men. This is an incorrect myth. Although there are some effeminate-behaving men and masculine-behaving women in the homosexual population, most homosexual men and women define themselves as satisfied with their gender and social role. They simply have a persistent desire to be with members of their own sex.

The origins of sexual orientation are still not understood. Biological theories describe heterosexuality and homosexuality in genetic terms and thus as determined at conception. These theories attribute sexual orientation to the genetic composition of the individual. Psychological theories emphasize that early learning experiences and cognitive processes determine sexual orientation. Other theories acknowledge the influence of genetics and environment in the development of sexual-partner preference.

VARIATIONS IN SEXUAL EXPRESSION

Transsexuals are people whose sexual or gender identity is opposite the biological sex. A man may think of himself as a woman in a man's body, or a woman may describe herself as a man trapped in a woman's body. Such a feeling of being "trapped" is called **gender dysphoria.** Researchers do not clearly understand the nature or cause of this mismatch. Explanations include both biological and social-learning theories. Transsexuals do not see their sexual identities as a matter of choice. Their identification of themselves as sexual and social females or males is clear and persistent, often from early childhood.

A **transvestite** is usually a heterosexual man who periodically dresses like a woman for psychological and sexual relief. Transvestites generally do this in private, and their behavior is sometimes kept secret even from the people closest to them.

ATTITUDES TOWARD SEXUAL HEALTH

Attitudes toward sexual feelings and behavior change as people develop and as they grow older. These changes may become more traditional or liberal because of societal changes, feedback from others, and involvement in religious or community groups.

Because wellness includes sexual health, sexuality should be part of a health care program. Yet sexual assessment and interventions are not always included in health care. The area of sexuality can be emotional for nurses and clients. Lack of information, conflicting value systems, anxiety, or guilt may invalidate the best intentions of nurses to promote sexual health. Clients may not discuss certain sexual concerns because they feel such topics are "off limits" or they fear that nurses will be judgmental. Nurses may ignore clients' hints about sexual concerns because they are uncomfortable with sexuality. Words such as *masturbation, homosexuality, abortion,* and *orgasm* may have emotional connotations that can make people uncomfortable. On a more subtle level, the invasion of privacy, lack of regard for hospitalized clients' needs for time alone with sexual partners, or even the way nurses touch clients reflect attitudes toward sexuality.

Clients' Sexual Attitudes

All people have sexual value systems—personal beliefs and preferences concerning sexuality—acquired throughout life. These experiences can either make it easy for a client to deal with sexual concerns in a health care setting or can be obstacles to expression. Some clients may be confused about their own sexual value systems and thus experience ambiguous or distressing feelings when dealing with their sexuality.

Additionally, if clients believe in traditional gender-appropriate roles, they may perceive the "nurse" as female and subservient. The historical image of the nurse is one of discipline, purity, and cleanliness. Because nurses had the right to touch hospitalized clients' bodies and carry out clients' personal hygiene, they were expected to suppress their own sexuality. This bias may still be held by some clients. Moreover, as more males enter the nursing profession, clients and care providers may experience conflict in defining sex roles related to nursing practice.

However, the most common concern of clients is whether specific sexual attitudes, feelings, and actions are normal. Because society has not encouraged open talk about sexuality, such anxiety is understandable. Religion, society, the media, family, peers, and experience sometimes transmit conflicting messages about sexual normalcy.

Clients may be concerned about the effect of nursing interventions on their self-care abilities and sexual activities. An injury or illness can cause changes in how an individual expresses himself or herself sexually. A hospitalized client should be given privacy when visited by a sexual partner. This allows time for intimate discussion, holding, or kissing. In the home setting the nurse takes time to help the client adapt to any physical restrictions so that sexual activity can be maintained.

Nurses' Attitudes Toward Sexuality

Because health care professionals represent society and its diverse sexual attitudes and behavior, diversity is under-standable and expected among health care professionals. Nurses can deal with personal attitudes by accepting their existence, exploring their sources, and finding ways to work with them. Professional behavior does not have to compromise the personal sexual ethics of nurses or clients. Professional behavior must guarantee that clients receive the best health care possible without diminishing their self-worth.

Nurses may find it difficult to be nonjudgmental about a client's sexuality when the client's sexual orientation or values differ. Situations that seem strange or wrong to the nurse might seem normal and acceptable to the client. Attempting to change a client's sexual attitudes and behavior ignores the fundamental differences in attitudes among people. Promotion of sex education and honest examination of sexual values and beliefs can help in reducing sexual bias. Clients need accurate, truthful information about the effects of illness on sexuality and the ways that it can contribute to wellness. Nurses need to provide this information so that biases do not interfere with care.

SEXUAL ANATOMY AND PHYSIOLOGY

Female Sex Organs

The female genitalia comprise the external and internal sex organs. The external sex organs, collectively called the *vulva,* include the mons veneris, labia majora, labia minora, clitoris, and vaginal opening or introitus (Fig. 24-1). The vagina, uterus, fallopian tubes, and ovaries compose the internal sex organs (Fig. 24-2).

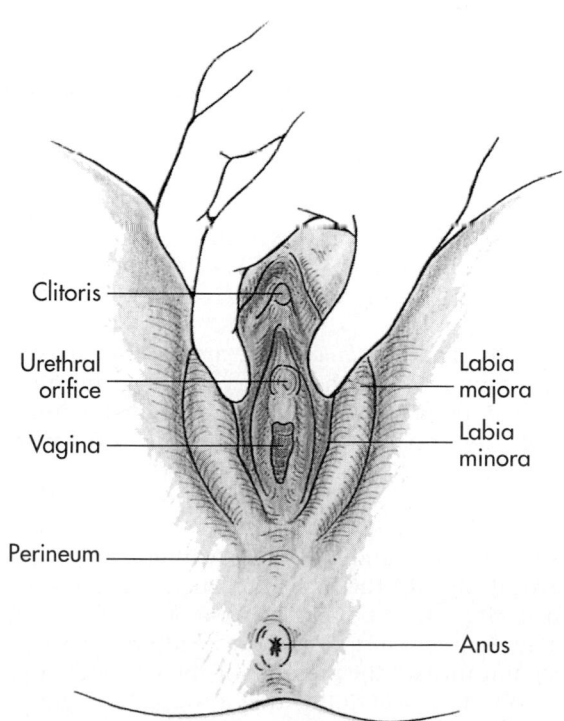

Fig. 24-1 External female genitalia.

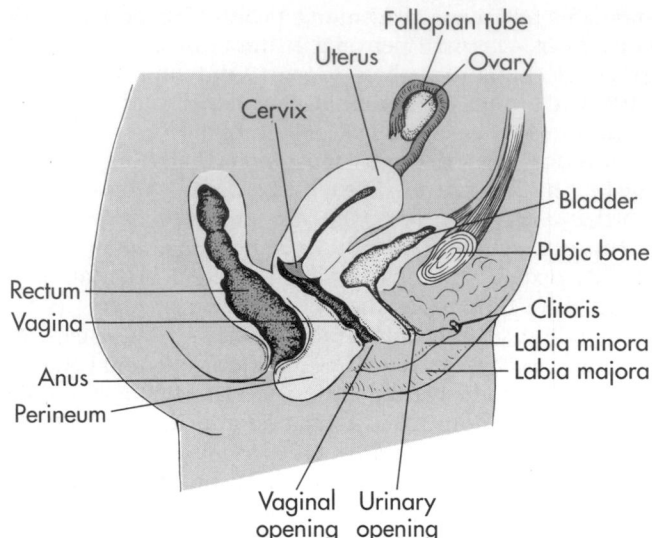

Fig. 24-2 Internal female genitalia.

EXTERNAL SEX ORGANS

Mons Veneris. The mons veneris (mons pubis) is a layer of fatty tissue that covers the pubic bone and is covered by pubic hair after puberty.

Labia. The two labia majora are fatty folds of skin that extend from the mons veneris and form the outer boundaries of the vulva. The labia majora cover and thereby protect the vaginal and urinary openings. They have sensory receptors that are sensitive to touch, pressure, pain, and temperature. The two labia minora, which are just inside the labia majora, are thin folds of pigmented skin that extend upward to form the clitoral hood. These inner folds possess many blood vessels and have many sensory nerve endings. Because of the number of blood vessels, the labia minora may display a significant color change during sexual arousal and are sometimes referred to as the *sex skin*.

Clitoris. When the clitoral hood is pulled back, the shaft and the glans of the clitoris are revealed. The clitoris is composed primarily of erectile tissue, has many nerve endings, and is very sensitive to touch, pressure, and temperature. It is the organ that is the most sensitive to stimulation and has a central role in sexual arousal and elevating feelings of sexual tension (Boston Women's Health Book Collective, 1992).

Vestibule. The *vestibule* is the area of the vulva inside the labia minora. Both the urinary opening (meatus) and the vaginal opening (introitus) are located within the vestibule. The urinary meatus lies midline in the vestibule between the clitoris and the vaginal opening. The vaginal opening or introitus is between the urethra and the anus. The hymen is a membranous fold of tissue that partially covers the introitus and has no known function. It usually remains intact until the first intercourse. At times the hymen in a virgin may be torn because of an athletic injury or, rarely, tampon insertion. Many cultures have placed great significance on the presence or absence of the hymen. A common misconception is that a woman's virginity can be proved or disproved by the pain or bleeding that may occur with initial coitus. Although discomfort and spotting

can sometimes occur with first intercourse, the hymen can be partial, flexible, or thin enough for there to be no discomfort or bleeding. Some women have intact hymens even after repeated intercourse, although this is rare.

INTERNAL SEX ORGANS

Vagina. The vagina is a thin-walled, muscular organ that tilts upward at a 45-degree angle toward the small of the back. The walls of the vagina consist of three layers of tissue:

1. A thin outer serosa, which is part of the membrane that lines the body cavity and covers its organs
2. A middle layer of smooth, involuntary muscle that is continuous with the muscle of the uterus
3. An inner layer of moist mucous membrane called *mucosa*

The vagina serves as a passageway for menstrual flow, childbirth, and sexual pleasure. The muscle layer is extremely distensible to allow sexual intercourse and childbirth. During sexual excitement, vasocongestion occurs. As a result the mucosal layer sweats and provides vaginal lubrication.

The *Bartholin's glands* are located on each side of the vaginal opening. They were once thought to be a source of lubrication during sexual arousal. Such a role is now questioned because the lubrication produced is minimal (Denney and Quadagno, 1992).

Uterus. The uterus is a thick-walled muscular organ located between the urinary bladder and rectum. It is about 7.6 cm (3 in) long and looks like a small pear turned upside down. The fallopian tubes enter the uterus on both sides near the top. The wide upper part of the uterus is known as the *body*. The bottom part, called the *cervix*, extends into the vagina. The external (vaginal) cervix is called the *ectocervix*, and the internal cervical canal is referred to as the *endocervix*. The junction of these areas is the site where squamous epithelium changes to columnar epithelial cells. Cells from this area are scraped and evaluated during a Papanicolaou (Pap) test (see Chapter 33) to assess for excessive precancerous or malignant growth.

The inner lining of the cervix contains many mucus-secreting glands. The constant downward flow of mucus protects the uterine cavity from bacterial invasion. Changes in the cervical mucus indicate when ovulation is taking place. The mucus is more readily penetrable by sperm at the time of ovulation.

The uterus is composed of a thin external connective tissue layer called the *perimetrium,* the middle layer of smooth muscle called the *myometrium,* and the inner mucous membrane called the *endometrium.* Muscle fibers of the myometrial layer enlarge during pregnancy to allow fetal growth. Contractions of these intertwining muscles and pressure from the presenting part of the fetus cause cervical effacement and dilation. Uterine muscle contractions and bearing-down movements expel the fetus. Contraction of uterine muscles also occurs during orgasm. Every month the endometrium thickens in preparation for possible implantation of a fertilized ovum.

Fallopian Tubes. The two fallopian tubes begin at the uterus and end in long, fingerlike fimbriae near the ovaries. Fallopian tubes function as a conduit for the passage of egg and sperm so that fertilization can occur. Fertilization usually occurs in the upper part of one of the fallopian tubes.

Ovaries. There are two walnut-sized ovaries, one on each side of the uterus. They secrete female hormones, including estrogens, progesterones, and small amounts of androgen, directly into the bloodstream. They also produce eggs that are released and transported through the fallopian tubes. The process of egg production begins in the female fetus and ends before birth. Every female is born with a total complement of ova. These eggs continue to undergo atresia (degeneration and resorption), so only about 400,000 remain at puberty. One egg undergoes maturation each month. The cycle continues until ovarian function ceases at menopause.

BREASTS

The breasts are not a part of the external or internal sex organs but rather are considered **secondary sex characteristics** (physical characteristics other than genitals that distinguish females from males). The breasts are composed internally of fatty tissue and milk-producing glands. Variations in breast size are due mainly to the amount of adipose tissue around the milk glands. Breasts are often not symmetrical in size or shape. Visible changes occur during development (see Chapter 29).

MENSTRUAL CYCLE

Between **menarche** and menopause, the female reproductive system undergoes cyclic changes termed the **menstrual cycle**. The average cycle lasts 28 days but may range from 21 to 40 days. Average length varies from cycle to cycle and from person to person. Menstrual flow consists of blood, mucus, and endometrial membranes that sometimes present as small clots. Average blood loss is about 6 to 8 ounces per cycle (Alexander and LaRosa, 1994). Again, individuals vary in the amount of blood loss per cycle. Menarche, the onset of a girl's first menstruation, usually occurs between 9 and 16 years of age.

During the menstrual cycle the uterine lining is prepared for implantation of a fertilized egg. If conception does not occur, the lining sloughs off and is expelled as menstrual flow. The cycle is controlled through a feedback loop involving hormones of the hypothalamus, pituitary, and ovaries. The hormones produce changes in the ovaries and uterine endometrium (Fig. 24-3). The hypothalamus regulates the pituitary hormones through gonadotropin-releasing hormone (Gn-RH) at the beginning of the cycle. Gn-RH stimulates the pituitary to release follicle-stimulating hormone (FSH) and luteinizing hormone (LH). These hormones stimulate the development of several ovarian primary follicles (immature eggs). Eventually, all but one follicle begins to regress. The remaining follicle grows rapidly and is known as the **Graafian follicle.** As it ripens, ovarian estrogen is produced and influences the pituitary to suppress FSH and increase production of LH. LH induces the ovum to rupture from the Graafian follicle; this is termed **ovulation** and occurs about day 14 of a 28-day cycle. The ova is transported through the fallopian tube to-

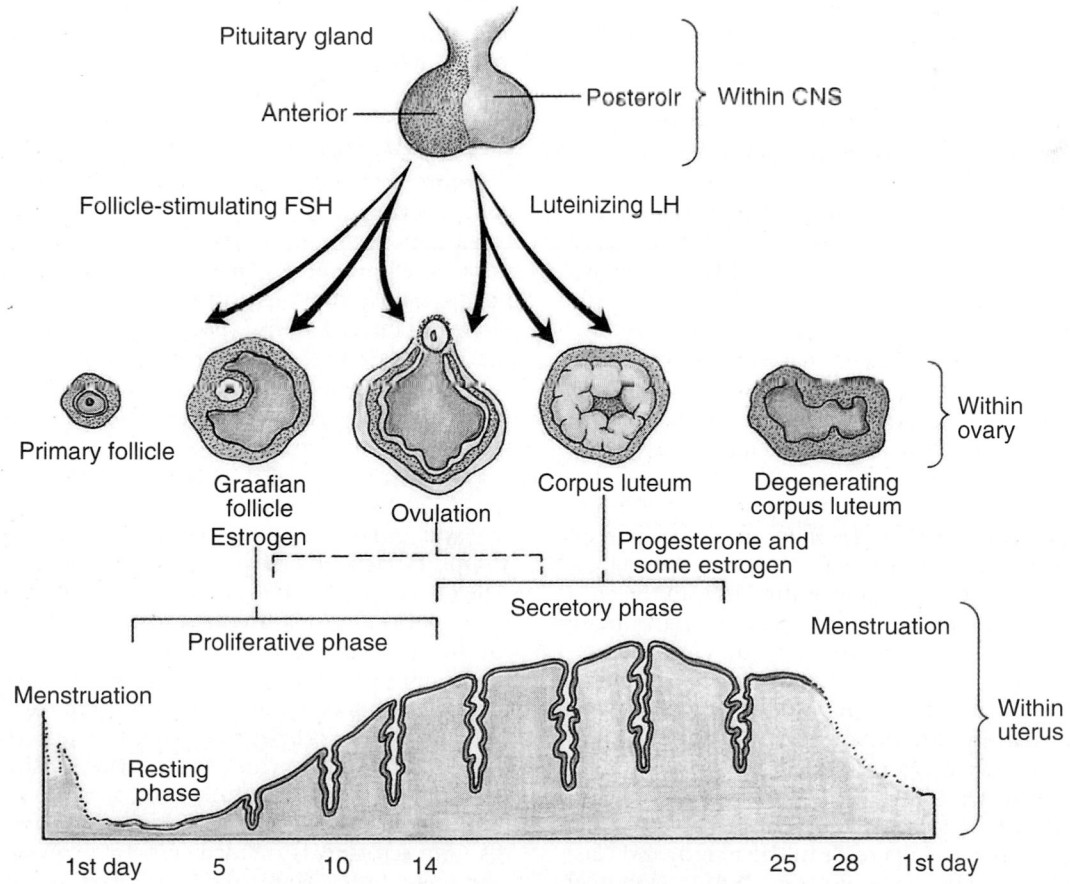

Fig. 24-3 Hormonal control of the menstrual cycle.

ward the uterus. After ovulation the ruptured follicle becomes known as the **corpus luteum**. It produces large amounts of progesterone. If pregnancy does not occur, LH levels decrease, progesterone levels fall, and menstrual flow begins about 14 days after ovulation.

The hormones that stimulate ovarian activities also cause uterine changes. The endometrial cycle consists of three phases. In the *proliferative* or preovulation phase, high levels of estrogen thicken the uterine endometrium and cervical mucus secretion increases and changes. These qualities of the mucus peak at ovulation and produce an environment receptive to the entrance of sperm for fertilization. (Noting these changes in the quality of cervical mucus is a helpful aid in fertility awareness for planning or preventing conception.)

The secretory phase of the menstrual cycle occurs after ovulation. Under the influence of high levels of progesterone and estrogen, the endometrium continues to thicken to prepare to nourish a fertilized egg. If pregnancy does not occur, estrogen and progesterone production decrease and trigger endometrium sloughing (shedding), which is the third, or menstrual phase. As hormone levels fall, the hypothalamus responds by stimulating the pituitary to release FSH; this initiates a new menstrual cycle.

Premenstrual Symptoms. Some women experience symptoms at ovulation or during the postovulatory phase. Some symptoms are partly due to the effects of estrogen or progesterone and may include lower abdominal pain or discomfort at ovulation, breast fullness or tenderness, weight gain, fluid retention, irritability, and depression. For some women these symptoms are more consistent and severe and cluster into the **premenstrual syndrome (PMS)**. The causes of PMS are not known but fluctuations in sex steroids and their effects on various organ systems are thought to be involved. Research about the nature, cause, and treatment of PMS lacks consistency and often has contradictory findings (Alexander and LaRosa, 1994).

Sex During Menstruation. There is no physiological reason for a woman to abstain from sexual activity during menstruation. However, excessive menstrual flow or physical discomfort may discourage a woman from sex while menstruating. Cultural attitudes or other factors may also inhibit sexual activity during menstruation. If a couple decides to abstain from genital sexual activity during menstruation, they can learn other ways of sharing intimacy until the woman is ready to resume sexual activity.

Menopause. One of the physiological responses to aging is the cessation of menstruation and fertility. **Menopause** takes place around 45 to 60 years of age. The ovaries cease production of estrogen and progesterone, although low levels remain in the bloodstream from the continued activity of the adrenal glands. Each woman's body responds to menopause in its own way. For some women the only symptom is the disappearance of menstruation. Other women report headaches, hot flashes, insomnia, and changes in breast and vaginal tissue. Hot flushes or flashes occur when blood vessels rapidly dilate as a result of fluctuating hormone levels. The decrease in hormone levels also may affect the skin, breasts, and genitalia, causing the tissue to thin. The resulting decrease in the length and elasticity of the vagina and decrease in vaginal lubrication may make intercourse uncomfortable or painful.

Menopause need not interfere with a woman's sexual capacity, and many women continue to be sexually active. Some women find that the lack of concern about pregnancy enhances their enjoyment of sex. Physical discomfort during penetration can be eased with water-based lubricants. Water-based lubricants are necessary so that they can easily be removed with soap and water; if they are not removed, they may provide a medium for bacterial growth and subsequent vaginitis and urethritis.

Hormone replacement therapy (HRT) is also frequently prescribed for menopausal symptoms. It usually consists of estrogen combined with progesterone. Combined hormone therapy has decreased the incidence of uterine cancer associated with prescribing estrogen alone to treat symptoms. Estrogen itself does appear to play a protective role in preventing heart disease and osteoporosis. However, not every woman needs HRT. Additionally, HRT is contraindicated for those women who have a history of breast or endometrial carcinoma or endometrial hyperplasia. Other medical conditions necessitate weighing the benefits versus the risks of HRT, for example, breast dysplasia, family history of breast cancer, previous heart attack, fibroids, or thromboembolic disease (Zawid, 1994).

Male Sex Organs

The male sex organs produce sperm and hormones and provide a system for conveying sperm from the testicles to outside the body. The external genitalia are the penis and scrotum. The male internal sex organs include the testicles, which produce hormones and sperm; the epididymis and ductus deferens, a system of ducts that transport sperm; and the prostate gland, seminal vesicles, and Cowper's glands, whose secretions become part of the ejaculated semen (Fig. 24-4).

EXTERNAL SEX ORGANS

Penis. The penis consists of the shaft and the glans and contains no muscle or bones. The shaft is composed of three parallel tubes of erectile tissue: two corpora cavernosa, which lie side by side, and beneath them a single corpus spongiosum, which surrounds the urethra. The erectile tissue resembles a dense sponge. During sexual excitement, the large vascular spaces or cavities between arteries and veins become engorged with blood, causing the penis to become stiff and erect. When the penis is flaccid, or not erect, the cavities contain little blood.

The anterior end of the corpus spongiosum that fits over the corpora cavernosa is called the *glans*. It has both erectile and sensory tissue. The area where the glans arises abruptly from the shaft is called the *corona*, meaning crown. The glans and especially the corona, which contains many nerve endings, are the most sensitive parts of the penis. If the male is uncircumcised, the skin of the shaft continues forward and forms a loose-fitting hood over the glans. This hood is the foreskin or prepuce. The undersurface of the glans is attached to the prepuce by a thin fold of skin, the frenulum, which is also very sensitive to touch.

Scrotum. The scrotum is a thin, loose sac of skin that protects the two testicles. It is located at the base of the penis. The scrotum is divided into two compartments; each contains a testis, epididymis, and part of the ductus deferens. The scrotum is responsive to temperature changes;

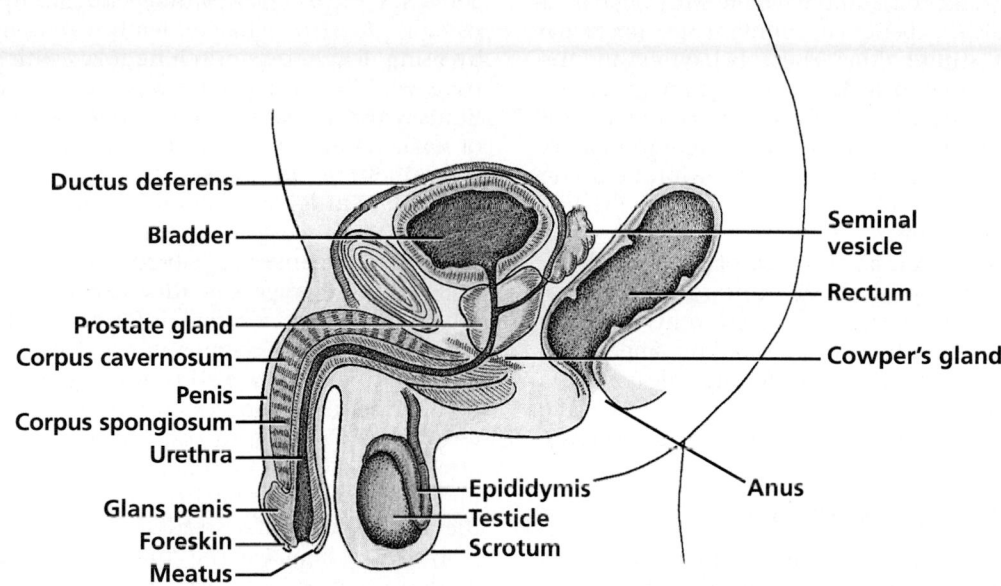

Fig. 24-4 External and internal male genitalia.

cold temperatures cause it to contract, pulling the testicles closer to the body. The temperature in the scrotum is slightly lower than body temperature so that spermatogenesis (formation of sperm) can occur.

INTERNAL SEX ORGANS

The male internal sex organs are the testicles (or testes), a system of ducts (epididymis, ductus or vas deferens, and urethra), and some accessory organs (seminal vesicles, prostate gland, and bulbourethral glands). The testes contain two specialized tissues: the seminiferous tubules, which produce the sperm, and the Leydig cells, which produce the male hormones, or *androgens*. Testosterone stimulates growth and development of the genital organs and contributes to growth and development of bones and muscles.

The sperm drain into the epididymis, a duct that lies just outside the testicle. Sperm take 2 to 4 weeks to travel from the epididymis to the ductus deferens. The ductus deferens is a long tube from each testicle that travels up and out of the scrotum. It curves around the urinary bladder and then turns downward and opens into the ampulla. The ampulla is a reservoir for sperm before they are discharged into the ejaculatory duct, which carries them through the prostate into the posterior urethra. The urethra continues from the bladder to the penis tip and carries urine or semen. These fluids are not carried simultaneously because of an internal bladder sphincter.

The seminal vesicles and prostate secrete seminal plasma. These secretions dilute and carry sperm and give ejaculate its characteristic odor. The seminal vesicles are glands secreting a portion of the ejaculate that contributes to the nutrition of the sperm. The prostate is about the size of a chestnut and is located beneath the bladder. The ejaculatory ducts and a portion of the urethra pass through it. In the prostate, prostatic secretions unite with the sperm and fluid from the seminal vesicles. This combined fluid is called *seminal fluid* and provides nutrients to the sperm passing into the urethra. The seminal fluid also buffers vaginal acidity to aid fertility.

The bulbourethral glands, sometimes referred to as the *Cowper's glands*, are located below the prostate on both sides of the penile urethra. They secrete a clear, alkaline lubricating fluid that sometimes appears at the tip of the penis soon after sexual arousal. This fluid removes urine from the urethra, neutralizes the acidity in the urethra and makes a suitable environment for sperm. It is also possible that the fluid from this gland may contain a small amount of sperm.

MALE CLIMACTERIC

Men do not experience the dramatic hormone changes or loss of fertility experienced by menopausal women. However, they do experience changes in sexual response or the **climacteric.** At 90, a man may be capable of spermatogenesis. However, the delayed erectile and ejaculatory ability experienced at 50 or 60 may cause significant concerns about potency and masculinity.

As they age, men experience a gradual increase in the length of time it takes to achieve full erection. Older men maintain erections for longer periods than when younger, resulting in delayed ejaculation. The ejaculatory phase usually becomes shorter and less intense. The refractory period (time it takes to achieve another erection) is lengthened, and the penis returns to its flaccid state much more quickly than in men younger than 60.

The aging man may continue to have a satisfying sex life. The changes in delayed erection and ejaculation may bring about a more mutually satisfying sexual relationship between partners. Both partners may benefit from extended foreplay, which may increase vaginal lubrication and aid full erection.

▮ SEXUAL DEVELOPMENT

Infancy

Both female and male infants are born with the capacity for sexual pleasure and response. Infant genitalia are sensitive to touch from birth. With stimulation the male infant responds with penile erection and the female with vaginal lubrication. Boys also experience spontaneous nocturnal erections without stimulation. These behaviors and responses are not associated with erotic psychological contact as in puberty or adulthood but rather are normal learning behaviors in forming a sense of self. Parental response to this exploratory behavior may set the tone for the child's sexual development, education, and comfort for dealing with sexuality in the home.

Parents should be encouraged to accept the infant's exploratory behavior as a positive step toward the development of a positive self-identity. Providing other forms of tactile stimulation through sucking, cuddling, and touching or stroking aids the infant in defining pleasant and comforting experiences through human interaction and from body contact. Touch and the human body begin to acquire a definition as "good."

Toddlerhood and Preschool

The child from age 1 to 5 or 6 solidifies the sense of gender identity and begins to differentiate socially defined, gender-appropriate behavior. This learning process occurs in the course of normal adult-child interactions from the toys given to the child, clothing worn, games played, and responses encouraged. The child also observes adult behavior, begins to imitate actions of the same-sex parent, and maintains or modifies behavior based on parental feedback.

Body exploration continues at this age. Exploration may include self-stroking; genital manipulation; cuddling of dolls, pets, or people; and other sensual experimentation. While learning that the body is good and that certain stimulation is pleasant, the child can also be taught the differences in private versus public behavior. Playmate sex games can be handled in a matter-of-fact manner. The parent can interpret the curiosity exhibited as an indication that the child is ready to learn the differences in and proper names for female and male genitalia.

Questions about where babies come from or sexual behavior the child observes should be addressed openly, honestly, and simply. Even if questions are not asked, learning opportunities should be offered through pointing out pregnant women or animal behavior at the zoo or through discussions of sexuality as a follow-up to stories or television programs that involve these topics.

School-Age Years

For children from 6 to 10 years of age, education about and reinforcement of sexuality come from parents and teachers but more significantly from the peer group. North American society defines a broad range of behavior acceptable to girls and boys (e.g., both sexes participate in cooking and woodworking activities). Parents and health care personnel can encourage socially acceptable behavior without applying labels of feminine or masculine.

School-age children will likely continue self-stimulating behavior. Parents and children can be informed that masturbation does not have any harmful physical or emotional effects. Explanations of times, places, and relationships appropriate for sexual expression can also be provided and given in the context of values and rationale on which these beliefs are based.

Children in this age group continue to have questions

about sex and assert their independence by testing the limits of appropriate behavior. Limit testing may be displayed by using dirty words or telling jokes with sexual connotations while watching adult reaction. The testing of sexual limits is also a means of identifying appropriate expressions of sexuality and an opportunity the parents can use to explore questions and concerns.

Children also have a desire and need for privacy. By the age of 10, many girls and some boys are already beginning some of the changes of puberty. As children enter puberty their bodies change and they experience increased modesty. They need accurate information from home and school about body changes during this period. This allows children to gain information and ask questions before they become personal concerns regarding normalcy and therefore too threatening to ask. The knowledge may also decrease the anxieties of puberty when an uninformed child may fear menstruation or nocturnal emission and view them as evidence of a dreadful disease.

By early school age, the child should also be given information to guard against sexual abuse potential. Many schools are beginning to include this content in their curriculum. Parents should be encouraged to view this material to approve of the content and provide follow-up. Very young children can be taught the differences between good touch and bad touch and that certain body parts are not usually touched by adults except at bath time or during physical examination. Children should be told that if they feel uncomfortable about how they are touched, they should say *no* and tell a trusted adult about the incident. Other ways to limit the potential for abuse include teaching children that families should not keep secrets (other than birthday surprises or other time-limited events), that adults are not always right, and that all people should have control over their bodies and can decide who may hug them.

If abuse occurs, a child who feels comfortable talking about his or her body will be able to accurately describe the incident. At these times the child should be assured that the adult abuser is the one who was wrong or did something bad and that the child is not responsible. Parental response can also be critical to how a child copes with the aftereffects of abuse. Parents should be encouraged to attempt controlled emotional expressions in front of the child and, as necessary, vent anger and frustration and find support with other adults.

Puberty and Adolescence

The onset of puberty in girls is usually signaled by the development of the breasts. After an initial growth of breast tissue, the nipple and areola increase in size. This process, which is in part controlled by heredity, may begin as early as age 8 and may not be complete until the late teens. Rising levels of estrogen also begin to affect the genitals. The uterus begins to enlarge, and increased vaginal lubrication occurs, either spontaneously or as a result of sexual arousal. The vagina lengthens, and pubic and axillary hair appears. Menarche varies widely. It may occur as early as age 8 or not until age 16 or later. Although the menstrual cycle is initially irregular and ovulation may not occur at first, fertility should always be assumed unless proved otherwise.

Rising testosterone levels in boys during puberty are

marked by an increase in size of the penis, testicles, prostate, and seminal vesicles. Boys and girls may experience orgasm before puberty, but ejaculation in boys does not occur until the sex organs begin to mature, around the age of 12 or 14. Ejaculation may first occur during sleep (nocturnal emission). This may be interpreted as an episode of bed-wetting and even in knowledgeable boys can be very embarrassing. Boys must understand that, although they may not produce sperm with their first ejaculations, they will soon be fertile. About the time genital development takes place, pubic, facial, and body hair begins to grow.

The emotional changes during puberty and adolescence are as dramatic as the physical ones. It is a period characterized by evolving responsibilities and assimilation of societal expectations. Adolescents are faced with many decisions and thus need accurate information on topics such as body changes, sexual relationships and activity, sexually transmitted diseases (STDs), and pregnancy. This factual information may come from home, school, books, or peers. Even with this information, adolescents may not integrate this knowledge into lifestyle. They have a present orientation and a sense of invulnerability. These characteristics may cause them to believe that pregnancy or disease cannot happen to them, and therefore precautions are not necessary. Health education must be provided within this developmental context.

More significant than the factual content is guidance in establishing a personal value or belief system to use as a framework for decision making. Much of this guidance has already been conveyed verbally and nonverbally by parents. Attitudes of parents regarding gender-appropriate roles and behavior influence the adolescent's career and family choices and may also affect decisions regarding sexual activity and parenting and partner/dating choices (Fig. 24-5).

This may be the age of identifying sexual orientation. Many adolescents have at least one homosexual experience with an individual or in a group. Adolescents may fear that this experience defines their total sexuality. This is not true; many individuals continue with a strictly heterosexual orientation after such experiences. However, some teens may recognize their preference as distinctly homosexual. This can be a frightening and confusing recognition for the ado-

lescent and family and requires a great deal of support. Support may come from a variety of sources such as school counselors, spiritual advisers, family, and mental health professionals.

Adolescence may be the first time the child seeks health care without parental accompaniment. To be effective in interventions with this age group, the health care provider needs to establish an environment of caring and trust and a willingness to listen. Issues of confidentiality must be clarified and respected. Nurses need to sort out personal values regarding teenage sexuality before they can be effective. Obtaining contraceptives or having an abortion without parental consent may be a legal issue in some states, but it is always an ethical issue. Those providing adolescent or reproductive health care must deal with these ethical concerns and legal concerns and have an in-depth knowledge of adolescent development.

Adulthood

The adult has gained physical maturation but continues to explore and define emotional maturation in relationships. Young adults are traditionally viewed in roles of childbearing and child rearing. This model represents the vast majority of adults. Intimacy and sexuality are also issues for adults who choose to abstain from sex, remain single by choice or circumstance while desiring sexual activity, are again single after leaving a relationship, are homosexual, are childless by choice, or are unable to bear children.

While developing intimate relationships, all sexually active adults must learn techniques of stimulation and sexual response that are satisfying to their partners. Some adults may only need permission to experiment with alternate behavior or assurance that sexual expression other than penile-vaginal intercourse is normal. Adults can be encouraged to verbalize to their partners the types of stimuli and sexual or affectionate acts perceived as pleasant. Mutual recognition of desires and preferences and negotiation of sexual practices provoke positive sexual expression. Religious teaching, family values, and attitudes influence acceptance of some forms of stimulation or may carry residual emotional effects such as guilt or anxiety and sexual dysfunction.

Later in the adult years, the individual adjusts to social and emotional changes as children move out. Renewed intimacy may be possible or needed between partners. However, one or both spouses may experience a threat to self-image as the body ages and may attempt to regain youth through sexual relationships with a much younger partner. If desired, couples can be helped to find novelty and new excitement in a long-standing, monogamous relationship through experimentation with sexual positions, techniques, and use of fantasy.

Older Adulthood

Sexuality in the aged shifts from an emphasis on procreation to emphasis on companionship, physical nearness, intimate communication, and a pleasure-seeking physical relationship (Ebersole and Hess, 1994). There is no reason people cannot remain sexually active as long as they choose. This can most effectively be accomplished by maintaining regular sexual activity throughout life. Particularly for the woman, regular intercourse helps maintain

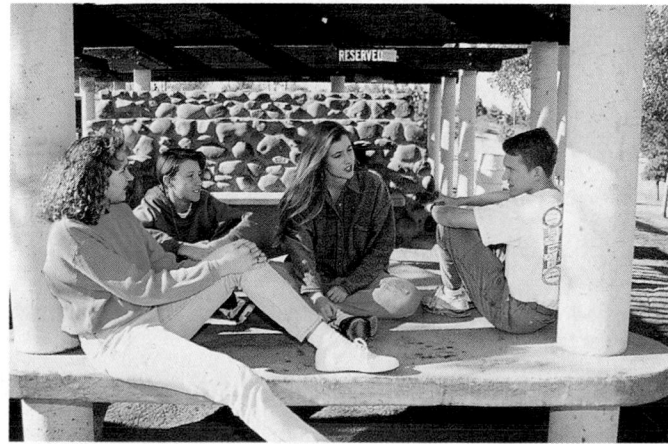

Fig. 24-5 Adolescents in group activities foster self-esteem.

vaginal elasticity, prevent atrophy, and maintain the ability to lubricate. Nonetheless, the aging process does affect sexual behavior. Physical changes that occur with aging need to be explained to older clients. Older people may also face health concerns that make it difficult for them to continue sexual activity. Aging adults may need to adjust sexual action and response to chronic illness, medications, aches and pains, or other health concerns.

SEXUAL RESPONSE

Sexual Response Cycle

Masters and Johnson (1966) have defined a **sexual response cycle** with the excitement, plateau, orgasm, and resolution phases. These phases are the result of vasocongestion and myotonia, which are the basic physiological responses of sexual arousal (Table 24-1). **Vasocongestion** is the pooling of blood in the genitals and female breasts during sexual arousal. In women this reaction leads to vaginal lubrication, **tumescence** (swelling) of the clitoris and the labia minora and majora, and engorgement of the outer third of the vagina. In men, vasocongestion leads to erection of the penis. **Myotonia**, or neuromuscular tension,

gradually increases throughout the body during the excitement and plateau phases. It peaks during orgasm, resulting in involuntary contractions of the woman's vagina and the man's ductus deferens and urethra. Both genders experience contractions of the arm, leg, facial, and gluteal muscles. Carpopedal spasms, or spastic contractions of the muscles of the hands and feet, may occur. After orgasm, the body returns to prearousal levels.

The phases described by Masters and Johnson are not absolute. Although these phases vary in duration and intensity, the female and male response patterns are more similar than different. They are strongly influenced by psychological and environmental factors such as fatigue and alcohol intake, and the timing and intensity of these phases vary among individuals.

PREGNANCY AND SEXUALITY

Women and men experience a variety of emotions with impending parenthood. Physical discomfort and fear of injury are major concerns limiting sexual activity (Zawid, 1994). Conversely, some couples are relieved because they no longer fear an untimely pregnancy, so sexual desire is increased. During the first trimester, women may have a de-

Table 24-1	Comparison of Sexual Response Cycle in Women and Men	
WOMEN	**MEN**
EXCITEMENT: GRADUAL INCREASE IN SEXUAL AROUSAL	
Vaginal lubrication: "sweating" of vaginal walls	Penile erection
Expansion of inner two thirds of vaginal barrel	Thickening and elevation of scrotum
Increased sensitivity and engorgement of clitoris and labia	Moderate elevation and enlargement of testicles
Nipple erection and increase in breast size	Nipple erection and tumescence
PLATEAU: HEIGHTENED RESPONSES OF EXCITEMENT PHASE	
Retraction of clitoris under clitoral hood	Increase in size of glans (tip) of penis
Formation of orgasmic platform: swelling of outer third of vagina and labia minora	Increase in intensity of glans color
Elevation of cervix and uterus: "tenting" effect	Elevation and 50% increase in size of testicles
"Sex skin": vivid color change in labia minora	Mucoid emission from Cowper's glands, possibly with sperm
Areolar and breast engorgement	Increase in muscle tension and breathing
Increase in muscle tension and breathing	Increase in heart rate, blood pressure, and respiratory rate
Increase in heart rate, blood pressure, and respiratory rate	
ORGASM: RELEASE OF POOLED BLOOD AND TENSION IN MUSCLES	
Involuntary contractions of orgasmic platform, uterus, rectal and urethral sphincters, and other muscle groups	Closing of internal urinary sphincter
Hyperventilation and increase in pulse rate	Sensation of ejaculatory inevitability
Peaking of heart rate, blood pressure, and respiratory rate	Contractions of ductus deferens, seminal vesicles, prostate, and ejaculatory duct
	Relaxation of external bladder sphincter
	Contractions of urethral and rectal sphincter muscles
	Peaking of heart rate, blood pressure, and respiratory rate
	Ejaculation
RESOLUTION: PHYSIOLOGICAL AND PSYCHOLOGICAL RETURN TO UNAROUSED STATE	
Gradual relaxation of vaginal walls	Loss of penile erection
Rapid color change of labia minora	Refractory period when continued stimulation is uncomfortable
Sweating	Sweating reaction
Gradual return to normal breathing, heart rate, blood pressure, and muscle tension	Descent of testicles
Often, ability to return to orgasm because women do not experience refractory period as often as men	Gradual return to normal of breathing, heart rate, blood pressure, and muscle tension

creased interest in sex because of nausea, vomiting, and fatigue. Often an increase in sexual interest and performance occurs in the second trimester because of a general sense of health and well-being and because pelvic and vulvar vasocongestion induces an almost constant state of semiarousal. Multiple orgasm may occur for the first time. During the third trimester, sexual intercourse often decreases, in part because of fatigue, size, position, and discomfort of pressure on the cervix from the penis and the fetal-presenting part. Couples who engage in intercourse after the second half of pregnancy should use positions that avoid having the woman flat on her back and placing uterine weight on the major blood vessels, which causes decreased maternal blood flow and therefore potential fetal hypoxia.

In general, studies have not shown a relationship between coital activity and premature labor. However, certain medical conditions do have the potential for causing premature labor. These include an incompetent cervical os (a cervix that is not fully closed), infections, bleeding, experiencing or being at risk for preterm labor, rupture of membranes, and excessive uterine contractions. The nurse may need to inform couples that sexual intercourse or nipple stimulation may prompt labor to begin or accelerate. Semen contains some prostaglandins and may encourage uterine contractions. Breast stimulation induces the release of natural oxytocin, which also stimulates uterine contractions. For this reason, some health care providers may warn against intercourse late in pregnancy.

Changes in sexuality also continue after birth. Some women may remain disinterested in or have diminished sexual responses for 6 months or longer. Hormonal changes, particularly decreased estrogen, decrease the amount of vaginal lubrication and may necessitate the use of water-soluble lubricants. Fatigue caused by infant feedings and sleep interruption and general changes in household chores and routines may negatively influence sexual desire in both partners. Fear of pain because of vaginal or episiotomy discomfort can also deter sexual activity. Physiologically, the couple should refrain from sexual intercourse until bleeding has stopped and episiotomy and vaginal discomfort subside. This often occurs 2 to 3 weeks after birth. During this early period and even with breastfeeding, the couple must consider contraceptives. The health care provider should discuss family planning options.

Lack of sexual desire and activity during pregnancy and after delivery is not uncommon. Nurses need to be sure that couples are aware of the possibility of this lack of desire so that the spouse does not interpret his wife's disinterest in intercourse as rejection. Other expressions of sexuality and affection can be encouraged. These activities may include cuddling, kissing, hand holding, and massage.

■ ISSUES RELATED TO SEXUALITY

Potential fertility is an issue for premenopausal women having sexual intercourse. Often the concern is prevention of conception. At times the choice may be to not use contraception. In this case, the couple may experience anxiety until the next menstrual period occurs. For a smaller percentage of couples, the issue may be infertility when children are desired.

An additional issue for sexually active individuals is the practice of safe sex. Practicing safe sex has gained increasing recognition in the last decade due to the fear of AIDS. The risks and consequences of STDs must always be considered.

Sexual intercourse and manipulation, although intended to provide pleasure for the participants, may be abusive in dysfunctional situations. Sexual abuse may include violence against women, sexual harassment, rape, pedophilia (sexual activity with children), child pornography, and incest.

The nurse's major roles related to these issues are reporting, teaching, and support. Nurses may also be involved in administering therapies and medications, providing assessment and evaluation of effectiveness, and providing public education regarding the facts, fiction, and importance of dealing with these issues in the family, school, and community.

Contraception

The ability to prevent a pregnancy or plan the time between pregnancies should be part of a client's health care plan. An unwanted pregnancy can affect health on many levels. The health of the parent, the child, and ultimately the community depends on adequate physical, emotional, and financial resources to care for the child. A client who is burdened with an unwanted child often enters the health care system with stress-related complaints. The unwanted child may suffer neglect or even abuse.

There are ways of preventing unwanted pregnancy. It would seem a simple process then to control pregnancy with an appropriate method of **contraception**. Yet the numbers of pregnancies among teenagers, abortions in all age groups, and unwanted children indicate that the decision to use contraceptives is much more complex.

FACTORS INFLUENCING USE OF CONTRACEPTION

The nurse considers three major factors when exploring the reasons that clients do not use contraception effectively. The first factor involves clients' abilities to take meaningful action. Some clients truly do not believe that they can control conception and often view themselves as controlled by events or other people. Some may fail to use contraceptive measures because they lack knowledge about contraception or the implications of pregnancy to health or lifestyle. Shame, guilt, and denial can affect the ability to use contraception effectively. Other clients may lack the intellectual capacity to understand and correctly use contraceptives or may have a problem with literacy. It is the nurse's responsibility to assess the client's mental status and level of understanding.

Adolescents fail to use contraceptives for a variety of reasons. Reasons identified include lack of awareness that pregnancy could occur with intercourse, lack of knowledge on availability of contraceptives, partner objection to use, fear of losing partner, unplanned intercourse, unavailability of contraceptives at the time of intercourse, perception that contraception is a woman's problem, and trust that the partner would take care of it (Brown, Cromer, and Fischer, 1992; Stotland, 1994). Characteristics of adolescents who use contraceptives effectively include high socioeconomic status, knowledge of a parent or sibling who uses contraceptives, and personal experience or a close friend who has experienced a pregnancy scare (Flick, 1986; Brown, Cromer, and Fischer, 1992).

A second factor influencing the effective use of contraception is an individual's environment. The family, community, or religion may disapprove of or prohibit contraception. Clients may have been reared in family environments in which they were taught that sex for pleasure rather than procreation is wrong. People also learn about contraception from peers, health care providers, and public health agencies. Good contraception education requires a health care system and an educational system that can deliver such education to the community, but not all communities can afford or support that kind of education.

Finally, the method of contraception must be appropriate for the client. The effectiveness of contraception is related to its safety, comfort, expense, availability, and ease of use. When discussing contraception with clients, the nurse should remember that each method has a theoretical effectiveness and an actual effectiveness. The former is based on the ideal circumstances under which the method could be used. The latter considers all personal and environmental factors and may be considerably lower if the client does not use the method regularly or properly.

The decision to use or not use a contraceptive method must be made by the client. The nurse can help the client clarify values (see Chapter 18) about contraception by providing accurate information.

BIOLOGICAL METHODS

For the purpose of this chapter, biological methods of contraception include any method not using chemical, mechanical, or surgical means to prevent pregnancy. The most effective means of preventing pregnancy is abstinence. This method is often overlooked when discussing options for pregnancy prevention with young, unmarried individuals. National campaigns promoting "say no" to smoking, alcohol, and drugs and the fear of AIDS, may help to make abstinence more common and socially acceptable for adolescents.

Coitus interruptus, or withdrawal, is a method of contraception often used by adolescents, but it is one of the least effective means of pregnancy prevention. Although the penis is withdrawn from the vagina before ejaculation, sperm are usually present in the preejaculation fluid discharged. Douching immediately after intercourse is also an ineffective means of contraception sometimes used by adolescents. Sperm travel into the cervix far too rapidly for douching to wash away all possibility of pregnancy. Pressure from douching may also aid in propulsion of sperm higher into the uterus or vagina.

Other biological methods of contraception involve the timing of sexual intercourse to points in the menstrual cycle when conception is least likely to occur. *Contraceptive methods based on the menstrual cycle* include the calendar method, the mucus method, and the basal body temperature method. Such methods are popular among clients who reject the idea of putting anything foreign into their bodies, who want a method with no side effects or health risks, or whose religious practices and beliefs prohibit the use of contraceptive agents. All three of the methods require that the client thoroughly understand the reproductive cycle of the body and be aware of its subtle signs and signals during the cycle.

Effective use of these methods requires consistent, accurate record keeping for 6 or more months before use as contraception and to determine least fertile days. All methods are not practical for women with irregular or recently established menstrual cycles. These methods also necessitate a degree of control because intercourse must be postponed during fertile days.

The calendar or rhythm method tries to predict fertile days based on information from past menstrual cycles. Because few, if any, women have consistently regular cycles, this method frequently fails. Bad experiences with it have led many women to discount "natural" birth control methods (Boston Women's Health Book Collective, 1992).

More accurate and scientific methods of predicting ovulation have been developed, however. They are based on the body changes produced by hormones. One method requires the woman to record basal body temperature (BBT) the first thing each morning. Just after ovulation, body temperature rises 0.4° to 0.8° F due to progesterone influence. The woman is no longer considered fertile after 2 to 3 full days of increased temperature. Because sperm survive several days, the individual may conceive if she has sexual intercourse 1, 2, or more days before the temperature rises. Effectiveness is also reduced when temperature fluctuates because of illness and schedule changes.

A method often combined with the BBT system monitors the quality of cervical mucus to predict ovulation. Just before ovulation the amount of mucus increases, and just after ovulation it becomes more clear, viscous (thick), and stringy or elastic. Days of wet, abundant, slippery, stretchable, clear cervical mucus are the most fertile. Use of spermicidal gels or creams, lubricants, douching, or checking mucus just after intercourse may affect the perceived quality of cervical mucus and decrease effectiveness of this contraceptive method.

CHEMICAL METHODS

One of the most effective methods of pregnancy prevention is the oral contraceptive pill (OCP). The OCP combines various concentrations of estrogen and progestin. A progestin-only "minipill" is also available. OCPs suppress the release of FSH and LH, thereby preventing ovulation. The pills must be prescribed and may be contraindicated for women with histories of thrombophlebitis, liver disease, hypertension, and diabetes, or for those who smoke and are over 35 years of age. The pills are costly and should be prescribed only under ongoing health supervision that includes an annual physical examination and Pap test. The OCP is started on the fifth day of the menstrual cycle and is taken daily for 21 days. A menstrual period occurs usually within 2 or 3 days of stopping the hormones.

Side effects of OCPs include weight gain, spotting between periods, headaches, nausea, breast tenderness, depression, and vaginal yeast infections. Side effects are mostly related to estrogen concentrations and may be minimized by adjusting the prescription to find the OCP with the proper combination of hormones. Serious reactions that should be promptly reported to the health care provider are severe chest pain, abdominal or leg pain, shortness of breath, severe headaches, blurred vision, and loss of vision.

Norplant is a long-lasting (5 years) progestin-only contraceptive that is implanted under the skin of a woman's arm. It inhibits ovulation and thickens cervical mucus to inhibit sperm penetration. Norplant's effectiveness is 99.5%, the highest of any birth control option (Zawid, 1994).

Depo-Provera or DMPA (medroxyprogesterone acetate) is an injectable progestin that acts in the same manner as Norplant. DMPA was approved for use as a contraceptive in the United States in 1992. A 150-mg intramuscular injection offers 3 months of protection. Quarterly injections provide an effectiveness comparable to sterilization (Mastroianni and Robinson, 1994). Advantages include long-acting efficacy and convenience, reduction in risk of ovarian and endometrial cancer, and relief of heavy menstrual flow, menstrual cramps, and premenstrual syndrome (PMS). The most frequently reported side effects are irregular bleeding and amenorrhea. In addition, a return to fertility is delayed and takes 10 months on the average (Wyeth-Ayerst Laboratories, 1994).

Spermicidal creams and jellies used alone are not as effective as when combined with a barrier method of condom or diaphragm. Spermicidal products are sold over the counter and are relatively inexpensive. They act by providing a barrier at the cervical opening to prevent ejaculate from entering the uterus. A disadvantage is that the spermicide needs to be inserted into the vagina close to the time of intercourse and therefore may interrupt foreplay.

MECHANICAL METHODS

Other forms of contraception, which ideally combine barrier and spermicide, are diaphragms and condoms. Some couples dislike them since they can interrupt sexual spontaneity. The **diaphragm** provides a barrier by covering the cervical os. It must be fitted and prescribed by a health care provider. The diaphragm should be replaced yearly and must be refitted after a weight change of 10 pounds and after childbirth. Before each use the woman should check the diaphragm for tears and punctures.

The diaphragm is used by placing spermicidal gel on the diaphragm, inserting it over the cervix, and inserting additional spermicidal gel into the vagina. The process should take place 30 minutes or less before intercourse, and the diaphragm should be left in place 6 to 8 hours after intercourse but not more than 24 hours. The risk of toxic shock syndrome (TSS) is present with this method. Allergic reactions to the rubber of the diaphragm or the spermicide may occur. Effectiveness is less than that of OCPs but more than that of spermicide or a diaphragm alone. Diaphragms provide the added benefit of some protection against STDs.

The cervical cap is a barrier similar to the diaphragm. It fits only over the cervix. The advantages and disadvantages are the same as for the diaphragm. Fewer providers are trained in the more precise fitting necessary to effectively use this method.

The condom provides the most effective protection against STDs for men and women while providing a contraceptive alternative to abstinence. **Condoms** are latex sheaths that cover the penis and contain the ejaculate. The condom should be placed on the erect penis with a pocket or reservoir at the tip to collect the ejaculate. To prevent leakage, the base end of the condom should be held in place as the penis is removed from the vagina. Use with spermicide increases the effectiveness. Condoms are the only readily available form of contraception used by men.

Intrauterine devices (IUDs) became less available in the late 1980s because of fear of litigation related to side effects. However, a progesterone containing IUD is still available and some women may have other IUDs in place. The IUD is an object, which may contain hormones or copper, that is inserted into and retained in the uterus. It is thought that the IUD body causes endometrial inflammation, which prevents implantation.

SURGICAL METHODS

The two surgical methods of contraception are male and female **sterilization**. Sterilization has become more popular because of improved surgical methods and increased societal approval. It is the most effective contraception method other than abstinence. Newer surgical techniques can reverse surgical sterilization procedures. However, when choosing this method the client needs to understand the permanence of this procedure.

Female sterilization or **tubal ligation** involves cutting and tying the fallopian tubes. It is usually done with a laparoscope through a surgical incision in the abdominal wall, usually at the umbilicus. The procedure involves only the fallopian tubes; no other part of the woman's sexual or hormonal system is affected.

In male sterilization, or **vasectomy**, the ductus deferens that carries the sperm away from the testicles is cut and tied. Using a local anesthetic, the surgeon makes an opening in the scrotal sac and removes a segment of the ductus deferens, tying off or cauterizing the ends to prevent them from rejoining.

There is a scarcity of male contraceptive research and techniques in general. While it seems appropriate for heterosexual partners to share the contraceptive burden, society has placed the responsibility on the woman; the consequences of unprotected sexual intercourse fall on the woman. In addition, though vasectomies are far less expensive and medically complicated than tubal ligations, the latter greatly outnumber the former (Stotland, 1994). This, too, underscores the fact that it is women who become pregnant and who have few other reliable means of establishing control over their vulnerability.

Infertility

Family planning is generally thought of in terms of pregnancy prevention. One group with special needs that receives little public attention is adults who want to conceive but cannot.

Infertility is generally thought of as a female problem. In reality, an equal percentage of women and men have problems that contribute to difficulties bearing children. The evaluation of fertility must include both partners. Health care evaluation is usually recommended if pregnancy does not occur after 1 year of regular, unprotected intercourse with the same partner. In couples over 30, this evaluation may be recommended if pregnancy does not occur in 6 months.

Evaluation of potentially infertile couples includes physical examinations to determine general health, review of sexual activity, and understanding of the physiological concepts of conception. Specific procedures related to infertility include semen analysis for men, postcoital testing for mucus and sperm compatibility, endometrial biopsy, hysterosalpingogram (x-ray study) to evaluate uterine and tubal structures, and possibly laparoscopy.

Causes of infertility may be altered levels of sperm motility and lowered quantity or abnormal formation of sperm. The woman may have reduced tubal patency because of endometriosis or pelvic infections, abnormal uterine anatomy, or hormonal alterations that affect endometrial changes during the menstrual cycle or the quality of the cervical mucus. Depending on the causes of infertility, treatment may be hormonal to stimulate ovulation or surgical to restore tubal patency through microsurgery. Other available but controversial forms of treatment include artificial insemination using the husband's sperm or donor sperm, in vitro fertilization, and surrogate motherhood and embryo transfer.

The stress of fertility testing, the pain and continuing routine of therapies, and excessive cost produce a tense environment. Support groups are available for couples coping with these stressors. A percentage of couples remain infertile regardless of treatments used. These individuals need to work through a grief process for the loss of their potential children. Couples also need to be able to deal with the advice and misconceptions of friends and family. Support groups such as RESOLVE can assist. Contrary to community beliefs, recommendations such as "just relax" or "adopt a child and then you'll get pregnant" are not means of increasing fertility.

With advances in reproductive technology, the dilemmas that infertile couples face are multifaceted and can involve religious and ethical values and financial constraints. The decision to pursue adoption or medical assistance with fertilization or to remain childless is one the couple must make based on values regarding family and parenthood. The number of children available for adoption has decreased because of improved contraceptive technology, increased abortions, and fewer decisions to give newborns up for adoption. Couples deciding on adoption may require support to decide to parent children who have physical handicaps or who are of multiple ethnic origin. Adoptions of South American, Korean, and European children have been a satisfying decision made by many couples. Support groups are available to assist these couples in continued integration of multiethnic families. North American infants are also available for adoption.

Abortion

Abortion is an issue that stimulates heated discussions of morality, women's rights to control their bodies and reproduction, and the beginning of life. Abortions have been performed since ancient times. The safety and availability of abortions in the United States have improved since the 1973 Supreme Court decision, *Roe v. Wade.* Abortions are also safer and less costly when performed in the early weeks of pregnancy. This is possible with improved pregnancy testing and more accurate early diagnosis. The availability of abortions, however, remains tenuous and uncertain. Community opinions relating to the right to life, results of elections or appointments to political offices or positions, advocacy by "pro-life" and "pro-choice" groups, and the increasing use of violence against women and workers in abortion clinics are all forces that could reshape federal and state laws.

Rationales for abortion are varied and may include a decision to terminate an untimely pregnancy or a choice to abort a fetus that has a defect. Clients who decide to abort a pregnancy may experience guilt and grief. The guilt may surface immediately after the procedure or may be more covert and manifest as sexual dysfunction or inappropriate perceptions (e.g., a woman who later develops cervical cancer viewing the condition as punishment for this wrongdoing). Some of these beliefs may be assessed before the procedure and should be evaluated by those counseling women experiencing unwanted pregnancies. The woman who has an abortion may experience a sense of loss and should be prepared for and supported through the necessary grief period. The male partner may also experience this loss and grief.

RU 486, or *mifepristone* as it will be called in the United States, could be available to American women in 1996 upon completion of a current ongoing clinical trial. Commonly called the *morning after pill,* it is used together with prostaglandins for early termination of pregnancy. RU 486 is a progesterone inhibitor; as such it causes the uterine lining to break down and shed and the fertilized egg to separate from the uterine wall. The purpose of the prostaglandin, which causes uterine contractions, is to assure expulsion of the egg. While the addition of prostaglandin has the advantage of increasing the effectiveness from 85% to 96% to 99%, it is also associated with more side effects such as cramping and nausea than RU 486 alone. RU 486 has an excellent record of effectiveness, safety, and acceptability in France, where it has been used since 1989. It has also been approved in Great Britain and Sweden (Bass, 1994). Controversy over its use in the United States centers primarily on women's reproductive rights (Bass, 1994).

Sexually Transmitted Diseases

Sexually transmitted diseases (STDs) have been a concern almost as long as individuals have engaged in sexual intercourse. Although human immunodeficiency virus (HIV) is an STD, it affects a much smaller group and is a different epidemic than the epidemic of all other STDs. Therefore, for the purposes of this section, it will be categorized and discussed separately.

As the name implies, STDs are transmitted from infected individuals to partners during intimate sexual contact. The site of transmission is usually genital, but may also be oral-genital or anal-genital. One in six Americans claim they have had a sexually transmitted disease at least once in their lives (Michael et al, 1994). Those persons most likely to be infected share one key characteristic: unprotected sex with multiple partners. Four of the diseases discussed here are caused by bacteria and can usually be cured with antibiotics: gonorrhea, chlamydia, syphilis, and pelvic inflammatory disease. All clients need to understand that antibiotics need to be taken for the full course of treatment. An emerging concern, however, is that some of these bacterial infections (e.g., gonorrhea and syphilis) are now developing antibiotic-resistant strains. Two of the diseases discussed are caused by viruses and cannot be cured: genital herpes and genital warts.

A major problem in dealing with STDs is finding and treating the people who have them. Some people may not even know that they are infected because symptoms are absent or go unnoticed. Because sexual behavior may include the whole body rather than just the genitalia, many parts of the body are potential sites for STD. The ears, mouth, throat, tongue, nose, and eyelids can be used for sexual pleasure. The perineum, anus, and rectum are also frequently included in sexual activity. Furthermore, any contact with another person's body fluids around the head or an open lesion on the skin, anus, or genitalia can transmit an STD.

Sometimes people do not seek treatment because they are embarrassed. They may also hesitate to talk about their sexual behavior if they feel it is not "normal." Oral-genital sex, anal-genital sex, or any sexual behavior that embarrasses the client may hinder the detection of an STD. Specific STDs of the throat and intestine can thus go undetected at great cost to the client.

The most valuable tool the nurse can develop for providing care in areas of sexuality is communication skills. By questioning and talking with the client in a caring manner that evokes trust, the nurse can pick up valuable clues about an STD that the client may have missed. The nurse can also begin to assess the client's attitudes toward sexuality and adjust the intervention to make it acceptable to the client's sexual value system.

BACTERIAL SEXUALLY TRANSMITTED DISEASES

Gonorrhea and Chlamydia. Although gonorrhea and chlamydia are separate diseases and require different antibiotic treatments, they have similar symptoms, consequences, and concerns. Men are more likely to be diagnosed with gonorrhea than women, whereas more women than men have chlamydia. Chlamydia is now the most common STD (Michael et al, 1994).

Symptoms occur in 90% of affected males within a few weeks of exposure. Symptoms are burning or itching on urination and a discharge of pus from the penis. Women with these diseases experience symptoms in only 25% to 30% of cases. These symptoms include burning on urination and vaginal discharge. With anal or oral transmission, the primary symptom is burning or soreness of the anus and rectum or throat, respectively.

Gonorrhea and chlamydia are diagnosed through a culture or "smear" from the affected organ. The individual should be treated and considered capable of transmitting the disease until symptoms are resolved. Untreated or inadequately treated, these diseases progress to infect reproductive organs, which may result in scarring of the tissue and permanent sterility.

Infants born to mothers with active gonorrhea are at risk for blindness. Routine newborn eye treatment with antibiotic ointment is required to prevent this infection. Chlamydia in mothers can result in pneumonia and eye infections in infants after birth. Treatment during pregnancy is easier than efforts to cure either disease in infants.

Pelvic Inflammatory Disease. Pelvic inflammatory disease (PID) is an infectious disorder causing inflammation, abscess, and scarring of ovaries, fallopian tubes, and other pelvic structures. The disorder is often caused by progressive unrecognized or untreated gonorrhea or chlamydia. PID usually produces pelvic pain, tenderness, and fever. Depending on the severity of symptoms, antibiotic treatment may be given intravenously in the hospital or through home nursing care. Severe cases of PID often necessitate surgery to remove abscesses, infected tubes, or ovaries and at times to perform a hysterectomy with removal of ovaries and tubes. This is a serious illness, requiring comprehensive, prolonged treatment. Ectopic pregnancies and scarring and sterility can occur, even when surgery is unnecessary. The client may experience guilt and depression resulting from prior sexual activity, the disease, and possible subsequent sterility. Therefore, besides administering and monitoring antibiotic therapy and providing education, the nurse also needs to create a climate for providing comfort and emotional support.

Syphilis. Symptoms of the disease may take up to 3 months after exposure to become evident. The initial symptom is a small, painless lesion known as a *chancre,* which occurs at the site of transmission. It spontaneously heals in a few weeks to months.

Without treatment, syphilis advances to a more systemic secondary phase. Secondary syphilis exhibits influenza-like symptoms of fever, muscle aches, and sore throat. The hallmark feature is a generalized rash that may last for several months. Syphilis is curable in the primary and secondary phases. Without treatment the infected individual is contagious to sex partners throughout this time.

If completely untreated, syphilis can advance to a nontreatable third phase. Tertiary syphilis includes central nervous system and cardiac effects. Although the organism is not transmittable at this phase, the damage is irreversible.

The fetus may contract syphilis in utero and be born with secondary syphilis. Routine prenatal care involves a blood test for syphilis so that appropriate prenatal treatment can be initiated.

VIRAL SEXUALLY TRANSMITTED DISEASES

Herpes Simplex Virus. The herpes simplex virus (HSV) is abundant in the environment. The specific organism of concern is HSV type II, the usual cause of genital herpes. The common cold sore is usually caused by HSV type I, and it is not a STD; however, cross infection can occur to produce genital HSV type I and oral HSV type II. For this reason, intimate sexual contact should be avoided with anyone with a lesion.

A herpetic lesion may occur a few days to weeks after exposure. Herpes appears as a small cluster of blisters that ulcerate and heal usually in several weeks. The lesions are quite painful. In addition to the local lesion, initial exposure to HSV often produces general influenza-like symptoms.

Generally, HSV should be considered a lifelong problem. The disease does not progress but recurs as blistery clusters that ulcerate and heal. Recurrences are more likely at times of illness and stress but may decrease in frequency over years. Most individuals come to recognize early signs of tingling, pain, or itching at the area of infection. This precedes lesion development by several hours to days. Clients should be considered capable of transmitting the virus from the time early symptoms appear until lesions are healed. During the intervening period, HSV cannot be transmitted. Medications, such as acyclovir, are available to decrease the discomfort of lesions and decrease the frequency of recurrence. If maternal genital lesions are present near term, the infant may contract HSV during vaginal birth. Herpes is a very serious and possibly fatal virus in the newborn. At term, the health care provider will check for genital lesions; if they are present, a cesarean delivery will be recommended.

Genital Warts. Venereal or genital warts, or condyloma acuminata, are caused by the human papilloma virus (HPV). The condition may be asymptomatic or cause a soft, flesh-color lesion at the area of sexual contact. HPV is the most common viral infection and the second most common of all STDs (Michael et al, 1994).

Genital warts may occur up to 6 months after exposure and can be difficult to treat. Treatment includes repeated application of medication such as podophyllum, or lesions may need to be removed through cryosurgery or lasers. HPV infections have also been linked to increased incidence of cancer, especially in women.

In women, the Pap test often identifies atypical cervical cells or dysplasia (abnormal development) that require further investigation. Colposcopy is a procedure that allows examiners to view the cervix through magnification and identify and then biopsy suspicious areas. Often, no warts or lesions are seen until acetic acid is applied to highlight abnormal cellular growth. After identification of dysplasia the woman should have repeated Pap tests to observe for progression of cellular changes. In cases of severe dysplasia or early cancerous changes, the woman may need surgery to remove lesions, abnormal cells, or portions of the cervix. Untreated cervical dysplasia may progress over several years to invasive cervical cancer.

HUMAN IMMUNODEFICIENCY VIRUS

HIV or acquired immunodeficiency syndrome (AIDS) is also spread through sexual contact. Although HIV is present in a majority of body fluids, it is really a blood-borne pathogen. For transmission to occur, therefore, some exchange of body fluid, particularly blood, must occur. Primary routes of transmission include contaminated IV needles; anal intercourse, vaginal intercourse, and oral-genital sex; and transfusion of blood and blood products. However, the majority of blood products are now safe.

Those primarily vulnerable to HIV infections, therefore, are gay men; intravenous drug users, their partners, and their children; and hemophiliacs and others who have received contaminated blood. As with other STDs, those het-

erosexual persons who have unprotected sex with multiple partners or who have a partner with multiple other partners are also at risk. Research reports disagree as to whether HIV is an epidemic or not and present conflicting results and opinions about the spread of HIV to the general heterosexual population (Michael et al, 1994). However, of increasing concern is the transmission of the virus in heterosexual women and, therefore, in utero, resulting in increasing numbers of children with HIV (Driscoll et al, 1994) (see the box below, left). Teens, especially females, are becoming one of the highest risk groups for AIDS (Zawid, 1994). Consequently they are a crucial target for interventions concerning HIV/AIDS (see the box below).

Odds of transmission of HIV increase with frequent unprotected sex with an infected partner. Transmission of HIV may produce AIDS. Some individuals may have no symptoms, whereas others may develop AIDS-related complex (ARC). AIDS may take as long as 7 to 10 years to present. It is also important for health care providers to know that women with HIV/AIDS have different symptoms than men. As a result of the initial focus on gay men and IV drug users, researchers and practitioners have only recently begun to understand and diagnose AIDS in women. Most health care workers are unable to diagnose HIV/AIDS in women until the disease is significantly advanced. The average death after diagnosis of AIDS is 30 months for a man but only 15 months for a woman (Rosser, 1994). Much remains to be learned about this virus, the disease, and those who have no symptoms or do not display the full range of symptoms. There is no cure for the disease, which is usually fatal. Treatments and vaccines are being investigated.

RESEARCH HIGHLIGHT

RESEARCH ABSTRACT

Many AIDS clients in their 20s likely became infected as teenagers since the average incubation period of HIV is 8 years. Adolescent sexual activity frequently occurs without protection, and adolescents become prime candidates for AIDS prevention and education strategies. The 30-minute magic show described in this pilot study was designed to reach 11- to 14-year-olds in an informative, visual, and interactive manner to provide information about AIDS, dispel misconceptions about transmission, practice refusing sex, and to teach skills to practice safer sex. The show has been seen by 281 students. Preliminary analysis suggests that perceived self-efficacy has significantly improved in refusing sex and putting on condoms.

IMPLICATIONS FOR PRACTICE

▶ Knowledge alone is not sufficient to change sexual behavior.

▶ Interactive, creative, and humorous education programs that seek and reinforce correct participant input can increase self-confidence and improve perceived self-efficacy in practicing safe sex. Self-efficacy is a better predictor of behavioral change than knowledge possession.

REFERENCE

Lustig SL: The AIDS prevention magic show: avoiding the tragic with magic, *Public Health Reports* 109:2, March-April, 1994.

CULTURAL ASPECTS OF CARE

In the United States, 57% of women report IV drug use as the primary source of HIV infection. However, globally, heterosexual contact is the major vehicle of transmission (Driscoll et al, 1994). In South Africa, for example, the pattern of AIDS shifted in 1986 from white homosexual and bisexual men to urban heterosexuals of both sexes and appears to be approaching the levels in central, east, and southern Africa. In these areas more women than men are affected and 25% of children born to HIV-positive mothers develop the disease. Women in Africa, as elsewhere around the globe, are dependent on male partner condom use. This is often widely resisted in a patriarchal society (Sanders, Nash, and Hoffman, 1994).

DISEASE PREVENTION

Safe sex is a phrase used to describe responsible sexual practices aimed at minimizing STD transmission, particularly AIDS. Safe sex is responsible sex and includes knowing sex partners, having a relationship with open communication that enables the partners to discuss current health status and disease exposure, and using protective devices. Additional measures include limiting the number of sex partners, avoiding sexual contact with intravenous drug users, and using condoms properly. Condoms provide a barrier between body fluids only with sexual activity involving the penis. No protection is provided for oral-genital contact, for example, and therefore these practices should be avoided. The only 100% effective method of avoiding contracting an STD is abstinence.

A controversial issue related to safe sex for adolescents is the placement of condom dispensers in public restrooms in places frequented by teenagers, particularly in schools. Those in favor of this program state that teenagers cannot be stopped from having sex; therefore adults should promote health through ensuring a means to minimize pregnancy and STDs. Those opposed believe that providing condoms implies approval for teenage sexual activity. The fact is that the rate of adolescent pregnancy and STD incidence continue to increase.

Discussion of limiting risks of STDs should be included with all sexually active clients. Middle-age and older adults may be engaged in relations with more than one partner and not realize the risk of STDs. Assessment should be comprehensive and not based on stereotypes or assumptions.

Sexual Abuse

Sexual abuse occurs far more often than reported. The known cases of woman abuse, incest, and child molestation probably represent only the tip of the iceberg. Abuse within dating relationships is a growing problem and "date" rape accounts for a substantial proportion of adolescent pregnancy. Incidents such as these have a traumatic effect on the victim and may cause physical and psychological problems and later sexual dysfunction.

Violence against women is a major health problem in the United States. It is the leading cause of female trauma (Campbell, 1993). One in four women experiences physical violence, sexual assault, or battering by a current or former partner. Injuries from such episodes account for 22% to 35% of women's visits to emergency rooms (Warshaw, 1994). Many of women's chronic health problems relate to these violent experiences.

There are also consequences to the children of abused women. Partner abuse during pregnancy has been associated with low birth weight. Child abuse is also associated with abuse of the mother. Abused children are at risk for health, emotional, and school performance problems; increased aggressiveness may occur and become adult violence (Campbell, 1993).

When abuse is recognized, support needs to be mobilized for the victims and families. Suspected abuse must be reported to proper authorities. Health care facilities must have procedures in place for reporting incidents of suspected child abuse. All family members may require long-term therapy to promote healthy interactions and relationships. Victims may need to work through the crises before

feeling comfortable with intimate expressions of affection. Partners may need support in understanding and altering the process of abuse and cycle of violence. Children and women who have been sexually molested or abused need to understand that they are not at fault for the incident. Nurses who come in contact with abused clients need to be aware of sources for referral and support in the community (e.g., rape crisis centers and women's self-help centers). Providers must understand the importance of their responses to the victim's reactions and adaptations and refrain from applying personal values and stereotypes to the victims and their families, for example, blaming the victim for provoking the violent attack or for not being "strong" enough to get out of the abusive situation. Providers also need to acknowledge their own feelings since the capacity for caring and empathy depends on knowing and understanding the self.

Effects of Illness on Sexuality

Illness can directly or indirectly influence any or all of the dimensions of human sexuality. The nurse helps the client integrate the physical, psychological, and social systems during the course of the illness. The degree to which any nursing intervention involving sex is successful depends on the attitudes and beliefs of the nurse and client and their understanding of the effects of the illness and its treatment on sexual functioning. Viewing sexuality in terms of a continuum rather than as being present or absent may be a helpful concept for the client.

PHYSIOLOGICAL AND PSYCHOLOGICAL CHANGES AND ILLNESS

The genitals and other soft body tissues that respond to sexual arousal require uninterrupted neural pathways and an adequate supply of blood. Hormones influence sexual moods and physiological functioning in sexual expression. Joints and muscles must bend and stretch as the body gives expression to sexual feelings. A change in any one of these systems can have an effect on the others. To accommodate to changes in these systems, the client may have to learn new sexual behavior. Changes in body functions and structures as a result of illness may not directly influence sexuality but may affect the client's feelings and perceptions of desirability and arousal.

Chronic illness may interfere with sexuality. A client or partner providing extended home care and attention may have little energy left for sexual feelings or activity. For a client with a highly debilitating illness such as chronic lung disease, only very limited sexual activity may be possible. Diabetes not only necessitates changes in daily habits but may also lead to changes in sexuality (see the box on p. 428). Vascular and neurological changes may cause lack of or change in orgasmic response and erectile dysfunction (Zawid, 1994). Spinal cord injuries sever nerve pathways and remove genital sensation. Self-esteem is usually lowered with the accompanying change in body image, gender identity, and altered ability to perform sex-role behavior. Chronic pain and limited range of movement present obstacles to sexual activity. Cancer can also interfere with sexuality. Medical and surgical treatments alter body image. Alopecia (loss of hair), severe nausea, and fatigue from chemotherapy may temporarily remove all sexual desires.

▶ RESEARCH HIGHLIGHT

RESEARCH ABSTRACT
This qualitative study explored sexuality in adults with insulin-dependent diabetes mellitus (IDDM). Data were collected from interviews of 11 diabetic women and men and analyzed to describe the process of changes in sexuality that occurred as a result of the effects and treatment of the illness. Individualized changes occurred in two subcategories: how the subjects valued themselves as sexual beings and how they met intimacy needs in their relationships.

IMPLICATIONS FOR PRACTICE
▶ Information can be used to develop a knowledge base in assessing and planning interventions to meet the sexual health care needs of adults with IDDM.
▶ Information-seeking questions and counseling should not focus solely on sexual performance; but also on how the client feels about self since diagnosis, how well the illness is accepted, and how the client feels about relationships with significant others.
▶ Teaching sessions can be used to discuss the correlation between diabetes control and the effects of IDDM on penile erection, vaginal lubrication, mucous membrane infections, and sexual desire.

REFERENCE
LeMone P: Human sexuality in adults with insulin-dependent diabetes mellitus, *IMAGE* 25(2):101, 1993.

The client's spouse or partner will need to deal with grief and beliefs to respond sexually.

For all of these clients, the nurse has an essential role in easing their adjustments. Initiating discussions of sexual topics or concerns, helping clients learn effective communication skills and explore altered expressions of affection and sexual stimulation, and encouraging them to experiment with new positions for sexual activity may be necessary.

EFFECTS OF MEDICATION ON SEXUALITY

The effect of medications on sexual feelings and functioning is complex. Medications can interfere with sexual desire and all phases of the sexual response cycle.

Antihypertensives such as methyldopa, propranolol, and clonidine often cause erectile dysfunction. Thiazide diuretics, also used to treat hypertension, cause erectile dysfunction, decreased vaginal lubrication, and decreased **libido** (sexual drive) (Seidel et al, 1991). Methyldopa has also been known to decrease libido. Depression usually causes diminished desire. Antidepressant medication may produce an increased libido but may also cause delayed female orgasms and delayed or failed ejaculation. Chemotherapeutic agents, with the psychological effects caused by alopecia and nausea, may also result in decreased libido, impotence, **amenorrhea** (absence of menstruation), decreased spermatogenesis, and sterility. Young men interested in becoming fathers can freeze sperm before chemotherapy or radiation treatment. The sexual effects of all medications must be considered and included as appropriate teaching content.

HOSPITALIZATION

Upon entering a hospital, clients leave their home and its security and privacy and enter a more public and intrusive environment. The hospital room is open to the nurse at all times, and privacy is represented only by a cubicle curtain. Hospital clothing is scant. Even carrying out activities of personal hygiene may be beyond the client's ability. Often, sexual behavior and feelings may diminish or vanish. The need to have some power over life and the powerlessness of being hospitalized may become crucial issues.

Nurses can assist clients in learning to meet sexual needs in the hospital. Simply acknowledging the openness of the setting lets a client know that the nurse understands. Knocking or signaling before entering the client's space is a basic courtesy and provides a needed sense of privacy. The use of a do-not-disturb sign offers the client some feeling of control over the privacy of the environment.

Some hospitalized clients may act out sexually through use of obscene language, pinching or other suggestive contact with the nurse, or consistent nudity or exposure of genitals when the nurse enters the room. This behavior may be a means of exerting control over the clinical environment or an attempt to validate continued identity as a sexual being. It may also be a means of attracting attention or testing limits. Assessment and intervention to deal with persistent sexual acting out is a challenge that benefits from the psychiatric nurse specialist's expertise. Consistency in approach to the client and attention and reinforcement for desirable behavior are essential to minimize the problem.

Surgery not only changes body structures and functions but also influences body image. Surgical clients may experience loss of self-esteem and feelings of loss involving their masculinity or femininity. They may blame themselves for needing surgery and consider the surgical consequences a punishment. Alteration or removal of the internal or external genitalia can make conventional and accustomed sexual activities uncomfortable or impossible. The client is then faced with not only the loss or alteration of body parts but also the necessity of having to learn new sexual behavior that may seem strange or repugnant. Prostatectomies, hysterectomies, mastectomies, and ostomies have the potential for creating sexual problems for clients and their partners.

After a heart attack or heart surgery, clients often have a decline in sexual activity. This is true even after they are evaluated as fit and able to resume normal activities of daily living. These clients typically fear having another attack or dying while masturbating or having intercourse (Zawid, 1994). The client's partner is often anxious about initiating sex because of fear of contributing to another attack. Such anxieties are cultivated through misunderstanding, misinformation, or lack of information. Clear, accurate, and honest information is needed at every stage of rehabilitation.

Sexual Dysfunction

The causes of **sexual dysfunction** may be physiological or psychological. Sometimes the cause of a dysfunction cannot be identified or is a combination of several factors. About 10% to 20% of sexual dysfunctions are caused by physiological factors (Kolodny, Masters, and Johnson, 1979). In another 15% of cases, physiological problems contribute to the sexual dysfunction but are not its sole cause (Masters, Johnson, and Kolodny, 1982). In most instances a sexual assessment should include a complete physical examination to identify or rule out physiological conditions that might contribute to sexual dysfunction.

PSYCHOLOGICAL FACTORS

In many instances, sexual dysfunction can be traced to a lack of knowledge about sexuality, ignorance of sexual techniques, or general misinformation about sexuality. For example, unsatisfactory lovemaking can be the result of a lack of information about sexual anatomy. Some segments of society still place strong prohibitions on discussions of sexual behavior. Children may receive some information at home and in school, although sharing among peers may still be a major source of misinformation. Open discussion of sex, even between partners, traditionally has not been encouraged, and the result has been feelings of distance or alienation.

Another psychological factor is the destructive belief that the ability to perform sexually is inherently developed by the time a person reaches adulthood. Sexual performance is often perceived as instinctual and mysteriously understood when a person comes of age. Thus ignorance and silence about sexual matters prevail because a person who lacks knowledge about sexual function seldom realizes that this information needs to be taught.

The psychological forces that prevent violation of sexual rules in many cultures are guilt and anxiety. When guilt and anxiety become associated with early sexual learning, the person develops a pattern of inhibited sexual response. For instance, a woman may be actively discouraged from sexual stimulation in early childhood. As an adult, she may find that she now has to learn to enjoy sexual stimulation and overcome negative feelings associated with her sexual self-concept.

Other sources of sexual anxiety, such as fear of failure, demand for performance, and rejection, can be destructive to sexual functioning. Anticipation of the inability to perform is a cause of erectile dysfunction and, perhaps to some extent, of orgasmic dysfunction. People who have experienced episodes of failure may have increased fears of its recurrence. Anticipatory anxiety related to sexual performance can start a self-defeating cycle of fear that escalates from a single failure into serious chronic dysfunction.

Fear of rejection by one's partner or an excessive need to please may also generate anxiety. To wish to give enjoyment and share pleasure with a partner is desirable and healthy. When this becomes a compulsive need, the emotion becomes dysfunctional.

Poor communication is frequently associated with sexual dysfunction. A person with communication problems may be unable to discuss sex, have limited knowledge, or have restrictive standards of acceptable sexual behavior. In this situation partners perpetuate ignorance, lack of understanding, and misinformation about their sexual and emotional needs. To communicate effectively about sex, they must openly share information about their interests, desires, and wishes. Negotiation, compromise, and satisfaction result from effective communication patterns.

A history of sexual abuse usually has an impact on sexual functioning. Anger, guilt, and a need for control are emotional sequelae to abuse and often underlie the development of sexual problems, including inhibited desire and avoidance of sexual contact. Researchers have begun to examine the variables associated with molestation that contribute to adult sexual adjustment. These include the person's age at the time of molestation, the frequency and duration of molestation, and the negative feelings associated with molestation. These findings help explain variations in sexual functioning that exist among people with histories of abuse. Further investigation is needed to help nurses understand and effectively treat the population of abused persons who seek counseling for sexual difficulties. Tables 24-2 and 24-3 summarize the most common female and male sexual dysfunctions, their possible causes, and intervention strategies.

PHYSIOLOGICAL FACTORS

Orgasmic dysfunction in women is seldom caused by physiological factors. However, severe chronic illness (e.g., diabetes mellitus), kidney disease, alcoholism, neurological problems, hormone deficiencies, and some pelvic disorders resulting from infection or surgery may impair or hinder sexual desire or orgasmic response. **Vaginismus**, an intense contraction of the perineal and vaginal musculature that closes the vaginal introitus, is only occasionally associated with painful genital conditions. Instead, it is most often a psychological response and frequently associated with rape or childhood sexual abuse (Zawid, 1994). **Dyspareunia**, or painful intercourse, on the other hand, is more likely the result of physical disorders such as infections, surgical scarring, diabetes, vaginal dryness from hormonal changes, or use of drugs (e.g., antihistamines, tranquilizers, and marijuana).

Physiological factors that may cause erectile dysfunction in men include neurological disorders such as spinal cord injury or multiple sclerosis, vascular insufficiency problems, hormonal deficiencies, and genital infections or injuries. Diabetes and alcoholism are the two most common physiological causes of erectile dysfunction. Prescription medications and street drugs sometimes cause erection problems. Physiological problems rarely cause premature ejaculation, but delayed ejaculation is sometimes the result of neurological disorders. About 10% of cases of delayed ejaculation are due to drug abuse and alcoholism (Masters, Johnson, and Kolodny, 1982).

The distinction between physiological and psychological causes of sexual dysfunction is not always clear. Physiological interventions sometimes clear up the problem. At other times, psychological concerns have been masked by a physiological condition. It is important to monitor the client's progress carefully, even when it seems that only a physiological condition is involved. An understanding of the possible psychological and physiological causes of sexual dysfunction is needed before the nurse can determine whether further assessment and intervention are necessary.

■ SEXUALITY AND THE NURSING PROCESS

 Assessment

Ideally, sex is a natural, spontaneous act that culminates in satisfaction for both partners. After sexual activity, there

Table 24-2	Common Female Sexual Dysfunctions		

DESCRIPTION	POSSIBLE CAUSES	INTERVENTIONS
Preorgasmic (primary) orgasmic dysfunction: impaired ability of woman to have orgasm	Religious prohibitions Restrictive learning environment Fear of losing control Poor communication with partner Inadequate clitoral stimulation Excessive drug or alcohol use Past negative sexual experiences	Provide information on sexual prohibitions and restrictions Teach sensate focus exercises* Suggest genital play Teach Kegel exercises† Suggest directed masturbation Encourage nondemand intercourse Initiate referral to sex therapist Initiate referral to preorgasmic support group
Secondary orgasmic dysfunction: impaired ability of woman to have orgasm currently but with history of ability to have orgasm	Low sexual interest Attitude toward partner Causes listed for primary orgasmic dysfunction	Discuss attitude toward partner Provide information on sexual prohibitions Teach sensate focus exercises* Suggest nondemand intercourse Suggest genital play Teach Kegel exercises† Suggest directed masturbation Encourage partner communication Initiate referral to sex therapist
Vaginismus: involuntary constriction of outer third of vagina, making vaginal penetration impossible	Religious prohibitions Sexual prohibitions Experience of sexual assault Painful intercourse Painful pelvic examinations Alcohol abuse Traumatic early experiences with sex Fear of pregnancy, venereal disease, or cancer	Legitimize existence of spasm Suggest use of vaginal dilators in graduated sizes Teach Kegel exercises† Encourage improvement of partner communication Initiate referral to sensitive, experienced health care provider
Dyspareunia: painful intercourse	Negative attitude toward partner Strong religious prohibitions Sexual prohibitions Genital sensitivity Physical problems (e.g., tears, infections, trauma, spasms, lack of lubrication) Roughness during intercourse Lack of arousal	Initiate referral to sensitive, experienced health care provider Treat physical problems Provide sufficient lubrication Discuss sexual attitudes Discuss comfortable positions
Lack of desire: loss of interest in being sexual	Strong negative emotions Illness Fatigue Drug or alcohol use Avoidance response because of feeling sexually pressured Unresolved anger or fear Depression History of sexual abuse or incest Pain associated with intercourse	Discuss attitude toward partner Provide information on sexual prohibitions and restrictions Teach sensate focus exercises* Teach Kegel exercises† Encourage genital play Encourage resolution of conflicts between partners Initiate referral to mental health professional or sex therapist

*Series of pleasurable touching exercises that are focused on sensual (not sexual) activities with partner.
†Exercises for pubococcygeus muscle to increase sensation and maintain muscle tone of pelvic floor.

should be a period of "afterglow" in which both partners experience a sense of warmth, well-being, and closeness. In reality, this is often the exception rather than the rule, as demonstrated by the number of self-help sexual enhancement books available in bookstores. Nurses can expect to encounter clients who have problems with one or more of the stages of sexual behavior, including the feeling of wanting sex, the physiology and emotions of having sex, and the feelings experienced after sex. Clients may uncon-

sciously provide the nurse with clues to their sexual problems. The nurse must provide the opportunity for clients to discuss sex by initiating the topic at the time of assessment.

Many nurses are uncomfortable talking about sexuality with clients, but they can reduce their discomfort using several methods. First, they can build a sound knowledge base and understanding of the dimensions of healthy sexuality and the most common areas of sexual alteration or dysfunction. Second, nurses can assess their own comfort

Table 24-3	Common Male Sexual Dysfunctions	
DESCRIPTION	**POSSIBLE CAUSES**	**INTERVENTIONS**
Primary erectile dysfunction: inability of man to penetrate during sexual contact and to sustain an erection to point of penetration (Man may masturbate to ejaculation.)	Extreme religious prohibitions Traumatic initial failure Performance anxiety and fears	Relieve pressure of goal-oriented sexual performance Discuss sexual prohibitions and restrictions Provide accurate information Teach sensate focus exercises Restrict intercourse Encourage female superior position with lubrication Encourage options to intercourse (e.g., manual stimulation, oral-genital sex) Initiate referral to sex therapist
Secondary erectile dysfunction: Inability of man to maintain or perhaps even experience erection but with a history of penetration at least one time (Man has experienced erectile failure during at least 25% of sexual opportunities.)	Interference with central nervous system caused by drugs, alcohol, stress, fatigue, diseases, or surgical procedures Performance anxiety Poor communication with partner Depression	Relieve pressure of goal-oriented sexual performance Discuss sexual prohibitions and restrictions Provide accurate information Teach sensate focus exercises Teach Kegel exercises to female partner Initiate referral to urologist
Premature ejaculation: consistent premature ejaculation	Fast ejaculation patterning during adolescence Failure to attend to internal cues of approaching ejaculation Lack of sensual self-awareness Performance anxiety	Provide accurate information Encourage communication with partner Teach sensate focus exercises Teach Kegel exercises to female partner Explain stop-start technique Encourage different positions Teach retraining of ejaculatory response Relieve pressure of performance anxiety Suggest changing tempo of thrusting during intercourse Initiate referral to sex therapist
Delayed ejaculation: inability to ejaculate during penetration	Religious restrictions Fear of impregnating Lack of physical interest Active dislike for partner Past traumatic sexual event Infidelity Punishment for masturbation as child Excessive drug or alcohol use	Relieve pressure of goal-oriented sexual performance Discuss sexual prohibitions and restrictions Provide accurate information Teach sensate focus exercises Teach Kegel exercises to female partner Encourage communication with partner Initiate referral to mental health professional or sex therapist

levels and limitations in discussing sexuality and sexual functioning. Practicing the pronunciation of terms related to sex and sexuality in both professional and lay language is one way of increasing the comfort level. Finally, nurses can learn to recognize sexual problems that are outside the realm of their expertise and refer the client for help.

FACTORS AFFECTING SEXUALITY

Sexual desire varies among individuals: some people want and enjoy sex every day, whereas others want sex only once a month, and still others have no sexual desire and are quite comfortable with that fact. Sexual desire becomes an issue if the client simply wants to feel sexual desire more often, if the client believes it is necessary to measure up to some cultural norm, or if a discrepancy in the sexual desires of partners causes conflict.

Physical Factors. A client may experience a decrease in sexual desire for physical reasons. Sexual activity may bring on pain or discomfort. Even imagining that sex could hurt can lessen sexual desire. Minor illness and fatigue are reasons a person may not feel sexual. Medications can affect sexual desire. Poor body image, particularly when magnified by feelings of rejection or by body-altering surgery, can turn off a client sexually.

Relationship Factors. Issues in a relationship can distract a person from wanting sex. After the initial glow of the relationship has faded, couples may find that they are faced with major differences in their values or lifestyles. The degree to which they still feel close to each other and interact on an intimate level depends on their ability to negotiate and compromise. Thus communication skills play a crucial role when dealing with sexual desire in a relationship. Decreased interest in sexual activity can result just from the anxiety of having to tell a partner what sexual behavior is acceptable or pleasurable.

Lifestyle Factors. Lifestyle factors, such as the use or abuse of alcohol or the lack of time to devote to a relationship, can influence sexual desire. Traditionally associated with sexual behavior, particularly in advertisements, alcohol can induce a false sense of well-being or seductiveness in the initial stages of sex. However, ample evidence now shows that alcohol's negative effects on sexuality far outweigh the euphoria it may initially produce.

Finding the time for sexual activity is another lifestyle factor. Some clients do not know how to structure work and home time to include sexual behavior. Working parents, for example, may feel so overburdened that they perceive sexual advances from a partner as an additional demand on them. Such clients often describe their need to be alone to think and rest as more important than sex. Other individuals may not have sex partners.

Self-Esteem Factors. The client's level of self-esteem can also lead to conflicts involving sexuality. If sexual self-esteem has not been nurtured by developing a strong sense of a sexual self and by learning sexual skills, sexuality may cause negative feelings or lead to the suppression of sexual feelings. Sexual self-esteem can be lowered in many ways. Rape, incest, and physical or emotional abuse leave deep scars. Lowered sexual self-esteem can also result from lack of adequate sex education, negative role models, and attempts to live up to unrealistic personal or cultural expectations.

It may be appropriate to explore physical, relationship, lifestyle, and self-esteem factors in more depth depending on other aspects of the assessment.

SEXUAL HEALTH HISTORY

Every nursing history, whether taken in a clinic, hospital, or practitioner's office should include a few sex-related questions to determine whether the client has any sexual concerns. These questions can be incorporated in the review of systems and addressed in a routine manner. The nurse must understand the reasons for the question and be able to provide this rationale to the client on request. Asking for information for the sake of curiosity is never appropriate. An opening statement such as "Sex is an important part of life and can be affected by our health status and vice versa. To better understand your health, it is useful to know . . ." is a good example to use. Other questions for adults follow:

1. How do you feel about the sexual part of your life?
2. Have you noticed any changes in the way you feel about yourself as a man, woman, husband, or wife?
3. How has your illness, medication, or surgery affected your sex life?
4. It is not unusual for people with your condition to be experiencing some sexual problems. Has that been a concern to you at all?

Questions that may be addressed to a child's parents include the following:

1. Have you noticed your child exploring his body, for example, touching his penis?
2. Has your child begun to ask questions about where babies come from?
3. Have you talked with your child about sex, pregnancy, and contraception?

Adolescents may best respond to a question such as the following:

1. Many adolescents have questions about STDs or whether their bodies are developing at the right rate. Do you have any questions about sex or other things?

Some clients may be too embarrassed or do not know how to ask sexual questions directly. Thus they may be very subtle in asking for information. The nurse must be aware of cues that indicate a question or problem. Such cues might include the following:

1. Talking about going home from the hospital and being afraid of their partner's thoughts or expectations of them
2. Asking direct easy questions and then seeming hesitant about the next question
3. Joking of a sexual nature
4. Asking questions that suggest concerns about achieving orgasms such as "When my episiotomy was repaired, could the doctor have sewn it up too tight?"
5. Making self-conscious comments such as, "Well, I'm just not as young as I used to be."
6. Using euphemisms such as, "I just want to be a good partner."
7. Looking down when asked a question about sexuality, blushing, and changing the topic
8. Asking questions about normal behavior such as, "Is it normal for a man not to ejaculate when he gets older?"

Observing and listening to clients' concerns about sexuality takes practice. The nurse clarifies and paraphrases or asks questions that will help clients be more direct about sexual concerns. If sexual concerns are identified, the nurse may wish to pursue a sexual health history in more detail. By including sexuality in the discussion, the nurse indicates that sexuality is an important component of health care and acknowledges the need for clients to discuss these concerns. When taking a sexual history, the nurse can use interview strategies to promote comfort (see Chapters 7 and 14).

A brief sex history would include answers to the following questions:

1. What do clients see as their sexual concerns?
2. When did these sexual concerns begin and how have they changed over time?
3. What do the clients see as the cause of the concerns?
4. What sorts of treatment have clients sought to help alleviate this concern?
5. How would clients like this concern to be resolved, and what are their goals for treatment?

The discussion between nurse and client might include questions such as the following:

1. How does the method work?
2. What are the risks involved in using the method?
3. Are there contraindications that rule out particular methods?
4. How will it affect lovemaking?
5. Does the partner object to it?
6. Will it cause any discomfort?
7. Is it readily available, affordable, and easy to use?
8. Will either partner feel embarrassed using it?
9. Is the risk of pregnancy acceptable?
10. Are there other alternatives?

As indicated by age, sex, and review of systems, the history should include other aspects related to sexual assessment. The history should include concerns about STDs such as known exposure, genital discharge, and multiple partners. The adequacy of or need for contraception is an appropriate point of questioning for all men and premenopausal women who are sexually active.

Determining whether clients, particularly females, are in abusive relationships is also important. A question such as "Are you in a relationship in which someone is hurting you?" may open the door for a client to reveal present or previous abuse. An additional question such as "Has anyone ever forced you to have sex you did not wish to participate in?" may more specifically inform the client of the option to discuss concerns at the time of questioning or later during further contact with the health care provider.

A detailed assessment of long-standing sexual problems or concerns such as erectile dysfunction or vaginismus is outside the realm of general nursing practice. These clients should be referred to health providers specializing in areas of sex therapy. Often, however, the nurse may identify a sex concern related to medication, lack of knowledge, or fear of abnormality. Interventions aimed at these concerns are appropriate to nursing practice in any setting.

PHYSICAL ASSESSMENT

The physical examination is important in evaluating the cause of sexual concerns or problems and may be the best opportunity to teach the client about sexuality. The techniques of inspection and palpation are used in this examination (see Chapter 33). The nurse assesses the client's breasts and external and internal genitalia. The nurse has the opportunity to assess the client's reaction, answer questions, and provide information about the examination or anatomical and physiological structures.

The female client can learn to perform a breast self-examination during physical assessment (see Chapter 33). In addition, the nurse may choose to teach the client Kegel exercises (see the box below, left). These exercises strengthen the pubococcygeus muscle. Toning of the muscle decreases because of stretching during childbirth and loss of general elasticity during aging. Maintaining good tone helps prevent bladder or rectal prolapse into the vagina (cystocele or rectocele), reduces problems with later urinary incontinence, and can enhance sexual enjoyment through and beyond menopause.

Male clients can learn to perform testicular self-examination during physical assessment (see Chapter 33). Knowledge of normal scrotal anatomical structures aids the client in detecting signs of testicular cancer.

Nursing Diagnosis

Altered sexuality patterns and sexual dysfunction are recognized as approved nursing diagnoses (Kim, McFarland, and McLane, 1995) (see the nursing diagnoses box below). The difference in diagnosing sexual dysfunction or altered sexuality patterns depends on whether the client perceives problems in achieving sexual satisfaction or expresses concern regarding sexuality. When client concern is expressed, the diagnosis is altered sexuality patterns. When making diagnoses of sexual problems, the nurse must assess anatomical, physiological, sociocultural, ethical, and situational issues (see the diagnostic process box on p. 434).

Clustering of defining characteristics yields accurate nursing diagnoses. In addition to nursing diagnoses that

CLIENT TEACHING
for Kegel Exercises

OBJECTIVE
- Client will demonstrate ability to tighten pubococcygeus muscle and will verbalize methods to assess correct procedures and increasing strength.

TEACHING STRATEGIES
- Explain method to identify proper muscle contraction by sitting on toilet with knees far apart and tighten muscles to stop the flow of urine.
- After muscle is identified, instruct client to contract muscle for a count of 3, hold and release for a count of 3 and repeat this 10 times. Client should do this about 5 times a day.
- Explain that within first week of exercises, client should assess if proper muscle contraction is occurring by placing two fingers in vagina to identify if tightening can be felt or asking partner to identify during sexual intercourse when muscle is tightened.

EVALUATION
- Ask client if she has identified pubococcygeus muscle via finger insertion or partner response.
- During vaginal bimanual examination, ask client to do exercises and assess muscle tone.

Examples of NANDA Nursing Diagnoses for Alterations in Sexual Health

Altered sexuality patterns *related to:*
- Fear of pregnancy
- Effects of antihypertensives
- Marital conflicts or stressors
- Depression over death of or separation from spouse

Sexual dysfunction *related to:*
- Spinal cord injury
- Chronic illness
- Pain
- Anxiety regarding placement in a nursing home

Rape-trauma syndrome *related to:*
- Inability to discuss past rape experience

Body-image disturbance *related to:*
- Effects of recent mastectomy or colostomy
- Sexual dysfunction
- Postpartum changes

Self-esteem disturbance *related to:*
- Perceived vulnerability after myocardial infarction
- Patterns of abuse as a child

Knowledge deficit *related to:*
- Sexual inexperience
- Age-related changes in sexual response

Decisional conflict *related to:*
- Premarital sexual activity
- Use of contraceptives

Sample Nursing Diagnostic Process for Altered Sexuality Patterns

ASSESSMENT ACTIVITIES	DEFINING CHARACTERISTICS	NURSING DIAGNOSIS
Observe readiness to discuss sex using verbalization (e.g., "When can I return to life as normal?" or "There goes my love life") or behavior (e.g., exhibitionism). Ask client and spouse about previous level and method of sexual expression (e.g., frequency, initiator). Observe for affectionate behavior (e.g., touching, hand holding, kissing). In privacy, ask spouse about perceptions of recovery and return to full functioning. Observe for anxiety (e.g., hand wringing).	Client verbalizes concern that sexual activity may cause another myocardial infarction or death. Client's spouse exhibits reluctance to touch client. Verbalizes concern that client will need continuous care, attention, and protection.	**Altered sexuality patterns** related to fear of recurrent myocardial infarction or death during intercourse

pertain to sexual problems, the client may experience additional problems resulting from sexual dysfunction. For example, altered body image may be a problem when a client is unable to perform sexually.

Based on the definition of sexuality, anything affecting physical, psychological, or emotional health or sociocultural or ethical attitudes and beliefs may have an impact on sexual functioning. These are areas for assessment, potential diagnosis of alterations or dysfunction, and intervention.

Planning

Goals for the client experiencing actual or potential alterations in sexual functioning include the following:

1. Obtains knowledge of sexual development and functioning of women and men
2. Attains or maintains biologically and emotionally healthy sexual practices
3. Establishes or maintains sexual satisfaction for self and partner if appropriate
4. Attains, maintains, or enhances positive self-esteem with integration of cultural, religious, and ethical beliefs; past and present sexual practices; and situational realities
5. Regains, maintains, or attains sexual functions sufficient to relieve anxiety

When planning interventions appropriate to the client's needs, the nurse must choose the appropriate diagnosis. Referrals may be necessary to physicians such as gynecologists or urologists for physical impediments to sexual functioning (e.g., severe pelvic discomfort with intercourse or inability to obtain an erection). Sexual conflict in a marriage or trauma over past sexual assault or incest requires intensive treatment with mental health professionals or a sex therapist.

When planning interventions, the nurse should involve the client and, with permission, the sex partner. The client must wish to achieve the goals. Because of the interpersonal nature of sexuality, goals must be regularly reevaluated to determine whether they remain realistic and of mutual interest.

Any plan should include referrals to resources to promote achievement of goals after contact with the health care provider is discontinued. Many community resource groups exist for self-help or peer support. The client experiencing diabetes, respiratory problems, cancer, and other physical problems may benefit from interaction with individuals with the same problem. They can share concerns and successes related to all aspects of coping with the disease, including sexual consequences. Self-help centers support women who experience abuse. Parents Without Partners and single adult groups appropriately deal with issues of sexuality such as STDs. Groups for older adults or community residents may be a source of help in confirming continuing sexual needs, issues of limited male partners, and raising concerns of safe sex for those again beginning sexual contact after widowhood. All plans should consider this type of community follow-up.

After a diagnosis is established and goals are set, expected outcomes should be established to serve as guides during the course of care. For example, the nurse hoping to help a client achieve sexual satisfaction in light of diabetic vascular changes will need to identify steps to indicate progress. Outcomes such as discussion between client and spouse regarding satisfying behavior, satisfaction expressed after nonintercourse stimulation, and verbalization of possible delay in excitement or orgasm resulting from vascular changes indicate that interventions are proceeding as planned. When outcomes are not met by established dates, the nurse must evaluate interventions and goals to determine where modifications are necessary.

A sample care plan is provided on p. 435. Expression and recognition of the values and preferences of both partners are critical to achieving successful interventions. Goals will not be achieved if recommended interventions fail to match the client's sexuality (i.e., gender identity, sex role, and partner preference).

Sample Nursing Care Plan for Altered Sexuality Patterns

NURSING DIAGNOSIS: **Altered sexuality patterns** related to fear of MI or death with intercourse
DEFINITION: Altered sexuality patterns is the state in which an individual expresses concern regarding his/her sexuality (Kim, McFarland, McLane, 1995).

GOALS	EXPECTED OUTCOMES	INTERVENTIONS	RATIONALE
Client and spouse will resume intimate expression of affection by 2 wk after myocardial infarction (MI).	Spouse will touch client by second visiting day. Client and spouse will progress to hand holding, hugging, or previous level of nonsexual affection by 2 wk.	Involve spouse in care; have spouse assist with bathing, shaving, and hair combing. Invite spouse to hug or kiss client goodbye. Schedule periods of ambulation to coincide with visiting hours.	Touch is basic form of communication and is basis of affection and sexual expression (Ebersole and Hess, 1994). Promoting intimacy while improving activity tolerance reinforces client's capacity (Seidel et al, 1991).
Client and spouse will regain positive adult level interaction by 5 wk.	Client and spouse will speak in terms of their abilities in positive gender-appropriate terms by 5 wk. Spouse will describe fears of loss and proceed to acceptance of necessary lifestyle changes for heart health by 3 wk.	Guide client in imagery exercise to visualize self as healthy and performing daily routines and sexual function. Refer to myocardial infarction support group for spouse and client. Discuss grief-adaptation process and allow privacy and permission to share fears and tears. Encourage weekly private opportunity for spouse to share concerns.	Client can verbalize fears and recognition that others experience same feelings. Support group provides contact with similar clients to provide evidence of progress.
Client will resume sexual relationship by 8 wk.	Client and spouse will experiment with sensate pleasure exercises by 5 wk. Client and spouse will express satisfaction of sexual activity by 8 wk.	Discuss alternative sexual expression (e.g., fondling, cuddling) as satisfying, not just as foreplay. Define realistic low-pressure expectation for gradual return to intercourse.	Spouse's stress, marital satisfaction, and sexual comfort influence recovery process of client (Beach et al, 1992). Sexual expression in continuum and sensate exercise provide low-stress, positive sexual experience and removes the pressure to perform (Seidel et al, 1991).

Implementation

The nurse's role includes the promotion of sexual health as a component of overall wellness. The nurse can promote sexual health by helping clients gain insight into their problems and explore methods to deal with them effectively.

HEALTH PROMOTION

Exploring and discussing values and levels of satisfaction and providing sex education require good communication skills. The environment and timing should be structured to provide privacy, uninterrupted time, and client comfort. For example, when discussing methods of contraception with a woman, the nurse provides comfortable chairs in an office rather than discussing this in the examination room when the client is only partially clothed.

Topics of education vary, depending on the defining characteristics and related factors (see the box on p. 436). Education may provide guidelines for normal development; for example, the nurse might talk to a toddler's mother regarding a new baby, a school-age child regarding appearance of pubic hair, or a 60-year-old man regarding delayed ejaculation. Details of physiological changes should be provided as a part of general health care. This also gives permission for clients to raise questions or concerns regarding personal functioning.

Discussions of healthy sex should always include contraception when talking with clients of childbearing age. Men should not be excluded from discussions of contraception.

CLIENT TEACHING for Resuming Sexual Activity After Myocardial Infarction

OBJECTIVE
- Client will identify factors related to activity intolerance and cardiovascular stressors during intercourse.

TEACHING STRATEGIES
- Provide privacy for client and spouse and sufficient time for uninterrupted discussion.
- Resume or initiate exercise and sex at a gradual rate.
- Discuss MET (metabolic equivalent) needs for sexual intercourse compared with other daily activities; excitement involves 3 to 4 METs and orgasm 4 to 5 METs, the equivalent of climbing 2 flights of stairs at a brisk rate.*
- Discuss evidence of activity tolerance:
  - Heart rate increase of less than 20 beats/min
  - Heart rate returning to baseline within 3 min
  - Blood pressure increase of less than 40 mm Hg systolic or 20 mm Hg diastolic
  - Lack of angina, dizziness, shortness of breath, tachycardia
  If during activities any of these appear, discontinue activity and call physician.
- Discuss environmental factors to decrease cardiovascular stress:
  - Room and bath/shower temperature: not too hot or cold
  - Refraining from food and alcohol for 3 hr before sexual activity
  - Use usual position during intercourse
  - Selection of a time of day when client feels rested (e.g., morning)
- Provide opportunity within next 3 days to follow up on teaching and answer questions.
- In private, inform client that sexual relations in new or extramarital relationship increase cardiac stress.

EVALUATION
- Client and spouse verbalize:
  - Evidence of activity tolerance
  - Signs and symptoms of intolerance
  - Methods to decrease environmental costressors
- If possible, follow up after discharge to evaluate satisfaction with sexual activity.

*Data from Seidel et al, 1991.

The discussion may include desire for children, usual sexual practices, and acceptable methods of contraception. Factors that need to be considered when educating clients about contraceptives include scheduling or frequency of sex, comfort with genital touching, and comfort with interruption of sexual acts. All methods of contraception should be reviewed to provide necessary information for an informed client choice. The best method is the one that the client will use consistently.

Individuals having more than one sex partner or whose partner has other sexual experiences need to learn more about safe-sex practices. As discussed earlier, information should be provided on STD transmission and symptoms, use of condoms, and risky sexual activities (e.g., trauma from penile-anal sex). Safe sex may also consider the client's emotional risks within a relationship. Role play may be a useful educational tool so that the client can learn to say *no* or negotiate with a partner to use a condom.

ACUTE CARE

Nursing interventions that address client alterations in sexual patterns or sexual dysfunction generally raise awareness, assist clarification of issues or concerns, and provide information. Nurses who have pursued specialized education in sexual functioning and counseling may provide more intensive sex therapy. Nurses should recognize when a client's needs exceed their expertise and provide appropriate referral. Most clients encountered in clinics or hospitals may benefit from the discussion and teaching provided by the nurse generalist.

The initial intervention often includes exploring present sexual practices with the client. The client should be encouraged to investigate and acknowledge social and ethical values and analyze the role of sexuality in self-concept. When there is significant discrepancy between values and past or present practices, the client may need referral for more intensive counseling.

Major developmental crises (e.g., puberty, climacteric, or menopause) should prompt education about effects on sexuality. Situational crises such as a life change with pregnancy, illness, extreme financial stress, placement of a spouse in a nursing home, or loss and grief affect sexuality. The effect may last for days, months, or years or may even generate performance anxieties that lead to continued sexual dysfunction. If a client is prepared for possible changes in sexual functioning, performance anxieties may be minimized. The client feels comfortable raising concerns about sexuality as they occur when a professional relationship has been established.

Illness and surgery are situational stressors. Clients may experience major physical changes, effects of drugs or treatments, and the emotional stress of prognosis, future functioning, and separation and hospitalization. Sexuality, as a component of personality, may be affected by all components of illness. The nurse should never assume that sexual functioning is not a concern merely because of an individual's age or severity of prognosis. After concerns are assessed and identified, they can be addressed in the context of the individual's value system.

In response to identified concerns the nurse may initiate discussion of methods of sexual stimulation, the sexual response cycle, or the use of creativity and fantasy in sexual relations. It may be appropriate to discuss sexual practices such as oral-genital sex or mutual masturbation as methods of expressing intimate affection when penile-vaginal intercourse is contraindicated. A partner experiencing joint pain may appreciate a discussion of various positions for intercourse. Use of fantasy or a sense of playfulness may add new romance or stimulation to a long-term relationship. A couple may need confirmation or assurance that the thoughts and acting out of nonharmful fantasy is normal and healthy.

RESTORATIVE CARE

When sexual dysfunctions are identified and pose lifestyle or health problems, the nurse should provide ap-

Sample Evaluation of Interventions for Altered Sexuality Patterns

GOALS	EVALUATIVE MEASURES	EXPECTED OUTCOMES
Client and spouse will resume intimate expression of affection 2 weeks after MI	Observe interaction between client and spouse.	Spouse will touch client. Client and spouse will progress in physical interaction.
Client and spouse will regain positive, adult-level interaction by week 5	Observe client's nonverbal behavior (e.g., use of personal clothing, personal toiletries, and grooming aids). Listen to client's description of self, abilities, discharge plans, and interactions with visitors. Observe for signs of cheerfulness, description of self in positive terms, talk of future plans, and independent actions.	Client will describe self in terms of abilities and in positive gender-appropriate terms.
	Ask spouse in privacy about feelings about myocardial infarction and lifestyle and role changes required.	Spouse will describe fears of loss and proceed to acceptance of life with necessary lifestyle changes for heart health.
Client will resume sexual relationship by week 8	Ask client and spouse about expression of intimacy and feelings related to these behaviors.	Client and spouse will experiment with sensate pleasure exercises.

propriate referrals such as counseling or evaluation by a gynecologist or genitourinary specialist. Clients may still require support to follow through with a referral and reinforcement of explanations of procedures, treatments, or exercises. To be effective with any intervention, the nurse must be comfortable with sexuality and aware of personal values and biases. Referral may also be necessary when a client's values or needs conflict with those of the nurse.

Evaluation

Individuals have a right to understand their body functions and to predict developmental changes. Clients should understand development of the body, the manner of male and female sexual response, and changes that normally occur with aging and life stresses. Illness results in challenges to many bodily functions, and sexuality should be addressed as one area of concern. The sample evaluation box (see the evaluation box above) shows the process of measuring actual versus expected outcomes.

Client or spouse verbalizations determine whether goals and outcomes have been achieved. Sexuality is felt more than observed, and sexual expression requires an intimacy not amenable to observation. Clients can be asked to verbalize concerns, share activities and satisfaction, and relate risk factors. The nurse can then observe for behavioral cues such as eye contact, posture, and extraneous hand movements that indicate comfort or suggest continued anxiety or concern. As outcomes are evaluated, the client, spouse, and nurse may need to modify expectations or establish more appropriate time frames to achieve the target goals. All people involved may need to be reminded of the individual nature of sexual expression and the multiple factors that affect perceptions and responses.

Sexual wellness is not an absolute. An individual must define what is acceptable and satisfying. The partner's level of sexual satisfaction must also be considered. Sexual performance is seldom the exclusive focus of sexual satisfaction. Open communication and positive self-esteem are essential factors in effectively resolving concerns.

▪ KEY CONCEPTS ▪

► Sexuality is related to all dimensions of health; therefore sexual concerns or problems should be addressed as a part of nursing care.

► Sexuality is a component of personality and includes biological sex, gender identity, gender role, and sexual partner preference.

► Attitudes toward sexuality vary widely and are influenced by religious beliefs, society's values, the media, the family, and other factors.

► Nurses' attitudes toward sexuality also vary and may differ from clients'; nurses should be sensitive to clients' sexual preferences and needs.

► The four-phase sexual response cycle is one way of understanding the physiological changes of sexual response during excitement, the plateau phase, orgasm, and resolution.

► Sexual development is a process beginning in infancy and involves some level of sexual behavior or growth in all developmental stages.

► The physiological sexual response changes with aging, but aging does not lead to diminished sexuality.

► Sexual health involves physical and psychosocial aspects and contributes to an individual's sense of self-worth and positive interpersonal relationships.

► Clients' problems involving sexuality include personal and emotional conflicts, the effects of illness on sexuality, and sexual dysfunction.

► Specific sexual dysfunctions result from psychological and physiological factors.

► Interventions for sexual dysfunctions depend on the condition and the client; interventions often include giving information, teaching specific exercises, and improving communication between partners.

► Concerns regarding acquired immunodeficiency syndrome and other sexually transmitted diseases should promote the use of condoms, but sexual transmission can be prevented only by abstinence.

► Choice and use of effective contraception methods are affected by sexual biases, comfort with touching genitalia, desire for future fertility, financial status, ability to plan sexual contact, and ability to communicate with sex partner regarding sensitive issues.

► A brief review of sexuality should be included in every nursing assessment of a client's level of wellness.

► Most nursing interventions to enhance a client's sexual health involve providing information and education.

► Evaluation is primarily determined through observation of client and partner expressions of satisfaction in meeting personal goals for sexual functioning.

▪ KEY TERMS ▪

Amenorrhea, p. 428
Bisexual, p. 412
Climacteric, p. 417
Coitus interruptus, p. 422
Condom, p. 423
Contraception, p. 421
Corpus luteum, p. 416
Diaphragm, p. 423
Dyspareunia, p. 429
Gay, p. 412
Gender identity, p. 412
Gender dysphoria, p. 412
Gender role, p. 412
Graafian follicle, p. 415
Heterosexual, p. 412
Homophobia, p. 412
Homosexual, p. 412
Lesbian, p. 412
Libido, p. 428
Menarche, p. 415
Menopause, p. 416
Menstrual cycle, p. 415
Myotonia, p. 420
Ovulation, p. 415
Premenstrual syndrome (PMS), p. 416
Secondary sex characteristics, p. 415
Sex, p. 410
Sexual dysfunction, p. 428
Sexual health, p. 410
Sexual orientation, p. 412
Sexual response cycle, p. 420
Sexuality, p. 410
Sexually transmitted diseases (STDs), p. 424
Sterilization, p. 423
Transsexuals, p. 412
Transvestite, p. 412
Tubal ligation, p. 423
Tumescence, p. 420
Vaginismus, p. 429
Vasectomy, p. 423
Vasocongestion, p. 420

■ CRITICAL THINKING EXERCISES ■

1. Suzie is an 18-year-old student. She has had one elective abortion as the result of an unplanned pregnancy. Her current relationship is with her third sexual partner, and she is seeking a "good type of birth control."

   a. What factors would you need to consider in order to help Suzie explore her contraceptive options?

   b. Suzie is at risk for developing sexually transmitted diseases. What assessment data support this conclusion?

   c. What would you teach Suzie about limiting her risk for STDs?

2. Mrs. Smith talks with you, an office nurse. She is 52 and has recently missed two menstrual periods. She is concerned also because her sexual response has lately been diminished. She appears depressed and shares that her youngest son has just left for college.

   a. What further assessment data would you collect before developing a response to Mrs. Smith's concerns?

   b. If she is menopausal, what would you counsel her to expect?

3. John is 22 years old. He is scheduled to have back surgery and expresses some concern over possible neurological injuries. He shares his concern about possible effects on sexual functioning because he is engaged to be married in 6 months. As you explore his concerns, John reveals that at 14 he had a sexual encounter with a man and carries feelings of guilt and fear that he may really be a latent homosexual.

   a. How would you respond to John's concerns?

   b. What assumptions are a part of your response?

REFERENCES

Alexander LL, LaRosa JH: *New dimensions in women's health,* Boston, 1994, Jones and Bartlett.

Bass M: Birth-control business, *The Women's Review of Books,* 11(10-11):19, 1994.

Beach EK et al: The spouse: a factor in recovery after acute myocardial infarction, *Heart & Lung* 21(1):30, 1992.

Boston Women's Health Book Collective: *The new our bodies, ourselves: a book by and for women,* New York, 1992, Simon & Schuster.

Brown RT, Cromer BA, Fischer R: Adolescent sexuality and issues in contraception, *Obstetric and Gynecologic Clinics of North America* 19(1):177, 1992.

Campbell JC: Women abuse and public policy: potential for nursing action, *AWHONN's Clinical Issues* 4(3):503, 1993.

Chodorow N: Family structure and feminine personality. In Rosalo M, Lamphere L, editors: *Women, culture and society,* Stanford, Calif, 1974, Stanford University.

Denney NW, Quadagno D: *Human sexuality,* ed 2, St Louis, 1992, Mosby.

Driscoll M et al: Women and HIV. In Dan A, editor: *Reframing women's health: multidisciplinary research and practice,* Thousand Oaks, Calif, 1994, Sage.

Ebersole P, Hess P: *Towards health aging: Human needs and nursing responses,* St Louis, 1994, Mosby.

Flick, LH: Paths to adolescent parenthood: implications for prevention, *Public Health Rep* 101(2):122, 1986.

Gilligan C: *In a different voice: psychological theory and women's development,* Cambridge, Mass, 1982, Harvard University.

Kim MJ, McFarland GK, McLane AM: *Pocket guide to nursing diagnosis,* ed 6, St Louis, 1995, Mosby.

Kolodny R, Masters W, Johnson V: *Textbook for sexual medicine,* Boston, 1979, Little, Brown.

Kopelman LM: Female circumcision/genital mutilation and ethical relativism, *Second Opinion* 20(2):55, 1994.

LeMone P: Human sexuality in adults with insulin-dependent diabetes mellitus, *Image* 25(2):101, 1993.

Lustig SL: The AIDS prevention magic show: avoiding the tragic with magic, *Public Health Reports* 109(2):162, 1994.

Mackey T et al: Factors associated with long-term depressive symptoms of sexual assault victims, *Archives of Psychiatric Nursing* 6(1):10, 1992.

Masters W, Johnson V: *Human sexual response,* Boston, 1966, Little, Brown.

Masters W, Johnson V, Kolodny R: *Human sexuality,* Boston, 1982, Little, Brown.

Mastroianni L, Robinson JC: Contraception in the 1990s, *Patient Care* 28(1):107, 1994.

Michael RT et al: *Sex in America: a definitive survey,* New York, 1994, Little, Brown.

Rosser SV: Gender bias in clinical research: the difference it makes. In Dan A, editor: *Reframing women's health: multidisciplinary research and practice,* Thousand Oaks, Calif, 1994, Sage.

Sanders HR, Nash E, Hoffman M: Women and health. In Lessing M, editor: *South African women today,* Cape Town, 1994, Maskew Miller Longman.

Seidel A et al: Understanding the effects of myocardial infarction on sexual functioning: a basis for sexual counselling, *Rehabilitation Nursing* 16(5):255, 1991.

Stotland N: Contraception and abortion: challenges now and for the next century. In Dan A, editor: *Reframing women's health: multidisciplinary research and practice,* Thousand Oaks, Calif, 1994, Sage.

Toubia N: Female circumcision as a public health issue, *New Eng J of Med* 331(11):712, 1994.

Warshaw C: Domestic violence: challenges to medical practice. In Dan A, editor: *Reframing women's health: multidisciplinary research and practice,* Thousand Oaks, Calif, 1994, Sage.

World Health Organization: Education and treatment in human sexuality: the training of health professionals, *WHO Tech Rep Ser 572,* Geneva, 1975, WHO.

Wyeth-Ayerst Laboratories and the Association of Women's Health, Obstetric, and Neonatal Nurses: *Issues in contraceptive method selection: contemporary studies in women's health,* Fair Lawn, NJ, 1994, MPE Communications.

Zawid CS: *Sexual health: a nurse's guide,* Albany, NY, 1994, Delmar.

ADDITIONAL READINGS

Billhorn DR: Sexuality and the chronically ill older adult, *Geriatric Nursing* 15:106, 1994.

Campbell JA: A review of nursing research on battering. In Sampselle CM, editor: *Violence against women: nursing research, education, and practice issues,* New York, 1992, Hemisphere.

Kaplan HS: A neglected issue: the sexual side effects of current treatments for breast cancer, *J of Sex and Marital Therapy* 18(1):3, 1992.

Lavee Y: Western and non western human sexuality: implications for clinical practice, *J of Sex and Marital Therapy* 17(3):203, 1991.

Lewis S, Bor R: Nurses' knowledge of and attitudes towards sexuality and the relationship of these with nursing practice, *J of Advanced Nursing* 20:251, 1994.

MacKinnon, CA: *Toward a feminist theory of the state,* Cambridge, Mass, 1989, Harvard University.

Smith LL, Lathrop LM: AIDS and human sexuality, *Canadian J of Public Health* 84(suppl 1):S14, 1993.

Taylor P: Beating the taboo . . . stoma and sexual difficulty, *Nursing Times* 90(13):51, 1994.

Vandevyer C: Homosexuals and AIDS: a new approach to the illness, *J of Homosexuality* 25(3):319, 1993.

Villeneuve MJ, Ozolins PH: Sexual counselling in the neuroscience setting: theory and practical tips for nurses, *Axone* 12(3):63, 1991.

Whitehead TL: Sexual health promotion of the patient with burns, *J of Burn Care Rehabilitation* 14:221, 1993.

Woods NF: Toward a holistic perspective of human sexuality: alterations in sexual health and nursing diagnosis, *Holistic Nurs Pract* 1(4):1, 1987.

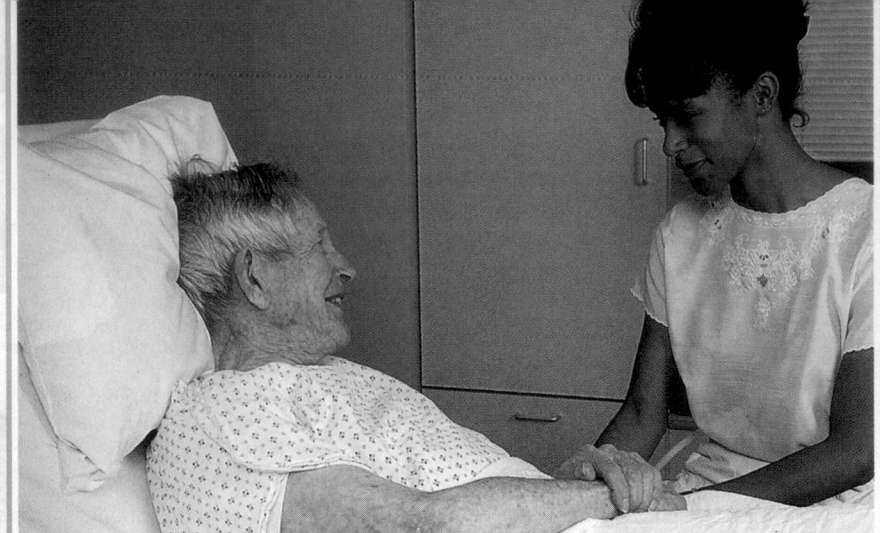

 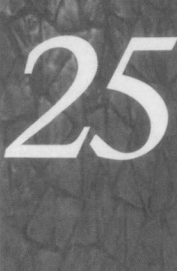

## Chapter 25

Spiritual Health

Objectives

Mastery of content in this chapter will enable the student to:

▶ Define the key terms listed.

▶ Compare and contrast the concepts of spirituality and religion.

▶ Discuss the relationship of the spiritual dimension to the totality of a person's being.

▶ Describe a spiritually healthy person.

▶ Explain the relationship of intuition to understanding a person's spirituality.

▶ Describe life experiences that may affect a client's spiritual health.

▶ Discuss the categories for spiritual assessment.

▶ Explain the importance of nurses being able to understand their own spiritual dimension before helping clients effectively understand theirs.

▶ Discuss nursing interventions designed to promote spiritual health.

▶ Evaluate attainment of spiritual health.

A value that shapes and influences our lives is that of wholeness and health. A person's health depends on a balance of physical, psychological, sociological, cultural, developmental, and spiritual variables. Nurses have traditionally approached health promotion through a holistic perspective. The basic assumption of holism is the belief that individuals cannot be broken down into component parts; the whole individual is greater than the sum of the parts (Mansen, 1993).

Spiritual well-being is an integrating aspect of human wholeness, characterized by meaning and hope (Clark et al, 1991). **Spirituality** gives a broad dimension to the holistic view of humanity. For nurses to give quality care, they must support clients as they identify and explore what is meaningful in their lives and as they find ways to adapt to the pain and suffering of illness. Nursing requires skills in spiritual care. Each nurse must have an understanding of spirituality and how spiritual beliefs influence every person's life.

SPIRITUALITY AND RELIGION

The need for meaning runs deep in each person. This deep need for meaning is connected to spirituality. Spirituality is hard to define. Words used to describe spirituality include *meaning, transcendent, hope, love, quality, relationship,* and *existence* (Emblen, 1992). Farran et al. (1989) suggest that the definition of spirituality, or the spiritual dimension, will be unique to each individual. Individuals' definitions of spirituality are influenced by their own culture, development, life experiences, and ideas about life. Perhaps the ambiguity in defining spirituality reveals its significance. Even though spirituality is difficult to define, there are two important characteristics of spirituality about which most authors agree: (1) It is a unifying theme in our lives and (2) It is a state of being. Farran et al. (1989) use a functional definition of spirituality—"an individual's ultimate commitment, most comprehensive principle of order, or final value that is the most powerful argument offered for the choices made in our lives."

Many nurses have had difficulty differentiating spirituality from **religion.** The two terms are frequently used interchangeably and certainly there is a relationship. A person may follow certain religious rituals or practices to express an aspect of spirituality. However, the two concepts are not the same. Religion is commonly associated with the "state of doing" or a specific unified system of practices associated with a particular denomination or form of worship. Emblen (1992) defines religion as a system of organized beliefs and worship that a person practices to outwardly demonstrate his or her spirituality. Religion serves different purposes in people's lives. For some, religion is a set of rules and rituals to worship a supreme being. For others, religion is a way of life providing profound nourishment and a connectedness to all of life. Organized religion can provide a framework for understanding the meaning of existance and a structure for worship. However, not all people recognize or participate in an organized religion. For example, a person claiming to be agnostic believes that it is *impossible for a person to know if God or any supreme being exists.* People who do not see themselves as connected to a religion may still feel very spiritually fulfilled.

One of the problems of interchanging spirituality and religion is that the nurse may merge the spiritual dimension with the psychosocial dimension. This can result in the nurse being unable to recognize spiritual hopes, needs, or problems that are masked by a person's emotions (Stoll, 1979). A nurse might diagnose a client's needs as being psychosocial, when instead the needs are related to spiritual health or function. Equating spirituality with religion can diminish the holistic perspective of the client by limiting the nurse's view of this dynamic aspect of life. Also when the spiritual dimension is reduced to include only religion, interventions can become standardized and will not address a client's actual needs (Mansen, 1993).

A broad view of spirituality is essential for nurses to make a more meaningful contribution to a person's overall well-being. It is important to recognize myths and fears. Nurses often hesitate to discuss spiritual concerns of clients because they believe it is inappropriate for them to share their own philosophical or spiritual beliefs with clients who may have debilitating symptoms (Peterson and Nelson, 1987). This hesitancy to discuss spirituality prevents the nurse from understanding the client's spiritual needs. For example, merely assessing a client's religious practices will not give the nurse the information needed to understand the set of beliefs a person applies for dealing with an illness.

A key to successfully providing spiritual care and support is gaining an understanding of one's own spiritual dimension. This requires a certain level of maturity and the ability to be nonjudgmental when another's beliefs differ form those of the nurse. It also requires recognition of personal biases. Heliker (1992) urges each nurse to look beyond himself or herself and commit to others so as to share and recognize the other person's spiritual dimension.

The Spiritual Dimension

Traditionally, nursing's holistic model of health has included the following dimensions: physical, psychological, cultural, developmental, social, and spiritual. One model, or option, for viewing the spiritual dimension is an integrated one (Fig. 25-1). Each dimension relates to the other,

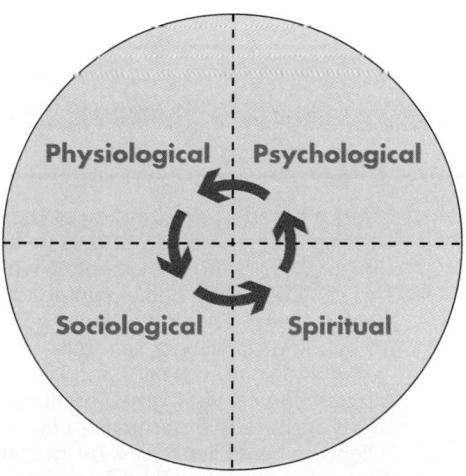

Fig. 25-1 The spiritual dimension: an integrated approach. *(Redrawn from Farran CJ et al: Development of a model for spiritual assessment and intervention,* J Religion Health *28(3):185, 1989.)*

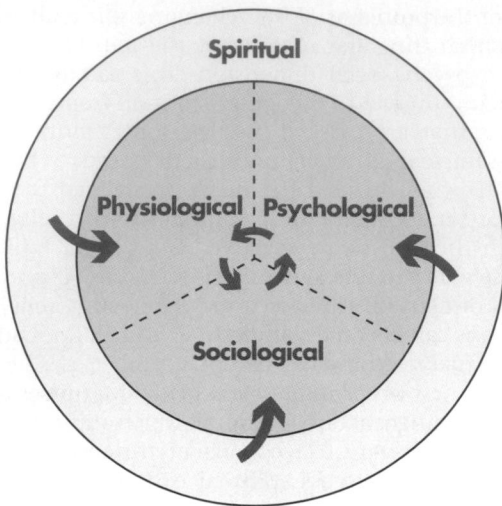

Fig. 25-2 The spiritual dimension: the unifying approach. *(Redrawn from Farran CJ et al: Development of a model for spiritual assessment and intervention,* J Religion Health *28(3):185, 1989.)*

while containing unique features or characteristics. An optional model that better demonstrates the significance of spirituality as an integrating theme in our lives is the unifying approach developed by Farran et al. (1989) (Fig. 25-2). In this model, spirituality represents the totality of one's being and serves as the overriding perspective that unifies the various aspects of the individual. Clark et al. (1991) stress how the spiritual dimension spreads throughout all other dimensions, whether or not a person acknowledges or develops it. Persons are energized through their "spirit," resulting in movement toward wellness. The influence of spirituality is particularly important during times of illness. When illness, loss, or pain affects a person, energy is depleted, and one's spirit is affected. How this influences a person's motivation to get well, participation in recovery, and ability to change is often underestimated.

Farran et al. (1989) have further defined their unifying

model for spirituality by summarizing various theoretical views of spirituality. These views help form a comprehensive approach for assessment and intervention in situations where clients need spiritual support. Each theoretical view helps the nurse better understand the spiritual dimension (Table 25-1). In addition, the unifying model includes a developmental aspect of spirituality. Spiritual growth likely occurs across the life span (Farran et al, 1989). Individuals reach different stages of spiritual development, depending on their individual characteristics and interpretations of life experiences and questions. This concept of spiritual development is important in understanding a client's spirituality and how the nurse's spiritual maturity affects his or her ability to initially meet clients, form relationships, and then assist clients with their health care needs.

Critical Thinking and Spirituality

Benner (1984) has described the helping role as an important domain of nursing practice. Clients look to nurses for a different kind of help than that sought from other professionals. Expert nurses acquire the unique ability to know the personal issues affecting clients' abilities to receive and seek help. The expert nurse embraces a holistic philosophy and caring that enables him or her to offer a level of comfort and support that is often intuitive.

Young (1987) defines clinical intuition as a process whereby the nurse knows something about a client that cannot be verbalized, is verbalized with difficulty, or for which a source of knowledge is not known. Intuition is an aspect of critical thinking (Chapter 6), which involves analyzing and sensing different cues, memories, and feelings to help the nurse have a better awareness of a client's needs. To be effective in offering spiritual care, nurses must learn the spiritual cues that clients exhibit during times of recovery, change, illness and loss. Intuition sometimes occurs without concrete information about a client. It is knowledge about the essence of something (Rew, 1989). Benner's description of the healing relationship between nurse and client is based in part on a nurse's intuitive abilities. The healing relationship happens when nurses have hope for

Table 25-1	Theoretical Views of Spirituality
THEORY	**APPLICATION TO NURSING**
Philosophy	Offers a broad understanding of the spiritual dimension. From a philosophical view, nurses can examine the essence, origin, nature, and value of a person's spiritual beliefs. Philosophy helps one examine a person's beliefs for their logic and the extent to which spirituality is a way of life.
Theology	This view helps the nurse gain an understanding of a person's beliefs about the nature of God or acknowledged higher being. Theology shapes a person's beliefs about life and the meaning of these experiences.
Physiology	A physiological view of spirituality helps the nurse to understand the interactions that occur among the body, mind and spirit in health and illness.
Psychology	A psychological view gives the nurse an understanding of a person's mental processes, experiences, and emotions and the role spirituality plays in his or her expression. Nurses must reflect on what gives life meaning for clients, where clients look for guidance, and from what sources clients gain courage and hope.
Sociology	All persons are influenced by the society or groups in which they live. This views helps the nurse understand the importance an individual and group place on fellowship with persons who share similar beliefs. This view also reveals the importance and meaning that rituals and practices have for individuals and groups.

Modified from Farran CJ et al: Development of a Model for Spiritual Assessment and Intervention, *J Religion Health* 28(3):185, 1989.

themselves and their clients; find an acceptable understanding of their clients' needs; and assist clients in using social, emotional, and spiritual support (Benner, 1984). It is important that intuition not replace logical judgment. Making assumptions, for example, about a client's spiritual beliefs can be a mistake. If the nurse senses something about a client, the thought or idea should be confirmed so that the nurse is dealing with accurate information.

Rew (1989) describes a relationship between spirituality and intuition. Nurses' intuitive experiences happen when they feel especially close to a client or a client's family. Intuition comes from a sense of relatedness to the client. It is a sense of warmth or empathy from within. The ability of a nurse to use intuition is vital to expert care. Often it is intuition and the associated sense of caring that helps nurses and clients come together to make the right decisions about the client's care.

Spiritual Health

Spiritual health or well-being is a "sense of harmonious interconnectedness between the self and others, nature, and an ultimate being" (Hungelmann et al, 1985). It is achieved when a person finds a balance between his or her life values, goals, and belief systems and their relationship within themselves and with others. In times of stress, illness, recovery, or loss, a person may turn to older ways of responding or adjusting to a situation. Often these coping styles lie within the person's basic beliefs or values. These beliefs are often grounded in the person's spirituality. Throughout life an individual may grow more spiritual, becoming increasingly aware of the meaning, purpose, and values of life.

Spirituality begins as children learn about themselves and their relationships with others. Many adults experience spiritual growth by entering into lifelong relationships. An ability to care meaningfully for others and the self is evidence of a healthy spirituality. Older adults often turn to important relationships and the giving of themselves to others as spiritual tasks.

Establishing a connection with a supreme being, beings, or value is one way a person can develop spiritually. Children often begin with a concept of a supreme being or value as presented to them by their home or religious community. Adolescents often reconsider their childlike concept of a spiritual power and, in the search for identity, may either question practices and values or find the spiritual power as the motivation to seek a clearer meaning to life.

As people mature they often turn inward to enduring values and to a concept of a supreme being that has been sustaining and meaningful. A healthy spirituality in older people is one that gives peace and acceptance of the self and that is often based on a lifelong relationship with a supreme being. Illness and loss can threaten and challenge the spiritual developmental process.

Spiritual Problems

When illness, loss, grief or pain affects a person, spiritual strengths either help a person move to recovery or spiritual needs and concerns develop. During illness or loss, for example, individuals often become less able to care for themselves and are more dependent on others for care and support. **Spiritual distress** may develop as a person seeks to

find meaning in what is happening, which may result in the person feeling alone and isolated from others. Individuals may question their spiritual values, raising questions about their whole way of life, purpose for living, and source of meaning.

ACUTE ILLNESS

Sudden, unexpected illnesses, which pose both an immediate and a long-term threat to a client's life, health, and well-being, can create significant spiritual distress. For example, the 40-year-old man who has a heart attack, the 20-year-old who is a victim of a motor vehicle accident, or the 32-year-old woman with breast cancer all face crises that may threaten their spiritual health. The illness or injury can be seen as a form of punishment, with clients blaming themselves for poor health habits, failure to follow safety precautions, or avoiding routine health screenings. Conflicts can develop around a person's beliefs and the meaning of life. The individual may have difficulty seeing the future and can become immobilized by grief.

Anger is not uncommon, and clients may express it against God, their families, and/or themselves. The strength of a client's spirituality influences how he or she copes with sudden illness and how quickly he or she can move to recovery. Yim (1994) has developed a spiritual healing critical pathway for coronary artery bypass clients. The pathway is based on the spiritual dynamics that can maximize a client's recovery. Hope arising from intimacy with an ally or partner, the ability to speak about life values and gain meaning from illness, and finding purpose and worth to move forward and recover are components that influence movement on Yim's pathway.

CHRONIC ILLNESS

Persons with chronic illness often suffer debilitating symptoms that alter the ability to continue their normal lifestyles. Independence can be seriously threatened, causing fear, anxiety, and an overall dispiritedness (Fig. 25-3). Dependence on others for routine self-care measures can create a feeling of powerlessness and a perception of decreased inner strength. One may feel a loss of a sense of

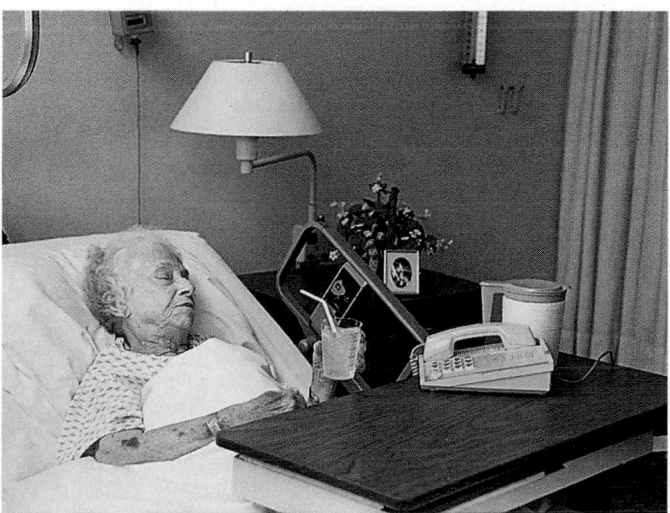

Fig. 25-3 Dispiritedness can affect one's adjustment to illness.

purpose in life that affects the inner strength needed to deal with alterations in functioning. The strength of a person's spirituality can be a significant factor in how a person adapts to the changes resulting from chronic illness. Successfully adapting to changes associated with chronic illness can strengthen a person spiritually. A reevaluation of life may occur. Those who are spiritually strong will reestablish a self-identity and live to their potential.

TERMINAL ILLNESS

Terminal illness commonly causes fears of physical pain, the unknown, dying, and the threat to integrity (Turner et al, 1995). Clients may have an uncertainty about what death means and thus be susceptible to spiritual distress. There are also clients who have a spiritual sense of peace that enables them to face death without fear.

Individuals experiencing a terminal illness will often find themselves reviewing their life and questioning its meaning. Common questions asked might include, "Why is this happening to me" or "What have I done?" Family and friends can be affected just as much as the client. Terminal illness causes members of the family to ask important questions about its meaning and how it will affect their relationship with the client (see Chapter 26).

Fryback (1992) conducted a study to learn how people with a terminal illness describe health (see the box below). Clients in the study identified the following three domains of health: mental-emotional, spiritual, and physical (Fig. 25-4). The spiritual domain was seen as being essential for health and included having a relationship with a higher power, recognizing one's mortality, and striving for self-actualization. Although many of the participants in the study either attended church or stated a desire to, others found spirituality was not dependent on a religion or church. They associated health with belief in a higher power that gave them faith and the ability to love (Fryback, 1992). The study revealed that when terminally ill clients have a perception of being unhealthy, it was not due to the disease but to being unable to live their lives fully and do the things they desired.

INDIVIDUATION

As persons live their lives, often the quest for finding and understanding the self as distinct yet also in relationship with others, occurs. Psychologist Carl Jung (Storr, 1983) describes this process as one of **individuation**. Also described as *midlife crisis*, individuation is common for individuals in middle age. It may be preceded by a sense of a vacuum in life or lack of ability to be self-motivated. Individuation is a common human experience characterized by confusion, conflict, despair, and a feeling of emptiness. One's spirituality needs to be sustained, since individuation seems to cause a person to fight the positive, life-asserting aspects of the personality. Events such as stress, success or lack of success in work, marital conflict, or loss of health can cause people to seek greater self-understanding.

▶ **RESEARCH HIGHLIGHT**

RESEARCH ABSTRACT

This study involved interviews with people with cancer and people with AIDS. The research question was "What is health?" as defined by people with potentially fatal diseases. Ten English-speaking white men and women were interviewed in-depth over a period of 60 to 90 minutes. The interviews were taped so that the researcher could code the concepts and themes revealed by the participants. Themes were combined into broader concepts, eventually revealing a framework for the data. The following three domains of health were defined: mental-emotional, spiritual, and physical. Each domain included main concepts and subconcepts for health (Fig. 25-4). The findings from the study support Newman's model of health, particularly the sense that disease was a part of the participant's health. When one's life becomes disorganized, the only way to achieve harmony or to expand one's consciousness is through sickness or disease. Facing disease caused the participants to rethink life's priorities and as a result, interpersonal relationships became more important.

IMPLICATIONS FOR PRACTICE

▶ Support a client's hope. This does not mean to deny pain, anger, or sadness. Clients will have short-term (e.g., relief of symptoms) and long-term goals (e.g., returning home or seeing a child get married), which the nurse must understand and foster.
▶ Help clients make their own decisions. Clients need to make informed choices about their care.
▶ Treat clients with respect.
▶ Learn about and value clients' spirituality and find a way for them to discuss their attitudes about life and death, the reason for their illness, and their life at the moment.

REFERENCE

Fryback PB: Health for people with a terminal diagnosis, *Nurs Sci* Q 6(3):147, 1992.

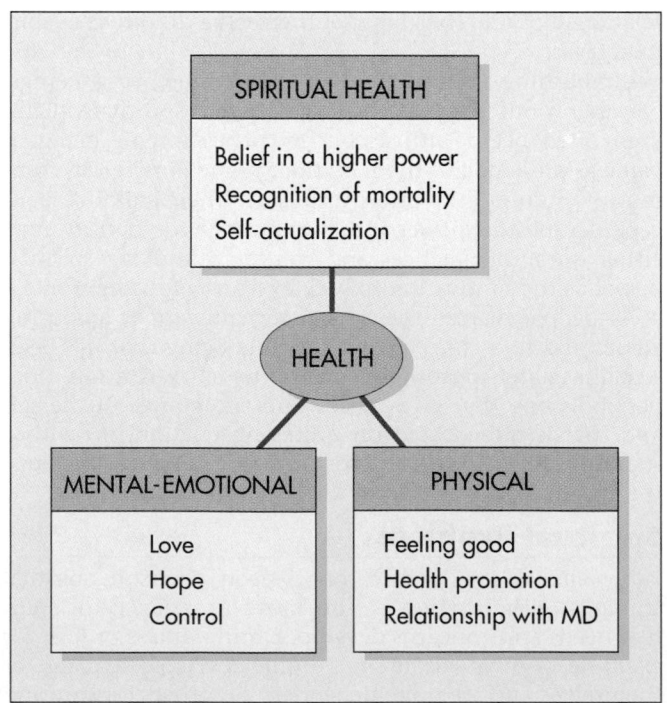

Fig. 25-4 Domains of health based on client perceptions.

NEAR-DEATH EXPERIENCE

Nurses may encounter clients who have had a **near-death experience (NDE).** A NDE has been identified as a psychological phenomenon of people who have either been close to clinical death or may have recovered after being declared dead. It is not associated with a mental disorder (Basford, 1990). Persons who experience a NDE after cardiopulmonary arrest, for example, often tell the same story of feeling themselves rising above their bodies and watching care givers initiate lifesaving measures. Most individuals describe passing through a tunnel to a bright light, encountering people who had preceded them in death, and feeling an inner tranquility and peace. Instead of moving toward the light, often they learn it is not time for them to die and they return to life.

Clients who have an NDE are often reluctant to discuss it, thinking family or care givers will not understand. Isolation and depression can occur as a result of not sharing the experience or experiencing others' judgment when they do share. However, individuals experiencing an NDE, and who can discuss it with family or care givers, find openness to the power of their experience as it is reported. They consistently report positive aftereffects, including a positive attitude, value changes, and spiritual development (Turner, 1995). After a client has survived cardiopulmonary arrest it is important for the nurse to remain open and give him or her a chance to explore what happened.

Religious Problems

A client's religious problems can influence his or her spirituality. Customary religious practices, if interrupted or changed, may affect the structure or support that religion contributed to the person's sense of well-being.

CHANGE IN DENOMINATIONAL MEMBERSHIP OR RELIGIOUS CONVERSION

Marrying a person with a different religious background or moving to a new community that does not have a branch of a particular religious group, will create loss for an individual. Of course, it can also open up new options. If a loss is felt, the individual experiences separation from a previously valued religious community (Turner et al, 1995). The extent of the loss will be influenced by the choice the individual had in the change and how flexible the person's religious expression of the spiritual self is.

INTENSIFICATION OF ADHERENCE TO BELIEFS

Turner et al. (1995) note that the voluntary intensification of religious practice may cause problems when a person either does not feel free or does not know how to talk about the religious aspects of the change. A person often intensifies religious practices to deal with guilt or to cope with a difficult trauma or loss. Becoming more deeply involved in religious practices or expressing one's beliefs more freely may be a way to find meaning in a distressing event or to exercise the person's spriritual development.

LOSS OR QUESTIONING OF FAITH

Faith is defined by Studzinski (1986) as more than a set of beliefs. It is a way of relating to one's self, one's community, and a higher power and a way of integrating our past, present, and future with a higher power at the center. A person often finds a way to express his or her faith through

religious practices. Faith develops over time, along with a person's spiritual growth. Persons who are at an early stage of development of their faith or find their faith challenged by a significant life event, may become vulnerable to loss of or doubt about their faith (Turner, 1995). This can occur when one is shunned by his or her religious community (e.g., a Jehovah's Witness who elects to have a heart transplant requiring a blood transfusion) or when one seriously questions the stand his or her religious denomination takes on an important public issue (e.g., abortion or euthanasia). A loss or questioning of faith can cause serious guilt and even a sense of loneliness.

■ NURSING PROCESS AND SPIRITUALITY

At the core of nursing is the commitment to caring. Care for others is an individualized, interactive process by which individuals help each other grow and become actualized (Clark et al, 1991). An element of quality health care is to exhibit caring for the client so that a relationship of trust forms. Trust is strengthened when the care giver acknowledges and supports the client's spiritual well being.

Application of the nursing process from the perspective of a client's spiritual needs is not simple. It goes far beyond just assessing a client's religious practices and rituals. Understanding a client's spirituality and then appropriately identifying the level of support and resources needed requires a new, broader perspective. Heliker (1992) describes this as the realm of shared community and compassion. *Compassion* comes from the Latin words *pati* and *cum,* meaning "to suffer with." Community is derived from the Latin word meaning "fellowship." To be compassionate is to "enter into places of pain, to share in brokenness with other human beings" (Heliker, 1992). To practice compassion as a nurse requires awareness of the tie between clients and a healing community. The nurse must remove from the assessment and plan any personal biases or misconceptions and learn to be available. This means the nurse has a willingness to share and discover another person's meaning and purpose in life, sickness, and health. A nurse learns to look beyond a personal view when establishing a client relationship. This means identifying the common values that make us human. Love, trust, hope, forgiveness, meaning, and community are spiritual needs we all have (Carson, 1989). Learning to share those needs or at least be aware of their commonality helps the nurse find a way to give clients spiritual care and support.

Another important aspect of spiritual care is recognizing that a client does not have to have a spiritual problem. Clients bring certain spiritual strengths that the nurse can use as resources to help them assume healthier lifestyles, recover from illness, or face a peaceful death. Nurses must learn to understand the positive aspects of a client's spirituality rather than thinking that in times of illnes spirituality will always be threatened. Supporting and recognizing the positive side of a client's spirituality will go a long way in delivering effective, individualized nursing care.

 ## Assessment

Clearly, a nurse's ability to gain a reliable picture of a client's spiritual dimension may be limited by the setting in which one practices. This is true if nurses have limited contact with clients or fail to build relationships. But once a trusting relationship is established, the nurse and client reach a point of learning together, and spiritual caring occurs. The question is not what kind of spiritual support can be given but how consciously is the nurse integrating spiritual care into the nursing process. Nurses must not use the excuse of "not enough time" to avoid recognizing the value spirituality holds for a client's health.

Farran et al. (1989) have developed a model for spiritual assessment that can provide a reliable picture of a client's spiritual dimension. The model is designed to reveal aspects of spirituality most likely to be influenced by life experiences, events, and questions in the event of illness and hospitalization. The assessment can reveal the opportunities nurses have in supporting or strengthening the client's spirituality. The assessment, itself, can be therapeutic because it conveys a level of caring and support. The nurse who understands the overall conceptual approach to spiritual assessment will be most successful. The essence of a person's spirituality is in the whole not just in the parts revealed through each assessment category.

Belief and Meaning

It can be important to learn about an individual's philosophy of life, his or her perspective of spirituality, and whether he or she views spirituality as a part of the whole being. Asking the client, "Can you tell me your philosophy of life," "Describe for me what is most important in your life," or "Tell me what it is that gives your life meaning or significance" may help to assess what gives the person's life meaning. This information can help a nurse to recognize the client's spiritual focus and the impact of illness or disability on that person's life. If a person's health (as defined by the client) is the most significant aspect of his or her life, obviously illness has tremendous implications. An understanding of belief and meaning reflects the spiritual resources the person brings in dealing with a stressful or traumatic event.

Fryback (1992) was able to better understand the spiritual domain by asking clients with AIDS or cancer to answer the question, "What is Health?" Beliefs about health can influence an individual's view of life and how he or she respond when illness occurs. Depending on a client's religious practices, views about health and the response to illness may influence how nurses and other care givers provide support (Table 25-2).

Authority and Guidance

Each individual has some source of authority and guidance in his or her life. It is that inner voice or outer authority that leads one to choose and act on his or her beliefs. The authority can be a supreme being, a specific religious leader, family or friends, oneself, or a combination of sources. An authority guides a person in exercising beliefs and experiencing growth. Knowing a person's source of authority and guidance can provide direction in interacting with the person. The nurse can assess a person's source of authority and guidance by asking a client, "What gives you your inner strength" or "To what or whom do you look to for guidance in life?"

Table 25-2	Religious Beliefs about Health	
RELIGION	HEALTH CARE BELIEFS	RESPONSE TO ILLNESS
Hinduism	Accepts modern medical science	Illness is caused by past sins Prolonging life is discouraged
Sikhism	Accepts modern medical science	Females to be examined by females Removing the undergarment will cause great distress
Buddhism	Accepts modern medical science	May refuse treatment on Holy Days Nonhuman spirits invading the body cause illness May want a Buddhist priest May permit withdrawal of life support Does not practice euthanasia
Shinto	Accepts modern medical treatments along with ancient traditions	Will not allow treatments that "appear" to injure the body
Islam	Must be able to practice the Five Pillars of Islam (see p. 447) May have a fatalistic view of health	Uses faith healing Family members are a comfort Group prayer is strengthening May permit withdrawal of life support Does not practice euthanasia
Judaism	Believes in the sanctity of life God and medicine must have a balance Observance of the Sabbath is important May refuse treatments on the Sabbath	Visiting the sick is an obligation They are obligated to seek care Euthanasia is forbidden Life supports are discouraged
Christianity	Accepts modern medical science	Uses prayer, faith healing Appreciates visits from clergy Some will use laying on of hands Holy Communion is commonly used

It is also important to learn if there is a religious source for guidance that conflicts with medical treatments. This can significantly affect the options nurses and other health care providers give to clients. For example, if a client looks to the Jehovah's Witnesses as a source of authority, blood products cannot be accepted as a form of treatment. Christian scientists and older members of the Church of the Nazarene may also refuse blood transfusions. Frequently, clients who embrace the beliefs of Christian Scientist refuse medical intervention, believing that their faith will heal them. Refusal of treatment may extend even to acceptance of vaccines.

Experience and Emotion

Farran et al. (1989) recommend spiritual assessment to include a review of a person's history with and capacity for religious experiences and whether the experiences have been sudden or gradual. Near death experiences, perceptions of being with a spiritual power, or psychic events, can create powerful feelings. The nurse may ask, "Have you ever had a religious or spiritual experience that made a difference in how you live your life?" The nurse explores the emotions or moods such as joy, peace, anger, hope, guilt, or shame that are associated with the religious experiences. The information can reveal the significance spirituality holds and whether feelings are incorporated into or rejected by the client's beliefs. If they are incorporated into a person's beliefs, access to those experiences can become tools in recovery.

Another important area of assessment is the impact current illness or hospitalization has upon religious experiences and emotion. A nurse might ask, "Is there something that threatens your spirituality as a result of your illness?" or "Has there been a change in those emotions or feelings you associate with your spirituality?" This may help a client discuss any inner conflicts or reveal if their relationship with a higher being or sense of meaning has changed.

Fellowship and Community

Fellowship is the relationship an individual has with other persons (Farran et al, 1989), including the client's immediate family, close personal friends, associates at work or school, fellow members of a church or community society, and neighbors. More specifically, this includes the extensiveness of the community of shared faith between clients and their support networks. A community of shared faith can create a strong bond. When a client knows that others of similar faith care, they become a source for hope. Hope is related to trust and a sense of presence (Clark et al, 1991).

The nurse's holistic assessment explores the extensiveness of a person's support networks and their relationship with the client. Does the client have one significant fellowship or several? What is the level of support received from this community? How does the community express feelings of concern and fellowship? Do they visit, say prayers, support the client's immediate family members? The nurse wants to learn whether openness exists between the client and those persons with whom he or she has formed a fellowship. Can the client express needs to those persons that are most likely to offer support and caring, and does the client perceive their support?

Ritual and Practice

The most common criteria nurses assess for spirituality are customary religious rituals and practices. Rituals include participation in group or private worship, prayer (Fig. 25-5), sacraments such as baptism or communion, singing, icons, use of a rosary, meditating, scripture reading, and making offerings or sacrifices. Different religions have established various rituals for certain life events (Table 25-3). The nurse examines whether a client's usual rituals or practices have been interrupted as a result of illness or hospitalization. A ritual can provide a client with structure and support during difficult times. Does this continue to be true, or are changes needed as a result of illness? Clients may also have requests for particular rituals. For example, Muslims practice the "Five Pillars of Islam" (see the box below) with the second pillar requiring a person to pray five times a day, facing east

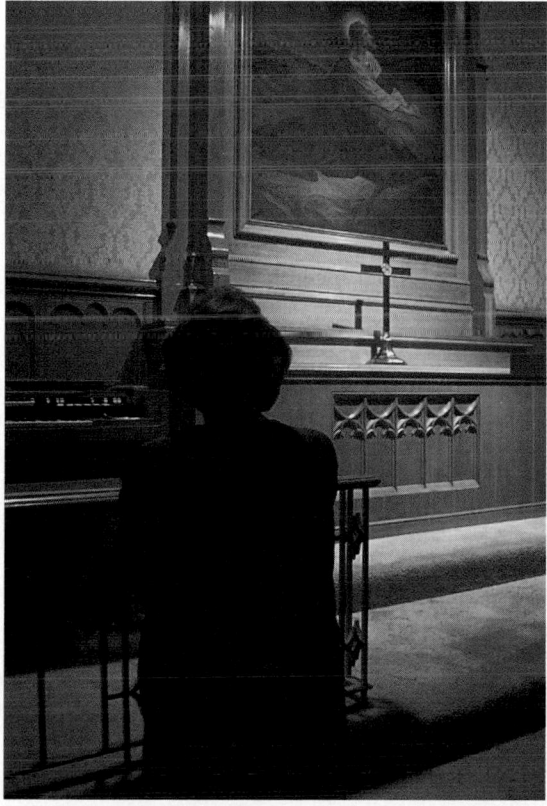

Fig. 25-5 Prayer offers an inner sense of calm.

Five Pillars of Islam

1. There is no god but God (Allah, the one GOD).
2. The formal prayer *(Salat)* is done five times per day; dawn, noon, midafternoon, sunset, and evening. The prayer is to be done facing east, toward Mecca.
3. To help the poor, through tax or charity.
4. To fast from dawn until sunset each day during the months of Ramadan, following the lunar calendar (usually June and July).
5. *Hajj,* or a pilgrimage, to Mecca, which must be made once in a lifetime, unless health or poverty precludes it.

Table 25-3	Religious Practices Related to Birth and Death	
RELIGION	**BIRTH RITUALS**	**DEATH RITUALS**
Hinduism	No special rituals	The dying may want to lie on the floor A priest will tie a thread around the neck or wrist *(do not remove)* A priest will pour water in the client's mouth Family will wash the body before cremation
Sikhism	Allow mother and child to remain together	The deceased will need the five Ks: *Kesh,* uncut hair; *Kangra,* wooden comb; *Kara,* wrist band; *Kirpan,* sword; *Kach,* shorts
Buddhism	No special rituals Baptism later in childhood	A priest should be called Last rites and chanting at bedside Burial or cremation is acceptable
Shinto	No special rituals	All jewelry should be removed, and the body is washed and dressed in a white kimono and straw shoes
Islam	A prayer is said into the infant's ear	The dying must confess their sins The body is washed and wrapped in white cloth The head is turned toward right shoulder The body faces east, toward Mecca A prayer called *Kalima* is said
Judaism	Circumcision on day 8 for Orthodox and Conservative Jews	Body is washed by burial society and someone needs to remain with the body for Orthodox and Conservative Jews
Christianity	Rituals vary Many will baptize	Rituals vary greatly among groups Many give last rites or Communion Prefers burial to cremation
Church of Jesus Christ of Latter-Day Saints (Mormon)	Baptism by immersion	Many give last rites or Communion Prefers burial to cremation

(toward Mecca, their holy city). Islamic clients may wish to incorporate their prayer ritual into the health care routine. When the death of a client is near, it is very important to know if religious practices need to be arranged to ensure peace of mind for the client and his or her family.

Courage and Growth

Farran et al. (1989) recommend an assessment of sources that have provided a sense of courage (hope) in the past for the client. The assessment includes reviewing whether the client can let old beliefs die in the hope that other beliefs will emerge. This is important since loss of hope can cause dispiritedness. For instance, a person's physical ability to remain independent and functional may be the source of courage or hope to face any difficulties. If illness makes a person more dependent, can a new source of hope emerge? For example, one option would be to learn what sense of identity or meaning in life was served by the client's autonomy. Autonomy could be realized through the client's ability to make decisions rather than dependence on physical integrity.

Hope has been identified as an essential component of health by clients with AIDS or cancer (Fryback, 1992). Hope motivates a person to achieve. It is future oriented and a state of anticipation of continued good. The common elements of hope include a future, action toward the future, and positive outcomes (Fryback, 1992). Even in the face of terminal illness, hope is important for a person to face the challenges in life.

Vocation and Consequences

Individuals express their spirituality on a daily basis in life routine, work, relationships, and other areas. It can be their vocation in life and part of their identity. The nurse tries to determine if illness or hospitalization has altered the person's ability to express his or her spirituality. Expressing one's spirituality is different than practicing rituals. Expression of spirituality includes showing an appreciation for life in the variety of things people do, living in the moment and not worrying about tomorrow, appreciating nature, and expressing love toward other individuals. The nurse assesses whether, in the face of illness, the client loses the ability to express a sense of relatedness to something greater than the self (Fryback, 1992). If illness is seen as a sacrifice or threat and prevents one from exercising his or her vocation, what are the implications psychologically, socially, and spiritually?

 ## Nursing Diagnosis

When reviewing a spiritual assessment and integrating the information into appropriate nursing diagnoses, the nurse should consider the client's current health status from a holistic perspective, with spirituality as the unifying principle. Nurses will encounter clients in a variety of settings and during times of health and illness. During events such as birth, illness, pain, suffering, daily life activities, and death, persons have experiences that create options. Life options are interrelated with a person's spirituality (Farran

Sample Nursing Diagnostic Process for Health Needs Related to Spirituality

ASSESSMENT ACTIVITIES	DEFINING CHARACTERISTICS	NURSING DIAGNOSES
Ask client to describe what gives meaning to life Ask how client feels about his or her illness Determine if illness has changed how client follows religious rituals	Expresses concern with meaning of life as a result of terminal illness Client states, "God is punishing me." Cries when asked about illness Reports that he or she prays more often but does not feel that God is forgiving	**Spiritual distress** related to challenged beliefs from suffering
Ask client to describe who makes up her support system Has their response to the client changed since the loss? Determine if client has had any physical symptoms following loss Ask client what the meaning of loss has to her view of life	Client reports a close relationship with spouse and younger sister The sister has been unable to provide comfort; grief has caused her to avoid client Husband is sole source of support Client has insomnia and loss of appetite Loss of her child is viewed as being unfair; she no longer can find meaning in her life	**Coping, ineffective individual** related to feelings of loss after death of child

et al, 1989). Some of the options lead to expanded functioning (increased understanding of life or an expansion of life's meaning). Other options result in the maintenance of one's spiritual development and practical understanding of spirituality. Finally, there are options that lead to altered functioning such as the inability to find meaning in life events, broken fellowship, and loss of hope. To support clients the nurse needs to focus not only on the alterations in functioning, but also on the options that provide strength, hope, and encouragement during times of illness.

A relatively new nursing diagnosis, *spiritual well-being, potential for enhanced,* is based on defining characteristics that show a pattern of well-being and the interconnectedness that comes from inner strengths (Kim et al, 1995). When the nurse's assessment reveals that the client has inner hope and faith, believes in a higher power, has a defined purpose and meaning in life, and expresses a harmony with self and others, spiritual well-being is a likely diagnosis. The presence of this state of being shows the client has resources to draw on when faced with other nursing diagnoses such as chronic pain, decreased cardiac output, sensory/perceptual alterations, or body image disturbance.

As a nurse identifies the diagnoses that apply to clients, it is important to recognize the significance that spirituality has for all types of health problems. Almost any nursing diagnosis has implications for a client's spirituality. Pain, anxiety, fear, impaired mobility, and self-care deficit are just examples of fairly common nursing diagnoses that will require the nurse to incorporate spiritual care principles.

There may be situations in which the nurse will gather defining characteristics from the assessment database and find patterns that reflect a client's dispiritedness (see the diagnostic process box above). Critical thinking requires a review of concrete data (e.g., religious practices and sources of fellowship) as well as an assessment of previous client experiences, the nurse's own spiritual consciousness, and the intuitive sense of the client's spiritual strengths. Defining characteristics must be validated and clarified with the

Examples of NANDA Nursing Diagnoses for Spirituality

Spiritual well-being, potential for enhanced *related to:*
- Recovery from acute illness
- Near-death experience
- Coping with chronic illness

Spiritual distress *related to:*
- Value conflict
- Isolation by others
- Fear resulting from diagnosis of AIDS
- Separation from religious denomination

Coping, ineffective individual *related to:*
- Lack of support system
- Individuation
- Symptoms of chronic illness

Anxiety *related to:*
- Threat of death
- Change in health status

Hopelessness *related to:*
- Loss of belief in God
- Abandonment by family

Self-esteem disturbance *related to:*
- Drug addiction
- Loss of independence

Modified from Kim MJ, McFarland GK, McLane AM: *Pocket guide to nursing diagnoses,* ed 6, St. Louis, 1995, Mosby.

client before a plan of care is made. With spiritual care, the importance of the nurse's own spiritual aspirations, inspiration, and perception cannot be overemphasized. The nurse avoids imposing his or her personal beliefs on the client. Each diagnosis must have an accurate related factor so that resulting interventions can be purposeful and direct (see the nursing diagnoses box on p. 449).

Planning

When the nurse and client identify that a client has spiritual needs, it is important for both to collaborate closely on a plan of care. Compassion and caring must clearly be communicated between the nurse and client. This can begin with a well-designed assessment, but the nurse-client relationship must continue to be based on caring and trust for interventions to be effective. Communication will be an integrated theme for whatever nursing interventions are chosen. The personal nature of spirituality requires the client to be able to speak openly with the nurse and recognize the nurse's interest in his or her needs.

Significant others, such as spouses, siblings, parents, and friends, need to be involved, as appropriate, to lend support. This means that the nurse learns from the assessment what individuals or groups have formed a relationship with the client. These individuals may become involved in all levels of the nurse's plan. The client's support network may assist in giving physical care, providing emotional comfort, and sharing spiritual support.

If the client participates in a formal religion, members of the clergy or members of the church, temple, mosque, or synagogue may need to be involved in the plan of care. De-

Sample Nursing Care Plan for Spiritual Well-Being

NURSING DIAGNOSIS: **Spiritual well-being, potential for enhanced** related to renewed appreciation of life following terminal illness diagnosis.

DEFINITION: The process of an individual's developing or unfolding of mystery through harmonious interconnectedness that springs from inner strengths (Kim et al, 1995).

GOALS	EXPECTED OUTCOMES	INTERVENTIONS	RATIONALE
Client will renew relationships with family members in 1 month.	Client will dedicate the evening hours, 5 days during the week, to build relationship with husband and children (to be met in 2 weeks).	Have client modify evening schedule 5 days during the week to provide time to build relationship with family. Have client use story telling to reminisce with family about family experience that was positive and enlightening.	Scheduling quality time with family gives individual opportunity to help family see individual's need for renewing relationship. Story telling allows a pattern to emerge that describes client's way of life filled with meaning. Helps family understand one another's needs (Heliker, 1992).
	Client will be able to express openly with family her love and appreciation for each of them (to be met in 1 month).	Have client discuss with family the meaning life now has for her, following a diagnosis of breast cancer. Encourage client to discuss how illness has changed her need to show the love she holds for her family.	Situations seen from the individual's point of view will enhance understanding and sensitivity on the part of the family. Clients facing terminal illness find that loving others and letting other people love them is a part of health (Fryback, 1992).
Client will gain greater self-awareness.	Client is able to set goals for her life (to be met in 1 month).	During clinic visit, have client discuss the meaning health has in her life and the implications of illness. Use discussion to help client find new avenues to the known meaning in her life.	Gaining greater self-awareness involves having an awareness of self, living up to one's potential, and finding meaning in life (Fryback, 1992). Gaining an awareness of the meaning of one's illness and learning how to move forward enables one to reset priorities and achieve better self-awareness.
		Use listening skills and direct questions to allow time for a reflection of how illness has influenced client's values and philosophy of life.	Listening allows one to enter into another person's frame of reference, see his or her view of the world, and develop an empathic relationship with him or her (Burnard, 1987).
		Have client establish realistic goals that maximize her potential and that involve family members.	Attempts to achieve understanding and acceptance of one's diagnosis often causes terminally ill clients to reestablish goals that foster interpersonal relationships (Fryback, 1992).

pending on the client's health status and needs, part of the plan will involve a continuation of appropriate religious rituals. The nurse must make sure that any icons or religious materials such as a Bible or prayer book be made available (see the care plan on p. 450).

In establishing a plan of care, there are three goals for spiritual caregiving (Munley, 1983):

1. The client will sense a feeling of trust in care givers.
2. The client will be able to bond with members of a support system.
3. The client's personal quest for meaning will be enhanced.

 ## Implementation

If a client experiences spiritual distress or has a health problem that causes dispiritedness, loneliness can occur. A client can feel isolated from the people that normally offer support. Regardless of the variety of interventions a nurse might choose for the client, a compassionate and understanding relationship is very important. Both the client and nurse must feel free to let go and discover together the meaning illness poses for the client and the impact it has on the meaning and purpose of life. Achieving this level of understanding with a client enables the nurse to deliver care in a sensitive, creative, and appropriate manner.

Establishing Presence

Clients have reported that the presence of nurses and their caregiving activities contributes to a sense of well-being and provides hope for recovery (Clark et al, 1991). Specific caregiving behaviors that established the nurse's presence included giving attention, answering questions, and having a positive and encouraging (but realistic) attitude. The ability to establish presence is part of the art of nursing. It is not simply performing procedures in rapid-fire fashion or sharing technical information with a client that may not be meaningful. Benner (1984) clarifies that presencing involves "being with" a client versus "doing for" a client. Presencing is being able to offer a closeness with the client, physically, psychologically, and spiritually.

A nurse can convey a caring presence in a variety of subtle ways: providing a backrub with a soothing, gentle touch; carefully repositioning a client without eliciting pain; gently administering mouth care; and working with a client to slowly and cautiously move from the bedside to a chair. Providing a soothing and supportive touch, displaying self-confidence, and taking time with a client as therapies are administered help establish presence. The client who is ill experiences a loss of control and looks for someone to offer direction and competent care. The nurse's artful use of hands, encouraging words of support, and calm and decisive approach establishes a presence that builds trust and well-being.

Trust is fundamental to any relationship. The attitude a nurse conveys when entering a client's room sets the tone for interaction. The nurse must prove that he or she is reliable and dependable. Careful attention to any client request, no matter how trivial, is important to clients. Demonstrating presence, showing a caring attitude, and performing competently communicates to the client the trust needed for a strong nurse-client relationship.

Supporting a Healing Relationship

An expert nurse learns to look beyond isolated client problems and recognizes the broader picture of a client's needs. This is applying a holistic view toward a client's health problems. For example, the nurse does not simply look at a client's back pain as a problem to solve with quick remedies, but rather how the pain influences the client's ability to function and achieve goals established in life. A holistic view enables the nurse to establish a helping role, described by Benner (1984) as one of the domains of nursing practice. A competency that nurse's acquire within the helping domain is learning to establish a healing relationship.

Benner (1984) defines three steps that are evident when a healing relationship develops between nurse and client:

1. Mobilizing hope for the nurse as well as for the client
2. Finding an acceptable interpretation or understanding of the illness, pain, fear, anxiety, or other stressful emotion
3. Assisting the client to use social, emotional, or spiritual support

Central to a healing relationship is mobilizing the client's hope. Hope is a motivator to arm people with the strategies needed to face any challenges in life. The nurse can help a client find things to hope for. A terminally ill client may hope to attend a daughter's graduation or to live each day to the fullest. A client who has undergone abdominal surgery for a bowel obstruction may hope for pain relief and a quick return to home.

Hope has both short- and long-term implications in a client's care. It is future oriented and helps a client work toward recovery. To help clients achieve hope, the nurse and client work together to find an interpretation of the situation that is acceptable to both. Then the nurse helps the client use the resources available to him or her. This might include a client's positive attitude toward life, a desire to be informed and make decisions, or a willingness to try different therapies. For example, the client with abdominal pain may be able to accept the fact that the pain will likely be short term because of the healing process. If the client is normally one who is independent and feels a need to be in control, the nurse offers several therapeutic options for pain management and has the client make informed choices.

To further support a healing relationship the nurse must remain aware of the client's spiritual strengths and needs. It always remains important for a client to be able to express and exercise his or her beliefs. Nurses who respect a client's faith and recognize the influence spirituality has on his or her recovery are perceived by clients as a source for hope (Clark et al, 1991). When illness or treatments create confusion or uncertainty for the client, the nurse must recognize the possible effect this can have on a client's well-being. What spiritual resources can be strengthened? The nurse may begin by first learning what the client wants to know and then providing the best information to relieve the client's uncertainties. The client may also require the presence of family or friends to maintain the fellowship that is needed for recovery.

Support Systems

In a study involving Jewish and Christian clients, Clark et al. (1991) learned that support systems provided them with the greatest sense of well-being during hospitalization. Support systems serve as a human link connecting the client, the nurse, and the client's lifestyle before the illness. Part of the client's caregiving environment is the regular presence of those family and friends viewed by the client as supportive. The nurse plans care with the client and the client's support network to promote the interpersonal bonding that is critical for recovery. The support system often provides the source of faith that renews the client's spiritual being. Family and friends may also become important resources in conducting the customary religious rituals on which a client relies.

After assessing the function family and friends play in a client's life, the nurse can encourage them to visit the client regularly. If family and friends are found to be a spiritual resource to a client, they can be an excellent source of therapy. The nurse's encouragment to family to be themselves can facilitate the family's ability to provide the spiritual comfort that they are capable of sharing. Often illness and the treatment environment create so many unknowns that family and friends become intimidated. The nurse can be very effective in helping the family feel welcome and know that their support and presence is an important part of the client's healing. Including family members in a prayer service is a thoughtful gesture if this is appropriate to the client's religion, and family members are comfortable participating. Encouraging the family to bring meaningful religious symbols can be a source of consolation and spiritual support.

Another important resource to clients are spiritual advisors and members of the clergy. The nurse should ask clients if they would like to have their spiritual advisor notified of their hospitalization. All spiritual advisors should be made welcome in nursing units. When requested by clients or families, the nurse should keep spiritual advisors informed of physiological, psychosocial, and spiritual concerns. This helps in providing holistic health care. The nurse shows respect for clients' spiritual values and needs by willingly cooperating with others giving spiritual care and by facilitating the administration of sacraments, rites, and rituals.

Providing privacy for the client and spiritual advisor is a thoughtful and sensitive gesture. If the nurse is unsure about the proper routine in a client's religion, asking the spiritual advisor, family, or client is appropriate. Often a client within the hospital may want to discuss spiritual concerns late in the evening or in the middle of the night, when support services such as clergy and social services are not available. The nurse can do a great deal to meet the clients needs, if only by listening.

Prayer

The act of prayer is a form of "self-dedication" that allows an individual to commune with God or a higher being (McCullough, 1995). It gives an individual the opportunity to renew his or her faith and belief in a higher being in a more formal way. For many, prayer is an opportunity to review personal shortcomings they perceive and to make a commitment to a better life. Clients may participate in private prayer or pursue opportunities for group prayer with family, friends, or clergy.

Prayer is being found to be an effective resource for persons to cope with pain, stress, and distress. A study by Turner and Clancy (1986) identified that increased praying and hoping by clients with chronic low back pain was related to decreased intensity of pain. There have also been studies suggesting that prayer may involve cardiovascular changes and muscle relaxation. Often prayer leads a person to feel an improvement in mood and a sense of peace and calm. During assessment the nurse learns whether prayer is a ritual important to the client and then determines if interventions are needed so that prayer can be practiced. Interventions may include establishing privacy, encouraging visits from clergy, or praying with the client.

Diet Therapies

Food and nutrition are important aspects of nursing care. Food is also an important component of religious observances. As with many aspects of a particular culture or religion, food and the rituals surrounding the preparation and serving of food can be an important part of one's spirituality.

Hindus have many dietary restrictions. Some sects are vegetarians, believing that killing any living creature is a crime. Many Buddhists also are vegetarians. Most members of the Buddhist religion practice moderation and do not use alcohol, tobacco, or drugs and will fast on special religious days.

Eating pork and consuming alcohol is prohibited by Muslims. As mentioned before, Ramadan is a month of daylight fasting. The sick, pregnant women, and nursing mothers are exempt from fasting rituals. Orthodox, Conservative, and some Reformed Jews strictly observe kosher dietary laws, which prohibit eating pork and shellfish. In addition, meat and milk, or milk products, must not be eaten within 6 hours of each other. Jews also have regulations about food preparation to keep foods "kosher," or blessed.

Some Christian traditions, such as Seventh-Day Adventists, have dietary laws. Other groups, such as Evangelicals, discourage the use of alcohol, caffeine, and tobacco. Some Seventh-Day Adventists may refuse meat products. Jehovah's Witnesses may avoid foods prepared with or containing blood, such as sausages or blood pudding. Many Roman Catholics, over the age of 7 and under 65 years, health permitting, fast or abstain from meat on Ash Wednesday (which marks the beginning of Lent, usually in late February) and Good Friday (the Friday before Easter). Greek Orthodox Catholics may fast during Lent and may abstain from meat and dairy products on Wednesdays and Fridays. Several branches of Christianity may fast 1 to 6 hours before Communion. Most fasting rituals are suspended for illness, pregnancy, or nursing (Table 25-4).

The nurse can integrate the client's dietary preferences into daily care. This will require consultation with the health care institution's dietitian. In the event that a hospital or nursing home kitchen cannot prepare food in the preferred way, the family can be encouraged to bring meals fitting into any dietary restrictions posed by the client's condition.

Supporting Rituals

For many clients, the ability to exercise religious rituals is an important coping resource. This is especially true for older adults (see the box on p. 453). Nurses in acute and

Table 25-4	Religious Dietary Regulations Affecting Health Care
RELIGION	**DIETARY PRACTICES**
Hinduism	Some sects are vegetarians. The belief is not to kill *any* living creatures.
Buddhism	Some are vegetarians, and many will not use alcohol or tobacco and may hesitate to use drugs. Many will fast on Holy Days.
Islam	Eating pork and consuming alcohol are prohibited. Fasting is done during the month of Ramadan.
Judaism	Some observe the kosher dietary restrictions of avoiding pork and shellfish and preparing and eating milk and meat at the same time.
Christianity	Some Baptists, Evangelicals, and Pentecostals discourage the use of alcohol, caffeine, and tobacco. Some Roman Catholics may fast during Lent, Ash Wednesday, Good Friday, and 1 hour before receiving communion.
Jehovah's Witnesses	Members may avoid food prepared with or containing blood.
Mormonism	Members abstain from alcohol, caffeine, and tobacco.
Baha'i	Members abstain from alcohol, caffeine, and tobacco.

long-term care settings can become active in their clients' spiritual care by becoming familiar with hospital policies concerning visitations, church services, and such things as the use of candles for prayer. In addition, nurses can consult with physicians and the pharmacy about the client's use of personal medication, home remedies, or herbal medications, when appropriate. Because a visit to the hospital chapel or attendance at services can be important to the hospitalized client and family, directions to the chapel should be included during orientation to the medical facility. Arrangements may need to be made with the pastoral care department for the client and family to receive the sacraments. The nurse plans personal care, therapies, or tests to allow for church services, religious reading, or spiritual visitations.

In the home setting, the nurse may need to find a way to incorporate a religious service. Many churches produce weekly audiotapes of the religious service for homebound members. Family members can plan a prayer session or an organized reading of scriptures on a regular basis. Clergy will routinely offer to make home visits for persons unable to attend religious services. Taped meditations and religious music and televised religious services provide another effective option.

Evaluation

Attainment of spiritual health can be considered a lifelong goal. Clients will experience the need to clarify values (Chapter 18), reshape philosophies, and live those experiences that help to shape one's purpose in life. When caring for clients, the nurse evaluates whether nursing interventions help strengthen a client's spirituality. The nurse compares the client's level of spiritual health with the behaviors and needs noted in the nursing assessment (see the evaluation box on p. 454). The client should be experiencing emotions appropriate to the situation; developing a strong, realistic self-image; and experiencing warm, open interpersonal relationships. Family and friends with whom the

GERONTOLOGICAL PRINCIPLES for Nursing

Older adults often feel that religion is more important to them than their younger counterparts.

Consideration and a belief in the afterlife increases as adults grow older. Visits from clergy, social work, lawyers, and even financial advisors can be made available so the client feels prepared.

Leaving a legacy (tangible or intangible asset) to another person prepares one to leave the world with a sense of meaning. Legacies may include oral histories, works of art, publications, photographs, or some other object of significance (Ebersole and Hess, 1994).

Assist an older adult to develop their legacy by discovering their lifelong interests, recording their stories or words, identify the recipients.

client has fellowhip can be a source of evaluative information. The client should also be maintaining a sense of mission in life and, for some individuals, a confidence and trust in a supreme being or beings.

For clients with a serious or terminal illness, evaluation focuses on success at helping the client retain hope. The nurse may need to evaluate the quality of the nurse-client relationship. Does the client express trust and confidence in the nurse? Is the client able to discuss those things important in life? For clients with continued anxiety, fears, and questions, there may be a need to readjust the plan of care. Additional resources such as spiritual advisors or members of a church congregation may become necessary. Eventually, a client whose spiritual needs are met may become peaceful, even while experiencing a severe illness.

If the client is comfortable expressing spiritual needs and hopes to the nurse, then an effective healing relationship has been developed. The accompanying evaluation box summa-

Sample Evaluation Intervention for Spiritual Well-Being

GOAL	EVALUATIVE MEASURES	EXPECTED OUTCOMES
Client will renew relationships with family members in 1 month	Have client keep personal journal of each evening activity with family Include a description of discussion topics and feelings client had afterward Ask client to describe quality of relationship with husband and children Observe client interaction with family members, noting subjects they are able to discuss together	Client will dedicate the evening hours, 5 days during the week, to build relationship with husband and children Client will be able to express openly with family her love and appreciation for each of them

rizes examples of evaluative measures used to achieve outcomes in a spiritual plan of care.

Holistic nursing care integrates interventions that support a client's spirituality. To provide spiritual care, the nurse must understand the dimensions of spiritual health and be able to recognize the spiritually healthy person. Likewise, each nurse must be able to understand his or her own spirituality so that he or she feels free and enabled to support a client with spiritual needs.

The development of a caring nurse-client relationship is central to providing spiritual care. Achieving a presence and openness with a client enables the nurse to deliver care in a sensitive, creative, and appropriate manner. The nurse also learns to mobilize the client's hope, while establishing a healing relationship. This helps clients become future oriented and able to work toward healing and recovery.

▪ KEY CONCEPTS ▪

► Spiritual well-being is an integrating aspect of human wholeness.

► Religion is commonly associated with a "state of doing," while spirituality is associated with "a state of being."

► The spiritual dimension is not the same as that of the psychosocial dimension.

► Understanding a client's spirituality requires maturity and a non-judgmental approach on the part of the nurse.

► Spirituality represents the totality of one's being and serves to unify a person's other dimensions.

► Spiritual health is achieved when one finds balance among life values, goals, belief systems, and one's relationship within self and others.

► Acute and chronic illness, terminal illness, individuation, and near-death experience can create spiritual problems for clients.

► Learning to practice compassion helps a nurse discover a client life's values and meaning.

► Assessing a client's capacity for religious experiences determines the significance spirituality holds for a person.

► Fellowship with other persons can be a source of hope for a client.

► Common religious rituals include private worship, prayer, singing, use of a rosary, and scripture reading.

► A nurse's assessment should focus not only on alterations in functioning but also on spiritual options, which provide strength, hope, and encouragment during times of illness.

► The personal nature of spirituality requires open communication between nurse and client.

► Establishing presence involves giving attention, answering questions, having an encouraging attitude, and conveying a sense of trust.

► Development of a healing relationship mobilizes hope for the client and helps the client find an acceptable understanding of illness.

► Part of a client's caregiving environment can be the regular presence of family, friends, and spiritual advisors.

► Prayer gives a person the opportunity to renew his or her faith in a higher being in a more formal way.

► Older adults value the ability to exercise religious rituals.

▪ KEY TERMS ▪

Faith, p. 445

Individuation, p. 444

Near-death experience, p. 445

Religion, p. 441

Spiritual distress, p. 443

Spiritual health, p. 443

Spirituality, p. 441

∎ CRITICAL THINKING EXERCISES ∎

1. Jan is a new graduate nurse, caring for Mr. Kline for the first time. He is experiencing acute pain and has had a sleepless night. Mr. Kline reveals a fear that he is not going to recover from whatever illness he has. A diagnosis has not as yet been made. How can Jan contribute to Mr. Kline's sense of well-being?

2. Mrs. Lucas is an 86-year-old woman with a below-the-knee amputation of the left leg. She is receiving visits from the home health nurse because of her need for dressing changes for a diabetic foot ulcer on the right leg. Recently, her close friend and neighbor died. Mrs. Lucas regularly attended church with her friend. How might the nurse help Mrs. Lucas continue excercising religious rituals.

3. Mr. Rossini has been diagnosed with terminal cancer. As the nurse assesses the client's spiritual health, he reveals that he is an atheist. He also shares that the terminal diagnosis has made him rethink his priorities. He always valued his health but now speaks of the value of the relationships he has with his family. How can the nurse support Mr. Rossini spiritually?

REFERENCES

Basford TK: *Near death experience: an annotated bibliography,* New York, 1990, Garland.

Benner P: *From novice to expert,* Menlo Park, 1984, Addison Wesley.

Burnard P: Spiritual distress and the nursing response: theoretical considerations and counseling skills, *J Adv Nurs* 12:377, 1987.

Carson V: *Spiritual dimensions of nursing practice,* Philadelphia, 1989, WB Saunders.

Clark CC et al: Spirituality:Integral to quality care, *Holistic Nurs Pract* 5(3):67-76, 1991.

Ebersole P, Hess P: *Toward healthy aging: human needs and nursing responses,* ed 4, St Louis, 1994, Mosby.

Emblen JD: Religion and spirituality defined according to current use in nursing literature, *J Prof Nurs* 8(1):41, 1992.

Farran CJ et al: Development of a model for spiritual assessment and intervention, *J Religion Health* 28(3):185, 1989.

Fryback PB: Health for people with a terminal diagnosis, *Nurs Sci Q* 6(3):147, 1992.

Heliker D: Reevaulation of a nursing diagnosis: spiritual distress, *Nurs Forum* 27(4):15, 1992.

Hungelmann J et al: Spiritual well-being in older adults: harmonious interconnectedness, *J Religion Health* 24(2):147, 1985.

Kim MJ, McFarland GK, McLane AM: *Pocket guide to nursing diagnosis,* ed 6, St Louis, 1995, Mosby.

Mansen TJ: The spiritual dimension of individuals: conceptual development, *Nurs Diagnosis* 4(4):140, 1993.

McCullough ME: Prayer and health: conceptual issues—research review, and research agenda, *J Psych Theol* 23(1):15, 1995.

Munley A: *The hospice alternative: a new context for death and dying,* New York, 1983, Basic Books.

Peterson E, Nelson K: How to meet your client's spiritual needs, *J of Psychosoc Nurs and Mental Health Services* 25(5):34, 1987.

Rew L: Intuition: nursing knowledge and the spiritual dimension of persons, *Holistic Nurs Pract* 3(3):56, 1989.

Storr A: *Jung: selected writings,* London, 1983, Fontana.

Stoll R: Guidelines for spiritual assessment, *Am J Nurs* 79:1574, 1979.

Studzinski R: Adult faith is regard for long life, *Envoy* 15(2):4, 1986.

Turner JA, Clancy S: Strategies for coping with chronic low back pain: relationship to pain and disability, *Pain* 24:355, 1986.

Turner RP et al: Religious or spiritual problem: a culturally sensitive diagnostic category in the DSM-IV, *J Nerv Ment Dis* 183(7):435, 1995.

Yim R: CABG Spiritual Healing CarePaths, Presentation at 4th annual expert user forum, Center for Case Management Inc., San Antonio, Texas, February 3, 1994.

Young CE: Intuition and the nursing process, *Holistic Nurs Pract* 1(3):52, 1987.

ADDITIONAL READINGS

Benner P, Wrubel J: *The primacy of caring,* Menlo Park, Calif., 1989, Addison-Wesley.

Carson V et al: Hope and spiritual well-being: essentials for living with AIDS, *Perspect Psychiatr Care* 26(2):28, 1990.

Dobmeier T: Professionalizing spiritual care, *J Christian Nurs* 7(1):32, 1990.

Emblen JD, Halstead L: Spiritual needs and interventions: comparing the views of patients, nurses, and chaplains, *Clin Nurs Specialist* 7(4):175, 1993.

Karns P: Building a foundation for spiritual care, *J Christian Nurs* 8(3):10, 1991.

Kirkwood NA: *A hospital handbook on multi-culturalism and religion,* 1993, Millennium Books.

Miller WR: Spirituality: the silent dimension in addiction research, *Drug Alcohol Rev* 9:259, 1990.

Newman M: The spirit of nursing, *Holistic Nurs Pract* 3(3):1, 1989.

Reed PG: An emerging paradigm for the investigation of spirituality in nursing, *Res Nurs Health* 15:349, 1992.

Shaffer J: Spiritual distress and critical illness, *Crit Care Nurs* 11:42, 1991.

Stepnick A, Perry B: Preventing spiritual distress in the dying client, *J Christian Nurs* 30(1), 17, 1992.

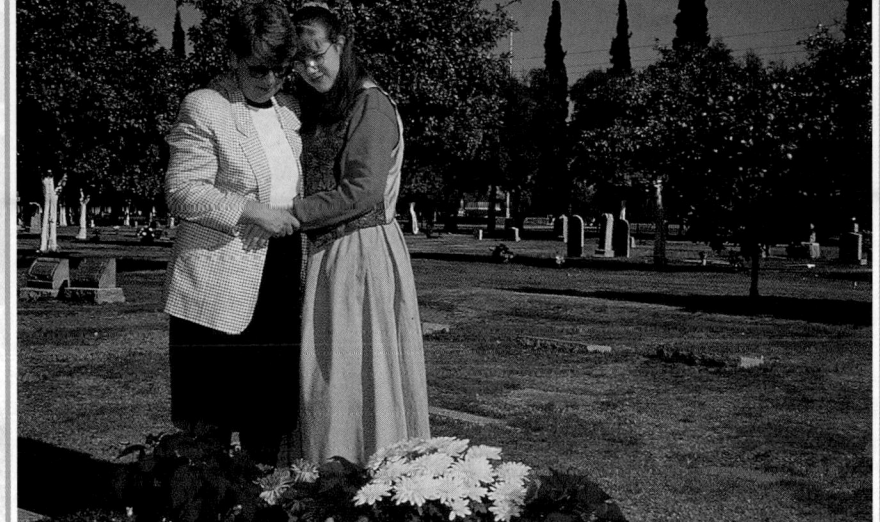
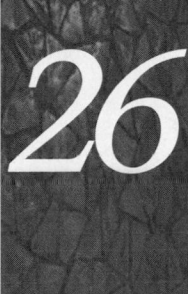

## Chapter 26

Coping With Loss, Death, and Grieving

Objectives

Mastery of content in this chapter will enable the student to:

▶ Define the key terms listed.

▶ Identify the nurse's role in helping clients with problems related to loss, death, and grief.

▶ Describe and compare the phases of grieving from Engel, Kübler-Ross, and Rando.

▶ Discuss five basic categories of loss.

▶ List factors influencing a client's reaction to loss and ability to cope.

▶ Describe characteristics of a person experiencing grief.

▶ Compare and contrast grief after loss, anticipatory grief, and accommodated grief.

▶ Develop a care plan for a client or family experiencing grief.

▶ Implement interventions for grieving clients to provide sensitive caring that supports the client and family in their grief work.

▶ Describe how a nurse meets a dying client's need for comfort and caring.

▶ Explain ways for the nurse to assist a family in caring for a dying client.

▶ Discuss the role of hospice in meeting the needs of a dying client and the family.

▶ Discuss important factors in caring for the body after death.

▶ Discuss the role of the nurse's own loss experience as it influences care of the grieving.

▶ Identify two ways nurses can meet their needs related to loss.

Loss and death are universal and individually unique events of the human experience. Life is a series of losses and gains. A child beginning to walk gains independence with mobility. An older person with visual and hearing changes may lose self-reliance. Illness and hospitalization often involve multiple losses.

A nurse works with many clients who experience different types of loss. Coping mechanisms influence people's ability to face and accept loss. Grief is a natural response to loss. It is important to note that whatever is said here about the process of grief and loss exists within a social and historical perspective that may change over time and circumstance. The nurse helps clients to understand and accept loss within the context of their culture so that life can continue. In the Western culture, when clients do not do grief work after a profound loss, serious emotional, mental, and social problems can occur.

Humans can anticipate death. This can cause many reactions including anxiety, planning, denial, love, loneliness, achievement, and lack of achievement. Death can be an overwhelming experience that affects dying persons and their families, friends, and care givers. The way a person dies reflects the person's style of living, cultural background, beliefs, and attitudes about life and death.

■ LOSS, DEATH, GRIEF, AND NURSING

Loss and death are frequent realities in many nursing care settings. Most nurses interact daily with clients and families experiencing loss and grief. It is critical that nurses understand loss and grief. While caring for clients and their families, nurses also experience personal loss as client-family-nurse relationships end through transfer, discharge, recovery, or death. When a person becomes terminally ill, nurses can be reminded of their own mortality. Nurses may find that it is easier to relieve physical symptoms of illness and death than to become involved in meaningful interpersonal relationships to support a person who is suffering or dying. Personal feelings, values, and experiences influence the extent to which nurses can support clients and families during loss or death. Self-assessment—exploring personal attitudes, feelings, and values—is necessary before nurses can respond with a genuine, sensitive, therapeutic approach to others. Developing the art of being with the grieving and dying requires an inner strength that arises from knowledge of and a positive belief in one's self. Development of a philosophy of life helps nurses function supportively during difficult times.

There are many variations in grief and mourning. This chapter will use a framework drawn from the context of our Western culture. Nurses must be open to learning from their clients about their experiences and ways of making sense of the world. The nurse can best help the client by bringing an attitude of "not knowing" to each unique encounter with the client and family and together exploring how grief and meaning unfold (Hepburn, 1994). The nurse utilizes knowledge of the concepts of loss and grief to creatively apply interventions to promote health, prevent illness, and support dying clients.

Loss

Personal loss is any significant loss that requires adaptation through the grieving process. Loss occurs when something or someone can no longer be seen, felt, heard, known, or experienced. The type of loss influences the degree of distress. For example, the loss of an object might not generate the same distress as the loss of a significant other. However, individuals respond to loss differently. The death of a family member would be expected to cause more distress than the loss of a pet, but for a person living alone the death of a pet that has been a constant companion would possibly cause more emotional distress than that of a relative who had not been seen for years. The type of loss is significant to the grieving process; yet the nurse must recognize that each person's interpretation of a loss is highly individualized.

Losses may be actual or perceived. Actual losses are easily identified, as with the child whose playmate moves away or the adult who loses a marriage partner through divorce. Perceived losses are less tangible and can be misunderstood, such as the loss of confidence or prestige. The more invested in what is lost, the greater the feeling of loss. The client may experience **maturational loss** (loss resulting from normal life transitions such as a child going off to school for the first time), **situational loss** (loss occurring suddenly in response to a specific external event such as the sudden death of a loved one), or both. The child learning to walk loses the infantlike body image, the woman experiencing menopause loses the ability to bear children, and the unemployed man may lose self-esteem.

Losses may be grouped into five categories: loss of external objects, loss of a known environment, loss of a significant other, loss of an aspect of self, and loss of life. Nurses may care for clients who have experienced more than one type of loss, such as the hospitalized client who has experienced many losses, including health, independence, control over one's environment, and financial security. Loss threatens self-concept, self-esteem, security, and sense of worth. The nurse must recognize the meaning of each loss to a client and its impact on physical and psychological functioning.

LOSS OF EXTERNAL OBJECTS

Loss of an external object involves any possession that is worn out, misplaced, stolen, or ruined by disaster. For a child the object may be a toy or a blanket; for an adult it may be jewelry or an article of clothing. The extent of grieving a person feels for a lost object depends on its value, the sentiment the person attaches to it, and the object's usefulness.

LOSS OF A KNOWN ENVIRONMENT

The loss associated with separation from a known environment includes leaving a familiar setting for a period or relocating permanently. Examples include moving to a new city, taking a new job, or hospitalization. Loss through separation from a known environment may occur through *maturational* circumstances, for example, when an older adult is moved into a nursing home, or *situational* circumstances, for example, the loss of a home due to disaster or through injury or illness.

Confinement within an institution results in isolation from routine events. The rules of a hospital create an environment that is often impersonal and demoralizing. The loneliness of an unfamiliar setting may threaten self-esteem and make grieving more difficult.

LOSS OF A SIGNIFICANT OTHER

Significant others include parents, spouses, children, siblings, teachers, clergy, friends, neighbors, and work associates. Entertainment figures and well-known athletes may be significant others for young people. Research shows that many people regard pets as significant others. Loss occurs as a result of separation, moving, running away, promotion at work, and death.

LOSS OF AN ASPECT OF SELF

The loss of an aspect of self may include a body part, physiological function, or psychological function. Loss of a body part may include a limb, eye, hair, teeth, or breast. Loss of physiological function includes loss of urinary or bowel control, mobility, strength, or sensory function. Loss of psychological function includes loss of memory, humor, self-esteem, self-confidence, power, respect, or love. The loss of these aspects of self may result from illness, injury, or developmental and situational changes. Such a loss can lessen the individual's well-being. A person not only experiences grief over the loss but also may experience permanent changes in body image and self-concept (see Chapter 23).

LOSS OF LIFE

Persons who face death continue to live, feel, think, and respond to events and people around them until the moment of death. The primary concern is often not about death itself but about pain and loss of control. Although most people are afraid of and anxious about death, the same issues will not be equally important to each person.

Each person responds differently to death. People who have lived alone and suffered long terminal illnesses may experience death as a relief. Some perceive death as an entry into an afterlife to be reunited with loved ones in paradise. Others fear separation, abandonment, loneliness, or mutilation. The threat of death often causes individuals to become dependent. The helplessness and shame of dependence experienced by some clients create a challenge for the nurse.

Doka (1993) describes responses to life-threatening illness in four phases. A *prediagnostic phase* occurs when the client's symptoms or risk factors of illness are recognized. An *acute phase* centers around the crisis of diagnosis. The client is faced with a series of decisions, including medical, psychological, and interpersonal, as to how to cope initially with the crisis of illness. In the *chronic phase* the client struggles with the illness and its treatment, which often involves a series of related crises. Finally there is a *recovery* or *terminal phase*. Sometimes in the acute or chronic phase a person may experience recovery. The client has reached the terminal phase when death is no longer merely possible, but likely. At each of these illness points the client and family are faced with various and changing losses.

Grief, Mourning, and Bereavement

Bereavement is the state of thought, feeling, and activity that follows loss. It includes grief and mourning. **Grief** is the process of experiencing the psychological, social and physical reactions to the perception of loss (Rando 1991). These responses often include helplessness, loneliness, hopelessness, sadness, guilt, and anger. **Mourning** is the process that follows a loss and includes working through grief. The processes of grief and mourning are intense, internal, painful, and lengthy. The terms *grief, mourning,* and *bereavement* are often used interchangeably.

Grief involves thoughts, feelings, and behaviors. Its purpose is to achieve more effective functioning by integrating the loss into the client's life experience. This takes time and work. The term "grief work" comes from the psychiatrist Erich Lindemann (1965) to describe the tasks and processes that must be completed successfully in order to resolve grief. The grieving person tries a variety of strategies to cope. Worden (1982) outlined four tasks of grief that facilitate healthy adjustment to loss, and Harper (1987) arranged the tasks in the acronym "TEAR":

1. T—To accept the reality of the loss
2. E—Experiencing the pain of loss
3. A—Adjustment to an environment that no longer includes the lost person, object, or aspect of self
4. R—Reinvesting emotional energy into new relationships

These tasks do not occur in a specified order. In fact, grieving people may work on all four tasks simultaneously, or only one or two may be priorities. Nurses can assist clients and families in understanding and working through these tasks as they apply to their unique situation (Fig. 26-1).

Society often discourages openness during grief or loss. Unhappy children may be told not to cry when playmates move away; awkward adolescents are told not to be embarrassed about sudden growth spurts, and dying persons are

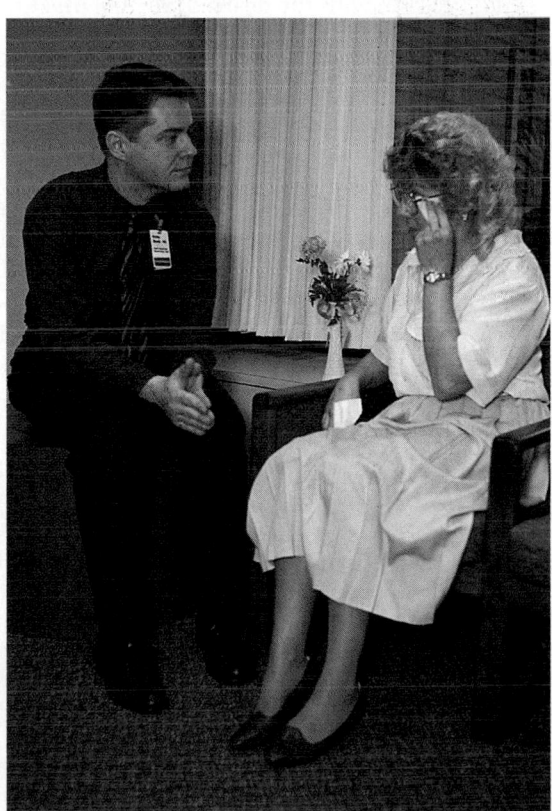

Fig. 26-1 Nurses assist family members in finding resources to help with the grieving process.

encouraged to remain calm and dignified. Recent changes in attitudes, beliefs, and values have promoted more open expressions of grief. However, many persons still hesitate to reveal their thoughts, fears, and feelings of grief, especially older adults. Nurses are learning to seek support from peers to express their concerns about dealing with terminally ill clients. Similarly, family members more often seek support from care givers to express anger and fear over loss. Grieving can lead to new understandings that promote growth. A person can grow from experiences of loss through openness, encouragement of others, and adequate support.

SPECIAL GRIEF RESPONSES: ANTICIPATORY GRIEF AND DISENFRANCHISED GRIEF

Anticipatory grief includes the processes of mourning, coping, interaction, planning, and psychosocial reorganization. These begin in response to the awareness of an impending loss and the recognition of associated losses in the past, present, and future. Anticipatory grief occurs in those who receive a diagnosis that has long-term effects on body function, as in systemic lupus erythematosis. The client may be feeling reasonably well at the time of diagnosis but begins grieving in response to information about future losses associated with the disease. In these situations anticipatory grief may extend over a long time and be open-ended. Anticipatory grief for the dying client involves the letting go of hopes, dreams, and expectations of a long-term future. Continued involvement with the dying client and the goal of maximizing the possibility of whatever living is possible is not inconsistent with the experience of anticipatory grief. Anticipatory grief for the dying has a definitive end. It ceases with the death of the client; although grief will continue, it will no longer be anticipatory. The client, the family, and the nurse are faced with a series of adaptational tasks in the process of anticipatory grief (Rando, 1986).

Disenfranchised grief occurs when persons experience a loss that is not or cannot be openly acknowledged, publicly mourned, or socially supported. The concept recognizes that societies have sets of norms regarding "grieving rules" that attempt to specify who, when, where, how, how long, and for whom people should grieve. Grief may be disenfranchised in those situations in which the relationship between the bereaved and the deceased is not based on recognized kin ties. These can include close friends, care givers, and co-workers or nontraditional relationships, such as extramarital affairs or homosexual relationships and those whose relationships existed in the past, such as ex-spouses.

In other cases the loss itself is not socially defined as significant, such as perinatal death, abortion, or adoption. Loss of a pet may not be viewed as significant. One can also speak of "psychological" deaths in which the personality of someone has changed so significantly that the family perceives the person, as previously existing, as dead, for example, in the case of chronic, debilitating mental illnesses (Doka, 1993).

Nurses often work with these situations at one time or another. The uniqueness of disenfranchised grief creates a situation in which the nurse often becomes a social and familial substitute for the client. It also requires that nurses focus on their own issues of concern and acceptance

around painful, potentially frightening, and embarrassing lifestyles and resulting loss experiences. When nurses get in touch with their own feelings and reactions, genuine support is possible.

Concepts and Theories of the Grieving Process

Grief is a normal response to any loss. Behaviors and feelings associated with the **grieving process** occur in individuals suffering losses such as physical deformities or deaths of close friends. They also occur when individuals face their own deaths. The person undergoing loss, the family, and other social supports experience grief.

There is no right way to grieve. The concept and theories of grief are only tools that can be used to anticipate the emotional needs of clients and families and plan interventions to help them understand their grief and deal with it.

It is important to consider several theories of grief (Table 26-1). Whether discussing stages, phases, or tasks, it is important to note that these do not occur in a fixed, predictable order. The goal is not to classify the client's grief; that is, the nurse should not identify a client as experiencing a certain stage of grief. The nurse's role is to observe grieving behaviors, recognize the influence of grief on behavior, and provide empathetic support.

ENGEL'S THEORY

Engel (1964) proposed that the grieving process has three phases that can be applied to grieving and dying persons.

In the first phase the individual denies reality of the loss and may withdraw, sit motionless, or wander aimlessly. It may seem to the observer that the person has not realized what the loss means. Physical reactions may include fainting, diaphoresis, nausea, diarrhea, rapid heart rate, restlessness, insomnia, and fatigue.

In the second phase the individual begins to feel the loss acutely and may experience desperation. Suddenly, anger, guilt, frustration, depression, and emptiness occur. Crying is typical as the individual becomes preoccupied with the loss.

In the third phase the reality of the loss is acknowledged. Anger or depression is no longer needed. The loss is clear to the individual, who begins to reorganize life. By experiencing these phases a person moves from a lower to a higher level of emotional and intellectual functioning. New self-awareness is developed.

Table 26-1	Comparison of Three Theories of the Grieving Process	
ENGEL (1964)	**KÜBLER-ROSS (1969)**	**RANDO (1991)**
Shock and disbelief	Denial	Avoidance
	Anger	
	Bargaining	
Developing awareness	Depression	Confrontation
Reorganization and restitution	Acceptance	Accommodation

KÜBLER-ROSS'S STAGES OF DYING

The framework provided by Kübler-Ross (1969) focuses on behavior and includes five stages. In the denial stage the individual acts as though nothing has happened and may refuse to believe that a loss has occurred. Statements such as "No, that can't be so," and "It can't be happening to me!" are common.

In the anger stage the individual resists the loss and may "act out" to everyone and everything in the environment. In the bargaining stage there is postponement of the reality of the loss. The individual may attempt to make a deal in a subtle or an overt way to prevent the loss. The client frequently seeks opinions of others during this stage. A hospitalized client may show model behavior because of a belief that the staff will find a cure if he or she is a "good client."

The depression stage occurs when the loss is realized and

Table 26-2	Nursing Implications of Rando's Phases of Grief and Kübler-Ross's Stages of Dying
BEHAVIORS	**NURSING IMPLICATIONS**
AVOIDANCE **Denial** Denial is immediate response to news of loss or impending loss. Physiological responses may include muscular weakness, tremors, deep sighs, flushed or cold and clammy skin, diaphoresis, anorexia, and discomfort. Individuals avoid accepting reality of situation by not making decisions; they may attempt activities that they are no longer able to do, fail to comply with treatment, search for evidence that loss has not or will not occur, and appear artificially happy. Mood swings are common. Individuals isolate themselves from sources of accurate information or reject offers of comfort and support.	Support emotional needs without reinforcing denial. Offer to remain with clients, without discussing reasons for behavior or need to cope, unless they bring it up. Offer basic care, such as food, drink, oxygenation, comfort, and safety.
Anger Individuals may express anger and retaliate against family, staff, physicians, or supreme being. Bereaved may express anger toward deceased. Individuals become demanding and accusing. Anger may precipitate guilt and lead to anxiety and lowered self-esteem. Individuals may feel resentful and jealous of others who still have lost object or loved one. Individuals may be reluctant to share feelings and thoughts.	Provide anticipatory guidance about feelings and their intensity experienced as part of grief; focus especially on anger. Do not take anger personally. Meet needs that cause angry response. Encourage client and family to express their feelings.
Bargaining Individuals are willing to do anything to avoid loss or change prognosis or fate. Individuals make bargains with supreme being. Individuals accept new forms of therapy.	Provide information needed for decision making.
CONFRONTATION **Depression** Reality and permanence of loss become recognized. Confusion, lack of motivation, disinterest, indecision, and crying are common. Withdrawal from relationships and activities occurs. Individuals may become quiet and noncommunicative. Feelings of loneliness surface. Reminiscence about past and lost object begins. Individuals may lose interest in appearance. Individuals may become suicidal or cope by beginning unhealthy behaviors such as excess drug use.	Provide support and empathy. Support crying by offering touch that communicates caring. Listen attentively. Assess risk of harm to self and refer to mental health professional if needed.
ACCOMMODATION **Acceptance** Individuals accept terms of loss and death and begin plans for it. Individuals can share feelings about loss. Reminiscence about past occurs. Periods of depression and well-being occur. Good times begin to outweigh bad. Life begins to stabilize.	Offer opportunities to share feelings verbally, in writing or art, or by tape recordings. Allow and encourage review as often as clients want to talk. Show acceptance of lability of feelings. Assist in discussing future plans.

the full impact of its significance is apparent. A person may feel overwhelming loneliness and withdrawal. The depression stage provides an opportunity to work through the loss and begin problem solving.

In the fifth stage acceptance is reached. Physiological reactions cease, and social interactions resume. Kübler-Ross defines *acceptance* as coming to terms with the situation rather than submitting to resignation or hopelessness.

RANDO'S PHASES OF GRIEVING

Although the grieving process has a generally predictable course and distinctive symptoms, no two persons progress through it in the same way or over the same time. A person progresses and then regresses until the loss is finally resolved. Rando (1993) refined the grieving responses into three categories: *avoidance,* in which there is shock, denial and disbelief; *confrontation,* which is a highly charged, and emotional state when clients repeatedly confront their loss and their grief is most intense and felt most acutely; and *accommodation,* when there is a gradual decline of acute grief and the beginning of an emotional and social reentry into the everyday world in which clients learn to live with their loss. To expect clients to progress in some specified manner over a specified time would be incorrect, inappropriate, and possibly harmful. Nursing implications based on Kübler-Ross's stages of dying and Rando's phases of grief can be seen in Table 26-2.

■ NURSING PROCESS AND GRIEF

Assessment

During assessment the nurse should not assume how or if the client or family experiences grief. The nurse should avoid assuming that a particular behavior indicates grief but allow persons to share what is happening in their own ways.

Assessment of the client and family begins by exploring the meaning of the loss to them. The nurse interviews the client and family, using honest, open communication; emphasizing listening skills; and observing responses and behaviors. Impressions are validated with the client and family so that nursing diagnoses and effective interventions can be developed.

The nurse assesses how the client *is* reacting rather than how the client *should be* reacting. Sequences of behavior or phases of grief may occur in order, they may be skipped, or they may recur. Many variables affect grief. Consideration of these variables gives the nurse a broad database from which to individualize care.

Several factors influence the way any individual responds to loss. Personal characteristics including age, sex, socioeconomic status, and education influence the response to loss. The nature of the relationship to the lost object, the characteristics of the loss, cultural and spiritual beliefs, support systems, and the potential for goal achievement affect the response to loss.

PERSONAL CHARACTERISTICS

Age. Age plays a role in the recognition and reaction to loss. Children's responses vary with age, previous experi-

---

Children's Responses to Death

BIRTH TO 2 YEARS
Lacks conception of death
Can experience a sense of loss and grief
These experiences lay a foundation for developing a conception of loss and grief

2 TO 5 YEARS
Denies death as a normal process
Sees death as reversible
Has unlimited faith in his or her ability to make things happen
May react with anger or displaced anger
Gives responses that may differ little from those of his or her parents

5 TO 8 YEARS
Sees death as final; does not see it will happen to him or her
Sees death as scary
Seeks to isolate what causes death and what death means
Feels the vulnerability that accompanies death
May take on more "adultlike" care giver roles in the family or become "self-reliant"

8 TO 12 YEARS
Views death as final and inevitable
May be unable to accept the finality of the loss
Realizes the possibilities of his or her own death; may develop fears of own mortality
Develops affective responses to death, as well as the defenses to handle his or her feelings (i.e., denial, avoidance, displacement, and reaction formation)
May create stories or jokes about death to hide fears
Experiences egocentric and magical thinking
Is aware of what this death will mean for his or her future

ADOLESCENTS
Understanding surrounding death resembles that of adulthood
Must face personal implications of death
Demonstrates risk-taking behaviors
Seriously seeks the meaning of life
More anxious about the future

Modified from Raphael B: *The anatomy of bereavement,* London, 1983, Hutchinson; and from Schaefer D, Lyons C: *How do we tell the children? Helping children understand and cope when someone dies,* New York, 1986, Newmarket; and from Wheeler SR, Pike MM. In Fawcett CS, editor: *Family psychiatric nursing,* St Louis, 1993, Mosby.

---

ence with loss, relationship with the deceased, personality, perceptions surrounding the loss, the particular meaning the loss has to them, and most important, their family's response to the loss (see the box above).

Although children may not understand the concept of death because of their age, they do develop perceptions of what loss means to them. They are especially perceptive to changes in differences in their parent's behavior. Parents may choose to avoid discussing the loss, but they cannot hide their grief. They may hide their tears, but they cannot hide their emotions at having to cope with their loss. Parents who keep their grief from their children may leave the false impression that the loss of a loved one did not matter.

Factors Influencing Grief in Older Adults
■ Physical changes accompanying aging
■ Loss of employment
■ Loss of social respect
■ Loss of relationships
■ Loss of self-care capabilities
■ Fear of loss of control
■ Sense of fulfillment and contributions made
■ Personality traits
■ Feelings of self-worth
■ Functional ability retained

▶ **RESEARCH HIGHLIGHT**

RESEARCH ABSTRACT

One of the most profound losses experienced by humans is the death of a spouse. The purposes of this report were to describe the grief experiences of older adults over the first 2 years after the death of their spouse and to compare these experiences with those of younger bereaved spouses. Emotional responses to the loss were similar. Two differences were noted: younger widows experienced a deep despair that was not described by older spouses; and younger spouses experienced feelings of disorganization accompanied by feelings of diminished capacity and fear of emotional breakdown that older spouses did not describe. Perhaps older spouses felt it was acceptable to acknowledge shock and sadness, but despair or fear of breakdown may have had different, more threatening meanings for them. Recommendations for how nurses can meet the needs of bereaved older adults were made.

IMPLICATIONS FOR PRACTICE

▶ Older bereaved spouses present a unique challenge to nurses, owing to the catastrophic nature of the loss and the complexities of the concerns facing older people in general.

▶ Acknowledgment of persistent, painful emotions months and years after the loss legitimizes these feelings and may enhance self-acceptance if the feelings are recognized as normal.

▶ An awareness that older people may be more reluctant to discuss their feelings suggests that nurses must encourage clients to do so by giving permission and making themselves available to the bereaved.

REFERENCE

Anderson KL, Dimond MF: *J Adv Nurs* 22:308, 1995.

Children at any age may feel responsible for the death. Their capacity of "magical thinking" can make them believe their thoughts, feelings, or behaviors toward their loved one might have caused the death. Children may feel guilty for being alive, being well, or having wished the death of their loved one (Wheeler and Pike, 1993).

The young adult relates loss to its significance for status, role, and lifestyle. A loss of job or economic well-being, divorce, or a physical impairment causes much grief and threatens success. A young adult's concept of death is largely a product of religious and cultural beliefs. The death of a young adult is seen as especially tragic by society because it is the loss of a life at the brink of realized potential.

A middle-age person begins to realize that youthfulness and physical fitness cannot be taken for granted. The adult begins to reexamine life to consider the options available to gain fulfillment. The person becomes sensitive to the physical changes of aging. Any loss in physical function can create grief. Loss of significant others creates a significant threat to lifestyle. The career-oriented adult has usually reached a professional peak. Any loss of job or ability to perform a job causes considerable grief. The middle-age adult knows that time is at a premium and life is finite. Adults often take time to consider life and death.

Older adults often experience as much life satisfaction as their juniors. It is a myth that usefulness and the enjoyment of life end at a certain age. It is also true that the longer a person lives and forms loving attachments, the more there is to lose. An older adult experiences accumulated grief as a result of many changes (see the boxes above). Older adults often fear events surrounding death more than death itself. They may perceive loneliness, isolation, loss of social role, prolonged illness, and loss of self-determination and dignity as worse than death (Rando, 1986, Kastenbaum, 1991).

Sex Roles. Reaction to loss is influenced by social expectations of male and female roles. In many cultures in the United States and Canada, it is generally more difficult for men than for women to express grief openly. The nurse must be alert to this and validate with the client feelings, reactions, and the personal meaning attached to a loss. Men and women attach different significance to body parts, functions, interpersonal relationships, and objects.

Education and Socioeconomic Status. Loss is universal, experienced by everyone, regardless of socioeconomic status. Assessment of a client's socioeconomic status is essential because it influences the client's ability to use options and supports when coping with loss. Generally, a lack of financial resources, education, or occupational skills magnifies the demands on the griever.

NATURE OF RELATIONSHIPS

The characteristics of the lost relationship and the functions that the deceased person performed in the griever's life are critical variables to assess in the grief experience. It has been said that to lose your parents is to lose your past, to lose your spouse is to lose your present, and to lose your child is to lose your future. The literature supports the belief that the loss of a child creates the most intense grief response (Saunders, 1992). A child's death is often traumatic because it is premature. Parents often feel guilt and blame themselves.

The reaction to the loss of a parent depends on the quality of the relationship. The death of a parent who was the most nurturing, or when the survivor is an only child, is likely to cause the greatest grief for a child. The loss of a parent in adulthood is influenced by the psychological relationship and degree of attachment.

The meaning of the relationship to the griever will influence the grief response, whether the loss is due to death, separation, or divorce. Those who strongly depend on the lost person often have more problems than others as they try to part with the lost relationship and establish new ones. A relationship characterized by extreme ambivalence is more difficult to resolve than one that is not.

One of the most stressful events in life is loss of a spouse. If marital partners usually divided household responsibilities, the loss of one may leave the other with incomplete skills in the face of total responsibility. If children still live at home, the remaining parent may become emotionally overloaded with extra responsibilities. The loss of a sexual partner may affect the remaining spouse's perception of sexuality and desire for sex. The loss of a spouse also makes it difficult for the survivor to establish new friendships or to maintain previously established relationships that were couple based.

The family will have to integrate the experience of a family member's illness into their ongoing life. Throughout the illness, the family will need to continue to function and develop, to cope with all the continuing tasks of life, and to interact with all the issues and needs that existed prior to the diagnosis. Families, just like the client, will have to cope with a series of tasks throughout all phases of life-threatening illness, and they will have varying degrees of success in coping with the variety of problems they face (Doka, 1993).

SOCIAL SUPPORT SYSTEM

Social support can influence the client's response to grief. The visibility of a loss, such as the loss of a home resulting from disaster, often brings support from unexpected sources. The visibility of a loss, such as a facial deformity, may cause the loss of support from family or friends, thus adding to its severity. Persons experiencing less visible or invisible losses, such as early miscarriage, or losses that are often considered socially unacceptable, such as the imprisonment of a family member or the death of a gay partner, often experience less support from family or friends. When clients do not receive nonjudgmental compassion and support, they lose the vital aid that allows them to handle grief. Lack of support usually leads to difficulty in successful grief resolution (Rando, 1991).

The timing of social support is crucial. Support must be available as the griever advances through the mourning process. Active sharing by the bereaved individual and the supporters is useful in order for needed support to be available. However, even when offered, it is common for grievers not to utilize the support offered (Rando, 1984).

NATURE OF THE LOSS

The ability to resolve grief depends on the meaning of the loss and the situation surrounding it. The ability to accept help influences whether the bereaved will be able to cope with the loss. The visibility of the loss influences the support received. The duration of a change (i.e., whether it is temporary or permanent) affects the amount of time spent in reestablishing physical, psychological, and social equilibrium.

Rando (1984) coined the term *death surround* to describe factors that influence the survivor's ability to do grief work. This includes the location, type, and reason for the death and degree of the preparation for it. Ideally the survivor feels that the circumstances are appropriate; for example,

the deceased had a fulfilled life and died in familiar surroundings, and the mourner had the chance and time to prepare for the loss and complete unfinished business. However, sudden, unexpected loss can lead to slower recovery from grief. Deaths by violence through suicide, homicide, or self-neglect are even more difficult to accept. A prolonged, painful illness may leave the survivor emotionally exhausted (Rando, 1984). Other studies show that survivors of clients who were ill 6 months or less had a greater need for dependency on others, isolated themselves more, and had increased feelings of anger and hostility.

CULTURAL AND SPIRITUAL BELIEFS

Values, attitudes, beliefs, and customs are cultural aspects that influence reaction to loss, grief, and death. Cultural background and family dynamics influence expressions of grief. Culture influences each person differently (see Chapter 21). A nurse avoids stereotyping clients by culture and uses self-assessment so that judgmental or prejudicial reactions can be avoided.

Spiritual beliefs include practices, rites, and rituals (see Chapter 25). An individual may find support, comfort, and meaning in losses through spiritual beliefs. Frequently a grieving person turns to formal religion for strength and support. The nurse should be alert to the significance of religious practices, not only for the client but also for the family. Using words and actions, the nurse can be sensitive to these needs. Through openness in responses, the nurse can determine coping mechanisms that are used and plan appropriate interventions.

For some clients loss triggers questions about the meaning of life, personal values, and beliefs. Typically this is shown by the "why me?" response. Internal conflicts concerning religious beliefs may also occur. Nurses willing to do what they can to meet the dying client's spiritual needs will rely on compassion and caring coupled with a sense of what is necessary to maintain spiritual integrity (Stepnick and Perry, 1992).

LOSS OF PERSONAL LIFE GOALS

Any change in a person's ability to achieve personal goals can be a significant loss. It is critical to understand the client's goals in relation to the loss experienced. Important goal characteristics include the number of goals, how central to the client's life plan the goal is, number of pathways to goal achievement, compatibility of goals, and change in goal characteristics (temporary or permanent). The more goals a person has, the more likely the person is to be able to adapt to the loss of only one. The more central the goal, the greater the grief; for example, the amputation of the leg of a woman who has worked her whole life to become a ballerina can seem more devastating than death. If a client has many pathways or options to achieving goals, the client has more than one coping strategy. If one is not available, the client can use another. Goals shift with loss and change; for clients to make this shift, they must have hope.

HOPE

Hope is a multidimensional, changing life force. It is characterized by a confident, yet uncertain expectation of achieving a goal (Dufault and Martocchio, 1985). Hope is not a single act but a complex series of thoughts, feelings, and actions that change often. The hope of grief lies in our ability to grow. Hope usually exists throughout the experience of life-threatening illness. Hope can enhance coping skill and even influence survival (Doka, 1993). Herth (1989) found that active participation in treatment might signify both hope and coping. Clients facing terminal illness or serious loss, as well as their families, experience different dimensions of hope. At a time when the client may not be concerned about growing, they are given countless opportunities to do just that. When they are torn from a most significant relationship, they are presented with the possibility of learning more about compassion and love (Saunders, 1992). The nurse listens carefully to what the clients say their expectations for life—present and future—are, as a way of assessing their hopefulness.

Throughout the course of illness the focus of hope may change. Before the diagnosis is confirmed, hope usually centers on the symptoms either disappearing or having no serious effect. During the acute phase of illness the hope may center on the most optimistic outcome: that the illness will not be life threatening. Hope of cure or remission may continue throughout the chronic phase. In the latter periods of that phase hope may center on a slowed rate of deterioration or on a lessening of pain. In the terminal phase hope may center on surviving beyond significant milestones or events or on the relief of symptoms or pain, or may focus on an afterlife and promise of a "better place."

PHASES OF GRIEF

Observation of grieving clients allows the nurse to develop sensitivity to how loss affects people. People do not grieve in exactly the same way. However, there are patterns; for example, people in shock and disbelief act differently from those who achieve reorganization. Clients may move back and forth through phases of grief until final adjustment to life occurs without the lost object.

The ability to recognize behaviors characteristic of grieving helps the nurse make nursing diagnoses and identify means of communicating with and supporting clients and families.

GRIEF OF DYING CLIENTS AND THEIR FAMILIES

The meaning of death varies widely for individuals. Nurses primarily care for dying clients in hospitals and outpatient settings. However, as hospice organizations develop, nurses increasingly work with the terminally ill in their homes. Nurses observe client behaviors toward staff and families.

The intensity of coping and the rate at which clients pass through grief are influenced by the time between their first awareness that they are going to die and the moment of death. In an intensive care unit, clients generally recover or die quickly. Death is sudden and unexpected, and clients and families have little time for expressing grief. In contrast, the process of dying is usually more gradual in units that care for terminally ill clients. Clients have more time to work through anticipatory grief issues.

Dying clients and their significant others experience many emotions. Each emotion serves a purpose. The nurse must not identify a client's grief phase on the basis of a single behavior or emotion. However, the client's responses suggest techniques the nurse can use to relate to the client. For example, as the client and family begin to confront death, the nurse can encourage the client to discuss feelings about leaving family members behind. This would not work if the client is expressing feelings of anguish and despair.

The nurse observes for behaviors and physical symptoms that may indicate grief. Gastrointestinal tract disturbances such as indigestion, nausea and vomiting, anorexia, or a recent change in weight may indicate grieving. Persons experiencing bereavement also may complain of sleep difficulty. Fatigue and a reduced activity level may also be present. A single physical symptom, as with behaviors, does not lead to a nursing diagnosis related to grief.

The client's death takes place in a social context. Even during the dying phase, the family begins to reorganize itself; the client is no longer available to fulfill the same number and types of roles. The nurse assesses the family's grief process, recognizing that they may be dealing with different aspects of grief than the client is.

RISK FACTORS IN SURVIVORS

Numerous risk factors influence whether a person in grief will suffer psychological or physical illness during bereavement. Early identification of risk factors and appropriate nursing interventions can improve a survivor's ability to grieve effectively. Rando (1991, 1993) lists the following risk factors for survivors. High-risk factors include those associated with the specific death, such as sudden, unexpected death (especially when traumatic, violent, mutilating, or random); death from an overly lengthy illness; loss of a child; and the mourner's perception of the death as preventable. The second category includes prior and subsequent variables: a relationship with the deceased that was markedly angry, ambivalent, or dependent; accumulated unresolved losses, mourner stressors, and mental health problems; and the mourner's perceived lack of social support.

NURSES' GRIEF

Nurses may also grieve when working with clients, especially with dying clients; as a result, their roles in supporting grieving clients and family can become complicated. Nurses who are not aware of their own grief issues have more difficulty in relating to clients as unique individuals. For example, a dying client may remind the nurse of a beloved grandparent, and the nurse may become emotionally involved. The nurse working with dying clients is challenged to come to grips with mortality, understand the grief process and appreciate the experience of the dying client, use effective listening skills, acknowledge personal limits, and know when there is a need to get away and take care of the self.

 Nursing Diagnosis

The nurse gathers data to make a nursing diagnosis regarding grief or a client's reaction to it (see the diagnostic process box on p. 466). Clustering of client or family behaviors, actual or potential losses (such as loss of a significant other), and data involving the loss (such as a fatal illness) leads to an individualized nursing diagnosis (see the

Examples of NANDA Nursing Diagnoses Related to Grieving

Anticipatory grieving *related to:*
Perceived potential loss of significant other
Perceived potential loss of physiopsychosocial well-being
Perceived potential loss of personal possessions
Dysfunctional grieving *related to:*
Actual or potential object loss
Thwarted grieving response
Absence of anticipatory grieving
Chronic terminal illness
Loss of significant other
Impaired adjustment *related to:*
Incomplete grieving
Altered nutrition: less than body requirements *related to:*
Depressed grief response
Ineffective family coping: compromised *related to:*
Temporary preoccupation by a significant person who is
  trying to manage emotional conflicts and personal

suffering (anticipatory grieving) and is unable to perceive
  or act effectively in regard to client's needs
Altered family processes *related to:*
Situational transition or crisis
Hopelessness *related to:*
Failing or deteriorating physiological condition
Long-term stress
Loss of belief in transcendent values or supreme being
Social isolation *related to:*
Inadequate personal resources
Spiritual distress (distress of the human spirit) *related to:*
Separation from religious and cultural ties
Sleep pattern disturbance *related to:*
Stress of grief response

Sample Nursing Diagnostic Process for Grieving

ASSESSMENT ACTIVITIES	DEFINING CHARACTERISTICS	NURSING DIAGNOSES
Observe client's nonverbal behavior when discussing loss.	Client becomes silent and looks away when topic of loss is raised.	**Dysfunctional grieving** related to loss of health and terminal illness
Ask client and family to discuss their understanding of loss situation.	Client and family believe that illness is minor and client will fully recover.	
Observe client's behavior related to treatment.	Client attempts activities prohibited by physical condition and refuses to follow prescribed treatment.	
Assess daily activity level.	Client reports difficulty in sleeping, decreased appetite, and difficulty in concentrating.	
Assess ability to perform roles	Client withdraws from usual decision-making role in family.	
Ask client to discuss future goals and plans.	Client sighs and says, "I have no future."	**Hopelessness** related to failing physical condition
Observe client's nonverbal behavior.	Client becomes passive with little affect and turns away from speaker.	
Offer client choices and observe responses.	Client shrugs and says, "What does it matter?"	
Assess activity level.	Client refuses to eat. Client sleeps all the time, keeping blinds pulled and lights out. Client refuses to participate in care.	

nursing diagnoses box above). Identification of defining characteristics forms the basis for an accurate diagnosis as well as development of interventions in the care plan.

Behavioral signs of **dysfunctional grief** include the following:

1. Overactivity without a sense of loss
2. Alteration in relationships with friends and family
3. Hostilities against specific persons

4. Agitated depression with tension, agitation, insomnia, feelings of worthlessness, extreme guilt, and even suicidal tendencies
5. Diminished participation in religious and ritual activities related to the client's culture
6. Inability to discuss the loss without crying (particularly more than a year after the loss)
7. False sense of well-being

Sample Nursing Care Plan for Grieving

NURSING DIAGNOSIS: **Dysfunctional grieving** related to loss of health and terminal illness
DEFINITION: Dysfunctional grieving is the state in which actual or perceived object loss (object loss is used in the broadest sense) exists. Objects include people, possessions, a job, status, home, ideals, and parts and processes of the body (Kim, McFarland, and McLane, 1995).

GOAL	EXPECTED OUTCOMES	INTERVENTIONS	RATIONALE
Client will experience relief of dysfunctional grieving or evidence of absence of delayed emotional reactions within 2 months.	Client will acknowledge awareness of loss in 1 week.	Acknowledge client's grief through empathetic presence.	Accepting client's feelings as valid allows gradual acceptance of reality and all feelings of grief (Rando, 1986).
	Client will express thoughts and feelings related to loss within 2 weeks.	Listen to client and encourage sharing of emotions, such as anger, guilt, or depression, in ways most comfortable for client (e.g., verbal or nonverbal, in writing, or through art).	Expression of feelings is unique to individual. Listening to client without judgment promotes development of therapeutic relationship that will support further trust and sharing (Rando, 1984).
		Arrange meetings with others who share same experience as client.	Sharing with those experiencing similar situations decreases feelings of isolation (Lewis et al, 1989).
	Client will participate in decision making and cooperate with recommended treatments within 1 month.	Offer family time to be with client as possible and assist with care as they wish.	Encouraging time for family to be with and participate in care promotes opportunities for sharing of feelings and completion of unfinished business (Rando, 1984).
		Offer as many choices and opportunities for decision making as possible.	It is important to client's self-esteem to continue making decisions as long as possible (Leavitt et al, 1989).

Exaggerated or prolonged grief responses should be identified. It is important for the nurse to identify the appropriate related factors for the diagnosis. For example, dysfunctional grieving related to loss of a spouse will require different interventions than dysfunctional grieving related to the loss of a job (see the care plan above) (Kim et al, 1995).

The nurse may also diagnose health problems common to a grieving client (e.g., sleep pattern disturbance). These may be significant enough to require close attention and the development of a separate plan of care to address the problem.

Dying clients require special consideration when nursing diagnoses are formulated. The need to grieve is only one of these clients' many problems. Clients with terminal illnesses that cause deformities or physical disabilities are likely to undergo alterations in body image or self-concept. Examples are clients with leukemia who receive drugs that cause loss of hair and clients with bone cancer who become disabled because of chronic pain. As the clients' conditions worsen, the nurse makes diagnoses relevant to basic needs such as alterations in comfort, alterations in elimination, ineffective breathing, or sensory alterations. Because of the nature and severity of terminal illness, physical assessment data are collected frequently and can be used to validate diagnoses.

 Planning

Grieving is the natural response to loss. Grieving has a therapeutic value, enabling people to work through their losses, recollect their thoughts and feelings, and resume life with new insights and direction.

Goals for a client dealing with loss include accommodating grief, accepting the reality of the loss, regaining a sense of self-esteem, and renewing normal activities or relationships. Physiological, developmental, and spiritual needs must also be met.

When caring for dying clients, the nurse's responsibilities include considering physical needs and unique psychological and social needs. The nurse must be tolerant and willing to spend more time with dying clients, to listen to expressions of grief, and to maintain their quality of life. Additional goals for dying clients include the following:
1. Gaining and maintaining comfort
2. Maintaining independence in daily activities
3. Maintaining hope
4. Achieving spiritual comfort
5. Gaining relief from loneliness and isolation

The three most crucial needs of the dying client are control of pain, preservation of dignity and self-worth, and love and affection (Rando, 1984). Nurses are in a unique position to address these needs. Their presence can bring comfort and reduce anxiety. They can structure schedules and surroundings so that the client has a sense of security and control over life and the environment. Nurses can support the client's self-esteem by asking for opinions regarding care. Nurses encourage families to participate in decisions with the client; they encourage mutual decision making. This may help prepare the family for when the client may not be able to make choices. As circumstances and the illness change, the client changes as well. Each client and family should be treated as unique, with recognition that their needs, fears, hopes, expectations, and concerns will change throughout the illness. Continuing reevaluation and planning are mandatory.

The dying client may be concerned with the circumstances and grief of those left behind. In addition to needing help with problems related to the illness and its emotional stresses, clients often need assistance with financial problems, changes in social and sexual relationships, and difficulties in dealing with the hospital. The formation of an interdisciplinary team is critical. The team may include the client, family, physicians, nurses, psychologists, social workers, clergy, pharmacists, physical and occupational therapists, dietitians, and volunteers. Using an interdisciplinary perspective, the nurse can address many potential practical problems before they become overwhelming.

 ## Implementation

A sensitivity to the client is most important in order for the nurse to function effectively. Nurses will also need to be sensitive to the culture, ethnicity, lifestyle, or social class of the client and family. They will need to be sensitive to the limits and nature of their own roles. They will need to intervene sensitively and skillfully when appropriate. If nurses wish to avoid the awesome emotional costs that can be experienced when one forms a bond with clients engaged in a life-and-death struggle, they will need to be sensitive to their own needs (Doka, 1993).

THERAPEUTIC COMMUNICATION

Nursing care of the grieving client begins with establishing the significance of the loss. This is difficult if the client is unwilling to express feelings or is experiencing shock or denial. The nurse observes the response to loss and then attempts to identify the client's strengths in dealing with it. The nurse uses open-ended questions and reflective statements such as "You appear concerned about your brother's condition" or "When the doctor informed you about the test results, you appeared frightened. What were you thinking?" These responses are respectful and give importance to the person's feelings. The nurse must schedule adequate private time with the client and family to promote open communication. Open communication tries to accomplish the following goals: (1) It lets the client set the pace and tone. (2) It is reflective: it allows clients to find the answers to their own questions. (3) It provides reassurance that any topic is open to consideration (Doka, 1993). The nurse shows acceptance of all grief reactions. For example, if a client begins to cry, the nurse quietly remains ready to offer comfort, rather than abandoning the client at the time of greatest need. Acknowledging grief through touch and concern promotes trust.

If clients choose not to share feelings or do not wish to be touched, the nurse can offer a willingness to be available when needed. It is also important to recognize clients' normal styles of dealing with difficult situations. If they do not normally talk about their feelings, they are unlikely to discuss feelings regarding loss. It is helpful to ask clients how they normally deal with difficult situations.

When considering a client's potential reactions to loss, the nurse is alert to expressions of denial, anger, depression, or guilt. Initial denial is normal. If the nurse encourages the client to face the loss too soon, the nurse may cause the client to feel depressed, upset, and confused or to further withdraw from reality.

The nurse often becomes the target of client or family anger. Because it is difficult not to take anger personally, the nurse may respond by avoiding the client and family. To deal effectively with anger, the nurse must examine personal feelings and responses to anger. With increased awareness of personal responses to anger, the nurse is better able to encourage the client's expression of anger. The nurse lets the client and family know that such expressions are normal. For example, the nurse might say "You are obviously upset. So are most people in this situation. I just want to let you know I'm available to talk if you'd like."

The nurse should not erect barriers to communication (see Chapter 14). Communication is blocked by denying the client's grief, providing false reassurance, or avoiding discussion of the problem. For example, when a client expresses anger about a terminal illness, the nurse avoids making statements such as "Don't worry, you'll probably outlive us all" or "Since you're upset, why don't we discuss something else?" Instead the nurse should support the client's expressions of anger by staying close and making statements such as "It doesn't seem fair" or "Go ahead and let your feelings out, I'll stay with you."

The nurse also avoids giving advice or analyzing possible causes for loss or behavior. Statements such as "It was God's will" or "You'd feel better if you interacted more with others" do not convey understanding of the client's sorrow and pain. The nurse must avoid giving false reassurance. Although the purpose may be encouragement, a statement such as "At least you still have your mother" can discount a client's true feelings.

No topic that a dying client wishes to discuss should be avoided. The client is more likely to talk about death with someone who listens and expresses sincere concern and caring. The client may initially test the nurse by offering a statement that does not express true concerns. For example, the client may make an open-ended statement such as "My doctor talked with me today," hoping that the nurse will respond.

Many times issues that arise in care giving will be affected by treatment goals, that is, whether the goal is aggressive treatment with the hope of recovery or palliative when there is no chance of recovery. When the expectations of the client and families differ from those of the health care team, the nurse must tread carefully. An ill person's hopes may be explored and should be what sets the pace. A person's sense of hope and defenses ought not be assaulted to obtain agreement with the treatment team's goals. The client's hope should not expire before he or she dies (Doka, 1993).

Table 26-3	**Promoting Comfort in the Terminally Ill Client**

CHARACTERISTICS OR CAUSES	NURSING IMPLICATIONS
PAIN Pain can be acute or chronic. Pain from progressive cancer is usually chronic and constant.	Administer narcotic analgesics on regular schedule (see Chapter 43). Use relaxation, guided imagery, distraction, and peripheral nerve stimulators to provide relief. Use combinations of analgesics or other therapies as client's needs change. Administer narcotics as ordered. (Oral route for narcotics is preferred, but rectal suppositories, injections, continuous intravenous infusions, and intrathecal infusions are available.)
Any source of physical irritation may worsen pain.	Minimize irritants through skin care, including daily baths, lubrication of skin, frequent repositioning, and dry, clean bed linens.
As client approaches death, mouth remains open, tongue becomes dry and edematous, and lips become dry and cracked. Blinking reflexes diminish near death, causing drying of cornea.	Provide frequent oral care every 2 to 4 hours. Use soft toothbrushes or foam swabs for frequent mouth care. Apply light film of petroleum jelly to lips and tongue (see Chapter 40). Remove crusts from eyelid margins and provide eye care. Reduce corneal drying with artificial tears.
NAUSEA AND VOMITING Nausea and vomiting result from disease process (e.g., gastric cancer), complications (e.g., bowel obstruction), or medications.	Confer with physician about changing medications when possible. Administer antiemetic before meals. Ask physician about providing relief from obstruction with bowel decompression with insertion of nasogastric tube. Provide mouth care and promptly clean up emesis.
FATIGUE Metabolic demands of cancerous tumor cause weakness and fatigue.	Set mutual goals with client after identifying valued or desired tasks, and conserve client's energy for only those tasks. Provide frequent rest periods in quiet environment. Time and pace nursing activities to conserve client's energy.
CONSTIPATION Narcotic medications and immobility slow peristalsis. Lack of bulk in diet or reduced fluid intake may occur with appetite changes.	Provide preventive care, including increasing fluid intake (e.g., bran, whole grain products, and fresh vegetables in diet) and encouraging exercise.
DIARRHEA Diarrhea results from disease process (e.g., colon cancer) and complications of treatment or medications.	Assess for fecal impaction. Confer with physician to change medication if possible. Provide low-residue diet (see Chapter 41).
URINARY INCONTINENCE Urinary incontinence results from progressive disease (e.g., involvement of spinal cord or reduced level of consciousness).	Protect skin from irritation or breakdown using absorbent pads and clean linen. Prepare for possible use of indwelling urinary or condom catheter.
INADEQUATE NUTRITION Nausea and vomiting can decrease appetite. Depression from grieving may cause anorexia.	Suggest that smaller portions and bland foods may be more palatable (see Chapter 41). Allow home-cooked meals, which may be preferred by client and gives family chance to participate.
DEHYDRATION As disease progresses, client is less willing or able to maintain oral fluid intake. Certain forms of cancer cause obstruction to portions of gastrointestinal tract.	Provide relief of thirst by using ice chips, sips of fluids, or moist cloth to lips. Provide frequent mouth care (see Chapter 40).
INEFFECTIVE BREATHING PATTERNS Causes include disease progression involving lung tissue capacity, pneumonia, and pulmonary edema. Clients may also be severely anemic, causing reduced oxygen capacity.	Position client upright to improve breathing capacity. Administer supplemental oxygen as ordered. Administer bronchodilator as ordered. Administer narcotics as ordered to suppress cough and ease breathing and apprehension. Suction accumulated secretions from mouth and throat (see Chapter 44).

From Marino L: *Cancer nursing*, St Louis, 1981, Mosby.

When a client loses all hope, there may be premature psychological and then physical surrender to death. This depends on the client's perception of self-worth and effectiveness. The nurse supports hope by helping the client retain control, dignity, and self-esteem. This is done by focusing on the present and immediate future, by emphasizing remaining potentials and abilities, and by structuring life events to render a sense of predictability and continuity. The nurse looks for ways to foster accomplishments that cause satisfaction and anticipation. The nurse encourages the client and family to reminisce about previous joys and fulfillments.

Refusal to die or accept the feeling of helplessness is a motivator. Clients who remain confident and determined, despite severe illness, are better able to tolerate the side effects of treatment and often live longer than predicted. By teaching and helping clients and families to identify the early signs of hopelessness and despair (such as asking few questions about treatment, avoiding discussions of the client's condition, refusing to eat, or ignoring efforts to maintain personal hygiene), the nurse can help the client assume healthier behaviors.

The nurse has limitations when attempting to provide appropriate interventions for grieving clients. The nurse may not have the time to address all the needs of terminally ill clients. In this case it is important to use other resources within the health care setting and community. When other professionals are needed, the nurse explores with the client and family alternatives in selecting resource persons, community agencies, or groups to enhance grief work. Self-help, bereavement, widow-to-widow, and parent groups are available in some communities. Signs of unresolved grief and pathological grieving may require referral to a psychologist, psychiatrist, or counselor.

MAINTENANCE OF SELF-ESTEEM

Nursing interventions focus on promoting a sense of identity, dignity, and self-esteem (see Chapter 23). The nurse can help by listening, responding quickly and positively to requests, maintaining confidentiality, and providing comfort and support. The quality and quantity of the time spent with the client create a therapeutic environment for the grieving process. Measures that provide comfort and support should be implemented in a caring, pleasant manner to reinforce the client's feelings of self-worth and dignity and to decrease the fear of rejection, isolation, and sense of hopelessness.

Self-esteem and dignity complement each other. Dignity is the ability to maintain self-concept. The disabilities of dying clients may threaten dignity. Care givers often take control of these clients' lives. Taking away the right to make decisions about care fosters hopelessness and feelings of despair, and clients may lose their will to live. To maintain self-esteem, clients must believe that their opinions are valuable in decisions that affect their dying.

The nurse can promote self-esteem by giving attention to the client's appearance. Cleanliness, a lack of body odors, attractive clothing, and personal grooming (shaving or well-groomed hair) promote sense of worth. The nurse who manages the client's body functions must show an attitude of respect and helpfulness rather than encourage dependence or guilt.

PROMOTION OF RETURN-TO-LIFE ACTIVITIES

As clients and their families begin to confront their losses, it is important for the nurse to encourage a return to their normal lifestyles within the limits of the situation. If clients and families are able to express grief openly and progress through the grief process with support and understanding, adjustment to their losses is easier. Depending on the nature of the loss, many demands may be placed on family resources.

CARE OF DYING CLIENTS AND THEIR FAMILIES

Nursing care of the terminally ill client can be demanding and stressful. However, helping a dying person retain dignity can be one of nursing's greatest rewards. A client may experience many symptoms for months before death occurs. The nurse can share the dying client's suffering and intervene in a way that improves the quality of life. A dying client must be cared for with respect and concern.

Promotion of Comfort. Comfort for dying clients includes acknowledgment of and relief of psychobiological distress (Oncology Nursing Society and the American Nurses Association, 1979). The nurse provides a variety of comfort measures for terminally ill clients (Table 26-3). Pain control is important because pain alters sleep, appetite, mobility, and psychological function. Fear of pain is common in cancer clients. The sooner dying clients obtain pain relief, the more energy they have for participating in quality-of-life activities. Providing comfort for terminally ill clients also involves controlling the symptoms of disease or the therapies administered.

Personal hygiene is a routine part of keeping the terminally ill client comfortable. The client may eventually depend on the nurse or family for basic needs. The client may be embarrassed by this dependence. When possible, clients make their own decisions about care.

Maintenance of Independence. An important choice for a dying client is choosing a location of care. There are options other than the acute care hospital. Hospice care (see later section) allows comprehensive care in the home. The nurse should inform clients about these options.

Most dying clients want to be as self-sufficient as possible. Allowing the client to perform simple tasks such as bathing, putting on eyeglasses, and eating maintains dignity and sense of worth. When a client becomes physically unable to perform self-care, the nurse encourages participation in decision making to give a sense of control. The nurse looks for nonverbal cues that suggest unwillingness to participate in care. The nurse should not force participation, particularly if physical limitations make it difficult. Families, in their concern, often have a tendency to take over for the client. The nurse can encourage the family to allow the client to make decisions. When care occurs in the home, normal routines may be established to help create a sense of control.

Prevention of Loneliness and Isolation. If the nurse is detached and avoids discussion of the situation, dying clients may experience overwhelming loneliness. It takes caring and experience for a nurse to respond effectively to dying clients. Often a nurse who has not cared for dying clients finds it difficult to provide the necessary support for those who die. Death symbolizes failure for many health care providers. Furthermore, the process of dying may cause clients to be unpleasant. If conditions cause offensive odors, incontinence, confusion, or combativeness, nurses may avoid clients. In hospitals, dying persons are often confined to private rooms to avoid exposing others to suffering. The room may be dimly lit, the curtains may be drawn, and sounds are reduced. Without meaningful sensory stimulation, dying people may feel abandoned and isolated.

To prevent loneliness and sensory deprivation, the nurse intervenes to improve the quality of the environment. Dying clients should not be routinely placed in private rooms in out-of-the-way locations. Clients feel a sense of involvement when sharing a room and watching the nurse's activities. The client can then also share conversation and companionship with roommates and visitors. When the client dies, however, the nurse should give attention to the roommate because watching a person die can be frightening.

Providing meaningful environmental stimulation comforts the client. Rooms in the hospital or home should be well lit and attractively decorated and should offer a stimulating view. Pictures, cherished objects, cards or letters from family members, and live plants console the client.

Perhaps most important in preventing loneliness is the client's involvement with family members and friends. Family and friends can more easily interact with the client in the home. In a hospital or extended care facility, visitors should be allowed to remain with the dying client at any time. If the client shares a room, however, the nurse should be sure that visitors do not disturb the roommate. If several family members visit or want to stay with the client, a private room may be necessary. The dying client becomes particularly lonely at night and may feel more secure if someone stays at the bedside. The nurse should know how to contact family members if a visit is requested or the client's condition worsens.

Clients should have someone be with them at the time of death. Nurses should not feel guilty if they cannot always provide this support. However, care may require long intervals of time with the client. The nurse should try to stay with dying clients when needed and show concern and compassion. To provide the care needed by the dying client, it may be necessary to ask for help from other nurses. It is also important to encourage and support the family or significant others to stay with the client.

Promotion of Spiritual Comfort. Providing spiritual comfort means much more than asking spiritual advisers to visit (see Chapter 25). The nurse can support the client in the expression of a philosophy of life. As death approaches, the client often seeks comfort by analyzing values and beliefs related to life and death. The nurse and family can assist the client by listening and encouraging expressions of beliefs and values. A dying client may seek to find purpose and meaning to life before surrendering to death. Dying clients may feel guilt if their lives are perceived as unfulfilled. The client may seek forgiveness, either from a supreme being or family members. Additional spiritual needs are hope and love. Love can best be expressed through kind, compassionate care.

The nurse or family can provide spiritual comfort by using therapeutic communication skills, expressing empathy, praying with the client, reading inspirational literature, and playing music. Prayer should be offered only at the request of the client or family. Reciting prayers or praying as a means to close a discussion does not address the client's feelings (Stepnick and Perry, 1992).

Support for the Grieving Family. Family members must be supported through the dying and death of their loved one and, at the same time, be encouraged to provide support. In an institutional setting families often have greater difficulty giving support (see the box below). The nurse must recognize the value of family members as resources and assist them in being with the dying person (see the box on p. 472).

Acknowledging grief is the nurse's first step in developing a supportive relationship with the family. When the family senses the nurse's concern, they are often more willing to share feelings. When the client is in a hospital, the nurse can ease family anxieties and fears by explaining equipment that is used. Most families want to know where a tube or equipment is located in the body, whether it hurts, why is it needed, and when it will be removed (Doka, 1993).

Before using family members as resources, the nurse must determine whether they want to be involved. Some do not. The nurse assesses the family's role as observer, comforter, or care giver. Their roles may change often.

Suggestions for Involving the Family in the Care of a Dying Client

- Assist in planning a visitation schedule for family members to prevent client and family from becoming fatigued.
- Allow young children to visit a dying parent when the client is able to communicate.
- Be willing to listen to family complaints about the client's care and feelings about the client.
- Help family members learn to interact with the dying person (e.g., using attentive listening, avoiding false reassurances, conducting conversations about normal family activities or problems).
- Allow family members to help with simple care measures such as feeding, bathing, and straightening bed linen. Recognize that family members are often more successful than nursing staff in persuading the client to eat.
- When the family becomes fatigued with care activities, relieve them from their duties so that they can acquire needed rest and support. Refer them to resources for meals and lodging.
- Support the act of grieving between client and family. Provide privacy when preferred. Do not discourage open expression of grief between family and client.
- Provide information daily with regard to the client's condition. Prepare the family for sudden changes in the client's appearance and behavior.
- Communicate news of impending death when the family is together, if possible. Remember that members can provide support for one another. Convey the news in a private area, and be willing to stay with the family.
- As death nears, help the family stay in communication with the dying person through short visits, caring silence, touch, and telling the client of their love.
- After death, assist the family with decision making, such as selection of a mortician, transportation of family members, and collection of the client's belongings.

CLIENT TEACHING
for the Dying Client's Family

OBJECTIVE
- The family will be able to demonstrate basic client care measures.

TEACHING STRATEGIES
- Describe and demonstrate feeding techniques and selection of foods to facilitate ease of chewing and swallowing.
- Demonstrate bathing, mouth care, and other hygiene measures, and allow family to perform return demonstration.
- Show video on simple transfer techniques to prevent injury to themselves and the client; help family to practice.
- Instruct family on need to enforce rest periods.
- Teach family to recognize signs and symptoms to expect as the client's condition worsens and information on whom to call in an emergency.
- Discuss ways to support the dying person and listen to needs and fears.
- Solicit questions from family and provide information as needed.

EVALUATION
- Family will perform client care independently.
- Observe the family and client interacting using effective communication skills.

Tissues and Organs Used for Transplant

NONVITAL TISSUES	VITAL ORGANS*
■ Corneas	■ Heart
■ Skin	■ Liver
■ Long bones	■ Lungs
■ Middle ear bones	■ Kidneys
	■ Pancreas

*These organs are recovered after a client is pronounced clinically dead or brain dead; circulatory and ventilatory support is maintained to perfuse the organs before removal.

In the home the family becomes closely involved in the client's care. They need to know what to expect. A terminal illness places heavy demands on social and financial resources. The emotional strain often disrupts normal communication channels. The family may become afraid to interact with the client. Benoliel (1985) describes circumstances that make it difficult for families to cope with demands of terminal illness. These include a lengthy period of dying, symptoms that are difficult to control, unpleasant sights and smells, limited coping resources, and poor relationships with care givers.

Hospice Care. Hospices were well established as early as the fifth century A.D. but almost disappeared until the 1800s. A desire to change traditional care for the dying has led to the reestablishment of hospice programs. A hospice program is family-centered care designed to help terminally ill clients be comfortable and maintain a lifestyle as close to normal as possible throughout the process of dying. Most clients in hospice programs have 6 months or less to live. Hospice programs began in Ireland in 1879, were then established in England, and reached the United States and Canada in the 1970s (Kastenbaum, 1991).

There are several types of hospice programs. Acute care hospitals and long-term care facilities often have separate units or designated beds for hospice care. A trained interdisciplinary team works with clients and families. The home care component of a hospice is operated by a hospital or separate home health care agency. In addition to hospice programs affiliated with hospitals and long-term care

facilities, there are those which care for clients in their homes. Pitorak (1985) describes the following components of hospice care:

1. Coordinated home care with available inpatient beds under hospital administration
2. Control of symptoms (physical, sociological, psychological, and spiritual)
3. Physician-directed services
4. Provision of an interdisciplinary care team of physicians, nurses, spiritual advisers, social workers, and counselors
5. Medical and nursing services available at all times
6. Client and family as the unit of care
7. Bereavement follow-up after a client's death
8. Use of trained volunteers as a part of the team
9. Acceptance into the program on the basis of health care needs rather than ability to pay

A hospice program emphasizes **palliative treatment**, which is the control of symptoms rather than curative treatment of disease. The client and family participate in care. Client care is coordinated between the home and inpatient setting. Efforts are directed at keeping the client at home as much as possible. The family becomes the primary care giver, administering medication and treatment, and the interdisciplinary team provides psychological and physical resources needed for family support.

CARE AFTER DEATH

In most states the physician is responsible for certifying a death in the medical record by recording the time of death and a description of therapies or actions taken. The physician may request permission from the family for an **autopsy.** Autopsies are required in circumstances of unusual death (e.g., violent trauma or unexpected death in the home).

Federal legislation requires hospitals to formulate policies and procedures for the identification and referral of potential donors to procurement agencies or tissue banks (see the box above). Hospital policies are meant to ensure that families of appropriate potential donors are provided the option of organ, eye, or tissue donation. Discussions of donations should be performed in a sensitive, caring manner. A trained staff member, often a nurse, discusses donation with families or guardians, making certain that they understand that donation is an option and that it is all right not to donate.

The nurse may be the best person to care for the client's body after death because of the therapeutic nurse-client relationship developed during the illness phase; thus the nurse may be more sensitive to the need of caring for the client's body with dignity and sensitivity. After death the body undergoes a number of physical changes (Table 26-4). The body should be cared for as soon as possible after death to prevent tissue damage or disfigurement. If the family requests organ donation, appropriate measures must be taken immediately.

The nurse offers the family the opportunity to view the body. It may help to suggest that this is an opportunity to say "good-bye" to their loved one, especially if they were not present at the time of death. If the family hesitates, the nurse lets them think about it. If they decide not to view the body, the nurse accepts their decision without judgment. If the family decides to view the body, they are assured that they will not be alone. The nurse will be glad to accompany them or will arrange for whomever they would like to be with them. The nurse spends as much time as possible assisting the grieving family and offers to contact other support services, such as social services and the spiritual adviser. The family now becomes the client.

Before the family views the body the nurse prepares it and the room to minimize the stress of the experience (see Table 26-4). The nurse removes supplies and equipment from sight. Tubes remaining in the body are removed, clamped, or cut to within 2.5 cm (1 inch) of the skin and taped in place. Care of tubes and specimens depends on agency policy, as well as on whether an autopsy will be performed. Dirty linen and other clutter should be removed. A spray deodorizer eliminates unpleasant odors.

The nurse prepares the body by making it look as natural and comfortable as possible. It is placed in a supine position with arms at the sides, palms down, or across the abdomen. The nurse places a small pillow or folded towel under the head to prevent discoloration from blood pooling. The eyelids usually remain closed if gently held down for a few seconds. If this does not work, a moistened cotton ball will hold them in place.

The nurse should insert the client's dentures to maintain normal facial features. A rolled-up towel under the chin will keep the mouth closed. The nurse washes soiled body parts, dresses the body in a clean gown, combs or brushes the hair, and covers the body to the shoulders with clean linen. The family may want to participate in this process and should be given the opportunity. Most shroud kits contain absorbent pads placed under the perineal and rectal area to collect oozing feces or urine from relaxed sphincter muscles. The nurse removes jewelry and presents it and other valuables to the family. In some agencies wedding bands may be left in place as long as they are taped securely to the finger.

After the body is prepared, the family is invited into the room. Generally, family members cope best if they are not alone. The nurse or another family member should be there to provide emotional support. The nurse can model loving acceptance of the body by calling it by name, gently stroking the head or holding the hand and saying "Good-bye John, we'll really miss you," or whatever is appropriate to the situation. It is important not to rush the family while they spend time with the deceased.

After the family leaves, according to specific hospital policy, the nurse places tags containing name and other information on the deceased client's wrist and ankle or toe. The gown is removed, and the body is wrapped completely in a shroud, a large bag or rectangular piece of plastic or cotton material. Another identification tag is placed on the shroud. If a client had a transmissible infection, special labeling is used to alert those who move and store the remains. The body is then transported to the morgue, or the mortician picks it up from the client's room. Methods for transporting the body through hallways vary between institutions.

Nurses are also responsible for disposing of the deceased's personal belongings and noting this in the medical record. The nurse can check with the client's family about taking the belongings or ensure that they are transported with the deceased. If the family or friends have left, the nurse contacts a supervisor. No clothing, dentures, plants, gifts, hairpieces, or other personal items are discarded.

Table 26-4	**Physiological Changes After Death**	
CHANGE	**RELATED INTERVENTIONS**
Stiffening of body (rigor mortis), developing 2 to 4 hours after death (involves contraction of skeletal and smooth muscle from lack of adenosine triphosphate)	Before rigor mortis develops, position body in normal anatomical alignment, close eyelids and mouth, and insert dentures in mouth.
Reduction in body temperature with loss of skin elasticity (algor mortis)	Remove tape and dressings gently to avoid tissue breakdown. Avoid pulling on skin or body parts.
Purple discoloration of skin (livor mortis) in dependent areas from breakdown of red blood cells	Elevate head to prevent facial discoloration.
Softening and liquifying of body tissues by bacterial fermentation	Store body in cool place in hospital morgue or other designated area.

Sample Evaluation of Interventions for Grieving

GOALS	EVALUATIVE MEASURES	EXPECTED OUTCOMES
Client will experience relief or dysfunctional grieving or evidence of absence of delayed emotional reaction within 2 months.	Observe client discussing loss with significant other.	Client will acknowledge awareness of loss in 1 week.
Client will gain sense of self-esteem within 2 months.	Observe client's behaviors. Ask client to talk about feelings of loss. Observe client's appearance and grooming habits.	Client will express thoughts and feelings related to loss within 2 weeks. Client will maintain neat, well-groomed appearance.
	Observe client's willingness to interact with others.	Client will initiate discussion with nurse and family about future.
Client will return to routines of daily living within 2 weeks.	Observe client's involvement in self-care activities. Ask client to discuss plans.	Client will resume self-care activities. Client will verbalize decisions about care.
	Evaluate client's level of participation in social activities with family.	Client will participate in more social activities.

CARING FOR THE NURSE

Nurses working with critically or terminally ill clients also experience grief (Fig. 26-2). Grief is the natural response to loss, and each loss needs to be grieved. When nurses experience multiple losses and fail to adequately process them, they can experience bereavement overload. They experience frustration, anger, guilt, sadness, helplessness, anxiety, depression, and feelings of being overwhelmed. Self-care is critical to survival. Nurses need to do for themselves what they do for their clients and families. They need to mourn their losses. This is done on an individual basis and as part of a larger group caring for the client. Nurses need to develop personal support systems that allow time away from the care giving setting; opportunities to share feelings in nonjudgmental, open relationships; and use of stress management techniques that restore energy (see Chapter 22).

Sometimes the institution provides opportunities for staff to get together for mutual support and for closure and grieving over the loss of a client. Nurses' roles in the care of the dying and bereaved are filled with experiences that bring grief and stress. They must attend to the need for relief from these demands. Unrelieved grief and stress can lead to diminished well-being and inability to care for others.

Evaluation

Although completion of grief work may require months or years, most clients are under a nurse's care only a short time. The nurse may become frustrated when, just as the client or family begins to express grief, the client leaves the health care institution or dies. Grieving is an individual process, and resolution of loss does not follow a set schedule. It is important for the client to discuss or share the experience with significant others. The goals established with the client and family become the bases for evaluation; for example, if one of the goals is for the client to communicate love and caring to the family, the nurse would evaluate whether this has occurred in verbal or written form. The nurse also observes the quality of interactions (see the evaluation box on above).

The care of the dying client requires the nurse to evaluate the client's level of comfort with illness and quality of life. The success of the evaluation depends partly on the bond formed with the client. Unless the client trusts the nurse, expression of true feelings and concerns is unlikely. The client's level of comfort is evaluated on the basis of outcomes such as a reduction in pain, control of symptoms, maintenance of functioning body systems, accomplishment of unfinished tasks, and emotional comfort.

Fig. 26-2 Nurses benefit from support of colleagues during their time of loss.

■ KEY CONCEPTS ■

▶ The grieving process involves a set of emotional, cognitive, and behavioral responses to an actual or perceived loss.

▶ Grieving integrates and accommodates loss to achieve more effective functioning.

▶ Individuals experience different aspects of the grieving process at different times.

▶ The phases of the grieving process vary among theories but progress from distress and shock to resolution and accommodation.

▶ Losses may lead to a grief response similar to that occurring following a death.

▶ A nurse's support of a client's hope can help relieve grieving associated with a loss.

▶ During assessment the nurse considers physical and behavioral characteristics that suggest the client is grieving.

▶ Risk factors (e.g., physical health) indicate the possibility that a person in grief will suffer psychological or physical illness during bereavement.

▶ Nursing diagnoses focus on the type of grief experienced by clients or health-related problems common to grieving clients.

▶ Therapeutic communication helps the nurse assist the grieving and the dying client in coping with loss.

▶ Nursing care of the grieving and dying client should promote a sense of identity, dignity, and self-esteem.

▶ Nursing interventions to promote return-to-life activities assist the client in accommodating grief and accepting the loss.

▶ Nursing care of the terminally ill client focuses on promoting comfort and improving the quality of remaining life.

▶ As death approaches, a client reviews and analyzes values and beliefs pertinent to the meaning of life and death.

▶ A nurse assesses whether family members are willing to be involved in a dying client's care before using them as resources.

▶ Care after death includes caring for the body with dignity and sensitivity.

▶ The evaluation of nursing care for the grieving and dying client is based on identifiable behavioral changes through the grieving process.

▶ The nurse's own loss history influences responses to client losses.

▶ Nurses who work with critically or terminally ill clients experience loss and grief.

▶ Nurses need to be aware of and mourn their own losses on an ongoing basis to avoid bereavement overload.

■ KEY TERMS ■

Anticipatory grief, p. 460

Autopsy, p. 472

Bereavement, p. 459

Disenfranchised grief, p. 460

Dysfunctional grief, p. 466

Grief, p. 459

Grieving process, p. 460

Hope, p. 464

Maturational loss, p. 458

Mourning, p. 459

Palliative treatment, p. 472

Situational loss, p. 458

■ CRITICAL THINKING EXERCISES ■

1. You are caring for a 16-year-old male accident victim, who lost his right leg in the accident. It has been 2 weeks since the accident, and you notice that he has become progressively withdrawn. He refuses to do physical therapy or anything for himself. You suspect that he is grieving but are not sure. Describe how you would approach the client and what you would assess.

2. Your 65-year-old client, Mrs. White, has been acting depressed. When you ask her what is happening, she tells you that she lost her husband of 50 years 6 months before. Her children have been telling her that she should sell her house and get on with her life. She says there must be something wrong with her because she "just can't forget" her husband. What would your response be, and what would you teach her about the grieving process?

3. You have been spending a lot of time with Mr. Charles. Your instructor says you spend far too much time with him. His condition has progressively deteriorated, and you find yourself thinking about him all the time. You do not trust anyone else to get him the care you know he needs. Your instructor comments on your attachment to the client and asks you to reflect on what is influencing your response to the client. What might be some factors that would influence a nurse to become overly attached to a client, and how would you recommend dealing with this situation?

REFERENCES

Anderson KL, Dimond MF: The experience of bereavement in older adults, *J Adv Nurs* 22:308, 1995.

Benoliel JQ: Loss and terminal illness, *Nurs Clin North Am* 20:439, 1985.

Doka KJ: *Living with life-threatening illness: a guide for patients, their families, and caregivers,* New York, 1993, Lexington.

Dufault K, Martocchio BC: Hope: its spheres and dimensions, *Nurs Clin North Am* 20:379, 1985.

Engel GL: Grief and grieving, *Am J Nurs* 64:93, 1964.

Harper JM: Plateaus of acceptance: pits of pain. In Corr CA, Stillion JM, Ribar MC, editors: *Creativity in death education and counseling*, Hartford, Conn, 1983, Forum for Death Education and Counseling, pp 91-104.

Hepburn A: What do we really know about grief counseling? Exploring the contemporary challenges of multiculturalism, postmodernism, and imaginal psychology, *Forum Newslett* 20(6):7, 1994.

Herth KA: The relationship between level of hope and level of coping response and other variables in patients with cancer, *Oncol Nurs Forum* 16(1):67, 1989.

Kastenbaum RJ: *Death, society and human experience*, ed 4, New York, 1991, Macmillan.

Kim MJ, McFarland GK, McLane AM: *Pocket guide to nursing diagnoses*, ed 6, St Louis, 1995, Mosby.

Kübler-Ross E: *On death and dying*, New York, 1969, Macmillan.

Leavitt PF et al: The patient who is dying. In Lewis S et al: *Manual of psychosocial nursing interventions: promoting mental health in medical-surgical settings*, Philadelphia, 1989, Saunders.

Lindemann E: Symptomatology and management of acute grief. In Parad H, editor: *Crisis intervention*, New York, 1965, Family Association of America.

Lewis S et al: *Manual of psychosocial nursing interventions: promoting mental health in medical-surgical settings*, Philadelphia, 1989, Saunders.

Marino L: *Cancer nursing*, St Louis, 1981, Mosby.

Oncology Nursing Society and the American Nurses Association: *Outcome standards for cancer nursing practice*, Kansas City, Mo, 1979, The Association.

Pitorak EF: Establishing a medicare-certified inpatient unit, *Nurs Clin North Am* 20:311, 1985.

Rando TA: *Grief, dying and death*, Champaign, Ill, 1984, Research.

Rando TA: *How to go on living when someone you love dies*, New York, 1991, Bantam.

Rando TA: *Loss and anticipatory grief*, Lexington, Mass, 1986, Lexington.

Rando TA: *Treatment of complicated mourning*, Champaign, Ill, 1993, Research.

Raphael B: *The anatomy of bereavement*, New York, 1983, Basic.

Saunders CM: *Surviving grief and learning to live again*, New York, 1992, John Wiley & Sons.

Schaefer D, Lyons C: *How do we tell the children? Helping children understand and cope when someone dies*, New York, 1986, Newmarket.

Stepnick A , Perry T: Preventing spiritual distress in the dying client, *J Psychosoc Nurs* 30(1):17, 1992.

Wheeler SR, Pike MM: Families' responses to the loss of a child. In Fawcett CS, editor: *Famly psychiatric nursing*, St Louis, 1993, Mosby.

Worden JW: *Grief counseling and grief therapy*, New York, 1982, Springer.

ADDITIONAL READINGS

Bateman A et al: Dysfunctional grieving, *J Psychosoc Nurs* 30(12):5, 1992.

Cowles KV, Rodgers BL: The concept of grief: a foundation for nursing research and practice, *Res Nurs Health* 14:119, 1991.

DeSpelder LS, Strickland AL: *The last dance: encountering death and dying*, Mountain View, Calif, 1987, Mayfield.

Ebersole P, Hess P: *Toward healthy aging: human needs and nursing responses*, ed 3, St Louis, 1990, Mosby.

Ellison V: Grief, bereavement and hope, *Forum Newslett* 20 (3):7, 1994.

Grollman EA: *Straight talk about death for teenagers: how to cope with losing someone you love*, Boston, 1993, Beacon.

Irish DP et al: *Ethnic variations in dying, death, and grief: diversity in universality*, Washington, DC, 1993, Taylor and Francis.

Jacob SR: An analysis of the concept of grief, *J Adv Nurs* 18:1787, 1993.

Johnston NE: Culturally relevant care in mental health. In Bauman A, Johnston NE, Antai-Ontong D, editors: *Decision making in psychiatric and psychosocial nursing*, Philadelphia, 1990, BC Decker.

Johnston J: Organ and tissue transplantation: what's in it for the donor family? *Forum Newslett* 20(3):7, 1994,

Musgrave CF: The ethical and legal implications of hospice care: an international overview, *Cancer Nurs* 10:183, 1987.

O'Connor AP: Understanding the cancer patient's search for meaning, *Cancer Nurs* 13:167, 1990.

Perryman JP: Providing the option to donate, *Forum Newslett* 13:6, 1989.

Rawlins RP, Heacock PE: *Clinical manual of psychiatric nursing*, ed 2, St Louis, 1993, Mosby.

Redmond LM: *Surviving when someone you love was murdered: a professional's guide to group grief therapy for families and friends of murder victims*, Clearwater, Fla, 1990, Psychological Consultation and Education Services.

Sperle K: Will I lose him again? *Forum Newslett* 20(2):5, 1994.

Steele LL: The death surround: factors influencing the grief experience of survivors, *Oncol Nurs Forum* 17(2):235, 1990.

Stroebe W, Stroebe MS: Is grief universal? Cultural variations in the emotional reaction to loss. In Fulton R, Bendiksen R, editors: *Death and identity*, ed 3, Philadelphia, 1994, Charles.

Wegmann JA: Hospice home death, hospital death, and coping abilities of widows, *Cancer Nurs* 10:148, 1987.

Werner-Beland JA: *Grief response of long-term illness and disability*, Reston, Va, 1980, Reston.

Wolfelt AD: Understanding the trend toward deritualization of the funeral, *Forum Newlett* 20(6):1, 1994.

Zisook S, editor: *Biopyschosocial aspects of bereavement*, Washington, DC, 1987, American Psychiatric Press.

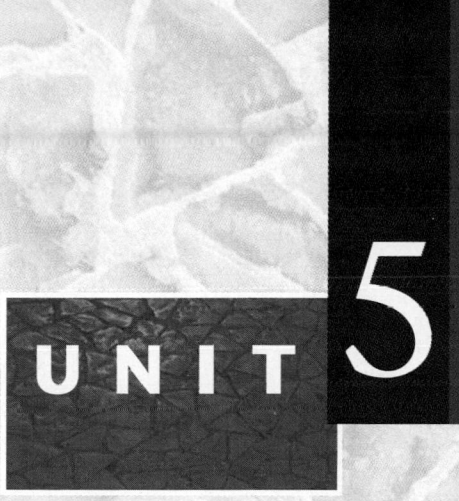

UNIT 5

Promoting Wellness Throughout the Lifespan

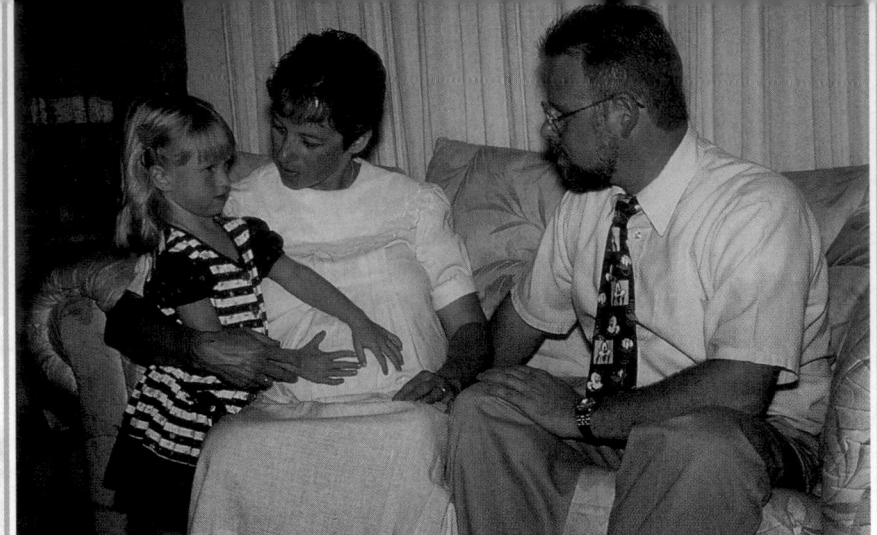

## Chapter 27

Basic Human Needs: Individual and Family

Objectives

Mastery of content in this chapter will enable the student to:

▶ Define the key terms listed.

▶ Discuss each component of Maslow's hierarchy of needs.

▶ Describe assessment techniques for identifying unmet needs.

▶ Describe relationships among the different levels of needs.

▶ State factors that influence individual need priorities.

▶ Describe current trends in the American family.

▶ Describe theoretical approaches to the study of families.

▶ Describe how family can be defined to reflect family diversity.

▶ Explain how family structure and patterns of functioning affect the health of family members and the family as a whole.

▶ Discuss the way family members influence one another's health.

▶ Describe external and internal factors that promote family health.

▶ Compare family as context to family as client, and explain the way that these perspectives influence nursing practice.

▶ Describe the use of all components of the nursing process as applied to family needs.

THE INDIVIDUAL

Basic human needs are matters such as food, water, safety, and love that are necessary for survival and health. Although each person has additional, unique needs, everyone has the same basic human needs. The extent to which basic needs are met determines a person's level of health and position on the health-illness continuum (see Chapter 1).

Maslow's **hierarchy of basic human needs** is a theory that nurses can use to understand the relationships among basic human needs when providing care. According to this theory, certain human needs are more basic than others; that is, some needs must be met before others. For example, a starving person is more likely to seek food than to engage in activities that increase self-esteem.

The hierarchy of human needs arranges the basic needs in five levels of priority (Fig. 27-1). The most basic, or first, level includes **physiological needs** such as air, water, and food. The second level includes **safety and security needs**, which involve physical and psychological security. The third level contains **love and belonging needs**, including friendship, social relationships, and sexual love. The fourth level encompasses **esteem and self-esteem needs**, which involve self-confidence, usefulness, achievement, and self-worth. The final level is the need for **self-actualization**, the state of fully achieving potential and having the ability to solve problems and cope realistically with life's situations.

Through life experiences an individual's basic human needs may be unmet, partially met, or wholly fulfilled. According to this theory, a person whose needs are all met is healthy, and a person with one or more unmet needs is at risk for illness or may be unhealthy in one or more of the human dimensions.

Clients and their families can have unmet needs, or they may be unable to continue meeting their needs. A person brought to an emergency room experiencing cardiac arrest has an unmet need for air, the most basic physiological need. An older woman in a high-crime area may be concerned about physical safety and, while hospitalized, may have a need for psychological security from fear that her home will be burglarized. A widowed homemaker whose children have moved away may feel that she does not belong or is not loved. Nurses in all practice settings encounter clients whose needs might be unmet. Nursing care includes helping clients and, often, the family meet these needs.

PHYSIOLOGICAL NEEDS

Physiological needs have the highest priority in Maslow's hierarchy. An individual who has several unmet needs generally seeks first to fulfill physiological needs (Maslow, 1970). For example, a person who lacks food, safety, and love usually searches for food before seeking love. Physiological needs are necessary or important for survival. Humans have eight such needs: oxygen, fluid, nutrition, temperature, elimination, shelter, rest, and sex.

The very young, very old, poor, ill, and handicapped clients frequently depend on others for meeting basic physiological needs. The nurse often has a role in helping these clients meet those needs.

Oxygen

Oxygen is the most essential physiological need. The body depends on oxygen for moment-to-moment survival. Some tissues, such as skeletal muscle, can survive for a time without oxygen through **anaerobic metabolism**, a process by which these tissues provide their own energy in the absence of oxygen. Tissues that carry out only **aerobic metabolism**, the process of providing energy in the presence of oxygen, depend totally on oxygen for survival.

Oxygen must be adequately delivered from the environment to the lungs, the bloodstream, and the tissues. At any point in their lives, clients are at risk for not meeting their oxygen needs. The need can be acute, as with a cardiac arrest, or chronic, as with the disease emphysema. Nursing measures to meet oxygen needs range from emergency cardiopulmonary resuscitation for cardiac arrest to supportive measures such as administration of oxygen to clients with pulmonary disease during exercise. Chapter 44 discusses in detail measures necessary for meeting oxygen needs of clients.

Fluids

The human body requires a balance between intake and output of fluids. Fluids are taken in by mouth, or parenterally, and fluids leave the body from the intestines, lungs, skin, and kidneys. Clients of any age can have unmet fluid needs, but the very young and very old have the greatest risk. Severely ill, traumatized, or handicapped clients are also more likely to have unmet fluid needs.

Dehydration and edema indicate unmet fluid needs. Dehydration may result from excessive and prolonged fever, vomiting, diarrhea, trauma, or any condition that causes a rapid fluid loss. Edema is also accompanied by a disturbance of electrolytes and may occur in a nutritional, cardiovascular, renal, malignant, traumatic, or other disorder that results in a rapid accumulation of fluids.

When the nursing assessment reveals findings consistent with fluid imbalances, nursing actions are directed toward restoring this balance to normal. Chapter 45 describes in detail the knowledge and techniques the nurse needs for restoring fluid, electrolyte, and acid-base balances.

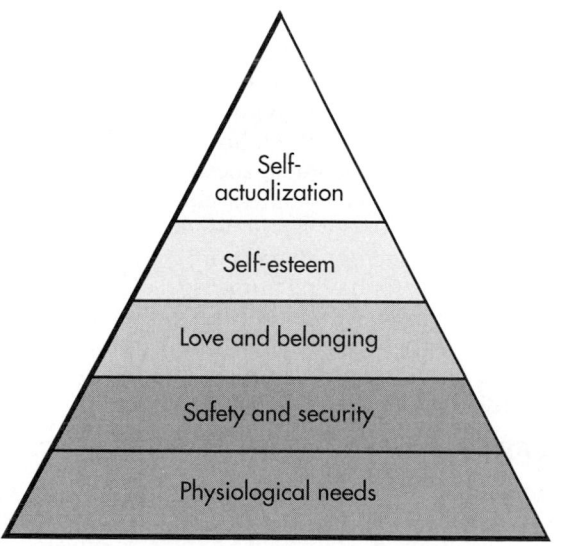

Fig. 27-1 Maslow's hierarchy of needs.

Nutrition

The human body has an essential need for nutrients, although it can survive without food longer than without fluids. Like other physiological needs, nutritional needs may be unmet in a person of any age.

The body's metabolic processes control digestion, storage of nutrients, and elimination of waste products. Digestion and storage of nutrients are essential in meeting the body's nutritional demands.

Sometimes a nurse assists in meeting nutritional needs through teaching. For example, an adult with *altered nutrition: more than body requirements* and recently diagnosed insulin-dependent diabetes mellitus needs to be taught to balance nutritional needs, insulin intake, and exercise habits.

To help clients meet their nutritional needs, the nurse must understand the digestive and metabolic processes of the body. The nurse may use various nutritional supplements and techniques to correct nutritional deficits. Chapter 41 discusses in detail nursing measures related to the nutritional needs of clients.

Temperature

The body can function normally within only a narrow temperature range, 37° C (98.6° F) ±1° C. Body temperatures outside this range can result in injuries, permanent effects such as brain damage, or death (see Chapter 32).

The body can temporarily regulate temperature by certain mechanisms. For example, a person shivers when moving from a warm environment to one of 55° F. This adaptive response can temporarily increase body temperature.

Prolonged exposure to heat increases the body's metabolic activity and increases tissue oxygen demand. Extreme or prolonged heat exposure can also have specific physiological effects. Local exposure to heat can result in first-, second-, or third-degree burns. Overexposure to the sun can lead to sunstroke, which is characterized by high fever, convulsions, and coma. Older persons living in poorly ventilated homes without air conditioning are at risk for heatstroke during prolonged hot weather.

Elimination

The elimination of waste materials is one of the body's metabolic processes. Waste products are eliminated by the lungs, skin, kidneys, and intestines.

The lungs primarily eliminate carbon dioxide, a gas formed during tissue metabolism. Most carbon dioxide is carried to the lungs by the venous system and excreted through breathing (see Chapter 44). The skin eliminates water and sodium, most noticeably as sweat. This also assists in temperature regulation because evaporation of sweat lowers body temperature (see Chapter 32).

The kidneys are the body's primary means of excreting excess body fluids, electrolytes, hydrogen ions, and acids. Urinary elimination normally depends on fluid intake and circulatory blood volume; if either is decreased, urinary output decreases. Urinary output is also changed in persons with kidney disease, which affects the quantity of urine and the content of waste products within the urine. Kidney disease can be life threatening (see Chapter 46).

The intestines eliminate solid waste products and some fluid from the body. The elimination of solid waste by bowel evacuation usually becomes a pattern at 30 to 36 months of age (see Chapter 47).

Shelter

Although most people have some kind of shelter, sometimes it is substandard and does not offer full protection. Disasters such as floods, fire, and tornadoes can render an entire community homeless. Disaster agencies such as the Red Cross and health care services such as Visiting Nurses Association, Public Health Nursing Clinics, and homeless shelters are resources in helping clients obtain permanent shelter.

When assessing whether a client is meeting shelter needs, the nurse identifies risk factors for illness or injury (see Chapter 36). Environments that are dirty may attract insects or rodents, which can increase the risk for illness. If a home is poorly lit or cluttered, there is an increased risk of accidental injury. In addition, overcrowding and lack of cleanliness are predisposing factors to communicable diseases.

Rest

Every person has a basic physiological need for regular rest. The amount of sleep needed varies, depending on the person's quality of sleep, health status, activity patterns, lifestyle, and age.

A client with chronic disease requires more rest than a healthy person of the same age. Pregnancy, lactation, and health status changes such as surgery also increase the need for rest. Physical and emotional stress may also increase a client's need for rest. Rest and sleep often provide temporary relief from stress. However, rest can also be a nonproductive method for resolving stress; a client may depend on it as an escape.

Frequently rest patterns are changed by illness or pain. The nurse uses specific methods to promote comfort and relieve pain so that the client's need for rest can be anticipated and met (see Chapters 42 and 43). If the client is unable to sleep and rest because of other factors, such as lifestyle or chronic stress, the nurse directs care at resolving the cause while helping meet these needs.

Sex

Sex is considered by Maslow (1970) to be a basic physiological need that generally takes priority over higher-level needs. Sexual needs and the manner in which they are met are influenced by age, sociocultural background, ethics, values, self-esteem, and level of wellness.

Health professionals are giving increasing attention to human sexuality. Sexuality involves more than physical sex. It may involve emotional, social, and spiritual needs. Sexuality can be affected by illness, chronic conditions, and hospitalization.

Clients experiencing depression, grief, or lifestyle changes are at risk for having unmet sexual needs. For some clients the meeting of sexual needs is only temporarily interrupted. For others, especially those with severe depression, sexual needs are unmet longer and may resolve only with counseling (see Chapter 24).

■ SAFETY AND SECURITY NEEDS

Next in priority after the client's physiological needs are needs for physical and psychological safety and security.

Physical Safety

An infant enters the world totally dependent on others for needs and physical safety. As the infant grows and develops, greater independence is gradually achieved. Adults are generally able to provide for their physical safety, but the ill and handicapped may need help.

Maintaining physical safety involves reducing or eliminating threats to body or life (see Chapter 36). The threat may be illness, accident, danger, or environmental exposure. When ill, a client may be vulnerable to complications such as infection and therefore depends on professionals in the health care system for protection.

Meeting physical safety needs sometimes takes precedence over meeting a physiological need. For example, a nurse may need to protect a disoriented client from falling out of bed before providing care to meet nutritional needs.

Psychological Safety

To be safe and secure psychologically, a person must understand what to expect from others, including family members and health care professionals. The person must also know what to expect from procedures, new experiences, and encounters within the environment. Everyone feels some threat to psychological safety with new and unfamiliar experiences. A student entering college may feel insecure, a person starting a new job may feel threatened by having to interact with unfamiliar people, and a client about to undergo a diagnostic test may be threatened by the technology involved. In such cases, people generally do not directly state that their psychological safety is threatened, but their conversation may indirectly reveal their feelings.

Healthy adults are generally able to meet physical and physiological safety needs without help from health care professionals. However, ill or handicapped people are more susceptible to threats to physical and emotional well-being, so the nurse intervenes to help protect them from harm.

▍ LOVE AND BELONGING NEEDS

The next priority after physiological and safety needs is the need for love and belonging. People generally need to feel that they are loved by their family and that they are accepted by peers and the community. This need generally arises after physiological and safety needs are met because only when individuals feel safe and secure do they have the time and energy to seek love and belonging and to share that love with others.

Even a person who is generally able to meet needs for love and belonging is often unable to fulfill them when illness or injury occurs. It becomes even more difficult in the hospital. The client is forced to adapt to aspects of the health care delivery system such as organization, routines, environmental limitations, and visiting hours. As a result, there is little time or energy left to meet the needs for love and belonging with family or significant others.

Finally, the nurse works with clients and families to adapt care plans to help clients meet their needs for love and belonging. The more actively involved clients are in developing care plans and the more control they have over the environment while receiving care, the easier it is for them to meet these needs.

▍ ESTEEM AND SELF-ESTEEM NEEDS

People need a stable sense of self-esteem, as well as the feeling that they are held in regard by others. The need for self-esteem is linked to the desire for strength, achievement, adequacy, competence, confidence, and independence. People also need recognition or appreciation from others. When both of these needs are met, a person feels self-confident and useful. If needs for self-esteem and esteem of others are unfulfilled, a person may feel helpless and inferior (Maslow, 1970).

If clients' self-concepts are changed by illness or injury, nursing care involves improving self-concept and body image. Specific nursing actions depend on clients' support systems and personalities, the cause of altered self-concept, and available resources (see Chapter 23). If clients' levels of self-esteem are so low that they fail to care for themselves, the nurse may have to help meet other needs, such as those for nutrition and safety, while taking steps to increase self-esteem.

▍ NEED FOR SELF-ACTUALIZATION

Self-actualization is the highest level of needs in Maslow's hierarchy of human needs. Theoretically, when people have met all the lower-level needs, it is by self-actualization that they achieve their fullest potential (Maslow, 1970).

Self-actualized people have a mature, multidimensional personality. Frequently they are able to assume and complete multiple tasks, and they achieve fulfillment from the pleasure of a job well done. They do not totally depend on the opinions of others about appearance, quality of work, or problem-solving methods. Although they may have failings and doubts, they generally deal with them realistically.

Present needs, environment, and stressors depend on how well people meet their need for self-actualization. Self-actualization is possible when there is a balance among the client's needs, stressors, and ability to adapt to changes of the body and environment.

The client's need for privacy must be respected and met. When in good health, the self-actualized person generally has a strong need for privacy. An illness, especially in a hospital setting, can greatly reduce privacy. Nurses can help meet this need by planning health care so that privacy will not be interrupted during specific times.

▍ APPLICATION OF BASIC NEEDS THEORY

Maslow's theory of human needs can provide a basis for nursing care of clients of all ages and in a variety of health care settings. When the nurse applies this theory in practice, however, the focus is on the needs of the individual rather than rigid adherence to Maslow's hierarchy. Maslow's hierarchy is a generalization about the need priorities of most but not all people. In all cases an emergency physiological need takes precedence over a higher-level need. With one client the need for self-esteem may be a higher priority than a long-term nutritional need, whereas for another client, this may be reversed. To provide the most effective care, the nurse needs to understand relationships among different needs for the individual. Furthermore, although the hierarchy of needs suggests that one need should be met before another, nursing care often addresses two or more at the same time.

Relationships Among Needs

In some nursing situations it is unrealistic to expect client's basic needs to be fulfilled in the fixed hierarchical order. For example, a client enters the health care system with a chronic respiratory infection. While providing care, the nurse learns that the client has not eaten adequately, slept well, or maintained social relationships since his wife died 2 years earlier. In this case the client has several unmet needs, including the physiological needs for nutrition and rest and needs for love and a sense of belonging. For the client, these separate needs are closely related. Nursing care in this situation would not simply be directed to helping the client meet the higher-priority needs for nutrition and rest because these needs in part occurred because the client was not meeting lower-priority needs. Nursing care focuses also on assisting this client through the grief process (see Chapter 26) so that, after grief and loneliness have been resolved, former eating and sleeping habits will be regained and thus these physiological needs will be met.

An opposite relationship among similar needs may be true of a different client. For example, a woman is receiving treatment for severe arthritis and often feels pain or discomfort during certain activities. Because of this, she has changed her habits and no longer visits family members and friends. The nurse realizes that the woman also has unmet needs for love and belonging. These two sets of needs are clearly related, and the nurse provides care directed at meeting both. In this situation, however, the priority is to provide relief from pain, which will then allow the woman to return to former activities that meet the lower-priority needs.

For different individuals, needs on different levels may be related in different ways. Some people may give sexual need a higher priority than the need for love, whereas for others, sexual need is deferred until the need for love is met. Similarly, people with unmet needs for self-esteem may be unable to seek fulfillment of the need for love if their self-esteem is so low that they feel inferior and fear rejection. In these and many other ways, needs on different levels may be closely related for individuals. When assessing needs and planning care, the nurse must not assume that a lower-level need always takes priority. As with all other aspects of providing care, the nurse individualizes the nursing care plan to provide for unique needs and desires.

Simultaneous Meeting of Needs

The nurse provides care for clients with many needs because illness often disrupts the ability to meet needs on different levels. After identifying clients' specific needs the nurse generally has to set priorities to help them meet these needs. However, setting priorities does not mean that the nurse provides care for only one need at a time. For example, the nurse does not simply begin with the first need in the hierarchy and move up only after the first has been met. In emergency situations, of course, physiological needs take precedence, but even then the nurse is aware of other needs. Even in an emergency, the nurse considers clients' higher-level needs. For example, a young man who is hospitalized with paraplegia resulting from a severed spinal cord needs assistance in meeting physiological needs. However, he may also have low self-esteem related to his condition. The nurse is faced with the challenge of simultaneously meeting his physiological needs and need for self-esteem because he may not eat properly or participate in physical care if he does not feel good about himself. The nurse should not offer the client false hope about future re-

covery. However, while planning care to meet physiological needs, the nurse can include measures that will help restore self-esteem.

Factors Influencing Need Priorities

Ideally nursing care can be directed at the simultaneous meeting of several needs. In practice, though, one need often takes precedence over another, and priorities must be determined so that care can be more focused and effective. Life-threatening situations always take priority, and unmet physiological needs that pose a threat to life certainly have a high priority. In other situations the nurse considers factors that influence the priority of needs for an individual.

A person's personality and mood affect the perception of and ability to meet a particular need. A depressed person may react negatively to a suggestion for an activity that could increase self-esteem, although in another mood the person might respond with enthusiasm. Thus when providing care to help meet several needs, the nurse can adjust the care plan to correspond most effectively to the client's personality and mood.

Some needs must be deferred until the client is in better health. A client recovering from an acute gastrointestinal tract infection should not be encouraged to resume physical activities related to needs for self-esteem until needs for physical safety and security have been met by achieving full health. Similarly, a diabetic client whose condition is unstable may have to defer other needs until nutritional needs related to insulin therapy are satisfied.

The client's perception of needs varies among socioeconomic and cultural groups (see Chapter 21). In addition, the client's perception of some needs, such as sexual needs, varies between the sexes and within different developmental levels. The nurse considers the client's perception of needs when planning care and does not impose personal perceptions about priorities.

The client's family structure can influence the way needs are satisfied. For example, a mother may place the needs of an infant before her own, such as when she interrupts a meal or sleep to feed the child.

When setting priorities, the nurse considers that basic needs are interrelated. Physiological functioning is closely related to body systems, environment, values, ethics, and culture. One need does not occur independently of others. For example, if nutritional needs are unmet for a long time, a person begins to show signs of malnutrition, the body deteriorates, weakness occurs, and the client is unable to recognize or meet the lower-priority needs of safety, love, and self-esteem. Needs are interrelated in unique ways for each person, and the nurse considers such relationships in planning care. Rather than simply following the hierarchy of the human needs theory, the nurse involves the client and family in planning so that priorities are not neglected.

▌ THE FAMILY

A few decades ago sociologists predicted that the family was in a state of decline with less influence on its individual members. Rapid social change and an increasingly mobile population would cause psychological and physical distancing of family members. However, it was also felt that family members would remain committed to each other and close family ties would continue. Major changes have occurred since these predictions were made, but it is evident that the family remains the central institution in American society. The current general assumption is that, although the family is in transition and may look very different from the families of the 1950s, it is here to stay. It is true that contemporary families face many challenges; they are, however, characterized by three important attributes: durability, resiliency, and diversity (Fine, 1992).

Current Trends

Although the institution of the family remains strong, the family itself is changing. The "typical" family (two biological parents and children) is no longer the norm (Fig. 27-2). Married couples with at least one child make up only 26% of contemporary families (U.S. Bureau of the Census, 1991).

People are marrying later, women are delaying childbirth, and couples are choosing to have fewer children or none at all. The number of people living alone is expanding rapidly and represents approximately 25% of all households. Divorce rates have tripled since the 1950s, and if current rates continue, half of all marriages will end in divorce. Some research suggests that the divorce rate may reach as high as 60% for recent marriages (Demo and Ganong, 1994). About 90% of young Americans are likely to marry, and between 66% and 75% of those who divorce remarry. The median interval between divorce and remarriage is about 3 years. Men are more likely to remarry than women, younger persons are more likely to remarry than older persons, and divorcees are more likely to remarry than widows or widowers (Crosbie-Burnet, 1994). Remarriage often results in a **blended family** with a complex set of relationships among step-parents, step-children, half brothers and sisters, and extended family members.

Marital roles are also more complex as families increasingly comprise two wage earners. The majority of women work outside the home, and about 63% of mothers are in the work force (Nichols, 1994). Balancing employment and family life creates a variety of challenges in terms of child care and household work. Concerns that maternal employment would prove to be detrimental for children are unsubstantiated. However, finding quality substitute child

care is a major issue for parents. Managing household tasks can also be a major issue. Research demonstrates that, although equal division of labor receives verbal approval, the majority of household tasks remains "women's work." There is some evidence that the fathering role is changing. Fathers are now expected to participate more fully in the day-to-day parenting responsibilities. However, studies of child rearing show that fathers currently do relatively little child care as compared with mothers (Atkinson, 1993).

The number of **single-parent families** has increased dramatically since the 1970s and makes up about 29% of all families with children. Although 90% of single-parent families are headed by mothers, father-only families are on the rise (Meyer and Garaskey, 1993). Twenty-seven percent of babies are born to unwed mothers (U.S. Bureau of the Census, 1991), many of these the result of an adolescent pregnancy. "Children having children" is an ever-increasing concern. The majority of these adolescents (between 65% to 85%) continue to live with their families. A teen pregnancy tends to have long-term consequences for the mother and often severely stresses family relationships and resources (Hanson, 1992).

Many individuals structure their lives very differently from their parents. The number of cohabitating couples has increased fivefold since the 1970s (Manning, 1993). Some who choose to cohabit view it as an alternative to marriage, whereas others view it as a pretrial to marriage.

Although unable to marry by law, many homosexual couples define their relationship in family terms. Approximately half of all gay male couples live together, compared with three fourths of lesbian couples. They have become more open about their sexual preferences and more vocal about their legal rights. Some homosexual families include children either through adoption or artificial insemination, or from prior relationships. The number of children parented by gay men or women is estimated to range from 6 million to 14 million (Hare and Richards, 1993).

The fastest-growing age-group is 65 years of age and over. For the first time in history the average American has more living parents than children, and children are more likely to have living grandparents and even great-grandparents. Only a few decades ago, long-term generational ties were the exception rather than the rule. Currently it is not unusual for families to include four or five generations. This "graying" of America has an impact on the family life cycle, perhaps most significantly for the middle generation. (see the box on p. 484). These individuals are finding that they must balance the needs of their offspring and the needs of their aging parents. This balance often occurs at the expense of their own well-being and resources, earning them the title of the "sandwiched generation." Caring for a frail or chronically ill relative is a primary concern for a growing number of families, and it is not uncommon for people in their 60s and 70s to be the major care givers of their own elderly parents (Taylor et al, 1993).

Grandparents are also increasingly being called on to raise their grandchildren. This parenting responsibility is due to a number of societal factors: the increase in divorce rate, dual-income families, and single parenthood. Most often it is the consequence of legal intervention when parents are deemed unfit or renounce their parental obligations (Kelley, 1993).

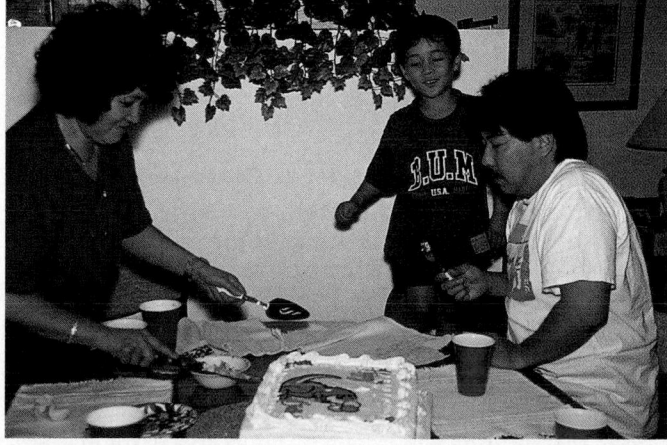

Fig. 27-2 Family celebrations and traditions strengthen the role of family.

GERONTOLOGICAL PRINCIPLES
for Families

- Members in later-life families may have more difficulty with role reversal and/or taking on new tasks, since roles were learned during a more traditional era.
- Nurse must consider care giver strain; care givers are usually spouses who are also older, who may have declining physical stamina, or middle-age children, who often have other responsibilities.
- Later-life families may have a different social network than younger families, since friends and same-generation family members may have died or be ill themselves. These families may need to look for social support within the community and church affiliation.
- As in other stages of life, members of later-life families need to be working on developmental tasks (see Chapter 31).
- Elder abuse in families occurs across all social classes at a rate of about 20 per 1000 individuals; spouses are the most frequent abusers (Gelles, 1994). Unexplained bruises and skin trauma should not be ignored.

RESEARCH HIGHLIGHT

RESEARCH ABSTRACT
A three-way panel study conducted during 1990 examined the relationship of childhood abuse to maternal depressive symptoms in 206 low-income single mothers. A retrospective report of the mother's physical abuse in childhood was obtained using a seven-item version of the Violence Scale of Conflict Tactics. Report of childhood sexual abuse was measured by two yes or no questions, and current depressive symptoms were measured with the 20-item CES-Depression Scale. Both severe physical abuse and sexual abuse in childhood were associated with high levels of depressive symptoms. Women who experienced violent sexual abuse were almost four and one-half times as likely to report high levels of depressive symptoms, compared with the women who were not sexually abused.

IMPLICATIONS FOR PRACTICE
▶ A history of childhood abuse indicates a higher than usual risk for mental health problems; nurses can have a significant impact by early identification of these problems and preventive and therapeutic interventions.
▶ The combination of the stress of caring for children, a history of abuse, and a maternal depressive state puts the children at risk; the nurse must be particularly alert for signs of child neglect and/or abuse.

REFERENCE
Hall LA, Sachs B, Rayens MK et al: *Image J Nurs Sch* 25(4):317, 1993.

In addition to family challenges related to divorce, changing structures and roles, and the aging of its older members, there are four further trends that social scientists identify as threats or concerns facing the family: (1) changing economic status, (2) homelessness, (3) family violence, and (4) human immunodeficiency virus (HIV).

CHANGING ECONOMIC STATUS

Making ends meet is a daily concern because of the declining economic status of families. Although two-income families have become the norm, real family income has not increased since 1973 (Levy and Michel, 1991). Families at the lower end of the income scale have been particularly affected, and single-parent families are especially vulnerable. Persistent or intermittent poverty characterizes the lives of approximately 6 million children in the United States (Allen, 1994), and families with children are the fastest-growing group within our nation's homeless population.

HOMELESSNESS

During the 1980s a new homeless population became apparent. While formerly homeless persons were primarily men residing in "skid row," the "new homeless" became increasingly women and families. Being homeless affects all aspects of family life. Finding food and shelter is the focus of daily existence; family relationships, physical health, and emotional stability are severely strained. The National Coalition for the Homeless estimates that about 43% of homeless children are able to attend school. Obstacles such as residency requirements, transportation, and poor nutrition can be overwhelming, however, and dropout rates are high and performance tends to be poor. Homeless children are at serious risk for developing long-term health, psychological, and socioeconomic problems, thus posing a major challenge for our entire society (Lindsey, 1994).

FAMILY VIOLENCE

The statistics regarding family violence are even more alarming. The inflicting of emotional and/or physical pain on family members occurs in more than half of all households in the United States (Gelles, 1994). Emotional, physical, and sexual abuse occurs toward spouses, children, and the elderly and across all social classes. Two decades of research has demonstrated that the cause of family violence is complex and multidimensional. Factors associated with violence include stress, poverty, social isolation, psychopathology, and learned family behavior (Andrews, 1994). Although abuse may end when one leaves a specific family environment, negative long-term physical and emotional consequences are often evident (see the box above).

HUMAN IMMUNODEFICIENCY VIRUS

The statistics regarding HIV are becoming more alarming. In 1992 it was estimated that between 1 and 1.5 million people in the United States are currently infected (Jurich and Adams, 1992). Finding that one is HIV positive is devastating not only for the individual, but for the family and friends as well. As with all serious illnesses, caring for a family member who develops active HIV is emotionally and financially devastating. A diagnosis of HIV often carries the additional burdens of guilt, social stigma, lifestyle conflicts, and isolation, which touch all family members (Durham, 1994).

Definition: What is a "Family"?

Defining "family" would at first appear to be a simple undertaking. However, different definitions have resulted in heated debates among social scientists and legislators.

The choice of a definition is not an insignificant matter. It determines who is included on health insurance policies, who has access to children's school records, who can file joint tax returns, and who has eligibility for sick-leave benefits or public programs (Fine, 1993). The **family** can be defined biologically, legally, or as a social network with personally constructed ties and ideologies.

A popular conception exists about what the family is or, at least, what it "should" be. This traditional model envisions the **nuclear family** as a unit consisting of a father, mother, and their children and exhibiting a sexual division of labor (i.e., the mother cooks, cleans, and is responsible for child rearing, and the father works outside the home). Families are often portrayed in a Norman Rockwell–type fashion: with adults and children living together in a contented, compatible environment. Families are, however, as diverse as the individuals that compose them. Nurses, like all people, have feelings and values rooted deeply in their family, which influence their definition of family. Unless nurses recognize these values, they may inhibit their understanding and acceptance of the client's perspective.

To effectively provide care, nurses must understand that individual attitudes about family are deeply ingrained and deserve respect. To some clients, family may include only persons related by marriage, birth, or adoption. To others, aunts, uncles, close friends, and cohabiting persons are defined as family. The nurse's personal beliefs do not have to coincide with those of the client. To provide individualized care, the nurse understands that families take many forms and have diverse cultural and ethnic orientations. Thus the nurse must think of family as defined by each individual. In other words, the nurse can think of the family as a set of relationships that the *client* identifies as family or as a network of individuals who influence each other's lives.

Family Forms

Family forms are patterns of people considered by family members to be included in the family (see the box below). Although all families have some things in common, each family form has unique problems and strengths. The nurse needs to have an open mind about family forms so that potential resources and concerns are not overlooked.

■ THEORETICAL APPROACHES: AN OVERVIEW

There are a number of different perspectives that can be applied when working with or studying families. Family scholars often look at families from three general perspectives.

Functional Theory or Functionalism

Functionalism is considered a "conservative" theory that emphasizes stability and harmony. The family is viewed as a universal, necessary, social institution that fulfills the needs of individuals and society.

Social Conflict Approach

As opposed to stability and harmony, this theory assumes that conflict and change are expected features of life. The family is assumed to consist of two kinds of power imbalances, those based on gender and those based on age.

Symbolic Interaction

This approach is based on the assumption that all interactions have different meanings to different individuals in different situations and that individuals interact only in re-

---

Family Forms

NUCLEAR FAMILY
This family consists of husband and wife and perhaps one or more children.
The presence of children affects family's time and economic resources.
The absence of children may lead husband and wife to seek counseling and health care.

EXTENDED FAMILY
This family includes relatives (aunts, uncles, grandparents, and cousins), in addition to nuclear family.
The closer the extended family, the more influence it has on health care.
This family can provide a diverse support base for members needing health care.

SINGLE-PARENT FAMILY
This family is formed when one parent leaves the nuclear family because of death, divorce, or desertion, or when a single person decides to have or adopt a child.
Circumstances of separation influence its impact on the family; it is most commonly the result of divorce today.
Reduced financial and emotional resources affect the health of single-parent families.

BLENDED FAMILY
This family is formed when parents bring unrelated children from prior relationships into a new, joint living situation.
The nature of prior living situations and rate of adapting to the change affect health.
Stress of newly formed family patterns can affect the mental health of family members.

ALTERNATE PATTERNS OF RELATIONSHIPS
Multiadult households
"Skip-generation" families (grandparents caring for grandchildren)
Communal groups with children
"Nonfamilies" (adults living alone)
Cohabiting partners
Homosexual couples
Health concerns focus on the specific needs integral to each form but may include the stability of the relationships, child-rearing practices, and availability of community resources.

lation to other people. According to this approach, a family can be understood only by knowing about its past experiences and the *meaning* that the individual members place on former and current situations.

Other approaches to the family include general systems theory and developmental theory. Both of these perspectives are more fully incorporated in this chapter, and their concepts provide the foundation for family assessment.

GENERAL SYSTEMS THEORY

Family as an Open Social System

The family is viewed as an open social system that exists in and interacts with the larger systems (suprasystems) of the community (e.g., political, religious, school, and health care systems). The family system consists of interrelated parts (family members) that form a variety of interaction patterns (subsystems). As with all systems, the family system has both implicit and explicit goals, which vary according to the stage in the family life cycle, family values, and individual concerns of the family members.

Structure

Families also have a structure and a way of functioning. Structure and function are closely related and continually interact with one another. Structure is based on *organization*, that is, the ongoing membership of the family and the pattern of relationships. Relationships can be numerous and complex. For example, a woman's relationships may include wife-husband, mother-son, and mother-daughter, each with different demands, roles, and expectations. Patterns of relationships form power and role structures within the family. These structures can be determined by observing family behavior and asking questions that identify who and how decisions are made (power structure) and who performs which tasks (role structure).

Structure may enhance or detract from the family's ability to respond to stressors. Very rigid or very flexible structures can impair functioning. A rigid structure specifically dictates who is permitted to accomplish a task, and it may also limit the number of persons outside the immediate family who are allowed to assume these tasks. For example, the mother might be considered the only acceptable person to provide emotional support for the children, or the husband the only one to provide financial support. A change in the health status of the person responsible for a task places a burden on the family because no other person is available or considered acceptable to assume that task.

An extremely open structure can also present problems for the family. Consistent patterns of behavior that lead to automatic action do not exist, and enactment of roles are overly flexible. A common example is an inconsistent parenting role. The parent is at one time a strict authoritarian figure and at another time treats the child as a "best friend and confidant." This type of conduct can cause family members to become confused about what behavior is appropriate and who can be relied on for support. A general feeling of instability is created. During a crisis or rapid change, family members do not have a defined structure to "fall back on," and family disintegration can be the result.

Function

Friedman (1992) describes functioning as what the family does. Family functioning focuses on the *processes* used by the family to achieve its goals. These processes include communication among family members, goal setting, conflict resolution, nurturing, and use of internal and external resources. The reproductive, sexual, economic, and educational goals that were once considered universal family goals no longer apply to all families. Although many families pursue these goals at various times during their development, they provide psychological support to their members throughout the life span. When the psychological needs of family members are not met, symptoms of family dysfunction are the usual consequence.

Family goals are more easily achieved when communication is clear and direct. Clear communication enhances problem solving and conflict resolution and can facilitate coping with life-threatening stressors (see the box at left). Another family process facilitating goal achievement includes the ability to nurture and promote growth. Families must have available, and must be able to use, internal and external resources. A social network is useful as an external resource. Social relationships within the community act as buffers, particularly during times of stress, and reduce a family's vulnerability.

DEVELOPMENTAL STAGES

Families, like individuals, change and grow over time. Although families are far from identical to one another, they tend to go through certain stages. Each developmental stage has its own challenges, needs, and resources and includes tasks that need to be completed before the family can successfully move on to the next stage. Societal changes and an aging population have precipitated changes in the stages and transitions in the family life cy-

---

▶ **RESEARCH HIGHLIGHT**

RESEARCH ABSTRACT
The communication patterns of 41 couples in which the woman was newly diagnosed with stage 1 or 2 breast cancer were investigated. Family interviews were done at five points, from the time of diagnosis to 1 year later. Three major types of couple discussion patterns about fears, doubts, and emotional issues were seen. The most facilitative pattern of communication was open but selective. The couples that had problems in coping also had problems communicating. The author concludes that providing opportunities for sharing can improve family communication and thereby facilitate adjustment.

IMPLICATIONS FOR PRACTICE
Open communication can encourage coping in life-threatening situations.
▶ The nurse needs to provide an opportunity to share concerns with other family members and health care professionals.
▶ The nurse can encourage participation in support groups.

REFERENCE
Hilton BA: *West J Nurs Res* 16(4):366, 1994.

Table 27-1	Stages of the Family Life Cycle	
FAMILY LIFE CYCLE STAGE	**EMOTIONAL PROCESS OF TRANSITION: KEY PRINCIPLES**	**CHANGES IN FAMILY STATUS REQUIRED TO PROCEED DEVELOPMENTALLY**
Between families: unattached young adult	Accepting parent-offspring separation	Differentiating self in relation to family of origin Developing intimate peer relationships Establishing self in work
Joining of families through marriage: newly married couple	Commitment to new system	Forming marital system Realigning relationships with extended families and friends to include spouse
Family with young children	Accepting new generation of members into system	Adjusting marital system to make space for children Taking on parenting roles Realigning relationships with extended family to include parenting and grandparenting roles
Family with adolescents	Increasing flexibility of family boundaries to include children's independence	Shifting parent-child relationships to permit adolescents to move in and out of system Refocusing midlife marital and career issues Beginning shift toward concerns for older generation
Launching children and moving on	Accepting multitude of exits from and entries into family system	Renegotiating marital system as dyad Developing adult-to-adult relationships between grown children and parents Realigning relationships to include in-laws and grandchildren Dealing with disabilities and death of parents (grandparents)
Family in later life	Accepting shifting of generational roles	Maintaining own and/or couple functioning and interests in face of physiological decline; exploration of new familial and social role options Supporting a more central role for middle generation Making room in system for wisdom and experience of older adults; supporting older generation without overfunctioning for them Dealing with loss of spouse, siblings, and other peers and preparation for own death; dealing with view and integration

From McGoldrick M, Carter E, In Henslin I, editor: *Marriage and family in a changing society,* New York, 1985. Free Press, and Walsh F. *Normal family processes,* New York, 1982, Guilford.

cle. For example, adult children are not leaving the nest as predictably or as early as in the past and many are returning home. In addition, more people are living into their 80s and 90s. Sixty-five is now considered the "backside of middle-age," and the length of the midlife stage in the family life cycle has increased, as has the later stage in family life (Estess, 1994).

McGoldrick and Carter (1985) have developed a model of family life stages based on expansion, contraction, and realignment of family relationships that support the entry, exit, and development of the members. This model provides the nurse with the emotional aspects of transition and the changes and tasks necessary for the family to proceed developmentally (Table 27-1). Thus the nurse can promote behaviors to achieve essential tasks and help families prepare for later transitions. It should be noted that this model does not address diverse family forms such as blended families, single-parent families, or cohabitating partners.

Family and Health

The health of the family is influenced by its relative position in society. Although American families exist within the same culture, they live in very different ways. The struc-

ture, function, and health of any family are a reflection and result of many variables. These variables include social class, economic resources, and racial and ethnic background. For some minority groups and the poor, patterned differences in family living are consequences of inequalities deeply rooted in society. Class and ethnicity can produce differences in the access of families to society's resources and rewards, and this access creates differences in family life, most significantly in different life chances for its members (Zinn and Eitzen, 1993). Distribution of wealth greatly affects the capacity to maintain health. "Low education, poverty, and low support feed on each other, magnify each other's impact *on* sickness in the family, and magnify the impact of sickness *in* the family" (Ross, 1990). Economic stability increases a family's access to adequate health care, creates more opportunity for education and sound nutrition, and decreases stress.

"The family is the primary social context in which health promotion and disease prevention take place" (Campbell, 1994). The family strongly influences health behaviors of its members; in turn, the health status of each individual influences how the family unit functions and its ability to achieve goals. When the family satisfactorily meets its goals through adequate functioning, its members tend to feel positive about themselves and their family. Conversely, when they do not meet goals, families view themselves as ineffective.

Good health may not be highly valued; in fact, detrimental practices may be accepted. In some cases a family member may provide mixed messages about health. For example, a parent may continue to smoke while telling children that smoking is bad for them. Family environment is crucial because health behavior reinforced in early life has a strong influence on later health practices. In addition, family environment can be a crucial factor in an individual's adjustment to a crisis. Although relationships can be strained when confronted with illness, research indicates that family members have the potential to be a primary force for coping (Hough, 1991).

Attributes of "Healthy" Families

Ruebin Hill's classic work (1958) noted that it is possible to explain the reactions of crisis-proof and crisis-prone families. The crisis-proof or effective family is able to integrate the need for stability with the need for growth and change. This family has a flexible structure that allows adaptable performance of tasks and acceptance of help from outside the family system. The structure is flexible enough to allow adaptability but not so flexible that the family lacks cohesiveness and a sense of stability. The effective family has control over the environment and exerts influence on the immediate environs of home, neighborhood, and school. The ineffective family may lack or believe it lacks control over these environs.

Recently health promotion research has started to focus on the stress-moderating effect of **"hardiness"** as a factor that contributes to long-term health (Bigbee, 1992). Danielson et al. (1993) define family hardiness as "the internal strengths and durability of the family unit; characterized by a sense of control over the outcome of life events and hardships, a view of change as beneficial and growth-producing, and as an active rather than passive orientation in responding to stressful life events."

▌ FAMILY NURSING

Although the past and present health care system tends to emphasize the individual, nursing's attempt to include families when providing care dates back to Florence Nightingale (Whall, 1991). A family-focused approach has been most evident when caring for children because of the recognition that the family is central in a child's life. Family nursing is based on the assumption that *all* people—regardless of age—are a member of some type of family group. The goal of the family nurse is to help the family and its individual members reach and maintain maximum health.

Nursing scholars have proposed different approaches for family nursing practice. Friedemann (1992) suggests three focuses: (1) the individual with family as context, (2) relationships within the family (relational), and (3) processes within the family (transactional) (Hanson et al, 1992). A very similar approach is offered by Wright and Leahy: a focus on (1) the individual within the context of the family, (2) the family with the individual as context, and (3) the whole family as the unit of care (Vosburgh and Simpson, 1993). The perspective that one uses is related to the clinical setting, the clinical problem, and realistic and practical considerations. Dealing with very complex family system problems often requires an interdisciplinary approach. The nurse must always be aware of the parameters of nursing practice and make referrals when appropriate.

For the purposes of this chapter, family nursing practice is conceptualized as having two levels of approaches, family as context and family as client, which includes both relational and transactional concepts. If only one family member is receptive to nursing care, it is realistic and practical to view the family as context. When all family members are involved in the day-to-day care of one another, nursing intervention with one individual necessitates some change in the activities of the others. Both approaches—family as context and family as client—can be useful in providing effective nursing care.

Family as Context

When the nurse views the **family as context**, the primary focus is the health and development of an individual member existing within a specific environment (i.e., the client's family). Although the nursing process concentrates on the individual's health status, the nurse also assesses the extent to which the family provides the individual's basic needs. These needs vary, depending on the individual's developmental level and situation. Families provide more than just material essentials, so their ability to help the client meet psychological needs must also be considered. Family members may need direct interventions themselves.

Family as Client

When **family as client** is the approach, family processes and relationships are the primary focuses of nursing care. Family patterns versus individual characteristics are studied. For example, a single, 25-year-old, Native American man lives at home with his mother, older brother, and two younger sisters. He has borderline hypertension and is overweight. The nurse at the neighborhood clinic is helping him with his diet and to cope with job stress and family obligations. If the family is viewed as context, the nurse focuses on the client as an individual. The nurse might assess the client's knowledge of high-sodium and high-fat foods, how or whether his cultural identity affects his eating patterns and strategies for making improvements in his food intake. The nurse also assesses realistic opportunities to reduce the number and extent of perceived stressors in work and family environments and knowledge and skill in stress management, such as biofeedback techniques. If the family is viewed as client, the nurse would assess the family's current dietary patterns, its cultural significance, and the family's desire and resources for changing the patterns. The nurse also determines the demands placed on the hypertensive family member and explores the potential for redistributing the demands among other family members. The family's capabilities to support the hypertensive member's development and use of stress management are also assessed.

It is important to understand that although theoretical and practical distinctions can be made between the two approaches, they are not necessarily mutually exclusive and both are often used simultaneously.

NURSING PROCESS FOR THE FAMILY

Nurses interact with families in a variety of community-based and clinical settings, including acute and extended care facilities, nursing homes, day-care centers, schools, and clients' homes. Family nursing process is the same, regardless of the setting or whether the focus is on family as context or as client. It is also the same process as that used with individual clients. Three beliefs underlie the family approach to the nursing process:

1. That all individuals must be viewed within their family context

2. That families have an impact on individuals
3. That individuals have an impact on families

 Assessment

Family assessment is an essential component of the nursing process (see the box below). Although the family as a whole differs from individual members, the measure of family health is more than a summation of the health of all members. Areas included in family assessment are the form, structure, and function of the family; its developmental

---

Family Assessment Tool

The family assessment tool is used when the beginning student interviews family members and observes family interaction. It is only a *guideline* and is not meant to be all inclusive. The student must also assume that individual health histories accompany this assessment.

FAMILY FORM AND STRUCTURE
Names of adults _____ Ages _____
Relationship _____
Names of children _____ Ages _____
_____
_____

Others living in home (include age, sex, relationship) _____
_____
Cultural background (include any pertinent health beliefs, child-rearing practices, related health concerns) __
_____
Developmental stage _____
Progress toward accomplishment of developmental tasks _____
Concerns related to developmental stage _____

RESOURCES
Significant relatives and friends not occupying immediate residence _____
Strengths and coping skills _____
Ways the family obtains health services _____
Membership in community groups (e.g., church affiliation) _____
Education (formal and informal) _____
Finances (ability to meet current and future needs) _____

FAMILY PATTERNS
Persons working outside the home _____
Type of work _____ Number of hours _____
Satisfaction with work _____
Ways the housekeeping tasks are accomplished _____
Family members' satisfaction with the way tasks are divided _____
Ways that child-rearing responsibilities are divided _____
Person who makes the major decisions in the family _____
Person who makes day-to-day decisions _____
Family members' satisfaction with the way decisions are made _____

FAMILY FUNCTION
Goals
Long term _____
Short term _____
Individual family members' goals _____
Are individual and family goals appropriate, considering their current health problem and status? _____
How are individual family members and the family as a whole coping with their current health problem and status? _____
_____

Communication
Do husband and wife communicate regularly and effectively with each other? _____
Are family members able to communicate openly and honestly with each other? _____
Is conflict openly expressed and discussed? _____
Do family members respect each other's point of view? _____
Do family members offer emotional support to each other? _____

stage; and its progress toward or accomplishment of developmental tasks.

The nurse begins assessment by determining the client's definition of and attitude toward family and the extent to which the family can be incorporated into the nursing process. To determine family form and membership, the nurse can ask whom the client considers family or with whom the client shares strong emotional feelings. If the client is unable to express a concept of family, the nurse can ask with whom the client lives, spends time, and shares confidences and then ask whether the client considers them to be family or like family. To further assess the family structure, the nurse asks questions that determine the power structure and patterning of roles and tasks (e.g., "Who decides where to go on vacation?" or "Who usually prepares the meals?").

The nurse assesses family functions such as the ability to provide emotional support for members, the ability to cope with its current health problem or situation, and the appropriateness of its goal setting and progress toward achievement of developmental tasks (Fig. 27-3). The nurse also assesses whether the family is able to provide and allocate sufficient economic resources and whether its social network is extensive enough to provide support.

Cultural background is an important variable when assessing the family because race and ethnicity can affect structure, function, health beliefs, values, and the way events are perceived (see the box on p. 491). The United States is increasingly more diverse. A large number of immigrants enter the country daily, adding both to the number and variety of the many ethnic groups that make up the population. American health care institutions tend to operate from a white, middle-class perspective, and immigrant populations may have particular difficulty understanding and "fitting into" the system. Congress (1994) encourages the use of a "culturagram" that assesses and empowers culturally diverse families and encourages "ethnic-sensitive" practice. This tool assesses a variety of factors such as language spoken in the home, impact of crisis events, and values regarding family, education, and work.

Drawing conclusions based on cultural backgrounds requires critical thinking and careful consideration; it is imperative to remember that categorical generalizations can be misleading. As Congress (1994) cautions, "Overgeneralizations in terms of racial and ethnic group characteristics does not lead to greater understanding of the culturally diverse family." Culturally different families can vary in meaningful and significant ways; however, neglecting to examine similarities can lead to inaccurate assumptions and stereotyping (Fine, 1993); some studies reveal a lack of cultural differences in certain family processes. For example, a study by Julian et al. (1994) indicated more similarities than differences in parenting behaviors between white, African-American, Hispanic, and Asian-American parents. To illustrate the nursing process using a family approach, consider the following scenario.

CASE STUDY Mr. and Mrs. Smith, a European-American couple in their 70s, have recently celebrated their fiftieth wedding anniversary and have been living in Florida since Mr. Smith retired 10 years ago. They have two married sons living in Iowa. Mr. and Mrs. Smith's marriage has been very traditional, with Mrs. Smith performing all the household tasks. They have many friends and are active in various church groups. Both have been comparatively healthy until 5 weeks ago, when Mrs. Smith suffered a stroke that left her with left-sided weakness. After 3 weeks in the hospital and 2 weeks in a rehabilitation center Mrs. Smith was discharged home, and Mr. Smith is expected to provide care and take over the household tasks. Discharge planning included physical therapy three times a week and home visits by the nurse to assess and monitor the Smiths' adjustment to their new situation.

During the initial home visit the nurse was able to talk to Mr. and Mrs. Smith together and separately. Mr. Smith's statements and behavior indicated to the nurse that he had unrealistic expectations of his wife's current and future abilities. For example, he became impatient with her slowness when she was trying to drink a glass of water and stated that he expects her to "be her old self" in a week or so. Mrs. Smith stated that their relationship is "strained" and that her husband often tells her that she is "just not trying hard enough to get well."

This older couple exemplifies a common case: the need for one member of the family to take on the role of care giver. The most common care giver for the elderly are spouses who themselves are also elderly (Browning and Schwirian, 1994). This case also points out how an illness can disrupt well-established patterns in a family and the necessity of careful long-term planning. ■

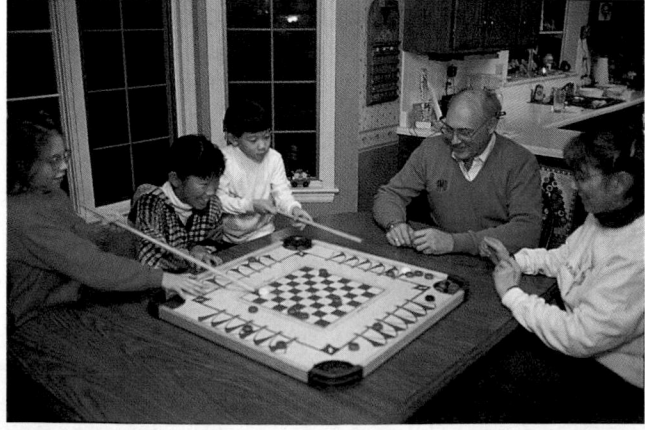

Fig. 27-3 Observing family interactions assists in understanding family functions.

Nursing Diagnosis

Nursing assessment results in clustering pertinent data that support a nursing diagnosis and identifies inadequate or deficient functioning and interventions that are needed. The diagnostic label may include the family's health needs, current and potential health problems, level of wellness, or a combination of these. In addition, the diagnostic statement should indicate possible causes and origins (see the box on p. 491).

The nursing diagnoses often focus on the family's ability to cope with its current situation, whether it is an acute illness, an anticipated developmental transition, or negative behaviors that are threatening short-term or long-term health. Appropriate use of external and internal resources

CULTURAL ASPECTS OF CARE

FAMILY CARE

Perception of certain events can vary across cultural groups and have particular impact on families. For example, the death of a grandparent may take on greater significance in families whose culture emphasizes veneration of older family members. Stressors such as rape may have an especially devastating effect on Hispanic women and their families, since great importance is placed on female virginity (Congress, 1994).

Intergenerational support and patterns of living arrangements can be related to cultural background. For example, older Chinese, Afro-American, Japanese, and Hispanic persons are more likely to live in extended family households than are their white counterparts (Kamo, Zhou, 1994; Taylor et al, 1993).

Health beliefs differ among various cultures, which may affect the decision of a family and its members about when and where to seek help. For example, Asians rarely consider symptoms as psychological and are not likely to go to mental health clinics (Congress, 1994).

Examples of NANDA Nursing Diagnoses for a Family with Adult Members

Altered family processes *related to:*
- Change in roles related to sudden, unexpected illness
- Financial concerns
- Inability to problem solve
- Inadequate communication

Fear (individual family members) *related to:*
- Hospitalization
- Knowledge deficit

Powerlessness (individual family members) *related to:*
- Unplanned hospitalization
- Knowledge deficit

Ineffective family coping: compromised or disabled *related to:*
- Effects of chronic illness
- Family disorganization

Impaired home maintenance management *related to:*
- Dysfunctional grieving
- Alteration in communication skills

Care giver role strain *related to:*
- Physical/emotional demands of role
- Perceived isolation of care giver

allows the family to cope with day-to-day stressors and with unexpected occurrences that threaten health. Coping strategies can be adaptive or maladaptive. During times of acute illness the family can become extremely distressed and focus solely on the ill member, neglecting the needs of the other members (McClowery, 1992). The needs of other family members can be easily overlooked unless the nurse consistently employs a family nursing perspective. For example, the diagnosis of care giver role strain should always be considered a possibility when long-term care of a family member is necessary.

"Nursing diagnosis involves a data base regulated by the family and the nurse's identification and evaluation of potential stressors that pose a threat to the stability of the family unit" (Berkey and Hanson, 1993). Identifying the correct related factors is essential to choosing the appropriate plan of action (see the diagnostic process box on p. 492). In the preceding clinical situation, during the assessment phase the nurse concluded that Mr. Smith was not providing Mrs. Smith with adequate emotional and physical support, thus threatening Mrs. Smith's well-being, their relationship, and their overall family functioning. Without intervention it is unlikely that this family would be able to reach their optimal level of wellness. The nurse also concluded that inadequate support was related to Mr. Smith's lack of understanding of his wife's long-term physical limitations. Drawing accurate conclusions through critical thinking allowed the nurse to plan interventions directed at the underlying cause.

Planning

When nursing diagnoses have been formulated, the next step is to plan a course of action with the family (see the care plan on p. 492). Planning includes setting goals and expected outcomes, identifying potential internal and external resources, choosing effective approaches, and setting priorities. The plan of care must be clearly understood by the family, and they must agree to it. Goal setting must be a mutual endeavor. Goals must also be concrete and realistic, compatible with the developmental stage, and acceptable to family members. Each goal includes the day when goals are to be achieved.

Collaboration with family members is an essential component during this stage. A positive collaborative relationship is based on mutual respect and trust (Danielson et al, 1993) and is facilitated by allowing the family to feel as "in control" as possible. For example, offering alternative actions and asking family members for their own ideas and suggestions can reduce feelings of powerlessness. Collaboration also extends to other health care professionals. As Danielson et al. (1993) point out, it is impossible to be all things to all families. Collaborating with other disciplines increases the likelihood of a comprehensive care plan and can provide for continuity of care. Using other disciplines is particularly important for discharge planning, since referrals are often necessary to ensure that long-term goals will be attained.

Goals for a care plan that incorporate a family approach may include those that view the family as client. For example, goals of care would be to have the family functional at an optimal level or that the family understands and copes with the health problems of its members. In addition, the goals may be established for the family as context. For example, the goal is that the client accomplishes appropriate developmental tasks within the family context. Also, the goals can include a combination of these two. The client situation and availability of family members dictate the type of goals that are feasible.

Sample Nursing Diagnostic Process for a Family With Adult Member

ASSESSMENT ACTIVITIES	DEFINING CHARACTERISTICS	NURSING DIAGNOSIS
Observe wife and husband interact during care activity.	Basic human needs of wife are neglected. Husband displays facial tension, poor eye contact, and quivering voice while interacting with wife.	**Ineffective family coping: compromised** related to husband's inadequate understanding of wife's physical limitations
Have husband describe personal reaction to wife's illness.	Husband expresses guilt over wife's illness. Husband describes inadequate understanding of wife's illness.	

Sample Nursing Care Plan for Ineffective Family Coping: Compromised

NURSING DIAGNOSIS: **Ineffective family coping: compromised** related to husband's inadequate understanding of wife's physical limitations

DEFINITION: Ineffective family coping: compromised is defined as insufficient, ineffective, or compromised support, comfort, or assistance—usually by a supportive primary person (family member or close friend); client may need it to manage or master adaptive tasks related to his/her health challenge (Kim, McFarland, McLane, 1995)

GOALS	EXPECTED OUTCOMES	INTERVENTIONS	RATIONALE
Husband will gain improved understanding of wife's physical limitations by end of home visits (3/25).	Husband will be able to identify activities appropriate for his wife to perform and activities with which he will have to assist her (3/21).	Discuss with husband long-term effects of stroke and provide reading material designed for family members of clients with strokes.	Accurate information will assist husband in interpreting wife's limitations (Browning and Schwirian, 1994).
Husband will accept wife's physical limitations (3/30).	Husband will not demonstrate impatient behavior (such as telling his wife to "hurry up") while she performs activities (3/27).	Provide list of care giver support groups.	Group support allows care giver to share experiences, stresses, and coping methods.

Sample Evaluation of Interventions for Ineffective Family Coping: Compromised

GOAL	EVALUATIVE MEASURES	EXPECTED OUTCOMES
Husband will gain improved understanding of wife's physical limitations by end of home visits (3/25).	Observe husband and wife interact.	Husband will be able to identify activities with which he will need to assist her by second home visit.
	Ask husband about activities wife will be able to perform and activities that will require assistance.	Husband will be able to identify activities that his wife will be able to perform on her own by second home visit.

Examples of *family as client* expected outcomes include the following:

- Communication between family members is appropriate direct, and clear.
- Family members are able to confront and resolve conflict in a healthy way.
- Family members use external and internal resources as needed.
- The family is able to meet the needs of all its individual members.

Examples of *family as context* expected outcomes include the following:

- The client uses external and internal resources as appropriate.
- The client communicates needs and goals appropriately to family members.

In Mr. and Mrs. Smith's case, planning must include actions that will help Mr. Smith better understand the chronic effects of stroke and to recognize his wife's limitations. Long-term planning focuses on new adaptive patterns so that the couple can reach their maximal individual health and family functioning. The nurse is aware that the multiple roles of primary care giver put Mr. Smith at risk; observation and evaluation of his physical and mental health need to be a part in the long-term plan of care.

Mr. Smith has had to assume the majority of household tasks and essentially change roles with Mrs. Smith. The nurse observes that this is difficult for both of them and decides that collaboration with a family therapist or family social worker, or both, would provide additional perspectives and suggestions. During the planning stage the nurse keeps in mind the couple's long marital history, their developmental stage, and the limitations and strengths inherent in both.

 Implementation

After goals and actions have been defined, implementation begins. Interventions are strategies that help families adjust goals or are the processes by which the family attains them. Family interventions include nursing actions that increase members' abilities in a certain area, remove barriers to health care, and do things that the family cannot do for itself (Friedman, 1992). The nurse guides the family in problem solving, provides practical service, and conveys a sense of acceptance and caring by listening carefully to family members concerns and suggestions.

Health Promotion

Identifying attributes that contribute to healthy, resilient families has been a focus of ongoing research for at least three decades. "Strong" families that adapt to expected transitions and unexpected crises and change tend to be characterized by clear communication, problem-solving skills, a commitment to each other and to the family unit, and a sense of cohesiveness and spirituality. Prevention programs aimed at enhancing these activities are available for families and children in many communities. The nurse must be aware of family-oriented offerings so that families can be referred as needed. Health promotion behaviors that the nurse needs to encourage are often tied to the developmental stage of the family (e.g., adequate prenatal care for the child-bearing family, effective parenting, and adherence to immunization schedules for the child-rearing family).

One approach for meeting goals and promoting health is the use of family strengths. Families do not look at their own system as one that has inherent, positive components. The nurse can help the family become aware of its own unique strengths, thereby increasing its potential and capabilities. Family strengths include clear communication, adaptability, healthy child-rearing practices, support and nurturing among family members, and the use of crisis for growth. The nurse can help the family focus on these strengths instead of its problems and weaknesses. For example, the nurse can point out that the Smiths' 50-year marriage must have endured many crises and transitions. Therefore they are likely to have the capabilities to adapt to this latest challenge.

 Evaluation

When family as context is the focus, evaluation emphasizes attainment of client needs. The response of the client is compared with predetermined outcomes. When the family receives care as the client, the measure of family health is more than a summation of the health of all family members. For example, the family's attainment of family developmental tasks may be a useful criterion. The nurse evaluates the family's change in functioning and its satisfaction with the new level of functioning. Evaluation is an ongoing process. Goals and interventions are modified as needed (see the evaluation box on p. 492).

Examples of *family as client* evaluative measures include the following.

- Observe interactions between family members.
- Note effective and ineffective communication patterns.
- Ask family members to describe how conflicts are resolved in their family.
- Ask family members what specific internal and external resources they are using to maintain optimal family functioning.
- Observe family members' abilities to maintain appropriate roles and relationships.
- Note members' awareness and willingness to facilitate the meeting of each others' needs.

Examples of *family as context* evaluative measures include the following:

- Ask clients what internal and external resources they are using to maintain optimal functioning within the family unit.
- Observe client's interaction with family members.
- Note client's ability to define and meet needs within the family context.

■ KEY CONCEPTS ■

▶ Basic human needs are the needs for things such as oxygen, food, water, safety, and love that are required to survive and be healthy.

▶ The very young, very old, chronically ill, and handicapped are generally less able than others to meet needs without assistance.

▶ The highest priority is given to physiological needs.

▶ Safety and security needs include physical and psychological safety and the need to prevent complications.

▶ Clients in the health care system may be unable to meet their needs for love and belonging because of changes in relationships with others and the separation often imposed by illness.

▶ People need self-esteem and the esteem of others. Illness, role changes, and changes in body image may threaten the ability to meet these needs.

▶ To apply basic needs theory in practice, the nurse considers the relationships among the client's specific needs, sets priorities by considering the client's priorities, and assists the client in simultaneously meeting needs on different levels.

▶ The family influences the lives of its members.

▶ Family members influence one another's health beliefs, practices, and status.

▶ Because the concept of family is highly individual, the nurse should base care on the client's attitude toward family rather than on an inflexible definition of the family.

▶ The family's structure, functioning, and relative position in society significantly influence its health and ability to respond to health problems.

▶ The nurse can view the family as an important context for the individual family member or can view the family unit as the client.

▶ Measures of family health involve more than a summation of individual members' health.

▶ The family's health is influenced by its social class, economic stability, and racial and ethnic background.

■ KEY TERMS ■

Aerobic metabolism, p. 479

Anaerobic metabolism, p. 479

Basic human needs, p. 479

Blended family, p. 483

Esteem and self-esteem needs, p. 479

Extended family, p. 485

Family, p. 485

Family as client, p. 488

Family as context, p. 488

Hardiness, p. 488

Hierarchy of basic human needs, p. 479

Love and belonging needs, p. 479

Nuclear family, p. 485

Physiological needs, p. 479

Safety and security needs, p. 479

Self-actualization, p. 479

Single-parent family, p. 483

■ CRITICAL THINKING EXERCISES ■

1. After your assessment, you note that Mr. Jones has recently become unemployed, his wife has chronic health problems, and there are two school-age children at home. What are the potential threats to the family from these stressors? What anticipatory interventions can be designed to minimize these threats?

2. Mrs. Weber is 31 years old and newly widowed with three children under the age of 10. What resources can nurses use to assist this mother in adapting to the abrupt transition to being a single parent?

3. Mr. and Mrs. Kline are in their mid-40s with two teenage children. Both sets of the Klines' parents are in their 80s and have chronic health problems. How can you assist Mr. and Mrs. Kline in developing extended resources to aid in caring for their parents and at the same time maintain the responsibilities of their own family unit?

REFERENCES

Allen CE: Families in poverty, *Nurs Clin North Am* 29(3):377, 1994.

Andrews AB: Developing community systems for the primary preventions of family violence, *Fam Community Health*, 16(4):1, 1994.

Atkinson MP: Fathering in the 20th century, *J Marriage Fam* 55(4):975, 1993.

Berkey KM, Hanson SM: *Family assessment and intervention*, St Louis, 1993, Mosby.

Bigbee JL: Family stress, hardiness, and illness: a pilot study, *Fam Relations* 41(2):212, 1992.

Campbell TL: Physical illness. In Mchenry PC, Price SJ, editors: *Families and change: coping with stressful events*, London, 1994, Sage.

Congress EP: The use of culturagrams to assess and empower culturally diverse families, *Fam Soc J Contemp Human Services* 23:531, 1994.

Crosbie-Burnet M: Remarriage and recoupling. In McHenry PC, Price SJ, editors: *Families and change: coping with stressful events*, London, 1994, Sage.

Danielson CB, Hamell-Bissell B, Winstead-Fry P: *Family health and illness*, St Louis, 1993, Mosby.

Demo DH, Ganong LH: *Divorce*. In McHenry PC, Price SJ, editors: *Families and change: coping with stressful events*, London, 1994, Sage.

Durham JD: The changing HIV/AIDS epidemic, *Nurs Clin North Am* 29(1):9, 1994.

Estess PS: When kids don't leave, *Modern Maturity* November-December, p 56, 1994.

Fine MA: Families in the United States: their current and future prospects, *Fam Relations* 41(4):430, 1992.

Fine MA: Family diversity: current approaches to understanding family diversity, *Fam Relations* 42(3):235, 1993.

Friedman M: *Family nursing: theory and assessment,* ed 3, New York, 1992, Appleton Century Crofts.

Gelles RJ: *Contemporary families: a sociological view,* Thousand Oaks, Calif, 1994, Sage.

Hall LA, Sachs B, Rayens MK et al: Childhood and sexual abuse: their relationship with depressive symptoms in adulthood, *Image J Nurs Sch* 25(4):317, 1993.

Hanson S: Involving families in programs for teen: consequences for teens and their families, *Fam Relations* 41(4):303, 1992.

Hanson S, Helms M, Julian D: Education for family health care professionals: nursing as a paradigm, *Fam Relations* 41(1):49, 1992.

Hare J, Richards L: Children raised by lesbian couples, *Fam Relations* 42(3):249, 1993.

Hough EE: Family response to mother's chronic illness, *West J Nurs Res* 13(5):568, 1991.

Hill R: Generic features of families under stress, *Social Casework* 39:145, 1958.

Hilton BA: Family communication patterns in coping with early breast cancer, *West J Nurs Res* 16(4):366, 1994.

Julian TW, McHenry PC, McKelvey MW: Cultural variations in parenting, *Fam Relations* 43(1):30, 1994.

Jurich JA, Adams RA, Schlenberg JE: Factors related to behavior change in response to AIDS, *Fam Relations* 41(1):97, 1992.

Kamo Y, Zhou M: Living arrangements of elderly Chinese and Japanese in the United States, *J Marriage Fam* 56(3):544, 1994.

Kelley SJ: Caregiver stress in grandparents raising grandchildren, *Image J Nurs Sch* 25(4):331, 1993.

Kim MJ, McFarland GK, McLane AM: *Pocket guide to nursing diagnoses,* ed 6, St Louis, 1995, Mosby.

Levy F, Michel R: *The economic future of American families,* Washington, DC, 1991, Urban Institute.

Lindsey EW: Homelessness. In McHenry PC, Price SH, editors: *Families and change: coping with stressful events,* London, 1994, Sage.

Manning WD: Marriage and cohabitation following premarital conception, *J Marriage Fam* 55(4), 1993.

Maslow AH: *Motivation and personality,* ed 2, New York, 1970, Harper & Row.

McClowry SG: Family functioning during a critical illness, *Crit Care Nurs Clinic Am* 4(4):559, 1992.

McGoldrick M, Carter E: The stage of the family life cycle. In Henslin J, editor: *Marriage and family in a changing society,* New York, 1985, Free Press.

Meyer DR, Garaskey S: Custodial fathers: myths, realities and child support policies, *J Marriage Fam* 55(1):73, 1993.

Nichols SY: Work and family stress. In McHenry PC, Price SJ, editors: *Families and change: coping with stressful events,* London, 1994, Sage.

Ross CE: Impact of family on health, *J Marriage Fam* 52(4):1059, 1990.

Taylor RJ, Chatters LM, Jackson JS: A profile of familial relations among three-generation black families, *Fam Relations* 42(3):332, 1993.

US Bureau of the Census: *Statistical abstract of the United States: 1987,* ed 108, Washington, DC, 1991, US Government Printing Office.

Vosburgh D, Simpson P: Linking family theory and practice, *Image J Nurs Sch* 25(3):231, 1993.

Whall A: *Family theory development in nursing: state of the science and art,* Philadelphia, 1991, FA Davis.

Zinn MB, Eitzen DS: *Diversity in American families,* ed 3, New York, 1993, Harper & Row.

ADDITIONAL READINGS

Ahmann, E: Family centered care: shifting orientation, *Pediatr Nurs* 20(2):113, 1994.

Browning JS, Schwirian PM: Spousal caregivers' burden: impact of care recipient health problems and mental status, *J Gerontol Nurs* 20(4):17, 1994.

D'Avanzo CE, Frye B, Froman R: Stress in Cambodian refugee families, *Image J Nurs Sch* 26(2):101, 1994.

Feetham SL, Meister SB, Bell JM et al, editors: *The nursing of families: theory, research, education, practice,* Newbury Park, Calif, 1992, Sage.

Fisher L, Lieberman MA: Alzheimer's disease: the impact of the family on spouses, offspring, and in-laws, *Fam Process* 33:305, 1994.

Harvath TA, Archibold PG, Stewart BJ: Establishing partnerships with family caregivers, *J Gerontol Nurs* 20(2):29, 1994.

Kissman K, Allen JA: *Single-parent families,* Newberry Park, Calif, 1993, Sage.

McHenry PS, Price SJ: *Families and change: coping with stressful events,* London, 1994, Sage.

Owen MT, Mulvihill BA: Benefits of a parent education program and support program in the first three years, *Fam Relations* 42(2):206, 1994.

Pruchno R, Burant C, Peters ND: Family mental health: marital and parent-child consensus as predictors, *J Marriage Fam* 56(3):747, 1994.

Reinhard SC: Perspectives on the family's caregiving experience in mental illness, *Image J Nurs Sch* 26(1):70, 1994.

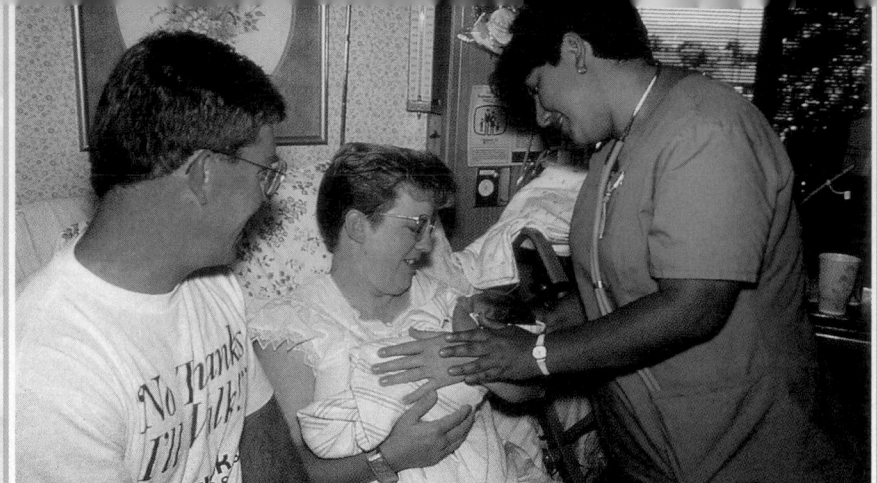

 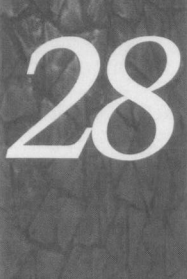
Conception Through Preschool

Objectives

Mastery of content in this chapter will enable the student to:

▶ Define the key terms listed.

▶ Identify the basic principles of growth and development.

▶ Discuss factors influencing growth and development.

▶ Compare and discuss theories of growth and development.

▶ Discuss physiological and psychosocial health concerns during the transition of the child from intrauterine to extrauterine life.

▶ Explain the concept of critical periods of development and identify factors that can disturb or promote optimal development of the child.

▶ Describe characteristics of the physical growth of the unborn child, infant, toddler, and preschooler.

▶ Describe cognitive and psychosocial development from birth to 6 years.

▶ Explain the interactions that occur between parent and child.

▶ Describe variables influencing how children learn about and perceive their health status.

▶ Identify areas in which parents of both well and hospitalized children can benefit from the nurse's anticipatory guidance.

▶ Describe the use of the nursing process to individualize the nursing care plan for the hospitalized child.

▶ Identify routine newborn screening tests for inborn errors of metabolism and the significance of their detection to the child's well-being.

▶ Explain the role of play in the development of the child.

▶ Discuss nursing interventions to effectively handle the fears of children.

Understanding children and their growth and development is essential to promoting health and establishing healthful patterns. The nurse must have a clear understanding of normal or expected growth and behavior in early developmental stages to guide and promote normalcy and to detect and prevent abnormalities. For example, without the knowledge that the average 8 month old is able to sit alone without support, the nurse may not promote the development of this skill at an appropriate age.

Nursing practice based on principles of growth and development is organized and directed at helping children and their families adapt to changing internal and external conditions. This chapter discusses principles and concepts of growth and development and their application to health promotion from conception through preschool. It also demonstrates that a good understanding of growth and development is essential for individualizing the care of ill children.

GROWTH AND DEVELOPMENT THEORY

Human growth and development are orderly, predictable processes beginning with conception and continuing until death. All persons progress through definite phases of growth and development, but the pace and behavior of this progression are highly individual. Children must learn to walk before they can run, but one child may walk at 10 months, and another may not walk until 15 months.

The ability to progress through each developmental phase influences the holistic health of the individual. The success or failure experienced within a phase affects the ability to complete subsequent phases. If an individual experiences repeated developmental failures, inadequacies result. However, if the individual experiences repeated successes, competencies that maintain and promote health result. A child not learning to walk by 18 or 20 months, for example, demonstrates delayed gross motor ability that slows exploration and manipulation of the environment. A child walking by 10 months is able to explore and find stimulation in the environment, thereby enhancing learning.

Understanding the growth and development process, its theories and principles, its stages, and factors that influence it allows the nurse to assess the individual's progress, and provides a foundation for the delivery of health care to persons of all ages. A developmental approach allows the nurse to organize knowledge about human behavior into common patterns that can be applied to individuals. Recognition that the stress of trauma or illness and hospitalization has the ability to impair the child's development motivates the nurse to plan care that maintains or promotes the child's development.

A developmental perspective helps the nurse understand *why* commonalities and variations exist and how they influence health. With this knowledge the nurse can provide care in a manner that addresses the client's unique needs and developmental level.

Definitions

Growth and development are synchronous processes that are interdependent in the healthy individual. A person experiences quantitative and qualitative changes in growth and development.

PHYSICAL GROWTH

Physical **growth** is the quantitative, or measurable, aspect of an individual's increase in physical measurements as a result of an increase in cell number. Measurable growth indicators include changes in height, weight, teeth, skeletal structures, and sexual characteristics. For example, children generally double their birth weight by 6 months of age and their birth height by 36 months.

DEVELOPMENT

The qualitative, or behavioral, aspects of progressive adaptation to the environment are called **development**. An example of these qualitative changes is increased functioning capacity resulting from mastery of several smaller skills. For instance, a significant qualitative and observable change for preschoolers is participating in telephone conversations with their parents. Before developing this capacity, they must develop a small vocabulary, learn to put words together in phrases and sentences, and develop a cognitive understanding of **object permanence** (that a person or object out of sight still exists).

MATURATION

Maturation is the process of becoming fully developed and grown. It involves an individual's biological ability, physiological condition, and desire to learn more mature behavior. To mature, the individual may have to relinquish previous behavior and learning, integrate new patterns into existing behavior, or both. Maturation influences the sequence and timing of the changes associated with growth and development. For example, the infant relinquishes crawling for walking because walking permits more extensive investigation of the environment and more learning. However, the infant cannot walk until the biological ability and structures to perform the action (i.e., increased muscle cells and tone) have developed.

CRITICAL PERIODS OF DEVELOPMENT

Stages of growth and development involve the concept of "critical periods of development." A **critical period** is a specific span of time during which the environment has its greatest impact on the individual (Papalia and Olds, 1992). During these critical periods some form of sensory stimulation is necessary for developmental progression. Without stimulation, task completion is difficult or unattainable. For example, the toddler who has not been encouraged to learn to walk during a set time may have difficulty learning to walk at another time. Therefore developmental progression depends on the timing and degree of stimulation, as well as on the readiness to be stimulated by the environment. A stimulus provided too early may not be useful. For example, an 18-month-old child cannot learn to write, regardless of the intensity of the stimuli.

PRINCIPLES OF GROWTH AND DEVELOPMENT

Some principles of growth and development are true for all people. These commonalities are expressed by the following concepts:

1. Individuals have an adaptive potential for qualitative and quantitative changes by receiving stimuli from and giving stimuli to the environment.

2. Individuals derive uniqueness from the interaction of heredity and environment.

3. The primary goal of development is achievement of potential (self-realization or self-actualization).

The basic principles of growth and development follow:

1. Development is orderly and follows a set sequence.

2. Development is directional and proceeds in the following manner:
   a. Cephalocaudal, in which growth proceeds from the head to the lower parts of the body;
   b. Proximodistal, in which development proceeds from the central (proximal) areas of the body to the outer (distal);
   c. Differentiation, in which development proceeds from simple to complex.

3. Development is complex, yet predictable, occurring with a consistent pattern and chronology.

4. Development is unique to individuals and their genetic potential, and each individual tends to seek a maximum potential for development.

5. Development occurs through conflict and adaptation, and different aspects develop at different rates, creating periods of equilibrium and disequilibrium.

6. Development involves challenges for individuals in the form of certain tasks specific to age and ability.

7. Developmental tasks require practice and energy, the focus of which varies with each developmental stage and task accomplished.

■ STAGES OF GROWTH AND DEVELOPMENT

Human growth and development are continuous and intricate, complex processes that are often divided into stages organized by age groups. Although this chronological division is arbitrary, it is based on the timing and sequence of developmental tasks that the individual must accomplish to progress to another stage. Developmental periods are listed in the box below.

Major Factors Influencing Growth and Development

The human being is a complex, open system influenced by natural forces from within and from the environment. Interaction between these forces affects development. In general, natural factors set the limits for development, whereas external factors present opportunities for achieving that potential (Table 28-1).

■ THEORIES OF HUMAN DEVELOPMENT

Research into human growth and development has led to several developmental theories. These theories vary in the way humans are viewed and in the aspect of development emphasized. Some theories view development as a continuous process, moving from the simple to the more complex. Others consider it as discontinuous, with alternating periods of relative equilibrium and disequilibrium. Health

---

Developmental Age Periods

PRENATAL PERIOD: CONCEPTION TO BIRTH
Germinal: Conception to approximately 2 weeks
Embryonic: 2-8 weeks
Fetal: 8-40 weeks (birth)
A rapid growth rate and total dependency make this one of the most crucial periods in the developmental process. The relationship between maternal health and certain manifestations in the newborn emphasizes the importance of adequate prenatal care to the health and well-being of the infant.

INFANCY PERIOD: BIRTH TO 12 OR 18 MONTHS
Neonatal: Birth to 28 days
Infancy: 1 to approximately 12 months
The infancy period is one of rapid motor, cognitive, and social development. Through mutuality with the care giver (parent), the infant establishes a basic trust in the world and the foundation for future interpersonal relationships. The critical first month of life, although part of the infancy period, is often differentiated from the remainder because of the major physical adjustments to extrauterine existence and the psychological adjustment of the parent.

EARLY CHILDHOOD: 1-6 YEARS
Toddler: 1 to 3 years
Preschool: 3 to 6 years
This period, which extends from the time children attain upright locomotion until they enter school, is characterized by intense activity and discovery. It is a time of marked physical and personality development. Motor

development advances steadily. Children at this age acquire language and wider social relationships, learn role standards, gain self-control and mastery, develop increasing awareness of dependence and independence, and begin to develop self-concepts.

MIDDLE CHILDHOOD: 6-11 OR 12 YEARS
Frequently referred to as the "school age," this period of development is one in which the child is directed away from the family group and is centered around the wider world of peer relationships. There is steady advancement in physical, mental, and social development, with emphasis on developing skill competencies. Social cooperation and early moral development take on more importance with relevance for later life stages. This is a critical period in the development of self-concept.

LATE CHILDHOOD: 11-21 YEARS
Preadolescence: 10-13 years
Adolescence proper: 13-18 years
Late adolescence: 18-21 years
The tumultuous period of rapid maturation and change known as *adolescence* is considered a transitional period that begins at the onset of puberty and extends to the point of entry into the adult world, which may occur after high school graduation, college graduation, or later. Biological and personality maturation are accompanied by physical and emotional turmoil, and there is a redefining of the self-concept. In late adolescence the child begins to internalize all previously learned values and focus on an individual, rather than a group, identity.

Modified from Wong DL: *Whaley and Wong's nursing care of infants and children*, ed 5, St Louis, 1995, Mosby.

Table 28-1	Major Factors Influencing Growth and Development	

FACTORS	RELEVANT INFLUENCES
FORCES OF NATURE	
Heredity	Genetic endowment determines sex, race, hair and eye color, physical growth, stature, and to some extent psychological uniqueness.
Temperament	Temperament is characteristic psychological mood with which the child is born and includes behavioral styles of easy, slow-to-warm, and difficult. It influences interactions between the individual and environment.
EXTERNAL FORCES	
Family	Family purpose is to protect and nurture its members.
	Family functions include means for survival, security, assistance with emotional and social development, assistance with maintenance of relationships, instruction about society and world, and assistance in learning roles and behaviors.
	Family influences through its values, beliefs, customs, and specific patterns of interaction and communication.
	Ordinal position and sex influence individual's interaction and communication in family.
Peer group	Peer group provides new and different learning environment.
	Peer group provides different patterns and structures of interaction and communication, necessitating different style of behavior.
	Functions of peer group include allowing individual to learn about success and failure; to validate and challenge thoughts, feelings, and concepts; to receive acceptance, support, and rejection as unique person apart from family; and to achieve group purposes by meeting demands, pressures, and expectations.
Life experiences	Life experiences and learning processes allow individual to develop by applying what has been learned to what needs to be learned.
	Learning process involves series of steps: recognition of need to know task; mastery of skills to perform task; mastery of task; expertise in performing task, which expands capabilities; integration into whole functioning; and use of accumulated skills and experiences to develop repertoire of effective behavior.
Health environment	Level of health affects individual's responsiveness to environment and responsiveness of others to the individual.
Prenatal health	Preconception (e.g., genetic and chromosomal factors, maternal age, health) and postconception (e.g., nutrition, weight gain, use of tobacco and alcohol, medical problems, use of prenatal services) factors affect fetal growth and development.
Nutrition	Growth is regulated by dietary factors. Adequacy of nutrients influences whether and how physiological needs, as well as subsequent growth and development needs, are met.
Rest, sleep, and exercise	Balance between rest or sleep and exercise is essential to rejuvenating body. Disturbances diminish growth, whereas equilibrium reinforces physiological and psychological health.
State of health	Illness or injury potentially hampers growth and development. Nature and duration of health problem influences its impact. Prolonged injury or illness may cause inability to cope and respond to demands and tasks of developmental stages.
Living environment	Factors affecting growth and development include season, climate, home life, and socioeconomic status.

care professionals often use different theoretical frameworks as a basis for care. Because theories differ it is important to communicate effectively with other health professionals when providing coordinated health care, and the nurse must be familiar with the common developmental theories (Table 28-2). No one framework addresses all developmental areas.

According to Freud, pleasure shifts from one erogenous zone of the body to another. A child's maturation level determines when this shift occurs. If gratification is excessive or denied, the child may become emotionally stuck (fixated) at a particular stage.

According to Erikson (1963), each stage has a personality crisis involving a major conflict that is critical at that time. The developing ego is greatly affected by societal and cultural influences, and the successful outcome of each crisis includes development of a particular virtue. The successful mastery of each conflict is built on satisfactory completion of the previous core conflict. This theory recognizes the importance of heredity and environment and has an epigenetic basis. Development is predetermined by genetic principles and proceeds along an age-stage pathway.

Maslow's theory of human needs (1970) describes a hierarchy of needs that motivate human behavior. When the most basic needs have been fulfilled, a person strives to satisfy those needs on the next level and so forth. The highest level, achieved by only a few, represents realization of one's potential.

Piaget (1952) views the development of the mind as occurring through adaptation to the environment. The child

Table 28-2	Summary of Development According to Stage Theorists	
STAGES AND AGES	**CHARACTERISTICS OF STAGES**	**THEORY ADDENDUM**
FREUD'S PSYCHOSEXUAL THEORY		
Oral-sensory (birth to 12-18 mo) (infancy)	Activities involving mouth such as sucking, biting, and chewing are chief source of pleasure.	Child deprived of sufficient sucking might attempt to satisfy this need later in life through activities such as gum chewing, smoking, and overeating.
Anal-muscular (12-18 mo to 3 yr) (toddlerhood)	Sensual gratification is derived from retention and expulsion of feces. Smearing is common activity.	External conflicts may be encountered when toilet training is attempted and later result in behaviors such as constipation, tardiness, or stinginess.
Phallic-locomotion (3-6 yr) (preschool)	Manipulation of genitalia results in pleasurable sensations. Masturbation begins and sexual curiosity becomes evident.	Emergence of Oedipus and Electra complexes for males and females respectively, occurs. Brashness, bashfulness, and timidity may be expressions of fixation at this stage.
Latency (6 yr to puberty) (school-age)	This is tranquil period when Freud believed sexual drives were dormant; however, child may engage in erogenous activities with same-sex peers.	Child's use of coping and defense mechanisms emerge at this time; any sexual interest may be sublimated through vigorous play and skill acquisition.
Genital (puberty through adulthood) (adolescence and adulthood)	Genitalia become center of sexual tension and pleasure. Sexual hormone production stimulates development of heterosexual relationships.	This is the time of biological upheaval, when immature emotional interactions often occur in early phase. In time, ability to give and receive mature love develops.
ERIKSON'S PSYCHOSOCIAL THEORY		
Trust versus mistrust (birth to 1 yr) (infancy) Mode: taking in and getting Virtue: hope	Care giver's satisfaction of infant's basic needs for food and sucking, warmth and comfort, and love and security in consistent and sensitive manner results in trust.	When basic needs of infant are not met or are met inadequately, infant becomes suspicious, fearful, and mistrusting. This is evidenced by poor eating, sleeping, and elimination behaviors.
Autonomy versus doubt and shame (1-3 yr) (toddlerhood) Mode: holding on and letting go Virtue: will	Child develops beginning independence while gaining control over bodily functions of undressing and dressing, walking, talking, feeding self, and toileting. Self-control begins.	If toddler's developing independence is discouraged by parents, child may doubt personal abilities; if child is made to feel bad when attempts to be autonomous fail, child develops shame.
Initiative versus guilt (3-6 yr) (preschool) Mode: intrusive attack and conquest Virtue: purpose	Child develops initiative when planning and trying out new things. Behavior of child is characterized as vigorous, imaginative, and intrusive. Conscience and identification with same-sex parent develop.	Parental restrictiveness may prevent child from developing initiative. Guilt may arise when child undertakes activities in conflict with those of parents. Child must learn to initiate activities without infringing on rights of others.
Industry versus inferiority (6-12 yr to puberty) (school-age) Mode: doing and producing Virtue: competence	Child wins recognition by demonstration of skill and production of things and develops self-esteem through achievements. Child is greatly influenced by teachers and school.	Feelings of inferiority may occur when adults perceive child's attempt to learn how things work through manipulation to be silly or troublesome. Lack of success in school, development of physical skills, and making of friends also contribute to inferiority.
Identify versus role confusion or diffusion (puberty to 18-21 yr) (adolescence) Virtue: fidelity	Individual develops integrated sense of "self." Peers have major influence over behavior. Major decision is to determine vocational goal.	Failure to develop sense of personal identity may lead to role confusion, which often results in feelings of inadequacy, isolation, and indecisiveness. Psychosocial moratorium provides extra time for making vocational decision.
Intimacy versus isolation (18-21 to 40 yr) (young adulthood) Mode: loving Virtue: love	Task is to develop close and sharing relationships with others, which may include sexual partner.	Individual unsure of self-identity will have difficulty developing intimacy. Person unwilling or unable to share self will be lonely.
Generativity versus self-absorption or stagnation (40-65 yr) (middle adulthood) Mode: nurturing Virtue: care	Mature adult is concerned with establishing and guiding next generation. Adult looks beyond self and expresses concern for future of world in general.	Self-absorbed adult will be preoccupied with personal well-being and material gains. Preoccupation with self leads to stagnation of life.

Table 28-2	Summary of Development According to Stage Theorists—cont'd	
STAGES AND AGES	**CHARACTERISTICS OF STAGES**	**THEORY ADDENDUM**

ERIKSON'S PSYCHOSOCIAL THEORY—CONT'D

Ego integrity versus despair (65 yr to death) (older adulthood) Mode: acceptance Virtue: wisdom	Older adult can look back with sense of satisfaction and acceptance of life and death.	Unsuccessful resolution of this crisis may result in sense of despair in which individual views life as series of misfortunes, disappointments, and failures.

MASLOW'S THEORY OF HUMAN NEED

Physiological needs	Physiological needs include food, beverages, and sleep.	Theory of motivation depicts individual driven to fulfill potential, capacities, and talents to become unique being. Person moves up and down hierarchy as life situations change.
Safety needs	Satisfying safety needs allows individual to feel safe and secure.	
Belongingness and love needs	Belongingness allows individual to affiliate with and be accepted by others.	
Esteem needs	Esteem allows individual to gain approval of others.	
Self-actualization	Self-fulfillment potential is recognized.	

PIAGET'S THEORY OF COGNITIVE DEVELOPMENT

Sensorimotor (Birth to 2 yr)	Child learns about world through sensory and motor activities.	Child slowly develops concept that people and objects have permanence, even though they are no longer visible.
Reflex activities (birth to 1 mo)	Child exercises inborn reflexes and gains some control over them.	Modified reflexes become more efficient. Sucking is more effective and selective.
Primary circular reactions (1-4 mo)	Infant repeats pleasurable actions that first occur by chance. Activities focus on body of infant; coordination begins.	Eye, eye-ear, and hand-mouth coordination develop, and activities such as thumb sucking and bottle sucking become more intentional and proficient.
Secondary circular reactions (4-8 mo)	Child attempts to reproduce interesting, pleasant events in environment. Interest goes beyond body.	Infant searches for object dropped and recognizes partially hidden object. Child begins to associate two behaviors such as cradle position and feeding.
Coordination of secondary schemas (8-12 mo)	Child puts together skills used earlier to reach goal in new situation.	Child will crawl across room to get desired toy and search for hidden objects where they were previously hidden.
Tertiary circular reactions (12-18 mo) ("trial and error")	Child actively explores world and varies actions to see novelty of object, event, or situation. Trial and error are used to problem solve.	Child might try to get toy out of small opening of container with hand first and then turn it upside down and hit it so that toy falls out. Child comprehends series of object displacements if visible.
Invention of new means through mental combinations (18-24 mo) ("representation")	Toddler begins creating mental images and thus can devise new ways to deal with environment. Child begins to think about events without resorting to action.	Child attains true object permanence and will search for objects he or she has not seen hidden; for example, toddler will look many places for bottle. Insight is demonstrated by looking for bottle in refrigerator.
Preoperational (2-7 yr)	Child develops representational system and uses symbols such as words to represent people, places, and objects.	Preoperational concepts are limited by ability to focus on only one aspect at time (centration), and thought often seems illogical because child reasons from one specific to another (e.g., car hit dog because boy was mad at it).
Preconceptual (2-4 yr)	Child is primarily egocentric. Perceptual-bound and transductive thinking begin; child is animistic.	Deferred imitation (imitation of observed action after time has passed) demonstrates use of symbolism.
Intuitive (4-7 yr)	Child begins to figure things out but cannot explain them rationally. Child is unable to consider parts as composing whole.	Intuitive concepts allow classification of items by one attribute, usually color or shape (e.g., inability to focus on more than one characteristic at time).

Continued.

Table 28-2	Summary of Development According to Stage Theorists—cont'd	
STAGES AND AGES	**CHARACTERISTICS OF STAGES**	**THEORY ADDENDUM**
PIAGET'S THEORY OF COGNITIVE DEVELOPMENT—CONT'D		
Concrete Operations (7-11 yr)	Ability to understand law of conservation results in logical thought patterns and mental operations such as reversibility, decentering, seriation, transformation, classification of two or more attributes, and inductive and deductive reasoning.	Limitations are inability of child to understand abstractions. Child's thinking is restricted to immediate and physical. School-ager can reason about what is but cannot hypothesize about what may be and thus cannot think about future problems (e.g., ability to play game of checkers).
Formal Operations (Develops 11-15 yr, Used Throughout Life)	Ability to think in abstract manner develops, and scientific reasoning emerges. Initially, thought is rigid, but it becomes adaptable and flexible.	Adolescent may confuse ideal with practical but, when confronted with problem (real or hypothetical), can suggest number of solutions. Ability to consider moral and political issues from variety of perspectives is present.
KOHLBERG'S THEORY OF MORAL REASONING		
Premoral Level (Birth to 9 yr)	There is little awareness of what is socially acceptable moral behavior. Control is external.	Infant defers to power and authority. Life is valued for number and power of possessions.
Punishment and obedience orientation (birth to 6 yr)	Rules of others are followed to avoid punishment.	Child integrates labels of *good* and *bad* and *right* and *wrong* into behavior in terms of the consequences of actions.
Naively egoistic orientation (6-9 yr)	Child conforms to rules out of self-interest; child reasons that reward or favor will be earned.	Elements of bargaining, equal sharing, and fairness are evident. Life is valued for how child can satisfy needs of others.
Conventional Morality (9-13 yr)	Efforts are made to please other persons. Control is becoming internal.	Child is loyal and concerned with maintaining family expectations regardless of consequences.
"Good boy, nice girl" (9-10 yr)	Desire to please and help others is foremost. Child conforms to avoid rejection.	Life is valued for how good interpersonal relationships are (identify with emotionally important persons).
Authority maintaining morality	Child does duty to avoid criticism by authorities.	Identification shifts to religious or social institutions such as school.
Postconventional Level of Morality (13 yr to Death)	Individual attains true morality. Conduct control is internal.	Attainment of true morality occurs after formal operations have been reached. Not everyone reaches this level.
Contractual and legalistic orientation	Individual selects moral principles by which to live and obeys laws.	Individual is careful not to violate rights and wills of others. Moral and legal views conflict. Person will work to change laws.
Universal ethical-principle orientation	Individual behaves in way that respects dignity of all.	This stage is rarely attained. If internal set of ideas is violated, guilt results.

assimilates (fits) new information into existing cognitive structures (schema) and accommodates (changes) the schema to deal with new information. Striving for balance (equilibration) occurs through these two processes. Piaget also incorporated the epigenetic principle into his theory. This principle states that development depends on a person's genetic programming and that each aspect or part has its own time for ascendancy. The constant interplay of genetics, maturation, experience, and interaction results in cognitive development. This theory places humans in an active learning role and is important for understanding how children learn.

Kohlberg (1968) contends that cognitive development underlies the progression of a person's morality from level to level. These stages occur in the same order, regardless of culture. Individuals differ in how quickly and how far they progress through these stages.

■ SELECTING A DEVELOPMENTAL FRAMEWORK FOR NURSING

Providing nursing care to clients of all developmental stages is easier when planning is based on a theoretical framework. An organized, systematic approach ensures that client needs are assessed and met by the plan of care. If nursing care is delivered only as a series of isolated actions, some of the client's developmental needs may be overlooked. A developmental approach encourages organized care directed at the client's current level of functioning to motivate self-direction and health promotion. For example, understanding an adolescent's need to be independent should prompt the nurse to establish a contract about the care plan and its implementation.

The developmental approach also has advantages for clients. Their capabilities are used, and they are actively involved in their own care. Total health is also promoted, because the nurse is aware of clients' developmental stages and the directions in which they are headed. Therefore the nurse can focus on activities that foster developmental task completion. For example, nurses might encourage toddlers to feed themselves to advance their developing independence and thus promote their sense of autonomy.

CONCEPTION

From the moment of conception, human development proceeds at a rapid rate. Intrauterine health problems are caused by both genetic and environmental factors. During the prenatal period, the embryo grows from a single cell to a complex, physiological being. All major organ systems develop in utero, with some functioning before birth. The psychosocial being also begins to emerge during gestation.

Intrauterine Life

Intrauterine life generally lasts 9 calendar or 10 lunar months. The organism's life begins after sexual intercourse has occurred, when the ovum is penetrated by one sperm. Fertilization usually takes place in the fallopian tube within 12 to 24 hours after the release of the ovum from the ovary. The ovum and sperm fuse, and the material from both cell nuclei unites. The organism then has its full genetic complement in one pair of sex chromosomes and 22 pairs of autosomal chromosomes. The ovum and the sperm each contribute one chromosome to each pair. It is through this mechanism that genetically programmed diseases (such as Down syndrome) and genetically determined characteristics (such as eye color) are transmitted from parent to child.

The fertilized ovum, or **zygote**, passes through the fallopian tube to the uterus within 4 days. During this time the zygote continues to divide. By the third day a solid ball of cells, the **morula**, has formed. This solid ball soon develops a central cavity, or **blastocyst**. Even at this early stage, cells begin to differentiate in structure and function. Cells at one end of the blastocyst develop into the **embryo**, and those at the opposite end form the **placenta**. By day 4 the embryo has traveled through the fallopian tube and has begun its implantation into the uterine wall.

Before implantation the embryo is relatively protected from the external environment, but with implantation it becomes more vulnerable to the larger maternal environment via exchange of materials through the placenta. The placenta produces essential hormones that help maintain the pregnancy and that permit transfer of material between the embryo and mother, including oxygen, carbon dioxide, nutrients, and waste products. Because the placenta is extremely porous, noxious materials such as viruses and drugs can also pass from mother to child. The effect of noxious agents on the unborn child depends on the developmental stage in which exposure takes place.

The period of gestation is frequently divided into three periods called *trimesters*. Because the developing baby, or **fetus**, is in a different stage of development in each trimester, interference with the development process has different outcomes in each.

Physical Development

FIRST TRIMESTER

The first trimester is the first 3 calendar months. After implantation, fetal cells continue to differentiate and develop into essential organ systems. These processes of cellular change (differentiation) and staged organ change (development) occur at different rates and times, and each organ is extremely vulnerable to environmental insult. Interference with growth can cause the congenital absence of an organ system or extensive structural or functional alterations. Because several organ systems develop at the same time, disruption of one system often occurs with disruption of others. The nurse should consider this simultaneous development when conducting the initial newborn nursing assessment. Fig. 28-1 shows the approximate times of critical differentiation for some of the major organ systems and their overlapping of development.

Health Promotion. Agents capable of producing adverse effects in the fetus are called **teratogens**. Some teratogens produce defects only if the fetus is exposed to the agent when the vulnerable organ is developing. The nurse educates the mother about avoiding exposure to teratogenic agents. One such teratogen is the rubella or German measles virus, which can cause spontaneous abortion, stillbirth, or birth defects of the eyes, ears, and heart; primarily when exposure is in the first trimester.

Many drugs are teratogenic during rapid organ growth (**organogenesis**) in the first trimester. Barbiturates, anticoagulants, anticonvulsants, antimicrobials, alcohol, cancer chemotherapeutics, and hydantoin anticonvulsants are only a few of the chemical agents associated with fetal abnormalities, and many other agents are still under investigation. Benefits of any drug needed to maintain the mother's health must be weighed against potential harm to the fetus. Abuse of drugs such as cocaine and LSD results in preterm labor and chromosomal breakage, respectively. Smoking has been shown to reduce birth weight and increase the incidence of fetal and neonatal death (Bobak, 1993). Although the effect on the fetus of maternal caffeine usage is controversial, the safest policy is to avoid it. With this knowledge, the nurse should explore lifestyle changes that can help a pregnant woman maintain abstinence from tobacco, alcohol, and medications.

The diet of a woman both before and during pregnancy has a significant effect on the development of the infant in utero. It has been repeatedly demonstrated that mothers who eat well have fewer complications of pregnancy and childbirth and bear healthier babies than those with inferior nutritional intake (Bobak, 1993). The consequences of maternal malnutrition on fetal development make the improvement of the nutritional state of pregnant women a worthy nursing aim (see the box on p. 505).

SECOND TRIMESTER

During the second trimester, months 3 through 6, some organ systems continue basic development while the functional capabilities of others are refined. By the end of the sixth month, most organ systems are complete and can function. The fetus is therefore considered viable, or capa-

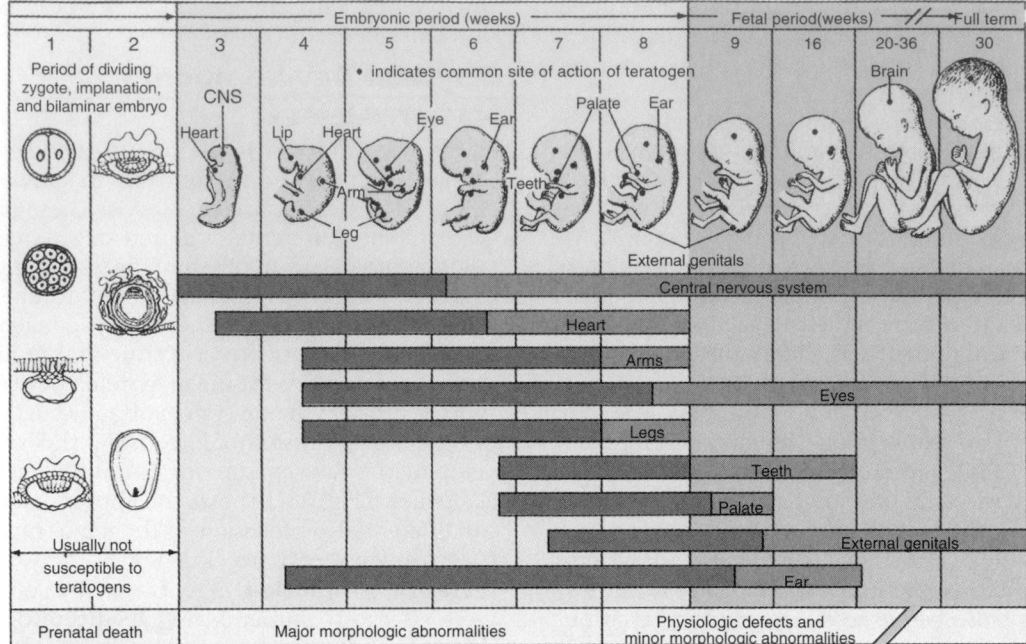

Fig. 28-1 Periods of organ differentiation. *(From Moore KL, Pernaud TV:* The developing human: clinically oriented embryology, *ed 5, Philadelphia, 1993, WB Saunders.)*

ble of life outside the uterus, if given intensive environmental support. The fetus weighs about 0.7 kg (1½ lb) and is approximately 30 cm (12 inches) long. Fingers and toes are differentiated, a rudimentary kidney functions, and the sex of the fetus can be determined. The fetus is covered with **vernix caseosa**, a cheeselike substance coating the skin. **Lanugo**, or fine hair, covers most of the body. These substances protect the thin, fragile skin and decrease in amount as the pregnancy nears its completion; thus infants born before 38 weeks gestation have more of these protective coverings than full-term infants.

Health Promotion. In the second trimester the fetal heart beat becomes audible to stethoscope auscultation, and the mother becomes aware of fetal movement. Both events are highly significant to the parents because they provide tangible evidence of the pregnancy and reassure them that the fetus is alive. Therefore the nurse should focus on these events during prenatal care.

Changes in maternal behavior during this period include planning for the birth, concern for personal safety, and preoccupation with health and appearance. The nurse can help the woman adapt to these changes and plan for the impending birth. This is often a good time for education about gestational events and appropriate maternal rest and nutrition. Discussing birth alternatives and providing support and reassurance about the pregnancy's progression are appropriate nursing actions at this stage.

THIRD TRIMESTER

During the last 3 months of intrauterine life the fetus grows to approximately 50 cm (19 to 20 inches) in length. Subcutaneous fat is stored, and weight increases to between 3.2 and 3.4 kg (7 to 7½ lb). The skin thickens, lanugo begins to disappear, and the fetal body becomes rounder and fuller.

A tremendous spurt in brain growth begins during this trimester and lasts well into the first few years of life. The central nervous system has established its total number of neurons and connections between neurons, and myelination of nerve fibers progresses at a rapid rate. Exposure to noxious agents and the absence of essential nutrients are the most common causes of damage to the central nervous system during this trimester. The nurse can teach the woman about these factors, particularly through nutritional counseling.

At the end of the third trimester the normal fetus is physically able to make the transition from intrauterine to extrauterine life. The cardiac system can change its circulation to end bypassing of the lungs. The lungs are capable of maintaining the inflated state for gas exchange. The primitive temperature maintenance systems, reflexes, and sensory organs are ready for use.

Health Promotion. Exposure to noxious agents and the absence of essential nutrients can cause damage to the central nervous system and result in alteration of high-level cognitive functions. The nurse can increase the mother's awareness of these dangers through counseling and help her evaluate the quality of her nutritional intake. Thoughts of delivering a healthy infant are foremost in the mother's mind as she focuses on preparing her mind and body for the delivery. Parents often seek information regarding the childbirth process and breast-feeding.

Cognitive Development

Relationships between prenatal events and cognitive development are difficult to establish. However, periods of diminished oxygen (anoxia) during fetal life are known to cause deficits in later cognitive functioning, and inadequate prenatal nutrition has been associated with lower brain weight. The large volume of research on develop-

CLIENT TEACHING on Folic Acid (Folacin) for Females Capable of Becoming Pregnant

OBJECTIVE
- Client will consume 0.4 mg of folic acid (Vitamin B₉) every day.

TEACHING STRATEGIES
- Educate women between the ages of 14 and 44 about the benefit of folic acid to a developing unborn child, particularly during the first month of pregnancy.
- Discuss the fact that the woman does not always know the moment of conception so she should have a daily intake of folic acid. (This water-soluble vitamin is readily excreted in the urine.)
- Encourage females capable of becoming pregnant to consume 0.4 mg of folic acid every day (recommendation of U.S. Public Health Service). It is possible to do this through daily food sources of folic acid but studies have shown that adolescent girls in particular have inadequate folacin status, with serum levels and dietary intake decreasing with increasing age. The deficiency is not related to family income (Williams, 1993).
- Discuss including rich food sources of folacin in the daily diet, such as green leafy vegetables, asparagus, kidney, and liver. Other poorer sources are milk, poultry, and eggs.
- Assist clients to develop menus containing a variety of sources of folacin.
- Recommend that clients take a daily multivitamin to supplement dietary intake.

EVALUATION
- Review client's food intake diary.

RATIONALE
- It can help to protect the developing unborn baby against birth defects of the spine and brain. Folic acid requirements are particularly high in rapidly growing cells such as fetal tissues, and when taken before or just after conception it can reduce the risk of neural tube defects.

mental outcomes in low-birth-weight (LBW) infants indicates these infants have an increased risk for learning disorders, school failures, temperament problems, neurological and motor impairment, and developmental delays. Recent research demonstrates a positive relationship between a supportive home environment and cognitive development in LBW infants (Feingold, 1994). The implication of this research is that families of LBW infants must be assessed for need of nursing interventions that may facilitate a supportive home environment for optimal cognitive outcomes.

Psychosocial Development

Little information is available about the relationship between prenatal experiences and the child's psychosocial development. Some authorities believe that the biochemical environment of the uterus can significantly influence later psychosocial development. Because the biochemical environment is influenced by the mother, her emotional and physical states may have significant psychosocial consequences for the unborn child. Furthermore, the mother's emotional state may influence her behavior after childbirth, whch in turn influences the child's psychosocial development.

▮ TRANSITION FROM INTRAUTERINE TO EXTRAUTERINE LIFE

The transition from intrauterine to extrauterine life requires rapid changes in the neonate. The nurse assesses the neonate's ability to make these changes and intervenes if necessary to ensure success. Gestational age, exposure to depressant drugs before or during labor, and the neonate's own behavioral style influence adjustment to the external environment. Therefore initial assessment encompasses a variety of physical and psychosocial elements. The nurse also provides opportunities for the parents and child to develop close emotional ties.

Physical Health Concerns

An immediate assessment of the neonate's condition is performed because the first concern is the physiological functioning of the major organ systems. Nursing care is then directed at maintaining an open airway, stabilizing body temperature, and protecting the neonate from infection.

Airway patency is best ensured by removing nasooropharyngeal secretions with suction or a bulb syringe. After the airway is open, the nurse stabilizes body temperature. Wrapping the neonate in small, soft blankets usually provides adequate heat preservation. For neonates unable to sustain body temperature, isolettes and incubators, which supply radiant heat, can be used.

Prevention of infection is a major concern in the care of the neonate, whose immune system is immature. Good handwashing technique is the most important factor in protecting the neonate and nurse from infection. Cover gowns do not need to be worn while providing care for the healthy newborn once the blood and amniotic fluid have been removed from the infant's skin. The Centers for Disease Control and Prevention (CDC) recommends that health care workers wear gloves when touching mucous membranes or nonintact skin such as in a new wound (i.e., fresh circumcision) and when drawing blood (e.g., heel stick).

The most commonly used prophylactic treatment against ophthalmia conjunctivitis is erythromycin (0.5%) because it prevents *Neisseria gonorrhoea* and other infections, which can be transmitted during passage through an infected vaginal canal. The traditional use of 1% silver nitrate solution is uncommon today because of chemical irritation to the eyes and its more narrow action against bacteria.

The stump of the umbilical cord is an excellent medium for bacterial growth and should be swabbed with an antibacterial agent such as triple dye shortly after birth. Stump drying is encouraged by application of alcohol at each diaper change and folding the diaper away from it.

The nurse is frequently responsible for assessing the newborn's physiological functioning. The most widely used assessment tool is the **Apgar score**, which rates heart rate, respiratory effort, muscle tone, reflex irritability, and color to determine overall status. The Apgar assessment is generally conducted at 1 and 5 minutes after birth and may be repeated until the newborn's condition stabilizes. Table

Table 28-3	Apgar Scoring			
SIGN	**SCORE 0**	**SCORE 1**	**SCORE 2**
Heart rate	Absent	Slow (below 100)	Over 100
Respiratory effort	Absent	Slow, irregular, hypoventilation	Good, crying lustily
Muscle tone	Flaccid	Some flexion of extremities	Active motion, well flexed
Reflex irritability	No response	Crying, some motion	Vigorous cry
Color	Blue, pale	Pink body, blue hands and feet	Completely pink

Modified from Wong DL: *Whaley and Wong's nursing care of infants and children,* ed 5, St Louis, 1995, Mosby.

28-3 outlines the scoring criteria of physiological functioning. A total score of 0 to 3 signifies severe distress, a score of 4 to 6 represents moderate difficulty, and a score of 7 to 10 indicates little difficulty in adjusting to extrauterine life. The nurse can use the Apgar score to determine areas requiring further assessment and careful observation. In addition, the nurse monitors the neonate's body temperature and continues to closely monitor vital signs until they stabilize.

Psychosocial Concerns

After immediate physical evaluation and application of identification bracelets, the nurse assesses the parents' and newborn's needs for close physical contact. Early parent-child interaction encourages parent-child attachment. Physical factors (e.g., fatigue, hunger, and health) and emotional factors (e.g., happiness and needs for affection and touch) are assessed.

Merely placing the family together does not promote closeness. The parents and neonate must be capable and desirous of exploring and responding to each other. Most healthy neonates are awake and alert for the first half hour after birth, and if the parents are receptive, this is an opportune time for parent-child interaction to begin. Close body contact, often including breast-feeding, is a satisfying way for most families to start. If immediate contact is not possible, the nurse incorporates it into the care plan as early as possible, which may mean bringing the newborn to an ill parent or bringing the parents to an ill or premature child.

Bonding occurs when parents and newborn elicit reciprocal and complementary behavior. Parental bonding behaviors include attentiveness and physical contact. Neonate bonding behavior involves maintenance of contact with the parent. Preterm and ill neonates and their parents have more difficulty forming this bond if separation is prolonged. The bonding process is further complicated if parents are unable to care for the usual infant needs. The nurse should give the parents support throughout the early attachment process, particularly if the newborn is ill or separated from the parents.

■ HEALTH PROMOTION FOR THE NEONATE

The **neonatal period** is the first month of life. During this stage the newborn's physical functioning is mostly reflexive, and stabilization of major organ systems is the body's primary task. Behavior greatly influences interaction between the newborn and the environment and care givers. For example, the average 2 week old smiles spontaneously and is able to regard the mother's face. The impact of these reflexive behaviors is generally a surge of maternal feelings of love that prompt the mother to cuddle the baby.

Nurses can apply their knowledge of this stage of growth and development to promote newborn and parental health. If the nurse understands, for example, that the newborn's cry is generally a reflexive response to an unmet need (such as hunger), parents can be assisted in identifying ways to meet those needs, such as counseling the parents to feed their baby on demand rather than on a rigid schedule.

Physical Development

A comprehensive nursing assessment is performed as soon as the neonate's physiological functioning is stable, generally within a few hours after birth. At this time the nurse measures height, weight, head circumference, temperature, pulse, and respirations and observes general appearance, body functions, sensory capabilities, and responsiveness.

The average newborn weighs 3400 g (7 lb, 8 oz), is 50 cm (20 inches) in length, and has a head circumference of 35 cm (14 inches). Up to 10% of birth weight is lost in the first few days of life, primarily through fluid losses by respiration, urination, defecation, and decreased intake. Birth weight is usually regained by the second week of life, and a gradual pattern of increase in weight, height, and head circumference is evident. During the first month, these increases average 4 to 8 oz in weight per week, 0.6 to 2.5 cm (¼ to 1 inch) in length, and 2 cm in head circumference.

The neonate's heart rate gradually decreases from the fetal rate of 130 to 160 beats per minute to 120 to 140 beats per minute. Systole and diastole are of shorter duration, greater intensity, and higher pitch. The average blood pressure is 74/46 mm Hg. The newborn's respiratory movements are primarily abdominal and vary in rate and rhythm, but the average rate is 30 to 50 breaths per minute. Because a neonate breathes through the nose, it is important to keep the nasal passages clear. Their axillary temperature ranges from 36° to 37.5° C (97.7° to 99.5° F) and generally stabilizes within 24 hours after birth.

Normal physical characteristics include the continued presence of lanugo on the skin of the back; cyanosis of the hands and feet, especially during activity; and a soft, protuberant abdomen. Skin color varies according to racial and

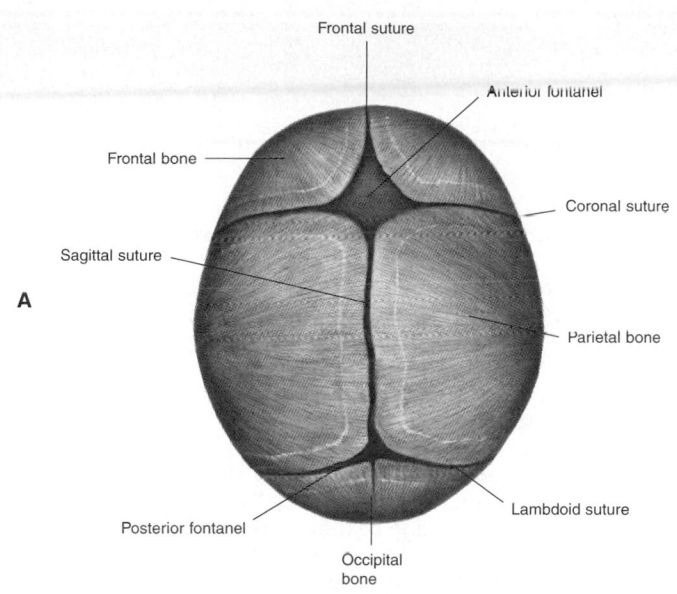

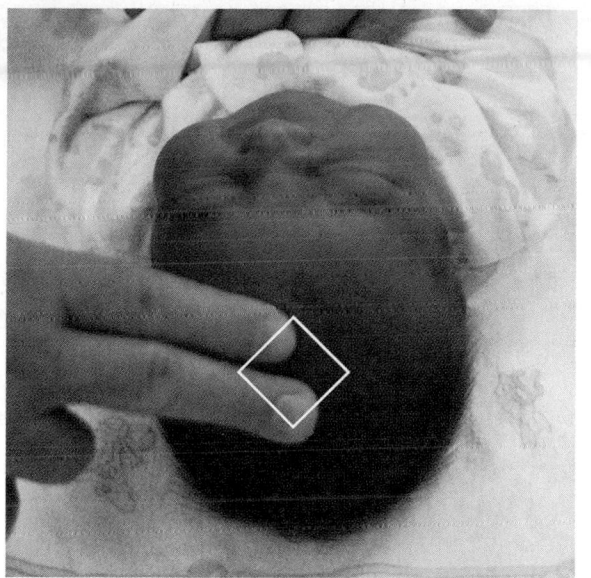

Fig. 28-2 Fontanels and suture lines. *(From Wong DL:* Whaley and Wong's nursing care of infants and children, *ed 5, St Louis, 1995, Mosby.)*

genetic heritage and gradually changes during infancy. **Molding,** or overlapping of the soft skull bones, is common during birth. The bones readjust in a few weeks, producing a more rounded appearance. The linear breaks, sutures, and fontanels, are usually palpable at birth. The diamond shape of the anterior fontanel and the triangular shape of the posterior fontanel between the unfused bones of the skull are shown in Fig. 28-2.

Neurological function is assessed by observing the neonate's level of activity, alertness, irritability, and responsiveness to stimuli and the presence and strength of reflexes. Normal reflexes include blinking in response to bright lights and startling in response to sudden, loud noises. Table 28-4 describes other commonly evaluated reflexes. Their absence indicates possible trauma or central nervous system complications. Because the newborn depends largely on reflexes for response to environment, assessment of these characteristic responses is vital.

Normal behavioral characteristics of the newborn include periods of sucking, crying, sleeping, and activity. Movements are generally sporadic, but they are symmetrical and involve all four extremities. The relatively flexed position of intrauterine life continues as the neonate attempts to maintain an enclosed, secure feeling. Newborns normally watch the care giver's face, reflexively smile, and respond to sensory stimuli, particularly the primary care giver's face, voice, and touch.

The first hour of the unmedicated newborn's life is spent in a primarily quiet alert state with wide open eyes and vigorous sucking activity. Then infants sleep almost continuously for the next 2 to 3 days to recover from the exhausting birth process. Thereafter sleep periods vary from 20 minutes to 6 hours with little day-night differentiation (Fig. 28-3). Infant behavior is characterized by five distinct states that are highly influenced by environmental stimuli. It is important for parents to understand these states (summarized in Table 28-5) and their implications for parental in-

teraction. Infants who are put down for sleep should be positioned on their side or back according to the American Academy of Pediatrics (see the box on p. 510).

The nurse coordinates screening tests and other laboratory tests as indicated by the neonate's state of health. Blood tests can be used to determine inborn errors of metabolism (IEM). This term applies to genetic disorders caused by the absence or deficiency of a substance, usually an enzyme, essential to cellular metabolism that results in abnormal protein, carbohydrate, or fat metabolism. Although IEM are rare, they account for a significant proportion of health problems in children. Neonatal screening can detect phenylketonuria (PKU), hypothyroidism, and galactosemia and thus allow appropriate treatment that can prevent permanent mental retardation and other health problems. This testing is mandatory in most of the United States.

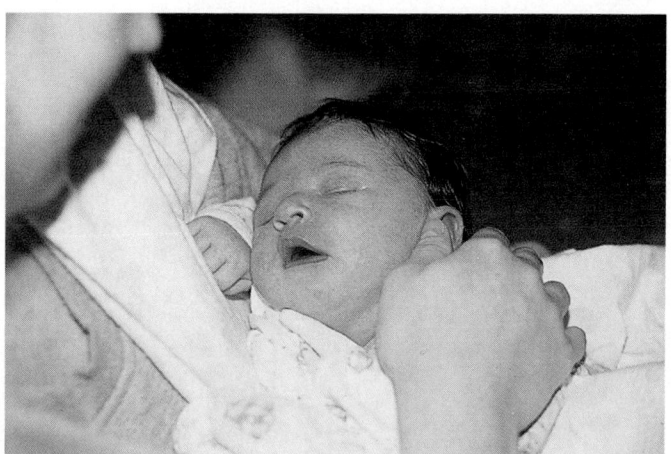

Fig. 28-3 Newborn sleep periods have little day-night differentiation.

Table 28-4	Assessment of Common Reflexes in the Newborn
REFLEXES	**EXPECTED BEHAVIORAL RESPONSES**

LOCALIZED

Eyes

Blinking or corneal reflex	Infant blinks at sudden appearance of bright light or at approach of object toward cornea. Reflex persists throughout life.
Doll's eye	As head is moved slowly to right or left, eyes lag behind and do not immediately adjust to new position of head. Reflex disappears as fixation develops. Persistent occurrence indicates neurological damage.

Nose

Sneeze	Nasal passages respond spontaneously to irritation or obstruction. Reflex persists throughout life.
Glabellar	Tapping briskly on glabella (bridge of nose) causes eyes to close tightly.

Mouth and Throat

Sucking	Infant begins strong sucking movements of circumoral area in response to stimulation. Reflex persists throughout infancy, even without stimulation, such as during sleep.
Gag	Stimulation of posterior pharynx by food, suction, or passage of tube causes infant to gag. Reflex persists throughout life.
Rooting	Touching or stroking cheek along side of mouth causes infant to turn head toward that side and begin to suck. Reflex should disappear at about age 3-4 mo but may persist up to 12 mo.
Extrusion	When tongue is touched or depressed, infant responds by forcing it outward. Reflex disappears by 4 mo.
Cough	Irritation of mucous membranes of larynx or tracheobronchial tree causes coughing. Reflex persists throughout life and is usually present first day after birth.
Swallowing	Appropriate swallowing of liquid introduced into mouth. Can also be elicited by directing a puff of air at infant's face.

Extremities

Grasp	Touching palms of hands or soles of feet near base of digits causes flexion of hands and toes. Palmar grasp lessens after 3 mo and is replaced by voluntary movement. Plantar grasp lessons by 8 mo.
Babinski	Stroking outer sole of foot upward from heel and across ball of foot causes toes to hyperextend and hallux to dorsiflex. Reflex disappears after age 1 yr (see the illustration below).

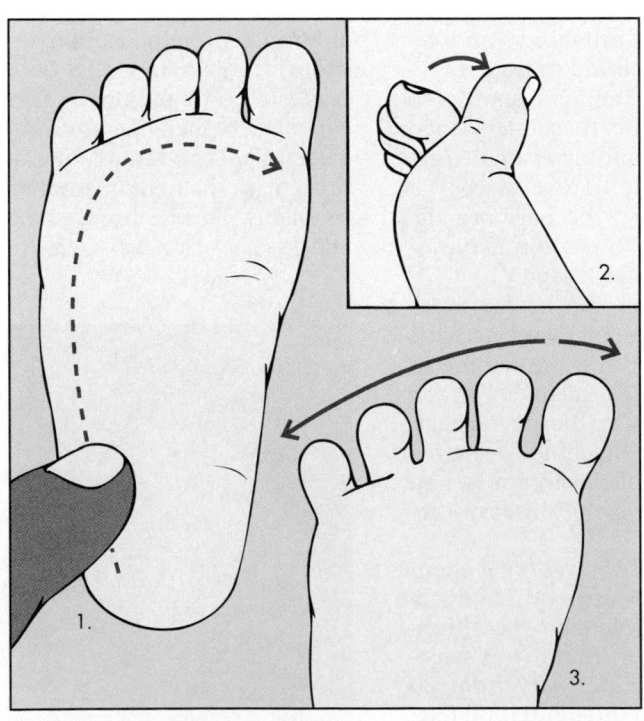

Modified from Wong DL: *Whaley and Wong's nursing care of infants and children*, ed 5, St Louis, 1995, Mosby.
Illustration redrawn from Wong DL: *Whaley and Wong's nursing care of infants and children*, ed 5, St Louis, 1995, Mosby.

Table 28-4	Assessment of Reflexes in the Newborn—cont'd

REFLEXES	EXPECTED BEHAVIORAL RESPONSES
Mass	
Moro	Sudden jarring or change in equilibrium causes sudden extension and abduction of extremities and fanning of fingers, with index finger and thumb forming C shape, followed by flexion and adduction of extremities. Legs may weakly flex. Infant may cry. Reflex disappears after 3-4 mo and is usually strongest during first 2 mo.
Startle	Sudden, loud noise causes abduction of arms with flexion of elbows. Hands remain clenched. Reflex disappears by 4 mo.
Dance or step	If infant is held so that sole of foot touches hard surface, there is reciprocal flexion and extension of leg, stimulating walking. Reflex disappears after 3-4 wk and is replaced by deliberate movement.
Crawl	When placed on abdomen, infant makes crawling movements with arms and leg. Reflex disappears at about 6 wk.
Placing	When infant is held upright under arms and dorsal side of foot is briskly placed against hard object, such as table, leg lifts as if foot is stepping on table. Age of disappearance varies.

Table 28-5	States of Sleep and Activity

STATE/BEHAVIOR	DURATION	IMPLICATIONS FOR PARENTING
REGULAR SLEEP Closed eyes Regular breathing Occasional body jerks	4-5 hours/day 10-20 minute sleep cycles	Not aroused by external stimuli Can continue usual house noises Leave infant alone even for brief cries
IRREGULAR SLEEP Closed eyes Irregular breathing Slight muscle twitching of body	12-15 hours/day 20-45 minute sleep cycles	External stimuli may arouse infant Periodic groaning or crying is usual; not an indication of discomfort
DROWSINESS Eyes may be open Irregular breathing Active body movement	Variable	Most stimuli arouse infant Pick infant up during this time rather than leave in crib
ALERT INACTIVITY Responds to environment by active body movement and staring at close-range objects	2-3 hours/day	Satisfy infant's needs such as hunger Place infant in area of activity Place toys/objects within infant's view
WAKING AND CRYING May begin with whimpering and slight body movements Progresses to strong, angry cry and uncoordinated thrashing of extremities	1-4 hours/day	Remove intense internal/external stimuli Repeat activities that were effective during alert inactivity Rock and swaddle to decrease crying

Cognitive Development

Early cognitive development begins with innate behavior, reflexes, and sensory functions. Newborns initiate reflex activities, assimilate new objects into behavior, and accommodate these behaviors to achieve their desires. For example, neonates learn to turn to the nipple. Although the infants behave of their own volition, activities learned are limited to reflex and sensory function.

Sensory functions contribute to cognitive development in the newborn. At birth, children can focus on objects about 8 to 10 inches from their faces and can perceive forms. A preference for the human face is apparent. Auditory and vestibular systems function from birth. These sensory capabilities allow neonates to elicit stimuli rather than simply receive it. Parents should be taught the importance of providing sensory stimulation, such as talking to their babies and holding them to see their faces. This allows infants to seek or take in stimuli, thereby enhancing learning and promoting cognitive development.

It is debatable whether infant crying is the precursor of

▶ **RESEARCH HIGHLIGHT**

RESEARCH ABSTRACT

Sudden Infant Death Syndrome (SIDS) is the sudden, un-expected, and unexplained death of a seemingly healthy infant. It appears to be a multi-etiological phe-nomenon with a statistically increased incidence among infants who sleep in the prone position. The findings of medical research regarding the association of infant po-sitioning with SIDS resulted in the American Academy of Pediatrics issuing the April 6, 1992 recommendation that normal infants, when put down for sleep, be posi-tioned on their side or back.

The majority of infants who sleep prone obviously do not die of SIDS; however, studies from various locales have demonstrated that in areas where infants have been placed in side-lying or supine position for sleep the inci-dence of SIDS has significantly decreased. Several hy-potheses exist for the biological explanation of this in-creased risk associated with the prone sleeping position. The two main hypotheses are airway obstruction due to compression of the pliable nasal cartilage or occlusion of the oropharynx and hyperthermia as a result of com-promised heat loss from the head due to excessive con-tact of face with underbedding and excessive clothing.

IMPLICATIONS FOR PRACTICE

▶ Position infant for sleep in side-lying or supine posi-tion. (Side-lying is recommended only until the infant is able to turn self to a prone position. Swaddling of the in-fant up to the shoulders with the feet covered first helps maintain this position and prevents the blanket from covering the face.) Once infants have learned to turn themselves completely over, parents should not be con-cerned about their sleeping position.

▶ Recognize that many parents will be concerned about infants vomiting and aspirating in the supine position. Share with them that in cultures where supine sleeping is the norm, aspiration is rare and does not appear to be a problem.

▶ Avoid thick beddings such as sheepskins, waterbeds, and mattresses, cushions, or "beanbags" filled with poly-styrene foam beads.

▶ Keep room where infant sleeps comfortably warm and limit amount of heavy bedding used.

▶ Certain babies, such as those born preterm, those with Pierre-Robin Syndrome, or those with severe gas-troesophageal reflux will continue to be medically ad-vised to sleep in the prone position.

REFERENCE

Herda JA: Nursing interventions aimed at reducing risks of SIDS, *Pediatr Nurs* 18(5):531, 1992.

refined language. However, crying elicits a response, and care givers discriminate cry patterns. Crying therefore has significance to newborns and parents. For neonates, crying is a means of communication. They cry for a reason, al-though at times this reason is difficult to determine. Some babies cry because their diapers are wet or they are hungry or want to be held. Others cry just to make noise or because they need a change in position or activity. Their crying may frustrate the parents if they cannot see an apparent cause. With the nurse's help, parents can learn to recognize infants' cry patterns and take appropriate action when necessary.

Psychosocial Development

During the first month of life, parents and newborns nor-mally develop a strong bond that grows into a deep **at-tachment**. Interactions during routine care enhance or de-tract from the attachment process. Feeding, hygiene, and comfort measures consume much of infants' waking time. These interactive experiences provide a foundation from which deep attachments form. Neonates are active partici-pants in this process.

If parents or children experience health complications after birth, bonding may be compromised. Infants' behav-ioral cues may be weak or absent. Care and care giving are less mutually satisfying. Tired, ill parents have difficulty in-terpreting and responding to their infants. Children who have congenital anomalies are often too weak to be re-sponsive to parental cues and require special supportive nursing care. For example, infants born with heart defects may tire easily during feedings. They may rest frequently after several bursts of sucking and fall asleep after taking 1 to 1½ oz. Infants may awaken after 1½ hours, crying be-cause they are hungry again. Mothers, not understanding that the crying is a physiologically dictated sequence of events, may think that the infants are being fussy or that they are inadequate. Both infants and mothers derive de-creasing pleasure from feeding experiences. In this case, however, bonding is not enhanced and may even be re-duced unless nursing intervention breaks the sequence of events.

▌ HEALTH PROMOTION FOR THE INFANT

Infancy, the period from 1 month to 1 year of age, is char-acterized by rapid physical growth and change. Psychoso-cial development advances, aided by the progression from reflexive to more purposeful behavior. Interaction between infants and the environment is greater and more meaning-ful. Infants who giggle and roll over in response to tickling are interacting more with their social environments and are displaying a greater response than when they merely smile in response to a hug. During this first year of life the nurse can easily observe the adaptive potential of infants because qualitative and quantitative changes in growth and devel-opment occur so rapidly.

Physical Development

Steady and proportional growth of the infant is more im-portant than absolute growth values. Charts of normal age- and sex-related growth measurements enable the nurse to compare growth with norms for a child's age. Using growth charts, the nurse can also evaluate growth patterns by recording measurements of weight, length, and head cir-cumference at intervals. Measurements recorded over time are the best way to monitor growth and identify problems. For example, an infant with a growth problem may be gen-erally below the expected norms at all intervals or may ex-perience an acute, brief interference with growth.

Size increases rapidly during the first year of life; birth weight doubles before 6 months and triples by 12 months. Height increases an average of 1 inch during each of the

Table 28-6	Milestones in Infant Motor Development				
MONTH 3	**MONTH 6**	**MONTH 9**	**MONTH 12**	**MONTH 15**	
GROSS MOTOR					
Lifts head 90 degrees when prone	Rolls completely over	Attains sitting position independently	Walks holding onto walls and furniture (cruising)	Walks alone	
Sits with support	Good head control in sitting position	Creeps on all four extremities	Stands alone		
	Crawls on abdomen with arms	Pulls self to standing position	Takes 1-2 steps		
FINE MOTOR					
Grasps and briefly holds objects and takes them to mouth	Uses palm grasp with fingers encircling object	Crude thumb-finger pincer grasp	Places tiny object, such as raisin, into container	Scribbles with crayon	
	Transfers cube from hand to hand	Bangs hand-held cubes together	Makes marks with crayon	Builds tower of two cubes	

Modified from Frankenburg WK et al: The Denver II: a major revision and restandardization of the Denver Developmental Screening Test, *Pediatrics* 89(1):91, 1992.

first 6 months and ½ inch the next 6 months. This 50% increase in birth height occurs primarily in the trunk, with the chest diameter approximating that of the head by the first birthday (Wong, 1995). The fontanels become smaller; the posterior fontanel closes at about 2 months.

Physiological functioning stabilizes, and by the end of the first year, the heart rate is 80 to 130 beats per minute, the blood pressure is 72 to 110/38 to 72 mm Hg, and respiratory rate is 30 to 35 breaths per minute. Patterns of body function also stabilize, as evidenced by predictable sleep, elimination, and feeding routines. Motor development proceeds steadily in a head-to-foot direction. Table 28-6 identifies milestones in gross motor and fine motor development.

NUTRITION

The quality and quantity of nutrition influence the infant's growth and development. The nurse helps parents select and provide a nutritionally adequate diet for their infant. The nurse must understand that nutrition is influenced by many variables (i.e., family culture, food preferences, slow eating, or food allergies) and that no diet is effective for all children or for one age group.

Feeding Alternatives. Supplying essential nutrients to the infant is the nurse's and parents' goal. Breast-feeding is recommended for infants because it contains the essential nutrients of protein, fats, carbohydrates, and immunoreactive proteins that bolster the ability to resist infection. However, milk other than human milk may be successfully used. Commercially prepared formulas are popular because they are convenient, contain standard ingredients, and are fortified with vitamins and minerals. The nurse supports the parents' choice of feeding methods and helps them feed the infant successfully. Unmodified cow's milk is not recommended in the first year because it often results in gastrointestinal bleeding, the renal solute load is too heavy for the immature infant kidneys to handle, and it is low in iron and high in calcium and phosphorus, which interferes with the absorption of iron (Williams, 1993).

The 1-month-old infant takes *approximately* 28 oz of milk per day. This amount increases slightly during the first 6 months and then drops to about 24 oz per day by the end of the first year as the baby begins to eat food. The addition of solid foods is not recommended before the age of 6 months because the gastrointestinal tract is not sufficiently mature to handle these complex nutrients and infants are exposed to food antigens that may produce food allergies. The introduction of cereals, fruits, vegetables, and meats during the second 6 months of life provides iron and additional sources of vitamins. These become especially important when children are taken off breast milk or formula and begun on whole cow's milk after the first birthday. Well-cooked table foods are also tolerated by 1 year. The amount and frequency of feedings vary among infants, so the nurse should discuss differing feeding patterns with parents.

Supplementation. The need for dietary vitamin and mineral supplements depends on the infant's diet. Full-term infants are born with some iron stores. The breast-fed infant absorbs adequate iron from breast milk during the first 4 to 6 months of life. After 6 months, iron-fortified cereal is generally considered an adequate supplemental source. Because iron in formula is less readily absorbed than that in breast milk, formula-fed infants should receive iron-fortified formula throughout the first year. Adequate concentrations of fluoride to protect against dental caries are not available in human milk, and therefore fluoridated water or supplemental fluoride is generally recommended. The presence of fluoride in formula depends on the type of formula and the source of water used in preparing the concentrated forms, and supplementation may be necessary.

The association between overfeeding, infant obesity, and later adult obesity is still controversial. However, early feeding experiences can influence later eating habits. The nurse should therefore emphasize balanced nutrition and good dietary habits through feeding experiences mutually satisfying for the parents and infant.

DENTITION

The average age for the first tooth to erupt is 7 months, but there is considerable variation among infants because of their genetic endowment. An occasional infant is born with a tooth while others remain toothless at 1 year. The order of tooth eruption is fairly predictable with the lower central incisors being first to appear, closely followed by the upper central incisors. Most 1 year olds have six teeth.

Teething may result in considerable discomfort for some infants and little or none for others. The inflammation of the gums as the tooth prepares to emerge may result in a low grade fever and irritability. The use of a frozen teething ring or ice cube wrapped in a washcloth is soothing. Over-the-counter teething medications to rub on the inflamed gums and appropriate doses of acetaminophen are helpful when the infant is irritable and has difficulty eating or sleeping.

Most dentists recommend that parents cleanse their infant's teeth after each feeding. This can be accomplished very simply and quickly with a wet washcloth and the parent's finger.

IMMUNIZATIONS

The widespread use of immunizations has resulted in the dramatic decline of infectious diseases over the past 50 years and is therefore a most important factor in health promotion during childhood. Although most immunizations can be given to persons of any age, it is recommended that their administration be begun soon after birth and be completed during early childhood except for the "boosters." See Table 28-7 for the 1994 CDC Recommended Schedule for Routine Active Vaccination of Infants and Children (Selekman, 1994).

The newest addition to the list of childhood immuniza-

| Table 28-7 | Recommended Childhood Immunization Schedule—United States |

					AGE					
VACCINE	**BIRTH**	**1 Mo**	**2 Mos**	**4 Mos**	**6 Mos**	**12 Mos**	**15 Mos**	**18 Mos**	**4-6 Yrs**	**11-12 Yrs**	**14-16 Yrs**
Hepatitis B[1,2]		Hep B-1									
			Hep B-2			Hep B-3				Hep B[2]	
Diphtheria, tetanus, pertussis[3]			DTP	DTP	DTP	DTP[3](DTaP at 15+ m)			DTP or DTaP	Td	
H. influenzae type b[4]			Hib	Hib	Hib[4]	Hib[4]					
Polio[5]			OPV[5]	OPV		OPV			OPV		
Measles, mumps, rubella[6]						MMR			MMR[6]	or MMR[6]	
Varicella zoster virus vaccine[7]						Var				Var[7]	

From *Pediatrics* 97(1):143, 1996.
Approved by the Advisory Committee on Immunization Practices (ACIP), the American Academy of Pediatrics (AAP), and the American Academy of Family Physicians (AAFP).
Vaccines are listed under the routinely recommended ages. Bars indicate range of acceptable ages for vaccination. Shaded bars indicate *catch-up vaccination:* at 11-12 years of age, hepatitis B vaccine should be administered to children not previously vaccinated, and Varicella Zoster Virus vaccine should be administered to children not previously vaccinated who lack a reliable history of chickenpox.
[1]*Infants born to HBsAg-negative mothers* should receive 2.5 µg of Merck vaccine (Recombivax HB) or 10 µg of SmithKline Beecham (SB) vaccine (Engerix-B). The 2nd dose should be administered ≥1 mo after the 1st dose.
Infants born to HBsAg-positive mothers should receive 0.5 mL Hepatitis B Immune Globulin (HBIG) within 12 hr of birth, and either 5 µg of Merck vaccine (Recombivax HB) or 10 µg of SB vaccine (Engerix-B) at a separate site. The 2nd dose is recommended at 1-2 mos of age and the 3rd dose at 6 mos of age.
Infants born to mothers whose HBsAg status is unknown should receive either 5 µg of Merck vaccine (Recombivax HB) or 10 µg of SB vaccine (Engerix-B) within 12 hr of birth. The 2nd dose of vaccine is recommended at 1 mo of age and the 3rd dose at 6 mos of age.
[2]Adolescents who have not previously received 3 doses of hepatitis B vaccine should initiate or complete the series at the 11-12 year-old visit. The 2nd dose should be administered at least 1 mo after the 1st dose, and the 3rd dose should be administered at least 4 mos after the 1st dose and at least 2 mos after the 2nd dose.
[3]DTP4 may be administered at 12 mos of age, if at least 6 mos have elapsed since DTP3. DTaP (diphtheria and tetanus toxoids and acellular pertussis vaccine) is licensed for the 4th and/or 5th vaccine dose(s) for children aged ≥15 mos and may be preferred for these doses in this age group. Td (tetanus and diphtheria toxoids, adsorbed, for adult use) is recommended at 11-12 years of age if at least 5 years have elapsed since the last dose of DTP, DTaP, or DT.
[4]Three *H. influenzae* type b (Hib) conjugate vaccines are licensed for infant use. If PRP-OMP (PedvaxHIB [Merck]) is administered at 2 and 4 mos of age, a dose at 6 mos is not required. After completing the primary series, any HIB conjugate vaccine may be used as a booster.
[5]Oral poliovirus vaccine (OPV) is recommended for routine infant vaccination. Inactivated poliovirus vaccine (IPV) is recommended for persons with a congenital or acquired immune deficiency disease or an altered immune status as a result of disease or immunosuppressive therapy, as well as their household contacts, and is an acceptable alternative for other persons. The primary 3-dose series for IPV should be given with a minimum interval of 4 wks between the 1st and 2nd doses and 6 mos between the 2nd and 3rd doses.
[6]The 2nd dose of MMR is routinely recommended at 4-6 yrs of age or at 11-12 yrs of age, but may be administered at any visit, provided at least 1 mo has elapsed since receipt of the 1st dose.
[7]Varicella zoster virus vaccine (Var) can be administered to susceptible children any time after 12 months of age. Unvaccinated children who lack a reliable history of chickenpox should be vaccinated at the 11-12 year-old visit.

tions is the single dose vaccination for chicken pox, which the American Academy of Pediatrics began recommending during the spring of 1995. All children without a history of chicken pox should be vaccinated between the ages of 12 and 18 months. Older children (up to 13 years) who have not had chicken pox should also be immunized.

Complacency and unwarranted fears regarding the side effects of vaccines, especially DTP, have resulted in large numbers of children not receiving appropriate immunizations during recent years. This attitude has resulted in measles epidemics and national laws designed to provide fair compensation for children who are inadvertently injured (The National Childhood Vaccine Injury Act of 1986 and the Vaccine Compensation Amendments of 1987). Researchers are beginning to investigate the problem of inadequate immunization of preschool children (see the box at right).

Cognitive Development

The infant learns much by experiencing and manipulating the environment. Developing motor skills and increasing mobility expand an infant's environment and, with developing visual and auditory skills, enhance cognitive development. For these reasons Piaget (1952) named his first stage of cognitive development, which extends until around the second birthday, the *sensorimotor period*. The characteristics of each of the four subphases of this period that occur during the first year of life are described in Table 28-2. Before the acquisition of language the extraordinary development of the mind occurs through the child's developing senses and motor abilities. For example, a 1 month old can follow the path of a moving object. Improved visual acuity and eye-hand coordination allow grasping and exploration of objects. In addition, rudimentary color vision begins by 2 months and improves throughout the first year, making the environment more interesting to see and explore. The infant's hearing also progresses, allowing localization and discrimination of sounds.

Speech is an important aspect of cognition that develops during the first year. Infants proceed from crying, cooing, and laughing to imitating sounds, comprehending the meaning of simple commands, and repeating words with knowledge of their meaning. By 1 year, infants not only recognize their own names but also have two- or three-word vocabularies including *Da-Da*, *Ma-Ma*, and *no*. The nurse can promote language development by encouraging mothers to name objects on which their infants' attention is focused.

Infants need opportunities to develop and use their senses. Nurses must evaluate the appropriateness and adequacy of these opportunities. For example, ill or hospitalized infants may lack the energy to interact with their environments, thereby slowing their cognitive development. On the other hand, continuous stimulation can overwhelm and confuse infants. Infants need to be stimulated according to their temperament, energy, and age. Visual, sensory, and tactile stimulation are as necessary for healthy development as food. The nurse uses stimulation strategies that maximize the development of infants while conserving their energy and orientation. An example of this is the nurse talking to and encouraging an infant to suck on a pacifier while administering the infant's tube feeding.

RESEARCH HIGHLIGHT

RESEARCH ABSTRACT
A community survey was conducted to assess the immunization status of 2-year-old children and barriers to immunization. The 299 respondents were more affluent and well-educated than the general population. Eighty-three percent of the respondents received immunizations from private physicians. Only 31.3% of the children were age-appropriately immunized, with deficiencies primarily in receiving the 18-month dosages of diphtheria-tetanus-pertussis (DTP) and polio. Parents reported multiple barriers and beliefs about immunization amenable to change by health providers. A profile of risk factors differentiating nonimmunized from immunized children was developed.

IMPLICATIONS FOR PRACTICE

▶ First Barrier: A high percentage of families receiving immunizations through regular checkups in conjunction with the low level of follow-up activity suggest parents are relying on providers to monitor immunizations and that this system is breaking down during the toddler years.

Strategies
- Development of a tracking system
- Helping parents with reminders
- Informing parents about the schedule for immunizations.

▶ Second Barrier: Parental fears about the effects of immunization

Strategies
- Parents must be educated about the risks of the disease relative to possible side effects of the vaccines.

▶ Nurses must be sensitive to these parental problems and address them at every opportunity.

REFERENCE
Salsberry PJ, Nickel JT, Mitch R: Inadequate immunization among 2-year-old children: a profile of children at risk, *J Pediatr Nurs* 9(3):158, 1994.

Psychosocial Development

During their first year, infants begin to differentiate themselves from others as separate beings capable of acting on their own. Initially, infants are unaware of the boundaries of self, but through repeated experiences with the environment, they learn where the self ends and the external world begins. As infants determine their physical boundaries, they begin to respond to others (Fig. 28-4). Two- and three-month-old infants begin to smile responsively rather than reflexively. Similarly, they can recognize differences in people when their sensory and cognitive capabilities improve. By 8 months, most infants can differentiate a stranger from a familiar person and respond differently to the two. Close attachment to the primary care givers, most often parents, is usually established by this age. Infants seek out these persons for support and comfort during times of stress. The ability to distinguish self from others allow infants to interact and socialize more within their environments. By 9 months, for example, infants play simple social games such

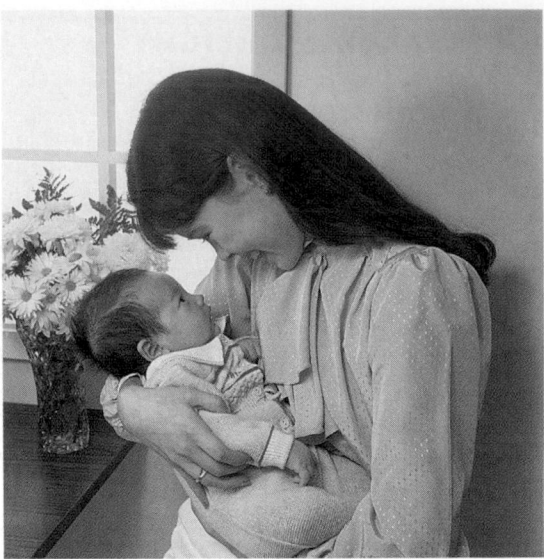

Fig. 28-4 Smiling at and talking to an infant encourages the infant to respond, which increases interaction with parent or care giver.

as pat-a-cake and peek-a-boo. More complex interactive games such as hide-and-seek involving objects are possible by age 1.

Erikson (1963) describes the psychosocial developmental crisis for the infant as *trust versus mistrust.* He explains that the quality of parent-infant interactions determines development of trust or mistrust. Parents who meet needs for warmth and comfort, love and security, and food when infants express these needs promote a sense of trust, whereas those that meet the needs of infants at their own convenience or not at all allow a sense of mistrust to develop.

The nurse assesses the availability and appropriateness of experiences contributing to psychosocial development. Hospitalized infants may have difficulty establishing physical boundaries because of repeated bodily intrusions and painful sensations. Limiting these negative experiences and providing pleasurable sensations are interventions that support early psychosocial development. Extended separations from parents complicate the attachment process and increase the number of care givers with whom the infant must interact. Ideally, the parents should provide the majority of care during hospitalization. When parents are not present, an attempt should be made to limit the number of care givers who have contact with the infant and to follow the parents' directions for care. These interventions will foster the infant's continuing development of trust.

Play is a meaningful set of activities through which individuals interact with their environment and relate to others. Play provides opportunities for the infant to develop many motor skills. Much of infant play is exploratory as they use their senses to observe and examine their own bodies and objects of interest in their surroundings. Activities such as the infant's placement of his toes in his mouth help provides him with pleasure, information about his own body, and help form his early self-concept. Play becomes manipulative as the child learns control of the hands. Adults can facilitate infant learning by planning ac-

tivities that promote the development of milestones and providing toys that are safe for the infant to explore with the mouth and manipulate with the hands, such as rattles, wooden blocks, plastic stacking rings, squeezable stuffed animals, and busy boxes. Infants most frequently engage in solitary (one-sided) play but do enjoy watching others, particularly the antics of their siblings. Infants need to be played with and stimulated through interactions with others. They delight in such activities as peek-a-boo and body games such as here's your nose.

Perception of Health

The foundation for children's perceptions of their health status is laid early in life. Internal body sensations and experiences with the outside world affect self-perceptions. The nature of this influence and the value of nursing interventions to alter later perceptions are unknown. It is known, however, that parents tend to label children who are ill in early life as more vulnerable than their siblings and that this labeling may affect the children's perceptions of their own health. In addition, because infants and children depend on others for their health care, their experiences with care givers influence their health attitudes and behavior. The nurse has a responsibility to educate parents and other care givers about health-promotion behavior that will positively affect perception of health and self.

■ HEALTH PROMOTION FOR THE TODDLER

Toddlerhood ranges from the time when children begin to walk independently until they walk and run with ease, which is approximately from 12 to 36 months. The toddler is characterized by increasing independence bolstered by greater physical mobility and cognitive abilities. Toddlers are increasingly aware of their abilities to control and are pleased with successful efforts with this new skill. This success leads them to repeated attempts to control their environments. Unsuccessful attempts at control may result in negative behavior and temper tantrums. These behaviors are most common when parents thwart the initial independent action. Parents cite these as the most problematic behaviors during the toddler years and at times express frustration with trying to set consistent and firm limits while simultaneously encouraging independence.

Physical Development

The rapid development of motor skills allows the child to participate in self-care activities such as feeding, dressing, and toileting. In the beginning the toddler walks in an upright position with a broad-stanced gait, protuberant abdomen, and arms out to the sides for balance. Soon the child begins to navigate stairs, using a rail or the wall to maintain balance while progressing upward, placing both feet on the same step before continuing. Success provides courage to attempt the upright mode for descending the stairs in the same manner. Locomotion skills soon include running, jumping, standing on one foot for several seconds, and kicking a ball. Most toddlers can ride tricycles, climb ladders, and run well by their third birthday. Fine motor capabilities move from scribbling spontaneously to drawing circles and crosses accurately. By 3 years the child draws simple stick people and can usually stack a tower of small blocks. Increased locomotion skills, the ability to undress, and development of sphincter control allow toilet training if the toddler has developed the necessary cognitive abilities. Parents often consult nurses for an assessment of readiness for toilet training. The nurse needs to remind parents that patience, consistency, and a nonjudgmental attitude, in addition to the child's readiness, are essential to successful toilet training.

The cardiopulmonary system becomes stable in the toddler years. The heart and respiratory rates slow to an average of 110 beats and 25 breaths per minute, respectively, and the blood pressure varies slightly from infancy with a slight increase in the diastolic. The normal range of blood pressure is 70-110 systolic and 40-70 diastolic.

The anterior fontanel closes between 12 and 18 months of age, ending the period of most rapid growth of the skull and brain. Routine measurement of head circumference should be done until 3 years of age.

The rate of increase in weight and length slows. By 2 years the child weighs 4 times the birth weight. Height during toddlerhood increases 3 to 5 inches a year, mainly as a result of increases in leg length. Slowed growth rates are accompanied by decreased caloric need and smaller food intake (**physiological anorexia**), which leads some parents to worry about the adequacy of dietary intake. Parents need encouragement to offer the child appropriate servings of food from the food pyramid and to avoid force feeding or allowing the child to fill up on foods that are high in fat and sugar. The nurse can reassure parents that the child's nutrition is adequate by demonstrating the child's satisfactory status on a growth grid.

Most toddlers change from breast milk or formula to cow's milk, consuming three to four 8-oz servings per day. Nutritional requirements are increasingly met by solid foods from the food pyramid. Because the consumption of more than a quart of milk per day usually decreases the child's appetite for these essential solid foods and results in inadequate iron intake, the nurse should advise parents to limit milk intake to 28 oz per day. Children are usually not offered low-fat or skim milk until age 2 because they need the fat for satisfactory physical and intellectual growth. The healthy toddler requires the daily intake of the foods in Table 28-8. Because parents frequently overestimate the size of a normal serving for their child, the nurse can reduce their anxiety about inadequate intake by pointing out the normal serving size.

Children who are ill, are undergoing surgery, or have diseases involving ingestion, absorption, or use of nutrients require special dietary considerations. Alterations in the type of foods and caloric requirements may be necessary. Children on strict vegetarian diets also require careful planning to ensure adequate, balanced protein intake. Regardless of children's health status, several basic principles of nutrition apply. Mealtime has psychosocial and physical significance. If the parents struggle to control toddlers' dietary intake, problem behavior and conflicts may result. Toddlers often develop "food jags" or the desire to eat one food repeatedly. Rather than becoming disturbed by this behavior, parents should be encouraged by the nurse to offer a variety of nutritious foods at meals and to provide only nutritious snacks between meals. Serving finger foods to toddlers allows them to eat by themselves and to satisfy their need for independence and control. Small, *reasonable* servings allow toddlers to eat all of their meals.

Cognitive Development

Toddlers' completion of the development of object permanence, their ability to remember events, and their beginning ability to put thoughts into words at about 2 years of age signal their transition from Piaget's sensorimotor stage of cognitive development to the **preoperational thought** stage (Piaget, 1952). Table 28-2 outlines the basic characteristics of the three subphases of cognitive development through which toddlers move between 12 and 36 months. Toddlers recognize that they are separate beings from their mothers, but they are unable to assume the view of another. They use symbols to represent objects, places, and persons. This function is demonstrated when children imitate the behavior of another that they viewed earlier (e.g., pretend to shave like daddy), pretend one object is another (use a finger as a gun), and use language to stand for absent objects (e.g., request bottle).

The 18-month-old child uses approximately 10 words. The 24-month-old child has a vocabulary of up to 300 words and is generally able to speak in short sentences. "Who's that?" and "What's that?" typify questions asked during this period. Verbal expressions such as "me do it" and "that's mine" demonstrate the 2-year-old child's use of pronouns and desire for independence and control. Despite the expanded vocabulary of an older toddler, most parents comment that their child's favorite word is *no* until well into the third year.

Table 28-8	Sample Menu for Toddlers Based on Food Guide Pyramid*
Breakfast	½ cup dry, unsweetened cereal
	½ cup orange juice
	4 oz low-fat milk
Snack	½-1 whole banana
Lunch	1 tbsp peanut butter
	2 tsp all-fruit preserves
	1 slice whole-wheat bread
	2 tbsp peas
	4 oz low-fat milk
Snack	2 graham crackers
	4 oz low-fat milk
Dinner	1 chicken leg, roasted without skin
	¼-½ cup macaroni and cheese
	2 tbsp green beans, cooked
	2 tbsp carrots, cooked
	4-6 oz low-fat milk
Snack	½ cup frozen yogurt
TOTAL SERVINGS	
Bread, cereal, rice, pasta	6-7
Vegetable	3
Fruit	3-4
Milk, yogurt, cheese	2-3
Meat, poultry, fish, dried beans, eggs, nuts	2

From Wong DL: *Whaley and Wong's nursing care of infants and children,* ed 5, St Louis, 1995, Mosby.
*Use fats, oils, and sweets sparingly. Increase fluids with servings of water. Serving sizes are minimums for nutritional adequacy.

Because children's moral development is closely associated with their cognitive abilities, the moral development of toddlers is only beginning and is also egocentric. Toddlers do not understand concepts of right and wrong. However, they do grasp the fact that some behaviors bring pleasant results (positive reinforcement) and others elicit unpleasant results (negative reinforcement). Therefore until toddlers achieve a higher level of cognitive function, they behave simply to avoid the unpleasant and seek out the pleasant.

Psychosocial Development

According to Erikson (1963), a sense of autonomy emerges during toddlerhood. Children strive for independence by using their developing muscles to do everything for themselves and become the master of their bodily functions. Their strong wills are frequently exhibited in negative behavior when care givers attempt to direct their actions. Temper tantrums may result when toddlers are frustrated by parental restrictions. Parents need to provide toddlers with graded independence, allowing them to do things that do not result in harm to themselves or others. This prevents them from doubting their ability to do things that they are capable of learning or feeling a sense of shame for those things they have done. Firm limits, patience, and support allow toddlers to develop socially acceptable behavior, which is the goal of parental guidance. Young toddlers who want to learn to hold their own cups may benefit from two-handled cups with spouts and plastic bibs with pockets to collect the milk that spills during the learning process.

Socially, toddlers remain strongly attached to their parents and fear separation from them. In their presence they feel safe, and their curiosity is evident in their exploration of the environment. Mothers of toddlers are rarely allowed any bathroom privacy because closing of the door results in incessant crying until the door is opened.

The child continues to engage in solitary play during toddlerhood but also begins to participate in parallel play, which is playing beside rather than with another child. An example is two toddlers sitting beside each other, each playing with his or her own doll in his or her own independent fashion. Toddlers who are just learning what belongs to them are often possessive of their toys. They learn the joy of sharing when they offer parents toys to hold and the parents express pleasure.

The newly developed locomotion abilities and insatiable curiosity of toddlers make them a danger to their own well-being. Toddlers need close supervision at all times and particularly when in environments that have not been "child-proofed." Poisonings occur frequently because children near 2 years of age are interested in placing any object or substance in their mouths to learn about it. Fortunately, these ingestions do not always result in death, but they do have many negative consequences such as chemical pneumonia. The wise parent removes or locks up all possible poisons, including plants, cleaning materials, and medications (see Chapter 36). These parental actions create a safer environment for exploratory behavior. Toddlers' lack of awareness regarding the danger of water and their newly developed walking skills combine to make drowning a major cause of accidental death in this age group. Limit setting

is extremely important for toddlers' safety. Automobile safety requires toddlers to remain in car seats, even though they say (often loudly) that they would prefer to move freely about the car. Children often learn to release the car restraints, and parents must be firm in their resolve not to drive unless the children are securely restrained. Toddlers completely depend on their parents for physical safety.

Perception of Health

Toddlers' perceptions of their own health are limited by their cognitive capabilities. Children increasingly recognize internal body sensations but have difficulty pinpointing their location. Therefore children often associate generalized responses with illness. Children who deviate radically from their usual patterns of eating, sleeping, or playing require assessment to determine whether these alterations result from illness.

During this stage, children begin to internalize the labels that parents or health care professionals give to the somatic states. That is, if the parents label particular sensations, such as abdominal discomfort, an "illness," children begin to label related sensations similarly. At the same time, children observe and mimic parents' health care practices. Health beliefs and practices are therefore being significantly shaped, even in these early years.

■ HEALTH PROMOTION FOR THE PRESCHOOLER

The **preschool period** refers to those years between 3 and 6. Children refine the mastery of their bodies and eagerly await the beginning of formal education. Many people consider these the most intriguing years of parenting because children are less negative, can more accurately share their thoughts, and can more effectively interact and communicate. Physical development continues to slow, whereas cognitive and psychosocial development are rapid.

Physical Development

Several aspects of physical development continue to stabilize in the preschool years. Heart and respiratory rates decrease only slightly to approximately 90 beats and 22 to 24 breaths per minute. Blood pressure rises slightly to an average of 95/58 mm Hg. Children gain about 5 lb per year; the average weight at 5 years is about 42 lb, approximately 6 times the birth weight. Preschoolers grow 2 to 3 inches per year, double their birth length around 4 years, and stand an average of 43 inches tall by their fifth birthday. The elongation of the legs results in more slender appearing children. The head has attained 90% of its adult size by the sixth birthday. Little difference exists between the sexes, although boys are slightly larger with more muscle and less fatty tissue. The most common nutritional deficiencies in children under 6 years of age are vitamins A and C and iron. Ingestion of large amounts of carbohydrates and fats from junk foods may result in overweight and undernourished preschoolers. Parents and health care providers need to make a conscious effort to help preschoolers develop healthy eating habits that prevent deficiencies and excesses.

Large and fine muscle coordination improves. Preschoolers run well, walk up and down steps with ease, and learn to hop. By 6 years they can usually skip and throw and catch balls. Improving fine motor skills allow intricate manipulations. They learn to copy circles, crosses, squares, and triangles. These skills make printing of letters and numbers possible.

Children need opportunities to learn and practice these physical skills. Nursing care of healthy and ill children includes an assessment of the availability of these opportunities. Although children with acute illnesses benefit from rest and exclusion from usual daily activities, children who have chronic conditions or who have been hospitalized for long periods need ongoing exposure to developmental opportunities. The parents and nurse weave these opportunities into the children's daily experiences, depending on their abilities, needs, and energy level.

Cognitive Development

Preschoolers continue to master the preoperational stage of cognition. The first phase of this period, known as **preconceptual thought** (2 to 4 years), is characterized by perceptual-bound thinking, in which children judge persons, objects, and events by their outward appearance or what seems to be (Piaget, 1952). For example, children may determine that an 8-oz glass full of fluid contains more than a 10-oz glass that also contains 8 oz of fluid because they center their thoughts on the fullness of the glass. Even if they watch the 8 oz of fluid from the full glass being poured into the 10-oz glass and the 8-oz glass refilled, they will still assert that the full 8-oz glass contains more because they cannot attend to the transfer. Thinking is hindered by their limited attention and attending skills. **Artificialism**, the misconception that everything in the world has been created by humanity, may result in children asking questions such as who built the mountains. Another misconception of preschool thinking, **animism**, the attribution of life to inanimate objects, often results in statements such as "Trees cry when their branches are broken." A third misconception is a type of reasoning called **immanent justice**, the notion that the world is equipped with a built-in code of law and order. It may result in children's beliefs that they were burned by matches because they were not supposed to handle them.

Around the age of 4 years, the intuitive phase of preoperational thought develops and children's ability to think more complexly is demonstrated by their ability to classify objects according to size or color and questions such as "Why do they call it the thirty-first day of the month instead of the thirty last?" Egocentricity persists, but during these 3 years, it begins to be replaced with social interaction, as is illustrated by the 5-year-old child who offers a bandage to a child with a cut finger. Children become aware of cause-and-effect relationships, as illustrated by the statement "The sun sets because people want to go to bed." Early causal thinking is also evident in preschoolers' transductive thoughts (reasoning occurs from one particular to another). If two events are related in time or space, children link them in a causal fashion. The hospitalized child, for example, may reason, "I cried last night, and that's why the nurse gave me the shot." As children near age 5, they begin to use or can be taught to use rules to understand causation. They then begin to reason from the general to the particular. This forms the basis for more formal logical thought. The child can now reason, "I get a shot twice a day, and that's why I got one last night."

Preschoolers' knowledge of the world remains closely linked to concrete (perceived by the senses) experiences. Even their rich fantasy life is grounded in the perception of reality. The mixing of the two aspects can lead to many childhood fears and may be misinterpreted by adults as lying when children are actually presenting reality from their perspective.

The greatest fear of this age group appears to be that of bodily harm, and it can be seen in children's fear of the dark, animals, thunderstorms, and medical personnel. This fear often interferes with their willingness to allow nursing interventions such as measurement of vital signs. They may cooperate if they are allowed to help the nurse measure the blood pressure of a parent.

The preschooler's moral development expands to include a beginning understanding of behaviors considered socially right or wrong. The child continues to be motivated, however, by the wish to avoid punishment or the desire to obtain a reward. The primary difference between this stage of moral development and that of a toddler is that a preschooler is better able to identify behaviors that elicit rewards or punishment and begins to label these behaviors as *right* or *wrong*.

Preschoolers' vocabularies continue to increase rapidly, and by the age of 5 children have more than 2000 words that they can use to define familiar objects, identify colors, and express their desires and frustrations. Language is more social, and questions expand to "Why?" and "How come?" in the quest for information. Phonetically similar words such as *die* and *dye* or *wood* and *would* may confuse preschool children. The nurse avoids such words when preparing children for procedures and assesses comprehension of explanations.

Psychosocial Development

The world of preschoolers expands beyond the family into the neighborhood where children meet other children and adults. Their curiosity and developing initiative lead to the active exploration of the environment, the development of new skills, and the making of new friends. Preschoolers have a surplus of energy that permits them to plan and attempt many activities that may be beyond their capabilities, such as pouring milk from a gallon container into their cereal bowls. Guilt arises within children when they overstep the limits of their abilities and feel they have not behaved correctly. Children who in anger have wished their sibling were dead experience guilt if that sibling becomes ill. Children need to be taught that "wishing" for something to happen does not make it occur. Erikson (1963) recommends that parents help their children strike a healthy balance between initiative and guilt by allowing them to do things on their own while setting firm limits and providing guidance.

During times of stress or illness, preschoolers may revert to bedwetting or thumbsucking and want the parents to feed, dress, and hold them. These dependent behaviors are often confusing and embarrassing to parents, who can benefit from the nurse's reassurance that they are the child's normal coping behaviors. The nurse should provide experiences that these children can master. Such successes help children return to their prior level of independent functioning.

The play of preschool children becomes more social after

the third birthday as it shifts from parallel to associative play. All participants engage in similar if not identical activity; however, there is no division of labor, and all children do as they wish. Most 3-year-old children are able to play with one other child in a cooperative manner in which they make something or play designated roles such as mother and baby. By age four, children play in groups of two or three, and by 5 years the group has a temporary leader for each activity.

In many play activities, preschoolers display awareness of social context. Sex-role identification is strengthening, and children most often assume roles of persons of their own sex. Children frequently mimic or repeat social experiences. This tendency is especially significant for the nurse working with hospitalized children. Through play, children may express questions, fears, anger, and misunderstanding about their illnesses and care. The nurse should be alert to such clues and ensure that children can play within energy limits. Play can provide a healthy outlet for frustration when children have been subjected to painful or restrictive experiences against their will.

Pretend play involving imaginary situations depends on children's ability to retain images of things they have seen or heard. This sociodramatic play involving other children occupies about a third of 5-year-old children's playtime. Pretending allows children to learn to understand other's points of view, develop skills in solving social problems, and become more creative. Children who watch a great deal of television engage less frequently in imaginative play, possibly because they develop the habit of passively absorbing images rather than generating their own.

Perception of Health

Little research has explored preschoolers' perceptions of their own health. Parental beliefs about health, children's bodily sensations, and their ability to perform usual daily activities help children develop attitudes about their health. Preschoolers are usually quite independent in washing, dressing, and feeding. Alterations in this independence can influence their feelings about their own health.

▌ HOSPITALIZATION AND ILLNESS

For children, hospitalization and illness are stressful experiences, primarily because of separation from the normal environment and significant others, a limited selection of coping behaviors, and altered states of health. An important nursing goal is to make the experience a positive one.

▌ NURSING PROCESS AND THE CHILD

 Assessment

A child's reaction to illness and hospitalization is based on developmental age, previous experiences with hospitalization, available support persons, coping skills, and the seriousness of the diagnosis (Wong, 1995). Table 28-9 identifies areas to assess and information to obtain. Thorough assessment of factors in each of these areas assists nurses in providing care that promotes resolution of illness and the general well-being of children and their families.

Nurses in many hospitals that care for children have as-

Table 28-9	Assessment of Hospitalized Child
ASSESSMENT AREA	**ASSESSMENT AIMS**
Development	Identify current developmental level and skills achieved.
Observation of response to hospitalization	Identify current coping behaviors and their intensity.
History of previous illness, hospitalization, and separation	Identify previous patterns of coping and their effects.
Medical history	Identify seriousness of problem and its effect on developmental abilities.
Perception of illness	Identify child's current understanding of illness and reason for hospitalization.
Available support systems	Identify availability and willingness of family to participate in care and provide support.

sessment tools that assist them to elicit, observe, and record data regarding the child's present and past health status, level of development, daily routines, and family situation, concerns, and interest in participating in care. Use of such a tool/checklist ensures that essential data are collected in an efficient manner.

DEVELOPMENTAL ASSESSMENT

Developmental assessment identifies specific attributes of the child so that the nurse can individualize the care plan and enhance the child's coping abilities. Examination of the child's motor skills reveals the amount of assistance the child needs with eating, brushing teeth, bathing, dressing, elimination, and ambulation. If during assessment the nurse identifies that the toddler is accustomed to climbing out of the crib at home, special measures should be taken to prevent a fall during hospitalization. When doing the sensory assessment, the nurse can identify and label any aids that the child uses such as hearing aids or eyeglasses.

Determination of the child's eating, sleeping, and elimination habits is an important assessment. Parents are reassured that nurses are interested in their child's individual needs when they ask about the child's appetite, favorite foods and drinks, use of bottle and favored utensils, and frequency of feedings, because distinct preferences become more important to the child at times of stress. Toileting habits and special words for urine and stool need to be clarified. Sleep assessment should include frequency of naps, bedtime, sleeping positions, security items, and occurrence of any night terrors or nightmares.

The Denver II, the 1990 revision of The Denver Developmental Screening Test, is a widely used screening tool for children from birth through 6 years. It assesses personal-social, fine motor adaptive, language, and gross motor skills. This tool was designed for use with well children, and the nurse may find that interventions such as intravenous fluids and casts, as well as children's illnesses, interfere with performance level. Although assessment at this time may not be a true picture of children's abilities, it can indicate how illness and hospitalization interfere with their achievement or display of expected development. Findings from the assessment provide the nurse with a basis on which to plan care that maintains and promotes development.

OBSERVATION OF RESPONSE TO HOSPITALIZATION

Separation anxiety, loss of control, fear of bodily harm, and pain are the primary causes of behavioral reactions of hospitalized children. Age dictates the specific manifestation, as evidenced by infants who loudly cry and protest separation from parents and toddlers who kick, bite, and/or hit to protest loss of autonomy. Loss of control behaviors are more apparent in toddlers and preschoolers, who may have frequent temper tantrums or exhibit regressive behaviors. Fear of bodily harm and pain occur in all children, including newborns. Infants react to pain with body rigidity, thrashing, and facial grimacing, whereas preschoolers loudly protest and can become physically and verbally aggressive (Wong, 1995).

Temperament, or how a child behaves or responds to a situation, is a key element in the child's coping style. The nurse assesses temperament by asking the parents questions about the child's usual activity level, general mood, persistence, and general response to new situations. When there is congruence between temperament and environment, the best possible development occurs. The difficult child who seeks activity during stress will have more of a problem adjusting to immobility than the child who is an avid reader and seeks to be alone during stress.

Behaviors such as crying for parents, being uncooperative, and regressing in toileting habits are reactions to an interruption in the preschool child's achieved developmental tasks. The observation of various behavioral reactions to hospitalization allows the nurse to identify coping behaviors and plan care accordingly.

HISTORY OF PREVIOUS ILLNESS, HOSPITALIZATION, AND SEPARATION

The nurse gathers data about the way a child coped with a previous hospitalization (specific behavior reactions such as protests, withdrawal, aggression, and regression). The nurse also determines the effect that the hospitalization had on subsequent behavior (negative behaviors after discharge such as nightmares, aloofness, clinging, and temper tantrums).

MEDICAL HISTORY

From the medical history the nurse should determine the seriousness of the health problem and its effect on development and nursing care. The nurse should also determine the effects of therapies on developmental achievements. For example, toddlers whose activities are severely restricted because of their illnesses or therapies (e.g., spica casts) will have difficulty maintaining their independence. Restricting or limiting movement interferes with exploration needed to develop a sense of autonomy.

PERCEPTION OF ILLNESS

Determining what children know and are able to comprehend about their illness is the first step in helping them understand the reason for their hospitalization. Children's degree of understanding is somewhat constrained by their specific experiences. Children's awareness of health and illness concepts probably reflects their access to relevant information as much as it does their level of cognitive maturity. Ascertaining any misconceptions children have about their illness and working to modify them is an important strategy in facilitating their accurate illness concepts (Yoos, 1994).

AVAILABLE SUPPORT PERSONS

The availability and willingness of families to participate in the care of their children are determined at admission. Parents are encouraged to remain with young children as much as possible so that separation behaviors are minimized. Parents' willingness to stay depends on their involvement with children at home, their work situations, their degree of comfort with the hospital, and the amount of support that they receive from extended family members and friends in meeting the needs of other family members. Based on the information that the parents give, the nurse helps families plan their support of the child during hospitalization.

Nursing Diagnosis

Assessment reveals how the child copes with hospitalization and whether this experience will result in other health problems (see the nursing diagnoses box on p. 520). The following case study provides an example.

> **CASE STUDY**   Assessment data for a 3-year-old on the second day of hospitalization reveal that she continues to cry for her parents in their absence, is not eating, has relinquished her normal toilet habits, and does not respond favorably to attention from the nurse. The parents found it impossible to spend the night because of the needs of their 3-month-old twins. The maternal grandmother lives nearby and made it possible for the mother to visit during the evening. The father visited in the morning on his way home from work. ■

The diagnostic process for the hospitalized child (see the diagnostic process box on p. 521) demonstrates how analysis of data from the assessment activities identifies the defining characteristics of two nursing diagnoses. The diagnostic statements identify the problems and their probable causes. This identification allows the nurse to plan specific interventions for resolution.

Planning

After identifying nursing diagnoses, the nurse develops a care plan (see the care plan on p. 521). The determination of goals and expected outcomes of care for each nursing diagnosis is the first step. Because the child often cannot articulate feelings and needs, it is essential to also involve the parents and sometimes other family members in the establishment of these goals. Goals of care for a hospitalized child should consider developmental needs and include the following:

1. Minimizing separation anxiety

Examples of NANDA Nursing Diagnoses for Hospitalized Young Children

Altered nutrition: less than body requirements *related to:*
- Separation from family during hospitalization
- Effect of illness
- Prescribed dietary restrictions
- Cultural food practices
- Pain

Risk for infection *related to:*
- Break in skin
- Decreased body defenses from chemotherapy
- Insufficient knowledge to avoid pathogens

Risk for injury *related to:*
- Change in environment
- Broken skin integrity
- Nosocomial agents
- Altered mobility

Social isolation *related to:*
- Separation from significant others
- Effects of illness
- Interruption of developmental task progress
- Schedule of hospitalization routines

Altered family processes *related to:*
- Hospitalization
- Effects of chronic illness

Activity intolerance *related to:*
- Conditions of illness
- Hospitalization

Sleep pattern disturbance *related to:*
- Unfamiliar environment
- Separation from family

- Procedure and therapies
- Pain

Diversional activity deficit *related to:*
- Effects of illness
- Pain

Altered growth and development *related to:*
- Effect of illness
- Pain
- Separation from family
- Multiple care givers

Powerlessness *related to:*
- Unfamiliar environment

Knowledge deficit *related to:*
- Cognitive limitations of age
- Lack of information
- Limited experiences

Fear *related to:*
- Separation from significant care givers
- Potentially threatening situation of hospital

Pain *related to:*
- Physical response of injury
- Trauma from invasive procedures therapies

Anxiety *related to:*
- Unfamiliar environment
- Strange care givers

Ineffective individual coping *related to:*
- Inadequate support system
- Strange environment of hospital
- Vulnerability of age

2. Establishing trust
3. Reducing fear
4. Minimizing physical discomfort
5. Fostering normal growth and development
6. Incorporating play and diversional activity into daily care

Children's and parents' responses to illness and hospitalization help the nurse determine priorities among goals. In situations in which family members do not remain with their children, who refuse to eat or play and sleep poorly, priority must be given to the goal that deals with minimizing separation anxiety. In the home setting parents may need assistance in achieving this goal, which focuses on maintaining the child's independence. Often the nurse can assist the parents in considering alternatives and mobilizing their resources.

Implementation

Implementation of interventions is performed by nurses, the child, or the family. When children are hospitalized or receive care in an outpatient facility or in their home, the nurse tries to ensure that the experience is positive for the child and family. This can be accomplished by remembering that each child is unique and by being sensitive to individual responses to nursing measures.

The nurse's organization and management of the child's care can acknowledge the individuality of the child and family by allowing them to have some control over preparation for tests, bath time, menus, bedtime, and certain procedures. For instance, the child who is accustomed to taking a bath at bedtime or having a nighttime snack of cereal should be allowed to maintain this ritual in the hospital unless contraindicated by a necessary medical regimen. Bath time is a good time to continue assessment of the child and family. It is also often an appropriate time for teaching the child or family about the child's care (see the box on p. 522) or to do anticipatory guidance. In a clinic setting the nurse can let the child decide where to sit. The child may feel more secure and less fearful sitting on a parent's lap rather than sitting on the examination table.

MINIMIZING SEPARATION ANXIETY

Parents are more likely to remain with their young hospitalized child when the nurse makes them feel comfortable and describes the accommodations the hospital has provided for them. When parents cannot continuously be with their child at the hospital, the nurse and parents need to plan together to make this situation more tolerable for the child. Appropriate guidelines include the following:

1. Parents should tell the child when they are leaving and when they will return in terms that the child can comprehend, such as "when daddy comes home from work." Then they should leave quickly.

Sample Nursing Diagnostic Process for the Hospitalized Young Child

ASSESSMENT ACTIVITIES	DEFINING CHARACTERISTICS	NURSING DIAGNOSIS
Observe child's behavior in response to hospital room and bed.	Insists on being held Protests strongly with cries and struggle	**Fear** related to threatening hospital environment and separation from parents.
Observe behavior as mother leaves child's side to use bathroom.	No exploratory activity Uncooperative with blood pressure measurement, even with mother's help	
Observe child in playroom with toys.	Regressive behaviors	**Ineffective individual coping** related to strange environment and care givers and vulnerability of age
Observe child's sleep behavior.	Child awoke sobbing at 2 AM	
Note child's ability to control bowel and bladder.	Wet bed during night	
Note child's eating behavior.	Refused to eat breakfast until father arrived and then allowed him to feed her	

Sample Nursing Care Plan for Fear

NURSING DIAGNOSIS: Fear related to threatening hospital environment and separation from parents.
DEFINITION: Fear is feeling a dread related to an identifiable source that the person validates (Kim MJ, McFarland GK, McLane AM, 1995).

GOAL	EXPECTED OUTCOMES	INTERVENTIONS	RATIONALE
Child will cope effectively with fear associated with hospitalization before discharge.	One parent will remain with child (4/2). Parents will participate in child's feeding, hygiene, and play activities each day.	Encourage parent to room-in or have other family member with child. Ask parents how they wish to participate in child's care. Anticipate parents' need for assistance and guidance. Orient parents to nursing division and supplies. Provide appropriate items for these activities.	Parent provides security and prevents development of mistrust. Object permanence is not complete until 2 yr of age. Parental anxiety will decrease. Strange environment undermines confidence of parents and results in fatigue. Parents who know events to expect experience less anxiety (Schepp, 1991). Provision of articles gives parents incentive to proceed.
	Child will use coping and defense mechanisms daily to combat fear (4/4).	Accept regressive behavior. Ask parent to bring to hospital items comforting to child (e.g., pacifier, blanket). Explain normalcy of this behavior to parents. Encourage information-seeking activities.	Comfortable earlier behaviors provide sense of security. Child should have access to familiar items that bring comfort and security. People of all ages combat fear and anxiety with regression after crisis behavior disappears.
	Child's use of regressive behavior will decrease (4/2).	Provide child with opportunities to "play out" fears, feelings, and concerns.	Explanation allows parents to know that this is coping behavior (Ritchie et al, 1988). Play is medium through which child can express inner feelings.

CLIENT TEACHING
for Car-Seat Safety

OBJECTIVE
- Child will ride correctly restrained in the car and be protected from injury and death.

TEACHING STRATEGIES
- Discuss these measures with parents.
- Tell parents that motor vehicle accidents are the most common cause of death in children.
- Inform parents that the younger the child, the greater the risk of death from automobile accidents. This is because the child is often held by the mother in the front seat and the child's proportionally large head and higher center of gravity cause him or her to be propelled head-first into the dashboard or windshield.
- Demonstrate how an infant rides facing the rear in a semireclining position.
- Demonstrate the use of convertible car seat model, which allows infant to ride in a rear-facing position and a toddler in a forward-facing position. Tell the parents that the child is switched to forward position when weight nears 20 lb.

- Tell parents that a preschool child who outgrows the convertible restraint should ride in a booster seat until the midpoint of the head is higher than the back of the vehicle seat.
- Encourage parents to purchase a crash-tested, government-approved car seat and follow manufacturer's directions carefully to achieve maximal protection. Some communities have resources that loan car seats to families who cannot afford to purchase them.
- Inform parents that the child should ride in car seats until they are outgrown. The child can use the regular car restraint system when weight reaches 40 lb or height reaches 40 inches.
- Explain that the car should not be started until everyone is properly restrained.
- Tell parents to ensure that child remains in car seat and that cooperative behavior should be rewarded.

EVALUATION
- Observe how parents place child in car seat when leaving hospital.

From US Preventive Services Task Force: Counseling to prevent household and environmental injuries, *Ann Fam Pract* 42(1):136, 1990.

2. The primary nurse should be with the child when the parents leave to provide some support and distraction.
3. The nurse should explain to the parents that protest is normal behavior and demonstrates a strong relationship with the parents.
4. Parents should leave some item that the child knows belongs to them because it will assure the child that they will return and provide comfort.
5. A child should have favorite toys from home or familiar objects such as a "special blanket" that provides comfort.
6. Parents should be encouraged to tape pictures of family members where the child can easily see them. Health care providers can discuss the photographs with the child.
7. Telephone calls from family members provide a link between home and hospital.
8. The child might be comforted by cassette tape recordings of family members reading stories, singing, or talking.

ESTABLISHING TRUST

The nurse's establishment of a trusting relationship with the child and family requires careful planning. The nurse who is friendly and informative, listens well to the concerns of the family, and is not threatening to the child has laid the foundation for a positive relationship. A few suggestions for nonthreatening communication techniques for the young child include the following:

1. Allow the child to observe friendly interaction between the parents and nurse before directly approaching the child.
2. Approach the child at eye level.
3. Communicate through a stuffed animal or doll before directly addressing the child.

4. Allow the child to become accustomed to the nurse through some type of play activity, such as balloon play, before touching the child.
5. Avoid gestures such as broad smiles and extended eye contact.
6. Speak in a clear manner that is unhurried and confident.
7. Incorporate parents into initial assessment activities such as vital sign measurement.

The parent's trust of the nurse will be enhanced by the efforts made to make their child comfortable. Parents often appreciate the opportunity to complete an assessment form that describes their child's eating, sleeping, toileting, and play routines. Providing parents with frequent opportunities to ask questions assures them of the nurse's interest in keeping them well informed and allows the trusting relationship to develop.

REDUCING FEAR

The nurse who is serious about reducing the fears of pediatric clients must be familiar with the fears' origins. These fears, which are based on cognitive and perceptual development, vary considerably at different ages. The most common fears among age groups are:

1. Infants from birth to 3 months: sudden movements, loud noises, and loss of physical support
2. Infants from 4 to 12 months: strangers, strange objects, heights, and anticipation of previous uncomfortable situations
3. Toddlers from 1 to 3 years: the dark, being alone, separation from parent, some animals such as barking dogs, and loud machines
4. Preschoolers from 3 to 6 years: body mutilation, supernatural beings, monsters, ghosts, unfamiliar routines, separation from trusted adults, and abandonment

► RESEARCH HIGHLIGHT

RESEARCH ABSTRACT
Young hospitalized children find many aspects of the experience stressful and respond to these events with distress reactions. Clinical observations and empirical evidence suggest that children who believe in their ability to master their hospital experiences exhibit fewer stress-related behaviors (e.g., excessive crying, fear). Children should receive training to develop their coping skills and parents should be incorporated into the teaching/learning process.

IMPLICATIONS FOR PRACTICE
► Nursing interventions during stressful events need to focus on providing the mode of support that will enhance children's feelings of control.
► Provide opportunities that encourage children to take direct action in stressful events such as allowing them to assist the nurse or doctor during a procedure.
► Teach children to use positive self-talk during a procedure (e.g., "I will be all better in a little while" and "Everything will be OK").
► Encourage young children to practice their treatment on a doll client.

REFERENCE
LaMontagne L: Bolstering personal control in child patients through coping interventions, *J Pediatr Nurs* 19(3):235, 1993.

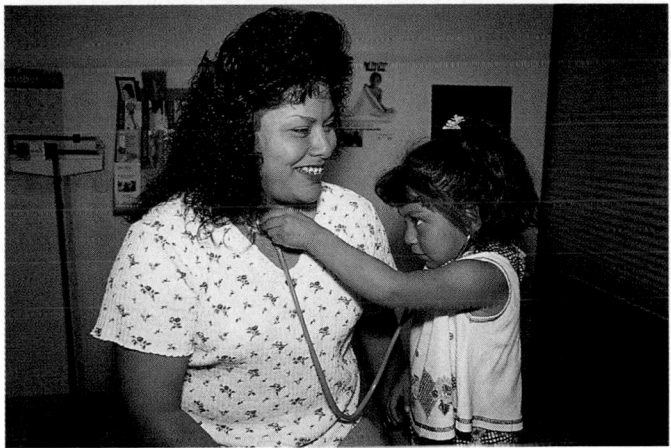

Fig. 28-5 Letting the child use the stethoscope on parent or health care provider helps to reduce the child's fear.

Some fears are associated with health care; these include being stuck with needles; having to take bad-tasting medications; experiencing invasive procedures (those that violate body surfaces) such as ear, nose, and throat examinations; being forced to lie down; and being subjected to the unknown such as x-ray procedures, electrocardiograms, and electroencephalograms.

Many appropriate methods for reduction of fear have already been discussed. However, the nurse should plan to use the following additional measures to reduce fear in the hospitalized young child:

1. Assist child to cope with fear/stress by helping the child to gain control (see the box above).
2. Allow the child to sit up for assessments and procedures whenever possible.
3. Demonstrate the exact steps of a procedure on a doll, another nurse, or parent before beginning the procedure on the child.
4. Allow the child to see and handle equipment or use it on a doll (e.g., a stethoscope) (Fig. 28-5).
5. Describe sensations that the child will experience such as "The x-ray table will be hard and cold when you lie on it."
6. Encourage parents' presence during procedures and treatments.
7. Provide the child with the opportunity to "play through" experiences and release pent-up feelings of anger and frustration in an acceptable fashion (e.g., syringe play, pounding toys, substances to be molded, and percussion instruments).
8. Allow the child to assist with the procedure (e.g., cleansing the skin with an alcohol wipe before an injection).
9. Plan for therapeutic play sessions.

MINIMIZING PHYSICAL DISCOMFORT

Children of all ages, including newborns, experience pain. The nurse is often unable to prevent pain but can do much to reduce the physical discomfort. The expression of pain is influenced by the children's culture and parents' child-rearing practices. Children's perception of pain varies according to their pain threshold and degree of anxiety regarding it.

Pain in infants can be differentiated from hunger and general discomfort by crying that does not decrease with comfort measures, increased restlessness, and increased random movements. Toddlers who still perceive sensations in generalized ways cannot indicate clearly where pain is felt. In addition, toddlers find anything that is intrusive or causes pressure to be painful. Infants and toddlers respond to restraint in the same manner as physical pain because they have difficulty using motor activity as a means of releasing tension. Forcing children of any age to lie down is threatening to their sense of control and results in protest. Preschoolers can point to the area of pain but have insufficient vocabulary to discuss or describe it. In addition, they associate a great deal of anxiety and fear with pain and may perceive that the pain is a punishment for some misdeed or "bad" thought. Nurses should use the following guidelines to minimize children's physical discomfort:

1. Keep periods of restraint or immobility to a minimum. This can be facilitated by having at the bedside a care giver whose watchfulness prevents the accidental removal of catheters and tubes.
2. Comfort infants and toddlers by talking in a soft voice or singing and with physical contact such as holding and rocking, hugging, cuddling, and caressing.
3. Provide young children with items that provide security and comfort (e.g., special blanket, favorite toy, or mother's scarf).
4. Reassure children that it is OK to cry, and emphasize the helpful things they do, such as keeping their arms very still during shots.

5. Allow choices that are acceptable such as which finger to stick for a blood glucose test or which bandage to put on afterward.
6. Encourage participation in a procedure that may result in discomfort, which is exaggerated by anxiety (e.g., removing the tape when intravenous fluids are being discontinued).
7. Provide incentives that encourage cooperation with uncomfortable nursing actions (e.g., allowing children to choose surprises from a special box each time they cooperate with finger sticks for blood sugar measurement).
8. Use a pain assessment tool that allows children to use faces to describe the degree of pain.
9. Use a variety of techniques such as positioning, distraction, relaxation, and rhythmic breathing with imagery to alleviate pain.
10. Provide adequate analgesic control of pain to provide comfort and promote cooperation with painful procedures such as coughing, turning, and deep breathing.

FOSTERING NORMAL GROWTH AND DEVELOPMENT

Illness and hospitalization of children have a disrupting effect on their development. When the illness is mild and hospitalization is short, the effect may be minimal, but a serious illness can have a more significant impact. The illness is often accompanied by physical restrictions, enforced dependency, and interruption of daily routines for eating, sleeping, elimination, and play. Regression to earlier behaviors that provide security is the most common defense mechanism used by young children to cope with these stresses. Use of the following guidelines will help the nurse plan for fostering of normal growth and development:

1. Provide an environment of acceptance for regressive behavior.
2. Provide favorite toys from home.
3. Encourage participation in self-care activities such as bathing, dressing, and feeding self.
4. Provide intermittent auditory and visual stimulation (e.g., take children for rides in wheelchairs or wagons, play sing-along records, read to children, and look at picture books with children).
5. Provide opportunities for children to socially interact with other children (e.g., take children to playroom in wagons or wheelchairs, encourage sibling visits, and have other clients visit children).
6. Provide toys and play equipment that promote development of fine and gross motor activities.
7. Encourage development of new vocabulary by learning names for hospital items and personnel.
8. Encourage participation in assessment and procedures.
9. Discuss the effects of hospitalization on growth and development with parents and explain how they can help children regain and attain optimal levels of growth and development.
10. Consider effect of children's cultural background on their development (see the box at left).

INCORPORATION OF PLAY AND DIVERSIONAL ACTIVITY INTO CARE

For children, play is work. It can be one of the most effective tools for managing hospitalized children. Play in the hospital brings a normalcy to the strange and sometimes hostile-appearing environment and provides an avenue for the release of tension. Diversional play allows children to focus their attention on pleasurable experiences and to downplay situations that result when a child combines reality with imagination.

Play helps children deal with strains and stresses, develop their capacities, and strengthen their defenses. The nurse may find the following guidelines helpful when planning play for the hospitalized child:

1. Incorporate play into the daily activities of bathing, dressing, feeding, and measurement of vital signs.
2. Provide opportunities for all children, especially those who are immobilized, to go to the playroom or engage in play with other children.
3. Keep the playroom as a "safe" area by prohibiting the administration of medications or performance of any procedures there.
4. Provide materials that encourage creativity (e.g., paper, paint, paste, play dough, crayons, and other art materials).

CULTURAL ASPECTS OF CARE

HISPANIC TODDLER WITH SEPARATION ANXIETY

Hospitalized Hispanic toddlers and their mothers need nursing interventions that are culturally sensitive and developmentally appropriate to help them tolerate separation anxiety. The role of the mother is idealized and her self-image is closely related to her nurturing role. Both the mother and the child are very stressed when the combination of hospitalization and home responsibilities results in their separation. Hispanic toddlers are less pressured to become autonomous and develop self-mastery; consequently, weaning, toilet training, and self-dressing skills are slower to develop than in white or black children. Hispanic toddlers may have an increased expression of separation anxiety due to the closely dependent attached relationship to their mothers. Loranger (1992) suggests that the problem of separation anxiety for the Hispanic toddler can be somewhat alleviated through the transcultural intervention of play. If the child does not speak English, the nurse needs to use words that are familiar to the child to initiate play. Names and pronunciation of favorite toys can be listed in Spanish on a poster in the child's room. Demonstration of all procedures on a doll or teddy bear helps children understand what the nurse will do to them. Tape-recordings of the mother reading stories may be comforting to the child. Pictures of family members and objects belonging to the mother (e.g., sweater) may also bring solace. The mother's visualization of the individualized care for her child helps her to become more trusting of the nurses and their willingness to meet the needs of her child. Play helps to bridge the gap between language and cultural barriers.

5. Provide sense-pleasure play that allows infants and young children to enjoy sound, movement, smells, tastes, touch, and color through activities and objects such as water play, mobiles, and stuffed toys.
6. Promote motor development through skill play such as putting objects in a container and dumping them out.
7. Promote cognitive development through activities such as reading, hiding and seeking of objects, and counting games.
8. Plan special activities for children whose activities are limited by their health problems or medical regimen. For example, have children with eye patches identify familiar objects by feel or provide a sense of mobility to children in traction by playing a game of ring toss.
9. When children are confined to their rooms by isolation, have parents select toys and games from the playroom to take to their child.
10. Request visits by volunteers or the child life worker when children are confined.
11. Prepare children for procedures through play with hospital equipment.
12. Use children's cognitive levels and past experiences as basis for choosing appropriate play activities for teaching purposes.
13. Provide for judicious television watching.

Collaboration with other health team members is often an important step in providing optimal care for the child. If the preschooler is having difficulty cooperating with the respiratory therapist for a breathing treatment, the nurse might request that the therapist leave the mask with the child for examination and play between treatments. If the toddler refuses to keep the nasal prongs in place and continuously fights a mask, the nurse and respiratory therapist might discuss the situation with the physician and decide that a Croupette would be a more satisfactory delivery system for oxygen.

 ## Evaluation

It is necessary to evaluate the response of the child and family to nursing interventions to determine whether the goals of care have been met. The establishment of expected outcomes (see the evaluation box below) provides a standard by which to use evaluative measures to determine the response to interventions. For instance, a goal may have been the active participation of the parents in the care of the child. The nurse's evaluation revealed the outcome of the mother demonstrating no interest or initiative in bathing the child. The nurse must review the goals and interventions to determine whether and how they should be revised. Modification of the care plan should reflect input from the child and parents. For example, infusion of intravenous fluids might have caused the mother to feel inadequate or afraid to disturb the child, and as a result she was inhibited from participating in the bath and needed further support from the nurse to do so.

Each health care agency has its own guidelines for recording and exchanging information about clients, but regardless of the methods used, it's important to always include the following:
1. Assessments and nursing actions related to nursing diagnoses
2. The child's and parents' response to teaching
3. Questions asked by the child or parents and the nurse's response
4. Social behavior of the child

In addition, the nurse incorporates principles of growth and development into the evaluation of care. Whether care is provided in the home, outpatient, or hospital setting, the child's progression with normal growth and development tasks must be evaluated. Growth and development are essential health promotion activities and are consistently part of the evaluation of nursing care of the child.

 ## Sample Evaluation of Interventions for Fear

GOAL	EVALUATIVE MEASURES	EXPECTED OUTCOMES
Child will cope effectively with anxiety associated with hospitalization before discharge.	Observe presence of and activity of family in child's room.	Parent or significant other will remain with child.
		Parent will participate in child's feeding, hygiene, and play each day.
	Observe child's use of self-comforting measures.	Child will use coping and defense mechanisms daily to combat fear.
	Observe child for evidence of regressive behavior.	Child's use of regressive behavior diminishes.
	Observe child's play.	

■ KEY CONCEPTS ■

▶ Growth and development are orderly, directional, predictable, interdependent, and complex processes that continue throughout life.

▶ People progress through similar chronological stages of growth and development but at an individual pace and with individual behaviors.

▶ A developmental perspective helps the nurse understand commonalities and variations in each stage and the impact they have on the client's health.

▶ During critical periods of development, a multitude of factors can foster or hinder optimal physical, cognitive, and psychosocial development.

▶ Growth and development are influenced by the inner forces of heredity and temperament and the outer forces of family, peers, life experiences, and environmental elements.

▶ The inner forces set the limits for development and the external forces provide opportunities for achieving that potential.

▶ Because the embryo and fetus grow and develop throughout the intrauterine period, genetic factors and environmental factors (teratogens) may result in impairments in any body system in utero.

▶ Physiological health concerns during childbirth include adequate functioning of all systems and prevention of infection.

▶ A psychosocial health concern that begins at childbirth is the establishment of parent-child attachment.

▶ Physiological, cognitive, and psychosocial development continue throughout the neonate, infant, toddler, and preschool periods, and the nurse must be familiar with normal parameters to determine potential problems and promote normal development.

▶ The nurse recognizes that the child's perception of health and health behaviors begin early and assists the parent and child in establishing healthful patterns that will continue for the entire life span.

▶ The developmental theories of Freud, Erikson, Maslow, Piaget, and Kohlberg help explain the individual aspects of development for each client.

▶ The nursing care plan for the hospitalized child is based on assessment of development, response to illness and hospitalization, previous experiences with separation, medical history, perceptions of illness, and available support systems.

▶ Nursing strategies of the child include incorporating the parents into the child's care and fostering the child's continued development.

■ KEY TERMS ■

Animism, p. 517

Apgar score, p. 505

Artificialism, p. 517

Attachment, p. 510

Blastocyst, p. 503

Bonding, p. 506

Critical period, p. 497

Development, p. 497

Embryo, p. 503

Fetus, p. 503

Growth, p. 497

Immanent justice, p. 517

Infancy, p. 510

Lanugo, p. 504

Maturation, p. 497

Molding, p. 507

Morula, p. 503

Neonatal period, p. 506

Object permanence, p. 497

Organogenesis, p. 503

Physiological anorexia, p. 515

Placenta, p. 503

Preconceptual thought, p. 517

Preoperational thought, p. 515

Preschool period, p. 516

Temperament, p. 519

Teratogens, p. 503

Toddlerhood, p. 514

Vernix caseosa, p. 504

Zygote, p. 503

■ CRITICAL THINKING EXERCISES ■

1. Two-day-old Sally has been admitted to the hospital because she has had a seizure. Newborns have very poor resistance to infection. What measures should the nurses take to be sure that Sally does not develop an infection during hospitalization?

2. Six-month-old Jimmy has been admitted to the hospital because of bronchiolitis. His parents wish to participate in his care when they are present but will not be able to be with him continuously. The mother plans to spend the late evening and night at the hospital but will continue to work during the day. The father will visit on his way home from work in the evening. Identify nursing measures that will assist Jimmy to continue developing his sense of trust.

3. Two-year-old Johnny has been admitted to the hospital for periorbital cellulitis of his right eye and is receiving intravenous antibiotic therapy. What strategies can the nurse use in his daily care to promote his developing autonomy? Since Johnny's mother will not be able to spend the night at the hospital with him, identify measures the nurse and mother could take to comfort him and help him cope with this separation.

REFERENCES

Bobak ID: *Maternity and gynecologic care: the nurse and the family*, ed 5, St Louis, 1993, Mosby.

Centers for Disease Control and Prevention: General recommendations on immunization: recommendations of the Advisory Committee on Immunization Practices (ACIP). *MMWR* 43(No RR-1), p 1, 1994.

Erikson EH: *Childhood and society*, ed 2, New York, 1963, Norton.

Feingold C: Correlates of cognitive development in low-birth-weight infants from low-income families, *J Pediatr Nurs* 9(2):91, 1994.

Frankenburg WK et al: The Denver II: a major revision and re-standardization of the Denver Developmental Screening Test, *Pediatrics* 89(1):91, 1992.

Herda JA: Nursing interventions aimed at reducing risks of SIDS, *Pediatr Nurs* 18(5):531, 1992.

Kim MJ, McFarland GK, McLane AM: *Pocket guide to nursing diagnoses*, ed 5, St Louis, 1995, Mosby.

Kohlberg L: The child as a moral philosopher, *Psychology Today* 2(4):25, 1968.

LaMontagne L: Bolstering personal control in child patients through coping interventions, *J Pediatr Nurs* 19(3):235, 1993.

Loranger N: Play intervention strategies for the Hispanic toddler with separation anxiety, *Pediatr Nurs* 18(6):571, 1992.

Maslow AH: *Motivation and personality*, ed 2, New York, 1970, Harper & Row.

Papalia DC, Olds SW: *Human development*, ed 5, St Louis, 1992, McGraw-Hill.

Piaget J: *The origins of intelligence in children*, New York, 1952, International Universities Press.

Ritchie JA et al: Coping behaviors of hospitalized preschool children, *Matern Child Nurs J* 17(3):153, 1988.

Salsberry PJ, Nickel JT, Mitch R: Inadequate immunization among 2-year-old children: a profile of children at risk, *J Pediatr Nurs* 9(3):158, 1994.

Schepp KG: Factors influencing the coping efforts of hospitalized children, *Nurs Res* 40(1):42, 1991.

Selekman J: The guidelines for immunizations have changed again, *Pediatr Nurs* 20(4),1994.

Williams SR: *Nutrition and diet therapy*, ed 7, St Louis, 1993, Mosby.

Wong DL: *Whaley and Wong's nursing care of infants and children*, ed 5, St Louis, 1995, Mosby.

Yoos HL: Children's illness concepts: old and new paradigms, *Pediatr Nurs* 20(2):134, 1994.

ADDITIONAL READINGS

Bergmann T, Freud A: *Children in the hospital*, New York, 1965, International Universities Press.

Bremman A: Caring for children during procedures: a review of the literature, *Pediatr Nurs* 20(5):451, 1994.

Clatworthy S: Therapeutic play: effects on hospitalized children, *Child Health Care* 9(4):108, 1981.

Forrest DC: The cocaine-exposed infant. I. Identification and assessment, *J Pediatr Health Care* 8(1):3, 1994.

Forrest DC: The cocaine-exposed infant. II. Intervention and teaching, *J Pediatr Health Care* 8(1):7, 1994.

Jones HE: Prevention of childhood injuries: Part II, *Pediatr Nurs* 18(6):619, 1992.

Kelley SJ, Walsh JH, Thompson IC: Birth outcomes, health problems, and neglect with prenatal exposure to cocaine, *Pediatr Nurs* 17(2):130, 1991.

Kramer NA: Comparison of therapeutic touch and casual touch in stress reduction of hospitalized children, *Pediatr Nurs* 16(5):483, 1990.

Le Vieux-Anglen L, Sawyer E: Incorporating play interventions into nursing care, *Pediatr Nurs* 19(5):459, 1993.

Robertson J: *Young children in hospital*, ed 2, London, 1970, Tavistock Publications.

Schepp KG: Factors influencing the coping effort of mothers of hospitalized children, *Nurs Res* 40(1):42, 1991.

Sewell KH, Gaines SK: A developmental approach to childhood safety education, *Pediatr Nurs* 19(5):619, 1993.

Wilson PD, Testani-Dufour L: Bicycle safety programs: targeting injury prevention through education, *Pediatric Nurs* 19(4):343, 1993.

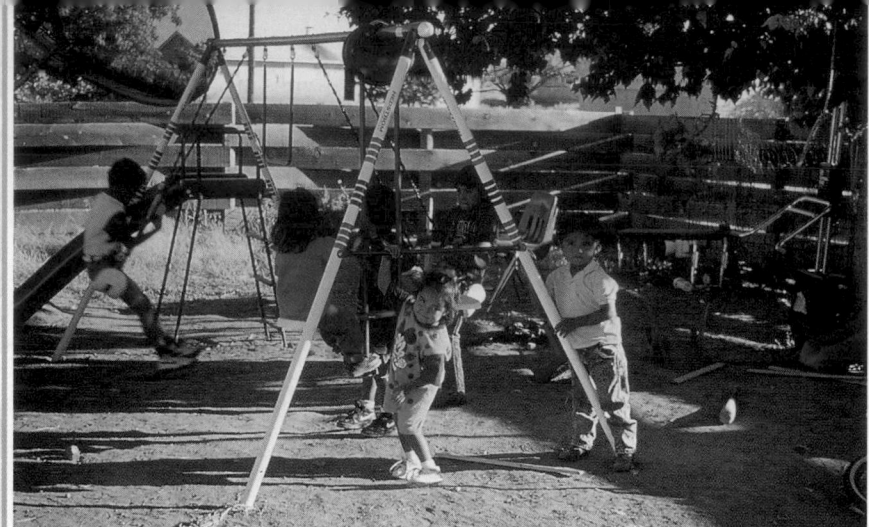

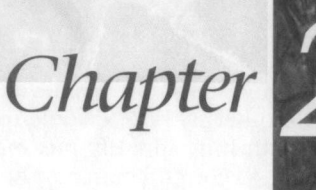

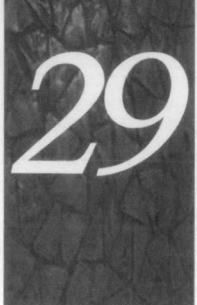

Chapter 29

School Age
Through Adolescence

Objectives

Mastery of content in this chapter will enable the student to:

▶ Define the key terms listed.

▶ Describe the normal physical changes that occur during the school-age years and adolescence.

▶ Discuss behaviors reflecting psychosocial and cognitive development of the school-age child and adolescent.

▶ Contrast the cognitive abilities of the school-age child and adolescent.

▶ Identify factors that contribute to self-esteem in youth.

▶ Describe the influence of the school environment on the development of the school-age child and adolescent.

▶ Discuss ways in which the nurse can help parents meet their children's developmental needs.

▶ Compare and contrast the ways by which a school-age child and adolescent develop moral values.

▶ Discuss the development of identity in the adolescent.

▶ Explain the significance of Erikson's psychosocial moratoriums to the adolescent.

▶ Identify health concerns of the school-age child and adolescent.

▶ Describe nursing interventions to promote optimal health in the school-age child and adolescent.

▶ Use the nursing process to individualize the nursing care of youth.

▶ Plan culturally appropriate health promotion activities for minority adolescents.

School-age children and adolescents lead demanding, challenging lives. The developmental changes between ages 6 and 18 are diverse and span all areas of growth and development. Physical, psychosocial, cognitive, and moral skills are developed, expanded, refined, and synchronized so that the individual may become an accepted and productive member of society. The environment in which the individual develops skills also expands and diversifies. Instead of the principal limits of family and close friends, the environment may include the school, community, and church. Because of expectations for development, increasing skill and knowledge base, and environmental expansion, the individual experiences new difficulties and dilemmas. With age-specific assessment, the nurse must review the appropriate developmental expectations for each age group. For example, before assessing risk-taking behaviors, the nurse recognizes that adolescents normally strive to achieve a sense of identity while developing a moral code compatible with society.

The nurse needs to direct school-age children and adolescents toward normal developmental behaviors, assisting them in maximizing their abilities and using them to cope. By helping children and adolescents achieve a necessary developmental balance, the nurse promotes health. Table 29-1 provides an overview of developmental behavior typical of school-age children and adolescents. The nurse must also increasingly involve the child or adolescent in charting a developmental course. Because preadolescents have increased cognitive and social skills, they are better able to plan developmental activities. Not only can they describe their feelings about the changes, but they can also think through these changes. Problem solving becomes more purposeful and sophisticated and results in the achievement of the outcomes that they desire. This paced, active participation may initiate a style of involvement in lifelong self-care.

School-age children and adolescents must cope with changes involving all areas of development. For example, 6-year-old children are confronted with new authority figures, teachers, as well as new rules and restrictions. They need to cooperatively work and play with a large group of children of various cultural backgrounds. School-age children must meet the challenge of developing cognitive skills that enhance their reasoning and allow them to learn to read, write, and manipulate numbers.

Because of the stress of these changes, a child may develop physical and psychosocial health problems (e.g., increased susceptibility to upper respiratory infections, school maladjustment, inadequate peer relationships, or learning disorders). The nurse designs health promotion interventions that are based on the child's developmental stage.

■ SCHOOL-AGE CHILD

During these "middle years" of childhood, the foundation for adult roles in work, recreation, and social interaction is laid. In industrialized countries this period begins when the child starts elementary school around the age of 6 years. Puberty, around 12 years of age, signals the end of middle childhood. Great developmental strides are made during these years when children develop competencies in physical, cognitive, and psychosocial skills. During these years children become "better" at things; for example, they can run faster and farther as proficiency and endurance develop.

The school or educational experience expands the child's world and is a transition from a life of relatively free play to a life of structured play, learning, and work. The school and home influence growth and development, requiring adjustment by the parents and child. The child must learn to cope with rules and expectations presented by the school and peers. Parents must learn to allow their child to make decisions, accept responsibility, and learn from life's experiences.

While the child goes through this adjustment, the nurse assists in promoting health. This is done by helping the parents and child to identify potential stressors and by designing interventions to minimize stress and the child's stress response. Interventions must include parent, child, and teacher for maximal success. Table 29-2 provides an overview of stressors commonly encountered by school-age children and appropriate nursing interventions.

Physical Development

HEIGHT AND WEIGHT

The rate of growth during these early school years is slower than any time since birth but continues steadily. A particular child may not follow the pattern precisely. The school-age child appears slimmer than the preschooler, as a result of changes in fat distribution and thickness (Edelman and Mandle, 1994). Growth accelerates at different times for different children. The average increase in height is 2 inches per year, and weight, which is more variable, increases by 4 to 7 pounds per year. Many children double their weight during these middle childhood years.

School provides children with the opportunity to compare themselves with large numbers of children of the same age. The physical examination usually required for the first grade is an excellent opportunity for the nurse to discuss with the child and parents the influences of genetic endowment, nutrition, and exercise on height and weight. Annual measurement of height and weight may reveal alterations in growth that are symptoms of the onset of a variety of childhood diseases.

Boys are slightly taller and heavier than girls during these early school years. Approximately 2 years before puberty, children experience a rapid acceleration in skeletal growth. Girls, who reach puberty first, begin to surpass boys in height and weight, which causes embarrassment to both sexes. These changes may begin as early as 9 years in girls but do not usually occur in boys before 12 years.

CARDIOVASCULAR FUNCTIONING

Cardiovascular functioning is refined and stabilized during the school-age years. The heart rate averages 70 to 90 beats per minute, the blood pressure normalizes to approximately 110/70 mm Hg, and the respiratory rate stabilizes to 19 to 21 breaths per minute. Lung growth is minimal and respirations become slower, deeper, and more regular. However, by the end of this period the heart is 6 times the size it was at birth and has generally reached its adult size.

NEUROMUSCULAR FUNCTIONING

School-age children become more graceful during the school years because their large muscle coordination improves and strength doubles. Most children practice the basic gross motor skills of running, jumping, balancing,

Table 29-1	Developmental Behaviors of School-Age Children and Adolescents

SCHOOL-AGE CHILDREN	ADOLESCENTS

RELATIONSHIPS WITH PARENTS

Children gradually learn that parents are less than perfect; they can be disillusioned with them and wish that friends' parents were their own. Sometimes they believe that they must be adopted. They rely on parents for unconditional love, security, guidance, and nurturing.

Adolescents' desire for increasing independence and autonomy and continuing need for some dependence and limit setting by parents place strain on their relationship. Effective communication and democratic parenting are best tools for meeting this challenge.

RELATIONSHIPS WITH SIBLINGS

School-agers seem to be at odds with one another at home; yet they are each others' best defenders away from home. Younger children often idolize older siblings, and this frequently leads to competition. Older children may envy attention that younger siblings require and be quite bossy and somewhat abusive.

Younger siblings rarely understand their adolescent siblings' need for privacy to think, dream, and talk with peers. Adolescents often enjoy interacting with and guiding younger brothers and sisters when timing is convenient for them and they can remain in control.

RELATIONSHIPS WITH PEERS

During primary grades (6-7 years), children of both sexes play together, depending on who is available and interested. Around age 8, social groupings of same-sex peers form. These "gangs" allow children to declare their independence from parental rules and establish their own secret codes or languages and rules of membership and behavior. This period is often referred to as *secret society* of childhood. Preadolescent (10-12 years) friendships are characterized by having best friend of same sex. These relationships may be transient, but they are intense and allow discussion of all areas of life. Some interest in heterosexual relationships develops but they usually are not reciprocal.

Peer group is factor of critical influence to adolescents, who have increasing need for recognition and acceptance. Companionship offered by peer groups provides secure environment for individuals to try out new ideas and share similar feelings and attitudes. Adolescents often form cliques with peers from same socioeconomic group with similar interests. Cliques, which are highly exclusive, help their members, who have strong emotional bonds, develop their identities. The crowd, which is more impersonal than clique, offers opportunities for heterosexual interaction and social activities. The crowd also maintains rigid membership requirements; clique membership is usually prerequisite for crowd membership.

SELF-CONCEPT

Children's feelings of competence regarding mastery of tasks are key elements in forming self-esteem. Children need to receive positive feedback from teachers and parents regarding their efforts. It is important for children to develop skills in at least one area such as reading, music, or swimming. Pets that require children's care and attention reward them with unconditional love and promote feelings of self-worth.

Formal and informal peer groups are primary force in shaping self-concept of group members. Popularity and recognition within peer group enhance self-esteem and reinforce self-concept. Total immersion in peer group may make it appear that adolescents have no original thoughts and are incapable of making decisions. Adolescents who withdraw from peers into isolation struggle with developing identity.

FEARS

There is decline in fears related to body safety such as storms, dogs, darkness, noises, scrapes, and scratches. Fears of supernatural such as ghosts and witches persist and decline slowly. New fears related to school and family occur. They fear ridicule from teachers and friends and disapproval and rejection of parents. They also become frightened about death and items that they hear on news such as war and destruction of environment.

Fears in this age group center around peer group acceptance, body changes, loss of self-control, and emerging sexual urges. Adolescents constantly examine their bodies for changes and signs of imperfection. Any defect, real or imagined, is cause of endless worry. Adolescents' developing awareness of economic and political problems may result in fear of going to war with its resulting death and destruction.

COPING PATTERNS

To deal with stress, school-agers use problem solving and defense mechanisms including regression, denial, aggression, and suppression. Several categories of coping behaviors of hospitalized school-agers include inactivity (total silence, lack of activity, and apathy), orientation or precoping (looking and listening, walking around and exploring, and asking questions), cooperation (compliance with care), resistance (attempt to get away from the situation by turning away or making physical or verbal attacks), and controlling (assuming responsibility for self-care and suggesting how things could be done).

Repertoire of coping behaviors has expanded with experiences adolescents have gained from life and from developing cognitive maturity. By age 15, most use full range of defense mechanisms, including rationalization and intellectualization. Adolescents' problem-solving abilities have matured, and they can reason through philosophical discussions and complex situations that require abstract thinking and proposition of hypotheses. Some adolescents use avoidance coping strategies in which the problem is denied or repressed and an attempt is made to reduce tension by engaging in chemical abuse or avoiding people.

Table 29-1	Developmental Behaviors of School-Age Children and Adolescents—cont'd

SCHOOL-AGE CHILDREN	ADOLESCENTS
MORALS Children learn rules from parents, but their understanding of rules or reasons for them is limited until about 10 years. Before that, they are concerned with own needs first and may cheat to win. After 10, justice is based on "eye for an eye," and punishment should correct situation (e.g., if children break something, they should pay to have it fixed).	According to Kohlberg (1964), as youths approach adolescence they reach conventional level where internalization of expectations of their family and society begins. Initially there is considerable conformity to rules to win praise or approval from others and to avoid social disapproval or rejection; later, they seek to avoid criticism from persons of authority in institutions.
DIVERSIONAL ACTIVITY School-agers play cooperatively in group activities such as jumping rope, hopscotch, soccer, and baseball. Play becomes competitive, and children often have difficulty learning to lose. Teasing, insults, dares, superstitions, and increased sensitivity are characteristics of this age.	Many teenagers develop special interests in certain sports and concentrate on developing maximal skills therein. Recreational activities are often determined by what is popular with peers and what can provide independence from parents (e.g., computers, cars).
NUTRITION Children have definite likes and dislikes. Few nutritional deficiencies occur in this age group. Children have voracious appetites after school and need quality snacks such as fruit and sandwiches to avoid empty calorie foods such as chips and candy.	Total nutritional needs become greater during adolescence. Girls' caloric needs decrease, and their need for protein increases slightly. Iron needed by adolescents is almost twice that of adult men, and growth spurt increases calcium demand.

throwing, and catching during play, resulting in refinement of neuromuscular function and skills. Individual differences in the rate of mastering skills and ultimate skill achievement become apparent. Individual differences in motor skills are established by participation in activities and games requiring coordinated muscle movements and innate ability.

Fine motor skills lag behind gross motor skills but progress at approximately the same rate. As control is gained over fingers and wrists, children become proficient in a wide range of activities.

Most 6-year-old children can hold a pencil adeptly and print letters and words, but by age 12 the child can make detailed drawings and write sentences in script. Painting, drawing, playing computer games, and modeling allow children to practice and improve newly refined skills. Nurses should encourage children and have parents encourage them to pursue these activities. Table 29-3 de-

Table 29-2	Potential School-Related Stressors

STRESSOR	NURSING INTERVENTION
Meeting teacher's behavioral expectations	Encourage parents to share information with teachers that will help them understand the child better Encourage unhurried communication about school expectations, events
Maintaining self-concept	Be positive on daily basis to foster child success
Separation; school adjustment	Assist child in identifying physical set-up of school and daily routines
Testing out new ideas	Encourage originality by helping children make their own projects from discarded or other available materials
Integrating peer values into behavior	Reinforce positive peer activities and interactions
Assuming responsibility for own learning	Encourage use of problem solving by child
Meeting cognitive requirements	Demonstrate interest in what child is learning Take advantage of situations that support and reinforce school learning Provide well-lit study area that is free of interruptions Share an interest in reading
Behavioral standard development	Promote good conduct through praise and example
Participation in school events	Assist parent in realizing need for extracurricular activities Assist child to select activity in which he or she is likely to be successful

Modified from Wong DL: *Whaley and Wong's nursing care of infants and children*, ed 5, St Louis, 1995, Mosby.

Table 29-3	Motor Development in the School-Age Child	
6-7 Years	**8-10 Years**	**11-12 Years**

FINE MOTOR SKILLS

6-7 Years	8-10 Years	11-12 Years
Uses knife to butter bread and learns to cut tender meat.	Uses knife and fork simultaneously.	Learns to peel apples and potatoes.
Cuts, folds, and pastes paper.	Learns to thread needle and tie knot.	Sews simple garments on machine.
Prints with pencil.	Uses hammer, saw, and screwdriver.	Builds simple objects like birdhouse.
Draws man with 12-16 details.	Becomes proficient at writing cursive.	Enjoys using decorative script.
Copies triangle at 6 years and diamond by 7 years.	Uses symbols in drawing (e.g., bird, star).	Begins to use creative and artistic talents.
Colors within line of picture.	Builds simple models of cars and planes and does simple handcrafts.	Builds complex models of cars and planes and does complex handcrafts.
Needs assistance to clean teeth thoroughly.	Learns to play jacks and marbles.	Learns to play musical instrument.
	Can learn to floss teeth effectively and be independent in tooth care.	Becomes proficient in caring for teeth with braces and other appliances.

GROSS MOTOR SKILLS

6-7 Years	8-10 Years	11-12 Years
Remains in constant motion.	Can catch, throw (70 feet), and hit baseball.	Can do standing broad jump of 5 feet.
Moves more cautiously at 7 years than at 6 years.	Engages in alternate rhythmic hopping in 2-2, 2-3, or 3-3 pattern.	Can do standing high jump of 3 feet.
Hops and jumps into small squares.	Engages in complex styles of skipping rope accompanied by verbal jingles.	Plays games involving simultaneous use of two or more complex motor skills such as roller skating, ice hockey, or dance skating.
Learns to roller skate, skip rope, ride bicycle, and swim.		

SELF-CARE

6-7 Years	8-10 Years	11-12 Years
Takes bath without supervision.	Learns to clean bathroom after bath.	Dusts, vacuums, and straightens own room.
Often returns to finger feeding.	Enjoys fixing own snacks and sack lunch.	Learns to cook simply prepared foods.
Learns to brush and comb hair in acceptable fashion without help.	Learns to part hair and insert hair ribbons and barrettes.	Washes, dries, and fixes own hair in braids, curls, and ponytails.
Puts on most clothes but may need assistance with shirttails, sashes, and final adjustments.	Dresses self completely and can help younger siblings with clothes.	Learns to sort, wash, dry, and press own clothing.
	Can make own bed.	Learns to care for fingernails and toenails.

scribes specific gross motor and fine motor skills and their use in self-care activities.

The improved fine motor capabilities of youngsters in middle childhood allow them to become very independent in bathing, dressing, and taking care of other personal needs. They develop strong personal preferences in the way these needs are met. Illness and hospitalization threaten children's control in these areas. Therefore it is important to allow them to participate in care and maintain as much independence as possible. Children whose care demands restriction of fluids cannot be allowed to decide the amount of fluids they will drink in 24 hours, but they can help decide the type of fluids and keep an accurate record of intake.

Assessment of neurological development is often based on fine motor coordination. This assessment may include penmanship, stacking ability, and performance of sequential, rapid, alternating movements such as touching the finger to the nose and then to the examiner's finger (smooth movement without tremors is the normal response). Fine motor coordination is critical to success in the typical American school, where children must be able to hold pencils and crayons and use scissors and rulers. The opportunity to practice these skills through school work and play is essential to the acquisition of coordinated, complex behaviors.

NUTRITION

The school-age period is one with relatively few nutritional problems. When deficiencies exist, they are usually in iron, vitamin A, or calcium. Obesity may become a problem because children often rush into the home after school or play and eat the most easily obtainable and appealing foods. Unfortunately, these foods are often nutritionally poor and calorie laden. Providing nutritious snacks is often the best way for a parent to ensure good nutritional intake. Parents should provide ready access to fresh fruit, raw vegetables, cheese, popcorn, and high-protein snacks such as skim-milk pudding and hot chocolate. Children can learn a great deal about the food pyramid and a balanced diet by helping to prepare their own lunches and snacks (see the box on p. 533). Nurses should encourage parents to provide children with a variety of foods in adequate amounts to support growth and energy for play. Activity levels vary from day to day, and children's appetites and consumption of food vary accordingly. When children are overweight, they should be encouraged to increase their expenditure of calories through exercise and vigorous play. Children who become overweight have lower self-esteem, have difficulty in keeping up with other children in physical activities, and are often rejected by their peers. Nurses should help families and children prevent obesity.

CLIENT TEACHING
on Nutrition for the School-Age Child

OBJECTIVE
- The school-age child will plan and select healthful meals and snacks that are well-balanced and adhere to dietary guidelines for fat

TEACHING STRATEGIES
- Define the food pyramid and indicate number of servings of each
- Discuss how a balanced diet contains essential vitamins and minerals
- Review the importance of eating breakfast every day
- Review family meal patterns and stress the importance of mealtime as a social time to be enjoyed by all family members
- Relate the role of exercise in maintaining ideal weight and improving cardiovascular stamina and flexibility
- Assist the school-age child in developing an appropriate menu for lunch that restricts dietary fat intake to 30% of calories or less and saturated fat intake to less than 10% of calories
- Discuss examples of snacks that are considered healthy and noncariogenic
- Encourage the child to ask for particular foods for after-school snacks such as raw vegetable sticks, frozen fruit juices, cereal with low-fat milk

EVALUATION
- Observe meal selections made by the child for the next day
- Observe participation in physical activity

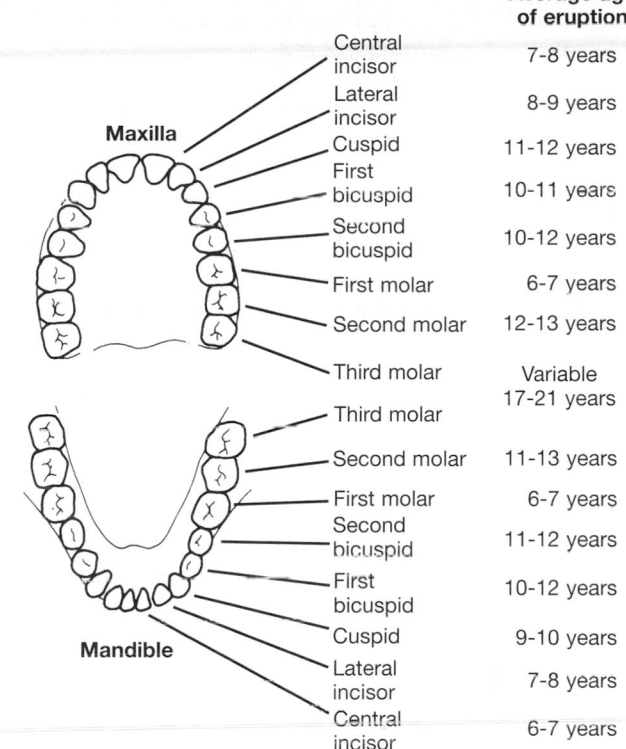

	Average age of eruption
Maxilla	
Central incisor	7-8 years
Lateral incisor	8-9 years
Cuspid	11-12 years
First bicuspid	10-11 years
Second bicuspid	10-12 years
First molar	6-7 years
Second molar	12-13 years
Third molar	Variable 17-21 years
Mandible	
Third molar	
Second molar	11-13 years
First molar	6-7 years
Second bicuspid	11-12 years
First bicuspid	10-12 years
Cuspid	9-10 years
Lateral incisor	7-8 years
Central incisor	6-7 years

Fig. 29-1 Sequence of eruption of secondary teeth. *(From Wong DL: Whaley and Wong's nursing care of infants and children, ed 5, St Louis, 1995, Mosby.)*

Today's families may often eat in fast-food restaurants where the food is high in fat, calories, and salt. Nurses need to encourage these restaurants to offer meats that are not breaded and are broiled, shakes that are made with low-fat yogurt or skim milk, and fruits and vegetables that are fresh or prepared in a low-calorie manner.

OTHER CHANGES

Other physical changes take place during the school-age years. Steady skeletal growth in the trunk and extremities occurs, and small- and long-bone ossification is present but not complete by age 12. Facial bones grow and remodel, as indicated by the presence of frontal sinuses by age 8 or 9. Dental growth is prominent during the school-age years. By 12 years, all primary teeth have been shed, and the majority of permanent teeth have erupted. Fig. 29-1 illustrates the pattern and timing of dental shedding and eruption. Infrequent or inadequate dental care remains a persistent need of many American children.

As skeletal growth progresses, body appearance and posture change. Earlier posture, which was characterized by a stoop-shouldered, slightly lordotic stance and prominent abdomen, changes to a more erect posture. It is essential that children, especially girls after the age of 12 years, be evaluated for scoliosis, the lateral curvature of the spine.

Eye shape alters because of skeletal growth. This improves visual acuity, and normal adult 20/20 vision is achievable. Screening for vision and hearing problems is easier, and re-

sults are more reliable because school-age children can more fully understand and cooperate with the test directions. The school nurse typically assesses the dental, visual, and auditory status of school-age children biannually and refers those with possible deviations to a pediatrician.

Cognitive Development

Cognitive changes provide the school-age child with the ability to think in a logical manner about the here and now but not about abstraction. The thoughts of school-age children are no longer dominated by their perceptions, and thus their ability to understand the world greatly expands. Around 7 years of age, children enter Piaget's third stage of cognitive development, known as **concrete operations**, in which they are able to use symbols to carry out operations (mental activities) in thought rather than in action. They begin to use logical thought processes with concrete materials (objects, people, and events they can touch and see). Table 28-2, p. 501, contains a summary of each stage of cognitive development according to Piaget.

Children in the concrete operational stage are considerably less egocentric than younger children and develop the ability to **decenter**, which enables them to concentrate on more than one aspect of a situation. Decentering has developed when children can look at two lines of dots unequal in length and recognize that they have the same number of dots even though the spaces in between dots differ (. . . . and ....). They also develop **reversibility**, the ability to trace their line of thinking back to its origin. An example would be the recognition that not only does 3 + 2 = 5 but that 5 − 3 = 2 and 5 − 2 = 3.

Decentering and reversibility allow the child to use **conservation**, the ability to recognize that the amount or quantity of a substance remains the same even when its shape or appearance changes. For instance, two balls of clay of equal size remain the same amount of clay even when one is flattened and the other remains in ball shape.

Seriation, the ability to place objects in order according to their increasing or decreasing size, develops by 7 or 8. This is easily measured by asking the child to arrange a group of pencils according to their length. The younger child usually aligns the tops of the pencils, whereas the child of 7 or 8 uses a methodical approach to line them up from the longest to the shortest.

The mental process of **classification** becomes more complex during the school years. The young child can separate objects into groups according to shape or color, but the school-age child understands that the same element can exist in two classes at the same time. For example, the school-age child could be shown a group of 16 wooden green beads and 4 wooden red beads and asked if there were more green beads or more wooden beads. The school-age child would recognize there were three classes of beads (red, green, and wooden) and would answer there were more wooden beads, whereas the preschool child would recognize only two classes of beads and answer green.

Middle childhood youngsters can use their newly developed cognitive skills to solve problems. Some individuals are better than others at problem solving because of native intelligence, education, and experience, but all children can improve these skills. Middle school-age children who are good problem solvers demonstrate the following characteristics: a positive attitude that the problem can be solved with persistence, a concern for accuracy, the ability to divide the problem into parts for study, and the ability to avoid guessing while searching for facts. Techniques that adults can use to help children improve their problem-solving strategies include helping them define the problem and its nature, plan their solution carefully, and evaluate their plan and the solution (Dacey and Travers, 1991). Nurses can use these strategies to help school-age children understand their illness and assume responsibility for their general health.

LANGUAGE DEVELOPMENT

Language growth is so rapid during middle childhood that it is no longer possible to match age with language achievements. The average 6-year-old child has a vocabulary of about 3000 words that quickly expands with exposure to peers and adults and reading ability. Children improve their use of language and expand their structural knowledge. They become more aware of the rules of **syntax**, the rules for linking words into phrases and sentences. They can also identify generalizations and exceptions to rules. They accept language as a means for representing the world in a subjective manner and realize that words have arbitrary, rather than absolute, meanings. They can use different words for the same object or concept, and they understand that a single word may have many meanings. Many school-agers use "bad language" to gain peer status

and to shock adults. It often begins with bathroom language and progresses to sexual or genital words. By the end of this period their use of language is similar to adults.

Psychosocial Development

The developmental task for school-age children is industry versus inferiority. During this time, children strive to acquire competence and skills necessary for them to function as adults. School-age children who are positively recognized for success feel a sense of worth. Those faced with failure can feel a sense of mediocrity or unworthiness, which may result in withdrawal from school and peers.

MORAL DEVELOPMENT

The need for a moral code and social rules becomes more evident as school-age children's cognitive abilities and social experiences increase. For example, 12-year-old children are able to consider what society would be like without rules because of their ability to reason logically and their experiences with group play. They view rules as necessary principles of life, not just dictates from authorities. In the early school years, children strictly interpret and adhere to rules. As they develop, they make more flexible judgments and evaluate rules for applicability to a given situation. School-age children consider motivations and the actual behavior when making judgments about the way that their behaviors affect themselves and others. The ability to be flexible when applying rules and to take the perspective of others is essential in developing moral judgments. These abilities are present at times in earlier years but are more consistently displayed in later school years.

PEER RELATIONSHIPS

Group and personal achievements become important to the school-age child. Success is important in physical and cognitive activities. Play involves peers and the pursuit of group goals. Although solitary activities are not eliminated, they are overshadowed by group play. Learning to contribute, collaborate, and work cooperatively toward a common goal becomes a measure of success (Fig. 29-2).

The school-age child prefers same-sex peers to opposite-sex peers. This strong gender identity is evidenced by the

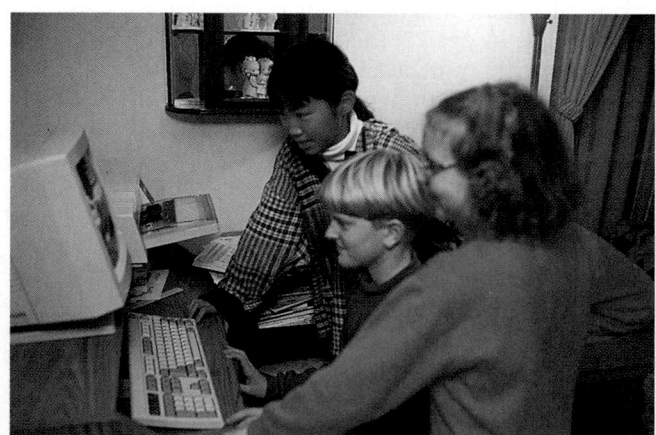

Fig. 29-2 School-age children gain a sense of achievement when playing with peers.

close network of same-sex companions that a child maintains, often referred to as the *gang*. In general, girls and boys view the opposite sex negatively. Peer influence becomes quite diverse during this stage of development. Conformity is evidenced in mannerisms, clothing styles, and speech patterns, which are reinforced and influenced by contact with peers. Group identity increases as the school-age child approaches adolescence.

SEXUAL IDENTITY

Freud described middle childhood as the *latency period* because he felt that children of this period had little interest in their sexuality (see Chapter 24). Today many researchers believe that school-agers have a great deal of interest in their sexuality. Some may engage in sex play and masturbation but hide it because of adult disapproval. Children's curiosity about adult magazines or meanings of sexually explicit words are also examples of their sexual interest.

Date _____

Child's first name _____

Child's age _____ Grade _____

Lifestyle Questionnaire for School-Age Children*

Activities that promote health	Yes	No	Sometimes
1. I sleep at least 8 hours every night.			
2. I brush my teeth twice a day.			
3. I visit the dentist every year.			
4. I watch less than 2 hours of TV every day.			
5. I exercise (running, biking, swimming, active sports) one hour every day.			
6. I eat fruits.			
7. I eat vegetables.			
8. I limit my intake of salty snacks and high-sugar snacks.			
9. I have a physical examination every 2 or 3 years.			
10. I stay away from cigarettes.			
11. I stay away from alcohol.			
Injury prevention	**Yes**	**No**	**Sometimes**
12. I wear a seat belt in an automobile.			
13. I look both ways when crossing streets.			
14. I follow bike safety rules.			
15. I stay away from lighters or matches.			
16. I never ride ATVs (all-terrain vehicles).*			
17. I wear a helmet when I go on bike trips.			
18. I swim with a buddy.			
19. I wear a life jacket when I ride in a boat.			
20. I take medicine only with my parent's permission.			
21. I stay away from real guns.			
22. I tell my parents where I am going.			
23. I say "no" to drugs.			
24. Our home has a smoke detector that works.			
25. Our home has a fire extinguisher.			
26. If there is a fire, I know a safe way out of my house.			
Feelings	**Yes**	**No**	**Sometimes**
27. I think it is okay to cry.			
28. I enjoy my family.			
29. It is easy for me to fall asleep at night.			
30. My appetite is good.			
31. I like myself just the way I am.			

*The American Academy of Pediatrics recommends that children do not ride on these vehicles.

Fig. 29-3 Lifestyle questionnaire for school-age children. *(From Antwerp CV, Spaiolo AM: MCN 16(3):144, 1991.)*

SELF-CONCEPT AND HEALTH

During the school-age years, identity and self-concept become stronger and more individualized. Perception of wellness is based on readily observable facts such as presence or absence of illness and adequacy of eating or sleeping. Functional ability is the standard by which personal health and the health of others are judged.

Antwerp and Spaniolo (1991) have developed a questionnaire that can be used as a tool to assess and promote healthy lifestyles among school-agers (Fig. 29-3). This tool increases children's and parents' awareness of activities that promote health and prevent injury. It also provides data that allow the nurse or health educator to assess the health education needs of children.

Specific Health Concerns of the School-Age Child

Accidents and injuries are a major health problem affecting school-age children. Motor vehicle accidents and accidents related to recreational activities or equipment are the leading causes of death or injury. These unintentional injuries account for nearly half of all childhood deaths.

Although falls account for a major portion of pediatric hospital admissions, they account for less than 5% of pediatric deaths resulting from injury. More children die from automobile accidents than from all major preventable childhood diseases. The rates of injury and death have begun to decrease with the institution of automobile child-restraint laws.

School-age children are also significantly affected by cancer, birth defects, homicide, and heart disease (U.S. Dept. of Health and Human Services (DHHS), 1989). In this age group, these problems have a relatively low mortality rate but a high morbidity rate compared to accidents. Infections account for nearly 80% of all childhood illnesses; respiratory infections are the most prevalent. The common cold remains the chief illness of childhood. Certain groups of children are more prone to disease and disability, often as a result of barriers to health care. Mental retardation, learning disorders, sensory impairments and malnutrition are far more prevalent among children living in poverty (U.S. DHHS, 1992). Involvement with social reform, environmental change, and the method of delivery of health care is necessary if the nurse wants to positively influence the health of children. Children's developing cognitive and psychomotor skills make it possible for them to become more involved in health promotion and the management of chronic illness.

HEALTH PROMOTION DURING THE SCHOOL-AGE PERIOD

The school-age period is a crucial period for the acquisition of behaviors and health practices for a healthy adult life. Since cognition is advancing during the period, effective health education must be developmentally appropriate. Promotion of good health practices is a nursing responsibility. Programs directed at health education are frequently organized and conducted in the school. Pender (1993) identifies the critical functions of school-based health promotion programs (see the box above).

During these programs, the nurse focuses on the development of behaviors that positively affect children's health

---

Critical Functions of School-Based Health Promotion Program

- Promote acquisition of knowledge and skills for competent self-care and informed decision making about health.
- Reinforce positive health attitudes.
- Structure environment and social influences to support health promoting behaviors.
- Facilitate growth and self-actualization.
- Sensitize students to aspects of the environment and Western culture that are detrimental to health and well-being.

Modified from Pender N: *Health promotion in nursing practice*, ed 3, Norwalk, Conn, 1993, Appleton & Lange.

---

status. Examples of topics that encourage positive behaviors by children are dental health and treatment for a cold. A comprehensive list of health-promotion topics is presented in Table 29-4.

Since accidents are the leading cause of death and injury in the school-age period, safety is a priority health teaching consideration. Nurses can contribute to the general health of children by educating them about safety measures to prevent accidents (see Table 29-4). At this age, children should be encouraged to take responsibility for their own safety.

Nurses can contribute to meeting national policy goals by promoting healthy lifestyle habits, including nutrition. School-age children should participate in educational programs that enable them to plan, select, and prepare healthy meals and snacks. These foods should be consistent with nutritional guidelines limiting fat intake to 30% of calories and saturated fat intake to less than 10% of calories (U.S. DHHS, 1992). Additionally, nurses need to promote an increase in the number of children involved in daily physical activity.

School-age children should receive age-appropriate HIV education that begins in the fourth grade (McGinnis and DeGraw, 1991). Other topic areas for elementary health education curricula that are consistent with Healthy People 2000 include tobacco and alcohol use prevention (U.S. DHHS, 1992).

Nurses also instruct parents regarding health promotion appropriate for the school-ager. Parents need to recognize the importance of annual health maintenance visits for immunizations, screenings, and dental care. When their school-ager reaches 10 years of age, parents need to begin discussions in preparation for upcoming pubertal changes. Topics should include introductory information regarding menstruation, sexual intercourse, and reproduction. Nurses should provide age-appropriate written materials to aid parents in their efforts.

The settings where health promotion activities for school-agers can occur are varied. These include the classroom, school nurse's office, school-based clinic, community-based clinic, or in the community itself.

▌ PREADOLESCENT

Today's children experience more emotional and social pressures than youngsters 30 years ago. As a result, children

Table 29-4	Health Promotion in the School-Age Period

SCHOOL-AGE HEALTH CONCERNS	HEALTH PROMOTION INTERVENTIONS
Unintentional injuries	Teach injury prevention-use of safety belts, smoke detectors, bicycle helmets
	Teach basic street safety principles—crossing the street, obeying traffic lights, safe bicycling in traffic
	Teach swimming and boating safety; basic life saving, CPR, use of life vests
	Encourage parents to teach children how to react in case of fire and review appropriate escape route
	Encourage parents to have smoke detectors in the home that are in working order
	Ensure that sporting and playground equipment meet safety standards
	Orient children to the use of any new equipment
	Teach children the importance of wearing appropriate protective equipment when involved in sporting activities
	Encourage parents to evaluate safety of fireworks, BB guns, air rifles; provide adult supervision for use
Nutrition	Provide nutrition education that promotes healthy lifestyle:
	Food Guide Pyramid; limiting fat intake to 30% of calories, saturated fat to 10% of calories
Oral hygiene	Provide examples of low cariogenic snacks
	Review mechanics of dental hygiene: brushing, flossing
	Stress importance of biannual dental check-ups
Infections	Provide immunization information and follow-up
	Teach infection prevention practices (handwashing, care of minor skin injuries)
	Teach concepts of viral and bacterial illness
Tobacco, alcohol, and drug use	Provide tobacco use prevention programs
	Provide information regarding the hazards of drug use
Human sexuality	Provide information about sexual maturation and reproduction in age-appropriate manner
	Encourage parents to view their child's sexual curiosity as part of the developmental process
	Discuss with parents the learning needs of their child regarding sexuality
	Provide age-appropriate HIV education

10 to 12 years old are now having experiences that were once unique to 13- and 14-year-old youths. This transitional period between childhood and adolescence is often referred to as **preadolescence** by professionals in behavioral science. Others have referred to this period as *late childhood, early adolescence, and pubescence.* Physically it refers to the beginning of the second skeletal growth spurt, when physical changes such as the development of pubic hair and female breasts begin. These physical changes that announce the approach of puberty begin about 2 years earlier in girls than boys. In addition, children become much more social, and their behavioral patterns become much less predictable. This preparatory period often includes experimentation with makeup by girls and an interest in music and performers that are popular among older adolescents. Both sexes usually develop "best friends" with whom they share intimate feelings. New interest in the opposite sex develops, but little activity other than talk usually occurs. Youths of both sexes often develop a friendship with adults other than their parents (ego ideal), which allows them to acquire information about grown-ups.

ADOLESCENT

Adolescence is the period of development during which the individual makes the transition from childhood to adulthood, usually between 13 and 20 years. The term *adolescent* usually refers to psychological maturation of the individual, whereas *puberty* refers to the point at which reproduction becomes possible. The hormonal changes of puberty result in changes in the appearance of the young person, and mental development results in the ability to hypothesize and deal with abstractions. Adjustments and adaptations are needed to cope with these simultaneous changes and the attempt to establish a mature sense of identity. In the past, many have referred to adolescence as a stormy and stressful period filled with inner turmoil, but today it is recognized that most teenagers successfully meet the challenges of this period. Adaptations required push the adolescent to develop coping mechanisms and styles of behavior that will be used or adapted throughout life. These challenges may cause the adolescent to be moody and difficult.

The nurse's understanding of development provides a unique perspective for helping teenagers and parents anticipate and cope with the stresses of adolescence. Nursing activities, particularly education, can promote healthy development. These activities occur in a variety of settings and can be directed at the adolescent, parents, or both. For example, the nurse can conduct seminars in a high school to provide practical suggestions for solving problems of concern to a large group of students, such as treating acne or making responsible decisions about drugs or alcohol use. Similarly, a group education program for parents about how to cope with teenagers would promote parental understanding of adolescent development. These programs can be held in the school, clinic, private office, or community center. To learn more about specific topics or problems, the nurse must identify teenagers' needs and desires. Involvement produces more active, interested learners.

Physical Changes and Sexual Maturation

Physical changes occur rapidly in adolescence. Sexual maturation occurs with the development of primary and secondary sexual characteristics. Primary characteristics are physical and hormonal changes necessary for reproduction, and secondary characteristics externally differentiate males from females. Four main focuses of the physical changes are:

1. Increased growth rate of skeleton, muscle, and viscera
2. Sex-specific changes, such as changes in shoulder and hip width
3. Alteration in distribution of muscle and fat
4. Development of the reproductive system and secondary sex characteristics

Wide variation exists in the timing of physical changes associated with puberty, and girls tend to begin their physical changes earlier than boys. Cultural variations exist in rapidity of growth. For example, African American youths obtain a greater proportion of their adult stature earlier.

WEIGHT AND SKELETAL CHANGES

Height and weight increases usually occur during the prepubertal growth spurt. The growth spurt for girls generally begins between 8 and 14 years of age. Height increases 2 to 8 inches, and weight increases by 15 to 55 lb. The male growth spurt usually takes place between 10 and 16 years of age. Height increases approximately 4 to 12 inches, and weight increases by 15 to 65 lb.

Girls attain 90% to 95% of their adult height by **menarche** (the onset of menstruation) and reach their full height

by 16 to 17 years of age, whereas boys continue to grow taller until 18 to 20 years of age. Fat is redistributed into adult proportions as height and weight increase, and gradually the adolescent torso takes on an adult appearance.

Although there are individual and sex differences, growth follows a similar pattern for both sexes. Growth in the length of the extremities occurs earliest, making the hands and feet appear very large and the legs very long; the individual often appears awkward and clumsy. At the same time the lower jaw and nose become longer and the forehead higher and wider as the baby face of childhood disappears. Next the thighs widen; then the shoulders broaden, and growth of the trunk proceeds. Widening of the female hips and broadening of the male shoulders continue throughout adolescence.

Personal growth curves help the nurse assess physical development. The individual's sustained progression along the curve, however, is more important than a comparison to the norm. The nurse charts growth measurements during routine health assessments to evaluate changes.

EFFECTS OF PHYSICAL CHANGES ON PEER INTERACTION

Adolescents are sensitive about physical changes that make them different from peers. For this reason they are generally interested in the normal pattern of growth and their personal growth curves. Consequently, the nurse should share this information to reassure adolescents that their own patterns are normal.

The number of eating disorders is on the rise in adolescent girls, and knowledge of growth progression may be a way to discourage radical weight-reduction activities. If an adolescent deviates radically from the usual pattern, further assessment is necessary to identify the cause. Weight extremes resulting from excessive or inadequate caloric intake

Table 29-5	Average Sequence of Physiological Changes in Adolescence		
CHARACTERISTICS		**GIRLS***	**BOYS***
Beginning of skeletal growth spurt		8-14½ (peak: 12)	10½-16 (peak: 14)
Beginning of breast development		8-13	
Enlargement of testes and scrotal sac			10-13½
Appearance of straight, pigmented pubic hair, which gradually becomes curly		8-14	10-15
Early voice changes (cracks)			11-14½
Enlargement of penis and prostate gland			11-14½
Menarche		10-18 (average: 12¼)	
Spermatogenesis (ejaculation of sperm)			11-17 (average: 13½)
Ovulation and completion of breast development		14-18 (average: 15½)	
Appearance of downy facial hair			12-17
Appearance of axillary (underarm) hair and increased output of oil and sweat-producing glands, which may lead to acne		10-16	12-17
Widening and deepening of female pelvis, with deposition of subcutaneous fat that gives rounded appearance to body		10-18	
Increase in shoulder width			11-21
Deepening of voice in males, with appearance of coarse and pigmented facial hair and appearance of chest hair			16-21

*Age range is in years.

are common during the adolescent years. Allowing the adolescent to see when and how the weight curve changed can be a first step in identifying the problem and implementing dietary changes.

PUBERTY

Timing. Wide variation exists between the sexes and within the same sex as to when the physical changes of **puberty** begin. This variation is more pronounced in boys.

Boys who mature early have been shown by some research to be more poised, relaxed, good-natured, skilled in athletic activities, and more likely to be school leaders than boys who mature late. In contrast, girls who mature early have been found to be less sociable and more shy and introverted, perhaps from feeling so conspicuous (Edelman and Mandle, 1994).

Sequence. The sequence of pubertal growth changes is the same in most individuals (Table 29-5). The ranges of *normal* are stressed. As with increases in height and weight, the pattern of sexual changes is more significant than their time of onset. Large deviations from normal frames require investigation. Being like peers is extremely important for adolescents (Fig. 29-4). Any deviation in the timing of the physical changes can be extremely difficult for them to accept. The nurse should therefore provide emotional support for adolescents undergoing assessment of early or delayed puberty. Even adolescents whose physical changes are

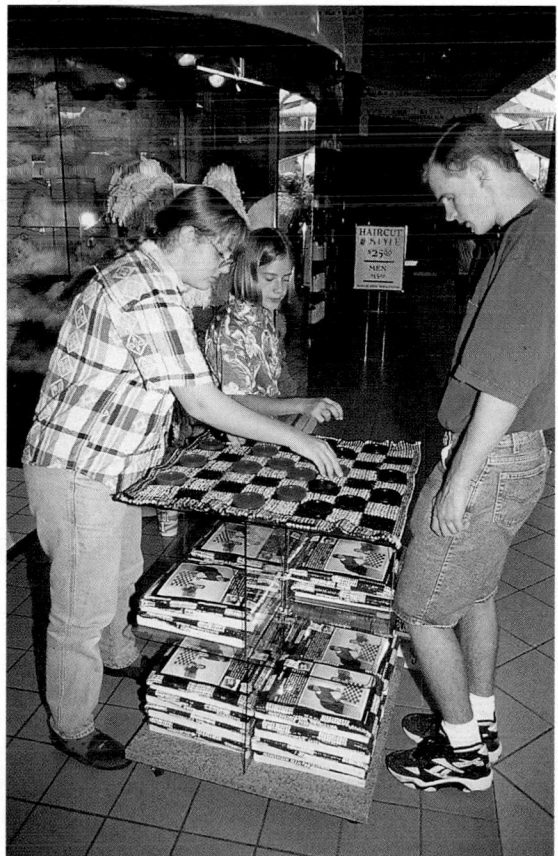

Fig. 29-4 Interacting with peers aids to increase self-esteem during puberty.

occurring at the normal times may seek confirmation of and reassurance about their normalcy.

Hormonal Changes. Visible and invisible changes take place during puberty. All of these changes are created by hormonal changes within the body when the hypothalamus begins to produce gonadotropin-releasing hormones, which signal the pituitary to secrete gonadotropic hormones. Gonadotropic hormones stimulate ovarian cells to produce **estrogen** and testicular cells to produce **testosterone.** These hormones contribute to the development of secondary sex characteristics such as hair growth and voice changes and play an essential role in reproduction. The changing concentrations of these hormones are also linked to acne and body odor. Understanding these hormonal changes enables the nurse to reassure adolescents and educate them about body care needs.

Cognitive Development

Changes that occur within the mind and the widening social environment of the adolescent result in formal operations, the highest level of intellectual development, according to Piaget (see Chapter 28). Without an appropriate educational environment, young persons who possess sufficient neurological development to reach this stage may not attain it and those who are guided toward rational thinking may reach this stage early.

The adolescent develops the ability to solve problems through logical operations. The teenager can think abstractly and deal effectively with hypothetical problems. When confronted with a problem, the teenager can consider an infinite variety of causes and solutions. For the first time the young person can move beyond the physical or concrete properties of a situation and use reasoning powers to understand the abstract. School-agers think about what is, whereas adolescents can imagine what might be. These newly developed abilities allow the individual to have more insight and skill in playing games such as checkers and *Clue* and to learn new board or computer games that require abstract thinking and deductive reasoning about many possible strategies. A teenager can even solve problems requiring simultaneous manipulation of several abstract concepts. Development of this ability is important in the pursuit of an identity. For example, newly acquired cognitive skills allow the teenager to define appropriate, effective, and comfortable sex-role behaviors and to consider their impact on peers, family, and society. The ability to think logically about these behaviors and their outcomes encourages the adolescent to develop personal thoughts and means of expressing sexual identity. In addition, a higher level of cognitive functioning makes the adolescent receptive to more detailed and diverse information about sexuality and sexual behaviors. For example, sex education can include an explanation of physiological sexual changes and birth control measures.

By mid-adolescence there is an introspective quality emerging with regard to cognition. At this time adolescents believe an "imaginary audience" (Elkind, 1984) provides them with an evaluative means and a sense of being unique. This concept may account for some typical adolescent behaviors, including self-consciousness and the desire for privacy.

Elkind (1984) also describes another characteristic of cognitive function, the personal fable. This is a story created by the adolescent that is not true. This concept may account for many undesirable risk-taking behaviors, since the adolescent believes he or she is immune from negative consequences.

The complex development of thought during this period leads adolescents to question society and its values. Although adolescents have the capability to think as well as an adult, they do not have experiences on which to build. It is common for teenagers to consider their parents too narrow minded or too materialistic. Cognitive abilities and performance vary greatly among adolescents. In fact, an adolescent may perform at different levels in different situations based on their past experiences, formal education, and motivation in the use of logic and effective deductive reasoning.

LANGUAGE SKILLS

Language development is fairly complete by adolescence, although vocabulary continues to expand. The primary focus becomes communication skills that can be used effectively in various situations. Adolescents need to communicate thoughts, feelings, and facts to peers, parents, teachers, and other persons of authority. The skills used in these diverse communication situations are varied. Adolescents must select the person with whom to communicate, decide on the exact message, and choose the way to transmit the message. For example, the way teenagers tell parents about failing grades is not the same as the way that they tell friends. Adolescents develop different skills and styles of communication and learn how and when to use them most effectively. These diverse communication skills are used and refined throughout life. Good communication skills are critical so that adolescents can overcome peer pressures to participate in nonhealthy behaviors.

Psychosocial Development

The search for personal identity is the major task of adolescent psychosocial development. Teenagers must establish close peer relationships or remain socially isolated. Erikson sees identity (or role) confusion as the prime danger of this stage and suggests that the cliquishness and intolerance of differences seen in adolescent behavior are defenses against identity confusion (Erikson, 1968). Adolescents work at becoming emotionally independent from their parents, while retaining family ties. In addition, they need to develop their own ethical systems based on personal values. Choices about vocation, future education, and lifestyle must be made. The various components of total identity evolve from these tasks and comprise an adult personal identity that is unique to the individual.

Behaviors indicating negative resolution of the developmental task for this age are indecisiveness and the inability to make an occupational choice.

SEXUAL IDENTITY

Achievement of sexual identity is enhanced by the physical changes of puberty. In Freud's view, these physiological changes of puberty reactivate the libido, the energy source that fuels the sex drive (see Chapter 24). This is evidenced by the teenager's interest in heterosexual relationships with partners outside of the family and the practice of mastur-

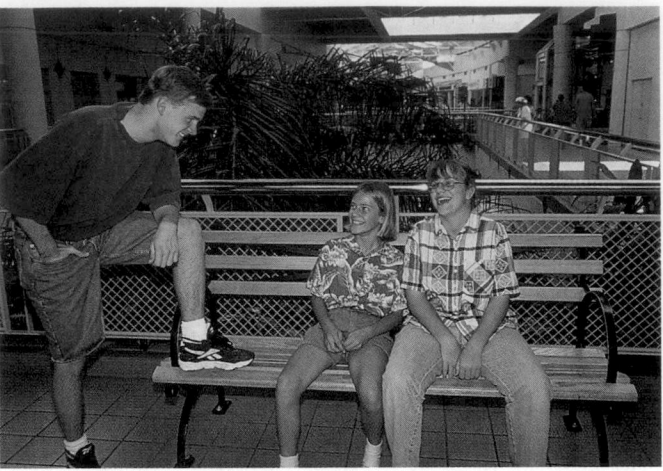

Fig. 29-5 Adolescents acquire sexual identity during social interactions.

bation. The physical evidence of maturity encourages the development of masculine and feminine behaviors. If these physical changes involve deviations, the person has more difficulty developing a comfortable sexual identity. Adolescents depend on these physical clues because they want assurance of maleness or femaleness and because they do not wish to be different from peers (Fig. 29-5). Without these physical characteristics, achieving sexual identity is difficult. Other influences are cultural attitudes and expectations of sex-role behavior and available role models. The masculine and feminine behaviors that teenagers see affect the way that they express sexuality. Adolescents master age-appropriate sexuality after feeling comfortable with sexual behaviors, choices, and relationships.

GROUP IDENTITY

Adolescents seek a group identity because they need esteem and acceptance. Similarity in dress or speech is common in teenage groups. Popularity is a major concern. Trends in the desire for popularity have not changed much in recent years. Girls of middle-class status, more than any other group, regard popularity as particularly important. Peer groups provide the adolescent with a sense of belonging, approval, and the opportunity to learn acceptable behavior. Popularity with opposite-sex and same-sex peers is important. The strong need for group identity seems to conflict at times with the search for personal identity. It is as though adolescents require close bonds with peers so that they can later redefine themselves against this group identity.

FAMILY IDENTITY

The movement toward stronger peer relationships is contrasted with adolescents' movements away from parents. Although financial independence for adolescents is not the norm in American society, many adolescents work part-time, using their income to bolster independence. When adolescents cannot have a part-time job because of studies, school-related activities, and other factors, parents can provide allowances for clothing and incidentals, which encourage adolescents to develop decision-making and budgeting skills.

Some adolescents and families have more difficulty during these years than others. Adolescents need to make choices, act independently, and experience the consequences of actions. This testing, however, is best done against a firm, supportive, family foundation. The family needs to allow independence while providing a haven in which adolescents can contemplate actions. Families unable to provide this support complicate movement toward identity formation. Support to the family and adolescent may be essential to their success.

Nurses can assist families to consider ways that are appropriate for them to foster the independence of their adolescent while maintaining family structure. Many of these discussions often involve curfews, jobs, and participation in family chores. Emancipation from the immediate family is most successful when accomplished gradually, resulting in separation from the family and family ties that last a lifetime.

VOCATIONAL IDENTITY

The selection of an occupation or a vocational direction in life provides a goal for adolescents. Because of society's changing needs, adolescents must be future oriented when making these choices. However, adolescents do not know which jobs will be available or which jobs will be rewarding 10 or 20 years in the future, so selecting a career is a complicated task. The nurse should provide emotional support during this process and should help adolescent clients select courses of action that promote self-satisfaction, identity, and continued opportunity for growth.

HEALTH IDENTITY

Another component of personal identity is perception of health. This component is of specific interest to health care providers. Healthy adolescents evaluate their own health according to feelings of well-being, ability to function normally, and absence of symptoms.

Research indicates that adolescents participate in health-related self-care practices (see the box at right). Interventions to improve health perception might, therefore, concentrate on the adolescent period. The rapid changes during this period make health promotion programs especially crucial. Adolescents try new roles, begin to stabilize their identity, and acquire values and behaviors from which their adult lifestyle will evolve.

MORAL IDENTITY

The development of moral judgment depends heavily on cognitive and communication skills and peer interaction. Although moral development begins in early childhood, it is consolidated in adolescence because of the presence of certain skills. Adolescents learn to understand that rules are cooperative agreements that can be modified to fit the situation, rather than absolutes. Regarding rules, adolescents learn to use their own judgments rather than use the rules to avoid punishment as in earlier years.

Kohlberg (1964) explains moral development in terms of stages (see Chapter 9). At the highest level, morality is derived from individual principles of conscience. Adolescents judge themselves by internalized ideals, which often leads to conflict between personal and group values. Group values become less significant in later adolescence.

RESEARCH HIGHLIGHT

RESEARCH ABSTRACT

A study based on Orem's Self-Care Model was conducted to determine health care practices of the healthy adolescent and to identify the relationship between self-concept and health-related practices in adolescents. The study examined self-concept and conditioning factors, such as age, gender, and sociocultural characteristics. The sample included 160 15- and 16-year-olds.

The Information Profile sought information relative to basic conditioning factors: age, gender, developmental status, health state, family and sociocultural characteristics. Sociocultural characteristics were assessed by responses to questions regarding educational level of parents, race, etc. The Self-Concept Scale was used to evaluate how subjects felt about themselves. The Denyes Self-Care Practice Instrument (DSCPI) measured self-care action and self-care requisites of adolescents. Results were consistent with the theoretical proposition of a link between self-concept and self-care. Sociocultural influences of race and religion were found to be important predictors of self-care agency and self-care practices of the individual. These results suggested adolescents are engaging in self-care practices.

IMPLICATIONS FOR PRACTICE

▶ Health promotion and prevention of disease should be the key to adolescent health care (see Table 29-6).
▶ Knowledge of adolescent health care practices should be incorporated into appropriate educational programs.
▶ Health care programs should be provided that enhance the adolescents' self-concept within school, church, and community settings.
▶ Nurses working in schools, clinics, and the community should consider cultural and religious factors when assessing self-care activities and health behaviors in the adolescent client.

REFERENCE

McCaleb A, Edgil A: Self-concept and self-care practices of healthy adolescents, *J Pediatr Nurs* 9(4):233, 1994.

Not all adolescents attain the same level of moral development. There is, however, a general forward movement through the stages of moral development, and the sequence of the stages is similar for all individuals even when their time of achievement varies.

PSYCHOSOCIAL MORATORIUM

According to Erikson (1968), adolescence provides a "time-out period" when society allows the physically mature teenager to delay the assumption of adult responsibilities. This is time for youth to try a variety of ideological and vocational roles before making a commitment. This **psychosocial moratorium** ends in the selection of values and a consolidation of identity.

Specific Health Concerns of the Adolescent Period

Accidents remain the leading cause of death in adolescence (about 70%). Motor vehicle accidents, which are the most common cause of death, result in almost half the fatalities of 16- to 19-year-olds (Edelman and Mandel, 1994). Such accidents are often associated with alcohol intoxication or drug abuse. Other frequent causes of accidental death in teenagers are drowning and firearms. Feelings of being indestructible lead to risk-taking behavior.

Substance abuse is in fact a major concern to those who work with adolescents. Adolescents may believe that mood-altering substances create a sense of well-being or improve level of performance. All adolescents are at risk for experimental or recreational substance use, but those who have unconventional values or come from unstable homes are more at risk for chronic use and physical dependency. Some adolescents believe that substance use makes them more mature.

Suicide is the third leading cause of death in adolescents between 15 and 24 years of age (Hawton, 1990); accidents and homicide are the leading causes. Depression and social isolation commonly precede a suicide attempt, but suicide probably results from a combination of several factors. Nurses should be alert to the following warning signs, which often occur for at least a month before suicide is attempted (Mattsson, 1992):

1. Decrease in school performance
2. Withdrawal
3. Loss of initiative
4. Loneliness, sadness, and crying
5. Appetite and sleep disturbances
6. Verbalization of suicidal thoughts

Immediate referrals to mental health professionals need to be made when assessment suggests that adolescents may be considering suicide. Guidance can help them focus on the positive aspects of life and strengthen coping abilities.

Another area of concern is the formation of healthy habits of daily living. Emphasis on exercise, sleep, nutrition, and stress-reduction habits is increasing. The nurse must recognize the importance of these habits and identify ways to adapt them to each adolescent. To do this the nurse must assess the individual's positive and negative habits and attitudes about health. Accidents and the formation of healthy habits have psychological and physical components and effects. Extensive and long-term follow-up is required if individualized interventions are to succeed. The nurse needs to be aware of the prevalence of these problems and make assessments accordingly.

Sexual experimentation is common among adolescents. Peer pressure, physiological and emotional changes, and societal expectations contribute to early heterosexual and homosexual relations. According to the Centers for Disease Control and Prevention (1993), 54% of adolescents between grades nine and twelve have admitted to having sexual intercourse at least once. The degree of sexual activity among teenagers may not change significantly, but the degree of informed, consenting participation can. Data from the Centers for Disease Control and Prevention (1991) indicate that 22% of teenagers report having sexual relations with at least four partners. Two prominent consequences of adolescent sexual activity are sexually transmitted disease and pregnancy.

Sexually transmitted disease (STD) annually afflicts around 10 million persons under the age of 25 years. This high degree of incidence makes it imperative that sexually active adolescents be screened for STDs, even when they have no symptoms (see Chapter 24). The annual physical examination of a sexually active adolescent should include careful examination of the genitalia so that condylomata acuminata (genital warts), herpes, *Phthirus pubis* (crab lice), primary syphilitic chancres, and other STDs are not missed. Recommended tests for women include Papanicolaou (Pap) smears, cervical cultures for gonorrhea and *Chlamydia* species, and syphilis tests; for men, urethral cultures for gonorrhea and *Chlamydia* species and syphilis tests are recommended. If men have participated in homosexual activities, rectal and pharyngeal cultures also need to be taken to check for gonorrhea.

The human immunodeficiency virus (HIV), which causes AIDS, is transmitted through unprotected sexual intercourse, the use of shared needles, and through infected blood products. Therefore, the risk-taking behaviors of adolescent sexual activity and drug use make adolescents vulnerable to the threat of AIDS. Approximately 30,000 HIV-infected adolescents live in the United States today; AIDS is the sixth leading cause of death among individuals between 15 and 24 years of age (CDC, 1994). Adolescents who have placed themselves at risk for AIDS should be tested for HIV.

Adolescent pregnancy is a common occurrence in the United States; 1 of every 10 women under the age of 20 years gets pregnant, and many choose to keep their babies. Pregnancy does not pose a physical risk to teenage mothers unless they are under 16 years of age or do not receive thorough prenatal care.

HEALTH PROMOTION DURING THE ADOLESCENT PERIOD

Community and school-based health programs for adolescents are focused on health promotion and illness prevention. Nurses are involved in community health through screening and teaching programs. Through their efforts in the school and community, nurses can make a contribution in meeting the Healthy People 2000 Objectives (U.S. DHHS, 1992). Appropriate topics for adolescents are listed in Table 29-6.

The services provided to adolescents must be easily accessed and confidential. Nelson (1995) finds that in order for adolescents to reveal intimate information about their risk-taking behaviors, they must first feel comfortable and respected as individuals.

Nurses can play an important role in preventing accidental deaths by supporting organizations that promote responsible behavior, including Mothers Against Drunk Driving (MADD) and Drug Abuse Resistance Education (DARE), and encouraging students to participate in Students Against Drunk Driving (SADD). Stimulating adolescents to discuss alternatives to driving when under the influence of drugs or alcohol prepares them to consider alternatives when such an occasion arises.

The nurse must identify those adolescents at risk for abuse, provide education to prevent accidents related to substance abuse, and provide counseling to those in rehabilitation.

The nurse must provide sex education and counseling. Nurses play a key role in counseling teenagers on ways to avoid pregnancies. After pregnancy has occurred, the nurse can assist them in obtaining thorough medical care and de-

Table 29-6	Health Promotion During the Adolescent Period

ADOLESCENT HEALTH CONCERNS	HEALTH PROMOTION INTERVENTION
Unintentional injuries	Advise adolescent to take driver's education course and to wear seat belts
	Inform the adolescent of risk associated with drinking and driving; use of drugs
	Promote helmet use by adolescent bicyclists and motorcyclists
	Ensure adolescent receives proper orientation to the use of all sports equipment
	Encourage adolescent to swim with a "buddy"
Firearm use and violence	Teach conflict resolution skills
Tobacco, alcohol, and drug use	Screen for tobacco (including smokeless), alcohol, and drug use and inform of the risks of use
Suicide	Offer suicide information
	Teach methods to deal with a suicidal peer
	Promote suicide alternatives
Sexually transmitted diseases	Provide adolescent with information regarding disease, mode of transmission, and related symptoms
	Encourage abstinence from sexual activity; or if sexually active, the use of condoms
	Provide accurate information about the consequences of sexual activity

veloping skills that will enhance their infants' development.

Extensive educational efforts to prevent the spread of AIDS and other STDs in this age group are a nursing responsibility.

Health Promotion: Minority Adolescents. An examination of 1990 census figures indicates that demographic changes are taking place in the nation. According to the U.S. Department of Commerce (1992), minority groups make up approximately 20% of the U.S. population. By the next century, it is expected that minorities as a group will become the majority. Minority adolescents have been identified as experiencing a greater percentage of health problems and barriers to health care.

Issues of concern for these adolescents living in a high-risk environment include learning or emotional difficulties, death related to violence, unintentional injuries, increased rate for adolescent pregnancy, STDs, and AIDS.

Poverty is a major factor negatively affecting the lives of minority adolescents. Limited access to health services is common. Nurses can make a significant contribution to improving access to appropriate health care for adolescents.

Nurses must be able to identify effective coping strategies that enable minority adolescents to overcome stresses inherent in their environment (Ryan-Wenger and Copeland, 1994). Health promotion initiatives must be based on topics of concern for these adolescents.

Nurses working in the community must adopt culturally sensitive interventions to meet the needs of minority adolescents and their families (Spector, 1991). They must be able to communicate in another language by speaking it or using an interpreter. Teaching materials need to be written in the appropriate language. Information regarding health beliefs and healing practices must be assessed.

With knowledge about various cultures and the means to care for minority adolescents, the nurse acts as an advocate to ensure accessibility of appropriate services.

NURSING PROCESS

The nursing process can be readily applied to the care of children, regardless of age. To illustrate the use of the nurs-

ing process in organizing and documenting the care of children and adolescents, an example will be provided from the case of a 14-year-old female with poor dietary practices and complaints of low energy level and frequent infections. She is being seen in a community health clinic setting.

CASE STUDY In the sample care plan, the 14-year-old female has a history of missed clinic appointments. Her past medical history reveals that she was treated for iron deficiency anemia as a toddler.

She weighs 128 pounds and is 62 inches tall. Her present history indicates that she eats breakfast once per week, has lunch in the school cafeteria "if she has the money," and prefers to eat at fast food restaurants for dinner. She rarely exercises and does not participate in sports activities. She expresses a concern that she often "overeats" during periods of stress. She smokes one-half a package of cigarettes per day. ■

 Assessment

Nursing assessment of the school-age child and adolescent includes developmental level, response to care, history of prior health care, medical history, and available support persons. Assessment provides information about the ability of the child to understand, cooperate with, and assume limited responsibility for immediate and long-term care. It focuses on cognitive, motor, and psychosocial abilities and limitations. In a primary care setting, cognitive and psychosocial information might initially be assessed directly from the adolescent, as well as from the parent. Motor abilities can be assessed by observing the adolescent unbuttoning a coat or removing pieces of clothing in preparation for the physical examination. Cognitive assessment might be based on the report of school grades, favorite activities, ability to describe the onset of illness, and responses to questions from parents and health care providers. A history of prior health care improves the nurse's understanding of the adolescent's response to current care.

The nurse needs to obtain a detailed diet history in order to determine adequacy of caloric intake. In addition, the nurse will focus the history to determine whether the adolescent recently experienced any weight or appetite changes and dietary problems. Other relevant information includes the adolescent's physical activity level, the size and number of her usual meals, as well as snacking patterns. Data about food preferences or allergies are obtained.

The nurse must determine a true picture of the adolescent's perspectives on her health status in order to plan health-promotion activities. The use of a health-risk appraisal, lifestyle assessment, and a stress assessment tool will assist in this process.

Data about the availability of supportive significant others and the adolescent's ability to use this support are critical. For instance, the verbal and nonverbal interaction between the client and her parent during the history may indicate the type of parent-daughter relationship and degree of closeness that exists. This information guides the selection of strategies that can maximize the support that this parent can offer. Sharing these observations with the parents can lessen their feelings of helplessness, which are related to the adolescent's ability to participate in her plan of care. It is also useful to identify the internal supports that the child believes are effective. For example, the adolescent might find exercising with friends or listening to favorite music helpful. School-age children and adolescents can often be helped to identify their internal support systems and taught to use them at appropriate times.

Data must also be collected to establish factors that are contributing to the adolescent's present condition, including the presence of personal crises or stressors, lack of financial resources, and peer pressure.

Nursing Diagnosis

The nursing diagnoses box at right lists examples of potentially relevant nursing diagnoses for the adolescent client. Any or all of the nursing diagnoses may be applicable to a youth in a variety of settings. The diagnostic process box below selects one of these diagnoses, states related factors, and gives examples of pertinent assessment activities and defining characteristics. Altered health maintenance represents a primary diagnosis for

Examples of NANDA Nursing Diagnoses for Promoting Health in an Adolescent

Risk for injury *related to:*
- Lifestyle choices
- Alcohol, tobacco, or drug use
- Participation in athletic competition, or recreational activities
- Sexual activity

Risk for infection *related to:*
- Sexual activity
- Malnutrition
- Impaired immunity

Altered health maintenance *related to:*
- Lack of adequate nutrients to support growth
- Skipping meals; food faddism
- Fast-food intake, use of convenience foods or vending machines
- Poverty
- Effects of alcohol or drug use

Knowledge deficit *related to:*
- Inexperience with unfamiliar recreational equipment
- Lack of information in school-related curriculum

Body image disturbance *related to:*
- Negative feelings about body
- Maturational changes associated with adolescent growth spurt

the adolescent in this case study. No one exhibits all of the possible defining characteristics for any particular nursing diagnosis but instead displays a combination of the defining characteristics.

Planning

The nursing care plan demonstrates further application of the nursing process for altered health maintenance and provides goals with related nursing interventions and expected outcomes. Their focus and content clearly relate them to the nursing diagnostic statement.

Sample Nursing Diagnostic Process for an Adolescent

ASSESSMENT ACTIVITIES	DEFINING CHARACTERISTICS	NURSING DIAGNOSIS
Weigh and measure the adolescent; obtain anthropometric measurements Assess body frame size Assess typical 24-hour dietary pattern Assess contributing factors: Stress Assessment Tool	Weight above the ideal standard for frame size Low energy level Food fads Strong peer influence Smoking Lack of physical exercise Easy fatigability	**Altered Health Maintenance** related to increased food consumption associated with stress and inadequate physical exercise for age

This plan is based on the nurse's prior knowledge of nursing care, physiology, pathophysiology, human development, and the assessment of the adolescent and family. Health maintenance activities are essential to the quality of the adolescents' life in the future. Thus the nurse plans interventions to increase adolescents' knowledge of sound nutritional principles, the importance of physical activity, and the benefits of smoking cessation (see the care plan below).

The planning phase must directly involve the adolescent and her parent in goal setting. This will ensure their willingness to carry out the activities planned for increasing awareness of nutrition principles and healthy lifestyle habits. The nurse must determine readiness and motivation on the part of the adolescent and her parent before proceeding. In addition, the nurse must determine whether the adolescent's goals are realistic and measurable.

Planning must also show consideration for social and psychological nursing problems that accompany physical nursing problems. An example of a psychosocial nursing problem in the sample scenario is ineffective individual coping. When planning care, the nurse structures the care plan to address inadequate coping strategies utilized. Therefore, efforts must be initiated to strengthen support systems and undertake activities to increase problem-solving ability.

A knowledge deficit may exist with the adolescent in the current situation. Planning often needs to include information that is developmentally appropriate; for example, the adolescent needs to obtain the caloric requirements for her

Sample Nursing Care Plan for Altered Health Maintenance

NURSING DIAGNOSIS: **Altered health maintenance** related to increased food consumption associated with stress and inadequate physical exercise for age

DEFINITION: A state in which the individual is unable to identify, manage, and/or seek out help to maintain health (Kim, McFarland, and McLane, 1995)

GOALS	EXPECTED OUTCOMES	INTERVENTIONS	RATIONALE
Adolescent will maintain weight within 10% of ideal standard within 6 months	Decreases daily caloric intake by 10% within 1 week Consumes a well-balanced diet: 2200-2400 calories; 50-60 g protein, 3 g calcium, 400 units vitamin D Describes Food Guide Pyramid and appropriate nutritional guidelines Describes the long-term effects of tobacco use	Assist menu selection for three meals and snacks that reflect decreased dietary fat intake to an average of 30% of calories or less and average saturated fat intake to less than 10% of calories Encourage adolescent to dine with family in a relaxed atmosphere Review the nutritional requirements with the adolescent and family including the Food Guide Pyramid (USDA, 1992) Recommend foods high in calcium and iron such as: cheeseburger, orange juice fortified with calcium	Inadequate income serves as barrier to food procurement (Wong, 1995) Current nutritional principles consistent with Healthy People 2000 Objectives (U.S. DHHS, 1992) Aids in mealtime pleasure; promotes optimal environment for nutritional health Increased caloric and nutrient needs are related to rapid physical growth and sexual maturation of this age Calcium needs are high in children, due to increase in skeletal mass; iron losses evident in adolescent girls are associated with menstruation (Dwyer, 1993)
Adolescent will seek appropriate help as needed to maintain health within 6 months	Identifies stressors and effective coping methods within 1 month Participates in exercise or recreational activity within 2 weeks	Encourage the adolescent to participate in preferred exercise or recreational activity: plan daily walking program schedule 3-5 times per week for minimum of 20 min Inform the adolescent about school and community resources supportive of health care practices Discuss the benefits of quitting tobacco use including increased stamina, decreased potential for addiction and improved breath and teeth	Nutrient metabolism and utilization are enhanced by activity Establishes lifelong habit to ensure cardiovascular function, weight maintenance at appropriate levels, and flexibility (Dwyer, 1993) Provides reinforcement of healthy lifestyle practices Smoking linked to disease

Sample Evaluation of Interventions for an Adolescent With Altered Health Maintenance

GOALS	EVALUATIVE MEASURES	EXPECTED OUTCOMES
Adolescent will maintain weight within 10% of ideal standard within 6 months	Weigh adolescent on a monthly basis and compare to ideal standard for frame	Decreases caloric intake by 10% Consumes a well-balanced diet: 2200-2400 calories; 50-60 g protein; 3 g calcium; 40 units vitamin D Describes Food Guide Pyramid and appropriate nutritional guidelines
Adolescent will seek appropriate help, as needed, to maintain health within 6 months	Evaluate presence of effective coping strategies; adolescent reports decreased episodes of overeating; adolescent states positive aspects of appearance	Identifies stressors and effective coping methods Participates in exercise or recreational activity

age and sex. She needs to understand the importance of dietary calcium to the adolescent who is increasing skeletal mass during this period.

Implementation

Implementation of the care plan must be highly individualized. In the sample care plan for the adolescent with altered health maintenance activities, the nurse must carry out activities to correct any nutrition misinformation, to emphasize the role of physical activity and risks of cigarette smoking. These activities may directly serve to contribute to the improvement of another nursing diagnosis, risk for infection, which is listed in the diagnosis box. The primary-care setting is directly involved not only in the screening of individuals for disease states, but also in the support and education of the family to promote adaptive coping and effective health management.

The nurse should serve as a model for health promotion. In order to do so, the nurse needs to develop an individual plan for a healthy lifestyle and follow through with health promotion strategies. This may serve to sensitize the nurse

to the difficulties encountered with behavior changes. Clients are more likely to work effectively with a nurse who has had first-hand experience with changing to a more healthy lifestyle.

Evaluation

The nursing process is incomplete unless a continuing evaluation is performed as a basis for revision of the care plan. The evaluation box above suggests evaluative measures and expected outcomes that the nurse can use to determine the success of the interventions. In this case, the effectiveness of the nursing interventions is indicated by the adolescent's maintenance of her ideal weight and her participation in health maintenance activities. If these expected outcomes are not attained, the nurse modifies the care plan. It may be appropriate to consult with the dietician regarding the planning of nutritionally sound meals and snacks. Further teaching regarding the importance of eating meals with the family might be necessary to gain the adolescent's cooperation. New interventions are often developed as a response to the evaluative process.

■ KEY CONCEPTS ■

► The major psychosocial developmental task of the school-age child is the development of a sense of industry, which is gained through personal achievements and results in positive self-esteem.

► School provides a new cultural environment for the child, with a new authority figure, new rules and restrictions, and a greater need to cooperate with numerous peers.

► Cognitively, the young school-age child develops conservation, the mental operation that allows thought processes to become more logical.

► Language development is very rapid during middle childhood; reading greatly increases vocabulary and the understanding of syntax.

► Physical growth during the school years is slow and steady until the skeletal growth spurt just before puberty.

► The prepubertal growth spurt usually occurs 2 years earlier in girls than in boys; during this time, development of secondary sexual changes begins.

► Development of muscle strength and coordination allows the school-ager to participate in complex gross and fine motor activities.

► The school-age child continues to develop the idea of what is morally right and wrong.

► Preadolescents move forward to the last stage of cognitive development, formal operations, in which they begin to think in an abstract manner, reflect on thought processes, and plan for the future.

► The adolescent is able to solve complex mental problems, use deductive reasoning, and hypothesize about the future.

► Adolescence begins with puberty, when primary sexual characteristics begin to develop and secondary sexual characteristics complete development.

► The physical changes of puberty do not occur at the same time among members of the same sex.

► The adolescent's rapid change in physical appearance heightens self-consciousness and concerns regarding body image.

► Motor vehicle accidents are the major cause of accidental death in adolescence.

► Sexually transmitted diseases are the most common communicable diseases among adolescents.

► The adolescent's sense of right and wrong evolves from the application of moral rules to daily decision making.

► Peer relationships are very important to the adolescent's psychosocial development and to the development of self-esteem.

► Adolescents begin the long process of emancipation from their parents and need parental support to accomplish this in a timely manner.

■ KEY TERMS ■

Adolescence, p. 537

Classification, p. 534

Concrete operations, p. 533

Conservation, p. 534

Decenter, p. 533

Estrogen, p. 539

Menarche, p. 538

Preadolescence, p. 537

Puberty, p. 539

Psychosocial moratorium, p. 541

Reversibility, p. 533

Seriation, p. 534

Sexually transmitted disease (STD), p. 542

Syntax, p. 534

Testosterone, p. 539

■ CRITICAL THINKING EXERCISES ■

1. Seven-year-old Carlos has been admitted to the hospital with an asthma attack and is receiving aminophylline intravenously and oxygen through nasal prongs. Therefore he is confined to his room and spends most of the time in bed. Considering his illness and his development (physical, psychosocial, and cognitive dimensions), choose at least six play activities and explain why they are appropriate for this 7 year old.

2. Ten-year-old Jim is brought to the pediatric clinic for a physical examination. He is obese and his blood pressure is elevated. What nursing strategies can be used to enable this school-age child to lose weight, lower his blood pressure, and build his self-esteem?

3. Sixteen-year-old Jane is in skeletal traction with a fractured femur. Discuss ways to meet Jane's needs for diversional activity.

REFERENCES

Antwerp CV, Spaniolo AM: Checking out children's lifestyles, *MCN* 16(3):144, 1991.

Centers for Disease Control and Prevention: *Survey: teen health and sex habits,* Atlanta, 1991, The Centers.

Centers for Disease Control and Prevention, Health Resources and Services Administration, *Facts about adolescents and HIV/AIDS,* Atlanta, 1993, The Centers.

Centers for Disease Control and Prevention: *HIV/AIDS Surveillance report,* Atlanta, 1994, The Centers.

Dacey J, Travers J: *Human development across the lifespan,* Dubuque, Iowa, 1991, William C Brown.

Dwyer J: Nutrition in the adolescent. In Suskind R, Lewinder-Suskind D: *Textbook of pediatric nutrition,* New York, 1993, Raven.

Edelman C, Mandle C, editors: *Health promotion throughout the life span,* ed 3, St Louis, 1994, Mosby.

Elkind D: *All grown up and no place to go,* Reading, Mass, 1984, Addison-Wesley.

Erikson EH: *Identity: youth and crises,* New York, 1968, Norton.

Hawton K: *Suicide and attempted suicide among children and adolescents,* 1990, Sage.

Kim MJ, McFarland GK, McLane AM: *Pocket guide to nursing diagnoses,* ed 6, St Louis, 1995, Mosby.

Kohlberg L: Development of moral character and moral ideology. In Hoffman ML, Hoffman LNW, editors: *Review of child development research,* vol 1, New York, 1964, Russell Sage Foundation.

Mattsson A: Adolescent depression and suicide. In Hoekelman R et al, editors: *Primary pediatric care,* ed 2, St Louis, 1992, Mosby.

McCaleb A, Edgil A: Self-concept and self-care practices of healthy adolescents, *J Pediatr Nurs* 9(4):233, 1994.

McGinnis J, DeGraw C: Healthy Schools 2000: creating partnerships for the decade, *J School Health* 61:292, 1991.

Nelson J: HIV in adolescents, *MCN* 20:34, 1995.

Pender N: *Health promotion in nursing practice,* ed 3, Norwalk, Conn, 1993, Appleton & Lange.

Ryan-Wenger NM, Copeland SG: Coping strategies used by Black school-age children from low-income families, *J Pediatr Nurs* 9(1):33, 1994.

Schreiner B, Brondham L: Nutrition in pediatric primary care, *Nurse Practitioner Forum* 5:13, 1994.

Spector R: *Cultural diversity in health and illness,* Norwalk, Conn, 1991, Appleton and Lange.

US Department of Commerce: *Statistical abstract of the United States,* Washington, DC, 1992, US Department of Commerce.

US Department of Health and Human Services: *Health, United States, 1989 and prevention profile,* DHHS Pub No (PHS) 89-1232, Hyattsville, Md, 1989, US Department of Human Services, National Center for Health Statistics.

US Department of Health and Human Services: *Healthy People 2000: national health promotion and disease prevention objectives,* Boston, 1992, Jones and Bartlett.

Williams SR, Worthington-Roberts B: *Nutrition throughout the life cycle,* ed 2, St Louis, 1992, Mosby.

Wong DL: *Whaley and Wong's nursing care of infants and children,* ed 5, St Louis, 1995, Mosby.

ADDITIONAL READINGS

Children's Safety Network: a data book of child and adolescent injury, Washington, DC, 1991, National Center For Education in Maternal and Child Health.

Feldman S, Elliot G, editors: *At the threshold: the developing adolescent,* Cambridge, Mass, 1990, Harvard University Press.

Knollmueller R, editor: *Prevention across the life span: healthy people for the 21st century,* Washington, DC, 1993, American Nurses Publishing.

Morgan I: Recognizing depression in the adolescent, *MCN* 19:6, 1994.

Ostrum G: Sports-related injuries in youths - prevention is the key- and nurses can help, *Pediatr Nurs* 19(4):333, 1993.

Sewell K, Gaines S: A developmental approach to childhood safety education, *Pediatr Nurs* 19(5):464, 1993.

Smith M: Pediatric sexuality: promoting normal sexual development in children, *Nurse Practitioner* 18(8):37, 1993.

US Department of Health and Human Services, *Healthy Children 2000: national health promotion and disease prevention objectives relate to infants, children, adolescents and youth,* Boston, 1992, Jones and Bartlett.

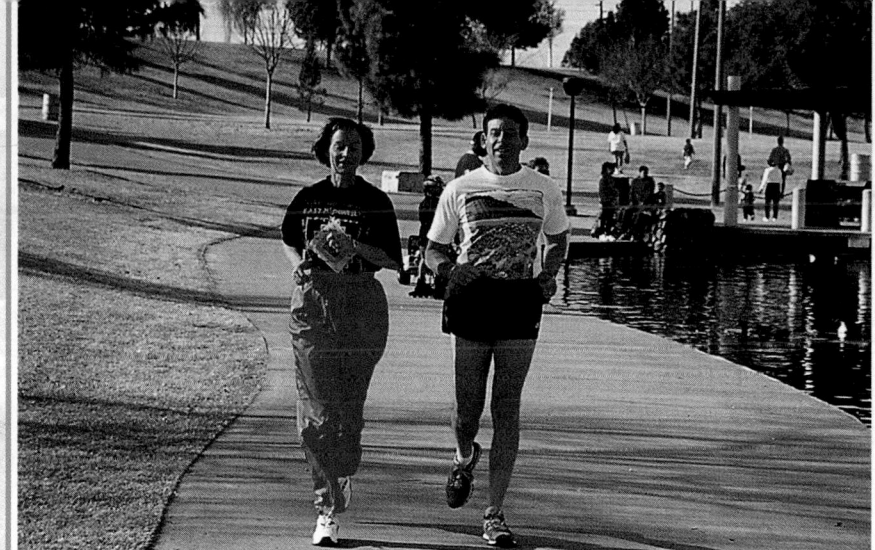

## Chapter 30

Young and Middle Adult

Objectives

Mastery of content in this chapter will enable the student to:

▶ Define key terms listed.

▶ Discuss developmental theories of young and middle adults.

▶ List and discuss major life events of young and middle adults and the childbearing family.

▶ Describe developmental tasks of the young adult, the childbearing family, and the middle adult.

▶ Discuss the significance of family in the life of the adult.

▶ Describe normal physiological changes in young and middle adulthood and in pregnancy.

▶ Discuss cognitive and psychosocial changes occurring during the adult years.

▶ Describe health concerns of the young adult, the childbearing family, and the middle adult.

▶ Identify nursing diagnoses related to the developmental needs of young and middle adults.

▶ Apply the nursing process to administer care to young and middle adults.

Young and middle adulthood is a period of challenges, rewards, and crises. Challenges may include the demands of work and raising families, although adults can also be rewarded by successes in their career endeavors and in their personal lives. Also, adults face such crises as caring for their aging parents, the possibility of job loss in a changing economic environment, and dealing with their own developmental needs as well as those of their family members.

Adult development involves orderly changes in characteristics and attitudes. Developmental changes are based on earlier characteristics that help shape subsequent behavior and characteristics. Each person's development, however, is a unique process (Haber et al, 1992). The changes experienced by young adults include the natural processes of maturation and socialization. Young adults pass through alternating periods of stability and change. During periods of stability, they make certain choices and build structures around them. In periods of change, they reevaluate these choices and consider new alternatives (Erikson, 1968, 1982).

Young adulthood is the period between the late teens and the mid- to late thirties (Edelman and Mandle, 1994). Young adults comprise approximately 26% of the population. During young adulthood, individuals increasingly separate from their families of origin, establish career goals, and decide whether to marry and begin families or remain single. Young adults are active and must adapt to new experiences. The transition into middle age occurs when young persons become aware that changes in reproductive and physical abilities signify the beginning of another stage in life. Middle age is a time of continuing transitions when individuals may reassess their goals in life and add new goals. In 1990, almost 84 million persons in the United States were between the ages of 35 and 64, or approximately 34% of the U.S. population were middle-age adults (U.S. Dept. of Commerce, 1992).

■ MATURITY AND ADULTHOOD

People are said to have reached **maturity** when they have reached a balance of growth in physiological, psychosocial, and cognitive areas. Mature individuals feel comfortable with the abilities, knowledge, and responses that they have developed over the years. They look at the world with a broad view, based on a blend of insight, emotion, and imagination. They take on problems that can be solved but recognize and learn to live with unsolvable problems.

Mature people are open to suggestions and can accept constructive criticism without a major loss of self-esteem. They weigh other persons' input and recommendations when making decisions but are not overly influenced or intimidated by others. Above all, mature people develop by learning from their own and others' experiences.

Other characteristics of maturity are related to interpersonal communication and behavior. Mature persons acknowledge accomplishments and shortcomings. Mature adults confront tasks openly, use decision-making techniques to solve problems, and are accountable and responsible for their actions.

■ YOUNG ADULT

Theories of Young Adulthood

Many theorists have attempted to describe the phases of young adulthood and related developmental tasks. Three theorists, Levinson, Gilligan, and Diekelmann, are presented in this section. Classic research by Levinson has identified the following phases of young and middle adult development (Levinson et al, 1978):

1. Early adult transition (ages 18 to 20), when the person separates from the family and desires independence
2. Entrance into the adult world (ages 21 to 27), when the person prepares for and tries out careers and lifestyles
3. Transition (ages 28 to 32), when the person may greatly modify life activities and thinks about future goals
4. Settling down (ages 33 to 39), when the person experiences greater stability
5. The payoff years (ages 40 to 65), a time for maximal influence, self-direction, and self-appraisal

Theorists propose that intellectual and moral development differ between men and women. According to Gilligan (1993), women struggle with the issues of care and responsibility, and in turn their relationships progress toward a maturity of interdependence. As women progress toward adulthood the moral dilemma changes from how to exercise their rights without interfering in the rights of others to "how to lead a moral life," which includes obligations to themselves and their families and people in general (Gilligan, 1993).

As women entered professional arenas, they hoped to develop the caring and nurturing roles in their male colleagues (Gordon, 1991). Women have long recognized that, without caring, the perceived quality of life is changed. As a result women maintained caring in the home and educational and work environments. However, women became frustrated in their development because the responsibility of caring was not shared, and frequently nurturing became a gender-specific responsibility.

In many cultures familial authority has historically been associated with the male. Men have traditionally assumed the overwhelming majority of positions of power (Finsterbusch and McKenna, 1992). Boys learn how to be men by absorbing messages about "manliness" from parents, siblings, peers, teachers, television, and action movies. These messages encourage boys to be competitive, focus on external success, rely on their intellect, withstand physical pain, and repress their vulnerable emotions. Traditional masculine roles include providing and protecting. Recently, however, men have been characterized as moving into greater disequilibrium. Faced with a societal structure that differs greatly from the norms of 20 years ago, many men are challenged with determining what it means to be a man and how to feel good about it in today's society (Sheehy, 1995). As a provider, for example, a man is traditionally viewed as the primary supporter of the family. More women, however, have been successful in entering the work force and pursuing careers, and in some age groups, men's incomes have declined, as much as 24% among young adult men. In fact, in the 1980s the driving force in the U.S. economy was earnings by women (Sheehy, 1995).

Another theory for young adult development has been proposed by Diekelmann (1976). Diekelmann suggests that young adults experience the following developmental tasks:

1. They achieve independence from parental controls.
2. They begin to develop strong friendships and intimate relationships outside the family.
3. They establish a personal set of values.
4. They develop a sense of personal identity.
5. They prepare for life work and develop the capacity for intimacy.

These theories, along with the works of Erikson (1963, 1982), provide nurses with a basis for understanding the life events and developmental tasks of the young adult. Each young adult, however, brings unique characteristics and needs to this developmental stage. A client in this developmental stage presents challenges to nurses who themselves may be young adults coping with the demands of this period. Young adult nurses must be careful to recognize the needs of a young adult client even if they are not experiencing the same challenges and events.

MIDDLE ADULT

In middle adulthood, the individual makes lasting contributions through involvement with others. Generally the middle adult years begin around the early to mid-30s and last through the late 60s (Edelman and Mandle, 1994) corresponding with Levinson's developmental phases of "settling down" and the "payoff years." During this period, personal and career achievements have often already been experienced. Many middle adults find particular joy in assisting their children and other young people to become productive and responsible adults. They may also begin to help aging parents. Using leisure time in satisfying and creative ways is a challenge that, if met satisfactorily, enables middle adults to prepare for retirement.

While most middle adults have achieved socioeconomic stability, recent trends in corporate downsizing have left many middle adults either jobless or forced to accept lower paying jobs with little or no fringe benefits. Fewer employers are offering or sharing the cost of health insurance plans that include coverage for dependents. As a result, a greater proportion of the population is currently unable to afford adequate health insurance coverage. Figures released in 1994 indicate that a growing number of families lack even the most basic health insurance coverage (Children's Defense Fund, 1995).

Men and women must adjust to inevitable biological changes. As in adolescence, middle adults use considerable energy to adapt self-concept and body image to physiological realities and changes in physical appearance. High self-esteem, a favorable body image, and a positive attitude toward physiological changes are fostered when adults engage in physical exercise, balanced diets, adequate sleep, and good hygiene practices that promote vigorous, healthy bodies.

Theories of Middle Adulthood

ERIKSON'S THEORY

According to Erikson's developmental theory, the primary developmental task of the middle years is to achieve generativity (Erikson, 1968, 1982). Generativity is the willingness to care for and guide others. Middle adults can achieve generativity with their own children or the children of close friends or through guidance in social interactions with the next generation. If middle adults fail to achieve generativity, stagnation occurs. This is shown by excessive concern with themselves or destructive behavior toward their children and the community. For example, the National Committee to Prevent Child Abuse indicated that in 1993 there were 3 million reported cases of abuse or neglect; and although recent media coverage has reinforced the increase in youth violence, federal statistics indicate that greater than 80% of the increase in violent crime since the early 1980s is attributable to adults (Children's Defense Fund, 1995).

HAVIGHURST'S THEORY

Havighurst's developmental theory has been summarized in terms of seven developmental tasks for the middle adult (Havighurst, 1972). These include achieving adult civic social responsibility; establishing and maintaining a standard of living; helping teenage children become responsible and happy adults; developing leisure activities; relating to one's spouse as a person; accepting and adjusting to the physiological changes of middle age; and adjusting to aging parents. Aging parents pose a unique challenge for middle adults in today's society. While most older adults are still able to function independently, increased age increases the need for assistance (Fawcett, 1993). Divorce and the increased childbearing by single women have increased the prevalence of single-parent families, and these changes in family structure may complicate caregiving for aging parents by the current generation of middle adults.

THE NURSING PROCESS AND YOUNG AND MIDDLE ADULTHOOD

 Assessment

When assessing young and middle adults, the nurse must consider their respective developmental tasks as well as differing stages and consequences of both psychosocial and biological development.

Young Adult

PHYSIOLOGICAL DEVELOPMENT

The young adult has completed physical growth by the age of 20. An exception to this is the pregnant or lactating woman. The physical, cognitive, and psychosocial changes and the health concerns of the pregnant woman and the childbearing family are extensive.

Young adults are usually quite active, experience severe illnesses less commonly than older age groups, tend to ignore physical symptoms, and often postpone seeking health care. Physical characteristics of young adults begin to change as middle age approaches. Unless clients have illnesses, assessment findings are generally within normal limits.

Nonetheless, clients in this developmental stage may benefit from a personal lifestyle assessment (see Chapter 1). A personal lifestyle assessment can help nurses and clients identify habits that increase the risk for cardiac, malignant, pulmonary, renal, or other chronic diseases. A personal lifestyle assessment of the young adult includes assessment of general life satisfaction; hobbies and interests; habits such as diet, sleeping, exercise, sexual habits and use of caffeine, alcohol and illicit drugs; home conditions including housing, economic condition, type of health insurance, and pets; and occupational environment including type of work, exposure to hazardous substances, and physical or mental strain. Military records including dates and geographical area of assignments may also be useful in assessing the young adult for risk factors.

COGNITIVE DEVELOPMENT

Rational thinking habits increase steadily through the young and middle adult years. Formal and informal educational experiences, general life experiences, and occupational opportunities dramatically increase the individual's conceptual, problem-solving, and motor skills.

Identifying preferred occupational areas is a major task of young adults. When people know their educational preparation, skills, talents, and personality characteristics, occupational choices are easier, and they are generally more satisfied with their choices. Many young adults, however, either lack the resources or the support systems to facilitate further education or the development of skills necessary for many positions in the work place. As a result, some young adults may have limited occupational choices.

An understanding of how adults learn assists the nurse in developing teaching plans (see Chapter 15). Adults enter the teaching-learning situation with a background of unique life experiences, including illness. Therefore, the nurse always views adults as individuals. Their compliance with regimens such as medications, treatments, or lifestyle changes such as smoking cessation, involves decision-making processes. When determining the amount of information that the individual needs to make decisions about the prescribed course of therapy, the nurse should consider those factors that may affect the individual's compliance with the regimen including educational level, socioeconomic factors, and motivation and desire to learn.

Because young adults are continually evolving and adjusting to changes in the home, work place, and personal lives, their decision-making processes should be flexible. The more secure young adults are in their roles, the more flexible and open they are to change. Insecure persons tend to be more rigid in making decisions.

PSYCHOSOCIAL DEVELOPMENT

The emotional health of the young adult is related to the individual's ability to address and resolve personal and social tasks. The young adult is usually caught between wanting to prolong the irresponsibility of adolescence and wanting to assume adult commitments. Certain patterns or trends, however, are relatively predictable. Between the ages of 23 to 28, the person refines self-perception and ability for intimacy. From 29 to 34 the person directs enormous energy toward achievement and mastery of the surrounding world. The years from 35 to 43 are a time of vigorous examination of life goals and relationships. Alterations are made in personal, social, and occupational lives. Often the stresses of this reexamination result in a "midlife crisis" in which marital partner, lifestyle, and occupation may change.

During the young adult years, people generally give more attention to occupational and social pursuits. During this period individuals attempt to improve their socioeconomic status. Upward mobility is sought through career choices. Recent trends toward corporate downsizing, however, are leading to fewer high-level positions. Subsequently, many young adults are facing the added stress of greater competition in the work place for fewer positions. For many young adults, a dual-income family is also needed to achieve and maintain middle-class status. Career and personal counseling can help individuals identify career choices and set realistic goals.

Ethnic and gender factors have a sociological and psychological influence in an adult's life, and these factors can pose a distinct challenge for nursing care. Each person holds culture-bound definitions of health and illness. Nurses and other health professionals bring with them distinct practices for the prevention and treatment of illness. Knowing too little about a client's self-perception or beliefs regarding health and illness may create conflict between the nurse and the client. An understanding of ethnicity, race, and gender differences enables the nurse to provide individualized care (see Chapter 21).

Support from the nurse, access to information, and appropriate referrals provide opportunities for achievement of a client's potential. Because health is not merely the absence of disease but involves wellness in all human dimensions, the holistic, humanistic nurse acknowledges the importance of the young adult's psychosocial needs and needs in other dimensions.

The young adult must make decisions concerning career, marriage, and parenthood. Although each person makes these decisions based on individual factors, the nurse should understand the general principles involved in these aspects of psychosocial development to assess the young adult's psychosocial status.

Career. Young men and women hope to have careers that will enable them to realize the occupational dreams of their childhood. They may formulate short- and long-term goals in traditional or nontraditional careers. A successful vocational adjustment is important in the lives of most men and women. Successful employment not only ensures economic security but also leads to friendships, social activities, support, and respect from co-workers.

Two-career marriages are increasing. The two-career marriage has benefits and liabilities. In addition to increasing the family's financial base, the person who works outside the home is able to expand friendships, activities, and interests. However, stress may occur in a two-career family. These stressors can result from a transfer to a new city; increased expenditures of physical, mental, or emotional energy; child care demands; or household needs. While working mothers originally were assumed to be responsible for numerous social ills involving children, studies show little or no difference between children of working and nonworking mothers with respect to behaviors such as aggression, obedience, self-reliance, sensitivity, or sociability (Rosenfeld, 1992).

Male and female stereotypes of the past are decreasing. Men are becoming more involved in child-rearing and homemaking duties. Women are becoming active in house and automobile maintenance. To avoid stress in a two-career family, neither partner can assume all responsibilities. For some families a solution may be to limit recreational expenses and instead hire someone to do routine housework. Others may set up an equal division of household, shopping, and cooking duties.

Sexuality. The development of secondary sexual characteristics occurs during the adolescent years (see Chapter 29). Physical development is accompanied by the ability to perform sexual acts. The young adult usually has emotional maturity to complement the physical ability and is therefore able to develop mature sexual relationships. Young adults who have failed to achieve the developmental task of personal integration may, however, develop relationships that are superficial and stereotyped (Haber et al, 1992).

Masters and Johnson (1970) have contributed important information about the physiological characteristics of the adult sexual response. Detailed discussion of the sexual response occurs in Chapter 24.

The psychodynamic aspect of sexual activity is as important as the type or frequency of sexual intercourse to young adults. Psychological beliefs and expectations give feelings of pleasure and satisfaction to adults. To maintain total wellness, adults should be encouraged to explore various aspects of their sexuality and be aware that their sexual needs and concerns evolve. As the rate of early initiation of sexual intercourse continues to increase, young adults are at risk for sexually transmitted diseases. Consequently, they need education regarding the mode of transmission, prevention, and symptom recognition and management.

Childbearing Cycle. Conception, pregnancy, birth, and the puerperium are major phases of the childbearing cycle. The changes during these phases are complex. Whall and Fawcett (1991) and Ruchala and Halstead (1994) have demonstrated that women perceive significant changes in physiological condition, emotion, and body image during the second trimester of pregnancy and during the early puerperium.

Education such as Lamaze classes can prepare pregnant women, their partners and other support persons to participate in the birthing process (Fig. 30-1). Social support has also been reported to have an impact on pregnant women and their families. Coffman, Levitt, and Brown (1994) reported that couples who knew they could rely on one another were found to have more positive relationship satisfaction and parenting attitudes. In this study, confirmation of support expectations was more important to women than to men. Another study indicated that social support may have a significant impact on the duration of labor (Pascoe, 1993). A current trend in some health care agencies is to provide a lay **doula** or support person to be present during labor to assist women who have no other source of support.

Lactation, or the process of breast-feeding, offers many advantages to both the new mother and baby. For the inexperienced mother, breast-feeding may also be a source of anxiety and frustration. Women who have had no contact with other mothers who breast-feed and who have had little or no contact with newborns require assistance to breast-feed successfully (Lawrence, 1994). The nurse must be alert for signs that the mother needs information and as-

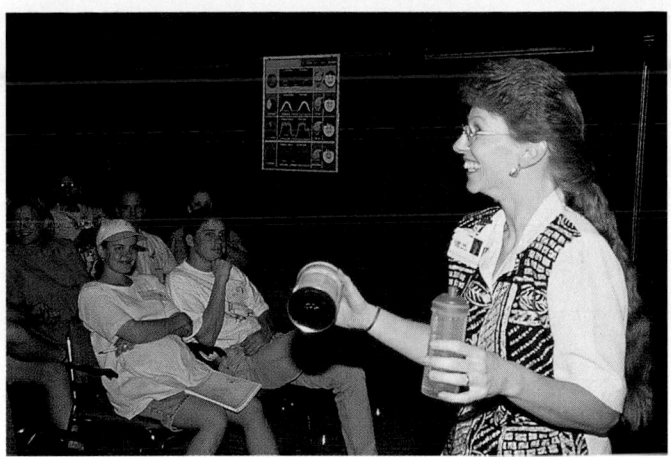

Fig. 30-1 Nurse providing Lamaze class for expectant young adults.

sistance. Direct observation of the breast-feeding mother-infant dyad alerts the nurse to such problems as proper positioning of either the mother and infant or ineffective sucking by the infant.

The personal and social changes occurring in the lives of a couple after the birth of a baby cannot be underestimated (Fig. 30-2). The nursing assessment of the couple's response to the birthing experience and parent-child bonding are detailed in a later section of this chapter.

Types of Families. During young adulthood most individuals experience singlehood and the opportunity to be on their own. Those who eventually marry experience several changes as they take on new responsibilities. Many married couples choose to become parents. Middle adults who remain single experience unique challenges and opportunities as well.

Singlehood. Social pressure to get married is not as great as it once was. Today it is socially acceptable for a young adult to leave home and live in an apartment or to own a home without marrying first. For young adults who remain single, parents and siblings become the nucleus for a family, although the single young adult maintains independence from parental controls. Close friends and associates of the single young adult may also be viewed as the individual's "family."

One cause for the increased single population is the expanding career opportunities for women. Women enter the job market with greater career potential and have greater opportunities for financial independence. It is also becoming more socially acceptable for single individuals to live together outside of marriage as well as for single young adults to become parents either biologically or through adoption. Similarly, it has become more socially acceptable for married couples to separate or divorce if they find their marital situation unsatisfactory.

Marriage. Every couple's relationship is unique. Although no rules guarantee a successful marriage, some guidelines are useful for building a happy marriage. Before marriage the couple ideally should complete five tasks. First, they should make certain that their emotions are based on love rather than physical or sexual attraction. Sec-

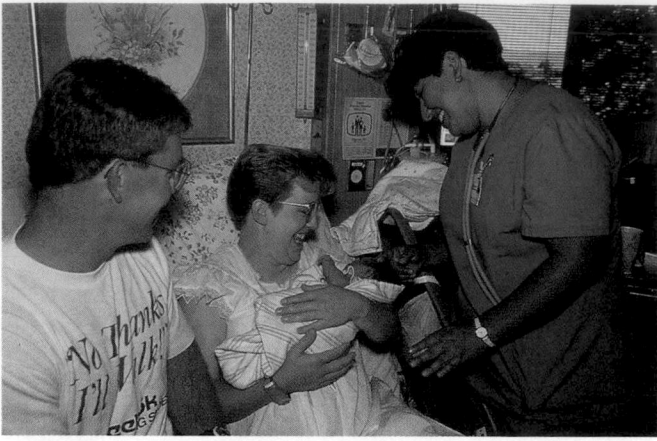

Fig. 30-2 Parent-child nurturing is important in adapting to a newborn.

Ten Hallmarks of Emotional Health

- A sense of meaning and direction in life
- Successful negotiation through transitions
- Absence of feelings of being cheated or disappointed by life
- Attainment of several long-term goals
- Satisfaction with personal growth and development
- When married, feelings of mutual love for partner; when single, satisfaction with social interactions
- Satisfaction with friendships
- Generally cheerful attitude
- No sensitivity to criticism
- No unrealistic fears

Modified from Stanhope M, Lancaster J: *Community health nursing: process and practice for promoting health,* ed 4, St Louis, 1996, Mosby.

ond, both partners should explore their motivation for wanting to marry. Third, they should focus on developing clear communication. Fourth, they should understand that any annoying behavior patterns and habits are unlikely to change after marriage. Last, they should determine their compatibility in important beliefs and values.

When establishing a household and family, the married couple must begin to work as a team. They have the following tasks:

1. Establishing an intimate relationship
2. Deciding on and working toward mutual goals
3. Establishing guidelines for power and decision-making issues
4. Setting standards for extrafamily interactions
5. Finding companionship with other people for a social life
6. Choosing morals, values, and ideologies acceptable to both

These major tasks of adults require considerable maturity and self-esteem. When accomplished, however, they provide the foundation for a stable relationship. Growth in marriage extends over many years. Success in solving the challenging problems that occur in any marriage offers marital partners insight into each other.

A marital relationship involves different developmental stages. The establishment stage begins at the wedding and continues as the couple attempts to function as a dyad (pair). They learn patterns of sexual expression and ways to live intimately with each other. They must learn styles of conflict resolution, decision making, and role patterns. In addition, each partner may experience a sense of loss of individuality and self in the transition from *me* to *we*.

The family orientation stage is directed at childbearing and child-rearing activities. Parenting roles must be defined and practiced. Nurturing and socialization needs of the children can put pressure on the couple's intimate relationship. In addition, parents' images of the "perfect parent" conflict with reality.

Parenthood. The availability of contraception makes it easier for today's couples to decide when and if to start a family. One factor influencing this decision is the reason for wanting a child. Social pressures may encourage a couple to have a child or may influence them to limit the number of children they have. Economic considerations frequently enter into the decision-making process because having and bringing up children are expensive. General health status and age are also considerations in decisions about parenthood because couples are getting married later and are postponing pregnancies.

Hallmarks of Emotional Health. Most young adults have the physical and emotional resources and support systems to meet the many challenges, tasks, and responsibilities they face. During psychosocial assessment of young adults, the nurse can assess for 10 hallmarks of emotional health (see the box above) that indicate successful maturation in this developmental stage.

HEALTH CONCERNS

Physiological Concerns. Young adults are generally active and have a minimum of major health problems. However, their lifestyles may put them at risk for illnesses or disabilities during their middle or older adult years. Young adults may also be genetically susceptible to certain chronic diseases such as diabetes mellitus and familial hypercholesterolemia (Price and Wilson, 1992). Crohn's disease, a chronic inflammatory disease of the small intestine, most commonly occurs between 15 and 35 years of age. The incidence of infertility has also increased in recent years, affecting 15% to 20% of otherwise healthy adults; many infertile clients are young adults (Bobak and Jensen, 1993).

Risk Factors. Risk factors for the young adult's health originate in the community, lifestyle, and family history. These risk factors fall into the following categories:

1. Violent death and injury
2. Substance abuse
3. Unwanted pregnancies
4. Sexually transmitted diseases
5. Environmental or occupational factors

Violence is the greatest cause of mortality and morbidity in the young adult population. Death and injury can occur from physical assaults, motor vehicle or other accidents, and suicide attempts. In 1992, the death rate (per 100,000 population) for 25- to 44-year-olds in the U.S. due to homicide was 14.3; the death rate for motor vehicle accidents was 17.1; and the death rate for suicide in this age group was 14.8 (U.S. DHHS, 1995).

While recent media attention has focused on the increase in violent crime among youth, adults still commit the majority of crimes. Eighty-four percent of all arrests for murder and 77% of all arrests for weapons violations in 1993 involved adults (Children's Defense Fund, 1995). Assessment of factors that may predispose to violence, with subsequent injury or death, include poverty, family breakdown, child abuse and neglect, repeated exposure to violence, and ready access to guns. It is important that the nurse perform a thorough psychosocial assessment, including such factors as behavior patterns, history of physical abuse and substance abuse, education, work history, and social support systems, to detect personal and environmental risk factors for violence.

Substance abuse directly or indirectly contributes to mortality and morbidity in young adults. Intoxicated young adults may be severely injured in motor-vehicle accidents that may result in death or permanent disability to other young adults as well.

Dependence on stimulant or depressant drugs can result in death. Overdose of a stimulant drug ("upper") can stress the cardiovascular and nervous systems to the extent that death occurs. The use of depressants ("downers") can lead to an accidental or intentional overdose and death.

Substance abuse is not always diagnosable, particularly in its early stages. Nonjudgmental questions about use of legal drugs (prescribed drugs, tobacco, and alcohol), use of soft drugs (marijuana), and use of more problematic drugs (cocaine or heroin) should be a routine part of any physical assessment. Important information may be obtained by making specific inquiries about past medical problems, changes in food intake or sleep patterns, or problems of emotional lability. Reports of arrests because of driving while intoxicated, wife or child abuse, or disorderly conduct should alert the health care provider to probe the possibility of drug abuse more carefully (Winger, Hofmann, and Woods, 1992).

Unplanned pregnancies, although more common among adolescents, account for 55% of pregnancies in young and middle adult women (Alan Guttmacher Institute, 1994). Unplanned pregnancies can have long-term physical and emotional effects in the young adult years. Unplanned pregnancies are a continual source of stress. Often young adults have educational and career goals that take precedence to family development. Interference with these goals can affect future relationships and affects later parent-child relationships.

Determination of situational factors that may affect the progress and outcome of an unplanned pregnancy is important. Exploration of problems such as financial, career, and living accommodations; family support systems; potential parenting disorders; depression; and coping mechanisms is important in assessing the woman with an unplanned pregnancy.

Sexually transmitted diseases (STDs) include syphilis, chlamydia, gonorrhea, genital herpes, and AIDS. Sexually transmitted diseases have immediate effects such as discharge, discomfort, and infection. They may also lead to chronic disorders, which can result from genital herpes; infertility, which can result from gonorrhea; or even death,

which results from AIDS. These diseases may occur in sexually active persons, and it is estimated that approximately two thirds of all cases of STDs occur in individuals between 15 and 24 years of age (Killion, 1994). Recently, sexual activity with multiple partners has decreased. Many young adults are seeking to establish meaningful relationships before engaging in sexual activity (see Chapter 24). In addition, partners are encouraged to know one another's previous sexual history and sexual practices (Bradley-Springer, 1994; Killion, 1994). The nurse should be alert for STDs when clients come to clinics with complaints of urological or gynecological problems (see Chapter 33). Young adults should be assessed for their knowledge of genital self-exams.

A common environmental or occupational risk factor is exposure to airborne particles, which may cause lung diseases and cancer. Such lung diseases include silicosis from inhalation of talcum and silicon dust and emphysema from inhalation of smoke. Cancers resulting from occupational exposures may involve the lung, liver, brain, blood, or skin (Table 30-1). Questions regarding occupational exposure to hazardous materials should be a routine part of the nurse's assessment.

Lifestyle. Lifestyle habits such as smoking, stress, lack of exercise, and poor personal hygiene increase the risk of future illness. Family history of cardiovascular, renal, endocrine, or neoplastic disease increases the risk of illness as well. The nurse's role in health promotion is to identify factors that increase the young adult's risk for health problems. Research has demonstrated that changing unhealthy lifestyle behaviors reduces selected risk factors (see the box on p. 556).

Those lifestyle habits that activate the stress response (see Chapter 22), increase the risk of illness. Smoking is a

Table 30-1	Occupational Hazards Associated With Cancers	
OCCUPATIONAL CHEMICAL	**CANCER**
Asbestos	Mesothelioma (pleural and peritoneal)
	Lung cancer
Vinyl chloride (plastics)	Liver cancer (hemangiosarcoma)
	Brain cancer
	Lung cancer
Benzene	Leukemia, predominantly acute myelogenous
Bischloromethane ether	Oat cell carcinoma of the lungs
Chromium	Cancer of nasal or paranasal sinus, lung, larynx
Arsenic	Lung cancer
Coal tar pitch, coke oven emissions	Cancer of lung, larynx, skin
Iron oxide	Cancer of lung, larynx
Nickel	Lung cancer
Petroleum distillates	Cancer of lung, larynx

From Stanhope M, Lancaster J: *Community health nursing: process and practice from promoting health,* ed 4, St Louis, 1996, Mosby.

RESEARCH HIGHLIGHT

RESEARCH ABSTRACT

The purpose of this study was to determine when, in the adult life span, health-related goals become dominant. Data collected from 171 young and middle-age adults showed that health-related issues became more predominant in midlife. In addition, both young and middle-age adults reported more fear in relation to future health state than what they hoped for in the realm of future health. Perceived self-efficacy and number of goal-oriented activities to avoid the feared health states were significant predictors of health behaviors. The results demonstrated that fear of future poor quality of health may be a motivating factor to change unhealthy lifestyle behaviors.

IMPLICATIONS FOR PRACTICE

▶ Health-related goals become more predominant in midlife; nurses should encourage and assist middle-age adults in developing health-related goals. Also, nurses should target young adults for health promotion and establishment of healthy lifestyles.

▶ Young and middle adults reported fear of future health state; nurses should encourage and support young and middle adults in their endeavors to change unhealthy lifestyles to promote a more healthy future.

▶ Perceived self-efficacy and number of goal-oriented activities were predictors of health behaviors; nurses should assist young and middle adults in developing realistic plans for accomplishment of healthy lifestyle behaviors.

REFERENCE

Hooker K, Kaus CR: Health-related possible selves in young and middle adulthood, *Psychology & Aging* 9(1):126, 1994.

well-documented risk factor for pulmonary, cardiac, and vascular diseases in smokers and the individuals who receive second-hand smoke. Inhaled cigarette pollutants increase the risk of lung cancer, emphysema, and chronic bronchitis. The nicotine in tobacco is a vasoconstrictor that acts on the coronary arteries, increasing the risk of angina, myocardial infarction, and coronary artery disease. Nicotine also causes peripheral vasoconstriction and may lead to vascular problems.

Prolonged stress increases wear and tear on the body's adaptive capacities. Stress-related diseases such as ulcers, emotional disorders, and infections can occur (see Chapter 22).

Exercise patterns can affect health status. Exercise that produces a sustained increase in the pulse rate for 15 to 20 minutes three times a week improves cardiopulmonary function by decreasing blood pressure and heart rate. In addition, exercise decreases fatigability, insomnia, tension, and irritability. The nurse should conduct a thorough musculoskeletal assessment, including joint mobility and muscle tone, and psychosocial assessment for improved tolerance to stress to determine the effects of exercise.

As in all age groups, personal hygiene habits in the young adult can be risk factors. Sharing eating utensils with a person who has a contagious illness increases the risk of

illness. Poor dental hygiene increases the risk of periodontal disease. Gingivitis (inflammation of the gums) and periodontitis (loss of tooth support) can be avoided through oral hygiene (see Chapter 40).

A familial history of a disease may put a young adult at risk for developing it in the middle or older adult years. For example, a young man whose father and paternal grandfather had myocardial infarctions (heart attacks) in their 50s has a risk for a future myocardial infarction. The presence of certain chronic illnesses in the family increases the family members' risk of developing a disease. This family risk is distinct from hereditary disease.

Poor adherence to routine screening examinations can put the client at risk for severe illnesses because of failed early detection. Clients should be encouraged to perform monthly breast self-examination (BSE) or genital self-examination (see Chapter 33). The nurse's role is extremely important in educating female clients about BSE and the current breast screening recommendations since breast cancer is the most common major cancer among women in the United States with a steadily increasing incidence (Edge and Miller, 1994). Routine assessment of the skin for recent changes in color or presence of lesions and changes in their appearance should be encouraged. Prolonged exposure to ultraviolet rays of the sun by the adolescent and young adult can increase the risk for development of skin cancer later in life.

Infertility. **Infertility** is a man's, woman's, or couple's involuntary inability to conceive. To most health professionals, it is the inability to conceive after a year or more of regular sexual intercourse. An estimated 15% to 20% of otherwise healthy adults are infertile (Bobak and Jensen, 1993). However, about half of the couples evaluated and treated in infertility clinics become pregnant. In about 10% to 20% of couples the cause of infertility is unknown and they remain infertile. In the remaining 30% the cause of the infertility is diagnosed but the couples remain infertile because of endometriosis, blocked fallopian tubes, or decreased sperm motility.

Research shows that among infertile couples, males and females may have different perceptions about childbearing (Halman, Andrews, and Abbey, 1994). This study determined that women experienced more stress from tests and treatment than men, placed greater importance on having children, were more accepting of indicated treatment, and wanted more children. For some infertile couples the nurse may be the first resource identified. Nursing assessment of the infertile couple should include comprehensive histories of both the male and female partners to determine factors that may have affected fertility as well as pertinent physical findings.

PSYCHOSOCIAL CONCERNS

The psychosocial health concerns of the young adult are often related to stress, such as job or family stress. As noted in Chapter 22, stress can be valuable because it motivates a client to change. However, if the stress is prolonged and the client is unable to adapt to the stressor, health problems can develop.

Job Stress. Job stress can occur every day or from time to time. Most young adults are able to handle day-to-day crises (Fig. 30-3). Situational job stress may occur when a

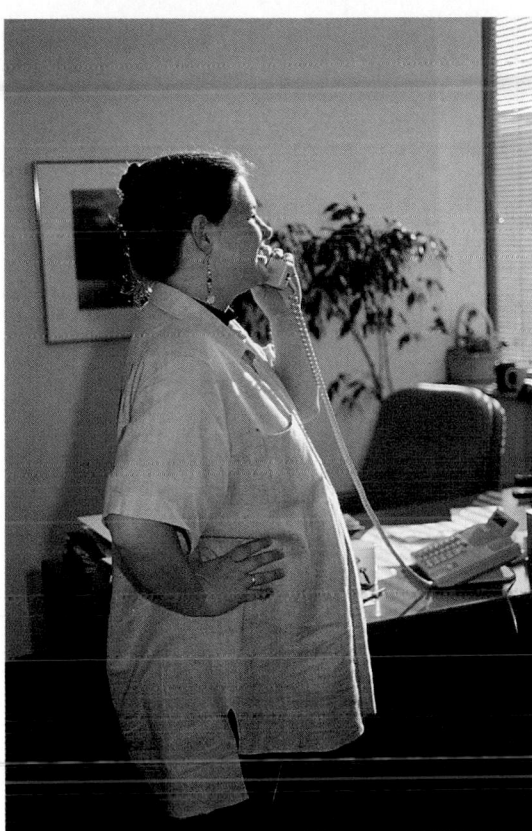

Fig. 30-3 The ability to handle day-to-day challenges at work minimizes stress.

new boss enters the workplace, a deadline is approaching, or the worker is given new or greater numbers of responsibilities. A recent trend in today's business world and risk factor for job stress is corporate downsizing, leading to increased responsibilities for employees with fewer positions within the corporate structure. Job stress also occurs when a person becomes dissatisfied with a job or responsibilities. Because individuals perceive jobs differently, the types of job stressors vary from client to client. The nurse's assessment of the young adult should include a description of the usual work performed and present work if different. Job assessment also includes conditions and hours, duration of employment, changes in sleep or eating habits, and evidence of increased irritability or nervousness.

Family Stress. Family stressors can occur at any time in family life (see Chapter 27). Family life has peaks, when everyone in the family works together, and valleys, when everyone appears to pull apart. Situational stressors occur during events such as births, deaths, illnesses, marriages, and job losses. When a client seeks health care and presents stress-related symptoms, the nurse should assess for the occurrence of a life change event.

Each family has certain predictable roles or jobs for members. These roles enable the family to function and be an effective part of society. One necessary role is the family leader. In most families one parent is the leader, or both parents act as coleaders. In single-parent families the parent or occasionally a member of the extended family is the family leader. When this changes as a result of illness, a sit-

uational crisis may occur. The nurse should assess environmental and familial factors including support systems and coping mechanisms commonly used by family members.

PREGNANT WOMAN AND CHILDBEARING FAMILY

A developmental task for most young adult couples is the decision to begin a family. Although the physiological changes of pregnancy and childbirth occur only in the woman, cognitive and psychosocial changes and health concerns affect the entire childbearing family, including the husband, siblings, and grandparents.

Physiological Changes. Women who are anticipating pregnancy benefit from good health practices before conception; these include a balanced diet, exercise, dental checkups, avoidance of alcohol, and cessation of smoking. Women trying to become pregnant should not try weight-reduction diets. The physiological changes and needs of the pregnant woman vary with each trimester (Table 30-2).

Prenatal Care. **Prenatal care** is the routine examination of the pregnant woman by an obstetrician, nurse practitioner, or certified nurse-midwife. Prenatal care includes assessment of the pregnant woman's weight; blood pressure; urine for glucose, acetone, and protein; and measurement of the fundus. Information should be provided from the beginning regarding sexually transmitted diseases, other vaginal infections, and urinary infections that could adversely affect the fetus. In addition, the pregnant woman may be counseled about exercise patterns, diet, and child care. Regular health care can address health concerns such as preeclampsia, eclampsia, excessive weight gain, and the high-risk infant.

First Trimester. All women experience some physiological changes in the first trimester, but some changes affect only certain women. These changes include morning sickness, increased urination, lack of energy, and changes in nutritional intake. The nurse must be familiar with these physiological changes, their causes, and helpful interventions.

During this period signs of pregnancy are usually not observable by others. If a woman frequently has **morning sickness**, however, her family, friends, and co-workers may suspect that she is pregnant. The newly pregnant woman needs routine prenatal care.

Second Trimester. During the second trimester, growth of the uterus and fetus results in some of the physical signs of pregnancy. Morning sickness has usually disappeared, and the woman's energy level is restored if her nutritional intake has caught up with her metabolic demands. The urinary frequency ceases, and she is able to sleep through the night.

If this is the woman's first pregnancy she may be able to see and feel the enlarged uterus. However, it is common for her abdomen to stay relatively flat. In subsequent pregnancies she may "show" as early as the beginning of the second trimester.

Third Trimester. During the third trimester increases in **Braxton Hicks contractions** (irregular, short contractions), fatigue, and urinary frequency occur. Close to the onset of labor, the woman may experience a burst of energy during which she cleans house and prepares for the baby by shopping for baby supplies. This period is called **nesting**. Many experts in obstetrics and seasoned veterans of pregnancy

Table 30-2	Major Physiological Changes During Pregnancy	

SIGNS AND SYMPTOMS	CAUSES
FIRST TRIMESTER	
Amenorrhea	Fertilization of egg by sperm
Morning sickness	Increased serum hormone levels
Breast changes:	Increased estrogen levels
Enlargement	
Tenderness	
Darkened and enlarged nipples	
Urinary frequency	Pressure of uterus on bladder
Fatigue	Increases in hormone levels
	Increased nutritional demands
	Decreased nutritional intake resulting from morning sickness
SECOND TRIMESTER	
Integumentary changes	Increased levels of melanocyte-stimulating hormone
Pigmented nipple and breast	
Hyperpigmentation of abdominal line (linea nigra)	
Mottling of cheeks or forehead (chloasma or "mask of pregnancy")	
Local or generalized pruritus	
Hypertrophy of gums causing gingival swelling and bleeding	Proliferation of interdental papillary blood vessels, resulting in local inflammation and hyperplasia
Increasing size of uterine fundus	Growth of fetus
Sensation of movement or gaslike movements (quickening)	Fetal movement
Braxton Hicks contractions	Expanding uterus and preparation of uterus for labor
THIRD TRIMESTER	
Increased colostrum	Hormonal influence; preparation of breasts for lactation
Increased urinary frequency	Pressure on bladder from enlarged fetus

Data from Bobak IM, Jensen MD: *Maternity and gynecologic care*, ed 5, St Louis, 1993, Mosby; and Dickason EJ, Silverman BL, Schult MO: *Maternal-infant nursing care*, St Louis, 1994, Mosby.

believe that nesting indicates a rapidly approaching time of delivery.

Puerperium. The **puerperium** is a period of approximately 6 weeks after delivery. During this time the woman's body reverts to its prepregnant physical status. The nurse should assess the woman's knowledge of and ability to care for both herself and for her newborn baby. Assessment of parenting skills and maternal-infant interactions is particularly important.

Cognitive Changes. Cognitive changes during pregnancy, primarily involving sensory perception and needs for education, affect both parents and may occur gradually or quickly.

Sensory Perception. The pregnant woman generally experiences changes in sensory perception. Temporary changes occur in visual and hearing acuity, taste, and smell. Many pregnant women frequently stroke the abdomen, possibly because of a change in the sensation of touch or other sensory need. The woman may be using the sensation of touch to initiate bonding with her child (Bobak, 1995).

Needs for Education. The entire childbearing family needs education about pregnancy, labor, delivery, breast-feeding, and integration of the newborn into the family structure. Traditionally, childbirth classes help parents plan for the

birth of the child and focus on the normal physiological changes of pregnancy, the processes of labor and delivery, methods of pain control, symptoms of impending labor, and care of the newborn. Many health care centers also have sibling and grandparent preparation classes. Not all pregnant women, however, attend childbirth classes for a variety of reasons. Childbirth education classes may not be accessible to women of all socioeconomic classes, and women may choose not to attend due to cultural beliefs about childbirth or lack of knowledge about the importance of childbirth education.

Psychosocial Changes. Like the physiological changes of pregnancy, psychosocial changes may occur at various times during the 9 months of pregnancy and in the puerperium. The major categories of psychosocial changes involve body image, role, sexuality, coping mechanisms, and stresses during the puerperium. Table 30-3 summarizes these psychosocial changes and implications for nursing intervention.

Health Concerns. The pregnant woman and her partner have many health questions. For example, they may wonder whether the pregnancy and baby will be normal. The majority of the health needs related to pregnancy can be met with proper prenatal care (Fig. 30-4).

Table 30-3	Major Psychosocial Changes During Pregnancy
CATEGORY	**IMPLICATIONS FOR NURSING**
Body image	Morning sickness and fatigue may contribute to poor body image.
	Client may feel big, awkward, and unattractive during third trimester when fetus is growing more rapidly.
	Increase in breast size may make the the woman feel more feminine and sexually appealing.
	May take extra time with hygiene and grooming, trying new hairstyles and makeup.
	Begins to "show" during the second trimester and starts to plan maternity wardrobe.
	General feeling of well-being when woman can feel the baby move and hear the heartbeat.
Role changes	Both partners think about and can have feelings of uncertainty about impending role changes.
	May have feelings of ambivalence about becoming parents and concern about ability to be parents.
Sexuality	Need reassurance that sexual activity will not harm fetus.
	Desire for sexual activity may be influenced by body image.
	May desire cuddling and holding rather than sexual intercourse.
Coping mechanisms	Need reassurance that childbirth and child rearing are natural and positive experiences, but can also be stressful.
	Often unable to cope with particular stressors such as finding new housing, preparing the nursery, or participating in childbirth classes.
Stresses during puerperium	May return home from hospital fatigued and unfamiliar with infant care.
	May experience physical discomfort or feelings of anxiety or depression.
	May be necessary for woman to return to work soon after delivery with subsequent feelings of guilt, anxiety, or, possibly, sense of freedom or relief.

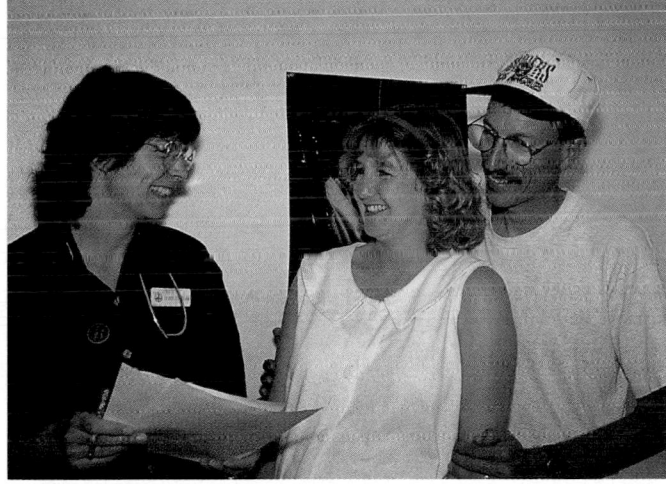

Fig. 30-4 Ongoing prenatal care reduces complications of pregnancy.

Middle Adult

PHYSIOLOGICAL DEVELOPMENT

Major physiological changes occur between 40 and 65 years of age. Table 30-4 summarizes these normal developmental changes that the nurse considers when conducting a physical examination.

The most visible changes are graying of the hair, wrinkling of the skin, and thickening of the waist. Balding commonly begins during the middle years, but it may also occur in young male adults. Decreases in hearing and visual acuity are often noted during this period. In 1992, approx-

imately 23% of all visits to office-based physicians by adults aged 44 to 64 were for a primary diagnosis of glaucoma (U.S. DHHS, 1995a). Often these physiological changes have an impact on self-concept and body image. The most significant physiological changes during middle age are menopause in women and the climacteric in men.

Menopause. Menstruation and ovulation occur in a cyclical rhythm in the woman from adolescence into middle adulthood. **Menopause** is the disruption of this cycle, primarily because of the inability of the neurohumoral system to maintain its periodic stimulation of the endocrine system. The ovaries no longer produce estrogen and progesterone, and the blood levels of these hormones drop markedly. Menopause typically occurs between 45 and 60 years of age (see Chapter 24). Approximately 10% of women have no symptoms of menopause other than cessation of menstruation, 70% to 80% are aware of other changes but have no problems and approximately 10% experience changes severe enough to interfere with activities of daily living (Edge and Miller, 1994).

Climacteric. The **climacteric**, or andropause, occurs in men in their late 40s or early 50s (see Chapter 24). It is caused by decreased levels of androgens. Throughout this period and thereafter, a man is still capable of producing fertile sperm and fathering a child. However, penile erection is less firm, ejaculation is less frequent, and the refractory period is longer.

COGNITIVE DEVELOPMENT

Changes in the cognitive function of middle adults are rare except with illness or trauma. The middle adult can learn new skills and information. Some middle adults enter educational or vocational programs to prepare themselves for entering the job market or changing jobs.

Table 30-4	Physiological Changes in the Middle Adult as Found During Physical Assessment

BODY SYSTEM	FINDINGS
Integument	Intact condition
	Appropriate distribution of pigmentation
	Slow, progressive decrease in skin turgor
	Graying and loss of hair (Baldness patterns in males and established by age 55; hair loss after this time might have other causes.)
Head and neck	Symmetry of scalp, skull, and face
	Normal accessory organs of vision
Eyes	Visual acuity by Snellen chart that is less than 20/50
	Pupillary reaction to light and accommodation
	Normal visual fields and extraocular movements
	Normal retinal structures
Ears	Normal auditory structures and acuity
Nose, sinuses, and throat	Patent nares and intact sinuses, mouth, and pharynx
	Location of trachea at midline
	Nonpalpable lateral thyroid lobes
Thorax and lungs	Increased anteroposterior diameter
	Respiratory rate 16-20 breaths per minute and regular
	Ratio of respiratory rate to heart rate: 1:4
	Normal tactile fremitus, resonance, and breath sounds
Heart and vascular system	Normal heart sounds
	Systole: S1 less than S2 at base
	Diastole: S1 greater than S2 at apex
	Point of maximal impulse: at fifth intercostal space in midclavicular line and 2 cm or less in diameter
	Vital signs
	Temperature: 36.7°-37.6° C (97°-99.6° F)
	Pulse: 60-100 (conditioned athlete ≈ 50)
	Blood pressure: 95-140/60-90 mm Hg
	All pulses palpable
Breasts	Decreased size resulting from decreased muscle mass
	Normal nipples
Abdomen	No tenderness or organomegaly
	Decreased strength of abdominal muscles
Female reproductive system	Change in menstrual cycle and in duration and quality of menstrual flow
	"Hot flashes"
	Change in cervical mucosa
Male reproductive system	Normal penis and scrotum
	Prostatic enlargement in some individuals
Musculoskeletal system	Decreased muscle mass
	Decreased range of joint motion
Neurological system	Appropriate effect, appearance, and behavior
	Lucidity and appropriate level of cognitive ability
	Intact cranial nerves
	Adequate motor responses
	Responsive sensory system

PSYCHOSOCIAL DEVELOPMENT

The psychosocial changes in the middle adult may involve expected events, such as children moving away from home, or unexpected events, such as a marital separation or the death of a close friend. These changes may result in stress that can affect the middle adult's overall level of health. Nurses should assess the major life changes occurring in the middle adult and the impact that the changes have on that person's state of health. Nursing assessment should also include individual psychosocial factors such as coping mechanisms and sources of social support.

In the middle adult years, as children depart from the household, the family enters the postparental family stage. Time and financial demands on the parents decrease, and the couple faces the task of redefining their own relationship. As grandchildren arrive, grandparenting styles must be chosen. It is during this period that many middle-age adults begin to take on a healthier lifestyle. Although not advisable to wait until this stage in life to think about health promotion, "better late than never" does apply. Assessment of health promotion needs for the middle adult include adequate rest, leisure activities, regular exercise, good nutrition, reduction or cessation in the use of tobacco or alcohol, and regular screening examinations. Assessment of the middle adult's social environment is also important, including relationship concerns; communication and relationships with children, grandchildren, and aging parents; and care giver concerns with their own aging or disabled parents.

Career Transition. Career changes may occur by choice or as a result of changes in the work place or society. In recent decades, middle adults more often change occupations for a variety of reasons including limited upward mobility, decreasing availability of jobs, and to seek an occupation that is more challenging to the individual. In some cases technological advances or other changes force middle adults to seek new jobs. Such changes, particularly when unanticipated, may result in stress that can affect health, family relationships, self-concept, and other dimensions.

Sexuality. After the departure of their last child from the home, many couples recultivate their relationships and find increased marital and sexual satisfaction during middle age. The onset of menopause and the climacteric can affect the sexual health of the middle adult. A woman may desire increased sexual activity because pregnancy is no longer possible.

During middle age a man may notice changes in the strength of his erection and a decrease in his ability to experience repeated orgasm. Other factors influencing sexuality during this period include work stress, diminished health of one or both partners, and the use of prescription medications, for example, antihypertensive agents, with side effects that may influence sexual desire or functioning. Both partners may experience stresses related to sexual changes or a conflict between their sexual needs and self-perceptions and social attitudes or expectations (see Chapter 24).

Family Types. Psychosocial factors involving the family may include the stresses of singlehood, marital changes, transition of the family as children leave home, and the care of aging parents.

Singlehood. In 1990, 10% of adults between the ages of 35 to 59 years of age in the United States had never been married (U.S. Dept. of Commerce, 1992). Many of those are college-educated people who have embraced the philosophy of choice and freedom, have delayed marriage, and have delayed parenthood. Some middle-age adults who have chosen to remain single, however, have also opted to become parents either biologically or through adoption. Many single middle-age adults may have no relatives but share a family-type relationship with close friends or work associates. Consequently, some single middle-age adults may feel isolated during traditional "family" holidays such as Thanksgiving or Christmas. In times of illness, middle-age adults who have chosen to remain single and childless may have to rely on other relatives or friends, increasing caregiving demands of those family members who may also have other care giving responsibilities. Nursing assessment of single middle-age adults should include a thorough assessment of psychosocial factors including the individual's definition of family and available support systems.

Marital Changes. Marital changes that may occur during middle age include death of a spouse, separation, divorce, and the choice of remarrying or remaining single. A widowed, separated, or divorced client goes through a period of grief and loss in which it is necessary to adapt to the change in marital status. Normal grieving progresses through a series of phases, and resolution of grief may take a year or more. The nurse should assess effective coping of the middle-age adult to the grief and loss associated with certain life changes.

If a single middle-age adult decides to marry, the stressors of marriage are similar to those for the young adult. In addition, the couple may have to cope with the social expectations and pressures related to marriage.

Family Transitions. The departure of the last child from the home may be a stressor. Many parents welcome freedom from child-rearing responsibilities, whereas others feel lonely or without direction because of this change. Eventually parents must reassess their marriage and are able to resolve conflicts and plan for the future. Occasionally this readjustment phase may lead to marital conflicts, separation, and divorce (Fawcett, 1993).

Care of Aging Parents. Increasing life spans in the United States and Canada have led to increased numbers of older adults in the population. Therefore greater numbers of middle-age adults must address the personal and social issues confronting their aging parents. As many middle adults find themselves in the "sandwich generation" caught between the responsibilities of caring for dependent children as well as for aging and ailing parents, the needs of the care givers is an area that continues to grow.

Housing, employment, health, and economic realities have changed the traditional social expectations between generations in families. The middle adult and the older adult parent may have conflicting priorities related to their relationship while the older adult strives to remain independent. Negotiations and compromises help in defining and resolving problems. Nurses deal with middle and older adults in the community, long-term care facilities, and hospitals. The nurse can help identify the health needs of both groups and can assist the multigenerational family in determining the health and community resources available to them as they make decisions and plans. The nurse should also assess family relationships to determine family members' perceptions of responsibility and loyalty in relation to caring for older adult members. Assessment of environmental resources (e.g., number of rooms in the house, stairwells) in relation to the complexity of health care demands for the older adult is also important.

HEALTH CONCERNS

Physiological Concerns. Physiological concerns for the middle adult include stress, chronic illnesses, level of wellness, and the formation of positive health habits.

Stress. Because middle adults are experiencing physiological changes and face certain health realities, their perceptions of health and health behaviors are often important factors in maintaining health. Today's complex world makes individuals more prone to stress-related illnesses such as heart attacks, hypertension, migraine headaches, ulcers, colitis, autoimmune disease, backache, arthritis, and cancer. In 1992, the death rate (per 100,000 population) attributable to heart attacks was 9.7 for 35 to 44 year olds; 42.7 for 45 to 54 year olds; and 131.1 for 55 to 64 year olds. For the same year and age groups, the death rates attributable to hypertensive heart disease were 0.1, 0.3, and 1.1, respectively (U.S. DHHS, 1995a).

When adults seek health care, the nurse's focus on the goal of wellness can guide clients to evaluate health behaviors, lifestyle, and environment. Attention to risk factors that can be altered to improve the client's health, such as stress, obesity, use of tobacco, excessive alcohol consumption, poor nutrition, and unsafe sexual practices, can increase the quality of life and add years to it.

Existence of Chronic Illnesses. Chronic illnesses such as diabetes mellitus, hypertension, rheumatoid arthritis, chronic obstructive pulmonary disease, or multiple sclerosis may affect the roles and responsibilities assumed by the middle adult. Strained family relationships, modifications in family activities, increased health care tasks, increased financial stress, the need for housing adaptation, social isolation, medical concerns, and grieving may all result from chronic illness. The degree of disability and the client's perception of both the illness and the disability determine the extent to which lifestyle changes will occur. A few examples of the problems experienced by clients who develop debilitating chronic illness during adulthood include role reversal, changes in sexual behavior, and alterations in self-image. Along with the current health status of the chronically ill middle adult, the nurse must assess the knowledge base of both the client and family regarding the medical course of the illness and the prognosis for the client; the coping mechanisms of the client and family; adherence to treatment and rehabilitation regimens; and the need for community and social services along with appropriate referrals.

Levels of Wellness. The nurse must be able to assess the health status of the middle adult client. Such assessment offers direction for planning nursing care and is useful in evaluating the effectiveness of nursing interventions. Table 30-4, which shows the physiological changes of the middle adult, can be used with other standard assessment techniques as a guide for physical assessment (see Chapter 33).

Forming Positive Health Habits. A habit is a person's usual practice or manner of behavior. This behavior pattern is reinforced by frequent repetition until it becomes the individual's customary way of behaving. Some habits support health, such as exercise and brushing and flossing the teeth each day. Other habits involve risk factors to health, such as smoking or eating foods with little or no nutritional value.

During assessment the nurse frequently obtains data indicating positive and negative health behaviors by the client. Examples of positive health behaviors include regular exercise; adherence to good dietary habits; avoidance of excess consumption of alcohol; participation in routine screening and diagnostic tests (lab work for serum cholesterol, mammography) for disease prevention and health promotion; and lifestyle changes to reduce stress. In the planning, implementation, and evaluation phases, the nurse helps the client maintain habits that protect health and offers healthier alternatives to poor habits.

Psychosocial Concerns. Two common psychosocial health concerns of the middle adult are anxiety and depression.

Anxiety. Anxiety is a critical maturational phenomenon related to change, conflict, and perceived control of the environment (Haber et al, 1992). Adults often experience anxiety in response to the physiological and psychosocial changes of middle age. Such anxiety can motivate the adult to rethink life goals and can stimulate productivity. For some adults, however, this anxiety precipitates psychosomatic illness and preoccupation with death. In this case the middle adult views life as being half or more over and thinks in terms of the time left to live.

Clearly, a life-threatening illness, marital transition, or job stressor increases the anxiety of the client and family. The nurse may need to use crisis-intervention or stress-management techniques to help the client adapt to the changes of the middle adult years (see Chapter 22).

Depression. Depression is a mood disorder that manifests itself in many ways. Although the most frequent age of onset is between ages 25 to 44, it is common among adults in the middle years and may have many causes (Haber et al, 1992). The risk factors for depression include being female, disappointments or losses at work, school or in family relationships, departure of the last child from the home, and family history. In fact, the incidence of depression in women is twice that of men (Haber et al, 1992). Persons experiencing mild depression describe themselves as feeling sad, blue, downcast, down in the dumps, and tearful. Other symptoms include alterations in sleep patterns such as difficulty in sleeping (insomnia) or sleeping too much (hypersomnia), irritability, feelings of social disinterest, and decreased alertness. Physical changes such as weight loss or weight gain, headaches, or feelings of fatigue regardless of the amount of rest may also be depressive symptoms. Depression that occurs during the middle years is commonly characterized by moderate-to-high anxiety and physical complaints. Mood changes and depression are common phenomena during menopause (Sheehy, 1992). Depression may be worsened by the abuse of alcohol or other substances. Nursing assessment of the depressed middle adult includes focused data collection regarding individual and family history of depression, mood changes, cognitive changes, behavioral and social changes, and physical changes. Assessment data should be collected from both the client and the client's family, since family data may be particularly important depending on the level of depression being experienced by the middle adult.

Nursing Diagnosis

The nursing assessment of the young or middle adult reveals clusters of defining characteristics that indicate potential or actual nursing diagnoses (see the diagnostic process box on p. 563). A diagnostic statement cannot be made without appropriate defining characteristics that provide the rationale for the nursing diagnosis (see the diagnoses box on p. 563). The nursing diagnostic statement should include expected or anticipated causes or etiologies for the statement. For example, the assessment of two clients and their families revealed distinct stressors that were causing each family to experience abrupt changes in lifestyle and daily activities. This resulted in the identification of *ineffective individual coping*. However, in one family the stressor was the death of a spouse, but in the second family the stressor was a new baby within the home. The inclusion of the etiology statement enables the nurse to quickly target specific goals and interventions for causative

Examples of NANDA Nursing Diagnoses for Young and Middle Adults

Impaired adjustment *related to:*
- Changes in physical appearance
- Changes in body image

Ineffective family or individual coping *related to:*
- Infertility
- Feelings about death of spouse
- Adjustment to baby
- Loss of job

Altered family processes *related to:*
- Chronic or acute illness
- Feelings about death of spouse
- Marital problems
- Financial problems

Altered sexuality patterns *related to:*
- Infertility
- Pregnancy
- Menopause or climacteric

Altered health maintenance *related to:*
- Risk factors (e.g., smoking, substance abuse)
- Lack of knowledge of positive health behaviors

factors for each diagnostic statement. The nurse uses critical thinking to develop a plan that focuses on removing the etiology of the problem through nursing interventions.

Planning

The identification and formulation of nursing diagnoses are followed by the development of a nursing care plan (see the care plan on p. 564). When providing nursing care for young and middle adults, the nurse must recognize that the needs of clients, families, and communities are interconnected. For example, culture, ethnicity, and psychosocial, spiritual, and biological characteristics are variables to consider when planning care. The manner in which the individual and the surrounding community view these variables may influence the individual's response to the plan of care.

For each diagnosis, the nurse partners with the client and family to identify the goal of care and expected outcomes. In the case of the family with a newborn baby, the goal for ineffective coping might be to assume supportive parental roles. The expected outcomes provide stepping stones for evaluating the family's progress. For example, the mother and newborn will jointly participate in nurturing and the father will participate in infant care. Nursing interventions are designed to achieve the expected outcomes so that goals will be met. Throughout the client's care, the expected outcomes become the nurse's focus for evaluating success of the plan of care.

Nursing interventions are individualized for the client and are modified accordingly for primary, acute, or restorative nursing care. While developing a plan, the nurse must also consider the client's developmental needs. A middle-age adult, for example, will want to be very independent, make his or her own decisions, and return to a functional status as soon as possible.

General nursing goals for young or middle adults reflect their reactions to day-to-day life events as opposed to nursing goals that result from their responses to specific illnesses or physiological, psychosocial, emotional, or spiritual needs. The goals of nursing for the young or middle adult can include the following:

1. Improved knowledge about the impact of risk factors on level of health
2. Improved health-promotion activities
3. Improved communication within their family structures
4. Fewer experiences of illnesses and inability to problem solve

Sample Nursing Diagnostic Process for Young and Middle Adults

ASSESSMENT ACTIVITIES	DEFINING CHARACTERISTICS	NURSING DIAGNOSES
Ask client about diet, exercise, and self-examination patterns	Lack of knowledge regarding basic health practices Poor diet	**Altered health maintenance** related to excessive alcohol use
Ask client about use of alcohol, nonprescription drugs, and tobacco	Verbalizes need for alcohol daily	
Review previous medical record	Motor vehicle accident with minor trauma (high blood alcohol level) Hospitalizations for alcohol abuse	
Observe family's interaction with ill family member	Family system unable to meet physical, emotional, social, or spiritual needs of members	**Altered family processes** related to chronic illness of spouse
Listen to family discussion	Family unable to adapt	
Observe nonverbal interactions	Poor communication	

Sample Nursing Care Plan for Altered Health Maintenance

NURSING DIAGNOSIS: **Altered health maintenance** related to excessive use of alcohol
DEFINITION: Altered health maintenance is the inability to identify, manage, and/or seek help to maintain health (Kim, McFarland, McLane, 1995).

GOALS	EXPECTED OUTCOMES	INTERVENTIONS	RATIONALE
Client will verbalize impact of alcohol excess on level of health by next home visit	Client will state three physiological, emotional, and psychosocial effects of alcohol excess (2/21)	Provide client with accurate information regarding the adverse health consequences of prolonged excessive alcohol use	Accurate information encourages further clarification of the client's problem, and may assist the client in making informed choices or decisions
		Encourage client to discuss the impact that excessive alcohol use has had on his own life and family	Consequences of alcoholism include physical health problems as well as disruption of family life and lowered self-esteem (Haber et al, 1992)
Client will modify behavior and remain free of alcohol by 6 months	Client will initiate actions to modify his behavior regarding alcohol use (8/31)	Provide client with information on 12-step program	Accurate information will assist client in making informed choices or decisions
		Encourage family involvement and support of client through program	12-Step self-help groups help the client develop an identity around the disease and acknowledge that recovery built on abstinence is a daily process and requires peer support (Haber et al 1992)

CLIENT TEACHING
for Positive Health Habits

OBJECTIVE
■ Client will increase exercise patterns to include three 1-mile walks per week to assist weight loss and improve cardiopulmonary functions.

TEACHING STRATEGIES
■ Review with client the daily work schedule and identify potential times for exercise.
■ Inform client about the effect of exercise on weight control and improved cardiac function.
■ Demonstrate how to calculate target heart rate and assess pulse correctly.
■ Provide warm-up and cool-down exercises and demonstrate how to do them.
■ Instruct client about support shoes for walking exercises.

EVALUATION
■ Have client keep log of exercise periods.
■ Have client demonstrate pulse measurement.
■ Have client demonstrate warm-up and cool-down exercises.
■ Inspect client's feet for blisters or sores.

Implementation

Nursing interventions for the young or middle adult are generalized into changing health habits and teaching health promotion and stress management. For some young and middle adults, the nurse may be the first resource identified to assist them in pursuing a healthier lifestyle.

Changing Health Habits

Health teaching and health counseling are often directed at improving health habits (see the box at left). The more fully the nurse understands the dynamics of behavior and habits, the more likely interventions will help the client to achieve or reinforce health-promoting behaviors.

To help clients form positive health habits the nurse becomes a teacher and facilitator. By providing information about how the body functions and how habits are formed and changed, the nurse raises clients' levels of knowledge regarding the potential impact of behavior on health. A nurse cannot change clients' habits. Clients have control of and are responsible for their own behaviors. The nurse can explain psychological principles of changing habits and offer information about health risks. The nurse can also offer positive reinforcement (such as praise and rewards) for health-directed behaviors and decisions. Such reinforcement increases the likelihood that the behavior will be repeated. Ultimately, however, the client decides which behaviors will become habits of daily living.

The nurse may assist young and middle adults in considering factors such as prevention of STDs, substance abuse, and accident prevention, in relation to decreasing health

<table>
<tr><td colspan="2">

Barriers to Change

EXTERNAL BARRIERS
- Lack of facilities
- Lack of materials
- Lack of social supports

INTERNAL BARRIERS
- Lack of knowledge
- Lack of motivation
- Insufficient skills to effect change in health habits
- Undefined short- and long-term goals

</td></tr>
</table>

risks. For example, clients should be provided with factual information on sexually transmitted disease causes, symptoms, and transmission. The nurse should discuss methods of protection during sexual activity with the client in an open and nonjudgmental manner and reinforce the importance of practicing "safe sex" (see Chapter 24). The nurse can provide counseling and support for clients seeking treatment for substance abuse. The nurse can assist clients to recognize and alter unsafe habits and potential health hazards (see Chapter 36). The nurse should also encourage clients to express their feelings to promote problem solving as well as recognition of risk factors by clients themselves.

Barriers to change do exist (see the box above). Unless these barriers are minimized or eliminated, it is futile to encourage the client to take actions that are going to be blocked.

Health Promotion

Community health programs for young and middle adults are designed to prevent illness, promote health, and detect disease in the early stages. Nurses can make valuable contributions to the community's health by taking an active part in the planning of screening and teaching programs.

Family planning, birthing, and parenting skills are program topics in which adults might be interested. Health screening for diabetes, hypertension, eye disease, and cancer is a good opportunity for the nurse to perform assessment and provide health teaching and health counseling.

Health education programs can promote changes in behavior and lifestyle. The nurse as health teacher offers in-

formation that enables the client to make decisions about health practices. Changes to more positive health practices during young and middle adulthood may lead to fewer or less complicated health problems as an older adult. During health counseling the nurse and client design a plan of action that addresses the client's health and well-being. Through objective problem solving, the nurse helps the client grow and change.

Regardless of the age of its members and its structure, the family faces certain health tasks. The nurse as health teacher and counselor understands the autonomy of the family and supports it while promoting family health.

Nursing roles include community-centered care, hospital-based acute care, and restorative care. Participation in community health programs for the adult or family often requires many nursing roles and skills.

Stress Reduction

Throughout life, people are exposed to many stressors (see Chapter 22). After these stressors are identified, the client and nurse can work together to intervene and modify the stress response. Specific interventions for stress reduction can fall into three categories. First, the frequency of stress-producing situations is minimized. Together the nurse and client identify approaches to prevent stressful situations, such as habituation, change avoidance, time blocking, time management, and environmental modification. The second category is psychophysiological preparation to increase stress resistance, such as increasing self-esteem, improving assertiveness, redirecting goal alternatives, and reorienting cognitive appraisal. Last, the physiological response to stress is avoided. The nurse uses relaxation techniques (see Chapter 43), imagery, and biofeedback to recondition the client's response to stress. Chapter 22 explains these general interventions in greater detail.

 ## Evaluation

Each young or middle adult has different health goals. The success of the nurse and client in achieving these goals is determined during evaluation (see the evaluation box below). Therefore, when the nurse evaluates the plan of care it is important to determine whether the desired client behaviors or responses (outcome criteria) that were identified in the goal statement have been accomplished.

 ## Sample Evaluation of Interventions for Altered Health Maintenance

GOALS	EVALUATIVE MEASURES	EXPECTED OUTCOMES
Client will verbalize impact of alcohol excess on level of health by next home visit	Ask client to describe his understanding of the effects of excessive alcohol use	Client will state three physiological, emotional, and psychosocial effects of alcohol excess
Client will modify behavior and remain free of alcohol by 6 months	Client will supply proof of attendance at 12-step self-help group such as Alcoholics Anonymous or other alcohol-abstinence support group	Client will initiate actions to modify his behavior regarding alcohol use

If outcomes have not been met, revision to the plan or a reassessment of the client's nursing diagnosis becomes necessary.

The plan of care for a client diagnosed with a sexually transmitted disease might include the goal "The client will understand the cause of the condition and how to prevent further infection." When evaluating the plan of care for this client, the nurse observes that the client is able to describe how the infection occurred (through unprotected sexual activity) and methods for minimizing the risk of future infection (using condoms during future sexual relations). The nurse evaluates that the goal has been achieved since the client was able to verbalize understanding of how he or she became infected and how to prevent further infection, both of the responses are outcome criteria specified in the original goal statement.

When evaluating therapies designed to assist clients in adjusting or coping with adult life difficulties, good communication skills are essential. Evaluation requires listening, empathy, and an accurate appraisal of the client's behaviors. A caring approach will assist in determining the client's views about the direction and success of the nurse's plan of care.

■ KEY CONCEPTS ■

► Adult development involves orderly and sequential changes in characteristics and attitudes that adults experience over time.

► Many changes experienced by the young adult are related to the natural process of maturation and socialization.

► Maturity is reached when the young adult attains a balance of growth in the physiological, psychosocial, and cognitive areas.

► Young adults are in a stable period of physical development, except for changes related to pregnancy.

► Cognitive development continues throughout the young and middle adult years.

► Emotional health of young adults is correlated with the ability to address and resolve personal and social problems.

► Young adults must choose a career and decide whether to remain single or marry and begin a family.

► Pregnant women need to understand physiological changes occurring in each trimester.

► Cognitive and psychosocial changes and health concerns during pregnancy and the puerperium affect the parents, the siblings, and often the extended family.

► Prenatal care reduces maternal and fetal mortality and morbidity.

► Midlife transition begins when a person becomes aware that physiological and psychosocial changes signify passage to another stage in life.

► Erikson and Havighurst have described the primary developmental tasks of the middle adult.

► Two significant physiological changes of the middle years are menopause in women and the climacteric in men.

► Cognitive changes are rare in middle age except in cases of illness or physical trauma.

► Psychosocial changes for middle adults may be related to career transition, sexuality, marital changes, family transition, and care of aging parents.

► Health concerns of middle adults commonly involve stress-related illnesses, health assessment, and adoption of positive health habits.

■ KEY TERMS ■

Braxton Hicks contractions, p. 557

Climacteric, p. 559

Doula, p. 553

Infertility, p. 556

Lactation, p. 553

Maturity, p. 550

Menopause, p. 559

Morning sickness, p. 557

Nesting, p. 557

Prenatal care, p. 557

Puerperium, p. 558

■ CRITICAL THINKING EXERCISES ■

1. You are providing health education to a couple in their mid-30s. What information do you need to obtain during your initial assessments to determine the general health risks and the risks that are specific to their developmental stage?

2. Your client confides that she wants to get pregnant. However, before getting pregnant she wants to modify her lifestyle to include more positive health habits. What do you need to know before you can intervene and assist this client in changing her lifestyle habits?

3. You suspect that your middle-age client is having difficulty adjusting to the fact that the children are out on their own and that both he and his wife are retiring. What do you need to know before designing a care plan to ease these role transitions?

REFERENCES

Alan Guttmacher Institute: *Sex and America's teenagers*, New York, 1994, Alan Guttmacher Institute.

Bobak IM: *Maternity nursing*, ed 4, St Louis, 1995, Mosby.

Bobak IM, Jensen MD: *Maternity & gynecologic care*, ed 5, St Louis, 1993, Mosby.

Bradley-Springer LA: Reproductive decision-making in the age of AIDS, *Image J Nurs Sch* 26(3):241, 1994.

Children's Defense Fund: *The state of America's children yearbook,* Washington, DC, 1995, Children's Defense Fund.

Coffman S, Levitt MJ, Brown L: Effects of clarification of support expectations in prenatal couples, *Nurs Res* 43(2):111, 1994.

Dickason EJ, Silverman BL, Schult MO: *Maternal-infant nursing care,* St Louis, 1994, Mosby.

Diekelmann JL: The young adult: the choice is health or illness, *Am J Nurs* 76:1276, 1976.

Edelman CL, Mandle CL: *Health promotion throughout the lifespan,* ed 3, St Louis, 1994, Mosby.

Edge V, Miller M: *Women's health care,* St Louis, 1994, Mosby.

Erikson EH: *Childhood and society,* ed 2, New York, 1963, Norton.

Erikson EH: *Identity: youth and crisis,* New York, 1968, Norton.

Erikson EH: *The life cycle completed: a review,* New York, 1982, Norton.

Fawcett CS: *Family psychiatric nursing,* St Louis, 1993, Mosby.

Finsterbusch K, McKenna G: *Taking sides: clashing views on controversial social issues,* ed 7, Guilford, Conn, 1992, Dushkin.

Gilligan C: *In a different voice,* Cambridge, Mass, 1993, Harvard University Press.

Gordon S: *Prisoners of men's dreams: striking out for a new feminine future,* Boston, 1991, Little, Brown.

Haber J et al: *Comprehensive psychiatric nursing,* St Louis, 1992, Mosby.

Halman LJ, Andrews FM, Abbey A: Gender differences and perceptions about childbearing among infertile couples, *J Obst Gyn Neonatal Nurs* 23(7):593, 1994.

Havighurst RJ: Successful aging. In Williams RH, Tibbits C, Donahue W, editors: *Process of aging,* vol 1, New York, 1972, Atherton.

Hooker K, Kaus CR: Health-related possible selves in young and middle adulthood, *Psychology & Aging* 9(1):126, 1994.

Killion C: Pregnancy: A critical time to target STDs, *Amer J Maternal-Child Nurs* 19(3):156, 1994.

Kim MJ, McFarland GK, McLane AM: *Pocket guide to nursing diagnoses,* ed 6, St Louis, 1995, Mosby.

Lawrence RA: *Breastfeeding: a guide for the medical profession,* ed 4, St Louis, 1994, Mosby.

Levinson D et al: *The seasons of a man's life,* New York, 1978, Knopf.

Masters WH, Johnson VE: *Human sexual response,* Boston, 1970, Little, Brown.

Pascoe JM: Social support during labor and duration of labor: a community-based study, *Public Nurs Journal* 10(2):97, 1993.

Price SA, Wilson LM: *Pathophysiology,* ed 4, St Louis, 1992, Mosby.

Rosenfeld J: Maternal work outside the home and its effect on women and their families, *J Am Med Women's Assoc* 7:47, 1992.

Ruchala PL, Halstead LK: The postpartum experience: a time of adjustment and change, *Mat Child Nurs J* 22(3):83, 1994.

Sheehy G: *The silent passage: menopause,* New York, 1992, Random House.

Sheehy G: *New passages: mapping your life across time,* New York, 1995, Random House.

Stanhope M, Lancaster J: *Community health nursing: process and practice for promoting health,* ed 4, St Louis, 1996, Mosby.

U.S. Department of Commerce: *1990 Census of population: general population characteristics, United States,* Washington, DC, 1992, Bureau of the Census.

U.S. DHHS, Public Health Service: *Monthly vital statistics report: advance report of final mortality statistics, 1992* 43(6), Supplement, Hyattsville, Md, 1995, Centers for Disease Control and Prevention, National Center for Health Statistics.

U.S. DHHS, Public Health Service: *Advance data: office visits for glaucoma: United States, 1991-92,* 262, Hyattsville, Md, 1995a, Centers for Disease Control and Prevention, National Center for Health Statistics.

Whall AL, Fawcett J: *Family theory development in nursing: state of the science and art,* Philadelphia, 1991, Davis.

Winger G, Hofmann FG, Woods JH: *A handbook on drug and alcohol abuse,* New York, 1992, Oxford University Press.

ADDITIONAL READINGS

Bernhard LA, Sheppard L: Health, symptoms, self-care, and dyadic adjustment in menopausal women, *J Obst Gyn Neonatal Nurs* 22(5):456, 1993.

Burns CM: Toward Healthy People 2000: the role of the nurse practitioner and health promotion, *J Amer Academy Nurs Practitioners* 6(1):29, 1994.

Gjerdingen DK, Chaloner KM: The relationship of women's postpartum mental health to employment, childbirth, and social support, *J Family Practice* 38(5):465, 1994.

Hartweg DL: Self-care actions of healthy middle-aged women to promote well-being, *Image J Nurs Sch* 42(4):221, 1993.

## Chapter 31

Older Adult

Objectives

Mastery of content in this chapter will enable the student to:

▶ Define the key terms listed.

▶ Describe common myths and stereotypes about older adults.

▶ Discuss nurses' attitudes toward older adults.

▶ Discuss biological and psychosocial theories of aging.

▶ State and discuss developmental tasks of the older adult.

▶ Describe physiological changes of aging.

▶ Describe cognitive changes of dementia and delirium found in some older adults.

▶ Describe common causes of dementia and delirium.

▶ Discuss psychosocial changes of retirement, social isolation, sexuality, housing, and death, to which older adults must adjust.

▶ Discuss physical and psychosocial health concerns of older adults and related nursing interventions.

▶ Describe community-based and institutional health care services available to older adults.

▶ Formulate a plan of care and interventions for an older adult with selected nursing diagnoses.

▶ Evaluate the plan of care and interventions for an older adult with selected nursing diagnoses.

Older adulthood traditionally begins after retirement, usually between 65 and 75 years of age. The number of people in this age group is increasing at a dramatic rate, and demographers project a continuing increase in the older adult population well into the next century (Fig. 31-1). Health professionals are spending increasingly more time with older adults in all health care settings, therefore they must focus on identifying and meeting their special needs. Older adults are seeking greater participation in identification, definition, and resolution of issues affecting them. A greater incidence of chronic health problems, technological advances, and contemporary economic, social, ethical, and health issues has prompted health care professionals to focus on improving the duration and quality of life (Stanhope and Lancaster, 1992).

Increased life expectancy and a relatively high birth rate during the early twentieth century has contributed to the increase of this "graying" population. Not only are large numbers of people living to reach age 65, but they are living longer. The nearly three million people over age 85 represent the fastest growing subset, with a growth rate of nearly 3 times that of the overall older population. The life expectancy at birth for men born in the urban United States is 72.7 years; for women it is 79.6 years (Ebersole and Hess, 1994). The older adult population is expanding in all cultural and ethnic groups in the United States and Canada. In the United States, African Americans compose approximately 8% of persons 65 years and older. This is expected to increase to 11% by 2000 (Stanhope and Lancaster, 1992). Population growth of other races (primarily Asian, Pacific Islander, and Native Americans) is rapid. This group has tripled in number since 1970 and is expected to be 50% of the population or larger by 2000 (U.S. Bureau of the Census, 1993). Older adults are distributed among the states in the same pattern as the total population. However, concentrations are found in some larger states, as well as the northeast and northcentral regions (Fig. 31-2).

Nursing care of older adults poses special challenges because of the diversity in physiological, cognitive, and psychosocial health. Older adults vary in their levels of functional ability. The majority are active, involved, productive members of their communities. A smaller number have lost the ability to care for themselves, are confused or withdrawn, and are unable to make decisions concerning their needs.

Nursing assessment of an older adult is a complex and challenging process that must take into account the following points to ensure an age-specific approach (Lueckenotte, 1994):

1. *The interrelationship between physical and psychosocial aspects of aging.* For the older person, a reduced ability to respond to stress, the increased frequency and multiplicity of loss, and the physical changes associated with normal aging may combine to place the person at high risk. Although the interaction of these physical and psychosocial factors can be serious, the nurse should not assume that all older adults have signs, symptoms, or behaviors representing decrement and decline. The older client's strengths and abilities must also be identified. Careful consideration then of the interrelationship between physical and psychosocial factors in every client situation is essential.

2. *The effects of disease and disability on functional status.* Aging does not necessarily equate with disease and disability. Most older people remain functionally independent despite the increasing prevalence of chronic disease with

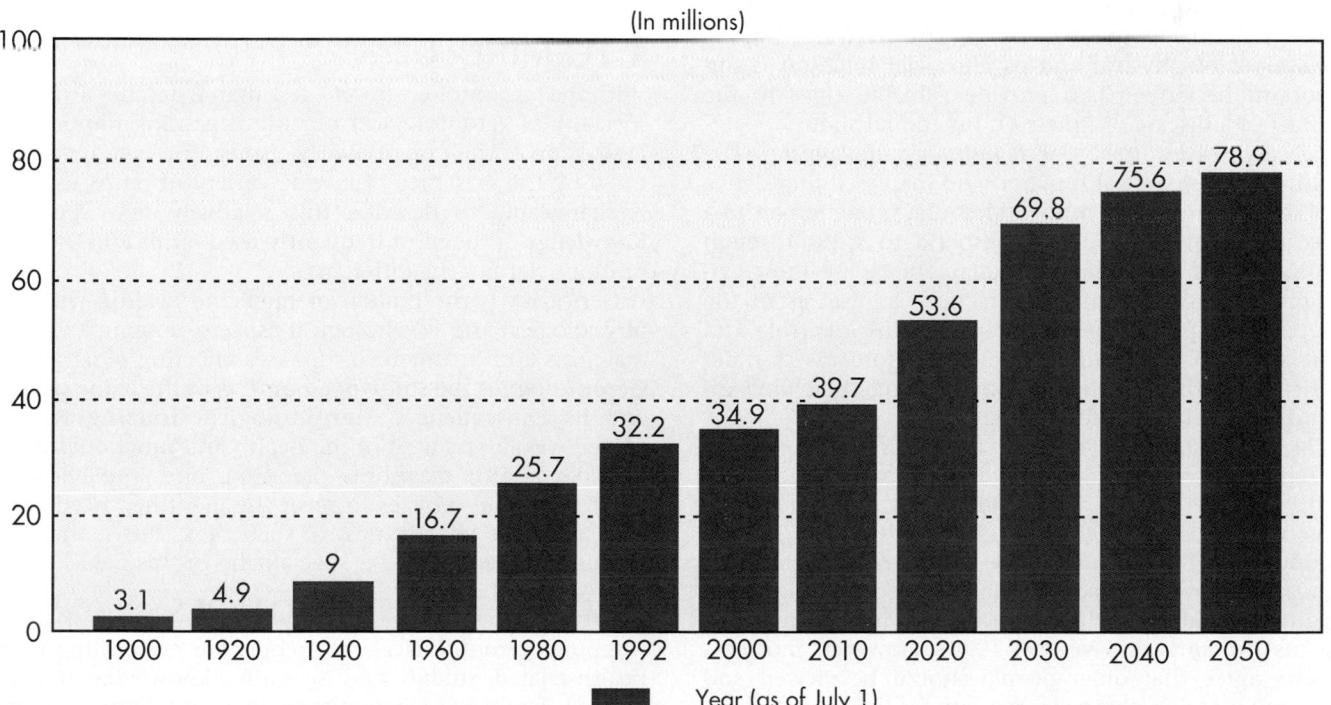

(In millions)

Fig. 31-1 Population growth and projections for older adults. *(Modified from Lueckenotte A: Textbook of gerontologic nursing, St Louis, 1996, Mosby.)*

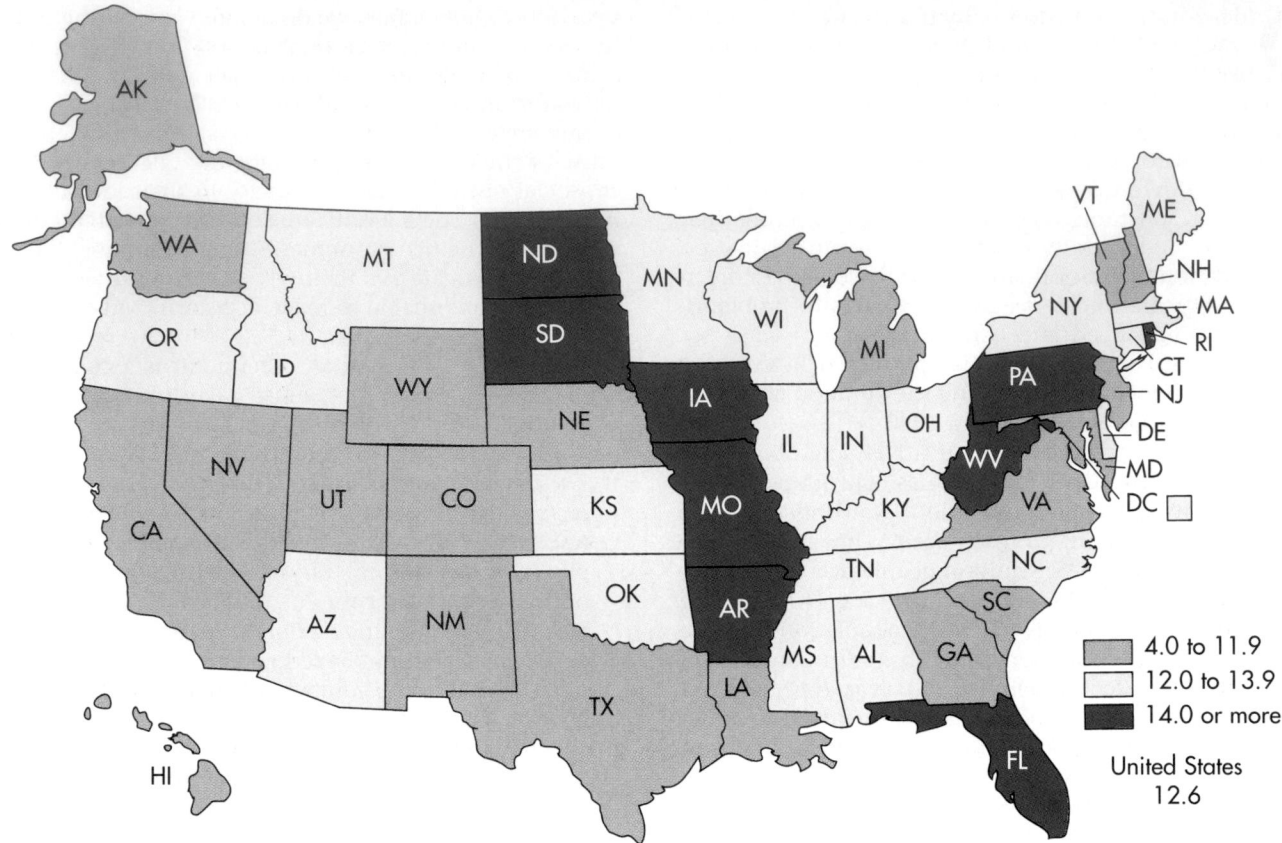

Fig. 31-2 Percentage of total state population 65 years and older: 1990. *(Modified from Lueckenotte A:* Textbook of gerontologic nursing, *St Louis, 1996, Mosby.)*

advancing age. However, studies support that chronic disease increases the older adult's vulnerability to functional decline (Guralnik, 1994). Therefore nursing assessment of physical and psychosocial function is important because it can provide valuable clues to the effect of a disease or illness on functional status.

3. *The decreased efficiency of homeostatic mechanisms.* Declining physiological function and increased prevalence of disease, especially in the oldest old, is due in part to a reduction in the ability to respond to stress through homeostasis. The deficits in adaptability are most evident in neuroendocrine interaction, as well as in the separate responses of these two systems (Ebersole and Hess, 1994). The nurse should therefore assess older clients for the presence of stressors and their physical and emotional manifestations.

4. *The lack of standards for health and illness norms.* The established norms for diagnostic testing, pathological conditions, and growth and development in older people are constantly changing as more scientific studies are conducted. But because of the lack of research in these areas, disagreement persists among experts on aging regarding what constitutes "normal" in any of the above areas (Abrams and Berkow, 1990). However, most experts agree that older people should be viewed and treated individually to compensate for the lack of definitive standards. The nurse can then compare the older person's own previous patterns of health and function

with the current status in determining the overall plan of care.

■ TERMINOLOGY

With the "gerontology boom" less than 2 decades away, the specialty of gerontological nursing is gaining importance. Discussion of the care of older persons, however, is complicated by the existence of a wide variety of terms used interchangeably to describe this relatively new specialty. Knowledge of the most frequently used terms and their definitions clarifies the differences.

Geriatrics is the branch of medicine dealing with the physiological and psychological aspects of aging and with diagnosis and treatment of diseases affecting older adults. **Gerontology** is the study of all aspects of the aging process and its consequences. **Gerontological nursing** is concerned with assessment of the health and functional status of older adults; diagnosis, planning, and implementing health care and services to meet the identified needs; and evaluating the effectiveness of such care. This is the term most often used by nurses specializing in this field.

■ MYTHS AND STEREOTYPES

Although gerontological researchers are performing more health-related studies and scientific knowledge has expanded, many false stereotypes persist. Some persons believe that older persons lack understanding and are forgetful, rigid, bored, and unpleasant. Furthermore, older adults are often stereotyped as ill, crippled, hard of hearing, and bald. Many people believe that most older adults are institutionalized. In fact, only about 5% of the older adult population resides in institutional settings (AARP, 1992).

Although financial constraints on older adults are significant, 87% of people 65 years and older have incomes above poverty level (AARP, 1992). However, it should be noted that the incomes of most older persons are fixed or do not rise as quickly as inflationary increases in the cost of basic necessities.

Many people incorrectly believe that older adults have decreased learning ability. As a result, health care professionals often fail to provide health education opportunities for them because they wrongly assume that older clients cannot learn to care for themselves (Stanhope and Lancaster, 1992). Theis (1991) noted that older people have a decrease in fluid intelligence, which includes the basic components of information processing and reasoning, but compensate with an increase in crystallized intelligence, the content and contextual elaboration of reasoning and knowledge. Additionally, a significant learning difference for older people is the increasing time required for acquiring knowledge or skill and retrieving information from memory (Ebersole and Hess, 1990). Therefore the nurse educating older clients should (1) provide more trials to transfer newly learned material to long-term memory, (2) give opportunities for frequent rehearsing of newly learned material, and (3) use a self-paced approach (Weinrich, Boyd, and Nussbaum, 1989).

There are many common misconceptions concerning older adults and sex (see the box below). Kain, Reilly, and Schultz (1990) report that society's views about sex and older people is primarily negative and that the persistence of such views inhibits the expression of sexuality among older adults. But the landmark study of Masters and Johnson (1986) demonstrated that older adults continued to enjoy sexual relationships throughout each decade of life.

Nurses too are susceptible to the myths and anxieties held by society toward the sexuality of older people (Wallace, 1996). Nurses must realize that the need to express sexuality continues among older adults, but because of disabling medical conditions, treatments, and normal aging changes, that expression may be difficult or even impossible. Additionally, the availability of mates, privacy, and living arrangements may also alter sexual activity. Nurses are in an ideal position to assess the above factors and intervene to prevent or correct sexual problems or concerns.

As people age, their contributions become less appreciated. Our society values attractiveness, energy, and youth. Some people believe that older adults become worthless after they leave the workforce. These notions have led to the concept of **ageism**, which is discrimination against people because of increasing age, just as people who are racists and sexists discriminate because of skin color and gender. However, sexists and racists never become concerned about changing their attitudes because neither their own gender nor skin color will change. In contrast, an ageist will eventually become old. This realization produces anxiety and a reluctance to accept aging as a normal process.

Unfortunately, when a youth image dominates society, the most diversified segment of our population is ignored. Older adults have a unique perspective on social, economic, and technological developments. In 100 years, society has progressed from riding horse-drawn carriages to space shuttle flights. Older adults may have experienced two world wars, the Spanish civil war, and the Korean, the Vietnam, and the Gulf wars.

In regard to health care, older adults have lived from the era of the family doctor into the age of specialization. They have seen the establishment of our first national health insurance, the Medicare and Medicaid systems, and are currently living with the changes imposed by health care reform.

▌ NURSES' ATTITUDES TOWARD OLDER ADULTS

It is important for nurses to assess their attitudes toward aging because these attitudes influence nursing care. To provide effective care, nurses must foster positive attitudes toward the aged (Fig. 31-3). Negative attitudes may result in a reduction in clients' sense of security, adequacy, and well-being. Furthermore, such attitudes may lead to a decline in the quality of care. Clients in long-term care facilities present a special challenge to nurses. These clients often view themselves as losers, and may be viewed that way by society as well. The nurse can promote independence and self-esteem of clients who feel that life is not worth living.

Common Myths and Misconceptions About Sex and Aging

- Sex does not matter. The later years are supposed to be (and usually are) sexless.
- Interest in sex is abnormal for older people.
- It is all right for older men to seek younger women as sex partners, but it is ridiculous for older women to be sexually involved with younger men.
- In institutions, older people should be separated according to sex to avoid problems for the staff and criticism by families and the community.
- Emission of semen during sexual activity weakens men and therefore should be avoided in old age.
- Masturbation is a childish activity that should not continue after adolescence.

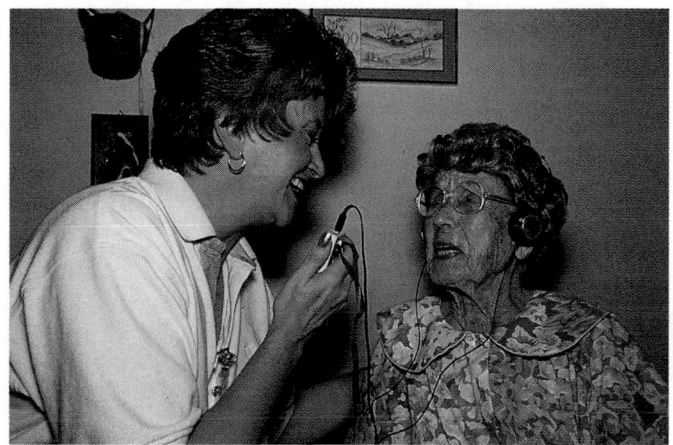

Fig. 31-3 Positive, supportive relationships with older adults foster therapeutic nurse-client interactions.

The nurse must clarify personal attitudes and values about older adults to provide the most effective care (see Chapter 18). A nurse's age, education, employment experience, and employing institution influence stereotypes. Personal experiences with older adults such as family members can also affect attitudes. Because older adults are becoming more prevalent in health care settings, it is imperative for the nurse to develop a positive approach to care for older clients.

■ THEORIES OF AGING

Theorists have tried to describe the complex biopsychosocial process of aging. No theory fully explains the aging process; all of these theories are in various stages of development and have limitations. However, nurses can use them to understand phenomena affecting the health and well-being of aged clients.

Aging is not a simple progression, so there is no universally accepted theory that can predict and explain the complexities of older adults. The nurse must be aware of uncertainties about aging, the scientific attempts to explain these phenomena, and the many environmental factors involved.

Biological Theories

FREE RADICAL THEORY

Free radicals are products of cellular metabolism that are highly reactive parts of molecules. These molecules have a strong extracellular charge that can create a reaction with proteins, changing their shape and nature; they can also react with lipids found in cell membranes, affecting their permeability, or they can bind to cell organelles (Christiansen and Grzybowski, 1993).

The process of oxygen metabolism is considered to be the greatest source of free radicals (Hayflick, 1987). Specifically, the oxidation of fat, protein, and carbohydrates within the body leads to free radical formation. Environmental pollutants are external sources of free radicals (Ebersole and Hess, 1994). The theory suggests that aging is caused by the accumulation of irreversible damage resulting from these oxidizing compounds. Research is being conducted on the role that free radicals play in aging. As a result, there has been considerable interest in recent years in the use of vitamins such as A, C, E, and niacin to counteract the effects of free radicals and extend life.

CROSS-LINK THEORY

The cross-link and connective tissue theory asserts that the molecules of collagen and elastin, connective tissue components, form bonds over time that increase cell rigidity. Cross-linkage is thought to result from chemical reactions that create bonds between normally separate molecules (Ebersole and Hess, 1994). When collagen fibers are initially deposited in soft tissue, the molecules are loosely associated and the tissue is flexible. As time passes, however, active sites on adjacent collagen molecules result in more closely associated molecules; thus tissue becomes more rigid (Christiansen and Grzybowski, 1993). Aging skin is an example of the cross-linkage of elastin. Examples of age-related connective tissue cross-linkage include the decrease in arterial wall tensile strength, loose teeth, and dry, fibrous tendons (Ebersole and Hess, 1994). Research efforts are directed at the factors that cause, reduce, and impede cross-linkage.

IMMUNOLOGICAL THEORY

Some theorists suggest that declines or alterations in the effectiveness of the immune system are responsible for aging. Erratic cellular mechanisms are thought to cause attacks on body tissues through autoaggression or immunodeficiencies (Ebersole and Hess, 1994). The body loses its ability to distinguish its own proteins from foreign ones; the immune system attacks and destroys its own tissues at a gradually increasing rate.

With advancing age, the ability of the immune system to destroy bacteria, viruses, and fungi is slowed; in fact, this system may not begin its attack until mutated cells have reproduced several times. Destruction of large blocks of tissue can occur before an immune response is initiated. This immune system dysfunction is thought to be a factor in the development of chronic diseases such as cancer, diabetes, and cardiovascular disease, as well as infections. Studies in immunoengineering attempt to control, to moderate, or to eliminate the effects of autoimmunity and immunodeficiency.

Psychosocial Theories

In the past, psychosocial theories of development have focused primarily on the child and adolescent. There is no adequate evidence to support theories about aspects of psychosocial aging. Researchers have demonstrated that genetics is not the primary determinant of longevity. People age along dimensions beyond the biological, including the psychological and social.

DISENGAGEMENT THEORY

The disengagement theory of Cummings and Henry (1961) states that aging people withdraw from customary roles and engage in more introspective, self-focused activities. This theory includes four basic concepts (Maddox, 1974):

1. Aging persons and society mutually withdraw from each other.
2. Disengagement is biologically and psychologically intrinsic and inevitable.
3. Disengagement is considered necessary for successful aging.
4. Disengagement is beneficial for older adults and society.

The disengagement theory remains controversial because it does not indicate whether society or the aging person initiates disengagement or whether personality, health, culture, and other factors influence disengagement.

ACTIVITY THEORY

The activity theory disagrees with the disengagement theory and asserts that the continuation of middle-adult activities is necessary for successful aging. The classic work by Lemon et al (1972) proposed that socially active older people are more likely to adjust well to aging. Studies since then have shown that older adults with greater social involvement have higher morale and life satisfaction, and more positive adjustment and mental health than those with less social involvement.

Critics, however, note that aging is too complex to be characterized in such a simple manner. They argue that this theory assumes that older adults have the same needs as middle-aged persons. In addition, this theory does not address the impact of biopsychosocial changes or the presence of multiple losses on the ability of older people to continue to replace activities. The general consensus of the critics is that there are many other variables affecting responses to aging, which this theory does not adequately explain.

CONTINUITY THEORY

The continuity or developmental theory (Neugarten, 1964) states that personality remains the same and behavior becomes more predictable as people age. Personality and behavior patterns developed during a lifetime determine the degree of engagement and activity in older adulthood. According to this theory personality is a critical factor in determining the relationship between role activity and life satisfaction. This psychosocial theory is viewed by some as a promising one because it addresses the complexities of the aging process and people's adaptive ability. Critics argue that it too is simplistic and does not consider the many factors that affect one's response to the aging process.

▌ GROWTH AND DEVELOPMENT

As in other stages of life, older adults have specific developmental tasks. These are described by Burnside (1979), Duvall (1977), and Havighurst (1953) and include seven major categories (see the box below).

The older adult must adjust to physical changes. As each body system ages, changes in appearance and functioning occur. These are not associated with a disease but are normal. Structural and functional changes associated with aging are described in the section on physiological development.

Older adults are commonly retired from full-time employment and therefore may need to adjust and make transitions because of the loss of the work role. However, because retirement is usually anticipated, persons can plan ahead to (1) participate in consultation or volunteer activities, (2) pursue new interests and hobbies, and (3) continue their education. Although most older adults are above the poverty level, financial resources clearly affect retirement pursuits.

The majority of older adults are faced with the deaths of spouses, friends, and sometimes children. These losses are often difficult to resolve. By assisting older adults through the grieving process the nurse can help them adjust to the loss (see Chapter 26). When grieving has ended, clients may need help in identifying resources to fill the void.

Some older adults find it difficult to accept themselves as

Developmental Tasks of the Older Adult

- Adjusting to decreasing health and physical strength
- Adjusting to retirement and reduced or fixed income
- Adjusting to death of a spouse
- Accepting self as aging person
- Maintaining satisfactory living arrangements
- Redefining relationships with adult children
- Finding ways to maintain quality of life

---

aging. They may demonstrate their inability to cope by denying functional declines, requesting that their grandchildren not call them "Grandma" or "Grandpa," or refuse to ask for assistance with tasks that place their safety at great risk. This is different from merely remaining active and can pose a threat to health if physical and psychosocial limitations are exceeded.

An older adult may have to change living arrangements. For example, physical impairments may require relocation to a smaller, single-level home. Severe health problems may require the older adult to live with relatives or friends. A change in living arrangements for the older adult may require an extended period of adjustment during which assistance and support from health care professionals and family are needed.

Older adults often need to redefine relationships with adult children. The issues of role reversal, dependence, conflict, guilt, and loss require recognition and resolution. Frequently, adult children must cope with guilt if they feel that they should have "come sooner" or should have had older parents move into their homes. Adult children need to be made aware that some of the unusual behaviors shown by their aging parents could be symptoms of illness rather than mean-spirited actions.

Older adults must learn to acquire new activities and interests to maintain their quality of life. People who were socially active throughout life may find it relatively easy to meet new people and acquire new interests. However, people who were somewhat introverted, with limited socialization, may have difficulty meeting new people during retirement.

These developmental tasks are common to older adults. The way that older adults adjust to the changes of aging, however, depends on the individual. For some, adaptation and adjustment are relatively easy. For others, each developmental task requires nursing intervention. Many of these tasks are associated with loss, which occurs with greater frequency in older adulthood. The most common losses are health, income, usefulness, socialization, loved ones, and independent living. The nurse must be sensitive to the effect of such losses on the older adult and be prepared to offer support.

▌ COMMUNITY-BASED AND INSTITUTIONAL HEALTH CARE SERVICES

General health care services are described in Chapter 2. However, four services are frequently used by the older population.

Home Care

Home health care and homemaker services prevent or delay institutionalization for older adults who need assistance with daily living. These agencies may be governmental, private, or voluntary. Some home health care is reimbursed by Medicare and health insurance. Care is provided by professional nurses and therapists or nonprofessional staff, such as homemaker aides.

Day Care

Day care provides an alternative to institutionalization, offering health and rehabilitative services. Day-care center clients are usually not seriously ill, although they may have chronic conditions or disabilities that limit independence. A typical participant lives with a family member who must be away during the day. Day care thus enables the family to maintain employment and other activities (Stanhope and Lancaster, 1992).

Respite Care

Respite care is temporary relief for the primary care giver of a dependent older adult. Service is provided in the home or institution. Respite care enables the care giver to be away from home for a few hours. The continual demand for care of a seriously ill or dependent family member can create emotional and physical stress. Studies indicate that respite services reduce care giver stress.

Long-Term Care

Declining health, decreased physical and human resources, and increased dependence may require an older adult to stay in a long-term care facility. Such a facility provides extended nursing care, medical care, and personal or psychosocial services. The nursing home is the usual setting in which long-term care is provided.

Nursing home residents can be classified into two groups according to length of stay: short-term and long-term residents. Growth of the subacute care industry and managed care are market forces that have changed the face of the traditional nursing home population, increasing the number of short-term residents. Typically, long-term residents reside in nursing homes for a period greater than six months and remain there until they die. They also tend to

Table 31-1	Normal Physical Changes of Aging
SYSTEM	**NORMAL FINDINGS**
Integument	
Skin color	Spotty pigmentation in areas exposed to the sun; pallor even in absence of anemia
Moisture	Dry, scaly condition
Temperature	Cooler extremities; decreased perspiration
Texture	Decreased elasticity; wrinkles; folding, sagging condition
Fat distribution	Decreased amount on extremities; increased amount on abdomen
Hair	Thinning and graying on scalp; often, decreased amount of axillary and pubic hair and hair on extremities; decreased facial hair in men; possible chin and upper lip hair in women
Nails	Decreased growth rate
Head and neck	
Head	Sharp and angular nasal and facial bones; loss of eyebrow hair in women; bushier eyebrows in men
Eyes	Decreased visual acuity; decreased accommodation; reduced adaptation to darkness; sensitivity to glare
Ears	Decreased pitch discrimination; diminished light reflex; diminished hearing acuity
Nose and sinuses	Increased nasal hair; decreased sense of smell
Mouth and pharynx	Use of bridges or dentures; decreased sense of taste; atrophy of papillae of lateral edges of tongue
Neck	Nodular thyroid gland; slight tracheal deviation resulting from muscle atrophy
Thorax and lungs	Increased anteroposterior diameter; increased chest rigidity; increased respiratory rate with decreased lung expansion; increased airway resistance
Heart and vascular system	Significant increase in systolic pressure with slight increase in diastolic pressure; usually insignificant changes in heart rate at rest; common diastolic murmurs; easily palpated peripheral pulses; weaker pedal pulses and colder lower extremities, especially at night
Breasts	Diminished breast tissue; pendulous, flabby condition
Gastrointestinal system	Decreased salivary secretions, which may make swallowing more difficult; decreased peristalsis; decreased production of digestive enzymes, including hydrochloric acid, pepsin, and pancreatic enzymes; constipation; reduced motility
Reproductive system	
Female	Decreased estrogen; decreased uterine size; decreased secretions; atrophy of epithelial lining of vagina
Male	Decreased levels of testosterone; decreased sperm count; decreased testicular size
Urinary system	Decreased renal filtration and renal efficiency; subsequent loss of protein from kidney; nocturia; decreased bladder capacity; increased incontinence
Female	Urgency and stress incontinence resulting from decrease in perineal muscle tone
Male	Urinary frequency and retention resulting from prostatic enlargement
Musculoskeletal system	Decreased muscle mass and strength; bone demineralization (more pronounced in women); shortening of trunk as result of intervertebral space narrowing; decreased joint mobility; decreased range of joint motion; enhanced bony prominences
Neurological system	Decreased rate of voluntary or automatic reflexes; decreased ability to respond to multiple stimuli; insomnia; shorter sleeping periods

Modified from Ebersole P, Hess P: *Toward healthy aging: human needs and nursing response,* ed 4, St Louis, 1994, Mosby.

be older and have greater cognitive deficits and functional impairments.

As life expectancy increases, so does the probability of entering a nursing home. The decision for such care is not easily made, and the older adult and family require much support. In addition, a nurse's help may be needed in locating a proper facility. When possible, the facility should be close to the client's and family's home to make visiting easier.

▮ THE NURSING PROCESS AND OLDER ADULTS

Assessment

Gerontological nursing offers creative approaches for maximizing the potential of older clients. With comprehensive assessment information regarding the older client's strengths, resources, and limitations, the nurse identifies client needs and problems and selects interventions that maintain the client's physical abilities and create an environment for psychosocial and spiritual well-being. A thorough assessment requires the nurse to actively engage the client and provide the client time to share important information about his or her health. The nurse assesses for changes in physiological development, cognition, and psychosocial behavior.

PHYSIOLOGICAL CHANGES

Perception of well-being can define quality of life. Understanding the older adult's perceptions about health status is essential for accurate assessment and development of clinically relevant interventions. Older adults' concepts of health generally depend on personal perceptions of functional ability. Therefore older adults engaged in activities of daily living usually consider themselves healthy, whereas those whose activities are limited by physical, emotional, or social impairments may perceive themselves as ill.

Physiological changes vary with each client. Table 31-1 describes general physiological changes anticipated in older adults. These physiological changes are not pathological processes. They occur in all persons but at different rates and depend on circumstances in life. The nurse should know about these changes to provide appropriate care for older adults and to assist them in adapting to the changes.

The nurse should also consider potential sensory changes that may influence data gathering. For example, the nurse must consider visual problems from cataracts or hearing impairments from nerve deafness when choosing communication techniques. If clients are unable to understand the nurse's visual or auditory cues, assessment data may be inaccurate. For example, if clients have difficulty hearing the nurse's questions, inappropriate responses may lead the nurse to believe that they are confused (Table 31-2).

Some older clients may experience all of these changes, and others experience only a few. The body changes continuously with age, but the effects on clients depend on health, lifestyle, stressors, and environmental conditions.

General Survey. The general survey begins during the initial nurse-client encounter and includes a concise written description of a quick but careful head-to-toe scan of

Table 31-2	Techniques for Assessing Older Adults With Sensory Problems
SENSORY ALTERATION	**ASSESSMENT TECHNIQUE**
Visual disturbance	Position self in full view of client
	Provide diffuse, bright light; avoid glare
	Make sure client's glasses are worn and in good working order
	Face client when speaking; do not cover mouth
Hearing deficit	Speak directly to client in clear, low tones at a moderate rate; do not cover mouth
	Articulate consonants with special care
	Restate if client does not understand question initially
	Speak toward "good" ear
	Reduce background noises
	Make sure client's hearing aid is worn and is working properly

the client. An initial inspection of an older adult might reveal eye contact and facial expression appropriate to the situation, facial wrinkles, gray hair, loss of tissue on the extremities, and an increase in tissue and fat on the trunk.

Integumentary System. The skin loses resilience and moisture in older adulthood. The epithelial layer thins, and elastic collagen fibers shrink and become rigid. Wrinkles of the face and neck reflect lifetime patterns of muscle activity and facial expressions, the pull of gravity on tissue, and diminished elasticity.

Spots and lesions may also be present on skin. Smooth, brown, irregularly shaped spots (age spots, or **senile lentigo**) initially appear on the backs of the hands and on forearms. Small, round, red or brown cherry angiomas may be found on the trunk. Seborrheic lesions or keratoses may appear as irregular, round or oval, brown, watery lesions.

Pressure ulcers are common in this population because they have many of the predisposing factors that lead to their development. Multiple factors play a role in pressure ulcer formation, including mobility and activity, sensory perception, moisture, friction and shearing, nutritional status, and arteriolar pressure (see Chapter 38).

Head and Neck. The facial features of the older adult become more pronounced from loss of fat and skin elasticity. Facial features may appear asymmetrical because of missing teeth or improperly fitting dentures. In addition, changes in voice pitch (usually a rise) occur from decline in power and range.

The older adult's visual acuity declines (see Chapter 39). This may be the result of retinal damage, reduction in pupillary diameter, reduction in opacity of the lens, or loss of lens elasticity. **Presbyopia**, a decline in the ability of the eyes to accommodate for close, detailed work, is common. Presbyopia begins early in the fourth decade and continues throughout life. The older adult also has a reduced ability to see in darkness, and glare can cause pain and limit the ability to see.

Auditory changes are subtle and may be noted as difficulty in hearing (see Chapter 39). Age-related changes in auditory acuity are called **presbycusis**. It affects ability to hear high-pitched sounds and sibilant consonants such as *s, sh,* and *ch.* The assessment of an older client's hearing is best accomplished using a tuning fork with frequencies of 500 to 1000 cycles per second (cps) to screen for high-frequency losses.

Taste buds atrophy and lose efficiency. The older adult is unable to discern salty, sweet, sour, and bitter tastes as acutely. Sense of smell is also decreased, further reducing taste. Salivary secretion is reduced.

Thorax and Lungs. Because of changes in the musculoskeletal system, the configuration of the thorax sometimes changes. There is an increase in the anteroposterior diameter. Kyphosis is a subtle, progressive change in the vertebral structure that is permanent when accompanied by osteoporosis. Calcification of the costal cartilage can cause decreased mobility of the ribs.

Decreased muscle mass and tone lead to decreased lung expansion. Decreased elasticity of lung alveoli results in emphysematous changes in the lungs, and hyperresonance may be present on percussion. If kyphosis or chronic obstructive lung disease is present, breath sounds are distant.

Heart and Vascular System. Decreased contractile strength of the myocardium results in a decreased cardiac output. The decrease is significant when the older adult is stressed by anxiety, excitement, illness, or strenuous activity. The body tries to compensate for decreased cardiac output by increasing the heart rate during exercise. However, after exercise, it takes longer for the client's rate to return to baseline.

Frequently the older adult's baseline blood pressure rises. This is the result of vascular changes and the accumulation of sclerotic plaques along the walls of the vessels, causing an overall stiffening of the vasculature. Peripheral pulses are palpable but frequently weaker in the lower extremities. The lower extremities may be cold, particularly at night.

Breasts. Decreased muscle mass, tone, and elasticity result in smaller breasts in older women. In addition, the breasts sag. Atrophy of glandular tissue, coupled with more fat deposits, results in a slightly smaller, less dense, and less nodular breast.

Gastrointestinal System and Abdomen. Aging leads to an increase in the amount of fatty tissue in the trunk and abdomen. As a result, the abdomen increases in size. Because muscle tone and elasticity decrease, it also becomes more protuberant.

The older adult also experiences changes in gastrointestinal function. Some changes may be slight, such as the sudden development of intolerance to certain foods. Because of decreased peristalsis, an older adult experiences delayed gastric emptying and may be unable to consume large meals. Decreased peristalsis also affects emptying of the colon, resulting in constipation.

Reproductive System. Changes in the structure and function of the reproductive system occur as the result of hormonal alterations. Female menopause is related to a reduced responsiveness of the ovaries to pituitary hormones and a resultant decrease in estrogen and progesterone levels. In men, there is no definite cessation of fertility associated with aging. Spermatogenesis begins to decline during the fourth decade but continues into the ninth. The changes in reproductive structure and function, however, do not affect libido. Less frequency of sexual activity can result from illness, death of a sexual partner, decreased socialization, or loss of sexual interest.

Urinary System. Hypertrophy of the prostate gland may develop in older men. This hypertrophy enlarges the gland, and pressure is displaced to the neck of the bladder. As a result, urinary tract infections, frequency, incontinence, and retention of urine occur. In addition, prostatic hypertrophy can result in difficulty initiating and maintaining a stream.

Older women, particularly those who have had children, can experience stress incontinence, in which an involuntary release of urine occurs when they cough, sneeze, or lift an object. This is a result of a weakening of the perineal and bladder muscles. In addition, older women notice urgency in voiding.

Musculoskeletal System. Older adults who exercise regularly do not lose as much bone and muscle mass or tone as those who are inactive. Muscle fibers are reduced in size, and muscle strength diminishes in proportion to the decline in muscle mass. Postmenopausal women have a greater rate of bone demineralization than older men. Women who maintain calcium intake throughout life and into menopause have less bone demineralization than those who do not.

Neurological System. The number of neurons in the nervous system begins to decrease in the middle of the second decade. These neurons do not regenerate, and decrease or damage can lead to functional changes. The changes can affect the special senses described earlier. In addition, the client may experience a decreased sense of balance or uncoordinated motor responses.

The sleep-wake cycle is also influenced by the brain (see Chapter 42). Characteristically, older adults do not sleep through the night. This disruption has the following causes:

1. The sleep cycle is shortened.
2. Sleep disruption can be the result of frequent bladder emptying, pain, or psychological upsets.
3. Medication may affect the sleep-wake cycle.

COGNITIVE CHANGES

Much of the psychological and emotional trauma of older adulthood arises from the misconception that older adults have cognitive impairments. However, the structural and physiological changes occurring in the brain during aging do not necessarily affect adaptive and functional abilities (Ebersole and Hess, 1994).

Neurophysiological cellular changes vary among individuals. Even with obvious cellular loss, some older adults do not demonstrate mental deterioration. Furthermore, some clients with significant cerebral cell loss respond well to the various psychotherapies and pharmacological treatments.

Occasionally when cerebral dysfunction is present, preexisting behavioral tendencies are magnified. Therefore persons who were compulsive as young and middle adults become more compulsive when older. Cognitive changes occur in older adults when cerebral dysfunction or trauma is present. The nurse must understand these changes so that clients can be helped to maintain optimal functioning.

A nurse who cares for an older adult with a cognitive impairment is challenged to meet physical needs and improve or maintain cognitive functioning. To achieve this, the nurse may use the specific techniques of reality orientation, resocialization, and remotivation, in addition to a repertoire of nursing interventions aimed at the etiology of the impairment.

Dementia. Dementia is a generalized impairment of intellectual functioning that interferes with social and occupational functioning. It is a syndrome characterized by irreversible, progressive cerebral dysfunction. Senile dementia of the Alzheimer type (SDAT), or **Alzheimer's disease**, the prototype of the dementias, is characterized by brain atrophy and the development of senile plaques and neurofibrillary tangles in the cerebral hemispheres. The cause of the disease is not known, and although several theories are being studied, none are definitive. It is an irreversible state characterized by decreased intellectual function, personality change, impairment of judgment, and often change in affect caused by permanently altered cerebral metabolism.

The progression of Alzheimer's disease has been divided into three stages (Brady, 1993). In the early stage the primary symptom is memory loss. The middle stage involves impaired language skills, motor activity, and object recognition. Urinary and fecal incontinence, inability to ambulate, and a complete loss of language skills are the classic features of the final or terminal stage.

Nursing management of clients with Alzheimer's disease is complex. Limited mobility increases the client's risk for hazards of immobility (see Chapter 37). Therefore the nurse must continually meet the client's physical needs. Confusion usually increases at night, and wandering through the home or hospital may increase. As the client progresses through the three stages, communication becomes more difficult. The client may easily misperceive the environment and feel threatened. Typical behavioral responses of the client who feels threatened include aggressive gestures or acts, increased voice volume, restlessness, agitation, and hostility. Nursing care objectives are individualized to help this client use remaining functional abilities.

Delirium and depression, both reversible disorders, are often mistaken for irreversible dementia in the older adult because widespread cerebral dysfunction and global cognitive impairment occur with these conditions as well. Consequently, older clients with such disorders may not be appropriately assessed and treated, and a reversible dementia may become irreversible.

Multiinfarct dementia is the second most common cause of dementia, accounting for 10% to 20% of cases. Although clients with this form of dementia may display symptoms of SDAT, multiinfarct dementia is distinguished by periods of remission, preservation of personality, insight, lability of emotion, and epileptoid attacks. Multiinfarct dementia may be related to vascular disorders within the brain and may result from conditions such as stroke and severe hypertension.

The causes of multiinfarct dementia are not known, but may have the same risk factors as heart disease and stroke. These may include high blood pressure, a high-cholesterol diet, obesity, smoking, and lack of exercise. Nursing management of clients is similar to that described in the box on p. 588.

 CULTURAL ASPECTS OF CARE

Normal and abnormal behaviors are culturally determined. Although it may not be understood by the nurse, people of all cultures have reasons for their behavior. Culture influences the presentation, recognition, labeling, and explanations for physical and psychological illness as well as its treatments and healers. For example, hallucinations, illusions, and even drug intoxication may be judged to be normal or abnormal, according to the cultural context. Some cultural groups may even encourage altered states of consciousness that nurses and other health care providers would consider a serious mental disturbance. Although mental disorders occur in every society, the nurse must develop a cultural tolerance for variations in human behavior.

Delirium. Delirium, or an acute confusional state, is a brain syndrome resembling irreversible dementia, but it is distinguished clinically by the presence of a clouded state of consciousness or, more precisely, altered attention and wakefulness (American Psychiatric Association, 1994). Other features include attentional deficits, illusions, hallucinations, occasional incoherent speech, disturbed sleep-wake cycle, and disorientation (see the box above). The onset of delirium is typically sudden, and there are rapid fluctuations in symptoms and severity. Delirium can resemble an irreversible dementia; however, its cause can usually be treated, and recovery is possible. The box on p. 578 summarizes frequent causes of delirium.

Substance Abuse and Cognitive Impairment. The abuse of alcohol and other drugs occurs in the older adult population. The incidence is difficult to determine. Studies of substance abuse in older adults indicate that it can be a long-standing or recent problem, making it difficult to determine prevalence. However, most studies indicate that it is a serious problem in older adults because of the stress and loss associated with aging, such as retirement, loss of spouse, and loneliness.

Long-term abuse of alcohol and drugs can affect cognitive functioning. After 15 to 20 years of alcohol abuse, tolerance for drinking declines. Prolonged use of large amounts of alcohol creates cerebral, cerebellar, sensory, and peripheral nervous system damage. Many chronic alcoholics also have vitamin B_1 deficiency. A prolonged deficiency can cause neuropathy, myopathy, and encephalopathy, exhibited as Wernicke's syndrome or Korsakoff's syndrome. **Wernicke's syndrome** is present in advanced stages of vitamin B_1 depletion and is characterized by nystagmus, pupillary abnormalities, ataxia, tremor, and stupor. **Korsakoff's syndrome** is a psychosis characterized by disorientation of time, place, and person; amnesia for recent events; and confabulation. **Confabulation** is a defense mechanism in which the person fabricates experiences or situations and recounts them in a detailed and plausible way to fill in memory gaps.

The effects of prolonged drug abuse on the older adult have not been clearly described, but cognitive impairments like those associated with alcohol abuse may occur. In ad-

Reversible Causes of Delirium

PHYSIOLOGICAL

A. Primary cerebral disease
Stroke
Subdural hematoma
Vascular occlusion
Transient ischemic attacks
Meningitis
Neurosyphilis
Brain abscess
Tumors: primary and metastatic
Concussion or contusion
Normal pressure hydrocephalus

B. Extracranial disease
Decreased cardiac output states: myocardial infarction (MI), congestive heart failure (CHF), arrhythmias, cardiogenic shock
Vascular occlusion: disseminated intravascular coagulation (DIC) emboli
Increased or decreased peripheral vascular resistance
Inadequate gas exchange states: pulmonary disease, alveolar hypoventilation
Bacterial or viral infections: tuberculosis, pneumonia, endocarditis, pyelonephritis, cystitis, diverticulitis, cholecystitis
Electrolyte abnormalities: hypercalcemia, hypo- and hypernatremia, hypo- and hyperkalemia, hypo- and hyperchloremia, hyperphosphatemia
Anemia
Hypo- and hyperglycemia
Acidosis/alkalosis

Azotemia or renal failure (dehydration, diuretics, obstruction, hypokalemia)
Volume depletion: hemorrhage, inadequate fluid intake, diuretics
Liver failure
Therapeutic drug intoxication
Substance abuse
Chemical intoxications: heavy metals (arsenic, lead, mercury), carbon monoxide
Hypo- and hyperthyroidism
Accidental hypothermia; hyperthermia

PSYCHOLOGICAL
Severe emotional stress: relocation, hospitalization, surgical procedure
Depression
Anxiety
Acute or chronic pain
Grief
Fatigue
Sensory-perceptual deficits: vision and hearing loss, noise
Paranoia

ENVIRONMENTAL
Unfamiliar environment creating a lack of meaning
Sensory deprivation or environmental monotony creating a lack of meaning
Sensory deprivation/overload
Immobilization: therapeutic, physical, or pharmacological
Sleep deprivation
Lack of temperospatial reference points

Modified from Foreman MD: Acute confusional states in hospitalized elderly: a research dilemma, *Nurs Res* 35(1):34, 1986.

dition, a drug overdose may cause cerebral impairment, so cognitive impairment may result from a decrease of oxygen to the brain.

PSYCHOSOCIAL CHANGES

The older adult must adapt to psychosocial changes that occur with aging. Although these vary, some are common to the majority of older adults.

Retirement. Retirement is often mistakenly associated with passivity and seclusion. In actuality, it is a stage of life characterized by transition and role changes, which can lead to psychosocial stresses. These include role changes with the spouse or family and problems of social isolation (see next section).

Mandatory retirement age varies. For example, in a state civil service job, it may be 65, whereas a federal employee may not be required to retire until 70. In private industry the mandatory retirement age is usually between 62 and 70. It is also possible to retire at age 55. More companies are developing early retirement plans to provide advancement for younger employees. One popular program is the "30 and out" plan, which allows workers to retire with full pension, and in some cases large bonuses, after 30 years.

Preretirement planning is advisable during middle age and essential in late middle age (see Chapter 30). People who plan retirement activities generally adjust better. For example, an individual may plan volunteer work, home re-

modeling, travel, or other activities. Meaningful retirement planning is critical because retirement can last for 30 or more years.

Retirement also has an impact on the spouse. For example, tension can occur because of role changes in the relationship and because a homemaker may feel that the workload is increased.

The most powerful factors that influence the retired person's satisfaction with life are health status, the option to continue working, and sufficient income (Ebersole and Hess, 1994). The nurse can help the client and family prepare for retirement by asking questions that may help them make decisions. The nurse should particularly ask the following questions:

1. Will retirement offer a satisfying lifestyle? Is the current job depleting health and energy or causing stress? Is the job important for friendship networks, self-esteem, or sense of achievement?
2. What provisions have they made for retirement income? Will these financial resources be enough to meet necessities—5 years, 10 years, or indefinitely?
3. What retirement activities are available after retirement? On what abilities, skills, and interests can the client draw (Fig. 31-4)? Will any of these be a source of income?
4. What living arrangements may be needed? Is the present home too large, difficult to maintain, or expen-

sive? Should relocation be considered? Ideally the client should spend several months in a new location before making a commitment.

5. What preparations have been made for role changes? Have the marriage partners discussed how they will spend time together? Will they divide household tasks, spend more time with grandchildren, or become involved in volunteer activities?

6. What provisions have been made to meet health care needs? How will the retired couple meet exercise, nutrition, and other health needs?

7. How will the retired person attend to legal affairs? Estate planning, education in legal affairs, and ability to cope with bureaucratic procedures are essential. Community colleges, offices on aging, and legal aid services may provide guidance.

Social Isolation. Many older adults experience social isolation, which increases as they age. The types of social isolation are attitudinal, presentational, behavioral, and geographical. Some older adults may be affected by all four; others are affected by only one (Ebersole and Hess, 1990).

Attitudinal isolation occurs because of personal or cultural values. Ageism is a prevailing attitude that stigmatizes the older adult. It is a bias against and rejection of older people. Therefore attitudinal social isolation occurs when the older adult is not easily accepted into social interactions because of society's bias. A vicious circle may result. As the older adult is increasingly rejected, self-esteem may diminish, leading to fewer attempts to socialize.

Presentational isolation results from an unacceptable appearance or other factors involved in presenting the self to others. Contributing factors are body image, hygiene, and visible signs of illness or functional loss (Ebersole and Hess, 1990). The person becomes isolated because of rejection by others or because little interaction is sought as a result of self-consciousness.

Behavioral isolation results from unacceptable behaviors. In all age groups and particularly with older adults, socially unacceptable behaviors cause others to withdraw. Behaviors commonly associated with isolation of older adults include confusion, dementia, alcoholism, eccentricity, and incontinence. The nurse can use behavior-modification techniques to help decrease the frequency of these behaviors in older adults (Ebersole and Hess, 1990).

Geographical isolation occurs because of distance from family, urban crime, and institutional barriers. In today's mobile society, it is common for children to live great distances from parents. Thus the opportunity to visit children decreases. This leads to even further isolation when parents have physical limitations or experience the death of a spouse.

In urban areas a high crime rate can deter older adults from socializing. Living in a high-crime area may result in unwillingness to leave home because it might be vandalized or robbed while unoccupied.

One institutional barrier is lack of easy access for persons who use wheelchairs, walkers, canes, or crutches. Also, when older adults require institutional care, segregation from friends occurs. Social interaction depends on those who come to visit.

The nurse can assist lonely older adults in rebuilding social networks. One resource is outreach programs designed to make contact with isolated older adults. The program may meet nutritional needs, such as Meals on Wheels; socialization needs, such as daily telephone calls by volunteers; or need for activities, such as outings. In addition, the nurse can investigate networks within older adults' communities (see the box below). These increase the opportunity to meet people with similar activities, interests, and needs.

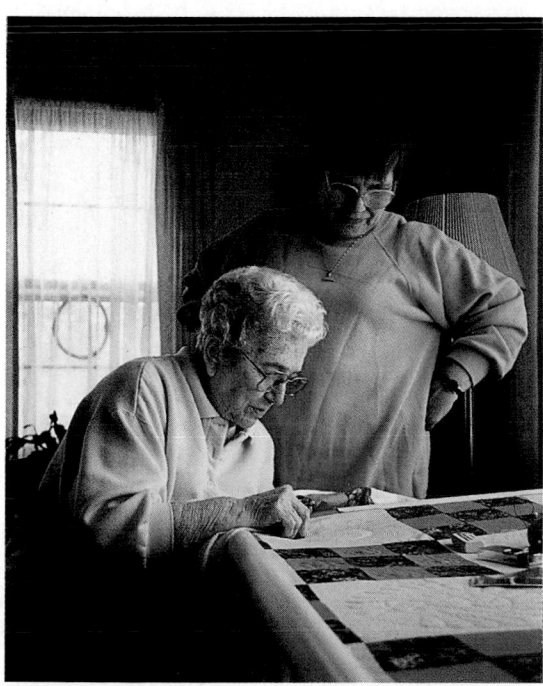

Fig. 31-4 Quilting is this older adult's favorite activity.

Contacts for Increasing Social Networks of the Older Adult

FORMAL
- Church
- Grandparenting
- Foster Grandparents
- Vista
- Peace Corps
- Retired Senior Volunteer Program
- National Retired Teachers Association
- Unions
- Friends of the Library
- Volunteers
- Public school
- Senior centers
- Title VII nutrition sites
- Involvement in social issues for seniors

INFORMAL
- Neighbors
- Maids, waitresses
- Beauty salons, restaurants, bars, service personnel, shops, laundromats
- Sports
- Buses for older adults
- Special tours
- Education, arts and crafts courses
- Trailer courts
- Retirement communities
- Pets
- Dancing
- Physicians' offices, clinics
- Nursing home—social corridor
- General social touching
- Radio shows

Modified from Ebersole P, Hess P: *Toward healthy aging: human needs and nursing response,* ed 3, St Louis, 1990, Mosby.

Sexuality. Sexuality is increasingly recognized as important in the care of older adults. All older adults, whether healthy or frail, need to express sexual feelings. Sexuality involves love, warmth, sharing, and touching, not just the act of intercourse. Sexuality is linked with identity and validates the belief that people can give to others and have the gift appreciated.

The nurse ensures that care is directed at helping the client maintain sexual health. It requires integration of somatic, emotional, intellectual, and social aspects of the sexual being. The older adult's expressions of sexuality can serve to promote communication with trust, caring, sharing, and pleasuring (Billhorn, 1994).

To help the older adult achieve or maintain sexual health, the nurse needs to understand the physical changes in sexual response. Knowledge of the changes described in Table 31-3, as well as the physical changes in male and female genitalia, enables the nurse to educate the older adult about changes in sexual functioning.

The client's libido does not decrease, although frequency of sexual activity may decline. An older woman who does not understand physical changes affecting sexual activity may be concerned that her sex life is nearly over with the onset of menopause. The older man may feel the same when he discovers a change in the firmness of his erection, has a decreased need for ejaculation with each orgasm, or has a longer recovery period between episodes of intercourse.

In addition to physical changes affecting sexual functioning, many older adults are prescribed medications that depress sexual activity, such as antihypertensives, antidepressants, sedatives, or hypnotics. Some drugs increase libido in older adults. Phenothiazines increase sexual desire in women, and levodopa has a similar effect in men.

The nurse assists older adults in achieving sexual health. However, a counselor for one or both partners may be needed to describe methods for sexual satisfaction. In addition, the nurse may help other health care professionals understand the sexual behavior of older adults. Not all nurses feel comfortable counseling clients about sexual health. The nurse need not feel obligated to do so. However, the nurse should recognize the need for assistance. If the nurse is uncomfortable with discussing sexuality, another health care professional should be consulted.

While considering the older adult's need for sexual expression, the nurse must not ignore the equally important need to touch and be touched. Touch is an overt expression with many meanings and is an important part of sexuality. Touch can complement traditional sexual methods or serve as an alternative sexual expression when physical intercourse is not desired or possible, and thus can serve as an important method of achieving intimacy (Wallace, 1996). The nursing student needs to recognize that knowledge of clients' sexual and intimacy needs will increase with professional growth. As information about the client is gained, the nurse will be able to incorporate this information into the nursing care plan (see Chapter 24).

Table 31-3	Physical Changes in Sexual Response in the Older Adult	
FEMALE		**MALE**
EXCITATION		
Diminished vaginal lubrication (1-3 min may be required for adequate amounts to appear)		Less intense and slower erection (which can be maintained longer without ejaculation)
Diminished flattening and separation of labia majora		Less vasocongestion of scrotal sac
Disappearance of elevation of labia majora		Less pronounced elevation and congestion of testicles
Decreased vasocongestion of labia minora		Decreased muscle tension
Decreased elastic expansion of vagina (depth and breadth)		
Slower and less prominent uterine elevation or tenting		
Decreased muscle tension		
PLATEAU		
Decreased capacity for vasocongestion		Less frequent nipple erection and sexual flush
Decreased areolar engorgement		Lack of color change at coronal edge of penis
Less evident labial color change		Decrease or absence of secretory activity (lubrication) by Cowper's gland before ejaculation
Less intense swelling or orgasmic platform		
Decreased secretions of Bartholin's glands		
ORGASM		
Fewer contractions of orgasmic platform		Fewer penile contractions
Rectal sphincter contractions with severe tension only		Fewer rectal sphincter contractions
		Decreased force of ejaculation with decreased amount of semen (seepage of semen with long ejaculation)
RESOLUTION		
Observably slower subsidence of nipple erection		Slow subsidence of vasocongestion of nipples and scrotum
Quicker subsidence of vasocongestion of clitoris and orgasmic platform		Loss of erection and descent of testicles shortly after ejaculation
		Extended refractory time (time before another erection: several to 24 hr, occasionally longer)

Modified from Ebersole P, Hess P: *Toward healthy aging: human needs and nursing response,* ed 4, St Louis, 1994, Mosby.

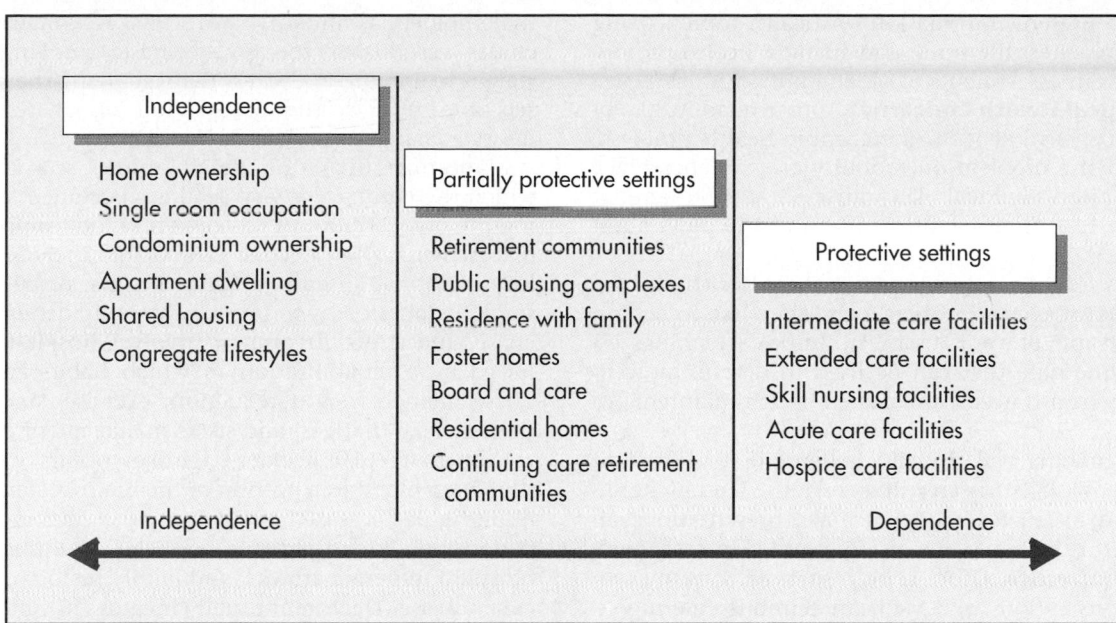

Fig. 31-5 Continuum of housing security. *(Redrawn from Ebersole P, Hess P:* Toward healthy aging: human needs and nursing response, *ed 3, St Louis, 1990, Mosby.)*

Alternative sexual practice. Although little information is available regarding the older adult homosexual, the reader is referred to the work by Berger (1982) on older homosexual men, and Kehoe (1988) on older lesbians. This subject is one that is in need of more research. Alternative sexual practices, as well as sexuality of older adults, is often difficult for some people to support or understand (Wallace, 1996). Nurses need to be aware of their own beliefs and the impact those beliefs may have on their ability to assist older homosexuals with meeting their sexual needs.

Housing and Environment. Changes in social roles, family responsibilities, and health status influence older clients' living arrangements. Some choose to live with family members. Others prefer their own homes or apartments near their families. Leisure or retirement communities provide older people with living and social opportunities in a one-generation setting. Federally subsidized housing, where available, offers apartments with communal, social, and, in some cases, eating arrangements. Housing most appropriate for older adults depends on their level of independence (Fig. 31-5).

When assisting older adults with housing needs, the nurse should assess their activity level, financial status, access to public transportation and community activities, environmental hazards, and support systems. In addition, the nurse should help clients determine the length of the arrangement. For example, an older adult with recently diagnosed angina may not be able to live in a second-floor apartment and should be advised to find one on the first floor.

Housing and environment are important because they can have a major impact on the health of older adults. The environment can support or hinder physical and social functioning, enhance or drain energy, and complement or tax existing physical changes such as vision and hearing. For example, red, orange, and yellow are easiest for older adults

to see; pastels, green, blue, violet, white, and dark colors are the most difficult. Some older adults in health care settings have difficulty finding their rooms, but painting the door frames a bright color to contrast with the wall helps them see it at a distance. Painting a stripe along the bottom of a wall makes the boundaries of a hall or room visible. The glare of highly polished floors should be eliminated.

Furniture should be comfortable and address musculoskeletal changes of older adults. It should be easy to get into and out of and should provide back support. Dining room chairs should be tested for comfort during meals and for height in relation to the table. Older clients should examine furniture carefully for size, comfort, and function before purchasing it.

The nurse assesses environmental needs of older adults in the home and institution. The environment should be modified to increase independence and functional ability and thus the quality of life.

Death. Birth and death are universal, but they are also unique events in life. A common misconception is that the death of an older adult is a blessing and the culmination of a full life. Many dying older adults still have goals, and they are not emotionally prepared to die. Families and friends are often unable to cope with the dying and loss of a loved one. With knowledge and skills the nurse can help make the dying process a time of fulfillment and growth while enlisting the support, understanding, and assistance of family and friends of the dying client (see Chapter 26).

HEALTH MAINTENANCE

Older adults particularly value good health. A state of wellness provides energy, vitality, and a zest for life. The nurse is in a unique position to establish health maintenance programs that promote older adults' wellness. Senior citizens' centers, churches, schools, shopping malls, libraries, and hospital lobbies can be used to conduct screening tests and present information on health topics. Using creative approaches, the nurse can include health-promotion activities in assessments of older adults.

Physiological Health Concerns. Approximately 80% of adults over 65 have at least one chronic health problem. The effect of the problem on mobility and independence depends on the individual. The nurse should be familiar with chronic health problems common in the older adult population.

Most older adults are interested in their health and are capable of taking charge of their lives. They like to remain independent and prevent disability. Initial screenings establish baseline data that can be used to determine wellness, identify health needs, and design health-maintenance programs.

Nursing students will find it challenging to test their knowledge and skills in screening sessions. Under the direction of an instructor, students make presentations on nutrition, arthritis, hypertension, foot and skin care, medications, and exercise. Other topics, such as consumer affairs, safety precautions, and Medicare reimbursement policies, are also of interest. Nurses can significantly improve the quality of life and health of older adults by health promotion, teaching, advising, and counseling.

The use of self-help strategies is appropriate because of older adults' limited financial and social resources. Many older adults monitor their own or their spouses' blood pressures, attend health fairs, plan special diets, and care for spouses with chronic disease. The self-help network of older adults is extensive. For example, while shopping, older adults may exchange information about the best physician for cataract surgery, a hospital that provides the best care, and nursing homes to avoid.

As part of health screening, the nurse encourages older adults to complete a stress inventory scale. Individuals at risk for illness resulting from stress should receive teaching. The nurse needs to know about relaxation and stress-reduction techniques (see Chapters 43 and 22) to assist the client in selecting the best one.

Cardiovascular problems. Cardiovascular problems frequently associated with aging are hypertension, angina pectoris, myocardial infarction, and cerebrovascular accident. Hypertension is diagnosed when repeated blood pressure measurements of 90 mm Hg or greater diastolic and 140 mm Hg or greater systolic are present. Risk factors include smoking, obesity, lack of exercise, and stress. Isolated systolic hypertension, the most prominent form of hypertension in older adults, is defined as a systolic blood pressure of 140 mm Hg or greater with a diastolic pressure of less than 90 mm Hg (National Heart, Lung, & Blood Institute, 1993). African Americans are at a greater risk than European Americans, and men are at greater risk than women. Treatment of hypertension includes weight reduction, decreased salt intake, exercise, stress management, and drugs (Stanhope and Lancaster, 1992). The nurse can teach the client about medications prescribed for hypertension, including drug action and adverse effects, and can evaluate the response to prescribed therapy.

Angina pectoris is a paroxysmal thoracic pain caused most often by coronary artery disease. Attacks are often induced by exertion, emotional stress, or exposure to cold. Risk factors include family history of heart disease, obesity, hyperlipidemia, smoking, and stress. Treatment usually includes vasodilator therapy, exercise, smoking cessation, weight reduction, and stress management. The nurse counsels and teaches the older adult about recommended lifestyle changes.

Myocardial infarction (heart attack) is a condition in which the coronary artery becomes occluded, thus depriving the myocardium of oxygen and blood supply. Myocardial ischemia then occurs. Risk factors include family history of cardiac disease, angina pectoris, diabetes mellitus, smoking, obesity, hypertension, hyperlipidemia, lack of exercise, and stress. Treatment involves hospitalization, followed by a rehabilitation in which habits are modified. These include weight reduction, exercise, smoking cessation, dietary changes, and stress management.

Cerebrovascular accident (stroke) occurs when vessels supplying blood to a portion of the brain become occluded, resulting in decreased circulation. Risk factors include hypertension, hyperlipidemia, diabetes mellitus, history of transient ischemic attacks, and family history of cardiovascular disease. Treatment usually includes hospitalization for days or months, depending on the degree of brain damage.

Cancer. Malignant neoplasms are the second most common cause of death among older adults. The nurse can develop programs to educate clients about early detection, treatment, and risk factors. Examples include encouraging smoking cessation, teaching female clients to perform breast self-examination and have routine Papanicolaou (Pap) smears, and encouraging all clients to have annual screening for fecal occult blood. It is also important to educate clients about the signs of cancer. Detection is not easy because symptoms may be mistakenly identified as part of the normal aging process.

Arthritis. Approximately 44% of older adults have arthritis. It is more common in women than in men (Stanhope and Lancaster, 1992). The degree to which the mobility of older adults is impaired depends on the extent of the disease and joints affected. Arthritis has no cure, but recently developed pharmacological agents can decrease pain and swelling and therefore increase joint motion. Treatment depends on the nature of the degeneration and deformity. Nursing interventions are aimed at promoting comfort, functional ability, and safety. Education about self-care, exercise, and socialization is also important.

Sensory impairments. The older adult usually has changes in vision, hearing, taste, and smell that are a result of normal aging. The nurse can help the older client identify resources to help correct visual and auditory problems (see Chapter 39). Seasonings can help make food more palatable. Depending on the degree of impairment, the consequences of age-related sensory alterations can be serious. The goal of nursing care is to help the client achieve an optimal level of sensory stimulation.

Reports of age-related changes in pain perception are controversial, and both health care professionals and lay persons believe that pain is a natural part of aging and disease (Ferrell and Rivera, 1996). This misperception results in under-reporting of pain and prevents appropriate use of pain relief measures in older adults. Frequent causes of pain according to these authors include arthritis, cancer, postherpetic neuralgia, polymyalgia rheumatica, atherosclerotic peripheral vascular disease, and temporal arteritis.

Many factors influence the management of pain for these and other conditions in this population, and are beyond the scope of this chapter. Nurses caring for older clients are challenged to advocate for appropriate and effective pain management.

Dental problems. Dental problems are common in older adults. When present, there can also be changes in taste and a decrease in nutritional intake. Because of missing teeth or poorly fitting dentures, the older adult may eat only soft foods. The nurse can help prevent dental and gum disease through education about routine dental care (see Chapter 40). The nurse can also help the client find dental services that offer reduced rates.

Mortality. Common causes of death in older adults are heart disease, malignant neoplasms, cerebrovascular disease, and chronic obstructive pulmonary disease (Table 31-4). Health screenings and fairs can identify older adults at risk so that prevention can be initiated. In addition, older adults, especially those with chronic disease, should be encouraged to obtain a yearly influenza shot. Older adults with chronic conditions and those with a history of pneumonia should be encouraged to get the Pneumovax vaccine, which provides lifelong immunity against pneumococcal pneumonia.

Drug Effects. As a group, adults over 65 are the greatest users of medications, accounting for nearly 40% of all prescribed medications (Hogstel, 1992). The most commonly prescribed medications are cardiovascular drugs, antiinfectives, antipsychotic drugs, antidepressants, and diuretics (Ebersole and Hess, 1994).

Medications may interact with one another, adding or negating the effect of another drug. In addition, prescription medications may cause confusion; affect balance and mobility; cause dizziness, nausea, and vomiting; or promote constipation, urinary frequency, or incontinence. Some older adults are unwilling to take prescribed drugs because of side effects. The nurse's role with an older client undergoing drug therapy is to ensure the greatest therapeutic benefit with the least amount of harm.

Sedatives and tranquilizers may cause acute confusion. Ironically, these drugs are frequently administered to confused older clients. Confusion that varies with time is referred to as **sundown syndrome** and occurs most frequently in an institutional setting. Older clients with clear mental status by day suddenly become disoriented at night. Drugs used to manage this behavior should be carefully administered, taking into account age-related changes in body systems that can affect the drugs' pharmacokinetic activity. In addition, the nurse can use creative measures, such as making the environment more meaningful, providing adequate light, encouraging use of prostheses, or even making telephone calls to friends or family members to let clients hear reassuring voices.

Nutrition. Minimum nutritional needs for the older adult are the same as those of younger adults, except that greater amounts of calcium, vitamin C, and vitamin A are required. Total caloric intake usually declines in response to illness, changes in metabolic rate, and physical activity. Nutritional needs of older adults are described in Chapter 41.

Exercise. The older adult should be encouraged to maintain physical exercise and activity. The primary benefits of exercise include maintaining and strengthening functional ability and promoting a sense of enhanced well-being. A study by Lord, Caplan, and Ward (1993) found that exercise may play a role in improving a number of sensorimotor systems that contribute to stability (balance, reaction time, muscular strength) and may help prevent falls in older women. In addition, a host of physiological benefits are associated with exercise. Before beginning a formal exercise program, the client should have a physical examination, which may include a stress cardiogram or stress test. This provides information about cardiovascular function during sustained exercise. The nurse should plan an exercise program that meets physical needs while allowing for physical impairments. Regular exercise to promote functional ability can be incorporated into the older adult's activities of daily living. For example, arm circles and leg circles can be performed while watching television.

Psychosocial Health Concerns. Psychosocial health concerns vary among older adults. The nurse assesses role transitions that occur between middle age and older adulthood. Because of the cognitive, social, and physical effects of aging, many older adults require assistance to maintain psychosocial health (see p. 578).

 Nursing Diagnosis

Data are systematically collected during assessment. Assessment is essential in gerontological nursing, because client status changes often. Data regarding the physiological, cognitive, and psychosocial status of the older adult lead to actual or at risk problems (see the nursing diagnoses box on p. 584). Any nursing diagnosis can have a variety of related factors. Identification of the related factor or probable cause for each diagnosis gives direction in developing nursing interventions. For example, interventions for constipation are different if the probable cause is a medication rather than immobility.

Analysis of data requires consideration of individual strengths and limitations, as well as the older client's perception of health status. Validation of data with family, friends,

Table 31-4	**Most Common Causes of Death Among Persons 75 and Older**			
	MEN	WOMEN	MEN	WOMEN
	75-84*		85 AND OLDER*	
Heart disease	3239	2122	7830	6810
Malignancies	1861	982	2528	1292
Cerebrovascular accident (CVA)	603	523	1625	1738
Chronic obstructive pulmonary disease (COPD)	504	197	777	245
Pneumonia and flu	352	199	1428	1006
Accidents	143	84	375	225
Diabetes	127	123	229	219
Suicide	57	7	60	5
Liver disease	44	25	34	14

From Ebersole P, Hess P: *Toward healthy aging: human needs and nursing response,* ed 4, St Louis, 1994, Mosby.
*Per 100,000.

Examples of NANDA Nursing Diagnoses for the Older Adult

Impaired physical mobility *related to:*
- Pain and discomfort
- Musculoskeletal impairment

Pain *related to:*
- Progressive degenerative musculoskeletal condition
- Bladder inflammation

Activity intolerance *related to:*
- Pain and stiffness secondary to musculoskeletal condition

Self-care deficit: bathing/hygiene, dressing/grooming, toileting *related to:*
- Decreased strength and endurance secondary to pain of musculoskeletal condition

Altered urinary elimination *related to:*
- Bladder inflammation

nursing colleagues, other health professionals, and client records may be necessary. Assessment data contain subjective and objective characteristics necessary for validation of a nursing diagnosis. Accurate assessment is essential because care is built on this foundation. The diagnostic process box below includes examples with related factors relevant to the situation described in the case study on p. 586.

Planning

The older adult client often has multiple physical and psychosocial problems. Accurate identification of these in the form of a nursing diagnosis is followed by development of a nursing care plan (see the care plan on p. 586).

A care plan for the older adult focuses on activities to prevent, improve, reduce, or eliminate problems (Fig. 31-6). Priorities of care are established, client goals and expected outcomes are determined, and appropriate interventions are selected. This is done with the client's participation so

Sample Nursing Diagnostic Process for the Older Adult

ASSESSMENT ACTIVITIES	DEFINING CHARACTERISTICS	NURSING DIAGNOSES
Determine onset, duration, and time sequence of pain; location; severity; quality.	Fairly constant moderate to severe aching in bilateral hips and knees, worse with any activity that requires walking or weight bearing; also frequently occurs after a night's rest BP 156/94, P 82, R 20	**Pain** related to progressive degenerative musculoskeletal condition
Note physical signs and symptoms: vital signs, facial and body movements, vocalizations, degree of social interaction.	Slight moaning as she describes her pain and rubs her knees and hips. Ambulates slowly and deliberately with a quad cane; moves cautiously from stand to sit and back to stand; rubbing knees	
Determine influence of pain on activities of daily living: hygiene, dressing and grooming, toileting, feeding, and usual social activities.	No longer able to bathe in a bathtub; able to dress independently but with difficulty; able to cook and feed herself, but relies increasingly on frozen dinners and foods. Stopped attending senior center three times/wk or Sunday church services because of difficulty boarding van	
Identify relief measures used to date and their effectiveness.	Has tried Tylenol 2 tablets at HS, but with little relief; uses Ben Gay® on knees and hips daily, but notes little relief from this either	
Observe appearance, stature, and posture. Observe body alignment, gait, and flexibility of movement while sitting, standing, and walking.	Ambulates slowly with stooped posture; reacts uncomfortably with position changes, and without flexibility or agility, relies on cane and assistance of niece	**Impaired physical mobility** related to pain and discomfort
Check range of motion of knees and hips.	Hip flexion, extension, abduction, and adduction all extremely limited; internal and external rotation considerably reduced; knee flexion and extension moderately limited; all movements performed with difficulty secondary to pain; no joint instability noted	
Inspect and palpate affected joints for swelling, redness, or deformity; listen and feel for crepitation with movement.	Slight swelling of knee joints, without redness or obvious deformity; right knee with some bony enlargement, crepitation, and tenderness	

Geriatric Outpatient Program CareMap®

Last Update: 05/94

Lakes Region General Hospital-Behavioral Health Services

Author: _____   Diagnosis _____

Interventions	Date: _____ **Visit One**	Initials
Assessments	1. CNS initiates Geriatric Assessment Form 2. MSW initiates psychosocial HX when indicated.	
Consults	CNS determines the need for consults and initiate the process per policy	
Specimens/ Tests	Health Screen 1	
	B12	
	Folate	
	EKG and CXR if not done in the past 6 months unless otherwise ordered by MD.	
	CNS reviews all recent lab results and notifies the medical director if indicated.	

Treatments	Data obtained during this visit discussed with
	    the appropriate discipline and with the medical
	    director to draw a plan of action for a treatment	

	Patient, family members, primary physician or the agency notified.	
Medications	All medications are brought to the CNS and documented.	
Nutrition	CNS determines the need for dietary consults.	
Activity/ Safety	CNS determines the need for consults.	

	If indicated, CNS discusses issues related to safety
	    and activity with the patient, family members, primary
	    physician or the agency.	

Teaching	CNS assesses the learning needs of the patient and significant others and draws a plan of action as appropriate.	

Transfer/ Discharge Coordination	Based on initial data, CNS determines the extent
	    of the role of the appropriate discipline in drawing a plan
	    of action and/or possibly convening a discharge meeting.	

	Signatures	
Check, initial and sign. Note detours (deviations from normal) on reverse side.	MD	
	ARNP	
	MSW	
	OTHER	

The Center for Case Management is the owner of the CareMap trademark and concept.   May 1992: The Center for Case Management, 6 Pleasant Street, South Natick, MA 01760.

NOTE: Acceptable medical practice generally does include a variety of responses to a particular clinical problem.

Fig. 31-6 Geriatric outpatient program CareMap®. *(Courtesy Lakes Regional General Hospital, Laconia, NH, and The Center for Case Managment, South Natick, MA.)*

Sample Nursing Care Plan for Impaired Physical Mobility

NURSING DIAGNOSES: **Impaired physical mobility** related to pain and discomfort
DEFINITION: The state in which an individual experiences a limitation of ability for independent physical movement (Kim, McFarland, McLane, 1995)

GOALS	EXPECTED OUTCOMES	INTERVENTIONS	RATIONALE
Client will experience relief of pain by end of week.	Client self-administers prescribed antiinflammatory medication on scheduled basis. Client reports hip and knee pain as 3 or less on a 10-point scale over a 24-hour period.	Instruct client on appropriate use and action of antiinflammatory agents. Apply warm, moist heat to affected joints for 10-15 minutes at least 4 times a day and prn. Take warm shower/bath on arising. Teach use of progressive relaxation exercises as an adjunct to pain medication.	Medication is most effective when used on a consistent, regular schedule to maintain adequate serum levels (McCaffery, 1989). Avoid hot water to reduce risk of thermal injury and increased fatigue. Moist heat is more penetrating than dry heat. Relief of pain is essential to promoting and maintaining maximum joint mobility and muscle function (McCaffery, 1989).
Client will achieve optimum level of physical mobility by end of month.	Client will be able to perform self-care activities without experiencing uncontrollable joint pain or joint movement limitations.	Ensure correct application of physical exercise program recommended by physical therapist, and balance of rest therapy with exercise program. Instruct in correct use of assistive devices and energy-saving techniques while performing daily self-care.	Slow, gradual exercise promotes joint strength and function and minimizes fatigue (Guralnik, 1994). Rest stabilizes and decreases stress on affected joints and promotes muscle relaxation. The use of devices and techniques promotes the client's sense of control over the disability, enhances self-esteem, and lessens pain and decreases joint stress (Ebersole and Hess, 1994).

CASE STUDY   Mrs. Moore is an 87-year-old woman who lives alone in her own home, independently managing most of her self-care needs. A niece and her husband who live nearby do Mrs. Moore's grocery shopping, housecleaning, and yard work. Her major medical diagnoses include hypertension and degenerative joint disease (DJD).

Because of new onset urinary symptoms of frequency, burning, urgency, and nocturia, Mrs. Moore made an appointment with her nurse practitioner. During the visit, the nurse practitioner also determined that Mrs. Moore's joint pain and stiffness, especially in her knees, hips, and shoulders, have become increasingly worse over the last 6 to 8 weeks, limiting her ability to perform even basic activities of daily living (ADLs). The following medications were prescribed: Septra DS 1 PO bid for 10 days for treatment of an *Escherichia coli* urinary tract infection, and ibuprofen 400 mg after meals and at bedtime with food or milk for joint pain and stiffness.

The niece expresses concern to the nurse that, because of the urinary and joint symptoms, Mrs. Moore has become increasingly dependent and limited in her ability to meet her own needs. Because she has not felt well in recent weeks, her appetite and energy level have decreased. Mrs. Moore wants to remain at home as long as possible and her niece agrees, but the urinary tract infection and DJD exacerbation seem to have seriously affected her functional ability, and both are concerned about the long-term effects of these problems on her overall health and independence. ■

that the interventions are understood and conflicts in approaches or priorities can be avoided. Consideration by the nurse of the experiences of a lifetime, as well as values and sociocultural patterns developed, should serve as the basis for planning individual care.

Goals of care established with the older adult should reflect consideration of factors that influence normal aging, maintain independence as much as possible, and facilitate an optimal level of comfort and coping. Although it is sometimes more time consuming and difficult, including the older client in the care planning process and allowing maximal independence in self-care activities can promote physical and psychosocial health.

In cases where the client's cognitive status prevents participation in establishing goals and outcomes and planning interventions, families must be included. Families and friends are rich sources of data when developing individualized care plans because they knew the client before the impairment. Frequently, they can provide explanations for clients' behaviors and suggest methods of management.

Implementation

Nursing interventions for older adults can encompass health promotion and maintenance, psychosocial support, home safety, self-medication, adjustment, and preservation. It is important to incorporate the client's routines or rituals when possible. The older adult feels more secure when rituals are continued. Interventions generally are aimed at facilitating independence and supporting self-care abilities. Care activities require more time because of slower responses, the number of problems, and the close relationship between physical and psychosocial aspects of aging.

Health Promotion

The efficacy of health promotion with the older adult population still raises controversy. Increasing scientific evidence suggests that lifestyle choices influence overall health status and longevity, even when changes are made in late life (Hogstel, 1994).

When a client has impaired physical mobility, the nurse's role is to promote optimal mobility, comfort, and safety by creating an environment that supports and compensates for the altered functioning. The degree of assistance required depends on the degree of limitation, but the nurse should be careful not to do more for the client than the condition warrants. Preservation of ability is crucial to the client's self-esteem.

The nurse also cares for families of older adults with physical impairments and disabilities. Care-giving family members can experience much distress and may need support, assistance with problem solving, and education about the client's care needs. This can be accomplished through support groups, in family meetings, or in a nurse-client interaction.

Home Safety

The home care nurse in the above situation observes the client's home environment to ensure there are no hazards present that would place the client at risk for injury in view of impaired mobility. The following list of environmental factors should be addressed to promote the client's safety in the home:

- Adequate lighting on stairs, in entry ways, and at night
- Pathways clear of clutter and free of loose mats/rugs and electrical cords/wire
- Convenient arrangements for kitchen and bathroom
- Stable, nonskid footwear
- Chairs and other furniture with sufficient support and at appropriate height for sitting down and getting up
- Skid-proof strips or mat in tub or shower
- Supportive handrails for stairs and bathroom

In addition, the nurse assesses the client's safe and correct use of the quad cane to prevent a fall or other injury.

Psychosocial Support

Interventions for psychosocial health of older adults resemble those for other age groups. However, some interventions are more crucial for older adults experiencing social isolation, cognitive impairment, or other psychosocial problems. These interventions include therapeutic communication, touch, reality orientation, resocialization, validation therapy, reminiscence, and interventions to improve body image.

Therapeutic communication. With therapeutic communication the nurse perceives and respects the client's uniqueness. The nurse who communicates effectively will be accepted as one who shares a genuine concern for the client's

welfare. The nurse cannot simply enter a client's environment and immediately establish a therapeutic relationship, but must first be knowledgeable and skilled in communication techniques. The nursing student can practice these techniques with other students (see Chapter 14).

Touch. Touch is the first sense to become functional. It provides knowledge about others throughout life. In all cultures, gentle touch conveys affection and friendliness. Often, older adults who are victims of social isolation are deprived of the touching that was an important part of earlier life.

Touch is a therapeutic tool that nurses can use to help comfort the older adult. It can provide sensory stimulation, relax the client, provide physical and emotional comfort, orient the person to reality, convey warmth, and communicate interest. It is a powerful physical expression of a relationship.

An older adult who is isolated, dependent, or ill; who fears death; or who lacks self-esteem has a greater need for touch. The client may invite touch by reaching for a nurse's hand. Often, older men are wrongly accused of sexual advances when they demonstrate this need. The nurse should recognize that the client may be suffering from touch deprivation. Nurses should not use touch in a condescending way, however, such as a pat on the head or a gentle pinch. Touch should convey respect and sensitivity. The nurse should not be surprised if the client reciprocates because of an unmet need for intimacy.

Reality orientation. Reality orientation, first described by Taulbee and Folsom in 1966, is a communication technique used to make a client aware of time, place, and person. The purposes of reality orientation include restoring a sense of reality; improving the level of awareness; promoting socialization; elevating independent functioning; and minimizing confusion, disorientation, and physical regression.

The nurse can use reality-orientation techniques anywhere. The older adult experiencing a change in environment, surgery, illness, or emotional stress is at risk for becoming disoriented. Environmental changes, such as the bright lights and lack of windows in specialized units of a hospital, often lead to disorientation and confusion. The environment and nursing personnel often change in a hospital, so the client's environment is unstable. This makes adaptation difficult. For this reason, many older clients lose track of time and become confused while in the hospital. The problem is compounded by sedatives, tranquilizers, anesthesia, and restraints that take away dignity.

The nurse should anticipate and monitor for disorientation and confusion as possible consequences of hospitalization, relocation, surgery, loss, or illness and incorporate reality orientation into the care plan. These interventions are based on seven principles (see the box on p. 588). Though not a remedy, reality orientation can diminish moderate confusional states when used with other therapies (Burnside, 1986).

Resocialization. Resocialization helps older adults to expand their social networks. It is especially beneficial to older adults whose social interaction depended primarily on employment. Similarly, resocialization is important for older adults whose spouses or close friends have died.

The key to resocialization is knowing resources easily

Guidelines for Reality Orientation

REALISM
- Use reality information such as time, date, place, and name in conversation.
- Refer clients to clocks and other reality-orientation props when necessary.
- Do not reinforce delusions or hallucinations.
- Direct clients back to reality-oriented endeavors if they ramble in conversation or talk unrealistically.
- If erratic behavior is shown, such as picking at clothes, give clients purposeful things to do.

INDEPENDENCE
- Express confidence in clients' ability to be self-directing.
- Encourage clients to perform tasks and make decisions, assisting only when necessary.
- Make sure clients have needed aids, such as glasses, dentures, and hearing aids, and that they work.
- Provide bowel and bladder training when necessary.
- Provide speech or physical therapy when necessary.
- Reduce medication to a minimum.

INDIVIDUALIZATION
- Keep reality-orientation classes small to permit individual attention.
- Allow clients to keep familiar treasures and objects.
- Encourage meaningful object relationships.

REINFORCEMENT
- Watch for small changes in behavior that indicate progress, and reward them.
- Reward correct behavior with verbal praise, touch, or smiles.
- Reinforce achievement with increased responsibility.
- Encourage special talents or interests.

REPETITION
- Repeat information, directions, statements, and questions as necessary.
- Be patient and allow time for responses or replies.
- Give clues to the answer when asking a question; if clients are unable to answer, provide the correct response and allow them to repeat it.

CLARITY
- Enunciate clearly and speak slowly.
- Reword statements and questions if necessary.
- Give directions in clear, simple, short statements.

CONSISTENCY
- Maintain continuity of care.
- Adhere to scheduling.
- Use the same personnel when possible.

From Ebersole P, Hess P: *Toward healthy aging: human needs and nursing response,* ed 4, St Louis, 1994, Mosby.

Table 31-5   Reminiscence Group Strategies

	COGNITIVELY IMPAIRED	PSYCHOLOGICALLY DISTURBED	DEPRESSED
CLIENT SELECTION	Choose no more than five members of same age but both sexes.	Choose 10 members of varied ages and both sexes.	Choose 8 to 10 members of both sexes. Choose persons with similar problems (e.g., grieving, retirement).
STRUCTURE	Choose consistent place and time. Conduct frequent, 30-min meetings. Use coleaders.	Choose consistent place and time. Conduct biweekly. 1-hr meetings. Use one leader consistently.	Choose varied meeting places. Meet weekly, for 1 hr. Vary leaders.
PROCESS	Connect specific events, things, and places common to group.	Connect members through shared feelings and survival strategies.	Focus on successful coping during life span; encourage mutuality.
GOALS	Stimulate memory, enhance identity, raise self-esteem, and increase socialization skills.	Recognize feelings and meaning of suppressed conflicts, enlarge coping strategies, integrate self-view, and promote universality.	Reduce feelings of hopelessness, restore personal control, increase affectual responsiveness, develop sense of integrity and acceptance of life as lived, and promote caring between members.
NURSE'S FUNCTION	Provide comfortable, mildly stimulating environment. Select props that will stimulate memories. Assist members by giving specific information, reminders, and clues. Give praise and recognition for participation.	Establish private meeting and closed group. Focus on specific developmental stages or critical life events. Accept and validate all expressions of feeling. Clarify multiple meanings of events. Reduce anxiety.	Provide comfortable, stimulating environment. Appeal to sensory memories. Focus on evidence of caring and sharing. Demonstrate caring attitude. Allow time to complain.

From Ebersole P, Hess P: *Toward healthy aging: human needs and nursing response,* ed 4, St Louis, 1994, Mosby.

available to clients. Many older adults eagerly participate in senior citizens' groups, foster grandparent programs, or hospital volunteer work. However, they may not know how to make the initial contact. The nurse can provide older adults with names or can personally contact the agency. The nurse and clients must work together for effective re-socialization.

Developing secondary relationships. Just as socialization is important for older adults who are at risk for isolation, secondary relationships are important for those who maintain primary relationships. Family and friends provide long-term support for many older adults. However, reliable secondary relationships with peers must be developed to provide a social group not bound by emotions frequently experienced in families. For example, older persons in a senior center enjoy socializing with peers and younger staff. They share their experiences and concerns but are related only by common feelings or ideas.

The nurse can help form secondary relationships by promoting discussion on topics of mutual interest at day-care centers, nutrition program sites, or long-term care centers. For example, clients with arthritis may benefit from discussing ways to maintain activity. The following are guidelines for conducting discussion sessions:

1. Select a small, quiet room that is well lit and has comfortable furniture. Consider visual, hearing, or musculoskeletal impairments.
2. Keep meetings short enough to promote learning and reduce exhaustion (20 minutes).
3. Choose participants who are able to participate.
4. Consider older adults' sensory deficits when using visual aids (such as brightly colored posters with large print).
5. Present one topic for discussion at each meeting.
6. Make it clear that participation is voluntary.

Peer group meetings allow participants to develop secondary relationships. Older adults learn to share ideas and solve problems without dwelling on physical ailments or feelings of hopelessness.

Validation therapy. **Validation therapy** is a technique used with severely confused and disoriented older adults. The goal is to provide a sense of dignity and self-worth and to validate clients' feelings. Clients are not confronted with their inappropriate behaviors. Rather, the nurse attempts to meet older adults in their reality and find the meaning behind the behaviors. Confused older adults gain a positive sense of self because the nurse validates their feelings.

Reminiscence. **Reminiscence** is recalling the past to assign new meanings to experiences. It is an adaptive function of older adults. As a therapy, reminiscence is an elaboration of the natural way that older adults revive their past to give meaning or to reconcile conflicts and disappointments as they prepare for death (Butler, 1963). Reminiscing contributes to successful adaptation by maintaining self-esteem, reaffirming identity, and working through loss (see the box above).

Reminiscence can be used for impaired, disturbed, or depressed older adults. The nurse organizes the group and selects strategies. The group's size, structure, process, goals, and activities are adapted to meet its members' needs. Table 31-5 details the techniques of reminiscence.

▶ RESEARCH HIGHLIGHT

RESEARCH ABSTRACT
The purpose of this study by Bramlett and Gueldner was to investigate the usefulness of reminiscent storytelling as a therapeutic modality to enhance the sense of power in well older persons. A quasi experimental pre- and posttest design was used to measure clients' sense of personal power. Subjects in the experimental group (n = 34) and the control group (n = 41) were pretested on the same schedule. The experimental group subjects participated in three 1-hour reminiscence sessions during a 1-week period; the control group subjects received no treatment. All participants were tested immediately after the third reminiscence session, and again at a 5-week interval. There were no significant differences between experimental and control groups at pretest, 1-week posttest, or 5-week posttest. Both groups experienced a small, insignificant decrease in power between the pretest and 1-week posttest. Both groups then showed a significant increase in power between 1-week posttest and 5-week posttest. Although the value of reminiscence as a therapeutic modality was not supported by these study findings, in light of the positive results of other studies of reminiscence as a treatment, it is recommended that more research be conducted on this topic. Today's health care system holds few opportunities for older persons to have human contact and genuine caring and consideration. Unique modalities such as reminiscence, which enables human exchange, may provide a useful strategy for meeting this challenge within the delivery system.

IMPLICATIONS FOR PRACTICE
▶ Reminiscing with clients supports a caring attitude
▶ Reminiscence may help clients become more involved in interaction with others

REFERENCE
Bramlett MH, Gueldner SH: Reminiscence: a viable option to enhance power in elders, *Clin Nurse Specialist* 7(2):68, 1993.

Body-image interventions. The way that older adults present themselves has a significant impact on body image and feelings of isolation. Some physical characteristics of older adulthood are socially desirable, such as distinguished-looking gray hair. Other features are also impressive, such as a lined face that displays character or wrinkled hands that convey a lifetime of hard work. Too often, however, society sees older people as incapacitated, deaf, obese, or shrunken in stature. When older adults have acute or chronic illnesses, the related physical dependence makes it difficult for them to maintain body image. A nurse with stereotypes about the appearance of older adults may give little attention to grooming or hygiene. Consequences of illness and aging that threaten the older adult's body image include invasive diagnostic procedures, pain, surgery, prosthesis, loss of sensation in a body part, skin changes, dependence on life-sustaining medication, denture odor, loss of scalp hair, and incontinence.

The nurse has a direct influence on the client's appearance. The importance to the older adult of presenting a socially acceptable image must be considered. It takes little effort to assist the client with combing hair, cleaning dentures, shaving, or changing clothing. The older adult does not choose to have an objectionable appearance. The nurse should also be sensitive to odors in the environment. Odors created by urine and some illnesses are often present. By controlling odors, the nurse may prevent visitors from shortening their stay or not coming at all.

Medication Use

Managing medications is a very important component of maintaining and promoting good health in old age. The nurse works collaboratively with the client to assure safe and appropriate use of all medications. The client should be taught the names of all drugs being taken, when and how to take them, and the desirable and undesirable effects of the drugs. The nurse also teaches how to avoid adverse effects and/or interactions of drugs, and how to establish and follow an appropriate self-administration pattern (see the box at right).

Additional strategies for reducing the risk of an adverse medication reaction in the older adult include the following:

- Reviewing the medications with the client at each visit
- Examining for potential interactions with food or other drugs
- Simplifying and individualizing the drug regimen
- Taking every opportunity to inform the client and family about all aspects of medication use
- Encouraging the client to question the physician, advanced practice nurse, and/or pharmacist about all prescribed drugs (Hogstel, 1994).

For some older adults on large numbers of medications, safely managing medications can be a complex activity that can easily become overwhelming. Nurses can provide valuable assistance to their older adult clients as they carry out this important self-care activity.

CLIENT TEACHING
for Medication Use

OBJECTIVE
- Client will correctly identify side effects of prescribed nonsteroidal antiinflammatory drug (NSAID).

TEACHING STRATEGIES
- Explain the drug classification, NSAID.
- Explain the significant and reportable side effects of NSAID therapy: nausea and vomiting, indigestion, epigastric pain, heartburn, diarrhea, abdominal distress, constipation, fullness of gastrointestinal tract (bloating and flatulence), dizziness, rash and/or pruritis, tinnitus.
- Explain correct administration methods to reduce/avoid side effects: take with food or milk, take only as directed.

EVALUATION
- Client will correctly identify possible side effects of NSAID therapy and ways to take medication to reduce/avoid their occurrence.

 Evaluation

Evaluation measures the degree to which the plan and interventions were effective in meeting the expected outcomes. The nurse determines whether goals have been met and what changes have occurred in the client's status as a result of the interventions. Goals may be revised or eliminated, or new goals may be developed. Implementation may be affected as goals change. Just as the client and family were included in developing the care plan, their input in evaluating outcomes of care should be sought.

 Sample Evaluation of Interventions for Impaired Physical Mobility

GOALS	EVALUATIVE MEASURES	EXPECTED OUTCOMES
Client will experience relief of pain by end of week.	Check client's diary of self-medication administration at home. Assess client's self-report of pain. Observe facial expressions and general body movements for evidence of discomfort while the client is sitting, standing, walking, and performing various self-care tasks.	Client correctly self-administers antiinflammatory medication on scheduled basis. Client reports hip and knee pain as 3 or less on a 10-point scale over a 24-hr period. Client exhibits and reports no discomfort during performance of daily activities.
Client will achieve optimum level of physical mobility by end of month.	Assess client's ability to perform self-care activities in the home: bathing, dressing, cooking, and toileting. Observe client's use of assistive devices and energy-saving techniques while performing various self-care activities. Assess clients joint ROM during exercise.	Client will be able to perform self-care activities without uncontrollable joint pain or joint movement limitations.

The frequency of evaluation with an older adult is highly individual. Change is often slow and subtle, thus infrequent or frequent evaluations may be performed. The type of problems, goals established, and interventions used determine the frequency of evaluation. For example, if the goal is for the client to be free from the skin complications of immobility, evaluation should be frequent and regular. If the intervention is a weight-reduction diet, evaluation of the client should be weekly. The nurse plays a major role in encouraging the older adult to participate in evaluating the plan, interventions, and progress. The evaluation box on p. 590 includes such measures as related to the case study on p. 586.

■ KEY CONCEPTS ■

▶ Myths and stereotypes portray older adults as ill, rigid in thinking, institutionalized, poor, unable to learn, and without sexual needs.

▶ A nurse's attitudes toward older adults can affect the quality and level of care.

▶ Physiological and biological theories of aging provide explanations for the aging process.

▶ The psychosocial theories of aging, which include the disengagement, activity, and continuity theories, attempt to describe the effects of lifestyle, personality, and environmental factors on longevity.

▶ The older adult must adjust to physical changes in body systems.

▶ The older adult must adjust to retirement and acquire new activities and interests to maintain quality of life.

▶ The death of a spouse, a friend, or children affects adaptation to aging.

▶ Realignment of relationships between older adults and their children is necessary.

▶ Physiological changes are a normal part of aging and are not the result of illness.

▶ Characteristics of dementia include decreased intellectual function, personality change, impaired judgment, and change in affect.

▶ Cognitive impairment includes acute, potentially reversible disorders and chronic, irreversible, progressive disorders.

▶ Classic symptoms of delirium include sudden onset, altered attention and wakefulness, disturbed sleep-wake cycle, attention deficits, illusions, hallucinations, and disorientation.

▶ Cognitive impairment can result from chemical substance abuse.

▶ Psychosocial changes affecting the older adult include retirement, social isolation, change in housing, death, and sexual changes.

▶ Sexuality is linked with identity and validates the belief that a person can give to others and have the gift appreciated.

▶ In addition to physical changes, drugs prescribed for the older adult may affect sexual functioning.

▶ Changes in social roles, family responsibility, and health status influence the choice of living arrangements appropriate for the older adult.

▶ The older adult and family require nursing interventions to help them cope with the dying process.

▶ The major health problems of the older adult include arthritis, hypertension, heart disease, cerebrovascular accident, cancer, diabetes, sensory impairments, and dental problems.

▶ The four leading causes of death in the older population are heart disease, malignant neoplasms, cerebrovascular disease, and chronic obstructive pulmonary disease.

▶ Nursing interventions for psychosocial problems should be individualized; they include therapeutic communication, touch, reality orientation, resocialization, validation therapy, reminiscence, and interventions to improve body image.

▶ Health care services for older adults are available in the community-based and institutional settings.

■ KEY TERMS ■

Ageism, p. 571

Alzheimer's disease, p. 577

Attitudinal isolation, p. 579

Behavioral isolation, p. 579

Confabulation, p. 577

Delirium, p. 577

Dementia, p. 577

Geographical isolation, p. 579

Geriatrics, p. 570

Gerontological nursing, p. 570

Gerontology, p. 570

Korsakoff's syndrome, p. 577

Presbycusis, p. 576

Presbyopia, p. 575

Presentational isolation, p. 579

Reality orientation, p. 587

Reminiscence, p. 589

Resocialization, p. 587

Senile lentigo, p. 575

Sundown syndrome, p. 583

Validation therapy, p. 589

Wernicke's syndrome, p. 577

■ CRITICAL THINKING EXERCISES ■

1. Mr. Stein, a 78-year-old client who was admitted through the emergency room after a fall at home, had surgery yesterday to repair a hip fracture. While giving his morning care, the nurse observes that Mr. Stein is acutely confused. Identify three possible causes of his delirium. List six possible interventions aimed at promoting his safety and feelings of security.

2. An older female client comes to the clinic with 11 medications prescribed by her primary physician and two specialists. She complains of not feeling well, despite taking the medications as prescribed. What actions should the nurse take in counseling this client about her medications?

3. You are planning a health screening fair for an area senior center. Identify three possible screenings you could offer, including appropriate health-teaching strategies.

4. You are conducting a physical examination on a 73-year-old woman who has noted a gradual decrease in mobility in recent years. What musculoskeletal system changes will you expect to find?

REFERENCES

Abrams WB, Berkow R: *The Merck manual of geriatrics,* Rahway, NJ, 1990, Merck, Sharp, and Dohme Research Laboratories.

American Association of Retired Persons: *A profile of older Americans, 1992,* Washington, DC, 1992, The Association.

American Psychiatric Association: *Diagnostic and statistical manual of mental disorders (DSM-IV-R),* Washington, DC, 1994, The Association.

Berger R: *Gay and gray: the older homosexual man,* Urbana, Illinois, 1982, The University of Illinois Press.

Billhorn D: Sexuality and the chronically ill older adult, *Geriatr Nurs* 15(2):106, 1994.

Brady BF: Mental health of the aging. In Johnson B, editor: *Psychiatric-mental health nursing: adaptation and growth,* ed 3, Philadelphia, 1993, Lippincott.

Burnside IM: Transition to later life: developmental theories and research. In Burnside IM, Ebersole P, Monea HE, editors: *Psychosocial caring through the life span,* New York, 1979, McGraw-Hill.

Burnside IM: *Working with the elderly: group process and techniques,* ed 2, Boston, 1986, Jones & Barlett.

Butler R: Life review: an interpretation of reminiscence in the aged, *Psychiatry* 26:65, 1963.

Christiansen JL, Grzybowski JM: *Biology of aging,* St Louis, 1993, Mosby.

Cummings E, Henry WE: *Growing old: the process of disengagement,* New York, 1961, Basic Books.

Diekelman N: Pre-retirement counseling, *Am J Nurs* 78:1337, 1978.

Duvall EM: *Family development,* ed 5, Philadelphia, 1977, Lippincott.

Ebersole P, Hess P: *Toward healthy aging: human needs and nursing response,* ed 3, St Louis, 1990, Mosby.

Ebersole P, Hess P: *Toward healthy aging: human needs and nursing response,* ed 4, St Louis, 1994, Mosby.

Ferrell BR, Rivera L: Pain. In Lueckenotte AG, editor: *Textbook of gerontologic nursing,* St Louis, 1996, Mosby.

Guralnik JM: Understanding the relationship between disease and disability, *J Am Geriatr Soc* 42:1128, 1994.

Havighurst RJ: *Human development and education,* New York, 1953, David McKay.

Hayflick L: Biologic aging theories. In Maddox G, editor: *The encyclopedia of aging,* New York, 1987, Springer.

Heyman A: Differentiation of Alzheimer's disease from multi-infarct dementia. In Katzman R, Terry RD, Bick KL, editors: *Alzheimer's disease: senile dementia and related disorders,* New York, 1978, Raven.

Hogstel M: *Clinical manual of gerontological nursing,* ed 2, St. Louis, 1992, Mosby.

Hogstel M: *Nursing care of the older adult,* ed 3, Albany, New York, 1994, Delmar.

Kain CD, Reilly N, Schultz ED: The older adult, a comparative assessment, *Nurs Clin North Am* 25:833, 1990.

Kehoe M: Have you ever seen a lesbian over 60? *The Aging Connection* 4(4):4, 1988.

Kim MJ, McFarland GK, McLane AM: *Pocket guide to nursing diagnoses,* ed 4, St Louis, 1993, Mosby.

Lemon BW et al: An exploration of the activity theory of aging: activity types and life satisfaction among in-movers to a retirement community, *J Gerontol* 27:511, 1972.

Lemon BW, Bengston VL, Peterson JA: An exploration of the activity theory of aging: activity types and life satisfaction among in-movers to a retirement community, *J Gerontol* 27:516, 1992.

Lord SR, Caplan GA, Ward JA: Balance, reaction time, and muscular strength in exercising and non-exercising older women: a pilot study, *Arch Phys Med Rehabil* 74(8):837, 1993.

Lueckenotte A: *Pocket guide to gerontologic assessment,* ed 2, St Louis, 1994, Mosby.

Lueckenotte A: *Textbook of gerontologic nursing,* St Louis, 1996, Mosby.

Maddox GL: Disengagement theory: a critical evaluation, *Gerontologist* 4:80, 1974.

Masters, WH: Sex and aging . . . expectations and reality, *Hosp Pract* 8:175, 1986.

McCaffery M, Beebe A: *Pain: clinical manual for nursing practice,* St Louis, 1989, CV Mosby.

National High Blood Pressure Education Program; National Heart, Lung, & Blood Institute; National Institutes of Health: *The fifth report of the Joint National Committee on Detection, Evaluation, and Treatment of High Blood Pressure,* NIH Pub No 93-1088, Bethesda, Md, 1993, NIH.

Neugarten BL: *Personality in middle and late life,* New York, 1964, Atherton.

Rawlins R et al: *Mental health–psychiatric nursing,* ed 3, St Louis, 1993, Mosby.

Stanhope M, Lancaster J: *Community health nursing: process and practice for promoting health,* ed 3, St Louis, 1992, Mosby.

Taulbee LA, Folsom JC: Reality orientation for geriatric patients, *Hosp Community Psychiatry* 17(5):133, 1966.

Theis SL: Using previous knowledge to teach elderly clients, *J Gerontol Nurs* 17(8):34, 1991.

United States Bureau of the Census: *Statistical abstract of the United States,* Washington, DC, 1993, The Bureau.

Wallace M: Intimacy and sexuality. In Lueckenotte AG, editor: *Textbook of gerontologic nursing,* St Louis, 1996, Mosby.

Weinrich SP, Boyd M, Nussbaum J: Continuing education: adapting strategies to teach the elderly, *J Gerontol Nurs* 15(11):17, 1989.

ADDITIONAL READINGS

Bramlett M, Gueldner S: Reminiscence: A viable option to enhance power in elders, *Clin Nurs Specialist* 7(2):68, 1993.

Butler R: *Why survive? Being old in America,* New York, 1975, Harper and Row.

Evans LK, Strumpf NE: Myths about elder restraint, *Image J Nurs Sch* 22(2):124, 1990.

Kreidler M et al: Community elderly: a nursing center's use of change theory as a model, *J Gerontol Nurs* 20(1):25, 1994.

Lorig K: Self-management of chronic illness: a model for the future, *Generations,* 17(3):11, 1993.

McCracken A, Gerdsen L: Sharing the legacy: hospice care principles for terminally ill elders, *J Gerontol Nurs* 17(12):4, 1991.

Pascucci M: Measuring incentives to health promotion in older adults. *J Gerontol Nurs* 18(3):16, 1992.

Stolley J: When your patient has Alzheimer's disease, *Amer J Nurs* 94(8):34, 1994.

Sullivan-Marx E: Delirium and physical restraint in the hospitalized elderly, *Image J Nurs Sch* 26(4);295, 1994.

Wanich C et al: Functional status outcomes of a nursing intervention in hospitalized elderly, *Image J Nurs Sch* 24(3), 1992.

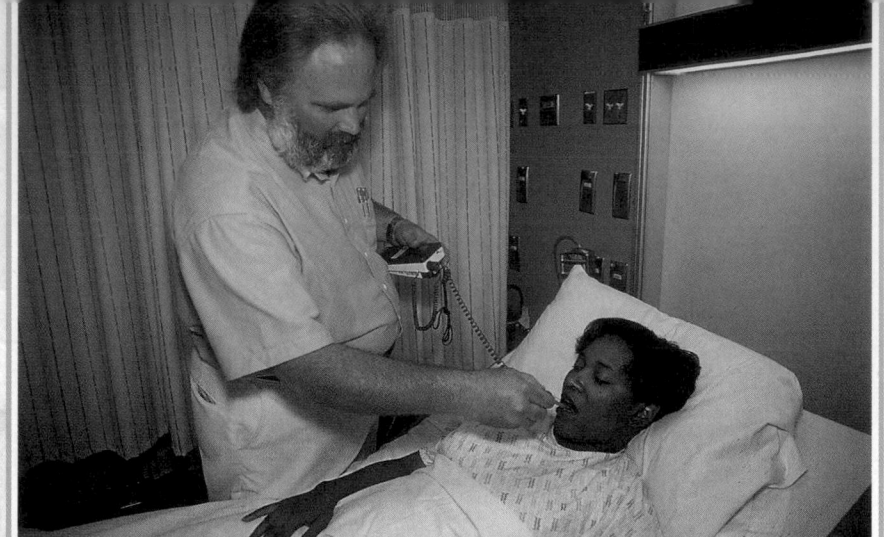

## Chapter 32

Vital Signs

Objectives

Mastery of content in this chapter will enable the student to:

► Define the key terms listed.

► Explain the principles and mechanisms of thermoregulation.

► Describe nursing measures that promote heat loss and heat conservation.

► Discuss physiological changes associated with fever.

► Accurately assess tympanic, oral, rectal, and axillary temperatures.

► Discuss the rationale for care plan interventions for a client with a fever.

► Accurately assess pulse, respirations, oxygen saturation, and blood pressure.

► Explain the physiology of normal regulation of blood pressure, pulse, oxygen saturation, and respirations.

► Describe factors that cause variations in body temperature, pulse, oxygen saturation, respirations, and blood pressure.

► Identify normal vital sign values for an infant and an adult.

► Explain variations in technique used to assess an infant's, child's, and adult's vital signs.

► Describe the benefits and precautions involving self-measurement of blood pressure.

► Identify when vital signs should be taken.

► Accurately record and report vital sign measurements.

The most frequent measurements obtained by health practitioners are those of temperature, pulse, blood pressure, respiratory rate, and oxygen saturation. As indicators of health status, these measures indicate the effectiveness of circulatory, respiratory, neural, and endocrine body functions. Because of their importance they are referred to as **vital signs.** Many factors, such as the temperature of the environment, physical exertion, and the effects of illness, cause vital signs to change, sometimes outside the normal range. Measurement of vital signs provides data to determine a client's usual state of health (baseline data), as well as response to physical and psychological stress and medical and nursing therapy. A change in vital signs can indicate a change in physiological function. An alteration in vital signs may signal the need for medical or nursing intervention.

Vital signs are a quick and efficient way of monitoring a client's condition or identifying problems and evaluating the client's response to intervention. The basic techniques of inspection, palpation, and auscultation are used to determine vital signs (see Chapter 33). These skills are simple but should not be taken for granted. Vital signs and other physiological measurements are the basis for clinical problem solving. Assessment of vital signs allows the nurse to identify nursing diagnoses, to implement planned interventions, and to evaluate success when vital signs have returned to acceptable values. When the nurse learns the physiological variables influencing vital signs and recognizes the relationship of vital sign changes to other physical assessment findings, precise determinations of the client's health problems can be made. Vital sign assessment is an essential ingredient when nurses and physicians collaborate to determine the client's health status. Careful measurement techniques ensure accurate findings.

GUIDELINES FOR TAKING VITAL SIGNS

Vital signs are a part of the data base that a nurse collects during assessment. The box below is a reference for normal values in the adult client. The nurse assesses vital signs whenever a client enters a health care agency. Vital signs are included in a complete physical assessment (see Chapter 33) or obtained individually to assess a client's condition. Establishing a data base of vital signs during a routine physical examination serves as a control for future occasions. The client's needs and condition determine when, where, and how vital signs are measured. The nurse must be able to measure vital signs correctly, understand and interpret the values, communicate findings appropriately, and begin interventions as needed. The following guidelines assist the nurse to incorporate vital sign measurement into nursing practice:

1. The nurse caring for the client is responsible for assessing vital signs. The nurse should obtain the vital signs, interpret their significance, and make decisions about interventions.
2. Equipment should be functional and appropriate. Equipment used to measure vital signs (e.g., a thermometer) must work properly to ensure accurate findings.
3. Equipment should be selected based on the client's condition and characteristics (e.g., an adult-size blood pressure cuff should not be used for a child).
4. The nurse knows the client's normal range of vital signs. A client's normal values may differ from the standard range for that age or physical state. The client's normal values serve as a baseline for comparison with later findings. Thus a nurse can detect a change in condition over time. Changes in vital signs help the nurse detect deviations from normal.
5. The nurse knows the client's medical history, therapies, and prescribed medications. Some illnesses or treatments cause predictable vital sign changes. Some medications affect at least one of the vital signs.
6. The nurse controls or minimizes environmental factors that may affect vital signs. Assessing the client's temperature in a warm, humid room may yield a value that is not a true indicator of the client's condition.
7. The nurse uses an organized, systematic approach when taking vital signs. Each procedure requires a step-by-step approach to ensure accuracy. Organization facilitates efficiency (e.g., respirations can be assessed while taking an oral temperature).
8. The manner of approach to the client can alter the vital signs. The nurse approaches the client in a calm, caring manner while demonstrating proficiency in handling the supplies needed for vital sign measurement.
9. Based on the client's condition, the nurse collaborates with the physician to decide the frequency of vital sign assessment. In the hospital the physician orders a minimum frequency of vital sign measurements for each client. Following surgery or treatment intervention, vital signs are measured frequently to detect complications. In a clinic or outpatient setting, vital signs are taken before the practitioner examines the client and after any invasive procedures.
10. The nurse develops a teaching plan to instruct the client or care giver in vital sign assessment.
11. The nurse analyzes the results of vital sign measurement. The nurse is often in the best position to assess

---

Vital Signs: Normal Ranges for Adults

TEMPERATURE RANGE: 36° TO 38°C (96.8° TO 100.4°F)

Average oral:	C = 37°	F = 98.6° (Range ± 1°F)
Average rectal:	C = 37.5°	F = 99.5°
Average axilla:	C = 36.5°	F = 97.7°

PULSE
60-100 beats/min

RESPIRATIONS
12-20 breaths/min

BLOOD PRESSURE
Average: 120/80 mm Hg
Hypertension: Systolic above 140 mm Hg
                 Diastolic above 90 mm Hg
Hypotension: Systolic below 90 mm Hg with signs of dizziness and increased pulse
Orthostatic hypotension: Fall in systolic blood pressure of 25 mm Hg systolic and 10 mm Hg diastolic accompanied by signs and symptoms of inadequate cerebral perfusion when arising from lying position to sitting or standing position

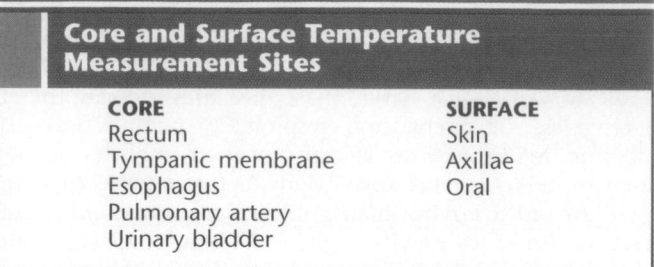

When to Take Vital Signs
When the client is admitted to a health care facility
In a hospital or care facility on a routine schedule according to the physician's order or the institution's standards of practice
Before and after a surgical procedure
Before and after an invasive diagnostic procedure
Before and after the administration of medications that affect cardiovascular, respiratory, and temperature-control function
When the client's general physical condition changes (as with loss of consciousness or increased intensity of pain)
Before and after nursing interventions influencing a vital sign (e.g., before a client previously on bed rest ambulates or before a client performs range of motion exercises)
When the client reports nonspecific symptoms of physical distress (e.g., feeling "funny" or "different")

Core and Surface Temperature Measurement Sites	
CORE	**SURFACE**
Rectum	Skin
Tympanic membrane	Axillae
Esophagus	Oral
Pulmonary artery	
Urinary bladder	

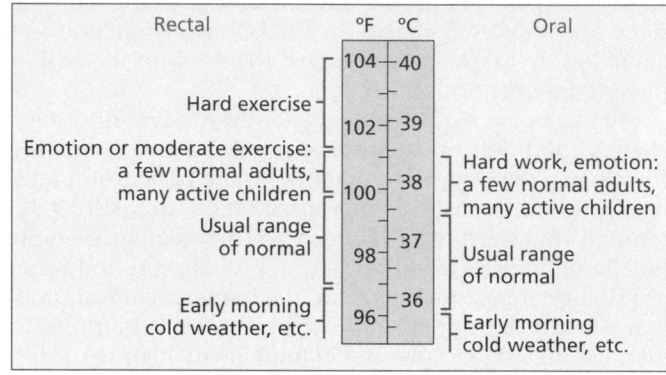

Fig. 32-1 Ranges of rectal and oral temperatures found in normal persons. *(Redrawn from Mountcastle VB: Medical physiology, vol 2, ed 14, St Louis, 1980, The CV Mosby Co; based on Dubois EF: Fever and regulation of body temperature, Springfield, Ill, 1948, Charles C Thomas.)*

all clinical findings about a client. Vital signs are not interpreted in isolation. The nurse must also know other physical signs or symptoms and be aware of the client's ongoing health status.

12. The nurse verifies and communicates significant changes in vital signs. Baseline measurements allow a nurse to identify changes in vital signs. When vital signs appear abnormal, it may help to have another nurse or a physician repeat the measurement. The nurse informs the physician or nurse in charge of abnormal vital signs. Vital signs are documented and communicated to the nurse assuming care of the client.

The nurse uses vital sign assessment to determine indications for medication administration. The physician may order certain cardiac drugs to be given only within a range of pulse or blood pressure. The nurse does not administer these drugs if vital sign assessment is outside of these limits.

Regardless of the environment, the nurse is responsible for judging whether more frequent assessments are needed (see the box above). Taking vital signs as a basis for determining changes and trends is useful in making therapeutic decisions. As a client's physical condition worsens, it may be necessary to monitor vital signs as often as every 5 to 10 minutes.

■ BODY TEMPERATURE
Physiology

Temperature is the "hotness" or "coldness" of a substance. The body temperature is the difference between the amount of heat produced by body processes and the amount of heat lost to the external environment.

HEAT PRODUCED – HEAT LOST = BODY TEMPERATURE

Despite extremes in environmental conditions and physical activity, temperature-control mechanisms of human beings keep the body's **core temperature** or temperature of deep tissues relatively constant (Fig. 32-1). However, surface temperature fluctuates depending on blood flow to the skin

and the amount of heat lost to the external environment. Because of these surface temperature fluctuations, the acceptable temperature of human beings ranges from 36°C to 38°C (96.8°F to 100.4°F). The body's tissues and cells function best within the relatively narrow temperature range.

The site of temperature measurement (oral, rectal, axillary, tympanic membrane, esophageal, pulmonary artery, or even urinary bladder) is one factor that determines the client's temperature within this narrow range. For healthy young adults the average oral temperature is 37°C (98.6°F). In clinical practice, nurses learn the temperature range of individual clients. No single temperature is normal for all people.

The measurement of body temperature is aimed at obtaining a representative average temperature of core body tissues. Average normal temperatures vary depending on the measurement site. Sites reflecting core temperatures are more reliable indicators of body temperature than sites reflecting surface temperatures (see the box above). The pulmonary artery offers the most representative readings because of the blood mix from all regions of the body. Measurement of the pulmonary artery temperature is the standard against which all other sites are judged for accuracy.

Regulation

The balance of body temperature is precisely regulated by physiological and behavioral mechanisms. For the body temperature to stay constant and within the normal range, the relationship between heat production and heat loss must be maintained. This relationship is regulated by neurological and cardiovascular mechanisms. A nurse applies knowledge of temperature control mechanisms to promote temperature regulation.

NEURAL AND VASCULAR CONTROL

The **hypothalamus**, located between the cerebral hemispheres, controls body temperature the same way a thermostat works in the home. A comfortable temperature is the "set point" at which a heating system operates. In the home a fall in environmental temperature activates the furnace, whereas a rise in temperature shuts the system down. The hypothalamus senses minor changes in body temperature. The anterior hypothalamus controls heat loss, and the posterior hypothalamus controls heat production.

When nerve cells in the anterior hypothalamus become heated beyond the set point, impulses are sent out to reduce body temperature (Fig. 32-2). Mechanisms of heat loss include sweating, vasodilation (widening) of blood vessels, and inhibition of heat production. Blood is redistributed to surface vessels to promote heat loss. If the posterior hypothalamus senses the body's temperature is lower than the set point, heat conservation mechanisms are instituted. Vasoconstriction (narrowing) of blood vessels reduces blood flow to the skin and extremities. Compensatory heat production is stimulated through voluntary muscle contraction and muscle shivering. When vasoconstriction is ineffective in preventing additional heat loss, shivering begins. Lesions or trauma to the hypothalamus or to the spinal cord, which carries hypothalamic messages, can cause serious alterations in temperature control.

HEAT PRODUCTION

Heat is produced in the body by metabolism, which is the chemical reaction in all body cells. Food is the primary fuel source for metabolism. **Thermoregulation** requires the normal function of heat-production processes. Cellular chemical reactions require energy in the form of adenosine triphosphate (ATP). The amount of energy used for metabolism is the metabolic rate. Activities requiring additional chemical reactions increase the metabolic rate. As metabolism increases, additional heat is produced. When metabolism decreases, less heat is produced. Heat production occurs during rest, voluntary movements, involuntary shivering, and nonshivering thermogenesis.

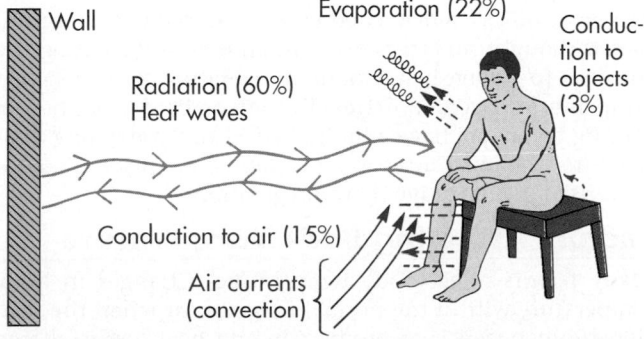

Fig. 32-2 Mechanisms of heat loss from the body. *(Modified rom Guyton AC: Textbook of medical physiology, ed 8, Philadelphia, 1991, WB Saunders.)*

1. Basal metabolism accounts for the heat produced by the body at absolute rest. The average **basal metabolic rate (BMR)** depends on the body surface area. Thyroid hormones also affect the BMR. By promoting the breakdown of body glucose and fat, thyroid hormones increase the rate of chemical reactions in almost all cells of the body. When large amounts of thyroid hormones are secreted, the BMR can increase 100% above normal. Absence of thyroid hormones can cut the BMR in half, causing a decrease in heat production. Stimulation of the sympathetic nervous system by norepinephrine and epinephrine also increases the metabolic rate of body tissues. These chemical mediators cause blood glucose levels to fall, which stimulates cells to manufacture glucose. The male sex hormone testosterone increases BMR. Men have a higher BMR than women.

2. Voluntary movements such as muscular activity during exercise require additional energy. The metabolic rate can increase up to 2000 times normal. Heat production can increase up to 50 times normal.

3. **Shivering** is an involuntary body response to temperature differences in the body. The skeletal muscle movement during shivering requires significant energy. Shivering can increase heat production 4 to 5 times greater than normal. Heat is produced to equalize body temperature.

HEAT LOSS

Heat loss and heat production occur simultaneously. The skin's structure and exposure to the environment result in constant, normal heat loss through radiation, conduction, convection, and evaporation.

Radiation. Radiation is the transfer of heat from the surface of one object to the surface of another without actual contact between the two (Thibodeau and Patton, 1993). Heat transfers through electromagnetic waves. Blood flows from the core internal organs carrying heat to skin and surface blood vessels. The amount of heat carried to the surface depends on the extent of vasoconstriction and vasodilation regulated by the hypothalamus. Heat radiates from the skin to any surrounding cooler object. Radiation increases as the temperature difference between the objects increases.

Peripheral vasodilation increases blood flow to the skin to increase radiant heat loss. Peripheral vasoconstriction minimizes radiant heat loss. Up to 85% of the human body's surface area radiates heat to the environment. However, if the surroundings are warmer than the skin, the body absorbs heat through radiation.

The nurse increases heat loss through radiation by removing clothing or blankets. The client's position enhances radiation heat loss (e.g., standing exposes a greater radiating surface area and lying in a fetal position minimizes heat radiation). Covering the body with dark, closely woven clothing also reduces the amount of radiation heat lost.

Conduction. Conduction is the transfer of heat from one object to another with direct contact. When the warm skin touches a cooler object, heat is lost. When the temperatures of the two objects are the same, conductive heat loss stops. Heat conducts through solids, gases, and liquids.

Conduction normally accounts for a small amount of heat loss. The nurse increases conductive heat loss when applying an ice pack or bathing a client with cool water. Applying several layers of clothing reduces conductive loss. The body gains heat by conduction when contact is made with materials warmer than skin temperature.

Convection. Convection is the transfer of heat away by air movement. Heat is first conducted to air molecules directly in contact with the skin. Air currents carry away the warmed air. As the air current velocity increases, convective heat loss increases. An electric fan promotes heat loss through convection. Convective heat loss increases when moistened skin comes into contact with slightly moving air.

Evaporation. Evaporation is the transfer of heat energy when a liquid is changed to a gas. During evaporation, approximately 0.6 of a **calorie** of heat is lost for each gram of water that evaporates (Guyton, 1991). The body continuously loses heat by evaporation. About 600 to 900 ml a day evaporates from the skin and lungs, resulting in water and heat loss. This normal loss is considered insensible water loss and does not play a major role in temperature regulation.

By regulating perspiration or sweating, the body promotes additional evaporative heat loss. Millions of sweat glands located in the dermis of the skin secrete sweat through tiny ducts on the skin's surface. When body temperature rises, the anterior hypothalamus signals the sweat glands to release sweat. Sweat evaporates from the skin surface, resulting in heat loss. During exercise and emotional or mental stress, sweating is one way to lose excessive heat produced by the increased metabolic rate. Excessive evaporation can cause skin scaling and itching, as well as drying of the nares and pharynx.

Diaphoresis is visual perspiration of the forehead and upper thorax. Sweat glands lie deep below the dermis of the skin. The glands secrete sweat, a watery solution containing sodium and chloride, which passes through tiny ducts on the skin's surface. The glands are controlled by the sympathetic nervous system. When the body's temperature rises, sweat glands release sweat, which evaporates from the skin to promote heat loss. A lowered body temperature inhibits sweat gland secretion. Diaphoresis is less efficient when air movement is minimal or when the humidity of the air is high. People who have a congenital absence of sweat glands or who have a serious skin disease that impairs diaphoresis are unable to tolerate warm temperatures because they cannot cool themselves adequately.

SKIN IN TEMPERATURE REGULATION

The skin's roles in temperature regulation include insulation of the body, vasoconstriction (which affects the amount of blood flow and heat loss to the skin), and temperature sensation. The skin, subcutaneous tissue, and fat keep heat inside the body. When blood flow between skin layers is reduced, the skin alone is an excellent insulator. Persons with more body fat have more natural insulation than do slim and muscular people.

The way that the skin controls body temperature is similar to the way that an automobile radiator controls engine temperature. The engine of an automobile generates a great deal of heat. Water is pumped through the engine's system to collect the heat and carry it to the radiator, where a fan transfers the heat from the water to the outside air. The radiator and fan keep the engine's temperature within safe limits to prevent damage from overheating. In the human body the internal organs produce heat, and during exercise or increased sympathetic stimulation, the amount of heat produced is greater than the normal core temperature. Blood flows from the internal organs, carrying heat to the body surface. The skin is well supplied with blood vessels. In the most exposed areas of the body—the hands, feet, and ears—blood can flow directly from arteries to veins. Blood flow through the more vascular areas of the skin may vary from minimal flow to as much as 30% of the blood ejected from the heart (Guyton, 1991). Heat transfers from the blood, through vessel walls, to the skin's surface and is lost to the environment through the heat-loss mechanisms. The body's core temperature remains within safe limits.

The degree of vasoconstriction determines the amount of blood flow and heat loss to the skin. If the core temperature is too high, the hypothalamus inhibits vasoconstriction. As a result, blood vessels dilate, and more blood reaches the skin's surface. On a hot, humid day the blood vessels in the hands are dilated and easily visible. In contrast, if the core temperature becomes too low, the hypothalamus initiates vasoconstriction and blood flow to the skin lessens. Thus body heat is conserved.

The skin is well supplied with heat and cold receptors. Because cold receptors are more plentiful, however, the skin functions primarily to detect cold surface temperatures. When the skin becomes chilled, its sensors send information to the hypothalamus, which initiates shivering to increase body heat production, inhibition of sweating, and vasoconstriction.

BEHAVIORAL CONTROL

Humans voluntarily act to maintain comfortable body temperature when exposed to temperature extremes. The ability of a person to control body temperature depends on (1) the degree of temperature extreme, (2) the person's ability to sense feeling comfortable or uncomfortable, (3) thought processes or emotions, and (4) the person's mobility or ability to remove or add clothes. Body temperature control is difficult if any of these abilities are absent or lost. Infants can sense uncomfortable warm conditions but need assistance in changing their environment. Older adults may need help in detecting cold environments and minimizing heat loss. Illness, a decreased level of consciousness, or impaired thought processes result in an inability to recognize the need to change behavior for temperature control. When temperatures become extremely hot or cold, health promoting behaviors have a limited effect on controlling temperature. The nurse assesses for variables that place clients at high risk for ineffective thermoregulation.

Factors Affecting Body Temperature

Many factors affect body temperature. Changes in body temperature within the normal range occur when the relationship between heat production and heat loss is altered by physiological or behavioral variables. The nurse must be aware of these factors when assessing temperature variations and evaluating deviations from normal.

AGE

At birth the newborn leaves a warm, relatively constant environment and enters one in which temperatures fluctuate widely. Temperature-control mechanisms are immature. An infant's temperature may respond drastically to changes in the environment. Extra care is needed to protect the newborn from environmental temperatures. Clothing must be adequate, and exposure to temperature extremes must be avoided. A newborn loses up to 30% of body heat through the head and therefore needs to wear a cap to prevent heat loss. When protected from environmental extremes, the newborn's body temperature is maintained within 35.5° to 39.5°C (96° to 99.5°F). Heat production steadily declines as the infant grows into childhood. Individual differences of 0.25° to 0.55°C (0.5° to 1° F) are normal (Whaley and Wong, 1995).

Temperature regulation is unstable until children reach puberty. The normal temperature range gradually drops as individuals approach older adulthood. The older adult has a narrower range of body temperatures than the younger adult. Oral temperatures of 35°C (95°F) are not unusual for older adults in cold weather. However, the average body temperature of older adults is approximately 36°C (96.8°F). Older adults are particularly sensitive to temperature extremes because of deterioration in control mechanisms, particularly poor vasomotor control (control of vasoconstriction and vasodilation), reduced amounts of subcutaneous tissue, reduced sweat gland activity, and reduced metabolism.

EXERCISE

Muscle activity requires an increased blood supply and an increased carbohydrate and fat breakdown. This increased metabolism causes an increase in heat production. Any form of exercise can increase heat production and thus body temperature. Prolonged strenuous exercise, such as long-distance running, can temporarily raise body temperatures up to 41°C (105.8°F).

HORMONE LEVEL

Women generally experience greater fluctuations in body temperature than men. Hormonal variations during the menstrual cycle cause body temperature fluctuations. Pro-

gesterone levels rise and fall cyclically during the menstrual cycle. When progesterone levels are low, the body temperature is a few tenths of a degree below the baseline level. The lower temperature persists until ovulation occurs. During ovulation, greater amounts of progesterone enter the circulatory system and raise the body temperature to previous baseline levels or higher. These temperature variations can be used to predict a woman's most fertile time to achieve pregnancy.

Body temperature changes also occur in women during menopause (cessation of menstruation). Women who have stopped menstruating may experience periods of intense body heat and sweating lasting from 30 seconds to 5 minutes. This is due to the instability of the vasomotor controls for vasodilation and vasoconstriction (Bobak, 1993).

CIRCADIAN RHYTHM

Body temperature normally changes 0.5° to 1°C (0.9° to 1.8°F) during a 24-hour period. However, temperature is one of the most stable rhythms in humans. The temperature is usually lowest between 1:00 and 4:00 AM (Fig. 32-3). During the day, body temperature rises steadily, until about 6:00 PM, and then declines to early morning levels. Interestingly, temperature patterns are not automatically reversed in people who work at night and sleep during the day. It takes 1 to 3 weeks for the cycle to reverse. In general, the circadian temperature rhythm does not change with age. Research indicates, however, that temperature peaks at an earlier time of the day in older adults (Lenz, 1984).

STRESS

Physical and emotional stress increase body temperature through hormonal and neural stimulation. These physiological changes increase metabolism, which increases heat production. The client who is anxious about entering a hospital or a physician's office may register a higher-than-normal temperature (see Chapter 22).

ENVIRONMENT

Environment influences body temperature. If temperature is assessed in a very warm room, a client may be unable to regulate body temperature by heat-loss mechanisms, and the body temperature will be elevated. If the client has just been outside in the cold without warm clothing, body temperature may be low because of extensive radiant and conductive heat loss. Infants and older adults are most likely to be affected by environmental temperatures because their temperature-regulating mechanisms are less efficient.

Temperature Alterations

Changes in body temperature outside the normal range affect the hypothalamic set point. These changes can be related to excess heat production, excessive heat loss, minimal heat production, minimal heat loss, or any combination of these alterations. The nature of the change affects the type of clinical problems a client experiences.

FEVER

Hyperpyrexia or **fever** occurs because heat loss mechanisms are unable to keep pace with excess heat production,

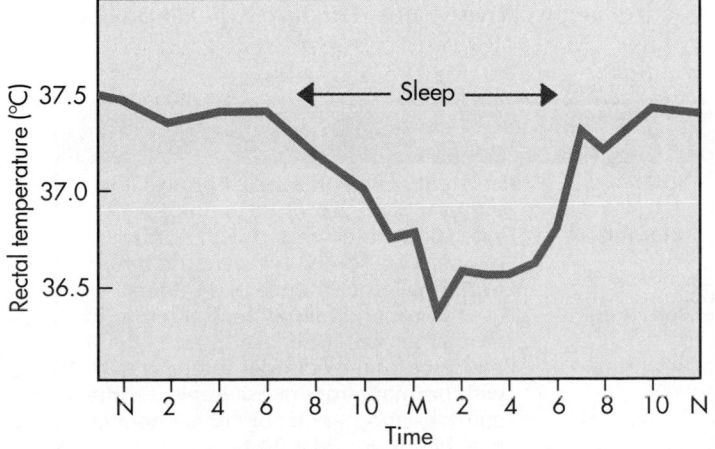

Fig. 32-3 Temperature cycle for 24 hours.

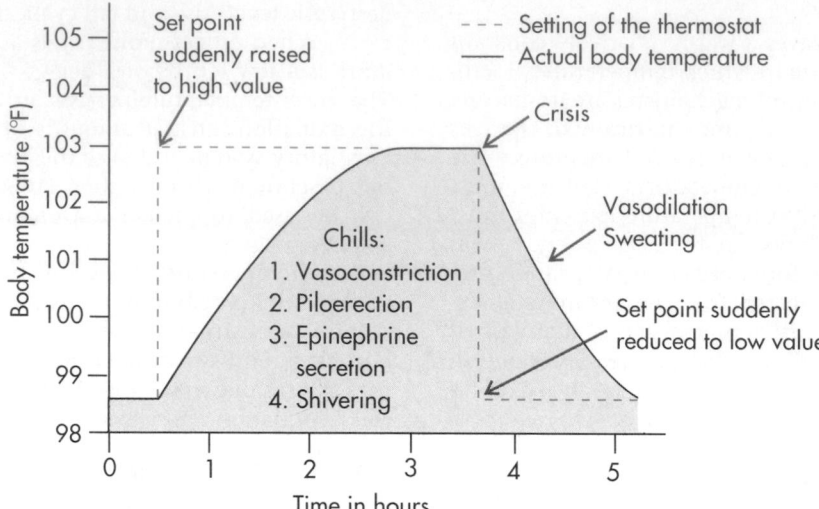

Fig. 32-4 Effects of changing the set point of the hypothalamic temperature control during a fever. *(Modified from Guyton AC: Textbook of medical physiology, ed 3, Philadelphia, 1992, WB Saunders.)*

resulting in an abnormal rise in body temperature. The level at which a fever threatens health is often a source of disagreement among health care providers. A fever is usually not harmful if it stays below 39°C (102°F). A single temperature reading may not indicate a fever. Davis and Lentz (1989) recommend determining a fever based on several temperature readings at different times of the day compared with the normal for that person at that time, in addition to physical signs and symptoms of infection.

A true fever results from an alteration in the hypothalamic set point. **Pyrogens** such as bacteria and viruses cause a rise in body temperature. When they enter the body, pyrogens act as antigens, triggering the immune system. More white cells are produced to help promote the body's defense against infection. In addition, hormone-like substances are released to further defend against infection. These substances also trigger the hypothalamus to raise the set point. To meet the new higher set point, the body produces and conserves heat. Several hours may pass before the body temperature reaches the new set point. During this period the person experiences chills, shivers, and feels cold, even though the body temperature is rising (Fig. 32-4). The chill phase resolves when the new set point, a higher temperature, is achieved. During the next phase, the plateau, the chills subside and a person feels warm and dry. If the new set point has been "overshot," or the pyrogens are removed (e.g., destruction of bacteria by antibiotics), the third phase of a **febrile** episode occurs. The hypothalamus set point drops, initiating heat-loss responses. The skin becomes warm and flushed because of vasodilation. Diaphoresis assists in evaporative heat loss. When the fever "breaks," the client become **afebrile**.

Fever is an important defense mechanism. Mild temperature elevations up to 39°C (102.2°F) enhance the body's immune system. During a febrile episode, white blood cell production is stimulated. Increased temperature reduces the concentration of iron in the blood plasma, suppressing the growth of bacteria. Fever also fights viral infections by stimulating interferon, the body's natural virus-fighting substance.

Fevers also serve a diagnostic purpose. Fever patterns differ depending on the causative pyrogen (see the box below). The increase or decrease in the amount of pyrogens results in fever spikes and declines at different times of the day. The duration and degree of fever depends on the pyrogen's strength and the ability of the individual to respond. The term *fever of unknown origin* (FUO) refers to a fever whose etiology (cause) cannot be determined.

During a fever, cellular metabolism increases and oxygen consumption rises. The body's metabolism increases 7% for every degree of temperature elevation. Heart and respiratory rates increase to meet the metabolic needs of the body for nutrients. The increased metabolism uses energy that produces additional heat. If the client has a cardiac or respiratory problem, the stress of a fever can be great. A prolonged fever can weaken a client by exhausting energy stores. Increased metabolism requires additional oxygen. If the demand for additional oxygen cannot be met, cellular hypoxia (inadequate oxygen) occurs. Myocardial hypoxia produces angina (chest pain). Cerebral hypoxia produces

Patterns of Fever	
Sustained	Persistent elevation over 24 hours varying by 1°C to 2°C (1.8° to 3.6° F)
Intermittent	Fever spikes interspersed with normal temperature levels. Temperature returns to normal at least once in 24 hours.
Remittent	Fever spikes and falls without a return to normal temperature levels.
Relapsing	Periods of febrile episodes interspersed with normal temperature levels. Febrile episodes and periods of normothermia may be longer than 24 hours.

confusion. Interventions during a fever may include oxygen therapy. The regulatory mechanism used to compensate for fever places a client at risk for fluid volume deficit. Water loss through increased respiration and diaphoresis can be excessive. Dehydration can be a serious problem for older adults and children with low body weight. Maintaining optimum fluid volume status is an important nursing action (see Chapter 45).

HEAT EXHAUSTION

Heat exhaustion occurs when profuse diaphoresis results in excess water and electrolyte loss. Caused by environmental heat exposure, the signs and symptoms of fluid volume deficit are common during heat exhaustion. First aid includes transporting the client to a cooler environment and restoring fluid and electrolyte balance.

HYPERTHERMIA

An elevated body temperature related to the body's inability to promote heat loss or reduce heat production is **hyperthermia.** Any disease or trauma to the hypothalamus can impair heat loss mechanisms. **Malignant hyperthermia** is a hereditary condition of uncontrolled heat production, occurring when susceptible persons receive certain anesthetic drugs.

HEATSTROKE

Prolonged exposure to the sun or high environmental temperatures can overwhelm the body's heat loss mechanisms. Heat also depresses hypothalamic function. These conditions cause **heatstroke**, a dangerous heat emergency with a high mortality rate. Clients at risk include those who are very young or very old and those who have cardiovascular disease, hypothyroidism, diabetes, or alcoholism. Also at risk are those who take medications that decrease the body's ability to lose heat (e.g., phenothiazines, anticholinergics, diuretics, amphetamines, and beta-adrenergic receptor antagonists) and those who exercise or work strenuously (e.g., athletes, construction workers, and farmers). Signs and symptoms of heatstroke include giddiness, confusion, delirium, excess thirst, nausea, muscle cramps, visual disturbances, and even incontinence. The most important sign of heatstroke is hot, dry skin.

Victims of heatstroke do not sweat because of severe electrolyte loss and hypothalamic malfunction. Heatstroke with a temperature greater than 40.5°C (105°F) produces tissue damage to the cells of all body organs. Vital signs reveal a body temperature sometimes as high as 45°C (113°F), tachycardia, and hypotension. The brain may be the first organ affected because of its sensitivity to electrolyte imbalances. As the condition progresses, a client becomes unconscious with fixed, unreactive pupils. Permanent neurological damage occurs unless cooling measures are rapidly started.

HYPOTHERMIA

Heat loss during prolonged exposure to cold overwhelms the body's ability to produce heat, causing **hypothermia.** Hypothermia is classified by core temperature measurements (Table 32-1). It can be accidental or unintentional, such as falling through the ice of a frozen lake. Hypothermia may be intentionally induced during surgical procedures to reduce metabolic demand and the body's need for oxygen.

Table 32-1	Classification of Hypothermia	
	CENTIGRADE	**FAHRENHEIT**
Mild	33°–36°	(91.4°–96.8°)
Moderate	30°–33°	(86.0°–91.4°)
Severe	27°–30°	(80.6°–86.0°)
Profound	<30°	<80.6°

Accidental hypothermia usually develops gradually and may go unnoticed for several hours. When skin temperature drops to 35°C (95°F), the client suffers uncontrolled shivering, loss of memory, depression, and poor judgment. As the body temperature falls below 34.4°C (94°F), heart, respiratory rates, and blood pressure fall. The skin becomes cyanotic. If hypothermia progresses, a client experiences cardiac dysrhythmias, loss of consciousness, and unresponsiveness to painful stimuli. In cases of severe hypothermia a person may demonstrate clinical signs similar to death (e.g., lack of response to stimuli and extremely slow respirations and pulse). The assessment of core temperature is critical when hypothermia is suspected. A special low-reading thermometer may be required because standard devices do not register below 35°C (95°F).

Frostbite occurs when the body is exposed to subnormal temperatures. Ice crystals forming inside the cell can result in permanent circulatory and tissue damage. Areas particularly susceptible to frostbite are the earlobes, tip of the nose, and fingers and toes. The injured area is white, waxy, and firm to the touch. The client loses sensation in the affected area. Intervention includes gradual warming measures, analgesia, and protection of the injured area.

■ NURSING PROCESS AND THERMOREGULATION

Knowledge of the physiology of body temperature regulation helps the nurse to assess the client's response to temperature alterations and to intervene safely. Independent measures can be implemented to increase or minimize heat loss, to promote heat conservation, and to increase comfort. These measures add to the effects of medically ordered therapies during illness. Many measures can also be taught to family members, parents of children, or other care givers.

 ## Assessment

SITES

There are several sites for measuring core and surface body temperature. The core temperatures of the pulmonary artery, esophagus, and urinary bladder are used in intensive care settings. These measurements require the use of continuous invasive devices placed in body cavities or organs. These devices obtain accurate readings quickly and continually display readings on an electronic monitor.

Text continued on p. 608.

PROCEDURE 32-1

Measuring Body Temperature

STEPS	RATIONALE

PREPARATION FOR MEASURING BODY TEMPERATURE

1. Assess for signs and symptoms of temperature alterations and for factors that normally influence body temperature.

   Physical signs and symptoms may indicate abnormal body temperature. Nurse can accurately assess nature of temperature variations.

2. Explain how temperature is to be taken and importance of maintaining proper position until reading is complete.

   Clients are often curious as to what their temperatures are and should be cautioned against prematurely removing thermometer to read results.

3. When taking oral temperature, wait 20 to 30 min before measuring temperature if client has smoked or ingested hot or cold liquids or foods.

   Smoking and hot or cold substances can cause false temperature readings in oral cavity.

4. Prepare needed equipment and supplies:
   a. Appropriate thermometer
   b. Soft tissues
   c. Lubricant (for rectal glass thermometer only)
   d. Pen, flow sheet or record form
   e. Disposable gloves
   f. Plastic sleeve or disposable probe cover

   Chosen on basis of preferred site for temperature measurement.

5. Wash hands.

   Reduces transmission of microorganisms.

ORAL TEMPERATURE— ELECTRONIC THERMOMETER

1. Complete preparation steps 1-5.

2. Assist client in assuming position of comfort that provides easy access to mouth.

   Ensures comfort and accuracy of temperatue reading.

3. Apply disposable gloves (optional).

   Gloves should be worn if there is risk of handling items soiled with body fluids (e.g., saliva) (Garner, 1996).

4. Remove thermometer pack from charging unit. Be sure oral probe (blue tip) is attached to thermometer unit. Grasp top of probe stem, being careful not to apply pressure to ejection button.

   Ejection button releases plastic cover from probe.

5. Slide disposable plastic probe cover over thermometer probe until it locks in place.

   Soft plastic cover will not break in mouth and prevents transmission of microorganisms between clients.

6. Ask client to open mouth and gently place probe under tongue in posterior sublingual pocket lateral to center of lower jaw (see the illustration below).

   Heat from superficial blood vessels in sublingual pocket produces temperature reading. With electronic thermometer, temperatures in right and left posterior sublingual pocket are significantly higher than in area under front of tongue.

7. Ask client to hold thermometer with lips closed.

   Maintains proper position of thermometer during recording.

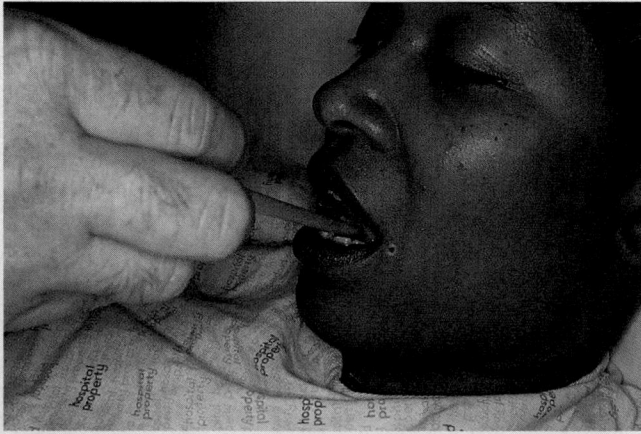

Step 6

Measuring Body Temperature—cont'd

STEPS	RATIONALE

ORAL TEMPERATURE— ELECTRONIC THERMOMETER, cont'd

8. Leave probe in place until audible signal occurs. Temperature appears on digital display.

Probe must stay in place until signal occurs to ensure accurate reading.

9. Remove probe from under tongue and inform client of temperature reading.

Promotes participation in care and understanding of health status.

10. Push ejection button on probe to discard plastic probe cover directly into proper receptacle.

Reduces transmission of microorganisms.

11. Return probe to storage well of recording unit.

Protects probe from damage. Automatically causes digital reading to disappear.

12. Remove and dispose of gloves. Wash hands.

Reduces transmission of microorganisms.

13. Return thermometer to charger.

Maintains battery charge.

14. Perform completion steps 1-3.

ORAL TEMPERATURE— GLASS THERMOMETER

1. Complete preparation steps 1-5.

2. Assist client in assuming comfortable position that provides easy access to mouth.

Ensures comfort and accuracy of temperature reading.

3. Apply disposable gloves.

Gloves should be worn for handling items soiled with body fluids (e.g., saliva) (Garner, 1996).

4. Hold color-coded end (blue tip) of glass thermometer with fingertips.

Reduces contamination of thermometer bulb.

5. If thermometer is stored in disinfectant solution, rinse in cold water before using.

Removes solution irritating to oral mucosa. Hot water can cause mercury to expand and break bulb.

6. Take soft tissue and wipe thermometer bulb end toward fingers in rotating fashion. Dispose of tissue.

Reduces contamination of bulb end.

7. Read mercury level while holding thermometer horizontally and gently rotating it.

Mercury level should be below 35.5° C (96° F). Thermometer reading must be below body temperature before use.

8. If mercury is above desired level, securely grasp tip and stand away from solid objects. Sharply flick wrist downward as though cracking a whip. Continue shaking until reading is below 35.5° C (96° F).

Brisk shaking lowers mercury level in glass tube. Standing in open spot avoids breakage of thermometer.

9. Insert thermometer into plastic sleeve

Protects nurse from contact with saliva.

10. Ask client to open mouth and gently place thermometer under tongue in posterior sublingual pocket lateral to center of lower jaw (see the illustration below).

Heat from lingual arteries in sublingual pocket produces temperature reading.

11. Ask client to hold thermometer with lips closed. Caution against biting down.

Maintains proper position of thermometer during recording. Breakage of thermometer may injure mucosa and cause mercury poisoning.

12. Leave thermometer in place for 3 min or according to agency policy.

Studies about proper length of time for recording vary. Holtzclaw (1992) recommends 3 min.

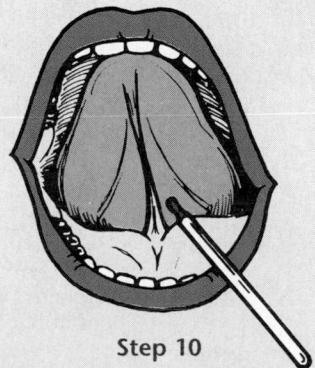

Step 10

Continued.

Measuring Body Temperature—cont'd

STEPS	RATIONALE

ORAL TEMPERATURE— GLASS THERMOMETER—cont'd

13. Carefully remove thermometer and remove and discard plastic sleeve. Read at eye level while holding thermometer horizontally.

Ensures accurate reading.

14. Inform client of temperature reading.

Promotes participation in care and understanding of health status.

15. Wipe secretions from thermometer with soft tissue. Wipe in rotating fashion from fingers toward bulb. Dipose of tissue. Store thermometer at bedside in proper container.

Wipe from area of least contamination to area of most contamination.

16. Remove and dispose of gloves. Wash hands.

Reduces transmission of microorganisms.

17. Perform completion steps 1-3.

RECTAL TEMPERATURE— ELECTRONIC THERMOMETER

1. Complete preparation steps 1-5.

2. Draw curtain around bed and/or close room door. Keep client's upper body and lower extremities covered with sheet or blanket.

Maintains privacy, minimizes embarrassment, and promotes comfort.

3. Assist client in assuming Sims' position with upper leg flexed. Move aside bed linen to expose only anal area.

Exposes anal area for correct thermometer placement.

4. Remove thermometer pack from charging unit. Be sure rectal probe (red tip) is attached to thermometer unit. Grasp top of probe stem, being careful not to apply pressure to ejection button.

Ejection button releases plastic cover from probe.

5. Slide disposable plastic cover over thermometer probe until it locks in place.

Probe cover prevents transmission of microorganisms between clients.

6. Apply disposable gloves.

Gloves should be worn for handling items soiled with body fluids (e.g., feces) (Garner, 1996).

7. With nondominant hand, separate buttocks to expose anus.

Fully exposes anus for thermometer insertion.

8. Ask client to breathe slowly and relax.

Relaxes anal sphincter for easier thermometer insertion.

9. Gently insert probe into anus in direction of umbilicus. Insert 1.2 cm ($^1/_2$ in) for infant and 3.5 cm ($1^1/_2$ in) for adult. Do not force thermometer.

Ensures adequate exposure against blood vessels in rectal wall.

   a. If resistance is felt during insertion, withdraw thermometer immediately. Never force it.

Prevents trauma to mucosa.

10. Hold probe until audible signal occurs. Read temperature on digital display.

Reading occurs within seconds after insertion.

11. Carefully remove probe from rectum and inform client of temperature reading.

Promotes participation in care and understanding of health status.

12. Push ejection button to discard plastic probe cover into receptacle.

Reduces transmission of microorganisms.

13. Return probe to storage well of recording unit.

Protects probe from damage. Automatically causes digital reading to disappear.

14. Wipe anal area to remove feces. Remove and dispose of gloves.

Provides comfort. Reduces transmission of microorganisms.

15. Help client return to comfortable position.

Restores comfort.

16. Wash hands.

Reduces transmission of microorganisms.

17. Perform completion steps 1-3.

RECTAL TEMPERATURE— GLASS THERMOMETER

1. Complete preparation steps 1-5.

2. Draw curtain around bed and/or close room door. Keep client's upper body and lower extremities covered with sheet or blanket.

Maintains privacy, minimizes embarrassment, and promotes comfort.

Measuring Body Temperature—cont'd

STEPS	RATIONALE

RECTAL TEMPERATURE—
GLASS THERMOMETER—cont'd

3. Assist client in assuming Sims' position with upper leg flexed. Move aside bed linen to expose only anal area.

Exposes anal area for correct thermometer placement.

4. Prepare thermometer as described under "oral temperature—glass thermometer," steps 4-8.

Mercury must be below temperature level before insertion.

5. Squeeze liberal portion of lubricant onto tissue. Dip thermometer's tapered end into lubricant, covering 2.5 to 3.5 cm (1 to 1$\frac{1}{2}$ in) for adult or 1.2 to 2.5 cm ($\frac{1}{2}$ to 1 in) for child.

Lubrication minimizes trauma to rectal mucosa during insertion. Tissue avoids contamination of all lubricant in container.

6. Apply disposable gloves.

Gloves should be worn for handling items soiled by body fluids (e.g., feces) (Garner, 1996).

7. With nondominant hand, separate buttocks to expose anus.

Fully exposes anus for thermometer insertion.

8. Ask client to breathe slowly and relax.

Relaxes anal sphincter for easier thermometer insertion.

9. Gently insert thermometer into anus in direction of umbilicus. Insert 1.2 ($\frac{1}{2}$ in) for child and 3.5 cm (1$\frac{1}{2}$ in) for adult. Do not force thermometer (see the illustration below).

Ensures adequate exposure against blood vessels in rectal wall.

   a. If resistance is felt during insertion, withdraw thermometer immediately. Never force it.

Prevents trauma to mucosa. Glass thermometers can break.

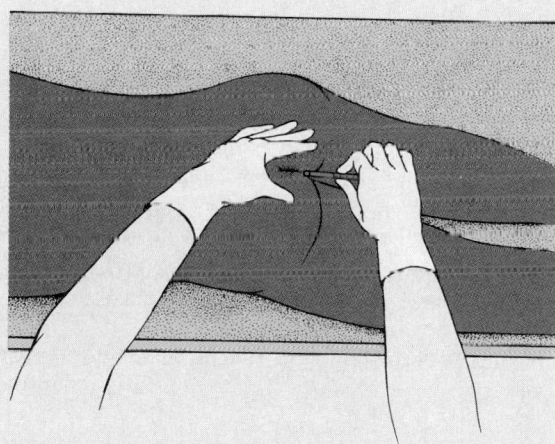

Step 9

10. Hold thermometer in place for 3 min or according to agency policy.

Prevents injury to client. Studies as to proper length of time for recording vary. Stephen and Sexton (1987) concluded that changes after 3 min had little significance.

11. Carefully remove thermometer and wipe off secretions with tissue. Wipe in rotating fashion from fingers toward bulb. Dispose of tissue.

Avoids contact with microorganisms. Wipe from area of least contamination to area of most contamination.

12. Read thermometer at eye level.

Ensures accurate reading.

13. Inform client of temperature reading.

Promotes participation in care and understanding of status.

14. Wipe anal area to remove lubricant or feces.

Provides comfort.

15. Help client return to comfortable position.

Restores comfort.

16. Wash thermometer in lukewarm soapy water, rinse in cool water, dry, and replace in storage container.

Mechanically removes organic material that can harbor microorganisms and hinder action of disinfectant. Storage container prevents breakage.

17. Dispose of gloves. Wash hands.

Reduces transmission of microorganisms.

18. Perform completion steps 1-3.

Continued.

Measuring Body Temperature—cont'd

STEPS	RATIONALE

AXILLARY TEMPERATURE—ELECTRONIC THERMOMETER

1. Complete preparation steps 1-5.
2. Draw curtain around bed and/or close room door.
3. Position client in supine or sitting position.
4. Move clothing or gown away from shoulder and arm.
5. Attach rectal probe (red) to thermometer unit. Prepare electronic thermometer as described under "rectal temperature—electronic thermometer," steps 4 and 5.
6. Insert probe into center of axilla, lower arm over thermometer, and place arm across client's chest.
7. Hold probe in place until audible signal occurs. Read temperature on digital display.
8. Remove probe from axilla and inform client of temperature reading.
9. Push ejection button to discard plastic probe into proper receptacle.
10. Return electronic probe to storage well.

11. Assist client in replacing clothing or gown.
12. Wash hands.
13. Perform completion steps 1-3.

Rationale (right column):

Provides privacy and minimizes embarrassment.
Provides easy access to axilla.
Provides optimal exposure of axilla.
Probe cover prevents transmission of microorganisms between clients.

Maintains proper position of thermometer against blood vessels in axilla.
Reading occurs within seconds after insertion.

Promotes participation in care and understanding of health status.
Reduces transmission of microorganisms.

Protects probe from damage. Automatically causes digital reading to disappear.
Restores comfort.
Reduces transmission of infection.

AXILLARY TEMPERATURE—GLASS THERMOMETER

1. Complete preparation steps 1-5.
2. Draw curtain around bed or close door.
3. Position client lying supine or sitting.
4. Move clothing or gown away from shoulder and arm.
5. Prepare glass thermometer as described under "oral temperature—glass thermometer," steps 4-8.
6. Insert thermometer into center of axilla, lower arm over thermometer, and place arm across client's chest (see the illustrations below).
7. Hold thermometer in place for 5-10 min or according to agency policy.

Rationale (right column):

Provides privacy and minimizes embarrassment.
Provides easy access to axilla.
Provides optimal exposure of axilla.
Mercury must be below temperature level before insertion.

Maintains proper position of thermometer against blood vessels in axilla.

Recommended time varies among institutions. Eoff and Joyce (1981) recommend 5 min for children.

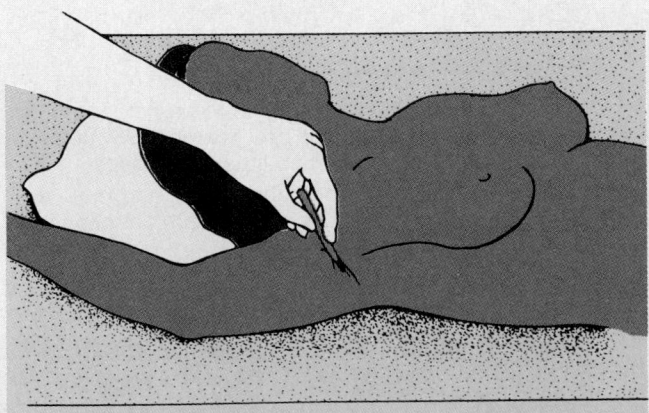 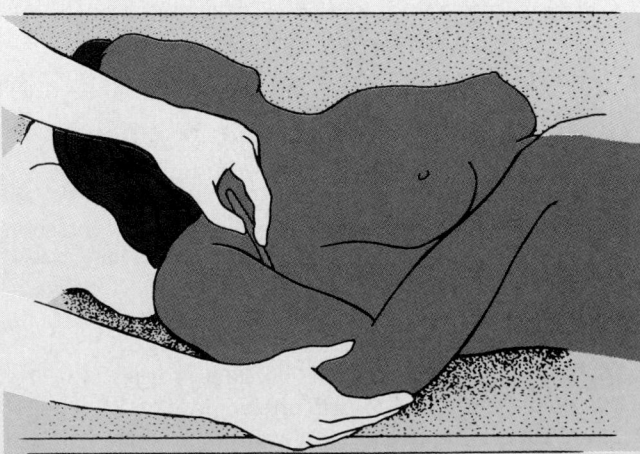

Step 6

Measuring Body Temperature—cont'd

STEPS	RATIONALE

AXILLARY TEMPERATURE— GLASS THERMOMETER—cont'd

8. Remove thermometer and wipe off any moisture with tissue. Wipe in rotating fashion from fingers toward bulb. Dispose of tissue.

Avoids contact with microorganisms. Wipe from area of least contamination to area of most contamination.

9. Read thermometer at eye level.

Ensures accurate reading.

10. Inform client of temperature reading.

Promotes participation in care and understanding of health status.

11. Wash thermometer in lukewarm soapy water, rinse in cool water, dry, and replace in storage container.

Mechanically removes organic material that can harbor microorganisms and hinder action of disinfectant. Storage container prevents breakage.

12. Assist client in replacing clothing or gown.

Restores sense of well-being.

13. Wash hands.

Reduces transmission of microorganisms.

14. Perform completion steps 1-3.

TYMPANIC MEMBRANE THERMOMETER

1. Complete preparation steps 1-5.

2. Assist client in assuming comfortable position with head turned toward side, away from nurse.

Ensures comfort and exposes auditory canal for accurate temperature reading.

3. Remove thermometer handheld unit from charging base, being careful not to apply pressure to ejection button.

Base provides battery power. Removal of hand unit from base prepares it to measure temperature. Ejection button releases plastic speculum cover.

4. Slide disposable plastic speculum cover over otoscope-like tip until it locks in place.

Reduces transmission of microorganisms.

5. Follow manufacturer's instructions for tympanic probe positioning.
   a. Pull ear pinna upward and back for an adult.
   b. Pull ear pinna down and back for a child.
   c. Move thermometer in a figure-eight pattern.
   d. Fit probe snug into canal. Do not move.
   e. Point toward nose, following manufacturer's positioning recommendations.

Correct positioning of the probe with respect to ear canal ensures accurate readings. The ear tug straightens the external auditory canal, allowing maximum exposure of the tympanic membrane.

6. Depress scan button on hand unit. Temperature appears on digital display.

Depression of scan button causes infrared energy to be measured. Probe must stay in place until signal occurs to ensure accurate reading.

   a. Carefully remove sensor from auditory meatus and inform client of reading.

Promotes participation in care and understanding of health status.

   b. Push release button to eject plastic speculum cover.

Reduces transmission of microorganisms.

   c. Discard into appropriate receptacle.

   d. Return hand unit to charging base.

Protects probe from damage. Automatically causes digital reading to disappear.

7. Assist client in assuming a comfortable position.

Restores comfort.

8. Wash hands.

Reduces transmission of microorganisms.

9. Perform Completion steps 1-3.

COMPLETION FOR MEASURING BODY TEMPERATURE

1. Compare temperature reading with baseline and normal temperature range for client's age-group.

Normal body temperature fluctuates within narrow range. Comparison reveals presence of abnormality.

2. If temperature is abnormal, repeat measurement. If indicated, select an alternative site or instrument.

Improper placement or movement of thermometer can cause inaccuracies. Second reading confirms initial finding of abnormal body temperature.

3. Record temperature on vital sign flow sheet or nurses' notes and report abnormal findings to nurse in charge or physician.

Vital sign measurements should be recorded promptly on flow sheets to avoid omissions from record. Abnormalities may require immediate therapy.

Advantages and Disadvantages of Select Temperature Measurement Sites

TYMPANIC

Advantages

Easily accessible site

Minimal client repositioning required

Provides accurate core reading

Very rapid measurement (2–5 sec)

Can be obtained without disturbing or waking client

Less emotionally invasive for children and adolescents who are developing sexual identity and body image

Disadvantages

Hearing aids must be removed before measurement

Should not be used with clients who have had surgery of the ear or tympanic membrane

Requires disposable probe cover

Cerumen impaction and otitis media may distort temperature measurement

Measurement accuracy in newborns and children under 3 years old has been questioned (Davis, 1993)

Variability of measurement exceeds those of other core temperature devices (Erickson and Kirklin, 1993)

RECTAL

Advantages

Argued to be more reliable when oral temperature cannot be obtained

Reflects core temperature

Disadvantages

Lags behind core temperature measurements during rapid temperature changes

Should not be used with clients who have had rectal surgery, a rectal disorder, pain in the rectal area, or bleeding tendencies

Requires positioning and may be source of client embarrassment and anxiety

Risk of body fluid exposure

Requires lubrication

Contraindicated in newborns

ORAL

Advantages

Accessible—requires no position change

Comfortable for client

Provides accurate surface temperature reading

Disadvantages

Affected by ingestion of fluids or foods, smoking, and oxygen delivery (Neff et al, 1988)

Should not be used if client is mouth breather (Kresovich-Wendler et al, 1989)

Should not be used with clients who have had oral surgery, trauma, history of epilepsy, or shaking chills

Should not be used with infants, small children, crying children, or confused, unconscious, or uncooperative clients

Risk of body fluid exposure

AXILLA

Advantages

Safe and noninvasive

Preferred route for newborns and uncooperative clients

Disadvantages

Long measurement time

Requires continuous positioning by nurse

Measurement lag behind core temperature during rapid temperature changes

Requires exposure of thorax

SKIN

Advantages

Inexpensive

Provides continuous reading

Safe and noninvasive

Disadvantages

Lags behind other sites during temperature changes, especially during hyperthermia

Diaphoresis or sweat can impair adhesion

The sites used most commonly for temperature measurement are also invasive but can be used intermittently. These include the tympanic membrane, mouth, rectum, and axillary sites. Noninvasive chemically prepared thermometer patches can also be applied to the skin. Oral, rectal, axillary, and skin temperature sites rely on effective blood circulation at the measurement site. The heat of the blood is conducted to the thermometer probe. Tympanic temperature relies on the radiation of body heat to an infrared sensor. Because the tympanic membrane shares the same arterial blood supply as the hypothalamus, tympanic temperature is considered a core temperature.

To ensure accurate temperature readings, each site must be measured correctly (Procedure 32-1). The temperature obtained varies depending on the site used, but should be between 36°C (96.8°F) and 38°C (100.4°F). Research findings from numerous studies are contradictory; however, it is generally accepted that rectal temperatures are usually 0.5°C (0.9°F) higher than oral temperatures, and axillary temperatures are usually 0.5°C (0.9°F) lower than oral temperatures (Pontious et al., 1994). Each of the common temperature measurement sites has advantages and disadvantages (see the box above). The nurse chooses the safest and most accurate site for the client. The same site should be used when repeated measurements are necessary.

Thermometers. The three types of thermometers used for determining body temperature are mercury-in-glass, electronic, and disposable. The nurse is responsible for being knowledgeable and skilled in the use of the selected measurement device. The level of inservice education can influence the accuracy and reliability of temperature readings (Pontious et al., 1994). Each device measures temperature using the centigrade or Fahrenheit scale. Electronic thermometers allow the nurse to convert scales by activating a switch. When it is necessary to convert temperature readings, the following formulas can be used:

1. To convert Fahrenheit to centigrade, subtract 32 from the Fahrenheit reading and multiply the result by $\frac{5}{9}$.

   $C = (F - 32°) \times \frac{5}{9}$ Example: $40°C = (104°F - 32°F) \times \frac{5}{9}$

2. To convert centigrade to Fahrenheit, multiply the centigrade reading by $\frac{9}{5}$ and add 32 to the product.

   $F = (\frac{9}{5} \times C) + 32°$ Example: $104°F = (\frac{9}{5} \times 40°C) + 32°$

MERCURY-IN-GLASS THERMOMETER

The mercury-in-glass thermometer is the most familiar, having been in use since the 15th century. It is a glass tube sealed at one end with a mercury-filled bulb at the other. Exposure of the bulb to heat causes the mercury to expand and rise in the enclosed tube. The length of the thermometer is marked with Fahrenheit or centigrade calibrations. The farthest point reached by the mercury in the tube is the temperature reading. The mercury will not fluctuate or fall unless the thermometer is shaken vigorously.

The nurse reads a mercury thermometer by using the fingertips to hold it horizontally, with the bulb pointed to the left (Fig. 32-5). By rotating the thermometer slowly, the column of silver mercury appears. The calibrated line at the end of the mercury column is the temperature reading. The bulb should not be touched. Touching it might affect the temperature reading or bring the fingers into contact with the client's body secretions. Disposable plastic sleeves may be available to cover the body of the thermometer. Observe standard precautions, including gloves, when using a glass thermometer because of potential contact with body fluids.

Three types of glass thermometers are the oral (slim tip), the stubby, and the rectal (pear-shaped tip) (Fig. 32-6). The oral thermometer tip is slender, allowing for greater exposure of the bulb against the blood vessels in the mouth. An oral thermometer usually has a blue tip. The stubby thermometer is shorter and thicker than the oral type. It can be used to measure temperature at any site. The rectal thermometer has a blunt or tapered end designed to prevent trauma to the rectal tissues during insertion. It is usually recognized by a red tip.

The time delay for recordings and breakability are disadvantages of mercury-in-glass thermometers. Mercury is a hazardous material if not properly contained. Accidental breakage of a mercury-in-glass thermometer is a health hazard to the client, nurse, and health care workers. Mercury is highly permeable through skin and mucous membranes; inhaled vapors diffuse rapidly into the blood and are transported to body tissues including the brain. The contents of two mercury-in-glass thermometers in a closed room exceed the permissible exposure limit established by the Occupational Safety and Health Administration (OSHA) (Material Safety Data Sheet, 1989). Steps to take in the event of a mercury spill are presented in the box below.

Advantages of mercury-in-glass thermometers are the low price, wide availability, and reliability. The accuracy of mercury-in-glass thermometers depends on the length of time they have been stored without being used. Generally these thermometers should not be stored more than 8 months.

Electronic thermometer. The electronic thermometer consists of a rechargeable battery-powered display unit, a thin wire cord, and a temperature-processing probe covered by a disposable plastic sheath (Fig. 32-7). One form of electronic

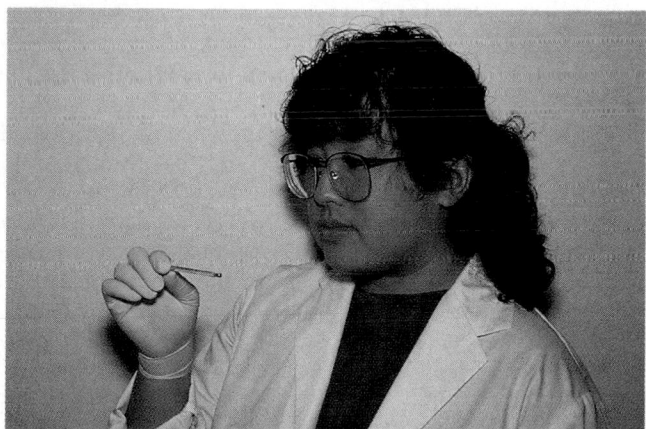

Fig. 32-5 Reading a glass thermometer.

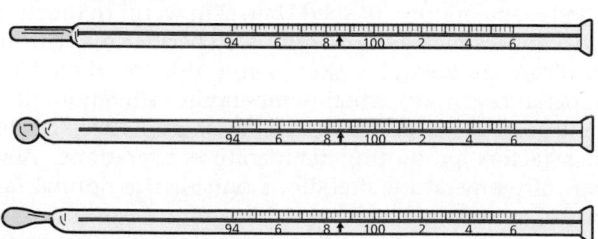

Fig. 32-6 Comparison of oral, stubby, and rectal thermometers (top to bottom).

Steps to Take in the Event of a Mercury Spill

1. Do NOT touch spilled mercury droplets. If skin contact has occurred, immediately flush area with water for 15 min.
2. If possible, remove client from immediate contaminated environment.
3. Change any clothing or linen that has been contaminated with mercury. Wash hands thoroughly after changing. Wash clothing before re-use.
4. Notify the Environmental Services Department or obtain a mercury spill kit if available.
5. Follow procedures for mercury removal as directed by Material Safety Data Sheet (MSDS). Spills are removed using special absorbent materials, filtered vacuum equipment, and protective clothing.
6. Promote exhaust ventilation to reduce concentration of mercury vapors.
7. Complete occurrence report as directed by institution procedure.

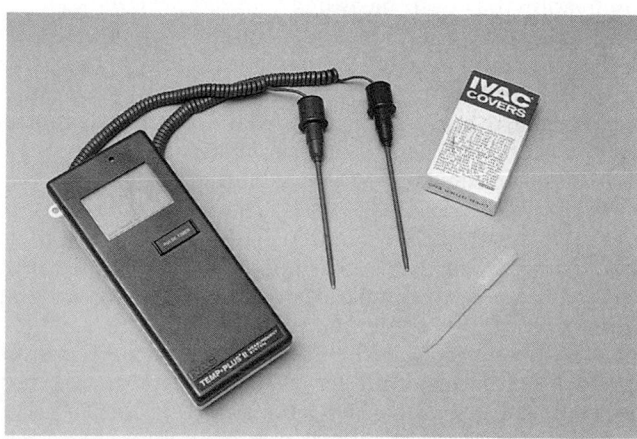

Fig. 32-7 Electronic thermometer.

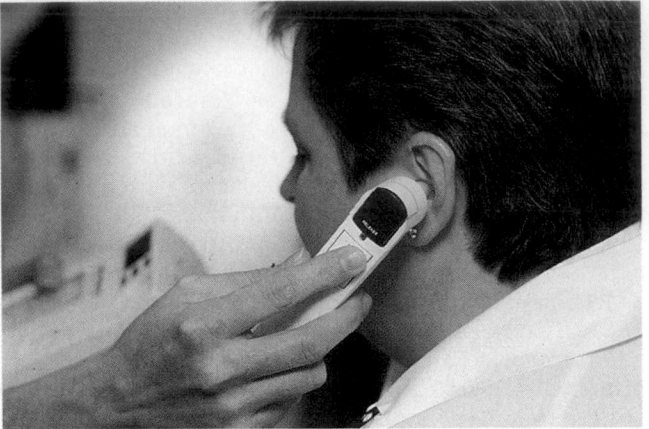

Fig. 32-8 Tympanic thermometer inserted in auditory canal.

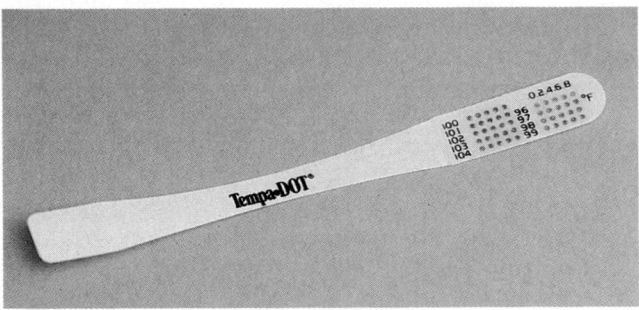

Fig. 32-9 Disposable, single-use thermometer strip.

![research highlight marker] **RESEARCH HIGHLIGHT**

RESEARCH ABSTRACT
Twenty-four stable postoperative cardiac clients participated in a study to determine the best peripheral method of measuring core body temperature. Ten measures of temperature were compared with temperatures from a pulmonary artery (PA) catheter. Temperatures compared included two tympanic infrared thermometers, electronic thermometers for oral, axillary, and rectal measurements, mercury-in-glass thermometers for oral axillary and rectal measurements, and chemical indicator thermometer strips for oral and axillary temperatures. Results indicated no significant difference between PA and aural temperatures. The oral chemical indicator thermometer temperatures had lower correlations with PA temperatures than did oral electronic or mercury. Axillary temperatures were significantly lower than PA temperatures. Rectal temperature measurements were significantly higher than PA temperatures but had an excellent correlation with PA temperatures.

IMPLICATIONS FOR PRACTICE
▶ Oral chemical thermometers should be used for screening and not diagnostic and treatment decisions.
▶ A single temperature device should be used consistently to track changes in a client's temperature.

REFERENCE
Henker R, Coyne C: Comparison of peripheral temperature measurements with core temperature, *AACN Clin Issues* 6(1):21, 1995.

thermometer uses a pencil-like probe. Separate nonbreakable probes are available for oral and rectal use. The oral probe can also be used for axillary temperature measurement. Within 20 to 50 seconds of insertion, a reading appears on the display unit. A sound signals when the peak temperature reading has been measured.

Another form of electronic thermometer is used exclusively for tympanic temperature (Fig. 32-8). An otoscope-like speculum with an infrared sensor tip detects heat radiated from the tympanic membrane. Within 2 to 5 seconds of placement in the auditory canal, a reading appears on the display unit. A sound signals when the peak temperature reading has been measured.

An electronic thermometer using an oral probe is not necessarily more accurate than a mercury-in-glass thermometer. For example, variables that alter oral temperature measurements affect all types of thermometers. The greatest advantages of electronic thermometers are that they can be inserted immediately, their readings appear within seconds, and they are easy to read. The plastic sheath is unbreakable and ideal for children. Their expense is a major disadvantage. Electronic thermometer devices measuring axillary temperatures have been reported as less accurate than mercury-in-glass devices.

Disposable thermometers. Disposable, single-use thermometers are thin strips of plastic with a temperature sensor at one end. The sensor consists of a matrix of dotlike indentations that contain chemicals that melt and change color at different temperatures. They are used for oral or axillary temperatures, particularly with children (Fig. 32-9). They are inserted the same way as an oral or axillary thermometer and used only once. Only 60 seconds is needed to register a temperature. (Erickson et al, 1996). The thermometer is removed and read after waiting about 10 seconds for the change to stabilize.

Another form of disposable thermometer is a temperature-sensitive patch or tape. Applied to the forehead or abdomen, the patch changes color at different temperatures.

Both forms of disposable thermometers are useful for screening temperatures, especially with newborns (see the box above). However, glass or electronic thermometers are preferred for their accuracy.

◐ Nursing Diagnosis

The nurse identifies assessment findings and clusters defining characteristics to form a nursing diagnosis (see the diagnostic process box on p. 611). For example, an increase in body temperature, flushed skin, skin warm to touch, and tachycardia indicate the diagnosis, hyperthermia. The nursing diagnosis identifies the client's risk for altered body temperature or an actual temperature alteration. If the client possesses risk factors, the nurse minimizes or eliminates factors promoting temperature alterations. Assessment of temperature alterations outside the normal range leads to a nursing diagnosis.

Once a diagnosis is determined, the nurse must accurately select the related factor or etiology (see the nursing diagnoses box on p. 612). The related factor allows the nurse to select appropriate nursing interventions. In the ex-

Sample Nursing Diagnostic Process for Thermoregulation

ASSESSMENT ACTIVITIES	DEFINING CHARACTERISTICS	NURSING DIAGNOSES
Obtain vital signs, including temperature, pulse, respirations.	Increased body temperature above normal range Tachycardia Tachypnea	**Hyperthermia** related to infectious process
Palpate skin. Observe client's appearance and behavior while talking and resting.	Warm skin Restlessness Flushed appearance	
Assess temperature, pulse, capillary refill, and blood pressure for changes.	Increased body temperature Tachycardia Hypotension	**Fluid volume deficit** related to hyperthermia
Observe mucous membranes in mouth, nose, eyes, skin for dryness. Assess skin turgor by gently pinching skin for slow, elastic recoil. Closely monitor intake and output levels for intake less than output. Evaluate laboratory values for alterations in sodium, potassium, chloride levels.	Dry skin and mucous membranes Thirst Decreased skin turgor Reduced fluid intake Concentrated urine Altered electrolyte values	

ample of hyperthermia, a related factor of vigorous activity will result in much different interventions than a related factor of inability to perspire.

Planning

Clients at high risk for alterations in body temperature require an individualized care plan directed at maintaining normothermia and reducing risk factors. Expected outcomes are established to gauge progress toward returning the body temperature to a normal range. For example, the outcome of intake equalling output is important to establish as the nurse provides fluids to manage the client's risk for fluid and electrolyte imbalance.

Education is important so clients can participate in maintaining normothermia. This is particularly the case for parents who need to know how to take action at home when an infant or child develops a temperature alteration. The care plan for clients with actual temperature alterations focuses on restoring normothermia, minimizing complications, and promoting comfort (see the care plan on p. 612). Often, other medical problems complicate the care plan. For instance, alterations in body temperature affect the body's requirements for fluids. Clients with heart problems may have difficulty tolerating required fluid replacement therapy.

The severity of a temperature alteration and its effects, together with the client's general health status, will influence the nurse's priorities in the care of a client.

Implementation

Hyperthermia

The procedures used to intervene and treat an elevated temperature depend on the fever's cause, its adverse effects,

and its strength, intensity, and duration. The physician may try to determine the cause of the fever by isolating the causative pyrogen. The nurse obtains necessary culture specimens for laboratory analysis such as urine, blood, sputum, and wound sites (see Chapter 34). Collecting these specimens requires strict aseptic technique to avoid introducing any outside organisms that might affect the culture results. The physician will order antibiotic medications to be given after the cultures have been obtained. Administering antibiotics destroys pyrogenic bacteria and eliminates the body's stimulus for fever. The nurse administers antibiotics promptly and educates the client regarding the importance of taking and continuing the antibiotic as directed until the course of treatment is complete.

Viral infections cannot be identified by cultures. Most fevers in children are of a viral origin, last only briefly, and have limited effects. However, children still have immature temperature control mechanisms and temperatures can rise rapidly. Dehydration and febrile seizures occur in rapidly rising temperatures of children younger than 5 years of age. Some researchers believe the rate of rise is more important than absolute temperature in precipitating a seizure (Leung and Robson, 1991). Children are at particular risk for fluid volume deficit because they can quickly lose large amounts of fluids in proportion to their body weight. The nurse maintains accurate intake and output records and encourages fluids.

The temperature of older adults is normally at the lower end of the temperature range. However, they are very sensitive to slight changes in temperature. The nurse must be aware that a temperature within the normal range may actually be considered a fever in an older adult.

Overall physical condition influences a client's ability to tolerate the increased heart rate, increased respiratory rate, decreased fluid volume, and increased metabolic oxygen demands of fever. Older adults, debilitated clients, and clients with severe burns, neoplastic disease, or a compromised immune system are at high risk for fever-induced complications. Temperatures higher than 39°C (102°F) serve little physiological purpose. As core temperature approaches 40°C (104°F), intervention is essential to avoid irreversible damage to cells.

A fever may be a hypersensitivity response to a drug. Drug fevers can be accompanied by other allergy symptoms such as rash or pruritus (itching). Treatment involves withdrawing the medication.

Fever therapy reduces heat production, increases heat loss, and prevents complications. **Antipyretics**, drugs that reduce fever, include corticosteroids and nonsteroidal compounds. Corticosteroids are not used to treat a fever; however, the nurse must be aware of their effect on suppressing the immune system and increasing the client's risk for developing a fever. Clients taking steroids can develop infections without the classic signs appearing. Nonsteroidal drugs such as acetaminophen, salicylates, indomethacin, and ketoralac reduce fever by increasing heat loss. These drugs are commonly prescribed for temperature control.

Nonpharmacological therapy for fever uses methods that increase heat loss by evaporation, conduction, convection, or radiation. Traditionally nurses have used tepid sponge baths, bathing with alcohol-water solutions, applying ice packs to axillae and groin areas, and cooling fans. Recent research has not demonstrated any advantage of these

Examples of NANDA Nursing Diagnoses for Thermoregulation

Risk for altered body temperature *related to:*
- Inappropriate clothing
- Central nervous system injury
- Environmental exposure (hot/cold)
- Compromised thermoregulatory systems

Ineffective thermoregulation *related to:*
- Immaturity
- Physiological changes of aging
- Central nervous system injury
- Environmental temperature

Hypothermia *related to:*
- Decreased metabolic rate
- Inadequate clothing
- Exposure to cold environment
- Inability to shiver
- Drug/alcohol consumption
- Inactivity
- Aging

Hyperthermia *related to:*
- Increased metabolic rate
- Inappropriate clothing
- Exposure to hot environment
- Inability to perspire
- Medications
- Vigorous activity
- Infectious process (bacterial/viral)

Sample Nursing Care Plan for Hyperthermia

Nursing Diagnosis: Hyperthermia related to infectious process
Definition: Hyperthermia is a state in which an individual's body temperature is elevated above his/her normal range.

GOAL	EXPECTED OUTCOMES	INTERVENTIONS	RATIONALES
Client will regain normal range of body temperature by 3/21.	Body temperature will decline at least 1°C (1.8°F) after therapy (by 3/19).	Keep room temperature at 21°C (70°F) unless shivering develops.	Ambient room temperature can elevate body temperature. However, shivering should be avoided because it increases body temperature (Guyton, 1991).
	Body temperature will remain between 36°-38°C (96.8° to 100.4°F) for at least 24 hr (by 3/20).	Administer acetaminophen as ordered for temperature higher than 39°C (102°F).	Antipyretics reduce set point.
Fluid electrolyte balance will be maintained by 3/21.	Intake will equal output by 3/20. No evidence of postural hypotension during ambulation on 3/22.	Encourage PO fluids of client choice q 4 h.	Fluids lost through insensible water loss require replacement.
Client will attain sense of comfort and rest by 3/21	Client will verbalize increased satisfaction with rest and sleep patterns on 3/21. Client will be able to rest or sleep quietly by 3/21.	Limit physical activity and source of emotional stress while hyperthermia exists. Reduce external covering on client's body. Keep clothing and bed linen dry.	Activity and stress increase metabolic rate requiring additional energy. Excessive or wet clothing prevents radiation, convection, and conductive heat loss. Excessive cooling from evaporation may produce shivering.
		Provide frequent mouth care as requested for comfort.	Mucous membranes dry easily from dehydration.

methods over antipyretic medications (Morgan, 1990). Blankets cooled by circulating water delivered by motorized units increase conductive heat loss. The nurse must follow manufacturer's instructions for applying these hypothermia blankets because of the risk for skin breakdown and "freeze burns." Placing a bath blanket between the client and the hypothermia blanket and wrapping distal extremities (fingers, toes, genitalia) is recommended (Holtzclaw, 1990).

Nursing measures to enhance body cooling must avoid the stimulation of shivering (Giuffre et al., 1991). Shivering is counterproductive because of the heat produced by muscle activity. Shivering intensity ranges from palpable but not visible to violent extremity contractions. Wrapping the client's extremities has been recommended to reduce the incidence and intensity of shivering (Holtzclaw, 1990). A dependent nursing intervention for shivering may involve

---

Nursing Measures for Clients With a Fever

ASSESSMENT

Obtain core temperature during each phase of febrile episode.
Assess for contributing factors such as dehydration, infection, or environmental temperature.
Identify physiological response to temperature.
- Obtain all vital signs.
- Observe skin color.
- Assess skin temperature.
- Observe for shivering and diaphoresis.
- Assess client comfort and well being.
Determine phase of fever: chill, plateau, fever break.

INTERVENTION (UNLESS CONTRAINDICATED)

Obtain blood cultures when ordered. Blood specimens are obtained to coincide with temperature spikes when the antigen-producing organism is most prevalent.
Initiate therapies to minimize heat production.
- Reduce the frequency of activities that increase oxygen demand such as excessive turning and ambulation. Allow rest periods.
- Limit physical activity.
Initiate therapies to maximize heat loss.
- Reduce external covering on client's body to promote heat loss through radiation and conduction. Do not induce shivering.
- Keep clothing and bed linen dry to increase heat loss through conduction and convection.
Initiate therapies to meet requirements for increased metabolic rate.
- Provide supplemental oxygen therapy as ordered to improve oxygen delivery to body cells.
- Provide measures to stimulate appetite and offer well-balanced meals.
- Provide fluids (at least 3 L per day for client with normal cardiac and renal function) to replace fluids lost through insensible water loss and sweating.
Initiate therapies to promote client comfort.
- Encourage oral hygiene because oral mucous membranes dry easily from dehydration.
- Control temperature of the environment without inducing shivering.
Identify onset and duration of febrile episode phases.
Examine previous temperature measurements for trends.
Initiate health teaching as indicated.

---

giving medications (e.g., meperidine, Stadol) that can reduce shivering (Vogelsang and Hayes, 1992).

Independent nursing measures enhance comfort, reduce metabolic demands, and provide nutrients to meet increased energy needs. These measures are listed in the box below.

Heatstroke

The best treatment for heatstroke is prevention. The nurse teaches clients to avoid strenuous exercise in hot, humid weather; to drink fluids such as clear fruit juices before, during, and after exercise; to wear light, loose-fitting, light-colored clothing; to avoid exercising in areas with poor ventilation; to wear protective covering over the head when outdoors; and to expose themselves to hot climates gradually.

First aid treatment for heatstroke includes moving the client to a cooler environment, reducing clothing covering the body, placing wet towels over the skin, and using oscillating fans to increase convective heat loss. Emergency medical treatment may include intravenous fluids and hypothermia blankets.

Hypothermia

Prevention is the key for clients at risk for hypothermia and frostbite. Prevention involves educating clients, family members, and friends. Clients most at risk include the very young, the very old, and persons debilitated by trauma, stroke, diabetes, drug or alcohol intoxication, sepsis, and Raynaud's disease. Mentally ill or handicapped clients may fall victim to hypothermia because they are unaware of the dangers of cold conditions. Fatigue, skin color (blacks are more susceptible), malnutrition, and hypoxemia also contribute to the risk of frostbite. Persons without adequate home heating, those with a poor diet, or those lacking warm clothing are also at risk.

The priority treatment for hypothermia is to prevent a further decrease in body temperature. The nurse removes wet clothes, provides dry ones, and wraps the client in blankets. In emergencies away from a health care setting, the client lies under blankets next to a warm person. A conscious client benefits from drinking hot liquids such as soup. Placing the client near a fire or in a warm room or placing heating pads next to areas of the body (head and neck) that lose heat the quickest help. When the client reaches an emergency department, treatment depends on the severity of the condition. Warmed intravenous fluids, heating blankets, and warm fluids may be used. Clients are monitored closely for cardiac irregularities and electrolyte imbalances.

 Evaluation

All nursing interventions are evaluated by comparing the client's actual response to the expected outcomes of the care plan (see the evaluation box on p. 614). Does the client's current status, at the time of evaluation, compare with what has been projected? This reveals whether goals of care have been met or if a revision to the plan is needed. After any intervention the nurse measures the client's temperature to evaluate for change. In addition, the nurse uses other evaluative measures such as palpation of the skin and

Sample Evaluation of Interventions for Hyperthermia

GOALS	EVALUATIVE MEASURES	EXPECTED OUTCOMES
Client will regain normal body temperature range by 3/21.	Monitor body temperature after intervention (e.g., antipyretic medications). Monitor body temperature every 4 hr.	Body temperature will decline at least 1° C (1.8° F) after therapy. Body temperature will remain between 36° and 38° C (96.8° to 100.4°F) for at least 24 hr by 3/20.
Fluid electrolyte balance will be maintained by 3/21. Client will attain sense of comfort and rest by 3/21.	Monitor serum electrolyte values. Measure intake and output levels. Question how client feels. Observe for restlessness, fatigue.	Electrolyte level will remain in normal range. Intake will equal output by 3/20. Client will verbalize increased satisfaction with rest and sleep. Client will be able to rest or sleep quietly.

assessment of pulse and respirations. If therapies are effective, body temperature will return to a normal range, other vital signs will stabilize, and the client will report a sense of comfort.

PULSE

The pulse is the palpable bounding of blood flow noted at various points on the body. It is an indicator of circulatory status. Circulation is the means by which cells receive nutrients and remove waste products of metabolism. For cells to function normally, there must be a continuous blood flow and an appropriate volume and distribution of blood to cells that need nutrients.

Physiology and Regulation

Blood flows through the body in a continuous circuit. Electrical impulses originating from the sinoatrial (SA) node travel through heart muscle to stimulate cardiac contraction. Approximately 60 to 70 ml (**stroke volume**) of blood enters the aorta with each ventricular contraction. With each stroke volume ejection, the walls of the aorta distend, creating a pulse wave that travels rapidly toward the distal ends of the arteries. The pulse wave moves 15 times faster through the aorta and 100 times faster through the small arteries than the ejected volume of blood (Guyton, 1991). When a pulse wave reaches a peripheral artery, it can be felt by palpating the artery lightly against underlying bone or muscle. The pulse is the palpable bounding of the blood flow in the peripheral artery. The number of pulsing sensations occurring in 1 minute is the pulse rate.

The volume of blood pumped by the heart during 1 minute is the **cardiac output**, the product of heart rate and the ventricle's stroke volume. In an adult the heart normally pumps 5000 ml of blood per minute. A change in heart rate or stroke volume does not always change the heart's output or the amount of blood in the arteries. For example, if a person's heart rate is 70 beats per minute and the stroke volume is 70 ml, the cardiac output is 4900 ml per minute. What happens if the heart rate drops to 60 beats per minute and the stroke volume rises to 85 ml? (See the box at right.)

Mechanical, neural, and chemical factors regulate the strength of heart contractions and its stroke volume. But when mechanical, neural, or chemical factors are unable to alter stroke volume, a change in heart rate will result in a change in blood pressure. As heart rate increases, there is less time for the heart to fill. As heart rate increases without a change in stroke volume, blood pressure will decrease. As the heart rate slows, filling time is increased and blood pressure increases. The inability of blood pressure to respond to increases or decreases in heart rate may indicate a health deviation and is reported to the physician.

The cause of an abnormally slow, rapid, or irregular pulse may alter cardiac output. The nurse assesses the heart's ability to meet the demands of the body's tissue for nutrients by palpating a peripheral pulse or by using a stethoscope to listen to heart sounds (apical rate).

Assessment of Pulse

Any artery can be assessed for pulse rate, but the radial and carotid arteries are easily palpated peripheral pulse sites. When a client's condition suddenly worsens, the carotid site is the best for quickly finding a pulse. The heart will continue delivering blood through the carotid artery to the brain as long as possible. When cardiac output declines significantly, peripheral pulses weaken and are difficult to palpate.

The radial and apical locations are the most common sites for pulse rate assessment (Fig. 32-10). They are used by persons learning to monitor their own heart rates (e.g., athletes, persons taking heart medications, and clients starting a prescribed exercise regimen). If the **radial pulse** at the wrist is abnormal or intermittent resulting from dysrhythmias, or if it is inaccessible because of a dressing, cast, or other encumbrance, the apical pulse is assessed. When a client takes medication that affects the heart rate, the apical pulse may provide a more accurate assessment of heart

Cardiac Output Determination

Pulse rate × Stroke volume = Cardiac output

70 beats/min × 70 ml/beat = 4.9 L/min

60 beats/min × 85 ml/beat = 5.1 L/min

function. The apical pulse is the best site for assessing an infant's or young child's pulse because the peripheral pulses are deep and difficult to palpate accurately.

Assessment of other peripheral pulse sites such as the brachial or femoral artery is unnecessary when routinely obtaining vital signs. Other peripheral pulses are assessed when a complete physical is conducted, when surgery or treatment has impaired blood flow to a body part, or when there are clinical indications of impaired peripheral blood flow (see Chapter 33). Table 32-2 summarizes pulse sites and criteria for measurement. Procedure 32-2 outlines pulse rate assessment.

USE OF A STETHOSCOPE

When assessing the apical rate the nurse uses a stethoscope (Fig. 32-11). The five major parts of the stethoscope are the earpieces, binaurals, tubing, bell chestpiece, and diaphragm chestpiece.

The plastic or rubber earpieces should fit snugly and comfortably in the nurse's ears. The binaurals should be an-

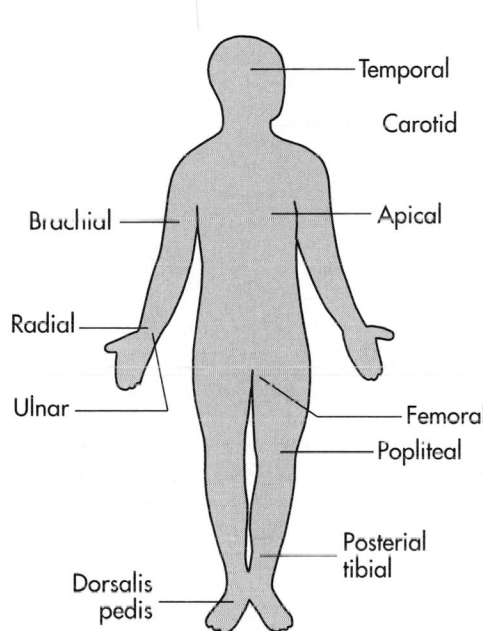

Fig. 32-10 Location of pulse points in the body.

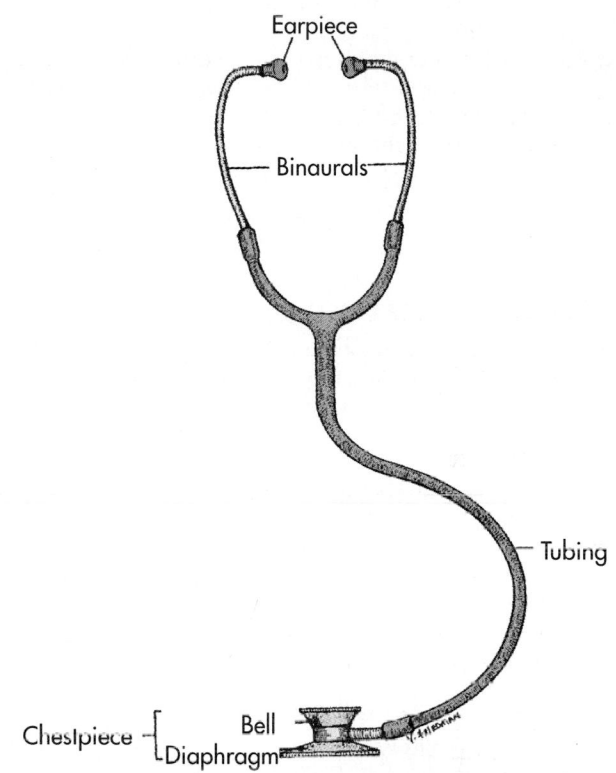

Fig. 32-11 Parts of a stethoscope.

Table 32-2	Pulse Sites	
SITE	**LOCATION**	**ASSESSMENT CRITERIA**
Temporal	Over temporal bone of head, above and lateral to eye	Easily accessible site used to assess pulse in children
Carotid	Along medial edge of sternocleidomastoid muscle in neck	Easily accessible site used during physiological shock or cardiac arrest when other sites are not palpable
Apical	Fourth to fifth intercostal space at left midclavicular line	Site used to auscultate for apical pulse
Brachial	Groove between biceps and triceps muscles at antecubital fossa	Site used to assess status of circulation to lower arm Site used to auscultate blood pressure
Radial	Radial or thumb side of forearm at wrist	Common site used to assess character of pulse peripherally and assess status of circulation to hand
Ulnar	Ulnar side of forearm at wrist	Site used to assess status of circulation to hand. Site also used to perform Allen test
Femoral	Below inguinal ligament, midway between symphysis pubis and anterior superior iliac spine	Site used to assess character of pulse during physiological shock or cardiac arrest when other pulses are not palpable; used to assess status of circulation to leg
Popliteal	Behind knee in popliteal fossa	Site used to assess status of circulation to lower leg
Posterior tibial	Inner side of ankle, below medial malleolus	Site used to assess status of circulation to foot
Dorsalis pedis	Along top of foot, between extension tendons of great and first toe	Site used to assess status of circulation to foot

PROCEDURE 32-2

Assessing Pulse Rate

STEPS	RATIONALE

PREPARATION FOR ASSESSING PULSE RATE

1. Before measuring pulse, consider factors that normally influence pulse character (e.g., age, exercise, and postural changes).

Allows nurse to accurately assess presence and significance of pulse alterations.

2. Explain that pulse or heart rate is to be assessed. Encourage client to relax and not speak. (If client has been active, wait 5 to 10 min.)

Activity and anxiety can elevate the heart rate. Client's voice interferes with nurse's ability to hear sound when apical pulse is measured.

3. Prepare equipment and supplies:

  a. Stethoscope, alcohol swab

  b. Pen, pencil, vital signs flow sheet or record form

  c. Wristwatch with second hand or digital display

Stethoscope used for apical rate assessment. Alcohol swab used as needed to cleanse stethoscope earpieces and diaphragm.

4. Wash hands.

Reduces transmission of microorganisms.

MEASURE RADIAL PULSE

1. Complete preparation steps 1-4.

2. If client is supine, place forearm across lower chest or alongside torso with wrist slightly flexed and palm facing down (see the illustration below). If client is sitting, bend elbow 90 degrees and support lower arm on chair or on nurse's arm. Slightly flex wrist with palm facing down.

Permits full exposure of artery to palpation.

3. Place tips of first two fingers of hand over groove along radial or thumb side of client's inner wrist (see the illustration below).

Fingertips are the most sensitive parts of hand to palpate arterial pulsation. Nurse's thumb has pulsation that may interfere with accuracy.

4. Lightly compress against radius, obliterate pulse initially, and then relax pressure so that pulse becomes easily palpable.

Pulse is more accurately assessed with moderate pressure. Too much pressure occludes pulse and impairs blood flow.

5. After pulse can be felt regularly, look at watch's second hand and begin to count rate; when sweep hand hits number on dial, start counting with *zero,* then *one,* and so on (see the illustration on p. 617).

Rate is determined accurately only after assessor is assured pulse can be palpated. Timing begins with zero. Count of one is first beat palpated after timing begins.

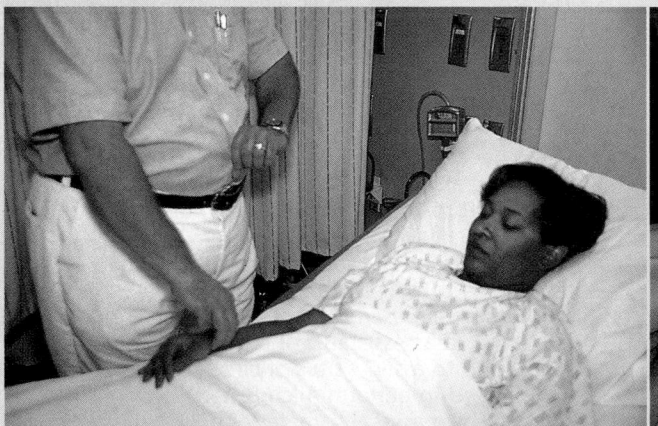

Step 2

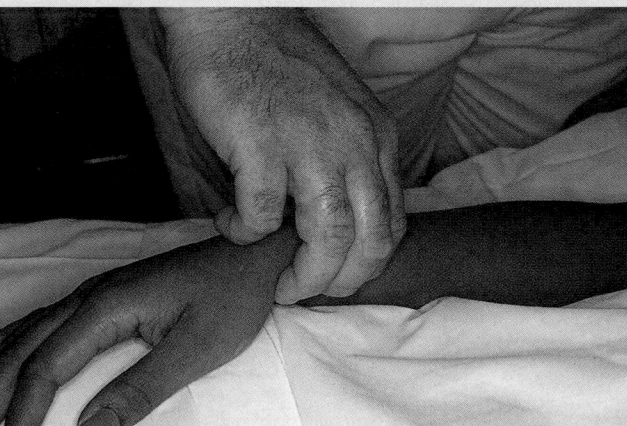

Step 3

Assessing Pulse Rate—cont'd

STEPS	RATIONALE

MEASURE RADIAL PULSE—cont'd

6. If pulse is regular, count rate for 30 sec and multiply total by 2.

A 30-sec check is adequate for rapid, slow, or regular heart rates.

7. If pulse is irregular, count rate for 60 sec. Assess frequency and pattern of irregularity.

Inefficient contraction of heart fails to transmit pulse wave, interferes with cardiac output, and results in irregular pulse. Longer time period ensures accurate count. Irregular pulse necessitates assessment for pulse deficit.

8. Determine strength of pulse. Note thrust of vessel against fingertips.

Strength reflects volume of blood ejected against arterial wall with each heart contraction.

9. Assist client in returning to comfortable position.

Promotes sense of well-being.

10. Discuss findings with client.

Promotes participation in care and understanding of health status.

11. Wash hands.

Reduces transmission of microorganisms.

12. Perform completion steps 1-2.

MEASURE APICAL RATE

1. Complete preparation steps 1-4.

2. Clean earpieces and diaphragm of stethoscope with alcohol swab as needed.

Ensures clean instrument and promotes auscultation.

3. With client in supine or sitting position, turn down bed linen and raise gown to expose sternum and left side of chest.

Exposes portion of chest wall for selection of auscultatory site.

4. Palpate angle of Louis, located just below suprasternal notch at point where horizontal ridge is felt along body of sternum. Place finger just to left of client's sternum and palpate second intercostal space. Place next finger in intercostal space below and proceed downward until fifth intercostal space is located. Move finger horizontally along fifth intercostal space to left midclavicular line (see the illustration below). Palpate point of maximal impulse (PMI).

Use of anatomical landmarks allows nurse to place stethoscope over apex of heart, which lies under fifth intercostal space along left midclavicular line. This position enhances ability to hear heart sounds clearly. PMI is normally over apex of heart.

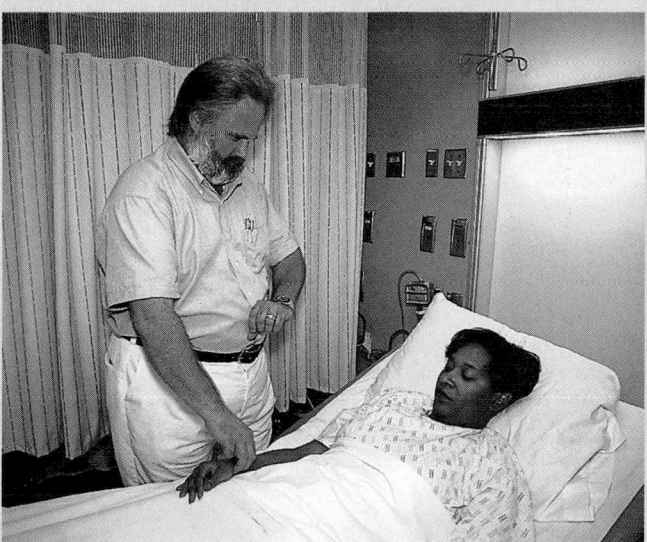

Step 5, p. 616

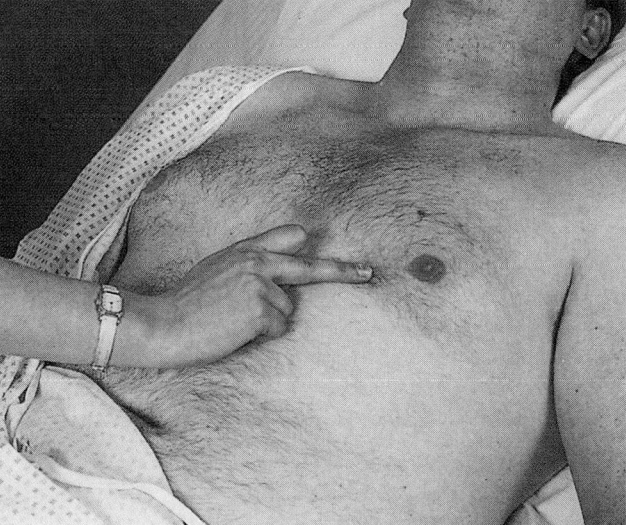

Step 4

Continued.

Assessing Pulse Rate—cont'd

STEPS	RATIONALE

MEASURE APICAL RATE

5. Place diaphragm of stethoscope in palm of hand for 5 to 10 seconds.

Warming of diaphragm prevents client from being startled and promotes comfort.

6. Place diaphragm over PMI and auscultate for normal S_1 and S_2 heart sounds (heard as "lub-dub") (see the illustration below).

Heart sounds are caused by movement of blood through heart valves.

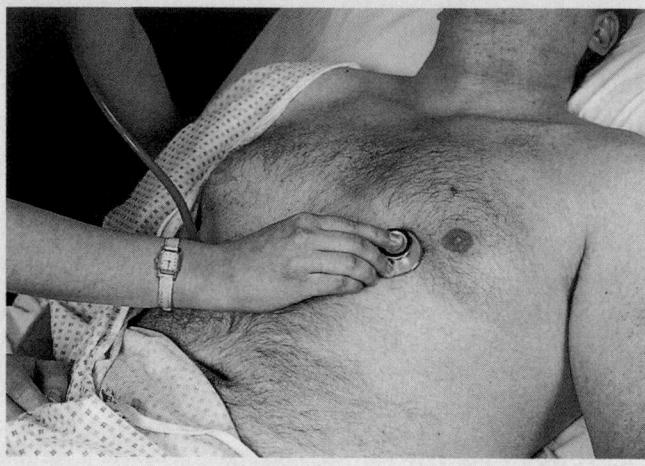

Step 6

7. After occurrence of S_1 and S_2 can be heard with regularity, use watch's second hand and begin to count rate; when sweep hand hits number on dial, start counting with *zero,* then *one,* and so on. Each "lub-dub" equals one heartbeat.

Rate is determined accurately only after nurse is able to auscultate sounds clearly.

8. If heart rate is regular, count for 30 sec and multiply by 2.

Regular apical rate can be assessed within 30 sec.

9. If heart rate is irregular, count for 60 sec. Assess frequency and pattern of irregularity.

Regular occurrence of irregularity may precipitate compromised cardiac output. Longer time period ensures more accurate count.

10. Replace gown and bed linen. Assist client in returning to comfortable position.

Maintains comfort.

11. Discuss findings with client.

Promotes participation in care and understanding of health status.

12. Wash hands, clean diaphragm with alcohol swab.

Reduces transmission of microorganisms.

13. Perform completion steps 1 and 2.

COMPLETION FOR ASSESSING PULSE

1. Compare peripheral pulse rate with apical rate and note discrepancy.

Differences between measurements indicate pulse deficit and may warn of cardiovascular compromise.

2. Record pulse characteristics on vital signs flow sheet or nurses' notes and report abnormal findings to nurse in charge or physician.

Vital sign measurements should be recorded promptly on flow sheet to avoid omissions to record. Abnormalities may require immediate therapy.

gled and strong enough so the earpieces stay firmly in the ears without causing discomfort. To ensure the best reception of sound, the earpieces follow the contour of the ear canal pointing toward the face when the stethoscope is in place.

The polyvinyl tubing should be flexible and 30 to 40 cm (12 to 18 inches) in length. Longer tubing decreases the transmission of sound waves. The tubing should be thick walled and moderately rigid to eliminate transmission of environmental noise and prevent the tubing from kinking, which distorts sound-wave transmission. Stethoscopes can have single or dual tubes. Dual tubes promote sound clarity by minimizing the number of turns the sound wave makes before reaching the earpiece.

The bell and diaphragm compose the stethoscope chestpiece. The diaphragm is the circular, flat portion of the chestpiece covered with a thin plastic disk. It transmits high-pitched sounds created by the high-velocity movement of air and blood. Bowel, lung, and heart sounds are auscultated using the diaphragm. The nurse positions the diaphragm to make a tight seal against the client's skin (Fig. 32-12). Enough pressure is exerted to leave a temporary red ring on the client's skin when the diaphragm is removed.

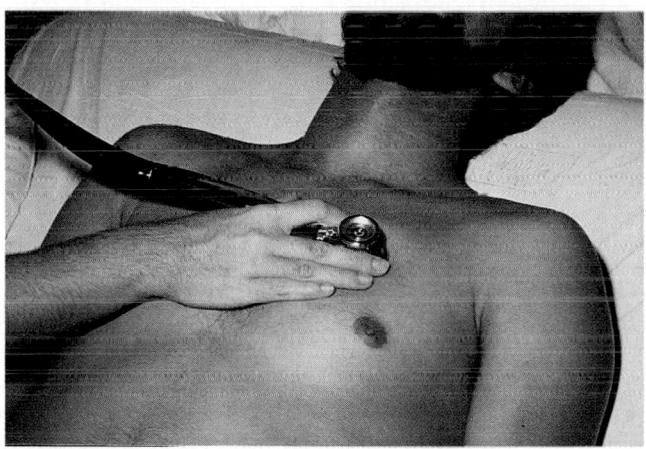

Fig. 32-12 Positioning the diaphragm of the stethoscope.

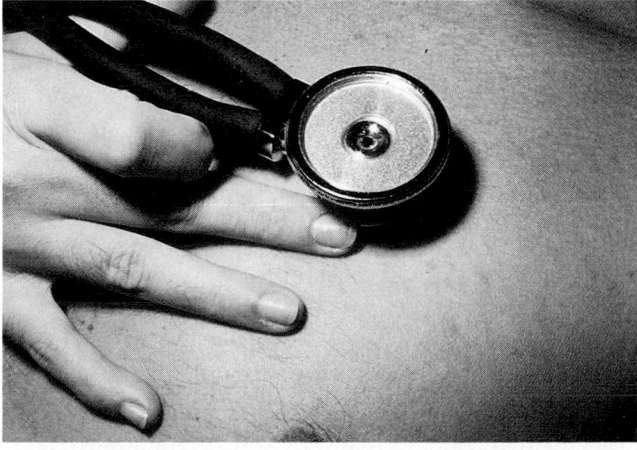

Fig. 32-13 Positioning the bell of the stethoscope.

The bell is the bowl-shaped chestpiece usually surrounded by a rubber ring. The ring avoids chilling the client with cold metal when placed on the skin. The bell transmits low-pitched sounds created by the low-velocity movement of blood. Heart and vascular sounds are auscultated using the bell. The nurse applies the bell lightly, resting the chestpiece on the skin (Fig. 32-13). Compressing the bell against the skin reduces low-pitched sound amplification and creates a "diaphragm of skin." The bell and diaphragm are rotated into position on the chestpiece, depending on which part the nurse chooses to use. The diaphragm or bell must be in proper position during use for the nurse to hear sounds through the stethoscope. To test, lightly tap to determine which side is functioning.

The stethoscope is a delicate instrument and requires proper care for optimal function. The earpieces should be removed regularly and cleaned of cerumen (ear wax). The bell and diaphragm are cleaned of dust, lint, and body oils. The tubing should be kept away from the nurse's body oils. Avoid draping the stethoscope around the neck next to the skin. Cleaning the tubing with alcohol can dry and crack the material and is not recommended. Mild soap and water are preferred.

Character of the Pulse

Assessment of the radial pulse includes measurement of the rate, rhythm, strength, and equality. When auscultating an apical pulse, the nurse assesses rate and rhythm only.

RATE

Before measuring a pulse, the nurse reviews the client's baseline rate for comparison (Table 32-3). Some practitioners prefer to make baseline measurements of the pulse rate as the client assumes a sitting, standing, and lying position. Postural changes cause changes in pulse rate because of alterations in blood volume and sympathetic activity. The heart rate temporarily increases when a person changes from a lying to a sitting or standing position.

When assessing the pulse, the nurse must consider the variety of factors influencing the pulse rate (Table 32-4). A combination of these factors may cause significant changes. If the nurse detects an abnormal rate while palpating a peripheral pulse, the next step is to assess the apical rate. The apical rate provides a more accurate assessment of cardiac contraction.

Table 32-3	Normal Heart Rate	
AGE	**HEART RATE (BEATS/MIN)**	
Infants	120-160/min	
Toddlers	90-140/min	
Preschoolers	80-110/min	
School agers	75-100/min	
Adolescent	60-90/min	
Adult	60-100/min	

Modified from Hazinski MF: Children are different. In Hazinski MF, editor: *Nursing care of the critically ill child*, St Louis, 1984, Mosby; and Kinney MR, et al: *AACN's clinical reference for critical care nursing*, ed 3, St Louis, 1993, Mosby.

Table 32-4	Factors Influencing Pulse Rates	
FACTOR	**INCREASE PULSE RATE**	**DECREASE PULSE RATE**
Exercise	Short-term exercise	A conditioned athlete who participates in long-term exercise will have a lower heart rate at rest
Temperature	Fever and heat	Hypothermia
Emotions	Acute pain and anxiety increase sympathetic stimulation, affecting heart rate	Unrelieved severe pain increases parasympathetic stimulation, affecting heart rate; relaxation
Drugs	Positive chronotropic drugs such as epinephrine	Negative chronotropic drugs such as digitalis
Hemorrhage	Loss of blood increases sympathetic stimulation	
Postural changes	Standing or sitting	Lying down
Pulmonary conditions	Diseases causing poor oxygenation	

The nurse assesses the apical rate by listening for heart sounds (see Chapter 33). The nurse tries to identify the first and second heart sounds (S_1 and S_2). At normal slow rates, S_1 is low pitched and dull, sounding like a "lub." S_2 is higher pitched and shorter, creating the sound, "dub." Each set of "lub-dub" is counted as one heart beat. Using the diaphragm or bell of the stethoscope, the nurse counts the number of lub-dubs occurring in 1 minute.

Peripheral and apical pulse rate assessment may reveal variations in heart rate. Two common abnormalities in pulse rate are tachycardia and bradycardia. **Tachycardia** is an abnormally elevated heart rate, above 100 beats per minute in adults. **Bradycardia** is a slow rate, below 60 beats per minute in adults.

RHYTHM

Normally a regular interval occurs between each pulse or heart beat. An interval interrupted by an early or late beat or a missed beat indicates an abnormal rhythm or **dysrhythmia.** A dysrhythmia threatens the heart's ability to provide adequate cardiac output, particularly if it occurs repetitively. The nurse identifies a dysrhythmia by palpating an interruption in successive pulse waves or auscultating an interruption between heart sounds. If a dysrhythmia is present, the regularity of its occurrence should be assessed. Dysrhythmias may be described as regularly irregular or irregularly irregular.

To document dysrhythmia, a physician may order an electrocardiogram, Holter monitor, or telemetry. An electrocardiogram records the electrical activity of the heart for a 12-second interval. This test requires placement of electrodes across the client's chest followed by recording of the heart rhythm. The Holter monitor records 24 hours of electrical activity in a small tape recorder that the client wears. Access to the information recorded is not available until after the 24 hours have passed and the data are printed for review. Cardiac telemetry provides continuous monitoring of the heart's electrical activity transmitted to a stationary monitor. Telemetry permits observation of heart rhythm during all of the client's daily activities and thus allows for immediate treatment if the rhythm becomes erratic or unstable.

Children often have a sinus dysrhythmia, which is an irregular heart beat that speeds up with inspiration and slows down with expiration. This is a normal finding and can be verified by having the child hold his breath; the heart rate should then become regular.

An inefficient contraction of the heart that fails to transmit a pulse wave to the peripheral pulse site creates a **pulse deficit.** To assess a pulse deficit the nurse and a colleague assess radial and apical rates simultaneously and then compare rates. The difference between the apical and radial pulse rates is the pulse deficit. For example, an apical rate of 92 with a radial rate of 78 leaves a pulse deficit of 14 beats. Pulse deficits are frequently associated with dysrhythmias.

STRENGTH

The strength or amplitude of a pulse reflects the volume of blood ejected against the arterial wall with each heart contraction and the condition of the arterial vascular system leading to the pulse site. Normally the pulse strength remains the same with each heart beat. Pulse strength may be graded or described as strong, weak, thready, or bounding. It is included during assessment of the vascular system (see Chapter 33).

EQUALITY

Pulses on both sides of the peripheral vascular system should be assessed. The nurse assesses both radial pulses to compare the characteristics of each. A pulse in one extremity may be unequal in strength or absent in many disease states (e.g., thrombus [clot] formation, aberrant blood vessels, cervical rib syndrome, or aortic dissection). All symmetrical pulses can be assessed simultaneously except for the carotid pulse. The carotid pulse should *never* be measured simultaneously because excessive pressure may occlude blood supply to the brain.

■ NURSING PROCESS AND PULSE DETERMINATION

Pulse assessment determines the general state of cardiovascular health and the response to other system imbalances. Tachycardia, bradycardia, and dysrhythmias are defining

Examples of NANDA Nursing Diagnoses Using Pulse Assessment Data as Defining Characteristics

Activity intolerance	Fluid volume excess
Altered tissue perfusion	Hyperthermia
Anxiety	Hypothermia
Decreased cardiac output	Impaired gas exchange
Fear	Pain
Fluid volume deficit	

characteristics of many nursing diagnoses and are considered along with other assessment data. For example, the defining characteristics of an abnormal heart rate, exertional dyspnea, and a client's verbal report of fatigue lead to a diagnosis of activity intolerance (see the nursing dianoses box above). The nursing care plan includes interventions based on the nursing diagnosis identified and the related factor. The nurse evaluates client outcomes by assessing the pulse rate, rhythm, strength, and equality following each intervention.

▌ RESPIRATION

Human survival depends on the ability of oxygen (O_2) to reach body cells and for carbon dioxide (CO_2) to be removed from the cells. Respiration is the mechanism the body uses to exchange gases between the atmosphere and the blood and the blood and the cells. Respiration involves **ventilation** (the movement of gases in and out of the lungs), **diffusion** (the movement of oxygen and carbon dioxide between the alveoli and the red blood cells), and **perfusion** (the distribution of red blood cells to and from the pulmonary capillaries). They can be assessed independently. The rate, depth, and rhythm of ventilatory movements indicate the quality and efficiency of ventilation. Diagnostic tests that measure O_2 and CO_2 levels in arterial blood offer useful information about both diffusion and perfusion. However, analyzing respiratory efficiency requires integrating assessment data from all three processes. The processes are interdependent. Ventilatory adequacy can affect diffusion and perfusion, which in turn will affect ventilation. Respiration can be affected by various factors (see the box above, right).

Physiological Control

Breathing is generally a passive process. Normally a person thinks little about it. The respiratory center in the brain stem regulates the involuntary control of respirations. Adults normally breathe smoothly and uninterrupted, 12 to 20 times a minute.

Ventilation is regulated by levels of CO_2, O_2, and hydrogen ion concentration (pH) in the arterial blood. The most important factor in the control of ventilation is the level of CO_2 (carbia) in the arterial blood. An elevation in the P_{CO_2} causes the respiratory control system in the brain to increase the rate and depth of breathing. The increased ventilatory effort removes excess CO_2 during exhalation. Hypercarbia, a chronic excess of CO_2 in arterial blood, can eventually depress ventilation.

Factors Influencing Character of Respirations

EXERCISE
Exercise increases rate and depth to meet the body's need for additional oxygen.

ACUTE PAIN
Acute pain increases rate and depth as a result of sympathetic stimulation.
Client may inhibit or splint chest wall movement when pain is in area of chest or abdomen. Breaths become shallow.

ANXIETY
Anxiety increases rate and depth as a result of sympathetic stimulation.

SMOKING
Chronic smoking changes the lung's airways, resulting in an increased rate.

ANEMIA
Decreased hemoglobin levels lower the amount of O_2 carried in the blood. A person breathes faster to increase O_2 delivery.

BODY POSITION
A straight, erect posture promotes full chest expansion. A stooped or slumped position impairs ventilatory movement.

MEDICATIONS
Narcotic analgesics and sedatives depress rate and depth.
Amphetamines and cocaine may increase rate and depth.

BRAIN STEM INJURY
Injury to the brain stem impairs the respiratory center and inhibits respiratory rate and rhythm.

Chemoreceptors in the carotid artery and aorta are sensitive to **hypoxemia**, or low levels of arterial O_2. If arterial oxygen levels fall, these receptors signal the brain to increase the rate and depth of ventilation. Hypoxemia helps to control ventilation in clients with chronic lung disease. Hypercarbia is constant in clients with chronic lung disease. Once an elevated CO_2 level fails to increase the rate and depth of breathing, hypoxemia, also present in these clients, becomes the stimulus to increase ventilation. Because low levels of arterial O_2 provide the stimulus that allows the client to breathe, administration of high oxygen levels can be fatal for clients with chronic lung disease.

Mechanics of Breathing

Although breathing is normally passive, muscular work is involved in moving the lungs and chest wall. Inspiration is an active process. During inspiration the respiratory center sends impulses along the phrenic nerve, causing the diaphragm to contract. Abdominal organs move downward and forward, increasing the length of the chest cavity to move air into the lungs. The diaphragm moves approximately 1 cm ($\frac{4}{10}$ inch), and the ribs retract upward from the body's midline approximately 1.2 to 2.5 cm ($\frac{1}{2}$ to 1 inch). During a normal, relaxed breath, a person inhales 500 ml of air. This amount is referred to as the **tidal volume.** During expiration the diaphragm relaxes and the abdominal organs return to their original positions. The lung and chest wall return to a relaxed position (see Fig. 32-14). Expiration is a passive process. The normal rate and depth of ventilation, **eupnea,** is interrupted by sighing. The sigh, a prolonged deeper breath, is a protective physiological mechanism for expanding small airways and alveoli not ventilated during a normal breath.

The accurate assessment of respirations depends on the nurse's recognition of normal thoracic and abdominal movements. During quiet breathing the chest wall gently rises and falls. Contraction of the intercostal muscles between the ribs or contraction of the muscles in the neck and shoulders, the accessory muscles of breathing, is not visible. During normal quiet breathing, diaphragmatic movement causes the abdominal cavity to rise and fall slowly.

When breathing requires greater effort, the intercostal and accessory muscles work actively to move air in and out. The shoulders may rise and fall, and the accessory muscles of ventilation in the neck visibly contract. Diaphragmatic movement becomes less noticeable as costal breathing increases. Certain clinical conditions such as chest wall pain, pneumothorax, emphysema, and neuromuscular disease affect ventilatory movement.

Assessment of Respirations

Respirations are the easiest of all vital signs to assess, but they are often the most haphazardly measured. A nurse must not estimate respirations. Accurate measurement requires observation and palpation of chest wall movement.

A sudden change in the character of respirations may be important. Because respiration is tied to the function of numerous body systems, the nurse must consider all variables when changes occur. For example, a drop in respirations occurring in a client after head trauma may signify injury to the brain stem. Abdominal trauma may injure the phrenic nerve, which is responsible for diaphragmatic contraction. The nurse must understand the extent of the injury and the implications for the respiratory system.

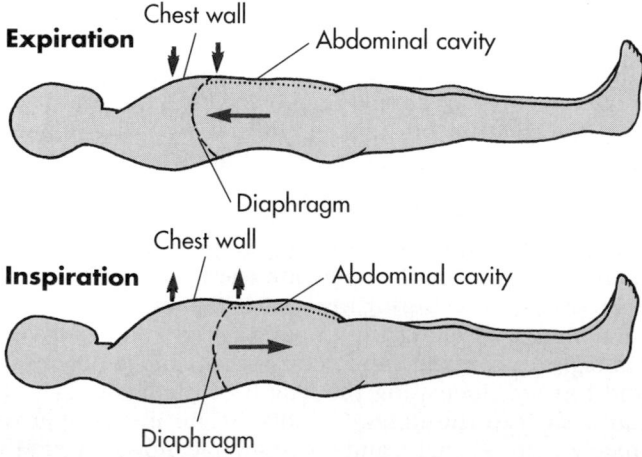

Fig. 32-14 Illustration of diaphragmatic movement during inspiration and expiration.

A skillful nurse does not let a client know that respirations are being assessed. A client aware of the nurse's intentions may consciously alter the rate and depth of breathing. Assessment can best be done immediately after measuring pulse rate, with the nurse's hand still on the client's wrist as it rests over the chest or abdomen. When assessing a client's respirations, the nurse should keep in mind the client's normal ventilatory rate and pattern, the influence any disease or illness has on respiratory function, the relationship between respiratory and cardiovascular function, and the influence of therapies on respirations. The objective measurements of an assessment of respiratory status include the rate and depth of breathing and the rhythm of ventilatory movements (Procedure 32-3).

RESPIRATORY RATE

The nurse observes a full inspiration and expiration when counting ventilation or respiration rate. The respiratory rate varies with age (Table 32-5). The normal respiratory rate declines throughout life.

A respiratory monitoring device that aids the nurse's assessment is the apnea monitor. This device uses leads attached to the client's chest wall that sense movement. The absence of chest wall movement is interpreted by the monitor as apnea and triggers an alarm. Apnea monitoring is used frequently with infants in the hospital and at home to observe for prolonged apneic events. Noninvasive monitoring provides information that helps the nurse assess the rate, depth, and rhythm of respiration more knowledgeably.

VENTILATORY DEPTH

The depth of respirations is assessed by observing the degree of excursion or movement in the chest wall. The nurse subjectively describes ventilatory movements as deep, normal, or shallow. A deep respiration involves a full expansion of the lungs with full exhalation. Respirations are shallow when only a small quantity of air passes through the lungs and ventilatory movement is difficult to see. More objective techniques are used if the nurse observes that chest excursion is unusually shallow (see Chapter 33). Table 32-6 summarizes types of respiratory alterations.

VENTILATORY RHYTHM

With normal breathing a regular interval occurs after each respiratory cycle. Infants tend to breathe less regularly. The young child may breathe slowly for a few seconds and then suddenly breathe more rapidly. While assessing respirations, the nurse estimates the time interval after each respiratory cycle. Respiration is regular or irregular in rhythm.

Table 32-5	Normal Average Respiratory Rates by Age	
AGE		**RATE**
Newborn		35-40
Infant (6 months)		30-50
Toddler (2 years)		25-32
Child		20-30
Adolescent		16-19
Adult		12-20

Assessing Respirations

STEPS	RATIONALE
1. Assess for factors that normally influence character of respirations.	Allows nurse to accurately assess for presence and significance of respiratory alterations.
2. If client has been active, wait 5 to 10 minutes.	Exercise increases respiratory rate and depth.
3. Be sure client is in comfortable position, preferably sitting or lying with head of bed elevated 45 to 60 degrees.	Discomfort causes client to breathe more rapidly. Erect, sitting position promotes full ventilation.

4. Prepare equipment and supplies:
  a. Watch with second hand or digital display
  b. Pen, vital sign flow sheet, or record form	

5. Draw curtain or close door. Wash hands.	Maintains privacy. Prevents transmission of microorganisms.
6. Be sure client's chest is visible. If necessary, move clothing or gown away from chest.	Ensures clear view of chest wall and abdominal movements.
7. Place client's arm in relaxed position that does not block visualization of client's chest, or place nurse's hand directly over client's upper abdomen (see the illustration below).	A similar position is used during pulse assessment, allowing respiratory rate assessment to be inconspicuous. A client aware of respiratory assessment may intentionally or unintentionally alter rate and depth of breathing.

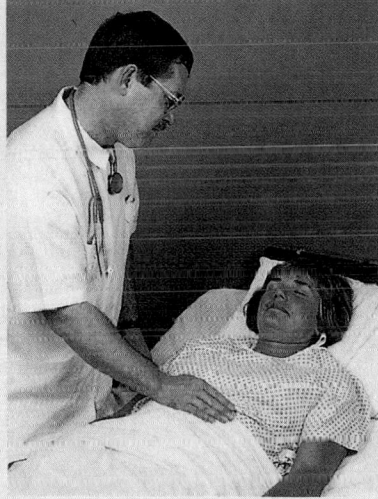

Step 7

STEPS	RATIONALE
8. Observe complete respiratory cycle (one inspiration and one expiration).	Rate is accurately determined only after nurse has viewed respiratory cycle.
9. After observing cycle, look at second hand or digital display on watch and count rate: begin counting *one* with first full respiratory cycle.	Timing begins with count of *one*. Respirations occur more slowly than pulse; thus timing does not begin with *zero*.
10. If rhythm is regular in adult, count number of respirations in 30 sec and multiply by 2. In infant or young child, count respirations for full minute.	Respiratory rate is equivalent to number of respiratory cycles per minute. Young infants and children normally breathe irregularly.
11. In an adult, if rhythm is irregular or rate is less than 12 or more than 20, count for 60 sec.	Suspected irregularities require assessment for at least 1 min.
12. Note depth, assessed subjectively by observing degree of chest wall movement while counting rate. Objectively assess depth by palpating chest wall excursion (see Chapter 33) after rate is counted.	Character of ventilatory movements may reveal specific alterations or disease status.
13. Note rhythm of respiratory cycle.	Character of ventilations can reveal specific types of alterations. Normal breathing is regular and uninterrupted.
14. Assist client in replacing clothing or gown.	Restores comfort, promotes sense of well-being.
15. Wash hands.	Reduces transmission of microorganisms.
16. Discuss findings with client as needed.	Promotes participation and understanding of health status.
17. Compare respirations to baseline and/or normal respiratory rate for age-group.	Allows nurse to assess for change in condition and for respiratory alterations.
18. Record respiratory rate and character on vital sign flow sheet and report abnormal findings to nurse in charge or physician.	Vital signs/measurements should be recorded promptly on flow sheet to avoid omissions from record. Abnormalities may require immediate therapy.

Table 32-6	Alterations in Breathing Pattern
ALTERATION	**DESCRIPTION**
Bradypnea	Rate of breathing is regular but abnormally slow (less than 12 breaths per min).
Tachypnea	Rate of breathing is regular but abnormally rapid (greater than 20 breaths per min).
Hyperpnea	Respirations are labored, increased in depth, and increased in rate (greater than 20 breaths per min). Occurs normally during exercise.
Apnea	Respirations cease for several seconds. Persistent cessation results in respiratory arrest.
Hyperventilation	Rate and depth of respirations increase. Hypocarbia may occur.
Hypoventilation	Respiratory rate is abnormally low and depth of ventilation may be depressed. Hypercarbia may occur.
Cheyne-Stokes respiration	Respiratory rate and depth are irregular, characterized by alternating periods of apnea and hyperventilation. Respiratory cycle begins with slow, shallow breaths that gradually increase to abnormal rate and depth. The pattern reverses, breathing slows and becomes shallow, climaxing in apnea before respiration resumes.
Kussmaul respiration	Respirations are abnormally deep, regular, and increased in rate.
Biot's respiration	Respirations are abnormally shallow for two to three breaths followed by irregular period of apnea.

ASSESSMENT OF DIFFUSION AND PERFUSION

The respiratory processes of diffusion and perfusion can be evaluated by measuring the oxygen saturation of the blood. Blood flow through the pulmonary capillaries provides red blood cells for oxygen attachment. After oxygen diffuses from the alveoli into the pulmonary blood, most of the oxygen attaches to hemoglobin molecules in red blood cells. Red blood cells carry the oxygenated hemoglobin molecules through the left side of the heart and out to the peripheral capillaries, where the oxygen detaches, depending on the needs of the tissues.

The percent of hemoglobin that is bound with oxygen in the arteries is the percent of saturation of hemoglobin (or Sao_2). It is normally between 95% and 100%. Sao_2 is affected by factors that interfere with ventilation, perfusion, or diffusion (see Chapter 44). The saturation of venous blood (Svo_2) is lower because the tissues have removed some of the oxygen from the hemoglobin molecules. A normal value for Svo_2 is 70%. Svo_2 is affected by factors that interfere with or increase the tissue's need for oxygen.

Measurement of Arterial Oxygen Saturation. The recent development of a reliable device, a pulse oximeter, allows for the indirect measurement of oxygen saturation in the client's vital sign data base (Procedure 32-4). The pulse oximeter is a probe with a light-emitting diode (LED) and photodetector connected by cable to an oximeter (Fig. 32-15). The LED emits light wavelengths that are absorbed by the oxygenated and deoxygenated hemoglobin molecules. The light reflected from the hemoglobin molecules is processed by the oximeter, which calculates pulse saturation (Spo_2). Spo_2 is a reliable estimate of Sao_2.

The measurement of Spo_2 is affected by factors that affect light transmission or peripheral arterial pulsations. An awareness of these factors allows the nurse's accurate interpretation of abnormal Spo_2 measurements (see the box on p. 626).

■ NURSING PROCESS AND RESPIRATORY VITAL SIGNS

Vital sign measurement of respiratory rate, pattern, and depth, along with Spo_2, allows the nurse to assess ventilation, diffusion, and perfusion. The nurse may also conduct other assessments to measure respiratory status (see Chapter 33). Each measurement can provide clues in determining the nature of a client's problem. Respiratory assessment data are defining characteristics of many nursing diagnoses and are considered with other assessment data. For example, the defining characteristics of tachypnea, changes in depth of respirations, use of accessory muscles, cyanosis and a decline in Spo_2 lead to a diagnosis of impaired gas exchange (see the nursing diagnoses box on p. 626). The nursing care plan includes interventions based on the nursing diagnosis identified and the related factor (see Chapter 44). The nurse evaluates client outcomes by assessing the respiratory rate, ventilatory depth, rhythm, and Spo_2 following each intervention.

■ BLOOD PRESSURE

Blood pressure is the lateral force on the walls of an artery by the pulsing blood under pressure from the heart. Sys-

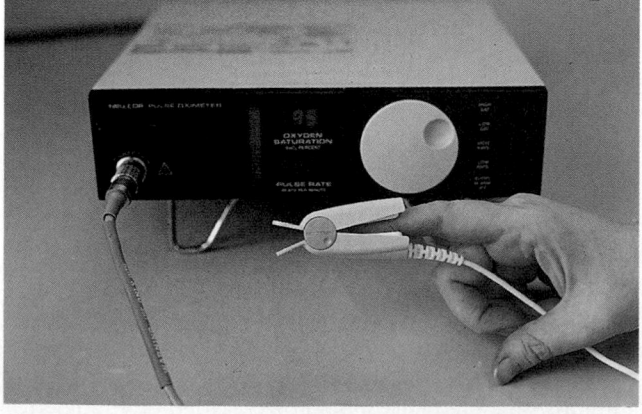

Fig. 32-15 Pulse oximeter.

Assessment of Oxygen Saturation With Pulse Oximeter

PROCEDURE 32-4

STEPS	RATIONALE
1. Assess for signs and symptoms of alterations in respiratory status, hypoxia, and factors that influence SpO_2.	Physical signs and symptoms may indicate abnormal arterial saturation.
2. Assess factors that influence client's respiratory status (e.g., oxygen therapy, hemoglobin level, temperature).	Early identification of clients at risk for unstable oxygen status prevents complications. Nurse can accurately assess nature of variations.
3. Review client's medical record for physician's order for pulse oximetry.	Medical order is required to assess oxygen saturation.
4. Prepare equipment and supplies and make sure they are in working order: a. Oximeter b. Oximeter probe appropriate for client and recommended by manufacturer c. Pen, vital sign flow sheet, or record form d. Acetone or nail polish remover	Mixing probes from different manufacturers can result in burn injury to client. Clip-on probes are convenient, quicker to apply, but more susceptible to movement interference. Adhesive probes suitable for pediatric use are less susceptible to motion artifact and can be taped to the skin.
5. Explain that SpO_2 is to be assessed; instruct client to breathe normally.	Clients are often curious about measurements. Prevents large fluctuations in minute ventilation and possible error in SpO_2 measurement.
6. Assess best site for obtaining SpO_2 measurement (e.g., finger, toe, earlobe, nose, palm, or foot).	Site selected must include a pulsating vascular bed. Changes in SpO_2 are reflected in the circulation of finger capillary bed within 30 sec and the capillary bed of earlobe within 5 to 10 sec. Peripheral vasoconstriction can interfere with SpO_2 determination.
7. If necessary, remove nail polish with acetone from digit to be assessed.	Ensures accurate readings. Opaque coatings decrease light transmission; nail polish containing blue pigment can absorb light emissions.
8. Assist client in assuming a comfortable sitting or supine position that provides easy access to measurement site.	Ensures comfort and accuracy of SpO_2 measurement. Movement can interfere with signal transmission between LED and photodetector.
9. Measure SpO_2: a. Apply oximeter probe and turn on oximeter by activating power. Observe pulse waveform/intensity display and audible beep. Correlate oximeter pulse rate with client's radial pulse.	Pulse waveform/intensity display enables detection of valid pulse or presence of interfering signal. Pitch of audible beep is proportional to SpO_2. Double checking pulse rate ensures oximeter accuracy.
b. Leave probe in place until oximeter readout reaches constant value and pulse display reaches full strength during each cardiac cycle.	Reading may take 10 to 30 sec, depending on site selected.
c. Read SpO_2 on digital display and inform client of reading.	Promotes participation in care and understanding of health status.
d. Remove probe and turn oximeter power off.	Batteries can be depleted if oximeter left on.
e. Assist client in returning to comfortable position.	Restores comfort, promotes sense of well-being.
f. Wash hands.	Reduces transmission of microorganisms.
10. Compare SpO_2 readings with baseline.	Comparison reveals presence of abnormality.
11. Record SpO_2 on vital sign flow sheet or nurses notes and report abnormal findings to nurse in charge or physician.	Vital sign measurement should be recorded promptly on flow sheets to avoid omissions from record. Abnormalities may require immediate therapy.

temic or arterial blood pressure, the blood pressure in the system of arteries in the body, is a good indicator of cardiovascular health. Blood flows throughout the circulatory system because of pressure changes. It moves from an area of high pressure to an area of low pressure. The heart's contraction forces blood under high pressure into the aorta. The peak of maximum pressure when ejection occurs is the **systolic** blood pressure. When the ventricles relax, the blood remaining in the arteries exerts a minimum or **dias**-tolic pressure. Diastolic pressure is the minimal pressure exerted against the arterial walls at all times.

The standard unit for measuring blood pressure is millimeters of mercury (mm Hg). The measurement indicates the height to which the blood pressure can raise a column of mercury. Blood pressure is recorded with the systolic reading before the diastolic (e.g., 120/80). The difference between systolic and diastolic pressure is the **pulse pressure**. For a blood pressure of 120/80, the pulse pressure is 40.

Factors Affecting Determination of Pulse Oxygen Saturation (SpO₂)

INTERFERENCE WITH LIGHT TRANSMISSION

Outside light sources can interfere with the oximeter's ability to process reflected light.

Carbon monoxide (caused by smoke inhalation or poisoning) artificially elevates SpO₂ by absorbing light similar to oxygen.

Client motion can interfere with the oximeter's ability to process reflected light.

Jaundice may interfere with the oximeter's ability to process reflected light.

Intravascular dyes (methylene blue) absorb light similar to deoxyhemoglobin and artificially lower saturation.

REDUCTION OF ARTERIAL PULSATIONS

Peripheral vascular disease (Raynaud's, atherosclerosis) can reduce pulse volume.

Hypothermia at assessment site decreases peripheral blood flow.

Pharmacological vasoconstrictors (epinephrine, neosynephrine, dopamine) will decrease peripheral pulse volume

Low cardiac output and hypotension decrease blood flow to peripheral arteries.

Peripheral edema can obscure arterial pulsation.

Examples of NANDA Nursing Diagnoses Using Respiratory Assessment Data as Defining Characteristics

Activity intolerance	Impaired gas exchange
Altered tissue perfusion	Ineffective airway clearance
Anxiety	Ineffective breathing
Dysfunctional ventilatory weaning response	pattern
	Pain

Physiology of Arterial Blood Pressure

Blood pressure reflects the interrelationships of cardiac output, peripheral vascular resistance, blood volume, blood viscosity, and artery elasticity. A nurse's knowledge of hemodynamic variables helps in the assessment of blood pressure alterations.

CARDIAC OUTPUT

A person's cardiac output is the volume of blood pumped by the heart (stroke volume) during 1 minute (heart rate):

$$CO = HR \times SV$$

The blood pressure (BP) depends on the cardiac output (CO) and peripheral vascular resistance (R):

$$BP = CO \times R$$

When volume increases in an enclosed space, such as a blood vessel, the pressure in that space rises. Thus, as cardiac output increases, more blood is pumped against arterial walls, causing the blood pressure to rise. Cardiac output can increase as a result of an increase in heart rate, greater heart muscle contractility, or an increase in blood volume. Changes in heart rate can occur faster than changes in muscle contractility or blood volume. An increase in heart rate without changes in contractility or blood volume results in a decrease in blood pressure.

PERIPHERAL RESISTANCE

Blood circulates through a network of arteries, arterioles, capillaries, venules, and veins. Arteries and arterioles are surrounded by smooth muscle that contracts or relaxes to change the size of the lumen. The size of arteries and arterioles changes to adjust blood flow to the needs of local tis-

sues. For example, when more blood is needed by a major organ, the peripheral arteries constrict, decreasing their supply of blood. More blood becomes available to the major organ because of the resistance change in the periphery. Normally, arteries and arterioles remain partially constricted to maintain a constant flow of blood. Peripheral vascular resistance is the resistance to blood flow determined by the tone of vascular musculature and diameter of blood vessels. The smaller the lumen of a vessel, the greater peripheral vascular resistance to blood flow. As resistance rises, arterial blood pressure rises. As vessels dilate and resistance falls, blood pressure drops.

BLOOD VOLUME

The volume of blood circulating within the vascular system affects blood pressure. Most adults have a circulating blood volume of 5000 ml. Normally the blood volume remains constant. However, if volume increases, more pressure is exerted against arterial walls. For example, the rapid, uncontrolled infusion of intravenous fluids elevates blood pressure. When circulating blood volume falls, as in the case of hemorrhage or dehydration, blood pressure falls.

VISCOSITY

The thickness or viscosity of blood affects the ease with which blood flows through small vessels. The **hematocrit**, or percentage of red blood cells in the blood, determines blood viscosity. When the hematocrit rises and blood flow slows, arterial blood pressure increases. The heart must contract more forcefully to move the viscous blood through the circulatory system.

ELASTICITY

Normally the walls of an artery are elastic and easily distensible. As pressure within the arteries increases, the diameter of vessel walls increases to accommodate the pressure change. Arterial distensibility prevents wide fluctuations in blood pressure. However, in certain diseases, such as arteriosclerosis, the vessel walls lose their elasticity and are replaced by fibrous tissue that cannot stretch well. With reduced elasticity there is greater resistance to blood flow. As a result, when the left ventricle ejects its stroke volume, the vessels no longer yield to pressure. Instead, a given volume of blood is forced through the rigid arterial walls, and the systemic pressure rises. Systolic pressure is more significantly elevated than diastolic pressure as a result of reduced arterial elasticity.

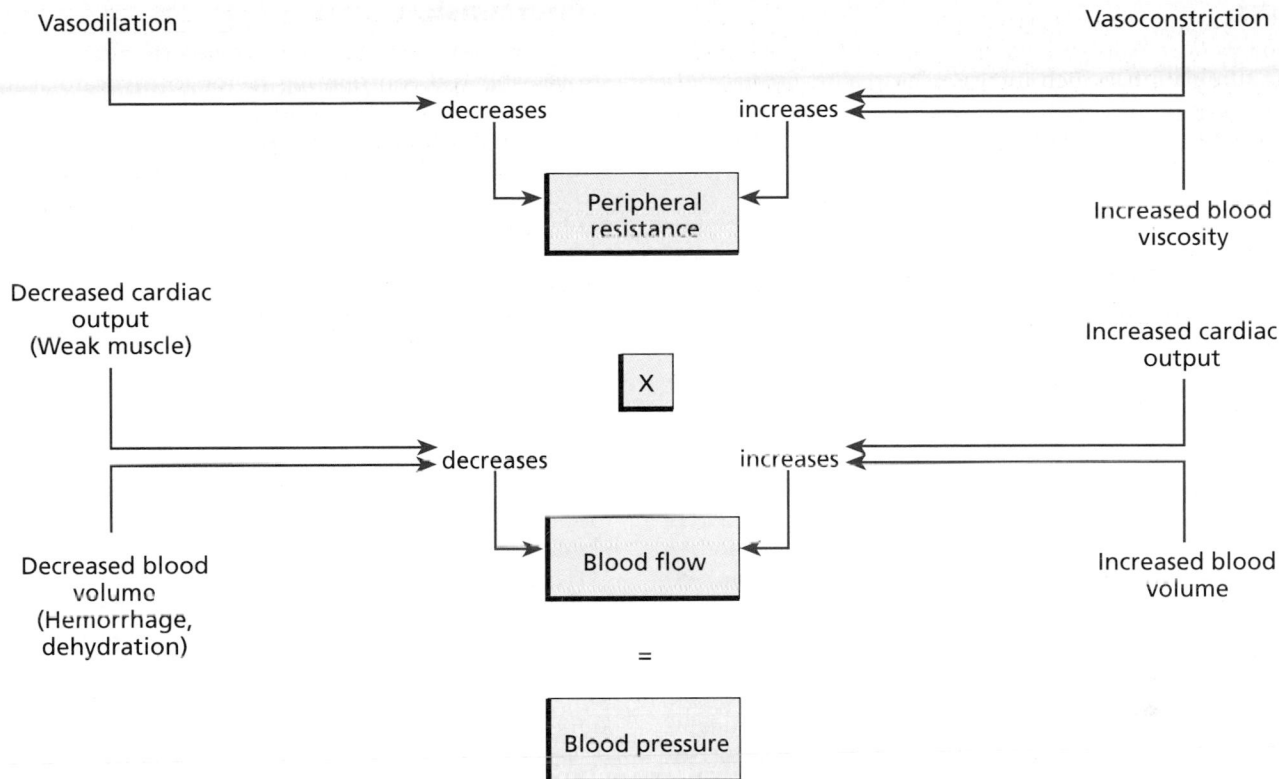

Fig. 32-16 Hemodynamic factors that affect blood pressure.

Each hemodynamic factor significantly affects the others. For example, as arterial elasticity declines peripheral vascular resistance increases. The complex control of the cardiovascular system normally prevents any single factor from permanently changing the blood pressure. For example, if the blood volume falls, the body compensates with an increased vascular resistance. Fig. 32-16 illustrates how hemodynamic variables can affect blood pressure.

Factors Influencing Blood Pressure

Blood pressure is not constant but is continually influenced by many factors during the day. One blood pressure measurement cannot adequately reflect a client's blood pressure. Even under the best conditions, blood pressure changes from heart beat to heart beat. Blood pressure trends, not individual measurements, guide nursing interventions. Understanding these factors ensures a more accurate interpretation of blood pressure readings.

AGE

Normal blood pressure levels vary throughout life (see Table 32-7). They increase during childhood. The level of a child's or adolescent's blood pressure is assessed with respect to body size and age (Task Force on Blood Pressure Control in Children, 1987). An infant's blood pressure ranges from 65-115/42-80. The normal blood pressure for a 7-year-old is 87-117/48-64. Larger children (heavier and/or taller) have higher blood pressures than smaller children of the same age.

During adolescence, blood pressure continues to vary according to body size. However, the normal range for 10- to 19-year-olds at the 90th percentile is 124-136/77-84 for boys and 124-127/63-74 for girls.

An adult's blood pressure tends to increase with advancing age. The standard norm for a healthy, middle-age adult is 120/80. However, the National High Blood Pressure Education Program (1993) lists <130/<85 as the accepted norm (see Table 32-9). Older adults have a rise in systolic pressure related to a decreased vessel elasticity. The older adult's blood pressure normally is 140/90.

Table 32-7	Average Normal Blood Pressure
AGE	**BLOOD PRESSURE (MM HG)**
Newborn (3000 g [6.6 lb])	40 (mean)
1 month	85/54
1 year	95/65
6 years	105/65
10-13 years	110/65
14-17 years	120/75
Middle adult	120/80
Older adult	140/90

From National High Blood Pressure Education Program; National Heart, Lung, and Blood Institute; National Institutes of Health: *The fifth report of the Joint National Committee on Detection, Evaluation, and Treatment of High Blood Pressure.* NIH Pub No 93-1088, Bethesda, Md, NIH, January 1993.

STRESS

Anxiety, fear, pain, and emotional stress result in sympathetic stimulation, which increases heart rate, cardiac output, and peripheral vascular resistance. The effects of sympathetic stimulation increase blood pressure.

RACE

The rate of **hypertension** (high blood pressure) is higher in urban African Americans than in European Americans. Hypertension-related deaths are also higher among African Americans. The tendency for this population to have hypertension is believed to be genetically and environmentally related.

MEDICATIONS

Some medications can directly or indirectly affect blood pressure. During blood pressure assessment, the nurse asks whether the client is receiving antihypertensive medications, which lower blood pressure (Table 32-8). Another class of medications affecting blood pressure is narcotic analgesics, which can lower blood pressure.

DIURNAL VARIATION

Blood pressure levels vary over the course of a day. Blood pressure is typically lowest in the early morning, gradually rises during the morning and afternoon, and peaks in late afternoon or evening. No two persons have the same pattern or degree of variation. Students may find it interesting to have their blood pressure checked by a friend at intervals during 24 hours.

GENDER

There is no clinically significant difference in blood pressure levels between boys and girls. After puberty, males tend to have higher blood pressure readings. After menopause, women tend to have higher levels of blood pressure than men of similar age.

Hypertension

Hypertension is a major factor underlying deaths from strokes and is a contributing factor to myocardial infarctions (heart attacks). The condition is the most common alteration in blood pressure. Hypertension is an often asymptomatic disorder characterized by persistently elevated blood pressure. The diagnosis of hypertension in adults is made when an average of two or more diastolic readings on at least two subsequent visits is 90 mm Hg or higher or when the average of multiple systolic blood pressures on two or more subsequent visits is consistently higher than 140 mm Hg. Categories of hypertension have been developed and determine medical intervention (Table 32-9).

One elevated blood pressure measurement does not qualify as a diagnosis of hypertension. However, if the nurse assesses a high reading during the first blood pressure measurement (e.g., 150/90 mm Hg), the client should be encouraged to return for another checkup within 2 months (Table 32-10).

Hypertension is associated with the thickening and loss of elasticity in the arterial walls. Peripheral vascular resistance increases within thick and inelastic vessels. The heart must continually pump against greater resistance. As a result, blood flow to vital organs such as the heart, brain, and kidney decreases.

Persons with a family history of hypertension are at significant risk. Obesity, cigarette smoking, heavy alcohol consumption, high blood cholesterol levels, and continued exposure to stress are also linked to hypertension. The incidence of hypertension is greater in older persons and in blacks. When clients are diagnosed with hypertension, the nurse helps to educate them about blood pressure values, long-term follow-up care and therapy, the usual lack of symptoms (the fact that it may not be "felt"), therapy's ability to control but not cure hypertension, and a consistently followed treatment plan that can ensure a relatively normal lifestyle (Joint National Committee on Detection, Evaluation, and Treatment of High Blood Pressure, 1993).

Table 32-8	Antihypertension Medications	
MEDICATION TYPE	**NAMES**	**ACTION**
Diuretics	Furosemide (Lasix), spironolactone (Aldactone), metolazone, polythiazide, benzthiazide	Lower blood pressure by reducing reabsorption of sodium and water by the kidneys, thus lowering circulating fluid volume.
Beta-adrenergic blockers	Atenolol (Tenormin), nadolol (Corgard), timolol maleate (Blocadren), propranalol (Inderal)	Combine with beta-adrenergic receptors in the heart, arteries, and arterioles to block response to sympathetic nerve impulses. Reduce heart rate and thus cardiac output.
Vasodilators	Hydralazine hydrocholoride (Apresoline), minoxidil (Loniten)	Act on arteriolar smooth muscle to cause relaxation and reduce peripheral vascular resistance.
Calcium channel blockers	Verapamil hydrochloride (Calan), nifedipine (Procardia)	Reduce peripheral vascular resistance by systemic vasodilation.
Angiotensin converting enzyme (ACE) inhibitors	Captopril (Capoten), enalapril (Vasotec), lisinopril (Prinivil)	Lower blood pressure by blocking the conversion of angiotensin I to angiotensin II, preventing vasoconstriction. Reduce aldosterone production and fluid retention, lowering circulating fluid volume.

Table 32-9	Classification of Blood Pressure for Adults Age 18 Years and Older*	
CATEGORY	SYSTOLIC (MM HG)	DIASTOLIC (MM HG)
Normal†	<130	<85
High normal	130-139	85-89
Hypertension‡		
STAGE 1 (Mild)	140-159	90-99
STAGE 2 (Moderate)	160-179	100-109
STAGE 3 (Severe)	180-209	110-119
STAGE 4 (Very Severe)	≥210	≥120

Modified from National High Blood Pressure Education Program; National Heart, Lung and Blood Institute; National Institutes of Health: *The fifth report of the Joint National Committee on Detection, Evaluation and Treatment of High Blood Pressure.* NIH Pub No 93-1088, Bethesda, Md., NIH, January 1993.

*Not taking antihypertensive drugs and not acutely ill. When systolic and diastolic pressures fall into different categories, the higher category should be selected to classify the individual's blood pressure status. For instance, 160/92 mm Hg should be classified as Stage 2, and 180/120 mm Hg should be classified as Stage 4. Isolated systolic hypertension (ISH) is defined as SBE ≥ 140 mm Hg and DBP < 90 mm Hg and staged appropriately (e.g., 170/85 mm Hg is defined as Stage 2 ISH).

†Optimal blood pressure with respect to cardiovascular risk is SBP < 120 mm Hg and DBP < 80 mm Hg. However, unusually low readings should be evaluated for clinical significance.

‡Based on the average of two or more readings taken at each of two or more visits following an initial screening.

Note: In addition to classifying stages of hypertension based on average blood pressure levels, the clinician should specify presence or absence of target-organ disease and additional risk factors. For example, a patient with diabetes and a blood pressure of 142/94 mm Hg plus left ventricular hypertrophy should be classified as "Stage 1 hypertension with target-organ disease (left ventricular hypertrophy) and with another major risk factor (diabetes)." The specificity is important for risk classification and management.

Hypotension

Hypotension is generally considered present when the systolic blood pressure falls to 90 mm Hg or below. Although some adults have a low blood pressure normally, for the majority of people, low blood pressure is an abnormal finding associated with illness.

Hypotension occurs because of the dilation of the arteries in the vascular bed, the loss of a substantial amount of blood volume (e.g., hemorrhage), or the failure of the heart muscle to pump adequately (e.g., myocardial infarction). Hypotension associated with pallor, skin mottling, clamminess, confusion, increased heart rate, or decreased urine output is life-threatening and should be reported to a physician immediately.

Assessment of Blood Pressure

Arterial blood pressure may be measured either directly (invasively) or indirectly (noninvasively). The direct method requires the insertion of a thin catheter into an artery. Tubing connects the catheter with electronic monitoring equipment. The monitor displays a constant arterial pressure waveform and reading. Because of the risk of sudden blood loss from an artery, invasive blood pressure monitoring is used only in intensive care settings. The more common noninvasive method requires use of the sphygmomanometer and stethoscope. The nurse measures blood

Table 32-10	Recommendations for Follow-up Based on Initial Set of Blood Pressure Measurements for Adults Age 18 and Older	
INITIAL SCREENING BLOOD PRESSURE (MM HG)*		
SYSTOLIC	DIASTOLIC	FOLLOW-UP RECOMMENDED†
<130	<85	Recheck in 2 years
130-139	85-89	Recheck in 1 year‡
140-159	90-99	Confirm within 2 months
160-179	100-109	Evaluate or refer to source of care within 1 month
180-209	110-119	Evaluate or refer to source of care within 1 week
≥210	≥120	Evaluate or refer to source of care immediately

*If the systolic and diastolic categories are different, follow recommendations for the shorter time follow-up (e.g., 160/85 mm Hg should be evaluated or referred to source of care within 1 month)

†The scheduling of follow-up should be modified by reliable information about past blood pressure measurements, other cardiovascular risk factors, or target-organ disease.

‡Consider providing advice about life-style modifications. From National High Blood Pressure Education Program; National Heart, Lung and Blood Institute; National Institutes of Health: *The fifth report of the Joint National Committee on Detection, Evaluation, and Treatment of High Blood Pressure.* NIH Pub No 93-1088, Bethesda, Md., NIH, January 1993.

pressure indirectly by auscultation or palpation. Auscultation is the most widely used technique (Procedure 32-5).

BLOOD PRESSURE EQUIPMENT

Before assessing blood pressure the nurse must be comfortable using a sphygmomanometer and stethoscope. A **sphygmomanometer** comprises a pressure manometer, an occlusive cuff that encloses an inflatable rubber bladder, and a pressure bulb with a release valve to inflate the cuff. The two types of sphygmomanometers are the aneroid and the mercury (Fig. 32-17). The aneroid manometer has a glass-enclosed circular gauge containing a needle that registers millimeter calibrations. A metal bellows within the gauge expands and collapses in response to pressure variations in the inflated cuff.

Aneroid manometers have the advantages of being lightweight, portable, and compact. Because metal parts in the aneroid model are subject to temperature expansion or contraction, the aneroid instrument is less reliable than the mercury type. Before using the aneroid model, the nurse must be sure that the needle points to zero and that the manometer is correctly calibrated. Aneroid sphygmomanometers require biomedical calibration at routine intervals to verify their accuracy.

Mercury manometers are more accurate than aneroid manometers. Repeated calibrations are not necessary. The mercury manometer is an upright tube containing mercury. Pressure created by the inflation of the compression cuff moves the column of mercury upward against the force of gravity. Millimeter calibrations mark the height of the mer-

Assessing Blood Pressure by Auscultation

STEPS	RATIONALE
1. Assess for factors that influence blood pressure.	Allows nurse to accurately assess blood pressure and the significance of pressure changes.
2. Assess best site for obtaining blood pressure measurement. Avoid applying cuff to arm when intravenous catheter is in antecubital fossa and intravenous fluids are infusing; when client has arteriovenous shunt (a surgically created vessel for hemodialysis); when breast or axillary surgery has been performed on that side; when arm or hand has been traumatized or diseased; when client has lower arm cast or bulky bandage.	Inappropriate site selection may result in poor amplification of sounds, causing inaccurate readings. Application of pressure from inflated bladder can temporarily impair and compromise blood flow in extremity that already has impaired circulation.
3. Prepare equipment and supplies and make sure they are in working order:	
a. Sphygmomanometer: control valve should be clear and freely adjustable; when closed, valve should hold mercury constant; when released, valve allows controlled fall in mercury level; air vent at top of mercury manometer should be patent; rubber tubing connecting bladder to manometer should be at least 80 cm (32 in) long and with airtight connections.	Used to measure arterial blood pressure indirectly. Accurate measurements depend on functional equipment.
b. Bladder and cuff: bladder should completely encircle arm without overlapping; cuff should be long enough to encircle arm several times.	Secure cuff and proper-sized bladder are needed to exert equal pressure around artery being auscultated. Bladder too narrow causes false high reading.
c. Stethoscope	Amplifies sound vibration produced by arterial pressure waves.
d. Pen, vital sign flow sheet, or record form	Provide for timely documentation of findings.
4. Encourage client to avoid caffeine and smoking for 30 minutes before assessment (Joint National Committee on Detection, Evaluation, and Treatment of High Blood Pressure, 1993).	Can cause false elevations in blood pressure.
5. Have client assume sitting or lying position. Be sure room is warm and quiet.	Maintains comfort.
6. Explain procedure to client and have client rest at least 5 minutes before measurement.	Reduces anxiety that can falsely elevate readings. Blood pressure readings taken at different times can be objectively compared when assessed with client at rest.
7. Wash hands.	Reduces transmission of microorganisms.
8. With client sitting or lying, position client's bare upper arm (support if needed) at heart level with palm turned up (see the illustration on p. 631).	If arm is unsupported, client may perform isometric exercise that can increase diastolic pressure 10%. Placement of arm above heart causes false low reading.
9. Expose upper arm fully by removing any constricting clothing.	Ensures proper cuff application.
10. Palpate brachial artery (see the illustration on p. 631, top). Position cuff 2.5 cm (1 in) above site of brachial pulsation (antecubital space). Center bladder of cuff above artery (see the illustration on p. 631, bottom).	Inflating bladder directly over brachial artery ensures proper pressure is applied during inflation.
11. With cuff fully deflated, wrap cuff evenly and snugly around upper arm (see the illustration on p. 631).	Loose-fitting cuff causes false high readings.
12. Be sure manometer is positioned vertically at eye level. Observer should be no further than 1 m (approximately 1 yd) away.	Ensures accurate reading of mercury level.
13. Palpate brachial or radial artery with fingertips of one hand while inflating cuff rapidly to pressure 30 mm Hg above point at which pulse disappears. Slowly deflate cuff and note point when pulse reappears.	Identifies approximate systolic pressure and determines maximal inflation point for accurate reading. Prevents ausculatory gap.
14. Deflate cuff fully and wait 30 seconds.	Prevents venous congestion and false high readings.
15. Place stethoscope earpieces in ears and be sure sounds are clear, not muffled.	Each earpiece should follow angle of ear canal to facilitate hearing.

Assessing Blood Pressure by Auscultation—cont'd

STEPS	RATIONALE

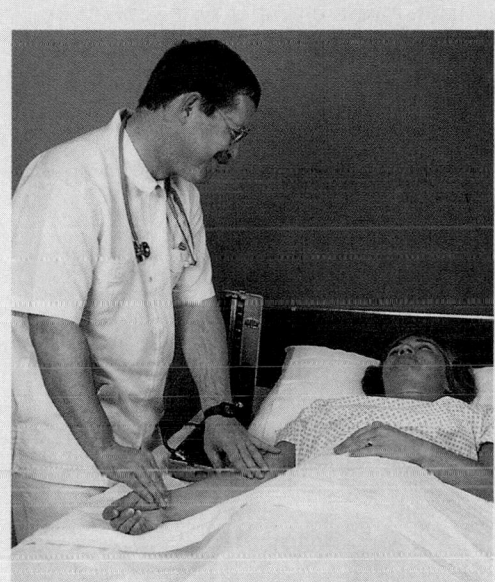

Step 8

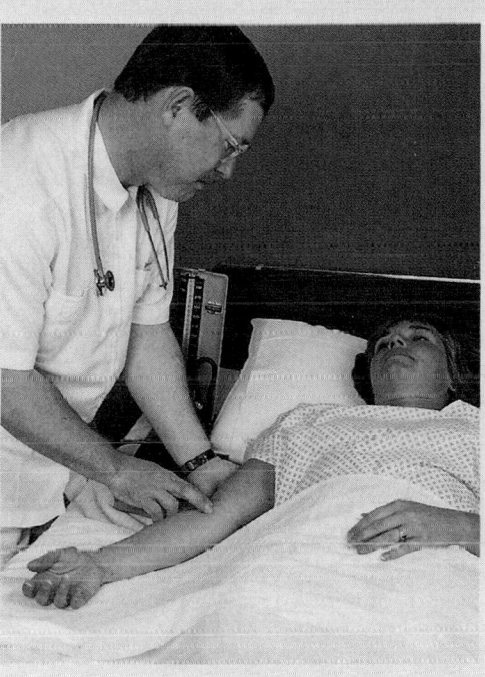

Step 10

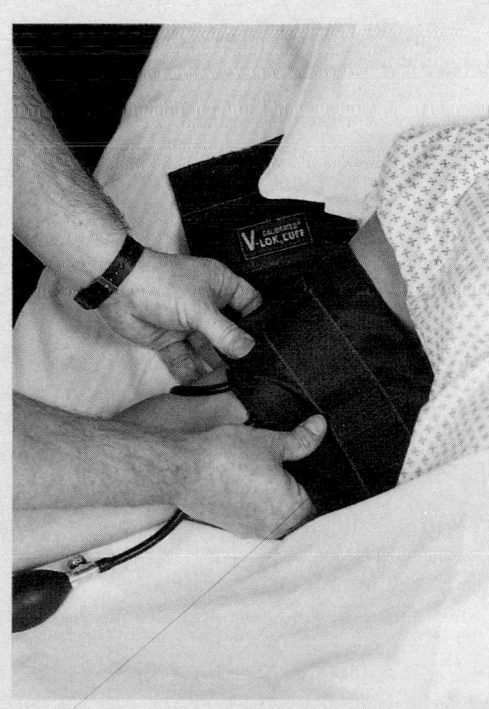

Step 10

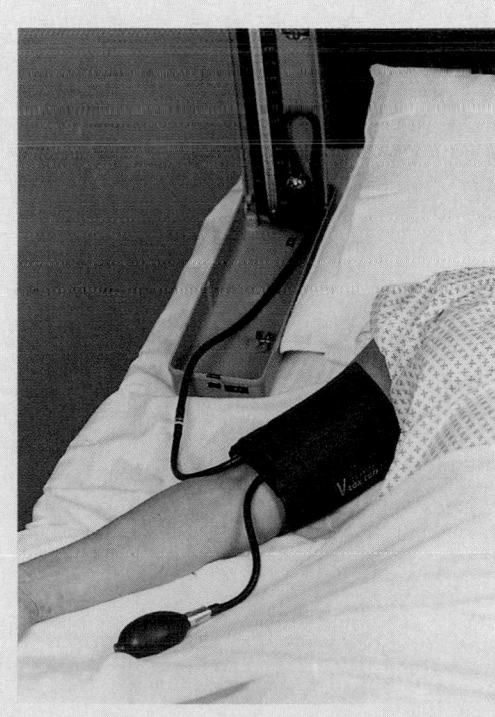

Step 11

Assessing Blood Pressure by Auscultation—cont'd

STEPS	RATIONALE

16. Relocate brachial artery and place bell or diaphragm chestpiece over it. Do not allow chestpiece to touch cuff or client's clothing (see the illustration below).

Ensures optimal sound reception. Stethoscope improperly positioned causes muffled sounds that often result in false low systolic and false high diastolic readings.

17. Close valve of pressure bulb clockwise until tight.

Prevents air leak during inflation.

18. Inflate cuff to 30 mm Hg above palpated systolic pressure (see the illustration below).

Ensures accurate measurement of systolic pressure.

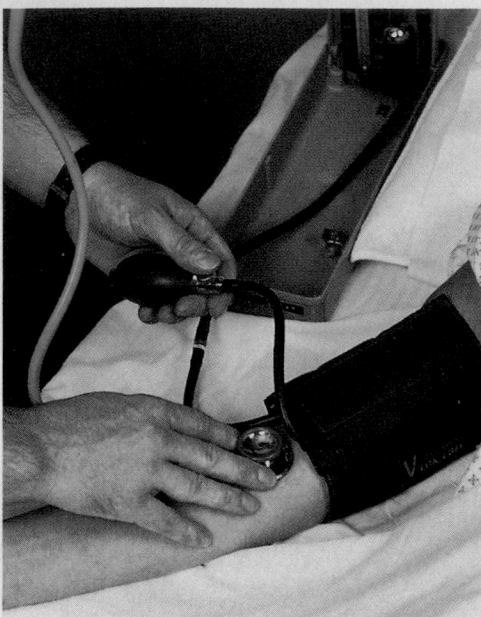

Step 16

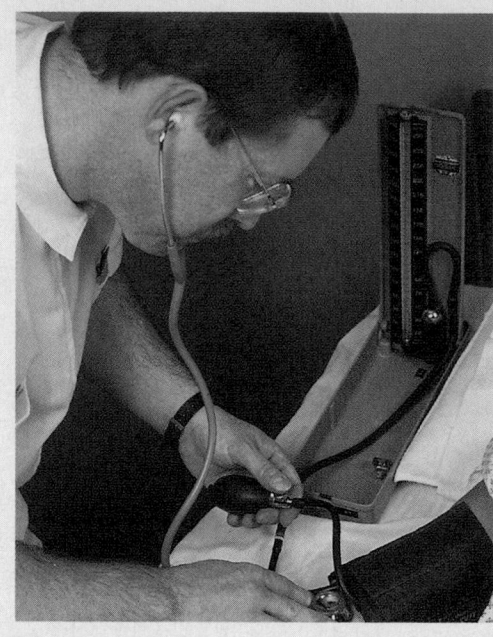

Step 18

19. Slowly release valve and allow mercury to fall at rate of 2 to 3 mm Hg per sec.

Too rapid or slow a decline in mercury level can cause inaccurate readings.

20. Note point on manometer when first clear sound is heard.

First Korotkoff sound indicates systolic pressure.

21. Continue to deflate cuff, noting point at which muffled or dampened sound appears.

Fourth Korotkoff sound involves distinct muffling of sounds and is recommended by the American Heart Association (AHA) as indication of diastolic pressure in children.

22. Continue cuff deflation, noting point on manometer to nearest 2 mm Hg at which sound disappears.

AHA (1987) recommends recording fifth Korotokoff sound as diastolic pressure in adults.

23. Deflate cuff rapidly and completely. Remove cuff from arm unless planning to repeat.

Continuous cuff inflation causes arterial occlusion, resulting in numbness and tingling of arm.

24. If this is first assessment of client, repeat procedure on other arm.

Comparison of pressure in both arms serves to detect any circulatory problems. Normal systolic difference of 5 to 10 mm Hg exists between arms.

25. Assist client in returning to comfortable position and cover upper arm.

Restores comfort.

26. Inform client of reading.

Promotes participation in care and understanding of health status.

27. Wash hands.

Prevents transmission of microorganisms.

28. Compare reading with previous baseline and/or normal average pressure for client's age.

Evaluates for change in condition and alterations.

29. Inform client of value and need for periodic reassessment.

Makes client accountable for follow-up assessment.

30. Record blood pressure on nurses' notes or vital sign flow sheet and report abnormal findings to nurse in charge or physician.

Vital sign measurements should be recorded promptly on flow sheet to avoid omissions from record. Abnormalities may require immediate therapy.

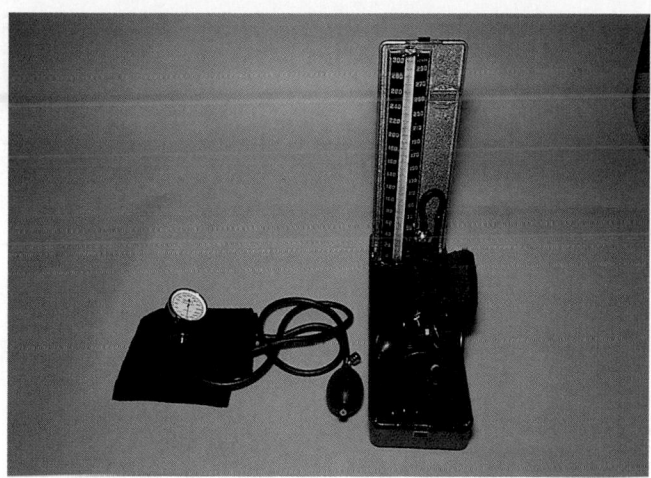

Fig. 32-17 Sphygmomanometers: *Right*, mercury manometer. *Left*, aneroid manometer.

cury column. To ensure accurate readings, the mercury column should fall freely as pressure is released and should always be at zero when the cuff is deflated. Mercury manometers may be wall mounted or portable. Accurate readings are obtained by looking at the meniscus of the mercury at eye level. This is the point where the crescent-shaped top of the mercury column aligns with the manometer scale. Looking up or down at the mercury results in distorted readings. The disadvantages of the mercury manometer are the potential for breakage and the release of mercury. Mercury is a health hazard if not properly contained. Steps to take in the event of a mercury spill are presented in the box on p. 609.

Cloth or disposable vinyl compression cuffs used with the sphygmomanometer come in several sizes. The size selected is proportional to the circumference of the limb being assessed. Ideally, the width of the cuff should be 40% of the circumference (or 20% wider than the diameter) of the midpoint of the limb on which the cuff is to be used (American Heart Association, 1987). The bladder, enclosed by the cuff, should encircle at least two thirds of the arm of an adult and the entire arm of a child (Joint National Committee on Detection, Evaluation and Treatment of High Blood Pressure, 1993). In children the lower edge of the cuff should be above the antecubital fossa, allowing room for placement of the stethoscope bell or diaphragm. An improperly fitting cuff causes inaccurate blood pressure measurement.

Before using a sphygmomanometer the nurse should inspect the parts of the release valve and the pressure bulb. The valve should be clean and freely movable in either direction. If it sticks or becomes too tightly closed, the deflation of the pressure cuff will be hard to regulate. The pressure bulb is made of tough rubber and should be free of leaks.

AUSCULTATION

The best environment for blood pressure measurement by auscultation is a quiet room at a comfortable temperature. Although the client may lie or stand, sitting is the pre-ferred position. In most cases blood pressure readings obtained with the client in the supine, sitting, and standing positions are similar. In some clients, however, blood pressure changes with position. The nurse may compare sitting and standing blood pressure readings to determine whether a change occurs. **Orthostatic** or **postural hypotension**, the lowering of blood pressure when the client moves from a sitting to a standing position, is frequently accompanied by dizziness, light-headedness, and even syncope (fainting). Orthostatic hypotension may be a symptom of fluid volume deficit or inadequate neurovascular control.

Antihypertensive medications may cause orthostatic blood pressure changes. Blood pressure should always be measured before administering such medications. When recording orthostatic blood pressure measurements, the nurse records the client's position in addition to the blood pressure measurement. For example: 140/80 supine, 132/72 sitting, 108/60 standing. The readings are obtained 1 to 3 minutes after the client changes position.

The client's position during routine blood pressure determination should be the same during each measurement to permit a meaningful comparison of values. Before assessment the nurse should attempt to control factors responsible for artificially high readings, such as pain, anxiety, or exertion. The client's perceptions that the physical or interpersonal environment is more or less stressful will affect the blood pressure measurement (Thomas et al., 1993). Blood pressure measurements taken at the client's place of employment or in a physician's office are higher than those taken at the client's home. Blood pressure is higher when measured by a physician than other health care providers.

During the initial assessment the nurse should obtain and record the blood pressure in both arms. Normally there is a difference of 5 to 10 mm Hg between the arms. In subsequent assessments the blood pressure should be measured in the arm with the higher pressure. Pressure differences greater than 10 mm Hg indicate vascular problems in the arm with the lower pressure.

The nurse asks the client to state his normal blood pressure. If the client does not know, the nurse informs him after measuring and recording the blood pressure. This is a good opportunity to educate a client about normal blood pressure, the risk factors for developing hypertension, and dangers of hypertension.

Indirect measurement of arterial blood pressure works on a basic principle of pressure. Blood flows freely through an artery until an inflated cuff applies pressure to tissues and causes the artery to collapse. After the cuff pressure is released, the point at which blood flow returns and sound appears through auscultation is the systolic pressure.

Korotkoff, a Russian surgeon, first described the sounds heard over an artery during cuff deflation in 1905. The first Korotkoff sound is a clear rhythmical tapping corresponding to the pulse rate that gradually increases in intensity. *Onset of the sound corresponds to the systolic pressure.* With the second Korotkoff sound a murmur or swishing sound occurs as the cuff continues to deflate. As the artery distends, there is a turbulence in blood flow. The third Korotkoff sound is a crisper and more intense tapping. The fourth Korotkoff sounds become muffled and low pitched as the cuff is further deflated. Cuff pressure falls below the pressure within the vessel walls; *this sound is the diastolic pressure*

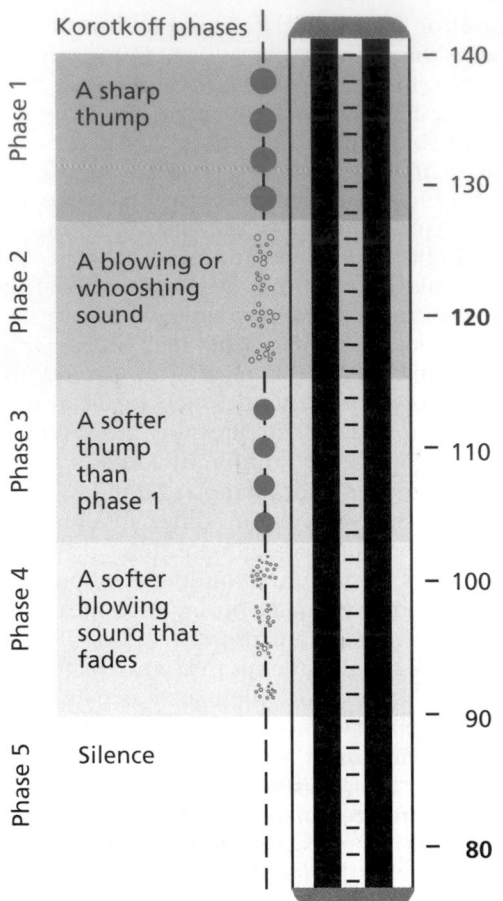

Korotkoff phases

Phase 1 — A sharp thump

Phase 2 — A blowing or whooshing sound

Phase 3 — A softer thump than phase 1

Phase 4 — A softer blowing sound that fades

Phase 5 — Silence

Fig. 32-18 The sounds auscultated during blood pressure measurement can be differentiated into five Korotkoff phases. In this example blood pressure is 140/90.

Table 32-11	Common Mistakes in Blood Pressure Measurement
ERROR	**EFFECT**
Bladder or cuff too wide	False low reading
Bladder or cuff too narrow	False high reading
Cuff wrapped too loosely	False high reading
Deflating cuff too slowly	False high diastolic reading
Deflating cuff too quickly	False low systolic and false high diastolic reading
Stethoscope that fits poorly or impairment of the examiner's hearing, causing sounds to be muffled	False low systolic and false high diastolic reading
Inaccurate inflation level	False low systolic reading
Multiple examiners using different Korotkoff sounds for diastolic readings	Inaccurate interpretation of systolic and diastolic readings

in infants and children. The fifth Korotkoff sound is an absence of sound. *In adolescents and adults, this sound corresponds with the diastolic pressure* (Fig. 32-18).

The American Heart Association (1987) recommends recording two numbers for a blood pressure measurement: the point on the manometer when the first sound is heard for systolic and the point on the manometer when the fifth sound is heard for diastolic. Some institutions recommend recording the point when the fourth sound is heard as well, especially for clients with hypertension. The numbers are divided by slashed lines (e.g., 120/80 or 120/100/80), and the arm used to measure the blood pressure is noted (e.g., RA 130/70). Many practitioners also record the client's position when the pressure is assessed. This is particularly useful when recording orthostatic hypotension.

Potential Errors in Auscultation. Several causes exist for error in blood pressure readings if auscultation is not performed correctly. Table 32-11 summarizes common mistakes in measurement. When a nurse is unsure of a reading, a colleague should reassess the blood pressure.

ULTRASONIC STETHOSCOPE

If a nurse is unable to auscultate sounds because of a weakened arterial pulse, an ultrasonic stethoscope can be used (see Chapter 33). This stethoscope allows the nurse to hear low-frequency systolic sounds and is commonly used when measuring the blood pressure of infants, children, and low blood pressure in adults.

PALPATION

The indirect palpation technique is useful for clients whose arterial pulsations are too weak to create Korotkoff sounds. Severe blood loss and decreased heart contractility are examples of conditions that result in blood pressures too low to auscultate accurately. Only the systolic blood pressure can be assessed by palpation (see the box on p. 635). The diastolic pressure is difficult to determine by palpation. A subtle change in sensation, usually in the form of a thin, snapping vibration, marks the diastolic level. When the palpation technique is used, the systolic value and the manner in which it was measured are recorded (e.g., RA 90/-, palpated).

The palpation technique is used with auscultation in some instances. In some hypertensive clients, the sounds usually heard over the brachial artery when the cuff pressure is high disappear as pressure is reduced and then reappear at a lower level. This temporary disappearance of sound is the **auscultatory gap.** It typically occurs between the first and second Korotkoff sounds. The gap in sound may cover a range of 40 mm Hg and thus may cause an underestimation of systolic pressure or overestimation of diastolic pressure. The examiner must be certain to inflate the cuff high enough to hear the true systolic pressure before the auscultatory gap. Palpation of the radial artery helps to determine how high to inflate the cuff. The examiner inflates the cuff 30 mm Hg above the pressure at which the radial pulse was palpated. The range of pressures in which the auscultatory gap occurs is recorded (e.g., "BP RA 180/94 with an auscultatory gap from 180 to 160).

ASSESSMENT OF LOWER EXTREMITIES

Dressings, casts, intravenous catheters, arteriovenous fistulas or shunts, and axillary lymph node dissection can make the upper extremities inaccessible. Blood pressure must then be measured in the lower extremities. Comparing upper extremity blood pressure with that in the legs is also necessary for clients with certain blood pressure abnormalities. The popliteal artery, palpable behind the knee in the popliteal space, is the site for auscultation. The cuff is positioned with the bladder over the posterior aspect of the midthigh. The cuff must be wide and long enough to allow for the larger girth of the thigh. Placing the client in a prone position is best. If such a position is impossible, the client should be asked to flex the knee slightly for easier access to the artery. The procedure is identical to brachial artery auscultation. Systolic pressure in the legs is usually higher by 10 to 40 mm Hg than in the brachial artery, but the diastolic pressure is the same.

AUTOMATIC BLOOD PRESSURE DEVICES

Many electronic devices can determine blood pressure automatically (Fig. 32-19). Once the blood pressure cuff is applied, the nurse can program the device to obtain and record blood pressure readings at preset intervals. Alarm limits can be programmed to alert the nurse if the blood pressure measurement is outside desired parameters. The system includes either a microphone or a pressure sensor built into the inflatable cuff. The microphone or acoustic system hears Korotkoff sounds and registers diastolic and systolic readings. The pressure sensor or ultrasonic system responds to the pressure waves generated by the movement of blood through the artery. The advantages of automatic devices are the ease of use and efficiency when repeated or when frequent measurements are indicated. The ability to use a stethoscope is not required. However, automatic devices are more sensitive to outside interference and are susceptible to error. The microphone or pressure sensor must be positioned directly over the artery for proper function. Client movements or vibration or outside noise can interfere with the microphone or sensor signal. Most automatic blood pressure devices are unable to process sounds or vibrations of low blood pressure. The range of device sophistication also can make blood pressure measurement comparisons difficult. The use of automatic blood pressure devices permits assessment of blood pressure during interpersonal interactions. However, the nurse should avoid speaking to the client for at least a minute before initiating a blood pressure recording. Talking to a client when the blood pressure is being assessed increases readings 10% to 40% (Thomas et al., 1993).

SELF-MEASUREMENT OF BLOOD PRESSURE

More people measure their own blood pressures because of improved technology in home monitoring devices and a

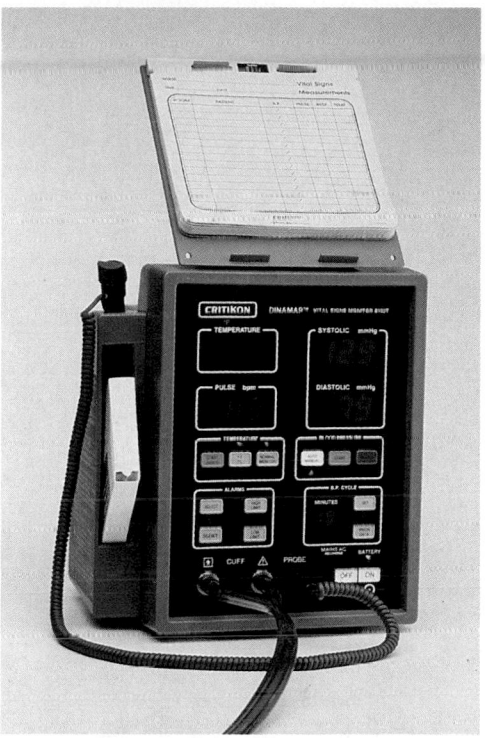

Fig. 32-19 The Dinamapp® automatic blood pressure monitor reports systolic, diastolic, and mean blood pressure. (Dinamapp Vital Signs Monitor® is a trademark of Critikon, Inc. Photo Courtesy Critikon, Inc., Tampa, FL.)

greater interest in health promotion. Two of the more common devices used by the general public include portable home sphygmomanometers and stationary automatic blood pressure machines.

The portable home devices include the mercury and aneroid sphygmomanometers and electronic digital readout devices that do not require use of a stethoscope. The electronic devices inflate and deflate cuffs with the push of a button. The electronic devices may be easier to manipulate but can easily become inaccurate and require recalibration more than once a year. Because of their sensitivity, improper cuff placement or movement of the arm can cause electronic devices to give incorrect readings.

Stationary automatic blood pressure devices can be found in public places such as grocery stores, fitness clubs, banks, airports, or work sites. Users simply rest their arms within the machine's inflatable cuff, which contains a pressure sensor. The cuff fits over clothing. A visual display tells users their blood pressure within 60 to 90 seconds. The reliability of the stationary machines is limited. Blood pressure values may vary by 5 to 10 mm Hg or more (for both systolic and diastolic values) compared with pressures taken with a manual sphygmomanometer.

The National High Blood Pressure Education Program Coordinating Committee (Hunt et al., 1985) has identified the following benefits of blood pressure self-measurement:

1. Self-administered blood pressure measurement can detect elevated blood pressure in persons previously unaware of a problem.
2. When persons have borderline hypertension, self-

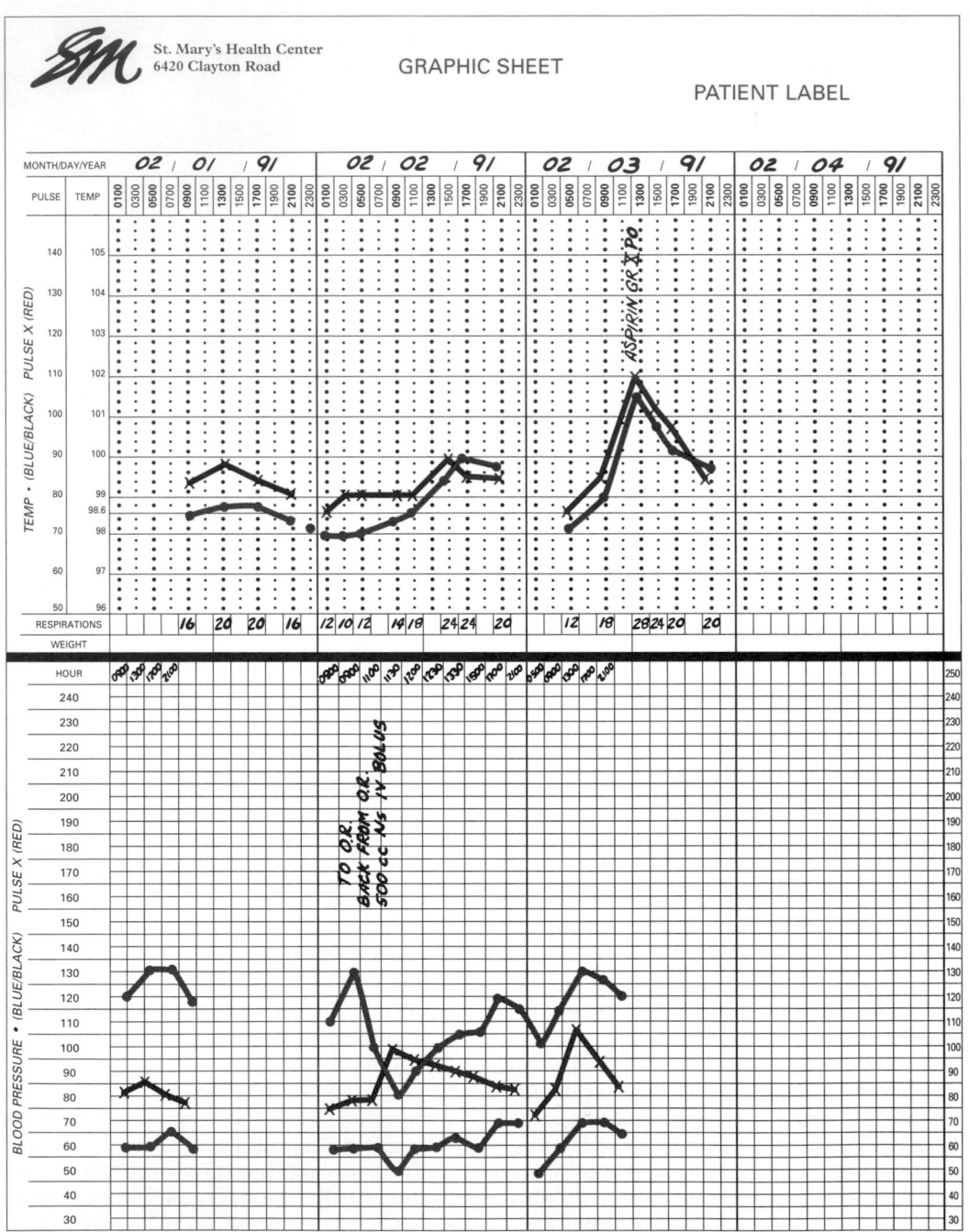

Fig. 32-20 Vital signs graphic flow sheet. *(Courtesy St Mary's Health Center, St Louis.)*

measurement can provide information about the pattern of blood pressure values.

3. Clients with hypertension can benefit from participating actively in their treatment through self-monitoring.

4. For some clients undergoing treatment for hypertension, visual evidence of blood pressure control may help compliance with treatment.

The Coordinating Committee (Hunt et al., 1985) also cites the following concerns about self-measurement of blood pressure:

1. There is the possibility that persons will be inadequately trained in using the devices. Printed instructions accompanying the equipment may be incomplete or written at an inappropriate reading level.

2. One elevated reading is not enough to diagnose hypertension and only indicates that further evaluation is needed by health care personnel. Thus a client may be needlessly alarmed.

3. Clients with hypertension may become overly conscious of their blood pressures and make inappropriate self-adjustment of medications.

Consumers can learn to use self-measurement devices if they have the information needed to perform the procedure correctly and if they know when to seek medical attention. The nurse can advise clients of possible inaccuracies in the blood pressure devices, help clients understand the meaning and implications of readings, and teach them proper measurement techniques.

Examples of NANDA Nursing Diagnoses Using Blood Pressure Data as Defining Characteristics

Activity intolerance	Fluid volume deficit
Altered tissue perfusion	At risk for injury
Anxiety	Pain
Decreased cardiac output	

NURSING PROCESS AND BLOOD PRESSURE DETERMINATION

The assessment of blood pressure along with pulse assessment is used to evaluate the general state of cardiovascular health and responses to other system imbalances. Hypotension, hypertension, and narrow or wide pulse pressures are defining characteristics of certain nursing diagnoses and are considered along with other assessment data. For example, the defining characteristics of hypotension, dizziness, pulse deficit, and dysrhythmia lead to a diagnosis of decreased cardiac output (see the nursing diagnoses box below). The nursing care plan includes interventions based on the nursing diagnosis identified and the related factor (see Chapter 44). The nurse evaluates client outcomes by assessing the blood pressure following each intervention.

RECORDING VITAL SIGNS

Special graphic flowsheets exist for recording vital signs (Fig. 32-20). The nurse identifies the institution's procedure for documenting on the graphic or vital sign flowsheet. In addition to the actual vital sign values, the nurse records in the nurses' notes any accompanying or precipitating symptoms such as chest pain and dizziness with abnormal blood pressure, shortness of breath with abnormal respirations, cyanosis with hypoxemia, or flushing and diaphoresis with elevated temperature. The nurse documents any interventions initiated as a result of vital sign measurement such as administration of oxygen therapy or an antihypertensive medication.

Client's being managed on critical paths or CareMaps® may have vital sign values listed as outcomes (see Chapter 11). If a vital sign value is above or below the anticipated outcomes, a variance note is written to explain the nature of the variance and the nurse's course of action. For example, a CareMap® for a client who has undergone a thoracotomy may have an outcome during the postoperative period of "afebrile." If the client has a fever, the nurse's variance note may address possible sources of fever (e.g., retained pulmonary secretions) and nursing interventions (e.g., increased suctioning, postural drainage, or hydration).

■ KEY CONCEPTS ■

▶ Vital signs include the physiological measurement of temperature, pulse, blood pressure, respirations, and oxygen saturation.

▶ Vital signs are measured as part of a complete physical examination or in a review of a client's condition.

▶ The nurse assesses vital sign changes with other physical assessment findings using clinical judgment to determine measurement frequency.

▶ Knowledge of the factors influencing vital signs assists the nurse in determining and evaluating abnormal values.

▶ Vital signs provide a basis for evaluating response to nursing interventions.

▶ Vital signs are best measured when the client is inactive and the environment is controlled for comfort.

▶ The nurse assists the client in maintaining body temperature by initiating interventions that promote heat loss, production, or conservation.

▶ A fever is one of the body's normal defense mechanisms.

▶ The tympanic route is the most accessible and acceptable site for core temperature measurement.

▶ Rectal temperature measurements should not be performed on newborn infants or adults with rectal alterations.

► To assess cardiac function, pulse rate and rhythm are most easily measured using the radial or apical pulse.

► Respiratory assessment includes determining the effectiveness of ventilation, perfusion, and diffusion.

► Assessment of respirations involves observing ventilatory movements throughout the respiratory cycle.

► Oxygen saturation is influenced by variables affecting ventilation, perfusion, and diffusion.

► Several hemodynamic variables contribute to blood pressure determination.

► Hypertension is diagnosed only after an average of readings made during two or more subsequent visits reveal an elevated blood pressure.

► Errors in blood pressure measurement can be made by selecting and applying the cuff improperly.

► Changes in one vital sign can influence characteristics of the other vital signs.

■ KEY TERMS ■

Afebrile, p. 600

Antipyretics, p. 612

Auscultatory gap, p. 634

Basal metabolic rate (BMR), p. 597

Bradycardia, p. 620

Calorie, p. 598

Cardiac output, p. 614

Conduction, p. 597

Convection, p. 598

Core temperature, p. 596

Diaphoresis, p. 598

Diastolic, p. 625

Diffusion, p. 621

Dysrhythmia, p. 620

Eupnea, p. 622

Evaporation, p. 598

Febrile, p. 600

Fever, p. 599

Frostbite, p. 601

Heat exhaustion, p. 601

Heatstroke, p. 601

Hematocrit, p. 626

Hypertension, p. 628

Hyperthermia, p. 601

Hypotension, p. 629

Hypothalamus, p. 597

Hypothermia, p. 601

Hypoxemia, p. 621

Malignant hyperthermia, p. 601

Orthostatic hypotension, p. 633

Perfusion, p. 621

Postural hypotension, p. 633

Pulse deficit, p. 620

Pulse pressure, p. 625

Pyrogens, p. 600

Radial pulse, p. 614

Radiation, p. 597

Shivering, p. 597

Sphygmomanometer, p. 629

Stroke volume, p. 614

Systolic, p. 625

Tachycardia, p. 620

Thermoregulation, p. 597

Tidal volume, p. 622

Ventilation, p. 621

Vital signs, p. 595

■ CRITICAL THINKING EXERCISES ■

1. A 77-year-old male is being admitted to the medical unit of the acute care hospital with a diagnosis of bilateral pneumonia. He has a medical history of diabetes and peripheral vascular disease. The nursing assistant reports that his oral temperature is 98.6°F using a mercury-in-glass thermometer, respirations of 28, and a pulse rate of 124. However, she states it was difficult to accurately count his pulse. What are your anticipated follow-up activities for this client?

2. A 3-month-old infant is brought into the clinic with otitis media. The father relates that the child has been fussing and crying for the past 4 hours. The child is currently quietly resting in the father's arms. What techniques and in what order would you use to assess the vital signs for this client?

3. A 65-year-old postmenopausal client takes the following medications: furosemide 80 PO bid, lanoxin 0.25 mg PO qd, nifedipine 10 mg PO tid. During a visit to the wellness center she tells you she has been very dizzy lately, especially in the morning when she gets out of bed. How should the client's medication regimen expect to affect vital signs? How would you assess blood pressure? Provide a nursing diagnosis with a care plan for this client.

4. The certified nurse's aid (CNA) reports she just obtained a client's blood pressure at rest of 110/90 in the right arm. You attempt to verify this measurement within 5 minutes with the client still resting and obtain a blood pressure of 120/75 in the right arm. Explain the possible reasons for the differences between the two readings. What action would you take to avoid this problem in the future?

REFERENCES

American Heart Association: *Recommendations for human blood pressure determination by sphygmomanometers,* pub no 701005, Dallas, 1987, The Association.

Bobak J: *Maternity and gynecologic care,* ed 5, St Louis, 1993, Mosby.

Centers for Disease Control: Update: universal precautions for prevention of transmission of human immunodeficiency virus, hepatitis B virus, and other blood borne pathogens in health care settings, *MMWR* 37(24):377, 1988.

Davis C, Lentz MJ: Circadian rhythms; charting oral temperatures to spot abnormalities, *J Gerontol Nurs* 15(4):34, 1989.

Davis K: The accuracy of tympanic temperature measurement in children, *Pediatr Nurs* 19(3):267, 1993.

Eoff M, Joyce B: Temperature measurement in children, *Am J Nurs* 81:1010, 1981.

Erickson RS et al: Accuracy of chemical dot thermometers in critically ill adults and young children, *Nurs Res* 28(1):23, 1996.

Erickson RS, Kirklin SK: Comparison of ear-based, bladder, oral and axillary methods for core temperature measurement, *Crit Care Med* 21(10):1528, 1993.

Garner JS: Hospital infection control practices advisory committee. Guidelines for isolation precautions in hospitals, *Infect Control Hosp Epidemiol* 17:53, 1996.

Guiffre M et al: Rewarming postoperative patient: lights, blankets or forced warm air, *JOPAN* 6(6):387, 1991.

Guyton AC: *Textbook of medical physiology,* ed 8, Philadelphia, 1991, WB Saunders.

Henker R, Coyne C: Comparison of peripheral temperature measurements with core temperature, *AACN Clinical Issues* 6(1):21, 1995.

Holtzclaw B: Effects of extremity wraps to control drug-induced shivering: a pilot study, *Nurs Res* 39:280, 1990.

Holtzclaw B: The febrile response in critical care: state of the science, *Heart Lung* 21(5):482, 1992.

Hunt JC et al: Devices used for the self-measurement of blood pressure: revised statement of the National High Blood Pressure Education Program, *Arch Intern Med* 145:2231, 1985.

Joint National Committee on Detection, Evaluation and Treatment of High Blood Pressure: *The fifth report of the Joint National Committee on Detection, Evaluation and Treatment of High Blood Pressure,* NIH Pub No 93-1088, Bethesda MD, NIH, Jan 1993.

Kresovich-Wendler K, Levitt MA, Yearly L: An evaluation of clinical predictors to determine need for rectal temperature measurement in the emergency department, *Am J Emerg Med* 7(4):391, 1989.

Lenz M: *Circadian phase relationships of sleep-wake cycle and body temperature rhythm in aging,* unpublished doctoral dissertation, Seattle, 1984, University of Washington.

Leung AK, Robson WL: Febrile convulsions: how dangerous are they? *Postgrad Med* 89(5):217, 1991.

Lobban M, Tredre B: Diurnal rhythms of renal excretion and of body temperature in aged subjects, *Proc Phys Soc* 188:48P, 1988.

Material Safety Data Sheet: *Mercury,* Houston, TX, 1989, Curtin Matheson Scientific.

Morgan SP: Comparison of three methods of managing fever in the neurologic patient, *J Neurosci Nurs* 132:19, 1990.

Mountcastle VB: *Medical physiology,* vol 2, ed 14, St Louis, 1980, CV Mosby.

National High Blood Pressure Education Program; National Heart, Lung and Blood Institute; National Institutes of Health: *The fifth report of the Joint National Committee on Detection, Evaluation and Treatment of High Blood Pressure,* NIH Pub No 93-1088, Bethesda, Md, 1993, NIH.

Neff J et al: Effect of respiratory rate, respiratory depth and open versus closed mouth breathing on sublingual temperature, *Res Nurs Health,* 12:195, 1992.

Neff T: Routine oximetry: a fifth vital sign? *Chest* 94:227, 1988.

Norman E, Gadaleta D, Griffing CC: An evaluation of three blood pressure methods in a stabilized acute trauma population, *Nurs Res* 40(2):86, 1991.

Pontious S, Kennedy AG, Shelley S, et al: Accuracy and reliability of temperature measurement by instrument and site, *J Pediatr Nurs* 9(2):114, 1994.

Stephen SB, Sexton PR: Neonatal axillary temperatures: Increases in readings over time, *Neonatal Network* 5:25, 1987.

Task Force on Blood Pressure Control in Children: Report of Second Task Force on Blood Pressure Control in Children—1987, *Pediatrics* 79:1, 1987.

Terndrup TE, Allegra JR, Kealy JA: A comparison of oral, rectal, and tympanic membrane-derived temperature changes after ingestion of liquids and smoking, *Am J Emerg Med* 7:150, 1987.

Thibodeau GA, Patton KT: *Anatomy and physiology,* ed 2, St Louis, 1993, CV Mosby.

Thomas SA, Leihr P, DeKeyser F, et al: Nursing blood pressure research, 1980-1990: A bio-psycho-social perspective, *Image J Nurs Sch* 25(2):157, 1993.

Vogelsang J, Hayes S: Butorphanol tartrate relieves postanesthesia shaking more effectively than meperidine or morphine, *J Post Anesthesia Nurs* 7(2):94, 1992.

Whaley LF, Wong DL: *Nursing care of infants and children,* ed 5, St. Louis, 1995, Mosby.

ADDITIONAL READINGS

Anderson F, Cunningham S, Maloney J: Indirect blood pressure measurement: A need to reassess, *Am J Crit Care* 2(4):272, 1993.

Carrol P: Clinical application of pulse oximetry, *Pediatr Nurs* 19(2):150, 1993.

Eoff M, Joyce B: Temperature measurements in children, *Am J Nurs* 81:1010, 1981.

Erickson R, Yount S: Comparison of tympanic and oral temperatures in surgical patients, *Nurs Res* 40(2):90, 1991.

Fulbrook P: Core temperature measurement in adults: a literature review, *J Adv Nurs* 18:1451, 1995.

Guiffre M et al: The relationship between axillary and core body temperatures, *Appl Nurs Res* 3(2):52, 1990.

Hill M, Grim C: How to take a precise blood pressure, *Am J Nurs* 91(2):38, 1991.

Hollerbach AD, Sneed NV: Accuracy of radial pulse assessment by length of counting interval, *Heart Lung* 19(3):258, 1990.

Holtzclaw B: Monitoring body temperature, *Clin Issues CCN* 4(1):44, 1993.

Hunter L: Measurement of axillary temperatures in neonates, *West J Nurs Res* 13(3):324, 1991.

Longman A et al: Research utilization: an evaluation and critique of research related to oral temperature measurement, *Appl Nurs Res* 3(1):14, 1990.

Root R, Petersdorf RC: Alteration in body temperature. In Wilson JD et al, eds: *Harrison's principles of internal medicine,* ed 12, New York, 1991, McGraw-Hill.

Severinghaus J, Kelleher J: Recent developments in pulse oximetry, *Anesthesiology* 76(6):1018, 1992.

The National High Blood Pressure Education Program Coordination Committee: National high blood pressure education program working group report on ambulatory blood pressure monitoring, *Arch Intern Med* 150:2270, 1990.

Webster H, Chellis M: Physiologic monitoring of infants and children, *Clin Issues CCN* 4(1):180, 1993.

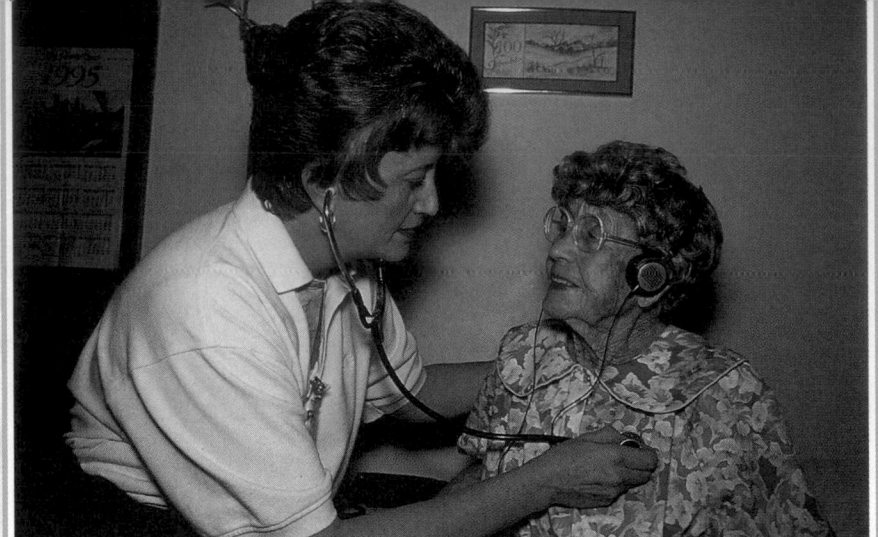

Chapter 33

Physical Examination and Health Assessment

Objectives

Mastery of content in this chapter will enable the student to:

▶ Define the key terms listed.

▶ Discuss the purposes of physical assessment.

▶ Describe the techniques used with each physical assessment skill.

▶ Discuss the importance of understanding cultural diversity as it influences the approach to health assessment.

▶ Describe the proper position for the client during each phase of the examination.

▶ List techniques used to prepare a client physically and psychologically before and during an examination.

▶ Describe interview techniques used to enhance communication during history taking.

▶ Make environmental preparations before an examination.

▶ Identify information to collect from the nursing history before an examination.

▶ Discuss normal physical findings in a young and middle-age adult compared with an older adult.

▶ Discuss ways to incorporate health teaching into the examination.

▶ Use physical assessment skills during routine nursing care.

▶ Conduct physical assessments in an organized and proper fashion.

▶ Describe physical measurements made in the assessment of each body system.

▶ Identify self-screening examinations commonly performed by clients.

▶ Document findings on a physical examination form.

Nurses are most often the first to detect changes in clients' conditions, regardless of the setting. For this reason the ability to critically think and interpret the meaning of client behaviors and presenting physiological changes is very important. The skills of physical assessment and examination provide nurses with powerful tools to detect subtle as well as obvious changes in a client's health. Physical assessment enables the nurse to assess patterns reflecting health problems and to evaluate the client's progress following therapy.

The nurse works in a variety of settings, seeking information about clients' health status. The nurse conducts health assessments at health fairs, at screening clinics, in physician's offices, or in hospitals. Health screenings involve measurement of specific physical functions or diagnostic tests to detect persons with high probabilities of having a characteristic (Larson, 1986). For example, blood pressure screenings detect the risk for high blood pressure. A tuberculin skin test identifies persons exposed to tuberculosis. Information from health screenings determines the need for more comprehensive examinations.

A complete health assessment involves a more detailed review of a client's condition. The nurse collects a nursing history (see Chapter 7) and performs a behavioral and physical examination. The health history involves a lengthy interview with a client to gather subjective data about any presenting conditions. The interview is an opportunity for the nurse to establish a relationship with the client that promotes sharing of information. A physical examination is a head-to-toe review of each body system that offers objective information about the client and allows the nurse to make clinical judgments. The client's condition and response affect the extent of the examination. The accuracy of a physical assessment influences the choice of therapies a client receives and the determination of the response to those therapies. Continuity in health care improves when the nurse makes ongoing, objective, and comprehensive assessment.

■ PURPOSES OF PHYSICAL EXAMINATION

An examination should be designed for the client's needs. If a client is acutely ill, the nurse recognizes the presenting symptoms and may choose to assess only the involved body systems. A more comprehensive examination is conducted when the client feels more at ease, and the nurse then learns about the client's total health status. A complete physical examination is performed for routine screening to promote wellness behaviors and preventive health care measures; for determination of eligibility for health insurance, military service, or a new job; and for admission to a hospital or long-term care facility. The nurse uses physical assessment for the following reasons:

1. To gather baseline data about the client's health
2. To supplement, confirm, or refute data obtained in the nursing history
3. To confirm and identify nursing diagnoses
4. To make clinical judgments about a client's changing health status and management
5. To evaluate the physiological outcomes of care

Gathering a Health History

The main objective of interacting with clients is to find out what is central to their concerns and to help find solutions. It is important for the nurse to pay attention to clients' worries and to direct an interview and examination so that a clear picture is created of their condition. This means that collection of a health history and a physical examination require patience and a dedication to thoroughness and detail.

There are some basic principles that can help in conducting a successful health history (see Chapter 7) and in laying the groundwork for a well-organized physical examination. Let the interview allow you to form a partnership with the client so that the interview is oriented to the client and not a disease. Know your own idiosyncrasies, for example, wanting to be liked, fear of harming the client or catching a disease. Do not allow the resultant feelings to harm the relationship with the client.

Developing Nursing Diagnoses and a Care Plan

The nursing health history allows the nurse to gather a complete and detailed data base about the client's health status. After collecting a history, the nurse conducts a physical assessment to refute, confirm, or supplement the existing data base. The nurse critically thinks about the information provided by the client, applies knowledge from previous clinical care, and methodically conducts an examination to create a clear picture of the client's status. For example, a client may complain of back pain. The nurse asks several questions to clarify the nature of the pain. During the examination the nurse carefully looks for the source of the pain, for example, discomfort when changing position or a bruise across the client's back, to rule out a variety of potential ailments.

One assessment finding cannot conclusively reveal the nature of an abnormality. A complete assessment is needed to form a definitive diagnosis. The nurse learns to group significant findings into patterns of data that reveal actual or high-risk nursing diagnoses. In addition, each abnormal finding directs the nurse to gather additional information. Information gathered during an initial physical assessment provides a baseline of a client's functional abilities. The baseline is not necessarily the normal range of physical findings but rather the pattern of findings identified when the client was first assessed. This baseline serves as a comparison for future assessment findings. During a subsequent assessment, the nurse can determine whether the client's condition has changed.

The accuracy of the data base allows the nurse to develop individualized nursing diagnoses (Table 33-1). Physical assessment findings help determine the etiology of diagnoses so that the nurse can select the correct type of interventions for the care plan. Physical assessment is ongoing, and thus the care plan changes with the client's condition. The nurse monitors the client's progress and responses to therapies to review existing diagnoses and identify new problems.

Managing Client Problems

When caring for clients, the nurse makes many observations and performs a variety of therapies. Yet the nurse's success in giving care depends on the ability to recognize change in status and to modify therapies so that clients

Table 33-1	Development of Individualized Nursing Diagnoses		
ASSESSMENT METHOD	**FINDINGS**	**PATTERNS**	**NURSING DIAGNOSIS**
Inspection of skin	Skin along sacral area is intact. There is 3-cm area of redness around coccyx; skin blanches on palpation. No skin lesions are observed.	There is pressure area around coccyx.	Risk for impaired skin integrity
Palpation of skin	Skin is moist from diaphoresis. There is tenderness to palpation around sacral area. There is good skin turgor.	Skin moisture promotes maceration.	
Historical data	Client suffered fractured left leg. Client is immobilized due to left leg traction.	Continued pressure is exerted over sacrum.	

gain the most desirable outcome. Physical assessment skills allow the nurse to judge the status of the client's health and direct the management of care. For example, the nurse inspects the skin during a routine bath and finds it excessively dry. The nurse does not use soap and applies body lotion to the skin. The nurse revises the written care plan so that other nurses know the type of skin care to provide. Instruction is also given to the client about skin care. Performing the mechanics of physical assessment is relatively simple. The more difficult challenge lies in using findings to make decisions.

Evaluating Nursing Care

Nurses become accountable for their nursing care by evaluating the results of nursing interventions. Physical assessment skills enhance the evaluation of nursing measures through monitoring physiological and behavioral outcomes of care. The same physical assessment skills used to assess a condition (e.g., palpation of the client's pulse) can be used as an evaluation measure after care is administered (e.g., an evaluation of a client's tolerance to an exercise plan).

Nurses make accurate, detailed, objective measurements through physical assessment. The measurements determine whether the expected outcomes of care are met. The nurse does not rely solely on intuition when physical assessment can be used to evaluate effectiveness of care.

■ CULTURAL SENSITIVITY

As is the case with any other aspect of nursing, a physical examination must be performed with the nurse respecting the cultural differences of clients. How members of different cultures behave influences their willingness to assume responsibility for their health and their tendency to seek professional health care. This is important for the nurse to remember before attempting to conduct a physical examination. A client's health beliefs, use of alternative therapies, nutritional habits, relationships with family, and comfort with the nurse's physical closeness during an exam must be considered during examination and history taking.

It is extremely important for nurses to remain culturally

aware and to avoid stereotyping on the basis of gender or race. There is a sharp difference between distinguishing cultural characteristics and distinguishing physical characteristics. It is important for nurses to learn common disorders of those ethnic populations within the nurse's community. For example, Navaho Indians often have ear anomalies, Polynesians often suffer clubfoot, and many African Americans experience sickle cell disease. Similarly, it is important to known variations in physical characteristics such as in the skin and musculoskeletal system that are related to cultural variables. Recognition of cultural diversity helps the nurse to respect a client's uniqueness and to provide care of a higher quality.

■ INTEGRATION OF PHYSICAL ASSESSMENT WITH NURSING CARE

Whether a complete or partial physical assessment is performed, an examination should be integrated into routine care. For example, the nurse can assess the condition of the skin and other body parts during a bed bath. When a client undergoes oral hygiene, the nurse can carefully assess oral cavity structures. As a client ambulates down the hall, the nurse assesses range of motion and gait. This practice makes more efficient use of time. The nurse also learns that physical assessment should become an automatic behavior when nurse and client interact. Physical assessment skills enable the nurse to gather more comprehensive and relevant assessment findings.

■ SKILLS OF PHYSICAL ASSESSMENT

Chapter 7 briefly describes the skills of inspection, palpation, percussion, and auscultation. This chapter provides a more detailed description of those skills and their application in the physical examination.

Inspection

Inspection is the process of observation. The nurse inspects body parts to detect normal characteristics or significant physical signs. An experienced nurse learns to make several observations, almost simultaneously, while becoming very perceptive of early warnings of abnormalities. The secret to inspection is to always pay attention to the client. Watch all movements and look very carefully at any body part or area being inspected.

It helps to know normal physical characteristics before trying to distinguish abnormal findings. It is especially important to know normal characteristics of clients of different ages. Dry, wrinkled, inelastic skin is normal in an older but not in a young adult. Experience is needed to recognize normal variations among clients, as well as ranges of normal in an individual. Inspection is a simple technique, but it is often under used. For example, when hurrying to complete a bath, a nurse may fail to inspect all skin surfaces and overlook a rash under the client's arm. The quality of an inspection depends on the nurse's willingness to spend time doing a thorough job. To use inspection effectively, the nurse observes the following principles:

1. Make sure good lighting is available.
2. Position and expose body parts so that all surfaces can be viewed.
3. Inspect each area for size, shape, color, symmetry, position, and abnormalities.
4. If possible, compare each area inspected with the same area on the opposite side of the body.
5. Use additional light (e.g., a penlight) to inspect body cavities.
6. Do not hurry inspection. Pay attention to detail.

After inspection of a body part is completed, findings may indicate further examination. Palpation is often used with or after visual inspection.

Palpation

Further assessment of body parts is made through the sense of touch. Through palpation the hands can make delicate and sensitive measurements of specific physical signs, including resistance, resilience, roughness, texture, and mobility (Table 33-2). The nurse uses different parts of the

hand when touching the skin to detect characteristics such as texture and temperature.

The client should be relaxed and positioned comfortably because muscle tension during palpation impairs its effectiveness. For example, tension of the abdominal muscles makes palpation of underlying organs impossible and mimics muscle rigidity. Asking the client to take slow deep breaths enhances muscle relaxation. Tender areas are palpated last. The nurse asks the client to point out the more sensitive areas and notes any nonverbal signs of discomfort.

Clients appreciate warm hands, short fingernails, and a gentle approach. Palpation may be either light or deep and is controlled by the amount of pressure applied with the fingers or hand. Light palpation always precedes deep palpation. The nurse applies tactile pressure slowly, gently, and deliberately. Light palpation of structures such as the abdomen is performed to determine areas of tenderness. The nurse's hand is placed on the part to be examined and depressed about 1 cm ($\frac{1}{2}$ inch). Tender areas are examined further. The sensation of touch is best preserved with light, intermittent pressure. Heavy, prolonged pressure causes a loss of sensitivity in the nurse's hand.

After palpation has been applied, deeper palpation is used to examine the condition of organs, such as those in the abdomen (Fig. 33-1). The nurse depresses the area being examined approximately 2 to 4 cm (1 to 2 inches) (Seidel et al, 1995). Caution is the rule. A nursing student should not

Table 33-2	Examples of Characteristics Measured by Palpation
Area Examined	**Criteria Measured**
Skin	Temperature
	Moisture
	Texture
	Turgor and elasticity
	Tenderness
	Thickness
Organs (e.g., liver and intestine)	Size
	Shape
	Tenderness
	Absence of masses
Glands (e.g., thyroid and lymph)	Swelling
	Symmetry and mobility
Blood vessels (e.g., carotid or femoral artery)	Pulse amplitude
	Elasticity
	Rate
	Rhythm
Thorax	Excursion
	Tenderness
	Fremitus

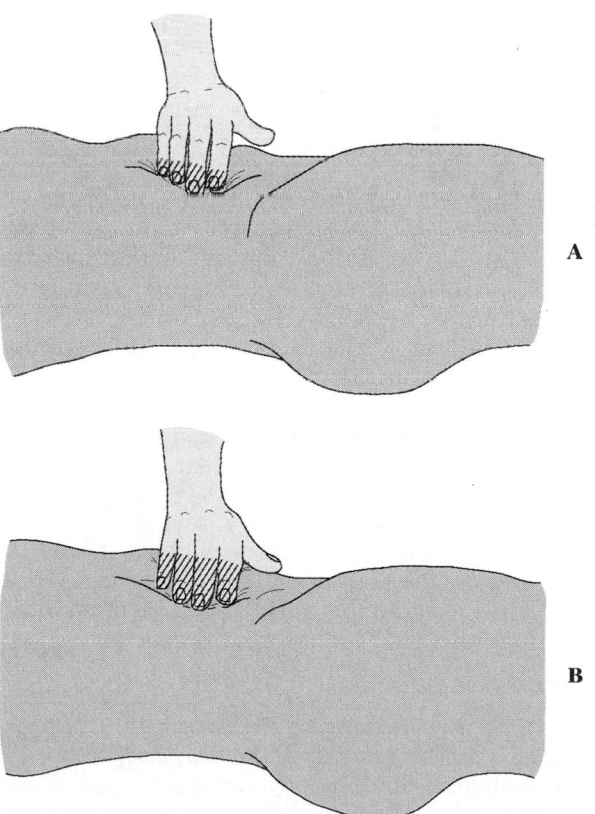

Fig. 33-1 A, During light palpation, gentle pressure against underlying skin and tissues can detect areas of irregularity and tenderness. **B,** During deep palpation, the nurse depresses tissue to assess the condition of underlying organs.

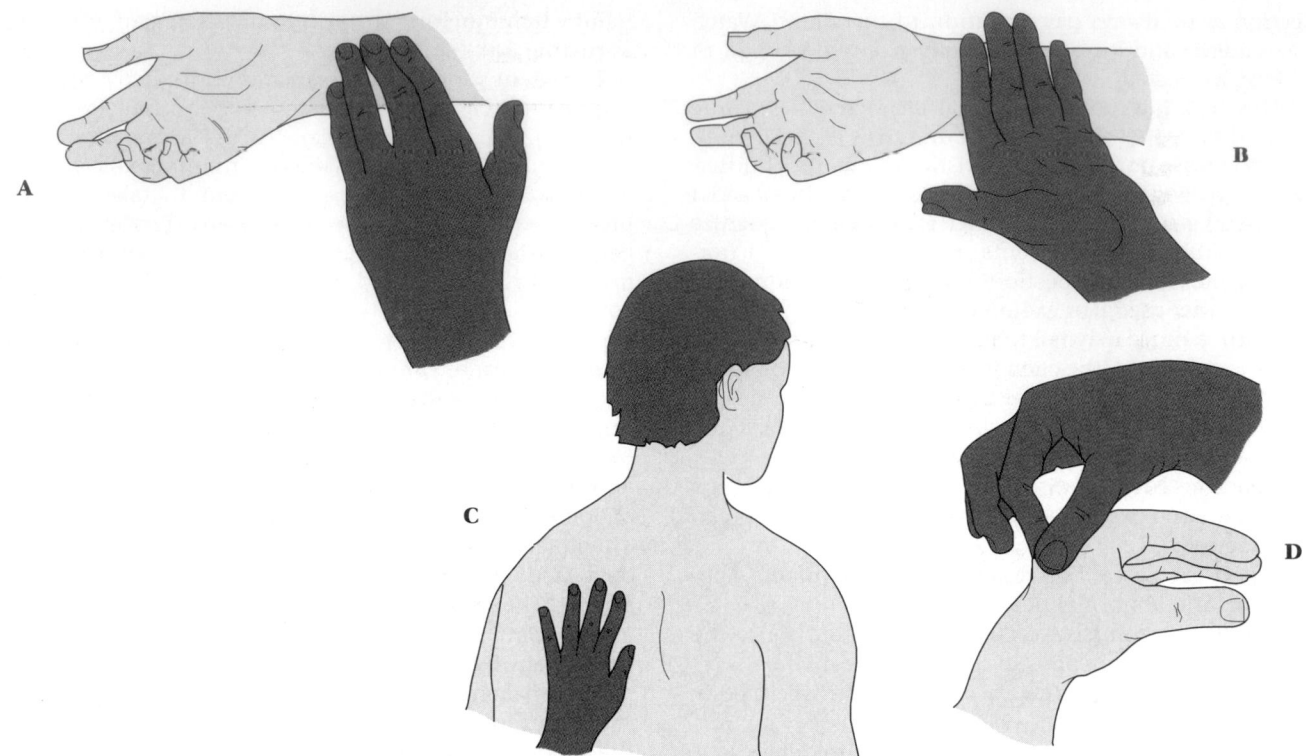

Fig. 33-2 A, The radial pulse is detected with the pads of the fingertips, the most sensitive part of the hand. **B,** The dorsum of the hand allows the nurse to detect temperature variations in skin. **C,** The nurse uses the bony part of the palm at the base of the fingers to detect vibration. **D,** The nurse grasps the skin with the fingertips to assess turgor.

attempt deep palpation without the assistance of a qualified instructor because prolonged pressure could cause internal injury.

The most sensitive parts of the hand, the palmar surface of the fingers and finger pads, are used to assess position, texture, size, consistency, form of a mass, and pulsation (Fig. 33-2, *A*). Temperature is best measured using the dorsum or back of the hand (Fig. 33-2, *B*) and fingers, where the skin is thinnest. The palm or ulnar surface of the hand (Fig. 33-2, *C*) is more sensitive to vibration. The nurse measures position, consistency, and turgor by lightly grasping the body part with the fingertips (Fig. 33-2, *D*). The nurse must not palpate without considering the client's condition. For example, if the client has a fractured rib, extra care is used to locate the painful area. A vital artery is not palpated with pressure that obstructs blood flow. The nurse also considers the body area being palpated and the reason for using palpation and must be able to discriminate and interpret the significance of what is sensed.

Percussion

Percussion involves tapping the body with the fingertips to evaluate the size, borders, and consistency of body organs and to discover fluid in body cavities. It requires considerable skill. It is perhaps the least-used assessment skill; however, it can help to confirm other assessment findings. Through percussion, the location, size, and density of an underlying structure are determined. Percussion helps verify abnormalities reported from x-ray studies or assessed

through palpation and auscultation. For example, if the nurse hears abnormal breath sounds when auscultating the lungs, percussion may rule out the presence of consolidated fluids or air in the pleural space.

Percussion involves striking one object against another, thus producing vibration and subsequent sound waves. When the examiner strikes the body's surface with a finger, vibration is transmitted through the body tissues. Sound waves are heard as percussion tones arising from vibrations 4 to 6 cm deep in body tissue (Seidel et al, 1995). The character of the sound depends on the density of the underlying tissue. For example, the normal lung transmits sounds with high intensity and low pitch, whereas the more solid liver transmits a high-pitched sound of soft intensity. By knowing the way that densities influence sound, the nurse can locate organs or masses, map their boundaries, and determine their size. An abnormal sound suggests a mass or substance such as air or fluid within an organ or body cavity.

The two methods of percussion are direct and indirect. The direct method involves striking the body surface directly with one or two fingers. The indirect technique is performed by placing the middle finger of the nondominant hand (called the *pleximeter*) firmly against the body surface, keeping the palm and remaining fingers off the skin. The tip of the middle finger of the dominant hand (called the *plexor*) strikes the base of the distal joint of the pleximeter (Fig. 33-3). The examiner uses a quick, sharp stroke with the plexor finger, keeping the forearm stationary. The wrist remains relaxed to deliver the proper blow.

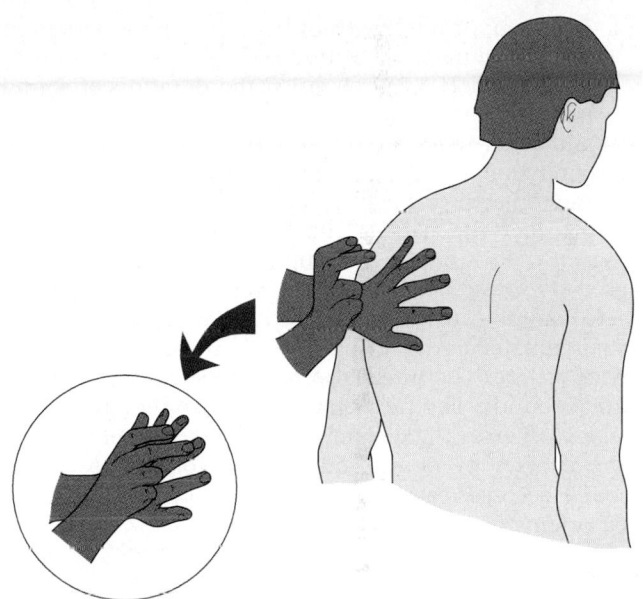

Fig. 33-3 To perform indirect percussion, the nurse places the middle finger of the nondominant hand against the body's surface. The tip of the middle finger of the dominant hand strikes the top of the middle finger of the nondominant hand.

Once the finger has struck, the wrist snaps back. If the blow is not sharp, if the pleximeter is held loosely, or if the palm rests on the body surface, the sound is dampened or softened, preventing transmission of sound to underlying structures. The same force must be applied to each area so that an accurate comparison of sounds can be made. A light, quick blow usually produces the clearest sound. Use of direct versus indirect percussion or firm versus light percussion can lead to different interpretation of results.

Percussion produces five types of sounds: tympany, resonance, hyperresonance, dullness, and flatness. Each sound is created by certain types of underlying tissues and is judged by its intensity of pitch, duration, and quality (Table 33-3).

Percussion takes practice. Seidel et al. (1995) suggest using a partially full milk carton to practice the skill. Percussion over the air-filled space of the carton creates a resonant type sound. As you percuss downward, the sound changes as you percuss over the milk. The same principle applies to body tissues.

Auscultation

Auscultation is listening to sounds produced by the body. Some sounds can be heard with the unassisted ear, although most sounds can be heard only through a stethoscope. To auscultate correctly, listen in a quiet environment. Listen for the presence of sound as well as its characteristics.

A student must first learn the normal sounds created by the cardiovascular, respiratory, and gastrointestinal systems, such as the passage of blood through an artery. Abnormal sounds can be recognized only after normal variations are learned. The nurse becomes more successful in auscultation by knowing the types of sounds arising from each body structure and the location in which they can most easily be heard. Likewise, the nurse becomes familiar with the areas that normally do not emit sounds.

To auscultate correctly the nurse needs good hearing acuity, a good stethoscope, and knowledge of how to use the stethoscope properly. Nurses with hearing disorders should purchase stethoscopes with greater sound amplification or ask colleagues to check findings through auscultation. Always place the stethoscope on naked skin, because clothing obscures sound.

Chapter 32 describes the parts of the acoustic stethoscope and the general use of the bell and diaphragm. The bell is best for low-pitched sounds, such as vascular and certain heart sounds, and the diaphragm is best for high-pitched sounds, such as bowel and lung sounds.

A nurse must become familiar with the stethoscope before attempting to use it on a client. It helps to practice using it with a friend. A number of extraneous sounds created by movement of the tubing or chestpiece interfere with auscultation of body organ sounds. By deliberately producing these sounds, the nurse learns to recognize and disregard them during the actual examination (see the box on p. 646). Through auscultation, the nurse notes the following characteristics of sounds:

1. Frequency, or the number of sound wave cycles generated per second by a vibrating object. The higher the frequency, the higher the pitch of a sound and vice versa.
2. Loudness, or the amplitude of a sound wave. Auscultated sounds are described as *loud* or *soft*.
3. Quality, or sounds of similar frequency and loudness from different sources. Terms such as *blowing* or *gurgling* describe the quality of sound.

Table 33-3	**Sounds Produced by Percussion**				
SOUND	**INTENSITY**	**PITCH**	**DURATION**	**QUALITY**	**COMMON LOCATION**
Tympany	Loud	High	Moderate	Drumlike	Enclosed, air-containing space; gastric air bubble, puffed-out cheek
Resonance	Moderate to loud	Low	Long	Hollow	Normal lung
Hyperresonance	Very loud	Very low	Longer than resonance	Booming	Emphysematous lung
Dullness	Soft to moderate	High	Moderate	Thudlike	Liver
Flatness	Soft	High	Short	Flat	Muscle

Exercises to Increase Familiarity with the Stethoscope

- Ensure that the earpiece follows the contour of the ear canal. Learn what fit is best for you by comparing amplification of sounds with the earpieces in both directions.
- Place the earpieces in your ears with the tips of the earpieces turned toward the face. *Lightly* blow into the diaphragm. Again place the earpieces in your ears, this time with the ends turned toward the back of the head. *Lightly* blow into the diaphragm. After you have learned the right fit for the loudest amplification, wear the stethoscope the same way each time.
- Put on the stethoscope and *lightly* blow into the diaphragm. If the sound is barely audible, *lightly* blow into the bell. Sound is carried through only one part of the chestpiece at a time. If the sound is greatly amplified through the diaphragm, the diaphragm is in position for use. If the sound is barely audible through the diaphragm, the bell is in position for use. Rotation of the diaphragm and bell places the chestpiece in the desired position. Leave the diaphragm in position for the next exercise.
- Place the diaphragm over the anterior part of your chest. Ask a friend to speak in a normal conversational tone. Environmental noise seriously detracts from hearing the noise created by body organs. When a stethoscope is used, the client and the examiner should remain quiet.
- Put the stethoscope on and gently tap the tubing. It is often difficult to avoid stretching or moving the stethoscope's tubing. The examiner should be in a position so that the tubing hangs free. Moving or touching the tubing creates extraneous sounds.

4. Duration, or the length of time that sound vibrations last. The duration of sound is short, medium, or long. Layers of soft tissue dampen the duration of sounds from deep internal organs.

Auscultation requires concentration and practice. Closing your eyes may help to focus on a particular sound. Taking time to listen to a sound is important. The nurse must also consider the part of the body auscultated and the causes of the sounds. For example, the first heart sound is caused by closure of the mitral valve. The nurse learns where sounds can best be heard. The first heart sound is best auscultated at the fifth intercostal space along the midclavicular line. The nurse also learns the characteristics of normal sounds. The first heart sound has the quality of a loud *lub,* whereas the second sound is a *dub.* After the cause and character of normal auscultated sounds are understood, it becomes easier to recognize abnormal sounds and their origins.

Olfaction

While assessing a client, the nurse should be familiar with the nature and source of body odors (Table 33-4). Olfaction helps the nurse detect abnormalities that cannot be recognized by any other means. For example, a client with a cast is expected to experience discomfort after an injury. However, the nurse who notes a strong odor will suspect that the discomfort may also be related to wound infection. The discomfort alone does not reveal the presence of infection. Findings from olfaction and other assessment skills allow the nurse to detect serious abnormalities. If a nurse notices an unfamiliar odor, a colleague may be able to identify the problem.

■ PREPARATION FOR EXAMINATION

Proper preparation of the environment, equipment, and client ensures a smooth physical examination with few interruptions. A disorganized approach when preparing for a physical examination can cause errors and incomplete findings.

Table 33-4	Assessment of Characteristic Odors		
ODOR	**SITE OR SOURCE**	**POTENTIAL CAUSES**
Alcohol	Oral cavity	Ingestion of alcohol, diabetes
Ammonia	Urine	Urinary tract infection
Body odor	Skin, particularly in areas where body parts rub together (e.g., under arms, and breasts)	Poor hygiene, excess perspiration (hyperhidrosis), foul-smelling perspiration (bromidrosis)
Feces	Wound site	Wound abscess
	Vomitus	Bowel obstruction
	Rectal area	Fecal incontinence
Foul-smelling stools in infant	Stool	Malabsorption syndrome
Halitosis	Oral cavity	Poor dental and oral hygiene, gum disease
Sweet, fruity ketones	Oral cavity	Diabetics acidosis
Stale urine	Skin	Uremic acidosis
Sweet, heavy, thick odor	Draining wound	*Pseudomonas* (bacterial) infection
Musty odor	Casted body part	Infection inside cast
Fetid, sweet odor	Tracheostomy or mucus secretions	Infection of bronchial tree (*Pseudomonas* bacteria)

Infection Control

During an examination the nurse may find clients with open skin lesions or weeping wounds. Examination techniques cause the nurse to contact body fluids and discharge. Standard precautions should be used throughout the examination (see Chapter 34). Gloves should be worn during palpation and percussion to reduce contact with microorganisms. If a client presents with excessive drainage from a wound, the examiner may need to wear a gown.

Environment

A physical examination requires privacy. A well-equipped examination room is preferable. However, in hospitals the examination usually occurs in the client's room, where it may be necessary to use room curtains or dividers around the bed. In the home, the nurse may perform an examination in the client's bedroom.

Any examination room should be well equipped for all necessary procedures. Adequate lighting is needed for proper illumination of body parts. Primary lighting can be either daylight or artificial, as long as the light is direct enough to reveal skin characteristics without distortion from shadows. Ideally an examination room is soundproofed so that clients feel comfortable discussing their conditions. The nurse eliminates sources of noise such as televisions or radios, takes steps to prevent interruptions from others, and makes sure the room is warm enough for the client's comfort.

Sometimes it is difficult to examine clients who are in beds or on stretchers. Special examination tables make clients easily accessible and help them assume special positions. The tables are high and narrow. The nurse must carefully assist clients so that they do not fall while getting on and off them. A confused, combative, or uncooperative client should not be left unsupervised on an examination table.

Examination tables are often hard and uncomfortable. When the client lies supine, the head of the table can be raised about 30 degrees. The client may also be given a small pillow. When examining a client in bed, the nurse can raise the bed to reach body parts more easily.

Equipment

Handwashing is done before equipment preparation and the examination. Handwashing reduces the transmission of microorganisms. The equipment needed for an examination should be clean, readily available, and arranged in order for easy use (Fig. 33-4). It should be kept warm as appropriate. The diaphragm of the stethoscope may be briskly rubbed between the hands before it is applied to the skin. Warm water should be run over the vaginal speculum. All equipment must be checked to see that it functions properly. The ophthalmoscope and otoscope require good batteries and light bulbs. Equipment typically used is listed in the box below.

Client

PHYSICAL PREPARATION

The client's physical comfort is vital for a successful examination. Before starting, the nurse asks if the client needs to use the toilet. An empty bladder and bowel facilitate examination of the abdomen, genitalia, and rectum and provide the opportunity to collect urine for fecal specimens. The nurse explains the proper method for collecting specimens and ensures that each specimen is properly labeled.

Physical preparation involves being sure the client is dressed and draped properly. A client in the hospital will likely be wearing only a simple gown. In an outpatient set-

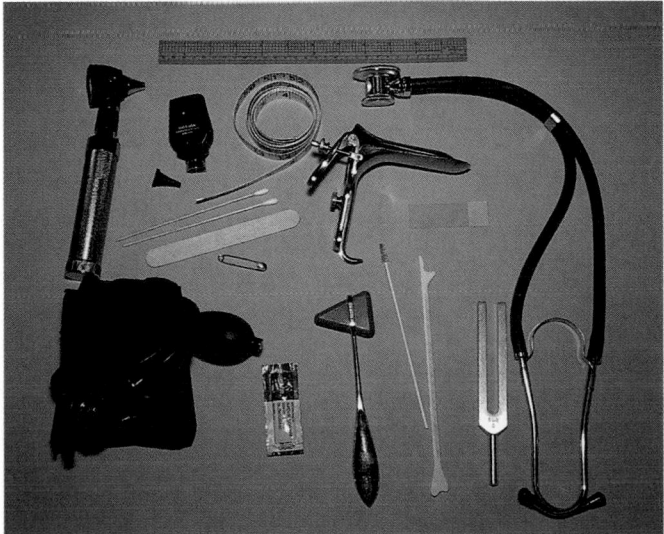

Fig. 33-4 Equipment used during a physical examination.

Equipment and Supplies for Physical Assessment

- Cotton applicators
- Cytobrush
- Disposable pad
- Drapes
- Eye chart (e.g., Snellen chart)
- Flashlight and spotlight
- Forms (e.g, physical, laboratory)
- Gloves (sterile or clean)
- Gown for client
- Water-soluble lubricant
- Ophthalmoscope
- Otoscope
- Papanicolaou smear slides
- Paper towels
- Percussion hammer
- Ruler
- Safety pin
- Scale with height measurement rod
- Specimen containers and microscope slides
- Sphygmomanometer and cuff
- Stethoscope
- Swabs or sponge forceps
- Tape measure
- Thermometer
- Tissues
- Tongue depressor
- Tuning fork
- Vaginal speculum
- Wristwatch with second hand or digital display

Table 33-5	Positions for Examination		
POSITION	**AREAS ASSESSED**	**RATIONALE**	**LIMITATIONS**
Sitting	Head and neck, back, posterior thorax and lungs, anterior thorax and lungs, breasts, axillae, heart, vital signs, and upper extremities	Sitting upright provides full expansion of lungs and provides better visualization of symmetry of upper body parts.	Physically weakened client may be unable to sit. Examiner should use supine position with head of bed elevated instead.
Supine	Head and neck, anterior thorax and lungs, breasts, axillae, heart, abdomen, extremities, pulses	This is most normally relaxed position. It provides easy access to pulse sites.	If client becomes short of breath easily, examiner may need to raise head of bed.
Dorsal recumbent	Head and neck, anterior thorax and lungs, breasts, axillae, heart, abdomen	Position is used for abdominal assessment because it promotes relaxation of abdominal muscles.	Clients with painful disorders are more comfortable with knees flexed.
Lithotomy*	Female genitalia and genital tract	This position provides maximal exposure of genitalia and facilitates insertion of vaginal speculum.	Lithotomy position is embarrassing and uncomfortable, so examiner minimizes time that client spends in it. Client is kept well draped.
Sims'	Rectum and vagina	Flexion of hip and knee improves exposure of rectal area.	Joint deformities may hinder client's ability to bend hip and knee.
Prone	Musculoskeletal system	This position is used only to assess extension of hip joint.	This position is poorly tolerated in clients with respiratory difficulties.
Lateral recumbent	Heart	This position aids in detecting murmurs.	This position is poorly tolerated in clients with respiratory difficulties.
Knee-chest*	Rectum	This position provides maximal exposure of rectal area.	This position is embarrassing and uncomfortable.

*Clients with arthritis or other joint deformities may be unable to assume this position.

ting, instruct the client to undress and apply a light cover gown. If the examination is limited to certain body systems, it may be unnecessary for the client to undress completely. The client should have privacy during undressing and plenty of time to finish. Walking into the room as the client undresses causes embarrassment. Drapes and gowns are made of linen or disposable paper. After clients have undressed and donned the gown, they should sit or lie down on the examination table with the drape over the lap or lower trunk. The examiner makes sure that the client stays warm by eliminating drafts, controlling room temperature, and providing warm blankets. A seriously ill client or older adult is more susceptible to chills. The nurse should ask if the client is comfortable. The client may become more relaxed if offered a pillow, sip of water, or tissue.

Positioning. During the examination, the nurse asks clients to assume proper positions so that body parts are accessible and clients stay comfortable. Table 33-5 lists the preferred positions for each part of the examination and contains figures illustrating these positions. Clients' abilities to assume positions will depend on their physical strength, mobility, age, and degree of wellness. Many of the positions, such as the lithotomy and knee-chest, are embarrassing and uncomfortable. Therefore clients should be kept in these positions no longer than necessary. The examiner explains the positions and assists clients in attaining them. The drapes are adjusted to be sure that the area to be examined is accessible and that no body part is unnecessarily exposed. More than one position can be assumed for the same part of an examination (e.g., supine and sitting for assessment of the anterior thorax), so the nurse first chooses the position that provides greater accessibility and accuracy in assessing body parts (sitting for anterior thorax). However, if clients are too weak or are physically unable to assume a position, the nurse may choose an alternative position. The nurse uses extra care to position older adults where they may avoid looking into the source of light, which can cause discomfort from glare.

PSYCHOLOGICAL PREPARATION

Clients are easily embarrassed when forced to answer sensitive questions about bodily functions or when body parts are exposed and examined. The possibility that the examiner will find something abnormal also creates anxiety, so reduction of this anxiety may be the nurse's highest priority before the examination. The nurse should convey an open, receptive, professional approach. A stiff, formal demeanor may inhibit the client's ability to communicate, but a too casual style may fail to instill confidence (Seidel et al, 1995). A thorough explanation lets clients know what to expect and what to do so that they can cooperate. The nurse first explains the examination in general terms.

Nurse: Ms. Bryce, I'm going to do a complete physical examination so that I can have a good idea of whether you have any health problems. As we go along, I'll explain to you exactly what I'll be doing. Feel free to ask any questions. If you become uncomfortable, please tell me.

Then as the nurse examines each body system, a more detailed explanation is given.

Nurse: As I examine your breasts, I want you to relax lying down. First I want to look at the color, size, and shape of your breasts. Then I'll gently use my hands to feel the breast tissue itself.

The nurse uses simple terms when describing steps of the examination. Complicated terminology confuses clients and adds to their fears. The nurse's manner should be professional. Yet, voice tone and facial expressions should be relaxed to put clients at ease. The nurse encourages clients to ask questions and mention discomfort they feel during the assessment. When the client and nurse are of opposite gender, it is necessary to have a third person of the client's gender in the room, especially when examination of the sexual organs is required. The presence of a third person assures the client that the examiner will behave ethically, and the third person acts as a witness to the examiner's proper conduct.

During the examination, the nurse watches the client's emotional responses. The nurse observes whether the client's facial expression conveys fear or concern and whether body movements reveal anxiety, such as frequently pulling the drape around the body or tensing up as the examiner touches the body. The nurse must remain calm and clearly explain each step of the assessment. It may be necessary to stop the examination and ask whether the client feels anxious, afraid, or uncomfortable. The client should not be forced to continue. Postponing the examination until a later time may be advantageous because the findings may be more accurate when the client can cooperate and relax. If the fears result from misconceptions, the nurse clarifies the purpose of the examination and how it is to be performed.

Assessment of Age Groups

The nurse uses different interview styles and approaches to physical examination for clients of different age groups. When assessing children, the nurse must be sensitive and anticipate the child's reaction to the examination as a strange and unfamiliar experience. Routine pediatric examinations have a focus on health promotion and illness prevention, particularly for the care of well children who receive competent parenting and have no serious health problems (Wong, 1995). The focus of an examination is on growth and development, sensory screening, dental examination, and behavioral assessment. Children who are chronically ill, disabled, foster children, or foreign-born adopted may require additional examination visits. When examining children, the following tips assist in data collection:

1. When obtaining histories on infants and children, gather all or part of the information from parents or guardians.
2. Perform the examination in a nonthreatening area and provide time for play to become acquainted.
3. Because parents may think they are being tested by the examiner, offer support during the examination and do not pass judgment.
4. Call children by their first name, and address the parents as "Mr. and Mrs." rather than by their first names.
5. Use open-ended questions to allow parents to share more information and describe more of the children's problems.
6. Interview older children to allow observation of parent-child interactions.

7. Interview older children, who can often provide details about their health history and severity of symptoms.

8. Treat adolescents as adults and individuals because they tend to respond best when treated as such.

9. Remember that adolescents have the right to confidentiality. After talking with parents about historical information, speak alone with adolescents.

A comprehensive health assessment and examination of older adults should include physical data as well as a review of growth and development, family relationships, group involvement, and religious and occupational pursuits (Ebersole and Hess, 1994). An important part of health assessment involves analysis of basic activities of daily living (dressing, bathing, toileting, feeding, and continence) that are fundamental to independent living. In addition, the more complex instrumental activities of daily living (using telephone, preparing meals, managing money) are also assessed. Any examination of an older adult should also include an evaluation of mental status.

Throughout an examination the nurse must recognize that with advancing age the body does not respond vigorously to injury or disease. Therefore, older persons do not always exhibit the expected signs and symptoms (Lueckenotte, 1994). Characteristically, older adults present more blunted or atypical signs and symptoms.

Principles to follow during examination of an older adult include:

1. Do not stereotype aging clients. Most are able to adapt to change and to learn about their health. Similarly, they are reliable historians.

2. Recognize that sensory or physical limitations can affect how quickly you are able to interview older adults and conduct examinations. Plan for more than one examination session. Sometimes it helps to give clients an initial health questionnaire before they come to a clinic or office (Ebersole and Hess, 1994).

3. Perform the examination with adequate space, this is especially important for clients with mobility aids such as a cane or walker.

4. During the examination use patience, allow for pauses, and observe for details. Recognize normalities of later life that would be abnormal in a younger client.

5. Older clients may find giving certain types of health information stressful. Illness is seen as a threat to independence and a step toward institutionalization.

6. Perform the examination near bathroom facilities. The client may experience an urgent need to void.

7. Be alert to signs of increasing fatigue such as sighing, grimacing, irritability, leaning against objects for support, and drooping of head and shoulders.

ORGANIZATION OF THE EXAMINATION

Regardless of the age of a client, a basic physical examination follows a similar approach. A physical examination is composed of individual assessments for each body system. The extent of an examination depends on its purpose and a client's condition. A client who comes to a clinic with symptoms of a severe chest cold will not routinely require a neurological assessment. A client entering the emergency room with an acute illness requires assessment of body systems most at risk for being abnormal. When a client is admitted to the hospital, a complete examination is usually performed. Clients with specific symptoms or needs often require only portions of an examination. The nurse's judgment is needed to ensure that an examination is relevant and includes the correct observations.

The performance of a complete health assessment follows the format of the nursing history (see Chapter 7). The nurse uses information from the history to focus attention on specific parts of the examination. For example, if the history reveals symptoms of abdominal discomfort, the nurse examines the abdomen carefully. If the client reports difficulties in performing basic activities of daily living, the nurse carefully examines musculoskeletal and neurological function. Findings from the history generally reveal a pattern of related signs and symptoms. The physical examination supplements information from the history to confirm or refute the data.

The examination should be systematic and well organized so that important assessments are not omitted. A head-to-toe approach includes all body systems and helps the nurse anticipate each step. In an adult, the nurse begins by assessing the head and neck area, progressing methodically down the body to incorporate all body systems. The following tips help the nurse keep an examination well organized:

1. Compare both sides of the body for symmetry. A degree of asymmetry is normal (e.g., the biceps muscles in the dominant arm may be more developed than the same muscles in the nondominant arm).

2. If a client is seriously ill, first assess the systems of the body more at risk for being abnormal. For example, a client with chest pain should undergo a cardiovascular assessment first.

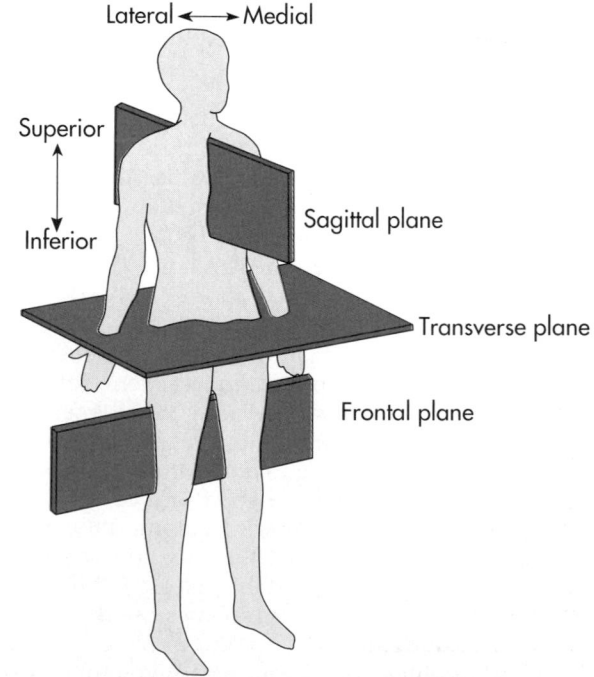

Fig. 33-5 The nurse describes assessment findings in terms of the anatomical position within body planes.

3. If a client becomes fatigued, offer rest periods between assessments.
4. Perform painful procedures near the end of the examination.
5. Record results of the examination in specific anatomical and scientific terms so that any professional can interpret the findings (Fig. 33-5).
6. Use common and accepted medical abbreviations to keep notes brief and concise.
7. Record quick notes during the examination to avoid keeping the client waiting. Complete any observations at the end of the examination.
8. A physical assessment form allows recording of information in the same sequence it is gathered.

∎ GENERAL SURVEY

Assessment begins when the nurse first meets the client. The nurse determines the reason the client is seeking health care. Initial data from the general survey begins with a review of the client's primary health problems. The nurse makes mental notes of the client's behavior and appearance. The examination begins with a general survey that includes observation of general appearance and behavior, vital signs, and height and weight measurements. The survey provides information about characteristics of an illness, a client's hygiene and body image, emotional state, recent changes in weight, and the client's developmental status. If abnormalities or problems are found, the affected body system is closely assessed later. For example, if a client's ap-

pearance is unkempt, the nurse later inspects the skin and nails for adequacy of hygiene.

General Appearance and Behavior

Assessment of appearance and behavior begins while the nurse prepares the client for the examination. The review of general appearance and behavior includes the following:

1. Gender and race. A person's gender affects the type of examination performed and the manner in which assessments are made. Different physical features are related to gender and race. Certain illnesses are more likely to affect a specific gender or race (Table 33-6) (American Cancer Society, 1995).
2. Age. Age influences normal physical characteristics. The ability to participate in some parts of the examination is also influenced by age.
3. Signs of distress. There may be obvious signs or symptoms indicating pain, difficulty in breathing, or anxiety. These signs establish priorities regarding what to examine first.
4. Body type. The nurse observes if a client appears trim and muscular, obese, or excessively thin. Body type can reflect level of health, age, and lifestyle.
5. Posture. Normal standing posture is an upright stance with parallel alignment of hips and shoulders. Normal sitting posture involves some degree of rounding of the shoulders. Observe whether the client has a slumped, erect, or bent posture. Posture may reflect mood or presence of pain. Many older adults assume a stooped,

Table 33-6	Reported Cancer Deaths for Black, American Indian, Chinese, Japanese, and Hispanic Persons, United States, 1991					
CANCER SITE	**BLACK MALES**	**BLACK FEMALES**	**AMERICAN INDIAN**	**CHINESE**	**JAPANESE**	**HISPANIC***
All sites	32,094	25,827	1,454	1,632	1,099	14,689
Oral cavity	933	341	31	62	16	224
Esophagus	1,465	522	20	25	23	233
Stomach	1,422	916	53	102	110	824
Colon & rectum	2,787	3,243	143	184	156	1,399
Liver & other biliary	784	621	81	206	67	860
Pancreas	1,379	1,554	77	94	79	810
Lung (male)	10,545	—	241	274	135	1,879
Lung (female)	—	4,656	130	145	82	848
Melanoma of skin	52	67	8	4	1	89
Breast (female)	—	4,809	84	99	85	1,264
Cervix uteri	—	983	42	17	10	292
Other uterus	—	921	14	16	13	207
Ovary	—	1,067	34	29	41	369
Prostate	5,299	—	71	32	47	833
Bladder	471	370	22	17	12	221
Kidney	578	399	61	19	17	399
Brain & CNS†	350	331	26	23	15	429
Lymphoma	780	664	41	58	47	750
Leukemia	869	740	41	46	35	714
Multiple myeloma	767	813	26	20	7	314

*Persons classified as of Hispanic origin on death may be of any race. Hispanic origin reporting, however, may be incomplete on death certificates in some states. These numbers are believed to include over 90% of cancer deaths in Hispanics in 1991.
†CNS = Central nervous system.
From American Cancer Society: *Cancer facts and figures,* Atlanta 1995, American Cancer Society.

forward-bent posture, with hips and knees somewhat flexed and arms bent at the elbows, raising the level of the arms.

6. Gait. Observe the client walk into the room or at the bedside (if client is ambulatory). Note if movements are coordinated or uncoordinated. A person normally walks with arms swinging freely at the sides, with the head and face leading the body.
7. Body movements. Observe whether movements are purposeful and note if there are any tremors involving the extremities. Determine if any body parts are immobile.
8. Hygiene and grooming. The client's level of cleanliness is noted by observing the appearance of the hair, skin, and fingernails. Observe if the client's clothes are clean. Grooming may depend on the activities being performed just before the examination as well as the client's occupation. Also note the amount and type of cosmetics used.
9. Dress. Culture, lifestyle, socioeconomic level, and personal preference affect the type of clothes worn. Note if the type of clothing worn is appropriate for temperature and weather conditions. Depressed or mentally ill persons may be unable to choose proper clothing. An older adult tends to wear extra clothing because of the sensitivity to cold.
10. Body odor. An unpleasant body odor may result from physical exercise, poor hygiene, or certain disease pathologies. Poor oral hygiene may cause bad breath.
11. Affect and mood. Affect is a person's feelings as they appear to others. Mood or emotional state is expressed verbally and nonverbally. Note if verbal expressions match nonverbal behavior and observe if mood is appropriate for the situation. For example, the mood is inappropriate if the client seems unusually happy after recently being diagnosed with cancer. Observe facial expressions as questions are asked.
12. Speech. Normal speech is understandable and moderately paced and shows an association with the person's thoughts. Note if the client talks rapidly or slowly. An abnormal pace may be caused by emotions or neurological impairment. Also note if the client speaks in a normal tone with clear inflection of words.
13. Client abuse. Abuse of children, women, and older adults is a growing and serious health problem. It may be first suspected in clients who have suffered obvious physical injury or neglect (e.g., evidence of malnutrition or presence of bruising on the extremities or

Clinical Indicators of Abuse

CHILD SEXUAL ABUSE
Physical Findings
Vaginal or penile discharge
Blood on underclothing
Pain or itching in genital area
Genital injuries
Difficulty sitting or walking
Pain while urinating
Foreign bodies in rectum, urethra, or vagina
Venereal disease

Behavioral Findings
Problem in sleeping or eating
Fear of certain people or places
Play activities recreate the abuse situation
Regressed behavior
Sexual acting out
Knowledge of explicit sexual matters
Preoccupation with other's or own genitals

DOMESTIC ABUSE
Physical Findings
Injuries and trauma are inconsistent with reported cause
Multiple injuries involving head, face, neck, breasts, abdomen, and genitalia (black eyes, orbital fractures, broken nose, fractured skull, lip lacerations, broken teeth, strangulation marks)
X-rays show old and new fractures in different stages of healing
Burns
Human bites

Behavioral Findings
Attempted suicide
Eating or sleeping disorders
Anxiety
Panic attacks
Pattern of substance abuse (follows physical abuse)
Low self-esteem
Depression
Sense of helplessness
Guilt
Increased forgetfulness

OLDER ADULT ABUSE
Physical Findings
Injuries and trauma are inconsistent with reported cause (cigarette burn, scratch, bruise, or bite)
Hematomas
Bruises at various stages of resolution
Bruises, chafing, excoriation on wrist or legs (restraints)
Burns
Fractures inconsistent with cause described
Dried blood
Prolonged interval between injury and medical treatment

Behavioral Findings
Dependent on caregiver
Physically and/or cognitively impaired
Combative
Wandering
Verbally belligerent
Minimal social support

trunk). Assess for the client's fear of the spouse or partner, care giver, parent, or adult child. Note if the partner or care giver has a history of violence, alcoholism, or drug abuse. Is the person unemployed, ill, or frustrated in caring for the client? Most states mandate a report to a social service center if abuse or neglect is suspected. When abuse is suspected, interview the client in private. It is difficult to detect abuse since victims often will not complain or report that they are in an abusive situation (Haviland and O'Brien, 1989). Clients are much more likely to reveal any problems to a nurse when the suspected abuser is absent from the room. Clinical indicators for abuse are summarized in the box on p. 652.

14. Substance Abuse. Health care providers' recognition of clients who abuse alcohol, prescribed medications, or illegal drugs, is typically poor. Studies have shown that only about 10% of clients who meet criteria for drug abuse are identified by primary health care providers (Caulker-Burnett, 1994). The problem affects all socioeconomic groups. A single visit to a clinic may not reveal the problem. Several visits often reveal behaviors that can be confirmed with a well-focused history and physical exam. The nurse must approach the client in a caring and nonjudgmental way, since issues of substance abuse involve both emotional and lifestyle issues. Clients to suspect for substance abuse include those listed in the box below. When abuse is suspected it is recommended that the nurse or examiner ask the following questions: Have you ever felt the need to CUT DOWN on your drinking or drug use? Have people ANNOYED you by criticizing your drinking or drug use? Have you ever felt bad or GUILTY about your drinking or drug use? Have you ever used or had a drink first thing in the morning as an EYE-OPENER to steady your nerves or feel normal? If two or more of the CAGE questions are positive, the nurse should strongly suspect abuse and consider how to motivate the client to seek treatment.

Vital Signs

Assessment of vital signs (see Chapter 32) should be the first part of the physical examination. Positioning or moving the client during the examination can interfere with obtaining accurate values. However, it is also appropriate for the nurse to measure specific vital signs during assessment of individual body systems. For example, the pulse can be assessed during examination of the peripheral pulses or the heart and respirations during examination of the thorax. Body temperature is always measured during the general survey.

Height, Weight, and Circumference

A person's general level of health can be reflected in the ratio of height to weight. Weight is a routine measure during health screenings and visits to physicians' offices or clinics. Both measures are routine when clients are admitted to a health care setting. A nurse measures infants' and children's height and weight to assess growth and development. In the elderly, height and weight coupled with a nutritional assessment are important in determining cause and treatment for chronic disease, and in assessing the older adult who has difficulty with feeding and other functional activities (see the box below). The nurse should look for overall trends in height and weight changes.

A client's weight will normally vary daily because of fluid loss or retention. Progressive weight gain is expected during pregnancy. A downward trend in a frail older adult may indicate serious reduction in nutritional reserves (Dwyer et al, 1993). The assessment screens for abnormal weight changes. The nursing history can help to focus on possible causes for change in weight (Table 33-7). Before measure-

---

Red Flags for Suspicion of Substance Abuse

- Clients who frequently miss appointments
- Clients who frequently request written excuses for work
- Clients who have chief complaints of insomnia, "bad nerves," or pain that does not fit a particular pattern
- Clients who often report lost prescriptions (e.g., tranquilizers or pain medications) or ask for frequent refills
- Clients who make frequent emergency room visits
- Clients who have a history of changing doctors or who bring in medication bottles prescribed by several different providers.
- Clients with histories of gastrointestinal bleeds, peptic ulcers, pancreatitis, cellulitis, or frequent pulmonary infections
- Clients with frequent sexually transmitted diseases, complicated pregnancies, multiple abortions, or sexual dysfunction
- Clients who complain of chest pains or palpitations or who have histories of admissions to rule out myocardial infarctions
- Clients who give histories of activities that place them at risk for human immunodeficiency virus (HIV) infections; (multiple sexual partners, multiple rapes)
- Clients with family history of addiction, history of childhood sexual, physical, or emotional abuse, social and financial or marital problems.

Modified from Master S, Terpstra JK: Recognition and diagnosis. In Schnoll SH, Horvatich PK, Terpstra JK: *Prescribing drugs with abuse liability*, Richmond, VA, 1992, DSAM, MCV-VCU.

Dietary History for Older Adults

- Does the older adult need or have help in preparing meals?
- Are meals ever skipped?
- Are the four food groups represented in the daily diet? (milk, two servings; meats, two to three servings; cereals, four servings; fruits and vegetables, four or more servings).
- Does the older adult take nutritional supplements such as multivitamins?
- Does the older adult take any medication affecting appetite or absorption of nutrients?
- Does the older adult have a special diet or does the client's diet contain an unusual amount of alcohol, sweets, or fried food?

Modified from Dwyer JT et al: Assessing nutritional status in elderly patients, *Am Family Physician* 47(3):613, 1993.

Table 33-7	**Nursing History for Weight Assessment**
ASSESSMENT CATEGORY	**RATIONALE**
Ask about total weight lost or gained; compare with usual weight; note time period for loss (e.g., gradual, sudden, desired, or undesired).	Determines severity of problem and may reveal if related to disease process, change in eating pattern, or pregnancy.
If weight loss desired; ask about eating pattern, diet plan followed, usual daily calorie intake, appetite.	Helps to determine appropriateness of diet plan followed.
If weight loss undesired; ask about anorexia, vomiting, diarrhea, thirst, frequent urination, change in lifestyle or activity.	Focuses on pathologies that may cause weight loss, e.g., gastrointestinal problems.
Assess if client has noted changes in social aspects of eating; more meals in restaurants, or rushing to eat meals; stress at work, missing meal time.	Lifestyle changes can contribute to weight changes.
Assess if client takes chemotherapy, diuretics, insulin, psychotropics, steroids, nonprescription diet pills, or laxatives.	Weight gain or loss can be side effect of these medications.

ment, the nurse asks clients their current height and weight. Standardized height and weight tables can help reveal the normal expected weight for a client at a given height (see Appendix). A weight gain of 5 lbs or 2.3 kg in a day may indicate fluid retention problems. If the client has lost more than 5% of body weight in a month or 10% in 6 months, the loss is significant.

Clients should be weighed at the same time of day, on the same scale, and in the same clothes to allow an objective comparison of subsequent weights. While body weight may seem routine, care should be taken to be certain of accuracy since medical and nursing decisions (e.g., drug dosage determinations, lifting and positioning) are made on weight changes. Clients capable of bearing their own weight use a standing scale. The nurse calibrates a standard platform scale by moving the large and small weights to *zero*. The balance beam should be made level and steady by adjusting the calibrating knob. Electronic scales are automatically calibrated each time they are used. The client stands on the scale platform and remains still (Fig. 33-6). The nurse moves the largest weight to the 50-lb or 10-kg increment under the client's weight. Then the smaller weight is adjusted to balance the scale at the nearest $1/4$ lb or 0.1 kg (Seidel et al, 1995). Electronic scales automatically display weight within seconds (Fig. 33-7).

Stretcher and chair scales are available for clients unable to bear weight. After being transferred to the scale, the client is lifted above the bed by a hydraulic device and the weight is measured on a balance beam or digital display. Caution must be used when transferring clients to and from the scales.

Infants can be weighed in baskets or on platform scales. The nurse removes clothing and weighs infants in dry, disposable diapers to ensure accurate readings. The weight can later be adjusted for the weight of the diaper. The room should be warm to prevent chills. A light cloth or paper placed on the scale's surface prevents cross-infection from urine or feces. The nurse places infants in baskets or on platforms and holds a hand lightly above them to prevent accidental falls. Weight is measured in ounces and grams.

Different techniques exist for measuring the height of weight-bearing and non–weight-bearing clients. Clients able to stand remove their shoes. A paper towel can be placed on the scale platform or floor so that the client's feet remain clean. A measuring stick or tape is attached vertically to the weight scales or wall. The nurse asks clients to stand erect, exercising good posture. On a standing scale a metal rod, which is attached to the back of the scale, swings out and over the crown of the head (Fig. 33-8). A measuring stick or flat book can also be placed on the head when a scale is unavailable. With the rod or stick placed level horizontally at a 90-degree angle to the measuring stick, the nurse measures height in inches or centimeters.

A non–weight-bearing client (such as an infant) is positioned supine on a firm surface. There are portable devices available that provide a reliable means to measure height. The nurse places the infant on the device, having the parent hold the infant's head against the headboard. With the infant's legs straight at the knees, the footboard is placed against the bottom of the infant's feet (Fig. 33-9). The infant's length is recorded to the nearest 0.5 cm or $1/4$ inch.

A more detailed assessment of infants and children requires measurement of circumference of head and chest. The nurse uses a paper measuring tape to record the infant's measurements at each health visit until 2 years of age, and then measures the child's head circumference until 6 years of age (Seidel et al, 1995).

Accurate measurements require placement of the measuring tape at the correct anatomical location. The nurse wraps the tape snugly around the child's head at the occipital protuberance and supraorbital prominence. This is the location of the largest circumference. The nurse records the nearest 0.5 cm or $1/8$ inch measurement. Growth charts indicate the appropriate circumference for the child's age.

A chest circumference can be compared with the head circumference to rule out problems in head or chest size. The nurse firmly wraps the measuring tape around the infant's chest at the nipple line without causing a skin indentation. Measurement is taken midway between inspiration and expiration and read to the nearest 0.5 cm or $1/8$ inch.

SKIN, HAIR, AND NAILS

The skin provides the body's external protection, regulates body temperature, and acts as a sensory organ for pain,

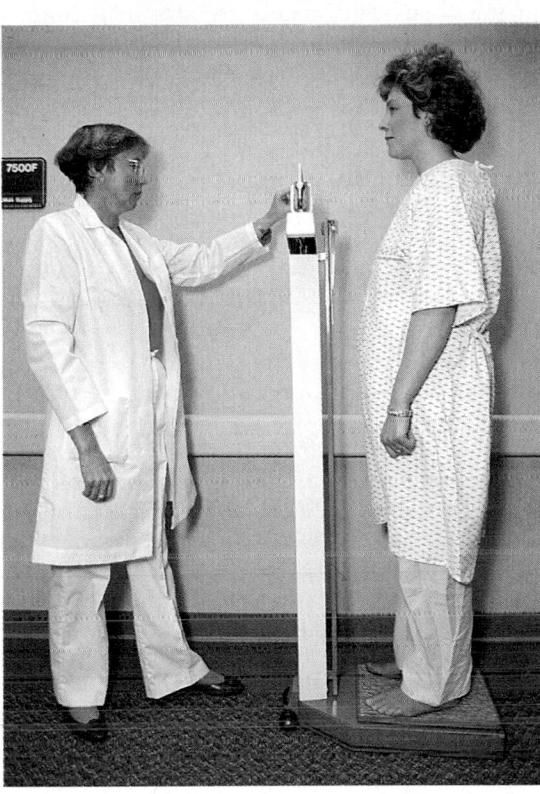

Fig. 33-6 The client stands on the scale as the nurse adjusts the balance.

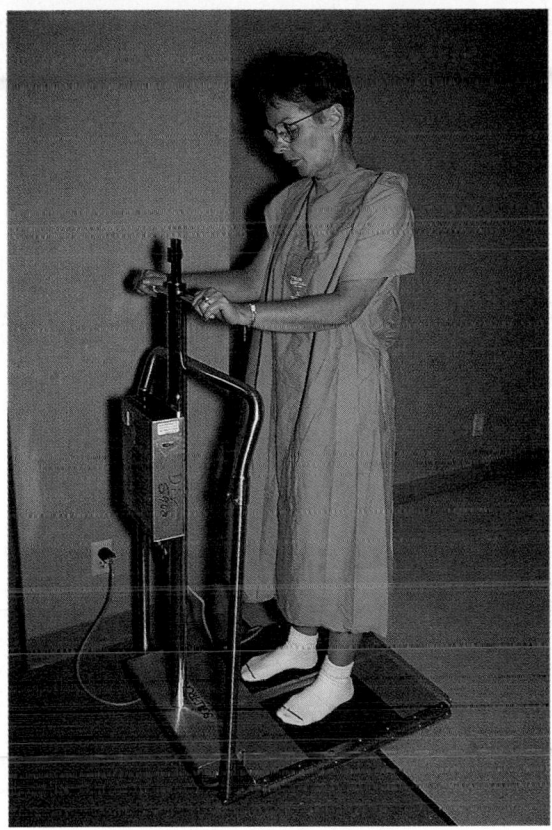

Fig. 33-7 Client stands on electronic scale.

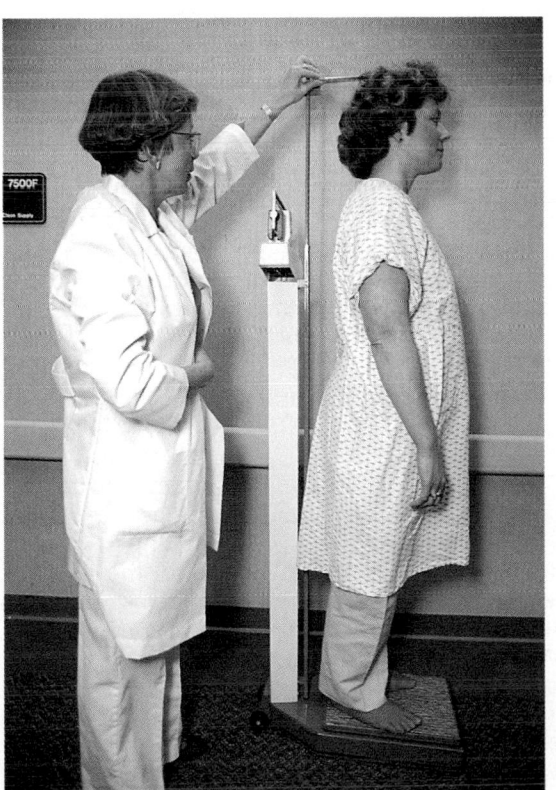

Fig. 33-8 The client stands erect to permit accurate measurement of height.

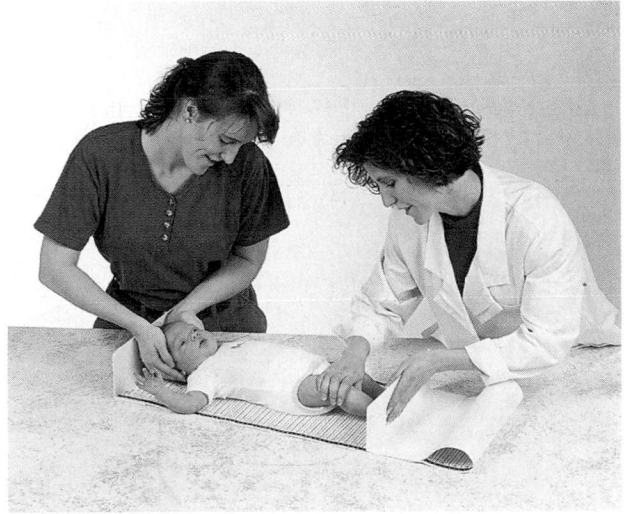

Fig. 33-9 Measurement of infant length. *(From Seidel HM et al: Mosby's guide to physical examination, ed 3, 1995, Mosby.)*

temperature, and touch. Assessment of the **integument** includes the skin, hair, scalp, and nails. The nurse may initially inspect all skin surfaces or may assess the skin gradually while other body systems are examined. The physical assessment skills of inspection, palpation, and olfaction are used to assess the integument's function and integrity.

Skin

Assessment of the skin can reveal a variety of conditions including changes in oxygenation, circulation, nutrition, local tissue damage, and hydration. In a hospital setting the majority of clients are older adults, debilitated clients, or young but seriously ill. As a result there are significant risks for skin lesions resulting from trauma to the skin while administering care, from exposure to pressure during immobilization, or from reaction to various medications used in treatment. Clients most at risk are the neurologically impaired, chronically ill, the orthopedic client, and clients with diminished mental status, poor tissue oxygenation, low cardiac output, and inadequate nutrition. In nursing homes and extended care facilities, clients may be at risk for many of the same problems depending on their level of mobility and presence of chronic illness. Nurses must routinely assess the skin to look for primary or initial lesions that may develop. Without proper care, primary lesions can quickly deteriorate to become secondary lesions that require more extensive nursing care. The development of a pressure ulcer, for example, can lengthen a hospital stay unless it is prevented or discovered early and treated properly (see Chapter 38).

The incidence of **melanoma**, an aggressive form of skin cancer, has increased about 4% every year since 1973 (ACS,

1995). In addition, the incidence of highly curable basal cell and squamous cell cancers are also increasing. Cutaneous malignancies are the most common neoplasms seen in clients (Smoller and Smoller, 1992). The nurse must incorporate a thorough skin assessment for all clients and educate them about self-examination (see the box below).

The condition of the client's skin reveals the need for nursing intervention. The nurse uses assessment findings to determine the type of hygiene measures required to maintain integrity of the integument (see Chapter 40). Adequate nutrition and hydration become goals of therapy if the nurse identifies alterations in the integument's status (see Chapter 41).

Adequate illumination of the skin is required during assessment. If open, moist, or draining skin lesions are present, disposable gloves are needed for palpation. Although the nurse observes each part of the body during an examination, it helps to make a brief but careful overall visual sweep of the entire body (Seidel et al, 1995). This gives the nurse a good idea of the distribution and extent of any lesions and to note overall symmetry in skin color. Because the nurse inspects all skin surfaces, the client must assume several positions. The nursing history for skin assessment is outlined in Table 33-8. If abnormalities are seen during an examination, the nurse palpates the involved areas. Skin odors are usually noted in the skin folds, such as the axilla or under the female client's breasts. Fig. 33-10 illustrates a normal cross section of the skin.

COLOR

Skin color varies from body part to body part and from person to person. Despite individual variations, skin color

---

CLIENT TEACHING
During Skin Assessment

OBJECTIVES
- Client will perform a monthly self-examination of the skin.
- Client will identify factors that increase the risk of skin cancer.
- Client will follow hygiene practices aimed at maintaining skin integrity.

TEACHING STRATEGIES
- Instruct client to conduct a complete monthly self-examination of the skin, noting moles, blemishes, and birthmarks. Tell client to inspect all skin surfaces. Cancerous melanomas start as small, molelike growths that increase in size, change color, become ulcerated, and bleed. A simple ABCD rule (American Cancer Society, 1995) outlines warning signals:
  - A is for **A**symmetry
  - B is for **B**order irregularity, edges are ragged, notched, or blurred.
  - C is for **C**olor, pigmentation is not uniform.
  - D is for **D**iameter; greater than 6 mm.
- Tell client to report to a physician or care provider any change in skin lesions or a sore that does not heal.
- Instruct client to prevent skin cancer by avoiding overexposure to the sun: wear wide-brimmed hats and long

sleeves, apply sunscreens with SPF of 15 or greater approximately 20 minutes before going into the sun and after swimming or perspiring, avoid tanning under the direct sun at midday (10 AM to 3 PM), and do not use indoor sunlamps, tanning parlors, or tanning pills. Medications such as oral contraceptives and antibiotics can make the skin more sensitive to the sun. Special care should be taken to protect children from the sun.
- Instruct client to report any lesion that bleeds or fails to heal to a physician. Especially instruct older adults, who tend to have delayed wound healing.
- To treat "winter itch," tell client to avoid hot water, harsh soaps, and drying agents such as rubbing alcohol. Use a superfatted (Dove) soap, pat rather than rub the skin.
- Tell client to apply lotion and moisturizers (mineral oil) to the skin regularly to reduce itching and drying, and wear cotton clothing (Hardy, 1990)

EVALUATION
- Observe client perform skin assessment.
- Have client describe signs of skin cancer and measures to take to prevent skin cancer.
- Ask client to describe methods for keeping the skin lubricated and supple.

Table 33-8	Nursing History for Skin Assessment

ASSESSMENT CATEGORY	RATIONALE
Ask client about history of changes in the skin: dryness, pruritus, sores, rashes, lumps, color, texture, odor, lesion that does not heal.	Client is best source to recognize change. Skin cancer may first be noticed as a localized change in skin color.
Consider if the client has the following history: Age (over 50); male; fair, freckled, ruddy complexion; light-colored hair or eyes; tendency to burn easily.	Characteristics are risk factors for skin cancer.
Determine whether client works or spends excessive time outside. If so, ask whether a sunscreen is worn and the level of protection.	Exposed areas such as face and arms will be more pigmented than rest of body. Use of sunscreen is recommended by the American Cancer Society (1995).
Determine whether client has noted lesions or changes in skin.	Most skin changes do not develop suddenly. Change in character of lesion might indicate cancer. Bruising indicates trauma or bleeding disorder.
Question client about frequency of bathing and type of soap used.	Excessive bathing and use of harsh soaps can cause dry skin.
Ask if client has had recent trauma to skin.	Injury can cause bruising and changes in skin texture.
Determine whether client has history of allergies.	Skin rashes commonly occur from allergies.
Ask if client uses topical medications or home remedies on skin.	Incorrect use of topical agents may cause inflammation or irritation.
Ask if client goes to tanning parlors, uses sun lamps, or takes tanning pills.	Overexposure of skin to these irritants can cause skin cancer.
Ask if client has family history of serious skin disorders such as skin cancer or psoriasis.	Family history may reveal information about client's condition.
Determine if client works with creosote, coal tar, and/or petroleum products.	Exposure to these agents creates risk for skin cancer.

is usually uniform over the body. Table 33-9 lists common variations. Normal skin pigmentation ranges in tone from ivory or light pink to ruddy pink in white skin; light to deep brown or olive in dark skin. Sundarkened or darker skin is common around knees and elbows. **Basal cell carcinomas** are most commonly seen in sun-exposed areas and frequently occur in a background of sun-damaged skin (Smoller and Smoller, 1992). In older adults, **pigmentation** increases unevenly, causing discolored skin. While inspecting the skin the nurse must be aware that color may be masked by cosmetics or tanning agents.

The assessment of color first involves areas of the skin not exposed to the sun, such as the palms of the hands. The nurse notes if the skin is unusually pale or dark. Areas exposed to the sun, such as the face and arms, will be darker. It is more difficult to note changes such as pallor or cyanosis in clients with dark skin. Usually color hues are best seen in the palms, soles of the feet, lips, tongue, and nail beds. Areas of increased color (hyperpigmentation) and decreased color (hypopigmentation) are common.

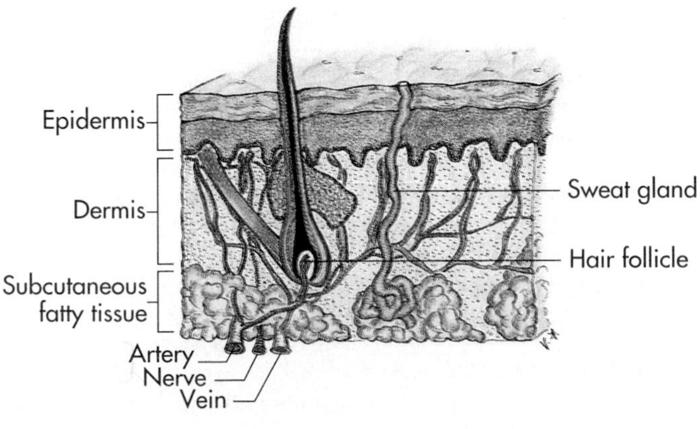

The nurse focuses inspection on sites where abnormalities are more easily identified. For example, pallor is more easily seen in the face, buccal (mouth) mucosa, conjunctiva, and nail beds. **Cyanosis** (bluish discoloration) is best observed in the lips, nail beds, palpebral conjunctivae, and palms. The best site to inspect for **jaundice** (yellow-orange discoloration) is the client's sclera. Normal reactive hyperemia, or redness, is most often seen in regions exposed to pressure such as the sacrum, heels, and greater trochanter.

The nurse inspects for any patches or areas of skin color variation. Localized skin changes, such as pallor or **erythema** (red discoloration), may indicate circulatory changes. For example, an area of erythema may be due to localized vasodilation resulting from a sunburn or fever. An area of an extremity that appears unusually pale may result from arterial occlusion or edema. It is important to ask if the client has noticed any changes in skin coloring. The client usually knows whether a change has occurred.

A pattern of findings that is becoming more common is that associated with clients who are chemically dependent and are IV drug abusers. Usually clients are in denial about their disease and it may be difficult to recognize signs and symptoms after just one physical exam (Caulker-Burnett, 1994). A client who takes repeated intravenous injections

Fig. 33-10 A cross section of the skin reveals three layers: epidermis, dermis, and subcutaneous fatty tissues.

Table 33-9	Skin Color Variations		
COLOR	**CONDITION**	**CAUSES**	**ASSESSMENT LOCATIONS**
Bluish (cyanosis)	Increased amount of deoxygenated hemoglobin (associated with hypoxia)	Heart or lung disease, cold environment	Nail beds, lips, mouth, skin (severe cases)
Pallor (decrease in color)	Reduced amount of oxyhemoglobin	Anemia	Face, conjunctivae, nail beds, palms of hands
	Reduced visibility of oxyhemoglobin resulting from decreased blood flow	Shock	Skin, nail beds, conjunctivae, lips
Loss of Pigmentation	Vitiligo	Congenital or autoimmune condition causing lack of pigment	Patchy areas on skin over face, hands, arms
Yellow-orange (jaundice)	Increased deposit of bilirubin in tissues	Liver disease, destruction of red blood cells	Sclera, mucous membranes, skin
Red (erythema)	Increased visibility of oxyhemoglobin caused by dilation or increased blood flow	Fever, direct trauma, blushing, alcohol intake	Face, area of trauma, sacrum, shoulders, other common sites for pressure ulcers
Tan-brown	Increased amount of melanin	Suntan, pregnancy	Areas exposed to sun: face, arms; areolae, nipples

---

Physical Findings of the Skin Indicative of Substance Abuse

BODY SYSTEM	COMMONLY ASSOCIATED DRUG
Diaphoresis	Sedative hypnotic (including alcohol)
Spider angiomas	Alcohol, stimulants
Burns (especially fingers)	Alcohol
Needle marks	Opioids
Contusion, abrasions, cuts, scars	Alcohol, other sedative hypnotics
"Homemade" tatoos	Cocaine, IV opioids, (prevents detection of injection sites)
Increased vascularity of face	Alcohol

Modified from Caulker-Burnett I: Primary care screening for substance abuse, *Nurse Practitioner* 19(6):42, 1994.

may have edematous, reddened, and warm areas along the arms and legs. This pattern suggests recent injections. Evidence of old injection sites appears as hyperpigmented and shiny or scarred areas. The box above summarizes additional physical findings associated with substance abuse.

MOISTURE

Moisture in the skin is directly related to the degree of client hydration and the condition of the outer lipid layer of the skin surface (DeWitt, 1990). The hydration of skin and mucous membranes helps reveal body fluid imbalances, changes in the integument's environment, and regulation of body temperature. *Moisture* refers to wetness and oiliness. The skin is normally smooth and dry. Minimal perspiration or oiliness should be present (Seidel et al, 1995). Increased perspiration may be associated with activity, warm environment, obesity, anxiety, or excitement.

Skin folds such as the axillae are normally moist. Excessively dry skin is common in older adults and persons who use excessive amounts of soap during bathing.

The nurse uses ungloved fingertips to palpate the skin surface and observes mucous membranes for dullness, dryness, crusting, and flaking. Flaking is the appearance of dandruff-like flakes when the skin surface is lightly rubbed. Scaling is fishlike scales that are easily rubbed off the skin's surface. Both flaking and scaling are believed to be valid indicators for abnormally dry skin (Hardy, 1990). The client is asked about itching. "Winter itch" is a common condition found in climates with low humidity during the winter season (DeWitt, 1990). This excessive dryness can worsen existing skin conditions such as **eczema** and **dermatitis**.

TEMPERATURE

The temperature of the skin depends on the amount of blood circulating through the dermis. Increased or decreased skin temperature indicates an increase or decrease in blood flow. Normally the skin temperature ranges from cool to warm to the touch. Temperature is more accurately assessed by palpating the skin with the dorsal surface of the hands or fingers. Skin temperature may be the same throughout the body or may vary in one area, such as the localized warmth at an infected wound site or the coldness of fingers resulting from reduced blood flow. The nurse looks for bilateral symmetry. Assessment of skin temperature is a basic assessment when the client is at risk for having impaired circulation (e.g., after application of a cast or tight bandage or after vascular surgery). In addition, a nurse can identify a stage I pressure ulcer early when noting warmth and erythema of an area of the skin.

TEXTURE

The character of the skin's surface and the feel of deeper portions are its texture. The nurse determines whether the client's skin is smooth or rough, thin or thick, tight or supple, and **indurated** (hardened) or soft by stroking it and palpating it lightly with the fingertips. The texture of the skin is normally smooth, soft, even and flexible in children and adults. However, the texture is usually not uniform throughout. The palms of the hand and soles of the feet tend to be thicker. In older adults, the skin becomes wrinkled and leathery because of a decrease in collagen, subcutaneous fat, and sweat glands.

Localized changes may result from trauma, surgical wounds, or lesions. When irregularities in texture such as scars or hardening are found, the nurse asks if the client has had a recent injury to the skin. Deeper palpation may reveal irregularities such as tenderness or localized areas of induration commonly caused by repeated intramuscular or subcutaneous injections. If the client has diabetes or receives vitamin B_{12} or iron injections, indurated areas are common.

TURGOR

Turgor is the skin's elasticity, which can be diminished by edema or dehydration. Normally the skin loses its elasticity with age. To assess the skin turgor, a fold of skin on the back of the forearm or sternal area is grasped with the fingertips and released (Fig. 33-11). Normally the skin lifts easily and snaps back immediately to its resting position. The back of the hand is not the best place to test for turgor as the skin is normally loose and thin (Seidel et al, 1995). The skin stays pinched when turgor is poor. The nurse notes the ease with which the skin moves and the speed at which it returns to place. Failure of the skin to reassume its normal contour or shape indicates dehydration. The client with poor skin turgor does not have a resilience to the normal wear and tear on the skin. The skin tends to stay pinched or tented when turgor is poor. A decrease in turgor predisposes the client to skin breakdown.

VASCULARITY

The circulation of the skin affects color in localized areas and the appearance of superficial blood vessels. With aging, capillaries become fragile. Localized pressure areas, found after a client has lain or sat in one position, appear reddened, pink, or pale (see Chapter 38). **Petechiae** are tiny, pinpoint-sized, red or purple spots on the skin caused by

small hemorrhages in the skin layers. Petechiae may indicate serious blood-clotting disorders, drug reactions, or liver disease.

EDEMA

Areas of the skin become swollen or edematous from a buildup of fluid in the tissues. Direct trauma and impairment of venous return are two common causes of **edema**. Edematous areas should be inspected for location, color, and shape. For the client with dependent edema caused by poor venous return, typical sites of edema are the feet, ankles, and sacrum. The formation of edema separates the skin's surface from the pigmented and vascular layers, masking skin color. Edematous skin looks stretched and shiny. The nurse palpates areas of edema to determine mobility, consistency, and tenderness. When pressure from the examiner's fingers leaves an indentation in the edematous area, it is called *pitting edema*. To check the degree of pitting edema the nurse presses the edematous area firmly with the thumb for 5 seconds and releases. The depth of pitting, recorded in millimeters (Seidel et al, 1995) determines the degree of edema. For example, 1+ edema equals 2 mm depth.

LESIONS

During palpation the nurse may locate skin lesions, which are any pathological skin change or occurrence (Seidel and others, 1995). The skin is normally free of lesions, except common freckles or age-related changes such as skin tags, **senile keratosis** (thickening of skin), **cherry angiomas** (ruby red papules), and atrophic warts. Lesions may be primary (occurring as initial spontaneous manifestations of a pathological process), such as the wheal of an insect bite, or secondary (resulting from later formation or trauma to a primary lesion), such as a pressure ulcer.

When a lesion is detected, it is inspected for color, location, texture, size, shape, type, grouping (clustered or linear), and distribution (localized or generalized). Any exudate is observed for color, odor, amount, and consistency. The size is best measured by using a small, clear, flexible ruler, divided in centimeters. Comparing a lesion to a household measure such as a coin or eraser, is not reliable (Seidel et al, 1995). Lesions should be measured in centimeters in all dimensions (height, width, depth) when possible.

Palpation determines the lesion's mobility, contour (flat, raised, or depressed), and consistency (soft or indurated). Certain types of lesions present a characteristic pattern. For example, a tumor is usually an elevated, solid lesion larger than 2 cm. Primary lesions such as macules and nodules arise from some stimulus to the skin (see the box on p. 660). Secondary lesions such as ulcers occur as alterations in primary lesions.

After it is identified, a lesion is closely inspected with good illumination. The lesion is palpated gently, covering its entire area. If the lesion is moist or draining fluid, gloves are worn during palpation to prevent contact or spread of infectious organisms.

It helps to ask clients if they have noticed any lesions, their causes, and any recent changes in their character (see the box on p. 656). Further questioning as to how a lesion bothers a client and what has been done to care for it may reveal how a client feels about the disorder. Many clients re-

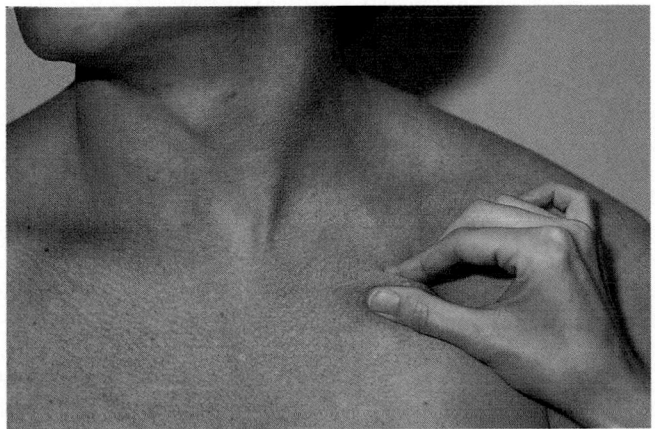

Fig. 33-11 Assessment for skin turgor. *(From Seidel HM et al: Mosby's guide to physical examination, ed 3, 1995, Mosby.)*

Types of Primary Skin Lesions

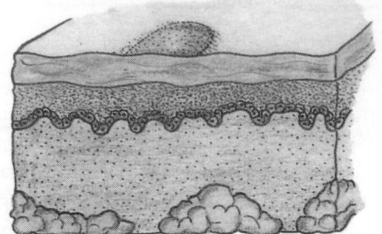

Macule: flat, nonpalpable change in skin color, smaller than 1 cm (e.g., freckle, petechia)

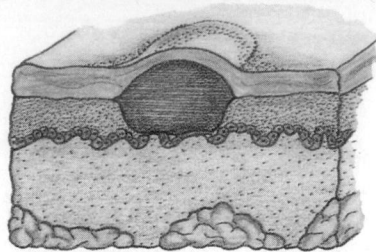

Papule: palpable, circumscribed, solid elevation in skin, smaller than 0.5 cm (e.g., elevated nevus)

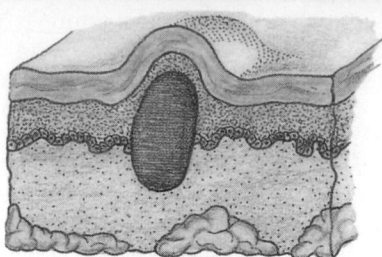

Nodule: elevated solid mass, deeper and firmer than papule, 0.5-0.2 cm (e.g., wart)

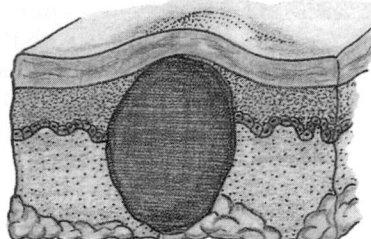

Tumor: solid mass that may extend deep through subcutaneous tissue, larger than 1-2 cm (e.g., epithelioma)

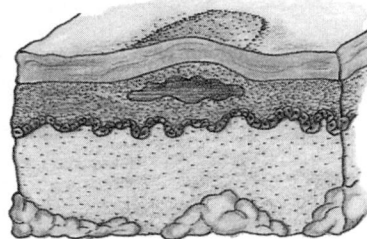

Wheal: irregularly shaped, elevated area or superficial localized edema, varies in size (e.g., hive, mosquito bite)

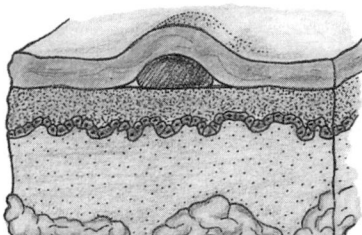

Vesicle: circumscribed elevation of skin (filled with serous fluid, smaller than 0.5 cm (e.g., herpes simplex, chickenpox)

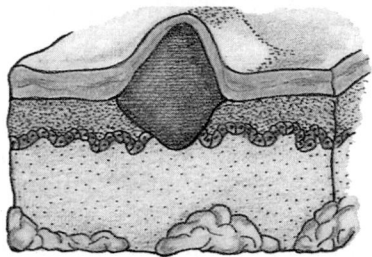

Pustule: circumscribed elevation of skin similar to vesicle but filled with puss, varies in size (e.g., acne, staphylococcal infection)

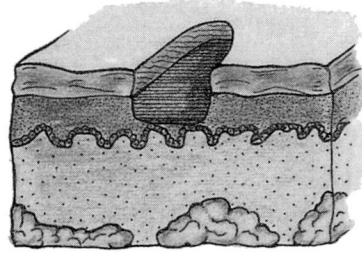

Ulcer: deep loss of skin surface that may extend to dermis and frequently bleeds and scars, varies in size (e.g., venous stasis ulcer)

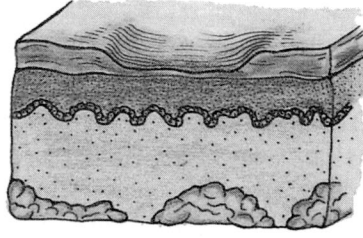

Atrophy: thinning of skin with loss of normal skin furrow with skin appearing shiny and translucent, varies in size (e.g., arterial insufficiency)

---

act with fear and anxiety to rashes or other lesions. Cancerous lesions frequently undergo changes in color and size (see the box on p. 661). Abnormal lesions are reported to the physician because further examination may be required.

Hair and Scalp

The following types of hair cover the body: terminal hair (long, coarse, thick hair easily visible on the scalp, axillae, pubic areas, and in the beard of males) and vellus hair (small, soft, tiny hairs covering the whole body except for palms and soles). Good lighting allows the nurse to inspect the condition and distribution of hair and integrity of the scalp. Assessment of the hair occurs during all portions of the examination. The nurse assesses the distribution, thick-

ness, texture, and lubrication of the hair. In addition, the nurse inspects for infection or infestation of the scalp.

INSPECTION

Clients are sensitive about personal appearance. During inspection explain the need to separate parts of the hair to detect problems. If lesions or lice are probable, the nurse wears disposable gloves to avoid infection. Table 33-10 describes the nursing history for a hair and scalp assessment.

The nurse begins inspection by noting the color, distribution, quantity, thickness, texture, and lubrication of body hair. Scalp hair may be coarse or fine, curly or straight, and should be shiny, smooth, and pliant. While separating sections of scalp hair the nurse observes characteristics of

Skin Malignancies in the Older Adult

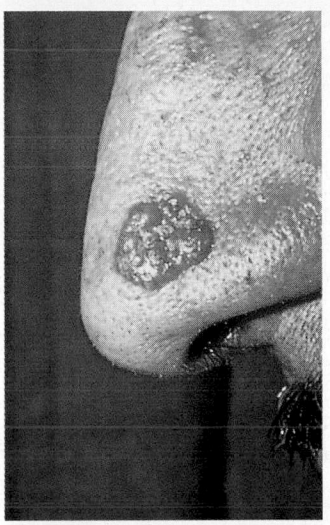

BASAL CELL CARCINOMA
0.5 cm to 1.0 cm crusted lesion that may be flat or
 raised, and may have a rolled somewhat scaly border.
Frequently there are underlying, widely dilated blood vessels that can be seen clinically within the lesions.

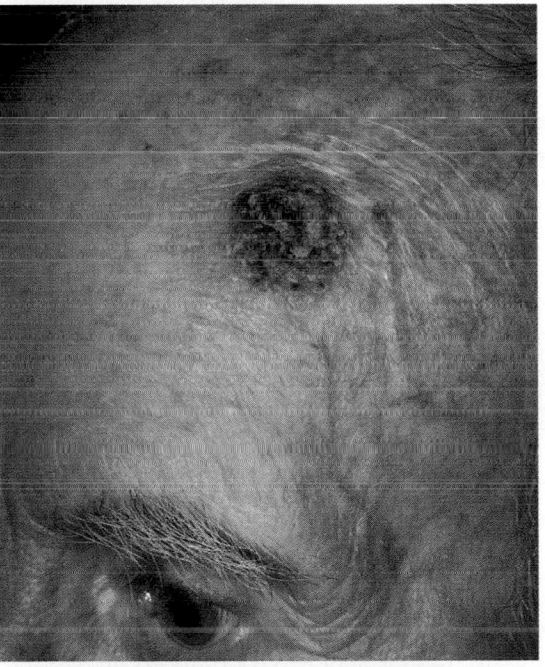

SQUAMOUS CELL CARCINOMA
Occurs more often on mucosal surfaces and nonexposed
 areas of skin, compared to basal cell.
0.5 cm to 1.5 cm scaly lesions, may be ulcerated or
 crusted. Frequently appear and grow more rapidly than
 basal cell.

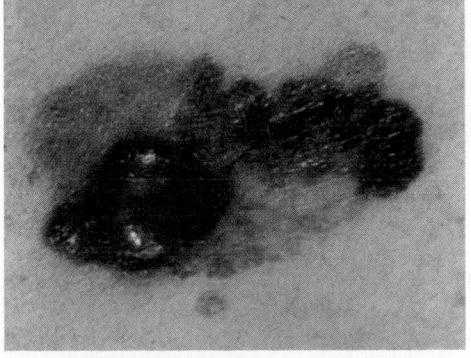

MELANOMA
0.5 cm to 1.0 cm brown, flat lesions that may arise on
 sun-exposed or nonexposed skin. Variegated pigmentation, irregular borders, and indistinct margins.
Ulceration, recent growth, or recent change in long-
 standing mole are ominous signs.

Modified from Smoller J, Smoller BR: Skin malignancies in the elderly: diagnosable, treatable, and potentially curable, *J Geront Nurs* 18(5):19, 1992). Illustrations from Belcher AE: *Cancer nursing*, St Louis, 1992, Mosby; Habif TP: *Clinical dermatology*, ed 3, St Louis, 1996, Mosby; and Zitelli B, Davis H: *Atlas of
pediatric physical diagnosis*, ed 2, St Louis, 1991, Mosby.

Table 33-10	Nursing History for Hair and Scalp Assessment	
ASSESSMENT CATEGORY	**RATIONALE**	
Ask client if wig or hairpiece is being worn and request that it be removed.	Wigs or hairpieces interfere with inspection of hair and scalp. (Client may request to omit this part of examination.)	
Determine if client has noted change in growth or loss of hair.	Change may occur slowly over time.	
Identify type of shampoo, other hair care products, and curling irons used for grooming.	Excessive use of chemical agents and burning of hair causes drying and brittleness.	
Determine if client has recently taken chemotherapy (if hair loss noted) or vasodilator (Minoxidil) if hair growth noted.	Chemotherapeutic agents kill cells that rapidly multiply, such as tumor cells and normal hair cells. Minoxidil causes excessive hair growth	
Has client noted changes in diet or appetite.	Nutrition can influence condition of hair.	

CLIENT TEACHING
During Hair and Scalp Assessment

OBJECTIVE
- Client will perform proper hygiene practices for care of the hair and scalp.

TEACHING STRATEGIES
- Instruct client about basic hygiene practices for care of the hair and scalp (see Chapter 40).
- Instruct clients who have head lice to shampoo thoroughly with pediculicide (shampoo available at drug stores) in cold water, comb thoroughly with fine-tooth comb (following product directions), and discard comb.
- After combing remove any detectable nits or nit cases with tweezers or between the fingernails. A dilute solution of vinegar and water may help loosen nits.
- Instruct clients and parents about ways to reduce transmission of lice:
  - Do not share personal care items with others.
  - Vacuum all rugs, car seats, pillows, furniture, and flooring thoroughly and discard vacuum bag.
  - Seal nonwashable items in plastic bags for 14 days if parents are unable to afford dry-cleaning and do not have vacuum (Clore, 1989).
  - Use thorough handwashing.
  - Launder all clothing, linen, and bedding in hot soap and water and dry in hot dryer for at least 20 minutes. Dry-clean nonwashable items (Wong, 1995).
- Instruct the client that his or her partner must be notified if lice were sexually transmitted.

EVALUATION
- Have client describe methods used to care for hair and scalp.
- Have client explain steps taken to reduce lice transmission in the home.

color and coarseness. Color varies from very light blond to black to gray and may show alterations from rinses or dyes. In older adults, the hair becomes dull gray, white, or yellow. It also thins over the scalp, axillae, and pubic areas. Older men lose facial hair, whereas older women may develop hair on the chin and upper lip.

Much of the information gathered about characteristics of hair growth comes from the client. The nurse needs to be aware of the normal distribution of hair growth in a man and a woman. At puberty a change in the amount and distribution of hair growth occurs. A client with hormone disorders may experience an unusual distribution and growth. A woman with **hirsutism** has hair growth on the upper lip, chin, and cheeks, with vellus hair becoming coarser over the body. A change in hair growth can negatively affect body image and emotional well-being.

Changes may occur in the thickness, texture, and lubrication of scalp hair. Disturbances such as a febrile illness or scalp disease can result in hair loss. Conditions such as thyroid disease can alter the condition of the hair, making it fine and brittle. Hair loss (**alopecia**), or thinning of the hair, is usually related to genetic tendencies and endocrine disorders such as diabetes, thyroiditis, and even menopause (DeWitt, 1990). Poor nutrition can cause stringy, dull, dry, and thin hair. The hair is lubricated from the oil of sebaceous glands. Excessively oily hair is associated with androgen hormone stimulation. Dry, brittle hair occurs with aging and with excessive use of shampoo or other chemical agents.

The amount of hair covering the extremities may be reduced as a result of aging and arterial insufficiency and is most commonly seen over the lower extremities. In women, loss of hair should not be confused with shaven legs.

When inspecting the scalp, the nurse asks if the client has noticed anything unusual. The scalp is normally smooth and inelastic, with even coloration. By carefully separating strands of hair the nurse can thoroughly examine the scalp for lesions, which can easily go unnoticed in thick hair. The nurse notes the characteristics of any scalp lesion. If lumps or bruises are found, the nurse asks if the client has experienced recent trauma to the head. Moles on the scalp are common. The nurse should warn the client that combing or brushing can cause a mole to bleed. Scaliness or dryness of the scalp is frequently caused by dandruff or psoriasis.

Careful inspection of hair follicles on the scalp and pubic areas may reveal lice or other parasites. The three types of lice are *Pediculus humanus capitis* (head lice), *Pediculus humanus corporis* (body lice), and *Pediculus pubis* (crab lice). Head and crab lice attach their eggs to hair. The tiny eggs look like oval particles of dandruff. The lice themselves are difficult to see. Head and body lice are very small with grayish white bodies. Crab lice have red legs. The nurse looks for bites or pustular eruptions in the hair follicles and in areas where skin surfaces meet, such as behind the ears and in the groin. The discovery of lice requires immediate treatment (see the box above).

Nails

The condition of the nails can reflect an individual's general state of health, state of nutriton, occupation, and level

Table 33-11	Nursing History for Nail Assessment
ASSESSMENT CATEGORY	**RATIONALE**
Ask if client has experienced recent trauma or changes in nails (splitting, breaking, discoloration, thickening, etc.).	Trauma may change shape and growth of nail. Systemic conditions cause changes in color, growth, and shape. Alterations may occur slowly over time.
Has the client had other symptoms of pain, swelling, presence of systemic disease with fever, psychological or physical stress?	Can help to indicate if change in nails is due to local or systemic problem
Question client's nail care practices.	Chemical agents can cause drying of nails. Improper care may damage nails and cuticles.
Determine if client has risks for nail or foot problems (e.g., diabetes, older adulthood, obesity).	Vascular changes associated with diabetes reduce blood flow to peripheral tissues; foot lesions and thickened nails are common. Older adult may have trouble performing foot and nail care because of poor vision, uncoordination, or inability to bend over. Obese clients have difficulty bending over.

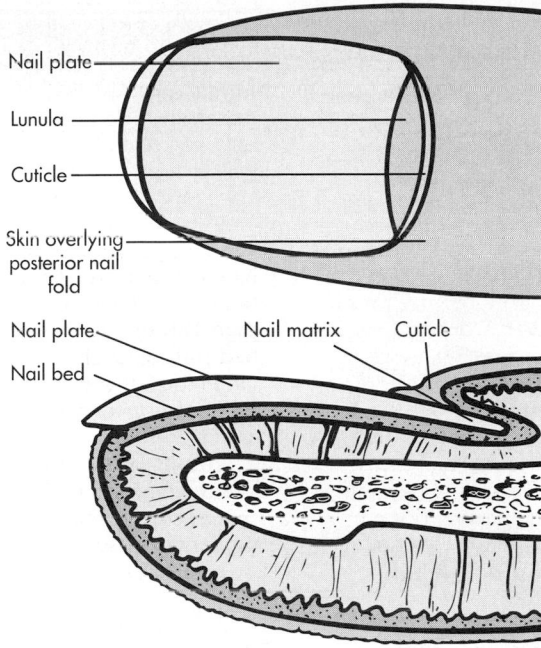

Fig. 33-12 Components of the nail unit. *(From Thompson SM et al: Mosby's manual of clinical nursing, ed 2, St Louis, 1989, Mosby–Year Book.)*

of self-care. Even a person's psychological state may be revealed by evidence of nail biting. Before assessing the nails the nurse gathers a brief history (Table 33-11). The most visible portion of the nails is the nail plate, the transparent layer of epithelial cells covering the nail bed (Fig. 33-12). The vascularity of the nail bed creates the nail's underlying color. The semilunar, whitish area at the base of the nail bed is called the *lunula,* from which the nail plate develops.

INSPECTION AND PALPATION

The nurse inspects the nail bed color, cleanliness, length, thickness and shape of the nail plate, texture of the nail, angle between the nail and the nail bed, and condition of the lateral and proximal nail folds aorund the nail. The nurse also palpates the nail base.

Upon first look, the nurse can obtain a quick sense about the client's hygiene practices. The nails are normally transparent, smooth, well rounded, and convex, with a nail bed angle of about 160 degrees. The surrounding cuticles are smooth, intact, and without inflammation. If the nails are ragged, dirty, and poorly kept, there is a good indication that either the client practices infrequent nail care or is physically unable to perform care. Jagged, bitten, or broken nail edges or cuticles can predispose a client to localized infection. Abnormalities such as erythema or swelling should be reported.

In whites the nail beds are pink with translucent white tips. In clients with dark skin, brown or black pigmentation is normally present in longitudinal streaks (Fig. 33-13). Splinter he-

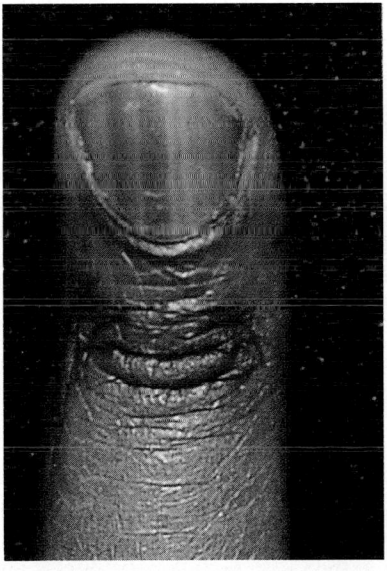

Fig. 33-13 Pigmented bands in nail of client with dark skin. *(From Seidel HM et al: Mosby's guide to physical examination, ed 3, 1995, Mosby.)*

morrhages can be caused by trauma, cirrhosis, diabetes mellitus, and hypertension. Vitamin, protein, and electrolyte changes can also cause lines or bands in the nail beds.

Nails normally grow at a constant rate, but direct injury or generalized disease can impair growth. With aging, the nails of the fingers and toes develop longitudinal striations and grow at a slower rate (Cornell, 1986). Because of insufficient calcium, nails may turn yellow in older adults

Abnormalities of the Nail Bed

160 degrees — Normal nail: Approximately 160 degree angle between nail plate and nail

180 degrees — Clubbing: Change in angle between nail and nail base (eventually larger than 180 degrees); nail bed softening, with nail flattening; often, enlargement of fingertips

180 degrees — *Causes:* Chronic lack of oxygen: heart or pulmonary disease

Beaus's lines: Transverse depressions in nails indicating temporary disturbance of nail growth (Nail grows out over several months.)
Causes: Systemic illness such as severe infection, nail injury

Koilonychia (spoon nail): Concave curves
Causes: Iron deficiency anemia, syphilis, use of strong detergents

Splinter hemorrhages: Red or brown linear streaks in nail bed
Causes: Minor trauma, subacute bacterial endocarditis, trichinosis

Paronychia: Inflammation of skin at base of nail
Causes: Local infection, trauma

CLIENT TEACHING
During Nail Assessment

OBJECTIVE
■ Client will be able to properly care for fingernails, feet, and toe nails.

TEACHING STRATEGIES
■ Instruct client to cut nails only after soaking them about 10 minutes in warm water.
■ Instruct client to avoid use of over-the-counter preparations to treat corns, calluses, or ingrown toenails.
■ Tell clients to cut nails straight across and even with the tops of the fingers or toes. If client has diabetes, tell client to file, not cut, nails.
■ Instruct client to shape nails with a file or emery board.
■ If client is diabetic:
  ■ Wash feet daily in warm water. Inspect the feet each day in a place with good lighting: looking for dry places and cracks in the skin. Soften dry feet by applying a cream or lotion such as Nivea, Eucerin, or Alpha Keri.
  ■ Do not put lotion between the toes.
  ■ Caution client against using sharp objects to poke or dig under the toenail or around the cuticle.
  ■ Have client see a podiatrist for treatment of ingrown toenails and nails that are thick or tend to split.

EVALUATION
■ Inspect nails during next home visit.
■ Have client explain steps to take to avoid injury.

---

turn promptly indicates circulatory insufficiency. An ongoing bluish or purplish cast to the nail bed occurs with cyanosis. A white cast or pallor results from anemia.

Calluses and corns are commonly found on the toes or fingers. A callus is flat and painless. It results from a thickening of the epidermis. Corns are caused by friction and pressure from shoes and can usually be seen over a bony prominence. During the examination, the nurse instructs clients about proper nail care (see the box above).

■ HEAD AND NECK

An examination of the head and neck includes assessment of the head, eyes, ears, nose, mouth, pharynx, and neck (lymph nodes, carotid arteries, thyroid gland, and trachea). The carotid arteries can also be assessed during assessment of peripheral arteries. Assessment of the head and neck uses inspection, palpation, and auscultation, with inspection and palpation often used simultaneously.

Head

INSPECTION AND PALPATION

The nursing history will screen for intracranial injury and local or congenital deformities (Table 33-12). The nurse begins by inspecting the client's head position and facial features. The head is normally held upright and still. Holding the head tilted to one side may be an indication of unilateral hearing or visual loss.

The nurse also notes the client's facial features, looking at the eyelids, eyebrows, nasolabial folds, and mouth for shape and symmetry. It is normal for slight asymmetry to

---

(Berman, Haxby, and Pomerantz, 1988). Also with age the cuticle becomes less thick and wide.

Inspection of the angle between the nail and nail bed normally reveals an angle of 160 degrees (see the box above). A larger angle and softening of the nail bed can indicate chronic oxygenation problems. The nurse palpates the nail base to determine firmness and the condition of circulation. The nail base is normally firm.

To palpate, the nurse gently grasps the client's finger and observes the color of the nail bed. Next, gentle, firm, quick pressure is applied with the thumb to the nail bed and released. As the pressure is applied, the nail bed appears white or blanched; however, the pink color should return immediately on release of pressure. Failure of the pinkness to re-

Table 33-12	Nursing History for Head Assessment
ASSESSMENT CATEGORY	**RATIONALE**
Determine if client experienced recent trauma to the head. If so, assess state of consciousness after injury (immediately upon return and 5 minutes later, duration of unconsciousness), and predisposing factors e.g., seizure, poor vision, blackout.	Trauma is major cause for lumps, bumps, cuts, bruises, or deformities of scalp or skull. Loss of consciousness following head injury indicates possible brain injury.
Ask if client has history of headache; note onset, duration, character, pattern, and associated symptoms.	Character of headache can help to reveal causative factors such as sinus infection, migraine, or neurological disorders.
Determine length of time client has experienced neurological symptoms.	Duration of signs or symptoms may reveal severity of problem.
Review the client's occupational history for use of safety helmets.	Nature of client's occupation can create a risk for head injury.
Ask if the client participates in contact sports, cycling, rollerblading, or skateboarding.	Activities require use of safety helmets.

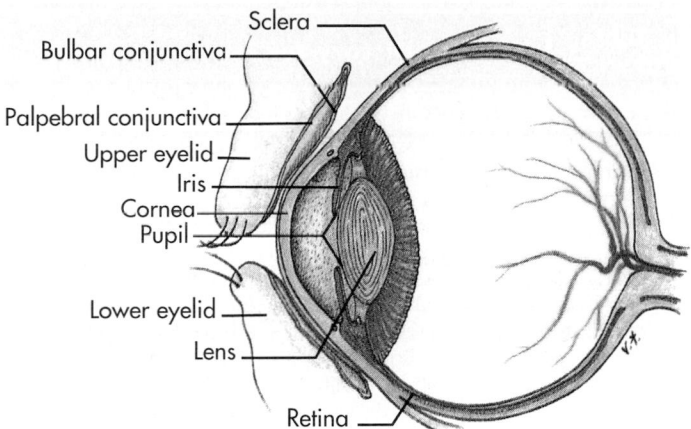

Fig. 33-14 Cross section of the eye.

exist. If there is facial asymmetry, the nurse notes if all features on one side of the face are affected or if only a portion of the face is involved. Various neurological disorders such as facial nerve paralysis affect different nerves that innervate muscles of the face.

Examination continues with the nurse noting the size, shape, and contour of the skull. The skull is generally round with prominences in the frontal area anteriorly and the occipital area posteriorly. Local skull deformities are typically caused by trauma. In infants, large heads may result from congenital anomalies or the buildup of cerebrospinal fluid in the ventricles (**hydrocephalus**). Adults may have enlarged jaws and facial bones resulting from **acromegaly**, a disorder caused by excessive secretion of growth hormone. The nurse palpates the skull for nodules or masses. Gentle rotation of the fingertips down the midline of the scalp and then along the sides of the head reveals abnormalities.

Eyes

Examination of the eyes includes assessment of visual acuity, visual fields, extraocular movements, and external and internal eye structures. Fig. 33-14 shows a cross section of the eye. The assessment detects visual alterations and determines the level of assistance clients require when ambulating or performing self-care activities. Clients with visual problems may also need special aids for reading teaching materials or instructions (e.g., medication labels). Table 33-13 reviews the nursing history for an eye examination. The box on p. 666 describes common types of visual problems.

Fig. 33-15 Assessment of visual acuity using a projection screen with an *E* chart.

VISUAL ACUITY

The assessment of visual acuity, the ability to see small details, tests central vision. The easiest way to assess near vision is to ask clients to read printed material under adequate lighting. If clients wear glasses, they should wear them during the exam. The nurse should know the language clients speak and whether they are literate and able to read. Asking clients to read aloud can help determine literacy. If the client has difficulty reading, move to the next step.

Assessment of distant vision requires use of a Snellen chart (paper chart or projection screen). The chart should be well lighted. Always test vision without corrective lenses first. The nurse has the client sit or stand 20 feet (6.1 m) away from the chart and try to read all of the letters beginning at any line—once with both eyes open and then with each eye separately (with opposite eye covered by an index card or eye cover (Fig. 33-15). Have the client avoid applying pressure to the eye. The nurse notes the smallest line in which the client can read all of the letters correctly and records the visual acuity for that line. Repeat the test with the client wearing corrective lenses. Do the test rapidly

Table 33-13	Nursing History for Eye Assessment

ASSESSMENT CATEGORY	RATIONALE
Determine if client has history of eye disease, eye trauma, diabetes, hypertension, or eye surgery.	Some diseases or trauma can cause risk for partial or complete visual loss. Surgery may have been performed for a visual disorder.
Determine problems that prompted client to seek health care. Ask client about eye pain, photophobia (sensitivity to light), burning, itching, excess tearing or crusting, diplopia (double vision), blurred vision, awareness of a "film" over field of vision, floaters (small, black spots that seem to float across the field of vision), flashing lights, or halos around lights.	Common symptoms of eye disease indicate need for physician referral.
Determine whether there is family history of eye disorders or diseases.	Certain eye problems such as glaucoma or retinitis pigmentosa are inherited.
Assess client's occupational history and recreational hobbies; are safety glasses worn?	Performance of close, intricate work can cause eye fatigue. Working with computers may cause eye strain. Certain occupational tasks (e.g., working with chemicals) and recreational activity (e.g., fencing or motorcycle riding) place persons at risk for eye injury unless precautions are taken.
Ask client if glasses or contacts are worn; how often?	Glasses or contacts should be worn during certain portions of examination for accurate assessment.
Determine when client last visited ophthalmologist or optometrist.	Date of last eye examination reveals level of preventive care taken by client.
Assess medications client is taking, including eye drops or ointment.	Determines need to assess client's knowledge of medications. Certain medications can cause visual symptoms.

Common Eye and Visual Problems

HYPEROPIA
Hyperopia is farsightedness, a refractive error in which rays of light enter the eye and focus behind the retina. Persons are able to clearly see distant objects but not close objects.

MYOPIA
Myopia is nearsightedness, a refractive error in which rays of light enter the eye and focus in front of the retina. Persons are able to clearly see close objects but not distant objects.

PRESBYOPIA
Presbyopia is impaired near vision in middle-age and older adults, caused by loss of elasticity of the lens and associated with the aging process.

ASTIGMATISM
Astigmatism is a condition in which parallel light rays do not focus on a single point on the retina. An uneven curvature of the cornea or lens causes light to be focused on different points.

RETINOPATHY
Noninflammatory eye disorder resulting from changes in retinal blood vessels. Leading cause of blindness.

STRABISMUS
Strabismus is a congenital problem in which the eyes appear crossed. The muscles controlling movement of the eyes are not coordinated.

CATARACTS
A cataract is an increased opacity of the lens, which blocks light rays entering the eye. Cataracts may develop slowly and progressively after age 35 or suddenly after trauma. Cataracts are one of the most common eye disorders. By age 70, most older adults have some evidence of visual impairment from cataracts.*

GLAUCOMA
Glaucoma is intraocular structural damage resulting from elevated intraocular pressure. It is caused by obstruction of the outflow of aqueous humor. Without treatment the disorder can cause blindness.

MACULAR DEGENERATION
Macular degeneration is blurred central vision often occurring suddenly caused by a progressive degeneration of the center of the retina. It is the most common cause of blindness in older adults. There is no cure.

*Data from Kirton M, Richardson M: *Ophthalmic nursing,* ed 3, Philadelphia, 1987, Bailliere-Tindall.

enough so that the client does not memorize the chart (Seidel et al, 1995).

If a client is unable to read, the nurse uses an *E* chart or one with pictures of familiar objects. Instead of reading letters, clients tell the nurse which direction each *E* is pointing or the name of the object. The visual acuity score is recorded for each eye and both eyes.

The Snellen chart has standardized numbers at the end of each line of the chart. The numerator is the number 20 or the distance the client stands from the chart. The denominator is the distance from which the normal eye can read the chart. Normal vision is 20/20. The larger the denominator, the poorer the client's visual acuity. For example, a value of 20/40 means the client, standing 20 feet away, can read a line that a person with normal vision can read from 40 feet away. The nurse records visual acuity as s̄c (without correction) or c̄c (with correction), depending on whether clients wear glasses or contact lenses.

If clients cannot read even the largest letters or figures of a Snellen chart, the nurse tests their ability to count upraised fingers or distinguish light. The nurse holds a hand 30 cm (1 foot) from the face and instructs clients to count the upraised fingers. To check light perception, the nurse shines a penlight into the eye and then turns the light off. If clients note when the light is turned on or off, light perception is intact.

Near vision can be assessed by asking the client to read a hand-held card containing a vision screening chart. Instruct the client to hold the card a comfortable distance (about 14 inches, 5 to 6 cm) from the eyes. The client reads the smallest line possible.

EXTRAOCULAR MOVEMENTS

Six small muscles guide the movement of each eye. Both eyes move parallel to each other in each of the eight directions of gaze (Fig. 33-16). The client sits or stands 2 feet away, facing the nurse. The nurse holds a finger at a comfortable distance (6 to 12 inches or 15 to 30 cm) in front of the client's eyes. The client keeps the head in a fixed position facing the nurse and follows the movement of the finger with the eyes only. The client looks to the right, to the left, up, down, and diagonally up and down to the left and right. The nurse's finger moves smoothly and slowly within the normal field of vision.

As the client gazes in each direction, the nurse observes for parallel eye movement, the position of the upper eyelid

in relation to the iris, and the presence of abnormal movements. As the eyes move through each direction of gaze, the upper eyelid only covers the iris slightly. By periodically stopping movement of the finger the nurse can assess **nystagmus**, an involuntary, rhythmical oscillation of the eyes. The nurse can also often initiate nystagmus in clients with normal eye movements by having them gaze to the far left or right. Disturbances in eye movement reflect local injury to eye muscles and supporting structures or a disorder of the cranial nerves innervating the muscles.

The nurse can also check the alignment of the eyes by assessing the corneal light reflex. A weakness or imbalance of the extraocular muscles can cause a misalignment. The nurse shines a penlight onto the bridge of the client's nose from 60 to 90 cm (2 to 3 feet) away in a darkened room. The client looks straight ahead. Normally light reflects on the cornea in the same spot on both eyes. If an abnormality is present, the light shines on a different spot on each eye.

VISUAL FIELDS

As a person looks straight ahead, all objects in the periphery can normally be seen. To assess visual fields the nurse has the client stand or sit 60 cm (2 feet) away, facing the nurse at eye level. The client gently closes or covers one eye (such as the left) and looks at the nurse's eye directly opposite. The nurse closes the opposite eye (in this case the right) so that the field of vision is superimposed on that of the client. The nurse moves a finger equidistant from the nurse and client outside the field of vision, then slowly brings it back into the visual field. The client is asked to tell when the nurse's finger is seen. If the nurse sees the finger before the client does, a portion of the client's visual field is reduced. To test temporal field vision, the object should be slightly behind the client. (NOTE: The nurse can see the finger.) The procedure is repeated for each field of vision for the other eye. Clients with visual field problems may be at risk for injury because they cannot see all objects in front of them. Older adults commonly have loss of peripheral vision caused by changes in the lens.

EXTERNAL EYE STRUCTURES

To inspect external eye structures, the nurse stands directly in front of the client at eye level and asks the client to look at the nurse's face.

Position and Alignment. The nurse assesses the position of the eyes in relation to one another. The eyes are normally parallel to each other. Bulging (**exophthalmos**) is usually caused by hyperthyroidism when both eyes are involved. Crossing of eyes (strabismus) results from neuromuscular injury or inherited abnormalities. Tumors or inflammation of the orbit can cause abnormal eye protrusion.

Eyebrows. The eyebrows are normally symmetrical. The eyebrows are inspected for size, extension, texture of hair, alignment, and movement. A loss or absence of hair may indicate a hormonal disturbance or is a result of waxing or plucking. Aging causes loss of the lateral third of the eyebrows. The brows should raise and lower symmetrically. Paralysis of the facial nerve exists if a client cannot move the eyebrows.

Eyelids. The nurse inspects the eyelids for position, color, condition of the surface, condition and direction of eyelashes, and the client's ability to open, close, and blink.

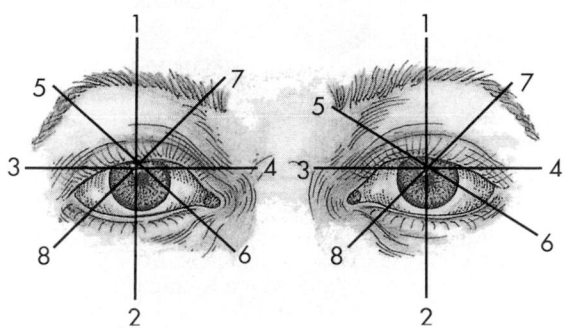

Fig. 33-16 The eight directions of gaze. The nurse directs the client to follow the finger movement through each gaze.

When the eyes are open in a normal position, the lids do not cover the pupil, and the sclera cannot be seen above the iris. The lids are also close to the eyeball. An abnormal drooping of the lid over the pupil is called **ptosis** (pronounced "toe-sis") and is caused by edema or impairment of the third cranial nerve. Defects in the position of the lid margins may also be observed. An older adult frequently has lid margins that turn out (**ectropion**) or in (**entropion**). An entropion may lead to the lid's lashes irritating the conjunctiva and cornea, increasing risk of infection. The eyelashes are normally distributed evenly and curved outward away from the eye.

To inspect the surface of the upper lids, the nurse asks clients to close their eyes and raises both eyebrows gently with the thumb and index finger to stretch the skin. The lids are normally smooth and the same color as the skin. Redness indicates inflammation or infection. Lid edema may be due to allergies or heart and kidney failure. Edema of the eyelids prevents them from closing. Lesions are inspected for typical characteristics and discomfort or drainage. Gloves should be worn if drainage is present.

The lids normally close symmetrically. Failure of the lids to close exposes the cornea to drying. This condition is common in unconscious clients or those with facial nerve paralysis.

The nurse asks the client to open the eyes for inspection of the lower lids. The same characteristics noted for the upper lids are assessed. Normally a person blinks involuntarily and bilaterally up to 20 times a minute. The blink reflex helps lubricate the cornea. The nurse reports absent or infrequent, rapid, or monocular (one-eyed) blinking.

Lacrimal Apparatus. The anterior surface of the eye, made up of the sensitive cornea and conjunctivae, is moistened or lubricated by tears secreted from the lacrimal gland (Fig. 33-17). The gland is located in the upper outer wall of the anterior part of the orbit. Tears flow from the gland across the eye's surface to the lacrimal duct, which is located in the nasal corner or inner canthus of the eye. The lacrimal gland can be the site of tumors or infections. The area of the gland is inspected for edema and redness, and it is palpated gently to detect tenderness. Normally the gland cannot be felt.

The nasolacrimal duct may become obstructed, blocking the flow of tears. If the client complains of excess tearing, the nurse looks for evidence of edema in the inner canthus. Mild palpation of the duct at the lower eyelid just inside the lower orbital rim, not on the side of the nose, may cause a regurgitation of tears.

Conjunctivae and Sclerae. The bulbar conjunctiva covers the exposed surface of the eyeball up to the outer edge of the cornea, and the palpebral conjunctiva is the delicate membrane lining the eyelids. Normally the conjunctiva is transparent, enabling the examiner to view the tiny underlying blood vessels that give it a light pink color. The sclera is seen under the bulbar conjunctiva and normally has the color of white porcelain in whites and light yellow in African Americans.

Care must be taken when inspecting the conjunctivae. For adequate exposure of the bulbar conjunctivae, the eyelids must be retracted without placing pressure directly on the eyeball. Both lids are gently retracted, with the thumb and index finger pressed against the lower and upper bony orbits. The client is asked to look up, down, and side to side. Many clients begin to blink, making the examination difficult. The nurse inspects for color, texture, and lesions. Normally the conjunctivae are free of erythema. Presence of redness may indicate an allergic or infectious **conjunctivitis**. Bright red blood in a localized area surrounded by normal appearing conjunctiva usually indicates subconjunctival hemorrhage.

To inspect the palpebral conjunctiva the nurse must evert the lower eyelids (Fig. 33-18). The lower lid is gently depressed with the thumb or index finger. Often the client can depress the eyelid to facilitate examination. The conjunctiva's color and edema or lesions are noted. A pale conjunctiva results from anemia, whereas a fiery red appearance is the result of inflammation (conjunctivitis). Conjunctivitis is a highly contagious infection. The crusty drainage that collects on eyelid margins can easily spread from one eye to the other. The nurse should wear gloves during the examination. Thorough handwashing is necessary before and after the examination.

A special technique is used to inspect the upper palpebral conjunctiva lining the upper eyelids (Fig. 33-19). The technique is only performed when a foreign body is suspected

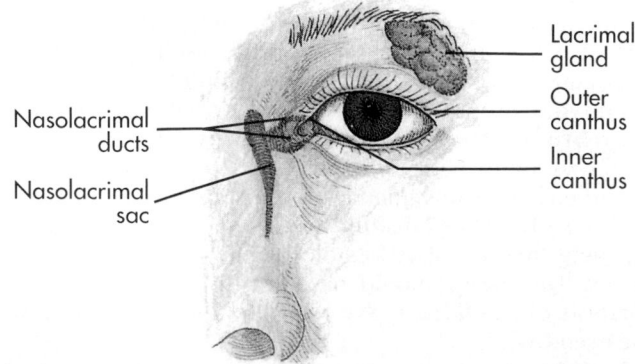

Fig. 33-17 The lacrimal apparatus secretes and drains tears, which moisten and lubricate eye structures.

Lacrimal gland

Outer canthus

Inner canthus

Nasolacrimal ducts

Nasolacrimal sac

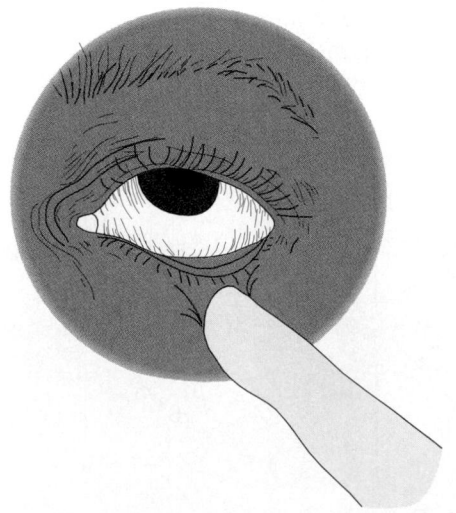

Fig. 33-18 Technique for retracting the lower eyelid.

and should not be attempted the first time without qualified assistance. The client is asked to look down, relax the eyes, and avoid any sudden movement. The upper lid is gently grasped with a gloved hand, and the lashes are pulled down and forward. The end of a cotton applicator is placed 1 cm (¹/₂ inch) above the lid margin. The nurse pushes down on the upper eyelid, turning it inside out. A light grasp on the upper lashes keeps the lid inverted. After inspection the eyelashes are gently pulled forward, and the client is instructed to look up. The eyelid will return to its normal position. If a foreign body appears to be embedded in the eye, the nurse should *not* attempt to remove it and should notify a physician immediately.

Corneas. The cornea is the transparent, colorless portion of the eye covering the pupil and iris. From a side view, the cornea looks like the crystal of a wristwatch. As the client looks straight ahead, the nurse inspects the cornea for clarity and texture while shining a penlight obliquely across the cornea's entire surface. The cornea is normally shiny, transparent, and smooth. However, in an older adult the cornea loses its luster. Any irregularity in the surface may indicate an abrasion or tear that warrants immediate examination by a physician. Both conditions are very painful. The color and details of the underlying iris should be easy to see. In an older adult the iris becomes faded. A thin, white ring along the margin of the iris, called an **arcus senilis**, is common with aging but is abnormal in anyone under age 40. To test for the corneal blink reflex, see the cranial nerve test section of this chapter.

Pupils and Irises. The nurse observes the pupils for size, shape, equality, accommodation, and reaction to light. The pupils are normally black, round, regular, and equal in size (3 to 7 mm in diameter, see Fig. 33-20). The iris should be clearly visible.

Cloudy pupils indicate cataracts. Dilated pupils can result from glaucoma, trauma, neurological disorders, eye medications (e.g., atropine), and withdrawal from opioids.

Constricted pupils may be caused by inflammation of the iris, use of drugs (e.g., pilocarpine, morphine, or cocaine). Pinpoint pupils are a common sign for opioid intoxication (Caulker-Burnett, 1994). When a beam of light is shined through the pupil and onto the retina, the third cranial nerve is stimulated and innervates the muscles of the iris to constrict. Any abnormality along the nerve pathways from the retina to the iris alters the ability of the pupils to react to light. Changes in intracranial pressure, lesions along the nerve pathways, locally applied ophthalmic medications, and direct trauma to the eye may alter pupillary reaction.

Pupillary reflexes (to light and accommodation) should be tested in a dimly lit room. As the client looks straight ahead, the nurse brings a penlight from the side of the client's face, directing the light onto the pupil (Fig. 33-21). If the client looks at the light, there will be a false reaction

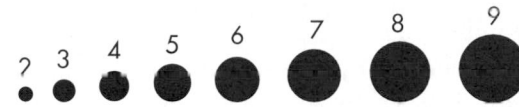

Fig. 33-20 Chart depicting pupillary size in millimeters.

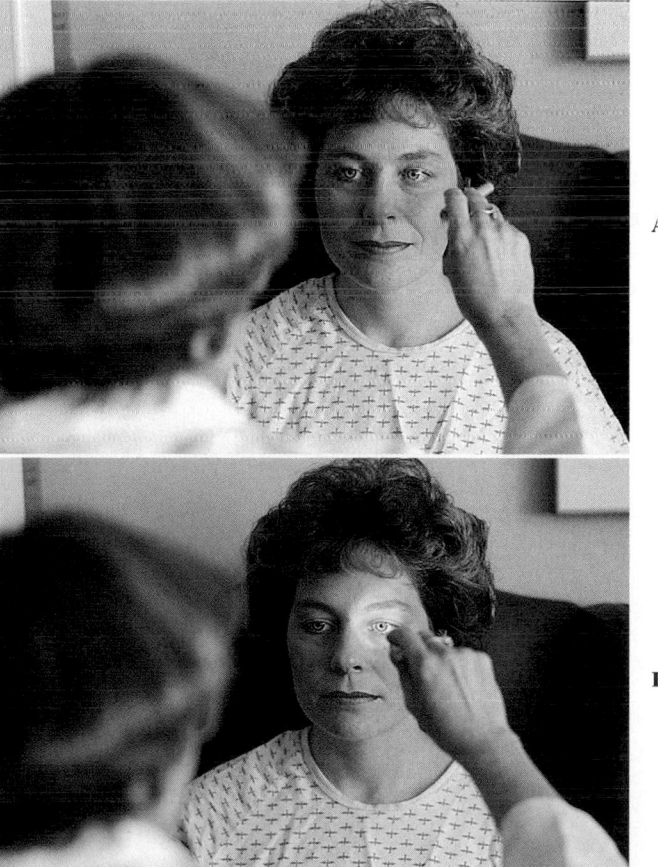

Fig. 33-21 **A,** To check pupil reflexes the nurse first holds the penlight to the side of the client's face. **B,** Illumination of the pupil causes pupillary constriction.

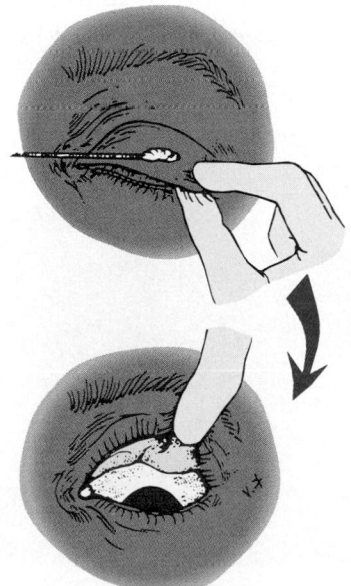

Fig. 33-19 Technique for inspecting the upper palpebral conjunctiva.

to accommodation. A directly illuminated pupil constricts, and the opposite pupil constricts consensually. The nurse observes the quickness and equality of the reflex. The exam is repeated for the opposite eye.

To test for accommodation, the client is asked to gaze at a distant object (the far wall) and then at a test object (finger or pencil) held by the nurse approximately 10 cm (4 inches) from the bridge of the client's nose. The pupils normally converge and accommodate by constricting when looking at close objects. The pupil responses are equal. Testing for accommodation is only important if the client has a defect in the pupillary response to light (Seidel et al, 1995). If assessment of pupillary reaction is normal in all tests, the nurse records the abbreviations, **PERRLA** (pupils equal, round, reactive to light, and accommodation).

INTERNAL EYE STRUCTURES

The internal eye cannot be observed without an instrument to illuminate its structures. The **ophthalmoscope** is used to inspect the fundus, which includes the retina, choroid, optic nerve disc, macula, fovea centralis, and retinal vessels. Clients in greatest need of an examination are those with diabetes, hypertension, and intracranial disorders. The nurse should feel competent in using an ophthalmoscope before attempting this examination.

The ophthalmoscope has a battery tube light source, two dials or disks, and a keyhole viewer (Fig. 33-22). The dial at the top of the battery tube changes the light image. Five lenses are available, but the large white light is used for general examination. The dial at the top of the viewer rotates clockwise for selection of lens, which adjusts the focus for the examiner.

The nurse should practice holding the ophthalmoscope in each hand, using the index finger to rotate the lens dial.

The nurse turns the white light on, rotates the lens dial to *0*, and looks through the keyhole, focusing on near objects such as the palm of the hand. Reading the newspaper with the ophthalmoscope is useful practice. During an examination the nurse keeps both eyes open when looking through the keyhole.

The examination is done in a darkened room. The nurse and client stand or sit in comfortable positions facing each other with their eyes at the same height. The client removes eyeglasses, but contact lenses may be left in place. The ophthalmoscope's light is switched on and the lens rotated to *0*. The index finger is kept on the lens dial to refocus the ophthalmoscope.

The examiner's right hand and eye are used to examine the client's right eye, and the left hand and eye are used for the client's left eye. The ophthalmoscope is held comfortably against the nurse's face. As the client gazes straight ahead with both eyes open, the examiner at a distance of approximately 25 cm (10 inches) from the client and 25 degrees lateral to the client's central line of vision, shines the light on the pupil (Fig. 33-23). A bright, orange glow in the pupil, called the *red reflex*, can then normally be seen. The light from the ophthalmoscope causes the pupil to constrict. The light is slowly moved toward the pupil while the nurse keeps it focused on the red reflex. The nurse must relax and keep both eyes open. As the light approaches the pupil, the nurse begins to see structures of the fundus. Rotating the lens dial brings the internal structures into focus. The examiner inspects the size, color, and clarity of the disc; integrity of vessels; presence of retinal lesions; and appearance of the macula and fovea (Fig. 33-24). Normally the following structures are observed:

1. A clear, yellow optic nerve disc
2. Reddish-pink retina (whites) or darkened retina (African Americans)
3. Light red arteries and dark red veins
4. A 3:2 vein to artery ratio in size proportion
5. The avascular macula

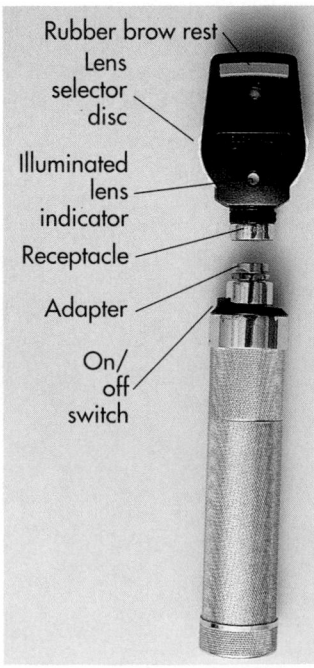

Fig. 33-22 An ophthalmoscope. *(From Seidel HM et al: Mosby's guide to physical examination, ed 3, St Louis, 1995, Mosby.)*

Rubber brow rest
Lens selector disc
Illuminated lens indicator
Receptacle
Adapter
On/ off switch

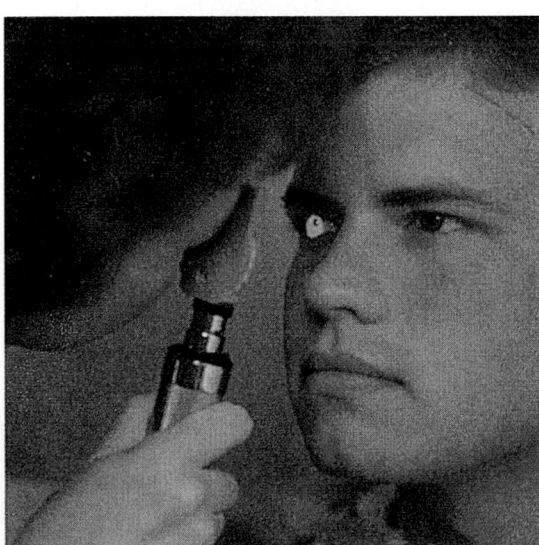

Fig. 33-23 To visualize internal eye structures, the nurse moves in toward the pupil with the ophthalmoscope's light focused on the red reflex.

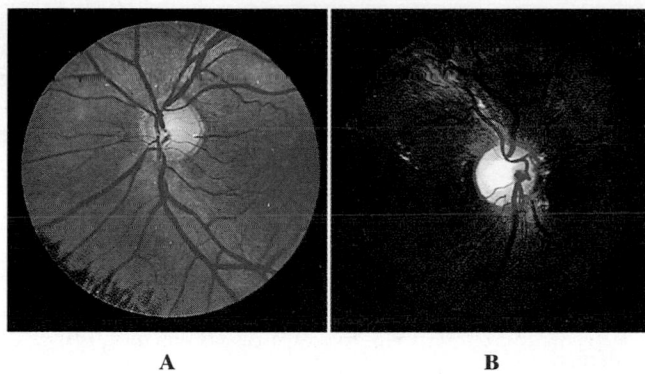

Fig. 33-24 Normal fundus. **A,** White adult. **B,** African American adult. *(From* Selected topics in ophthalmology, *Medcom clinical lecture guides, Garden Grove, Calif, 1973, Medcom.)*

If any abnormalities are observed, the client should be examined by an ophthalmologist (see the box at right). The client's fundus should not be illuminated for extended periods. The bright light of the ophthalmoscope is very irritating and can cause discomfort and tearing. During the examination, the nurse assesses the client for discomfort.

Ears

The ears are easy to examine because of their accessibility. The three parts of the ear are the external, middle, and inner ear (Fig. 33-25). The nurse inspects and palpates external ear structures, inspects middle ear structures with an otoscope, and tests the inner ear by measuring hearing acuity. External ear structures consist of the auricle, outer ear canal, and tympanic membrane (eardrum). The ear canal is normally curved and approximately 1 inch (2.5 cm) long in an adult. It is lined with skin containing fine hairs, nerve endings, and glands secreting cerumen. The middle ear is an air-filled cavity containing the three bony ossicles

CLIENT TEACHING
During Eye Assessment

OBJECTIVES
- Client will follow recommendations for regular eye examinations.
- Client will be able to recognize warning signs and symptoms of eye disease.
- Client will take appropriate safety precautions for visual deficits.

TEACHING STRATEGIES
- Tell client that persons under age 40 should have complete eye examination every 3 to 5 years (or more often if family histories reveal risks such as diabetes or hypertension).
- Tell client that persons over age 40 should have eye examinations every 2 years to screen for glaucoma.
- Tell client that persons over age 65 should have yearly eye examinations.
- Describe the typical symptoms of eye disease (see the box on p. 666).
- Instruct older adult to take the following precautions because of normal visual changes: avoid or use caution while driving at night, increase lighting in the home to reduce risk of falls, and paint the first and last steps of a staircase and the edge of each step in between a bright color to aid depth perception.

EVALUATION
- Ask client or family member to report on most recent visit to ophthalmologist.
- Have client describe when to have an eye examination.
- Ask client to describe common symptoms of eye disease.
- Observe the home environment of a client with visual deficits.

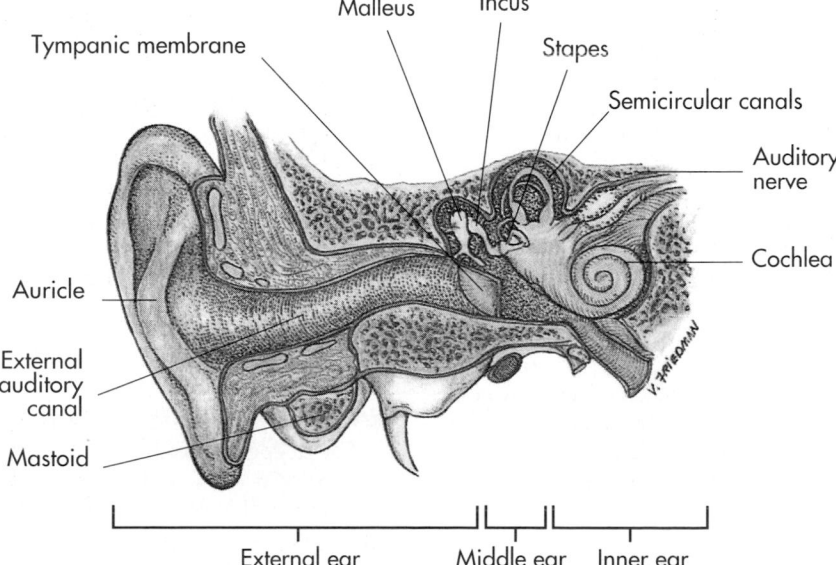

Fig. 33-25 The structures of the external, middle, and inner ear.

Table 33-14	**Nursing History for Ear Assessment**

ASSESSMENT CATEGORY	RATIONALE
Ask if client has experienced ear pain, itching, discharge, vertigo, tinnitus (ringing in ears), or change in hearing.	These signs and symptoms indicate infection or hearing loss.
Assess risks for hearing problem.	Risk factors predispose client to permanent hearing loss. It may be difficult to assess infant's hearing status with examination only.
Infants/children: hypoxia at birth, meningitis, birth weight less than 1500 g, family history of hearing loss, congenital anomalies of skull or face, nonbacterial intrauterine infections (rubella, herpes)	
Maternal drug use, excessively high bilirubin, head trauma.	
Adults: Exposure to industrial or recreational noise, genetic disease (Ménière disease), neurodegenerative disorder.	
Determine client's exposure to loud noises at work and availability of protective devices.	Prolonged noise exposure can cause temporary or permanent hearing loss.
Note behaviors indicative of hearing loss such as failure to respond when spoken to, requests to repeat comments, leaning forward to hear, and child's inattentiveness or use of monotonous voice tone.	Persons with hearing loss cope with sensory deficit through variety of behavioral cues.
Assess if client takes large doses of aspirin or other ototoxic drugs, e.g., aminoglycosides, furosemide, streptomycin, cisplatin, ethacrynic acid.	Medications have side effects of hearing loss.
Determine whether client uses hearing aid.	Determination allows nurse to assess ability to care for device and allows nurse to adjust voice tone to communicate.
If client had recent hearing problem, note onset, contributing factors, affected ear, and effect on activities of daily living.	Nature and severity of hearing problem are determined.
Determine whether client has repeated history of cerumen buildup in ear.	Cerumen impaction is common cause for conduction deafness.

(malleus, incus, and stapes). The eustachian tube connects the middle ear to the nasopharynx. Pressure between the outer atmosphere and middle ear is stabilized through the eustachian tube.

The inner ear contains the cochlea, vestibule, and semicircular canals. The nurse assesses the ears to determine the integrity of ear structures and the condition of hearing. Nursing history data (Table 33-14) aid in identifying risks for hearing disorders.

Understanding the mechanisms for sound transmission helps the nurse identify the nature of hearing disorders. Sound travels through the ear by air and bone conduction; the following explains the steps of hearing:

1. Sound waves in the air enter the external ear, passing through the outer ear canal.
2. The sound waves reach the tympanic membrane, causing it to vibrate.
3. Vibrations are transmitted through the middle ear by the bony ossicular chain to the oval window at the opening of the inner ear.
4. The cochlea receives the sound vibration.
5. Nerve impulses from the cochlea travel to the auditory (eighth cranial) nerve and to the cerebral cortex.

Disorders of the ear result from several types of problems, including mechanical dysfunction (blockage by ear wax or foreign body), trauma (foreign bodies or noise exposure), neurological disorders (auditory nerve damage), acute illnesses (viral infection), and toxic effects of medications.

AURICLES

With the client sitting comfortably the nurse inspects the auricle's size, shape, symmetry, landmarks, position, and color (Fig. 33-26). The auricles are normally level with each other. The upper point of attachment is in a straight line with the lateral canthus, or corner of the eye. The position of the auricle should also be almost vertical. Ears that are low set or at an unusual angle are a sign of chromosome abnormality (e.g., Down's syndrome). The color should be the same as that of the face, without moles, cysts, deformities, or nodules. Redness is a sign of inflammation or fever. Extreme pallor can indicate frostbite.

The nurse palpates the auricles for texture, tenderness, and skin lesions. The auricle is normally smooth without lesions. If the client complains of pain, the nurse gently pulls the auricle and presses on the tragus and palpates behind the ear over the mastoid process. If palpating the external ear increases the pain, an external ear infection is likely. If palpation of the auricle and tragus does not influence the pain, the client may have a middle ear infection. Tenderness in the mastoid area can indicate mastoiditis.

The nurse inspects the opening of the ear canal for size and discharge. Discharge may be accompanied by an odor. The meatus should not be swollen or occluded. A yellow, waxy substance called **cerumen** is common. Yellow or green, foul-smelling discharge may indicate infection or a foreign body.

EAR CANALS AND EARDRUMS

The deeper structures of the external and middle ear can be observed only with an **otoscope**, which is an ophthalmoscope with a special ear speculum attached to the battery tube. Speculums come in different sizes to conform to the size of ear canals. For best visualization the largest speculum that fits comfortably into the ear canal should be used.

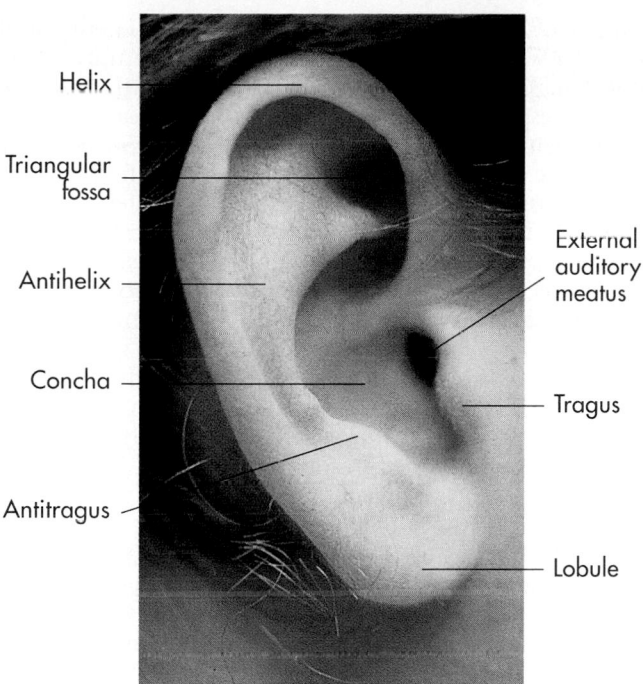

Fig. 33-26 Anatomical structures of the auricle. *(From Seidel HM et al: Mosby's guide to physical examination, ed 3, St Louis, 1995, Mosby.)*

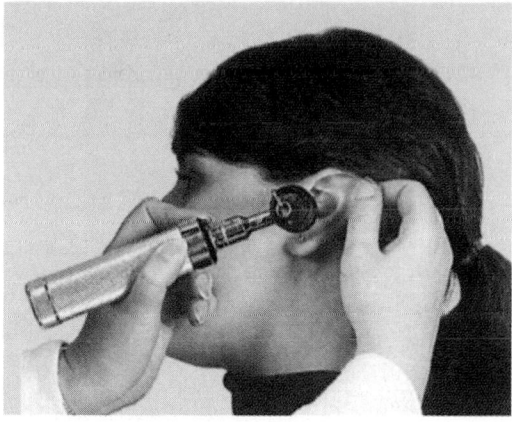

Fig. 33-27 Otoscopic examination. *(From Seidel HM et al: Mosby's guide to physical examination, ed 3, St Louis, 1995, Mosby.)*

CLIENT TEACHING
During Ear Assessment

OBJECTIVES
- Client will use proper technique for cleansing the ears.
- Client will follow preventive guidelines for screening of hearing loss.
- Client with hearing loss will communicate effectively.

TEACHING STRATEGIES
- Instruct client about the proper way to clean outer ear (see Chapter 40), avoiding use of cotton-tipped applicators and sharp objects such as hairpins.
- Tell client to avoid inserting pointed objects into the ear canal.
- Encourage clients over 65 to have regular hearing checks. Explain that a reduction in hearing is a normal part of aging (see Chapter 39).
- Instruct family members of clients with hearing losses to avoid shouting, speaking instead in low tones, and to be sure the client can see the speaker's face.

EVALUATION
- Ask client to explain the proper technique for cleansing the ears.
- In a follow-up visit, question client about frequency of hearing checks.
- Observe client with hearing loss interact with family members.

Before inserting the speculum, the examiner checks for foreign bodies in the opening of the auditory canal. Clients must not move their heads during the examination to avoid damage to the canal and tympanic membrane. Infants and young children often need to be restrained. Infants should lie supine with their heads turned to one side and their arms held securely at their sides. Young children can sit on their parents' laps with their legs held between the parents' knees.

The nurse turns on the otoscope by rotating the dial at the top of the battery tube. To insert the speculum properly the nurse asks the client to tip the head slightly toward the opposite shoulder. The nurse holds the handle of the otoscope in the space between the thumb and index finger, supported on the middle finger. This leaves the ulnar side of the hand to rest against the client's head, stabilizing the otoscope as it is inserted into the canal (Seidel et al, 1995). Two grips on the otoscope may be used. In one, the nurse holds the battery tube along the client's face with the fingers against the face or neck. In the other grip, the inverted otoscope is lightly braced against the side of the client's head or cheek. This grip, used with children, prevents accidental movement of the otoscope deeper into the ear canal. The nurse inserts the scope while pulling the auricle upward and backward in the adult and older child (Fig. 33-27). Pulling the auricle gently up, back, and slightly out in the adult or older child straightens the ear canal. In infants the nurse pulls the auricle back and down.

The nurse inserts the speculum slightly down and forward 1.0 or 1.5 cm ($^1/_2$ inch) into the ear canal. Care is taken not to abrade the sensitive lining of the ear canal, as this can be painful. The skin has little subcutaneous fat between it and the underlying bone. The canal normally has little cerumen and is uniformly pink with tiny hairs in the outer third of the canal. The nurse observes for color, discharge, scaling, lesions, foreign bodies, and cerumen. Normally cerumen is dry (light brown to grey and flaky) or moist (dark yellow or brown) and sticky. Dry cerumen occurs in Orientals and Native Americans about 85% of the time (Ibraimov, 1991; Seidel et al, 1995). A reddened canal with discharge is a sign of inflammation or infection. During the examination the examiner asks about methods that the client uses to clean the ear canal (see the box above).

The light from the otoscope allows visualization of the tympanic membrane. The nurse must be familiar with the common anatomical landmarks and their appearances (Fig.

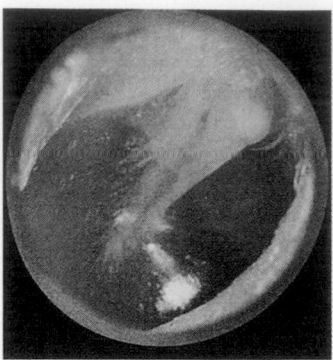

Fig. 33-28 Normal right tympanic membrane. *(Courtesy Dr. Richard A Buckingham, Abraham Lincoln School of Medicine, University of Illinois, Chicago; From Malasanos L et al, 1990.)*

33-28). This takes practice. The otoscope is slowly moved to see the entire tympanic membrane and its periphery. Because the tympanic membrane is angled away from the ear canal, the light from the otoscope appears as a cone rather than a circle. A ring of fibrous cartilage surrounds the oval membrane. The umbo is near the center of the membrane, and the attachment of the malleus is behind it. A knoblike structure at the top of the tympanic membrane is created by the underlying short process of the malleus. The nurse should check carefully to be sure there are no tears or breaks in the membrane. The normal tympanic membrane is translucent, shiny, and pearly gray. It is free from tears or breaks. A pink or red bulging membrane indicates inflammation. A white color reveals pus behind it. The membrane is taut, except for the small triangular pars flaccida near the top. If the tympanic membrane is blocked by cerumen, a warm water irrigation will safely remove the wax.

HEARING ACUITY

Often the nurse can tell whether the client has a hearing loss from a response to conversation. The three types of hearing loss are conduction, sensorineural, and mixed. A conduction loss interrupts sound waves as they travel from the outer ear to the cochlea of the inner ear because the sound waves are not transmitted through the outer and middle ear structures. Examples of causes of a conduction loss are swelling of the auditory canal or tears in the tympanic membrane. A sensorineural loss involves the inner ear, auditory nerve, or hearing center of the brain. Sound is conducted through the outer and middle ear structures, but the continued transmission of sound becomes interrupted at some point beyond the bony ossicles. A mixed loss involves a combination of conduction and sensorineural loss.

Clients working or living around loud noises are at risk for hearing loss. Older adults experience an inability to hear high-frequency sounds and consonants (e.g., *S, Z, T,* and *G*). Deterioration of the cochlea and a thickening of the tympanic membrane causes older adults to gradually lose hearing acuity. They are especially at risk for hearing loss due to **ototoxicity** (injury to auditory nerve) resulting from high maintenance doses of antibiotics, for example, the aminoglycosides.

To begin a hearing assessment, the nurse has the client remove any hearing aid that is worn. The nurse notes the client's response to questions. Normally the client should respond without excess requests to have the nurse repeat questions. If hearing loss is suspected, the nurse checks the client's response to the whispered voice. One ear is tested at a time, while the client occludes the other ear with a finger. The nurse asks the client to gently move the finger up and down during the test. While standing 1 to 2 feet (30 to 60 cm) from the ear being tested, the nurse covers the mouth so that the client is unable to read lips. After exhaling fully, the nurse first whispers softly toward the unoccluded ear, reciting random numbers with equally accented syllables such as *nine-four-ten.* If necessary, the nurse gradually increases voice intensity until the client correctly repeats the numbers. The other ear is then tested for comparison. Seidel et al. (1995) report that clients normally hear numbers clearly when whispered, responding correctly at least 50% of the time. A ticking watch may also be used to test hearing acuity, but the spoken word allows for more accuracy and control in testing.

If a hearing loss is present, there are tests that can be performed utilizing a tuning fork or audiometry. A tuning fork of 256 to 512 hertz (Hz) is most commonly used. The tuning fork allows for comparison of hearing by bone conduction with that of air conduction. The nurse holds the base of the tuning fork with one hand without touching the tines. The fork should be lightly tapped against the palm of the other hand, setting the fork in vibration (Table 33-15).

Nose and Sinuses

The nurse uses inspection and palpation to assess the nose and sinuses. The client sits during the exam. A penlight allows for gross examination of each naris. A more detailed examination requires use of a nasal speculum to inspect the deeper nasal turbinates. A student should not use a speculum unless a qualified practitioner is present. Table 33-16 lists components of the nursing history.

NOSE

When inspecting the external nose, the nurse observes for shape, size, skin color, and presence of deformity or inflammation. The nose is normally smooth and symmetric and the same color as the face. Recent trauma may have caused edema and discoloration. If swelling or deformities exist, the nurse gently palpates the ridge and soft tissue of the nose by placing one finger on each side of the nasal arch and gently moving fingers from the nasal bridge to the tip. The nurse notes any tenderness, masses, and underlying deviations. Nasal structures are usually firm and stable.

Air normally passes freely through the nose as a person breathes. To assess patency of the nares the nurse places a finger on the side of the client's nose and occludes one naris. The client is asked to breathe with the mouth closed. The exam is repeated for the other naris.

While illuminating the anterior nares, the nurse inspects the mucosa for color, lesions, discharge, swelling, and evidence of bleeding. If discharge is present, gloves should be worn. Normal mucosa is pink and moist without lesions. Pale mucosa with clear discharge indicates allergy. A mucoid discharge indicates rhinitis. A sinus infection results in yellowish or greenish discharge. Habitual use of intranasal cocaine and opioids can cause puffiness and increased vascularity of the nasal mucosa (Master and Terpstra, 1992).

Table 33 15	Tuning Fork Tests

TESTS AND STEPS / **RATIONALE**

WEBER'S TEST (LATERALIZATION OF SOUND)

Hold fork at its base and tap it lightly against heel of palm.

Place base of vibrating fork on midline vertex of client's head or middle of forehead (see the illustration at right).

Ask client if sound is heard equally in both ears or better in one ear.

Client with normal hearing hears sound equally in both ears or in midline of head. In conduction deafness, sound is heard best in impaired ear. In unilateral sensorineural hearing loss, sound is identified only in normal ear.

RINNE TEST (COMPARISON OF AIR AND BONE CONDUCTION)

Place stem of vibrating tuning fork against client's mastoid process (see the illustration below, left).

Begin counting the interval with your watch.

Ask client to tell you when sound is no longer heard, note number of seconds. Quickly place the still vibrating tines 1 to 2 cm (½ to 1 inch) from the ear canal, and ask client to tell you when the sound is no longer heard (see the illustration below, right).

Continue counting time the sound is heard by air conduction.

Compare number of seconds sound is heard by bone conduction versus air conduction.

Air-conducted sound should be heard twice as long as bone-conducted sound. In conduction deafness, bone-conducted sound can be heard longer. In sensorineural loss, sound is reduced and heard longer through air.

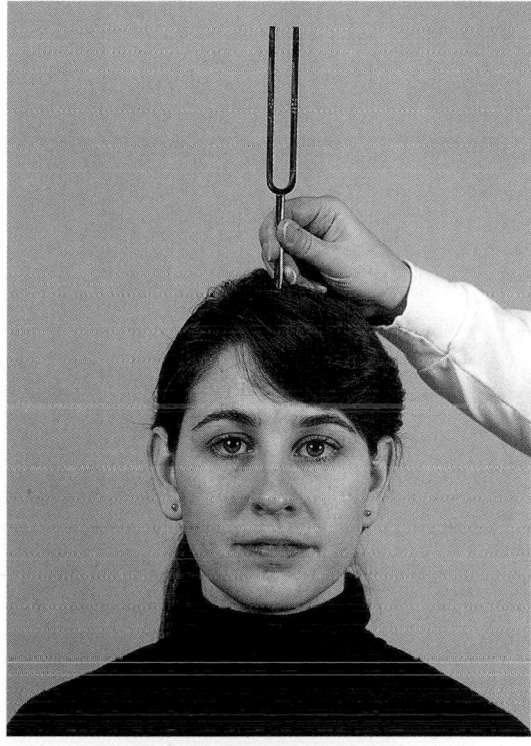

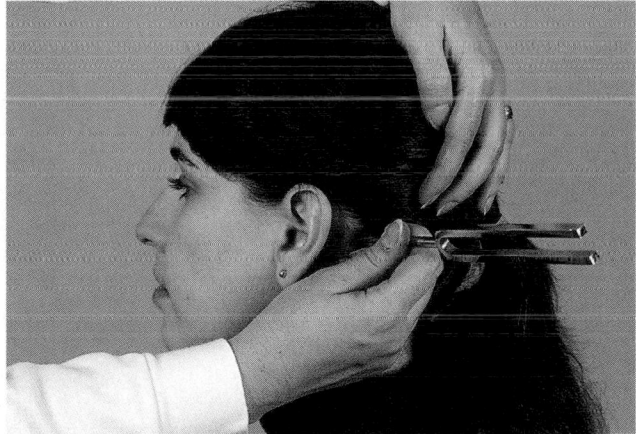

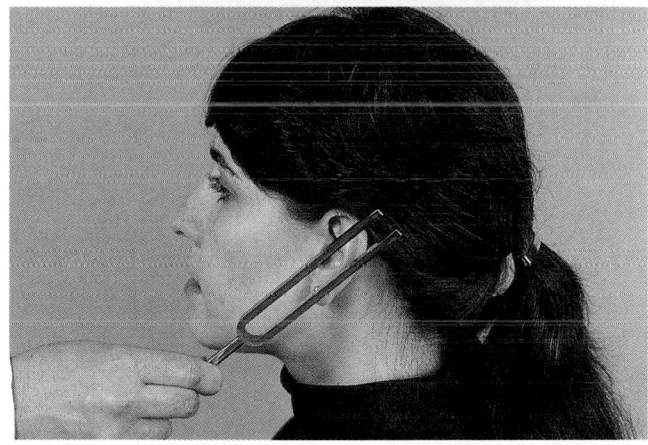

Illustrations from Seidel HM et al: *Mosby's guide to physical examination*, ed 3, St Louis, 1995, Mosby.

For the client with a nasogastric or nasopharyngeal tube, the nurse routinely checks for local skin breakdown (**excoriation**) of the naris, characterized by redness and sloughing of the skin.

To view the septum and turbinates, the client tips the head back slightly to give the nurse a clear view. The septum is inspected for alignment, perforation, or bleeding. Normally the septum is close to midline, and thicker anteriorly than posteriorly. The turbinates are covered with mucous membranes that warm and moisten inspired air. The mucosa is pink and moist, with clear mucus. A deviated septum can obstruct breathing and interfere with passage of a nasogastric tube. Perforation of the septum can occur after repeated use of intranasal cocaine. The nurse notes any **polyps** (tumorlike growth) or purulent drainage.

SINUSES

Examination of the sinuses involves palpation and transillumination. In cases of allergies or infection, the interior of the sinuses become inflamed and swollen. The most ef-

Table 33-16	Nursing History for Nose and Sinus Assessment	
ASSESSMENT CATEGORY		**RATIONALE**

ASSESSMENT CATEGORY	RATIONALE
Ask if client has had trauma to the nose.	Trauma can cause septal deviation and assymetry of external nose.
Ask if client has a history of allergies, nasal discharge, epistaxis (nose bleeds), or postnasal drip.	History is useful in determining source or nature of nasal and sinus drainage.
If there is a history of nasal discharge assess character, amount, odor, duration, and associated symptoms, e.g., sneezing, nasal congestion, obstruction or mouth breathing.	Can help to rule out presence of infection, allergy, or drug use.
Assess for history of nosebleed including site, frequency, amount of bleeding, treatment, and difficulty stopping bleeding.	Characteristics may reveal trauma, medication use, excessive dryness, etc., as causative factors.
Ask if client uses nasal spray or drops.	Overuse of over-the-counter nasal preparations can cause physical change in mucosa.
Ask if client snores at night or has difficulty breathing.	Difficulty with breathing or snoring may indicate septal deviation or obstruction.

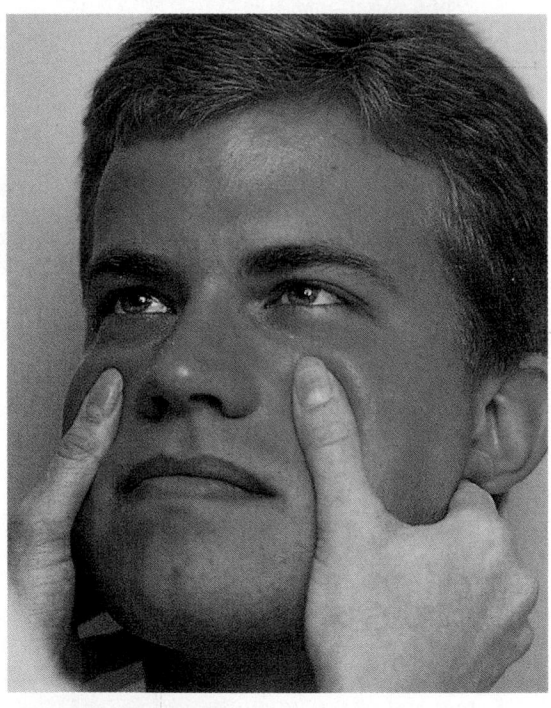

Fig. 33-29 Palpation of maxillary sinuses.

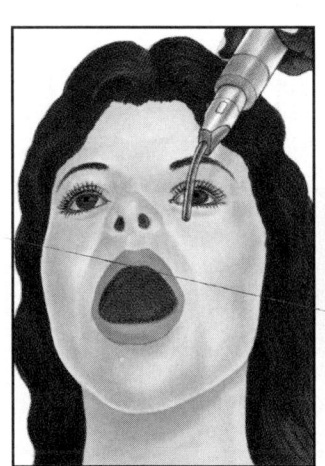
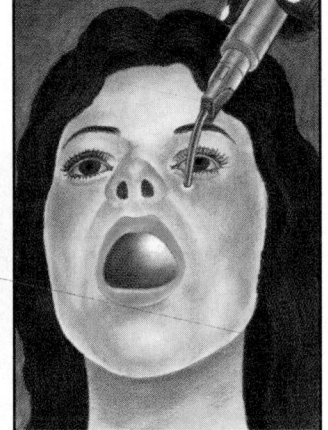
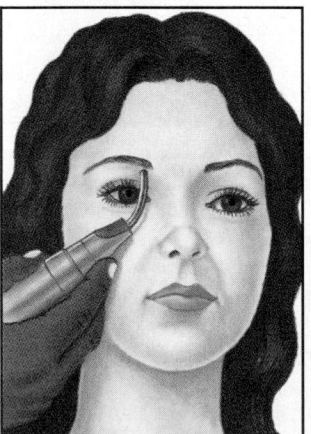
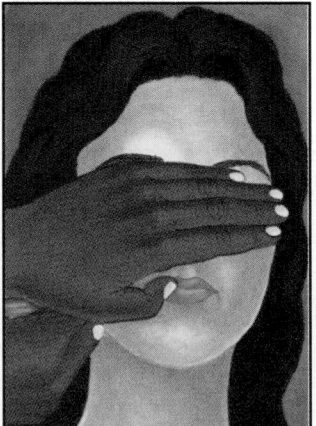

A

B

fective way to assess for tenderness is by externally palpating the frontal and maxillary facial areas (Fig. 33-29). The frontal sinus is palpated by exerting pressure with the thumb up and under the client's eyebrow. Gentle, upward pressure elicits tenderness easily if sinus irritation is present and reveals the severity of sinus irritation. Pressure should not be applied to the eyes.

If sinus tenderness is present or infection is suspected, transillumination is a technique to detect air or fluid in the sinuses. The examination must be done in a darkened room using a sinus transilluminator or small bright light. To view maxillary sinuses, the nurse places the light lateral to the client's nose, just beneath the medial aspect of the eye (Seidel

Fig. 33-30 Transillumination of the sinuses: placement of the light and expected area of transillumination A, Maxillary sinus. B, Frontal sinus. (*Modified from Seidel HM et al: Mosby's guide to physical examination, ed 3, St Louis, 1995, Mosby.*)

CLIENT TEACHING
During Nose and Sinus Assessment

OBJECTIVES
- Client will safely use over-the-counter nasal sprays.
- Parents will take proper measures to stop a child's nosebleed.
- Older adult will take safety precautions for loss of olfaction.

TEACHING STRATEGIES
- Caution client against overuse of over-the-counter nasal sprays, which can lead to "rebound" effect causing excess nasal congestion.
- Instruct parents on care of child with nosebleeds: have child sit up and lean forward to avoid aspiration of blood, apply pressure to anterior nose with thumb and forefinger as child breathes through mouth, and apply ice or cold cloth to bridge of nose if pressure fails to stop bleeding.
- Instruct older adults to install smoke detectors on each floor of home.
- Instruct older adults to always check dated labels on food to ensure against spoilage.

EVALUATION
- Have client explain proper use of over-the-counter nasal sprays.
- Have parents demonstrate and describe technique for stopping a nosebleed.
- Inspect client's home during visit and look for smoke detectors. Ask to check some food items in refrigerator.

Table 33-17	Nursing History for Mouth and Pharynx Assessment
ASSESSMENT CATEGORY	**RATIONALE**
Determine if client wears dentures or retainers and if they are comfortable.	Dentures must be removed to visualize and palpate gums. Ill-fitting dentures chronically irritate mucosa and gums.
Determine if client has had recent change in appetite or weight.	Symptoms may result from painful mouth conditions or poor hygiene.
Determine if client smokes or chews tobacco.	Tobacco users have greater risk for mouth and throat cancers than nonusers (ACS, 1995).
Review history for alcohol consumption.	Heavy drinkers appear to have greater risk for oral cancer. Effects of alcohol are independent of tobacco use (Franco, 1991).
Assess dental hygiene practices including use of fluoride toothpaste, frequency of brushing and flossing, and frequency of dental visits.	Assessment reveals client's need for education and/or financial support. Periodontal disease has a higher prevalence in older adults who have history of high plaque buildup, use tobacco, and visit the dentist infrequently (Rozier and Beck, 1991).
Ask if client has pain from chewing or eating. If so, ask if mouth lesions are present including duration and associated symptoms.	May be associated with broken tooth, tooth grinding, or temporomandibular joint problems. Extra care needed during oral hygiene administration.

et al, 1995). As the client opens the mouth the nurse looks to see if the hard palate is illuminated (Fig. 33-30). To view the frontal sinuses, the nurse places the light against the medial aspect of each supraorbital rim. A dim red glow of light should be transmitted just above the eyebrow. Absence of a glow in the sinus indicates either the sinus contains secretions or it never developed. Normally, sinuses show different degrees of illumination. The box above describes teaching guidelines during nose and sinus assessment.

Mouth and Pharynx

The nurse assesses the mouth and pharynx to detect signs of overall health, determine oral hygiene needs, and develop nursing therapies for clients with dehydration, restricted intake, oral trauma, or oral airway obstruction. To assess the oral cavity the nurse uses a penlight and tongue depressor or single gauze square. Gloves should be worn during the examination. The client may sit or lie during the examination. Assessment of the oral cavity can be made during administration of oral hygiene (see Chapter 40). Table 33-17 describes the nursing history.

LIPS

The lips are inspected for color, texture, hydration, contour, and lesions. With the client's mouth closed, the nurse views the lips from end to end. Normally they are pink, moist, symmetrical, and smooth (Fig. 33-31). Female clients

should remove their lipstick before the exam. Pallor of the lips can be caused by anemia, with cyanosis caused by respiratory or cardiovascular problems. Any lesions such as nodules or ulcerations can be related to infection, irritation, or skin cancer.

BUCCAL MUCOSA, GUMS, AND TEETH

The nurse begins inspection by having the client clench the teeth and smile. The maneuver allows assessment of teeth occlusion. The upper molars should rest directly on the lower molars with the upper incisors slightly overriding the lower incisors. A symmetrical smile reveals normal facial nerve function.

The quality of dental hygiene is easily determined by inspecting the teeth (see the box on p. 678). The position and alignment of teeth are noted. To examine the posterior surface of the teeth the nurse has the client open the mouth with lips relaxed. A tongue depressor may be needed to retract the lips and cheeks, especially when viewing the molars. Tartar along the base of the teeth, dental **caries** (cavities), extraction sites, and tooth color should be noted. Normal, healthy teeth are smooth, white, and shiny. A chalky white discoloration of the enamel is an early indication of caries formation. Brown or black discolorations indicate formation of caries. In the older adult, loose or missing teeth are common because bone resorption increases. An older adult's teeth often feel rough when tooth enamel

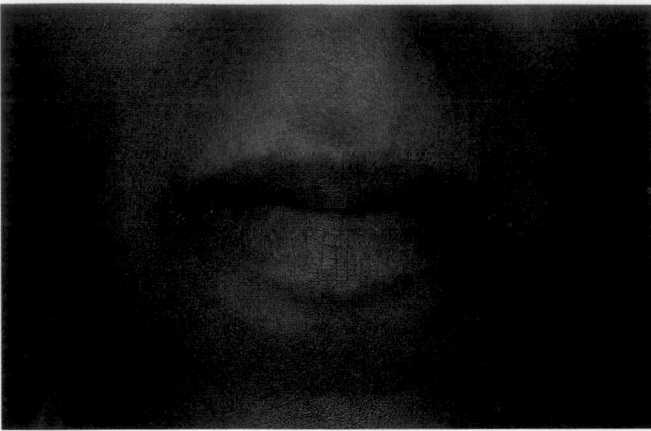

Fig. 33-31 The lips are normally pink, symmetrical, smooth, and moist.

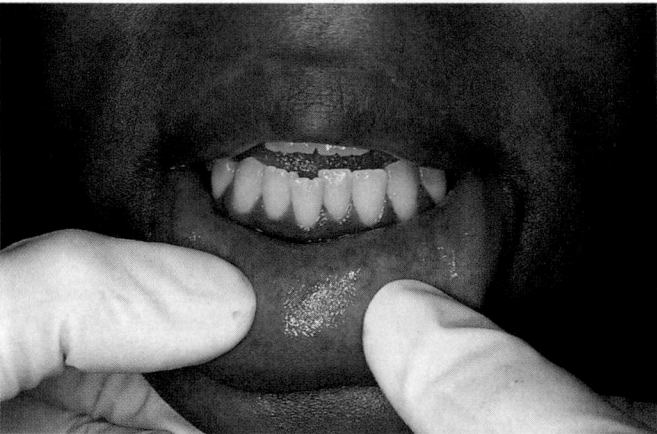

Fig. 33-32 Inspection of inner oral mucosa of lower lip.

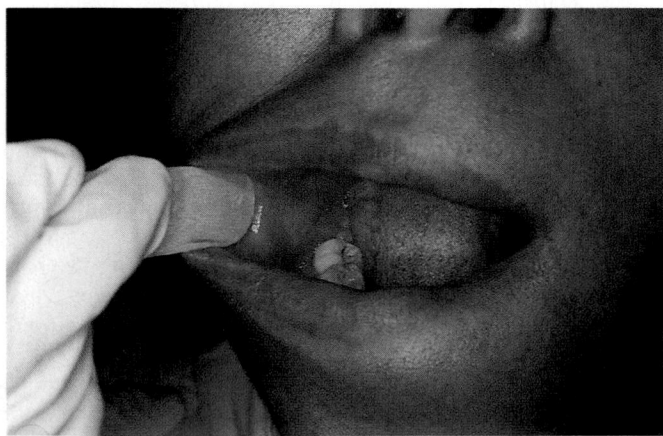

Fig. 33-33 Retraction of the buccal mucosa allows for clear visualization.

CLIENT TEACHING
During Mouth and Pharynx Assessment

OBJECTIVES
- Client will practice proper oral hygiene measures and dental care.
- Client will describe warning signs of oral cancer.
- Older adult will maintain normal solid food intake.

TEACHING STRATEGIES
- Discuss proper techniques for oral hygiene, including brushing and flossing (see Chapter 40).
- Explain the early warning signs of oral cancer, including a sore that bleeds easily and does not heal, a lump or thickening, and a red or white patch on the mucosa that persists.* Difficulty chewing or swallowing are late changes.
- Encourage a yearly dental examination for each child and adult. Inquire whether client's dentist uses dental sealants. Rozier and Beck (1991) report a significant decline in oral caries related to use of sealants.
- An older adult should visit a dentist every 6 months.
- Identify older client that has difficulty in chewing and changes in the teeth. Teach client to eat soft foods and cut food into small pieces.

EVALUATION
- Ask client to demonstrate brushing.
- Have client identify when to have regular dental checkups.
- Have client identify warning signs of oral cancer.
- Ask older adult to keep diet record for 3 days.

*Data from American Cancer Society: *1995 Cancer facts and figures,* New York, 1995, The Society.

calcifies. Yellow or darkened teeth are also common in the older adult because of the general wear and tear that exposes the darker, underlying dentin.

To view the mucosa and gums, the nurse asks the client to first remove any dental appliance. The nurse views the inner oral mucosa by having the client open and relax the mouth slightly and then gently retracts the client's lower lip away from the teeth (Fig. 33-32). This process is repeated for the upper lip. The mucosa is inspected for color, hydration, texture, and lesions such as ulcers, abrasions, or cysts. Normal mucous membrane is pinkish red, smooth, and moist. Small, yellow-white raised lesions commonly seen on the buccal mucosa and lips are Fordyce spots, ectopic sebaceous glands (Seidel et al, 1995). If lesions are present, the nurse palpates them gently with a gloved hand for tenderness, size, and consistency.

To visualize the buccal mucosa, the nurse asks the client to open the mouth and then gently retracts the cheeks with a tongue depressor or gloved finger covered with gauze (Fig. 33-33). The surface of the mucosa must be viewed from right to left and top to bottom. A penlight illuminates the most posterior portion of the mucosa. Normal mucosa is glistening, pink, soft, moist, and smooth. An increase in color or hyperpigmentation is normal in 10% of whites after age 50 and up to 90% of African Americans by the same age. For clients with normal pigmentation the buccal mucosa is a good site to inspect for jaundice and pallor. In older adults the mucosa is normally dry because of reduced salivation. Thick, white patches (**leukoplakia**) can be seen in heavy smokers and alcoholics. Leukoplakia should be reported because it can also be a precancerous lesion. The nurse palpates the cheek with one finger along the inner mucosa and the thumb along the outside cheek to check for deep-seated lumps or ulcerations.

While the nurse retracts the cheeks, the gums or gingivae are inspected for color, edema, retraction, bleeding, and lesions. The gums around the back molars should be viewed because this is a difficult area to reach when cleaning teeth. Healthy gums are pink, smooth, and moist with a tight margin at each tooth. African Americans may have patchy pigmentation. In older adults the gums are usually pale. Using gloves, the nurse palpates the gums to assess for lesions, thickening, or masses. There should be no tenderness on palpation. Spongy gums that bleed easily indicate periodontal disease and vitamin C deficiency. If the client has loose or mobile teeth, swollen gums, or pockets containing debris at tooth margins, periodontal disease or gingivitis can be expected.

TONGUE AND FLOOR OF MOUTH

The tongue is carefully inspected on all sides, and the floor of the mouth is checked. The client first relaxes the mouth and sticks the tongue out halfway. The nurse notes any deviation, tremor, or limitation in movement. This tests hypoglossal nerve function. If the client protrudes the tongue too far, the gag reflex may be elicited. When the tongue protrudes, it lies midline. To test for tongue mobility the nurse asks the client to raise the tongue up and move it side to side. The tongue should move freely.

Using the penlight for illumination, the nurse examines the tongue for color, size, position, texture, and coatings or lesions. The tongue should be medium or dull red in color, moist, slightly rough on the top surface and smooth along lateral margins. The undersurface of the tongue and the floor of the mouth are highly vascular (Fig. 33-34). Extra care is taken to inspect these areas, common sites for oral cancer lesions. The client lifts the tongue by placing its tip on the palate behind the upper incisors. The nurse looks for color, swelling, and lesions such as nodules or cysts. The ventral surface of the tongue is pink and smooth with large veins between the frenulum folds. To palpate the tongue,

the nurse explains the procedure and then asks the client to protrude the tongue. The nurse grasps the tip with a gauze square and gently pulls it to one side. With a gloved hand the nurse palpates the full length of the tongue and the base for any areas of hardening or ulceration. **Varicosities** (swollen, tortuous veins) may be seen. Varicosities rarely cause problems but are common in the older adult.

PALATE

The client should extend the head backward, holding the mouth open so that the nurse can inspect the hard and soft palates for color, shape, texture, and extra bony prominences or defects (Fig. 33-35). The hard palate or roof of the mouth is located anteriorly. The whitish hard palate should be dome shaped. The soft palate, best seen while depressing the tongue with a tongue blade, extends posteriorly toward the pharynx. It is normally light pink and smooth. A bony growth, or **exostosis**, between the two palates is common.

PHARYNX

The pharynx can be a site for infection, inflammation, or lesions. Before examining the pharynx the nurse explains the procedure to the client. The client tips the head back slightly, opens the mouth wide, and says "ah." The nurse places the tip of a tongue depressor on the middle third of the tongue, taking care not to press the lower lip against the teeth. If the tongue depressor is placed too far anteriorly, the posterior part of the tongue mounds up, obstructing the view. The gag reflex is elicited when the tongue depressor touches the posterior tongue.

With a penlight, the nurse inspects the uvula and soft palate (Fig. 33-36). Both structures, which are innervated by the tenth cranial (vagus) nerve, should rise centrally as the client says "ah." The nurse also inspects the arch formed by the anterior and posterior pillars, soft palate, and uvula. The tonsils can be viewed in the cavities between the anterior and posterior pillars and are oval with infoldings of tissue. The posterior pharynx is behind the pillars. The pharyngeal tissues are normally pink and smooth. Edema, ulceration, or inflammation indicates infection or abnormal lesions. Clients with chronic sinus problems frequently exhibit a clear exudate that drains along the wall of the posterior pharynx. Yellow or green exudate indicates infec-

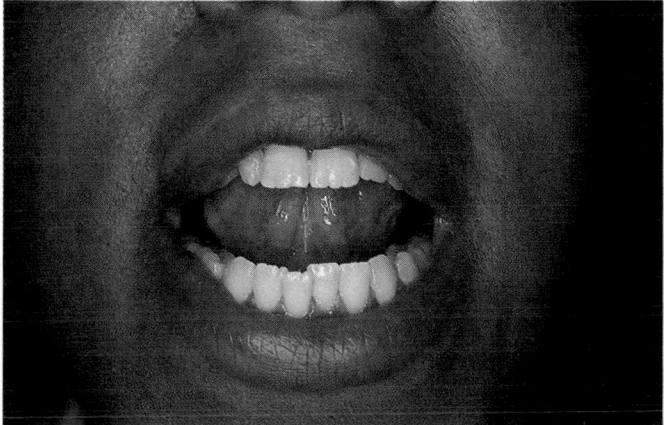

Fig. 33-34 The undersurface of the tongue is highly vascular.

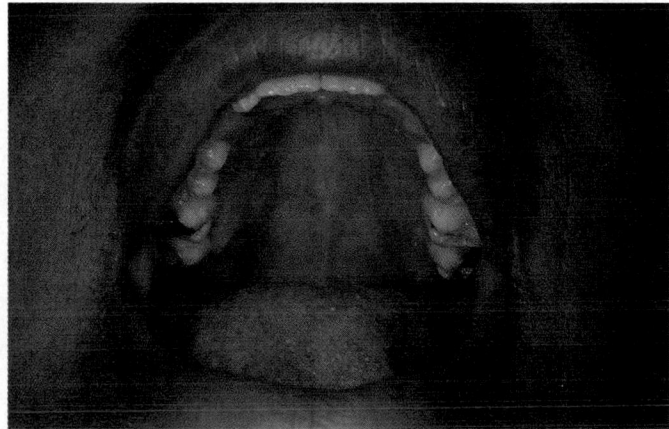

Fig. 33-35 The hard palate is located anteriorly in the roof of the mouth.

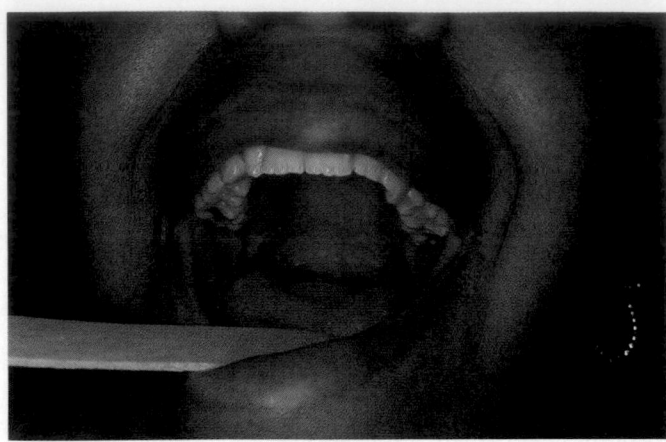

Fig. 33-36 A tongue depressor allows the nurse to visualize the uvula and posterior soft palate.

tion. A client with a typical sore throat has a reddened and edematous uvula and tonsillar pillars with the possible presence of yellow exudate.

Neck

The neck muscles, lymph nodes of the head and neck, carotid arteries, jugular veins, thyroid gland, and trachea are located within the neck (Fig. 33-37). An examination of the jugular veins and carotid arteries can wait until assessment of the vascular system. The nurse inspects and palpates the neck to determine the integrity of neck structures and to examine the lymphatic system. Remember that the lymphatic system is examined region by region during the assessment of other body systems (head and neck, breast, genitalia, and extremities). An abnormality of superficial lymph nodes may reveal an infection or malignancy. Examination of the thyroid gland and trachea also aids in ruling out malignancies. Examination is best performed with the client sitting. Areas of the neck are outlined by the sternocleidomastoid and trapezius muscles, which divide each side of the neck into two triangles. The anterior triangle contains the trachea, thyroid gland, carotid artery, and anterior cervical lymph nodes. The posterior triangle contains the posterior lymph nodes. Table 33-18 reviews the nursing history for the head and neck examination.

NECK MUSCLES

The nurse begins the examination by inspecting the neck in the usual anatomical position, in slight hyperextension. Inspect for bilateral symmetry of the neck muscles. To test the function of the sternocleidomastoid muscle, the nurse asks the client to flex the neck with the chin to the chest. Then the client hyperextends the neck backward so that the nurse can check for trapezius muscle function. Movement of the head sideways so that the ear moves toward the shoulder further tests function of the sternocleidomastoid muscle. The neck should move freely without discomfort or dizziness. Other tests for muscle strength and function can be performed during assessment of the musculoskeletal system.

LYMPH NODES

An extensive system of lymph nodes collects lymph from the head, ears, nose, cheeks, and lips (Fig. 33-38). The immune system protects the body from foreign antigens, re-

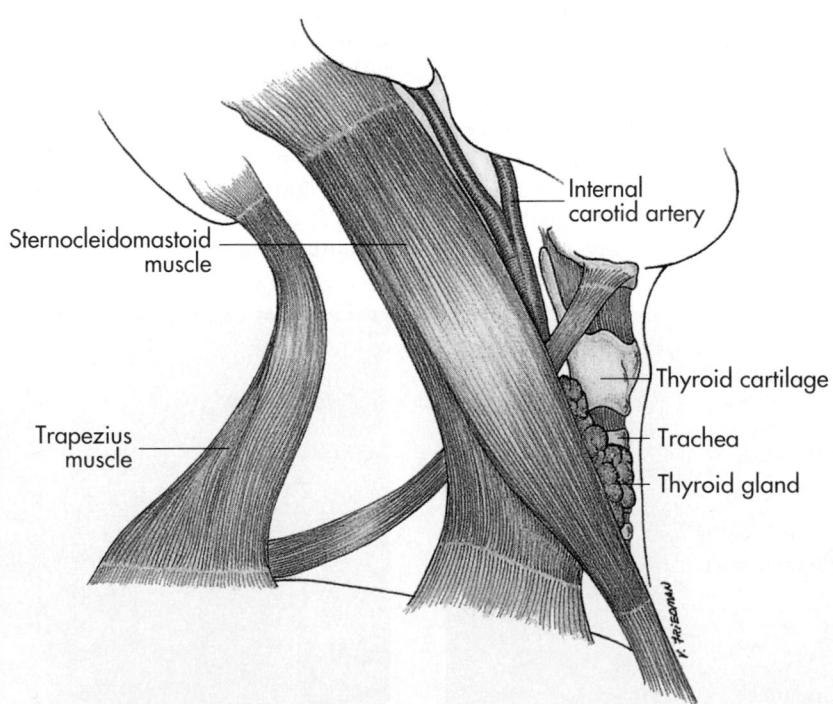

Fig. 33-37 Anatomical position of major neck structures. Note the triangles formed by the sternocleidomastoid muscle, lower jaw, and anterior neck anteriorly and sternocleidomastoid muscle, trapezius muscle, and lower neck posteriorly.

Table 33-18	Nursing History for Neck Assessment	
ASSESSMENT CATEGORY	**RATIONALE**	
Assess for history of recent cold or infection.	Colds or infections can cause temporary or permanent lymph node enlargement. These are risk factors for HIV infection.	
If there is an enlarged lymph node consider reviewing history of IV drug use, hemophilia, sexual contact with persons infected with HIV, history of blood transfusion, multiple and indiscriminate sexual contacts, or male with homosexual or bisexual activities.		
Ask if client has had history of neck pain with restriction in movement.	May indicate muscle strain, head injury, local nerve injury, or enlarged or swollen lymph node.	
Ask if client has had change in temperature preference (more or less clothing); swelling in neck; change in texture of hair, skin, or nails; or change in emotional stability.	Symptoms indicative of thyroid disease.	
Ask if client has history of thyroid problem or takes thyroid medication.	Disease or medications may influence tissue growth of gland.	
Review medical history of pneumothorax (collapsed lung) or bronchial tumor.	Conditions place client at risk for tracheal displacement or lateral deviation.	

moves damaged cells from the circulation, and provides a partial barrier to growth of malignant cells within the body. The nurse should become particularly competent in assessing the lymph nodes when caring for clients with suspected immunoincompetence, which can be linked to allergies, HIV infection, autoimmune disease such as lupus erythematosus, or serious infection.

With the client's chin raised and head tilted slightly, the nurse first inspects the area where lymph nodes are distributed and compares both sides. This position stretches the skin slightly over any possible enlarged nodes. Visible nodes are inspected for edema, erythema, or red streaks. Nodes are not normally visible.

A methodical approach is used to examine the lymph nodes to avoid overlooking any single node or chain. The client relaxes with the neck flexed slightly forward and, if needed, toward the nurse. This maneuver relaxes tissues and muscles. Both sides of the neck are inspected and palpated for comparison. During palpation the nurse faces or stands to the side of the client for easy access to all nodes. Using the pads of the middle three fingers of the hand, the nurse palpates gently in a rotary motion for superficial lymph nodes (Fig. 33-39). Each node is checked methodically in the following sequence: occipital nodes at base of skull, postauricular nodes over the mastoid, preauricular nodes just in front of the ear, retropharyngeal nodes at angle of the mandible, submaxillary nodes, and submental nodes in the midline behind the mandibular tip. The nurse tries to detect enlargement and notes the location, size, shape, surface characteristics, consistency, mobility, tenderness, and warmth of the nodes. If the skin is mobile, the

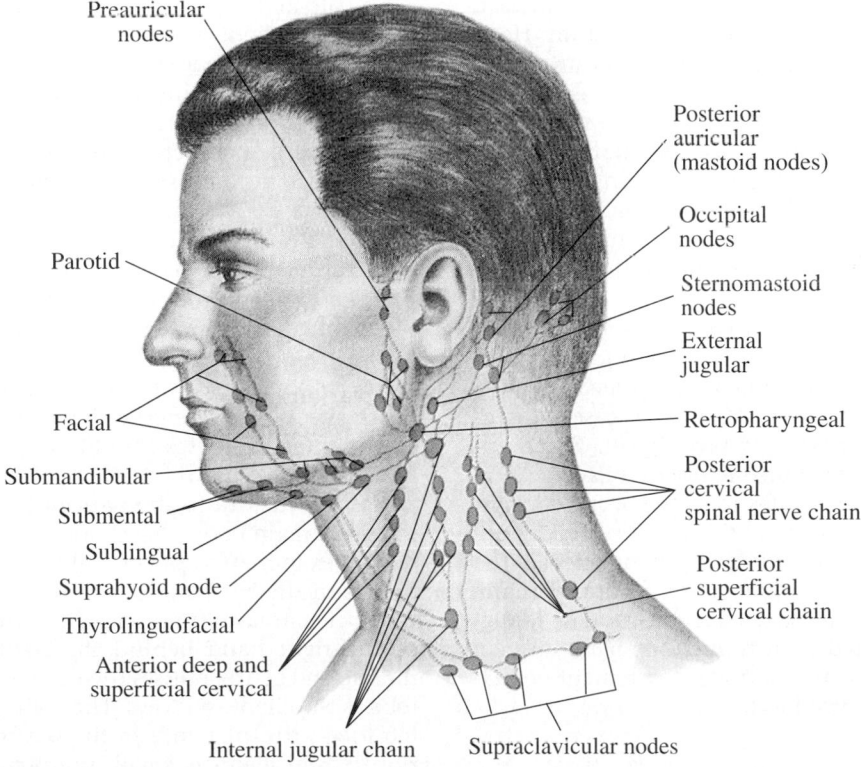

Fig. 33-38 Head and neck lymphatic system. *(From Seidel HM et al: Mosby's guide to physical examination, ed 3, St Louis, 1995, Mosby.)*

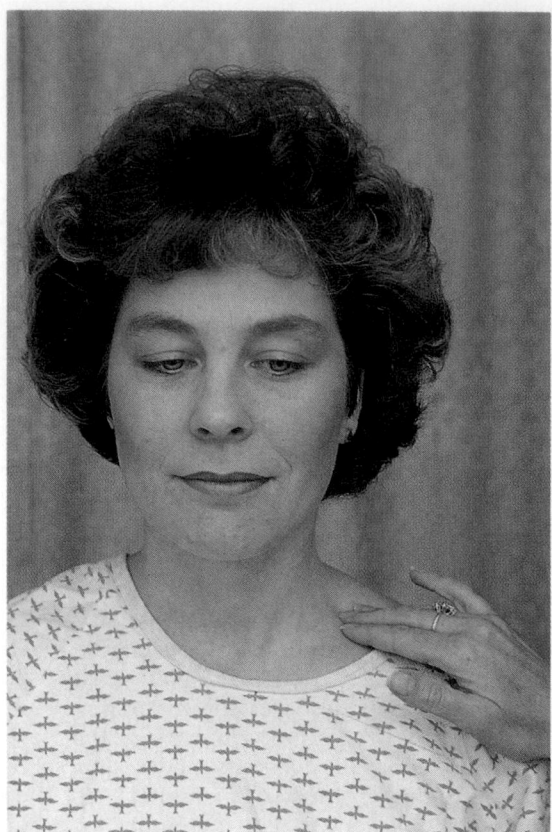

Fig. 33-39 Palpation of cervical lymph nodes.

CLIENT TEACHING
During Neck Assessment

OBJECTIVE
■ Client will take proper preventive action if mass is noted in neck.

TEACHING STRATEGIES
■ Instruct client about the lymph nodes and how infection can commonly cause node tenderness.
■ Instruct client to call the physician when an enlarged lump or mass is noted in the neck.
■ Teach client risk factors for HIV infection (see Table 33-18).

EVALUATION
■ Have client explain when to notify a physician about a neck mass.

nurse moves the skin over the area of the nodes (Seidel et al, 1995). It is important to press underlying tissue in each area and not simply move the fingers over the skin. However, if excessive pressure is applied, small nodes are missed and palpable nodes are obliterated.

To palpate supraclavicular nodes the nurse asks the client to bend the head forward and relax the shoulders. The nurse may have to hook the index and third finger over the clavicle, lateral to the sternocleidomastoid muscle, to palpate these nodes. The deep cervical nodes can be palpated only with the nurse's fingers hooked around the sternocleidomastoid muscle.

Normally lymph nodes are not easily palpable. However, small, mobile, nontender nodes are common. Lymph nodes that are large, fixed, inflamed, or tender indicate a problem such as local infection, systemic disease, or neoplasm (Seidel et al, 1995) (see the box above). When enlarged nodes are found the nurse explores adjacent areas and regions drained by the nodes for signs of infection or malignancy. Tenderness is usually the result of inflammation. Noting which nodes are enlarged may help locate the site of an infection. For example, ear infections usually drain to the preauricular or deep cervical nodes. Malignancy is usually associated with nontender, hard, discrete nodes. After a serious infection a node may remain permanently enlarged but may not be tender.

THYROID GLAND

The thyroid gland lies in the anterior lower neck, in front of and to both sides of the trachea. The gland is fixed to the

trachea with the isthmus overlying the trachea and connecting the two irregular, cone-shaped lobes (Fig. 33-40). The nurse assesses the gland by inspection, palpation, and auscultation.

The nurse stands in front of the client and inspects the area of the lower neck overlying the thyroid gland for visible masses, symmetry, and any subtle fullness at the base of the neck. Asking the client to hyperextend the neck helps tighten the skin for better visualization. The nurse offers the client a glass of water and then has the client swallow, while noting whether there is a bulging of the gland. Normally the thyroid cannot be visualized.

To palpate the gland, the examiner stands in front of or behind the client. Light, gentle palpation is needed in order to feel any abnormalities. Seidel et al. (1995) recommend allowing the fingers to drift over the gland. For both the anterior and posterior approach the client flexes the neck forward and laterally toward the side being examined to relax the neck muscles. The client holds a cup of water and takes a sip to swallow once instructed by the nurse.

For the posterior approach, the nurse has the client sit with the neck at a comfortable level. Both of the nurse's hands are placed around the neck, with two fingers of each hand on the sides of the trachea just beneath the cricoid cartilage. As the client swallows the nurse feels for movement of the thyroid isthmus. The thyroid should move beneath the fingers when the client swallows. Enlargement of the isthmus as it rises should be noted. To examine each lobe, the nurse has the client swallow while the nurse displaces the trachea to the right or left. The nurse then palpates the main body of each lobe (Fig. 33-41). For example, during examination of the right lobe the nurse moves the fingers of the left hand between the trachea and the right sternocleiodmastoid muscle. Then the nurse places fingers of the right hand behind the right sternocleidomastoid muscle and gently presses the hands together to palpate the lobe as the client swallows. The approach is repeated for the left lobe with the hands in the reverse positions. Normally the thyroid gland is small, smooth, and free of nodules. However, in extremely thin individuals the thyroid is more easily palpable. Enlargement is a manifestation of thyroid

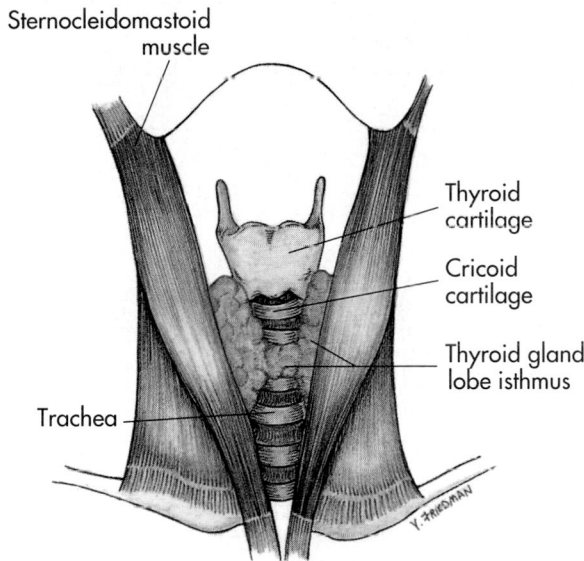

Fig. 33-40 Anatomical position of the thyroid gland.

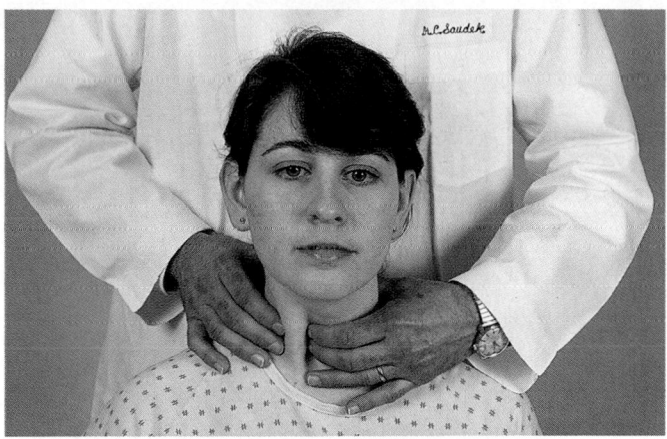

Fig. 33-41 Palpation of the right thyroid lobe from behind the client. *(From Seidel HM et al: Mosby's guide to physical examination, ed 3, St Louis, 1995, Mosby.)*

dysfunction. Masses or nodules may be signs of malignant disease. However, not all nodules are malignant.

The anterior approach requires the client to sit as the nurse stands to the side. Using the pads of the index and middle finger, the nurse palpates the left lobe with the right hand and the right lobe with the left hand as the client swallows. Gentle displacement of the trachea allows palpation of the main body of each thyroid lobe. It helps to move the skin medially over the sternocleidomastoid muscle and to reach under its anterior borders while the fingers stay beneath the cricoid cartilage.

When the gland appears enlarged, the nurse places the diaphragm of the stethoscope over the thyroid. If the gland is enlarged, blood flow through the thyroid arteries increases and causes a fine vibration. The nurse can auscultate the vibration, which is heard as a soft, rushing sound, or bruit.

CAROTID ARTERY AND JUGULAR VEIN

This portion of the examination is described under examination of the vascular system (see later section).

TRACHEA

The trachea can be directly palpated and is normally located in the midline of the neck, above the suprasternal notch. Masses in the neck or mediastinum and pulmonary abnormalities can cause displacement laterally. The client may sit or lie down during palpation. The position of the trachea is determined by palpating at the suprasternal notch, slipping the thumb and index fingers to each side. Forceful pressure must not be applied because this action may elicit a cough.

■ THORAX AND LUNGS

Accurate physical assessment of the thorax and lungs requires review of the ventilatory and respiratory functions of the lungs. If the lungs are affected by disease, other body systems will reflect alterations. For example, reduced oxy-

genation can cause changes in mental alertness because of the brain's sensitivity to lowered oxygen levels. The alert nurse uses the data from all body systems to determine the nature of pulmonary alterations.

Before assessing the thorax and lungs, the nurse must be familiar with the landmarks of the chest (Fig. 33-42). These landmarks help the nurse locate findings and use assessment skills correctly. For example, by knowing the position of underlying organs in relation to the landmarks, the nurse can anticipate where to percuss or auscultate the chest wall. The client's nipples, angle of Louis, suprasternal notch, costal angle, clavicles, and vertebrae are key landmarks that provide a series of imaginary lines for sign identification. The lungs and thorax are assessed posteriorly, laterally (on both sides), and anteriorly, with the nurse using landmarks to record localized findings.

During the examination the nurse keeps a mental image of the location of the lobes of the lung and the position of each rib (Fig. 33-43). Locating the position of each rib is critical to visualizing the lobe of the lung being assessed. To begin, the nurse locates the angle of Louis at the manubriosternal junction. The angle is a visible and palpable angulation of the sternum and point at which the second rib articulates with the sternum. The nurse counts the ribs and intercostal spaces (between the ribs) from this point. The number of each intercostal space corresponds to that of the rib just above it. The spinous process of the third thoracic vertebra and the fourth, fifth, and sixth ribs help to locate the lung's lobes laterally. The lower lobes project laterally and anteriorly (Fig. 33-44). Posteriorly the tip or inferior margin of the scapula lies approximately at the level of the seventh rib (Fig. 33-45). After identifying the seventh rib the examiner can count upward to locate the third thoracic vertebra and align it with the inner borders of the scapula to locate the posterior lobes.

Examination of the lungs and thorax requires the client to be undressed to the waist. Good lighting is essential. The nurse should assess clients at risk for pulmonary problems, such as the client confined to bed rest or the client with chest pain who cannot fully expand the lungs. The examination begins with the client sitting for assessment of the

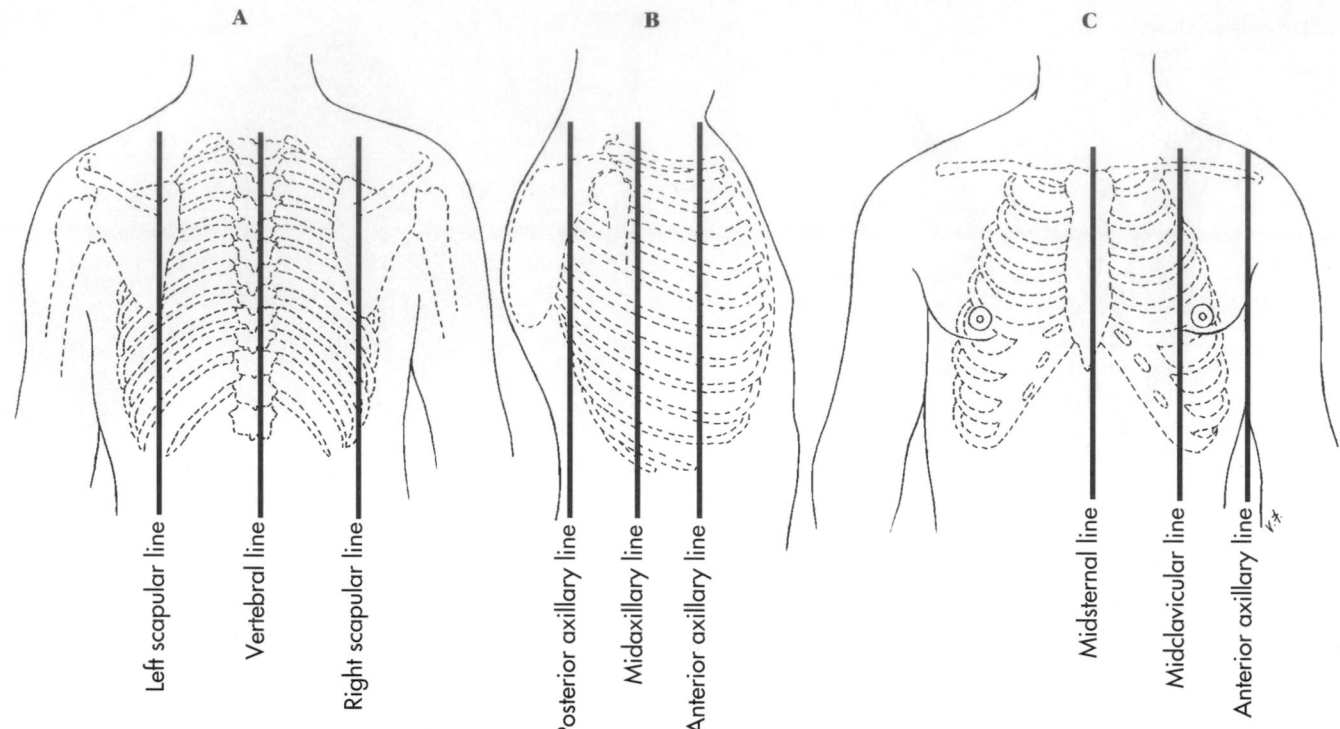

Fig. 33-42 Anatomical chest wall landmarks. **A,** Posterior chest landmarks. **B,** Lateral chest landmarks. **C,** Anterior chest landmarks.

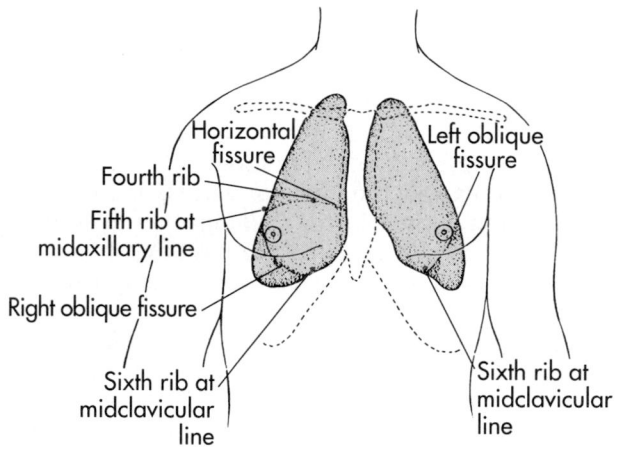

Fig. 33-43 Anterior position of lung lobes in relation to anatomical landmarks.

posterior and lateral chest. For assessment of the anterior chest, the client sits or lies. Table 33-19 reviews the nursing history for lung examination.

Posterior Thorax

The nurse first inspects the shape and symmetry of the client's chest from the back and front. The anteroposterior diameter is noted. Shape or posture can significantly impair ventilatory movement. Normally the chest contour is symmetrical with the anteroposterior diameter $^1/_3$ to $^1/_2$ of the transverse or side-to-side diameter. Aging and chronic lung disease are characterized by a barrel-shaped chest (anteroposterior diameter equals transverse). Infants have an almost round shape. Abnormal contours are caused by congenital and postural alterations. A client may assume a posture such as leaning over a table or splinting the side of the chest as a result of a breathing problem. Splinting or holding the chest wall as a result of localized pain causes a client to bend toward the side affected. Such a posture impairs ventilatory movement.

Standing at a midline position behind the client, the nurse looks for deformities, position of the spine, slope of the ribs, retraction of the intercostal spaces during inspiration, and bulging of the intercostal spaces during expiration. The scapulae are normally symmetrical and closely attached to the thoracic wall. The normal spine is straight without lateral deviation. Posteriorly, the ribs tend to slope across and down. The ribs and intercostal spaces are easier to see in a thin person. Normally, no bulging or active movement occurs within the intercostal spaces during breathing. Bulging indicates that the client is using great effort to breathe.

The nurse may also inspect the posterior thorax to determine the rate and rhythm of breathing (see Chapter 32). The thorax as a whole is observed. The entire thorax normally expands and relaxes regularly with equality of movement. In healthy adults the normal respiratory rates vary from 12 to 20 respirations per minute.

Palpation of the posterior thorax assesses further characteristics and confirms or supplements assessment findings. The thoracic muscles and skeleton are palpated for lumps, masses, pulsations, and unusual movement. If pain or ten-

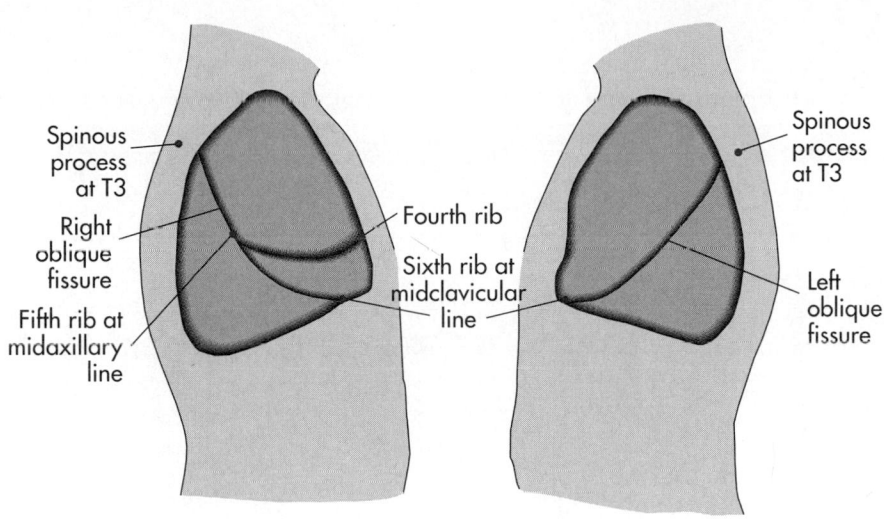

Fig. 33-44 Lateral position of lung lobes in relation to anatomical landmarks.

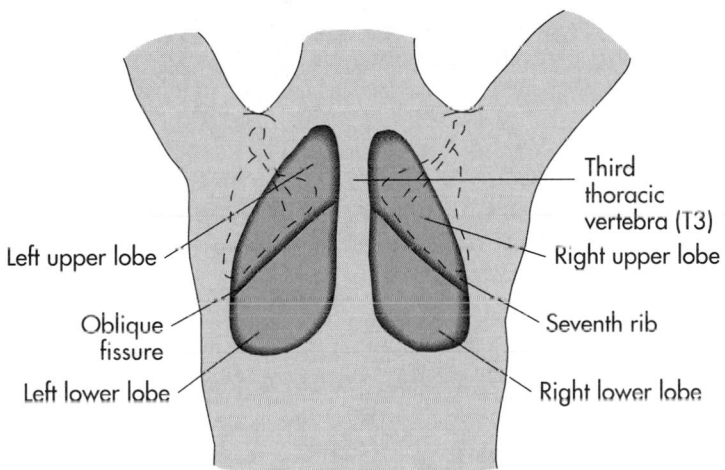

Fig. 33-45 Posterior position of lung lobes in relation to anatomical landmarks.

Table 33-19	Nursing History for Lung Assessment

ASSESSMENT CATEGORY	RATIONALE
Assess history of tobacco or marijuana use, including type of tobacco, duration and amount (pack years = number of years smoking × number of packs per day), age started, and efforts to quit.	Smoking is a risk factor for lung cancer, heart disease, and emphysema or bronchitis. Cigarette smoking accounts for a significant percentage of all cancer deaths.
Ask if client has had a *persistent cough* (productive or nonproductive), *sputum production, chest pain,* shortness of breath, orthopnea, dyspnea during exertion, poor activity tolerance, and *recurrent attacks of pneumonia or bronchitis.*	Symptoms of respiratory alterations may help nurse localize objective physical findings. (Warning signals for lung cancer are in italic type.)
Determine if client works in environment containing pollutants, (e.g., asbestos, arsenic, coal dust) or requiring exposure to radiation. Does client have exposure to sidestream cigarette smoke?	These risk factors increase chance for various lung diseases.
Review history for known or suspected HIV infection, substance abuse, low-income, and residence in nursing home (ATS, 1992).	These are risk factors for tuberculosis.
Ask if client has history of cough, hemoptysis, weight loss, fatigue, night sweats, and fever.	Risk factors for both tuberculosis and HIV infection.
Does client have history of chronic hoarseness?	May indicate laryngeal disorder or abuse of cocaine, opioids (sniffing).
Assess history of allergies to pollens, dust, or other airborne irritants and to foods, drugs, or chemical substances.	Symptoms such as choking feeling, bronchospasm with respiratory stridor, wheezes on auscultation and dyspnea may be caused by allergic response.
Review family history for cancer, tuberculosis, allergies, or chronic obstructive pulmonary disease.	Conditions place client at risk for lung disease.

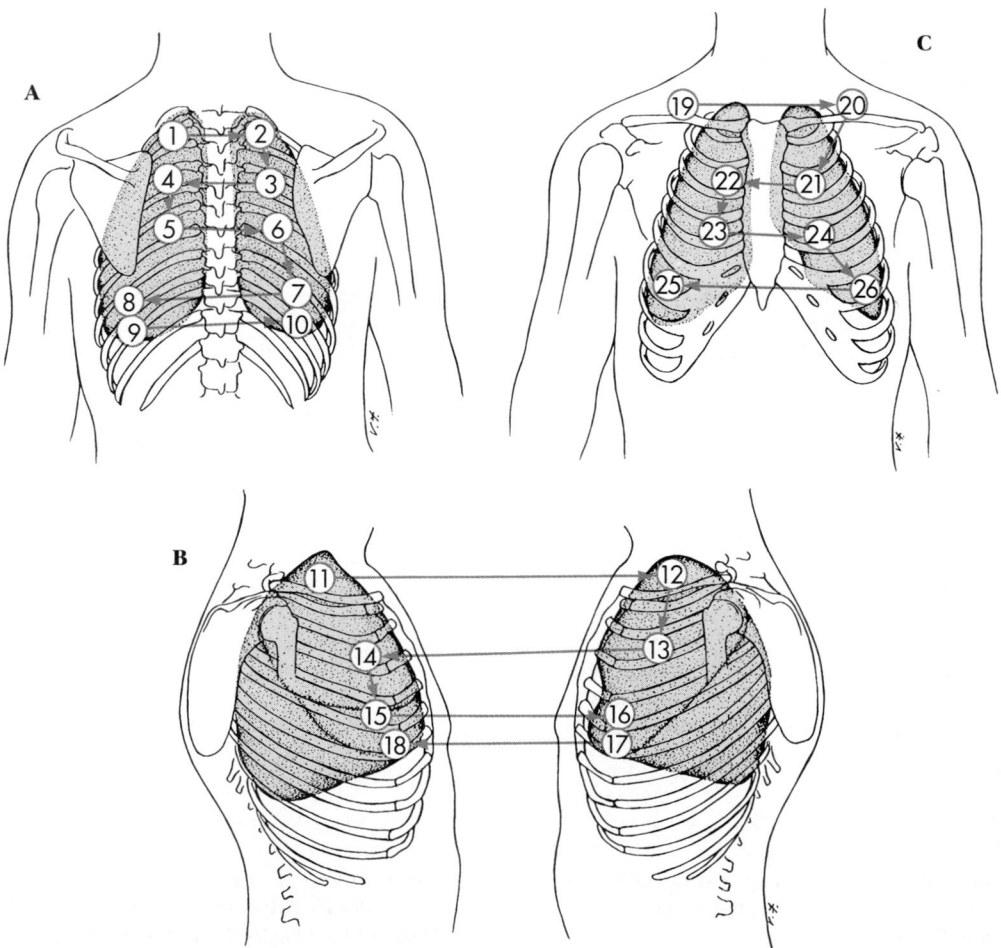

Fig. 33-46 A, Position of nurse's hands for palpation of posterior thorax excursion. **B,** As the client inhales, the movement of chest excursion separates the nurse's thumbs.

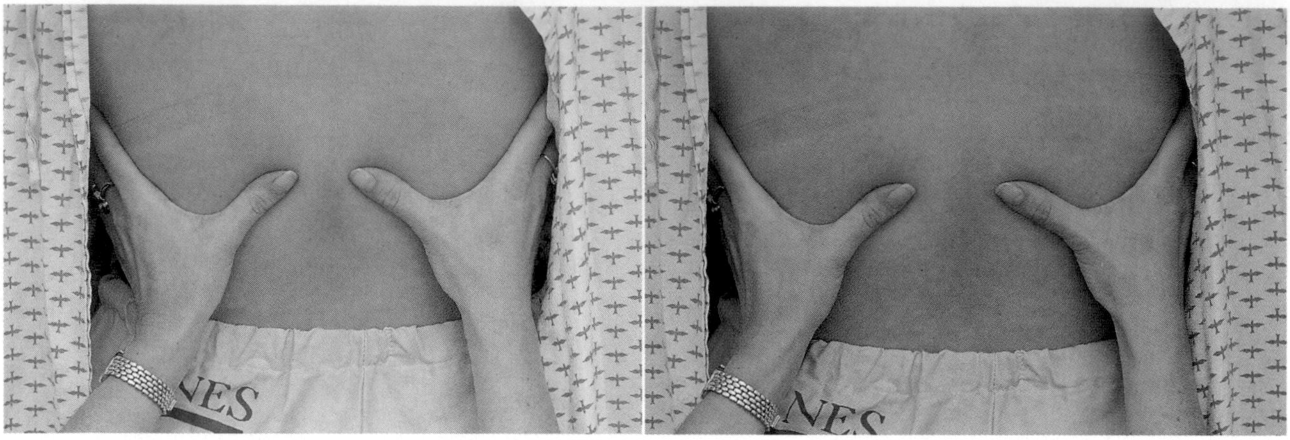

Fig. 33-47 A to **C,** the nurse follows a systematic pattern (posterior-lateral-anterior) when comparing fremitus, percussion notes, and auscultation.

derness is noted, the nurse avoids deep palpation. Fractured rib fragments could be displaced against vital organs. Normally the chest wall is not tender. If a suspicious mass or swollen area is detected, it is lightly palpated for size, shape, and the typical qualities of a lesion.

To measure chest excursion or depth of breathing, the nurse stands behind the client and places the thumbs along the spinal processes at the tenth rib, with the palms lightly contacting the posterolateral surfaces. The nurse's thumbs should be about 2 inches (5 cm) apart, pointing toward the spine and fingers pointing laterally (Fig. 33-46, *A*). The hands are pressed toward the spine so that a small skinfold appears between the thumbs. The nurse does not slide the hands over the skin. The nurse instructs the client to take a deep breath after exhaling. The nurse notes movement of the thumbs (Fig. 33-46, *B*). Chest excursion should be symmetric, separating the thumbs $1^{1}/_{4}$ to 2 inches (3 to 5 cm). Reduced chest excursion may be caused by pain, postural deformity, or fatigue. In the older adult, chest movement declines because of costal cartilage calcification and respiratory muscle atrophy.

During speech the sound created by the vocal cords is transmitted through the lung to the chest wall. The sound waves create vibrations that can be palpated externally. These vibrations are called **vocal** or **tactile fremitus.** The accumulation of mucus, the collapse of lung tissue, or the presence of lung lesions can block the vibrations from reaching the chest wall.

To palpate for tactile fremitus, the nurse places the ball or lower palm of the hand over symmetric intercostal spaces, beginning at the lung apex (Fig. 33-47, *A*). A firm light touch is best. The nurse asks the client to repeat the words *ninety-nine* or *one-one-one*. Normally there is a faint vibration as the client speaks. Both sides of the thorax are compared, moving from top to bottom. Only one hand is used to ensure accuracy. If fremitus is faint, it may be necessary to ask the client to speak in a louder or lower tone of voice. Symmetry of fremitus is normal. Vibrations are strongest at the top, near the level of the tracheal bifurcation. It is easy to assess for tactile fremitus in a crying infant because strong vibrations can be felt through the chest wall.

Percussion of the chest wall is a difficult assessment technique that determines whether underlying lung tissue is filled with air or fluid or is solid. Percussion reaches only 5 to 7 cm (2 to 3 inches) into the chest wall and thus cannot detect deep lesions. The client folds the arms forward across the chest with head bent forward. This position separates the scapulae further to expose more lung to assessment. Using the indirect technique, the nurse percusses in the intercostal spaces over symmetrical areas of the lungs. Fig. 33-47 shows how following a systematic pattern starting posteriorly and then moving laterally and anteriorly allows the nurse to compare percussion notes for all lung lobes. Resonance, the sound created by air-filled lungs, is normally heard over the posterior thorax. Percussion over the scapula, ribs, or spine is dull. The chest is normally more resonant in the child than in the adult. A lung mass causes a flat sound.

Auscultation assesses the movement of air through the tracheobronchial tree and detects mucus or obstructed airways. Normally air flows through the airways in an unobstructed pattern. Recognizing the sounds created by normal

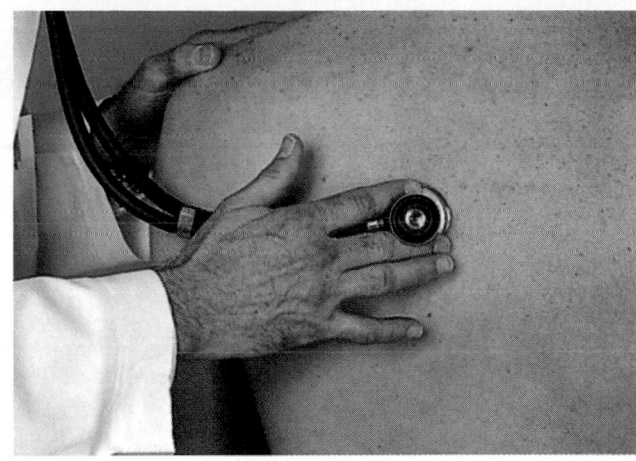

Fig. 33-48 In an adult the nurse uses the diaphragm of the stethoscope to auscultate breath sounds. *(From Seidel HM et al: Mosby's guide to physical examination, ed 3, St Louis, 1995, Mosby.)*

airflow allows the nurse to detect sounds caused by obstruction.

In an adult the diaphragm of the stethoscope is placed firmly on the skin, over the posterior chest wall between the ribs (Fig. 33-48). The client sits upright (if possible) and folds the arms in front of the chest and keeps the head bent forward while taking slow deep breaths with the mouth slightly open. It helps to demonstrate for the client. The nurse listens to an entire inspiration and expiration at each position of the stethoscope. If sounds are faint, as in the obese client, the client should be asked to breathe harder and faster. Breath sounds are much louder in children because of the thinness of the chest wall. In children the bell works best because of a child's small chest.

A systematic pattern throughout should be used when comparing the right and left sides (Fig. 33-47, *A*). An inexperienced student may attempt to auscultate all of the left side and then return to the right side. This is incorrect. The examiner compares lung sounds in one region on one side of the body with sounds in the same region on the opposite side. It is impossible to remember the quality of all sounds noted on one side of the body and then compare them with the other side.

The nurse auscultates for normal breath sounds and abnormal or **adventitious sounds.** Normal breath sounds differ in character, depending on the area of lungs being auscultated. Sounds normally heard over the posterior thorax include bronchovesicular and vesicular sounds (Table 33-20).

Abnormal sounds result from air passing through moisture, mucus, or narrowed airways; from alveoli suddenly reinflating, or from an inflammation between the lung's pleural linings. Adventitious or added sounds often occur superimposed over normal sounds. The four types of adventitious sounds include crackles (previously called *rales*), rhonchi, wheezes, and pleural friction rub. Each sound is caused by a specific entity and is characterized by typical auditory features (Table 33-21). The location and characteristics of the sounds should be noted, as should the absence

Table 33-20	**Normal Breath Sounds**		
DESCRIPTION	**LOCATION**	**ORIGIN**	
VESICULAR Vesicular sounds are soft, breezy, and low pitched. Inspiratory phase is 3 times longer than expiratory phase.	Best heard over lung's periphery (except over scapula)	Created by air moving through smaller airways	
BRONCHOVESICULAR Bronchovesicular sounds are medium-pitched and blowing sounds of medium intensity. Inspiratory phase is equal to expiratory phase.	Best heard posteriorly between scapulae and anteriorly over bronchioles lateral to sternum at first and second intercostal spaces	Created by air moving through large airways	
BRONCHIAL Bronchial sounds are loud and high pitched with hollow quality. Expiration lasts longer than inspiration (3:2 ratio).	Best heard over trachea	Created by air moving through trachea close to chest wall	

of breath sounds (found in clients with collapsed or surgically removed lobes).

If the nurse assesses abnormalities in tactile fremitus, percussion, or auscultation, another test is performed for spoken and whispered voice sounds. With the stethoscope placed over the same locations used to assess breath sounds, the client says *ninety-nine* or *eee* in a normal voice tone. Normally the sounds are muffled. If fluid is compressing the lung, vibrations from the client's voice are transmitted to the chest wall and the sounds become clear (**bronchophony**). The nurse then asks the client to whisper *ninety-nine*. The whispered voice is usually faint and indistinct. Certain lung abnormalities may cause the whispered voice to become clear and distinct (**whispered pectoriloquy**).

Lateral Thorax

The client sits during examination of the lateral chest. Usually the nurse extends the assessment of the posterior thorax to the lateral sides of the chest. The client is asked to raise the arms, which improves access to lateral thoracic structures. The nurse uses all four assessment skills to methodically examine the lateral thorax (Fig. 33-47, *B*). Excursion cannot be assessed laterally. Normally, percussion notes are resonant, and breath sounds are vesicular.

Anterior Thorax

The anterior thorax is inspected for the same features as the posterior thorax. The client sits or lies down with head elevated. The nurse observes the accessory muscles of breathing: sternocleidomastoid, trapezius, and abdominal mus-

CLIENT TEACHING
During Lung Assessment

OBJECTIVES
- Client will describe warning signs of lung disease.
- Older adult will receive influenza and pneumonia vaccines annually.
- Client with chronic obstructive pulmonary disease (COPD) will clear airways more effectively and report less shortness of breath.

TEACHING STRATEGIES
- Explain the risk factors for chronic lung disease and lung cancer, including cigarette smoking, history of cigarette smoking for over 20 years, exposure to certain industrial substances (e.g., arsenic, asbestos), and radiation exposure from occupational, medical, and environmental sources. Residential radon exposure may increase risk for lung cancer, especially in cigarette smokers.*
- Share brochures on lung cancer from American Cancer Society with client and family.

- Discuss the warning signs of lung cancer, such as a persistent cough, sputum streaked with blood, chest pains, and recurrent attacks of pneumonia or bronchitis.
- Counsel older adult on benefits from receiving annual influenza and pneumonia vaccinations because of a greater susceptibility to respiratory infection.
- Instruct client with COPD in coughing and pursed-lip breathing exercises.

EVALUATION
- Have client describe risk factors for lung disease and cancer.
- Ask client to identify any known risks for cancer.
- Ask client to name warning signs for cancer.
- In a follow-up visit, review client's immunization record.
- Observe client perform breathing exercises and coughing.

*Data from American Cancer Society: *1995 cancer facts and figures,* New York, 1995, The Society.

Table 33-21	Adventitious Sounds		
SOUND	**SITE AUSCULTATED**	**CAUSE**	**CHARACTER**
Crackles (previously called *rales*)	Are most commonly heard in dependent lobes: right and left lung bases	Random, sudden reinflation of groups of alveoli*; disruptive passage of air	Fine crackles are high-pitched fine, short, interrupted crackling sounds heard during end of inspiration, usually not cleared with coughing* Moist crackles are lower, more moist sounds heard during middle of inspiration; not cleared with coughing
Rhonchi	Are primarily heard over trachea and bronchi; if loud enough, can be heard over most lung fields	Muscular spasm, fluid, or mucus in larger airways, causing turbulence	Are loud, low-pitched, rumbling coarse sounds heard most often during inspiration or expiration; may be cleared by coughing
Wheezes	Can be heard over all lung fields	High-velocity air flow through severely narrowed bronchus	Are high-pitched, continuous musical sounds like a squeak heard continuously during inspiration or expiration; usually louder on expiration, do not clear with coughing†
Pleural friction rub	Is heard over anterior lateral lung field (if client is sitting upright)	Inflamed pleura, parietal pleura rubbing against visceral pleura	Has dry, grating quality heard best during inspiration; does not clear with coughing, heard loudest over lower lateral anterior surface

*Data from Forgacs P: *Chest* 73:399, 1978.
†Data from Wilkins RL, Hodgkin JE, Lopez B: *Lung sounds: a practical guide,* St Louis, 1988, Mosby—Year Book.

cles. The accessory muscles move little with normal passive breathing. When a client requires effort to breathe as a result of strenuous exercise or disease (e.g., chronic obstructive pulmonary disease), the accessory muscles and abdominal muscles contract (see the box on p. 688). Some clients produce a grunting sound.

The nurse observes the width of the costal angle. It is usually larger than 90 degrees between the two costal margins. The nurse observes the breathing pattern. Normal breathing is quiet and barely audible near the open mouth. Respiratory rate and rhythm are more often assessed anteriorly (see Chapter 32). A man's respirations are usually diaphragmatic, whereas a woman's are more costal. Accurate assessment occurs as a client breathes passively.

The examiner palpates anterior thoracic muscles and skeleton for lumps, masses, tenderness, or unusual movement. The sternum and xiphoid are relatively inflexible. To measure chest excursion anteriorly, the nurse places the hands over each lateral rib cage, with the thumbs approximately 2.5 cm (2 inches) apart and angled along each costal margin (Fig. 33-49, *A*). The thumbs are pushed toward the midline to create a fold of skin between the thumbs. As the client inhales deeply, the thumbs should normally separate approximately 2.5 to 5 cm (1 to 2 inches), with each side expanding equally (Fig. 33-49, *B*).

Tactile fremitus is assessed over the chest wall. Anterior findings differ from posterior findings because of the heart and female breast tissue. Fremitus is best felt next to the

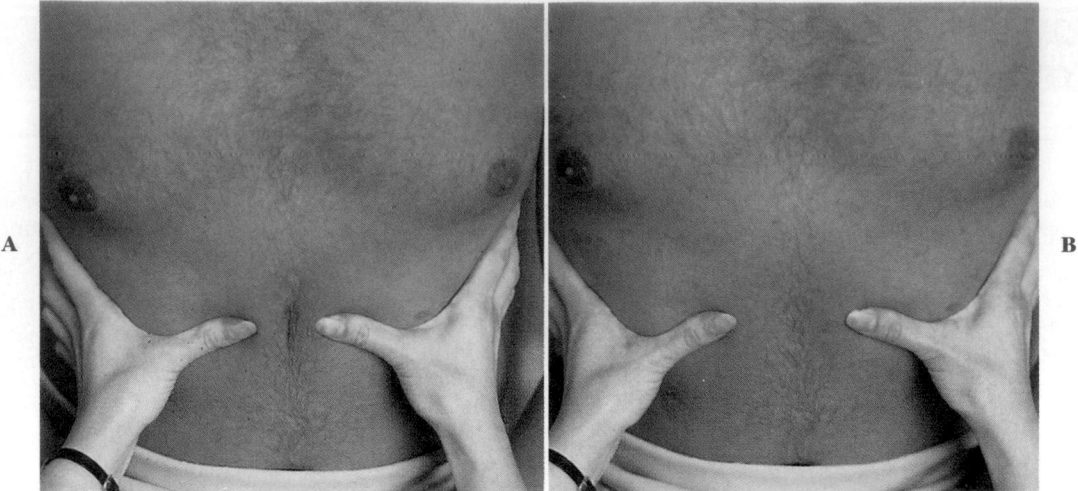

Fig. 33-49 A, Position of nurse's hands before excursion of the anterior chest wall. **B,** As the client inhales, the nurse's hands normally separate 3 to 5 cm (1½ to 2 inches).

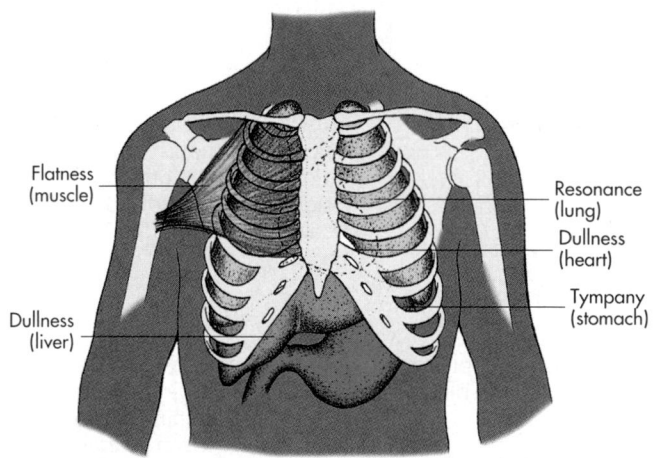

Flatness (muscle)

Dullness (liver)

Resonance (lung)

Dullness (heart)

Tympany (stomach)

Fig. 33-50 Variations in percussion notes in the normal thorax and upper abdomen.

sternum at the second intercostal space, at the level of the bronchial bifurcation. It is decreased over the heart, lower thorax, and breast tissue. The nurse will not be able to sense vibrations over breast tissue and thus must retract the breasts gently during palpation. If the breasts are large, this portion of the examination may be omitted.

Percussion of the anterior thorax follows a systematic pattern. The nurse must imagine the location of all internal organs anteriorly accessible to examination. The underlying liver, heart, and stomach create percussion notes characteristically different from those of the lung (Fig. 33-50). Percussion may be conducted with the client in a sitting or lying position. However, the procedure is easier if the client lies down. The nurse starts above the clavicles and moves across and then down. The female breasts are displaced as needed. The normal lung is resonant. As the examiner proceeds downward, the areas of heart and liver dullness and the tympanic gastric air bubble will be detectable.

Auscultation of the anterior thorax follows the same pattern as percussion (see Fig. 32-47, *C*). The client should sit if possible to maximize chest expansion. Special attention should be paid to the lower lobes, where mucous secretions commonly gather. Bronchovesicular and vesicular sounds are heard above and below the clavicles and along the lung periphery. An additional normal breath sound, the bronchial sound, can be heard over the trachea. It is loud, high pitched, and hollow sounding, with expiration lasting longer than inspiration (3:2 ratio).

HEART

The assessment of heart function involves a review of signs and symptoms from the nursing history, pulse assessment, and direct examination of the heart. A client who has signs or symptoms of heart (cardiac) problems (e.g., chest pain and irregular heart rate) may be suffering a life-threatening condition requiring immediate attention. In this case, the nurse acts quickly and decides on the portions of the examination that are absolutely necessary. When a client's condition is stable, a more thorough assessment can reveal baseline heart function and any risks for heart disease. Abnormal findings require a physician's attention. The nurse performing a cardiac assessment compares findings with those made in the vascular examination (see later section). The nursing history (Table 33-22) provides data that help the nurse interpret physical findings.

Assessment of cardiac function is performed through the anterior thorax. The nurse forms a mental image of the heart's exact location (Fig. 33-51). In the adult, it is in the center of the chest (precordium), behind and to the left of the sternum, with a small section of the right atrium extending to the sternum's right. The base of the heart is the upper portion, and the apex is the bottom tip. The surface of the right ventricle composes most of the heart's anterior surface. A section of the left ventricle shapes the left anterior side of the apex. The apex actually touches the anterior chest wall at approximately the fourth to fifth intercostal space just medial to the left midclavicular line. This loca-

Table 33-22	**Nursing History for Heart Assessment**

ASSESSMENT CATEGORY	RATIONALE
Determine history of smoking, alcohol intake, use of drugs, exercise habits, and dietary patterns and intake (including fat and sodium intake).	Smoking, alcohol ingestion, cocaine use, lack of regular exercise, and intake of foods high in carbohydrates, fats, and cholesterol are risk factors for cardiovascular disease.
Determine if client is taking medications for cardiovascular function (e.g., antidysrhythmics, antihypertensives) and if client knows their purpose, dosage, and side effects.	Knowledge allows nurse to assess compliance with drug therapies. Medications may affect vital sign values.
Assess for chest pain, palpitations, excess fatigue, cough, dyspnea, leg pain or cramps, edema of feet, cyanosis, fainting, and orthopnea. Ask if symptoms occur at rest or during exercise.	These are key symptoms of heart disease. Cardiovascular function may be adequate during rest but not during exercise.
If client reports chest pain, determine if it is cardiac in nature. Anginal pain is usually a deep pressure or ache that is substernal and diffuse, radiating to one or both arms, neck, or jaw.	Determines nature of pain and need to initiate care immediately.
Determine whether client has a stressful lifestyle. What physical demands or emotional stress exists.	Repeated exposure to stress may increase risk for heart disease.
Assess family history for heart disease, diabetes, high cholesterol levels, hypertension, stroke, or rheumatic heart disease.	Factors increase risk for heart disease.
Ask client about history of heart trouble (e.g., congestive heart failure, congenital heart disease, coronary artery disease, dysrhythmias, murmurs).	Knowledge reveals client's level of understanding of condition. Preexisting condition influences examination techniques used by nurse, as well as findings to expect.
Determine whether client has preexisting diabetes, lung disease, obesity, or hypertension.	These disorders may alter heart function.
Determine whether client drinks excessive amounts of coffee, tea, other caffeine-containing soft drinks, or chocolate.	Caffeine can cause heart dysrhythmias.

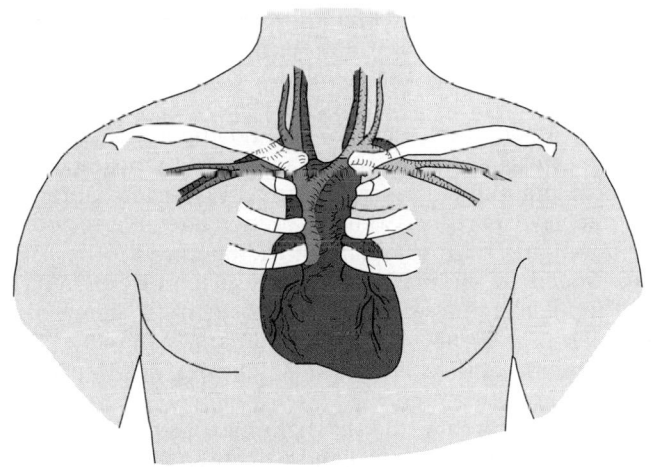

Fig. 33-51 Anatomical position of heart.

tion is known as the **apical impulse** or **point of maximal impulse (PMI)**.

An infant's heart is positioned more horizontally and has a larger diameter compared with that of an adult. The apex of the heart in an infant is at the third or fourth intercostal space, just to the left of the midclavicular line. By the age of 7 a child's PMI is in the same location as the adult's.

In tall slender persons the heart hangs more vertically and is positioned more centrally. In persons who are stocky and short, the heart tends to lie more to the left and horizontally (Seidel et al, 1995).

To understand the significance of assessment findings,

the nurse must first understand timing in relation to the cardiac cycle (Fig. 33-52). The heart normally pumps blood through its four chambers in a methodical, even sequence. Events on the left side occur just before those on the right. As blood flows through each chamber, the valves open and close, the pressures within chambers rise and fall, and the chambers contract. Each event creates a physiological sign that can be detected by an examiner. Both sides of the heart function in a coordinated fashion.

There are two phases to the cardiac cycle: systole and diastole. During systole the ventricles contract and eject blood from the left ventricle into the aorta and from the right ventricle into the pulmonary artery. During diastole the ventricles relax and the atria contract to move blood into the ventricles and fill the coronary arteries.

Events occurring on the left side of the heart have the most dramatic effect on assessment findings. Pressure is greatest on the left side, so longer and louder sounds are created. Events on the left side slightly precede those on the right. When the left ventricle is at rest (diastolic phase), the pressure in the left atrium exceeds that in the ventricle, creating a pressure gradient that moves blood through the opened mitral valve. During ventricular filling, pressure rises in the ventricle to exceed the pressure in the left atrium. Just before the ventricle contracts, the mitral valve closes to prevent regurgitation of blood into the atrium, creating the first heart sound (S_1), often described as "lub." Ventricular pressure builds, causing the aortic valve to open as the ventricle contracts (systolic phase). Blood flows into the aorta, elevating aortic pressure. When the ventricle empties, pressure within the chamber falls. To prevent regurgitation from the aorta into the left ventricle, the aortic

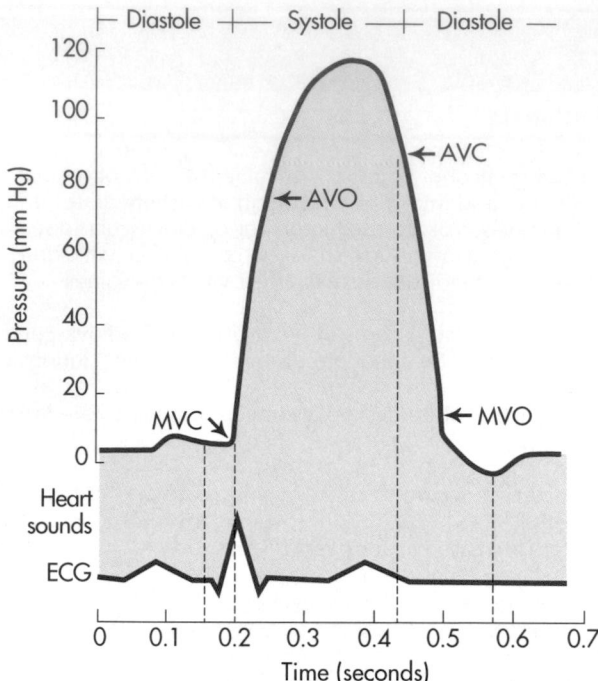

Fig. 33-52 Cardiac cycle. *MVC,* Mitral valve closes; *AVO,* aortic valve opens; *AVC,* aortic valve closes; *MVO,* mitral valve opens.

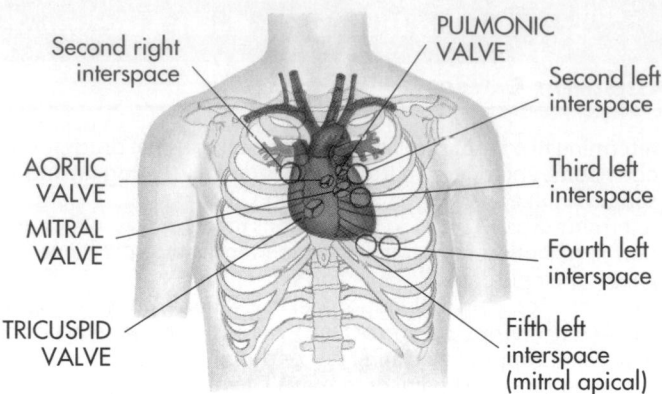

Fig. 33-53 Areas for auscultation of the heart. *(From Seidel HM et al:* Mosby's guide to physical examination, *ed 3, St Louis, 1995, Mosby.)*

valve closes, creating the second heart sound (S₂), described as "dub." As ventricular pressure continues to fall, it drops below that of the left atrium. The mitral valve reopens to again allow ventricular filling. The rapid filling of the ventricle may create a third heart sound (S₃), heard more often in children and young adults. An S₃ can also be heard as an abnormality in adults over 30 years of age. When the atria contract to enhance ventricular filling, a fourth heart sound (S₄) is produced. The S₄ is not normally heard in adults, but may be heard in healthy older adults, children, and athletes. Because it may also indicate an abnormal condition, it should be reported to a physician.

Inspection and Palpation

Before beginning the examination, the nurse ensures that the client is relaxed and comfortable. An anxious or uncomfortable client can have mild tachycardia that may lead the nurse to misinterpret the findings. Findings from the examination of other body systems, such as signs of heart failure (crackles in the lungs) influence judgments made during cardiovascular assessment. The nurse must be able to successfully examine the client but also integrate and interpret findings correctly.

The nurse uses inspection and palpation simultaneously. The examination begins with the client in the supine position or with the upper body elevated 45 degrees because clients with heart disease frequently suffer shortness of breath while lying flat. The nurse stands at the client's right side. The client must not talk, especially when the nurse auscultates heart sounds. Good lighting in the room is essential.

During inspection and palpation the nurse will methodically look for visible pulsations and exaggerated lifts and palpate for the apical impulse and any source of vibrations (thrills). It helps to follow an orderly sequence beginning with assessment of the base of the heart and moving toward the apex. First the nurse inspects the angle of Louis, which lies between the sternal body and manubrium and can be felt as a ridge in the sternum approximately 2 inches below the sternal notch. The nurse can slip the fingers along the angle on each side of the sternum to feel adjacent ribs. The intercostal spaces are just below each rib. The second intercostal space allows identification of the first two anatomical landmarks (Fig. 33-53), the second right and left interspace. The third and fourth left interspaces can be found by progressing down along the left side of the sternum, palpating each intercostal space. Deeper palpation is required to feel the spaces in obese clients or those with well-developed chest muscles. To find the apical area the nurse locates the fifth intercostal space just to the left of the sternum and moves the fingers laterally, just medial to the left midclavicular line. Some examiners are able to locate the apical area with the palm of the hand, but others use their fingertips. Normally at the apical impulse there is a light tap felt in an area 1 to 2 cm (¹/₂ inch) in diameter at the apex (Fig. 33-54). Another landmark is the epigastric area at the tip of the sternum. It is typically used to palpate for aortic abnormalities.

As the nurse locates the six anatomical landmarks of the heart, each area is inspected and palpated. The nurse looks for the appearance of pulsations, viewing each area over the chest at an angle to the side. Normally, no pulsations can be seen except perhaps at the PMI in thin clients or at the epigastric area as a result of abdominal aorta pulsation. Palpation for pulsations is best done using the proximal halves of the four fingers together and then alternating with the ball of the hand. The nurse touches the areas gently to allow movements to lift the hand. Normally no pulsations or vibrations can be felt in the second, third, or fourth intercostal spaces. A vibration is caused by loud murmurs. If pulsations or vibrations are palpated, the nurse times their occurrence in relation to systole or diastole by auscultating heart sounds simultaneously.

If the PMI cannot be found with the client in the supine position, the nurse asks the client to roll onto the left side, which moves the heart closer to the chest wall. The nurse

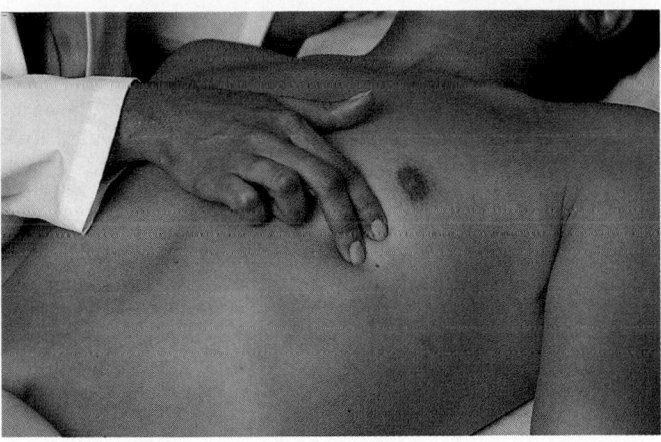

Fig. 33-54 Palpation of PMI at the fourth to fifth intercostal space along the midclavicular line. *(From Canobbio MM: Cardiovascular disorders, St Louis, 1990, Mosby.)*

estimates the heart's size by noting the diameter of the PMI and its position relative to the midclavicular line. In cases of serious heart disease, the cardiac muscle enlarges, with the PMI found to the left of the midclavicular line. The PMI may be difficult to find in the older adult because the chest deepens in its anteroposterior diameters. It may also be difficult to locate in a client who is very muscular or overweight. The PMI of an infant can usually be found near the third or fourth intercostal space. It is easy to palpate the child's PMI because of the thin chest wall.

Auscultation

Auscultation of the heart detects normal heart sounds, extra heart sounds, and murmurs. The nursing student should first become skilled in detecting normal heart sounds. These low-intensity sounds created by the closing of the valves are often difficult to hear, especially if breath sounds are noisy. Concentration is needed when detecting heart sounds. To begin auscultation the nurse eliminates all sources of room noise and explains the procedure to relieve the client's anxiety. The nurse follows a pattern during auscultation moving systematically and inching the stethoscope across each of the anatomical sites (see Fig. 33-53). It is important to hear heart sounds clearly at each location. Then the sequence is repeated using the bell of the stethoscope. The client may be asked to assume three different positions during the examination (Fig. 33-55): sitting up and leaning forward (good position to hear all areas and to hear high-pitched murmurs), supine (good for all areas), and left lateral recumbent (good for all areas and best position to hear low-pitched sounds in diastole).

The nurse usually must lift the female client's left breast to listen better to the chest wall. The nurse learns to identify the first (S_1) and second (S_2) heart sounds. At normal rates, S_1 occurs after the long diastolic pause and preceding the short systolic pause. S_1 is high pitched, dull in quality, and heard best at the apex. If the nurse has difficulty hearing S_1, it can be timed in relation to the carotid pulse. It occurs just before the carotid pulsation. S_2 follows the short systolic pause and precedes the long diastolic pause. It is heard best at the aortic area.

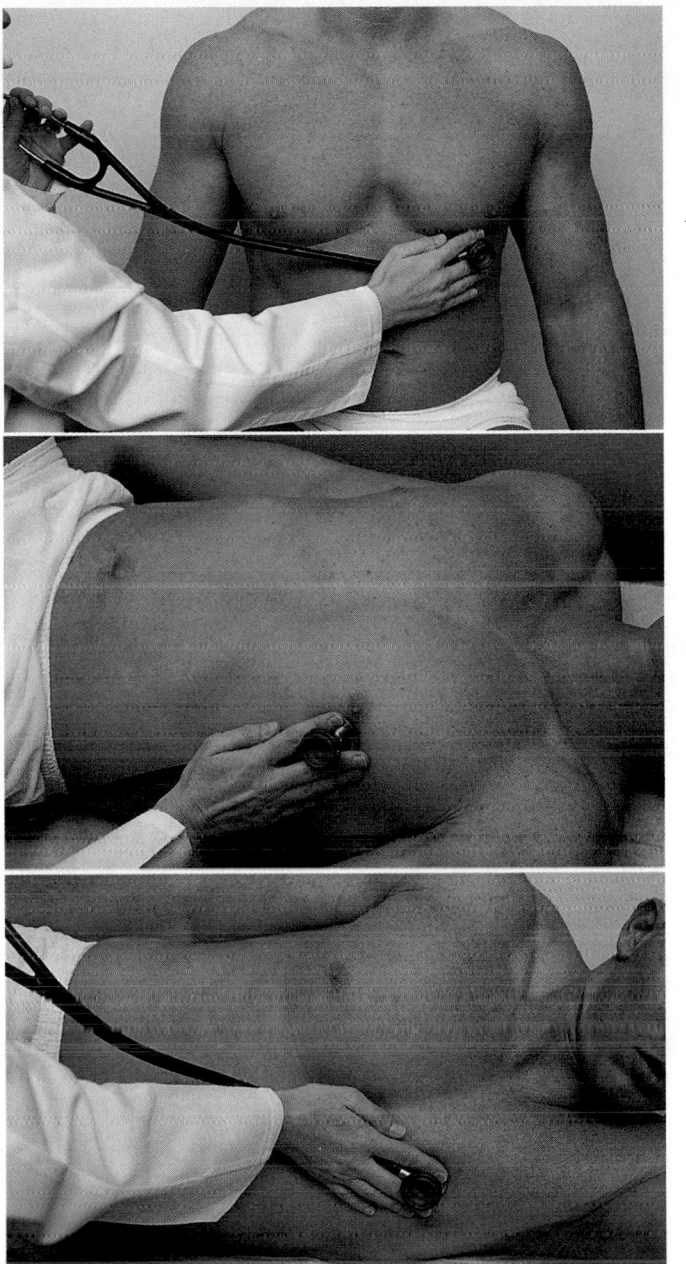

Fig. 33-55 Sequence of client positions for heart auscultation **A.** Sitting, **B.** Supine, **C.** Left lateral recumbent *(From Seidel HM et al: Mosby's guide to physical examination, ed 3, St Louis, 1995, Mosby.)*

The nurse auscultates for rate and rhythm after both sounds can be heard clearly. Each combination of S_1 and S_2 or "lub-dub" counts as one heartbeat. The nurse counts the rate for 1 minute and listens for the interval between S_1 and S_2 and then the time between S_2 and the next S_1. A regular rhythm involves regular intervals of time between each sequence of beats. There is a distinct silent pause between S_1 and S_2. Failure of the heart to beat at regular successive intervals is a **dysrhythmia**. Some dysrhythmias can be life-threatening.

When the heart rhythm is irregular, the nurse compares

apical and radial pulse rates to determine if a pulse deficit exists. Auscultate the apical pulse first and then immediately palpate the radial pulse (one examiner technique). When two examiners are available, the apical and radial rates are assessed at the same time. The nurse compares the two rates. When a client has a **pulse deficit**, the radial pulse is slower than the apical because ineffective contractions fail to send pulse waves to the periphery. A difference in pulse rates is reported to the physician immediately.

The nurse also learns to assess for extra heart sounds at each auscultatory site. Using the bell of the stethoscope, the nurse listens for low-pitched extra heart sounds such as S_3 and S_4 gallops, clicks, and rubs. Auscultate over all anatomical areas. S_3, or a **ventricular gallop**, occurs just after S_2 at the end of ventricular diastole. It may be caused by a premature rush of blood into a ventricle that is stiff or dilated due to heart failure and hypertension. Some examiners describe the combination of S_1, S_2, and S_3 as sounding like the word "Ken-tuck-ky."

S_4, or an atrial gallop, occurs just before S_1 or ventricular systole. The sound of an S_4 is similar to that of "Tennessee." Physiologically it may be due to an atrial contraction pushing against a ventricle that is not accepting blood because of heart failure or other alterations. One can often hear extra heart sounds more easily with the client lying on the left side and the stethoscope at the apical site.

Further auscultation may reveal clicks and rubs. Clicks are short, high-pitched, extra heart sounds created by mitral valve prolapse, aortic stenosis, or prosthetic valves. In contrast, rubs result from a rubbing of inflamed visceral and parietal layers of the pericardium against one another. Myocardial infarction and infection of the pericardium can predispose to inflammation of the tissues surrounding the heart.

The final portion of the examination includes assessment for heart murmurs. **Murmurs** are sustained swishing or blowing sounds heard at the beginning, middle, or end of the systolic or diastolic phase. They are caused by increased blood flow through a normal valve, forward flow through a stenotic valve or into a dilated vessel or heart chamber, or backward flow through a valve that fails to close. A murmur can be asymptomatic or a sign of heart disease (see the box below). Murmurs are common in children. The nurse keeps the following factors in mind when auscultating to detect murmurs:

1. When a murmur is detected, the nurse auscultates the mitral, tricuspid, aortic, and pulmonic valve areas for its place in the cardiac cycle (timing), place it is heard best (location), radiation, loudness, pitch, and quality.
2. If a murmur occurs between S_1 and S_2, it is a systolic murmur. If it occurs between S_2 and the next S_1, it is a diastolic murmur.
3. The location of a murmur is not necessarily directly over the valves. With experience, a nurse can learn where each type of murmur is best heard. For example, mitral murmurs are heard best at the apex of the heart.
4. To assess for radiation the nurse listens for a murmur over areas besides where it is heard best. Murmurs can also sometimes be heard over the neck or back.
5. Intensity or loudness is related to the rate of blood flow through the heart or the amount of blood regurgitated. In serious murmurs the nurse may feel a thrust or intermittent palpable sensation at the auscultation site. A **thrill** is a continuous palpable sensation like the purring of a cat. Intensity is recorded in the following grades:

CLIENT TEACHING
During Heart Assessment

OBJECTIVES
■ Client will know risks of heart disease and take appropriate steps to eliminate risks from lifestyle.
■ Client with risk for heart disease will seek support from appropriate care givers.

TEACHING STRATEGIES
■ Explain the risk factors for heart disease, including high dietary intake of saturated fat or cholesterol, lack of regular aerobic exercise, smoking, excess weight, stressful lifestyle, hypertension, and family history of heart disease.
■ Refer client (if appropriate) to resources available for controlling or reducing risks (e.g., nutritional counseling, exercise class, stress-reduction programs).
■ Explain that research shows clinical benefit from reducing dietary intake of cholesterol and saturated fats. Tell client that about 70% to 75% of saturated fatty acids come from meats, poultry, fish, and dairy products and that the one-step diet recommended by the National Institutes of Health includes an intake of total fat less than 30% of calories, saturated fatty acids less than 10% of calories, and cholesterol less than 300 mg/100 ml.*

■ Encourage client to have regular measurement of total blood cholesterol levels and triglycerides. Desirable levels are 150-200 mg/100 ml.† More than one cholesterol measurement is needed to assess the blood cholesterol level accurately. Low-density lipoprotein (LDL) cholesterol is the major component of atherosclerotic plaques. Separate measurement of LDL cholesterol is wise in a client with high total blood cholesterol levels. An LDL cholesterol level of 160 mg/dl or higher is high risk.
■ Clients who have known angina may benefit from taking a daily low dose of aspirin. Consult physician before starting therapy.

EVALUATION
■ Ask client to identify risk factors for heart disease.
■ Have client develop a meal plan low in saturated fat and cholesterol.
■ Check client's cholesterol level during follow-up appointments at clinic or physician's office.

---

*Data from Ernst ND: *Fam Community Health* 12(1):23, 1989.
†Data from Bullock B, Rosenthal PP: *Pathophysiology: adaptation and alteration,* ed 3, Philadelphia, 1992, Lippincott.

Grade 1   Barely audible
Grade 2   Audible immediately but faint
Grade 3   Loud, without thrust or thrill
Grade 4   Loud, with thrust or thrill
Grade 5   Very loud, with thrust or thrill; audible with stethoscope only partially applied
Grade 6   Louder, may be heard without stethoscope

6. A murmur may be low, medium, or high in pitch, depending on the velocity of blood flow through the valves. A low-pitched murmur is heard best with the bell of the stethoscope. If it is heard best with the diaphragm, a murmur is high pitched.

The quality of a murmur refers to its characteristic pattern and sound. A crescendo murmur starts softly and builds in loudness. A decrescendo murmur starts loudly and then becomes less intense.

∎ VASCULAR SYSTEM

Examination of the vascular system includes measurement of the blood pressure (see Chapter 32) and a thorough assessment of the integrity of the peripheral vascular system. Table 33-23 reviews the nursing history data collected before the examination. The nurse may perform portions of the vascular examination during assessment of other body systems. For example, the carotid pulse may be checked after palpation of cervical lymph nodes. As the nurse inspects the skin, signs and symptoms of arterial and venous insufficiency are noted. An experienced nurse integrates vascular assessment with other portions of the examination if it is important to minimize time spent in the total examination.

Blood Pressure

The nurse auscultates the blood pressure at the brachial artery site in both arms. Most examiners use the diaphragm of the stethoscope to auscultate blood pressure but the bell is more effective in transmitting the low-pitched Korotkoff sounds. Readings between the arms may vary by as much as 10 mm Hg and tend to be higher in the right arm (Seidel et al, 1995). Always record the higher reading. Systolic read-

ings that differ by 15 mm Hg or more suggest atherosclerosis or disease of the aorta.

The nurse also compares the blood pressure with the client in the lying position with that in the sitting or standing position. This maneuver assesses for orthostatic (postural) hypotension (see Chapter 32). Ordinarily as a client changes position from supine to standing there is a slight or no drop in systolic pressure and a slight rise in diastolic pressure. A fall in systolic blood pressure greater than 15 mm Hg (Seidel et al, 1995) and a fall in diastolic pressure signifies postural hypotension. Clients most at risk include those who have just donated blood, have autonomic nervous system disease, or have stayed a prolonged time in a recumbent position.

Carotid Arteries

When the left ventricle pumps blood into the aorta, pressure waves are transmitted through the arterial system. Pressure waves are manifested as pulses that are palpable in arteries close to the skin or that lie over bones. The carotid arteries reflect heart function better than peripheral arteries because they are positioned closest to the heart and thus their pressure correlates with that of the aorta.

The carotid arteries supply oxygenated blood to the head and neck (Fig. 33-56) and are protected by the overlying sternocleidomastoid muscle. To examine the carotid arteries, the nurse has the client sit or lie supine with the head of the bed elevated 30 degrees. One carotid artery is examined at a time. If both arteries were occluded during palpation, the client could lose consciousness as a result of inadequate circulation to the brain. The carotids must not be vigorously palpated or massaged. The carotid sinus is located at the bifurcation of the common carotid arteries in the upper third of the neck. The sinus sends impulses along the vagus nerve. Its stimulation can cause a reflex drop in heart rate and blood pressure, which causes **syncope** or circulatory arrest. This can be a particular problem for older adults.

The neck is first inspected for obvious pulsation of the artery. The client turns the head slightly away from the artery being examined. Sometimes the wave of the pulse

Table 33-23	**Nursing History for Vascular Assessment**
ASSESSMENT CATEGORY	**RATIONALE**

Determine if client experiences leg cramps, numbness or tingling in the extremities, sensation of cold hands or feet, pain in the legs, or swelling or cyanosis of the feet, ankles, or hand.	These signs and symptoms indicate vascular disease.
If client experiences leg pain or cramping in lower extremities, ask if it is relieved or aggravated by walking or standing for long periods or during sleep.	Relationship of symptoms to exercise can clarify whether problem is vascular or musculoskeletal. Pain caused by vascular condition tends to increase with activity. Musculoskeletal pain is not usually relieved when exercise ends.
Ask women if they wear tight-fitting garters or hosiery and sit or lie in bed with legs crossed.	Tight hosiery around lower extremities and crossing legs can impair venous return.
Reconsider previous heart risk factors, e.g., smoking, exercise, nutritional problems.	These predispose to vascular disease.
Assess medical history for heart disease, hypertension, phlebitis, diabetes, or varicose veins.	Circulatory and vascular disorders influence findings gathered during examination.

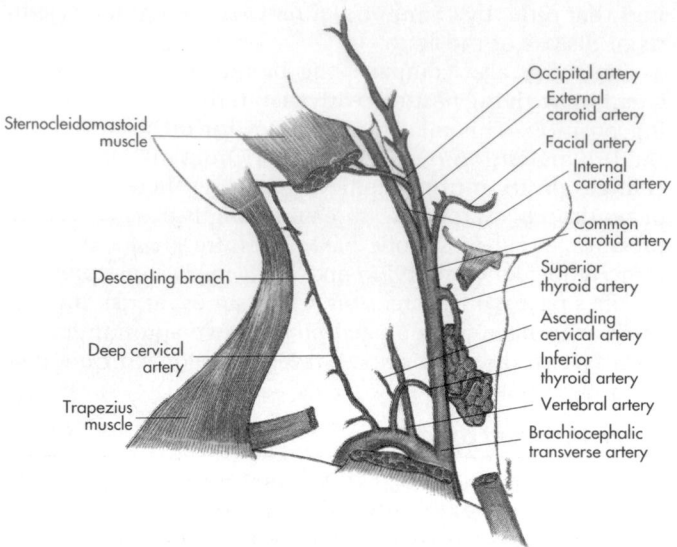

Fig. 33-56 Anatomical position of the carotid artery.

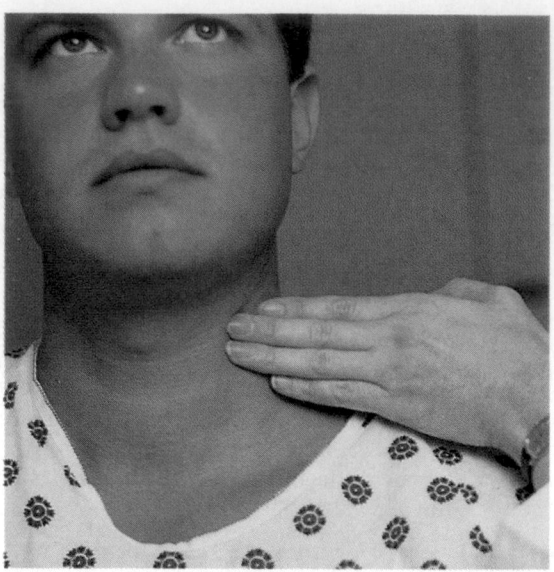

Fig. 33-57 Palpation of internal carotid artery along the margin of the sternocleidomastoid muscle.

can be seen. The carotid is the only site for assessing the quality of a pulse wave. Only an experienced assessor can evalute the quality of the wave in relation to systole and diastole of the cardiac cycle. An absent pulse wave can indicate arterial **occlusion** (blockage) or **stenosis** (narrowing).

For palpation of the pulse, the client turns the head slightly toward the side being examined. This maneuver relaxes the neck muscles for easier palpation. The nurse slides the tips of the index and middle fingers around the medial edge of the sternocleidomastoid muscle. Gentle palpation avoids occlusion of circulation (Fig. 33-57).

The normal carotid pulse is localized rather than diffuse. A strong pulse, the carotid has a thrusting quality. As the client breathes, no change occurs during inspiration or expiration. Rotation of the neck or a shift from a sitting to a supine position does not change the carotid's quality. Both carotid arteries should be equal in pulse rate, rhythm, and strength and should be equally elastic. Diminished or unequal carotid pulsations can indicate **atherosclerosis** or aortic arch disease.

The carotid is the most commonly auscultated pulse. (Others might include the jugular, temporal, femoral, renal, and abdominal arteries). Auscultation is especially important for middle-age clients, older adults, or clients suspected of having cerebrovascular disease manifested by carotid artery obstruction. When the lumen of a blood vessel is narrowed, its blood flow is disturbed. As blood passes through the narrowed section, a turbulence is created, causing a blowing or swishing sound. The blowing sound is called a **bruit** (pronounced "brew-ee") (Fig. 33-58).

The bell of the stethoscope is placed over the carotid artery at the lateral end of the clavicle and the posterior margin of the sternocleidomastoid muscle. The client turns the head slightly away from the side being examined (Fig. 33-59). The nurse asks the client to hold the breath for a moment so that breath sounds do not obscure a bruit. Normally no sound is heard during carotid auscultation. If a bruit is heard, the nurse palpates the artery lightly for a thrill (palpable bruit).

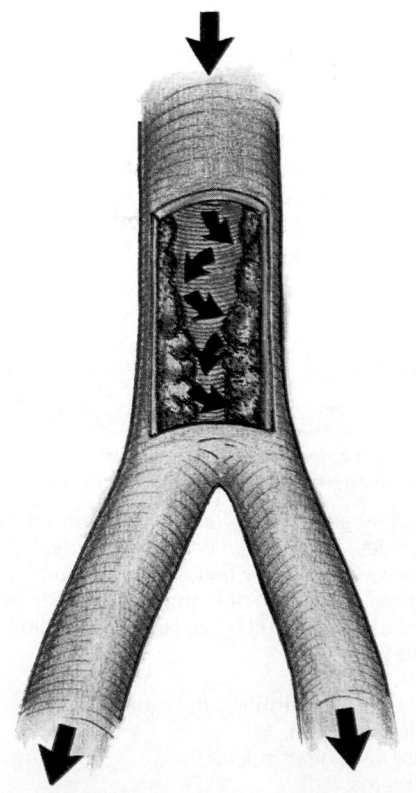

Fig. 33-58 Occlusion or narrowing of the carotid artery disrupts normal blood flow. The resultant turbulence creates a sound (bruit) that the nurse can auscultate.

Jugular Veins

The most accessible veins are the internal and external jugular veins in the neck. Both veins drain bilaterally from the head and neck into the superior vena cava. The external jugular lies superficially and can be seen just above the clavicle. The internal jugular lies deeper, along the carotid artery.

It is best to examine the right internal jugular because it follows a more direct anatomical path to the right atrium

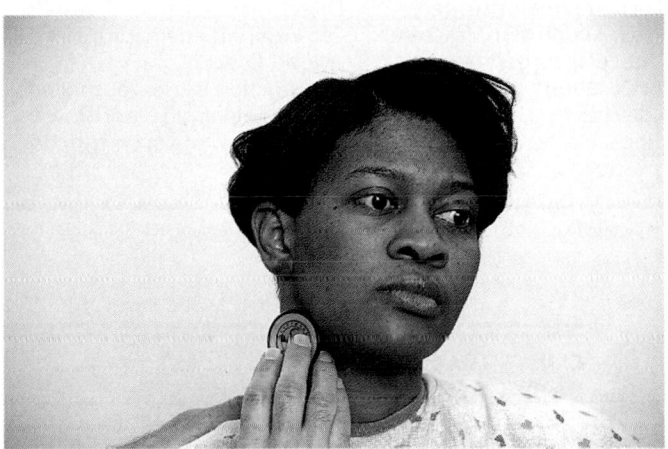

Fig. 33-59 Auscultation for carotid artery bruit. *(From Seidel HM et al: Mosby's guide to physical examination, ed 3, St Louis, 1995, Mosby.)*

of the heart. The column of blood inside the internal jugular serves as a manometer, reflecting pressure in the right atrium. The higher the column, the greater the venous pressure. Raised venous pressure reflects right-sided heart failure.

Normally when a client lies in the supine position the external jugular distends and becomes easily visible. In contrast the jugular veins normally flatten when the client is in a sitting position. A client with heart disease, however, may have distended jugular veins when sitting.

The jugular veins are inspected to measure venous pressures, which are influenced by blood volume, the capacity of the right atrium to receive blood and send it to the right ventricle, and the ability of the right ventricle to contract and force blood into the pulmonary artery. Any factor resulting in greater blood volume within the venous system results in elevated venous pressure. The nurse assesses venous pressure by using the following steps:

1. Have the client lie supine with head elevated 30 to 45 degrees (semi-Fowler's position).
2. Be sure the neck and upper thorax are exposed. Use a pillow to align the head. Avoid neck hyperextension or flexion to ensure that the vein is not stretched or kinked (Fig. 33-60).
3. Usually pulsations are not evident with the client sitting up. As the client slowly leans back into a supine position, the level of venous pulsations begins to rise above the level of the manubrium as much as 1 or 2

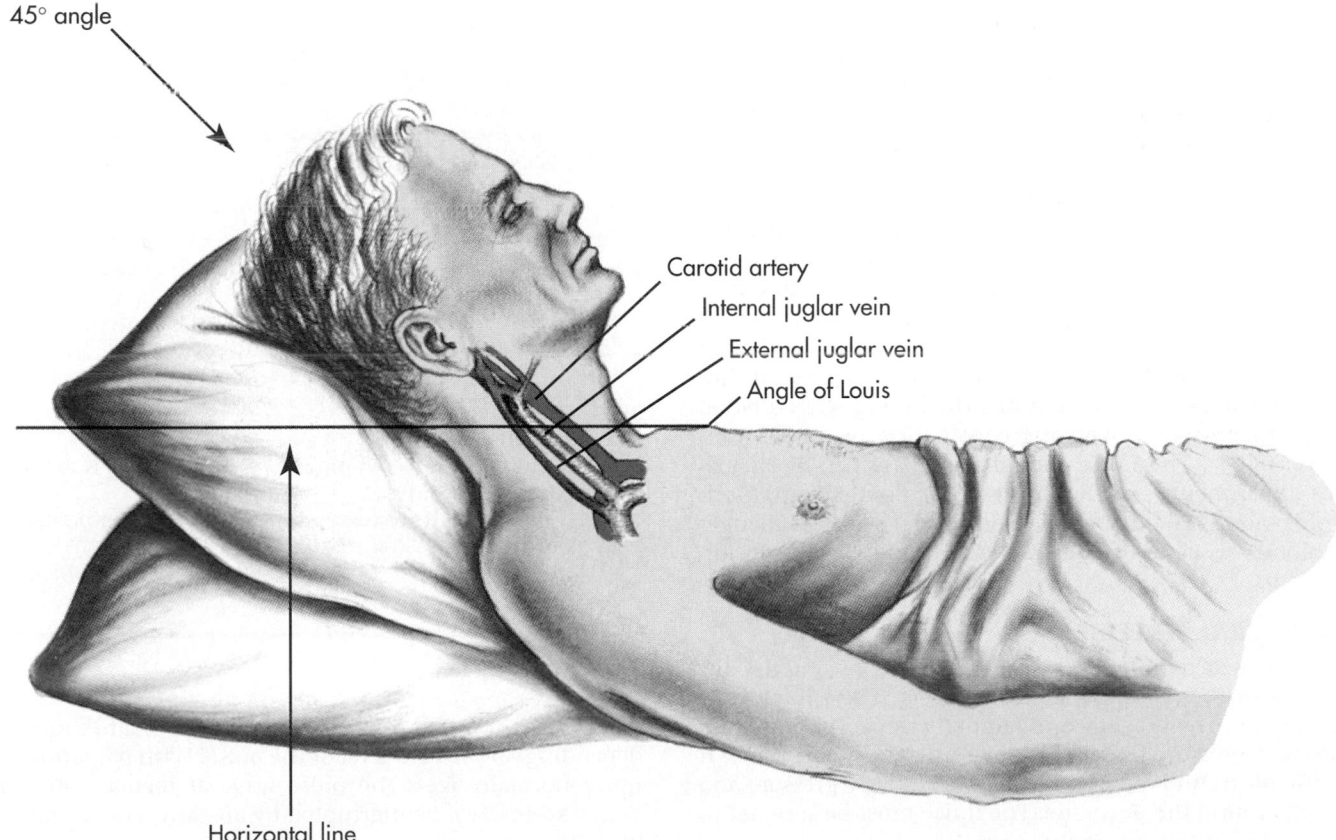

45° angle

Carotid artery
Internal juglar vein
External juglar vein
Angle of Louis

Horizontal line

Fig. 33-60 Position of client to assess jugular vein distention. *(From Thompson JM et al: Mosby's manual of clinical nursing, ed 3, St Louis, 1993, Mosby.)*

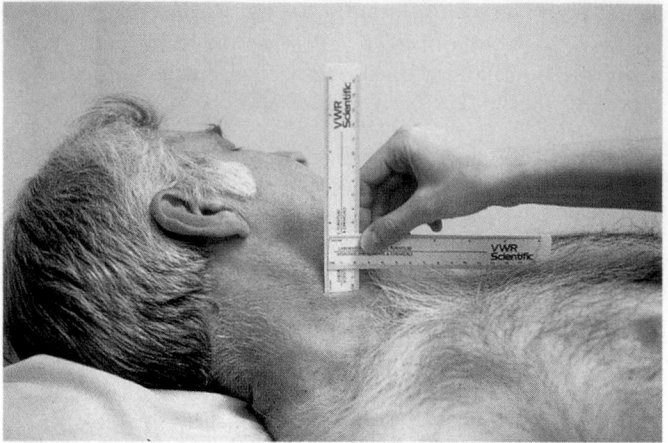

Fig. 33-61 Measurement of jugular vein distention. *(From Seidel HM et al: Mosby's guide to physical examination, ed 2, St Louis, 1991, Mosby.)*

Table 33-24	Indicators for Assessing Local Blood Flow
INDICATOR	**RATIONALE**
Systemic diseases (e.g., arteriosclerosis, atherosclerosis, diabetes)	Diseases result in changes in integrity of walls of arteries and smaller blood vessels.
Coagulation disorders (e.g., thrombosis, embolus)	Blood clot causes mechanical obstruction to blood flow.
Local trauma or surgery (e.g., contusion, fracture, vascular surgery)	Direct manipulation of vessels or localized edema impairs blood flow.
Application of constricting devices (e.g., casts, dressings, elastic bandages, restraints)	Constriction causes tourniquet effect, impairing blood flow to areas below site of constriction.

cm as the client reaches a 45 degree angle. Measure venous pressure by measuring the vertical distance between the angle of Louis and the highest level of the visible point of the internal jugular vein pulsation.

4. Use two rulers. Line up the bottom edge of a regular ruler with the top of the area of pulsation in the jugular vein. Then take a centimeter ruler and align it perpendicular to the first ruler at the level of the sternal angle. Measure in centimeters the distance between the second ruler and the sternal angle (Fig. 33-61).
5. Repeat the same measurement on the other side. Bilateral pressures higher than 2.5 cm (1 inch) are considered elevated and are a sign of right-sided heart failure. One-sided pressure elevation can be caused by obstruction.

Peripheral Arteries and Veins

To examine the peripheral vascular system the nurse first assesses the adequacy of blood flow to the extremities by measuring arterial pulses and inspecting the condition of the skin and nails. The integrity of the venous system is also assessed, with attention given to determining whether the client has abnormalities. A number of factors can impair circulation to the extremities, including altered blood vessel integrity and overlying constriction on vessel walls (Table 33-24). The nurse should anticipate risk of circulatory impairment (see the box at right). Some clients, such as older adults and diabetic persons, suffer physical changes in blood vessel walls that increase the risk of perfusion problems.

PERIPHERAL ARTERIES

The nurse examines each peripheral artery using the distal pads of the second and third fingers. The thumb may help anchor the brachial and femoral artery. The nurse applies firm pressure but avoids occluding the pulse. When it is difficult to find a pulse, it is helpful to vary pressure and feel all around the pulse site. The nurse must be sure not to palpate his or her own pulse.

Routine vital signs usually include assessment of the rate and rhythm of the radial artery because it is easily accessible.

CLIENT TEACHING
During Vascular Assessment

OBJECTIVES
■ Client will know normal blood pressure range for age and compare it with own blood pressure readings to identify normalcy of blood pressure.
■ Client with vascular insufficiency will avoid activities that worsen circulatory status.

TEACHING STRATEGIES
■ Tell the client the blood pressure reading. Explain the normal reading for the client's age. Discuss implications of abnormalities.
■ Instruct the client with risk or evidence of vascular insufficiency in the lower extremities to avoid tight clothing over the lower body or legs, to avoid sitting or standing for long periods, to walk regularly, and to elevate feet when sitting.
■ Advise client to avoid cigarette smoking because nicotine causes vasoconstriction.
■ Identify older adult with hypertension who may benefit from regular monitoring of blood pressure (daily, weekly, or monthly). Teach client how to use home monitoring kits (see Chapter 32).

EVALUATION
■ Ask client to identify if blood pressure reading is within normal limits for age.
■ Have client with vascular insufficiency describe precautions to take to avoid further circulatory deficiency.
■ Have older adult demonstrate self-monitoring of blood pressure.

The pulse is counted for either 30 seconds or a full minute, depending on the character of the pulse. With palpation the nurse normally feels the pulse wave at regular intervals. When an interval is interrupted by an early, late, or missed beat, the pulse rhythm is irregular. In emergencies, the carotid artery is chosen because it is accessible and most useful in evaluating heart activity. To check local circulatory status of tissues, the nurse palpates peripheral arteries long enough to note that a pulse is present.

The nurse assesses each peripheral artery for elasticity of the vessel wall, strength, and equality. A systematic technique is useful, starting with the temporal arteries in the head and moving down to the arteries in the upper and lower extremities. The wall of an artery is normally elastic, making it easily palpable. After the artery is depressed, it will spring back to shape when pressure is released. An abnormal artery may be described as hard, inelastic, or calcified.

The strength of a pulse is a measurement of the force at which blood is ejected against the arterial wall. Some examiners use a scale rating from *0* to *4+* for the strength of a pulse (Seidel et al, 1995):

0   Absent, not palpable.
1+   Pulse is diminished, barely palpable, easy to obliterate.
2+   Easily palpable, normal pulse.
3+   Full pulse, increased.
4+   Strong, bounding pulse, cannot be obliterated.

All peripheral pulses are measured for equality and symmetry. The left radial pulse is compared with that of the right, the left brachial pulse is compared with the left ra-

dial, and so on. An inequality may indicate localized obstruction or an abnormally positioned artery.

In the upper extremities the primary artery is the brachial, which channels blood to the radial and ulnar arteries of the forearm and hand. If circulation in this artery becomes blocked, the hands will not receive adequate blood flow. If circulation in the radial or ulnar arteries becomes impaired, the hand will still receive adequate perfusion. An interconnection between the radial and ulnar arteries guards against arterial occlusion (Fig. 33-62).

The nurse should practice locating pulses on a friend. To locate pulses in the arm and hand, the nurse has the client sit or lie dow. The radial pulse is found along the radial side of the forearm, at the wrist. In a thin individual, a groove is formed lateral to the flexor tendon of the wrist. The radial pulse can be felt with light palpation in the groove (Fig. 33-63). The ulnar pulse is on the opposite side of the wrist and tends to feel less prominent than the radial pulse (Fig. 33-64). An examiner palpates the ulnar pulse only when arterial insufficiency to the hand is expected.

The **Allen's test** can be performed to assess collateral circulation. The client makes a fist as the ulnar and radial arteries are compressed simultaneously. The client then opens the hand, and the nurse releases the ulnar artery. The hand should quickly turn pink if the ulnar artery is patent. The test may be repeated by releasing only the radial artery.

To palpate the brachial pulse, the nurse finds the groove between the biceps and triceps muscles above the elbow at the antecubital fossa (Fig. 33-65). The artery runs along the medial side of the extended arm. The nurse palpates the artery with the fingertips of the first three fingers in the muscle groove.

The femoral artery is the primary artery in the leg, delivering blood to the popliteal, posterior tibial, and dorsalis pedis arteries (Fig. 33-66). It is one of the strongest arteries in an infant or small child. An interconnection between the posterior tibial and dorsalis pedis arteries guards against local arterial occlusion.

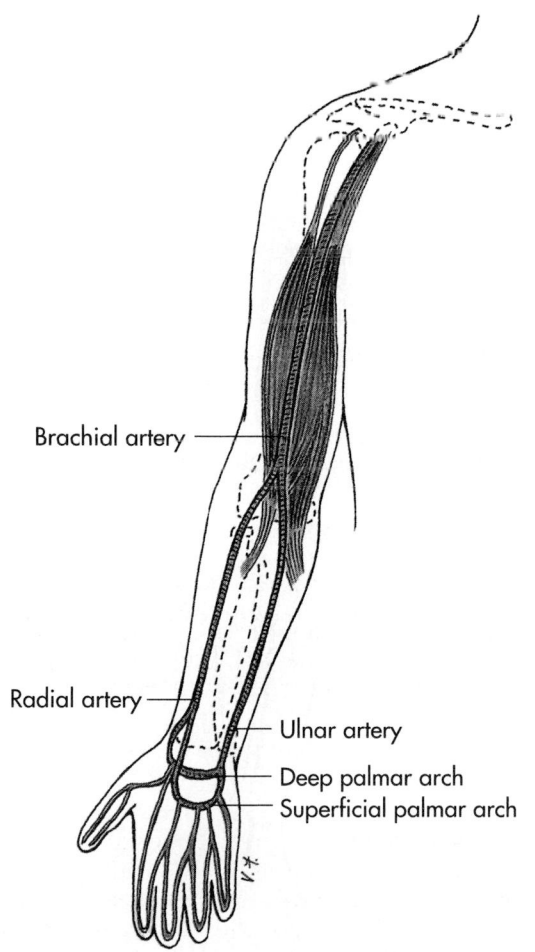

Fig. 33-62 Anatomical positions of brachial, radial, and ulnar arteries.

Brachial artery

Radial artery

Ulnar artery

Deep palmar arch

Superficial palmar arch

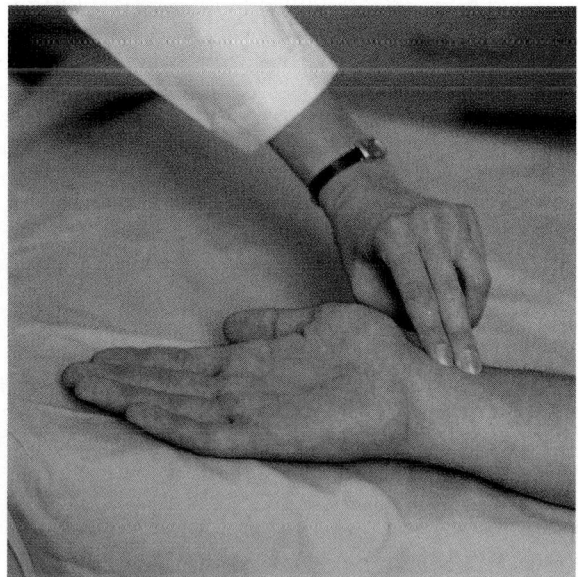

Fig. 33-63 Palpation of radial pulse.

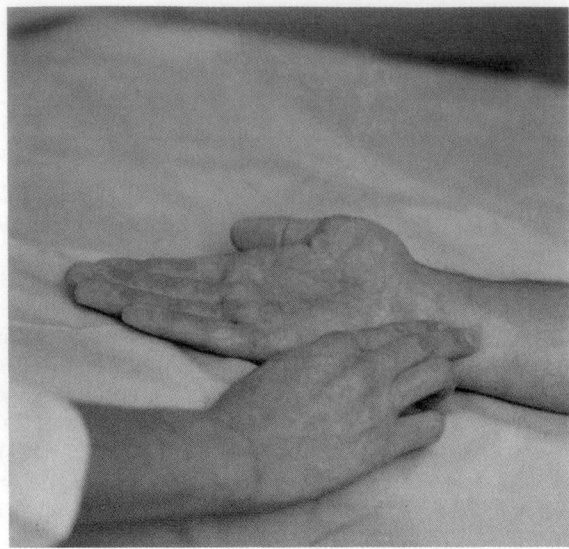

Fig. 33-64 Palpation of ulnar pulse.

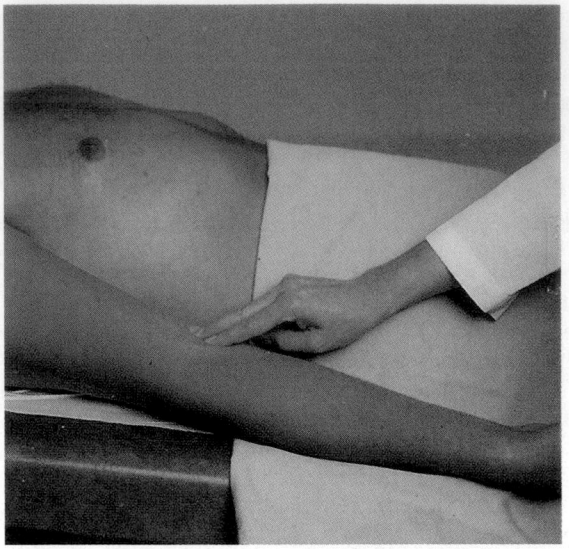

Fig. 33-65 The nurse palpates brachial pulse.

The femoral pulse is found best with the client lying down with the inguinal area exposed (Fig. 33-67). The femoral artery runs below the inguinal ligament, midway between the symphysis pubis and the anterosuperior iliac spine. Deep palpation may be required to feel the pulse. Bimanual palpation is effective in obese clients. This technique differs from the previous description of bimanual palpation. The nurse places the fingertips of both hands on opposite sides of the pulse site. A pulsatile sensation can be felt as the fingertips are pushed apart by arterial pulsation.

The popliteal pulse is found behind the knee. The client should slightly flex the knee, with the foot resting on the examination table, or assume a prone position with the knee slightly flexed (Fig. 33-68). The client is instructed to keep leg muscles relaxed. The nurse palpates with the fingers of both hands deeply into the popliteal fossa, just lateral to the midline. The popliteal pulse is difficult to locate.

With the client's foot relaxed the nurse locates the dorsalis pedis pulse. The artery runs along the top of the foot in line with the groove between the extensor tendons of the great toe and first toe (Fig. 33-69). Often an examiner finds the pulse by placing the fingertips between the great and first toe and slowly inching up the foot. This pulse may be congenitally absent.

The posterior tibial pulse is found on the inner side of each ankle (Fig. 33-70). The nurse places the fingers behind and below the medial malleolus (ankle bone). The artery is easily located with the foot relaxed and slightly extended.

Ultrasound Stethoscopes. If a nurse cannot palpate a pulse, an ultrasound stethoscope is a useful tool that amplifies sounds of a pulse wave. Factors that may weaken a pulse or make palpation difficult include obesity, reduction in the heart's stroke volume, diminished blood volume, or arterial obstruction. A thin layer of transmission gel is first applied to the client's skin at the pulse site or directly onto the transducer tip of the probe. The nurse then turns the volume control to "on" and places the tip of the probe at a 45 to 90 degree angle on the skin (Fig. 33-71). The nurse

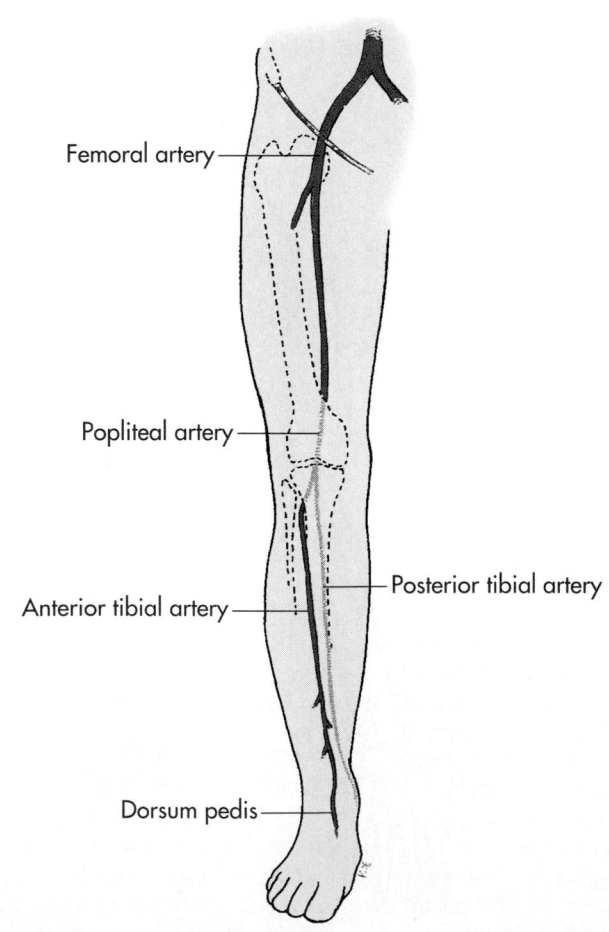

Fig. 33-66 Anatomical position of femoral, popliteal, dorsalis pedis, and posterior tibial arteries.

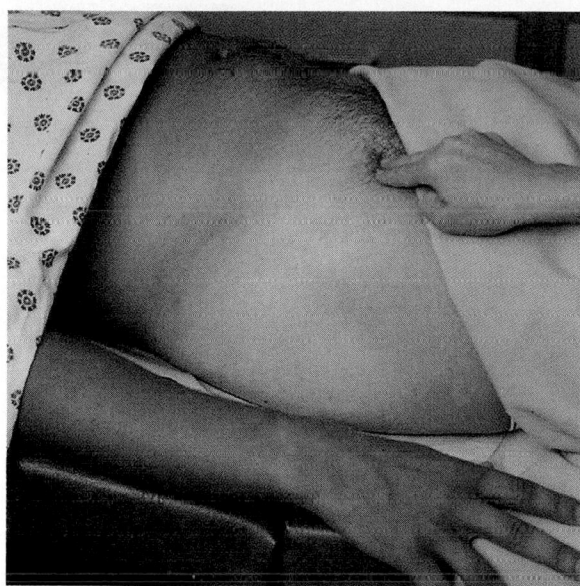

Fig. 33-67 Palpation of femoral pulse.

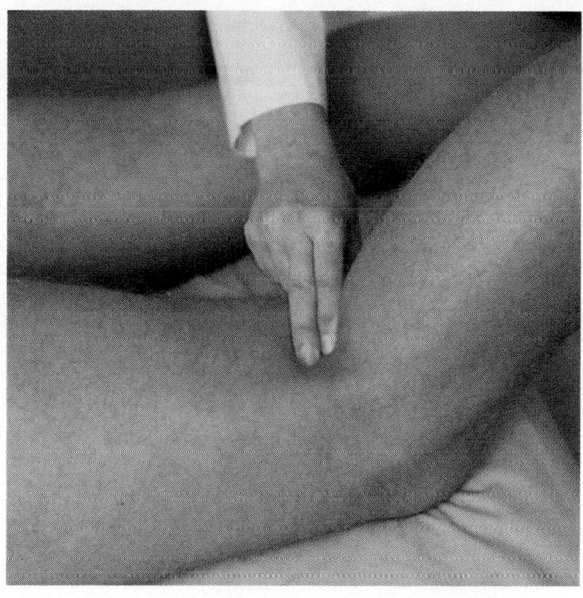

Fig. 33-68 Palpation of popliteal pulse.

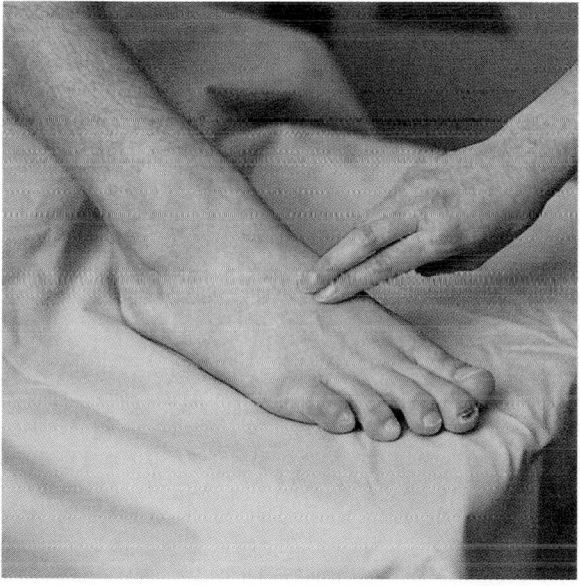

Fig. 33-69 Palpation of dorsalis pedis pulse.

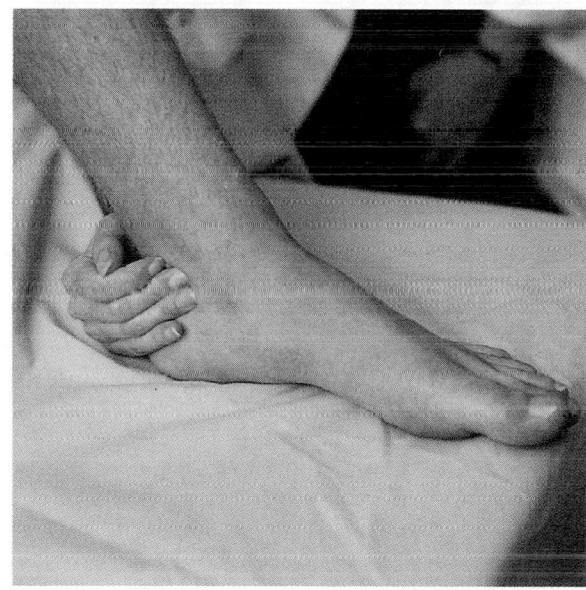

Fig. 33-70 Palpation of posterior tibial pulse.

moves the probe until a pulsating "whooshing" sound is heard that indicates arterial blood flow is present.

Tissue Perfusion. The condition of the skin, mucosa, and nail beds offers useful data about the status of circulatory blood flow. The nurse first examines the face and upper extremities, looking at the color of the skin, mucosa, and nail beds. The presence of cyanosis requires special attention. Central cyanosis, which indicates poor arterial oxygenation, may be due to heart disease. It can be noted by a bluish discoloration of the lips, mouth, and conjunctivae. Peripheral cyanosis, which indicates peripheral vasoconstriction, is noted by blue lips, earlobes, and nail beds. When cyanosis is present, the nurse refers to available lab-

oratory data on oxygen saturation to determine the severity of the problem. Examination of the nails involves inspection for **clubbing**, a bulging of the tissues at the nail base. Clubbing is due to insufficient oxygenation at the periphery resulting from conditions such as chronic emphysema and congenital heart disease.

The nurse inspects the lower extremities for changes in color, temperature, and condition of the skin indicating either arterial or venous alterations (Table 33-25). This is a good time to ask the client about history of pain in the legs. If an arterial occlusion is present, the client has signs resulting from an absence of blood flow. Pain will be distal to the occlusion. The *three P's* characterize an occlusion—*pain,*

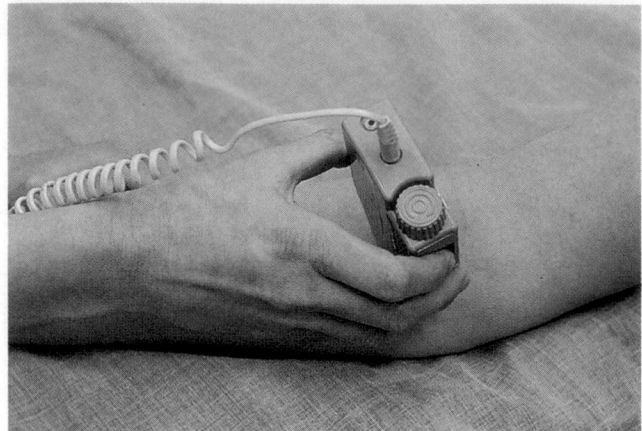

Fig. 33-71 Ultrasound stethoscope in position on brachial artery.

Table 33-25	Signs of Venous and Arterial Insufficiency	
ASSESSMENT CRITERION	**VENOUS**	**ARTERIAL**
Color	Normal or cyanotic	Pale; worsened by elevation of extremity; dusky red when extremity lowered
Temperature	Normal	Cool (blood flow blocked to extremity)
Pulse	Normal	Decreased or absent
Edema	Often marked	Absent or mild
Skin changes	Brown pigmentation around ankles	Thin, shiny skin; decreased hair growth; thickened nails

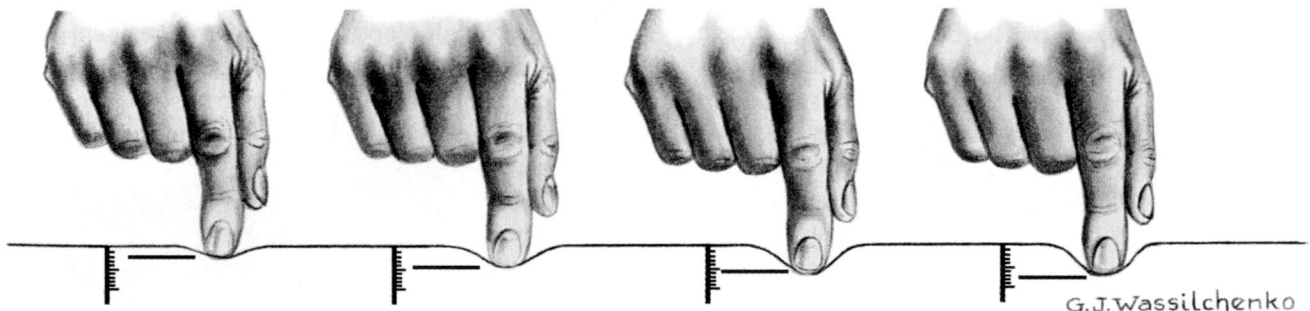

Fig. 33-72 Assessing for pitting edema. *(From Seidel HM et al: Mosby's guide to physical examination, ed 3, St Louis, 1995, Mosby.)*

*p*allor, and *p*ulselessness. Venous congestion causes tissue changes indicating an inadequate circulatory flow back to the heart.

During examination of the lower extremities, the nurse also inspects skin and nail texture; hair distribution on the lower legs, feet, and toes; venous pattern; and scars, pigmentation, or ulcers. The absence of hair growth over the legs may indicate circulatory insufficiency. The nurse should not be misled by shaven lower legs. Also, many men have less hair around the calves due to tight fitting dress socks. Chronic recurring ulcers of the feet or lower legs are a serious sign of circulatory insufficiency and require a physician's intervention.

PERIPHERAL VEINS

The nurse assesses the status of the peripheral veins by asking the client to assume sitting and standing positions. Assessment includes inspection and palpation for varicosities, peripheral edema, and phlebitis. Varicosities are superficial veins that become dilated, especially when the legs are in a dependent position. They are common in older adults because the veins normally fibrose, dilate, and stretch. They are also common in people who stand for prolonged periods. Varicosities in the anterior or medial part of the thigh and the posterolateral part of the calf are abnormal.

Dependent edema around the area of the feet and ankles can be a sign of venous insufficiency and right-sided heart failure. Dependent edema is common in older adults and persons who spend a lot of time standing (e.g., waitresses, security guards, or nurses). To assess for pitting edema, the nurse uses a thumb to press firmly 1 to 2 seconds and then release over the medial malleolus or the shins. A depression left in the skin indicates edema. The severity of the edema is characterized by grading 1+ through 4+ (Fig. 33-72).

Phlebitis is an inflammation of a vein that occurs commonly after trauma to the vessel wall, infection, prolonged immobilization, and prolonged insertion of intravenous catheters (see Chapter 45). Phlebitis promotes clot formation, a potentially dangerous situation because a clot within a deep vein of the leg can become dislodged and travel through the heart, causing a pulmonary embolus. To assess for phlebitis the nurse inspects the calves for localized redness, tenderness, and swelling over vein sites. Gentle palpation of calf muscles reveals tenderness and firmness of the muscle. The nurse may also check for Homans' sign by supporting the leg while flexing the foot upward. If phlebitis is present in the lower leg, forceful dorsiflexion of the foot often causes pain in the calf.

LYMPHATIC SYSTEM

Assessment of the lymphatic drainage of the lower extremities is performed during examination of the vascular

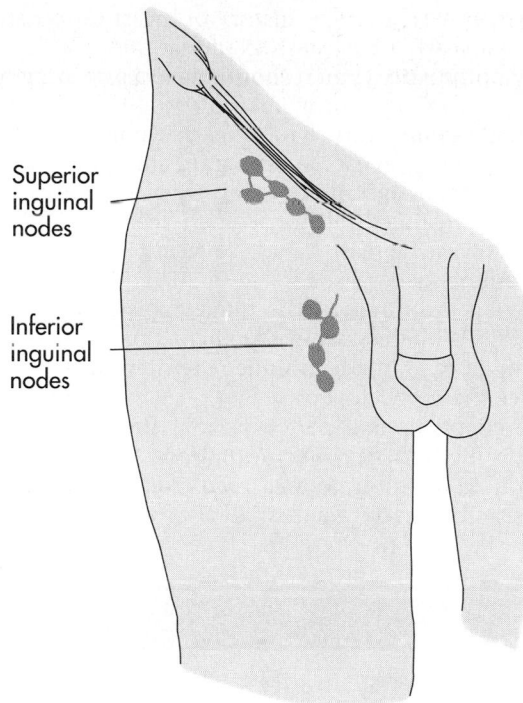

Superior
inguinal
nodes

Inferior
inguinal
nodes

Fig. 33-73 Inguinal lymph nodes.

system. The nurse may also perform this examination just before the female or male genital examination. The legs are drained by superficial and deep nodes, but only the two groups of superficial nodes are palpable. The nurse palpates the area of the superficial inguinal nodes (Fig. 33-73), beginning in the groin area and moving down toward the inner thigh. The vertical group of nodes lies close to the upper portion of the great saphenous vein. The horizontal group lies below the inguinal ligament. The nurse uses a firm but gentle pressure when palpating over each lymphatic chain. Multiple nodes are not normally palpable, although a few soft, nontender nodes are not unusual. Enlarged, hardened, tender nodes can reveal potential sites of infection or metastatic disease. An infection site can be identified by drainage collected by the nodes. For example, the horizontal group drains lymph from the skin of the lower abdominal wall, the external genitalia, anal canal, and lower vagina.

BREASTS

It is important to examine the breasts of female and male clients. A small amount of glandular tissue, a potential site for the growth of cancer cells, is located in the male breast. In contrast, the majority of the female breast is glandular tissue.

Female Breasts

Breast cancer will affect an estimated 182,000 (approximately one in every nine) women in the United States in 1995 (American Cancer Society, 1995). The disease is second to lung cancer as the leading cause of death in women with cancer. Early detection is the key to cure. Fibrocystic breast disease is a benign condition involving a variety of

---

▶ RESEARCH HIGHLIGHT

RESEARCH ABSTRACT

Women who are at risk for breast cancer should routinely perform breast self-examinations. This study attempted to determine the breast cancer screening practices of older women at increased risk for breast cancer and to determine whether education about early detection practices would improve the women's screening behaviors. Subjects were identified through women with known breast cancer. The researchers asked these women to identify female first degree (mother or sister) relatives. The 755 women identified with breast cancer yielded 1327 first degree female relatives, 470 women 50 years and older participated in the study. Participants were interviewed about their health practices, including cancer screening practices.

The average age of the sample was 63.4 years and were predominantly Caucasian (94.7%). Over 75% had at least a high school diploma. Over 81% of the sample reported ever practicing breast self-exam. The proportion of women over 70 years of age who had examined their breasts (31%) was smaller. Frequency of practice was varied. Slightly less than 30% performed breast self-exam monthly. Only 17.8% of women 70 years and older examined their breasts monthly. Even though less than 25% of the sample initiated breast self-exam under the age of 40, it was interesting to find that 18% had initiated self-breast examination after reaching 70 years. The study found that women in general were not negative about a breast self-exam. However, a good number of women (38.5%) were afraid of finding a lump. Older women were more likely to perceive the examination as unpleasant. Ninety-four percent of the sample knew the importance of regular examination when women were at risk. However, 16% reported self-exams were not important if physicians performed exams. The study also suggested that few subjects performed the exam correctly. Interestingly, nearly 42% of those who began self-examination at age 50 or older learned through the media, and not through a health care provider.

IMPLICATIONS FOR PRACTICE

▶ Older women should be approached to learn breast self-exam as they are likely to adopt new screening behaviors.
▶ Health providers should assess the accuracy of breast self-exam for women educated through the media, as this method does not ensure accuracy.
▶ Health providers should reeducate older women on screening practices regularly.

REFERENCE

Dunbar J et al: Breast self-examination compliance among older high risk women, *Patient Education Counseling* 18:223, 1991.

breast changes observed in premenopausal women: cysts, adenosis, fibrosis, and fibroadenoma (Hockenberger, 1993). Over 50% of women of childbearing age have a form of fibrocystic disease (Norwood, 1990). A major responsibility for nurses is to teach clients health behavior such as breast self-examination (BSE). Studies suggest that a minority of women actually perform BSE. Nurses should know factors that increase the likelihood of a woman performing BSE (see the box on p. 703). Incorporating these interventions into teaching strategies may improve the likelihood of a client detecting breast cancer early (Champion, 1989). The American Cancer Society (1995) recommends the following guidelines for the early detection of breast cancer:

1. BSE should be performed monthly by women 20 years of age and older.
2. An examination by a physician should be performed every 3 years from ages 20 to 40, and after 40, the examination should be performed every year.
3. Women with a family history of breast cancer should have a yearly physician's examination.
4. Asymptomatic women should have a screening mammogram by age 40; women 40 to 49 should have a mammogram every 1 to 2 years; women age 50 and over should have a mammogram annually.
5. For women age 40 or over with a family history of breast cancer and for women age 35 or over with a history of breast cancer, a yearly examination is recommended.

During an examination the nurse explains how to perform a BSE. While assessing the client's breasts, the nurse uses many of the same techniques the client will use in the home (see the box below).

If the client already performs BSE, the nurse can ask about the method she uses and times she does the examination in relation to her menstrual cycle. The best time for a BSE is on the last day of the menstrual pe-

---

Breast Self-Examination

Instruct client on BSE. All women 20 years and older should perform this self-examination monthly using the following steps:

■ Stand before a mirror. Look at both breasts for anything unusual, such as discharge from the nipples, puckering, dimpling, or scaling of the skin.
■ To note changes in the shape of the breasts, perform the following measures (see the illustration):
   ■ Watch in the mirror while raising the arms above the head.
   ■ Press hands firmly on the hips and bow slightly toward the mirror when pulling the shoulders and elbows forward.

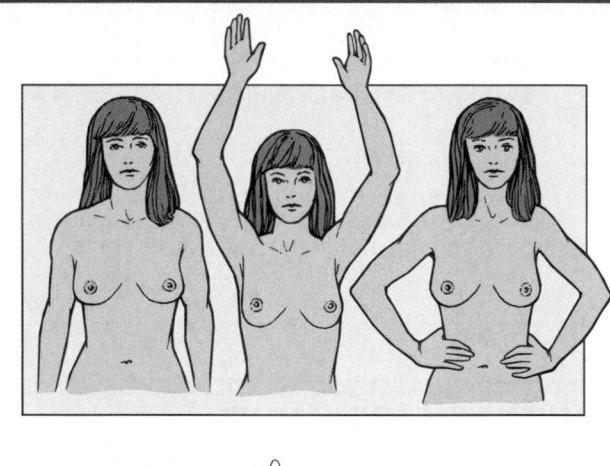

■ In the shower or in front of the mirror, palpate each breast. Raise the right arm and use three or four fingers of the left hand to explore the breast carefully (see the illustration). Then start at the outer edge, pressing the flat part of the fingers in small circles, moving the circles slowly around the breast, gradually working toward the nipple (see the illustration). Pay close attention to the area between the breast and armpit and feel for unusual lumps or masses. Repeat the process for the left breast.
■ Gently palpate each nipple, looking for discharge (see the illustration). Caution against pinching.

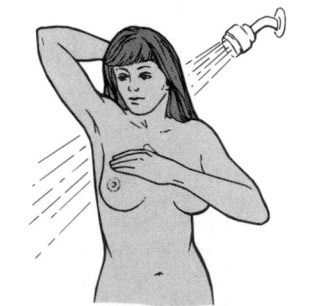
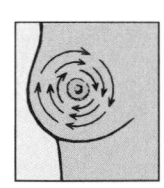
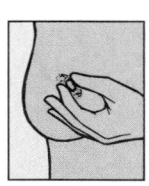

■ Repeat the third and fourth steps lying down. Lie flat on the back with the right arm over the head and a small pillow under the right shoulder. Palpate the right breast (see the illustration). Repeat the process on the left breast.
■ Call your physician if you find a lump.

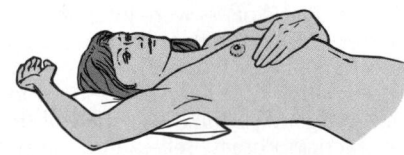

Illustrations from Payne WA, Hahn DB: *Understanding your health,* ed 2, St Louis, 1989, Mosby—Year Book.

riod, when the breast is no longer swollen or tender from hormone elevations. If the woman has already experienced menopause, she should check her breasts the same time each month. The pregnant woman also must check her breasts monthly.

Older women may require special attention when reviewing the need for regular BSE. Many older women are limited by fixed incomes and thus fail to pursue regular clinical breast examination and mammography. Unfortunately, many older women ignore changes in their breasts, assuming that they are a part of aging. In addition, physiological factors can affect the ease at which older women can

perform a BSE. Musculoskeletal limitations, diminished peripheral sensation, reduced eyesight, and changes in joint range of motion can limit palpation and inspection abilities. The nurse should find resources for older women, including free screening programs. Often family members can be taught to perform examinations.

The client's history (Table 33-26) should alert the nurse to any signs of breast disease and normal developmental changes. Because of its glandular structure, the breast undergoes changes during a woman's life. Knowledge of these changes (see the box below) helps the nurse complete an accurate assessment.

Table 33-26	Nursing History for Breast Assessment

ASSESSMENT CATEGORY	RATIONALE
Determine if woman is over age 40, has a personal or family history of breast cancer, early onset menarche (before age 12), or late age menopause (after age 50), has never had children or gave birth to first child after age 30, or has not breastfed.	These are risk factors for breast cancer
Ask if client (both sexes) has noticed lump, thickening, pain, or tenderness of breast; discharge, distortion, retraction, or scaling of nipple; or change in size of breast.	Potential signs and symptoms of breast cancer allow nurse to focus on specific areas of breast during assessment.
Ask if client performs monthly BSE. If so, determine time of month she performs examination in relation to menstrual cycle. Have client describe or demonstrate method used.	Nurse's role is to educate client about breast cancer and techniques for BSE.
Determine if client is taking oral contraceptives, digitalis, diuretics, steroids, or estrogen hormones. Determine the client's caffeine intake.	Medications may cause nipple discharge. Hormones and caffeine may cause fibrocystic changes in breast. Studies conflict over association of caffeine intake and breast cancer (Folsom et al, 1993).
If client reports a breast mass ask about length of time since lump first noted, does lump come and go or is it always present, have there been changes in the lump, e.g., size, relationship to menses, and are there associated symptoms.	Helps to determine nature of mass.

Normal Changes in the Breast During a Woman's Life Span

PUBERTY (8 TO 20 YEARS)*
Breasts mature in five stages. One breast may grow more rapidly than the other. The ages of which changes occur and rate of developmental progression vary.
Stage 1 (Preadolescent)
- This stage involves elevation of the nipple only.
Stage 2
- The breast and nipple elevate as a small mound, and the areolar diameters enlarge.
Stage 3
- There is further enlargement and elevation of the breast and areola, with no separation of contour.
Stage 4
- The areola and nipple project into the secondary mound above the level of the breast. (May not occur in all girls.)
Stage 5 (Mature Breast)
- Only the nipple projects, and the areola recedes (may vary in some women).

YOUNG ADULTHOOD (20 TO 30 YEARS)
- Breasts reach full (nonpregnant) size. Shape is generally symmetrical. Breasts may be unequal in size.

PREGNANCY
- Breast size gradually enlarges to 2 to 3 times the previous size. Nipples enlarge and may become erect. Areolae darken and diameters increase. Superficial veins become prominent. A yellowish fluid (colostrum) may be expelled from the nipples.

MENOPAUSE
- Breasts shrink. Tissue becomes softer, sometimes flabby.

OLDER ADULTHOOD
- Breasts become elongated, pendulous, and flaccid as a result of glandular tissue atrophy. The skin of the breasts tends to wrinkle, appearing loose and flabby.
- Nipples become smaller flatter and lose erectile ability.[†]

*Wong D: *Whaley and Wong's Nursing care of infants and children,* ed 5, St Louis, 1995, Mosby.
[†]Seidel HM et al: *Mosby's guide to physical examination,* ed 3, St Louis, 1995, Mosby.

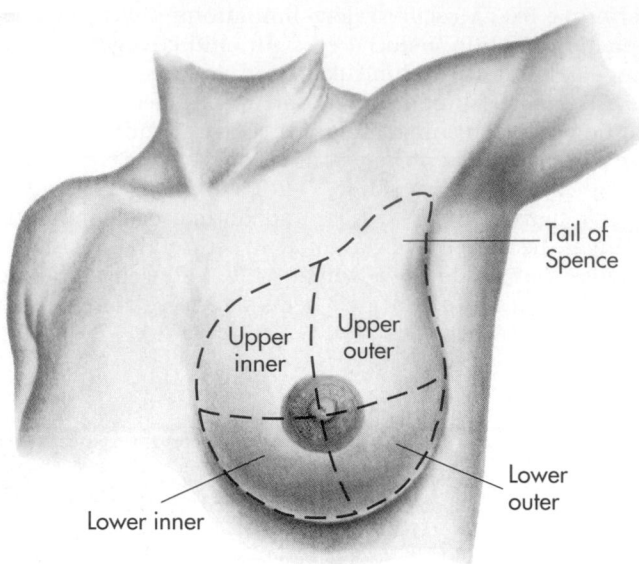

Fig. 33-74 Quadrants of the left breast and axillary tail of Spence. *(From Seidel HM et al:* Mosby's guide to physical examination, *ed 3, St Louis, 1995, Mosby.)*

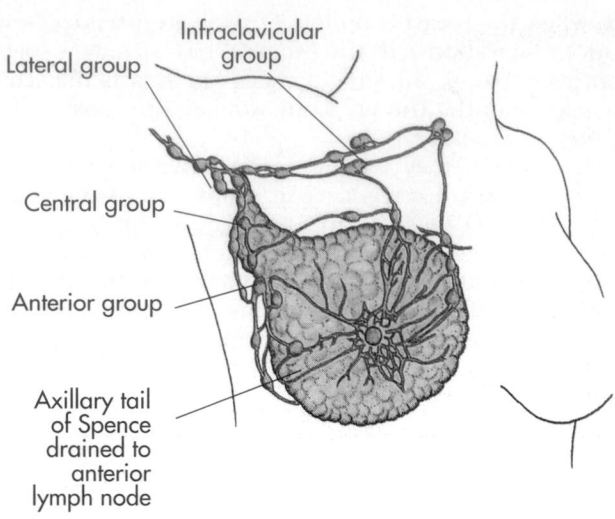

Fig. 33-75 Anatomical position of axillary and clavicular lymph nodes.

INSPECTION

The client removes the top gown or drape to allow simultaneous visualization of both breasts. The client may stand or sit with arms hanging loosely at her sides. If possible, the nurse places a mirror in front of the client so that she can see what to look for when performing a BSE. To recognize abnormalities, the client must be familiar with the normal appearance of her breasts.

The nurse describes observations or findings in relation to imaginary lines that divide the breast into four quadrants and a tail. The lines cross at the center of the nipple. Each tail extends outward from the upper outer quadrant (Fig. 33-74).

The breasts are inspected for size and symmetry. The breasts usually extend from the third to the sixth ribs, with the nipple at the level of the fourth intercostal space. One breast is commonly larger than the other. However, a difference in size may be caused by inflammation or a mass. As the woman becomes older, the ligaments supporting the breast tissue weaken, causing the breasts to sag and the nipples to lower (see the box on p. 705).

The nurse observes the contour or shape of the breasts and notes masses, flattening, retraction, or dimpling. Breasts vary in shape from convex to pendulous or conical. Retraction or dimpling results from invasion of underlying ligaments by tumors. The ligaments become fibrotic and pull the overlying skin inward toward the tumor. Edema also changes the breasts' contour. To bring out retraction or changes in the shape of breasts, the nurse asks the client to assume three positions: raise arms above the head, press hands against the hips, and extend arms straight ahead while sitting and leaning forward. Each maneuver causes a contraction of the pectoral muscles, which will accentuate retraction.

The overlying skin is carefully inspected for color and venous pattern. Venous patterns are more easily seen in thin clients or pregnant women. Presence of lesions, edema, or inflammation is also noted. The nurse lifts each breast when necessary to observe lower and lateral aspects for color and texture changes. The breasts are the color of neighboring skin and venous patterns are the same bilaterally. For women with large breasts the nurse should be sure to look carefully at the undersurface, a common site for redness and excoriation caused by rubbing of skin surfaces.

The nurse inspects the nipple and areola for size, color, shape, discharge, and the direction the nipples point. The normal areolae are round or oval and nearly equal bilaterally. Color ranges from pink to brown. In light-skinned women the areola turns brown during pregnancy and remains dark. In dark-skinned women the areola is brown before pregnancy (Seidel et al, 1995). Normally the nipples point in symmetrical directions, they are everted, and without drainage. Their surface may be either smooth or wrinkled. If the nipples are inverted, the nurse asks if this has been a lifetime history. A recent inversion or inward turning of the nipple may indicate an underlying growth. Rashes or ulcerations are not normal on the breast or nipples. Bleeding or discharge from the nipple is noted. Clear yellow discharge 2 days after childbirth is common. While inspecting the breasts, the nurse explains the characteristics observed. The client must be taught the significance of abnormal signs or symptoms.

PALPATION

Palpation allows the nurse to determine the condition of underlying breast tissue and lymph nodes. Breast tissue consists of glandular tissue, fibrous supportive ligaments, and fat. Glandular tissue is organized into lobes that end in ducts that open onto the nipple's surface. The largest portion of glandular tissue is in the upper outer quadrant and tail of each breast. Suspensory ligaments connect to skin and fascia underlying the breast to support the breast and maintain its upright position. Fatty tissue is located superficially and to the sides of the breast.

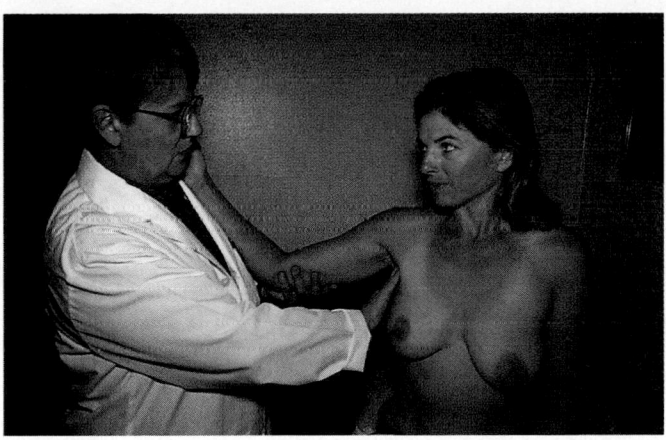

Fig. 33-76 The nurse supports the client's arm and palpates axillary lymph nodes.

A large portion of lymph from the breasts drains into axillary lymph nodes. If cancerous lesions **metastasize** (spread), the nodes are commonly involved. The nurse learns the location of supraclavicular, infraclavicular, and axillary nodes (Fig. 33-75). The axillary nodes drain lymph from the chest wall, breasts, arms, and hands. A tumor of one breast may also involve nodes on the opposite side.

The lymph nodes are best palpated when the client sits, although the examination can be performed with the client supine. Easy access is gained to the axillary nodes with the client's arms at her sides and muscles relaxed. While facing the client and standing on the side being examined, the nurse supports the client's arm in a slightly flexed position and abducts the arm away from the chest wall. Then the nurse places the free hand against the client's chest wall and high in the axillary hollow. With the fingertips the nurse presses gently down over the surface of the ribs and muscles. The axillary nodes are palpated with the fingertips gently rolling soft tissue (Fig. 33-76). Four areas of the axilla are palpated:

1. The edge of the pectoralis major muscle along the anterior axillary line
2. The chest wall in the midaxillary area
3. The upper part of the humerus
4. The anterior edge of the latissimus dorsi muscle along the posterior axillary line

Normally lymph nodes are not palpable. Each area must be assessed carefully because enlarged nodes are easily missed. The nurse notes their number, consistency, mobility, and size. One or two small, soft, nontender nodes may be normal. A palpable node feels like a small mass that may be hard, tender, and immobile. The nurse also palpates along the upper and lower clavicular ridges. The procedure is reversed for the other side.

It may be difficult for the client to learn to palpate for lymph nodes. Lying down with the arm abducted makes the area more accessible. The client is instructed to use her left hand for the right axillary and clavicular areas. The nurse can take the client's fingertips and move them in the proper circular fashion. The client then uses her right hand to palpate left-side nodes.

Palpation of breast tissue is best performed with the

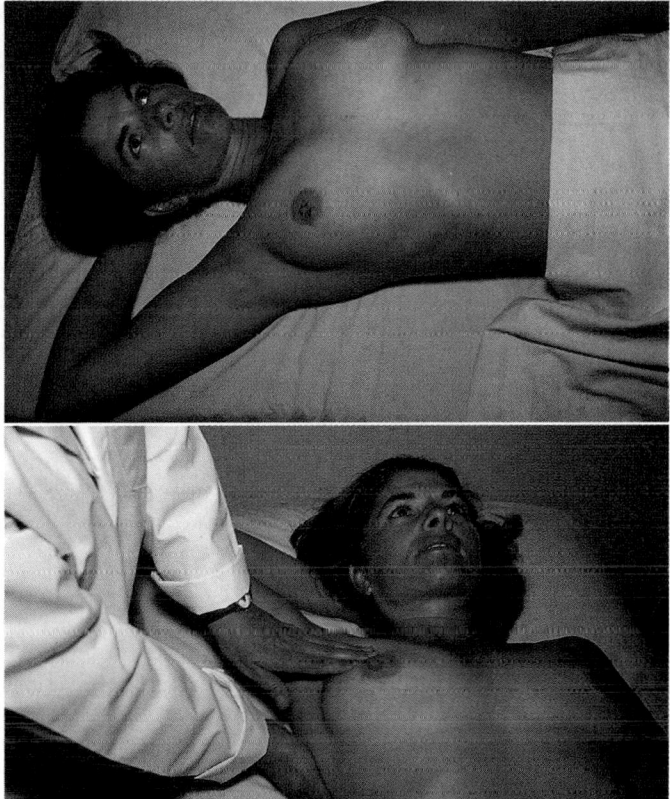

Fig. 33-77 The client lies flat with arm abducted and hand under head to help flatten breast tissue evenly over the chest wall.

client lying supine and one arm behind the head (alternating with each breast). The supine position allows the breast tissue to flatten evenly against the chest wall. The client should raise her hand and place it behind the neck to further stretch and position breast tissue evenly (Fig. 33-77). The examiner often places a small pillow or towel under the shoulder blade to further position breast tissue.

The consistency of normal breast tissue varies widely. The breasts of a young client are firm and elastic. In an older client the tissue may feel stringy and nodular. The client's familiarity with the texture of her own breasts is very important. This familiarity is gained through monthly BSE (see the box on p. 708).

If the client complains of a mass, the nurse examines the opposite breast first to ensure an objective comparison of normal and abnormal tissue. The nurse uses the pads of the first three fingers to compress breast tissue gently against the chest wall, noting tissue consistency. Palpation is performed systematically in one of two ways: clockwise or counterclockwise, forming small circles with the fingers along each quadrant and the tail, or a back-and-forth technique with the fingers moving up and down each quadrant (Fig. 33-78). Whatever approach is used, the nurse must be sure to cover the entire breast and tail, directing attention to any areas of tenderness.

When palpating large, pendulous breasts, the nurse uses

a bimanual technique. The inferior portion of the breast is supported in one hand while the nurse uses the other hand to palpate breast tissue against the supporting hand.

During palpation the nurse notes the consistency of breast tissue. It normally feels dense, firm, and elastic. In fibrocystic disease, a common problem in women, tissue feels lumpy, but it is found bilaterally. With menopause, breast tissue shrinks and becomes softer. The lobular feel of glandular tissue is normal. The lower edge of each breast may feel firm and hard. This is the normal inframammary ridge and not a tumor. It may be helpful to move the client's hand so that she can feel normal tissue variations. Abnormal masses are palpated to determine the following:

1. Location in relation to quadrants
2. Diameter in centimeters
3. Shape (e.g., round or discoid)
4. Consistency (soft, firm, or hard)
5. Tenderness
6. Mobility
7. Discreteness (whether boundaries of mass are clear or unclear)

Cancerous lesions are hard, fixed, nontender, and irregular in shape. A common benign condition of the breast is **fibrocystic breast disease.** This condition is characterized by lumpy painful breasts and sometimes nipple discharge. Symptoms are more apparent during the menstrual period. When palpated, the cysts (lumps) are soft, well differentiated, and movable. Deep cysts may feel hard.

As the nurse or client continues the examination, special attention is given to gentle palpation of the entire surface of the nipple and areola. The thumb and index finger com-

CLIENT TEACHING
During Female Breast Assessment

OBJECTIVES
- Client will perform BSE (see the box on p. 704).
- Client will have screening mammography performed at recommended intervals.
- Client will identify signs and symptoms of breast cancer.
- Client will identify signs and symptoms of fibrocystic disease.
- Client will follow a low-fat diet.

TEACHING STRATEGIES
- Have client perform return demonstration of BSE and offer the opportunity to ask questions.
- Explain recommended frequency of mammography and BSE by a health care provider.
- Discuss signs and symptoms of breast cancer.
- Discuss signs and symptoms of fibrocystic disease.
- Inform a woman who is obese or who has a family history of breast cancer that she is at higher risk for the disease.* Encourage dietary changes, including limiting meat consumption to well-trimmed, lean beef, pork, or lamb; removing skin from cooked chicken before eating it; selecting tuna and salmon packed in water and not oil; and using low-fat dairy products.
- Encourage client to reduce intake of caffeine and theophyllines. Although this approach is controversial, it may reduce symptoms of fibrocystic disease.

EVALUATION
- Have client demonstrate BSE.
- During follow-up visit, determine whether client has had mammography performed.
- Ask client to explain frequency of mammography.
- Have client describe signs and symptoms of breast cancer compared with fibrocystic disease.

*Data from Willett W et al: Dietary fat and the risk of breast cancer, *N Engl J Med* 316:22, 1987.

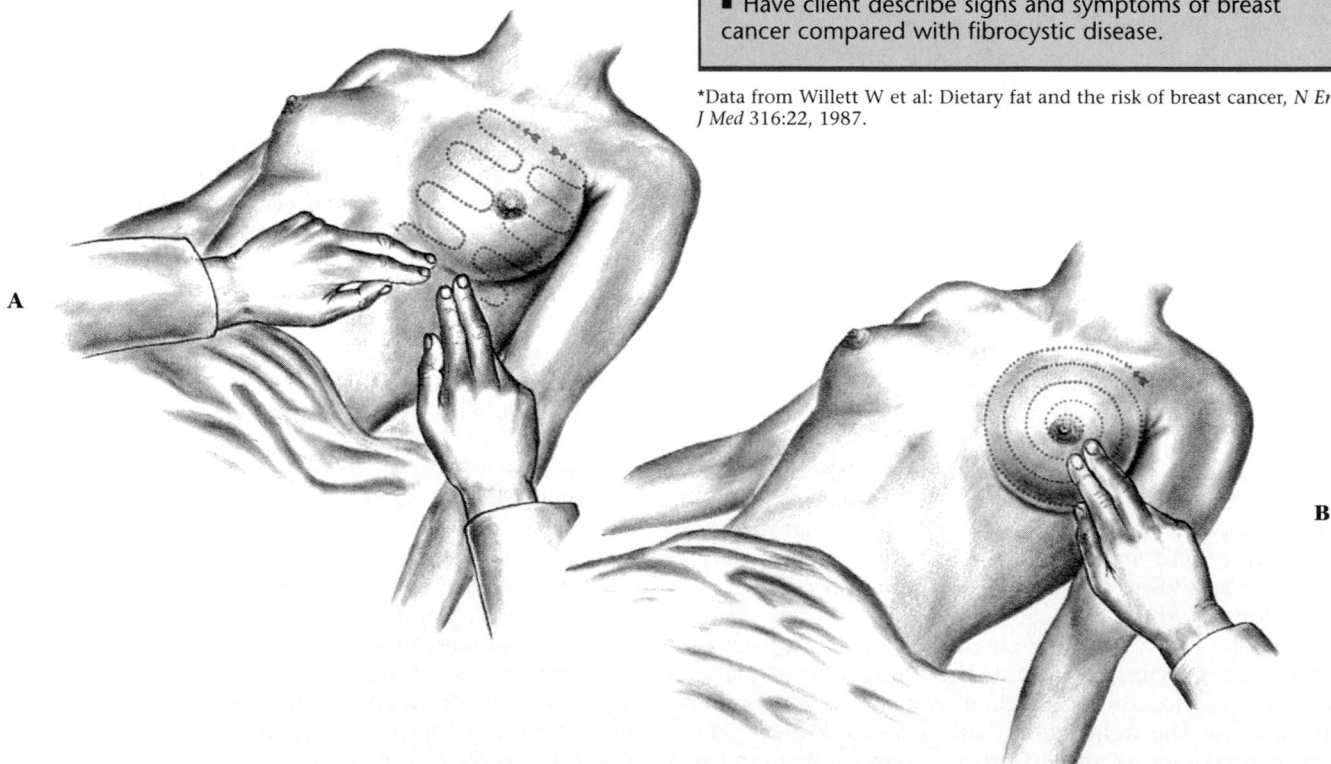

Fig. 33-78 Methods for breast palpation **A,** Back and forth. **B,** Concentric circles. *(From Seidel HM et al: Mosby's guide to physical examination, ed 3, St Louis, 1995, Mosby.)*

press the nipple gently, and the nurse notes any discharge. As the nurse examines the nipple and areola, the nipple may become erect with wrinkling of the areola. These changes are normal.

After the nurse completes the examination, the client can demonstrate self-palpation. Observing the client's technique helps the nurse emphasize the importance of a systematic approach. The client is urged to see her physician if she discovers an abnormal mass during routine monthly BSE. She should also know all signs and symptoms of breast cancer.

Male Breasts

Examination of the male breast is relatively easy. The nipple and areola are inspected for nodules, edema, and ulceration. An enlarged male breast may result from obesity or glandular enlargement. Breast enlargement in young males may be indicative of steroid use. Fatty tissue feels soft, whereas glandular tissue is firm. Any masses are palpated for the same characteristics as the female breast. Because breast cancer in men is relatively rare, routine self-examinations are unnecessary.

▋ ABDOMEN

The abdominal examination can be complex because of the organs located within and near the abdominal cavity. A thorough nursing history (Table 33-27) helps the nurse interpret physical signs. The examination includes an assessment of structures of the lower gastrointestinal (GI) tract in addition to the liver, stomach, uterus, ovaries, kidneys, and bladder. Abdominal pain is one of the most common symptoms clients report when seeking medical care. An accurate assessment requires matching client history data with a careful assessment of the location of physical symptoms.

Landmarks help the nurse map out the abdominal region. The xiphoid process (tip of the sternum) marks the upper boundary of the abdominal region, and the symphysis pubis delineates the lower boundary. By dividing the abdomen into four imaginary quadrants (Fig. 33-79, *A*) the nurse can refer to assessment findings and record them in relation to each quadrant. For example, the nurse may determine that the client is experiencing tenderness over the left lower quadrant (LLQ) with normal bowel sounds present. Posteriorly the kidneys, located from the T12 to L3 vertebrae, are protected by the lower ribs and heavy back mus-

Table 33-27	Nursing History for Abdomen Assessment

ASSESSMENT CATEGORY	RATIONALE
If client has abdominal or low back pain, assess character of pain in detail (location, onset, frequency, precipitating factors, aggravating factors, type of pain, severity, course).	Pattern of characteristics of pain helps determine its source.
Carefully observe client's movement and position, including lying still with knees drawn up, moving restlessly to find comfortable position, and lying on one side or sitting with knees drawn to chest.	Positions assumed by client may reveal nature and source of pain, including peritonitis, renal stone, and pancreatitis.
Assess normal bowel habits and stool character.	Data compared with physical findings can help identify cause and nature of elimination problems.
Determine if client has had abdominal surgery, trauma, or diagnostic tests of GI tract.	Surgical or traumatic alterations of abdominal organs may cause changes in expected findings (e.g., position of underlying organs). Diagnostic tests may change character of stool.
Assess if client has had recent weight changes or intolerance to diet (e.g., nausea, vomiting, cramping, especially in last 24 hours).	Data may indicate alterations in upper gastrointestinal tract (stomach or gallbladder) or lower colon.
Assess for difficulty in swallowing, belching, flatulence, bloody emesis (hematemesis), black or tarry stools (melena), heartburn, diarrhea, or constipation.	These characteristic signs and symptoms indicate gastrointestinal alterations.
Ask if client takes antiinflammatory medication (e.g., aspirin, ibuprofen, or steroids) or antibiotics.	Pharmacological agents may cause GI upset or bleeding.
Ask client to locate tender areas.	Nurse assesses painful areas last to minimize discomfort and anxiety.
Inquire about family history of cancer, kidney disease, alcoholism, hypertension, or heart disease.	Data may reveal risk for alterations identifiable during examination.
Determine if female client is pregnant; note last menstrual period.	Pregnancy causes changes in abdominal shape and contour.
Assess client's usual intake of alcohol.	Chronic alcohol ingestion can cause gastrointestinal and liver problems.
Review client's history for the following factors: health care occupation, hemodialysis, IV drug user, household or sexual contact with hepatitis B virus (HBV) carrier, heterosexual person with more than one sex partner in previous 6 months, sexually active homosexual or bisexual male, international traveler in area of high HBV infection rate.	Risk factors for hepatitis B virus exposure (Reece, 1993).

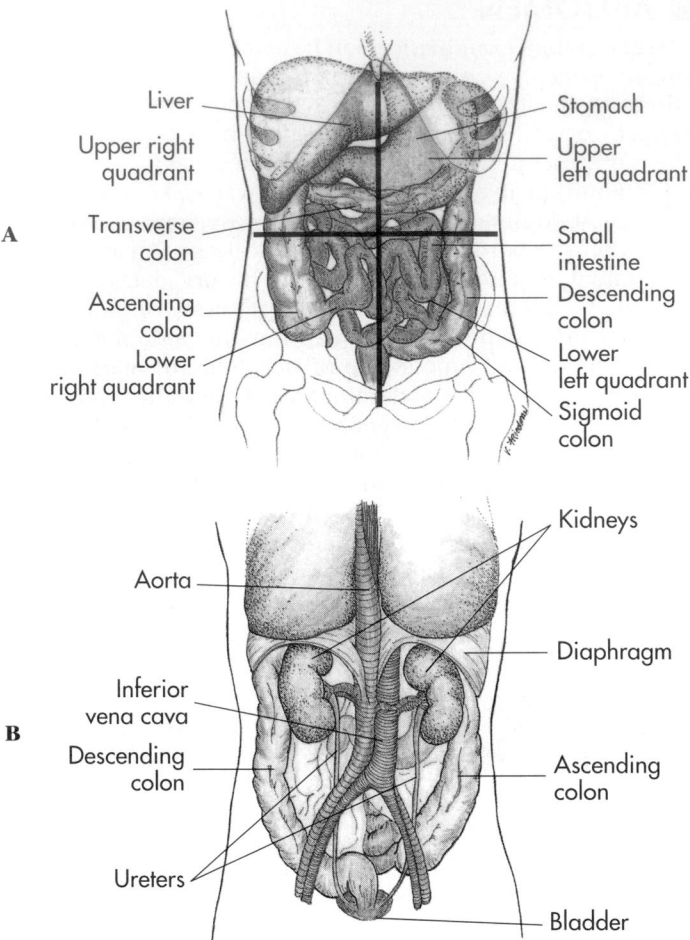

A

Liver
Upper right quadrant
Transverse colon
Ascending colon
Lower right quadrant

Stomach
Upper left quadrant
Small intestine
Descending colon
Lower left quadrant
Sigmoid colon

B

Aorta
Inferior vena cava
Descending colon
Ureters

Kidneys
Diaphragm
Ascending colon
Bladder

Fig. 33-79 A, Anterior view of abdomen divided by quadrants. **B,** Posterior view of abdominal sections.

cles (Fig. 33-79, *B*). The costovertebral angle formed by the last rib and vertebral column is a landmark used during kidney palpation.

Clients must be relaxed for abdominal examinations. A tightening of abdominal muscles hinders accuracy with palpation and auscultation. The nurse asks the client to void before beginning. The room should be warm and the client's upper chest and legs draped. The client lies supine or in a dorsal recumbent position with the arms at the sides and knees slightly bent. Small pillows can be placed beneath the knees (McConnell, 1990). If the client places the arms under the head, the abdominal muscles may tighten. The examiner proceeds calmly and slowly, being sure there is adequate lighting. The abdomen is exposed from just above the xiphoid process down to the symphysis pubis. Warm hands and stethoscope further promote relaxation. Maintaining conversation except during auscultation helps to distract clients. Clients should be asked to report pain and point out tender areas. Tender areas are assessed last.

The order of an abdominal examination differs slightly from previous assessments. The nurse begins with inspection and then follows with auscultation. It is important to auscultate before palpation and percussion because palpation and percussion may alter frequency and character of

bowel sounds. The nurse also needs a tape measure and marking pen.

Inspection

The nurse may be able to observe the client during routine care activities. The nurse notes the client's posture and looks for evidence of abdominal splinting, lying with the knees drawn up, or moving restlessly in bed. A client free from abdominal pain will not stoop or splint the abdomen. To inspect the abdomen for abnormal movement or shadows, the nurse stands on the client's right side and inspects from above the abdomen. By sitting down to look across the abdomen, the nurse assesses contour. The examination light is directed over the abdomen.

SKIN

The nurse inspects the skin over the abdomen for color, scars, venous patterns, lesions, and **striae** (stretch marks). The skin is subject to the same color variations as the rest of the body. Venous patterns are normally faint, except in thin clients. Striae result from stretching of tissue by obesity or pregnancy. An artificial opening may indicate a drainage site resulting from surgery (see Chapter 48) or an ostomy (see Chapters 46 and 47). Scars indicate past trauma or surgery that may have created permanent changes in underlying organ anatomy. Bruising may indicate accidental injury, physical abuse, or a type of bleeding disorder. Ask if the client self-administers injections (e.g., heparin or insulin). Unexpected findings include generalized color changes such as jaundice or cyanosis. A glistening taut appearance indicates ascites.

UMBILICUS

The position, shape, color, and signs of inflammation, discharge, or protruding masses are noted. Normally the umbilicus is a flat or concave hemisphere positioned midway between the xiphoid process and symphysis pubis. The color is the same as that of the surrounding skin. Underlying masses can cause displacement of the umbilicus. An everted (pouched out) umbilicus usually indicates distention. **Hernias** (protrusions of abdominal organs through the muscle wall) cause upward protrusion of the umbilicus. Normally no discharge is emitted from the umbilical area.

CONTOUR AND SYMMETRY

The nurse inspects for contour, symmetry, and surface motion of the abdomen, noting any masses, bulging, or distention. A flat abdomen forms a horizontal plane from the xiphoid process to the symphysis pubis. A round abdomen protrudes in a convex sphere from the horizontal plane. A concave abdomen appears to sink into the muscular wall. Each of these findings is normal if the abdomen's shape is symmetrical. In older adults there is often an overall increased distribution of adipose tissue. The presence of masses on only one side, or asymmetry, may indicate an underlying pathological condition.

Intestinal gas, tumor, or fluid in the abdominal cavity may cause **distention** (swelling). When distention is generalized, the entire abdomen protrudes. The skin often appears taut, as if it were stretched over the abdomen. When gas causes distention, the flanks do not bulge. However, if fluid is the source of the problem, the flanks bulge. The client should be asked to roll onto one side. A protuberance forms on the dependent side if fluid is the cause of the distention. The nurse asks the client if the abdomen feels unusually tight. The nurse must be careful not to confuse distention with obesity. In obesity the abdomen is large, rolls of adipose tissue are often present along the flanks, and the client does not complain of tightness in the abdomen. If abdominal distention is expected, the nurse may choose to measure the abdomen's girth by placing a tape measure around the abdomen at the level of the umbilicus. Consecutive measurements will show any increase or decrease in distention. A marking pen is used to indicate where the tape measure was applied.

ENLARGED ORGANS OR MASSES

While observing the abdominal contour, the nurse asks the client to take a deep breath and hold it. The contour should remain smooth and symmetric. This maneuver forces the diaphragm downward and reduces the size of the abdominal cavity. Any enlarged organs in the upper abdominal cavity (e.g., liver or spleen) may descend below the rib cage to cause a bulge. Closer examination can be performed with palpation.

To evaluate the abdominal musculature, the nurse has clients raise their heads. This position causes superficial abdominal wall masses, hernias, and muscle separations to become more apparent.

MOVEMENT OR PULSATIONS

The nurse should remember that a man breathes abdominally and a woman breathes more costally. If the client has severe pain, respiratory movement is diminished, and the client tightens abdominal muscles to guard against the pain. On closer inspection the nurse may see peristaltic movement and aortic pulsation by looking across the abdomen from the side to detect movement. It may take several minutes to see a peristaltic wave. In contrast, aortic pulsations occur with each beat of systole and appear in the midline above the umbilicus (epigastric area).

Auscultation

The nurse auscultates the abdomen to listen to the bowel sounds of intestinal motility and to detect vascular sounds. Clients are asked to not talk. If a client has a nasogastric or intestinal tube connected to intermittent suction, it should be momentarily turned off. Sound from the suction obscures bowel sounds.

BOWEL MOTILITY

Peristalsis, or intestinal motility, is a normal function of the small and large intestine. Bowel sounds are the audible passage of air and fluid created by peristalsis. The warmed diaphragm of the stethoscope is placed lightly over each of the four quadrants. Normally air and fluid move through the intestines creating soft gurgling or clicking sounds that occur irregularly 5 to 35 times per minute (Seidel et al, 1995). Sounds may last $\frac{1}{2}$ second to several seconds. It normally takes 5 to 20 seconds to hear a bowel sound. However, it may take 5 minutes of continuous listening before deciding bowel sounds are absent. Auscultate all four quadrants to be sure no sounds are missed. The best time to auscultate is between meals. When the nurse auscultates just

CLIENT TEACHING
During Abdomen Assessment

OBJECTIVES
- Client will maintain normal bowel elimination.
- Client will achieve pain relief.
- Clients at high risk for HBV will receive immunization.

TEACHING STRATEGIES
- Explain factors such as diet, regular exercise, limited use of over-the-counter drugs causing constipation, establishment of regular elimination schedule, and a good fluid intake that promote normal bowel elimination (see Chapter 47). Stress importance for older adults.
- Caution clients about dangers of excessive use of laxatives or enemas.
- If client has chronic pain, explain measures used for pain relief (e.g., relaxation exercises, positioning) (see Chapter 43).
- If client has acute pain, explain activities or positions to avoid.
- If client is a health care worker or has contact with blood or fluids of affected persons, encourage to receive the series of three vaccine doses.

EVALUATION
- Reassess client's bowel elimination pattern and stool character after therapies are started.
- Observe client use pain-relief measures and reassess character of pain.
- During follow-up clinic or office visit, check client's compliance with HBV vaccine schedule.

after meals or long after the client eats, bowel sounds tend to be increased. Sounds are generally described as normal, audible, absent, hyperactive, or hypoactive. Absent sounds indicate a cessation of gastrointestinal motility that may result from late-stage bowel obstruction, **paralytic ileus**, or **peritonitis**. Hyperactive sounds are loud, "growling" sounds called **borborygmi**, which indicate increased gastrointestinal motility. Inflammation of the bowel, anxiety, diarrhea, bleeding, excess ingestion of laxatives, and reaction of the intestines to certain foods cause increased motility (see the box above).

VASCULAR SOUNDS

Bruits indicate narrowing of major blood vessels and disruption of blood flow. Presence of bruits in the abdominal area can reveal aneurysms or stenotic vessels. The nurse uses the stethoscope's bell to auscultate in the epigastric region and each of the four quadrants. Normally there are no vascular sounds over the aorta (midline through the abdomen), or femoral arteries (lower quadrants). Renal artery bruits can be heard by placing the stethoscope over each upper quadrant anteriorly or the costovertebral angle posteriorly (which can be done when the client sits). A bruit should be reported immediately to a physician.

Percussion

Percussion of the abdomen maps out underlying organs, bone, and masses and helps reveal the presence of air in the stomach and intestines. The beginning student uses this skill in a limited fashion. Practice is needed to ensure accuracy.

ORGANS AND MASSES

The nurse systematically percusses each quadrant to assess areas of tympany and dullness. Potentially painful areas are always percussed last. Tympany usually predominates because of air in the stomach and intestines. A dull percussion note is a medium-to-high-pitched short sound heard over solid masses such as the liver, spleen, pancreas, kidneys, and distended bladder. In addition, a dull note may indicate a tumor. When dullness is noted, it may be useful to also use palpation to complete a detailed assessment.

LIVER SIZE

Percussion allows the nurse to identify borders of the liver to detect organ enlargement. The nurse starts at the right iliac crest and percusses upward along the right midclavicular line. The percussion note changes from tympanic to dull at the liver's lower border, which is usually at the right costal margin. Extension beyond the right costal margin should be reported immediately. The nurse may mark the lower border on the client's abdomen with a water-soluble pencil. The upper border is found by percussing down from the clavicle along the intercostal spaces at the midclavicular line. This time the note changes from resonant to dull (Fig. 33-80). The liver's upper border is usually found in the fifth, sixth, or seventh intercostal space. The distance between the upper and lower liver borders should be 6 to 12 cm (2½ to 5 inches) at the right midclavicular line. Diseases such as **cirrhosis**, cancer, and **hepatitis** cause liver enlargement.

KIDNEY TENDERNESS

With the client sitting or standing erect, the nurse uses direct or indirect percussion to assess for kidney inflammation. With the ulnar surface of the partially closed fist, the nurse percusses posteriorly the costovertebral angle at the scapular line. If the kidneys are inflamed, the client feels tenderness during percussion.

Palpation

With palpation, nursing students are primarily concerned with detecting areas of abdominal tenderness and noting the quality of abnormal distentions or masses. As students become more skilled, they learn to palpate for specific organs such as the liver. Light and deep palpation are used.

After rubbing the hands together, the nurse uses light palpation over each quadrant. The nurse waits to palpate painful areas last. The nurse lays the palm of the hand with fingers extended and approximated lightly on the abdomen. The nurse keeps the palm and forearm horizontal (Fig. 33-81). The pads of the fingertips depress approximately 1.3 cm (½ inch) in a gentle dipping motion. The nurse avoids quick jabs and uses smooth coordinated movements. If the client is ticklish, it may help to place the client's hand on the abdomen with the nurse's hand on the client's. This continues until the nurse can gradually remove the client's hand.

A systematic palpation of each quadrant assesses for muscular resistance, distention, tenderness, and superficial organs or masses. While palpating the nurse observes the client's face for signs of discomfort. The abdomen is normally smooth with consistent softness and nontender without masses. The older adult often lacks abdominal tone. If the nurse palpates a sensitive area, guarding or muscle tenseness may occur. If tightening remains after the client is helped to relax, peritonitis, acute **cholecystitis**, or appendicitis may be the cause. A distended bladder is easy to detect with light palpation. Normally the bladder lies below the umbilicus and above the symphysis pubis. The

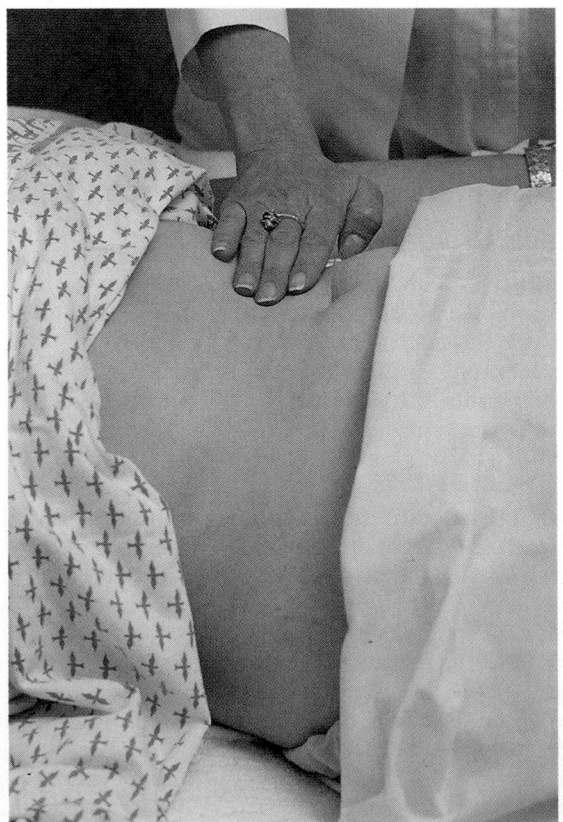

Fig. 33-81 Light palpation of abdomen.

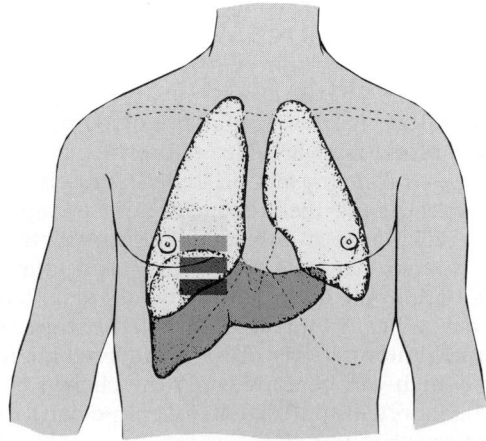

Fig. 33-80 To locate the liver's upper border, the nurse percusses downward, noting the change in sound from resonance (lung) to dullness (liver).

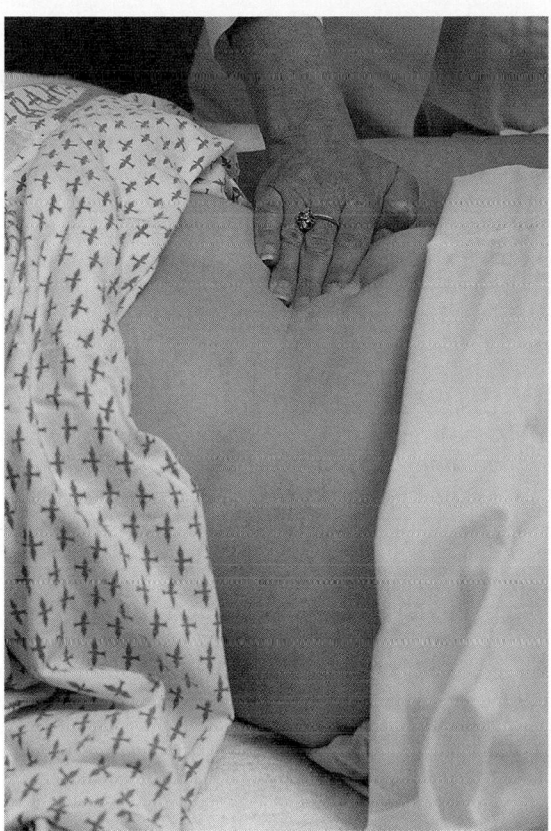

Fig. 33-82 Deep palpation of abdomen.

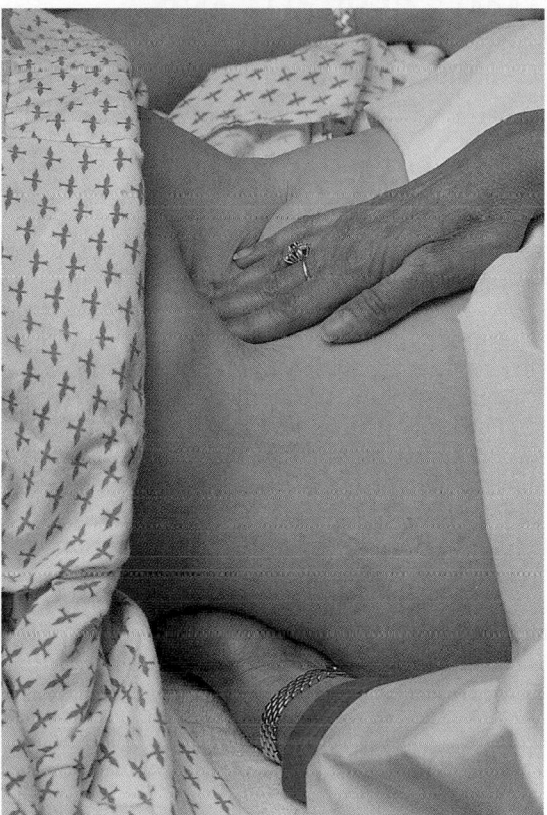

Fig. 33-83 The nurse's left hand is placed under the client's posterior thorax at the eleventh and twelfth ribs. The nurse's right hand palpates in and up to feel the liver's edge as the client inhales.

nurse routinely checks for a distended bladder if a client has been unable to void (e.g., due to anesthesia or sedation), has been incontinent, or if an indwelling urinary catheter is not draining well.

With experience the nurse can perform deep palpation to delineate abdominal organs and to detect less obvious masses. Short fingernails are needed. It is important for the client to be relaxed as the nurse's hands are depressed approximately 2.5 to 7.5 cm (1 to 3 inches) into the abdomen (Fig. 33-82). Deep palpation is never used over a surgical incision or over extremely tender organs. It is also unwise to use palpation on abnormal masses. Deep pressure may cause tenderness in the healthy client over the cecum, sigmoid colon, aorta, and in the midline near the xiphoid process (Seidel et al, 1995).

Each quadrant is surveyed systematically. Masses palpated are assessed for size, location, shape, consistency, tenderness, pulsation, and mobility. If tenderness is found, the examiner checks for rebound tenderness. With this test the examiner presses a hand slowly and deeply into the involved area and then lets go quickly. If pain is elicited with the release of the hand, the test is positive. Rebound tenderness occurs in clients with peritoneal irritation such as in appendicitis, **pancreatitis**, or any peritoneal injury causing bile, blood, or enzymes to enter the peritoneal cavity.

LIVER

The liver lies in the right upper quadrant under the rib cage. The nurse uses deep palpation to locate the liver's lower edge. This technique detects liver enlargement. To palpate the liver, the nurse places the left hand under the client's right posterior thorax at the eleventh and twelfth ribs and then applies upward pressure. This maneuver makes it easier to feel the liver anteriorly. With the fingers of the right hand pointing toward the right costal margin, the nurse places the hand on the right upper quadrant well below the liver's lower border. As the nurse presses gently in and up (Fig. 33-83), the client takes a deep abdominal breath. As the client inhales, the nurse tries to palpate the liver's edge as it descends. A normal liver may not be palpable. However, it is nontender and has a firm, regular, and sharp edge. If the liver is palpable, the nurse traces its edge medially and laterally by repeating the maneuver.

AORTIC PULSATION

To assess aortic pulsation, the nurse palpates with the thumb and forefinger of one hand deeply into the upper abdomen, just left of the midline. Normally a pulsation is transmitted forward. If there is enlargement of the aorta from an **aneurysm** (localized dilation of a vessel wall), the pulsation expands laterally. In obese clients it may be necessary to palpate with both hands, one on each side of the aorta.

FEMALE GENITALIA AND REPRODUCTIVE TRACT

An examination of the female genitalia can be embarrassing for many women unless the nurse uses a calm and relaxed approach. The gynecological examination is one of the most difficult experiences for adolescents. Cultural background may further add to apprehension. The lithotomy position assumed during the examination is an added source of embarrassment. Comfort is established through correct positioning and draping. Each portion of the examination is explained in advance so that clients can anticipate the nurse's actions. Adolescents may choose to have parents present in the examination room. Delays that might aggravate embarrassment should be avoided.

The client may require a complete examination of the female reproductive organs, which includes assessment of external genitalia and a vaginal examination. Most nurses do not perform a vaginal examination until they become nurse practitioners with extensive experience. However, it is important for the nurse to understand the procedure because a physician will require the nurse's assistance. An examination should be part of each woman's preventive health care because uterine cancers have a high incidence rate and ovarian cancer causes more deaths than any other cancer of the female reproductive system (ACS, 1995). Frequently a client will undergo an examination of external

genitalia during routine hygiene measures or urinary catheter care.

Adolescents and young adults should be examined because of the growing incidence of sexually transmitted diseases (STD). The average age of menarche among young girls has declined and the majority of male and female teenagers are sexually active by age 19 (Wong, 1995). As the nurse collects a history (Table 33-28) it is also important to assess the client's level of anxiety. Ask if the client has ever had a vaginal examination before. Rectal and anal assessment are easily combined with this examination because the client can assume a lithotomy or dorsal recumbent position.

Preparation of the Client

If a complete examination will be performed, the following special equipment will be needed: Examination table with stirrups, vaginal speculum of correct size, adjustable light source, sink, clean disposable gloves, glass microscopic slides and coverslips, plastic spatula and/or cytobrush, and specimen bottles with fixative spray (hairspray).

Equipment must be ready before the examination begins. The client is asked to empty her bladder so that urine is not accidentally expelled during the examination and so as to perform any urine screening tests. Assist the client to the lithotomy position, in bed or on an examination table for an external genitalia assessment. Assist the client into

---

Table 33-28	**Nursing History for Female Genitalia and Reproductive Tract Assessment**

ASSESSMENT CATEGORY	RATIONALE
Determine if client has had previous illness or surgery involving reproductive organs, including sexually transmitted disease.	Illness or surgery can influence appearance and position of organs being examined.
Review menstrual history, including age at menarche, frequency and duration of menstrual cycle, character of flow (e.g., amount, presence of clots), presence of dysmenorrhea (painful menstruation), pelvic pain, dates of last two menstrual periods.	This information helps to reveal level of reproductive health, including normalcy of menstrual cycle.
Ask client to describe obstetrical history, including each pregnancy and history of abortions or miscarriages.	Observed physical findings will vary, depending on woman's history of pregnancy.
Ask client to describe current and past contraceptive practices and problems encountered. Determine whether client uses safe sex practices. Discuss risk of STDs and HIV infection.	Use of certain types of contraceptives may influence reproductive health (e.g., sensitivity reaction to spermicidal jelly). Sexual history reveals risk for and understanding of sexually transmitted disease.
Assess if client has signs and symptoms of vaginal discharge, painful or swollen perianal tissues, or genital lesions.	These signs and symptoms indicate sexually transmitted disease.
Determine if client has symptoms or history of genitourinary problems, including burning during urination, frequency, urgency, nocturia, hematuria, incontinence, or stress incontinence (see Chapter 46).	Urinary problems may be associated with gynecological disorders, including sexually transmitted diseases.
Ask if client has had signs of bleeding outside of normal menstrual period or after menopause or has had unusual vaginal discharge.	These are warning signs for cervical cancer and endometrial cancer.
Determine if client is between ages of 40 to 50 and has history of condyloma cuminatum infection, herpes simplex, or cervical dysplasia; has multiple sex partners, smokes, has had multiple pregnancies, or was young at first intercourse.	These are risk factors for cervical cancer.
Determine if client is between ages of 40 to 60 and has history of ovarian dysfunction, cancer of the breast or endometrium, irradiation of pelvic organs, endometriosis, has a family history of ovarian or breast cancer, or has history of infertility or nulliparity.	These are risk factors for ovarian cancer.
Determine if client is postmenopausal, obese, infertile, had early menarche (before age 12), had late menopause (after age 50), has history of hypertension, diabetes, liver disease, or has family history of endometrial, breast, or colon cancer.	These are risk factors for endometrial cancer.

stirrups if a speculum examination is to be performed. Have the woman stabilize each foot in a stirrup and then have her slide her buttocks down to the edge of the examining table. The nurse places a hand at the edge of the table and instructs the client to move until touching the hand. The client's arms should be at her sides or folded across the chest to prevent tightening of abdominal muscles.

A woman suffering pain or deformity of the joints may be unable to assume a lithotomy position. In this situation it may be necessary to have the client abduct only one leg or to have another nurse assist in separating the client's thighs. The side-lying position may also be used with the client on the left side and right thigh and knee drawn up to her chest.

A square drape or sheet is given to the client. She holds one corner over her sternum, the adjacent corners fall over each knee, and the fourth corner covers the perineum. Once the examination begins, the drape over the perineum is lifted. A nurse often asks a colleague to be in attendance during the examination to allay the client's anxiety. Adolescents being examined for the first time tend to prefer a female examiner.

External Genitalia

The perineal area must be well illuminated. The nurse gloves both hands to prevent contact with infectious organisms. The perineum is extremely sensitive and tender. The area is not touched suddenly without warning the client. It is best to touch the neighboring thigh first before advancing to the perineum.

To assess sexual maturity, quantity and distribution of hair growth is noted. A preadolescent has no pubic hair except for fine body hair like that on the abdomen. During adolescence, hair grows along the labia, becoming darker, coarser, and curlier as it spreads over the pubic symphysis. Hair growth eventually forms a triangle over the female perineum and along the medial surfaces of the thighs. Hair growth should not spread up over the abdomen. Hair should be free of nits and lice. The underlying skin should be free of inflammation, irritation, or lesions.

The nurse inspects surface characteristics of the labia majora. The skin of the perineum is smooth, clean, and slightly darker than other skin. The mucous membranes appear dark pink and moist. The labia majora may be gaping or closed and appear dry or moist. They are usually symmetric. After childbirth the labia majora are separated, causing the labia minora to become more prominent. When a woman reaches menopause, the labia majora become thinned, and with advancing age, they become atrophied. The labia majora are normally without inflammation, edema, lesions, or lacerations.

To inspect the remaining external structures, the nurse gently places the thumb and index finger of the nondominant hand inside the labia minora and retracts the tissues outwardly (Fig. 33-84). The nurse should have a firm hold to avoid repeated retraction against the sensitive tissues. The nurse uses the other hand to palpate the labia minora between the thumb and second finger. On inspection the labia minora are normally thinner than the labia majora and one side may be larger. The tissue should feel soft on palpation and without tenderness. The size of the clitoris is variable. However, it normally is about 2 cm ($^4/_5$ inch) or

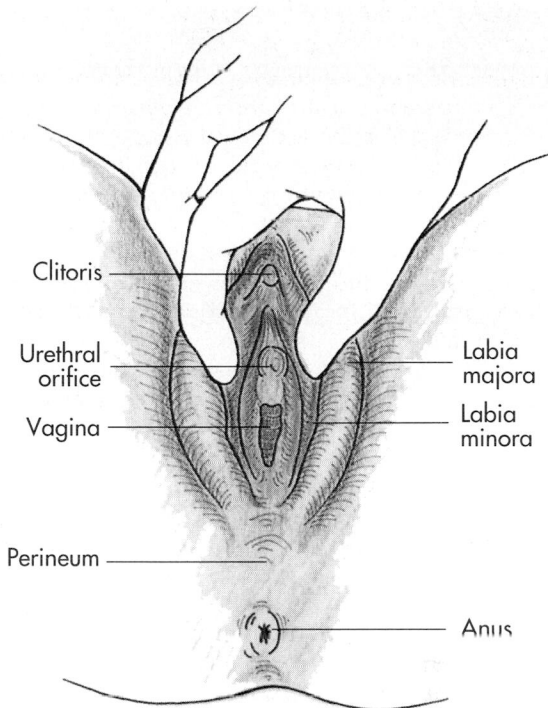

Fig. 33-84 Female external genitalia.

less in length and 0.5 cm ($^1/_5$ inch) in width. The nurse looks for atrophy, inflammation, or adhesions. If inflamed, the clitoris will be a bright cherry red. In young women it is a common site for syphilitic lesions or **chancres**, which appear as small open ulcers that drain serous material. Older women may have malignant changes that result in dry, scaly, nodular lesions.

The urethral orifice is carefully observed for color and position. It is normally intact without inflammation. The urethral meatus is anterior to the vaginal orifice and is pink. At times it is difficult to locate. It may appear as a small slit or pinhole opening just above the vaginal canal. In women who have had several vaginal childbirths, the opening to the vaginal canal often extends upward, interfering with the view of the urethra. The nurse notes any discharge, polyps, or fistulas.

When inspecting the vaginal orifice (introitus), the nurse inspects for inflammation, edema, discoloration, discharge, and lesions. Normally the introitus is a thin vertical slit or a large orifice. The tissue is moist. The hymen is just inside the introitus. In the virgin the hymen may restrict the opening of the vagina. Only remnants of the hymen remain after sexual intercourse.

With the labia still retracted, the nurse examines the Skene and Bartholin's glands. Tell the client you are going to insert one finger in her vagina and that she will feel pressure. With the palm facing upward, the nurse inserts an index finger of the examining hand into the vagina as far as the second joint. Exerting upward pressure, the nurse milks the Skene glands by moving the finger outward. Discharge and tenderness are abnormal. The exam is done on both sides of the urethra and then directly on the urethra (Fig. 33-85). The technique may cause discharge to appear. If so, the nurse notes the color, odor, and consistency and ob-

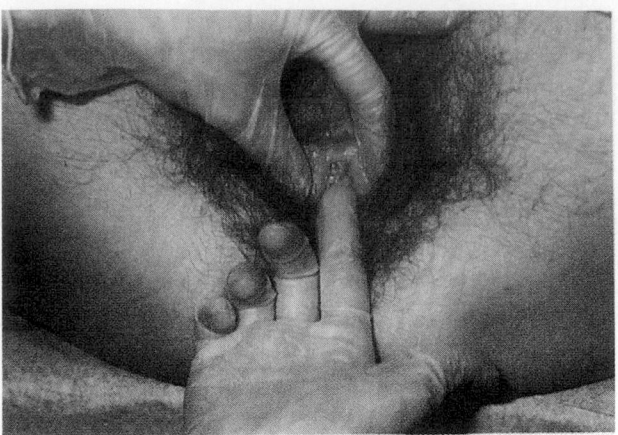

Fig. 33-85 Milking the urethra and paraurethral glands.

tains a culture. The nurse then changes into a new pair of gloves.

If inflammation and edema are found near the posterior end of the introitus, the Bartholin's glands may be infected. The glands cannot normally be palpated. To attempt palpation the nurse places a thumb and index finger between the labia majora and introitus and palpates one side at a time.

With the gloved index and middle fingers in the vaginal orifice, the nurse asks the client to strain downward as if she were voiding. If the client lacks adequate muscular support, the vaginal walls bulge, blocking the introitus. A portion of the vaginal wall and bladder may prolapse or fall into the orifice anteriorly; this is a **cystocele**. Bulging of the posterior wall may be caused by prolapse of the rectum (**rectocele**). Normally when a client is asked to constrict or close the vaginal orifice, the nurse palpates tension in the muscles. A woman who has undergone vaginal childbirth has less muscle tone than one who has not.

The nurse may also inspect the anus at this time, looking for lesions and hemorrhoids (see section on rectal examination). If the nurse performs only the external examination, the examination gloves are disposed of at this time. The client is then offered perineal hygiene if the skin is soiled with secretions.

Clients who are at risk for contracting a sexually transmitted disease (STD) should learn to perform a genital self-examination (GSE) (see the box at right). The purpose is to detect any signs or symptoms of STD. Many persons do not know they have an STD and some STDs can remain undetected for years.

Speculum Examination of Internal Genitalia

An examination of the internal genitalia requires much skill and practice. Usually it is performed only by advanced nurse practitioners or nurse midwives. Beginning students will more than likely only observe the procedure or assist the examiner.

The examination involves use of a plastic or metal speculum. Consisting of two blades and an adjustable thumbscrew, the speculum is inserted into the vagina to assess the internal genitalia for cancerous lesions and other abnormalities. During the examination a **Papanicolaou (Pap) smear** is collected to test for cervical and vaginal cancer.

CLIENT TEACHING During Female Genitalia and Reproductive Tract Assessment

OBJECTIVES
- Client will pursue routine gynecological examinations based on her level of risk for cervical cancer.
- Client with a sexually transmitted disease will follow safe sexual practices.
- Client will use measures to prevent acquisition and transmission of sexually transmitted disease.

TEACHING STRATEGIES
- Instruct client about purpose and recommended frequency of Pap smears and gynecological examinations.
- Counsel client with sexually transmitted disease about diagnosis and treatment.
- Instruct on genital self-examination (GSE): Using a mirror, position self in order to examine the area covered by the pubic hair. Spread the hair apart, looking for bumps, sores, or blisters. Also, look for any warts, which may appear as small, bumpy spots and then enlarge to fleshy, cauliflower-like lesions. Next, spread the outer vaginal lips apart and look at the clitoris for bumps, blisters, sores, or warts. Also look at both sides of the inner vaginal lips. The area around the urinary and vaginal opening should be inspected for bumps, blisters, sores, or warts.
- Explain warning signs of STD: pain or burning on urination, pain in pelvic area, bleeding between menstruation, an itchy rash around vagina, and vaginal discharge (different from usual).
- Teach measures to prevent sexually transmitted disease, including preventive measures (e.g., male partner's use of condoms, restricting number of sexual partners, avoiding sex with persons who have several other partners, perineal hygiene measures).
- Tell client with sexually transmitted disease that they must inform sexual partner of the need for an examination.
- Reinforce the importance of perineal hygiene (as appropriate).

EVALUATION
- Ask client to explain when she should routinely have a gynecological examination and Pap smear.
- Have client describe ways to prevent transmission of sexually transmitted diseases.
- For client with sexually transmitted disease, determine during follow-up visit if safe sexual practices have been followed (use nonthreatening inquiry).

To assist an examiner, the nurse makes sure the client is comfortably positioned in the stirrups. A variety of speculum sizes (small, medium, large) should be available so that the examiner may select the appropriate size for the client. The smallest size will fit a virgin. If the woman is sexually active, a medium-sized speculum is best. For women who have had children vaginally, the examiner uses a medium-to-large speculum.

In addition, the nurse will have gloves, specimen slides, and a spatula and/or cytobrush close at hand. Water-soluble lubricant is only used when specimens are not being collected. Most examiners lubricate the speculum with warm water.

CERVIX

The first portion of the examination involves careful insertion of the speculum until the examiner can fully visualize the cervix (Fig. 33-86). The examiner sits on a stool facing the client's perineum. The adjustable light is placed over the examiner's shoulder, directed at the examination site. The examiner holds the speculum in the dominant hand and explains the procedure to the client. If the woman has never been examined, two fingers are gently inserted into the vagina to explore for abnormalities. Then with two fingers the examiner presses down on the perineal body just inside the introitus. After checking to be sure that the speculum blades are closed, the examiner introduces the closed speculum obliquely (rotated 50 degrees counterclockwise from the vertical position) past the fingers. The speculum is inserted downward at a 45-degree angle toward the examination table to avoid trauma to the urethra (this maneuver corresponds with the normal downward slope of the vaginal canal). Care is taken to avoid pulling the pubic hair or pinching the labia.

After the wide portions of the blades have passed the introitus, the speculum is rotated so that the blades are horizontal. The blades are opened slowly after full insertion and the speculum is moved to visualize the cervix. When the cervix is in full view, the blades are locked in the open position.

The examiner inspects the cervix for color, appearance of the os or opening, position, size, surface characteristics, and discharge. The normal cervix is glistening pink, smooth, and round. Its diameter is about 1 inch (2.5 to 3 cm) in a young woman and smaller in an older adult. The cervix should be midline and without lesions.

PAPANICOLAOU SMEAR

The surface of the cervix at the cervical canal opening is lined with layers of vaginal squamous cells. The cells meet a different group of cells, columnar cells. The columnar cells secrete mucus and line the passageway that leads up into the central cavity of the uterus. The squamous cells have a protective role for the cervix, and the columnar cells have a reproductive role (helping sperm to enter the uterus for fertilization). A Pap smear is a painless screening test for cervical cancer. Specimens are taken from the endocervix and ectocervix (Table 33-29). The test is simple and has no side effects. It should be performed annually with a pelvic exam in women who are, or have been, sexually active, and in women who have reached the age of 18. After three or more consecutive annual exams with normal findings, the

A

B

C

Fig. 33-86 A, Angle of speculum insertion. **B,** View of cervix. **C,** Vaginal speculum in place with cervix in full view.

Table 33-29	Methods for Obtaining Pap Smears
LOCATION	**TECHNIQUE**
Outer cervix	Use plastic spatula. Place tip of longer arm in os. Rotate spatula, scraping outer surface of cervix. Apply cells to glass slide. Apply fixative solution and label slide. 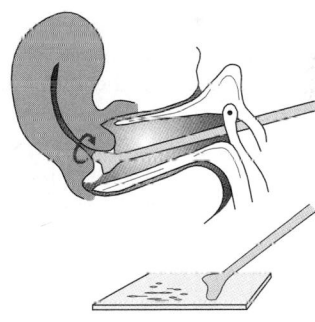
Endocervical	Use cervical brush (cytobrush). WARNING: Do *not* use on pregnant clients. Gently insert brush through os. Rotate brush 180 to 360 degrees. Apply cells by rolling and twisting brush on glass slide. Apply fixative solution and label slide. 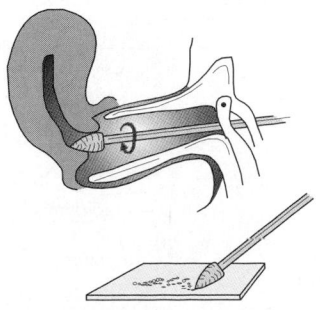

Pap test may be done less often at the discretion of the physician. Women at high risk for cervical cancer and those over 40 should have annual checkups.

The examiner first collects a sample of the outer cervix or ectocervix. A plastic spatula is rotated 360 degrees against the cervical surface. Once the spatula is withdrawn, the examiner spreads the specimen lightly over a glass slide. The nurse assisting sprays the specimen with cytological fixative and labels the slide. The examiner next uses a cytobrush to collect endocervical cells. The cytobrush is inserted into the cervical os and rotated one full turn. The specimen is then spread across the slide by rolling the brush with moderate pressure. Again the specimen is sprayed and the slide is labeled. At the end of the procedure the nurse warns the client that blood spotting is normal for a few hours.

There is also a paintbrush device (Cervex-brush) that can be used to collect both specimens at the same time. It uses flexible plastic bristles, which reportedly cause less blood spotting (Seidel et al, 1995).

VAGINA

Once specimens are collected the examiner views the vaginal walls as the speculum is slowly withdrawn. As the speculum leaves the cervix the thumbscrew is loosened, but the blades are kept open with the thumb. During the withdrawal the examiner notes the color, surface characteristics, and secretions. The vaginal walls are normally pink throughout and free from discharge and lesions. The surface should be moist and smooth or rugated. Normal secretions are thin, clear or cloudy, and odorless. Women commonly acquire yeast infection, causing thick, white, patchy, malodorous, curdlike discharge.

After speculum withdrawal the nurse assists the client to a sitting position and allows the client to dress and perform hygiene. In a hospital setting the client may need assistance with perineal hygiene. The nurse makes sure the gloves, speculum, and other disposable equipment are appropriately discarded in a receptacle. The client is informed that Pap smear results will be available in 3 to 4 days (check agency policy).

❙ MALE GENITALIA

An examination of the male genitalia includes assessment of the external genitalia (Fig. 33-87) and the inguinal ring

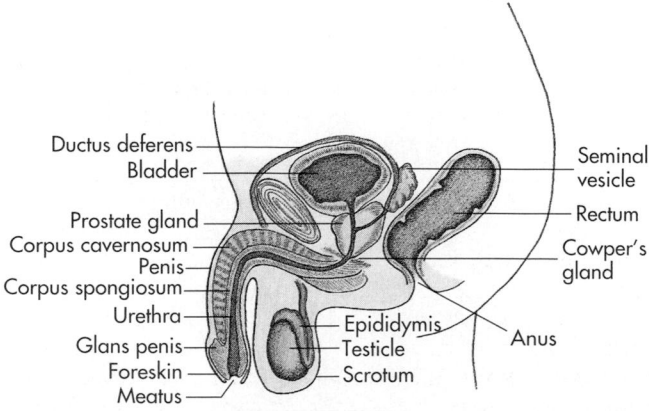

Ductus deferens
Bladder
Prostate gland
Corpus cavernosum
Penis
Corpus spongiosum
Urethra
Glans penis
Foreskin
Meatus

Seminal vesicle
Rectum
Cowper's gland
Epididymis
Testicle
Scrotum
Anus

Fig. 33-87 External and internal male sex organs.

and canal. Because the incidence of sexually transmitted disease in adolescents and young adults is high, an assessment of the genitalia should be a routine part of any health maintenance examination for this age group (see the box on p. 720). The examination begins with the client lying supine with the chest, abdomen, and lower legs draped. Inspection and palpation are used. The nurse applies disposable gloves to prevent the chance of cross-infection from urethral discharge.

The nurse must learn to relax and to help the client relax during the exam to avoid any embarrassment or anxiety for the client. Often adolescents and men are fearful of having an erection during the examination. Boys and adolescents may worry about their genitals being "normal" (Seidel et al, 1995). The nurse should limit discussion of the client's sexual activity during the examination because the client might perceive this as evaluative or judgmental (see the box below). The client's modesty must be preserved. It may help to provide teaching after the examination. Do not joke or use nonverbal expressions that may convey concern or worry. The genitalia are gently manipulated to avoid causing erection or discomfort. A thorough nursing history (Table 33-30) prior to the examination ensures the assessment will be complete.

Sexual Maturity

The nurse begins by assessing the sexual maturity of the client, noting the size and shape of the penis and testes, the color and texture of the scrotal skin, and the character and distribution of pubic hair. The first sign of puberty, an increase in genital and pubic hair development, is variable

CLIENT TEACHING
During Male Genitalia Assessment

OBJECTIVES
- Client will describe methods to prevent transmission of sexually transmitted diseases
- Client will perform genital self-exam
- Client with sexually transmitted disease will follow safe sex practices

TEACHING STRATEGIES
- Counsel client with sexually transmitted disease about diagnosis and treatment.
- Teach measures to prevent sexually transmitted diseases:
  - Use of condoms
  - Avoiding sex with partner who becomes infected
  - Restricting number of sexual partners
  - Avoiding sex with persons who have multiple partners
  - Using regular perineal hygiene
- Tell clients with sexually transmitted disease that sexual partners must be informed of the need to have an examination
- Instruct client on how to perform genital exam (see the box on p. 720)

EVALUATION
- Ask client to describe methods for treating and preventing sexually transmitted disease
- During a follow-up visit, determine whether client with sexually transmitted disease has used safe sexual practices.

Table 33-30	Nursing History for Male Genitalia Assessment
ASSESSMENT CATEGORY	**RATIONALE**
Review normal urinary elimination pattern including frequency of voiding; history of nocturia; character and volume of urine; daily fluid intake; symptoms of burning, urgency, frequency; difficulty starting stream; hematuria (see Chapter 46).	Urinary problems can be directly associated with genitourinary problems because of anatomical structure of men's reproductive and urinary systems.
Assess client's sexual history and use of safe sex habits; (multiple partners, infection in partners, failure to use condom).	Sexual history reveals risk for and understanding of sexually transmitted disease.
Determine if client has had previous surgery or illness involving urinary or reproductive organs, including sexually transmitted disease.	Alterations resulting from disease or surgery may be responsible for symptoms or changes in organ structure or function.
Ask if client has noted penile pain or swelling, genital lesions, or urethral discharge.	These signs and symptoms indicate sexually transmitted disease.
Determine if client has noticed heaviness or painless enlargement of testis, irregular lumps.	These signs and symptoms are early warning sign for testicular cancer.
If client reports an enlargement in inguinal area assess if it is intermittent or constant, associated with straining or lifting, painful, and whether pain is affected by coughing, lifting, or straining at stool.	Signs and symptoms reflect potential inguinal hernia.

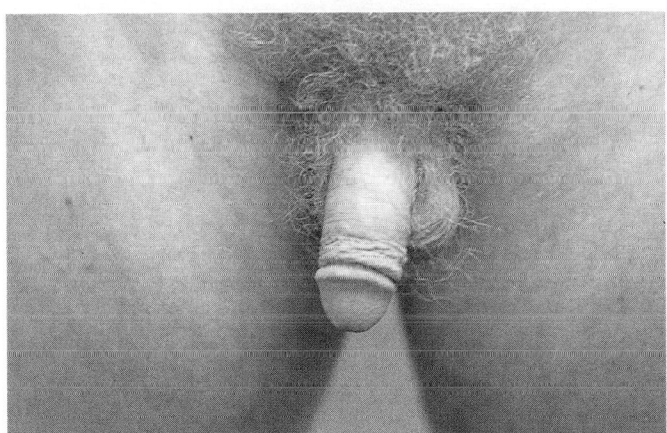

Fig. 33-88 Normal male genitalia (circumcised). *(From Seidel HM et al: Mosby's guide to physical examination, ed 3, St Louis, 1995, Mosby.)*

but generally does not start before 9.5 years of age. During the preadolescent stage there is no pubic hair except for the fine body hair found on the abdomen. By puberty the pubic hair extends from the base of the penis over the symphysis pubis and becomes coarse and curly. The testes and penis develop with the scrotal skin darkening and becoming thinner and more wrinkled in texture. The penis slowly lengthens, eventually reaching to the bottom of the scrotum (Fig. 33-88). The nurse inspects the skin covering the genitalia for lice, rashes, excoriations, or lesions.

Penis

The nurse inspects the structures of the penis, including the shaft, corona, prepuce (foreskin), glans, and urethral meatus. The dorsal vein should be apparent on inspection. In uncircumcised males the foreskin is retracted to reveal the glans and urethral meatus. The foreskin should retract eas-

ily. A small amount of thick, white secretion between the glans and foreskin is normal. If there is evidence of abnormal discharge, a culture is usually obtained. The urethral meatus is slitlike and should be positioned on the ventral surface just millimeters from the tip of the glans. In some congenital conditions the meatus is displaced along the penile shaft. Gentle compression of the glans between the nurse's thumb and index finger opens the urethral meatus to allow inspection for discharge. The opening should be glistening and pink. The meatus is also inspected for lesions, edema, and inflammation.

The glans is carefully checked around its entire circumference for lesions. The area between the foreskin and glans is a common site for venereal lesions. Any lesion is palpated gently to note tenderness, size, consistency, and shape.

The nurse continues to inspect the entire shaft of the penis, including the undersurface, looking for lesions, scars, and edema. The shaft is palpated between the thumb and first two fingers to detect any localized areas of hardness and tenderness. When inspection and palpation of the penis is completed, the foreskin is pulled down to its original position. It is important for any male client to learn to perform a genital self-examination in order to detect signs or symptoms of a sexually transmitted disease. Many people who have an STD do not know it. A self-examination should be a routine part of self-care (see the box on p. 720).

Scrotum

The nurse must be particularly cautious when inspecting and palpating the scrotum because the structures lying within the scrotal sac are very sensitive. The scrotum is a saclike structure divided internally into two halves. Each half contains a testicle, epididymis, and the vas deferens, which travels upward into the inguinal ring. Normally the left testicle is lower than the right. The nurse inspects the scrotum's size, shape, and symmetry while observing for lesions or edema. The scrotum is usually more deeply pig-

Male Genital Self-Examination

All men 15 years and older should perform this examination monthly using the following steps:

GENITAL EXAM

Perform the examination after a warm bath or shower when the scrotal sac is relaxed.

Stand naked in front of a mirror and hold the penis in your hand and examine the head. Pull back the foreskin if uncircumcised.

Inspect and palpate the entire head of the penis in a clockwise motion, looking carefully for any bumps, sores, or blisters. Look also for any bumpy warts (see the illustration).

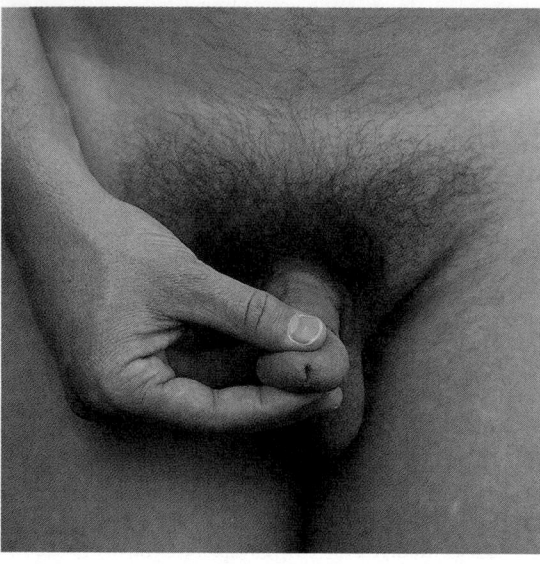

Look at the opening at the end of the penis for discharge.

Look along the entire shaft of the penis for the same signs.

Be sure to separate pubic hair at the base of the penis and carefully examine the skin underneath.

TESTICULAR SELF-EXAM

Look for swelling or lumps in the skin of the scrotum while looking in the mirror.

Use both hands, placing the index and middle fingers under the testicles and the thumb on top (see the illustration).

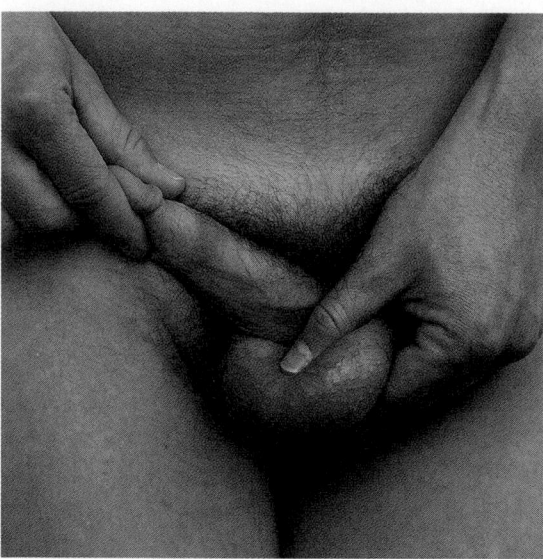

Gently roll the testicle, feeling for lumps, thickening, or a change in consistency (hardening).

Find the epididymis (a cordlike structure on the top and back of the testicle; it is not a lump).

Feel for small, pea-sized lumps on the front and side of the testicle. The lumps are usually painless and are abnormal.

Call your physician if you find a lump.

Illustrations from Seidel HM et al: *Mosby's guide to physical examination*, ed 3, St Louis, 1995, Mosby.

mented than the body skin and the surface is coarse. It is gently lifted to view the posterior surface. The scrotal skin is usually loose. A tightening of the skin may reveal edema. The scrotum's size normally changes with temperature variations as the dartos muscle contracts in cold and relaxes in warm temperatures.

Testicular cancer has become a common solid tumor among young men aged 18 to 34 years. Early detection is critical, and thus clients must learn to perform testicular self-examinations (TSE) (see the box above). The nurse can explain the technique while examining the client. The underlying testicles are normally ovoid and approximately 2 to 4 cm ($4/_5$ to $1^3/_5$ inches) in size. The testicles and epididymis are gently palpated between the nurse's thumb and first two fingers. They should be sensitive to gentle compression but not tender, and feel smooth and rubbery and free of nodules. The most common symptoms of testicular cancer are a painless enlargement of one testis and appearance of a palpable small, hard lump, about the size of a pea,

on the front or side of the testicle. The size, shape, and consistency of the organs are noted. In the older man the testicles decrease in size and are less firm during palpation. The client should be asked about any unusual tenderness. The nurse continues palpating the vas deferens separately as it forms the spermatic cord toward the inguinal ring, noting the presence of nodules or swelling.

Inguinal Ring and Canal

The external inguinal ring provides the opening for the spermatic cord to pass into the inguinal canal. The canal forms a passage through the abdominal wall, a potential site for hernia formation. An intestinal loop may even enter the scrotum. The client stands during this portion of the examination.

Both inguinal areas are inspected for signs of obvious bulging. During inspection the client is asked to strain or bear down. The maneuver helps make a hernia more visible.

The nurse completes an examination by palpating for inguinal lymph nodes. Small, nontender, mobile horizontal nodes may be normally found. Normally the nodes are not palpable. Any abnormality may indicate local or systemic infection or metastatic disease.

RECTUM AND ANUS

A good time to perform the rectal examination is after the genital examination. Usually the examination is not performed in young children or adolescents. The examination can detect colorectal cancer in its early stages. In men the rectal examination can also detect prostatic tumors. The nurse collects a thorough history (Table 33-31) to detect risk for bowel or rectal disease or prostatic disease.

The rectal examination can be uncomfortable and embarrassing, so the nurse uses a calm, slow-paced, gentle approach. Explanation of steps of the procedure helps clients to relax and lessens discomfort during the digital examination. Women can be examined immediately after examination of genitalia while still in dorsal recumbent positions. Otherwise the left lateral side-lying (Sims') position is preferred. Men are best examined by having the client bend over forward with his hips flexed and upper body resting across the examination table. A nonambulatory client can be examined in the Sims' position. Clients are draped with only the anal area exposed. The nurse applies disposable gloves for the examination.

Inspection

The nurse begins by inspecting the perianal and sacrococcygeal areas. The skin should be smooth and uninterrupted. The nurse looks for lumps, rashes, inflammation, excoriation, and scars. Fungal infection can cause perianal irritation.

Using the nondominant hand, the nurse gently retracts the buttocks apart to inspect the anus. Anal tissues are normally moist and hairless compared with perianal skin. The tissue is coarser and more darkly pigmented. The anus is held closed by the voluntary external muscle sphincter. The nurse inspects anal tissue for skin lesions, external **hemorrhoids** (dilated veins that appear as reddened protrusions), fissures and fistulas, inflammation, rashes, or discoloration. Next, the nurse asks the client to bear down as though having a bowel movement. Any internal hemorrhoids, fistulas, fissures, or polyps will appear at this time. Normally the anal lining is intact.

Digital Palpation

Some institutions do not permit nurses to perform digital examinations. When policy permits, the nursing student should have a qualified examiner present during the first examination.

The nurse lubricates the index finger of the gloved dominant hand. The procedure is explained, and then the client is asked to bear down gently as if having a bowel movement. As the anal sphincter relaxes, the nurse's fingertip is gently slipped into the anal canal in a direction toward the umbilicus. Normally the client feels as though stool is being passed. The nurse never forces digital insertion, so mucosal tissues are not injured.

The anal canal is the distal portion of the gastrointestinal tract. The canal extends in a line toward the umbilicus before turning into the mucus-lined rectum. The anus contains a rich supply of sensory nerve fibers. Thus digital manipulation can be painful. At the junction of the anal canal and rectum, the rectum balloons out and turns posteriorly into the hollow of the coccyx and sacrum.

Initially the nurse notes the tone of the anal sphincter as the muscle closes snugly around the finger. After asking the client to tighten the sphincter around the finger, the nurse notes sphincter tone. The sphincter should tighten evenly without discomfort. A weak sphincter may indicate a neurological problem. Acute rectal pain is not normal. Irrita-

Table 33-31	Nursing History for Rectum and Anus Assessment	
ASSESSMENT CATEGORY	**RATIONALE**
Determine whether client has experienced bleeding from rectum, black or tarry stools (melena), rectal pain, or change in bowel habits (constipation or diarrhea).	These are warning signs of colorectal cancer or other gastrointestinal alterations.
Determine whether client has personal or family history of colorectal cancer, polyps, or inflammatory bowel disease. Ask if client is over age 40.	These are risk factors for colorectal cancer.*
Assess dietary habits for high-fat intake or deficient fiber content.	Bowel cancer may be linked to dietary intake of fat or insufficient fiber intake.*
Determine whether client has undergone screening for colorectal cancer (digital examination, stool blood slide test, proctosigmoidoscopy).	Undergoing this screening reflects understanding and compliance with preventive health care measures.
Assess medication history for use of laxatives or cathartic medications.	Repeated use can cause diarrhea and eventual loss of intestinal muscle tone.
Assess for use of codeine or iron preparations.	Codeine causes constipation. Iron turns the color of feces black and tarry.
Ask male client if weak or interrupted urine flow, inability to urinate, difficulty in starting or stopping urine flow, polyuria, nocturia, hematuria, or dysuria has been experienced. Does client have continuing pain in lower back, pelvis, or upper thighs?	These are warning signs of prostatic cancer.* Symptoms also can suggest infection or prostate enlargement.

*Data from American Cancer Society: *1995 cancer facts and figures,* New York, 1995, The Society.

tion, fissures, inflamed hemorrhoids, or rock hard constipation can be the source of discomfort.

Beyond the anal canal the nurse palpates each side of the rectal wall for tenderness, irregularities, polyps, masses, or nodules. The wall should feel even and smooth. After the finger is advanced fully the client is asked to bear down again. High lesions within the rectum will descend against the fingertip (see the box above).

In men, the nurse turns the hand so that the finger palpates the anterior rectal wall. Warn the client that he may feel the urge to urinate, but that he will not. The prostate gland is palpable anteriorly as a rounded, heart-shaped structure about 2.5 to 4 cm (1 to 1$^1/_2$ inches) in diameter with less than 1 cm (1 inch) protrusion into the rectum (Fig. 33-89). A small medial groove separates the gland into two lateral lobes. The nurse palpates the size, shape, and consistency of the prostate. The gland normally is firm, without bogginess, tenderness, or nodules. Hardness or nodules may indicate presence of a cancerous lesion. Prostate enlargement is classified by the amount of projection into the rectum: grade I is 1 to 2 cm protrusion; grade II, 2 to 3 cm; grade III, 3 to 4 cm; grade IV, more than 4 cm (Seidel et al, 1995).

In women, it may be possible to palpate the cervix through the anterior rectal wall. It is common to mistake the cervix or an inserted tampon for a rectal tumor.

After palpation is completed the nurse gently withdraws the finger and observes it for feces. Feces are normally brown. The presence of mucus, blood, or black, tarry stool should be reported. A sample of the feces is tested for occult blood (see Chapter 47). For women suspected of having sexually transmitted disease, a rectal culture may be taken to rule out cross-infection from vaginal discharge. The nurse cleans the perianal area before continuing to the next part of the examination.

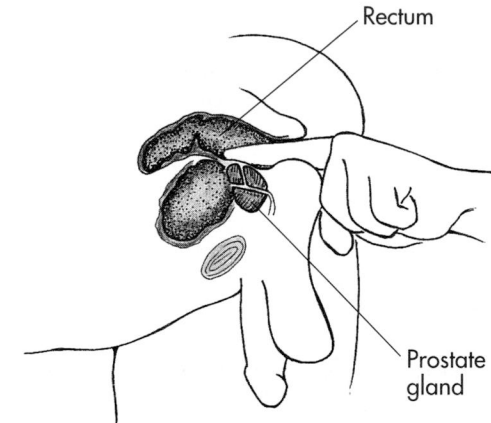

Fig. 33-89 Palpation of prostate gland during rectal examination.

■ MUSCULOSKELETAL SYSTEM

The nurse can learn to integrate portions of the musculoskeletal assessment when the client walks, moves in bed, or performs any type of physical activity. The assessment of musculoskeletal function focuses on determining range of joint motion, muscle strength and tone, and joint and muscle condition. Assessment of musculoskeletal integrity is especially important when the client reports pain or loss of function in a joint or muscle. Frequently muscular disorders are manifestations of neurological disease. For this reason a neurological assessment is often conducted simultaneously.

It is important to review the anatomy of bone and muscle placement and joint structure (see Chapter 37). Joints vary in their degree of mobility. Some, as in the knee, are

Table 33-32	Nursing History for Musculoskeletal System Assessment

ASSESSMENT CATEGORY	RATIONALE
Determine if client is involved in competitive sports (particularly involving collision and contact), fails to warm up adequately, is in poor physical condition, or had had a rapid growth spurt (adolescents).	These are risk factors for sports injury.
Review client history for heavy alcohol use, cigarette smoking, constant dieting, calcium intake less than 500 mg daily, thin and light body frame, nulliparous, menopause before age 45, postmenopause, family history of osteoporosis, or is Caucasian, Asian, or Native American.	These are risk factors for osteoporosis.
Ask client to describe history of alteration in bone, muscle, or joint function (e.g., recent fall, trauma, lifting of heavy objects, history of bone or joint disease with sudden or gradual onset, location of alteration).	History assists in assessing nature of musculoskeletal problem.
Assess nature and extent of pain, including location, duration, severity, predisposing and aggravating factors, relieving factors, and type.	Alterations in bone, joints, or muscle are frequently accompanied by pain, which has implications for not only comfort but also ability to perform activities of daily living.
Determine how alteration influences ability to perform activities of daily living (e.g., bathing, feeding, dressing, toileting, and ambulating) and social functions (e.g., household chores, work, recreation, sexual activities).	Level of nursing care will be determined by extent to which client is able to perform self-care.
	Type and degree of restriction in continuing social activities influence topics for client education and ability of nurse to identify alternative ways to maintain function.
Assess height loss of woman over age 50 by subtracting current height from recall of maximum adult height.*	Measurement may be useful screening tool to predict osteoporosis. In study by Reed and Birge,* 75% of clients who had lost 2 inches or more in height were later found to have osteoporosis on x-ray films.

*Data from Reed AT, Birge SJ: Screening for osteoporosis, *J Gerontol Nurs* 14(7):18, 1988.

freely movable. The spinal vertebrae are examples of slightly movable joints.

The examination uses inspection and palpation. The muscles and joints should be exposed and free to move. Depending on the muscle groups assessed the client assumes a sitting, supine, prone, or standing position. Table 33-32 lists the information gathered in the nursing history.

General Inspection

The nurse observes gait and the anterior, posterior, and lateral aspects of the client's posture as the client walks into and stands in the examination room. When the client is unaware of the nature of the observations, gait is more natural. Later a more formal test involves having the client walk in a straight line away from the nurse and then return. The nurse looks for foot dragging, limping, shuffling, and the position of the trunk in relation to the legs. Normally the client walks with arms swinging freely at the sides and the head and face leading the body. An older adult often walks with smaller steps and a wider base of support.

The normal standing posture is an upright stance with parallel alignment of the hips and shoulders (Fig. 33-90). There should be an even contour of the shoulders, level scapulae and iliac crests, alignment of the head over the gluteal folds, and symmetry of extremities. Looking sideways at the client, the nurse notes the normal cervical, thoracic, and lumbar curves. The head is held erect. As the client sits, some degree of rounding of the shoulders is normal. Older adults tend to assume a stooped, forward-bent posture, with hips and knees somewhat flexed and arms bent at the elbows, raising the level of the arms (Ebersole and Hess, 1994).

Common postural abnormalities include lordosis, kyphosis, and scoliosis (Fig. 33-91). **Kyphosis**, or hunchback, is an exaggeration of the posterior curvature of the thoracic spine. This postural abnormality is common in the older adult. **Lordosis**, or swayback, is an increased lumbar curvature. A lateral spinal curvature is called **scoliosis** (see the box on p. 724). Loss of height is frequently the first clinical sign of **osteoporosis**, in which height loss occurs in the trunk as a result of vertebral fracture and collapse (Reed and Birge, 1988). Although a small amount of height loss is to be expected with aging, if the amount of loss is greater than expected, osteoporosis is likely (see Chapter 37).

During general inspection the nurse looks at the extremities for overall size, gross deformity, bony enlargement, alignment, and symmetry. There should be bilateral symmetry in length, circumference, alignment, and position and number of skin folds (Seidel et al, 1995). A general review pinpoints areas requiring specialized assessment.

Palpation

The nurse applies gentle palpation to all bones, joints, and surrounding muscles in a complete examination. In the case of a focused assessment, only an involved area needs to be examined. The nurse notes any heat, tenderness, edema, or resistance to pressure. The client should feel no discomfort when palpation is applied. Muscles should be firm.

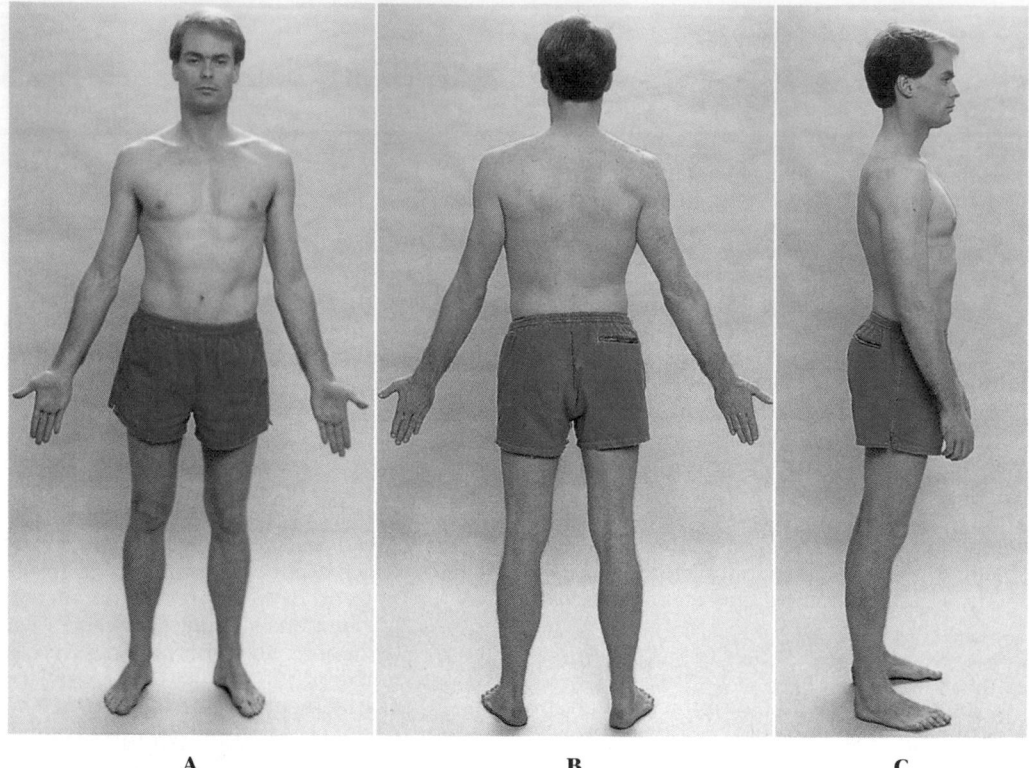

Fig. 33-90 Inspection of overall body posture **A,** Anterior view. **B,** Posterior view. **C,** Lateral view. *(From Seidel HM et al:* Mosby's guide to physical examination, *ed 3, St Louis, 1995, Mosby.)*

CLIENT TEACHING
During Musculoskeletal Assessment

OBJECTIVES
- Female client will follow measures to prevent or minimize osteoporosis.
- Client will assume proper body posture.
- Client will be able to perform self-care measures.

TEACHING STRATEGIES
- Instruct client about correct postural alignment. Consult with physical therapist to provide client with exercises for improving posture.
- To reduce bone demineralization, instruct older client about a proper exercise program (e.g., walking) to be followed 3 or more times a week. Also encourage intake of calcium to meet the recommended daily allowance. Increased vitamin D will aid calcium absorption. Recommendations for daily calcium supplements are 1000 mg before and 1500 mg after menopause.
- Explain to clients with low back pain that they can benefit from modification of worker risk factors (e.g., lifting heavy weights, use of protective equipment), regular aerobic exercise, exercises that strengthen the back and increase trunk flexibility, and learning how to lift properly.

Use of nonsteroidal antiinflammatory drugs and muscle relaxants has questionable value (Malter, 1994).
- For client with osteoporosis, instruct on proper body mechanics (see Chapter 43) and range of motion and moderate-weight-bearing exercises (swimming and walking) to minimize trauma and subsequent fracture of bones.
- When client is unable to perform self-care, instruct on use of assistive devices (e.g., zippers on clothing instead of buttons, elevation of chairs to minimize bending of knees and hips).
- Instruct older client to pace activities to compensate for loss in muscle strength.

EVALUATION
- Observe client's posture.
- Ask client to describe therapies for preventing osteoporosis.
- Observe client perform range of motion exercises.
- Have client keep log of regular weight-training exercises.
- Ask client or family members to describe client's use of self-care aids.

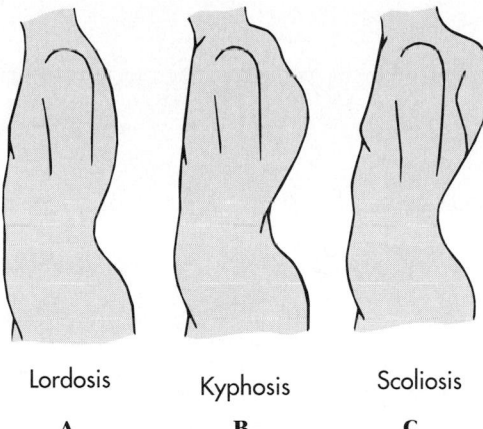

Fig. 33-91 Common postural abnormalities. **A,** Lordosis. **B,** Kyphosis. **C,** Scoliosis.

Range of Joint Motion

The nurse asks the client to put each major joint through active and passive full range of motion (see Chapter 37). It is important to have plenty of room for the client to fully move each extremity. The nurse assesses range of motion passively by gently supporting and moving the extremities through their range of movement. The nurse must learn the correct terminology for the movements that the joints are capable of making (Table 33-33) and instruct the client on how to move through each range of motion. It also helps to demonstrate range of motion to the client when possible. The same body parts are compared for equality in movement. Fig. 33-92 shows an example of range of motion positions for the hand and wrist.

When assessing range of motion the nurse does not force a joint if there is pain or muscle spasm. The nurse must know the joint's normal range and the extent to which it can be moved. Range of motion should be equal between contralateral joints. Ideally the normal range is assessed to determine a baseline for assessing later change.

A **goniometer** measures the precise degree of motion in a particular joint and is used mainly in clients who have a suspected reduction in joint movement. The instrument has two flexible arms with a 180-degree protractor in the center. The center of the protractor is positioned at the center of the joint being measured (Fig. 33-93). The arms extend along the body parts on each side of the protractor. A measurement is taken of the joint angle before moving the joint. After taking the joint through a full range of motion the nurse measures the angle again to determine the degree of movement. The reading is compared with the normal degree of joint movement.

When putting each joint through its range of motion the nurse makes a number of basic observations, noting pain, limited mobility, spastic movement, joint instability, stiffness, and contracture. Normal joints are nontender, without swelling, and move freely. In older adults, joints often become swollen and stiff with reduced range of motion resulting from cartilage erosion and fibrosis of synovial membranes (see Chapter 37).

Muscle Tone and Strength

The nurse may assess muscle strength and tone during measurement of range of motion. Findings are integrated with those from the neurological assessment. Tone is the slight muscular resistance felt by the examiner as the relaxed extremity is passively moved through its range of motion.

The client is asked to allow an extremity to relax or hang limp. This is often difficult, particularly if the client feels pain in the extremity. The extremity is supported, and each limb grasped, moving it through the normal range of motion (Fig. 33-94). Normal tone causes a mild, even resistance to movement through the entire range.

If a muscle has increased tone, or **hypertonicity,** any sudden passive movement of a joint is met with considerable resistance. Continued movement eventually causes the muscle to relax. A muscle that has little tone (**hypotonicity**) feels flabby. The involved extremity hangs loosely in a position determined by gravity.

For assessment of muscle strength the client assumes a stable position. The client performs maneuvers demonstrat-

Table 33-33	**Terminology for Normal Range of Motion Positions**	
TERM	**RANGE OF MOTION**	**EXAMPLES OF JOINTS**
Flexion	Movement decreasing angle between two adjoining bones; bending of limb	Elbow, fingers, knee
Extension	Movement increasing angle between two adjoining bones	Elbow, knee, fingers
Hyperextension	Movement of body part beyond its normal resting extended position	Head
Pronation	Movement of body part so that front or ventral surface faces downward	Hand, forearm
Supination	Movement of body part so that the front or ventral surface faces upward	Hand, forearm
Abduction	Movement of extremity away from midline of body	Leg, arm, fingers
Adduction	Movement of extremity toward midline of body	Leg, arm, fingers
Internal rotation	Rotation of joint inward	Knee, hip
External rotation	Rotation of joint outward	Knee, hip
Eversion	Turning of body part away from midline	Foot
Inversion	Turning of body part toward midline	Foot
Dorsiflexion	Flexion of toes and foot upward	Foot
Plantar flexion	Bending of toes and foot downward	Foot

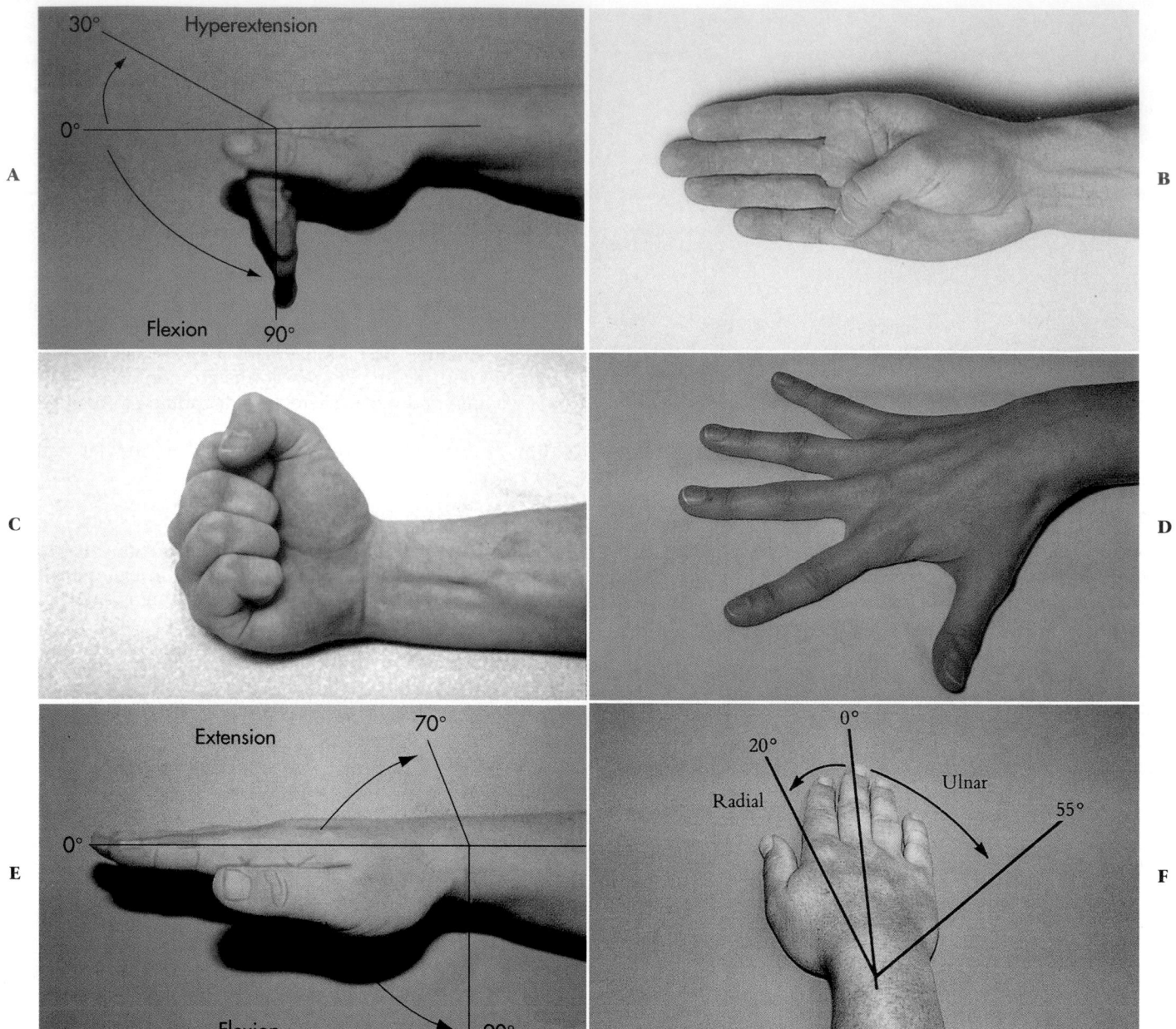

Fig. 33-92 Range of motion of the hand and wrist. **A,** Meta-carpophalangeal flexion and hyperextension. **B,** Finger flexion: thumb to each fingertip and to the base of the little finger. **C,** Finger flexion, first formation. **D,** Finger abduction. **E,** Wrist flexion and hyperextension. **F,** Wrist radial and ulnar movement. *(From Seidel HM et al: Mosby's guide to physical examination, ed 3, St Louis, 1995, Mosby.)*

ing strength of major muscle groups (Table 33-34). Symmetrical muscle pairs are compared (Table 33-35). The arm on the dominant side is normally stronger than the arm on the nondominant side. In the older adult a loss of muscle mass causes bilateral weakness, but muscle strength remains greater in the dominant arm or leg.

Each muscle group is examined. The nurse asks the client to first flex the muscle to be examined and then to resist when the nurse applies opposing force against that flexion.

It is important to not allow the client to move the joint. The nurse gradually increases pressure to a muscle group (e.g., elbow extension). The client resists the pressure applied by the nurse by attempting to move against resistance (e.g., elbow flexion). The client resists until instructed to stop. As the examiner varies the amount of pressure applied, the joint moves.

If a weakness is identified, the muscle's size is compared to its opposite counterpart by measuring the muscle body's

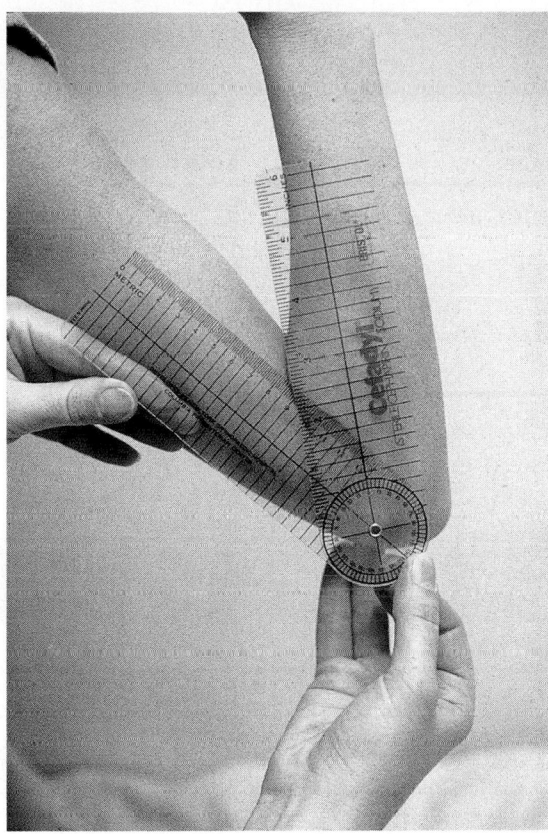

Fig. 33-93 After the client flexes the arm the goniometer measures the degree of joint flexion. *(From Seidel HM et al:* Mosby's guide to physical examination, *ed 2, St Louis, 1991, Mosby.)*

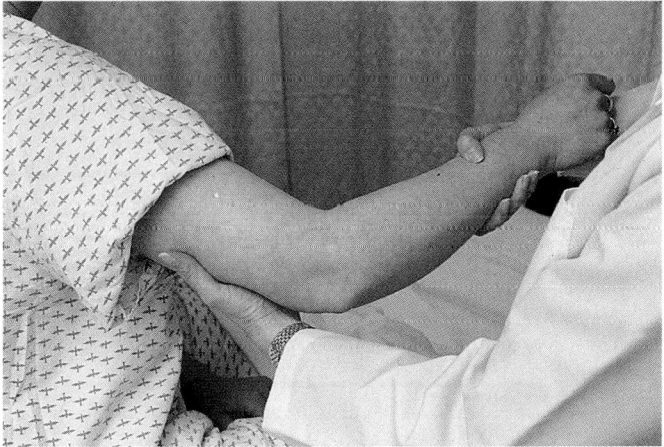

Fig. 33-94 The nurse assesses muscle tone.

Table 33-34	Maneuvers to Assess Muscle Strength
MUSCLE GROUP	**MANEUVER**
Neck (sternocleidomastoid)	Place hand firmly against client's upper jaw. Ask client to turn head laterally against resistance.
Shoulder (trapezius)	Place hand over midline of client's shoulder, exerting firm pressure. Have client raise shoulders against resistance.
Elbow	
Biceps	Pull down on forearm as client attempts to flex arm.
Triceps	As client's arm is flexed, apply pressure against forearm. Ask client to straighten arm.
Hip	
Quadriceps	When client is sitting, apply downward pressure to thigh. Ask client to raise leg up from table.
Gastrocnemius	Client sits, holding shin of flexed leg. Ask client to straighten leg against resistance.

circumference with a tape measure. A muscle that has **atrophied** (reduced in size) may feel soft and boggy when palpated.

∎ NEUROLOGICAL SYSTEM

The neurological system is responsible for many functions, including initiation and coordination of movement, reception and perception of sensory stimulii, organization of thought processes, control of speech, and storage of memory. A close integration exists between the neurological system and all other body systems. For example, urine production relies in part on the adequacy of blood flow to the kidneys, and the size of arterioles supplying the kidneys is under neural control.

An assessment of neurological function can be time consuming. An efficient nurse integrates neurological measurements with other parts of the physical examination. For example, cranial nerve function can be tested during the survey of the head and neck. Mental and emotional status is observed as the nursing history is collected.

Many variables must be considered when deciding the extent of the examination. A client's level of consciousness influences the ability to follow directions. A person's general physical status influences tolerance to assessment. For example, an inability to walk makes a detailed assessment of coordination difficult. The client's chief complaint also helps determine the need for a thorough neurological assessment. If the client complains of headache or a recent loss of function in an extremity, a complete neurological review is needed. Table 33-36 reviews the data collected in the nursing history. For a complete examination, the following special equipment will be needed:

1. Reading material
2. Vials containing aromatic substances (e.g., vanilla and coffee)
3. Opposite tip of cotton swab or tongue blade broken in half
4. Snellen chart
5. Penlight
6. Vials containing sugar or salt
7. Tongue blade

Table 33-35	Muscle Strength			
		SCALES		
MUSCLE FUNCTION LEVEL		**GRADE**	**% NORMAL**	**LOVETT SCALE**
No evidence of contractility		0	0	0 (zero)
Slight contractility, no movement		1	10	T (trace)
Full range of motion, gravity eliminated*		2	25	P (poor)
Full range of motion with gravity		3	50	F (fair)
Full range of motion against gravity, some resistance		4	75	G (good)
Full range of motion against gravity, full resistance		5	100	N (normal)

From Barkauskas VH et al: *Health and physical assessment*, St Louis, 1994, Mosby.
*Passive movement.

Table 33-36	Nursing History for Neurological System Assessment

ASSESSMENT CATEGORY	RATIONALE
Determine if client is taking analgesics, antipsychotics, antidepressants, or nervous system stimulants.	These medications can alter level of consciousness or cause behavioral changes.
Assess client's use of alcohol or sedative-hypnotics.	Abuse can cause tremors, ataxia, and changes in peripheral nerve function.
Determine if client has recent history of seizures/convulsions: clarify sequence of events (aura, fall to ground, motor activity, loss of consciousness), character of any symptoms, relationship of seizure to time of day, fatigue, or emotional stress.	Seizure activity often originates from central nervous system alteration. Characteristics of seizure help determine its origin.
Screen client for headache, tremors, dizziness, vertigo, numbness or tingling of body part, visual changes, weakness, pain, or changes in speech.	These symptoms frequently originate from alterations in central nervous system or peripheral nervous system function. Identification of specific patterns may aid in diagnosis of pathological condition.
Discuss with spouse, family members, or friends any recent changes in client's behavior (e.g., increased irritability, mood swings, memory loss, change in energy level).	Behavioral changes may result from intracranial pathological states.
Assess client for history of change in vision, hearing, smell, taste, or touch.	Major sensory nerves originate from brainstem. These symptoms may help to localize nature of problem.
If an older adult client displays sudden acute confusion (delirium), review history for drug toxicity (anticholinergics, diuretics, digoxin, cimetidine, sedatives, antihypertensives, antiarrhythmics), serious infections, metabolic disturbances, heart failure, and severe anemia.	One of the commonest mental disorders in older persons. Condition is always potentially reversible (see the box on p. 730).
Review past history for head or spinal cord injury, hypertension, or psychiatric disorders.	Factors may cause neurological symptoms or behavioral changes to develop, focusing assessment on possible cause.

8. Two test tubes, one filled with hot water and the other with cold water
9. Cotton balls or cotton-tipped applicators
10. Tuning fork
11. Reflex hammer

Mental and Emotional Status

A great deal can be learned about mental capacities and emotional state by simply interacting with a client. A nurse can ask questions throughout an examination to gather data and observe the appropriateness of emotions and ideas. There are special assessment tools designed to assess a client's mental status. Kahn's (1960) mental status questionnaire (MSQ) is a ten item instrument and a widely used tool. Folstein et al. (1975) developed the Mini–Mental State (MMS) to measure orientation and cognitive function (see the box on p. 729).

To ensure an objective assessment the nurse considers the client's cultural and educational background, values, beliefs, and previous experiences. Such factors influence the client's response to questions. An alteration in mental or emotional status may reflect a disturbance in cerebral functioning. The cerebral cortex controls and integrates intellectual and emotional functioning. Primary brain disorders, medication, and metabolic changes are examples of factors that may change cerebral function.

Folstein's Mini–Mental State

"MINI–MENTAL STATE"
Maximum
Score
ORIENTATION
5 ( ) What is the (year) (season) (date) (day) (month)?
5 ( ) Where are we: (state) (county) (town) (hospital) (floor).
REGISTRATION
3 ( ) Name 3 objects: 1 second to say each. Then ask the patient all 3 after you have said them. Give 1 point for each correct answer. Then repeat them until he learns all 3. Count trials are record.
ATTENTION AND CALCULATION
5 ( ) Serial 7's. 1 point for each correct. Stop after 5 answers. Alternatively spell "world" backwards.
RECALL
3 ( ) Ask for the 3 objects repeated above. Give 1 point for each correct.
LANGUAGE
9 ( ) Name a pencil, and watch (2 points)
Repeat the following "No ifs, ands or buts," (1 point)
Follow a 3-stage command:
"Take a paper in your right hand, fold it in half, and put it on the floor" (3 points)
Read and obey the following:
CLOSE YOUR EYES (1 point)
Write a sentence (1 point)
Copy design (1 point)
_____ Total score
ASSESS level of consciousness along a continuum

| Alert | Drowsy | Stupor | Coma |

INSTRUCTIONS FOR ADMINISTRATION OF MINI–MENTAL STATE EXAMINATION
ORIENTATION
(1) Ask for the date. Then ask specifically for parts omitted, e.g., "Can you also tell me what season it is?" One point for each correct.
(2) Ask in turn "Can you tell me the name of this hospital?" (town, county, etc.). One point for each correct.

REGISTRATION
Ask the patient if you may test his memory. Then say the names of 3 unrelated objects, clearly and slowly, about one second for each. After you have said all 3, ask him to repeat them. This first repetition determines his score (0–3) but keep saying them until he can repeat all 3, up to 6 trials. If he does not eventually learn all 3, recall cannot be meaningfully tested.
ATTENTION AND CALCULATION
Ask the patient to begin with 100 and count backwards by 7. Stop after 5 subtractions (93, 86, 79, 72, 65). Score the total number of correct answers.
If the patient cannot or will not perform this task, ask him to spell the word "world" backwards. The score is the number of letters in correct order. E.g., dlrow = 5, dlorw = 3.
RECALL
Ask the patient if he can recall the 3 words you previously asked him to remember. Score 0-3.
LANGUAGE
Naming: Show the patient a wrist watch and ask him what it is. Repeat for pencil. Score 0-2.
Repetition: Ask the patient to repeat the sentence after you. Allow only one trial. Score 0 or 1.
3-Stage command: Give the patient a piece of plain blank paper and repeat the command. Score 1 point for each part correctly executed.
Reading: On a blank piece of paper print the sentence "Close your eyes", in letters large enough for the patient to see clearly. Ask him to read it and do what it says. Score 1 point only if he actually closes his eyes.
Writing: Give the patient a blank piece of paper and ask him to write a sentence for you. Do not dictate a sentence, it is to be written spontaneously. It must contain a subject and verb and be sensible. Correct grammar and punctuation are not necessary.
Copying: On a clean sheet of paper, draw intersecting pentagons, each side about 1 in., and ask him to copy it exactly as it is. All 10 angles must be present and 2 must intersect to score 1 point. Tremor and rotation are ignored. Estimate the patient's level of sensorium along a continuum, from alert on the left to coma on the right.

From Folstein MF, Folstein S, McHugh PR: Mini–Mental State; a practical method for grading the cognitive state of patients for the clinician, *J Psychiatric Res* 12:189, 1975.

A common mental disorder affecting older adults is delirium. It is an acute mental disorder characterized by confusion, disorientation, and restlessness. The acute condition is often misdiagnosed as a form of dementia, a more progressive, organic mental disorder such as Alzheimer's disease. Thus the underlying cause of the condition is missed. When it occurs many nurses and physicians think it is common older adult's behavior. Delirium is often overlooked in older adults because of a failure to adequately assess mental status (Barry, 1993). The condition can fortunately be reversed when correctly assessed. Frequently clients who develop delirium are labeled with "sundowner's syndrome" because the delirium frequently worsens at night. Many practitioners mistake this as common with old age. The nurse should obtain a good history of the client's behavior before delirium develops so as to recognize the condition early. Family can usually be a good resource. The box on p. 730 summarizes clinical criteria for delirium.

LEVEL OF CONSCIOUSNESS

The level of consciousness exists along a continuum, from full awakening, alertness, and cooperation to unresponsiveness to any form of external stimuli. A fully conscious client responds to questions spontaneously. As consciousness lowers, a client may show irritability, a shortened attention span, or an unwillingness to cooperate. To avoid ambiguity in the assessment of the level of consciousness, the Glasgow coma scale (GCS) measures consciousness by an objective numerical scale (Table 33-37). Caution is needed in using the scale with clients who have sensory losses. For example, a client may not respond to a nurse's presence if both sight and hearing are impaired.

Clinical Criteria for Delirium

Definition: An acute disturbance of consciousness that is accompanied by a change in cognition. It cannot be accounted for by a preexisting or evolving dementia. Delirium develops over a short period of time, usually hours to days, and tends to fluctuate during the course of the day. Usually a direct physiological consequence of a general medical condition.

- Reduced clarity of awareness of the environment
- Impaired ability to focus, sustain, or shift attention (questions must be repeated)
- Person is easily distracted by irrelevant stimuli
- There is an accompanying change in cognition (memory impairment, disorientation, or language disturbance)
- Recent memory most commonly affected
- Disorientation is usually shown with client disoriented to time or place
- Language disturbance may involve impaired ability to name objects or ability to write; speech may be rambling
- Perceptual disturbances may include misinterpretations, illusions, or hallucinations

Modified from American Psychiatric Association: Diagnostic and statistical manual of mental disorders, ed 4, Washington, DC, 1994, American Psychiatric Association.

Table 33-37 **Glasgow Coma Scale**

ACTION	RESPONSE	SCORE
Eyes open	Spontaneously	④
	To speech	3
	To pain	2
	None	1
Best verbal response	Oriented	⑤
	Confused	4
	Inappropriate words	3
	Incomprehensible sounds	2
	None	1
Best motor response	Obeys commands	⑥
	Localized pain	5
	Flexion withdrawal	4
	Abnormal flexion	3
	Abnormal extension	2
	Flaccid	1
	Total Score	⑮

As consciousness deteriorates, a client becomes disoriented to name, time, and place. The nurse asks short, to-the-point questions regarding information that the client knows (e.g., "Tell me your name," "What's the name of this place?" and "What day is this?"). The client's ability to understand and answer questions has a direct effect on the nurse's ability to perform a complete examination. The client must be aroused to full alertness before the assessment can be conducted.

A client may be unable to follow simple commands such as "Squeeze my finger" or "Move your toes." At this lowered level of consciousness the client often is responsive only to painful stimuli. The nurse tests the client by applying firm pressure with the thumb over the root of the fingernail. The client should withdraw the hand from the painful stimulus. In cases of serious neurological impairment a client exhibits abnormal posturing in response to pain. A flaccid response indicates an absence of muscle tone in the extremities and severe injury to brain tissue.

The GCS allows the nurse to evaluate a client's neurological status over time. The higher the score, the more improved or normal the level of functioning.

BEHAVIOR AND APPEARANCE

Behavior, moods, hygiene, grooming, and choice of dress reveal pertinent information about mental status. The nurse must be perceptive of mannerisms and actions during the entire physical assessment. The nurse notes nonverbal as well as verbal behavior. Does the client respond appropriately to directions? Does the client's mood vary with no apparent cause? Does the client show concern about appearance? Is the client's hair clean, neatly groomed, and are the nails trim and clean? The client should behave in a manner expressing concern and interest in the examination. The client should make eye contact with the nurse and express appropriate feelings that correspond to the situation. Normally the client will show some degree of personal hygiene.

Choice and fit of clothing may reflect socioeconomic background or personal taste rather than deficiency in self-concept or self-care. The nurse avoids being judgmental and focuses assessment on the appropriateness of clothing for the weather. Older adults may neglect their appearance because of a lack of energy, finances, or reduced vision.

LANGUAGE

The ability of an individual to understand spoken or written words and to express the self through writing, words, or gestures is a function of the cerebral cortex. The nurse assesses the client's voice inflection, tone, and manner of speech. The client's voice should have inflections, be clear and strong, and increase in volume appropriately. Speech should be fluent. When communication is clearly ineffective (e.g., omission or addition of letters and words, misuse of words, hesitations), the nurse assesses for **aphasia.** An injury to the cerebral cortex may result in aphasia.

The two types of aphasia are sensory (or receptive) and motor (or expressive). With receptive aphasia a person cannot understand written or verbal speech. With expressive aphasia a person understands written and verbal speech but cannot write or speak appropriately when trying to communicate. A client may suffer a combination of receptive and expressive aphasia, depending on the portion of the cerebral cortex involved. The nurse assesses language capabilities when it is clear that communication with the client is ineffective. Some simple assessment techniques include the following:

1. Asking the client to name a familiar object to which the nurse points
2. Asking the client to respond to simple verbal and written commands such as "Stand up" or "Sit down"
3. Asking the client to read simple sentences out loud

Normally a client names objects correctly, follows commands, and reads sentences correctly.

Intellectual Function

Intellectual function includes memory (recent, immediate, and past), knowledge, abstract thinking, association, and judgment. Each aspect of intellectual function is tested through a specific technique. However, because cultural and educational background influence the ability to respond to test questions, the nurse should not ask questions related to concepts or ideas with which the client is unfamiliar.

MEMORY

The nurse assesses immediate recall and recent and remote memory. Often a problem with memory becomes apparent when the nurse takes the nursing history. To assess immediate recall the nurse has the client repeat a series of numbers (e.g., 7, 4, 1) in the order they are presented or in reverse order. The nurse gradually increases the number of digits (e.g., 7, 4, 1, 8, 6) until the client fails to repeat the digits correctly. Normally an individual is able to repeat a series of 5 to 8 digits forward and 4 to 6 digits backward.

The nurse asks if the client's memory can be tested. Then the nurse says clearly and slowly the name of three unrelated objects. After the nurse says all three, the client is asked to repeat each. This is continued until the client is successful. Then, later in the assessment, the nurse asks the client to repeat the three words again. The client should be able to identify the three words. Another test for recent memory involves asking the client to recall events occurring during the same day (e.g., what was eaten for breakfast). Information may need to be validated with a family member.

To assess past memory the nurse can ask the client to recall the mother's maiden name, a birthday, or special date in history. It is best to ask open-ended questions rather than simple yes/no questions. A client should have immediate recall of such information. With older adults a nurse should not interpret a hearing loss as confusion. Good communication techniques are necessary throughout the examination to ensure the client clearly understands all directions and testing.

KNOWLEDGE

The nurse can assess knowledge by asking clients what they know about their illnesses or the reason for seeking health care. By assessing knowledge the nurse determines clients' abilities to learn or understand. If an opportunity to teach exists, the nurse can test mental status by asking for feedback during a follow-up visit.

ABSTRACT THINKING

Interpreting abstract ideas or concepts reflects the capacity for abstract thinking. A higher level of intellectual functioning is required for an individual to explain such phrases as "A stitch in time saves nine" or "Don't count your chickens before they're hatched." The nurse notes whether the client's explanations are relevant and concrete. The client with altered mentation will likely interpret the phrase literally or merely rephrase the words.

ASSOCIATION

Another higher level of intellectual function involves finding similarities or associations between concepts: a dog is to a beagle as a cat is to a Siamese. The nurse names related concepts and asks the client to identify their associa-

tions. Questions should be appropriate to the client's level of intelligence. It is sufficient to use simple concepts.

JUDGMENT

Judgment requires a comparison and evaluation of facts and ideas to understand their relationships and to form appropriate conclusions. The nurse attempts to measure the ability to make logical decisions. By assessing judgment the nurse also measures the ability to organize thought processes. The nurse may choose to ask clients why they decided to seek health care or how they plan to adjust to limitations after returning home. A simpler test would involve asking what the clients would do if placed in a situation such as being locked out of their homes or suddenly becoming ill when alone at home.

Cranial Nerve Function

The nurse may assess all 12 cranial nerves or test a single nerve or related group of nerves. A test of the oculomotor nerve measures pupillary response. Assessment of the glossopharyngeal and vagus nerves reveals integrity of the gag reflex. Measurements used to assess the integrity of organs within the head and neck also assess cranial nerve function. For example, the cochlear branch of the eighth cranial nerve is tested during a hearing assessment. The function of the ninth and tenth nerves can be assessed during examination of the pharynx. A dysfunction in any nerve reflects an alteration at some point along the cranial nerve's distribution. Cranial nerve assessment is easy after the nurse is familiar with the nerve's normal functions. To remember the order of the 12 nerves the nurse can use this simple phrase, "On old Olympus' towering tops, a Finn and German viewed some hops." The first letter of each word in the phrase is the same as the first letter of the names of the cranial nerves (Table 33-38).

Sensory Function

The sensory pathways of the central nervous system conduct sensations of pain, temperature, position, vibration, and crude and finely localized touch. Different nerve pathways relay the sensations. For most clients a quick screening of sensory function is sufficient unless there are symptoms of reduced sensation, motor impairment, or paralysis.

Normally a client has sensory responses to all stimuli that are tested. Sensations along the body's surface are felt equally on both sides of the face, trunk, and extremities. A nurse can assess the major sensory nerves by knowing the sensory dermatome zones (Fig. 33-95). Some areas of the skin are innervated by specific dorsal root cutaneous nerves. For example, if the nurse notes reduced sensation when checking for light touch along an area of the skin (e.g., the lower neck), the nurse can determine, in general, where a neurological lesion may exist (e.g., fourth cervical spinal cord segment).

All sensory testing is performed with the client's eyes closed so that the client is unable to see when or where a stimulus strikes the skin (Table 33-39). Stimuli are applied in a random, unpredictable order to maintain the client's attention and prevent detection of a predictable pattern. The client is asked to tell the nurse when, what, and where each stimulus is felt. The nurse compares symmetrical areas of the body while applying stimuli to the client's arms, trunk, and legs.

Table 33-38	Cranial Nerve Function and Assessment			
NUMBER	**NAME**	**TYPE**	**FUNCTION**	**METHOD**
I	Olfactory	Sensory	Sense of smell	Ask client to identify different nonirritating aromas such as coffee and vanilla.
II	Optic	Sensory	Visual acuity	Use Snellen chart or ask client to read printed material while wearing glasses.
III	Oculomotor	Motor	Extraocular eye movement	Assess directions of gaze.
			Pupil constriction and dilation	Measure pupil reaction to light reflex and accommodation.
IV	Trochlear	Motor	Upward and downward movement of eyeball	Assess directions of gaze.
V	Trigeminal	Sensory and motor	Sensory nerve to skin of face	Lightly touch cornea with wisp of cotton. Assess corneal reflex. Measure sensation of light pain and touch across skin of face.
			Motor nerve to muscles of jaw	Palpate temples as client clenches teeth.
VI	Abducens	Motor	Lateral movement of eyeballs	Assess directions of gaze.
VII	Facial	Sensory and motor	Facial expression	As client smiles, frowns, puffs out cheeks, and raises and lowers eyebrows look for asymmetry.
			Taste	Have client identify salty or sweet taste on front of tongue.
VIII	Auditory	Sensory	Hearing	Assess ability to hear spoken word.
IX	Glossopharyngeal	Sensory and motor	Taste	Ask client to identify sour or sweet taste on back of tongue.
			Ability to swallow	Use tongue blade to elicit gag reflex.
X	Vagus	Sensory and motor	Sensation of pharynx	Ask client to say "ah." Observe palate and pharynx movement.
			Movement of vocal cords	Assess speech for hoarseness.
XI	Spinal accessory	Motor	Movement of head and shoulders	Ask client to shrug shoulders and turn head against passive resistance.
XII	Hypoglossal	Motor	Position of tongue	Ask client to stick out tongue to midline and move it from side to side.

Motor Function

An assessment of motor function includes the same measurements made during the musculoskeletal examination. In addition, cerebellar function is assessed. The cerebellum coordinates muscular activity by producing smooth, steady, and efficient movements of muscle groups. The maintenance of balance and equilibrium is also a function of the cerebellum. Sensory impulses from the vestibular portion of the inner ear travel to the cerebellum, where impulses are relayed to proper motor nerves to maintain body equilibrium. The cerebellum also controls posture.

COORDINATION

It is difficult for the nurse to explain the tests used to measure coordination. To avoid confusion the nurse demonstrates each maneuver and then has clients repeat it after determining that their mobility is normal and they are physically able to make the necessary movements. The nurse observes the smoothness and balance of movements

(see the box on p. 734). In older adults a slow reaction time may cause movements to be less rhythmical.

To assess fine motor function the nurse has the client extend the arms out to the sides and touch each forefinger alternately to the nose (first with eyes open, then with eyes closed). Normally the client alternately touches the nose smoothly. Performing rapid, rhythmical, alternating movements demonstrates coordination in the upper extremities. While sitting, the client begins by patting the knees with both hands. Then the client alternately turns up the palm and back of the hands while continuously patting. The maneuver should be done smoothly and regularly with increasing speed.

An additional maneuver for upper extremity coordination involves touching each finger with the thumb of the same hand in rapid sequence. The client moves from the index finger to the little finger and back with one hand tested at a time. The client's dominant hand is slightly less

Table 33-39	Assessment of Sensory Nerve Function		
FUNCTION	**EQUIPMENT**	**METHOD**	**PRECAUTIONS**
Pain	Broken tongue blade or wooden end of cotton applicator	Ask client to voice when dull or sharp sensation is felt. Alternately apply sharp and blunt ends of tongue blade to skin's surface. Note areas of numbness or increased sensitivity.	Remember that areas where skin is thickened, such as heel or sole of foot, may be less sensitive to pain.
Temperature	Two test tubes, one filled with hot water and other with cold	Touch skin with tube. Ask client to identify hot or cold sensation.	Omit test if pain sensation is normal.
Light touch	Cotton ball or cotton-tip applicator	Apply light wisp of cotton to different points along skin's surface. Ask client to voice when sensation is felt.	Apply at areas where skin is thin or more sensitive (e.g., face, neck, inner aspect of arms, top of feet and hands).
Vibration	Tuning fork	Apply stem of vibrating fork to distal interphalangeal joint of fingers and interphalangeal joint of great toe, elbow, and wrist. Have client voice when and where the vibration is felt.	Be sure client feels vibration and not merely pressure.
Position		Grasp finger or toe, holding it by its sides with thumb and index finger. Alternate moving finger or toe up and down. Ask client to state when finger is up or down. Repeat with toes.	Avoid rubbing adjacent appendages as finger or toe is moved. Do not move joint laterally; return to neutral position before moving again.
Two-point discrimination	Two broken tongue blades	Lightly apply one or both tongue blade tips simultaneously to skin's surface. Ask client if one or two pricks are felt. Find the distance at which client can no longer distinguish two points.	Apply blade tips to same anatomical site (e.g., fingertips, palm of hand, or upper arms). Minimum distance at which client can discriminate two points varies (2 to 8 mm on fingertips).

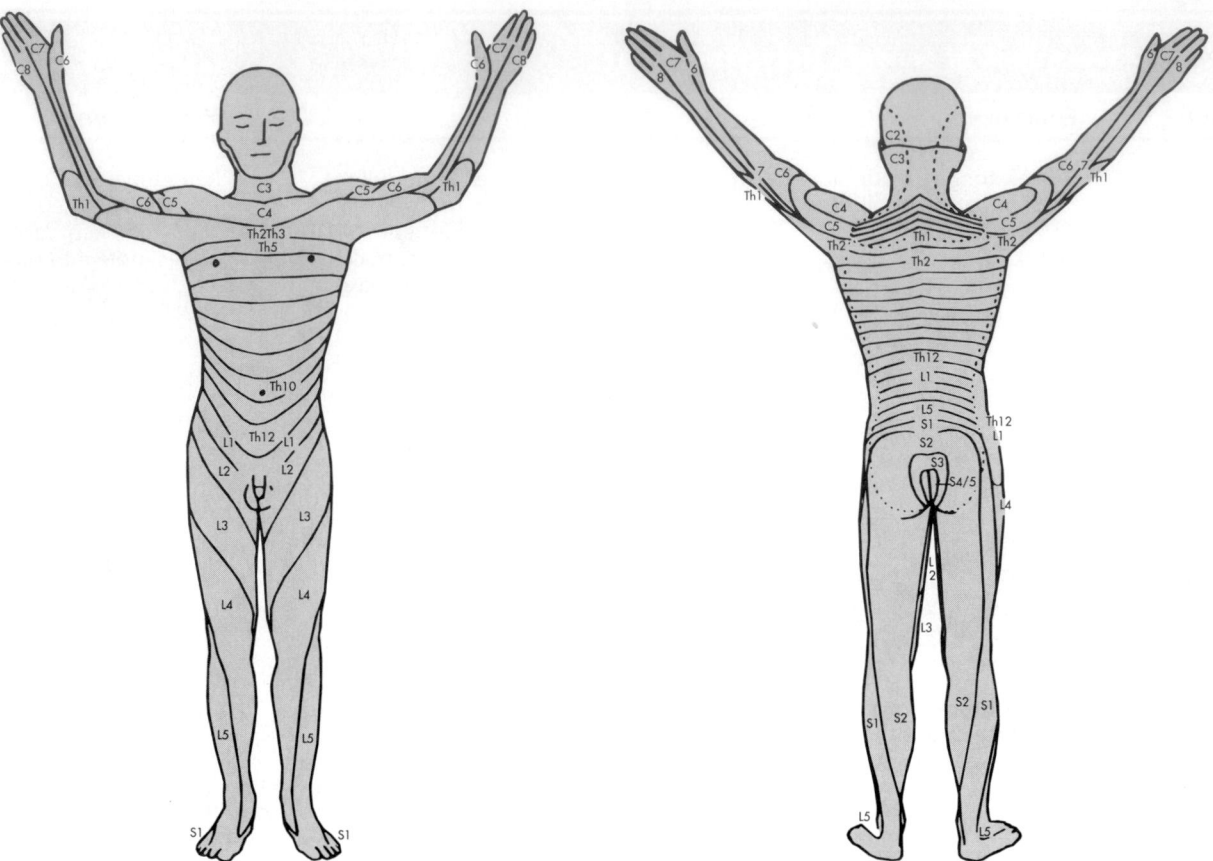

Fig. 33-95 Sensory dermatome areas overlying the human body. *(From Thelan LA, Dane JK, Urden LD:* Textbook of critical care nursing: diagnosis and management, *St Louis, 1990, Mosby.)*

CLIENT TEACHING
During Neurological Assessment

OBJECTIVES
- Client's family will understand relationship of client's behavioral and mental changes to physical status.
- Client with sensory or motor impairment will select safety measures for self-care.
- Older adult will routinely inspect skin for injuries.

TEACHING STRATEGIES
- Explain to family or friends the neurological implications of any behavioral or mental impairment shown by the client.
- If the client has sensory or motor impairments, explain measures to ensure safety (e.g., use of ambulation aids or safety bars in bathrooms or stairways).
- Teach the older adult to plan enough time to complete tasks because reaction time is slowed.
- Teach older adult to observe skin surfaces for areas of trauma because perception of pain is reduced.

EVALUATION
- Ask family to discuss client behaviors that result from neurological impairments.
- Have client explain safety measures used to avoid injury from sensory and motor limitations.
- Have older client explain reason for inspecting skin surface routinely.

awkward when performing this movement. Movement should be smooth and in succession.

Lower extremity coordination is tested with the client lying supine, legs extended. The nurse places a hand at the ball of the client's foot. The client taps the nurse's hand with the foot as quickly as possible. Each foot is tested for speed and smoothness. The feet do not move as rapidly or evenly as the hands.

BALANCE

The nurse may use one or two of the following tests to assess balance and gross motor function:
1. Have the client perform a Romberg test by standing with feet together, arms at the side, both with eyes open and eyes closed. While protecting the client's safety by standing at the side, observe swaying. Slight swaying is normal. The client normally does not have to break the stance.
2. Have the client close the eyes, with arms held straight at the sides, and stand on one foot and then the other. Normally balance is maintained for 5 seconds with slight swaying.
3. Ask the client to walk a straight line by placing the heel of one foot directly in front of the toes of the other foot.

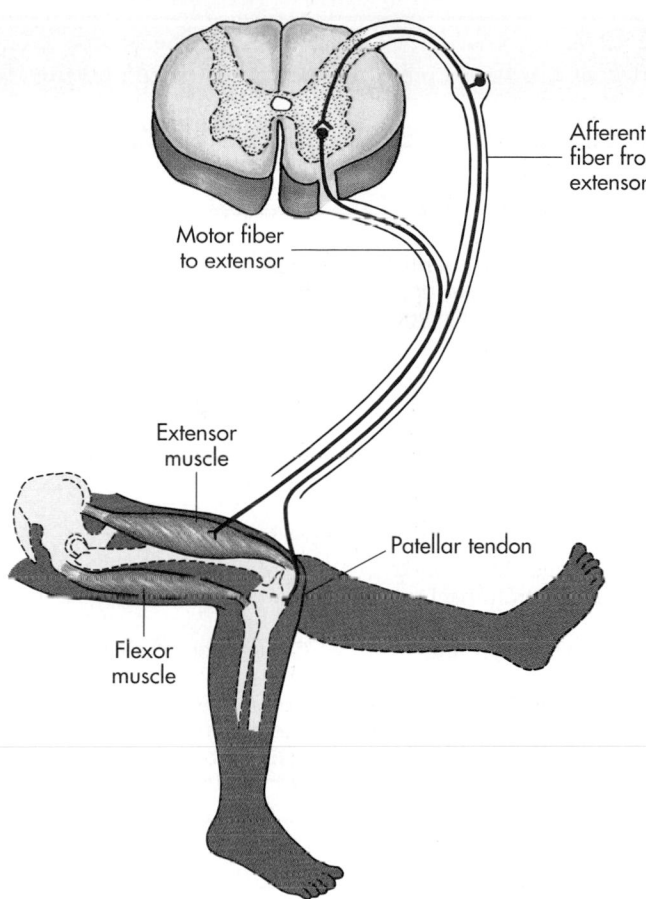

Fig. 33-96 Pathway of the reflex arc.

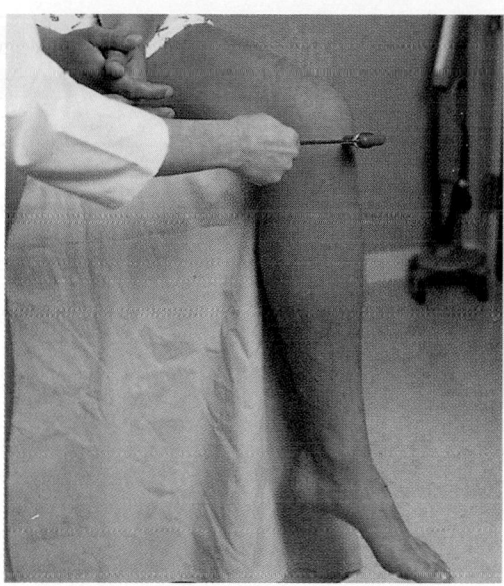

Fig. 33-97 Position for eliciting the patellar tendon reflex. The lower leg normally extends.

Reflexes

Eliciting reflex reactions allows the nurse to assess the integrity of sensory and motor pathways of the reflex arc and specific spinal cord segments. Assessment of reflexes does not determine higher neural center functioning. Fig. 33-96 traces the pathway of the reflex arc. Each muscle contains a small sensory unit called a *muscle spindle*, which controls muscle tone and detects changes in the length of muscle fibers. By tapping a tendon with a reflex hammer, the nurse stretches the muscle and tendon, lengthening the spindle. The spindle sends nerve impulses along afferent nerve pathways to the dorsal horn of the spinal cord segment. Within milliseconds the impulses reach the spinal cord and synapse to travel to the efferent motor neuron in the spinal cord. A motor nerve sends the impulses back to the muscle, causing the reflex response.

The two categories of normal reflexes are deep tendon reflexes, elicited by mildly stretching a muscle and tapping a tendon, and cutaneous reflexes, elicited by stimulating the skin superficially. Reflexes are graded as follows:

0	No response
1+	Low normal with slight muscle contraction
2+	Normal with visible muscle twitch and movement of the arm or leg
3+	Brisker than normal; may not indicate disease
4+	Hyperactive and very brisk; often associated with spinal cord disorders

When reflexes are being assessed the client should relax as much as possible to avoid voluntary movement or tensing of muscles. The nurse positions the limbs to slightly stretch the muscle being tested. The reflex hammer is held loosely between the nurse's thumb and fingers so that it can swing freely and tap the tendon briskly (Fig. 33-97). The nurse compares the symmetry of the reflex from one side of the body to the other. In the older adult, reflexes are normally slowed. Reflexes can be hyperactive in clients with alcohol, cocaine, or opioid intoxication (Caulker-Burnett, 1994). Practitioners often use stick figures to record reflexes. Table 33-40 summarizes common deep tendon and cutaneous reflexes.

■ AFTER THE EXAMINATION

The nurse may choose to record findings from the physical assessment during the examination or at the end. Most institutions have special forms that make it easy to record examination data (see Chapter 12). The nurse reviews all findings before assisting the client with dressing, in case there is a need to recheck any information or gather additional data. Findings from physical assessment are integrated into the plan of care.

After completing the assessment the nurse assists the client in dressing if necessary. The hospitalized client may need a new gown and help in returning to bed and assuming a comfortable position. The client in the home may only need time to dress and join the nurse in the living room or kitchen. When the client is comfortable it helps to share a summary of the assessment findings. If the findings have revealed serious abnormalities such as a mass or highly irregular heart rate, the client's physician should be consulted before any findings are revealed. It is the physician's responsibility to make definitive medical diagnoses. The nurse can explain the type of abnormality found and the need for the physician to conduct an additional examination.

The nurse has a technician clean the examination area, store all reusable equipment, and dispose of materials that

Table 33-40	Assessment of Common Reflexes	
TYPE	**PROCEDURE**	**NORMAL REFLEX**
DEEP TENDON REFLEXES		
Biceps	Flex client's arm up to 45 degrees at elbow with palms down. Place your thumb in antecubital fossa at base of biceps tendon and your fingers over the biceps muscle. Strike triceps tendon with reflex hammer.	Flexion of arm at elbow
Triceps	Flex client's arm at the elbow, holding arm across chest, or hold upper arm horizontally and allow lower arm to go limp. Strike triceps tendon just above elbow.	Extension at elbow
Patellar	Have client sit with legs hanging freely over side of table or chair or have client lie supine and support knee in a flexed 90-degree position. Briskly tap patellar tendon just below patella.	Extension of lower leg
Achilles	Have client assume same position as for patellar reflex. Slightly dorsiflex client's ankle by grasping toes in palm of your hand. Strike Archilles tendon just above heel at the ankle malleolus.	Plantar flexion of foot
CUTANEOUS REFLEXES		
Plantar	Have client lie supine with legs straight and feet relaxed. Take handle end of reflex hammer and stroke lateral aspect of sole from heel to ball of foot, curving across ball of foot toward big toe.	Plantar flexion of all toes
Gluteal	Have client assume side-lying position. Spread buttocks apart and lightly stimulate perineal area with cotton applicator.	Contraction of anal sphincter
Abdominal	Have client stand or lie supine. Stroke abdominal skin with base of cotton applicator over lateral borders of rectus abdominus muscle toward midline. Repeat test in each abdominal quadrant.	Contraction of rectus abdominus muscle with pulling of umbilicus toward stimulated side

cannot be reused. Infection-control practices are used in removing materials or instruments soiled with potentially infectious wastes. If the client's bedside was the examination site, staff clears away soiled items from the table and makes sure the bed linen is dry and clean. The client may appreciate a clean gown and the opportunity to wash the face and hands.

The nurse checks to be sure the recording of the assessment is complete. If entry of items into the assessment form was delayed, the nurse records them at this time to avoid forgetting any important information. If entries were made periodically during the examination, they are re-

viewed for accuracy and thoroughness. Significant findings are communicated to appropriate medical and nursing personnel, either verbally or in the written care plan.

The client often needs a number of ancillary examinations such as x-ray examinations, laboratory tests, or ultrasonography after a physical examination. These tests provide additional screening information to rule out the presence of abnormalities and help in the diagnosis of specific abnormalities found during the examination. The nurse explains the purpose of these tests and the sensations that the client can expect.

■ KEY CONCEPTS ■

▶ Baseline assessment findings reflect the client's functional abilities when the nurse first assesses the client and serve as the basis for comparison with subsequent assessment findings.

▶ Assessment data are used to make nursing diagnoses, select appropriate nursing interventions, and evaluate the outcomes of nursing care.

▶ Physical assessment of a child or infant requires the nurse to apply principles of physical growth and development.

▶ The nurse recognizes that the normal process of aging affects physical findings collected from an older adult.

▶ Client teaching should be integrated throughout the examination to help clients learn about health promotion and disease prevention.

▶ The nurse can use time more efficiently by integrating physical assessment with routine nursing care.

▶ Inspection requires good lighting, full exposure of the body part, and a careful comparison of the part with its counterpart on the opposite side of the body.

▶ A good stethoscope should have earpieces that fit snugly, flexible thick-walled tubing of the proper length, and a chestpiece with a bell and diaphragm.

▶ A physical examination should be performed only after

proper preparation of the environment and equipment and after preparing the client physically and psychologically.

▶ Throughout the examination the nurse should keep the client warm, comfortable, and informed of each step of the process.

▶ The client assumes various positions during the physical examination to provide greater accessibility to body parts and to increase accuracy in assessment.

▶ The nurse uses a systematic approach when conducting a physical assessment.

▶ When assessing a seriously ill client the nurse concentrates on the body systems most likely to be affected.

▶ Information from the nursing history helps the nurse focus on examining body systems likely to be affected.

▶ Accuracy in assessing the thorax, heart, and abdomen is enhanced by creating a mental image of internal organs in relation to external anatomical landmarks.

▶ When assessing heart sounds the nurse imagines events occurring during the cardiac cycle.

▶ The carotid arteries should never be palpated simultaneously.

▶ When examining a woman's breasts, the nurse explains the techniques for breast self-examination.

▶ The abdominal assessment differs from other portions of the examination in that auscultation follows inspection.

▶ During assessment of the genitalia, the nurse explains the techniques for genital self-examination.

▶ Assessment of musculoskeletal function can easily be conducted when observing the client ambulate or participate in other active movements.

▶ The nurse assesses mental and emotional status by interacting with the client throughout the examination.

∎ KEY TERMS ∎

Acromegaly, p. 665

Adventitious sounds, p. 687

Allen's test, p. 699

Alopecia, p. 662

Aneurysm, p. 713

Aphasia, p. 730

Apical impulse, p. 691

Arcus senilis, p. 669

Atherosclerosis, p. 696

Atrophied, p. 727

Basal cell carcinoma, p. 657

Borborygmi, p. 711

Bronchophony, p. 688

Bruit, p. 696

Caries, p. 677

Cerumen, p. 672

Chancres, p. 715

Cherry angiomas, p. 659

Cholecystitis, p. 712

Cirrhosis, p. 712

Clubbing, p. 701

Conjunctivitis, p. 668

Cyanosis, p. 657

Cystocele, p. 716

Dermatitis, p. 658

Distention, p. 710

Dysrhythmia, p. 693

Ectropion, p. 668

Eczema, p. 658

Edema, p. 659

Entropion, p. 668

Erythema, p. 657

Excoriation, p. 675

Exophthalmos, p. 667

Exostosis, p. 679

Fibrocystic breast disease, p. 708

Goniometer, p. 725

Hemorrhoids, p. 721

Hepatitis, p. 712

Hernias, p. 710

Hirsutism, p. 662

Hydrocephalus, p. 665

Hypertonicity, p. 725

Hypotonicity, p. 725

Indurated, p. 659

Integument, p. 656

Jaundice, p. 657

Kyphosis, p. 723

Leukoplakia, p. 679

Lordosis, p. 723

Melanoma, p. 656

Metastasize, p. 707

Murmurs, p. 694

Nystagmus, p. 667

Occlusion, p. 696

Ophthalmoscope, p. 670

Osteoporosis, p. 723

Otoscope, p. 672

Ototoxicity, p. 674

Pancreatitis, p. 713

Papanicolaou (Pap) smear, p. 716

Paralytic ileus, p. 711

Peristalsis, p. 711

Peritonitis, p. 711

PERRLA, p. 670

Petechiae, p. 659

Phlebitis, p. 702

Pigmentation, p. 657

Point of maximal impulse (PMI), p. 691

Polyps, p. 675

Ptosis, p. 668

Pulse deficit, p. 694

Rectocele, p. 716

Scoliosis, p. 723

■ CRITICAL THINKING EXERCISES ■

1. While turning a client in bed the nurse notices the right heel is reddened. What assessment is made and what might be the contributing cause for the redness?

2. When assisting a client in setting up a meal tray and preparing for a meal, identify four different body systems you might choose to assess during this time.

3. A 70-year-old client entering the neighborhood health clinic reports a 3-day history of flulike symptoms; cough, fever, generalized aching, and loss of appetite. What focused assessments should the nurse conduct?

4. Two body systems are assessed when determining the nature of edema; identify each.

5. What physical examination measures would you use to evaluate application of a warm moist pack to the lower back, ambulation down a hallway, and application of a cast?

6. An elderly woman with reduced visual acuity would have difficulty performing what aspect of a breast self-examination?

REFERENCES

American Cancer Society: *1995 Cancer facts and figures,* New York, 1995, The Society.

American Psychiatric Association: DSM-IV, *Diagnostic and statistical manual of mental disorders,* ed 4, Washington, DC, 1994, American Psychiatric Assoc.

Barkauskas VH et al: *Health and physical assessment,* St Louis, 1994, Mosby.

Barry PP: Differentiating confusion: delirium or dementia? *Emerg Med* 25(6):96, 1993.

Belcher AE: *Cancer nursing,* St Louis, 1992, Mosby.

Berman R, Haxby JV, Pomerantz RS: Physiology of aging. I. Normal changes, *Patient Care* 22:20, 1988.

Bullock B, Rosenthal PP: *Pathophysiology: adaptation and alteration,* ed 3, Philadelphia, 1992, Lippincott.

Caulker-Burnett I: Primary care screening for substance abuse, *Nurse Practitioner* 19(6):42, 1994.

Champion VL: Effect of knowledge, teaching method, confidence and social influence on breast self-examination behavior, *Image J Nurs Schol,* 21(2)76, 1989.

Clore ER: Dispelling the common myths about pediculosis, *J Pediatr Health Care* 3:28, 1989.

Cornell RC: Aging and the skin: what is normal aging, *Geriatric Med Today,* Part XX 5:24, 1986.

DeWitt S: Nursing assessment of the skin and dermatologic lesions, *Nurs Clin North Am* 25(1):235, 1990.

Dunbar J et al: Breast self-examination compliance among older high risk women, *Pt Educ and Counseling* 18:223, 1991.

Dwyer JT et al: Assessing nutritional status in elderly patients, *Am Family Physician* 47(3):613, 1993.

Ebersole P, Hess P: *Toward healthy aging,* ed 4, St Louis, 1994, Mosby.

Ernst ND: The national cholesterol education program's recommendations for treatment of high blood cholesterol, *Fam Community Health* 12(1):23, 1989.

Folsom AR et al: No association between caffeine intake and postmenopausal breast cancer incidence in the Iowa women's health study, *Am J Epidemiology* 138(6):380, 1993.

Folstein MF, Folstein S: Mini-mental state: a practical method for grading the cognitive state of patients for the clinician, *J Psychiatr Res* 12:82, 1975.

Forgacs P: The functional basis of pulmonary sounds, *Chest* 73:399, 1978.

Franco EL: Multiple cancers of the upper aero-digestive tract: the challenge of risk factor identification, *Cancer Letters* 60:1, 1991.

Habif TP: *Clinical dermatology,* ed 3, St Louis, 1996, Mosby.

Hardy MA: A pilot study of the diagnosis and treatment of impaired skin integrity: dry skin in older persons, *Nurs Diag* 1(2):57, 1990.

Haviland S, O'Brien J: Physical abuse and neglect of the elderly: assessment and intervention, *Orthopaedic Nurs* 8(4):11, 1989.

Hockenberger SJ: Fibrocystic breast disease: every woman is at risk, *Plast Surg Nurs* 13(1)37, 1993.

Ibraimov AL: Cerumen phenotypes of certain populations of Eurasia and Africa, *Am J Phys Anthropol* 84(2) 209, 1991.

Kahn RL, Goldfarb AI, et al: Brief objective measures for the determination of mental status of the aged, *Am J Psychiatr* 117:326, 1960.

Kirton M, Richardson M: *Ophthalmic nursing,* ed 3, Philadelphia, 1987, Bailliere-Tindall.

Larson E: Evaluating validity of screening tests, *Nurs Res* 35:186, 1986.

Lueckenotte A: *Pocket guide to gerontologic assessment,* ed 2, St Louis, 1994, Mosby.

Malter LA et al: The effectiveness of four interventions for the prevention of low back pain, *JAMA* 272(16):1286, 1994.

Master S, Terpstra JK: Recognition and diagnosis. In Schnoll SH, Horvatich PK, Terpstra JK: *Prescribing drugs with abuse liability,* Richmond, Va, 1992, DSAM, MCV-VCU.

McConnell E: Auscultating bowel sounds, *Nurs 90* 20:106, 1990.

Moss VA, Taylor WK: Domestic violence: identification, assessment, intervention, *AORN Journal* 53(5):1158, 1991.

Norwood SL: Fibrocystic breast disease: an update and review, *JOGNN* 19(2):116, 1990.

Payne WA, Hahn DB: *Understanding your health,* ed 2, St Louis, 1989, Mosby–Year Book.

Reece SM: Immunization strategies for the elimination of hepatitis B, *Nurs Prac* 18:2, 1993.

Reed AT, Birge SJ: Screening for osteoporosis, *J Gerontol Nurs* 14(7):18, 1988.

Rozier RG, Beck JD: Epidemiology of oral diseases, *Current Opinion in Dentistry* 1:308, 1991.

Seidel HM et al: *Mosby's guide to physical examination,* ed 3, St Louis, 1995, Mosby.

Smoller J, Smoller BR: Skin malignancies in the elderly: diagnosable, treatable, and potentially curable, *J Geront Nurs* 18(5):19, 1992.

Stanley SR: Child sexual abuse: recognition and nursing intervention, *Orthopaedic Nurs* 8(1):33, 1989.

Thompson JM et al: *Mosby's manual of clinical nursing,* ed 3, St Louis, 1993, Mosby.

Wilkins RL, Hodgkin JE, Lopez B: *Lung sounds: a practical guide,* St Louis, 1988, Mosby–Year Book.

Willett W et al: Dietary fat and the risk of breast cancer, *N Engl J Med* 316:22, 1987.

Wong DL: *Whaley and Wong's nursing care of infants and children,* ed 5, St Louis, 1995, Mosby.

Zitelli B, Davis H: *Atlas of pediatric physical diagnosis,* ed 2, St Louis, 1991, Mosby.

ADDITIONAL READINGS

Barger SE: The delivery of early and periodic screening, diagnosis and treatment program services by NPs in a nursing center, *Nurse Prac* 18(6):65, 1993.

Beck JD et al: Prevalence and risk indicators for periodontal attachment loss in a population of older community dwelling blacks and whites, *J Peridontol* 61:521, 1990.

Carlson KJ et al: Screening for ovarian cancer: recommendations and rationale, *Annals Internal Medicine* 121(2):141, 1994.

Catalona WJ et al: Comparison of digital rectal examination and serum prostate specific antigen in the early detection of prostate cancer: results of a multicenter clinical trial of 6,630 men, *Journal of Urology* 151:1283, 1994.

Ernst ND: The national cholesterol education program's recommendations for treatment of high blood cholesterol, *Fam Community Health* 12(1):23, 1989.

Haid M et al: Digital rectal examination, serum prostate specific antigen, and prostatic ultrasound: how effective is this diagnostic triad? *J Surg Onc* 56:32, 1994.

Ismail AI et al: Natural history of periodontal disease in adults; findings from the Tecumseh periodontal disease study 1959-1987, *Je Dent Res* 69:430, 1990.

Lierman L et al: Predicting breast self-examination using the theory of reasoned action, *Nurs Res* 39(2):97, 1990.

Metersky ML, Catanzaro A: A rapid tuberculosis screening program for new mothers who have had no prenatal care, *Chest* 103(2):364, 1993.

McHugh J, McHugh W: How to assess deep tendon reflexes, *Nurs 90* 20:62, 1990.

Morra ME, Blumberg BD: Women's perceptions of early detection in breast cancer: how are we doing? *Seminars in Onc Nurs* 7(3):151, 1991.

National Cholesterol Education Program: Recommendations regarding public screening for measuring blood cholesterol, *Arch Intern Med* 149:2650, 1989.

National Institutes on Aging: *Constipation; Age Page, National Institutes on Aging,* Bethesda, Md, 1991, U.S. Dept. of Health and Human Services, Public Health Service, National Institutes of Health.

Nokes KM et al: Development of an HIV assessment tool, *IMAGE* 26(2):133, 1994.

Phipps W et al: *Medical-surgical nursing: concepts and clinical practice,* ed 5, St Louis, 1995, Mosby.

Weaver MG et al: Differences in blood pressure levels obtained by auscultatory and oscillometric methods, *AJDC* 144:911, 1990.

Weinrich SP et al: Timely detection of colorectal cancer in the elderly: implications of the aging process, *Cancer Nurs* 12(3):170, 1989.

Yacone-Morton LA: Cardiac assessment: perfecting the art, *RN* 54:28, 1991.

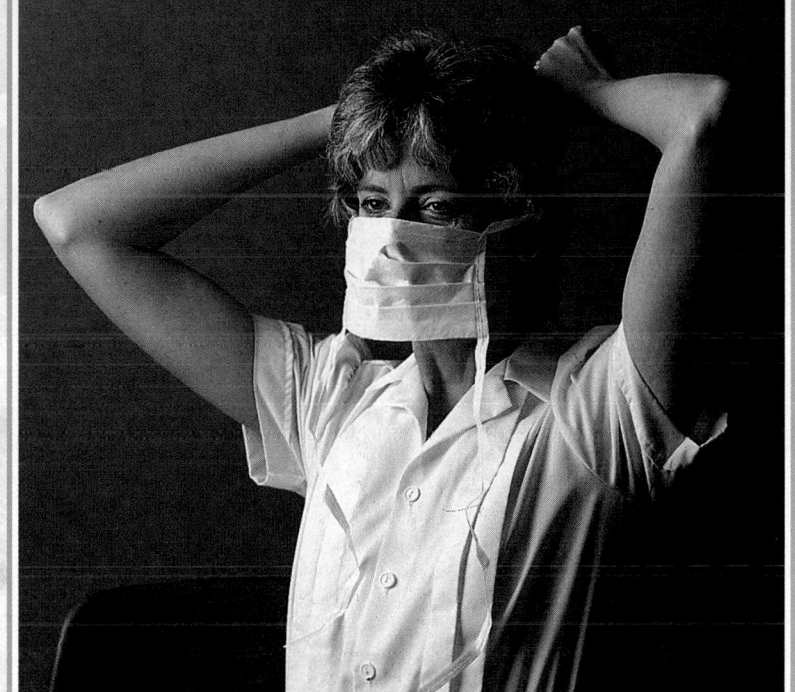

## Chapter 34

Infection Control

Objectives

Mastery of content in this chapter will enable the student to:

▶ Define the key terms listed.

▶ Explain the relationship of the chain of infection to transmission of infections.

▶ Identify the body's normal defenses against infection.

▶ Discuss the events in the inflammatory response.

▶ Explain the difference between cell-mediated and humoral immunity.

▶ Describe the signs/symptoms of a localized and systemic infection.

▶ Identify clients most at risk for infection.

▶ Explain conditions that promote the transmission of nosocomial infections.

▶ Explain the difference between medical and surgical asepsis.

▶ Give an example for preventing infection for each element of the infection chain.

▶ Explain the rationale for standard precautions.

▶ Perform proper procedures for handwashing.

▶ Explain how infection-control measures may differ in the home versus the hospital.

▶ Properly apply a surgical mask, sterile gown, and sterile gloves.

Good health depends in part on a safe environment. Practices or techniques that control or prevent transmission of infection help to protect clients and health care workers from disease. Clients in all health care settings are at risk for acquiring infections because of lower resistance to infectious **microorganisms**, increased exposure to numbers and types of disease-causing microorganisms, and invasive procedures. In acute care or ambulatory care facilities, clients can be exposed to new or different microorganisms, some of which may be resistant to most antibiotics. By practicing infection prevention and control techniques, the nurse can avoid spreading microorganisms to clients.

In all settings, clients and their families must be able to recognize sources of infections and be able to institute protective measures. Client teaching should include information concerning infections, modes of transmission, and methods of prevention.

Health care workers can protect themselves from contact with infectious material or exposure to a **communicable** disease by having knowledge of the infectious process and appropriate barrier protection. Diseases such as hepatitis B, AIDS, and tuberculosis have caused a greater emphasis on infection control techniques.

‖ NATURE OF INFECTION

An infection is an invasion of the body by **pathogens**, or microorganisms capable of producing disease. If the microorganisms fail to cause serious injury to cells or tissues, the infection is **asymptomatic**. Disease results if the pathogens multiply and cause an alteration in normal tissue. If the infectious disease can be transmitted directly from one person to another, it is a communicable or contagious disease.

Chain of Infection

The presence of a pathogen does not mean that an infection will begin. Development of an infection occurs in a cycle that depends on the following elements:
1. An infectious agent or pathogen
2. A reservoir or source for pathogen growth
3. A portal of exit from the reservoir
4. A mode of transmission
5. A portal of entry to a host
6. A susceptible host

An infection will develop if this chain remains intact (Fig. 34-1). Nurses use infection prevention and control practices to break the chain so that infection will not develop.

INFECTIOUS AGENT

Microorganisms include bacteria, viruses, fungi, and protozoa (Table 34-1). Microorganisms on the skin may be resident or transient flora. Resident organisms are normally present and stable in number. They survive and multiply on the skin. Most are found in superficial skin layers, but about 10% to 20% inhabit deep epidermal layers (Garner and Favero, 1986). Resident organisms are not easily removed by handwashing with plain soaps and detergents unless considerable friction is used. Resident microorganisms in deep skin layers are usually killed only by handwashing with products containing antimicrobial ingredients.

Transient microorganisms attach to the skin when a person has contact with another person or object during normal activities of living. For example, when a nurse touches a bedpan or a contaminated dressing, transient bacteria adhere to the nurse's skin. The organisms attach loosely to the skin in dirt and grease or under fingernails. These organisms may be readily transmitted unless removed by handwashing (Larson, 1995).

The potential for microorganisms or parasites to cause disease depends on the following factors:
1. Sufficient number of organisms
2. **Virulence**, or ability to produce disease
3. Ability to enter and survive in the host
4. Susceptibility of host

Some resident skin microorganisms are not virulent and cause only minor skin infections. However, they can cause serious infection when surgery or other **invasive** procedures allow them to enter deep tissues or when a client is severely **immunocompromised** (impaired immune system).

RESERVOIR

A reservoir is where a pathogen can survive but may or may not multiply. For example, hepatitis A virus survives in shellfish, but does not multiply; *Pseudomonas* survives and multiplies in nebulizer reservoirs used in the care of clients with respiratory alterations. The most common reservoir is the human body. A variety of microorganisms live on the skin and within the body cavities, fluids and discharges. The presence of microorganisms does not always cause a person to be ill. **Carriers** are persons or animals who show no symptoms of illness but who have pathogens on or in their bodies that can be transferred to others. For example, a person can be a carrier of hepatitis B virus without having signs or symptoms of infection. Animals, food, water, insects, and inanimate objects can also be reservoirs for infectious organisms. Shellfish can become contaminated with *Vibrio cholerae*, the bacterium that causes cholera. *Clostridium botulinum* toxin survives in improperly processed foods (e.g., home canned green beans) to cause bot-

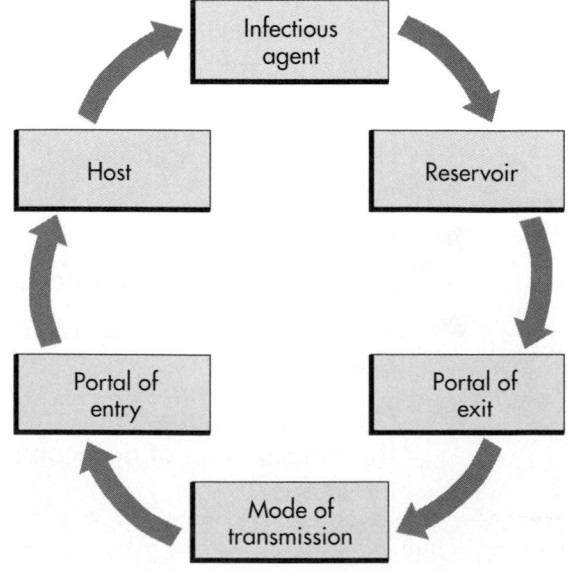

Fig. 34-1 Chain of infection.

Table 34-1	Common Pathogens and Some Infections or Diseases They Produce	
ORGANISM	**MAJOR RESERVOIR(S)**	**MAJOR INFECTIONS/DISEASES**
BACTERIA		
Escherichia coli	Colon	Gastroenteritis, urinary tract infection
Staphylococcus aureus	Skin, hair, anterior nares	Wound infection, pneumonia, food poisoning, cellulitis
Streptococcus (beta-hemolytic group A) organisms	Oropharynx, skin, perianal area	"Strep throat," rheumatic fever, scarlet fever, impetigo, wound infection
Streptococcus (beta-hemolytic group B) organisms	Adult genitalia	Urinary tract infection, wound infection, postpartum sepsis, neonatal sepsis
Mycobacterium tuberculosis	Droplet nuclei from lungs	Tuberculosis
Neisseria gonorrhoeae	Genitourinary tract, rectum, mouth	Gonorrhea, pelvic inflammatory disease, infectious arthritis, conjunctivitis
Rickettsia rickettsii	Wood tick	Rocky Mountain spotted fever
Staphylococcus epidermidis	Skin	Wound infection, bacteremia, line infection
VIRUSES		
Hepatitis A virus	Feces	Hepatitis A
Hepatitis B virus	Blood and body fluids	Hepatitis B
Hepatitis C virus	Blood	Hepatitis C
Herpes simplex virus (type I)	Lesions of mouth or skin, saliva, genitalia	Cold sores, aseptic meningitis, sexually transmitted disease, herpetic whitlow
Human immunodeficiency virus (HIV)	Blood, semen, vaginal secretions (also isolated in saliva, tears, urine, (AIDS) breast milk but not proven to be sources of transmission)	Acquired immunodeficiency syndrome (AIDS)
FUNGI		
Aspergillus organisms	Soil, dust, mouth, skin, colon, genital tract	Aspergillosis, pneumonia, sepsis
Candida albicans	Mouth, skin, colon, genital tract	Candidiasis, pneumonia, sepsis
PROTOZOA		
Plasmodium falciparum	Blood	Malaria

ulism. The bacterium *Legionella pneumophila,* which causes legionnaires' disease, lives in contaminated water and water systems. To thrive, organisms require a proper environment, including food, oxygen, water, appropriate temperature, and pH, and light.

Food. Microorganisms require nourishment. Some, such as *Clostridium perfringens,* the microbe that causes gas gangrene, thrive on organic matter. Others, such as *E. coli,* consume undigested foodstuff in the bowel. Carbon dioxide and inorganic material such as soil provide nourishment for other organisms.

Oxygen. Aerobic bacteria require oxygen for survival and for multiplication sufficient to cause disease. Aerobic organisms tend to cause more infections in humans. Examples of aerobic organisms are *Staphylococcus aureus* and strains of *Streptococcus* organisms.

Anaerobic bacteria thrive where little or no free oxygen is available. Infections deep within the pleural cavity, in a joint, or in a deep sinus tract are typically caused by anaerobes. Bacteria that cause tetanus, gas gangrene, and botulism are anaerobes.

Water. Most organisms require water or moisture for survival. For example, a favorite place of microorganisms is the moist drainage from a surgical wound. The spirochete that causes syphilis, *Treponema pallidum,* lives only in a moist environment. Some bacteria assume a form, called a *spore,* which is resistant to drying. These spore-forming bacteria, such as those that cause anthrax, botulism, and tetanus, can live without water.

Temperature. Microorganisms can live only in certain temperature ranges. However, some can survive temperature extremes that would be fatal to humans. Some viruses (e.g., the AIDS virus) are resistant to boiling water. Cold temperatures tend to prevent growth and reproduction of bacteria (**bacteriostasis**). A temperature that destroys bacteria is **bacteriocidal.**

pH. The acidity of an environment determines the viability of microorganisms. Most microorganisms prefer an environment within a pH range of 5 to 8. Bacteria in particular thrive in urine with an alkaline pH. Most organisms cannot survive the acid environment of the stomach.

Light. Microorganisms thrive in dark environments such as those under dressings and within body cavities. Ultraviolet light may be effective in killing certain forms of bacteria.

PORTAL OF EXIT

After microorganisms find a site to grow and multiply, they must find a portal of exit if they are to enter another host and cause disease. Microorganisms can exit through a variety of sites, such as skin and mucous membranes, respiratory tract, urinary tract, gastrointestinal tract, reproductive tract, and blood.

Skin and Mucous Membranes. Normally the skin is considered a portal of entry because any break in the integrity of skin and mucous membranes can lead to an infection. However, many times the body responds to a pathogenic organism with the creation of **purulent** drainage. For example, *S. aureus* causes a characteristic yellow drainage, whereas *Pseudomonas aeruginosa* causes a greenish drainage. This drainage is a potential portal of exit.

Respiratory Tract. Pathogens such as *Mycobacterium tuberculosis* that reside in the respiratory tract can be released from the body when an infected person sneezes, coughs, talks, or even breathes. Microorganisms exit through the mouth and nose in normal clients. In clients with artificial airways such as tracheostomy or endotracheal tubes (see Chapter 44), organisms easily exit the respiratory tract through these devices.

Urinary Tract. Normally urine is sterile. However, when a client has a urinary tract infection, microorganisms exit during urination or through urinary diversions such as ileostomies and suprapubic drains (see Chapter 46).

Gastrointestinal Tract. The mouth is one of the most bacterially contaminated sites of the body, although most of the organisms are normal flora, bacteria that reside within the body and defend against infection. However, organisms that are normal flora in one person can be pathogens in another. Organisms, for example, exit when a person expectorates saliva. Kissing can also provide a means of exit. Bowel elimination, drainage of bile via surgical wounds or drainage tubes, and escape of gastric contents during vomiting are additional portals of exit.

Reproductive Tract. Organisms such as *Neisseria gonorrhoeae* and human immunodeficiency virus (HIV) may exit through a man's urethral meatus or a woman's vaginal canal. In the man, semen may be the vehicle of pathogens. Discharge and vaginal fluid from the woman's vaginal canal may carry pathogens.

Blood. The blood is normally sterile; but in the case of infectious diseases such as hepatitis B or C, it becomes a reservoir for infectious organisms. A break in the skin allows pathogens to exit the body. Care givers can easily become exposed unless precautions are taken.

MODES OF TRANSMISSION

There are many modes for transmission of microorganisms from the reservoir to the host. Table 34-2 summarizes common modes of transmission. Certain infectious diseases tend to be transmitted more commonly by specific

Table 34-2	Modes of Transmission	
ROUTES AND MEANS		**EXAMPLES OF ORGANISMS**
I. CONTACT		
A. Direct	Person-to-person (fecal, oral) or physical contact between source and susceptible host (e.g., touching client)	Hepatitis A virus, *Shigella, Staphylococcus,* Herpes simplex
B. Indirect	Personal contact of susceptible host with contaminated inanimate object (e.g., needles or sharps, dressings)	Hepatitis B virus, *Staphylococcus,* Respiratory syncytial virus (RSV)
C. Droplet	Large particles that travel up to 3 feet and come in contact with susceptible (e.g., coughing, sneezing, or talking)	Measles virus, Influenza virus, Rubella virus
II. AIR		
A. Droplet nuclei, or residue or evaporated droplets suspended in air (e.g., coughing, sneezing) or carried on dust particles		*Mycobacterium tuberculosis* (TB), Varicella zoster virus (chicken pox), *Aspergillus*
III. VEHICLES		
A. Contaminated items	Water	*Vibrio cholerae*
	Drugs, solutions	*Pseudomonas*
	Blood	Hepatitis C virus
B. Food (improperly handled, stored, or cooked, fresh or thawed meats		Salmonella, *Escherichia coli, Clostridium botulinum*
IV. VECTOR		
A. External mechanical transfer (flies)		*Vibrio cholerae*
B. Internal transmission such as parasitic conditions between vector and host such as:	Mosquito	*Plasmodium falciparum* (malaria)
	Louse	*Rickettsia typhi*
	Flea	*Yersinia pestis* (plague)

modes. However, the same microorganisms may be transmitted by more than one route. For example, herpes zoster may be spread by the airborne route in droplet nuclei or by direct contact.

Although the major mode of transmission of microorganisms is the hands of the health care worker, almost any object within the environment (e.g., a stethoscope or thermometer) can become a means of transmitting pathogens. All hospital personnel providing direct care (e.g., nurses, physical therapists, and physicians) and performing diagnostic and support services (e.g., laboratory technicians, respiratory therapists, and dietary workers) must follow practices to minimize the spread of infection. Each group follows procedures for handling equipment and supplies used by a client. For example, respiratory therapists wash their hands before working with each client and dispose of soiled therapy equipment in a prescribed manner. Certain medical devices and diagnostic procedures provide avenues for spread of pathogens. Invasive procedures such as cystoscopy (visualization of the bladder) facilitate diagnosis of problems but also increase the risk of transmitting infection. Because so many factors can promote the spread of infection to a client, all health care workers must be conscientious in using infection-control practices, such as proper handwashing and ensuring that equipment has been adequately disinfected or sterilized.

PORTAL OF ENTRY

Organisms can enter the body through the same routes they use for exiting. For example, when a contaminated needle pierces a client's skin, organisms enter the body. Any obstruction to the flow of urine from a urinary catheter allows organisms to travel up the urethra. Mishandling of sterile bandages over an open wound permits pathogens to enter exposed tissues. Factors that reduce the body's defenses enhance the chances of pathogens entering the body.

SUSCEPTIBLE HOST

Whether a person acquires an infection depends on susceptibility to an infectious agent. **Susceptibility** depends on the individual degree of resistance to a pathogen. Although everyone is constantly in contact with large numbers of microorganisms, an infection will not develop until an individual becomes susceptible to the strength and numbers of those microorganisms. The more virulent an organism, the greater the likelihood of a person's susceptibility. Acute care settings are seeing more virulent organisms appearing. This is believed to be associated with the frequent use of third-generation cephalosporins, to which the organisms become resistant. A person's natural defenses against infection, as well as a number of other factors, influence resistance. A person's resistance to an infectious agent is enhanced by vaccines or actually contracting the disease.

■ THE INFECTIOUS PROCESS

By understanding the chain of infection, the nurse can intervene to prevent infections from developing. When the client acquires an infection, the nurse is able to observe signs and symptoms of infection and take appropriate actions to prevent its spread. Infections follow a progressive

---

Course of Infection by Stage

INCUBATION PERIOD
■ Interval between entrance of pathogen into body and appearance of first symptoms (e.g., chickenpox, 2-3 weeks; common cold, 1-2 days; influenza, 1-3 days; mumps, 18 days)

PRODROMAL STAGE
■ Interval from onset of nonspecific signs and symptoms (malaise, low-grade fever, fatigue) to more specific symptoms. (During this time, microorganisms grow and multiply, and client is more capable of spreading disease to others).

ILLNESS STAGE
■ Interval when client manifests signs and symptoms specific to type of infection (e.g., common cold manifested by sore throat, sinus congestion, rhinitis; mumps manifested by earache, high fever, parotid and salivary gland swelling).

CONVALESCENCE
■ Interval when acute symptoms of infection disappear. (Length of recovery depends on severity of infection and client's general state of health; recovery may take several days to months.)

---

course (see the box above). The severity of the client's illness depends on the extent of the infection, the **pathogenicity** of the microorganisms, and susceptibility of the host.

If infection is **localized** (i.e., a wound infection), proper care controls the spread and minimizes the illness. The client may experience localized symptoms such as pain and tenderness at the wound site. An infection that affects the entire body instead of just a single organ or part is **systemic** and can become fatal.

The course of an infection influences the level of nursing care provided. The nurse is responsible for properly administering antibiotics and monitoring the response to drug therapy (see Chapter 35). Supportive therapy includes providing adequate nutrition and rest to bolster defenses against the infectious process. The complexity of care further depends on body systems affected by the infection.

Regardless of whether infection is localized or systemic, the nurse plays a critical role in minimizing its spread. The organism causing a simple wound infection can spread to involve an intravenous (IV) needle insertion site if the nurse uses improper technique during an IV dressing change. Nurses who have breaks in their own skin can also acquire infections from clients if their techniques for controlling infection transmission are inadequate.

Defenses Against Infection

The body has normal defenses against infection. Normal body flora that reside inside and outside of the body protect a person from several pathogens. Each organ system has defense mechanisms that defend against exposure to infectious microorganisms. The **inflammatory response** is a protective vascular and cellular reaction that neutralizes pathogens and repairs body cells. Normal flora, body system defenses, and inflammation are all nonspecific defenses that protect against microorganisms regardless of prior exposure. The immune system is composed of separate cells and molecules that help the body resist disease. Certain responses of the immune system are nonspecific, whereas others are specific defenses against specific pathogens. If any of the body's defenses fail, an infection can quickly progress to a serious health problem.

NORMAL FLORA

The body normally contains microorganisms that reside on the surface and deep layers of skin, in the saliva and oral mucosa, and in the gastrointestinal tract. A person normally excretes trillions of microbes daily through the intestines. The skin also has a large population of resident flora. Normal flora do not usually cause disease but instead participate in maintaining health.

Normal flora of the large intestine exist in large numbers without causing injury. These bacterial flora compete with disease-producing microorganisms for food. Normal flora also secrete antibacterial substances within the intestine's walls. The skin's normal flora exert a protective action by inhibiting multiplication of organisms landing on the skin. The mouth and pharynx are also protected by flora that impair growth of invading microbes. The mass of normal flora maintains a sensitive balance with other microorganisms to prevent infection. Any factor that disrupts this balance places a person at increased risk for acquiring an infectious disease. For example, the use of **broad-spectrum antibiotics** for the treatment of infection can lead to suprainfection. Normal bacterial flora are eliminated, allowing disease-producing microorganisms to multiply.

BODY SYSTEM DEFENSES

A number of the body's organ systems have unique defenses against infection (Table 34-3). The skin, respiratory tract, and gastrointestinal tract are easily accessible to microorganisms. Pathogenic organisms easily adhere to the skin's surface, are inhaled into the lungs, or are ingested

Table 34-3	Normal Defense Mechanisms Against Infection	
DEFENSE MECHANISMS	**ACTION**	**FACTORS THAT MAY ALTER DEFENSE**
SKIN		
Intact multilayered surface (body's first line of defense against infection)	Provides barrier to microorganisms	Cuts, abrasions, puncture wounds, areas of maceration
Shedding of outer layer of skin cells	Removes organisms that adhere to skin's outer layers	Failure to bathe regularly
Sebum	Contains fatty acid that kills some bacteria	Excessive bathing
MOUTH		
Intact multilayered mucosa	Provides mechanical barrier to microorganisms	Lacerations, trauma, extracted teeth
Saliva	Washes away particles containing microorganisms	Poor oral hygiene, dehydration
	Contains microbial inhibitors (e.g., lysozyme)	
RESPIRATORY TRACT		
Cilia lining upper airway, coated by mucus	Trap inhaled microbes and sweep them outward in mucus to be expectorated or swallowed	Smoking, high concentration of oxygen and carbon dioxide, decreased humidity, cold air
Macrophages	Engulf and destroy microorganisms that reach lung's alveoli	Smoking
URINARY TRACT		
Flushing action of urine flow	Washes away microorganisms on lining of bladder and urethra	Obstruction to normal flow by urinary catheter placement, obstruction from growth or tumor, delayed micturition
Intact multilayered epithelium	Provides barrier to microorganisms	Introduction of urinary catheter, continual movement of catheter in urethra
GASTROINTESTINAL TRACT		
Acidity of gastric secretions	Chemically destroys microorganisms incapable of surviving low pH	Administration of antacids
Rapid peristalsis in small intestine	Prevents retention of bacterial contents	Delayed motility resulting from impaction of fecal contents in large bowel or mechanical obstruction by masses
VAGINA		
At puberty, normal flora causing vaginal secretions to achieve low pH	Inhibit growth of many microorganisms	Antibiotics and oral contraceptives disrupting normal flora

with food. Each organ system has defense mechanisms physiologically suited to its structure and function. For example, the lungs cannot completely control the entrance of microorganisms. However, the airways are lined with hair-like projections, or cilia, that rhythmically beat to move a blanket of mucus and adherent organisms up to the pharynx to be exhaled. Conditions that impair an organ's specialized defenses increase susceptibility to infection.

INFLAMMATION

The body's cellular response to injury or infection is inflammation. Inflammation is a protective vascular reaction that delivers fluid, blood products, and nutrients to interstitial tissues in an area of injury. The process neutralizes and eliminates pathogens or dead (**necrotic**) tissues and establishes a means of repairing body cells and tissues. Signs of inflammation may include swelling, redness, heat, pain or tenderness, and loss of function in the affected body part. When inflammation becomes systemic, other signs and symptoms develop, including fever, leukocytosis, malaise, anorexia, nausea, vomiting, and lymph node enlargement.

The inflammatory response may be triggered by physical agents, chemical agents, or microorganisms. Mechanical trauma, temperature extremes, and radiation are examples of physical agents. Chemical agents include external and internal irritants such as harsh poisons or gastric acid. Microorganisms may trigger this response, as previously discussed.

After tissues are injured, a series of well-coordinated events occurs. The inflammatory response includes the following:
1. Vascular and cellular responses
2. Formation of inflammatory exudate
3. Tissue repair

Vascular and Cellular Responses. Acute inflammation is an immediate response to cellular injury. Arterioles supplying the infected or injured area dilate, allowing more blood into local circulation. The increase in local blood flow causes the characteristic redness of inflammation. The symptom of localized warmth results from a greater volume of blood at the inflammatory site. Local vasodilation delivers blood and white blood cells (WBCs) to injured tissues.

Injury causes tissue necrosis, and as a result the body releases histamine, bradykinin, prostaglandin, and serotonin. These chemical mediators increase the permeability of small blood vessels. Fluid, protein, and cells enter interstitial spaces. Accumulated fluid appears as localized swelling (**edema**).

Another sign of inflammation is pain. The swelling of inflamed tissues increases pressure on nerve endings, causing pain. Chemical substances such as histamine stimulate nerve endings. As a result of physiological changes occurring with inflammation, the involved body part usually undergoes a temporary loss of function. For example, a localized infection of the hand causes the fingers to become swollen, painful, and discolored. Joints may become stiff as a result of swelling, but function of the fingers returns when inflammation subsides.

The cellular response of inflammation involves WBCs arriving at the site. WBCs pass through blood vessels and into the tissues. Through the process of **phagocytosis**, special-

ized WBCs, called *neutrophils* and *monocytes,* ingest and destroy microorganisms or other small particles. As inflammation becomes systemic, other signs and symptoms develop. **Leukocytosis**, or an increase in the number of circulating WBCs, is the body's response to WBCs leaving blood vessels. A serum WBC count is normally 5000 to 10,000/mm^3 but may rise to 15,000 to 20,000/mm^3 during inflammation. Fever is caused by phagocytic release of pyrogens from bacterial cells that cause a rise in the hypothalamic set point (see Chapter 32). Other systemic signs and symptoms include malaise, anorexia, and lymph node enlargement.

Inflammatory Exudate. Accumulation of fluid and dead tissue cells and WBCs forms an **exudate** at the site of inflammation. Exudate may be **serous** (clear like plasma), **sanguineous** (containing red blood cells), or purulent (containing WBCs and bacteria). Eventually the exudate is cleared away through lymphatic drainage. Platelets and plasma proteins such as fibrinogen form a meshlike matrix at the site of inflammation to prevent its spread.

Tissue Repair. When there is injury to tissue cells, healing involves the defensive, reconstructive, and maturative stages (see Chapter 49). Damaged cells are eventually replaced with healthy new cells. The new cells undergo a gradual maturation until they take on the same structural characteristics and appearance as the previous cells. If inflammation is chronic, tissue defects may fill with fragile **granulation tissue**. Granulation tissue is not as strong as tissue collagen and assumes the form of scar tissue.

IMMUNE RESPONSE

When an invading microorganism enters the body, it is first attacked by monocytes. Remnants of the microorganism then trigger the immune response. The remaining foreign material (**antigen**) causes a series of responses that changes the body's biological makeup so that reactions to future exposures are different from the first reaction. These altered responses are known as **immune responses**. In a normal immune response, the antigen is neutralized, destroyed, or eliminated.

Antigens are usually composed of proteins that are not normally found in a person's body. Often, antigens exist as part of the structure of a bacterium or virus. After an antigen enters the body, it travels in the blood or lymph and initiates cell-mediated or humoral immunity.

Cell-Mediated Immunity. There are two classes of lymphocytes; T lymphocytes (CD4T) and B lymphocytes (B cells). T lymphocytes play a major role in cell-mediated immunity. There are antigen receptors on the surface membranes of CD4T lymphocytes. When an antigen meets the cell whose surface receptors fit the antigen, a binding occurs. This binding activates the CD4T lymphocyte to divide rapidly to form sensitized cells. Sensitized CD4T lymphocytes travel to the area of inflammation or injury, bind with antigens, and release chemical compounds called **lymphokines**. The lymphokines attract macrophages and stimulate them to attack antigens. Eventually the antigens are killed. The cell-mediated response is altered by the HIV, which causes AIDS (Fig. 34-2).

Humoral Immunity. Stimulation of B cells triggers the humoral immune response, causing synthesis of immunoglobulins or antibodies that destroy antigens. After a

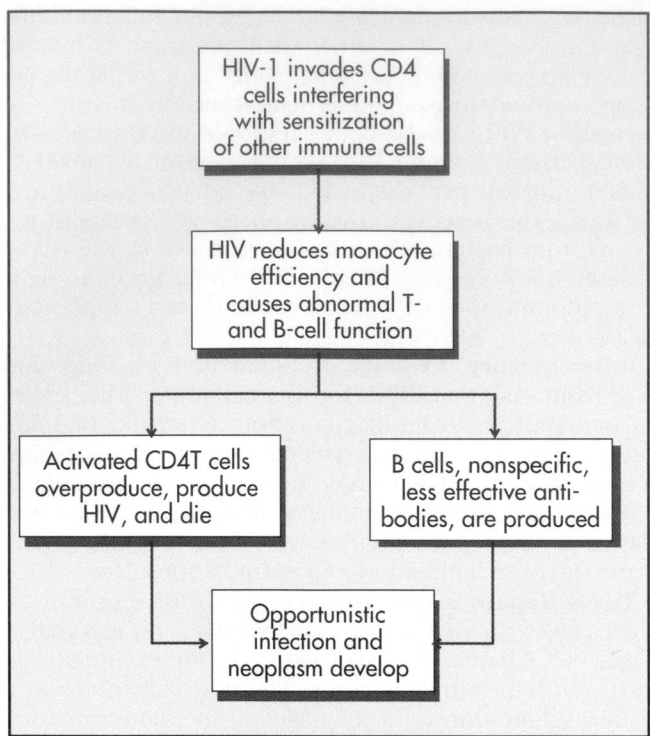

Fig. 34-2 The pathologic responses of HIV.

B cell binds with an antigen, it causes formation of plasma and memory B cells. Plasma cells synthesize and secrete large amounts of antibodies, which are proteins normally found in the body that provide general immunity. Memory B cells prepare the body against future antigen invasion. Thus when an antigen enters the body again, antibodies form more rapidly than during the first exposure, and immunoglobulin levels remain high to attack the antigen.

Antibodies are large protein molecules. There are five classes of antibody **immunoglobulins,** which are identified by the letters M, G, A, E, and D. Immunoglobulin M (IgM) is the predominant early antibody formed after initial contact with an antigen. This initial contact is the primary immune response, and presence of IgM denotes current infection. The most abundant circulating antibody is IgG, which is formed after subsequent contacts with antigens or during the secondary immune response, and its presence denotes past infections.

Formation of antibodies is the basis of immunization against disease and can be either a natural or artificially-induced event. **Natural immunity** results after having a certain disease, such as measles, and usually lasts a lifetime. Artificial immunity follows the receipt of a vaccine such as polio vaccine. The duration is variable and may or may not require a booster. **Passive immunity** is usually of short duration and is the type that can be obtained transplacentally.

Complement. A **complement** is an inactive protein compound found in blood serum. It is activated when an antigen and antibody bind together. After a complement is activated, a rapid sequence of catalytic activity changes the shape of antigenic cells. The foreign bacteria, for example, assume the shape of a doughnut. The complement actually makes a hole through the antigen's cell membrane. Ions

Modified from Crow S: *Crit Care Nurs* Q 11(4):11, 1989.

and water enter the cell, causing it to burst. This process is called **cytolysis.**

Interferon. When certain cells are invaded by viruses, they synthesize the protein interferon. **Interferon** interferes with the ability of viruses to multiply and protects body cells from simultaneous infection with other viruses. Classified as a biological response modifier, interferon also directly inhibits the growth and division of tumor cells (Grimes and Grimes, 1994).

Nosocomial Infections

Clients in health care settings may have an increased risk of acquiring infections. **Nosocomial infections** result from delivery of health services in a health care facility. A hospital is one of the most likely places for acquiring an infection because it harbors a high population of virulent strains of microorganisms that may be resistant to antibiotics. The intensive care unit (ICU) is one area in the hospital where the risk of acquiring a nosocomial infection is especially high (see the box above). Unfortunately, most nosocomial infections are transmitted by health care workers.

Iatrogenic infections are a type of nosocomial infection resulting from a diagnostic or therapeutic procedure. A urinary tract infection that develops after catheter insertion is an example of an iatrogenic nosocomial infection. The incidence of nosocomial infections can be reduced if nurses use critical thinking when practicing aseptic techniques. The nurse should always consider the client's risks for infection and anticipate how the approach to care may increase or decrease the chances of infection transmission.

Nosocomial infections may be exogenous or endogenous. An **exogenous infection** arises from microorganisms external to the individual, which do not exist as normal flora; examples are *Salmonella* organisms and *Clostridium tetani.* An **endogenous infection** can occur when part of the client's flora becomes altered and an overgrowth results. Examples are infections caused by enterococci, yeasts, and streptococci. When sufficient numbers of microorgan-

---

Risk of Nosocomial Infection in ICUs

■ Nurses working in ICUs should be particularly conscious of aseptic practices. Clients are at risk for infection for the following reasons:
■ ICU clients are critically ill and often have more underlying disease than other clients.
■ More invasive devices such as intravenous or intraarterial lines are used in ICUs.
■ More invasive procedures are performed in the ICU than other general-care areas.
■ Often, surgical procedures are performed in the ICU instead of the operating room because of a client's critical condition.
■ Overuse of broad-spectrum antibiotics causes the formation of resistant microorganisms that later cause infection.
■ The pace of activities in an ICU can often cause nurses and other health care providers to become less diligent with aseptic technique.

isms normally found in one body cavity or lining are transferred to another body site, an endogenous infection develops. For example, transmission of enterococci, normally found in fecal material, from the hands to the skin is a common cause of wound infections. The number of microorganisms needed to cause a nosocomial infection depends on the virulence of the organism, the host's susceptibility, and the site affected.

The number of health care employees having direct contact with a client, type and number of invasive procedures, therapy received, and length of hospitalization influence the risk of infection. Major sites for nosocomial infection include the urinary tract, surgical or traumatic wounds, respiratory tract, and bloodstream (see the box below).

Nosocomial infections significantly increase costs of health care. Extended stays in health care institutions, increased disability, increased costs of antibodies, and prolonged recovery times add to the expenses of the client, as well as the health care institution and funding bodies (e.g., Medicare). Often, costs for nosocomial infections are not reimbursed; as a result, prevention has a beneficial financial impact and is an important part of managed care.

■ CONCEPT OF ASEPSIS

The nurse's efforts to minimize the onset and spread of infection are based on the principles of aseptic technique. **Asepsis** is the absence of disease-producing pathogens. Aseptic technique is the effort to keep a client as free from microorganisms as possible (Crow, 1989). The two types of aseptic technique are medical and surgical asepsis.

Medical asepsis, or clean technique, includes procedures used to reduce and prevent the spread of microorganisms. Handwashing, changing a client's bed linen, and using clean medication cups are examples of medical asepsis. Principles of medical asepsis are commonly followed in the home, as in washing hands before preparing food.

Surgical asepsis, or sterile technique, includes procedures used to eliminate microorganisms from an area. Sterilization destroys all microorganisms and their spores (Ru-

tala, 1990). Sterile technique should be practiced during invasive procedures.

After an object becomes unsterile or unclean, it is contaminated. In medical asepsis an area or object is considered contaminated if it contains or is suspected of containing pathogens. For example, a used bedpan, the floor, and a wet piece of gauze are contaminated. In surgical asepsis an area or object is considered contaminated if touched by any object that is not sterile. For example, a tear in a surgical glove exposes the outside of the glove to the skin surface, thus contaminating it.

The nurse is responsible for providing the client with a safe environment. The effectiveness of infection-control practices depends on the nurse's conscientiousness and consistency in using effective aseptic technique. It is easy to forget key procedural steps or, when hurried, to take shortcuts that break aseptic procedures. However, the nurse's failure to be meticulous will place the client at risk for an infection that can seriously impair recovery.

■ THE NURSING PROCESS IN INFECTION CONTROL

 Assessment

The nurse assesses the client's defense mechanisms, susceptibility, and knowledge of infections. A review of disease history with the client and family may reveal an exposure to a communicable disease. A thorough review of the client's clinical condition may detect signs and symptoms of infection. An analysis of laboratory findings provides information about a client's defense against infection. By knowing the factors that increase susceptibility or risk for infection, the nurse is better able to plan preventive therapy that includes aseptic technique. By recognizing early signs and symptoms of infection, the nurse can alert others on the health care team to the potential need for therapy and initiate supportive nursing measures.

Sites and Causes for Nosocomial Infections

URINARY TRACT
- Insertion of urinary catheter
- Open drainage system
- Catheter and tube becoming disconnected
- Drainage bag port touching contaminated surface
- Improper specimen collection technique
- Obstruction or interference with urinary drainage
- Urine in catheter or drainage tube being allowed to reenter bladder (reflux)
- Improper handwashing technique
- Repeated catheter irrigations with solutions

SURGICAL OR TRAUMATIC WOUNDS
- Improper skin preparation (shaving and bathing) before surgery
- Improper handwashing technique
- Failure to cleanse skin surface properly
- Failure to use aseptic technique during dressing changes
- Use of contaminated antiseptic solutions

RESPIRATORY TRACT
- Contaminated respiratory therapy equipment
- Failure to use aseptic technique while suctioning airway
- Improper disposal of mucous secretions
- Improper handwashing technique

BLOODSTREAM
- Contamination of intravenous fluids by tubing or needle changes
- Insertion of drug additives to intravenous fluid
- Addition of connecting tube or stopcocks to intravenous system
- Improper care of needle insertion site
- Contaminated needles or catheters
- Failure to change intravenous access site when inflammation first appears
- Improper technique during administration of multiple blood products
- Improper care of peritoneal or hemodialysis shunts
- Improper handwashing technique

Status of Defense Mechanisms

A review of physical assessment findings and the client's medical condition reveals the status of normal defense mechanisms against infection. For example, any break in the skin or mucosa is a potential site for infection. Similarly, a chronic smoker is at greater risk for acquiring a respiratory tract infection after general surgery because the cilia of the lung are less likely to be active and able to propel retained mucus from the lung's airways. Any reduction in the body's primary or secondary defenses against infection places a client at risk (see the box below).

CLIENT SUSCEPTIBILITY

Many factors influence susceptibility to infection. The nurse gathers information about each factor through the client's and family's history.

Age. Throughout the life span, susceptibility to infection changes. An infant has reduced defenses against infection. Born with only the antibodies provided by the mother, the infant's immature immune system is incapable of producing the necessary immunoglobulins and WBCs. However, breastfed infants have greater immunity than bottle-fed infants, because they receive the mother's antibodies through the breast milk. As the child grows, the immune system matures, but the child is still susceptible to organisms that cause the common cold, intestinal infections, and infectious diseases such as mumps and measles.

The young or middle-aged adult has refined defenses against infection. Normal flora, body system defenses, inflammation, and the immune response provide protection against invading microorganisms. Viruses are the most common cause of infectious illness in young or middle-aged adults.

Defenses against infection may change with aging (Smith and Rusnak, 1991). The immune response, particularly cell-mediated immunity, declines. Older adults also undergo alterations in the structure and function of the skin, urinary tract, and lungs. For example, the skin loses its turgor and the epithelium thins. As a result, the skin is more easily abraded or torn. This increases exposure to pathogens (Table 34-4).

Alterations in the immune system may even trigger the aging process. Cells of the immune system such as lymphocytes become more diversified with age, and the body undergoes a progressive loss of cellular regulation. When viruses or other antigens and corresponding antibodies lodge in sites such as the kidney and arteries, factors injurious to the tissues are released, and deterioration begins. With aging and autoimmune diseases (alterations of the immune system), cellular changes such as depletion of lymphoid tissues occur. The basic mechanism for the aging process is not understood. However, it is known that immunity to infection decreases with advancing age.

Nutritional Status. When protein intake is inadequate as a result of poor diet or debilitating disease, the rate of protein breakdown exceeds that of tissue synthesis (see Chapter 41). A reduction in the intake of protein and other nutrients such as carbohydrates and fats reduces the body's defenses against infection and impairs wound healing (see Chapter 49).

Clients with illnesses or problems that increase protein requirements are at further risk. These problems include traumatic injury, extensive burns, and conditions causing fever. Clients who have had surgery also have this problem.

The nurse assesses clients' dietary intakes and abilities to tolerate solid foods. Clients who have difficulty with swallowing, who experience alterations in digestion, or who are too confused or weak to feed themselves are at risk for inadequate dietary intake. A dietitian may be called to assist in calculating the calorie count of foods ingested. In preparation for discharge, the nurse evaluates the client's and family's understanding of nutritional needs.

Stress. The body responds to emotional or physical stress by the general adaptation syndrome (see Chapter 22). During the alarm stage, the basal metabolic rate increases as the body uses energy stores. Adrenocorticotropic hormone (ACTH) acts to increase serum glucose levels and decrease unnecessary antiinflammatory responses through the release of cortisone. If stress continues or becomes intense, elevated cortisone levels result in decreased resistance to infection. Continued stress leads to exhaustion, wherein energy stores are depleted and the body has no resistance to invading organisms. The same conditions that increase nutritional requirements such as surgery or trauma also increase physiological stress.

Heredity. Certain hereditary conditions impair an individual's response to infection. The client's history of preexisting medical problems should reveal known hereditary disorders. For example, agammaglobulinemia is a rare inherited or acquired disorder characterized by the absence of serum antibodies. The client with this disorder has virtually no ability to initiate defenses against infection, such as the formation of antibodies.

Disease Process. Clients with diseases of the immune system are at particular risk for infection. Leukemia, AIDS, lymphoma, and aplastic anemia are conditions that compromise a host by weakening defenses against infectious organisms. Clients with leukemia are unable to produce enough WBCs to ward off infection.

Victims of chronic disease such as diabetes mellitus and multiple sclerosis are also more susceptible to infection because of general debilitation and nutritional impairment. Diseases that impair body system defenses, such as pulmonary emphysema and bronchitis (which impair ciliary action and thicken mucus), cancer (which alters the im-

---

Risk Factors for Infection

INADEQUATE PRIMARY DEFENSES
- Broken skin or mucosa
- Traumatized tissue
- Decreased ciliary action
- Obstructed urine outflow
- Altered peristalsis
- Change in pH of secretions
- Decreased mobility

INADEQUATE SECONDARY DEFENSES
- Reduced hemoglobin level
- Suppression of WBCs (drug or disease related)
- Suppressed inflammatory response (drug or disease related)
- Low WBC count (leukopenia)

Table 34-4	Assessing the Risk of Infection in Older Adults	
COMPONENT	**POSSIBLE CHANGES WITH AGE**	**OUTCOME**
Skin	Thinner dermal and epidermal layers, decreased collagen strength, decreased skin elasticity, decreased sweat	Pressure ulcers
Peripheral nerves	Reduced sensitivity, particularly in clients with history of alcohol abuse, vitamin B_{12} deficiency, and diabetes mellitus	Pressure ulcers, ignored trauma leading to infection
Circulation	Congestive heart failure, calcified mitral and aortic valves	Pneumonia, bacterial endocarditis
Peripheral circulation	More elastic veins, less effective venous valves, blood pooling in lower extremities	Venous stasis ulcers
Mouth	Dehydration, loss of saliva production, functional inability to maintain oral hygiene	Parotid gland infection, peridontal disease, localized abscess, bacteremia
Gastrointestinal tract	Loss of ability to secrete stomach acid in 30% of persons over 70	Salmonellal diarrhea
Pulmonary system	Increased colonization of oropharynx, impaired mucociliary clearance, decreased macrophage function, decreased cough reflex	Viral and bacterial pneumonia
Urinary tract	Prostatic hyperplasia, urethral strictures, age-related hormonal changes in vaginal wall, pelvic floor relaxation, ureterocele or cystocele, degeneration of nerves leading to neurogenic bladder, use of tricyclic antidepressants, dehydration	Asymptomatic bacteriuria, cystitis, pyelonephritis
Nutrition	Malnutrition, vitamin deficiency (vitamin A, pyridoxine, and riboflavin), protein and caloric malnutrition	Impaired immune response to infection
Drug therapy	Corticosteroid and cytotoxic drugs	Impaired immune response to infection
Nursing home residency	Exposure to nosocomial infections, including influenza, *Proteus* and *Providencia* organisms with an indwelling catheter, turberculosis, and wound infections. (Incidence of bacteremia after admission is 50%.)	Frequent serious infection, increased risk of pneumonia

Modified from Tideiksaar R: *Physician Assist* 11(2):17, 1987.

mune response), and peripheral vascular disease (which reduces blood flow to injured tissues), increase susceptibility to infection. Burn clients have a very high susceptibility to infection because of the damage of skin surfaces. The greater the depth and extent of the burns, the higher the risk for infection.

Medical Therapy. Some drug and medical therapies compromise immunity to infection. The nurse assesses the client's history to determine whether the client takes medications at home that increase infection susceptibility. A review of therapies received within the health care setting further reveals risks. Adrenal corticosteroids, prescribed for several conditions, are antiinflammatory drugs that cause protein breakdown and impair the inflammatory response against bacteria and other pathogens. Cytotoxic or antineoplastic drugs attack cancer cells but cause side effects of bone marrow depression and normal cell toxicity. With bone marrow depression the body is unable to produce lymphocytes and sufficient WBCs. When normal cells become altered by antineoplastic agents, cellular defenses against infection fail. Cyclosporine and other immunosuppressant drugs, which decrease the body's immune response, are commonly taken by clients who are organ transplant recipients. The immunosuppressants prevent organ and tissue rejection; yet they increase susceptibility to infection.

Cancer clients receiving radiotherapy are also at risk for infection. The massive doses of radiation, which destroy cancerous cells, can also depress the bone marrow and destroy normal cells.

Clinical Appearance

The signs and symptoms of infection may be local or systemic. Localized infections are most common in areas of skin or mucous membrane breakdown such as surgical and traumatic wounds, pressure ulcers, and mouth lesions. Infections also develop locally in cavities beneath the skin; an example is an abscess.

To assess an area for localized infection, the nurse first inspects the area for redness and swelling caused by inflammation. Because there may be drainage from open lesions or wounds, the nurse wears gloves. Infected drainage may be yellow, green, or brown, depending on the pathogen. The nurse asks the client about pain or tenderness around the site. The client may complain of tightness caused by edema. If the infected area is large enough, movement of a body part may be restricted. Gentle palpation of an infected area usually results in some degree of tenderness.

Systemic infections cause more generalized symptoms than local infection. They usually result in fever, fatigue, and malaise. Lymph nodes that drain the area of infection often become enlarged, swollen, and tender during palpation. For example, an abscess in the peritoneal cavity may cause enlargement of lymph nodes in the groin. An infection of the upper respiratory tract may cause cervical lymph node enlargement. If an infection is serious and widespread, all major lymph nodes may enlarge. Systemic infections commonly cause a loss of appetite, nausea, and vomiting.

Systemic infections often develop after treatment for localized infection has failed. The nurse should be alert for changes in the client's level of activity and responsiveness. As systemic infections develop, the client may become lethargic and complain of a loss of energy. An elevation in body temperature may lead to episodes of increased heart and respiratory rates. Involvement of major body systems may produce specific signs. For example, a pulmonary infection may result in a productive cough with purulent sputum. A urinary tract infection may result in cloudy, foul-smelling urine.

An infection in older adults may not present with typical signs and symptoms. Often older adults have advanced infection before it is identified. This is because of their reduced inflammatory and immune responses. Normally older adults have diminished pain sensitivity. A reduced or absent fever response may occur from chronic use of aspirin or nonsteroidal antiinflammatory drugs. Atypical symptoms such as confusion, incontinence, or agitation may be the only symptoms of an infectious illness (Tideik-saar, 1987). An example is pneumonia, the main complication of influenza. As many as 20% of older adults with pneumonia do not have the typical signs and symptoms of fever, shaking, chills, and rusty productive sputum. The only symptoms may be an increased, unexplained heart rate or generalized fatigue.

Laboratory Data

A review of test results may reveal infection (Table 34-5). Laboratory values, however, are not enough to detect infection. Other clinical signs must be assessed. Factors other than infection may alter test values. For example, trauma and physical stress can cause an elevation in the number of neutrophils.

Clients With Infection

A client with infection may have a variety of health problems. The nurse assesses ways the infection affects the client's and family's needs. These may be physical, psychological, social, or economical. For example, a client with a chronic disease such as AIDS may experience serious psychological problems as a result of self-imposed isolation or rejection by family and friends (see the box on p. 753). Clients or their families may not be able to afford the cost of medical care. The nurse, using a case management approach, determines the client's and family's ability to adjust to the disease and the available resources needed for managing health care challenges (Grimes and Grimes, 1994).

 Nursing Diagnosis

During assessment, the nurse gathers objective findings, such as an open incision or a reduced caloric intake, and subjective data, such as a client's complaint of tenderness over a surgical wound site. Then the nurse interprets the data carefully, looking for clusters of defining characteristics or risk factors that create a pattern suggesting a specific nursing diagnosis (see the nursing diagnoses box on p. 753). It may be necessary for the nurse to validate data (e.g., by inspecting the integrity of a wound more carefully). Like-

Table 34-5	Laboratory Tests to Screen for Infection	
LABORATORY VALUE	**NORMAL (ADULT) VALUES**	**INDICATION OF INFECTION**
WBC count	5000-10,000/mm³	Increased in acute infection, decreased in certain viral or overwhelming infections
Erythrocyte sedimentation rate	Up to 15 mm/hr for men and 20 mm/hr for women	Elevated in presence of inflammatory process
Iron level	60-90 g/dl	Decreased in chronic infection
Cultures of urine and blood	Normally sterile, without microorganism growth	Presence of infectious microorganism growth
Cultures of wound, sputum, and throat	Possible normal flora	Presence of infectious microorganism growth
DIFFERENTIAL COUNT (PERCENTAGE OF EACH TYPE OF WBC)		
Neutrophils	55%-70%	Increased in acute suppurative infection, decreased in overwhelming bacterial infection (older adult)
Lymphocytes	20%-40%	Increased in chronic bacterial and viral infection, decreased in sepsis
Monocytes	2%-8%	Increased in protozoal, rickettsial, and tuberculosis infections
Eosinophils	1%-4%	Increased in parasitic infection
Basophils	0.5%-1%	Normal during infection

RESEARCH HIGHLIGHT

RESEARCH ABSTRACT

More than 1 million people in the United States are estimated to be infected with HIV, the causative agent of AIDS. Nurses who remain in the profession will eventually be expected to care for HIV clients. The purpose of the study was to assess nurses' reaction to the possibility of working with HIV clients. Using a sentence-completion format, nurses were asked to respond to a statement root, "When I think of caring for patients with HIV infection or AIDS, I . . . ." The survey was sent to 2,434 randomly selected nurses, with 502 (20.6%) returning a completed tool for a total of 3,180 responses. Card sorting was used to discover themes that included positive, neutral, or negative reaction. The thematic categories that evolved from the data were: caring (899 or 28%), care as usual (1,198 or 37.6%), and avoidance (1,083 or 34%). The qualitative research revealed that nurses, when confronted with an anticipation of caring for HIV-infected clients, have a variety of opinions and concerns.

IMPLICATIONS FOR PRACTICE

▶ Nurses should evaluate their own reactions to caring for an HIV client.

▶ Nurse manager and educator should promote positive attitudes for nurses caring for HIV clients.

▶ Nurses should have current knowledge concerning HIV disease transmission.

▶ Nurses who have negative reactions to caring for clients with HIV should attend focus groups that deal with such issues.

REFERENCE

Springer L et al: Anticipated care for HIV-infected clients: nurses' reactions, *J Assoc nurses in AIDS Care* 5(1):29, 1994.

Examples of NANDA Nursing Diagnoses for Infection

Risk for infection *related to:*
- Altered immunity
- Tissue destruction
- Malnutrition

Risk for injury *related to:*
- Altered immunity

Impaired tissue integrity *related to:*
- Altered circulation
- Exposure to irritants

Altered oral mucous membrane *related to:*
- Traumatic irritation of nasogastric tube
- Ineffective oral hygiene

Altered nutrition: less than body requirements *related to:*
- Poor diet habits
- Altered gastrointestinal function

Risk for impaired skin integrity *related to:*
- Shearing force
- Physical immobilization
- Exposure to skin irritants

Social isolation *related to:*
- Misconceptions about sexually transmitted disease

Body image disturbance *related to:*
- Client's aversion to open wound
- Self-perception regarding sexually transmitted disease

---

wise, additional data such as laboratory findings may help. The selection of appropriate nursing diagnoses depends on analyzing and organizing data correctly (see the diagnostic process box on p. 754).

The diagnosis must have the appropriate etiological factor in order for the nurse to establish an appropriate and well–thought-out plan. For example, *risk for infection related to broken skin* requires good hygiene measures and wound care. *Risk for infection related to malnutrition* requires good nutritional support and fluid balance.

The nurse may diagnose a risk for infection or make diagnoses that result from the effects of infection on health status. The nurse's success in planning appropriate nursing interventions depends on the accuracy of the diagnosis and the ability to meet the client's needs.

Planning

The client's care plan is based on each nursing diagnosis and related factor. The nurse's aim is to develop a plan that sets attainable outcomes so that interventions are purposeful and directed. The nurse caring for the client with *risk for infection related to broken skin* implements skin care and

measures to promote healing. The expected outcomes of "reduction in wound size by 1 cm" and "absence of drainage" set targets for measuring the client's improvement. Once outcomes are met, the goal of "skin intact and without drainage" can be reached. Interventions are selected in collaboration with the client, the family, and others on the health care team. The nurse directs the care in the acute care setting and may involve the dietitian or respiratory therapist in assisting with instruction of procedures that need to be followed after discharge. Common goals of care may include the following:

1. Preventing exposure to infectious organisms
2. Controlling or reducing the extent of infection
3. Maintaining a resistance to infection
4. The client and family learn about infection control techniques

The nurse establishes priorities for the goals of care. For example, a client has developed an open wound, suffers a debilitating disease such as cancer, and has been unable to tolerate solid foods. The priority of administering therapies that promote wound healing exceeds the goal of educating the client to assume self-care therapies at home. When the client's condition improves, the priorities will change, and client education becomes an essential intervention (JCAHO, 1995).

The development of a care plan (see the care plan on p. 754) includes infection prevention practices. The nurse may include appropriate referrals such as a dietitian, infection-control professional, or home health care nurse. When care is being administered in the home, the nurse

Sample Nursing Diagnostic Process for Infection

ASSESSMENT ACTIVITIES	DEFINING CHARACTERISTICS	NURSING DIAGNOSES
Check results of laboratory tests.	WBC count 5000/mm³	**Risk for infection** related to lowered immunity
Review current medications.	Client receiving azathioprine (Imuran), an immunosuppressant	
Identify potential sites of infection.	Intravenous catheter in right forearm, in place for 3 days Foley catheter draining amber-colored urine	
Inspect condition of dependent pressure points.	Area 2 cm in diameter, superficial broken skin over sacrum	**Impaired skin integrity** related to pressure and exposure to fecal irritants
Observe for skin contamination.	Client incontinent (semiliquid stool)	

Sample Nursing Care Plan for Risk for Infection

NURSING DIAGNOSIS: **Risk for infection** related to lowered immunity
DEFINITION: Risk for infection is the state in which an individual is at increased risk for being invaded by pathogenic organisms (Kim, McFarland, McLane, 1995)

GOAL	EXPECTED OUTCOMES	INTERVENTIONS	RATIONALE
Client will remain free of nosocomial infection.	Intravenous needle site will not become infected. Client will remain afebrile during hospitalization.	Change intravenous peripheral catheters every 48-72 hr; cover site with sterile dressing. When moisture or blood accumulates on dressing, change it and cleanse site with an antiseptic.	Replacement of peripheral venous catheters every 48-72 hr reduces nosocomial septicemia. Visible moisture or blood beneath IV dressing is risk factor for catheter-related infection (Maki, Ringer, 1987).
	Client's urine will remain clear, without bacterial growth during hospitalization.	Provide daily perineal hygiene with soap and water. Anchor urinary catheter to avoid up-and-down movement within urethra. Keep junction between catheter and drainage bag sealed.	Regular periurethral cleansing and reduced urethral manipulation may decrease migration of bacteria up urethra. Break in integrity of system can allow introduction of microorganisms and bladder colonization (Classen et al, 1991).

plans to be sure the environment promotes good infection-control practices. For example, if a client does not have running water, even simple handwashing is difficult to achieve.

Implementation

In all health care settings, the nurse's primary goals are preventing the onset and spread of infection and administering measures for treatment of infection. By recognizing and assessing a client's risk factors and implementing appropriate measures, the nurse can reduce the risk of infection.

Disease Prevention

Through critical thinking, the nurse may prevent an infection from developing or spreading by minimizing the numbers and kinds of organisms transmitted to potential infection sites. Eliminating reservoirs of infection, controlling portals of exit and entry, and avoiding actions that transmit microorganisms prevent bacteria from finding a site to grow. Proper use of sterile supplies, barrier protection, and proper handwashing are examples of methods that the nurse may use to control the spread of microorganisms. A final preventive measure is to strengthen a potential host's defenses against infection. Nutritional support, rest, maintenance of physiological protective mechanisms, and immunization protect a client from invasion by pathogens. Having an infection-control conscience helps the nurse apply good medical-surgical aseptic practices at the right time and the right clinical situation. When a client develops an infection, the nurse continues preventive care so that health care personnel and other clients are not exposed to the infection. Clients with communicable diseases may require isolation precautions that control the environment by forming barriers against transmission of infection.

Acute Care Measures

Treatment of an infectious process includes eliminating the infectious organisms and supporting the client's defenses. The nurse collects specimens of body fluids or drainage from infected body sites for cultures. When the disease process or causative organism has been identified, the physician prescribes the treatment most effective for the situation. The nurse properly administers antibiotics and other treatments, watching for adverse reactions and assessing the progress of the infection.

Systemic infections require measures to prevent complications of fever (see Chapter 32). Maintaining intake of fluids prevents dehydration resulting from diaphoresis. The client's increased metabolic rate requires an adequate nutritional intake. Rest preserves energy for the healing process.

Localized infections often require measures to facilitate removal of debris to promote healing. The nurse applies principles of wound care to remove infected drainage from wound sites and support the integrity of healing wounds. Special dressings can be applied to facilitate removal of infectious drainage and promote healing of wound margins. Drainage tubes may be inserted to remove infected drainage from body cavities. The nurse uses medical and surgical aseptic techniques to manage wounds and ensures correct handling of all drainage or body fluids.

During the course of infection the nurse supports the client's body defense mechanisms. For example, if a client has infectious diarrhea, the nurse must maintain skin integrity to prevent breakdown and the entrance of microorganisms. Other routine hygiene measures such as cleansing the oral cavity and bathing protect the skin and mucous membranes from organism spread.

Medical Asepsis

The nurse follows certain principles and procedures to prevent infection and control its spread. During daily routine care the nurse uses basic medical aseptic techniques to break the infection chain. Because infections are readily transmissible between clients and care givers, the nurse follows isolation precautions as appropriate.

CONTROL OR ELIMINATION OF INFECTIOUS AGENTS

Proper cleansing, disinfection, and sterilization of contaminated objects significantly reduce and often eliminate microorganisms. In health care centers a central supply department disinfects and sterilizes reusable supplies. However, the nurse may encounter situations that require use of these techniques. Many principles of cleaning and disinfection also apply to the home.

Cleaning. Cleaning is the removal of all foreign materials such as soil and organic material from objects (Rutala, 1990). Generally, cleaning involves use of water and mechanical action with or without detergents. When an object comes in contact with infectious or potentially infectious material, the object is contaminated. If the object is disposable, it is discarded. Reusable objects must be cleaned thoroughly before reuse and either disinfected or sterilized.

When cleaning equipment that is soiled by organic material such as blood, fecal matter, mucus, or pus, the nurse applies a mask, protective eyewear, and waterproof gloves. These barriers provide protection from infectious organisms. A stiff-bristled brush and detergent or soap are needed for cleaning. The following steps ensure that an object is clean:

1. Rinse a contaminated object or article with cold running water to remove organic material. Hot water causes the protein in organic material to coagulate and stick to objects, making removal difficult.
2. After rinsing, wash the object with soap and warm water. Soap or detergent reduces the surface tension of water and emulsifies dirt or remaining material. Few household detergents, however, have disinfectant properties. Rinse the object thoroughly to remove the emulsified dirt.
3. Use a brush to remove dirt or material in grooves or seams. Friction dislodges contaminated material for easy removal. Open hinged items.
4. Rinse the object in warm water.

Items Requiring Disinfection or Sterilization

CRITICAL ITEMS
Items that enter sterile tissue or the vascular system present a high risk of infection if the items are contaminated with microorganisms, especially bacterial spores. *Critical items* must be *sterile.* Some of these items follow:
- Surgical instruments
- Intravascular catheters
- Urinary catheters
- Needles

SEMICRITICAL ITEMS
Items that come in contact with mucous membranes or skin that is not intact also present risks. These objects must be free of all microorganisms (except bacterial spores). *Semicritical items* must be *disinfected* or *sterilized.* Some of these items follow:
- Respiratory suction tubing and catheters
- Endotracheal tubes
- Gastrointestinal endoscopes
- Thermometers

NONCRITICAL ITEMS
Items that come in contact with intact skin but not mucous membranes must be clean. *Noncritical items* must be *disinfected.* Some of these items follow:
- Bedpans
- Blood pressure cuffs
- Linens
- Stethoscopes

5. Dry the object and prepare it for disinfection or sterilization.
6. The brush, gloves, and sink in which the equipment is cleaned should be considered contaminated and should be cleansed.

Disinfection and Sterilization. **Disinfection** describes a process that eliminates many or all microorganisms, with the exception of bacterial spores, from inanimate objects (Rutala, 1995). This is generally accomplished by the use of a chemical disinfectant or wet pasteurization (used for respiratory therapy equipment). Examples of disinfectants are alcohols, chlorines, glutaraldehydes, and phenols. These chemicals can be caustic and toxic to tissues.

Sterilization is the complete elimination or destruction of all microorganisms, including spores. Steam under pressure, ethylene oxide (ETO) gas, and chemicals are the most common sterilizing agents.

Whether an item is to be disinfected or sterilized depends on the degree of risk of infection involved with the use of the item. There are three categories of device classification (see the box on p. 755). Nurses should be familiar with agency policy and procedures for cleaning, handling, and delivering care items for eventual disinfection and sterilization. Workers especially trained in disinfection and sterilization should perform most of the procedures. Selection of a method for disinfecting or sterilizing is made after considering the following factors:

1. Concentration of solution and duration of contact. A weakened concentration or shortened exposure time may lessen effectiveness.
2. Type and number of pathogens. Certain organisms are killed more easily than others by disruption. The greater the number of pathogens on an object, the longer the required disinfecting time.
3. Surface areas to treat. All dirty surfaces and areas must be fully exposed to disinfecting and sterilizing agents.
4. Temperature of environment. Disinfectants tend to work best at room temperature.
5. Presence of soap. Soap may cause certain disinfectants to be ineffective. Thorough rinsing of an object is necessary before disinfecting.
6. Presence of organic materials. Disinfectants can become inactivated unless blood, saliva, pus, or body excretions are washed off. Table 34-6 lists processes for disinfection and sterilization and their characteristics.

CONTROL OR ELIMINATION OF RESERVOIRS

To control or eliminate reservoir sites for infection, the nurse eliminates sources of body fluids, drainage, or solutions that might harbor microorganisms. The nurse also carefully discards articles that become contaminated with infectious material (see the box on p. 757). The Occupational Safety and Health Act of 1991 set standards for minimizing occupational exposure to blood-borne pathogens or other potentially infectious materials (OSHA, 1991). All health care institutions must have guidelines for the disposal of infectious waste material according to local and state regulations.

CONTROL OF PORTALS OF EXIT

The nurse follows prevention and control practices to minimize or prevent infectious organisms from exiting the body. To control organisms exiting via the respiratory tract, the nurse should avoid talking directly into clients' faces or talking, sneezing, or coughing directly over surgical wounds or sterile dressing fields. The nurse should cover the mouth or nose when sneezing or coughing. The nurse is also responsible for teaching clients to protect others

Table 34-6	**Examples of Disinfection and Sterilization Processes**
CHARACTERISTICS	**EXAMPLES OF USE**
MOIST HEAT Moist heat includes steam (moist heat under pressure). When exposed to high pressure, water vapor can attain temperature above boiling point to kill pathogens and spores.	Autoclave is used to sterilize surgical instruments, parenteral solutions, and surgical dressings.
RADIATION Ionizing radiation penetrates deeply into objects for effective sterilization and disinfection.	Radiation is used in sterilizing drugs, foods, and other heat-sensitive items.
CHEMICALS Chemicals are effective disinfectants because they attack all types of microorganisms, act rapidly, work with water, retain no order, are stable in light and heat, are inexpensive are not harmful to body tissues, do not destroy article being disinfected, and are not inactivated by organic material.	Chemicals are used for disinfection of instruments and equipment such as glass thermometers. Chlorine is useful for disinfecting water and for housekeeping purposes.
ETHYLENE OXIDE GAS This gas destroys spores and microorganisms by altering cells' metabolic processes. Fumes are released within an autoclave-like chamber. Ethylene oxide gas is toxic to humans and aeration time varies with products.	This gas sterilizes some rubber and plastic items.
BOILING WATER Boiling is least expensive for use in home. Bacterial spores and some viruses resist boiling. It is not used in hospitals.	The items (e.g., glass baby bottles) should be boiled for at least 15 minutes.

Infection Control to Reduce Reservoirs of Infection

BATHING
- Use soap and water to remove drainage, dried secretions, or excess perspiration.

DRESSING CHANGES
- Change dressings that become wet and/or soiled (see Chapter 49).

CONTAMINATED ARTICLES
- Place tissues, soiled dressings, or soiled linen in moisture-resistant bags for proper disposal.

CONTAMINATED NEEDLES
- Place syringes and uncapped hypodermic needles and intravenous needles in puncture-proof containers, which should be located in client rooms or treatment areas so that exposed, contaminated equipment need not be carried a distance (see Chapter 35).
- Do not recap needles or attempt to break them.

BEDSIDE UNIT
- Keep table surfaces clean and dry.

BOTTLED SOLUTIONS
- Do not leave bottled solutions open for prolonged periods.
- Keep solutions tightly capped.
- Date bottles when opened and discard according to facility policy.

SURGICAL WOUNDS
- Keep drainage tubes and collection bags patent to prevent accumulation of serous fluid under the skin surface.

DRAINAGE BOTTLES AND BAGS
- Empty and dispose of drainage suction bottles according to facility policy.
- Empty all drainage systems on each shift unless otherwise ordered by a physician.
- Never raise a drainage system (e.g., urinary drainage bag) above the level of the site being drained unless it is clamped off.

---

when they sneeze or cough and for providing clients with disposable wipes or tissues to control the spread of microorganisms.

A nurse who has a mild cold and continues to work with clients should wear a mask, especially when changing a dressing or performing a sterile procedure. The same nurse should refrain from working with clients who are highly susceptible to infection.

Another way of controlling the exit of microorganisms is the careful handling of exudate (i.e., urine, feces, emesis, and blood). Contaminated fluids can easily splash while being discarded in toilets or hoppers. The nurse should always wear disposable gloves when handling exudate. Masks, gowns, and eye wear are worn if there is a high probability of splashing and contact with any fluids. The nurse appropriately bags and disposes of soiled items. Laboratory specimens from all clients are handled as if they were infectious.

CONTROL OF TRANSMISSION

Effective control of infection requires a nurse to remain aware of the modes of transmission and ways to control them. In the hospital, home, or extended care facility a client should have a personal set of care items. Sharing bedpans, urinals, bath basins, and eating utensils can easily lead to transmission of infection. Glass thermometers, even when individually used, warrant special care. Because the client's own mucus can become a source for microorganism growth, after each use the glass thermometer is washed in soap and water and dried.

To prevent transmission of microorganisms through indirect contact, soiled items and equipment must be kept from touching the nurse's clothing. A common error is to carry dirty linen in the arms against the uniform. Fluid-resistant linen bags should be used, or soiled linen should be carried with hands held out from the body. Laundry hampers should not be allowed to overflow.

Handwashing. The most important and most basic technique in preventing and controlling transmission of infections is handwashing. **Handwashing** is a vigorous, brief rubbing together of all surfaces of hands lathered in soap, followed by rinsing under a stream of water (Larson, 1995). The purpose is to remove soil and transient organisms from the hands and to reduce total microbial counts over time.

Contaminated hands are a prime cause of cross-infection. For example, a nurse caring for a client who has excessive pulmonary excretions assists the client in expectorating mucus and disposes of the tissues in a bedside container. The client's roommate asks the nurse to open containers of food on the meal tray. The nurse then leaves the client's room to pour a dose of medication due in 5 minutes. If the nurse fails to wash hands before each of these actions, organisms from the first client's mucus could easily be transmitted to the roommate's food and to the medication container.

The decision regarding when handwashing should occur depends on the following: the intensity of contact with clients or contaminated objects; the degree or amount of contamination that could occur with that contact; the susceptibility of the client or the health care worker to infection; and the procedure or activity to be performed (Larson and Lusk, 1985; Ayleffe et al, 1992). For example, if a nurse touches an object that is not visibly soiled, handwashing is not required. In contrast, prolonged and intense contact with a client's wound drainage would require thorough handwashing. Larson (1995) recommends that nurses wash hands in the following situations:

1. When visibly soiled
2. Before and after client contact
3. After contact with a source of microorganisms (blood or body fluids, mucous membrane, nonintact skin, or inanimate objects that might be contaminated)
4. Before the performance of invasive procedures such as placement of intravascular catheters or indwelling catheters (antimicrobial soap recommended)
5. After removing gloves

The Centers for Disease Control (CDC) and Public Health Service note that washing times of at least 10 to 15 seconds (Garner and Favero, 1986) will remove most transient microorganisms from the skin. If hands are visibly soiled, more time may be needed. The frequency of washing also affects the type and number of bacteria on the hands. Larson and Lusk (1985) have found that nurses who washed

Handwashing

STEPS	RATIONALE
1. Use easy-to-reach sink with warm running water, plain soap or antimicrobial soap, paper towels or air dryer.	Running water facilitates removal of organisms. Paper towels are easy to discard.
2. Push wristwatch and long uniform sleeves above wrists. Avoid wearing rings. If worn, remove during washing.	Provides complete access to fingers, hands, wrists. Wearing of rings increases number of microorganisms on hands (Meeker, Rothrock, 1995).
3. Keep fingernails short and filed.	Most microbes on hands come from subungual region (beneath fingernails).
4. Inspect surface of hands and fingers for breaks or cuts in skin and cuticles. Report such lesions when caring for highly susceptible clients.	Open cuts or wounds can harbor high concentrations of microorganisms and may serve as portals of exit, increasing client's exposure to infection, or as portals of entry, increasing nurse's risk of acquiring infection.
5. Stand in front of sink, keeping hands and uniform away from sink surface. (If hands touch sink during handwashing, repeat).	Inside of sink is contaminated area. Reaching over sink increases risk of touching edge, which is contaminated.
6. Turn on water. Press pedals with foot to regulate flow and temperature (see the illustration below) or push knee pedals laterally to control flow and temperature.	When hands contact faucet, they are contaminated. Organisms spread easily from hands to faucet.
7. Avoid splashing water against uniform.	Microorganisms travel and grow in moisture.
8. Regulate flow of water so that temperature is warm.	Warm water removes less of the protective oils than hot water.
9. Wet hands and lower arms thoroughly under running warm water. Keep hands and forearms lower than elbows during washing.	Hands are most contaminated parts to be washed. Water flows from least to most contaminated area, rinsing microorganisms into sink.

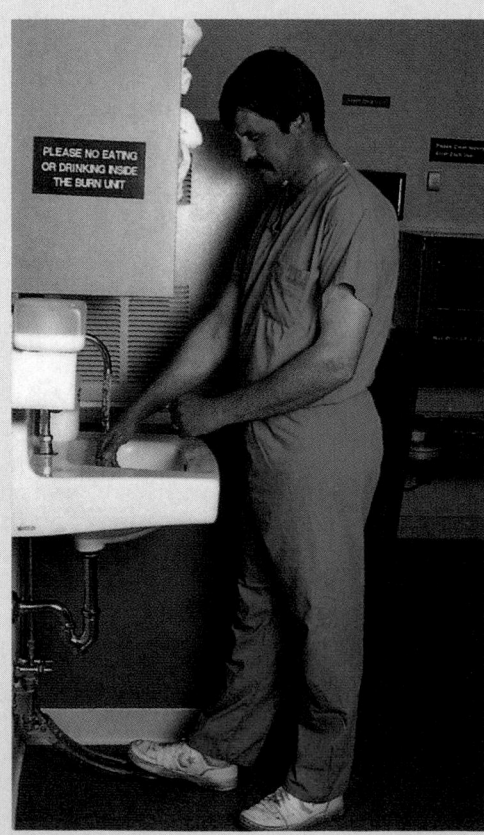

Step 6

Handwashing—cont'd

STEPS	RATIONALE
10. Apply small amount regular or antimicrobial liquid soap to hands, lathering thoroughly. Soap granules and leaflet preparations may be used.	Too much soap can be drying and irritating to skin.
11. Rub hands briskly using friction for at least 10 to 15 sec. Interlace fingers and rub palms and back of hands with circular motion at least five times each (see the illustration below). Keep fingertips pointed down to facilitate removal of microorganisms.	Soap cleanses by emulsifying fat and oil and lowering surface tension. Friction and rubbing mechanically loosen and remove dirt and transient bacteria. Interlacing fingers and thumbs ensures that all surfaces are cleansed.
12. If areas underlying fingernails are soiled, clean them with fingernails of other hand and additional soap or clean orangewood stick. Do not tear or cut skin under or around nail.	

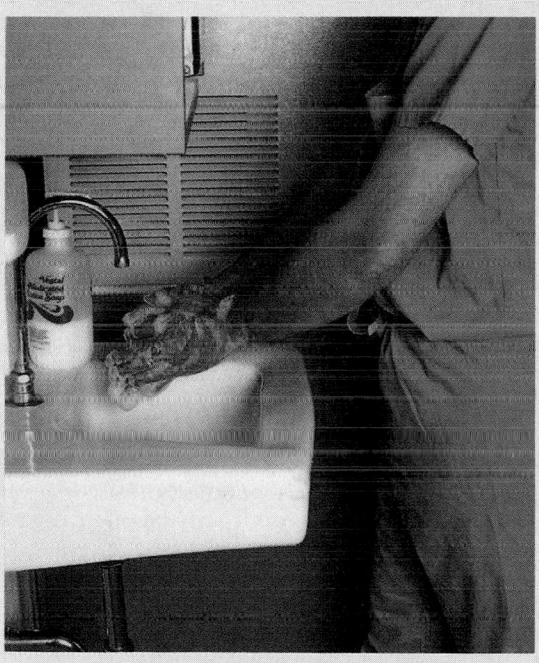

Step 11

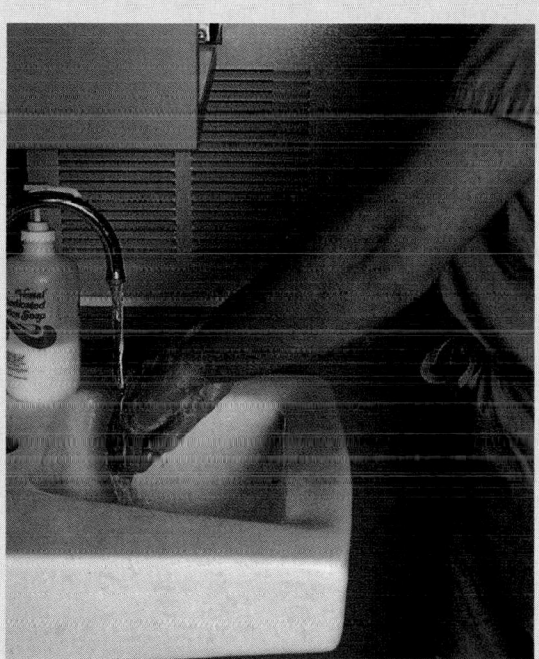

Step 13

13. Rinse hands and wrists thoroughly, keeping hands down below elbows (see the illustration above).	Rinsing mechanically washes away dirt and microorganisms.
14. Optional: repeat steps 10 through 12 but extend period of washing to 1, 2, and 3 min.	Greater the likelihood of hands being contaminated, greater the need for thorough handwashing.
15. Dry hands thoroughly from fingers to wrists and forearms with paper towel or air dryer.	Drying from cleanest (fingertips) to least clean area avoids contamination. Drying hands prevents chapping and roughened skin.
16. If used, discard paper towel in proper receptacle.	Prevents transfer of microorganisms.
17. Turn off water with foot and knee pedals. To turn off hand faucet, use clean, dry paper towel.	Wet towel and hands allow transfer of pathogens by capillary action.

their hands eight times a day were less likely to carry gram-negative bacteria on their hands. Routine handwashing may be performed with soap in any convenient form (bar, leaflets, liquid, or powder).

Use of antimicrobial soap is encouraged when nurses need to reduce total microbial counts on hands. These include situations where nurses are in contact with older adults and clients who are immunosuppressed or have damage to their integumentary system (e.g., wounds or bruises). Additionally, an antimicrobial soap should be used prior to performing an invasive procedure such as care or insertion of an intravascular catheter. There are a number of effective antimicrobial soaps, including chlorohexidine gluconate (CHG), alcohols, and iodophors. Certain antimicrobial soaps can irritate the skin, and the need for antimicrobial soap must be evaluated against potential skin irritation. Procedure 34-1 lists the steps for handwashing.

Plain soap with water can be used for general handwashing; but if it is necessary to kill or inhibit microorganisms such as in a surgical procedure, antiseptic agents should be used (Larson, 1995). Additional alcohol-based handrubs are recommended for use in settings where handwashing facilities are inadequate or inaccessible and hands are not heavily soiled (Larson, 1995).

The nurse instructs clients and visitors about the proper technique and times for handwashing. Teaching handwashing is particularly important if health care is to continue at home. Clients should wash their hands before eating or handling food; after handling contaminated equipment, linen, or organic material; and after elimination. Visitors are encouraged to wash their hands before eating or handling food, after coming in contact with infected clients, and after handling contaminated equipment or organic material.

CONTROL OF PORTALS OF ENTRY

Many measures that control the exit of microorganisms likewise control the entrance of pathogens. Maintaining the integrity of skin and mucous membranes reduces the chances of microorganisms reaching a host. The client's skin should be kept well lubricated by using hand lotion as appropriate. Immobilized and debilitated clients are particularly susceptible to skin breakdown. Clients should not be positioned on tubes or objects that might cause breaks in the skin. Dry, wrinkle-free linen also reduces the chances of skin breakdown. Turning and positioning are needed before a client's skin becomes reddened. Frequent oral hygiene prevents drying of mucous membranes. A water-soluble ointment keeps the client's lips well lubricated.

After elimination, a woman should clean the rectum and perineum by wiping from the urinary meatus toward the rectum. Cleansing in a direction from the least to the most contaminated area helps reduce genitourinary infections.

Clients, health care personnel, and even housekeepers are at risk for acquiring infections from accidental needle sticks. After administering an injection or inserting an intravenous catheter, the nurse should carefully dispose of uncapped needles in a puncture-resistant box (see Chapter 35). A stray needle lying in bed linen or carelessly thrown into a wastebasket is a prime source for blood-borne pathogens. Hepatitis B and hepatitis C are the infections most commonly transmitted by contaminated needles. A

Hepatitis B Vaccination and Follow-up After Exposure

- Health care employers shall make available the hepatitis B vaccine and vaccination series to all employees who may have occupational exposures. Evaluation and follow-up care will be available to all employees who have been exposed.
- All medical evaluations and procedures, including the vaccine and vaccination series and evaluation after exposure (prophylaxis) are made available at no cost to at-risk employees.
- A confidential written medical evaluation will be available to employees with exposure incidents.
- Hepatitis B vaccinations will be made available to employees within 10 working days of assignment.

From Occupational Safety and Health Act of 1991, Federal Register, 1991.

---

needle stick should be reported immediately. Health care agencies require the victim of a needle stick to complete an injury report and seek appropriate treatment (see the box above).

Another cause for entrance of microorganisms into a host is improper handling and management of urinary catheters and drainage sets (see Chapter 46). The point of connection between a catheter and drainage tube should remain closed and intact. As long as such systems are closed, their contents are considered sterile. Outflow of spigots on drainage bags should also remain closed and cleansed to prevent entrance of bacteria. Movement of the catheter at the urethra should be minimized to reduce chances of microorganisms ascending the urethra into the bladder.

The nurse may care for clients with closed drainage systems that collect wound drainage, bile, or other body fluids. In each example the site from which a drainage tube exits should remain clear of excess moisture or accumulated drainage. All tubing should remain connected throughout use. Drainage receptacles should only be opened when it is necessary to discard or measure volume of drainage.

At times the nurse obtains specimens from drainage tubes or inserts needles into intravenous tubing ports. The nurse disinfects tubes and ports by wiping outward with alcohol or an iodine solution before entering the system. Temporarily placing squares of sterile gauze around the ends of an opened drainage tube such as a urinary catheter adds further protection against bacteria. However, keeping drainage tubes closed and secure is the best practice.

A final method for reducing the entrance of microorganisms is the technique for cleansing wounds (see Chapter 49). The wound itself is considered to be sterile. To prevent entrance of microorganisms into the wound, the nurse should clean outward from a wound site. When applying a disinfectant or cleaning with soap and water, the nurse wipes around the wound edge first and then cleans outward. A clean gauze should be used for each revolution around the wound's circumference.

PROTECTION OF THE SUSCEPTIBLE HOST

A client's resistance to infection improves as the nurse protects normal body defenses against infection. The nurse

Infection Control: Protecting the Susceptible Host

PROTECTING NORMAL DEFENSE MECHANISMS

- Regular bathing removes transient microorganisms from the skin's surface. Lubrication helps keep the skin hydrated and intact.
- Regular oral hygiene removes proteins in the saliva that attract microorganisms. Flossing removes tartar and plaque that can cause germ infection.
- Maintenance of adequate fluid intake promotes normal urine formation and a resultant outflow of urine to flush the bladder and urethral lining of microorganisms.
- For physically dependent or immobilized clients, the nurse encourages routine coughing and deep breathing to keep lower airways clear of mucus.
- The nurse encourages proper immunization of children or adult clients who become exposed to certain infectious microorganisms. Children are vaccinated for smallpox, measles, mumps, rubella, and diphtheria. Adults should have tetanus-diphtheria boosters every 10 years. Influenza vaccines are recommended for health care workers. Older adults should regularly receive influenza and pneumococcal vaccines.

MAINTAINING HEALING PROCESSES

- The nurse promotes intake of adequate fluids and a well-balanced diet containing essential proteins, vitamins, carbohydrates, and fats. The nurse also uses measures to increase the client's appetite.
- The nurse promotes a client's comfort and sleep so that energy stores are replaced daily.
- The nurse assists the client in learning techniques to reduce stress.

also intervenes to maintain the body's normal reparative processes (see the box above).

Isolation Practices The risk of transmitting nosocomial infection or infectious disease among clients is high. When a client has a potential or known source of infection, health care workers become alerted and follow infection-control practices. However, health care workers may not be aware that clients have infections. The majority of organisms causing nosocomial infections are found in the **colonized** body substances of clients regardless of whether a culture has confirmed infection and a diagnosis has been made (Jackson and Lynch, 1991). Body substances such as feces, urine, mucus, and wound drainage always contain potentially infectious organisms.

Isolation or barrier precautions include the appropriate use of gowns, gloves, masks, eyewear, and other protective devices or clothing. Barrier protection is indicated for use with all clients because the risk for infection transmission can be unknown. Due to the increased attention to the prevention of blood-borne pathogens and tuberculosis, the Centers for Disease Control and Prevention (CDC) and the Occupational Safety and Health Administration (OSHA) have stressed the importance of barrier protection.

In 1983, CDC published guidelines for isolation that required decision making on the part of the user. Hospitals were given the choice of selecting between two systems: category-specific or disease-specific isolation. The need for a private room also was based on the decision of the user

(Garner and Simmons, 1984). Some clients were "over isolated" while others were "under isolated." As new information regarding disease transmission became available, CDC updated the guidelines. For example, CDC has modified the recommendations for barrier protection for prevention of tuberculosis transmission (CDC, 1994a).

In 1988, the Body Substance Isolation (BSI) system was developed and stressed generic precautions for all clients (Jackson and Lynch, 1992). This system emphasizes the potential infectiousness of moist body substances. Jackson and Lynch (1990) explained that BSI could prevent transmission of colonized body substances as a source of infection.

Another system, Universal Precautions (UP), recommended that barriers and procedures be used to limit an individual's exposure to blood-borne pathogens. In 1991, OSHA published regulations that required employers to use UP as a minimum standard of practice (OSHA, 1991). However, other types of isolation were needed. For example, clients with respiratory illness would also have to be in respiratory isolation. Additionally, there was considerable confusion regarding which body fluids or substances were required under BSI or UP. There was a continual lack of agreement about the importance of handwashing and the use of gloves.

CDC recognized the need for new isolation guidelines that combined the major features of UP and BSI and updated the previous category-specific isolation into a transmission-based precaution. With this in mind, the CDC issued new isolation guidelines that contain two tiers of approach (Garner, 1996). The first and most important tier contains precautions designed to care for all clients in health care facilities regardless of their diagnosis or presumed infectiousness. This new isolation will be called Standard Precautions and combines the major features of UP and BSI. These precautions apply to (1) blood; (2) all body fluids, secretions, and excretions *except sweat* regardless of whether they contain blood; (3) nonintact skin; and (4) mucous membranes. These precautions promote handwashing and use of gloves, masks, eye protection, or gowns when appropriate for client contact (Table 34-7).

The second tier condenses the old disease-specific and categories approach to isolation into new transmission categories: airborne, droplet, and contact precautions. These precautions are designed for specific clients with highly transmissible or epidemiologically important pathogens.

The CDC further recommends the use of Standard Precautions for all immunocompromised clients. In addition, transmission-based precautions may be needed to reduce infection risks for these clients. Users of the Isolation Guidelines are referred to additional CDC documents to prevent nosocomial aspergillosis and Legionnaire's disease in immunocompromised clients (CDC, 1994a) and vancomycin-resistant organisms (HICPAC, CDC, 1995).

With the increase of numbers of reported cases of tuberculosis (TB) in the United States, CDC (1990) issued guidelines for prevention of transmission of TB in health care facilities. These and latter revisions (CDC, 1994a) stress the early identification and treatment of persons with known or suspected TB, facility risk assessment for TB exposures, engineering control, and proper isolation techniques. In addition, OSHA (1993) issued a mandate requiring health

Table 34-7	CDC Isolation Guidelines

STANDARD PRECAUTIONS (TIER ONE)

Standard precautions apply to blood, all body fluids, secretions, excretions (except sweat), nonintact skin, and mucous membranes.

Hands are washed between client contacts; after contact with blood, body fluids, secretions, and excretions and after contact with equipment or articles contaminated by them; and immediately after gloves are removed.

Gloves are worn when touching blood, body fluids, secretions, excretions, nonintact skin, mucous membranes, or contaminated items. Gloves should be removed and hands washed between client care.

Masks, eye protection, or face shields are worn if client care activities may generate splashes or sprays of blood or body fluid.

Gowns are worn if soiling of clothing is likely from blood or body fluid. Wash hands after removing gown.

Client care equipment is properly cleaned and reprocessed and single-use items are discarded.

Contaminated linen is placed in leak-proof bag and handled as to prevent skin and mucous membrane exposure.

All sharp instruments and needles are discarded in a puncture-resistant container. CDC recommends that needles be disposed or uncapped or use a mechanical device for recapping.

A private room is unnecessary unless the client's hygiene is unacceptable. Check with an Infection Control Professional.

TRANSMISSION CATEGORIES (TIER TWO)

CATEGORY	DISEASE	BARRIER PROTECTION
Airborne precautions	Droplet nuclei smaller than 5 microns; measles; chicken pox (Varicella); disseminated varicella zoster; pulmonary or laryngeal TB	Private room, negative airflow of at least six exchanges per hour, mask or respiratory protection device* (see CDC TB Guidelines)
Droplet precautions	Droplets larger than 5 microns, Diphtheria (pharyngeal); Rubella; Streptococcal pharyngitis, pneumonia, or scarlet fever in infants and young children; Pertussis; mumps; mycoplasma pneumonia; meningococcal pneumonia or sepsis; pneumonic plague	Private room or cohort clients; mask
Contact precautions	Direct client or environmental contact; colonization or infection with multidrug-resistant organism; respiratory syncytial virus; shigella and other enteric pathogens; major wound infections; herpes simplex; scabies, varicella zoster (disseminated)	Private room or cohort clients; gloves, gowns

Modified from Garner JS: Guidelines for isolation precautions for hospitals, *Infect Control Hosp Epidemiol* 17(1):54, 1996.

care facilities to follow CDC guidelines and required that health care workers (HCW) be offered free TB skin test screening programs and respiratory protective devices. Airborne precautions are required for TB in addition to the following:

1. Single-client room maintained under negative pressure
2. Door must be kept closed except when entering or exiting room
3. Negative pressure should be monitored daily (smoke tube or differential pressure-sensing devices)
4. Minimum of six air exchanges per hour (existing facilities) and minimum of 12 air exchanges (new construction facilities)
5. Possible use of ultraviolet germicide irradiation or HEPA filter, which may reduce the number of droplet nuclei
6. Personal respiratory protective devices capable of filtration of $\geq 95\%$ efficiency when entering AFB room (Fig. 34-3)
7. Ability to qualitatively or quantitatively fit-test to obtain a face-seal leakage of $\leq 10\%$
8. Client known or suspected of having TB should wear a mask when out of room

Regardless of the type of isolation system, the nurse must follow the following basic principles:

1. Nurse should wash hands thoroughly before entering and leaving the room of a client in isolation.
2. Contaminated supplies and equipment should be disposed of in a manner that prevents spread of microorganisms to other persons as indicated by the mode of transmission of the organism.
3. Knowledge of a disease process and the mode of infection transmission should be applied when using protective barriers.
4. All persons who might be exposed during transport of a client outside the isolation room must be protected.

Psychological Implications of Isolation. When a client requires isolation in a private room, a sense of loneliness may develop because normal social relationships become disrupted. This situation can be psychologically harmful, especially for children.

As a result of the infectious process, clients' body images are altered. They may feel unclean, rejected, lonely, or guilty. Infection prevention and control practices further intensify these beliefs of difference or undesirability. Isolation in a private room limits sensory contact. Unless the nurse acts to minimize feelings of psychological and physical isolation, clients' emotional states can interfere with recovery.

Before isolation measures are instituted, the client and family must understand the nature of the disease or condi-

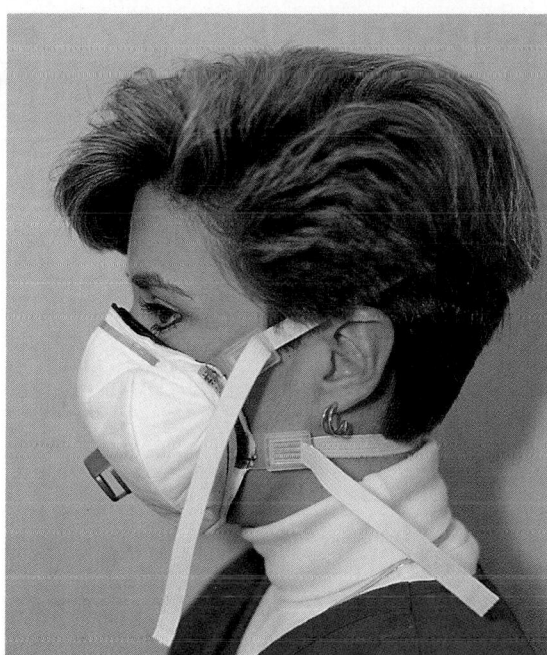

Fig. 34-3 Disposable HEPA air-purifying respirator.

tion, the purposes of isolation, and steps for carrying out specific precautions. If they are able to participate in maintaining infection prevention, the chances of reducing the spread of infection are increased. The client and family should be taught to wash hands and use barrier protection if appropriate. Each procedure should be demonstrated, and the client and family should be given an opportunity for practice. It is also important to explain how infectious organisms can be transmitted so that the client understands the difference between contaminated and clean objects.

The nurse also takes measures to improve the client's sensory stimulation during isolation. The room environment should be clean and pleasant. Drapes or shades should be opened, and excess supplies and equipment removed. The nurse must listen to the client's concerns or interests. If the nurse rushes through care or shows a lack of interest, the client will feel rejected and even more isolated. Mealtime is a particularly good opportunity for conversation. Providing comfort measures such as repositioning, a back massage, or a tepid sponge bath increases physical stimulation. If the client's condition permits, the nurse should encourage the client to walk and sit up in a chair.

The nurse must explain to family the client's risk of depression or loneliness. Visiting family members should be encouraged to avoid expressions or actions that convey revulsion or disgust. The nurse discusses ways to provide meaningful stimulation.

Protective Environment. When precautions are in place because of a respiratory infection, a private room serves to control microorganisms within the environment. Private rooms used for isolation may have negative-pressure air flow to prevent infectious particles from flowing out of the room. There are also special rooms with positive-pressure air flow that are used for highly susceptible clients such as transplant recipients. On the door or

wall outside the room, the nurse posts a card listing precautions for the client's isolation category. The card is a handy reference for health care personnel and visitors and alerts anyone who might enter the room accidentally that special precautions must be followed.

The isolation room or an adjoining anteroom should contain handwashing, bathing, and toilet facilities. Soap and antiseptic solutions are made available. Personnel and visitors should wash their hands before coming to the client's bedside and again before leaving the room.

The nurse makes certain that each isolation room contains a impervious bag for soiled or contaminated linen, as well as a trash container with plastic liners. Impervious receptacles prevent transmission of microorganisms by preventing seepage to and soiling of the outside surface. A disposable impervious container should be available in the room to discard used needles, syringes, and sharp objects.

The nurse must remain aware of infection prevention and control techniques while working with clients in protected environments. The nurse should feel comfortable performing all procedures and yet remain conscious of infection-control principles. Depending upon the microorganism and the mode of transmission, the nurse must evaluate what articles or equipment can be taken into an isolation room. For example, CDC has recommended the dedicated use of noncritical items such as stethoscopes, sphygmomanometers, or rectal thermometers in the room of a client infected or colonized with vancomycin-resistent enterococci (VRE). If these devices are used on other clients, they must first be adequately cleaned and disinfected (HICPAC, CDC, 1995). If after bringing any article into the room, the nurse exposes an article to infected material and then touches or removes the article, the risk of transmitting infection to other clients or personnel is increased. Procedure 34-2 describes the procedures commonly performed in an isolation room.

PROTECTION FOR PERSONNEL

Barrier protections should be readily available for personnel entering an isolation room. Sometimes a special anteroom or an isolation cart in the hallway holds supplies of gowns, masks, and gloves.

Gowns. The primary reason for gowning is to prevent soiling clothes during contact with the client. Gowns protect health care personnel and visitors from coming in contact with infected material and blood or body fluid. Gowns are required for contact isolation. Some gowns are reusable and some are disposable.

Reusable isolation gowns open at the back and have ties at the neck and waist to keep them closed and secure. Gowns should be long enough to cover all outer garments. Long sleeves with tight-fitting cuffs provide added protection. There is no special technique required for applying clean gowns as long as they are fastened securely. However, the nurse must carefully remove gowns to minimize contamination of the hands and uniform and then discard them after removal (Procedure 34-2).

Masks. Masks should be worn when splashing or spraying of blood or body fluid into the face is anticipated. Additionally, the mask protects the nurse from inhaling microorganisms from a client's respiratory tract and prevents transmission of pathogens from the nurse's respiratory tract

PROCEDURE 34-2

Caring for a Client Under Isolation Precautions

STEPS	RATIONALE
1. Review the precautions for isolation.	Mode of transmission for infectious microorganisms determines types and degree of precautions followed.
2. Explain purpose of isolation and precautions necessary to client, family, visitors, offering opportunity for questions.	Improves client's ability to participate in care and minimizes anxiety.
3. Wash hands.	Reduces transmission of microorganisms.
4. Apply gown, mask, gloves, and goggles as appropriate.	Barrier protection prevents transmission of organisms from nurse to client and protects nurse from contact with infectious pathogens.
a. Apply gown, being sure it covers all outer garments. Pull sleeves down to wrist. Tie securely at neck and waist (see the illustration below).	
b. Apply disposable gloves. If worn with gown, bring cuffs over edge of gown sleeves.	
c. Apply surgical mask around mouth and nose; tie securely.	
d. Apply goggles to fit snugly around face and eyes.	Goggles are worn when exposure to splashing or spray of body fluids is likely.
5. Assess if items can be brought into a client's room.	If organism transmission can occur from inanimate objects, use dedicated equipment.
6. Enter client's room. Arrange supplies and equipment. (If equipment will be removed from room for reuse, place on clean paper towel.)	Prevents contamination of items.
7. Assess vital signs:	
a. If equipment remains in room, proceed to assess vital signs by routine procedures. Avoid contact of stethoscope or blood pressure cuff with infective material.	Helps avoid contact of clean items with contaminated environment in isolation room.

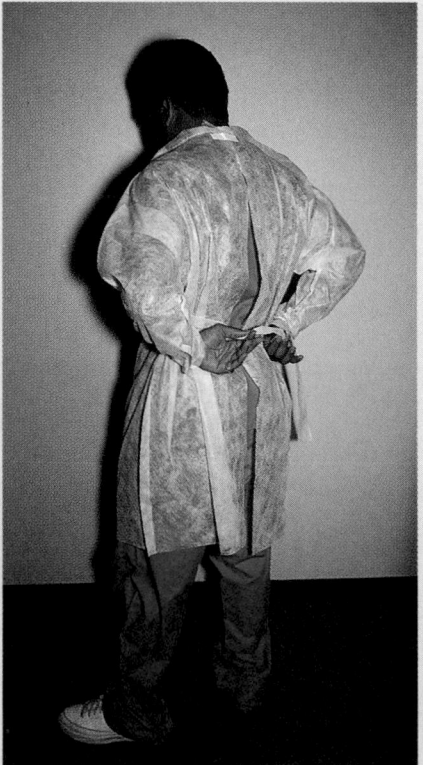

Step 4a

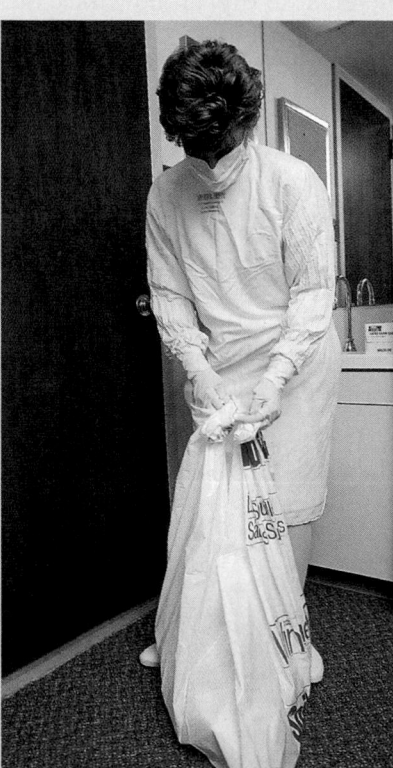

Step 12b

Caring for a Client Under Isolation Precautions—cont'd

STEPS	RATIONALE
b. If stethoscope is to be reused, clean diaphragm or bell with alcohol. Set aside on clean surface.	
c. Individual or disposable thermometers should be used.	
8. Administer medication (see Chapter 35):	
a. Give oral medication in wrapper or cup.	Supplies are handled and discarded to minimize transfer of microorganisms.
b. Dispose of wrapper or cup in plastic-lined receptacle.	
c. Administer injection, being sure gloves are worn.	
d. Discard syringe and uncapped needle into special container. If reusable syringe (e.g., Carpuject) is used, dispose of inner cartridge and needle in special container.	
9. Administer hygiene (see Chapter 40):	
a. Avoid allowing your gown to become wet, carry washbasin outward away from gown, avoid leaning against wet table top.	Moisture allows organisms to travel through gown to uniform.
b. Assist client in removing gown; discard in impervious linen bag.	
c. Remove linen from bed; if excessively soiled, avoid contact with your gown. Dispose in special linen bag.	Linen soiled by client's body fluids is disposed of to prevent contact with clean items
d. Provide clean bed linen and set of towels.	
e. Change gloves if they become excessively soiled and further care is necessary.	
10. Collect specimens:	
a. Place specimen containers on clean paper towel in client's bathroom.	Specimens of blood and body fluids are placed in well-constructed containers with secure lids to prevent leaks during transport.
b. Follow procedure (Table 34-8) for collecting specimens of body fluids.	
c. Transfer specimen to container without soiling outside of container. Place container in plastic bag.	
d. Check label on specimen for accuracy. Send to laboratory (warning labels may be used, depending on hospital policy).	

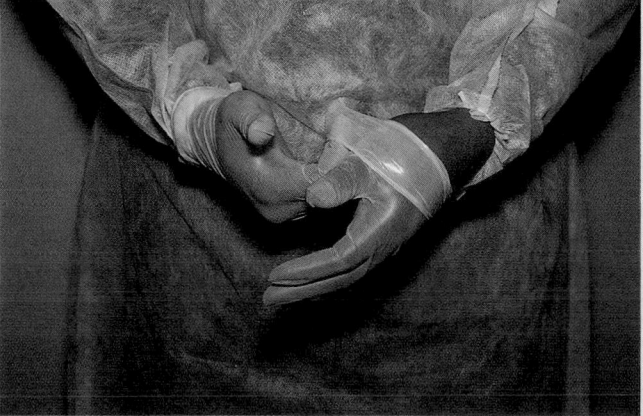

Step 14b

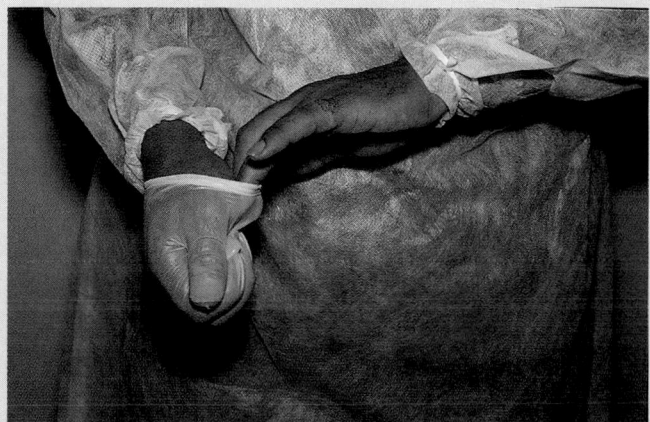

Step 14b

Continued.

PROCEDURE 34-2

Caring for a Client Under Isolation Precautions—cont'd

STEPS	RATIONALE
11. Explain to client when you plan to return to room.	Includes client in care plan.
12. Dispose of linen and trash bags as they become full:	Linen or refuse should be totally contained to prevent exposure of personnel to infective material.
a. Use single bags to contain soiled articles if they are impervious to moisture and are sturdy.	
b. Tie bags securely at top in knot (see the illustration on p. 764).	
13. Resupply room as needed.	Limited trips of personnel into and out of room reduce your and client's exposure to microorganisms.
14. Leave isolation room:	
a. Remove eyewear or goggles.	
b. Untie gown at waist. Remove one glove by grasping cuff and pulling glove inside out over hand (see the illustration on p. 765). Discard glove. With ungloved hand, tuck finger inside cuff of remaining glove and pull it off, inside out (see the illustration on p. 765).	Gloves and gown are removed by avoiding contamination of hands.
c. Untie mask strings, drop mask into trash receptacle.	
d. Untie neck strings of gown. Allow gown to fall from shoulders. Remove hands from sleeves, without touching outside of gown. Hold gown inside at shoulder seams and fold inside out (see the illustration below). Discard in laundry bag.	
e. Wash hands minimum of 10 sec.	
f. Leave room and close door, if necessary.	Door should be closed if client in negative airflow room.

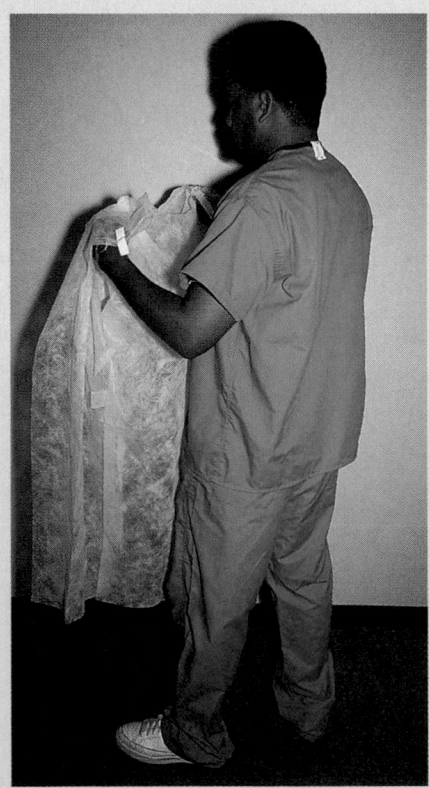

Step 14d

Applying a Surgical Mask

PROCEDURE 34-3

STEPS	RATIONALE

1. Find top edge of mask (usually has thin, metal strip along edge).

   Pliable metal fits snugly against bridge of nose.

2. Hold mask by top two strings or loops. Tie two top ties at top of back of head with ties above ears (see the illustration below) (alternative: slip loops over each ear).

   Position of ties at top of head provides tight fit. Ties over ears may cause irritation.

3. Tie two lower ties snugly around neck with mask well under chin (see the illustration below).

   Prevents escape of microorganisms through sides of mask as you talk or breathe.

4. Gently pinch upper metal band around bridge of nose.

   Prevents microorganisms from escaping around nose.

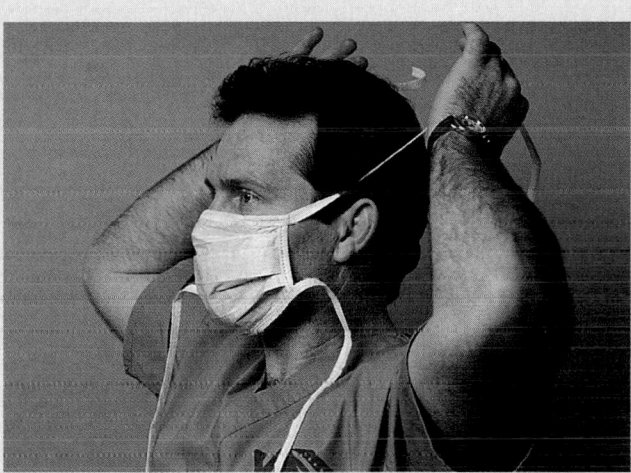

Step 2

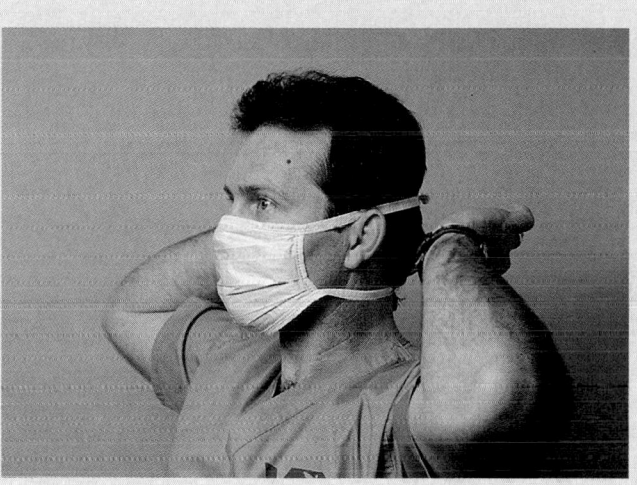

Step 3

to the client. The surgical mask protects a wearer from inhaling large-particle aerosols that travel short distances (3 feet) and small-particle droplet nuclei that remain suspended in the air and travel longer distances. At times a client who is susceptible to infection wears a mask to prevent inhalation of pathogens. Clients in droplet or airborne precautions who are transported outside of their rooms, should wear masks to protect other clients and personnel.

According to the CDC, masks may prevent transmission of infection by direct contact with mucous membranes (CDC, 1994a). A mask discourages the wearer from touching the eyes, nose, or mouth.

A properly applied mask fits snugly over the mouth and nose so that pathogens and body fluids cannot enter or escape through the sides (Procedure 34-3). If a person wears glasses, the top edge of the mask fits below the glasses so that they will not cloud over as the person exhales. Talking should be kept to a minimum while wearing a mask to reduce respiratory air flow. A mask that has become moist does not provide a barrier to microorganisms and thus is ineffective. It should be discarded. A mask should not be reused. Clients and family members should be warned that a mask can cause a sensation of smothering. If family members become uncomfortable, they should leave the room and discard the mask.

Special respiratory protective devices or masks are required when caring for a client with known or suspected tuberculosis (CDC, 1994a; OSHA, 1994). The nurse should be aware of agency policy regarding the type of respiratory protective device required.

Gloves. Gloves prevent the transmission of pathogens by direct and indirect contact. The CDC (Williams, 1983) cites the following reasons for wearing gloves:

1. Reduces possibility of personnel coming in contact with infectious organisms that infect clients (e.g., handling contaminated dressings or cleaning an incontinent client with hepatitis)
2. Reduces likelihood that personnel will transmit their own endogenous flora to clients
3. Reduces possibility that personnel will become transiently colonized with microorganisms that can be transmitted to other clients (Transient colonization can usually be prevented with handwashing.)

Nurses apply gloves when there is risk of exposure to infected material. Specifically, gloves are recommended when nurses have scratches or breaks in the skin, when performing venipuncture or finger or heel sticks, when they are at risk for spilling blood or other body fluids on the hands, and when they are inexperienced (CDC, 1988). The CDC further recommends gloves be worn only once and then discarded. In most cases, disposable, single-use gloves are worn. When full protective apparel is needed, the nurse first applies a mask, washes and dries hands, applies a gown and then applies gloves. Disposable gloves are easily applied and designed to fit either hand. The glove's thin rubber, however, can be easily torn. The glove cuffs should be pulled up over the wrists or cuffs of a gown. Larson (1989) stresses that hands must be washed after removing gloves.

After coming in contact with any infected material, the nurse should change gloves if care is not completed. If the nurse does not plan to have more contact with the client, reapplying gloves is unnecessary. Researchers have determined that repeated manipulations of gloved hands can allow bacteria to pass through the rubber.

Family members often believe that they can touch any object after they have applied gloves. The nurse should explain that gloves can also become contaminated after touching infected material or another contaminated object. It is very important to wash hands after removing gloves.

Protective Eyewear. When participating in an invasive procedure that creates droplets or splashing or spraying of blood or other body fluids, a nurse must wear protective eyewear, mask, or face shield (Garner, 1996). Examples of invasive procedures include irrigation of a large abdominal wound or insertion of an arterial catheter in which the nurse assists a physician. Eyewear may be available in the form of plastic glasses or goggles (Fig. 34-4). The eyewear should fit snugly around the face so that fluids cannot enter between the face and glasses.

Specimen Collection. Many laboratory studies may be required when a client is suspected of having an infectious disease. Body fluids and secretions suspected of containing infectious organisms are collected for culture and sensitivity tests. The specimen is placed in a medium that promotes growth of organisms. A laboratory technologist then identifies the microorganisms growing in the culture. Additional test results indicate antibiotics to which the organisms are resistant or sensitive. Sensitivity reports determine the antibiotics used in treatment.

The nurse obtains all culture specimens using disposable

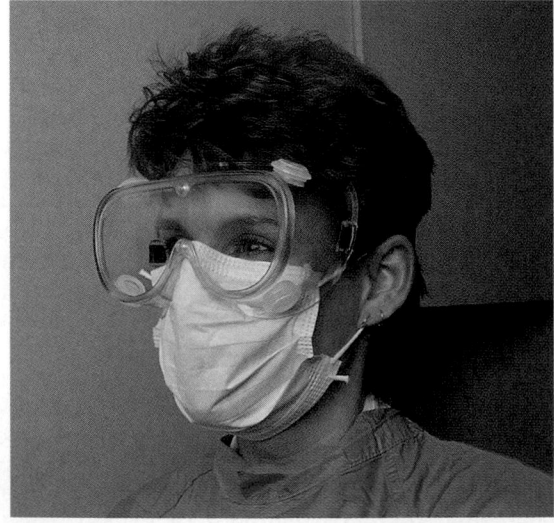

Fig. 34-4 Nurse wearing protective goggles and mask.

gloves and sterile equipment. Collecting fresh material from the site of infection, such as in the case of wound drainage, ensures that the specimen is not contaminated by neighboring microbes. All specimen containers should be sealed tightly to prevent spillage and contamination of the outside of the container. Table 34-8 describes techniques for collecting specimens from the client with a suspected infection.

Bagging Articles or Linen. Nurses use special bagging procedures for removing contaminated items from the client's environment. Bagging articles prevents accidental exposure of personnel to contaminated articles and prevents contamination of the surrounding environment.

The CDC recommends a single bag for discarding or wrapping items if the bag is impervious and sturdy and if the article can be placed in the bag without contaminating the outside of the bag. The CDC suggests the following guidelines (Weinstein et al, 1989) for handling isolation linen:

1. Soiled linen should be placed in an impervious laundry bag in the client's room.
2. The bag should be labeled, or it should be a specific color.
3. Linen requires less handling if the bag is soluble in hot water. However, such a bag may need to be double bagged because it punctures or tears easily.

The CDC recommends double bagging if it is impossible to prevent contamination of the bag's outer surface. Double bagging is not routine in hospitals. Studies have shown that this procedure is not necessary to control infection (Maki et al, 1986; Weinstein et al, 1989). Use of one standard-sized linen bag that is not overfilled, is tied securely, and if intact is adequate to prevent infection transmission. The same rule applies to trash bags.

Transporting Clients. Clients infected with airborne organisms should leave their rooms only for essential purposes such as diagnostic procedures or surgery. Before transferring clients to wheelchairs or stretchers, the nurse gives them clean gowns to serve as robes. Clients infected by organisms transmitted via the respiratory tract must also wear masks. Personnel transporting these clients should also wear barrier protection as needed.

At times a client being transported may drain body fluids onto a stretcher or wheelchair. When this occurs, the nurse must be sure to have the equipment cleaned after the client returns to the room. An extra layer of sheets may be used to cover the stretcher or seat of the wheelchair.

Personnel in diagnostic or procedural areas or the operating room should be notified that the client is on isolation precautions. The nurse explains ways the client can help prevent transmission of infection during transport. A client on respiratory isolation is given tissues and a bag to allow proper disposal of secretions. The nurse records the type of isolation on the client's chart.

Role of the Infection Control Professional

Many hospitals employ professionals, most of whom are nurses, who are specially trained in infection prevention and control. These individuals are responsible for advising hospital personnel in prevention and control practices and for monitoring infection outbreaks within the hospi-

Table 34-8	Specimen Collection Techniques	
AMOUNT NEEDED*	COLLECTION DEVICE*	SPECIMEN COLLECTION AND TRANSFER
WOUND CULTURE		
As much as possible (after cleaning skin to remove flora)	Cotton-tipped swab or syringe	Place clean test tube or culturette tube on clean paper towel. Wearing gloves, swab center of wound site, grasp collection tube by holding it with paper towel. Carefully insert swab without touching outside of tube. After washing hands and securing tube's top, transfer labeled tube into bag for transport to laboratory.
BLOOD CULTURE		
10 ml per culture bottle, from two different venipuncture sites (Volume may differ based on collection containers and institutional policy)	Syringes and culture media bottles	Perform venipuncture at two different sites to decrease likelihood of both specimens being contaminated by skin flora. Inject 10 ml of blood into each bottle. Wash hands. Secure tops of bottles, label specimens, and send to laboratory.
STOOL CULTURE		
Small amount, approximately size of a walnut	Clean cup with seal top (not necessary to be sterile) and tongue blade	Place cup on clean paper towel in client's bathroom. Wearing gloves, collect needed amount of feces from bedpan. Using tongue blade, transfer feces to cup without touching cup's outside surface. Wash hands and place seal on cup. Transfer specimen cup into clean bag for transport to laboratory.
URINE CULTURE		
1-5 ml	Syringe and sterile cup	Place cup or tube on clean towel in client's bathroom. Use syringe to collect specimen if client has an indwelling catheter. Have client follow procedure to obtain clean-voided specimen (see Chapter 46) if not catheterized. Wearing gloves, transfer urine into sterile container by injecting urine from syringe or pouring it from used container. Wash hands and secure top of labeled container. Transfer labeled specimen into clean bag for transport to laboratory.

*Agency policies may differ on type of containers, amount of specimen material required, and bagging.

tal. Duties of an infection control professional include the following:

1. Provide staff education on infection prevention and control
2. Develop and review infection prevention and control policies and procedures
3. Recommend appropriate isolation procedures
4. Screen client records for community-acquired infections
5. Consult with employee health departments concerning recommendations to prevent and control the spread of infection among personnel, such as tuberculosis testing
6. Gather statistics regarding the **epidemiology** of nosocomial infections
7. Notify public health department of incidences of communicable diseases
8. Confer with all hospital departments to investigate unusual events or clusters of infection
9. Educate clients and families
10. Identify infection-control problems with equipment
11. Monitor antibiotic-resistant organisms in the institution

An infection control professional can be a valuable resource for controlling nosocomial infections.

Infection Prevention and Control for Hospital Personnel

Health care workers are continually at risk for exposure to infectious microorganisms. The Occupational Safety and Health Act of 1991 established rules and regulations to protect employees from infectious hazards in the workplace (OSHA, 1991). The OSHA guidelines are incorporated into the policies and procedures of health care institutions. Elements of the OSHA guidelines include the following:

1. Exposure-control plan. Institutions must have exposure-control plans designed to eliminate or minimize employee exposure. The plan must be accessible to all employees. The plan also describes how to avoid exposure to infectious agents, such as when to use protective equipment.
2. Compliance with standard precautions. Employees are to follow precautions to prevent contact with blood or other infectious materials during the routine care of clients. Personal protective equipment must be provided at no cost to employees who are at risk for exposure.
3. Housekeeping. Workplaces are to be maintained in a clean and sanitary condition. Routine cleaning and decontamination procedures are established.
4. High-risk exposure. If health care workers have par-

enteral (needle stick) or mucous membrane exposure to blood or other infectious body fluids, the incident should be reported immediately. Evaluation and preventive treatment for hepatitis B and HIV are critical.

5. Training. Employers will ensure that all employees with risk of occupational exposure participate in a training program. The program will present the exposure-control plan for the institution and specifically explain the measures to be taken by employees for their safety. Written policies and guidelines must be provided for all personnel with respect to infection prevention and infection control activities (JCAHO, 1995).

Client Education

Often clients must learn to use infection-control practices at home (see the box below). Preventive technique becomes almost second nature to the nurse who practices it daily. However, the client is less aware of factors that promote the spread of infection or ways to prevent its transmission. The home environment does not always lend itself to infection prevention. Often a nurse must help a client adapt with the resources available to maintain hygienic techniques. Generally clients in a home care setting have a decreased risk of infection because of decreased exposure to resistant organisms and fewer invasive procedures.

After clients are at home, nurses determine their compli-

CLIENT TEACHING
for Infection Control

OBJECTIVE
- Client will assume self-care using proper infection-control techniques.

TEACHING STRATEGIES
- Instruct client about cleaning equipment using soap and water and disinfecting with an appropriate disinfectant.
- Demonstrate proper handwashing, explaining that it should be done before and after all treatments and when infected body fluids are contacted.
- Instruct client about signs and symptoms of wound infection.
- For clients who receive tube feedings at home, explain the importance of preparing enough formula for only 8 hours (commercially prepared) or 4 hours (home prepared). Tell client that contaminated enteral feeding can cause infections. Rinse feeding bag and tubing with mild soap and water daily and dry.
- Instruct client to place contaminated dressings and other disposable items containing infectious body fluids in impervious plastic bags. Place needles in metal containers such as soda cans and tape the openings shut.
- Clean noticeably soiled linen separate from other laundry. Wash in water that is as hot as the fabric will tolerate. Add 1 cup of bleach to detergent. Set dryer temperature as high as fabric will allow.

EVALUATION
- Ask client or family member to describe techniques used to reduce transmission of infection
- Have client demonstrate select techniques.
- Ask client to explain risks for infection based on the condition.

ance with infection-control practices. The nurse educates clients about infection and techniques to prevent or control its spread. Topics the nurse can discuss in a teaching session include the following:

1. Clients' susceptibility to infection
2. The chain of infection with specific reference to means of transmission
3. Hygienic practices that minimize organism growth and spread
4. Preventive health care (e.g., diet, immunizations, and exercise)
5. Proper methods for handling and storage of food
6. Family members who are at risk for acquiring infection

Family members caring for such a client must be involved in the teaching plan. The nurse teaches clients and family members a common sense approach to controlling and preventing infection.

Surgical Asepsis

Surgical asepsis or sterile technique requires a nurse to use different precautions from those of medical asepsis. Surgical asepsis requires the absence of all microorganisms, including pathogens and spores, from an object. The nurse working with a sterile field or with sterile equipment must understand that the slightest break in technique results in contamination. The nurse also practices surgical asepsis to keep microorganisms away from an area (see the box below).

Although surgical asepsis is commonly practiced in the operating room, labor and delivery area, and major diagnostic areas, the nurse may also use surgical aseptic techniques at the client's bedside. This includes, for example, inserting intravenous or urinary catheters, suctioning the tracheobronchial airway, and reapplying sterile dressings. A nurse in an operating room follows a series of steps to maintain sterile technique, including applying a mask, protective eyewear, and a cap; performing a surgical handwashing; and applying a sterile gown and gloves. In contrast, a nurse performing a dressing change at a client's bedside may only wash hands and apply sterile gloves. See the principles of surgical asepsis below.

CLIENT PREPARATION

Because surgical asepsis requires exact techniques, the nurse must have the client's cooperation. Therefore the nurse must prepare the client before any procedure. Certain clients may fear moving or touching objects during a sterile procedure, whereas others may even try to assist. The nurse explains how a procedure is to be performed and what the client can do to avoid contaminating sterile items, including the following:

Indications for Using Sterile Technique

- During procedures that require intentional perforation of a client's skin (e.g., insertion of intravenous catheters, administration of injections)
- When the skin's integrity is broken due to trauma, surgical incision, or burns
- During procedures that involve insertion of catheters or surgical instruments into sterile body cavities

1. Avoid sudden movements of body parts covered by sterile drapes
2. Refrain from touching sterile supplies, drapes, or the nurse's gloves and gown
3. Avoid coughing, sneezing, or talking over a sterile area

Certain sterile procedures may last a long time. The nurse must assess the client's needs and anticipate factors that may disrupt a procedure. If a client is in pain, the nurse tries to administer analgesics no more than half an hour before a sterile procedure begins. The nurse allows the client to have elimination needs met. Often clients must assume relatively uncomfortable positions during sterile procedures. The nurse helps the client assume the most comfortable position possible. Finally, the client's condition may result in actions or events that contaminate a sterile field, such as the client with a respiratory infection who transmits organisms by coughing or breathing. The nurse anticipates such a problem and offers the client a mask.

PRINCIPLES OF SURGICAL ASEPSIS

When beginning a surgically aseptic procedure, the nurse follows certain principles to ensure maintenance of asepsis. Failure to follow principles places clients at risk for infection. The following principles are important:

1. A sterile object remains sterile only when touched by another sterile object. This principle guides the nurse in placement of sterile objects and how to handle them.
   a. Sterile touching sterile remains sterile; for example, sterile gloves are worn, or sterile forceps are used to handle objects on a sterile field.
   b. Sterile touching clean becomes contaminated; for example, if the tip of a syringe or other sterile object touches the surface of a clean disposable glove, the object is contaminated.
   c. Sterile touching contaminated becomes contaminated; for example, when the nurse touches a sterile object with an ungloved hand, the object is contaminated.
   d. Sterile touching questionable is contaminated; for example, when a tear or break in the covering of a sterile object is found, it is discarded regardless of whether the object itself appears untouched.
2. Only sterile objects may be placed on a sterile field. All items are properly sterilized before use. Sterile objects are kept in clean, dry storage areas. The package or container holding a sterile object must be intact and dry. A package that is torn, punctured, wet, or open is unsterile.
3. A sterile object or field out of the range of vision or an object held below a person's waist is contaminated. Nurses never turn their backs on a sterile tray or leave it unattended. Contamination can occur accidentally by a dangling piece of clothing, falling hair, or an unknowing client touching a sterile object. Any object held below waist level is considered contaminated because it cannot be viewed at all times. Sterile objects should be kept in front with hands as close together as possible.
4. A sterile object or field becomes contaminated by prolonged exposure to air. The nurse avoids activities that may create air currents, such as excessive movements or rearranging linen after a sterile object or field becomes exposed. When sterile packages are being opened, it is important to minimize the number of people walking into the area. Microorganisms also travel by droplet through the air. No one should talk, laugh, sneeze, or cough over a sterile field or when gathering and using sterile equipment. A nurse with a cold or other respiratory ailment should never perform sterile procedures unless a double mask is worn. Microorganisms traveling through the air can fall on sterile items or fields if the nurse reaches over the work area. When opening sterile packages, the nurse holds the item or piece of equipment as close as possible to the sterile field without touching the sterile surface. Minimal movement or rearranging of sterile items also reduces contamination by air transmission.
5. When a sterile surface comes in contact with a wet, contaminated surface, the sterile object or field becomes contaminated by capillary action. If moisture seeps through a sterile package's protective covering, microorganisms travel to the sterile object. When stored sterile packages become wet, the nurse discards the objects immediately or sends the equipment for resterilization. When working with a sterile field or tray, the nurse may have to pour sterile solutions. Any spill can be a source of contamination unless the object or field rests on a sterile surface that cannot be penetrated by moisture. Urinary catheterization trays contain sterile supplies that rest in a sterile, plastic container. In this example, sterile solutions spilled within the container will not contaminate the catheter or other objects. In contrast, if a nurse places a piece of sterile gauze in its wrapper on a client's bedside table and the table surface is wet, the gauze is considered contaminated.
6. Fluid flows in the direction of gravity. A sterile object becomes contaminated if gravity causes a contaminated liquid to flow over the object's surface. To avoid contamination during a surgical hand scrub, the nurse holds the hands above the elbows. This allows water to flow downward without contaminating the nurse's hands and fingers. The principle of water flow by gravity is also the reason for drying from fingers to elbows with hands held up, after the scrub.
7. The edges of a sterile field or container are considered to be contaminated. Frequently a nurse places sterile objects on a sterile towel or drape. Because the edge of the drape touches an unsterile surface, such as a table or bed linen, a 2.5-cm (1 inch) border around the drape is considered contaminated. The edges of sterile containers become exposed to air after they are open and are thus contaminated. After a sterile needle is removed from its protective cap or after forceps are removed from a container, the objects must not touch the container's edge. The lip of an opened bottle of solution also becomes contaminated after it is exposed to air. When pouring a sterile liquid, the nurse first pours a small amount of solution and discards it. The solution washes away microorganisms on the bottle lip. Then the nurse pours a second time on the same side to fill a container with the desired amount of solution.

PERFORMING STERILE PROCEDURES

All the equipment that will be needed should be assembled before a procedure. Thus the nurse avoids having to leave a sterile area unattended because equipment is missing. A few extra supplies should be available in case objects accidentally become contaminated. Before the sterile procedure, each step should be explained so that the client can cooperate fully. If an object becomes contaminated during the procedure, the nurse should not hesitate to discard it immediately.

Donning and Removing Caps, Masks, and Eyewear. For sterile procedures on a general nursing division, the nurse may wear a surgical mask and eyewear without a cap. Eyewear is worn as a part of standard precautions if there is a risk of fluid or blood splashing into the nurse's eyes. For sterile surgical procedures in the operating room, the nurse first applies a clean cap that covers all of the hair and then the surgical mask and eyewear.

A mask must fit snugly around the face and nose to prevent contamination by droplet nuclei. After a mask is worn for several hours, the area over the mouth and nose often becomes moist. Moisture promotes the spread of microorganisms. The nurse in the operating room must apply a second mask over the first because removing a mask in a surgical area results in immediate contamination of surrounding objects. Procedure 34-3 describes the steps for applying a mask.

Protective glasses or goggles should fit snugly around the forehead and face to fully protect the eyes. Eyewear needs to be worn only for procedures that create the risk of body fluids splashing into the eyes. Before removing a mask, eyewear, and cap, the nurse removes sterile gloves to prevent contamination of the hair, neck, and facial area. After untying the mask, the nurse holds it by the ties and discards it with the cap. Eyewear is removed and cleaned later for reuse. After removing all protective wear, the nurse washes hands thoroughly.

Opening Sterile Packages. Sterile items such as syringes, gauze dressings, or catheters are packaged in paper or plastic containers impervious to microorganisms as long as they are dry and intact. Some institutions wrap reusable supplies in a double thickness of linen or muslin. Packages are permeable to steam and thus allow for steam autoclaving. A disadvantage of paper wrappers is that they tear or puncture relatively easily. Sterile items are kept in clean, enclosed storage cabinets and are separated from dirty equipment.

Sterile supplies have dated labels or chemical tapes that indicate the date when the sterilization period expires. The tapes change color during the sterilization process. Failure of the tapes to change color means the item is not sterile. A sterile supply should never be used if the integrity of the packaging is compromised. Most health care facilities use event-related rather than expiration date, but check with your facility's policies regarding outdates.

Before opening a sterile item the nurse washes hands thoroughly. The nurse assembles the supplies in the work area such as the bedside table or treatment room before opening packages. A bedside table or counter top provides a large, clean working area for opening items. The work area should be above waist level. Sterile supplies should not be opened in a confined space where a dirty object might fall on or strike them.

Opening a Sterile Item on a Flat Surface. Sterile packaged items can be opened without contaminating the contents. Commercially packaged items are usually designed so

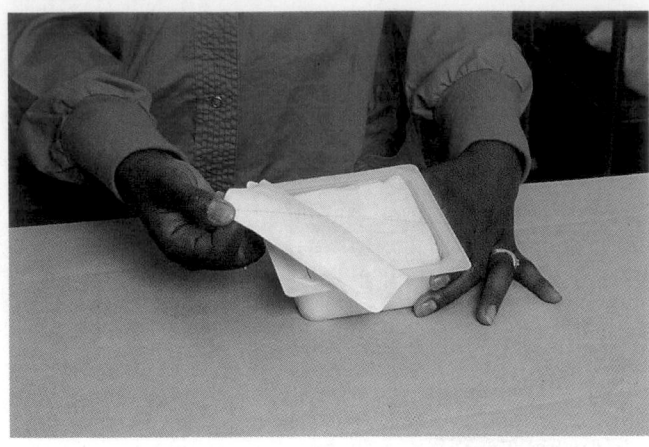

Fig. 34-5 When opening a commercially packaged sterile item, the nurse tears the wrapper away from the body.

that the nurse only has to tear away or separate the paper or plastic cover. The item is held in one hand while the wrapper is pulled away with the other (Fig. 34-5). Care is then taken to keep the inner contents sterile before use. When opening items packed in linen, the nurse uses the following steps:

1. Place the item flat in the center of the work surface.
2. Remove the tape or seal indicating the sterilization date.
3. Grasp the outer surface of the tip of the outermost flap.
4. Open the outer flap away from the body, keeping the arm outstretched and away from the sterile field (Fig. 34-6, *A*).
5. Grasp the outside surface of the first side flap.
6. Open the side flap, allowing it to lie flat on the table surface. Keep the arm to the side and not over the sterile surface (Fig. 34-6, *B*). Do not allow flaps to spring back over the sterile contents.
7. Grasp the outside surface of the second side flap and allow it to lie flat on table surface (Fig. 34-6, *C*).
8. Grasp the outside surface of the last and innermost flap.
9. Stand away from the sterile package and pull the flap back, allowing it to fall flat on the surface (Fig. 34-6, *D*).
10. Use the inner surface of the linen package (except for the 1 inch border around the edges) as a sterile field to add additional sterile items. The 1 inch border can be grasped to maneuver the field on the table surface.

If the sterile supplies are not to be used immediately, the nurse can close the sterile package. In this case the nurse should touch only the wrapper's outside surface. To close a package the order of unwrapping is reversed and the nurse does not touch the inside contents or reach over the field.

Opening a Sterile Item While Holding It. To open small, sterile items, the package is held in the nondominant hand while the top flap is opened and pulled away from the nurse. Using the dominant hand the nurse carefully opens the sides and top flaps away from the enclosed

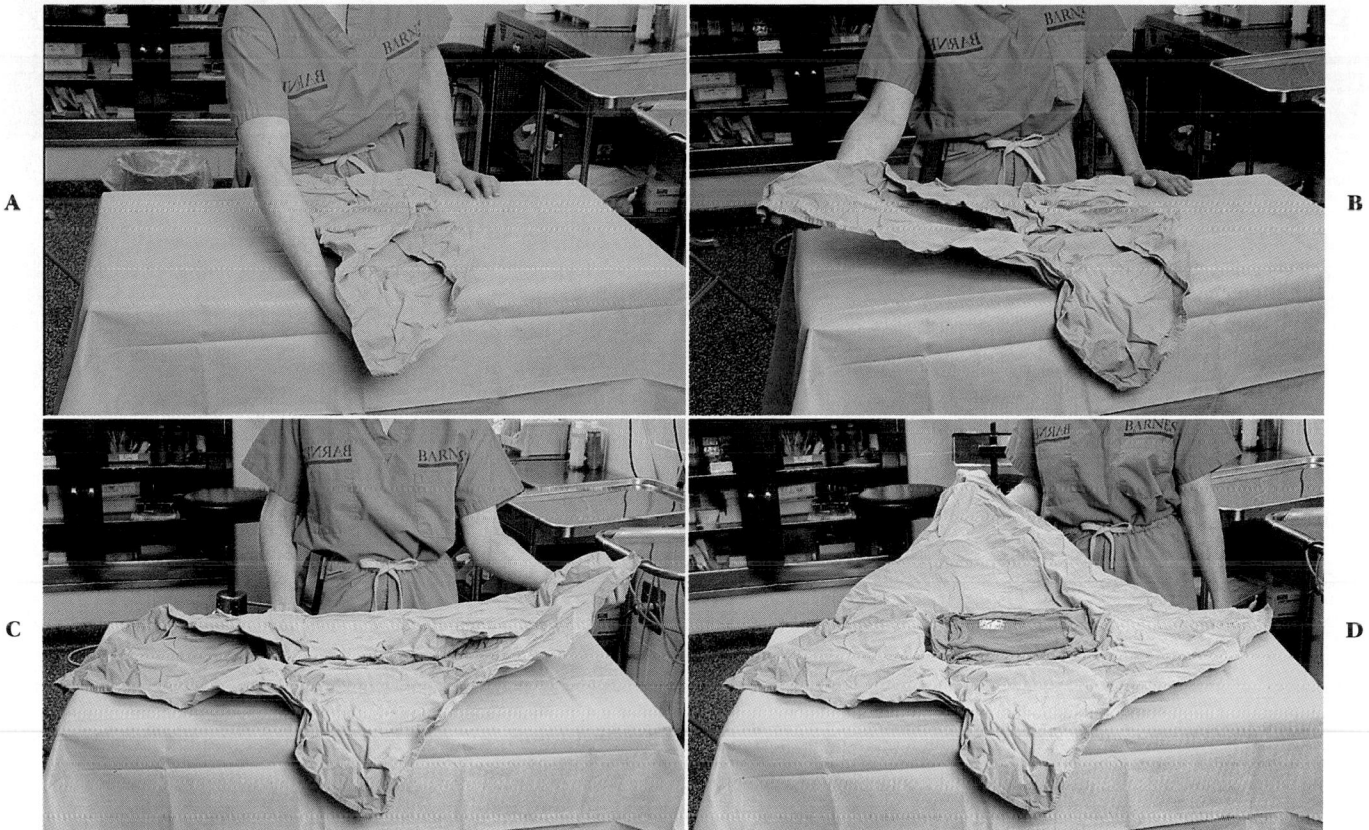

Fig. 34-6 Opening sterile packaged items on a flat surface. **A,** Nurse opens the top flap away from the body. **B,** The nurse's arm is kept out away from the sterile field while opening a side flap. **C,** The second side flap is opened. **D,** The back flap is opened.

sterile item in the same order previously mentioned. The nurse opens items in a hand so that the item can be handed to a person wearing sterile gloves or transferred to a sterile field.

Preparing a Sterile Field. When performing sterile procedures, the nurse needs a sterile work area that provides room for handling and placing of sterile items. A **sterile field** is an area free of microorganisms and prepared to receive sterile items. The field may be prepared by using the inner surface of a sterile wrapper as the work surface or by using a sterile drape. Procedure 34-4 describes preparation of a sterile field. After the surface for the field is created, the nurse adds sterile items by placing them directly on the field or by transferring them with a sterile forceps. When transferring sterile items, the nurse must carefully place objects onto the sterile field. An object that comes in contact with the 1 inch border must be discarded.

The nurse may choose to wear sterile gloves while preparing items on the field. If this is done, the nurse can touch the entire drape, but sterile items must be handed over by an assistant. The nurse's gloves cannot touch the wrappers of sterile items.

Pouring Sterile Solutions. Often the nurse must pour sterile solutions into sterile containers. A bottle containing

a sterile solution is sterile on the inside and contaminated on the outside; the bottle's neck is also contaminated, but the inside of the bottle cap is considered sterile. After a cap or lid is opened, it is held in the hand or placed sterile side (inside) up on a clean surface. This means that the inside of the lid can be seen as it rests on the table surface. A bottle cap or lid should never rest on a sterile surface, even though the inside of the cap is sterile. The outer edge of the cap is unsterile and would contaminate the surface. Likewise, placing a sterile cap down on an unsterile surface increases the chances of the inside of the cap becoming contaminated.

The bottle should be held with its label in the palm of the hand to prevent the possibility of the solution wetting and fading the label. Before pouring the solution into the container, the nurse pours a small amount (1 to 2 ml) into a disposable cap or plastic-lined waste receptacle. The discarded solution cleans the lip of the bottle. The edge of the bottle is kept away from the edge or inside of the receiving container. The nurse pours the solution slowly to avoid splashing the underlying drape or field. The bottle should never be held so high above the container that even slow pouring will cause splashing. The bottle should be held outside the edge of the sterile field.

Preparing a Sterile Field

STEPS	RATIONALE
1. Prepare sterile field just before planned procedure. Supplies are to be used immediately.	Prevents exposure of sterile field and supplies to air and contamination.
2. Select clean work surface above waist level.	Sterile object held below waist is contaminated.
3. Assemble necessary equipment: a. Sterile drape b. Assorted sterile supplies	Preparation of equipment in advance prevents break in technique.
4. Check dates or labels on supplies for sterility of equipment.	Equipment stored beyond expiration date is considered unsterile.
5. Wash hands thoroughly.	Prevents transmission of infection.
6. Place pack containing sterile drape on work surface and open as described on p. 772.	Ensures sterility of packaged drape.
7. With fingertips of one hand, pick up folded top edge of sterile drape.	One inch border around drape is unsterile and may be touched.
8. Gently lift drape up from its outer cover and let it unfold by itself without touching any object. Discard outer cover with your other hand.	If sterile object touches any other nonsterile object, it becomes contaminated.

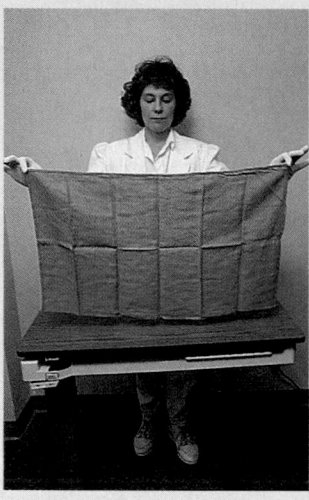

Step 9

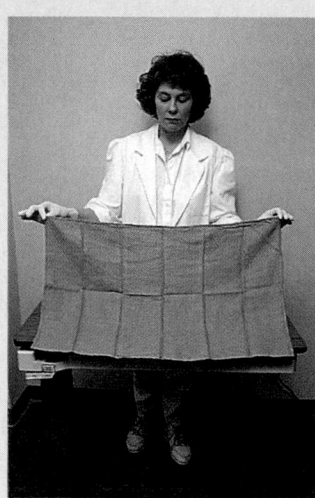

Step 10

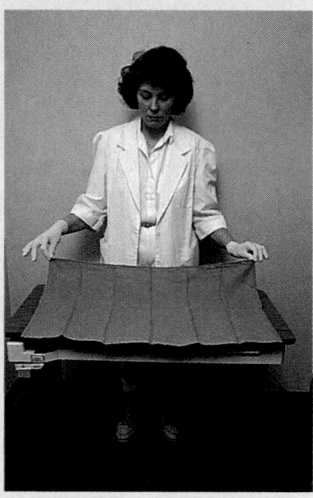

Step 11

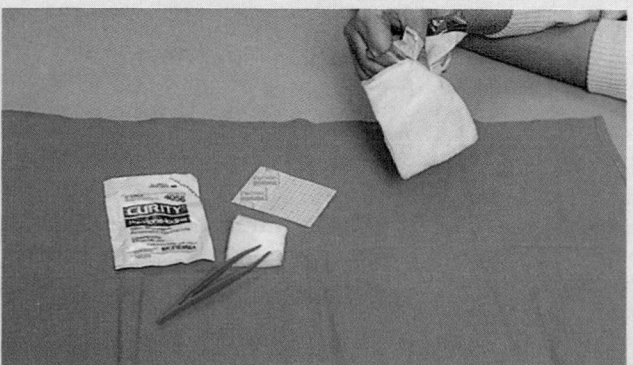

Step 14

Preparing a Sterile Field—cont'd

STEPS	RATIONALE
9. With other hand, grasp adjacent corner of drape and hold it straight up and away from your body (see the illustration on p. 774).	Drape can now be properly placed while using two hands. Drape must be held away from unsterile surfaces.
10. Holding drape, first position the bottom half over intended work surface (see the illustration on p. 774).	Prevents nurse from reaching over sterile field.
11. Allow top half of drape to be placed over work surface last (see the illustration on p. 774).	Creates flat, sterile work surface.
ADDING STERILE ITEMS	
12. Open sterile item (following package directions) while holding outside wrapper in nondominant hand.	Frees dominant hand for unwrapping outer wrapper.
13. Carefully peel wrapper onto nondominant hand.	Item remains sterile. Inner surface of wrapper covers hand, making it sterile.
14. Being sure wrapper does not fall down on sterile field, place item onto field at angle. Do not hold arm over sterile field (see the illustration on p. 774).	Prevents reaching over field and contaminating its surface.
15. Dispose of outer wrapper.	Prevents accidental contamination of sterile field.
16. Perform procedure using sterile technique.	Prevents transmission of infection to client.

Surgical Scrub. Clients undergoing operative procedures are at an increased risk for infection. Nurses working in operating rooms perform surgical hand scrubs to decrease and suppress the growth of skin microorganisms in case of glove tears (AORN, 1994).

During surgical handwashing, the nurse scrubs from fingertips to elbows with an antimicrobial soap or detergent before each operation. The optimum duration of the surgical hand scrub is unclear, although research indicates that it may be dependent on type of antimicrobial product (Pereira et al, 1990; O'Shaughnessy et al, 1991; Hingst et al, 1992). The traditional scrub time in the United States for both the initial and subsequent scrub has been 5 minutes (Meeker and Rothrock, 1995). Larson (1995) recommends that at least 2 minutes of friction be used for surgical handwashing. The nurse should follow the agency's policy for length of scrub time.

For maximum elimination of bacteria, all jewelry should be removed and nails kept clean and short (AORN, 1994). Artificial nails should not be worn as they may harbor a greater number of bacteria (Pottinger et al, 1989). Nurses who have active skin infections, open lesions or cuts, or respiratory infections should be excluded from the surgical team. In scrubbing, light friction is effective in removing microorganisms; too much brushing may remove the outer layer of epidermis, thereby exposing bacterial flora in the deeper skin layers (Meeker and Rothrock, 1995). Procedure 34-5 describes the steps for surgical scrub.

Applying Sterile Gloves. Sterile gloves are an additional barrier to bacterial transfer. There are two gloving methods: open and closed. Nurses who work on general nursing divisions use open gloving before procedures such as dressing changes or urinary catheter insertions. The closed gloved method, which is performed after nurses apply sterile gowns, is practiced in operating rooms and special treatment areas. Procedures 34-6 and 34-7 review the steps of each gloving technique.

The proper glove size should be selected; the glove should not stretch so tightly that it can easily tear; yet it should be tight enough that objects can be picked up easily.

Donning a Sterile Gown. Nurses must wear sterile gowns in the operating room and delivery room so that sterile objects can be comfortably handled with less risk of contamination. The sterile gown acts as a barrier to decrease shedding of microorganisms from skin surfaces into the air and thus prevents wound contamination. Nurses caring for clients with large open wounds or assisting physicians during major invasive procedures (e.g., inserting an arterial catheter) may also wear sterile gowns.

Nurses do not apply sterile gowns until after applying masks and surgical caps and performing surgical handwashing. Nurses pick up the gown from sterile packs or have gowned assistants hand them the gowns. Only a certain portion of the gown—the area from the anterior waist to but not including the collar and the anterior surface of the sleeves—is considered sterile. The back of the gown, the area under the arms, the collar, the area below the waist, and the underside of the sleeves are not sterile because the nurse cannot keep these areas in constant view and ensure their sterility. Procedure 34-6 reviews the steps for applying a gown.

Text continued on p. 784.

Surgical Scrub: Preparing for Gowning

1. Remove all jewelry. Ensure that fingernails are short and that cuticles are in good condition.	Minimizes number of resident and transient micro-organisms.
2. Use deep sink with foot pedals or knee controls for dispensing soap and controlling water temperature and flow.	Minimizes risk of hands and lower arms touching dirty surface.
3. Use approved antimicrobial agent such as CHG or iodophor.	Broad-spectrum antimicrobial agents maximally reduce number of microorganisms on hands.
4. Have two disposable hand brushes or sponges and disposable nail file available.	Brushes or sponges are used to enhance mechanical friction during handwashing.
5. Apply cap, covering hair completely. Contain pierced earrings within cap.	Microorganisms reside on hair. Hair and earrings would act as foreign bodies if allowed to enter operative wound.
6. Apply face mask and eyewear, making certain to cover nose and mouth snugly with mask.	Mask prevents escape of microorganisms into air, which can contaminate hands. Eyewear protects nurse from splashes in operative unit.

HANDWASHING

7. Adjust water flow to comfortable temperature. (Most sinks have automatic knee or foot controls.)	Hot water removes protective oils from skin and increases sensitivity to soap.
8. Wet hands and forearms liberally, keeping arms and hands above elbow level during entire procedure. NOTE: Scrub uniform must be kept dry.	Water runs by gravity from fingertips to elbows. Hands become cleanest part of upper extremity. Keeping hands elevated allows water to flow from least to most contaminated area.
9. Dispense liberal amounts of soap (2 to 5 ml) into hands and lather hands and arms to 5 cm (2 in) above elbows.	Washing wide area reduces risk of contaminating overlying gown that is later applied.
10. Clean nails with file under running water (see the illustration below). Discard file.	Removes dirt and organic material that harbor large numbers of microorganisms.

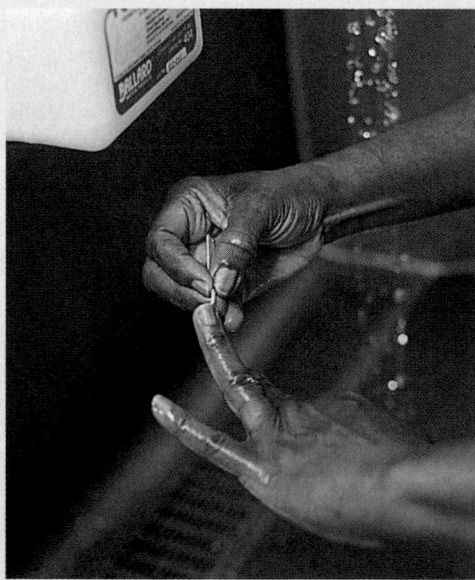

Step 10

Surgical Scrub: Preparing for Gowning—cont'd

STEPS	RATIONALE

11. Wet brush and apply antimicrobial soap. If an impregnated brush or sponge is used, it should be first moistened. The number of strokes is usually 30 strokes to nails and 20 strokes to each area of the skin (Meeker and Rothrock, 1995). Scrub fingertips, hands, and arms in the following manner:
  a. Scrub nails vigorously while brush is held perpendicular to them.
  b. Scrub each side of digit including web space between fingers.
  c. Scrub palm and back of hand.
	Loosens resident bacteria that adhere to skin surfaces.

12. Rinse brush thoroughly. Reapply soap.	Rinsing of brush removes microorganisms and avoids contamination of arms.
13. Mentally divide arms into thirds. Scrub each surface of lower forearm with circular motion (see the illustration below); scrub middle and upper forearms in same manner. Discard brush.	Removes microorganisms over wide area.
14. With arms flexed, rinse thoroughly from fingertips to elbow in one motion, allowing water to run off at elbow (see the illustration below).	Allows water to flow from least to most contaminated area.
15. Repeat Steps 11 through 14 for second arm.	
16. Keeping arms flexed, discard brush. Turn off water with knee or foot control. Proceed to operating room with elbows flexed and held up.	After touching skin, brush is contaminated. Rinsing removes resident bacteria.
17. Pick up sterile towel found on top of sterile gownpack. Be sure no one is within arm's reach.	Dry from cleanest to least clean area. Drying prevents chapping, facilitates application of gloves, and prevents contamination of gown.
18. Open towel full length, holding one side away from scrub attire.	Avoids contact with microorganisms on scrub gown.
19. Dry each hand separately. To dry one arm, hold towel in opposite hand; using rotating motion, draw towel from fingers up to elbow.	Drying hands first prevents contaminating hands from areas proximal to elbows.
20. Carefully reverse towel and dry other hand and arm.	
21. Discard towel. Prevents accidental contamination.	
22. Proceed with sterile gowning (see Procedure 34-6).	

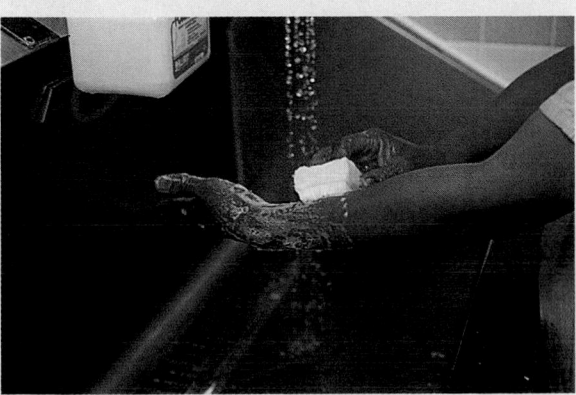

Step 13

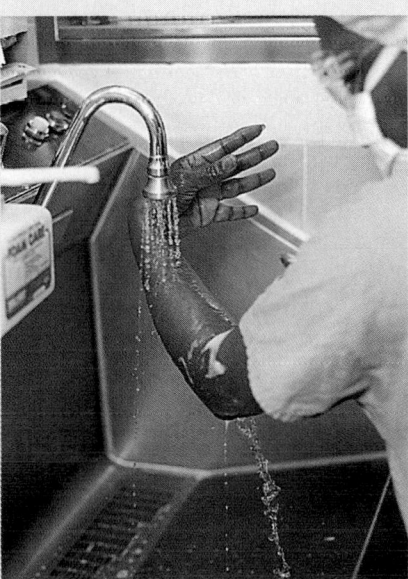

Step 14

PROCEDURE 34-6

Applying a Sterile Gown and Performing Closed Gloving

STEPS	RATIONALE

GOWNING

1. Before entering operating room or treatment area, apply cap, face mask, and eyewear. Foot covers are also required in operating room.

Prevents hair and air droplet nuclei from contaminating sterile work areas. Eyewear protects mucous membranes of eye. Foot covers are paper or cloth and fit over work shoes.

2. Perform thorough surgical handwash (see Procedure 34-5).

Removes transient and resident bacteria from fingers, hands, forearms.

3. Ask circulating nurse to assist by opening sterile pack containing sterile gown (folded inside out).

Gown's outer surface remains sterile.

4. Have circulating nurse prepare glove package by peeling outer wrapper open while keeping inner contents sterile. Inner glove package is then placed on sterile field created by sterile outer wrapper.

Keeps gloves sterile and allows nurse who has scrubbed to handle sterile items.

5. Reach down to sterile gown package (see the illustration below); lift folded gown directly upward and step back away from table (see the illustration below).

Provides wide margin of safety, avoiding contamination of gown.

6. Holding folded gown, locate neckband. With both hands, grasp inside front of gown just below neckband.

Clean hands may touch inside of gown without contaminating outer surface.

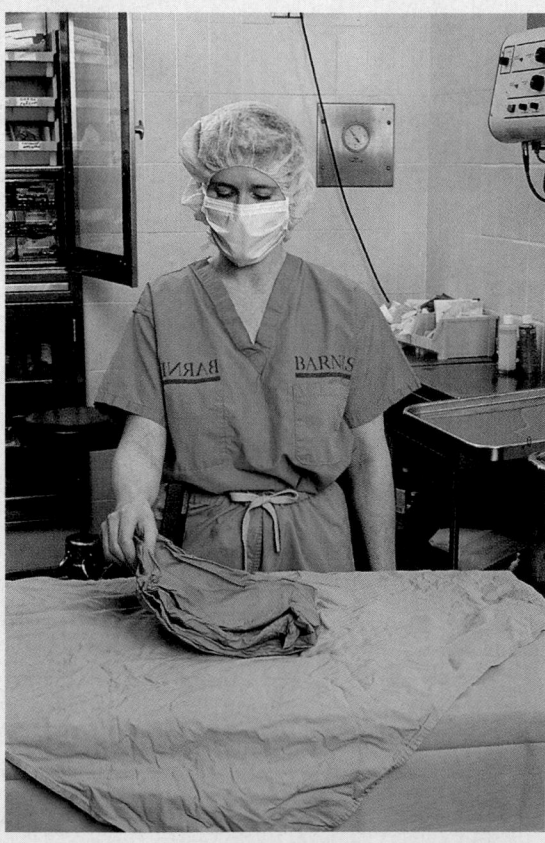

Step 5

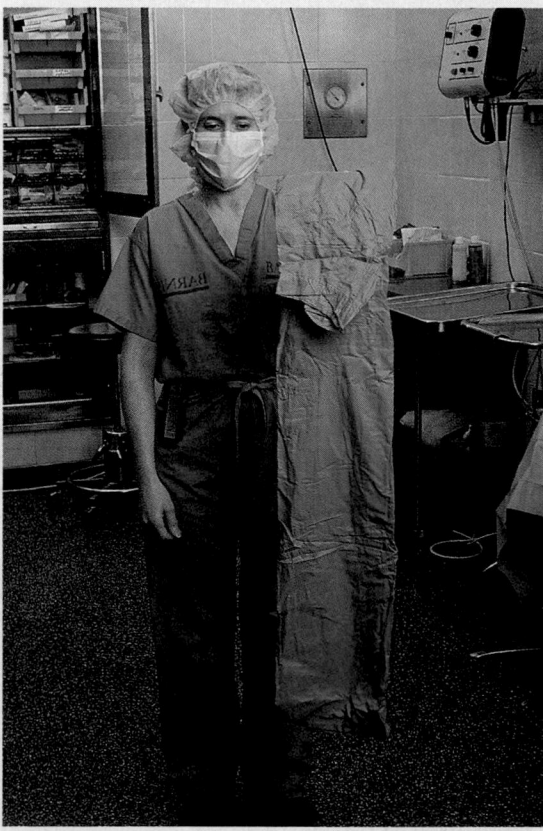

Step 5

Applying a Sterile Gown and Performing Closed Gloving—cont'd

STEPS	RATIONALE
7. Allow gown to unfold, keeping inside of gown toward body. Do not touch outside of gown with bare hands (see the illustration below).	Outside of gown will be sterile surface.
8. With hands at shoulder level, slip both arms into arm-holes simultaneously (see the illustration below). Ask circulating nurse to bring gown over shoulders by reaching inside to arm seams. Gown is pulled on, leaving sleeves covering hands (see the illustration on p. 780).	Careful application prevents contamination. Gown covers hands to prepare for closed gloving.
9. Have circulating nurse securely tie back of gown at neck and waist. (If gown is a wraparound style, sterile flap to cover gown is not touched until the nurse has gloved).	Gown must completely enclose underlying garments.

CLOSED GLOVING

1. With hands covered by gown sleeves, open inner sterile glove package.	Hands remain clean. Sterile gown cuff will touch sterile glove surface.
2. With nondominant hand inside gown cuff, pick up glove for the dominant hand by grasping folded cuff.	Sterile gown touches sterile glove.

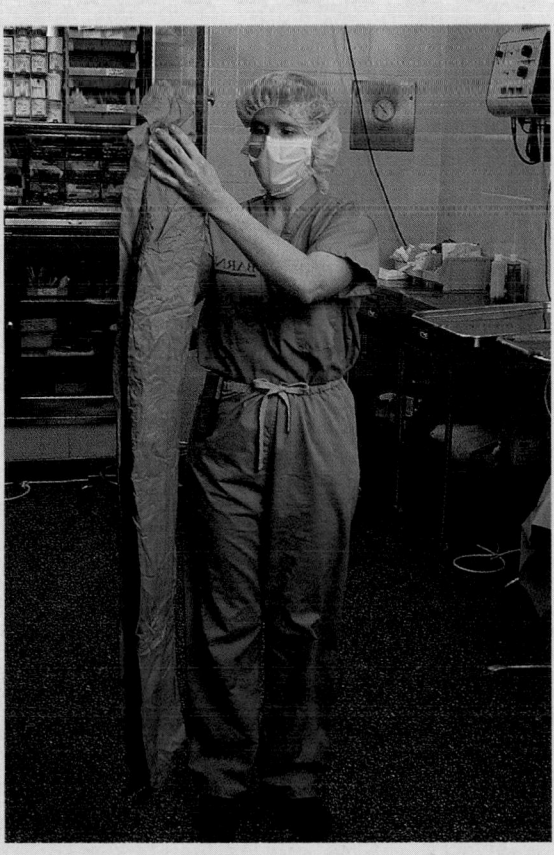

Step 7

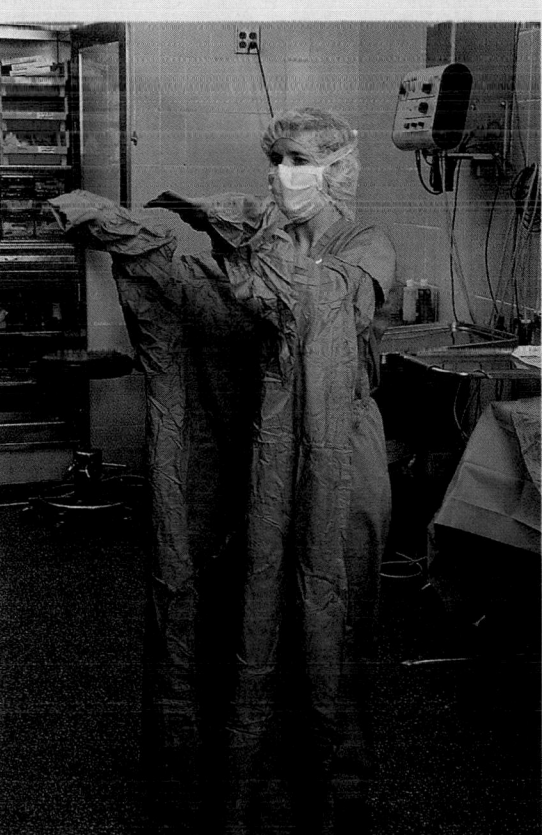

Step 8

Continued.

Applying a Sterile Gown and Performing Closed Gloving—cont'd

STEPS	RATIONALE
3. Extend dominant forearm with palm up and place palm of glove against palm of dominant hand. Glove fingers will point toward elbow.	Positions glove for application over cuffed hand, keeping glove sterile.
4. Grasp back of glove cuff with nondominant hand and turn glove cuff over end of dominant hand and gown cuff (see the illustration on p. 781).	
5. Grasp top of glove and underlying gown sleeve with covered nondominant hand. Carefully extend fingers into glove, being sure glove's cuff covers gown's cuff.	Seal created by glove cuff over gown prevents exit of microorganisms over operative sterile field.
6. Glove nondominant hand in same manner, reversing hands (see the illustration on p. 781). Used gloved dominant hand to pull on glove. Keep hand inside sleeve (see the illustration on p. 781).	Sterile touches sterile.
7. Be sure fingers are fully extended into both gloves.	Ensures that nurse has full dexterity while using gloved hand.

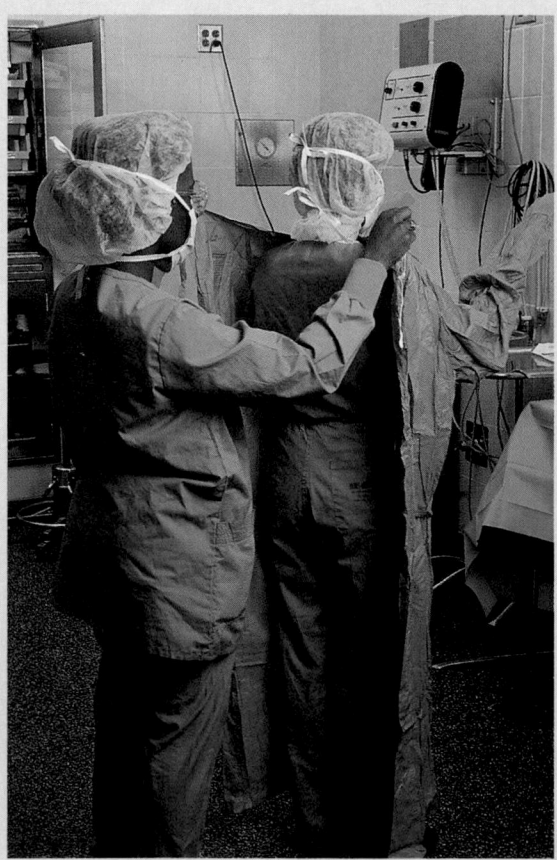

Step 8, p. 779

Applying a Sterile Gown and Performing Closed Gloving—cont'd

STEPS	RATIONALE
8. For wraparound sterile gowns: take gloved hand and release fastener or ties in front of gown.	Front of gown is sterile.
9. Hand tie to sterile team member who stands still. Allowing margin of safety, turn around to the left, covering back with extended gown flap. Take back tie from team member and secure tie to gown.	Contact with team member could contaminate gown and gloves. Gown must enclose undergarments.

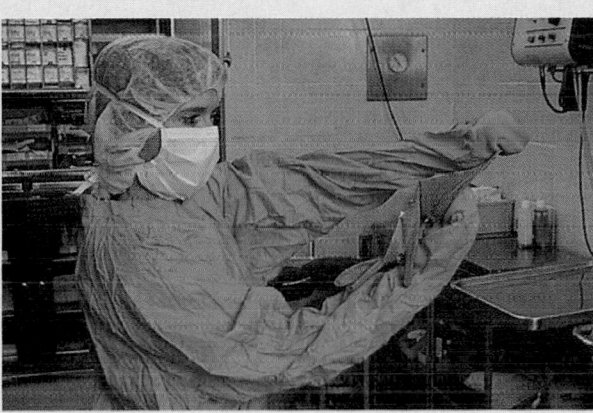

Step 4

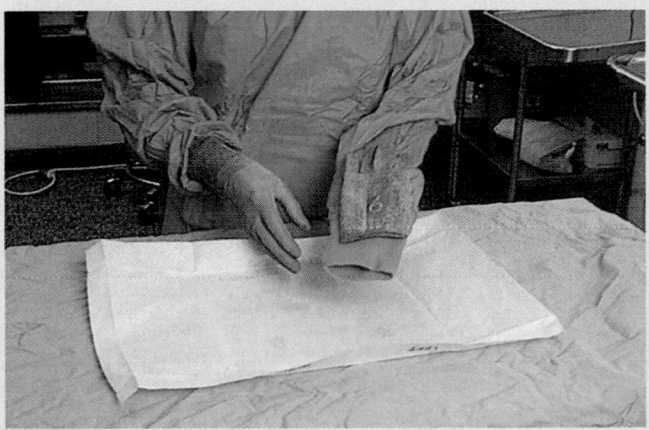

Step 6

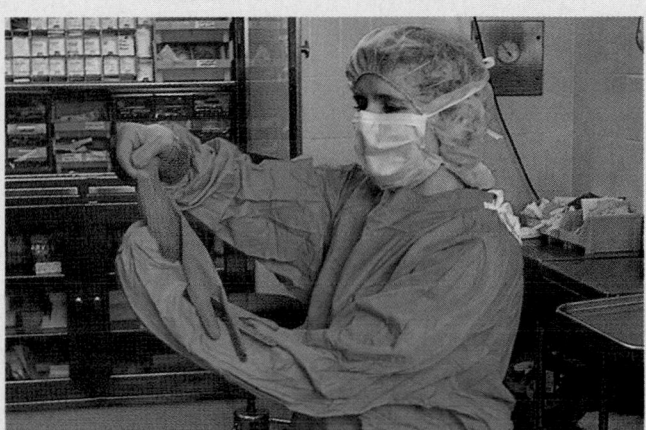

Step 6

Performing Open Gloving

STEPS	RATIONALE
1. Have package of proper-sized sterile gloves at treatment area.	
2. Perform thorough handwashing.	Removes bacteria from skin surfaces and reduces transmission of infection.
3. Remove outer glove package wrapper by carefully separating and peeling apart sides.	Prevents inner glove package from accidentally opening and touching contaminated objects.
4. Grasp inner package and lay it on clean, flat surface just above waist level. Open package, keeping gloves on wrapper's inside surface.	Sterile object held below waist is contaminated. Inner surface of glove package is sterile.
5. If gloves are not prepowdered, take packet of powder and apply lightly to hands over sink or wastebasket.	Powder allows gloves to slip on easily. (Some staff members do not use powder for fear of promoting growth of micro-organisms.)
6. Identify right and left glove. Each glove has cuff approximately 5 cm (2 inches) wide. Glove dominant hand first.	Proper identification of gloves prevents contamination by improper fit. Gloving of dominant hand first improves dexterity.
7. With thumb and first two fingers of nondominant hand, grasp edge of cuff of glove for dominant hand. Touch only glove's inside surface.	Inner edge of cuff will lie against skin and thus is not sterile.
8. Carefully pull glove over dominant hand (see the illustration below), leaving cuff and being sure cuff does not roll up wrist. Be sure thumb and fingers are in proper spaces (see the illustration below).	If glove's outer surface touches hand or wrist, it is contaminated.
9. With gloved dominant hand, slip fingers underneath second glove's cuff (see the illustration on p. 783).	Cuff protects gloved fingers. Sterile touching sterile prevents glove contamination.
10. Carefully pull second glove over nondominant hand. Do not allow fingers and thumb of gloved dominant hand to touch any part of exposed nondominant hand. Keep thumb of dominant hand abducted back (see the illustration on p. 783).	Contact of gloved hand with exposed hand results in contamination.

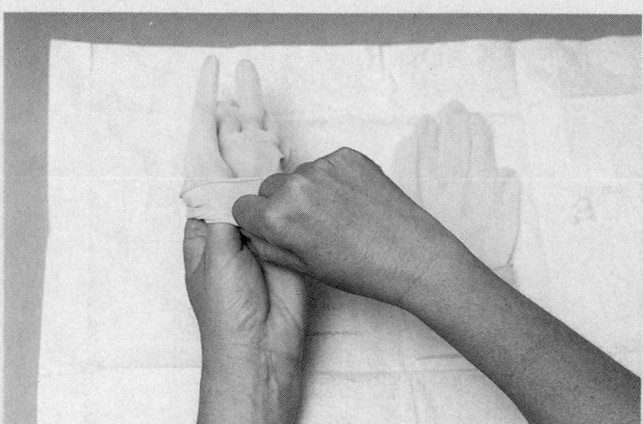

Step 8

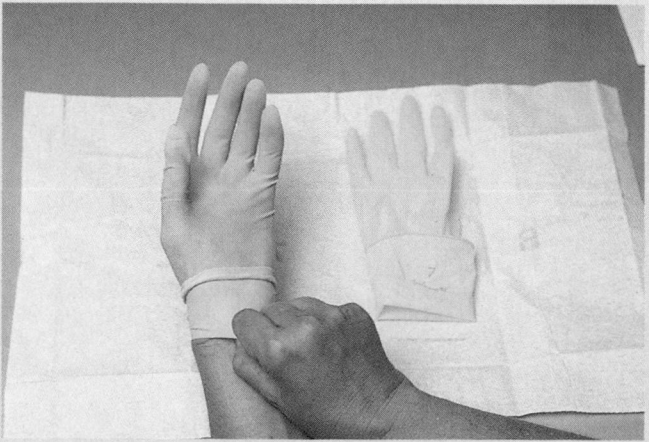

Step 8

Performing Open Gloving—cont'd

STEPS	RATIONALE
11. After second glove is on, interlock hands. The cuffs usually fall down after application. Be sure to touch only sterile sides (see the illustration below).	Ensures smooth fit over fingers.

GLOVE DISPOSAL

12. Grasp outside of one cuff with other gloved hand; avoid touching wrist.	Minimizes contamination of underlying skin.
13. Pull glove off, turning it inside out. Discard in receptacle.	Outside of glove does not touch skin surface.
14. Take fingers of bare hand and tuck inside remaining glove cuff. Peel glove off, inside out. Discard in receptacle.	

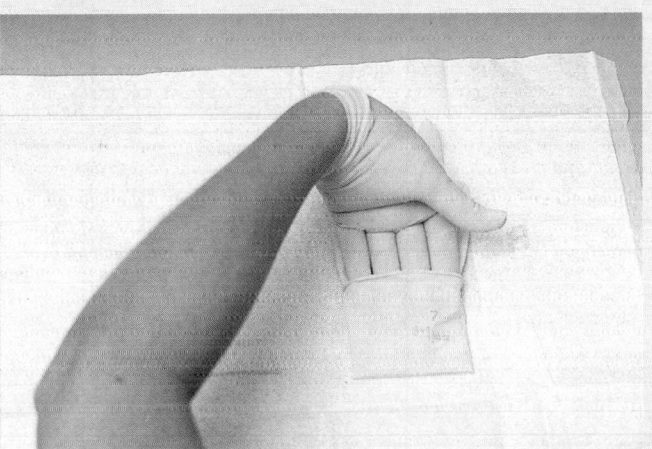

Step 9

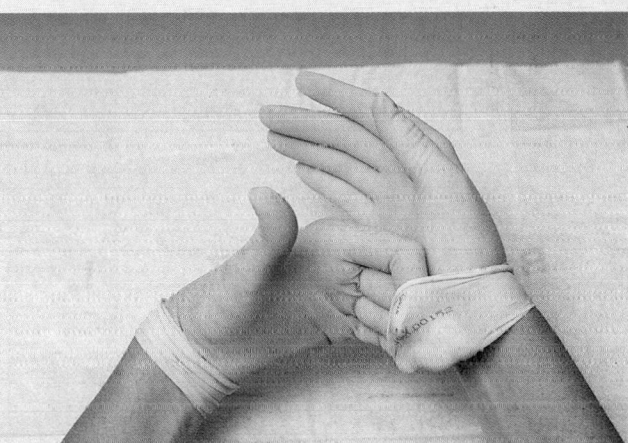

Step 10

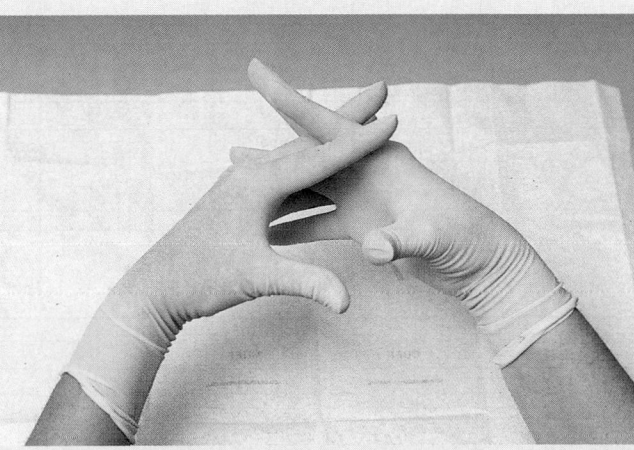

Step 11

Evaluation

The success of the nurse who practices infection-control techniques is measured by determining whether the goals for reducing or preventing infection are achieved. A comparison of the client's response, such as absence of fever or development of wound drainage, with expected outcomes determines the success of nursing interventions (Fig. 34-7). Similarly, a determination is made about whether interventions should be revised or eliminated. The ability to correctly assess wounds for healing and conduct a physical assessment of body systems (see Chapter 33) are important

---

SEPSIS WITH NEUTROPENIA

DRG # 416
Target LOS 9 days

	DATE	DATE	DATE
Hosp day	**HOSPITAL DAY 1**	**HOSPITAL DAY 2**	**HOSPITAL DAY 3**
CONSULTS	Notify Radiation Therapy if applicable	Dr. Clements if ordered Social Service Dietician	
TESTS	CBC, SMA 18, Magnesium, Creatinine Blood cultures X 2 sites before antibiotics started Chest Xray Type and Screen	CBC Blood cultures for chills or temp > 101 No more than 3 sets in 24 hours	CBC - > - >
SPECIMENS	U/A for c&s before antibiotics started Sputum for c&s if productive cough	- >	- >
TREATMENTS	O2 at 2L by NC if Hgb < 8 Mouth care every 4 hours per protocol	- > - >	- > - >
VITAL SIGNS	Every 4 hours	- >	- >
I & O	Every 8 hours	- >	- >
DIET	Neutropenic DAT until WBC > 1.5	- >	- >
IVs	Fluids as ordered Antibiotics as ordered	Check w/MD re: fluid changes Continue antibiotics as ordered until d/c'd	Continue until d/c'd - >
MEDS	ID home meds and check with MD Check those that are ordered: ——Tylenol gr X po temp > 101 ——Pain PRN ——Sleeper ——Antidiarrhea ——Antiemetic ——Antianxiety	Check those that are ordered: ——Tylenol gr X po temp > 101 ——Pain PRN ——Sleeper ——Antidiarrhea ——Antiemetic ——Antianxiety	Check those that are ordered: ——Tylenol gr X po temp > 101 ——Pain PRN ——Sleeper ——Antidiarrhea ——Antiemetic ——Antianxiety
ACTIVITY	Up as tolerated	- >	- >
MISC	Protective Isolation	- >	Continue until WBC > 1.5
TEACHING	Instruct pt to report any: bleeding, diarrhea, N&V, pain.	Dietician to teach re: neutropenic diet. Mouth Care	Instruct re: personal hygiene
DISCHARGE PLANNING	Evaluate need for d/c planning.	Social services called if appropriate	Determine d/c destination

	Shift	Shift	Shift
Nurse signature	_____ / ____	_____ / ____	_____ / ____
Nurse signature	_____ / ____	_____ / ____	_____ / ____
Nurse signature	_____ / ____	_____ / ____	_____ / ____

Authored by Janie Barnett, RN; Lucy Wallace, LPN

Fig. 34-7 First 3 days of 9-day CareMap® for sepsis with neutropenia. *(Courtesy Baptist Hospital, Pensacola, Fla, and The Center for Case Management, South Natick MA.)*

skills in evaluation. The nurse closely monitors clients, especially those at risk, for signs and symptoms of infection. The evaluation box on p. 786 describes criteria used in evaluating the effects of infection-control techniques.

The client at risk for infection must understand the measures needed to reduce or prevent microorganism growth and spread. Providing clients or family members the opportunity to discuss infection-control measures or to demonstrate procedures will reveal their ability to comply with therapy. The nurse may determine that clients require new information or that previously instructed information needs reinforcement.

The nurse documents the client's response to therapies for infection control. A clear description of any signs and symptoms of systemic or local infection is necessary to give all nurses a baseline for comparative evaluation. The efficacy of any intervention in reducing infection must also be reported.

SUMMARY
PATIENT PROBLEMS/OUTCOME CRITERIA

Sepsis w/Neutropenia   **Target LOS 9 days**

Date	Initial	Nsg Diagnosis/Problem	Outcome Criteria/Goal	Date d/c	Initial
		1. Activity intolerance re: disease process.	1. PT will be able to perform own hygeine care by d/c.		
		2. Altered Nutrition re: less than body requirements re: anorexia, illness, dehydration.	2a Patient will be able to eat at least 1/3 of their ordered diets by d/c. 2b Patient will identify at least 3 food items that they find appealing 2c 1500cc po flds q 24 by d/c		
		3. Hyperthermia re: increase in metabolic rate and illness.	3. Pt. will be afebrile by day 5.		
		4. Potential knowledge deficit re: s/s to report neutropenic diet, personal hygeine, activity restrictions	4. Prior to d/c, the pt/s.o. will be able to demonstrate competency and/or verbalize understanding of instructions provided		

Signature   Title

_____   _____

_____   _____

_____   _____

_____   _____

_____   _____

Fig. 34-7, cont'd First 3 days of 9-day CareMap® for sepsis with neutropenia.

Sample Evaluation of Interventions for Risk for Infection

GOALS	EVALUATIVE MEASURES	EXPECTED OUTCOMES
Client will remain free of nosocomial infection.	Inspect intravenous puncture site for erythema swelling, purulent drainage. Palpate site for tenderness. Measure client's body temperature.	Intravenous needle site will not become infected. Client will remain afebrile during hospitalization. WBC count will remain normal.
Client will practice infection-control techniques at home.	Review laboratory test results. Ask client to describe basic infection control measures used in the home. Observe client performing medical aseptic procedures.	Client will identify examples of infection control (e.g., handwashing before meal preparation) appropriate to home. Client will correctly perform procedures such as dressing change and self-administration of injections.

■ KEY CONCEPTS ■

▶ Handwashing is the most important technique in preventing and controlling transmission of infection.

▶ The potential for microorganisms to cause disease depends on number of organisms, virulence, ability to enter and survive in a host, and susceptibility of the host.

▶ Normal body flora helps to resist infection by releasing antibacterial substances and inhibiting multiplication of pathogenic microorganisms.

▶ The signs of local inflammation and infection are identical.

▶ An infection can develop as long as the six elements composing the infection chain are uninterrupted.

▶ Microorganisms are transmitted by direct and indirect contact, by airborne spread, and by vectors and contaminated vehicles.

▶ Increasing age, poor nutrition, stress, inherited conditions, chronic disease, and treatments or conditions that compromise the immune response may increase susceptibility to infection.

▶ The major sites for nosocomial infections include the urinary and respiratory tracts, bloodstream, and surgical or traumatic wounds.

▶ Invasive procedures, medical therapies, long hospitalization, and contact with health care personnel increase a hospitalized client's risk for acquiring a nosocomial infection.

▶ Clients within an intensive care unit have a higher risk for infection than clients who are not in this area due to increased exposure to invasive procedures.

▶ Isolation practices may prevent personnel and clients from acquiring infections and may prevent transmission of microorganisms to other persons.

▶ Body Substance Isolation uses generic infection-control precautions for all clients.

▶ Proper cleansing requires mechanical removal of all foreign material from an object or area.

▶ Standard Precautions combine the features of universal precautions and BSI to prevent the spread of organisms in blood, all other body fluids, nonintact skin, and mucous membranes.

▶ A client in isolation is subject to sensory deprivation because of the restricted environment.

▶ An infection-control professional monitors the incidence of infection within an institution and provides educational and consultative services to maintain infection prevention.

▶ Surgical asepsis requires more stringent techniques than medical asepsis and is directed at eliminating microorganisms.

▶ If the skin is broken or if the nurse performs an invasive procedure into a body cavity normally free of microorganisms, surgical aseptic practices are followed.

■ KEY TERMS ■

Aerobic, p. 743

Anaerobic, p. 743

Antibodies, p. 748

Antigen, p. 747

Asepsis, p. 749

Asymptomatic, p. 742

Bacteriocidal, p. 743

Bacteriostasis, p. 743

Broad-spectrum antibiotics, p. 746

■ CRITICAL THINKING EXERCISES ■

1. It is a busy day on 6300, a general surgery nursing unit. Joe Thomas, RN, enters Mr. Willis' room to administer his 8:00 AM dose of antibiotic. The physician has ordered a blood test on Mr. Willis, so Joe obtains a blood specimen. While in the room, Joe also prepares the bath water for Mr. Willis to begin morning hygiene. Joe next visits Ms. Marshall, who underwent colon surgery. Her dressing shows drainage, so Joe removes the soiled gauze and applies a new dressing. While in the room, Joe measures Ms. Marshall's temperature. Finally, Joe is called to check Mr. Skiles, who requests a pain medication. Joe prepares an injection and administers it to Mr. Skiles. Which of the activities in the above clinical situation required Joe to use clean, disposable gloves? When should Joe be washing his hands?

2. The infection chain consists of six elements. Identify the elements of the infection chain, then describe which part of the chain may be broken by the introduction of an intravenous catheter into a client. Explain the potential risks to the client. What barriers should the nurse use to protect and prevent transmission of microorganisms from the client to the nurse?

3. Mrs. Lacson became ill suddenly with fever, chills, and malaise. Her doctor diagnosed viral influenza. Describe the phase of the immune response in which the viral cells are attacked by the body. What class of immunoglobulins would be measured at this time?

4. Mrs. Niles is 83 years old and lives alone. She has difficulty walking and relies on a church volunteer group to deliver lunches during the week. Her fixed income limits her ability to buy food. Last week, Mrs. Niles' 79-year-old sister died. The two sisters had been very close. As a home health care nurse, explain the factors that might increase Mrs. Niles' risk for infection.

REFERENCES

Association of Operating Room Nurses: *Standards and recommended practices for perioperative nursing,* Denver, 1994, The Association.

Ayleffe G et al: *Control of hospital infections: a practical handbook,* ed 3, London, 1992, Chapman and Hall.

Centers for Disease Control: Update: universal precautions for prevention of transmission of human immunodeficiency virus, Hepatitis B virus, and other bloodborne pathogens in health care settings, *MMWR* 37(24):377, 1988.

Centers for Disease Control and Prevention: Guidelines for preventing the transmission of tuberculosis in the health care setting, with special focus on HIV-related issues, *MMWR* 39(RR-17):1, 1990.

Centers for Disease Control and Prevention: Guideline for preventing the transmission of mycobacterium tuberculosis in health-care facilities, *Federal Register* 59(208):54242, 1994a.

Centers for Disease Control and Prevention: Recommendations for prevention of nosocomial pneumonia, *Am J Infect Control* 22(4):247, 1994b.

Centers for Disease Control and Prevention: Draft guideline for isolation precautions in hospitals, *Federal Register* 59(214):55552, 1994.

Classen DC et al: Prevention of catheter-associated bacteriuria: clinical trial of methods to block three known pathways of infection, *Am J Infect Control* 19(3):136, 1991.

Crow S: Asepsis: an indispensable part of the patient's care plan, *Critical Care Nursing Q* 11(4):11, 1989.

Garner J, Favero M: CDC guidelines for handwashing and hospital environmental control, *Infect Control* 7:231, 1986.

Garner JS: Guidelines for isolation precautions in hospitals, *Infect Control Hosp Epidemiol* 17(1):54, 1996.

Garner JS, Simmons BP: CDC guidelines for the prevention and control of nosocomial infections: guidelines for isolation precautions in hospitals, *Am J Infect Control* 12:103, 1984.

Grimes D, Grimes R: *AIDS and HIV infections,* St Louis, 1994, Mosby.

Hingst V et al: Evaluation of the efficacy of surgical hand disinfection following a reduced application time of 3 instead of 5 minutes, *J Hosp Infect* 20:79, 1992.

Hospital Infection Control Practices Advisory Committee (HICPAC), Centers for Disease Control and Prevention: Recommendations for preventing the spread of vancomycin resistance, *Am J Infect Control* 23(2):87, 1995.

Jackson M, Lynch P: An attempt to make an issue less murky: a comparison of four systems for infection precautions, *Infect Control & Hosp Epidemiology* 12:448, 1991.

Jackson M, Lynch P: Body substance isolation, *Infect Control & Hosp Epidemiology* 13(4):191, 1992.

Joint Commission on Accreditation of Health Care Organizations: *Comprehensive accreditation manual for hospitals*, Oakbrook Terrace, Ill, 1995, The Commission.

Kim MJ, McFarland, McLane: *Pocket guide to nursing diagnoses*, ed 6, St Louis, 1995, Mosby.

Larson E: APIC guidelines for use of topical antimicrobial agents, *Amer J Infect Control* 16(6):253, 1988.

Larson E: Handwashing: it's essential even when you use gloves, *Amer J Nursing* 89:934, 1989.

Larson E: APIC guidelines for handwashing and hand antisepsis in health care setting, *Amer Infect Control* 23:4, 1995.

Larson E, Lusk E: Evaluating handwashing technique, *J Advance Nursing* 10:547, 1985.

Lynch P, Jackson M: Implementing and evaluating a system of generic infection precautions: body substance isolation, *Amer J Infect Control* 18:1, 1990.

Maki DG, Ringer M: Evaluation of dressing regimens for prevention of infection with peripheral intravenous catheters, *JAMA* 258(17):2396, 1987.

Maki DG et al: Double-bagging of items from isolation rooms is unnecessary as an infection control measure: a comparative study of surface contamination with single and double-bagging, *Infect Control* 7(11):535, 1986.

Meeker M, Rothrock J: *Alexander's care of patient in surgery*, ed 10, St Louis, 1995, Mosby.

Occupational Safety and Health Administration, Occupational Safety and Health Act of 1991: Blood-borne pathogens, *Federal Register* 56(235):64175, 1991.

Occupational Safety and Health Administration: Respiratory protection: proposed rule, *Federal Register* 59(219):58884, 1994.

O'Shaughnessy M et al: Given H.F. optimum duration of surgical scrub time, *Brit J Surgery* 78:685, 1991.

Pereira LJ et al: The effect of surgical handwashing routines on the microbial counts of operating room nurses, *Amer J Infect Control* 18:354, 1990.

Pottinger J et al: Bacterial carriage by artificial versus natural nails, *Amer J Infect Control* 17(6):340, 1989.

Rutala W: APIC guideline for selection and use of disinfectant, *Amer J Infect Control* 18(2):99, 1990.

Rutala W: *Chemical germicides in health care*, Washington, DC, 1995, APIC.

Smith P, Rusnak P: APIC guideline for infection prevention and control in the long-term care facility, *Amer J Infect Control* 19(4):198, 1991.

Springer L et al: Anticipated care for HIV-infected clients: nurses' reactions, *J Assoc Nurses in AIDS Care* 5(1):29, 1994.

Tideiksaar R: Infections in the elderly. I. Diagnosis and treatment, *Physician Assist* 11(2):17, 1987.

Weinstein SA et al: Bacterial surface contamination of patient's linen: isolation precautions versus standard care, *Am J Infect Control* 17(5):264, 1989.

Williams WW: CDC guidelines for infection control in hospital personnel, *Infect Control* 4(4):325, 1983.

ADDITIONAL READINGS

Banick B: Light at the end of a decade, *AJN* 90:37, 1990.

Benenson A: *Control of communicable disease in man*, Washington, DC, 1990, APHA.

Choudhuri M et al: Efficiency of skin sterilization for a venipuncture with the use of commercially available alcohol or iodine pads, *Am J Infect Control* 18(2):82, 1990.

Department of Labor: Joint advisory notice: Department of Labor and Department of Health and Human Services, *HBV/HIV* Oct 30, 1987, p 52.

Ebersole P, Hess P: *Toward healthy aging*, ed 4, St Louis, 1994, Mosby.

Forrester DA: AIDS-related risk factors, medical diagnosis, do-not-resuscitate orders and aggressiveness of nursing care, *Nurs Res* 39(6):350, 1990.

Grimes D, Grimes B: *Infectious disease*, St Louis, 1995, Mosby.

Health Services and Promotion Branch: *Infection control guidelines for isolation precautions*, Ottawa, 1990, Department of National Health and Welfare.

Jackson M et al: *The body substance isolation system, infection prevention and control manual*, San Diego, 1987, University of California, San Diego Medical Center.

MMWR update: Universal precautions for prevention of transmission of HIV, hepatitis B virus and other bloodborne pathogens in health care settings, *MMWR* 37(24):378, 1988.

Pagana KD, Pagana TJ: *Diagnostic testing and nursing implications*, ed 4, St Louis, 1994, Mosby.

Thibodeau GA, Patton K: *Anatomy and physiology*, ed 2, St Louis, 1993, Mosby.

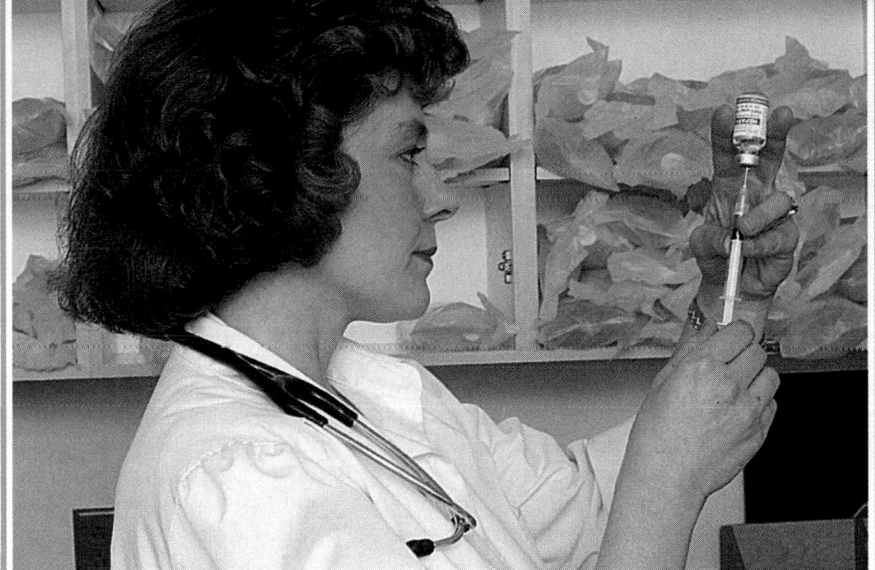

Chapter 35

Administration of
Medications

Objectives

Mastery of content in this chapter will enable the student to:

▶ Define the key terms listed.

▶ Discuss the nurse's legal responsibilities in drug prescription and administration.

▶ Describe the physiological mechanisms of drug action, including absorption, distribution, metabolism, and excretion.

▶ Differentiate among toxic, idiosyncratic, allergic, and side effects of drugs.

▶ Discuss developmental factors that influence drug pharmacokinetics.

▶ Discuss factors that influence drug actions.

▶ Discuss methods of promoting and maintaining a client's health through medication teaching.

▶ Describe the roles of the pharmacist, physician, and nurse in drug administration.

▶ Describe factors to consider in choosing routes of administration.

▶ Correctly calculate a prescribed drug dosage.

▶ Assess the client's need for and response to drug therapy.

▶ List the "five rights" of drug administration.

▶ Correctly prepare and administer subcutaneous, intramuscular, and intradermal injections and intravenous medication; insulin injections; oral medications; topical skin preparations; eye, ear, and nose drops; vaginal instillations; rectal suppositories; and inhalants.

▶ Identify educational preparation for the client receiving home IV therapy.

The safe and accurate administration of medications is one of the nurse's most important responsibilities. Drugs are a primary means of therapy by which physicians treat clients with health problems. Although drugs benefit clients in many ways, any drug can have serious side effects or has the potential for causing harmful effects when administered improperly. The nurse is responsible for understanding a drug's action and its side effects, administering it correctly, monitoring the client's response, and helping the client self-administer drugs correctly and knowledgeably.

In addition to knowing about a specific drug's action, the nurse must also understand the client's previous and current health problems to determine whether a particular medication is safe to give. The nurse's judgment is critical for proper and safe drug administration.

■ DRUG NOMENCLATURE AND FORMS

A drug, or **medication**, is a substance used in the diagnosis, treatment, cure, relief, or prevention of disease. Health care personnel use the terms *drugs* and *medications* interchangeably. Lay persons commonly refer to medications as *medicines*.

Physicians and dentists prescribe the majority of medications in the United States and Canada. However, in a few states, nurse practitioners and physician assistants may prescribe selected medications, under the supervision of a physician.

Names

A single medication may have as many as four different names. The *chemical name* provides an exact description of the drug's composition. An example of a chemical name is acetylsalicylic acid, commonly known as *aspirin*. The generic name is given by the manufacturer who first develops the drug before it receives FDA approval, and it is protected by law. *Aspirin* and *verapamil hydrochloride* are examples of generic names. Federal legislation in 1962 mandated that there be one official name for each drug. The official name of a drug is the name under which the drug is listed in official publications such as the *United States Pharmacopeia (USP)*. A drug's generic name often becomes its official name, as in the case of aspirin.

The *trade name, brand name,* or *proprietary name* is the name under which a manufacturer markets a drug. A generic drug may have many different trade names. For example, aspirin is known by the trade name *Bufferin,* and verapamil hydrochloride is known by the trade names *Calan* and *Isoptin.* The trade name has the symbol ® at the upper right of the name, indicating that the drug has been registered. Manufacturers try to choose trade names that are easy to pronounce and spell to help the lay person recognize and remember the medications more readily. Because many companies may produce the same drug, similarities in trade names can be confusing. The nurse encounters medications under a variety of different nomenclatures, or names, and must be careful to obtain the exact name and spelling for a particular drug.

Classification

Care givers categorize medications with similar characteristics by their classifications. Drug classification indicates the effect on a body system, the symptoms relieved, or the desired effect. Each class contains drugs prescribed for similar types of health problems. The physical and chemical composition of drugs within a class is not necessarily the same. A drug may also belong to more than one class. For example, aspirin is an analgesic, an antipyretic, and an antiinflammatory.

Nurses should know the general characteristics of medications in each class. Each class has nursing implications for proper administration and monitoring. For example, nursing implications related to diuretic administration include monitoring intake and output, weighing the client daily, assessing the development of edema in body tissues, and monitoring serum electrolyte levels. Nursing implications for all drugs within a class provide guidelines for safe and effective care.

Drug Forms

Drugs are available in a variety of forms, or preparations (Fig. 35-1). The form of the drug determines its route of administration. For example, a capsule is taken orally, and a solution may be given intravenously. The composition of a drug is designed to enhance its absorption and metabolism within the body. Many drugs are available in several forms such as tablets, capsules, elixirs, and suppositories. When administering a medication, the nurse must be certain to give the medication in the proper form (Table 35-1).

■ DRUG LEGISLATION AND STANDARDS

Drug Standards

In 1906, the U.S. government set standards for drug quality and purity as a result of the Pure Food and Drug Act. Official publications, such as the *USP* and the *National Formulary*, set standards for drug strength, quality, purity, packaging, safety, labeling, and dosage form. In Canada the *British Pharmacopoeia (BP)* sets similar standards. Physicians, nurses, and pharmacists depend on these standards to ensure that clients receive pure drugs in safe and effec-

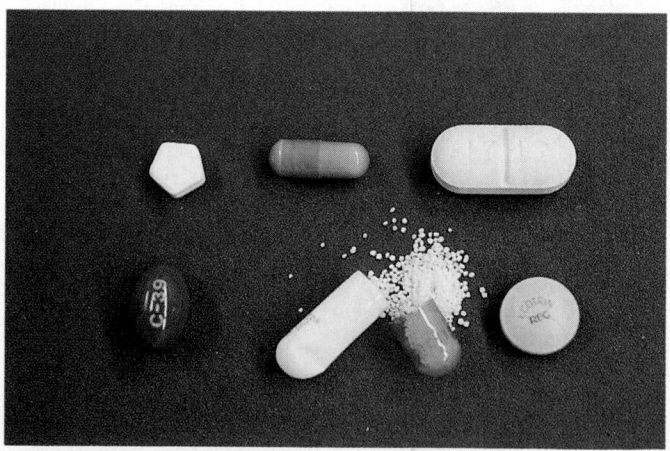

Fig. 35-1 Forms of oral medications: *(top row)* uniquely shaped tablet, capsule, scored tablet; *(bottom row)* gelatin-coated liquid, extended-release capsule, enteric-coated tablet.

	Table 35-1	Forms of Medication

FORM	DESCRIPTION
Caplet	Solid dosage form for oral use; shaped like capsule and coated for ease of swallowing
Capsule	Solid dosage form for oral use; medication in powder, liquid, or oil form and encased by gelatin shell; capsule colored to aid in product identification
Elixir	Clear fluid containing water and/or alcohol; designed for oral use; usually has sweetener added
Enteric-coated tablet	Tablet for oral use coated with materials that do not dissolve in stomach; coatings dissolve in intestine, where medication is absorbed
Extract	Concentrated drug form made by removing active portion of drug from its other components (e.g., fluid extract is drug made into solution from vegetable source)
Glycerite	Solution of drug combined with glycerin for external use; contains at least 50% glycerin
Intraocular disk	A small, flexible oval consisting of two soft, outer layers and a middle layer containing medication. When moistened by ocular fluid, it releases medication for up to 1 week.
Liniment	Preparation usually containing alcohol, oil, or soapy emollient that is applied to skin
Lotion	Drug in liquid, suspension applied externally to protect skin
Ointment (salve)	Semisolid, externally applied preparation, usually containing one or more drugs
Paste	Semisolid preparation, thicker and stiffer than ointment; absorbed through skin more slowly than ointment
Pill	Solid dosage form containing one or more drugs, shaped into globules, ovoids, or oblong shapes; true pills rarely used because they have been replaced by tablets
Solution	Liquid preparation that may be used orally, parenterally, or externally; can also be instilled into body organ or cavity (e.g., bladder irrigations); contains water with one or more dissolved compounds; must be sterile for parenteral use
Suppository	Solid dosage form mixed with gelatin and shaped in form of pellet for insertion into body cavity (rectum or vagina); melts when it reaches body temperature, releasing drug for absorption
Suspension	Finely divided drug particles dispersed in liquid medium; when suspension is left standing, particles settle to bottom of container; commonly oral medication and not given intravenously
Syrup	Medication dissolved in concentrated sugar solution; may contain flavoring to make drug more palatable
Tablet	Powdered dosage form compressed into hard disks or cylinders; in addition to primary drug, contains binders (adhesive to allow powder to stick together), disintegrators (to promote tablet dissolution), lubricants (for ease of manufacturing), and fillers (for convenient tablet size)
Transdermal disk or patch	Medication contained within semipermeable membrane disk or patch, which allows medications to be absorbed through skin slowly over long period
Tincture	Alcohol or water-alcohol drug solution
Troche (lozenge)	Flat, round dosage form containing drug, flavoring, sugar, and mucilage; dissolves in mouth to release drug

tive dosages. Accepted standards must be met in the following areas:

1. Purity. Manufacturers must meet purity standards for the type and concentration of other substances allowed in drug products.
2. Potency. The concentration of active drug in the preparation affects strength, or potency.
3. Bioavailability. The ability of a drug to be released from its dosage form and dissolved, absorbed, and transported by the body to its site of action is its **bioavailability.**
4. Efficacy. Detailed laboratory studies can help determine a drug's effectiveness.
5. Safety. All drugs should be continually evaluated to determine their side effects.

Legislation and Control

In the United States, drug legislation began with the Pure Food and Drug Act of 1906. The act focused attention on the purity of food but also set official standards for drugs. Manufacturers were required to label drugs accurately and ensure that the strength and purity of drugs conformed to their claims. Since that time, federal law has extended and refined government controls on drug sales and distribution;

drug testing, naming, and labeling; and the regulation of controlled substances (Tables 35-2 and 35-3).

State drug laws must conform with federal legislation. States can also impose additional controls, including control of substances not regulated by the federal government. For example, local governments can regulate the sale and use of alcohol and tobacco.

Health care institutions establish policies that conform to federal, state, and local regulations. The size of an institution, the types of services it provides, and the types of professional personnel it employs influence policies for drug control, distribution, and administration. Institutional policies are often more restrictive than government controls. An institution is primarily concerned with preventing health problems resulting from drug use. For example, a common institutional policy is the automatic discontinuation of antibiotic therapy after a set number of days. Although a physician may reorder an antibiotic, this policy helps to control unnecessarily prolonged drug therapy, which may lead to sensitivity or toxic reactions.

Federal, state, and local legislation governs nursing practice, including the administration of medications. State nurse practice acts define and set limits on the scope of a nurse's professional functions and responsibilities. These

Table 35-2	Federal Drug Laws in the United States	
DATE	**TITLE OF LAW**	**PROVISIONS**
1906	Pure Food and Drug Act	Designated official standards for drugs (*USP* and the *National Formulary*); specified standards for drug labeling
1912	Sherley Amendment	Prohibited manufacturers from making fraudulent claims about drug efficacy and therapeutic effects
1914	Harrison Narcotic Act	Legally classified drugs believed to be habit forming as *narcotics;* regulated importation, manufacture, sale, and use of narcotic substances
1938	Federal Food, Drug, and Cosmetic Act	Added the *Homeopathic Pharmacopeia of the United States* as a third drug standard; required that drug preparation be approved as safe by the Food and Drug Administration (FDA) before marketing; further outlined criteria for drug labeling
1945	Amendment to the Food and Drug Act	Provided for certification of biological products used as drugs (e.g., insulin, antibiotics) on batch basis; allowed for direct supervision and inspection of drug production
1952	Durham-Humphrey Amendment	Distinguished between prescription ("legend") and nonprescription drugs
1962	Kefauver-Harris Amendment	Authorized FDA to supervise drug production to ensure safety and efficacy and to establish official drug names; specified greater controls on investigational drugs
1970	Comprehensive Drug Abuse Prevention and Control Act (Controlled Substances Act)	Set strict controls on manufacture and distribution of controlled drugs (possession of controlled substances unlawful without prescription); established government programs to promote prevention and treatment of drug dependence

Table 35-3	Canadian Drug Legislation	
DATE	**TITLE OF LAW**	**PROVISIONS**
1908	Proprietary or Patent Medicine Act	Set standards to protect consumers from unsafe and ineffective nonprescription drugs
1953	Canadian Food and Drug Act	Prohibited sale of contaminated, unsafe drugs and of improperly labeled drugs; designated official standards (*Pharmacopoeia Internationalis, BP,* and *Canadian Formulary*); defined certain controlled drugs; prohibited advertising of prescription and controlled drugs to general public; set standards for labeling
1961	Canadian Narcotic Control Act	Restricted sale, possession, and use of narcotics; set guidelines for reporting loss of theft of narcotics; set standards for labeling and record keeping

acts are joint policy statements made by nursing, medical, and hospital associations in a state. Institutions and agencies may interpret specific actions allowed under the acts, but they cannot modify, expand, or restrict the act's intent. The nurse practice acts protect the public from unskilled, undereducated, and unlicensed nurses.

Nurses must know the regulations affecting drug administration in their practice areas. When moving from one state to another, nurses may discover significant differences in the laws governing drug administration. For example, laws vary concerning the prescription and administration of drugs. In the past, only physicians prescribed medications. Today, several states have recognized the expanding role of the nurse and have revised nurse practice acts to include the prescribing of medications by nurses in advanced practice. In most cases, this privilege is limited to certified nurse practitioners, clinical nurse specialists, nurse anesthetists and nurse midwives who collaborate with a physician.

Before assuming the responsibility of administering IV medications, the nurse should be aware of the administrative policies of the employing institution related to them. Because IV injection of medications may cause serious adverse effects, nurses who perform this function must be qualified through proper training, education, and experience.

The nurse is responsible for following legal provisions when administering **controlled substances** (drugs that affect the mind or behavior), which can be dispensed only with a prescription. Violations of the Controlled Substances Act are punishable by fines, imprisonment, and loss of nurse licensure. Hospitals and other health care institutions have policies for the proper storage and distribution of controlled substances, including **narcotics** (see the box on p. 793, left).

Nontherapeutic Drug Use

Despite legislative controls, some people use drugs for purposes other than their proper one. The indiscriminate use of drugs poses serious health problems for users, families,

---

Guidelines for Safe Narcotic Administration and Control

- Store all narcotics in a locked, secure cabinet or container. (Computerized, locked cabinets are now available.)
- Nurses in charge carry a set of keys (or a special computer entry code) for the narcotics cabinet.
- During an institution's change-of-shift, the nurse going off duty counts all narcotics with the nurse coming on duty. Both nurses sign the narcotic record to indicate that the count is correct.
- Discrepancies in narcotic counts are reported immediately.
- A special inventory record is used each time a narcotic is dispensed.
- The record is used to document the client's name, date, time of drug administration, name of drug, dosage, and signature of nurse dispensing the drug.
- The form provides an accurate ongoing count of narcotics used and remaining.
- If only one part of a premeasured dosage of a controlled substance is given, a second nurse witnesses disposal of the unused portion and documents such on the record form.

Terms Associated with the Nontherapeutic Use of Drugs

ABUSE
A maladaptive pattern of substance use indicated by at least one of the following in a 12-month period:
- Recurrent substance use resulting in a failure to fulfill major role obligations at work, school, or home (e.g., repeated absences or poor work performance)
- Recurrent substance use in situations in which it is physically hazardous (e.g., driving an automobile or operating a machine when impaired by substance use)
- Recurrent substance-related legal problems (e.g., arrests for substance-related disorderly conduct)
- Continued substance use despite having persistent or recurrent social or interpersonal problems caused or exacerbated by the effects of the substance (e.g., arguments with spouse about consequences of intoxication, physical fights)

DEPENDENCE
At least three of the following in a 12-month period:
- Substance often taken in larger amounts of over a longer period than the person intended
- Persistent desire or one or more unsuccessful efforts to cut down or control substance use
- A great deal of time spent in activities necessary to get the substance, taking the substance, or recovering from its effects
- Frequent intoxication or withdrawal symptoms when expected to fulfill major role obligations at work, school, or home
- Important social, occupational, or recreational activities given up or reduced because of substance use
- Continued substance use despite knowledge of having a persistent or recurrent social, psychological, or physical problem caused or exacerbated by the use of the substance
- Marked tolerance, need for markedly increased amounts of the substance to achieve intoxication or desired effect, or markedly diminished effect with continued use of the same amount

Modified from American Psychiatric Association: *Diagnostic and statistical manual of mental disorders (DSM-IV)*, rev 4, Washington, DC, 1994, The Association.

---

and communities. In the past, the misuse or abuse of medications was related to use for therapeutic qualities, such as the relief of pain or reduction in anxiety. Today, factors such as peer pressure, curiosity, and the pursuit of pleasure are motivators for nontherapeutic drug use. Problems with drug use are not limited to heroin, cocaine, and other "hard" drugs. Millions of people in the United States and Canada consume alcohol daily. Our society is drug conscious, as shown by the frequent advertisements for pain relievers, decongestants, and antacids on television.

Nurses have ethical and legal obligations to understand the problems of persons using drugs improperly. When caring for clients with suspected **drug abuse** or **drug dependence**, nurses must be aware of their own values and attitudes about the willful use of potentially harmful substances. Nurses cannot develop therapeutic relationships with clients if personal values interfere with acceptance or understanding of their needs. Knowing the physical, psychological, and social changes resulting from drug abuse allows nurses to identify clients with drug problems.

A problem involving the misuse of drugs by health professionals also exists. Stress in the work place, personal problems, and the strong desire to perform well are some of the factors that may cause nurses to rely on drugs. Nurses must recognize and understand the problems of colleagues who suffer from drug abuse (see the box above, right). Today, many programs are available to assist these nurses toward recovery. These programs may be offered through the institution's Employee's Assistance Program, the state board of nursing, or community agencies.

■ NATURE OF DRUG ACTIONS

Medications act to produce therapeutically useful effects. A drug does not create a function in a tissue or organ but rather alters physiological functions. Drugs may protect cells from the influence of other chemical agents, promote cell function, or accelerate or slow cell processes. A medication may replace a substance that is missing (e.g., insulin, thyroid hormone, or estrogen).

Mechanisms of Action

Drugs produce actions by altering body fluids or cell membranes or by interacting with receptor sites. The drug aluminum hydroxide gel alters the chemical properties of a body fluid (specifically by neutralizing the stomach's acid contents). Drugs such as general anesthetic gases interact with cell membranes. After properties of the cells become altered, the drug exerts its effects. The most common mechanism of drug action is binding to a cell's receptor sites. Receptors localize drug effects. Sites on the receptors interact with drugs because of similar chemical shapes. The drug and receptor bind together like a lock and key. When receptors and drugs lock together, the therapeutic effects are realized. Each tissue or cell in the body possesses a unique group of receptors. For example, receptors in the myocardial cells respond to digitalis preparations.

Pharmacokinetics

Pharmacokinetics is the study of how drugs enter the body, reach their site of action, are metabolized, and exit the body. The physician and nurse use the knowledge of pharmacokinetics when timing drug administration, selecting the route of administration, judging the risk for alterations in drug action, and observing client response.

Absorption

Absorption is the passage of drug molecules into the blood. Most drugs, except those applied topically for local effects, must enter the systemic circulation to exert a therapeutic effect. Factors influencing drug absorption include route of administration, ability of the drug to dissolve, and conditions at the site of absorption.

Each route has a different influence on drug absorption, depending on the physical structure of the tissues. The skin is relatively impermeable to chemicals, making absorption slow. The mucous membranes and respiratory airways allow quick drug absorption because of the high vascularity of mucosal and alveolar-capillary surfaces. Because orally administered drugs must pass through the gastrointestinal tract to be absorbed, the overall rate of absorption may be slowed. IV injection produces the most rapid absorption because this route provides immediate access to the systemic circulation.

The ability of an oral medication to dissolve after ingestion depends largely on its forms or preparation. Solutions and suspensions already in a liquid state are absorbed more readily than tablets or capsules. Solid dosage forms must first disintegrate to expose the chemical to gastric and intestinal secretions. Acidic drugs pass through the gastric mucosa rapidly. Drugs that are basic are not absorbed before reaching the small intestine.

Conditions at the site of absorption influence the ease with which medications enter the systemic circulation. When skin is abraded, topical drugs are absorbed easily. Topical substances normally prescribed for local effect can cause serious reactions when absorbed through the skin's layers. The formation of edema in mucous membranes slows drug absorption because medications take longer to diffuse to blood vessels. The absorption of parenterally administered medications depends on the blood supply of the tissues. Before administering a drug by injection, the nurse should assess for local factors, such as edema, bruising, or scarring, which might impair the absorption of the medication. Because muscles have a richer blood supply than subcutaneous (SQ) tissues, a drug given intramuscularly is absorbed more quickly than one injected subcutaneously. In some instances a delayed SQ absorption is preferable because it produces long-lasting drug effects. If a client's tissue perfusion is poor, as in the case of circulatory shock, the IV route is best. IV administration provides the most rapid and dependable absorption.

Oral medications are absorbed more easily when administered between meals. When the stomach is filled with food, the contents are emptied slowly into the duodenum, thus slowing drug absorption. Certain foods and antacids cause drugs to bind into complexes that cannot pass through the gastrointestinal tract lining. For example, milk interferes with the absorption of iron and tetracycline. Some drugs are destroyed by the increased acidity of gastric contents and protein digestion during a meal. Enteric coatings on certain tablets resist dissolution in gastric juices and prevent certain medications from being digested in the upper gastrointestinal tract. The coating also protects the stomach lining from irritation by the medication.

The route of drug administration is prescribed by the health care provider. Nurses may need to request that a medication be given by an alternate route or in a different form, based on physical assessment of the client. For example, a client may not be able to swallow tablets; therefore the nurse would request the medication be an elixir or syrup. Knowledge of factors that alter or impair drug absorption helps the nurse administer drugs correctly. Food in the gastrointestinal tract can affect the pH, motility, and emptying of drugs into the GI tract. The rate of absorption and extent of absoprtion may also be affected by foods. The nurse should be aware of the nursing implications for each medication given. For example, drugs such as aspirin, iron, and phenytoin sodium (Dilantin) irritate the gastrointestinal tract and should be administered with or immediately after a meal. However, food may interfere with the absorption of drugs such as cloxacillin sodium and penicillin; therefore they should be given 1 to 2 hours before meals or 2 to 3 hours afterward. Before administering any drug, the nurse should consult nursing drug books, package inserts or the hospital pharmacist regarding drug-nutrient interactions.

Distribution

After a drug is absorbed, it is distributed within the body to tissues and organs and ultimately to its specific site of action. The rate and extent of distribution depend on the physical and chemical properties of the drug and the physiological makeup of the person taking the drug.

■ BODY WEIGHT AND COMPOSITION

A direct relationship exists between the amount of drug administration and the amount of body tissue in which it is distributed. Most medications are prescribed based on the average adult weight and body composition. Changes in body composition can significantly affect distribution of drugs. An example of this can be found in the older client. With aging, the amount of body water decreases. Therefore drugs that are water-soluble are not distributed as well, and their concentration is elevated in the older client's blood. An increase in the percentage of body fat, commonly found in the older client, causes a longer duration of drug action because of slower distribution throughout the body. The less a client weighs, the greater the concentration of a drug in his or her tissues, and the more powerful the drug's effects. The older adult experiences a reduction in both tissue mass and height and often requires a lower drug dose than a younger client.

■ CIRCULATORY DYNAMICS

Drugs pass more easily from interstitial to intravascular spaces than between body compartments. Blood vessels are permeable to most dissolved substances unless drug particles are large or bound to serum proteins. The concentration of a drug at a specific site depends on the number of blood vessels in tissues, the degree of local vasodilation or vasoconstriction, and the rate of blood flow to a tissue site. Exercise, warming, and chilling alter local circulation. For example, if a client applies a warm compress to an intra-muscular (IM) injection site, the resultant vasodilation increases drug distribution.

Biological membranes may serve as barriers to passage of drugs. The blood-brain barrier allows only fat-soluble drugs to pass into the brain and cerebrospinal fluid. Central nervous system infections require treatment with antibiotics injected directly into the subarachnoid space in the spinal cord. Older clients may experience adverse effects (e.g., confusion) as a result of a change in the permeability of the blood-brain barrier, with easier passage of fat-soluble drugs. The placental membrane is a nonselective barrier to drugs. Fat- and nonfat-soluble agents may cross the placenta and produce fetal deformities, respiratory depression and, with narcotic abuse, withdrawal symptoms. Women need to know the hazards of drug use during pregnancy.

PROTEIN BINDING

The degree to which drugs bind to serum protein, such as albumin, affects drug distribution. Most medications bind to this protein to some extent. When drug molecules are bound to albumin, they cannot exert any pharmacological activity. Unbound or "free" drug is the active form of the drug. Older adults have a decreased albumin level in the bloodstream, probably caused by a change in liver function. The same is true for clients with liver disease or malnutrition. Because of this, older adults may be at risk for an increase in drug activity, toxicity, or both.

Metabolism

After a drug reaches its site of action, it is metabolized into an inactive form that is more easily excreted. This **biotransformation** occurs under the influence of enzymes that detoxify, degrade (break down), and remove biologically active chemicals. Most biotransformation occurs within the liver, although the lungs, kidneys, blood, and intestines also metabolize drugs.

The liver is especially important because its specialized structure oxidizes and transforms many toxic substances. The liver degrades many harmful chemicals before they are distributed to the tissues. The decrease in liver function that occurs with aging or with liver disease influences the rate at which a drug is eliminated from the body. The resultant slowing of metabolism causes the drug to accumulate in the body. Thus a client would be at greater risk for drug toxicity. If any of the organs that participate in drug metabolism are altered, a client is at risk for drug toxicity.

Excretion

After drugs are metabolized, they exit the body through the kidneys, liver, bowel, lungs, and exocrine glands. The chemical makeup of a drug determines the organ of excretion. Gaseous and volatile compounds such as ether, nitrous oxide, and alcohol exit through the lungs. Deep breathing and coughing help the postoperative client eliminate anesthetic gases more rapidly.

The exocrine glands excrete lipid-soluble drugs. When medications exit through sweat glands, the skin may become irritated. The nurse assists the client in good hygiene practices to promote cleanliness and skin integrity. If a drug exits through the mammary glands, a nursing infant may absorb the chemicals. Nursing mothers should check on the safety of each drug. The risk to the infant receiving the drug and the risk of the mother not taking the drug must be given careful consideration.

The gastrointestinal tract is another route for drug excretion. Many drugs enter the hepatic circulation to be broken down by the liver and excreted into the bile. After chemicals enter the intestines through the biliary tract, they may be reabsorbed by the intestines. Factors increasing peristalsis, such as laxatives and enemas, accelerate drug excretion through the feces, whereas factors slowing peristalsis, such as inactivity and improper diet, may prolong a drug's effects.

The kidneys are the main organs for drug excretion. Some drugs escape extensive metabolism and exit relatively unchanged in the urine. Others undergo biotransformation in the liver before they are excreted by the kidney. If renal function declines, a common change in aging, the risk for drug toxicity increases. If the kidneys cannot adequately excrete a drug, it may be necessary to reduce the dosage. Maintenance of a normal fluid intake promotes proper elimination of drugs.

Because of its chemical makeup and physiological action, a drug may produce more than one effect.

Therapeutic Effects

The **therapeutic effect** is the intended or predicted physiological response that a drug causes. Each drug has a desired therapeutic effect for which it is prescribed. For example, the nurse administers codeine phosphate to create analgesia and gives theophylline to dilate narrowed respiratory bronchioles. A single medication may have many therapeutic effects. For example, aspirin is an analgesic, antipyretic, and antiinflammatory, and it reduces platelet aggregation (clumping).

Side Effects

Predictably a drug will cause unintended, secondary effects. These **side effects** may be harmless or injurious. For example, with codeine phosphate, a client may also experience constipation, and theophylline may cause headache and dizziness; these side effects may be considered harmless. However, digoxin may cause cardiac dysrhythmias that could be lethal. If the side effects are serious enough to negate the beneficial effects of a drug's therapeutic action, the physician may discontinue it. Because of side effects, clients often stop taking medications without consulting their health care providers.

Toxic Effects

Generally, **toxic effects** develop after prolonged intake of high doses of medication, after prolonged use of a drug intended for external application, or after a drug accumulates in the blood because of impaired metabolism or excretion. *One* dose of medication can have toxic effects for some clients. Excess amounts of a drug within the body may have lethal effects, depending on the drug's action. For example, morphine, a narcotic analgesic, relieves pain by depressing the central nervous system. However, toxic levels of morphine cause severe respiratory depression and death.

Idiosyncratic Reactions

Medications may cause unpredictable effects such as an **idiosyncratic reaction**, in which a client overreacts, underreacts, or has an abnormal reaction to a drug. For example, a child receiving an antihistamine (e.g., Benadryl) may become extremely agitated or excited instead of drowsy. It is impossible to predict which client will have an idiosyncratic response.

Allergic Reactions

An **allergic reaction** is another unpredictable response to a drug. Allergic reactions account for 5% to 10% of all drug reactions. A client can become sensitized immunologically to the initial dose of a medication. With repeated administration the client develops an allergic response to the drug, its chemical preservatives, or a metabolite. In this case the drug or chemical acts as an antigen, triggering the release of antibodies.

A drug allergy may be mild or severe. Allergic symptoms vary, depending on the individual and the drug; for example, antibiotics cause many allergic reactions. Common allergy symptoms are summarized in Table 35-4. Severe or anaphylactic reactions are characterized by sudden constriction of bronchiolar muscles, edema of the pharynx and larynx, and severe wheezing and shortness of breath. The client may also become severely hypotensive, requiring emergency resuscitation. A client with a known history of allergy to a particular medication should avoid reexposure and should wear an identification bracelet or medal that alerts nurses and physicians to the allergy if the client is unconscious when receiving medical care.

Drug Tolerance

Some clients who receive drugs for long periods may require higher doses to produce the same effect. Clients that are taking various pain medications may develop a tolerance over time. Frequently, clients require increasing doses of pain medications over time to relieve pain.

Drug Interactions

When one drug modifies the action of another, a **drug interaction** occurs. Drug interactions are common in individuals taking several medications. A drug may potentiate or diminish the action of other drugs and may alter the way in which another drug is absorbed, metabolized, or eliminated from the body.

Table 35-4	Mild Allergic Reactions
SYMPTOM	**DESCRIPTION**
Urticaria	Raised, irregularly shaped skin eruptions with varying sizes and shapes; eruptions have reddened margins and pale centers
Rash	Small, raised vesicles that are usually reddened; often distributed over entire body
Pruritus	Itching of skin; accompanies most rashes
Rhinitis	Inflammation of mucous membranes lining nose; causes swelling and clear, watery discharge

When two drugs are given simultaneously, they can have a synergistic or addictive effect. With a **synergistic effect**, the physiological action of the two drugs in combination is greater than the effect of the drugs when given separately. Alcohol is a central nervous system depressant that has a synergistic effect on antihistamines, antidepressants, barbituates and narcotic analgesics.

A drug interaction is not always undesirable. Often a physician orders combination drug therapy to create a drug interaction for therapeutic benefit. For example, a client with moderate hypertension may receive combination drug therapy, such as diuretics and vasodilators, that act together to keep the blood pressure at a desirable level.

Drug Dose Responses

After the nurse administers a drug, it undergoes absorption, distribution, metabolism, and excretion. Except when administered intravenously, drugs take time to enter the bloodstream. The quantity and distribution of a drug in different body compartments change constantly.

When a medication is prescribed, the goal is to achieve a constant blood level within a safe therapeutic range. Repeated doses are required to achieve a constant therapeutic concentration of a medication because a portion of a drug is always being excreted. When absorption ceases, only metabolism, excretion, and distribution continue. The highest **serum concentration** (peak concentration) of the drug usually occurs just before the last of the drug is absorbed. After peaking, the serum concentration falls progressively. With IV drug infusions, the peak concentration occurs quickly, but the serum level also begins to fall immediately.

All drugs have a **serum half-life**, or the time it takes for excretion processes to lower the serum concentration by half. To maintain a therapeutic plateau, the client must re-

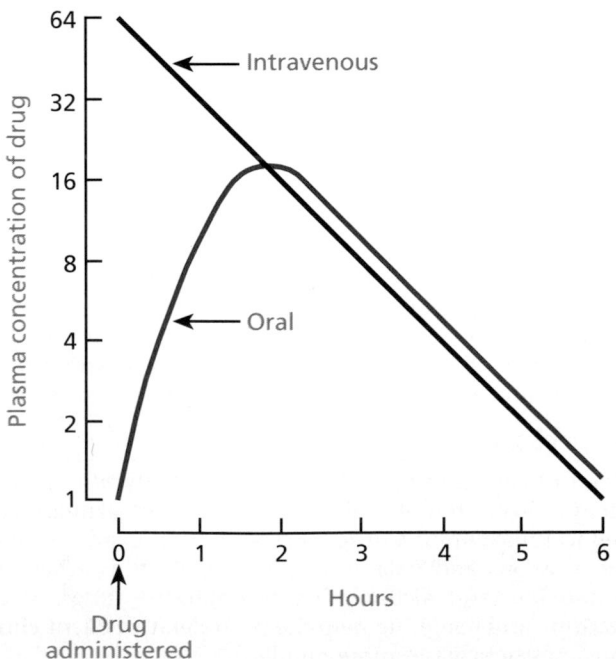

Fig. 35-2 Curve showing therapeutic blood levels. *(From Clark J, Queeners S, Karb V: Pharmacological basis of nursing practice, ed 4, St. Louis, 1993, Mosby.)*

ceive regular, fixed doses. After an initial medication dose the client receives each successive dose when the previous dose reaches its half-life (Fig. 35-2). In this way an almost constant therapeutic drug concentration is maintained.

The client and nurse must follow regular dosage schedules and adhere to prescribed doses and dosage intervals. Knowledge of the following time intervals of drug action also helps to anticipate a drug's effect:

1. Onset of drug action. The time it takes after a drug is administered for it to produce a response.
2. Peak action. The time it takes for a drug to reach its highest effective concentration.
3. Duration of action. The length of time during which the drug is present in a concentration great enough to produce a response.
4. Plateau. Blood serum concentration reached and maintained after repeated, fixed doses of the medication.

The ideal way to achieve a constant therapeutic drug level is by using continuous IV infusions, which eliminate the fluctuating effects of intermittent dosages.

FACTORS INFLUENCING DRUG ACTIONS

Because of differences in the manner in which drugs act and their types of action, responses to medications vary considerably. Factors other than characteristics of the medication also influence drug actions. A client may not respond in the same way to each successive dose of a medication. Likewise, the same drug dosage may cause very different responses in different clients.

Genetic Differences

Genetic makeup affects the manner in which biotransformation of drugs occurs. Metabolic patterns are often similar within families. Genetic factors determine whether naturally occurring enzymes are present to assist in drug degradation. As a result, members of a family may share a sensitivity to a medication.

Physiological Variables

Hormonal differences between men and women alter the metabolism of certain drugs. Hormones and drugs compete with each other in biotransformation because they are degraded by the same metabolic processes. Diurnal variations in estrogen secretion may be responsible for the cyclic fluctuations in drug reactions experienced by women.

Age has a direct effect on drug action. Infants lack many of the enzymes necessary for normal drug metabolism. A number of physiological changes accompanying the aging process influence the response to drug therapy (Table 35-5). Body systems undergo functional and structural changes that alter the influence of drugs. The nurse initiates actions that minimize a drug's harmful effects and promote the client's remaining functional capacities.

If a client's nutritional status is poor, proper cell function for biotransformation cannot occur. Like all body functions, drug metabolism relies on adequate nutrition for enzyme and protein formation. Most drugs bind with proteins before being distributed to their sites of action.

Any disease state that impairs the function of organs responsible for normal pharmacokinetics also impairs drug action. Altered skin integrity, reduced gastrointestinal absorption or motility, and impaired renal or hepatic function are just some of the disease-related conditions that can reduce a drug's efficacy or place a client at risk for drug toxicity.

Environmental Conditions

A client's exposure to severe physical and emotional stress triggers a hormonal response that eventually may interfere with drug metabolism. Ionizing radiation creates a similar effect by altering the rate of enzyme activity.

Exposure to heat and cold can affect responses to drugs. Hypertensive clients receive vasodilators to control blood pressure. In hot weather, it may be necessary to reduce vasodilator dosages because the temperature adds to the medication's effects. Cold weather tends to promote vasoconstriction, necessitating an increase in vasodilator dosage.

A reaction to a medication may vary, depending on the setting in which it is taken. Clients in protective isolation often receive less pain relief from an analgesic than clients in rooms where their families can visit them. Similarly, when drinking alcohol alone, persons may only become sleepy. However, drinking with a group of friends can cause people to become playful and outgoing.

Psychological Factors

A number of psychological factors influence the use of drugs and response to a medication. A person's attitude about drugs may stem from early experiences or familial influences. Seeing a parent use medications frequently may cause a child to accept drugs as a normal part of life.

The meaning or significance that a drug or taking a drug has for clients influences their response to therapy. A drug may serve as a means for overcoming feelings of insecurity. In this situation, clients depend on drugs as a means of coping with life. In contrast, if clients resent their physical conditions, anger and hostility may result in adverse reactions to medications. Medications often provide a sense of security. The regular use of nonprescription medications, or **over-the-counter drugs**, such as vitamins, laxatives, and aspirin, gives many people a sense of control over their health.

The nurse's behavior when administering a drug can have a significant impact on the client's response to a medication. If the nurse conveys a sense that the medication can be helpful, it is more likely that the drug will have a positive effect. If the nurse seems uncaring when the client experiences discomfort, the medication administered may prove relatively ineffective.

Diet

Drug and nutrient interactions can alter a drug's action or the effect of a nutrient. For example, vitamin K (found in green leafy vegetables) is a nutrient that antagonizes the effect of warfarin sodium (Coumadin), decreasing its effect on blood-clotting mechanisms. Mineral oil decreases the absorption of fat-soluble vitamins. Clients may be required to take nutritional supplements when taking drugs that reduce a nutrient's effect. Similarly, withholding certain nutrients may ensure a drug's therapeutic effect.

ROUTES OF ADMINISTRATION

The route chosen for administering a drug depends on its properties and desired effect as well as the client's physical

Table 35-5	Influence of Drug Actions in Older Adults		
PHYSIOLOGICAL CHANGE	**DRUG ACTION/CLIENT RESPONSE**	**NURSING INTERVENTIONS**
GASTROINTESTINAL TRACT **Oral Cavity** Loss of elasticity in oral mucosa, which becomes dry and easily abraded	Difficulty in swallowing tablets or capsules; sensitivity to drugs that cause dryness of mouth; susceptibility to gum disease and dental caries	Rinse client's oral cavity frequently with tepid clear water. Floss daily. Brush teeth and gums gently. Use substitute saliva.
Esophagus Delayed esophageal clearance because of weakened contractions and failure of lower esophageal sphincter to relax	Difficulty in swallowing large tablets or capsules; tissue erosion caused by drugs such as aspirin and uncoated potassium chloride	Position client upright. Administer full glass of liquid with drug. Crush tablets and mix with food (if gastric pH does not affect absorption).
Stomach Decrease in gastric acidity and peristalsis	Potentiation of irritating effects of highly acidic drugs (e.g., aspirin); alteration of solubility of certain drugs	Have client drink full glass of water and take medication with nonfat snack to reduce gastric distress.
Large Intestine Reduced colon muscle tone; loss of defecation reflex; decreased intestinal blood flow	Slowing of drug excretion; overuse and abuse of laxatives by client; delayed drug absorption	Provide normal fluid intake. Instruct client to eat bulk-forming foods and avoid use of constipating drugs.
SKIN AND VASCULAR SYSTEM Reduced SQ skin fold thickness in extremities (less body fat); reduced elasticity in skin and vascular system	Fragile blood vessels; client prone to bleeding after injection	Avoid using veins in hand for IV injections. Apply pressure to injection sites after administration. Observe injection sites for bleeding.
LIVER Reduced liver size; decline in hepatic blood flow	Longer biotransformation time; longer-than-normal duration of drug action; greater risk for drug sensitivity and toxicity	Monitor for signs of liver impairment (jaundice, pruritus, dark urine). Question dosages for clients with known liver disease.
KIDNEYS Reduced glomerular filtration; decreased tubular function and renal blood flow	Risk of drug accumulation and toxicity	Prevent urinary retention (keep catheters free flowing and observe frequency of urination). Monitor for signs of renal impairment (reduced output and difficulty in urinating). Question dosages for clients with renal disease.

and mental condition (Table 35-6). Because the nurse is constantly involved in caring for clients, he or she frequently is involved in judging the best route for a medication in collaboration with physicians.

Oral Routes

ORAL ADMINISTRATION

The oral route is the easiest and the most commonly used route. Medications are given by mouth and swallowed. Orally administered medications are less expensive than many other preparations. They have a slower onset of action and a more prolonged effect. Clients generally prefer the oral route.

SUBLINGUAL ADMINISTRATION

Sublingual drugs are designed to be absorbed readily after being placed under the tongue to dissolve. A drug given sublingually should not be swallowed. Otherwise the desired effect will not be achieved. Nitroglycerin is commonly

given sublingually. Liquids should not be taken by the client until the drug is completely dissolved.

BUCCAL ADMINISTRATION

Administration of a drug by the **buccal** route involves placing the solid medication against the mucous membranes of the cheek until the drug dissolves. Clients should be taught to alternate cheeks with each subsequent dose to avoid mucosal irritation. Clients are also warned not to chew or swallow the drug or to take liquids with it. A buccal medication acts locally on the mucosa or systemically as it is swallowed in saliva.

Parenteral Routes

Parenteral administration involves giving a drug by a route through injection into body tissues. Parenteral administration of medication involves the following four major types of injections:

Table 35-6	Factors Influencing Choice of Administration Routes
ADVANTAGES	**DISADVANTAGES OR CONTRAINDICATIONS**

ORAL, BUCCAL, SUBLINGUAL ROUTES

Routes are convenient and comfortable for client. Routes are economical. Medications may produce local or systemic effects. Routes rarely cause anxiety for client.	These routes are avoided when client has alterations in gastrointestinal function (e.g., nausea, vomiting), reduced motility (after general anesthesia or bowel inflammation, and surgical resection of portion of gastrointestinal tract. Some drugs are destroyed by gastric secretions. Oral administration is contraindicated in clients unable to swallow (e.g., clients with neuromuscular disorders, esophageal strictures, mouth lesions). Oral medications cannot be given when client has gastric suction and are contraindicated in clients before some tests or surgery. Unconscious or confused client is unable or unwilling to swallow or hold medication under tongue. Oral medications may irritate lining of gastrointestinal tract, discolor teeth, or have unpleasant taste.

SQ, IM, IV, INTRADERMAL ROUTES

Routes provide means of administration when oral drugs are contraindicated. More rapid absorption occurs than with topical or oral routes. IV infusion provides drug delivery when client is critically ill or long-term therapy is required. If peripheral perfusion is poor, IV route is preferred over injections.	There is risk of introducing infection and drugs are expensive. Clients must experience repeated needlesticks. The SQ, IM, and intradermal routes are avoided in clients with bleeding tendencies. There is risk of tissue damage with SQ injections. IM and IV routes are dangerous because of rapid absorption. These routes cause considerable anxiety in many clients, especially children.

SKIN

Topical

Topical skin applications primarily provide local effect. Route is painless. Limited side effects occur.	Extensive applications may be bulky and cause difficulty in maneuvering. Clients with skin abrasions are at risk for rapid drug absorption and systemic effects.

Transdermal

Transdermal applications provide prolonged systemic effects, with limited side effects.	Application leaves oily or pasty substance on skin and may soil clothing

MUCOUS MEMBRANES*

Therapeutic effects are provided by local application to involved sites. Aqueous solutions are readily absorbed and capable of causing systemic effects. Mucous membranes provide route of administration when oral drugs are contraindicated.	Mucous membranes are highly sensitive to some drug concentrations. Insertion of rectal and vaginal medication often causes embarrassment. Client with ruptured eardrum cannot receive irrigations. Rectal suppositories are contraindicated if client has had rectal surgery or if active rectal bleeding is present.

INHALATION

Inhalation provides rapid relief for local respiratory problems. Route provides easy access for introduction of general anesthetic gases.	Some local agents can cause serious systemic effects.

*Includes eyes, ears, nose, vagina, rectum, buccal, and sublingual routes.

1. **Subcutaneous (SQ).** Injection into tissues just below the dermis of the skin.
2. **Intradermal (ID).** Injection into the dermis just under the epidermis.
3. **Intramuscular (IM).** Injection into a muscle body.
4. **Intravenous (IV).** Injection into a vein.

Some medications are administered into body cavities other than the four types listed above. In some institutions nurses may or may not be responsible for the administration of medications through these advanced techniques.

Whether or not the nurse actually administers the drug by these routes, the nurse often remains responsible for monitoring the integrity of the system of medication delivery, understanding the therapeutic value of the medication, and evaluating the client's response to the therapy. The following are advanced techniques of medication administration for which the nurse may be responsible:

1. **Epidural.** Drugs are administered in the epidural space via a catheter, which has been placed by a nurse anesthetist or an anesthesiologist. This technique of

drug administration is most commonly used for the administration of analgesia postoperatively (see Chapter 43). Specially trained nurses can administer drugs in bolus form (see Procedure 35-6) or by continuous infusion.

2. **Intrathecal.** Intrathecal drugs are administered through a catheter that has been placed into the subarachnoid space or into one of the ventricles of the brain. Intrathecal administration is often associated with long-term drug administration through catheters that have been surgically implanted. In most institutions a physician usually injects drugs into intrathecal catheters. However, specially trained nurses may also do this.

3. **Intraosseous.** This method of drug administration involves the infusion of medication directly into the bone marrow. It is most commonly used in infants and toddlers who have poor access to their intravascular space. This method is most popular when an emergency arises and IV access is impossible. The physician inserts an intraosseous infusion needle into the bone, usually the tibia, for the administration of medication by the nurse.

4. **Intraperitoneal.** Drugs are administered into the peritoneal cavity where they are absorbed into the circulation. Chemotherapeutics and antibiotics are commonly administered in this fashion. One method of dialysis also uses the peritoneal route for the removal of fluid, electrolytes, and waste products. Oncology nurses usually instill chemotherapeutics into the peritoneal cavity. General nurses often initiate and teach clients how to manage peritoneal dialysis.

5. **Intrapleural.** Drugs are administered through the chest wall and directly into the pleural space. This may be done through an injection or through a chest tube that has been inserted by the physician. Chemotherapeutics are the most common medications administered via this method. Doctors also instill drugs that help resolve persistent pleural effusion. This is called *pleuradesis*. This technique promotes adhesion between the visceral and parietal pleura. Increasingly newer indications of this method of drug delivery are being used. One such indication is for the instillation of analgesic agents through specially designed intrapleural catheters (Martin and Mehery, 1994).

6. **Intraarterial.** This method calls for drugs to be administered directly into the arteries. Intraarterial infusions are common in clients who have arterial clots. The nurse will manage a continuous infusion of clot-dissolving agents. The nurse must carefully monitor the integrity of this infusion so as to prevent inadvertent disconnection of the system and subsequent bleeding.

Other methods of drug administration that are usually limited to physician administration are **intracardiac**, injection of a drug directly into cardiac tissue, and **intraarticular**, injection of a drug into a joint.

Topical Administration

Drugs applied to the skin and mucous membranes principally have local effects. The **topical** medication is applied to the skin by painting or spreading it over an area, applying moist dressings, soaking body parts in a solution, or giving medicated baths. Systemic effects can occur if a client's skin is thin, if the drug concentration is high, or if skin contact is prolonged.

Drugs are applied topically by a transdermal disk or patch (e.g., nitroglycerin, scopolamine, fentanyl, and estrogens). The disk secures the medicated ointment to the skin. This method of drug delivery ensures that the client receives a continuous level of medication in his or her blood rather than a discontinuous level that may occur with oral or injectable forms of these drugs. These topical medications may be applied for as little as 24 hours or up to 7 days.

Drugs can also be applied to mucous membranes. They are usually absorbed rather quickly when applied in this manner. The nurse uses the following methods for applying medications to mucous membranes:

1. Direct application of liquid (e.g., having the client gargle, swabbing the throat).
2. Insertion of the drug into a body cavity (e.g., placing a suppository in the rectum or vagina or inserting medicated packing into the vagina).
3. **Instillation** (slow introduction) of fluid into a body cavity (e.g., instilling eardrops, nose drops, and bladder and rectal fluids).
4. **Irrigation** (washing out) of body cavity (e.g., flushing the eye, ear, vagina, bladder, or rectum with medicated fluid).
5. Spraying (e.g., instilling medication into nose and throat).

Inhalation

The deeper passages of the respiratory tract provide a large surface area for drug absorption. Drugs can be administered through the nasal passage, oral passage, or tubes that have been placed into the trachea. Inhaled medications may have local effects. Drugs such as oxygen and general anesthetics create general systemic effects.

NASAL INHALATION

Drugs are inhaled through the nose by a device that delivers the medications. You may be familiar with spray type devices, like phenylephrine (Neo-Synephrine) that produce the local effect of vasoconstriction in the nasal passages. Other drugs administered in this fashion are local anesthetics, steroids, and oxygen.

ORAL INHALATION

Oral inhalation is most commonly used to deliver medication to targeted cells or organisms in lung parenchyma. The drugs are always delivered by a machine held in the client's hands. Drugs administered with hand-held inhalers are dispersed through an aerosol spray, mist, or powder that penetrates lung airways. Metered dose inhalers (MDI) facilitate the delivery of medications to the pulmonary parenchyma. Drugs to treat pulmonary infections such as *pneumocystis carinii* can by delivered as nebulized drugs.

When clients are receiving drugs as oral inhalants, it is very important that the nurse monitor the technique that the client uses, particularly with the very young or older client. These devices have several complex steps and to ensure accuracy of medication delivery, modifications may need to be made if the client cannot carry out the activities properly (see Procedure 35-14).

ENDOTRACHEAL OR TRACHEAL ADMINISTRATION

In an emergency, when a client does not have an intravenous line, several emergency drugs can be given via tubes that have been placed into the client's trachea. Nurses who participate in resuscitative efforts have special training to deliver drugs in this manner.

Intraocular

Intraocular drug delivery involves inserting a medication disk, similar to a contact lens, into the client's eye. The eye medication disk has two soft outer layers that have medication enclosed in them. The disk is inserted into the client's eye, much like a contact lens. The disk can remain in the client's eye for up to 1 week. Pilocarpine, a medication used to treat glaucoma, is the most common medication disk seen. Other drugs such as DHPG, used to treat a common fungal eye infection, may soon become available for intraocular delivery.

■ SYSTEMS OF DRUG MEASUREMENT

The proper administration of medication depends on the nurse's ability to compute drug dosages accurately and measure medications correctly. A careless mistake in placing a decimal point or adding a zero to a dosage can lead to a fatal error. The nurse is responsible for checking the dose before giving a drug and for teaching clients about prescribed doses.

The metric, apothecary, and household systems of measurement are used in drug therapy. Most nations of the world, including Canada, use the metric system as their standard of measurement. Although the U.S. Congress has not officially adopted the metric system, most health professionals in the United States use both it and the apothecary system. Prescriptions to be self-administered are often written in household measures for clients.

Metric System

Because it is a decimal system, the **metric system** is the most logically organized of the measurement systems. Metric units can easily be converted and computed through simple multiplication and division. Each basic unit of measurement is organized into units of 10. Multiplying or dividing by 10 forms secondary units. In multiplication, the decimal point moves to the right; in division, the decimal moves to the left. For example,

$$10.0 \text{ mg} \times 10 = 100 \text{ mg}$$

$$10.0 \text{ mg} \div 10 = 1.00 \text{ mg}$$

The basic units of measurement in the metric system are the meter (length), liter (volume), and gram (weight). For drug calculations the nurse uses primarily volume and weight units. In the metric system, small and large letters are used to designate the basic units (e.g., gram = g or Gm; liter = l or L). Small letters are abbreviations for subdivisions of major units (e.g., milligram = mg; milliliter = ml).

The following system of Latin prefixes designates subdivision of the basic units: *deci-* (1/10 or 0.1), *centi-* (1/100 or 0.01), and *milli-* (1/1000 or 0.001). The following Greek prefixes designate multiples of the basic units: *deka-* (10), *hecto-* (100), and *kilo-* (1000). When writing drug dosages in metric units, physicians and nurses use fractions or multiples of a unit. Fractions are always in decimal form (e.g., 500 mg or 0.5 g, *not* ½ g and 10 ml or 0.01 L, *not* 1/100 L). When fractions are used, a zero is always placed in front of the decimal to prevent error.

Apothecary System

The **apothecary system** of measurement is familiar to most people in the United States and Canada. The standards for measurement are commonly used in the home; for example, milk is bottled in pints and quarts, a yardstick has inches and feet, and a bathroom scale weighs in pounds.

The basic unit of weight is a grain. In colonial days the grain represented the weight of one grain of wheat. Units of weight derived from the grain are the dram, ounce, and pound. The apothecary unit for volume of fluid measurement is the minim. The minim is the approximate quantity of water that weighs a grain. The fluidram, fluid ounce, pint, quart, and gallon are measures derived from the minim.

In the apothecary system, the following small letters or symbols are used for measurement units: grain = gr, ounce = oz or ℥ fluid ounce = f℥, minim = ♏, and dram = ʒ. Lowercase Roman numerals designate the quantities of the apothecary units. The Roman numeral follows the unit of measure (e.g., 3 grains = gr iii). Physicians often use fractions and symbols with apothecary units (e.g., 2½ fluid ounces = f℥ iiss and ½ fluid ounce = f℥ ½ or f℥ ss).

Although the apothecary system has been around for a long time, its safety in clinical practice has recently been questioned. Cohen (1993) reports that the apothecary system is imprecise, and in many cases the metric equivalents are estimated or need to be calculated. Moreover, serious medication errors have occurred when units or measurements in the apothecary system have been confused with units of measurements in the metric system. Examples of this are the dram symbol, which looks like a 3; the abbreviations for grains and grams ("gr" and "g") can be mistaken for each other, and the minim symbol resembles "ml."

Household Measurements

Household units of measurement are also familiar to most people. Household measures include drops, teaspoons, tablespoons, and cups for volume and ounces and pounds for weight. Although pints and quarts are considered household measures, they are also used in the apothecary system. The disadvantage with household measures is their inaccuracy. Household utensils such as teaspoons and cups often vary in size. Scales to measure pints or quarts are often not well calibrated.

The advantage of household measurements is their convenience and familiarity. When accuracy is not critical, it is safe to use household measures. For example, many over-the-counter drugs, such as laxatives, antacids, and cough syrups, can safely be measured by using household measurements. Table 35-7 gives common equivalents from each measurement unit.

Table 35-7	Equivalents of Measurement		
METRIC	**APOTHECARY**	**HOUSEHOLD**	
1 ml	15-16 minims (m)	15 drops (gtt)	
4-5 ml	fluidram (f3)	1 teaspoon (tsp)	
16 ml	4 fluidrams (f3)	1 tablespoon (tbsp)	
30 ml	1 fluid ounce (f3)	2 tablespoons (tbsp)	
240 ml	8 fluid ounces (f3)	1 cup (c)	
480 ml (approximately 500 ml)	1 pint (pt)	1 pint (pt)	
960 ml (approximately 1 L)	1 quart (qt)	1 quart (qt)	
3840 ml (approximately 5 L)	1 gallon (gal)	1 gallon (gal)	

Solutions

In clinical practice the nurse uses solutions of various concentrations for injections, irrigations, and infusions. The nurse should understand terms that describe concentrations of solutions. A **solution** is a given mass of solid substance dissolved in a known volume of fluid or a given volume of liquid dissolved in a known volume of another fluid. When a solid is dissolved in fluid, the **concentration** is in units of mass per units of volume (e.g., g/ml, g/L, mg/ml). A concentration may also be expressed as a percentage. A 10% solution, for example, is 10 g of solid dissolved in 100 ml of solution. A proportion also expresses concentrations. A 1:1000 solution is a solution containing 1 g of solid in 1000 ml of liquid or 1 ml of liquid with 1000 ml of another liquid.

■ CONVERTING MEASUREMENT UNITS

A pharmacist does not always dispense a medication in the unit of measure in which it is ordered. Drug companies package and bottle certain standard equivalents. For example, the physician may order 250 mg of a medication that is available only in grams. The nurse is responsible for converting available units of volume and weight to the desired dosages. The nurse must know the standardized equivalents in all of the major measurement systems.

Drug administration is not the only function in which nurses use conversions (see the box above, right). They are used in many nursing activities.

Conversions Within One System

Converting measurements within one system is relatively easy. In the metric system the nurse simply divides or multiplies. To change milligrams to grams the nurse divides by 1000, moving the decimal 3 points to the left (e.g., 1000 mg = 1 g and 350 mg = 0.35 g). To convert liters to milliliters the nurse multiplies by 1000 or moves the decimal 3 points to the right (e.g., 1 L = 1000 ml and 0.25 L = 250 ml).

Common Reasons for Drug Conversions
■ Converting fluid ounces to milliliters for measurement of intake and output ■ Converting body weight from pounds to kilograms and vice versa ■ Converting volume equivalents to calculate IV flow rates and prepare wound irrigation solutions, enemas, or bladder irrigations

To convert units of measurement within the apothecary or household system, the nurse must consult a conversion table. For example, when converting fluid ounces to quarts, the nurse must first know that 32 ounces is the equivalent of 1 quart. To convert 8 ounces to a quart measurement, the nurse divides 8 by 32 to get the equivalent, ¼ or 0.25 quart.

Conversion Between Systems

Frequently the nurse must determine the proper dosage of a medication by converting weights or volumes from one system of measurement to another. Commonly, apothecary and metric units must be converted to equivalent household measures for use at home. When the time comes to make actual drug calculations, it is necessary to work with units in the same measurement system. Tables of equivalent measurements are available in all health care institutions. The pharmacist is also a good resource.

Before making a conversion, the nurse compares the measurement system available with that ordered. For example, a physician orders, "Morphine gr ⅙ IM." The medication is available only in milligrams. To convert grains to milligrams, the nurse must know the equivalents, 1 mg = $\frac{1}{60}$ gr or 60 mg = 1 gr. Therefore by converting gr ⅙ to milligrams, the nurse has the measurements needed to make the eventual dosage calculation. The nurse divides by 6:

$$60 \text{ mg} \div 6 = \text{⅙ gr}$$

$$10 \text{ mg} = \text{⅙ gr}$$

After calculating that the physician's order for "morphine gr ⅙" is the same as 10 mg of morphine, the nurse can accurately prepare the medication based on the available dosage.

Dosage Calculations

The nurse can use a simple formula in many types of dosage calculations. The following formula can be applied when preparing solid or liquid forms of medications:

$$\frac{\text{Dose ordered}}{\text{Dose on hand}} \times \text{Amount on hand} = \text{Amount to administer}$$

The dose ordered is the amount of pure drug that the physician prescribes for a client. The dose on hand is the weight or volume of drug available in units supplied by the pharmacy; it may be expressed on the drug label as the contents of a tablet or capsule or the amount of drug dissolved per unit volume of liquid. The amount on hand is the basic unit or quantity of the drug containing the dose on hand. For solid drugs the amount on hand may be 1 tablet or capsule; the amount of liquid on hand may be a milliliter or liter. The amount to administer is always expressed in the same unit as the amount on hand.

The following example illustrates how to apply the formula. The physician orders the client to receive Versed 2.5 mg IM. Thus the *dose ordered* is 2.5 mg. The medication is available in ampules containing 5 mg per 1 ml. Thus the *dose on hand* is 5 mg in an *amount on hand* of 1 ml. The formula is applied as follows:

$$\frac{2.5 \text{ mg}}{5 \text{ mg}} \times 1 \text{ ml} = \text{Volume to administer in milliliters}$$

To simplify the fraction, divide numerator and denominator by 2.5:

$$\frac{1}{2} \times 1 \text{ ml} = 0.5 \text{ ml to administer}$$

Another example demonstrates how the formula applies with solid dosage forms. The physician orders 0.125 mg PO of digoxin. The drug is available in tablets containing 0.25 mg.

$$\frac{0.125 \text{ mg}}{0.250 \text{ mg}} \times 1 \text{ tablet} = \text{Number of tablets to administer}$$

The fraction 0.125/0.250 equals ½ or 0.5. Therefore:

$$0.5 \times 1 \text{ tablet} = 0.5 \text{ or half a tablet to be administered}$$

Many tablets come with scores, or indentations, across the center of the tablet. A scored tablet is easy to break for divided dosages. The nurse should never attempt to estimate the amount of medication in a broken, unscored tablet because the potential for giving a dangerously low or high dose of medication is likely.

Liquid medications often come prepared in volumes greater than 1 ml. In this situation the formula still applies. For example, the medication order is, "Erythromycin suspension 250 mg PO." The pharmacy delivers 100-ml bottles with the labels stating, "5 ml contains 125 mg of erythromycin."

$$\frac{250 \text{ mg}}{125 \text{ mg}} \times 5 \text{ ml} = \text{Volume to administer}$$

The fraction 250/125 equals 2. Therefore:

$$2 \times 5 \text{ ml} = 10 \text{ ml to administer}$$

In this situation the nurse does not use the total volume of medication available in the bottle and instead uses the dosage values noted on the label. If the nurse calculated the dosage on the basis of 100 ml available, the following error would occur:

$$\frac{250 \text{ mg}}{125 \text{ mg}} \times 100 \text{ ml} = 200 \text{ ml to administer}$$

On the basis of this calculation the client would receive 20 times the desired dosage. The nurse should always double check calculations or check with another professional if the answer seems unreasonable.

Pediatric Dosages

Calculating a child's drug dosages requires special caution. A child is unable to metabolize many drugs as readily as an adult. The child's body size also necessitates smaller dosages. In most cases physicians calculate the safe dosage for a child before ordering the medication. However, nurses should be aware of the formula used to calculate pediatric dosages and recheck all dosages before administration. Most drug references list the normal ranges for pediatric dosages.

The most accurate method of calculating pediatric dosages is based on body surface area. Body surface area is estimated on the basis of weight. Standard nomograms, or charts, list body surface area by weight and approximate age (Fig. 35-3). The formula is a ratio of the child's body surface area compared with the body surface area of an average adult (1.7 square meters, or 1.7 m²).

$$\text{Child's dose} = \frac{\text{Surface area of child}}{1.7 \text{ m}^2} \times \text{Normal adult dose}$$

For example, a physician orders ampicillin for a child weighing 12 kg, but the normal single adult dose is 250 mg. The nomogram chart shows that a child weighing 12 kg has a surface area of 0.54 m².

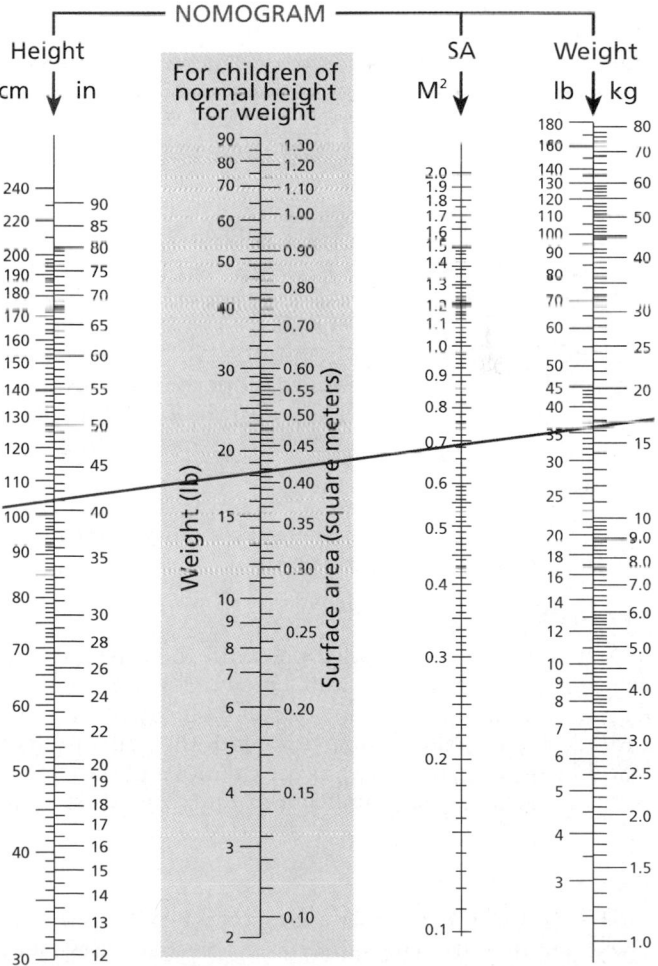

Fig. 35-3 West nomogram for estimation of surface areas in children. A straight line is drawn between height and weight. The point where the line crosses the surface area column is the estimated body surface area. *(From Behrman RE, Vaughan VC, editors: Nelson textbook of pediatrics, ed 13, Philadelphia, 1987, Saunders; modified from data of Boyd E, by West CD.)*

$$\text{Child's dose} = \frac{0.54\text{m}^2}{1.7\text{m}^2} \times 250 \text{ mg}$$

The m² units cancel out and can be ignored.

$$\text{Child's dose} = \frac{0.54}{1.7} \times 250 \text{ mg}$$

$$\frac{0.54}{1.7} = 0.3$$

Child's dose = 0.3×250 mg = 75 mg

ADMINISTERING MEDICATIONS

The nurse does not bear sole responsibility for drug administration. The physician and pharmacist play key roles in ensuring that the right medication gets to the right client. However, the nurse giving the medications bears responsibility and accountability for accuracy of the five rights.

Physician's Role

The physician prescribes medications (unless a state's nurse practice act allows advanced practice nurses to prescribe in specific situations). The physician writes an order on a designated form in the client's medical record, in a physician's order book, or on a legal prescription pad. In some situations a physician may also order a medication by telephone or by giving the nurse a verbal order. The nurse enters and signs all telephone and verbal orders by writing the time, date, and name of the physician ordering the drug, and later has the physician countersign the order. Most institutions require a physician's signature within 24 hours after the order is given. Institutional policies vary as to which personnel can take verbal or telephone orders. Generally, nursing students cannot take medication orders. *No* medication is given without an order.

Common abbreviations (see inside back cover) are used when writing orders. The abbreviations indicate dosage frequencies or times, routes of administration, and special information for the nurse to follow in giving the drug.

Types of Orders

The four common types of medication orders are based on the frequency of drug administration.

STANDING ORDERS

A standing order is carried out until the physician cancels it by another order or until a prescribed number of days elapse. A standing order may have a final date. Many institutions have policies for automatically discontinuing standing orders. The following are examples of standing orders: "tetracycline 500 mg PO q6h" and "Decadron 10 mg qd × 5 days."

PRN ORDERS

The physician may order a drug on a PRN basis (when a client requires it). The nurse uses objective assessments, subjective assessments, and discretion in determining the client's need. Often the physician sets minimal intervals for the time of administration. This means that a drug cannot be given any more often than what is prescribed. Examples of PRN orders are "morphine sulfate 2 mg SQ q3 to 4h PRN for incisional pain" and "Maalox 30 ml PRN for gastric dis-

comfort." When medications are administered, the nurse documents the assessment made and the time of drug administration. The nurse should make frequent evaluation of the effectiveness of the drug and record findings in the appropriate place. This may be on the medication administration record or in the client's medical record.

SINGLE (ONE-TIME) ORDERS

A physician may order a drug to be given only once at a specified time. This is common for preoperative drugs or drugs given before diagnostic examinations. Examples include the following: "Valium 10 mg PO at 0900" and "Stadol 4 mg IM on call to OR."

STAT ORDERS

A STAT order signifies that a single dose of a medication is to be given immediately and only once. Often stat orders are written for emergencies when a client's condition changes suddenly, for example, "Give Apresoline 10 mg IV stat."

Some conditions change the status of a client's medication orders. Surgery automatically cancels all preoperative medications (see Chapter 48). Because the client's condition is generally changed after surgery, the physician must write new orders. When a client is transferred to another health care agency or a different medical service within a hospital or is discharged, the physician should review the medications and rewrite them to reflect the medication regimen desired. Various institutions have policies regarding the frequency and circumstances under which medications must be reviewed and reordered.

Prescriptions

The physician writes prescriptions for clients to take medications outside the hospital. The prescription includes more detailed information than a regular order because the client must understand how to take the medication and when to refill the prescription if necessary (Fig. 35-4). Parts of a prescription include the following:

1. Superscription. The client's name, address, and age and the date are given for identification purposes. The symbol ℞ ("take thou") is at the top of the form.
2. Inscription. This is the drug name, strength, and dose.
3. Subscription. Directions about the number of tablets or the amount to be dispensed are given to the pharmacist.
4. Signature. Information to be written on the label, such as directions to the client (for example, take with full glass of water or take between meals), directions for refilling the prescription, and whether the drug name should be on the label, is included.
5. Personal data. The physician signs the prescription. If the drug is a controlled substance, the physician includes his or her registration number and address.

Pharmacist's Role

The pharmacist prepares and distributes prescribed drugs. Pharmacists may also promote optimal drug therapy through assessment of the drug plan and evaluation of the client's medication-related needs (American Pharmaceutical Association, 1994). The pharmacist is responsible for filling prescriptions accurately and for being sure that prescriptions are valid. If there is any question that a prescrip-

Saint Louis University
Health Center/Doctor's Offices
3660 Vista Avenue
St. Louis, Missouri 63110

Arlene Casey
1010 First Street
St. Louis, Missouri
October 8, 19___ ___

Phone: 577-6100

Department of Internal Medicine
Division of General Internal Medicine
DEA #

Rx: *AMOXICILLIN 500 mg*
    ī TABLET
    3 TIMES A DAY FOR 10 DAYS
    DISPENSE 30 TABLETS

Refills: 0 1 2 3 4 5 6   Check here if easy-
                                   open top requested ☐

Signed: *Douglas Keithley, M.D.*
        SUBSTITUTION PERMITTED   DISPENSE AS WRITTEN

Fig. 35-4 Example of a medication prescription. *(Courtesy of St Louis University Medical Center, St Louis.)*

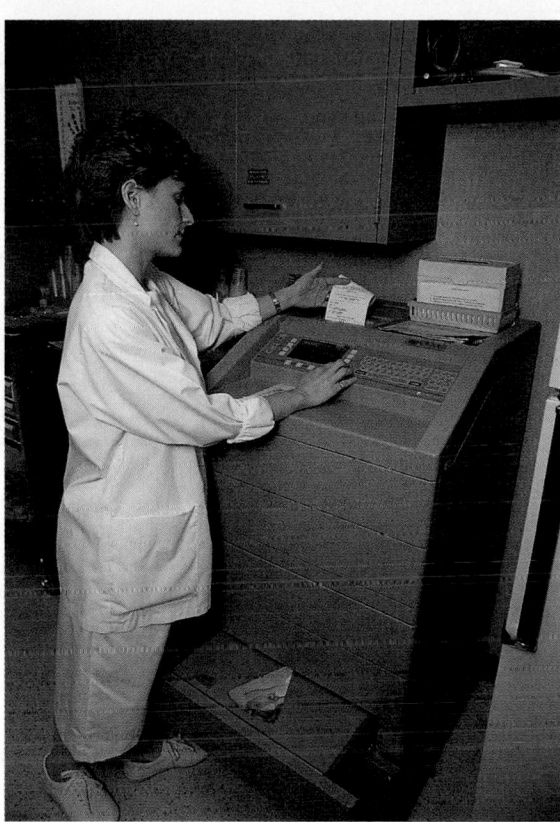

Fig. 35-5 Nurse using computer-controlled dispensing system.

tion is forged or that the prescribing physician is unlicensed, the pharmacist will not fill the prescription. The pharmacist calls the physician if an ordered dose seems outside the safe therapeutic range.

The pharmacist in a health care agency today rarely has to mix compounds or solutions except in the case of IV additive solutions. Most drug companies deliver drugs in a form ready for administration. Dispensing the correct drug, in the proper dosage and amount, with an accurate label is the pharmacist's chief responsibility. The pharmacist can also provide information about drug side effects, toxicity, interactions, and incompatibilities.

Distribution Systems

Systems for the storage and distribution of medications vary among health care agencies. Institutions providing nursing care have a designated area for stocking and dispensing drugs. Special medication rooms, portable locked carts, and individual storage units adjacent to clients' rooms are some of the facilities used. Nurses should keep a close watch on the supply of medications, making sure that storage areas are locked when unattended.

STOCK SUPPLY

With a stock system, medications are available in quantity in stock containers. A nurse prepares individual doses from a large stock supply container. The system is time-consuming and costly. This type of system of medication delivery has been associated with a high rate of medication errors and is not commonly used today (Perini and Vermeulen, 1994). Narcotics are often provided in stock supply.

UNIT-DOSE SYSTEM

The unit-dose system consists of a drawer with a 24-hour supply of medications for each client. The unit-dose is the ordered dose of medication the client receives at a prescribed hour. At a designated time each day the pharmacist refills the drawers with a fresh supply of individually wrapped medications. Included are limited amounts of PRN medications. Use of the unit-dose system reduces the number of medication errors and saves steps in dispensing drugs. The nurse and pharmacist are more likely to identify missed doses earlier.

COMPUTER-CONTROLLED DISPENSING SYSTEMS

Computer-controlled dispensing systems are being used successfully throughout the country (Fig. 35-5). The system is especially useful for the delivery and control of **narcotics**. Each nurse has a security code that allows access to the unit. The client's name or hospital identification number is then entered. The nurse then selects the desired drug, dose, and route. The system delivers the medication to the nurse, records it, and charges it to the client. For example, the following narcotics are entered into the computer for Mr. Svoda:

1. Morphine 2 mg IM q3h*
2. Morphine 5 mg IM q3h
3. Percodan II PO q4h
4. Halcion 0.125 mg PO HS†

*q, Every.
†HS, Hour of sleep.

The nurse first enters the security code number and the client's identification number and then reviews the orders. The nurse may then enter 1, and a single unit-dose of Morphine 2 mg for IM injection would open up in a drawer on the system, ready for preparation and administration.

Computers can also facilitate medication administration. Nurses may also scan bar codes to identify the client, drug, and nurse administering the drug (Abdoo, 1992). This information is then automatically recorded into a database for viewing, retrieving, and printing.

Nurse's Role

The nurse is the most appropriate health care worker to administer medications, spending most of the time with the client. This puts nurses in the ideal position to monitor clients' responses to medication, provide education to the client and family about the medication regimen and inform the physician when medications are effective, ineffective, or no longer necessary. The nurse's role extends beyond simply giving drugs to a client. The nurse must determine whether a client should receive a drug at a given time and assess the client's ability to self-administer drugs. The nurse uses the nursing process to integrate drug therapy into care.

■ NURSING PROCESS AND MEDICATIONS

 ## Assessment

To determine the need for and potential response to drug therapy, the nurse assesses many factors.

MEDICAL HISTORY

A medical history provides indications or contraindications for drug therapy. Disease or illness may place clients at risk for adverse drug effects. For example, if a client has a gastric ulcer or bleeding tendency, compounds containing aspirin or anticoagulants will increase the likelihood of bleeding. Long-term health problems such as diabetes or arthritis, which require medication, suggest to the nurse the type of drugs a client is taking. A client's surgical history may indicate the use of medications. For example, after a thyroidectomy a client may require hormone replacement. From this history, nurses may need to request orders for drugs the client takes routinely (for example, Synthroid and antihypertensives) if they are not ordered on admission.

HISTORY OF ALLERGIES

If the client has a history of allergies to medication, the nurse informs other members of the health care team. Food allergies should also be carefully documented because many drugs have ingredients found in food sources. One example is shellfish. If clients are allergic to shellfish, the client may be sensitive to any product containing iodine. In a hospital, clients wear identification bands listing medications to which they are allergic. All allergies should be noted on the nurse's admission notes, medication records, and physician's history.

DRUG DATA

The nurse assesses information about each drug, including action, purpose, normal dosages, routes, side effects, and nursing implications for administration and monitoring. Common questions to think about include the following: "Is this the smallest possible dose ordered" (a question pertinent to older adults), "Can a certain drug interact with other drugs being used," and "Are there special instructions for administering the drug?"

Often, several resources must be consulted to gather needed information. Pharmacology textbooks, nursing journals, the *Physicians' Desk Reference (PDR)*, drug package inserts, and the pharmacist are valuable resources. The nurse is responsible for knowing as much as possible about each drug given. Many nursing students prepare or purchase cards and/or books containing drug data to use as a quick resource.

DIET HISTORY

A diet history reveals the client's usual eating patterns and food preferences. The nurse can then plan the dosage schedule more effectively and advise the client to avoid foods that may interact with medications.

CLIENT'S CURRENT CONDITION

The ongoing physical or mental status of a client may affect whether a drug is given or how it is administered. The nurse should assess a client carefully before giving any drug. For example, the nurse checks blood pressure before giving an antihypertensive. If the client is nauseated, it is unlikely that a tablet can be swallowed. Assessment findings can also serve as a baseline in evaluating the effects of drug therapy.

CLIENT'S PERCEPTUAL OR COORDINATION PROBLEMS

For a client with perceptual or coordination limitations, self-administration may be difficult. The nurse must assess the client's ability to prepare dosages and take medications correctly. If the client is unable to self-administer drugs, the nurse learns whether family members or friends are available to assist.

CLIENT'S ATTITUDE ABOUT THE USE OF DRUGS

The client's attitude about drugs may reveal the level of drug dependence. Clients are often reluctant to express feelings about drugs, particularly if drug dependence is a problem. To assess attitudes, the nurse may have to observe the client's behavior for evidence of drug dependence.

CLIENT'S KNOWLEDGE AND UNDERSTANDING OF DRUG THERAPY

The client's knowledge and understanding of drug therapy influence his or her willingness or ability to follow a drug regimen. Unless a client understands a drug's purpose, the importance of regular dosage schedules and proper administration methods, and the possible side effects, compliance is unlikely. When assessing knowledge of a drug, the nurse asks the client the following questions:

1. What is it for?
2. How and when is it taken?

3. What side effects have there been?
4. Have you ever stopped taking doses?
5. Is there anything else you do not understand and would like to know about the drug?

When the client has a history of poor compliance, the nurse should also review resources available for purchase of medications.

CLIENT'S LEARNING NEEDS

By assessing the client's level of knowledge about a medication, the nurse determines the need for instruction. It may be necessary for the nurse to explain the action and purpose of the drug, expected side effects, correct administration techniques, and ways to remember the drug schedule. If a client has been placed on a newly prescribed drug, instruction may need to be more involved. It may be necessary to involve a friend or family member.

 ## Nursing Diagnosis

Assessment provides data on the client's condition, ability to self-administer drugs, and drug use patterns, which can be used to determine actual or potential problems with drug therapy (see the nursing diagnoses box at right). The nurse clusters together defining characteristics to make accurate nursing diagnoses. For example, a client's admission of missing a dosage, evidence that a medication has not reversed symptoms, and evidence that the client has not progressed indicates noncompliance regarding a drug regimen. Once a diagnosis is selected, the nurse chooses the appropriate related factors. The related factor of inadequate resources versus lack of knowledge will require different interventions. To resolve noncompliance, the nurse thinks critically, to interpret assessment data so that the right diagnoses are chosen (see the diagnostic process box below). If the nurse diagnoses knowledge deficit or factors interfering with drug therapy compliance, client education becomes a part of the nursing care plan. If the client has physical limitations that interfere with drug administration, the nurse plans strategies to ensure safety.

 ## Examples of NANDA Nursing Diagnoses for Drug Therapy

Knowledge deficit regarding drug therapy *related to:*
- Lack of exposure and inexperience
- Cognitive limitations
- Unfamiliarity with information resources

Noncompliance regarding drug therapy *related to:*
- Limited economic resources
- Health beliefs
- Cultural influences

Impaired physical mobility *related to:*
- Decreased strength
- Pain and discomfort

Sensory/perceptual alterations: visual *related to:*
- Blurred vision

Anxiety *related to:*
- Threat to or change in health status
- Threat to or change in socioeconomic status
- Threat to or change in interaction patterns

Impaired swallowing *related to:*
- Neuromuscular impairment
- Irritated oral cavity
- Limited awareness

Ineffective management of therapeutic regimen *related to:*
- Complexity of drug therapy
- Knowledge deficit

 ## Planning

The nurse organizes care activities to ensure that safe administrative techniques are used. Hurrying to give clients medications can lead to errors. The nurse can also plan to use time during drug administration to teach clients about their medications.

In situations in which clients learn to self-administer medications, the nurse plans to use all available teaching re-

 ## Sample Nursing Diagnostic Process for Drug Therapy

ASSESSMENT ACTIVITIES	DEFINING CHARACTERISTICS	NURSING DIAGNOSES
Ask client about previous use of prescribed medication.	Client denies use. Inquires about purpose of medication	**Knowledge deficit regarding drug therapy** related to newly prescribed medication
Check client's medical record for new orders.	New drug ordered in morning No previous history of taking prescribed medication	
Observe client swallow medication.	Coughs when attempting to swallow capsule	**Impaired swallowing** related to right facial paralysis
Ask if client is able to perceive food in the mouth.	Food retained in mouth after eating	
Perform neurological assessment of ninth and tenth cranial nerves (see Chapter 33).	Reduced gag reflex	

Components of Drug Orders

A medication order is incomplete unless it has the following parts:

- Client's full name. The client's full name distinguishes the client from other persons with the same last name.
- Date that the order is written. The day, month, year, and time must be included. Designating the time that an order is written helps clarify when certain orders are to stop automatically. If an incident occurs involving a medication error, it is easier to document what happened when this information is available.
- Drug name. The physician will order a generic or trade-name drug. Correct spelling is essential in preventing confusion with drugs with similar spelling.
- Dosage. The amount or strength of the medication is included.
- Route of administration. The physician uses common abbreviations for drug routes. Accuracy is important because some drugs are administered by more than one route.
- Time and frequency of administration. The nurse needs to know when to initiate drug therapy. Orders for multiple doses establish a routine schedule for drug administration.
- Signature of physician, nurse practitioner, or physician assistant. Signature makes the order a legal request.

sources. Inclusion of family members or friends in instruction is very important. Family members will often reinforce the impact of drug regimens in the home setting. When clients are hospitalized, it is important for the nurse to not postpone instruction until the day of discharge. For the client to understand medications and self-administration, early discharge planning is needed. The nurse should make comprehensive client assessments identifying physical, psychological, economic, or social factors that may make the client unable to consistently self-administer medications. For example, the client may have disabling arthritis that may make it difficult to travel to the pharmacy. The nurse, with the assistance of other health care workers, works to resolve these issues before discharge. When there is little time for instruction, brochures or pamphlets can be used to reinforce information reviewed with clients. The nursing unit or education department may have videos that the client can view. If clients have been newly diagnosed and require a medicine such as insulin, a home health referral is an important option of the care plan. Home health nurses can assist clients in establishing medication schedules to fit home routines.

Whether a client attempts self-administration or the nurse assumes responsibility for administering medications (see the care plan below), the following goals should be met:

1. Absence of complications related to the route of administration
2. Achievement of the therapeutic effect of the prescribed medications safely while maintaining the client's comfort
3. Client and family understanding of drug therapy
4. Safe self-administration of medications

Sample Nursing Care Plan for Knowledge Deficit

NURSING DIAGNOSIS: **Knowledge deficit regarding drug therapy** related to newly prescribed medication
DEFINITION: Knowledge deficit is the state in which specific information is lacking (Kim, McFarland, McLane, 1995).

GOAL	EXPECTED OUTCOMES	INTERVENTIONS	RATIONALE
Client will correctly self-administer insulin by day of planned discharge (2/18).	Client will correctly prepare proper insulin dose (2/16). Client will state rationale for rotating injection sites (2/17).	Provide syringe and allow client to manipulate parts. Explain and demonstrate aseptic technique for preparing dosage from vial.	Client becomes familiar with working parts of syringe. Explanation provides learner with clear mental image of how skill is performed; demonstration is method most suited for teaching psychomotor skill (Redman, 1993).
	Client will correctly state rationale and implications for insulin dose (2/16). Client will correctly self-administer subcutaneous insulin 3 times before discharge 2/18.	Discuss importance of proper dosage. Explain and demonstrate method for administering subcutaneous injection (have client stand behind nurse).	Insulin can create serious side effects if improper dosage is administered. Demonstration provides image of injection technique; over-the-shoulder view provides clear image of how to do action (Redman, 1993).

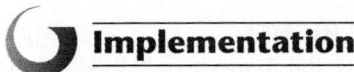

Implementation

CORRECT TRANSCRIPTION AND COMMUNICATION OF ORDERS

The nurse's interventions focus on safe and effective drug administration. This includes careful drug preparation, correct administration, and client education.

The nurse or a designated unit secretary writes the physician's complete order (see the box on p. 808) on the appropriate medication forms or tickets (Fig. 35-6). The transcribed order includes the client's name, room, and bed number; drug name, dosage, and time; and route of administration.

Each time a drug dosage is prepared, the nurse refers to the medication form or ticket. With the unit-dose system, only one transcription is necessary, limiting the opportunity for errors. When transcribing orders, the nurse should be sure that names, dosages, and symbols are legible. The nurse should recopy any smudged or illegible transcriptions.

In some institutions a computer printout lists all currently ordered medications with dosage information. Orders are entered directly into the computer, preventing the need for transcription of orders. The same printout may be used to record medications given.

A registered nurse checks all transcribed orders against the original order for accuracy and thoroughness. If an order seems incorrect or inappropriate, the nurse consults the physician. The nurse who gives the wrong medication or an incorrect dosage is legally responsible for the error.

ACCURATE DOSAGE CALCULATION AND MEASUREMENT

When measuring liquid drugs, the nurse uses standard measuring receptacles. The procedure for drug measurement is systematic, to lessen the chance of error. The nurse calculates each dose when preparing the drug, pays close attention to calculation, and avoids interference from other nursing activities.

CORRECT ADMINISTRATION

The nurse uses aseptic technique and proper procedures when handling and giving medications. Certain drugs require the nurse to perform assessments at the time of administration, such as assessing heart rate before giving antiarrhythmic medications.

RECORDING DRUG ADMINISTRATION

To avoid having another nurse give a medication without knowing that the client had already received a dose, the nurse documents medications at the time of administration. If a nurse forgets to record medications, double doses could easily be given. Agency policy determines whether a nurse should document while preparing the medication for a client or immediately after administering the medications. If the nurse records a drug, but the medication is not given because of client refusal or physical assessment findings contraindicating drug use, the medication record must include this information.

The recording of a drug includes the name of the drug, dosage, route, and exact time of administration. Often the drug forms are prepared in advance, and the nurse needs to record only the time. Agency policies may also require that the nurse record the location of an injection.

If a client refuses a drug or is undergoing tests or procedures that result in a missed dose, the nurse explains in the nurses' notes the reason that the drug was not given. Some agencies require the nurse to circle and initial the prescribed administration time on the drug record when a dose is missed.

ALLERGIES: *Codeine*							
RECORDED BY INITIALS L.T.			**RN SIGNATURE** *Ben Wilson, R.N.*				
BARNES HOSPITAL — PATIENT ROUTINE MEDICATION RECORD		**NITES**	*M. Soerrer R.N.*	*M. Soerrer R.N.*	*M. Soerrer R.N.*		
		DAYS	*P. Little R.N.*	*P. Little R.N.*	*P. Little R.N.*		
		EVES	*D. Gail R.N.*	*D. Gail R.N.*			
ORDER DATE / EXP DATE	**INT**	**ROUTINE MEDICATION** Name of drug, strength, and frequency	**RTE**	**SCHEDULE**	**SHIFT**	2/6/--	2/7/--	2/8/--
2/6	PL	Lanoxin 0.25 mg qd.	PO	10	NITES			
					DAYS	0950 PL	1000 PL	1010 PL
					EVES			
2/7	DG	Lasix 40 mg b.i.d.	PO	10 / 16	NITES			
					DAYS			1010 PL
					EVES		1545 DG	
2/7	DG	Ancef GmT q6°	IVP B	06 12 18-24	NITES			06 MD
					DAYS		1215 PL	1200 PL
					EVES		1800 2345 DG	
2/8	PL	Nitro Paste 1 inch q8°	Top	06 14 22	NITES			
					DAYS			1410 PL
					EVES			
2/8	PL	Neosporin Opthalmic Oint. OD	Top	10 22	NITES			
					DAYS			1010 PL
					EVES			

Fig. 35-6 Example of medication record.
(Courtesy Barnes-Jewish Hospital, St Louis, Mo.)

HEALTH PROMOTION THROUGH CLIENT TEACHING

Client teaching is a very important role ascribed to the nurse. Medication teaching is one type of teaching that the nurse renders (see Chapter 15). Sometimes clients may require medications for the rest of their lives. An example of this is the diabetic client. To prevent complications related to diabetes, the nurse teaches the client how to monitor glucose therapy and how to self-administer insulin injections. Complications of diabetes are also minimized through diet and exercise, both of which must be taught to the client newly diagnosed with diabetes. Through medication and client teaching, the nurse helps clients in modifying their lifestyles to achieve optimal wellness.

Unless clients are properly informed about drugs, they may take the drugs incorrectly or not at all. The nurse provides information about the purpose of medications and their actions and effects. Many health care institutions offer easy-to-read leaflets on specific types of drugs. The nurse must be certain to assess the reading level of the client before providing these pamphlets to the client.

Clients must know the way to take drugs properly and the effects if they fail to do so. For example, a client receiving a prescription for an antibiotic must understand the importance of taking the full prescription. Failure to do this can lead to a worsening of the condition, as well as the development of bacterial resistance to the drug.

Nurses teach proper self-administration of drugs to clients who depend on daily injections. The client learns to prepare and administer injections correctly using aseptic technique. Family members should be taught to give injections in case clients become ill or physically unable to handle syringes. For clients with visual alterations, nurses can provide specially designed equipment such as syringes with enlarged calibrated scales for easier reading or Braille-labeled medication vials. Many older clients are responsible for self-medication, so instructions should include detailed information about medications and dosage schedules that help them remember to take medications regularly.

Clients must be aware of the symptoms of drug side effects or toxicity. For example, clients taking anticoagulants learn to notify the physician immediately when bleeding or frequent bruising develops. Family members should be informed of drug side effects, such as changes in behavior, because they are often the first persons to recognize such effects. Clients are better able to cope with problems caused by drugs if they understand how and when to act. All clients should learn the following basic guidelines for drug safety in the home:

1. Keep each drug in its original, labeled container.
2. Be sure labels are legible.
3. Discard any outdated medications.
4. Always finish a prescribed drug unless otherwise instructed. Never save a drug for future illnesses.
5. Dispose of drugs in a sink or toilet. Do not place drugs in the trash within reach of children.
6. Do not give a family member or friend a drug prescribed for another.
7. Refrigerate medications that require it.
8. Read labels carefully, and follow all instructions.

MAINTAINING CLIENTS' RIGHTS

In 1992 the American Hospital Association issued a revision to the Patient's Bill of Rights (see Chapter 4), a comprehensive statement defining the rights and responsibilities for a broad area of medical and nursing practice. The Patient's Bill of Rights helps clarify the rights of clients in an area of practice such as medication administration. Because of the potential risks related to drug administration, a client has the right to:

1. Be informed of the drug name, purpose, action, and potential undesired effects
2. Refuse a medication, regardless of the consequences
3. Have qualified nurses or physicians assess a drug history, including allergies
4. Be properly advised of the experimental nature of any drug therapy and give written consent for its use
5. Receive labeled medications safely without discomfort in accordance with the "five rights" of drug administration (see p. 811)
6. Receive appropriate supportive therapy in relation to drug therapy
7. Not receive unnecessary medications

The nurse must be aware of these rights and handle all inquiries by clients and families courteously and professionally. A nurse should not become defensive if a client refuses drug therapy. The nurse must have the knowledge and skill to satisfy the responsibilities of safe and effective drug administration.

Evaluation

The nurse monitors a client's response to medications on an ongoing basis. To do this the nurse knows the therapeutic action and common side effects of each medication. A change in a client's condition can be physiologically related to health status, may result from medications, or both. The nurse must be alert for reactions when a client takes several medications.

The goal of safe and effective drug administration involves a careful evaluation of technique and the client's response to therapy and ability to assume responsibility for self-care. To evaluate the effectiveness of nursing interventions when meeting established goals of care, the nurse uses evaluative measures to identify actual outcomes. Examples of evaluative measures for determining the absence of complications related to the route of administration include the following, in addition to those listed in the evaluation box on p. 811:

1. Observing injection sites for bruises, inflammation, localized pain, or bleeding
2. Questioning the client about localized numbness or tingling at injection sites
3. Assessing the client for gastrointestinal disturbances, including nausea, vomiting, and diarrhea
4. Inspecting IV sites for phlebitis, including fever, swelling, and localized tenderness

Examples of evaluative measures for determining whether the therapeutic effect of prescribed medication has been achieved safely include the following:

1. Questioning the client for expected response to the drug (e.g., pain relief or reduction in symptoms)

Sample Evaluation of Interventions for Knowledge Deficit

GOALS	EVALUATIVE MEASURES	EXPECTED OUTCOMES
Client will correctly self-administer insulin by day of planned discharge (2/18).	Observe client perform return demonstration of preparing dose in syringe. Ask client to describe ordered insulin dosage and implications of receiving incorrect dose. Observe client perform return demonstration of self-administration of injections.	Client will correctly prepare proper insulin dose. Client will correctly state rationale and implications for insulin dose. Client will correctly self-administer subcutaneous insulin. Client will state rationale for rotating injection sites.
Client will not experience complication related to route of administration.	Inspect injection sites for localized tenderness, inflammation, hardness, or bruising. Inspect IV sites for redness, swelling, tenderness, or cool or warm skin. Ask client if gastric distress follows oral intake of medication.	Injection sites will have no inflammation and minimal bruising. IV sites will have no signs of phlebitis or infiltration. Client will deny symptoms of gastric distress.
Client will achieve therapeutic effect of prescribed medications.	Monitor or have client monitor desired effect of medication (e.g., relief of discomfort after analgesic, lowering of body temperature after antipyretic, lowering or maintenance of blood pressure after antihypertensive).	Medication will exert measurable therapeutic effect.
Client will be safe and comfortable.	Note positioning of client before administration (e.g., sitting up for oral medication ingestion, lying on side before ventrogluteal injection). Monitor IV infusion rate regularly. Observe for potential side or toxic effects.	When sitting, client will be able to swallow oral medications without difficulty, or when lying on side, injection will be given correctly in proper tissue. IV medication will infuse over prescribed time. Client will deny side effects, and no adverse effects will be observed.
Client will understand drug therapy.	Ask client or family member to explain purpose of medication and all pertinent information related to drug administration.	Client or family member will explain information needed to demonstrate understanding of drug regimen.

2. Monitoring client's physical response to medication (e.g., antiarrhythmic medication, regular heart rhythm; hypertension medication, lowered blood pressure; diuretics, increased urine output)

Examples of evaluative measures for maintaining the client's safety and comfort include the following:
1. Monitoring the client for potential side or toxic effects, allergic reactions, or interactions
2. Evaluating the client for up to 30 minutes after administration of medications for symptoms of discomfort

Examples of evaluative measures for understanding drug therapy include the following:
1. Asking the client to explain the drug's purpose, action, dosage, schedule of administration, and possible side effects
2. Asking the client to describe when each medication is taken during the day

Examples of evaluative measures for determining the client's ability to self-administer medications safely include the following:
1. Observing the client preparing an ordered dose of medication
2. Observing the client administering the ordered dose of medication

▌MEDICATION DELIVERY
Preparing and administering medications requires accuracy by the nurse. The nurse must pay full attention to preparing medications and must not attempt to do other tasks simultaneously. The nurse uses the "five rights" of drug administration, to ensure safe drug administration (see the box below).

Right Drug
When drugs are first ordered, the nurse compares the medicine ticket or unit-dose recording form with the physi-

> **Five "Rights" for Administration of Medication**
> - Right drug
> - Right dose
> - Right client
> - Right route
> - Right time

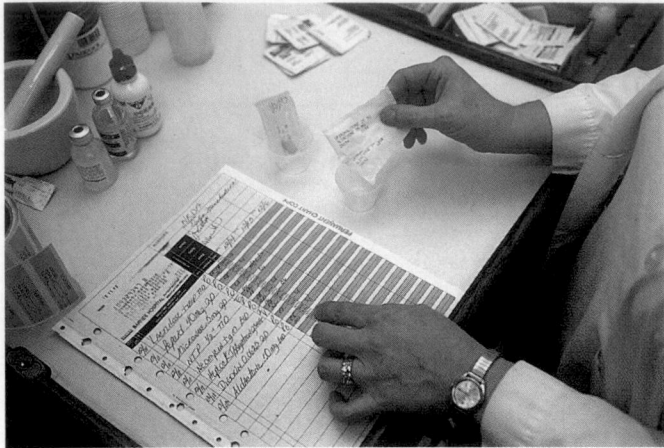

Fig. 35-7 The nurse checks the label of the medication against the transcribed medication order.

cian's written orders. When administering drugs, the nurse compares the label of the drug container with the form or medicine ticket. The nurse does this at the following three times: (1) before removing the container from the drawer or shelf, (2) as the amount of drug ordered is removed from the container, and (3) before returning the container to storage. With single-dose, prepackaged drugs, the nurse checks the label with the medicine ticket or form three times even though the medication is not being taken from a bulk container (Fig. 35-7). Nurses administer *only* the drugs they prepare. If an error occurs, the nurse administering the drug is responsible for its effects.

If a client questions the medication, the nurse does not ignore these concerns. An alert client will know whether a drug is different from those received before. In most cases the drug order has been changed. However, the client's questions might reveal an error. The nurse should withhold the drug until it can be rechecked against physician's orders. Clients who self-administer drugs should keep them in their original labeled containers, separate from other drugs, to avoid confusion.

The nurse never prepares medications from unmarked containers or containers with illegible labels. If a client refuses a drug, the nurse should never return the medication to the original container or transfer the drug to another container. Single-dose, prepackaged drugs can be returned to storage areas if they are unopened.

Right Dose

The unit-dose system of drug distribution minimizes errors because most medications come prepared in proper doses. When a medication must be prepared from a larger or smaller volume or strength than needed, or when a physician orders a system of measurement different from what the pharmacist supplies, the chance of error increases. In these situations, a nurse should check another nurse's dosage calculations. For example, some institutions require two nurses to check all insulin and anticoagulant dosages.

After calculating dosages, the nurse prepares the medication by using standard measurement devices. For example, many liquid pediatric medications come with a scaled

dropper. Graduated cups, syringes, and specially designed spoons can be used to measure medications accurately. In the home, clients should use standard kitchen measuring spoons rather than flatware teaspoons and tablespoons, which vary in volume.

To break a scored tablet, the nurse makes sure that the break is even. A tablet may be cut in half by using a knife edge or by folding a tissue over the tablet and breaking it with the fingers. Any tablets that do not break evenly are discarded. After a tablet is split, the nurse may give the two halves in successive doses, but only if the second half has been repackaged and labeled.

Often a nurse prepares a tablet by crushing it in a special tablet crusher so that it can be mixed in food. This may be done when a client has difficulty swallowing, and an injection is unnecessary or undesirable. The crusher should always be cleaned completely before the tablet is crushed. Remnants of previously crushed drugs may increase a drug's concentration or result in the client receiving a portion of an unprescribed drug. Crushed medications should be mixed with very small amounts of food or liquid. The nurse should make accurate assessments about the chosen food and the client's medical conditions. Some suggestions are jelly, syrup, and chocolate syrup or other ice cream toppings, which must be sugar free for diabetic persons.

Right Client

An important step in administering drugs safely is being sure that the medication is given to the right client. The nurse working in a hospital or extended care setting is frequently responsible for administering drugs to several clients. Clients often have similar last names, and it is difficult to remember every name and face, especially if a nurse has been off duty for several days. To identify clients correctly, the nurse checks the medicine tickets, forms, or printouts against clients' identification bracelets (Fig. 35-8) and asks clients to state their names.

If an identification bracelet becomes smudged or illegible, the nurse should replace it with a new one. When asking for a name, the nurse should not speak the name and then assume that the response indicates that the client is the right person. Instead, the nurse asks the client to state a full name. This is vital even if the nurse has been caring for a client for several days. To avoid making the client feel uneasy, the nurse simply says that the routine for giving a medication requires identification by name.

Clients who self-administer medications at home should be cautioned to never give a family member or friend one of their medications. A physician should be consulted before one person uses a prescription meant for another because a drug that is safe for one person can be dangerous for another.

Right Route

If a medication order does not designate a route of administration, the nurse consults the physician. Likewise, if the specified route is not the recommended route, the nurse should alert the physician immediately.

When administering injections (see p. 827), it is especially important that the route be correct. It is also important to prepare injections only from preparations designed for parenteral use. The injection of a liquid designed for

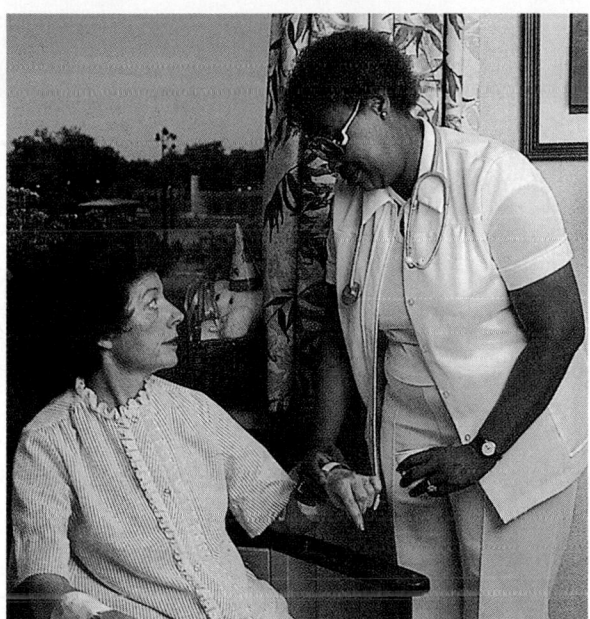

Fig. 35-8 Before administering any medication, the nurse checks the client's identification and allergy bracelet.

oral use can produce local complications such as a sterile abscess or fatal systemic effects. Drug companies label parenteral drugs for "injectable use only."

Right Time

The nurse must know why a drug is ordered for certain times of the day and whether the time schedule can be altered. For example, two drugs are ordered, one q8h (every 8 hours) and the other tid (3 times a day). Both medications are given 3 times within 24 hours. The physician intends the q8h medication to be given around the clock to maintain therapeutic blood levels of the drug. In contrast, the tid medication is given during the waking hours. Each institution has a recommended time schedule for medications ordered at frequent intervals. For example, qid (4 times a day) medications may be given at 0800, 1200, 1600, and 2000; tid medications may be given at 0800, 1400, and 2000.

The physician often gives specific instructions about when to administer a medication. A preoperative medication to be given on call means that the nurse is to administer the drug when the operating room notifies the nursing division. A drug ordered pc (after meals) is to be given within half an hour after a meal, when the client has a full stomach. A STAT medication is to be given immediately.

When a nurse is responsible for administering several medications, drugs that must act at certain times are given priority. For example, insulin should be administered at a precise interval before a meal. All routinely ordered medications should be given within 30 minutes of the times ordered.

Some medications require the nurse's clinical judgment in determining the proper time for administration. A prn sleeping medication should be administered when the client is prepared for bed. Many hospitalized clients prefer to go to sleep earlier than they might normally at home.

However, if the nurse is aware that a procedure might interrupt the client's sleep, it is appropriate to withhold the drug until a time when the client can gain full benefit from the medication. A nurse also uses judgment in administering prn analgesics. When a client's order reads, "q3 to 4h," the nurse may give the medication as often as every 3 hours. The nurse assesses the client's level of pain to determine the degree of discomfort. If a client is made to wait until the pain becomes severe, the analgesic effect may not be sufficient. The nurse may need to obtain an order from the physician to supplement the prn analgesic. (For more about analgesia, see Chapter 43.)

In the home a client may have to take several medications throughout the day. The nurse can help plan medication schedules based on the preferred drug intervals and the client's daily schedule. For example, the schedule for drugs to be given around mealtime can be easily adjusted to client preferences. For clients who have difficulty remembering when to take medications, the nurse can make a chart that lists the times when each drug is to be taken.

▌ MEDICATION ERRORS

A medication error is any event that could cause or lead to a client receiving inappropriate drug therapy or failing to receive appropriate drug therapy (Edgar, Lee, Cousins, 1994). Medication errors can occur by anyone involved in the prescribing, transcribing, preparation, dispensing, and administration of medications. Hospital medication delivery systems should be designed so that there is a system of checks and balances. This will help reduce medication errors. Consider this example:

CASE STUDY The physician writes an order for a drug. The nurse receives the order and checks for completeness and appropriateness (see the box on p. 808). The nurse may question the order, for example: if the written order is illegible, the dose seems unusually low or high, or the medication seems inappropriate for the client's condition. The order is sent to the pharmacy where it may be read by a pharmacy technician and may be prepared by the technician. The pharmacist checks the technician's work, that the drug is the appropriate dosage, and for drug interactions and drug allergies. When a medication order seems inappropriate, for example, a drug order written for 2000 mg when the proper dosage calls for 200 mg, the pharmacist may call the nurse for physician clarification (or the pharmacist may call the physician directly). When the order is appropriate, the medications are sent to the nursing unit. The nurse receives the drug and checks the administration record against what the pharmacy has sent and the physician order. Before administration, the nurse performs the five rights of drug administration. The nurse allows the client to be the final check by reviewing the name of the drug, the dosage, and why he or she is receiving the drug. ▪

The above example illustrates the important role that nurses play in the prevention of drug errors. The nurse is crucial as the essential link in the prevention of drug errors. Unfortunately, most medication errors are made by nurses and occur when a nurse fails to follow routine procedures (Table 35-8). When an error occurs, it should be acknowledged immediately and reported to the appropriate hospital personnel. The nurse has the ethical and professional obligation to report the error to the physician and the

Table 35-8	**Ways to Prevent Drug Administration Errors**
PRECAUTION	**RATIONALE**
Read drug labels carefully.	Many products come in similar containers, colors, and shapes.
Question administration of multiple tablets or vials for single dose.	Most doses are one or two tablets or capsules or one single-dose vial. Incorrect interpretation of order may result in excessively high dose.
Be aware of drugs with similar names.	Many drug names sound alike (e.g., digoxin and digitoxin, Keflex and Keflin, Orinase and Ornade).
Check decimal point.	Some drugs come in quantities that are multiples of one another (e.g., Coumadin in 2.5 and 25 mg tablets, Thorazine in 30 and 300 mg spansules).
Question abrupt and excessive increases in dosages.	Most dosages are made gradually so that physician can monitor therapeutic effect and response.
When new or unfamiliar drug is ordered, consult resource.	If physician is also unfamiliar with drug, there is greater risk of inaccurate dosages being ordered.
Do not administer drug ordered by nickname or unofficial abbreviation.	Many physicians refer to commonly ordered medications by nicknames or unofficial abbreviations. If nurse or pharmacist is unfamiliar with name, wrong drug may be dispensed and administered.
Do not attempt to decipher illegible writing.	When in doubt, ask physician. Unless nurse questions order that is difficult to read, chance of misinterpretation is great.
Know clients with same last names. Also have clients state their full names. Check name bands carefully.	It is common to have two or more clients with same or similar last names. Special labels on Kardex or medication book can warn of potential problem.
Do not confuse equivalents.	When in hurry, it may be easy to misread equivalents (e.g., milligram instead of milliliter).

nurse manager. The physician may decide to counteract the effects of the error, by administering an antidote when the wrong drug is given, withholding a dose when a previous medication has been given too soon, or monitoring the effects when an unusually high dosage is given. Attempts should not be made to hide the medication error. There should be a notation in the client's record as to what was administered to the client, the notification of the physician, the observed side effects in the client as a response to the error and the events undertaken to counteract the drugs, for example, the administration of an antidote.

The nurse is also responsible for completing a report describing the nature of the incident. The incident report is not an admission of guilt or the basis for punishment and is not a part of the client's legal medical record. The report provides an objective analysis of what went wrong and is a means for the institution's risk management team to monitor such occurrences. Incident reports assist interdisciplinary committees in identifying errors and solving hospital system problems contributing to medication errors.

■ SPECIAL CONSIDERATIONS FOR ADMINISTERING MEDICATIONS TO SPECIFIC AGE GROUPS

A client's developmental level is a factor in the way in which nurses administer medications. Knowledge of a client's developmental needs helps the nurse anticipate responses to drug therapy.

Infants and Children

Children vary in age, weight, body surface area, and the ability to absorb, metabolize, and excrete medications. Children's dosages are lower than those of adults, so special caution is needed in preparing medications for them. Drugs are usually not prepared and packaged in standardized dosage ranges for children. Preparing an ordered dosage from an available amount requires careful calculation.

A child's parents are valuable resources for learning the best way to give a child medications. Sometimes it is less traumatic for the child if a parent gives the drug and the nurse supervises.

All children require special psychological preparation before receiving medications. Supportive care for the child is needed if a child is expected to cooperate. The nurse explains the procedure to a child, using short words and simple language appropriate to the child's level of comprehension. The young child who refuses to cooperate or resists consistently despite explanation and encouragement may require physical coercion. If so, it is carried out quickly and carefully (Wong, 1995). If it is possible to involve the child and the child's parent, the nurse may have greater success giving a medication. For example, saying "It's time to take your pill now. Do you want it with water or juice?" allows a child to make a choice. The nurse *never* gives the child the option of not taking a medication. After a drug is given, the nurse praises the child and may even offer a simple reward such as a star or token. Depending on the route of administration, the nurse can use several tips described in the box on p. 815, left, when administering drugs to children.

Older Adults

Older adults also require special consideration during drug administration. In addition to the physiological changes of aging, behavioral and economic factors will influence an older person's use of drugs.

Individuals over the age of 65 are the largest users of drugs (Ebersole, Hess, 1994). The nurse who administers drugs to older clients should be aware of five patterns of drug use by the elderly client as identified by Ebersole and Hess (1994).

1. **Polypharmacy.** This means that the client is taking

Tips for Administering Drugs to Children

ORAL MEDICATIONS

- Liquid forms are safer to swallow to avoid aspiration.
- Juice, a soft drink, or a frozen juice bar is offered after a drug is swallowed.
- Carbonated beverages poured over finely crushed ice reduce nausea.
- When mixing drugs with palatable flavorings such as syrup or honey, the nurse uses only a small amount. The child may refuse to take all of a larger mixture. The nurse avoids mixing a drug with foods or liquids that the child is taking well because the child may in turn refuse them.
- A plastic, disposable syringe is the most accurate device for preparing liquid dosages, especially those less than 10 ml. (Cups, teaspoons, and droppers are inaccurate.)
- When administering liquid drugs, a spoon, plastic cup, or oral syringe (without needle) are useful.

INJECTIONS

- The nurse is very careful when selecting IM injection sites. Infants and small children have underdeveloped muscles.
- Children can be unpredictable and uncooperative. Someone should be available to restrain a child if needed.
- The nurse always awakens a sleeping child before giving an injection.
- Distracting the child with conversation or a toy may reduce pain perception.
- The nurse gives the injection quickly and does not fight with the child.

GERONTOLOGICAL PRINCIPLES for Administration of Medications

- Take a complete medication history including:
  - Past medications
  - Present medications (prescription and OTC)
  - Allergies of all kinds
  - Client's understanding of medications being taken (name, purpose, dosage, method, times)
- Space oral medications so that not more than one or two are taken at one time
- Have client drink a little fluid *before* taking oral medications (to ease swallowing)
- Encourage the client to drink at least 5 to 6 ounces of fluid after taking medications (to assure that the medications have left the esophagus and are in the stomach and to speed absorption of the medication)
- Do not routinely give analgesics for pain every 4 hours. Because of delayed absorption and distribution and the half-life of the medication, there may be an adverse cumulative effect
- If the client has difficulty swallowing a large capsule or tablet, ask the physician to substitute a liquid medication if possible (cutting the tablet in half or crushing it and placing it in applesauce or fruit juice may distort the action of some medications, reduce the dose, or cause choking or aspiration of particles of medication or applesauce)
- Teach alternatives to medications, such as the following:
  - Proper diet instead of vitamins
  - Exercise instead of laxatives
  - Bedtime snacks instead of hypnotics
  - Decrease in weight, salt, fats, stress, and smoking and increased exercise instead of hypertensive agents (if approved by the physician)

Modified from Ebersole P, Hess P: *Toward health aging: human needs and nursing response,* ed 4, St Louis, 1994, Mosby.

many medications, prescribed or not, in an attempt to treat several disorders simultaneously. When this occurs, there is a high risk of drug interactions with other drugs and with foods. There is also an increased risk of the client having an adverse reaction to the medications.

2. Self-prescribing of medications. A variety of symptoms can be experienced by older adult clients, for example, pain, constipation, insomnia, and indigestion. All these symptoms are amenable to over-the-counter medications. Older adults often attempt to seek relief from the problems by using over-the-counter preparations, folk medicines, and herbs.

3. Over-the-counter (OTC) medications. It is known that OTC drugs are used by 75% of the aged to relieve symptoms. Many of these OTC preparations have ingredients that, when used inappropriately, may cause undesirable side effects, adverse reactions or may be contraindicated in the client's condition.

4. Misuse of drugs. Forms of misuse by the elderly include: overuse, underuse, erratic use, and contraindicated use.

5. Noncompliance. Nonconpliance is defined as *a deliberate misuse of medication.* Of older adults, 75% intentionally do not adhere to their drug regimen either by altering the dose because of ineffectiveness or uncomfortable side effects.

The nurse uses the nursing process to identify patterns of drug use in the elderly client. Medication administration

time gives the nurse the opportunity to carry out education or reinforcement of previous medication teaching. The box above outlines tips for administering medications to the older client.

ORAL DRUG ADMINISTRATION

The most desirable way to administer medications is by mouth (Procedure 35-1). Unless the client has impaired gastrointestinal functioning or is unable to swallow, an oral medication is the safest and easiest to give.

Most tablets and capsules should be swallowed and administered with an adequate amount of fluid, providing an opportunity for the nurse to increase a client's fluid intake. For clients with nasogastric feeding tubes, liquid medications are preferred. However, some tablets can be crushed and capsules opened to mix in a solution for administration (see the box on p. 819, left).

When administering medications orally, the nurse must protect the client against possible aspiration. Positioning the client in a sitting or side-lying position will prevent the accumulation of a liquid or a solid medication in the back of the throat. A client who swallows slowly should not be forced to take a large amount of liquid with each swallow.

PROCEDURE 35-1

Administering Oral Medications

STEPS	RATIONALE
1. Assess for contraindications to client receiving oral medication, including difficulty in swallowing, nausea or vomiting, bowel inflammation or reduced peristalsis, recent gastrointestinal surgery, reduced or absent bowel sounds, gastric suction, decreased level of consciousness.	Alterations in gastrointestinal function interfere with drug distribution, absorption, and excretion. When gastric suction is in place, medication can be suctioned out before it can be absorbed. Clients with lowered consciousness are prone to aspiration.
2. Determine client's preferences and tolerances for fluids.	Offering fluids can increase fluid intake unless it is contradicted by heart, lung, or renal diseases.
3. Prepare needed supplies and equipment:	
a. Medication cards, record forms, or printout	
b. Medication cart or tray	
c. Disposable medication cups	
d. Glass of water, juice, or preferred liquid	
e. Drinking straw	
f. Pill crush device (optional)	Used to crush tablets for clients who have difficulty in swallowing.
g. Paper towels	
4. Check accuracy and completeness of each medication card, form, or printout with physician's written medication order. Check client's name and drug name, dosage, route of administration, and time for administration. Report discrepancy in order to charge nurse or physician.	Physician's order is most reliable source and only legal record of drugs client is to receive.
5. Prepare drug:	
a. Wash hands.	Reduces transfer of microorganisms from your hands to medications and equipment.
b. Arrange medication tray and cups in medicine room or move medication cart to position outside client's room.	Saves time and reduces error.
c. Unlock medicine drawer or cart (see the illustration below, left). (Narcotics are generally stored in double-locked box separate from medicine drawers or carts.) (Computerized cart systems are accessed by electronic number entry).	Medications are safeguarded when locked in cabinet or cart.
d. Prepare medications for one client at a time. Keep medication tickets or forms for each client together.	Prevents preparation errors.
e. Select correct drug from stock supply or unit-dose drawer. Compare label of medication with medication form, card, or printout.	Reduces error.

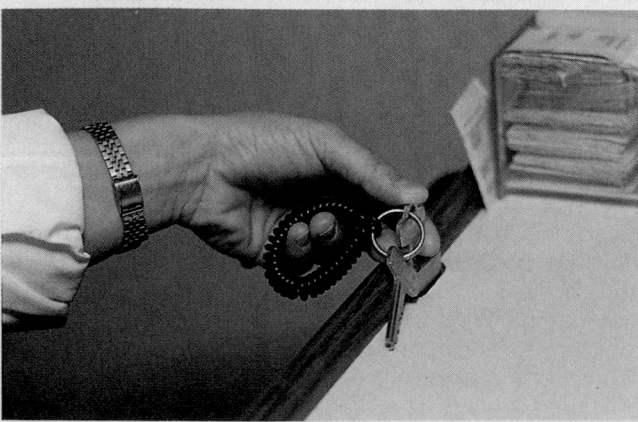

Step 5c

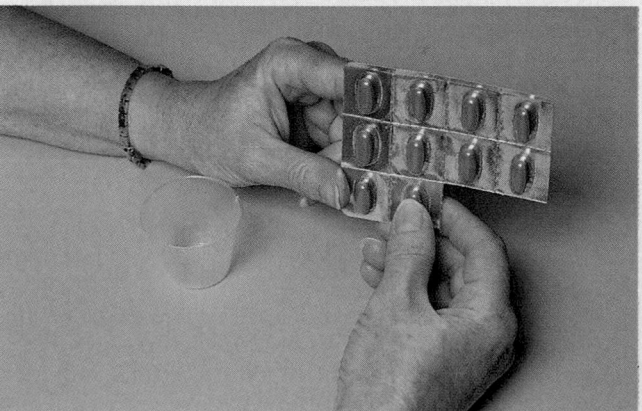

Step 5h

Administering Oral Medications—cont'd

STEPS	RATIONALE

5. Prepare drug—cont'd

  f. Calculate correct drug dose. Take time. Double check calculation.

     Calculation is more accurate when information from drug label is at hand.

  g. To prepare tablet or capsules from bottle, pour required number into bottle cap and transfer to medication cup. Do not touch with fingers. Extra tablets or capsules may be returned to bottle.

     Maintains cleanliness of drugs.

  h. To prepare unit-dose tablets or capsules, place packaged tablet or capsule directly into medicine cup. (Do not remove wrapper.) (See the illustration on p. 816, right.)

     Wrappers maintain cleanliness and identification of medications. Unopened medications may be returned to pharmacy if they are refused.

  i. Place all tablets or capsules given at same time in one cup except for those requiring preadministration assessments (e.g., pulse rate or blood pressure).

     Keeping medications that require preadministration assessments separate from others makes it easier for you to withhold drugs as necessary.

  j. Scored tablets can be broken with gloved hands or cut with a cutting device (see the illustration below, left). Discard unused portions of divided tablets.

  k. If client has difficulty in swallowing, grind tablets in pill crusher. Place tablet in bottom of crusher and grind. Continue to crush fragments until smooth powder remains. Mix crushed tablet in small amount of soft food, such as custard or applesauce. CAUTION: Do not crush enteric-coated or sustained-action medications.

     Large tablets can be difficult to swallow. Ground tablet mixed with palatable soft food is usually easy to swallow. Verify that medication can be crushed before doing so; enteric-coated medications are not designed to be absorbed in stomach.

  l. Prepare liquids:

    1. Thoroughly mix before administering. Check and discard those that have turned cloudy or changed color

      (1) Remove bottle cap from container and place cap upside down.

         Prevents contamination of inside of cap.

      (2) Hold bottle with label against palm of hand while pouring.

         Spilled liquid will not soil or fade label.

      (3) Hold medication cup at eye level and fill to desired level on scale (see the illustration below, right). (Scale should be even with fluid level at its surface or base of meniscus, not edges.)

         Ensures accuracy of measurement.

      (4) Discard excess liquid in cup into sink. Wipe lip of bottle with paper towel.

         Prevents contamination of bottle's contents and prevents bottle cap from sticking.

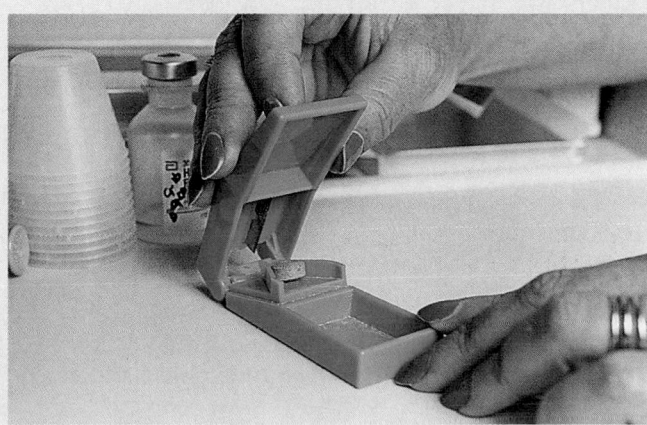

Step 5j

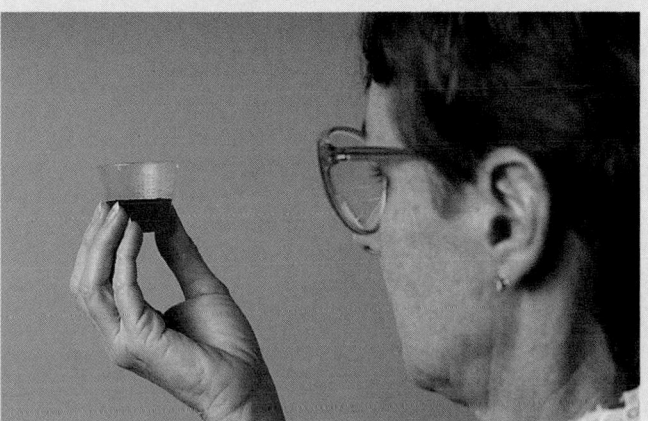

Step 5l(3)

Continued.

Administering Oral Medications—cont'd

STEPS	RATIONALE

5. Prepare drug—cont'd

(5) Some liquid medications are in unit dose containers (see the illustration at right). Draw volumes of less than 10 ml in syringe **(without needle).**

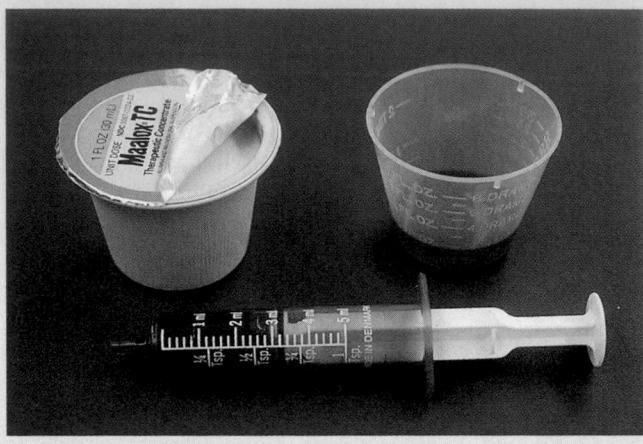

m. When preparing narcotic, check narcotic record for previous drug count, compare with supply available, remove drug, and complete necessary information on narcotic form and sign.

Controlled substance laws require careful monitoring of dispensed narcotics.

n. Compare medication form, card, or printout with prepared drug and container.

Reading label second time reduces error.

o. Return stock containers or unused unit-dose medications to shelf or drawer and read label again.

Third check of label reduces errors.

p. Place medications and cards, forms, or printouts together on tray or cart.

Drugs are labeled at all times for identification.

q. Do not leave drugs unattended.

Nurse is responsible for safekeeping of drugs.

6. Administer medications:

a. Take medications to client at correct time.

Medications are given within 30 min before or after prescribed time to ensure intended effect. Stat or single-order medications should be given at time ordered.

b. Identify client by comparing name on card, form, or printout with name on client's identification bracelet. Ask client to state full name.

Identification bracelets are made at same time of client's admission and are most reliable source of identification. Missing or faded bracelets are replaced to avoid errors.

c. Perform necessary preadministration assessment for specific medications (e.g., blood pressure or pulse).

Assessment data determine whether specific medications should be given at that time.

d. Explain purpose of each medication and its action to client. Allow client to ask questions about drugs.

Client has right to be informed, and understanding of medication improves compliance with therapy.

e. Assist client to sitting or side-lying position.

Prevents aspiration during swallowing.

f. Administer drugs properly:

(1) Ask if client wishes to hold solid medications in hand or cup before placing in mouth.

Client can become familiar with medications by seeing each drug.

(2) Offer full glass of water or juice with drugs to be swallowed.

Choice of fluid promotes comfort and can improve fluid intake.

(3) For sublingual administered drugs, have client place medication under tongue and allow it to dissolve completely. Caution client against swallowing.

Drug is absorbed through blood vessels of undersurface of tongue. If swallowed, drug is destroyed by gastric juices or is so rapidly detoxified by liver that therapeutic blood levels are not attained.

(4) Mix powdered medications with liquids at bedside and give to client to drink.

When prepared in advance, powdered drug forms may thicken and even harden, making swallowing difficult.

(5) Caution client against chewing or swallowing lozenges.

Drug acts through slow absorption through oral mucosa, not gastric mucosa.

(6) Give effervescent powders and tablets immediately after dissolving.

Effervescence helps improve unpleasant taste of drug and often has therapeutic value for gastrointestinal problems.

Administering Oral Medications—cont'd

STEPS	RATIONALE
6. Administer medications—cont'd	
g. If client is unable to hold medications, place medication cup to lips and gently introduce each drug into mouth, one at a time. Do not rush.	Prevents contamination of medications. Administering single tablet or capsule eases swallowing and prevents aspiration.
h. If tablet or capsule falls to floor, discard it and repeat preparation.	Drug is contaminated when it touches floor.
i. Stay with client until each medication has been swallowed. If uncertain whether medication has been swallowed, ask client to open the mouth.	Nurse assumes responsibility for ensuring that client receives ordered dosage. If left unattended, client may not take dose or may save drugs, causing risk to health.
j. For highly acidic medications (e.g., aspirin), offer nonfat snack (e.g., crackers).	Reduces gastric irritation.
k. Assist client in returning to comfortable position.	Maintains comfort.
l. Dispose of soiled supplies and wash hands.	Reduces transmission of microorganisms.
m. Return medication cards, forms, or printouts to appropriate file for next administration time.	Cards, forms, and printouts are used as reference for when next dose is due. Loss can lead to administration error.
n. Replenish stock such as cups and straws, return cart to medicine room, and clean work area.	Clean working space assists other staff in completing duties efficiently.
7. Record actual time that each drug was administered on medication record or computer. Include initials or signature (see Fig. 35-6).	Prompt documentation prevents errors such as repeated doses. Signature establishes accountability for administration.
8. Return within 30 min to evaluate response to medications.	Used to assess drug's therapeutic benefit and detect onset of side effects or allergic reactions.

Likewise, a client should swallow only one pill or capsule at a time. If a client begins to cough while taking a medication, the nurse should withhold the remaining portion of the drug until the client can breathe more easily. If the client has difficulty swallowing tablets, other forms of the medication, such as a suppository should be considered. After the administration of medications, if the client is having intake recorded, record the amount of liquid used to administer the medication.

Guidelines for Giving Drugs Through a Nasogastric Tube, J-Tube, G-Tube, or Small-Bore Feeding Tube

- Administer medications in a liquid form (suspension, elixir, or solution) when possible to prevent tube obstruction.
- Read medication labels carefully before crushing a tablet or opening a capsule.
- Do *not* crush buccal or sublingual tablets.
- Do not crush enteric-coated or sustained-action medications.
- Dissolve crushed tablets and powders in warm water.
- Dissolve soft, gelatin capsules in warm water.
- Irrigate the tube before and after all medication is given with 50-150 ml of water.
- Do not use pigtail vent for irrigation or instillation of fluid.
- Avoid giving syrups or medications with a pH of less than 4.
- Do not attempt to give whole or undissolved medications.

Modified from Petrosin BM et al: *Crit Care Nurs* Q 12:1, 1989

■ ADMINISTRATION OF INJECTIONS

Administering an injection is an invasive procedure that must be performed using aseptic technique (see the box below). After a needle pierces the skin, the risk of infection exists. The nurse administers drugs parenterally by the SQ, IM, ID, and IV routes. Each type of injection requires certain skills to ensure that the drug reaches the proper location. The effects of a parenterally administered drug can develop rapidly, depending on the rate of drug absorption. The nurse closely observes the client's response.

Equipment

A variety of syringes and needles are available, and each is designed to deliver a certain volume of a drug to a specific

---

Preventing Infection During an Injection

- To prevent contamination of solution, draw medication from ampule quickly. Do not allow it to stand open.
- To prevent needle contamination, avoid letting needle touch contaminated surface (e.g., outer edges of ampule or vial, outer surface of needle cap, nurse's hands, counter top, table surface).
- To prevent syringe contamination, avoid touching length of plunger or inner part of barrel. Keep tip of syringe covered with cap or needle.
- To prepare skin, wash skin soiled with dirt, drainage, or feces with soap and water and dry. Use friction and a circular motion while cleaning with an antiseptic swab. Swab from center of site, and move outward in a 2-inch radius.

type of tissue. The nurse exercises judgment when determining which syringe or needle will be the most effective.

Syringes

Syringes consist of a cylindrical barrel with a tip designed to fit the hub of a hypodermic needle and a close-fitting plunger. Syringes, in general, are classified as being *Luer-lok* or *nonLuer-lok*. This nomenclature is based on the design of the syringe's tip. Luer-lok syringes (Fig. 35-9, *A*) require special needles, which are twisted onto the tip and lock themselves in place. This design prevents the inadvertent re-

moval of the needle. NonLuer-lok (Fig. 35-9, *B-D*) syringes require needles that slip onto the tip. Most health care institutions use disposable, single-use plastic syringes that are inexpensive and easy to manipulate. The syringes are packaged separately, with or without a sterile needle in a paper wrapper or rigid, plastic container.

The nurse fills a syringe by aspiration, pulling the plunger outward while the needle tip remains immersed in the prepared solution. The nurse may handle the outside of the syringe barrel and the handle of the plunger. To maintain sterility the nurse avoids letting any unsterile object touch the tip or inside of the barrel, the hub, the shaft of the plunger, or the needle (Fig. 35-10).

Syringes come in a number of sizes, from 0.5 to 60 ml. It is unusual to use a syringe larger than 5 ml for a SQ or IM injection. A 2- to 3-ml syringe is usually adequate. A larger volume creates discomfort. Larger syringes are used to prepare IV drugs. The 2.5- or 3-ml hypodermic syringe often comes packaged with a needle attached. However, the nurse may change needle sizes. The hypodermic has two scales on the barrel. One scale is divided into minims and the other into tenths of a milliliter.

Insulin syringes (see Fig. 35-9, *C* and *D*) hold 0.5 to 1 ml and are calibrated in units. Insulin syringes that hold 0.5 ml are known as *low-dose syringes* (50 μ per 0.5 ml) and are easier to read. Insulin syringes in the United States and Canada are U-100s, designed for use with U-100 strength insulin. Each milliliter of solution contains 100 units of insulin.

The tuberculin syringe (see Fig. 35-9, *B*) has a long, thin barrel with a preattached thin needle. The syringe is calibrated in sixteenths of a minim and hundredths of a milliliter and has a capacity of 1 ml. The nurse uses a tuberculin syringe to prepare small amounts of potent drugs. A tuberculin syringe is useful in preparing small, precise doses for infants or young children.

The nurse uses large hypodermic syringes to administer certain IV drugs and add medications to IV solutions.

Needles

Needles come packaged in individual sheaths to allow flexibility in choosing the right needle. Some needles are preattached to standard-size syringes. Most are made of stainless steel and are disposable.

The needle has three parts: the hub, which fits onto the

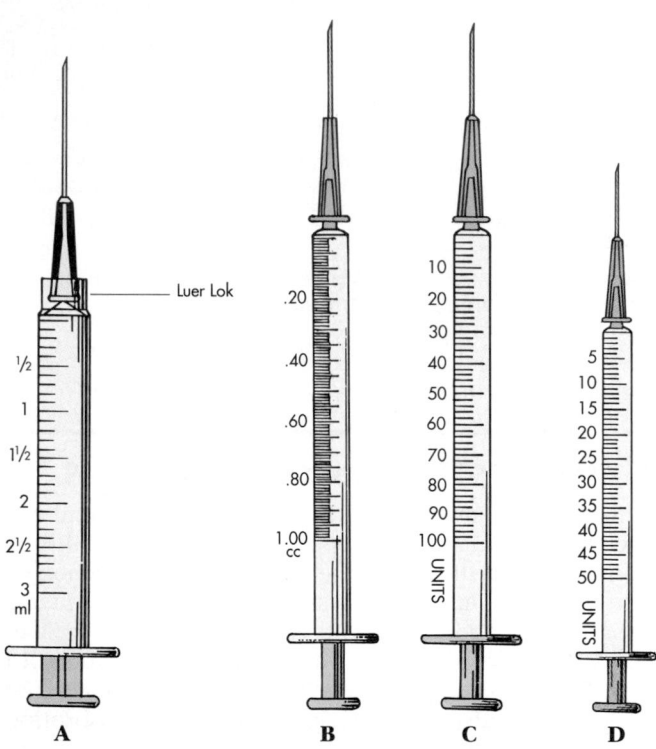

Fig. 35-9 Types of syringes. **A,** A Luer-lok syringe marked in 0.1 tenths. **B,** Tuberculin syringe marked in 0.01 (hundredths) for doses of less than 1 ml. **C,** Insulin syringe marked in units (100). **D,** Insulin syringe marked in units (50).

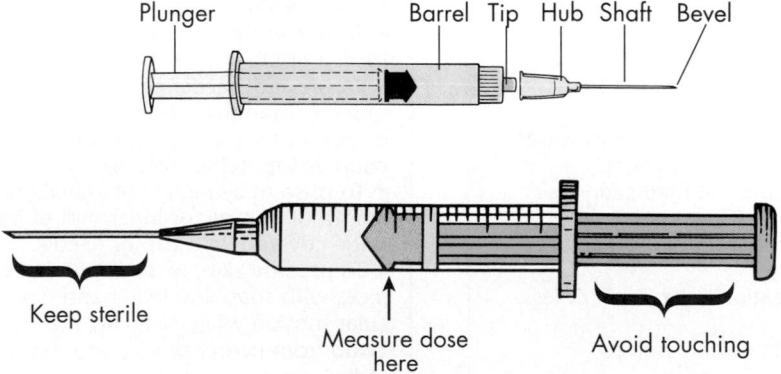

Fig. 35-10 Parts of a syringe.

tip of a syringe; the shaft, which connects to the hub; and the bevel, or slanted tip (see Fig. 35-10).

Each needle has three characteristic features: the slant of the bevel, the length of the shaft, and the needle gauge or diameter. Long bevels are sharper, which minimizes discomfort caused by SQ and IM injections. Needles vary in length from ¼ to 5 inches. The nurse chooses needle length according to client size and weight and the type of tissue into which the drug is to be injected. A child or a slender adult generally requires a shorter needle. The nurse uses a longer needle (usually 1 to 1½ inches) for IM injections and a shorter needle (usually ⅜ to ⅝ inch) for SQ injections.

The smaller the gauge, the larger the needle diameter (Fig. 35- 11). The selection of a gauge depends on the viscosity of the fluid to be injected or infused. An IM injection usually requires a 19- to 23-gauge needle, depending on the viscosity of the medication. SQ injections require smaller diameter needles, such as a 25-gauge. For an ID injection a 26-gauge needle is used.

Disposable Injection Units

Disposable, single-dose, prefilled syringes are available for many medications. The nurse must be careful to check the medication and concentration because all prefilled syringes appear very similar.

The Tubex and Carpuject injection systems include reusable plastic mechanisms that hold prefilled, disposable, sterile cartridge-needle units (Fig. 35-12). The nurse slips the cartridge into the mechanism, secures it (following package directions), and checks for air bubbles in the syringe. The nurse advances the plunger to expel the medication as in a regular syringe. These systems are designed to

decrease the chance of accidental needlesticks if used according to the manufactures' recommendations.

Preparing an Injection From an Ampule

Ampules contain single doses of medication in a liquid and are available in several sizes, from 1 ml to 10 ml or more (Fig. 35-13, *A*). An ampule is made of glass with a constricted neck that must be snapped off to allow access to the medication. A colored ring around the neck indicates

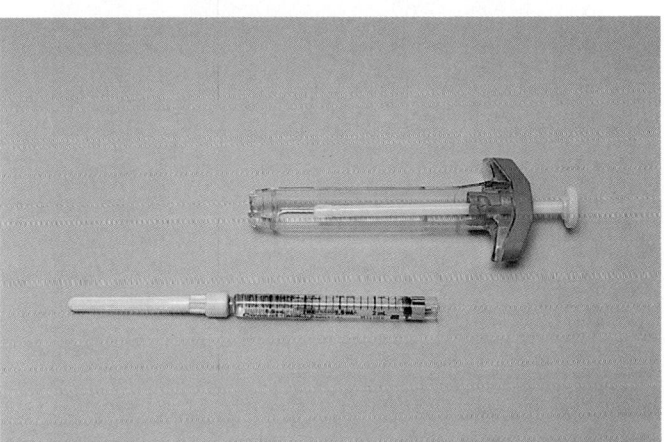

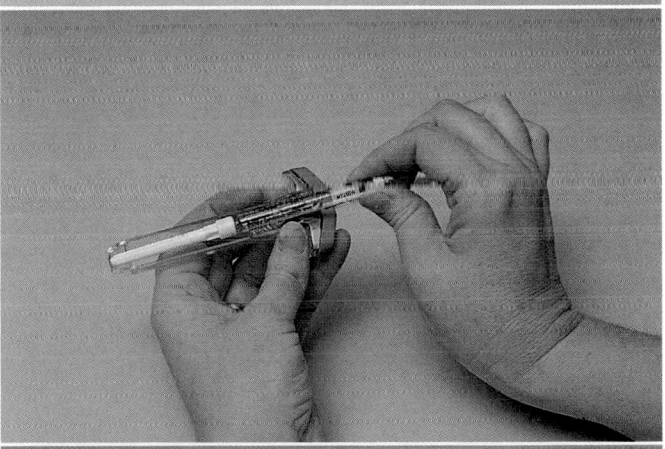

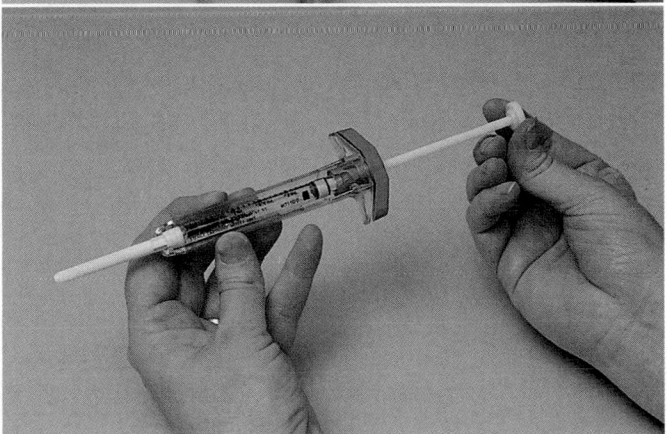

Fig. 35-12 A, Carpujet syringe and prefilled sterile cartridge with needle. **B,** Assembling the Carpujet. **C,** The cartridge slides into the syringe barrel, turns, and locks at the needle end. The plunger then screws into the cartridge end.

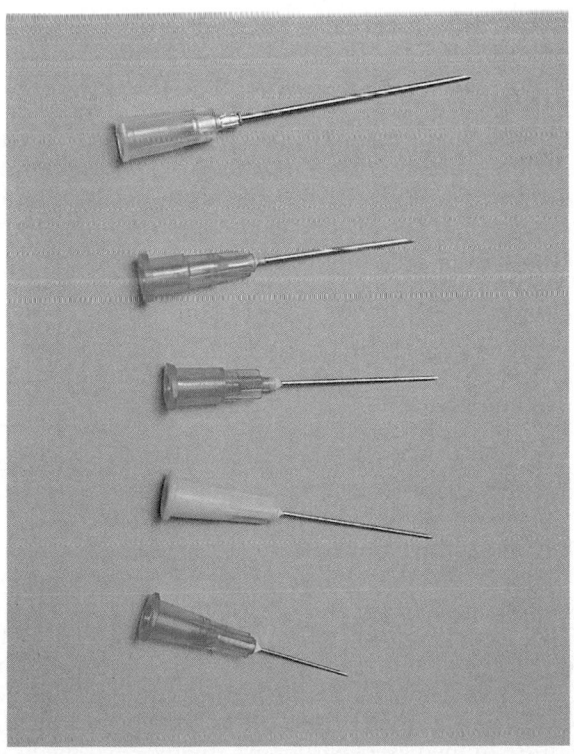

Fig. 35-11 Hypodermic needles arranged in order of gauge (G). Top to bottom 19 G, 20 G, 21 G, 23 G, and 25 G.

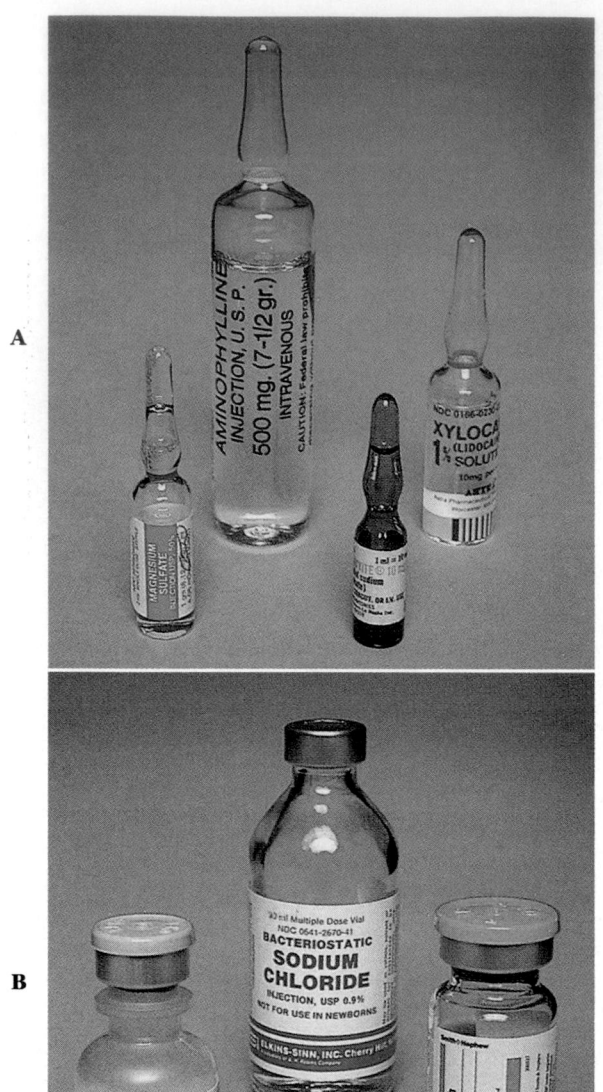

Fig. 35-13 **A,** Ampules. **B,** Vials.

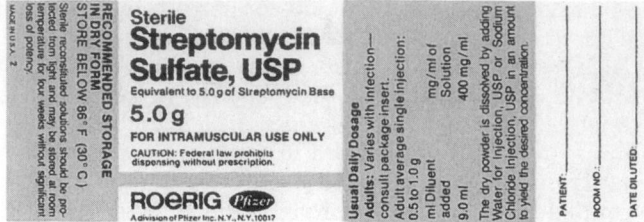

Fig. 35-14 Medication label for powdered drug. *(From Gray D: Calculate with confidence, St Louis, 1994, Mosby.)*

solution (solvent) used to dissolve the drug and the amount needed to prepare a desired drug concentration (Fig. 35-14). Normal saline and sterile distilled water are solutions commonly used to dissolve drugs.

Unlike the ampule, the vial is a closed system, and air must be injected into it to permit easy withdrawal of the solution. Failure to inject air before withdrawing the solution leaves a vacuum within the vial that makes withdrawal difficult (Procedure 35-2).

To prepare a powdered drug, the nurse draws up the amount of solvent recommended on the vial's label (see the box on p. 827). The nurse injects the solvent into the vial in the same manner as when injecting air into the vial. Most powdered drugs dissolve easily, but it may be necessary to withdraw the needle to mix the contents thoroughly. Gently shaking or rolling the vial between the hands will dissolve the powdered drug. The needle is reinserted to draw up the dissolved medication. After mixing multidose vials the nurse makes a label that includes the date of mixing and concentration of drug per milliliter. Multidose vials may require refrigeration after the contents are reconstituted.

Mixing Medications

If two drugs are compatible, it is possible to mix them together into one injection if the total dosage is within the accepted limits. A client will appreciate not having to receive more than one injection at a time. Most nursing units have charts that list common compatible drugs. If there is any uncertainty about drug compatibilities, a pharmacist should be consulted.

Mixing Medications From Two Vials

Follow these principles when mixing medications from two vials:

1. Do not contaminate one medication with another.
2. Ensure that the final dosage is accurate.
3. Maintain aseptic technique.

Only one syringe is needed to mix medications from two vials (Fig. 35-15). The nurse takes a syringe and aspirates the volume of air equivalent to the first drug's dosage (vial A). The nurse injects air into vial A, making sure that the needle does not touch the solution. The nurse withdraws the needle, aspirates air equivalent to the second drug's dose (vial B), and then injects the volume of air into vial B. The nurse immediately withdraws the required medication from vial B into the syringe. At this point the drug from vial A has not contaminated vial B.

where the ampule is prescored to break easily. Aspiration of the drug into a syringe may require that the nurse use a filter needle. The nurse should check institutional policy for withdrawal of medication from ampules. The procedure for withdrawal of medications from ampules is outlined in Procedure 35-2.

Preparing an Injection From a Vial

A vial is a single-dose or multidose glass container with a rubber seal at the top (Fig. 35-13, *B*). A metal or plastic cap protects the seal until it is ready for use. Vials contain liquid and/or dry forms of medications. Drugs that are unstable in solution are packaged dry. The vial label specifies the

Preparing Injections From Ampules and Vials

STEPS	RATIONALE
1. Wash hands.	Reduces transmission of infection.
2. Prepare needed equipment and supplies:	
a. Ampules:	
(1) Ampule containing medication	
(2) Syringe and needle	
(3) Small gauze pad or alcohol swab	
(4) Container for disposing of glass	
b. Vials:	
(1) Vial with medication	
(2) Syringe and needle	
(3) Alcohol swab	
(4) Solvent (e.g., normal saline or sterile water)	Used to dissolve drugs in dry form.
c. Medication cards, forms, or printouts	Verifies order.
3. Assemble supplies at work area in medicine room.	Makes procedure orderly.
4. Check each medication card, form, or computer printout against label on each ampule or vial.	Ensures that right drug and dosage are prepared.
5. Prepare injection from ampule:	
a. Tap top of ampule lightly and quickly with finger until fluid leaves neck (see the illustration below, left).	Dislodges fluid that collects above neck. All solution moves into lower chamber.
b. Place small gauze pad or dry alcohol swab around neck of ampule.	Protects your fingers from trauma as glass tip is broken off.
c. Snap neck quickly and firmly away from hands (see the illustration below, middle).	Prevents shattering glass toward or in your fingers or face.
d. Draw up medication quickly. Hold ampule upside down or set it on flat surface. Insert syringe needle into center of ampule opening (see the illustration below, right). Do not allow needle tip or shaft to touch rim of ampule.	Broken rim of ampule is considered contaminated. As long as needle tip or shaft does not touch rim, solution does not dribble out.
e. Aspirate medication into syringe by gently pulling back on plunger.	Withdrawal of plunger creates negative pressure within syringe barrel, which pulls fluid into syringe.

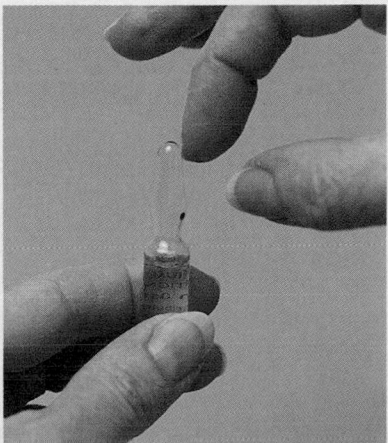

Step 5a

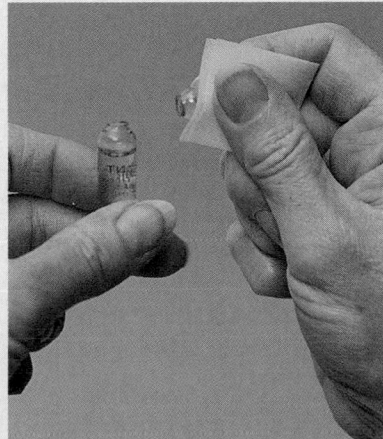

Step 5c

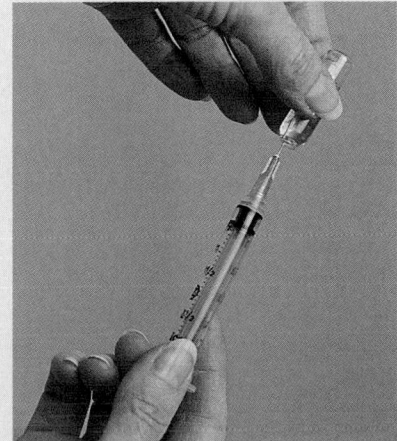

Step 5d

Continued.

PROCEDURE 35-2

Preparing Injections From Ampules and Vials—cont'd

5. Prepare injection from ampule—cont'd

  f. Keep needle tip below surface of liquid. Tip ampule to bring all fluid within reach of needle (see the illustration below, left).

Prevents aspiration of air bubbles.

  g. If air bubbles are aspirated, do not expel air into ampule.

Air pressure may force fluid out of ampule, and medication will be lost.

  h. To expel excess air bubbles, remove needle. Hold syringe with needle pointing up. Tap side of syringe to cause bubbles to rise toward needle (see the illustration below, middle). Draw back slightly on plunger, and push plunger upward to eject air. *Do not eject fluid.*

Withdrawing plunger too far will pull it from barrel. Holding syringe vertically allows fluid to settle in bottom of barrel. Pulling back on plunger allows fluid within needle to enter barrel so that fluid is not expelled. Air at top of barrel and within needle is then expelled.

  i. If syringe contains excess fluid, use sink for disposal. Hold syringe vertically with needle tip up and slanted slightly toward sink. Slowly eject excess fluid into sink. Recheck fluid level in syringe by holding it vertically.

Medication is safely dispersed into sink. Position of needle allows medication to be expelled without flowing down needle shaft. Rechecking fluid level ensures proper dose.

  j. Cover needle with sheath or cap. Change needle on syringe. Ensure that needle is securely seated to the syringe.

Prevents contamination of needle and protects you from needlestick. Changing needle is required if you suspect that medication is on needle shaft. New needle prevents tracking medication through skin and SQ tissues.

  k. Dispose of soiled supplies. Place broken ampule in special container for glass.

Controls transmission of infection. Proper disposal of glass prevents accidental injury to personnel.

6. Prepare injection from vial:

  a. Remove metal cap covering top of unused vial. Expose rubber seal.

Vial comes packaged with cap to prevent contamination of rubber seal.

  b. Wipe off surface of rubber seal with alcohol swab, if vial had been previously opened.

Removes dust or grease but does not sterilize surface.

  c. Take syringe. Ensure that needle is securly seated to the syringe. Remove needle cap. Pull back on plunger to draw amount of air into syringe equivalent to volume of medication to be aspirated from vial (see the illustration below, right).

To prevent buildup of negative pressure on vial when aspirating medication, air must first be injected into vial.

  d. Insert tip of needle, with bevel pointing up, through center of rubber seal (see the illustration on p. 825, left). Apply pressure to tip of needle during insertion.

Center of seal is thinner and easier to penetrate. Keeping bevel up and using firm pressure prevents cutting rubber core from seal.

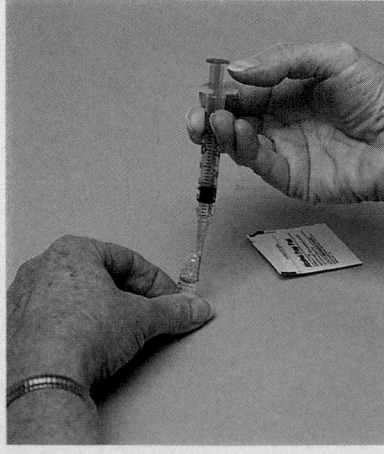

Step 5f

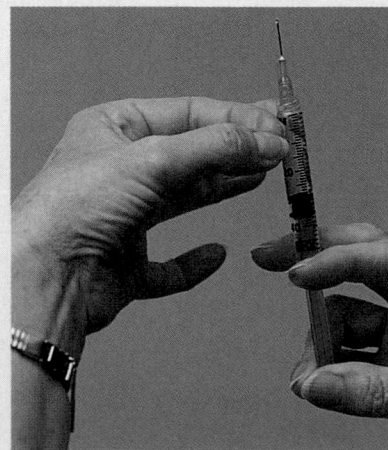

Step 5h

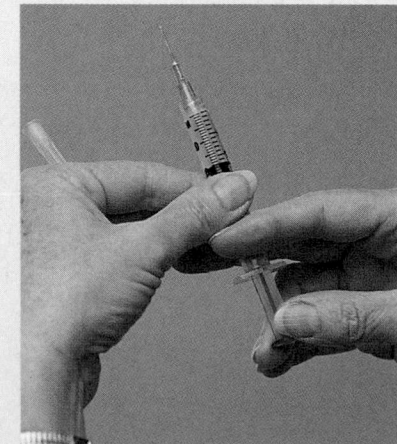

Step 6c

Preparing Injections From Ampules and Vials—cont'd

STEPS	RATIONALE

6. Prepare injection from vial—cont'd

e. Inject air into vial, holding on to plunger.

Air must be injected before aspirating fluid. Plunger may be forced backward by air pressure within vial.

f. Invert vial while keeping firm hold on syringe and plunger. Hold vial between thumb and middle fingers of nondominant hand. Grasp end of syringe barrel and plunger with thumb and forefinger of dominant hand.

Inverting vial allows fluid to settle in lower half of container. Position of hands prevents movement of plunger and permits easy manipulation of syringe.

g. Keep tip of needle below fluid level.

Prevents aspiration of air.

h. Allow air pressure to fill syringe gradually with medication (see the illustration below, middle). Pull back slightly on plunger if necessary.

Positive pressure within vial forces fluid into syringe.

i. Tap side of syringe barrel carefully to dislodge air bubbles. Eject air remaining at top of syringe into vial.

Forcefully striking barrel while needle is inserted in vial may bend needle. Accumulation of air displaces medication and causes errors.

j. After correct volume is obtained, remove needle from vial by pulling back on barrel of syringe.

Pulling plunger rather than barrel causes separation from barrel and loss of medication.

k. Remove remaining air from syringe by holding it and needle upright. Tap barrel to dislodge air bubbles (see the illustration below, right). Draw back slightly on plunger, and then push plunger upward to eject air. Do not eject fluid.

Holding syringe vertically allows fluid to settle in bottom of barrel. Pulling back on plunger allows fluid within needle to enter barrel so that fluid is not expelled. Air at end of barrel and within needle is then expelled.

l. Change needle and cover.

Inserting needle through rubber stopper may blunt bevel. New needle is sharper, and because no fluid is along shaft, it will not track medication through tissues.

m. For multidose vial, make label that includes date of mixing, concentration of drug per milliliter, and your initials.

Ensures that future doses will be prepared correctly. Certain drugs should be discarded after set number of days after mixing of vial.

n. Dispose of soiled supplies in proper containers.

Reduces transmission of microorganisms.

7. Clean work area. Wash hands.

Reduces transmission of microorganisms.

8. Check fluid level in syringe and compare with desired dose.

Ensures that accurate dose has been prepared.

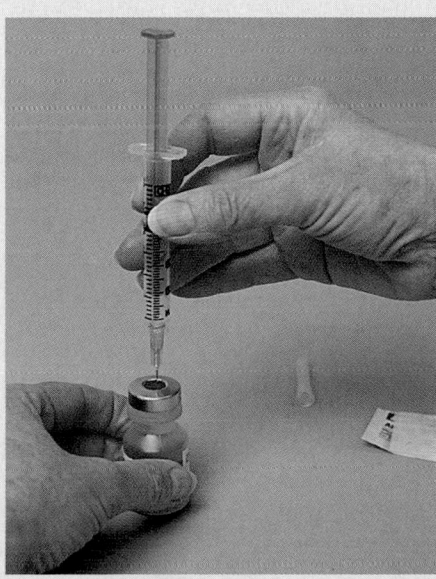

Step 6d

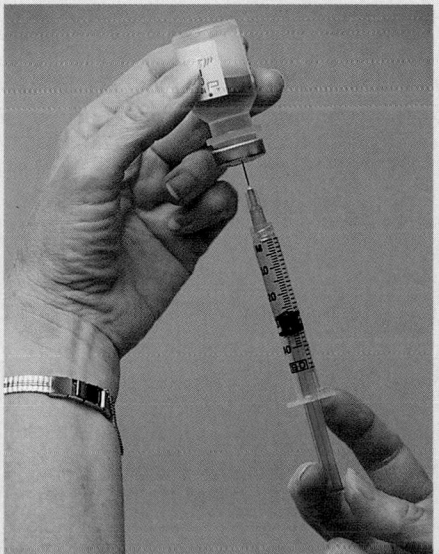

Step 6h

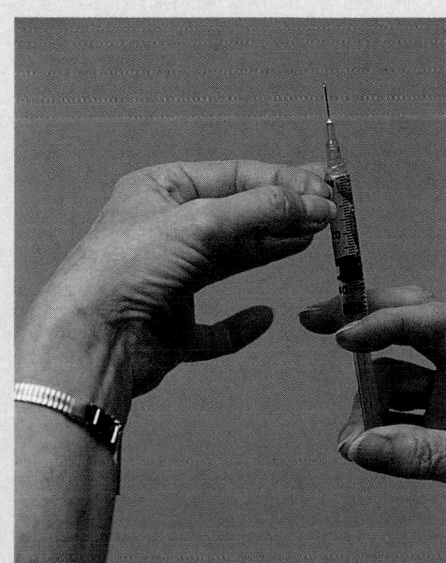

Step 6k

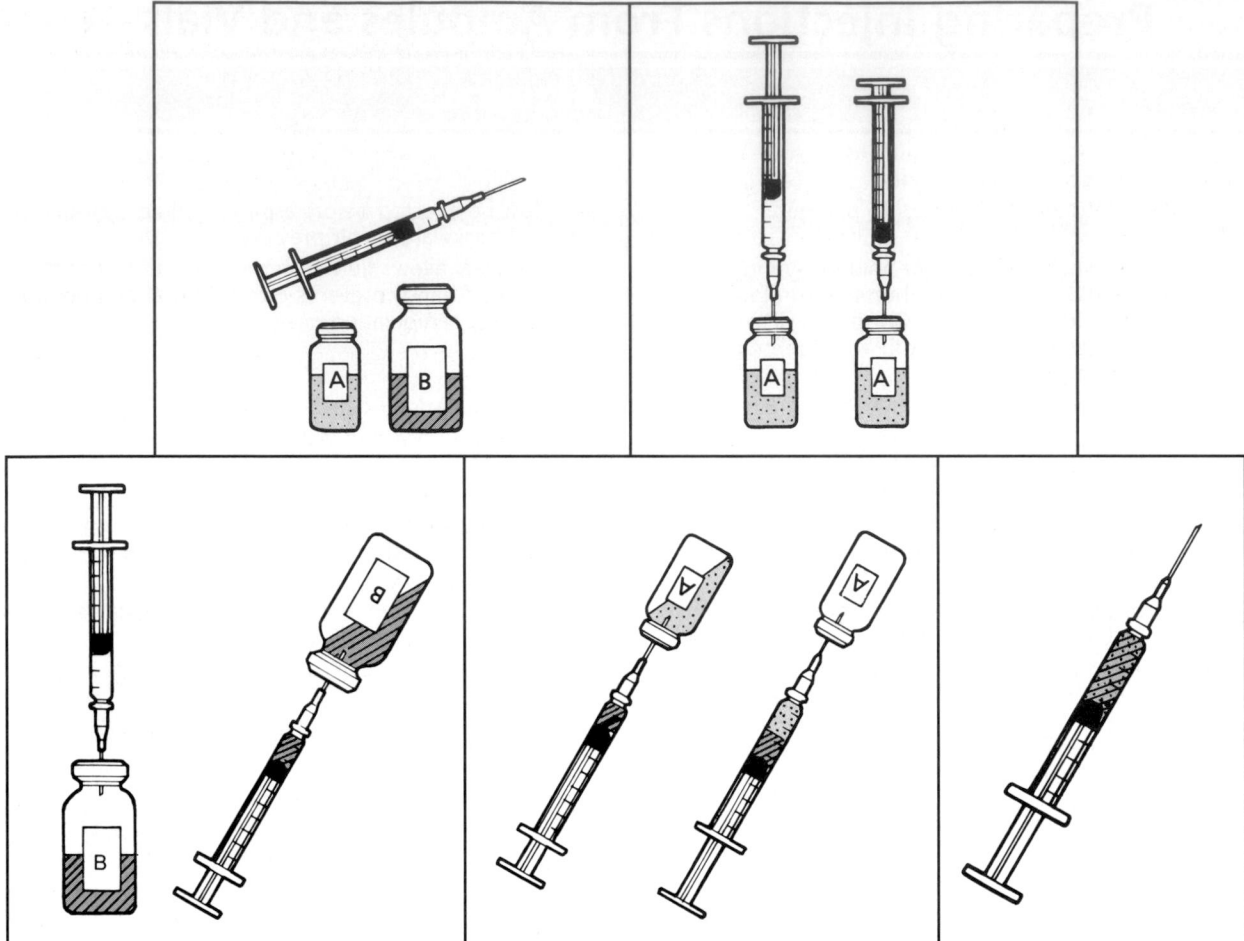

Fig. 35-15 Steps in mixing medications form two vials.

The nurse applies a new, sterile needle to the syringe and inserts it into vial A, being careful not to push the plunger and expel the drug within the syringe into the vial. The nurse then withdraws the desired amount of drug from vial A into the syringe. If a vial has excess positive pressure, the plunger may begin to move before the nurse is ready. This can cause an accidental withdrawal of too much of the drug. After withdrawing the necessary amount of solution, the nurse withdraws the needle, applies a new needle, and sheaths the syringe.

Mixing Medications From One Vial and One Ampule

Mixing medications from a vial and an ampule is simple because it is unnecessary to add air to withdraw medication from an ampule. The nurse prepares medication from the vial first and then, using the same syringe and needle, withdraws medication from the ampule. This technique prevents contamination of solutions from the needle.

Preparing Insulin

Insulin is the hormone used to treat diabetes. The drug must be administered by injection because it is a protein and therefore would be digested and destroyed in the gastrointestinal tract. Most clients with diabetes requiring in-

sulin learn to self-administer injections. In the United States and Canada, insulin comes in 100 units (U) per milliliter of solution. A 100-unit scaled syringe is used to prepare 100-unit insulin.

Insulin is classified by its rate of action as *rapid, intermediate,* and *long acting.* Each type has a different onset, peak, and duration of action. A client with diabetes may require more than one type of insulin. For example, by receiving a rapid-acting (regular) insulin and an intermediate-acting insulin (Isophane [NPH Insulin]), a client receives more sustained control of blood glucose levels over a 24-hour period.

Regular, unmodified insulin is a clear solution that can be given subcutaneously or intravenously. The other types of insulin are cloudy solutions because of the addition of a protein, which slows absorption. These slower acting, modified types of insulin can only be given subcutaneously.

Insulin can be stored safely for about 1 month at room temperature, but it requires refrigeration for longer periods (Clark, Queener, Karb, 1993). The drug should not be administered cold but should be allowed to warm to room temperature.

Before mixing different types of insulin, each vial should be rotated for at least 1 minute between both hands. This resuspends the modified insulin preparations and helps warm the medication. The nurse should not shake insulin

► **RESEARCH HIGHLIGHT**

RESEARCH ABSTRACT

The purpose of this study was to determine the necessity of alcohol disinfection of the rubber stopper after removing the cap on a single-dose vial and to compare the efficacy of different methods of stopper disinfection before needle penetration on the multiple-dose vials. Controversy exists about whether disinfection of the rubber stopper is necessary before initial needle aspiration of fluid from single-dose vials. The researchers surveyed nurses and found variability in whether they disinfected the stopper of single-dose vials before needle aspiration. On multiple dose vials, two disinfection techniques are used before needle penetration. These methods include swabbing the stopper with alcohol only or with povidone-iodine and alcohol. The researchers cultured 5 rubber stoppers of single-dose vials from 20 plastic-wrapped packages (n=100). They also cultured 87 multiple-dose vials that had been previously opened and had been routinely used. Of the single dose vials 99% of the vial stopper surfaces were sterile. One culture returned positive and this was thought to be due to air contamination during the culturing procedure. Of the multiple-dose vials using povidone-iodine and alcohol 95% of the vials were sterile. Of the multiple-dose vials using the alcohol, only technique, all 100 of the surface cultures were sterile. The authors concluded that it is unnecessary to wipe the stopper surface of a single-dose vial after removing the cap. For multiple-dose vials the authors concluded that alcohol swab before disinfection is sufficient.

IMPLICATIONS FOR PRACTICE

► This time-honored nursing practice has been passed on without scientific justification. This study provides a scientific rationale for this procedure.

► Although the savings realized by the change in procedure may be minimal, all levels of practice must be examined for their potential benefit

REFERENCE

Buckley T, Dudley S, Donowitz L: Defining unnecessary disinfection procedures for single-dose and multiple dose vials, *Am J Crit Care* 3(6):448, 1994.

Example of Sliding Scale Insulin Order

Give Regular insulin SQ:
2 U for glucose 200 - 240
4 U for glucose 241 - 250
6 U for glucose 251 - 300
For glucose ≥300, call M.D.

(NPH) insulin (cloudy vial). Do not touch tip of needle to the solution.

2. Remove the syringe from the vial of modified insulin.
3. With the same syringe, inject air equal to the dose of insulin to be withdrawn into the vial of unmodified (regular) insulin (clear vial). Then withdraw the correct dose.
4. Remove the syringe from the unmodified (regular) insulin. Carefully remove air bubbles in the syringe.
5. Return to the vial of modified (NPH) insulin, and withdraw the correct dose.
6. Administer mixture of insulins within 5 minutes of preparation. Regular insulin binds with the modified (NPH) insulin, and the action of the regular insulin is reduced.

Always prepare the unmodified (regular) insulin first. This prevents adding modified insulin to the unmodified (regular) vial. If two modified forms are mixed, it makes no difference which vial is prepared first.

Administering Injections

Each injection route is unique with regard to the type of tissues into which the medication is injected. The characteristics of the tissues influence the rate of drug absorption and thus the onset of drug action. Before injecting a drug, the nurse should know the volume of the drug to administer, the drug's characteristics and viscosity, and the location of anatomical structures underlying injection sites (Procedure 35-3).

Serious consequences may occur if an injection is administered incorrectly. Failure to select an injection site in relation to anatomical landmarks can result in nerve or bone damage during needle insertion. If the nurse fails to aspirate the syringe before injecting a drug, the drug may accidentally be injected directly into an artery or vein. Injecting too large a volume of medication for the site selected can cause extreme pain and may result in local tissue damage.

Many clients, particularly children, fear injections. Clients with serious or chronic illness often are given multiple injections daily. The nurse can attempt to minimize discomfort in the following ways:

1. Use a sharp, beveled needle in the smallest suitable length and gauge.
2. Position the client as comfortably as possible to reduce muscular tension.
3. Select the proper injection site, using anatomical landmarks.
4. Apply ice to the injection site to create local anesthesia before needle insertion.
5. Divert the client's attention from the injection through conversation.

---

vials. Shaking causes foaming and bubbles to form, which may trap particles of insulin and alter the dosage. Insulin is ordered by specific dosages at select times or by a sliding scale. (Only regular insulin is used for sliding scales.) With a sliding scale order, the physician orders different insulin doses based on a client's blood glucose reading (see the box above, right). Several doses may thus be given throughout the day. The following are some simple guidelines for mixing two kinds of insulin in the same syringe:

1. Regular insulin can be mixed with any other type of insulin.
2. Insulin zinc suspensions (Lente Insulin) can be mixed with each other and with regular insulin. They should not be mixed with other types of insulin.

To prepare insulin from two vials, the nurse or client follows these steps:

1. With a syringe and needle, inject air equal to the dose of insulin to be withdrawn into the vial of modified

6. Insert the needle smoothly and quickly to minimize tissue pulling.
7. Hold the syringe steady while the needle remains in the tissues.
8. Massage the injected area gently for several seconds, unless contraindicated.

Subcutaneous Injections

Subcutaneous (SQ) injections involve placing medication into the loose connective tissue under the dermis (Procedure 35-3). Because SQ tissue is not as richly supplied with blood as the muscles, drug absorption is somewhat slower than with IM injections. However, drugs are absorbed completely if circulatory status is normal. Because subcutaneous tissue contains pain receptors, the client may experience some discomfort.

The best sites for SQ injections include vascular areas around the outer aspect of the upper arms, the abdomen from below the costal margins to the iliac crests, and the anterior aspect of the thighs. These areas are easily accessible, especially for clients with diabetes who self-administer insulin. The site most frequently recommended for heparin injections is the abdomen (Fig. 35-16). Other sites include the scapular areas of the upper back and the upper ventral or dorsal gluteal areas. The injection site chosen should be free of infection, skin lesions, scars, bony prominences, and large underlying muscles or nerves. Clients with diabetes regularly rotate daily injection sites to prevent hypertrophy (thickening) of the skin and **lipodystrophy** (atrophy of the tissue). No injection site should be used more than every 6 to 7 weeks. An injection diagram allows nurses and clients to record daily injections to be sure that sites are rotated (Fig. 35-17).

Only small doses (0.5 to 1 ml) of water-soluble medication should be given by the SQ route. SQ tissue is sensitive to irritating solutions and large volumes of medication. Collection of medication within the tissues can cause sterile abscesses, which appear as hardened, painful lumps under the skin.

Body weight indicates the depth of the SQ layer. Therefore the nurse must choose the needle length and angle of insertion based on the client's weight. Generally, a 25-gauge ⅝-inch needle inserted at a 45-degree angle (Fig. 35-18) de-posits medication into the SQ tissue of a normal-size client. A child may require a ½-inch needle (Wong, 1995). If the client is obese, the nurse pinches the tissue and uses a needle long enough to insert through fatty tissue at the base of the skinfold. The preferred needle length is half the width of the skinfold. With this method the angle of insertion may be between 45 and 90 degrees.

Thin, cachectic clients may have insufficient tissue for SQ injections. The upper abdomen is the best site for injection with this client. Insulin syringes usually come with 26-gauge needles. To ensure that the insulin reaches SQ tissue, the nurse follows this simple rule: If 2 inches of tissue can be grasped, the needle should be inserted at a 90-degree angle, and if 1 inch of tissue can be grasped, the needle should be inserted at a 45-degree angle.

Intramuscular Injections

The intramuscular (IM) route provides faster drug absorption than the SQ route because of a muscle's greater vascularity. The danger of causing tissue damage is less when drugs enter deep muscle, but there is the risk of inadvertently injecting drugs directly into blood vessels. The nurse uses a longer and larger gauge needle to pass through SQ tissue and penetrate deep muscle tissue (Procedure 35-3). However, weight influences selection of needle size. For example, a client weighing 100 pounds may only require a needle 1¼ to 1½ inches long, whereas a child weighing 50

Text continued on p. 833.

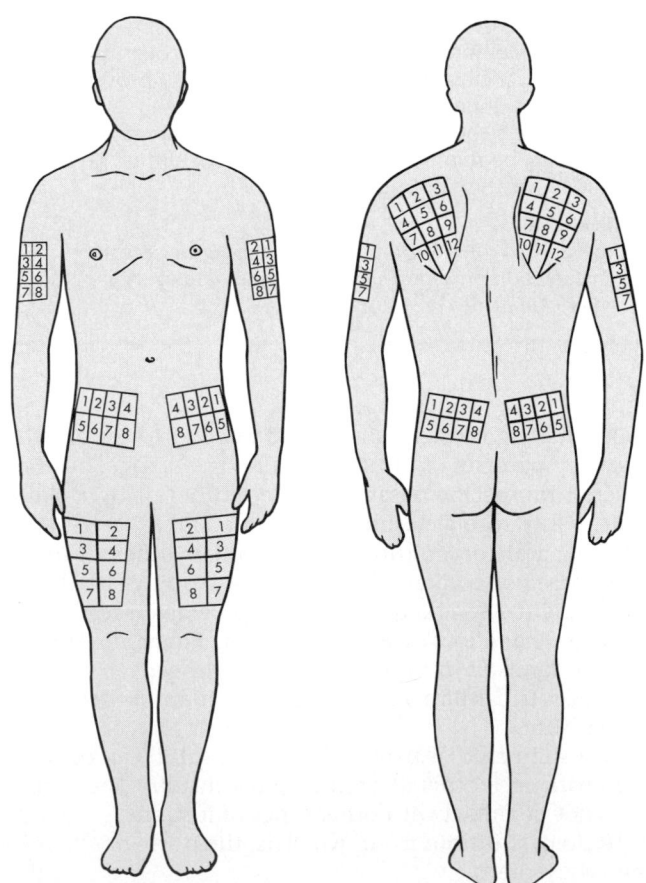

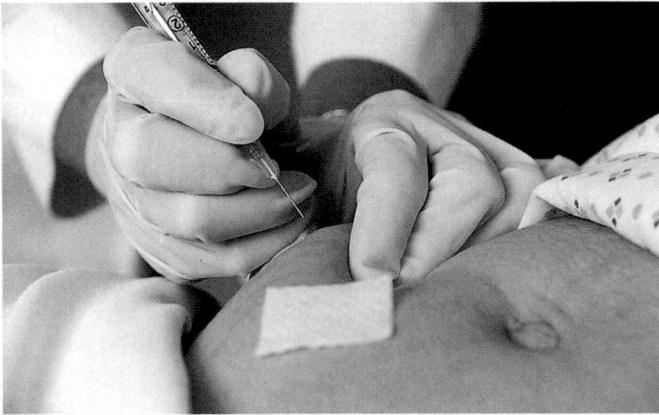

Fig. 35-16 Injecting subcutaneous heparin in the abdomen.

Fig. 35-17 Common site for subcutaneous injections. Note how sites may be rotated.

Administering Subcutaneous, Intramuscular, and Intradermal Injections

STEPS	RATIONALE
1. Assess indications for proper route for medication.	Ensures proper drug absorption and distribution through tissues to enhance drug action. Ensures proper route appropriate for client per physician orders.
2. Assess medical history and history of allergies.	Alerts nurse to any precautions to observe for during administration. History of allergies may cancel order for drug.
3. Observe verbal and nonverbal responses toward receiving injection.	Injections can be painful. Clients may have anxiety, which can increase pain.
4. Wash hands.	Reduces transmission of microorganisms.
5. Prepare needed equipment and supplies:	
a. Proper-size syringe:	Volume injected should be compatible with tissue type.
(1) SQ: 1 ml, 100 U insulin	
(2) IM: 2 to 5 ml for adult, 1 to 2 ml for child	
(3) ID: 1-ml tuberculin	
b. Proper-size needle:	Prevents client injury and ensures drug distribution.
(1) SQ: 25- to 27-gauge and $^3/_8$ to $^5/_8$ inches in length	
(2) IM: 19- to 23-gauge and 1 to $1^1/_2$ inches in length for adults, 25- to 27-gauge and $^1/_2$ to 1 inches in length for child and $^5/_8$ inches for newborn (Wong, 1995)	
(3) ID: 26- to 27-gauge	
c. Antiseptic swab (Betadine or alcohol)	Used to cleanse skin.
d. Disposable gloves	
e. Medication ampule or vial	
f. Medication card, forms, or printouts	Identifies medication dose ordered and client's name.
6. Check medication order.	Ensures accuracy.
7. Prepare correct medication dose from ampule or vial (see Procedure 35-2). Check carefully. Be sure all air is expelled. (For IM medications that are particularly irritating to tissues, draw 0.2 ml of air into syringe, being careful not to expel drug dose. See air-lock technique (p. 836).	Ensures that medication is sterile. Preparation techniques differ for ampule and vial. Injection of a small volume of air clears the needle of medication and prevents tracking of the drug.
8. For IM injection, change needle if medication is irritating to SQ tissue.	Prevents tracking of irritating substance through tissues as needle passes into muscle.
9. Apply disposable gloves.	Injections could cause mild seepage of blood at injection site. Gloves reduce risk of exposure.
10. Identify client by checking identification armband and asking name.	Ensures that correct client is receiving prescribed medication.
11. Explain procedure to client and proceed in calm, confident manner.	Helps client anticipate actions. Calm approach minimizes anxiety.
12. Close room curtains or door.	Provides for privacy.
13. Keep sheet or gown draped over body parts not requiring exposure.	Proper selection of injection site may require exposure of body parts.
14. Select appropriate injection site. Inspect skin surface over sites for bruises, inflammation, or edema:	Injection sites should be free of anormalities that may interfere with drug absorption. Site used repeatedly can become hardened from lipohypertrophy (increased growth in fatty tissue). ID site should be clear so that results of skin test can be seen and interpreted correctly.
a. SQ: palpate sites for masses or tenderness. For daily insulin rotate site daily. Be sure needle is correct size by grasping skinfold at site with thumb and forefinger. Measure fold from top to bottom. Needle should be one-half this length.	
b. IM: note integrity and size of muscle and palpate for tenderness or hardness. If injections are given frequently, rotate sites.	
c. ID: note lesions or discolorations of forearm. Select site three to four finger widths below antecubital space and hand width above wrist.	

Continued.

Administering Subcutaneous, Intramuscular, and Intradermal Injections—cont'd

STEPS	RATIONALE
15. Assist client to comfortable position:	
a. SQ: have client relax arm, leg, or abdomen, depending on site chosen.	Relaxation of site minimizes discomfort.
b. IM: have client lie flat, on side, or prone or have client sit, depending on site chosen.	Reduces strain on muscle and minimizes discomfort of injections.
c. ID: have client extend elbow and support it and forearm on flat surface.	Stabilizes site for easiest accessibility.
Talk with client about subject of interest.	Distraction reduces anxiety.
16. Relocate site using anatomical landmarks.	Accurate injection requires insertion in correct site to avoid injury to underlying tissues, blood vessels, nerves, or bone.
17. Cleanse site with antiseptic swab. Apply swab at center of site and rotate outward in circular direction for about 5 cm (2 in) (see the illustration below, left).	Mechanical action of swab removes secretions containing microorganisms.
18. Keep swab close to hand.	Swab remains readily accessible when needle is withdrawn.
19. Remove cap from needle by pulling it straight off.	Prevents contamination.
20. Hold syringe correctly between thumb and forefinger of dominant hand:	Quick, smooth injection requires proper manipulation of syringe parts.
a. SQ: hold as dart (see the illustration below, right), palm down	
b. IM: hold as dart, palm down.	
c. ID: hold bevel of needle pointing up.	With bevel up, medication will less likely be deposited into tissues below dermis.

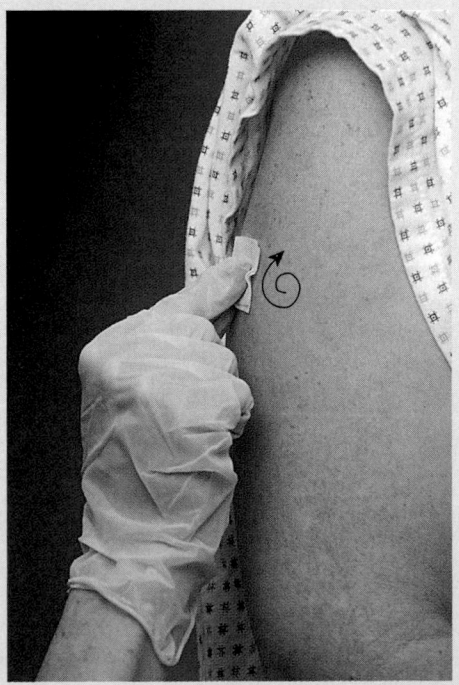

Step 17

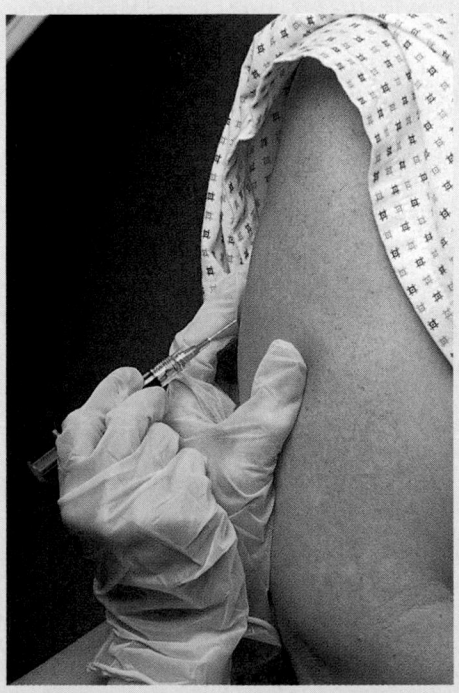

Step 20a

Administering Subcutaneous, Intramuscular, and Intradermal Injections—cont'd

STEPS	RATIONALE

21. Administer injection:

a. Subcutaneous

(1) For average-size client use nondominant hand to spread skin tightly across injection site or grasp tissue, creating a roll of $\frac{1}{2}$ inch.

Needle penetrates tight skin easier than loose skin. Pinching skin elevates SQ tissue and may desensitize area.

(2) Inject needle quickly and firmly at 45- to 90-degree angle. (Then release skin, if pinched.)

Quick, firm insertion minimizes discomfort. (Injecting medication into compressed tissue irritates nerve fibers.)

(3) For obese client, pinch skin at site and inject needle below tissue fold.

Obese clients have fatty layer of tissue above SQ layer. Pinching skin elevates the SQ tissue for injection.

(4) Grasp lower end of syringe barrel with nondominant hand to end of plunger. Avoid moving syringe while slowly pulling back on plunger to aspirate drug (see the Illustration below, left). If blood appears in syringe, remove needle, discard medication and syringe, and repeat procedure. Exception: Do not aspirate when giving heparin.

Properly performed injection requires smooth manipulation of syringe parts. Movement of syringe may displace needle and cause discomfort. Aspiration of blood into syringe indicates IV placement of needle. SQ and IM injections are not for IV use (dermis is relatively vascular).

Aspiration of heparin injection may cause the needle to move, creating tissue damage and bleeding.

(5) Inject medication slowly.

b. Intramuscular

(1) Position nondominant hand at proper anatomical landmarks and spread skin tightly. Inject needle quickly at 90-degree angle into muscle.

Speeds insertion and reduces discomfort.

(2) If client's muscle mass is small, grasp body of muscle between thumb and other fingers.

Ensures that medication reaches muscle mass.

(3) If medication is irritating, use Z-track method (see section on Z-track method, p. 835).

Used to prevent tracking of drug through SQ tissue.

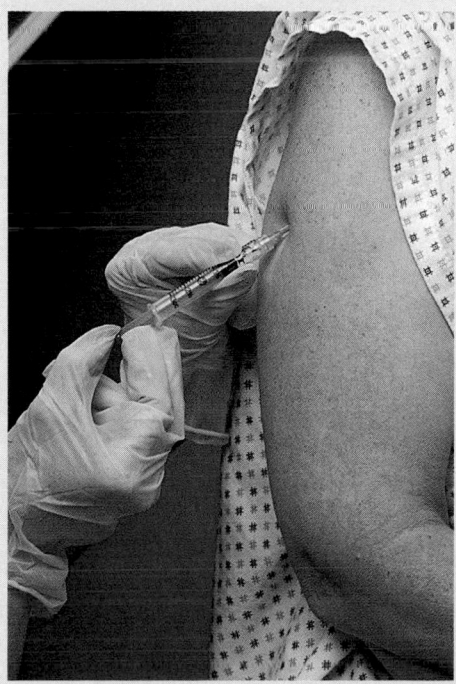

Step 21a(4)

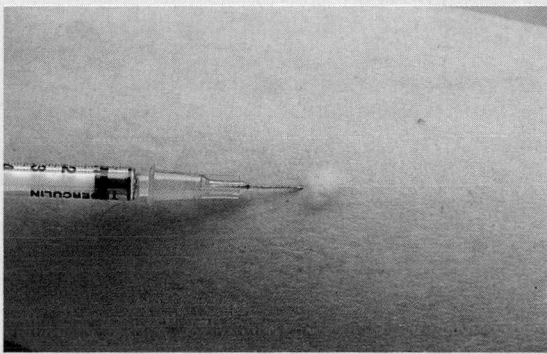

Step 21c(4)

Continued.

PROCEDURE 35-3

Administering Subcutaneous, Intramuscular, and Intradermal Injections—cont'd

STEPS	RATIONALE
21. Administer injection—cont'd	
b. Intramuscular—cont'd	
(4) Aspirate as in step 21a(4).	
(5) Inject medication slowly.	
c. Intradermal	
(1) With nondominant hand, stretch skin over site with forefinger or thumb.	Needle pierces tight skin more easily.
(2) With needle almost against client's skin, insert it slowly at 5- to 15-degree angle until resistance is felt. Then advance needle through epidermis to approximately 3 mm ($^1/_8$ in) below surface. Needle tip can be seen through skin.	Ensures that needle tip is in dermis.
(3) Inject medication slowly (it is normal to feel resistance; if not, needle is too deep and should be withdrawn).	Dermal layer is tight and does not expand easily. It is not necessary to aspirate, since dermis is relatively avascular.
(4) While injecting medication, a light-colored bleb resembling a mosquito bite approximately 6 mm ($^1/_2$ in) in diameter forms at site and then disappears (see the illustration on p. 831, right).	Indicates medication is deposited in dermis.
22. Withdraw needle while applying alcohol swab gently above or over injection site.	Supports tissues around injection site to minimize discomfort during needle withdrawal.
23. For SQ or IM injections, massage skin lightly. Do not massage after SQ injection of heparin or insulin. OP-TIONAL: Apply bandage. For ID injections, *do not massage site.*	Stimulates circulation and improves drug distribution. Massage of site after heparin injection may cause bleeding, and may increase absorption rate of insulin. Massage of ID site may disperse medication into underlying tissue layers and alter test results (e.g., tuberculin test).
24. Assist client to comfortable position.	Gives client sense of well-being.
25. Discard an uncapped needle or needle enclosed in safety shield and attached syringe in appropriately labeled receptacle. When nurse is unable to leave client's bedside, a one-handed technique can be done to recap a needle (see Procedure 35-4).	CDC and OSHA mandate that needles not be re-capped for prevention of needlesticks and disease transmission.
26. Remove disposable gloves. Wash hands.	Reduces transmission of microorganisms.
27. For ID injection, draw circle around perimeter of injection site with skin pencil or ink pen.	Site must be read at various intervals to determine test results.
28. For SQ and IM injections, chart medication dose, route, and site and time and date given in medication record. Correctly sign according to institutional policy.	Timely documentation prevents administration errors.
29. For ID injections, record area of injection, amount and type of testing substance, and date and time on medication record.	Timely documentation prevents administration errors and allows for follow-up assessment.
30. Return to room and ask if client feels acute pain, burning, numbness, or tingling at injection site. Observe for allergic reaction after ID injection.	Continued discomfort may indicate injury to underlying bones or nerves. Anaphylactic reaction may occur suddenly after ID injection because of drug's toxicity.
31. Return to evaluate response to medication in 10 to 30 min.	IM medications absorb quicker than SQ; undesired effects may also develop rapidly. Observations determine efficacy

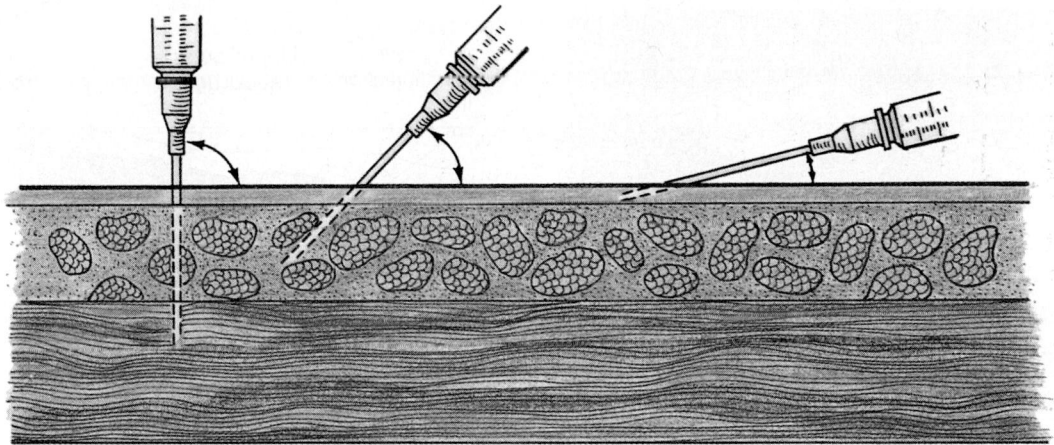

Fig. 35-18 Comparison of the angles of insertion of IM (90 degrees), SQ (45 degrees), and ID (15 degrees) injections.

pounds usually requires a 1-inch needle. The angle of insertion for an IM injection is 90 degrees (see Fig. 35-18). Muscle is less sensitive to irritating and viscous drugs. A normal, well-developed client can safely tolerate as much as 3 ml of medication in larger, more developed muscles such as the dorsogluteal or vastus lateralis. Smaller muscles can tolerate only smaller amounts of medication without severe muscle discomfort. Children, older adults, and thin clients tolerate less than 2 ml of medication. Wong (1995) recommends giving no more than 1 ml to small children and older infants.

The nurse assesses the integrity of a muscle before giving an injection. The muscle should be free of tenderness. Repeated injections in the same muscle cause considerable discomfort. By asking the client to relax, the nurse can palpate the muscle to rule out the presence of hardened lesions. Normally a muscle feels soft when relaxed and firm when tense. The nurse can minimize discomfort during an injection by helping the client assume a position that will help reduce the strain on the muscle.

▌ SITES

When selecting an IM site, the nurse assesses the following:
1. Is the area free of infection or necrosis?
2. Are there local areas of bruising or abrasions?
3. What is the location of underlying bones, nerves, and major blood vessels?
4. What volume of medication is to be administered?

Vastus Lateralis Muscle

The thick, well-developed vastus lateralis muscle is a preferred injection site for adults, children, and infants. The muscle is located on the anterior lateral aspect of the thigh and extends in an adult from a handbreadth above the knee to a handbreath below the greater trochanter of the femur (Fig. 35-19, *A*). The middle third of the muscle is the best site for injection (Fig. 35-19, *B*). In width the site extends from the midline of the thigh's top to the midline of the thigh's outer side.

With young children or cachectic clients, it helps to grasp the body of the muscle during injection to be sure that the drug is deposited in muscle tissue. To help relax the

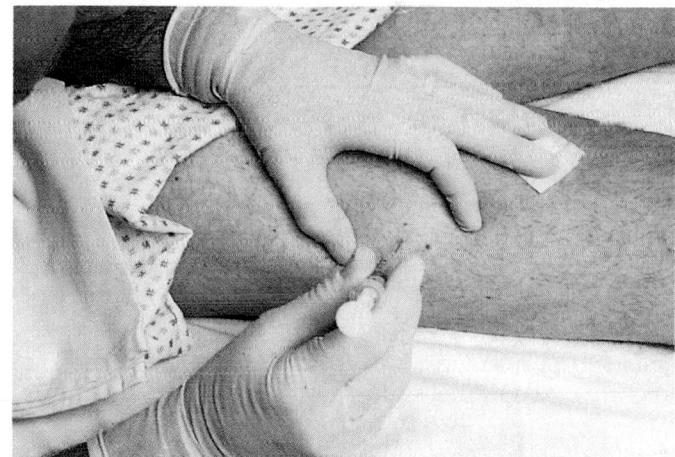

A

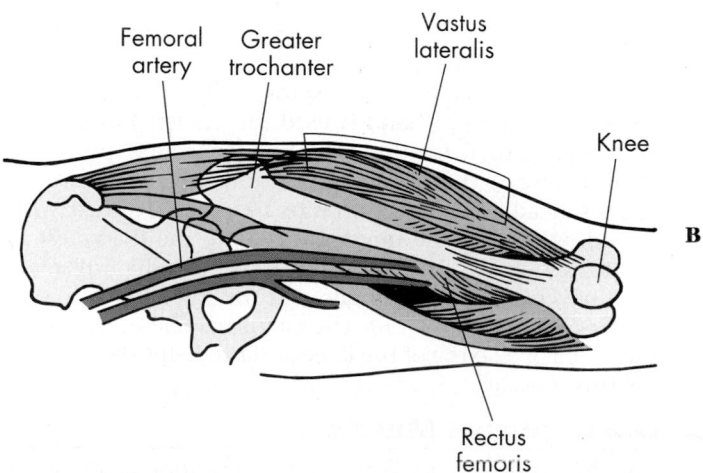

B

Fig. 35-19 A, Injection site into the vastus lateralis muscle. **B,** Anatomical view of the site for IM injection into the vastus lateralis muscle.

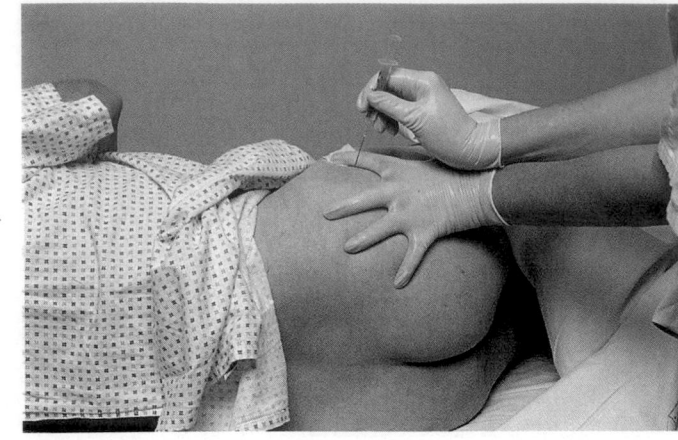

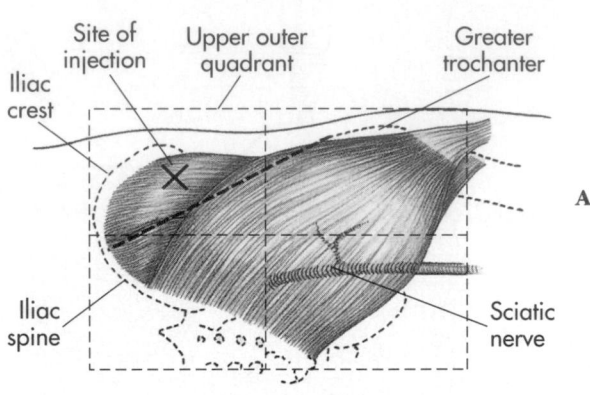

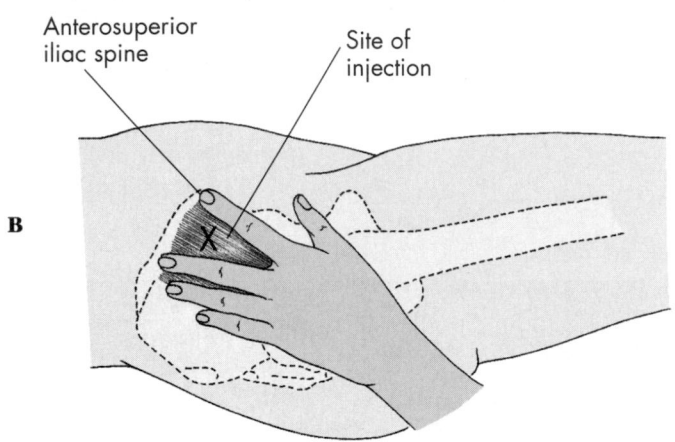

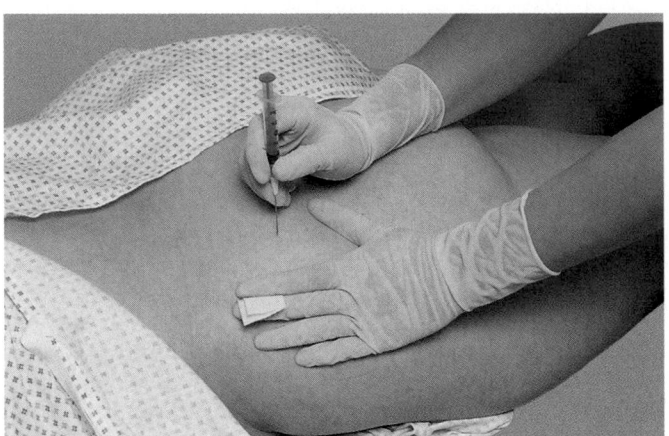

Fig. 35-20 **A,** Injection site into ventrogluteal muscle avoid major nerves and blood vessels. **B,** Anatomical view of ventrogluteal muscle injection site.

Fig. 35-21 **A,** Landmark for dorsogluteal site. **B,** Giving IM injection in left dorsogluteal site (client is prone).

muscle, the nurse asks the client to lie flat with the knee slightly flexed or in a sitting position.

Ventrogluteal Muscle

The ventrogluteal muscle involves the gluteus medius and minimus. The client lies on either side with knee bent, and the nurse locates the muscle by placing the palm of the hand over the greater trochanter and index finger on the anterior superior iliac spine of the client's hip (Fig. 35-20, *A*). The right hand is used for the left hip, and the left hand is used for the right hip. The nurse points the thumb toward the client's groin and fingers toward the client's head. The injection site becomes exposed while spreading the middle finger back along the iliac crest toward the buttock. The index finger, the middle finger, and the iliac crest form a triangle, and the injection site is the center of it (Fig. 35-20, *B*). The client may lie on his or her side or back. Flexing of the knee and hip helps the client relax this muscle.

Dorsogluteal Muscle

The dorsogluteal muscle has been a traditional site for IM injections. However, accidental insertion of a needle into the sciatic nerve can cause permanent or partial paralysis of the involved leg. Major blood vessels and bone are also

near the site. In clients with flabby, sagging tissues, the site is difficult to locate.

The dorsogluteal site is located in the upper outer aspect of the upper outer quadrant of the buttock, approximately 5 to 8 cm (2 to 3 in) below the iliac crest. Clients may lie in the prone position with toes turned medially or in a sidelying position with the upper leg flexed at the hip and knee. To locate the dorsogluteal site, the nurse palpates the posterosuperior iliac spine and the greater trochanter of the femur. An imaginary line is drawn between the two anatomical landmarks. The sciatic nerve runs parallel and below the line. The injection site is above and lateral to the line (Fig. 35-21). Nurses may use the dorsogluteal injection site in adults and children (at least 3 years of age) with well-developed gluteal muscles.

Deltoid Muscle

In some adults, infants, and most children, the deltoid muscle is not well developed. The radial and ulnar nerves and brachial artery lie within the upper arm along the humerus. The nurse rarely uses the deltoid site unless other injection sites are inaccessible because of dressings, casts, or other obstructions.

To locate the deltoid muscle the nurse has the client fully expose the upper arm and shoulder. The nurse should not

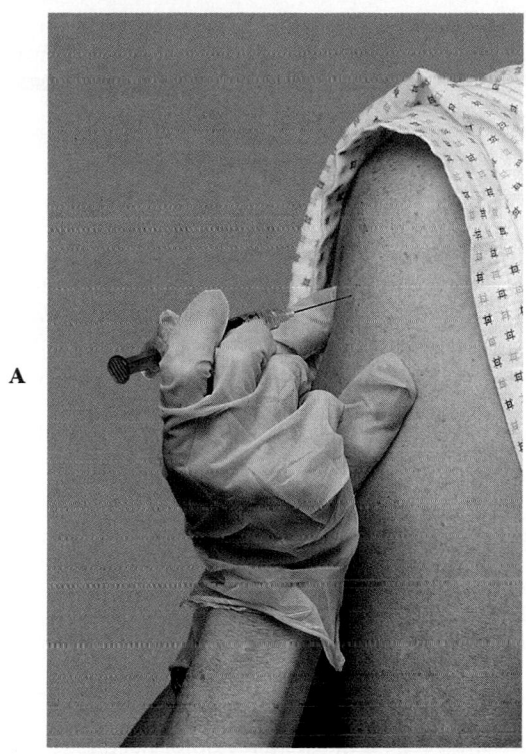

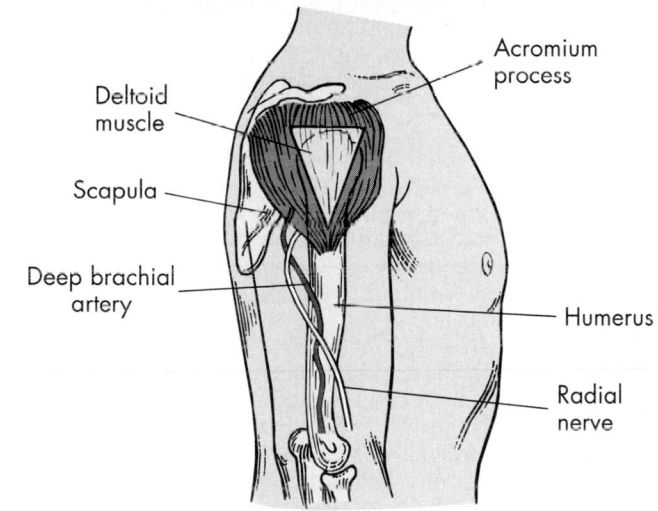

Fig. 35-22 A, Site of IM injection into the deltoid muscle. **B,** Site of deltoid muscle injection below the acromion process.

try to roll up a tight-fitting sleeve. The nurse has the client relax the arm at the side and flex the elbow (Fig. 35-22, *A*). The client may sit, stand, or lie down. The nurse palpates the lower edge of the acromion process, which forms the base of a triangle in line with the midpoint of the lateral aspect of the upper arm (Fig. 35-22, *B*). The injection site is in the center of the triangle, about 2.5 to 5 cm (1 to 2 in) below the acromion process. The nurse may also locate the site by placing four fingers across the deltoid muscle, with the top finger along the acromion process. The injection site is then three fingerbreadths below the acromion process.

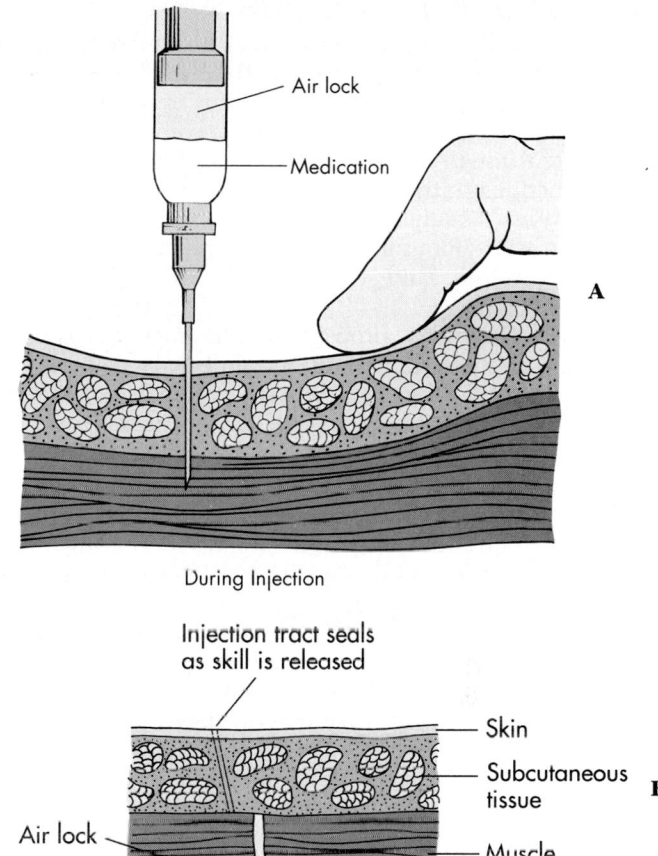

Fig. 35-23 A, Pull on overlying skin during IM injection moves tissues to prevent later tracking. **B,** The Z-track left after injection prevents the deposit of medication through sensitive tissue.

▮ Z-TRACK METHOD

When irritating preparations (for example, iron) are given intramuscularly, the **Z-track method** of injection minimizes tissue irritation by sealing the drug within the muscle tissues. The nurse selects an IM site, preferably in larger, deeper muscles such as the ventrogluteal muscle. A new needle must be applied to the syringe after preparing the drug so that no solution remains on the outside needle shaft. The nurse draws up 0.2 ml of air to create an air lock. After preparing the site with an antiseptic swab, the nurse pulls the overlying skin and SQ tissues approximately 2.5 to 3.5 cm (1 to 1½ in) laterally to the side (Fig. 35-23, *A*). Holding the skin taut with the nondominant hand, the nurse injects the needle deep into the muscle. With practice the nurse learns to hold the syringe and aspirate with one hand. The nurse injects the drug and air slowly if there is no blood return on aspiration. The needle remains inserted for 10 seconds to allow the medication to disperse evenly. The nurse releases the skin after withdrawing the needle, which leaves a zigzag path that seals the needle track wherever tissue planes slide across each other (Fig. 35-23, *B*). The drug cannot escape from the muscle tissue.

AIR-LOCK TECHNIQUE

IM injections using the **air-lock technique** are less irritating to SQ tissues during needle withdrawal. When a small volume of air is injected behind a bolus of medication, the air clears the needle of medication, preventing tracking of the drug through SQ tissues. This technique is specifically recommended in the drug information insert of only a few medications. Examples include Inferon, Wyeth's vaccines prepared with aluminum adjuvant, diphtheria and tetanus toxoid vaccines, and the pertussis (whooping cough) vaccine.

After preparing the proper dose, the nurse draws up 0.2 ml of air. The needle then must be injected downward at a 90-degree angle so that the air rises to the top of the drug toward the plunger (Fig. 35-24). As the nurse injects the drug into the muscle, the air follows the medication, creating an air lock. If the nurse administers the drug with the needle at an angle less than 90 degrees, the air collects along the barrel of the syringe and enters the muscle too soon. Medication can then easily leak back into SQ tissues.

Intradermal Injections

The nurse typically gives intradermal (ID) injections for skin testing (e.g., tuberculin screening and allergy tests). Because these medications are potent, they are injected into the dermis, where the blood supply is reduced and drug absorption occurs slowly. A client may have a severe anaphylactic reaction if the medications enter the circulation too rapidly. For clients with a history of numerous allergies, the physician often performs skin testing.

Skin testing requires the nurse to be able to clearly see the injection sites for changes in color and tissue integrity. ID sites should be free of lesions and relatively hairless. The inner forearm and upper back are ideal locations.

The nurse uses a tuberculin or small hypodermic syringe for skin testing. The angle of insertion is 5 to 15 degrees (see Fig. 35-18). As the nurse injects the drug, a small bleb resembling a mosquito bite should appear on the skin's surface (see Procedure 35-3). If a bleb does not appear or if the site bleeds after needle withdrawal, there is a good chance the medication entered SQ tissues. In this case, skin test results will not be valid.

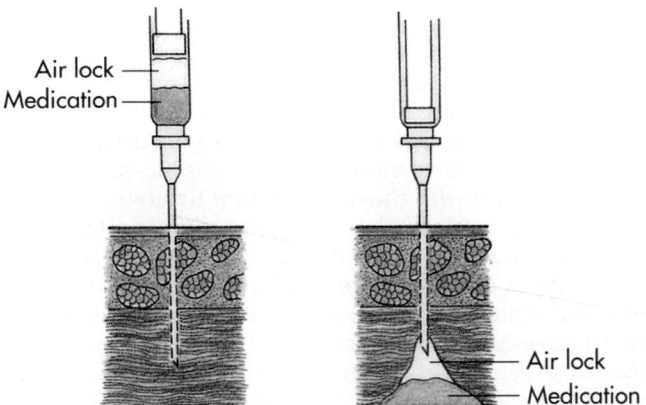

Fig. 35-24 Administering IM injection by the air-lock technique prevents tracking of medication through SQ tissue.

Data from an ID injection include a description of the precise location and time of administration. The injected site must be "read" within a prescribed time, for example 48 hours after a PPD injection.

SAFETY IN ADMINISTERING MEDICATIONS BY INJECTION

Injury to the nurse from a needlestick is a significant problem in health care institutions today. It is estimated that over one million needlesticks are incurred annually by health care workers (Jagger, 1992). When the nurse sticks himself or herself with a needle that has entered the tissue of clients, the nurse is at risk for at least 20 potential pathogens. The two most problematic pathogens are the hepatitis B virus (HBV) and the human immunodeficiency

▶ RESEARCH HIGHLIGHT

RESEARCH ABSTRACT

The researchers compared the proportion of recapped needles, found in disposable boxes on two different types of hospital units, both before and after an intervention. The number of recapped needles (which should not be found) would be an indicator for needlestick injury risk. The first type of hospital unit was a medical-surgical unit that had existing mounted in-bathroom needle disposable boxes, and the second type was an intensive care unit that had unmounted needle disposable boxes in the room but not necessarily near the client's bedside. The intervention by the researchers consisted of installing, in the medical-surgical unit only, mounted needle disposal boxes on the wall near the client's bed. There was no change to the boxes in the location of the boxes in the intensive care unit. However, the researchers did change the type of needle disposal unit. Before the intervention, the recapping rates in the medical-surgical units and in the intensive care units were similar, approximately 32% to 34%. Following the intervention (placing the disposal boxes mounted on the wall near the client's bedside), the proportion of recapped needles was significantly reduced, down to 18% to 27%, in the disposal containers adjacent to the bedsides in medical-surgical units. In the intensive care units, which merely had a brand of box changed, there was no significant change in the rate of recapping.

IMPLICATIONS FOR PRACTICE

▶ An environmental change alone is an effective means of altering the risk to health care workers for needlestick injuries.

▶ Environmental changes may also create a behavioral change in hospital workers.

▶ Despite improvements in needle disposal systems, needlesticks to health care workers continue to occur at unacceptably high rates.

▶ Easy access to protective equipment may improve utilization.

▶ The disposal system appeared to pose no greater risk of infection to clients, and nurses preferred it for its reduced risk of potential needlestick injuries.

REFERENCE

Mafofsky D, Cone JE: *Infect Control Hosp Epidemiol* 14(3):140, 1993.

virus (HIV) (see Chapter 34). Miller (1994) reports that you are likely to receive a needlestick injury in one of the following six ways:

1. You miss the needle as you're trying to recap it and stick your opposite hand.
2. You recap the needle, and the needle pierces the cap.
3. The cap falls off a recapped needle.
4. You injure yourself as you are gathering debris for disposal which contains a sharp instrument.
5. You attempt to dispose of too many sharps at one time.
6. You are stuck by a protruding sharp instrument from an overfilled sharps disposal container as you are disposing of a sharp instrument (see the box on p. 836).

Needles and other instruments considered "sharps" are always disposed of into clearly marked, appropriate containers (Fig. 35-25). Containers should be puncture and leak proof. *A needle should never be forced by anyone into a full needle disposable receptacle.* Used needles and syringes are never placed in any wastebaskets, in the nurse's pocket, a client's meal tray, or at the client's bedside.

▌ PROTECTING YOURSELF FROM NEEDLESTICK INJURIES

In 1987, the Centers for Disease Control issued comprehensive guidelines called *Universal Precautions* (see Chapter 34) which include, but are not limited to, recommendations for the safe use and disposal of sharp instruments. These served merely as guidelines for institutions and were not enforce-

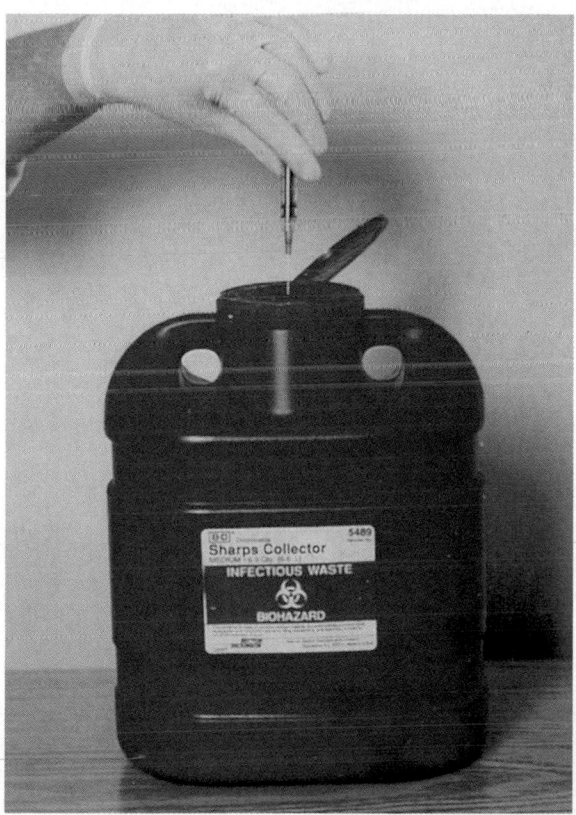

Fig. 35-25 Special containers are available in patient rooms and in nursing units for the disposal of contaminated needles and sharps.

able by law. In 1991, the Occupational Safety and Health Administration (OSHA) issued a mandate that makes Universal Precautions enforceable. Universal Precautions are now incorporated into what is described as *standard precautions* (see Chapter 34). Included in this mandate are regulations that state institutions must provide, for the employee, protective equipment to prevent the transmission of blood-borne pathogens. Since the most frequent route of exposure to blood-borne disease is from needlesticks (Bohony, 1993), many institutions now supply "safety syringes" for the nurse to use when giving injections. A safety syringe is equipped with a plastic guard shield that slips over the needle as it is withdrawn from the skin.

Giving Medications With a Safety Syringe

After preparing the medication dose, the nurse injects the medication either SQ, IM, or ID. Once the medication is completely injected, the nurse grabs the protective sheath and slides the needle out of the client. This causes the protective sheath to cover the needle and lock into place. Once the sheath is in place, it is not meant to be removed (Fig. 35-26). Depending on the manufacturer, there may be modifications to this technique. The nurse should read the manufacturer's instruction for proper use of the equipment. Many institutions train nurses in the handling of this special equipment.

If the nurse must ever recap a needle, one-handed needle recapping technique as outlined in Procedure 35-4 should be used.

IV Administration

The nurse administers drugs intravenously by the following methods:

1. As mixtures within large volumes of IV fluids
2. By injection of a bolus, or small volume, of medication through an existing IV infusion line or heparin lock
3. By "piggyback" **infusion** of a solution containing the prescribed drug and a small volume of IV fluid through an existing IV line

In all three methods the client has an existing IV infusion line or an IV access site such as a heparin lock. In most institutions, policies and procedures list persons who may give IV medication and the situations in which they may be given. These policies are based on the drug, capability and availability of staff, and the type of monitoring equipment available.

Chapter 45 describes the technique for performing venipuncture and establishing continuous IV fluid infusions. Medication administration is only one reason for supplying IV fluids. IV fluid therapy is used primarily for fluid and electrolyte replacement in clients unable to take oral fluids.

When using any method of IV drug administration, the nurse must observe clients closely for symptoms of adverse reactions. After a drug enters the bloodstream, it begins to act immediately, and there is no way to stop its action. Thus the nurse takes special care to avoid errors in dosage calculation and preparation. The nurse should double-check the "five rights" of safe drug administration and know the desired action and potential side effects. If the

PROCEDURE 35-4

One-Handed Needle Recapping Technique

STEPS	RATIONALE

1. *Needles should never be recapped.* Use this procedure only when a sharps disposal box is unavailable and you cannot leave the client's room.

Needlestick injuries place the health care worker at risk for blood-borne pathogens. After using a needle, the health care worker should dispose of the sharp in the nearest designated container.

2. Before giving the injection, place the needle cover on a solid, immovable object such as the rim of a bedside table. The open end of the cap should face the nurse and be within reach of the nurse's dominant, or injection, hand.

This readies the nurse to carry out the rest of the procedure in a safe manner.

3. Give the injection.

This ensures medication delivery.

4. Place the tip of the needle at the entrance of the cap. *Gently* slide the needle into the needle cover (see the illustrations below).

Forcing the needle into the cover may result in a bent needle.

5. Once the needle is inside the cover, use the object's resistance to completely cover the needle (see illustration below).

Use slow maneuvers, and never force needle into place.

6. Dispose of the needle at the first opportunity.

This ensures a safe environment for both client and nurse.

7. Wash hands.

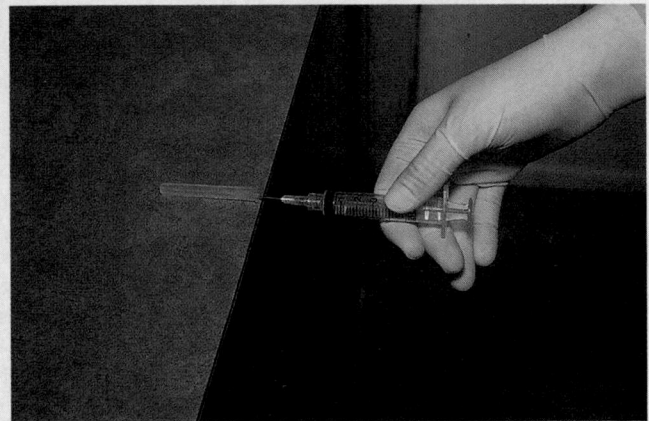 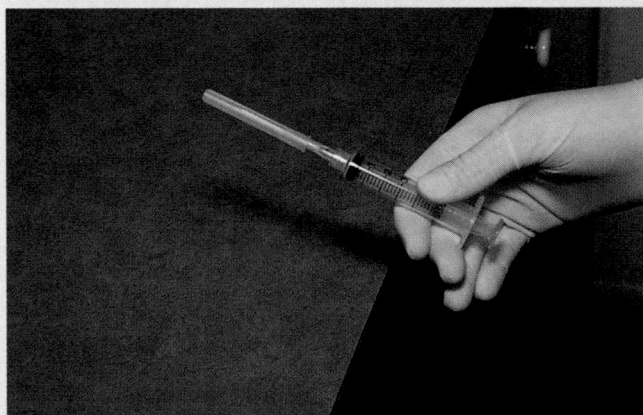

Step 4

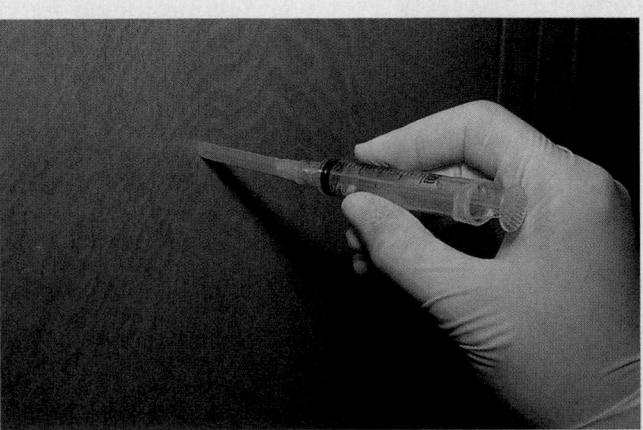

Step 5

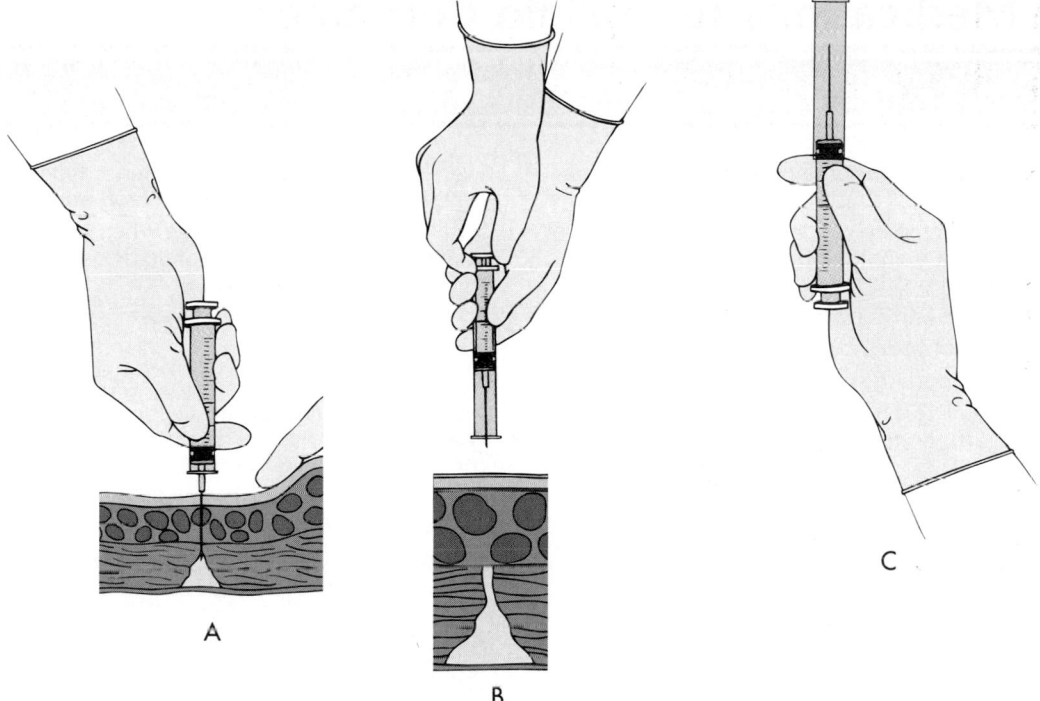

Fig. 35-26 A, Administering an IM injection with a safety syringe. **B,** After the medication has been infused, grasp the protective sheath and withdraw the needle from the injection site. The protective sheath should be pulled forward until it clicks. **C,** The shield is now firmly into place and ready for disposal into the proper receptacle.

drug has an antidote, the nurse must have it available during administration. When administering potent drugs, the nurse assesses vital signs before, during, and after infusion.

Administering drugs by the IV route has advantages. In emergencies when a fast-acting drug must be delivered quickly, the IV route is most desirable. The IV route is also best when constant therapeutic blood levels must be established. Some medications are highly alkaline and irritating to muscle and SQ tissue. Therefore giving these drugs intravenously causes less discomfort.

LARGE-VOLUME INFUSIONS

Of the three methods of administering IV medications, mixing a drug in a large volume of fluid is the safest and easiest. Drugs are diluted in large volumes (500 ml or 1000 ml) of compatible IV fluids such as normal saline or Ringer's lactate solution. In most institutions the pharmacist adds drugs to the primary container of IV solution to ensure asepsis. Because the drug is not in a concentrated form, the risk of side effects or fatal reactions is lessened. Vitamins and potassium chloride are two types of drugs commonly added to IV fluids. The danger with continuous infusion is that the client may suffer circulatory fluid overload if the IV fluid is infused too rapidly (see Chapter 45 and Procedure 35-5).

INTRAVENOUS BOLUS

An **IV bolus** involves introducing a concentrated dose of a drug directly into systemic circulation (Procedure 35-6).

The IV bolus is used during emergencies, with critically unstable clients, and as a route of administration when rapid and predictable responses are required (Burman, Berkowitz, 1986). An IV bolus may be introduced directly into a vein; into an existing IV line, through an injection port; or through a heparin lock.

Because only a small amount of fluid is required to deliver a drug, use of a bolus is an advantage when the amount of fluid the client can take is restricted. The IV bolus is the most dangerous method for administering drugs because there is no time to correct errors. In addition, a bolus may cause direct irritation to the lining of the blood vessels. Before administering a bolus, the nurse confirms placement of the IV line. This involves obtaining a blood return through the IV catheter or needle. The inability to obtain a blood return may suggest that the needle or catheter is in the tissues or resting against the vein wall. A drug should never be given intravenously if the insertion site appears puffy or edematous or the IV fluid cannot flow at the proper rate. Accidental injection of a medication into the tissues surrounding a vein can cause pain, sloughing of tissues, and abscesses, depending on the drug's composition.

The rate of administration of an IV bolus medication is usually determined by the amount of drug that can be given each minute. The nurse should look up each medication to be given to determine the maximum concentration and rate of administration recommended. The standard rate is 1 ml/min if no specific rate of administration is recommended (Burman, Berkowitz, 1986). The purpose for

Text continued on p. 847.

Adding Medications to IV Fluid Containers

STEPS	RATIONALE
1. Check physician's order for type of IV solution, medication, and dose.	Overall physical condition determines type of solution to use. Ensures safe and accurate drug administration.
2. When more than one medication is to be added to solution, assess for drug compatability. Check the compatibility of the drug with the IV fluid.	Certain drugs are incompatible when mixed. May result in clouding or crystallization of fluids or cause drug interaction that is not visible.
3. Prepare equipment and supplies:	
a. Vial or ampule of prescribed medication	
b. Syringe of appropriate size (5 to 20 ml)	
c. Sterile needle (1 to 1$^1/_2$ in, 19- to 21-gauge) with special filters (optional)	Larger needle gauge ensures easy aspiration of drugs from vial or ampule. Filter prevents particles from entering syringe and thus avoids transfer to fluid container.
d. Correct diluent (e.g., sterile water or normal saline)	Certain IV medications are prepared in dry powder form. Solvent must be added for mixing.
e. Sterile IV fluid container (bag or bottle, 500 to 1000 ml in volume)	Solution bags are kept sterile by being stored in separate intact plastic bag. Bottles have plastic or metal seal over bottle cap.
f. Alcohol or antiseptic swab	
g. Label to attach to IV bag or bottle	Continuously infusing medication must be labeled properly for all nurses to observe.
4. Wash hands thoroughly.	Reduces transfer of microorganisms when handling sterile equipment.
5. Assemble supplies in medication room.	Ensures that procedure will be orderly with less likelihood of contaminating supplies.
6. Prepare prescribed medication from vial or ampule (Procedure 35-2). (If filter needle is used, replace it with regular needle before injecting medication into IV fluid container.)	Different techniques are used for each type of container.
7. Identify client by reading identification band and asking name.	Ensures that correct client receives ordered medication.
8. Prepare client by explaining that medication is to be given through existing IV line or one to be started. Explain that no discomfort should be felt during infusion. Encourage client to report symptoms of discomfort.	Allows client to understand procedure and minimizes anxiety. Most IV medications will not cause discomfort when diluted. However, potassium chloride can be irritating. Pain at insertion site may be early indication of infiltration.
9. Add medication to new container.	
a. Locate medication injection port on IV solution bag:	
(1) Remove plastic cover over port. Port has small rubber stopper at end. Do not select port for IV tubing insertion or air vent.	Medication injection port is self-sealing to prevent introduction of microorganisms after repeated use.
b. Locate injection site on IV solution bottle:	
(1) Remove metal or plastic cap and rubber disk. Place cap upside down on counter top.	Cap seals bottle to maintain sterility. Inside of cap may remain sterile for reuse.
(2) Locate medication injection site on bottle's rubber stopper. Site is usually marked by X, circle, or triangle.	Accidental injection of medication through main tubing port or air vent can alter pressure within bottle and cause fluid leaks through air vent.
c. Wipe off port or injection site with alcohol or antiseptic swab (see the illustration on p. 841, left).	Reduces risk of introducing microorganisms into bag during needle insertion.
d. Remove needle cap from syringe and insert needle of syringe through center of injection port or site, and inject medication (see the illustration on p. 841, middle).	Injection of needle into sides of port may produce leak and lead to fluid contamination.
e. Withdraw syringe from bag or bottle.	
f. Mix medication and IV solution by holding bag or bottle and turning it gently end to end.	Allows medication to be distributed evenly.
g. Complete medication label with name and dose of medication, date, time, and your initials. Stick it upside down on bottle or bag (see the illustration on p. 841, right).	Label can be easily read during infusion of solution. Informs nurses and physicians of contents of bag or bottle.
h. Spike bag or bottle with IV tubing and hang (see Chapter 45). Regulate infusion at ordered rate.	Prevents rapid infusion of fluid.

Adding Medications to IV Fluid Containers—cont'd

STEPS	RATIONALE

10. Add medication to existing container:

   a. Prepare vented IV bottle or plastic bag: — Proper volume is needed to dilute medication adequately.

     (1) Check volume of solution remaining in bottle.

     (2) Verify dilution of medication desired (amount of medication per milliliter).

     (3) Close off IV infusion clamp. — Prevents medication from directly entering circulation as it is injected into bag or bottle.

     (4) Wipe medication port with alcohol or antiseptic swab. — Mechanically removes microorganisms that could enter container during needle insertion.

     (5) Lower bag or bottle from IV pole. Insert syringe needle through injection port and inject medication. — Injection port is self-sealing and prevents fluid leaks.

     (6) Gently mix bottle or bag. — Ensures that medication is evenly distributed.

     (7) Rehang bag and regulate infusion to desired rate. — Prevents rapid infusion of fluid.

   b. Complete medication label and stick it to bag or bottle. — Informs nurses and physicians of contents of bag or bottle.

11. Properly dispose of equipment and supplies. Wash hands. — Reduces transmission of microorganisms.

12. Record solution and medication added to parenteral fluid on appropriate form. — Information used to monitor type of solutions client receives and fluid intake over 24 hours.

13. Report side effects (e.g., change in pulse rate, noisy respirations, or change in blood pressure) to nurse in charge or physician. — Reaction may require therapeutic intervention.

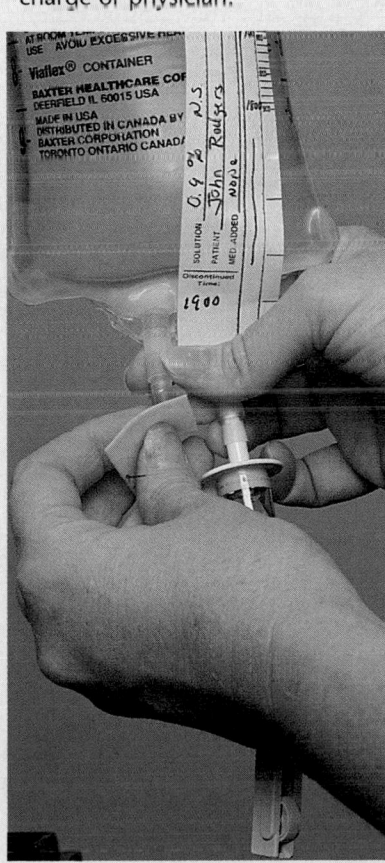

Step 9c

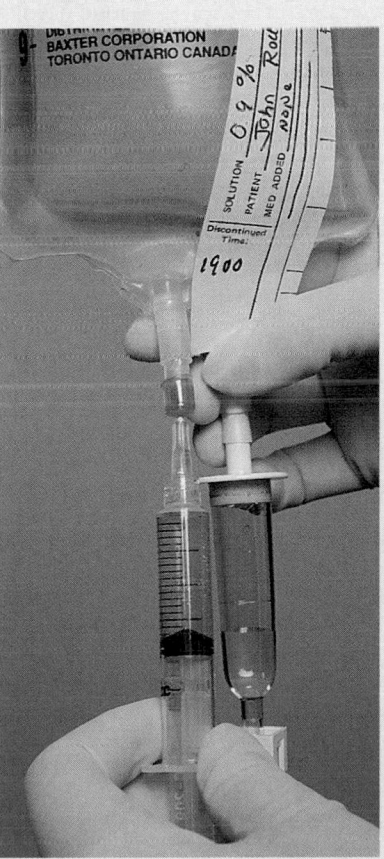

Step 9d

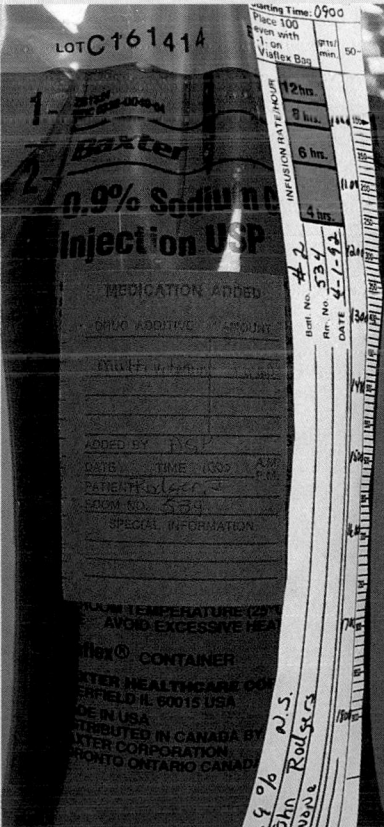

Step 9g

Administering Medication by IV Bolus (Push)

STEPS	RATIONALE
1. Check the physician's order for type of medication to be administered, dosage, and route.	This ensures safe and accurate drug administration.
2. Assess IV or heparin (saline) lock insertion site for signs of infiltration or phlebitis (see Chapter 45)	Confirming the placement of the IV catheter and the integrity of the surrounding tissue ensures that the medication is administered safely.
3. If medication is to be pushed into an IV line, assess the patency of the line by noting infusion rate.	The IV line must be patent, and fluids must infuse easily for medication to reach venous circulation effectively.
4. Prepare equipment and supplies:	
a. IV push (existing line)	
(1) Medication in vial or ampule	
(2) Syringe (3 to 5 ml)	
(3) Sterile needles (19- to 21-gauge)	
(4) Antiseptic swab	
(5) Watch with second hand or digital readout	
b. IV push (IV lock)	
(1) Medication in vial or ampule	
(2) Syringe (3 to 5 ml)	This is used for medication preparation.
(3) Syringe (3 ml)	This is used for heparin flush or saline solution.
(4) Vial of heparin flush solution (1ml =100 units or 1ml = 10 units) or vial of normal saline. Refer to agency policy (some agencies are using only saline flush to clear IV catheter, see p. 847)	
(5) Sterile needles (21 gauge)	Large-gauge needles are used to draw up medications. Small gauge needles are used to insert through Y port of tubing.
(6) Antiseptic swab	
(7) Watch with second hand or digital readout.	
c. Disposable gloves.	
5. Prepare ordered medication from vial or ampule (see Procedure 35-2). Read package directions carefully for proper IV dilution of medications.	
6. After drawing up medications, apply a small-gauge needle to the syringe.	Used to insert through IV line with needle system.
7. Wash hands. Apply gloves.	Reduces transmission of infection. During IV bolus administration, risk of blood exposure is low. However, nurse may manipulate IV dressing or expose site while completing other activities. Gloves reduce exposure.
8. Check client's identification by looking at armband and asking name.	Ensures that drug is administered to correct client.
9. Administer medications by IV push (existing line):	
a. Select injection port of IV tubing closest to client. (Circle on port may indicate site for needle insertion.) If add on 0.22 μ filter is used, give medication below filter next to client.	Allows for easier fluid aspiration to obtain blood return. Injection ports are self sealing and will not leak.
b. Clean off injection port with antiseptic swab. Allow to dry.	Prevents introduction of microorganisms during needle insertion.
c. Connect syringe to IV line.	
(1) Needle system Insert small-gauge needle of syringe containing prepared drug through center of injection port (see the illustration on p. 843).	Prevents damage to port's diaphragm and subsequent leakage.
(2) Needleless system Remove cap of needleless injection port. Connect tip of syringe directly (see the illustration on p. 843).	

Administering Medication by IV Bolus (Push)—cont'd

STEPS	RATIONALE

9. Administer medications by IV push (existing line)—cont'd

d. Occlude IV line by pinching tubing just above injection port (see the illustration below). Pull back gently on syringe's plunger to aspirate blood return.

Final check that medication is being delivered into the bloodstream.

e. After noting blood return, continue to occude tubing and inject medication slowly over several minutes (read directions on drug package). Use watch to time administration (see the illustration below).

Ensures safe drug infusion. Rapid injection of IV drug can prove fatal.

f. After injecting medication, release tubing, withdraw syringe, and recheck fluid infusion rate.

Injection of bolus may alter rate of fluid infusion. Rapid fluid infusion can cause circulatory overload.

h. If using a needleless system, replace injection port cap with new sterile cap.

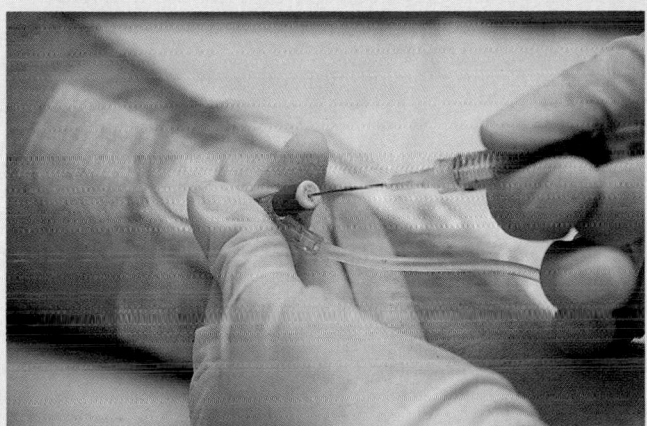

Step 9c(1)

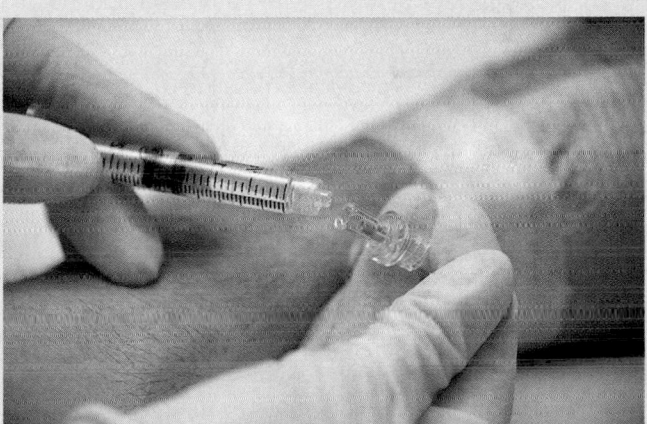

Step 9c(2)

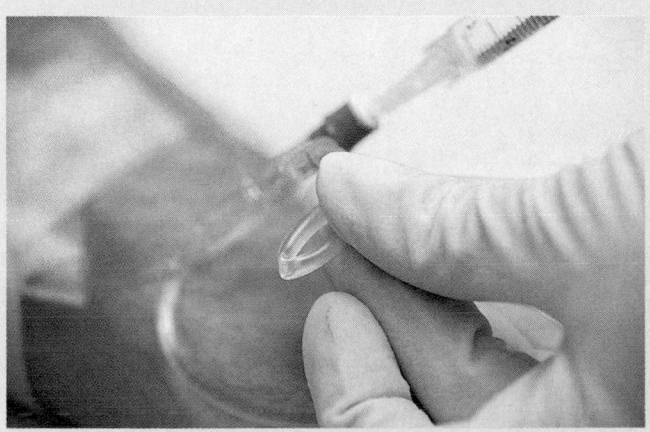

Step 9d

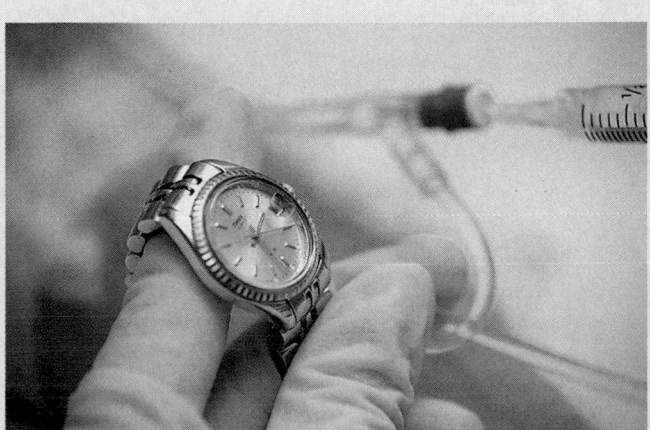

Step 9e

Continued.

PROCEDURE 35-6

Administering Medication by IV Bolus (Push)—cont'd

STEPS	RATIONALE

10. Administering medications by IV push (IV lock or a needleless system)

a. Prepare flush solutions according to hospital policy.

  (1) Flushing with heparin

    (a) Prepare syringe with 1 ml of heparin flush solution — *Flush solution keeps heparin lock patent after drug is administered.*

    (b) Prepare 2 syringes with 1 ml of normal saline

  (2) Flushing with saline only

    (a) Prepare 2 syringes with 1 ml of normal saline each

b. IV lock

  (1) Clean lock's rubber diaphragm with antiseptic swab. — *Prevents introduction of microorganisms during needle insertion.*

  (2) Insert needle of syringe containing normal saline through center of diaphragm.

  (3) Pull back gently on syringe plunger and look for blood return. — *Determines whether IV needle or catheter is positioned in vein. (At times heparin lock will not yield blood return even though it is patent.)*

  (4) Flush reservoir with 1 ml saline by pushing slowly on plunger. — *Clears needle and reservoir of blood.*

  (5) Remove needle and saline-filled syringe.

  (6) Clean lock's diaphragm with antiseptic swab. — *Prevents transmission of infection.*

  (7) Insert needle of syringe containing prepared drug through center of diaphragm (see the illustration below). — *Using center of diaphragm prevents leakage.*

  (8) Inject medication bolus slowly over several minutes. (Each medication has recommended rate for bolus administration. Check package directions). Use watch to time administration. — *Rapid injection of IV drug can result in death.*

  (9) After administering bolus, withdraw syringe.

  (10) Clean lock's diaphragm with antiseptic swab. — *Prevents transmission of microorganisms.*

  (11) Repeat injection of 1 ml of normal saline. — *Flushes reservoir and needle of medication.*

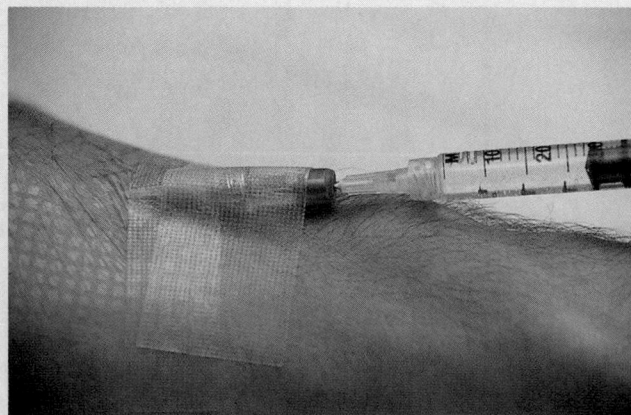

Step 10b(7)

Administering Medication by IV Bolus (Push)—cont'd

STEPS	RATIONALE

10. Administering medications by IV push (IV lock or a needleless system)—cont'd

   b. IV lock—cont'd

      (12) *Heparin flush:* Insert needle of syringe containing heparin through diaphragm. Inject heparin slowly, and remove syringe.
          Saline only: If using only saline to flush reservoir, use 1 ml of saline before and after each use of IV lock.
— Maintains patency of needle by inhibiting clot formation.

   c. IV needleless valve cap

      (1) Remove protective cap from needleless port.

      (2) Insert syringe containing normal saline into the valve.

      (3) Flush reservoir with 1 ml saline by pushing slowly on plunger. — Clears reservoir of any blood.

      (4) Remove the syringe.

      (5) Insert syringe containing prepared drug into the valve.

      (6) Inject medication slowly over several minutes. Follow precautions in step 10b(8) (see the illustration on p. 844). — Rapid injection of IV drug can result in death.

      (7) After administering bolus, withdraw syringe.

      (8) Repeat injection of 1 ml of normal saline.

      (9) See step 10b(12) above.

      (10) Replace sterile cap over valve.

11. IV push by epidural route (given by specially trained nurses only)

   a. Check physician's order for type of medication to be administered and dosage. — Ensures safe and accurate drug administration. Narcotics, such as morphine or fentanyl, are the only drugs administered by the epidural route.

   b. Prepare equipment and supplies:

      (1) Preservative free medication in vial or ampule — Preservative-free drugs are used because preservative may be neurotoxic and cause severe spinal cord injury.

      (2) Syringe (3 ml) — Used for catheter aspiration.

      (3) Syringe (5 ml or larger) — Used for administering narcotic. A large syringe lessens the force of fluid as it exits catheter. This reduces pain which can occur because of the forward pressure of the solution against nerve roots in the epidural space (Wild, Coyne, 1992).

      (4) Large-gauge needle (19 to 21 gauge) — Used to aspirate medication from vial or ampule.

      (5) Two small-gauge needles (23 to 25 gauge) — Used to verify catheter placement and to inject medication into epidural catheter.

      (6) Preservative free normal saline

      (7) Povidone-iodine swabs

      (8) Sterile gauze

      (9) Disposable gloves

   c. Using a 5 ml syringe or larger, draw up the narcotic. *Verify hospital policy if filter needle is required when aspirating medication from ampule.* — See Procedure 35-2, Preparing Injections From Ampules and Vials.

   d. Check client's identification by looking at armband and asking name. — Ensures that the correct drug is administered to correct client.

   e. Assess client's sedation using standardized scale (see Chapter 37). — Oversedation may lead to respiratory depression and death.

Continued.

Administering Medication by IV Bolus (Push)—cont'd

STEPS	RATIONALE

11. IV push by epidural route (given by specially trained nurses only)—cont'd

   f. Remove protective cap from needleless port. Swab the client's injection cap with povidone-iodine. Swab cap with sterile gauze (see the illustrations below).

   Prevents the transmission of microorganisms into the epidural space. Swabbing with gauze prevents the injection of povidone-iodine into epidural space.

   g. Using 3 cc syringe, insert the syringe into the needleless port and aspirate. If more than 1 cc of clear fluid or bloody fluid is aspirated terminate procedure and notify the nurse anesthetist or anesthesiologist *(do not reinject aspirate)*. If less than ½ ml fluid returns continue with procedure (see the illustration below).

   More than 1 ml of clear fluid indicates that catheter may be in intrathecal space. A bloody return indicates that the catheter may have punctured an epidural vein.

   h. Insert medication syringe into needleless port. Inject drug slowly and steadily. Reduce rate of injection if client complains of pain.

   See step 10c(6).

12. Dispose of equipment properly.

   Reduces accidental needlesticks.

13. Remove and dispose of gloves. Wash hands.

   Reduces the transmission of microorganisms.

14. Observe client closely for adverse reaction as drug is administered and for several minutes thereafter.

   IV medications act rapidly.

15. Record drug, dose, route and time administered on medication form (Fig. 35-6).

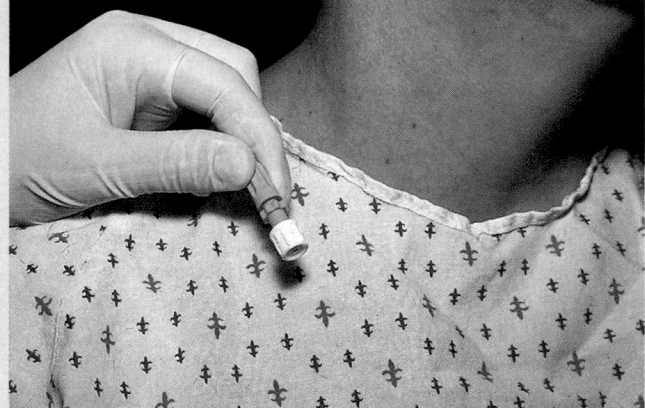 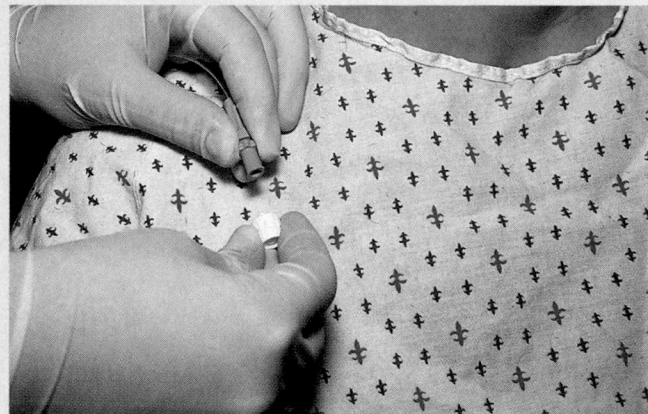

Step 11f

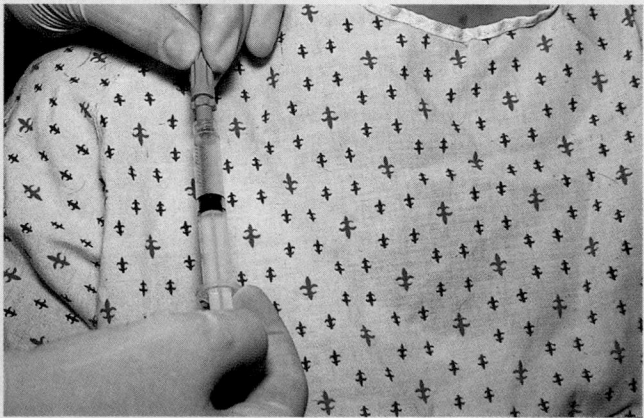

Step 11g

which a drug is prescribed and any potential adverse effects related to the rate or route of administration must be considered when a nurse gives a drug IV push

∎ VOLUME-CONTROLLED INFUSIONS

Another way of administering IV medications is through small amounts (50 to 100 ml) of compatible IV fluids. The fluid is within a secondary fluid container separate from the primary IV fluid bag. The container connects directly to the primary IV line or to a separate tubing that inserts into the primary IV line. Three types of containers are volume-control administration sets (e.g., Volutrol or Pediatrol), piggyback sets, and miniinfusers (see Chapter 45). There are several advantages to using volume-controlled infusions, including the following:

1. Reduces risk of rapid-dose infusion by IV push; IV medications are diluted and infused over longer time intervals (e.g., 30 to 60 minutes)
2. Allows administration of drugs that are incompatible with drugs in the primary IV solution
3. Allows administration of drugs (e.g., antibiotics) that are stable for a limited time in solution
4. Allows control of IV fluid intake

Volume-control administration sets are small (100 to 150 ml) containers that attach just below the primary infusion bag or bottle (Procedure 35-7). The set is attached and filled in a manner similar to that used to a regular IV infusion (see Chapter 45). However, the priming, or filling, of the set is different, depending on the type of filter (floating valve or membrane) within the set. Package directions should be followed during priming, or the set will not function properly.

∎ PIGGYBACK IV ADMINISTRATION

Piggyback sets are small (50 or 100 ml) IV bags or bottles connected to short tubing lines that connect to the upper Y-port of a primary infusion line or an intermittent venous access. The piggyback tubing is a microdrip or macrodrip system. Because of the risk of needlestick injuries, nurses should avoid using needles when connecting a secondary infusion. Commercially available connectors can be used for the safe connection of secondary lines to primary infusion lines (see Procedure 35-7, Step 8E). There are institutions that continue to use needles when connecting lines. Extreme caution is necessary.

∎ INTERMITTENT VENOUS ACCESS

An intermittent lock (sometimes referred to as *sterile injection cap*, **heparin lock**, *saline lock*, or *med-lock*) is an IV infusion device with a special connector called a *male adapter*, traditionally covered by a rubber diaphragm (Fig. 35-27). To reduce the risk of needlestick injuries some hospitals use a needleless valve device instead of the diaphragm. An intermittent lock is inserted into an intravenous catheter and used only on an intermittent or emergency basis for the infusion of medication. Advantages to an intermittent venous access device include the following:

1. Increased mobility, safety, and comfort for the client
2. Convenience to the nurse by eliminating constant monitoring of flow rates
3. Cost savings resulting from the omission of continuous IV therapy

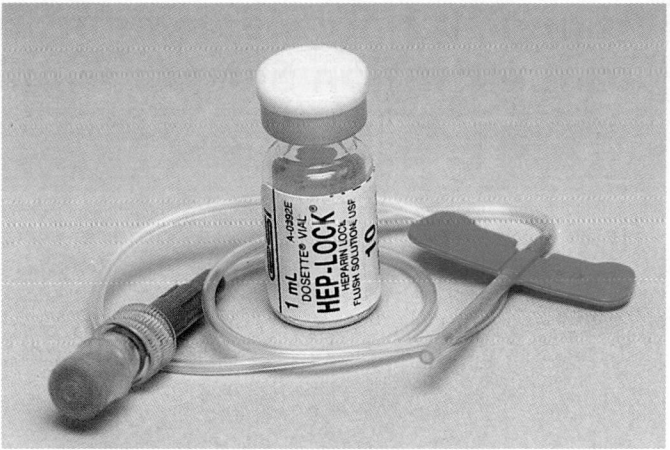

Fig. 35-27 Intermittent lock covered with a rubber diaphragm. Requires a needle to flush.

After an IV bolus or piggyback medication has been administered through an intermittent lock, the lock must be flushed with a solution to keep it patent (free of clots). Traditionally heparin has been used. Peterson and Kirchoff (1991) analyzed 13 studies that compared heparin as a flush solution, as compared with normal saline, and found that there is no significant difference between heparin and saline flush procedures in peripheral intravenous catheters. The most obvious benefit of using saline as a flush solution rather than heparin is a cost saving to the institution.

∎ TOPICAL DRUG APPLICATIONS

Skin Applications

Because many locally applied drugs such as lotions, pastes, patches, and ointments can create systemic and local effects, the nurse should apply these drugs using gloves and applicators. Sterile technique is important, especially if the client has an open wound.

Skin encrustations and dead tissues harbor microorganisms and block contact of medications with the tissues to be treated. Simply applying new medications over previously applied drugs does little to prevent infection or offer therapeutic benefit. Before applying medications, the nurse cleans the skin thoroughly by washing the area gently with soap and water, soaking an involved site, or locally debriding tissue.

When applying ointments or pastes, the nurse spreads the medication evenly over the involved surface and covers the area well without applying an overly thick layer. Opaque ointments prevent visualization of underlying skin. Physicians often order a gauze dressing to be applied over the medication to prevent soiling of clothes and wiping away of the drug.

Each type of medication—ointment, lotion, powder, and patches—should be applied a specific way to ensure proper penetration and absorption. The nurse applies lotions and creams by smearing them lightly onto the skin's surface. Rubbing may cause irritation. A liniment is applied by rubbing it gently but firmly into the skin. A powder is dusted lightly to cover the affected area with a thin layer. The

Administering Medications by Piggyback, Volume Administration Sets, or Miniinfusors (Syringe Pump)

STEPS	RATIONALE
1. Check physician's order to determine type of medication, dosage of medication and type of solution to be used.	Client's overall physical condition determines types of solutions used. Ensures safe and accurate drug administration.
2. Assess patency of existing IV infusion line by noting infusion rate of main IV line.	IV line must be patent and fluids must infuse easily for medications to reach venous circulation effectively.
3. Assess insertion site for signs of infiltration or phlebitis (see Chapter 45).	Confirmation of placement of catheter and integrity of surrounding tissue ensures that medication is administered safely.
4. Prepare following equipment and supplies: a. Piggyback setup:	
(1) Medication prepared in a 50 to 100 ml, labeled infusion bag with IV line, microdrip or macrodrip infusion tubing set with "needleless" connector or 21- or 23-gauge needle.	Used for piggyback administration. Most piggybacks are prepared by pharmacy. Medication is "piggybacked" or connected to main infusion line by commercially available needleless connector. Needles can be used but are not recommended because of risk of needlestick injury.

(2) Adhesive tape (optional)
  (3) Antiseptic swab
  (4) Metal or plastic hook (optional)
	Used to lower primary infusion bag below smaller infusion bag (only if tubing is shorter than primary tubing).

(5) Disposable gloves b. Volume-control administration set:	
(1) Volutrol, Pediatrol, Buretrol set.	Graduated container connects to main IV solution.

(2) Syringe (5 to 20 ml)
  (3) Needle (1 to ½ inch, 21- or 23-gauge)
  (4) Vial or ampule of ordered medication
  (5) Medication label
  c. Miniinfusor (syringe pump):	

(1) Miniinfusor (syringe pump)	Electronic device used to drive a syringe's plunger for infusion of medication.
(2) Infusion tubing (3) Sterile 20-gauge needle or needleless connector	Used to "piggyback" medicated syringe to primary infusion line.

(4) Syringe with medication
  (5) Alcohol swabs
  (6) Adhesive tape (optional)	

5. Prepare medication in medication area. a. Piggyback set:	
(1) Medication in 50 to 100 ml bag. Verify the bag's medication label against physician order. If medication is not pre-mixed, inject medication into a 50 to 100 ml bag.	Medications for "piggybacking" may come premixed from the pharmacy.
b. Volume-control administration set (1) Prepare medication in syringe (see Procedure 35-2).	
c. Miniinfusor/syringe pump (1) Prepare medicated syringe (5 to 60 ml) according to manufacturer's recommendation and hospital policy.	Most medicated syringes come pre-mixed and prelabeled from the pharmacy. Not all drugs can be infused in this manner. The nurse uses the pharmacist as a resource to identify which medication can and those that cannot be infused by the miniinfusor.
6. Check client's identification by looking at identification bracelet and asking name.	Ensures that correct client receives medication.

Administering Medications by Piggyback, Volume Administration Sets, or Miniinfusors (Syringe Pump)—cont'd

STEPS	RATIONALE
7. Wash hands and apply gloves.	Reduces transfer of microorganisms when handling sterile equipment. During connection of piggybacking of medications, the risk of blood exposure is low. However, nurse may manipulate IV dressing or expose site while completing other activities.
8. Administer medications by piggyback set:	
a. Connect infusion tubing to medication bag (see Chapter 45). Allow solution to fill tubing by opening regulator flow clamp.	Infusion tube should be filled with solution and free of air bubbles to prevent air embolus.
b. Hang medication bag at or above level of main fluid bag. Hook may be used to lower main bag.	Height of fluid affects rate of flow to client.
c. Connect covered sterile needle or needleless device to end of infusion tubing.	Cover keeps needle or device sterile before connecting it to main line.
d. Clean injection Y-port of main line with antiseptic swab.	Prevents introduction of microorganisms during connection.
e. **Needle:** Remove cover and insert needle of secondary piggyback line through insertion port of main line away from client (see the illustration below, left). Secure with strip of adhesive tape if necessary.	Establishes route for medication to enter main IV line. Tape prevents needle from slipping out of port.
f. **Needleless device:** Use needle-lock device to secure needle of secondary piggyback line through injection port of main line (see the illustrations below, right).	Needleless devices are designed to lock-in place. Use of needleless devices reduce the risk of needlestick injury to health care workers.

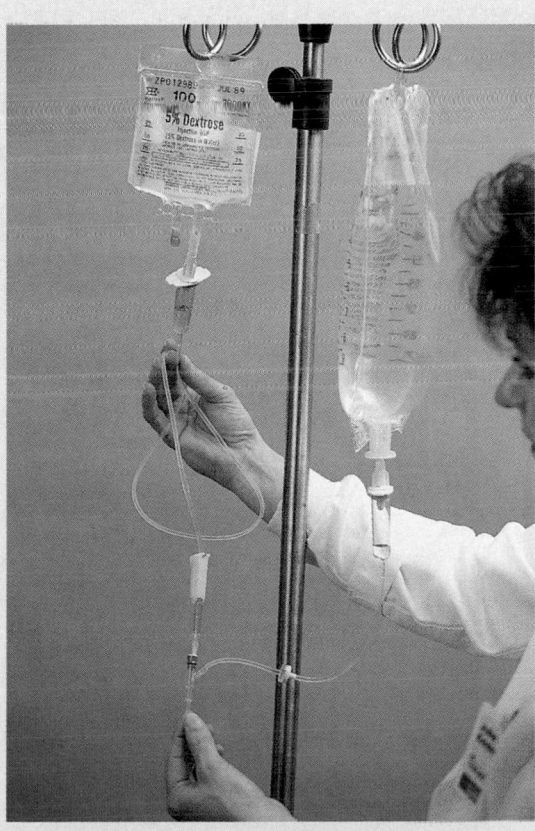

Step 8e

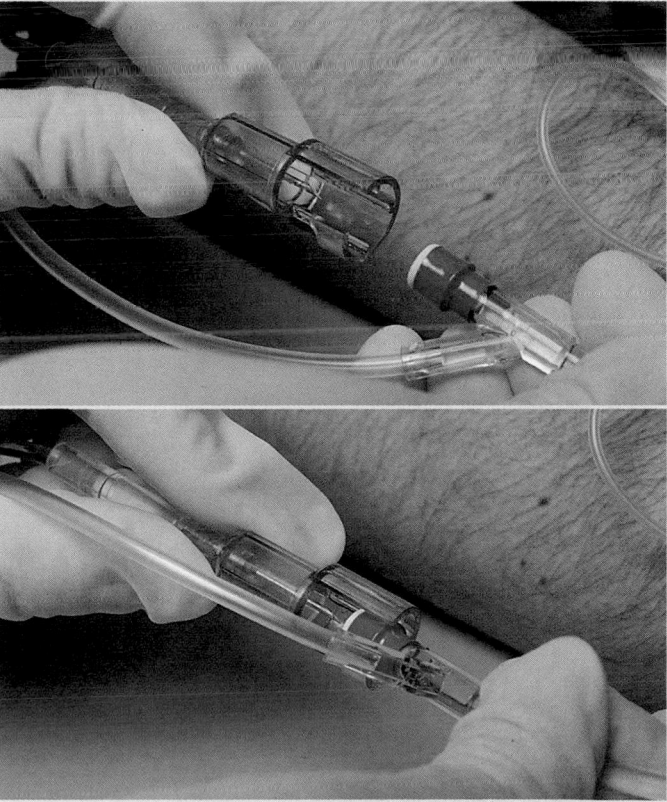

Step 8f

Continued.

Administering Medications by Piggyback, Volume Administration Sets, or Miniinfusors (Syringe Pump)—cont'd

STEPS	RATIONALE

8. Administer medications by piggyback set—cont'd

  g. Regulate flow rate appropriate or as ordered by physician.

Intermittent infusion of medication maintains therapeutic blood levels. For optimal effect, drug should infuse in prescribed time interval.

  h. After medication has infused, check flow regulator on primary infusion. Piggyback set hung at level of primary bag has backcheck valve that automatically stops flow of primary infusion until medication infuses. Primary infusion should automatically begin to flow after piggyback is empty.

Valve prevents backup of medication into infusion line. Checking flow rate ensures proper administration of fluids.

  i. Regulate main infusion line to desired rate, if necessary.

Infusion of piggyback may interfere with main line infusion rate.

  j. Leave secondary bag, tubing, and inserted needle in place for future drug administration or discard in appropriate container (check hospital policy).

Establishment of secondary line produces route for microorganisms to enter main line. Repeated changes in tubing or needles increase risk of infection transmission.

9. Administer medication by volume control administration set (e.g., Volutrol):

  a. Fill Volutrol with desired amount of fluid (50 to 100 ml) by opening clamp between Volutrol and main IV bag (see the illustration below, left).

Fluid dilutes medication and reduces risk of too rapid infusion.

  b. Close clamp and check to be sure clamp in air vent of Volutrol chamber is open.

Prevents additional leakage of fluid into Volutrol. Air vent allows fluid in Volutrol to exit at regulated rate.

  c. Clean injection port on top of Volutrol with antiseptic swab.

Prevents introduction of microorganisms during needle insertion.

  d. Remove needle cap and insert syringe needle through port, and then inject medication (see the illustration below, right). Gently rotate Volutrol between hands.

Rotating mixes medication with solution in Volutrol to ensure equal distribution.

  e. Regulate IV infusion rate appropriate for medication. Follow physician, manufacturer's recommendations for infusion rates.

For optimal therapeutic effect, drug should infuse in prescribed time interval.

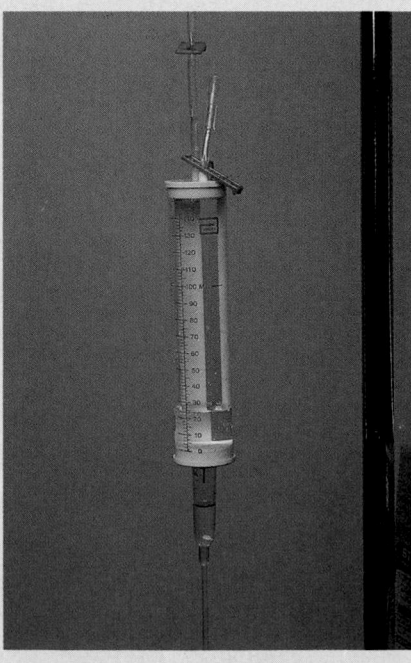

Step 9a

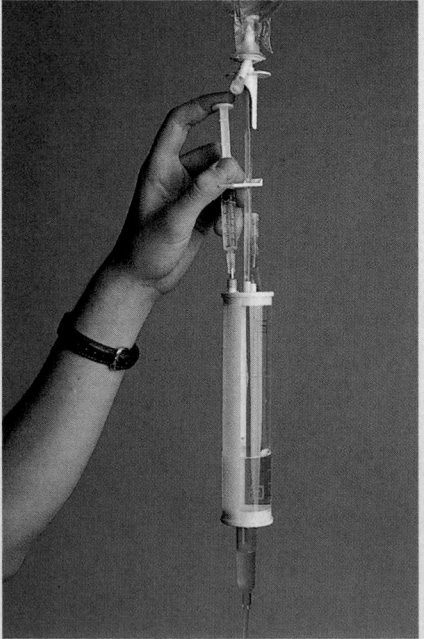

Step 9d

Administering Medications by Piggyback, Volume Administration Sets, or Miniinfusors (Syringe Pump)—cont'd

STEPS	RATIONALE
9. Administer medication by volume control administration set (e.g., Volutrol)—cont'd	
f. Label Volutrol with name of drug, dose, total volume including diluent, and time of administration.	Alerts nurses to drug being infused. Prevents other medications from being added to Volutrol.
g. Dispose of uncapped needle and syringe in proper container.	Prevents accidental needlesticks.
10. Administer medication by miniinfusor (syringe-pump).	Following manufacturer's recommendation ensures accurate delivery of medication to be infused.
a. Attach microbore tubing to medicated syringe. Prime tubing and attach needle with cap or needleless device.	
b. Prepare equipment to accept syringe according to manufacturer's recommendation. Snap syringe barrel into syringe holder of the miniinfusor pump according to manufacturer's recommendation (see the illustration at right).	
c. Set timing function to infuse medication as ordered by physician or as recommended.	
d. Connect microbore tubing to IV lock or Y-port of main line with needle or needleless device.	

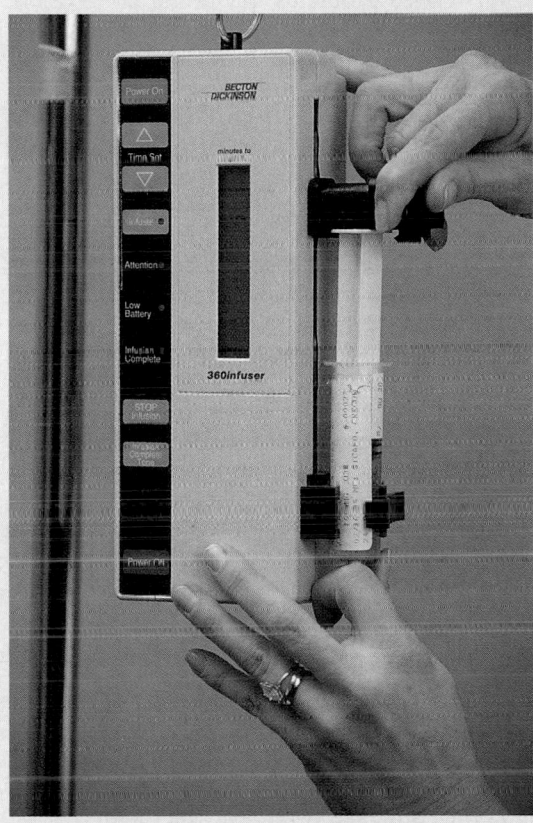

Step 10b

STEPS	RATIONALE
e. Start miniinfusor. Observe for proper functioning.	Use of certain piggyback ports with miniinfusor may result in retrograde flow or continuation of the primary line. When infusing into a Y site, the volume of the primary set may cause either a delay of the drug infusion or a bolus effect depending on the speed of infusion flow.
f. When infusion is complete, turn miniinfusor off, disconnect microbore tubing. Maintain sterility of microbore tube with a clean needle. If using IV lock for infusion flush IV lock according to agency policy (see Procedure 35-6).	
11. Remove and dispose of gloves.	Prevents the transmission of microorganisms.
12. During infusion, periodically check infusion rate and condition of IV site.	IV line must remain patent for proper drug administration. Development of infiltration necessitates discontinuing infusion.
13. Record drug, dose, route, and time administered on medication form (Fig. 35-6). Record volume of syringe on intake and output form.	Timely documentation prevents medication errors. Fluid balance is regulated and monitored on basis of total intake.

nurse applies transdermal medication (patches) to any clean, dry, hairless area on the body with the exception of the extremities below the knee or elbow. The nurse ensures that the patch is adhered firmly to the skin. During any skin application, the nurse should assess the skin thoroughly. To record administration the nurse notes the area applied, name of medication, and condition of skin.

Eye Applications

A common medication used by clients is eye drops and ointments, including over-the-counter preparations such as artificial tears and vasoconstrictors (e.g., Visine and Murine). However, many clients receive prescribed ophthalmic drugs for eye conditions such as glaucoma and for treatment after procedures such as cataract extraction. A large percentage of clients receiving eye medications are older adults. Age-related problems, including poor vision, hand tremors, and difficulty in grasping or manipulating containers, affect the ease with which older adults can self-administer eye medications. The nurse instructs clients and family members about the proper techniques for administering eye medications. Donnelly (1987) suggests showing clients each step of the procedure for instilling eye drops to improve compliance. Procedure 35-8 reviews the steps for administering eye medications. The following principles can be followed when administering eye medications:

1. The cornea of the eye is richly supplied with pain fibers and thus is very sensitive to anything applied to it. As a result the nurse avoids instilling any form of eye medication directly onto the cornea.
2. The risk of transmitting infection from one eye to the other is high. The nurse avoids touching the eyelids or other eye structures with eye droppers or ointment tubes.
3. The nurse uses eye medication only for the affected eye.
4. The nurse never allows one person to use another's eye medications.

Some medications are administered intraocularly. Medications delivered this way resemble a contact lens. The nurse places the medication into the conjuctival sac where it remains in place for up to 1 week. Currently, medications such as pilocarpine are administered this way. Experiments are underway to evaluate other medications that may be delivered in this form. The client receiving medications in this way requires teaching about monitoring for adverse reactions to the disk. Clients will also need to be taught how to insert and remove the disk. Procedure 35-8 reviews the steps the nurse uses for administering intraocular drugs.

Ear Instillations

Internal ear structures are very sensitive to temperature extremes. Failure to instill ear drops or irrigating fluid at room temperature may cause vertigo (severe dizziness) or nausea. Although the structures of the outer ear are not sterile, it is wise to use sterile drops and solutions in case the eardrum is ruptured. Entrance of nonsterile solutions into middle ear structures could result in infection. With ear drainage, the nurse can also check with the physician to be sure that the client does not have a ruptured eardrum. A nurse should never occlude the ear canal with the dropper or irrigating syringe. Forcing medication into an occluded ear canal creates pressure that may injure the eardrum.

The external ear structures of children are different from those of adults. When instilling drops or irrigating the canal (Procedure 35-9; see Procedure 35-14), the nurse must straighten the ear canal. In infants and young children the nurse straightens the cartilaginous canal by grasping the auricle of the ear and pulling it gently *down* and backward. In adults the ear canal is longer and composed of underlying bone and is straightened by pulling the auricle *upward* and backward. Failure to straighten the canal properly may prevent medicinal solutions from reaching the deeper external ear structures.

Nasal Instillations

Clients with nasal sinus alterations may receive drugs by spray, drops, or tampons (Procedure 35-10). The most commonly administered form of nasal instillation is decongestant spray or drops, which are used to relieve symptoms of sinus congestion and colds. Clients must be cautioned to avoid overuse because it can lead to a rebound effect in which the nasal congestion worsens. When excess decongestant solution is swallowed, serious systemic effects may also develop, especially in children. Saline drops are safer as a decongestant for children than nasal preparations that contain sympathomimetics (e.g., Afrin or Neo-Synephrine).

It is easier to have the client self-administer sprays. In the supine position with the head tilted back, the client holds the tip of the container just inside the nares. The client inhales as the spray enters the nasal passages. For clients who use nasal sprays repeatedly, the nurse checks the nares for irritation. In children, nasal sprays should be given with the head in an upright position so that excess spray will drip anteriorly from the nostrils and not be swallowed.

Nasal drops are effective in treating sinus infections. The nurse learns the proper way of positioning clients to permit the medication to reach the affected sinus. Severe nose bleeds are usually treated with packing or tampons. Tampons are treated with epinephrine, which causes peripheral vasoconstriction, to reduce blood flow. Usually a physician places nasal tampons.

Vaginal Instillations

Vaginal medications are available as suppositories, foam, jellies, or creams. Suppositories come individually packaged in foil wrappers. Storage in a refrigerator prevents the solid, oval-shaped suppositories from melting. After a suppository is inserted into the vaginal cavity, body temperature causes it to melt and be distributed and absorbed. Foam, jellies, and creams are administered with an inserter or applicator (Procedure 35-11). A suppository is given with a gloved hand. Client's often prefer administering their own vaginal medications and should be given privacy. After instillation, the client may wish to wear perineal pads to collect excess drainage. Because vaginal medications are frequently given to treat infection, any discharge may be foul smelling. Good aseptic technique should be followed, and clients should be offered frequent opportunities to maintain perineal hygiene (see Chapter 40).

Rectal Instillations

Rectal suppositories differ in shape from vaginal suppositories; they are thinner and bullet shaped. The rounded end prevents anal trauma during insertion. Rectal suppositories

Text continued on p. 857.

Administering Ophthalmic Medications

STEPS	RATIONALE
1. Review physician's medication order, including client's name, drug name, concentration, number of drops (if liquid), time, and eye (right or left) to receive medication.	Ensures correct administration of medication.
2. Wash hands.	Reduces transmission of microorganisms.
3. Prepare equipment and supplies:	
a. Drops or ointment	Ophthalmic drops come in plastic or glass bottles.
(1) Medication bottle with sterile eye dropper or ointment tube	Ointments are prepared in small tubes.
(2) Eye patch and tape (optional)	
(3) Medication card, form, or printout	
(4) Cotton ball or tissue	
(5) Wash basin filled with warm water and wash cloth	
(6) Disposable gloves	
b. Intraocular disk	
(1) Medicated disk	
(2) Medication card, form, or printout	
(3) Disposable gloves	
4. Check client's identification by looking at identification bracelet and asking name.	Ensures that correct client receives medication.
5. If eye patch is present, remove it.	
6. Assess condition of external eye structure (see Chapter 33).	Provides baseline to later determine whether local response to medications occurs. Also indicates need to clean eye before drug application.
7. Check if client has an allergy to latex. If so, use non-latex gloves.	Clients will have a hypersensitivity response if gloves touch mucous membranes.
8. Explain procedure to client.	Clients often becomes anxious about medication being instilled into eye because of potential for discomfort.
9. Arrange supplies at bedside and apply gloves.	Ensures smooth, orderly procedure. Gloves reduce exposure to infectious drainage.
10. Ask client to lie supine or sit back in chair with head slightly hyperextended.	Provides easy access to eye for medication instillation and minimizes drainage through tear duct.
11. If crust or drainage are present along eyelid margins or inner canthus, gently wash away. Soak crusts that are dried and difficult to remove by applying damp washcloth or cotton ball over eye for few minutes. Always wipe from inner to outer canthus.	Crust and drainage harbor microorganisms. Soaking allows easy removal, thus preventing pressure from being applied directly over eye. Cleansing from inner to outer canthus avoids entrance of microorganisms into lacrimal duct.
12. Instill drops, ointment, or disk.	
a. If instilling drops or ointment, hold cotton ball or clean tissue in non-dominant hand on client's cheekbone just below lower eyelid.	Cotton or tissue absorbs medication that escapes eye.
b. If instilling drops or ointment, with tissue or cotton resting below lower lid, gently press downward with thumb or forefinger against bony orbit.	Technique exposes lower conjunctival sac. Retraction against bony orbit prevents pressure and trauma to eyeball and prevents fingers from touching eye.
c. Ask client to look at ceiling.	Action retracts sensitive cornea up and away from conjunctival sac and reduces stimulation of blink reflex.
d. Instill eye drops:	
(1) With dominant hand resting on client's forehead, hold filled medication eye dropper approximately 1 to 2 cm (½ to ¾ in) above conjunctival sac (see the illustration on p. 854).	Helps prevent accidental contact of eyedropper with eye structures, thus reducing risk of injury to eye and transfer of infection to dropper. Ophthalmic medications are sterilized.
(2) Drop prescribed number of drops into conjunctival sac.	Conjunctival sac normally holds 1 to 2 drops. Applying drops to sac provides even distribution across eye.
(3) If client blinks or closes eye or if drops land on outer lid margins, repeat procedure.	Therapeutic effect is obtained only when drops enter conjunctival sac.

Continued.

Administering Ophthalmic Medications—cont'd

STEPS	RATIONALE

12. Instill drops, ointment, or disk—cont'd

d. Instill eye drops—cont'd

(4) When administering drugs that cause systemic effect, protect your fingers with clean tissue and apply gentle pressure to client's nasolacrimal duct for 30 to 60 sec.

    Prevent overflow of medication into nasal and pharyngeal passages. Prevents absorption into systemic circulation.

(5) After instilling drops, ask client to close eye gently.

    Helps distribute medication. Squinting or squeezing of eyelid forces medication from conjunctival sac.

e. Instill eye ointment:

(1) Holding ointment applicator above lid margin, apply thin stream of ointment evenly along inside edge of lower eyelid on conjunctiva (see the illustration below, right).

    Distributes medication evenly across eye and lid margin.

(2) Ask client to look down.

    Reduces blinking reflex during ointment application.

(3) Apply thin stream of ointment along upper lid margin on inner conjunctiva.

    Distributes medication evenly across eye and lid margin.

(4) Have client close eye and rub lid lightly in circular motion with cotton ball.

    Further distributes medication without traumatizing eye.

(5) If excess medication is on eyelid, gently wipe it from inner to outer canthus.

    Promotes comfort and prevents trauma to eye.

(6) If client has eye patch, apply clean one by placing it over affected eye so that entire eye is covered. Tape securely without applying pressure to eye.

    Reduces chance of infection.

f. Apply intraocular disk

(1) Open the package containing the medication disk. Gently press your fingertip against the disk so that it adheres to your finger. Position the convex part of the disk on your fingertip (see the illustration on p. 855).

    Allows the nurse to inspect the disk for damage or deformity prior to administration.

(2) With your other hand, pull the client's lower eyelid away from his eye. Ask the client to look up while you are doing this.

    Prepares the conjunctival sac for receiving the medicated disk.

(3) Place the disk in the conjunctival sac, so that it floats on the sclera between the iris and lower eyelid (see the illustration on p. 855).

    Ensures delivery of medication.

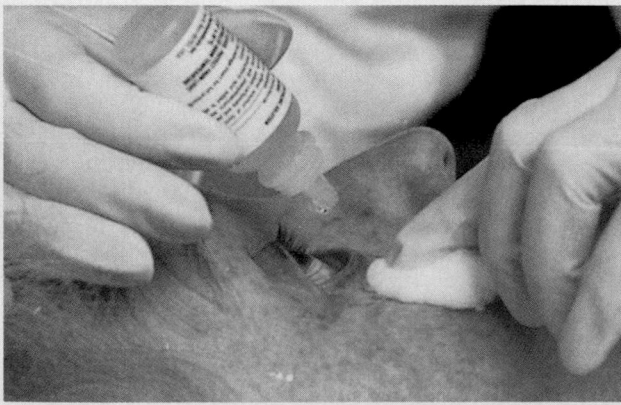

Step 12d(1), p. 853

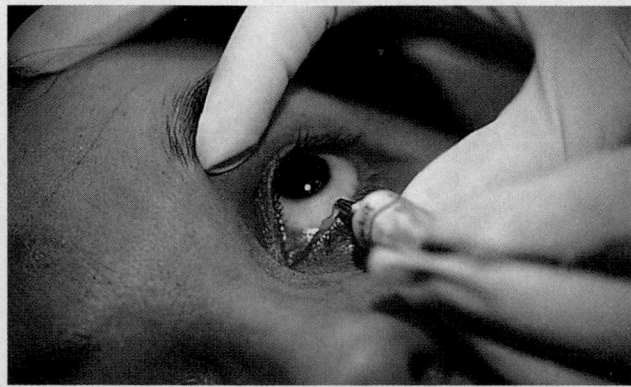

Step 12e(1)

Administering Ophthalmic Medications—cont'd

STEPS	RATIONALE
12. Instill drops, ointment, or disk—cont'd	
f. Apply intraocular disk—cont'd	
(4) Pull the client's lower eyelid out and over the disk. You should not be able to see the disk at this time. Repeat this step if you can see the medication disk (see the illustration below).	Ensures accurate delivery of medication.
13. Remove intraocular disk	
a. Wash hands and don gloves.	Reduces the transmission of microorganisms.
b. Explain the procedure to the client.	Prepares the client for the procedure.
c. Gently pull on the client's lower eyelid to expose the disk.	
d. Using your forefinger and thumb of your opposite hand, pinch the medication disk and lift it out of the client's eye (see the illustration below).	
14. Dispose of soiled supplies in proper receptacle. Remove and dispose of gloves. Wash hands.	Maintains neat environment at bedside and reduces transmission of microorganisms.
15. Observe client's response to the medication, noting signs and symptoms of potential systemic effects and condition of eye.	Evaluates reaction to medication.
16. Record drug concentration, number of drops or disk, time of administration, and eye (left, right, or both) that received medication.	Timely documentation prevents drug errors (e.g., repeated or missed doses).

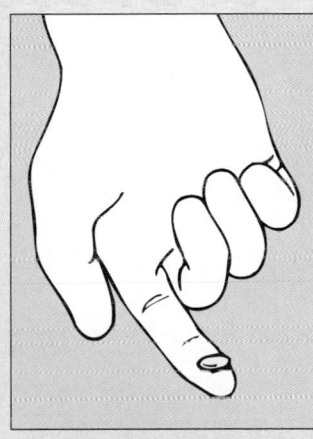

Step 12f(1)

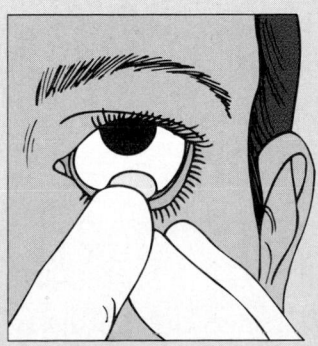

Step 12f(3)

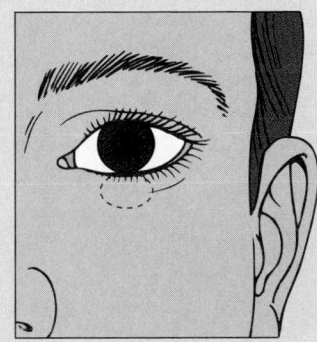

Step 12f(4)

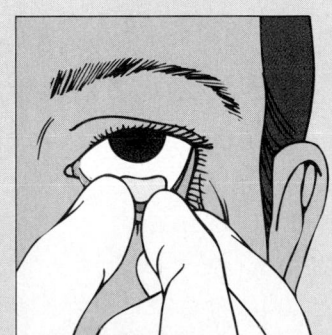

Step 13d

PROCEDURE 35-9

Administering Eardrops

STEPS	RATIONALE
1. Review physician's medication order for client's name, drug name, concentration, time of administration, number of drops to instill, and ear (right or left) to receive medication.	Ensures safe and correct administration of medication.
2. Wash hands.	Reduces transmission of miroorganisms.
3. Prepare equipment and supplies: a. Medication bottle and dropper b. Medication card, form, or printout c. Cotton-tipped applicator d. Tissue e. Cotton ball (optional) f. Disposable gloves (optional)	Used to remove cerumen or drainage.
4. Identify client by reading identification bracelet and asking name.	Ensures that correct client receives medication.
5. Apply gloves.	Reduces exposure to microorganisms.
6. Assess condition of external ear structures and canal (see Chapter 33).	Provides baseline to determine whether local response to medication occurs, client's condition improves, or cleansing will be necessary before instillation.
7. Explain procedure to client.	Reduces anxiety.
8. Arrange supplies at bedside.	Ensures smooth procedure.
9. Have client assume side-lying position with ear to be treated facing up.	Provides easy access to ear for instillation of medication. Ear canal is in position to receive medication.
10. If cerumen or drainage occludes outermost portion of ear canal, wipe out gently with cotton-tipped applicator. Do *not* force wax inward to block or occlude canal.	Cerumen and drainage harbor microorganisms and can block distribution of medication into canal. Occlusion of canal interferes with normal sound conduction.
11. Straighten ear canal by pulling auricle down and back (children) or upward and outward (adult).	Straightening of ear canal provides direct access to deeper external ear structures.
12. Instill prescribed drops holding dropper 1 cm ($\frac{1}{2}$ in) above ear canal (see the illustration below).	Forcing drops into occluded canal can cause injury to eardrum.
13. Ask client to remain in side-lying position 2 to 3 min. Apply gentle massage or pressure to tragus of ear with finger.	Allows complete distribution of medication. Pressure and massage move medication inward.

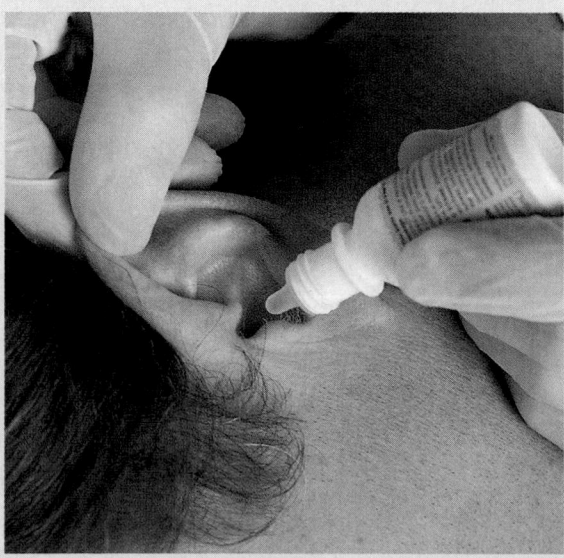

Step 12

Administering Eardrops—cont'd

STEPS	RATIONALE
14. At times, physician orders placement of cotton ball into outermost part of canal. Do not press cotton into innermost part of canal.	Inserting cotton into outer canal prevents escape of medication when client sits or stands. Cotton should not block canal to impair hearing.
15. Remove cotton in 15 min.	Promotes drug distribution and absorption.
16. Dispose of soiled supplies and gloves and wash hands.	Keeps bedside neat. Reduces transmission of infection.
17. Assist client to comfortable position after drops are absorbed.	Restores comfort.
18. Evaluate condition of external ear between drug instillations.	Determines response to medication.
19. Record drug, concentration, number of drops, time administered, and ear into which drops were instilled on medication form.	Timely documentation prevents drug errors (e.g., repeated doses).
20. Record condition of ear canal in nurses' notes.	Documents client's status and response to therapy.

contain medications that exert local effects, such as promoting defecation, or systemic effects, such as reducing nausea and lowering body temperature. They are particularly useful when clients are unable to tolerate oral medications. Rectal suppositories are stored in the refrigerator until they are administered.

During administration the nurse must place the suppository past the internal anal sphincter and against the rectal mucosa (Procedure 35-12). Otherwise the suppository may be expelled before it can dissolve and be absorbed into the mucosa. With practice, a nurse learns to recognize the sensation of the sphincter relaxing around the finger. The suppository should not be forced into a mass of fecal material. It may be necessary to clear the rectum with a small cleansing enema before a suppository can be inserted.

■ ADMINISTERING DRUGS BY INHALATION

Clients who receive drugs by inhalation frequently suffer chronic respiratory disease such as chronic asthma, emphysema, or bronchitis. Drugs given by inhalation provide these clients with control of airway obstruction, and because these clients depend on medications for disease control, they must learn about them and their safe administration.

A metered dose inhaler (MDI) (Procedure 35-13) delivers a measured dose of drug with each push of a canister. To activate the aerosol the client must push approximately 5 to 10 pounds of pressure. This is important for the nurse to know because hand strength diminishes with age and from the effects of chronic respiratory disease. The nurse evaluates whether clients have enough hand strength to use the MDI appropriately. Statz (1984) found that MDI works best when clients use a three-point or lateral hand position to activate canisters. Manufacturers indicate that the two-point hand position is least effective.

Irrigations

Medications may be used to irrigate or wash out a body cavity and are delivered through a stream of solution. Irriga-

tions are most commonly performed with sterile water, saline, or antiseptic solutions on the eye, ear, throat, vagina, and urinary tract. When there is a break in the skin or mucosa, the nurse uses aseptic technique to perform an irrigation. When the cavity to be irrigated is not sterile, as in the case with the ear canal (Procedure 35-14), vagina, or eye, clean technique is acceptable. In health care settings, however, sterile solutions are used. An irrigation can be used to cleanse an area or apply a medication or heat or cold to injured tissue. When performing irrigations, the nurse follows the following principles:

1. Avoid further injury to tissue
2. Prevent the transmission of infection
3. Maintain the client's comfort

■ RESTORATIVE CARE: TEACHING CLIENTS TO ADMINISTER INTRAVENOUS THERAPY AT HOME

Sometimes clients may be discharged from an acute care setting and receive intravenous therapy in the home setting. Medications such as antibiotics, chemotherapy, total parenteral nutrition, pain medications and blood transfusion may be given in the home. Most clients who receive home intravenous therapy will have a central venous catheter (see Chapter 44) inserted before being discharged home. Begin your client education by teaching clients how to identify complications of infections such as erythema, swelling, and fever. Teach the client to report any problems with infusion such as the inability to infuse the solution and how to respond to alarms if electronic equipment is in use. The client will also need to learn how to flush the catheter with a heparinized solution and change the catheter dressing.

Clients who are sent home with intravenous therapy should be carefully assessed in their ability to manage this therapy at home. Most institutions require that the client and a care giver be taught how to care for home IV therapy.

Administering Nasal Drops and Sprays

STEPS	RATIONALE
1. Review physician's medication order for client's name, drug name, concentration of solution, number of drops, and time of administration.	Ensures safe and correct administration of medication.
2. Refer to medical record to determine which sinus is affected.	Will affect positioning that client assumes during drug instillation.
3. Wash hands.	Reduces transmission of microorganisms.
4. Prepare equipment and supplies:	
a. Prepared medication with clean dropper	Dropper or applicator need not be sterile but should be clean.
b. Medication card, form, or printout	
c. Facial tissue	
d. Small pillow (optional)	Used in positioning client.
e. Washcloth (optional)	Used to clean nares.
5. Check client's identification by reading identification bracelet and asking name.	Ensures that correct client receives medication.
6. Apply gloves. Inspect condition of nose and sinuses (see Chapter 33). Palpate sinuses for tenderness.	Findings provide baseline to monitor effect of medication. Discharge will interfere with drug absorption.
7. Explain procedure regarding positioning and sensations to expect, such as burning or stinging of mucosa or choking sensation as medication trickles into throat.	Helps reduce anxiety.
8. Arrange supplies and medications at bedside.	Ensures smooth, orderly procedure.
9. Instruct client to blow nose unless contraindicated (e.g., risk of increased intracranial pressure or nose bleeds).	Removes mucus and secretions that can block distribution of medication.
10. Administer nasal drops:	
a. Assist client to supine position.	Position provides access to nasal passages.
b. Position head properly:	Position allows medication to drain into affected sinus.
(1) Posterior pharynx—tilt client's head backward.	
(2) Ethmoid or sphenoid sinus—tilt head back over edge of bed or place pillow under shoulder and tilt head back (see the illustration below).	

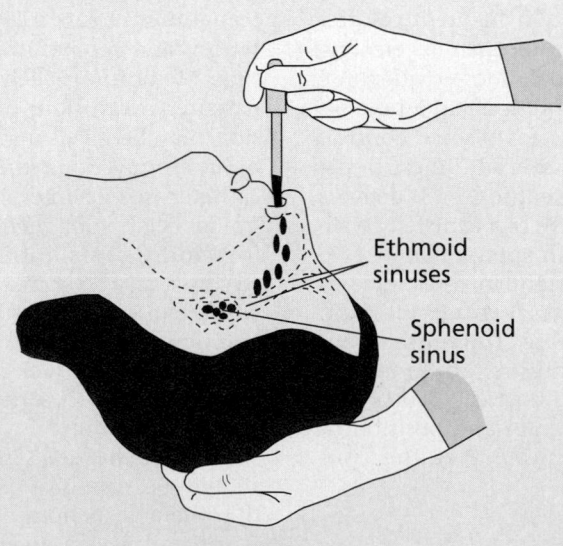

Ethmoid sinuses

Sphenoid sinus

Step 10b(2)

Administering Nasal Drops and Sprays—cont'd

STEPS	RATIONALE
10. Administer nasal drops—cont'd	
b. Position head properly—cont'd	
(3) Frontal and maxillary sinus—tilt head back over edge of bed or pillow with head turned toward side treated (see the illustration below).	
Support client's head with nondominant hand.	Prevents straining of neck muscles.
c. Instruct client to breathe through mouth.	Reduces chance of aspirating nasal drops into trachea and lungs.
d. Hold dropper 1 cm ($^1/_2$ in) above nares and instill prescribed number of drops toward midline of ethmoid bone.	Avoids contamination of dropper. Instilling toward ethmoid bone facilitates distribution of medication over nasal mucosa.
e. Have client remain in supine position 5 min.	Prevents premature loss of medication through nares.
f. Offer facial tissue to blot runny nose, but caution against blowing nose for several minutes.	Allows maximum amount of medication to be absorbed.
11. Administer nasal spray.	
a. Assist client to supine position.	Position provides access to nasal passages
b. Position head properly:	
(1) Tilt client's head backward.	Position allows medication to reach nasal passages.
(2) Support client's head with nondominant hand.	Prevents straining of neck muscles.
(3) For children, keep head in upright position.	Prevents swallowing of spray.
c. Hold tip of container just inside nares.	Position provides best access for spray to reach nasal passages.
d. Instruct client to inhale as the spray enters the nasal passages.	Promotes maximum amount of medication to reach nasal passages.
12. Assist client to a comfortable position after drug has been absorbed.	Restores comfort.
13. Remove gloves and dispose of soiled supplies in proper container. Wash hands.	Maintains neat, orderly environment. Reduces spread of microorganisms.
14. Record medication administration, including drug name, concentration, number of drops, nostril into which drug was instilled, and time of administration.	Timely documentation prevents drug errors (e.g., repeated doses).
15. Observe client for side effects 15 to 30 min after administration.	Drugs absorbed through mucosa can cause systemic reaction.

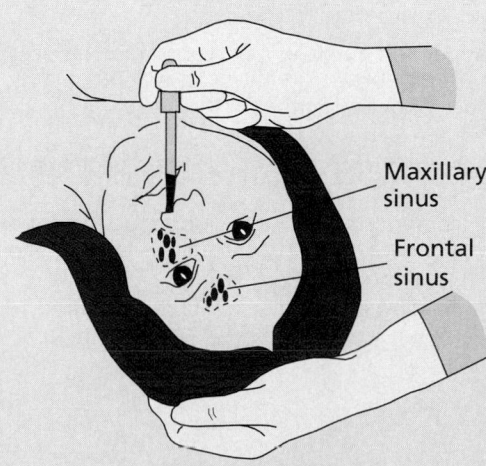

Maxillary sinus

Frontal sinus

Step 10b(3)

Administering Vaginal Medications

STEPS	RATIONALE
1. Review physician's order including client's name, drug name, form (cream or suppository), route, dosage, and time of administration.	Ensures safe and correct administration of medication.
2. Wash hands.	Reduces transfer of microorganisms.
3. Prepare supplies:	
a. Suppository insertion:	
(1) Vaginal suppository	Stored in refrigerator to maintain solid shape.
(2) Clean, disposable gloves	
(3) Lubricating jelly	Eases insertion of suppository.
(4) Clean facial tissues	
(5) Perineal pad (optional)	
(6) Medication ticket, form, or printout	
b. Cream or foam instillation:	
(1) Vaginal cream or foam	Prepared in plastic tube or can.
(2) Plastic applicator	
(3) Clean, disposable gloves	
(4) Paper towel	
(5) Perineal pad (optional)	
(6) Medication ticket, form, or printout	
4. Check client's identification by reading identification bracelet and asking name.	Ensures that correct client receives medication.
5. Inspect condition of external genitalia and vaginal canal (see Chapter 33).	Findings provide baseline to monitor effect of medication.
6. Assess client's ability to manipulate applicator or suppository and to position self to insert medication.	Mobility restriction indicates level of assistance required from nurse.
7. Explain procedure to client. Be specific if client plans to self-administer medication.	Promotes understanding. Will enable client to self-administer drug if physically able.
8. Arrange supplies at bedside.	Ensures smooth procedure.
9. Close room curtain or door.	Provides privacy.
10. Assist client to lie in dorsal recumbent position.	Provides easy access to and good exposure of vaginal canal. Also allows suppository to dissolve without escaping through orifice.
11. Keep abdomen and lower extremities draped.	Minimizes embarrassment.
12. Apply disposable gloves.	Prevents transmission of infection between you and client.
13. Be sure vaginal orifice is well-illuminated by room light or gooseneck lamp.	Proper insertion requires visualization of external genitalia.
14. Insert suppository with gloved hand:	
a. Remove suppository from foil wrapper and apply liberal amount of petroleum jelly to smooth or rounded end. Lubricate gloved index finger of dominant hand.	Lubrication reduces friction against mucosal surfaces during insertion.
b. With nondominant gloved hand, gently retract labial folds.	Exposes vaginal orifice.
c. Insert rounded end of suppository along posterior wall of vaginal canal entire length of finger (7.5 to 10 cm or 3 to 4 in) (see the illustration on p. 861, left).	Proper placement ensures equal distribution of medication along walls of vaginal cavity.
d. Withdraw finger and wipe away remaining lubricant from around orifice and labia.	Maintains comfort.

Administering Vaginal Medications—cont'd

STEPS	RATIONALE

15. Apply cream or foam:

　a. Fill cream or foam applicator following package directions.

Dosage is prescribed by volume in applicator.

　b. With nondominant gloved hand, gently retract labial folds.

Exposes vaginal orifice.

　c. With dominant gloved hand, insert applicator approximately 5 to 7.5 cm (2 to 3 in). Push applicator plunger to deposit medication into vagina (see the illustration below, right).

Allows equal distribution of medication along vaginal walls.

　d. Withdraw applicator and place on paper towel. Wipe off residual cream from labia or vaginal orifice.

Residual cream on applicator may contain microorganisms.

16. Remove gloves by pulling them inside out and discard in appropriate receptacle. Wash hands.

Reduces transfer of microorganisms.

17. Instruct client to remain on back for at least 10 min.

Medication will be distributed and absorbed evenly throughout vaginal cavity and not be lost through orifice.

18. If applicator is used, wash with soap and warm water, rinse, and store for future use.

Vaginal cavity is not sterile. Soap and water assist in removal of bacteria and residual cream.

19. Offer client perineal pad when she resumes ambulation.

Provides comfort.

20. Inspect condition of vaginal canal and external genitalia between applications.

Evaluates whether vagial medication effectively reduced irritation or inflammation of tissues.

21. Record drug name, dosage, route, and time of administration on medication record.

Timely recording prevents drug errors.

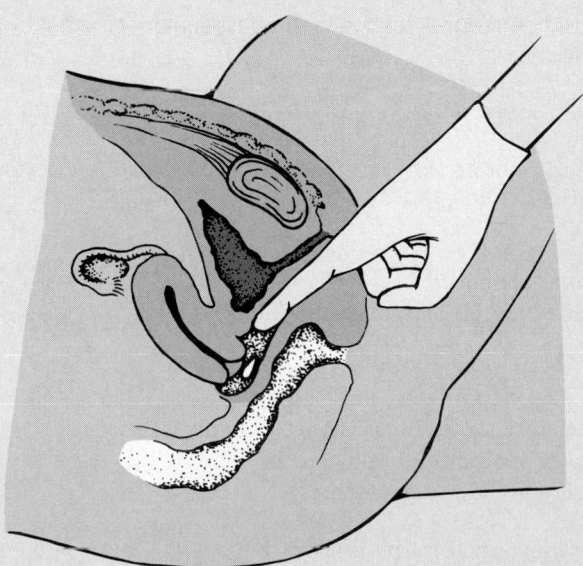

Step 14c

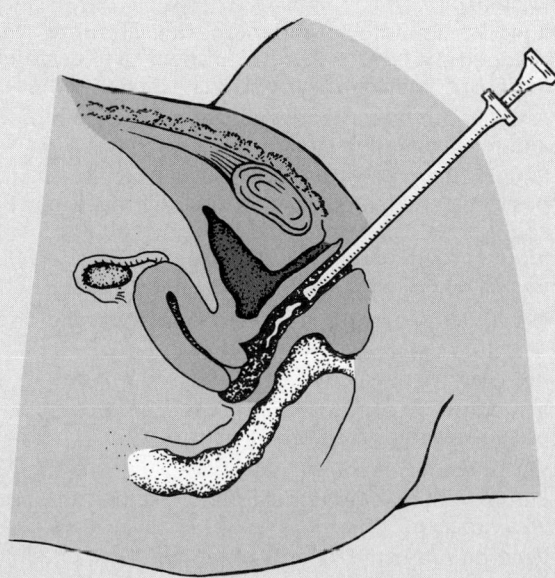

Step 15c

PROCEDURE 35-12

Administering Rectal Suppositories

STEPS	RATIONALE
1. Review physician's order, including client's name, drug name, form, route, and time of administration.	Ensures safe and correct administration of medication.
2. Review medical record for rectal surgery or bleeding.	Conditions contraindicate use of suppository.
3. Wash hands.	Reduces transfer of microorganisms.
4. Prepare equipment and supplies: a. Rectal suppository b. Water-soluble lubricant c. Clean, disposable gloves d. Tissue e. Medication form or printout	

Step 13

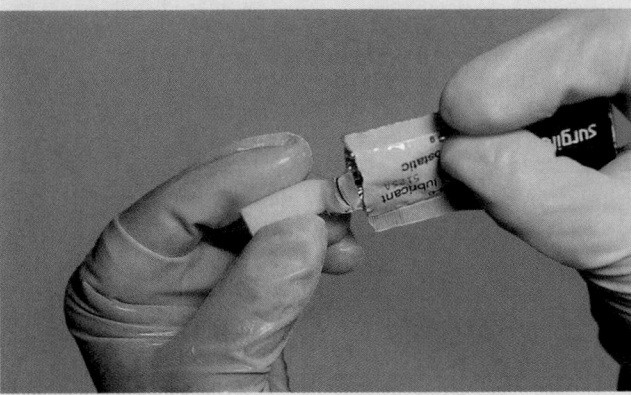

5. Apply disposable gloves.	Prevents contact with infected fecal material.
6. Check client's identification by reading identification bracelet and asking name.	Ensures that correct client receives medication.
7. Explain procedure. Be specific if client wishes to self-administer drug.	Promotes understanding and cooperation. Will enable client to self-administer drug if physically able.
8. Arrange supplies at bedside.	Ensures smooth procedure.
9. Close room curtain or door.	Maintains privacy and minimizes embarrassment.
10. Assist client in assuming Sims' position. Keep client draped with only anal area exposed.	Exposes anus and helps client relax external anal sphincter. Maintains privacy and facilitates relaxation.
11. Examine condition of anus externally and palpate rectal walls as needed (see Chapter 33). If gloves become soiled, dispose of them by turning them inside out and placing them in proper receptacle.	Determines presence of active rectal bleeding. Palpation determines whether rectum is filled with feces, which may interfere with suppository placement. Reduces transmission of infection.
12. Apply disposable gloves (if previous gloves were discarded).	Minimizes contact with fecal material and reduces transmission of microorganisms.
13. Remove suppository from wrapper and lubricate rounded end (see the illustration above). Lubricate index finger of dominant hand with a water-soluble lubricant.	Lubrication reduces friction as suppository enters rectal canal.
14. Ask client to take slow deep breaths through mouth and relax anal sphincter.	Forcing suppository through constricted sphincter causes pain.
15. Retract buttocks with nondominant hand. Insert suppository gently through anus, past internal sphincter and against rectal wall, 10 cm (4 in) in adults, 5 cm (2 in) in children and infants.	Suppository must be placed against rectal mucosa for eventual absorption and therapeutic action.
16. Withdraw finger and wipe anal area with tissue.	Provides comfort.
17. Discard gloves by turning them inside out, and dispose of them in appropriate receptacle.	Reduces transfer of microorganisms.
18. Ask client to remain flat or on side for 5 min.	Prevents expulsion of suppository.
19. If suppository contains laxative or fecal softener, place call light within reach.	Provides client with sense of control over elimination. Allows client to obtain assistance to bedpan or toilet.
20. Wash hands.	Reduces risk of transfer of infection.
21. Return within 5 min to determine whether suppository was expelled.	Reinsertion may be necessary.
22. Record drug name, doage, route, and time of administration on medication record.	Timely recording prevents errors.
23. Observe for effects of suppository (e.g., bowel movement, relief of nausea) 30 min after administration.	Evaluates effectiveness of medication and relief of client's symptoms.

Using Metered-Dose Inhalers

STEPS	RATIONALE
1. Review physician's medication order, including client's name, drug name, dosage, number of inhalations, and time of administration.	Ensures safe and correct administration of medication.
2. Assess client's ability to hold and manipulate inhaler.	Impairment of grasp, muscle strength, or tremors of hands interfere with ability to depress inhaler canister.
3. Assess drug schedule and number of inhalations prescribed for each dose.	Influences explanations nurse provides for use of inhaler.
4. Have client prepare equipment and supplies:	
a. MDI with medication canister	
b. Facial tissues (optional)	
c. Wash basin or sink with warm water	Used to clean inhaler.
d. Paper towel	
5. Instruct client in comfortable environment by sitting in chair in hospital room or at kitchen table in home.	Client will be more likely to remain perceptive of explanation.
6. Allow client to manipulate inhaler and canister. Explain and demonstrate how canister fits into inhaler.	Client must be familiar with how to use equipment.
7. Explain *metered dose* and warn client about overuse of inhaler, including drug side effects.	Client must not arbitrarily decide to administer excessive inhalations because of risk of serious side effects. If given in recommended doses, side effects are uncommon.
8. Explain steps used to administer inhaled dose of medication. (Demonstrate steps when possible.)	Use of simple, step-by-step explanations allows client to ask questions at any point during procedure. Nurse demonstrates depression of canister without self-administering drug dose.
a. Remove cap and hold inhaler upright, grasping it with thumb and first two fingers.	
b. Shake inhaler.	Mixes medication evenly within solution so that aerosol drug concentration is even.
c. Tilt head back slightly and breathe out.	Maximizes airway exposure to medication from inhaler.
d. Position inhaler in one of following ways:	
(1) Open mouth with inhaler 0.5 to 1 cm (1 to 2 in) away from mouth (see the illustration below, left).	Avoids rapid influx of inhaled medication and subsequent airway irritation.
(2) OPTION: attach spacer to mouthpiece of inhaler (see the illustration below, right).	Eliminates rapid influx of particles from inhaled drugs, which reduces irritant properties and tendency to cough. Spacer is recommended for young children (National Heart, Lung, and Blood Institute, 1991).
(3) Place mouthpiece of inhaler or spacer in mouth (see the illustration on p. 864).	

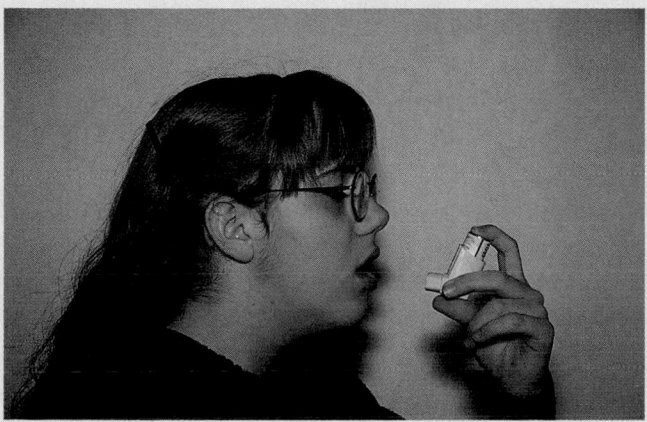

Step 8d(1)

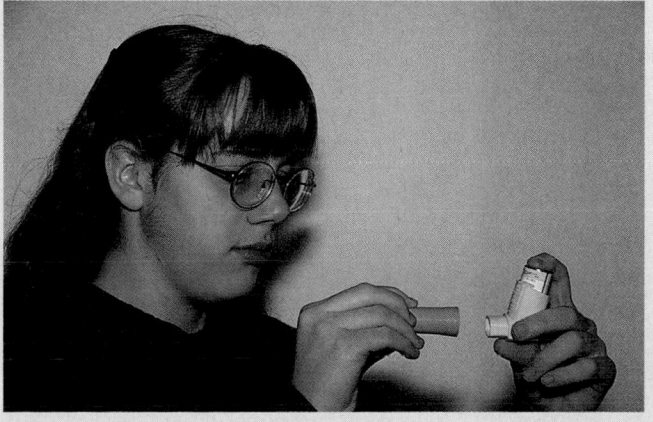

Step 8d(2)

Continued.

PROCEDURE 35-13

Using Metered-Dose Inhalers—cont'd

STEPS	RATIONALE
8. Explain steps used to administer inhaled dose of medication. (Demonstrate steps when possible.)—cont'd	
e. Press down on inhaler to release medication (one puff) while inhaling slowly.	Medication is distributed to airways during inhalation. Inhalation through mouth rather than nose draws medication more effectively into airways.
f. Breathe in slowly for 2 to 3 sec.	As client inhales, particles of medication are delivered to airway (National Heart, Lung, and Blood Institute, 1991).
g. Hold breath for approximately 10 sec.	Allows tiny drops of aerosol spray to reach deeper branches of airways.
h. Repeat puffs as ordered, waiting 1 min between puffs.	Allows maximal airway effect from first puff of medication. Therefore airways are more open for second delivery. Thus more particles are delivered directly to airways.
9. If two inhaled medications are prescribed, wait 5 to 10 min between inhalations or as ordered by physician.	Drugs must be inhaled sequentially. Usually bronchodilator are given first to maximize airway opening, followed by other inhaled medications such as steroids.
10. Explain that client may feel gagging sensation in throat caused by droplets of medication on pharynx or tongue.	Results when inhalant is sprayed and inhaled incorrectly.
11. Instruct client in removing medication canister and cleaning inhaler in warm water.	Accumulation of spray around mouthpiece can interfere with proper distribution during use. Accumulation at mouthpiece increases risk of microorganism accumulation and oral infections.
12. Teach client to measure amount of medication remaining in canister by immersing in large bowel of water	
13. Ask if client has questions.	Allows clarification of misconceptions or misunderstanding.
14. Have client demonstrate use of inhaler and explain drug schedule.	Provides feedback for measuring learning. Improves likelihood of compliance with therapy (Redman, 1993).
15. Instruct client against repeating inhalations before next scheduled dose.	Drugs are prescribed at intervals during day to provide constant bronchodilation and minimize side effects.
16. Describe in nurses' notes content of skill taught and client's ability to perform skill.	Provides continuity to teach plan so that other members of nursing staff will not teach same material.

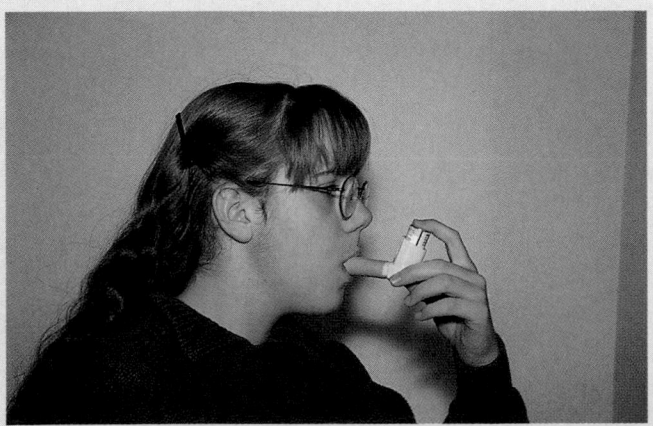

Step 8d(3)

Ear Irrigations

STEPS	RATIONALE
1. Review physician's order for client name, purpose of irrigation, type of irrigant ordered, and time of administration.	Ensures safe and correct administration of irrigation.
2. Check client's identification by reading identification bracelet and asking name.	Ensures that correct client receives irrigation.
3. Wash hands. Apply gloves.	Reduces transfer of microorganisms.
4. Assess condition of external ear structures and canal for redness, swelling, and discharge (see Chapter 33).	Evidence of signs of infection serves as baseline data in determining effectiveness of irrigation.
5. Determine whether client is experiencing localized tenderness or discomfort.	Indicates inflammation of outer ear structures.
6. Prepare equipment and supplies:	
a. Container of sterile irrigating solution warmed to room temperature	Warmed solution minimizes chance of causing client to feel dizzy when solution comes in contact with tympanic membrane.
b. Irrigating syringe (rubber bulb or Asepto)	Used to introduce solution under low pressure.
c. Kidney-shaped basin	Used to collect irrigating solution.
d. Towel	
e. Applicator swab and cotton balls	Used to clean and dry ear canal.
7. Explain procedure. Warn that irrigation may cause sensation of dizziness, fullness, and warmth.	Prepares client to anticipate effects of irrigation and promotes cooperation.
8. Arrange supplies at bedside.	Ensures smooth procedure.
9. Close curtain or room door.	Maintains privacy.
10. Assist client to assume sitting or lying position with head tilted or turned toward affected ear. Place towel under client's head and shoulder and have client hold basin under affected ear.	Position minimizes leakage of fluids around neck and facial area for comfort. Solution will flow from ear canal to basin.
11. Gently clean auricle and ear canal with cotton applicator. Do not force drainage or cerumen into ear canal.	Prevents infected material from reentering ear canal.
12. Fill irrigating syringe with solution (approximately 50 ml).	Enough fluid is needed to provide steady irrigating stream.
13. Gently grasp auricle and straighten ear canal by pulling it down and back (children) or upward and outward (adult).	Allows fluid to flow length of canal.
14. Slowly instill irrigating solution by holding tip of syringe 1 cm ($^1/_2$ inch) above opening of ear canal. Allow fluid to drain out during instillation. Continue until canal is cleansed or all solution is used.	Slow instillation prevents buildup of pressure in ear canal and ensures contact of medication with all of canal surfaces.
15. Do *not* occlude canal with tip of syringe.	Buildup of fluid in canal under forced pressure could cause rupture of tympanic membrane.
16. Dry off outer ear canal with cotton ball. Leave cotton loosely in place for 5 to 10 min.	Maintains comfort. Absorbs excess moisture in ear canal.
17. Assist client to sitting position.	Maintains comfort.
18. Remove gloves and wash hands. Dispose of supplies.	Reduces transmission of infection.
19. Record and report irrigation solution used, character of ear structures, appearance of fluid return or discharge, and client's response.	Documents response to therapy.

■ Key Concepts ■

▶ Learning drug classifications improves the understanding of nursing implications for administering drugs with similar characteristics.

▶ Nurse practice acts define and set limits on the scope of a nurse's professional functions and responsibilities in giving medications.

▶ All controlled substances are handled according to strict procedures that account for each drug.

▶ The nurse applies understanding of the physiological action of drug action when timing administration, selecting routes, initiating actions to promote drug efficacy, and observing responses to drugs.

▶ Clients with alterations in organs that metabolize or excrete drugs are at risk for drug toxicity.

▶ The older adult's body undergoes structural and functional changes that alter drug actions and influence the manner in which nurses provide drug therapy.

▶ Children's drug dosages are computed on the basis of body surface area.

▶ Repeated doses of a drug are required to achieve constant therapeutic blood levels.

▶ Drugs given parenterally are absorbed more quickly than drugs administered by other routes.

▶ Each drug order should include the client's name, order date, drug name, dosage, route and frequency of administration, and physician's signature.

▶ A teaching plan for drug therapy should include guidelines for drug safety.

▶ The "five rights" of drug administration ensure accurate preparation and administration of drug dosages.

▶ Nurses administer only medications they prepare.

▶ The nurse never administers a drug without accurately identifying a client.

▶ Drugs should be charted immediately after administration.

▶ A nurse uses clinical judgment in determining the best time to administer PRN medications.

▶ The nurse reports a drug error immediately.

▶ When preparing medications, the nurse checks the drug container label against the medication card, form, or printout three times.

▶ The nurse never leaves a prepared medication unattended.

▶ The nurse rotates injection sites when giving repeated parenteral administrations.

▶ Failure to select injection sites by anatomical landmarks may lead to tissue, bone, or nerve damage.

■ Key Terms ■

Absorption, p. 794
Air-lock technique, p. 836
Allergic reaction, p. 796
Apothecary system, p. 801
Bioavailability, p. 791
Biotransformation, p. 795
Buccal, p. 798
Concentration, p. 802
Controlled substances, p. 792
Drug abuse, p. 793
Drug dependence, p. 793
Drug interaction, p. 796
Epidural, p. 799
Heparin lock, p. 847
Idiosyncratic reaction, p. 796
Infusion, p. 837
Instillation, p. 800
Intraarterial, p. 800
Intraarticular, p. 800
Intracardiac, p. 800
Intradermal (ID), p. 799
Intramuscular (IM), p. 799
Intraosseous, p. 800
Intraperitoneal, p. 800
Intrapleural, p. 800
Intrathecal, p. 800
Intravenous (IV), p. 799
Irrigation, p. 800
IV bolus, p. 839
Lipodystrophy, p. 828
Medication, p. 790
Metric system, p. 801
Narcotics, p. 805
Over-the-counter drugs, p. 797
Parenteral, p. 798
Pharmacokinetics, p. 794
Piggyback sets, p. 847
Polypharmacy, p. 814
Serum concentration, p. 796
Serum half-life, p. 796
Side effects, p. 795
Solution, p. 802
Subcutaneous (SQ), p. 799
Sublingual, p. 798
Synergistic effect, p. 796
Therapeutic effect, p. 795

Topical, p. 800

Toxic effects, p. 795

Z-track method, p. 835

∎ CRITICAL THINKING EXERCISES ∎

1. During assessment, you note that your client is taking two types of antihypertensive medications prescribed by two different physicians. What actions do you need to take?

2. You are preparing to give a parenteral injection of preoperative atropine. You check the order and calculate the dose. You note that your calculations result in a 3-ml dose. You recognize that this is an excessive dose, and you recalculate the dose and obtain the same answer. You check the dosing information against the physician's order and realize that the order is excessive. You verify this information with the charge nurse, who says "The order is okay." What action do you take at this point?

3. You need to give an injectable pain medication to a client with metastatic cancer. The client's pain increases with change of position, the client is cachexic and is receiving multiple injections. What information do you need to prepare the medication, the syringe, and the needle and to determine the site of injection?

4. You are caring for a septic client, and the physician writes two new intravenous antibiotic orders in addition to the two intravenous antibiotics the client is already receiving. In planning care, you and the physician agree that there could be potential drug interactions with these antibiotics. What do you do to reduce the risk of drug interactions for this client?

REFERENCES

Abdoo YM: Designing a patient care medication and recording system that uses code technology, *Comput Nurs* 10(3): 116, 1992.

American Pharmaceutical Association: Summary of the final report of the scope of pharmacy practice project, *Am J Hosp Pharm* 51:2179, 1994.

American Psychiatric Association: *Diagnostic and Statistical manual of mental disorders (DSM-IV)*, rev 4, Washington, DC, 1994, The Association.

Bohony J: Fighting the needlestick battle without needles, *Med Surg Nurs* 2(6):469, 1993.

Buckley T, Dudley S, Donowitz L: Defining unnecessary disinfection procedures for single-dose and multiple dose vials, *Am J Crit Care* 3(6):448, 1994.

Burman R, Berkowitz H: IV bolus: effective but potentially hazardous, *Crit Care Nurs* 6(1):22, 1986.

Clark JB, Queener SF, Karb GB: *Pharmacologic basis of nursing practice,* ed 4, St Louis, 1993, Mosby.

Cohen M: Do we still need the apothecary system? *Nurs* 23(2):57, 1993.

Donnelly D: Instilling eye drops: difficulties experienced by clients following cataract surgery, *J Adv Nurs* 12:235, 1987.

Ebersole P, Hess P: *Toward health aging: human needs and nursing response,* ed 4, St Louis, 1994, Mosby.

Edgar TA, Lee DS, Cousins DD: Experience with a national medication error reporting program, *Am J Hosp Pharm* 51:1335, 1994.

Jagger J: *Preventable needlesticks, preventable HIV infections, preventable deaths among health care workers.* Testimony before Rep. Ron Wyden Hearings in Washington, DC, 1992.

Kim MJ, McFarland GK, McLane AM: *Pocket guide to nursing diagnosis,* ed 5, St Louis, 1994, Mosby.

Mafofsky D, Cone JE: *Infect Control Hosp Epidemiol* 14(3):140, 1993.

Martin M, Mehery D: Intrapleural analgesia: a new technique, *Crit Care Nurs* 14(5):31, 1994.

Miller T: How you can reduce your risk of a needle's stick, *Crit Care Choices 94* 1994, Springhouse Corporation.

National Heart, Lung, and Blood Institute: *Guidelines for the diagnosis and management of asthma,* National Asthma Education Program, Expert Panel Report, Pub No 91-3042, Bethesda, Md, 1991, The Institute

Perini V, Vermeulen LC: Comparison of automated medication-management systems, *Am J Hosp Pharm* 51:1883, 1994.

Peterson FY, Kirchoff KT: Analysis of the research about heparinized versus nonheparinized intravascular lines, *Heart Lung* 20(6):631, 1991.

Petrosin BM et al: Implications of selected problems with nasoenteral tube feedings, *Crit Care Nurs Q* 12:1, 1989.

Redman BK: *The process of client education,* ed 7, St Louis, 1993, Mosby.

Statz E: Hand strength and metered dose inhalers, *Am J Nurs* 84:800, 1984.

Wild L, Coyne C: The basics and beyond: Epidural analgesia, *Am J Nurs* 92:4, 1992.

Wong DL: *Essentials of pediatric nursing,* ed 4, St Louis, 1993, Mosby.

Wong DL: *Whaley & Wong's nursing care of infants and children* ed 5, St Louis, 1995, Mosby.

ADDITIONAL READINGS

Adams KS, Zehrer CL, Thomas W. Comparison of a needleless system with conventional heparin locks, *Am J Infect Control* 21(5):263, 1993.

Beecroft PC, Kongelbeck S: How safe are intramuscular injections, *AACN Clin Issues* 5(2):207, 1994.

Brown M, Mulhound J: *Drug calculations,* ed 5, 1995, St Louis, Mosby.

Cohen MR, Senders J, Davis N: 12 ways to prevent medications errors, *Nurs* 24(2):34, 1994

Doan L, Fischer L, McDonald T: How to give peritoneal chemotherapy, *Am J Nurs* 90(4):59, 1990.

Estoup M: Approaches and limitations of medication delivery in clients with enteral feeding tubes, *Crit Care Nurs* 14(1):68, 1994.

Jurb JB: Evaluating needless products, *Med Surg Nurs* 3(3):176, 1994.

Lyons M, Stuart T: Epidural narcotics for general care units, *Nurs Manage* 22:33, 1991.

Martin M, Mehery D: Intrapleural analgesia: a new technique, *Crit Care Nurs* 14(5):31, 1994.

Naber L, Jones G, Halm M: Epidural analgesia for effective pain control, *Crit Care Nurs* 14(5):69, 1994.

Newhouse J: Opening your eyes to intraocular drug administration, *Nurs* 24 (6):44, 1994.

Owens SE, Fraser VJ: Needles and needle protection devices: a second look at efficacy and selection, *Infect Control Hosp Epidemiol* 14(11):657, 1993.

Rettig FM, Southby JR: Using different body positions to reduce discomfort from dorsogluteal injection, *Nurs Res* 31:219, 1982.

Woodridge JB, Jackson JG: Evaluation of bruises and areas of induration after two techniques of subcutaneous heparin injection, *Heart Lung* 17:476, 1988.

Willens JB: Giving fentanyl for pain outside the OR, *Am J Nurs* 94(2):24, 1994.

Shepherd MJ, Swearingen P: Z-track injections, *Am J Nurs* 84:746, 1984.

UNIT 7

Providing a Safe Environment

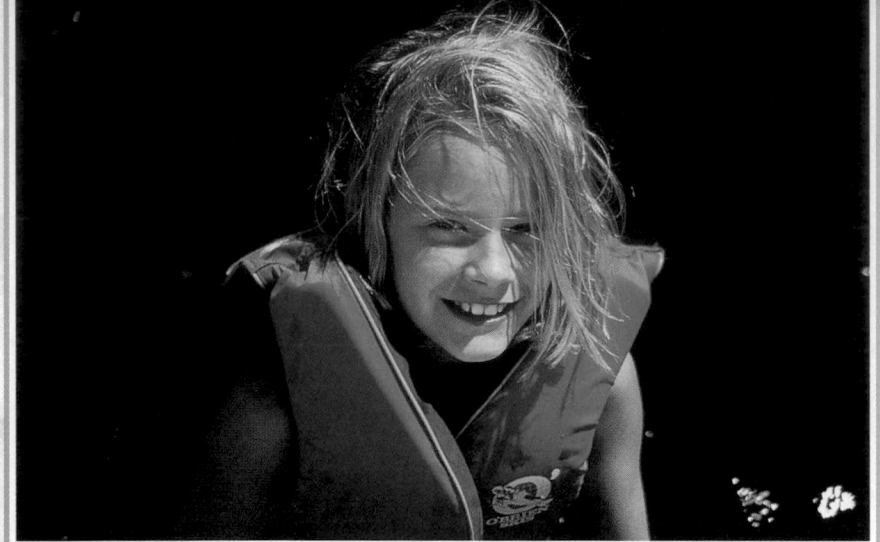

## Chapter 36

Safety

Objectives

Mastery of content in this chapter will enable the student to:

▶ Define the key terms listed.

▶ Describe how unmet basic physiological needs of oxygen, fluids, nutrition, and temperature can threaten clients' safety.

▶ Discuss methods to reduce physical hazards.

▶ Describe current methods to reduce the transmission of pathogens.

▶ Describe present methods of pollution control.

▶ Discuss the specific risks to safety related to developmental age.

▶ Describe the four categories of risks in a health care agency.

▶ Describe assessment activities designed to identify clients' physical, psychosocial, and intellectual status as it pertains to their safety status.

▶ State nursing diagnoses associated with risks to safety.

▶ Develop a care plan for clients whose safety is threatened.

▶ Describe nursing interventions specific to clients' age for reducing risk of falls, fires, poisonings, and electrical hazards.

▶ Describe methods to evaluate interventions designed to maintain or promote safety.

Safety, often defined as freedom from psychological and physical injury, is a basic human need that must be met. Safe health care and community environment are essential for a client's survival. The nurse must assess the client and the environment for hazards that threaten safety, and then intervene when necessary. By doing this, the nurse is an active participant in illness prevention, health maintenance, and health promotion.

ENVIRONMENTAL SAFETY

A client's **environment** includes all of the many physical and psychosocial factors that influence or affect the life and survival of that client. This broad definition of environment incorporates all of the settings in which the nurse and client interact; for example, the home, community center, clinic, hospital, and long-term care facility. Safety in these settings reduces the incidence of illness and injury, shortens the length of treatment and/or hospitalization, improves or maintains a client's functional status, and increases the client's sense of well-being. A safe environment affords protection to the staff as well, and allows them to function at their optimal level.

A safe environment is one in which basic needs are met, physical hazards are reduced, transmission of pathogenic organisms is reduced, sanitation is maintained, and pollution is controlled.

Basic Needs

Physiological needs, including oxygen, optimum humidity, nutrition, and optimum temperature, influence a person's safety. Meeting basic physiological human needs is necessary for achieving safety and security needs (see Chapter 27).

OXYGEN

The nurse must be aware of factors in a client's environment that decrease the amount of available oxygen. A common environmental hazard in the home is an improperly functioning heating system. A furnace that is not properly vented may introduce carbon monoxide into the environment. **Carbon monoxide** is a colorless, odorless, poisonous gas produced by the combustion of carbon or organic fuels. Carbon monoxide binds strongly with hemoglobin, preventing the formation of oxyhemoglobin and thus reducing the supply of oxygen delivered to tissues (see Chapter 44). Seasonal inspections of heating systems and appliances should be done in private homes as well as institutions. Carbon monoxide detectors (Fig. 36-1) are available for home or institutional use at a reasonable cost.

Humidity

The relative humidity of the air in the environment may affect the client's health and safety. **Relative humidity** is the amount of water vapor in the air compared with the maximum amount of water vapor that the air could contain at the same temperature. The comfort zone for humidity varies from person to person, but most people are comfortable when the humidity is between 60% and 70%.

When the relative humidity is high, the skin's moisture evaporates slowly. Thus, during hot, humid weather, people feel uncomfortably hot and sticky. If the relative humidity is low, the skin's moisture evaporates quickly. This is why people feel cooler and more comfortable when the temperature is 32.2°C (90°F) with a relative humidity of 30% than when the temperature is 32.2°C (90°F) with a relative humidity of 85%.

Increasing the environmental humidity can have therapeutic benefits. Children and adults with upper respiratory tract infections usually experience improvement in their symptoms when a humidifier is placed in the room while they sleep. The humidifier increases the relative humidity of the inhaled air, which helps liquefy secretions and improve breathing. It is important to follow the manufacturer's directions regarding the cleaning of home humidifiers to reduce the contamination of the water.

NUTRITION

Meeting nutritional needs adequately and safely requires environmental controls and knowledge. In the home the client needs a refrigerator and a freezer compartment to keep perishable foods fresh. An adequate, clean water supply is needed to wash fresh produce and dishes. Provisions for garbage collection are necessary to maintain sanitary conditions.

Foods that are inadequately prepared or stored, or subject to unsanitary conditions, increase the client's risk for food infections and food poisoning. Bacterial food infections result from eating food contaminated by bacteria such as salmonellosis, shigellosis, and listeriosis. **Food poisoning** is caused by ingestion of bacterial toxins produced in food; staphylococcal and clostridial bacteria are the most common causes. Although most foodborne diseases are bacterial, the hepatitis A virus is spread by fecal contamination of food, water, or milk (Williams, 1994).

For illnesses caused by bacterial contamination, the onset of symptoms may be very rapid or may take a week or longer. The incubation period for hepatitis A is from 2 to 6 weeks (Pagana and Pagana, 1995). Assessments for suspected food infections or poisoning include obtaining a client's history, conducting an examination of gastrointestinal (GI) and central nervous system (CNS) function, observing for a fever, and analyzing cultures of feces and vomitus. Suspected food and water sources are also studied. Preventive measures include thorough handwashing prior to handling food, adequate cooking, and proper storage and refrigeration of perishable foods.

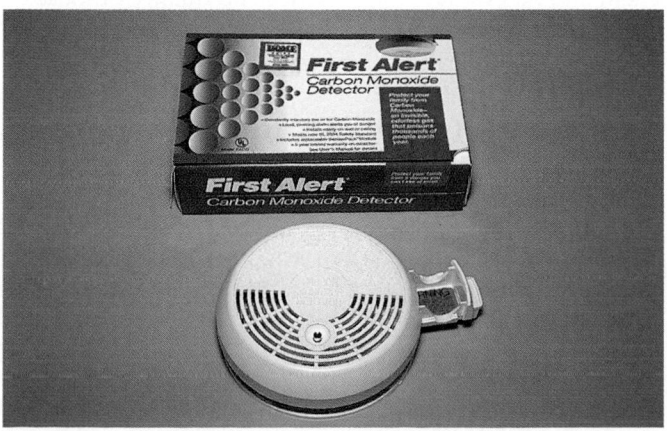

Fig. 36-1 Carbon monoxide detector.

To protect consumers, commercially processed and packaged foods are subject to **Food and Drug Administration (FDA)** regulations and usually contain a minimal amount of contaminants. The FDA is a federal agency responsible for the enforcement of federal regulations regarding the manufacture, processing, and distribution of food, drugs, and cosmetics to protect consumers against the sale of impure or dangerous substances.

Temperature. The comfort zone for environmental temperature varies among individuals, but the usual comfort range is between 18.3° and 23.9°C (65° and 75°F). Temperature extremes that frequently occur during the winter and summer affect not only comfort and productivity but also safety.

Exposure to severe cold for prolonged periods causes frostbite and accidental hypothermia. Frostbite occurs when a surface area of the skin freezes due to exposure to extremely cold temperatures. **Hypothermia** occurs when the core body temperature is 35°C (95°F) or below. A faint, irregular heart rate; slow and shallow respirations; pallor; and mild shivering may be observed. Death may ensue if the condition is not corrected.

Older adults, the young, clients with cardiovascular conditions, clients who have ingested drugs or alcohol in excess, and the homeless are at high risk for hypothermia.

Exposure to extreme heat can result in heatstroke or heat exhaustion. Heat exhaustion causes profuse diaphoresis, hypotension, changes in mental status, muscle cramps, and nausea. Heatstroke is a life-threatening condition with severe changes in mental status, including coma; hyperpyrexia with hot dry skin; and rectal temperatures in excess of 40.5°C (105°F). Chronically ill clients, older adults, and infants are at greatest risk for injury from extreme heat (see Chapter 32).

Reduction of Physical Hazards

Physical hazards in the community and health care settings place clients at risk for injury. Of accidental deaths, motor vehicle accidents rank first, followed by falls, poisonings, drownings, fires, and burns. Falls are the major cause of accidental death in clients 75 years of age and older (Accident Facts, 1993). Up to 40% of persons over 65 fall at least once a year, with 1% to 6% incurring serious injuries (Loew, 1993). Many physical hazards, especially those contributing to falls, can be minimized through adequate lighting, reduction of obstacles, control of bathroom hazards, and security measures.

ENSURING ADEQUATE LIGHTING

Adequate lighting reduces physical hazards by illuminating areas in which the client moves and works. Outside the home, there should be adequate lighting on all walkways. Outdoor lighting also helps protect the home and its inhabitants from crime. Well-lighted garages, walkways, and doorways discourage intruders from entering the premises or hiding in shadows.

Inside the house, halls, staircases, and individual rooms should be adequately lighted so that residents can safely carry out activities of daily living. Night-lights in dark halls, bathrooms, and the rooms of children and older adults help maintain safety by reducing the risk of falls. A night-light in a guest room can help orient an overnight guest who needs to get up in the middle of the night. Artificial lighting should be soft and nonglaring, because glare is a major problem for older adults (Ebersole and Hess, 1994).

DECREASING OBSTACLES

Injuries in the home frequently result from objects, including small rugs on the stairs and floor, wet spots on the floor, and clutter on bedside tables, closet shelves, the top of the refrigerator, and bookshelves. The risk of falls from obstacles is present for all age groups; however, it is greatest for older adults. Falls are usually the result of a combination of intrinsic risk factors, such as illness, drug therapy, and alcohol use, and extrinsic or environmental factors. In some cases, an obstacle or extrinsic factor may be the only cause of a fall. Intrinsic factors may be difficult to modify or eliminate, but usually extrinsic ones are not.

To reduce the risk of injury, all obstacles should be removed from halls and other heavily traveled areas. Necessary objects such as clocks, glasses, tissues, or medications should remain on bedside tables within reach of the client but out of the reach of children in the home. Care should also be taken to ensure that end tables are secure and have stable, straight legs. Nonessential items should be placed in drawers to eliminate clutter.

If small area rugs are used, they should be secured with a nonslip pad or skid-resistant adhesive strips. Area rugs and runners should not be used on stairs. Any carpeting on the stairs should be secured with carpet tacks.

CONTROLLING BATHROOM HAZARDS

Accidents, such as falls, burns, and poisoning, frequently occur in the bathroom. Secure, easily seen grab bars and nonslip, colored adhesive tape on the bottom of the tub are useful in reducing falls in the bathtub. A raised toilet seat with armrests and nonslip strips on the floor in front of the toilet are also helpful (Tideiksaar, 1989). Care should be taken to lower the thermostat setting on the water heater to reduce the risk of burns. In the medicine cabinet, medications should be clearly marked and out of the reach of children. Medication not in use or out-of-date should be discarded by flushing it down the toilet.

SECURING THE HOME

Clients need to take precautions to secure their homes from intruders. When assessing the home for safety, the client should evaluate the presence and quality of locks on doors and windows. Clients should be encouraged to join block associations and work closely with law enforcement personnel to reduce crime in their neighborhoods.

Reduction of Transmission of Pathogens

A **pathogen** is any microorganism capable of producing an illness. One of the most effective methods for limiting the transmission of pathogens is the medical aseptic practice of handwashing (see Chapter 34). Clients must be instructed in proper handwashing technique and encouraged to use it frequently in the home and hospital.

The transmission of disease from person to person can also be reduced and in some cases prevented by immunization. **Immunization** is the process by which resistance to an infectious disease is produced or augmented. Active immunity is acquired by injecting a small amount of attenuated (weakened) or dead organisms or modified toxins from the organism (toxoids) into the body. Passive immunity occurs when antibodies produced by other persons or animals can be introduced into a person's bloodstream for protection against a pathogen (Phipps et al, 1995).

The **human immunodeficiency virus (HIV)**, the pathogen that causes AIDS, and the hepatitis B virus are transmitted through blood and certain other body fluids. Drug abusers frequently share syringes and needles, which increases the risk of acquiring these viruses. Safe sexual practices, including the correct use of condoms and elimination of casual sexual activities, reduce the risk for both of these diseases as well as for other sexually transmitted diseases (STDs). Nurses utilize standard precautions when caring for all clients in order to protect themselves from contact with blood and body fluids (see Chapter 34).

The transmission of disease is also controlled by adequate disposal of human waste through proper construction and repair of sewers and drains. Insect and rodent control is also necessary to reduce the transmission of disease.

Pollution Control

A healthy environment is free of pollution. A **pollutant** is a harmful chemical or waste material discharged into the water, soil, or air. People commonly think of pollution only in terms of air, land, or water pollution, but noise can also be a form of pollution that presents health risks.

Air pollution is the contamination of the atmosphere. Prolonged exposure to air pollution increases the risk of pulmonary disease. In urban areas, industrial waste and vehicle exhaust are common contributors to air pollution. In the home, school, or workplace, cigarette smoke is the primary cause of air pollution. **Land pollution** of soil can be caused by improper disposal of radioactive and bioactive waste products such as dioxin.

Water pollution is the contamination of lakes, rivers, and streams, usually by industrial pollutants. Water-treatment facilities filter harmful contaminants from the water, but these systems may contain flaws. If water becomes contaminated, the public is notified to boil water used for drinking and cooking. Flooding frequently causes damage to water-treatment stations and also requires the boiling of drinking and cooking water.

Noise pollution occurs when the noise level in an en-

vironment becomes uncomfortable to the inhabitants of the environment. Noise levels are measured in units of sound intensity called decibels. Noise-level tolerance varies from individual to individual and is influenced by health status. Occupational noise–induced hearing loss, an irreversible injury, is among the 10 leading causes of occupational diseases in the United States and Canada (Yassi et al, 1991). Clients working in environments with high noise levels need to wear protective devices to reduce hearing loss (Fig. 36-2).

A health care agency such as an intensive care unit can also be polluted by noise. The sounds of machines, people talking, and intercoms can create increased noise levels. Even when the noise level is not high enough to affect hearing acuity, it may produce a syndrome called sensory overload. Sensory overload is a marked increase in the intensity of auditory and visual stimuli. It disrupts processing of information and the client no longer perceives the environment in a meaningful way (see Chapter 39).

∎ NURSING PROCESS AND SAFETY

Assessment

Nurses provide care to clients and families in their communities and health care settings. To ensure a safe environment, the nurse needs to understand what contributes to a safe home, community, or health care environment, and then assess the client and environment for threats to safety. Assessment of the client includes history and physical examination. Assessment of the environment, including the client's home and the health care setting, involves inspection of the facilities (see the box on p. 874). The following section on assessment discusses risk factors to clients in the community and in health care agencies.

COMMUNITY

Risks at Developmental Stages. Threats to safety within the community are influenced by clients' developmental stage, lifestyle, mobility status, sensory impairments, and safety awareness.

Infant, Toddler, and Preschooler. Injuries are the leading cause of death in children over age 1 and cause more death and disabilities than do all diseases combined. The nature of the injury sustained is closely related to normal growth and development behavior. For example, lead poisoning, which is usually caused by the ingestion of paint chips that contain lead, is highest in late infancy and toddlerhood because of the increased level of oral activity and the growing ability to explore the environment (Wong, 1995). Accidents involving children are largely preventable, but parents need to be aware of specific dangers at each stage of growth and development (Table 36-1). Accident prevention thus requires health education for parents and the removal of dangers whenever possible.

School-Age Child. When a child enters school, the environment expands to include the school, transportation to and from school, school friends, and after-school activities. Through discussions with examples, parents, teachers, and nurses must instruct the child in safe practices to follow at school or play.

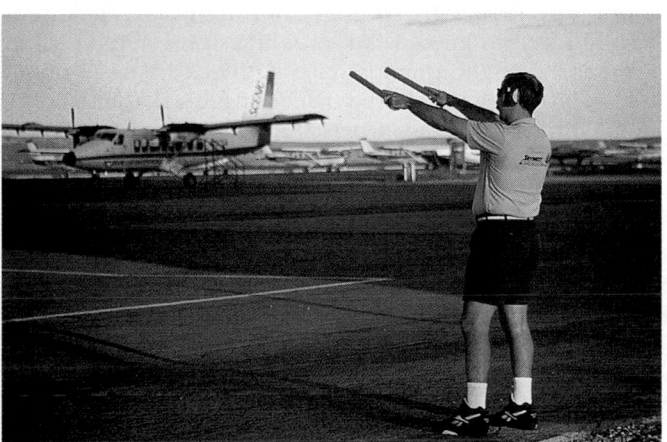

Fig. 36-2 Protective device to reduce hearing loss.

Home Hazard Assessment

HOME EXTERIOR
Are sidewalks uneven?
Are steps in good repair?
Do steps have securely fastened handrails?
Is there adequate lighting?
Is outdoor furniture sturdy?

HOME INTERIOR
Do all rooms, stairways, and halls have adequate lighting?
Are night-lights available?
Are area rugs secured?
Are wooden floors nonslippery?
Is furniture placed appropriately to permit mobility?
Is furniture sturdy enough to provide support for getting
  up and down?
Is temperature and humidity within normal range?
Are there any steps or thresholds that may pose a hazard?
Are all steps in good repair?
Are step edges clearly marked with colored tape?
Are handrails available and secure?

KITCHEN
Are handwashing facilities available?
Is the pilot light on and the area clean on a gas stove?
Are the dials on the stove readable?
Are storage areas within easy reach?
Are cleaning fluids, bleach, etc., in original containers
  and stored safely?
Are cleaning fluids stored out of the reach of children?
Is the water temperature within normal range (115°F to
  145°F)?
Are there clean areas for food storage and preparation?
Is refrigeration adequate?

BATHROOM
Are handwashing facilities available?
Are there skidproof strips or surfaces in the tub/shower?
Are bath mats secured?

Does the client need grab bars near the bathtub and
  toilet?
Does the client need an elevated toilet seat?
Is the medicine cabinet well lighted?
Are all medications current and in original containers?
Are medications out of children's reach?
Are two doses of syrup of ipecac available in homes with
  children?
Is the poison control phone number visible and next to a
  phone?

BEDROOM
Are beds of adequate height to allow getting on and off
  easily?
Is day and night lighting adequate?
Are floor coverings nonskid?
Does the client have a telephone nearby?

ELECTRICAL AND FIRE HAZARDS
Are all appliances in good working order?
Is equipment grounded?
Are electrical cords in good condition?
Are extension cords used only when necessary?
Are the correct number of appliances plugged into one
  outlet?
Are electrical appliances kept away from the sink, tub, or
  shower?
Are the heating/cooling units and fireplace inspected
  annually?
Is there a guard or screen in front of the fireplace?
Are combustible materials stored properly?
Are there smoke, fire (Fig. 36-3) and carbon monoxide
  detectors (Fig. 36-1)?
Is the emergency number for police and fire departments
  visible near the phone?
Has the family discussed and practiced an escape plan in
  case of fire?

Modified from Tideiksaar, 1989; Wong, 1995; Top, 1987; Ebersole and Hess, 1994; and Beck, 1993.

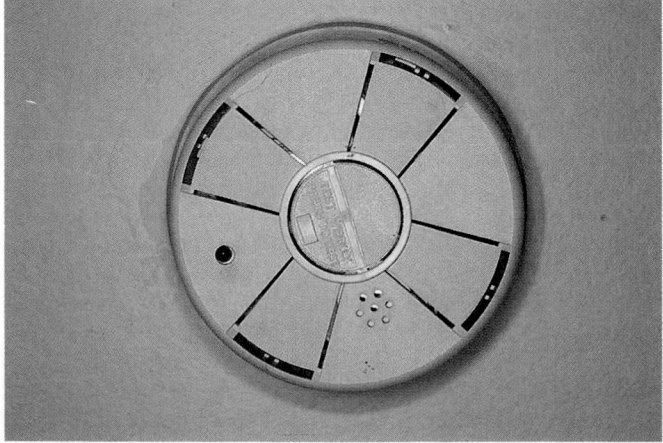

Fig. 36-3 Smoke and fire detector.

Because school-age children are participating in more activities outside their home and neighborhood environments, they are at greater risk of injury from strangers. Therefore the child should be warned repeatedly not to accept candy, food, gifts, or rides from strangers. In addition, a child needs to know what to do if a stranger approaches. Frequently neighborhoods have a "block home" or "safe house." In these homes the owner ensures that an adult is home during the times when children are walking to and from school. If a stranger approaches a child, the child can run to that home, and the adult will protect the child and call the proper authorities. Nurses can work with school systems or neighborhoods to initiate such a system to protect children.

Sports safety is stressed in school sports, but parents and health professionals can reinforce these safety tips by insisting that children wear protective gear while participating in sports at home. For example, schools provide hard batting helmets for baseball games, and parents should also provide this equipment when children are playing baseball in their own backyards.

Table 36-1	Motor Development Changes that Increase Risk of Injury in Infants and Toddlers*	

AGE	MOTOR DEVELOPMENT	HAZARD
1 mo	Baby can hold head midline and parallel to body but is unable to hold head erect.	If not supported, infant's head flops forward or backward.
2 mo	Grasp reflex is present; infant grasps and holds object for few moments or longer.	Child can grasp electrical cords and other dangerous items on floor.
3 mo	Child may begin to roll from back to abdomen and bears weight on forearms.	There is increased risk of falling off bed, changing table, and counter.
4 mo	Increased grasping ability is present. Child explores new objects with mouth.	Infant is able to pick up small objects, which usually are placed immediately into mouth.
	Child possesses increased ability to roll from abdomen and from side to side and to move in rocking motion.	There is increased risk of falling from surfaces.
5 mo	Ability of locomotion increases by rocking, rolling, and twisting.	Infant is able to move purposefully toward objects that may be dangerous.
	Child is able to grasp bottle but should not be left unattended.	Risk of choking on contents increases. Drinking from bottle in supine position can increase risk of ear infections and dental caries in baby and permanent teeth.
	Ability to grasp small objects increases.	There is increased risk of choking on small objects.
6 mo	Infant creeps by propelling self on abdomen, steering with arms and legs.	Child is able to move to potential dangers, such as electrical outlets and household cleaners.
7 mo	Child may be crawling and is able to sit alone for short periods of time.	Infant can move rapidly from one spot to another. Risk of ingesting lead-based paint chips is posed by child's increased mobility.
8 mo	Infant may be able to pull self to standing position and can sit unsupported.	Child can easily fall unless helped back to sitting or lying position.
9 mo	Child begins to crawl up stairs and can stand and move by using furniture for support. (Walking may occur any time after 8 mo.)	Infant can lose balance and fall down stairs, can lose balance with wobbly furniture, and can bruise self on sharp corners of tables and bookcases.
10 mo	Infant climbs up and tries to climb down from chairs and is able to change from prone to sitting position.	Child may fall from chair or open window and is unable to judge distances or limits.
11 mo	Interest in feeding self begins.	Unless foods are cut into small pieces, choking may result.
12 mo	Child may climb out of crib.	There is increased risk of falling out of crib or play pen.
	Infant takes cover off plastic screwtop containers.	Child can open and possibly taste harmful substances.*
15 mo	Child walks with help but cannot walk around corners or stop suddenly without losing balance.	Infant loses sense of balance and falls easily.*
18 mo	Child runs clumsily and falls often.	Child may injure head from severe falls.
	Infant moves furniture and climbs on it.	Infant may pull furniture over on self or fall off furniture.
24 mo	Child is able to turn door knobs.	Child can independently open closed door and may ingest harmful products stored in cabinet, closet, or bathroom. Child may wander to backyard swimming pool.*

Data from Wong DL: *Whaley and Wong's Nursing care of infants and children*, ed 5, St. Louis, 1995, Mosby.
*Data from US Preventive Services Task Force: *Ann Family Pract* 42(1):136, 1990

Bicycle-related injuries are a major cause of death and disability among children, accounting for more than 600 deaths and thousands of emergency room visits each year (Child Health Alert, 1993). Bikes should be in good working order and be the proper size for the child. The child should be taught the rules of the road and cautioned not to engage in dangerous stunts or activities while bike riding. Among the children who die from bicycle accidents, 85% die from head injuries. Researchers estimate that 75% of these deaths could be prevented by wearing a bicycle helmet. Many states are implementing laws requiring bike helmets, and federal legislation is being considered (Child Health Alert, 1993).

Adolescent. As children enter adolescence, they develop greater independence and begin to develop a sense of identity and their own values. In addition, adolescents begin to separate emotionally from their families, and peer groups begin to have a stronger influence.

The struggle toward identity may cause the teenager to experience shyness, fear, and anxiety, with resulting dysfunction at home, at school, or within the peer group. In an attempt to relieve the tensions associated with the physical and psychosocial changes, as well as peer pressures, adolescents may turn to drugs. In addition to the health risks posed by drugs, the ingestion of drugs, including alcohol, increases the incidence of other types of accidents such as drowning and motor vehicle accidents. Accidental injuries are the leading cause of death for adolescents, and approximately 40% of these injuries are related to alcohol use. Alcohol is also related to a significant percent of adolescent homicides and suicides (U.S. Public Health Service, 1994).

When adolescents learn to drive, their environment expands and so does their potential for injury. The young driver must be taught and expected to comply with rules and regulations regarding use of a car. Not using a seat belt is a major risk factor for injury. Many states have mandatory seat belt laws. Common rules include proper use of seat belts, abstinence from alcohol, not riding in a car when the driver is under the influence of alcohol or drugs, and setting a time to be home with the car.

Because adolescence is a time when mature sexual physical characteristics develop, adolescents may begin to have physical relationships with others. They need prompt, correct instruction about abstinence and/or safe sexual practices and birth control.

An emerging problem in the adolescent and young adult population is violence. In 1991, nearly half of the nation's homicide victims were males aged 15 to 34 years. Among males in this age group, homicide was the second leading cause of death. The statistics indicate that this group was responsible for most homicides as well. Between 1985 and 1991, arrest rates for murder and non-negligent manslaughter increased 127% for males 15 to 19, and 43% for males 20 to 24 (CDC, 1994).

Adult. The threats to an adult's safety are frequently related to lifestyle habits. For example, the client who uses alcohol excessively is at greater risk for motor-vehicle accidents. The long-term smoker has a greater risk of cardiovascular or pulmonary disease as a result of the inhalation of smoke into the lungs and the effect of nicotine on the circulatory system. Likewise, the adult experiencing a high level of stress is more likely to have an accident or illness such as headaches, GI disorders, and infections (see Chapter 22).

Older Adult. The physiological changes that occur during the aging process increase the client's risk for falls and other types of accidents such as burns and car accidents (see the box above). Older clients are more likely to fall in the bedroom, bathroom, and kitchen, and outside due to ice on walkways or obstacles in the garden. These falls most often occur while transferring from beds, chairs, and toilets; getting into or out of bathtubs; tripping over carpet edges or doorway thresholds; slipping on wet surfaces; and descending stairs (Tideiskaar, 1989).

Other Risk Factors. Other risk factors include lifestyle, mobility, sensory impairments, and safety awareness.

Lifestyle. Lifestyle can increase safety risks. At greater risk of injury are people who drive or operate machinery while under the influence of chemical substances, who work at inherently dangerous jobs, and who are risk-takers. In addition, people experiencing stress, anxiety, fatigue, or alcohol or drug withdrawal, or those taking prescribed medications may be more accident prone. Because of these factors, clients may be too preoccupied to notice the source of potential accidents such as cluttered stairs or a stop sign.

Mobility. Impaired mobility due to muscle weakness, paralysis, or poor coordination or balance is a major factor in client falls. Immobilization predisposes the client to ad-

---

Physical Assessment Findings in the Older Adult That Increase the Risk of Accidents

MUSCULOSKELETAL CHANGES
Muscle strength and function decreases
Joints become less mobile
Posture changes, some kyphosis is common
Range of motion limited

NERVOUS SYSTEM CHANGES
All voluntary or automatic reflexes slower
Decreased ability to respond to multiple stimuli
Kinesthetic sense less efficient

SENSORY CHANGES
Peripheral vision and lens accommodation decrease
Lens may develop opacity
Stimuli threshold for light touch and pain increases
Hearing impaired as high-frequency tones are less perceptible

GENITOURINARY
Increased nocturia
Increased occurrence of incontinence

Modified from Ebersole P, Hess P: *Toward health aging: human needs and nursing respones,* ed 4, St Louis, 1994, Mosby.

---

ditional physiological and emotional hazards, which in turn can further restrict mobility and independence (see Chapter 37).

Sensory Impairments. Clients with visual, hearing, or communication impairments, such as aphasia and language barriers, are at greater risk for injury in the community. Such clients may not be able to perceive a potential danger or to express their need for assistance (see Chapter 39).

Safety Awareness. Some clients are unaware of safety precautions, such as keeping medicine away from children or reading the expiration date on food products. A complete nursing assessment including home inspection should help the nurse identify the client's level of knowledge regarding home safety so that deficiencies can be corrected with an individualized nursing care plan.

HEALTH CARE AGENCY

The basic types of risks to a client's safety within the health care environment are falls, client-inherent accidents, procedure-related accidents, and equipment-related accidents. The nurse must assess for these four potential problem areas and, considering the developmental level of the client, take steps to prevent or minimize accidents in the agency.

An accident necessitates the filing of an incident report, a confidential document that completely describes any client accident occurring on the premises of a health care agency (see Chapter 12). It documents the accident, client assessment, and interventions carried out for the client. In addition to completing the incident report, the nurse must document the accident in the client's medical record.

Falls. Falls account for up to 90% of all reported incidences in hospitals. The risk for falling is significantly higher in older clients. In addition to age, a history of previous falls, gait and mobility problems, postural hypoten-

Seizure Precautions

STEPS	RATIONALE
1. Assess seizure history, noting frequency of seizures, presence of an aura, and sequence of events if known. Assess medical and surgical conditions that may lead to seizures or exacerbate an existing seizure condition.	This allows the nurse to anticipate impending seizure activity.
2. Assess medication history.	Seizure medication must be taken as prescribed and not stopped suddenly as this may precipitate seizures (Shantz and Spitz, 1993).
3. Have the following equipment available: airway (see the illustration below, left) padding for siderails, headboard (see the illustration below, right) suction machine, and oral suction equipment.	Ensures prompt, organized intervention.

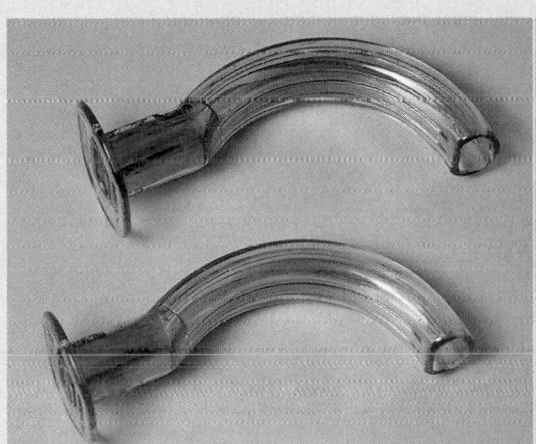 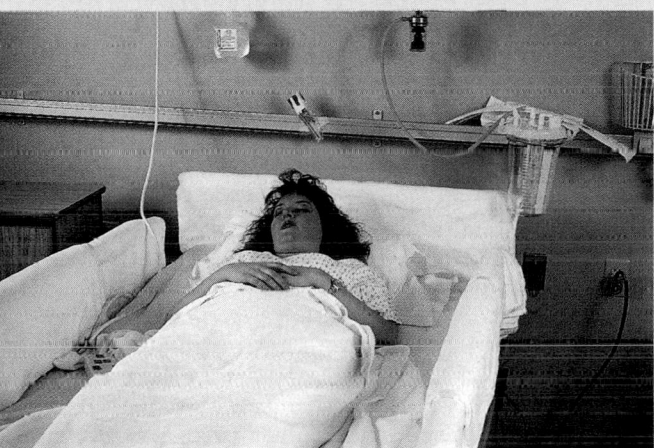

STEPS	RATIONALE
4. When a seizure begins, position client safely. If standing or sitting at the time of the seizure, guide the client to floor and protect head by cradling it in your lap or placing a pillow under head. Clear surrounding area of furniture. If the client is in bed, raise siderails and put bed in low position.	Protects client from traumatic injury.
5. If possible, turn client on the side, with head flexed slightly forward.	This position prevents the tongue from blocking the airway and promotes drainage of secretions, thus reducing the risk of aspiration (Seizure Recognition and Observation, 1992).
6. Do not restrain client. Loosen clothing.	Restraining clients can result in musculoskeletal injury.
7. Do not place any objects in the client's mouth.	Injury to the oral cavity may result from forcible insertion of a hard object. Soft objects may break or come apart and be aspirated (Ziemba, 1995).
8. Have a staff member provide privacy.	Clients may feel embarrassed following a seizure, especially if there were onlookers.
9. Observe the onset, duration, and sequence of the seizure activity. Note aura, if any, level of consciousness, posture, color, movements of extremities, incontinence, and sleep patterns or confusion afterwards.	Accurate observation and reporting assists in the diagnosis and treatment of the seizure disorder.
10. Stay with the client after the seizure, explaining what happened and offering support.	

STATUS EPILEPTICUS

STEPS	RATIONALE
11. Insert airway when jaw is relaxed between seizure activity (see Chapter 44).	An open airway needs to be maintained.
Do not place fingers in the client's mouth.	The nurse could suffer injury from a bite.
12. Obtain oxygen and suction equipment. Prepare for IV insertion (see Chapters 44 and 45).	Status Epilepticus is a medical emergency. Medications should be given intravenously, the client should be suctioned, and oxygen is often needed.
13. Pad side rails and headboard.	Traumatic injury will be avoided.
14. Document seizure activity and all interventions.	Documentation may assist diagnosis and treatment of the condition.

sion, sensory impairment, urinary and bladder dysfunction, and certain medical diagnostic categories such as cancer and cardiovascular, neurological and cerebrovascular diseases increase the risk. Drug use and drug interactions are also implicated in falls (Brady and Chester, 1993).

Client-Inherent Accidents. Client-inherent accidents are accidents other than falls in which the client is the primary factor. Examples of client-inherent accidents are self-inflicted cuts, injuries, and burns; ingestion or injection of foreign substances; self-mutilation or fire setting; and pinching fingers in drawers or doors.

A client-inherent accident may occur as a result of a **seizure.** A seizure is characterized by a cry, loss of consciousness with falling if upright, tonicity (rigidity), and clonicity (jerking). The client may have shallow breathing, cyanosis, and possibly loss of bladder and bowel control. Following the seizure there is a postictal phase, where the client has amnesia, confusion, and may fall into a deep sleep (Seizure Recognition and Observation, 1992). Prior to a convulsive episode, a few clients may report an aura, a warning or sense that a seizure is about to occur. An aura may be a bright light, smell, or taste (Shatz and Spitz, 1993). Seizures that last longer than 5 minutes or are followed quickly by subsequent seizures are called status epilepticus. This condition is a medical emergency and requires intensive monitoring and treatment.

It has been found that significant injury to the client's oral cavity is rare, even during the most violent seizures (Ellis, 1993). Injury may occur from forcing an object into the mouth and from the teeth biting down on a hard object. Soft objects may break in the mouth during a seizure and be aspirated. Therefore, the Epilepsy Foundation of America, in its recommendations for seizure first aid, includes avoiding the insertion of objects into the mouth (Seizure Recognition and Observation, 1992). Clients experiencing a seizure are never restrained, but are placed on **seizure precautions** and need to be adquately protected from traumatic injury (Procedure 36-1).

Procedure-Related Accidents. Procedure-related accidents occur during therapy. They include medication and fluid administration errors, improper application of external devices, and accidents related to improper performance of procedures, such as dressing changes.

The nurse can prevent many procedure-related accidents. For example, strictly following the procedure for administering medications will prevent medication errors. Proper administration of intravenous (IV) fluids prevents fluid overload or deficit. The potential for infection is reduced when surgical asepsis is used for sterile dressing changes or any invasive procedure, such as insertion of a Foley catheter. Finally, correct use of body mechanics and transfer techniques reduces the risk of injuries when moving and lifting clients.

Equipment-Related Accidents. Equipment-related accidents result from the malfunction, disrepair, or misuse of equipment or from an electrical hazard. To avoid injury, the nurse should not operate monitoring or therapy equipment without instruction.

A checklist should be used to assess potential electrical hazards to reduce the risk of electrical fires, electrocution, or injury from faulty equipment (see the box on p. 874). In health care settings, the engineering staff make regular safety checks of equipment.

Examples of NANDA Nursing Diagnoses for Safety Risks

Risk for injury *related to:*
- Altered mobility
- Design of physical environment in the home

Risk for poisoning *related to:*
- Chemical contamination of food or water
- Accessibility of medications to children
- Reduced vision

Risk for suffocation *related to:*
- Reduced motor abilities
- Pillow placed in infant's crib
- Improperly vented heaters

Risk for trauma *related to:*
- Contact with extreme cold
- Obstructed stairways

Altered thought processes *related to:*
- Loss of memory
- Sleep deprivation
- Side effect of medication

Impaired home maintenance management *related to:*
- Insufficient finances
- Impaired cognitive functioning

Knowledge deficit *related to:*
- Information misinterpretation
- Unfamiliarity with safety precautions for children

Risk for altered body temperature *related to:*
- Exposure to extreme hot or cold environments
- Immature temperature control mechanisms

Nursing Diagnosis

Assessment reveals clusters of data that indicate when a client has an actual or potential risk to safety (see the nursing diagnoses box above). When developing the nursing diagnostic statement, the nurse must ensure that the appropriate defining characteristics are present in the assessment data base (see the diagnostic process box on p. 879, top). The nursing diagnostic statement identifies the related or risk factors; for example, impaired vision, substance abuse, or side effects of prescribed medications.

Planning

The nurse plans therapeutic interventions for clients with actual or high risks to safety (see the care plan on p. 879, bottom). The overall goal for a client with a threat to safety is that the client will remain free from injury. The nurse plans individualized interventions based on the severity of risks to the client, the client's developmental stage, level of health, and lifestyle. Nursing interventions are designed to provide care in a safe and efficient manner. The following are potential goals focusing on the client's need for safety:

- Modifiable hazards are reduced in the home environment.
- Client will correctly use medications and equipment, and carry out treatments.
- Client identifies and avoids risks within the community.

Sample Nursing Diagnostic Process for Safety Risks

ASSESSMENT ACTIVITIES	DEFINING CHARACTERISTICS	NURSING DIAGNOSIS
Observe client's mobility in the home. Ask client about visual acuity. Observe client's home for hazards and obstacles.	Uncoordinated gait Reports difficulty seeing at night Reports frequent "tripping" over furniture Reports frequent use of step ladder to reach items Home has poor lighting Rooms are cluttered with furniture and personal items Rugs are not secure	**Risk for injury** related to poorly lighted and cluttered home environment.

Sample Nursing Care Plan for Risk for Injury

NURSING DIAGNOSIS: **Risk for injury** related to poorly lighted and cluttered home environment.
DEFINITION: Risk for injury is the state in which an individual is at risk for injury as a result of environmental conditions interacting with the individual's adaptive and defensive resources (Kim, 1995).

GOAL	EXPECTED OUTCOMES	INTERVENTIONS	RATIONALE
Client will have a safe home environment within 6 mos.	Client will list hazards within home by end of third teaching session.	Give three 20-min teaching sessions on identifying and avoiding hazards or falls and injuries, and increasing safety.	Counseling and teaching sessions increase client's awareness of hazards (Loew, 1993).
	After 3 mo, client will modify hazards by 50%. After 6 mo, client will modify 100% of hazards.	Have client complete a home safety check to identify potential risk to safety.	Thorough review of potential hazards can increase client's knowledge of risk preventions (Loew, 1993).
		Secure safety bars on bathtub and shower area.	Grab bars and nonslick surfaces reduce risk of falls (Ebersole and Hess, 1994).
		Place at least 75-watt bulbs in all fixtures.	Improving lighting changes environmental hazards and reduces risk of falling (Ebersole and Hess, 1994).

It is important to consider the client's home when planning therapies to maintain or improve the level of safety. Planning care also involves an understanding of the client's need to maintain independence. The nurse and the client work together to establish ways of maintaining client involvement to create a safe environment in the hospital and home. Education of the client and family is a major nursing intervention to decrease accidents.

Implementation

Nursing interventions are directed at promoting and maintaining the client's safety. Because most nursing measures are applicable in all environments, the interventions are presented in two sections: developmental considerations and environmental protection. The first category of interventions includes those specifically for reducing risks for each developmental age group. Environmental interventions are developed to modify the environment so that present or potential hazards are eliminated or minimized.

DEVELOPMENTAL CONSIDERATIONS

Infant, Toddler, and Preschooler. Infants, toddlers, and preschoolers depend on adults to protect them from injury. Growing children are curious and completely trusting of their environment and do not perceive themselves to be in danger.

Nurses are frequently in a position to educate parents or

Table 36-2	Nursing Interventions to Promote Safety	
INTERVENTION	**RATIONALE**

INFANTS, TODDLERS, AND PRESCHOOLERS

Use large, soft toys without plastic eyes, nose, or mouth.	Small parts can be dislodged by baby, and accidental aspiration can occur.
If playpen with mesh sides is used, do not leave one side down.	Baby's head can become wedged between playpen pad and lowered mesh side, and asphyxiation can occur.
Never leave sides of crib down or turn away from baby on changing table.	Child can suddenly roll and fall from crib or changing table.
Hold baby at feeding time; do not prop bottle.	This increases bonding with parent and reduces risk of choking.
If formula is used, be sure to read instructions. Most formulas must be diluted with water.	Using undiluted formula can cause fluid and electrolyte imbalances in newborn.
Discontinue use of infant seat at 3 mo, or earlier if infant is very mobile.	A 3 mo, active infants may be able to propel themselves out of seat and fall.
Baby-proof house for small objects, sharp objects, and toxic and poisonous substances.	Babies explore their world with their hands and mouth, and ingestion of small objects can result in choking. Toxic and poisonous substances require prompt action.
Cover electrical outlets with protective covers (see Fig. 35-4)	Electrical wall outlets are at baby's eye level and stimulate curiosity. Crawling baby will frequently attempt to play with electrical wall plates regardless of number of toys available.
Use guardrails at top and bottom of stairs and at doorway of rooms considered off-limits to crawling or walking toddler.	This prevents child from falling down stairs or being exposed to rooms with unguarded dangers.
Use windowguards for all windows.	This prevents child from falling out of window.
Never leave baby unattended in infant seat, walker, stroller, or high chair.	Active child can easily slide out of these devices and fall.
Never leave baby or child unattended in bath or wading pool.	Accidental drowning may occur.
Never attach pacifier to child with string around neck.	String can easily become tangled, and strangulation can result.
Restrain child in back seat of automobile. Child under 4 should be in approved car seat (see Fig. 36-5). Older children should be restrained with seat belt.	In event of sudden stop or auto accident, unrestrained child is bounced against hard, sharp surfaces of the vehicle's interior, and injuries result.
Plastic bags, such as those for storing fruit or dry cleaning, should be removed from home.	If child places these items over head, air supply decreases, and child suffocates.
Install on doors strong dead-bolt locks well beyond toddler's reach, even when child is standing on chair.	This prevents child from leaving home without parents' knowledge, reducing danger of child getting lost, freezing to death, falling into swimming pool, or being abducted.
Use the words *no* and *don't* to convey that object or action increases child's risk of injury, such as playing with matches.	Improperly using these words renders them meaningless to child.
Teach child to swim at early age, but always provide supervision.	Child is able to enjoy the water safely. Child who knows how to swim can still encounter difficulty in water and needs supervision.
Teach child to cross street and to walk in parking lots.	This provides child with self-protection against dangers from automobiles.
Teach child not to talk to or accept anything from stranger and to notify parents or responsible adult if approached by stranger.	This reduces risk of injury or abduction by stranger. Reporting stranger's presence helps law-enforcement personnel investigate and remove threat.
Do not allow child to run with sucker or popsicle in mouth.	Child may fall and stick from sucker or popsicle can cause puncture injury or foreign body in airway.
Impress on child not to eat anything found on street or in grass.	Substance may be poisonous and can cause severe illness.
Use back burners on stoves and get into habit of turning pot handles toward wall.	This reduces risk of child pulling down pot of hot liquid and being burned.
Remove doors from unused refrigerators and freezers, and instruct child not to hide in these items.	Door may latch and on older models cannot be released from inside; as result, asphyxiation can occur.

SCHOOL-AGE CHILD*

Teach child the safe use of equipment for play and work activities.	Child needs to learn that some equipment is for play and other equipment is for work and that improper use can result in injury.
Teach child to ride bicycle safely and responsibilities that go with bicycling.	If bicycling is prohibited on sidewalks, child must learn to obey traffic signals and ride with traffic patterns or identify safe locations for bicycle riding.
Teach child to wear protective helmet and knee and elbow pads when roller skating.	When roller skating, child often falls; protective devices reduce risk of serious injury.
Never allow child to operate appliances while alone.	If electrical mishap occurs, no one would be available to help child.

Modified from Wong DL: *Whaley and Wong's Nursing care of infants and children,* ed 4, St Louis, 1995, Mosby.

Table 36-2	**Nursing Interventions to Promote Safety—cont'd**
INTERVENTION	**RATIONALE**
If parent chooses to have firearms in house, teach parent to keep them unloaded, locked up, and out of reach.	This prevents injury from accidental discharge or improper use.
ADOLESCENT Encourage enrollment in driver's education classes.	Many injuries are auto related at this age. Adolescents need to learn the rules of the road, seat belt laws, and the effects of alcohol and other drugs on their ability to drive safely.
Provide information about the use of alcohol and drugs.	Adolescents are subject to the effects of peer pressure.
Provide sex education, emphasizing safe sex practices.	Many adolescents begin sexual relationships. Pregnancy and transmission of HIV must be avoided.
Refer adolescents to community and school-sponsored activities.	The adolescent needs adult supervision, yet needs time to socialize safely with peers.
Listen to adolescents and observe for changes in behavior.	Adolescents can suffer from depression and have a high suicide rate.
ADULTS Refer clients to stress-management classes and instruct in necessary lifestyle changes.	The effects of stress and lifestyle patterns can pose significant risks to safety of adult clients.
OLDER ADULTS Assist clients to conduct a home hazard appraisal (see the box on p. 874).	Extrinsic, physical hazards pose safety risks to older adults. Falls are associated with increasing age; accidental poisoning may occur due to poor vision; reduced mobility, vision, and hearing increase the risks of fire, electrical shocks, and car accidents.
Encourage clients to have periodic vision and hearing tests.	This may decrease car and pedestrian accidents.
Encourage client to enroll in an exercise class and to keep as active as possible.	Exercise maintains muscle strength and flexibility.

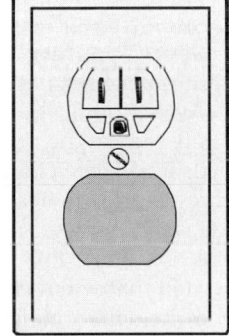

Fig. 36-4 Safety covers for electrical outlets.

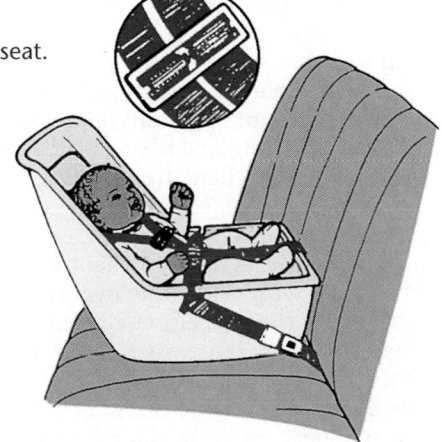

Fig. 36-5 Infant car seat.

guardians about reducing risks of injuries for young children. Nurses working in prenatal clinics can easily incorporate safety into the care plan of the childbearing family. Community health nurses can assess the home and show parents how to promote safety in their homes (Table 36-2 and Figs. 36-4 and 36-5).

School-Age Child. School-age children increasingly explore their environment. They have friends outside their immediate neighborhood, and they become more active in school, church, and community activities. The school-age child needs specific teaching regarding safety in school and at play (Fig. 36-6). Some nursing interventions help guide the parent to provide for the safety of the school-age child (see Table 36-2).

Adolescent. Risks to the adolescent's safety involve many factors outside the home environment. Adults serve as role models for adolescents and, through example and education, can help adolescents minimize risks to their safety. This age group has a high incidence of suicide because of feelings of decreased self-worth and hopelessness. The nurse must be aware of the risks posed at this time and be prepared to teach adolescents and their parents measures to prevent accidents and injury (see Table 36-2).

Adult. Risks to young and middle-age adults frequently result from lifestyle factors such as childrearing, high-stress states, inadequate nutrition, excessive alcohol intake, and substance abuse. Adults need to be taught that their safety is threatened and as a result their lifestyle needs to be modified.

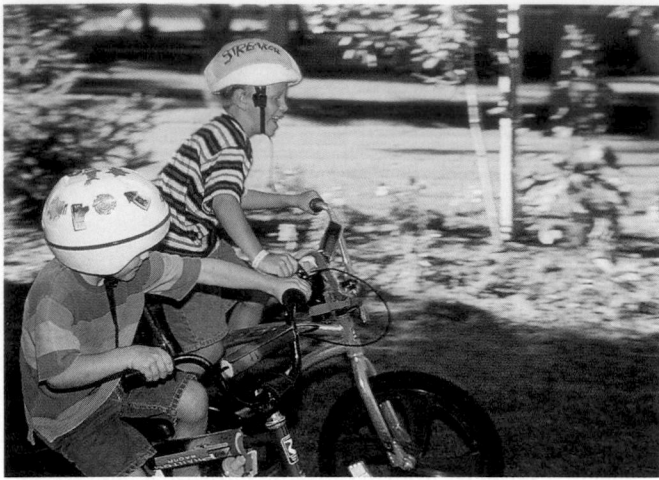

Fig. 36-6 Proper bike safety equipment for school-age children.

GERONTOLOGICAL PRINCIPLES
for Accident Prevention

The older adult experiences alterations in vision and hearing. The nurse should encourage yearly vision and hearing exams as a means to prevent falls, burns, and car accidents.

Range of motion, flexibility, and strength are decreased. The nurse should teach the older client to seek assistance with household tasks as needed and to store items within easy reach.

Reflexes are slowed and the ability to respond to multiple stimuli is reduced. The nurse must provide adequate, meaningful stimuli, but prevent sensory overload in the older client.

Nocturia and incontinence are more frequent in older adults. The nurse should implement a toileting schedule and assist the client to adhere to it. At night, lighting should be adequate for the client who needs to go to the bathroom and assistance should be provided. Give diuretics in the morning.

Stress-management centers (see Chapter 22) and health-promotion activities (see Chapter 3) have been incorporated into many community service programs and hospitals. In addition, neighborhood centers, community clinics, and outpatient clinics are equipped to assist the adult in modifying lifestyle habits (e.g., smoking, overeating, lack of exercise, and alcoholism) that present risks to health.

Older Adult. Nursing interventions for older adults are designed to reduce the risk of falls and other accidents and to compensate for the physiological changes of aging (see Table 36-2 and the box above).

Older adults are more likely to have automobile accidents because of three specific physiological changes. First, changes in visual acuity and depth perception prevent the client from quickly observing situations in which an accident is likely to occur. Second, decreased hearing acuity alters older clients' abilities to hear emergency vehicle sirens or car and truck horns. Third, because of decreased nervous system response, older adults may be unable to react as quickly as they once could to avoid an accident (Ebersole and Hess, 1994).

Pedestrian accidents can be reduced for older adults and for all other age groups by persuading people to wear reflectors on garments when walking at night, to stand on the sidewalk and not in the street when waiting to cross a street, to always cross at corners and not in the middle of the block (particularly if the street is a major one), to cross with the traffic light and not against it, and to look left, right, and left again before entering the street or crosswalk.

Burns and scalds are also more apt to occur with older people, whose risk is increased by several factors. Older people may forget and leave hot water running or become confused when turning the dials on a stove. Nursing measures for preventing burns are designed to minimize the risk from impaired vision and hearing.

ENVIRONMENTAL CONSIDERATIONS

General Preventive Measures. Nurses can contribute to a safer environment by helping the client meet basic physiological and psychosocial needs. To prevent infection,

nurses utilize aseptic practices. Medical asepsis, which includes handwashing and environmental cleanliness, reduces the transfer of organisms. Surgical asepsis, or sterile technique, provides an environment free of all organisms, including spores. Parents of infants should be taught the importance of having their children immunized. All clients should receive immunization boosters at scheduled intervals (see Chapter 28). In the home, awareness of methods of food handling helps reduce the risk of pathogen transmission through contaminated food.

Specific Safety Concerns. Specific safety concerns include falls, fires, poisoning, electrical hazards, and radiation.

Falls. Modifications in the health care environment can easily reduce the risk of falls. Safety bars in toilets, locks on beds and wheelchairs, and call bells are several safety features found in health care settings (Figs. 36-7 and 36-8). Measures nurses can implement to prevent falls are listed in the box on p. 883, left. In addition, research has demonstrated that when clients' needs are met in a timely fashion, the incidence of falls decreases (see the box on p. 883, right).

A client experiencing a seizure is at particular risk for injury related to falling. Procedure 36-1 describes the nursing interventions when caring for a client experiencing a seizure.

Side Rails. Chapter 37 discusses side rails as a device for increasing the client's mobility and stability when in bed or when moving from bed to chair. Side rails also help prevent the unconscious client from falling out of bed or from a stretcher (Fig. 36-9). However, the use of side rails for a disoriented client may cause more confusion and further injury. Frequently a confused client who is determined to get out of bed attempts to climb over the side rail or climbs out at the foot of the bed. Either attempt usually results in a fall. Whenever side rails are used, the bed should be maintained in the lowest position possible.

Restraints. In extreme cases, a client who is at risk for injury may need to be restrained. A **restraint** is any one of

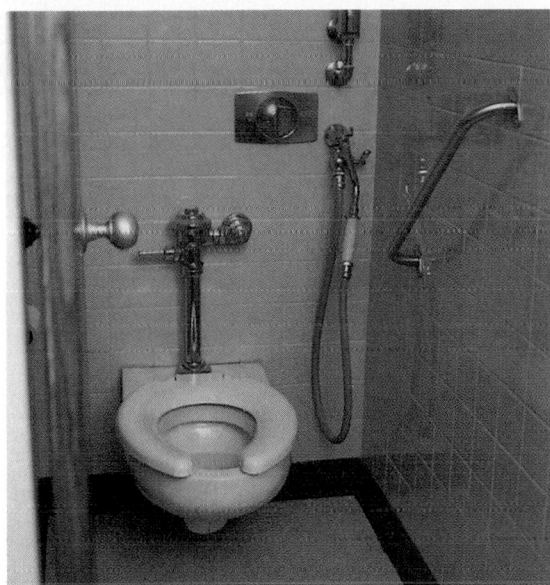

Fig. 36-7 Safety bars around toilets and showers.

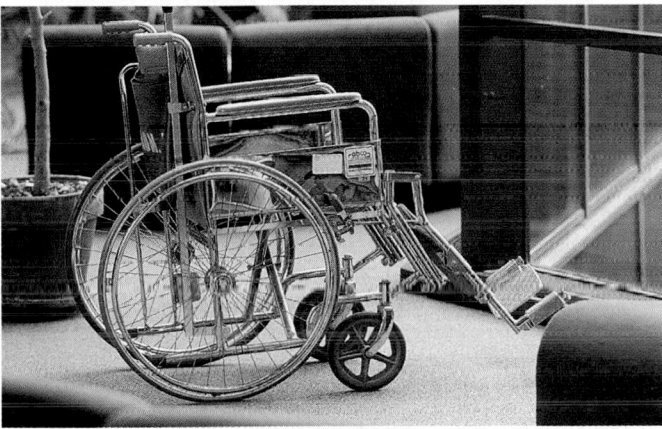

Fig. 36-8 Safety locks on wheelchairs.

Measures to Prevent Falls in the Health Care Agency

Orient client to physical surroundings.
Explain use of call bell system.
Assess client's risk for falling.
Assign clients at risk for falling to rooms near the nurses' station.
Alert all personnel to the client's risk for falling.
Instruct client and family to seek assistance when getting up.
Answer client's call bell promptly.
Keep bed in the low position with side rails up if needed.
Keep personal items within reach.
Eliminate clutter in client's room.
Lock all beds, wheelchairs, and stretchers.
Maintain client's toileting schedule throughout the day.
Observe client frequently; reorient as necessary.
Encourage family participation in client's care.

numerous devices used to immobilize a client. Physical restraints are any manual method or mechanical device, material, or equipment attached or adjacent to a client's body that the client cannot easily remove and that restricts freedom of movement or normal access to one's body. The Omnibus Budget Reconciliation Act (OBRA) of 1987 defines clients' rights and choices regarding use of restraints. Under these guidelines, reasons for use of physical restraint are to be clearly stated. The use of restraints must be part of the client's medical treatment, all less restrictive interventions must be tried first, other disciplines must be used, and supporting documentation must be provided (Health Care Financing Administration, 1990).

Restraints do not necessarily prevent falls or injury. In fact, it has been shown that clients incur less severe injuries if left unrestrained. It is reported that devices such as belts, jackets, and limb or extremity restraints are used on approximately 500,000 Americans each day (Weick, 1992). This is an alarming statistic, considering that restraints are associated with many complications. Almost all types of restraints have been implicated in client deaths, the majority associated with suffocation using the vest or jacket type (Weick, 1992). The Food and Drug Administration, which regulates restraints as medical devices and requires manufacturers to label them "prescription only," estimates that hundreds of restraint-related injuries occur each year, with at least 100 deaths taking place in nursing homes, hospi-

RESEARCH HIGHLIGHT

RESEARCH ABSTRACT

This article describes efforts to decrease the incidence of geriatric falls in a rehabilitation center. In order to establish a baseline regarding client falls, a retrospective chart review was done. The fallers were generally in the 70- to 79-year-old age group, and most falls occurred in the client's room or bathroom. Clients were trying to get to the bathroom, leaning forward in their chairs, or transferring in and out of bed when the falls occurred. The need to toilet, rest, or obtain nutrition and hydration were activities most commonly cited in the falls. The highest percentage of falls occurred during the day shift, with 15% occurring between 2:00 and 3:00 PM. With these data in mind, a proactive falls-prevention protocol was devised. A comparison between falls occurring during the monitor period of the falls prevention program and 2 previous years showed an 80% and 88% decrease in falls, respectively. This supported the belief that clients whose needs are anticipated and met fall less.

IMPLICATIONS FOR PRACTICE

▶ Assess cognitive, sensory, and motor status of the client during each shift.
▶ Timed interventions for hygiene, nutrition, and toileting reduce unsafe client activities and result in fewer falls and less restraint use.
▶ Planning interventions throughout the shift allows for better time management for staff.

REFERENCE

Brady R, Chester F, et al: Geriatric falls: prevention strategies for the staff, *J Gerontol Nurs* 19(9):26, 40, 1993.

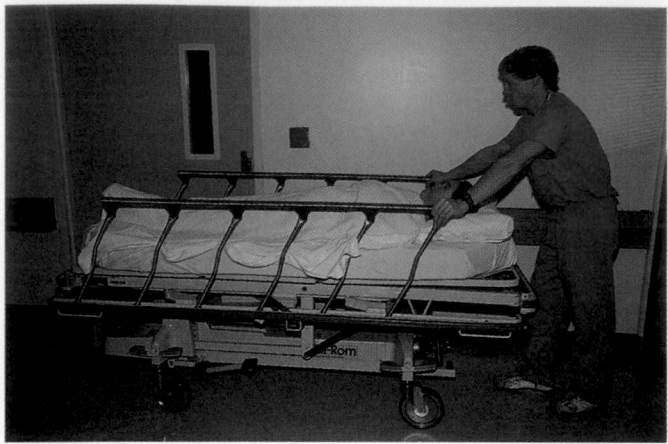

Fig. 36-9 Side rails in the *up* position on a stretcher.

tals, and private homes (Lambert, 1992). In addition, the immobility imposed by restraining a client can lead to pressure ulcer formation, hypostatic pneumonia, constipation, urinary and fecal incontinence, and urinary retention. Contractures, nerve damage, and circulatory impairment are also potential hazards. Loss of self-esteem, humiliation, fear, and anger can also result (Weick, 1992). Therefore nurses have a responsibility to utilize all alternatives before restraining a client.

Establishing a Restraint-Free Environment. Nurses have an obligation to assess clients and carefully plan for their safety needs without the use of restraints. The box above provides information for establishing a restraint-free environment.

One device designed to reduce the use of restraints as well as the number of falls in health care agencies is **AMBULARM.** This device, which is secured to the client's thigh, emits an intermittent sound when the leg assumes a dependent angle of 45 degrees, such as when the client's leg is over the edge of the bed.

When restraints are necessary, the doctor's order should state the type of restraint, specific client behaviors for which restraints are to be used, and a limited time frame. These orders should be renewed within a specific time frame according to the agency's policy. Restraints are not to be ordered PRN ("as needed"). The reason for the restraint should be given to the client and family, and their permission should be sought whenever possible. Procedure 36-2 describes the proper application of restraints. Assessment of clients who are restrained must be ongoing. Proper documentation, including the behaviors that necessitated the application of restraints, the procedure used in restraining, and the evaluation of the client response is essential. Clients should also be given a "trial release." Clients periodically have their restraints removed and the nurse assesses them to determine if the restraints are needed.

Fires. The home and hospital are always at risk for fires. Accidental home fires typically result from smoking in bed, extinguishing of cigarettes in trash cans, grease fires, or electrical fires resulting from faulty wiring or appliances. Insti-

---

Alternatives to Restraints

Orient clients and families to surroundings; explain all procedures and treatments to them.

Encourage family and friends to stay or utilize sitters for clients who need supervision.

Assign confused or disoriented clients to rooms near the nurses' station. Observe these clients frequently.

Provide appropriate visual and auditory stimuli; for example, family pictures, clocks, and a radio.

Eliminate bothersome treatments as soon as possible. For example, discontinue tube feedings and begin oral feedings as quickly as the client's condition allows.

Use relaxation techniques, such as massage.

Institute exercise and ambulation schedules as clients' conditions allow.

Maintain toileting routines.

Consult with physical and occupational therapists to enhance clients' abilities to carry out activities of daily living.

Evaluate all medications clients are receiving to determine if the medication is having the desired therapeutic effect.

Conduct ongoing assessment and evaluation of clients' care and their response to care.

Modified from Stolley J: Freeing your patients from restraints, *Am J Nurs* 95(2):27, 1995.

Fire-Containment Guidelines for Nurses Working in Agencies

Know the telephone number for reporting fires. Make sure the number is visible near the phone.

Know the agency's fire drill and evacuation plan.

Know the location of all fire alarms, exits, and extinguishers (see Table 36-3).

Report a fire before attempting to extinguish it, regardless of its size.

Close doors and windows when a fire is detected.

Never use the elevator in the event of a fire.

Turn off oxygen and appliances in the vicinity of the fire.

Remember the acronym RACE to set priorities:
  R rescue
  A alarm
  C confine
  E extinguish

---

tutional fires typically result from an electrical or anesthetic-related fire.

The interventions described here are directed toward fires occurring in health care agencies, but the same principles apply for fires in the home. Homes should be equipped with smoke and fire alarms. It is important to have a plan of action in the event of fire (see the box above).

If a fire occurs in a health care agency, the nurse protects clients from injury, reports the location of the fire, and contains the fire. One helpful acronym for priorities in a fire is

RACE: rescue, alarm, confine, and extinguish. Rescue and remove all clients from *immediate* danger. Use the alarm procedure to report the location of the fire. After clients are out of danger and the fire has been reported, personnel must take measures to confine or extinguish the fire (e.g., closing doors and windows, turning off oxygen and electrical equipment, and using a fire extinguisher).

The three basic types of fires for which extinguishers are used are paper and rubbish (type A), grease and anesthetic gas (type B), and electrical (type C). The appropriate extinguisher must be used for each type (Table 36-3).

Clients who are close to the fire, regardless of its size, are at risk of injury and should be moved to another area. If a client is receiving oxygen but not life support, the nurse discontinues the oxygen, which is combustible and can fuel an existing fire. If the client is on life support, the nurse may need to maintain the client's respiratory status manually with an Ambu-bag (see Chapter 44) until the client is moved away from the threat of fire. Ambulatory clients can be directed to walk by themselves to a safe area and in some cases may be able to assist in moving clients in wheelchairs. Bedridden clients are generally moved from the scene of a fire by a stretcher, their bed, or a wheelchair. If none of these methods is appropriate, clients must be carried from the area. If a client must be carried, the nurse should be careful not to overextend physical limits for lifting because injury to the nurse can result in further injury to the client. If fire department personnel are on the scene, they can help evacuate the clients.

Poisoning. A poison is any substance that impairs health or destroys life when ingested, inhaled, or otherwise absorbed by the body. Specific antidotes or treatments are available for only some types of poisons. The capacity of body tissue to recover from the poison determines the reversibility of the effect. Poisons can impair the respiratory, circulatory, central nervous, hepatic, GI, and renal systems of the body.

The toddler, preschooler, and young school-age child must be protected from accidental poisoning. Using child-resistant caps, placing medications and cleaning fluids and powders out of the reach of children, leaving potentially poisonous materials in original containers, and removing poisonous plants from the home prevent accidental ingestion of poisonous materials. In older adults, diminished eyesight and impaired memory may result in accidental ingestion of poisonous substances or an overdose of prescribed medications. Although the majority of children's ingestions are accidental, most drug overdoses in adults are intentional, the result of a suicide attempt or drug abuse (McKenry and Salerno, 1992).

The Poison Control Center phone number should be visible on the telephone itself in homes with young children. In all cases of suspected poisoning, this number should be called immediately (Procedure 36-3).

Electrical Hazards. Electrical equipment must be maintained in good working order and should be **grounded**. The third longer prong in an electrical plug is the ground (Fig. 36-10). Theoretically the ground prong carries any stray electrical current back to the ground, hence its name. The other two prongs carry the power to the piece of electrical equipment.

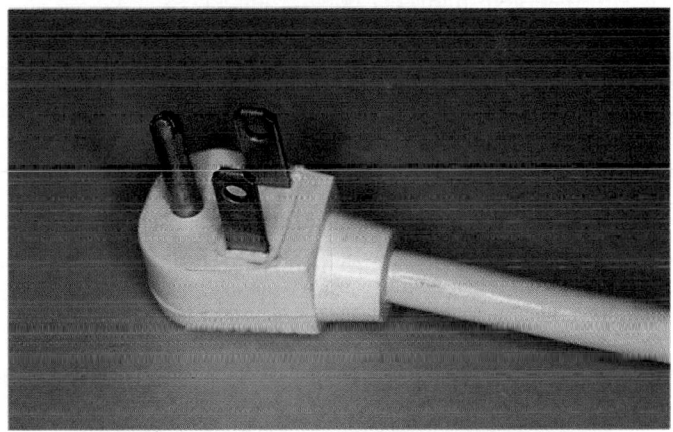

Fig. 36-10 Three-pronged grounded plug.

Table 36-3	Types of Fire Extinguishers and Their Uses		
TYPE	**CLASS OF FIRE**	**HOW TO USE**	**PRECAUTIONS**
Carbon dioxide	Grease, electrical	Direct carbon dioxide into flame, cutting off fire's oxygen supply.	
Soda and acid (water extinguisher)	Paper and rubbish, wood	Turn canister upside down, mixing soda and acid. Carbon dioxide is then produced, releasing water extinguisher under pressure. To stop flow, turn canister right side up.	Ineffective against grease and electrical fires because it causes grease spatter, spreading fire, and because water conducts electricity
Dry chemical	Rubbish, electrical	Pull pin or press lever on extinguisher, blanketing fire with foam and cutting off fire's oxygen supply.	Ineffective against grease because it causes grease to spatter, spreading fire
Water pump	Rubbish, wood	Pump handle while pointing nozzle toward fire.	Ineffective against grease and electrical fires because grease can spatter, spreading fire, and because water conducts electricity
Antifreeze or water	Rubbish, wood, grease, anesthetics	Pull pin and handle of extinguisher and direct extinguisher toward fire.	Ineffective against electrical fires because water conducts electricity

PROCEDURE 36-2

Applying Restraints

STEPS	RATIONALE
1. Identify clients whose behavior places them at risk for injury: confused or disoriented clients; clients who are combative; clients awakening from sedation.	Restraints are used to *reduce risk* of client falling out of bed, chair, or wheelchair; to prevent interruption of therapy such as traction, intravenous infusions, or nasogastric tube feedings; to prevent confused or combative client from injuring self by removing Foley catheter, surgical drain, or life support equipment; and to reduce risk of injury to others by client.
2. Check physician's order for time that restraint is to be applied, rationale for restraint, and assess type of restraint to be used.	Physician's order protects nurse from liability.
3. Explain carefully to client and family reasons restraint is necessary, type of restraint selected, and anticipated duration of restraint.	Restraints can increase confusion or combativeness in client. In addition, family may express anger about restraint. Explanation and reinforcement can reduce or even prevent some of these negative perceptions.
4. Prepare equipment: a. Proper restraint	Nurse is able to complete restraining procedure without having to leave client partially restrained.
b. Padding to protect bony prominences	Padding protects circulation to distal portion of extremity if wrist or ankle restraints are selected.

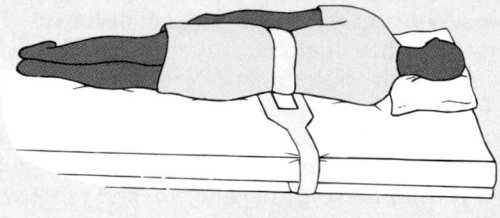

Step 7b

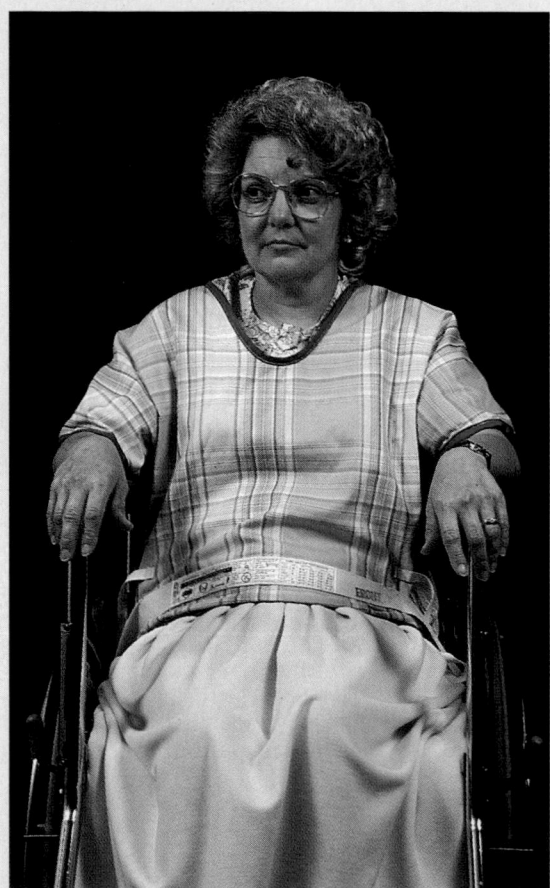

Step 7a

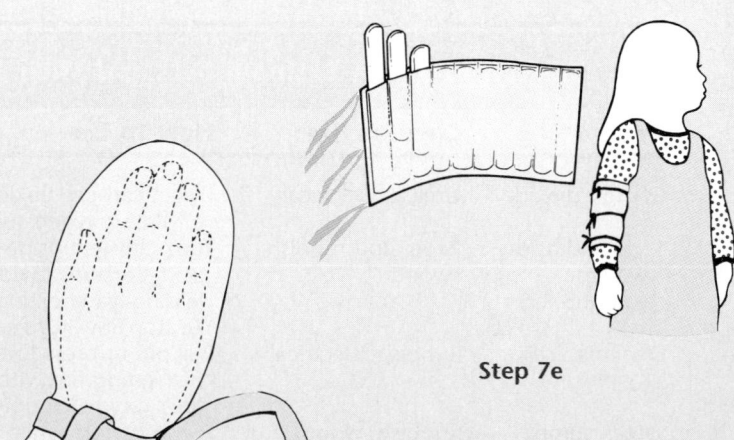

Step 7e

Step 7d

Applying Restraints—cont'd

STEPS	RATIONALE

5. Wash hands.

6. Pad bony prominences before applying restraint.

7. Apply selected restraint (follow manufacturer's guidelines):

a. **Jacket restraint:** Poncho-type garment that crosses or closes in back of client (see manufacturer's directions) (see the illustration on p. 886).

b. **Belt restraint:** Device that secures client on stretcher (see the illustration on p. 886). Avoid placing belt too tightly across client's chest or abdomen.

c. **Extremity restraints (ankle or wrist):** Designed to immobilize one or all extremities. Commercially available limb restraints are composed of sheepskin and foam pad that comes in contact with skin. Restraints are designed so that client can pull against it without device tightening against extremity. (Use manufacturer's directions for application.)

d. **Mitten restraint:** Thumbless mitten devices (see the illustration on p. 886) to restrain hands.

Reduces transmission of microorganisms.
Padding decreases injury to underlying skin.

Restrains client while lying or reclining in bed or sitting in chair or wheelchair. Are useful in home care settings but should not be used unless other methods have failed.
Restrains center of gravity and prevents client from rolling off or sitting up while on stretcher.

Maintains immobilization of extremity to protect client from injury from fall or accidental removal of therapeutic device such as an intravenous tube or Foley catheter.

Prevents clients from dislodging invasive equipment, removing dressings, or scratching.

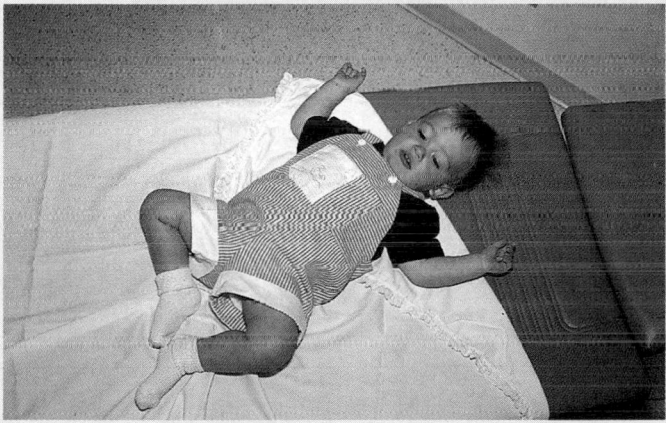

Step 7f

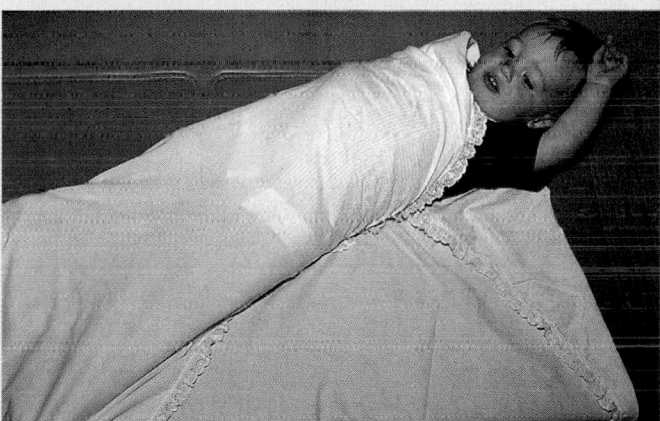

Step 7f

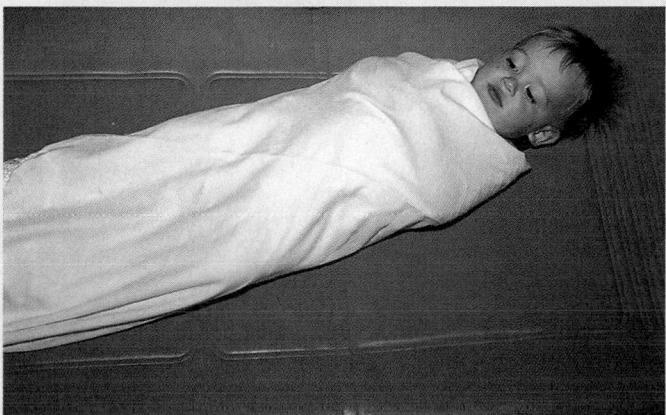

Step 7f

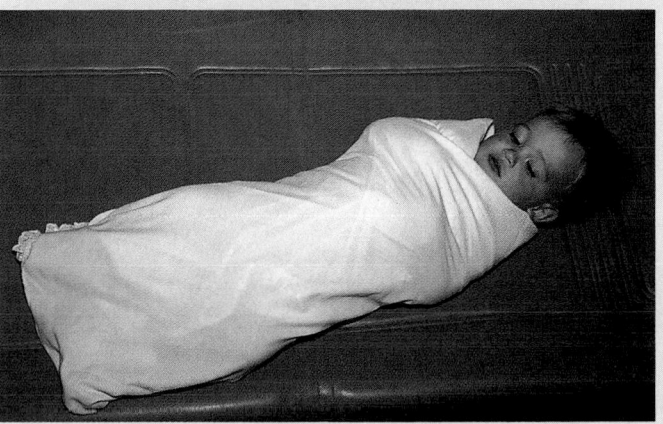

Step 7f

Continued.

Applying Restraints—cont'd

PROCEDURE 36-2

STEPS	RATIONALE

e. **Elbow restraint:** Piece of fabric with slots in which tongue blades are placed so that elbow joint remains rigid (see the illustration on p. 886).

Used with infants and children to prevent elbow flexion.

f. **Mummy restraint:** Blanket or sheet is opened on bed or crib with one corner folded toward center. Child is placed on blanket with shoulders at fold with feet toward opposite corner (see the illustration on p. 887). With child's right arm straight down against the body, right side of blanket is pulled firmly across right shoulder and chest and secured beneath left side of body (see the illustration on p. 887). Left arm is placed straight against side, and left side of blanket is brought across shoulder and chest and locked beneath child's body on right side (see the illustration on p. 887). Lower corner is folded and brought over body and tucked or fastened securely with safety pins (see the illustration on p. 887) (Wong, 1995).

Maintains short-term restraint of small child or infant for examination or treatment involving head and neck. Effectively controls movement of torso and extremities.

8. Secure ties of jacket or extremity restraints by wrapping them around stable parts of the bed, bed frame, or chair (legs or under frame of wheelchair) (see the illustrations below). Never tie to side rail.

When client is able to undo restraint, purpose of restraint is negated. Client may be injured if side rail is lowered with restraint in place.

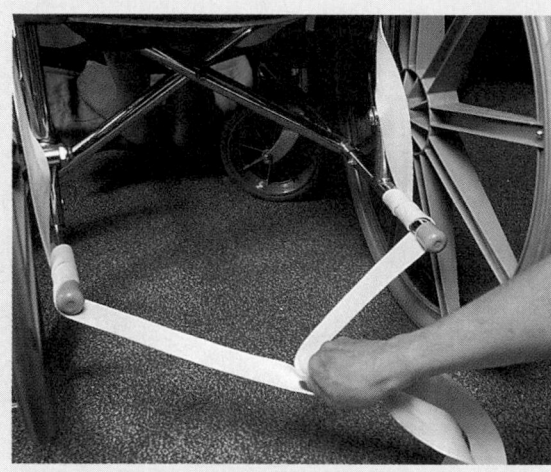

Step 8

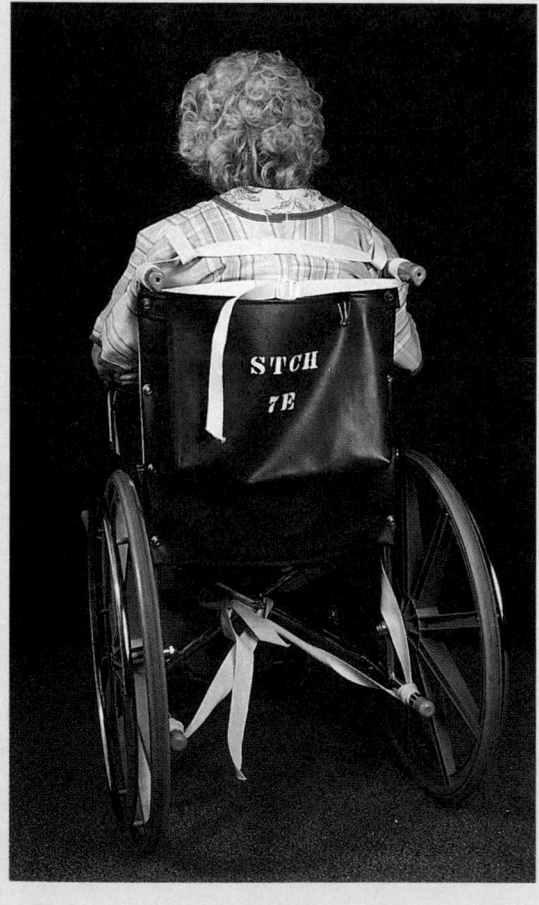

Step 8

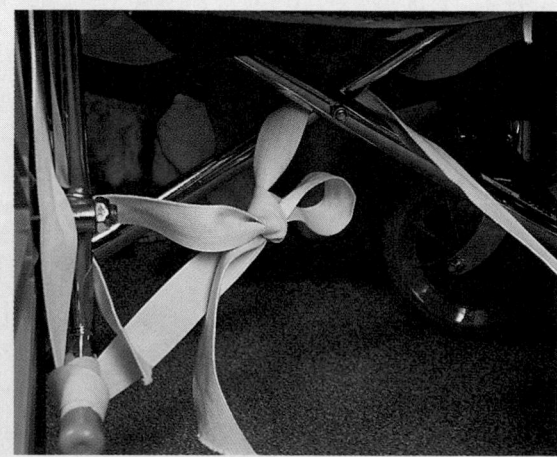

Step 9

Applying Restraints—cont'd

STEPS	RATIONALE
9. Do not tie the end of a restraint in a knot. Use a quick release tie for all restraints (see the illustration on p. 888).	A client can become improperly positioned in a restraint—requiring immediate release.
10. Wash hands.	Reduces transmission of microorganisms.
11. Completely remove restraints briefly at least every 2 hr and document in nurse's notes. Client should not be left unattended. Observe color of extremity and palpate pulses below extremity. Have client move extremity.	Provides opportunity to assess circulation, range of motion, and respiration, and to provide skin care and assist the client with elimination. Timely assessment enables nurse to routinely observe musculoskeletal system and prevent complications from restraint device.
12. Observe for correct application of restraint every hour.	Incorrect application of restraints can result in injury to client.
13. Attempt a trial release when client's orientation and behavior begin to improve.	A trial release is a period when the nurse reassesses client to determine if continued use of restraint is needed.
14. Record in nurse's notes nursing assessment before and after restraints were used and if any restraint alternatives were attempted focusing on client's safety, level of orientation, type of restraint selected, response to restraint	Documents that client's physical safety was at risk and that specific restraint was warranted.

Improperly grounded or malfunctioning electrical equipment increases the risk of electrical injury and fire. Educating both the client and family can reduce the risk for electrical hazards in the home environment (see the box at right).

If a client receives an electrical shock, the nurse should immediately determine whether the client has a pulse. If the client has no pulse, cardiopulmonary resuscitation (CPR) should be initiated and emergency personnel should be notified (see Chapter 44). If the client has a pulse and remains alert and oriented, the nurse should quickly obtain vital signs and assess the skin for signs of thermal injury. The client's physician must be notified. If an electrical shock occurs in the home, the nurse follows the same procedure but has the client go to the emergency room and then notifies the client's physician.

Radiation. Radiation is a health hazard in the health care setting and the community. Radiation and radioactive materials are utilized in the diagnosis and treatment of clients. Hospitals have guidelines on the care of clients who are receiving radiation and radioactive materials. The nurse must be familiar with established agency protocols. To reduce the nurse's exposure to radiation, time near the source should be limited, distance from the source should be as great as possible, and shielding devices such as lead aprons should be used.

The community may be at risk for radiation exposure because of incorrect disposal and transportation of radioactive waste products. Community health agencies and the Environmental Protection Agency (EPA) establish specific, strict guidelines for the disposal of radioactive waste. If a radioactive leak occurs, these agencies institute measures to prevent exposure of surrounding neighborhoods, to clean up radioactive leaks as quickly as possible, and to ensure that injured parties receive prompt medical care.

CLIENT TEACHING for Prevention of Electrical Hazards

OBJECTIVE
- Client will recognize electrical hazards in the home and take steps to eliminate them.

TEACHING STRATEGIES
- Discuss the method of grounding appliances and other equipment.
- Provide examples of common hazards: frayed cords, visibly damaged equipment, overloaded outlets.
- Discuss guidelines to prevent electrical shocks:
  - Use extension cords only when absolutely necessary and tape to ground with electrical tape.
  - Never run electrical wiring under carpets.
  - Never pull a plug using the cord, always grasp the plug itself.
  - Never use electrical appliances near sinks, bathtubs, or other water sources.
  - Never operate unfamiliar equipment.
  - Always disconnect before cleaning equipment or appliances.

EVALUATION
- Have client list hazards currently existing in the home.
- Review steps client intends to take to eliminate hazards.
- Observe client's home within 1 week of teaching session.

PROCEDURE 36-3

Intervening in Poisoning

STEPS	RATIONALE
1. Remove materials from mouth, eyes, etc.	This will limit amount of poison client receives.
2. Identify the type and amount of substance ingested.	Will help to determine correct type and amount of antidote needed for victim.
3. Call poison control center before attempting intervention.	Centers have information needed to treat poisoned client or to offer referral to treatment centers.
4. If instructed to induce vomiting: a. Infants up to 12 months: ipecac administered only under direction of a physician b. Children (1 to 12 years): 1 tablespoon (15 ml) of ipecac c. Adults: 2 tablespoons (30 ml) of ipecac	Households should keep syrup of ipecac in easily accessible place. Ipecac causes vomiting and emptying of stomach, rather than gagging or retching. Experts recommend these doses and do not advise inducing vomiting with substances other than ipecac. Vomiting should be induced only under physician's instruction and is not induced with ingestion of gasoline or other caustic poisons.
5. Give oral fluids to assist vomiting: a. Children (1 to 12 years): 5 to 15 ml/kg, up to 8 oz of water b. Adults: 16 oz of water	Assists in emptying of stomach and further avoids gagging and retching.
6. If requested to do so, save vomitus and deliver to poison control center.	Laboratory analysis can determine further treatment.
7. Place victim with head turned to side.	Reduces the risk of aspiration.
8. Vomiting is never induced for the following substances: lye, household cleaners, grease or petroleum products, and furniture polish.	Vomiting can increase area of internal burns (in case of lye) and risk of aspiration.
9. Vomiting is never induced in an unconscious victim.	Vomiting increases risk of aspiration.
10. If instructed by poison control center to take person to emergency room, call ambulance.	Ambulance personnel will be able to provide emergency measures if needed. In addition, parent or guardian may be too upset to drive safely.

Evaluation

The plan of care, which was designed to reduce the client's risk for injury, is evaluated by comparing outcome criteria to the goals established during the planning phase (see the evaluation box below). If the goals have been met, the nursing interventions can be considered effective and appropriate. If not, the nurse determines whether new risks to the client have developed or whether previous risks remain. The client and family need to participate to find permanent ways to reduce risks to safety. The nurse continually as-

sesses the client's and family's need for additional support services such as home health care, physical therapy and counseling, and further teaching.

A safe environment is essential to promoting, maintaining and restoring health. Using the nursing process, the nurse assesses the client and the environment to determine risk factors for injury, clusters risk factors, formulates a nursing diagnosis, and plans specific interventions, including client education. The expected outcomes include a safe physical environment, a client knowledgeable about safety factors and precautions, and a client free of injury.

Sample Evaluation of Interventions for Risk for Injury

GOAL	EVALUATIVE MEASURES	EXPECTED OUTCOMES
Client will have a safe home environment within 6 months.	Ask client to state potential hazards. Inspect client's safe use of home appliances, medications, and health care equipment. Observe home environment after intervention.	Client will list hazards within the home by end of third teaching session. After 3 months, client will modify hazards by 50%. After 6 months, modifiable hazards in the home will be reduced by 100%.

■ KEY CONCEPTS ■

► In the community, a safe environment is one in which basic needs are achievable, physical hazards are reduced, transmission of pathogens is reduced, pollution is controlled, and sanitation is maintained.

► In a health care agency, a safe environment is one which minimizes falls, client-inherent accidents, procedure-inherent accidents, and equipment-related accidents.

► A factor that reduces atmospheric oxygen is the presence of high carbon monoxide levels, which may result from an improperly functioning furnace.

► Prolonged exposure to extreme environmental temperatures can cause client injury or even death.

► Reduction of physical hazards in the environment includes providing adequate lighting, decreasing clutter, and securing the home.

► The transmission of pathogens is reduced through medical and surgical asepsis, immunization, adequate food sanitation, insect and rodent control, and appropriate disposal of human wastes.

► Children under 5 years of age are at greatest risk for home accidents that may result in severe injury and death.

► The school-age child is at risk for injury at home, at school, and while traveling to and from school.

► Adolescents are at risk for injury from automobile accidents and substance abuse.

► Threats to an adult's safety are frequently associated with lifestyle habits.

► Risks of injury for older clients are directly related to the physiological changes of the aging process.

► Risks to client safety within a health care agency include falls and client-inherent, procedure-related, and equipment-related accidents.

► Nursing interventions for promoting safety are individualized for developmental stage, lifestyle, and environment.

► Nursing interventions are developed to modify the environment for protection from falls, fires, poisonings, and electrical hazards.

■ KEY TERMS ■

■ CRITICAL THINKING EXERCISES ■

1. During the nurse's home visit to a client with Alzheimer's disease, the client's wife comments that she is worried about her husband's safety because he "wanders around" during the night. Describe the assessment needed, as well as appropriate interventions to maintain this client's safety.

2. Describe the home assessment that parents of 2-year-old twins should conduct to eliminate the risk of poisoning. Develop a teaching plan for the parents about interventions in case of poisoning.

3. While working in a long-term care facility, the nurse is assigned to a client who becomes confused at times. What plans can the nurse initiate to avoid a client fall and the use restraints?

REFERENCES

Accident facts, Itasca, IL, 1993, National Safety Council.

Beck N: *The complete book of home inspection,* ed 2, Pennsylvania, 1993, TAB Books.

Brady R, Chester F, et al: Geriatric falls: prevention strategies for the staff, *J Gerontol Nurs* 19(9):26, 40, 1993.

Centers for Disease Control: Homicides among 15- to 19-year-old males—United States 1963-1991, *MMWR* 43(40):735, 1994.

Child Health Alert: Bicycle safety: what care-givers believe—and what do they do?, 11(9):2, 1993.

Ebersole P, Hess P: *Toward healthy aging: human needs and nursing response,* ed 4, St Louis, 1994, Mosby.

Ellis C: Nursing assessment and intervention for the patient experiencing seizures: a structured approach, *Clin Nurs Pract Epilepsy,* 1(2):4, 1993.

Health Care Financing Administration: *Federal Register* 54(21):1, 1990.

Kim MJ, McFarland GK, McLane AM: *Pocket guide to nursing diagnoses,* ed 6, St Louis, 1995, Mosby.

Lambert V: Patient restraints, *FDA Consumer* 26(8):9, 1992.

Loew F: The elderly can avoid falls, *World Health* 1(2):10, 1993.

McKenry L, Salerno E: *Pharmacology in nursing,* ed 18, St Louis, 1992, Mosby.

Pagana K, Pagana T: *Diagnostic and laboratory test reference,* ed 2, St Louis, 1995, Mosby.

Phipps W, Cassmeyer V, et al: *Medical-surgical nursing, concepts and clinical practice,* ed 5, St Louis, 1995, Mosby.

Seizure recognition and observation, a guide for allied health professionals, ed 2, Maryland, 1992, Epilepsy Foundation of America.

Shantz D, Spitz M: What you need to know about seizures, *Nurs 93* 23(11):34, 1993.

Stolley J: Freeing your patients from restraints, *Am J Nurs,* 95(2):27, 1995.

Tideiksaar R: Home safe home: practical tips for fall-proofing, *Geriatr Nurs* 11(6):280, 1989.

Top D: *Insuring electrical safety in the critical care setting,* New York, 1987, American Journal of Nursing Educational Services Division.

U.S. Public Health Service: Alcohol and other drug abuse in adolescents, *Am Fam Physician* 2(50):1737, December 1994.

Weick M: Physical restraints: an FDA update, *Am J Nurs* 92(11):74, 1992.

Williams SR: *Essentials of nutrition and diet therapy,* ed 6, St Louis, 1994, Mosby.

Wong DL: *Whaley and Wong's Nursing care of infants and children,* ed 5, St Louis, 1995, Mosby.

Yassi A, Gaborieau D, et al: The noise hazard in a large health care facility, *J Occup Environ Med* 33(10):1067, 1991.

Ziemba S: Clinical snapshot: seizures, *Am J Nurs,* 95(2):32, 1995.

ADDITIONAL READINGS

Corr K, Corr D: Taking the gloves off: caring for confused patients without using restraints, *Nursing* 24(9):70, 1994.

Cutchins C: Blueprint for restraint-free care, *Am J Nurs* 91(7)36, 1991.

Fletcher K: Restraints should be a last resort, *RN* 53(1):52, 1990.

Goodner B: *The OSHA handbook: interpretive guidelines for the bloodborne pathogen standard,* El Paso, 1993, Skidmore-Roth.

Houston K, Lach H: Restraints: how do you score?, *Geriatr Nurs* 11(5):231, 1990.

Leger-Krall S: When restraints become abusive, *Nurs 94* 24(3):55, 1994.

Magee R, Hyatt E, et al: Institutional policy: use of restraints in extended care and nursing homes, *J Gerontol Nurs* 19(4):31, 1993.

O'Brien K: Managing the seizure patient, *Nurs 91* 21(1):63, 1991.

Strumpf N, Evans L, Schwartz D: Restraint-free care: from dream to reality, *Geriatr Nurs* 11(3):122, 1990.

Watzke J, Wister A: Staff attitudes: monitoring technology in long-term care, *J Gerontol Nurs* 19(11):23, 1993.

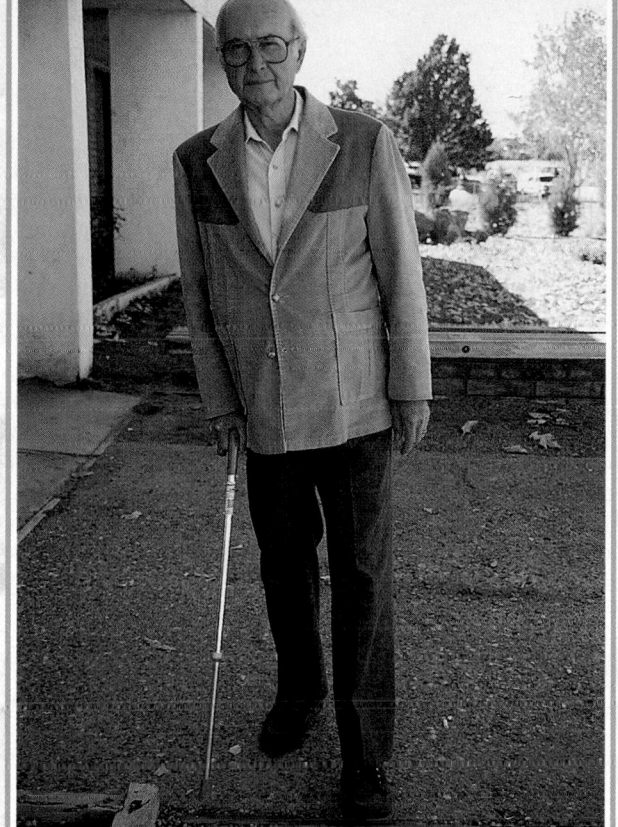

Mobility and Immobility

Objectives

Mastery of content in this chapter will enable the student to:

▶ Define the key terms listed.

▶ Describe the roles of the skeleton, skeletal muscles, and nervous system in the regulation of movement.

▶ Discuss physiological and pathological influences on body alignment and joint mobility.

▶ Identify changes in physiological and psychosocial function associated with immobility.

▶ Assess for impaired body alignment and mobility.

▶ State correct nursing diagnoses for impaired body alignment and mobility.

▶ Write nursing care plans for impaired body alignment and mobility.

▶ Describe essential techniques when assisting a client to move up in bed, repositioning a helpless client, assisting a client to a sitting position, and transferring a client from a bed to a chair or a bed to a stretcher.

▶ Describe active/passive range of motion exercises.

▶ Describe essential techniques when assisting a client to safely use crutches.

▶ Evaluate the nursing plan for maintaining body alignment and mobility.

Clinical nursing requires the nurse to incorporate knowledge and skills into practice. One component of knowledge and skill is *body mechanics,* a broad term used to describe coordinated efforts of the musculoskeletal and nervous systems.

Body mechanics includes knowing how and why certain muscle groups are used to safely produce and maintain motion. To use proper body mechanics the nurse needs to understand the regulation of movement, including how coordinated body motion involves integrated functioning of the skeletal system, skeletal muscle, and nervous system. In addition, certain muscle groups are used primarily for movement and others primarily for posture.

Mobility serves many purposes, such as expression of an emotion with a nonverbal gesture, self-defense, satisfaction of basic needs, the activities of daily living, and recreational activities. To maintain optimal physical mobility, the nervous, muscular, and skeletal systems of the body must be intact and functioning.

■ OVERVIEW OF BODY MECHANICS

Body mechanics are the coordinated efforts of the musculoskeletal and nervous systems to maintain balance, posture, and body alignment during lifting, bending, moving, and performing activities of daily living. Use of proper body mechanics reduces risk of injury to the musculoskeletal system. Proper mechanics also facilitates body movement, which allows physical mobility without muscle strain and excessive use of muscle energy.

Body Alignment

Body alignment and *posture* are analogous terms and refer to the positioning of the joints, tendons, ligaments, and muscles while in the standing, sitting, and lying positions. Correct body alignment reduces strain on musculoskeletal structures, maintains adequate muscle tone, and contributes to balance.

Body Balance

Body alignment contributes to body balance. Without this balance, the **center of gravity** is displaced, which increases the force of gravity, consequently creating a risk for falling and receiving an injury. Body balance is achieved when a wide base of support exists, the center of gravity falls within the base of support, and a vertical line can be drawn from the center of gravity through the base of support. Body balance also is enhanced by posture and lowering the center of gravity, which can be achieved by a squatting position. The more aligned the posture, the greater the balance (Perry and Potter, 1994).

Balance is required for maintaining a position, remaining stable while moving from one position to another, performing acts of daily living, and moving freely in the community. The ability to balance can be compromised by disease, a toddler's unsteady gait, pregnancy, medications, and the processes of aging. Impairment of this ability poses a threat to physical safety and can lead to a fear for one's safety with self-imposed restrictions on activity (Berg et al, 1992).

Coordinated Body Movement

Weight is the force exerted on a body by gravity. When an object is lifted, the lifter must overcome the object's weight and know its center of gravity. In symmetrical objects the center of gravity is located at the exact center of the object. Because people are not geometrically perfect, their centers of gravity are usually at 55% to 57% of standing height and are located in the midline. The force of weight is always directed downward, which is why an unbalanced object falls. Clients who are unsteady fall because, as their centers of gravity become unbalanced, the gravitational force of their weight eventually causes them to fall. Therefore the nurse needs to design nursing interventions that protect such clients from falling and ensure their safety (see Chapter 36).

Friction is a force that occurs in a direction to oppose movement. As the nurse turns, transfers, or moves a client up in bed, friction must be overcome. A nurse can reduce friction by following some basic principles. The greater the surface area of the object to be moved, the greater the friction. If a client is unable to assist in moving up in bed, the client's arms should be placed across the chest. This decreases surface area and reduces friction.

A passive or immobilized client produces greater friction to movement. Thus, whenever possible, the nurse should use some of the client's strength and mobility when lifting, transferring, or moving the client up in bed. This can be done by explaining the procedure and telling the client when to move. The result should be a synchronized movement in which the client can then participate and friction is decreased.

Friction can also be reduced by lifting rather than pushing a client. Lifting has an upward component and decreases the pressure between the client and the bed or chair. The use of a pull sheet reduces friction because the client is more easily moved along the bed's surface.

■ REGULATION OF MOVEMENT

Coordinated body movement involves integrated functioning of the skeletal system, skeletal muscle, and nervous system. Because these three systems cooperate so closely in mechanical support of the body, they can be considered as a single functional unit.

Skeletal System

The skeleton is the body's supporting framework and comprises four types of bones: long, short, flat, and irregular. **Long bones** contribute to height (e.g., the femur, fibula, and tibia in the leg) and length (e.g., the phalanges of the fingers and toes). **Short bones** occur in clusters and, when combined with ligaments and cartilage, permit movement of the extremities. Two examples of short bones are the carpal bones in the foot and the patella in the knee. **Flat bones** provide structural contour, such as bones in the skull and the ribs in the thorax. **Irregular bones** make up the vertebral column and some bones of the skull, such as the mandible.

The skeleton provides attachments for muscles and ligaments. These attachments allow movement of parts of the skeleton, such as opening and closing the mouth or extending an arm or a leg. The skeleton also protects vital organs. For example, the skull protects the brain, and the ribs protect the heart and lungs. Bones assist in regulation of calcium balance. Bones can store calcium and release it into the circulation as needed. Clients with altered calcium regulation and metabolism are at risk for developing osteoporosis and **pathological fractures** (fractures caused by weakened bone tissue), which can occur in all bones, but are most common in the ribs and weight-bearing bones. In addition, the internal structure of bones contains bone marrow, participates in red blood cell (RBC) production, and acts as a reservoir for blood. Clients with altered bone marrow function or diminished RBC production are usually weakened and fatigue easily, which decreases mobility and places clients at risk of falling.

CHARACTERISTICS OF BONE

The characteristics of bone include firmness, rigidity, and elasticity. Firmness results from inorganic salts, such as calcium and phosphate, that are laid down in the bone matrix. Firmness is related to the bone's rigidity, which is necessary to keep long bones straight, and enables bones to withstand weight bearing. In addition, bones have a degree of elasticity and skeletal flexibility that changes with age. For example, the newborn has a large amount of cartilage and is highly flexible but is unable to support weight. The toddler's bones are more pliable than those of an older person and are better able to withstand falls.

JOINTS

Joints are the connections between bones. Each joint is classified according to its structure and degree of mobility. There are four classifications of joints: synostotic, cartilaginous, fibrous, and synovial.

The **synostotic joint** refers to bones jointed by bones. No movement is associated with this type of joint, and the bony tissue that forms between the bones provides strength and stability. The classic example of this type of joint is the sacrum, in which vertebrae are joined (Fig. 37-1, *A*).

The **cartilaginous joint**, or synchondrodial joint, has little movement but is elastic and uses cartilage to unite body surfaces. Cartilaginous joints are found when bones are exposed to constant pressure, such as the costosternal joints between the sternum and ribs (Fig. 37-1, *B*).

The **fibrous joint**, or syndesmodial joint, is a joint in which two bony surfaces are united by a ligament or mem-

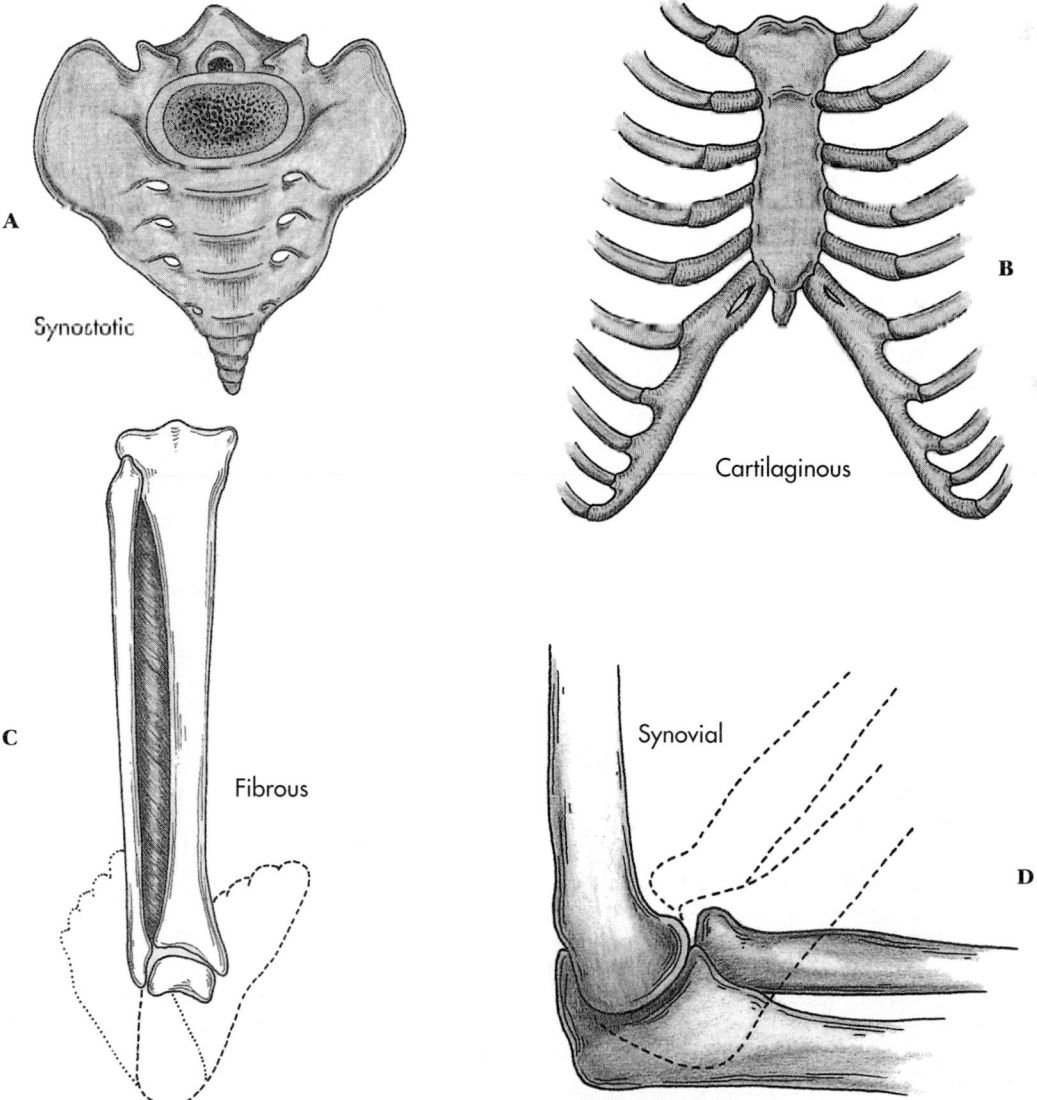

Fig. 37-1 Joint types.

brane. The fibers of ligaments are flexible and stretch, permitting a limited amount of movement. For example, the paired bones of the lower leg (tibia and fibula) are syndesmotic joints (McCance and Huether, 1994) (Fig. 37-1, *C*).

The **synovial joint**, or true joint, is a freely movable joint in which contiguous bony surfaces are covered by articular cartilage and connected by ligaments lined with a synovial membrane. Joining of the humeral radius and ulna by cartilage and ligaments forms a pivotal joint (Fig. 37-1, *D*). Other types of synovial joints are ball-and-socket joints, such as the hip joint, and hinge joints, such as interphalangeal joints of fingers.

LIGAMENTS

Ligaments are white, shiny, flexible bands of fibrous tissue binding joints together and connecting bones and cartilages. Ligaments are elastic and aid joint flexibility and support (Fig. 37-2). In addition, some ligaments have a protective function. For example, ligaments between the vertebral bodies, nonelastic ligaments, and the ligamentum flavum prevent damage to the spinal cord during movement of the back.

TENDONS

Tendons are white, glistening, fibrous bands of tissue that connect muscle to bone. Tendons are strong, flexible, and inelastic, and occur in various lengths and thicknesses. The Achilles tendon (tendo calcaneus) is the thickest and strongest tendon in the body. It begins near the middle of the posterior of the leg and attaches the gastrocnemius and soleus muscles in the calf to the calcaneal bone in the back of the foot (Fig. 37-3).

CARTILAGE

Cartilage is nonvascular, supporting connective tissue located chiefly in the joints and thorax, trachea, larynx, nose, and ear. The fetus has a large amount of temporary cartilage, which is replaced by bone developed during infancy. Permanent cartilage is unossified except in advanced age and diseases such as osteoarthritis.

Joints, ligaments, tendons, and cartilage permit strength and flexibility of the skeleton. Strength enables the skeletal system to support the body. A person's flexibility is demonstrated through range of motion (ROM). However, strength and flexibility do not result entirely from these four structures. Adequate skeletal muscle is also necessary.

Skeletal Muscle

Movement of bones and joints involves active processes that must be carefully integrated to achieve coordination. Skeletal muscles, because of their ability to contract and relax, are the working elements of movement. Contractile elements of the skeletal muscle are enhanced by anatomical structure and attachment to the skeleton.

Muscle contraction is stimulated by an electrochemical impulse that travels from the nerve to the muscle across the myoneural junction. The electrochemical impulse causes the thin, actin-containing filaments to shorten, thus contracting the muscle. Removal of the stimulus results in muscle relaxation.

There are two types of muscle contractions: isotonic and isometric. In **isotonic contraction**, increased muscle tension results in muscle shortening. **Isometric contraction** causes an increase in muscle tension or muscle work but no shortening or active movement of the muscle; for example, instructing the client in quadricep set exercises. Voluntary

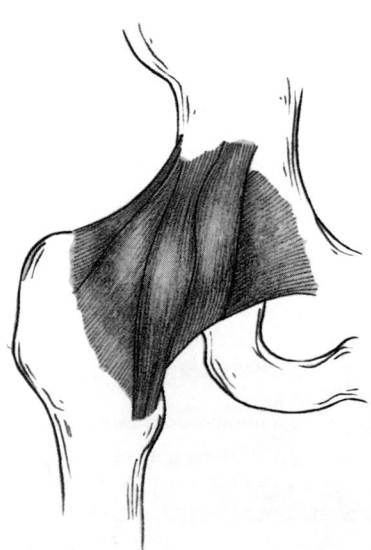

Fig. 37-2 Ligaments of the hip joint.

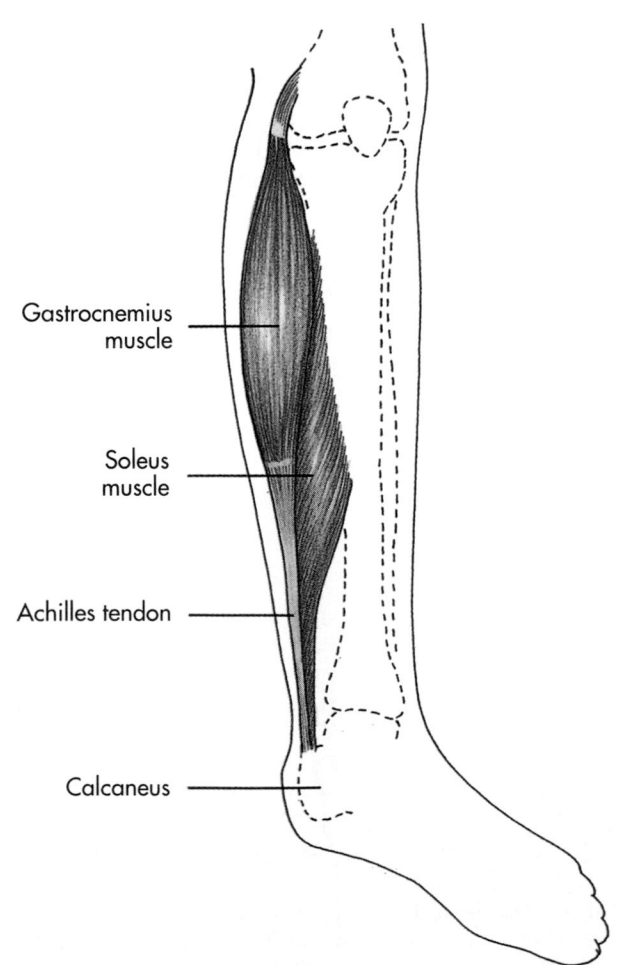

Gastrocnemius muscle

Soleus muscle

Achilles tendon

Calcaneus

Fig. 37-3 Tendons and muscles of the lower leg.

movement is a combination of isotonic and isometric contractions. For example, when the nurse lifts a client up in bed, the client's weight causes increased tension in the muscles of the nurse's arms until the tension (isometric) is equal to the weight to be lifted and the weight of the lower arm. When this equilibrium is reached, continued stimulation to the muscles results in muscle shortening (isotonic) and bending of the elbow (active movement), and the client is lifted off the bed.

Although isometric contractions do not result in muscle shortening, energy expenditure is increased. This type of muscle work is comparable to having a car in neutral with the driver continually depressing the accelerator and racing the engine. The driver is not going anywhere but expends a large amount of energy. The nurse must recognize the energy expenditure (increased respiratory rate, fluctuations in heart rate, blood pressure) associated with isometric exercises because they may be contraindicated in certain clients' illnesses (e.g., myocardial infarction or chronic obstructive pulmonary disease).

MUSCLES CONCERNED WITH MOVEMENT

Muscles concerned primarily with movement are located near the skeletal region where movement is caused by leverage. Leverage occurs when specific bones, such as the humerus, ulna, and radius, and the associated joints, such as the elbow joint, act together as a lever. Thus the force applied to one end of the bone to lift a weight at another point tends to rotate the bone in the direction opposite that of the applied force. Muscles that attach to bones of leverage provide necessary strength to move the object.

Leverage is characteristic of movements of the upper extremities. Arm muscles are parallel to one another and extend the full length of the bones. The long parallel muscles provide strength and work together with the bones and joints to enable lifting an object with the arms.

MUSCLES CONCERNED WITH POSTURE/BODY ALIGNMENT

Muscles associated primarily with maintaining posture are short and featherlike in appearance because they converge obliquely at a common tendon. Muscles of the lower extremities, trunk, neck, and back are concerned primarily with **posture** (the position of the body in relation to the surrounding space). These muscle groups work together to stabilize and support body weight standing or sitting, and they allow an individual to maintain a sitting or standing posture.

Muscle Regulation of Posture and Movement. Posture and movement can be reflections of personality and mood. For example, a person with a dramatic personality gestures with the hands, and a person who is fatigued or depressed may slouch.

Posture and movement also depend on the skeleton and the shape and development of skeletal muscles. Coordination and regulation of different muscle groups depend on muscle tone and activity of antagonistic, synergistic, and antigravity muscles.

Muscle Tone. **Muscle tone**, or tonus, is the normal state of balanced muscle tension. Tension is achieved by alternate contraction and relaxation, without active movement, of neighboring fibers of a specific muscle group. Muscle tone enables a body part to be maintained in a functioning position without muscle fatigue. In addition, muscle tone promotes venous return to the heart, as is the case with leg muscles.

Muscle tone is maintained through continual use of muscles. Activities of daily living require muscle action and help maintain muscle tone. As a result of immobility or prolonged bed rest, activity level and muscle tone decrease.

Muscle Groups. The antagonistic, synergistic, and antigravity muscle groups are coordinated by the nervous system and work together to maintain posture and initiate movement.

Antagonistic muscles work together to bring about movement at the joint. During movement, the active mover muscle contracts, and its antagonist relaxes. For example, when flexing the arm, the active biceps brachii contracts, and its antagonist, the triceps brachii, relaxes. During extension of the arm, the active triceps brachii contracts, and the new antagonist, the biceps brachii, relaxes.

Synergistic muscles contract together to accomplish the same movement. When the arm is flexed, the strength of contraction of the biceps brachii is increased by contraction of the synergistic muscle, the brachialis. Thus with synergistic muscle activity, there are two active movers, the biceps brachii and the brachialis, that contract while the antagonistic muscle, the triceps brachii, relaxes.

Antigravity muscles are specifically involved with stabilization of joints. These muscles continuously oppose the effect of gravity on the body and permit the maintenance of an upright or sitting posture. In an adult the antigravity muscles are the extensors of the leg, gluteus maximus, quadriceps femoris, soleus muscles, and muscles of the back.

Nervous System

Movement and posture are regulated by the nervous system. The major voluntary motor area, located in the cerebral cortex, is the precentral gyrus or motor strip. A majority of motor fibers descend from the motor strip and cross at the level of the medulla. Thus the motor fibers from the right motor strip initiate voluntary movement for the left side of the body, and motor fibers from the left motor strip initiate voluntary movement for the right side of the body.

During voluntary movement, impulses descend from the motor strip to the spinal cord. An impulse exits the spinal cord through efferent motor nerves and travels through the nerves to the muscles, where movement occurs. This impulse is controlled by synapses, which keep the impulse traveling in one direction.

Transmission of the impulse from the nervous system to the musculoskeletal system is an electrochemical event and requires a neurotransmitter. Basically, **neurotransmitters** are chemicals such as acetylcholine that transfer the electric impulse from the nerve across the myoneural junction to the muscle. The neurotransmitter reaches a muscle and stimulates it, causing movement.

Movement can be impaired by disorders that alter neurotransmitter production, transfer from the nerve to the muscle, or activation of muscle activity. Posture is also regulated by the nervous system. Posture requires coordination of proprioception and balance.

PROPRIOCEPTION

Proprioception is the sensation achieved through stimuli from within the body regarding spatial position and muscular activity. Proprioception in the body is monitored by proprioceptors, which are any nerve endings located in muscles, tendons, and joints.

As a person carries out activities of daily living, proprioceptors are continuously monitoring muscle activity and body position. For example, the proprioceptors on the soles of the foot contribute to correct posture while standing or walking. In standing, there is continuous pressure on the bottom of the feet. The proprioceptors monitor the pressure, communicating this information through the nervous system to the antigravity muscles. The standing person remains upright until deciding to change position. As a person walks, the proprioceptors on the bottom of the feet monitor pressure changes. Thus when the bottom of the moving foot comes in contact with the walking surface, the individual automatically moves the stationary foot forward. The proprioceptors allow people to walk without having to watch their feet.

BALANCE

Balance is the ability to attain and maintain an upright posture against gravity (sitting or standing) as well as to make adjustments in posture throughout skilled motor activities (Glick, 1992).

The cerebellum is responsible for reflexive, involuntary fine tuning of motor control and for maintaining balance and posture. Damage to the cerebellum is characterized by a loss of equilibrium, balance, and motor coordination (McCance and Huether, 1994).

Balance is also controlled by the inner ear. Within the inner ear are semicircular canals, three fluid-filled structures that assist in maintaining balance. Fluid within the canals has a certain inertia and, when the head is suddenly rotated in one direction, the fluid remains stationary for a moment while the canals turn with the head. This allows a person to change position suddenly without losing balance.

■ PRINCIPLES OF BODY MECHANICS

Proper body mechanics is important to the nurse and client. It affects their levels of wellness. Correct body mechanics is necessary for health promotion and prevention of disability.

The nurse uses a variety of muscle groups for each nursing activity, such as walking during nursing rounds, administering medications, lifting and transferring clients, and moving objects. The physical forces of weight and friction can influence body movement. Correctly used, these forces increase the nurse's efficiency. Incorrect use can impair the nurse's ability to lift, transfer, and position clients (Owen and Garg, 1991). The nurse also incorporates knowledge of physiological and pathological influences on mobility and body alignment. Table 37-1 lists principles of body mechanics that are useful in a variety of settings.

■ PATHOLOGICAL INFLUENCES ON BODY ALIGNMENT AND MOBILITY

Many pathological conditions affect body alignment and mobility. Although a complete description of each is beyond the scope of this chapter, tables and summaries provide baseline information about these pathological influences, four of which are presented here: postural abnormalities, impaired muscle development, damage to the central nervous system, and direct trauma to the musculoskeletal system.

Postural Abnormalities

Congenital or acquired postural abnormalities affect the efficiency of the musculoskeletal system, as well as body alignment, balance, and appearance. During physical assessment, the nurse observes body alignment and ROM (see Chapter 33). Postural abnormalities can impair alignment, **mobility**, or both.

Knowledge about the characteristics, causes, and treatment of common postural abnormalities (Table 37-2) is used first to improve the client's body alignment during lifting, transfer, and positioning. Because some postural ab-

Table 37-1	**Body Mechanics for Health Care Workers**

ACTION	RATIONALE
When planning to move a client, arrange for adequate help. Use mechanical aids if help is unavailable.	Two workers lifting together divide the workload by 50%.
Encourage client to assist as much as possible.	This promotes client's abilities and strength while minimizing workload.
Keep back, neck, pelvis, and feet aligned. Avoid twisting.	Reduces risk of injury to lumbar vertebrae and muscle groups (Owen and Garg, 1991). Twisting increases risk of injury.
Flex knees; keep feet wide apart.	A broad base of support increases stability.
Position self close to client (or object being lifted).	The force is minimized. Ten pounds at waist height close to body is equal to 100 pounds at arms' length.
Use arms and legs (not back).	The leg muscles are stronger, larger muscles capable of greater work without injury.
Slide client toward yourself using a pull sheet.	Sliding requires less effort than lifting. Pull sheet minimizes shearing forces, which can damage client's skin.
Set (tighten) abdominal and gluteal muscles in preparation for move.	Preparing muscles for the load minimizes strain.
Person with the heaviest load coordinates efforts of team involved by counting to three.	Simultaneous lifting minimizes the load for any one lifter.

Table 37-2	Postural Abnormalities		
ABNORMALITY	DESCRIPTION	CAUSE	TREATMENT
Torticollis	Inclining of head to affected side, in which sternocleidomastoid muscle is contracted	Congenital or acquired condition	Surgery, heat, support, or immobilization, depending on cause and severity
Lordosis	Exaggeration of anterior convex curve of lumbar spine	Congenital condition Temporary condition (e.g., pregnancy)	Spine-stretching exercises (based on cause)
Kyphosis	Increased convexity in curvature of thoracic spine	Congenital condition Rickets Tuberculosis of spine	Spine-stretching exercises, sleeping without pillows, using bed board, bracing, spinal fusion (based on cause and severity)
Kypholordosis	Combination of kyphosis and lordosis	Congenital condition	Similar to methods used in kyphosis or lordosis (based on cause)
Scoliosis	Lateral curvature of spine, unequal heights of hips and shoulders	Congenital condition Poliomyelitis Spastic paralysis Unequal leg length	Immobilization and surgery (based on cause and severity)
Kyphoscoliosis	Abnormal anteroposterior and lateral curvature of spine	Congenital condition Poliomyelitis Cor pulmonale	Immobilization and surgery (based on cause and severity)
Congenital hip dysplasia	Hip instability with limited abduction of hips and, occasionally, adduction contractures (head of femur does not articulate with acetabulum because of abnormal shallowness of acetabulum)	Congenital condition (more common with breech deliveries)	Maintenance of continuous abduction of thigh so that head of femur presses into center of acetabulum Abduction splints, casting, surgery
Knock-knee (genu valgum)	Legs curved inward so that knees knock together as person walks	Congenital condition Rickets	Knee braces, surgery if not corrected by growth
Bowlegs (genu varum)	One or both legs bent outward at knee, which is normal until 2 to 3 years of age	Congenital condition Rickets	Slowing rate of curving if not corrected by growth With rickets, increase of vitamin D, calcium, and phosphorus intake to normal ranges
Clubfoot	95%: medial deviation and plantar flexion of foot (equinovarus) 5%: lateral deviation and dorsiflexion (calcaneovalgus)	Congenital condition	Casts, splints such as Denis-Browne splint, and surgery (based on degree and rigidity of deformity)
Footdrop	Plantar flexion, inability to invert foot because of peroneal nerve damage	Congenital condition Trauma Improper position of immobilized client	None (cannot be corrected) Prevention through physical therapy
Pigeon-toes	Internal rotation of forefoot or entire foot, common in infants	Congenital condition Habit	Growth, wearing reversed shoes

Data from McCance KL, Huether SE: *Pathophysiology: the biologic basis for disease in adults and children,* ed 2, St Louis, 1994, Mosby.

normalities limit ROM in some joints, the nurse maintains maximum ROM in unaffected joints. Finally, the nurse designs nursing interventions to strengthen affected muscle and joint groups, improve the client's posture, and adequately use affected and unaffected muscle groups.

Impaired Muscle Development

The muscular dystrophies are a group of familial disorders that cause degeneration of skeletal muscle fibers. The most prevalent of the muscle diseases in childhood, the muscular dystrophies are characterized by progressive, symmetrical weakness and wasting of skeletal muscle groups, with increasing disability and deformity (McCance and Huether, 1994).

Damage to the Central Nervous System

Damage to any component of the central nervous system that regulates voluntary movement results in impaired body alignment and mobility. The motor strip in the cerebrum can be damaged by trauma from a head injury, ischemia from a cerebrovascular accident (stroke), or bacterial infection from meningitis. Motor impairment is directly related to the amount of destruction of the motor strip. For example, in the case of a person with a right-sided cerebral hemorrhage with complete necrosis, destruction of the right motor strip and left-sided hemiplegia are consequences. However, a person with a right-sided head injury will have cerebral edema and damage (but not destruction) of the motor strip, and with extensive physical therapy, voluntary movement may gradually return to the left side.

Because voluntary motor fibers descend from the motor strip in the cerebrum down the spinal cord, trauma to the spinal cord also impairs mobility. The most common trauma is transection of the spinal cord in which motor fibers are cut. This can cause a complete bilateral loss of voluntary motor control below the level of the trauma. Spinal cord trauma frequently results from diving or automobile accidents or gunshot or knife wounds to the neck and back.

Direct Trauma to the Musculoskeletal System

Direct trauma to the musculoskeletal system can result in bruises, contusions, sprains, and fractures. A **fracture** is a disruption of bone tissue continuity. Fractures most commonly result from direct external trauma, but they can also occur as a consequence of some deformity of the bone (e.g., pathological fractures of osteoporosis, Paget's disease, and osteogenesis imperfecta).

As the fracture heals, bone begins to repair. The fractured bone initiates a cellular process that results in bone formation. Young children are able to form new bone more easily than adults and, as a result, have few complications after a bone fracture. Treatment includes positioning the fractured bone in proper alignment and immobilizing it to promote healing and restore function. Immobilization results in some muscle atrophy, loss of tone, and joint stiffness.

Acquired or congenital conditions that affect the structure of the musculoskeletal or nervous system impair body alignment or joint mobility. Impairment can be temporary or permanent. Regardless of duration of the impairment, the nursing care plan includes interventions that maintain the present level of alignment and joint mobility and increase the client's level of motor function.

▌ IMPAIRED MOBILITY

Mobility refers to a person's *ability* to move about freely, and immobility refers to the *inability* to move about freely. Mobility and immobility are best understood as the endpoints of a continuum, with many degrees of partial immobility between. Some clients move back and forth on the mobility-immobility continuum, but for other clients, immobility is absolute and continues indefinitely (Perry and Potter, 1994).

Bed Rest

Bed rest is an intervention in which the client is restricted to bed for therapeutic reasons. Bed rest has different meanings among nurses, physicians, and other health care professionals. Clients with a wide variety of conditions are placed on bed rest. The duration of bed rest depends on the illness or injury and the client's prior state of health (see the box above).

The effects of muscular deconditioning associated with lack of physical activity may be apparent in a matter of days. The normal individual on bed rest loses muscle strength from baseline levels at a rate of 3% a day. Bed rest also is associated with cardiovascular, skeletal, and other organ changes. The term *disuse atrophy* has been used to describe the pathological reduction in normal size of muscle fibers after prolonged inactivity from bed rest, trauma, casting, or local nerve damage (McCance and Huether, 1994).

General Objectives of Bed Rest

- Reducing physical activity and the oxygen needs of the body
- Reducing pain, including postoperative pain, and the need for large doses of analgesics
- Allowing ill or debilitated clients to rest and regain strength
- Allowing exhausted clients the opportunity for uninterrupted rest

---

Immobility

Impaired physical mobility (**immobility**) is defined by the North American Nursing Diagnosis Association (NANDA) as a state in which the individual experiences or is at risk of experiencing limitation of physical movement (Kim et al, 1995).

Alterations in the level of physical mobility can result from prescribed restriction of movement in the form of bed rest, physical restriction of movement through the use of external devices (e.g., a cast or skeletal traction), voluntary restriction of movement, or impairment or loss of motor function.

PHYSIOLOGICAL EFFECTS

When there is an alteration in mobility, each body system is at risk for impairment. The severity of the impairment depends on the client's age and overall health and degree of immobility experienced. For example, older adults with chronic illnesses develop pronounced effects of immobility more quickly than do younger clients (Perry and Potter, 1994).

Metabolic Changes. The endocrine system, made up of hormone-secreting glands, helps to maintain and regulate vital functions such as (1) response to stress and injury, (2) growth and development, (3) reproduction, (4) ionic homeostasis, and (5) energy metabolism. When injury or stress occurs, the endocrine system triggers a series of responses aimed at maintaining blood pressure and preserving life. The endocrine system is important in maintenance of ionic homeostasis. Mammalian organisms live in an external environment that changes constantly. However, tissues and cells live in an internal environment that must remain constant. The endocrine system participates in the regulation of this internal environment through maintenance of sodium, potassium, water, and acid-base balance. Finally, the endocrine system acts as a regulator of energy metabolism. The basal metabolic rate (BMR) is increased by thyroid hormone, and energy is made available to cells through the integrated action of gastrointestinal and pancreatic hormones (Price and Wilson, 1992).

Immobility disrupts normal metabolic functioning, including metabolic rate; metabolism of carbohydrates, fats, and proteins; fluid and electrolyte imbalances; calcium imbalance; and gastrointestinal disturbances. However, in the presence of an infectious process, immobilized clients may have an increased BMR as a result of fever or wound healing. Fever and repair of wounds increase cellular oxygen requirements (McCance and Huether, 1994).

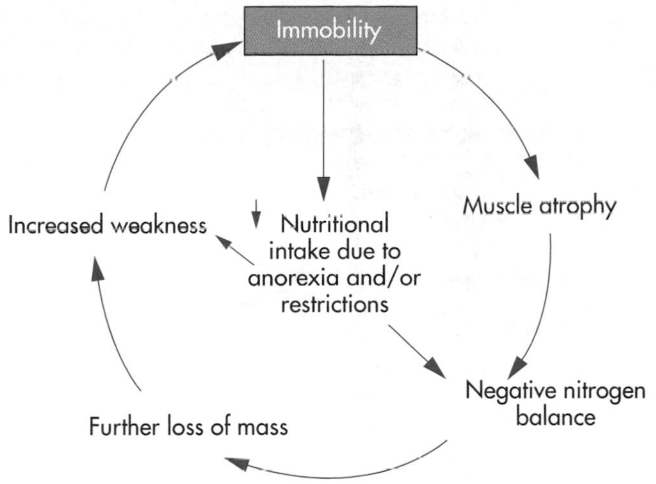

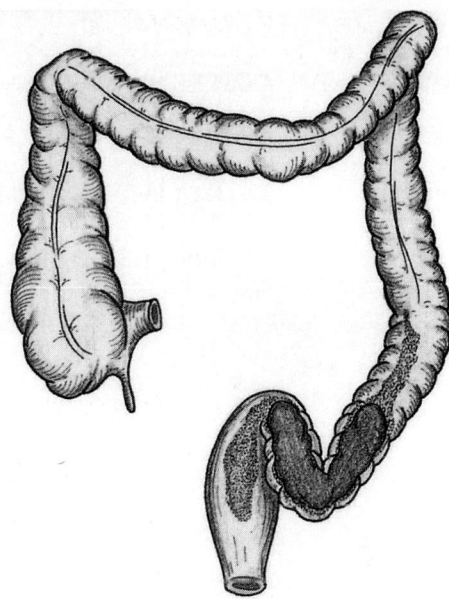

Fig. 37-4 Factors contributing to negative nitrogen balance associated with immobility. *(From Gröer MW, Shekleton ME:* Basic pathophysiology: a conceptual approach, *ed 3, St Louis, 1989, Mosby–Year Book.)*

Fig. 37-5 Fecal impaction with liquid stool passing around the impaction.

A deficiency in calories and protein is characteristic of clients with a decreased appetite secondary to immobility. Proteins are constantly being synthesized and broken down into amino acids in the body to be reformed into other proteins. Amino acids that are not used are excreted. The body can synthesize certain amino acids (nonessential) but depends on ingested proteins to supply the eight essential amino acids. When more nitrogen (the end product of amino acid breakdown) is excreted than is ingested in proteins, the body is said to have a **negative nitrogen balance** (Fig. 37-4), and weight loss, decreased muscle mass, and weakness result from tissue catabolism. Protein loss leads to decreased muscle mass, especially in the liver, heart, lungs, gastrointestinal (GI) tract, and immune system (Long et al, 1993).

Urinary excretion of calcium is increased through **bone resorption**. Immobility causes the release of calcium into the circulation. Normally the kidneys can excrete the excess calcium. However, if the kidneys are unable to respond appropriately, hypercalcemia results (Holm, 1989).

Impairments of GI functioning vary and result from decreased GI motility. Constipation is a common symptom. Diarrhea is frequently the result of a fecal impaction (Fig. 37-5). The nurse must be aware that this finding is not normal diarrhea, but rather liquid stool passing around the area of impaction. Left untreated, fecal impaction can result in a mechanical bowel obstruction that may partially or completely occlude the intestinal lumen, blocking normal propulsion of liquid and gas. The resulting fluid in the intestine produces distention and increases intraluminal pressure. Over time, intestinal function becomes depressed, dehydration occurs, absorption ceases, and fluid and electrolyte disturbances worsen.

Respiratory Changes. Postoperative and immobile clients are at high risk for developing pulmonary complications. The most common respiratory complications are atelectasis and hypostatic pneumonia. In atelectasis a bronchiole becomes blocked by secretions and the distal alveoli collapse as the existing air is absorbed, producing hypoventilation. A major bronchus or many small bronchioles may be involved. The extent of atelectasis is determined by the site of the blockage. Hypostatic pneumonia is inflammation of the lung from stasis of secretions. Both atelectasis and hypostatic pneumonia decrease oxygenation, prolong recovery, and add to the client's discomfort (Long et al, 1993).

At some point in the development of these complications, there is a proportional decline in the client's ability to cough productively. Ultimately the distribution of mucus in the bronchi increases, particularly when the client is in the supine, prone, or lateral position (Fig. 37-6). Mucus accumulates in the dependent regions of the airways (Fig. 37-7). Because mucus is an excellent medium for bacterial growth, hypostatic bronchopneumonia may result.

Cardiovascular Changes. The cardiovascular system is also affected by immobilization. The three major changes are orthostatic hypotension, increased cardiac workload, and thrombus formation.

Orthostatic hypotension is a drop of 25 mm Hg systolic and of 10 mm Hg diastolic in blood pressure when the client rises from a lying or sitting position to a standing position. In the immobilized client, decreased circulating fluid volume, pooling of blood in the lower extremities, and decreased autonomic response occur. These factors result in decreased venous return, followed by a decrease in cardiac output, which is reflected by a decline in blood pressure (McCance and Huether, 1994).

As the workload of the heart increases, its oxygen consumption does, too. The heart therefore works harder and less efficiently during periods of prolonged rest. As immobilization increases, cardiac output falls, further decreasing cardiac efficiency and increasing workload.

Clients are also at risk for thrombus formation. A **thrombus** is an accumulation of platelets, fibrin, clotting factors,

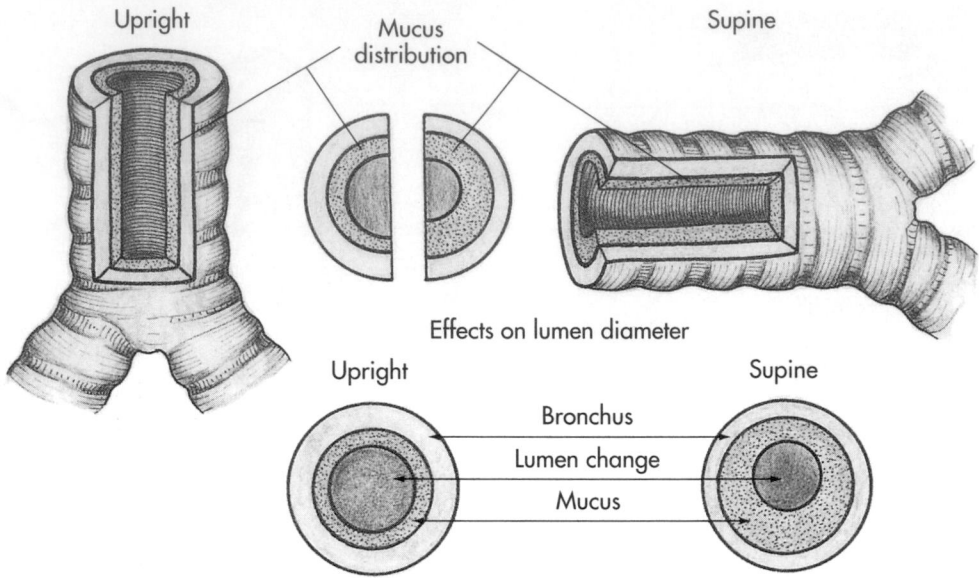

Fig. 37-6 Effect of recumbency and gravity on distribution of respiratory tract and diameter of bronchiolar lumen. *(From Gröer MW, Shekleton ME:* Basic pathophysiology: a conceptual approach, *ed 2, St Louis, 1989, Mosby–Year Book.)*

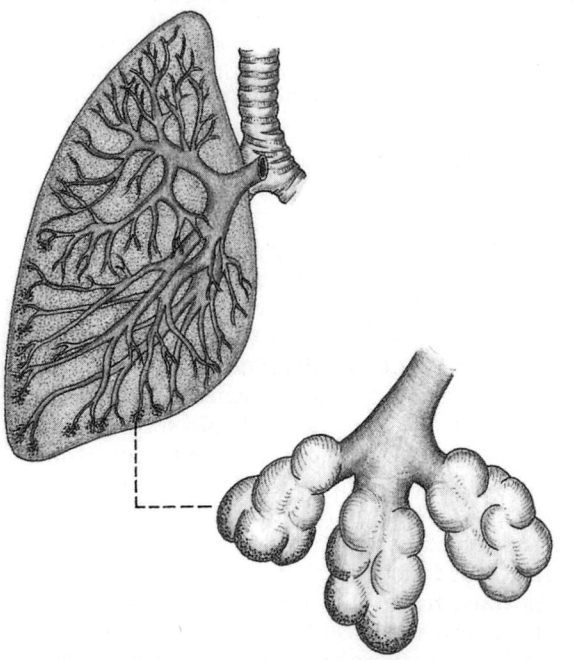

Fig. 37-7 Pooling of secretions in dependent regions of the lungs in the supine position.

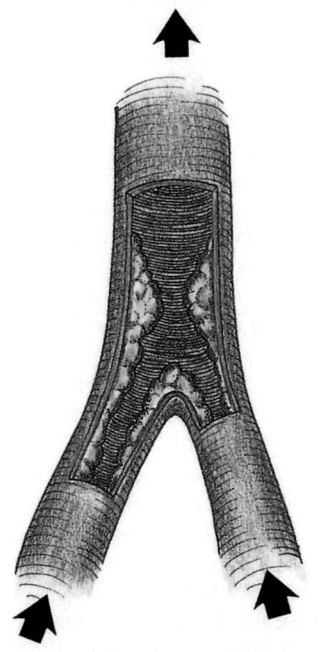

Fig. 37-8 Thrombus formation in a vessel.

and the cellular elements of the blood attached to the interior wall of a vein or artery, sometimes occluding the lumen of the vessel (Fig. 37-8).

There are three factors that can cause thrombus formation: (1) loss of integrity of the vessel wall (e.g., atherosclerosis), (2) abnormalities of blood flow (e.g., slow blood flow in veins associated with bed rest and immobility), and (3) alterations in blood constituents (e.g., a change in clot-

ting factors or increased platelet activity) (McCance and Huether, 1994).

Musculoskeletal Changes. The effects of immobility on the musculoskeletal system can include permanent impairment of mobility. Restricted mobility affects the client's muscles through loss of endurance, decreased muscle mass, atrophy, and decreased stability. Other effects of restricted mobility affecting the skeletal system are impaired calcium metabolism and impaired joint mobility.

Fig. 37-9 Contracture of the elbow resulting in permanent flexion of the joint. Normally the elbow is able to extend to a 90-degree angle *(dotted line)* and to a 180-degree angle (not illustrated).

Muscle Effects. Because of protein breakdown, the client loses lean body mass, which is composed partially of muscle. Therefore the reduced muscle mass is unable to sustain activity without increased fatigue. The muscle mass is decreased from metabolic causes and disuse. As immobility continues and the muscles are not exercised, there is continued decrease in mass.

Decreased mobility and movement result in gross musculoskeletal impairment, of which the primary pathophysiological alteration is atrophy. Atrophy is a phenomenon widely observed in response to illness and decreased activities of daily living, as well as in response to immobilization and bed rest (Kasper et al, 1993).

Decreased stability results from loss of endurance, decreased muscle mass, atrophy, and actual joint abnormalities. Therefore these clients are unable to move steadily, and their risk for falling increases.

Skeletal Effects. Immobilization causes two skeletal changes: impaired calcium metabolism and joint abnormalities. Because immobilization results in bone resorption, the bone tissue is less dense, and osteoporosis results (Holm, 1989). When osteoporosis occurs, the client is at risk for pathological fractures. Immobilization and non–weight-bearing activities increase the rate of bone resorption. Bone resorption also causes calcium to be released in the blood, and hypercalcemia results.

Immobility can lead to joint contractures. A **joint contracture** is an abnormal and usually permanent condition characterized by flexion and fixation of the joint. It is caused by disuse, atrophy, and shortening of the muscle fibers. When a contracture occurs, the joint cannot maintain full ROM. Unfortunately, contracture usually leaves the joint in a nonfunctional position (Lehmkuhl et al, 1990) (Fig. 37-9).

One common and debilitating contracture is footdrop (Fig. 37-10). When **footdrop** occurs, the foot is permanently fixed in plantar flexion. Ambulation is difficult with the foot in this position.

Integumentary Changes. A **pressure ulcer**, or decubitus ulcer, is the consequence of ischemia and anoxia to tissue. Tissues are compressed, blood diverted, and blood ves-

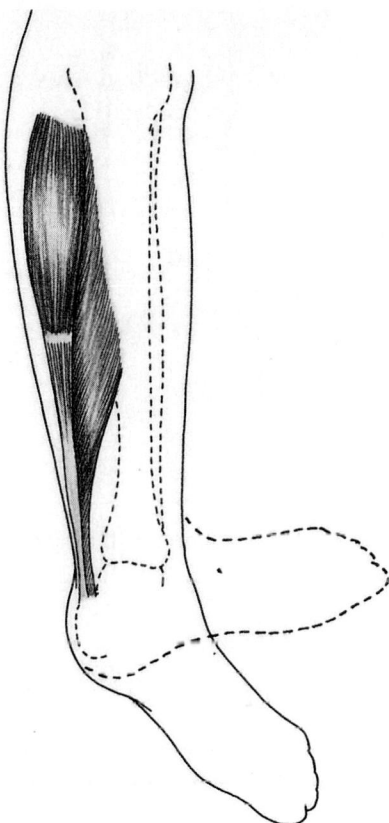

Fig. 37-10 Footdrop. Ankle is fixed in plantar flexion. Normally the ankle is able to flex *(dotted line)*, which eases walking.

sels forcibly constricted by persistent pressure on the skin and underlying structures; thus cellular respiration is impaired, and cells die (Ebersole and Hess, 1994). Pressure ulcers are one of the most common iatrogenic illnesses in health care that affect a specific client population—the elderly and the immobile (Alterescu and Alterescu, 1992). Impairments in skin integrity have significant impact on the level of wellness, nursing care, and length of hospital stay (see Chapter 38).

Urinary Elimination Changes. The client's urinary elimination is altered by immobility. In the upright position, urine flows out of the renal pelvis and into the ureter and bladder because of gravitational forces. When the client is recumbent or flat, the kidneys and the ureters move toward a more level plane. Urine formed by the kidney must enter the bladder against gravity. Because the peristaltic contractions of the ureters are insufficient to overcome gravity, the renal pelvis may fill before urine enters the ureters (Fig. 37-11). This condition is called **urinary stasis** and increases the risk of urinary tract infection and renal calculi (see Chapter 46).

Renal calculi are calcium stones that lodge in the renal pelvis and pass through the ureters (Fig. 37-12). Immobilized clients are at risk for calculi because of altered calcium metabolism and the resulting hypercalcemia (Holm, 1989).

As the period of immobility continues, fluid intake can diminish, and other causes, such as fever, increase the risk for dehydration. As a result, urinary output declines on or

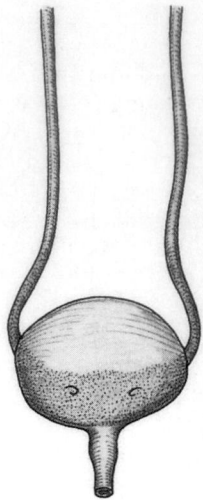

Fig. 37-11 Stasis of urine with reflux to ureters.

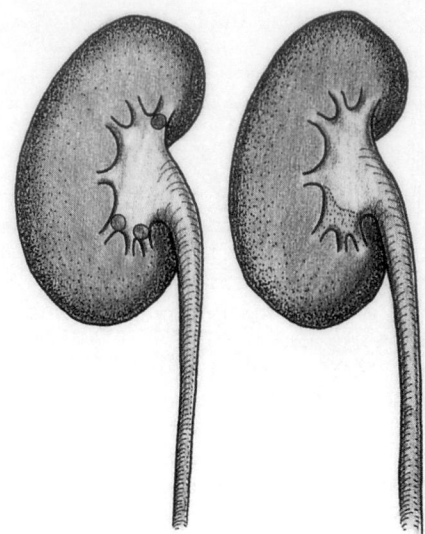

Fig. 37-12 Types of renal calculi in the renal pelvis.

about the fifth or sixth day. The urine that is produced is usually highly concentrated.

This concentrated urine increases the risk for calculi formation and infection. Poor perineal care after bowel movements, particularly in women, increases the risk of urinary tract contamination by *Escherichia coli* bacteria. Another cause of urinary tract infections in immobilized clients is the use of an indwelling urinary catheter.

PSYCHOSOCIAL EFFECTS

Immobilization may lead to emotional, intellectual, sensory, and sociocultural responses. Changes in emotional status usually occur gradually. However, the older adult may be more susceptible to these changes, so the nurse may observe them earlier. The most common emotional changes are depression, behavioral changes, changes in the sleep-wake cycle, and impaired coping.

■ DEVELOPMENTAL CHANGES

Throughout life, the body's appearance and functioning undergo change. The greatest impact is observed in childhood and old age.

Infants

The newborn infant's spine is flexed and lacks the anteroposterior curves of the adult. The first spinal curve occurs when the infant extends the neck from the prone position. As growth and stability increase, the thoracic spine straightens, and the lumbar spinal curve appears, which allows sitting and standing. The infant's musculoskeletal system is flexible. The extremities are flexed and joints have complete ROM. As the newborn matures, the musculoskeletal system becomes stronger, and the infant is able to resist movement and reach out and grasp objects (see Chapter 28). As the baby grows, musculoskeletal development permits support of weight for standing and walking. Posture is awkward because the head and upper trunk are carried forward. Because body weight is not evenly distributed along a line of gravity, posture is off balance, and falls occur often.

Toddlers

The toddler's posture—slightly swaybacked with a protruding abdomen—is awkward. As the child walks, the legs and feet are usually far apart and the feet are slightly everted. Toward the end of toddlerhood, posture appears less awkward, curves in the cervical and lumbar vertebrae are accentuated, and foot eversion disappears.

Preschool and School-Age Children

By the third year the body is slimmer, taller, and better balanced. Abdominal protrusion is decreased, the feet are not as far apart, and arms and legs have increased in length. The child also appears more coordinated. From the third year through beginning adolescence the musculoskeletal system continues to develop. Long bones in the arms and legs grow. Muscles, ligaments, and tendons become stronger, resulting in improved posture and increased muscle strength. Greater coordination enables the child to perform tasks that require fine motor skills (see Chapter 29).

Adolescents

The adolescence stage is usually initiated by a tremendous growth spurt (see Chapter 29). Growth is frequently uneven. As a result, the adolescent may appear awkward and uncoordinated. Adolescent girls usually grow and develop earlier than boys. Hips widen, and fat is deposited in the upper arms, thighs, and buttocks. The boy's changes in shape are usually the result of long-bone growth and increased muscle mass. Legs become longer and hips narrower. Muscular development increases in the chest, arms, shoulders, and upper legs.

Adults

An adult who has correct posture and body alignment feels good, looks good, and generally appears self-confident. The healthy adult also has the necessary musculoskeletal development and coordination to carry out activities of daily living (see Chapter 30). Normal changes in posture and body alignment in adulthood occur mainly in pregnant women.

These changes result from the body's adaptive response to weight gain and the growing fetus. The center of gravity shifts toward the anterior. The pregnant woman leans back and is slightly swaybacked. She may complain of backache.

Older Adults

A progressive loss of total bone mass occurs with the older adult. Some of the possible causes of this loss include physical activity, hormonal changes, and actual bone resorption. The effect of bone loss is weaker bones: vertebrae are softer and may become compressed, and long shaft bones are less resistant to bending (Lueckenotte, 1994). In addition, older adults experience functional status changes secondary to altered mobility status (see the box below).

Older adults may walk more slowly and appear less coordinated. They may also take smaller steps, keeping their feet closer together, which decreases the base of support. Thus body balance is unstable, and they are at greater risk for falls and injuries (see Chapter 31).

▌ NURSING PROCESS FOR IMPAIRED BODY ALIGNMENT AND MOBILITY

The use of the nursing process, critical application of anatomy and physiology, and experience with clients enables the nurse to develop individualized care plans for clients with preexisting mobility impairments and for those who are at risk. A care plan is designed to improve the client's functional status, promote self-care, maintain psychological well-being, and reduce the hazards of immobility.

 Assessment

Nursing assessment is presented in two sections, mobility and immobility. Both areas are usually assessed during the complete physical examination.

MOBILITY

Assessment of client mobility focuses on range of motion, gait, exercise and activity tolerance, and body alignment.

Range of Motion. Range of motion (ROM) is the maximum amount of movement possible at a joint in one of the three planes of the body: sagittal, frontal, and transverse (Fig. 37-13). The sagittal plane is a line that passes through the body from front to back, dividing the body into a left and a right side. The frontal plane passes through the body from side to side and divides the body into front and back. The transverse plane is a horizontal line that divides the body into upper and lower portions.

Joint mobility in each of the planes is limited by ligaments, muscles, and construction of the joint. However, some joint movements are specific to each plane. In the sagittal plane, movements are flexion and extension (fingers and elbows) and hyperextension (hip). In the frontal plane, movements are abduction and adduction (arms and legs) and eversion and inversion (feet). In the transverse plane, movements are pronation and supination (hands), internal and external rotation (knees), and dorsiflexion and plantar flexion (feet).

When assessing ROM, the nurse asks questions and makes observations to collect data about joint stiffness, swelling, pain, limited movement, and unequal movement. Clients whose joint mobility is restricted because of illness, disability, or trauma require exercise of joints to reduce the hazards of immobility. These exercises, performed by the nurse, are called passive ROM exercises. The nurse takes each affected joint through its complete ROM (Table 37-3).

Gait. The term **gait** is used to describe a particular manner or style of walking (Fish and Nielsen, 1993). The gait cycle begins with the heel strike of one leg and continues to the heel strike of the same leg. This interval equals 100% of

Text continued on p. 910.

Hazards of Hospitalization of the Older Adult

For many older persons, hospitalization results in functional decline, despite cure or repair of the condition for which they were admitted. Hospitalization can result in complications unrelated to the problem that caused admission or to its specific treatment and for reasons that are explainable and avoidable.

Usual aging is often associated with functional change, such as a decline in muscle strength and aerobic capacity; vasomotor instability; reduced bone density; diminished pulmonary ventilation; altered sensory continence, appetite, and thirst; and a tendency toward urinary incontinence. Hospitalization and bed rest superimpose factors such as enforced immobilization, reduction of plasma volume, accelerated bone loss, increased closing volume, and sensory deprivation. Any of these factors may thrust vulnerable older persons into a state of irreversible functional decline.

The relationships among physicians, nurses, and other health care professionals must reflect the importance of interdisciplinary care and the implementation of shared objectives.

Modified from Creditor MC: Hazards of hospitalization of the elderly, *Am Coll Phys* 118(3):219, 1993.

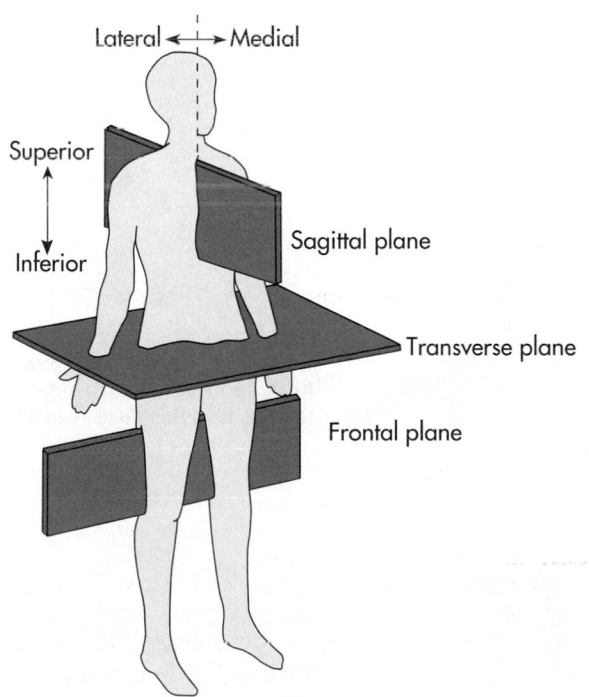

Fig. 37-13 Planes of the body.

Table 37-3	Range of Motion Exercises			
BODY PART	**TYPE OF JOINT**	**TYPE OF MOVEMENT**	**RANGE (DEGREES)**	**PRIMARY MUSCLES**
Neck, cervical spine	Pivotal	Flexion: bring chin to rest on chest	45	Sternocleidomastoid
		Extension: return head to erect position	45	Trapezius
		Hyperextension: bend head back as far as possible	10	Trapezius
		Lateral flexion: tilt head as far as possible toward each shoulder	40-45	Sternocleidomastoid
		Rotation: turn head as far as possible in circular movement	180	Sternocleidomastoid, trapezius
Shoulder	Ball and socket	Flexion: raise arm from side position forward to position above head	180	Coracobrachialis, biceps brachii, deltoid, pectoralis major
		Extension: return arm to position at side of body	180	Latissimus dorsi, teres major, triceps brachii
		Hyperextension: move arm behind body, keeping elbow straight	45-60	Latissimus dorsi, teres major, deltoid
		Abduction: raise arm to side to position above head with palm away from head	180	Deltoid, supraspinatus
		Adduction: lower arm sideways and across body as far as possible	320	Pectoralis major

Table 37-3	**Range of Motion Exercises—cont'd**			
BODY PART	**TYPE OF JOINT**	**TYPE OF MOVEMENT**	**RANGE (DEGREES)**	**PRIMARY MUSCLES**
		Internal rotation: with elbow flexed, rotate shoulder by moving arm until thumb is turned inward and toward back	90	Pectoralis major, latissimus dorsi, teres major, subscapularis
		External rotation: with elbow flexed, move arm until thumb is upward and lateral to head	90	Infraspinatus, teres major, deltoid
		Circumduction: move arm in full circle (Circumduction is combination of all movements of ball-and-socket joint.)	360	Deltoid, coracobrachialis, latissimus dorsi, teres major
Elbow	Hinge	Flexion: bend elbow so that lower arm moves toward its shoulder joint and hand is level with shoulder	150	Biceps brachii, brachialis, brachioradialis
		Extension: straighten elbow by lowering hand	150	Triceps brachii
Forearm	Pivotal	Supination: turn lower arm and hand so that palm is up	70-90	Supinator, biceps brachii
		Pronation: turn lower arm so that palm is down	70-90	Pronator teres, pronator quadratus
Wrist	Condyloid	Flexion: move palm toward inner aspect of forearm	80-90	Flexor carpi ulnaris, flexor carpi radialis
		Extension: move fingers so that fingers, hands, and forearm are in same plane	80-90	Extensor carpi ulnaris, extensor carpi radialis brevis, extensor carpi radialis longus
		Hyperextension: bring dorsal surface of hand back as far as possible	89-90	Extensor carpi radialis brevis, extensor carpi radialis longus, extensor carpi ulnaris
		Abduction (radial flexion): bend wrist medially toward thumb	Up to 30	Flexor carpi radialis, extensor carpi radialis brevis, extensor carpi radialis longus
		Adduction (ulnar flexion): bend wrist laterally toward fifth finger	30-50	Flexor carpi ulnaris, extensor carpi ulnaris

Continued.

Table 37-3		Range of Motion Exercises—cont'd		
Body Part	**Type of Joint**	**Type of Movement**	**Range (Degrees)**	**Primary Muscles**
Fingers	Condyloid hinge	Flexion: make fist	90	Lumbricales, interosseus volaris, interosseus dorsalis
		Extension: straighten fingers	90	Extensor digiti quinti proprius, extensor digitorum communis, extensor indicis proprius
		Hyperextension: bend fingers back as far as possible	30-60	
		Abduction: spread fingers apart	30	Interosseus dorsalis
		Adduction: bring fingers together	30	Interosseus volaris
Thumb	Saddle	Flexion: move thumb across palmar surface of hand	90	Flexor pollicis brevis
		Extension: move thumb straight away from hand	90	Extensor pollicis longus, extensor pollicis brevis
		Abduction: extend thumb laterally (usually done when placing fingers in abduction and adduction)	30	Abductor pollicis brevis
		Adduction: move thumb back toward hand	30	Adductor pollicis obliquus, adductor pollicis transversus
		Opposition: touch thumb to each finger of same hand		Opponeus pollicis, opponeus digiti minimi
Hip	Ball and socket	Flexion: move leg forward and up	90-120	Psoas major, iliacus, iliopsoas, sartorius
		Extension: move back beside other leg	90-120	Gluteus maximus, semitendinosus, semimembranosus
		Hyperextension: move leg behind body	30-50	Gluteus maximus, semitendinosus, semimembranosus

| Table 37-3 | Range of Motion Exercises—cont'd | | | |

BODY PART	TYPE OF JOINT	TYPE OF MOVEMENT	RANGE (DEGREES)	PRIMARY MUSCLES
		Abduction: move leg laterally away from body	30-50	Gluteus medius, gluteus minimus
		Adduction: move leg back toward medial position and beyond if possible	30-50	Adductor longus, adductor brevis, adductor magnus
		Internal rotation: turn foot and leg toward other leg	90	Gluteus medius, gluteus minimus, tensor fasciae latae
		External rotation: turn foot and leg away from other leg	90	Obturatorius internus, obutratorius externus
		Circumduction: move leg in circle		Psoas major, gluteus maximus, gluteus medius, adductor magnus
Knee	Hinge	Flexion: bring heel back toward back of thigh	120-130	Biceps femoris, semitendinosus, semimembranosus, sartorius
		Extension: return leg to the floor	120-130	Rectus femoris, vastus lateralis, vastus medialis, vastus intermedius
Ankle	Hinge	Dorsal flexion: move foot so that toes are pointed upward	20-30	Tibialis anterior
		Plantar flexion: move foot so that toes are pointed downward	45-50	Gastrocnemius, soleus
Foot	Gliding	Inversion: turn sole of foot medially	10 or less	Tibialis anterior, tibialis posterior
		Eversion: turn sole of foot laterally	10 or less	Peroneus longus, peroneus brevis
Toes	Condyloid	Flexion: curl toes downward	30-60	Flexor digitorum, lumbricalis pedis, flexor hallucis brevis
		Extension: straighten toes	30-60	Extensor digitorum longus, extensor digitorum brevis, extensor hallucis longus
		Abduction: spread toes apart	15 or less	Abductor hallucis, interosseus dorsalis
		Adduction: bring toes together	15 or less	Adductor hallucis, interosseus plantaris

the gait cycle and lasts, for comfortable walking, 1 second (Lehmann et al, 1992).

Assessing a client's gait allows the nurse to draw conclusions about balance, posture, safety, and ability to walk without assistance. The mechanics of human gait involve synchronization of the skeletal, neurological, and muscular systems of the human body (Fish and Nielsen, 1993).

Exercise and Activity Tolerance. Exercise is physical activity for conditioning the body, improving health, and maintaining fitness. It can also be used as therapy for correcting a deformity or restoring the overall body to a maximal state of health. When a person exercises, physiological changes occur in body systems (see the box below).

Assessment of the client's energy level includes the physiological effects of exercise and activity tolerance. **Activity tolerance** is the kind and amount of exercise or work that a person is able to perform. Assessment of activity tolerance is necessary when planning activity such as walking, ROM exercises, or activities of daily living for clients with acute or chronic illness. In addition, knowledge of the client's activity tolerance is needed to plan other nursing therapies.

Activity tolerance assessment includes data from physio-

logical, emotional, and developmental domains (see the box below). This assessment is applicable in all clinical settings and is quickly completed by the nurse.

The client who experiences changes in physiological function such as dyspnea or chest pain during exercise will not tolerate activity as well as the client who does not. Likewise, the weak or debilitated client is unable to sustain activity because the greater energy needed to complete the activity creates fatigue and generalized weakness.

People who are depressed, worried, or anxious are frequently unable to tolerate exercise. Depressed clients are usually not motivated to participate. Clients who are worried or anxious fatigue easily because they expend a great deal of energy in worry and anxiety. Thus they may experience physical and emotional exhaustion.

Developmental changes also affect activity tolerance. As the infant enters the toddler stage, the activity level increases and the need for sleep declines. The child entering nursery school, preschool, or primary grades expends mental energy in learning and may require more rest after school or before strenuous play. The adolescent going through puberty may require more rest because much of the body's energy is expended for growth and hormone changes.

A pregnant woman has fluctuations in her energy tolerance. During the first trimester she may have increased fatigue. Hormonal changes and fetal development use body energy, and the woman may be unable or unmotivated to carry out physical activities. The second trimester of preg-

---

Effects of Exercise

■ **CARDIOVASCULAR SYSTEM**
Increased cardiac output
Improved myocardial contraction, thus strengthening cardiac muscle
Decreased resting heart rate
Improved venous return

■ **PULMONARY SYSTEM**
Increased respiratory rate and depth followed by quicker return-to-rest rate
Improved alveolar ventilation
Decreased work of breathing
Improved diaphragmatic excursion

■ **METABOLIC SYSTEM**
Increased basal metabolic rate
Increased use of glucose and fatty acids
Increased triglyceride breakdown
Increased gastric motility
Increased production of body heat

■ **MUSCULOSKELETAL SYSTEM**
Improved muscle tone
Increased joint mobility
Improved muscle tolerance to exercise
Possible increase in muscle mass
Reduced bone loss

■ **ACTIVITY TOLERANCE**
Improved tolerance
Decreased fatigue

■ **PSYCHOSOCIAL FACTORS**
Improved tolerance to stress
Reports of "feeling better"
Reports of decrease in illness (e.g., colds and influenza viruses)

Modified from Gröer MW, Shekleton ME: *Basic pathophysiology: a conceptual approach*, ed 3, St Louis, 1989, Mosby–Year Book; and McCance KL, Huether SE: *Pathophysiology: the biologic basis for disease in adults and children*, ed 2, St Louis, 1994, Mosby.

Factors Influencing Activity Tolerance

■ **PHYSIOLOGICAL FACTORS**
Frequency of illness or surgery during past 12 mo
Types of illnesses or surgery during past 12 mo
Cardiopulmonary status (e.g., dyspnea, chest pain)
Musculoskeletal status (e.g., decreased muscle mass)
Sleep patterns
Presence of pain, pain control
Vital signs: respiratory and heart rates return to resting level within 5 minutes following exercise; blood pressure returns to baseline within 5 to 10 minutes following exercise
Type and frequency of exercise activity
Abnormality in laboratory studies, such as decreased arterial oxygen concentration, decreased hemoglobin level, abnormal electrolyte levels

■ **EMOTIONAL FACTORS**
Mood: depression, anxiety
Motivation
Chemical addictions (e.g., drugs, alcohol, nicotine)
Self-image

■ **DEVELOPMENTAL FACTORS**
Age
Sex
Pregnancy
Change in muscle mass because of developmental changes
Changes in skeletal system because of developmental changes

Physiological data from Gröer MW, Shekleton ME: *Basic Pathophysiology: a conceptual approach*, ed 3, St Louis, 1989, Mosby–Year Book.

nancy usually results in a return of activity tolerance to the prepregnancy state. In fact, some women feel their activity tolerance is greater during this period. During the last trimester, fetal development consumes a great deal of the mother's energy. In addition, because of the size and location of the fetus, the pregnant woman's ability to take a deep breath is decreased and less oxygen is available for physical activities.

As the person grows older, activity tolerance changes. Muscle mass is reduced, posture changes, and the composition of bones is altered. The individual may still exercise but will do it at a reduced intensity.

There is an overall improvement of physiological functioning as a result of exercise. All systems become stronger and function more efficiently. In nursing, certain interventions are directed at exercise. However, nurses often care for clients whose mobility is restricted and, as a result, must develop nursing therapies designed to reduce the hazards of immobility.

Body Alignment. Assessment of body alignment can be carried out with the client standing, sitting, or lying down. This assessment has the following objectives:

1. Determining normal physiological changes in body alignment resulting from growth and development
2. Identifying deviations in body alignment caused by poor posture
3. Providing opportunities for clients to observe their posture
4. Identifying learning needs of clients for maintaining correct body alignment
5. Identifying trauma, muscle damage, or nerve dysfunction
6. Obtaining information concerning other factors that contribute to poor alignment, such as fatigue, malnutrition, and psychological problems

The first step in assessing body alignment is to put clients at ease so that unnatural or rigid positions are not assumed. When the body alignment of an immobilized or unconscious client is assessed, pillows and positioning supports should be removed from the bed and the client placed in the supine position.

Standing. The nurse should focus assessment of body alignment for the standing client on the following points:

1. The head is erect and midline.
2. When observed posteriorly, the shoulders and hips are straight and parallel.
3. When observed posteriorly, the vertebral column is straight.
4. When the client is observed laterally, the head is erect and the spinal curves are aligned in a reversed S pattern. The cervical vertebrae are anteriorly convex, the thoracic vertebrae are posteriorly convex, and the lumbar vertebrae are anteriorly convex.
5. When observed laterally, the abdomen is comfortably tucked in and the knees and ankles are slightly flexed. The person appears comfortable and does not seem conscious of the flexion of knees or ankles.
6. The client's arms are comfortably at the sides.
7. Feet are placed slightly apart to achieve a base of support, and the toes are pointed forward.
8. When the client is viewed anteriorly, the center of gravity is in the midline, and the line of gravity is

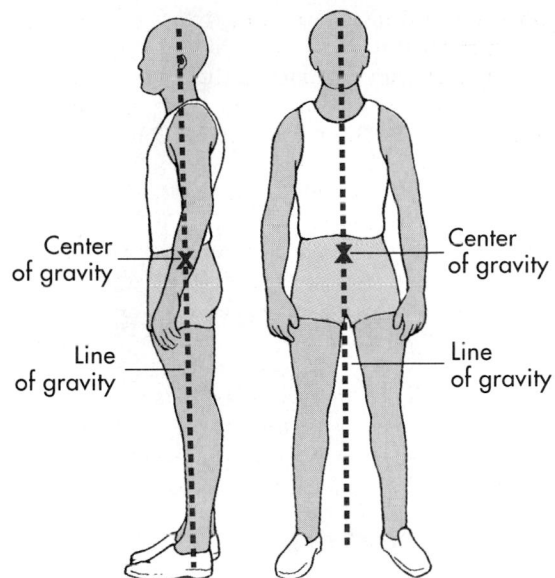

Fig. 37-14 Correct body alignment when standing.

from the middle of the forehead to a midpoint between the feet. Laterally the line of gravity runs vertically from the middle of the skull to the posterior third of the foot (Fig. 37-14).

Sitting. The nurse assesses alignment of the sitting client by the following observations:

1. The head is erect, and the neck and vertebral column are in straight alignment.
2. The body weight is evenly distributed on the buttocks and thighs.
3. The thighs are parallel and in a horizontal plane.
4. Both feet are supported on the floor (Fig. 37-15). With clients of short stature, a footstool is used and the ankles are comfortably flexed.
5. A 2- to 4-cm (1- to 2-in) space is maintained between the edge of the seat and the popliteal space on the posterior surface of the knee. This space ensures that there is no pressure on the popliteal artery or nerve to decrease circulation or impair nerve function.
6. The client's forearms are supported on the armrest, in the lap, or on a table in front of the chair.

It is particularly important to assess alignment when sitting if the client has muscle weakness, muscle paralysis, or nerve damage. Because of these alterations, the client has diminished sensation in the affected area and is unable to perceive pressure or decreased circulation. Proper alignment while sitting reduces the risk of musculoskeletal system damage in such a client.

Lying. People who are conscious have voluntary muscle control and normal perception of pressure. As a result, they usually assume the position of comfort when lying down. Because their range of motion, sensation, and circulation are within normal limits, they change positions when they perceive muscle strain and decreased circulation.

Assessment of body alignment while lying requires that the client be placed in the lateral position with all but one pillow and all positioning supports removed from the bed (Fig. 37-16). The body should be supported by an adequate mattress. The vertebrae should be in straight alignment

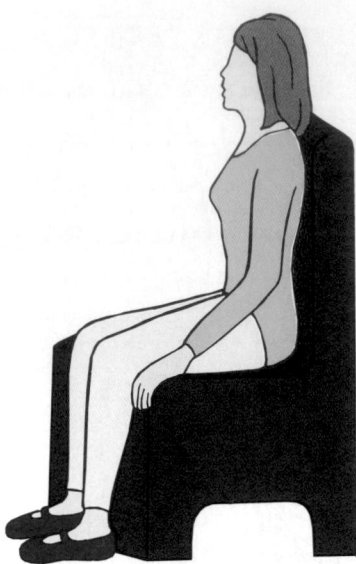

Fig. 37-15 Correct body alignment when sitting.

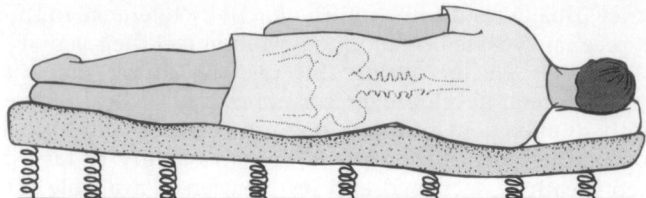

Fig. 37-16 Correct body alignment when lying down.

without observable curves. This assessment provides baseline data concerning the client's body alignment.

Conditions that create a risk of damage to the musculoskeletal system when lying down include clients with impaired mobility, such as those in traction or with arthritis; clients with decreased sensation, such as those with hemiparesis resulting from a stroke; clients with impaired circulation, such as those with diabetes; and clients with lack of voluntary muscle control, such as those with spinal cord injuries.

When assessment indicates that a client is at risk for damage to the musculoskeletal system while lying down, interventions are directed at maintaining proper body alignment while positioning the client (see p. 917).

IMMOBILITY

The nurse assesses the immobilized client for hazards of immobility by performing a head-to-toe physical assessment (see Chapter 33). In addition, the nursing assessment should focus on certain physiological areas, as well as the client's psychosocial and developmental dimensions.

Physiological Factors. The physiological hazards of immobility that may be identified during a nursing assessment are summarized in Table 37-4.

Metabolic System. When assessing metabolic functioning, the nurse uses anthropometric measurements to evaluate muscle atrophy, uses intake and output records and laboratory data to evaluate fluid and electrolyte status and serum protein levels, assesses wound healing to evaluate alterations in the exchange of nutrients, and assesses the client's food intake and elimination patterns to determine altered GI functioning.

Intake and output measurements assist the nurse in determining whether a fluid imbalance exists. Dehydration and edema can increase the rate of skin breakdown in an immobilized client. Laboratory measurement of serum electrolyte levels can also indicate an electrolyte imbalance (see Chapter 45).

If an immobilized client has a wound, the rate of healing

indicates how well nutrients are being delivered to tissues. Normal progression of healing indicates that metabolic needs of injured tissues are being met.

Anorexia occurs commonly in immobilized clients. The client's food intake should be assessed before the tray is removed to determine the amount eaten. Nutritional imbalances can be avoided if the nurse assesses the client's dietary patterns and food preferences early in immobilization (see Chapter 41).

Respiratory System. A respiratory assessment should be performed at least every 2 hours for clients with restricted activity. The nurse inspects chest wall movements during the full inspiratory-expiratory cycle. If a client has an atelectatic area, chest movement may be asymmetrical. In addition, the nurse auscultates the entire lung region to identify diminished breath sounds, crackles, or wheezes. Auscultation should focus on the dependent lung fields because pulmonary secretions tend to collect in these lower regions. A complete respiratory assessment identifies the presence of secretions and can be used to determine nursing interventions necessary for optimal respiratory function.

Cardiovascular System. Cardiovascular nursing assessment of the immobilized client includes blood pressure monitoring, evaluation of apical and peripheral pulses, and observation for signs of venous stasis (e.g., edema and poor wound healing). Because of the risk for orthostatic hypotension, the client's blood pressure should be measured, particularly when changing from a lying (recumbent) to a sitting or standing position. In this way, the ability to tolerate postural changes can be assessed before the client leaves the safety of the bed.

The nurse also assesses the apical and peripheral pulses. Recumbency increases cardiac workload and results in an increased pulse rate. In some clients, particularly older adults, the heart may not tolerate the increased workload, and a form of cardiac failure may develop. A third heart sound, heard at the apex, can be an early indication of congestive heart failure. Monitoring peripheral pulses allows the nurse to evaluate the heart's ability to pump blood. The absence of a peripheral pulse in the lower extremities, particularly one that was previously present, should be documented and reported to the client's physician.

Edema may indicate the heart's inability to handle the increased workload. Because edema moves to dependent body regions, assessment of the immobilized client should include the sacrum, legs, and feet. If the heart is unable to tolerate the increased workload, peripheral body regions, such as the hands, feet, nose, and earlobes, will be colder than central body regions.

Finally, the nurse assesses the venous system because deep vein thrombosis is a hazard of restricted mobility. A

Table 37-4	Physiological Hazards of Immobility	
SYSTEM	**ASSESSMENT TECHNIQUES**	**ABNORMAL FINDINGS**
Metabolic	Inspection	Slowed wound healing, abnormal laboratory data
	Inspection	Muscle atrophy
	Anthropometric measurements (mid–upper arm circumference, triceps skinfold measurement)	Decreased amount of subcutaneous fat
	Palpation	Generalized edema
Respiratory	Inspection	Asymmetrical chest wall movement, dyspnea
	Auscultation	Crackles, wheezes, increased respiratory rate
Cardiovascular	Auscultation	Orthostatic hypotension
	Auscultation, palpation	Increased heart rate, third heart sound, weak peripheral pulses, peripheral edema
Musculoskeletal	Inspection, palpation	Erythema, increased diameter in calf or thigh
	Palpation	Decreased ROM, joint contracture
	Inspection	Activity intolerance, muscle atrophy, joint contracture
Skin	Inspection, palpation	Break in skin integrity
Elimination	Inspection	Decreased urine output, cloudy or concentrated urine, decreased frequency of bowel movements
	Palpation	Distended bladder and abdomen
	Auscultation	Decreased bowel sounds

dislodged thrombus, called an *embolus,* may travel through the circulatory system to the lungs or brain and impair circulation. Emboli to the lungs or brain pose a threat to life.

To assess for a deep vein thrombosis, the nurse removes the client's elastic stockings and/or sequential compression devices (SCDs) every 8 hours and observes the calves for redness, warmth, and tenderness. Homan's sign, or calf pain on dorsiflexion of the foot, indicates a probable thrombus, but this sign is not always present (Beare and Myers, 1994). In addition, calf circumference should be measured daily. To do this the nurse marks a point on each calf 10 cm from the midpatella. The circumference is measured each day using the mark for placement of the tape measure. One-sided increases in calf diameter can be an early indication of thrombosis. Because deep vein thrombosis can also occur in the thigh, thigh measurements should be taken daily if the client is prone to thrombosis. In many clients, deep vein thrombosis can be prevented by active exercise and elastic stockings.

Musculoskeletal System. Major musculoskeletal abnormalities that may be identified during nursing assessment include decreased muscle tone, loss of muscle mass, and contractures. The anthropometric measurements described previously may indicate losses in muscle tone and muscle mass.

Assessment of ROM is important as a baseline against which later measurements can be compared to evaluate whether a loss in joint mobility has occurred. ROM is measured with a goniometer (see Fig. 37-30, p. 936).

Disuse osteoporosis cannot be identified by physical assessment. However, postmenopausal women and persons with increased serum and urine calcium levels probably have a greater risk for bone demineralization. The risk of disuse osteoporosis should be considered when planning nursing interventions. For example, rib percussion and vibration (see Chapter 44) should be done cautiously with a client with probable disuse osteoporosis because of the risk of rib fracture.

Integumentary System. The nurse must continually assess the client's skin for signs of breakdown. The skin should be observed when the client is turned, hygiene measures are performed, or elimination needs are provided. At the minimum, assessment should occur every 2 hours (see Chapter 38).

Elimination System. The client's elimination status should be evaluated on each shift, and total intake and output should be evaluated every 24 hours. The nurse should determine that the client is receiving the correct amount and type of fluids orally or parenterally (see Chapter 46).

Inadequate intake and output or fluid and electrolyte imbalances can increase the risk for renal system impairment, ranging from recurrent infections to kidney failure. Dehydration can also increase the risk for skin breakdown, thrombi formation, respiratory infections, and constipation. Such physical complications can decrease the overall level of mobility and increase duration and cost of care.

Assessment of elimination status should also include the frequency and consistency of bowel movements (see Chapter 47). Accurate assessment enables the nurse to intervene before constipation and fecal impaction occur.

HEALTH ASSESSMENT OF THE OLDER ADULT

Psychosocial Factors. Changes in the client's psychosocial status usually occur slowly and are often overlooked by health care personnel. The nurse should observe for changes in emotional status. The nurse should observe for several days before concluding that depression is the problem. Everyone becomes depressed at some time, especially hospitalized and immobilized clients, but not all depression requires nursing intervention. If the depression is caused by boredom or isolation, it can be alleviated by increasing bedside activities and occupational therapy.

The nurse also observes for behavioral changes, such as the cooperative client who becomes argumentative or the modest client who begins to expose genitalia repeatedly. The nurse should try to determine the reasons for such alterations to identify specific nursing therapies.

Unexplained changes in the sleep-wake cycle must be identified and corrected. Most can be prevented or minimized, such as those occurring because of nursing activities, a noisy environment, or discomfort. They may also occur because of medications such as analgesics, sleeping pills, or cardiovascular drugs (see Chapter 42).

Finally, the nurse should observe for changes in the client's use of normal coping mechanisms to adapt to immobilization (see Chapter 22). Decreasing coping ability may cause the client to become disoriented, confused, or depressed or to experience other behavioral changes.

Because psychosocial changes usually occur gradually, the nurse should observe the client's behavior on a daily basis. If behavioral changes occur, the nurse should determine the causes and evaluate the changes as short or long term. Identifying the cause helps the nurse design appropriate nursing interventions.

DEVELOPMENTAL FACTORS

Assessment of the immobilized client should include developmental considerations to ensure that the client's needs are identified. The nurse determines whether the young child can meet developmental tasks and is progressing normally. The child's development may regress or be slowed because of immobilization. By identifying a child's overall developmental needs, the nurse can design nursing therapies to maintain normal development. The nurse may also need to assure the parents that developmental delays are usually temporary.

Immobility can have a significant effect on the older adult's levels of health, independence, and functional status. Nursing assessment enables the nurse to determine the older client's ability to meet needs independently and to adapt to developmental changes such as declining physical functioning and altered family and peer relationships. A decline in developmental functioning needs prompt investigation to determine why the change occurred and what can be done to return to an optimal level of function as soon as possible. Mobility assessment also includes the client's home and community to identify factors that are risks to the client's mobility and safety (see Chapter 36).

HEALTH PROMOTION FOR THE OLDER ADULT

Health promotion classes/workshops are developing all over the United States and internationally (see the box above). The main goal is to enable older people to make decisions that will improve their health and to make use of services by providing information and encouragement. Older adults have much more of a thirst for knowledge about health conditions than younger people do. Older adults should never be treated as passive recipients of professional advice and care but as active partners in maintaining and improving their own health and fitness. Empowerment is the key to developing health care skills and having the confidence to seek access to professional services when required (Laurent, 1992).

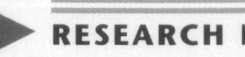

RESEARCH HIGHLIGHT

RESEARCH ABSTRACT

The purpose of this study was to determine if low-intensity aerobic exercises, specific to muscles of the knees and ankles, would improve muscle strength, flexibility, and balance among sedentary older adults, compared with elderly persons who did not participate in this intervention. Fifty-six older adults from two apartment complexes were randomly designated as either the experimental or comparison group. Subjects ranged in age from 65 to 88.

The procedure consisted of a 3-times-per-week exercise program. The 8-week, low-intensity aerobic exercise program produced significant differences between the experimental and comparison groups for flexibility of both ankles and the right knee, but not for muscle strength of the lower extremities. The experimental group experienced an increase in balance, whereas the comparison group did not. This research demonstrated that an exercise program of low-intensity aerobic exercise improved flexibility, and that inactive elders will exercise if the program is simple, safe, easy to do, and fits into their daily routine.

IMPLICATIONS FOR PRACTICE
▶ Prior to initiating exercise clients should consult their primary care provider.
▶ Older adults can access senior citizen centers for regular exercise.
▶ Encouraging older adults to have regular exercise has the potential to maintain independence.

REFERENCE
Mills EM: The effect of low-intensity aerobic exercise on muscle strength, flexibility, and balance among sedentary elderly persons, *Nurs Res* 43(4):207, 1994.

 ## Nursing Diagnosis

Nursing diagnoses identifying actual or potential alterations in body alignment and mobility are based on data collected during assessment. Analysis reveals clusters of data that indicate the presence or risk for a problem (see the nursing diagnoses box on p. 915, top).

Alterations in body alignment can result from developmental changes, postural abnormalities, abnormalities in bone formation, impaired muscle development, damage to the central nervous system, and direct trauma to the musculoskeletal system. Assessment data should contain appropriate defining characteristics to support the diagnostic label (see the diagnostic process box on p. 915, bottom).

Body alignment and mobility are interrelated. A person with poor body alignment may have reduced mobility. When identifying nursing diagnoses, the nurse designs nursing strategies that reduce or prevent hazards associated with poor body alignment or impaired mobility.

Often, the physiological dimension is the only focus of nursing care for clients with impaired mobility. Thus the psychosocial and developmental dimensions are neglected. Yet they are important to health. For example, during immobilization, social interaction and stimuli are decreased.

Examples of NANDA Nursing Diagnoses Related to Improper Body Mechanics and Impaired Mobility

Activity intolerance *related to:*
- Poor body alignment
- Decreased mobility

Risk for injury *related to:*
- Improper body mechanics
- Improper positioning
- Improper transfer techniques

Impaired physical mobility *related to:*
- Reduced ROM
- Bed rest
- Decreased strength

Ineffective airway clearance *related to:*
- Stasis of pulmonary secretions
- Improper body positioning

Ineffective breathing pattern *related to:*
- Decreased lung expansion
- Accumulation of pulmonary secretions
- Improper body positioning

Impaired gas exchange *related to:*
- Asymmetrical breathing patterns
- Decreased lung expansion
- Accumulation of pulmonary secretions

Impaired skin integrity or risk for impaired skin integrity *related to:*
- Restricted mobility
- Pressure on skin's surface
- Shearing force

Altered urinary elimination *related to:*
- Restricted mobility
- Risk for infection
- Urinary retention

Risk for infection *related to:*
- Stasis of pulmonary secretions
- Impaired skin integrity
- Stasis of urine

Total incontinence *related to:*
- Altered elimination patterns
- Restricted mobility

Risk for fluid volume deficit *related to:*
- Decreased fluid intake

Ineffective individual coping *related to:*
- Reduced activity level
- Social isolation

Sleep pattern disturbance *related to:*
- Restricted mobility
- Discomfort

Sample Nursing Diagnostic Process for Impaired Physical Mobility and Risk for Injury

ASSESSMENT ACTIVITIES	DEFINING CHARACTERISTICS	NURSING DIAGNOSES
Measure ROM during exercises of extremities.	Limited ROM with left shoulder Reluctance to attempt movement with left shoulder Impaired coordination while attempting to perform ROM with left shoulder	**Impaired physical mobility** related to left shoulder pain
Ask client about perception of pain. Ask client about endurance and activity tolerance.	Client complains of sharp pain in shoulder Client reports decreased muscle strength in left shoulder	
Inspect client's skin for degree of intactness around casted extremity. Observe client's gait and ability to move independently.	Abrasions on skin on the perimeter of the casted area Decreased ability to independently change body position	**Risk for injury** related to pressure from cast

Ultimately the client may become isolated, withdrawn, and bored. Such clients may frequently use the nurse's call bell to request minor physical attention, when their real need is greater socialization.

Planning

The nurse plans therapeutic interventions for clients with actual problems or risks to body alignment and mobility. The nurse plans therapies according to severity of risks to the client, and the plan is individualized according to the client's developmental stage, level of health, and lifestyle.

It is important to consider the client's home environment when planning therapies to maintain or improve body alignment and mobility. Planning care also involves an understanding of the client's need to maintain motor function and independence. The nurse and client work together to establish ways of maintaining client involvement in nursing care and to maintain optimal body alignment and mobility whether the client is in the hospital or at home.

Sample Nursing Care Plan for Impaired Physical Mobility

NURSING DIAGNOSIS: Impaired physical mobility related to left shoulder pain
DEFINITION: Impaired physical mobility is the state in which an individual experiences a limitation of ability for independent physical mobility (Kim et al, 1995).

GOAL	EXPECTED OUTCOMES	INTERVENTIONS	RATIONALE
Client will regain normal ROM (180 degrees flexion and extension) of left shoulder within 4 mo.	Client will maintain present ROM in upper extremity joints. Client will perform self-care activities using left arm within 2 days. Client will follow regular exercise program by discharge.	Offer analgesic 30 min before ROM exercises. Teach client specific ROM exercises to left shoulder and arm. Schedule active exercises between meals and hygiene.	Action of analgesic will peak as client begins exercises. Teaching provides client with opportunity and knowledge to maintain and increase ROM (Lehmkuhl et al, 1990). This promotes frequent exercise to affected joints and reduces risk of contracture development (Lehmkuhl et al, 1990).

Clients at risk for hazards associated with improper body alignment and impaired mobility require a care plan directed at actual or potential positioning and mobility needs (see the care plan above). A physical therapist is an excellent resource to the nurse in selecting ROM exercises. The care plan is based on one or more of the following client goals:

1. Maintains proper body alignment
2. Regains proper body alignment or optimal level of body alignment
3. Reduces injuries to the skin and musculoskeletal systems resulting from improper body mechanics or alignment
4. Achieves full or optimal ROM
5. Prevents contractures
6. Maintains a patent airway
7. Achieves optimal lung expansion and gas exchange
8. Mobilizes airway secretions
9. Maintains cardiovascular function
10. Increases activity tolerance
11. Achieves normal elimination patterns
12. Maintains normal sleep-wake patterns
13. Achieves socialization
14. Achieves independent completion of self-care activities
15. Achieves physical and mental stimulation

Maintaining body alignment is especially important for clients with actual or potential limitations in mobility. For example, a comatose client should be positioned with pillows and the position changed frequently to reduce the risk of poor alignment and future injury to the skin and musculoskeletal system. The frequency of turning is based on client assessment for risk of pressure ulcer development (see Chapter 38).

Implementation

BODY ALIGNMENT

To maintain proper body alignment the nurse correctly lifts the client, uses proper positioning techniques, and safely transfers clients from a bed to a chair or a bed to a stretcher. Procedures described in this section incorporate principles of body mechanics needed to maintain or restore body alignment.

Lifting Techniques. The rate of injuries in occupational settings has increased in recent years, and more than half are back injuries that are the direct result of improper lifting and bending techniques (Owen and Garg, 1991). The most common back injury is strain on the lumbar muscle group, which includes the muscles around the lumbar vertebrae (Owen and Garg, 1991). Muscle injury to these areas affects the ability to bend forward, backward, and side to side. In addition, the ability to rotate the hips and lower back is decreased.

The nurse is at risk for injury to lumbar muscles when lifting, transferring, or positioning the immobilized client. Before lifting, the nurse should assess ability to lift the client or object by determining the following basic lifting criteria:

1. Position of weight. The weight to be lifted should be as close to the lifter as possible. Positioning the object in such a manner uses the lifting force of the nurse because the object is in the same plane (Stamps, 1989).
2. Height of the object. The best height for lifting vertically is slightly above the level of the middle finger of a person with the arm hanging at the side (Owen and Garg, 1991).
3. Body position. When the lifter's body position varies with different lifting tasks, the following general rule is applicable to most lifting situations: The body is positioned with the trunk erect so that multiple muscle groups work together in a synchronized manner.
4. Maximum weight. Each nurse should know the maximum weight that is safe to carry—safe for the nurse and the client. An object is too heavy if its weight is 35% or more of a person's body weight. Therefore a nurse who weighs 130 lb (59.1 kg) should not try to lift an immobilized 100-lb (45.5-kg) person. Although the nurse may be able to do it, there is a risk of dropping the client or causing injury to the nurse's back.

Proper Lifting

STEPS	RATIONALE
1. Assess position of weight, height of object, body position, and maximum weight.	Determines whether you are able to do it yourself or require help (Stamps, 1989).
2. Lift object correctly from below center of gravity:	
a. Come close to object to be moved.	Moves center of gravity closer to object.
b. Enlarge your base of support by placing feet slightly apart.	Maintains better body balance, thus reducing risk of falling.
c. Lower your center of gravity to object to be lifted.	Increases body balance and enables muscle groups to work together in syncrohnized manner.
d. Maintain proper alignment of head and neck with vertebrae, keeping trunk straight.	Reduces risk of injury to lumbar vertebrae and muscle groups (Owen and Garg, 1991).
3. Lift object correctly from shelf above center of gravity:	
a. Use safe, stable step stool. Do not stand on top stair.	Raises center of gravity closer to object.
b. Stand as close to shelf as possible.	Increases body balance during the lift.
c. Quickly transfer weight of object from shelf to arms and over base of support.	Reduces danger of falling by moving lifted object close to center of gravity over base of support.

When lifting, the nurse should follow a procedure designed to protect the musculoskeletal system (Procedure 37-1).

Lifting an object from a high shelf increases risks because it is more difficult to maintain body balance. To reach an object overhead, people often stand on tiptoe with their feet together, thereby decreasing their base of support, elevating their center of gravity, and ultimately decreasing their balance.

Positioning Techniques. Clients with impaired nervous, skeletal, or muscular system functioning and increased weakness and fatigability often require help from the nurse to attain proper body alignment while in bed or sitting. Several devices are available for the nurse to maintain good body alignment for clients while they are being positioned (Table 37-5).

Pillows are readily available in hospitals or extended care facilities. However, when the client is at home, the supply may be limited. Before using a pillow, the nurse should determine whether it is the proper size. A thick pillow under the client's head increases cervical flexion. A thin pillow under body prominences may be inadequate to protect skin and tissue from damage caused by pressure. When additional pillows are unavailable or if they are an improper size, the nurse can fold sheets, blankets, or towels.

A footboard is placed perpendicular to the mattress, parallel to and touching the plantar surfaces of the client's feet. The **footboard** prevents footdrop by maintaining the feet in dorsiflexion. After placing it on the bed, the nurse needs to determine that it is correctly placed, with the client's feet placed firmly against the board. A Posey footguard is a device that uses foam structures to maintain the client's feet in the dorsiflexed position. Another commonly used technique is high-top tennis shoes.

The **trochanter roll** prevents external rotation of the legs when the client is in a supine position. To form a trochanter roll, a cotton bath blanket is folded lengthwise to a width that will extend from the greater trochanter of the femur to the lower border of the popliteal space (Fig. 37-17). The blanket is placed under the buttocks and then rolled counterclockwise until the thigh is in the neutral position or in inward rotation. When correct alignment of the hip is achieved, the patella faces directly upward.

Sandbags are sand-filled plastic tubes that can be shaped to body contours. Sandbags can be used in place of or in addition to trochanter rolls. They immobilize an extremity or maintain body alignment.

Hand rolls maintain the thumb in slight adduction and in opposition to the fingers. A hand roll maintains the hand, thumb, and fingers in a functional position. The nurse eval-

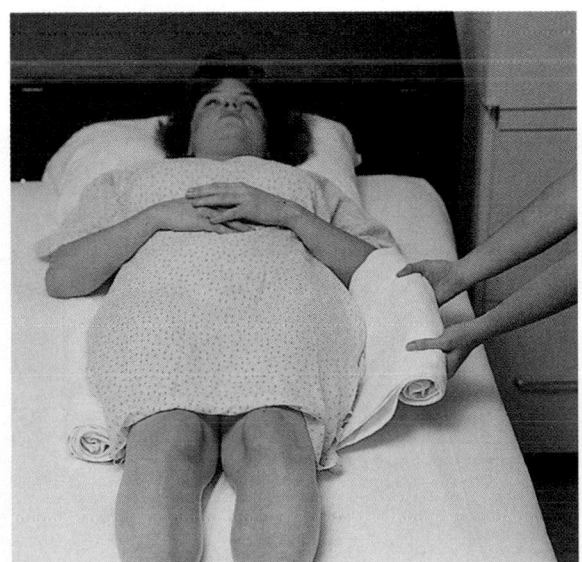

Fig. 37-17 Trochanter roll.

Table 37-5	Devices Used for Proper Positioning
DEVICE	**USES**
Pillow	Provides support of body or extremity; elevates body part; splints incisional area to reduce postoperative pain during activity or coughing and deep breathing
Footboard or Posey footguard	Maintains feet in dorsiflexion
Trochanter roll	Prevents external rotation of legs when client is in supine position
Sandbag	Provides support and shape to body contours; immobilizes extremity; maintains specific body alignment
Hand roll	Maintains thumb slightly adducted and in opposition to fingers; maintains fingers in slightly flexed position
Hand-wrist splint	Are individually molded for client to maintain proper alignment of thumb; are slightly adducted in opposition to fingers; maintains wrist in slight dorsal flexion
Trapeze bar	Enables client to raise trunk from bed; enables client to transfer from bed to wheelchair; allows client to perform exercises that strengthen upper arms
Side rail	Allows weak client to roll from side to side or to sit up in bed
Bed board	Provides additional support to mattress and improves vertebral alignment

uates the hand roll to make sure that the hand is indeed in a functional position (Fig. 37-18).

Hand-wrist splints are individually molded for the client to maintain proper alignment of the thumb (slight adduction) and the wrist (slight dorsiflexion). These splints should be used only by the client for whom the splint was made.

The **trapeze bar** is a triangular device that descends from a securely fastened overhead bar that is attached to the bed frame. It allows the client to pull with upper extremities to raise the trunk off the bed, to assist in transfer from bed to wheelchair, or to perform upper arm exercises (Fig. 37-19).

Restraints are devices used for immobilization, especially of confused or disoriented clients. A common jacket restraint is the Posey jacket (Fig. 37-20). When placing the jacket on the client, the nurse laps one side over the other across the client's back. The ties are placed under the loop on the jacket and secured to the bed, chair, or wheelchair frame. Restraints should *never* be tied to side rails because the client may be injured if a side rail is lowered with the restraint in place (see Chapter 36).

Side rails, bars positioned along the sides of the bed, en-sure client safety (see Chapter 36) and are also useful for in-creasing mobility. In addition, they allow the weak client to roll from side to side or sit up in bed.

Bed boards are plywood boards placed under the entire mattress. They are useful for increasing back support and alignment, especially with a soft mattress.

Although each procedure for positioning has specific guidelines, there are some universal steps the nurse should follow for clients who require positioning assistance (Proce-dure 37-2). Following the guidelines reduces the risk of in-jury to the musculoskeletal system when the client is sitting or lying. When joints are unsupported, their alignment is impaired. Likewise, if joints are not positioned in a slightly flexed position, their mobility is decreased. During posi-tioning, the nurse also assesses for pressure points. When ac-tual or potential pressure areas exist, nursing interventions involve removal of the pressure, thus decreasing the risk for development of pressure ulcers (see Chapter 38) and further trauma to the musculoskeletal system.

Supported Fowler's Position. In the supported Fowler's po-sition, the head of the bed is elevated 45 to 60 degrees and the client's knees are slightly elevated without pressure to restrict circulation in the lower legs. The angle of head and knee elevation and the length of time that the client should remain in the Fowler's position are influenced by the client's illness and overall condition. Supports must permit flexion of the hips and knees and proper alignment of the normal curves in the cervical, thoracic, and lumbar verte-brae. The following are common trouble areas for the client in the Fowler's position:

1. Increased cervical flexion because the pillow at the head is too thick and the head thrusts forward
2. Extension of knees, allowing the client to slide to the foot of the bed
3. Pressure on the posterior aspect of the knee, decreas-ing circulation to the feet
4. External rotation of hips
5. Arms hanging unsupported at the client's sides
6. Unsupported feet
7. Unprotected pressure points at the sacrum and heels

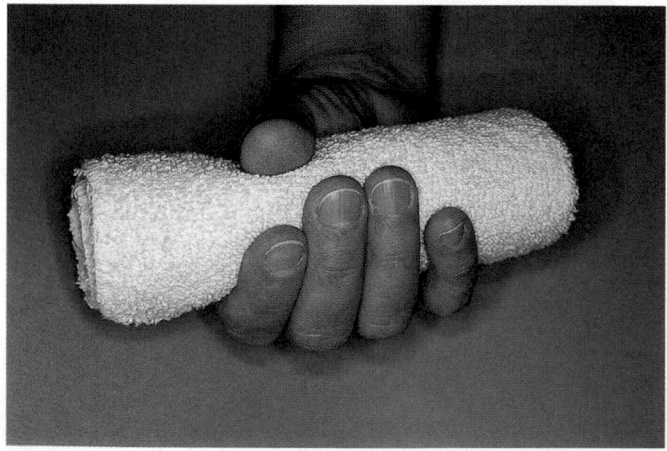

Fig. 37-18 Hand roll.

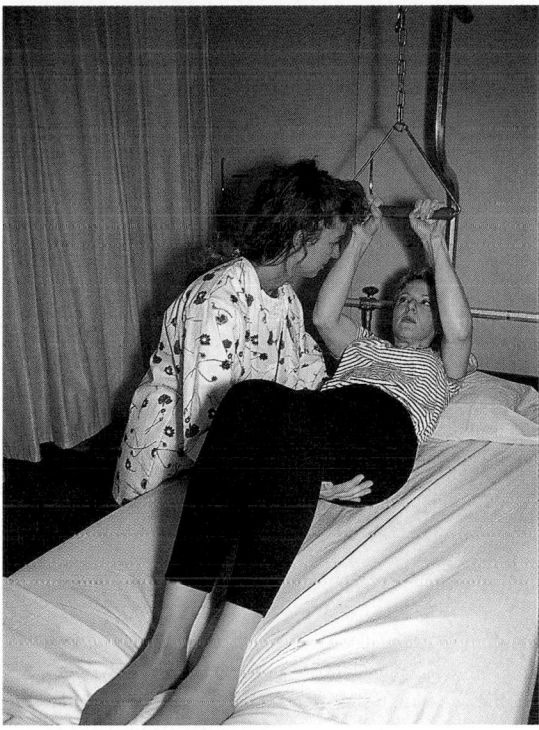

Fig. 37-19 Client using a trapeze bar.

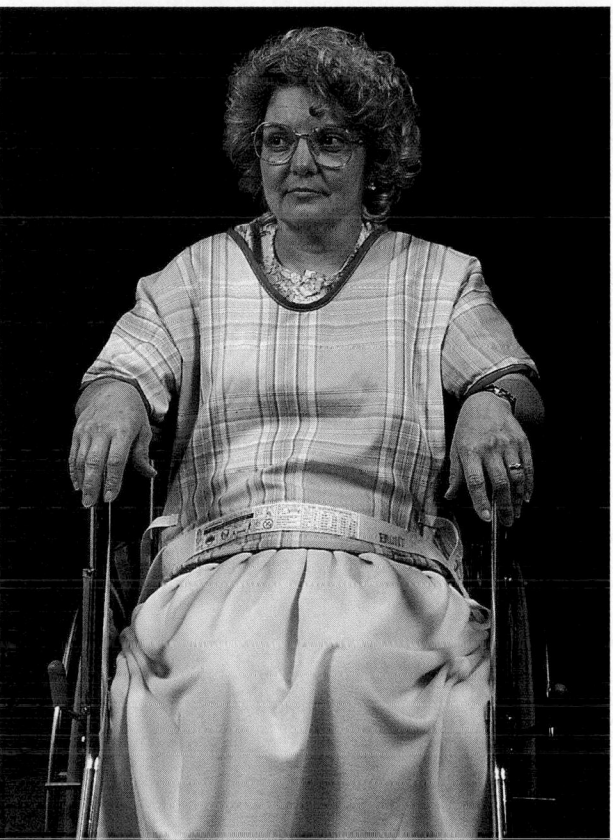

Fig. 37-20 Client restrained with Posey jacket.

Supine Position. The supine position, in which the client rests on the back, is also called the *dorsal recumbent position*. In the supine position the relationship of body parts is essentially the same as in good standing alignment except that the body is in the horizontal plane. Pillows, trochanter rolls, and hand rolls or arm splints are used to increase comfort and reduce injury to the skin or musculoskeletal system.

The mattress should be firm enough to support the cervical, thoracic, and lumbar vertebrae. Shoulders are supported and the elbows are slightly flexed to control shoulder rotation. A foot support is used to prevent footdrop and maintain proper alignment. The following are some common trouble areas for the supine position:

1. Pillow at the head too thick, increasing cervical flexion
2. Head flat on the mattress
3. Shoulders unsupported and internally rotated
4. Elbows extended
5. Thumb not in opposition to the fingers
6. Hips externally rotated
7. Unsupported feet
8. Unprotected pressure points at the occiput region of the head, lumbar vertebrae, elbows, and heels

Prone Position. The client in the prone position is lying face down. The pillow under the head should be thin enough to prevent cervical flexion or extension and maintain alignment of the lumbar spine. Placing a pillow under the lower leg permits dorsiflexion of the ankles and some knee flexion, which promotes relaxation. If a pillow is unavailable, the ankles should be in dorsiflexion over the end of the mattress. The nurse should assess for and correct any of the following potential trouble points:

1. Neck hyperextension
2. Hyperextension of the lumbar spine

3. Plantar flexion of the ankles
4. Unprotected pressure points at the chin, elbows, hips, knees, and toes

Side-Lying Position. In the side-lying (or lateral) position the client is resting on the side, with the major portion of body weight on the dependent hip and shoulder. Trunk alignment should be the same as in standing. For example, the structural curves of the spine should be maintained, the head should be supported in line with the midline of the trunk, and rotation of the spine should be avoided. The following trouble points are common in the side-lying position:

1. Lateral flexion of the neck
2. Spinal curves out of normal alignment
3. Shoulder and hip joints internally rotated, adducted, or unsupported
4. Lack of support for the feet
5. Lack of protection for pressure points at the ear, ilium, knees, and ankles

Sims' Position. The Sims' position differs from the side-lying position in the distribution of the client's weight. In the Sims' position the weight is placed on the anterior ilium, humerus, and clavicle. Trouble points common in the Sims' position include the following:

1. Lateral flexion of the neck
2. Internal rotation, adduction, or lack of support to the shoulders and hips
3. Lack of support for the feet
4. Lack of protection for pressure points at the ilium, humerus, clavicle, knees, and ankles

Text continued on p. 924.

Positioning Clients in Bed

STEPS	RATIONALE

PREPARATION FOR POSITIONING CLIENTS IN BED

STEPS	RATIONALE
1. Assess client's body alignment and comfort level while client is lying down.	Provides baseline data concerning client's body alignment and comfort level.
2. Prepare following equipment and supplies: a. Pillows e. Hand rolls b. Footboard f. Restraints c. Trochanter rolls g. Side rails d. Sandbags	Provides easy access to equipment necessary for proper positioning.
3. Raise level of bed to comfortable working height and remove pillows and devices used in previous position.	Raises level of work toward nurse's center of gravity, reduces interference from bedding during positioning procedure (Owen and Garg, 1991).
4. Obtain help as needed.	Provides for safety.
5. Explain procedure to client.	Helps decrease anxiety and increase cooperation.
6. Wash hands.	Reduces transmission of infection.
7. Provide for client privacy.	Ensuring client's mental comfort is important.
8. Put bed in flat position and move client to head of bed.	Provides easy access to client and allows nursing personnel to reposition client without working against gravity. Allows room for proper positioning. Helps maintain proper body alignment.

POSITION CLIENT IN SUPPORTED FOWLER'S POSITION

STEPS	RATIONALE
1. Complete preparation steps 1-8.	
2. Elevate head of bed 45-60 degrees.	Increases comfort, improves ventilation, and increases opportunity to socialize or relax.
3. Rest head against mattress or on small pillow.	Prevents cervical flexion contractures.
4. Use pillows to support arms and hand if client does not have voluntary control or use of hands and arms.	Prevents shoulder dislocation from effect of downward gravitational pull of unsupported arms, promotes circulation by preventing venous pooling, and prevents flexion contractures of arms and wrists.
5. Position pillow at lower back.	Supports lumbar vertebrae and decreases flexion of vertebrae.
6. Place small pillow or roll under thigh.	Prevents hyperextension of knee and occlusion of popliteal artery from pressure from body weight.
7. Place small pillow or roll under ankles.	Prevents prolonged pressure on heels from mattress.
8. Place footboard at bottom of client's feet (see the illustration below).	Maintains dorsal flexion and prevents footdrop.
9. Perform completion steps 1-4.	

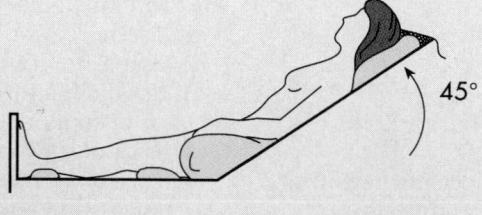

Step 8

POSITION HEMIPLEGIC CLIENT IN SUPPORTED FOWLER'S POSITION

STEPS	RATIONALE
1. Complete preparation steps 1-8.	
2. Elevate head of bed 45-60 degrees.	Increases comfort, improves ventilation, and increases opportunity to relax.
3. Sit client up as straight as possible.	Counteracts tendency to slump toward affected side. Improves ventilation, cardiac output; decreases intracranial pressure. Improves ability to swallow and helps prevent aspiration of food, liquids, or gastric secretions.

Positioning Clients in Bed—cont'd

STEPS	RATIONALE

POSITION HEMIPLEGIC CLIENT IN SUPPORTED FOWLER'S POSITION—cont'd

4. Position head with chin slightly forward.	Reduces risk of joint dislocation.
5. Provide support for involved arm and hand on overbed table in front of client; place arm away from client's side and support elbow on pillow.	Paralyzed muscles do not automatically resist pull of gravity as they do normally. As a result, shoulder subluxation, pain, or edema may occur.
6. Position *flaccid* hand in normal resting position with wrist slightly extended, arches of hand maintained, and fingers partially flexed; OPTION: use one section of rubber ball cut in half.	Maintains hand in functional position. Prevents contractures (Lehmkuhl et al, 1990).
7. Position *spastic* hand with wrist in neutral position or slightly extended; fingers should be extended with palm down or may be left in relaxed position with palm up.	Maintains hand in functional position. Inhibits flexor spasticity (Lehmkuhl et al, 1990).
8. Flex knees and hips by using pillow or folded blanket under knees.	Ensures proper alignment. Prevents prolonged hyperextension, which could impair joint mobility.
9. Support feet in dorsiflexion with soft pillow or footboard.	Prevents footdrop. Stimulation of ball of foot by hard surface has tendency to increase muscle tone in client with extensor spasticity of lower extremity.
10. Perform completion steps 1-4.	

POSITION CLIENT IN SUPINE POSITION

1. Complete preparation steps 1-8.	
2. Place client on back with head of bed flat.	Necessary for positioning in supine position.
3. Place small rolled towel under lumbar area of back.	Provides support for lumbar spine.
4. Place pillow under upper shoulders, neck, and head.	Maintains correct alignment and prevents flexion contractures of cervical vertebrae.
5. Place trochanter rolls or sandbags parallel to lateral surface of thighs.	Reduces external rotation of hip.
6. Place small pillow or roll under ankle to elevate heels.	Reduces pressure on heels, helping prevent pressure ulcers.
7. Place footboard or soft pillows against bottom of feet.	Maintains feet in dorsiflexion. Prevents footdrop.
8. Place pillows under pronated forearms, maintaining upper arms parallel to client's body (see the illustration below).	Reduces internal rotation of shoulder and prevents extension of elbows. Maintains correct body alignment.
9. Place hand rolls in hand.	Reduces extension of fingers and abduction of thumb. Maintains thumb slightly adducted and in opposition.
10. Perform completion steps 1-4.	

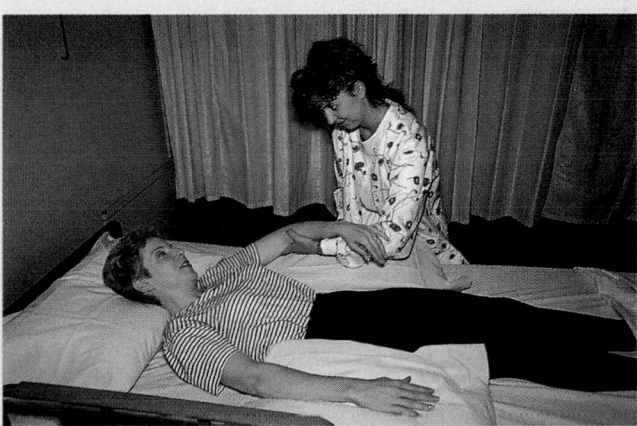

Step 8

Continued.

Positioning Clients in Bed—cont'd

STEPS	RATIONALE

POSITION HEMIPLEGIC CLIENT IN SUPINE POSITION

1. Complete preparation steps 1-8.

2. Place head of bed flat.

Necessary for positioning in supine position.

3. Place folded towel or pillow under shoulder of affected side.

Decreases possibility of pain, joint contracture, or subluxation. Maintains mobility in muscles around shoulder to permit movement patterns.

4. Keep affected arm away from body with elbow extended and palm up. OPTION: place arm out to side with elbow bent and hand toward head of bed.

Maintains mobility in arm, joints, and muscles around shoulder to permit normal movement patterns. (Counteracts limitation of ability of arm to rotate outward at shoulder [external rotation]. External rotation must be present to raise arm overhead without pain.)

5. Position affected hand in one of recommended positions for flaccid or spastic hand (see above).

Maintains hand in functional position.

6. Place folded towel under hip of involved side.

Diminishes effect of spasticity in entire leg by controlling hip position.

7. Flex affected knee 30 degrees by supporting it on pillow or folded blanket.

Slight flexion breaks up abnormal extension pattern of leg. Extensor spasticity is most severe when client is supine.

8. Support feet with soft pillows at right angle to leg.

Maintains foot in dorsiflexion and prevents footdrop. Soft pillows prevent stimulation to ball of foot by hard surface, which has tendency to increase muscle tone in client with extensor spasticity of lower extremity.

9. Perform completion steps 1-4.

POSITION CLIENT IN PRONE POSITION

1. Complete preparation steps 1-8.

2. Roll client over arm positioned close to body with elbow straight and hand under hip. Position on abdomen in center of bed with bed flat.

Positions client so that alignment can be maintained.

3. Turn client's head to one side and support with small pillow.

Reduces flexion or hyperextension of cervical vertebrae.

4. Place small pillow under abdomen below level of diaphragm.

Reduces pressure on breasts of some women. Decreases hyperextension of lumbar vertebrae and strain on lower back. Improves breathing by reducing mattress pressure on diaphragm.

5. Support arms in flexed position level at shoulders.

Maintains proper body alignment. Support reduces risk of joint dislocation.

6. Support lower legs with pillow to elevate toes (see the illustration below).

Prevents footdrop. Reduces external rotation of legs. Reduces mattress pressure on toes.

7. Perform completion steps 1-4.

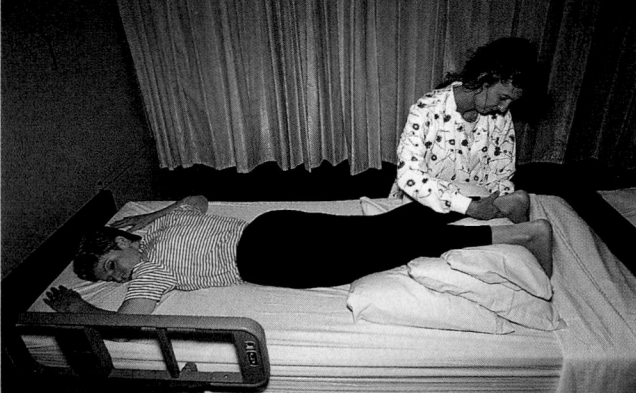

Step 6, above

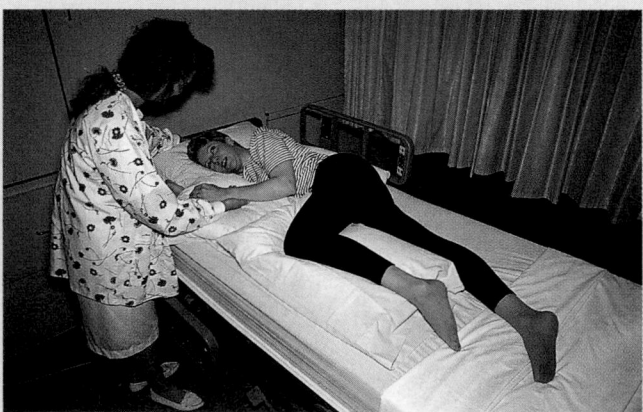

Step 9, p. 923

Positioning Clients in Bed—cont'd

STEPS	RATIONALE

POSITION HEMIPLEGIC CLIENT IN PRONE POSITION

STEPS	RATIONALE
1. Complete preparation steps 1-8.	
2. With head of bed flat, move client toward unaffected side.	Ensures proper client alignment in center of bed when rolled onto abdomen.
3. Roll client onto unaffected side:	
a. Place pillow against abdomen.	Prevents sagging of abdomen when client is rolled over. Decreases hyperextension of lumbar vertebrae and strain on lower back.
b. Roll client onto abdomen by positioning involved arm close to client's body with elbow straight and hand under hip. Roll client carefully over arm.	Prevents injury to affected side.
4. Turn head toward involved side.	Promotes development of neck and trunk extension, which is necessary for standing and walking.
5. Position involved arm out to side with elbow bent and hand toward head of bed, fingers extended if possible.	Counteracts limitation of arm's ability to rotate outward at shoulder (external rotation). External rotation must be present to raise arm over head without pain.
6. Flex both knees slightly by placing pillow under both legs from knees to ankles.	Prevents prolonged hyperextension, which could impair joint mobility.
7. Keep feet at right angles to legs by using pillow high enough to keep toes off mattress.	Maintains feet in dorsiflexion.
8. Perform completion steps 1-4.	

POSITION CLIENT IN LATERAL (SIDE-LYING) POSITION

STEPS	RATIONALE
1. Complete preparation steps 1-8.	
2. Lower head of bed completely or as low as client can tolerate.	Provides position of comfort for client and removes pressure from bony prominences on back.
3. Position client to side of bed.	Provides room for client to turn to side.
4. Turn client onto side:	
a. To turn helpless client onto side, flex client's knee that will not be next to mattress. Place one hand on client's hip and one hand on shoulder.	Prevents injury to joints as client is rolled to side. Leverage on hip makes turning easy.
b. Roll client onto side.	Rolling client toward you causes less trauma to tissues.
5. Place pillow under client's head and neck.	Maintains alignment. Reduces lateral neck flexion. Decreases strain on sternocleidomastoid muscle.
6. Bring shoulder blade forward.	Prevents weight from resting directly on shoulder joint.
7. Position both arms in slightly flexed position. Uppermost arm is supported by pillow level with shoulder.	Decreases internal rotation and adduction of shoulder. Protects joint. Ventilation is improved because chest can expand more easily.
8. Place tuck-back pillow behind client's back. (Make tuck-back pillow by folding pillow lengthwise. Smooth area is slightly tucked under back.)	Provides support to maintain client on side.
9. Place pillow under semiflexed upper leg level at hip from groin to foot (see the illustration on p. 922).	Prevents hyperextension of leg. Maintains leg in proper alignment. Prevents pressure on bony prominence.
10. Place sandbag parallel to plantar surface of dependent foot.	Maintains dorsiflexion of the foot. Prevents footdrop.
11. Perform completion steps 1-4.	

POSITION CLIENT IN SIMS' (SEMIPRONE) POSITION

STEPS	RATIONALE
1. Complete preparation steps 1-8.	
2. Place head of bed flat.	Provides for proper body alignment while client is lying.
3. Place client in supine position.	Prepares client for Sims' position.
4. Position client in lateral position lying partially on abdomen.	Client is rolled only partially on abdomen.

Continued.

Positioning Clients in Bed—cont'd

STEPS	RATIONALE

POSITION CLIENT IN SIMS' (SEMIPRONE) POSITION—cont'd

5. Place small pillow under head.

Maintains proper alignment and prevents lateral neck flexion.

6. Place pillow under flexed upper arm, supporting arm level with shoulder. Support other arm on mattress.

Prevents internal rotation of shoulder. Maintains proper alignment.

7. Place pillow under flexed upper legs, supporting leg level with hip (see the illustration below).

Prevents internal rotation of hip and adduction of leg. Prevents hyperextension of leg. Reduces mattress pressure on knees and ankles.

8. Place sandbags parallel to plantar surface of foot.

Maintains foot in dorsiflexion. Prevents footdrop.

9. Perform completion steps 1-4.

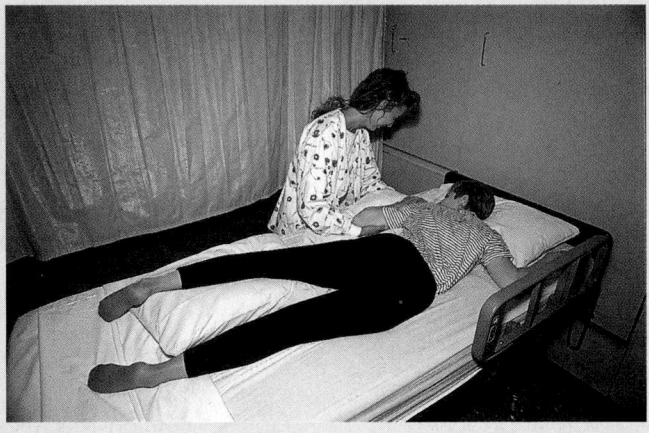

Step 6

COMPLETION FOR POSITIONING CLIENTS IN BED

1. Wash hands.

Reduces transmission of infection.

2. Lower bed.

Provides for client safety.

3. Observe body alignment position, level of comfort, and potential pressure points.

Determines effectiveness of positioning, maintenance of body alignment, and protection from pressure. Reduces risk of musculoskeletal injury related to improper positioning.

4. Record procedure in nurses' notes, including position assumed, frequency of turning, condition of skin, joint movement, use of supports or splints, client's ability to assist with repositioning, number of staff needed to complete procedure, and client comfort.

Documents effectiveness of nursing care. Provides for consistency among nursing staff.

Transfer Techniques. Nurses often provide care for immobilized clients whose position must be changed, who must be moved up in bed, or who must be transferred from a bed to a chair or a bed to a stretcher. Proper body mechanics enables the nurse to move, lift, or transfer clients safely and also protects the nurse from injury to the musculoskeletal system. Although nurses use many transfer techniques, the following general guidelines should be followed in any transfer procedure:

1. Raising the side rail on the side of the bed opposite the nurse to prevent the client from falling out of bed

2. Elevating the level of the bed to a comfortable height
3. Assessing the client's mobility and strength to determine assistance the client can offer during transfer
4. Determining the need for assistance
5. Explaining the procedure and describing what is expected of the client
6. Assessing for correct body alignment and pressure areas after each transfer

The nurse who is attempting transfer or moving techniques for the first time should request help to reduce the risk of injury to client and nurse. The nurse should also recognize

Moving a Client Up in Bed

STEPS	RATIONALE

PREPARATION FOR MOVING A CLIENT UP IN BED

1. Assess client's comfort level, activity tolerance, muscle strength, and mobility.
2. Raise level of bed to comfortable working height.
3. Remove pillows and devices used in previous position.
4. Get extra help as needed.
5. Explain procedure to client.
6. Pull curtains and close door.
7. Wash hands.
8. Put bed in flat position with wheels on bed locked.

Provides baseline data to determine client's ability to assist in moving.

Raises level of work toward your center of gravity.

Reduces interference from bedding.

Provides for safety.

Decreases client anxiety and increases cooperation.

Ensures client's mental comfort.

Reduces transmission of infection.

Provides easy access to client and allows you to reposition client without having to work against gravity.

MOVE HELPLESS CLIENT UP IN BED (ONE NURSE)

1. Complete preparation steps 1-7.
2. Place client on back with head of bed flat. Stand on one side of bed.
3. Place pillow at head of bed.
4. Begin at client's feet. Face foot of bed at 45-degree angle. Place feet apart with foot nearest head of bed behind other foot (forward-backward stance) (see the illustration below). Flex knees and hips as needed to bring your arms level with client's legs. Shift your weight from front to back leg and slide client's legs diagonally toward head of bed.
5. Move parallel to client's hips. Flex knees and hips as needed to bring your arms level with client's hips.
6. Slide client's hips diagonally toward head of bed.
7. Move parallel to client's head and shoulders. Flex knees and hips as needed to bring arms level with client's body.
8. Slide your arm closest to head of bed under client's neck, with your hand reaching under and supporting shoulder.
9. Place your other arm under client's upper back.

Enables you to assess body alignment. Reduces gravitational pull on client's upper body.

Prevents striking client's head against bed.

Positioning is begun at client's legs because they are lighter and easier to move. Facing direction of movement ensures proper balance. Shifting your weight reduces force needed to move load. Diagonal motion permits pull in direction of force. Flexing knees lowers your center of gravity and uses thigh muscles rather than back muscles.

Maintains your proper body alignment. Brings you closest to object to be moved and lowers center of gravity. Uses thigh muscles rather than back muscles.

Aligns client's hips and feet.

Maintains your proper body alignment. Brings you closer to object to be moved. Lowers your center of gravity. Uses thigh muscles rather than back muscles.

Supports client's head and neck, maintaining proper alignment and preventing injury during movement.

Supports client's body weight and reduces friction.

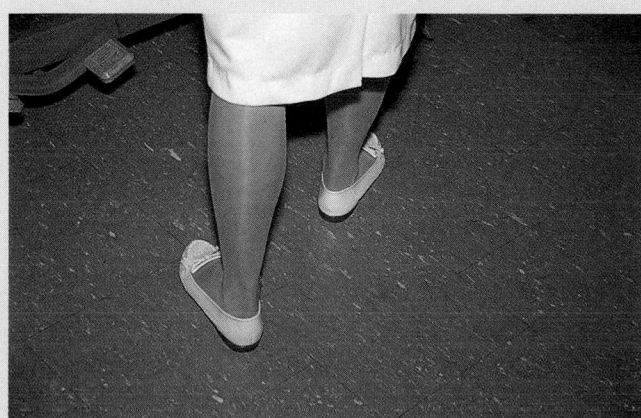

Step 4

Continued.

Moving a Client Up in Bed—cont'd

STEPS	RATIONALE

MOVE HELPLESS CLIENT UP IN BED (ONE NURSE)—cont'd

10. Slide client's trunk, shoulders, head, and neck diagonally toward head of bed.

Realigns client's body on one side of bed.

11. Elevate side rail. Move to other side of bed and lower side rail.

Protects client from falling out of bed.

12. Repeat procedure, switching sides until client reaches desired height in bed.

13. Center client in middle of bed, moving body in same three sections.

Maintains proper body alignment. Provides ample room for turning, positioning, or other nursing activities.

14. Raise side rails.

Provides for client safety.

15. Perform completion steps 1-5.

ASSIST CLIENT TO MOVE UP IN BED (ONE OR TWO NURSES)

1. Complete preparation steps 1-7.
2. Place client on back with head of bed flat.

Enables you to assess body alignment. Reduces gravitational pull on client's upper body.

3. Place pillow at head of bed.

Prevents striking client's head against bed.

4. Face head of bed.

   a. If two nurses assist client, each nurse should have one arm under client's shoulders and one arm under client's thighs.

   Facing direction of movement prevents twisting your body while moving client.

   b. *Alternate position:* Position one nurse at client's upper body. Nurse's arm nearest head of bed should be under client's head and opposite shoulder. Other arm should be under client's closest arm and shoulder. Position other nurse at client's lower torso. This nurse's arms should be under client's lower back and torso.

   Prevents trauma to client's musculoskeletal system by supporting shoulder and hip joints and evenly distributing weight.

5. Place feet apart with foot nearest head of bed behind other foot (forward-backward stance).

Wide base of support increases your balance. Forward-backward stance enables you to shift body weight as client is moved up in bed, thereby reducing force needed to move load.

6. Ask client to flex knees with feet flat on bed (see the illustration below).

Enables client to use femoral muscles during movement.

7. Instruct client to flex neck, tilting chin toward chest.

Prevents hyperextension of neck.

8. Instruct client to assist moving by pushing with feet on bed surface.

Reduces friction. Increases client mobility. Decreases your workload.

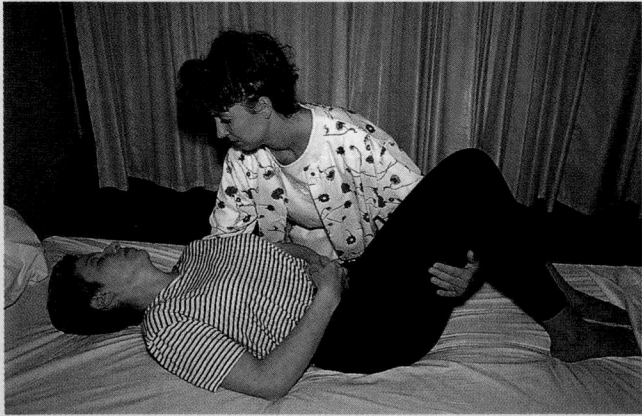

Step 6

Moving a Client Up in Bed—cont'd

STEPS	RATIONALE
9. Flex your knees and hips, bringing your forearms closer to level of bed.	Increases balance and strength by bringing your center of gravity closer to client—the "object" to be moved. Uses thigh muscles instead of back muscles.
10. Instruct client to push with heels and elevate trunk while breathing out, thus moving toward head of bed on count of 3.	Prepares client for move. Reinforces client's assistance in moving up in bed. Increases client cooperation. Breathing out avoids Valsalva maneuver.
11. On count of 3, rock and shift your weight from front to back leg. At same time, client pushes with heels and elevates trunk.	Rocking enables you to improve balance and overcome inertia. Shifting your weight counteracts client's weight and reduces force needed to move load. Client's assistance reduces friction and your workload.
12. Perform completion steps 1-5.	

COMPLETION FOR MOVING A CLIENT UP IN BED

1. Realign client in supported Fowler's, supine, prone, lateral, or Sims' position.	Maintains client's proper body alignment, preventing injury to skin and musculoskeletal system.
2. Wash hands.	Reduces transmission of infection.
3. Lower bed.	Provides for client safety.
4. Observe client's body alignment, position, level of comfort, and potential pressure points.	Maintains support to musculoskeletal system and reduces risk of injury related to improper movement or positioning.
5. Record procedure in nurses' notes, including position assumed, frequency of turning, condition of skin, joint movement, use of supports or splints, and client's ability to assist with moving and positioning.	Documents effectiveness of nursing care. Provides for consistency among nursing staff.

personal strength and its limits. Moving a completely immobilized client alone is difficult and dangerous.

Moving Clients. Clients require various levels of assistance to move up in bed, move to the side-lying position, or sit up at the side of the bed. For example, a young, healthy woman may need only a little support as she sits at the side of the bed for the first time after childbirth, whereas an older man may need help from one or more nurses to do the same task 1 day after an appendectomy.

To determine what the client is able to do alone and how many people are needed to help move the client in bed, the nurse assesses the client to determine whether the illness contradicts exertion (e.g., cardiovascular disease). Next, the nurse determines whether the client comprehends what is expected. For example, a client recently medicated for postoperative pain may be too lethargic to understand instruction, so to ensure safety, two nurses are needed to move the client in bed. The nurse then determines the comfort level of the client. The nurse also evaluates personal strength and knowledge of the procedure. Finally the nurse determines whether the client is too heavy or immobile for the nurse to complete the procedure alone. In doubtful cases the nurse should always request assistance from another person. Procedures 37-3 and 37-4 describe the steps commonly used in moving clients in bed and transferring them to a sitting position at the side of the bed.

Transferring a Client From a Bed to a Chair. Transfer of a client from bed to chair by one nurse requires assistance from the client and should not be attempted with a client who cannot help (Procedure 37-4). The nurse explains the procedure to the client before the transfer. The environment is also prepared by moving obstacles out of the way. The chair is placed next to the bed with the chair back in the same plane as the head of the bed. Placement of the chair allows the nurse to pivot with the client and to transfer the client's weight quickly.

A safe transfer is the first priority. The nurse who is doubtful about personal strength or the client's ability to help should request assistance. The client should sit and dangle the feet at the side of the bed for a minute before standing. Then the client should stand at the side of the bed for another minute so that the client can quickly be lowered back into it in case of dizziness or fainting.

When moving an immoblized client from bed to wheelchair both nurses must use proper body mechanics and, whenever possible, elicit as much cooperation as possible from the client (Fig. 37-21).

Transferring a Client From a Bed to a Stretcher. An immobilized client who must be transferred from bed to stretcher or bed to bed requires a three-person carry (see Procedure 37-4). This technique is best implemented when personnel who are doing the lifting are similar in height. If their centers of gravity are within the same plane, they can lift as a team. Another way to transfer a client is by using a lift sheet placed under the client (Fig. 37-22). The lift sheet serves as a "cradle" while the client is being transferred to the

Text continued on p. 932.

Transfer Techniques

STEPS	RATIONALE

PREPARATION FOR TRANSFER TECHNIQUES

1. Assess client's muscle strength, joint mobility, presence of paralysis or paresis, orthostatic hypotension, activity tolerance, level of consciousness, level of comfort, and ability to follow instructions.

Determines client's physiological and cognitive level for participating in transfer technique.

2. Prepare needed equipment and supplies:
   a. Transfer belt (if needed)

Reduces risk of injury. Should be used with all clients who require moderate-to-maximal assistance or have risk of falling or injury. Research (Owen and Garg, 1991) demonstrated that transfer belt was more readily and correctly used than mechanical devices.

   b. Wheelchair (Position chair at 45-degree angle to bed; lock brakes; remove footrests; lock bed brakes.)

Position of wheelchair or stretcher facilitates quick transfer from bed to wheelchair or bed to stretcher.

   c. Stretcher (position at 90-degree angle to bed; lock brakes on stretcher; lock brakes on bed.)

3. Explain procedure to client.

Promotes client cooperation and understanding of procedure and benefits of mobilization.

4. Close door or curtain.

Ensures privacy.

5. Wash hands.

Reduces transfer of infection.

ASSIST CLIENT TO SITTING POSITION IN BED

1. Complete preparation steps 1-5.
2. Place client in supine position.

Enables continual assessment of client's body alignment and administration of additional care, such as suctioning or hygiene needs.

3. Remove pillows from bed.

Decreases interference while sitting client up in bed.

4. Face head of bed.

Reduces twisting of your body when moving client.

5. Place feet apart with foot nearer bed behind other foot.

Improves your balance and allows transfer of body weight as client is moved to sitting position.

6. Place hand that is farther from client under shoulders, supporting head and cervical vertebrae.

Maintains alignment of head and cervical vertebrae and allows for even lifting of client's upper trunk.

7. Place other hand on bed surface.

Provides support and balance.

8. Raise client to sitting position by shifting your weight from front leg to back leg.

Improves your balance, overcomes inertia, and transfers weight in direction in which client is moved.

9. Push against bed using arm that was placed on bed surface.

Divides activity of raising client to sitting position between your arms and legs and protects back from strain. By bracing one hand against mattress and pushing against it as client is lifted, part of weight that would be lifted by your back muscles is transferred through arms onto mattress (Stamps, 1989).

10. Perform completion steps 1-4.

ASSIST CLIENT TO SITTING POSITION ON SIDE OF BED

1. Complete preparation steps 1-5.
2. Place client in side-lying position, facing you on side of bed on which client will be sitting.

Prepares client to move to side of bed and protects client from falling.

3. Raise head of bed to highest level client is able to tolerate.

Decreases amount of work needed by client and nurse to raise client to sitting position.

4. Stand opposite client's hips.

Places your center of gravity nearer client.

5. Turn on diagonal so that you are facing client and far corner of foot of bed.

Reduces twisting of your body because nurse is facing direction of movement.

6. Place feet apart with foot closer to head of bed in front of other foot.

Increases balance and allows you to transfer weight as client is brought to sitting position at side of bed.

7. Place arm nearer head of bed under client's shoulders, supporting the head and neck.

Maintains alignment of head and neck as you bring client to sitting position.

8. Place other arm over client's thighs (see the illustration on p. 929).

Supports hip and prevents client from falling backward during procedure.

Transfer Techniques—cont'd

STEPS	RATIONALE

ASSIST CLIENT TO SITTING POSITION ON SIDE OF BED—cont'd

9. Move client's lower legs and feet over side of bed. — Decreases friction and resistance.

10. Pivot toward your rear leg, allowing client's upper legs to swing downward. — Allows gravity to lower client's legs.

11. At same time, shift your weight to your rear leg and elevate client (see the illustration below). — Allows you to transfer weight in direction of motion.

12. Remain in front of client until balance is regained. — Reduces risk of falling.

13. Lower level of bed until client's feet touch floor. — Supports client's feet in dorsal flexion and allows client to easily stand at side of bed.

14. Perform completion steps 1-4.

TRANSFER CLIENT FROM BED TO CHAIR

1. Complete preparation steps 1-5.

2. Assist client to sitting position on side of bed. Have chair in position at 45-degree angle to bed. — Positions chair within easy access for transfer.

3. Apply transfer belt if necessary. — Allows you to maintain stability of client during transfer and reduces risk of falling.

4. Ensure that client has stable, nonskid shoes. — Decreases risk of slipping during transfer.

5. Spread your feet apart. — Ensures balance with wide base of support.

6. Flex your hips and knees, aligning your knees with client's. — Lowers your center of gravity to object to be raised and allows stabilization of knees when client stands.

7. Grasp transfer belt from underneath or reach through client's axillae and place hands on client's scapulae (see the illustration below). — Reduces pressure on axillae and maintains client stability.

8. Rock client up to standing on count of 3 while straightening your hips and legs, keeping knees slightly flexed (see the illustration below). — Gives client's body momentum and requires less muscular effort to lift client. Uses correct body mechanics to raise client to standing position.

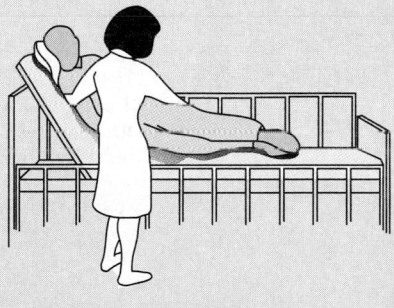

Step 8, p. 928

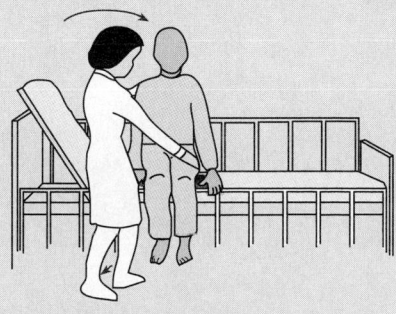

Step 11

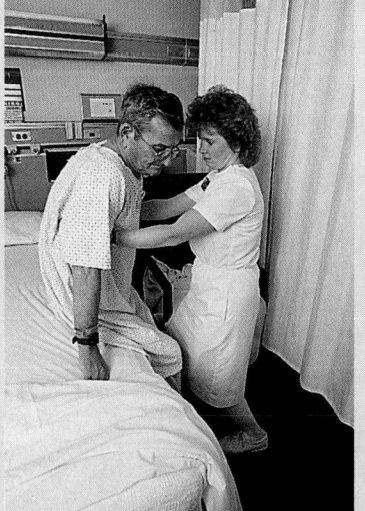

Step 7

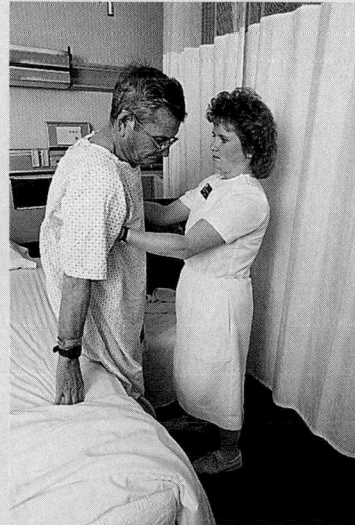

Step 8

Continued.

PROCEDURE 37-4

Transfer Techniques—cont'd

STEPS	RATIONALE
9. Maintain stability of weak or paralyzed leg with knee.	Ability to stand can often be maintained in paralyzed or weak limb with support of knee to stabilize.
10. Pivot on foot that is farther from chair (see the illustration below).	Maintains support of client while allowing adequate space for client to move.
11. Instruct client to use arm rests on chair for support.	Increases client stability.
12. Flex your hips and knees while lowering client into chair (see the illustration below).	Prevents injury resulting from poor body mechanics.
13. Assess client for proper alignment for sitting position.	Prevents injury to client from poor body alignment.
14. Perform completion steps 1-4.	

PERFORM THREE-PERSON CARRY

1. Complete preparation steps 1-5.	
2. Three nurses of nearly equal height stand side by side facing side of client's bed.	Prevents twisting of bodies. Client's alignment is maintained.
3. Each person assumes responsibility for one of three areas: head and shoulders, hips, and thighs and ankles.	Distributes client's body weight.

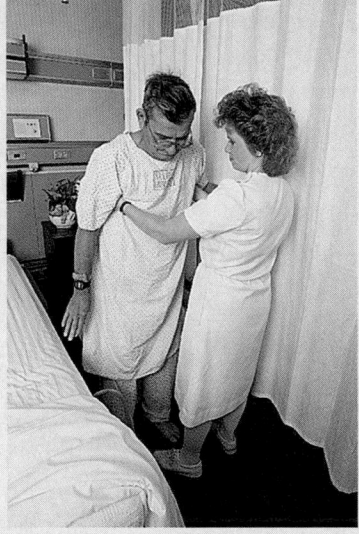

Step 10

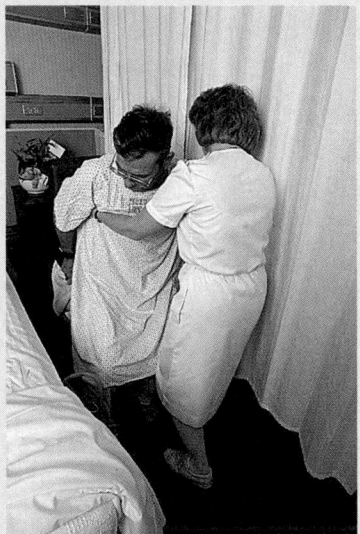

Step 12

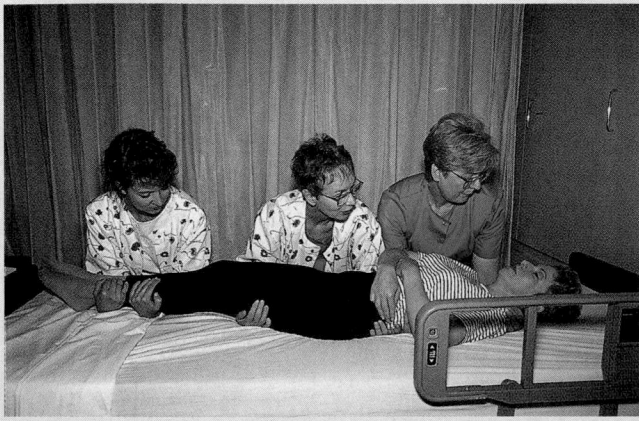

Step 5, p. 931

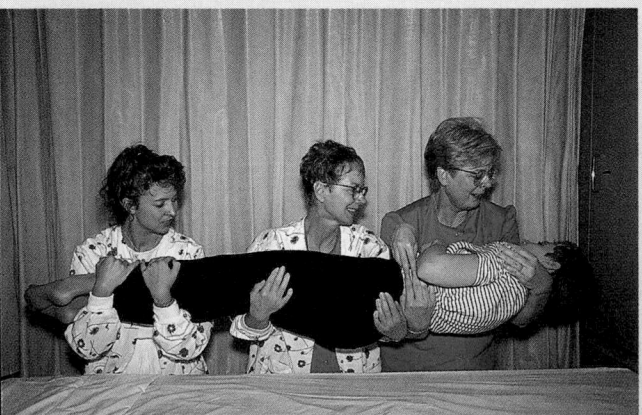

Step 6, p. 931

Transfer Techniques—cont'd

STEPS	RATIONALE

PERFORM THREE-PERSON CARRY—cont'd

4. Each assumes wide base of support with foot that is closer to stretcher in front, knees slightly flexed.

   Increases balance and lowers lifters' center of gravity.

5. Lifters' arms are placed under client's head and shoulders, hips, and thighs and lower legs, with their fingers securely around other side of client's body (see the illustration on p. 930).

   Distributes client's weight over lifters' forearms.

6. Lifters roll client toward their chests (see the illustration on p. 930).

   Moves workload over lifters' base of support.

7. On count of 3, client is lifted and held against nurses' chests.

   Enables lifters to work together and safely lift client.

8. On second count of 3, nurses step back and pivot toward stretcher, moving forward if needed.

   Transfers weight toward stretcher.

9. Nurses gently lower client onto center of stretcher by flexing their knees and hips until their elbows are level with edge of stretcher.

   Maintains alignment during transfer.

10. Nurses assess client's body alignment, place safety straps across client, and raise side rails.

    Reduces risk of injury from poor alignment or falling.

11. Perform completion steps 1-4.

COMPLETION FOR TRANSFERRING

1. Position client in selected position.

   Reduces risk of injury to musculoskeletal system from improper positioning.

2. Wash hands.

   Reduces transmission of infection.

3. Observe client to determine response to transfer. Observe for correct body alignment and presence of pressure points.

   Reduces risk of injury from subsequent transfers and positioning.

4. Record procedure in nurses' notes.

   Documents effectiveness of nursing care. Provides for consistency among nursing staff.

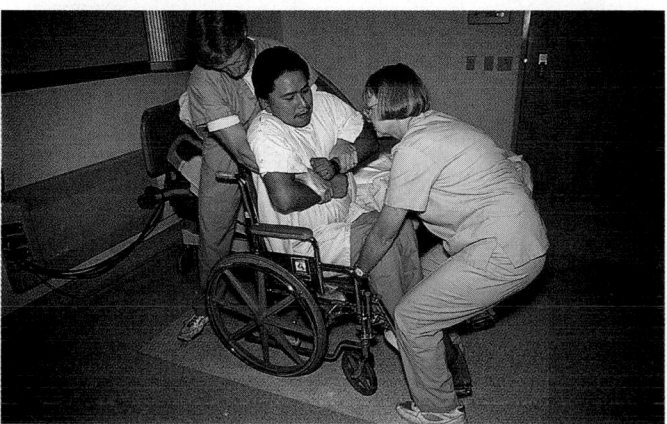

Fig. 37-21 Transferring an immobile client from bed to wheelchair.

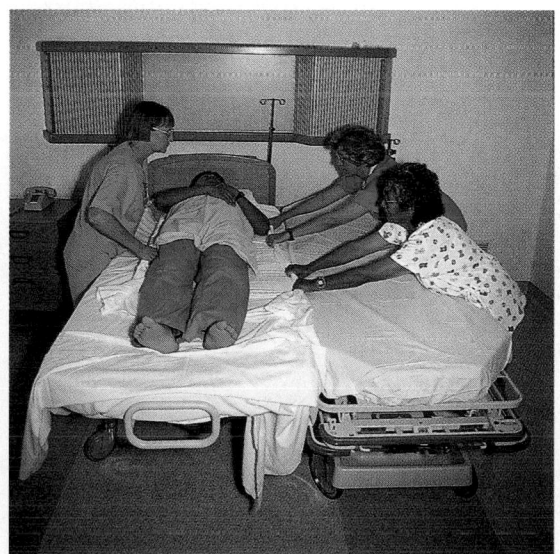

Fig. 37-22 Use of a draw or pull sheet to transfer a client from bed to stretcher.

stretcher. In this technique, nurses need to be on opposite sides of the bed and holding onto the lift sheet when transferring the client to the stretcher. The stretcher and the bed are placed side by side so that the client can be transferred quickly and easily using the lift sheet.

Caution is used when the client has spinal cord trauma. If the client must be moved, a transfer board should be placed under the client to maintain spinal alignment before transferring the client to a stretcher.

The client should be prepared for the transfer and asked to help when possible; for example, by folding the arms over the chest. The environment should be free from obstacles and unnecessary equipment should be removed from the bed. The stretcher should be placed at a right angle to the bed so that the lifters can pivot toward the stretcher and transfer the client quickly.

As with all procedures, safety is the priority. Safety is increased in the three-person carry if the lifters work together. Therefore one person should assume the leadership role.

JOINT MOBILITY

To ensure adequate joint mobility the nurse can teach the client about ROM exercises. When the client does not have voluntary motor control, the nurse institutes passive ROM exercises. Joint mobility is also increased by walking. Occasionally clients need to use mechanical devices such as crutches to help them walk.

ROM Exercises. Clients with restricted mobility are unable to perform some or all ROM exercises independently. This limitation can be identified in clients for whom one extremity has limited movement or in completely immobilized clients. When caring for clients with actual or potential impaired mobility, the nurse designs interventions directed at maintaining maximum joint mobility. One such nursing intervention is ROM exercises.

To ensure that clients routinely receive these exercises, the nurse should schedule them at specific times, perhaps with another nursing activity, such as during the client's bath. This enables the nurse to systematically assess and improve the client's ROM. In addition, bathing or receiving a bed bath usually requires that extremities and joints are put through complete ROM.

ROM exercises may be active (the client is able to move all joints through their ROM unassisted), passive (the client is unable to move independently and the nurse moves each joint through its ROM), or somewhere in between. With a weak client, for example, the nurse may merely provide support while the client performs most of the movement, or the client may be able to move some joints actively while the nurse passively moves others. The nurse first assesses the client's ability to engage in active ROM exercises and the need for assistance from the nurse. In general, exercises should be as active as health and mobility allow. Contractures may develop in joints not moved periodically through their full ROM.

Unless contraindicated, the care plan should include moving the client's extremities through the full ROM possible. Passive ROM exercises should begin as soon as the client's ability to move the extremity or joint is lost. Movements are carried out slowly and smoothly and should not cause pain. The nurse should never force a joint beyond its capacity. Each movement should be repeated 5 times during the session.

When performing passive ROM exercises, the nurse stands at the side of the bed closest to the joint being exercised. If an extremity is to be moved or lifted, the nurse places a cupped hand under the joint to support it (Fig. 37-23), supports the joint by holding the adjacent distal and proximal areas (Fig. 37-24), or supports the joint with one hand and cradles the distal portion of the extremity with the remaining arm (Fig. 37-25).

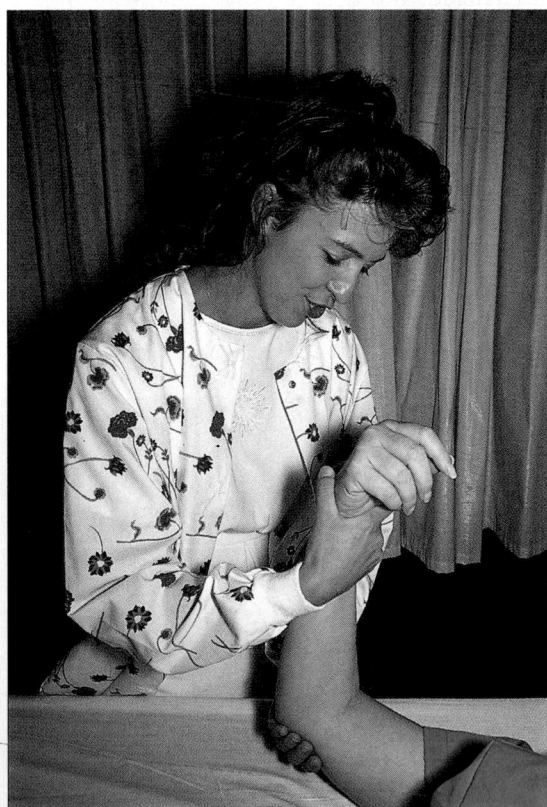

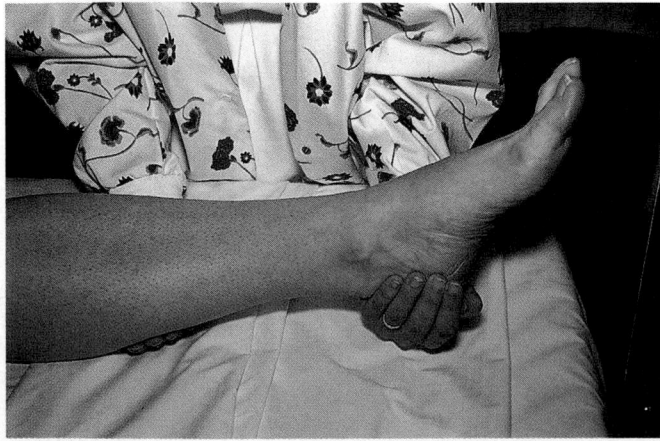

Fig. 37-23 Using a cupped hand to support a joint.

Fig. 37-24 Supporting the joint by holding the distal and proximal areas adjacent to the joint.

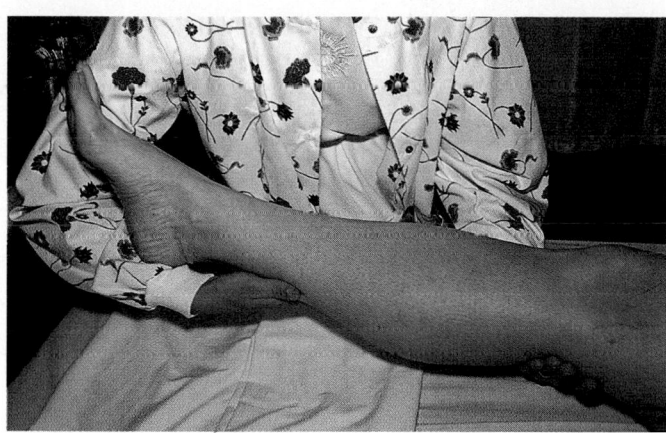

Fig. 37-25 Cradling the distal portion of an extremity.

The following sections describe specific movements for major joints in the body. Table 37-3 details ROM for each area and illustrates motion of each joint.

Neck. ROM for the neck is permitted by the flexibility of the cervical vertebrae and the pivotal connection between the head and neck. Unless contraindicated because of spinal surgery, spinal cord trauma, or other central nervous system trauma, ROM exercises should be performed by clients with limited neck mobility. When flexion contracture of the neck occurs, the client's neck is permanently flexed with the chin close to or actually touching the chest. Ultimately, the client's body alignment is altered, the visual field is changed, and the level of independent functioning is decreased.

Shoulder. One feature of the shoulder that sets it apart from other joints in the body is that the strongest muscle controlling it, the deltoid, is in complete elongation in the normal position. No other muscle exerts its full strength when in complete elongation. Thus exercising the shoulder effectively increases the power of the deltoid and ROM. To accomplish this, the shoulder must first be abducted.

The goal of action in the shoulder is full ROM. Shoulder movements include flexion, extension, hyperextension, abduction, adduction, internal and external rotation, and circumduction. The full ROM must be maintained or regained to avoid pain.

When caring for a client with limited mobility of the shoulder, the nurse should design interventions to place and support the shoulder in the adducted position. This can be achieved with slings when the client is standing or sitting or pillows when the client is in bed. Correctly positioning the shoulder prevents pain, joint dislocation, and further changes in body alignment.

Elbow. The elbow functions optimally at an angle of about 90 degrees. An elbow fixed in full extension is disabling and limits the client's independence.

Forearm. Most functions of the hand are best carried out with the forearm in moderate pronation. When the forearm is fixed in a position of full supination, the client's use of the hand is limited. For optimal functioning the forearm must be able to rotate from supination to pronation.

Wrist. The primary function of the wrist is to place the hand in slight dorsal flexion, the position of functioning.

Therefore full ROM is not as great a priority as maintaining the wrist in a functional position. When the wrist is fixed in even a slightly flexed position, grasp is weakened. In the immobilized client the functional position of the wrist can be achieved by using hand rolls and splints.

Fingers and Thumb. The ROM in fingers and the thumb enables the client to perform activities of daily living and activities requiring fine motor skills such as carpentry, needlework, drawing, and painting. The functional position of the fingers and thumb is slight flexion of the thumb in opposition to the fingers. In clients with restricted mobility, hand rolls help maintain this position.

Hip. Because the lower extremities are concerned chiefly with locomotion and weight bearing, stability of the hip joint may be more important than its mobility. For example, if one hip has no mobility but is fixed in a neutral position and fully extended, it is possible to walk without a significant limp.

However, contractures often fix the hip in positions of deformity. Excessive abduction makes the affected leg appear too long, whereas excessive adduction makes the affected leg appear too short. In either case the client has limited locomotion and walks with an obvious limp. Flexion contractures result in lordosis when the person is standing. Internal and external rotation contractures cause an abnormal and unbalanced gait.

Knee. A primary function of the knee is stability, which is achieved by ROM, ligaments, and muscles. However, knees cannot remain stable under weight-bearing conditions unless there is adequate quadriceps power to maintain the knee in full extension. ROM exercises should include pulling the knee into full extension.

An immobile knee joint can result in serious disability. The degree of disability depends on the position in which the knee is stiffened. If the knee is fixed in full extension, the person must sit with the leg thrust out in front. When the knee is flexed, the person limps while walking. The greater the flexion, the greater the limp. Complete flexion contractures prevent the person from walking without a walker or crutches.

Ankle and Foot. During walking, movement of the ankle joint is minimal. However, the joint must be stabilized and able to bear weight, or the person will fall. If joint mobility is diminished, the nurse should maintain the joint in a position in which walking can be carried out with a forward rolling motion from the heel onto the forefoot.

When the person relaxes as in sleep or coma, the foot relaxes and assumes a position of plantar flexion. This results from relaxation of the gastrocnemius and soleus muscles, which maintain dorsiflexion. If the foot remains in plantar flexion without support, these two muscles shorten and the dorsiflexion muscles try to compensate by overstretching. As a result the foot becomes fixed in plantar flexion (footdrop), which impairs the ability to walk.

Inversion and eversion must also be avoided to allow the foot to rest flat on the floor. The foot must be flat to allow weight bearing and proper walking.

Toes. Excessive flexion of the toes results in a clawing. When this is a permanent deformity, the foot is unable to rest flat on the floor and the client is unable to walk properly. Flexion contractures are the most common foot deformity associated with reduced joint mobility.

Adequate ROM gives the necessary mobility to carry out activities of daily living and exercise and to engage in relaxing activities. In addition, adequate ROM in the lower extremities allows walking.

WALKING

In the normal walking posture the head is erect; the cervical, thoracic, and lumbar vertebrae are aligned; the hips and knees have appropriate flexion; and the arms swing freely with the legs. Illness or trauma can reduce activity tolerance, so assistance in walking is required. In addition, temporary or permanent damage to the musculoskeletal and nervous systems may necessitate use of a mechanical device for walking.

Assisting a Client to Walk. Like other procedures, assisting the client to walk requires preparation. The nurse assesses the client's activity tolerance, strength, presence of pain, coordination, and balance to determine the amount of assistance needed.

The nurse explains how far the client should try to walk, who is going to help, when the walk will take place, and why walking is important. In addition, the nurse and client determine how much independence the client can assume.

The nurse also checks the environment to be sure that there are no obstacles in the client's path. Chairs, over-the-bed tables, and wheelchairs are cleared out of the way so that the client has ample room to walk safely.

Before starting, rest points should be established in case activity tolerance is less than estimated or the client becomes dizzy. For example, a chair might be placed in the hall for the client to rest if needed.

To prevent orthostatic hypotension, the client should be assisted to a position of sitting at the side of the bed and should rest for 1 to 2 minutes before standing. Likewise, after standing, the client should remain stationary for 1 to 2 minutes before moving. The client's balance must stabilize before walking. Thus the nurse can quickly ease a dizzy client back to bed. The longer the period of immobility, the greater the risk of hypotension when the client stands.

The nurse should provide support at the waist so that the client's center of gravity remains midline. This can be achieved when the nurse places both hands at the client's waist or uses a walking belt. A **walking belt** is a leather belt that encircles the waist and has handles attached for the nurse to hold. While walking, the client should not lean to one side because this alters the center of gravity, distorts balance, and increases the risk of falling.

The client who at any point appears unsteady or complains of dizziness should be returned to a close bed or chair. If the client faints or begins to fall, the nurse should assume a wide base of support with one foot in front of the other, thus supporting the body weight. Then the nurse should gently lower the client to the floor, protecting the head. Although lowering a client to the floor is not difficult, the student should practice this technique with a friend or classmate before attempting it in a clinical setting.

Clients with **hemiplegia** (one-sided paralysis) or **hemiparesis** (one-sided weakness) often need assistance to walk. The nurse always stands on the client's affected side and supports the client by holding one arm around the client's waist and the other arm around the inferior aspect of the client's upper arm so that the nurse's hand is under the client's axilla. Providing support by holding the client's arm is incorrect because the nurse cannot easily support the weight to lower the client to the floor if the client faints or falls. In addition, if the client falls with the nurse holding an arm, a shoulder joint may be dislocated.

A nurse who does not have a lot of strength and who is unable to ambulate a client alone should request help. The two-nurse method helps distribute the client's weight evenly. The two nurses stand on either side of the client. Each nurse's near arm is around the client's waist, and the other arm is around the inferior aspect of the client's arm so that both nurses' hands are supporting the client's axillae.

A second method requires that the nurses and client be of similar height. The nurses stand on either side of the client with their near arms slipped under the client's arms toward the back. The nurses then grasp each other's arms. The client's arms are placed over the nurses' shoulders, and the nurses stabilize the client's hands with their free hands. This technique is effective with weakened or heavy clients.

Using Assistive Devices for Walking. Walkers are extremely light, movable devices, about waist high, made of metal tubing. They have four widely placed, sturdy legs. The client holds the handgrips on the upper bars, takes a step, moves the walker forward, and takes another step (Fig. 37-26).

Canes are light, easily movable devices, about waist high, made of wood or metal. Two common types of canes are the single straight-legged cane and the quad cane (Fig. 37-27). The straight-legged cane is more common and is used to support and balance a client with decreased leg strength.

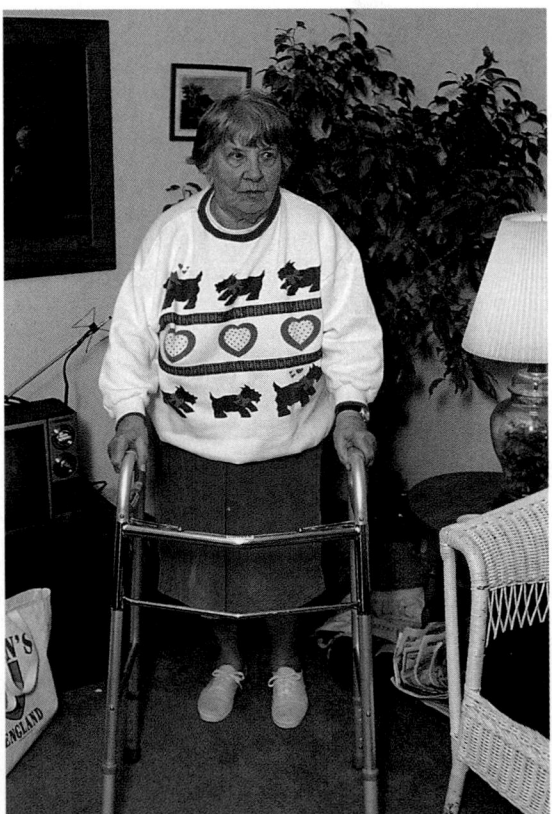

Fig. 37-26 Client using a walker.

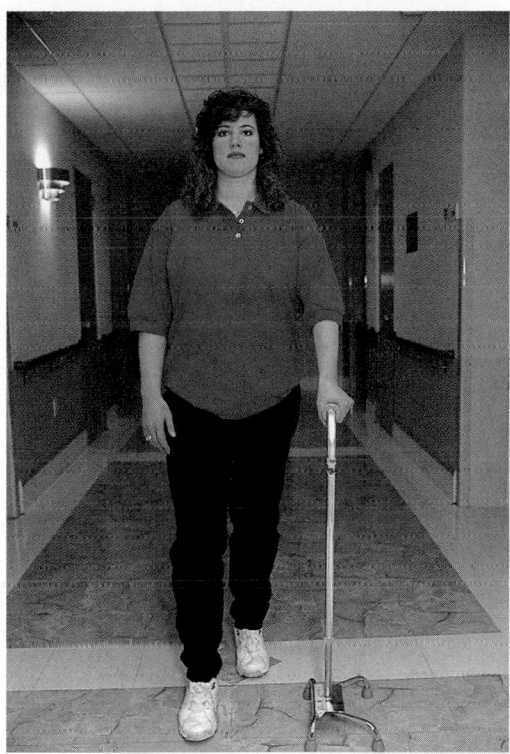

Fig. 37-27 Quad cane.

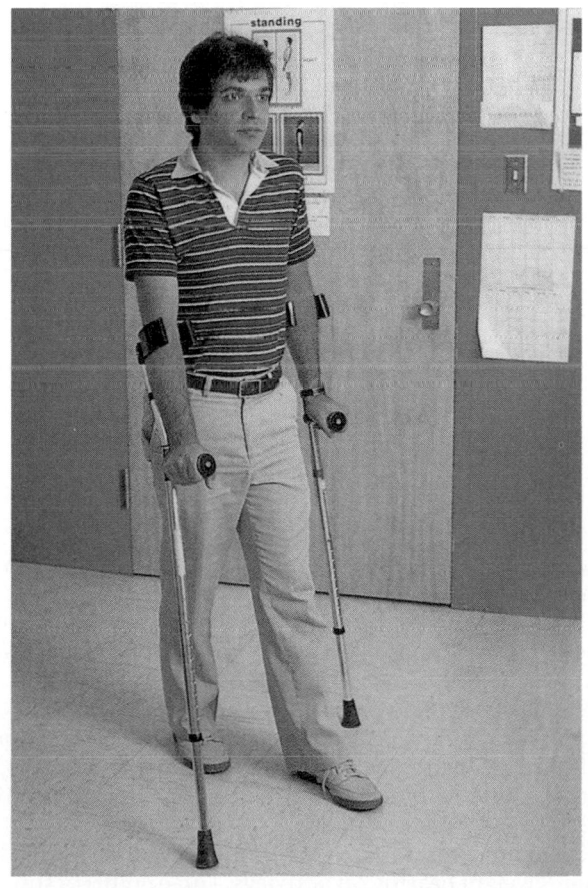

Fig. 37-28 Double adjustable Lofstrand or forearm crutches.

This cane should be kept on the stronger side of the body. For maximum support when walking, the client places the cane forward 15 to 25 cm (6 to 10 in), keeping body weight on both legs. The weaker leg is moved forward to the cane so that the body weight is divided between the cane and the stronger leg. The stronger leg is advanced past the cane so that the weaker leg and the body weight are supported by the cane and weaker leg. To walk, the client continually repeats these steps. The client is taught that two points of support, such as both feet or one foot and cane, are present at all times.

The quad cane provides the greater support and is used when there is partial or complete leg paralysis or hemiplegia. The same three steps used with the straight-legged cane are taught to the client.

Crutches are often needed to increase mobility. Their use may be temporary, such as after ligament damage to the knee. Crutches may be needed permanently (e.g., by the client with paralysis of the lower extremities). A crutch is a wooden or metal staff. There are two types of crutches, the double adjustable Lofstrand or forearm crutch (Fig. 37-28) and the axillary wooden crutch (used in Fig. 37-36, p. 938). The forearm crutch has a handgrip and a metal band that fits around the forearm. Both the metal band and the handgrip are adjusted to fit the client's height. The axillary crutch has a padded curved surface at the top, which fits under the axilla. A handgrip in the form of a crossbar is held at the level of the palms to support the body. Crutches must be measured for the appropriate length, and clients must be taught to use their crutches safely, to achieve a stable gait, to ascend and descend stairs, and to rise from a sitting position.

Measuring for Crutches. The axillary crutch is more commonly used. When preparing the client for crutches, the nurse must also teach crutch safety (see the box on p. 936) and correctly measure the client for crutches. Crutch measurement includes three areas: client's height, distance between crutch pad and axilla, and angle of elbow flexion. Measurements are taken by one of two methods, with the client supine or standing. Supine—Crutch tips should be positioned 6 inches (15 cm) lateral to client's heel (Fig. 37-29). Place the end of the tape measure three to four finger widths (1 to 2 inches or 4 to 5 cm) from the axilla and measure to the client's heel. Standing—Position crutches with crutch tips at a point 4 to 6 inches (14 to 15 cm) to side and 4 to 6 inches in front of client's feet. With either method, elbows should be flexed 15 to 30 degrees. Elbow flexion is verified with goniometer (Fig. 37-30). Crutch pads should be 3 to 4 fingerwidths (1 to 2 inches or 4 to 5 cm) under axilla (Fig. 37-31).

Teaching Crutch Gait. A **crutch gait** is assumed by alternately bearing weight on one or both legs and on the crutches. The gait used by the client is determined by

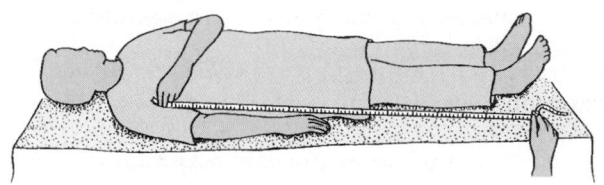

Fig. 37-29 Measuring crutch length.

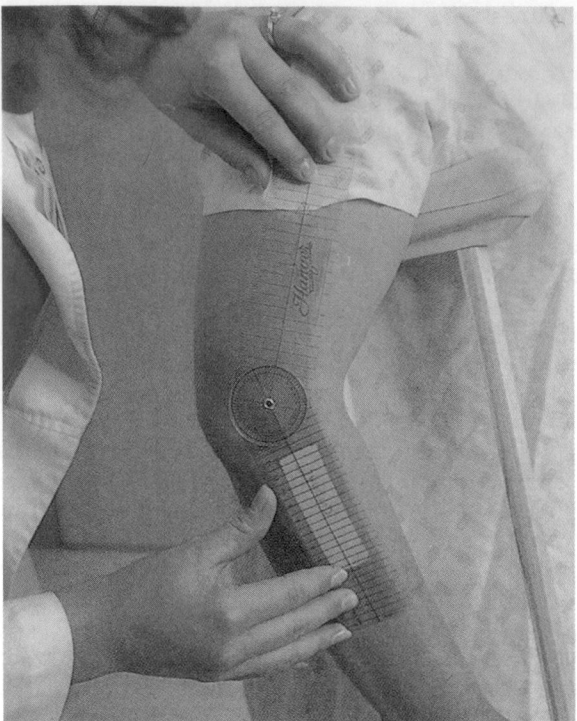

Fig. 37-30 Verifying correct elbow flexion with crutches. Measurement is obtained with a goniometer.

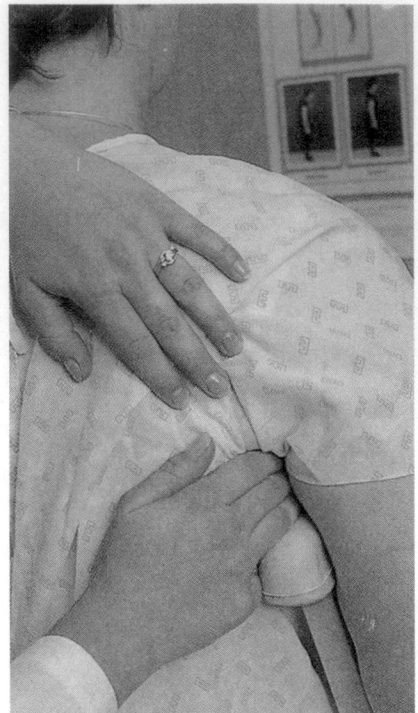

Fig. 37-31 Verifying correct distance between crutch pads and axilla.

CLIENT TEACHING
for Crutch Safety

OBJECTIVE
- Client will state and demonstrate safe crutch walking.

TEACHING STRATEGIES
- Teach client with axillary crutches about the dangers of pressure on the axillae, which occurs when leaning on the crutches to support body weight.
- Explain why client must use crutches that were measured for him or her.
- Show client how to routinely inspect crutch tips. Rubber tips should be securely attached to the crutches. When tips are worn, they should be replaced. Rubber crutch tips increase surface friction and help prevent slipping.
- Explain that crutch tips should remain dry. Water decreases surface friction and increases the risk of slipping.
- Show client how to dry the crutch tips if they become wet; client may use paper or cloth towels.
- Show client how to inspect the structure of the crutches. Cracks in a wooden crutch decrease its ability to support weight. Bends in aluminum crutches can alter body alignment.
- Provide client with a list of medical supply companies in the community for obtaining repairs, new rubber tips, handgrips, and crutch pads.
- Instruct client to have spare crutches and tips readily available.

EVALUATION
- Client states and demonstrates principles of crutch safety.

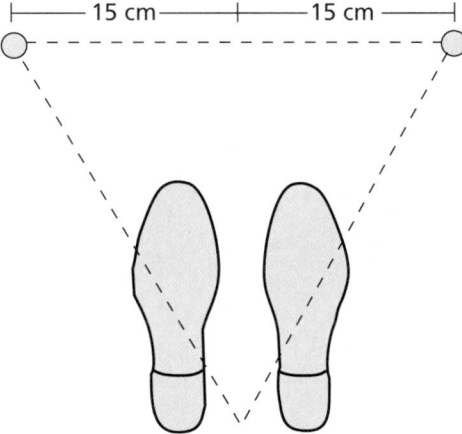

Fig. 37-32 Tripod position, the basic crutch stance.

the nurse's assessment of the client's physical and functional abilities and the disease or injury.

The basic crutch stance is the tripod position, formed when the crutches are placed 15 cm (6 in) in front of and 15 cm to the side of each foot (Fig. 37-32). This position improves balance by providing a wider base of support. Body alignment in the tripod position includes erect head and neck, straight vertebrae, and extended hips and knees. No weight should be borne by the axillae. The tripod position is used before crutch walking.

Four-point alternating or four-point gait gives stability but requires weight bearing on both legs. Three points of support are on the floor at all times (Fig. 37-33). The client first positions the crutch and then positions the opposite foot (e.g., right crutch and left foot). The client then repeats this sequence with the other crutch and foot, alternating this pattern (Lane and LeBlanc, 1990).

Three-point alternating or three-point gait requires the client to bear all of the weight on one foot. In a three-point gait, weight is borne on the uninvolved leg (Fig. 37-34) and then on both crutches, and the sequence is repeated. The affected leg does not touch the ground during the early phase of the three-point gait. Gradually the client progresses to touchdown and full weight bearing on the affected leg (Lane and LeBlanc, 1990).

The two-point gait requires at least partial weight bearing on each foot (Fig. 37-35). Each crutch is moved at the same time as the opposing leg so that crutch movements are similar to arm motion during normal walking (Lane and LeBlanc, 1990).

The swing-through or swing-to gait is frequently used by paraplegic clients who wear weight-supporting braces. With weight placed on their supported legs, these clients place the crutches one stride in front and then swing to or through the crutches while supporting their weight (Lane and LeBlanc, 1990).

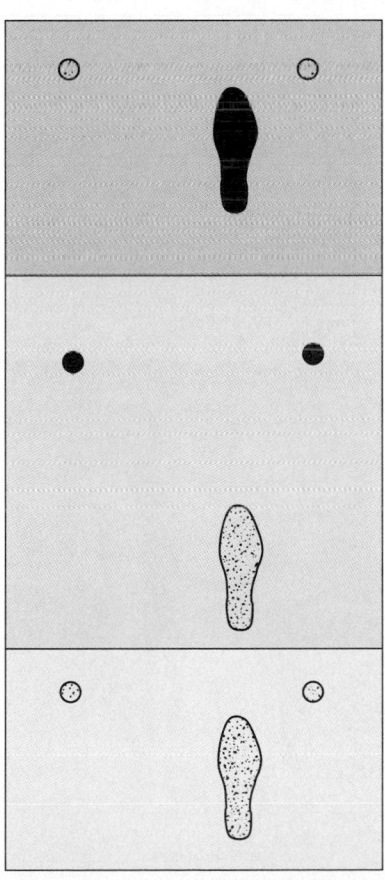

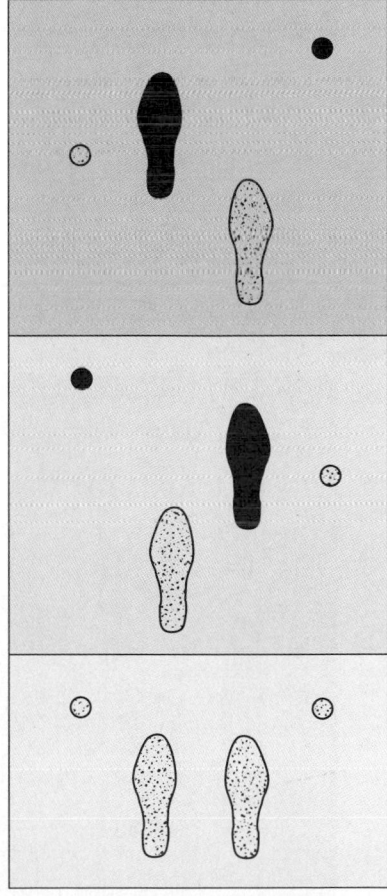

Fig. 37-33 Four-point alternating gait. Black foot and crutch tips show weight bearing in each phase of the gait.

Fig. 37-34 Three-point alternating gait, with weight borne on the uninvolved leg. Black foot and crutch tips show weight bearing in each phase of the gait.

Fig. 37-35 Two-point alternating gait, with weight borne partially on each foot and crutch advancing with the opposing leg. Black areas indicate leg and crutch tips bearing weight.

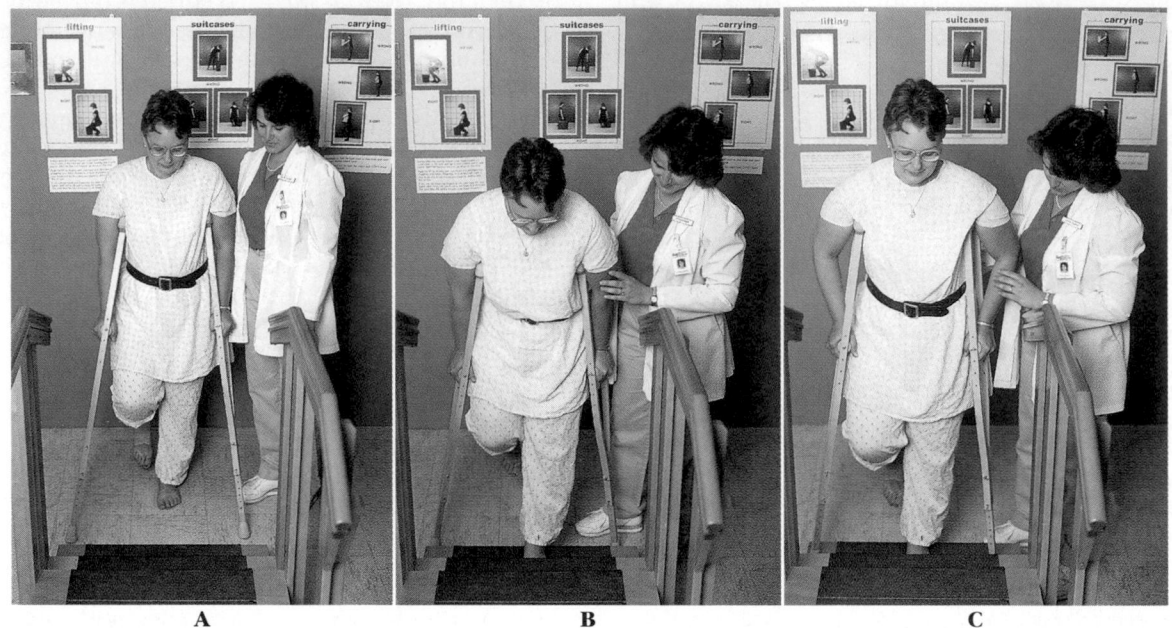

A B C

Fig. 37-36 Ascending stairs. **A,** Weight is placed on crutches. **B,** Weight is transferred from crutches to unaffected leg on the stairs. **C,** Crutches are aligned with unaffected leg on the stairs.

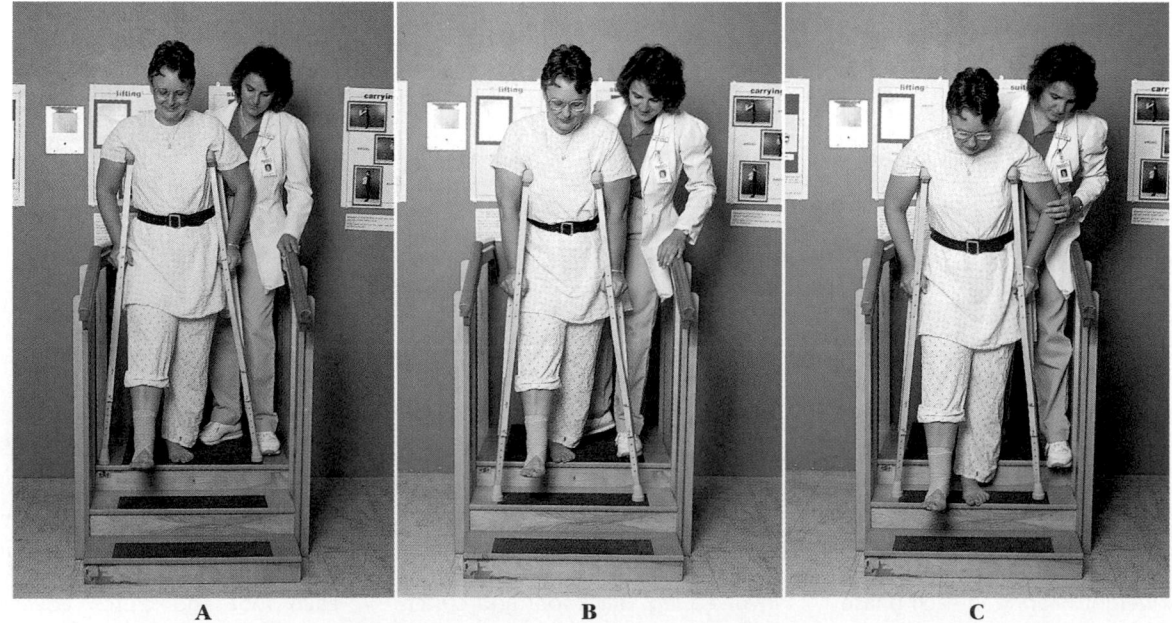

A B C

Fig. 37-37 Descending stairs. **A,** Body weight on unaffected leg. **B,** Body weight transferred to crutches. **C,** Unaffected leg aligned on stairs with crutches.

Teaching Crutch Walking on Stairs. When *ascending* stairs on crutches, the client usually uses a modified three-point gait (Fig. 37-36, *A*). First the client stands at the bottom of the stairs and transfers the body weight to the crutches. Second, the unaffected leg is advanced between the crutches to the stairs (Fig. 37-36, *B*). Then weight is shifted from the crutches to the unaffected leg (Fig. 37-36, *C*). Last, the client aligns both crutches on the stairs. This sequence is repeated until the client reaches the top.

To *descend* the stairs, a three-phase sequence is also used. First, the client transfers body weight to the unaffected leg (Fig. 37-37, *A*). Second, the crutches are placed on the stair and the client begins to transfer body weight to the crutches, moving the affected leg forward (Fig. 37-37, *B*). Last, the unaffected leg is moved to the stairs with the crutches (Fig. 37-37, *C*). Again, the client repeats the sequence until reaching the bottom.

Clients usually need to use crutches for some time, so they should be taught to use them on stairs before discharge. Instruction in stair climbing applies to all crutch-dependent clients, not only to those who have stairs in their homes.

Teaching Sitting With Crutches. The procedure for sitting in a chair requires the client to transfer weight. First, the client should be positioned at the center front of the chair with the posterior aspect of the legs touching the chair. Second, the client holds both crutches in the hand opposite the affected leg. If both legs are affected, as with a paraplegic client who wears weight-supporting braces, the crutches are held on the client's stronger side. With both crutches in one hand the client supports the body's weight on the unaffected leg and crutches (Fig. 37-38, *A*). While still holding the crutches, the client grasps the arm of the chair with the remaining hand (Fig. 37-38, *B*) and lowers the body

(Fig. 37-38, *C*). To stand, the procedure is reversed, and the client, when fully erect, should assume the tripod position before walking.

REDUCTION OF HAZARDS OF IMMOBILITY

Nursing interventions for an immobilized client should focus on preventing or minimizing the hazards of immobility. Interventions should therefore be directed at maintaining optimal function of all body systems.

Metabolic System. The immobilized client requires a high-protein, high-calorie diet with vitamin B and C supplements. Protein is needed to repair injured tissue and rebuild depleted protein stores. A high-calorie intake provides sufficient fuel to meet metabolic needs and to replace subcutaneous tissue. Supplementation with vitamin C is necessary to replace protein stores. Vitamin B complex is needed for skin integrity and wound healing.

If the client is unable to eat, nutrition must be provided parenterally or enterally. Enteral feedings include delivery through a nasogastric, gastrostomy, or jejunostomy tube of high-protein, high-calorie solutions with complete requirements of vitamins, minerals, and electrolytes (see Chapter 41). Total parenteral nutrition is delivery of nutritional supplements through a central or peripheral intravenous catheter.

Respiratory System. Nursing interventions for the respiratory system are aimed at promoting expansion of the chest and lungs, preventing stasis of pulmonary secretions, maintaining a patent airway, and promoting adequate exchange of respiratory gases.

Promoting Expansion of Chest and Lungs. The nurse promotes chest expansion with several interventions. Changing the position of the client at least every 2 hours allows the dependent lung regions to re-expand. Re-expansion

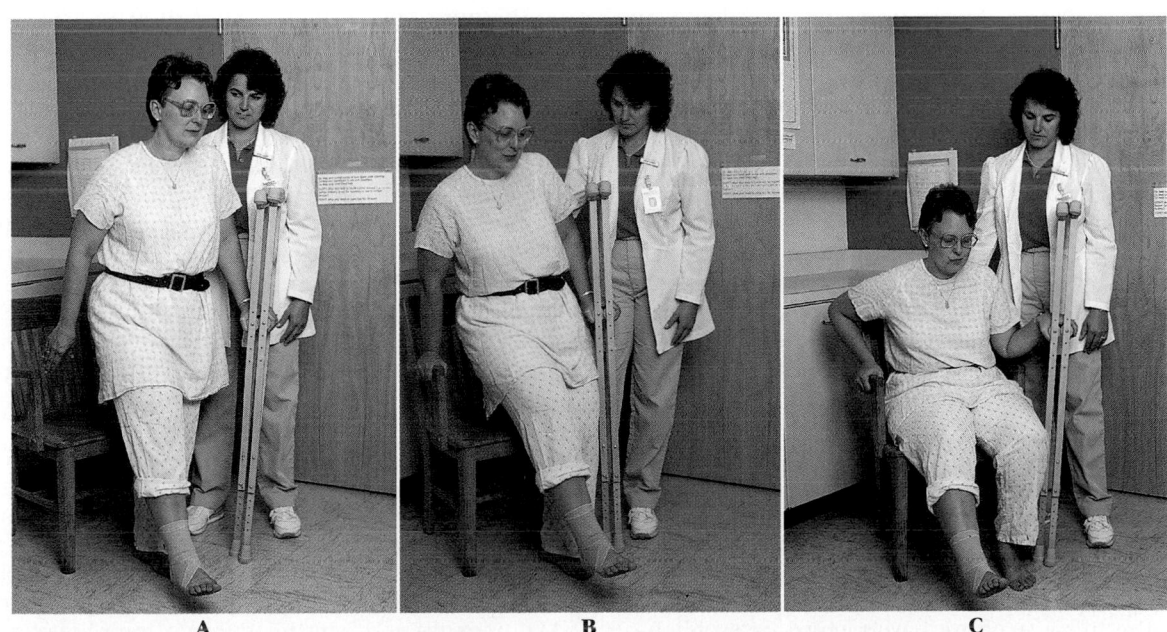

| A | B | C |

Fig. 37-38 Sitting in a chair. **A,** Both crutches are held by one hand. Client transfers weight to the crutches and the unaffected leg. **B,** Client grasps arm of the chair with the free hand and begins to lower herself into the chair. **C,** Client completely lowers herself into the chair.

maintains the elastic recoil property of the lungs and clears the dependent lung regions of pulmonary secretions.

The nurse should encourage the client to deep breathe and cough every 1 to 2 hours. Alert clients can be taught to deep breathe or yawn every hour. This action expands all lobes of the lungs and prevents atelectasis. Coughing reduces the stasis of pulmonary secretions. For unconscious clients with an artificial airway, the nurse can expand the chest and lungs by using an Ambu-bag (see Chapter 44).

The nurse uses caution when administering postoperative pain medications. These medications can depress the respiratory center, so the rate of respiration or expansion of the lungs is decreased. The nurse should ask a postoperative client who has received pain medication to deep breathe and cough at the peak effect of the analgesic, which is 20 to 30 minutes after administration. This reduces the respiratory-depressant action of the drug.

If abdominal binders and rib supports are required, they should be removed every 2 hours to allow the client to breathe deeply. Removal may be contraindicated, however, for the client who has just had surgery or has just suffered trauma.

Preventing Stasis of Pulmonary Secretions. Stagnant secretions accumulating in the bronchi and lungs may lead to growth of bacteria and subsequent development of pneumonia. Pulmonary infections still develop despite interventions to prevent them. Stagnation of secretions can be reduced by changing the client's position every 2 hours. This change repositions the dependent lung and mobilizes secretions.

Chest physiotherapy is an effective method of preventing pulmonary secretions. It uses positioning techniques to drain secretions from specific segments of the bronchi and lungs into the trachea. The client then expels secretions by coughing. Respiratory assessment findings help to identify areas of the lungs that require chest physiotherapy (see Chapter 44).

Maintaining a Patent Airway. Immobilized clients and those on bed rest are generally weakened. If weakness progresses, the cough reflex gradually becomes inefficient. If the client is too weak or is unable to cough up secretions, the nurse must maintain a patent airway using suctioning techniques. The stasis of secretions in the lungs may be life threatening for an immobilized client because hypostatic bronchopneumonia can easily develop. Assessment findings that indicate this condition include productive cough with greenish yellow sputum, fever, pain on breathing, and crackles, wheezes, and dyspnea. Dislodging and mobilizing the stagnant secretions reduce the risk of pneumonia.

In the immobilized client an obstructed airway is usually the result of a mucous plug. The nurse can implement several therapies to reduce the risk of mucous plugs and to maintain the patent airway.

First, the nurse can ask the client to deep breathe and cough every 1 to 2 hours. The nurse instructs the client to take in three deep breaths and cough with the third exhalation. This technique produces a more forceful, productive cough without excessive fatigue.

Second, the nurse may use nasotracheal or orotracheal suction to remove secretions in the upper airways of a client unable to cough productively. This procedure must be performed aseptically. The nurse places a suction catheter in the client's nose or through the mouth and applies suction.

Last, the nurse can suction secretions from an artificial airway such as an endotracheal or tracheal tube. The nurse inserts a catheter into the artificial airway in a sterile procedure. This removes pulmonary secretions from the upper and lower airways (see Chapter 44).

Cardiovascular System. The effects of bed rest or immobilization on the cardiovascular system include orthostatic hypotension, increased cardiac workload, and thrombus formation. Nursing therapies are designed to minimize or prevent these alterations.

Reducing Orthostatic Hypotension. Clients who have been on bed rest or who have been immobilized for an extended period of time are at risk for orthostatic hypotension. Orthostatic (or postural) hypotension is a severely disabling condition characterized by a decrease in blood pressure when the client assumes a standing position. It is associated with light-headedness, dizziness, weakness, fatigue, lack of energy, visual disturbances, dyspnea, head or neck discomfort, and near-syncope or even syncope (Gilden, 1993). Although not all of these clients experience orthostatic hypotension, clients should have their vital signs monitored during the first few attempts at sitting or standing.

When being moved from a supine position into a chair, the client should change positions gradually. When doing this procedure, the nurse should document any orthostatic changes. The nurse obtains baseline vital signs with the client in the supine position. The nurse then raises the client to a high-Fowler's position and measures the vital signs again to evaluate decreases in blood pressure or elevations in pulse. The nurse remains with the client, who should stay in the high-Fowler's position for a few moments to allow the body to adapt to any changes in vital signs. The nurse continually monitors the client for dizziness and light-headedness. The nurse also asks whether the client sees spots.

The nurse then has the client sit at the side of the bed with the feet on the floor. The client is instructed to lie down and tell the nurse if dizziness or faintness is felt. If there is no dizziness, the nurse assists the client to the chair.

Reducing Cardiac Workload. The nurse designs interventions to reduce cardiac workload, which is increased by immobility. The nurses' primary intervention is to discourage the client from using the Valsalva maneuver. When using this maneuver, the client holds his breath, which increases intrathoracic pressure. This decreases venous return and cardiac output, therefore cardiac workload increases.

Preventing Thrombus Formation. The most cost-effective way to address the deep vein thrombosis (DVT) problem is through an aggressive program of prophylaxis. It begins with identification of clients at risk, and continues throughout the time clients are immobile or otherwise at risk. This is clearly a collaborative role between nurses and physicians. Risk factors can be easily identified by the nurse during an admission nursing assessment; then the physician should order the appropriate prophylactic measures. Maintenance and administration of prophylaxis is a nursing role, and nurses can determine when the client is fully mobile postoperatively, decreasing continued risk for DVT (Carroll, 1993).

Applying Elastic Stockings

STEPS	RATIONALE
1. Identify need for elastic stockings: immobility, lower extremity edema, and varicose veins.	These conditions increase the risk of thrombus formation.

2. Prepare following equipment:
  a. Tape measure
  b. Stockings in proper size
  c. Talcum powder
	Stockings must be measured according to directions of specific manufacturer. Measure client's calf circumference length from foot to knee. For thigh-high elastic stockings, measure calf circumference, thigh circumference, and length from foot to thigh.

3. Explain procedure to client.	Relieves anxiety and increases cooperation.
4. Wash hands.	Reduces transmission of microorganisms.
5. Elevate bed to comfortable position, and assist client to supine position.	Promotes good body mechanics for nurse. Position eases stocking application.
6. After legs have been cleansed, apply small amount of talcum powder to each leg and foot.	Reduces friction and allows for easier application of stocking.
7. Turn elastic stocking inside out by placing one hand into sock, holding toe with other hand, and pulling (see the illustration below).	Prepares stocking for application.
8. Place client's toe into foot of elastic stocking, making sure that sock is smooth (see the illustration below).	Wrinkles in sock can impede circulation to lower region of extremity.
9. Slide remaining portion of sock over client's foot, ensuring that toes are covered. Sock will now be right side out (see the illustration below).	If toes remain uncovered, they will become constricted by elastic and their circulation can be reduced.
10. Slide sock over client's calf until it is completely extended. Be sure that sock is smooth and no ridges are present (see the illustration below).	Ridges impede venous return and can counteract purpose of elastic stocking.

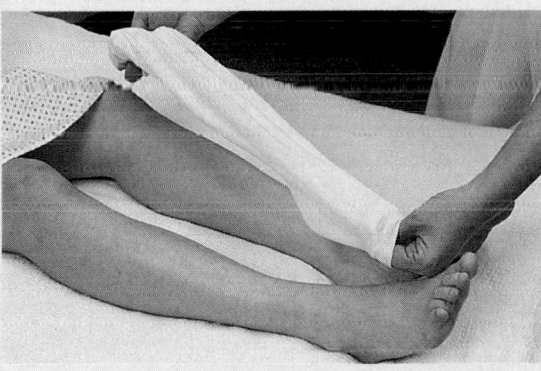

Step 7

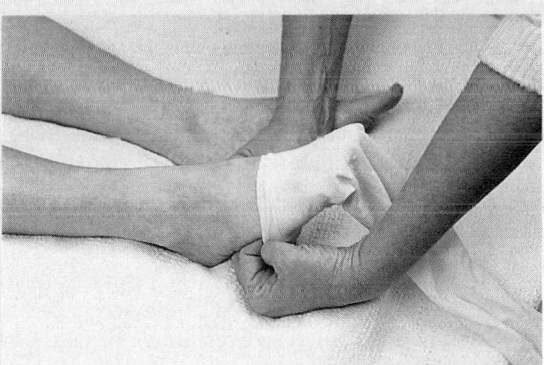

Step 8

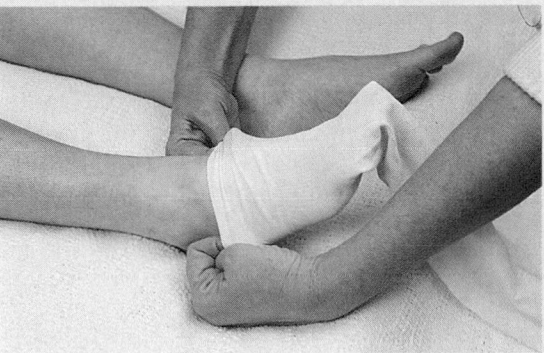

Step 9

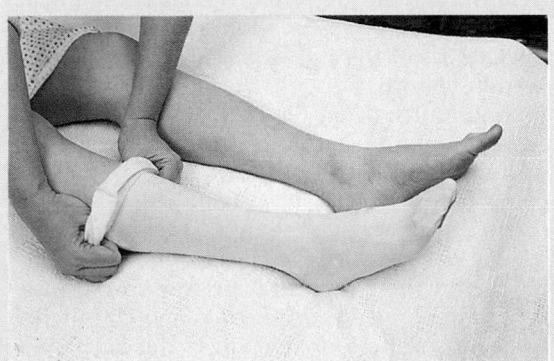

Step 10

Continued.

Applying Elastic Stockings—cont'd

STEPS	RATIONALE
11. Instruct client not to roll socks partially down.	Rolling the sock partially down will have constricting effect and impede venous return.
12. Reposition client for comfort.	Maintains body alignment and promotes comfort.
13. Wash hands.	Reduces transmission of microorganisms.
14. After 1 hr, observe stockings for wrinkles in binding and assess capillary refill in toes and palpate pulses in feet.	Wrinkles increase pressure to skin and impair circulation. Assessment ensures that circulatory status in lower extremities has not been compromised.
15. Remove stockings at least once a shift.	Provides for assessment of skin and circulatory status.
16. Record in nurses' notes date and time of stocking application and condition of skin before application, circulatory status of lower extremities, and stocking length and size.	Documents condition of lower extremities and performance of procedure.

Heparin is the most widely used drug in the prophylaxis of DVT. It has become the "gold standard" in this area because it has been well studied and validated. Common dosage for low-dose heparin (LDH) therapy is 5000 units subcutaneously 2 hours prior to surgery and continued until the client is fully mobile or discharged. Schedules of 8- and 12-hour dosing have both been found to be effective (Goucke, 1989). Heparin is an anticoagulant. Therefore it suppresses clot formation. Because of the action of this medication, the nurse must continually assess the client for signs of bleeding, such as increased bruising, guaiac positive stools, and bleeding gums. Although the majority of clients receiving LDH do not experience side effects, the risk remains present.

Intermittent pneumatic compression (IPC) devices (also referred to as sequential compression [SCD] devices) consist of garments, which can be called sleeves, made of fabric or plastic that are wrapped around the leg and secured with Velcro. The sleeves are then connected to a pump that alternately inflates and deflates the garment around the leg. A typical cycle is inflation for 10 to 15 seconds and deflation for 45 to 60 seconds. Inflation pressures average 40 mm Hg. IPC/SCDs of the legs decrease venous stasis by increasing venous return through the deep veins of the legs. For optimal results, begin IPC/SCDs as soon as possible. The system should be maintained until the client becomes fully ambulatory (Carroll, 1993).

Graded compression stockings can help prevent DVT, as long as the right clients receive the right size and the right regimen (Evans, 1991). Elastic stockings aid in maintaining external pressure on the muscles of the lower extremities and thus may promote venous return. When considering applying graded compression stockings, the nurse first needs to assess the client's suitability for wearing them. The stockings should not be worn if there is any local condition affecting the leg (e.g., any skin lesion, gangrenous

condition, or recent vein ligation), as it may compromise circulation (Evans, 1991). The stockings must be applied properly and they must be removed and reapplied (Procedure 37-5) at least twice a day. In addition, the stockings should always be clean and dry, and it may be useful for the client to have two pairs.

Positioning techniques aid in reducing pressure to the skin. Proper positioning used with other therapies (e.g., heparin or elastic stockings) aid in reducing the client's risk of thrombus formation. When positioning clients, the nurse uses caution to prevent pressure on the posterior knee and deep veins in the lower extremities.

ROM exercises are designed to reduce the risk of contractures, but these exercises also have beneficial effects in preventing thrombi. The exercise activity causes contraction of the skeletal muscles, which in turn exerts pressure on the veins and promotes venous return. Venous stasis is reduced.

When DVT is suspected, the nurse should report it immediately. The leg should be elevated with no pressure on the thrombus. The family, client, and all health care personnel should be instructed not to massage the area because of the danger of dislodging the thrombus.

Musculoskeletal System. The immobilized client must receive some exercise to prevent excessive muscle wasting, atrophy, and joint contractures. If the client is unable to move part or all of the body, the nurse must perform passive ROM exercises for all immobilized joints while bathing the client and at least 2 or 3 more times a day. If one extremity is paralyzed, the client can be taught to put each joint independently through its ROM.

Some orthopedic conditions require more frequent passive ROM exercises to restore the injured joint's function after surgery. Clients with such conditions may use automatic equipment for passive ROM exercises (Fig. 37-39). The equipment extends an extremity to a prescribed angle for a pre-

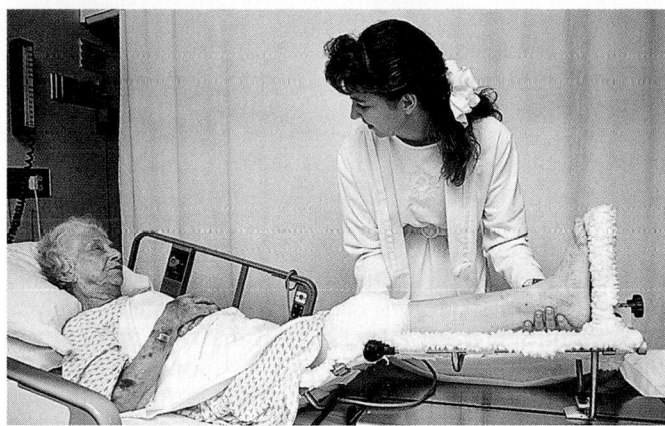

Fig. 37-39 Continuous passive range of motion machine.

scribed period. This is beneficial when the client must gradually increase the degree and duration of extension.

Clients on bed rest should have active ROM exercises incorporated into their daily schedules. They can perform these exercises during activities of daily living. The box at right, top, describes joint movements that occur with daily activities.

Active ROM exercises maintain function of the musculoskeletal system. The nurse should also plan interventions for the gradual return of mobility for clients who will be able to resume normal activity.

Progressive exercise programs are used for clients with musculoskeletal, neurological, cardiopulmonary, renal, and other chronic diseases. Before beginning the program, warm-up exercises should be performed, unless they are contraindicated (see the box at right, bottom, for exercise precautions for older adults).

Integumentary System. As discussed previously, the major risk to skin from restricted mobility is pressure ulcers. Nursing interventions therefore focus on prevention and treatment (see Chapter 38) (see the box on p. 944 for health promotion and prevention of pressure ulcers).

Elimination System. The nursing interventions for maintaining optimal urinary functioning are directed at keeping the client well hydrated without causing bladder distention and preventing urinary stasis, calculi, and infections.

Adequate hydration (e.g., 2000 to 3000 ml of fluids per day) helps prevent renal calculi and urinary tract infections. The well-hydrated client should void large amounts of dilute urine. If the client is also incontinent, the nurse should modify the care plan to meet the increased urinary elimination needs.

To prevent bladder distention, the nurse assesses the frequency and amount of urinary output. A client who continually dribbles urine and whose bladder is distended has overflow incontinence. If the immobilized client does not have voluntary control of urinary elimination, the nurse may have to insert a straight or indwelling catheter to prevent distention (see Chapter 46).

The nurse must also record the frequency and consistency of bowel movements. A diet rich in fruits, vegetables, and bulk can facilitate normal peristalsis. If a client is unable to

---

Incorporating Active Exercises into Activities of Daily Living

- Nodding head "yes" exercises *neck* (flexion and extension).
- Shaking head "no" exercises *neck* (rotation).
- Moving right ear to right shoulder exercises *neck* (lateral flexion).
- Moving left ear to left shoulder exercises *neck* (lateral flexion).
- Reaching to turn on overhead light exercises *shoulder* (flexion).
- Reaching to bedside stand for book exercises *shoulder* (abduction).
- Scratching back exercises *shoulder* (hyperextension and inward rotation).
- Rotating shoulders toward chest exercises *shoulder.*
- Rotating shoulders toward back exercises *shoulder.*
- Eating, bathing, shaving, and grooming exercise *elbow* (flexion, extension).
- All activities requiring fine motor coordination, such as writing and eating, exercise *fingers* and *thumb* (flexion, extension, abduction, adduction, opposition).
- Walking exercises *hip* (flexion, extension, hyperextension).
- Rolling toes inward exercises *hip* (internal rotation).
- Rolling toes outward exercises *hip* (external rotation).
- Walking exercises *knee* (flexion, extension).
- Walking exercises *ankle* (dorsiflexion, plantar flexion).
- Pointing toe toward head of bed exercises *ankle* (dorsiflexion).
- Pointing toe toward foot of bed exercises *ankle* (plantar flexion).
- Walking exercises *toes* (extension, hyperextension).
- Wiggling toes exercises *toes* (abduction, adduction)

Exercise Precautions for Older Adults

- Ensure low exercise intensity of 40% to 70% maximum predicted heart rate and very gentle exercise progression.
- Use perceived exertion versus exercise heart rate to monitor exercise intensity.
- Perform a gradual, extended exercise warm-up and cool-down to decrease risk of postural hypotension and cardiac arrhythmias.
- Use correct body mechanics, appropriate clothing, exercise-specific shoes, and sufficient hydration.
- Avoid sudden twisting movements, rapid movements, and rapid transitions from one movement to the next.
- Avoid exercises that tax vision and balance.
- Avoid sustained isometric contractions of greater than 10 sec.
- Avoid exercise during acute viral infections.
- Stop exercising if angina, premature ventricular contractions, or excessive breathlessness occurs.
- Obtain physician approval and written orders for specific exercise restrictions before onset of an exercise program.

Modified from Gillett PA et al: The nurse as exercise leader, *Geriatr Nurs* 14(3):135, 1993.

Health Promotion and Prevention of Pressure Ulcers

The goal in preventing pressure ulcers is to maintain and improve tissue tolerance to pressure. The following guidelines will assist the care giver in skin care and early treatment:

- All individuals at risk should have a systematic skin inspection at least once a day, paying particular attention to the bony prominences.
- Skin cleansing should occur at the time of soiling and at routine intervals.
- Minimize environmental factors leading to skin drying, such as decreased humidity and exposure to cold. Dry skin should be treated with moisturizers.
- Do not massage over bony prominences.
- Minimize skin exposure to moisture due to incontinence, perspiration, or wound drainage.
- Skin injury due to friction and shearing forces should be minimized through proper positioning, transferring, and turning techniques.
- When apparently well-nourished individuals develop an inadequate dietary intake of protein or calories, care givers should first attempt to discover the factors compromising intake and offer support with eating.
- If potential for improving mobility and activity status exists, rehabilitation efforts should be instituted if consistent with the overall goals of therapy.
- Interventions and outcomes should be monitored and documented.

Modified from Bergstrom N et al: How to predict and prevent pressure ulcers, *Am J Nurs* 92(7):54, 1992.

---

maintain regular bowel patterns, the physician may order stool softeners, cathartics, or enemas (see Chapter 47).

Psychosocial Changes. Assessment can identify effects of prolonged immobilization on the client's psychosocial dimension. People who have a tendency toward depression or mood swings are at greater risk for developing psychosocial effects during bed rest or immobilization. There are many nursing interventions to meet the client's psychosocial needs.

The nurse should anticipate changes in the client's psychosocial status. The nurse can provide routine and informal socialization. Nursing activities can be planned so that the client can talk and interact with staff. If possible the client should be placed in a room with others who are mobile and interactive. If a private room is required, staff members should be asked to visit at least once a shift.

The nurse also provides stimuli to maintain orientation. A daily newspaper helps the client keep track of events and time. Bedside chats at appropriate moments orient the client to nursing activities, meals, and visiting hours. Books help occupy the client when alone. The client can participate in craft activities. Radio, television, and videotapes provide stimulation and help pass the time.

Clients should be encouraged to wear their glasses or artificial teeth and to shave or apply makeup. These are activities through which people maintain their body images. Maintenance of body image can alleviate depression resulting from immobilization.

Clients should also be involved in their care whenever possible. For example, the nurse should encourage the client to determine when the bed should be made. Some clients rest better during the night when fresh sheets are put on in the evening rather than in the morning. The client should provide as much self-care as possible. Hygiene and grooming articles should be kept within easy reach.

In institutional-based health care settings, nursing care given between 10:00 PM and 7:00 AM should be scheduled to minimize interruptions of sleep. For example, the nurse may administer medications and assess vital signs at the time when the client is turned or receives special skin care.

The nurse should also observe the client's failure to cope with restricted mobility. If the nursing care plan is not improving coping patterns, a clinical nurse specialist, counselor, social worker, spiritual adviser, or other consultant may be needed. Their recommendations should be incorporated into the care plan.

Developmental Changes. Ideally, immobilized clients continue normal development. However, this is unrealistic for the very young or very old. Nursing interventions can help.

Nursing care should provide mental and physical stimulation, particularly for a young child. Play activities can be incorporated into the care plan. Completing puzzles, for example, helps a child to develop fine motor skills, and reading helps the child develop cognitively. An immobilized child should be placed with children of the same age who are not immobilized, unless a contagious disease is present. Nursing activities, such as dressing changes, cast care, and care of traction, can be designed to require participation of the child. The nurse must recognize significant changes from normal behavioral patterns. If these continue, the nurse should consult with a clinical nurse, counselor, or other health care professional whose specialty is children.

Restricted mobility of older clients presents unique nursing problems. Older clients may have chronic illnesses that place them at increased risk for the hazards of immobility.

Inactive older clients are at greater risk for confusion, depression, and disorientation, which result from immobilization, chronic illness, medications, and aging. To assist in maintaining orientation to time, a calendar and a clock with a large dial should be in the client's room (see Chapter 31). The calendar should be marked so that the client can immediately identify the correct day and date. Chapter 31 describes other measures to assist older clients in meeting developmental needs.

Nursing care should encourage older immobilized clients to perform as many activities of daily living as independently as possible. Clients should continue to perform personal grooming if they did so before their mobility was restricted.

The nurse must remember that older clients are extremely susceptible to the hazards of immobility. A care plan should be designed to prevent or minimize these hazards. Frail older clients may need position changes every hour instead of every 2 hours, and may need more frequent ROM exercises. Not only are older clients more susceptible to the hazards of immobility, but the consequences and severity of immobility are more rapid.

Sample Evaluation of Interventions for Impaired Physical Mobility

GOALS	EVALUATIVE MEASURES	EXPECTED OUTCOMES
Client will regain normal ROM (180-degree flexion and extension) of left shoulder within 4 months.	Observe client perform ROM to both extremities and compare with initial assessment findings. Ask client about muscle strength to affected extremity.	Client will maintain present ROM in upper extremity joints. Client will perform self-care activities using left arm within 2 days. Client will follow regular exercise program 3-4 times a day by discharge. Client will have full ROM in affected joint.
Optimal joint motion will be achieved Joint contractures will be prevented.	Observe joint through ROM. Palpate joint during ROM exercises. Measure ROM.	Joint contractures will be absent.

Evaluation

To evaluate outcomes and response to nursing care, the nurse measures the effectiveness of all interventions. The goals and outcomes are the client's ability to maintain or improve body alignment and joint mobility.

The nurse evaluates specific interventions designed to promote body alignment, improve mobility, and protect the client from the hazards of immobility. Client and family teaching to prevent future risks to body alignment and hazards of immobility is also evaluated. Last, the nurse investigates the client's and family's needs for additional support services (e.g., home health care, physical therapy, and counseling) and initiates the referral process.

Evaluation of nursing care for clients with altered body alignment and mobility is based on objective outcomes for each nursing goal (see the evaluation box above).

Maintaining good body alignment and mobility and preventing the hazards of immobility increase independence and overall mobility. A client with inadequate joint mobility must receive assistance to carry out activities of daily living. The best approach to problems with body alignment and joint mobility is prevention, which begins early in the care plan.

■ KEY CONCEPTS ■

▶ Body mechanics is the coordinated efforts of the musculoskeletal and nervous systems as the person moves, lifts, bends, stands, sits, lies down, and completes daily activities.

▶ Coordinated body movement requires integrated functioning of the skeletal system, skeletal muscles, and nervous system.

▶ The skeleton provides bony support structure for movement, attachment of ligaments and muscles, protection of vital organs, some of the regulation of calcium, and production of red blood cells.

▶ The nervous system provides initiation and voluntary control of movement.

▶ Muscles primarily associated with movement are located near the skeletal region, where movement results from leverage, which is characteristic of movements of the upper extremities.

▶ Coordination and regulation of muscle groups depend on muscle tone and activity of antagonistic, synergistic, and antigravity muscles.

▶ Balance is assisted through nervous system control by the cerebellum and inner ear.

▶ Body alignment is the condition of joints, tendons, ligaments, and muscles in various body positions.

▶ Body balance is achieved when there is a wide base of support, the center of gravity falls within the base of support, and a vertical line falls from the center of gravity through the base of support.

▶ Developmental stages influence body alignment and mobility; the greatest impact of physiological changes on the musculoskeletal system is observed in children and older adults.

▶ Normal physical mobility depends on intact and functioning nervous and musculoskeletal systems.

▶ The risk of disabilities related to immobilization depends on the extent and duration of immobilization.

▶ Immobility may result from illness or trauma or may be prescribed for therapeutic reasons. Immobility presents hazards in the physiological, psychological, and developmental dimensions.

▶ The nurse uses the nursing process to provide care for clients experiencing or at risk for the adverse effects of impaired body alignment and immobility.

▶ After identifying nursing diagnoses, the nurse plans and implements interventions to prevent or minimize the hazards and complications of impaired body alignment and immobilization.

▶ Clients with impaired body alignment require nursing interventions to maintain them in the supported Fowler's, supine, prone, side-lying, and Sims' positions.

▶ Range of motion exercises include one or all of the body joints.

▶ Mechanical devices to promote walking include canes, walkers, and crutches.

■ KEY TERMS ■

Activity tolerance, p. 910
Antagonistic muscles, p. 897
Antigravity muscles, p. 897
Bed rest, p. 900
Body mechanics, p. 894
Bone resorption, p. 901
Cartilage, p. 896
Cartilaginous joint, p. 895
Center of gravity, p. 894
Crutch gait, p. 935
Exercise, p. 910
Fibrous joint, p. 895
Flat bones, p. 894
Footboard, p. 917
Footdrop, p. 903
Fracture, p. 900
Friction, p. 894
Gait, p. 905
Hand rolls, p. 917
Hand-wrist splints, p. 918
Hemiparesis, p. 934
Hemiplegia, p. 934
Immobility, p. 900
Irregular bones, p. 894
Isometric contraction, p. 896
Isotonic contraction, p. 896
Joint contracture, p. 903
Joints, p. 895
Ligaments, p. 896
Long bones, p. 894
Mobility, p. 898
Muscle tone, p. 897
Negative nitrogen balance, p. 901
Neurotransmitters, p. 897
Orthostatic hypotension, p. 901
Pathological fractures, p. 895

Posture, p. 897
Pressure ulcer, p. 903
Proprioception, p. 898
Range of motion (ROM), p. 905
Renal calculi, p. 903
Restraints, p. 918
Short bones, p. 894
Synergistic muscles, p. 897
Synostotic joint, p. 895
Synovial joint, p. 896
Tendons, p. 896
Thrombus, p. 901
Trapeze bar, p. 918
Trochanter roll, p. 917
Urinary stasis, p. 903
Walking belt, p. 934

■ CRITICAL THINKING EXERCISES ■

1. You are caring for a client who is in bilateral leg traction. How do you determine what type of mobility this client can safely perform and how this mobility can be incorporated into the care plan?

2. When caring for a client with a spinal cord injury, you note that the client's extremity "stiffens" and resists motion occasionally when the client performs passive range of motion exercises. What do you do so that further injury does not occur to the musculoskeletal system?

3. Mrs. Miller's mobility is limited after a stroke that left her with hemiplegia. She has a history of chronic constipation. What measures can the nurse independently implement to reduce the hazards of immobility to the gastrointestinal system? What evaluative criteria determine that these nursing measures were effective?

4. You're caring for a 27-year-old mother who is immobilized after spinal cord trauma. You note that she is becoming increasingly depressed and withdrawn. What actions are important at this point in the client's care?

REFERENCES

Alterescu V, Alterescu KE: Pressure ulcers: assessment and treatment, *Orthop Nurse* 11(2):37, 1992.
Beare P, Myers J: *Principles and practice of adult health nursing,* ed 2, St Louis, 1994, Mosby.
Berg KO et al: Clinical and laboratory measures of postural balance in an elderly population, *Arch Phys Med Rehabil* 73(11):1073, 1992.
Bergstrom N et al: How to predict and prevent pressure ulcers, *Am J Nurs* 92(7):54, 1992.
Carroll P: Deep venous thrombosis: Implications for orthopaedic nursing, *Orthop Nurse* 12(3):36, 1993.
Ebersole P, Hess P: *Toward healthy aging: human needs and nursing response,* ed 4, St Louis, 1994, Mosby.
Evans A: Sensible stockings, *Nursing Times* 87(51):40, 1991.
Fish DJ, Nielsen JP: Clinical assessment of human gait, *J Prosthet Orthot* 5(2):39, 1993.
Gillett PA et al: The nurse as exercise leader, *Geriatr Nurs* 14(3):135, 1993.
Glick OJ: Interventions related to activity and movement, *Nurs Clin North Am* 27(2):541, 1992.

Gilden JL: Orthostatic hypotension: important clues in the evaluation and tips for management, *Consultant* 33(5):117, 1993.

Goucke CR: Prophylaxis against venous thromboembolism, *Anesth Intensive Care* 17(4):458-465, 1989.

Groer MW, Skekleton ME: *Basic pathophysiology: a conceptual approach,* ed 3, St Louis, 1989, Mosby.

Holm K: Immobility and bone loss in the aging adult, *Crit Care Nurs Q* 12(1):46, 1989.

Kasper CE et al: Alterations in skeletal muscle related to impaired physical mobility: an empirical model, *Res Nurs Health* 16(4):265, 1993.

Kim MH, et al: *Pocket guide to nursing diagnoses,* ed 6, St Louis, 1995, Mosby.

Lane PL, LeBlanc R: Crutch walking, *Orthop Nurse* 9(5):31, 1990.

Lehmann JF et al: Biomechanics of normal gait, *Phys Med Rehabil Clin North Am* 3(1):95, 1992.

Lehmkuhl LD et al: Multidimensional treatment of joint contractures in patients with severe brain injury, *J Head Trauma Rehabil* 5(4):23, 1990.

Long BC et al: *Medical-surgical nursing: a nursing process approach,* ed 3, St Louis, 1993, Mosby.

Lueckenotte A: *Pocket guide to gerontologic assessment,* ed 2, St Louis, 1994, Mosby.

McCance KL, Huether SE: *Pathophysiology: the biologic basis for disease in adults and children,* ed 2, St Louis, 1994, Mosby.

Mills EM: The effect of low-intensity aerobic exercises on muscle strength, flexibility, and balance among sedentary elderly persons, *Nurs Res* 43(4):207, 1994.

Owen BD, Garg A: Reducing risk for back pain in nursing personnel, *J Am Assoc Occup Health Nurs* 39(1):24, 1991.

Perry A, Potter, P: *Clinical nursing skills and techniques,* ed 3, St Louis, 1994, Mosby.

Price S, Wilson L: *Pathophysiology: clinical concepts of disease processes,* St Louis, 1992, Mosby.

Stamps JL: "Back" to basics, *Emerg Med Serv* 18(2):38, 1989.

ADDITIONAL READINGS

Fenske NA et al: Tips for treating aging skin, *Patient Care* 26(6):61, 1992.

Gehring PE: Physical assessment begins with a history, *RN* 54(11):27, 1991.

Gross CR: Clinical signs of dehydration in the elderly, *Emerg Med* 24(15):59, 1992.

Hall J, Clarke AK: An evaluation of crutches, *Physiotherapy* 77(3):156, 1991.

Kuhn JK, McGovern M: Respiratory assessment of the elderly, *J Gerontol Nurs* 18(5):40, 1992.

LeBlanc MA et al: A quantitative comparison of four experimental axillary crutches, *J Prosth Orthot* 5(1):20, 1993.

McCauley M: The effect of body mechanics instruction on work performance among young workers, *Am J Occup Ther* 44(4):402, 1990.

Mitchell PH et al: Perspectives on human response to health and illness, *Nurs Outlook* 39(4):154, 1991.

Neilson DH et al: Energy, cost, exercise intensity, and gait efficiency of standard versus rocker-bottom axillary crutch walking, *Phys Ther* 70(8):47, 1990.

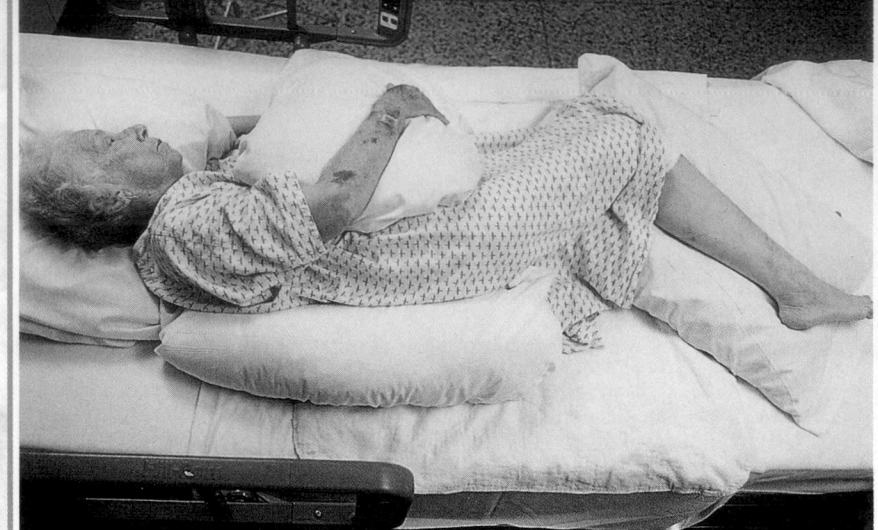

Chapter *38*

Skin Integrity

Objectives

Mastery of content in this chapter will enable the student to:

▶ Define the key terms listed.

▶ Describe the economic consequences of pressure ulcers.

▶ Describe four risk factors for pressure ulcer development.

▶ Discuss 10 contributing factors to pressure ulcer formation.

▶ Describe the different risk assessment tools used to identify clients at risk for developing pressure ulcers.

▶ Develop a nursing care plan for preventing the development of pressure ulcers.

▶ Discuss the pathogenesis of pressure ulcers.

▶ Define the four stages for classification of pressure ulcers.

▶ Complete an assessment for a client with impaired skin integrity.

▶ List nursing diagnoses associated with impaired skin integrity.

▶ Develop a nursing care plan for a client with impaired skin integrity.

▶ List appropriate nursing interventions for a client with impaired skin integrity.

▶ State evaluation criteria for a client with impaired skin integrity.

A major aspect of nursing care is the maintenance of skin integrity. Consistent, planned skin-care interventions are critical to ensuring high quality in care (Hoff, 1989). Nurses constantly observe their clients' skin for breaks or impairment in skin integrity. Impaired skin integrity occurs from prolonged pressure, irritation of the skin, or immobility, leading to the development of pressure ulcers.

A **pressure ulcer** is a localized area of tissue necrosis (death) that tends to develop when soft tissue is compressed between a bony prominence and an external surface for a prolonged period (National Pressure Ulcer Advisory Panel [NPUAP], 1989a, 1989b). Controversy exists over this definition, especially regarding stage I pressure ulcers. A new definition was proposed at the 4th National Conference of NPUAP (1995a). Margolis (1995) suggested "the best definition of a pressure ulcer is the disruption of normal anatomic structure and function of the skin that results from an external force associated with a bony prominence and that does not heal in an orderly and timely fashion. Further, these disruptions occur in an individual who is mostly chair- or bed-bound, often incontinent, malnourished or who has difficulty with self-feeding, and has an altered level of consciousness."

Nursing care interventions aimed at the prevention, assessment, and treatment of pressure ulcers ought to be based on research (AHCPR, 1992, 1994). A new research monograph published by NPUAP (1995b) has identified gaps in pressure ulcer research. It also lists suggested research questions that need further inquiry.

ECONOMIC CONSEQUENCES OF PRESSURE ULCERS

Pressure ulcers are a continual problem in acute and restorative care settings. Prevalence is the "number of cases present in a population at one point in time" (AHCPR, 1994). The prevalence rates vary among different client settings. Reported prevalence rates in the acute hospital setting range between 3% and 11% (Allman, 1989), 11% (Meehan, 1994), 14% (Langemo et al, 1989), and 20% (Leshem and Skelskey, 1994). Prevalence rates in the restorative and long-term care settings have ranged from 3.5% (Leshem and Skelskey, 1994), 5% (McKnight's Survey, 1992) to 23% (Langemo et al, 1989; Young, 1989). "The prevalence of pressure ulcers among persons cared for in the home without supervision

or assistance of professionals is not completely clear" (AHCPR, 1994). In the home care setting, prevalence rates have been reported to be 12.9% (Hentzen, Bergstrom, and Pozehl, 1993) and 19% (Hanson et al, 1993).

When a pressure ulcer occurs, the length of stay in a hospital and the overall cost of health care increase (AHCPR, 1994). The actual cost of treatment is difficult to approximate. Ranges are between $5000 and $27,000, depending on the number and severity of ulcers (Maklebust, 1987; Stotts, 1988; Hoff, 1989; Bryant, 1992). Although treatment of pressure ulcers is more costly than prevention (Oot-Giromini et al, 1989), the preventive measures themselves are expensive. Extra equipment, such as special beds and mattresses, and increased nursing time are needed to administer these measures. When an ulcer develops, the increased cost of nursing care alone is estimated at 50% (Maklebust, 1987).

The Agency for Health Care Policy and Research (AHCPR) has as its mission to develop clinical guidelines written by panels of multidisciplinary experts. The panels responsible for writing the two guidelines about pressure ulcers were both chaired by a nurse, Nancy Bergstrom, PhD, RN. The first guideline, *Pressure Ulcers in Adults: Prediction and Prevention Clinical Practice Guideline #3* (1992) recommended strategies for identifying at-risk individuals, implementing preventive measures, and treating early (stage I) pressure ulcers. The other guideline, *Treatment of Pressure Ulcers, Clinical Guideline #15* (1994), provides a comprehensive plan for treating stages II, III, and IV pressure ulcers in adults by clinicians who examine and treat individuals in all health care settings. The recommendations in both guidelines are supported by research, literature, or expert opinion.

Prediction and Prevention of Pressure Ulcers

RISK ASSESSMENT

Four instruments for assessing the risk of pressure ulcer development can readily identify clients at high risk. Clients with little risk for pressure ulcer development are spared the unnecessary and sometimes costly preventive treatments and the related risk of complications (Stotts, 1988). Prevention and treatment of pressure ulcers are major nursing priorities. The ability to identify clients at risk helps contain health care costs (Gosnell, 1973; Norton,

Table 38-1	Norton Scale				
		PHYSICAL CONDITION	**MENTAL CONDITION**	**ACTIVITY**	**MOBILITY**	**INCONTINENT**
Name	Date	Good 4 Fair 3 Poor 2 Very bad 1	Alert 4 Apathetic 3 Confused 2 Stupor 1	Ambulant 4 Walk/help 3 Chairbound 2 Bed 1	Full 4 Slightly limited 3 Very limited 2 Immobile 1	Not 4 Occasional 3 Usually/urine 2 Doubly 1	**Total score**

Modified from Centre for Policy on Ageing: London, England, 1962.

Table 38-2	Gosnell Scale: Pressure Sore Risk Assessment (Part 1)

I.D. _____   Medical Diagnosis: _____

Age _____ Sex _____   Primary _____

Height _____ Weight _____   Secondary _____

Date of Admission_____   Nursing Diagnosis: _____

Date of Discharge _____   _____

Instructions: Complete all categories within 24 hours of admission and every other day thereafter. Refer to the accompanying guidelines for specific rating details.

Date	MENTAL STATUS*	CONTINENCE*	MOBILITY*	ACTIVITY*	NUTRITION*	Total score
	1. Alert 2. Apathetic 3. Confused 4. Stuporous 5. Unconscious	1. Fully Controlled 2. Usually Controlled 3. Minimally Controlled 4. Absence of Control	1. Full 2. Slightly Limited 3. Very Limited 4. Immobile	1. Ambulatory 2. Walks with Assistance 3. Chairfast 4. Bedfast	1. Good 2. Fair 3. Poor	

PRESSURE SORE RISK ASSESSMENT MEDICATION PROFILE

MEDICATION	DOSAGE	FREQUENCY†	ROUTE	DATE BEGUN	DATE DISCONTINUED

*See Part 3, p. 952, for guidelines for rating.
†If PRN, record pattern past 48 hours.

et al, 1962). Several risk assessment scales developed by nurses enable them to systematically assess their clients. Each tool has a different number of risk factors (5 to 8 items) that are ranked by number. The client's risk assessment score is obtained by adding the individual number given for each risk factor. Interpretation of the meaning of the numerical score differs with each scale.

The first scale reported in the literature is the Norton Scale (1962) (Table 38-1). It scores five risk factors: physical condition, mental condition, activity, mobility, and incontinence. The total score ranges from 5 to 20; a total lower score indicates a higher risk for pressure ulcer development. A score of 16 is now considered to be the risk score (Norton, 1989).

Based on the Norton Scale, the original Gosnell Scale (1973) was developed from research on 30 clients in a nursing home. Nutrition replaced Norton's category of physical condition, and incontinence was renamed continence. Demographic data, clinical items, and narrative criteria guidelines were also added. The scale scores five factors: mental status, continence, mobility, activity, and nutrition (Table 38-2). The total score ranges from 5 to 20, a higher total score indicates risk for pressure ulcer development (Gosnell, 1987, 1989a, 1989b).

The Knoll Assessment Tool was developed based on risk factors of clients in a large acute care hospital. The eight risk factors include general state of health, mental status, activity, mobility, incontinence, oral nutrition intake, oral fluid intake, and predisposing diseases. The total score ranges from 0 to 33; a higher total score indicates a higher risk for pressure ulcer development. The at-risk score is 12 or greater.

The last instrument is the Braden Scale (Table 38-3), which was developed based on risk factors in a nursing

| Table 38-2 | Gosnell Scale: Pressure Sore Risk Assessment—cont'd (Part 2) | | | | | | | | | | | | | |

	VITAL SIGNS					**24-HOUR FLUID BALANCE**		**COLOR** 1. Pallor 2. Mottled 3. Pink 4. Ashen 5. Ruddy 6. Cyanotic 7. Jaundice 8. Other	**GENERAL SKIN APPEARANCE**			**INTERVENTIONS**		
									MOISTURE 1. Dry 2. Damp 3. Oily 4. Other	**TEMPERATURE** 1. Cold 2. Cool 3. Warm 4. Hot	**TEXTURE** 1. Smooth 2. Rough 3. Thin/Transp 4. Scaly 5. Crusty 6. Other			
Date	T	P	R	BP	Diet	Intake	Output					No	Yes	Describe

Vital signs: The temperature, pulse, respiration, and blood pressure to be taken and recorded at the time of every assessment rating.

Skin appearance: A description of observed skin characteristics: color, moisture, temperature, and texture.

Diet: Record the specific diet order.

24-hour fluid balance: The amount of fluid intake and output during the previous 24-hour period should be recorded.

Interventions: List all devices, measures, and/or nursing care activity being used for the purpose of pressure sore prevention.

Medications: List name, dosage, frequency, and route for all prescribed medications. If a PRN order, list the pattern for the period since last assessment.

Comments: Use this space to add explanation or further detail regarding any of the previously recorded data, patient condition, etc.
or
Describe anything that you believe to be of importance but not accounted for previously.

Note: For any item marked "other," please describe.

If any signs of pressure, etc., on bony prominences or other body parts are observed, please describe in detail the location, color, temperature, moisture, texture, and size and any other pertinent items.

Courtesy Davina Gosnell, RN, PhD.

Continued.

home population (Bergstrom et al, 1987). The Braden Scale is composed of six subscales: sensory perception, moisture, activity, mobility, nutrition, friction, and shear. The total score ranges from 6 to 23; a lower total score indicates a higher risk for pressure ulcer development (Braden and Bergstrom, 1989). Hospitalized adults with a score of 16 or below and older clients with a score of 17 or 18 are considered at risk (Braden and Bergstrom, 1994; Bryant, 1992).

This instrument is highly reliable for identifying clients at greatest risk for pressure ulcers (Bergstrom et al, 1987).

PREVENTION

The prevention of pressure ulcers is a priority in caring for clients and is not limited to clients with restrictions in mobility. Impaired skin integrity may not be a problem in healthy, immobilized individuals but is a serious and po-

Table 38-2	Gosnell Scale: Pressure Sore Risk Assessment—cont'd (Part 3)				

GUIDELINES FOR NUMERICAL RATING OF THE DEFINED CATEGORIES

RATING	1	2	3	4	5
MENTAL STATUS An assessment of one's level of response to the environment.	**ALERT** Oriented to time, place, and person. Responsive to all stimuli and understands explanations.	**APATHETIC** Lethargic, forgetful, drowsy, passive, and dull. Sluggish, depressed. Able to obey simple commands. Possibly disoriented to time.	**CONFUSED** Partial and/or intermittent disorientation to time, place and person. Purposeless response to stimuli. Restless, aggressive, irritable, anxious, and may require tranquilizers or sedatives.	**STUPOROUS** Total disorientation. Does not respond to name, simple commands, or verbal stimuli.	**UNCONSCIOUS** Nonresponsive to painful stimuli.
CONTINENCE The amount of bodily control or urination and defecation.	**FULLY CONTROLLED** Total control of urine and feces.	**USUALLY CONTROLLED** Incontinent of urine and/or of feces not more often than once every 48 hours or has Foley catheter and is incontinent of feces.	**MINIMALLY CONTROLLED** Incontinent of urine or feces at least once every 24 hours.	**ABSENCE OF CONTROL** Consistently incontinent of both urine and feces.	
MOBILITY The amount and control of movement of one's body.	**FULL** Able to control and move all extremities at will. May require the use of a device but turns, lifts, pulls, balances, and attains sitting position at will.	**SLIGHTLY LIMITED** Able to control and move all extremities but a degree of limitation is present. Requires assistance of another person to turn, pull, balance, and/or attain a sitting position at will but self-initiates movement or requests for help to move.	**VERY LIMITED** Can assist another person, who must initiate movement via turning, lifting, pulling, balancing, and/or attaining a sitting position (contractures, paralysis may be present).	**IMMOBILE** Does not assist self in any way to change position. Is unable to change position without assistance. Is completely dependent on others for movement.	
ACTIVITY The ability of an individual to ambulate.	**AMBULATORY** Is able to walk unassisted. Rises from bed unassisted. With the use of a device such as cane or walker is able to ambulate without the assistance of another person.	**WALKS WITH HELP** Able to ambulate with assistance of another person, braces, or crutches. May have limitation of stairs.	**CHAIRFAST** Ambulates only to a chair, requires assistance to do so or is confined to a wheelchair.	**BEDFAST** Is confined to bed during entire 24 hours of the day.	
NUTRITION The process of food intake.	Eats some food from each basic food category every day and the majority of each meal served or is on tube feeding.	Occasionally refuses a meal or frequently leaves at least half of a meal.	Seldom eats a complete meal and only a few bites of food at a meal.		

Table 38-3	Braden Scale for Predicting Pressure Sore Risk

Patient's Name _____ Evaluator's Name _____ Date of Assessment _____

SENSORY PERCEPTION Ability to respond meaningfully to pressure-related discomfort	1. Completely Limited Unresponsive (does not moan, flinch, or grasp) to painful stimuli due to diminished level of consciousness or sedation. OR Limited ability to feel pain over most of body surface.	2. Very Limited Responds only to painful stimuli. Cannot communicate discomfort except by moaning or restlessness. OR Has a sensory impairment which limits the ability to feel pain or discomfort over $\frac{1}{2}$ of body.	3. Slightly Limited Responds to verbal commands, but cannot always communicate discomfort or need to be turned. OR Has some sensory impairment that limits ability to feel pain or discomfort in 1 or 2 extremities.	4. No Impairment Responds to verbal commands. Has no sensory deficit that would limit ability to feel or voice pain or discomfort.	
MOISTURE Degree to which skin is exposed to moisture	1. Constantly Moist Skin is kept moist almost constantly by perspiration, urine, etc. Dampness is detected every time patient is moved or turned.	2. Very Moist Skin is often, but not always, moist. Linen must be changed at least once a shift.	3. Occasionally Moist Skin is occasionally moist, requiring an extra linen change approximately once a day.	4. Rarely Moist Skin is usually dry, linen only requires changing at routine intervals.	
ACTIVITY Degree of physical activity	1. Bedfast Confined to bed.	2. Chairfast Ability to walk severely limited or nonexistent. Cannot bear own weight and/or must be assisted into chair or wheelchair.	3. Walks Occasionally Walks occasionally during day, but for very short distances, with or without assistance. Spends majority of each shift in bed or chair.	4. Walks Frequently Walks outside the room at least twice a day and inside room at least once every 2 hours during waking hours.	
MOBILITY Ability to change and control body position	1. Completely Immobile Does not make even slight changes in body or extremity position without assistance.	2. Very Limited Makes occasional slight changes in body or extremity position but unable to make frequent or significant changes independently.	3. Slightly Limited Makes frequent though slight changes in body or extremity position independently.	4. No Limitations Makes major and frequent changes in position without assistance.	

Courtesy Barbara Braden and Nancy Bergstrom.   *Continued.*

tentially devastating problem in ill or debilitated clients (AHCPR, 1992).

■ PRESSURE ULCERS

Pressure ulcer, pressure sore, decubitus ulcer, and *bedsore* are terms used to describe impaired skin integrity. The most current terminology is *pressure ulcer* (Fig. 38-1), which is consistent with the NPUAP and the AHCPR's Pressure Ulcer Guidelines Panel (Margolis, 1995; Maklebust and Margolis, 1995; Maklebust, 1991a, 1991b; Lucas, 1991; Green and

Katz, 1991; Hastings, 1991; AHCPR, 1992). An ill client experiencing decreased mobility, impaired neurological functioning, decreased sensory perception, or decreased circulation is at risk for pressure ulcer development.

Tissues receive oxygen and nutrients and eliminate metabolic wastes via the blood. Any factor that interferes with this affects cellular metabolism and the function or life of the cell. Pressure affects cellular metabolism by decreasing or obliterating tissue circulation, resulting in tissue ischemia.

Tissue ischemia is the localized absence of blood or a

Table 38-3	Braden Scale for Predicting Pressure Sore Risk—cont'd			

Patient's Name _____   Evaluator's Name _____   Date of Assessment _____

NUTRITION *Usual* food intake pattern	1. Very Poor Never eats a complete meal. Rarely eats more than ⅓ of any food offered. Eats 2 servings or less of protein (meat or dairy products) per day. Takes fluids poorly. Does not take a liquid dietary supplement. OR Is NPO and/or maintained on clear liquids or IVs for more than 5 days.	2. Probably Inadequate Rarely eats a complete meal and generally eats only about ½ of any food offered. Protein intake includes only 3 servings of meat or dairy products per day. Occasionally will take a dietary supplement. OR Receives less than optimum amount of liquid diet or tube feeding.	3. Adequate Eats over half of most meals. Eats a total of 4 servings of protein (meat, dairy products) each day. Occasionally will refuse a meal, but will usually take a supplement if offered. OR Is on a tube feeding or total parenteral nutrition regimen that probably meets most of nutritional needs.	4. Excellent Eats most of every meal. Never refuses a meal. Usually eats a total of 4 or more servings of meat and dairy products. Occasionally eats between meals. Does not require supplementation.
FRICTION AND SHEAR	1. Problem Requires moderate to maximum assistance in moving. Complete lifting without sliding against sheets is impossible. Frequently slides down in bed or chair, requiring frequent repositioning with maximum assistance. Spasticity, contractures, or agitation leads to almost constant friction.	2. Potential Problem Moves feebly or requires minimum assistance. During a move skin probably slides to some extent against sheets, chair, restraints, or other devices. Maintains relatively good position in chair or bed most of the time but occasionally slides down.	3. No Apparent Problem Moves in bed and in chair independently and has sufficient muscle strength to lift up completely during move. Maintains good position in bed or chair at all times.	
			Total Score	

Characteristics of Intact Dark Skin

The following are characteristics of intact dark skin to include in a nursing assessment to identify a client's potential for development of pressure ulcers.*

- Appears darker than surrounding skin (purplish/bluish hue)
- May be taut, shiny, or indurated; edema may occur with induration of more than 15 mm in diameter.
- May have a purplish/bluish hue
- When first touched, will feel warm compared to surrounding skin. Later this will be replaced by an area of coolness, which is a sign of tissue devitalization.

*Data from Task Force for the implications for darkly pigmented intact skin and the prediction and prevention of pressure ulcers, Brooklyn, New York, 1995.
For further information contact the Task Force chairperson: M. Alisan Bennett, EdD, RN; Special Projects Coordinator; Woodhull Medical And Mental Health Center; 760 Broadway; Brooklyn, New York, 11206; 718-963-8000.

major reduction of blood flow resulting from mechanical obstruction (Pires and Muller, 1991). The reduction in blood flow causes blanching. **Blanching** is seen when the normal red tones of the light-skinned client are absent. Blanching does not occur with darkly pigmented–skin clients (Task Force for the Implications for Darkly Pigmented Intact Skin and the Prediction and Prevention of Pressure Ulcers, 1995). The Task Force has defined **darkly pigmented skin** as follows "the obvious color of intact dark skin remains unchanged (does not blanch) when pressure is applied over a bony prominence, irrespective of the client's race or ethnicity." Characteristics of intact dark skin that might alert nurses to the potential for pressure ulcers have been identified by this Task Force (see the box at left).

Tissue damage occurs when the pressure exerted on the capillaries is high enough to close the capillaries (capillary closing pressure). **Capillary closing pressure** is the pressure needed to close the capillaries (e.g., when the pres-

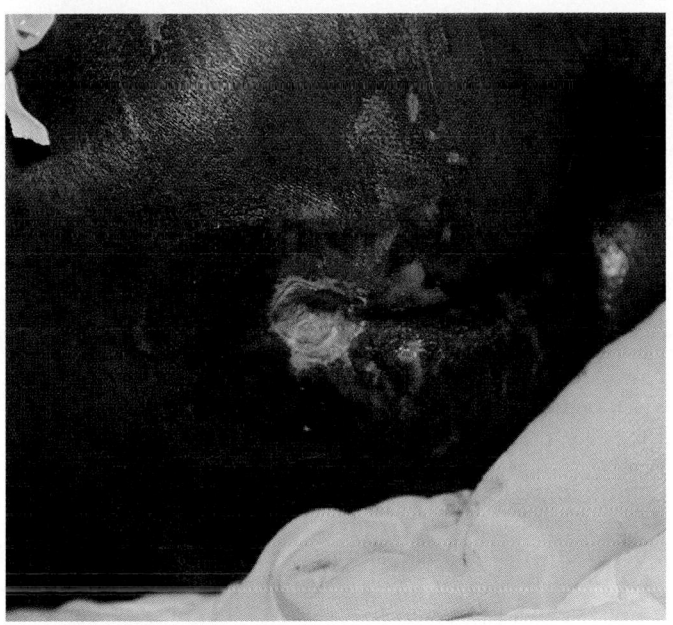

Fig. 38-1 Pressure ulcer with tissue necrosis.

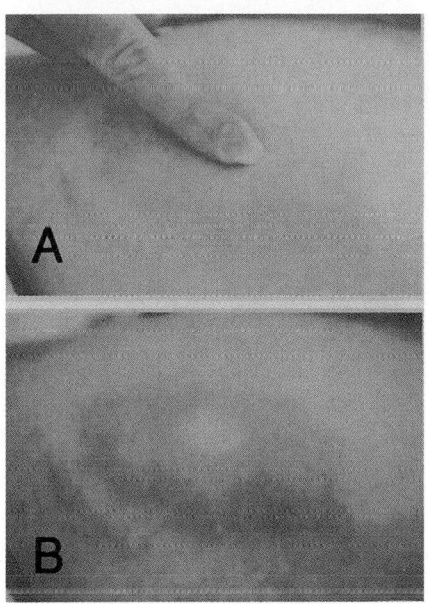

Fig. 38-2 A, Reactive hyperemia. **B,** Blanches with fingertip pressure. *(From Pires M, Muller A:* Progressions *3(3):3, 1991.)*

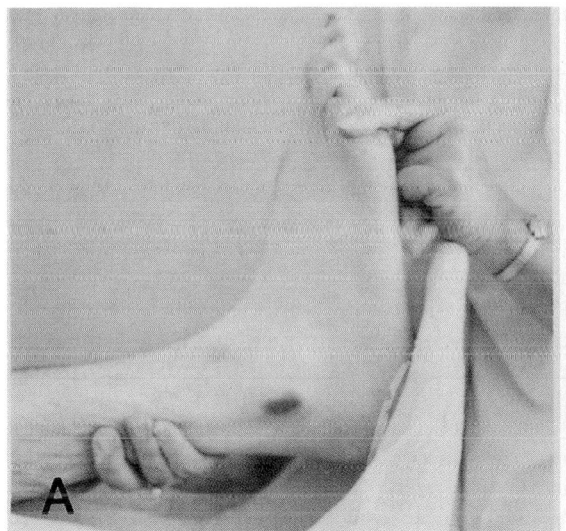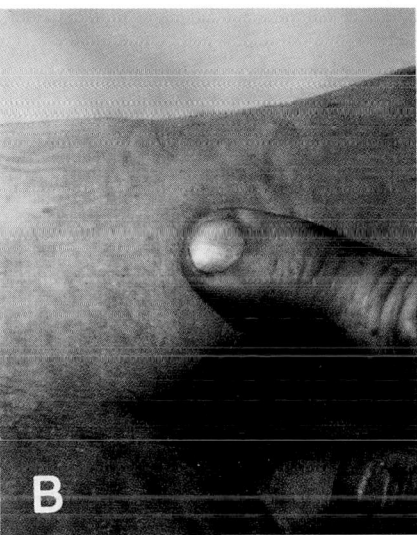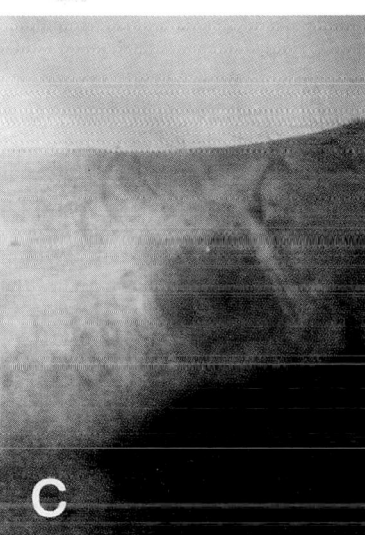

Fig. 38-3 A, Abnormal reactive hyperemia. **B** and **C,** In abnormal reactive hyperemia the area is much darker than the surrounding skin and does not blanch with fingertip pressure. *(From Pires M, Muller A:* Progressions *3 (3):3, 1991.)*

sure exceeds the normal capillary pressure range of 16 to 32 mm Hg) (Maklebust, 1987).

After a period of ischemia, light-toned skin can undergo one of two hyperemic changes. **Normal reactive hyperemia** (redness) is the visible effect of localized vasodilation, the body's normal response to lack of blood flow to the underlying tissue (Fig. 38-2, *A*). The area blanches with fingertip pressure (Fig. 38-2, *B*), and reactive hyperemia lasts less than 1 hour. **Abnormal reactive hyperemia** is an excessive vasodilation and induration in response to pressure. The skin appears bright pink to red. The **induration** is

an area of localized edema under the skin. Abnormal reactive hyperemia (Fig. 38-3) can last more than 1 hour up to 2 weeks after the removal of pressure (Pires and Muller, 1991).

When a client is lying or sitting, the body weight is placed on bony prominences. The longer the pressure is applied, the greater the risk of skin breakdown. Pressure causes a decrease in blood supply to the tissues, and ischemia occurs. When the pressure is removed, there is a period of reactive hyperemia, or a sudden increase in blood flow to the region. Reactive hyperemia is a compensatory response and is only effective if the pressure on the skin is removed before necrosis or damage occurs.

Risk Factors for Pressure Ulcer Development

A variety of factors can predispose a client to pressure ulcer formation.

IMPAIRED SENSORY INPUT

Clients with altered sensory perception for pain and pressure are at greater risk for impaired skin integrity than are clients with normal sensation. Clients whose sensory perception of pain and pressure is intact can feel when a portion of their body senses too much pressure or pain. In turn, when clients are alert and oriented, they can change positions or request assistance in changing positions.

IMPAIRED MOTOR FUNCTION

Clients unable to independently change positions are at greater risk for pressure ulcers. These clients can perceive the pressure but are unable to independently change positions to relieve it. Thus the chance of pressure ulcer development increases. In clients with spinal cord injuries, there is motor and sensory impairment. The incidence of pressure ulcers in clients with spinal cord injuries is estimated to be as high as 85%, and ulcers or ulcer-related complications are the cause of death in 8% of this population (Reuler and Cooney, 1981).

ALTERATIONS IN LEVEL OF CONSCIOUSNESS

Clients who are confused, disoriented, or have changing levels of consciousness are unable to protect themselves from pressure ulcers. Clients who are confused or disoriented may be able to feel the pressure, but they may not be able to understand how to relieve it. Clients who are in a coma may not perceive pressure and are unable to move voluntarily into a more protective position. In addition, clients whose levels of consciousness change may easily become confused. Some examples are clients in the operating room and intensive care units who are sedated.

CASTS, TRACTION, ORTHOTIC DEVICES, AND OTHER EQUIPMENT

Casts and traction reduce mobility of the client or of an extremity. A client with a cast has an increased risk of pressure ulcer development because of the mechanical external force of friction from the surface of the cast rubbing against the skin. A second mechanical force is the pressure exerted by the cast on the skin if the cast dries too tightly or if the extremity swells.

Orthotic devices such as cervical collars are used in the treatment of clients with fractures of the upper cervical spine. Pressure ulcers are a potential complication of these cervical collars. A study by Plaisier et al. (1994) examined the amount of pressure exerted on the scalp and face by four different cervical collars with the subjects in both the supine and upright positions. Results showed that for some of the cervical collars, the capillary closing pressure was exceeded. Nurses need to be aware of the risk of skin breakdown in clients wearing these cervical collars. Nurses must assess skin beneath cervical collars, braces, or other orthotic devices to observe for signs of skin breakdown.

Any equipment that exerts pressure on a client's skin can lead to the development of a pressure ulcer. Oxygen tubing and nasogastric tubes are just two common examples of equipment that may cause pressure ulcers. Appropriate nursing care for clients with such equipment includes frequent assessment of the client's skin beneath the tube to identify any signs of skin breakdown.

Contributing Factors to Pressure Ulcer Formation

Impaired skin integrity resulting in pressure ulcers is primarily the result of pressure. However, additional factors can further increase the client's risk for pressure ulcer development. These include shearing and friction forces, moisture, poor nutrition, anemia, infection, fever, impaired peripheral circulation, obesity, cachexia, and age.

Shearing force is the pressure exerted against the skin in a direction parallel to the body's surface (AHCPR, 1994). It can occur when a client is moved or repositioned in bed by being pulled or being allowed to slide down in bed while in a high-Fowler's position (Fig. 38-4). When a shearing force is present, the skin and subcutaneous layers adhere to the surface of the bed, and the layers of muscle and even the bones slide in the direction of body movement. The client's bone slides down into the skin and exerts a force onto the skin (Maklebust and Sieggreen, 1991). The underlying tissue capillaries are compressed and severed by the pressure. As a result, minute layers of bleeding and necrosis occur *deep* within the tissue layers. In addition, there is a decrease in capillary blood flow from the external pressure against the skin. Subcutaneous fat is more vulnerable to the effects of shearing and the resultant pressure from the underlying bony structure. Eventually a tract can open to the skin to allow drainage from the necrotic area. It is important to remember that shearing force injuries usually occur over bony prominences such as the sacral and coccygeal areas. These injuries involve deep tissue layers and are most often initially the size of the outline of the bone located beneath the destroyed tissue. Keeping the head of the bed below 30 degrees can avoid injuries from shearing forces (AHCPR, 1992, 1994). "It is not possible to have shear without friction" (Bryant et al, 1992).

Friction is "the mechanical force exerted when skin is dragged across a coarse surface such as bed linens" (AHCPR, 1994). Unlike shearing injuries, friction injuries affect the epidermis or *top* layer of the skin, which is rubbed away as the client is repositioned. They are frequently shallow abrasion injuries seen on the elbows or heels (Wysocki and Bryant, 1992). Because of the way these wounds occur, nurses often refer to them as "sheet burns" (Bryant et al,

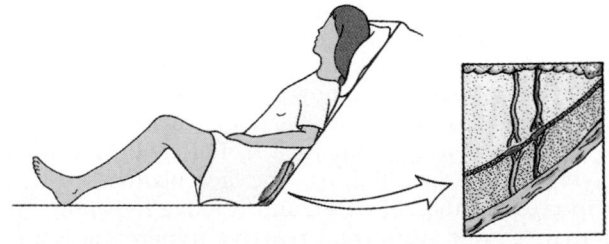

Fig. 38-4 Diagrammatic sketch of shearing force exerted against sacral area.

1992). They can occur in clients who are restless; those who have uncontrollable movements, such as spastic conditions; and those whose skin is dragged rather than lifted from the bed surface during position changes (Maklebust and Sieggreen, 1991). Nursing measures to prevent friction injuries include the following: proper transfer of clients using correct lifting techniques; using products on the elbows and heels such as sheepskin protectors, skin sealants, and transparent membrane or hydrocolloid dressings to protect the skin; and applying moisturizers to maintain the hydration of the epidermis.

The presence and duration of *moisture* on the skin increases the risk of ulcer formation. The presence of moisture increases the risk of pressure ulcer formation fivefold (Reuler and Cooney, 1981). Moisture reduces the skin's resistance to other physical factors such as pressure or shearing force.

Immobilized clients, who are unable to perform their own hygiene needs, depend on the nurse to keep the skin dry and intact. The nurse must therefore incorporate hygiene into the care plan. Moisture on the skin can originate from wound drainage, perspiration, condensation from humidified oxygen-delivery systems, vomitus, and incontinence. Certain body fluids (e.g., urine, stool, and wound drainage) cause skin erosion and, in the presence of pressure, the client's risk increases.

Clients with *poor nutrition* often experience serious muscle atrophy and decreases in subcutaneous tissue (see Chapter 41). Because of these changes, less tissue is present to serve as padding between the skin and underlying bone. Therefore the effects of pressure are increased on remaining tissue. Malnutrition is second only to excessive pressure in the etiology, pathogenesis, and nonhealing of pressure ulcers (Hanan and Scheele, 1991; NPUAP, 1989a, 1989b). The malnourished client can also have protein deficiency and negative nitrogen balance and have an inadequate intake of vitamin C (Shekleton and Litwack, 1991). Poor nutritional status may be overlooked if the client has a weight equal to or above the ideal body weight (IBW). The client with poor nutritional status frequently has hypoalbuminemia (serum albumin levels below 3 g/100 ml) and anemia (Natlow, 1983; Steinberg, 1990).

Albumin is a frequently measured variable used to evaluate the client's protein status. A client with a serum albumin level below 3 g/100 ml is at greater risk for pressure ulcers than a client with a higher albumin level. In addition, low albumin levels are associated with poor wound healing (Hanan and Scheele, 1991; Pinchcofsky-Devin and Kaminski, 1989). Although serum albumin levels are slow to reflect changes in visceral proteins, they are the best predictors of malnutrition in all age groups (Hanan and Scheele, 1991).

Total protein levels are also correlated with pressure ulcer development. Total protein levels below 5.4 g/100 ml decrease colloid osmotic pressure, which leads to interstitial edema and decreased oxygen to the tissues (Hanan and Scheele, 1991). Edema decreases the skin and underlying tissue's tolerance to pressure, friction, and shearing force. In addition, the decreased oxygen levels increase the speed of ischemic injury to the tissue.

Poor nutrition also alters fluid and electrolyte balance. In clients with severe protein loss, hypoalbuminemia leads to a shift of fluid from the extracellular fluid volume to the tissues, resulting in edema. **Edema** increases the affected tissue's risk for pressure ulcers. The blood supply to the edematous tissue is decreased, and waste products remain because of the changing pressures in the capillary circulation and capillary bed (Shekleton and Litwack, 1991).

Clients with **anemia** are at risk for pressure ulcer formation. Decreased levels of hemoglobin reduce the oxygen-carrying capacity of the blood and the amount of oxygen available to tissues. Anemia also alters cellular metabolism and impairs wound healing.

Cachexia is generalized ill health and malnutrition, marked by weakness and emaciation. It is usually associated with severe diseases such as cancer and end-stage cardiopulmonary diseases. This condition increases the client's risk for pressure ulcers. Basically the cachexic client has lost the adipose tissue necessary to protect bony prominences from pressure.

Obesity can accelerate pressure ulcer development. Adipose tissue in small quantities protects the skin by cushioning bony prominences against pressure. However, in moderate-to-severe obesity, adipose tissue is poorly vascularized, and the adipose and underlying tissues are more susceptible to ischemic damage.

Infection results from the presence of pathogens in the body. A client with an infection usually has a fever. Infection and *fever* increase the metabolic needs of the body, making already hypoxic (decreased oxygen) tissue more susceptible to ischemic injury (Shekleton and Litwack, 1991). In addition, fever results in diaphoresis (sweating) and increased skin moisture, which further predispose the client to skin breakdown.

Impaired peripheral circulation is also related to pressure ulcer development. With decreased circulation the tissue becomes hypoxic and more susceptible to ischemic damage. Impaired circulation occurs in clients who have peripheral vascular diseases, who are in shock, or who are receiving vasopressor-type medications.

Older adults have a more frequent occurrence of pressure ulcers. Studies by Stotts (1988) and by Kane, Ouslander, and Abrass (1989) note a greater incidence of ulcer development in people over 75 years of age. Some of the normal changes in aging skin account for the increased risk of pressure ulcers in the elderly (see Table 49-1 in Chapter 49).

Using the Web of Causation (Fig. 38-5), Oot-Giromini (1993) recently proposed a new conceptual framework with which to view the development of pressure ulcers. This model involves the concept where the whole is greater than the sum of its parts. This model also considers personal wellness (e.g., activities of daily living, medical diagnosis, coping abilities, attitudes, and the desire to participate in health regimens) and socioeconomic variables (e.g., living conditions, income, support systems, ability to purchase needed supplies, knowledge of care givers, availability and affordability of help outside the home, rural or urban setting, and personal value systems). The complex interrelationships among the multiple factors, rather than the individual factors themselves, are emphasized.

Pathogenesis of Pressure Ulcers

Three elements are the cornerstone of pressure ulcer development: (1) intensity of pressure and capillary closing pres-

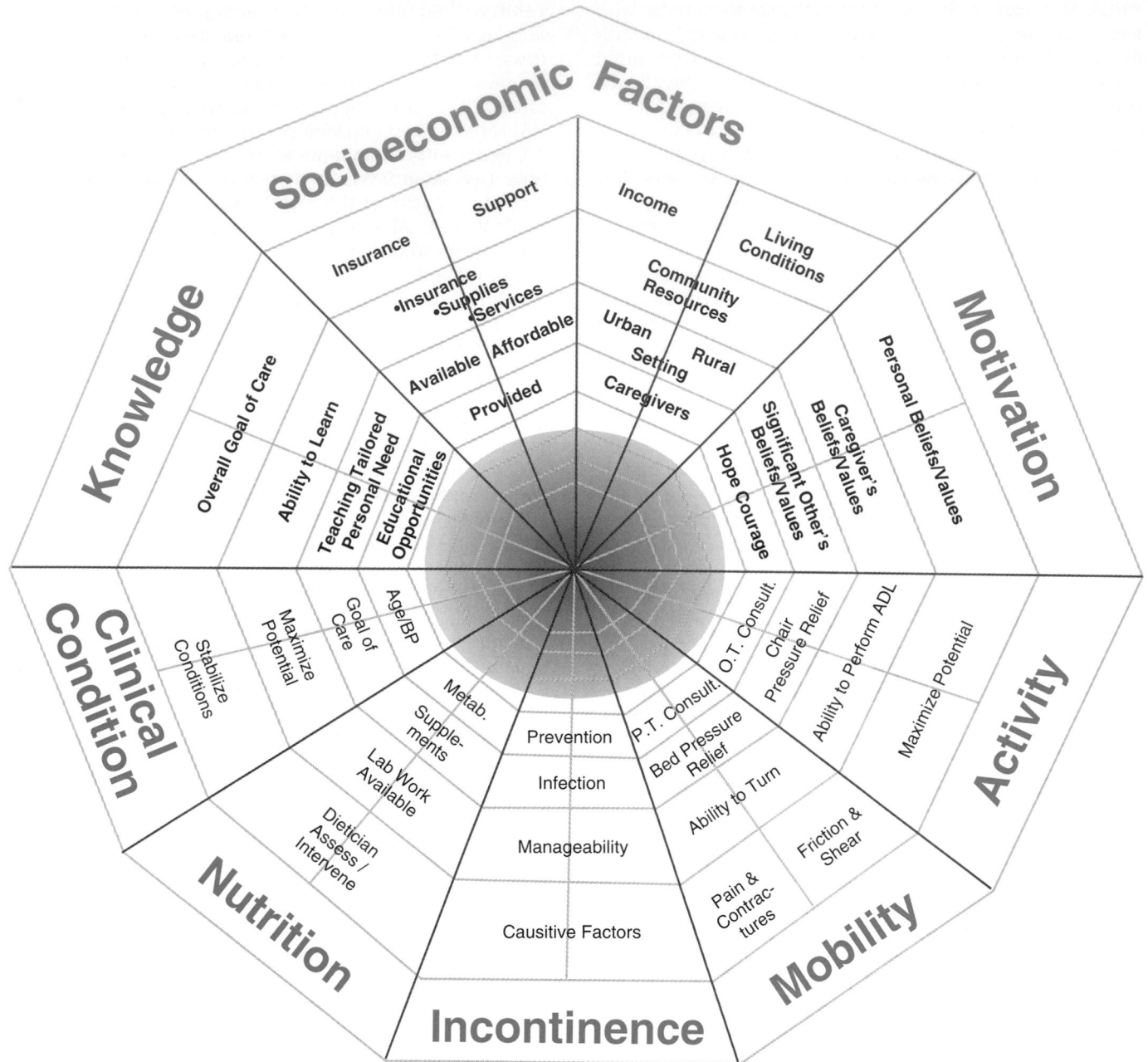

Fig. 38-5 Web of causation for pressure ulcers *(Courtesy Barbara Oot-Giromini.)*

sure (Landis, 1930); (2) duration and sustenance of pressure (Koziak, 1959); and (3) tissue tolerance (Husain, 1953; Trumble, 1930). Some of the most common sites that pressure ulcers develop are the sacrum, heels, elbows, lateral malleoli, greater trochanter, and ischial tuberosities (Meehan, 1994).

A pressure ulcer occurs as a result of a time-pressure relationship (Stotts, 1988). The greater the pressure and the duration of the pressure, the greater the incidence of ulcer formation. The skin and subcutaneous tissue can tolerate some pressure. However, externally applied pressure greater than the pressure in the capillary bed decreases or obliterates blood flow to adjacent tissues. These tissues become hypoxic, and ischemic injury results. If this pressure is

greater than 32 mm Hg and remains unrelieved to the point of hypoxia, the vessels collapse and thrombose (develop a clot) (Maklebust, 1987). If the pressure is relieved before the critical point, circulation to the affected tissues is restored through the physiological mechanism of reactive hyperemia. "Because the skin has greater ability to tolerate ischemia than does muscle, true pressure ulcers begin at the bone with pressure-related muscle ischemia eventually declaring itself at the epidermis" (Maklebust, 1995).

Pressure ulcers also form due to shearing force that occurs when moving the client up in bed. The sacral areas and heels are the most susceptible (Maklebust, 1987). The effect of pressure can also be increased by unequal distribution of body weight. Because of gravity, a person is subjected to constant pressures of the body against any surface on which it rests (Berecek, 1975). If the pressure is unevenly distributed on the body, a pressure gradient is increased on tissues receiving the pressure. The cellular metabolism of the skin is altered at the point of pressure.

The compensatory response of the tissues to ischemia—reactive hyperemia—permits ischemic tissue to be flooded with blood when pressure is removed. Increased blood flow increases delivery of oxygen and nutrients to tissue. The metabolic debt resulting from pressure can then be met. Healthy equilibrium is restored, and necrosis of the compressed tissue is avoided (Maklebust, 1991a, 1991b; Pires and Muller, 1991). Reactive hyperemia is effective only if pressure is removed before damage occurs. Some researchers feel that the interval before damage occurs can be between 1 and 2 hours. However, this is a subjective time interval, and it is not based on client assessment data.

CLASSIFICATION OF PRESSURE ULCERS—STAGING OR COLOR

One of the earliest ways to classify pressure ulcers was by using a grading or staging system. It was first proposed by Shea (1975) as a way to have a clear and consistent method of describing and classifying pressure ulcers. Staging systems for pressure ulcers are based on describing the depth of tissue destroyed (Maklebust, 1995). An ulcer that is covered with necrotic tissue such as eschar cannot be staged until it is debrided and the depth of the pressure ulcer can be observed (AHCPR, 1992, 1994). Orthopedic devices and braces can make assessment difficult (AHCPR, 1992, 1994).

There are several different staging systems that are used clinically (Shea, 1975; AHCPR, 1992, 1994; and NPUAP, 1989a, 1989b, 1992). It is important to note that the defin-

CULTURAL ASPECTS OF CARE

Detecting cyanosis in clients is an important clinical skill. Cyanosis is defined by "a slightly bluish grayish slate-like or dark purple discoloration of the skin due to the presence of at least 5 grams of reduced hemoglobin in arterial blood." Color differentiation of cyanosis varies according to skin pigmentation. In dark-skinned clients, the nurse needs to know the individual's baseline skin tone. The nurse should not confuse the normal hyperpigmentation of Mongolian spots that are seen on the sacrum of African, Native American, and Asian clients as cyanosis. The nurse should observe the client's skin in nonglare daylight and note any signs of dyspnea. The Gaskin's Nursing Assessment of Skin Color (GNASC) may be a useful tool for assessment.

IMPLICATIONS FOR PRACTICE
- Cyanosis is difficult but is possible to detect in the dark-skinned client.
- Nurses need to be aware of situations that produce cyanosis.
- Examine body sites with the least melanin for underlying color identification.
- The skin should be evaluated for cyanotic changes, color-specific to the pigmented skin.

Modified from Gaskin FC: Detection of cyanosis in the person with dark skin, *J Nat Black Nurses Assoc* 1:52, 1986.

itions are different for each of these staging systems. Therefore the same pressure ulcer could have a different stage number, depending on the staging system used. The stages below are from the National Pressure Ulcer Advisory Panel (NPUAP, 1989a, 1989b, 1992), and they are also used in the AHCPR Treatment Guidelines (1994). At the 1995 NPUAP Consensus Conference the need to change the stage I definition to reflect assessment characteristics of clients with dark skin tones was discussed (see the box below). Indicators other than skin color, such as temperature, "orange peel" pore appearance, firmness or tightness, hardness, and laboratory data, may be helpful when assessing clients with dark skin (Graves, 1990; Maklebust and Sieggreen, 1991). Bennett (1995) suggests that when assessing clients with darkly pigmented skin, proper lighting is important to accurately assess the skin. Either natural or a halogen light is recommended. This prevents the blue tones that are produced by fluorescent light sources on darkly pigmented skin, which can interfere with accurate assessment. A comparison of stage I pressure ulcer in light- and darkly pigmented skin can be seen in Fig. 38-6.

I   Nonblanchable erythema of the intact skin, the heralding lesion of skin ulceration. Discoloration of skin, warmth, or hardness also may be indicators (Fig. 38-7, *A*).

II   Partial-thickness skin loss involving epidermis and/or dermis. The ulcer is superficial and presents clinically as an abrasion, blister, or shallow crater (Fig. 38-7, *B*).

III   Full-thickness skin loss involving damage or necrosis of subcutaneous tissue that may extend down to, but not through, underlying fascia. The ulcer presents clinically as a deep crater with or without undermining of adjacent tissue (Fig. 38-7, *C*).

IV   Full-thickness skin loss with extensive destruction; tissue necrosis; or damage to muscle, bone, or supporting structures (e.g., tendon, joint capsules, etc.) (Fig. 38-7, *D*).

Some problems with the use of sequential numbers in staging systems were raised again at the 1995 NPUAP 4th National Conference. Pressure ulcers do *not* progress from a stage I to a stage IV (NPUAP, 1995). Maklebust (1995) cautions clinicians to remember that, although staging systems use sequential numbers to describe pressure ulcers, this does not mean that there is a progression in pressure ulcer severity. It is also erroneous to use staging numbers in

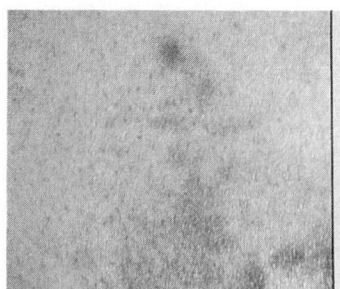

Fig. 38-6 Comparision of stage I pressure ulcers in light and darkly pigmented clients. *(Courtesy Convatec.)*

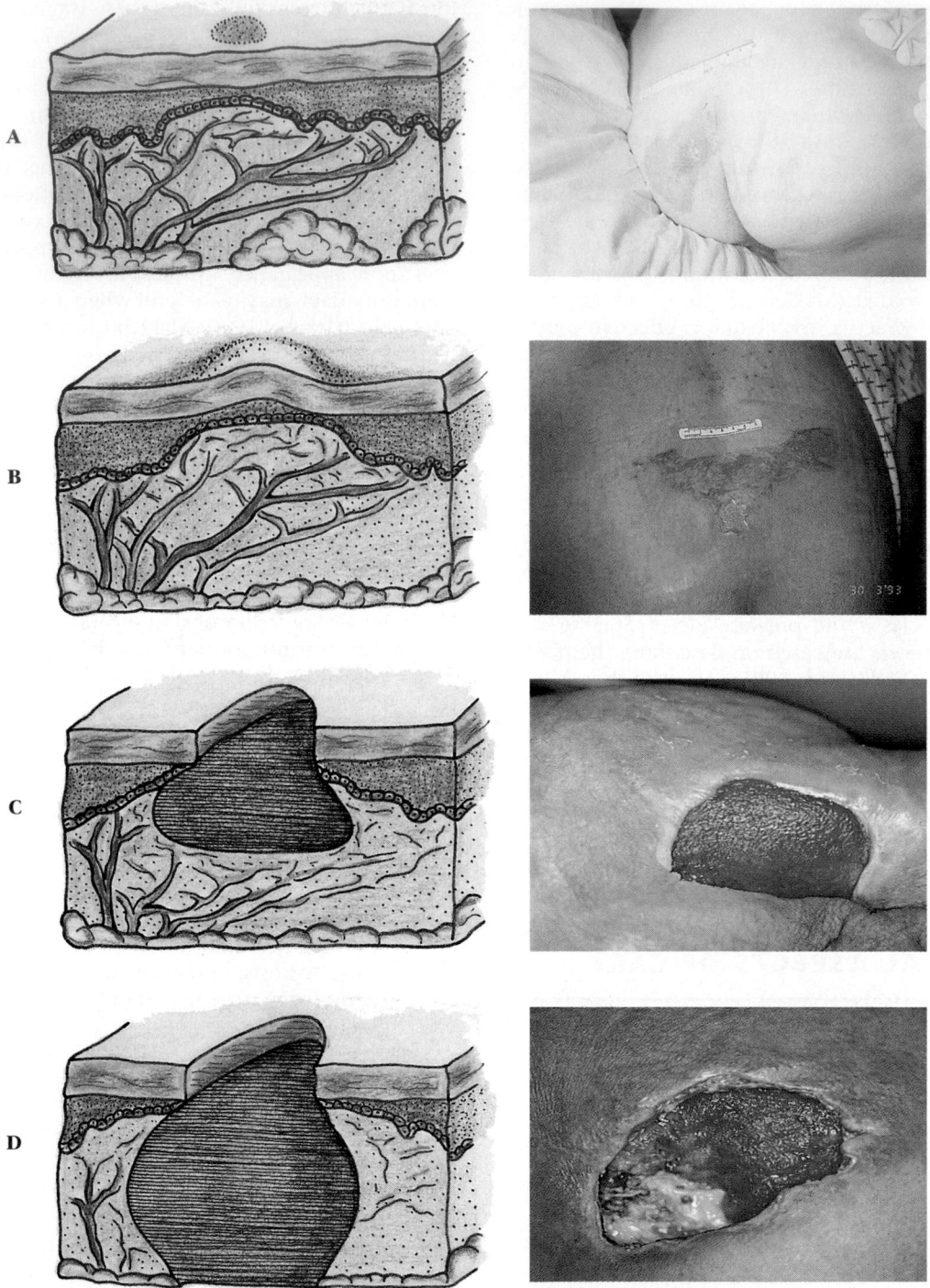

Fig. 38-7 Diagram of Stages. **A,** Stage I pressure ulcer. **B,** Stage II pressure ulcer. **C,** Stage III pressure ulcer. **D,** Stage IV pressure ulcer. *(Courtesy Laurel Wiersma, RN, MSN, Clinical Nurse Specialist, Barnes Hospital, St Louis, Mo.)*

reverse order to measure improvement in a pressure ulcer. In the literature this incorrect idea of using staging numbers to measure pressure ulcer healing is referred to as *downstaging*.

Another method of wound classification is by the color of the wound, which identifies its healing phase. Wounds that are necrotic are classified as black wounds (Fig. 38-8, *A*); wounds with exudate and yellow fibrous debris are classified

as yellow wounds (Fig. 38-8, *B*); and wounds that are in the active healing phase and are clean with pink to red granulation and epithelial tissue are classified as red wounds (Fig. 38-8, *C*). Wounds may be a mixture of colors; for example, 25% yellow and 75% red (Fig. 38-8, *D*). Clinicians may find this color method of classifying wounds to be quick and easy (Krasner, 1995).

There is no consensus about the best way to classify pres-

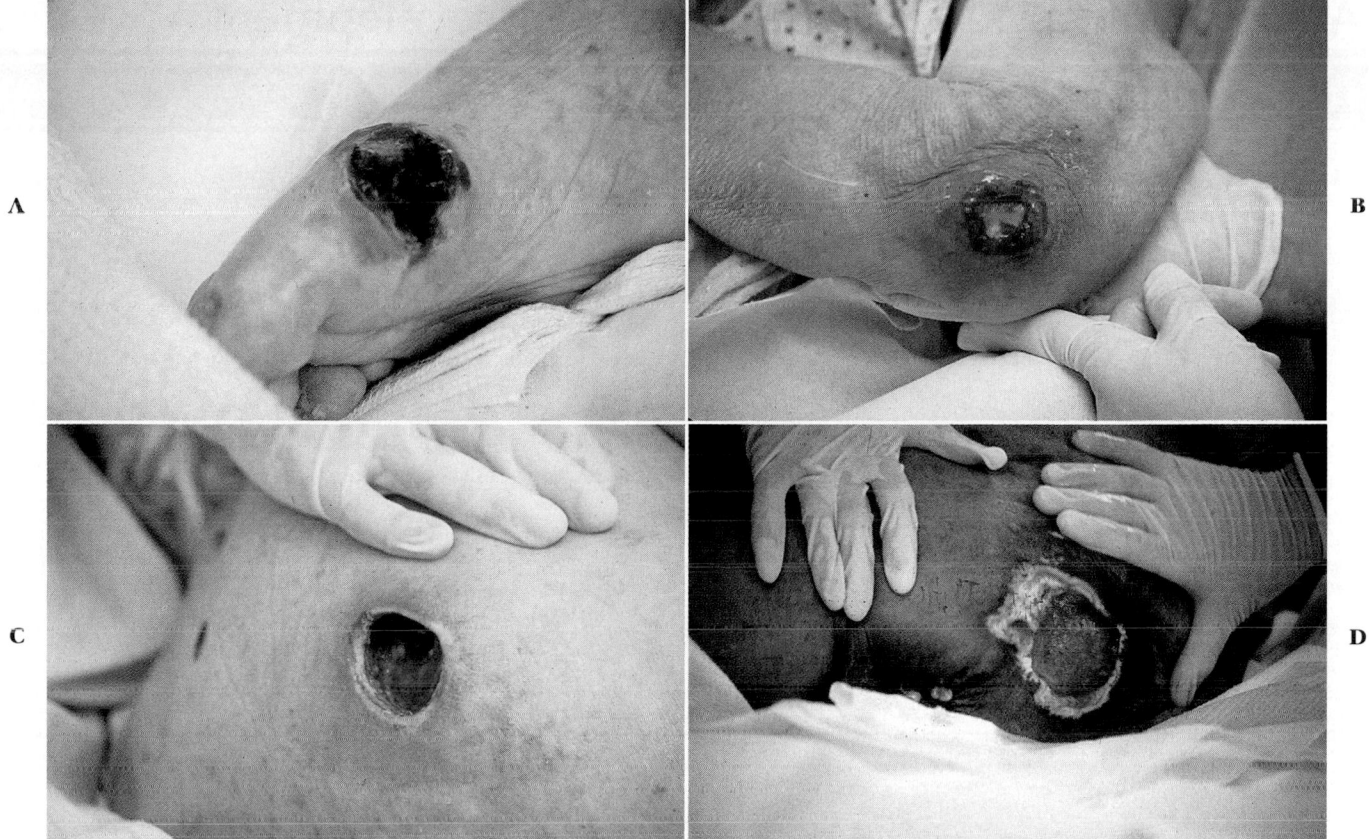

Fig. 38-8 Wounds classified by color assessment. **A,** A "black" wound. **B,** A "yellow" wound. **C,** A "red" wound. **D,** A mixed-color wound. *(Courtesy Scott Health Care—A Mölnlyche Company, Philadelphia, PA.)*

sure ulcers (NPUAP, 1995). However, it is generally agreed that more than staging or color classification should be used to fully describe the pressure ulcer and to give it a comprehensive description (NPUAP, 1995; Maklebust and Margolis, 1995; Cooper, 1995; Bates-Jensen, 1995; Rodeheaver and Stotts, 1995; Harding, 1995; Gentzkow, 1995).

NURSING PROCESS AND PRESSURE ULCERS

 ## Assessment

Baseline and continual assessment data provide critical information about the client's skin integrity and the increased risk for pressure ulcer development. Because pressure ulcers have multiple etiological factors, assessment for pressure ulcers (Procedure 38-1) is not limited to the skin. Therefore, the initial assessment of clients with pressure ulcers has several dimensions (AHCPR, 1994).

PREDICTIVE MEASURES

Upon admission to acute care and rehabilitation hospitals, nursing homes, home care programs, and other health care facilities, individuals should be assessed for risk of pressure ulcer development (AHCPR, 1992). Pressure ulcer risk assessment should be done systematically (AHCPR, 1992; NPUAP, 1989a, 1989b). An assessment tool that is validated for a specific type of client population is recommended (see p. 949). Interpretation of the meaning of the total numerical scores differs with each risk assessment scale. A *low* numerical score on the Braden or Norton scale indicates that a client is at high risk for skin breakdown. A *high* numerical score on the Gosnell or Knoll scale indicates high risk for skin breakdown.

A benefit of the predictive instruments is to increase the nurse's early detection of clients at greatest risk for ulcer development. Once these clients are identified, appropriate interventions are instituted to maintain skin integrity. Reassessment for pressure ulcer risk should be done periodically (AHCPR, 1992). Once a client is identified to be at risk for developing pressure ulcers, prevention strategies proposed by AHCPR (1992) and summarized by NPUAP (1992) in pressure points (see the box on p. 964) should be implemented.

SKIN

The nurse must continually assess the skin for signs of ulcer development. The neurologically impaired client; the

Assessment for Risk of Pressure Ulcer Development

STEPS	RATIONALE
1. Identify client's risk for pressure ulcer formation:	Determines need to administer preventive care and use topical agents for existing ulcers.
a. Paralysis or immobilization caused by restrictive devices	Client is unable to turn or reposition independently.
b. Sensory loss	Client feels no discomfort from pressure.
c. Circulatory disorders	Reduce perfusion of skin's tissue layers.
d. Decreased level of consciousness, sedation, or anesthesia	Client is unable to perceive pressure to turn or reposition independently.
e. Shearing force, friction	Causes skin and underlying subcutaneous layers to adhere to surface of bed. Trauma occurs to underlying tissues.
f. Moisture: incontinence, perspiration, wound drainage, or vomitus	Reduces skin's resistance to pressure from shearing force.
g. Malnutrition	Can lead to weight loss, muscle atrophy, and reduced tissue mass. Less tissue is available to pad between skin and underlying bone. Poor protein, vitamin, and caloric intake limit wound-healing capabilities.
h. Anemia	Decreased hemoglobin level reduces oxygen-carrying capacity of blood and amount of oxygen available to tissues.
i. Infection	Causes increase in metabolic demands of tissues. Accompanying diaphoresis leaves skin moist.
j. Obesity	Poorly vascularized excess adipose tissue is more susceptible to pressure.
k. Cachexia	Causes loss of adipose tissue that protects bony prominences from pressure.
l. Hydration: edema or dehydration	Edematous tissue has decreased blood supply and thereby is less tolerant of pressure, friction, and shearing force. Dehydrated skin is less elastic, and skin turgor is poor.
m. Older adulthood	Skin is less elastic and drier; tissue mass is reduced.
n. Existing pressure ulcers	Limits surfaces available for position changes, placing available tissues at increased risk.
2. Assess condition of skin over regions of pressure (see Fig. 38-9, *A*). Look for the following areas:	Body weight against bony prominences places underlying skin at risk for breakdown.
a. Normal reactive hyperemia	May indicate that tissue was under pressure. Normal reactive hyperemia is normal physiological response to hypoxemia. In dark-skinned persons, skin that was under pressure will appear darker than surrounding skin and may even take on purplish hue (Pires and Muller, 1991). Normal reactive hyperemia over pressure area lasts less than 1 hr. Affected area blanches at fingertip pressure (Pires and Muller, 1991). Abnormal reactive hyperemia lasts longer than 1 hr. Surrounding tissue does not blanch (Pires and Muller, 1991).
b. Blanching	Blanching is normal, expected response.
c. Induration	Localized edema beneath the skin surface, induration commonly occurs with abnormal reactive hyperemia (Pires and Muller, 1991).
d. Pallor and mottling	Persistent hypoxia in tissues that were under pressure is abnormal physiological response.
e. Absence of superficial skin layers	Represents early pressure ulcer formation.
f. Scabs, blisters, or pimples (see Fig. 38-9, *B*)	Early signs of skin damage, but damage to underlying tissue may be more progressive (Pires and Muller, 1991).

Assessment for Risk of Pressure Ulcer Development—cont'd

STEPS	RATIONALE
3. Assess client for additional areas of potential pressure:	Clients at high risk have multiple sites of pressure necrosis.
a. Nares	Site of nasogastric tube.
b. Tongue, lips	Skin and oral mucosa near oral airway and endotracheal tube are high-risk locations.
c. Intravenous sites (especially long-term access sites)	Stress occurs at catheter exit sites.
d. Drainage tubes	There is stress against tissue at exit site.
e. Foley catheter	There is pressure against labia, especially with edema.
4. Observe client for preferred positions when in bed or chair.	Weight of body will be placed on bony prominences. Contractures (flexion and fixation of joint) may result in pressure exerted in unexpected places. Phenomenon is best assessed through observation.
5. Observe client's mobility and ability to initiate and assist with position changes.	Potential for friction and shear increases when client is completely dependent for position changes.
6. Obtain risk score:	Risk score depends on instrument used and predicts client's need for preventive care (AHCPR, 1992).
a. Norton Scale	
b. Gosnell Scale	
c. Braden Scale	
7. Monitor length of time any area of redness persists:	Redness usually persists for half of time hypoxia occurred. For example, redness lasts 15 min, so hypoxia lasted approximately 30 min.
a. Determine appropriate turning interval, which should be turning interval − hypoxia time = suggested interval.	For example, turning interval is 2 hr, hypoxia time is 30 min. 2 hr − 30 min = 1½ hr suggested turning interval
b. Use pressure-relief device, if indicated.	Short turning intervals (e.g., 1-2 hr) may not be realistic. Therefore use of device is recommended.
8. Obtain nutritional assessment data, including serum albumin level, total protein level, hemoglobin level, and IBW percentage (see Chapter 41).	Poor nutritional status decreases skin's and underlying tissue's tolerance to pressure, friction, and shearing force (Hanan and Scheele 1991).
9. Assess client's and family's understanding of risks for pressure ulcers.	Provides opportunity to begin prevention education.
10. Document assessment findings.	Provides baseline data for skin integrity and risk of pressure ulcer development.

chronically ill client in long-term care; the client with diminished mental status; and the intensive care unit (ICU), oncology, hospice, and orthopedic client have increased potential for developing pressure ulcers.

Assessment for tissue pressure indicators includes visual and tactile inspection of the skin (Pires and Muller, 1991). Baseline assessment is performed to determine the client's normal skin characteristics and any actual or potential areas of breakdown. Assessment characteristics of a client's skin should be individualized, depending upon the client's skin tone. Assessment characteristics of darkly pigmented skin have been described in this chapter (see the boxes on pp. 954 and 959). The nurse pays particular attention to areas under casts, traction, splints, braces, collars, or other orthopedic devices. The frequency of pressure checks depends on the schedule of appliance application and the skin's response to the external pressure (Figs. 38-9 and 38-10).

When hyperemia is noted, the nurse documents location, size, and color and reassesses the area after 1 hour (Fig. 38-11, *A*). When abnormal reactive hyperemia is suspected, the nurse can outline the affected area with a marker to make reassessment easier. Another early warning sign of pressure damage is a blister or pimple over the weight-bearing area with possible hyperemia. Pires and Muller (1991) report that a frequently overlooked sign of early pressure is scabbing over of the weight-bearing areas in the absence of trauma (Fig. 38-11, *B*). All of these signs are very early indicators of impaired skin integrity, but damage to the underlying tissue may be more progressive (Fig. 38-11, *C*). Tactile assessment enables the nurse to use palpation to acquire further data about induration and the damage to the skin and underlying tissues.

The nurse palpates the tissue adjacent to the observed area of hyperemia, assessing for blanching with return to normal skin tones in clients with light-toned skin. In addition, the nurse palpates for induration, noting the size in millimeters or centimeters of the induration around the injured area. The nurse *also* notes changes in temperature of the surrounding skin and tissues (Pires and Muller, 1991).

The nurse includes visual and tactile inspection over the

Pressure Ulcer Prevention Points

I. Risk assessment
1. Consider all bed-bound or chair-bound persons, or those whose ability to reposition is impaired, to be at risk for pressure ulcers.
2. Select and use a method of risk assessment, such as the Norton Scale or the Braden Scale, that ensures systematic evaluation of individual risk factors.
3. Assess all at-risk clients at the time of admission to health care facilities and at regular intervals thereafter.
4. Identify all individual risk factors (decreased mental status, moisture, incontinence, nutritional deficits) to direct specific preventive treatments. Modify care according to the individual factors.

II. Skin care and early treatment
1. Inspect the skin at least daily, and document assessment results.
2. Individualize bathing frequency. Use a mild cleansing agent. Avoid hot water and excessive friction.
3. Assess and treat incontinence. When incontinence cannot be controlled, cleanse skin at time of soiling, use a topical moisture barrier, and select underpads or briefs that are absorbent and provide a quick drying surface to the skin.
4. Use moisturizers for dry skin. Minimize environmental factors leading to dry skin such as low humidity and cold air.
5. Do not massage over bony prominences.
6. Use proper positioning, transferring, and turning techniques to minimize skin injury caused by friction and shear forces.
7. Use dry lubricants (cornstarch) or protective coverings to reduce friction injury.
8. Identify and correct factors compromising protein/caloric intake, and consider nutritional supplementation/support for nutritionally compromised persons.
9. Institute a rehabilitation program to maintain or improve mobility/activity status.
10. Monitor and document interventions and outcomes.

III. Mechanical loading and support surfaces
1. Reposition bed-bound persons at least every 2 hours, chair-bound persons every hour.
2. Use a written repositioning schedule.
3. Place at-risk persons on a pressure-reducing mattress/chair cushion. Do not use donut-type devices.
4. Consider postural alignment, distribution of weight, balance and stability, and pressure relief when positioning persons in chairs or wheelchairs.
5. Teach chair-bound persons, who are able, to shift weight every 15 minutes.
6. Use lifting device (e.g., trapeze or bed linen) to move rather than drag persons during transfer and position changes.
7. Use pillows or foam wedges to keep bony prominences such as knees and ankles from direct contact with each other.
8. Use devices that totally relieve pressure on the heels (e.g., place pillows under the calf to raise the heels off the bed).
9. Avoid positioning directly on the trochanter when using the side-lying position (use the 30-degree lateral inclined position).
10. Elevate the head of the bed as little (maximum 30-degree angle) and for as short a time as possible.

IV. Education
1. Implement educational programs for the prevention of pressure ulcers that are structured, organized, comprehensive, and directed at all levels of health care providers, clients, family, and care givers.
2. Include information on:
   a. Etiology of and risk factors for pressure ulcers
   b. Risk assessment tools and their application
   c. Skin assessment
   d. Selection/use of support surfaces
   e. Development/implementation of individualized programs of skin care
   f. Demonstration of positioning to decrease risk of tissue breakdown
   g. Accurate documentation of pertinent data
3. Include built-in mechanisms to evaluate program effectiveness in preventing pressure ulcers.

Modified from National Pressure Ulcer Advisory Panel (NPUAP), 1989.

body areas most frequently at risk for pressure ulcer development (Fig. 38-12). When a client lays in bed or sits in a chair, body weight is heavily placed on certain bony prominences. Body surfaces subjected to the greatest weight or pressure are at greatest risk for pressure ulcer formation. Remember that "time wounds all heels" (Helt, 1991).

MOBILITY

Assessment includes documenting the level of mobility and the potential effects of impaired mobility on skin integrity. Assessment of mobility should also include obtaining data regarding the quality of muscle tone and strength. For example, the nurse determines whether the client can lift the weight off the ischial tuberosities and can roll the body to a side-lying position. The client may have adequate range of motion (ROM) to move independently into a more protective position. Finally the nurse notes the client's activity tolerance (see Chapter 37).

Mobility must be assessed as part of baseline data. If the client has some degree of independence in mobility, the nurse reinforces the frequency of position changes and measures to relieve pressure. The frequency of position changes is based on ongoing skin assessment and is revised as data change. The following case study illustrates this point.

CASE STUDY A nurse is caring for Calvin Jones, a 40-year-old, completely rehabilitated paraplegic who is hospitalized for a cholecystectomy. The nurse obtains baseline assessment data regarding skin integrity and mobility status, and notes that the client has intact skin, has never had a pressure ulcer, and is able to lift his body weight off his ischial tuberosities. The nurse also notes that the client routinely performs pressure-relieving exercises every 30 minutes for 15 seconds when sitting in his wheelchair at work and at home. ∎

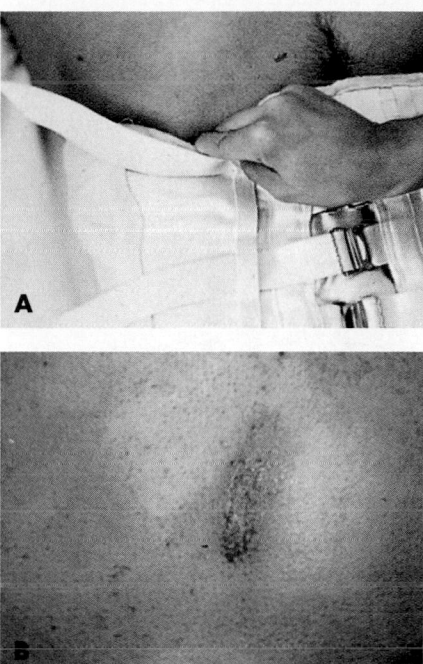

Fig. 38-9 Benign devices such as this corset, **A,** may result in scabbing or blistering, **B,** resulting from external pressure. *(From Pires M, Muller A: Progressions 3(3):3, 1991.)*

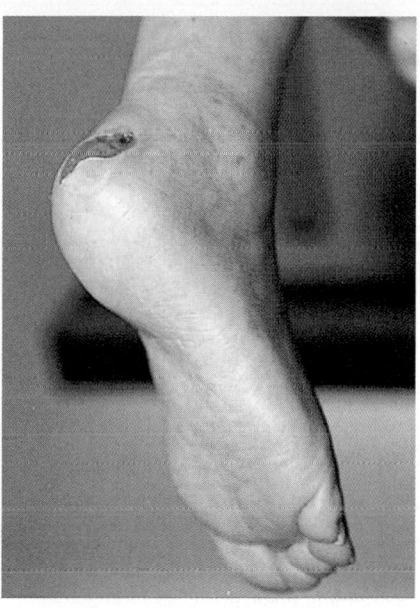

Fig. 38-10 Formation of pressure ulcer on heel resulting from external pressure from mattress of bed.

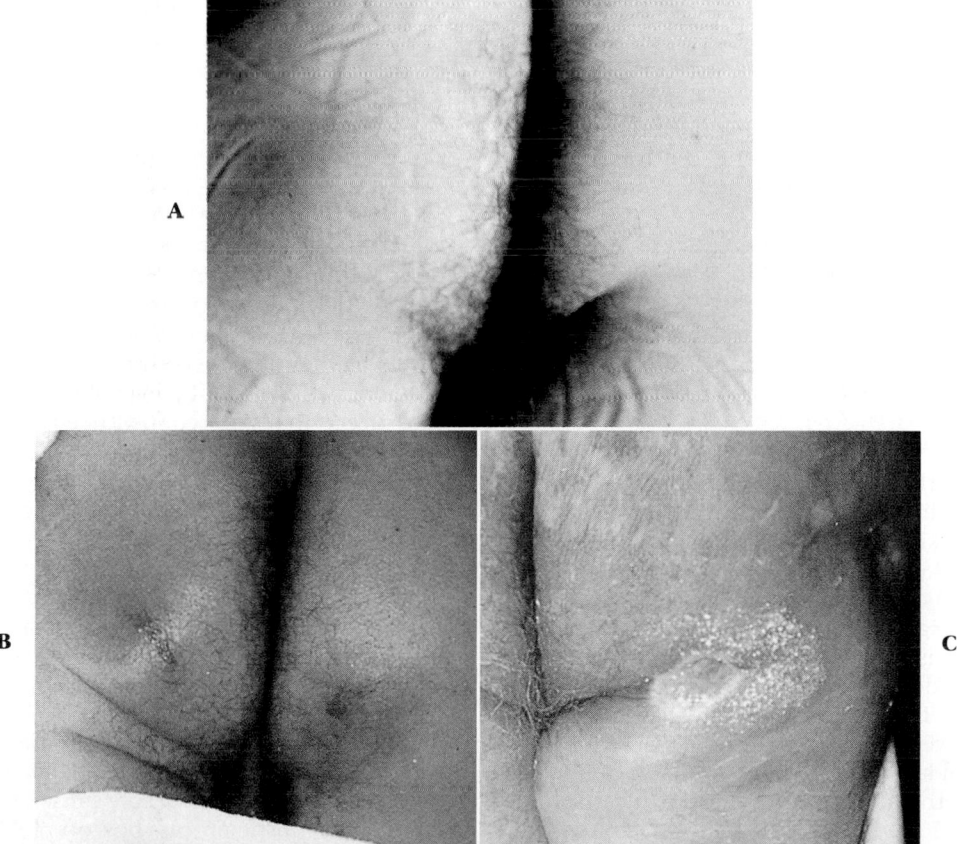

Fig. 38-11 A, Hyperemia on ischial tuberosities. **B,** Scabbing over bony prominences is a sign of excessive pressure. **C,** Deeper stages of ulceration. *(From Pires M, Mueller M: Progressions 3(3):3, 1991.)*

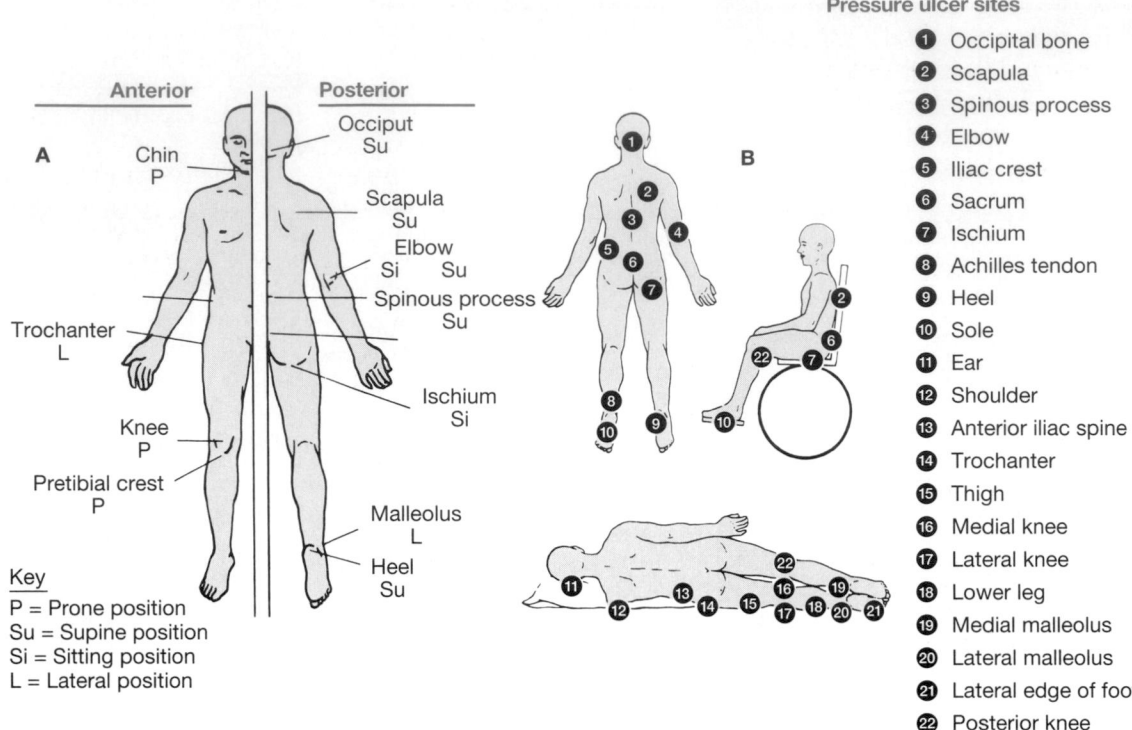

Pressure ulcer sites

❶ Occipital bone
❷ Scapula
❸ Spinous process
❹ Elbow
❺ Iliac crest
❻ Sacrum
❼ Ischium
❽ Achilles tendon
❾ Heel
❿ Sole
⓫ Ear
⓬ Shoulder
⓭ Anterior iliac spine
⓮ Trochanter
⓯ Thigh
⓰ Medial knee
⓱ Lateral knee
⓲ Lower leg
⓳ Medial malleolus
⓴ Lateral malleolus
㉑ Lateral edge of foot
㉒ Posterior knee

Fig. 38-12 A, Bony prominence most frequently underlying pressure ulcer. **B,** Pressure ulcer sites. *(From Trelease CC: Ostomy/Wound Manage 20:46, 1988.)*

Because Mr. Jones will have general anesthesia, his ability to perform pressure-relieving exercises will change, and the nursing care plan must include nursing measures designed to maintain skin integrity for this client. The nurse must be meticulous when assessing Mr. Jones' pressure sites. Normal reactive hyperemia must be present, because once abnormal reactive hyperemia occurs, it may take as long as 2 weeks of non–weight-bearing or total pressure relief to heal completely (Pires and Muller, 1991). As a result, if attention is not paid to skin integrity for this client, his lost work time can increase by an additional 2 weeks beyond the normal postoperative course of treatment.

NUTRITIONAL STATUS

An assessment of the client's nutritional status should be an integral part of the initial assessment data for clients at risk for impaired skin integrity (Breslow and Bergstrom, 1994; Finucane, 1995; Konstantinides and Lehmann, 1993; Walter et al, 1994). A client who is malnourished or cachexic and whose body weight is less than 90% of IBW or a client whose body weight is greater than 110% of IBW has an increased risk for the development of pressure ulcers (Hanan and Scheele 1991). The percentage of IBW alone is not a good predictor; however, when used with a low serum albumin or total protein level, the client's percentage of IBW can have an impact on the occurrence of pressure ulcers.

PAIN

Until recently, little has been written or researched about pain and pressure ulcers. AHCPR (1994) has recommended that the assessment and management of pain be included

in the care of clients with pressure ulcers. Additionally, AHCPR (1994) points out the need for research on pain in clients with pressure ulcers. One of the first studies to quantify the pain experience in hospitalized clients with pressure ulcers was done by Dallam et al. (1995). In this study, 59.1% of the clients reported the presence of pain using the visual analog scale; 68.2% reported the presence of pressure ulcer pain using the FACES pain rating scale. In sharp contrast to those reporting pain, pain medicine was used by 2.3% of clients. Some of the implications for practice suggested by the researchers (Dallam et al, 1995) are to add the evaluation of the client's level of pain to assessment of pressure ulcers, that pain control needs frequent reassessment to evaluate effectiveness, and that educational programs are needed to sensitize health care providers to the existence of pain associated with pressure ulcers.

 Nursing Diagnosis

Assessment reveals clusters of data that indicate whether an actual or a risk for impaired skin integrity exists. The nursing diagnosis is developed based on assessment data (see the nursing diagnoses box on p. 967). In addition, assessment data should contain appropriate defining characteristics to support the diagnostic label. The nursing diagnoses should also include a probable cause of the client's problem (see the diagnostic process box on p. 967).

A client may have one or more problems related to impaired skin integrity. Many alterations in physiological functioning are related to skin breakdown. For example, a client may develop a kidney infection, which produces

Examples of NANDA Nursing Diagnoses Related to Impaired Skin Integrity

Impaired physical mobility *related to:*
- Effects of bed rest
- Decreased strength
- Musculoskeletal impairment

Actual or risk for impaired skin integrity *related to:*
- Restricted mobility
- Pressure on skin's surface
- Shearing force
- Friction
- Moisture

Risk for infection *related to:*
- Open wound

Pain *related to:*
- Stage 2 pressure ulcer

---

fever and diaphoresis. The resulting increased skin moisture may then increase the potential for skin breakdown.

Planning

The nurse plans therapeutic interventions for clients with actual or potential risks to skin integrity. These therapies are designed according to severity of risks to the client, and the plan is individualized according to developmental stage, level of health, individual's wishes, and goals of overall health management (AHCPR, 1994).

Planning care also involves an understanding of the client's need to maintain independence. The nurse and client work together to establish ways of maintaining skin integrity. Clients at risk for hazards of pressure ulcers require a nursing care plan directed at meeting their actual or potential positioning, nutritional, and mobility needs (see the care plan on p. 968). The plan is based on one or more of the following client goals:

1. Maintaining vitality of the skin through hygiene and topical care
2. Reducing and preventing injuries to the skin and musculoskeletal system from pressure, friction, and shearing force
3. Improving nutritional intake
4. Improving mobility and activity
5. Improving or maintaining body alignment
6. Learning appropriate local wound care

These goals and the organization of the nursing intervention content are based on the AHCPR Pressure Ulcer Guidelines, 1992, 1994.

Implementation

When the client is immobile, the major risk to the skin is the formation of pressure ulcers. Nursing interventions focus on prevention or treatment of pressure ulcers.

PREVENTION

The first step in prevention is to assess the client's risk factors. The nurse then reduces environmental factors that accelerate pressure ulcer formation, such as high room temperature (causing diaphoresis), moisture, or wrinkled bed linen.

Early identification of clients at risk and their risk factors aids the nurse in preventing pressure ulcers. Procedure 38-1 identifies frequent pressure ulcer sites. Prevention minimizes the impact that risk factors or contributing fac-

---

Sample Nursing Diagnostic Process for Impaired Skin Integrity

ASSESSMENT ACTIVITIES	DEFINING CHARACTERISTICS	NURSING DIAGNOSIS
Observe skin over bony prominences or area under external pressure (e.g., casts, splints, cervical collars, braces, and other orthotic devices).	Blanching hyperemia Nonblanching hyperemia Scab formation Blister formation	**Actual** or **risk for impaired skin integrity** related to pressure
Palpate skin over bony prominences or areas under external pressure (e.g., casts, splints, cervical collars, braces, and other orthotic devices).	Induration Edema Tenderness Moisture Heat	
Observe skin for moisture.	Wound drainage Diaphoresis Vomitus Moisture from oxygen therapy equipment Incontinence	
Observe mobility and activity status.	Fatigue Immobility Restricted mobility	

NURSING DIAGNOSIS: **Actual or risk for impaired skin integrity** related to pressure on bony prominences
DEFINITION: Impaired skin integrity is the state in which an individual's skin is at risk of being adversely altered (Kim, McFarland, and McLane, 1995).

GOALS	EXPECTED OUTCOMES	INTERVENTIONS	RATIONALE
Injury to skin and underlying tissue resulting from pressure on bony prominences will be prevented.	Skin will remain intact (6/1). Normal reactive hyperemia will occur (6/1). Blanching will occur (6/1).	Instruct client to shift body weight every 15 min when sitting.	Redistribution of body weight every 15 min when sitting relieves the downward pressure on the ischial tuberosities (Pires and Muller, 1991).
		Reposition client every 90 min.	Repositioning removes pressure and allows normal hyperemic response. Frequency of turning is based on initial assessment (Maklebust, 1991b).
		Obtain oscillating air mattress for client's bed.	Distributes pressure over a greater area and away from bony pressure points.
Injury to skin and underlying tissue resulting from pressure on bony prominences will be reduced by 6/20.	Wound size will decrease (6/10). Wound drainage will decrease (6/20). Decreased hyperemia will be observed in affected areas (6/15).	Apply dressing to wound.	Dressings protect underlying skin and remove drainage from surface of wound (Maklebust, 1991b).
		Implement measures listed above to reduce risk of other pressure ulcer development.	Clients with pressure ulcer development are at greater risk for new ulcers and need meticulous preventive nursing measures to prevent more ulcers (NPUAP, 1989b).

Table 38-4	**A Quick Guide to Prevention**
RISK FACTOR	**NURSING INTERVENTIONS**
Immobility	Establish individualized turning schedule. Reduce shear and friction. Provide pressure-relief surface.
Inactivity	Provide assistive devices to increase activity.
Incontinence	Assess need for incontinence management. Clean and dry skin after soiling.
Malnutrition	Provide adequate nutritional and fluid intake. Consult dietitian for nutritional evaluation.
Diminished sensation, decreased mental status	Assess client's and family's ability to provide care. Educate care giver regarding pressure ulcer prevention.
Impaired skin integrity	Avoid pressure. Do not use donut-shaped cushions. Lubricate skin. Do not massage red areas. Do not use heat lamps.

Modified from Maklebust J, Sieggreen M: *Pressure ulcers: guidelines for prevention and nursing management,* West Dundee, Ill, 1991, S-N Publications.

tors may have on pressure ulcer development. The box on p. 964 and Table 38-4 outline some universal nursing interventions for the prevention of pressure ulcers. Three major areas of nursing interventions for prevention of pressure ulcers are skin care, which includes hygiene and topical skin care; mechanical loading and support surfaces, which include positioning and the use of therapeutic beds and mattresses; and education (AHCPR, 1992).

Hygiene and Skin Care. The nurse must keep the client's skin clean and dry. In this initial line of defense for preventing skin breakdown, the client's skin is continually assessed by nurses, rather than being delegated to other personnel. In addition, the types of products available for skin care are numerous, and their uses need to be matched to the specific needs of the client (Hess, 1995; Maklebust, 1991a, 1991b).

When the skin is cleaned, soaps and hot water are avoided (AHCPR, 1992). Soaps and alcohol-based lotions cause drying and leave an alkaline residue. The alkaline residue discourages the growth of normal skin bacteria, thus promoting an overgrowth of opportunistic bacteria, which can then enter an open wound (Barnes, 1987).

After the skin is cleansed and completely dried, protective moisturizer should be applied to keep the epidermis well lubricated but not oversaturated (AHCPR, 1992). Cornstarch is a dry lubricant and helps to reduce friction (Maklebust, 1991b). A & D, Unicare, and Pericare are some

Table 38-5	Measures to Reduce Risk of Pressure Ulcers: Practical Management of Loose Bowel Movements Related to Tube Feeding*	
POSSIBLE CAUSE(S)	**TREATMENT**	
Antibiotic use	Lactobacilli per feeding tube (2 packets tid × 3 doses)	
Lactose intolerance	Use lactose-free liquid diet	
Choleretic diarrhea	Questran, 1 g q6–8h and/or Titralac tabs, 2 q6–8h	
Mild enterotoxigenic pathogens	Pepto-Bismol, 30 ml q6–8h	
Severe enterotoxigenic pathogens with WBCs in stool-on Gram stain	Selected antibiotic per stool culture and sensitivity testing	
Insufficient fiber	Fiber supplement, 3 g q6–8h	
Idiopathic	Lomotil, Imodium, Paregoric (Warning: This may cause reactive constipation.)	

From Bergstrom N et al: *Treatment of pressure ulcers,* AHCPR pub no 95-0652, Rockville, Md, 1994, DHHS, PHS, AHCPR.
*Any or all treatments may be indicated. *tid,* Three times daily; *q,* every; *h,* hours; *WBCs,* white blood cells.

examples of bland, water-repellent ointments that protect the skin from moisture (AHCPR, 1992). In addition, these ointments are easily cleansed from the skin (Barnes, 1987). When using any water-repellent ointment, the nurse must completely clean the area on a routine basis. Ointment, when left in place too long, can be a medium for bacteria and can cause further skin problems, such as maceration, yeast, and other infections.

Efforts should be made to control, contain, or correct incontinence, perspiration, or wound drainage. Clinicians may find *AHCPR, Urinary Incontinence in Adults: Clinical Practice Guideline* (1992) helpful in assessing and managing urinary incontinence. Another resource from AHCPR (1994) is a table depicting management of loose bowel movements for clients receiving tube feedings in the pressure ulcer treatment guidelines (Table 38-5). When clients are incontinent, the area should be cleansed and a skin barrier applied. These barriers protect the skin from excessive moisture and toxins from urine or stool (Maklebust, 1991b).

The expertise of an enterostomal therapy (ET) nurse or a master's prepared nurse certified in continence nursing should be used in planning and implementing care for incontinent clients. Methods for controlling or containing incontinence vary. After an assessment by specially educated nurses as to the cause and type of incontinence, the most appropriate method to use for an individual client can be decided. Urinary incontinence can be treated with behavioral techniques, medication, and surgery. Behavioral techniques are used to help clients learn ways to control their bladder and sphincter muscles. Two examples are bladder training (also called bladder retraining), which is especially useful for clients with urge incontinence, and pelvic muscle exercises (also called Kegel exercises). Habit training (also called time voiding) and prompted voiding are other strategies used to treat urinary incontinence. Biofeedback, electrical stimulation, and alterations of the physical and social environment have all been used as part of the treatment plan for clients with incontinence. Although they should not be the first method considered, urinary collection devices may be used at times as part of the incontinence treatment plan. Condom catheters and penile clamps are some of the supportive devices attached exter-

nally that may be used on male clients. Clients can also be taught to do intermittent and/or self catheterization.

Use of absorbent pads and garments should be considered *only* after the above described incontinent treatment modalities have been unsuccessful. Although controversial, absorbent products (absorptive underpads and garments such as adult diapers or incontinence briefs) may be part of the treatment plan for some clients who are incontinent. The nurse must only use those products that drain moisture away from the client's skin (AHCPR, 1992). The absorptive garments have a quilted lining and contain a polymer filling. Disposable, plastic-lined underpads should not be placed directly under the client's skin because they do not drain moisture away from the client's skin. These products protect the bed, not the client. The plastic also causes diaphoresis, which can lead to skin maceration. Moist, macerated skin is more susceptible to pressure, friction, and the shearing force, so tissue breakdown occurs more rapidly. If these pads are necessary to absorb body fluids, they should be placed in pillowcases under a draw sheet. Proper use of these products, meticulous skin care, and frequent changes are all part of the client plan of care when absorptive products are used (AHCPR, 1992).

Positioning. Positioning interventions are designed to reduce pressure and shearing force to the skin. Keeping the head of the bed to 30 degrees or less will decrease the chance of pressure ulcer development from shearing forces (AHCPR, 1992). The immobilized client's position should be changed according to activity level, perceptual ability, and daily routines (Pajk et al, 1986; Bergstrom et al, 1987). Therefore a standard turning interval of 1½ to 2 hours may not prevent pressure ulcer development in some clients. AHCPR (1992) recommends that a written turning and positioning schedule be used. Clients should be repositioned at least every 2 hours. When doing full position changes, positioning devices should be used to protect bony prominences (AHCPR, 1992, 1994; Jacobs, 1994) (see Fig. 38-12). A 30-degree lateral position is recommended by AHCPR (1992) (Fig. 38-13). To prevent friction injuries, *lift* rather than *drag* the client when changing positions.

Clients able to sit in a chair should be limited to 2 hours or less. Again, the exact time is individualized, but the nurse should not allow the client to sit for a period longer

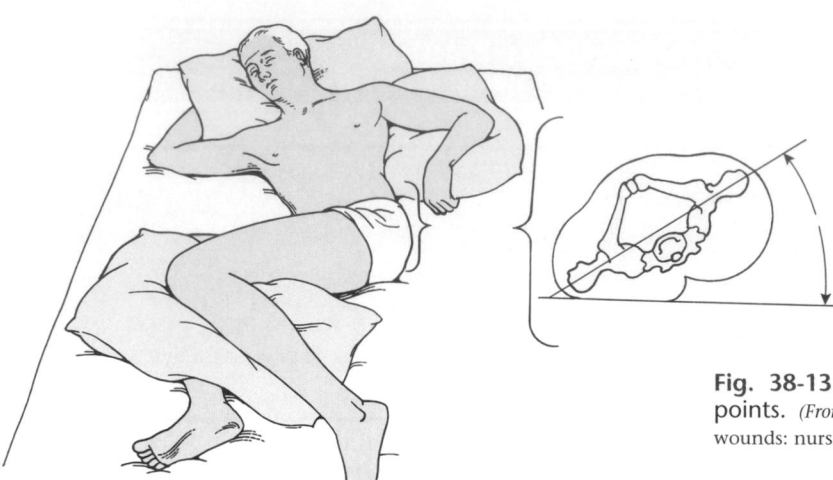

Fig. 38-13 Thirty-degree lateral position to avoid pressure points. *(From Bryant et al: Pressure ulcer. In Bryant RA, ed:* Acute chronic wounds: nursing management, *St Louis, 1992, Mosby.)*

than the recommended time that was calculated during assessment (see Procedure 38-1, p. 962). Thus if the interval is every 1½ hours, the client should remain in a sitting position less than 1½ hours. In the sitting position, the pressure on the ischial tuberosities is greater than when in the supine position (Pajk et al, 1986). In addition, a client at risk such as an individual with a spinal cord injury, sitting in a chair should be taught or assisted to shift weight every 15 minutes (AHCPR, 1992). Shifting weight provides short-term relief on the ischial tuberosities. A client should also sit on foam, gel, or an air cushion to redistribute weight so that it is not all on the ischium. Rigid and donut-shaped cushions are contraindicated because they reduce blood supply to the area, resulting in wider areas of ischemia (AHCPR, 1992, 1994; Maklebust, 1991a).

After the client is repositioned, the nurse reassesses the skin. Identifying characteristics that might indicate early signs of tissue ischemia in darkly pigmented skin can be found in the boxes on pp. 954 and 959. For clients with light-tone skin, the nurse observes for normal reactive hyperemia and blanching. The reddened areas should *never* be massaged. This change in practice is a result of nursing research (Maklebust, 1991a; AHCPR, 1992). Massaging the reddened areas increases breaks in the capillaries in the underlying tissues and increases the risk of pressure ulcer formation.

Support Surfaces (Therapeutic Beds and Mattresses). A variety of support surfaces, including specialty beds and mattresses, have been designed to reduce the hazards of immobility to the skin and musculoskeletal system. However, none eliminates the need for meticulous nursing care. No single device eliminates the effects of pressure on the skin. It is important to understand the difference between a pressure-*reducing* and a pressure-*relieving* support surface or device. A **pressure relieving** device reduces the interface pressure (the pressure between the body and the support surface) below 32 mm Hg (capillary closing pressure). **Pressure reducing** devices also reduce the interface pressure, but not necessarily below the capillary closing pressure (AHCPR, 1994).

When selecting specialty beds, the nurse must thoroughly assess clients' needs. A flow diagram (Fig. 38-14) and table of support surface characteristics (Table 38-6) as-

sists the nurse in clinical decision making. In selecting a support surface, the nurse should know its purpose. The Support Surface Consensus Panel identified three purposes of support surfaces: comfort, postural control, and pressure management (Krouskop and van Rijswijk, 1995). Furthermore, they identified nine parameters to use when evaluating support surfaces and their relationship to each of the three purposes: life expectancy, skin moisture control, skin temperature control, redistribution of pressure, product service requirements, fall safety, infection control, flammability, and client/product friction (Krouskop and van Rijswijk, 1995). A summary of AHCPR (1994) recommendations regarding the use of support surfaces is found in the box below. In addition, Table 38-7 lists the specific device, client assessment, and pertinent nurse alerts for using the equipment safely. Clients and families need to be taught the reason for and proper use of the beds or mat-

---

AHCPR 1994 Support Surface Recommendations

- Assess all clients with existing pressure ulcers to determine their risk for developing additional pressure ulcers. If the client remains at risk, use a pressure-reducing surface.
- Use a static support surface if a client can assume a variety of positions without bearing weight on a pressure ulcer and without "bottoming out."
- Use a dynamic support surface if the client cannot assume a variety of positions without bearing weight on a pressure ulcer, if the client fully compresses the static support surface, or if the pressure ulcer does not show evidence of healing.
- If a client has large stage III or stage IV pressure ulcers on multiple turning surfaces, a low–air-loss bed or an air-fluidized bed may be indicated.
- When excess moisture on intact skin is a potential source of maceration and skin breakdown, a support surface that provides air flow can be important in drying the skin and preventing additional pressure ulcers.

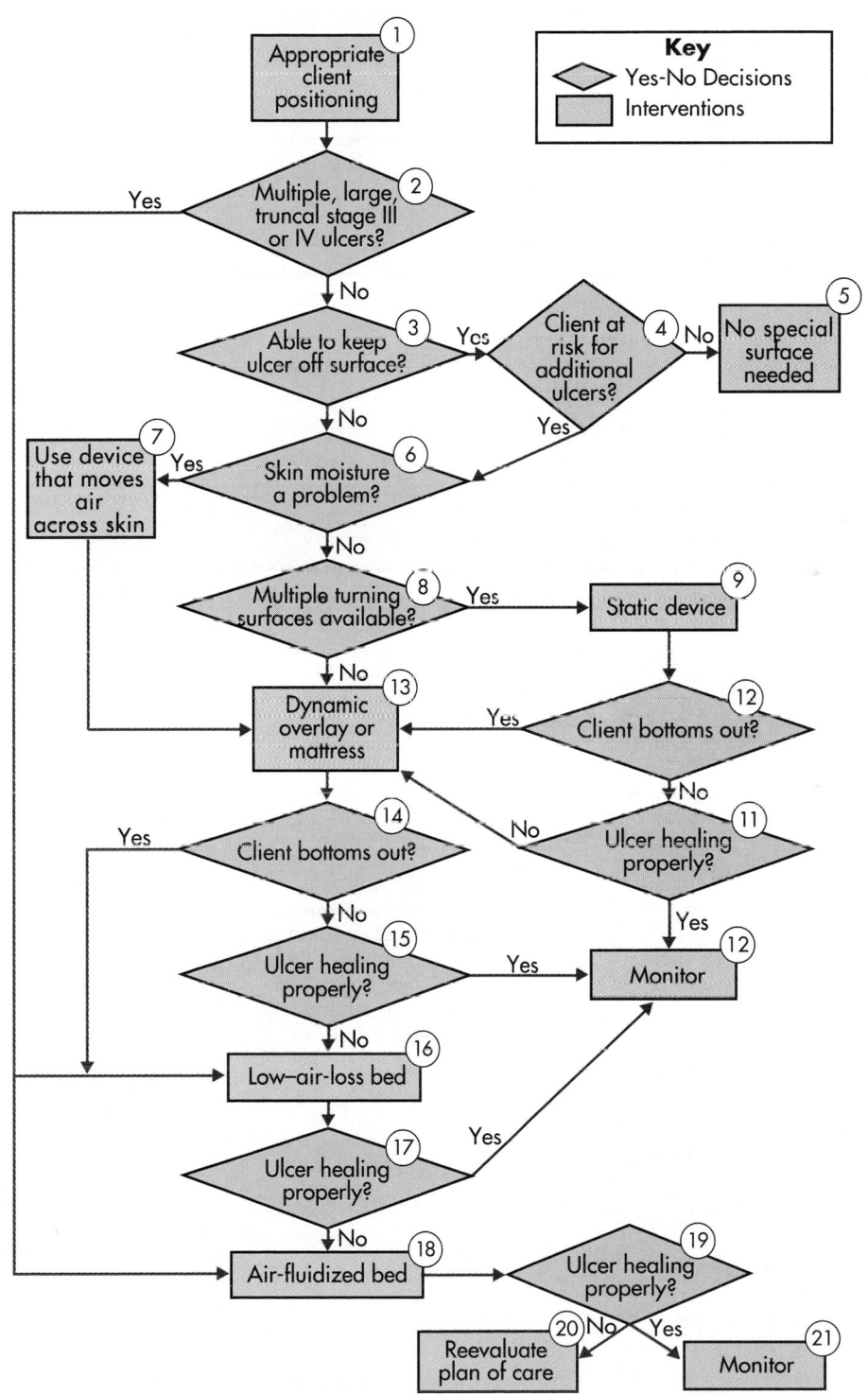

Fig. 38-14 Support surfaces flow diagram. (From AHCPR, 1994, *Clinical Guidelines,* p. 36.)

Table 38-6	Selected Characteristics for Classes of Support Surfaces					
	SUPPORT DEVICES					
PERFORMANCE CHARACTERISTICS	**AIR-FLUIDIZED**	**LOW–AIR-LOSS**	**ALTERNATING AIR**	**STATIC FLOTATION (AIR OR WATER)**	**FOAM**	**STANDARD MATTRESS**
Increased support area	Yes	Yes	Yes	Yes	Yes	No
Low moisture retention	Yes	Yes	No	No	No	No
Reduced heat accumulation	Yes	Yes	No	No	No	No
Shear reduction	Yes	?	Yes	Yes	No	No
Pressure reduction	Yes	Yes	Yes	Yes	Yes	No
Dynamic	Yes	Yes	Yes	No	No	No
Cost per day	High	High	Moderate	Low	Low	Low

From Bergstrom N et al: *Treatment of pressure ulcers,* AHCPR pub no 95 0652 Rockville, Md, 1994, DHHS, PHS, AHCPR.

Table 38-7	Support Beds and Mattresses		
BRAND NAMES	**MANUFACTURER**	**INDICATIONS**	**COMMENTS**
LOW–AIR-LOSS			
Flexicair	Support Systems International	Pressure relief in clients in whom repositioning is difficult or contraindicated	Nurse must consider need for built-in or underbed scales (may cost extra and be optional feature).
KinAir	Kinetic Concepts		Nurse should use only incontinence pads recommended by manufacturer.
Mediscus	Mediscus Group		Nurse cannot adjust temperature to cool feverish client.
OSCILLATING LOW–AIR-LOSS			
BioDyne	Kinetic Concepts	Hemodynamically unstable clients who cannot tolerate sudden changes in position	If client has small frame, it is difficult to prevent sliding, and there is higher risk of falls.
Pulmonair-40	Mediscus Group	Clients with documented pneumonia and unmanageable secretions requiring frequent position changes to mobilize secretions	Movement of bed may contribute to agitation or cause motion sickness in some clients.
Rescue	Support Systems International		Nurse cannot adjust temperature to cool feverish client. Nurse should use only incontinence pads recommended by manufacturer.
OSCILLATING SUPPORT SURFACE			
Keane Mobility System	Mediscus Group	Clients who require frequent turning but have unstable spines	Movement of bed raises risk of skin shearing on support surface.
RotoRest	Kinetic Concepts		Movement of bed may contribute to agitation or cause motion sickness in some clients.
Tilt and Turn Paragon 9000	Egerton Hospital Equipment, UK		Bed does not have built-in scales.
AIR-FLUIDIZED			
Air Plus Therapy System	Air Plus	Clients who require minimal movement to prevent skin damage by shearing forces (e.g., posterior grafts, flaps)	Several people or lift are required to transfer client to and from bed.
Clinitron	Support Systems International		Air flow increases evaporative water loss and can contribute to dehydration. Foam wedge is needed for head elevation.

Modified from Willey T: *Am J Nurs* 89:1142, 1989.

Table 38-7	Support Beds and Mattresses—cont'd		
BRAND NAMES	**MANUFACTURER**	**INDICATIONS**	**COMMENTS**
FluidAir	Kinetic Concepts		Bed requires routine cleaning of beads (check with manufacturer for frequency).
Skytron	Skytron		Nurse should use only incontinence pads recommended by manufacturer.
OBESE			
Burke Bariatric Treatment System	Kinetic Concepts	Clients over 300 lb	Pressure relief capabilities may vary from client to client.
MegaBed Paragon 8000/8500	Egerton Hospital Equipment, UK		
SPECIAL FUNCTION			
TheraPulse	Kinetic Concepts	Same as low–air-loss beds, plus pulsation	No evidence yet exists to support therapeutic effect of pulsation.
Rescue	Support Systems International	Clients needing low–air-loss therapy, oscillating therapy, or pulsation therapy	
FOAM			
Bio Gard	Bio Clinic	Reduction of pressure in clients at risk	Nurse should check with manufacturer regarding flammability of product and to determine whether flame retardation is removed with washing or sterilization.
Geo-Matt	Span-America	Adjunct to care of clients with established ulcer if client can be turned frequently and positioned off ulcer	
High Float	Pre-Foam		
STATIC AIR MATTRESS			
Clini-Care	Gaymar Industries		Nurse should avoid puncturing it (requires mattress replacement with some models).
Sof-Care	Gaymar Industries		Nurse follows manufacturer's instructions for checking inflation level (every 8 hr and as needed).
Roho (see the illustration below)	Roho		Nurse checks for increased perspiration because of plastic surface.
First Step	Kinetic Concepts		
KoalaKair	Pharmaseal		
ALTERNATING AIR MATTRESS			
Bio Flote	Bio Clinic		Nurse should follow manufacturer's instructions for proper functioning of equipment; it may require some assembly.
Grant PCA Systems	Grant		
WATER MATTRESS			
Lotus Water Flotation Mattress	Lotus		Nurse should avoid puncturing it (check every shift and as needed for water leakage).

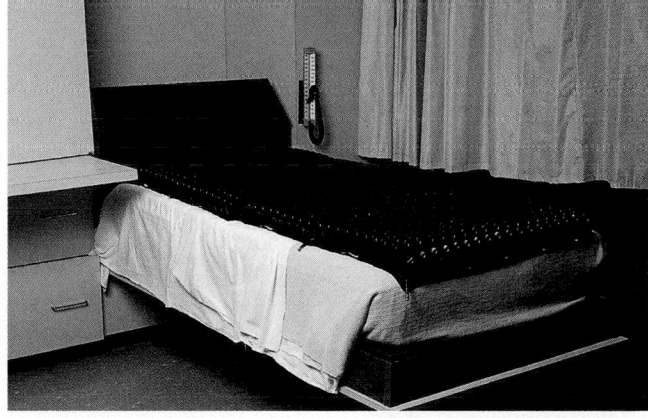

Placing a Client on a Support Surface Mattress

STEPS	RATIONALE
1. Assess condition of skin, especially over dependent sites and bony prominences.	Provides baseline to determine change in skin integrity or change in existing pressure ulcers.
2. Prepare necessary equipment and supplies:	
a. Flotation pad, foam mattress, air mattress, or sheepskin	
b. Two bed sheets	Used to cover certain types of support surfaces and bed mattresses.
c. Pillowcases (optional)	Used to cover flotation pads only.
d. Air flow pumping unit	Used only with alternating air-flow mattresses.
3. Explain purpose and application of mattress or pad.	Reduces client anxiety.
4. Wash hands.	Reduces transmission of microorganisms.
5. Close room door or bedside curtain.	Provides client privacy.
6. Apply support surface to bed (bed may be occupied or unoccupied).	Pressure-reducing devices can decrease the incidence of pressure ulcers but must be used with other prevention measures (AHCPR, 1992).
a. *Flotation pad:*	
(1) Apply foam pad over bed mattress by unrolling it fully.	Pad should lie flat to ensure smooth surface.
(2) Apply sheet over foam pad.	Minimizes soiling.
(3) Place flotation pad in center cut-out portion of foam pad.	Pad is designed to distribute pressure along greater trochanters of hip and sacrum.
b. *Foam mattress:*	
(1) Apply foam mattress over bed. (With egg crate variety, foam peaks should point up.)	Pad should lie flat to ensure smooth surface. Peaks distribute weight to more effectively relieve pressure.
(2) Apply bed sheet over mattress, being careful to avoid wrinkles.	Prevents soiling.
c. *Air mattress:*	
(1) Apply deflated mattress flat over bed mattress.	Provides smooth, even surface.
(2) Bring plastic strips or flaps around corners of bed mattress.	Secures air mattress in place.
(3) Attach connector on air mattress to inflation device.	Mattresses vary as to requiring one-time or continuous inflation cycle.
(4) Inflate mattress to proper air pressure determined by air pump or blower.	Manufacturer's directions indicate air pressure to distribute weight evenly.
(5) Place sheet over air mattress, being sure to eliminate all wrinkles.	Prevents soiling of mattress and reduces direct contact of skin against plastic surface.
(6) Check air pumps to be sure pressure cycle alternates.	Produces intermittent cycling, inflating only parts of mattress at any time. Intermittent cycle continually alternates pressure against skin and soft tissue.
7. Position client comfortably as desired over support surface. Reposition routinely.	Location of existing pressure ulcers might influence type of positioning. Regular turning is still required.
8. Wash hands.	Reduces transmission of microorganisms.
9. Inspect skin and bony prominences routinely.	Determines whether pressure sores develop or whether condition of existing sores changes.
10. Record transfer of client to support surface and related information in nurse's notes.	Documents safe completion of the procedure and records initial baseline data.

Placing a Client on a Clinitron Bed

STEPS	RATIONALE
1. Assess condition of client's skin, paying particular attention to potential pressure sites and skin lesions.	Data provide baseline to determine change in client's condition while on bed.
2. For client with severe to moderate pain, premedicate approximately 30 min before transfer.	Promotes client comfort and ability to cooperate.

3. Prepare necessary equipment and supplies:
  a. Clinitron bed
  b. Filter sheet
	Is permeable to rising air flow from mattress and downward flow of fluids (e.g., sweat, urine, or wound drainage).

4. Explain procedure and purpose of bed to client and family.	Reduces anxiety and promotes cooperation.
5. Obtain additional personnel needed to transfer client to bed.	Ensures client's safety.
6. Wash hands.	Reduces transmission of microorganisms.
7. Close client's room door or bedside curtain.	Maintains client privacy during transfer.
8. Transfer client to bed using appropriate transfer techniques (see Chapter 43).	Appropriate transfer techniques maintain alignment and reduce risk of injury during procedure.
9. Turn fluidization cycle on by depressing continuous or intermittent-mode switch. Regulate temperature in continuous mode.	Fluidization minimizes pressure against skin's surface and reduces friction and shearing force when client moves.
10. Position client and perform ROM exercises as appropriate.	Promotes comfort and reduces contracture formation. Bed reduces pressure on skin, but client must be turned and exercised to avoid joint deformity or contractures.
a. To turn clients, position bed pans, or perform other therapies, set intermittent-fluidization mode. After procedure is completed, set mode to continuous fluidization.	Intermittent fluidization provides firm, molded support that facilitates turning and handling client. Continuous fluidization provides permanent fluid support.
b. In emergencies when cardiopulmonary resuscitation is required, touch button to defluidize bed immediately.	Creates firm surface against which cardiopulmonary resuscitation can be performed.
11. Wash hands.	Reduces transmission of microorganisms.
12. Inspect condition of client's skin periodically.	Evaluates healing progress of existing lesions. Determines whether new pressure areas are forming.
13. Assess client for nausea.	Flotation effects of bed can cause sensation of nausea.
14. Measure client's level of consciousness.	Determines onset of perceptual changes.
15. Record transfer of client to bed, tolerance to procedure, and condition of skin in nurses' notes.	Documents safe completion of procedure and records initial baseline data.

tresses (see the box on p. 976). When used correctly, these mattresses and specialty beds assist in reducing pressure ulcers in clients at risk (see the boxes on p. 976; see Procedures 38-2 and 38-3.)

Research suggests that clients on air-fluidized beds may have increased fluid losses and decreased urinary nitrogen losses (Breslow, 1994; Breslow et al, 1993). Clients on air-fluidized beds should have increased amounts of fluids to prevent dehydration and may need increased protein intake (Breslow, 1994; Breslow et al, 1993).

TREATING PRESSURE ULCERS

Treatment of clients with pressure ulcers requires a holistic approach that uses the expertise of several multidisciplinary health care professionals (AHCPR, 1994; Olshansky, 1994). In addition to the nurse, this can include the physi-

cian, physical therapist, occupational therapist, nutritionist, and pharmacist (Rodeheaver et al, 1994). Aspects of pressure ulcer treatment include local care of the wound and supportive measures such as adequate nutrients and relief of pressure.

Upon discovery of a pressure ulcer, the wound should be assessed for location, stage, size, sinus tracts, undermining, tunneling, exudate, necrotic tissue, and the presence or absence of granulation tissue and epithelialization (AHCPR, 1994). Pressure ulcers should be reassessed at least daily (AHCPR, 1994). This may be modified in the home care setting (see the box on p. 977), as weekly assessment by health care providers may not always be feasible (AHCPR, 1994). "A clean pressure ulcer should show evidence of some healing within 2-4 weeks" (AHCPR, 1994).

A thorough description of the pressure ulcer provides the

basis for the decision-making tree for the treatment plan (AHCPR, 1994, Maklebust and Sieggreen, 1991). In the literature there are two tools that may provide a useful means for consistent assessment and reassessment of pressure ulcers. Exploration of the Bates-Jensen (1990) (Fig. 38-15) and Ayello (1992) (see the box on p. 977) tool may prove helpful. This would enhance communication and collaboration among team members for more focused treatment of these ulcers.

Skin. In addition to removing all pressure from the affected area and keeping pressure from the area, cleanliness of the ulcer area and all skin surfaces is essential (Procedure 38-4). Maintaining cleanliness may be extremely difficult with incontinent, feverish, or confused clients.

Moisture in and around an area of skin breakdown can cause further ulceration and infection. Many products are available for the care of pressure ulcers (Table 38-8). Before instituting treatment measures, the nurse must thoroughly assess the client's pressure ulcer and determine the correct dressing based on the stage of ulcer development.

Principles of local wound care include debridement, cleansing, and dressing application (Fig. 38-16). An ulcer that has necrotic tissue or eschar or shows signs of sloughing must be debrided. **Eschar** is the scab or dry crust that results from death of the skin. **Sloughing** is the shedding of dead tissue as the result of skin ulceration.

Debridement is the removal of necrotic tissue so that healthy tissue can regenerate. Removal of necrotic tissue is necessary to rid the ulcer of a source of infection, to enable visualization of the wound bed to accurately stage the ulcer, and to provide a clean base necessary for healing (Rodeheaver et al, 1994). An *exception* to the rule that all eschar be debrided is a dry necrotic heel pressure ulcer. AHCPR (1994) states that "heel ulcers with dry eschar need not be debrided if they do not have edema, erythema, flucturance, or drainage."

Text continued on p. 983

CLIENT TEACHING
for Therapeutic Beds and Mattresses

OBJECTIVE
- Client will demonstrate understanding of the purposes and basic operations of the therapeutic bed.

TEACHING STRATEGIES
- Explain to client the reasons for the therapeutic bed.
- Explain proper body mechanics while using the therapeutic bed.
- Educate family about the use and care of the therapeutic bed.
- Explain to client and family about additional pressure-relief measures.
- Give client and family a copy of each of the AHCPR client's prevention and treatment pressure ulcer booklets.

EVALUATION
- Client and family will state basic purposes for the therapeutic mattresses.
- Client and family will be able to describe function of therapeutic bed.

The 12 Commandments of Wound Care

1. Assess the wound thoroughly:
   - Measure the wound
   - Identify the wound type
   - Determine the nursing diagnosis
   - Assess the phase of the wound healing process
   - Stage a pressure ulcer
2. Outline a care plan.
3. Modify the plan as needed.
4. Keep the wound bed moist.
5. Keep the wound bed clean and debrided.
6. Protect healthy tissue.
7. Select dressings thoughtfully.
8. Eliminate dead space.
9. Evaluate and reevaluate the wound.
10. Control costs.
11. Know your limits and the limits of treatment.
12. Treat the whole client, not just the wound.

Modified from Krasner D: The twelve commandments of wound care, *Nurs '92*, 22(12):34, 1992.

Devices Used to Prevent or Treat Pressure Ulcers

DEVICES TO SUPPORT PRESSURE AREAS
- Flotation pads are pliable pads with a consistency like body fat, which disperse pressure over a larger area (see Procedure 38-2).
- Pillows and bridging techniques lift the pressure site off the mattress and separate two points of pressure.

DEVICES TO AID IN TURNING A CLIENT
- A Rotokinetic treatment table continuously rotates the client 270 degrees every 3 min.
- A Stryker wedge turning frame rotates the client horizontally from the prone to the supine position.

DEVICES TO MINIMIZE OR EQUALIZE PRESSURE
- Alternating air mattresses made of polyvinyl air cells are attached to a pump that inflates and deflates them every 3-7 sec, alternating pressure points (see Procedure 38-2).
- Water mattresses disperse and evenly distribute the client's body weight.
- A Clinitron bed decreases pressure and reduces shearing, friction, and maceration by distributing the client's weight through a gentle flow of temperature-controlled air forced upward through a mass of fine ceramic microspheres (see Procedure 38-3).
- An egg crate mattress is a foam rubber pad that rests on the bed mattress and disperses the client's body weight evenly over the mattress (see Procedure 38-2).

Home Care Recommendations from AHCPR, 1994

ASSESSMENT

- "Assessment and documentation [of the pressure ulcer] should be carried out at least weekly, unless there is evidence of deterioration, in which case both the pressure ulcer and the client's overall management must be reassessed immediately. In the home setting, this may require the assistance of the client and family because weekly assessment by health care providers is not always feasible."

PSYCHOSOCIAL ASSESSMENT AND MANAGEMENT

- Assess resources (e.g., availability and skill of care givers, finances, equipment) of individuals being treated for pressure ulcers in the home.
  - A successful treatment program requires adequate care-giver and equipment resources. Care givers need to be evaluated for their ability to comprehend and implement the treatment requirements. Care givers should also be evaluated for their level of strength and endurance. Economic factors should be considered, because they may limit the supply and availability of equipment as well as opportunities to relieve care givers.

ULCER CARE DRESSINGS

- Consider care giver time when selecting a dressing.
  - In the home setting, care givers may choose more expensive dressing materials to reduce the frequency of dressing changes.

INFECTION CONTROL

- Clean dressing may also be used in the home setting. Disposal of contaminated dressings in the home should be done in a manner consistent with local regulations.
  - Clean dressings, as opposed to sterile ones, are recommended for home use until research demonstrates otherwise. This recommendation is in keeping with principles regarding nosocomial infections and with past success of clean urinary catheterization in the home setting, and it takes into account the expense of sterile dressings and the dexterity required to apply them. The "no-touch" technique can be used for dressing changes. This technique is a method of changing surface dressings without touching the wound or the surface of any dressing that might be in contact with the wound. Adherent dressings should be grasped by the corner and removed slowly, whereas gauze dressings can be pinched in the center and lifted off.
- The Environmental Protection Agency recommends that soiled dressings be placed in securely fastened plastic bags before being added to other household trash. Local regulations vary, however, and home care agencies and clients are advised to follow procedures that are consistent with local laws.

Modified from AHCPR Panel for the Treatment of Pressure Ulcers: Treatment of pressure ulcers (AHCPR Publication No. 95-0652). Rockville, MD: Agency for Health Care Policy and Research, Public Health Service, U.S. Department of Health and Human Services. [Clinical Practice Guideline, Number 15], 1994).

Ayello's Assessment

A natomical location, age of wound	**A** Chronic wounds heal slower. Wounds near the anus need more frequent observation of dressings.
S ize, shape, stage	**S** taging of the wound will help in selecting the appropriate healing treatments and dressing. Measuring guides can assist in determining the length and width of the ulcer. A sterile cotton-tipped applicator can be used to measure the depth of the ulcer.
S inus tract	**S** Gently use a sterile cotton-tipped applicator to locate any sinus tracts. Use a clock as a reference to describe location.
E xudate	**E** Wound drainage must be contained to protect the surrounding skin. Note amount, color, and characteristic of the drainage.
S epsis	**S** All pressure ulcers are considered colonized. Wounds with bacterial counts $> 10^5$ are infected. Observe for S&S of local infection: purulent exudate, odor, erythema, warmth, tenderness, edema, pain, fever, and elevated white count. Systemic infection such as osteomyelitis must be treated. Routine swab culturing of all pressure ulcers is not recommended.
S urrounding skin	**S** Protect the surrounding skin from breakdown from moisture.
M argins, maceration	**M** Identify condition of wound margins and if they are contracting. Evaluate for maceration if present. Institute measures to protect skin.
E rythrema, epithelialization, eschar	**E** valuate for wound healing as evidenced by these changes in the ulcer, skin tone. Changes in dark-skinned clients are best assessed with good lighting.
N ecrotic, nose, neovascularization	**N** ecrotic tissue must be removed to stage and heal the ulcer. If an odor is present, more frequent cleansing and maybe debridement are needed.
T issue bed, tenderness to touch, tension	**T** Identify tissue bed and medicate for pain.

From Ayello EA, 1992 (revised 1995).

PRESSURE SORE STATUS TOOL   NAME_____

Complete the rating sheet to assess pressure sore status. Evaluate each item by picking the response that best describes the wound and entering the score in the item score column for the appropriate date.

Location: Anatomic site. Circle, identify right (**R**) or left (**L**) and use "**X**" to mark site on body diagrams:

_____ Sacrum & coccyx	_____ Lateral ankle
_____ Trochanter	_____ Medial ankle
_____ Ischial tuberosity	_____ Heel Other Site _____

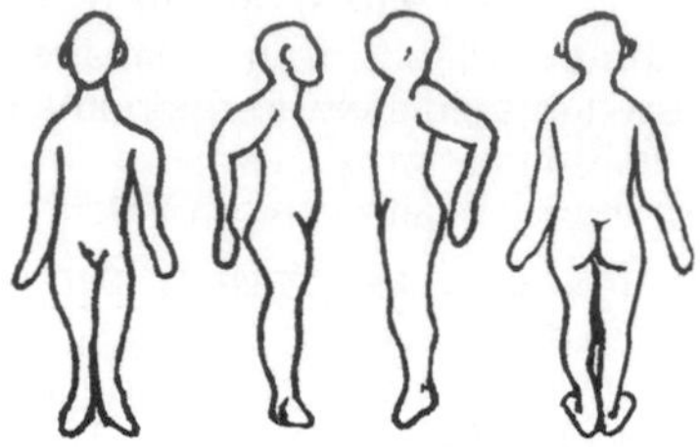

Shape: Overall wound pattern; assess by observing perimeter and depth.
Circle and <u>date</u> appropriate description:

_____ Irregular	_____ Linear or elongated
_____ Round/oval	_____ Bowl/boat
_____ Square/rectangle _____	Butterfly Other Shape _____

Item	Assessment	Date	Date	Date
		Score	**Score**	**Score**
1. Size	1 = Length x width < 4 sq cm 2 = Length x width 4 -16 sq cm 3 = Length x width 16.1 - 36 sq cm 4 = Length x width 36.1 - 80 sq cm 5 = Length x width > 80 sq cm			
2. Depth	1 = Non-blanchable erythema on intact skin 2 = Partial thickness skin loss involving epidermis &/or dermis 3 = Full thickness skin loss involving damage or necrosis of subcutaneous tissue; may extend down to but not through underlying fascia; &/or mixed partial & full thickness &/or tissue layers obscured by granulation tissue 4 = Obscured by necrosis 5 = Full thickness skin loss with extensive destruction, tissue necrosis or damage to muscle, bone or supporting structures			
3. Edges	1 = Indistinct, diffuse, none clearly visible 2 = Distinct, outline clearly visible, attached, even with wound base 3 = Well-defined, not attached to wound base 4 = Well-defined, not attached to base, rolled under, thickened 5 = Well-defined, fibrotic, scarred or hyperkeratotic			
4. Under-mining	1 = Undermining < 2 cm in any area 2 = Undermining 2-4 cm involving < 50% wound margins 3 = Undermining 2-4 cm involving > 50% wound margins 4 = Undermining > 4 cm in any area 5 = Tunneling &/or sinus tract formation			
5. Necrotic Tissue Type	1 = None visible 2 = White/grey non-viable tissue &/or non-adherent yellow slough 3 = Loosely adherent yellow slough 4 = Adherent, soft, black eschar 5 = Firmly adherent, hard, black eschar			
6. Necrotic Tissue Amount	1 = None visible 2 = < 25% of wound bed covered 3 = 25% to 50% of wound covered 4 = > 50% and < 75% of wound covered 5 = 75% to 100% of wound covered			

c 1990 Barbara Bates-Jensen

Fig. 38-15 Pressure sore status tool. *(Courtesy Barbara Bates Jensen.)*

Item	Assessment	Date	Date	Date
		Score	Score	Score
7. Exudate Type	1 = None or bloody 2 = Serosanguineous: thin, watery, pale red/pink 3 = Serous: thin, watery, clear 4 = Purulent: thin or thick, opaque, tan/yellow 5 = Foul purulent: thick, opaque, yellow/green with odor			
8. Exudate Amount	1 = None 2 = Scant 3 = Small 4 = Moderate 5 = Large			
9. Skin color Surrounding Wound	1 = Pink or normal for ethnic group 2 = Bright red &/or blanches to touch 3 = White or grey pallor or hypopigmented 4 = Dark red or purple &/or non-blanchable 5 = Black or hyperpigmented			
10. Peripheral Tissue Edema	1 = Minimal swelling around wound 2 = Non-pitting edema extends < 4 cm around wound 3 = Non-pitting edema extends ≥ 4 cm around wound 4 = Pitting edema extends < 4 cm around wound 5 = Crepitus &/or pitting edema extends ≥ 4 cm			
11. Peripheral Tissue Induration	1 = Minimal firmness around wound 2 = Induration < 2 cm around wound 3 = Induration 2-4 cm extending < 50% around wound 4 = Induration 2-4 cm extending ≥ 50% around wound 5 = Induration > 4 cm in any area			
12. Granulation Tissue	1 = Skin intact or partial thickness wound 2 = Bright, beefy red; 75% to 100% of wound filled &/or tissue overgrowth 3 = Bright, beefy red; < 75% & > 25% of wound filled 4 = Pink, &/or dull, dusky red &/or fills ≤ 25% of wound 5 = No granulation tissue present			
13. Epithelialization	1 = 100% wound covered, surface intact 2 = 75% to <100% wound covered &/or epithelial tissue extends >0.5cm into wound bed 3 = 50% to <75% wound covered &/or epithelial tissue extends to <0.5cm into wound bed 4 = 25% to < 50% wound covered 5 = < 25% wound covered			
TOTAL SCORE				
SIGNATURE				

PRESSURE SORE STATUS CONTINUUM

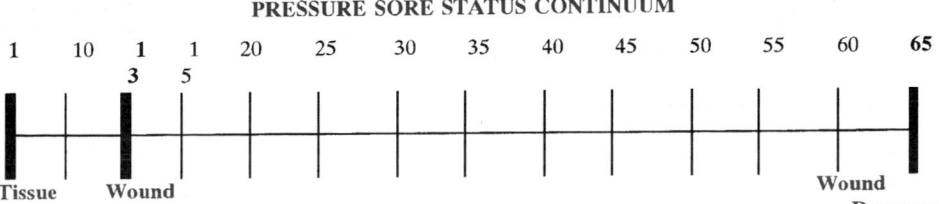

Plot the total score on the Pressure Sore Status Continuum by putting an "X" on the line and the date beneath the line. Plot multiple scores with their dates to see-at-a-glance regeneration or degeneration of the wound.

c 1990 Barbara Bates-Jensen

Fig. 38-15, cont'd Pressure sore status tool.

PRESSURE SORE STATUS TOOL

Instructions for use

General Guidelines:

Fill out the attached rating sheet to assess a pressure sore's status after reading the definitions and methods of assessment described below. Evaluate once a week and whenever a change occurs in the wound. Rate according to each item by picking the response that best describes the wound and entering that score in the item score column for the appropriate date. When you have rated the pressure sore on all items, determine the total score by adding together the 13-item scores. The HIGHER the total score, the more severe the pressure sore status. Plot total score on the Pressure Sore Status Continuum to determine progress.

Specific Instructions:

1. **Size**: Use ruler to measure the longest and widest aspect of the wound surface in centimeters; multiply length x width.

2. **Depth**: Pick the depth, thickness, most appropriate to the wound using these additional descriptions:
   1 = tissues damaged but no break in skin surface.
   2 = superficial, abrasion, blister or shallow crater. Even with, &/or elevated above skin surface (e.g., hyperplasia).
   3 = deep crater with or without undermining of adjacent tissue.
   4 = visualization of tissue layers not possible due to necrosis.
   5 = supporting structures include tendon, joint capsule.

3. **Edges**: Use this guide:

Indistinct, diffuse	=	unable to clearly distinguish wound outline.
Attached	=	even or flush with wound base, <u>no</u> sides or walls present; flat.
Not attached	=	sides or walls <u>are</u> present; floor or base of wound is deeper than edge.
Rolled under, thickened	=	soft to firm and flexible to touch.
Hyperkeratosis	=	callous-like tissue formation around wound & at edges.
Fibrotic, scarred	=	hard, rigid to touch.

4. **Undermining**: Assess by inserting a cotton tipped applicator under the wound edge; advance it as far as it will go without using undue force; raise the tip of the applicator so it may be seen or felt on the surface of the skin; mark the surface with a pen; measure the distance from the mark on the skin to the edge of the wound. Continue process around the wound. Then use a transparent metric measuring guide with concentric circles divided into 4 (25%) pie-shaped quadrants to help determine percent of wound involved.

5. **Necrotic Tissue Type**: Pick the type of necrotic tissue that is <u>predominant</u> in the wound according to color, consistency and adherence using this guide:

White/gray non-viable tissue	=	may appear prior to wound opening; skin surface is white or gray.
Non-adherent, yellow slough	=	thin, mucinous substance; scattered throughout wound bed; easily separated from wound tissue.
Loosely adherent, yellow slough	=	thick, stringy, clumps of debris; attached to wound tissue.
Adherent, soft, black eschar	=	soggy tissue; strongly attached to tissue in center or base of wound.
Firmly adherent, hard/black eschar	=	firm, crusty tissue; strongly attached to wound base <u>and</u> edges (like a hard scab).

c 1990 Barbara Bates-Jensen

Fig. 38-15, cont'd Pressure sore status tool.

6. **Necrotic Tissue Amount:** Use a transparent metric measuring guide with concentric circles divided into 4 (25%) pie-shaped quadrants to help determine percent of wound involved.

7. **Exudate Type:** Some dressings interact with wound drainage to produce a gel or trap liquid. Before assessing exudate type, gently cleanse wound with normal saline or water. Pick the exudate type that is <u>predominant</u> in the wound according to color and consistency, using this guide:

Bloody	=	thin, bright red
Serosanguineous	=	thin, watery pale red to pink
Serous	=	thin, watery, clear
Purulent	=	thin or thick, opaque tan to yellow
Foul purulent	=	thick, opaque yellow to green with offensive odor

8. **Exudate Amount:** Use a transparent metric measuring guide with concentric circles divided into 4 (25%) pie-shaped quadrants to determine percent of dressing involved with exudate. Use this guide:

None	=	wound tissues dry.
Scant	=	wound tissues moist; no measurable exudate.
Small	=	wound tissues wet; moisture evenly distributed in wound; drainage involves $\leq$ 25% dressing.
Moderate	=	wound tissues saturated; drainage may or may not be evenly distributed in wound; drainage involves > 25% to $\leq$ 75% dressing.
Large	=	wound tissues bathed in fluid; drainage freely expressed; may or may not be evenly distributed in wound; drainage involves > 75% of dressing.

9. **Skin Color Surrounding Wound:** Assess tissues within 4cm of wound edge. Dark-skinned persons show the colors "bright red" and "dark red" as a deepening of normal ethnic skin color or a purple hue. As healing occurs in dark-skinned persons, the new skin is pink and may never darken.

10. **Peripheral Tissue Edema:** Assess tissues within 4cm of wound edge. Non-pitting edema appears as skin that is shiny and taut. Identify pitting edema by firmly pressing a finger down into the tissues and waiting for 5 seconds, on release of pressure, tissues fail to resume previous position and an indentation appears. Crepitus is accumulation of air or gas in tissues. Use a transparent metric measuring guide to determine how far edema extends beyond wound.

11. **Peripheral Tissue Induration:** Assess tissues within 4cm of wound edge. Induration is abnormal firmness of tissues with margins. Assess by gently pinching the tissues. Induration results in an inability to pinch the tissues. Use a transparent metric measuring guide with concentric circles divided into 4 (25%) pie-shaped quadrants to determine percent of wound and area involved.

12. **Granulation Tissue:** Granulation tissue is the growth of small blood vessels and connective tissue to fill in full thickness wounds. Tissue is healthy when bright, beefy red, shiny and granular with a velvety appearance. Poor vascular supply appears as pale pink or blanched to dull, dusky red color.

13. **Epithelialization:** Epithelialization is the process of epidermal resurfacing and appears as pink or red skin. In partial thickness wounds it can occur throughout the wound bed as well as from the wound edges. In full thickness wounds it occurs from the edges only. Use a transparent metric measuring guide with concentric circles divided into 4 (25%) pie-shaped quadrants to help determine percent of wound involved and to measure the distance the epithelial tissue extends into the wound.

Fig. 38-15, cont'd Pressure sore status tool.

Treating Pressure Ulcers

PROCEDURE 38-4

STEPS	RATIONALE
1. Close door or bedside curtains.	Maintains privacy.
2. Position client comfortably with area of pressure ulcer and surrounding skin easily accessible.	Area should be accessible for cleansing of ulcer and surrounding skin.
3. Assemble supplies at bedside. Open sterile packages and topical solution containers.	Sterile supplies should be ready for easy application so that nurse can use them without contaminating them.
a. Wash basin, warm water, washcloth, and towel	Used to bathe surrounding skin.
b. Cleansing agent	
c. Prescribed topical agent: for *infected* or *necrotic* wounds. Do not use on CLEAN UNINFECTED WOUNDS.	
(1) Necrotic wounds Enzymes: collagenase, fibrinolysin, deoxyribonuclease or sutilains	Debride dead tissue to allow for granulation.
(2) Infected wounds	
(a) Antiseptics: providone-iodine (ointment or solution), merbromin (5% or 10% solution), or sodium hypochlorite (1:12 or 1:20 solution)	Reduce bacterial growth in the presence of necrotic tissue, pus, serum, or blood. Reduce infection in weeping ulcer.
(b) Oxydizing agents: benzoyl peroxide (20%) or hydrogen peroxide (half-strength)	Clean wounds, especially with anerobic bacteria. Decreases oxygen supply to devitalized tissues.
(c) Dextranomer beads: Debrisan	Clean wounds with heavy exudate. Absorb fluid, protein, fibrin, fibrinogen, and all products of tissue breakdown and bacterial infection.
d. Sterile dressing.	
e. Hypoallergenic tape or adhesive dressing sheet (Hypofx)	Used to apply gauze dressing. Prevents skin irritation and tearing.
f. Clean gloves	Reduces transmission of microorganisms.
g. Protective paste (e.g., zinc oxide [optional])	Protects nonaffected skin from irritating solutions.
h. Tools to measure wound size:	Used to provide objective measure to evaluate healing.
(1) Transparency film and marker	
(2) Metric ruler	
(3) Camera in some circumstances	Photography provides objective method to assess wound progression.
4. Remove bed linen and client's gown to expose ulcer and surrounding skin. Keep remaining body parts draped.	Prevents unnecessary exposure of body parts.
5. Wash hands. Apply clean disposable gloves.	AHCPR (1994) guidelines state that clean gloves rather than sterile may be used.
6. Assess pressure ulcer and surrounding skin:	
a. Note and document color and appearance of skin around ulcer.	Skin condition may indicate progressive tissue damage.
b. Measure diameter of pressure ulcer with ruler or transparency film.	Provides objective measure of wound size. May determine type of dressing chosen.
c. Measure depth of ulcer using sterile, cotton-tipped applicator or other device that will allow measurement of wound depth.	Depth measure is important for staging ulcer. Kundin scale is a three-dimensional (length, width, and depth) tool for wound volume calculations (Cooper, 1992).
d. Measure depth of undermining skin by lateral tissue necrosis. Use cotton-tipped applicator and gently probe under skin edges.	Undermining may indicate progressive tissue necrosis.
7. Wash skin around ulcer gently with warm water.	Reduces number of resident bacteria.
8. Rinse area thoroughly with water.	
9. Gently dry skin thoroughly by patting lightly with gauze.	Retained moisture causes maceration of skin layers.

Treating Pressure Ulcers—cont'd

STEPS	RATIONALE
10. Cleanse ulcer thoroughly with normal saline or wound cleansing agent:	Removes debris from wound from digested material. A 19-gauge needle and 35-cc syringe has a psi pressure of 8 and is safe to use for cleaning a pressure ulcer (AHCPR, 1994).
a. Use an irrigating system for deep ulcers that has a pressure between 4 and 15 psi.	
b. Use shower with hand-held shower head.	
c. Use whirlpool treatments to assist with wound cleansing and debridement.	
11. Apply topical agents, if prescribed:	
a. Enzymes:	
(1) Place small amount of enzyme ointment in wound or on gauze dressing.	Thin layer absorbs and acts more effectively. Excess medication can irritate surrounding skin.
(2) Soften medication by rubbing briskly in palm of hand.	Follow manufacturer's directions. Use of each brand of enzyme debriders is different.
(3) Apply thin, even layer of ointment over necrotic areas. Do not apply enzyme to surrounding skin.	Proper distribution ensures effective action. Enzyme can cause burning, paresthesia, and dermatitis to surrounding skin.
(4) Cover with dry gauze and tape securely in place.	Protects wound. Keeping ulcer surface moist reduces time needed for healing. Skin cells normally live in moist environment.
b. Dextranomer beads:	Absorbs wound exudate.
(1) Hold container of beads approximately 2.5 cm (1 in) above site and lightly sprinkle 5 mm diameter layer over wound.	
(2) Apply gauze dressing over ulcer.	Holds beads in place and protects wound.
c. Hydrocolloid beads/paste:	
(1) Fill wound to approximately half of the total depth with hydrocolloid beads or paste.	Assists in absorbing wound drainage. Highly draining wounds are best treated with hydrocolloid beads or granules.
(2) Cover with hydrocolloid dressing; extend dressing 1-1½ in beyond edges of wound.	Dressing maintains wound humidity. May be left in place up to 7 days.
d. Hydrogel agents:	
(1) Cover surface of ulcer with hydrogel using applicator or gloved hand. Some hydrogels are available as sponges and strips.	Provides maintenance of wound humidity while absorbing excess drainage. May be used as carrier for topical agents.
(2) Apply dry, fluffy gauze over gel to completely cover ulcer.	Holds hydrogel against wound surface. Used as absorbent.
12. Reposition client comfortably off ulcer.	Avoids accidental removal of dressings. Pressure on existing ulcers must be avoided.
13. Remove gloves and dispose of soiled supplies. Wash hands.	Prevents transmission of microorganisms.
14. Report worsening in ulcer's appearance to nurse in charge or physician.	Worsening of condition may indicate need for additional therapy.
15. Record appearance of ulcer in nurses' notes. Describe type of topical agent used, dressing applied, and response.	Documents status of ulcer and specific treatment. Response documents evaluation of treatment.

The method of debridement used should depend on which is most appropriate to the client's condition and care goals (AHCPR, 1994). It is important to remember that during the debridement process some normal wound observations that may occur are an increase in wound exudate, odor, and size. Pain that occurs with debridement needs to be assessed and prevented or effectively managed (AHCPR, 1994).

Methods of debridement include mechanical, autolytic, chemical/enzymatic, and surgical. Mechanical debridement may use wet to dry saline gauze dressings. The dressing must be allowed to dry thoroughly before the nurse "pulls" the gauze that has adhered to the tissue out of the pressure ulcer. This is a nonselective method of debridement as devitalized and viable tissue are *both* removed. It should *never* be used in a clean granulating wound. Other methods of mechanical debridement are wound irrigation, dextranomers, and whirlpool (AHCPR, 1994). Dextra-

Table 38-8	Dressing by Ulcer Stage
DRESSING	**COMMENTS***

STAGE I	
Film dressing (Tegadern, Bioclusive, Op-site, Uniflex)	Protects from shearing force May be left in place up to 7 days, if occlusive seal remains Will facilitate softening of eschar on deeper ulcers Traps serous exudate and provides moist wound environment
Hydrocolloid dressing (such as DuoDERM, Comfeel, IntraSite)	Is absorbent May be left in place up to 7 days, if occlusive seal remains (Nurse is unable to assess wound with dressing in place.) Reacts with wound fluid to create a soft gel that promotes granulation and epithelialization
STAGE II	
Hydrocolloid dressing	See stage I
Composite dressing (such as Viasorb, film dressing over Telfa)	Provides absorbent, nonadherent layer over wound with occlusive cover
Hydrogel dressing (such as Vigilon, Geliperm, J&J Gel)	Is absorbent for draining ulcers Usually requires gauze dressing cover
Absorptive dressing (such as Exu-dry, Bard absorption dressing)	Is absorbent and nonadherent Protects from shearing force May be used with topical agents Is not occlusive dressing Absorbs exudate and debris while maintaining moist environment*
STAGE III	
Polyurethane foam (Lyofoam, Allevyn)	Absorbs exudate Maintains moist wound environment*
Hydrocolloid dressing (see stage I)	Increases absorbency and wear time when hydrocolloid granules or paste is used Can cause damage because of frequent removal (every day or more often) (Recommend other dressing.)
Hydrogel dressing (see stage II)	May be used as carrier for topical agents, including topically applied growth factors
Absorptive dressing	See stage II
STAGE IV	
Hydrocolloid dressing (see stages I to III)	May be contraindicated because of location of ulcer, exposed bone, and amount of drainage
Hydrogel dressing	See stages II to III

Gauze dressing	*Kerlix type:*
	  Is absorbent but not occlusive
	  Generally requires dressing changes every 8 to 12 hr
	Dry gauze:
	  Removes drainage away from wound surface†
	Moist gauze:
	  Maintains moist wound environment while removing drainage away from surface†
	Moist-to-dry:
	  Debrides necrotic and healthy tissue nonselectively

*As with *all* occlusive dressing, wounds should *not* be clinically infected.
†Data from Maklebust J: *RN* 41(12):56, 1991.

nomers are highly hydrophilic dextran-polymer beads that are put into the pressure ulcer wound bed to absorb exudate, bacteria, and other wound debris (AHCPR, 1994). Whirlpool treatments are performed by physical therapists.

Autolytic debridement uses synthetic dressings over a wound to allow the eschar to be self-digested by the action of enzymes that are present in wound fluids (AHCPR, 1994). It can be accomplished by using some of the newer dressing materials over the pressure ulcer. Some examples

of dressings used are transparent synthetic membrane dressings or hydrocolloid dressings. The dressing will interact with the pressure ulcer tissue surface. Eschar is softened because the devitalized tissue is self-digested from the enzymes that are normally found in wound fluid. Autolytic debridement is contraindicated for infected wounds (AHCPR, 1994).

Enzymatic debridement is the application of topical debriding enzymes to the devitalized tissue on the wound sur-

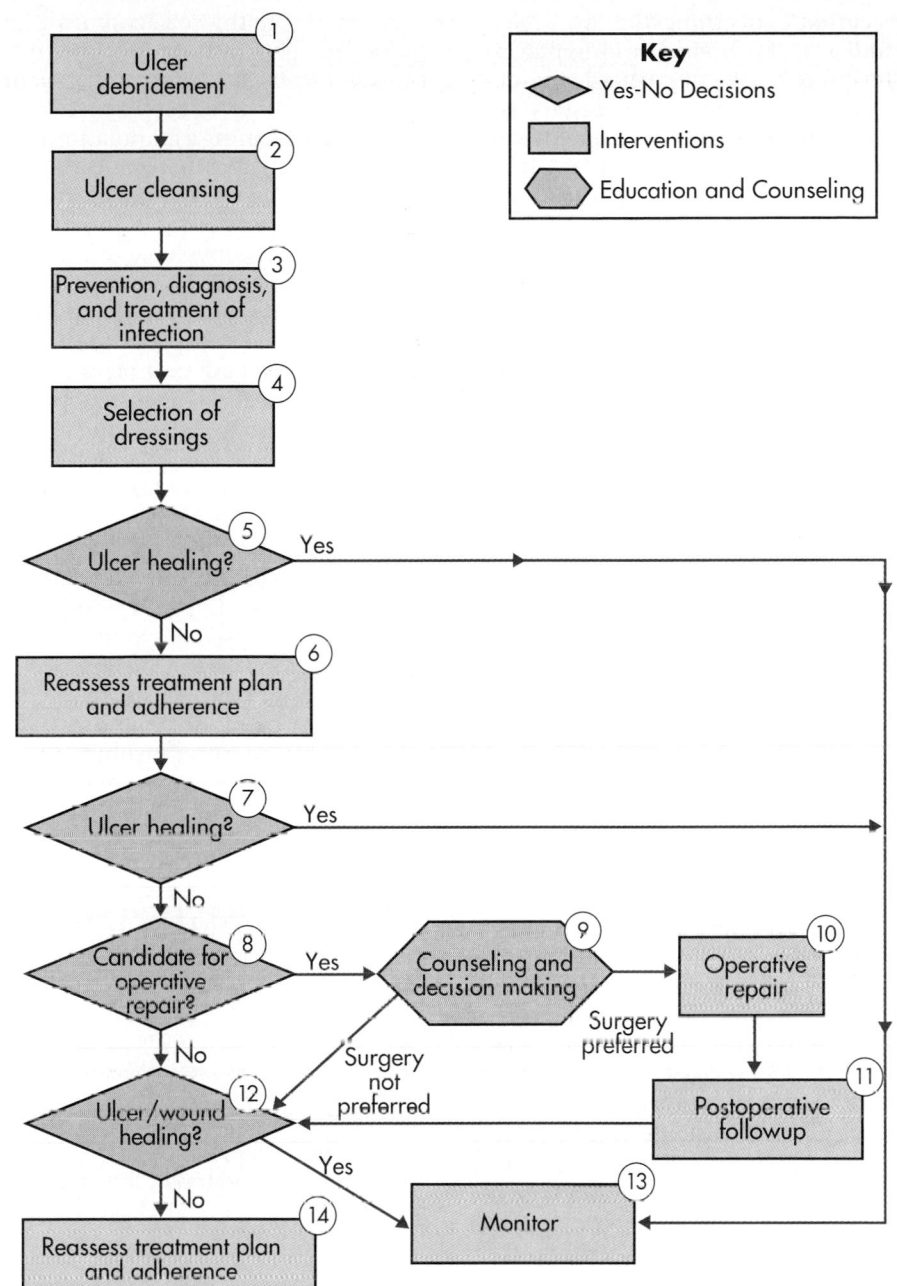

Fig. 38-16 Ulcer care. *(From AHCPR panel for the treatment of pressure ulcers [Publication No 95-0652, Rockville MD, 1994].)*

face. These drugs require a physician's order. It is important to remember that the techniques for use and the properties of each of the enzymatic debriding agents are different. Clinicians should follow the manufacturer's specific directions. Of all the enzymatic debriding agents, only collagenase (Santyl) is mentioned by AHCPR (1994) as promoting debridement and growth of granulation tissue.

Surgical debridement is the removal of devitalized tissue by using a scalpel, scissor, or other sharp instrument. Physicians and, in some states, specially educated nurses can perform surgical debridement of a pressure ulcer. Nurses should check the Nurse Practice Act for their state to see if surgical debridement is covered as a nursing function. It is

the quickest method of debridement. It is usually indicated when the client has signs of cellulitis or sepsis. Clean, dry dressings should be used for 8 to 24 hours after sharp debridement associated with bleeding. Afterward, moist dressings can be reinstituted to promote wound healing (AHCPR, 1994).

MOIST WOUND HEALING

In the past, choices for wound care management have been based on superstition and magic (Levine, 1992) and clinician preference (Doughty, 1992). Clinicians previously believed that a dry environment was necessary to heal a wound. Since the 1960s, a revolution led by the research of

Dr. G.D. Winter has occurred concerning the local management of wounds. Studies of the wound healing process have shown that a moist rather than a dry wound environment (e.g., when a heat lamp is used) is necessary for wound healing. A **moist wound-healing** environment is of prime importance for wound healing because it affects both the rate of epithelialization and the amount of scar formation. A moist wound-healing environment provides the optimum condition for rapid healing. Winter (1962) found that when the epidermis is lost, uncovered wounds can become dry, desiccated, and dehydrated. Epidermal cells must then migrate under the dry crusts or scabs and over the fibrous tissue probing for the "path of least resistance." As this rerouting of the epidermal cells is less efficient and increases the amount of time the cells must travel before they reach the other side of the wound, wound healing takes longer. When a barrier, such as a dressing, is placed over the wound (either semioccluded or occluded), the surface of the wound remains moist with wound fluid. This allows epidermal cells to migrate more readily and rapidly. A moist wound environment can be promoted with the use of appropriate dressings.

Once a pressure ulcer has been successfully debrided and has a *clean granulating* base, the goal of local care is to provide an appropriate environment for moist wound-healing and to support the newly formed granulation tissue. Wounds should be cleansed initially and at each dressing change (AHCPR, 1994). Pressure ulcers should be cleansed only with wound cleaners such as normal saline or some commercial wound cleansers that will not damage or kill (cytotoxic) cells, such as fibroblasts and healing tissue (AHCPR, 1994). Research has reported that some commercial wound cleansers are cytotoxic (Foresman et al, 1993; Wright and Orr, 1993) (see the box titled Toxicity for Wound and Skin Cleansers in Chapter 49). Skin cleaners are not the same as wound cleansers. *DO NOT CLEAN UNINFECTED OR NECROTIC ULCER WOUNDS WITH SKIN CLEANERS OR ANTISEPTIC AGENTS* (AHCPR, 1994). Some commonly used solutions that are cytotoxic and therefore should *not* be used to clean granulating wounds are Dakin's solution (sodium hypochlorite solution), acetic acid, povidone iodine, hydrogen peroxide, and some commercial wound cleansers.

Besides using the correct type of solution, it is important to use enough irrigation pressure to *clean* the pressure ulcer *without causing trauma* to the wound bed (Barr, 1995). AHCPR (1994) states that 4 to 15 psi is a safe and effective pressure for cleaning a granulating pressure ulcer. A 19-gauge needle or an angiocatheter and a 35-cc syringe delivers saline to a pressure ulcer at 8 psi (Fig. 38-17). A bulb syringe has an irrigation pressure below 4 psi and therefore will not adequately clean the pressure ulcer (AHCPR, 1994). A list of different types of systems used to clean pressure ulcers and a list of their pressures can be found in Table 38-9.

Next the cleansed pressure ulcer needs a dressing. The goal of dressings are to protect the pressure ulcer, to maintain a moist healing environment, and to prevent maceration of the surrounding wound skin. There are many dressings available today from which the clinician can choose to use on pressure ulcers (Baranoski, 1995; Krasner, 1992) (see Chapter 49 for a description of some of the different types of dressings currently in use). Some factors to consider when selecting a dressing are maintenance of a moist environment, prevention of wound desiccation (drying out), ability to absorb the wound drainage, location of the wound, elimination of dead space, amount of care giver time, cost, and clean versus sterile dressings. Studies of different types of moist wound dressings showed no differences in pressure ulcer healing outcomes (AHCPR, 1994).

Table 38-9	Irrigation Pressures Delivered by Various Devices	
DEVICE		**IRRIGATION IMPACT PRESSURE (PSI)**
Spray Bottle—Ultra Klenz™ [a] (Carrington Laboratories, Inc., Dallas, Tex)		1.2
Bulb Syrine[a] (Davol Inc., Cranston, RI)		2.0
Piston Irrigation Syringe (60-mL) with catheter tip (Premium Plastics, Inc., Chicago, IL)		4.2
Saline Squeeze Bottle (250-mL) with irrigation cap (Baxter Healthcare Corp., Deerfield, IL)		4.5
Water Pik® at lowest setting (#1) (Teledyne Water PIk, Fort Collins, CO)		6.0
Irrijet® DS Syringe with tip (Ackrad Laboratories, Inc., Cranford, NJ)		7.6
35-mL syringe with 19-gauge needle or angiocatheter		8.0
Water Pik® at middle setting (#3)[b] (Teledyne Water Pik, Fort Collins, CO)		42
Water Pik® at highest setting (#5)[b] (Teledyne Water Pik, Fort Collins, CO)		>50
Pressurized Cannister-Dey-Wash™[b] (Dey Laboratories, Inc., Napa, CA)		>50

From AHCPR Treatment guidelines, 1994.
[a]These devices may not delivery enough pressure to adequately cleanse wounds.
[b]These devices may cause trauma and drive bacteria into wounds. They are not recommended for cleansing of soft-tissue wounds.

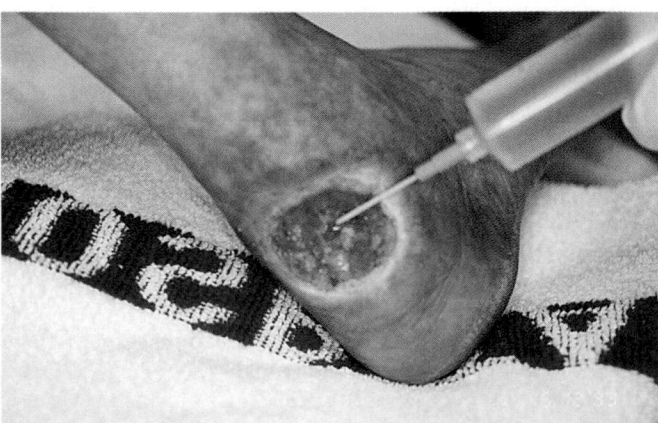

Fig. 38-17 Wound irrigation.

The treatment plan will change as the ulcer heals. For example, for a necrotic wound, a membrane dressing may be used initially to debride the wound by autolysis. Afterward, pressure ulcers stages (III or IV) that had large amounts of exudate require a dressing with absorptive ability. For reddened areas or areas of broken skin integrity, skin care products that lubricate and protect and promote wound healing are recommended. When the ulcer is pink with granulation tissue throughout, a dressing is indicated to promote healing. A clean, moist environment promotes migration of epithelial cells across the ulcer surface (Kloth, McCulloch, and Feedar, 1990; Winter, 1962).

There are many practice changes as a result of the AHCPR 1994 treatment guidelines. Clean dressings, especially in the home setting, can be used on pressure ulcers. Clean gloves can be used for pressure ulcer care. If a client has more than one pressure ulcer, one pair of clean gloves can be used to do all the dressing changes. The nurse must clean the *least* contaminated pressure ulcer first. For example, if a client has a pressure ulcer near the anus, it should be cleaned last. After the nurse completes all the dressing changes for a particular client, the nurse can remove the gloves, wash hands, and put on clean gloves to care for the next client's wounds. All pressure ulcers are considered contaminated or colonized with bacteria; therefore, routine swab cultures are not recommended. AHCPR (1994) recommends that quantitative swab cultures may be indicated in a clean pressure ulcer that is not healing. Stotts (1995) believes that quantitative bacterial cultures can be performed by either needle biopsy or quantitative swab culture. Furthermore, a standardized technique for performing these two types of cultures is recommended by Dr. Stotts (see the box below).

In addition to local wound treatment, other methods, such as electromagnetic energy, have been used to foster ulcer healing (Itoh et al, 1991). AHCPR (1994) recommends considering a course of treatment with electrotherapy for stages III and IV pressure ulcers that are unresponsive to conventional therapies. AHCPR (1994) states that other adjunctive therapies, such as hyperbaric oxygen; infrared, ultraviolet, and low-energy laser irradiation; ultrasound; platelet-derived growth factors; miscellaneous topical agents; and systemic drugs other than antibiotics, need more research before they can make a recommendation about the use of these therapies in the treatment of pressure ulcers.

Education. Education (Ayello, 1993, 1995; Maklebust and Magnan, 1992) of the client and care givers/family are important nursing functions. There are a variety of educational tools, including videotapes and written materials, that can be used by the nurse when teaching clients and care givers/family to prevent and treat pressure ulcers. Written materials are available on a variety of topics, including dressing changes, wound measuring guides, and client positioning charts. A step-by-step outline of practical pointers for nurses who will be developing their own client teaching materials has been written by Doak, Doak, and Root (1996). AHCPR (1992, 1994) has client booklets on pressure ulcer prevention and treatment that can be helpful when teaching clients and their care givers/family. These booklets are available in English and in Spanish. Teaching should be individualized for each client, especially for the elderly (see the box below). A review of these booklets with suggestions on how to use them in the teaching plan of clients can be found in the literature (Ayello, 1993, 1995).

Understanding and assessment of the experience of the client and support person are also important dimensions in the treatment of people with pressure ulcers (AHCPR, 1994). Clinicians are only just now exploring through research the care giver's perspective of the concerns and issues faced by frail elderly spouses caring for their loved ones with pressure ulcers (Baharestani, 1994) (see the box on p. 988). Interventions should be planned to meet the

---

Recommendations for Standardized Techniques for Wound Cultures

NEEDLE ASPIRATION PROCEDURE
- Clean intact skin with an antimicrobial solution. Allow it to dry.
- Insert the needle through the client's skin while maintaining adequate *negative* pressure in the syringe and while pulling back on the syringe.
- When performing the aspiration culture technique, it is essential to probe 2-4 areas when obtaining the culture.

QUANTITATIVE SWAB PROCEDURE
- Clean the wound surface with a nonantimicrobial solution. Allow it to dry.
- Swabbing of the wound should encompass 1- to 2-cm area. Enough pressure needs to be used so that fluid is expressed from the wound tissue.
- The culture can be processed during either a quantitative or semiquantitative method, depending on the microbiological expertise of the laboratory.

Modified from Stotts NA: Determination of bacterial burden in wounds. NPUAP Proceedings 1995, *Adv Wound Care* 8(4):28, 1995.

CLIENT TEACHING
for Impaired Skin Integrity

OBJECTIVE
- Risks for impaired skin integrity will be reduced.

TEACHING STRATEGIES
- Demonstrate measures to reduce pressure, moisture, and friction on the skin.
- Explain how to evaluate and select proper incontinence control devices.
- Provide written materials that explain skin care procedures in clear, easy to understand, nontechnical language.
- Explain to client whom to contact and what to do if a break in skin integrity occurs.

EVALUATION
- Observe client perform proper positioning and skin-care measures.
- Assess skin for breaks in integrity.
- Ask client how an incontinence control device was selected.
- Ask client what to do if a break in skin integrity occurs.

► RESEARCH HIGHLIGHT

RESEARCH ABSTRACT

The purpose of this study was to describe and gain understanding of the unexplored experiences of wives who were caring for their frail, homebound elderly husbands with pressure ulcers. The study consisted of six caucasian wives who ranged in age from 69 to 82 years. The husbands ranged in age from 73 to 88.5 years. All of the men experienced either total or intermittent fecal incontinence. Each husband had one or more stage III or IV pressure ulcers. The length of time that the women cared for their husbands ranged from 2 to 10 years.

Analysis of the interviews revealed five major themes: (1) difficult care giving (which was further delineated into the physical, emotional, safety, and financial realms), (2) frailty of the care giver, (3) limited socialization, (4) limited social support systems, and (5) limited care-giving knowledge. The two minor recurring themes were (1) fear regarding the future and (2) the symbolic meaning of the pressure ulcer.

IMPLICATIONS FOR PRACTICE

► More family education is needed.

► Innovative strategies to reach out to families and educate care givers could include:

■ Educational programming on TV

■ Attaching to social security checks toll-free numbers for obtaining home assistance, counseling, and free educational literature.

■ Marketing of home care nursing services and providing general care giving resource literature in grocery stores and in physician offices.

REFERENCE

Baharestani MM: The lived experience of wives caring for their frail, homebound, elderly husbands with pressure ulcers, *Adv Wound Care* 7(3):40, 1994.

Table 38-10	Oral and Cutaneous Signs of Vitamin or Mineral Deficiencies
CLINICAL SIGNS (BY SITE)	**DEFICIENCY(IES)**
ORAL CAVITY	
Cheilosis and angular stomatitis	Vitamin B_2
Glossitis (i.e., pink or magenta discoloration with loss of villi)	Multiple B vitamins
EYES	
Scleral changes	Vitamin A
Bitot's spots	Vitamin A
FACE	
Seborrhea-like dryness and redness of nasolabial fold and eyebrows	Zinc
UPPER EXTREMITIES	
Purplish blotches on lightly traumatized areas (due to capillary fragility and subepithelial hemorrhages)	Vitamin C
Extreme transparency of skin of hands ("cellophane skin")	Vitamin C
ABDOMEN/BUTTOCKS	
Waxy, perifollicular hyperkeratosis	Vitamin A
LOWER EXTREMITIES	
Superficial flaking of epidermis, large flakes of dandruff	Essential fatty acids
Cracks in skin between islands of hyperkeratosis:	
■ Pigmented	Nicotinamide (niacinamide)
■ Nonpigmented	Vitamin A

Note: These manifestations may be seen in disease processes other than vitamin deficiencies. If the cause is in fact a deficiency, clinical improvement should be evident 4 weeks after supplementation is begun.

From Bergstrom N, Bennett MA, Carlson CE, et al: *Treatment of pressure ulcers*. Clinical Practice Guideline, No. 15. Rockville, MD: U.S. Department of Health and Human Services. Public Health Service, Agency for Health Care Policy and Research. AHCPR Publication No. 95–0652. December 1994.

identified psychosocial needs of clients and their support persons (AHCPR, 1994).

Nutritional Status. Maintaining adequate protein intake and hemoglobin levels is important in the treatment of pressure ulcers (Kaminski and Pinchocofsky-Devin, 1989). An algorithm provided by AHCPR (1994) can be used to help clinicians meet the goals of nutritional assessment and management for clients with pressure ulcers. AHCPR (1994) recommends that an abbreviated nutritional assessment be done every 3 months for individuals at risk for malnutrition (see the box at right). This includes individuals who are unable to take food by mouth or who have experienced an involuntary change in weight. Parameters for clinically significant malnutrition have been defined by AHCPR (1994) (see the box on p. 989). The client's mouth and skin should be assessed for signs of nutritional deficiencies (Table 38-10). Vitamins and mineral supplements should be given if deficiencies are confirmed or suspected. The client's hydration status, especially the amount of fluids and the weight pattern, should also be assessed.

Protein Status. Clients with a potential for or actual decreased serum albumin levels or poor protein intake need a

Nutritional Assessment and Management of Pressure Ulcers AHCPR 1994 Treatment Guideline Recommendations

■ Ensure adequate dietary intake to prevent malnutrition to the extent that this is compatible with the individual's wishes.

■ Perform an abbreviated nutritional assessment, as defined by the Nutritional Screening Initiative, at least every 3 months for individuals who are unable to take food by mouth or who experience an involuntary change in weight.

■ Encourage dietary intake or supplementation if an individual with a pressure ulcer is malnourished. If dietary intake continues to be inadequate, impractical, or impossible, nutritional support (usually tube feeding) should be used to place the client into positive nitrogen balance (approximately 30 to 35 calories/kg/day and 1.25 to 1.50 of protein/kg/day) according to the goals of care.

■ Give vitamin and mineral supplements if deficiencies are confirmed or suspected.

Clinically Significant Malnutrition

- Serum albumin less than 3.5 mg/dL
- Total lymphocyte count is less than 1800/mm^3
- Body weight has decreased more than 15%

Modified from AHCPR Treatment Guidelines, 1994.

nutritional evaluation to ensure proper caloric intake (AHCPR, 1994; Maklebust, 1991a). A client can lose as much as 50 g of protein per day from an open, weeping pressure ulcer. This is a sizable amount of the daily recommended requirement of 60 g for women and 70 g for men (Kavchak-Keyes, 1977). Increased protein intake helps rebuild epidermal tissue. Increased caloric intake helps replace subcutaneous tissue. Increased intake of vitamin C promotes protein synthesis and tissue repair (Shekleton and Litwack, 1991).

Hemoglobin. A low hemoglobin level decreases delivery of oxygen to the tissues and leads to further ischemia. When possible, hemoglobin should be maintained at 12 g/100 ml.

Evaluation

Because each client has different risk factors for impaired skin integrity, nursing interventions must be individualized. Clients with minimal mobility impairments or relatively stable health status may need only a few measures.

Nursing interventions for reducing and treating pressure ulcers are evaluated by determining the client's response to nursing therapies and by determining whether each goal was achieved (see the evaluation box below).

To evaluate outcomes and responses to care, the nurse measures the effectiveness of interventions. This often occurs over an extended period of time, requiring the nurse to make careful ongoing measurements of an ulcer's condition. The nurse also evaluates specific interventions designed to promote skin integrity and to teach the client and family to reduce future threats to skin integrity.

Using the nursing process, the nurse collects data related to the client's skin integrity, exposure to risks, and physical condition. Nursing interventions are developed to promote skin integrity in the hospital and in the home or restorative care facility after discharge. The nurse makes referrals to other experts in pressure ulcers such as ET nurses and physical therapists (PTs) when indicated. The nurse also evaluates the client's and family's need for additional support services (e.g., home health care, physical therapy, and counseling) and initiates the referral process. Care of the client with a pressure ulcer requires a multidisciplinary team approach. The nurse is part of that team and consults with members of the team to provide a comprehensive approach to care of the client with a pressure ulcer. The nurse also recognizes personal limitations and makes referrals to other team members such as dietitians, pharmacists, physicians, PTs, and ET nurses, to name a few, whose expertise can enhance the care of clients with pressure ulcers.

Sample Evaluation of Interventions for Impaired Skin Integrity

GOALS	EVALUATION MEASURES	EXPECTED OUTCOMES
Injury to skin and underlying tissue resulting from pressure on bony prominences will be prevented.	Observe skin over bony prominences.	Skin will remain intact (6/1). Normal reactive hyperemia will occur (6/1).
	Palpate skin and underlying tissue over bony prominences.	Blanching will occur (6/1).
Injury to skin and underlying tissue resulting from pressure on bony prominences will be reduced by 6/20.	Measure perimeter and diameter of wound.	Wound size will decrease (6/10).
	Observe drainage.	There will be a decrease in wound drainage (6/20).
	Observe nonaffected areas.	
	Observe and time reactive hyperemic response in affected area.	There will be decreased hyperemia in affected areas (6/15).

■ KEY CONCEPTS ■

▶ Pressure ulcers remain a potential problem in acute and restorative care settings.

▶ Pressure ulcers increase length of stay in hospitals and extended care settings, as well as the overall cost of nursing care needed to manage the wound.

▶ The Agency for Health Care Policy and Research developed guidelines for future research directions and for the prevention and treatment of pressure ulcers.

▶ Prediction for development of pressure ulcers must focus on clients having the greatest risk for developing impaired skin integrity.

▶ Alterations in mobility, sensory perception, level of consciousness, and nutrition; the use of orthopedic devices such as casts; and the presence of severe infection or other debilitating diseases increase the risk for pressure ulcer development.

▶ External pressure, shearing force, moisture, impaired peripheral circulation, edema, and obesity are also contributing factors to the development of pressure ulcers.

▶ When the external pressure against the skin is greater than the pressure in the capillary bed, blood flow decreases to the adjacent tissues.

▶ Decreased circulation to the tissues results in tissue hypoxia; if untreated, tissue necrosis results.

▶ There are four stages of pressure ulcers.

▶ Meticulous assessment of the skin and underlying tissue and identification of risk factors are important in decreasing the opportunity for pressure ulcer development.

▶ In addition to assessing reactive hyperemia, the nurse must also palpate adjacent tissue for signs of induration.

▶ Preventive skin care is aimed at controlling external pressure on bony prominences and keeping the skin clean, well lubricated and hydrated, and free of excess moisture.

▶ Plastic-lined pads protect the bed, not the client's skin, because they do not remove moisture away from the client's skin.

▶ Proper positioning should reduce the effects of pressure and guard against the shearing force.

▶ Therapeutic beds and mattresses reduce the effects of pressure; however, selection is based on assessment data to identify the best bed for individual needs.

▶ Cleansing and topical agents used to treat pressure ulcers vary according to the stage of the pressure ulcer and condition of the wound bed. Assessment of the ulcer enables the nurse to select proper skin care agents.

▶ Nutritional interventions are directed at improving wound healing through increasing protein, calorie, and hemoglobin levels.

▶ The risk of impaired skin integrity related to immobilization depends on the extent and duration of immobilization.

■ KEY TERMS ■

Abnormal reactive hyperemia, p. 955

Anemia, p. 957

Blanching, p. 954

Cachexia, p. 957

Capillary closing pressure, p. 954

Darkly pigmented skin, p. 954

Debridement, p. 976

Edema, p. 957

Eschar, p. 976

Friction, p. 956

Induration, p. 955

Moist wound healing, p. 986

Normal reactive hyperemia, p. 955

Pressure ulcer, p. 949

Pressure reducing, p. 970

Pressure relieving, p. 970

Shearing force, p. 956

Sloughing, p. 976

Tissue ischemia, p. 953

■ CRITICAL THINKING EXERCISES ■

1. You are caring for a client with a spinal cord injury. What are your priorities for reducing the risk for pressure ulcers?

2. After changing a client's position, you observe redness over the bony prominences. What type of assessment must you perform to obtain correct information regarding pressure ulcer risk?

3. You have just admitted a client from a nursing home to your division. On initial assessment, you assess a stage III pressure ulcer. How do you determine the type of care and dressing to use with this particular pressure ulcer?

4. You are providing care to an elderly incontinent Hispanic male that is bed-bound. How will you assess for pressure ulcers in this client? What measures can you take to prevent his skin from breaking down?

REFERENCES

AHCPR Panel for the Prediction and Prevention of Pressure Ulcers in Adults: *Pressure ulcers in adults: prediction and prevention* (AHCPR Publication No. 92-0047). Rockville, MD: Agency for Health Care Policy and Research, Public Health Service, U.S. Department of Health and Human Services. (Clinical Practice Guideline, Number 3), (1992).

AHCPR Panel for the Treatment of Pressure Ulcers: *Treatment of pressure ulcers* (AHCPR Publication No. 95-0652). Rockville, MD: Agency for Health Care Policy and Research, Public Health Service, U.S. Department of Health and Human Services. (Clinical Practice Guideline, Number 15), (1994).

AHCPR Panel for Urinary Incontinence Guideline: *Urinary incontinence in adults* (AHCPR Publication No. 920038). Rockville, Md: Agency for Health Care Policy and Research, Public Health Service, U.S. Department of Health and Human Services. (Clinical Practice Guideline), (March, 1992).

Allman RM: Epidemiology of pressure sores in different populations, *Decubitus* 2(20):30, 1989.

Ayello EA: Teaching the assessment of patients with pressure ulcers, *Decubitus* 5(4):53, 1992.

Ayello EA: A critique of the AHCPR's "Preventing pressure ulcers—a patient's guide" as a written instructional tool, *Decubitus* 6(3):44, 1993.

Ayello EA: Critique of AHCPR's Consumer guide "Treating pressure sores," *Adv Wound Care* 7(5):18, 1995.

Baharestani MM: The lived experience of wives caring for their frail, homebound, elderly husbands with pressure ulcers, *Adv Wound Care* 7(3):40, 1994.

Baranoski S: Wound assessment and dressing selection, *Ostomy/Wound Manage* 41(7A):7S, 1995.

Barnes SH: Patient/family education for the patient with a pressure necrosis, *Nurs Clin North Am* 22:463, 1987.

Barr JE: Principles of wound cleansing, *Ostomy/Wound Manage* 41(7A):15S, 1995.

Bates-Jensen B: New pressure ulcer status tool, *Decubitus* 3(3):14, 1990.

Bates-Jensen B: Indices to include in wound healing assessment, NPUAP Proceedings 1995, *Adv Wound Care* 7(4):28, 1995.

Bennett MA: Characteristics of intact dark skin. *Report of the task force on the implications for darkly pigmented intact skin and the predictions and prevention of pressure ulcers*, Brooklyn, New York, 1995, Woodhull Medical and Mental Health Center.

Berecek KH: Etiology of decubitus ulcers, *Nurs Clin North Am* 10:157, 1975.

Bergstrom N, Demuth PJ, Branden B: A clinical trial of the Braden scale for predicting pressure sore risk, *Nurs Clin North Am* 22(2):417, 1987.

Bergstrom N et al: The Braden Scale for predicting pressure sore risk, *Nurs Res* 36:205, 1987.

Braden BJ, Bergstrom N: Clinical utility of the Braden Scale for predicting pressure sore risk, *Decubitus* 2:3, 1989.

Braden BJ, Bergstrom N: Predictive validity of the Braden Scale for pressure sore risk in a nursing home population, *Res Nurs Health* 17(6):459, 1994.

Breslow RA: Nutrition and air-fluidized beds: a literature review, *Adv Wound Care* 7(3):57, 1994.

Breslow RA, Bergstrom N: Nutritional prediction of pressure ulcers, *J Am Diet Assoc* 94(11):1301, 1994.

Breslow RA, Hallfrisch J, Guy DG et al: The importance of dietary protein in healing pressure ulcers, *J Am Geriatr Soc* 41(4):357, 1993.

Bryant RA, ed: *Acute and chronic wounds: nursing management*, St Louis, 1992, Mosby.

Bryant RA, Shannon ML, Pieper B, et al: Pressure ulcers. In Bryant RA, ed: *Acute and chronic wounds: nursing management*, St Louis, 1992, Mosby.

Cooper DM: Indices to include in wound assessment. NPUAP Proceedings 1995, *Adv Wound Care* 7(4):28, 1995.

Dallam L, Smyth C, Jackson B, et al: Pressure ulcer pain: assessment and quantification. Poster session presented at the National Pressure Ulcer Advisory Panel (NPUAP) Fourth National Conference on Pressure Ulcers, "Pressure Ulcer Healing: controversy to consensus, Assessment methods and outcomes, Washington, DC, February 24-25, 1995.

Doak CC, Doak LG, Root JH: *Teaching patients with low literacy skills*, ed 2, Philadelphia, 1996, Lippincott.

Doughty DB: Principles of wound healing and wound management. In Bryant RA, ed: *Acute and chronic wounds: nursing management*, St Louis, 1992, Mosby.

Ebersole P, Hess P: *Toward elderly aging: human needs and nursing responses*, St Louis, 1994, Mosby.

Finucane TE: Malnutrition, tube feeding and pressure sores: data are incomplete, *Am Geriatr Soc* 43(4):447, 1995.

Foresman PA, Payne DS, Becker D, et al: A relative toxicity index for wound cleansers, *Wounds* 5(5):226, 1993.

Gaskin FC: Detection of cyanosis in the person with dark skin, *J Natl Black Nurses Assoc* 1:52, 1986.

Gentzkow GD: Methods for measuring size in pressure ulcers. NPUAP Proceedings 1995, *Adv Wound Care* 7(4):28, 1995.

Gosnell DJ: An assessment tool to identify pressure sores, *Nurs Res* 22(1):55, 1973.

Gosnell DJ: Assessment and evaluation of pressure sores, *Nurs Clin North Am* 22(2):399, 1987.

Gosnell, DJ: Pressure sore risk assessment: a critique, part I, the Gosnell Scale, *Decubitus* 2:3, 1989.

Gosnell DJ: Pressure sore risk assessment part II: analysis of risk factors, *Decubitus* 2:3, 1989b.

Green E, Katz J: Practice guidelines for management of pressure ulcers, *Decubitus* 4(1):36, 1991.

Graves DJ: Stage I in ebony complexion. Letters to the editor, *Decubitus* 3(4):4, 1990.

Hanan K, Scheele L: Albumin vs. weight as a predictor of nutritional status and pressure ulcer development, *Ostomy/Wound Manage* 33:22, 1991.

Hanson D, Langemo D, Olson B, et al: The prevalence and incidence of pressure ulcers in home care: are patients at risk? *J Home Health Care* 5(3):25, 1993.

Harding KG: Methods for assessing change in ulcer status. NPUAP Proceedings 1995, *Adv Wound Care* 7(4):28, 1995.

Hastings KE: Legal aspects of the AHCPR pressure ulcer guidelines, *Decubitus* 4(2):36, 1991.

Helt J: Foot care and footwear to prevent amputation, *J Vasc Nurs* 9(4):2, 1991.

Hentzen B, Bergstrom N, Pozehl B: Prevalence and incidence of pressure ulcers and associated risk factors in rural-based home health population. Poster presentation at 17th Annual Midwest Nursing Research Society, March 28-30, Cleveland, Ohio, 1993.

Hess CT: *Nurse's clinical guide: wound care*, Philadelphia, 1995, Springhouse.

Hoff J: Effecting a change in nursing practice: pressure ulcer prevention, *J Nurs Qual Assur* 3(4):56, 1989.

Husain T: An experimental study of some pressure effects on tissues, with reference to the bedsore problem, *J Pathol Bacteriol* 66:347, 1953.

Itoh M, Montemayor JS Jr, Matsumoto E, et al: Accelerated wound healing of pressure ulcers by pulsed high peak power electromagnetic energy (Diapulse), *Decubitus* 4(1):24, 1991.

Jacobs BW: Working on the right moves, *Nurs 94* 58, 1994.

Kaminski MV, Pinchcofsky-Devin G, Williams JP: Nutritional management of decubitus ulcers in the elderly, *Decubitus* 2(4):20, 1989.

Kane RL, Ouslander JG, Abrass IB: *Essentials of clinical geriatrics*, ed 2, New York, 1989, McGraw-Hill.

Kavchak-Keyes MA: Four proven steps for preventing decubitus ulcers, *Nurs 77* 7:58, 1977.

Kim MJ, McFarland GK, McLane AM: *Pocket guide to nursing diagnoses*, ed 6, St Louis, 1995, Mosby.

Konstantinides NN, Lehmann S: The impact of nutrition on wound healing, *Crit Care Nurse* 25, 1993.

Koziak M: Etiology and pathology of ischemic ulcers, *Arch Phys Med Rehabil* 40:62, 1959.

Kloth LC, McCulloch JM, Feedar JA: *Wound healing: alternatives in management*, Philadelphia, 1990, FA Davis.

Krasner D: The twelve commandments of wound care, *Nurs 92* 22(12):34, 1992.

Krasner D: Wound care: how to use the red-yellow-black system, *Am J Nurs* 5:44, 1995.

Krouskop T, van Rijswijk L: Standardizing performance-based criteria for support surfaces, *Ostomy/Wound Manage* 41(1):34, 1995.

Landis EM: Micro-injection studies of capillary blood pressure in human skin, *Heart* 15:209, 1930.

Langemo DK, Olson B, Hunters S, et al: Incidences of pressure sores in acute care, rehabilitation, extended care, home health, and hospice in one locale, *Decubitus* 2(2):42, 1989.

Leshem OA, Skelskey C: Pressure ulcers: quality management, prevalence, and severity in a long-term care setting, *Adv Wound Care* 7(2):50, 1994.

Levine JM: Historical notes on pressure ulcers: the cure of Ambrose Pare, *Decubitus* 5(2):23, 1992.

Lucas MD: Research implications of the pressure ulcer guideline, *Decubitus* 4(2):52, 1991.

Maklebust J: Pressure ulcers: etiology and intervention, *Nurs Clin North Am* 22(2):359, 1987.

Maklebust J: Impact of AHCPR pressure ulcer guidelines on nursing practice, *Decubitus* 4(2):46, 1991a.

Maklebust J: Pressure ulcer update, *RN* 41(12):56, 1991b.

Maklebust J: Pressure ulcer staging systems. NPUAP Proceeding 1995, *Adv Wound Care* 7(4):28, 1995.

Maklebust J, Magnan MA: Approaches to patient and family education for pressure ulcer management, *Decubitus* 5(4):18, 1992.

Maklebust J, Margolis D: Pressure ulcers: definition and assessment parameters. NPUAP Proceedings 1995, *Adv Wound Care* 7(4):28, 1995.

Maklebust J, Sieggreen M: *Pressure ulcers: guidelines for prevention and nursing management.* West Dundee, IL, 1991, S-N Publications.

Margolis DJ: Definition of a pressure ulcer. NPUAP Proceedings 1995, *Adv Wound Care* 7(4):28, 1995

Meehan M: National Pressure Ulcer Prevalence Survey, *Adv Wound Care* 7(3):27, 1994.

National Pressure Ulcer Advisory Panel (NPUAP): Pressure ulcer prevalence, cost and risk assessment: consensus development conference statement, *Decubitus* 2(2):24, 1989a.

National Pressure Ulcer Advisory Panel (NPUAP): Pressure ulcers incidence, economics, risk assessment: consensus development conference statement, *Decubitus* 2(2):24, 1989b.

National Pressure Ulcer Advisory Panel (NPUAP): *Pressure ulcer research: etiology, assessment, and early intervention*, monograph, Buffalo, New York, NPUAP author, 1995a.

National Pressure Ulcer Advisory Panel (NPUAP): NPUAP proceedings of the Fourth National NPUAP Conference—pressure ulcer healing: controversy to consensus—assessment methods and outcomes, Washington, DC, February 24-25, 1995b.

Natlow AB: Nutrition in prevention and treatment of decubitus ulcers, *Top Clin Nurs* 5(2):39, 1983.

Norton D: Calculating the risk: reflections on the Norton Scale, *Decubitus* 2:3, 1989.

Norton D, McLaren R, Exon-Smith AN: *An investigation of geriatric nursing problems in hospital, 1962,* Edinburgh, reissue 1975, Churchill Livingstone.

Olshansky K: Essay on knowledge, caring and psychological factors in prevention and treatment of pressure ulcers, *Adv Wound Care* 7(3):64, 1994.

Oot-Giromini BA: Pressure ulcer prevalence, incidence and associated risk factors in the community, *Decubitus* 6(5):24, 1993.

Oot-Giromini BA, Bidwell FC, Heller NB, et al: Pressure ulcer prevention versus treatment: comparative product cost study, *Decubitus* 2(3):52, 1989.

Pajk M et al: Investigating the problem of pressure sores, *J Gerontol Nurs* 12(7):11, 1986.

Pinchcofsky-Devin GD, Kaminski MV: Correlation of pressure sores and nutritional status, *J Am Geriatr Soc* 34:435, 1989.

Pires M, Muller A: Detection and management of early tissue pressure indicators: a pictorial essay, *Progressions* 3(3):3, 1991.

Plaisier B, Gabram SGA, Schwartz RJ et al: Prospective evaluation of craniofacial pressure in four different cervical orthoses, *J Trauma* 37(5):714, 1994.

Reuler JB, Cooney TG: The pressure sore: pathophysiology and principles of management, *Ann Intern Med* 94(5):661, 1981.

Rodeheaver GT: Preface to the program of the National Pressure Ulcer Advisory Panel (NPUAP) Fourth National Conference—Pressure ulcer healing: controversy to consensus, NPUAP Proceedings 1995, *Adv Wound Care* 8(4):28, 1995.

Rodeheaver G, Baharestani M, Brabec ME, et al: Wound healing and wound management: focus on debridement, *Adv Wound Care* 7(1):22, 1994.

Rodeheaver GT, Stotts NA: Methods for assessing change in pressure ulcer status. NPUAP Proceedings 1995, *Adv Wound Care* 7(4):28, 1995.

Shea JD: Pressure sores: classification and management, *Clin Orthop* 112:89, 1975.

Shekleton ME, Litwack K: *Critical care nursing of the surgical patient*, Philadelphia, 1991, Saunders.

Steinberg J: Prevalence of decubitus ulcers: issues of concern, *Decubitus* 2(2):50, 1990.

Stotts NA: Determination of bacterial burden in wounds. NPUAP Proceedings 1995, *Adv Wound Care* 7(4):28, 1995.

Stotts NA: Predicting pressure ulcer development in surgical patients, *Heart Lung* 17(6):641, 1988.

Task Force for the implications for darkly pigmented intact skin and the prediction and prevention of pressure ulcers, Brooklyn, New York, 1995.

Trumble HC: The skin tolerance for pressure and pressure sores, *Med J Aust* 2:724, 1930.

van Rijswijk L: Frequency of reassessment of pressure ulcers. NPUAP Proceedings 1995, *Adv Wound Care* 7(4):28, 1995.

Walter MJ, Bartell TH, Paletta CE, et al: Wound healing and nutritional state in patients undergoing reconstruction of chronic wounds. *WOUNDS: a compendium of clinical research and practice* 6(4):128, 1994.

Winter GD: Formation of scab and the rate of epithelialization of superficial wounds in the skin of the domestic pig, *Nature*, 193:293, 1962.

Wright RW, Orr R: Fibroblast cytotocity and blood cell integrity following exposure to dermal wound cleaners, *Ostomy/Wound Manage* 39(7):33, 1993.

Young L: Pressure ulcer prevalence and associated patient characteristics in one long-term care facility, *Decubitus* 2(2):52, 1989.

ADDITIONAL READINGS

Beckett WS et al: Effect of prolonged bedrest on lung volume in normal individuals, *J Appl Physiol* 61(3):919, 1986.

Brown-Etris M: Measuring healing in wounds. NPUAP Proceedings 1995, *Adv Wound Care* 7(4):28, 1995.

Byrne N, Feld M: Overcoming the red menace: preventing and treating decubitus ulcers, *Nurs 84* 14:55, 1984.

Cassell BL: Treating pressure sores stage by stage, *RN* 36:41, 1986.

Kosiak M: Etiology of decubitus ulcers, *Arch Phys Med Rehabil* 42:19, 1961.

Linden O et al: Pressure distribution on the surface of the human body, *Arch Phys Med Rehabil* 46:378, 1965.

McCance KL, Huether SE: *Pathophysiology: the biologic basis for disease in adults and children*, ed 2, St Louis, 1994, Mosby.

Norton D, McLaren R, Exon-Smith A: Pressure sores. In Horsley JA, ed: *Preventing decubitus ulcers: CURN project,* New York, 1981, Grune & Stratton.

Rubin M: The physiology of bedrest, *Am J Nurs* 88:50, 1988.

Shannon ML: Five famous fallacies about pressure sores, *Nurs 84* 13:34, 1984.

Thomas C: Specialty beds: decision-making made easy, *Ostomy/Wound Manage* 23:51, 1989.

Trelease CC: Developing standards for wound care, *Ostomy/Wound Manage* 20:46, 1988.

Willey T: High tech beds and mattress overlays: a decision guide, *Am J Nurs* 89:1142, 1989.

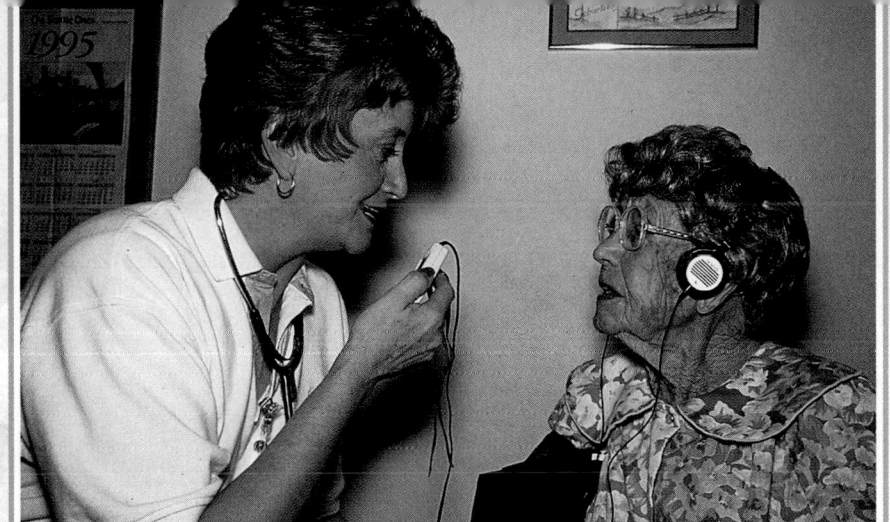
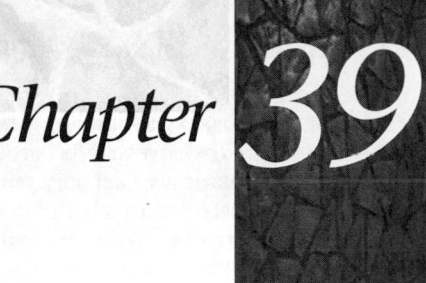

## Chapter 39

Sensory Alterations

Objectives

Mastery of content in this chapter will enable the student to:

▶ Define the key terms listed.

▶ Differentiate among the processes of reception, perception, and reaction to sensory stimuli.

▶ Discuss the relationship of sensory function to an individual's level of wellness.

▶ Discuss common causes and effects of sensory alterations.

▶ Discuss common sensory changes that normally occur with aging.

▶ Identify factors to assess in determining a client's sensory status.

▶ Identify nursing diagnoses relevant to clients with sensory alterations..

▶ Develop a plan of care for clients with visual, auditory, tactile, speech, and olfactory deficits.

▶ List interventions for preventing sensory deprivation and controlling sensory overload.

▶ Describe conditions in the health care agency or client's home that can be adjusted to promote meaningful sensory stimulation.

▶ Discuss ways to maintain a safe environment for clients with sensory deficits.

Imagine the world without sight, hearing, or the ability to feel objects or sense aromas around you. Human beings rely on a variety of sensory stimuli to give meaning and order to events occurring in their environment. The senses are tightly interwoven in forming the perceptual base of our world (Ebersole and Hess, 1994). Stimulation comes from many sources in and outside the body, particularly through the senses of sight (visual), hearing (**auditory**), touch (**tactile**), smell (**olfactory**), and taste (**gustatory**). The body also has a **kinesthetic** sense that enables a person to be aware of the position and movement of body parts without seeing them. **Stereognosis** is a sense that allows a person to recognize an object's size, shape, and texture. The ability to speak is not considered a sense, but it is similar in that the client may lose the ability to interact meaningfully with other human beings. Meaningful stimuli allow a person to learn about the environment and are necessary for healthy functioning and normal development. When sensory function is altered, the person's ability to relate to and function within the environment changes drastically.

Many clients seeking health care have preexisting sensory alterations. Others may develop sensory alterations as a result of medical treatment (e.g., hearing loss from antibiotic use). The environment of a health care setting (e.g., a noisy intensive care unit) can cause sensory alterations. Clients who have partial or complete loss of a major sense need to find alternative ways to function safely within the environment. If sensory alterations occur early in life, clients often have developmental and socialization problems because of difficulty in responding to people and the environment. A health care setting is often a place of unfamiliar sights, sounds, and smells and minimal contact with family and friends. If clients feel depersonalized and are unable to receive meaningful stimuli, serious sensory alterations can develop.

The nurse must understand and help meet the needs of clients with sensory alterations as well as recognize clients most at risk for developing sensory problems. The nurse helps clients learn to interact and react safely and effectively in their environment.

NORMAL SENSATION

Normally, the nervous system continually receives thousands of bits of information from sensory nerve organs, relays the information through appropriate channels, and integrates the information into a meaningful response. Sensory stimuli reach the sensory organs and can elicit an immediate reaction or present information to the brain to be stored for future use. The nervous system must be intact for sensory stimuli to reach appropriate brain centers and for the individual to perceive the sensation. After interpreting the significance of a sensation, the person can then react to the stimulus. Table 39-1 summarizes normal hearing and vision.

Reception, perception, and reaction are the three components of any sensory experience (see Chapter 43). Reception begins with stimulation of a nerve cell called a *receptor*, which is usually designed for only one type of stimulus, such as light or sound. In the case of special senses, the receptors are grouped close together or located in specialized organs (Thibodeau and Patton, 1993) such as the taste buds of the tongue or the retina of the eye. Once a nerve impulse is created it travels along pathways to the spinal cord or directly to the brain. For example, sound waves stimulate hair cell receptors within the organ of Corti, which causes im-

Table 39-1	Normal Hearing and Vision	
FUNCTION	**ANATOMY AND PHYSIOLOGY**
THE EAR Transmits to the brain an accurate pattern of all sounds received from the environment, the relative intensity of these sounds, and the direction from which they originate.	Two ears provide stereophonic hearing to judge sound direction. The external ear canal shelters the eardrum and maintains relatively constant temperature and humidity to maintain elasticity. The middle ear is an air-containing space between the eardrum and oval window. It contains three small bones (ossicles). The eardrum and ossicles transfer sound to the fluid-filled inner ear. Movement of the stapes in the oval window creates vibrations in the fluid that bathes the membranous labyrinth, which contains the end organs of hearing and balance. The union of the vestibular (balance) and cochlear (hearing) portions of the labyrinth explains the combination of hearing and balance symptoms of inner ear disorders. Vibration of the eardrum is transmitted through the bony ossicles. Vibrations at the oval window are transmitted in perilymph within the inner ear to stimulate hair cells that send impulses along the eighth cranial nerve to the brain.
THE EYE Transmits to the brain an accurate pattern of light reflected from solid objects in the environment and transformed into color and hue.	Light rays enter the convex cornea and begin to converge. Fine adjustment of light rays occurs as they pass through the pupil and through the lens. Change in the shape of the lens focuses light on the retina. The retina has a pigmented layer of cells to enhance visual acuity. The sensory retina contains the rods and cones, photoreceptor cells sensitive to stimulation from light. Photoreceptor cells send electrical potentials by way of the optic nerve to the brain.

pulses to travel along the eighth cranial nerve to the acoustic area of the temporal lobe. Sensory nerve pathways usually cross over to send stimuli to opposite sides of the brain. The actual perception or awareness of unique sensations depends on the receiving region of the cerebral cortex, where specialized brain cells interpret the quality and nature of sensory stimuli. When the person becomes conscious of the stimuli and receives the information, perception takes place. A person's level of consciousness influences how well stimuli are perceived and interpreted. Any factors lowering consciousness impair sensory perception. Perception includes integration and interpretation of the stimuli based on the person's experiences. If sensation is incomplete, such as blurred vision, or if past experience is inadequate for understanding stimuli such as pain, the person may react to the sensory stimulus inappropriately.

It is impossible to react to each of the multiple stimuli entering the nervous system. The brain prevents sensory bombardment by discarding or storing sensory information. A person will usually react to stimuli that are most meaningful or significant at the time. After continued reception of the same stimulus, however, a person stops responding and the sensory experience goes unnoticed. For example, a person concentrating on reading a good book may not be aware of music in the background. This adaptability phenomenon occurs with most sensory stimuli except for those of pain.

The balance between sensory stimuli entering the brain and those actually reaching a person's conscious awareness maintains a person's well-being. If an individual attempts to react to every stimulus within the environment or if there is insufficient variety and quality of stimuli, sensory alterations will occur.

SENSORY ALTERATIONS

Many factors change the capacity to receive or perceive sensations (see the box below), thus causing sensory alterations. The types of sensory alterations commonly seen by the nurse are sensory deficits, sensory deprivation, and sensory overload. When a client suffers from more than one sensory alteration, the ability to function and relate effectively within the environment is seriously impaired.

Sensory Deficits

A defect in the normal function of sensory reception and perception is a **sensory deficit**. A client may not be able to receive certain stimuli (e.g., blindness or deafness), or stimuli become distorted (e.g., blurred vision from cataracts). A sudden sensory loss can cause fear, anger, and feelings of helplessness. When senses are impaired, the sense of self is impaired. Initially a person may withdraw by avoiding communication or socialization with others in an attempt to cope with the sensory loss. It becomes difficult for the person to interact safely with the environment until new skills

---

Factors that Influence Sensory Function

AGE
- Infants are unable to discriminate sensory stimuli. Nerve pathways are immature.
- Visual changes during adulthood include presbyopia (inability to focus on near objects) and the need for glasses for reading (usually occurring from ages 40 to 50).
- Hearing changes, which begin at age 30, include decreased hearing acuity, speech intelligibility, pitch discrimination, and hearing threshold. Tinnitus often accompanies a hearing loss as a side effect of drugs. Older adults hear low-pitched sounds the best but have difficulty hearing conversation over background noise.
- Older adults have reduced visual fields, increased glare sensitivity, impaired night vision, reduced accommodation and depth perception, and reduced color discrimination.
- Older adults have difficulty discriminating the consonants (*f, s, th, ch*). Speech sounds are garbled, and there is a delayed reception and reaction to speech.
- Gustatory and olfactory changes include a decrease in the number of taste buds in later years and reduction of olfactory nerve fibers by age 50. Reduced taste discrimination and sensitivity to odors are common.
- **Proprioceptive** changes after age 60 include increased difficulty with balance, spatial orientation, and coordination.
- Older adults experience tactile changes, including declining sensitivity to pain, pressure, and temperature.

MEDICATIONS
- Some antibiotics (e.g., streptomycin, gentamicin) are ototoxic and can permanently damage the auditory nerve; chloramphenicol can irritate the optic nerve. Narcotic analgesics, sedatives, and antidepressant medications can alter the perception of stimuli.

ENVIRONMENT
- Excessive environmental stimuli (e.g., equipment noise and staff conversation in an intensive care unit) can result in sensory overload, marked by confusion, disorientation, and the inability to make decisions. Restricted environmental stimulation (e.g., with isolation) can lead to sensory deprivation. Poor quality of environment (e.g., reduced lighting, narrow walkways, background noise) can worsen sensory impairment.

COMFORT LEVEL
- Pain and fatigue alter the way a person perceives and reacts to stimuli.

PREEXISTING ILLNESSES
- Peripheral vascular disease can cause reduced sensation in the extremities and impaired cognition. Chronic diabetes can lead to reduced vision, blindness, or peripheral neuropathy. Strokes often produce loss of speech. Some neurological disorders impair motor function and sensory reception.

SMOKING
- Chronic tobacco use can atrophy the taste buds, lessening the perception of flavors.

NOISE LEVELS
- Constant exposure to high noise levels (e.g., on a construction job site) can cause hearing loss.

ENDOTRACHEAL INTUBATION
- Temporary loss of speech results from insertion of an endotracheal tube through the mouth or nose into the trachea.

Table 39-2	Common Sensory Deficits	
DEFICIT	**SENSORY CHANGE**	**INFLUENCE ON CLIENT**
VISUAL		
Presbyopia	Loss of accommodation of lens to focus light from near objects.	Person unable to see close objects clearly. Requires bifocal lens. Person compensates by holding objects to be viewed, farther away. Distant vision is unaffected.
Cataract	An opacity of the lens. This loss of transparency blocks light from reaching the retina.	Slow, painless, progressive loss of vision in one or both eyes. Most persons experience glare from bright lights. Lens on examination appears cloudy.
Glaucoma	An increase in intraocular pressure, which if unrelieved damages internal eye structures, including the optic nerve.	Condition is initially symptom free. Change in peripheral vision is first sign. This progresses and can cause loss of central vision. Pain occurs late.
HEARING		
Presbycusis	Progressive loss of hearing acuity that occurs with advancing age. Sensorineural hearing loss.	Condition alters ability to hear high-frequency sounds, initially. Deficit progresses to affect lower tones. Common sign is difficulty discriminating conversation.
External otitis	Infection of the skin in the external auditory canal.	Canal becomes blocked from swelling and buildup of drainage. Causes a temporary conduction deafness.
NEUROLOGICAL		
Cerebrovascular accident (stroke)	Clot, hemorrhage, or embolus obstructs blood flow in artery to the brain, causing ischemia to tissues supplied by blood vessel(s).	Loss of sensation and motor function occurs depending on location of stroke. Client may also lose proprioception, with incoordination and poor balance.
Peripheral neuropathy	Disorder of peripheral nerve lying outside spinal cord and brain. Damage to nerve can affect sensory and motor function.	Disorders lead to alterations in pain, touch, temperature, and motor function. Typically neuropathies affect a person's functional ability to use extremities.

relying on existing functions are learned. When a deficit develops gradually or when considerable time has passed since the onset of an acute sensory loss, the person learns to rely on unaffected senses. Some senses may even become more acute to compensate for an alteration. For example, a blind client often develops an acute sense of hearing.

Clients with sensory deficits may change behavior in adaptive or maladaptive ways. For example, one client with a hearing impairment may turn the unaffected ear toward a speaker to hear better, whereas another client may shun other people to avoid the embarrassment of not being able to understand their speech. Table 39-2 summarizes common sensory deficits and their influence on those affected.

Sensory Deprivation

The reticular activating system in the brain stem mediates all sensory stimuli to the cerebral cortex, so even in deep sleep, clients are able to receive stimuli. Sensory stimulation must be of sufficient quality and quantity to maintain a person's awareness. The most significant sensory deprivation that clients experience is reported to be lack of human touch (MacKellaig, 1986). Clients in ICUs are often exposed to physical touch, but it is usually associated with technical intervention rather than personal, comforting touch. When a person experiences an inadequate quality or quantity of stimulation such as monotonous or meaningless stimuli, **sensory deprivation** occurs. Three types of sensory deprivation are reduced sensory input (sensory deficit from

visual or hearing loss), elimination of order or meaning from input (e.g., exposure to strange environments), and restriction of the environment (e.g., bed rest or reduced environmental variation) that produces monotony and boredom (Ebersole and Hess, 1994).

Individuals at risk for sensory deprivation are commonly those living in the confines of a nursing home. Although most quality nursing homes offer meaningful stimulation through group activities, environmental design, and mealtime gatherings, there are exceptions. The older adult who is confined to a wheelchair, suffers from poor hearing and/or vision, has decreased energy, and avoids contact with others is at significant risk for sensory deprivation (Fig 39-1). If the environment creates monotony, the nursing home resident has a reduced capacity to learn and to think.

There are many effects of sensory deprivation (see the box on p. 997). The symptoms can easily cause nurses and physicians to believe a client is psychologically ill and confused, is suffering from severe electrolyte imbalance, or is under the influence of psychotropic drugs. Therefore the nurse must always be aware of the client's existing sensory function and the quality of stimuli within the environment.

Sensory Overload

When a person receives multiple sensory stimuli and cannot perceptually disregard or selectively ignore some stimuli, **sensory overload** occurs. Excessive sensory stimulation prevents the brain from appropriately responding to or ig-

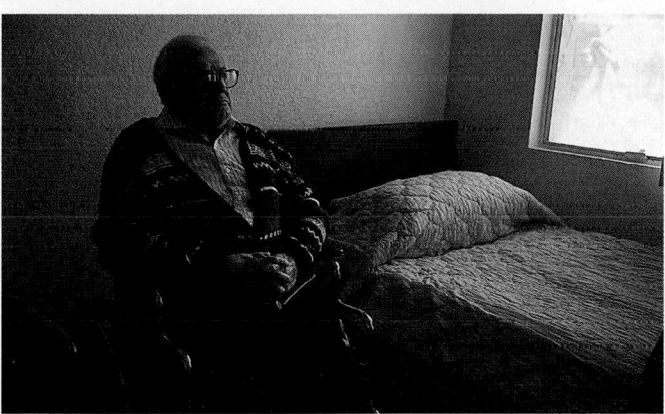

Fig. 39-1 Isolation contributes to sensory deprivation.

Effects of Sensory Deprivation

COGNITIVE
Reduced capacity to learn, inability to think or problem solve, poor task performance, disorientation, bizarre thinking, regression, and increased need for socialization. Mechanisms of attention are altered.

AFFECTIVE
Boredom, restlessness, increased anxiety, emotional lability, panic, and increased need for physical stimulation.

PERCEPTUAL
Perceptual disorganization occurs in visual/motor coordination, color perception, apparent movement, tactile accuracy, ability to perceive size and shape, and spatial and time judgment (Ebersole and Hess, 1994).

noring certain stimuli. Because of the multitude of stimuli leading to overload, the person no longer perceives the environment in a way that makes sense. Overload prevents meaningful response by the brain; the person's thoughts race, attention moves in many directions, and restlessness occurs. As a result, overload causes a state similar to that produced by sensory deprivation. However, in contrast to deprivation, overload is individualized. The amount of stimuli needed for healthy function varies with each individual. Persons may be more subject to environmental overload at one time than another. A person's tolerance to sensory overload may vary by level of fatigue, attitude, and emotional and physical well-being.

The acutely ill client may fall victim to sensory overload. The constant pain from the disease process, the nurse's frequent monitoring of vital signs, and the irritation from drainage tubes protruding from the body combine to cause overload. Even if the nurse offers a comforting word or provides a gentle back rub, clients may not benefit because their attention and energy are focused on more stressful stimuli. Another example is the client hospitalized in an intensive care unit. There the activity is constant. Lights are always on. Sounds can be heard from monitoring equipment, staff conversations, equipment alarms, and the activities of people entering the unit. Even at night an ICU can be very noisy.

The behavioral changes associated with sensory overload can easily be confused with mood swings or simple disorientation. The nurse must look for symptoms such as racing thoughts, scattered attention, restlessness, and anxiety. Intensive care clients sometimes resort to constantly fingering tubes and dressings. Constant reorientation and control of excessive stimuli become an important part of the client's care.

▌ NURSING PROCESS AND SENSORY ALTERATIONS

 ### Assessment

When assessing clients with or at risk for sensory alterations, the nurse considers all the factors influencing sensory function (see the box on p. 995), particularly age. The

nurse collects a history that also assesses the client's current sensory status and the degree to which a sensory deficit affects the client's lifestyle, psychosocial adjustment, self-care ability, and safety. The assessment must also focus on the quality and quantity of environmental stimuli.

Health Promotion Habits

It is important for the nurse to assess the daily routines clients follow to maintain sensory function. This can be a part of the nursing history (see Nursing History section). What type of eye and ear care is incorporated into daily hygiene? For those individuals who participate in sports (e.g., racquetball), recreational activities (e.g., motorcycle riding), or who work in a setting where eye injury is a possibility (e.g., chemical exposure, welding, glass or stone polishing), the nurse determines if safety glasses are worn. Do clients who use assistive devices such as eyeglasses, contact lenses, or hearing aids, know how to provide daily care (see Chapter 40)? Are the devices in proper working order?

The nurse also assesses a client's compliance with routine health screening. When was the last time a client had an eye examination or hearing evaluation? Recommended screening guidelines are usually structured on the basis of client age. When a client begins to show a hearing deficit, routine screening should be incorporated in regular examinations.

Persons at Risk

A nurse assesses sensory function for clients most at risk. Older adults are a high-risk group because of normal physiological changes involving sensory organs. The nurse must be careful to not automatically assume that an older adult's hearing problem is related to advancing age. Adult sensorineural hearing loss can be due to metabolic, vascular, and other systemic lesions. A client may benefit from a referral to an audiologist or otolaryngologist if the assessment reveals serious problems.

A person's occupation can place them at risk for visual, hearing, and peripheral nerve alterations (see the box on p. 998). Individuals who are exposed to loud noises at work or who have occupations involving risk of exposure to chemicals or flying objects should be screened for hearing and visual problems. Clients who use their hands in a repetitive fashion, causing trauma to the median nerve, can

---

Occupations and Leisure Activities that Pose Risk for Sensory Alterations

HEARING
Factory Worker
Airport Worker
Rock Musician
Construction worker using jackhammer

VISION
Exposure to irritating gases
Welder
Exposure to high-speed machinery
Racquetball, squash or fencing
Motorcycle riding
Power tools use

PERIPHERAL NERVE INJURY
Repetitive motion
Computer programmer
Manicurist
Factory worker

TRAUMA
Industrial equipment
Home wood working

Observations Indicating Hearing Loss

- Client seems inattentive to others
- Client responds with inappropriate anger when spoken to
- Client believes people are talking about him or her
- Client has trouble following clear directions
- Client asks to have something repeated
- Client has monotonous or unusual voice quality and speaks unusually loud or soft
- Client has TV unusually loud

Modified from Ebersole P, Hess P: *Toward healthy aging*, ed 4, St Louis, 1994, Mosby.

---

develop carpal tunnel syndrome. The condition is one of the most common industrial or work-related injuries.

A hospitalized client can be at risk for sensory alterations due to exposure to environmental stimuli or a change in sensory input. Clients who are immobilized due to bed rest or physical encumbrances (e.g., casts or traction) are at risk since they are unable to experience all the normal sensations of free movement. Another group at risk includes clients isolated in a health care setting or at home. For example, the client placed in isolation because of tuberculosis (see Chapter 34) is often restricted to a hospital room and is unable to enjoy normal interactions with visitors. A hospital environment is full of sensory stimuli. Therapeutic isolation, the sounds of electrical monitors and equipment, bright lighting, and the odors of body fluids are just some examples. A healthy person can change an environment or seek a different one. As a result of illness or hospitalization, a client is often confined to an unfamiliar and unresponsive environment. This does not mean that all hospitalized clients have sensory alterations. However, the nurse must assess more carefully those clients subjected to continued sensory stimulation (e.g., ICU clients, long term hospitalization, multiple therapies).

Nursing History

The nursing history allows assessment of the nature and characteristics of sensory alterations or any problem related to an alteration. It is important to remember that many older adults are sensitive about admitting losses and may hesitate to share information (Ebersole and Hess, 1994). The nurse begins by asking the client to describe the sensory deficit. For example:

Describe your hearing loss for me.
Describe how your vision is affected.
Explain how use of your hands has changed.

Knowledge about the onset and duration of the sensory alteration can be helpful. The nurse begins to learn how long the client has taken measures to adjust to the alteration.

How long have you had a visual problem?
When did you begin to feel numbness in your legs?
How long have you noticed being unable to hear conversations clearly?

It is also useful to assess the client's self-rating for a sensory deficit. Lewis-Cullinan and Janken (1990) found that a client's self-rating for hearing was one of the most important defining characteristics for the nursing diagnosis auditory sensory/perceptual alteration. The nurse can simply say:

"Rate your hearing as either excellent, good, fair, poor, or bad."

Based on a client's self-rating the nurse may explore more fully the client's perception of a sensory loss. This provides a more in-depth look at how the client's quality of life has been influenced. In the specific case of hearing problems there is a screening tool developed by Ventry and Weinstein (1986) that has been found to be effective in identifying clients needing audiological intervention. The screening version of the Hearing Handicap Inventory for the Elderly (HHIE-S) is a 5 minute, 10 item questionnaire (Fig 39-2) designed to assess how a client perceives the emotional and social effects of hearing loss (Weinstein, 1994).

A nursing history can also reveal any recent changes in a client's behavior. Frequently friends or family are the best resources for this information as the client may be unaware of any change.

Has the client shown any recent mood swings (e.g., outbursts of anger, nervousness, fear, or irritability)?
Have you noticed the client avoiding social activities?

Finally, the nurse must often rely on personal observation of the client to detect sensory alterations. Ebersole and Hess (1994) have identified some typical observations indicating hearing loss (see the box above).

Ability to Perform Self-Care

The nurse assesses clients' functional abilities in their home environments and health care settings, including feeding, dressing, grooming, and toileting activities. For example, the nurse assesses whether a client with altered vision can find items on a meal tray and can read directions on a prescription. The nurse also determines a visually impaired client's ability to perform daily routines such as reading bills and writing checks, differentiating money denomina-

Screening version of the Hearing Handicap Inventory for the Elderly (HHIE-S)

	ITEM	YES (4 pts)	NO (0 pts)	SOMETIMES (2 pts)
E-1	Does a hearing problem cause you to feel embarrassed when you meet new people?	_____	_____	_____
E-2	Does a hearing problem cause you to feel frustrated when talking to members of your family?	_____	_____	_____
S-3	Do you have difficulting hearing when someone speaks in a whisper?	_____	_____	_____
E-4	Do you feel handicapped by a hearing problem?	_____	_____	_____
S-5	Does a hearing problem cause you difficulty when visiting friends, relatives, or neighbors?	_____	_____	_____
S-6	Does a hearing problem cause you to attend religious services less often than you would like?	_____	_____	_____
E-7	Does a hearing problem cause you to have arguments with family members?	_____	_____	_____
S-8	Does a hearing problem cause you difficulty when listening to TV or radio?	_____	_____	_____
E-9	Do you feel that any difficulty with your hearing limits or hampers your personal or social life?	_____	_____	_____
S-10	Does a hearing problem cause you difficulty when in a restaurant with relatives or friends?	_____	_____	_____

RAW SCORE _____ (sum of the points assigned each of the items)

INTERPRETING THE RAW SCORE[6]
0 to 8 = 13% probability of hearing impairment (no handicap/no referral)
10 to 24 = 50% probability of hearing impairment (mild-moderate handicap)
26 to 40 = 84% probability of hearing impairment (severe handicap)

E = Emotional items
S = Social/situational items

Source: Reprinted with permission from Ventry I, Weinstien B. The Hearing Handicap Inventory for the Elderly: A new tool. Ear Hearing 1986: 3:133-4.

Fig. 39-2 Screening version of the Hearing Handicap Inventory for the Elderly (HHIE-S). *(Redrawn from Ventry I, Weinstein B. The hearing handicap inventory for the elderly: a new tool,* Ear Hearing *3:133, 1986.)*

tions, and driving a vehicle at night. If a client seems sensorially deprived, is concern shown for grooming? Does a client's loss of balance prevent rising from a toilet seat safely? Can the client with a stroke manipulate buttons or zippers for dressing? Any impairment in the ability to perform self-care has implications for planning discharge from a health care setting and in providing resources within the home.

Environment

The environment can either minimize or heighten sensory alterations. In some cases the environment (e.g., ICU set-

ting) is the cause of the problem. The nurse assesses the client's environment, both within the health care setting and the home, looking for factors that pose risks or that need adjustment to provide safety and more stimulation.

HAZARDS

A client with sensory alterations is at risk for injury if the living environment is unsafe. For example, a client with visual impairment cannot see potential hazards clearly. A client with proprioceptive problems may lose balance easily. In the home, the nurse carefully assesses the condition of all rooms in the house, including front and back entrances. Some of the hazards to look for include the following:

- Uneven, cracked walkways leading to front/back door
- Doormats with slippery backing
- Extension and phone cords in the main route of walking traffic
- Loose area rugs and runners placed over carpeting
- Bathrooms without shower or tub grab bars
- Water faucets unmarked to designate hot and cold
- Bathroom floor with slippery surface
- Absence of smoke detectors in rooms
- Unlit stairways
- Cluttered furniture, including foot stools
- Kitchen equipment (e.g., ovens, irons, toasters) with control knobs with hard-to-read settings

In the hospital environment, care givers often forget to re-arrange furniture and equipment to keep paths from the bed and chair to the bathroom and entrance clear. Walking into a client's room and looking for safety hazards can be a useful exercise:

Are IV poles on wheels, easy to move?

Are foot stools in the middle of the room?

Are suction machines, IV pumps, or drainage bags positioned so that a client can rise from a bed or chair easily?

An additional problem faced by the visually impaired is the inability to read medication labels and syringe gauges. The nurse asks the client to read a label to determine if the dosage and frequency can be determined. If a client has a hearing impairment, the nurse checks to see whether the sounds of a doorbell, telephone, smoke alarm, and alarm clock are easy to discriminate.

MEANINGFUL STIMULI

Meaningful stimuli reduce the incidence of sensory deprivation. The nurse observes the home environment for stimuli such as pets, a record player or television, pictures of family members, and a calendar and clock. The same type of items should be present in a nursing home. In a health care setting the nurse notes whether clients have roommates or visitors. The presence of others can offer positive stimulation. However, a roommate who constantly watches television, persistently tries to talk, or continuously keeps lights on can contribute to sensory overload. A client can become disoriented in a barren environment that gives few signals for normal sensory perception. The presence or absence of meaningful stimuli influences alertness and the ability to participate in care. In the home or health care setting the nurse checks the environment for bright colors, comfortable furnishings, adequate lighting, good ventilation, and clean surroundings.

AMOUNT OF STIMULI

Excessive stimuli in an environment can cause sensory overload. In an acute care setting the nurse assesses the level of care required. The frequency of observations and procedures performed may be stressful. If the client is in pain, has many tubes and dressings, or is restricted by casts or traction, overstimulation can be a problem. A client's room may be near repetitive or loud noises (e.g., an elevator, stairwell, or nurses station).

Socialization

The amount and quality of contact with supportive family members and significant others can influence the degree of isolation the client feels. The nurse assesses whether a client lives alone and whether family and friends frequently visit. The absence of visitors during hospitalization or residency in a nursing home or extended care facility can also affect sensory status. This is a common problem in hospital intensive care settings where visitation is often restricted. A pattern of social isolation can contribute to sensory changes. The ability to discuss fears or concerns with loved ones is an important coping mechanism for most people. The absence of meaningful conversation can cause a person to become sensorially deprived, and the nurse may not be alerted until behavioral changes occur.

Clients with hearing loss tend to decrease verbal communication, an important source of human intimacy (Chen, 1994). Often a client becomes embarrassed by continually asking another person to repeat what they have said. So instead, they initiate little communication. There have been studies of the relationship between hearing loss

▶ **RESEARCH HIGHLIGHT**

RESEARCH ABSTRACT

Eighty-eight adult subjects ranging in age from 65 to 90 who perceived a hearing loss participated in a study examining the relations among hearing handicap, loneliness, and self-esteem. Hearing loss was defined as a decrease of hearing acuity caused by aging. Hearing handicap was defined as the individual's response to the hearing loss, as it affected normal daily living functions. Each participant in the study was asked to complete four data instruments; a demographic form, the Hearing Handicap Inventory for the Elderly (Ventry and Weinstein, 1986), the UCLA Loneliness Scale (Russel et al, 1987), and the Rosenberg Global Self-Esteem Scale (Rosenberg, 1965). Statistical analysis showed a significant correlation between loneliness and low self-esteem, indicating that the higher the level of loneliness, the lower the self-esteem and vice versa. Hearing handicap tended to be related to loneliness and low self-esteem for women, but not for men. Social difficulties related to hearing loss tend to be related to low self-esteem for women and loneliness for men. The researcher suggested that hearing handicap might have a greater overall effect on women, but further studies were needed.

IMPLICATIONS FOR PRACTICE

▶ Hearing function should be routinely assessed in all older adult clients. Early detection is important.

▶ Nurses caring for clients with hearing impairment should assist them in learning to communicate more actively and instruct families on good communcation techniques.

▶ Special emotional support and attention may be needed for elderly women with hearing handicap.

REFERENCE

Chen H: Hearing in the elderly: relation of hearing loss, loneliness, and self-esteem, *J Geron Nurs* 20 (6):22, 1994.

and loneliness and self-esteem (see the box on p. 1000). Clients who find their lifestyles influenced by a hearing loss experience loneliness and lowered self-esteem. Social difficulties caused by hearing loss further contribute to the feeling of loneliness.

It is important for the nurse to know the client's social skills and level of satisfaction in the support given by family and friends. Is the client satisfied with the support made available from friends? Is the client able to solve problems with family members? Does the family offer the support needed when the client requires assistance as a result of a sensory loss? The long term effects of sensory alterations can influence family dynamics and a client's willingness to remain active in society.

Communication Methods

Clients with existing sensory deficits often develop alternative ways of communicating. The nurse must understand the client's method of communication to interact with the client and to promote interaction with others (Fig. 39-3). A deaf or hearing-impaired client may read lips, use sign language, listen with the help of a hearing aid, or read and write notes. Vision becomes almost a primary sense for the hearing impaired.

Visually impaired clients are unable to observe facial expressions and other nonverbal behaviors that clarify the content of spoken communication. Instead, they rely on voice tones and inflections to detect the emotional tone of communication. Clients with visual deficits often learn to read Braille.

Clients with **aphasia** may be unable to produce or understand language. **Expressive aphasia**, a motor type of aphasia, is the inability to name common objects or to express simple ideas in words or writing. For example, a client may understand a question but be unable to express an answer. Sensory or **receptive aphasia** is an inability to understand written or spoken language. The client may be able to express words but is unable to understand questions or comments of others. Global aphasia is the inability to understand language or communicate orally.

The temporary or permanent loss of the ability to speak is extremely traumatic to an individual. The nurse assesses a client's alternative communication method and whether it causes anxiety in the client. Clients who have undergone laryngectomies often write notes, use communication boards, speak with mechanical vibrators, or use esophageal speech. Clients with endotracheal or tracheostomy tubes have a temporary loss of speech. Most use a notepad to write their questions and requests. However, the client may become incapacitated and unable to write messages. The nurse needs to determine whether the client has developed a sign language or system of symbols to communicate needs.

To understand the nature of a communication problem, the nurse must know whether a client has trouble speaking, understanding, naming, reading, or writing. Depending on the nature of the problem, the nurse selects the best way to interact with the client.

Mental Status

Mental status assessment is an important component of any evaluation of sensory function (see the box below). Observation of the client during history taking, the physical examination, and care giving provides valuable data that can serve as the basis for evaluation of mental status.

Physical Assessment

To identify sensory deficits, the nurse assesses vision, hearing, olfaction, taste, and the ability to discriminate light touch, temperature, pain, and position (see Chapter 33). Table 39-3 summarizes assessment techniques for identifying sensory deficits. In all examples the nurse will gather more accurate data if the examination room is private, quiet, and comfortable for the client.

The typical physical tests used to screen for hearing impairment rely on an examiner's whispered voice or a tuning fork. The Welch Allyn audioscope is very effective for measuring hearing acuity. The hand-held instrument includes an ear speculum that is placed within the external ear

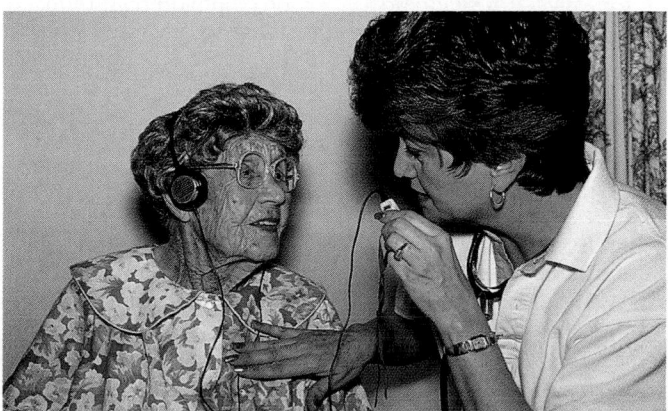

Fig. 39-3 The nurse must know how to communicate with clients who have hearing deficits.

Assessment of Mental Status

PHYSICAL APPEARANCE AND BEHAVIOR
- Motor activity
- Posture
- Facial expression
- Hygiene

COGNITIVE ABILITY
- Level of consciousness
- Abstract reasoning
- Calculation
- Attention
- Judgment
- Ability to carry on conversation
- Ability to read, write, and copy figures
- Recent and remote memory

EMOTIONAL STABILITY
- Agitation, euphoria, irritability, hopelessness, or wide mood swings
- Auditory, visual, or tactile hallucinations
- Illusions
- Delusions

Table 39-3	Assessment of Sensory Function		
ASSESSMENT		**BEHAVIOR INDICATING DEFICIT (CHILDREN)**	**BEHAVIOR INDICATING DEFICIT (ADULT)**
VISION Ask client to read newspaper, magazine, or lettering on menu. Measure visual acuity with Snellen chart (see Chapter 33). Assess visual fields and depth perception. Assess pupil size and accommodation to light. Ask client to identify colors on color chart or crayons.		Self-stimulation, including eye rubbing, body rocking, sniffing or smelling, arm twirling; hitching (using legs to propel while in sitting position) instead of crawling	Poor coordination, squinting, underreaching or overreaching for objects, persistent repositioning of objects, impaired night vision, accidental falls
HEARING Perform conventional assessment, including ticking watch, whisper, and tuning fork (see Chapter 33). Perform audiometry. Observe client conversing with others. Compare client's ability to recognize consonants with ability to distinguish vowels. Assess client's perception of hearing ability and history of tinnitus. Inspect ear canal for hardened cerumen.		Frightened when unfamiliar people approach, no reflex or purposeful response to sounds, failure to be awakened by loud noise, slow or absent development of speech, greater response to movement than to sound, avoidance of social interaction with other children	Blank looks, decreased attention span, lack of reaction to loud noises, increased volume of speech, positioning of head toward sound, smiling and nodding of head in approval when someone speaks, use of other means of communication such as lip reading or writing, complaints of ringing in ears
TOUCH Assess client for sensitivity to light touch and temperature (see Chapter 33). Check client's ability to discriminate between sharp and full stimuli. Assess whether client can distinguish objects (coin or safety pin) in the hand with eyes closed. Ask whether client feels unusual sensations.		Inability to perform developmental tasks related to grasping objects or drawing, repeated injury from handling of harmful objects (e.g., hot stove, sharp knife)	Clumsiness, overreaction or underreaction to painful stimulus, failure to respond when touched, avoidance of touch, sensation of pins and needles, numbness
SMELL Have client close eyes and identify several nonirritating odors (e.g., coffee, vanilla).		Difficult to assess until child is 6 or 7 years old, difficulty discriminating noxious odors	Failure to react to noxious or strong odor, increased body odor, increased sensitivity to odors
TASTE Ask client to sample and distinguish different tastes (e.g, lemon, sugar, salt). (Have client drink or sip water and wait 1 min between each taste.) Ask client if recent weight change has occurred.		Inability to tell whether food is salty or sweet, possible ingestion of strange-tasting things	Change in appetite, excessive use of seasoning and sugar, complaints about taste of food, weight change
POSITION SENSE Perform conventional tests for balance and position sense (see Chapter 33).		Clumsiness, extraneous movement, excessive arm swinging in those with hyperactivity or learning difficulty	Poor balance and spatial orientation, shuffling gait, reduced response to brace self when falling, more precise and deliberate movements

canal. The examiner can view the tympanic membrane to ensure that cerumen is not blocking the canal. A tonal sequence is initiated by pressing a button on the audioscope. The instrument is highly sensitive to detecting hearing loss.

An assessment of mental status is valuable if the nurse suspects sensory deprivation or overload. Observation of the client during history taking, physical examination, or during care can provide data that reveal key client behaviors. The nurse will observe the client's physical appearance and behavior, measure cognitive ability, and assess the client's emotional status. The MMSE (Mini-Mental Status Examination) is an example of a tool that can be used to measure disorientation, altered conceptualization and abstract thinking, and change in problem-solving abilities (see Chapter 33). For example, a client with severe sensory deprivation may not be able to carry on a conversation, remain attentive, or display recent or past memory. The nurse should remember that factors other than sensory deprivation or overload may cause impaired perception (e.g., medications, pain, and reduced oxygenation).

Examples of NANDA Nursing Diagnoses for Sensory Alterations

Sensory/perceptual alterations (visual) *related to:*
- Effects of aging
- Effects of temporary surgical eye patch

Sensory/perceptual alterations (auditory) *related to:*
- Drug side effects
- Strange/noisy environment of ICU

Sensory/perceptual alterations (kinesthetic) *related to:*
- Effects of bed rest

Sensory/perceptual alterations (gustatory) *related to:*
- Effects of aging
- Side effects of chemotherapy

Bathing/hygiene, dressing/grooming, or toileting self-care deficit *related to:*
- Visual loss
- Reduced tactile sensation

Risk for injury *related to:*
- Decreased depth perception
- Reduced sense of smell

Impaired verbal communication *related to:*
- Motor aphasia

Impaired adjustment *related to:*
- Sensory overload
- Sensory deficit

Impaired physical mobility *related to:*
- Altered balance

Social isolation *related to:*
- Expressive aphasia
- Inability to speak secondary to ET tube

Self-esteem disturbance *related to:*
- Hearing loss

Altered thought processes *related to:*
- Sensory overload

Nursing Diagnosis

After assessment, the nurse reviews all available data and critically looks for patterns and trends suggestive of a health problem relating to sensory alterations (see the diagnostic process box below). For example, the advanced age of a client, along with apathy, the client's inattentiveness during conversations, and the client's self-rating of hearing as "poor" are all defining characteristics for the nursing diagnosis, sensory/perceptual alterations (auditory) (Lewis-Cullinan and Janken, 1990). The nurse validates findings to ensure accuracy of the diagnosis. For example, the diagnosis of altered thought processes could mistakenly be made if the nurse does not confirm the client's hearing deficit and perception of poor hearing.

The nurse determines the factor that likely causes the client's health problem. In the previous example, impacted cerumen is the etiology for the client's hearing alteration. The etiology of a nursing diagnosis is a condition that can be affected by nursing interventions. The etiology must be accurate; otherwise nursing therapies will be ineffective. For a client with impacted cerumen, regular irrigations of the ear canal have the potential for improving auditory perception (Lewis-Cullinan and Janken, 1990). In contrast, if the client's auditory alteration was related to hearing loss from nerve deafness, nursing interventions for alternative communication methods would be necessary.

The client may also have health care problems for which sensory alteration is the etiology, such as risk for injury. The nurse may also select nursing diagnoses by predicting the way sensory alterations will affect a client's ability to function (e.g., self-care deficit). The nurse must recognize patterns of data that reveal health problems created by the client's sensory alteration (see the nursing diagnoses box at left).

Sample Nursing Diagnostic Process for Sensory Alterations

ASSESSMENT ACTIVITIES	DEFINING CHARACTERISTICS	NURSING DIAGNOSES
Assess client's visual acuity	Reduced ability to see objects clearly, needs brighter light to read. Has trouble distinguishing edges of stairs.	Risk for injury related to visual impairment from cataract formation
Visit home setting and inspect for any hazards that may pose risks to client	Lighting in rooms, hallways, and stairwells is very dim. Carpet in living room is old with edges curled up. Steps lead up to front entrance of home.	
Review medical record from clinic visit	Client diagnosed to have senile cataracts in both eyes.	
Review client's medical history	Therapeutically restricted environment: Length of stay in ICU equals 5 days.	Sensory/perceptual alterations (auditory) related to sensory overload
Assess client's orientation and recent memory	Confused as to date and time. Unable to recall reason for hospitalization.	
Observe client's behavior	Restlessness in bed, sudden frantic movement when nurse approaches bedside.	

Sample Nursing Care Plan for Sensory/Perceptual Alterations

NURSING DIAGNOSIS: **Risk for injury** related to visual impairment from cataract formation.
DEFINITION: The state in which an individual is at risk of injury as a result of environmental conditions interacting with the individual's adaptive and defensive resources (Kim, McFarland, and McLane, 1995)

GOAL	EXPECTED OUTCOMES	INTERVENTIONS	RATIONALE
Client's home environment is safe and free of hazards in 4 weeks	Client has proper lighting for illumination of stairways and to do close visual work in 2 weeks	Have family or home repair service install maximum wattage bulbs in fixture with frosted bulbs and indirect lighting.	Cataract causes glare or sensitivity to light, requiring use of indirect lighting. Due to aging the intensity of illumination needs to be 3 times as powerful. Some communities have organized repair services for older adults (Ebersole and Hess, 1994).
	Hazards obstructing free ambulation are removed in 1 week	Instruct client on importance of keeping walkways in rooms clear. Have family attach loose area rugs to the floor.	Cataracts cause blurring of vision, coupled with reduced depth perception of advancing age, prevents a person from seeing location of objects clearly (American Academy of Ophthalmology, 1993).
	Client able to identify potential hazard within home as a result of visual limitations in 4 weeks	Have client and family complete a home safety checklist to identify potential hazards in major living areas.	Finding dangers within the home allows the nurse to assist in making the environment safe (Ebersole and Hess, 1994).

 ## Planning

The plan of care (see the care plan above) depends on the nurse's assessment of the client's perception and acceptance of the sensory alteration. It also depends on the extent to which the client has adjusted to sensory loss. The nurse provides care that enables the client to adapt to the health care setting and to the home. The client must actively participate in selecting therapies for the plan of care. Clients who have sensory alterations at the time of entering a health care setting are usually most informed about how to adapt interventions to their lifestyles. The blind in particular need to control whatever part of their care they can.

Priorities of care must be set with regard to the extent a sensory alteration affects a client. Safety is a top priority. The client can help prioritize aspects of care. For example, the client may wish to learn ways to communicate more effectively or to participate in favorite hobbies.

Some sensory alterations are short term, for example, a client suffering sensory/perceptual alterations as a result of sensory overload in an intensive care unit. Appropriate interventions are thus likely to be only temporary, for example, frequent reorientation, or introduction of intimate and pleasant stimuli such as a backrub. Sensory alterations such as permanent visual loss require long-term goals of care. Sometimes it becomes necessary for the client to make major changes in self-care activities, communication, and socialization.

When developing a plan of care, the nurse considers all resources available to clients. The family can play a key role in providing meaningful stimulation and learning ways to help the client adjust to any limitations. The nurse may also refer the client to other health care professionals. Early referrals to occupational or speech therapists, for example, can speed a client's recovery. There are also numerous community-based resources (i.e., local chapter of the Society for the Blind and Visually Impaired, Area on Aging, and the National Council on Independent Living Programs). The nurse may be able to arrange a volunteer to visit a client or have printed materials made available that describe ways to cope with sensory problems.

The goals of care for a client with actual or potential sensory alterations may include the following:
1. Client maintains current functioning of existing senses
2. Client's environment contains meaningful sensory stimuli
3. Client interacts in a safe environment
4. Client experiences no additional sensory loss
5. Client communicates effectively with existing sensory alterations
6. Client is able to perform self-care
7. Client engages in regular social activities
8. Client understands the nature and implications of sensory loss

 ## Implementation

Nursing interventions involve the client and family so that a safe, pleasant, and stimulating sensory environment can be maintained. The most effective interventions enable the client with sensory alterations to function safely with existing deficits. The client generally is able to continue a normal lifestyle. Nursing interventions are chosen depending on the nursing diagnosis identified and the related factors contributing to the client's problem.

Health Promotion

Good sensory function begins with prevention. Almost everyone can be exposed to risks in the environment that may cause sensory alterations. When clients enter primary care settings the nurse can take the opportunity to review common sense approaches for reducing risk of sensory loss.

SCREENING

The prevention of visual impairment in children requires appropriate screening (Wong, 1995). There are three recommended interventions: screening for rubella or syphilis of women who are considering pregnancy; adequate prenatal care to prevent premature birth with the danger of exposure of the infant to excessive oxygen; and periodic screening of all children, especially newborn through preschoolers, for congenital blindness and visual impairment caused by refractive errors and **strabismus**.

Visual impairments are common during childhood. The most common visual problem is a **refractive error** such as nearsightedness. The nurse's role is one of detection and referral. Parents must know signs suggesting visual impairment, for example, failure to react to light and reduced eye contact from the infant. These signs should be reported to a physician immediately. Vision screening of school-age children and adolescents can detect problems early. The school nurse is usually responsible for vision testing.

Hearing impairment is one of the most common disabilities in the United States. It is estimated that over 24 million Americans have a hearing, speech, or language impairment (Silverstein et al, 1993). Children at risk include those with a family history of childhood hearing impairment, perinatal infection (rubella, herpes, cytomegalovirus), low birth weight, chronic ear infection, and Down's syndrome. Nurses should advise pregnant women of the importance of early prenatal care, avoidance of ototoxic drugs, and testing for syphilis or rubella.

Children with chronic middle ear infections—a common cause of impaired hearing—should receive periodic auditory testing. Parents must be warned of the risks and should seek medical care when the child has symptoms of earache or respiratory infection.

For adults, routine screening of visual and hearing function is imperative to detect problems early. This is especially true in the case of glaucoma, which if undetected, can lead to permanent visual loss. The American Academy of Ophthalmology (1993) recommends regular medical eye examinations every 3 to 5 years if a client is age 39 and over. Examinations should occur every 1 to 2 years if there is a family history of glaucoma, if the client is of African ancestry, if the client has had a serious eye injury in the past, or is taking steroid medications.

The guidelines for hearing screening for adults are less prescriptive. Generally, if a client works or lives in an environment where there is a high noise level, routine screening is highly recommended. The most important thing for adults to understand is to not accept hearing loss as a natural part of aging. Once hearing loss becomes acknowledged by a client, it is important to have regular hearing testing. Nurses should encourage older adults to follow through with recommendations for hearing aids.

PREVENTIVE SAFETY

Trauma is a common cause of blindness in children. Penetrating injury from propulsive objects such as firecrackers, slingshots, rocks, or penetrating wounds from sticks, scissors or toy weapons are just a few examples. Parents and children require counseling on ways to avoid eye trauma (see the box at left). Safety equipment can easily be found in most sports shops and large department stores.

Adults are at risk for eye injury when playing sports and working in jobs involving exposure to chemicals or flying objects. The Occupational Safety and Health Administration has guidelines for safety in the work place. Employers are required to have employees wear eye goggles and/or use equipment that reduces the risk of injury. Nurses in occupational health settings can reinforce use of protective devices.

Preventing hearing loss requires individuals to avoid exposure to continuous high noise levels and brief loud impulse noise. Protective devices should be worn by clients forced to work around noise. Earplugs and earphones are useful in blocking high decibel sounds.

Another means of prevention involves regular immunization of children against diseases capable of causing hearing loss (e.g., rubella, mumps, and measles). Nurses who work in physicians' offices, schools, and community clinics should reinforce the importance of early and timely immunization. When a child or an adult develops any type of health problem, caution should be used in prescribing drugs that are **ototoxic**.

HEALTH MAINTENANCE

Learning to adjust to sensory impairments can occur at an early age. However, every person begins to develop sensory changes as they age. There are measures to take to maintain sensory function at the highest level possible.

Tips for Preventing Eye Injury in Children

INFANTS AND TODDLERS
- Avoid toys with long pointed handles or projections.
- Do not allow child to walk or run with pointed object in hand.
- Keep pointed instruments and tools out of reach.

PRESCHOOLERS
- Supervise use of sharp or pointed objects such as scissors.
- Teach child to walk carefully when carrying pointed objects.
- Keep child away from projectile activities.
- Begin to teach respect for firearms and fireworks.

SCHOOL AGERS AND ADOLESCENTS
- Teach proper use of potentially dangerous equipment such as power tools, fireworks, and sports equipment (hockey sticks).
- Stress use of eye protection when playing ball and racquet sports, shooting, using power tools, or riding motorcycles.
- Warn children not to look directly at the sun even when wearing sunglasses.
- Be sure corrective lenses are made of safety glass, which is shatterproof.

Modified from Wong DL: *Whaley and Wong's nursing care of infants and children,* ed 5, St Louis, 1995, Mosby.

This ensures a stimulating environment for a client and an improved level of health.

Use of Assistive Devices. Health maintenance requires appropriate use of assistive aids and good, routine hygiene measures. A client who wears corrective contact lenses, eyeglasses, or hearing aids should make sure they are kept clean, accessible, and functional (see Chapter 40). It is helpful to have a family member or friend also know how to clean an assistive aid.

It is critical for contact lens wearers to frequently clean lenses (see Chapter 40) and to use the appropriate solutions for cleaning and disinfection. With the rise in use of soft contact lenses, particularly extended-wear lenses, there has been an increase in serious corneal infections (Cohen and Krachmer, 1992). Infrequent lens disinfection, contamination of lens storage cases and contact lens solutions, and use of homemade saline adds to a client's risk. Swimming while wearing lenses also creates a serious risk of infection.

Wearing a hearing aid no longer has to be a social stigma. There are a wide variety of aids that not only successfully enhance a person's hearing but can be cosmetically acceptable. Chapter 40 summarizes the type of hearing aids available and tips for proper care and use.

Cunningham and Ganzel (1991) identify three factors that determine a person's candidacy for a hearing aid: perceived need for hearing help, attitude toward the hearing problem, and motivation to seek solutions. Acknowledging a need to improve hearing is a person's first step. The nurse can give clients useful information on the benefits of wearing a hearing aid. It is also important to have a significant other available to assist with hearing aid adjustment. Federal regulations require medical clearance from a physician before a person can be fitted with a hearing aid (Ebersole and Hess, 1994). If a client has any of the following ear conditions a hearing aid cannot be purchased: visible congenital or traumatic deformity of the ear, active drainage in the last 90 days, sudden or progressive hearing loss within the last 90 days, acute or chronic dizziness, unilateral sudden hearing loss within last 90 days, visible cerumen accumulation or a foreign body in the ear canal, pain or discomfort in the ear, and an audiometric air-bone gap of 15 decibels or greater. The nurse can detect the first seven on physical exam and should refer the client to an **otolaryngologist** for further counseling (Ebersole and Hess, 1994).

Promoting Meaningful Stimulation. Life becomes much more enriching and satisfying when meaningful and pleasant stimuli exist within the environment. There are many ways the nurse can help clients make adjustments to their environment so that it becomes more stimulating. This is best done when the nurse considers the normal physiological changes that accompany sensory deficits.

Vision. As a result of the normal changes of aging, the pupil's ability to adjust to light is diminished. As a result, older adults can be very sensitive to glare. The nurse can suggest ways for the client to minimize glare by selecting satin and nongloss finishes for walls and countertops in the home and choosing sheer curtains, tinted windows, or adjustable shades to reduce outdoor light. Wearing sunglasses outside obviously can reduce the glare of direct sunlight.

The ability to read is important to everyone. Clients with reduced visual acuity may need more than corrective lenses. A pocket magnifier can help a client read most printed material. Telescopic lens eyeglasses are smaller, easier to focus, and have a greater range. There are also books and other publications available in larger print. If a client has a legal or other important document he or she wishes to read, standard copying machines have enlarging capabilities. There are now closed-circuit television magnifying units that enlarge written characters up to 45 times (Ebersole and Hess, 1994).

With aging, a person experiences a change in color perception. Perception of the colors blue, violet, and green usually declines. Brighter colors, such as red, orange, and yellow are easier to see. The nurse can offer suggestions of ways the client may decorate a room and paint hallways or stairwells so that differentiations can be made in surfaces and objects in a room.

Hearing. One way to help an older adult with a hearing loss is to ensure the problem is not impacted cerumen. With aging, cerumen thickens and builds up in the ear canal. Excessive cerumen occluding the ear canal can cause a **conductive hearing loss.** Irrigation of the canal with tepid water in a 60-ml syringe (see Chapter 40) will remove cerumen. Removal of cerumen can significantly improve the client's hearing ability. Lewis-Cullinan and Janken (1990) conducted a study involving 226 older adults. They found improvement in the hearing test scores in 75% of the ears after cerumen removal.

To maximize residual hearing function, the nurse suggests ways to modify the environment. Telephones and televisions can be amplified. Alarm clocks that shake the bed or activate a flashing light are useful adaptive devices. An innovative way to enrich the lives of the hearing impaired is recorded music. Music recorded in the low frequency sound cycles can be heard by clients with severe hearing loss.

Taste and smell. The nurse can easily promote the sense of taste by using measures to enhance remaining taste perception. Good oral hygiene keeps the taste buds well hydrated. Taste perception is heightened if foods are well seasoned, differently textured, and eaten separately. Vinegar or lemon juice can add tartness to food. The nurse should always ask the client what foods are the most taste appealing. If taste perception is improved, food intake and appetite will also improve.

Stimulation of the sense of smell with aromas such as brewing coffee and baking bread can heighten taste sensation. The client should avoid blending or mixing foods because these actions make it difficult to identify tastes. Older persons should chew food thoroughly to allow more food to contact remaining taste buds.

Smell can be improved by strengthening pleasant olfactory stimulation. A client's environment can be made more pleasant with smells such as cologne, mild room deodorizers, fragrant flowers, and sachets. The nurse also encourages clients to sniff food before eating. In a health care setting when the nurse assists clients with eating or sets up a meal tray, naming the foods may help clients imagine the aromas. The client is again an important resource. Certain aromas may actually cause clients to lose their appetites.

Removal of unpleasant odors improves the quality of a person's environment. The nurse should keep a client's room clean, empty bedpans or urinals, and keep bathroom doors closed.

Touch. Clients with reduced tactile sensation usually have the impairment over a limited portion of their bodies. The nurse can stimulate existing function by providing touch therapy. If the client is willing to be touched, hair brushing and combing, a backrub, and touching of the arms or shoulders are ways of increasing tactile contact. When sensation is reduced, a firm pressure may be necessary for the client to feel the nurse's hand. Turning and repositioning can also improve the quality of tactile sensation.

If a client is overly sensitive to tactile stimuli (hyperesthesia), the nurse must minimize irritating stimuli. Keeping bed linens loose to minimize direct contact with the client and protecting the skin from exposure to irritants are helpful measures.

ESTABLISHING SAFE ENVIRONMENTS

When sensory function becomes impaired, individuals become less secure and the world around them becomes smaller. Older adults in particular find it important to feel secure about their immediate environment. This is necessary for the person to have a sense of independence. Feeling safe allows a person to function within the home. The nurse can make recommendations to assist clients in making their living environment safer without restricting their independence. During a home visit or while completing an examination in the clinic, the nurse can offer several useful suggestions for home safety. The nature of the actual or potential sensory loss determines the safety precautions taken.

Adaptations for Visual Loss. Whether a visual alteration is a result of injury, eye disease, or the changes of aging, safety becomes a factor if visual acuity, peripheral vision, adaptation to the dark, and depth perception are permanently reduced. With reduced peripheral vision a client cannot see panoramically, as the outer visual field is less discrete. This creates a special hazard for driving. Older adults with reduced adaptation to the dark require three times as much light to see objects as they did as young adults. With reduced depth perception, a person cannot see how far away objects are located. This is a special danger as an older adult attempts to walk down stairs.

To create a safe environment the nurse begins by looking at the results of the home environment assessment. What hazards exist in the client's living areas? Clutter such as footstools, childrens' toys, and electrical cords in walking paths should be removed. Electrical cords should be placed under furniture, rugs, or carpeting. Furniture should be arranged so that a client can move about easily without fear of tripping or running into objects.

Because of reduced depth perception, an older adult can trip on throw rugs, runners, or the edge of stairs. All flooring or carpeting should be kept in good repair. The nurse can advise the client to use low pile rugs instead of shag. Thresholds between rooms should be level with the floor. Any stairwell should have a securely fastened banister or handrail extending the full length of the stairs.

Front and back entrances to the home, work areas, and stairwells can be dangerous if improperly lighted. The nurse encourages the client to have a repairman install light with higher wattage and wider illumination. Fluorescent lighting should be avoided. A light switch should be located at

<table>
<tr><td>**Driving Tips for Older Adults**</td></tr>
<tr><td>Drive in familiar areas
Do not drive during rush hour
Drive defensively
Avoid driving at dusk or night
Go slow, but not too slow
Look to travel with her always
Keep the car in good working condition</td></tr>
</table>

the top and bottom of stairwells. It is also important to be sure lighting on the stairs does not cast shadows. Be sure the client can clearly see the edge of each step, especially the first and last. When possible, steps inside and outside the home should be replaced with ramps.

Driving can be a particular safety hazard for older adults. The changes in the lens cause the older adult to be highly sensitive to glare during night driving. Reduced peripheral vision may prevent a driver from seeing a car in an adjacent lane. Vision is a primary consideration for safety but there are other factors as well. Older clients may have decreased reaction time, reduced hearing, and decreased strength in the legs and arms. All of these factors can affect an older adult's driving skills. The box above summarizes tips to give older adult clients who continue to drive.

The inability to see visual contrast can be a problem for an older adult. Sometimes settings on electrical appliances and equipment are only highlighted in black and white or shades of grey. Color contrasts help to distinguish settings. Colored tape, paint, or nail enamel can be used to color code appliance dials. Color can also be useful to highlight the edge of stairs. Painting the edge of stairs with bright orange paint or applying a broad strip of colored tape at the stair edge can help a person see the edges of stairs more clearly. The nurse can help the client tour the home to find opportunities for color coding.

If a client is partially or totally blind, fire hazards should be removed from the home. Flammable items such as paper and cloth should be kept away from the stove. A client who smokes must learn to discard ashes frequently into an ashtray. Water in the bottom of an ashtray helps ensure that cigarette butts are extinguished.

An added consideration for the visually impaired is the assurance that eye medications are administered safely. For conditions such as glaucoma, clients must closely adhere to regular medication schedules. Older adults may have some difficulty manipulating eye droppers. A friend or spouse should always be familiar with dosage schedules in case a client is unable to self-administer a medication. The nurse can share several useful guidelines to ensure safe eye medication administration (see the box on p. 1008).

Adaptations for Reduced Hearing. Important environmental sounds (e.g., doorbells and alarm clocks) may best be heard if amplified or changed to a more low-pitched, buzzerlike sound. There are also sound lamps that respond with light to sounds such as doorbells, burglar alarms, smoke detectors, and babies crying. These can be purchased from hearing aid dealers, telephone companies, and appliance stores (Ebersole and Hess, 1994). Signaling devices allow the deaf person greater independence. Family

CLIENT TEACHING for Use of Eye Medications in the Visually Impaired

OBJECTIVES
Client will follow eye medication regimen daily
Client will identify side effects of eye drops

TEACHING STRATEGIES
■ Include spouse or friend in medication instruction so that if client becomes ill, someone is able to give eye drops.
■ Warn client against changing or stopping medications without first calling the ophthalmologist.
■ Review common side effects of eye medications (common side effects include stinging, red eyes, blurred vision, and headaches).
■ Instruct client to take pills and drops regularly at prescribed intervals. Have client use a medication reminder system such as a daily calendar tear off or circling hours on a clock face to designate administration times.

EVALUATION
■ Have client and family member explain when eye medications are to be routinely taken
■ Have client keep a weekly log of medication administration and check during next clinic appointment
■ Ask client to describe common side effects of eye drops

members or anyone who calls the client regularly should learn to let the phone ring for a longer period. A telecommunications device for the deaf (TDD) is a computer and printer that transfers written words over the telephone to the hearing impaired. Both sender and receiver must have a TDD to complete a call (Walsh and Eldredge, 1989).

Adaptations for Reduced Olfaction. A reduced sensitivity to odors means the client may be unable to smell leaking gas, a smoldering cigarette or fire, and tainted food. The client should use smoke detectors and other alternative precautions such as checking ashtrays or placing cigarette butts in water. A client can learn to check dates on food packages and the color and texture of food. Pilot gas flames should be checked visually.

Adaptations for Reduced Tactile Sensation. When clients have reduced sensation in their extremities, they are at risk for injury from exposure to temperature extremes. The nurse should caution them on the use of water bottles or heating pads (see Chapter 49). The temperature setting on the home water heater should be no higher than 120 degrees. If a client also has a visual impairment, it is important to be sure water faucets are clearly marked "Hot" and "Cold."

PROMOTING COMMUNICATION

A sensory deficit can cause a person to feel isolated because of an inability to communicate with others. It is important for individuals to be able to interact with people whom they encounter. This problem can complicate a nurse's effectiveness in teaching clients information and skills. The nature of the sensory loss influences the meth-

ods and styles of communication (see the box on p. 1009) that nurses can use. Communication methods can also be taught to family members and significant others.

When beginning a conversation with a client who has a hearing deficit, it helps to reduce any background noise by turning off or lowering the volume of any TV, appliance, or radio. It is also helpful to have conversations in settings where floor coverings and drapes muffle extraneous background noises (Bernardini, 1985). The client with a hearing impairment may be able to speak normally. However, the deaf client's inability to hear self-spoken words may cause serious speech alterations. Clients may use sign language, lipreading, write with a pad and pencil, or learn to use a computer for communication. Special communication boards contain common terms used in nursing care and help clients express their needs.

Client instruction is one aspect of communication. There are teaching booklets available in large print for clients with visual loss. The client who is blind may require more frequent and detailed verbal descriptions of information. This is particularly true if there are no instructional booklets written in Braille. The visually impaired can learn by listening to audiotapes or the sound portion of a televised teaching session. Clients with hearing impairment may benefit from written instructional materials and visual teaching aids, for example, posters and graphs. Demonstrations by the nurse are very useful. Hospitals are required to make interpreters available to read sign language of deaf clients.

Managing Acute Sensory Deficits

When clients enter acute care settings for therapeutic management of sensory deficits or as a result of traumatic injury, the nurse uses approaches to maximize sensory function existing at the time. Safety again is an obvious priority until the client's sensory status is either stabilized or improved. For example, clients with sensory deficits have a high risk for falls in the acute care environment. It becomes very important to know the extent of any sensory impairment prior to the acute episode of illness so that the nurse can reinforce what the client already knows about self-care or plan for more instruction prior to and following discharge.

Another group of clients who are at risk for developing sensory alterations while hospitalized are those in intensive care units (ICUs) and the acutely ill. The constant activity within an ICU and the frequent monitoring of the acutely ill can easily cause clients to experience sensory overload. The nurse's main challenge becomes introducing regular, meaningful stimulation so that clients maintain a clearer perception of their immediate environment.

ORIENTATION TO THE ENVIRONMENT

The client with recent sensory impairment requires a complete orientation to the immediate environment. Reorientation to the institutional environment may be provided by ensuring name tags on uniforms are visible, addressing the client by name, explaining where they are (especially if they are transported to different areas for treatment), and using conversational cues to time or location. The tendency for clients to become confused can be

Communication Methods

CLIENTS WITH APHASIA
- Listen to the client and wait for the client to communicate.
- Do not shout or speak loudly (hearing loss is not the problem).
- If the client has problems with comprehension, use simple, short questions and facial gestures to give additional clues.
- Speak of things familiar and of interest to the client
- If the client has problems speaking, ask questions that require simple yes or no answers or blinking of the eyes. Offer pictures or a communication board so that the client can point.
- Give the client time to understand, be calm and patient.
- Do not pressure or tire the client.
- Avoid patronizing and childish phrases.

CLIENTS WITH AN ARTIFICIAL AIRWAY
- Use pictures, objects, or word cards so that the client can point.
- Offer a pad and pencil or magic slate for the client to write messages.
- Do not shout or speak loudly.
- Give the client time to write messages as they become easily fatigued.
- Provide an artificial voice box (vibrator) for the client with a laryngectomy to use to speak words and phrases.

CLIENTS WITH HEARING IMPAIRMENT
- Get the client's attention. Do not startle the client when entering the room. Do not approach a client from behind. Be sure the client knows you wish to speak.
- Face the client and stand or sit on same level. Be sure your face and lips are illuminated to promote lip reading. Keep hands away from mouth.
- If the client wears glasses, be sure they are clean so that your gestures and face can be seen. If the client wears a hearing aid, make sure it is in place and working.
- Speak slowly and articulate clearly. Older adults may take longer to process verbal messages. Use a normal tone of voice and inflections of speech. Refrain from speaking with something in your mouth.
- When you are not understood, rephrase rather than repeat the conversation.
- Use visible expressions. Speak with your hands, your face, and your eyes.
- Do not shout. Loud sounds are usually higher pitched and may impede hearing by accentuating vowel sounds and concealing consonants. If it is necessary to raise your voice, speak in lower tones.
- Talk toward the client's best or normal ear.
- Use written information to enhance the spoken word.
- Do not restrict a deaf client's hands. Never have intravenous lines in both of the client's hands if the preferred method of communication is sign language.
- Avoid eating, chewing, or smoking while speaking.
- Avoid speaking from another room or while walking away.

reduced by offering short and simple repeated explanations and reassurance. Family members and visitors can also help orient clients to the hospital surroundings.

A client with serious visual impairment must feel comfortable in knowing the boundaries of the immediate environment. Normally we see physical boundaries within a room. The blind or severely visually impaired must touch the boundaries to make them real (Norris, 1989). The client needs to walk through a room and feel the walls to establish a sense of direction. The nurse can help by explaining objects within the room such as furniture or equipment. It takes time for the client to absorb a room's arrangement. The client may need to reorient again with the nurse explaining the location of key items (e.g., call light, telephone, chair). It also helps to always approach a blind client from the front to avoid startling him or her.

It is important to keep all objects in the same position and place (Norris, 1989). After moving an object even a short distance, it no longer exists for a blind person. Simply moving a chair aside may create a dangerous safety hazard. The nurse should ask the client if any item should be arranged to make ambulation easier. Keep traffic patterns clear and avoid use of furniture with sharp edges. The blind client always needs extra time to perform any task. The client needs a detailed description of how to perform an activity and will move slowly in order to remain safe.

Bedridden clients are easy victims for sensory deprivation. Normally movement gives an integrated awareness of the self through vestibular and tactile stimulation. A person's sensory perception is influenced by movement patterns. The limited movement of bedrest changes how a person interprets the environment; surroundings seem different and objects seem to assume shapes different than normal. A person who is on bedrest requires routine stimulation through range of motion exercises, positioning, and participation in self-care activities (as appropriate). Comfort measures such as washing the face and hands and providing backrubs can help to improve the quality of stimulation and lessen the chance of sensory deprivation. Planning time to talk with clients is also essential. The nurse should explain unfamiliar environmental noises and sensations. A calm, unhurried approach during contact with a client gives the nurse quality time to help reorient and familiarize the client with care activities. The client who is well enough to read benefits from a variety of reading material.

SAFETY MEASURES

The client with recent visual impairment often requires help with walking. The presence of an eye patch, frequently instilled eye drops, or the swelling of eyelid structures following surgery are just a few factors that cause a client to need more assistance than usual. A sighted guide can give confidence to the visually impaired and ensure safe mobility. Ebersole and Hess (1994) list four suggestions for a sighted guide:

- Ask the blind client if he or she wants a "sighted guide."
- If assistance is accepted, offer an elbow or arm. Instruct the client to grasp your arm just above the elbow. If necessary, physically assist the person by guiding his or her hand to your arm or elbow (Fig. 39-4).
- Go one half step ahead and slightly to the side of the blind person. The shoulder of the person should be directly behind your shoulder. If the person is frail, place the hand on your forearm.
- Relax and walk at a comfortable pace. Warn the client when you approach doorways or narrow spaces.

While walking the client describe the course of movement and ensure that obstacles have been removed. A client with visual impairment should never be left standing alone in an unfamiliar area. For clients who undergo eye surgery, it is important to teach family members ambulation assist techniques.

A visually impaired client who spends considerable time in bed should have a call light nearby. Necessary objects should be placed in front of the client to prevent falls caused by reaching over the bedside. Side rails are also important in this regard. At night a nightlight with a red bulb can help reduce falls. The red light reduces the time required for the eyes to adapt to the dark and allows the client to see well enough to function without keeping the regular light on (Matteson and McConnell, 1988).

Nurses may rely on clients in health care settings to re-

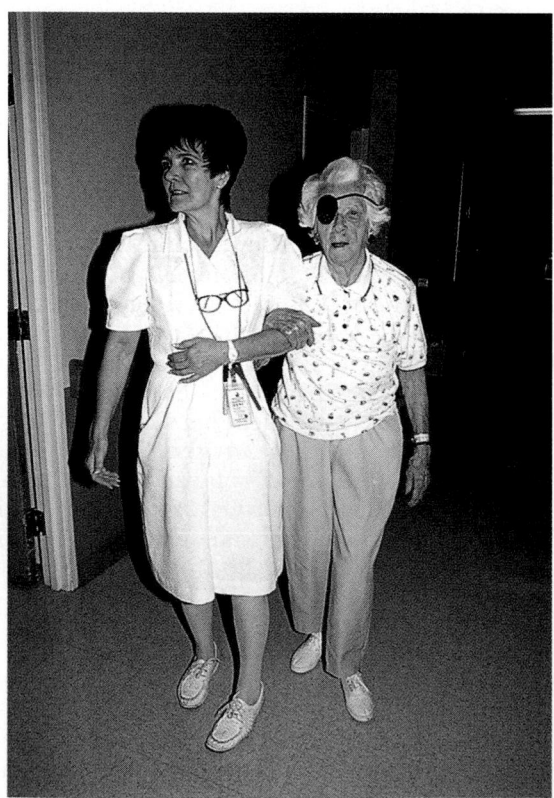

Fig. 39-4 Nurse assists in the ambulation of a client wearing an eye patch.

port unusual sounds, such as a suction apparatus running improperly or an intravenous pump alarm. However, the client with a hearing loss may not hear such sounds and thus requires more frequent visits by the nurse. The client can also benefit from learning to use vision to discover sources of danger. Never restrict both arms of deaf or hearing impaired clients with restraints, IV lines, etc., as they need their hands to communicate. It is wise to note on the intercom button and a client's chart if the client is deaf and/or blind.

A client lacking the ability to speak cannot call out for assistance. Clients with aphasia, a laryngectomy, or an artificial airway must have alternative means of communication such as message boards close at hand. In the hospital a call light should always be near the client.

Clients with reduced tactile sensation risk injury when their conditions confine them to bed because they are unable to sense pressure on bony prominences or the need to change position. These clients rely on nurses for timely repositioning, moving tubes or devices the client may lie on, and turning to avoid skin breakdown. When the ability to sense temperature variations is reduced, the nurse should use extra caution in applying heat and cold therapies (see Chapter 49) and preparing bath water. The nurse must frequently check the condition of the client's skin.

COMMUNICATION

The most common language disorder following stroke is aphasia. As a result of a disruption in blood flow to the brain, the speech center becomes damaged, altering a person's ability to either use or understand spoken words. Depending on the type of aphasia, the inability to communicate can be frustrating and frightening (see the box on p. 1009). The nurse should initially establish very basic communication and recognize that aphasia does not indicate intellectual impairment or degeneration of personality. The nurse explains situations and treatments that are pertinent to the client as he or she may understand (Ebersole and Hess, 1994). Because a stroke often causes partial or complete paralysis of one side of the client's body, an aphasic client may need special assistive devices. There are communication boards developed for several levels of disability. Sensitive pressure switches, activated by touch of an ear, nose, or chin can control electronic communication boards (Ebersole and Hess, 1994). Clients who have had a stroke usually acquire referrals to speech therapists to develop appropriate rehabilitation plans.

In acute care hospitals or long-term care facilities, nurses often care for clients with artificial airways (see Chapter 44). For example, an endotracheal tube is inserted into the oropharynx and down through the vocal cords of the larynx into the upper bronchus. The placement of the tube prevents a client from speaking. In this case the nurse must use special communication methods to facilitate the client's ability to express needs (see the box on p. 1009). The client may be completely alert and able to hear and see the nurse normally. Giving the client time to convey any needs or requests is very important.

CONTROLLING SENSORY STIMULI

The nurse controls excessive stimuli for clients at risk for sensory overload. Clients need time for rest and freedom from stress caused by frequent monitoring and repeated tests. The nurse can reduce sensory overload by organizing the care plan. Combining activities such as dressing changes, bathing, and vital sign measurement in one visit prevents the client from becoming overly fatigued. The client also needs scheduled time for rest and quiet. Planning for rest periods often requires cooperation from family and visitors. Coordination with laboratory and radiology departments may help minimize the number of procedures the client must undergo. The nurse may encourage a family member to sit quietly with a client or involve the client in an undemanding repetitive activity such as combing hair or brushing teeth. Helping clients to become as mobile and independent as possible within prescribed limits provides meaningful stimulation.

When clients experience sensory overload or deprivation, the resultant behavior can be difficult for family or friends to accept. The nurse encourages the family not to argue with or contradict the confused client but to calmly explain location, identity, and time of day. Engaging the client in a normal discussion about familiar topics may assist in reorientation. Prearranging tests and procedures with departments reduces the amount of time needed for tests and examinations. Anticipating client needs such as voiding helps reduce uncomfortable stimuli.

The nurse can also try to control extraneous noise in and around the client's room. It may be necessary to ask a roommate to lower the volume on a television or to move the client to a quieter room. Equipment noise should be kept to a minimum. Bedside equipment not in use, such as suction and oxygen equipment, should be turned off. The nurse also avoids abrupt loud noises such as clattering or rinsing of bedpans. Nursing staff should also try to control laughter or conversation at the nurses' station. Nurses should allow clients to close room doors.

When the client leaves an acute care setting for the home environment, nurses should communicate with colleagues in the home care setting about the interventions that helped the client adapt to sensory problems. Similarly, information describing the client's existing sensory deficits should be reported. Continuity of care is achieved when the client is required to make only minimal changes in the home setting.

Maintaining Healthy Lifestyles

After a client has experienced a sensory loss it becomes important to understand the implications of the loss and to make the adjustments needed to continue a normal lifestyle. Sensory impairments need not prevent a person from leading an active, rewarding life. Many of the interventions applicable to health promotion, such as adapting the home environment, can be used after a client leaves an acute care setting.

UNDERSTANDING SENSORY LOSS

Clients who have experienced a recent loss must understand how to adapt so that living environments can be safe and appropriately stimulating. All family members should understand the way a client's sensory impairment affects normal daily activities. Family and friends can be more supportive when they understand sensory deficits and the types of elements that worsen or lessen sensory problems.

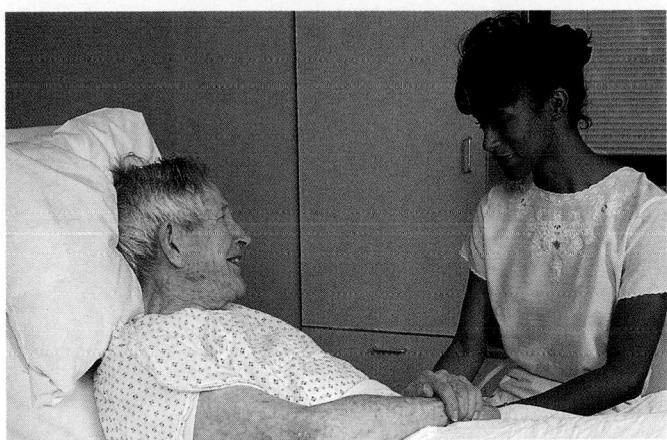

Fig. 39-5 Conversation with nurse can reduce loneliness and sense of isolation.

For example, family and friends need to learn how to communicate with someone who has a hearing loss. There are resources within a community that provide information that assists clients with personal management needs. The American Foundation for the Blind, American National Red Cross, and National Association for Speech and Hearing offer resource materials and product information.

SOCIALIZATION

The ability to communicate is gratifying. It tests our intellect, opens opportunities, and allows us to exchange the feelings we have about others (Fig. 39-5). When interactions are hindered by sensory alterations, a person can feel ineffective and lose self-esteem. If clients feel socially unaccepted they will perceive sensory losses as seriously impairing the quality of life.

Interacting with others can become a burden for many clients with sensory alterations. Asking people to continuously repeat what they say is both embarrassing and exhausting for a client with hearing loss. Many clients lose the motivation to engage in social situations. As a person withdraws from interaction a deep sense of loneliness can develop. The nurse can introduce therapies to reduce loneliness, particularly for older adult clients (see the box on p. 1012). In addition, family members must learn to focus on a person's ability to interact rather than their disability. It should not be assumed, for example, that a person who is hard of hearing does not wish to speak. A blind person can still enjoy a walk through a park with a companion describing the sights around them.

PROMOTING SELF-CARE

The ability to perform self-care is essential for self-esteem. Frequently, family members and nurses believe sensorially impaired persons require assistance, when in fact they can help themselves. Useful guidelines assist clients with visual or tactile impairment when help is required with activities of daily living.

A meal tray can be set up as though food on the tray and condiments and drinks around the tray are numbers on the face of a clock. The visually impaired client can easily be-

GERONTOLOGICAL PRINCIPLES for Reducing Loneliness

Spend time with a person in silence or conversation
Use physical contact; holding a hand, embracing a
 shoulder to convey caring
Help recommend alterations in living arrangements if
 physical isolation is a factor
Assist an older adult in keeping contact with people im-
 portant to them
Help obtain information about mutual help groups
Arrange for security escort services as needed
Bring a pet that is easy to care for into the home
Link a person with religious organizations attuned to the
 social needs of older adults

come oriented to the items after the nurse or family member explains each item's location.

If tactile sense is diminished, the client can dress more easily with zippers or velcro strips, pullover sweaters or blouses, and elasticized waists. If a client has partial paralysis and reduced sensation, the affected side should be dressed first. Family members responsible for selecting clothing for visually impaired clients should be encouraged to follow the client's preferences. Any sensory impairment has a significant influence on body image, and it is important for the client to feel well groomed and attractive. A client may also need assistance with basic grooming such as brushing, combing, and shampooing hair.

The client with visual problems needs assistance in reaching toilet facilities safely. Safety bars should be installed near the toilet. It may be helpful to have the bar a different color from the wall for easier visibility. Towels should never be placed on safety bars to interfere with a person's grasp. Toilet paper should be within easy reach.

Clients with proprioceptive problems may lose their balance easily. Bathrooms should have nonskid surfaces in the tub and shower. The nurse can instruct family members to supervise ambulation and sitting, make frequent checks to prevent falls, and caution the client against leaning forward.

Evaluation

When caring for a client with a sensory alteration, the nurse evaluates whether care measures improve or at least maintain a client's ability to interact and function within the environment. The nature of a client's sensory alteration influences the way the nurse evaluates care. The nurse adapts evaluation measures to the client's sensory deficit to determine whether actual outcomes are the same as expected outcomes. For example, the nurse uses proper communication techniques to evaluate whether a client with a hearing deficit has gained the ability to hear more effectively. Similarly the nurse uses large printed materials to test a visually impaired client's ability to read a prescription. When expected outcomes have not been achieved, there may be a need to change interventions or alter the client's environment. Family members may need to become more involved in support of the client.

If nursing care has been directed at improving sensory acuity, the nurse evaluates the integrity of the sensory organs and the client's ability to perceive stimuli. Any interventions designed to relieve problems associated with sensory alterations are evaluated on the basis of the client's ability to function normally without injury. When the nurse attempts to directly or indirectly (through education) alter the client's environment, evaluation is directed at observing whether the client makes environmental changes. When client teaching is designed to improve a client's sensory function, it is important to determine whether the client is following recommended therapies. Asking the client to explain or demonstrate self-care skills evaluates the level of learning that has occurred. It may be necessary to reinforce previous instruction if learning has not taken place. The evaluation box below demonstrates how the nurse evaluates success at meeting client goals.

Sample Evaluation of Interventions for Sensory/Perceptual Alterations

GOAL	EVALUATIVE MEASURES	EXPECTED OUTCOMES
Client's home environment is safe and free of hazards within 4 weeks	Tour home during scheduled follow-up visits; examine living areas for lighting and presence of obvious hazards Observe client walk through living area of home by next home visit (1 week) Ask client to identify hazards that should be removed to prevent injury	Client has proper lighting for illumination of stairways and to do close visual work within 2 weeks Hazards obstructing free ambulation are removed in 1 week Client able to identify hazards within the home as a result of visual limitations within 4 weeks

▪ KEY CONCEPTS ▪

► Sensory reception involves the stimulation of sensory nerve fibers and the transmission of impulses to higher centers within the brain.

► When sensory function is impaired, the sense of self is impaired.

► Sensory deprivation results from an inadequate quality or quantity of sensory stimuli.

► Aging results in a gradual decline of acuity in all senses.

► Clients in intensive care units are at risk for sensory deprivation as a result of the lack of personal, comforting touch.

► Clients who are older, immobilized, or confined in isolated environments are at risk for sensory alterations.

► The extent of support from family members and significant others can influence the quality of sensory experiences.

► Assessment of a client's health promotion habits helps to reveal risks for sensory impairment.

► An older adult often will not admit to a sensory loss.

► An assessment of hazards in the environment requires the nurse to tour living areas in the home and to look for conditions that increase the chances of injury such as falls.

► The plan of care for clients with sensory alterations should include participation by family members.

► Hearing loss should not be accepted as a natural part of aging.

► Clients with sensory deficits develop alternative ways of communicating that rely on other senses.

► Eye injuries can occur while participating in contact sports.

► Care of clients at risk for sensory deprivation includes introducing meaningful and pleasant stimuli for all senses.

► Sensory losses can impair a person's ability to socialize.

► To prevent sensory overload, the nurse controls stimuli and orients the client to the environment.

► To improve communication with the hearing impaired, the nurse speaks clearly, stands in front of the client, and makes sure that lip and facial movements are visible.

► Clients with artificial airways can communicate effectively with communication boards and written messages.

▪ KEY TERMS ▪

Aphasia, p. 1001

Auditory, p. 994

Conductive hearing loss, p. 1006

Expressive aphasia, p. 1001

Gustatory, p. 994

Kinesthetic, p. 994

Olfactory, p. 994

Otolaryngologist, p. 1006

Ototoxic, p. 1005

Proprioceptive, p. 995

Receptive aphasia, p. 1001

Refractive error, p. 1005

Sensory deficit, p. 995

Sensory deprivation, p. 996

Sensory overload, p. 996

Stereognosis, p. 994

Strabismus, p. 1005

Tactile, p. 994

▪ CRITICAL THINKING EXERCISES ▪

1. Mr. Wilcox is a 72-year-old man who comes to the clinic regularly for checkups. During an assessment of Mr. Wilcox you notice the following behaviors: He is inattentive to questions, fails to respond to a sudden noise in the hallway, and has trouble following directions when you explain the procedure for auscultation of the lungs. What further assessment might you make?

2. You learn that Mr. Wilcox has had a reduction in hearing for over a year. He currently lives alone. What would you assess about his living environment as it pertains to his safety?

3. Mrs. Garcia is a 70-year-old female confined to bed following a blood clot to her lung (pulmonary embolus). Her medical history reveals bilateral cataracts. What nursing considerations are important to support this client's sensory function?

4. Mrs. McCay is the daughter of the client Mr. Snead. He has a history of hearing loss in his right ear and has been fitted with a hearing aid in the past but does not wear it regularly. Mr. Snead was admitted to the ICU following a motor vehicle accident and has an endotracheal tube in place (which prevents him from speaking). Mrs. McCay wants to be able to communicate with her father, but she is frustrated. How can you advise her?

REFERENCES

American Academy of Ophthalmology: *Cataract,* San Francisco, 1993, American Academy of Ophthalmology.

Bernardini L: Effective communication as an intervention for sensory deprivation in the elderly client, *Top Clin Nurs* 6(4):72, 1985.

Chen H: Hearing in the elderly: relation of hearing loss, loneliness, and self-esteem, *J Geron Nurs* 20(6):22, 1994.

Cohen EJ, Krachmer JH: Red eyes and contact lenses, *Patient Care* 26:143, 1992.

Cunningham DR, Ganzel TM: Hearing aids: how they work and whom they help, *Hosp Med* 41:71, 1991.

Ebersole P, Hess P: *Toward healthy aging,* ed 4, St Louis, 1994, Mosby.

Kim MJ, McFarland GK, McLane AM: *Pocket guide to nursing diagnoses,* ed 6, St Louis, 1995, Mosby.

Lewis-Cullinan C, Janken JK: Effect of cerumen removal on the hearing ability of geriatric patients, *J Adv Nurs* 15:594, 1990.

MacKellaig JA: A study of psychological effects of intensive care with particular emphasis on patients in isolation, *Intensive Care Nurs* 2:176, 1986.

Matteson MA, McConnell ES: *Gerontological nursing: concepts and practice,* Philadelphia, 1988, Saunders.

Norris RM: Commonsense tips for working with blind patients, *AJN* 89:360, 1989.

Rosenberg M: *Society and the adolescent self-image,* Princeton, NJ 1965, Princeton University Press.

Russel D, et al: Loneliness and social support: same or different constructs? Paper presented at the IOWA conference on personal relationships, Iowa City, Iowa, 1987.

Silverstein H et al: Diagnosis and management of hearing loss, *Clinical Symposia* 44(3):2, 1993.

Thibodeau GA, Patton KT: *Anatomy and physiology,* ed 2, St Louis, 1993, Mosby.

Ventry I, Weinstein B: The hearing handicap inventory for the elderly, a new tool, *Ear Hearing* 3:133, 1986.

Walsh C, Eldredge N: When deaf people become elderly, *J Gerontol Nurs* 15(12):27, 1989.

Weinstein BE: Age related hearing loss: how to screen for it, and when to intervene, *Geriatrics* 49(8):40, 1994.

Wong DL: *Whaley and Wong's nursing care of infants and children,* ed 5, St Louis, 1995, Mosby.

ADDITIONAL READINGS

Brinkman K: Why can't your patient hear you? *RN* 54:46, 1991.

Mulrow CD: Screening for hearing impairment in the elderly, *Hospital Prac* 26:79, 1991.

Ney DF: Cerumen impaction, ear hygiene practices, and hearing acuity, *Geriatric Nurs* 14(2):70, 1993.

Palumbo MV: Hearing access 2000: increasing awareness of the hearing impaired, *J Gerontol Nurs* 16(9):26, 1990.

Primental PA: Alteration in communication. In Dudas S, Bukowski L, editors: Nursing care of the stroke patient, *Nurs Clin North Am* 21:321, 1986.

Basic Physiological Needs

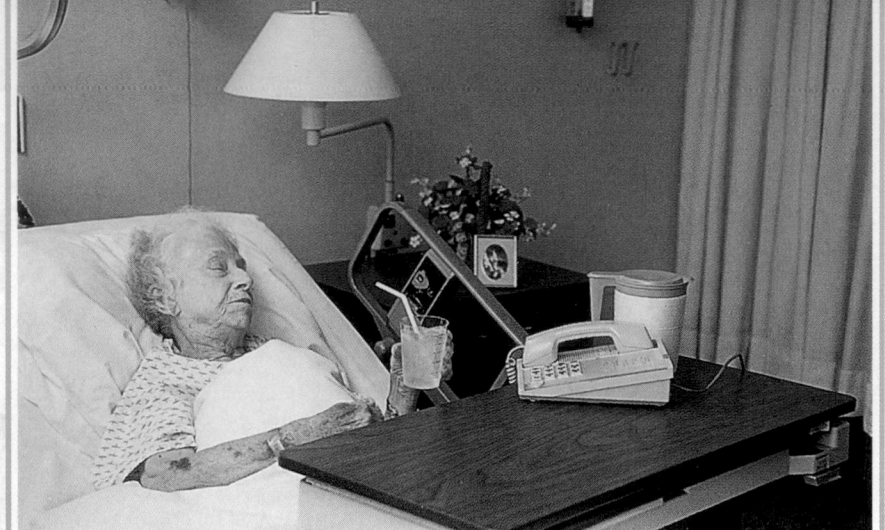

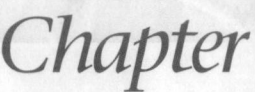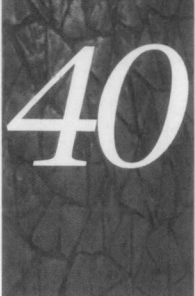

Hygiene

Objectives

Mastery of content in this chapter will enable the student to:

▶ Define the key terms listed.

▶ Identify common skin problems and related interventions.

▶ Describe factors that influence personal hygiene practices.

▶ Discuss conditions that may put a client at risk for impaired skin integrity.

▶ Describe the types of bathing techniques used for various physical conditions.

▶ Discuss the effect that different types of bathing techniques may have on the individual.

▶ Develop a care plan based on client preferences and hygienic practices.

▶ Describe techniques for providing hygiene to clients in the home setting.

▶ Perform a complete bed bath and back rub.

▶ Discuss factors that influence the condition of the nails and feet.

▶ Explain the importance of foot care for the diabetic client.

▶ Describe the methods used for cleaning and cutting the nails.

▶ Discuss conditions that may put a client at risk for impaired oral mucous membranes.

▶ Discuss measures used to provide special oral hygiene.

▶ Assist with or provide oral hygiene.

▶ List common hair and scalp problems and their related interventions.

▶ Offer hygiene to meet the needs of clients requiring eye, ear, and nose care.

▶ Successfully make an occupied, unoccupied, and surgical hospital bed.

Nurses work with a wide variety of clients who require assistance with personal hygiene or must learn proper hygienic techniques. **Hygiene** is the science of health. The self-care measures people use to maintain their health are called *personal hygiene*. Self-care measures may be complicated because of the physical condition or emotional state of the client.

Maintenance of personal hygiene is necessary for an individual's comfort, safety, and well-being. Whereas well people are capable of meeting their own hygienic needs, ill or physically challenged people may require the nurse's assistance to carry out routine hygienic practices. In addition, a variety of personal and sociocultural factors influence the client's hygienic practice. The nurse determines a client's ability to perform self-care and provides hygienic care according to the client's needs and preferences. In the home setting, the nurse assists the client and family members in adapting hygiene techniques and approaches. While providing routine hygienic care, the nurse assesses the client's physical and emotional state, and implements the nursing process for the client's total well-being. For example, complete assessment of the integument can be done during the client's bath, and the nurse can assess the client's psychosocial level as well.

Because hygienic care often requires close contact with the client, the nurse can use communication skills to promote a therapeutic relationship and to learn about the client's emotional needs (see Chapter 14). During hygienic care the nurse can also integrate other nursing strategies such as teaching health promotion practices or implementing range of motion exercises. The nurse must also consider clients' specific physical limitations, beliefs, values, and habits. Cultural preferences must also be respected. Unless the client's hygienic preferences significantly affect the client's health condition, they can usually be incorporated into the care plan. The nurse needs to preserve as much of the client's independence as possible, ensure privacy, convey respect, and foster the client's physical well-being. It is especially important to respect older adult clients while providing hygiene, since they may perceive a lack of respect and consideration from the care giver (Wagnild, Manning, 1985).

Hygiene practices are congruent with health promotion. The skin is the body's first line of defense against infection. By implementing hygiene measures for the client, or assisting family members to do so in the home setting, the nurse is adding to the level of wellness for the client. By teaching hygiene measures to the client, he or she will be playing an active part in promoting health and will be a participant in self-care whenever possible.

▌ FACTORS INFLUENCING HYGIENIC PRACTICE

The manner in which a person performs personal hygiene can be influenced by a number of factors. No two people perform hygienic care in the same way, and the nurse can provide individualized care only after knowing the client's unique hygienic practices.

Body Image

A client's general appearance may reflect the importance hygiene holds for that person. Body image is a person's subjective concept of his or her physical appearance. These images can change frequently. Body image affects the way in which hygiene is maintained. If a client is neatly groomed, the nurse considers the details of grooming when planning care and consults the client before making decisions about how hygienic care is to be provided. Clients who appear unkempt or uninterested in hygiene may require education about the importance of hygiene. The nurse should be sensitive in considering that the client's economic status may influence his or her ability to regularly maintain hygiene. The nurse must not convey feelings of disapproval or revulsion when caring for clients whose hygienic practices are different from the nurse's.

Because the client's body image may change as a result of surgery or a physical ailment, the nurse must make an extra effort to promote hygiene. For example, a client who has undergone a colostomy may be concerned about the appearance of the stoma and fecal odors. In addition to helping the client keep the stomal area clean, the nurse can discuss ways to reduce or eliminate odors (see Chapter 47).

Social Practices

The social groups to which a client relates can influence personal hygiene practices. During childhood, children acquire the hygiene practices of their parents. Family customs, the number of people in the house, and the availability of hot and/or running water are just a few of the factors influencing hygienic care. Teenagers may become more concerned with hygiene as their interest in dating increases. Later in life, friends and work groups shape the expectations people have about their personal appearance and the care taken to maintain adequate hygiene. Older adults' hygiene practices may change because of their living situation. For example, if they reside in a nursing home, they may not have the privacy in their new surroundings they may have had in their own home. They may not have the physical ability to bend to get in to and out of a bathtub unless the bathroom has been altered to accommodate their physical limitations.

Socioeconomic Status

A person's economic resources influence the type and extent of hygiene practices used. The nurse should determine whether the client can afford necessary supplies such as deodorant, shampoo, toothpaste, and cosmetics. The nurse should also determine if the use of these products is part of the social habits practiced by the client's social group.

In the home environment there may be a need to add devices that help clients maintain hygiene in a safe manner. Bars can be installed in the tub area or near the commode. This may not be possible if the client is on a fixed income. The nurse can demonstrate the use of a solid chair to aid in getting into or out of the tub or shower. An inexpensive but sturdy lawn chair placed on a rubber mat can be placed in the shower so the client can sit for stability.

Knowledge

Knowledge about the importance of hygiene and its implications for well-being influences hygiene practices. However, knowledge alone is not enough. The client also must be motivated to maintain self-care. Often, learning about an illness or condition encourages the client to improve hygiene. For example, when diabetic clients are aware of the effect of diabetes on circulation to the feet, they are more likely to learn proper techniques for foot care. Learning that certain practices are expected and beneficial in reducing health risks may motivate the person to comply with necessary care.

Cultural Variables

A client's cultural beliefs and personal values influence hygienic care. People from diverse cultural backgrounds follow different self-care practices (see Chapter 21). In North America, for example, many people take daily showers or tub baths. In Asia cleanliness is viewed as essential to well-being. In European countries, however, it is not unusual to bathe completely only once a week. When caring for clients with different hygienic practices, the nurse avoids being judgmental or trying to impose his or her own standards of hygiene.

Personal Preferences

Each client has individual desires and preferences about when to bathe, shave, and perform hair care. Clients select different products (for example, soap, shampoo, deodorant, and toothpaste) according to personal preferences and needs. Clients also have preferences regarding how hygiene is performed. For example, one man may prefer to shave

---

Hygiene Care Schedule

EARLY MORNING CARE
Nursing personnel on the night shift provide basic hygiene to clients getting ready for breakfast, scheduled tests, or early morning surgery. "AM care" includes offering a bedpan or urinal if the client is not ambulatory, washing the client's hands and face, and assisting with oral care.

MORNING, OR AFTER-BREAKFAST, CARE
In care performed after breakfast, the nurse assists by offering a bedpan or urinal to clients confined to bed; providing a bath or shower; providing oral, foot, nail, and hair care; giving a backrub; changing the client's gown or pajamas; changing the bed linens; and straightening the client's bedside unit and room. This is often referred to as "complete AM care."

AFTERNOON CARE
Hospitalized clients often undergo many exhausting diagnostic tests or procedures in the morning. In rehabilitation centers, clients may participate in physical therapy during the morning. Afternoon hygiene care includes washing the hands and face, assisting with oral care, offering a bedpan or urinal, and straightening bed linen.

EVENING, OR HOUR-BEFORE-SLEEP, CARE
Before bedtime the nurse offers personal hygiene care that helps a client relax to promote sleep. "PM care" may include changing soiled bed linens, gowns, or pajamas; assisting the client in washing the face and hands; providing oral hygiene; giving a back massage; and offering the bedpan or urinal to nonambulatory clients. Some clients may enjoy a beverage such as juice.

---

before a bath, whereas another may prefer to shave after taking a shower. Client preferences should help the nurse develop a more individualized care plan. The nurse does not attempt to change a client's preferences unless the client's health is affected. For example, clients with diabetes must carefully keep their feet clean to avoid the risk of infection. The nurse must explain and reinforce the need for good foot care if the client has repeated infections.

Physical Condition

People who suffer certain illnesses (for example, the late stages of cancer) or those who have undergone surgery often lack the physical energy or dexterity to perform personal hygiene. A client whose arm has been placed in a cast or who is in traction requires assistance in performing a complete bath. Serious cardiac, neurological, pulmonary, and metabolic conditions may exhaust or incapacitate clients and require the nurse to perform total hygienic care.

▌TYPES OF HYGIENIC CARE

The nurse provides a variety of hygienic measures throughout a day and can often schedule other care measures around the times that hygiene is planned. The box at left describes the types of hygienic care commonly performed at certain times of day in an acute care setting. However, these times may change because of factors affecting the nurse's organization and scheduling of care. These factors include client preferences and habits, the client's need for more hygiene (for example, soiling from a fever or infection), other scheduled activities or procedures, the nurse's other assignments, and the nurse-client ratio. In extended care facilities and nursing homes, the schedule for bathing is often less frequent.

▌CARE OF THE SKIN

The skin is an active organ with the functions of protection, secretion, excretion, temperature regulation, and sensation (Table 40-1). The skin has three primary layers: epidermis, dermis, and subcutaneous. The **epidermis** (outer layer) is composed of several thin layers of cells undergoing different stages of maturation. It shields underlying tissue against water loss and mechanical and chemical injury and prevents the entry of disease-producing microorganisms. The innermost layer of the epidermis generates new cells that migrate slowly toward the epidermal surface, or top layer (called the **stratum corneum**). These cells replace the dead cells that are continuously shed from the skin's outer surface. The epidermis also contains melanocytes, special cells that produce the melanin, or dark pigment, of the skin. Exposure to sunlight causes melanocytes to produce **melanin**, which gives some people a tan. Darker skinned races have more active melanocytes, which produce more melanin. The distribution of pigmentation in dark-skinned people varies widely.

Bacteria commonly reside on the skin's outer surface. These resident bacteria (for example, corynebacterium) are normal flora (see Chapter 34) that do not cause disease but instead inhibit the multiplication of disease-causing microorganisms.

The **dermis** is a thicker skin layer containing bundles of collagen and elastic fibers to support the epidermis. Nerve fibers, blood vessels, sweat glands, sebaceous glands, and

Table 40-1	Function of the Skin and Implications for Care	

FUNCTION/DESCRIPTION	IMPLICATIONS FOR CARE
PROTECTION Epidermis is relatively impermeable layer that prevents entrance of microorganisms. Although microorganisms reside on skin surface and in hair follicles, relative dryness of skin's surface inhibits bacterial growth. Sebum removes bacteria from hair follicles. Acidic pH of skin further retards bacterial growth.	Weakening of epidermis occurs by scraping or stripping its surface (e.g., use of dry razors, tape removal, or improper turning or positioning techniques). Excessive dryness causes cracks and breaks in skin and mucosa that allow bacteria to enter. Emollients soften skin and prevent moisture loss, soaking of skin improves moisture retention, and hydration of mucosa prevents dryness. However, constant exposure of skin to moisture causes maceration or softening, which interrupts dermal integrity and promotes ulcer formation and bacterial growth. Bed linen and clothing should be kept dry. Misuse of soap, detergents, cosmetics, deodorant, and depilatories can cause chemical irritation. Alkaline soaps neutralize protective acid condition of skin. Cleansing of skin removes excess oil, sweat, dead skin cells, and dirt that can promote bacterial growth.
SENSATION Skin contains sensory organs for touch, pain, heat, cold, and pressure.	Friction should be minimized to avoid loss of stratum corneum, which can result in development of pressure ulcers. Smoothing linen removes sources of mechanical irritation. Removing rings from fingers prevents nurse from accidentally injuring client's skin. Bath water should not be excessively hot or cold.
TEMPERATURE REGULATION Body temperature is controlled by radiation, evaporation, conduction, and convection.	Factors that interfere with heat loss can alter temperature control. Wet bed linen or gowns interfere with convection and conduction. Excess blankets or bed coverings can interfere with heat loss through radiation and conduction. Coverings can promote heat conservation.
EXCRETION AND SECRETION Sweat promotes heat loss by evaporation. Sebum lubricates skin and hair.	Perspiration and oil can harbor microorganisms. Bathing removes excess body secretions, although if excessive it can cause drying of skin.

hair follicles course through the dermal layer. Sebaceous glands secrete sebum, an oily, odorous fluid, into the hair follicles. Sebum lubricates the skin and hair to keep them supple and pliant. There are two types of sweat glands: eccrine and apocrine. The **eccrine glands** are distributed throughout the skin but are more abundant in the forehead, palms, and soles. Sweat excreted from the eccrine glands assists in temperature control through evaporation. The **apocrine glands** can be found in the axillary and genital areas. The bacterial decomposition of sweat from these glands is responsible for body odor. In the ears, ceruminous glands secrete **cerumen** into the external ear canal. This heavy, oily substance traps any foreign material entering the ear.

The subcutaneous tissue layer contains blood vessels, nerves, lymph, and loose connective tissue filled with fat cells. The fatty tissue serves as a heat insulator for the body. Subcutaneous tissue also provides support for upper skin layers, enabling it to withstand stresses and pressure without injury. Very little subcutaneous tissue can be found underlying the oral mucosa.

The skin exchanges oxygen, nutrients, and fluid with underlying blood vessels; synthesizes new cells; and eliminates dead, nonfunctioning cells. The cells of the integument require adequate nutrition and hydration to resist injury and disease. Adequate circulation is essential to maintain cell life. The skin often reflects a change in physical condition by alterations in color, thickness, texture, turgor, temperature, and hydration (see Chapter 33). As

long as the skin remains intact and healthy, its physiological function remains optimal.

■ THE NURSING PROCESS AND SKIN CARE

Assessment

Nursing assessment continues throughout hygienic care. First, the nurse must determine whether the client can tolerate hygienic procedures, which can often be exhausting. An assessment will then guide the nurse in identifying the type of care required by the client.

Most assessment occurs as the nurse provides for the client's hygienic needs. For example, during the bath, the condition of the skin can be observed. Hygienic care allows the nurse to make assessment findings for a variety of health care problems and thus helps set health care priorities.

PHYSICAL ASSESSMENT OF THE SKIN

While assisting a client with personal hygiene, the nurse assesses all external body surfaces. Using the skills of inspection and palpation (see Chapter 33), the nurse looks for alterations in the integument in addition to circulatory changes, determines the client's need for ongoing hygiene, and notes changes of the integument in response to nursing and medical therapies.

The nurse determines the condition of the skin by ob-

Table 40-2	Common Skin Problems	
CHARACTERISTICS	**IMPLICATIONS**	**INTERVENTIONS**
DRY SKIN Flaky, rough texture on exposed areas such as hands, arms, legs, or face	Skin may become infected if epidermal layer is allowed to crack.	Have client bathe less frequently and rinse body of all soap because residue left on skin can cause irritation and breakdown. Add moisture to air through use of humidifier. Increase fluid intake when skin is dry. Use moisturizing cream to aid healing. (Cream forms protective barrier and helps maintain fluid within skin.) Use cream such as Eucerin. Use creams to clean skin that is dry or allergic to soaps and detergents.
ACNE Inflammatory, papulo-pustular skin eruption, usually involving bacterial breakdown of sebum; appears on face, neck, shoulders, and back	Infected material within pustule can spread if area is squeezed or picked. Permanent scarring can result.	Wash hair and skin thoroughly each day with hot water and soap to remove oil. Use cosmetics sparingly because oily cosmetics or creams accumulate in pores and tend to make condition worse. Implement dietary restrictions, if necessary. (Foods that aggravate condition should be eliminated from diet.) Inform client that exposure to ultraviolet rays, either from sunshine or heat lamp, may help control acne. (Caution should be used to prevent burning of skin.) Use prescribed topical antibiotics for severe forms of acne.
HIRSUTISM Excessive growth of body and facial hair, especially in women	Hirsutism may cause negative body image by giving women a male appearance.	Use following to remove unwanted hair: depilatories (can cause infection, rashes, dermatitis), shaving (safest method), electrolysis (permanently removes hair by destroying hair follicles), tweezing (lasts only temporarily), bleaching of hair (lasts only temporarily), waxing (can cause ingrown hair).
SKIN RASHES Skin eruption that may result from overexposure to sun or moisture or from allergic reaction (may be flat or raised, localized or systemic, pruritic or nonpruritic)	If skin is continually scratched, inflammation and infection may occur. Rashes can also cause discomfort.	Wash area thoroughly and apply antiseptic spray or lotion to prevent further itching and aid in healing process. Apply warm or cold soaks to relieve inflammation, if indicated.
CONTACT DERMATITIS Inflammation of skin characterized by abrupt onset with erythema, pruritus, pain, and appearance of scaly oozing lesions (seen on face, neck, hands, forearms, and genitalia)	Dermatitis is often difficult to eliminate because person is usually in continual contact with substance causing skin reaction. Substance may be hard to identify.	Avoid causative agents (e.g., cleansers and soaps).
ABRASION Scraping or rubbing away of epidermis that may result in localized bleeding and later weeping of serous fluid	Infection occurs easily because of loss of protective skin layer.	Be careful not to scratch client with jewelry or fingernails. Wash abrasions with mild soap and water. Observe dressing or bandage for retained moisture because it could increase risk of infection.

> ### Normal Skin Characteristics
>
> - Skin is smooth and dry.
> - Skin is intact and has no abrasions.
> - Skin feels warm when palpated.
> - Localized changes in texture can be palpated across skin's surface. The skin is soft and flexible.
> - There is good turgor (elastic and firm), with skin generally smooth and soft.
> - Skin color varies from body part to body part, ranging from deep brown to rudy pink to light pink.

serving its color, texture, thickness, turgor, temperature, and hydration. Chapter 33 describes in detail the techniques for assessing each of these characteristics. The box above describes normal skin characteristics.

The nurse also assesses for skin problems influenced by hygienic measures (Table 40-2). The nurse notes areas of dry skin resulting from too many baths; excessive use of soap; or use of harsh, alkaline soaps. Areas of skin **maceration** (softening) may have formed as a result of improper drying. The nurse observes for calloused areas on the feet or hands that might benefit from soaking and the application of lotion. However, caution must be taken not to leave lotion between the toes, since this can lead to skin breakdown.

While inspecting the skin, the nurse notes the presence and condition of lesions (see Chapter 33). Certain types have implications for hygienic measures. When the nurse observes skin problems, it helps to explain proper skin care to the client. For example, a rash on the skin often indicates an allergic reaction. The nurse teaches the client about the significance of the rash and the proper use of medications prescribed for the rash and cautions against specific over-the-counter drugs that may prove useless or may even worsen the rash. Likewise, the nurse educates the client about avoiding irritants such as harsh soaps or cosmetics, which can aggravate the condition.

DEVELOPMENTAL CHANGES

Age influences the normal condition of the skin and the type of hygienic measures required. The neonate's skin is relatively immature. The epidermis and dermis are loosely bound together. The skin is extremely thin. Because any friction against the skin layers can cause bruising, the nurse must handle the neonate carefully during bathing. A break in the neonate's skin can easily lead to infection.

A toddler's skin layers are more tightly bound together. Thus the child has a greater resistance to infection and skin irritation. However, because of the child's more active play, and the absence of established hygienic habits, greater attention is needed from parents and care givers to provide thorough hygiene and to begin teaching good hygiene habits.

During adolescence the growth and maturation of the integument are increased. In girls, estrogen secretion causes the skin to become soft, smooth, and thicker, with increased vascularity. In boys, male hormones produce an increased thickness of the skin with some darkening in color. Sebaceous glands become more active, predisposing adolescents to **acne**. Eccrine and apocrine sweat glands become fully functional during puberty. Adolescents usually begin to use antiperspirants. More frequent bathing and shampooing also become necessary to reduce body odors. Sweating is usually more pronounced in boys. The growth of body hair increases during adolescence as a result of hormonal changes. The body hair has a characteristic pattern of distribution, which the nurse can assess (see Chapter 33). Pubic and axillary hair develops in both sexes. Beard and mustache hair grows in boys as a result of testicular androgens. Some girls and women have increased androgen levels causing **hirsutism**, the growth of facial hair.

The condition of an adult's skin depends on hygienic practices and exposure to environmental irritants. Normally the skin is elastic, well hydrated, firm, and smooth. With age, the skin loses its resiliency and moisture, and sebaceous and sweat glands become less active. The epithelium thins, and elastic collagen fibers shrink, making the skin fragile and subject to bruising and breaking. These changes warrant caution when turning and repositioning older adults. Typically the older person's skin is dry and wrinkled. Daily bathing as well as bathing with water that is too hot or soap that is harsh may cause the skin to become excessively dry.

SELF-CARE ABILITY

When a client becomes unable to bathe or perform personal skin care, the nurse either provides the necessary assistance or teaches family or friends how to provide hygiene. To determine whether a client requires a bed bath instead of a tub bath or shower, the nurse should assess the client's balance, activity tolerance, muscle strength, and coordination. The degree of assistance needed by a client during bathing may also depend on vision, the ability to sit without support, hand grasp, attached equipment, and the range of motion of the client's extremities. The client's health problem should also be considered when deciding what type of bathing to institute. If a client's cognitive function is impaired, the nurse's help probably will be needed. The nurse should also assess the home environment and its impact on the client's hygiene practices. The nurse must evaluate the physical condition of the client as well as what is available for the client when he or she returns to the home. Will there be barriers in the home that may affect the client's self-care activities pertaining to hygiene?

RISKS FOR SKIN IMPAIRMENT

The nurse looks for certain conditions that place a client at risk for impaired skin integrity (see Chapter 38).

Immobilization. A client who is unable to move freely as a result of illness or some external restraint is at risk for skin breakdown. The dependent body parts are exposed to pressure from underlying surfaces (for example, a mattress, a body cast, or a wrinkled layer of linen), reducing circulation to affected body parts. Chapter 38 describes how the impairment of circulation to dependent body parts can result in pressure ulcer formation. The nurse should be aware of clients who require assistance to turn and change positions. For example, it may be necessary to have a turning sheet on a bed to reduce straining while moving the client. Localized redness and tenderness are early signs of pressure on dependent body parts and, if left untreated, can result in pressure ulcers.

Reduced Sensation. Many clients are unable to sense an injury to the skin's surface. Clients with paralysis, circulatory insufficiency, or local nerve damage do not receive normal transmission of nerve impulses when excessive heat or cold, pressure, friction, or chemical irritants are applied to the skin. During the bath, the nurse can easily assess the status of sensory nerve function by checking for pain, tactile sensation, or temperature sensation (see Chapter 33).

Nutrition and Hydration Alterations. Adequate nutrients are essential for maintaining the normal integrity of the skin. Clients with limited caloric and protein intake have impaired tissue synthesis (see Chapter 41). The skin becomes thinner, less elastic, and smoother, with a subsequent loss of subcutaneous tissue, which can result in impaired or delayed tissue healing. Poor digestion and absorption of nutrients caused by inflammatory conditions of the bowel or bowel surgery; excessive protein metabolism caused by fever, burns, or surgery; and excessive loss of protein caused by blood loss, wound exudate, or burns place clients at risk for imbalances. An older adult with poorly fitting dentures may have difficulty meeting the nutritional needs necessary for healthy skin. A hospitalized client who is not permitted to eat is also a candidate for nutritional and hydration problems that can affect the integrity of the skin.

Secretions and Excretions on the Skin. Moisture on the skin's surface is a medium for bacterial growth and can cause local irritation, soften epidermal cells, and contribute to skin maceration. Perspiration, urine, watery fecal material, and wound drainage can accumulate on the skin's surface, resulting in breakdown and infection. The nurse gives particular attention to body areas, such as under a woman's breasts, the perineal area, or under the arms, where moisture may collect, and skin surfaces may rub against each other and cause friction.

Vascular Insufficiency. In peripheral vascular disease, the arterial blood supply to tissues is inadequate or venous return is impaired, causing decreased circulation to the extremities. Inadequate blood flow to the skin results in ischemia and breakdown. Clients with this disease have a

high risk of infection because delivery of nutrients, oxygen, and white blood cells to injured tissues is inadequate.

External Devices. When a client has some type of external device applied to or around the skin, the device can exert pressure or friction against the skin's surface. A cast, cloth restraint, bandage, dressing, or orthopedic brace can rub against the skin and cause breakdown. The nurse assesses all skin surfaces exposed to any external device.

 Nursing Diagnosis

The nurse's assessment reveals the condition of the client's skin and the client's need for and ability to meet personal hygiene needs. The nurse reviews all data gathered (e.g., risk for immobilization or altered sensation), considers previous clients cared for, reviews knowledge pertaining to

---

 Examples of NANDA Nursing Diagnoses for Skin Integrity

Impaired skin integrity *related to:*
- Pressure from cast
- Immobilizatiton
- Exposure to chemical irritants

Risk for impaired skin integrity *related to:*
- Immobilization
- Vascular insufficiency
- Inadequate nutritional intake

Altered peripheral tissue perfusion *related to:*
- Impaired arterial blood flow
- Impaired venous blood flow

Bathing/hygiene self-care deficit *related to:*
- Pain in hands
- Forced immobilization
- Musculoskeletal weakness

Impaired tissue integrity *related to:*
- Altered circulation
- Nutritional deficit
- Mechanical irritation

 Sample Nursing Diagnostic Process for Impaired Skin Integrity

ASSESSMENT ACTIVITIES	DEFINING CHARACTERISTICS	NURSING DIAGNOSES
Check to see if client is able to turn or move on own. Ask if client is experiencing discomfort over bony prominences. Inspect skin surfaces for redness, irritation, dryness, excessive perspiration, lesions, or open wounds.	Limited ability, to turn Erythema over coccyx with some tenderness Excess prespiration over skin	**Risk for impaired skin integrity** related to immobilization
Assess amount of assistance needed. Check to see if supplies are within client's reach. Determine whether client has physical or cognitive defects.	Inability to wash body or body parts Inability to get to water source Inability to regulate flow of water	**Bathing/hygiene self-care deficit** related to cast on right lower extremity

preexisting conditions, clusters defining characteristics, and then makes the nursing diagnosis specific to the client's actual or potential health problems (see the nursing diagnoses box on p. 1022, top). Accurate selection of a diagnosis requires critical thinking and ultimately ensures the appropriate choice of therapies.

Purposes of Bathing

CLEANSING THE SKIN
Cleansing removes perspiration, some bacteria, sebum, and dead skin cells, which minimizes skin irritation and reduces the chance of infection.

STIMULATION OF CIRCULATION
Good circulation is promoted through the use of warm water and gentle stroking of the extremities.

IMPROVED SELF-IMAGE
Bathing promotes relaxation and a feeling of being refreshed and comfortable.

REDUCTION OF BODY ODORS
Excessive secretion of sweat from apocrine glands located in the axillae and pubic areas causes unpleasant body odors. Bathing and use of antiperspirants minimize odors.

PROMOTION OF RANGE OF MOTION (ROM)
Movement of the extremities during bathing maintains joint function.

Whether a client has an alteration in skin integrity or is at high risk determines the focus of the nursing intervention. For example, if the client has the potential for skin breakdown, the nurse plans preventive measures. The related factors contributing to the problem determine the nurse's interventions (see the diagnostic process box on p. 1022, bottom). Skin breakdown resulting from chronic exposure to urine will require different therapies than breakdown related to irritation from a cast.

If the client has skin breakdown, the nurse must provide care that promotes healing of injured skin surfaces and prevents infection. The nurse also eliminates factors that may lead to further tissue injury.

 Planning

There are many reasons to provide skin care other than maintaining cleanliness. A bath or shower helps the client relax, stimulates circulation to the skin, provides exercise through range of motion during bathing, improves self-image, and stimulates the rate and depth of respirations (see the box at left). The interaction between nurse and client during bathing and skin care gives the nurse an opportunity to develop a meaningful relationship with the client.

Planning should focus on the methods of skin care that the nurse will deliver, the desired outcomes for improving the condition of the skin, and the variety of nursing care measures the nurse can perform as a client bathes. Teaching, providing emotional support, values clarification, and as-

---

 Sample Nursing Care Plan for Impaired Skin Integrity

NURSING DIAGNOSIS: Risk for impaired skin integrity related to immobilization
Definition: Risk for impaired skin integrity is the state in which an individual's skin is at risk of being adversely altered (Kim, McFarland, and McLane, 1995)

GOALS	EXPECTED OUTCOMES	INTERVENTIONS	RATIONALE
Client will have intact skin during hospitalization.	Skin will be without redness. Skin will be warm, soft, smooth, and well hydrated.	Bathe client daily.	Cleansing removes excess oil, sweat, dead skin cells, and dirt that promote bacterial growth.
	Odors will be reduced or eliminated.	Turn regularly (at least every 2 hr).	Longer pressure is applied, greater the risk of skin breakdown. Pressure decreases or obliterates circulation, depriving tissue of oxygen and nutrients (Pires, Mueller, 1991).
		Apply lotion to skin after bathing.	Emollients soften skin and prevent moisture loss.
Client will be free of odors during hospitalization.	Drainage or secretions will be reduced or absent.	Dry skin thoroughly after each cleansing.	Excess moisture causes skin maceration, which promotes bacterial growth (NPUAP, 1989).
		Give perineal care after each voiding and defecation.	Excessive secretion of sweat from apocrine glands in axillae and pubic areas causes unpleasant odors. Bathing minimizes odors. Secretions that accumulate on surface of skin around genitalia act as reservoir for infection.

sisting with range-of-motion exercises are just some of the types of interaction the nurse can include during hygiene.

The client's condition influences the plan for delivering hygiene. A seriously ill client usually needs a daily bath because body secretions accumulate, and the client is unable to maintain cleanliness (see the care plan on p. 1023). An older client at home may require a visit from the nurse to assist with a tub bath. Clients who are normally inactive during the day and have skin that tends to be dry, may need to bathe only twice a week. The nurse must plan for necessary assistance for clients who are weakened or possess poor muscle strength and coordination. For example, an obese client who has had difficulty getting out of a tub should have a tub chair, hand rails, or extra personnel available for help.

Timing is also important in planning hygienic care. Being interrupted in the middle of a bath to go to an x-ray examination can frustrate and embarrass a client. In the home, bathing may be planned to refresh the client before daily activities. The nurse should try to plan hygienic care around tests, procedures, and client needs. This can be difficult in a hospital because tests may not be scheduled for specific times. The home setting obviously allows clients more opportunity to decide in the plan of care.

Goals for clients receiving skin care include the following:
1. Clients will have intact skin free of body odors.
2. Client will maintain range of motion.
3. Client will achieve a sense of comfort and well-being.
4. Client will participate in and understand methods of skin care.

 ## Implementation

BATHING AN ADULT

Bathing a client is a part of total hygienic care. Baths can be categorized as cleansing or therapeutic (see the box below). A physician's order is necessary for baths designed for therapeutic purposes. The order designates the body part being treated (in the case of soaks), and any medicated solution used (for example, saline, sodium bicarbonate, or potassium permanganate).

The extent of the client's bath and the methods used for bathing depend on the client's physical capabilities and the degree of hygiene required. A complete bed bath is needed for clients who are totally dependent and require total hygienic care (Procedure 40-1). For older adults, the nurse may use and instruct older adults about use of soap that contains a moisturizer. If the older client has very dry skin, the nurse may recommend that soap only be used in the axilla, genital, and feet areas.

A **partial bed bath** involves bathing only body parts that would cause discomfort or odor if left unbathed (for example, hands, face, perineal area, and axillae). Dependent clients in need of only partial hygiene or self-sufficient bedridden clients who are unable to reach all body parts receive a partial bed bath. Nurses need to assess carefully to determine that clients can sufficiently bathe other body parts on their own.

The tub bath or shower can be used to give a more thorough bath than a bed bath. Washing and rinsing all body parts are easier. Safety is of primary concern because the surface of a tub or shower stall is slippery. Clients vary in how much help they will need. Some tubs are specially designed for dependent clients. The nurse should adhere to the following guidelines when clients receive or take baths:
1. Provide privacy. Close the door or pull room curtains around the bathing area. While bathing the client, expose only the areas being bathed.
2. Maintain safety. Keep side rails up while away from the client's bedside. This is particularly important for dependent or unconscious clients. Place the call light within the client's reach if it is necessary to leave the room temporarily.
3. Maintain warmth. The use of a bath blanket will conserve body heat, which may be lost during the bath.

Text continued on p. 1031.

Types of Therapeutic Baths

HOT WATER TUB BATH
Immersion in hot water helps relieve muscle soreness and spasm. However, a danger of causing burns exists. Water temperature should be 45° to 46° C (113°-114.8° F) for adults.

WARM WATER TUB BATH
Bathing in warm water relieves muscle tension. Water temperature should be 43° C (109.4° F).

COOL WATER BATH
Bathing in tepid water can help lower body temperature in cases where a child's body temperature is over 40° C (104° F). Tepid baths should not be used for common fevers as they are ineffective and cause discomfort (Newman, 1985). Water temperature should be tepid (37° C [98.6° F]) rather than cold to avoid chilling and to promote slow cooling; this avoids temperature fluctuations. This type of bath can be effective in reducing the body temperature of a small child. Start with warm water and gradually add cool water until the temperature

of 37° C (98.6° F) is reached to accustom child to lower temperature. The child is placed in the bath while water is squeezed over back and chest for 30 min.

SOAK
Local application of water or a medicated solution can remove dead tissue or soften encrusted secretions. An aseptic technique is necessary when cleansing open or abraded areas of the skin. Soaks are also useful in reducing pain and swelling of inflamed or irritated skin surfaces.

SITZ BATH
A sitz bath cleanses and reduces inflammation of the perineal and anal areas of a client who has undergone rectal or vaginal surgery or childbirth or who has local rectal irritation from hemorrhoids or fissures. Water temperature depends on the client's condition but should be 43° to 45° C (109.4°-113° F). Cold sitz baths are more effective in relieving pain in the postpartum period.

Bathing a Client

STEPS	RATIONALE
1. Assess client's preferences for bathing practices, frequency of bathing, time of day preferred, type of hygiene products used.	Promotes participation and sense of comfort.
2. Consider client's condition and review orders for precautions concerning client's movement or positioning.	Prevents accidental injury to client during bathing.
3. Explain procedure and ask client for suggestions or ways to prepare supplies. If partial bath is to be performed, ask how much of bath client wishes to complete.	Promotes client cooperation and participation.
4. If shower or tub bath is to be done, schedule use of facilities if private bath unavailable.	Prevents unnecessary waiting that can cause fatigue.
5. Adjust room temperature and ventilation, and close room doors and windows. Close curtains around bed.	Prevents rapid loss of body heat during bathing. Ensures privacy.
6. Prepare necessary equipment and supplies:	
a. Two bath towels	Separate towel and washcloth are used for client's face and for body to enhance feeling of cleanliness.
b. Two washcloths	
c. Washbasin (for complete or partial bed bath)	
d. Soap and soap dish	Bath blanket maintains client's warmth during procedure.
e. Bath blanket or top spread (for complete or partial bed bath)	
f. Clean gown or pajamas	
g. Hygienic aids, such as water repellant skin, ointment, skin moisturizer, deodorant, and powder	For client to use before bath.
h. Bedpan or urinal and toilet paper	
i. Linen hamper or laundry bag	
j. Disposable gloves	Prevents contact with potentially infected body secretions.
k. Bed linen (optional)	
COMPLETE OR PARTIAL BED BATH	
7. Offer client bedpan or urinal (see Chapter 46). Provide towel and washcloth for client.	Client will feel more comfortable after voiding. Prevents interruption of bath.
8. Wash hands. OPTION: Apply gloves if drainage on skin	Reduces transmission of microorganisms.
9. Lower side rail closest to you and assist client in assuming comfortable position maintaining body alignment.	Aids nurse's access to client. Maintains client comfort.
10. Bring client toward side closest to you. Place hospital bed in high position.	When you do not have to reach across bed, strain on back muscles is minimized.
11. Loosen top covers at foot of bed. Place bath blanket over top sheet. Fold and remove top sheet from under blanket. If possible, have client hold bath blanket while you withdraw sheet.	Removal of top linens prevents them from becoming soiled or moist during bath. Blanket provides warmth and privacy.
12. If top sheet is to be reused, fold it for replacement later. If not, dispose in laundry bag, taking care not to allow linen to contact your uniform.	Proper disposal prevents transmission of microorganisms.
13. Remove client's gown or pajamas while maintaining privacy. If extremity is injured or has reduced mobility, begin removal from unaffected side. If client has intravenous (IV) tube, remove gown from arm *without* IV first, and then lower IV container and slide gown covering affected arm over tubing and container. Rehang IV container and check flow rate (see the illustrations on p. 1026).	Provides full exposure of body parts during bathing. Undressing unaffected side first allows easier manipulation of gown over body part with reduced ROM.
14. Pull side rail up. Fill washbasin two-thirds full, with warm water. Have client place fingers in water to test temperature tolerance. OPTION: Place plastic container of bath lotion in bath water.	Raising side rail maintains safety as you leave bedside. Warm water promotes comfort and prevents chilling. Testing temperature prevents accidental burning of client's skin. Keeps lotion warm for application to skin.
15. Lower side rail. Remove pillow if allowed and raise head of bed 30-45 degrees. Place bath towel under client's head.	Removal of pillow makes it easier to wash client's ears and neck. Placement of towel prevents soiling of bed linen.

Continued.

Bathing a Client—cont'd

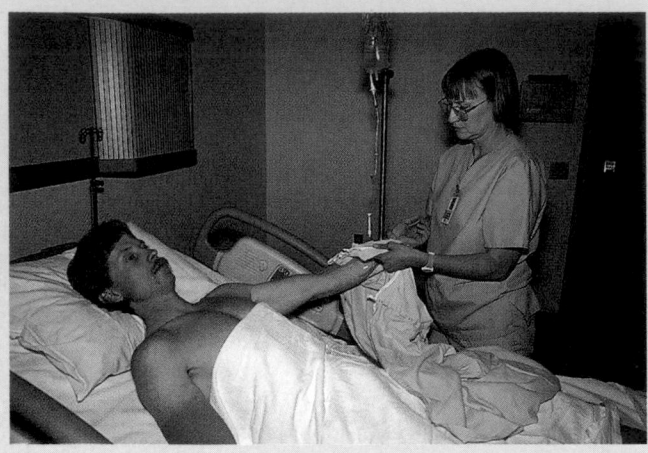 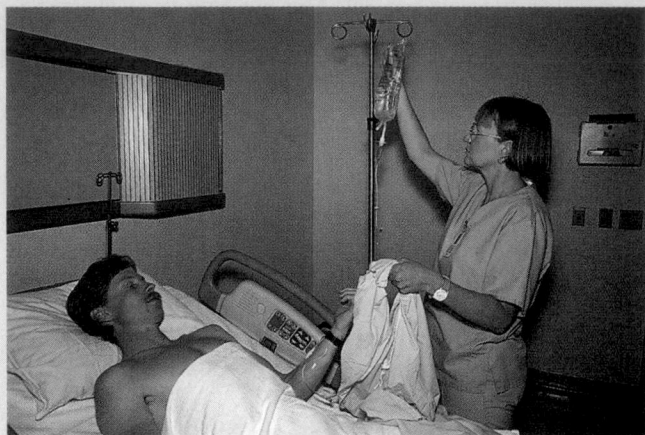

Step 13

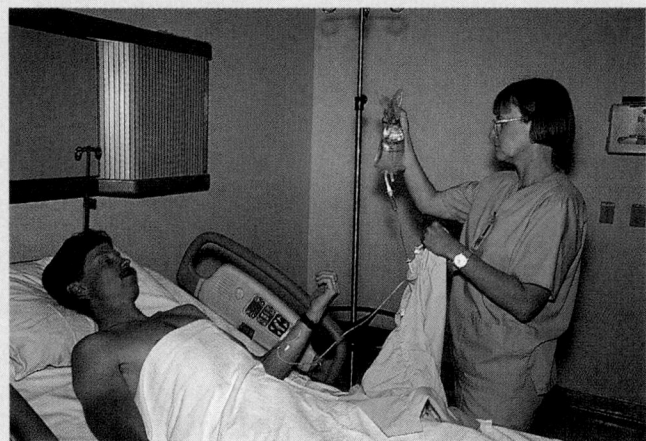 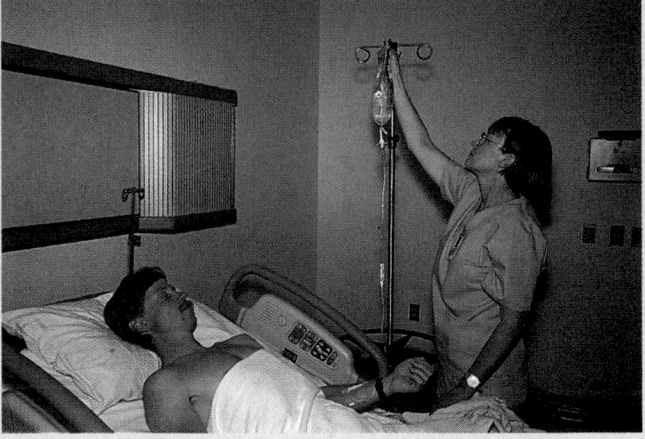

Step 13

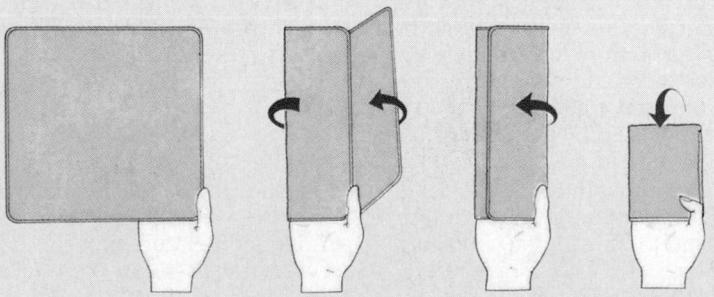

Step 17 *(From Sorrentino SA: Mosby's textbook for nursing assistants, ed 3, St Louis, 1995, Mosby.)*

Bathing a Client—cont'd

STEPS	RATIONALE

COMPLETE OR PARTIAL BED BATH—cont'd

16. Place bath towel over client's chest.

17. Fold washcloth around fingers of your hand to form a mitt (see the illustration on p. 1026). Immerse mitt in water and wring thoroughly.

18. Wash client's eyes with plain warm water. Use different section of mitt for each eye. Move mitt from inner to outer canthus (see the illustration below). Soak encrustations on eyelid for 2-3 min with damp cloth before attempting removal. Dry eye thoroughly but gently.

19. Ask client about preference for using soap on face. Wash, rinse, and dry well forehead, cheeks, nose, neck, and ears. (Men may wish to shave at this point or after bath.)

20. Remove bath blanket from over client's arm that is nearest you. Place bath towel lengthwise under arm.

21. Bathe arm with soap and water using long, firm strokes from distal to proximal areas (fingers to axilla). Raise and support arm above head (if possible) while thoroughly washing axilla (see the illustration below).

22. Rinse and dry arm and axilla thoroughly. If client prefers, apply deodorant or talcum powder.

23. Fold bath towel in half and lay it on bed beside client. Place basin on towel. Immerse client's hand in water. OPTION: Allow hand to soak for 3-5 min before washing hand and fingernails (Procedure 40-4). Remove basin and dry hand well. Raise side rail and go to other side of bed.

24. Lower side rail and repeat Steps 20-23 for other arm.

25. Check temperature of bath water and change water if necessary. (Do not leave side rail down if there is a risk of fall.)

26. Cover client's chest with bath towel and fold bath blanket down to umbilicus.

27. With one hand, lift edge of towel away from chest. With mitted hand, bathe chest using long, firm strokes. Take special care to wash skinfolds under female client's breasts, lifting breast if necessary. Keep chest covered between wash and rinse periods. Dry well.

RATIONALE

Prevents soiling of bath blanket, and easy access to towel.

Mitt retains water and heat better than loosely held washcloth, keeps cold edges from brushing against client, prevents splashing.

Soap irritates eyes. Use of separate sections of mitt reduces infection transmission. Bathing eye from inner to outer canthus prevents secretions from entering nasolacrimal duct. Pressure can cause internal injury.

Soap tends to dry face more quickly because it is exposed to air more than other body parts.

Prevents soiling of bed.

Soap lowers surface tension and facilitates removal of debris and bacteria when friction is applied during washing. Long, firm strokes stimulate circulation. Movement of arm exposes axilla and exercises joint's normal ROM.

Alkaline residue from soap discourages growth of normal skin bacteria (Barnes, 1987). Excess moisture causes skin maceration or softening. Deodorant controls body odor.

Soaking softens cuticles and calluses of hand and loosens debris beneath nails. Soaking also enhances feeling of cleanliness. Thorough drying removes moisture from between fingers.

Use of warm water maintains client's comfort.

Prevents unnecessary exposure of body parts.

Maintains warmth and privacy. Secretions and dirt collect easily in areas of tight skinfolds.

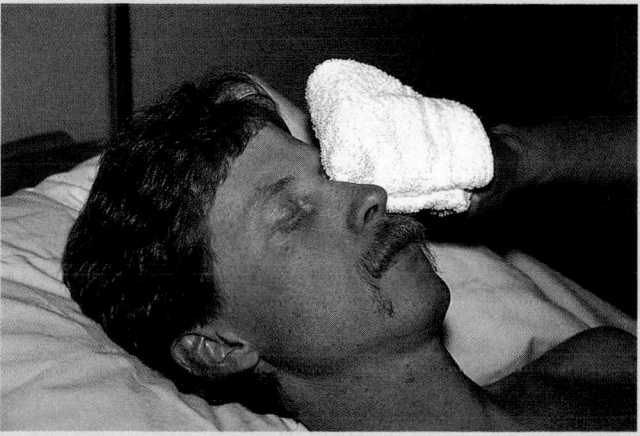

Step 18

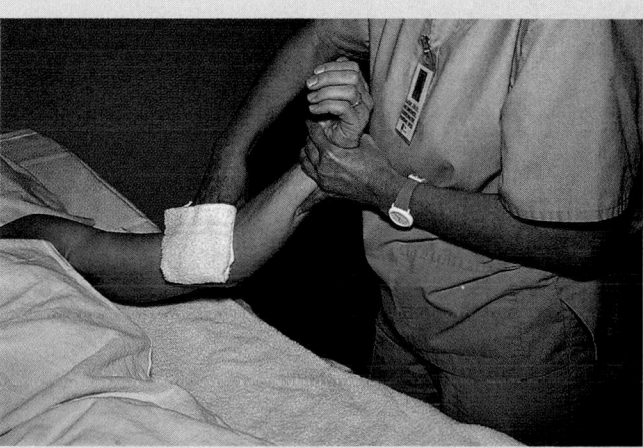

Step 21

Continued.

Bathing a Client—cont'd

STEPS	RATIONALE

COMPLETE OR PARTIAL BED BATH—cont'd

28. Place bath towel lengthwise over chest and abdomen. (Two towels may be needed.) Fold blanket down to just above pubic region.

Prevents chilling and exposure of body parts.

29. With one hand, lift bath towel. With mitted hand, bathe abdomen, giving special attention to bathing umbilicus and abdominal folds. Stroke from side to side. Keep abdomen covered between washing and rinsing. Dry well.

Moisture and sediment that collect in skinfolds predispose client to skin maceration and irritation.

30. Apply clean gown or pajama top. If one extremity is injured or immobilized, always dress affected side first. (This step may be omitted until completion of bath; gown should not become soiled during remainder of bath.)

Maintains client's warmth and comfort. Dressing affected side first allows easier manipulation of gown over body part with reduced ROM.

31. Cover chest and abdomen with top of bath blanket. Expose far leg by folding blanket over toward midline. Be sure perineum is draped.

Prevents unnecessary exposure.

32. Bend client's leg at knee by positioning your arm under leg. While grasping client's heel, elevate leg from mattress slightly and slide bath towel lengthwise under leg.

Prevents soiling of bed linen. Support of joint and extremity during lifting prevents strain on musculoskeletal structures.

33. Ask client to hold foot still. Place bath basin on towel on bed and secure its position next to foot to be washed.

Sudden movement by client could cause spillage of bathwater. (This step is omitted if client is unable to hold leg in basin.)

34. With one hand supporting lower leg at joints, raise it and slide basin under lifted foot. Make sure foot is firmly placed on bottom of basin. OPTION: Allow foot to soak while you wash leg (see the illustration below).

Proper positioning of foot prevents pressure from being applied from edge of basin against calf. Soaking softens calluses and rough skin. (NOTE: if client is unable to hold leg in basin, do not immerse; simply wash with washcloth.)

35. Unless contraindicated, use long, firm strokes in washing from ankle to knee and from knee to thigh. Dry well. Apply moisturizer to skin as needed.

Promotes venous return. Long, firm strokes would not be used for client with blood clots.
Keeps epidermis lubricated.

36. Cleanse foot, making sure to bathe between toes. Cleanse and clip nails as needed (Procedure 40-4). Dry well. If skin is dry, apply lotion.

Secretions and moisture may be present between toes. Lotion helps to retain moisture and soften skin.

37. Raise side rail and move to other side of bed. Lower side rail. Repeat Steps 31-36 for other leg and foot.

38. Cover client with bath blanket, raise side rail for client's safety, and change bathwater.

Drop in water temperature during bathing can cause chilling. Clean water reduces microorganism transmission.

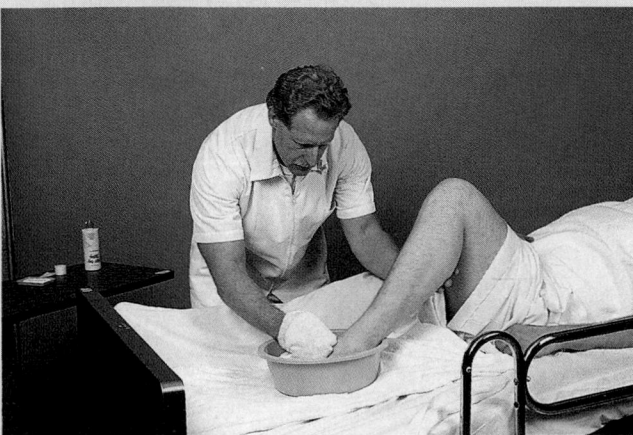

Step 34

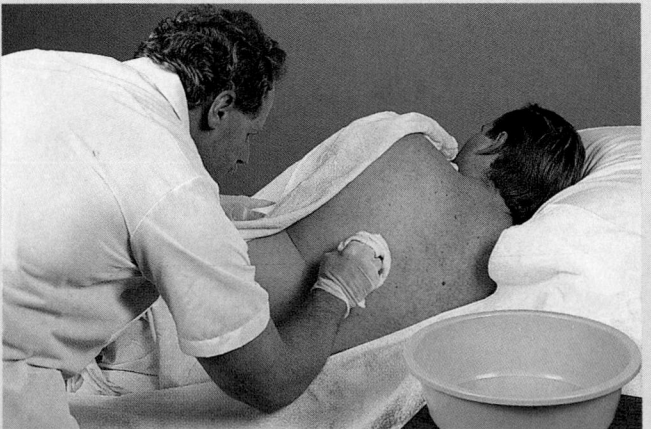

Step 42

Bathing a Client—cont'd

STEPS	RATIONALE

COMPLETE OR PARTIAL BED BATH—cont'd

39. Lower side rail. Assist client in assuming prone or side-lying position (as applicable). Place towel lengthwise along client's side.
Exposes back and buttocks for bathing.

40. Keep client draped by sliding bath blanket over shoulders and thighs.
Maintains warmth and prevents unnecessary exposure.

41. Apply disposable gloves (if not done in Step 8).
Prevents contact with microorganisms in body secretions.

42. Wash, rinse, and dry back from neck to coccyx using long, firm strokes (see the illustration on p. 1028). Pay special attention to folds of buttocks and anus. Give backrub (Procedure 40-3). Move from anterior to posterior.
This direction moves from clean to contaminated. Skinfolds near buttocks and anus may contain fecal secretions that harbor microorganisms.

43. Change bathwater and washcloth.
Prevents transfer of microorganisms from anal area to genitalia.

44. Assist client in assuming side-lying or supine position. Cover chest and upper extremities with towel and lower extremities with bath blanket. Expose only genitalia. (If client can help, covering entire body with bath blanket may be preferable.) Wash, rinse, and dry perineum (Procedure 40-2). Give special attention to skinfolds. Apply water repellant ointment to area exposed to moisture.
Maintains client's privacy. Clients capable of performing partial bath usually prefer to wash their own genitalia. Skinfolds are site for accumulation of secretions and moisture. Water repellant ointments (e.q., A&D, Pericare) protect the skin from moisture (AHCPR, 1992).

45. Dispose of gloves in receptacle and wash hands.
Prevents transmission of microorganisms.

46. Apply any additional body lotion or oil as desired.
Moisturizing lotion prevents dry, chapped skin.

47. Assist client in dressing.

48. Comb client's hair (see p. 1055). Women may want to apply makeup.
Maintains client's body image.

49. Make client's bed (Procedures 40-10 and 40-11).
Provides clean environment.

50. Remove soiled linen and place in dirty linen bag. Cleanse and replace bathing equipment. Replace call light and personal possessions. Leave room as clean and comfortable as possible.
Prevents transmission of infection. Clean environment promotes comfort. Keeping call light and articles of care within reach promotes safety.

51. Wash hands.
Reduces transmission of microorganisms.

52. Perform evaluation of bath techniques.

TUB BATH OR SHOWER

1. Preparation for bathing client. Assess client's preferences for bathing practices, frequency of bathing, time of day preferred, type of hygiene products used.
Promotes participation and sense of comfort.

2. Consider client's condition and review orders for precautions concerning client's movement or positioning.
Prevents accidental injury to client during bathing.

3. Explain procedure and ask client for suggestions or ways to prepare supplies. If partial bath is to be performed, ask how much of bath client wishes to complete.
Promotes client cooperation and participation.

4. If shower or tub bath is to be done, schedule use of facilities if private bath unavailable.
Prevents unnecessary waiting that can cause fatigue.

5. Adjust room temperature and ventilation, and close room doors and windows. Close curtains around bed.
Prevents rapid loss of body heat during bathing. Ensures privacy.

6. Prepare necessary equipment and supplies:
  a. Two bath towels
  b. Two washcloths
Separate towel and washcloth are used for client's face and for body to enhance feeling of cleanliness.
  c. Washbasin (for complete or partial bed bath)
  d. Soap and soap dish
  e. Bath blanket or top spread (for complete or partial bed bath)
Bath blanket maintains client's warmth during procedure.
  f. Clean gown or pajamas

Continued.

Bathing a Client—cont'd

TUB BATH OR SHOWER—cont'd

6. Prepare necessary equipment and supplies—cont'd:

   g. Hygienic aids, such as water repellant skin, ointment, skin moisturizer, deodorant, and powder

   h. Bedpan or urinal and toilet paper   For client to use before bath.

   i.   Linen hamper or laundry bag

   j.   Disposable gloves   Prevents contact with potentially infected body secretions.

   k. Bed linen (optional)

7. Check tub or shower for cleanliness. Use cleansing techniques according to agency policy. Place rubber mat on tub or shower bottom. Place disposable bathmat or towel on floor in front of tub or shower. — Prevents transmission of infection. Mats prevent slipping and falling.

8. Collect all hygienic aids, toiletry items, and linen requested by client. Place within easy reach (see the illustration below). — Prevents possible falls when client reaches for equipment.

9. Assist client to bathroom if necessary. Have client wear robe and slippers en route to bathroom. — Prevents accidental falls. Wearing robe and slippers prevents chilling.

10. Demonstrate to client how to use call signal for assistance when in hospital or extended care facility. NOTE: If safety is jeopardized, make arrangements for help during procedure. — Bathrooms are equiped with signaling devices in case client feels faint or weak or needs immediate assistance. Clients prefer privacy during bath if safety is not jeopardized.

11. Place "occupied" sign on bathroom door when in hospital or extended care facility. — Maintains privacy.

12. Fill bathtub halfway with warm water. Ask client to test water, and adjust water temperature if it is too warm or too cold. Explain which faucet controls hot water. If client is taking shower, turn shower on and adjust water temperature before client enters shower stall. — Adjusting water temperature prevents accidental burns. Older clients and clients with neurological alterations (e.g., spinal cord injury) are at high risk for burns resulting from reduced sensation.

13. Instruct client to use safety bars when getting in and out of tub or shower. — Prevents slipping and falls.

14. Caution client against use of bath oil in tub water. — Oil causes tub surfaces to become slippery, predisposing client to accidental falls.

15. Instruct client not to remain in tub longer than 20 min. Check on client every 5 min. — Prolonged exposure to warm water may cause vasodilation and pooling of blood, leading to lightheadedness or dizziness.

16. Return to bathroom when client signals, and knock before entering. — Provides privacy.

17. For client who is unsteady, drain tub of water before client attempts to get out of it. Place bath towel over client's shoulders. — Prevents accidental falls. Client may become chilled as water drains.

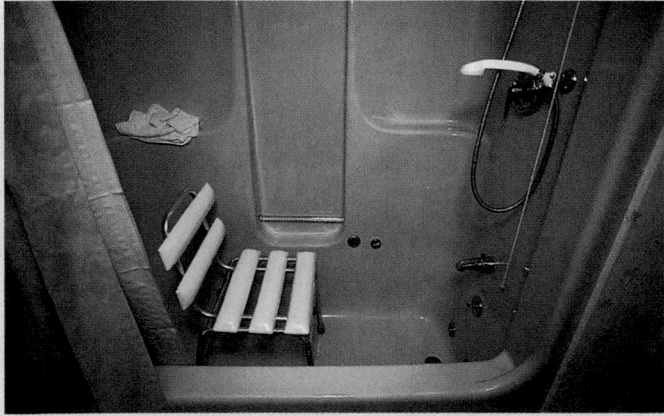

Step 8

Bathing a Client—cont'd

STEPS	RATIONALE
## TUB BATH OR SHOWER—cont'd	
18. Assist client in getting out of tub as needed and assist with drying.	Moisture may cause excessive softening of skin and promote spread of infection.
19. Assist client as needed in donning clean gown or pajamas, slippers, and robe. (In home and extended-care or long-term care facilities, the client may don regular clothing.)	Maintains warmth to prevent chilling.
20. Assist client to room and help client assume comfortable position in bed or chair.	Maintains relaxation gained from bathing.
21. Cleanse tub or shower according to agency policy. Remove soiled linen and place in dirty linen bag. Discard disposable equipment in proper receptacle. Place "unoccupied" sign on bathroom door. Return supplies to storage area.	Prevents transmission of infection through soiled linen and moisture.
22. Wash hands.	Reduces transfer of microorganisms.
23. Perform Evaluation of Bath Techniques	
## EVALUATION OF BATH TECHNIQUES	
1. Observe client's behavior and ask if fatigue or discomfort is felt.	Determines tolerance to bathing activities.
2. Note areas on skin that were previously soiled or reddened or showed early signs of breakdown.	Techniques used during bathing should leave skin clean and clear.
3. Record type of bath and client's tolerance of bathing. Also note condition of skin and any significant findings such as reddened skin areas or joint or muscle pain. Record level of assistance required by client.	Timely documentation maintains accuracy of client's record. Condition of skin documents response to therapy such as turning and positioning.

Keeping the room warm while the client is partially uncovered will reduce the occurrence of chilling. Control drafts; keep windows and bed curtains closed.

4. Promote the client's independence as much as possible during bathing activities. Offer assistance as needed.

PERINEAL CARE

Usually **perineal care** (pericare) (Procedure 40-2) is part of the complete bath. Clients most in need of meticulous perineal care are those at greatest risk for acquiring an infection (e.g., clients who have indwelling urinary catheters), are recovering from rectal or genital surgery, or have undergone childbirth. A client able to perform self-care should be allowed to do so. Nurses may become embarrassed about providing perineal care, particularly to clients of the opposite sex. It may help to have a nurse of the opposite sex present in the room when providing perineal care. Embarrassment should not cause the nurse to overlook the client's hygiene needs. A professional, dignified attitude can reduce embarrassment and put the client at ease.

If a client performs self-care, various problems such as vaginal or urethral discharge, skin irritation, and unpleasant odors may go unnoticed. The nurse must be alert for complaints of burning during urination or localized soreness, excoriation, or pain in the perineum. The nurse also inspects the client's bed linen for signs of discharge. Clients most at risk for skin breakdown in the perineal area are those with urinary or fecal incontinence, rectal and perineal surgical dressings, and indwelling urinary catheters.

BACK RUB

A back rub, or back massage, usually follows the client's bath (Procedure 40-3). It promotes relaxation, relieves muscular tension, and stimulates skin circulation. During the back rub, the nurse can assess the condition of the client's skin.

An effective back rub takes 3 to 5 minutes. The nurse should first ask whether the client would like a back rub because some clients dislike the physical contact. The nurse should also consult the client's medical record for any back rub contraindications before offering a massage to the client.

BATHING AN INFANT

An infant can be bathed in much the same way as an adult, by a sponge bath or in a small tub. However, the nurse should take special precautions. Because an infant's temperature control mechanisms are still immature, prolonged exposure of body parts may cause rapid cooling. When giving a sponge bath, the nurse keeps the infant covered as much as possible. When giving a tub bath, the nurse should work quickly and be sure the water temperature is warm enough to prevent chilling.

Text continued on p. 1036.

Perineal Care

STEPS	RATIONALE
1. Identify clients at risk for developing infection of genitalia, urinary tract, or reproductive tract (e.g., presence of indwelling catheter, fecal incontinence, or surgical incision).	Secretions that accumulate on surface of skin around female and male genitalia act as reservoir for infection. Traumatized tissues provide route for introduction of infectious organisms.
2. Explain procedure and purpose to client.	Helps minimize anxiety during procedure that is often embarrassing to you and client.
3. Prepare necessary equipment and supplies:	Used when administering a bed bath.
a. Washbasin	
b. Soap dish with soap	
c. Two or three washcloths	
d. Bath towel	
e. Bath blanket	Used for draping client.
f. Waterproof pad or bedpan	Prevents soiling of bed linen.
g. Toilet tissue	
h. Disposable gloves	Prevents contact with microorganisms in body secretions.
Additional supplies when pericare is given during times other than a bath:	
a. Cotton balls or swabs	Used for cleansing menstruating women or around indwelling catheters.
b. Solution bottle or container filled with warm water or prescribed rinsing solution	
c. Waterproof bag	For disposal of cotton balls.
4. Assemble supplies at bedside.	Ensures orderly procedure.
5. Wash hands	Reduces transmission of organisms.
6. Pull curtain around bed or close room door. Raise bed to comfortable working position.	Maintains client's privacy. Facilitates good body mechanics.
7. Lower side rail and assist client in assuming side-lying position, placing towel lengthwise along client's side and keeping client covered with bath blanket as much as possible.	If client is totally dependent, assistance is necessary to support client in side-position.
8. Apply disposable gloves	Prevents contact with body fluids
9. If fecal material is present, enclose in a fold of underpad or toilet tissue and remove with disposable wipes. Cleanse buttocks and anus washing from front to back (see the illustration). Cleanse and rinse thoroughly. Dry area completely. Remove and discard underpad and replace with clean one.	Cleansing reduces transmission of microorganisms from anus to urethra or genitalia.

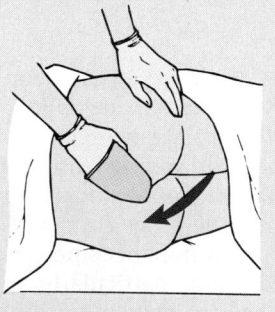

Step 9

STEPS	RATIONALE
10. Provide perineal care	
a. Female perineal care:	
(1) Change gloves if badly soiled	
(2) Position waterproof pad under client's buttocks with client supine. (OPTION: place bedpan under client)	Protects bed linen from soiling
(3) Assist client in assuming dorsal recumbent position.	Provides easy access to genitalia.
(4) Fold top bed linen down toward foot of bed and raise client's gown up above genital area.	Exposes perineal area for easy accessibility.

Perineal Care—cont'd

STEPS	RATIONALE

10. Provide perineal care—cont'd

 a. Female perineal care—cont'd

> (5) "Diamond" drape client by placing bath blanket with one corner between client's legs, one corner pointing toward each side of bed, and one corner over chest. Tuck side corners around legs and under hips (see the illustrations).

Prevents client from accidentally falling. Proper water temperature prevents burns to perineum.

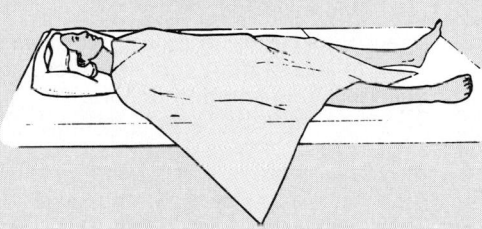 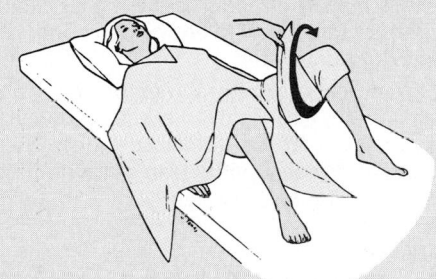

Step 10a(5) *(From Sorrentino SA:* Mosby's textbook for nursing assistants, *ed 3, St Louis, 1995, Mosby.)*

> (6) Raise side rail. Fill washbasin with warm water. Place on over bed table.

Prevents unnecessary exposure of body parts and maintains client's warmth and comfort.

> (7) Lower side rail and help client flex her knees and spread legs apart

Provides full exposure of female genitalia.

> (8) Fold lower corner of bath blanket up between client's legs onto abdomen.

Keeping client draped until procedure begins minimizes anxiety.

> (9) Wash and dry client's upper thighs.

Buildup of perineal secretions can soil surrounding skin surfaces.

> (10) Wash labia majora. Use nondominant hand to gently retract labia from thigh; with dominant hand, wash carefully in skinfolds. Wipe in direction from perineum to rectum. Repeat on opposite side, using separate section of washcloth. Rinse and dry area thoroughly

Skinfolds may contain body secretions that harbor microorganisms. Wiping from perineum to rectum reduces chance of transmitting fecal organisms to urinary meatus.

> (11) Separate labia with nondominant hand to expose urethral meatus and vaginal orifice. With dominant hand, wash downward from pubic area toward rectum in one smooth stroke (see the illustration). Use separate section of cloth for each stroke. Cleanse thoroughly around labia minora, clitoris, and vaginal orifice.

Cleansing method reduces transfer of microorganisms to urinary meatus. (For menstruating women or clients with indwelling urinary catheters, cleanse with cotton balls.)

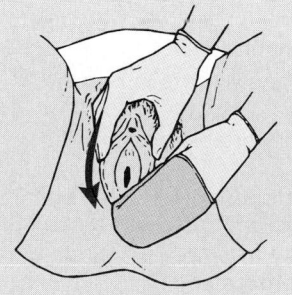

Step 10a(11)

> (12) If client is on bedpan, pour warm water over perineal area.

Rinsing removes soap and microorganisms more effectively than wiping.

> (13) Dry perineal area thoroughly.

Retained moisture harbors microorganisms.

> (14) Fold lower corner of bath blanket back between client's legs and over perineum. Ask client to lower legs and assume comfortable position.

Side-lying position provides access to anal area for cleansing.

Continued.

Perineal Care—cont'd

STEPS	RATIONALE

10. Provide perineal care—cont'd

  b. Male perineal care:

    (1) Change gloves if badly soiled

    (2) Lower side rail, Lower top edge of bath blanket below client's perineum. Gently raise penis and place bath towel underneath.

        Towel prevents moisture from collecting in inguinal area.

    (3) Gently grasp shaft of penis. If client is uncircumcised, retract foreskin. If client has erection, defer procedure until later.

        Gentle handling reduces chance of client having erection. Secretions capable of harboring microorganisms collect under foreskin.

    (4) Wash tip of penis at urethral meatus first. Using circular motion, cleanse from meatus outward and down the shaft (see the illustration). Discard washcloth and repeat with clean cloth until penis is clean. Rinse and dry gently.

        Direction of cleansing moves from area of least contamination to area of most contamination, preventing microorganisms from entering urethra.

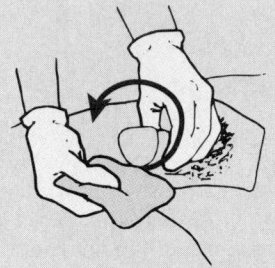

Step 10b(4)

    (5) Return foreskin to natural position.

        Retracted of foreskin can tighten around shaft of penis, causing local edema and discomfort.

    (6) Wash shaft of penis with gentle but firm downward strokes. Pay special attention to underlying surface of penis.

        Vigorous massage of penis can lead to erection, which can cause embarrassment for client and you. Underlying surface of penis may have greater accumulation of secretions.

    (7) Rinse and dry penis thoroughly. Instruct client to spread legs slightly.

        Abduction of legs provides easier access to scrotal tissues.

    (8) Gently cleanse scrotum. Lift it carefully and wash underlying skinfolds. Rinse and dry.

        Pressure on scrotal tissues can be very painful to client. Secretions collect between skinfolds. Underlying surface of scrotum may develop pressure sores.

    (9) Fold bath blanket back over perineum and assist client in turning to comfortable position

        Draping promotes comfort and minimizes anxiety. Side-lying position provides access to anal area.

11. If client has been incontinent of feces and/or urine, apply thin layer of skin barrier containing petrolatum or zinc oxide over anal and perineal skin.

    Protect skin from excess moisture and toxins from urine on stool (Maklebust, 1991)

12. Remove disposable gloves and dispose in proper receptacle.

    Moisture and body secretions on gloves can harbor microorganisms.

13. Assist client in assuming comfortable position and cover with sheet.

    Client's comfort minimizes emotional stress of procedure.

14. Remove bath blanket and dispose of all soiled bed linen. Return unused equipment to storage area.

    Reduces transmission of infection.

15. Raise side rail and lower bed to proper height. Return room to condition before procedure.

    Prevents client from accidentally falling. Clean environment enhances client's comfort.

16. Wash hands.

    Reduces transmission of infection.

17. Inspect surface of external genitalia and surrounding skin for redness, swelling, discharge or irritation, after cleansing.

    Thick secretions may cover underlying skin lesions or areas of breakdown. Evaluation can determine need for additional therapy.

18. If indwelling catheter is in place, make sure it is secured with tape (see Chapter 46).

19. Record procedure and of any abnormal findings (e.g., discharge or condition of genitalia).

    Ensures accurate and timely documentation of care.

Administering a Backrub

STEPS	RATIONALE

1. Identify factors or conditions such as rib or vertebral fractures, burns, reddened areas on the skin, or open wounds that contraindicate backrub.
2. For clients with history of hypertension or dysrhythmias, assess pulse and blood pressure.

Massage of sensitive tissues might lead to further tissue injury. Massaging reddened areas of skin increases breaks in capillaries in underlying tissues (AHCPR, 1992)

Massage may cause autonomic nervous system stimulation that induces changes in heart rate and blood pressure. Research has not shown consistent relationships between human touch and cardiac response of those being touched (Weiss, 1986).

3. Explain procedure and desired position to client.
4. Prepare necessary equipment and supplies:
   a. Bath blanket
   b. Bath towel
   c. Skin application (lotion, alcohol, powder)

Helps promote relaxation.

Lotion lubricates skin and prevents friction during massage. Alcohol cools skin but has drying effect. Powder reduces friction during massage.

5. Adjust bed to high, comfortable position.

Ensures proper body mechanics and prevents strain on back muscles.

6. Adjust light, temperature, and sound within room.
7. Lower side rail and help client assume prone or side-lying (Sims') position with back toward you. Close curtain around bed.

Environmental distractions can prevent client from relaxing.

Position makes it easier to apply necessary pressure to back muscles. Privacy promotes relaxation.

8. Expose client's back, shoulders, upper arms, and buttocks. Cover remainder of body with bath blanket. Lay towel alongside client's back.

Prevents unnecessary exposure of body parts and prevents excess lotion from touching linens.

9. Wash your hands in warm water. Warm lotion in your hands or by placing container under warm water. Place small amount of lotion in hands.

Cold causes muscle tension.

10. Explain to client that lotion will feel cool and wet.
11. Apply hands first to sacral area, massaging in circular motion. Stroke upward from buttocks to shoulders. Massage over scapulae with smooth, firm stroke. Continue in one smooth stroke to upper arms and laterally along sides of back down to iliac crests (see the illustration). Do not allow your hands to leave client's skin. Continue massage pattern for 3 min.

Warning client reduces startled response.

Gentle, firm pressure applied to all muscle groups promotes relaxation. Continuous contact with skin's surface is soothing and stimulates circulation to tissues.

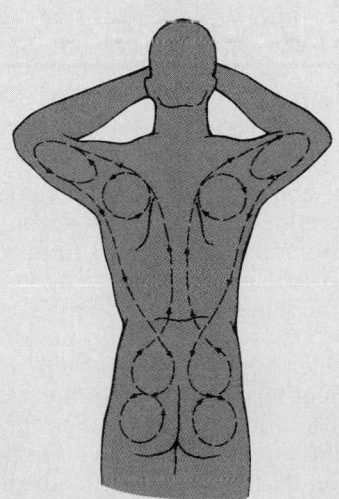

Step 11

Continued.

Administering a Backrub—cont'd

STEPS	RATIONALE
12. Knead skin by grasping tissue between your thumb and fingers (see the illustrations below). Knead upward along one side of spine from buttocks to shoulders and around nape of neck. Knead or stroke downward toward sacrum. Repeat along other side of back.	Kneading increases circulation. Motion is soothing and relieving.
13. End massage with long stroking movements and tell client you are ending massage.	Long stroking is most soothing.
14. If lying on side, ask client to turn to opposite side, and massage other hip.	
15. Wipe excess lubricant from client's back with bath towel. Retie gown or assist with pajamas. Help client to comfortable position. Raise side rails as needed, and open curtain. Lower bed.	Excess lotion can be irritant. Comfortable position enhances backrub's effects.
16. Dispose of soiled towel and wash hands.	Promotes infection control.
17. Ask client about comfort. Note any areas of muscle pain or tension.	Degree of relief gained depends on length of massage, client's ability to relax, and degree of discomfort before massage.
18. Reassess pulse and blood pressure.	Gentle back massage may increase heart rate and systolic blood pressure.
19. Record response to massage and condition of skin.	Describes response to therapy.

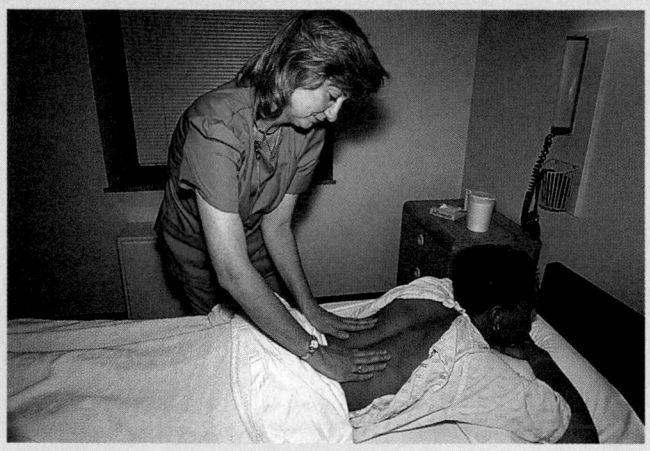 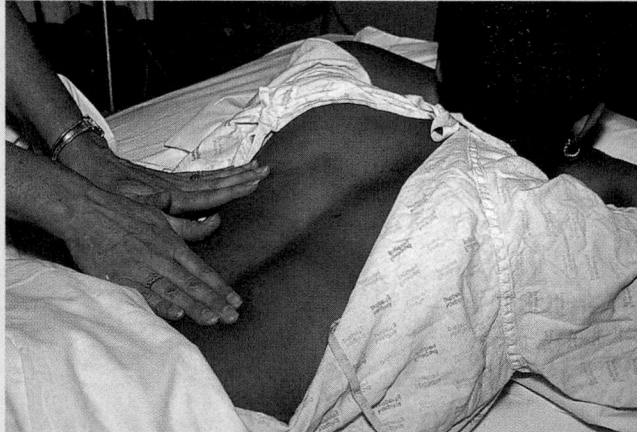

Step 12

The surface of an infant's skin has a pH of about 4.95 soon after birth (Wong, 1995). This acidic covering helps prevent the growth of bacteria on the skin's surface. Thus plain water is preferred for bathing. Alkaline soaps, such as Ivory, and oils, powder, and lotion can alter the skin's pH and provide a medium for bacterial growth.

Care of the umbilical cord is a special consideration for the newborn. The umbilical stump is an excellent medium for bacterial growth. Thus sponge baths are given until the cord falls off and the skin heals. Immersion of the umbilicus in a tub of water before the skin heals can result in a serious infection. Triple dye is used by many institutions to prevent infection. The daily application of alcohol to the base of the cord aids drying.

The nurse also gives special care to infants who have been circumcised. A small amount of bleeding normally occurs from the penis. The physician applies a sterile gauze dressing impregnated with petrolatum jelly around the circumcised area. The nurse may clean the penis periodically with moistened cotton balls until the dressing can be removed permanently (Wong, 1995).

In hospitals where there is rooming-in of the infant and mother, the infant's bath is an excellent opportunity to involve the parents in the child's care. The parents can examine the infant's body parts and learn about normal variations in skin characteristics. A parent may worry about minor birth injuries unless the nurse explains how they occur and when they will disappear.

Sponge Bath. Newborn infants are bathed after their vital signs have stabilized. Nurses wear gloves when initially handling infants whose skin has become soiled from the blood of the mother. Initial washing only involves cleaning blood from the face and head. The **vernix caseosa**, a grayish white, cheeselike substance covering the skin, may temporarily provide insulation and lubricating properties. The vernix caseosa dries and disappears within 24 to 48 hours.

Supplies for the bath include a shirt, a diaper (disposable or cloth), safety pins if using cloth diapers, a soft washcloth, cotton balls, a towel, and facial tissue. Plain water is used for bathing to minimize skin irritation from soap or oils. A mild unscented soap should be used only for soiled areas such as around the anus. Optional supplies include alcohol for cleansing the umbilical cord and petrolatum jelly to prevent diaper rash.

The nurse prepares a basin of warm water so that it feels comfortable when tested on the inside of the nurse's forearm. This prevents the infant from getting cold. The nurse washes the infant's face, eyes, ears, and scalp before removing the shirt and diaper. The towel may also be kept over the infant for warming.

The nurse cleanses the infant's eyes and ears with clean, moistened cotton balls or a washcloth. The eyes are gently wiped from the inner to the outer canthus, using a clean cotton ball with each stroke or turning the cloth so that only a clean part touches the eyes. While washing the face, the nurse inspects the nares for encrusted secretions. Cotton tipped swabs should not be used to cleanse the nares or ears because an infant may move suddenly, causing the swab to break and damage the eardrum or mucous membranes. A rolled wisp of dampened cotton or the twisted end of the washcloth works well for cleansing the external ear canal and pinna.

The infant's scalp can be cleansed by wiping off any secretions with a washcloth. However, if shampooing is necessary, the nurse secures the baby's head with one hand and positions it over the bath basin. A mild soap is best for shampooing. The nurse rinses the scalp by pouring water from a small cup or container over the infant's head into the basin. Thorough drying is necessary to prevent evaporative heat loss.

The nurse then undresses the infant for the remainder of the bath. The towel is again used to drape areas not being washed. Keeping the infant covered may be difficult because infants often kick and twist. Because of the infant's sensitive skin, little rubbing should be done when cleansing. However, the nurse gives special attention to the folds in the neck, axillae, and creases at joints. For example, neck creases often collect regurgitated food, which may cause a rash. The umbilical cord should be cleansed with mild soap and water and dried thoroughly. Alcohol may be applied to the umbilicus to help dry it and to reduce the chance of infection. Then the nurse dresses the infant in a shirt.

The nurse bathes the infant's genitalia before the buttocks. For a girl, it is important to retract the labia fully to remove the vernix caseosa after it has dried. If the vernix caseosa is thick and adherent, the nurse may choose to remove it gradually during successive diaper changes to avoid causing unnecessary irritation during one bath. The vulva is cleansed from front to back to prevent the spread of microorganisms from the anal area to the urethra. This technique should be explained to the parents. In male infants, the nurse washes carefully around the penis and scrotum. Noncircumcised infants should not have the foreskin retracted because it is often too tight. Later, after the foreskin loosens, the nurse should teach the parents to retract the foreskin, cleanse the area, and return the foreskin to its position. No special care is required around a circumcised penis. The nurse wipes off any blood with a clean cotton ball or washcloth. The original petrolatum jelly dressing remains in place for only a day.

The nurse bathes the buttocks last. Fecal material can be removed with facial tissue. The washcloth is moved from anterior to posterior to prevent moving fecal material toward the urethra. Using mild soap helps ensure thorough cleansing of the anal area. After thorough drying, the application of a thin layer of petrolatum jelly or ointment helps retain skin moisture and prevents diaper rash.

After the bath, the nurse applies a clean diaper, which should fit snugly around the thighs and abdomen to prevent the leakage of urine. If the child is circumcised, the diaper should fit loosely to prevent friction against the penis. The diaper should always be below the umbilical site until it is completely healed. The nurse fastens the diaper with the back overlapping the front to permit full hip flexion.

Tub Bath. Infants can be given a tub bath after the umbilicus has healed. The supplies for the tub bath are the same as those for a sponge bath. Supplies should be within easy reach. The face, neck, ears, eyes, and scalp are washed before the infant is undressed and immersed in the tub. The nurse lowers the infant slowly into the tub to avoid startling them. The child must always be held firmly with one hand (Fig. 40-1). A child is never left unattended in the bathinette. Often infants enjoy the sensation of being immersed in water, and older infants may enjoy playing dur-

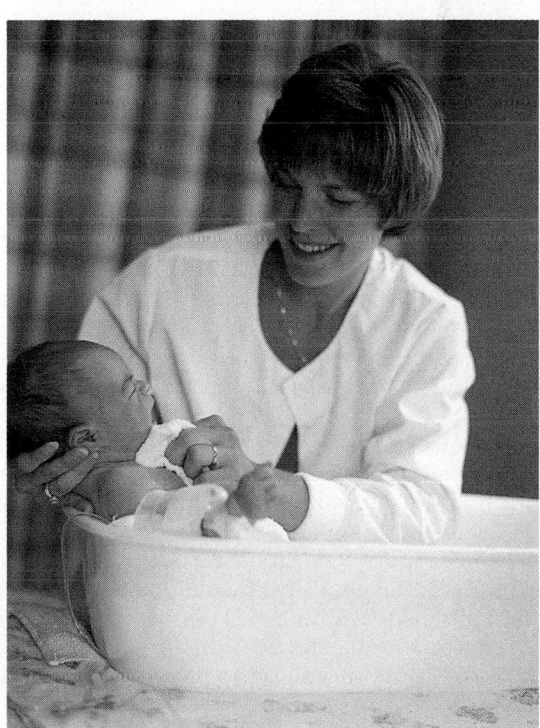

Fig. 40-1 Holding infant during tub bath.

Sample Evaluation of Interventions for Impaired Skin Integrity

GOALS	EVALUATIVE MEASURES	EXPECTED OUTCOMES
Client will have intact skin free of odors by discharge from hospital.	Inspect surfaces of skin after cleansing. Take time to note presence of obvious body odors.	Skin will be intact, warm, smooth, soft, well hydrated, and without redness.
	Exercise joint through ROM during bathing of body part.	Joints will move within same ROM as client's baseline. Normal joints will move freely without discomfort.
Client will maintain joint ROM by discharge from hospital.	Question client about level of comfort.	Client will verbalize less discomfort and will indicate sense of relaxation.
Client will achieve sense of comfort and well-being within 24 hours.	Observe client's body movements or gestures.	Client will be calm. Body movements will be purposeful and relaxed. Client will express positive statements about well-being.
	Observe client's initiation of and assistance with bathing activities.	Client will initiate hygiene measures or participate in bathing with nurse's assistance.
Client will participate in and understand methods of skin care by first home visit.	Observe if client asks questions regarding self-care measures. Ask client to explain proper technique to follow in bathing.	Client will describe proper hygienic methods to maintain skin integrity.

ing the bath. Body creases are much easier to cleanse and rinse in a tub bath. After the bath, the nurse wraps the infant completely in a towel and gently pats the infant dry, paying special attention to body creases. Application of body lotion to dry, cracked areas of the skin is soothing and provides important tactile stimulation.

Evaluation

During and at the completion of the client's bathing and skin care, the nurse evaluates the success of the interventions. The process is dynamic because the client's condition may change. The nurse must prepare to change the plan if outcomes are not met. For example, if the client's skin remains reddened over the sacrum, more frequent turning may be necessary. For each goal established in the care plan, the nurse evaluates the accomplishment of expected outcomes. Evaluation involves physical assessment measures, as well as questions that measure the client's knowledge of hygiene techniques (see the evaluation box above).

■ CARE OF THE FEET AND NAILS

The feet and nails often require special attention to prevent infection, odors, and injury to tissues. Care can be incorporated during bathing or at a separate time. Often, people are unaware of foot or nail problems until pain or discomfort occurs. Problems result from abuse or poor care of the feet and hands such as biting nails or trimming them improperly, exposure to harsh chemicals, and wearing poorly fitted shoes. Discomfort can lead to physical and emotional stress.

The feet are important to physical and emotional health. Foot pain can cause a person to walk differently, causing strain on different muscle groups. Many people must walk or stand comfortably to perform their jobs effectively.

■ NURSING PROCESS AND FOOT CARE

Assessment

PHYSICAL ASSESSMENT

Assessment of the feet involves a thorough examination of all skin surfaces; the shape, size, and number of toes; the shape of the foot; and the condition of the toenails. The nurse inspects the feet for lesions and notes whether areas of dryness, inflammation, or cracking are present. The areas between the toes should be checked carefully. The heels, soles, and sides of the feet are prone to irritation from poorly fitting shoes. The toes are normally straight and flat. The feet should be in straight alignment with the ankle and tibia. Table 40-3 reviews common types of foot and nail problems.

The nurse assesses the client's gait. Painful foot disorders can cause limping or an unnatural gait. The nurse asks whether the client has discomfort of the feet and determines factors that aggravate the pain. Foot problems may result from bone or muscular alterations rather than skin disorders.

Clients with peripheral vascular disease, such as those with diabetes, should be assessed for the adequacy of circulation to the feet. Chapter 33 describes the signs of arterial and venous insufficiency. Palpation of the dorsalis pedis and posterior tibial pulses indicates whether adequate blood flow is reaching peripheral tissues. Edema and

Table 40-3 — Common Foot and Nail Problems

CHARACTERISTICS	IMPLICATIONS	INTERVENTIONS
CALLUS Thickened portion of epidermis consists of mass of horny, keratotic cells. Callus is usually flat, painless, and found on undersurface of foot or on palm of hand. Problem is caused by local friction or pressure.	Condition may cause discomfort when wearing tight shoes.	Nurse advises client to wear gloves when using tools or objects that may create friction on palmar surfaces. Nurse encourages client to wear comfortable shoes. Nurse soaks callus in warm water and Epsom salts to soften cell layers. Applications of creams or lotions can reduce reformation. Encourage client to see podiatrist
CORNS Keratosis is caused by friction and pressure from shoes. It is seen mainly on toes, over bony prominence. Corn is usually cone shaped, round, and raised.	Conical shape compresses underlying dermis, making it thin and tender. Pain is aggravated when tight shoes are worn. Tissue can become attached to bone if allowed to grow. Client may suffer alteration in gait resulting from pain.	Surgical removal may be necessary, depending on severity of pain and size of corn. Nurse avoid use of oval corn pads, which increase pressure on toes and reduce circulation.
PLANTAR WARTS Fungating lesion appears on sole of foot and is caused by papilloma virus.	Warts may be contagious. They are painful and make walking difficult.	Treatment ordered by physician may include applications of salicyclic acid, electrodesiccation (burning with electrical spark), or freezing with solid carbon dioxide.
ATHLETE'S FOOT (TINEA PEDIS) Athlete's foot is fungal infection of foot; scaliness and cracking of skin occurs between toes and on soles of feet. Small blister containing fluid may appear. Problem is apparently induced by wearing of constricting footwear.	Athlete's foot can spread to other body parts, especially hands. It is contagious and frequently recurs.	Feet should be well ventilated. Drying feet well after bathing and applying powder help prevent infection. Wearing of clean socks or stockings reduces incidence. Physician may order application of griseofulvin, miconazole, or tolnaftate.
INGROWN NAILS Toenail or fingernail grows inward into soft tissue around nail. Ingrown nail often results from improper nail trimming.	Ingrown nails can cause localized pain when pressure is applied.	Treatment is frequent hot soaks in antiseptic solution and removal of portion of nail that has grown into skin. Instruct client on proper nail-trimming techniques and refer to podiatrist
RAM'S HORN NAILS Ram's horn nails are usually long curved nails.	Attempt by nurse to cut nails may result in damage to nail bed with risk of infection.	Nurse refers client to podiatrist.
PARONYCHIA Inflammation of tissue surrounding nail occurs after hangnail or other injury. It occurs in people who frequently have their hands in water and is common in diabetic clients.	Area can become infected.	Treatment is hot compresses or soaks and local application of antibiotic ointments. Paronychia can be prevented by careful manicuring.
FOOT ODORS Foot odors are result of excess perspiration promoting microorganism growth.	Condition may cause discomfort because of excess perspiration.	Frequent washing, use of foot deodorants and powders, and wearing clean footwear prevent or reduce problem.

changes in skin color, texture, and temperature can indicate that the client is in need of special hygienic care.

If a client is also diabetic, the nurse should check for **neuropathy**, which is a degeneration of the peripheral nerves characterized by a loss of sensation. This is done by checking the client's sensation to light touch, pin prick, and temperature (see Chapter 33). The nails of the feet and hands are assessed using inspection and palpation.

A normal, healthy nail is transparent, smooth, and convex with pink nail beds and translucent white tips. In African Americans, a brown or black pigmentation is normally present between the nail and nail base. In older adults, the nail may be thickened and yellow. The nail is surrounded by a cuticle, which slowly grows over the nail and must be regularly pushed back. The skin around the nail beds and cuticles should be smooth and without inflammation. The nurse should ask women whether they frequently polish their nails and use polish remover because chemicals in these products may cause excessive nail dryness. Disease can change the shape and curvature of nails (see Chapter 33). Inflammatory lesions of the nail bed cause the formation of thickened, horny nails, which can separate from the nail bed.

DEVELOPMENTAL FACTORS

The nurse's assessment considers the special needs of older adults, who are often unable to maintain proper foot and nail care. Noting the presence of poor vision, hand tremors, obesity, or the inability to bend over reveals the level of assistance required by the older client. If foot or nail problems stay unresolved, an older adult can easily become disabled. The nurse also assesses common problems of older adulthood. Changes occur with years of continuous stress and the degenerative diseases that accompany older adulthood. A thorough nursing assessment should integrate these changes with the symptoms of chronic diseases and treatable conditions.

Older adults often have dry feet because of a decrease in sebaceous gland secretion, dehydration of epidermal cells, and poor condition of footwear. Fissures that result in itching commonly develop. Common foot problems of the older adult include heel pain; metatarsalgia (pain beneath the metatarsal head); hammer toes and claw toes (flexion contractures); bunions, corns, and calluses; arthritis; loss of sensation; and pathological nail conditions (Osterman, Stuck, 1990). Fungal infections commonly occur under toenails, causing dirty yellow streaks or total discoloration. The nails can also become opaque, scaly, and hypertrophied.

If an older client has chronic foot problems, the nurse should assess the type of home remedies used. Many over-the-counter preparations, such as those used to treat corns, can damage normal skin layers. Burns or ulcerations resulting from these products increase the risk of infection.

FOOTWEAR

The types of footwear worn can predispose clients to foot and nail problems. Children or young adults who frequently fail to wear socks may have excess perspiration that promotes fungal growth. Tight or poorly fitting shoes, socks, garters, or knee-high nylon stockings may cause certain skin lesions and interfere with circulation in the feet. The nurse also assesses whether clients wear clean footwear daily because repeated use of soiled footwear can lead to infection. If the client has a health problem such as diabetes, it is extremely important that correct footwear be worn. Extra-wide and extra-depth shoes will accommodate bunions or claw toes. Cushioned inner soles help redistribute pressure on the metatarsal heads. Rocker bottom shoes help with ambulation (Young, Young, 1994).

KNOWLEDGE OF FOOT AND NAIL CARE PRACTICES

The nurse determines clients' knowledge about foot and nail care to assess educational needs. The nurse observes whether clients know how to cut nails or use over-the-counter products for nail care and grooming. It is especially important to assess the knowledge of diabetic clients because they must inspect their feet daily. If the client is unable to visualize the whole foot, someone else should perform this task daily. Because of vascular insufficiency and neuropathy, a diabetic is at risk for injury to the feet. Trauma to a diabetic's foot can easily lead to infection.

 ## Nursing Diagnosis

An assessment of the condition of a client's feet and nails reveals defining characteristics for the presence of actual or potential health problems (see the nursing diagnoses box below). The related factor causing a client's health problem (e.g., reduced circulation or poor hygiene practices) directs the nurse to perform supportive or preventive nursing care. Accurate identification of related factors ensures the nurse will select appropriate nursing interventions.

 ## Planning

The nurse may provide foot and nail care during the bed bath or at a separate time in the day, according to the client's preference. Many community home health nurses visit clients at home solely to provide foot and nail care.

If a client's nails are extremely hard or if a client is unable to perform personal nail care, a podiatrist can provide nail care. The podiatrist is trained in the treatment of nail and foot problems. Goals for clients receiving nail and foot care include the following:

1. Client will have smooth and intact skin and nail surfaces.
2. Client will achieve sense of comfort and cleanliness.

 ## Examples of NANDA Nursing Diagnoses for Foot and Nail Problems

Pain *related to:*
- Callus formation
- Ingrown toenails

Impaired physical mobility *related to:*
- Painful foot lesion

Bathing/hygiene self-care deficit *related to:*
- Visual disturbance
- Altered hand coordination

Impaired skin integrity *related to:*
- Impaired arterial perfusion
- Improper nail-cutting practices
- Friction of shoes
- Injury to nails

Risk for impaired skin integrity *related to:*
- Impaired arterial perfusion
- Poorly fitting footwear

Risk for infection *related to:*
- Broken or traumatized skin

Knowledge deficit about foot and nail care *related to:*
- Information misinterpretation
- Lack of exposure to information

Nail and Foot Care

STEPS	RATIONALE

1. Identify clients at risk for foot or nail problems, including the following:
   a. Older adults

      Changes in sensory and motor function with aging can impair self-care practices. Physiological changes of older adulthood alter condition of foot and nails.

   b. Clients with diabetes

      Vascular changes associated with diabetes can reduce blood flow to peripheral tissues.

   c. Clients with heart failure or renal disease

      These conditions can cause tissue edema and reduced blood flow to extremities.

   d. Clients who have had cerebrovascular accident (stroke).

      Residual paralysis or reduced sensation can cause abnormal walking patterns resulting in friction and pressure on feet.

2. Obtain physician's order for cutting nails if agency policy requires it.

   Client's skin may be accidentally cut. Certain clients are more at risk for infection, depending on medical condition.

3. Explain procedure to client, including fact that proper soaking requires several minutes.

   Client must be willing to place fingers and feet in basins for 10 to 20 min. Client may become anxious or fatigued.

4. Prepare necessary equipment and supplies:
   a. Washbasin   g. Emery board
   b. Emesis basin   h. Body lotion
   c. Washcloth   i. Disposable bath mat
   d. Bath or face towel   j. Paper towels
   e. Nail clippers   k. Disposable gloves
   f. Orange stick   (optional)

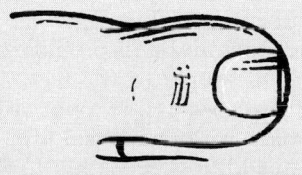

Step 15

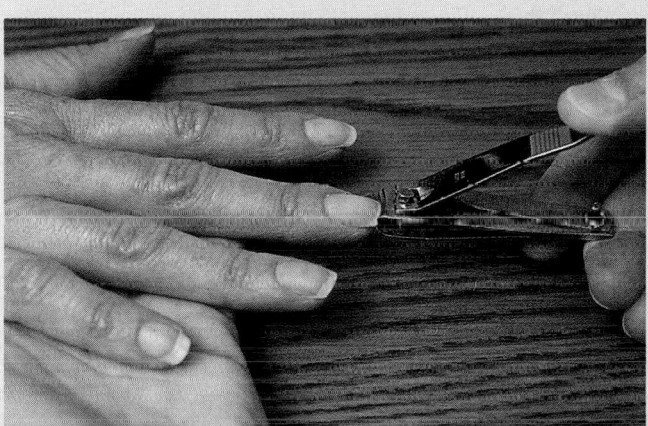

5. Wash hands. Arrange equipment on overbed table.

   Prevents delays. Reduces transmission of infection.

6. Pull curtain around bed or close room door (if desired).

   Maintaining client's privacy reduces anxiety.

7. Assist client to bedside chair if possible. Place disposable bath mat on floor under client's feet. Place call light within client's reach.

   Sitting in chair makes it easier to immerse feet in basin. Bath mat protects feet from exposure to soil or debris. Call light maintains safety of environment.

8. Fill wash basin with warm water. Test temperature of water.

   Warm water softens nails and thickened epidermal cells, reduces inflammation of skin, and promotes local circulation. Proper water temperature prevents burns of skin.

9. Place basin on bath mat and help client place feet in basin.

   Clients with muscular weakness or tremors may have difficulty positioning feet.

10. Adjust overbed table to low position and place it over client's lap.

    Easy access prevents accidental spills.

11. Fill emesis basin with warm water and place basin on paper towels on overbed table.

    Warm water softens nails and thickened epidermal cells.

12. Instruct client to place fingers in emesis basin and place client's arms in comfortable position.

    Prolonged positioning can cause discomfort unless normal anatomical alignment is maintained.

13. Allow client's feet and fingernails to soak 10 to 20 min. Rewarm water in 10 min if needed.

    Softening of corns, calluses, and cuticles ensures easy removal of dead cells and easy manipulation of cuticle.

14. Clean gently under fingernails with orange stick while fingers are immersed. Then remove emesis basin and dry fingers thoroughly.

    Orange stick removes debris under nails that harbors microorganisms. Thorough drying impedes fungal growth and prevents maceration of tissues.

15. With nail clippers, clip fingernails straight across and even with tops of fingers (see the illustrations above). Shape nails with emery board.

    Cutting straight across prevents splitting of nail margins and formation of sharp nail spikes that can irritate lateral nail margins. Filing prevents cutting nail too close to nail bed.

Continued.

Nail and Foot Care—cont'd

STEPS	RATIONALE
16. Push cuticle back gently with orange stick.	Reduces incidence of inflamed cuticles.
17. Move overbed table away from client.	Provide easier access to feet.
18. Apply disposable gloves and scrub calloused areas of feet with washcloth.	Prevents transmission of fungal infection. Friction removes dead skin layers.
19. Clean gently under nails with orange stick. Remove feet from basin and dry them thoroughly.	Reduces chances of infection.
20. Clean and trim toenails using procedures in Steps 15-16.	
21. Apply lotion to feet and hands and then assist client back to bed and into comfortable position.	Lubricates dry skin by helping retain moisture.
22. Remove disposable gloves and dispose in receptacle. Clean and return equipment and supplies to proper place. Dispose of soiled linen in hamper. Wash hands.	Prevents transmission of infection.
23. Inspect nails and surrounding skin after soaking and nail trimming.	Evaluates condition of skin and allows you to note any rough nail edges remaining.
24. Record procedure and observations. Report any breaks in skin.	Documents procedure and response. Abnormalities may pose risk of infection.

3. Client will walk and bear weight normally.
4. Client will understand and perform methods for foot and nail care correctly.

 ## Implementation

Foot and nail care involves soaking to soften cuticles and layers of horny cells, thorough cleansing, drying, and proper nail trimming. The nurse may provide the care in bed for an immobilized client or have the client sit in a chair (Procedure 40-4). The nurse must take time during the procedure to teach the client and family proper techniques for cleansing and nail trimming and provide tips on selecting proper footwear. By allowing the client to perform a part of foot and nail care, the nurse can stress principles related to promoting good circulation and preventing infection and tissue injury.

A diabetic client or one with peripheral vascular disease is at risk for foot and nail problems as a result of poor peripheral blood supply to the feet. Although ongoing foot care can help prevent toe amputation, studies show that many clients have not learned proper care (Christensen et al, 1991). In addition, sensation in the feet can be reduced. The nurse should observe for changes that would indicate peripheral neuropathy or vascular insufficiency (see the box at left).

Trauma to a diabetic's foot can often go unnoticed. With a break in the skin, infection can easily develop as a result of poor circulation. The nurse can advise these clients to use the following guidelines:

1. Inspect the feet daily, including the tops and soles of the feet, the heels, and the area between the toes. Use a mirror to help inspect the feet thoroughly, or ask a family member to check daily.
2. Wash and soak the feet daily using lukewarm water at no more than 37°C or 98.6°F. Have clients alone at home use a thermometer to measure the temperature of the water because their skin sensation may be impaired. Thoroughly pat the feet dry, and dry well between the toes. Apply a thin layer of moisturizer.
3. Do not cut corns or calluses or use commercial removers. Consult a physician or **podiatrist**. Apply moleskin to areas of the feet that are under friction. Wrap *small* pieces of lamb's wool around toes.
4. If the feet perspire, apply a bland foot powder. Wear shoes with porous uppers.
5. If dryness is noted along the feet or between the toes, apply lanolin, baby oil, or even corn oil and rub gently into the skin. Do not oversaturate.

Objective Signs of Peripheral Neuropathy or Vascular Disease

PERIPHERAL NEUROPATHY
Muscle wasting of lower extremities
Absence of deep tendon reflexes
Foot deformities
Abnormal gait
Decreased or absent vibratory sensation

VASCULAR INSUFFICIENCY
Decreased hair growth on legs and feet
Absent or decreased pulses
Infection in the foot
Shiny appearance of the skin
Blanching of the skin on elevation

From Harley JR: Preventing diabetic foot disease, *Nurs Pract* 18(10):37, 1993.

6. File the toenails straight across and square; do not use scissors or clippers. Consult a podiatrist as needed.
7. Do not use over-the-counter preparations to treat athlete's foot or ingrown toenails. Consult a physician or podiatrist.
8. Avoid wearing elastic stockings, knee-high hosiery, or constricting garters. Do not cross the legs. These impair circulation to the lower extremities.
9. Wear clean socks or stockings daily. Change socks twice a day if feet perspire heavily. Socks should be free of holes or darns that might cause pressure.
10. Do not walk barefoot.
11. Wear properly fitted shoes. The soles of the shoes should be flexible and nonslipping. Lamb's wool can be used between toes that rub or overlap. Shoes should be sturdy, closed in, and not restrictive to the feet. If a client has reduced sensation, check the inside of shoes daily for pebbles, foreign objects, or roughness.
12. Extra-deep and extra-wide shoes will accommodate deformed toes, and cushioned insoles will redistribute the pressure of prominent metatarsal heads (Young, Young, 1994).
13. Do not wear new shoes for an extended time. Wear them for short periods over several days to break them in.
14. Exercise regularly to improve circulation to the lower extremities. Walk slowly and elevate, rotate, flex, and extend the feet at the ankles. Dangle the feet over the side of the bed 1 min, and then extend both legs and hold them parallel to the bed while lying supine for 1 min, and, finally, rest 1 min (Jordan, Nickerson, 1982).
15. Do not apply hot water bottles or heating pads to the feet. Use warm soaks or extra coverings instead.
16. Immediately wash minor cuts and dry them thoroughly. Only mild antiseptics (e.g., Neosporin ointment) should be applied to the skin. Avoid iodine or Mercurochrome. Contact a physician to treat slow healing cuts or lacerations.

HEALTH PROMOTION

Clients, especially those with diabetes, need instruction on proper foot care (see the box above, right). Many complications can be avoided if clients are motivated to carry out proper foot and nail care as part of their daily hygiene.

To help clients follow guidelines for foot and nail care, it would be beneficial to include significant others in the teaching sessions, especially if the client is an older adult. Handouts outlining how to buy new shoes can be a simple yet effective way the nurse can help clients promote their own well-being. Proper care of the feet may help keep adults active, thereby allowing clients to participate in other health promoting activities.

 Evaluation

A client's response to nail and foot care is best evaluated over several days or weeks. If the client has any existing problems, it may take time for the alterations to improve. Evaluation based on expected outcomes requires the nurse to determine the success of interventions. For example, if

> **RESEARCH HIGHLIGHT**

RESEARCH ABSTRACT

This study investigated the effectiveness of a "hands-on" foot care teaching/learning approach for adults with diabetes. By random assignment, the control group received a lecture presentation on foot care, while the experimental group participated in a hands-on session on foot care in addition to the lecture presentation. Data concerning the subjects, including foot care knowledge and skills, the condition of their feet, and their level of HbAie, were gathered before and 6 months after foot care educational sessions.

No significant increases in knowledge about foot care were observed in the experimental group. The experimental group reported improvements in inspecting and washing their feet on a daily basis, and in care of the toenails. No significant differences were observed in the status of the subjects' feet over time. The HbAie readings were significantly improved for both the experimental and control groups.

IMPLICATIONS FOR PRACTICE

▶ At each visit, nurses must reinforce the materials taught to the client with diabetes to encourage continued self-care practices.

▶ Hands-on teaching does help clients with diabetes involve themselves with self-care foot activities, but it may be only temporary. Therefore teaching must be done on an ongoing basis.

▶ Long-term effects of self-care foot care must be studied and results documented.

REFERENCE

Kruger S, Guthrie D: Foot care: knowledge retention and self-care practices, *Diabetes Educ* 18:6, 1992

the client continues to have discomfort while walking, a different style of footwear may be needed. The nurse also instructs the client on ways to evaluate personal nail and foot care practices.

■ ORAL HYGIENE

The oral cavity is lined with mucous membrane continuous with the skin. The membrane is an epithelial tissue that lines and protects organs, secretes mucus to keep passageways of the digestive system moist and lubricated, and absorbs nutrients.

The oral, or **buccal**, cavity consists of the lips surrounding the opening of the mouth, the cheeks running along the side walls of the cavity, the tongue and its muscles, and the hard and soft palate forming the roof of the cavity. The oral mucosa is normally light pink and moist. The teeth are for chewing, or **mastication**. A normal tooth consists of three parts: crown, neck, and root (Fig. 40-2). The periodontal membrane lies just below the gum margins, surrounds a tooth, and holds it firmly in place. Healthy teeth appear white, smooth, shiny, and properly aligned.

Oral hygiene helps maintain the healthy state of the mouth, teeth, gums, and lips. Brushing cleanses the teeth of food particles, plaque, and bacteria; massages the gums; and relieves discomfort resulting from unpleasant odors

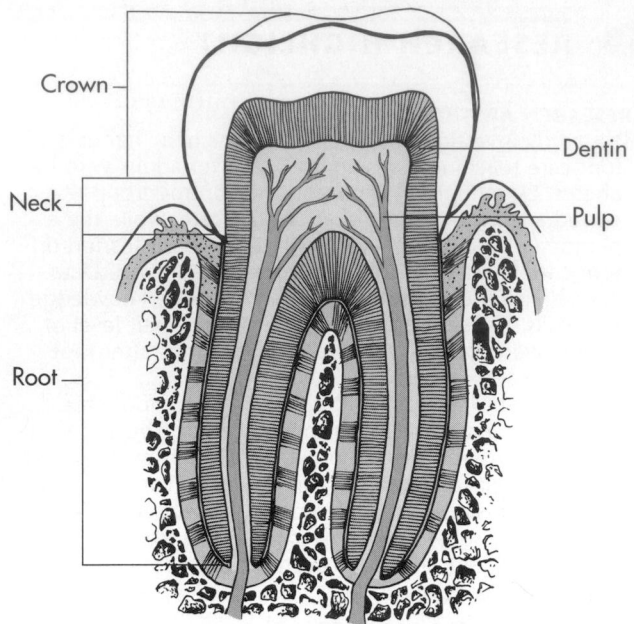

Fig. 40-2 A normal tooth.

and tastes. Flossing further helps remove plaque and tartar from between teeth to reduce gum inflammation and infection. Complete oral hygiene gives a sense of well-being and thus can stimulate appetite.

The nurse's responsibilities in oral hygiene are maintenance and prevention. This is of special importance if the client is going to receive radiation or chemotherapy as part of his or her medical regimen. The nurse can help clients maintain good oral hygiene by teaching them correct techniques or by actually performing hygiene for weakened or disabled clients. Often the nurse must make referrals to a dentist for problems requiring special care. Education about common gum and tooth disorders and methods of prevention can motivate clients to follow good oral hygiene practices.

Health Promotion for Teeth

The *Healthy People 2000* (see Chapter 3) hopes to improve the dental health of the population. The goals are to decrease tooth loss caused by tooth decay or periodontal disease for people ages 35 to 44; reduce the number of elderly who have lost their natural teeth; reduce the prevalence of gingivitis; and reduce destructive periodontal disease among individuals aged 35 to 44 (*Healthy People 2000*). Much work is needed, particularly in rural settings, to educate people as to the importance of dental health and overall well being.

■ NURSING PROCESS AND ORAL HYGIENE

 Assessment

PHYSICAL ASSESSMENT

Chapter 33 describes in detail the nurse's assessment of the client's lips, teeth, buccal mucosa, gums, palate, and tongue. The nurse inspects all of these areas carefully for color, hydration, texture, and lesions. Clients who do not follow regular oral hygiene practices may have receding gum tissue, inflamed gums, discolored teeth (particularly along gum margins), dental caries, missing teeth, and halitosis. Localized pain is a common symptom of a gum disease and certain tooth disorders. An infection of the mouth may involve organisms such as *Treponema pallidum, Neisseria gonorrhoeae,* and herpes virus hominis. As mentioned earlier, if the client is going to have radiation or chemotherapy, it is extremely important to gather baseline data concerning the state of the client's oral cavity. This serves as a basis for preventive care for clients as they are going through treatment (Greifzu,Radjeski, Winnick, 1990).

DEVELOPMENTAL CHANGES

Throughout a person's life span, physiological changes affect the condition and appearance of structures in the oral cavity (Table 40-4). The child may develop dental caries in the deciduous teeth because of eating patterns or lack of dental care. The adolescent's teeth are permanent and require regular attention to diet and dental care to prevent problems in later years. As a person grows older, oral hygiene practices change to further influence the teeth and mucosa. Age-related changes in the mouth, combined with chronic disease, physical disabilities, and prescribed medications that have side effects in the mouth, can result in poor oral care. Effects of inadequate care include dental caries and loss; periodontal disease; onset of systemic infections; and long-term effects on self-esteem, the ability to eat, and the maintenance of relationships (Danielson, 1988). Assessment of a client's developmental level helps in determining the types of hygienic problems to expect.

EATING PATTERNS

It is important to assess a client's current eating pattern to detect the presence of local irritation to gum or mucosal structures. Ask a client if any problems are noted with chewing, denture fit, or swallowing. The presence of an ulcer or irritation may impair chewing and cause a client to avoid eating. This is not uncommon in an older client with poorly fitting dentures.

HYGIENIC PREFERENCES AND PRACTICES

Because of the significant increase in the numbers of older adults and minorities, dental practice is facing new challenges. Data show a pattern of untreated dental caries in African Americans and Mexican Americans and a prevalence of gingivitis in Spanish Americans (Ismail, Szpunar, 1990). Therefore it is important that the nurse assess the client's oral hygiene practices to identify errors in technique, deficiencies in types of practices, and the client's knowledge level about dental care. Helpful questions include the following:

1. How often does the client brush the teeth?
2. What type of toothpaste or dentifrice is used?
3. Does the client have dentures? When and how are they cleansed?
4. Does the client use mouthwash or lemon-glycerin preparations?
5. Does the client floss? If so, how often?
6. When was the client's last dental visit? What were the results?

7. Has the client had dental sealants applied to teeth?
8. How often does the client visit a dentist?
9. Is the water the client drinks fluoridated?

Asking clients to demonstrate brushing and flossing techniques is useful when developing a teaching plan.

RISK FACTORS FOR ORAL HYGIENE PROBLEMS

Certain clients are at risk for oral problems because of a lack of knowledge about oral hygiene, an inability to perform oral care, or an alteration in the integrity of teeth and mucosa resulting from disease or treatments (Table 40-5).

Table 40-4	Physiological Development of the Mouth
DEVELOPMENTAL LEVEL	**CHANGES**
Infant	Deciduous teeth begin to erupt at about 5 mo of age. Solid food can be taken in mouth at 5-6 mo. Chewing begins by 6-8 mo.
18 mo-6 yr	Twenty deciduous teeth are present. By age 2, child can begin to brush teeth and learn hygienic practices from parents. Dental caries may become problem if dental hygiene is neglected. By age 6, "baby" teeth begin to fall out and are replaced by permanent teeth.
6-12 yr	Deciduous teeth are replaced by permanent teeth. Permanent teeth are present by age 12 except second and third molars. Definite food preferences become apparent. Dental caries and irregularity in spacing of teeth are significant health problems.
12-18 yr	All permanent teeth are present. Dental hygienic practices tend to improve because of increased awareness of body image.
18-40 yr	Third molars appear. Good oral hygiene and nutrition practices are needed to avoid problems in later years.
Pregnancy	Changes in female sex hormones may exaggerate reaction to irritants in dental plaque, causing gingivitis and increased risk of severe periodontal disease.*
40-65 yr	Although loss of teeth, usually a result of periodontal disease, is declining, about half of people over age 55 have lost some or all of their teeth because of poor oral care. Root caries and oral cancer occur with higher frequency.
65 yr and over	Aging teeth become brittle, drier, and darker in color. Teeth become uneven, jagged, and fractured after years of crushing and grinding. Gums lose vascularity and tissue elasticity, causing dentures to fit poorly. Eating habits often change, and malnutrition may be a problem. Diminished taste sensitivity, thinning of mucosa, and decreased mass and strength of muscles of mastication also occur.

*Data from de Liefde B, Ritchie GR: Evaluation in dental public health in New Zealand, *N Z Dent J* 80:8, 1984.

Table 40-5	Risk Factors for Oral Problems
TYPE OF CLIENT	**RISK FACTORS**
Clients who are paralyzed, seriously ill, or have physical restrictions to upper extremities (e.g., cast or dressing)	Client lacks upper extremity strength or dexterity needed to perform oral hygiene (Phipps, 1995).
Unconscious, confused, combative, or depressed clients	Client is unable or unwilling to attend to personal hygiene needs.
Diabetic clients	Client is prone to dryness of mouth, gingivitis, periodontal disease, and loss of teeth (Phipps, 1995).
Clients who cannot take anything by mouth or are on fluid restrictions, have nasogastric tubes, receive continuous nasal oxygen, or are mouth-breathers.	Client is prone to dehydration and drying of mucous membranes. Thick secretions develop on tongue and gums. Lips become cracked and reddened.
Clients undergoing radiation therapy	Radiation therapy causes soreness, mild erythema, swollen mucosa, dysphagia, dryness, taste changes, and possible oral infection.
Clients receiving chemotherapeutic drugs	Chemotherapeutic drugs cause ulcerations and inflammation of mucosa and possible oral infection.
Clients experiencing oral surgery, trauma to mouth, placement of oral endotracheal tubes or airways	Tissues in oral cavity become traumatized with swelling, ulcerations, inflammation, and possible bleeding.
Clients with immunosuppression (e.g., HIV, organ transplantation)	Immunosuppression and immunosuppressant drugs may increase risk for oral infection

COMMON ORAL PROBLEMS

It helps a nurse to be familiar with common oral problems. Each problem presents recognizable signs and symptoms and influences the type of hygiene care and teaching provided.

The two major types of problems are dental caries (cavities) and periodontal disease (**pyorrhea**). Dental caries is the most common oral problem of younger people. The development of cavities is a pathological process that involves the eventual destruction of the tooth enamel through decalcification. Decalcification is a result of an accumulation of mucin, carbohydrates, and lactic acid bacilli in the saliva normally found in the mouth, which forms a coating on the teeth called **plaque**. Plaque is transparent and adheres to the teeth, particularly near the base of the crown at the gum margins. The plaque prevents normal acid dilution and neutralization, preventing the dissolution of bacteria in the oral cavity. The acid eventually destroys the tooth enamel and, in severe cases, the pulp, or inner spongy tissue of the tooth. A cavity first begins as a chalky white discoloration of the tooth. As the cavity advances, the tooth takes on a brown or black discoloration.

For people over 35 years of age, the most common problem is pyorrhea. **Periodontal disease** is the disease of the tissues around a tooth, such as an inflammation of the periodontal membrane or periodontal ligament (Mosby, 1994). It is estimated that 25% to 75% of the adult population with natural teeth have some evidence of this disease (Coleman, Nelson, 1993). The progression of the disease involves the following: (1) a calculus deposit on teeth at the gum line; (2) gingivae become swollen and tender; (3) inflammation spreads, pockets develop between gums and gingivae, and gums recede; (4) alveolar bone is destroyed, and teeth loosen (Lewis, Collier, 1996).

Halitosis (bad breath) is a common problem of the oral cavity. It may be the result of poor oral hygiene, the ingestion of certain foods, or an infection or disease process. Proper oral hygiene can eliminate the odors unless the cause is a systemic condition such as liver disease or diabetes.

The nurse frequently encounters **cheilosis** in clients. The disorder involves cracking of the lips, especially at the angle of the mouth. Riboflavin deficiency, mouth breathing, and excess salivation may cause cheilosis. Lubrication of the lips helps retain moisture, and antifungal or antibacterial ointments discourage microorganism growth.

Symptoms of periodontal disease include bleeding gums; swollen, inflamed tissues; receding gumlines, with the formation of gaps or pockets between the teeth and gums, and the eventual loss of teeth. If proper oral care is not maintained, dead bacteria, called *tartar*, can collect along the gumline. The tartar attacks the gums and fibers attached to the teeth, resulting in the loss of teeth. The best preventive measures are regular flossing and brushing.

OTHER ORAL PROBLEMS

Stomatitis is an inflammatory condition of the mouth resulting from contact with irritants, such as tobacco; vitamin deficiency; infection by bacteria, viruses, or fungi; or the use of chemotherapeutic drugs. **Glossitis** is an inflammation of the tongue resulting from an infectious disease or injury, such as a burn or bite. **Gingivitis** is an inflammation of the gums, usually resulting from poor oral hy-

Examples of NANDA Nursing Diagnoses for Oral Hygiene Problems

Altered oral mucous membrane *related to:*
- Oral trauma
- Restricted fluid intake
- Ineffective oral hygiene
- Trauma associated with chemotherapy or radiation therapy to head and neck

Pain *related to:*
- Gingivitis
- Loose teeth

Altered nutrition: less than body requirements *related to:*
- Ill-fitting dentures
- Gingivitis

Bathing/hygiene self-care deficit (oral) *related to:*
- Altered level of consciousness
- Upper extremity weakness

Body-image disturbance *related to:*
- Halitosis
- Absence of teeth

Knowledge of deficit about oral-hygiene *related to:*
- Misunderstanding of hygienic practices

Risk for infection *related to:*
- Oral mucosa trauma

---

giene or occurring as a sign of leukemia, vitamin deficiency, or diabetes mellitus. Special oral care is a must if the client has any of these oral problems. The associated oral mucosal changes may easily lead to malnutrition, which is a major concern for clients who have cancer (Griefzu, Radjeski, Winnick, 1990).

Oral malignancies appear as lumps or ulcers in or around the mouth. They are commonly found in clients with a history of pipe smoking or who use chewing tobacco. The most common site is at the base of the tongue. Early detection is vital to the success of treatment. Any sore in the mouth that does not heal should be brought to the attention of a dentist.

Nursing Diagnosis

Assessment of the client's oral cavity may reveal actual or potential alterations in the integrity of mouth structures (see the nursing diagnoses box above). Pertinent nursing diagnoses may reflect problems or complications resulting from alterations of the oral cavity. The nurse's findings may also reveal a client's need for assistance with oral care because of a self-care deficit. The identification of an accurate diagnosis requires selection of the related factor causing the client's problem (see the diagnostic process box on p. 1047). Alterations to oral mucosa resulting from radiation exposure, for example, will require different interventions than mucosal damage from endotracheal tube placement.

Planning

Developing a care plan for clients in need of oral hygiene involves considering the client's personal preferences, emotional status, economic resources, and physical capabilities. The nurse must establish a good relationship with the client to assist with oral hygiene practices. Some clients are very sensitive about the condition of their mouths and are reluctant to let someone else care for them. In many cases, clients (such as those with diabetes and cancer) are also unaware that they are at risk for serious dental and periodontal disease and thus require extensive education (see the care plan below). Clients with existing oral mucosa alteration will likely require long-term care. Outcomes may not be met for several days or weeks. The family can play an important role in learning how to examine the client's oral cavity for changes and to provide hygiene. Goals for clients in need of oral hygiene include the following:

1. Client will have intact oral mucosa that is well hydrated.

Sample Nursing Diagnostic Process for Oral Hygiene

ASSESSMENT ACTIVITIES	DEFINING CHARACTERISTICS	NURSING DIAGNOSIS
Inspect condition of oral cavity. Ask if client has pain, burning, irritation. Ask if client has chewing difficulties. Check for proper-fitting dentures. Inspect oral cavity for redness, dryness, lesions, or ulcers and bleeding. Note client's breath for mouth odor. Review medical history (radiation therapy).	Coated tongue Stomatitis Oral or gum lesions Oral pain noted when chewing Decreased salivation Halitosis	**Altered oral mucous membranes** related to radiation of oral cavity

Sample Nursing Care Plan for Altered Oral Mucous Membranes

NURSING DIAGNOSIS: Altered oral mucous membrane related to radiation of oral cavity
DEFINITION: Altered oral mucous membrane is the state in which an individual experiences disruptions in the tissue layers of the oral cavity (Kim, McFarland, and McLane, 1995).

GOALS	EXPECTED OUTCOMES	INTERVENTIONS	RATIONALE
Client will have intact mucosa that is well hydrated at time of discharge.	Mucosa, tongue, and lips will be pink, moist, and intact. Inflammation, crusts, lesions, and hard debris will remain absent. Teeth will be free of food particles. Client will verbalize comfort and feeling of oral cleanliness. Client will swallow and talk without discomfort.	Establish mouth-care regimen after meals and at bedtime: ■ Brush with soft toothbrush using horizontal strokes. ■ Rinse with warm salt or baking soda solution ($^1/_2$ tsp to 1 pt of water). ■ Floss with unwaxed dental floss 2 times a day. Avoid vigorous flossing near gumline.	Consistent brushing improves gingival tissue, removes debris, and results in plaque control (Kahn, 1986). Soft toothbrush with horizontal strokes helps protect delicate gingival tissue and prevent bleeding (Crosby, 1989). Rinsing dilutes oral acids, removes debris; and helps relieve dry mouth (xerostomia) that occurs with therapy-induced drop in saliva production (Greifzu, Radjeski, Winnick, 1990).
Client will independently perform oral hygiene correctly by 9/12.	Oral hygiene techniques will be properly demonstrated.	Have client perform oral hygiene.	Soda and salt solutions promote healing and aid in formation of granulation tissue. They act as astringent and may repress bacterial growth (Pettigrew, 1989). Systematic flossing removes decay-producing bacteria growing on tooth surfaces and near gumline (Kahn, 1986). Using unwaxed floss and avoiding vigorous flossing prevent bleeding (Greifzu, Radjesk, Winnick, 1990).

2. Client will be able to independently perform correct oral-hygiene care.
3. Client will achieve sense of comfort.
4. Client will understand oral-hygiene practices.

 ## Implementation

ORAL HYGIENE

Good oral hygiene involves cleanliness, comfort, and the moisturizing of mouth structures. Proper care prevents oral disease and tooth destruction. Clients in hospitals or long-term care facilities often do not receive the aggressive care they need. Oral care must be provided on a regular and daily basis. The frequency of hygienic measures depends on the condition of the client's oral cavity.

Brushing, flossing, and irrigation are necessary for proper cleansing. Clients also benefit from a proper diet, which excludes foods promoting plaque formation and tooth decay and promotes healthy periodontal structures. Clients of all ages should have a dental checkup at least every 6 months.

DIET

To prevent tooth decay, clients may have to change their eating habits, reducing the intake of carbohydrates, especially sweet snacks between meals. Sweet or starchy food adheres to tooth surfaces. After eating sweets, a client should brush within 30 minutes to reduce the action of plaque. Eating acid-containing fruits (e.g., apples and fibrous foods such as fresh vegetables) also reduces plaque. The acidic quality of fruits eliminates bacteria that form on teeth. A well-balanced diet ensures the integrity of oral tissues.

For pregnant women, appropriate nutrients are essential for the development of primary teeth in the fetus. The recommended amount of daily calcium intake is 1200 mg for the pregnant adult and 1600 mg for the pregnant adolescent (Marshall, 1991). Four to six cups of milk a day meet the calcium requirement.

BRUSHING

Thorough brushing of the teeth at least four times a day (after meals and at bedtime) is basic to an effective oral hygiene program. A toothbrush should have a straight handle, and a brush should be small enough to reach all areas of the mouth. Toothbrushes should be replaced every 3 months. An older adult with reduced dexterity and grip may require an enlarged toothbrush handle that provides an easier grip. This can be accomplished by piercing a soft rubber ball and pushing the brush handle through or by gluing a short piece of plastic tubing around the handle. An even, rounded brushing surface with soft, multitufted, nylon bristles is best. Rounded soft bristles stimulate the gums without causing abrasion and bleeding. All tooth surfaces—inner, outer, and chewing should be brushed thoroughly. Unflavored oral care sponges are used with clients unable to tolerate brushing because of oral trauma or bleeding tendencies.

A fluoride toothpaste is preferred for brushing teeth. Most toothpastes are pleasant tasting. Lemon-glycerin sponges can have harmful effects on teeth and mucosa. Glycerin has an astringent effect, drying and shrinking gums and mucous membranes. The lemon, if used extensively, changes the natural pH of the oral cavity, exhausts

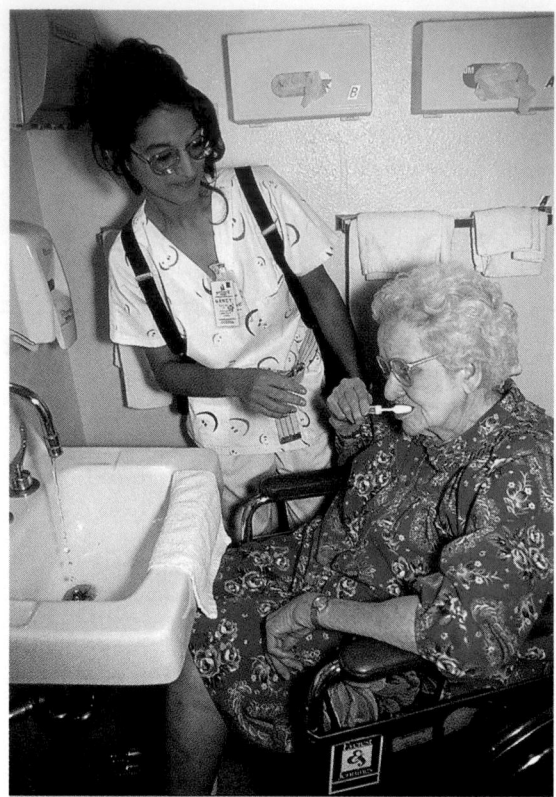

Fig. 40-3 The nurse observes client brushing teeth. During such observations, the nurse can determine how much assistance the client may need.

the salivary reflex through overstimulation and can erode tooth enamel (Pettigrew, 1989). Because swabbing fails to cleanse teeth adequately, plaque accumulates around the base of the teeth. The glycerin provides nourishment for bacteria. A swab containing an aqueous solution of sorbitol, sodium, carboxymethylcellulose, and electrolytes has been shown effective in treating dry mouth. Moi-Stir is a salivary supplement that improves moisture and texture of the tongue and mucous membranes (Poland, 1987).

Whether a brush or sponge is used, thorough rinsing after brushing is important to remove dislodged food particles and excess toothpaste. Some people enjoy using mouthwash for its pleasant taste. Used over a long period, however, mouthwash dries mucosa.

When teaching clients about mouth care, the nurse reminds them not to share toothbrushes at home and not to drink directly from a bottle of mouthwash. Cross-contamination occurs easily. The use of disclosure tablets or drops to stain the plaque that collects at the gumline can be useful for showing clients how effectively they brush.

The amount of assistance needed by the client in brushing the teeth may vary. Many clients can perform their own oral care and should be encouraged to do so. The nurse observes the client to be sure proper techniques are used (Fig. 40-3). Other clients need total assistance with hygiene.

SPECIAL ORAL HYGIENE

Some clients require special oral hygiene methods because of their level of dependence on the nurse or the presence of oral mucosa problems.

Performing Mouth Care for an Unconscious or Debilitated Client

STEPS	RATIONALE
1. Assess for presence of gag reflex. Position client in Sims' or side-lying position with head turned well toward dependent side.	Reveals client's risk for aspiration. Allows secretions to drain from mouth instead of collecting in back of pharynx and prevents aspiration.
2. Explain procedure to client.	Unconscious client may retain ability to hear.
3. Prepare necessary equipment and supplies:	
a. Antiinfective solution	Loosens encrustations and acts as antiinfective.
b. Sponge toothbrush or tongue blade wrapped in single layer of gauze; small toothbrush	Brush clean teeth most effectively. Sponge or swab stimulates and cleans gums and mucosa.
c. Padded tongue blade	Keeps mouth open and teeth separated during procedure without traumatizing oral structures.
d. Face towel	
e. Emesis basin	
f. Paper towels	
g. Water glass with cool water	
h. Water soluble jelly	Lubricates lips.
i. Portable suction machine (optional) with suction catheter	Removes retained oral secretions while oral cavity is cleansed.
j. Disposable gloves	Oral cavity contains highly infectious microorganisms.
4. Wash hands and apply disposable gloves.	Reduces transfer of microorganisms.
5. Place paper towels on overbed table and arrange equipment. Turn on suction machine and connect tubing to suction catheter.	Prevents soiling of table top. Equipment prepared in advance ensures smooth, safe procedure.
6. Pull curtain around bed or close room door.	Provides privacy.
7. Raise bed to highest horizontal level; lower side rail.	Use of good body mechanics with bed in high position prevents injury to you and client.
8. Bring client close to side of bed and near you; be sure client's head is turned toward mattress.	Proper positioning of head prevents aspiration.
9. Place towel under client's face and emesis basin under chin.	Prevents soiling of bed linen.
10. Carefully retract the client's upper and lower teeth with padded tongue blade by inserting blade quickly but gently between the back molars. Insert when client is relaxed, if possible (see the illustration).	Prevents client from biting down on fingers and provides access to oral cavity.

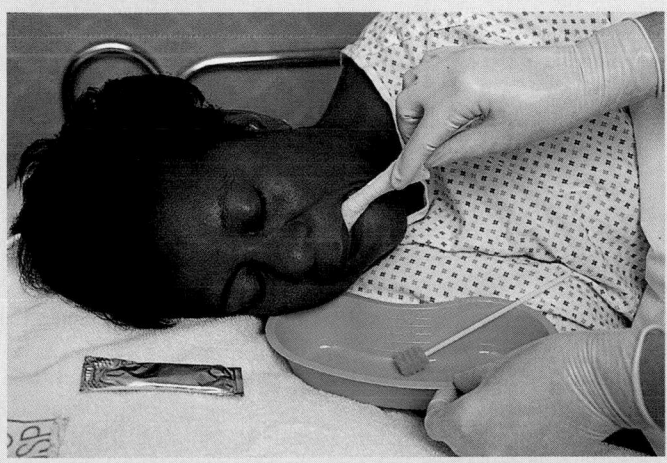

Step 10

Continued.

Performing Mouth Care for an Unconscious or Debilitated Client—cont'd

STEPS	RATIONALE
11. Clean mouth using brush or tongue blade moistened with Antifective and water. Have second nurse suction as secretions accumulate during cleansing. Clean chewing and inner tooth surfaces first (see the illustration below). Clean outer tooth surfaces. Swab roof of mouth and inside cheeks. Gently swab or brush tongue but avoid stimulating gag reflex (if present). Moisten clean swab or toothete with water to rinse. Repeat rinse several times. Suction any remaining secretions.	Brushing action removes food particles between teeth and along chewing surfaces. Swabbing helps remove secretions and encrustations from mucosa and moistens mucosa. Suction removes secretions and fluid that can collect in posterior pharynx. Repeated rinsing removes loose debris and peroxide that can be irritating to mucosa.
12. Apply thin layer of water soluble jelly to lips. (see the illustration below).	Lubricates lips to prevent drying and cracking.
13. Explain that procedure is completed.	Provides meaningful stimulation to unconscious or less responsive client.
14. Remove gloves and dispose in proper receptacle.	Prevents transmission of microorganisms.
15. Reposition client comfortably, raise side rail, and return bed to original position.	Maintains client's comfort and safety.
16. Clean equipment and return to its proper place. Place soiled linen in proper receptacle.	Proper disposal of soiled equipment prevents spread of infection.
17. Wash hands.	Reduces transmission of microorganisms.
18. Inspect oral cavity.	Determines efficacy of cleansing. After thick secretions are removed, underlying inflammation or lesions may be revealed.
19. Record procedure, including pertinent observation (e.g., bleeding gums, dry mucosa, ulcerations, or crusts on tonguge) and report any unusual findings to nurse in charge or physician.	Documents response of client to nursing therapy. Bleeding may indicate more serious systemic problems. Lesions of oral cavity can be cancerous.

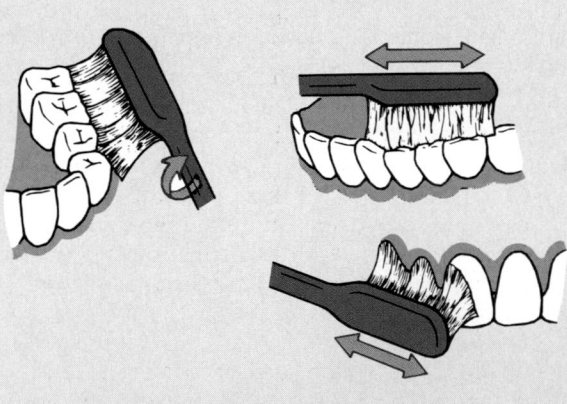

Step 11

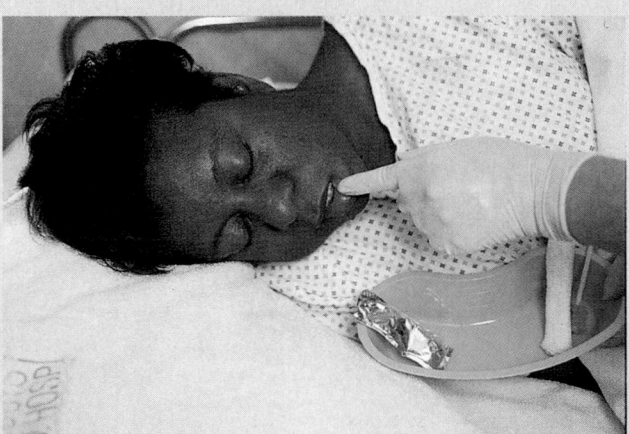

Step 12

Unconscious Clients. These clients are susceptible to drying of mucous-thickened salivary secretions because they are unable to eat or drink, frequently breathe through the mouth, and often receive oxygen therapy. The unconscious client also cannot swallow salivary secretions that accumulate in the mouth. These secretions often contain gram-negative bacteria that can cause pneumonia if aspirated into the lungs. Therefore the nurse must protect the client from choking and aspirating. Regular cleansing and rinsing of the oral cavity is critical (see the box on p. 1051). Procedure 40-5 describes mouth care for debilitated clients.

Clients at Risk for Stomatitis. Chemotherapy, radiation, and nasogastric tube intubation can cause stomatitis. Clients should rinse their mouths before and after each meal using a solution containing ½ to 1 tsp. of salt or baking soda to 1 pt of water (Greifzu, Radjeski, Winnick, 1990). To remove thick mucus, they should use 1 part hydrogen peroxide to four parts normal saline (Greifzu, Radjeski, Winnick, 1990).

► RESEARCH HIGHLIGHT

RESEARCH ABSTRACT

Hydrogen peroxide (H_2O_2) rinses have been advocated for oral hygiene. The results of this study indicated that when 1/4 and 1/2 strength dilutions of H_2O_2 were used, there were abnormal objective and subjective changes in the oral mucosa of healthy individuals. Using H_2O_2 may also alter the microflora of the mouth in a detrimental manner. Therefore it is recommended that hydrogen peroxide *not* be used in the oral care of clients, particularly for clients who may have impaired oral mucosa. Normal saline rinses may be a possible alternative agent because they are not associated with abnormal changes of the oral mucosa. In this study the responses of participants who used the saline rinses were neutral or positive. There should be further investigation using other oral agents such as tap water and solutions of sodium bicarbonate.

IMPLICATIONS FOR PRACTICE
► Based on this research, nurses should be educating their colleagues as to the detrimental effects of using H_2O_2 for oral care.
► Clients with impaired mucous membranes need oral care that will not change the tissues of the oral cavity and will provide comfort, such as normal saline.

REFERENCE
Tombes MB, Gallucci B: The effects of hydrogen peroxide rinses on the normal oral mucosa, *Nurs Res* 42:336, 1993.

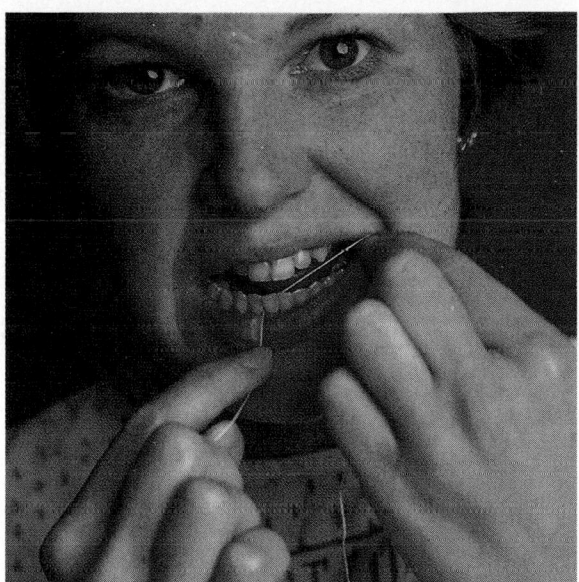

Fig. 40-4 Flossing.

Clients with Diabetes. Visits to the dentist are needed every 3 or 4 months. All tissues should be handled gently with a minimum of trauma. Clients should be taught to follow rigid cleansing schedules. The nurse may need to assist clients who have diabetes because they have an increased occurrence of periodontal disease (Smeltzer, Bare, 1992).

Clients with Oral Infections. The nurse notifies a physician when signs of an infection such as coated ulcerations; a red, dry, swollen tongue; halitosis; or coated tongue develops (Barkauskas, et al, 1994). Liquid topical antibiotics can be applied to mucosal surfaces with a soft sponge or by having clients rinse the oral cavity with the medication. Clients who wear dentures must remove them before using topical antibiotics.

FLUORIDE USE

In most communities the water supply contains fluoride. Rozier and Beck (1991) report a summary of epidemiological studies showing that water fluoridation has played a dominant role in the decline in tooth caries. People who do not have fluoridated water can obtain fluoride in the form of mouthwash, toothpaste, or supplements. Most toothpastes on the market today contain fluoride. Fluoride supplements can be given to children beginning at the age of 2 weeks. Supplements are available without a prescription and can be taken with water, juice, or milk. The family dentist should be consulted concerning the amount of fluoride to be given. Dental sealants can be applied to teeth to further prevent tooth decay.

Excessive fluoridation can result in a discoloration of tooth enamel. Clients should be advised to watch for this condition. Parents should keep fluoride supplements out of the reach of children.

FLOSSING

Dental flossing is necessary for effective removal of plaque and tartar between teeth. Flossing involves insertion of waxed or unwaxed dental floss between all tooth surfaces, one at a time (Mosby, 1994) (Fig. 40-4). The seesaw motion used to pull floss between teeth removes plaque and tartar from tooth enamel. To prevent bleeding, clients receiving chemotherapy or radiation should use unwaxed floss and avoid vigorous flossing near the gumline. If toothpaste is applied to the teeth before flossing, the fluoride can come in direct contact with tooth surfaces, aiding in cavity prevention. Flossing once a day is sufficient. Because it is important to clean all tooth surfaces thoroughly, the nurse should not rush to complete flossing. Placing a mirror in front of the client helps the nurse demonstrate the proper methods for holding the floss and cleansing between the teeth. Flossing is most easily done immediately after brushing.

DENTURE CARE

Clients should be encouraged to clean their own dentures as frequently as natural teeth to prevent gingival infection and irritation (Procedure 40-6). The nurse must assist with denture care if clients become disabled, incapacitated, or confused. Dentures are the client's personal property and should be handled with care because they can be easily broken. Dentures should be removed before going to bed to give the gums a rest and to prevent bacterial buildup and inflamed mucosa. To prevent warping, they should be kept in water when they are not worn. The nurse always stores dentures in an enclosed, labeled cup during soaking or when the dentures are not being worn. The client should be discouraged from wrapping dentures in facial or toilet tissue or placing them on meal trays because the dentures may be accidentally thrown away.

Cleaning Dentures

STEPS	RATIONALE
1. Ask client if dentures are loose fitting and if there is any gum or mucous membrane tenderness or irritation. After dentures are removed, inspect oral cavity and denture surfaces.	Ill-fitting dentures rub against gums and mucous membranes. Area of irritation may require special care.
2. Explain procedure and assure client that individual practice preferences will be used (when appropriate).	Promotes client understanding and cooperation.
3. Prepare necessary equipment and supplies:	
a. Soft-bristled toothbrush	Used to brush gums and tongue.
b. Denture toothbrush	
c. Emesis basin or sink	
d. Denture dentifrice or toothpaste	
e. Water glasses (for warm and cool water)	
f. Single 4 × 4 gauze	Used to remove dentures.
g. Washcloth	
h. Plastic denture cup	
i. Disposable gloves	Prevents contact with microorganisms in saliva.
4. Wash hands.	Reduces transmission of microorganisms.
5. Arrange supplies on bedside table or near sink.	Ensures smooth, organized procedure.
6. Pour emesis basin half full with tepid water or place washcloth in sink and run water until it is approximately 1-in deep.	Aids in distribution of dentifrice over denture surfaces. Cloth protects dentures against breakage. Hot water can cause warping or softening of dentures.
7. Apply disposable gloves.	Reduces transmission of infection.
8. Ask client to remove dentures and place them in emesis basin. If client is unable to remove dentures, grasp upper plate at front with thumb and index finger wrapped in gauze. Use steady, downward pull. Gently lift lower denture from jaw and rotate one side downward to remove from mouth. Place dentures in basin.	Gauze prevents accidental slipping while handling dentures. Rotating denture at angle reduces pulling of lips during removal.

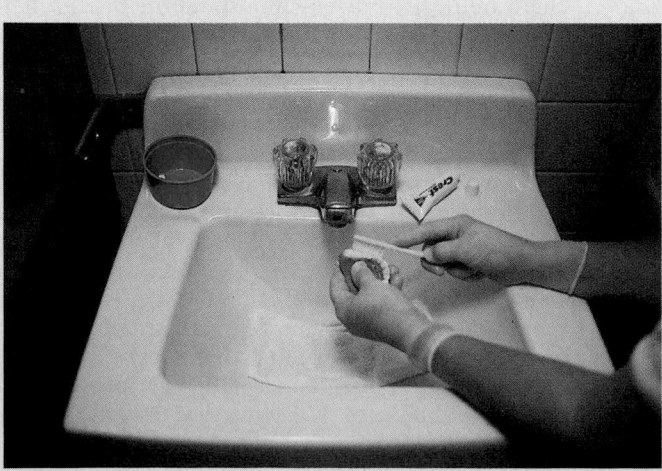

Step 9 *(From Sorrentino SA: Mosby's textbook for nursing assistants, ed 3, St Louis, 1995, Mosby)*

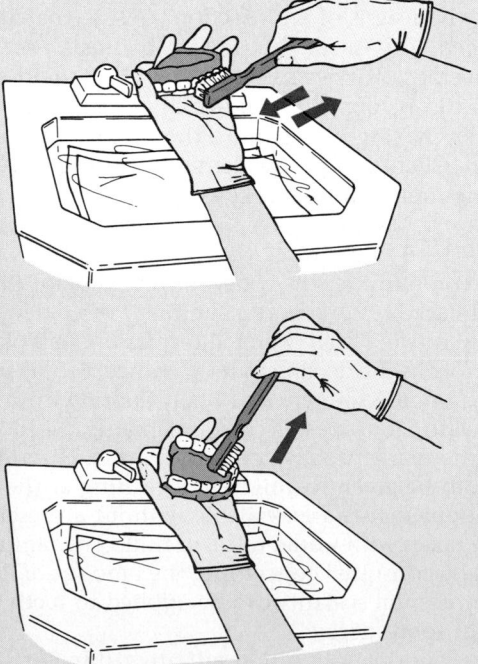

Cleaning Dentures—cont'd

STEPS	RATIONALE
9. Apply dentifrice to denture and brush surfaces of dentures. Hold dentures close to water (see the illustration on p. 1052). Hold brush horizontally and use back-and-forth motion to cleanse biting surfaces (see the illustration on p. 1052). Hold brush horizontally and use short strokes from top of denture to biting surfaces of teeth to clean outer tooth surface. Hold brush vertically and use short strokes to clean inner tooth surfaces (see the illustration on p. 1052). Hold brush horizontally and use back-and-forth motion to clean undersurface of dentures.	Prevents food and bacteria from collecting on denture surfaces and prevents odor and stain buildup. Holding dentures close to water reduces chance of breakage, because water will break fall if dentures slip.
10. Rinse dentures thoroughly in tepid water.	Warm water dilutes and rinses dentifrice more effectively than cool water.
11. Return dentures to client or store in tepid water in denture cup.	Storage protects dentures from breakage. Tepid water keeps dentures well moistened to make eventual insertion easier. Plastic dentures become brittle and warp if not kept moist.
12. Empty emesis basin and add fresh cool water. Apply toothpaste to soft toothbrush, and gently brush gums, palate, and tongue.	Helps stimulate circulation to gums and removes residual film of debris on gums and mucosa.
13. Have client rinse mouth thoroughly.	Rinsing removes all food particles and secretions.
14. Reinsert dentures if client desires, or allow client to do so. Begin by gently inserting moistened upper denture. Have client use finger to press denture firmly in place, then insert moistened lower denture.	Bulkier upper denture easier to insert first when client has both upper and lower plates. Moistening lubricates denture for easier insertion. Applying gentle pressure to upper denture seals it against palate.
15. Dispose of gloves in proper receptacle. Clean and store supplies. Wash hands.	Controls spread of infection.
16. Ask client if dentures feel comfortable.	Cleansing removes sources of irritation.
17. Record procedure on flowsheet or nurses' notes.	Accurate and timely documentation maintains accuracy of client's record.

Evaluation

The expected outcomes of oral hygiene may not be seen for several days. Repeated cleansing is often needed to remove thick encrustations of the tongue and to restore the mucosa's normal hydration. The nurse evaluates the success of interventions to maintain mucosa integrity or to prevent oral mucosal injury. The nurse anticipates the need to change interventions during evaluation. It takes many weeks of rigorous hygiene to reduce the incidence of dental caries. The evaluation box on p. 1054 outlines the evaluation of oral hygiene care.

▌HAIR CARE

A person's appearance and feeling of well-being often depend on the way the hair looks and feels. Illness or disability may prevent a client from maintaining daily hair care. An immobilized client's hair will soon become tangled. Dressings may leave sticky blood or antiseptic solutions on the hair. Brushing, combing, and shampooing are basic hygienic measures for all clients. Clients should also be permitted to shave when their conditions allow it.

Hair growth, distribution, and pattern can be indicators of general health status (see Chapter 33). Hormonal changes, emotional and physical stress, aging, infection, and certain diseases or drugs can affect characteristics of the hair. The hair shaft is an inert structure. Changes in its color or condition occur as a result of hormonal activity and nutrient supply to the follicle. Table 40-6 describes common hair and scalp problems and nursing interventions.

▌NURSING PROCESS AND HAIR CARE

Assessment

PHYSICAL ASSESSMENT

Before performing hair care, the nurse assesses the condition of the hair and scalp (see Chapter 33). Normally the hair is clean, shiny, and untangled, and the scalp is clear of lesions. The hair of black-skinned clients is usually thicker, drier, and curlier than the hair of lighter skinned clients. The loss of hair (**alopecia**) can result from improper hair care practices (Table 40-6) or the use of chemotherapy medications.

DEVELOPMENTAL CHANGES

Throughout life, changes in the growth, distribution, and condition of hair can influence the hygiene that a person requires (Table 40-7).

Sample Evaluation of Interventions for Oral Hygiene Problems

GOALS	EVALUATIVE MEASURES	EXPECTED OUTCOMES
Client will have intact and well hydrated oral mucosa at time of discharge.	Inspect condition of tongue, gums, and lining of cheeks. Observe condition of lips. Inspect tooth surfaces.	Mucosa, tongue, and lips will be moist, pink and intact. Inflammation, crusts, lesions, and hard debris will remain absent. Teeth will be free of food particles and plaque.
Client will independently perform oral-hygiene care correctly by 9/12.	Observe client perform brushing, flossing, and denture care. Ask client to describe oral-hygiene techniques.	Oral-hygiene techniques will be properly demonstrated. Client will correctly describe steps to follow in brushing, flossing, or denture care.

Table 40-6 — Hair and Scalp Problems

CHARACTERISTICS	IMPLICATIONS	INTERVENTIONS
DANDRUFF Scaling of scalp is accompanied by itching. In severe cases, dandruff is found on eyebrows.	Dandruff causes person embarrassment. If dandruff enters eyes, conjunctivis may develop.	Shampoo regularly with medicated shampoo. In severe cases, obtain physician's advice.
TICKS Small, gray-brown parasites burrow into skin and suck blood.	Ticks transmit several diseases to people. Most common are Rocky Mountain spotted fever, tularemia, and Lyme disease.	Do not pull ticks from skin because sucking apparatus remains and may become infected. Suffocate tick by placing a drop of oil or ether on tick or covering it with petrolatum jelly to ease removal.
PEDICULOSIS (LICE) Tiny, grayish-white parasite insects infest mammals.		
PEDICULOSIS CAPITIS (HEAD LICE) Parasite is found on scalp attached to hair strands. Eggs look like oval particles, similar to dandruff. Bites or pustules may be observed behind ears and at hairline.	Head lice are difficult to remove and may spread to furniture and other people if not treated.	Shampoo with Kwell shampoo and repeat 12-24 hr later. Change bed linens. Wash linens in hot water to kill lice
PEDICULOSIS CORPORIS (BODY LICE) Parasites tend to cling to clothing, so they may not be easily seen. Body lice suck blood and lay eggs on clothing and furniture.	Client itches constantly. Scratches seen on skin may become infected. Hemorrhagic spots may appear on skin where lice are sucking blood.	Bathe or shower thoroughly. After skin is dried, apply Kwell lotion. After 12-24 hr, take another bath or shower. Bag infested clothing or linen until laundered in hot water. Vacuum rooms thoroughly and throw away bag after completion
PEDICULOSIS PUBIS (CRAB LICE) Parasites are found in pubic hair. Crab lice are grayish white with red legs.	Lice may spread through bed linen, clothing, or furniture or between persons via sexual contact.	Shave hair off affected area. Cleanse as for body lice. If lice were sexually transmitted, notify partner.
HAIR LOSS (ALOPECIA) Alopecia occurs in all races. Balding patches are seen in periphery of hair line. Hair becomes brittle and broken. Condition is caused by use of hair curlers, hair picks, tight braiding, and use of hot comb.	Patches of uneven hair growth and loss alter client's appearance.	Stop hair-care practices that damage hair.

Table 40-7	Physiological Development of Hair Growth	
AGE	**CONDITION OF HAIR**
Infancy	Infants may have little or no scalp hair at birth. Scalp hair grows by first year. Fine body hair (lanugo) is present on forehead, cheeks, shoulders, and back.
Childhood	Scalp hair is lustrous, silky, strong, and elastic. Hair of black-skinned child is curlier and coarser.
Middle childhood to puberty	Androgenic hormones cause increase in thickening and darkening of scalp hair, growth of hair in axillae and pubic areas in both sexes, and growth of facial hair in boys.
Adolescence	Boys may acquire additional amounts of distribution of body hair, such as on chest. Increase in sebaceous gland activity causes hair to become oily.
Adulthood	Men with genetic tendency develop baldness.
Older adulthood	Axillary and pubic hair diminish in women. Scalp hair becomes thinner and depleted of melanin, causing gray coloring. Older women may develop chin and facial hair because of decreased estrogen production. Men may experience balding or receding hair line.

SELF-CARE ABILITY

The nurse assesses a client's physical ability to care for hair. Painful conditions of the upper extremities such as arthritis, a weakened hand grip, fatigue, and physical encumbrances (e.g., a cast or dressing) are just some of the conditions that impair a client's ability to perform hair care.

HAIR CARE PRACTICES

One way to assess a person's hair care practices is by observing the appearance of the hair. Dull, tangled, dirty hair indicates improper care. Unkempt hair may be the result of lack of interest, depression, or physical inability to care for the hair.

By assessing a client's preferred hairstyle, the nurse can attempt to arrange the client's hair in the same manner. Asking the client to assist or teach the nurse how to style the hair correctly gives the client a greater sense of independence and helps the nurse avoid making a mistake that can damage hair.

The nurse also assesses the type of hair care products a client uses, as well as the time of day when hair care is usually performed. Assessment of shaving products is necessary with all clients.

 Nursing Diagnosis

The problems most likely to be identified by the nurse after assessment of the hair and scalp center on comfort and grooming. If actual lesions or abnormalities involving the scalp are identified, nursing diagnoses focus on the integrity of the scalp (see the nursing diagnoses box at right).

 Planning

Good hair care practices must be done routinely to meet clients' hygienic needs. The nurse must remember that clients remain aware of their appearances at all times. Therefore an effective plan allows clients to initiate and participate in hygienic measures whenever possible. Select-

ing appropriate related factors influences the nurse's care plan. For example, the diagnosis "impaired skin integrity related to parasite infestation" requires action, such as shampooing and isolating bed linens, to remove the infestation. The diagnosis "impaired skin integrity related to scalp laceration" will require measures to promote healing, such as wound care.

Goals for clients in need of hair and scalp care include the following:

1. Client will have clean healthy hair and scalp.
2. Client will achieve a sense of comfort and self-esteem.
3. Client will participate in hair care practices.

 Implementation

BRUSHING AND COMBING

Frequent brushing helps keep hair clean and distributes oil evenly along hair shafts. Combing merely styles the hair

 Examples of NANDA Nursing Diagnoses for Hair and Scalp Care

Dressing/grooming self-care deficit *related to:*
- Altered level of consciousness
- Physical immobility or weakness

Impaired skin integrity *related to:*
- Scalp laceration
- Insect bite

Pain *related to:*
- Scalp lesion
- Accumulated secretions in hair

Body-image disturbance *related to:*
- Unkempt physical appearance

Risk for infection *related to:*
- Scalp laceration
- Insect bites

and prevents it from becoming tangled. Short-tooth combs are adequate for short hair, but large-tooth combs are preferable for curly hair. Combs with sharp, irregular teeth may scratch the scalp. The client able to perform self-care should be encouraged to maintain hair care daily. However, clients with limited mobility and poor coordination and those who are confused or seriously weakened by their illnesses require the nurse's help.

Long hair can easily become matted after a client has been confined to bed even for a short period. When lacerations or incisions involve the scalp, blood and topical medications can also cause tangling. Frequent brushing and combing keep long hair neatly groomed. However, braiding can help to avoid repeated tangles (Fig. 40-5). The nurse should ask the client's permission to braid hair. If braids are made too tightly, balding patches can develop.

To brush hair properly the nurse parts the hair into two sections and then separates each section into two more sections. Parting allows for ease in brushing smaller sections of hair. The nurse brushes from the scalp toward the hair ends. If tangles are present, the nurse uses the fingers to separate a small lock of hair, grasps it firmly near the scalp, and combs the loose end of the lock. Anchoring the tangled hair prevents painful pulling of the scalp during combing. If the hair is excessively tangled, the nurse should comb out only a few sections at a time. Moistening the hair with water or alcohol often frees tangles for easier combing. The nurse never cuts the client's hair without written consent.

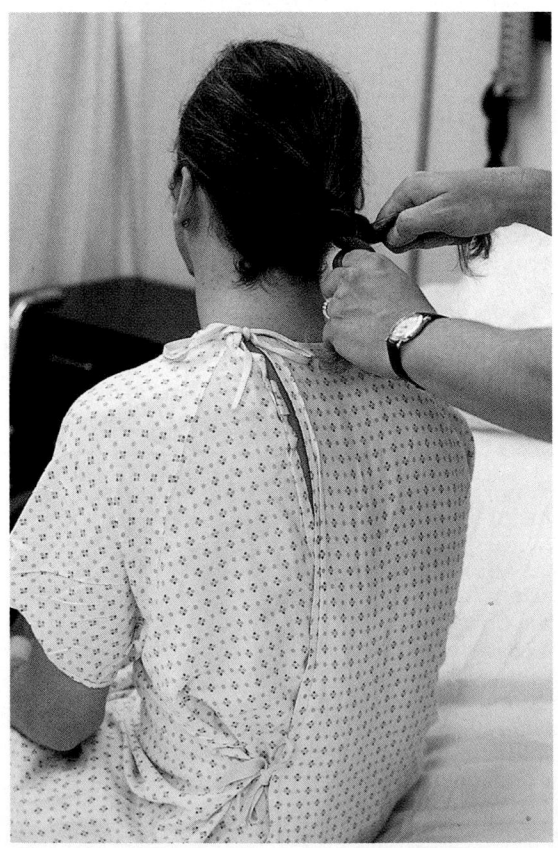

Fig. 40-5 Braiding a client's hair.

Clients who have curly hair usually comb their hair with a special comb that has long teeth spaced far apart. The open-toothed comb causes less pulling during combing. Wetting the client's hair with water before combing prevents trauma to the hair. To comb curly hair, the nurse starts at the client's neckline and slowly lifts and fluffs the hair outward until the forehead is reached. The nurse combs one side of the client's head at a time and then repeats on the other side.

African-American clients have thick, coarse, hair, which often becomes very dry and brittle. Because the hair and scalp have a tendency to be dry, daily combing, gentle brushing, and an application of a moisture product may be necessary (Andrews, Boyle, 1995). Thus the nurse should caution against the use of hair care practices that can damage hair. To braid daily is more damaging than to cornrow. The tight braids may cause balding patches. The use of a hot comb for straightening hair may cause chronic inflammation and permanent scarring of the scalp. Application of hair straighteners with alkaline chemicals may cause the hair to become brittle.

SHAMPOOING

Frequency of shampooing depends on a person's daily routine and the condition of the hair. The nurse should remind hospitalized clients that staying in bed, excess perspiration, or treatments that leave blood or solutions in the hair may require more frequent shampooing. For clients at home, the nurse's greatest challenge may be to find ways that the client can shampoo the hair without injury. For example, the older client may sit on a tub chair and use a handheld nozzle rather than leaning over to reach the faucet.

If clients are able to take showers or baths, the hair can usually be shampooed without difficulty. Shower chairs may be used for clients who are ambulatory but who become tired or faint. Handheld shower nozzles allow clients to wash their hair during a tub bath or shower. The hair of clients who are allowed to sit in a chair can usually be shampooed in front of a sink. If the client can sit only at the bedside, it is possible to shampoo the hair as the client leans forward over a washbasin. However, bending is limited or contraindicated in certain conditions (e.g., eye surgery and total hip replacement surgery). In these situations, the nurse needs to teach the client the degree of bending allowed.

If a client is unable to sit but can be moved, the nurse may transfer the client to a stretcher for transportation to a sink or shower equipped with a handheld nozzle. The nurse places a towel or small pillow under the client's head and neck, allowing the head to hang slightly over the stretcher's edge. Caution is needed with clients who have suffered neck injuries because hyperextension of the neck could cause further injury.

If the client is unable to sit in a chair or to be transferred to a stretcher, shampooing must be done with the client in bed. After shampooing (Procedure 40-7), clients may like having their hair rolled on curlers or styled. Most health care centers have portable hair dryers. Dry shampoos that reduce the need to wet the client's hair are also available.

Because the hair of African Americans has a natural tendency to be dry, daily shampooing is unnecessary. The

Shampooing Hair in Bed

STEPS	RATIONALE
1. Determine if any risks exist that might contraindicate shampooing or positioning. Review physician's orders to determine if medicated shampoo is ordered.	Certain medical conditions (e.g., total hip replacement, cervical neck injuries, open incisions, tracheostomy) may place client at risk of injury because of positioning, exposure to moisture, or manipulation of scalp. For conditions such as lice or dandruff, special shampoos may be ordered.
2. Explain procedure to client.	Client may be anxious about positioning or risk of water entering eyes.
3. Prepare necessary equipment and supplies:	
a. Two bath towels	
b. Face towel or washcloth	
c. Shampoo (OPTION: hair conditioner and cream rinse)	
d. Water pitcher	Used to pour water over hair.
e. Plastic shampoo trough	Diverts water to basin to prevent soiling bed linen.
f. Washbasin	
g. Bath blanket	
h. Waterproof pad	
i. Clean comb and brush	
j. Hair dryer	
k. Bottle of hydrogen peroxide (optional)	Cleanses hair matted with blood.
l. Disposible gloves (optional)	
4. Wash hands.	Reduces transmission of microorganisms.
5. Arrange equipment in convenient place, raise level of bed, and lower side rail.	Prevents interruption and facilitates body mechanics.

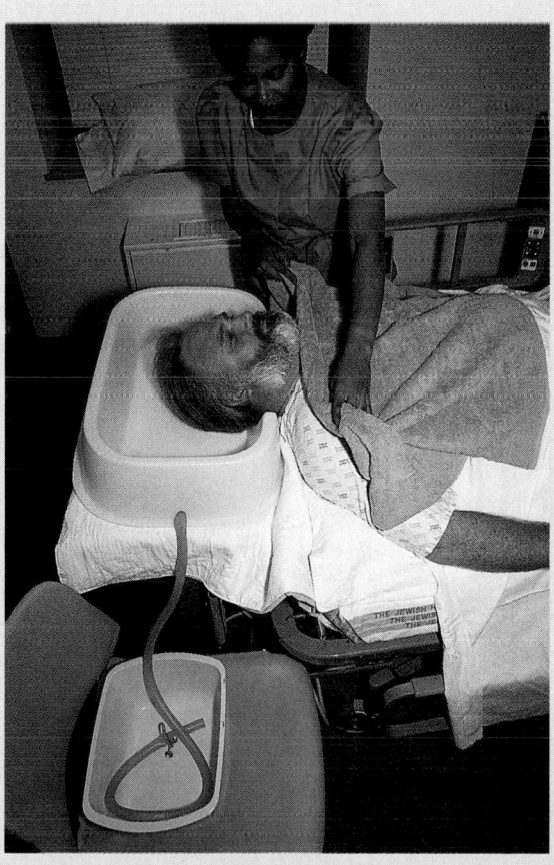

Step 7

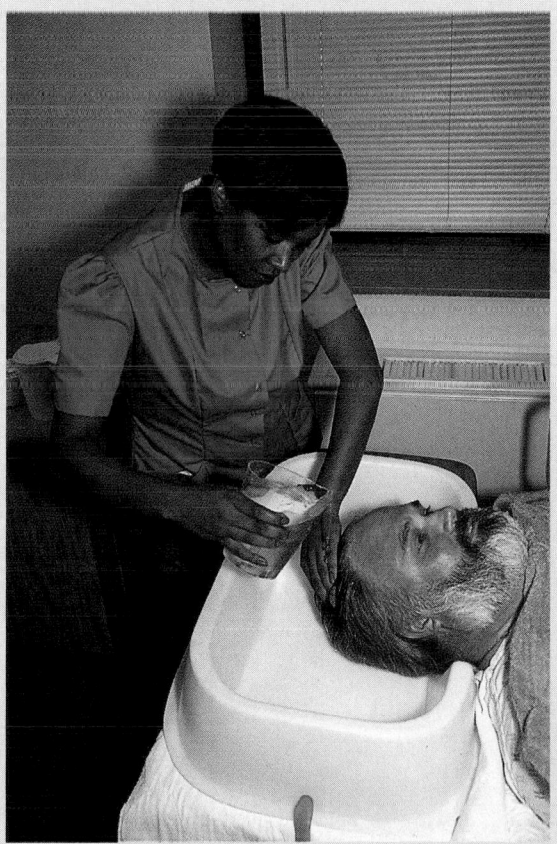

Step 12

Continued.

Shampooing Hair in Bed—cont'd

STEPS	RATIONALE
6. Place waterproof pad under client's shoulders, neck, and head. Position client supine with head and shoulders at top edge of bed. Place plastic trough under head and washbasin at end of trough, being sure that trough spout extends beyond edge of mattress and runs into washbasin.	Prevents soiling of bed linen.
7. Place rolled towel under neck and bath towel across shoulders (see the illustration on p. 1057).	Slight hyperextension of neck minimizes problem of water draining down back of neck.
8. Brush and comb hair.	Removing tangles results in more thorough cleansing.
9. Obtain warm water and fill pitcher. Check temperature by placing small amount of water on inner aspect of your forearm.	Prevents burns to face and scalp.
10. Apply gloves if client has lesions of scalp or presence of lice.	Prevents transmission of microorganisms.
11. Offer client option of holding face towel or washcloth over eyes.	Prevents shampoo or water for entering eyes.
12. With water pitcher, slowly pour water over hair until it is completely wet (see the illustration on p. 1057). Apply small amount of shampoo.	Water aids in distribution of shampoo suds or hair.
13. Work up lather with both hands. Start at hairline and work toward back of neck. Lift head slightly with one hand to wash back of head. Shampoo sides of head. Massage scalp by applying pressure with fingertips (see the illustration below).	Systematic progression over hair and scalp ensures thorough cleansing. Massage increases scalp circulation. Use of fingernails during massage can cause scratching of scalp.

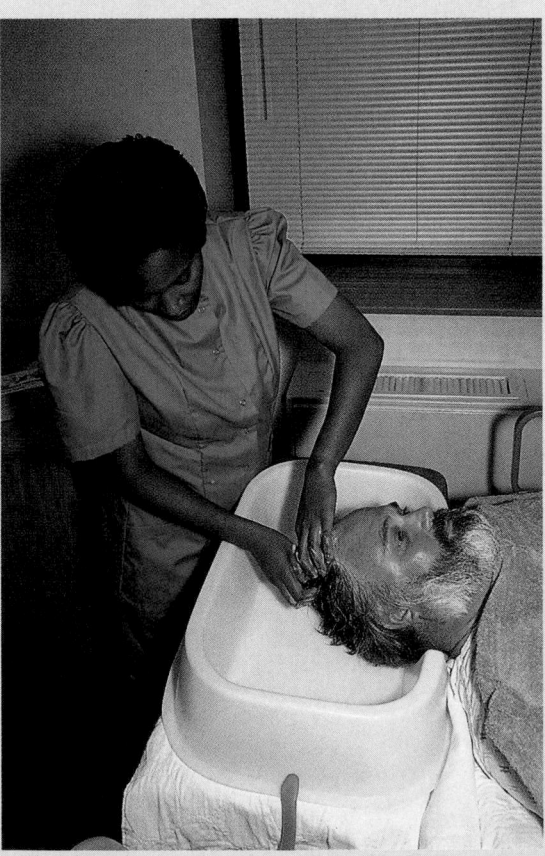

Step 13

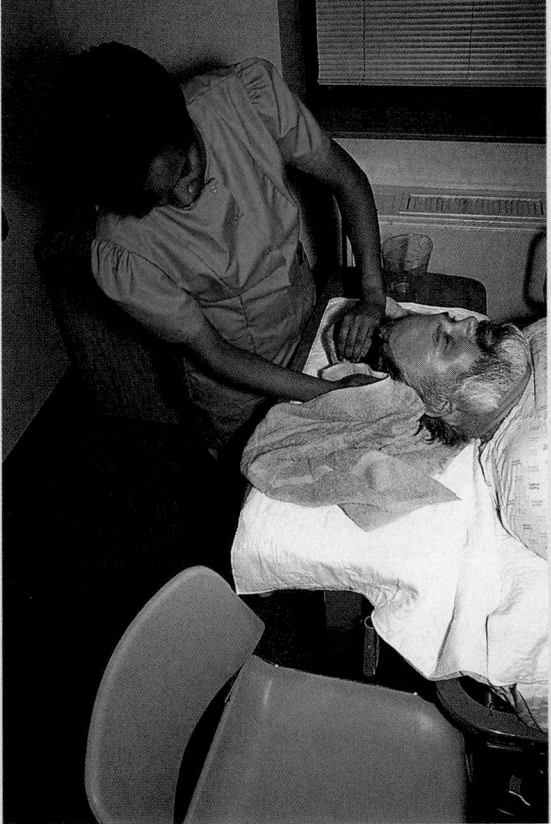

Step 17

Shampooing Hair in Bed—cont'd

STEPS	RATIONALE
14. Rinse hair with water. Make sure water drains into basin. Repeat rinsing until hair is free of shampoo. To speed drainage from trough, press down on its spout.	Retained shampoo leaves dull finish on hair. Dried shampoo may cause scalp irritation.
15. Repeat Steps 12-14.	Ensures thorough cleansing.
16. Apply conditioner or rinse if requested and rinse hair thoroughly.	Conditioner prevents excess drying. Cream rinse makes combing and brushing easier.
17. Wrap head in bath towel. Dry face with cloth used to protect eyes. Dry off moisture along neck or shoulders (see the illustration on p. 1058).	Retained moisture may cause cooling and chills.
18. Dry hair and scalp. Use second towel if first becomes saturated. Dispose of gloves if needed.	
19. Comb hair to remove tangles and dry with dryer or remaining towel as quickly as possible.	Drying prevents chilling.
20. Assist client to comfortable position and complete styling of hair.	Promotes client's sense of well-being.
21. Return equipment to its proper place. Discard soiled linen in linen hamper. Wash hands.	Maintains cleanliness of environment and controls transmission of infection.
22. Ask client how hair feels.	Client will experience sense of cleanliness after shampooing.
23. Inspect condition of hair.	Shampooing should leave hair in clean condition.
24. Record procedure and pertinent findings related to condition of hair or scalp.	Documents client's response to therapy and condition of hair or scalp should further treatment be necessary.

nurse asks the client how often shampooing is preferred. Normally, it is necessary for African Americans to shampoo their hair only once or twice a week, or only once a month. A client with cornrows can have the hair shampooed without undoing the braids (Andrews, Boyle, 1995). Water shampoos tend to make their hair curlier and harder to comb. A mild shampoo is preferred if they have had their hair straightened.

A client's hair becomes drier and more brittle with advanced age. Frequently older adults will shampoo only once a week. The nurse who works in an extended care facility or nursing home should be sure the client's hair is thoroughly combed and styled daily.

SHAVING

Shaving facial hair can be done after the bath or shampoo. Women may prefer to shave their legs or axillae during the bath. When assisting a client, the nurse should take care to avoid cutting the client with razor blades. Suicidal clients are not allowed to use razor blades. Clients prone to bleeding, such as those receiving anticoagulant medications (heparin or Coumadin), high doses of aspirin, or nonsteroidal antiinflammatory drugs, and those with bleeding disorders (hemophilia or leukemia) are instructed to use an electric razor. Before using an electric razor, the nurse checks for electrical hazards.

When a razor blade is used for shaving, the skin must be softened to prevent pulling, scraping, or cutting. For example, placing a warm washcloth over the male client's face for a few seconds, followed by the application of shaving cream or a lathering of mild soap, effectively soft-

ens the skin. If the male client is unable to shave his own face, the nurse may shave him. To avoid causing discomfort or razor cuts, the nurse holds the razor at a 45-degree angle to the skin and gently pulls the skin taut while using short, firm razor strokes in the direction that the hair grows. Short, downward strokes work best to remove hair over the upper lip. Often a client can explain the best way to move the razor across the skin. After the shave is completed, the nurse washes the client's face thoroughly to remove soap and hair. After drying the face, the nurse assists in applying powder or an aftershave lotion to the client's face.

MUSTACHE AND BEARD CARE

Male clients with mustaches or beards require daily grooming. Keeping these clean is important because food particles can easily collect in the hair. If clients are unable to care for themselves, the nurse should trim, comb, or wash beards or mustaches when needed or on request. The nurse never shaves off a mustache or beard without the client's consent.

 Evaluation

Evaluation of nursing care measures for the client's hair care are based on the expected outcomes (e.g., verbalizing a sense of comfort or demonstrating correct grooming), and goals of care. The nurse uses evaluative measures, such as having the client demonstrate hair care practices or reinspecting the condition of the hair and scalp, to determine the success of nursing interventions.

■ CARE OF THE EYES, EARS, AND NOSE

Special attention is given to the cleansing of the client's eyes, ears, and nose during the client's bath. However, clients may also have special problems that require cleansing of these organs throughout the day. Nursing care centers on preventing infection and maintaining the client's normal organ function.

Eyes

Normally no special care is required for the eyes because they are continually cleansed by tears, and the eyelids and lashes prevent the entrance of foreign particles. A person needs only to remove any dried secretions that have collected on the inner canthus or the eyelashes. Unconscious clients are at risk for eye injury because the blink reflex may be absent. In these clients, excessive drainage frequently collects along eyelid margins. Special attention is also needed for clients who have had eye surgery or an eye infection that can result in increased discharge or drainage. The nurse often assists clients in the care of eyeglasses, contact lenses, or artificial eyes.

Ears

Hygiene of the ears has implications for hearing acuity when wax or foreign substances collect in the external ear canal, and they interfere with sound conduction. Older adults are particularly susceptible to this problem. The nurse should be sensitive to any behavioral cues that might indicate a hearing impairment (see Chapter 39). When caring for a client with a hearing aid, the nurse instructs the client on proper cleansing and maintenance as well as communication techniques that promote hearing the spoken word.

Nose

The nose provides for the sense of smell but also controls the temperature and humidity of inhaled air and prevents the entrance of foreign particles into the respiratory system. The accumulation of encrusted secretions within the nares can impair olfactory sensation and breathing. Irritation of nasal mucosa can cause swelling, leading to obstruction of the nares. Typically, hygienic care of the nose is simple, but clients with nasogastric, enteral feeding, or endotracheal tubes that enter the nose may require special attention.

■ NURSING PROCESS AND EYES, EARS, AND NOSE CARE

Assessment

PHYSICAL ASSESSMENT

Chapter 33 describes the techniques used to assess the condition and function of the eyes, ears, and nose. Normally the eyes are free of infection and irritation. The sclerae are visible anteriorly as the white portion of the eye. The conjunctivae (the lining of the eyelids) are clear, pink, and without inflammation. The eyelid margins are in close approximation with the eyeball, and the lashes are turned outward. The lid margins are without inflammation, drainage, or lesions. The eyebrows should be symmetrical.

Assessing a Client's Use of Sensory Aids

EYEGLASSES
- Purpose for wearing glasses (e.g., reading, distance, or both)
- Methods used to clean glasses
- Presence of symptoms (e.g., blurred vision, photophobia, headaches, irritation)

CONTACT LENSES
- Type of lens worn
- Frequency and duration of time lenses are worn (including sleep time)
- Presence of symptoms (e.g., burning, excess tearing, redness, irritation, swelling, sensitivity to light)
- Techniques used by the client to cleanse, store, insert, and remove lenses
- Use of eyedrops or ointments
- Use of emergency identification bracelet or card that warns others to remove client's lenses in case of emergency

ARTIFICIAL EYE
- Method used to insert and remove eye
- Method for cleansing eye
- Presence of symptoms (e.g., drainage, inflammation, pain involving the orbit)

HEARING AID
- Type of aid worn
- Methods used to cleanse aid
- Client's ability to change battery and adjust hearing aid volume

---

Assessment of the external ear structures includes inspection of the auricle, external ear canal, and tympanic membrane. While performing hygienic measures, the nurse is most concerned with noting the presence of accumulated cerumen or drainage in the ear canal, local inflammation, or pain.

The nurse inspects the nares for signs of inflammation, discharge, lesions, edema, and deformity. The nasal mucosa is normally pink and clear and has little or no discharge. A clear, watery discharge may be the result of allergies. If clients have any form of tubing exiting the nose, the nurse should look at the nares surfaces that come in contact with the tubing for tissue sloughing, localized tenderness, inflammation, and bleeding.

USE OF SENSORY AIDS

If clients wear eyeglasses, contact lenses, artificial eyes, or hearing aids, the nurse assesses the client's knowledge, the methods used to care for the aids, and the presence of any problems caused by the aids. The box above outlines factors to assess clients using sensory aids. The nurse's findings have implications for client education.

SELF-CARE ABILITY

The nurse assesses a client's physical ability to perform eye, ear, and nose care, as well as to care for any sensory aids. Clients who are unable to grasp small objects, who have limited mobility in the upper extremities, who have reduced vision, or who are seriously fatigued require assistance from the nurse or a family member.

Nursing Diagnosis

Assessment may reveal an actual alteration in the function of sensory organs (Chapter 39), a problem in the client's ability to perform personal hygiene, or a deficit in the client's understanding of hygiene. Clustering defining characteristics such as reduced visual acuity, avoidance of activities, or irritation to the eyes helps the nurse form an accurate nursing diagnosis, for example *sensory perceptual/alteration, visual*. The critical thinking used to select diagnoses requires not only a review of the client's presenting problem but a consideration of previous clients with similar problems. This helps the nurse validate findings while pursuing a comprehensive assessment. The nursing diagnoses box below lists some common nursing diagnoses.

Planning

The client's personal preferences and habits are incorporated into the nurse's plan for hygienic care. Family members should be involved early, since they may be required to assist with hygiene measures. One principle to consider in planning care is that the eyes, ears, and nose are sensitive to irritating or painful stimuli. Extra care must be taken to avoid injury to tissues. The goals of care for the client include the following:

1. Client's eyes, ears, and nose will be free from infection.
2. Client will have normal sensory organ functioning.
3. Client will perform daily care for the eyes, ears, and nose.

Implementation

BASIC EYE CARE

Cleansing of the eyes is usually performed during the bath and involves washing with a clean washcloth moistened in water. Soap may cause burning and irritation and is

Examples of NANDA Nursing Diagnoses for Eye, Ear, and Nose Problems

Bathing/hygiene self-care deficit *related to:*
- Physical limitations
- Visual impairment

Knowledge deficit about personal hygiene *related to:*
- Lack of exposure to information
- Information misinterpretation

Pain *related to:*
- Physical irritation of eye
- Inflammation of ear canal
- Mechanical irritation of nares

Risk for infection *related to:*
- Poor hygienic practices

Sensory/perceptual alterations (visual, auditory, or olfactory) *related to:*
- Obstruction in ear canal
- Nasal obstruction
- Inflammation of eyes or local eye infection

usually omitted. The nurse wipes from the inner to the outer canthus of the eye to prevent secretions from draining into the lacrimal sac. A separate section of the washcloth is used each time to prevent the spread of infection. If a client has dried secretions that are not removed easily with wiping, the nurse may first place a damp cloth or cotton ball on the lid margins to loosen the secretions. Direct pressure should never be applied over the eyeball because it may cause serious injury.

The unconscious client may require more frequent eye care. Secretions may collect along the lid margins and inner canthus when the blink reflex is absent or when the eye does not close totally. The eyes may be cleansed with a sterile cotton ball moistened with sterile normal saline. Artificial tears may be required, and an order for them should be obtained from the physician. Caution must be used if a patch is applied to the eye because it may cause injury to the cornea (Smeltzer, Bare, 1992).

Cleaning Glasses. Glasses are made of hardened glass or plastic that is impact resistant to prevent shattering. Nevertheless, because of the cost, the nurse uses care when cleaning glasses and should protect them from breakage or other damage when not worn. Glasses should be put in their case and in a drawer of the bedside table when not in use.

Warm water is sufficient for cleansing glass lenses. A soft cloth is best for drying to prevent scratching. Plastic lenses may scratch easily and require special cleaning solutions and drying tissues.

Contact Lens Care. A contact lens is a small, round, transparent, and sometimes colored disk that fits directly over the cornea of the eye. The lens floats on the tear layer that lubricates the eye. Contact lenses are designed specifically to correct refractive errors of the eye or abnormalities in the cornea's shape. They are relatively easy to apply and remove. There are three types of contact lenses: hard, soft, and rigid gas permeable (RGP), also known as oxygen permeable.

Hard plastic lenses, introduced in the 1950s, are rigid, thick, durable, and optically precise. They are relatively easy to clean and handle. However, they can be uncomfortable and difficult to fit. Hard lenses have become obsolete.

The newer, more popular rigid gas permeable lenses provide clear vision but are more flexible and comfortable than the traditional hard lenses and allow oxygen through to the cornea. However, they are more likely to slip, causing blurred or distorted vision, or to pop out. They also are more readily scratched or chipped.

Soft contact lenses, introduced in the 1970s, are more comfortable because they are thinner, soft, and more pliable. Like rigid gas permeable lenses, they are less likely to cause corneal epithelial damage because they are oxygen permeable. Soft lenses are more pliable and flimsy because they consist primarily of water, 38% to 70% by weight (Rakow, 1990). Therefore soft lenses easily tear and are thus less durable. Disadvantages may include a higher initial cost and the need for frequent replacement. They are also more difficult to clean and maintain (Phipps, 1995). There are several varieties of soft lenses: bifocal, multifocal, tinted (to enhance or alter eye color), toric (for astigmatism), and extended wear. Soft disposables, worn as daily or extended wear lenses, are also available. The client may also be using the new disposable lens that is discarded after use.

The normal eye needs oxygen and receives most of it

through air and tears (OxyFlow, 1987). Although soft lenses and newer rigid lenses are gas permeable and allow oxygen to pass directly through the lens, all contact lenses still restrict the flow of oxygen to the eye's surface. Overwearing of contacts can cause edema and abrasion of the cornea (Phipps et al, 1995). A major difference between the types of lenses is the length of time each can be safely worn. Rigid and daily wear soft lenses should be removed overnight and should not be worn more than 12 to 14 hours daily. It is not recommended that extended wear soft lenses be left in place longer than 1 week (Phipps et al, 1995). Pain, tearing, discomfort, and redness of the conjunctiva may be symptomatic of lens overwear. The persistence of symptoms, even after lens removal, is abnormal, however, and may indicate serious ocular damage.

As contact lenses are worn by clients, they accumulate secretions and foreign matter. This material deteriorates and then irritates the eye, causing distorted vision and risk for infection. Once removed, contact lenses should be cleansed and thoroughly disinfected. A contact lens provides certain advantages over eyeglasses:

1. Improves clarity of vision
2. Is safer than eyeglasses during certain physical activities
3. Smooths optically irregular surfaces of the eye
4. Provides a more attractive appearance for the wearer

Clients who wear contact lenses generally care for them themselves. An eye specialist instructs clients on the proper techniques to care for the lens. Often, the nurse is responsible for removing contacts in an emergency and for reinforcing techniques of proper lens care. The box below lists some common guidelines for all contact lens wearers that the nurse can reinforce during hygienic care. Clients should also be aware of the symptoms or problems that may be related, directly or indirectly, to contact lens use (Table 40-8).

The basic steps of contact lens care include cleansing to remove the accumulation of deposits from tear film, rinsing to remove lens debris after cleaning, disinfecting to protect eyes from infection, and lubricating to replace water lost from lens and tears through evaporation. A variety of products is available for lens care, and each type of lens requires a different cleansing technique.

Some eye specialists also recommend periodic enzyme cleansing. The enzymes dissolve protein deposits on the lens surface. Some lenses can be cleansed with electrical heat disinfecting units.

Clients may require assistance with contact lens care, insertion, and removal. The nurse protects clients unable to care for their lenses properly. Prolonged wearing of contact lenses can cause serious corneal damage. Clients who become unconscious; who are restricted from moving their hands; or who lose clear judgment because of psychiatric illness, temporary mental confusion, or substance abuse should have their lenses removed immediately. Procedure 40-8 describes techniques for the care of contact lenses. Lenses for these clients need not be reinserted until they are more capable of caring for the lenses themselves.

Text continued on p. 1067.

Contact Lens Care

DO

- Wash and rinse hands thoroughly before handling a lens.
- Keep fingernails clean.
- At the time of lens insertion, thoroughly rinse the storage case with warm water and dry because microorganisms can grow in any water or solution.
- Remove extended wear lenses at least weekly for thorough cleaning and disinfection.
- When inserting lens, start with the same lens (right or left) each time.
- Use proper lens care products.
- Discard and replace disposable soft lenses weekly.
- Wear lenses daily, and follow the prescribed wearing schedule.
- Remove a lens if it becomes uncomfortable.
- Keep regular appointments with the eye specialist.
- Remove lenses during sunbathing, showering, or swimming.
- Report the following symptoms immediately: localized pain that radiates around the eyes, reduced visual acuity (recent onset), photophobia (sensitivity to light), and discharge from the eye.

DO NOT

- Use soaps that contain cream or perfume for cleaning lenses
- Let fingernails touch lenses
- Mix up lenses
- Exceed prescribed wearing time
- Use saliva to wet lenses
- Use homemade saline solution or tap water to wet or clean lenses
- Borrow or mix lens care solution
- Reuse disposable lenses

Table 40-8	Common Problems for Contact Lens Wearers	
PROBLEM	**CAUSE**
Uncomfortable lens	Dirty or damaged lens
	Dust on eyelash entering eye
	Eye infection
	Decreased eye moisture (tears)
Redness of eye	Lens overwear
	Sensitivity to lens care solution
	Allergy
	Eye infection
Blurred vision	Dirty or damaged lens
	Mix up of left with right lens
	Corneal irritation
	Wearing lens inside out (soft lenses only)
Excess tearing	Corneal irritation
	Lens overwear
	Eye infection
Corneal infection	Failure to remove extended wear lenses in time
	Contamination of lens storage case and cleaning solution
	Infrequent lens disinfection
	Use of homemade saline
	Swimming while wearing lens

Taking Care of Contact Lenses

STEPS	RATIONALE
1. Inspect the eye or ask client if contact lens is in place.	Lenses are usually comfortable to wear and client may forget they are in place.
2. Assess client's ability to manipulate and hold contact lens.	Determines level of assistance required in care.
3. After lenses are removed, inspect eye for signs of corneal irritation, excess tearing, redness, burning.	Signs of corneal irritation may require client to refrain from contact use.
4. Prepare necessary equipment and supplies for lens removal:	
a. Contact lens storage container (see the illustration below) labeled with client's name.	Separate cups labeled *R* for right lens and *L* for left lens protect against lens breakage. (Certain lenses are stored dry, whereas others are stored in solution.)
b. Lens suction cup (optional)	Used to remove hard lenses from unconscious or debilitated client.
c. Sterile saline solution	Used to moisten cornea before lens removal.
d. Bath towel	
5. Prepare equipment and supplies for cleansing and insertion:	
a. Lenses in clean storage container, labeled with client name	
b. Thermal disinfecting kit (optional)	Heats up to 80° C to sterilize soft lenses.
c. Surfactant cleaner	
d. Rinsing solution	
e. Sterile lens disinfectant and enzyme solution (see the illustration below)	Cleanses lens surfaces and reduces number of microorganisms present.
f. Sterile wetting solution for hard lenses	Allows lens to glide easily over cornea during insertion.
g. Cotton ball or cotton-tipped applicator	Used to spread lens cleaner over surface of rigid contact lens.
h. Bath towel	
i. Emesis basin	
j. Glass of warm tap water	
6. Discuss procedure with client.	Client can assist in planning by explaining technique that may aid removal and insertion. Client may be anxious as nurse retracts eye lids and manipulates lenses.
7. Have client assume supine or sitting position in bed or chair.	Provides easy access while retracting eyelids and manipulating lens.

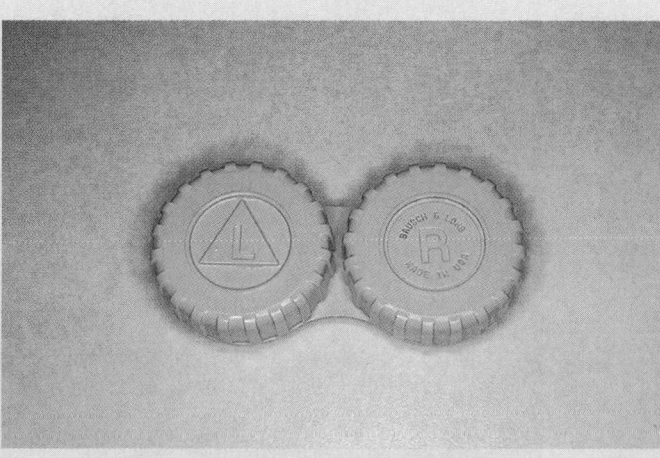

Step 4a

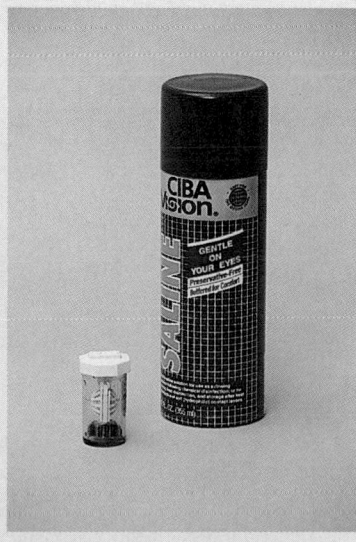

Step 5e

Continued.

Taking Care of Contact Lenses—cont'd

STEPS	RATIONALE

8. Removing soft lenses

a. Wash hands.

b. Place towel just below client's face.

c. Add few drops of sterile saline to client's eye.

d. Tell client to look straight ahead.

e. Using middle finger, retract lower eyelid.

f. With pad of index finger of same hand, slide lens off cornea onto white of eye.

g. Pull upper eyelid down gently with thumb of other hand and compress lens slightly between thumb and index finger.

h. Gently pinch lens and lift out without allowing lens edges to stick together.

i. If lens edges stick together, place lens in palm and soak thoroughly with sterile saline. Gently roll lens with index finger in back and forth motion. If gentle rubbing does not separate edges, soak lens in sterile solution.

j. Clean and rinse lens (see cleansing and disfecting). Place lens in proper storage case compartment: *R* for right lens and *L* for left lens. Be sure lens is centered.

k. Repeat Steps 8c-8j for other lens. Secure cover over storage case.

l. Dispose of towel and wash hands.

9. Removing rigid lenses

a. Wash hands.

b. Place towel just below client's face.

c. Be sure lens is positioned directly over cornea. If it is not, have client close eyelids, place index and middle fingers of one hand behind lens, gently but firmly massage lens back into place.

d. Place index finger on outer corner of eye and draw skin gently back toward ear (see the illustration below).

e. Tell client to blink. Do not release pressure on lids until blink is completed.

RATIONALE

Reduces transmission of microorganisms.

Catches lens if one accidentally falls from eye.

Lubricates eye to facilitate lens removal.

Eases tipping of lens during removal.

Exposes lower edge of lens.

Positions lens for easy grasping. Use of finger pad prevents injury to cornea and damage to lens.

Causes soft lens to double up. Air enters underneath lens to release suction.

Protects lens from damage. Prevents lens edges from sticking together.

Assist in returning lens to normal shape.

Ensures that proper lens will be reinserted into correct eye. Proper storage prevents cracking or tearing.

Proper storage prevents damage to lens.

Reduces transmission of infection. Reduces transmission of microorganisms.

Catches lens if one accidentally falls from eye.

Correct position of lens allows easy removal from eye.

Tightens lids against eyeball.

Maneuver should cause lens to dislodge and pop out. Lid margins must clear top and bottom of lens until blink.

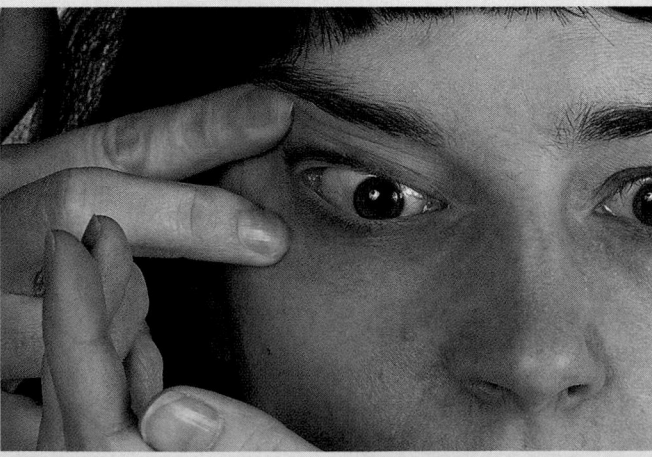

Step 9d

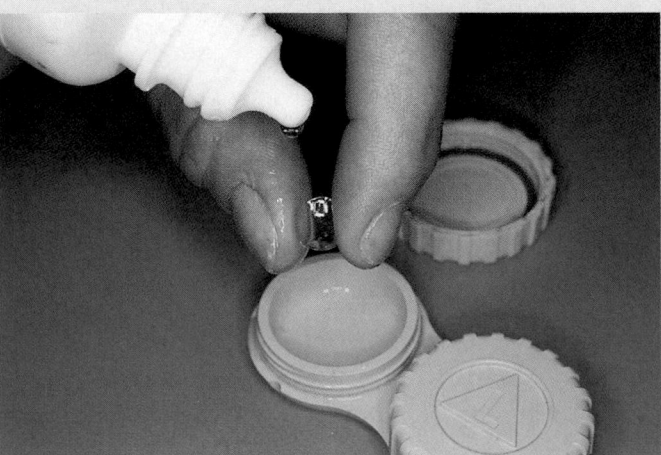

Step 11c

Taking Care of Contact Lenses—cont'd

STEPS	RATIONALE
9. Removing rigid lenses—cont'd	
f. If lens fails to pop out, gently retract eyelid beyond edges of lens. Press lower eyelid gently against lower edge of lens.	Pressure causes upper edge of lens to tip forward.
g. Allow eyelids to close slightly and grasp lens as it rises from eye. A suction cup can be used for confused or unconscious clients.	Maneuver causes lens to slide off easily.
h. Cup lens in your hand.	Protects lens from breakage.
i. Cleanse and rinse lens (see Step 9). Place lens in proper storage case compartment: *R* for right lens and *L* for left lens. Center lens in storage case, convex side down.	Both lenses may not have the same prescription. Proper storage prevents cracking, tearing, or chipping.
j. Repeat Steps 8c-8i for other lens. Secure cover over storage case.	Proper storage prevents damage to lens.
k. Dispose of towel and wash hands.	Reduces spread of infection and keeps environment neat.
10. Cleanse and disinfect contact lenses	
a. Wash hands.	Reduces transmission of microorganisms.
b. Assemble supplies at bedside.	Provides easy access to supplies.
c. Place towel over work area.	Towel helps prevent lens breakage.
d. Open lens container carefully, taking care not to flip lens caps open suddenly.	Prevents lenses from being accidentally spilled or flipped out of case.
e. After removal of lens from eye, apply 1-2 drops of cleaning solution on lens in palm of your hand (use cleaner recommended) by lens manufacturer or eye care practitioner).	Removes tear components, including mucus, lipid, and proteins that collect on lens.
f. Rub lens gently but thoroughly on both sides for 20-30 sec. Use index finger (soft lenses) or little finger or cotton tip applicator soaked with cleaner (rigid lenses) to clean inside lens. Be careful not to contact or scratch lens with fingernail.	It is easier to manipulate and clean lenses using fingertips. Cleanses all surfaces for microorganisms.
g. Holding lens over emesis basin, rinse thoroughly with manufacturer-recommended rinsing solution (soft lenses) or cold tap water (rigid lenses).	Removes debris and cleaning agent from lens surface.
h. Place lenses in storage case and fill with disinfecting solution recommended by manufacturer or eyecare practitioner. Center lens in storage case, convex side down, fill with solution	Disinfects lenses, removes residue, enhances wettability of lenses, and prevents scratches from dry case.
11. Insert rigid lenses	
a. Wash hands thoroughly with mild noncosmetic soap. Rinse well. Dry with clean, lint-free towel or paper towel.	Lint or film on hands from soaps containing perfumes, deodorants, or complexion creams can be transferred to lenses and cause eye irritation.
b. Place towel over client's chest.	Towel will catch dropped lens and prevent breakage, scratching, or tearing.
c. Remove right lens from storage case; attempt to lift lens straight up (see the illustration on p. 1064).	Sliding lens out of case can cause scratches on the surface.
d. Rinse with cold tap water.	Hot water causes lens to warp.
e. Wet lens on both sides using prescribed wetting solution.	Lubricates lens so that it slides easily over and adheres to cornea.
f. Place right lens concave side up on tip of index finger of dominant hand (see the illustration on p. 1066).	Proper manipulation of lens ensures easy insertion. Inner surface of lens should face up so that it is applied against cornea.
g. Instruct client to look straight ahead with eyes open wide while retracting lower eyelids; place lens gently over center of cornea (see the illustration on p. 1066).	Lenses are rigid and can be placed as client looks straight ahead. Retraction of lids promotes easy insertion between lid margins.
h. Ask client to close eyes briefly and avoid blinking.	Helps to secure position of lens.
i. Ask client to open eyes. Be sure lens is centered properly by asking client if vision is blurred.	If lens slips to side of cornea or into conjunctival sac, vision will blur.

Continued.

Taking Care of Contact Lenses—cont'd

STEPS	RATIONALE

11. Insert rigid lenses—cont'd

j. Repeat Steps 10c-10i for left eye.

k. Assist client to comfortable position. — Promotes client's comfort.

l. Discard soiled supplies, discard solution in storage case, rinse case thoroughly and allow to air dry, and wash hands. — Use of fresh solution daily prevents infection.

12. Insert soft lenses

a. Wash hands with mild, noncosmetic soap, rinse well, dry with clean lint-free or paper towel. — Lint or film left on hands from cosmetic or deodorant soaps can be transferred to lenses and irritate eye.

b. Place towel over client's chest. — Towel will catch dropped lens and prevent breakage, scratching, or tearing.

c. Remove right lens from storage case and rinse with recommended rinsing solution; inspect lens for foreign materials, tears, or other damage. — Removes disinfectant solution. Prevents irritation or damage to eye.

d. Check that lens is not inverted (inside out). — Soft lens is inverted if bowl has a lip; it is in proper position if curve is even from base to rim.

e. Using middle or index finger of opposite hand, retract upper lid until iris is exposed. — Soft lenses do not adhere as easily as hard lenses. Separating lids as much as possible allows room for lens to contact cornea without touching lids or lashes.

f. Use middle finger or hand holding lens to pull down lower lid.

g. Tell client to look straight ahead and "through" lens and finger. Gently place lens directly on cornea, and release lens slowly, starting with lower lid. — Ensures secure fit and comfort.

h. If lens is on sclera rather than cornea, tell client to slowly close eye and roll it toward lens. — Maneuver centers soft lens over cornea.

i. Tell client to blink a few times. — Ensures that lens is centered, free of trapped air, and comfortable.

j. Be sure lens is centered properly by asking client if vision is blurred. — If lens slips to side of cornea or into conjunctival sac, vision will blur.

k. If client's vision is blurred, retract eyelids, locate position of lens, ask client to look in direction opposite of lens and with your index finger, apply pressure to lower eyelid margin and position lens over cornea. Have client look slowly toward lens. — Repositions lens over center of cornea as client looks toward lens.

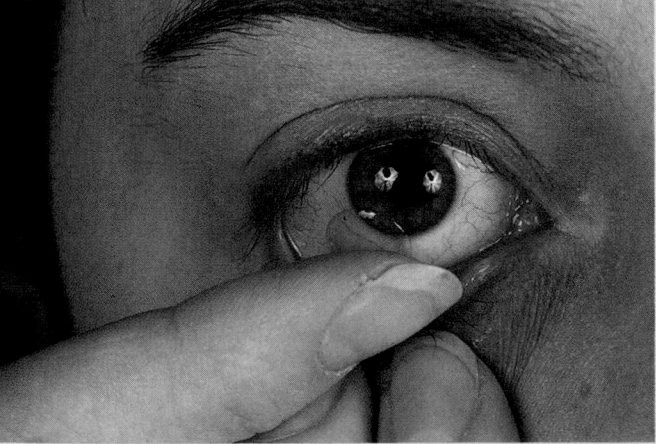

Step 11f

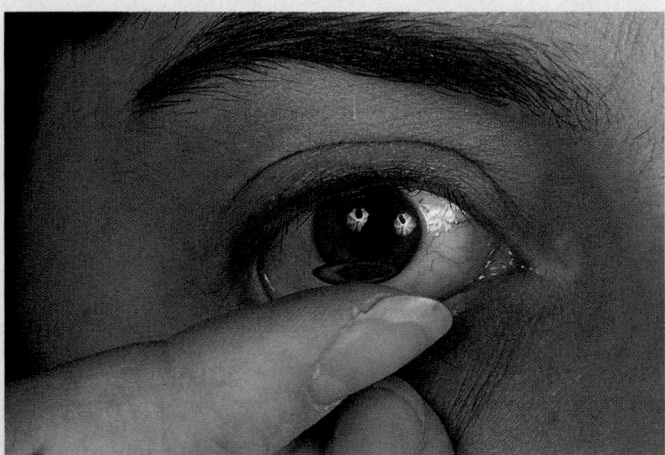

Step 11g

Taking Care of Contact Lenses—cont'd

STEPS	RATIONALE
12. Insert soft lenses—cont'd	
l. Repeat Steps 12c-12k for other eye.	Promotes client's comfort.
m. Assist client to comfortable position.	Prevents infection and maintains neat environment.
n. Discard soiled supplies, discard solution in storage case, rinse case thoroughly and allow to air dry, and wash hands.	
13. Ask client if lenses feel comfortable after reinsertion.	Determines whether debris is caught between lens and cornea.
14. Record or report any signs or symptoms of visual alterations noted during procedure.	May indicate eye injury or disease.
15. Record on nursing care plan or Kardex times of lens insertion and removal.	Determines safe period of time for insertion.

Artificial Eyes. Clients with artificial eyes have had an enucleation of an entire eyeball as a result of tumor growth, severe infection, or eye trauma. Some artificial eyes are permanently implanted. Others can be removed for routine cleaning. Clients with artificial eyes usually prefer to care for their own eyes. The nurse should respect the client's wishes and help by obtaining the necessary equipment.

For clients who are scheduled for surgery, are unconscious, or are unable to move their arms, head, or neck, the nurse assists with the removal and cleaning of artificial eyes. To remove an artificial eye, the nurse retracts the lower eyelid and exerts slight pressure just below the eye (Fig. 40-6). This action causes the artificial eye to rise from the socket because the suction holding the eye in place has been broken. The nurse may also use a small, rubber bulb syringe or medicine dropper bulb to create a suction effect. The suction created by placing the bulb tip directly over the eye and squeezing lifts the eye from the socket.

The artificial eye is usually made of glass or plastic. Warm normal saline cleanses the prosthesis effectively. The nurse also cleanses the edges of the eye socket and surrounding tissues with soft gauze moistened in saline or clean tap water. Signs of infection should be reported immediately because bacteria can spread to the neighboring eye, underlying sinuses, or underlying brain tissue. To reinsert the eye, the nurse retracts the upper and lower lids and gently slips the eye into the socket, fitting it neatly under the upper eyelid. An artificial eye may be stored in a labeled container filled with tap water or saline.

Vision Health Promotion. All clients benefit from learning the following simple guidelines for their visual health:

1. Clients under the age of 40 should have an eye examination every 3 to 5 years. Eye examination and routine testing for glaucoma are advised every 2 years for all adults over age 40. (See the box on p. 1068 for other strategies to preserve vision in older adults.)
2. Common symptoms of eye disorders include pain, photophobia, blurred vision, burning, itching, excess tearing, halos around lights, and floaters.

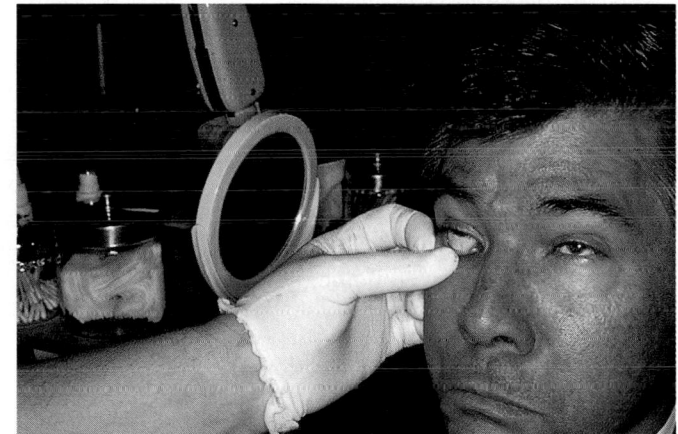

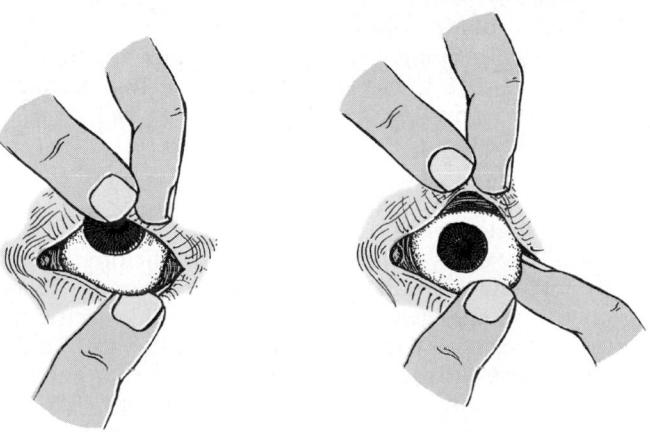

Fig. 40-6 Removal of prosthetic eye.

CLIENT TEACHING on Maintaining and Improving Eyesight in Older Adults

OBJECTIVE
- The older adult will state methods for maintaining and improving eyesight.

TEACHING STRATEGIES
- Encourage regular eye examinations. Stress its importance in preserving sight and preventing blindness.
- Discuss vision changes that occur naturally with aging, including presbyopia, a need for increased illumination, a delayed adaptation to darkness, increased light scatter, increased glare sensitivity and glare recovery, disturbance in hue discrimination, mild reductions in total visual field, and slowed visual interpretive reaction.
- Identify major eye diseases associated with aging such as glaucoma and cataracts.
- Discuss signs and symptoms of eye diseases.
- Determine whether any health or hereditary factors make the client more likely to develop vision problems.
- Ascertain whether the client needs and is able to make changes in environment and lifestyle to accommodate vision changes.
- Review prescribed medications and any visual side effects. If client is taking medications for eye problems, review purpose, action, dosage, and proper administration technique.
- Correct misinformation and misconceptions.
- Demonstrate proper eyedrop administration technique if necessary.

EVALUATION
- Listen to client's statements for correct information about normal eye changes, diseases, and medications.
- Reappraise accuracy of information after correcting misinformation and misconceptions.
- Observe eyedrop administration technique.

3. Clients should avoid home remedies for eye problems or injuries. Treatment for chemicals or dust that enter the eye includes flushing the eye continuously with tepid water for at least 10 minutes.
4. Clients should never try to remove foreign objects from the eye but should seek medical attention immediately.
5. Clients should wear eye goggles for protection when exposed to flying chemicals and/or dust in the work environment. In recreational sports, such as motorcycle riding, in-line hockey, or racquet ball, goggles should be worn.

CLEANING THE EARS

The nurse cleanses the client's ears as a routine part of a bed bath. The clean end of a moistened washcloth, rotated gently into the ear canal, works best for cleaning. When cerumen is visible, gentle, downward retraction at the entrance of the ear canal may cause the wax to loosen and slip out. The nurse instructs clients never to use sharp objects such as bobby pins or toothpicks to remove ear wax. The use of such objects can cause trauma to the ear canal and rupture of the tympanic membrane. Use of cotton tipped applicators should also be avoided because they can cause wax to become impacted within the canal.

Children and older adults commonly have impacted cerumen. Excessive or impacted cerumen can usually be removed only by irrigation. The procedure first involves instilling three drops of glycerine at bedtime to soften the wax, and three drops of hydrogen peroxide twice a day to loosen the wax (Phipps et al, 1995). Then the instillation of approximately 250 ml of warm water (37° C or 98.6° F) into the external ear canal mechanically washes away loosened wax. Cold or hot water causes nausea or vomiting.

The client may sit or lie on their side with the affected ear up. The nurse places a small curved basin under the affected ear to catch the irrigating solution. A Water Pik (set on No. 2 setting) or a bulb irrigating syringe can be used to irrigate the ear canal. The tip of the syringe or Water Pik should not occlude the ear canal to avoid exerting pressure against the tympanic membrane. Gentle irrigation directed at the top of the canal loosens the cerumen from the sides of the ear canal. After the canal is clear, the nurse wipes off any moisture from the client's ear and inspects the canal for remaining cerumen.

Hearing Aids. Chapter 39 discusses the need for and use of hearing aids. Hearing loss is a common health problem and an often forgotten disability that can affect the quality of a client's life. Hearing aids are instruments made up of miniature parts working together as a system to amplify sound in a controlled manner. The aid receives normal low-intensity sound inputs and delivers them to the client's ear as louder outputs. Older models of hearing aids created problems in noisy settings. The aid amplified foreground speech as well as background. A new class of hearing aid can reduce background noise interference. Hearing aids are used by both hard-of-hearing (slight or moderate hearing loss) and deaf persons (severe or profound hearing loss) (Phipps et al, 1995).

There are three popular types of hearing aids. An in-the-canal (ITC) aid is the newest, smallest, and least visible and fits entirely in the ear canal. It has cosmetic appeal, is easy to manipulate and place in the ear, does not interfere with wearing eyeglasses or using the telephone, and can be worn during most physical exercise. However, it requires adequate ear diameter and depth for proper fit. It does not accommodate progressive hearing loss, and it requires manual dexterity to operate, insert, remove, and change batteries. Also, cerumen tends to plug this model more than the others.

An in-the-ear (ITE or intraaural) aid (Fig. 40-7) fits into the external auditory ear and allows more fine tuning. It is more powerful and stronger and therefore is useful for a wider range of hearing loss than the ITC aid. It is also easy to position and adjust and does not interfere with eyeglass wearing. It is, however, slightly more noticeable than the ITC aid and is not recommended for persons with moisture or skin problems in the ear canal.

A behind-the-ear (BTE, or postaural) aid hooks around and behind the ear and is connected by a short, clear, hollow plastic tube to an ear mold inserted into the external auditory canal (Fig. 40-8). It also allows for fine tuning. It is the largest of the three and is useful for clients with rapidly progressive hearing loss or manual dexterity difficulties or those who find partial ear occlusion intolerable. Disadvan-

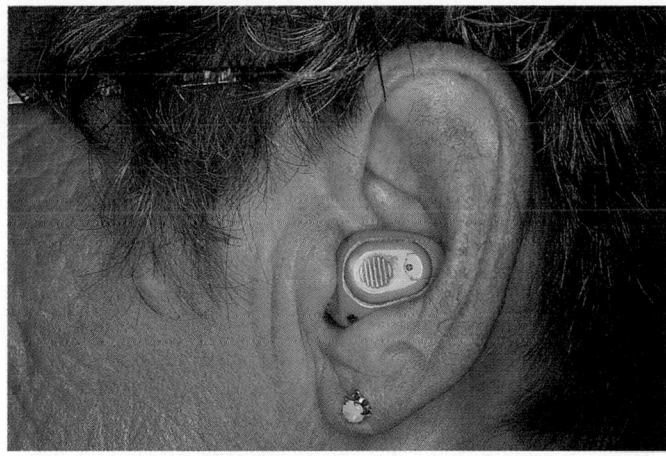

Fig. 40-7 In-the-ear hearing aid.

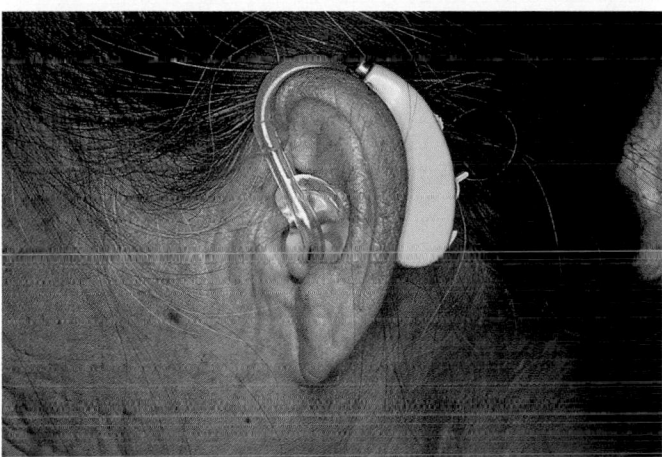

Fig. 40-8 Behind-the-ear hearing aid.

tages are that it is more visible (depending on hairstyle), may interfere with wearing eyeglasses and using the telephone, and is more difficult to keep in place during physical exercise. The care of a hearing aid involves routine cleaning, battery care, and proper insertion technique (Procedure 40-9). The box above summarizes tips for ongoing care and use.

NOSE CARE

The client can usually remove secretions from the nose by gently blowing into a soft tissue. This may be all the daily hygiene needed. The nurse cautions the client against harsh blowing that creates pressure capable of injuring the eardrum, nasal mucosa, and even sensitive eye structures. Bleeding from the nares is a key sign of harsh blowing, mucosal irritation, or dryness.

If the client cannot remove nasal secretions, the nurse assists by using a wet washcloth or a cotton tipped applicator moistened in water or saline. The applicator should never be inserted beyond the length of the cotton tip. Excessive nasal secretions can also be removed by suctioning. Nasal suctioning is contraindicated in nasal or brain surgery.

Care and Use of Hearing Aids
▪ Initially wear a hearing aid 15 to 20 minutes; then gradually increase time until 10 to 12 hours.   ▪ Once inserted, turn the aid slowly to one third to one half volume.   ▪ A whistling sound indicates incorrect ear mold insertion.   ▪ Adjust volume to a comfortable level for talking at a distance of 1 yard.   ▪ Do not wear aid under heat lamps; a hair dryer; or in very wet, cold weather.   ▪ Batteries last 1 week with daily wearing of 10 to 12 hours.   ▪ Remove or disconnect battery when not in use.   ▪ Replace ear molds every 2 or 3 years.

Modified from Ebersole P, Hess P: *Toward healthy aging*, ed 4, St Louis, 1995, Mosby.

When clients have feeding or suction tubes inserted through the nose, the nurse should change the tape anchoring the tube at least once a day (see Chapter 48). When the tape becomes moist from nasal secretions, the skin and mucosa can easily become macerated. The up-and-down movement of tubing causes tissue injury. The nurse should know how to tape tubing correctly to minimize tension or friction on the nares. When tissue injury occurs, it may be necessary to remove the tube and insert one through the other naris. The nurse should always cleanse the nares thoroughly around the tubing because secretions accumulate.

 ## Evaluation

Evaluation of eye, ear, and nose care must be individualized on the basis of the client's existing sensory function and desired outcomes. Hygienic care alone will not improve sensory function beyond a client's baseline level. Evaluation is ongoing. For example, for the diagnosis of bathing/hygiene self-care deficit, the expected outcome might include, "Client performs daily care for the eyes." After having the client attempt demonstration of eye care and finding the client has trouble manipulating equipment, the nurse may revise the plan and involve family members more directly.

CLIENT'S ROOM ENVIRONMENT

Attempting to make clients' rooms as comfortable as their home environments is one of the nurse's priorities. Clients with severe illnesses may be restricted to bed for many days. Likewise, clients immobilized by traction apparatus, casts, or monitoring equipment do not always enjoy the luxury of leaving their rooms as they wish. Clients hospitalized in semiprivate rooms must share the environment with other people. Chronically disabled persons living in nursing homes or skilled care facilities are often confined to rooms for long periods. Rooms should be comfortable, safe, and large enough to allow clients and visitors to move about freely. The nurse can control factors such as room temperature, ventilation, noise, and odors to create a more comfortable environment. Keeping rooms neat, clean, and orderly also contributes to a sense of well-being.

PROCEDURE 40-9

Care of a Behind-the-Ear Hearing Aid

STEPS	RATIONALE
1. Assess client's knowledge of and routines for cleansing and caring for hearing aid.	Determines client's understanding and need for health education. Adapts method of care to client's procedure.
2. Determine whether client can hear clearly with use of aid by talking slowly and clearly in normal voice tone.	Inability to hear may indicate faulty function of hearing aid.
3. Have client suggest any additional tips for care; explain that you are going to clean and replace hearing aid.	Client becomes uncomfortable when unable to hear clearly. Minimizes confusion and anxiety.
4. Assess whether hearing aid is working by removing from client's ear. Close battery case and turn volume slowly to high. Cup hand over earmold. If aid emits no sound, replace batteries and assess again.	Determines need for new battery. Feedback squeal will cause harsh whistling sound.
5. Check to be sure plastic connecting tube is not twisted or cracked.	Cracked or twisted tube prevents transmission of sound.
6. Check to see if earmold is cracked or has rough edges.	Can cause irritation to external ear canal.
7. Check for accumulation of cerumen around earmold and plugging of opening in mold.	Prevents clear sound reception and transmission.
8. Prepare necessary equipment and supplies:	
a. Emesis basin	Used to soak ear mold.
b. Mild soap and warm water	
c. Brush or wax loop	Used to clean plastic connecting tube.
d. Syringe needle (optional)	Used to clean opening in ear mold.
e. Soft towel	
f. Wash cloth	
g. Storage case	
h. Disposable gloves	
9. Clean hearing aid:	
a. Wash hands.	Reduces transmission of microorganisms.
b. Assemble supplies at bedside table or sink area.	Procedure can be performed without delays.
c. Wipe aid with soft wash cloth. Use wax loop or brush or tip of syringe needle to clean holes in aid. Do not jam wax into holes.	
d. Open battery door and allow it to air dry.	Increases battery life and allows moisture to evaporate (Shimon, 1992).
e. Wash ear canal with washcloth moistened in soap and water. Rinse and dry.	Removes cerumen and debris. Wax will prevent normal sound transmission. Soap may form residue that blocks opening in mold. Water droplets left in connecting tube could enter hearing aid and damage parts. Removes moisture and debris that can interfere with sound transmission and hearing aid function. Reassembly allows check of functioning.
f. If aid is to be stored, place in storage case labeled with client's name. If more than one aid, note right or left. Turn off when not in use.	
g. Store hearing aid in storage case if client is about to bathe, walk in rain, use hair dryer, sit under sun lamp or heat, go to surgery or major procedure, go to sleep, or is diaphoretic.	Protects hearing aid against damage and breakage.
10. Insert hearing aid:	
a. Check batteries (see Step 4); replace batteries as needed.	Necessary for proper sound amplification. Always change batteries over soft surface (e.g., towel or bed) to avoid breakage.
b. Turn aid off and turn volume control down.	Protects client from sudden exposure to sound.
c. Hold aid so that the bore—the long portion with the hole(s)—is at the bottom.	Proper fit ensures optimal sound transmission.
d. Insert bore into canal first. Use other hand to pull up and back on outer ear. Gently press and twist until mold feels snug.	

Care of a Behind-the-Ear Hearing Aid—cont'd

STEPS	RATIONALE
10. Insert hearing aid—cont'd	
e. Adjust volume gradually to comfortable level for talking to client in regular voice at a 1-1.25 m (3-4 ft) distance. Rotate volume control toward nose to increase volume.	Gradual adjustment prevents exposing client to harsh squeal or feedback. Client should hear nurse comfortably.
f. Remove soiled equipment from bedside. Dispose of used supplies. Wash hands.	Maintains clean environment and reduces risk of infection.
11. Return to client to assess whether hearing is clear or hearing aid is producing inappropriate feedback sound.	If earmold is not securely in place, it will squeal or not function.
12. Document that aid is removed and stored if client is going to surgery or special procedure.	Protects from liability of loss of hearing aid.
13. Report difficulties client has in communicating to nursing staff.	Improves continuity of care in communication techniques for client.
14. Note on nursing Kardex that client uses hearing aid.	Alerts personnel to hearing impairment.

Maintaining Comfort

In providing a comfortable environment, the nurse takes into account the client's age, the severity of his or her illness, and the client's level of normal daily activity. Depending on the client's age and physical condition, room temperature should be between 20° C and 23° C (68° F and 74° F). Infants, older adults, and the acutely ill may need a warmer temperature. However, some critically ill clients benefit from cooler temperatures to lower the body's metabolic demands. A client who is physically active will usually be more comfortable in a cool room.

A good ventilation system keeps stale air and odors from lingering in the room. Because drafts may occur as the air moves about the room, the nurse must protect acutely ill clients, infants, and older adults by ensuring that they are adequately dressed and covered with lightweight blankets. Clients who complain of excess drafts, despite the nurse's interventions, may need to be moved to a different room.

Good ventilation also reduces lingering odors caused by draining wounds, vomitus, bowel movements, and the failure to empty bedpans and urinals promptly. Body and breath odors may also be offensive to some people. Room deodorizers help by eliminating many unpleasant odors. Nurses should always empty and rinse bedpans or urinals promptly after use. Thorough hygienic measures are the best way to control body or breath odors. Hospitals are now required to maintain no-smoking policies on client care areas. The nurse should monitor visitors who attempt to smoke in clients' rooms. Only special orders by a physician will allow a client to smoke in a room. In such a situation, the client should have a private room.

Ill clients seem to be more sensitive to the noises commonly heard within a hospital environment, such as the clanging of metal equipment, wheelchairs or stretchers moving down halls, and loud talking and laughter at the nurse's station. The nurse should try to control the noise level by handling equipment properly, making sure that equipment is in proper working order, and controlling voice volume. The nurse also explains the source of any unfamiliar noises. Proper lighting is necessary for the safety and comfort of the client and health care workers. A brightly lit room is usually stimulating. When clients attempt to fall asleep, the nurse reduces lighting levels. Room lighting can be adjusted by closing or opening drapes, regulating overbed and floor lights, and closing or opening room doors.

Controlling stimuli within the room environment helps promote the client's feeling of security. A comfortable environment enhances the client's ability to gain needed rest and sleep so that all energy can be directed to recovery.

In the home environment, comfort as well as safety is important. Clients, having their own furniture and room decorations, are aided in promoting rest and needed sleep. If, however, the home environment is not conducive to rest and safety, the nurse should suggest ways to make it so. For example, removing throw rugs from the floors if clients have problems with their balance or sight.

Room Equipment

A typical room in a hospital or other health care facility (Fig. 40-9) contains certain basic pieces of furniture: overbed table, bedside stand, chairs, lights, and beds. Special equipment designed for comfort or positioning of clients includes special mattresses and foot boots. For some clients, foot boots may be necessary to keep the client's foot from developing foot drop or for the immobilization of an extremity (Fig. 40-10).

OVERBED TABLE

The overbed table rolls on wheels and can be adjusted to various heights over the bed or a chair. Usually, two storage areas are under the table top. The table provides ideal working space for the nurse performing procedures and also serves as a surface to place meal trays, toiletry items, and objects frequently used by the client.

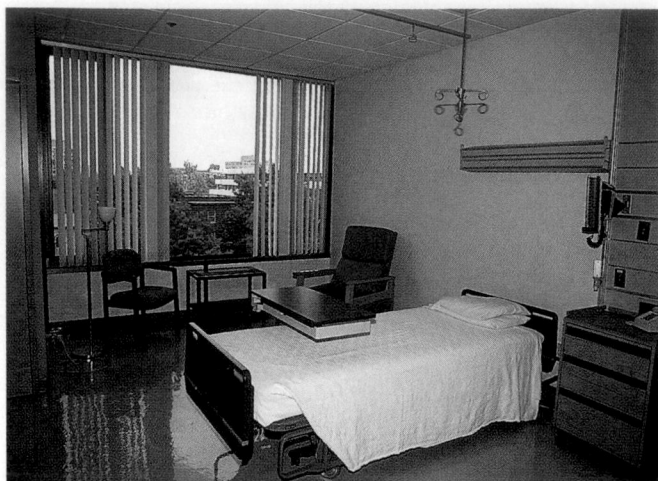

Fig. 40-9 Typical hospital room.

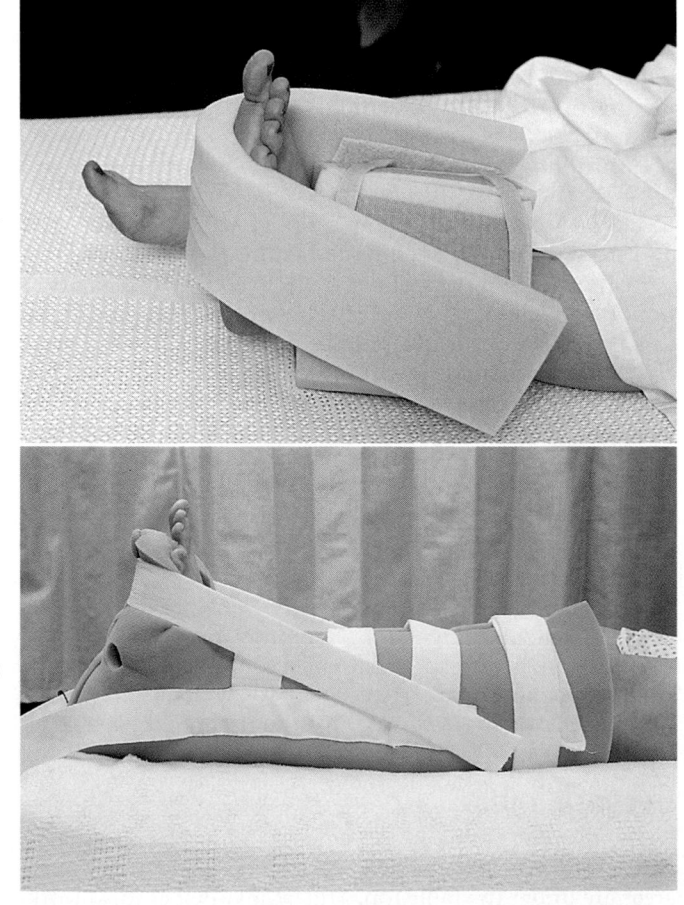

Fig. 40-10 A, Foot boot; **B,** foot boot with lower leg extension.

BEDSIDE STAND

The bedside stand is used to store the client's personal articles and hygienic equipment such as a bath basin, extra towels, and an emesis basin. The telephone, water pitcher, and drinking cup are commonly found on a bedside table.

CHAIRS

Most hospital rooms contain a straight-back chair and a lounge chair with arms. The lounge chair is used by the client and visitors and is placed at the foot of the bed or beside it. Straight-back chairs are convenient when temporarily transferring the client from the bed (e.g., during bedmaking). A straight-back chair is also more maneuverable than the larger lounge chair. Nurses often place clean linen on the chair or hang linen bags over the back.

LIGHTS

Each room usually has an overbed light and ceiling lights. Some may also have a floor or table lamp. Movable lights that extend over the bed from the wall should be positioned for easy reach but moved aside when not in use to prevent clients or staff from bumping their heads. Gooseneck or special examination lights are portable standing lights used to provide extra illumination during bedside procedures.

A call light is at each bedside (Fig. 40-11). When a client presses a button located on the side rail of the bed or at the end of an extension cord, a light goes on at the nurses' station or just outside the client's room. The call light signal indicates that a client needs assistance. The nurse should respond as soon as possible. In addition to call lights, most hospitals have intercoms that allow clients to talk to a staff person at the nurses' station. A few hospitals have beeper systems that relay calls from clients directly so that a digital message appears on the beeper attached to the nurse's uniform. Many hospitals also have emergency signal lights to call for assistance when clients are in trouble.

BEDS

Beds should be designed for comfort, safety, and adaptability for changing positions. The typical hospital bed con-

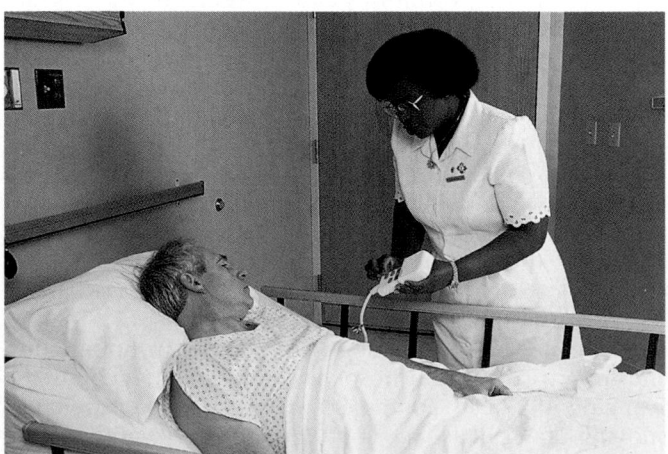

Fig. 40-11 Nurse instructing client on use of a call light.

Table 40-9	Common Bed Positions	
POSITION	**DESCRIPTION**	**USES**
Fowler's	Head of bed raised to angle of 45 degrees or more; semisitting position	Is preferred while client eats Is used during nasogastric tube insertion and nasotracheal suction Promotes lung expansion
Semi-Fowler's	Head of bed raised approximately 30 degrees; inclination less than Fowler's position	Promotes lung expansion
Trendelenburg's	Entire bed frame tilted with head of bed down	Is used for postural drainage Facilitates venous return in clients with poor peripheral perfusion
Reverse Trendelenburg's	Entire bed frame tilted with foot of bed down	Is used infrequently Promotes gastric emptying Prevents esophageal reflux
Flat	Entire bed frame horizontally parallel with floor	Is used for clients with vertebral injuries and in cervical traction Is used for clients who are hypotensive Is generally preferred by clients for sleeping

sists of a firm mattress on a metal frame that can be raised and lowered horizontally. The frame is divided into three sections, so the operator can raise and lower the head and foot of the bed, in addition to inclining the entire bed with the headboard up or down. Table 40-9 lists common bed positions. Most beds are powered by electrical motors, but some are run manually or by hydraulic power.

The position of a bed is usually changed by electrical controls on the side of the bed, at the foot of the bed, or in a bedside cable. Clients can thus raise or lower sections of the bed without expending much energy. Nurses instruct clients on the proper use of controls and caution them against raising the bed to a position that might cause harm. At its lowest level, a hospital bed is usually 65 to 70 cm (26 to 28 in) above the floor, whereas in the home, most beds are only 50 to 55 cm (20 to 22 in) high. The greater height of a hospital bed prevents undue musculoskeletal strain on the nurse and client. It is unnecessary for the nurse to reach across or bend down while caring for clients, and clients can move from the bed to a chair with minimal stress on

their hips and knees. The client's bed should never be left in a high position when the client is unattended.

Beds contain a number of safety features. Locks on the wheels or casters are used when the bed is stationary to prevent movement during the performance of a procedure. Side rails, located on both sides of a bed, protect clients from falls, help clients position themselves, and provide upper extremity support as a client gets out of bed. Side rails are adjustable, metal frames that raise and lower by pushing or pulling a knob. *The nurse never leaves the bedside when a side rail is lowered with the client in bed.* Each bed also has a special removable headboard. This is important when the medical team must have easy access to the client's head during cardiopulmonary resuscitation.

Most beds have firm, water-repellent mattresses. A mattress should have an even surface for comfort. Most mattresses have handles on the sides to be used when the mattresses are removed or turned over.

In the home, the clients may be using their standard bed or may need to alter it for their health needs. For example, to facilitate breathing, the client may have to insert a wedge under the head of the mattress, causing the head of the mattress to be elevated and assisting with respirations. In some cases, hospital style beds can be rented or purchased if there is a need.

Bedmaking. Making a bed is a responsibility of the nurse. The nurse keeps the bed clean and comfortable. This requires frequent inspections to be sure that linen is clean, dry, and wrinkle free. The nurse usually makes a bed after the client's bath, while the client is bathing and showering, or when the client is out of the room for tests or procedures. Throughout the day, the nurse straightens linen that becomes loose or wrinkled. The bed linen should also be checked for food particles after meals and for wetness or soiling. Linen that becomes wet or soiled should be changed.

When changing the bed linen, the nurse follows principles of asepsis by keeping soiled linen away from the uniform (Fig. 40-12). It is best to place soiled linen in special bags before discarding it in the hamper. To avoid air currents, which can spread microorganisms, the nurse never fans linen. Dirty linen should never be placed on the floor to prevent transmitting infection. If clean linen touches the floor, it is immediately discarded.

The nurse must use proper body mechanics during bedmaking. The bed should be raised to a comfortable working height toward the nurse's center of gravity before changing linen so that the nurse does not have to bend or stretch over the mattress. When making an occupied bed, the nurse should also use the principles of body mechanics while turning and repositioning the client (see Chapter 37).

The client's privacy, comfort, and safety are all important when making a bed. Using side rails, keeping call lights within the client's reach, and maintaining the proper bed position help promote comfort and safety. After making a bed, the nurse always returns it to the lowest horizontal position to prevent falls.

Whenever possible, the nurse should make the bed while it is unoccupied (Procedure 40-10). If the client is confined to bed, the nurse organizes bedmaking activities to conserve time and energy (Procedure 40-11). When making an unoccupied bed, the nurse follows the same basic principles as those for making an occupied bed.

An unoccupied bed can be open or closed. In an open bed, the top covers are folded back so that a client can easily get into bed. In a closed bed, the top sheet, blanket, and bedspread are drawn up to the head of the mattress and under the pillows. A closed bed is prepared in a hospital room before a new client is admitted to that room.

A surgical, recovery, or postoperative bed is a modified version of the unoccupied bed. The top bed linen is arranged for easy transfer of the client from a stretcher to the bed. The top sheets and spread are not tucked or mitered at the corners. Instead, the top sheets are folded to one side or fanfolded to the bottom third of the bed (Fig. 40-13). If a client is returning from surgery, the nurse always makes a complete linen change. After a client is discharged, all bed linen is sent to the laundry, the mattress and bed are cleansed by housekeeping personnel, and new bed linen is applied.

Linens. Before bedmaking, it is important to collect not only bed linens but also the client's personal items. Linens are pressed and folded to prevent the spread of microorganisms and to make bedmaking easier. Bed linens have a center crease that the nurse places in the center of the bed from the head to the foot. The linens unfold easily to the sides, with creases often fitting over the mattress edge. New linens are applied whenever there is soiling.

A complete linen change is not always necessary. The nurse may reuse the mattress pad, sheet, blanket, and bed pread for the same client if they are not wet or soiled.

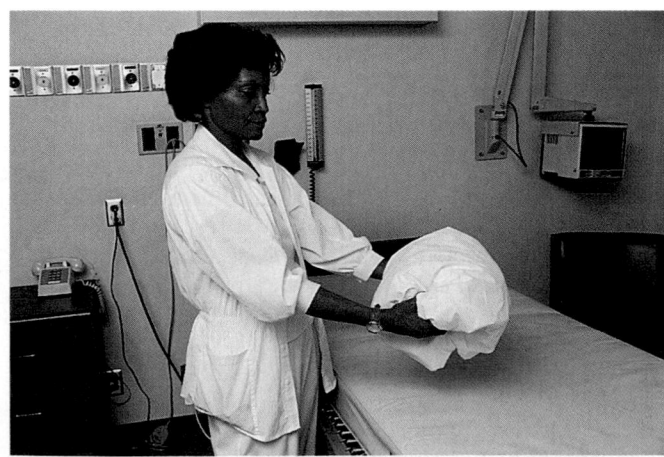

Fig. 40-12 Holding linen away from the uniform prevents contact with microorganisms.

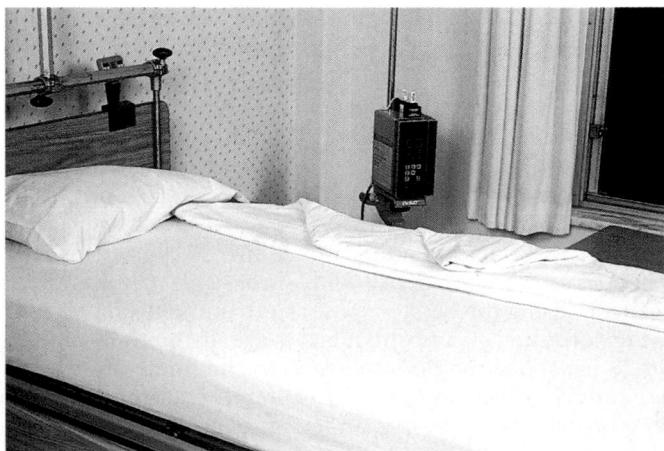

Fig. 40-13 Surgical or recovery bed.

Making an Unoccupied Bed

STEPS	RATIONALE
1. Assess potential for client being incontinent or having excess drainage on bed linen. Assess client's activity orders and physical mobility.	Determines need for protective waterproof pads or bath blankets on bed. Determines level of activity allowed, including whether client should be out of bed.
2. If client is in bed, explain that you wish to change bed while client is sitting up. Ask if client feels able to sit in chair. Assist client to chair if necessary.	Client should not feel inconvenienced by procedure. Client may feel anxious if uncomfortable or fatigued.
3. Prepare needed equipment and supplies:	
a. Linen bags	Collecting linen top to bottom in order of use makes it easier to make bed without delays.
b. Mattress pad (needs only be changed when soiled)	
c. Bottom sheet (flat or fitted)	
d. Drawsheet	Used to help lift or move client and to protect bottom sheet from soiling.
e. Top sheet (flat or fitted at foot)	
f. Blanket	
g. Bedspread	
h. Waterproof pads or bath blankets (optional)	Used to lay under client at points where drainage is expected. Reduces soiling of bed linen.
i. Pillow cases	
j. Bedside chair or table	Used to place linen on in order of use.
k. Disposable gloves (optional)	
4. Wash hands.	Reduces transmission of microorganisms.
5. Assemble equipment and arrange it on bedside chair or table. Remove all unnecessary equipment, such as overbed table.	Provides orderly procedure and ensures client comfort. Placing linen on clean surface minimizes spread of infection.
6. Lower side rail on your side of bed and remove call light. Adjust bed height to comfortable working position.	Provides easy access to bed. Minimizes strain on back and muscles.
7. On your side, loosen linen, starting at top of bed. Move along sides and then down toward foot. Move to other side of bed, lower side rail, and loosen all linen.	Makes linen easier to remove.
8. Remove bedspread and blanket separately by folding each into ball or folded square and discarding into linen bag if they are not to be reused. Do not allow uniform to come in contact with soiled linen. Avoid fanning or shaking linen.	Reduces transmission of microorganisms.
9. If spread or blanket is to be reused, fold each by grasping top edge with both hands, one hand at center, other hand at end. Fold top edge down, even with the bottom edge. Pick up spread at center and fold so that farthest side comes even with nearest side. Bring top and bottom edges together again. Place folded spread or blanket over back of chair.	Facilitates replacement and prevents wrinkling.
10. Remove soiled pillow cases by grasping closed end with one hand and slipping pillow out with other. Discard cases in linen bag and place pillows on table.	Pillows slide out easily, minimizing chance of contact with soiled linen.
11. Fold each piece of remaining bed linen into ball or folded square and discard into linen bag. Do not put linen on floor.	Attempting to fold all soiled linen at once creates bulky bundle that is difficult to discard and may easily come in contact with uniform.
12. Slide mattress toward head of bed. Wipe off any moisture on mattress with washcloth moistened in antiseptic solution; dry thoroughly.	If mattress slides toward foot of bed when head of bed is raised, it is difficult to tuck in linen. Reduces transmission of microorganisms.
13. Stand at side of bed where linen is placed. Spread mattress pad over mattress. Smooth out all wrinkles in pad.	Time is saved by making half of bed first and then moving to opposite side. Wrinkles or folds of linen are source of chronic irritation against client's skin.

Continued.

Making an Unoccupied Bed—cont'd

STEPS	RATIONALE

14. If using flat sheet as bottom sheet, unfold bottom sheet lengthwise and place vertical center crease of sheet lengthwise along center of bed. Fold sheet's top layer over toward opposite side of bed. Smooth bottom layer of sheet across mattress on your side; bring edge over side of mattress. Allow it to hang 25 cm (10 in) over mattress edge. Hem of bottom edge of sheet should lie seam down, even with bottom edge of mattress (see the illustration at right). Pull remaining top portion of sheet over top edge of mattress.

Method of unfolding linen saves time and energy. Making one side of bed at a time avoids excess movement. Proper placement of linen ensures that adequate length will be available to cover opposite side of bed. Keeping seam edge down eliminates source of irritation to client's skin. If bottom edge of sheet is not tucked in, it can later be changed without removing top linen.

15. While standing at head of the bed, miter top corner of bottom sheet:

Mitered corner is not loosened easily.

a. Face head of bed diagonally. Place hand that is away from head of bed under top corner of mattress near mattress edge and lift.

b. With other hand, tuck top edge of bottom sheet smoothly under mattress so that side edges of sheet above and below mattress would meet if brought together.

c. Face side of bed and pick up top edge of sheet approximately 45 cm (18 in) down from top of mattress (see the illustrations below).

d. Lift sheet and lay it on top of mattress to form neat, triangular fold, with lower base of triangle even with mattress side edge (see the illustration on p. 1077).

e. Tuck lower edge of sheet, hanging free below mattress, under mattress. Tuck with your palms down. Do this without pulling triangular fold (see the illustrations on p. 1077).

f. Hold portion of sheet covering side edge of mattress in place with one hand. With other hand, pick up top of triangular linen fold and bring it down over side of mattress. Tuck this portion of sheet under mattress (see the illustrations on p. 1077).

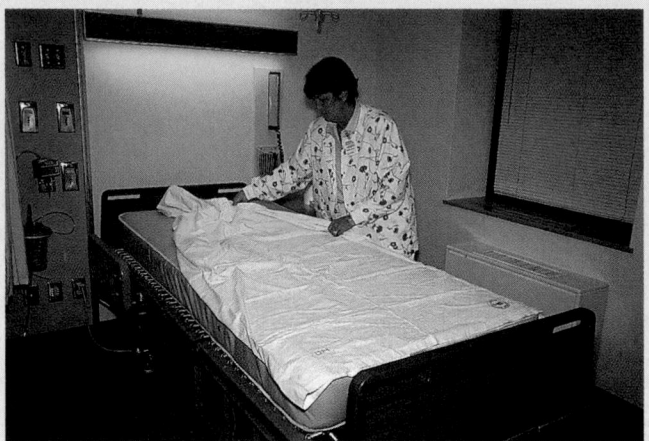

Step 14

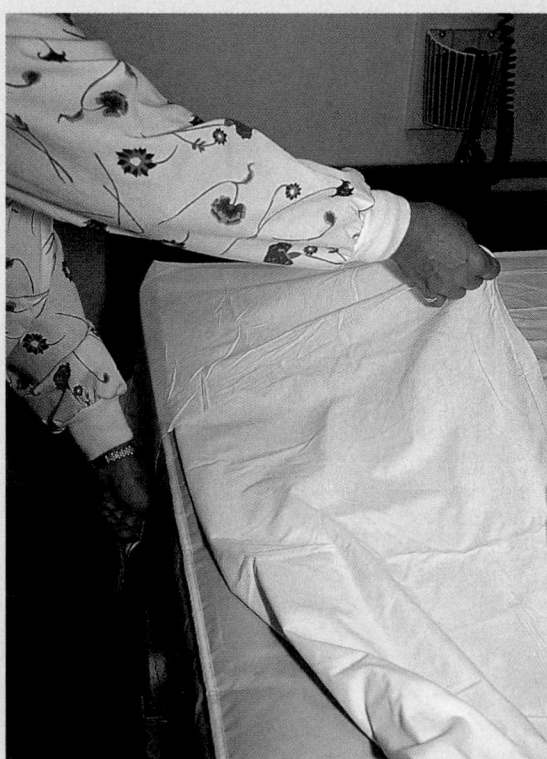

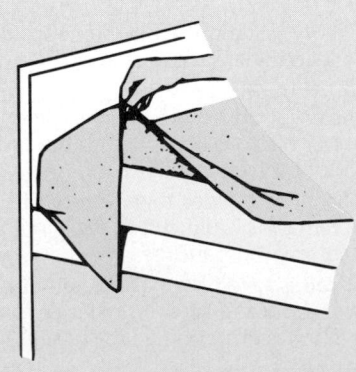

Step15c

Making an Unoccupied Bed—cont'd

STEPS	RATIONALE

16. Tuck remaining portion of sheet under mattress. Keep linen smooth (see the illustration below).

Folds of linen can irritate client's skin.

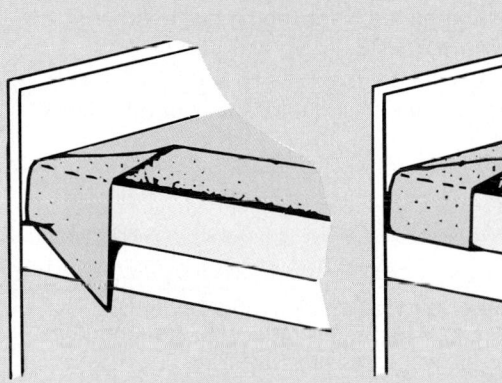
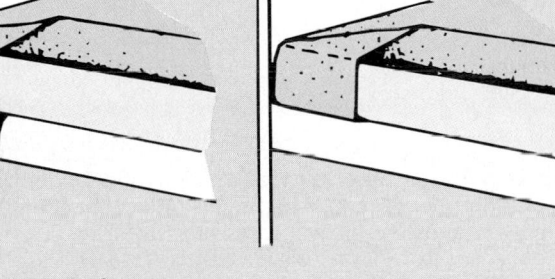

Step 15d

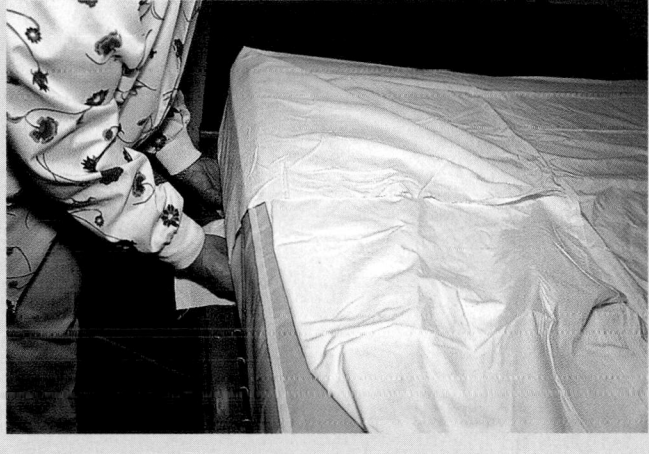

Step 15e

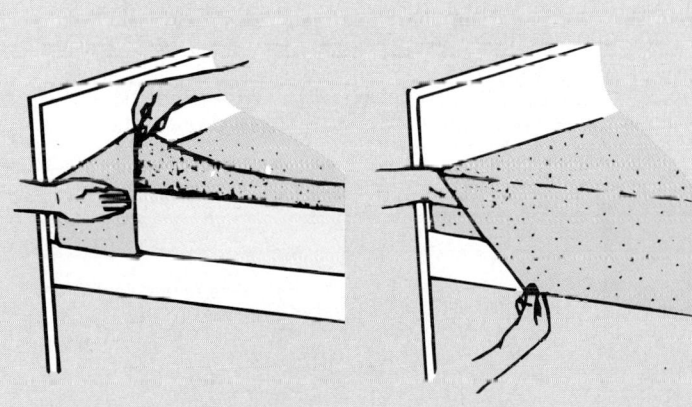

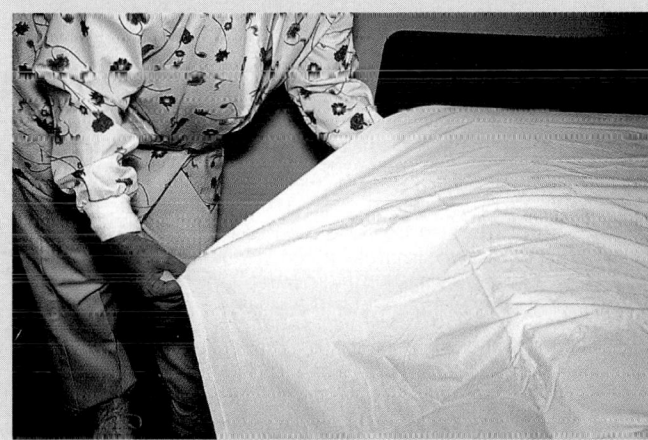

Step 15f

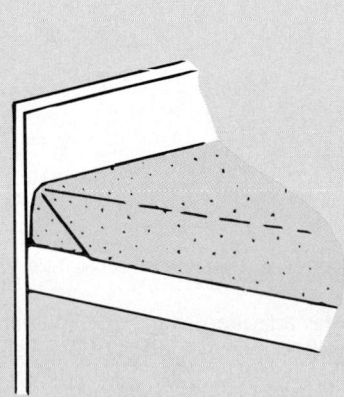

Step 15f

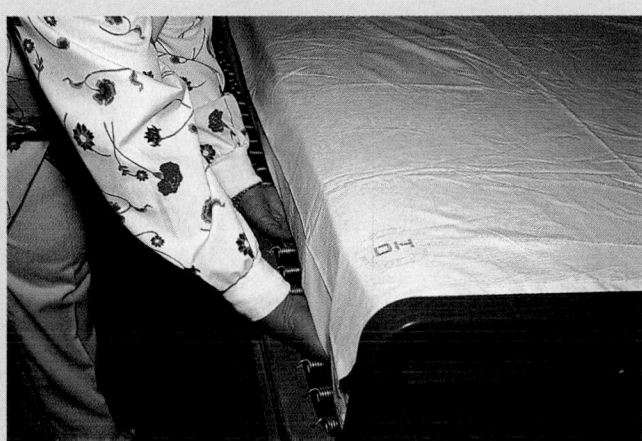

Step 16

Continued.

PROCEDURE 40-10

Making an Unoccupied Bed—cont'd

STEPS	RATIONALE

17. OPTIONAL: Open draw-sheet so that it unfolds in half. Lay center fold lengthwise along middle of the bed. Fanfold top layer at center of bed. Smooth bottom layer of draw-sheet out over mattress. Tuck excess edge under mattress, keeping palms down.

Draw-sheet is used to lift and reposition client. Placement under client's torso distributes most of body weight over sheet. Tucking excess under mattress anchors sheet in place to prevent sliding and wrinkling.

18. Move to opposite side of bed.

One side of bed is completed before you move to other side.

19. Spread fanfolded bottom sheet smoothly over edge of mattress from head to foot of bed.

Wrinkles can cause irritation.

20. Miter top corner of bottom sheet (see Step 15). When tucking corner, be sure sheet is taut.

Taut sheet eliminates wrinkles and folds that can rub client's skin.

21. Facing side of bed, grasp remaining edge of bottom sheet, lean back, keeping your back straight, and pull as you tuck excess linen tightly under mattress. Proceed from head to foot of bed. (Avoid lifting mattress during tucking to ensure tight fit.)

Proper use of body mechanics while tucking linen prevents injury.

22. Smooth folded draw-sheet over bottom sheet. Grasp edge of drawsheet with palms down, lean back, and tuck sheet under mattress. Tuck first at middle, then at top, and then at bottom

Tucking first at top or bottom may pull sheet sideways, causing poor fit. Loose bedsheets reduce friction and help prevent pressure ulcers (Rousseau, 1988).

23. If needed apply waterproof pad or bath blanket over draw-sheet.

Pad collects body secretions and drainage, protecting linen from becoming soiled.

24. Move to side of bed where linen is located. Place top sheet over bed with vertical center fold lengthwise down middle of bed. Open sheet out from head to foot, being sure top edge of sheet is seam up and even with top edge of mattress. Spread excess sheet over bottom edge of mattress. (Do not fan top sheet over bed.)

Placement ensures equal distribution of sheet over bed. Positioning sheet with seam up prevents irritation of client's skin. Fanning creates air currents, which can spread microorganisms throughout room.

25. OPTIONAL: Make horizontal toe pleat: stand at foot of bed and from fold in sheet 5-10 cm (2-4 in) across bed. Pull sheet up from bottom to make fold. Fold should be approximately 15 cm (6 in) from bottom edge of mattress (see the illustration).

Allows for free movement of client's feet and prevents friction against surface of toes.

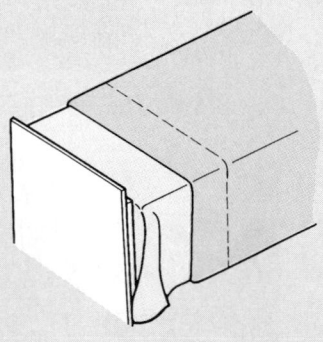

Step 25

26. Tuck in remaining portion of sheet on one side of foot of mattress (optional).

Anchors top sheet so that client can move freely.

27. Place blanket on bed, unfolding it so that crease runs lengthwise along middle of bed. Top edge should be parallel with edge of top sheet and 15-20 cm (6-8 in) down from mattress top edge. Bottom edge should hang over mattress. Spread blanket evenly over bed.

Blanket provides adequate warmth. Cuff will be formed with sheet folded over top edge of blanket and spread.

Making an Unoccupied Bed—cont'd

STEPS	RATIONALE
28. Place spread over bed according to Step 7. Be sure that top edge of spread extends about 2.5 cm (1 in) above blanket's edge. Then tuck top edge of spread over and under top edge of blanket.	Spread gives bed neat appearance and provides extra warmth.
29. Make cuff by running edge of top sheet down over top edge of blanket and spread.	Smooth cuff protects client's face from irritation.
30. Standing on one side at foot of bed, lift mattress corner slightly with one hand and with other hand tuck top sheet, blanket, and spread under mattress. Be sure you have not pulled out toe pleat of sheet so that linens are loose enough for client to move.	Pressure ulcers can develop on client's toes and heels if feet rub between tight-fitting bed sheets. Lifting mattress too high can loosen bottom linen.
31. Make modified mitered corner with top sheet, blanket and spread: pick up side edge of top sheet, blanket, and spread approximately 45 cm (18 in) up from foot of mattress. Lift linens to form triangular fold and lay it on bed. Tuck loose edge hanging down under side of mattress. Pick up triangular fold and bring it down over mattress, holding linen along side of mattress. Do not tuck tip of triangle (see the illustration).	Modified mitered corner secures top linen but keeps even edge of top sheet, blanket, and spread draped over mattress.

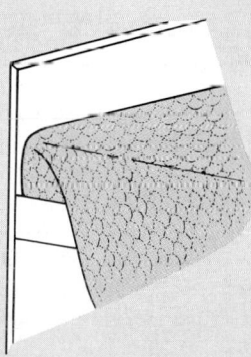

Step 31

STEPS	RATIONALE
32. Go to other side: spread sheet, blanket, and spread evenly. Fold top edge of spread over blanket and make cuff with top sheet (see Step 33). Make modified mitered corner at foot of bed (see Step 35).	Saves time and energy by completing one side of bed at time.
33. Apply clean pillowcase. With one hand, grasp pillowcase at center of closed end. Gather case, turning it inside out over hand holding it. With same hand, pick up middle of one end of pillow. Pull pillow case down over pillow with other hand. Be sure corners of case fit evenly over pillow.	Eases sliding of case smoothly over pillow.
34. Position pillows at center of head of bed.	Maintains neat appearance.
35. Place call light within client's reach and return bed to comfortable height.	Provides for client safety.
36. Fold back top covers to one side or fanfold them to bottom third of bed.	Eases client's return to bed.
37. Rearrange furniture and place personal items within easy reach.	Promotes sense of well-being.
38. Discard dirty linen in linen hamper or chute. Wash hands.	Prevents transmission of microorganisms.
39. Evaluate client's tolerance to sitting up in chair; compare heart rate to previous resting rate. Ask if client feels weak, dizzy, or fatigued; assess blood pressure if client complains of dizziness or weakness.	Client's inability to tolerate exertion, even low levels of exercise, may be reflected in changes in vital signs or subjective report of symptoms.
40. Assist client in returning to bed as necessary.	

Making an Occupied Bed

STEPS	RATIONALE
1. Determine potential for client being incontinent or having excess drainage on bed linen.	Determines need for protective waterproof pads or extra bath blankets on bed.
2. Check chart for orders or specific precautions for movement and positioning.	Ensures client safety and use of proper body mechanics.
3. Explain procedure to client, noting that client will be asked to turn on side to roll over linen.	Minimizes anxiety and promotes client cooperation.
4. Prepare needed equipment and supplies:	
a. Linen bags	Collecting linen top to bottom in order of use makes it easier to make bed without delays.
b. Bath blanket	Provides warmth.
c. Mattress pad (needs only be changed when soiled)	
d. Bottom sheet (flat or fitted)	
e. Draw-sheet	Used to help lift or move client at points where drainage is expected. Reduces soiling of bed linen.
f. Top sheet (flat or fitted at foot)	
g. Blanket	
h. Bedspread	
i. Pillow cases	
j. Waterproof pads (optional)	Lay under client at points where drainage is expected. Reduces soiling of bed linen.
k. Bedside chair or table	
l. Disposable gloves (optional)	
5. Wash hands.	Reduces transmission of microorganisms.
6. Assemble equipment and arrange it on bedside chair or table. Remove unnecessary equipment.	Assembling all equipment provides for smooth procedure and ensures comfort. Placing linen on clean surface minimizes spread of infection.
7. Draw room curtain around bed or close door.	Maintains client's privacy, thus promoting emotional and physical comfort.
8. Adjust bed height to comfortable working position. Lower side rail on your side of bed. Remove call light.	Minimizes strain on back. It is easier to remove and apply linen evenly to bed in flat position. Provides easy access to bed and linen.
9. Loosen top linen sheet at foot of bed.	Makes linen easier to remove.
10. Remove bedspread and blanket separately and place them in linen bag (if not to be reused). Do not allow linen to contact uniform. Do not fan or shake linen.	Reduces transmission of microorganisms.
11. If blanket and spread are to be reused, fold by bringing top and bottom edges together. Fold farthest side over onto nearer bottom edges. Bring top and bottom edges together again. Place folded linen over back of chair.	Folding method facilitates replacement and prevents wrinkles.
12. Cover client with bath blanket: unfold bath blanket over top sheet. Ask client to hold top edge of bath blanket. If client is unable to help, tuck top of bath blanket under shoulder. Grasp top sheet under bath blanket at client's shoulders and bring sheet down to foot of bed. Remove sheet and discard it in linen bag.	Provides warmth and keeps body parts covered during linen removal.
13. With assistance from another nurse, slide mattress toward head of bed.	If mattress slides toward foot of bed when head of bed is raised, it is difficult to tuck linen and is uncomfortable for client.
14. Position client on side on far side of bed, facing away. Adjust pillow under head. Be sure side rail is up.	Moving client to side provides space for placement of clean linen. Side rail ensures client's safety.
15. Loosen bottom linens, moving from head to foot.	Prepares for removal of all bottom linen simultaneously.
16. Remove bottom linen; fanfold bottom sheet and draw sheet toward client: first draw-sheet, then bottom sheet. Tuck edges of linen just under buttocks, back, and shoulders. Do not fanfold mattress pad if it is to be reused (see the illustration on p.1081).	Provides maximum work space for placing clean linen. Later, when client turns to other side, soiled linen can be easily removed.

Making an Occupied Bed—cont'd

STEPS	RATIONALE

17. Wipe off any moisture on the exposed mattress with towel and appropriate disinfectant.

Reduces transmission of microorganisms.

18. Apply clean linen to exposed half of bed:

a. Place clean mattress pad on bed by folding it lengthwise with center crease in middle of bed. Fanfold top layer over mattress. (If pad is reused, simply smooth out any wrinkles.)

Applying linen over bed in successive layers minimizes energy and time used in bedmaking.

b. Unfold bottom sheet lengthwise so that center crease is situated lengthwise along center of bed. Fanfold sheet's top layer toward center of bed alongside client. Smooth bottom layer of sheet over mattress and bring edge over near side of mattress (see the illustration below). Allow sheet's edge to hang about 25 cm (10 in) over mattress edge. Lower hem of bottom sheet should lie seam down and even with bottom edge of mattress.

Proper positioning of linen on one side ensures that adequate linen will be available to cover opposite side of bed. Keeping seam edges down eliminates irritation to client's skin.

19. Miter bottom sheet at head of bed:

a. Face head of bed diagonally. Place hand away from head of bed under top corner of mattress, near mattress edge, and lift.

Mitered corner cannot be loosened easily even if client moves about frequently in bed.

b. With other hand, tuck top edge of bottom sheet smoothly under mattress so that side edges of sheet above and below mattress would meet if brought together.

c. Face side of bed and pick up top edge of sheet at approximately 45 cm (18 in) from top of mattress.

d. Lift sheet and lay it on top of mattress to form neat triangular fold, with lower base of triangle even with mattress side edge.

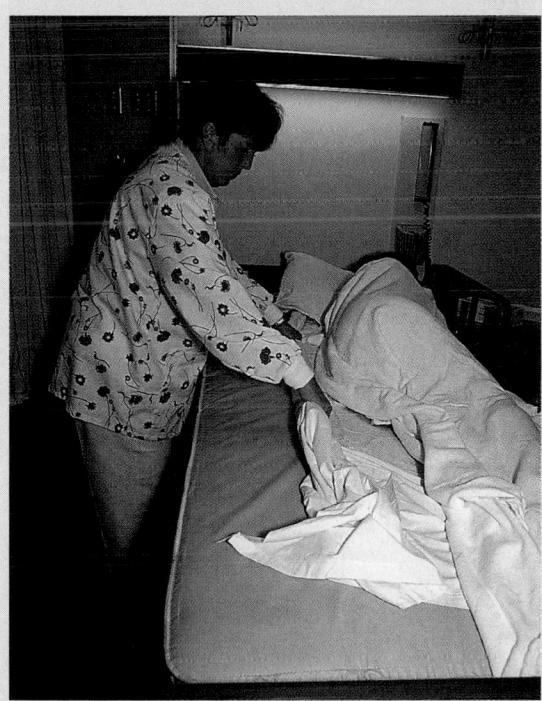

Step 16

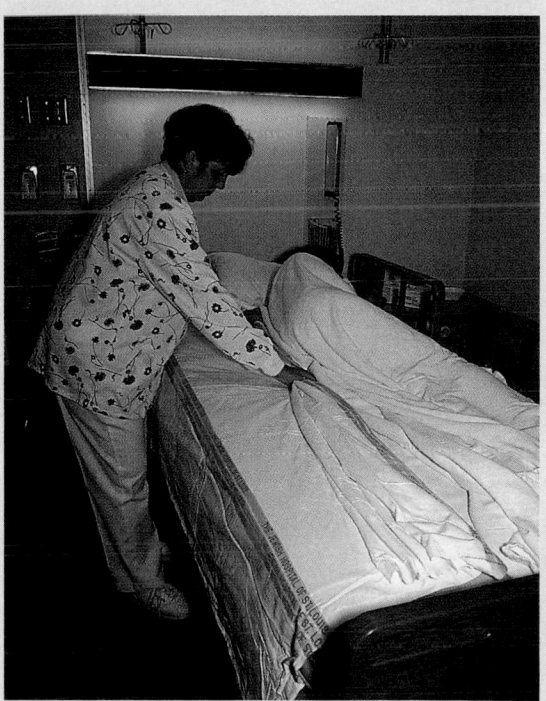

Step 18b

Making an Occupied Bed—cont'd

STEPS	RATIONALE

19. Miter bottom sheet at head of bed—cont'd

   e. Tuck lower edge of sheet, which is hanging free below mattress, under mattress. Tuck with palms down. Do this without pulling triangular fold.

   f. Hold portion of sheet covering side of mattress in place with one hand. With other hand, pick up top of triangular linen fold and bring it down over side of mattress. Tuck this portion under mattress.

20. Tuck remaining portion of sheet under mattress, moving toward foot of bed. Keep linen smooth (see the illustration below).   *Folds of linen are source of irritation.*

21. OPTIONAL: Open draw-sheet so that it unfolds in half. Lay center fold along middle of bed lengthwise and position sheet so that it will be under buttocks and torso (see the illustration below). Fanfold top layer toward client with edge along back. Smooth bottom layer out over mattress and tuck excess edge under mattress (keep palms down).   *Draw-sheet is used to lift and reposition client. Placement under client's torso distributes most of client's body weight over sheet.*

22. Place waterproof pad over draw-sheet with center fold against client's side. Fanfold far half toward client.   *Used to protect bed linen from soiling.*

23. Raise side rail on working side and go to other side.   *Maintains client's safety during turning.*

24. Lower side rail. Assist client to roll slowly onto other side, over folds of linen (see the illustration on p. 1083).   *Exposes opposite side of bed for removal of soiled linen and placement of clean linen.*

25. Loosen edges of soiled linen from under mattress.   *Makes linen easier to remove.*

26. Remove soiled linen by folding it into bundle or square, with soiled side turned in. Discard it in linen bag.   *Reduces transmission of microorganisms.*

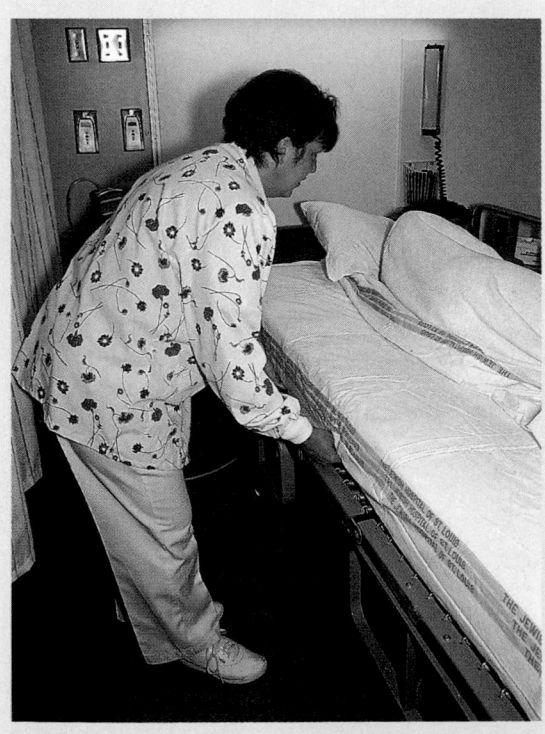

Step 20

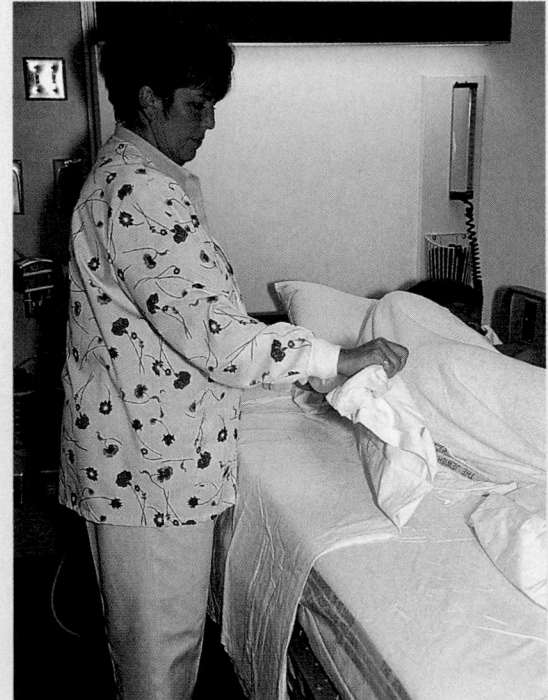

Step 21

Making an Occupied Bed—cont'd

STEPS	RATIONALE
27. Spread clean, fanfolded linen smoothly over edge of mattress from head to foot of bed (see the illustration below).	Smooth linen will not irritate client's skin.
28. Assist client in rolling back into supine position. Reposition pillow.	Maintains client's comfort.
29. Miter top corner of bottom sheet (see Step 19). When tucking corner, be sure sheet is smooth and free of wrinkles.	Wrinkles and folds can cause mechanical irritation to skin.
30. Facing side of bed, grasp remaining edge of bottom sheet. Lean back, keep back straight, and pull as you tuck excess linen under mattress. Proceed from head to foot of bed. (Avoid lifting mattress during tucking to ensure fit.)	Proper use of body mechanics while tucking linen prevents injury.
31. Smooth fanfolded draw-sheet out over bottom sheet. Grasp edge of sheet with palms down, lean back, and tuck sheet under mattress. Tuck from middle to top and then to bottom.	Tucking first at top or bottom may pull sheet sideways, causing poor fit.
32. Place top sheet over client with center fold lengthwise down middle of bed. Open sheet from head to foot and unfold it over client (see the illustration on p. 1084).	Sheet should be equally distributed over bed by correctly positioning center fold.
33. Ask client to hold clean top sheet, or tuck sheet around client's shoulders. Remove bath blanket and discard it in linen bag.	Sheet prevents exposure of body parts. Having client hold sheet encourages client participation in care.
34. Place blanket on bed, unfolding it so that crease runs lengthwise along middle of bed. Unfold blanket to cover client. Top edge should be parallel with edge of top sheet and 15-20 cm (6-8 in) from top sheet's edge.	Blanket should be placed to cover client completely and provide adequate warmth.

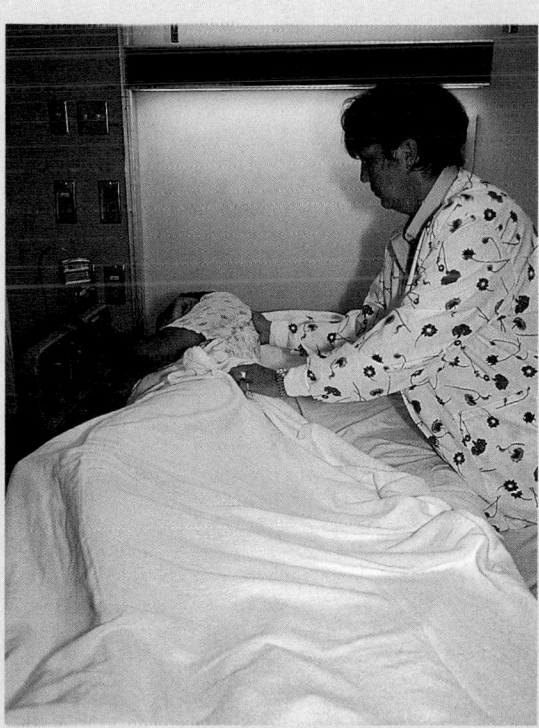

Step 24

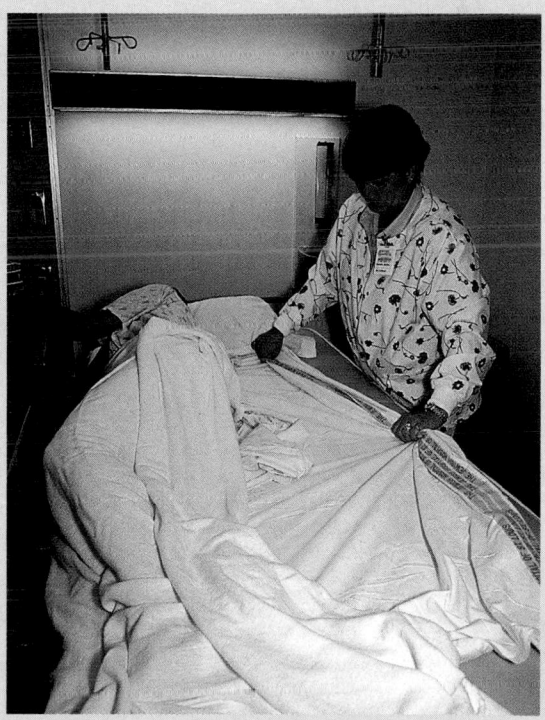

Step 27

Continued.

Making an Occupied Bed—cont'd

STEPS	RATIONALE

35. Place spread over bed according to Step 34. Be sure that top edge of spread extends about 2.5 cm (1 in) above blanket's edge. Tuck top edge of spread over and under top edge of blanket.

Gives bed neat appearance and provides extra warmth.

36. Make cuff by turning edge of top sheet down over top edge of blanket and spread.

Protects client's face from rubbing against blanket or spread.

37. Standing on one side at foot of bed, lift mattress corner slightly with one hand and tuck top linens under mattress. Top sheet and blanket are tucked under together. Be sure that linens are loose enough to allow movement of client's feet. (You may make horizontal toe pleat [Procedure 39-10, Step 39-10].)

Makes neat-appearing bed. Pressure ulcers can develop on client's toes and heels from feet rubbing between tight-fitting bed sheets.

38. Make modified mitered corner with top sheet, blanket, and spread:

a. Pick up side edge of top sheet, blanket, and spread approximately 45 cm (18 in) from foot of mattress. Lift linens to form triangular fold and lay it on bed.

Secures top linen but keeps even edge of blanket and top sheet draped over mattress.

b. Tuck lower edge of sheet, which is hanging free below mattress, under mattress. Do not pull triangular fold.

c. Pick up triangular fold and bring it down over mattress while holding linen in place along side of mattress. Do not tuck tip of triangle.

39. Raise side rail. Make other side of bed; spread sheet, blanket, and bedspread out evenly. Fold top edge of spread over blanket and make cuff with top sheet (see Step 37); make modified mitered corner at foot of bed (see Step 38).

Side rail protects client from accidental falls.

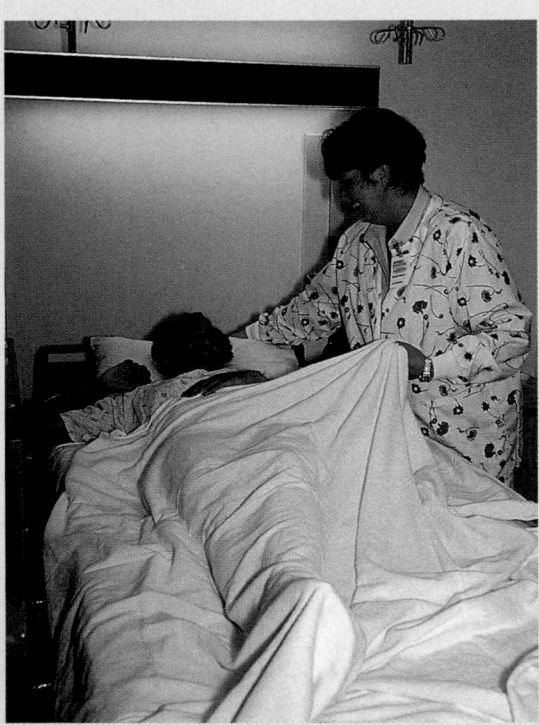

Step 32

Making an Occupied Bed—cont'd

STEPS	RATIONALE
40. Change pillowcase:	
a. Have client raise head. While supporting neck remove pillow. Allow client to lower head.	Support of neck muscles prevents injury during flexion and extension of neck.
b. Remove soiled case by grasping pillow at open end with one hand and pulling case over pillow with other hand. Discard case in linen bag.	Pillows slide out easily, thus minimizing contact with soiled linen.
c. Grasp clean pillowcase at center of closed end. Gather case, turning it inside out over hand holding it. With same hand pick up middle of one end of pillow. Pull pillowcase down over pillow with other hand.	Eases sliding of pillowcase over pillow.
d. Be sure pillow corners fit evenly in corners of pillowcase. Place pillow under client's head.	Poorly fitting case constricts fluffing and expansion of pillow. Promotes comfort.
41. Place call light within client's reach and return bed to comfortable position. Lower bed.	Ensures safety and comfort.
42. Open room curtains. Rearrange furniture. Place personal items within easy reach on overbed table or bedside stand. Return bed to comfortable height.	Promotes sense of well-being.
43. Discard dirty linen in hamper or chute; wash hands.	Prevents transmission of microorganisms.

■ KEY CONCEPTS ■

▶ Hygiene is a personal matter, and the nurse considers all factors influencing personal hygiene routine, be they in the health care setting or the home setting.

▶ The nurse assumes responsibility for providing clients' daily hygienic needs if they are unable to care for themselves adequately.

▶ Providing hygienic care gives the nurse the opportunity to assess all external body surfaces as well as the client's emotional state.

▶ The nurse must convey respect to the client during hygiene procedures by displaying a caring attitude.

▶ Assisting the client with daily hygienic needs or providing care for him or her allows the nurse to use teaching and communication skills to develop a meaningful, therapeutic relationship with the client.

▶ The client's personal preferences must always be considered as the nurse plans the client's daily hygienic care.

▶ The nurse must maintain the client's privacy and comfort when providing daily care.

▶ During assessment of the skin and oral mucosa, the nurse observes characteristics most influenced by hygienic measures.

▶ Clients who are immobilized, poorly nourished, and who have reduced sensation or peripheral circulation are at risk for altered skin integrity.

▶ Gloves should be worn by nurses during hygienic care when the risk of contacting body fluids is high.

▶ Techniques used during tepid sponging are designed to minimize the risk of a client chilling.

▶ Clients with diabetes require special consideration when a nurse provides skin, nail, and foot care.

▶ When administering oral care to unconscious clients, the nurse takes measures to prevent them from aspirating fluid into their lungs.

▶ Clients who wear contact lenses must learn proper self-care techniques to avoid corneal injury, or else this must be taught to a family member or significant other.

▶ The evaluation of hygienic care is based on the client's expression of a sense of comfort, relaxation, well-being, and an understanding of personal hygienic techniques.

▶ There may be need to evaluate and adapt the home environment to make sure hygienic outcomes are obtained.

▶ Meeting the hygienic needs of clients is a positive measure to promote health.

■ KEY TERMS ■

Acne, p. 1021

Alopecia, p. 1053

Apocrine glands, p. 1019

Buccal, p. 1043

Cerumen, p. 1019

Cheilosis, p. 1046

Dermis, p. 1018

Eccrine glands, p. 1019

Epidermis, p. 1018

Gingivitis, p. 1046

Glossitis, p. 1046

Halitosis, p. 1046

Hirsutism, p. 1021

Hygiene, p. 1017

Maceration, p. 1021

Mastication, p. 1043

Melanin, p. 1018

Neuropathy, p. 1039

Oral hygiene, p. 1043

Partial bed bath, p. 1024

Perineal care, p. 1031

Periodontal disease, p. 1046

Plaque, p. 1046

Podiatrist, p. 1042

Pyorrhea, p. 1046

Stomatitis, p. 1046

Stratum corneum, p. 1018

Vernix caseosa, p. 1037

■ CRITICAL THINKING EXERCISES ■

1. You are assigned to care for a 77-year-old woman who has been hit by a car while crossing the street. She has been admitted for a fractured pelvis and fractures of her left femur and humerus. She is a non-English-speaking Russian Jew who recently immigrated. Identify the factors you need to consider when planning hygienic care for this person. What additional information would you need before implementing care for her?

2. Mr. Johannson is a 43-year-old insulin-dependent diabetic who has been admitted for an infected ulcer on his right foot. Describe the nurse's assessment of Mr. Johannson's self-care practices. What should the nurse do, and why?

3. Mrs. Taylor, who is 83 years old, has been admitted to the hospital for a total hip replacement for a fracture of the femoral neck of her right femur. Her history reveals that she had a cerebrovascular accident 2 years before and has residual weakness on her left side. Given her age, history, and current condition, discuss how you would intervene postoperatively to prevent skin breakdown. Discuss the reasons for your decisions.

REFERENCES

Agency for Health Care Policy and Research (AHCPR): *Pressure ulcers in adults: prediction and prevention*, Pub No 92-0047, 92-0050. Rockville, Md, 1992, Public Health Service, US Department of Health and Human Services.

Andrews MM, Boyle JS: *Transcultural concepts in nursing care*, Philadelphia, 1995, Lippincott.

Barnes SH: Patient and family education for the patient with a pressure necrosis, *Nurs Clin North Am* 22:463, 1987.

Barkauskas V et al: *Health and physical assessment*, St Louis, 1994, Mosby.

Christensen MH et al: How to care for the diabetic foot, *Am J Nurs* 91(3):50, 1991.

Coleman GC, Nelson JF: *Principles of oral diagnosis*, St Louis, 1993, Mosby.

Crosby C: Methods in mouth care, *Nurs Times* 85(35): 38, 1989.

Danielson KH: Oral care and older adults, *J Gerontol Nurs* 14:6, 1988.

de Liefde B, Ritchie GR: Evaluation in dental public health in New Zealand, *NZ Dent J* 80:8, 1984.

Ebersole P, Hess P: *Toward healthy aging*, ed 4, St Louis, 1995, Mosby.

Graham K et al: Reducing the incidence of stomatitis using a quality assessment and improve approach *Cancer Nurs* 16(2):117, 1993.

Greifzu S, Radjeski D, Winnick B: Oral care is part of cancer care, *RN* 53:43, 1990.

Harley JR: Preventing diabetic foot disease, *Nurs Pract* 18(10):37, 1993.

Ismail AI, Szpunar SM: The prevalence of total tooth loss, dental caries, and periodontal disease among Mexican Americans, Cuban Americans, and Puerto Ricans: findings from HHANES 1982-1984, *Am J Public Health* 80(suppl):66, 1990.

Jordan J, Nickerson D: Hygiene. In Guthrie D, Guthrie R, editors: *Nursing management of diabetes mellitus*, ed 2, St Louis, 1982, Mosby–Year Book.

Kahn R: Renewing commitment to oral hygiene...teaching the elderly learner, *Geriatr Nurs* 7(5):244, 1986.

Kim MJ, McFarland GK, McLane AM: *Pocket guide to nursing diagnosis*, ed 6, St Louis, 1995, Mosby.

Kruger S, Guthrie D: Foot care: knowledge retention and self-care practices, *Diabetic Ed* 18:6, 1992.

Lewis MN, Collier I: *Medical-surg nurs*, ed 3, St Louis, 1996, Mosby.

Maklebust J: Pressure ulcer update, *RN* 41(12):56, 1991.

Marshall C: *From here to maternity*, Los Angeles, California, 1991, Prima Publishing.

Mosby's medical, nursing, and allied health dictionary, ed 4, St Louis, 1994, Mosby.

National Pressure Ulcer Advisory Panel (NPUAP): Pressure ulcer incidence, economics, risk assessment: consensus development conference statement, *Decubitus* 2(2):24, 1989.

Newman J: Evaluation of sponging to reduce body temperature in febrile children, *Can Med Assoc J*, 132:641, 1985.

Osterman HM, Stuck RM: The aging foot, *Orthop Nurs* 9:43, 1990.

OxyFlow EW: *Rigid permeable contact lens: instructions for wearers*, Little Rock, Ark, 1987, PDC Contact Lens Network.

Pettigrew D: Investing in mouth care, *Geriatr Nurs* 10:22, 1989.

Phipps W et al: *Medical surgical nursing concepts and clinical practice*, ed 5, St Louis, 1995, Mosby.

Pires M, Mueller A: Detection and management of early tissue pressure indications: a pictorial essay, *Progressions* 3(3):3, 1991.

Poland JM: Comparing Moi-Stir to lemon glycerine swabs, *Am J Nurs* 87:422, 1987.

Rakow PL: Where have all the dropouts gone? *J Ophthal Nurs Technol* 9:223, 1990.

Rousseau P: Pressure sores in the aged: a preventable problem? *Continuing Care* July:38, 1988.

Rozier RG, Beck JD: Epidemiology of oral diseases, *Curr Opin Dentistry*, 1:308, 1991.

Smeltzer S, Bare B: *Brunner and Suddarth's textbook of medical surgical nursing*, ed 7, Philadelphia, 1992, Lippincott.

US Department of Health and Human Services Public Health Service: *Healthy people 2000: summary report*, Boston, 1992, Jones & Bartlett.

Wagnild G, Manning R: Convey respect during bathing procedures, *J Gerontol Nurs* 11(12):6, 1985.

Weiss SJ: Psychophysiologic effects of care giver touch on incidence of cardiac dysrhythmias, *Heart Lung* 15(5):495, 1986.

Wong DL: Whaley and Wong's *nursing care of infants and children,* ed 5, St Louis, 1995, Mosby.

Young M, Young C: Footwork, *Nurs Times* 90(7):70, 1994.

ADDITIONAL READINGS

Barbour-Randall L: Assessment promotes proper oral care *Oncol Nurs Forum* 19(6):940, 1992.

Beltramba E: Nurse educators: link to community ophthalmic care, *J Am Society Opth RN* 18(4):10, 1993.

Brinkmann KL: Why can't your patient hear you? *RN* 54:46, 1991.

Centers for Disease Control and Prevention: Recommendations for prevention of HIV transmission in health care settings, *MMWR* 36(suppl 25):3s, 1987.

Evanski PM, Reinherz RP: Easing the pain of common foot problems, *Patient Care* 25:38, 1991.

Gerali PS: Preventing blindness, *J Ophthal Nurs Technol* 10:181, 1990.

Helt J: Foot care and footwear to prevent amputation, *J Vasc Nurs* 9(4):2, 1991.

Kenny SA: Effect of two oral care protocols on the incidence of stomatitis in hematology patients, *Cancer Nurs* 13:345, 1990.

Kupietsky A: Teaching kindergarten and elementary school children dental health: a practical approach *J Clin Pediatr Dentistry* 17(4):255, 1993.

Lloyd F: Eye care for ventilated unconscious patients, *Nurs Times* 86:36, 1990.

Palumbo MV: Hearing access 2000: increasing awareness of the hearing impaired, *J Gerontol Nurs* 16:26, 1990.

Rakow PL: Maintaining a healthy eye, *J Ophthal Nurs Technol* 9:112, 1990.

Rising C: The relationship of selected nursing activities to ICP *J Neurosci Nurs* 25(5):302, 1993.

Simon D: Coping with hearing loss and hearing aids, San Diego, 1992, Singular Publishing Group.

Sorrentino SA: *Mosby's textbook for nursing assistants,* ed 3, St Louis, 1992, Mosby.

Thibodeau GA, Patton K: *Anatomy and physiology,* ed 2, St Louis, 1993, Mosby.

Tombes MB, Gallucci: The effects of hydrogen peroxide rinses on the normal oral mucosa, *Nurs Res* 42(6):332, 1993.

Winkley G, Brown J, Stone T: Interventions to improve oral care: the nursing assistant's role, *J Geront Nurs* 19(11):47, 1993.

Winslow E, Smith J: Effects of basin baths, tub baths, and showers on cardiovascular response in 51 healthy men and women, *Cardiovasc Nurs* 27(5):25, 1991.

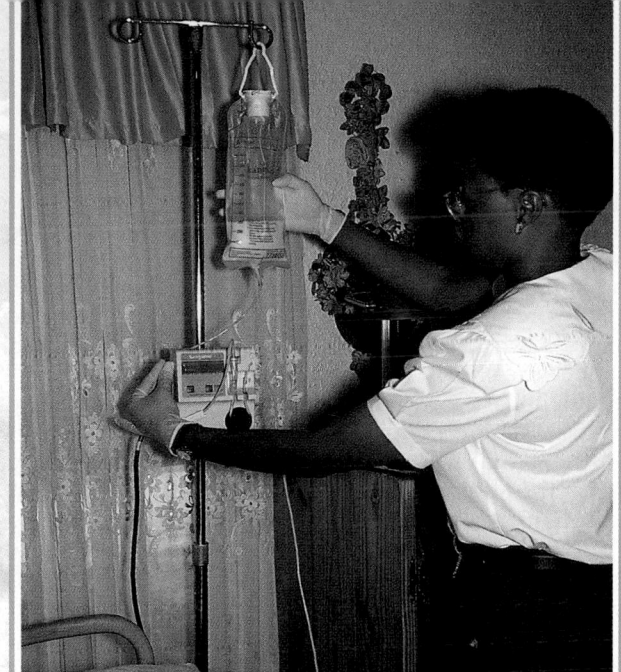

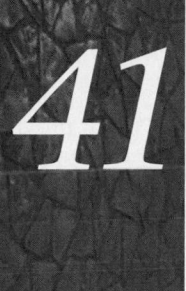

## Chapter 41

Nutrition

Objectives

Mastery of content in this chapter will enable the student to:

► Define the key terms listed.

► Explain why each major nutrient is necessary for nutrition.

► Explain the importance of a balance between energy intake and energy requirements.

► List the end products of carbohydrate, protein, and lipid metabolism.

► Explain the significance of saturated, unsaturated, and polyunsaturated lipids in nutrition.

► Describe the food guide pyramid and discuss its value in planning meals for good nutrition.

► Explain recommended daily allowances.

► List seven dietary guidelines for health promotion.

► Discuss the major methods of nutritional assessment.

► Identify three major nutritional problems and describe clients at risk for these problems.

► State the goals of enteral and parenteral nutrition.

► Describe the procedure for initiating and maintaining tube feedings.

► Describe methods to avoid complications associated with tube feedings.

► Describe methods to avoid complications associated with parenteral nutrition.

► Discuss the importance of diet counseling and client teaching.

Food provides sustenance and also holds symbolic meaning. The giving or taking of food is part of ceremonies, social gatherings, holiday traditions, religious events, the celebration of a birth, and the mourning of a death. The difficulty of the decision to withdraw food in a terminal illness, even food in the form of intravenous nutrients, is a testament to the symbolic power of food and feeding. Food products and herbs were an important part of early American folk medicine and Native American medicine. Grains, teas, botanicals, herbs, and spices were among the ingredients that formed a basis for folk remedies. Interestingly, many of these folk medicines are receiving renewed interest among modern naturopaths (Carper, 1993; Fuhrman, 1995). Folk medicines continue to be prevalent in some cultures or ethnic groups and can affect an individual's acceptance of "organized medicine" or have effects upon health status that can go unrecognized by practitioners. In the early nineteenth century, the description of a calorie as a unit of energy obtained from food and the development of a method to break foods down into protein, carbohydrate, and fat moved nutrition into the realm of a science (Stacey, 1994).

Florence Nightingale incorporated a diet kitchen into British medical hospitals in Turkey and stressed the nurse's role in the science and art of feeding during the mid-1800s (Grant and Kennedy-Caldwell, 1988). The nurse's role in nutrition and diet therapy has changed over the years. Before World War II, nursing schools provided instruction in nutrition and diet therapy, laboratory courses in food preparation, and clinical experiences in the preparation and serving of therapeutic diets. In the battlefield hospitals, the surgical, pharmacological, and medical technologies necessary to save the lives of many victims were developed. The use of diets adequate in carbohydrates, fats, and proteins was recognized to promote wound healing and reduce the rate of complications for soldiers recovering from injuries.

After World War II, knowledge about illnesses and trauma increased, and attitudes about hospitals changed. Hospitals that had been regarded as placement facilities for the terminally ill were now recognized as important in promoting the restoration of health.

Nursing curricula placed greater emphasis on the impact of nutrition on health promotion, disease prevention and health restoration. Nursing students were taught normal and therapeutic nutrition, nutrition in disease, and the role of a new member of the health care team, the clinical dietitian. During the late 1960s and early 1970s, nursing curricula integrated nutrition content into the curricula rather than having a separate course.

Nutrition is now recognized as an important treatment in any illness that places clients at risk for malnutrition. In some illnesses, such as non–insulin-dependent diabetes mellitus or mild hypertension, diet therapy may be the major treatment for disease control. Other conditions, such as inflammatory bowel disease, may require specialized nutrition support such as enteral tube feeding or parenteral nutrition (PN). Standards for the Joint Commission on Accreditation of Health Care Organizations (1996) require that health care practitioners collaborate with the client and each other to develop, implement, and evaluate a nutritional plan of care.

■ PRINCIPLES OF NUTRITION

The body requires fuel to provide energy for organ function and body movement, to maintain body temperature, and to provide raw materials for enzyme function, growth, and replacement and repair of cells. **Metabolism** refers to all the biochemical reactions within the cells of the body. Metabolic processes can be anabolic (building) or catabolic (breaking down). Food is ingested, digested, and absorbed to produce the energy needed for these reactions.

An individual's energy requirements are influenced by several factors. The energy requirement of a person at rest, called the **basal metabolic rate (BMR)**, is the energy needed at the lowest level of cellular function. An equation commonly used to estimate the **basal energy expenditure (BEE)** of adults and children over 6 years of age at rest is shown in the box below. A number of factors, such as activity, illness, injury, fever, infection, ingestion of food, and starvation can affect the BEE. Energy requirements for children under six are calculated based on weight and age. Energy requirements can also be estimated by measuring oxygen consumption and carbon dioxide production by means of a metabolic measurement cart.

In general, when energy requirements are completely met by calorie intake in food, body weight does not change. If the calories ingested exceed energy needs, a person gains weight. When the calories ingested fail to meet energy requirements, a person loses weight.

Nutrients are the elements necessary for body processes and function. The six categories of nutrients are water, carbohydrates, proteins, lipids, vitamins, and minerals. Energy needs are met by the metabolism of carbohydrates, proteins, and lipids. Water is a vital component of the body and acts as a solvent for nutrients. Vitamins and minerals do not provide energy, but are essential to metabolic processes and acid-base balance.

Foods are sometimes described according to their **nutrient density**, the proportion of essential nutrients to the number of calories. High nutrient density foods, such as fruits and vegetables, provide a large number of nutrients in relationship to calories. Low nutrient density foods, such as alcohol or sugar, are high in calories but are nutrient poor.

Carbohydrates

Carbohydrates are the main source of energy in the diet. Each gram of carbohydrate produces 4 kilocalories (kcal). Carbohydrates are obtained primarily from plant foods, except for lactose (milk sugar). Carbohydrates are classified according to their sugar units, or **saccharides**. Monosac-

---

> ### Calculation of the Basal Energy Expenditure (BEE)
>
> **Women:** BEE= 655 + (9.6 × *weight in kg*) + (1.7 × *height in cm*) − (4.7 × *age in years*)
> **Men:** BEE= 66 + (13.7 × *weight in kg*) + (5 × *height in cm*) − (6.8 × *age in years*)

From Harris JA, Benedict FG: *A biometric study of basal metabolism,* Washington, DC, 1919, Carnegie Institution of Washington.

charides such as glucose (dextrose) or fructose cannot be broken down into a more basic sugar unit. Disaccharides such as sucrose, lactose, and maltose are composed of two monosaccharides and water. Polysaccharides such as glycogen are composed of many sugar units. They are insoluble in water and are digested to varying degrees.

Plants store carbohydrates as starch. Starch is made up of granules enclosed by cell walls. When starch is cooked, the granules swell and burst their cellulose walls. Raw starch foods, such as potatoes, are more difficult to digest than the same foods after cooking because the freeing of the granules from the cellulose permits greater contact with digestive enzymes and more complete digestion. Starch digestion consists of several steps (Fig. 41-1). Dextrin is produced commercially and is used to increase the digestibility of foods such as baby foods, cereals, and toasted breads.

Some polysaccharides cannot be digested because humans do not have enzymes capable of breaking them down. Nevertheless, these polysaccharides have a role in human nutrition because they add fiber to the diet. **Fiber** has received attention as a dietary factor in disease prevention and treatment and in the prevention of diarrhea during tube feeding. Fibers classified as insoluble because they are largely indigestible include cellulose and lignins. Soluble fibers include hemicelluloses, pectins, gums, and mucilages. Current recommendations from the American Cancer Society include increasing fiber in the diet (American Cancer Society, 1993).

A small amount of carbohydrate is stored in the liver and muscles in the form of glycogen. Glycogen, which is synthesized from glucose, provides energy during brief periods of fasting. Excess carbohydrate calories are stored as fat. Carbohydrate metabolism consists of three main processes:

1. Catabolism of glycogen into glucose, carbon dioxide, and water **(glycogenolysis)**
2. Anabolism of glucose into glycogen for storage **(glycogenesis)**
3. Conversion of amino acids and glycerol into glucose for energy **(gluconeogenesis)**

A recommended range for carbohydrate intake in the diet is 50% to 60% of total calories, preferably in the form of complex carbohydrates, such as whole grain breads and cereals. Carbohydrate is the main source of fuel for the brain, skeletal muscle during exercise, erythrocytes and leukocytes, and the renal medulla.

Proteins

Although proteins provide a source of energy (4 kcal/g), they are essential for synthesis (building) of body tissue in growth, maintenance, and repair. The simplest form of protein is the **amino acid.** Essential amino acids are those that the body cannot synthesize, but must be provided in the diet. Other amino acids can be synthesized and are classified as nonessential. Amino acids can be linked together to form tripeptides and oligopeptides. Albumin and insulin are simple proteins because they contain only amino acids or their derivatives. The combination of a simple protein with a nonprotein substance produces a complex protein, such as lipoprotein, formed by a combination of a lipid and a simple protein.

Amino acids are anabolized (combined and changed) into tissues, hormones, and enzymes. Amino acids can also be converted to fat and stored as adipose tissue or catabolized (broken down) into energy via gluconeogenesis.

A complete protein contains all of the essential amino acids in sufficient quantity to support growth and maintain nitrogen balance. Complete proteins are also referred to as *high-biological value proteins.* Examples of foods containing complete or high-biological value proteins are meat, fish, poultry, milk, and eggs. Examples of foods that contain incomplete proteins are cereals, legumes (beans, peas), and vegetables. The combination of one incomplete protein with another incomplete protein (that contains the missing amino acids or increases the amount of amino acids) supplies the essential amino acids (Fig. 41-2) to support growth and maintain nitrogen balance. Incomplete proteins can also be made complete by the supplementation of syn-

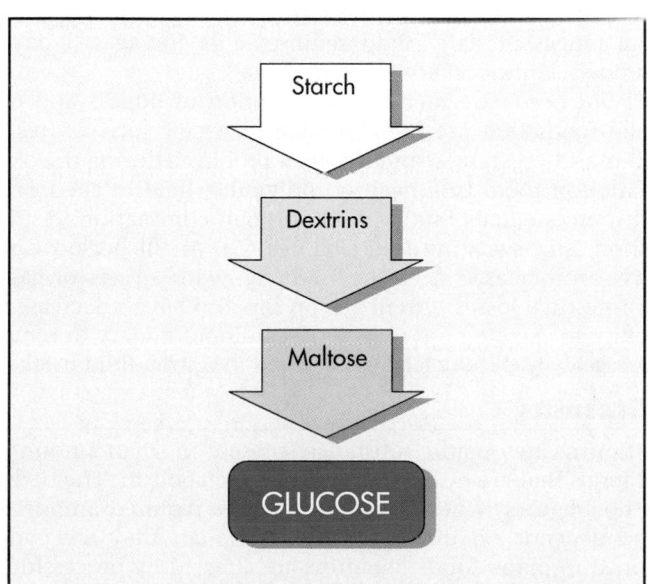

Fig. 41-1 Digestion of starch.

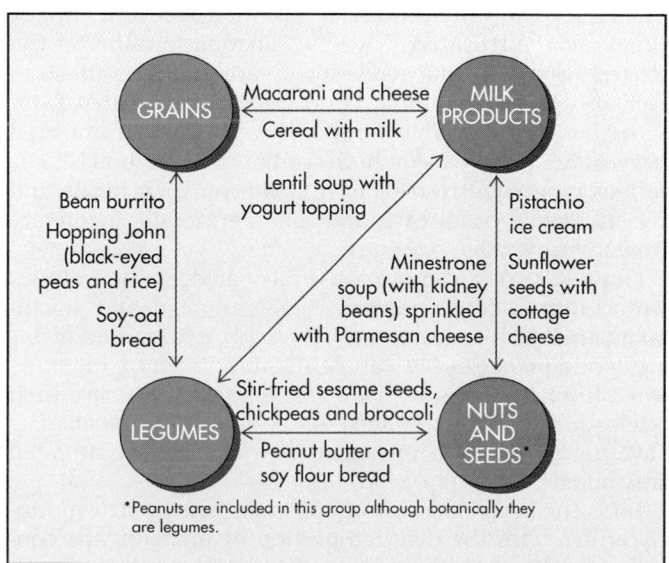

Fig. 41-2 Examples of complete and incomplete protein. *(From Moore MC: Pocket guide: nutrition and diet therapy, ed 2, St Louis, 1993, Mosby.)*

thetic amino acids. The addition of synthetic lysine to wheat is an example of amino acid supplementation.

Protein is 16% nitrogen and is the body's only source of nitrogen. The body is in **nitrogen balance** when the intake and output of nitrogen are equal. When the intake of nitrogen exceeds the output, the body is in positive nitrogen balance, which is required for growth, normal pregnancy, and wound healing. The nitrogen retained by the body is used for building, repair, and replacement of body tissues.

Negative nitrogen balance occurs when the body loses more nitrogen than it gains. The increased nitrogen loss is the result of body tissue destruction or loss of nitrogen containing body fluids. Negative nitrogen balance can occur with infection, burns, fever, starvation, and injury.

Protein can be used to provide energy, but because of protein's essential role in growth, maintenance, and repair, adequate calories should be provided in the diet from non-protein sources. Protein is spared as an energy source when there is sufficient carbohydrate in the diet to meet the energy needs of the body. Proteins can then be used in nitrogen balance and tissue building. The required daily allowance of protein for adults is shown in Table 41-7. Additional protein is required during pregnancy and lactation (Food and Nutrition Board, 1989).

Lipids

Lipids (fats) are the most calorically dense nutrient and they provide 9 kcal per gram. Lipids include fats that are solid at room temperature and oils that are liquid at room temperature. Lipids are composed of carbon, hydrogen, and oxygen, but the proportion of each element differs from that of carbohydrate.

Basic lipids are composed of **triglycerides** and **fatty acids**. Triglycerides circulate in the blood and are made up of three fatty acids attached to glycerol. Fatty acids are composed of chains of carbon atoms and hydrogen atoms with an acid group on one end of the chain and a methyl group at the other. The process during which fatty acids are synthesized is called **lipogenesis**. Fatty acids can be **saturated**, where each carbon in the chain has two attached hydrogen atoms, or **unsaturated**, where an unequal number of hydrogen atoms are attached and the carbon atoms attach to each other with a double bond. **Monounsaturated fatty acids** have one double bond, whereas **polyunsaturated fatty acids** have two or more carbon double bonds. The various types of fatty acids have significance for health and the incidence of disease and are mentioned in dietary guidelines.

Linoleic acid, an unsaturated fatty acid, is the only essential fatty acid in humans. Linolenic acid and arachidonic acid, also unsaturated fatty acids, are important for metabolic processes but can be manufactured by the body when linoleic acid is available. Most animal fats have high proportions of saturated fatty acids, whereas vegetable fats have higher amounts of unsaturated and polyunsaturated fatty acids.

Fat is the body's major form of stored energy. The monoglycerides from the digested portion of lipids can be converted to glucose by gluconeogenesis. All body cells except red blood cells and neurons can oxidize fatty acids for energy.

The metabolism of 1 g of lipid yields more than twice the

Table 41-1	Ranges of Daily Fluid Requirements		
Age	**Fluid Requirements***	**Age**	**Fluid Requirements***
3 days	80-100	6 yr	100-110
10 days	125-150	10 yr	90-100
3 mo	140-160	14 yr	50-60
6 mo	130-155	18 yr	40-50
9 mo	125-145	19-50 yr	50
1 yr	120-135		
2 yr	115-125		
4 yr	100-110		

Modified from Behrman RE, Vaughan VC, editors: *Nelson's textbook of pediatrics*, ed 3, Philadelphia, 1987, Saunders.
*In ml/kg/day.

energy provided by carbohydrates or proteins. Lipids typically account for 35% to 45% of the American diet. Current dietary guidelines established by a number of health organizations recommend a diet that contains no more than 30% of the total kilocalories as fat, and is low in saturated fat and cholesterol (American Cancer Society, 1993; U.S. Department of Health and Human Services, 1990). Diets high in fat and cholesterol have been associated with coronary artery disease and some types of cancer. Fat, however, has an important role in human nutrition and an intake below 10% in the diet can lead to deficiency.

Water

Water is a critical component of the body because cell function depends on a fluid environment. Water composes 60% to 70% of total body weight. The percent of total body water is greater for lean people than for obese people because muscle contains more water than any tissue except blood. Infants have the greatest percentage of total body weight as water, and older people have the least. When deprived of water, a person can survive for no more than a few hours in a desert or a few days in the most protected environment. The ranges of daily fluid requirements for ages 3 days through adulthood are listed in Table 41-1.

Fluid needs are met by consumption of liquids and of solid foods that are high in water content, such as fresh fruits and vegetables, and by water produced during the oxidation of food. In a healthy individual, fluid intake from all sources equals fluid output through elimination, respiration, and sweating (see Chapter 45). An ill person can have an increased need for fluid (e.g., with a fever or gastrointestinal losses). An ill person can also have a decreased ability to excrete fluid (e.g., with cardiopulmonary or renal disease), which may lead to the need to restrict fluid intake.

Vitamins

Vitamins are organic substances present in small amounts in foods that are essential to normal metabolism. The body is unable to synthesize vitamins in the required amounts and depends on dietary intake. Although they are contained in many foods, vitamins are affected by processing, storage, and preparation. Vitamin content is usually highest in fresh foods that are used quickly after minimal expo-

Table 41-2	Water-Soluble Vitamins		
FUNCTIONS	**EFFECTS OF DEFICIENCY***	**EFFECTS OF EXCESS**	**SOURCES**
Vitamin C (Ascorbic Acid) Production of collagen; integrity of capillary walls; formation of red blood cells; metabolism of amino acids; reduction of iron salts; protection of other vitamins from oxidation	Scurvy, poor wound healing, bleeding gums, loose teeth, bruising	Kidney stones, scurvy on withdrawal, urinary tract infection	Citrus fruits, potatoes, cabbage, tomatoes, broccoli, strawberries, cantaloupe, green peppers
VITAMIN B COMPLEX **Vitamin B₁ (Thiamine)** Component of enzymes; carbohydrate oxidation; oxidative conversion of pyruvic acid and hence citric acid cycle	Beriberi (rare), polyneuritis, mental confusion, muscular weakness, ataxia, cardiac rhythm disturbances, cardiac enlargement	Rapid pulse, headaches, weakness, irritability, insomnia	Pork, fish, eggs, poultry, dried beans, whole grains, wheat germ, oatmeal, bread, pasta
Vitamin B₂ (Riboflavin) Metabolism of nutrients; growth; oxidation and reduction of fat, carbohydrates, proteins	Ariboflavinosis: cracks at mouth corners, scaly desquamation of skin around mouth, eye irritation, glossitis (shiny tongue), photophobia (light sensitivity)	Ulcer, elevated blood glucose level, increased uric acid levels in blood	Milk, whole grains, green vegetables, liver
Niacin Protein utilization; glycolysis; fat synthesis; tissue repair	Pellagra: weakness, anorexia, indigestion; severe pellagra: dermatitis, diarrhea, dementia	Ulcer, liver dysfunction, elevated blood glucose level, increased blood uric acid levels, diarrhea, nausea, flushing	Meats, dairy products, whole grains, cereals, tuna
Vitamin B₆ (Complex of Pyridoxine, Pyridoxal, Pyridoxamine) Metabolism of nutrients, synthesis of nonessential amino acids; conversion of tryptophan to niacin; proper function of blood and central nervous system cells	Anemia, irritability, skin lesions, cracks at corners of mouth	Bloating, depression, fatigue, headache, nerve damage, irritability	Whole grains, liver, fish, poultry, green beans, nuts, meats, potatoes
Folacin, Folic Acid, Folate Metabolism of some amino acids; maturation of red blood cells; synthesis of purines and pyrimidines, which are necessary for ribonucleic acid (RNA) and deoxyribonucleic acid (DNA)	Macrocytic anemia	Diarrhea, insomnia, irritability, masking of vitamin B₁₂ deficiency	Liver, green leafy vegetables, meat, fish, poultry, whole grains
Vitamin B₁₂ (Cobalamin) Manufacture of enzymes essential to metabolism of nutrients, nucleic acid, folic acid; proper function of cells of bone marrow, gastrointestinal tract, and nervous system; formation of purines and thus RNA and DNA	Pernicious anemia and neurological disorders	None reported	Milk, eggs, cheese, meat, fish, poultry, foods of animal origin (Plant foods contain no vitamin B₁₂.)
Pantothenic Acid Metabolism of nutrients; synthesis of cholesterol and steroid hormones; activity of adrenal cortex	None known	Increased need for thiamin, occasional diarrhea, water retention	Meats, whole grain cereals, legumes
Biotin Synthesis of fatty acids; utilization of glucose; metabolism of protein; utilization of vitamin B₁₂ and folic acid	None known	None known	Liver, kidneys, dark green vegetables, egg yolk, green beans

From Grant JA, Kennedy-Caldwell C: *Nutritional support in nursing*, New York, 1988, Grune & Stratton; and Whitney EN, Cataldo CB, Rolfes SR: *Understanding normal and clinical nutrition*, ed 3, St Paul, 1991, West.
*For normal ranges, see Table 41-7. Normal range for pantothenic acid is 4-7 mg/day, and for biotin, it is 30-100 µg/day.

sure to heat, air, or water. Vitamins are classified as water soluble and fat soluble.

WATER-SOLUBLE VITAMINS

The water-soluble vitamins are vitamin C and vitamin B complex, which consists of eight different vitamins. Water-soluble vitamins cannot be stored in the body and must be provided in the daily food intake. **Hypervitaminosis**, a condition caused by excessive intake of a vitamin, is less likely to occur with water-soluble vitamins. However, megadoses of vitamin C and pyridoxine (B$_6$) can lead to toxicity. Vitamins are chemicals used as catalysts in biochemical reactions. When there is enough of any specific vitamin to meet the catalytic demands, the rest of the vitamin supply acts as a free chemical and may be toxic to the body. Table 41-2 lists the water-soluble vitamins, their major food sources, and signs and symptoms of deficiency and excess.

FAT-SOLUBLE VITAMINS

The fat-soluble vitamins—A, D, E, and K—can be stored in the body. With the exception of vitamin D, these vitamins are provided through dietary intake. Toxicity to some fat-soluble vitamins has been recognized for years. Toxicity can result from megadoses (intentional or unintentional) of synthetic vitamins, excessive amounts in fortified food, and diets that include a large intake of fish liver oils. The characteristics of fat-soluble vitamins are listed in Table 41-3.

Certain vitamins are currently of considerable interest in their role as antioxidants, substances that neutralize sub-

stances called *free radicals* that are thought to produce oxidative damage to body cells and tissues. These vitamins include beta carotene and vitamins A, C, and E (Malone, 1991; Hunter et al, 1993).

Minerals

Minerals are inorganic elements essential to the body as catalysts in biochemical reactions. Minerals are classified as macrominerals when the daily requirement is 100 mg or more and trace elements when less than 100 mg is needed daily. The characteristics of macrominerals are summarized in Table 41-4 and trace elements in Table 41-5. Silicon, vanadium, nickel, tin, cadmium, arsenic, aluminum, and boron may play as yet unidentified roles in human nutrition. Toxic effects of arsenic, aluminum, and cadmium have been identified.

▌ DIGESTION

Digestion of food consists of mechanical breakdown by chewing, churning, and mixing with fluid, and chemical reactions by which food is reduced to its simplest form. Each part of the gastrointestinal system has an important digestive or absorptive function. Enzymes are an essential component of the chemistry of digestion. **Enzymes** are proteinlike substances that act as catalysts to speed up chemical reactions. As catalysts, enzymes are not part of the end product of the reaction. Most enzymes have one specific function, although some enzymes are involved in several closely related reactions. Each enzyme functions best at a specific pH and is inactivated by major variations from

Table 41-3	Fat-Soluble Vitamins		
FUNCTIONS	EFFECTS OF DEFICIENCY*	EFFECTS OF EXCESS	SOURCES
VITAMIN A (RETINOL, RETINAL, RETINOIC ACID)			
Growth and maintenance of epithelial tissue; maintenance of visual acuity in dim light; immune functions, especially antigen recognition	Night blindness, rough scaly skin, dry mucous membranes, decreased resistance to infection, faulty tooth and bone development	Nausea, vomiting, abdominal pain, and growth failure in children; weight loss in adults; megadoses: hair loss, bone swelling and tenderness, joint pain, hepatomegaly, splenomegaly, headache	Whole milk, whole milk products, eggs, green leafy vegetables, yellow fruits and vegetables, fish liver oil, liver
VITAMIN D (CHOLECALCIFEROL, ERGOSTEROL)			
Absorption and utilization of calcium in bone and tooth development	Rickets and delayed dentition in children, osteomalacia (softening of bones) in adults	Megadoses: loss of appetite, vomiting, growth failure, weight loss, increased calcium deposits in soft tissue, blood vessels, and kidneys	Sunlight, fortified milk, fortified margarines, fish liver oils
VITAMIN E (TOCOPHEROL)			
Protection of vitamins A and C and polyunsaturated fatty acids from oxidation; synthesis of heme	Increased hemolysis of red blood cells and macrocytic anemia in premature infants	Interference with utilization of vitamins A and K, prolonged prothrombin time, intestinal irritability, headache, fatigue, dizziness	Vegetable oils, green leafy vegetables, milk, eggs, meats, cereals
VITAMIN K			
Prothrombin formation; blood clotting	Hemorrhagic disease of the newborn, prolonged clotting time in adults	Hyperbilirubinemia in infants, vomiting in adults	Green leafy vegetables, liver synthesis in gastrointestinal tract

From Grant JA, Kennedy-Caldwell C: *Nutritional support in nursing,* New York, 1988, Grune & Stratton; and Whitney EN, Cataldo CB, Rolfes SR: *Understanding normal and clinical nutrition,* ed 3, St Paul, 1991, West.
*For normal ranges, see Table 41-7.

Table 41-4	Macrominerals			

FUNCTIONS	EFFECTS OF DEFICIENCY*	EFFECTS OF EXCESS	SOURCES
CALCIUM			
Formation of teeth and bones; contraction of muscle fibers; transmission of nerve impulses; activation of enzymes; permeability of cell membranes; coagulation of blood; cardiac function	Tingling of fingers and area around mouth, muscle cramps, carpopedal (thumb or toe) spasm, tetany, convulsions, pathological fractures, stunted growth in children, bone loss in adults	Relaxed skeletal muscles, cardiac irregularities	Milk, milk products, leafy vegetables, fish, and small edible bones
MAGNESIUM			
Support of function of B vitamins; utilization of calcium, potassium, protein; maintenance of electrical activity in nerves and muscles	Neuromuscular irritability, confusion, hallucinations, growth failure	Lethargy, diarrhea	Whole grains, nuts, legumes, green vegetables
PHOSPHORUS			
Formation of bone and teeth; activation of B vitamins; transfer of energy in cells; promotion of muscle and nerve activity; metabolism of carbohydrates; regulation of acid-base balance; transmission of hereditary traits	Hemolytic anemia, defective white blood cell function, delayed clotting, bone pain, pathological fractures	Erosion of jaw, calcium loss	Pork, beef, dried peas and beans, milk and milk products

From Grant JA, Kennedy-Caldwell C: *Nutritional support in nursing,* New York, 1988, Grune & Stratton; Whitney EN, Cataldo CB, Rolfes SR: *Understanding normal and clinical nutrition,* ed 3, St Paul, 1991, West.
*For normal ranges, see Table 41-7.

Table 41-5	Trace Elements			

FUNCTIONS	EFFECTS OF DEFICIENCY*	EFFECTS OF EXCESS	SOURCES
COPPER			
Hemoglobin formation; synthesis of phospholipids; formation and activity of some enzymes; synthesis of prostaglandin	Abnormal blood cell development in infants, bone demineralization	Headache, dizziness, heartburn, weakness, nausea, vomiting, diarrhea, Wilson's disease	Liver, kidney, shellfish, nuts, raisins
FLUORIDE			
Formation of teeth; prevention of dental caries	Poor dental health	Mottling, pitting, and discoloration of tooth enamel	Fluoridated water, seafood, toothpaste, mouthwash
IODINE			
Basic component of thyroid hormones	Cretinism in infants, depressed thyroid activity	Toxic goiter	Iodized salt, seafood, food additives, dough oxidizers, dairy disinfectants, coloring agents
IRON			
Formation of hemoglobin; synthesis of vitamins, purines, and antibodies	Anemia, fatigue, weakness, lethargy, lowered immunity	Hemosiderosis, poisoning from accidental ingestion in infants and children: cramps, abdominal pain, nausea, vomiting, black stools, cirrhosis	Liver, lean meats, whole grains, enriched breads and cereals, green leafy vegetables
ZINC			
Connective tissue integrity; immune response; formation of enzymes and insulin	Impaired wound healing, decreased sensations of taste and smell, skin lesions, delayed growth	Anemia, fever, nausea, vomiting, diarrhea, muscle pain and weakness, decreased calcium absorption	Oysters, liver, meats, poultry, legumes, nuts

From Grant JA, Kennedy-Caldwell C: *Nutritional support in nursing,* New York, 1988, Grune & Stratton; Whitney EN, Cataldo CB, Rolfes SR: *Understanding normal and clinical nutrition,* ed 3, St Paul, 1991, West.
*For normal ranges, see Table 41-7. Normal range for copper is 1.5 to 3 mg/day, and for fluoride it is 1.5 to 4 mg/day.

that level. The secretions of the gastrointestinal tract have vastly different pH levels. For example, saliva is relatively neutral, gastric juice is highly acidic, and the secretions of the small intestine are alkaline.

The mechanical, chemical, and hormonal activities of digestion are interdependent. Enzyme activity depends on the mechanical breakdown of food to increase its surface area for chemical action. Hormones regulate the flow of digestive secretions needed for enzyme supply, and digestion may also be decreased or increased by strong emotional states. The secretion of digestive juice and motility of the gastrointestinal tract are regulated by physical, chemical, and hormonal factors, and they are intricately bound to psychological, emotional, and nervous system alterations.

Digestion begins in the mouth, where food is mechanically broken down by chewing. The food is mixed with saliva, which contains ptyalin (salivary amylase), an enzyme that acts on cooked starch to begin its conversion to maltose. The longer food is chewed, the more starch digestion occurs in the mouth. Proteins and fats are broken down physically but remain unchanged chemically because enzymes in the mouth do not react with these nutrients. Chewing reduces food particles to a size suitable for swallowing, and saliva provides lubrication to further ease swallowing of the food.

Swallowed food enters the esophagus and is moved along by wavelike muscular contractions (**peristalsis**). Food mass at the cardiac sphincter, located at the upper opening of the stomach, causes the sphincter to relax and allows food to enter the stomach.

In the stomach, pepsinogen is secreted and activated by hydrochloric acid to pepsin, a protein splitting enzyme. The stomach also secretes small amounts of lipase and amylase to digest fat and starch, respectively. The stomach's pyloric glands also secrete gastrin, a hormone that regulates the acid environment. The stomach acts as a reservoir and food remains in the stomach about 3 hours, with a range of 1 to 7 hours. The volume of food, fat content, oncotic pressure, and physical makeup of the food affect gastric motility.

Food leaves the stomach at the pyloric sphincter as an acidic, liquefied mass called **chyme.** Chyme flows into the duodenum and is quickly mixed with bile, intestinal juices, and pancreatic secretions. Bile emulsifies fat to permit enzyme action and holds fatty acids in solution.

Intestinal secretions contain seven enzymes: lipase for fat digestion; two peptidases for protein digestion; and amylase, sucrase, lactase, and maltase for carbohydrate digestion. Pancreatic secretions contain five enzymes: amylase to digest starch; lipase to break down emulsified fats; and trypsin, chymotrypsin, and carboxypeptidase to break down proteins.

Peristalsis continues in the small intestine, mixing the secretions with the chyme. The mixture becomes increasingly alkaline, inhibiting the action of the gastric enzymes and promoting the action of the duodenal secretions. The major portion of digestion occurs in the small intestine, producing glucose, fructose, and galactose from carbohydrates; amino acids and dipeptides from proteins; and fatty acids, glycerides, and glycerol from lipids.

ABSORPTION

The small intestine is the primary site of absorption of nutrients. It is lined with fingerlike projections called *villi,* which increase the surface area available for absorption.

Table 41-6	**Intestinal Absorption of Some Major Nutrients**			
NUTRIENT	**FORM**	**MEANS OF ABSORPTION**	**CONTROL AGENT OR REQUIRED COFACTOR**	**ROUTE**
Carbohydrate	Monosaccharides (glucose and galactose)	Competitive	—	Blood
		Selective	—	
		Active transport via sodium-potassium pump	Sodium	
Protein	Amino acids	Selective	—	Blood
	Some dipeptides	Carrier transport systems	Pyridoxine (pyridoxal phosphate)	Blood
	Whole protein (rare)	Pinocytosis (process by which cells absorb and digest nutrients)	—	Blood
Fat	Fatty acids	Fatty acid-bile complex (micelles)	Bile	Lymph
	Monoglyceride, diglyceride		—	Lymph
	Triclycerides (neutral fat)	Pinocytosis	—	Lymph
Vitamins	B_{12}	Carrier transport	Intrinsic factor	Blood
	A	Bile complex	Bile	Blood
	K	Bile complex	Bile	Large intestine to blood
Minerals	Sodium	Active transport via sodium pump	—	Blood
	Calcium	Active transport	Vitamin D	Blood
	Iron	Active transport	Ferritin mechanisms	Blood (as transferin)
Water	Water	Osmosis	—	Blood, lymph, interstitial fluid

From Williams SR: *Nutrition and diet therapy,* ed 7, St Louis, 1994, Mosby.

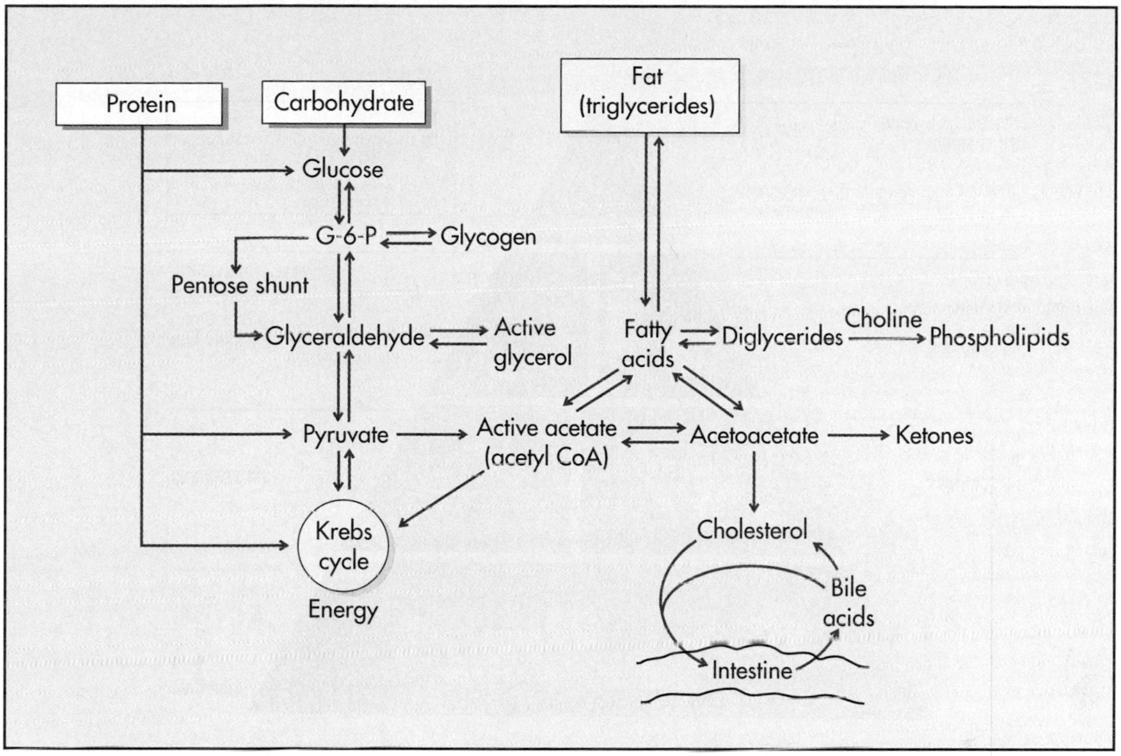

Fig. 41-3 Summary of metabolism of the nutrients. Note metabolic interrelationships of carbohydrate, protein, and fat. *(From: Williams SR: Nutrition and diet therapy, ed 7, St. Louis, 1993, Mosby.)*

Nutrients are absorbed by passive diffusion and osmosis, active transport, and pinocytosis. Table 41-6 describes the means and route of absorption of major nutrients.

The intestinal contents move by peristaltic action into the large intestine. Absorption of water is the main function of the colon. Approximately 1 to 2 L of water are absorbed from ileal fluid daily. In addition to water, electrolytes and minerals are absorbed, and bacteria in the colon synthesize vitamin K and some B complex vitamins. Finally, feces are formed in the colon for elimination. When intestinal motility is increased, as in diarrhea, the body loses nutrients and water that move through the small intestine too quickly for complete absorption.

Metabolism

Nutrients absorbed in the intestines, including water, are transported through the circulatory system to body tissues. Through the chemical changes of metabolism nutrients are converted into a number of substances required by the body. Carbohydrates, protein, and fat undergo metabolism to produce chemical energy and to maintain a balance between tissue build-up and breakdown. To carry out the body's work, the chemical energy produced by metabolism is converted to other types of energy by different tissues. Muscle contraction involves mechanical energy, nervous system function involves electrical energy, and the mechanisms of heat production involve thermal energy. All of these forms of energy originate in metabolism. The interrelationships of protein, carbohydrate, and fat metabolism are depicted in Fig. 41-3.

The two basic types of metabolism are anabolism and catabolism. **Anabolism** is the production of more complex chemical substances by synthesis of nutrients. **Catabolism** is the breakdown of chemical substances into simpler substances. Although catabolism produces some energy, both processes require energy, which must be provided from food or stored energy sources.

Storage

Some, but not all, of the nutrients required by the body are stored in body tissues. The body's major form of stored energy is fat, which is stored as adipose tissue. Glycogen is stored in small reserves in liver and muscle tissue, and protein is stored in muscle mass. When the body's energy requirements exceed the energy supplied by ingested nutrients, stored energy is used. Conversely, unused energy is stored, principally in fat.

ELIMINATION

The intestinal contents move through the various segments of the large intestine by peristalsis. As the material moves toward the rectum, water is absorbed into the mucosa. The longer the material stays in the large intestine, the more water is absorbed and the firmer the remaining solid material becomes. Feces contain cellulose and similar fibrous substances that the body is unable to digest, sloughed cells from the intestinal walls, mucus, digestive secretions, water, and microorganisms.

NUTRITION AND HEALTH PROMOTION

Today there is increased interest in the role of nutrition in health promotion and the prevention of disease. This interest has led to studies of the link between nutrition and

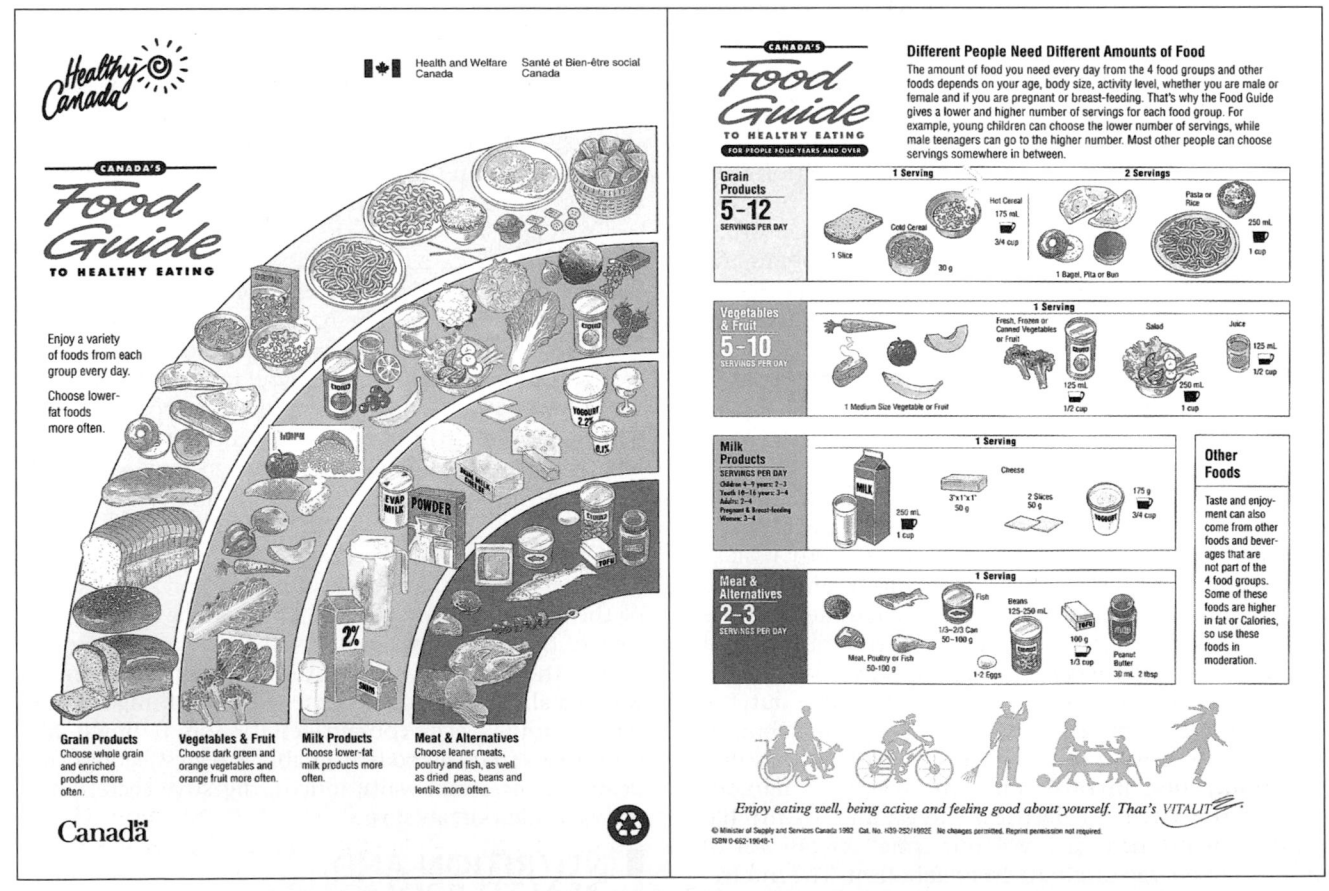

Fig. 41-4 A, U.S. food guide pyramid. **B,** Canada's food guide to healthy eating. *(From US Department of Agriculture:* USDA's food guide pyramid, *USDA Human Nutrition Information Pub No 249, Washington, DC, 1992, US Government Printing Office; and Health and Welfare Canada, Minister of Supply and Services Canada, Cat No. H39-252/1992E, Ottawa, 1992.)*

the onset of acute and chronic illnesses. Researchers are currently exploring the association between nutrition and a number of health problems, such as cancer and coronary heart disease. The use of specific nutrients to modulate the immune response and the response to trauma and illness is a new area of study, currently dubbed *nutriceutical therapy* (Zaloga, 1994). Current dietary guidelines are based upon available scientific evidence, meal planning to provide a nutritionally adequate diet, and levels of intake of specific nutrients to maintain health.

Food Guide Pyramid

The basic four food groups were first introduced by the U.S. Department of Agriculture in the late 1950s. The food groups were used to provide nutrition education and meal planning. In 1992, the United States and Canadian health organizations developed food guides designed to model a daily diet (Fig. 41-4). This basic plan provides for diets ranging from 1600 to 1800 kcal/day (USDA, 1992; Health and Welfare Canada, 1992). Additional foods to round out meals and meet energy requirements can be selected from enriched cereals, complex carbohydrates, and additional grains.

Recommended Daily Allowances

The Committee on Dietary Allowances of the Food and Nutrition Board of the National Academy of Sciences has published a list of **recommended daily allowances (RDAs)** since the 1940s. The RDAs are the level of intake of essential nutrients considered, in the judgment of the committee and on the basis of scientific knowledge, to be adequate to meet the nutritional needs of healthy people. The RDAs were originally designed as a guide for planning and securing food supplies for national defense during World War II. Now they are revised approximately every 5 years to incorporate changes and new knowledge based on current research (Table 41-7).

In 1990, Congress passed the Nutrition Labeling and Education Act (NLEA) to require mandatory nutrition labeling for most FDA-regulated foods. The final regulations were published in 1993 by the FDA and USDA. The NLEA replaced RDAs with daily reference values (DRVs) based in the percentages of 2000 kcal or the highest amount that is recommended. The label includes DRVs for carbohydrate, protein, total fat, saturated fat, fiber, cholesterol, sodium, and potassium. Serving sizes were set by the FDA and terms to describe food products, such as *low calorie, diet,* and *lite,* were changed to universal terms with legal definitions. Nurses should be familiar with the changes in food labeling and their meaning.

Other Dietary Guidelines

Dietary guidelines are published by other groups, such as the Nutrition Committee of the American Heart Association and the Committee on Diet, Nutrition, and Cancer of the National Institutes of Health (1991). These dietary guidelines use current research to recommend diets that attempt to reduce the risk of developing heart disease or cancer.

In 1990, the USDHHS and Public Health Service (PHS), after a 4-year consensus process, published *Healthy People 2000, National Health Promotion and Disease Prevention Objectives*. The report defines national goals or objectives to be

1990 Dietary Guidelines
Eat a variety of foods
Maintain a healthy weight
Choose a diet low in fat, saturated fat, and cholesterol
Choose a diet with plenty of vegetables, fruits, and grain products
Use sugar in moderation
Use salt and sodium in moderation
Drink alcoholic beverages in moderation, if at all

Data from USDA and USDHHS: *Nutrition and your health: dietary guidelines for Americans,* USDA/DHHS Home and Garden Bull No 232, Washington, DC, 1990, US Government Printing Office.

 CULTURAL ASPECTS OF CARE

FOOD CHOICES
Mrs. Nuyen, a 20-year-old Vietnamese woman, is 20 weeks pregnant when she is seen by the nurse during a home health visit. The nurse notes that Mrs. Nuyen is underweight and begins to take a dietary history with the help of Mrs. Nuyen's sister, who acts as an interpreter. The nurse discovers that Mrs. Nuyen has been underweight for several years and has gained only 2 pounds since she became pregnant. Her intake of grains and vegetables is sufficient, however, her intake of protein foods is slightly low, and of dairy foods is very low. Mrs. Nuyen explains that she does not drink milk because it causes diarrhea and cramping. Her diet contains many traditional Southeast Asian foods, such as rice, soy products, fish, bamboo shoots, and bananas. Mrs. Nuyen plans to breast-feed her infant. The nurse identifies that Mrs. Nuyen's diet is deficient in protein, calcium, phosphorus, and energy. Working with Mrs. Nuyen's traditional diet, the nurse suggests increased use of soy products such as tofu and soy milk to increase her protein intake. She also educates Mrs. Nuyen about using dairy products that are lower in lactose content or contain lactase and counsels her to ingest these products in small amounts over time. The nurse helps Mrs. Nuyen identify a pattern of eating that takes into account her traditional patterns with increased kilocalories per day. Mrs. Nuyen's sister offers to help her choose foods that will provide the nutrients needed for a healthy pregnancy. The nurse plans a follow-up home visit in 2 weeks to evaluate the effectiveness of the nutritional plan of care for this client.

met in this decade to increase the proportion of Americans who live long, healthy lives (see the box above).

All 21 nutrition-related goals for the year 2000 include baseline data. For example, one objective is to reduce the prevalence of overweight people to no more than 20% among people age 20 years and older, a decrease from the current baseline level of 26%. Other objectives are to reduce dietary fat intake to an average of 30% of total calories, down from the recent level of 36%, and to reduce saturated fat intake to less than 10%, down from the present 13%. Additional objectives include increasing intake of

| | | WEIGHT[b] | | HEIGHT[b] | | | | FAT-SOLUBLE VITAMINS | | | |
CATEGORY	AGE (YR) OR CONDITION	(KG)	(LB)	(CM)	(IN)	KCAL PER DAY	PROTEIN (G)	VITA-MIN A (μG RE)[c]	VITA-MIN D (μG)[d]	VITA-MIN E (MG α-TE)[e]	VITA-MIN K (μG)
Infants	0.0-0.5	6	13	60	24	650	13	375	7.5	3	5
	0.5-1.0	9	20	71	28	850	14	375	10	4	10
Children	1-3	13	29	90	35	1300	16	400	10	6	15
	4-6	20	44	112	44	1800	24	500	10	7	20
	7-10	28	62	132	52	2000	28	700	10	7	30
Men	11-14	45	99	157	62	2500	45	1000	10	10	45
	15-18	66	145	176	69	3000	59	1000	10	10	65
	19-24	72	160	177	70	2900	58	1000	10	10	70
	25-50	79	174	176	70	2900	63	1000	5	10	80
	over 51	77	170	173	68	2300	63	1000	5	10	80
Women	11-14	46	101	157	62	2200	46	800	10	8	45
	15-18	55	120	163	64	2200	44	800	10	8	55
	19-24	58	128	164	65	2200	46	800	10	8	60
	25-50	63	138	163	64	2200	50	800	5	8	65
	Over 51	65	143	160	63	1900	50	800	5	8	65
Pregnant						2200	60	800	10	10	65
Lactating:	1st 6 mo					2700	65	1300	10	12	65
	2nd 6 mo					2700	62	1200	10	11	65

Table 41-7 Recommended Dietary Allowances[a]

[a]The allowances, expressed as average daily intakes over time, are intended to provide for individual variations among most normal persons as they live in the United States under usual environmental stresses. Diets should be based on a variety of common foods to provide other nutrients for which human requirements have been less well defined.
[b]Weights and heights of Reference Adults are actual medians for the U.S. population of the designated age.
[c]Retinol equivalents. 1 RE = 1 μg retinol or 6 μg β-carotene. See text for calculations of vitamin A activity of diets as retinol equivalents.

fruits, vegetables, and grain products and reducing sodium consumption.

The remaining challenge is to motivate consumers to put these dietary recommendations into practice. Health professionals (e.g., nurses, registered dietitians, nutritionists, nutrition educators, physicians, teachers, and scientists) can play a key role in promoting healthy dietary habits.

Alternative Food Patterns

Long before recommended allowances and guidelines were issued, many people followed special patterns of food intake based on religion, cultural background (see the box on p. 1099), ethics, health beliefs, personal preference, or concern for the efficient use of land to produce food. Such special diets are not necessarily more or less nutritional than diets based on the basic four food groups or other nutritional guidelines because good nutrition depends on a balanced intake of all required nutrients. A common alternative dietary pattern is the vegetarian diet.

Vegetarianism is the consumption of a diet consisting predominantly of plant foods. Vegetarians may be lactoovovegetarian (avoid meat, fish, and poultry but eat eggs and milk), lactovegetarians (drink milk but avoid eggs), or vegans (consume only plant foods). Vegan, zen macrobiotic (eat only brown rice and herb tea), and fruitarian (eat only fruits, nuts, honey, and olive oil) diets are nutrient poor and can result in malnutrition. Otherwise, vegetarian diets can be nutritionally adequate if planned carefully.

■ DEVELOPMENTAL VARIABLES IN PROMOTING AND MAINTAINING HEALTHY NUTRITION

Infants

Infancy is marked by rapid growth and high protein, vitamin, mineral, and energy requirements. The average birth weight of an American baby is 3.2 to 3.4 kg (7 to 7½ lb). The infant usually doubles birth weight at 4 to 5 months and triples it at 1 year. An energy intake of approximately 108 kcal/kg of body weight is needed in the first half of infancy and 98 kcal/kg in the second half (Food and Nutrition Board, 1989). A full-term newborn is able to digest and absorb simple carbohydrates, proteins, and a moderate amount of emulsified fat. Amylase, the starch-splitting enzyme, is not present until approximately 2½ or 3½ months. Infants need about 100 to 150 ml/kg/day of fluid because a large portion of total body weight is water.

BREAST-FED INFANTS

Breast milk provides nutritional, antiviral, antibacterial, and psychosocial benefits to the infant (Fig. 41-5). Despite the fact that breast-feeding is promoted, only about 50% of mothers elect to breast-feed. Breast milk contains antibodies to protect against viruses and bacteria. Antiallergenic factors in human milk avoid common allergies in infancy. Breast-fed infants need supplemental vitamin D. Other possible supplements include vitamin K, iron and fluoride although their use is controversial.

Table 41-7	Recommended Dietary Allowances[a]—cont'd												

WATER-SOLUBLE VITAMINS							MINERALS						
VITA-MIN C (MG)	THIA-MIN (MG)	RIBO-FLAVIN (MG)	NIACIN (MG NE)[f]	VITA-MIN B_6 (MG)	FO-LATE (µG)	VITAMIN B_{12} (µG)	CAL-CIUM (MG)	PHOS-PHORUS (MG)	MAG-NESIUM (MG)	IRON (MG)	ZINC (MG)	IODINE (µG)	SELE-NIUM (µG) 35
30	0.3	0.4	5	0.3	25	0.3	400	300	40	6	5	40	10
35	0.4	0.5	6	0.6	35	0.5	600	500	60	10	5	50	15
40	0.7	0.8	9	1.0	50	0.7	800	800	80	10	10	70	20
45	0.9	1.1	12	1.1	75	1.0	800	800	120	10	10	90	20
45	1.0	1.2	13	1.4	100	1.4	800	800	170	10	10	120	20
50	1.3	1.5	17	1.7	150	2.0	1200	1200	270	12	15	150	40
60	1.5	1.8	20	2.0	200	2.0	1200	1200	400	12	15	150	50
60	1.5	1.7	29	2.0	200	2.0	1200	1200	350	10	15	150	70
60	1.5	1.7	19	2.0	200	2.0	800	800	350	10	15	150	70
60	1.2	1.4	15	2.0	200	2.0	800	800	350	10	15	150	70
50	1.1	1.3	15	1.4	150	2.0	1200	1200	280	15	12	150	45
60	1.1	1.3	15	1.5	180	2.0	1200	1200	300	15	12	150	50
60	1.1	1.3	15	1.6	180	2.0	1200	1200	280	15	12	150	55
60	1.1	1.3	15	1.6	180	2.0	800	800	280	15	12	150	55
60	1.0	1.3	13	1.6	180	2.0	800	800	280	10	12	150	55
70	1.5	1.6	17	2.2	400	2.2	1200	1200	320	30	15	175	65
95	1.6	1.8	20	2.1	280	2.6	1200	1200	355	15	19	200	75
90	1.6	1.7	20	2.1	260	2.6	1200	1200	340	15	16	200	75

From Food and Nutrition Board, National Academy of Sciences—National Research Council: *Recommended dietary allowances*, ed 10, Washington, DC, 1989, The Council.

[d]As cholecalciferol. 10 µg cholecalciferol = 400 U of vitamin D.
[e]Tocopherol equivalents. 1 mg d-α-tocopherol = 1 α-TE.
[f]Ne niacin equivalent = 1 mg of niacin or 60 mg of dietary tryptophan.

BOTTLE-FED INFANTS

Infant formulas are designed to contain approximately the nutrient composition of human milk. Protein in the formula is typically supplied as whey, soy, cow's milk base, casein hydrolysate, or elemental amino acids. The American Academy of Pediatrics (1985) has set standards for the levels of nutrients in infant formulas.

Regular cow's milk should not be used for infant formula because it may cause gastrointestinal bleeding and is too concentrated for the infant's kidneys to manage. Honey and corn syrup are potential sources of the botulism toxin and should not be used in the infant's diet. The toxin can be fatal in children under 1 year of age (Wardlaw, Insel, and Seyler, 1994).

INTRODUCTION TO SOLID FOOD

Breast milk or formula provides sufficient nutrition for the first 4 to 6 months of life. The development of fine motor skills of the hand and fingers parallels the infant's interest in food and self-feeding. Iron-fortified cereals are typically the first semisolid food to be introduced.

Table 41-8 presents a suggested sequence for introducing new foods (Whitney, Cataldo, and Rolfes, 1991). The addition of foods to an infant's diet should be governed by the infant's nutrient needs, physical readiness to handle different forms of foods, and the need to detect and control allergic reactions. New foods should be introduced one at a time.

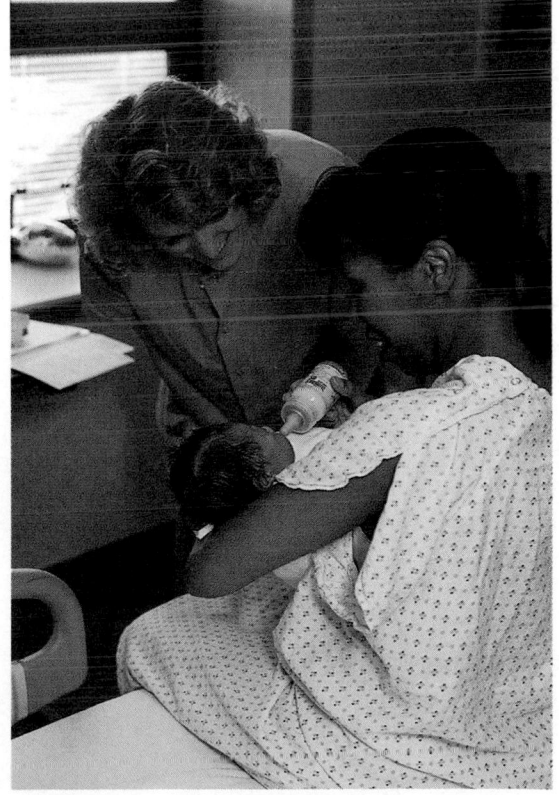

Fig. 41-5 Nurse assisting new mother with feeding the newborn.

Table 41-8	How to Feed Your Baby Step-By-Step

Food Group	Foods	Daily Servings	Suggested Serving Size	Feeding Tips
0-4 MO				
Milk	Breast milk or	8-12 or on demand		Nurse baby at least 5-10 min on each breast. Six wet diapers a day is good sign.
	Formula* 0-1 mo	6-8	2-5 oz	There is no need to force baby to finish bottle.
	1-2 mo	5-7	3-6 oz	Putting baby to bed with bottle could cause choking.
	2-3 mo	4-7	4-7 oz	Heating formula in microwave is not recommended.
	3-4 mo	4-6	6-8 oz	
4-6 MO				
Milk	Breast milk or	4-6		May need to start baby cereal (iron-fortified).
	Formula*	4-6	6-8 oz	Feed only one new cereal each week.
Grain	Baby cereal (iron-fortified)	2	1-2 tbsp	There is no need to add salt or sugar to cereal. Offer baby extra water. Use microwave with caution.
6-8 MO				
Milk	Breast milk or	3-5		Add strained fruits and vegetables at first. Add mashed or finely chopped fruits and cooked vegetables later on.
	Formula*	3-5	6-8 oz	
Grain	Baby cereal (iron-fortified)	2	2-4 tbsp	
	Bread, bagel, or bun	Offer	$^1/_2$	Feed only one new fruit or vegetable each week.
	Crackers		2 crackers	Take out of jar amount of food for one feeding. Refrigerate remaining food.
Fruit-vegetable	Fruit or vegetables	4	2-3 tbsp	Try giving baby fruit juice in cup.
	Baby fruit juice	1	3 oz (from cup)	Offer following foods only when baby has full set of teeth: apple chunks or slices, grapes, hot dogs, sausages, peanut butter, popcorn, nuts, seeds, round candies, hard chunks of uncooked vegetables. These foods can cause choking.
8-12 MO				
Milk	Breast milk,	3-4		Ask your doctor if baby is ready for whole milk.
	Formula,* or whole milk	3-4	6-8 oz	
	Cheese		$^1/_2$ oz	Add strained or finely chopped meats.
	Plain yogurt	Offer	$^1/_2$ cup	Feed only one new meat a week.
	Cottage cheese		$^1/_4$ cup	Wait until baby's first birthday to feed egg whites. Some babies are sensitive to egg white. It is okay to give egg yolks.
Grain	Baby cereal (iron-fortified)	2	2-4 tbsp	
	Bread, bagel, or bun	2	$^1/_2$	
	Crackers		2 crackers	Be patient. Babies make messes when they feed themselves.
Fruit-vegetable	Fruit or vegetables	4	3-4 tbsp	
	Baby fruit juice	1	3 oz (from cup)	Always test heated foods before serving them to baby.
Meat	Chicken, beef, pork Cooked, dried beans, or egg yolks	2	3-4 tbsp	
12-24 MO				
Milk	Whole milk, yogurt	3	$^1/_2$ cup	Add whole milk now.
	Cheese		$^1/_2$ oz	Offer small portions and never force toddler to eat.
	Cottage cheese		$^1/_4$ cup	
Grain	Cereal, pasta, or rice	4	$^1/_4$ cup	"Food jags" are common now. Don't make big deal out of them.
	Bread, muffins, bagels, rolls		$^1/_2$	
	Crackers		2 crackers	Respect toddler's likes and dislikes. Offer rejected foods again.
Fruit-vegetable	All fruits and vegetables:	4		
	Cooked, juice		$^1/_4$ cup	Make meals fun and interesting. Serve colorful foods that are crunchy, smooth, or warm.
	Whole		$^1/_2$ medium	
Meat	Fish, chicken, turkey, beef, pork	2	1 oz	Feed toddler at least three snacks every day.
	Cooked dried beans or peas		$^1/_4$ cup	
	Eggs		1	

From National Dairy Council: *Feeding guide for the first two years,* Rosemont, Ill, 1990. The Council.
Every baby is an individual. Do not worry if your baby eats a little more or less than this guide suggests. In fact, this is perfectly normal. The suggested serving sizes are only guidelines to help you get started.
*Ask your doctor which formula is best for your baby.

Toddlers and Preschoolers

The growth rate slows during toddler years (1 to 3). The toddler needs fewer calories but an increased amount of protein in relation to body weight. Calcium and phosphorus are important for healthy bone growth. Toddlers are more interested in their environments and increasing motor skills than in food.

The toddler needs a minimum of two servings (16 oz) daily from the milk group to supply protein, calcium, riboflavin, and vitamins A and B$_{12}$. Fortified milk provides vitamin D and additional vitamin A. Whole milk should be used until the toddler reaches 2 years of age to help ensure adequate intake of fatty acids. Half of the toddler's protein intake should consist of high-biological value proteins. Toddlers who consume more than 24 oz of milk daily instead of other foods may develop milk anemia. Whole grains, enriched cereals, and breads are good sources of iron in addition to meats. When meats are given to a toddler, the foods should be cut small to avoid the possibility of choking. Certain foods, such as hot dogs, candy, nuts, grapes, and popcorn are the foods most often implicated in choking deaths and should be avoided.

The toddler should receive four servings daily from the fruit and vegetable group. One serving should be a good source of vitamin C. Green leafy vegetables and deep yellow fruits and vegetables should be served frequently. Toddlers like bite-sized raw vegetables but should not be given raw carrots because of the danger of choking.

The toddler's four servings from the bread and cereal group should include whole grain or enriched breads, cereals, and pastas. Infant cereals may continue to be used because of their higher iron content. Toddlers often prefer dry cereals but sugar-coated cereals and sugar on cereals should be avoided. In addition to the basic four food groups, the toddler should have 1 to 2 tsp of margarine or butter for vitamin A.

Preschoolers need about 16 oz of milk daily, 1 to 3 oz from the meat group, four to five servings from the fruit and vegetable group (including a daily source of vitamin C and frequent servings of leafy green and deep yellow vegetables and fruits), three servings of whole grain or enriched foods from the bread and cereal group, and 3 to 4 tsp of margarine or butter.

School-Age Children

School-age children, 6 to 12 years old, grow at a slower and steadier rate, with a gradual decline in energy requirements per unit of body weight. The school-age child gains 3 to 5 kg (6½ to 11 lb) in weight and 6 cm (2½ inches) in height a year until puberty.

The appetites of school-age children are greater than those of younger children, and food intake is more varied. Recommended intake includes two servings from the milk group, 2 to 3 oz of meat group foods, four or more servings from the fruit and vegetable group (with a daily source of vitamin C and a source of vitamin A every other day), three to four servings from whole grain and enriched breads and cereals, and 1 to 2 tsp of margarine or butter.

Despite better appetites and more varied food intake, the diets of school-age children should be carefully assessed for adequate protein and vitamin A and C. Milk intake usually exceeds recommendations. However, school-age children frequently fail to eat a proper breakfast and have unsupervised intake at school; as a result, milk can provide a good source of nutrients. High fat, sugar, and salt can result from too liberal intake of snack foods.

Adolescents

During adolescence, physiological age is a better guide to nutritional needs than chronological age. Adolescence begins with the growth spurt of puberty at the end of childhood and ends with the completion of physical growth. Caloric needs are greatly increased to meet increased metabolic demands. Girls need approximately 2200 kcal/day; boys 2500 to 3000 kcal/day. Protein needs increase to a daily requirement of 45 to 59 g. Calcium is essential for the rapid bone growth of adolescence, and girls need a continuous source of iron to replace menstrual losses. Boys also need adequate iron for muscle development. Iodine supports increased thyroid activity, and B-complex vitamins support the heightened metabolic activity.

Adolescents' requirements from the basic groups include three or more servings from the milk group, two or more from the meat group, four or more from the vegetable-fruit group (with a daily source of vitamin C and a source of vitamin A every other day), four to six or more from the bread and cereal group (with emphasis on whole grains), and 1 to 2 tbsp of margarine or butter.

The adolescent's diet is influenced by many factors other than nutritional needs, including concern about body image and appearance, desire for independence, and fad diets. Nutritional deficiencies may occur in adolescent girls as a result of dieting and using oral contraceptives. The nutrients involved are folic acid, vitamin B$_6$, vitamin C, thiamine, riboflavin, and iron. The adolescent boy's diet may be inadequate in total calories, protein, iron, folic acid, B vitamins, and iodine.

Snacks provide approximately 25% of the teenager's total dietary intake (Whitney, Cataldo, and Rolfes, 1991). Skipping meals, or eating meals and the wrong choice of snacks contribute to obesity and nutrient deficits. Snack foods from the dairy and fruit-vegetable groups are good choices and contribute calcium, phosphorus, protein, zinc, vitamin A, vitamin C, and some of the B-complex vitamins.

Fast-food eating is common and adds extra salt, fat, and calories. Eating disorders such as anorexia nervosa or bulimia nervosa may emerge during adolescence. Adolescents who engage in sports and regular moderate to intense exercise require modification of their diets to meet increased energy needs. Carbohydrates, both simple and complex, should be the main source of energy, providing 55% to 60% of total daily kilocalories. Protein needs are not significantly increased and are met by ingestion of 1.0 to 1.5 g/kg per day. Fat needs are not increased. Adequate hydration is extremely important and ingestion of water before and during exercise is necessary to prevent dehydration, especially in younger athletes, and in hot, humid environments. Vitamin and mineral supplements are not required, but intake of iron-rich foods; such as dark green leafy vegetables, meats, and whole grains; is required to prevent anemia (see the box on p. 1104).

Pregnancy occurring within 4 years after menarche may place mother and fetus at risk because of anatomical and physiological immaturity. Malnutrition at the time of con-

CLIENT TEACHING on Nutrition for the Adolescent Athlete

OBJECTIVE
Client will plan a menu for daily intake that is sufficient in nutrients and fluid for an adolescent athlete

TEACHING STRATEGIES
Educate client about the basic food groups and daily kilocalorie and nutrient needs.
Discuss how vigorous exercise increases needs for kilocalories, fluid, and iron.
Discuss the need for increased carbohydrates in simple and complex form to meet increased kilocalorie needs.
Provide examples of simple and complex carbohydrate-containing foods.
Discuss fluid needs during exercise and the importance of adequate fluid.
Discuss examples of iron-rich foods to be included in the diet to prevent sports anemia.
Describe common myths about nutrition in sports (steak and eggs before competition, sports drinks, carbohydrate loading, high-fat meals).
Assist client to develop menu for 1 day.

EVALUATION
Ask client to plan a 1-week menu

---

ception increases the risk to the adolescent and her fetus. Most teenage girls do not want to gain weight. Counseling related to the nutritional needs of pregnancy may be very difficult, and suggestions are better than rigid directions. The diet of a pregnant adolescent is most often deficient in calcium, iron, and vitamins A and C.

Young and Middle Adults

The demands for most nutrients are reduced as the growth period ends. Mature adults need nutrients for energy, maintenance, and repair. Energy needs usually decline over the years. Obesity may become a problem because of decreased physical exercise, increased dining out, or the ability to afford more luxury foods.

Adult women who use oral contraceptives need extra folic acid, vitamin C, thiamin, riboflavin, vitamin B_6, and vitamin B_{12}. Iron and calcium intake are also necessary for all women.

Young and middle-age adults follow the same recommendations from the basic food groups: two or more servings each from the milk and meat groups, four or more from the vegetable-fruit group (with a daily source of vitamin C and three to four weekly servings of sources of vitamin A), four or more from the whole grain or enriched bread and cereal group, and 1 to 2 tbsp of margarine or butter.

PREGNANCY

Poor nutrition during pregnancy can cause low birth weight in infants and decreased chances of survival. Generally the fetus' needs are met at the expense of the mother. However, if nutrient sources are not available, both suffer. The nutritional status of the mother at the time of concep-

tion is important in terms of nutritional reserves and basic eating habits. Often significant aspects of fetal growth and development occur before pregnancy is even suspected.

The energy requirements of pregnancy are related to body weight and activity. An average weight gain of 11 to 14 kg (25 to 30 lb) occurs during pregnancy. Rigid recommendations about weight gain should be avoided. Women of normal weight and underweight women may need to gain slightly more than overweight women. Pregnant women should be cautioned against fasting as a method of weight control, because fasting leads to **ketoacidosis**, which can be dangerous to both the fetus and the mother.

The quality of nutrition during pregnancy is more important than weight gain per se or kilocalories consumed per day. Food intake in the first trimester should include balanced portions of essential nutrients with emphasis on quality. Protein intake throughout pregnancy is increased to 60 g (Food and Nutrition Board, 1989). High-risk mothers are advised to double their normal protein intake.

Calcium intake should be increased to 1200 mg/day. Calcium is needed for fetal tooth and bone development, muscle contraction, and blood clotting. Calcium intake is especially critical in the third trimester, when fetal bones are mineralized.

Pregnant women need 30 mg/day of iron, which is difficult to obtain from dietary sources, and, therefore, a supplement may be given. Iron is needed to correct preexisting deficiencies and to provide for increased maternal blood volume, for fetal blood storage, and for blood loss during delivery.

Iodine needs are increased by 25 mg (15% to 17%) because of increased activity of the thyroid gland. Vitamin A is needed for cell development, epithelial tissue maintenance, and tooth and bone development. Requirements are increased to 800 retinol equivalents (REs).

Pregnancy also increases requirements for B vitamins, which are needed for enzyme production necessitated by increased metabolic activity. Folic acid intake is particularly important for DNA synthesis and the growth of red blood cells. Inadequate intake may lead to megaloblastic anemia, a type of anemia seen in women who have had many pregnancies.

Vitamin C requirements are increased to 70 mg to provide the intercellular "cement" in connective and vascular tissue and to enhance the absorption of iron. Vitamin D needs are increased to 10 μg because this vitamin promotes the absorption of calcium and phosphorus needed for tooth and bone development.

The pregnant woman should have a minimum of three or more servings from the milk group; seven from the protein group including at least one vegetable protein; five to seven from the vegetable-fruit group (including a citrus fruit and a potato daily and leafy green or dark yellow vegetables three to four times a week); seven from the enriched or whole grain bread and cereal group; and three from the unsaturated fats group per day.

Pregnant women should increase their fluid intake by drinking at least eight glasses of water daily. They should avoid artificial sweeteners, alcohol, excessive caffeine, and all drugs not specifically ordered. Adequate fluid intake can prevent constipation, commonly associated with pregnancy.

LACTATION

The lactating woman needs 500 kcal above the usual allowance. The production of breast milk increases energy requirements. Protein requirements are increased to 65 g/day. The need for calcium remains the same as during pregnancy. There is an increased need for vitamins A and C.

The increased calories should be provided by leafy green vegetables, citrus fruits, whole grains, milk, meats, and poultry to provide vitamins A and C, niacin, riboflavin, and zinc. Daily intake of the water-soluble vitamins (B and C) is needed to ensure adequate levels in breast milk. Three servings from the milk group provide protein and calcium. Fluid intake should be adequate but need not be excessive. Caffeine, alcohol, and drugs are excreted in breast milk and should be avoided. Tobacco use can decrease milk production.

Older Adults

Adults 65 years and older have a decreased need for calories as the metabolic rate slows with age. The average allowance for men is 2300 kcal/day and for women is 1900 kcal/day. Vitamin and mineral allowances remain unchanged from middle adulthood levels.

Numerous factors influence the nutritional status of the older adult. Income is probably the most important because a fixed income may reduce the amount of money used to buy food. Health is another important influence. The older adult may be on a therapeutic diet or have difficulty eating because of physical symptoms, lack of teeth, or dentures, or be at risk of drug-nutrient interactions (see the box below). Food shopping and preparation may be difficult because of physical disability or lack of transportation. Living alone decreases the interest and pleasure of preparing and eating meals. The *Nutritional Screening Initiative* is a multidisciplinary effort to identify warning signs of malnutrition in older adults. Seven basic risk areas were identified and screening tools were designed for the nutritional assessment of older adults (Fig. 41-6).

GERONTOLOGICAL PRINCIPLES
for Drug-Nutrient Interactions

The older adult is at risk of nutrition problems related to the use of medications to treat chronic illnesses.
Older adults, as a group, are more likely to be taking medications for chronic illnesses than their younger counterparts.
Drugs can affect the absorption and metabolism of nutrients, and have effects upon appetite.
Nutrients can interact with drugs to increase or decrease their absorption and metabolism.
Drugs that increase appetite; such as prednisone, insulin, and lithium; can place the older adult at risk for obesity.
Drugs that decrease appetite, or alter taste and smell; such as captopril, digoxin, and penacillamine; can place the older adult at risk for malnutrition.

Nutrition Interventions Manual for Professionals Caring for Older Americans. Greer, Margolis, Mitchell, Grunwald & Associates, Inc. Nutrition Screening Initiative, 1010 Wisconsin Avenue NW, Suite 800, Washington, DC, 20007, 1992.

There are a number of physiological changes that can impede dietary intake. Taste acuity may decline with age. Dentures may increase bitter and sour taste sensations. A normal decline in gastric secretions results in less-efficient digestion. The thirst sensation may diminish leading to inadequate fluid intake.

The basic food group selections for older adults are the same as for younger adults, although the way that foods are prepared or the types of foods selected may need to be changed. Diets of older adults are typically low in protein foods and high in breads, cakes, and cereals. Meats may be avoided because of cost or because they are difficult to chew. Cheese, eggs, and peanut butter are useful in providing protein. Milk continues to be an important food, particularly for the older woman who needs adequate calcium to protect against osteoporosis (loss of calcium from bones). Whole grain cereals and breads should be encouraged. Cream soups and meat-based vegetable soups are good for the older adult with chewing problems. The diet of the older adult should contain choices from all food groups and may require vitamin supplements.

■ NUTRITION AND THE NURSING PROCESS

Nurses are in an excellent position to recognize signs of poor nutrition and to take steps to initiate change. Close daily contact with clients and their families enables nurses to make observations about their physical status, food intake, weight gain or loss, and responses to therapy. The nurse can identify actual or potential problems in nutritional status and implement appropriate nursing, medical, and nutritional therapies to reduce or reverse nutritional alterations.

 ### Assessment

Nurses collaborate with dieticians in conducting a comprehensive nutritional assessment. Because food and fluid are basic biological needs of all human beings, a nutritional assessment is essential. Nutritional assessment is particularly important for clients at risk for nutritional problems related to stress, illness, hospitalization, lifestyle habits, and other factors. Nutritional assessment centers around four major areas:

1. Physical measurements (height and weight) and anthropometry
2. Laboratory tests
3. Dietary history and health history
4. Clinical observations

PHYSICAL AND ANTHROPOMETRIC MEASUREMENTS

The client's height and weight measurements should be obtained on hospital admission or entry into any health care setting. If possible, the client should be weighed at the same time each day, on the same scale, and with the same clothing or linen. The client's height and weight can be compared to standards for height-weight relationships, such as the Metropolitan Life Insurance table (see Appendix). Recent weight changes should be documented.

If height cannot be measured with the client standing, the armspan, or distance from fingertip to fingertip with

The Warning Signs of poor nutritional health are often overlooked. Use this checklist to find out if you or someone you know is at nutritional risk.

Read the statements below. Circle the number in the yes column for those that apply. For each yes answer, score the number in the box. Total the nutritional score.

DETERMINE YOUR NUTRITIONAL HEALTH

	YES
I have an illness or condition that made me change the kind and/or amount of food I eat.	2
I eat fewer than 2 meals per day.	3
I eat few fruits or vegetables, or milk products.	2
I have 3 or more drinks of beer, liquor or wine almost every day.	2
I have tooth or mouth problems that make it hard for me to eat.	2
I don't always have enough money to buy the food I need.	4
I eat alone most of the time.	1
I take 3 or more different prescribed or over-the-counter drugs a day.	1
Without wanting to, I have lost or gained 10 pounds in the last 6 months.	2
I am not always physically able to shop, cook and/or feed myself.	2
TOTAL	

Total Your Nutritional Score. If it's –

0–2   **Good!** Recheck your nutritional score in 6 months.

3–5   **You are at moderate nutritional risk.** See what can be done to improve your eating habits and lifestyle. Your office on aging, senior nutrition program, senior citizens center or health department can help. Recheck your nutritional score in 3 months.

6 or more   **You are at high nutritional risk.** Bring this checklist the next time you see your doctor, dietitian or other qualified health or social service professional. Talk with them about any problems you may have. Ask for help to improve your nutritional health.

These materials developed and distributed by the Nutritional Screening Initiative, a project of:

AMERICAN ACADEMY
OF FAMILY PHYSICIANS

THE AMERICAN
DIETETIC ASSOCIATION

NATIONAL COUNCIL
ON THE AGING

Remember that warning signs suggest risk, but do not represent diagnosis of any condition.

Fig. 41-6 Nutrition screening tool for older adults. *(From the Nutrition Screening Initiative, a project of the American Academy of Family Physicians, the American Dietetic Association, and the National Council of the Aging, Inc. and funded in part by a grant from Ross Products Division, Abbott Laboratories.)*

arms fully outstretched at shoulder level, approximates height for the mature adult.

Anthropometry is a system of measurement of the size and makeup of the body and specific body parts. Anthropometric measurements that aid in identifying nutritional problems include the ratio of height to wrist circumference, mid-upper arm circumference (MAC), triceps skinfold (TSF), and mid-upper arm muscle circumference (MAMC).

Anthropometric measurements can have significant variation unless the examiner is skilled, has practiced these measurements, and has proper equipment. In addition, anthropometric measurements provide data that, in general, have more applicability in settings where multiple measurements can be made over time. A single measurement during a brief hospital stay is of limited applicability.

Wrist circumference is used to estimate the client's body frame. A tape measure is used to measure the smallest portion of the wrist distal to the styloid process. The nurse calculates the frame size by dividing the wrist circumference into the client's height (height [cm] ÷ wrist circumference [cm]). The result is the calculated *r* value. Body frame values for women are >11.0 (small), 10.1 to 11.0 (medium), and >10.1 (large). Frame sizes for men are >10.4 (small), 9.6 to 10.4 (medium), >9.6 (large) (Williams, 1993).

The MAC estimates skeletal muscle mass. The client's nondominant arm is relaxed, and the circumference is measured at the midpoint of the arm, between the tip of the acromial process of the scapula and the olecranon process of the ulna. Measurement of the nondominant arm prevents false recordings secondary to increased muscle mass from activities of daily living or employment.

Skinfold measurements are used to estimate fat content of subcutaneous tissue. TSF is the most common measurement. With the thumb and forefinger, a lengthwise fold of skin and fat is grasped about 1 cm above midpoint of the MAC. The jaws of a standard skinfold caliper are placed on either side of the fat fold. The average measurement is taken from three readings. Other anatomical areas for skinfold measurements include the biceps, scapula, and abdominal muscles.

The mid-upper arm muscle circumference (MAMC) is an estimation of skeletal muscle mass. It is calculated from the MAC and TSF anthropometric measures. The formula is MAMC = MAC − (TSF × 3.14).

Values for the MAC, TSF, and MAMC are compared to standards and calculated as a percentage of the standard. Changes in values for an individual over time are of greater significance than isolated measurements.

LABORATORY AND BIOCHEMICAL TESTS

No single laboratory or biochemical test is diagnostic for malnutrition. Tests are affected by numerous factors such as fluid balance, liver function, kidney function, and the presence of disease. Common laboratory tests used to study nutritional status include measures of plasma proteins such as albumin, transferrin, prealbumin, retinol binding protein, total iron binding capacity, and hemoglobin. The response time for changes in these proteins as a result of feeding ranges from hours to weeks. Most plasma proteins have a >7 day half-life and will not reflect changes in less than a week.

Other tests used to determine nutritional status include measures of immunity, such as delayed cutaneous sensitivity, and measures of protein metabolism, such as 24-hour urinary urea nitrogen and nitrogen balance studies.

DIETARY HISTORY AND HEALTH HISTORY

In addition to the general nursing history, the nurse obtains a more specific diet history to assess the client's actual or potential nutritional needs. The diet history focuses on the client's habitual intake of food and liquids, as well as information about preferences, allergies, problems, and other relevant areas, such as the client's ability to obtain food. During the nursing history the nurse also gathers information about the client's activity level to determine the energy need and compare it with food intake.

In outpatient settings, a 3- to 7-day diet history can be kept of the client's food intake. This history allows the nurse to calculate the client's nutritional intake and to compare it with recommended allowances to determine whether the client's usual dietary habits are providing all nutrients in required amounts.

An additional area for the nurse to assess is a set of factors that influence the client's dietary pattern and nutritional status (see the box on p. 1108). These factors include health status, cultural background, religion, socioeconomic status, personal preference, psychological factors, use of alcohol or drugs, and misinformation about food values.

Other tools used to collect a dietary assessment include a 24-hour food record and a food frequency questionnaire, which helps to establish food patterns over time. The nutritionist is a valuable resource to the nurse in planning and obtaining a dietary history.

CLINICAL OBSERVATIONS

Clinical observations can be among the most important aspects of a nutritional assessment. As in other kinds of nursing assessment, the nurse observes the client for signs of nutritional alterations. Because improper nutrition affects all body systems, clues to malnutrition may be observed during physical assessment (see Chapter 33). When the general physical assessment of body systems is complete, the nurse can recheck pertinent areas to evaluate the client's nutritional status. The clinical signs of nutritional status (Table 41-9) provide guidelines for observation during physical assessment.

CLIENTS AT RISK FOR NUTRITIONAL PROBLEMS

Any client with a condition that interferes with the ability to ingest, digest, or absorb adequate nutrients should be considered at risk. Congenital anomalies, excessive losses of gastrointestinal fluids, and surgical revisions of the gastrointestinal tract interfere with normal function. Clients who have an order for nothing by mouth (NPO) and who receive only standard IV fluids for more than 5 days are at nutritional risk. In addition, nutritional problems commonly occur in conditions such as AIDS, cancer, eating disorders, gastrointestinal disease, critical illness, malabsorption problems, metabolic diseases, obesity, renal disease, and diseases of the liver, pancreas, and gallbladder.

Postoperative Clients. The intake of food is often altered in the perioperative period. Preoperative preparation with diagnostic tests or bowel cleansing usually involves at least 8 hours of fasting. The resumption of food intake post-

Factors Influencing Dietary Patterns

HEALTH STATUS
- A good appetite is a sign of health.
- Anorexia (lack of appetite) is usually a symptom of disease or can be a side effect of drugs.
- Nutritional support is an essential part of recovery from any medical treatment.

CULTURE AND RELIGION
- Cultural, ethnic, and religious patterns and restrictions concerning food must be taken into account.
- Special foods and diets should be given when appropriate.
- Older clients are more apt to cling to ethnic food habits. This tendency may be increased during illness.

SOCIOECONOMIC STATUS
- Food expenses are not fixed, and spending varies according to the amount of money available.
- Whether someone is around to prepare food determines the amount of convenience foods used.

PERSONAL PREFERENCE
- Individual likes and dislikes are perhaps the strongest influence on diet.
- Foods associated with pleasant memories tend to become favorite foods. Foods associated with unpleasant memories tend to be avoided.
- Luxury foods may be used as status symbols.
- Individual preferences must be considered when planning a therapeutic diet.

PSYCHOLOGICAL FACTORS
- Individual motivations to eat balanced meals and individual perceptions about diet are strong influences.
- Food has strong symbolic value for many people (e.g., milk symbolizing helplessness and meat symbolizing strength).

ALCOHOL AND DRUGS
- Excess alcohol or drug use contributes to nutritional deficiencies because money may be spent on alcohol instead of food, and alcohol may replace part of the diet and depress appetite.
- Excess alcohol can also affect gastrointestinal organs.
- Drugs that depress appetite can lower the intake of essential nutrients.
- Drugs can also deplete nutrient stores and lessen their absorption in the intestines.

MISINFORMATION AND FOOD FADS
- Food myths can be the result of cultural background, popular interest in natural foods, peer pressure, or a desire to control diet choices.
- Food fads often involve erroneous beliefs that certain foods are especially healthy (e.g., yogurt being more nutritional than milk, oysters increasing sexual potency, or honey being healthier than sugar).
- Nurses must be careful not to be condescending when teaching a client that foods may not have the qualities attributed to them.

---

operatively depends upon the return of bowel function, the extent of the surgical procedure, the presence of any complications, and surgeon's preferences for when to initiate feeding (see Chapter 48).

Clients who have had oral and throat surgery must chew and swallow food in the presence of excision sites, sutures, or otherwise manipulated tissue. The ingestion of food causes discomfort, so clients are usually reluctant to eat or drink. Fluids are usually offered first. The use of a straw may help in some cases, but it is specifically contraindicated in others such as dental extractions, dental surgeries, and cleft palate repairs. Soft foods are sometimes easier to swallow than liquids. Hot fluids, tart juices, and coarse food that is difficult to chew should be avoided after throat and mouth surgery.

When surgery is performed on the stomach and intestines, an alternative method of food intake, such as parenteral nutrition (PN), may be prescribed when resumption of oral intake is not possible within about 5 days. Nasogastric suction is often used following gastrointestinal surgery to prevent distention and pressure on resected areas. When oral intake is restricted for a short period, fluids are usually given intravenously but these fluids are characteristically nutrient poor. Standard 5% dextrose solutions contain only 170 kcal/L. Gastric resections may limit the amount of food that can be ingested per meal if the remaining gastric pouch is small. Small frequent meals may be advised.

Intestinal surgery may interfere with absorption of nutrients or the amount of stool losses, if large portions of the intestine are resected or bypassed or if an ileostomy or mu-

cous fistula is created. Clients with ileostomies may also lose some of their ability to absorb vitamin B_{12} because the terminal ileum is the major site of absorption of this vitamin. Clients with ileostomies and colostomies require dietary counseling regarding the consistency of the ostomy output, the prevention of obstruction of the ostomy, and instruction about management of the ostomy appliance to prevent intestinal enzymes from causing skin irritation.

Immobilized Clients. Extended immobilization can result in deossification and osteoporosis of bones and in hypercalcemia (see Chapter 37). Hypercalcemia predisposes clients to kidney and bladder stones. It is a particular problem in children and adolescents because of their rapid bone growth. Ambulation is the best way to prevent demineralization of bone from immobility. When ambulation is not possible, adequate quantities of high-biological value proteins help prevent skin breakdown and infections, and high phosphorus intake in the early weeks of immobilization reduces blood calcium levels. Generous fluid intake also protects against kidney stones. Range of motion exercises for uninvolved joints provide some protection.

 Nursing Diagnosis

The nursing assessment enables the nurse to determine whether actual or potential nutritional problems exist (see the nursing diagnoses box on p. 1110). A deficit may occur when overall oral intake is significantly decreased or increased or when one or more nutrients are not ingested, are incompletely digested, or are incompletely absorbed. Spe-

Table 41-9	Clinical Signs of Nutritional Status	
BODY AREA	**SIGNS OF GOOD NUTRITION**	**SIGNS OF POOR NUTRITION**
General appearance	Alert: responsive	Listless, apathetic, cachexia, cachectic appearance
Weight	Weight normal for height, age, body build	Obesity or underweight appearance (special concern for underweight)
Posture	Erect posture; straight arms and legs	Sagging shoulders; sunken chest; humped back
Muscles	Well-developed, firm muscles; good tone; some fat under skin	Flaccid appearance, poor tone, underdeveloped tone; tenderness; edema; wasted appearance; inability to walk properly
Nervous system control	Good attention span; lack of irritability or restlessness; normal reflexes; psychological stability	Inattention; irritability; confusion; burning and tingling of hands and feet (paresthesia); loss of position and vibratory sense; weakness and tenderness of muscles (may result in inability to walk); decrease or loss of ankle and knee reflexes; absent vibratory sense
Gastrointestinal function	Good appetite and digestion; normal regular elimination; no palpable organs or masses	Anorexia; indigestion; constipation or diarrhea; liver or spleen enlargement
Cardiovascular function	Normal heart rate and rhythm; lack of murmurs; normal blood pressure for age	Rapid heart rate (above 100 beats/min), enlarged heart; abnormal rhythm; elevated blood pressure
General vitality	Endurance; energy, good sleep habits; vigorous appearance	Easily fatigued; lack of energy; falling asleep easily, tired and apathetic appearance
Hair	Shiny, lustrous appearance; firmness; strands not easily plucked, healthy scalp	Stringy, dull, brittle, dry, thin, and sparse, depigmented appearance; strands that can be easily plucked
Skin (general)	Smooth and slightly moist skin with good color	Rough, dry, scaly, pale, pigmented, irritated appearance; bruises; petechiae; subcutaneous fat loss
Face and neck	Uniform color; smooth, pink, healthy appearance; lack of swelling	Greasy, discolored, scaly, swollen appearance; dark skin over cheeks and under eyes; lumpiness or flakiness of skin around nose and mouth
Lips	Smoothness; good color; moist (not chapped or swollen) appearance	Dry, scaly, swollen appearance; redness and swelling (cheilosis); angular lesions at corners of mouth; fissures or scars (stomatitis)
Mouth, oral membranes	Reddish pink mucous membranes in oral cavity	Swollen, boggy oral mucous membranes
Gums	Good pink color; healthy and red appearance; lack of swelling or bleeding	Spongy gums that bleed easily; marginal redness, inflammation; receding gums
Tongue	Good pink or deep reddish color; lack of swelling; smoothness, presence of surface papillae; lack of lesions	Swelling, scarlet and raw appearance; magenta color, beefiness (glossitis); hyperemic and hypertrophic papillae; atrophic papillae
Teeth	Lack of cavities and pain; bright, straight appearance; lack of crowding; well-shaped jaw; clean appearance with no discoloration	Unfilled caries; absent teeth; worn surfaces; mottled (fluorosis), malpositioned appearance
Eyes	Bright, clear, shiny appearance; lack of sores at corner of membranes; eyelids; moist and healthy pink color; prominent blood vessels or lack of mound of tissue or sclera; lack of fatigue circles beneath eyes	Pale eye membranes (pale conjunctivas); redness of membrane (conjunctival injection); dryness; signs of infection; Bitot's spots, redness and fissuring of eyelid corners (angular palpebritis); dryness of eye membrane (conjunctival xerosis); dull appearance of cornea (corneal xerosis); soft cornea (keratomalacia)
Neck (glands)	Lack of enlargement	Thyroid enlargement
Nails	Firm, pink appearance	Spoon shape (koilonychia); brittleness; ridges
Legs, feet	Lack of tenderness, weakness, or swelling; good color	Edema; tender calf; tingling; weakness
Skeleton	Lack of malformations	Bowlegs; knock-knees; chest deformity at diaphragm; prominent scapulae and ribs

From Williams SR: Nutritional guidance in prenatal care. In Worthington-Roberts BS, Vermeersch JA, Williams SR: *Nutrition in pregnancy and lactation*, ed 5, St Louis, 1993, Mosby; Grant JA, Kennedy Caldwell C: *Nutritional support in nursing*, New York, 1988, Grune & Stratton.

Examples of NANDA Nursing Diagnoses for Altered Nutritional Status

Altered nutrition: less than body requirements *related to:*
- Increased metabolic rates
- Inadequate intake of nutrients in the diet
- Increased loss of nutrients via gastrointestinal fluids
- High energy needs related to excessive exercise

Altered nutrition: more than body requirements *related to:*
- Decreased metabolic rates
- Excessive intake of nutrients and kilocalories in the diet
- Inadequate exercise or activity

Altered nutrition: risk for more than body requirements *related to:*
- Dysfunctional pattern of food intake
- Disruption of relationship with significant other
- Impaired swallowing related to artificial airway

Modified from Kim MJ, McFarland GK, McLane AM: *Pocket guide to nursing diagnoses*, ed 6, St Louis, 1995, Mosby.

cific diagnoses are related to the actual nutritional deficiency (e.g., inadequate intake). The nursing diagnosis may also involve a general nutritional deficiency or problems that place the client at risk for nutritional deficiencies, such as oral trauma, severe burns or infections.

The nursing diagnostic statement is based on supporting diagnostic characteristics present in the assessment data base (see the diagnostic process box below). In addition, the suspected etiology of the diagnosis is stated. Identification of the cause further individualizes the nursing diagnostic statement and subsequent care plan.

Planning

Planning to maintain proper nutritional status provides a higher quality of care than correction of deficits once they have occurred (see the care plan below). The identification of clients at risk for nutritional problems should result in a care plan that will prevent or minimize nutritional problems. Nutritional education and counseling are important for clients on regular diets to prevent disease and promote health. Clients on therapeutic diets who understand the

---

Sample Nursing Diagnostic Process for Altered Nutritional Status

ASSESSMENT ACTIVITIES	DEFINING CHARACTERISTICS	NURSING DIAGNOSIS
Ask client about planned or unplanned changes in weight. Weigh client.	Unplanned weight loss Weight less than 20% of ideal body weight	**Altered nutrition less than body requirements** related to decreased intake
Ask client about food likes and dislikes. Inspect client's oral mucosa. Palpate abdomen.	Aversion to food Inflamed buccal mucosa Abdominal tenderness	

Sample Nursing Care Plan for Altered Nutrition: Less Than Body Requirements

NURSING DIAGNOSIS: Altered nutrition: less than body requirements.
DEFINITION: Altered nutrition: less than body requirements is the state in which an individual has decreased ability to voluntarily pass fluids and/or solids from the mouth to the stomach (Kim, McFarland, and McLane, 1995).

GOAL	EXPECTED OUTCOMES	INTERVENTIONS	RATIONALE
Client will return to within 10% of good weight-for-height range (based on a standard reference such as the Metropolitan Life Insurance Table) within 6 months	Client will gain ½ to 1 lb/wk on average	Customize diet for the client and use oral supplements as needed to achieve adequate energy and nutrient intake	Enteral nutrition is physiologically superior and less costly than parenteral nutrition, and may preserve intestinal structure and function (Mainous, Block, and Dietch, 1994)
	Laboratory parameters will show evidence of adequate hydration and improving nutritional parameters	Instruct client to drink water and noncaffeinated beverages at and between meals	Continued erosion in nutritional status places the client at risk for complications related to malnutriton, such as sepsis, dehydration, and electrolyte imbalances (Williams, 1993)

rationale for the diets are more likely to be compliant. For this group of clients the care plan is based on one or more of the following goals:

1. Client will return to within 10% of good body weight-for-height range.
2. Client will maintain fluid and electrolyte balance within normal limits.
3. Client will ingest or have administered a diet or nutritional therapy that, at a minimum, meets the RDAs.
4. No complications will result from nutritional therapies.

In the health care and home care settings, clients with physiological conditions that affect nutrition may require enteral or parenteral nutrition to meet fluid, electrolyte, and nutritional needs. When planning for complex nutritional needs, consultation with nutritionists helps to ensure adequate food sources. In addition, occupational therapists can work with the client and family to identify assistive devices to help the client eat or to rearrange the food preparation area to maximize the client's functional capacity (see Chapter 5).

Parenteral nutrition (PN) is a nutritionally adequate solution consisting of glucose, amino acids, lipids, minerals, and vitamins given through a peripheral or central intravenous catheter. A peripheral catheter can only be used for parenteral nutrition that contains no more than 10% dextrose because higher levels of dextrose are too hypertonic for peripheral vein administration. Clients who typically require PN are those who have gastrointestinal dysfunction that prevents enteral tube feeding, who require bowel rest, or in whom enteral access cannot be achieved. The nursing care plan for clients receiving PN is based on one or more of the following additional goals:

1. Clients will achieve positive nitrogen balance (a state where more nitrogen, as protein, is taken in than is lost) when illness prevents absorption of sufficient amounts of nutrients.
2. Essential nutrients for wound healing, metabolic processes, and restoration of body tissues will be achieved via the parenteral route.
3. Clients will receive enteral nutrition as soon as is physiologically possible either in combination with PN or by means of a transition to enteral nutrition.

 Implementation

Ill or debilitated clients often have poor appetites. The ketosis that accompanies starvation is an appetite suppressant, and surgical procedures and trauma cause pain. Deficiencies in certain vitamins and minerals can cause **anorexia.** Nurses can help clients to understand the factors that cause reduced appetite, use creative approaches to stimulate appetite, and assess clients for the need for pharmacological agents to stimulate appetite or to manage symptoms that reduce appetite.

One of the most disruptive influences on intake is diagnostic testing. Many laboratory and radiographical studies require the client to fast. Therefore, client's meals are withheld until the client returns from the test or testing is completed.

Stress also influences intake. Clients who are worried about their families, finances, employment, or illnesses are unable to eat or to eat enough to compensate for the effect of stress on their metabolism.

Medications can affect intake and the utilization of nutrients. Medications can affect the sensations of taste or smell causing unpleasant tastes or aversions to food odors. In addition, medications can cause gastrointestinal symptoms such as nausea or vomiting. Medications such as insulin and thyroid hormones can also affect metabolism. Interactions between nutrients and medications can affect the absorption, stability, or metabolism of drugs or nutrients.

STIMULATING APPETITE

A nurse can help stimulate the client's appetite through adaptation of the environment, consultation with a nutritionist, provision of special diets and food preferences, administration of appetite stimulant drugs, and counseling of the client and family.

Environment. Clients receive care in diverse settings, such as their homes, extended care facilities, community-based settings, and hospitals. In addition, some clients may receive all their meals in congregate meal sites such as senior centers. Wherever the setting, nurses are responsible for providing an environment conducive to eating. The client's room should be free of reminders of treatments. The environment should be free of odors. Mouth care should be provided prior to meals and whenever necessary to remove unpleasant tastes. The client needs to be positioned comfortably so that the meal can be more enjoyable. If the client has visitors or needs hygiene care before eating, sufficient time is given to permit anticipation and preparation for the meal.

Nutritionist. After a meal, the client's intake is evaluated and charted. The nurse shares responsibility with the nutritionist (dietitian) for evaluating food intake. The nutritionist's knowledge of normal and therapuetic nutrition assists the nurse in designing a plan that meets the client's nutritional goals. Sharing information about a client's concerns and response to diet therapy benefits the nurse, nutritionist, and client. The client's education about the therapeutic diet should be a shared responsibility. The nutritionist is the expert in diet therapy, and the nurse can relate dietary modifications to the client's overall condition and explain how the diet contributes to the care plan.

Therapeutic Diets and Diet Supplements. A regular diet contains approximately 2500 kcal and consists of appropriate servings from a variety of food groups. In some cases a diet is changed to reflect dietary recommendations of decreasing lipid content and increasing complex carbohydrate and fiber.

Modified diets or therapeutic diets address specific needs in disease processes. These modified diets are available in home care, extended care, and long-term care settings. Components of the diets that may be modified include the content of specific nutrients, the number of kilocalories, the texture of foods, or the seasoning of foods. Any therapeutic diet is only as good as the client's willingness to follow it. Meal plans should be individualized and developed in collaboration with the client.

Clients who have the ability to ingest food, and who have no or minimal problems with digestion or absorption, should have every chance to achieve an adequate oral diet. This may include the need for dietary supplements such as milk shakes, modular nutrients added to food, or commercial oral supplement products, or making meals more appealing.

DIET THERAPY IN DISEASE MANAGEMENT

Good nutrition is important in health and illness, but the specific dietary intake pattern that results in good nutrition must often be modified for clients with particular diseases. Diet modifications are necessary to correspond with the body's ability to metabolize certain nutrients, correct nutritional deficiencies related to the disease, and eliminate foods that may exacerbate disease symptoms. This section provides a summary of the dietary management of a variety of diseases.

Gastrointestinal Diseases. **Peptic ulcers** are controlled with regular meals and medications such as cimetidine. Cimetidine is one of a class of drugs that are histamine receptor antagonists that block secretion of hydrochloric acid. Clients are also encouraged to avoid foods that increase stomach acidity such as caffeine, decaffeinated coffee, frequent milk intake, citric acid juices, and certain seasonings (hot chili peppers, chili powder). Smoking and alcohol are discouraged.

The treatment of acute **inflammatory bowel disease** may include elemental diets (formula with the nutrients in their simplest form ready for absorption) or parenteral nutrition when symptoms such as diarrhea and weight loss are prevalent. In the chronic stage of the disease a regular highly nourishing diet is appropriate (Williams, 1993). Vitamins and iron supplements may be required to correct or prevent anemia. **Irritable bowel syndrome** is managed by increasing fiber, reducing fat, avoiding large meals, and avoiding lactose-containing or sorbitol-containing foods for susceptible individuals.

The treatment of **malabsorption syndromes**, such as celiac disease, includes a gluten-free diet. Gluten is present in wheat, rye, barley, and oats.

The treatment of **diverticulitis** is a moderate- or low-residue diet until the infection subsides. Afterward, a high-fiber diet is generally prescribed for chronic diverticulosis. Constipation often responds to increased dietary intake of whole grains and vegetables and fruits, adequate fluids, and increased activity. Chronic enema and laxative use should be discouraged.

Cardiovascular Diseases. The American Heart Association dietary guidelines to reduce risk factors for the development of coronary artery disease include maintenance of ideal body weight, reduction of dietary fats to 30% to 35% of total kilocalories and no more than 10% as saturated fats, an increase in carbohydrate to 50% to 55% of total kilocalories, use of protein in moderation with less animal protein, limitation of cholesterol to 300 mg or less, and limitation of sodium to 2 to 3 g/day (American Heart Association, 1993). Dietary therapy following an acute myocardial infarction includes initial reduction in kilocalories, soft textured foods, and fat and sodium contents that conform to the American Heart Association's guidelines.

Nutritional therapy for hypertension includes kilocalorie reduction to promote weight reduction as appropriate, decreased sodium intake, and potassium rich foods if potassium-wasting diuretics are used in treatment.

Diabetes. Non–insulin-dependent diabetes mellitus (NIDDM) or type II diabetes mellitus (DM) can usually be controlled by diet therapy. Insulin-dependent diabetes mellitus (IDDM) or type I DM requires insulin and dietary restrictions. In both cases the diet is individualized according to the client's age, build, weight, and activity level. Fats are moderately controlled (30% or less), and complex carbohydrates make up a higher percentage (50% to 60%) of the diet than simple carbohydrates. Foods that contain soluble fiber are recommended with a daily intake of 40 g fiber. Foods for dietary planning are classified in six exchange groups. Each item has about the same nutrient value as other foods in the same group. Meals are planned around balanced numbers of food exchanges, and foods may be exchanged within groups.

Renal Diseases. The dietary treatment of acute **glomerulonephritis** depends on the client's symptoms and is designed to maximize nutritional intake. Fluid, salt, and protein are not restricted unless indicated by symptoms such as edema, uremia, or oliguria.

The treatment of acute **renal failure** usually consists of fluid restriction to approximately 400 ml/day. Protein may be restricted and parenteral amino acids may be required. A balanced mixture of essential and nonessential amino acids is provided along with concentrated dextrose and lipids. If the gastrointestinal tract is functional, specially designed enteral tube feeding products are also available. Treatment of chronic renal failure typically consists of a diet that provides about 80 g/day of protein and restricted amounts of potassium, phosphate, sodium, calcium, and fluid. Adequate carbohydrate kilocalories prevent the use of protein for energy.

Dietary treatment for **renal stones** depends on the type of stones. For calcium phosphate stones the diet is low in calcium and high in acid ash. For uric acid stones the diet is low in purines. For calcium oxalate stones the diet avoids all foods high in calcium and oxalates.

Cancer and Cancer Treatment. Malignant cells compete with normal cells for nutrients, increasing the metabolic needs of the client. Clients with cancer typically complain of anorexia and taste distortions, and most cancer treatments cause nutritional problems. Malnutrition in the client with cancer is associated with increased morbidity and decreased length of survival. Enhanced nutritional status may improve the client's quality of life.

Radiation therapy is intended to destroy rapidly dividing malignant cells, however, other normal rapidly dividing cells, such as those in the gastrointestinal tract, can also be affected. Radiation therapy can cause anorexia, stomatitis, severe diarrhea, strictures of the intestine, and pain. Radiation treatment of the head and neck region can cause taste and smell disturbances, decreased salivation, and **dysphagia.** Nutritional management of the client with cancer focuses on maximizing intake of nutrients and fluids. The nurse should use creative approaches to manage alterations in taste and smell.

Human Immunodeficiency Virus (HIV). Human immunodeficiency virus (HIV) infected clients typically experience body wasting and severe weight loss. The wasting can be related to inadequate intake of nutrients and kilocalories, loss of nutrients in severe diarrhea, malabsorption of nutrients from disease of the gastrointestinal tract, alterations in metabolism, and factors that have not yet been identified.

Nutritional management in AIDS focuses upon maximization of kilocalories and nutrients. Fat intolerance related to malabsorption may pose a particular problem for clients with AIDS. Oral supplements that contain medium chain triglycerides may be better tolerated than safflower or soybean based products. Unproven nutritional regimens may interest clients with AIDS. The nurse should be supportive and attempt to assist the client to validate or investigate claims of "nutritional cures for AIDS". Each client's diet will need to be individualized.

Psychosocial Effects of Special Diets. Foods have symbolic meanings for clients and are closely related to lifestyle, habits, cultural background (see the box on p. 1099), and other aspects of the individual. Clients may have difficulty adjusting to special diets. Many clients consider mealtime a pleasurable period distinct from routines or an interlude from work activities. Alterations in the usual diet may affect the client's pleasure in eating. In addition, eating with others may have been a primary form of social interaction for the client who may now eat alone in a hospital room or cannot eat the same foods at home as other family members. Nurses and other health care professionals should recognize the client's response to dietary alterations and plan with the client to counteract negative effects. Suggest that the client: continue to have meals at usual meal times and with family members or significant others, vary the texture and temperature of foods to provide variety, creatively use herbs and spices to enhance flavor, and include a variety of foods in the diet to prevent taste fatigue.

SELF-FEEDING

Clients with disabilities that interfere with independent food intake should be allowed to do as much as possible for themselves. The nurse should prepare the tray, cutting food into bite-sized pieces, buttering bread, and pouring liquids. Special eating utensils should be provided if they contribute to clients' independence. Some disabled clients may become tired from their efforts to feed themselves. Clients who stop eating may still be hungry and may need assistance to finish their meals. The results of self-feeding should be evaluated on the basis of food intake and not neatness. Success should be recognized and commended. Small, frequent meals may be best to achieve adequate nutrition. The nurse who finds a way to aid disabled clients in eating more independently should share this information by incorporating it into the care plan.

Clients with visual impairment may need assistance from the nurse to feed themselves. If the visual impairment is new or temporary, the client may prefer to be fed. Clients with visual impairment can successfully feed themselves independently if the nurse describes the food and its location on the tray, places the tray within the client's reach, makes sure that cups of liquid are not excessively full, and orients the client to the location of each food by holding the client's hand and bringing it to the food's location.

CLIENT AND FAMILY COUNSELING

Clients discharged from a hospital with diet prescriptions often need dietary counseling to plan meals that meet specific diet requirements or general nutrition needs. Similarly, in other health care settings, clients with nutrition deficits or specific problems such as obesity may require assistance in menu planning and compliance with recommended diet therapies. The nurse's counseling role often includes families and information about community resources.

Meal planning must take into account the family's budget and differences in the preferences of family members. Specific foods are chosen on the basis of the dietary prescriptions or standard dietary guidelines such as the basic food groups. Meals should also provide a variety of foods and contrasting colors and consistencies. For families on limited budgets, substitutes can be used. For example, bean or cheese dishes can often replace meat in a meal, and evaporated or dry skim milk can be used for cooking. The method of preparation may also be modified when it is necessary to minimize certain substances. For example, baking rather than frying reduces fat intake, and lemon juice or spices can be used to add flavor to a low-sodium diet.

Planning menus a week in advance has several benefits. It helps ensure good nutrition or compliance with a specific diet and helps family members avoid impulse eating of less nutritional foods. Fruit and other nutritional items can be included in the plan for between-meal snacks. Careful advance planning can also help the family stay within the allotted budget because planned food buying is generally more economical. Last-minute shopping often includes more expensive processed and packaged foods. Often a simple tip can be of value in meal planning, such as advice to avoid grocery shopping when hungry, which can lead to spontaneous purchases of more expensive or less nutritional foods not included in meal plans.

Finally, the nurse can assist the client with referrals to community resources for assistance with dietary problems. Assistance in obtaining food is provided by several government programs such as food commodities; food stamps; the Women, Infant, Children (WIC) nutrition program; and school lunch programs. Private organizations such as Meals on Wheels provide assistance. Volunteer health agencies, such as the American Heart Association and the American Diabetes Association, provide nutrition consultation, diet information, and educational materials. Other community groups also offer planned menus and other nutritional guidelines. The American Dietetic Association, through its nutrition center, offers a wide range of materials. Detailed counseling can also be obtained from a registered or licensed dietitian.

ORAL FEEDINGS

Assisting Clients With Feeding. Being fed deprives clients of the independence they gained over their food intake as toddlers. At best, being fed is an unpleasant experience. Nurses can improve client feeding by carefully protecting clients' dignity and actively involving them in the process. Any material used to protect clothing should be referred to as a napkin, not a bib. The nurse should allow clients time to empty their mouths after every spoonful, attempting to match the speed of feeding to their readiness and asking frequently whether it is too fast or slow. The nurse should also allow clients to direct the order in which they wish to eat food items, and conversation about topics other than food should be an integral part of the process. The nurse who has several clients to feed should delegate feeding responsibility to other personnel so that all clients are fed in a timely, well-planned manner.

Administering Enteral Feedings via Gastrostomy or Jejunostomy Tube

STEPS	RATIONALE
1. Assess client's need for enteral tube feedings: NPO >5 days, functional GI tract, inability to ingest sufficient nutrients.	Identifying clients who need tube feedings before they become nutritionally depleted may prevent complications related to malnutrition.
a. Auscultate for bowel sounds before feeding.	Reflects presence of peristalsis. Changes in the frequency or character of bowel sounds may indicate changes in bowel motility.
b. Observe for abdominal distention.	Assists in recognizing delayed gastric emptying and reduces risk of regurgitation and pulmonary aspiration related to gastric distention (Petrosino, Christian, Becker, 1989).
c. While wearing gloves, assess gastrostomy or jejunostomy site for breakdown, irritation, drainage.	Infection, pressure from tube, or drainage of secretions can cause skin breakdown.
2. Verify physician's order for formula, rate, route, and frequency.	Tube feedings must be ordered by physician.
3. Wash hands and put on clean gloves.	Standard precautions.
4. Assemble equipment:	
a. Disposable feeding container and tubing.	
b. 60-ml syringe (catheter tip or Luer-lock)	Formula can be administered via syringe for intermittent gastrostomy feedings. Jejunostomy feedings usually require continuous infusion via a pump.
c. Formula	
d. Enteral feeding pump	Helps regulate flow of continuous feedings.
5. Explain procedure to client.	
6. Elevate head of bed at least 45° or assist client to sit in chair.	Reduces risk of aspiration.
7. Verify placement of tube:	
GASTROSTOMY TUBE	
a. Aspirate gastric secretions and check pH.	pH <4 indicates gastric placement. Tube should be flushed with 30 ml air before pH is measured.
b. Measure gastric residual.	Gastric residual of >150 ml may indicate delayed gastric emptying.
JEJUNOSTOMY TUBE	
a. Aspirate intestinal secretions and check pH.	pH >6 indicates intestinal placement. Tube should be flushed with 30 ml air before pH is measured.
8. Initiate feeding:	
a. Syringe feedings:	
(1) Pinch proximal end of gastrostomy tube.	Prevents air from entering stomach.
(2) Attach syringe to end of tube and fill syringe with formula.	
(3) Allow syringe to empty gradually. Refill until prescribed amount has been delivered to client.	Gradual emptying reduces risk of bloating and diarrhea induced by bolus tube feedings. Ideally, administration should occur over about 20 minutes, similar to ingesting a meal.
b. Continuous drip method:	This method is designed to deliver prescribed rate of feeding over 24 hours. Clients who receive these feedings into the stomach should have residuals checked every 4-6 hours or have periodic checks of the pH of secretions aspirated from the tube. The tube should be flushed with air before pH checks or after each residual check.
(1) Fill feeding container with enough formula for 4 hours of feeding.	
(2) Hang container on IV pole and clear tubing of air.	
(3) Thread tubing on pump according to manufacturer's directions.	
(4) Connect tubing to end of feeding tube.	
(5) Begin infusion at prescribed rate.	

Administering Enteral Feedings via Gastrostomy or Jejunostomy Tube—cont'd

STEPS	RATIONALE
9. Assess skin around tube exit site. The skin around the site should be cleansed daily with warm water and mild soap. Dressings around the exit site are not recommended.	Report any drainage, redness, swelling, or displacement of the tube to the physician.
10. Dispose of supplies and wash hands.	Prevents transmission of microorganisms.
11. Assess the client's tolerance of the feeding by checking residuals of gastric feedings, assessing bowel sounds, palpating the client's abdomen for distention or tenderness, and asking the client about symptoms such as nausea, bloating, or discomfort.	Determines that the client's gastrointestinal tract is digesting and absorbing nutrients.
12. Record amount, route, formula, assessment of tolerance, and client's response. Record amount of residual obtained or pH measurements.	Documents administration of tube feeding and communicates client's response.

ENTERAL NUTRITION AND TUBE FEEDING

Enteral nutrition (EN) refers to nutrients given via the gastrointestinal tract. This includes whole foods, blended whole foods, oral supplements, and tube feeding formulas. Enteral nutrition is the preferred method of meeting nutritional needs if the client's gastrointestinal tract is functioning by providing physiological, safe, and economical nutritional support. For clients with eating difficulties, enteral nutrition may be provided with nasogastric, jejunal, or gastric tubes. Enteral nutrition and tube feedings are easily given in home care settings by the nurse or by the family. Regardless of the setting, the principles in Procedure 41-1 for gastrostomy and jejunostomy enteral feedings must be maintained.

Studies have demonstrated a beneficial effect of enteral feedings as compared to parenteral nutrition, that of nourishing the gastrointestinal mucosa. Feeding by the enteral route may reduce sepsis, blunt the hypermetabolic response to trauma, and maintain intestinal structure and function (Mainous, Block, and Dietch, 1994).

EN has been used successfully within 24 to 48 hours after surgery or trauma to provide fluids, electrolytes, and nutritional support. Gastric ileus may prevent nasogastric feedings in cases where nasointestinal or jejunal tubes allow successful postpyloric feedings (Kudsk, 1994).

EN formulas vary in composition and nutrient density. General categories of EN formulas include standard whole protein formulas, elemental or peptide based formulas, and disease-specific formulas. Standard formulas are suitable for clients who do not have altered digestion or absorption, elemental and peptide formulas are used for clients who have impaired digestion or absorption, and disease-specific formulas have modifications in the content of specific nutrients or in caloric density. Nearly all tube feeding formulas are lactose free. Specialty enteral products tend to be very costly and their use is generally reserved for specific indications (Matarese, 1994). Current research is focusing on the effect of specific nutrients such as glutamine, arginine, nucleotides, and omega-3 fatty acids when added to enteral formulas (Kudsk, 1994).

Enteral Access Tubes. When the client is unable to ingest food but is still able to digest and absorb nutrients, enteral tube feeding is indicated. Feeding tubes can be inserted through the nose (nasogastric or nasointestinal), surgically (gastrostomy or jejunostomy), or endoscopically (percutaneous endoscopic gastrostomy or jejunostomy [PEG or PEJ]). Surgical or endoscopically placed tubes are preferred for long-term feeding to reduce the discomfort of a nasal tube and to provide a more secure and reliable access.

Nursing research has investigated the problems associated with feeding tube placement, type of feeding instilled, rate of feeding, and complications associated with tube feeding.

Large-bore rubber or plastic feeding tubes were initially used for nasogastric tube feedings. However, the problems associated with these tubes—local irritation, pharyngitis, otitis, sinusitis, and esophageal sphincter incompetence—led to the development of more flexible and comfortable small-bore feeding tubes (Metheny, Spies, and Eisenberg, 1988). For the adult, most of these tubes are 8 to 12 Fr and 36 to 43 inches long. A stylet is often used during insertion of a small-bore tube to stiffen it. The stylet is removed when the correct position of the feeding tube has been confirmed.

Chapter 48 discusses the placement, management, irrigation, and removal of the large-bore nasogastric tube, which is frequently placed during abdominal surgery for gastric decompression and irrigation. This section and the procedure described focus solely on the small-bore nasogastric, gastric, and jejunostomy enteral tubes for feeding (Fig. 41-7). Procedures 41-2 and 41-3 describe the procedure for inserting a small-bore nasoenteric tube and initiating enteral feedings. Critically ill clients often require placement of tubes beyond the stomach into the intestine because gastric emptying is often altered in this population (Minard, 1994).

Verification of the placement of small-bore feeding tubes

Inserting a Small-Bore Nasoenteric Tube for Enteral Feedings

STEPS	RATIONALE
1. Assess client for the need for enteral tube feeding: NPO or insufficient intake for >5 days, functional GI tract, unable to ingest sufficient nutrients.	Identifying clients who need tube feedings before they become nutritionally depleted may help to prevent complications related to malnutriton.
2. Assess client for appropriate route of administration:	Evaluates nares for patency.
a. Close each nostril alternately and ask client to breathe.	Nares may be obstructed. Assessment determines which nares to use.
b. Assess for gag reflex.	Identifies ability to swallow and risk of aspiration.
c. Review client's medical history for nasal problems and risk of aspiration.	Nurse may seek physician's order to change route of nutrition support or to place tube past the stomach into the intestine with increased risk of aspiration.
3. Review physician's order for type of tube and enteral feeding schedule.	Procedure and tube feedings require a physician's order.
4. Wash hands.	Reduces transfer of microorganisms.
5. Assemble equipment at bedside:	Organizes procedure and limits client discomfort.
a. Small-bore feeding tube (8-12 Fr)	
b. Large syringe: 30- to 60-ml Luer-lock or catheter tip syringe	Small syringe (<20 ml) may create enough pressure to rupture tube.
c. pH test strips	Used to measure gastric acidity and indicate placement of tube in stomach or intestine.
d. Hypoallergenic tape and tincture of benzoin	Tincture of benzoin increases adhesion of tape to nose.
e. Glass of water and straw	Client drinks to activate swallowing reflex, which aids in passing tube.
f. Emesis basin	Nasoenteric intubation may activate gag reflex and cause vomiting.
g. Tongue blade	Used to visualize posterior pharynx for tube placement.
h. Penlight or flashlight	
i. Towel	
j. Clean gloves	
k. Facial tissue	
l. Guidewire or stylet	Used to stiffen soft, flexible feeding tubes during insertion. Removed after placement of tube is confirmed.
m. Water-soluble lubricant	Used to lubricate tip of feeding tube for insertion.
n. Safety pin and rubber band	Used to attach tube to client's gown.
6. Explain procedure to client.	Reduces anxiety and helps client to assist in insertion.
7. Stand on same side of bed as nares for insertion and assist client to high Fowler's position unless contraindicated. Place pillow behind head and shoulders.	Allows easier manipulation of tube. Fowler's position reduces risk of aspiration and promotes effective swallowing.
8. Place bath towel over chest. Keep facial tissues within reach.	Prevents soiling of gown. Insertion of tube may produce tearing.
9. Determine length of tube to be inserted and mark with tape:	Length approximates distance from nose to stomach in 98% of clients. For duodenal or jejunal placement, an additional 20-30 cm is required (Grant, Kennedy-Caldwell, 1988).
a. Traditional method: measure distance from tip of nose to earlobe to xiphoid process of sternum (see the illustration on p. 1117).	
10. Instruct client to relax and breathe normally.	
11. Prepare for intubation:	
a. Do not ice plastic tubes.	Tubes will become stiff and inflexible and can cause trauma to mucous membranes.
b. Inject 10 ml of water from syringe into tube to activate lubricant.	Aids in guidewire insertion.
c. Insert guidewire or stylet into tube, making certain that it is securely in position and that guidewire and tube are securely fitted together.	Improperly positioned guidewire or stylet can cause trauma to nasopharynx, esophagus, or stomach.

Inserting a Small-Bore Nasoenteric Tube for Enteral Feedings—cont'd

STEPS	RATIONALE
11. Prepare for intubation—cont'd:	
d. Lubricate distal end of tube with water-soluble lubricant.	Ensures timely anchoring of tube once it has been passed.
e. Cut 10-cm (4-in) piece of tape. Split one end lengthwise 5 cm (2 in).	
12. Put on clean gloves.	Standard precautions.
13. Insert tube through nostril to back of throat. Client may gag. Direct tube back and toward ear.	Natural contours facilitate passage of tube.
14. Flex head toward chest after tube has passed through back of throat.	Closes off glottis and reduces risk of tube entering trachea.
15. Encourage clients who are able, to swallow by giving small sips of water or ice chips when possible. Advance tube as client swallows. Rotate tube 180 degrees while inserting and emphasize the need to mouth breathe and swallow.	Facilitates passage of tube down esophagus and can help to prevent coiling of tube in oropharynx. Small sips of water are usually allowed during tube insertion for clients who are NPO.
16. Advance tube each time client swallows until desired length is reached.	
a. Do not force the tube. When resistance is met, or the client starts to gag, choke, or become cyanotic, stop advancing the tube and pull back until symptoms subside. Check for position of tube in oropharynx with tongue blade and penlight.	Tube may be kinked or coiled in oropharynx. Tube may also pass into trachea.
17. Check placement of tube:	
a. Aspirate fluid with syringe.	Estimates proper postion before radiograph is taken.
b. Measure pH of aspirate with color-coded pH paper.	Gastric aspirates have acidic pH values: preferably value is 4 or less.
	Intestinal values are preferably 6 or more (Metheny et al, 1989) (see the illustation below).
18. Apply tincture of benzoin or skin prep on tip of nose and tube. Allow to dry.	Helps tape adhere better.

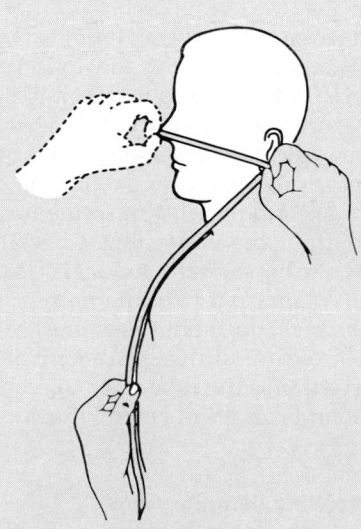

Step 9a

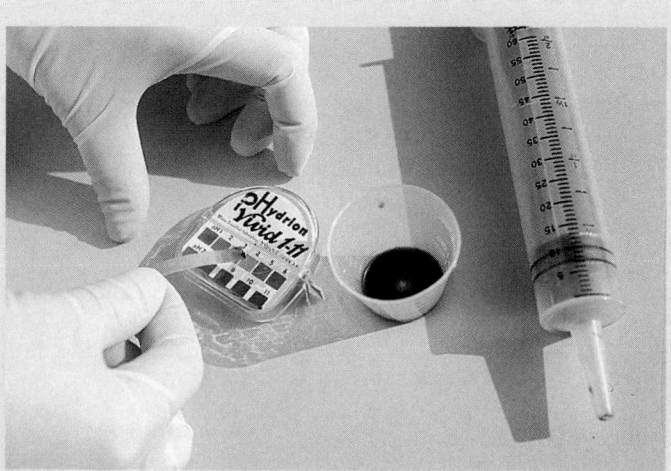

Step 17b

Continued.

Inserting a Small-Bore Nasoenteric Tube for Enteral Feedings—cont'd

STEPS	RATIONALE
19. Secure tube with tape and avoid pressure on nares.	Avoids development of necrosis from pressure on nose.
a. Take 10-cm piece of tape that was split. Place intact section of tape over bridge of nose. Carefully wrap split ends around tube.	Reduces friction on nares when client turns head.
b. Fasten end of tube to gown by looping rubber band around tube in slip knot. Pin rubber band to gown.	Guidewire or stylet may puncture gastrointestinal tract.
20. Leave stylet in place until correct position is verified. Never reinsert stylet or guidewire once it has been removed.	
21. Assist client to a comfortable position until x-ray is taken.	Enhances comfort.
22. Remove gloves, dispose of equipment, and wash hands.	Reduces transmission of microorganisms.
23. Record type and size of tube placed, color and amount of aspirate obtained, and client's response to insertion.	
24. Administer oral hygiene frequently (see Chapter 40).	

is unreliable except for x-rays. Historically, large-bore feeding tube placement was verified by withdrawing gastric contents from the tube, injecting air through the nasogastric tube while auscultating the stomach for a gurgling or bubbling sound, or asking the client to speak (Metheny, Spies, and Eisenberg, 1988). These methods do not apply as readily to small-bore nasogastric tubes and each has a high degree of inaccuracy. Nurses reported correct location in the stomach using the auscultatory method when the tube was actually in the esophagus, duodenum, jejunum, or stomach (Metheny, Spies, and Eisenberg, 1988). A number of clients have reportedly been able to speak despite tube placement in the respiratory tract (Rombeau and Barot, 1981).

Current bedside methods to test placement of small-bore feeding tubes are frequently ineffective. At present, the most reliable method is radiographic verification. This method is cost prohibitive. Therefore, new methods to test placement must be explored. The measurement of pH of secretions withdrawn from the feeding tube may help to differentiate the location of the tube (see the box on p. 1119). In the meantime, the nurse must have a high index of suspicion for tube displacement in clients at risk and use meticulous assessment skills.

Aspiration of gastric or intestinal fluid and pH testing of the fluid or use of a pH sensing feeding tube is an area of study that holds promise as a relatively reliable, cost effective, and simple method to confirm tube placement after the initial insertion (Berry et al, 1994; Metheny et al, 1994). For accurate pH measurements, 30 ml of air is injected into the tube prior to measurement, to flush out formula, medications, flush solutions, or other substances (Metheny et al, 1994).

Metheny, Spies, and Eisenberg (1986) examined nasoenteral feeding tube displacement and found that a sizable number of these tubes were found by radiological examination to be spontaneously displaced. That is, the distal tips of the tubes dislocated upwardly in the gastrointestinal tract, whereas the proximal external portion of the feeding tube remained taped in place. Displacement can occur with coughing, vomiting, and suctioning. Checking samples of fluid withdrawn from the tube for acidic (gastric) or alkaline (intestinal) values prior to intermittent feedings, and periodically during continuous feedings, is perhaps the most sensitive indicator of tube placement at this time. Air should be injected into the tube prior to each pH measurement. Major complications of enteral nutrition include the following:

1. Aspiration
2. Gastrointestinal complications
3. Problems with access devices, feeding tube, feeding pump, etc.
4. Electrolyte or metabolic complications

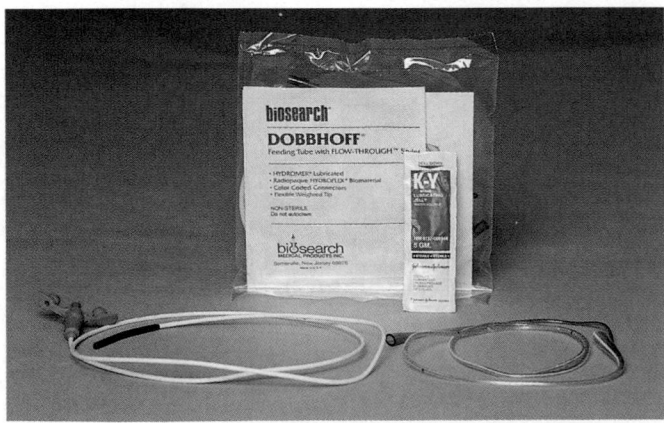

Fig. 41-7 Small-bore feeding tubes.

► **RESEARCH HIGHLIGHT**

RESEARCH ABSTRACT

The two most dreaded complications of nasoenteric tube feedings [are]: (1) introduction of feedings through tubes positioned in the respiratory tract, and (2) pulmonary aspiration. Bedside methods that lack reliability in ruling out inadvertent respiratory placement of feeding tubes include the auscultatory method, the bubbling under water method, and observing for respiratory symptoms. Testing the pH of aspirates from inserted feeding tubes when acidic values are properly obtained; further, migrated from the stomach to the intestine. Based on experience, the most frequently cited values for gastric residuals are 100 to 150 ml. In a recent small study, researchers concluded that the residual volume that should raise concern in clients with nasogastric tubes is 200 ml and in clients with gastrostomy tubes is 100 ml. Several recent studies indicate that although elevating the head of the bed 30 to 45 degrees does not prevent aspiration, it does reduce its frequency and severity. Because many studies described in this review have not been replicated, readiness of their findings for clinical application is variable. Many questions regarding methods to prevent respiratory complications in tube-fed clients remain unanswered, largely because it is difficult to design clinical studies with sufficient control of significant variables.

IMPLICATIONS FOR PRACTICE

► Traditional methods to test feeding tube placement, such as ascultation, assessment for respiratory distress, and checking for bubbling when the end of the tube is placed under water are unreliable and may fail to distinguish correct placement from placement in the pulmonary system.

► Measurement of the pH of fluid samples obtained through feeding tubes may help to distinguish pulmonary placement from gastric placement, when acidic readings are obtained.

► In general, there is a lack of research about the volume of residual feeding in the stomach that may pose the risk of aspiration.

► Studies have shown that raising the head of the bed during tube feeding does not prevent aspiration but may reduce its frequency and severity, therefore this practice should continue.

REFERENCE

Metheny N: Minimizing respiratory complications of nasoenteric tube feedings: state of the science, *Heart & Lung* 22:213, 1993.

Table 41-10 presents the most common complications of tube feeding, their possible causes, and nursing interventions. Electrolyte and metabolic complications are common with tube feeding and include those that are seen with parenteral nutrition.

PARENTERAL NUTRITION (PN)

PN is a form of specialized nutritional support in which nutrients are provided by the intravenous route. Although PN can effectively prevent malnutrition in clients who cannot be fed using the enteral route, PN can cause complications and requires skillful nursing management. Safe administration of this form of nutrition depends on an appropriate assessment of nutrition needs, meticulous management of the central venous catheter, and careful monitoring to prevent or treat metabolic complications. Parenteral nutrition is adminstered in a variety of settings, including the client's home. Regardless of the setting, the nurse adheres to the same priciples of asepsis and infusion management to ensure safe and correct nutritional support.

Clients who are unable to digest or absorb enteral nutrition are candidates for PN. PN is contraindicated when clients' gastrointestinal tracts are functional, when a trial of enteral nutrition has not been attempted in cases of partial gastrointestinal dysfunction, when clients have clearly indicated their wishes not to receive PN in terminal illness, and when the risks of therapy clearly outweigh the benefits.

PN solutions that contain greater than 10% dextrose are hypertonic and must be infused through a central vein to prevent thrombosis. The solution is tailored to the client's specific nutritional needs, and typical solutions consist of 12% to 25% dextrose, 3% to 6% amino acids, and may have lipid emulsion added. A solution that contains dextrose, animo acids, and lipids is called a *3-in-1 admixture* or *total nutrient admixture*. Solutions that contain 10% dextrose or less can be given by peripheral vein in combination with amino acids and lipids. Peripheral solutions are not as calorically dense, and therefore may be given for a limited period of time or be contraindicated for some clients. Electrolyte needs during PN vary with the client's fluid losses, organ dysfunction, and degree of malnutrition. Severely malnourished clients are at risk for electrolyte disturbances from "refeeding syndrome" as cations move intracellularly during PN (Jolly and Blank, 1994). PN for pediatric clients may also be administered by the peripheral route or the central route with a solution that contains an amino acid solution designed for the pediatric client.

Lipid Emulsions. **Lipid emulsions** provide supplemental calories and prevent essential fatty acid deficiencies. These emulsions can be administered through a separate peripheral line, through the central line by Y-connector tubing (see Chapter 45), or as an admixture to the PN solution. The addition of lipid emulsion to the PN solution as a 3-in-1 admixture is limited by the stability of the admixture. The admixture should not be used if oil droplets are observed or if an oil or creamy layer is observed on the surface of the admixture. This observation indicates that the emulsion has broken into large lipid droplets that can cause fat emboli if administered. Lipid emulsions are white and opaque like milk and care should be taken to avoid confusing enteral formula with parenteral lipids.

The recommended initial infusion rate for lipid emulsions is 1 ml/min for the first 30 minutes. Adverse reactions

Initiating Enteral Tube Feedings via Nasoenteric Tubes

STEPS	RATIONALE
1. Assess client for the need for tube feedings: NPO > 5 days, functional GI tract, inability to ingest sufficient nutrients.	Identifying clients who need tube feedings before they become nutritionally depleted may prevent complications related to malnutrition.
2. Verify physician's order.	Tube feedings must be ordered by physician. Order should include formula, route, and frequency.
3. Elevate head of bed to at least 45° or have client sit in chair.	Reduces risk of pulmonary aspiration from gastric reflux during or following administration of tube feeding.
4. Wash hands.	
5. Assemble the following equipment:	
a. Disposable tube feeding container and tubing	Ensures prompt efficient completion of feeding.
b. 60-ml syringe (catheter tip or Luer-lock)	Formula can be administered via syringe for intermittent feedings into the stomach.
c. Prescribed amount of formula	
d. Enteral feeding pump for continuous administration	Pump is necessary to regulate continuous feedings or for intestinal feedings.
e. Disposable gloves	
6. Put on gloves.	Standard precautions.
7. Determine placement of feeding tube (see Procedure 41-2, Step 17):	Verifies placement of tube in stomach or intestine.
a. Aspirate gastric secretions and check gastric residual in stomach.	Indicates the possibility of delayed gastric emptying (if >150 ml remains in stomach).
b. Aspirate intestinal secretions and measure pH to confirm intestinal placement.	Intestinal placement is indicated by pH values >6.
c. Flush tube with 30 ml water after pH or residual is measured.	Clumping of formula can occur with contact of acidic secretions.
d. Observe for abdominal distention and assess for abdominal discomfort.	Assists in recognizing delayed gastric emptying and reduces risk of regurgitation related to gastric distention (Petrosino, Christian, Becker, 1989).
8. Auscultate for bowel sounds.	Absence of bowel sounds when accompanied by other symptoms such as abdominal distention may indicate delayed or absent peristalsis.
9. Administer tube feedings.	
a. INTERMITTENT FEEDINGS WITH SYRINGE OR FEEDING CONTAINER	
(1) Pinch feeding tube below proximal end.	Prevents air from entering client's stomach.
(2) Attach syringe with plunger removed to end of tube.	
(3) Fill syringe with formula. Allow syringe to empty slowly refilling until prescribed amount has been delivered to client.	Gradual emptying reduces risk of bloating or diarrhea induced by bolus tube feedings. Ideally, administration should occur over about 20 minutes, similar to ingesting a meal.
(4) For feedings via a container, fill container with prescribed amount of formula and clear air from tubing. Hang container on an IV pole. Attach end of tubing to tube and regulate flow to infuse feeding over about 20 minutes (see the illustration on p. 1121).	
b. CONTINUOUS DRIP METHOD	
(1) Fill feeding container with enough formula for 4 hours of infusion.	This method is designed to deliver prescribed rate of feeding over 24 hours. Clients who receive these feedings into the stomach should have gastric residuals checked every 6-8 hours or have periodic checks of the pH of secretions aspirated from the tube. The tube should be flushed with water before pH checks or after each residual check.
(2) Hang container on IV pole.	
(3) Thread tubing on pump according to manufacturer's directions (see the illustration on p. 1121).	
(4) Connect tubing to end of feeding tube.	
(5) Begin infusion at prescribed rate.	

Initiating Enteral Tube Feedings via Nasoenteric Tubes—cont'd

STEPS	RATIONALE
10. Remove and dispose of gloves in proper receptacle. Wash hands.	Prevents transmission of microorganisms.
11. When tube feedings are not being administered, clamp or cap proximal end of feeding tube.	Prevents air from entering client's stomach or intestines between feedings.
12. Administer water via feeding tube as ordered with or between feedings.	Provides client with source of water to help maintain fluid and electrolyte balance.
13. Record amount, route, formula, and client's response. Record amount of residual obtained.	Documents administration of feeding.

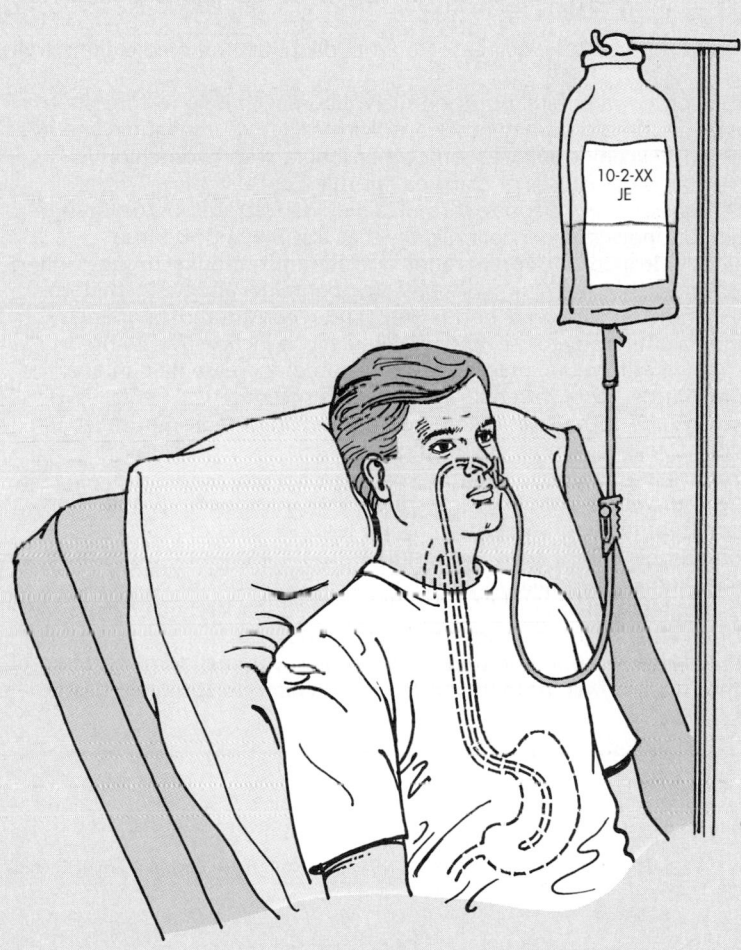

Step 9a(4)

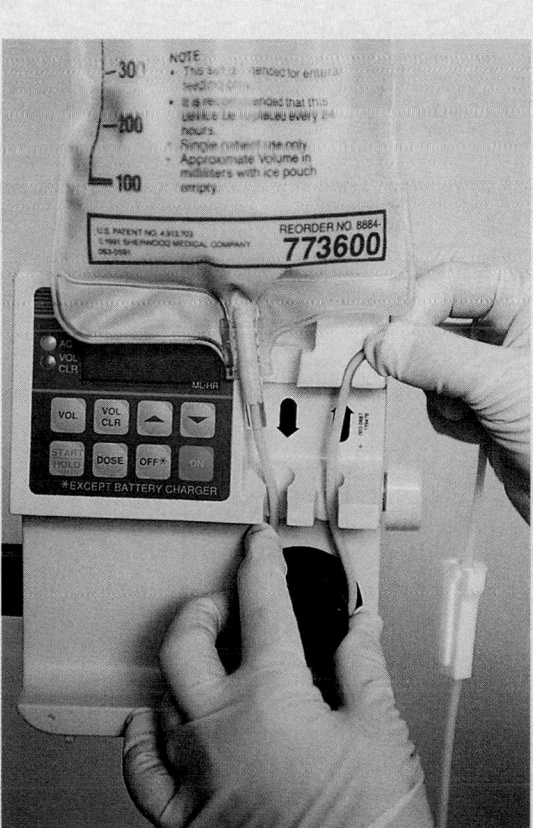

Step 9b(3)

Table 41-10	Preventing Complications of Enteral Nutrition	
COMPLICATION	**POSSIBLE CAUSE**	**INTERVENTION**
Pulmonary aspiration*	Feeding tube in esophagus or respiratory tract	Confirm proper placement of tube before administering any feeding; check placement (e.g., check pH of fluid aspirated from tube) at least every 4-8 hr during continuous feedings
	Regurgitation of formula	Aspiration is thought by some authorities to be less likely if feedings are administered below the pylorus; keep head elevated 30° during feedings; stop feedings temporarily during treatments such as chest physiotherapy; formula can be tinted with food coloring to make detection of formula in the respiratory tract easier
Diarrhea	Antibiotic therapy	Physician may order pectin (e.g., banana flakes) or kaolin and pectin (e.g., Kaopectate); lactobacillus-containing medications or dairy products (e.g., yogurt) are sometimes used in an effort to establish benign gut flora but are often ineffective
	Hypertonic formula or medications (e.g., KCl)	Deliver formula continuously, decrease volume; dilute enteral medications well
	Malnutrition/ hypoalbuminemia	Physician may order parenteral nutrition or IV albumin to help restore plasma oncotic pressure; physician may order antidiarrheals (e.g., diphenoxylate hydrochloride with atropine sulfate [Lomotil] or loperamide hydrochloride [Imodium]) if all other causes of diarrhea are ruled out
		It has been suggested that peptide formulas may be tolerated better than intact protein, but newer evidence indicates that this may not be true
	Bacterial contamination	Use scrupulously clean formula preparation and administration techniques; hang formula no longer than 4-8 hr and rinse feeding container and tubing before adding fresh formula; refrigerate home-prepared, reconstituted, or opened cans of formula until ready to use, and use all such products within 24 hr
Constipation	Lack of fiber	Use fiber-containing formula, unless contraindicated; increase fluid intake; physician may order stool softeners if problem is severe
Tube occlusion	Giving medications via tube	Irrigate feeding tube with water before and after giving medications; avoid crushed tablets and administer medications in elixir or suspension form whenever possible
	Sedimentation of formula	Irrigate tube with water† every 4-8 hr during continuous feedings and after every intermittent feeding‡; one study found less clogging of polyurethane than silicone rubber tubes; checking residuals from nasogastric tubes may cause precipitation of formula by gastric juices in the tube, so NG tubes should be irrigated well after residuals are measured; pancreatic enzyme has been reported effective in clearing some occlusions
Delayed gastric emptying	Serious illness, diabetic gastroparesis, prematurity	Physician may order temporary reduction in feeding volume, administration of feedings into small bowel, or metoclopramide (Reglan) to stimulate gastric emptying

From: Moore MC: Pocket guide: nutrition and diet therapy, ed 2, St Louis, 1993, Mosby.
*Signs and symptoms of pulmonary aspiration include tachypnea, shortness of breath, hypoxia, and infiltrate on chest x-ray films.
†Some nurses recommend fluids such as cranberry juice or Coca-Cola as an irrigant, but research has shown cranberry juice to be inferior to and Coca-Cola no better than water.
‡In one report commercial fiber-containing formulas were most likely to be associated with tube occlusion, tubes through which these formulas are delivered should be irrigated often.'

to lipid emulsion include dyspnea, cyanosis, allergy, nausea, vomiting, headache, chest pain, back pain, pressure over the eyes, and dizziness. The appearance of any of these symptoms warrants stopping the infusion and immediately notifying the physician. If the client tolerates the fat emulsion, the rate can gradually be increased as ordered by the physician.

Initiating PN. PN with concentrated dextrose requires a central venous catheter that is placed into a high flow central vein such as the superior vena cava. Nurses do not place central catheters inserted via the subclavian or jugular approach but assist in the procedure. Nurses who have special training do insert peripherally inserted central catheters (PICC) that are inserted via a vein in the forearm and threaded into the superior vena cava or subclavian vein. Insertion of a central venous catheter is a sterile procedure and requires that personnel at the client's bedside during the insertion wear masks and gowns.

When assisting with insertion of a central venous catheter, the nurse explains the procedure to the client and witnesses informed consent. The client is taught to perform the Valsalva maneuver, bearing down with mouth closed and holding a breath. This increases intrathoracic pressure and reduces the risk of an air embolism during catheter insertion. After the client has learned the technique satisfactorily, the catheter can be inserted.

The client is placed in Trendelenburg's position to dilate the central veins in the neck and shoulder. The physician drapes the venipuncture site with sterile barriers and cleanses the site with betadine followed by alcohol. Lidocaine is injected for local anesthesia and a mild sedative may also be administered. The physician performs a percutaneous venipuncture and obtains a nonpulsatile blood return. A pulsating blood return can indicate that an artery, not a vein, was punctured. A guidewire is placed through the needle that was used for the venipuncture and the needle is then removed. Whenever the physician must leave the needle or catheter open to air, the nurse instructs the client to do the Valsalva maneuver. The central venous catheter is inserted over the guidewire into the superior vena cava just above the right atrium and the guide wire is removed (Nussbaum and Fischer, 1994).

After placement of the catheter an intravenous infusion is connected to the hub of the catheter or the catheter is flushed with saline or heparin until the correct position is confirmed by radiograph. The physician sutures the catheter in place and covers the site with a sterile dressing. A chest x-ray identifies any complications such as malposition of the catheter, pneumothorax, or other complications. Infusion of the hypertonic PN solution does not begin until the correct position of the central venous catheter is confirmed.

The nurse carefully observes a client after insertion of a central venous catheter for signs of respiratory distress, which could indicate a pneumothorax, and for bleeding around the insertion site.

The catheter is used only for parenteral nutrition if it is a single lumen because multiple uses increase the risk of bacterial contamination. Multiple lumen central venous catheters enable infusion of medications and other infusions through any lumen that is not used for PN, however, all lumens of the central venous catheter require the same meticulous attention to asepsis.

Beginning an Infusion. Before beginning an infusion, the nurse compares the physician's order with the solution prepared by the pharmacy and checks the solution for particulate matter or a break in the lipid emulsion. PN is administered using an infusion pump.

Infusion Flow Rate. Clients initially receive PN solutions at a moderate rate such as 40 to 60 ml/hour. The rate is gradually increased each day until the target calories and rate are achieved.

Too-rapid administration of hypertonic dextrose can result in osmotic diuresis and dehydration (see Chapter 45). If an infusion falls behind schedule, the nurse should not increase the rate in an attempt to catch up. Sudden discontinuation of the solution can cause hypoglycemia. Usually, 5% to 10% dextrose is infused if the PN solution is suddenly discontinued.

Preventing Complications. Complications of PN include mechanical complications from insertion of the central venous catheter, infectious complications from the presence of the catheter, and metabolic complications related to the PN solution. A chest x-ray is used to assess placement of the catheter. The distal tip of the catheter should be located in the superior vena cava, proximal to the right atrium. The film can also show a pneumothorax (collapsed lung), which may occur if the needle punctures the pleura during insertion, allowing air to enter the pleural space and collapse the lung. Pneumothorax is often accompanied by

symptoms such as chest pain, dyspnea, and coughing; the rapidity of onset and the degree of symptoms depend on the severity. Pneumothorax can also be delayed. Air embolus can occur during insertion of the catheter or changing of the tubing. Air embolus can be prevented by having the client do the Valsalva maneuver whenever the central venous catheter is open to air and by placing the client in Trendelenburg's position for the insertion; however, if air embolism does occur, the client should be positioned side down.

To prevent infection, the infusion tubing should be changed every 24 to 48 hours. PN solutions with 3-in-1 admixtures should be changed every 24 hours. The procedure is the same as the procedure for changing intravenous infusion tubing. The nurse assesses the central venous catheter insertion site and the client for signs of infection (see Chapter 45).

The temperature of a client receiving PN should be monitored. Fever may be a sign of catheter infection. Hyperglycemia, leukocytosis, and erythema or drainage at the catheter exit site can also indicate infection.

The PN solution contains most major electrolytes and minerals. Without careful monitoring, electrolyte and mineral imbalances can occur. The administration of concentrated glucose, which is accompanied by increases in endogenous insulin production, causes cations to move intracellularly. The risk of hypokalemia, hypocalcemia, hypophosphatemia, and hypomagnesemia is greatest in the cachectic client and has been called *refeeding syndrome.*

Hyperglycemia is the most frequently occurring metabolic complication during PN and it occurs when the body's production of endogenous insulin is insufficient to manage the dextrose in the PN solution or when the rate of administration of dextrose exceeds the body's ability to oxidize this substrate. Risk factors for hyperglycemia include physiological stress, increased age, excessive or too rapid administration of dextrose, and renal, hepatic, and pancreatic disease. Hyperglycemia can cause polyuria, polydipsia, weakness, and lethargy. The risk of hyperglycemia can be reduced by giving the solution at a moderate rate such as 40 to 60 ml/hr in the first 24 hours of infusion and by using a moderate amount of dextrose such as 150 to 200 g/day. Checking the client's capillary blood glucose or urine for glucosuria can identify hyperglycemia. Clients who become hyperglycemic can be given subcutaneous insulin injections or have regular insulin added to the PN solution. When supplemental insulin is required during PN, blood glucose should be monitored to assess the adequacy of treatment or to recognize hypoglycemia with too aggressive treatment.

Hypoglycemia can also occur if PN is abruptly discontinued. The high glucose concentration of the PN solution stimulates the pancreas to secrete more insulin. Symptoms of hypoglycemia include occipital headaches, sweating, cold clammy skin, nervousness, dizziness, tachycardia, and tingling of the extremities and circumoral regions. Hypoglycemia can be prevented by maintaining an accurate infusion rate, assessing the effect of insulin supplementation, and gradually reducing the PN solution rate. The gradual reduction allows the pancreas time to adapt to the decreased glucose load. If the PN solution must be discontinued abruptly, a 5% or 10% glucose in water solution usually provides enough glucose to prevent rebound hypoglycemia (Grant and Kennedy-Caldwell, 1988).

Fluid overload causes an increase in extracellular fluid volume. If severe, fluid overload can result in pulmonary edema and congestive heart failure. Signs and symptoms include shortness of breath, tachycardia, weak pulse, hypertension or hypotension, confusion, decreased urine output, crackles, and pitting edema. Fluid overload can be prevented by maintaining an accurate rate of infusion, careful evaluation of intake and output, measuring changes in body weight, evaluating the client for edema, and monitoring central venous pressure. If signs of fluid overload are noted, the nurse notifies the physician before symptoms occur.

The major complications of PN and nursing interventions to prevent them are shown in Table 41-11.

Evaluation

Nutritional evaluation must be ongoing to evaluate the results of nursing interventions. Nutritional therapy, however, does not produce rapid results. A weight gain or loss of 5 pounds or more in a few days usually indicates fluid shifts, not gains or losses of lean body mass. Laboratory monitors of nutritional repletion, such as serum albumin and transferrin, do not reflect changes until about 20 days and 8 days, respectively (Curtas, Chapman, and Mequid,

1989). Early nutritional goals should concentrate on provision of estimated kilocalorie and protein needs.

Nutritional therapies, especially enteral nutrition, are frequently interrupted. Evaluation of ordered versus administered volumes will indicate whether the rate should be advanced to compensate for interruptions. If gradual weight gain is not observed, or if weight loss continues, the prescription may need to be increased. Changes in the client's condition may also indicate a need to change the nutritional plan of care. If PN is being used, the nurse should be alert to signs and symptoms to indicate that enteral nutrition would be tolerated. For example, if symptoms of pancreatitis subside; if bowel function returns as indicated by flatus, bowel sounds, and passage of stools; if an obstruction is relieved, or if stool losses decrease with enhanced absorption. Combined PN and EN therapy is becoming more commonplace, even when small volumes of EN are administered.

Care plans should reflect reasonable and achievable goals. Nurses should evaluate outcomes of nursing actions and be alert for signs that goals are being met (see the evaluation box on p. 1125). Adequate time should be allowed to test a nursing approach to a problem. The nurse collaborates with the nutritionist and physician to evaluate the effectiveness of nutrition support therapy.

Outcomes may result in changes in therapy. Whenever possible, the client should be an active participant in the planning and evaluation of care.

Table 41-11	Preventing PN Complications	
COMPLICATION	**SIGNS SYMPTOMS**	**INTERVENTION**
Catheter-related sepsis	Fever, chills, glucose intolerance, positive blood culture	Maintain an intact dressing, change if contaminated by vomitus, sputum, etc; use aseptic technique whenever handling catheter, IV tubing, and TPN solutions; hang a single bottle of TPN no longer than 24 hr, lipid emulsion no longer than 12 hr; use an in-line 0.22 μ filter with TPN to remove bacteria
Air embolism	Dyspnea, cyanosis, tachycardia, hypotension, possibly death	Use Luer-lock system or secure all connections well; Groshong catheter, which has valve at tip, may reduce risk of air embolism; use an in-line 0.22 μ air-eliminating filter; have client perform Valsalva's maneuver during tubing changes; if air embolism is suggested, place client in left lateral decubitus position and administer oxygen; immediately notify physician, who will attempt to aspirate air from the heart
Central venous thrombosis	Unilateral edema of neck, shoulder, and arm; development of collateral circulation on chest; pain in insertion site	Follow measures to prevent sepsis; repeated or traumatic catheterizations are most likely to result in thrombosis
Catheter occlusion or semiocclusion	No flow or sluggish flow through the catheter	Flush catheter with heparinized saline if infusion is stopped temporarily; if catheter appears to be occluded, attempt to aspirate the clot; if ineffective, physician may order thrombolytic agent such as streptokinase or urokinase instilled in the catheter
Hypoglycemia	Diaphoresis, shakiness, confusion, loss of consciousness	Do not discontinue TPN abruptly, taper rate over several hours; use pump to regulate infusion so that it remains ±10% of ordered rate; if hypoglycemia is suggested, administer oral carbohydrate; if oral intake is contraindicated or patient is unconscious, physician may order a bolus of IV dextrose
Hyperglycemia	Thirst, headache, lethargy, increased urination	Monitor blood glucose at least daily until stable; TPN is usually initiated at a slow rate or with a low dextrose concentration and increased over 2-3 days to avoid hyperglycemia; the client may require insulin added to the TPN if the problem is severe

Modified from Moore MC: *Pocket guide: nutrition and diet therapy*, ed 2, St Louis, 1993, Mosby.

Sample Evaluation of Interventions for Altered Nutritional Status

GOALS	EVALUATIVE MEASURES	EXPECTED OUTCOMES
Client will return to within 10% of good weight for height range.	Weigh client.	Weight will show appropriate gain of $1/2$-1 lb/wk (0.25-0.5 kg/wk).
	Observe client for signs of nutritional deficits.	Laboratory parameters will show evidence of adequate hydration and improving nutritional parameters.
	Observe client for signs of dehydration or overhydration.	
	Palpate skin for loss of turgor.	
	Palpate skin for signs of edema.	
	Monitor electrolyte levels and observe for electrolyte imbalance.	

∎ KEY CONCEPTS ∎

► Nutrients needed by the body to carry out vital functions are water, carbohydrates, proteins, lipids, vitamins, and minerals.

► Body weight is maintained when food intake equals energy requirements.

► Carbohydrates are anabolized into glycogen and adipose tissue or catabolized into energy.

► Proteins are anabolized into tissue, hormones, or enzymes, or catabolized into energy.

► Lipids may be anabolized into adipose tissue or catabolized into energy.

► Proteins are essential for growth, maintenance, and repair.

► The essential amino acids and the essential fatty acids must be supplied by dietary intake because the body is unable to synthesize them from other ingested substances.

► Through digestion, food is broken down into its simplest form for absorption. Digestion and absorption occur mainly in the small intestine.

► Recommended daily allowances, another basis for diet selection, were formulated for population groups, not individuals.

► Guidelines for dietary change advocate reduced intake of fat, saturated fat, salt, refined sugar, and cholesterol, and increased intake of complex carbohydrates and fiber.

► Age affects the requirements for essential nutrients. Periods of rapid growth increase the need for protein, vitamins, and minerals.

► Because improper nutrition can affect all body systems, nutritional assessment includes a review of the total physical assessment.

► Nurses can improve food intake of clients by thoughtful attention to the preparation of the client and environment before meals are served.

► Disabled clients should be supported in their efforts to eat as independently as possible.

► Proper feeding techniques can protect the dependent client from loss of dignity and self-esteem.

► Special diets alter the composition, texture, digestibility, and residue of foods to suit the client's particular needs.

► Tube feedings can be used for clients who are unable to ingest food but are able to digest and absorb foods.

► Enteral nutrition may protect intestinal structure and function and enhance immunity.

► Total parenteral nutrition supplies essential nutrients in appropriate amounts to support life through the introduction of a concentrated nutrient solution into a large central vein or the right atrium of the heart.

► Evaluation of the outcomes of nursing intervention in the area of nutritional support is essential to revise, update, or continue nursing activities.

∎ KEY TERMS ∎

■ CRITICAL THINKING EXERCISES ■

1. During a home visit to a mother and 3-month-old infant, the mother asks you how soon to begin solid foods. How would you instruct this client in the introduction of solid foods to her infant?

2. You are seeing a client who is HIV positive in a clinic visit. You note that she is underweight with noticeable muscle wasting. She relates problems associated with diarrhea following meals. Identify appropriate interventions to obtain a more complete nutritional assessment for this client.

3. Your client has a nasogastric feeding tube. During the morning he had a prolonged period of severe coughing. What measure would you take to determine that the tube is properly located?

4. Mr. Miller has been on PN for several weeks following extensive gastrointestinal surgery. During a physical exam and discussion with him, you note that he is passing stools, has bowel sounds, and states that he feels hungry. What interventions might be appropriate for Mr. Miller at this time?

REFERENCES

Amersican Academy of Pediatrics, Committee on Nutrition, Forbes GB, Woodruff CW, editors: *Pediatric nutrition handbook,* ed 2, Elk Grove, Ill, 1985, The Academy.

American Cancer Society: *Nutrition, common sense, and cancer,* No. 2096-LE, New York, 1993, American Cancer Society.

American Heart Association: *Dietary treatment for hypercholesterolemia: handbook for counselors,* vol 70-2001, Dallas, 1993, The Association.

Behrman RE, Vaughan VC, editors: *Nelson's textbook of pediatrics,* ed 3, Philadelphia, 1987, WB Saunders.

Berry S et al: Intestinal placement of pH-sensing nasointestinal feeding tubes, *JPEN* 18(1):67, 1994.

Bodinski LH: *The nurse's guide to diet therapy,* New York, 1982, Wiley.

Carper J: *Food-your miracle medicine,* New York, 1993, Harper Perennial.

Curtas S, Chapman G, Meguid M: Evaluation of nutritional status, *Nur Clin N Am* 24(2):301, 1989.

Food and Nutrition Board: *Recommended dietary allowances,* ed 10, Washington, DC, 1989, Nation Academy of Sciences.

Fuhrman J: *Fasting and eating for health,* New York, 1995, St Martin's Press.

Grant JA, Kennedy-Caldwell C: *Nutritional support in nursing,* New York, 1988, Grune & Stratton.

Hunter D et al: A prospective study of the intake of vitamins C, E, and A and the risk of breast cancer, *NEJM* 329(4):234, 1993.

Kim MJ, McFarland GK, McLane AM: *Pocket guide to nursing diagnoses,* ed 6, St Louis, 1995, Mosby.

Kudsk K: Clinical applications of enteral nutrition, *NCP* 9(5):165, 1994.

Mainous M, Block E, Deitch E: Nutritional support of the gut: how and why, *New Horizons* 2(3):193, 1994.

Malone WF: Studies evaluating antioxidants and B-carotene as chemopreventives, *Am J Clin Nutr* 53:305S, 1991.

Matarese LE: Rationale and efficacy of specialized enteral nutrition, *NCP* 9(2):58, 1994.

Metheny N: Minimizing respiratory complications of nasoenteric tube feedings: state of the science, *Heart-Lung* 22:213, 1993.

Metheny NM, Spies M, Eisenberg P: Frequency of nasoenteral tube displacement and associated risk factors, *Res Nurs Health* 9(3):241, 1986.

Metheny NM, Spies M, Eisenberg P: Measures to test placement of nasogastric and nasointestinal feeding tubes: a review, *Nurs Res* 37:324, 1988.

Metheny N et al: Effectiveness of pH measurements in predicting feeding tube placement, *Nurs Res* 38:280, 1989.

Metheny N et al: 1994.

Minard G: Enteral access, *NCP* 9(5):172, 1994.

Moore MC: *Pocket guide: nutrition and diet therapy,* ed 2, St Louis, 1993, Mosby.

National Dairy Council: *Feeding guide for the first two years,* Rosemont, Ill, 1990, The Council.

National Institutes of Health: *National cholesterol education program: report of the expert panel on blood cholesterol levels in children and adolescents,* DHHS Pub No 91-2732, Washington, DC, 1991, US Government Printing Office.

Nussbaum M, Fischer J: Parenteral nutrition. In Zaloga G, editor: *Nutrition in Critical Care,* St Louis, 1994, Mosby.

Nutrition Interventions Manual for Professionals Caring for Older Americans. Greer, Margolis, Mitchell, Grunwald, & Associates, Inc. Nutrition Screening Initiative, 1010 Wisconsin Ave NW, Suite 800, Washington, DC, 20007, 1992.

Petrosino BM, Christian BJ, Becker H: Implications of selected problems with nasoenteral tube feedings, *Crit Care Nurs Q* 12(3):1, 1989.

Pipes PL, Trahms CM: Nutrition in infancy and childhood, ed 5, St Louis, 1993, Mosby.

Public Law 101-535. *Nutrition Labeling And Education Act of 1990.* 103 STAT. 2353.21 USC 301, Nov 8, 1990.

Rombeau J, Barot L: Enteral nutritional therapy, *Surg Clin North Am* 61:605, 1981.

Stacey M: *Consumed—why Americans love, hate, and fear food,* New York, 1994, Simon & Schuster.

US Department of Agriculture: *USDA's food guide pyramid,* USDA Human Nutrition Information Service Pub No 249, Washington, DC, 1992, US Government Printing Office.

US Department of Agriculture and US Department of Health and Human Services: *Nutrition and your health: dietary guidelines for Americans,* USDA/DHHS Home and Garden Bull No 232, Washington, DC, 1990, US Government Printing Office.

US Department of Health and Human Services. *Healthy people 2000: national health promotion and disease prevention objectives,* DHHS Pub No (PHS) 91-50212, Washington, DC, 1990, US Government Printing Office.

Wardlaw GM, Insel PM, Seyler MF: *Contemporary nutrition: issues and insights,* ed 2, St Louis, 1994, Mosby.

Whitney EN, Cataldo CB, Rolfes SR: *Understanding normal and clinical nutrition,* ed 3, St Paul, Minn, 1991, West.

Williams SR: *Nutrition and diet therapy,* ed 7, St Louis, 1993, Mosby.

Williams SR: Nutritional guidance in prenatal care. In Worthington-Roberts BS, Vermeersch JA, Williams SR: *Nutrition in pregnancy and lactation,* ed 5, St Louis, 1993, Mosby.

Zaloga G: Frontiers in critical care nutrition, *New Horizons* 2(2):121, 1994.

ADDITIONAL READINGS

Baker DJ: 10 years of TPN at home, *Am J Nurs* 84:1248, 1984.

Food and Drug Administration, Department of Health and Human Services: *Federal Register* 55:5176, 1990.

Legislative Highlights: Update: the Nutrition Labeling and Education Act of 1990, *J Am Diet Assn* 91:1054, 1991.

National Academy of Sciences: *Report on nutrition labeling: issues and directions for the 1990s,* Washington, DC, 1990, National Academy Press.

National Institutes of Health: *National Cholesterol Education Program: report of the expert panel on population strategies for blood cholesterol reduction,* DHHS Pub No 90-3046, Washington, DC, 1990, US Government Printing Office.

National Research Council: *Estimated safe and adequate daily dietary intakes,* ed 10, Washington, DC, 1989, National Academy Press.

National Research Council Committee on Diet and Health of Food and Nutrition: *National Academy of Sciences Report: diet and health: implications for reducing chronic disease,* Washington, DC, 1989, National Academy Press.

Surgeon General's report on nutrition and health: summary and recommendations, DHHS (PHS) Pub No 88-50211, Washington, DC, 1988, US Government Printing Office.

Teasley-Strausburg KM et al: *Nutrition support handbook,* Cincinnati, 1992, Harvey Whitney Books.

Thomas PR, editor: *Improving America's diet and health: from recommendations to action,* Washington, DC, 1991, National Academy Press.

Worthington-Roberts BS, Williams SR: *Nutrition in pregnancy and lactation,* ed 5, St Louis, 1993, Mosby.

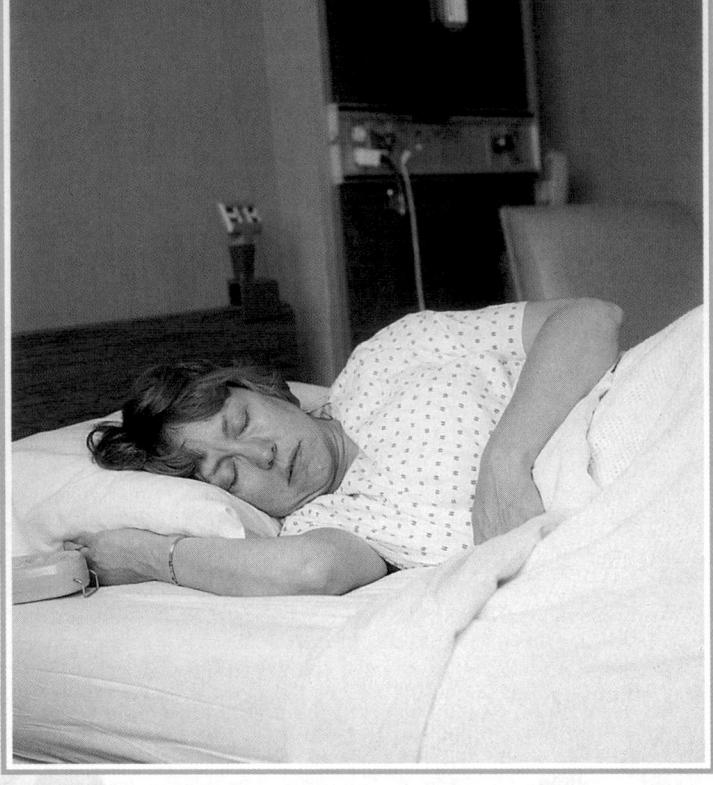

## Chapter 42

Sleep

Objectives

Mastery of content in this chapter will enable the student to:

▶ Define the key terms listed.

▶ Compare the characteristics of rest and sleep.

▶ Explain the effect the 24-hour sleep-wake cycle has on biological function.

▶ Discuss mechanisms that regulate sleep.

▶ Describe the stages of a normal sleep cycle.

▶ Explain the functions of sleep.

▶ Compare and contrast the sleep requirements of different age groups.

▶ Identify factors that normally promote and disrupt sleep.

▶ Discuss characteristics of common sleep disorders.

▶ Conduct a sleep history for a client.

▶ Identify nursing diagnoses appropriate for clients with sleep alterations.

▶ Identify nursing interventions designed to promote normal sleep cycles for clients of all ages.

▶ Describe ways to evaluate sleep therapies.

Proper rest and sleep are as important to good health as good nutrition and adequate exercise. Individuals need different amounts of sleep and rest. Physical and emotional health depend on the ability to fulfill these basic human needs. Without proper amounts of rest and sleep, the ability to concentrate, make judgments, and participate in daily activities decreases, and irritability increases.

Identifying and treating clients' sleep pattern disturbances is an important goal for a nurse. To help a client gain needed rest and sleep, a nurse must understand the nature of sleep, the factors influencing it, and the client's sleep habits. Clients require an individualized approach based on their personal habits and pattern of sleep as well as the particular problem that is influencing their sleep. Nursing interventions can be effective in resolving short- and long-term sleep disturbances.

One theory about the function of sleep is that it is associated with healing (Evans and French, 1995). Achieving the best possible sleep quality is important for the promotion of good health as well as the recovery of ill individuals. Nurses care for clients who often have preexisting sleep disturbances and for clients who develop sleep problems as a result of illness or hospitalization. Sometimes clients seek health care because they have a sleep problem that may have gone unnoticed for many years. Ill clients often require more sleep and rest than healthy clients. However, the nature of illness may prevent clients from gaining adequate rest and sleep. The institutional environment of a hospital or long-term care facility and the activities of health care personnel make sleep difficult.

■ SLEEP AND REST

When people are at rest they usually feel mentally relaxed, free from anxiety, and physically calm. Rest does not imply inactivity, although everyone often thinks of it as settling down in comfortable chairs or lying in bed. When people are at rest they are in a state of mental and physical activity that leaves them feeling refreshed, rejuvenated, and ready to resume the activities of the day. All persons have their own habits for obtaining rest and can find ways to adjust as best as possible to new environments or conditions that affect the ability to rest. Rest may be gained from reading a book, practicing a relaxation exercise (see Chapter 43), or taking a long walk.

Nurses frequently care for clients on bed rest in a variety of health care settings. This treatment confines clients to bed to reduce physical and psychological demands on the body. Such people do not necessarily feel rested. They still may have emotional worries that prevent complete relaxation. For example, concern over physical limitations or a fear of being unable to return to their usual lifestyle may cause such clients to feel stressed and unable to relax.

Sleep is a recurrent, altered state of consciousness that occurs for sustained periods. When people obtain proper sleep, they feel that their energy has been restored. Some sleep experts believe that these feelings of energy restoration imply that sleep provides time for the repair and recovery of body systems for the next period of wakefulness.

The usual rest and sleep patterns of persons entering a hospital or other health care facility can easily be affected by illness or unfamiliar health care routines. The extent of change in usual sleep and rest patterns depends on the clients' physiological and psychological states, and the physical environment, such as background noise and the work patterns of care givers. The nurse must always be aware of clients' needs for rest. A lack of rest for long periods can cause illness or worsening of existing illness. The nurse can help clients learn the importance of rest and ways to promote it at home or in the health care environment.

Promoting Rest

Many factors affect the ability to gain adequate rest. In community health and home settings the nurse helps clients develop behaviors conducive to rest and relaxation. This may include suggesting changes in the environment or certain lifestyle habits. For example, inadequate attention to sleep needs among working adults is a significant problem in our society. When faced with the often conflicting demands of work and parenthood, young adults may not attend properly to their own rest needs and compress the time allocated to their own relaxation activities. Adults faced with these circumstances may need assistance in examining their lifestyle and reprioritizing their activities so that they obtain adequate rest.

In home settings the nurse frequently cares for clients with chronic debilitating disease. The nursing care plan might include having clients set aside afternoons for rest in order to promote optimal health. The nurse helps adjust medication schedules, instructs clients to regularly void before rest periods and suggests unplugging the telephone so that rest periods are uninterrupted. In a health care setting the nurse promotes rest by using measures to control clients' physical symptoms and altering stressful factors in the environment. This can be difficult on a busy nursing unit. Loud or unfamiliar noises, loss of privacy, and frequency of therapeutic procedures can interfere with rest. Clients who are hospitalized for extensive diagnostic testing often have difficulty resting because of uncertainty about their state of health and the tiring procedures they may experience in this setting. A nurse can promote rest by allowing clients to determine the timing and methods of delivery of basic care measures. Providing information about the purpose and routines of all procedures also helps.

Conditions for Proper Rest

PHYSICAL COMFORT
- Eliminate sources of physical irritation.
- Control sources of pain.
- Control room temperature.
- Maintain proper anatomical alignment or positioning.
- Remove environmental distractions.
- Provide adequate ventilation.

FREEDOM FROM WORRY
- Make own decisions.
- Participate in personal health care.
- Have knowledge needed to understand health problems and implications.
- Practice restful activities regularly.
- Know that the environment is safe.

SUFFICIENT SLEEP
- Obtain hours of sleep needed to feel refreshed.
- Follow good sleep hygiene habits.

Giving clients' control over their health care minimizes uncertainty and anxiety. The box on p. 1129 lists conditions needed to promote proper rest.

PHYSIOLOGY OF SLEEP

Sleep is a cyclical physiological process that alternates with longer periods of wakefulness. The sleep-wake cycle influences and regulates physiological function and behavioral responses.

Circadian Rhythms

People experience cyclical rhythms as part of their everyday life. The most familiar rhythm is the 24-hour, day-night cycle known as the *diurnal* or **circadian rhythm** (derived from Latin: *circa,* "about," and *dies,* "day"). A woman's menstrual cycle is an **infradian rhythm**, one that occurs in a cycle longer than 24 hours. Biological cycles lasting less than 24 hours are called **ultradian rhythms**. Circadian rhythms influence the pattern of major biological and behavioral functions. The fluctuation and predictability of body temperature, heart rate, blood pressure, hormone secretion, sensory acuity, and mood depend on the maintenance of the 24-hour circadian cycle.

Circadian rhythms, including daily sleep-wake cycles, are affected by light and temperature as well as external factors such as social activities and work routines. All persons have **biological clocks** that synchronize their sleep cycles. Some people can fall asleep at 8 PM, whereas others go to bed at midnight or early in the morning. Different people also function best at different times of the day. Horne and Ostberg (1976) described two groups of people, morning and evening types. The morning person prefers to go to bed and get up early, performing best in the morning. The evening person prefers to go to bed and get up later, functioning best in the evenings.

Hospitals or extended-care facilities usually do not adapt care to an individual's sleep-wake cycle preferences. Typical routines cause interruptions in sleep or prevent clients from falling asleep at their usual time. If a person's sleep-wake cycle is altered significantly, a poor quality of sleep can result. Reversals in the sleep-wake cycle such as falling asleep during the day (or vice versa for people who work nights) can indicate a serious illness. Anxiety, restlessness, irritability, and impaired judgment are common symptoms of disturbances in the sleep cycle.

The biological rhythm of sleep frequently becomes synchronized with other body functions. Changes in body temperature, for example, correlate with sleep patterns. Normally, body temperature peaks in the afternoon, decreases gradually, and then drops sharply after a person falls asleep (see Chapter 32). When the sleep-wake cycle becomes disrupted (e.g., by working rotating shifts), other physiological functions may change as well. For example, the person may experience a decreased appetite and lose weight. Failure to maintain the individual's usual sleep-wake cycle can adversely influence the client's overall health.

Sleep Regulation

Sleep involves a sequence of physiological states maintained by highly integrated central nervous system (CNS) activity that is associated with changes in the peripheral nervous, endocrine, cardiovascular, respiratory, and muscular systems (Robinson, 1993). Each sequence can be identified by specific physiological responses and patterns of brain activity. Instruments such as the electroencephalogram (EEG), which measures electrical activity in the cerebral cortex, the electromyogram (EMG), which measures muscle tone, and the electrooculogram (EOG), which measures eye movements, provide information about some structural physiological aspects of sleep.

The control and regulation of sleep may depend on the interrelationship between two cerebral mechanisms that intermittently activate and suppress the brain's higher centers to control sleep and wakefulness. One mechanism causes wakefulness, whereas the other causes sleep.

The **reticular activating system (RAS)** is located in the upper brain stem. It is believed to contain special cells that maintain alertness and wakefulness. The RAS receives visual, auditory, pain, and tactile sensory stimuli. Activity from the cerebral cortex (e.g., emotions or thought processes) also stimulates the RAS. Wakefulness results from neurons in the RAS that release catecholamines such as norepinephrine (Sleep Research Society, 1993).

Sleep may be produced by the release of serotonin from specialized cells in the raphe sleep system of the pons and medial forebrain. This area of the brain is also called the **bulbar synchronizing region (BSR)**. Whether a person remains awake or falls asleep depends on a balance of impulses received from higher centers (e.g., thoughts), peripheral sensory receptors (e.g., sound or light stimuli), and the limbic system (emotions) (Fig. 42-1).

As people try to fall asleep, they close their eyes and assume relaxed positions. Stimuli to the RAS decline. If the room is dark and quiet, activation of the RAS further declines. At some point the BSR takes over, causing sleep.

STAGES OF SLEEP

EEG, EMG, and EOG electrical signals show that different levels of brain, muscle, and eye activity are associated with

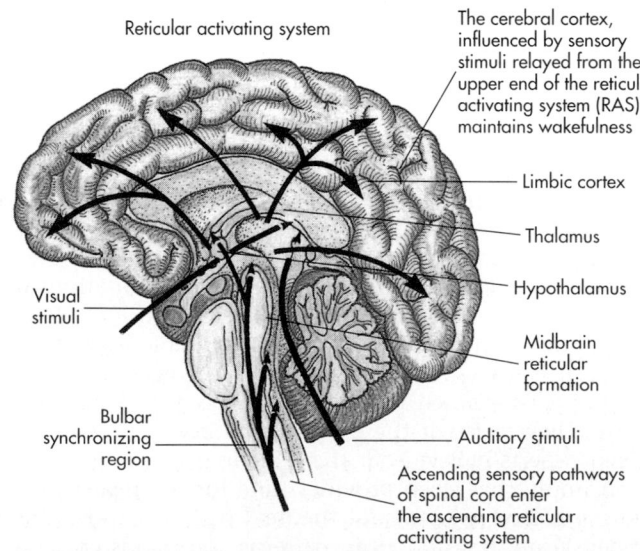

Fig. 42-1 RAS and BSR control sensory input, intermittently activating and suppressing the brain's higher centers to control sleep and wakefulness.

Stages of the Sleep Cycle

STAGE 1: NREM
- Stage includes lightest level of sleep.
- Stage lasts few minutes.
- Decreased physiological activity begins with gradual fall in vital signs and metabolism.
- Person is easily aroused by sensory stimuli such as noise.
- Awakened, person feels as though daydreaming has occurred.

STAGE 2: NREM
- Stage 2 is period of sound sleep.
- Relaxation progresses.
- Arousal is still relatively easy.
- Stage lasts 10 to 20 minutes.
- Body functions continue to slow.

STAGE 3: NREM
- Stage 3 involves initial stages of deep sleep.
- Sleeper is difficult to arouse and rarely moves.
- Muscles are completely relaxed.
- Vital signs decline but remain regular.
- Stage lasts 15 to 30 minutes.

STAGE 4: NREM
- Stage 4 is deepest stage of sleep.
- It is very difficult to arouse sleeper.
- If sleep loss has occurred, sleeper will spend considerable portion of night in this stage.
- Vital signs are significantly lower than during waking hours.
- Stage lasts approximately 15 to 30 minutes.
- Sleepwalking and enuresis may occur.

REM SLEEP
- Vivid, full-color dreaming may occur in REM. Less vivid dreaming may occur in other stages.
- Stage usually begins about 90 minutes after sleep has begun.
- It is typified by autonomic response of rapidly moving eyes, fluctuating heart and respiratory rates, and increased or fluctuating blood pressure.
- Loss of skeletal muscle tone occurs.
- Gastric secretions increase.
- It is very difficult to arouse sleeper.
- Duration of REM sleep increases with each cycle and averages 20 minutes.

---

different stages of sleep (Sleep Research Society, 1993). Normal sleep involves two phases: nonrapid eye movement (**NREM sleep**) and rapid eye movement (**REM sleep**) (see the box above). During NREM a sleeper progresses through four stages during a typical 90 minute sleep cycle. The quality of sleep from stage 1 through stage 4 becomes increasingly deep. Lighter sleep is characteristic of stages 1 and 2, and a person is more easily arousable. Stages 3 and 4 involve a deeper sleep called *slow-wave sleep* from which a person is more difficult to arouse. REM sleep is the phase at the end of each 90 minute sleep cycle. Memory consolidation (Karni et al, 1994) and psychological restoration may occur at this time. Different factors may promote or interfere with various stages of the sleep cycle. The nurse chooses therapies that foster sleep or attempts to eliminate factors that can disrupt it.

SLEEP CYCLE

Normally, in an adult the routine sleep pattern begins with a presleep period during which the person is aware only of a gradually developing sleepiness. This period normally lasts 10 to 30 minutes, but if a person has difficulty falling asleep, it may last an hour or more.

Once asleep, the person usually passes through four to six complete sleep cycles, each consisting of four stages of NREM sleep and a period of REM sleep. The cyclical pattern usually progresses from stage 1 through stage 4 of NREM, followed by a reversal from stage 4 to 3 to 2, ending with a period of REM sleep (Fig. 42-2). A person usually reaches REM sleep about 90 minutes into the sleep cycle.

With each successive cycle, stages 3 and 4 shorten, and the period of REM lengthens. REM sleep may last up to 60 minutes during the last sleep cycle. Not all people progress consistently through the usual stages of sleep. For example, a sleeper may fluctuate for short intervals between NREM stages 2, 3, and 4 before entering REM stage. The amount of time spent in each stage varies (Fig. 42-3). Shifts from stage to stage tend to accompany body movements, and shifts to light sleep tend to occur suddenly, whereas shifts to deep sleep tend to be gradual (Closs, 1988). The number of sleep cycles depends on the total amount of time that the client spends sleeping.

▌ FUNCTIONS OF SLEEP

The purpose of sleep remains unclear (Hodgson, 1991). Sleep is believed to contribute to physiological and psychological restoration (Oswald, 1984; Anch et al, 1988). According to one theory, sleep is a time of restoration and preparation for the next period of wakefulness. During NREM sleep, biological functions slow. A healthy adult's normal heart rate throughout the day averages 70 to 80 beats per minute or less if the individual is in excellent physical condition. However, during sleep the heart rate falls to 60 beats per minute or less. This means that the heart beats 10 to 20 fewer times in each minute during sleep or 60 to 120 fewer times in each hour. Clearly, restful sleep may be beneficial in preserving cardiac function.

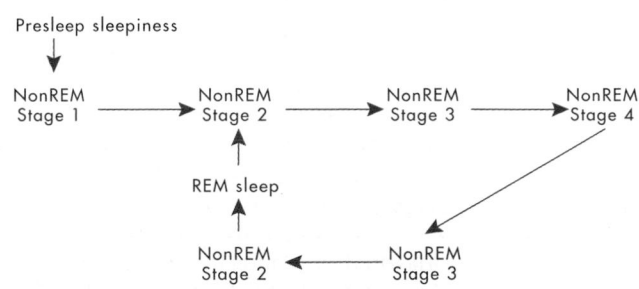

Fig. 42-2 The stages of the adult sleep cycle.

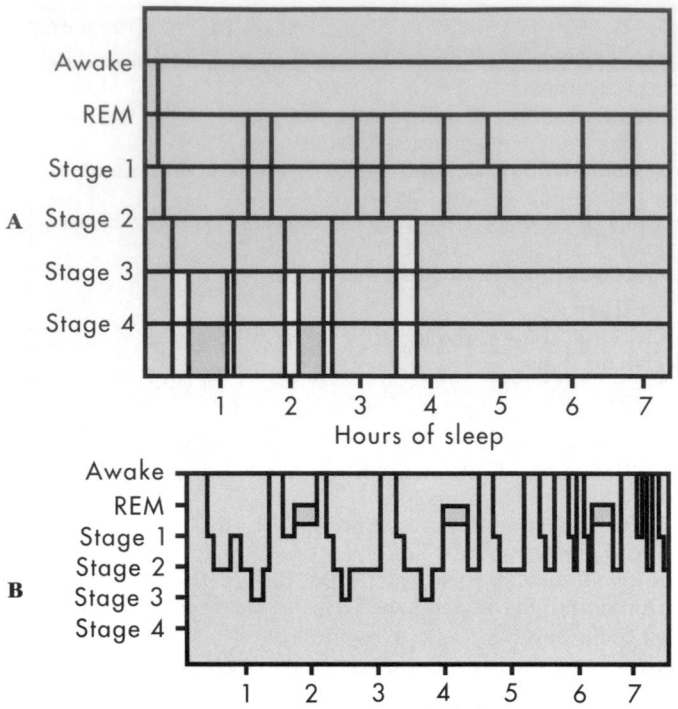

Fig. 42-3 Comparison of normal sleep patterns in a healthy young adult and older adult. **A,** The young adult has little awake time and moves through the sleep stages progressively. **B,** The older adult has frequent awakenings and more time spent in the lighter stages of sleep. *(Modified from Emra KL, Herrera CO: RN 52:79, 1989; Kavey NB, Anderson D: RN 49:16, 1986.)*

Sleep appears to be needed to routinely restore biological processes. During deep slow-wave (NREM stage 4) sleep, the body releases human growth hormone for the repair and renewal of epithelial and specialized cells such as brain cells (Horne, 1983; Mendleson, 1987; Born, Muth, and Fehm, 1988). However, Horne (1983) also argues that the usual role of growth hormone as a promoter of protein synthesis is limited because its release is unrelated to blood glucose levels and amino acids. Other studies have shown that protein synthesis and cell division for renewal of tissues such as the skin, bone marrow, gastric mucosa, or brain occur during rest and sleep (Oswald, 1984). NREM sleep may be especially important in children, who experience more stage 4 sleep.

Another theory about the purpose of sleep is that the body conserves energy during sleep. The skeletal muscles relax progressively, and the absence of muscular contraction preserves chemical energy for cellular processes. Lowering of the basal metabolic rate further conserves the body's energy supply (Anch et al, 1988).

REM sleep appears to be important for cognitive restoration. REM sleep is associated with changes in cerebral blood flow, increased cortical activity, increased oxygen consumption, and epinephrine release. This association may assist with memory storage and learning. During sleep, the brain filters stored information about the day's activities.

The benefits of sleep on behavior often go unnoticed until a person develops a problem resulting from sleep depri-

vation. A loss of REM sleep can lead to feelings of confusion and suspicion. No clear cause-and-effect relationship exists between sleep loss and a specific body dysfunction (Webster and Thompson, 1986). However, various body functions (e.g., motor performance, memory, and equilibrium) can be altered when prolonged sleep loss occurs. Some of the more recent industrial accidents, such as the Valdez oil spill in Alaska and the nuclear accident in Chernobyl, have been attributed to human error associated with sleep deprivation. Traffic, home, and work-related accidents due to falling asleep have been estimated to cost billions of dollars a year in the United States (Leger, 1994, 1995; Webb, 1995). Because of concern over an increased incidence of automobile accidents, six states in the United States have implemented guidelines regulating the driving privileges of people with narcolepsy and/or sleep apnea, disorders that cause excessive sleepiness and can affect driving performance (Pakola, Dinges, and Pack, 1995).

Dreams

While dreams occur during both NREM and REM sleep, the dreams of REM sleep are more vivid and elaborate and are believed to be functionally important to the consolidation of long-term memory. REM dreams may progress in content throughout the night from dreams about current events to emotional dreams of childhood or the past. Personality can influence the quality of dreams; for example, a creative person may have creative dreams, and a depressed person may dream of helplessness.

Most people dream about immediate concerns such as an argument with a spouse, plans for a wedding, or worries over work. Sometimes a person is unaware of fears represented in bizarre dreams. People with graduate level education related to the field of psychology may attempt to analyze the symbolic nature of dreams. For example, an apple may represent a forbidden object or a lion may symbolize rage. The ability to describe a dream and interpret its significance may help resolve personal concerns or fears.

Another theory suggests that dreams erase certain fantasies or nonsensical memories. Since most dreams are forgotten, many people have little dream recall and don't believe they dream at all. To remember a dream, a person must consciously think about it on awakening. People who recall dreams vividly usually awake just after a period of REM sleep.

Normal Sleep Requirements and Patterns

Sleep duration and quality vary among persons of all age groups. One person may feel adequately rested with 4 hours of sleep, whereas another requires 10 hours. Fig. 42-4 shows the change in the distribution of sleep stages during life.

NEONATES

The neonate up to the age of 3 months averages about 16 hours of sleep a day. The infant born of an unmedicated mother enters the world in a state of wakefulness. Eyes are wide open and sucking is vigorous. After about an hour the newborn becomes quiet and less responsive to internal and external stimuli. A period of sleep lasting a few minutes up to 2 to 4 hours follows (Wong, 1995). The infant then awakens again and often becomes overly responsive to

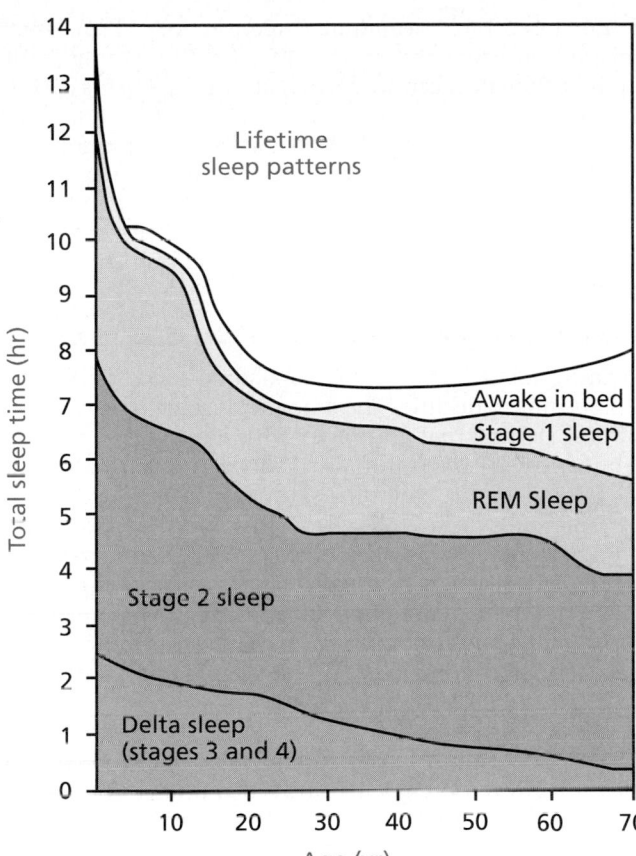

Fig. 42-4 Distribution of sleep stages over the life span. *(From Berman et al:* Patient Care *24:85, 1990.)*

stimuli. Hunger, pain, cold, or other stimuli frequently cause crying. For the first week the neonate sleeps almost constantly. Approximately 50% of this sleep is REM sleep, which stimulates the higher brain centers. This is thought to be essential for development because the neonate is not awake long enough for significant external stimulation. Table 42-1 describes behaviors seen in the newborn during sleep and wakefulness.

INFANTS

Infants usually develop a nighttime pattern of sleep by 3 months of age. The infant may take several naps during the day but usually sleeps an average of 8 to 10 hours during the night. About 30% of sleep time is spent in the REM cycle. Awakening commonly occurs early in the morning, although it is not unusual for an infant to awaken during the night. If awakening during the night becomes routine, the problem may be with diet because hunger frequently awakens the child. A breast-fed infant usually sleeps for shorter periods, with more frequent awakenings, than a bottle-fed infant (Wong, 1995). A large infant sleeps longer than a smaller one because of greater stomach capacity. An infant between 1 month and 1 year of age sleeps an average of 14 hours a day. Compared to older children, active (REM) sleep comprises a larger proportion of sleep. In contrast with newborns in whom sleep and wake alternate throughout a 24-hour period, by 3 months of age the longest sleep period appears at night.

TODDLERS

By the age of 2, children usually sleep through the night and take daily naps. Total sleep averages 12 hours a day. Naps may be eliminated at 3 years. It is common for toddlers to awaken during the night. The percentage of REM sleep continues to fall. During this period the toddler may be unwilling to go to bed at night. This unwillingness may be due to a need for autonomy, or a fear of separation. Tod-

Table 42-1	States of Sleep and Wakefulness in the Newborn*
STATE	**BEHAVIOR**
Active sleep (AS-REM)	Sucking movements present
	Fine twitches almost continuous with some bursts of muscle movement
	Grimaces, smiles, and tremors occur
	Limb movements and stretching of torso present
	Phasic eye movements and irregular respirations seen together
Quiet sleep (QS-NREM)	Minimal movement
	Muscle tone increased compared to active sleep
	Respiration = 25 breaths per minute or less
Indeterminate sleep	Clear criteria for either AS or QS are not met
Awake	Sustained muscle tone with bursts of activity
	Eyes open
	Respiration greater than 45 breaths per minute
	Noises are vocalized
	Sustained gross motor movements

*From Hoppenbrouwers T: Sleep in infants. In Guilleminault C, editor: *Sleep and its disorders in children,* New York, 1987, Raven Press; Sheldon SH, Spire JP, Levy HB: *Pediatric sleep medicine,* Philadelphia, 1992, Saunders.

dlers have a need to explore and satisfy their curiosity, which may explain why some of them try to delay bedtime.

PRESCHOOLERS

On average a preschooler sleeps about 12 hours a night (about 20% is REM.) By the age of 5, the preschooler rarely takes daytime naps (Wong, 1995) except in cultures where a siesta is the custom. The preschooler usually has difficulty relaxing or quieting down after long, active days. A preschooler also has problems with bedtime fears, waking during the night, or nightmares. Parents are most successful in getting a preschooler to bed by establishing a consistent ritual that includes some quiet time activity before bedtime. Ordinarily, experts do not recommend that a child be allowed to sleep with parents. However, in some cultures sharing a bed or room with parents is an accepted sleeping practice.

SCHOOL-AGE CHILDREN

The amount of sleep needed during the school years is individualized because of varying states of activity and levels of health. The school-age child usually does not require a nap. A 6-year-old averages 11 to 12 hours of sleep nightly, whereas an 11-year-old sleeps about 9 to 10 hours (Wong, 1995). The 6- or 7-year-old can usually be persuaded to go to bed by encouraging quiet activities. The older child often resists sleeping because of an unawareness of fatigue or a need to be independent. A school-age child will be tired the following day if allowed to stay up later than usual. An older child may seek a later bedtime as a symbol of dominance over a younger child. Parents are usually successful in getting the older child to bed by using a firm, consistent approach. The older school-age child may be allowed to go to bed later, but such a privilege may be dependent on the child going to bed promptly without complaints.

ADOLESCENTS

Typically, teenagers get about 7½ hours of sleep per night (Carskadon, 1990a). At a time when sleep needs actually increase, the typical adolescent is subject to a number of changes that often reduce the time spent sleeping (Carskadon, 1990b). Usually parents are no longer involved in setting a specific bedtime. School demands, after-school social activities, and part-time jobs may result in compressed time available for sleep. Teens go to bed later and rise earlier during the high school years. A common societal expectation is that adolescents require less sleep than preadolescents. However, laboratory data indicate that adolescents may have a physiological need for more sleep when compared to preadolescents (Carskadon, 1990b). Because of lifestyle demands that shorten the time available for sleep and probable physiological need, teens often experience excessive daytime sleepiness (EDS). Performance in school, vulnerability to accidents, and behavior and mood problems can be the result of EDS due to insufficient sleep. Parents, teachers, and teens themselves often lack knowledge about what is proper sleep. All may need education in order to improve what can be a significant health problem for teens.

YOUNG ADULTS

Most young adults average 6 to 8½ hours of sleep a night, but this can vary. Young adults rarely take regular naps. Approximately 20% of sleep time is spent in REM sleep, which remains consistent throughout life. Healthy young adults require adequate sleep to participate in the busy activities that fill their days. However, it is common for lifestyle demands to interrupt usual sleep patterns. The stresses of jobs, family relationships, and social activities may lead to insomnia (i.e., difficulties initiating and/or maintaining sleep) and the use of medication for sleep. Long-term use of such medications can disrupt sleep patterns and make the insomnia problem worse.

MIDDLE ADULTS

During mid-adulthood the total time spent sleeping at night begins to decline. The amount of stage 4 sleep begins to fall, a decline that continues with advancing age. Sleep disturbances are often initially diagnosed among people in this age range even when the symptoms of a disorder have been present for several years. Insomnia is particularly common, probably because of the changes and stresses of middle age. Sleep disturbances can be caused by anxiety, depression, or certain physical ailments. Women experiencing menopausal symptoms may have insomnia. Members of this age group may rely on sleeping medications.

OLDER ADULTS

The total amount of sleep does not change as age increases. However, the quality of sleep appears to deteriorate for many older adults (Bliwise, 1993). Episodes of REM sleep tend to shorten. There is a progressive decrease in stages 3 and 4 NREM sleep; some older adults have almost no stage 4, or deep sleep. An older adult awakens more often during the night, and it may take more time for an older adult to fall asleep. However, older adults who adapt successfully to the physiological and psychosocial changes in aging are more likely to preserve REM sleep and continuity in the sleep cycle that is similar to younger adults (Reynolds et al, 1993).

Variability in the sleep behaviors of older adults is common. Complaints about difficulties with nighttime sleep frequently occur among the elderly, often resulting from the presence of another chronic illness. For example, an older adult with arthritis may have difficulty sleeping due to painful joints. The tendency to nap seems to increase progressively with age. The increased daytime spent napping may occur due to the frequent wakenings experienced at night. Compared to the amount of time spent in bed, the time spent sleeping may be decreased by an hour or more (Evans and Rogers, 1994).

The changes in an older person's sleep pattern may be due to changes in the CNS that affect the regulation of sleep. Sensory impairment, common with aging, may reduce sensitivity to time cues that maintain circadian rhythms.

■ FACTORS AFFECTING SLEEP

A number of factors affect the quantity and quality of sleep. Often a single factor may not be the only cause for a sleep problem. Physiological, psychological, and environmental factors can alter the quality and quantity of sleep.

Physical Illness

Any illness that causes pain, physical discomfort (e.g., difficulty breathing), or mood problems, such as anxiety or depression, can result in sleep problems. Persons with such alterations may have trouble falling or staying asleep. Illnesses also may force clients to sleep in positions to which they are unaccustomed. For example, assuming an awkward position when an arm or leg has been immobilized in traction can interfere with sleep.

Respiratory disease often interferes with sleep. Clients with chronic lung disease such as emphysema are short of breath and frequently cannot sleep without two or three pillows to raise their heads. Asthma, bronchitis, and allergic rhinitis alter the rhythm of breathing and disturb sleep. A person with a common cold has nasal congestion, sinus drainage, and a sore throat, which impair breathing and the ability to relax.

Coronary heart disease often is characterized by episodes of sudden chest pain and irregular heart rates. Clients with this disease often experience frequent awakenings and stage changes during sleep (i.e., frequent shifts from stages 3 and 4 to lighter stage 2 sleep) as well as significant alterations in all stages of sleep, for example, suppressed REM sleep and stages 3 and 4 (Landis, 1988).

Hypertension often causes early morning awakening and fatigue. Hypothyroidism decreases stage 4 sleep, whereas hyperthyroidism causes persons to take more time to fall asleep.

Nocturia, or urination during the night, disrupts sleep and the sleep cycle. This condition is most common in older people with reduced bladder tone or persons with cardiac disease, diabetes, urethritis, or prostatic disease. After a person awakens repeatedly to urinate, returning to sleep may be difficult.

Older adults often experience "restless leg syndrome," which occurs prior to sleep onset. People experience recurrent, rhythmical movements of the feet and legs. An itching sensation is felt deep in the muscles. Relief comes only from moving the legs, which prevents relaxation and subsequent sleep. Depending upon how severely sleep is disrupted, restless leg syndrome may be a relatively benign condition. In contrast, people who have severe leg cramps during the night may have a problem with arterial circulation.

Persons with peptic ulcer disease often awaken in the middle of the night. Gastric acid levels reach a peak in the stomach around 1 to 3 AM (McNeil et al, 1986), causing stomach pain.

Drugs and Substances

Of drugs listed in the 1990 PDR, 584 prescription or over-the-counter drugs listed sleepiness as a side effect, 486 listed insomnia, and 281 listed fatigue (Buysse, 1991). Sleepiness and sleep deprivation are common side effects of medications (see the box above). Medications prescribed for sleep often cause more problems than benefits. Young and middle-age adults may rely on sleeping medications to deal with lifestyle stressors. Older adults often take a variety of drugs to control or treat chronic illness, and the combined effects of several drugs can seriously disrupt sleep. L-Tryptophan, a natural protein found in foods such as milk, cheese, and meats, may help a person sleep.

Lifestyle

A person's daily routine may influence sleep patterns. An individual working a rotating shift (e.g., 2 weeks of days followed by a week of nights) often has difficulty adjusting to the altered sleep schedule. The body's internal clock might

Drugs and Their Effects on Sleep
HYPNOTICS
▪ Interfere with reaching deeper sleep stages
▪ Provide only temporary (1-week) increase in quantity of sleep
▪ Eventually cause "hangover" during day: excess drowsiness, confusion, decreased energy
▪ May worsen sleep apnea in older adults
DIURETICS
▪ Cause nocturia
ANTIDEPRESSANTS AND STIMULANTS
▪ Suppress REM sleep
▪ Decrease total sleep time
ALCOHOL
▪ Speeds onset of sleep
▪ Disrupts REM sleep
▪ Awakens person during night and causes difficulty returning to sleep
CAFFEINE
▪ Prevents person from falling asleep
▪ May cause person to awaken during night
BETA-BLOCKERS
▪ Cause nightmares
▪ Cause insomnia
▪ Cause awakening from sleep
BENZODIAZEPINES
▪ Increase sleep time
▪ Increase daytime sleepiness
NARCOTICS (MORPHINE/DEMEROL)
▪ Suppress REM sleep
▪ Cause increased daytime drowsiness

be set at 11 PM, but the work schedule forces sleep at 9 AM instead. The individual may be able to sleep only 3 or 4 hours because the body's clock perceives that it is time to be awake and active. Difficulties with maintaining alertness during work time can result in decreased and even hazardous performance. After several weeks of working a night shift a person's biological clock usually does adjust. Other alterations in routine that can disrupt sleep patterns include performing unaccustomed heavy work, engaging in late-night social activities, and changing evening mealtime.

Usual Sleep Patterns and Excessive Daytime Sleepiness (EDS)

In the past century the amount of sleep obtained nightly by U.S. citizens has decreased over 20% (National Commission on Sleep Disorders Research, 1993), indicating that many Americans are sleep deprived and experience excessive sleepiness during the day. EDS often results in impairment of waking function, poor work or school performance, accidents while driving or using equipment, and behavioral or emotional problems. Feelings of sleepiness are usually most intense upon awakening from, or right before going to, sleep, and about 12 hours after the midsleep period.

Sleepiness becomes pathological when it occurs at times when individuals need or want to be awake. People who experience temporary sleep deprivation as a result of an active social evening or lengthened work schedule usually feel sleepy the next day. However, they may be able to overcome these feelings even though they have difficulty performing tasks and remaining attentive. Chronic lack of sleep is much more serious than temporary sleep deprivation and can cause serious alterations in the ability to perform daily functions. EDS tends to be most difficult to overcome during sedentary tasks. For example, single-vehicle accidents related to a driver falling asleep at the wheel occur most often between midnight and 4 AM due to the sleepiness that can occur when people are awake during what is their normal period of sleep (Mitler et al, 1988; Leger, 1994).

Emotional Stress

Worry over personal problems or situations can disrupt sleep. Emotional stress causes a person to be tense and often leads to frustration when sleep does not come. Stress may also cause a person to try too hard to fall asleep, to awaken frequently during the sleep cycle, or to oversleep. Continued stress may cause poor sleep habits.

Older clients frequently experience losses that lead to emotional stress. Retirement, physical impairment, death of a loved one, and loss of economic security are examples of situations that predispose older adults to anxiety and depression. Older adults, as well as other individuals who experience depressive mood problems, often also experience delays in falling asleep, earlier appearance of REM sleep, frequent awakening, increased total bed time, feelings of sleeping poorly, and early awakening (Bliwise, 1993).

Environment

The physical environment in which a person sleeps has a significant influence on the ability to fall and remain asleep. Good ventilation is essential for restful sleep. The size, firmness, and position of the bed can affect the quality of sleep. Hospital beds are often harder than those at home. If a person usually sleeps with another individual, sleeping alone can cause wakefulness. On the other hand sleeping with a restless or snoring bed partner can also disrupt sleep.

Sound also influences sleep. The level of noise needed to awaken people depends on the stage of sleep (Webster and Thompson, 1986). Low noises are more likely to arouse a person from stage 1 sleep, whereas louder noises awaken people in stage 3 or 4 sleep. Some persons require silence to fall asleep, whereas others prefer background noise such as soft music or television.

In hospitals and other in-patient facilities, noise creates a problem for clients. Noise in hospitals is usually new or strange. Thus clients are prone to awaken. This problem is greatest the first night of hospitalization, when clients often experience increased total wake time, increased awakenings, and decreased REM sleep and total sleep time (Agnew et al, 1966). The level of noise in hospitals can be very loud. Normal conversation measures about 50 decibels. Hilton (1987) found that an intravenous controller-alarm created noise at 44 to 80 decibels, a flushing toilet at 44 to 76 decibels and paper ripping at 41 to 81 decibels. Sounds become noise at 35 to 40 decibels. People-induced noises (i.e., nursing activities) are sources of increased sound lev-

> ▶ **RESEARCH HIGHLIGHT**
>
> **RESEARCH ABSTRACT**
> Williamson investigated the influence of ocean sounds on the subjective assessment of the night sleep pattern of postoperative coronary artery bypass graft clients. An experimental group (n = 30) listened to ocean sounds at their preferred volume while going to sleep for three nights after transfer to a progressive care unit. Four experimental subjects refused to continue in the study after listening to the sounds for one night because they found the sounds annoying and the sounds increased their discomfort. A control group (n = 30), subjected only to the usual hospital environmental sounds, served as a comparison. When pre- and post-scores on several self-reported sleep variables were compared between the two groups, the ocean sound group reported significantly better sleep depth and quality, fewer awakenings, and less difficulty in returning to sleep if they awakened.
>
> **IMPLICATIONS FOR PRACTICE**
> ▶ Ocean sounds can be effective in aiding sleep.
> ▶ Sounds may aid sleep by masking other noise, or providing a focus for attention while going to sleep.
> ▶ Professional judgment in the use of sound to improve perceived sleep quality needs to be used since some clients may feel that sound increases their discomfort.
>
> **REFERENCE**
> From Williamson J: The effects of ocean sounds on sleep after coronary artery bypass graft surgery, *Amer J Cri Care* 1:91, 1992.

els. Intensive care units are sources for high noise levels. Close proximity of clients, noise from confused and ill clients, the ringing of alarm systems and telephones, and disturbances caused by emergencies make the environment unpleasant. Strategies to control environmental noise or use pleasant sound to mask annoying sounds have been described (see the box above).

Light levels may affect the ability to fall asleep. Some clients may prefer a dark room, whereas others, such as children or older adults, may prefer keeping a soft light on during sleep. Clients also may have trouble sleeping based on the temperature of a room. A room that is too warm or too cold often causes a client to become restless.

Exercise and Fatigue

A person who is moderately fatigued usually achieves restful sleep, especially if the fatigue is the result of enjoyable work or exercise. Exercising 2 hours or more before bedtime allows the body to cool down and maintains a state of fatigue that promotes relaxation. However, excess fatigue resulting from exhausting or stressful work can make falling asleep difficult. This can be a common problem for grade school children and adolescents.

Food and Caloric Intake

People sleep better when they are healthy so that following good eating habits is important to proper health and sleep

(Hauri and Linde, 1990). Eating a large, heavy, and/or spicy meal at night may result in indigestion that interferes with sleep. Caffeine and alcohol consumed in the evening have insomnia-producing effects so a drastic reduction or avoidance of these substances is an important strategy that can be used to improve sleep. Food allergies may cause insomnia. In infants, nighttime waking and crying or colic may be caused by a milk allergy requiring that breast milk or a nonmilk formula be used. Besides milk, other foods that often result in an insomnia-producing allergy among both children and adults include corn, wheat, nuts, chocolate, eggs, seafood, red and yellow food dyes, and yeast (Hauri and Linde, 1990). Restoration of normal sleep may take up to 2 weeks when the particular food causing difficulty has been eliminated from the diet.

Weight loss or gain influences sleep patterns. When a person gains weight, sleep periods become longer with fewer interruptions. Weight loss can cause short and fragmented sleep. Certain sleep disorders may be the result of the semistarvation diets popular in a weight-conscious society.

▌SLEEP DISORDERS

Sleep disorders are conditions that, if untreated, generally cause disturbed nighttime sleep that results in one of three problems: insomnia; abnormal movements or sensation during sleep or when awakening at night; or excessive daytime sleepiness (Naylor and Aldrich, 1994). Many adults in the United States have significant sleep debts from inadequacies in either the quantity or quality of their nighttime sleep and experience hypersomnolence on a daily basis (National Commission on Sleep Disorders Research, 1993).

Sleep disorders have been classified into four major categories (Thorpy, 1994) (see the box below). The *dyssomnias* (Section I) are primary disorders that have their origin in different body systems and are subdivided into three major groups. The intrinsic sleep disorders include disorders of initiating and maintaining sleep, that is, various forms of insomnia and disorders of excessive sleepiness such as narcolepsy and obstructive sleep apnea. Extrinsic sleep disorders develop from external factors, which if removed, lead to resolution of the sleep disorder. The circadian rhythm sleep disorders arise from a misalignment between the timing of sleep and what is desired by the individual or is a societal norm. The *parasomnias* are undesirable behaviors that occur predominantly during sleep: arousal disorders, partial arousals, or during transitions in the sleep cycle or from sleep to wakefulness. Many *medical and psychiatric sleep disorders* are associated with sleep and wake disturbances. These sleep disturbances are divided into those associated with psychiatric, neurological, or other medical specialty disorders. The *proposed sleep disorders* are newly described disturbances for which inadequate information currently exists to substantiate their existence.

A careful, comprehensive health, social, family, and sleep history is obtained to gather detailed information about the sleep complaint (Naylor and Aldrich, 1994). Sleep laboratory studies are often used to diagnose a sleep disorder, including the use of a nighttime **polysomnogram** (PSG) and the Multiple Sleep Latency Test (MSLT) (Carskadon, 1994). PSG involves use of the EEG, EMG, and EOG to monitor stages of sleep and wakefulness during nighttime sleep. The MSLT provides objective information about sleepiness and selected aspects of sleep structure by measuring how rapidly individuals fall asleep during at least four napping opportunities spread throughout the day. Sleep-onset REM episodes are also noted since this abnormality is associated with several sleep disorders.

▌ Classification of Sleep Disorders

DYSSOMNIAS
Intrinsic sleep disorders
Psychophysiological insomnia
Narcolepsy
Obstructive sleep apnea syndrome
Periodic limb movement disorder
Extrinsic sleep disorders
Inadequate sleep hygiene
Insufficient sleep syndrome
Hypnotic-dependent sleep disorders
Alcohol-dependent sleep disorders
Circadian rhythm sleep disorders
Time-zone change (jet lag) syndrome
Shift-work sleep disorder
Delayed sleep phase syndrome

PARASOMNIAS
Arousal disorders
Sleepwalking
Sleep terrors
Sleep-wake transition disorders
Sleep talking
Nocturnal leg cramps

Parasomnias usually associated with REM sleep
Nightmares
REM sleep behavior disorder
Other parasomnias
Sleep bruxism (teeth-grinding)
Sleep enuresis (bed wetting)
Sudden infant death syndrome

SLEEP DISORDERS ASSOCIATED WITH MEDICAL/PSYCHIATRIC DISORDERS
Associated with psychiatric disorders
Mood disorders
Anxiety disorders
Associated with neurological disorders
Dementia
Parkinsonism
Associated with other medical disorders
Nocturnal cardiac ischemia
Chronic obstructive pulmonary disease

PROPOSED SLEEP DISORDERS
Menstruation-associated sleep disorders
Sleep choking syndrome

Modified from American Sleep Disorders Association: *The international classification of sleep disorders: diagnostic and coding manual,* Rochester, 1990, Allen Press.

Insomnia

Insomnia is a symptom experienced by clients who have chronic difficulty falling asleep, frequent awakenings from sleep, and/or a short sleep or nonrestorative sleep (Zorick, 1994). The insomniac complains of excessive daytime sleepiness as well as insufficient quantity and quality of sleep. Frequently, however, the client gets more sleep than is realized. Insomnia may signal an underlying physical or psychological disorder.

People may experience transient insomnia as a result of situational stresses such as family, work or school problems, jet lag, illness, or loss of a loved one. Insomnia may recur, but between episodes the client is able to sleep well. However, a temporary case of insomnia due to a stressful situation can lead to chronic difficulty in obtaining sufficient sleep, perhaps due to the worry and anxiety that develops about obtaining adequate sleep.

Insomnia is often associated with poor sleep habits. If the condition continues, the fear of not being able to sleep can be enough to cause wakefulness. During the day, a person with chronic insomnia may feel sleepy, fatigued, depressed, and anxious.

Because there are many causes of insomnia, management involves several approaches (Walsh, Hartman, and Kowall, 1994). As appropriate, it is important to treat underlying emotional or medical problems that may be causing this nighttime sleep problem. Treatment can also be symptomatic, including improved sleep hygiene measures, biofeedback, cognitive techniques, and relaxation techniques. When insomnia develops secondary to inappropriate health behaviors, treatment is directed at changing these behaviors. For example, in drug-dependence insomnia the client is unable to fall asleep because of excessive use of hypnotic medications. This client usually benefits from a gradual withdrawal of the hypnotics.

Sleep Apnea

Sleep apnea is a disorder characterized by the lack of airflow through the nose and mouth for periods of 10 seconds or longer during sleep. There are three types of sleep apnea: central, obstructive, and mixed apnea that has both a central and obstructive component.

The most common form, obstructive sleep apnea (OSA), occurs when muscles or structures of the oral cavity or throat relax during sleep. The upper airway becomes partially or completely blocked, and nasal airflow is diminished (hypopnea) or stopped (apnea) for as long as 30 seconds (Guilleminault, 1994). The person still attempts to breathe because chest and abdominal movement continue, which often results in loud snoring and snorting sounds. When breathing is partially or completely diminished, each successive diaphragmatic movement becomes stronger until the obstruction is relieved. Structural abnormalities such as a deviated septum, nasal polyps, or enlarged tonsils predispose a client to obstructive apnea. The effort to breathe during sleep results in arousals from deep sleep often to the stage 2 cycle. In severe cases, hundreds of hypopnea/apnea episodes can occur every hour resulting in severe interference with deep sleep. Excessive daytime sleepiness is the most common complaint of people with OSA. The National Commission on Sleep Disorders Research (1993) estimated that 18 million people in the United States meet the diagnostic criteria for OSA.

Obstructive apnea causes a serious decline in arterial oxygen level (see Chapter 44). Clients are at risk for cardiac dysrhythmias, right heart failure, pulmonary hypertension, anginal attacks, stroke, and hypertension. Middle-aged men are usually thought to be more frequently affected, particularly when they are obese. However, recent evidence is accumulating that postmenopausal women also relatively commonly experience obstructive sleep apnea that is also strongly related to hypertension (Gislason et al, 1993). The most frequent time of what appears to be naturally occurring or otherwise unexplained death is between 4 and 6 AM. Some researchers believe that sleep apneas are a cause for many of these types of death (Berman et al, 1990).

Central sleep apnea (CSA) involves dysfunction in the brain's respiratory control center. The impulse to breathe temporarily fails, and nasal airflow and chest wall movement cease. The oxygen saturation of the blood falls. The condition is seen in clients with brainstem injury, muscular dystrophy, and encephalitis as well as people who breathe normally during the day. Less than 10% of sleep apnea is predominantly central in origin. People with CSA tend to awaken during sleep and therefore complain of insomnia and EDS. Mild and intermittent snoring is also present.

The client with sleep apnea is often significantly deprived of deep sleep. In addition to complaints of excessive daytime sleepiness, sleep attacks, fatigue, morning headaches, and decreased sex drive are common. Treatment includes therapy for underlying cardiac or respiratory complications and emotional problems that arise as a result of the symptoms of this disorder. Sleep hygiene and a weight-loss program may help. One of the most effective therapies is use of a nasal continuous positive airway pressure (CPAP) device at night. CPAP requires a client to wear a mask over the nose. Room air is delivered through the mask at a high pressure. The air pressure prevents airway collapse. The CPAP device is portable and effective particularly for obstructive apnea. In cases of severe sleep apnea the tonsils, uvula, or portions of the soft palate may be surgically removed. Success with surgical procedures is variable.

Narcolepsy

Narcolepsy is a dysfunction of mechanisms that regulate the sleep and wake states. EDS is the most common complaint associated with this disorder. During the day a person may suddenly feel an overwhelming wave of sleepiness and fall asleep. REM sleep can occur within 15 minutes of falling asleep. **Cataplexy**, or sudden muscle weakness during intense emotions such as anger, sadness, or laughter, may occur at any time during the day. If the cataplectic attack is severe, the client may lose voluntary muscle control and fall to the floor. A person with narcolepsy may have vivid dreams that occur as the person is falling asleep that are difficult to distinguish from reality (called *hypnogic hallucinations*). Sleep paralysis, or the feeling of being unable to move or talk just before waking or falling asleep, is another symptom. Recent studies show a genetic link for narcolepsy (Mitler et al, 1990; Aldrich, 1992).

A significant problem for the person with narcolepsy is that the individual falls asleep uncontrollably at inappropriate times. Unless this disorder is understood, a sleep attack can easily be mistaken for laziness, lack of interest in activities, or drunkenness. Typically, the symptoms first begin to arise in adolescence and may be confused with the EDS that is thought to commonly occur in teens. Narcoleptics are treated with stimulants that may only partially increase wakefulness and reduce sleep attacks, and medications that suppress cataplexy and the other REM-related symptoms. Brief daytime naps no longer than 20 minutes may help reduce subjective feelings of sleepiness. Factors that increase a narcoleptic client's drowsiness (e.g., alcohol or exhausting activities) should be avoided.

Sleep Deprivation

Sleep deprivation is a problem many clients experience as a result of the dyssomnias. Causes may include illness (e.g., fever, difficulty breathing, or pain), emotional stress, medications, environmental disturbances (i.e., frequent nursing care), and variability in the timing of sleep due to shift work. Physicians and nurses may be particularly prone to sleep deprivation due to long work schedules and rotating shifts. Gold et al. (1992) found that nurses who worked rotating shifts reported sleeping less hours and were significantly more likely to report accidents or errors when compared to nurses who worked a straight day or evening shift.

Hospitalization, especially in intensive care units, makes clients particularly vulnerable to the extrinsic and circadian sleep disorders (Wood, 1992). Sleep deprivation involves decreases in the quantity and quality of sleep as well as inconsistency in the timing of sleep. When sleep becomes interrupted or fragmented, changes in the normal sequencing of the sleep cycles occur. A cumulative sleep deprivation develops.

A person's response to sleep deprivation is highly variable. Clients may experience a variety of physiological and psychological symptoms (see the box below). The severity of symptoms is often related to the duration of sleep deprivation. The most effective treatment for sleep deprivation is elimination or correction of factors that disrupt the sleep pattern. Nurses can play an important role in identifying treatable sleep deprivation problems.

Parasomnias

The parasomnias are sleep problems that are more common in children compared to adults. Sudden infant death syndrome (SIDS) is hypothesized to be related to apnea, hyp-

oxia, and cardiac arrhythmias caused by abnormalities in the autonomic nervous system that are manifested during sleep (Gillis and Flemons, 1994). Currently, the American Academy of Pediatrics recommends that apparently healthy infants be placed in the sidelying or supine positions during sleep due to an association between the prone position and the occurrence of SIDS (Long and Barron, 1992).

Parasomnias that occur among older children include somnambulism (sleepwalking), night terrors, nightmares, nocturnal enuresis (bedwetting), and tooth grinding (bruxism) (Mindell, 1993). When adults have these problems, it may indicate more serious disorders. Specific treatment for these disorders varies. However, in all cases it is important to support clients and maintain their safety. For example, sleepwalkers are unaware of their surroundings and are slow to react. Thus the risk of falls is great. A nurse should not startle sleepwalkers but instead gently awaken them and lead them back to bed.

■ NURSING PROCESS AND SLEEP

 Assessment

To promote a normal restful sleep for clients, the nurse assesses their sleep patterns using the nursing history to gather information about factors that usually influence sleep. If the client perceives that sleep is adequate, the nursing history can be brief.

Sleep is a subjective experience. Only the client can report whether or not it is sufficient and restful. If the client is satisfied with the quantity and quality of sleep received, it may be considered normal (Closs, 1988). If a client admits to, or the nurse suspects a sleep problem, a more detailed history is needed.

SLEEP ASSESSMENT

Most persons can provide a reasonably accurate estimate of their sleep patterns, particularly if any changes have occurred. One effective, brief subjective method for assessing sleep quality is the use of a visual analog scale (Closs, 1988). The nurse draws a straight horizontal line about 100 mm (4 inches) long. Opposing statements such as "best night's sleep" and "worst night's sleep" are at each end of the line. Clients are asked to place a mark on the horizontal line at the point corresponding to their perceptions of the previous night's sleep. The distance of the mark along the line can be measured in millimeters and offers a numerical value for satisfaction with sleep. The scale can be repeatedly administered to show change over time.

Assessment is aimed at understanding the characteristics of any sleep problem and the client's usual sleep habits so that ways for promoting sleep can be incorporated into nursing care. For example, if the nursing history reveals that a client always reads before falling asleep, it makes sense to offer reading material at bedtime.

Sources for Sleep Assessment. Usually, clients are the best resource for describing a sleep problem and the extent to which a problem represents a change from their usual sleep and waking patterns. Often the client knows the cause for sleep problems, such as a noisy environment or worry over a relationship.

Sleep Deprivation Symptoms

PHYSIOLOGICAL SYMPTOMS
- Ptosis, blurred vision
- Fine motor clumsiness
- Decreased reflexes
- Slowed response time
- Decreases in reasoning and judgment
- Decreased auditory and visual alertness
- Cardiac arrhythmias

PSYCHOLOGICAL SYMPTOMS
- Confusion and disorientation
- Increased sensitivity to pain
- Irritable, withdrawn, apathetic
- Excessive sleepiness
- Agitation
- Hyperactive
- Decreased motivation

Additionally, bed partners can provide information on the clients' patterns that may reveal the nature of certain sleep disorders. For example, partners of clients with sleep apnea often complain that their sleep is disturbed by clients' snoring. Often the partners must sleep in different beds or rooms in order to obtain adequate sleep. The nurse should ask bed partners whether the clients have pauses of breathing during sleep and how frequently the apneic attacks occur. Some partners mention becoming fearful when clients apparently stop breathing for periods during sleep.

When caring for children, the nurse needs to seek information about sleep patterns from parents since they are usually a good source of information about why their child is having trouble sleeping. Some parents may not realize that there is a wide variability in the sleeping patterns of infants and may need reassurance if their infant seems to sleep less than others but is otherwise healthy and thriving (Parkinson, 1994). Hunger, excessive warmth, and separation anxiety are factors that may contribute to an infant's difficulty with going to sleep or frequent wakenings during the night. Older children often are able to relate fears or worries that inhibit their ability to fall asleep. If children frequently awaken in the middle of bad dreams, parents can identify the problem but perhaps do not understand the meanings of the dreams. Parents can also describe the typical behavior patterns that foster or impair sleep. For example, excessive stimulation from active play or visiting friends may predictably impair sleep. With chronic sleep problems, parents can relate the duration of the problem, its progression, and children's responses. Parents of infants may need to keep a 24-hour log of their infant's waking and sleeping behavior for several days in order to determine what may be causing the problem. The infant's eating pattern and sleeping environment also need to be described since these may influence sleeping behavior.

SLEEP HISTORY

Clients may report that they enjoy adequate sleep. In this situation the sleep history can be brief (see the box below). A determination of usual bedtime, normal bedtime rituals, preferred environment for sleeping, and what time the client usually rises gives the nurse information for planning care conducive to sleep. When suspecting a sleep problem, the nurse assesses the quality and characteristics of sleep in greater depth.

Components of a Sleep History

- Description of client's sleep problem
- Prior usual sleep pattern
- Recent changes in sleep pattern
- Bedtime routines and sleeping environment
- Use of sleep and other prescription medications and OTC drugs
- Pattern of dietary intake and amount of substances (e.g., alcohol) that influence sleep
- Symptoms experienced during waking hours
- Concurrent physical illness
- Recent life events
- Current emotional and mental status

Description of Sleeping Problems. When a client admits to or the nurse suspects a sleep problem, the nursing history must be detailed so that therapeutic care can be provided. Open-ended questions help a client to describe a problem more fully. A general description of the problem followed by more focused questions usually reveals specific characteristics that can be used in planning therapies.

To begin, the nurse needs to understand the nature of the sleep problem, its signs and symptoms, its onset and duration, its severity, any predisposing factors or causes, and the overall effect on the client. Assessment questions might include the following:

1. *Nature of the problem:* Tell me what type of problem you have with your sleep. Tell me why you think your sleep is inadequate. Describe for me a recent typical night's sleep. How is this sleep different from what you are used to?

2. *Signs and symptoms:* Do you have difficulty falling asleep, staying asleep, or waking up? Have you been told that you snore loudly? Do you have headaches when awakening? Does your child awaken from nightmares?

3. *Onset and duration:* When did you notice the problem? How long has this problem lasted?

4. *Severity:* How long does it take you to fall asleep? How often during the week do you have trouble falling asleep? Tell me how many hours of sleep a night you got this week; compare that to what is usual for you. What do you do when you awaken during the night or too early in the morning?

5. *Predisposing factors:* Tell me what you do just before going to bed. Have you recently had any changes at work or at home? How is your mood and have you noticed any changes recently? What medications or recreational drugs do you take on a regular basis? Are you taking any new prescription or over-the-counter medications? How long have you been taking the medications? Do you eat foods (e.g., spicy or greasy foods) or drink substances (e.g., alcohol or caffeinated beverages) that could be interfering with your sleep? Do you have a physical illness that might be interfering with your sleep?

6. *Effect on client:* How has the loss of sleep affected you? (Ask a spouse or friend: Have you noticed any changes in behavior since the sleep problem started?) Do you feel excessively sleepy, irritable, or have trouble concentrating during waking hours? Do you have trouble staying awake or have you fallen asleep at inappropriate times, for example, while driving, sitting quietly in a meeting, or watching TV?

Proper questioning helps the nurse determine the type of sleep disturbance and the nature of the problem. Table 42-2 gives examples of additional questions to ask when specific sleep disorders are suspected.

As an adjunct to the sleep history, a client and bed partner may be asked to keep a sleep-wake log for 1 to 2 weeks (Douglas, Carskadon, and Houser, 1990). The sleep-wake log is completed daily to provide information on day-to-day variations in sleep-wake patterns over extended periods. Entries in the log often include 24-hour information about various waking and sleeping health behaviors such as physical activities, mealtimes, type and amount of intake (alcohol and caffeine), time and length of daytime naps, evening and bedtime routines, the time the client tries to fall asleep, nighttime awakenings, and the time of morning

Table 42-7	Questions to Ask to Assess for Sleep Disorders	
ASSESSMENT QUESTIONS		**RATIONALE**

INSOMNIA

How easily do you fall asleep?
Do you fall asleep and have difficulty staying asleep? How many times do you awaken?
Do you awaken early from sleep?
What time do you awaken for good? What causes you to awaken early?
What do you do to prepare for sleep? To improve your sleep?
What do you think about as you try to fall asleep?
How often do you have trouble sleeping?

Rationale: Determine nature and severity of insomnia.
Help in selection of sleep therapies.

SLEEP APNEA

Do you snore loudly?
Has anyone ever told you that you often stop breathing for short periods during sleep? (Spouse or bed partner/roommate may report this.)
Do you experience headaches after awakening?
Do you have difficulty staying awake during the day?

Rationale: Reveal presence of sleep apnea and severity of condition.

NARCOLEPSY

Are you tired during the day?
Do you fall asleep at inopportune times? (Friends or relatives may report this.)
Do you have episodes of losing muscle control or falling to the floor?
Have you ever had the feeling of being unable to move or talk just before falling asleep?
Do you have vivid lifelike dreams when going to sleep or waking up?

Rationale: Help diagnose narcolepsy and influence on daily activities.

awakening. A partner can help record the estimated times the client falls asleep or awakens. While the log is helpful, the client must be motivated to participate in its completion. Ordinarily it is not used with acutely ill clients who have short hospital stays.

Usual Sleep Pattern. Normal sleep is difficult to define because individuals vary in the quantity and quality of sleep that they perceive as adequate for them. It is important, however, to have clients describe their usual sleep pattern to determine the significance of the changes that may be being created by a sleep disorder. Knowing a client's usual, preferred sleep pattern allows a nurse to try to match sleeping conditions in a health care setting with those in the home. To determine the client's sleep pattern the nurse asks the following questions:

1. What time do you usually get in bed each night?
2. What time do you usually fall asleep? Do you do anything special to help you fall asleep?
3. How many times do you awaken at night? Why do you think you awaken? What do you do about awakening?
4. What time do you typically wake up in the morning?
5. What time do you get out of bed for good once you have awakened?
6. What is the average number of hours you sleep each night?

The nurse compares these data with the predominant pattern usually found for other clients of the same age.

Based on this comparison, the nurse begins to assess for identifiable patterns such as insomnia.

Clients with sleep problems may show patterns drastically different from their usual one, or the change may be relatively minor. Hospitalized clients usually need or want more sleep as a result of illness. However, some may require less sleep because they are less active. Clients who are ill may think that it is important to try to sleep more than what is usual for them, eventually making sleeping difficult. The St. Mary's Hospital Sleep Questionnaire is a brief instrument that can be used to evaluate the sleep of clients in health care settings (Fig. 42-5) (Leigh et al, 1988). The questionnaire is easily scored and provides information about the process and speed of going to sleep and the perceived quality of sleep.

Physical Illness. The nurse determines whether the client has any preexisting health problems that might interfere with sleep. A history of psychiatric problems may make a difference. A manic depressive client sleeps more when depressed than when manic. A depressed client often experiences an inadequate amount of sleep that is fragmented. Chronic diseases such as chronic obstructive pulmonary disease and painful disorders such as arthritis interfere with sleep. Children with attention deficit hyperactivity disorder may have difficulty obtaining adequate nighttime sleep. The nurse also assesses the client's medication history, including a description of over-the-counter and prescribed drugs. If a client takes medications

THE SMH SLEEP QUESTIONNAIRE

This questionnaire refers to your sleep over the past 24 hours. Please try to answer every question.

Name: _____

Today's date: _____

Age: _____Yrs.

Sex: Male/Female (delete whichever inapplicable).

At what time did you:

1. Settle down for the night? _____ Hrs. _____ Mins.
2. Fall asleep last night? _____ Hrs. _____ Mins.
3. Finally wake this morning? _____ Hrs. _____ Mins.
4. Get up this morning? _____ Hrs. _____ Mins.
5. Was your sleep: (tick below)
   1. Very light _____
   2. Light _____
   3. Fairly light _____
   4. Light average _____
   5. Deep average _____
   6. Fairly deep _____
   7. Deep _____
   8. Very deep _____
6. How many times did you wake up? (tick below)
   0. Not at all _____
   1. Once _____
   2. Twice _____
   3. Three times _____
   4. Four times _____
   5. Five times _____
   6. Six times _____
   7. More than six times _____

How much sleep did you have:

7. Last night? _____ Hr. _____ Mins.
8. During the day, yesterday? _____ Hrs. _____ Mins.
9. How well did you sleep last night? (tick below)
   1. Very badly _____
   2. Badly _____
   3. Fairly badly _____
   4. Fairly well _____
   5. Well _____
   6. Very well _____

If not well, what was the trouble? (e.g., restless, etc.)

1. _____
2. _____
3. _____

10. How clear-headed did you feel after getting up this morning? (tick below)
    1. Still very drowsy indeed _____
    2. Still moderately drowsy _____
    3. Still slightly drowsy _____
    4. Fairly clear-headed _____
    5. Alert _____
    6. Very alert _____
11. How satisfied were you with last night's sleep? (tick below)
    1. Very unsatisfied _____
    2. Moderately unsatisfied _____
    3. Slightly unsatisfied _____
    4. Fairly satisfied _____
    5. Completely satisfied _____
12. Were you troubled by waking early and being unable to get to sleep again? (tick below)
    1. No _____
    2. Yes _____
13. How much difficulty did you have in getting to sleep last night? (tick below)
    1. None or very little _____
    2. Some _____
    3. A lot _____
    4. Extreme difficulty _____
14. How long did it take you to fall asleep last night?
    _____ Hrs. _____ Mins.

Fig. 42-5 The St. Mary's Hospital Sleep Questionnaire. *(From Leigh TJ et al: Sleep 11:451, 1988.*

to aid sleep, the nurse gathers information about the type and amount of medication that is being used. The nurse may also assess daily caffeine intake.

If the client has recently undergone surgery the nurse can expect the client to experience some disturbance in sleep. The effect on sleep depends on the severity of pain experienced after surgery (Closs, 1992). Clients may awaken frequently during the first night after surgery and receive little deep or REM sleep. Depending on the type of surgery, it may take several days for a normal sleep cycle to return.

Current Life Events. The nurse learns whether the client is experiencing any changes in lifestyle that may be disrupting sleep. A person's occupation may offer a clue to the nature of a sleep problem. Changes in job responsibilities, rotating shifts, or long hours can contribute to a sleep disturbance. Questions about social activities, recent travel, or mealtime schedules help clarify the sleep assessment.

Emotional and Mental Status. If a client is anxious, excitable, or angry, mental preoccupations can seriously disrupt sleep. The client may be experiencing emotional stress related to illness or situational crises such as loss of job or a loved one. Thus the client's emotions may affect the ability to sleep. Clients with psychiatric disorders may need mild sedation for adequate rest. The nurse assesses the effectiveness of the medication and its effect on daytime function.

Bedtime Routines. The nurse asks about what the client does to prepare for sleep. For example, the client may drink a glass of milk, take a sleeping pill, eat a snack, or watch television. The nurse assesses habits that are beneficial compared with those that have been found to disturb sleep. Not all clients are alike. Watching television may promote sleep for one person, whereas another individual may be stimulated to stay awake while watching TV. Sometimes pointing out that a particular habit may be interfering with sleep can help clients to find ways to change or eliminate habits that may be disrupting sleep.

The nurse should pay special attention to a child's bedtime rituals. The parents can report whether it is necessary, for example, to read the child a bedtime story, rock the child to sleep, or engage in quiet play.

Bedtime Environment. The nurse asks the client to describe preferred bedroom conditions. The bedroom may be dark or light and the door to the room may be open or closed. The client may listen to the radio or watch television, or prefer a quiet environment since noise may prevent the client from falling asleep. The nurse also observes the bed and mattress for preferred type (e.g., soft). In addition, a child may require the company of a parent to fall asleep. The nurse may learn that changes in the home or institutional environment may be necessary to promote sleep. In a health care environment there may be environmental distractions that can interfere with sleep such as a roommate's television, an electronic monitor in the hallway, a noisy nurses' station, or another client who cries out at night. The nurse identifies factors that can be reduced or controlled.

Behaviors of Sleep Deprivation. Some clients may be unaware of how their sleep problems are affecting their behavior. The nurse observes for behaviors such as irritability, disorientation (similar to a drunken state), and slurred speech. If sleep deprivation has lasted a long time, psychotic behavior such as delusions and paranoia may develop. For example, a client may report seeing strange objects or colors in the room. The client may act afraid when the nurse enters the room.

Clients hospitalized in intensive care units for an extended time may show the "ICU syndrome" of sleep deprivation (Kido, 1992). Constant environmental stimuli within the ICU, such as strange noises from equipment, the frequent monitoring and care given by nurses, and everpresent lights, confuse clients. Soon a client cannot tell the difference between night and day. Repeated environmental stimuli and the client's poor physical status lead to sleep deprivation (Richards and Barnsfather, 1988).

 ## Nursing Diagnosis

Assessment reveals clusters of data that include defining characteristics for a sleep problem that results from disturbed sleep (Cohen and Merritt, 1992). If a sleep pattern disturbance is identified the nurse specifies the specific condition (see the nursing diagnoses box above). By specifying the nature of a sleep disturbance, the nurse can design more effective interventions. For example, the nurse uses specific therapies to help clients who are unable to fall asleep versus those with sleep apnea. The diagnostic process box on p. 1144 demonstrates how the identification of defining characteristics ensures an accurate nursing diagnosis.

Assessment should also identify the probable cause of the sleep disturbance, such as a noisy environment, a high intake of caffeinated beverages in the evening, or stress involving a marital relationship. These causes become the focus of interventions for minimizing or eliminating the problem. For example, if a client is experiencing insomnia as a result of a noisy health care environment, the nurse could offer some basic recommendations for helping sleep such as controlling the noise of hospital equipment, reduc-

Examples of NANDA Nursing Diagnoses for Sleep Disturbances

Sleep pattern disturbance (difficulty falling asleep) *related to:*
- Noisy environment
- Arthritis pain

Sleep pattern disturbance (frequent awakenings) *related to:*
- Concern over loss of job
- Barbiturate dependency

Risk for injury *related to:*
- Attacks of sleepwalking

Ineffective family coping: compromised *related to:*
- Spouse's poor understanding of narcolepsy

Self-esteem disturbance *related to:*
- Incidents of bed-wetting

Altered thought processes *related to:*
- Sleep deprivation

Impaired gas exchange during sleep *related to:*
- Altered oxygen supply

Ineffective breathing pattern *related to:*
- Tracheobronchial obstruction

ing interruptions, or keeping doors closed. If the insomnia is related to worry over a threatened marital separation, the nurse's actions involve introduction of coping strategies and creation of an environment for sleep. If the probable cause or related factors are incorrectly defined, the client may not benefit from care.

Sleep problems may affect clients in other ways. For example, a nurse may find that a client with sleep apnea has problems with a spouse who is tired and frustrated over the client's snoring. In addition, the spouse is concerned that the client is breathing improperly and thus is in danger. The nursing diagnosis of ineffective family coping indicates that the nurse must provide support to the client and spouse so that they can understand sleep apnea and obtain the medical treatment needed.

 ## Planning

After identifying each nursing diagnosis, the nurse develops a care plan (see the care plan on p. 1144). An individualized care plan can be developed only after the nurse understands the client's current sleep pattern (based on objective data), the client's perception of that sleep pattern, and the factors disrupting sleep. Together the nurse and client develop realistic interventions to promote rest and sleep in the home or health care setting. The client's bed partner may have useful suggestions.

It is important for the plan of care to include strategies that are appropriate for the client's living environment and lifestyle. An effective plan includes outcomes established over a realistic time that focus on the goal of improving the quality of sleep in the home. This type of plan may require many weeks to accomplish. The nurse partners closely with the client and significant others to ensure that any thera-

Sample Nursing Diagnostic Process for Sleep Disturbances

ASSESSMENT ACTIVITIES	DEFINING CHARACTERISTICS	NURSING DIAGNOSES
Ask client to explain nature of sleep problem.	Client reports difficulty in falling asleep, taking up to an hour. Client reports awakening two to three times nightly, with difficulty returning to sleep.	Sleep pattern disturbance, difficulty falling and/or remaining asleep related to worry over job loss
Observe client's behavior and ask bed partner if behavior changes have been noted.	Client admits to not feeling well rested. Spouse describes episodes of client being lethargic and irritable.	
Determine if client has had recent lifestyle changes.	Spouse reports client recently lost job; has concern over finding new position.	
Ask client and spouse to describe nature of sleep problem.	Client reports excessive sleepiness during the day with morning headaches. Spouse reports client snores loudly and often seems to stop breathing for several seconds.	Ineffective family coping: compromised related to spouse and client's poor understanding of sleep apnea
Ask client and spouse whether the sleep problem has affected their relationship.	Client admits to a decreased sexual drive, says spouse "doesn't understand." Spouse reports client is unwilling to talk about problem or seek help.	
Gather a sleep-wake log for a week.	Log indicates frequent awakenings from sleep, spouse moved to different bedroom day 4 due to loud snoring.	

Sample Nursing Care Plan for Sleep Pattern Disturbance

NURSING DIAGNOSIS: **Sleep pattern disturbance** (difficulty falling asleep) related to worry over job loss
DEFINITION: Sleep pattern disturbance is a disruption of sleep time that causes discomfort or interferes with desired lifestyle (Kim, McFarland, McLane, 1995).

GOAL	EXPECTED OUTCOMES	INTERVENTIONS	RATIONALE
Client will report that usual sleep pattern is reestablished within 1 month.	Client will fall asleep within 30 minutes of going to bed.	Suggest caffeine and alcohol be removed from client's diet in the evening. Have client follow bedtime ritual: go to bed at same time each night, drink glass of milk beforehand.	Caffeine and alcohol disrupt sleep cycle Milk contains L-tryptophan, natural amino acid that induces sleep (Ross et al, 1986).
	Client will use relaxation therapies each night before bedtime.	Establish time before client goes to bed for quiet relaxation, soothing bath, or progressive relaxation exercises.	Effect of relaxation requires further study. Insomniacs may have increase in sympathetic tone, and relaxation may help reduce it (Berman et al, 1990).
	Client will report feeling of restfulness after awakening each morning.	Control sources of environmental noise and be sure that bedroom is darkened and well ventilated.	Loud noises can disrupt and interfere with rest.

pies, such as a change in the sleep schedule or changes to the bedroom environment, are realistic and achievable.

In a health care setting the nurse plans treatments or routines so that the client will be able to rest. For example, in the intensive care unit, nurses check available electronic monitors to track trends in vital signs without awakening a client each hour. Other staff members should be aware of the care plan so that they can cluster activities at certain times to reduce awakenings. In a nursing home the focus of the plan may involve better planning of rest periods around the activities of other residents. Often the schedule of one roommate may not coincide with that of another.

The nature of a sleep disturbance determines whether referrals to additional health care providers are necessary. For example, if a sleep problem is related to a situational crisis or emotional problem, the nurse may refer the client to a psychiatric clinical nurse specialist, or clinical psychologist for counseling. When chronic insomnia is the problem, a medical referral or referral to a sleep center can be beneficial. If the nurse works in an in patient setting and the client is to receive a referral for continued care after discharge, offering information about the sleep problem will be useful to the home health care nurse.

The success of sleep therapy depends on an approach that fits the client's lifestyle and the nature of the sleep disorder. The goals of any care plan for a client needing sleep or rest include the following:

1. Client obtains a sense of restfulness and renewed energy following sleep.
2. Client establishes a healthy sleep pattern.
3. Client understands factors that promote or disrupt sleep.
4. Client assumes self-care behaviors to eliminate factors contributing to the sleep disturbance.

 Implementation

Nursing interventions designed to improve the quality of a person's sleep are largely focused on health promotion. Clients need adequate sleep and rest to maintain active and productive lifestyles. During times of illness, sleep promotion is important for recovery from physical illness. Nursing care in an acute-care setting differs from that provided in a client's home. The primary differences are in the environment and the nurse's ability to support normal sleep habits. The client's age also influences the type of therapies that are most effective (see the box below). Despite the cause or related factors for a sleep problem, the nurse performs specific interventions that promote normal sleep patterns.

ENVIRONMENTAL CONTROLS

All clients require a sleeping environment with a comfortable room temperature and proper ventilation, minimal sources of noise, a comfortable bed, and proper lighting. Infants sleep best when the room temperature is 18° to 21°C (65° to 69.8°F) at night. Cribs should be positioned away from open windows or drafts. The infant is covered with a light, warm blanket. Children and adults vary more in regards to comfortable room temperature. Some prefer to sleep without covers. Older adults often require extra blankets or covers. Many older clients sleep wearing socks.

Distracting noise needs to be eliminated so that the bedroom is as quiet as possible. In the home the TV or the intermittent chiming of a clock may disrupt a client's sleep. The family becomes an important part of the nurse's approach, especially if there are several family members, all with different schedules for going to sleep. At home it may require the cooperation of several people living with the

---

 GERONTOLOGICAL PRINCIPLES for Promoting Sleep

SLEEP-WAKE PATTERN
- Maintain a regular rising time.
- Eliminate naps unless they are a routine part of the schedule.
- If naps are used, limit to 20 minutes or less twice a day.
- Avoid extremes of sleep, that is, becoming excessively sleepy on the weekends.
- Go to bed when sleepy.
- Use relaxation techniques to promote sleep.
- If unable to sleep in 15 to 30 minutes, get out of bed.

ENVIRONMENT
- Sleep where you sleep best.
- Keep noise to minimum; use soft music to mask noise if necessary.
- Use nightlight and keep path to bathroom free of obstacles.
- Set room temperature to preference; use blankets and socks to promote warmth.

MEDICATIONS
- Use sedatives and hypnotics as last resort and then only short-term if absolutely necessary.
- Adjust medications being taken for other conditions and look for drug interactions that may cause insomnia or EDS.

DIET
- Limit alcohol, caffeine, and nicotine in late afternoon and evening.
- Consume carbohydrates or milk as a light snack before bedtime.
- Decrease fluids 2 to 4 hours before sleep.

PHYSIOLOGICAL/ILLNESS FACTORS
- Elevate head of bed and provide extra pillows as preferred.
- Use analgesics 30 minutes before bed to ease aches and pains.
- Use therapeutics to control symptoms of chronic conditions as prescribed.

client to reduce noise. It is also important to remember that some clients are used to sleeping with familiar inside noises, such as the hum of a fan.

In a hospital the nurse can control noise in several ways (see the box below). In addition, nurses should participate in product review and selection (e.g., intravenous pumps) to help equipment manufacturers become aware of the need for quiet in future product designs.

A bed and mattress should provide support and comfortable firmness. Bed boards can be placed under mattresses to add support. Sometimes extra pillows are important to help a person position comfortably in bed. The position of the bed in the room may also make a difference for some clients.

Infants' beds must be safe. To reduce the chance of suffocation, pillows or the ends of loose blankets should not be placed in cribs. Loose-fitting plastic mattress covers should not be used because infants might pull them over their faces and suffocate. Infants are usually placed on their back to prevent suffocation or sides to prevent aspiration of stomach contents.

For any client prone to confusion or falls, safety is critical. In the home a small nightlight might assist the client in orienting to the room environment before arising to go to the bathroom. Beds set lower to the floor may lessen the chance of a person falling when first standing. Clutter should always be removed from the path a client uses to walk from the bed to the bathroom. If a client needs assistance in ambulating from a bed to the bathroom, a small bell at the bedside can be used to call family members. In a health care setting a call light should always be placed within the client's easy reach. The nurse should be sure the client knows how to turn the light on correctly. Some hospital beds are equipped with an alarm that goes off when a client at risk for falling gets out of bed.

Clients vary in regard to the amount of light that they prefer at night. Infants and older adults sleep best in softly lit rooms. Light should not shine directly on their eyes. Small table lamps prevent total darkness. For older adults, this reduces the chance of confusion and prevents falls en route to the bathroom. If street lights shine through windows or when clients nap during the day, heavy shades, drapes, or slatted blinds are helpful. Nurses should close curtains between clients in semiprivate rooms. Lights on a hospital nursing unit can be dimmed at night.

PROMOTING BEDTIME ROUTINES

Bedtime routines relax clients in preparation for sleep. It is always important for persons to go to sleep when they feel fatigued or sleepy. Going to bed while fully awake and thinking about other things can cause insomnia and interfere with the bed as a stimulus for sleep.

Newborns and infants sleep through so much of the day that a specific routine is hardly necessary. However, quieting activities, such as holding them snugly in blankets, singing or talking softly, and gently rocking, help infants fall asleep.

A bedtime routine (e.g., same hour for bedtime, snack, or quiet activity) used consistently helps young children avoid delaying sleep. Toddlers and preschoolers may be too excited and full of energy to go to bed. Patterns of preparing for bedtime need to be reinforced. Reading stories, allowing children to sit in a parent's lap while listening to music, or listening to a prayer are routines that can be associated with preparing for bed. Quiet activities such as coloring and reading work well with school-age children.

Adults need to avoid excessive mental stimulation just before bedtime. Reading a light novel, watching a relaxing television program, or listening to music helps a person relax. Relaxation exercises can be useful at bedtime (see Chapter 43). Slow, deep breathing for 1 or 2 minutes induces calm. Rhythmic contraction and relaxation of muscles alleviates tension and prepares the body for rest (Hoch and Reynolds, 1986). Guided imagery and praying may also promote sleep.

At home a client should not try to finish office work or resolve family problems before bedtime. The bedroom should not be used as a place to work and should always be associated with sleep. Working toward a consistent time for sleep helps most clients gain a healthy sleep pattern and strengthens the rhythm of the sleep-wake cycle.

PROMOTING COMFORT

People fall asleep only after feeling comfortable and relaxed. The nurse can recommend and use several measures to promote comfort (see the box on p. 1147). Minor irritants can keep clients awake. Diapers should be changed before placing infants in bed. Soft cotton nightclothes keep infants or small children warm and comfortable. An extra blanket may be all that is needed to prevent a person from feeling chilled and being unable to fall asleep.

Compared with beds at home, hospital beds are often harder and of a different height, length, or width. Keeping beds clean and dry and in a comfortable position may help clients relax. Some clients suffer painful illnesses requiring special comfort measures such as application of dry or moist heat, use of supportive dressings or splints, and proper positioning before retiring (Fig. 42-6).

Providing for personal hygiene improves sense of comfort. A warm bath or shower before bedtime can be relaxing. Clients should void before retiring so they are not kept awake by a full bladder. Clients restricted to bed should be

---

Control of Noise in the Hospital

- Close doors to the client's room when possible.
- Keep doors to work areas on unit closed when in use.
- Reduce volume of nearby telephone and paging equipment.
- Wear rubber-soled shoes. Avoid clogs.
- Turn off bedside oxygen and other equipment that is not in use.
- Turn down alarms and beeps on bedside monitoring equipment.
- Turn off room TV and radio unless client prefers soft music.
- Avoid abrupt loud noise such as flushing a toilet or moving a bed.
- Keep necessary conversations at low levels, particularly at night.
- Conduct conversations and reports in a private area away from client rooms.

> ### Comfort Measures for Promoting Sleep
>
> - Administer hygiene measures for clients on bed rest.
> - Encourage clients to wear loose-fitting nightwear.
> - Remove or change any irritants against the client's skin such as moist dressings or drainage tubing.
> - Position and support dependent body parts to protect pressure points and aid muscle relaxation.
> - Provide caps and socks for older clients and those prone to cold.
> - Encourage client to void before going to sleep.
> - Administer analgesics or sedatives about 30 minutes before bedtime.
> - Offer a massage just before client goes to sleep.
> - Provide a comfortable mattress and keep bed clean and dry.

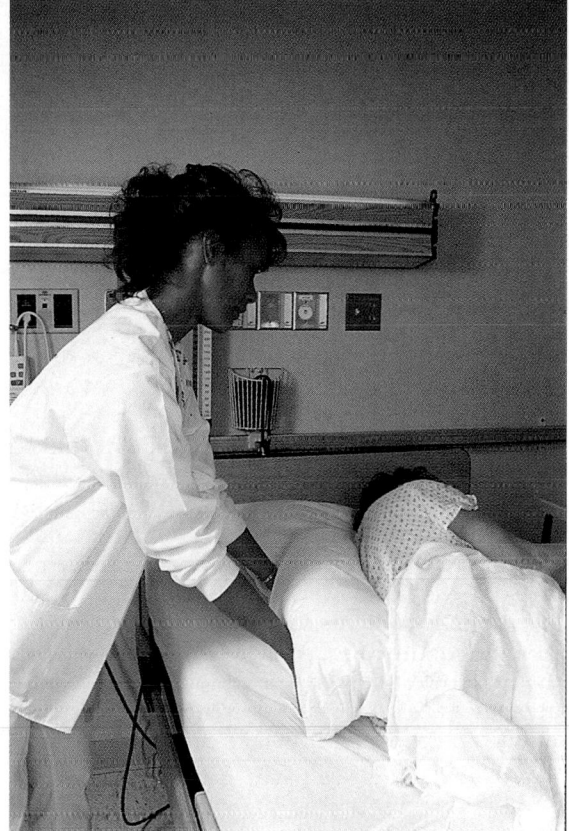

Fig. 42-6 Client position for sleep.

offered the opportunity to wash their face and hands. Toothbrushing and care of dentures also help to prepare the client for sleep.

ESTABLISHING PERIODS OF REST AND SLEEP

In the home it may help to encourage clients to stay physically active during the day so that they are more likely to sleep at night. Increasing daytime activity lessens problems with falling asleep. Rigorous exercise should always be planned at least several hours before bedtime.

While older adults get less deep nighttime sleep, some often take short naps during the day (Bliwise, 1993). This change in pattern associated with aging may not represent a decrease in need for sleep but a redistribution of sleeping behavior during a 24 hour period. Naps should be taken at the same time each day to maintain a consistent schedule.

In a hospital or extended-care setting it is difficult to provide clients with the time needed to rest and sleep. However, the nurse plans care to avoid awakening clients for nonessential tasks. The nurse can help by scheduling assessments, treatments, procedures, and routines for times when clients are awake. For example, if a client's physical condition has been stable, the nurse should avoid awakening the client to check vital signs. Blood should be drawn at a time when the client is awake. Unless maintaining a drug's therapeutic blood level is essential, medications should be given during waking hours. The nurse should work with the radiology department and other support services to schedule therapies at intervals that allow clients time for rest.

When the client's condition demands more frequent monitoring, the nurse can plan activities to allow extended rest periods. This means planning activities so that instead of a nurse returning to the room every few minutes, the client may have up to an hour or more to rest quietly. For example, if a client needs frequent dressing changes, is receiving intravenous therapy, and has drainage tubes from several sites, the nurse should not make a separate trip into the room to check each problem. Instead the nurse should use a single visit to change the dressing, regulate the intravenous system, and empty the drainage tubes. The nurse can become a client's advocate for promoting optimal sleep. This may mean becoming a gatekeeper by postponing or rescheduling visits by family, asking consultants to reschedule visits, or questioning the frequency of certain procedures.

CONTROLLING PHYSIOLOGICAL DISTURBANCES

For clients with physical illness, the nurse can help control symptoms that disrupt sleep. For example, a client with respiratory abnormalities should sleep with two pillows or in a semisitting position to ease the effort to breathe. The client may benefit from taking prescribed bronchodilators before sleep to prevent airway obstruction. A client with a hiatal hernia also needs special care. After meals the client may experience a burning sensation as a result of gastric reflux. To prevent sleep disturbances, the client should eat a small meal several hours before bedtime and sleep in a semisitting position. Clients with pain, nausea, or other recurrent symptoms should receive any symptom-relieving medication timed so that the drug takes effect at bedtime.

STRESS REDUCTION

Emotional stress can interfere with sleep. The inability to sleep can also make a person feel irritable and tense. When clients feel emotionally upset, they should be encouraged to try not to force sleep. Otherwise, insomnia frequently develops, and soon bedtime is associated with the inability to relax. A client who has difficulty falling asleep can be helped by getting up and pursuing a relaxing activity, such

CULTURAL ASPECTS OF CARE

Traditionally, experts recommend having infants and children sleep in their own beds. Cosleeping, in which children are allowed to sleep with parents or siblings, is a common practice among black, Hispanic, and Asian families. This approach lessens the child's anxiety and creates a strong sense of security.

as sewing or reading, rather than staying in bed and thinking about sleep.

In a health care setting a nurse on the night shift should take personal time to sit and talk with clients unable to sleep. This helps the nurse determine the factors keeping clients awake. Explaining procedures and the sources of noises or answering questions may give clients the peace of mind needed to fall asleep. Backrubs (see Chapter 40) can also be used to help clients relax more thoroughly. If a sedative is indicated, the nurse confers with the physician to be sure that the lowest dosage is used initially. Discontinuing a sedative as soon as possible prevents a dependence that can seriously disrupt the normal sleep cycle. Older adults can be vulnerable to the side effects of sedatives, hypnotics, or analgesics because the medications are metabolized slowly.

Children often have problems going to bed and falling asleep. Toddlers often become fearful due to separation from parents. Preschoolers commonly have difficulty falling asleep because of so much activity and stimulation during the day (Wong, 1995). Preschoolers also have bedtime fears (fear of the dark or strange noises), awaken during the night, or have nightmares. After nightmares, the nurse or parent should enter children's rooms immediately and talk to them briefly about fears to provide a cooling-down period. One approach is to comfort children and leave them in their own beds so that their fears are not used as excuses to delay bedtime. Keeping a light on in the room may also help. Cultural tradition may cause families to approach sleep practices differently (see the box above). The nurse should respect those that differ from traditional recommendations.

BEDTIME SNACKS

Some persons enjoy bedtime snacks, whereas others cannot sleep after eating. A dairy product snack such as warm milk or cocoa that contains *L*-tryptophan may be helpful in promoting sleep. A full meal before bedtime can often cause gastrointestinal upset and interfere with the ability to fall asleep.

Nurses should encourage clients to try to refrain from drinking or ingesting caffeine before bedtime. Coffee, tea, cola, and chocolate act as stimulants, causing a person to stay awake or awaken throughout the night. Alcohol can interrupt sleep cycles and reduce the amount of deep sleep. Coffee, tea, colas, and alcohol act as diuretics and may cause a person to awaken in the night to void.

Infants require special measures to minimize nighttime awakenings for feeding. It is common for children to have a need for middle-of-the-night bottle- or breast-feeding.

Wong (1995) recommends offering the last feeding as late as possible. Eventually it may help to gradually reduce the amount of formula or duration of breast-feeding. Infants should not be given bottles in bed.

PHARMACOLOGICAL APPROACHES TO PROMOTING SLEEP

The liberal use of drugs to manage symptoms is quite common in American culture. There are drugs commonly used that are associated with causing insomnia. Central nervous system stimulants such as amphetamines, nicotine, terbutaline, theophylline, and pemoline (Cylert), should be used sparingly and under medical management (McKenry and Salerno, 1995). In addition, withdrawal from CNS depressants such as alcohol, barbiturates, tricyclic antidepressants (amitriptyline, imipramine, and doxepin, and triazolam (Halcion), can cause insomnia and must be managed carefully.

Sleep medications can help a client if used correctly. However, long-term use of antianxiety, sedative, or hypnotic agents can disrupt sleep and lead to more serious problems. One group of drugs considered to be relatively safe are the benzodiazepines (Table 42-3). These medications do not cause general CNS depression like **sedatives** or **hypnotics** do. The benzodiazepines create relaxation, antianxiety, and hypnotic effects by facilitating the action of neurons in the CNS that suppress responsiveness to stimulation, therefore decreasing levels of arousal (Trevor and Way, 1995). Physicians prescribe this group of drugs because antianxiety effects occur at safe, nontoxic doses. The benzodiazepines are used cautiously with children under 12 years of age and contraindicated in infants under 6 months.

Pregnant clients should avoid benzodiazepines because their use is associated with risk of congenital anomalies. Nursing mothers should not receive the drugs because they are excreted in breast milk. Older adults are susceptible to side effects of any antianxiety or sedative agent because of physiological changes in metabolism. Short-acting benzodiazepines such as oxazepam, lorazepam, temazepam, alprazolam, and triazolam are usually recommended (Davison, 1994). Initial doses should be small, and increments are added gradually, based on client response, for a limited period of time. If older clients who were recently continent, ambulatory, and alert, become incontinent, confused, and/or demonstrate impaired mobility, the use of benzodiazepines should be considered as a possible cause.

The use of nonprescription sleeping medications is not advisable. Clients should learn the risks of such drugs, especially that, over the long term, these drugs can lead to further sleep disruption even when they initially seemed to be effective. The nurse can help clients use behavioral and proper sleep hygiene measures to establish sleep patterns that do not require the use of drugs.

Regular use of any sleep medication can lead to tolerance, and withdrawal can then cause rebound insomnia. Immediately administering a sleeping medication when a hospitalized client complains of being unable to sleep may be doing the client more harm than good. Alternative approaches must be considered. All clients should understand the possible side effects of sleep medications. Routine monitoring of client response to sleeping medications is important.

Table 42-3	Pharmacology of Antiinsomnia Agents			
GENERIC NAME	**TRADE NAME**	**ONSET OF ACTION (IN MINUTES)**	**ORAL DOSAGE* (MG)**	**INDICATIONS**
Alprazolam	Xanax	15-60	0.25-0.5 (3 times daily)	Anxiety
Diazepam	Valium	15-45	5-10 at bedtime	Sleep disorder
Flurazepam	Dalmane Apo-Flurazepam	15-45	15-30 at bedtime	Sleep disorder
Lorazepam	Ativan Apo-Lorazepam	15-60	1-4 at bedtime	Anxiety, sleep disorder
Oxazepam	Serax Zapex	45-90	10-30 (3-4 times daily)	Anxiety
Temazepam	Restoril	25-27	15-30 at bedtime	Sleep disorder
Triazolam	Halcion	15-30	.125-.25 at bedtime	Sleep disorder
Zolpidem	Ambien	15-45	10-20 at bedtime	Sleep disorder

* Smaller dosages may be prescribed for elderly clients.

HEALTH PROMOTION THROUGH CLIENT EDUCATION

To develop good sleep habits at home, clients and their bed partners should learn techniques that promote sleep and conditions that interfere with sleep (Zarcone, 1994) (see the box at right). Parents should also learn how to promote good sleep habits with their offspring.

Clients benefit most from instructions based on information about their homes and lifestyles. Similarly, they will more likely apply information that is useful and valued. For example, if the client lives near a busy airport, the use of another soft, monotonous noise may help block out the sounds of air traffic. A client who works a late afternoon shift should have time to relax once returning home and not feel pressured to go to sleep when other family members do. Any suggestions for relaxing bedtime activities should include activities that the client enjoys.

A client who takes sleep medications should know about their proper use as well as the risks and possible side effects. The hazards of habitual use of sleeping medications such as tolerance and drug-dependence insomnia need to be stressed so these side effects can be avoided. Nurses should caution clients against taking benzodiazepines with alcoholic beverages, opioid analgesics, or MAO and tricyclic antidepressants. CNS depression may result. The nurse also warns clients not to take more than the prescribed dose especially if the medication seems to become less effective after initial use.

Clients should also learn the effects of disease states on sleep. For example, a client with a hiatal hernia should learn to avoid eating large meals before bedtime. This prevents an irritating regurgitation of food into the esophagus that causes burning and keeps the person from being able to fall or stay asleep. Clients should learn about alternative measures for promoting sleep (e.g., relaxation and warm baths).

CLIENT TEACHING for Sleep Hygiene Habits

OBJECTIVE
- Client will follow proper sleep hygiene habits at home

TEACHING STRATEGIES
- Instruct client to try to exercise daily (e.g., walking, swimming, bicycling), preferably in morning or afternoon and to avoid vigorous exercise in the evening, within 2 hours of bedtime.
- Caution client against sleeping long hours during weekends or holidays to prevent disturbance of normal sleep-wake cycle.
- Explain that if possible, the bedroom should not be used for intensive studying, snacking, TV watching, or other nonsleep activity, besides sex.
- Explain that client should try to avoid worrisome thinking when going to bed and should use relaxation exercises.
- If client has trouble falling asleep, advise to get out of bed and do some quiet activity until feeling sleepy enough to go back to bed.
- Recommend client limit caffeine to morning coffee and limit alcohol intake (over 1 to 2 drinks a day can interrupt sleep cycle).
- Ask client to examine environment; keep room dark, well-ventilated, quiet, and at a comfortable temperature. Instruct that use of earplugs and eye shades is okay.
- Instruct client to avoid heavy meals for 3 hours before bedtime; a light snack may help.

EVALUATION
- Have client complete sleep-wake log for 1 week, and compare it with previous sleep-wake log.
- Ask client to periodically complete visual analog scale for perceptions of quality of sleep.

Sample Evaluation of Interventions for Sleep Disturbances

GOALS	EVALUATIVE MEASURES	EXPECTED OUTCOMES
Client will report that regular sleep pattern is reestablished within 1 month.	Observe client 30-60 minutes after bedtime (if in health care institution). Have client report on success in falling and staying asleep.	Client will fall asleep within 30 minutes of bedtime. Client will use relaxation therapies each night before going to sleep. Client will report feeling of restfulness after awakening each morning.
Client will experience less daytime sleepiness within 1 month.	Have client describe waking behaviors at work or home during the day. Observe waking nonverbal expressions and behaviors.	Client will describe fewer episodes of EDS within 2 weeks. Client will report being able to complete work-related responsibilities within 4 weeks.

Evaluation

Each client has a unique need for sleep and rest. For this reason the evaluation of therapies designed to promote sleep and rest must be individualized. Clients in relatively good health may not need as much sleep or require as many adjustments to their sleep patterns as clients whose physical conditions are poor.

The nurse determines whether expected outcomes have been met (see the evaluation box above). Evaluative measures may be used shortly after a therapy has been tried (e.g., observing whether a client falls asleep after reducing noise and darkening a room). Other evaluative measures may be used after a client awakens from sleep (e.g., asking a client to describe the number of awakenings during the previous night). The client and bed partner can usually provide accurate evaluative information. Over longer periods, the nurse may use assessment tools such as the visual analog scale to determine whether sleep has progressively improved or changed.

The nurse also assesses the level of understanding that clients or family members gain after receiving instruction on sleep habits. Compliance with these practices may best be measured during a home visit, when the environment can be observed.

When expected outcomes are not met, the nurse revises nursing measures based on the client's needs or preferences. Finding an effective therapy depends on the client's sleep disturbance, age, and normal sleep pattern. The nurse documents the client's response to sleep therapies so that a continuum of care can be maintained. The nurse is effective in promoting rest and sleep if the goals of care are met.

■ KEY CONCEPTS ■

▶ Rest is not inactivity but a feeling of physical calm and freedom from worry.

▶ Sleep is believed to provide physiological and psychological restoration.

▶ The 24-hour sleep-wake cycle is a circadian rhythm that influences physiological function and behavior.

▶ The control and regulation of sleep depends on a balance between central nervous system regulators.

▶ During a typical night's sleep a person passes through four to six complete sleep cycles. Each sleep cycle contains three NREM stages of sleep and a period of REM sleep.

▶ The number of hours of sleep needed by each person to feel rested is variable.

▶ Neonates, infants, children, and adolescents require more sleep than adults. Symptoms of various diseases may disrupt sleep.

▶ Long-term use of sleeping pills may lead to difficulty in initiating and maintaining sleep.

▶ The hectic pace of a person's lifestyle, emotional and psychological stress, and alcohol ingestion disrupt the sleep pattern.

▶ An environment with a darkened room, reduced noise, comfortable bed, and good ventilation promotes sleep.

▶ The most common type of sleep disorder is insomnia, which is characterized by the inability to fall asleep, remain asleep during the night, or go back to sleep after awakening earlier than is desired.

▶ If a client's sleep is adequate the nurse assesses the

client's usual bedtime, normal bedtime ritual, the preferred environment for sleeping, and usual, preferred rising time.

▶ Only a client can report whether sleep is restful.

▶ When a client has a sleep problem, the nurse conducts a complete sleep history.

▶ Diagnosing sleep problems depends on identifying factors that impair sleep.

▶ When using environmental controls to promote sleep, the nurse should consider the usual characteristics of the client's home environment and normal lifestyle.

▶ Noise can disrupt sleep and enhance pain perception.

▶ A bedtime routine of relaxing activities prepares a person physically and mentally for sleep.

▶ Pain or other symptom control is essential to promote the ability to sleep.

▶ One of the most important nursing interventions for promoting sleep is establishing periods for uninterrupted sleep and rest.

■ KEY TERMS ■

Biological clocks, p. 1130

Bulbar synchronizing region (BSR), p. 1130

Cataplexy, p. 1138

Circadian rhythm, p. 1130

Hypnotics, p. 1148

Infradian rhythm, p. 1130

Insomnia, p. 1138

Narcolepsy, p. 1138

Nocturia, p. 1135

NREM sleep, p. 1131

Polysomnogram, p. 1137

REM sleep, p. 1131

Reticular activating system (RAS), p. 1130

Sedatives, p. 1148

Sleep, p. 1129

Sleep apnea, p. 1138

Sleep deprivation, p. 1139

Ultradian rhythms, p. 1130

■ CRITICAL THINKING EXERCISES ■

1. Mrs. Wills visits the community health clinic for a routine visit. She is 78 years old. During a health history she tells you that she normally spends about 7 hours in bed at night. She complains of awakening as many as three times a night. She states that frequently it takes her a ½ hour or longer to fall asleep. Mrs. Wills is concerned. What would you as the nurse assess regarding her sleep-wake patterns? What counseling might be appropriate?

2. If a client has symptoms of insomnia, what type of sleep hygiene habits might you recommend?

3. When conducting an assessment of a client's sleep pattern, what information can be gathered from a bed partner?

What would be the differences when assessing the patterns of children versus adults?

4. Mr. John is a 55-year-old sheet-metal worker who works the evening shift. He typically drinks three to four beers before going to bed. He normally sleeps about 6 hours a night after he goes to bed around 1 AM. It is common for him to arise during the night to urinate. His favorite way to relax is watching television in bed. As the nurse, what would you assess regarding Mr. John's sleep history?

REFERENCES

Agnew HW et al: The first night effect: an EEG study of sleep, *Psychophysiology* 2:263, 1966.

Aldrich MS: Narcolepsy, *Neurology* 42(Suppl 6):34, 1992.

American Sleep Disorders Association: *The international classification of sleep disorders: diagnostic and coding manual*, Rochester, 1990, Allen Press.

Anch AM et al: *Sleep: a scientific perspective*, Englewood Cliffs, New Jersey, 1988, Prentice-Hall.

Berman TM et al: Sleep disorders: take them seriously, *Patient Care* 24:85, 1990.

Bliwise DL: Sleep in normal aging and dementia, *Sleep* 16(1):40, 1993.

Born J, Muth S, Fehm HL: The significance of sleep onset and slow wave sleep for nocturnal release of growth hormone (GH) and cortisol, *Psychoneuroendocrinology* 13:233, 1988.

Buysse DL: *Drugs affecting sleep, sleepiness and performance*. In Monk TH, editor: *Sleep, sleepiness and performance*, Pittsburgh, 1991, Wiley.

Carskadon MA: Patterns of sleep and sleepiness in adolescents, *Pediatrician* 17:5, 1990a.

Carskadon MA: *Sleep disturbances*. In Friedman SB, Fisher M, Schonberg SK, editors: *Comprehensive adolescent health care*, St Louis, 1990b, Mosby.

Carskadon MA: *Measuring daytime sleepiness*. In Kryger MH, Roth T, Dement WC, editors: *Principles and practice of sleep medicine*, ed 2, Philadelphia, 1994, Saunders.

Closs SJ: Assessment of sleep in hospital patients: a review of methods, *J Adv Nurs* 13:501, 1988.

Closs SJ: Post-operative patients' views of sleep, pain and recovery, *J Clin Nurs* 1(2):83, 1992.

Cohen FL, Merritt SL: *Sleep promotion*. In Bulechek GM, McCloskey JC, editors: *Nursing interventions: essential nursing interventions*, Philadelphia, 1992, Saunders.

Davison MA: *Sedative, hypnotic, and anxiolytic drugs*. In Kuhn MA, editor: *Pharmacotherapeutics: a nursing process approach*, ed 3, Philadelphia, 1994, FA Davis.

Douglas AB, Carskadon MA, Houser R: *Historical data base questionnaires, sleep and life cycle diaries*. In Laughton FM, Broughton RJ, editors: *Medical monitoring in the home and work environment*, New York, 1990, Raven Press.

Emra KL, Herrera CO: When your patient tells you he can't sleep, *RN* 52: 79, 1989.

Evans BD, Rogers AE: 24-Hour sleep/wake patterns in healthy elderly persons, *Appl Nurs Res*, 7(2):75, 1994.

Evans JC, French DG: Sleep and healing in intensive care settings, *Dimensions of critical care nursing* 14(4): 189, 1995.

Gillis AM, Flemons WW: *Cardiac arrhythmias during sleep*. In Kryger MH, Roth T, Dement WC, editors: *Principles and practice of sleep medicine*, ed 2, Philadelphia, 1994, Saunders.

Gislason R et al: Snoring, hypertension and the sleep apnea syndrome: an epidemiologic survey of middle-aged women, *Chest* 103(4):1147, 1993.

Gold DR et al: Rotating shift work, sleep, and accidents related to sleepiness in hospital nurses, *Amer J Pub Health* 82(7):1011, 1992.

Guilleminault C: *Clinical features and evaluation of obstructive sleep apnea*. In Kryger MH, Roth T, Dement WC, editors: *Principles and practice of sleep medicine*, ed 2, Philadelphia, 1994, Saunders.

Hauri P, Linde S: *No more sleepless nights*, New York, 1990, Wiley.

Hilton A: The hospital racket: how noisy is your unit? *Am J Nurs* 87:59, 1987.

Hoch C, Reynolds C III: Sleep disturbances and what to do about them, *Geriatr Nurs* 7:24, 1986.

Hodgson LA: Why do we need sleep: relating theory to nursing practice, *J Adv Nurs* 16:1503, 1991.

Hoppenbrouwers T: *Sleep in infants*. In Guilleminault C, editor: *Sleep and its disorders in children*, New York, 1987, Raven Press.

Horne JA: Human sleep and tissue restitution: some qualifications and doubts, *Clin Sci* 65:569, 1983.

Horne JA, Ostberg O: A self-assessment questionnaire to determine morningness-eveningness in human circadian rhythms, *Int J Chronobiology* 4:97, 1976.

Karni A et al: Dependence on REM sleep of overnight improvement of a perceptual skill, *Science* 265:679, 1994.

Kavey NB, Anderson D: Why every patient needs a good night's sleep, *RN* 49:16, 1986.

Kido LM: Sleep deprivation and intensive care unit psychosis, *Emphasis: Nursing* 4(1):23, 1992.

Kim MJ, McFarland GK, McLane AM: *Pocket guide to nursing diagnosis*, ed 6, St Louis, 1995, Mosby.

Landis CA: Arrhythmias and sleep pattern disturbances in cardiac patients, *Prog in Cardiovas Nurs* 3:73, 1988.

Leger D: The cost of sleep-related accidents: a report for the National Commission on Sleep Disorders Research, *Sleep* 17(1):84, 1994.

Leger D: The cost of sleepiness: a response to comments, *Sleep* 18(4):281, 1995.

Leigh TJ et al: Factor analysis of the St. Mary's Hospital Sleep Questionnaire, *Sleep* 11(5):448, 1988.

Long CA, Barron D: SIDS and infant positioning: implications for critical care, *Ped Nurs* 18(5):524, 1992.

McKenry LM, Salerno E: Mosby's pharmacology in nursing, ed 19, St Louis, 1995, Mosby.

McNeil BJ el al: Sleep questionnaire, *Am J Nurs* 86(1):261, 1986.

Mendleson WB: Neuroendocrinology and sleep. In *Human sleep: research and clinical care*, New York, 1987, Plenum Medical Book.

Mindell JA: Sleep disorders in children, *Health Psych* 12(2):151, 1993.

Mitler MM et al: Catastrophies, sleep and public policy: consensus report, *Sleep* 11:100, 1988.

Mitler MM et al: Narcolepsy, *J Clin Neurophysiol* 7(1):93, 1990.

National Commission on Sleep Disorders Research: *Wake up America: a national sleep alert*, vol 3, 1993.

Naylor MW, Aldrich MS: *Approach to the patient with disordered sleep*. In Kryger MH, Roth T, Dement WC, editors: *Principles and practice of sleep medicine*, ed 2, Philadelphia, 1994, Saunders.

Oswald I: *Good, poor, and disordered sleep*. In Priest RG, editor: *Sleep: an international monograph*, London, 1984, Update Books.

Pakola SJ, Dinges DF, Pack AI: Driving and sleepiness: review of regulations and guidelines for commercial and noncommercial drivers with sleep apnea and narcolepsy, *Sleep* 18(9):787, 1995.

Parkinson D: Strategies for helping parents: overcoming sleep problems in babies and toddlers, *Professional care of mother & child* 4:215, 1994.

Reynolds CF et al: REM sleep in successful, usual, and pathological aging: the Pittsburgh experience 1980-1993, *J Sleep Res* 2:203, 1993.

Richards KC, Barnsfather L: A description of night sleep patterns in the critical care unit, *Heart Lung* 18(1):35, 1988.

Robinson CR: Impaired sleep. In *Pathophysiological phenomena in nursing: human responses to illness*, ed 2, Philadelphia, 1993, Saunders.

Ross MS et al: When sleep won't come: helping our elderly clients, *Canad Nurs* 82:14, 1986.

Sheldon SH, Spire JP, Levy HB: *Pediatric sleep medicine*, Philadelphia, 1992, Saunders.

Sleep Research Society: *Brain mechanisms of sleep and wakefulness: basics of sleep behavior*, Rochester, Minn, 1993, UCLA & Sleep Research Society.

Thorpy M: Classification of sleep disorders. In Chokroverty S, editor: *Sleep disorders medicine: basic science, technical considerations and clinical aspects*, Boston, 1994, Butterworth-Heineman.

Trevor AJ, Way WL: *Sedative-Hypnotic drugs*. In BG Katzung, editor: *Basic & clinical pharmacology*, ed 6, Norwalk, Conn, 1995, Appleton & Lange.

Walsh JK, Hartman PG, Kowall JP: *Insomnia*. In Chokroverty S, editor: *Sleep disorders medicine: basic science, technical considerations and clinical aspects*, Boston, 1994, Butterworth-Heineman.

Webb WB: Technical comments: the cost of sleep-related accidents: a reanalysis, *Sleep* 18(4):276, 1995.

Webster RA, Thompson DR: Sleep in hospital, *J Adv Nurs* 11:447, 1986.

Williamson JW: The effects of ocean sounds on sleep after coronary artery bypass graft surgery, *Amer J Cri Care* 1(1):91, 1992.

Wong DL: *Whaley and Wong's nursing care of infants and children*, ed 5, St Louis, 1995, Mosby.

Wood AM: A review of literature relating to sleep in hospital with emphasis on the sleep of the ICU patient, *Inten Cri Care Nurs* 9:129, 1992.

Zarcone VP: *Sleep hygiene*. In Kryger MH, Roth T, Dement WC, editors: *Principles and practice of sleep medicine*, ed 2, Philadelphia, 1994, Saunders.

Zorick F: *Insomnia*. In Kryger MH, Roth T, Dement WC, editors: *Principles and practice of sleep medicine*, ed 2, Philadelphia, 1994, Saunders.

ADDITIONAL READINGS

Alward RR, Monk TH: *The nurse's shift work handbook*, Washington, DC, 1993, American Nurses Publishing.

American Nurses Association: *Integrating an understanding of sleep knowledge into your practice: parts 1-6*, New York, 1994-95, American Journal of Nursing.

Bootzin RR, Lahmeyer H, Lillie JK: *Integrated approach to sleep management: the healthcare practitioner's guide to the diagnosis and treatment of sleep disorders*, Belle Mead, NJ, 1994, Amer J of Medicine and Cahner Healthcare Communications.

Broughton RJ, Ogilvie RD, editors: *Sleep, arousal, and performance*, Boston, 1992, Birkhauser.

Chuman MA: The neurological basis of sleep, *Heart Lung* 12:177, 1983.

Foreman MD, Wykle M, NICHE Faculty: Nursing standard of practice protocol: sleep disturbances in elderly patients, *Geriatr Nurs* 16(2):1, 1995.

Fritz RF: *Sleep disorders: America's hidden nightmare*, Naperville, Ill, 1993, National Sleep Alert.

Monk TH, editor: *Sleep, sleepiness and performance*, New York, 1991, Wiley.

Spenceley SM: Sleep inquiry: a look with fresh eyes, *Image* 25(3):249, 1993.

## Chapter 43

Comfort

Mastery of content in this chapter will enable the student to:

- ▶ Define the key terms listed.
- ▶ Discuss common misconceptions about pain.
- ▶ Describe the physiology of pain.
- ▶ Identify components of the pain experience.
- ▶ Explain how the physiology of pain relates to selecting nursing therapies for pain relief.
- ▶ Describe the dimensions of pain assessment.
- ▶ Explain the different focus of pain assessment in acute care versus restorative care settings.
- ▶ Perform an assessment of a client experiencing pain.
- ▶ Explain how cultural factors influence the pain experience.

- ▶ Describe guidelines for selecting and individualizing pain therapies.
- ▶ Explain the difference in the pharmacological approach to treating acute versus chronic pain.
- ▶ Describe applications for use of nonpharmacological pain therapies.
- ▶ Discuss nursing implications for administering analgesics.
- ▶ Describe interventions for the relief of acute pain following operative or medical procedures.
- ▶ Describe the sequence of activities related to pain management in cancer clients.
- ▶ Evaluate a client's response to pain therapies.

Everyone has experienced some type or degree of **pain**. It is the most common reason people seek health care. Despite being one of the most common occurring symptoms in the medical world, pain is one of the least understood. A person in pain feels distress or suffering and seeks relief. The nurse uses a variety of interventions to bring relief or to restore comfort. However, the nurse cannot see or feel the client's pain. Pain is subjective; no two persons experience pain in the same way, and no two painful events create identical responses or feelings in a person. Pain is a source of frustration for clients and care givers alike. The International Association for the Study of Pain (IASP) defined pain as "an unpleasant, subjective sensory and emotional experience associated with actual or potential tissue damage, or described in terms of such damage" (IASP, 1979). Pain can be a major factor inhibiting the ability and willingness to recover from illness.

Nurses care for clients in many settings and situations in which interventions are provided to promote comfort. For example, the home health nurse cares for a terminal cancer client, the school nurse delivers first aid to an injured child, and a clinic nurse suggests therapies for chronic arthritic pain. Since the experience of pain is dynamic, the nurse has a responsibility to understand the pain experience. The nurse, client, family, and members of the health care team must collaborate to find the most effective approach to pain control. *Nurses are ethically responsible to manage pain and relieve suffering.* Effective pain management not only reduces physical discomfort but promotes earlier mobilization and return to work, fewer clinic visits, shortened hospital stays, and reduced health care costs.

■ COMFORT

Comfort is a concept central to the art of nursing. Donahue (1989) summarized "through comfort and comfort measures . . . nurses provide strength, hope, solace, support, encouragement, and assistance." A variety of nursing theorists refer to comfort as a basic client need for which nursing care is delivered.

The concept of comfort is as subjective as that of pain. Each individual brings physiological, social, spiritual, psychological, and cultural characteristics that influence how comfort is interpreted and experienced. Kolcaba (1992) defined comfort in a manner consistent with clients' subjective experiences. She defines comfort as the state of having met basic human needs for ease (contentment that promotes routine performance), relief (need being met), and transcendence (state in which one rises above problems or pain).

A holistic view of comfort helps to identify four contexts:
Physical—Pertaining to bodily sensations
Social—Pertaining to interpersonal, family, and societal relationships
Psychospiritual—Pertaining to internal awareness of self, including esteem, sexuality, and meaning in life
Environmental—Pertaining to the external background of human experience: light, noise, temperature, color, and natural elements

An appreciation of the context of comfort gives a nurse a larger range of choices when seeking pain-relief measures. This holistic view reinforces Mahon's (1994) concept that the pain experience must be understood as it is lived. It is important for the nurse to seek to understand the meaning of pain for the individual. Pain management is much more than administering analgesics. Given a more holistic view, nurses can develop better strategies in the successful management of pain.

■ NATURE OF PAIN

Pain is much more than a single sensation caused by a specific stimulus. Pain is subjective and highly individualized. The stimulus for pain can be physical and/or mental in nature, whereby damage may be to actual tissues or to a person's ego function (Mahon, 1994). According to McCaffery (1980): "Pain is whatever the experiencing person says it is, existing whenever he says it does." Mahon found four defining attributes for the pain experience: it is personal, unpleasant, a dominating force, and is endless in nature (1994). Pain is tiring and demands a person's energy. It can interfere with personal relationships and influence the meaning of life (Mahon, 1994). Pain cannot be objectively measured, such as with an x-ray or blood test. Although certain types of pain create predictable signs and symptoms, often the nurse can only assess pain by relying on the client's words and behavior. Only the client knows whether pain is present and what the experience is like. To help a client gain relief, the nurse must believe that the pain exists.

Pain is a protective physiological mechanism. When felt, pain changes how a person behaves. For example, a person with a sprained ankle avoids bearing full weight on the foot to prevent further injury. A client with a history of chest pain learns to stop all activity when pain develops. Pain is a warning of tissue damage, which should be the nurse's first consideration when assessing pain (Clancy and McVicar, 1992). Careful techniques must be used to assess for injury, such as in the case of a burned hand or a bruised chest wall. Clients who are unable to feel sensations, such as after spinal cord injury or stroke, are unaware of pain-inducing injuries. In these cases, the nurse must anticipate what sources of pain the client might have and learn to closely monitor physiological changes, such as in vital signs.

Pain is a leading cause of disability. As the average life span increases, more people have chronic disease in which pain is a common symptom. Medical advances have resulted in diagnostic and therapeutic measures that are often uncomfortable. Nurses care daily for clients in pain. One of the earliest fears of any client with a diagnosed illness is the concern over the pain that might be experienced.

Prejudices and Misconceptions

Health care personnel often hold prejudices against clients in pain. Unless clients have objective signs of pain, a nurse may not believe that they are uncomfortable. The attitudes many nurses have about pain are caused in part by the traditional medical model of illness. This model suggests that physical problems result from physical causes. Thus pain is viewed as a physical response to organic dysfunction. When no obvious source of pain can be found, nurses may stereotype pain sufferers as complainers or difficult clients.

Ryan et al. (1994) studied the attitudes of nurses toward management of cancer pain. Their study compared oncology nurses with nurses working in long-term care facilities, where a large number of cancer clients are eventually cared

> **Common Biases and Misconceptions about Pain**
>
> - Drug abusers and alcoholics overreact to discomforts.
> - Clients with minor illnesses have less pain than those with severe physical alterations.
> - Administering analgesics regularly will lead to drug dependence.
> - The amount of tissue damage in an injury can accurately indicate pain intensity.
> - Health care personnel are the best authorities on the nature of a client's pain.
> - Psychogenic pain is not real.
> - Chronic pain is psychological.
> - Clients should expect to have pain in a hospital.

for. Their study showed that oncology nurses, who specialize in the care of cancer clients, were no more liberal in their attitudes toward cancer-pain management than the long-term care nurses. However, both groups were rated as reasonably liberal in thinking. The most interesting finding was nurses' perceptions of barriers to optimal pain management. A significant number of nurses from both groups perceived a reluctance on the part of nurses to administer opioids, a reluctance on the part of clients to take opioids, and inadequate staff knowledge of pain management (Mahon, 1994).

The extent to which nurses make assumptions about clients in pain seriously limits their ability to offer pain relief. Unfortunately, all people are influenced by prejudices based on their culture, education, and experience. Too often, nurses allow misconceptions about pain (see the box above) to affect their willingness to intervene. Many nurses even avoid acknowledging a client's pain because of their own fear and denial.

To help a client gain comfort or relief, the nurse must view the experience through the client's eyes. Pain is tiring and demands energy from the person experiencing it (Mahon, 1994). It interferes with relationships and the individual's ability to maintain self-care. Acknowledging personal prejudices or misconceptions helps the nurse address the client's problem more professionally. The nurse who becomes an active, knowledgeable observer of a client in pain will make a more objective analysis of the pain experience. The client makes the diagnosis that pain is present, and the nurse works to apply techniques and skills that ultimately give relief.

PHYSIOLOGY OF PAIN

Pain is a complex mixture of physical, emotional, and behavioral reactions. To best understand the pain experience, it helps to describe its three physiological components: reception, perception, and reaction. A pain-producing stimulus sends an impulse across a peripheral nerve fiber. The pain fiber enters the spinal cord and travels one of several routes until ending within the gray matter of the spinal cord. There the pain message either interacts with inhibitory nerve cells, preventing the pain stimulus from reaching the brain, or it is transmitted uninhibited to the cerebral cortex. Once a pain stimulus reaches the cerebral cortex, the brain interprets the quality of pain and processes information about past experience, knowledge, and cultural associations in the perception of pain (McNair, 1990).

A client in pain cannot discriminate among the components. However, understanding each component helps the nurse recognize factors that can cause pain, symptoms that accompany pain, and the rationale and actions of select therapies.

Reception

All cellular damage caused by thermal, mechanical, chemical, or electrical stimuli results in the release of pain-producing substances. Exposure to hot or cold, pressure, friction, and chemicals release substances such as histamine, bradykinin, and potassium, which combine with receptor sites on **nociceptors** (receptors that respond to harmful stimuli) to initiate the neural transmission associated with pain (Clancy and McVicar, 1992). Table 43-1 summarizes the physical alterations that elicit pain-producing stimuli.

Not all tissues contain receptors that transmit pain signals. The brain and alveoli of the lung are examples of these tissues. Some receptors respond to only one type of pain stimulus, whereas others are also sensitive to temperature and pressure. When the combination with pain receptors reaches the threshold (minimum level of stimulus intensity required to evoke a nervous impulse), then activation of pain neurons occurs. Because of the variation in body shapes and sizes, the distribution of pain receptors in parts of the body varies. This explains anatomical subjectivity to pain (Clancy and McVicar, 1992). Certain body parts in different individuals are more or less sensitive to pain. In addition, individuals have different production capacities of pain-producing substances, which are controlled by the person's genes.

Nerve impulses resulting from the painful stimulus travel along afferent peripheral nerve fibers. Two types of peripheral nerve fibers conduct painful stimuli: the fast, myelinated A-delta fibers, and the very small, slow, unmyelinated C fibers. The A fibers send sharp, localized, and distinct sensations that localize the source of pain and detect pain intensity. They account for the immediate component on an acute injury (Jones and Cory, 1990). C fibers relay impulses that are poorly localized, visceral, and persistent (Puntillo, 1988). For example, after stepping on a nail, a person initially feels a sharp, localized pain, which is the result of A-fiber transmission. Within a few seconds pain becomes more diffuse and widespread until the whole foot aches because of C-fiber innervation. The C fibers remain exposed to the chemicals released when cells are damaged.

When A-delta and C fibers transmit impulses from peripheral nerve fibers, biochemical mediators that activate or sensitize the pain response are released. For example, potassium and **prostaglandins** are released when local cells are damaged. Transmission of the pain stimulus continues along the afferent nerve fibers until they end in the dorsal horn of the spinal cord. Within the dorsal horn, **neurotransmitters** such as substance P are released, causing a synaptic transmission from the afferent (sensory) peripheral nerve to spinothalamic tract nerves (Paice, 1991) (Fig.

Table 43-1	Examples of Physical Sources of Pain	
TYPE OF STIMULUS	**SOURCE**	**PATHOPHYSIOLOGICAL PROCESS**
Mechanical	Alteration in body fluids	Edema distending body tissues
	Duct distention	Overstretching of duct's narrow lumen (e.g., passage of kidney stone through ureter)
	Space-occupying lesion (tumor)	Irritation of peripheral nerves by growth of lesion within confined space
Chemical	Perforated visceral organ	Chemical irritation by secretions on sensitive nerve endings (e.g., ruptured appendix, duodenal ulcer)
Thermal	Burn (heat or extreme cold)	Inflammation or loss of superficial layers of epidermis, causing increased sensitivity of nerve endings
Electrical	Burn	Skin layers burned with muscle and subcutaneous tissue injury, causing injury to nerve endings

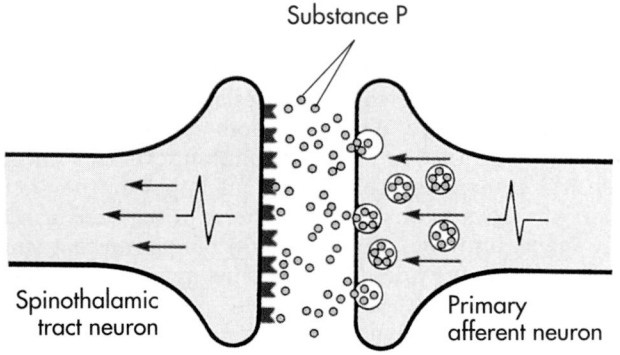

Fig. 43-1 Substance P and other neurotransmitters are released from primary afferent fibers that terminate in the dorsal horn of the spinal cord. *(From Paice JA:* Oncol Nurs Forum *18(5):843, 1991.)*

43-1). This allows the pain impulse to be transmitted further within the central nervous system. Pain stimuli travel through nerve fibers in the spinothalamic tracts that cross to the opposite side of the spinal cord. Pain impulses then travel up the spinal cord. Fig. 43-2 shows the normal pain reception pathway. After the pain impulse ascends the spinal cord, information is transmitted quickly to higher centers in the brain, including the reticular formation, limbic system, thalamus, and **sensory** and **association cortex**.

Along with transmission of pain stimuli, the body is able to adjust or vary pain reception. There are nerve fibers in the spinothalamic tract that end in the midbrain, stimulating regions to send stimuli back down to the dorsal horn of the spinal cord (Paice, 1991). These fibers are called the *descending pain system*, which acts by releasing neuroregulators that inhibit transmission of painful stimuli.

A protective reflex response also occurs with pain reception (Fig. 43-3). A-delta fibers send sensory impulses to the spinal cord, where they synapse with spinal motor neurons. The motor impulses travel via a reflex arc along efferent (motor) nerve fibers back to a peripheral muscle near

the site of stimulation. Contraction of the muscle leads to a protective withdrawal from the source of pain. For example, when a person accidentally touches a hot iron, a burning sensation is felt, but the hand also reflexively withdraws from the iron's surface. When superficial fibers in the skin are stimulated, a person moves away from the pain source. If internal tissues such as muscle or mucous membranes become stimulated, tightening and guarding of muscles occur.

Pain reception requires an intact peripheral nervous system and spinal cord. Common factors that can disrupt normal pain reception include trauma, drugs, tumor growth, and metabolic disorders.

NEUROREGULATORS

Neuroregulators, or substances that affect the transmission of nerve stimuli, play an important role in the pain experience. These substances are found at the site of a nociceptor, at nerve terminals within the dorsal horn of the spinal cord, and at receptor sites within the spinothalamic tract. Neuroregulators are divided into two groups: neurotransmitters and neuromodulators (see the box on p. 1158). Neurotransmitters such as substance P send electrical impulses across the synaptic cleft between two nerve fibers. They are excitatory or inhibitory. Neuromodulators modify neuron activity and adjust or vary the transmission of pain stimuli, without directly transferring a nerve signal through a synapse. They are believed to act indirectly by increasing and decreasing the effects of particular neurotransmitters. Endorphins are an example of a neuromodulator. Pharmacological therapy for pain is largely based on the influence select medications have on neuroregulators.

GATE CONTROL THEORY OF PAIN

Researchers know there is no specific pain center in the nervous system. Melzack and Wall's (1965) gate control theory suggests that pain impulses can be regulated or even blocked by gating mechanisms along the central nervous system. Gating mechanisms can be found in substantia gelatinosa cells within the dorsal horn of the spinal cord, thalamus, and limbic system (Clancy and McVicar, 1992).

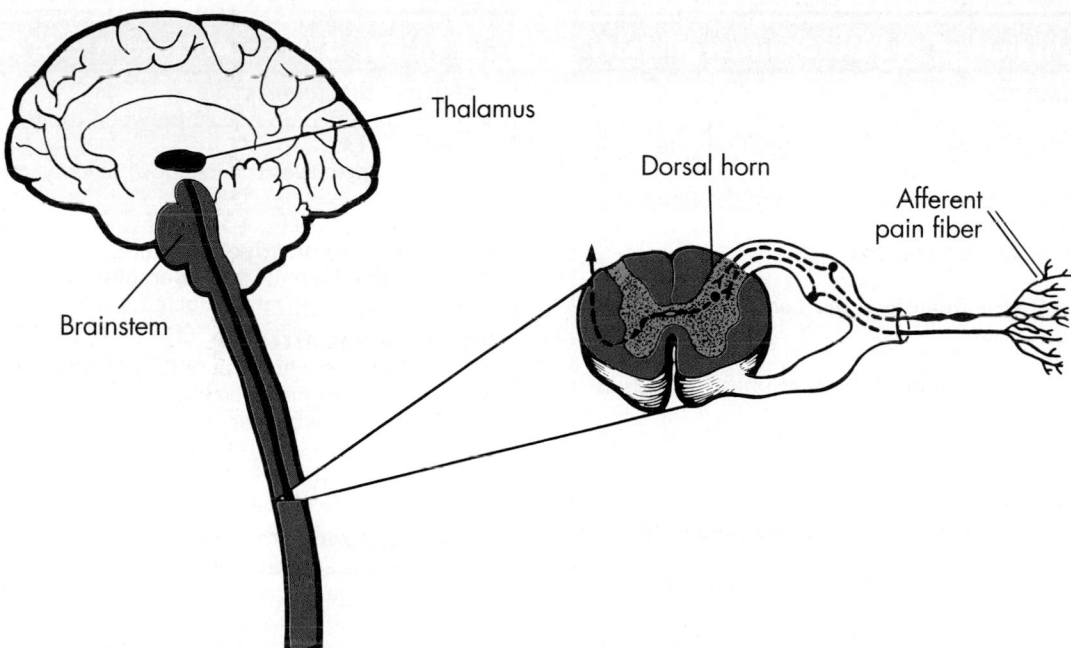

Fig. 43-2 Pain reception pathway. Pain is transmitted from primary afferent fibers to the dorsal horn of the spinal cord. The fibers synapse with spinothalamic tract neurons, which cross over and then ascend the spinal cord to the thalamus.

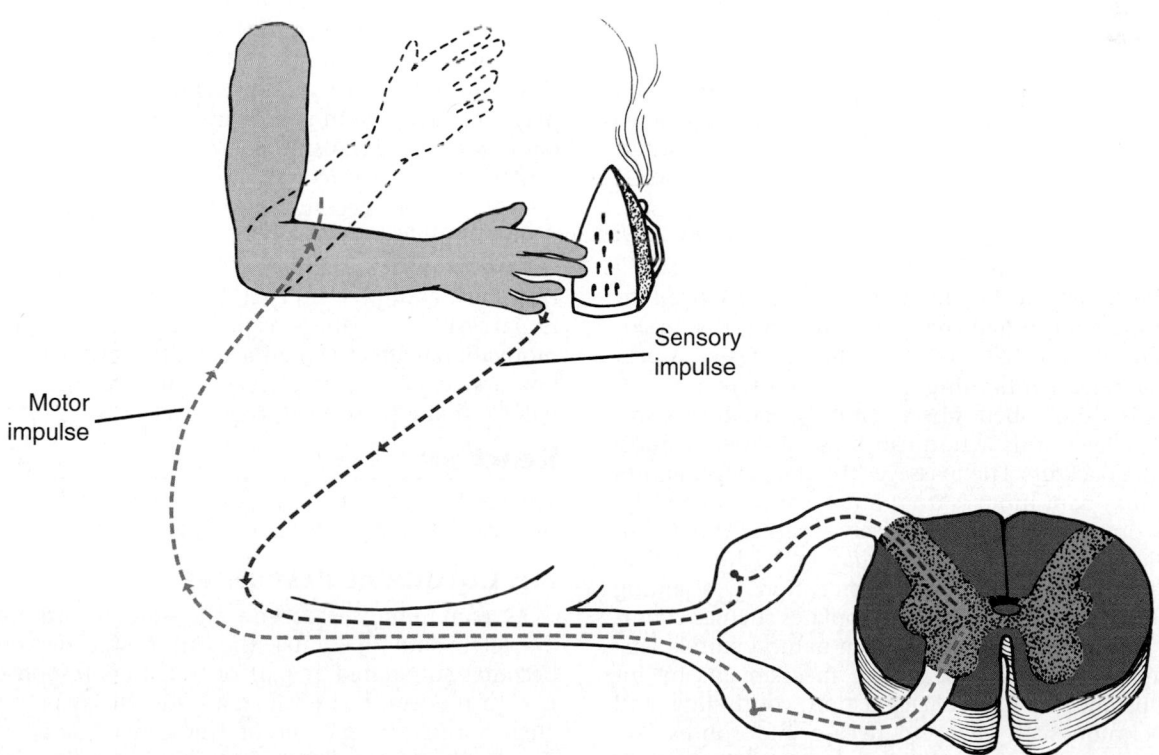

Fig. 43-3 Protective reflex to pain stimulus.

Neurophysiology of Pain: Neuroregulators

NEUROTRANSMITTERS

Substance P
- Is found in the pain neurons of the dorsal horn (excitatory peptide)
- Is needed to transmit pain impulses from the periphery to higher brain centers
- Causes vasodilation and edema

Serotonin
- Is released from the brainstem and dorsal horn to inhibit pain transmission

Prostaglandins
- Are generated from the breakdown of phospholipids in cell membranes
- Are believed to increase sensitivity to pain

NEUROMODULATORS

Endorphins and Dynorphins
- Are the body's natural supply of morphine-like substances
- Are activated by stress and pain
- Are located within the brain, spinal cord, and gastrointestinal tract
- Cause analgesia when they attach to opiate receptors in the brain
- Are present in higher levels in people who have less pain than others with a similar injury

Bradykinin
- Is released from plasma that leaks from surrounding blood vessels at the site of tissue injury
- Binds to receptors on peripheral nerves, increasing pain stimuli
- Binds to cells that cause the chain reaction producing prostaglandins

Possible Sources of Error in Pain Assessment

SENSORY-DISCRIMINATIVE
- Nerve transmission occurs between the thalamus and sensory cortex.
- A person perceives the location, severity, and character of pain.
- Factors that lower consciousness (e.g., analgesics, anesthetics, cerebral disease) decrease pain perception.
- Factors that increase the awareness of stimuli (e.g., anxiety, sleep deprivation) increase pain perception.

MOTIVATIONAL-AFFECTIVE
- Interaction between the reticular formation and limbic system results in pain perception.
- The reticular formation creates a defensive response, causing a person to interrupt or avoid pain stimuli.
- The limbic system controls emotional response and the ability to cope with pain.

COGNITIVE-EVALUATIVE
- Higher cortical centers in the brain influence perception.
- Culture, experience with pain, and emotions influence evaluation of the pain experience.
- This system helps a person to interpret the intensity and quality of pain so that action can be taken.

Perception

Perception is the point at which a person is aware of pain. Pain stimuli are transmitted up the spinal cord to the thalamus and midbrain. From the thalamus, fibers transmit the pain message to various areas of the brain, including the sensory cortex and association cortex (both in the parietal lobe), the frontal lobe, and the limbic system (Paice, 1991). There are cells within the limbic system believed to control emotion, particularly anxiety. Thus the limbic system may play an active role in processing the emotional reaction to pain. After nerve transmission ends within the higher brain centers, a person perceives the sensation of pain.

As a person becomes aware of pain, a complex reaction unfolds. Psychological and cognitive factors interact with neurophysiological ones in the perception of pain. Meinhart and McCaffery (1983) describe three interactional systems of pain perception as sensory-discriminative, motivational-affective, and cognitive-evaluative (see the box above). Perception gives awareness and meaning to pain so that a person can then react.

Reaction

The reaction to pain is the physiological and behavioral responses that occur after pain is perceived.

PHYSIOLOGICAL RESPONSES

As pain impulses ascend the spinal cord toward the brainstem and thalamus, the autonomic nervous system becomes stimulated as part of the stress response. Pain of low to moderate intensity and superficial pain elicit the "flight-or-fight" reaction of the general adaptation syndrome (see Chapter 22). Stimulation of the sympathetic branch of the autonomic nervous system results in physio-

By understanding what can influence these gates, nurses can gain a useful conceptual framework for pain management. The theory suggests that pain impulses pass through when a gate is open and impulses are blocked when a gate is closed. Closing the gate is the basis for pain-relief therapies.

A balance of activity from sensory neurons and descending control fibers from the brain regulate the gating process. The A-delta and C neurons release substance P to transmit impulses through the gating mechanisms. In addition, there are mechanoreceptor, thicker, faster A-beta neurons that release inhibiting neurotransmitters. If dominant input is from A-beta fibers, gating mechanisms will close. It is believed this action can be seen when a nurse gives a gentle backrub. The massage stimulates mechanoreceptors. If dominant input is from A-delta and C fibers, the gates likely open and the client perceives pain. Even if pain impulses flow to the brain, there may be higher cortical centers in the brain to modify pain perception. Descending neural pathways release endogenous opiates such as endorphins and dynorphins, the body's own natural pain killers. These neuromodulators close gating mechanisms by inhibiting substance P's release. Distraction, counseling, and placebo techniques are ways to release endorphins. Researchers do not know how persons can activate their endorphins.

Table 43-2	**Physiological Reactions to Pain**
RESPONSE	**CAUSE OR EFFECT**

SYMPATHETIC STIMULATION*	
Dilation of bronchial tubes and increased respiratory rate	Provides increased oxygen intake
Increased heart rate	Provides increased oxygen transport
Peripheral vasoconstriction (pallor, elevation in blood pressure)	Elevates blood pressure with shift of blood supply from periphery and viscera to skeletal muscles and brain
Increased blood glucose level	Provides additional energy
Diaphoresis	Controls body temperature during stress
Increased muscle tension	Prepares muscles for action
Dilation of pupils	Affords better vision
Decreased gastrointestinal motility	Frees energy for more immediate activity
PARASYMPATHETIC STIMULATION†	
Pallor	Causes blood supply to shift away from periphery
Muscle tension	Results from fatigue
Decreased heart rate and blood pressure	Results from vagal stimulation
Rapid, irregular breathing	Causes body defenses to fail under prolonged stress of pain
Nausea and vomiting	Causes return of gastrointestinal function
Weakness or exhaustion	Results from expenditure of physical energy

*Pain of low to moderate intensity and superficial pain.
†Severe or deep pain.

logical responses (Table 43-2). If the pain is continuous, severe, or deep, typically involving the visceral organs (such as with a myocardial infarction, colic from gallbladder or renal stones), the parasympathetic nervous system goes into action. Sustained physiological responses to pain could cause serious harm to an individual. Except in cases of severe traumatic pain, which may send a person into shock, most people reach a level of adaptation in which physical signs return to normal. Thus a client in pain will not always have physical signs.

BEHAVIORAL RESPONSES

Once pain is experienced, there begins a cycle of events that, if left untreated or unrelieved, can significantly alter the quality of a person's life. Mahon (1994) notes that pain can have a dominating nature, interfering with the ability to relate to and care for oneself. The component of pain reaction helps to explain why the management of pain can be such a challenge. Meinhart and McCaffery (1983) describe three phases of a pain experience: anticipation, sensation, and aftermath. The anticipation phase occurs before pain is perceived. A person knows pain will occur. The anticipation phase is perhaps most important, because it can affect the other two. In situations of traumatic injury or unforeseen painful procedures, a person will not anticipate pain.

Anticipation of pain allows a person to learn about pain and its relief. With adequate instruction and support, clients learn to understand pain and control anxiety before it occurs. Nurses play an important role in helping clients during the anticipatory phase. An example involves the nurse explaining the stinging sensation of a needle stick. Proper explanation helps clients reason and control their anxiety. In situations where clients are too fearful or anx-

ious, anticipation of pain can heighten the perception of pain severity.

Sensation of pain occurs when pain is felt. People react to pain in different ways. A person's **tolerance** of pain is the point at which there is an unwillingness to accept pain of greater severity or duration. Tolerance depends on attitudes, motivation, and values.

Pain threatens physical and psychological well-being. Clients may choose not to express pain if they believe such expression would inconvenience others or signal loss of self-control. The client with high pain tolerance is able to endure severe pain without assistance. Often a nurse must encourage such a client to accept pain-relieving measures so that activity or nutritional intake is not seriously curtailed. In contrast, a client with low pain tolerance may seek relief before pain occurs. For example, a client may request an aspirin in anticipation of a headache. The client's ability to tolerate pain significantly influences the nurse's perceptions of degree of the discomfort. Often the nurse is willing to attend to the client whose pain tolerance is high. Yet it is unfair to ignore the needs of the client who cannot tolerate even minor pain.

Typical body movements and facial expressions that indicate pain include clenching the teeth, holding the painful part, bent posture, and grimaces. A client may cry or moan, be restless, or make frequent requests of the nurse. The nurse soon learns to recognize patterns of behavior that reflect pain. However, lack of pain expression, as in the case of confused clients, does not necessarily mean that the client is not experiencing pain. Unless a client openly reacts to pain, it is difficult to determine the nature and extent of the discomfort. The nurse helps the client communicate the pain response effectively. Knowledge of the disease or illness helps the nurse to anticipate the

Table 43-3	Common Disorders and Pain Patterns
DISORDER	**PAIN PATTERN**
Kidney disease	Abdominal aching
Angina pectoris	Tenderness and pain in back area of costovertebral angle
	Crushing sensation in chest, often radiating down left shoulder and arm
Ruptured intravertebral disk	Low-back pain accompanied by pain radiating down leg
Gastric ulcer	Burning pain around umbilicus, referred pain in shoulder
Trigeminal neuralgia	Lightning-like or stabbing pain along distribution of trigeminal nerve, involving gums, lips, mouth, nose, and chin

client's pain. For example, a ruptured intravertebral disk in a lower lumbar vertebra typically causes severe low-back pain and pain that radiates or extends down the leg. Table 43-3 summarizes common disorders and the accompanying pattern of pain.

The aftermath phase of pain occurs when it is reduced or stopped. Even though the source of pain is controlled, a client may still require the nurse's attention. Pain is a crisis. After a painful experience clients may experience physical symptoms such as chills, nausea, vomiting, anger, or depression. If there are repeated episodes of pain, aftermath responses can become serious health problems. The nurse helps clients gain control and self-esteem to minimize fear of potential pain experiences.

■ ACUTE AND CHRONIC PAIN

Everyone experiences some level of pain throughout the day. Common examples include the ache of overexercised muscles, the burning discomfort from eye strain, and pressure from sitting in one position for too long. These minor discomforts rarely cause a person to seek health care.

The pain that nurses most often observe in clients includes three types: acute, chronic malignant, and chronic nonmalignant (National Institutes of Health [NIH], 1986). Acute pain follows acute injury, disease, or surgical intervention and has a rapid onset, varying in intensity (mild to severe) and lasting for a brief time (Meinhart and McCaffery, 1983; NIH, 1986). The function of acute pain is to warn persons of impending injury or disease. It eventually resolves with or without treatment after a damaged area heals.

Clients in acute pain are frightened and anxious, and they expect relief quickly. The time sequence of acute pain usually results in a willingness by health team members to treat acute pain aggressively. However, conflict between nurse and client may arise if the nurse does not provide quick relief. Acute pain is self-limiting and the client therefore knows an end is in sight.

Acute pain seriously threatens a client's recovery and should be one of the nurse's priorities of care. For example, acute postoperative pain hampers the client's ability to become active and increases the risk of complications from immobility (see Chapter 37). Rehabilitation may be delayed and hospitalization may be prolonged if acute pain is not controlled. There cannot be physical or psychological progress as long as it persists, because the client focuses all interests on pain relief. The nurse's efforts at teaching and motivating the client toward self-care will often be useless. After pain is relieved, the client and health care team can direct full attention toward recovery.

Chronic pain is prolonged, varies in intensity, and usually lasts more than 6 months (McCaffery, 1986). Chronic pain caused by uncontrolled cancer or its treatment, or other progressive disorders, is called **intractable pain** (malignant pain). It can last until death.

Chronic nonmalignant pain, such as low-back pain, results from nonprogressive or healed tissue injury. However, the pain is ongoing and often does not respond to treatment. Frequently the cause for nonmalignant pain is unknown. An injured area may have healed long ago, yet pain persists. In chronic pain, endorphins often cease to function (Meinhart and McCaffery, 1983).

Health care workers are usually less willing to treat chronic pain as aggressively as acute pain. However, the Agency for Health Care Policy and Research (AHCPR) reports that up to 90% of the 8 million Americans who have cancer can have their pain managed with relatively simple means (Jacox et al, 1994). Too often these clients are undertreated. Marzinski (1991) has described studies where nurses reported that if they assessed euphoria in clients receiving narcotics for chronic pain, they would decrease the amount of pain medication given. **Euphoria** is an expected and temporary side effect of proper analgesic control. If the cause of pain is unclear, care givers too often question the severity of a client's discomfort. For cancer sufferers, clients may be unwilling to take pain medications, and family members may be unwilling to give needed narcotics, for fear of causing side effects such as lethargy and drug dependence.

The client with chronic pain often has periods of **remissions** (partial or complete disappearance of symptoms) and **exacerbations** (increase in severity). The unpredictability of chronic pain frustrates the client, frequently leading to psychological depression. Flor et al. (1993) report that chronic pain clients had more pain-related negative self-statements and convictions of helplessness than did healthy clients. The pain becomes part of every aspect of life. Chronic pain is a major cause of psychological and physical disability, leading to problems such as loss of job, inability to perform simple daily activities, sexual dysfunction, and social isolation from family and friends.

The person with chronic pain often does not show overt symptoms and does not adapt to the pain, but seems to suffer more with time because of physical and mental exhaustion. Chronic pain creates an insecurity of never knowing how one will feel from day to day. Symptoms of chronic pain include fatigue, insomnia, anorexia, weight loss, depression, hopelessness, and anger.

The life of a person with chronic pain can be tragic. Often the person consults many physicians and therefore accumulates various medications and therapies. However, taking several medications may result in undesirable side effects. Clients desperate for pain relief may fall prey to quackery (e.g., special liniments, diets, or pain-relief devices). Alcohol abuse may become another alternative. Fortunately, pain clinics are available throughout the United States and Canada to help clients find more acceptable methods of pain control. Physicians and other health care providers in these clinics understand pain better and offer therapies other than pharmacological remedies, such as exercise and biofeedback.

Caring for the client with chronic pain is an unusual challenge. The nurse should not become frustrated when relief measures fail. Likewise, the nurse should not offer false hope for a cure. The nurse must minimize or reduce the client's perception of pain.

FACTORS INFLUENCING PAIN

Because pain is complex, numerous factors influence an individual's pain experience (Fig. 43-4). The nurse considers all factors that affect the client in pain. This is necessary to ensure a holistic approach to the assessment and care of the client in pain.

Age

Age is an important variable that influences pain, particularly in children and older adults. Developmental differences found among these age groups can influence how children and older adults react to pain. Young children have difficulty understanding pain and the procedures nurses administer that may cause pain. Young children who have not developed full vocabularies also have difficulty verbally describing and expressing pain to parents or care givers. Cognitively, toddlers or preschoolers are unable to recall explanations about pain or associate pain as experiences that can occur in various situations. With these developmental considerations in mind, the nurse must adapt

approaches for how to assess a child's pain (including what to ask and the behaviors to observe for) and how to prepare a child for a painful medical procedure.

Pain is not an inevitable part of aging. The presence of pain in an older adult requires aggressive assessment, diagnosis, and management. However, the aged are at high risk for pain-inducing situations (Ebersole and Hess, 1994). Because an older adult has lived longer, there is a greater likelihood of having developed a pathological condition that may be accompanied by pain. Once an older client suffers pain, there can be serious impairment of functional status. Mobility, self-care activities, socialization outside the home, and activity tolerance can all be reduced.

The ability of older clients to interpret pain can be complicated by the presence of multiple diseases with vague symptoms that may affect similar parts of the body. When older clients have more than one source of pain, a nurse must gather detailed assessments. The manifestations of different diseases can cause an atypical presentation of painful conditions. In other words, different diseases can cause similar symptoms. For example, chest pain does not always indicate a heart attack; it may be a symptom of arthritis of the spine or of an abdominal disorder. Older adults also often have different presentations of common illnesses, including "painless" intraabdominal emergencies (Bender, 1989). Not all older adults experience cognitive impairment. However, when an older adult experiences confusion, recalling pain experiences and providing detailed explanations is difficult.

Herr and Mobily (1991) note that older clients may not report pain for the following reasons:

1. Older clients may believe that pain is something they must accept. Because care givers and children believe

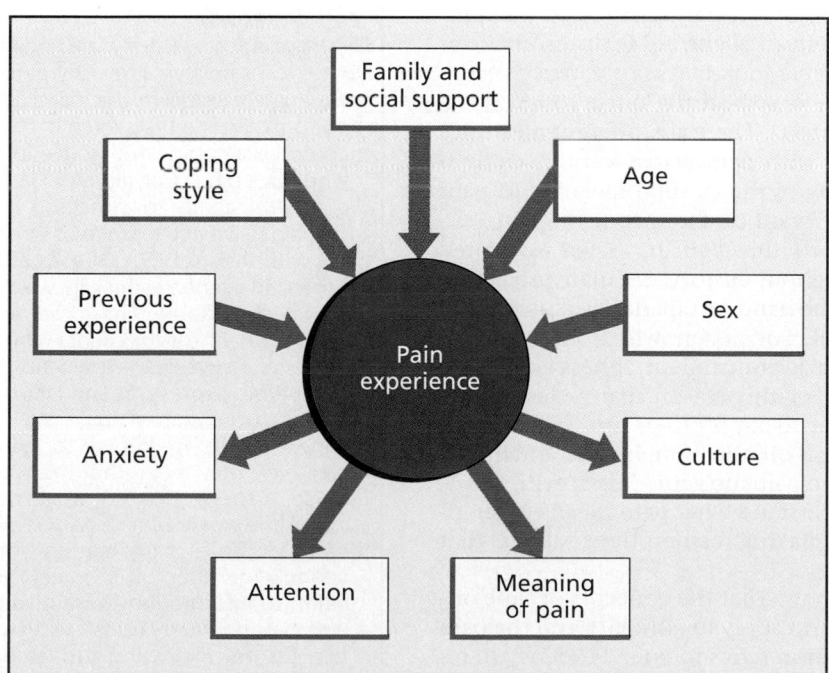

Fig. 43-4 Factors that influence the pain experience. *(From Gil K: Anesthesiol Report 2(2):246, 1990.)*

that pain is a natural result of aging, complaints are often ignored. This angers older clients, who in turn decide not to report pain.

2. Older clients may deny pain because of the fear of unknown consequences. They have considerable fear of the loss of independence. Admitting to pain can also lead to unpleasant and expensive diagnostic and therapeutic measures.

3. Older clients may choose not to admit having pain for fear of serious illness or death.

4. Older clients use different terminology to describe the pain experience. Terms such as *discomfort, ache,* or *hurt* are used instead to deny that pain exists.

5. Many older clients believe that it is not acceptable to show a response to pain. Often older clients use a variety of ways to distract attention from pain (McCaffery and Beebe, 1989).

Gender

Generally, men and women do not differ significantly in their responses to pain (Gil, 1990). It is doubtful whether gender alone is a factor in the expression of pain. There are cultural influences on gender (e.g., deeming it appropriate for a little boy to be brave and not cry, whereas a little girl in the same situation is allowed to cry). Pain tolerance has been the subject of research involving men and women. However, tolerance to pain is influenced by biochemical factors and is unique to each individual, regardless of sex.

Culture

Cultural beliefs and values affect how individuals deal with pain. Individuals learn what is expected and accepted by their culture; this includes how to react to pain (Calvillo and Flaskerud, 1991). Health care providers often assume that their ways and beliefs are equal to others. Thus they try to presume how clients will respond to pain. For example, if a nurse believes that crying and moaning indicate an inability to tolerate pain, resultant therapy may be inappropriate for a Mexican-American client. A Mexican-American who cries out in pain does not necessarily perceive the pain experience as severe or expect the nurse to intervene (Calvillo and Flaskerud, 1991). There are different meanings and attitudes associated with pain across various cultural groups. An understanding of the cultural meaning of pain helps the nurse design relevant care for people in pain.

Martinelli (1987) reports that pain has been associated with punishment throughout history. In many societies, pain, such as the slap of the hand or a spanking, is associated with obedience and guilt. For people who consciously or subconsciously view pain as punishment, illness is a way to atone for their wrongs. For this reason many clients may view chronic pain as a way to pay for their sins. In American society today, the emphasis on nutrition, health, and fitness leads people to believe "no pain, no gain" (Martinelli, 1987). Clearly a nurse must understand what pain means to an individual client before making assumptions about that client's behavior.

A review of research shows that the concepts of time orientation and expressiveness apply to ethnicity and the pain experience. Time orientation refers to one's tendency to focus on either the past, present, or future. Hispanics generally give preference to the present. They neither plan for the future nor hope that it will be better than the present or past (Martinelli, 1987). The Chinese have historically given preference to the past. Their attitude has been that nothing new happens in the present or will happen in the future—it had already happened in the past. Americans with Anglo-Saxon heritage place an emphasis on the future and are not content with the present. A client's time orientation will affect the pain experience. The person who is future oriented is more likely to be concerned with how the pain might affect future health, earning capabilities, or relationships. The pain itself may be secondary. In contrast, a present-oriented person would be concerned with the immediacy and actual sensation of pain, therefore becoming preoccupied with pain relief. A past-oriented person might accept pain as a part of life, a natural occurrence, and therefore something to tolerate (Martinelli, 1987)

How people express pain is another cultural trait (Martinelli, 1987). Some cultures believe it is natural to be demonstrative about pain. Others tend to exercise more introvertive behavior. Clancy and McVicar (1992) suggest that cultural socialization determines one's psychological behavior. This in turn may affect the physiological output of endogenous opiates and thus pain perception.

It is also important to know to what extent a member of a particular culture has assimilated into American society. For example, if several generations of a Hispanic's family have lived in the United States, the influence of the Spanish culture may be limited. In contrast, a client who has just recently come to the United States and who embraces the cultural norms of his ethnic group may have very different attitudes than an Anglo-Saxon American. Calvillo and Flaskerud (1991) report that Mexican women with a

---

 CULTURAL ASPECTS OF CARE

PAIN RESPONSE

First-generation, elderly, and newly arrived Mexican-Americans believe a healthy person is one who functions adequately and is free of pain. This means being able to perform routine tasks even in the presence of pain. Self-control is a common practice for Mexican-Americans who have pain (Calvillo and Flaskerud, 1991). This includes the ability to withstand stress in times of adversity, a passive acceptance of one's fate, or an active coping with the problem. Nurses often find that Mexican-American clients, especially women, moan when they are uncomfortable. These clients can be mistaken for "complainers" or for clients who cannot tolerate pain; however, in Mexican-American culture crying out is an acceptable expression and is not synonymous with an inability to tolerate pain.

Chinese clients are known to tell their family and physician how they feel rather than report pain to their nurse. A strong bond of trust must form between the client and nurse before pain is discussed freely (Walker et al, 1995). First-generation Chinese often delegate to a family member, often male, the gatekeeper role in relation to information to be given between the client and care providers. This can frustrate the nurse, who benefits from knowing subtle changes in a client's condition as soon as possible.

more intense adherence to the Mexican culture believe in the traditional folk beliefs of that culture (see the box on p. 1162).

Meaning of Pain

The meaning that a person associates with pain affects the experience of pain and how one adapts to it. This can be closely associated with the person's cultural background. A person will perceive pain differently if it suggests a threat, loss, punishment, or challenge. For example, a woman in labor will perceive pain differently from a woman experiencing pain from an injury inflicted by a spouse. The degree and quality of pain perceived by a client are related to the meaning of pain.

Attention

The degree to which a client focuses attention on pain can influence pain perception. Increased attention has been associated with increased pain, whereas distraction has been associated with a diminished pain response (Gil, 1990). This concept is one that nurses apply in various pain-relief therapies such as relaxation, guided imagery, and massage. By focusing a client's attention and concentration on other stimuli, the nurse places pain on the periphery of awareness. Usually, this results in an increased tolerance for pain that lasts only during the time of distraction.

Anxiety

The relationship between pain and anxiety is complex. Anxiety often increases the perception of pain, but pain may also cause feelings of anxiety. Autonomic arousal patterns are similar in pain and anxiety (Gil, 1990). It is difficult to separate the two sensations. Paice (1991) reported evidence that painful stimuli activate the portion of the limbic system believed to control emotion, particularly anxiety. The limbic system may process the emotional reaction to pain, aggravating or relieving it.

Emotionally healthy persons are usually able to tolerate moderate or even severe pain better than those whose emotions are less stable. Critically ill or injured clients who often perceive a lack of control over their environment and care may have high anxiety levels. This anxiety, if it has gone unnoticed in the high-tech environment of an intensive care unit (ICU), can lead to serious pain management problems. Unrelieved pain in these clients often causes psychosis and personality disorders.

Fatigue

Fatigue heightens the perception of pain. The sense of exhaustion intensifies pain and decreases coping abilities. This can be a common problem with any person experiencing a long-term illness. If fatigue occurs along with sleeplessness, the perception of pain may be even greater. Pain is often experienced less after a restful sleep than at the end of a long day.

Previous Experience

Each person learns from painful experiences. Previous experience does not necessarily mean that a person will accept pain more easily in the future. If a person has had frequent episodes of pain without relief or has had bouts of severe pain, anxiety or even fear may recur. In contrast, if a person has had repeated experiences with the same type of pain but the pain has been successfully relieved, it becomes easier to interpret the pain sensation. As a result, the client is better prepared to take necessary actions to relieve the pain.

When a client has had no experience with pain, the first perception of it can impair the ability to cope. For example, after abdominal surgery, it is common for a client to experience severe incisional pain for several days. Unless the client is aware of this, the onset of pain may be viewed as a serious complication. Rather than participate actively in postoperative breathing exercises (see Chapter 48), the client may lie immobile in bed and maintain shallow breathing because of fear that something has gone wrong. The nurse should prepare the client with a clear explanation of the type of pain that will be experienced and methods to reduce it.

Coping Style

The experience of pain can be lonely. When clients experience pain in health care settings such as hospitals, the loneliness can be unbearable. Frequently, clients feel a loss of control of the environment or the outcome of events. Coping style thus influences the ability to deal with pain.

Persons with internal loci of control perceive themselves as having personal control over their environments and the outcome of events, such as pain (Gil, 1990). In contrast, persons with external loci of control perceive other factors in their environments, such as nurses, as being responsible for the outcome of events. Individuals with an internal loci of control report less severe pain than those with external loci (Schultheis et al, 1987). This concept is applied in the use of patient-controlled analgesia (PCA). Clients who are able to self-administer small doses of intravenous pain medication during an acute episode successfully achieve pain control more quickly than those who rely on nurses to administer intermittent doses of pain medications.

Pain may cause partial or total disability. Clients often find various ways to cope with the physical and psychological effects of pain. It is important to understand a client's coping resources during a painful experience. These resources, such as communicating with a supportive family, exercise, or singing, can be used in the nurse's care plan to support the client and offer a degree of pain relief.

Family and Social Support

Another factor that can significantly affect pain response is the presence and attitudes of significant others. Persons of different sociocultural groups have different expectations of people to whom they complain about pain (Meinhart and McCaffery, 1983). People in pain often depend on family members or close friends for support, assistance, or protection. Although pain still exists, the presence of a loved one can minimize loneliness and fear. An absence of family or friends can often make the pain experience more stressful. The presence of parents is especially important for children experiencing pain.

■ NURSING PROCESS AND PAIN

Nurses need to approach pain management systematically to understand a client's pain and to provide appropriate therapy. The reporting of pain is a social transaction between nurse and client (AHCPR, 1992). Successful management of pain depends on establishing a positive relationship between the health care provider, client, and family. Clients can then become more active participants in their care. Pain management extends beyond pain relief, encompassing the client's quality of life and ability to work productively, to enjoy recreation, and to function normally in the family and society (Jacox et al, 1994).

Assessment

Accurate and factual pain assessment is needed to establish a baseline, to arrive at proper nursing diagnoses, to select the right therapies, and to evaluate the client's response to treatment. Although pain assessment is one of the most common activities a nurse performs, it is one of the most difficult. The nurse must explore the pain experience through the eyes of the client. Nurses cannot allow personal biases to prejudice their assessment of pain. It is important also to carefully interpret pain cues and to remember that psychological and physical components of pain influence the reaction to it. Benefits of assessment for clients include the facts that pain is identified, recognized as real, quantified and described, and used to evaluate care (McGuire, 1992). Appropriate assessment of pain allows care givers to be more knowledgeable of pain status, more responsible and accountable for care, and more collegial in managing pain.

AHCPR has established specific guidelines for assessing clients who are to have surgery or invasive procedures or who have experienced trauma. The focus is planning successful pain management therapies before pain is experienced. Because it involves a collaborative approach, the AHCPR pain treatment flow chart (Fig. 43-5) offers a useful conceptual approach to the control of acute pain. Clients must understand that informed reporting of pain is valuable and necessary if the health care team is to manage pain effectively.

When assessing pain, the nurse must be sensitive to the client's level of discomfort. If pain is acute or severe, it is unlikely that the client can provide a detailed description of the entire experience. During an episode of acute pain, the nurse primarily assesses how the client feels, determining physiological responses to pain and its location, severity, and quality. A more thorough pain assessment takes time and should be conducted when the client becomes more alert and attentive. It may help to reduce a client's anxiety before trying to quantify the client's perception of pain.

For clients with chronic pain, assessment may best be focused on affective, cognitive, and behavioral dimensions of the pain experience and on its history and context (NIH, 1986; McGuire, 1992). In the case of chronic nonmalignant pain, assessment should include level of function, because it may not be possible to achieve complete pain relief. The AHCPR recommends that families of cancer clients learn how to assess pain to promote continuity of effective pain management (Jacox et al, 1994). In the home care setting, family members are the assessors of pain. This collaborative approach empowers the client and family to exercise some control over the pain experience (see the box on p. 1165).

The nurse should be aware of possible errors in pain as-

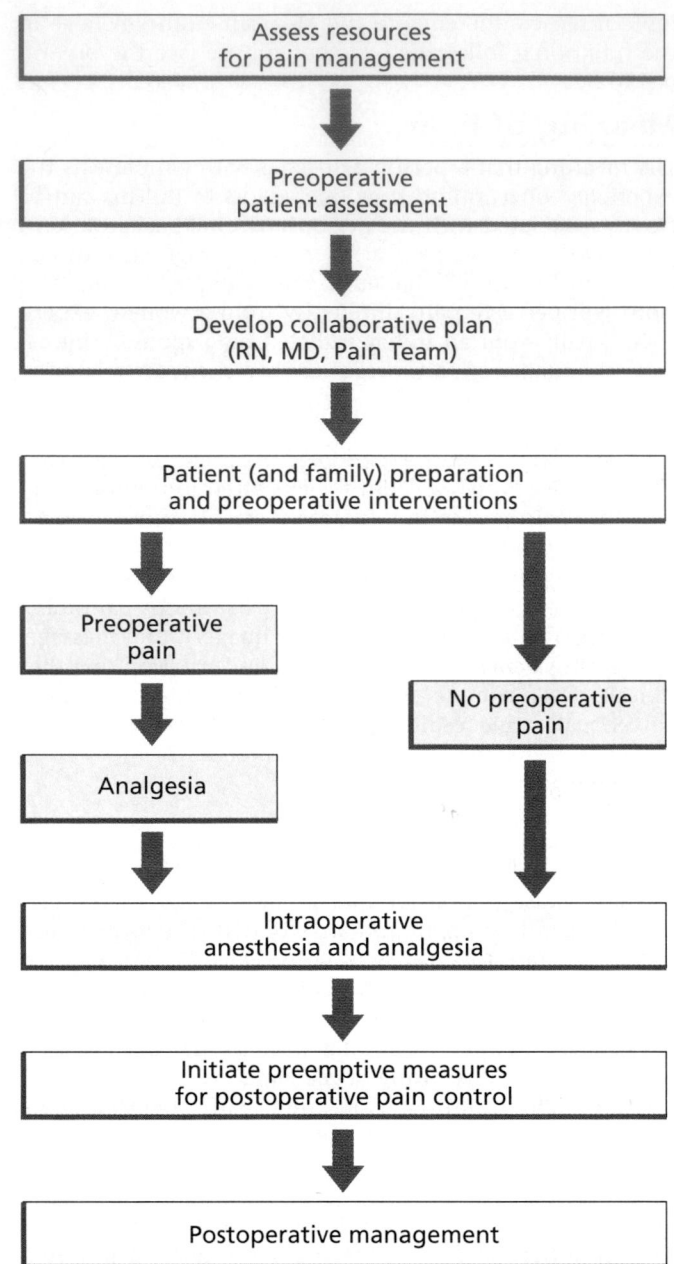

Fig. 43-5 Pain treatment flow chart: preoperative and intraoperative phases. *(From Acute Pain Management Guideline Panel: Acute pain management: operative or medical procedures and trauma. Clinical practice guideline, AHCPR Publication No 92-0032, Rockville, MD, 1992, Agency for Health Care Policy and Research, PHS, USDHHS.)*

sessment (see the box on p. 1165). Using the right tools and methods can help to avoid errors and to ensure that the right pain therapies are chosen (Harrison, 1991).

CLIENT'S EXPRESSION OF PAIN

Many clients fail to report or discuss discomfort. To complicate pain assessment, many nurses believe that clients will report pain if they have it. This is not always true. Clients must first perceive a need to report pain and then trust the nurse and perceive the nurse's willingness to help before discussing pain openly. If clients sense that the nurse

	Routine Clinical Approach to Pain Assessment and Management "ABCDE"
A	*Ask* about pain regularly.
	Assess pain systematically.
B	*Believe* the client and family in their report of pain and what relieves it.
C	*Choose* pain control options appropriate for the client, family, and setting.
D	*Deliver* interventions in a timely, logical, and coordinated fashion.
E	*Empower* clients and their families.
	Enable them to control their course to the greatest extent possible.

From Jacox A, Carr DB, Payne R, et al: *Management of cancer pain*, Clinical Practice Guideline No. 9, AHCPR Publication No. 94-0592, Rockville, Md, 1994, Agency for Health Care Policy and Research, US Department of Health and Human Services, PHS.

Possible Sources for Error in Pain Assessment

- Bias, which causes nurses to consistently overestimate or underestimate the pain that clients experience
- Vague or unclear assessment questions, which lead to unreliable assessment data
- Use of pain assessment tools that have not been proved reliable and valid with identical clients (a reliable assessment tool focuses only on pain cues that provide a reliable measure of relevant clinical changes)
- Clients who do not always provide complete, pertinent, and accurate pain information
- Clients who may lack sufficient medical knowledge to be able to select information to help medical and nursing staff make decisions about the pain

doubts that pain exists, they will share little information. The nurse must develop positive therapeutic relationships and give clients time to discuss pain. Positioning a client comfortably before asking questions may help clients sense the nurse's interest. The nurse avoids aggravating pain with a lengthy assessment.

The nurse should learn the verbal and nonverbal ways that clients communicate discomfort. Grimacing, splinting a body part, and unusual posturing are examples of nonverbal expressions of pain.

Clients unable to communicate effectively often require special attention during assessment. Children, persons who are developmentally delayed, clients who are psychotic, the critically ill, clients with dementia, and clients who do not speak English all require different approaches. Children's verbal statements are most important (Whaley and Wong, 1995). Young children may not know what the word "pain" means, and therefore assessment may require the nurse to use words such as "owie," "boo-boo," or "hurt." Cognitively impaired clients require simple assessment approaches involving close observation of behavior changes. A critically ill client who may have a clouded sensorium

and the presence of nasogastric tubes or artificial airways may require the nurse to ask specific directive questions that the client can answer with a nod of the head. If the client speaks a different language, pain assessment will be difficult. A family member or interpreter may be necessary to describe the client's feelings and sensations. Often a client in pain confides in only one person.

CLASSIFICATION OF THE PAIN EXPERIENCE

It can help to know the phase of pain clients are undergoing. The phase—anticipatory, sensation, or aftermath—influences not only clients' symptoms but also the types of therapies most likely to relieve pain. Clients in the anticipatory phase include those scheduled to undergo invasive diagnostic or therapeutic procedures or surgery and those with histories of recurring pain, such as the anginal pain of myocardial ischemia. These clients may be anxious or fearful, or they may ask questions about upcoming pain. Studies have shown that providing clients with physiological coping (positioning, deep breathing), sensory information (description of discomfort to be expected), and procedural information leads to clients with fewer complications who report less pain and use less analgesia (Fortin and Kirouac, 1976; Van Aernam and Lindeman, 1971; AHCPR, 1992)

Clients in the sensation phase generally demonstrate signs and symptoms of discomfort. Clients with traumatic injuries and clients who have had surgery are uncomfortable, so the nurse should not ask several detailed questions. Clients who are sensing pain, especially severe pain, want relief fast. After the pain has been relieved, the nurse must assess carefully for physical and psychological effects. Clients may later express apologies to the nurse for acting "improperly" during the pain experience.

The nurse assesses whether the client's pain is acute or chronic. If the pain is acute, a detailed assessment of pain characteristics is needed. With chronic pain the nurse determines whether it is intermittent, persistent, or of limited duration. After the phase or type of pain is assessed, findings direct the nurse to conduct further assessment for eventual selection of specific interventions.

CHARACTERISTICS OF PAIN

A client's self-report of pain is the single most reliable indicator of the existence and intensity of pain and any related discomfort (NIH, 1986). Pain is individualistic. Assessment of common characteristics of pain helps the nurse form an understanding of the pattern of pain and the type of therapies that may bring relief. Use of instruments to quantify the extent and degree of pain depends on a client being cognitively alert and able to understand a nurse's instructions.

Onset and Duration. The nurse asks questions to determine the onset, duration, and sequence of pain. When did the pain begin? How long has it lasted? Does it occur at the same time each day? How often does it recur?

It may be easier to diagnose the nature of pain by identifying time factors. For example, certain types of headaches can be characterized by the time of day when they occur. The onset of sudden and severe pain is easier to assess than is gradual, mild discomfort. An understanding of the time cycle of pain helps the nurse to know when to intervene before the pain occurs or worsens (Table 43-4).

Table 43-4	**Implications of Pain Assessment for Nursing Interventions**
ASSESSMENT CRITERIA	**NURSING INTERVENTIONS**
Onset and duration	Administer analgesics so that peak action occurs when pain is most acute (e.g., during dressing change or exercise therapy).
Location	Position client off affected area. Apply local treatments (e.g., elastic bandage and splinting) directly over painful site.
Severity	Change or revise interventions, depending on success of one intervention.
Precipitating or aggravating factors	Avoid activities that cause or aggravate pain. Teach client or family to avoid same activities.
Relief measures	Use measures that client uses to relieve pain, as long as they are safe and appropriate.

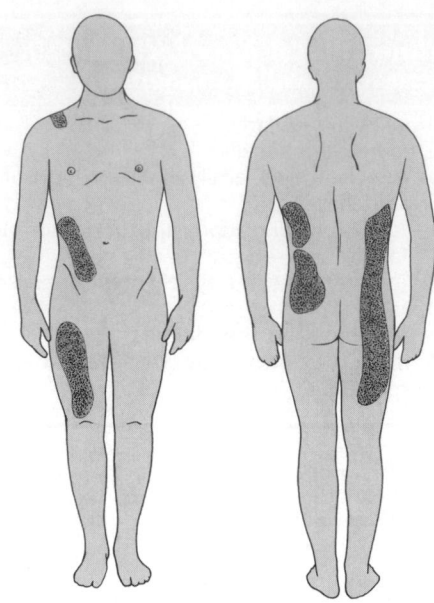

Fig. 43-6 Body diagrams to locate a client's pain.

Table 43-5	**Classification of Pain by Location**		
LOCATION		**CHARACTERISTICS**	**EXAMPLES OF CAUSES**
SUPERFICIAL OR CUTANEOUS Pain resulting from stimulation of skin		Pain is of short duration and is localized. It usually is sharp sensation.	Needlestick; small cut or laceration
DEEP VISCERAL Pain resulting from stimulation of internal organs		Pain is diffuse and may radiate in several directions. Duration varies but it usually lasts longer than superficial pain. Pain may be sharp, dull, or unique to organ involved.	Crushing sensation (e.g., angina pectoris); burning sensation (e.g., gastric ulcer)
REFERRED Common phenomenon in visceral pain because many organs themselves have no pain receptors; entrance of sensory neurons from affected organ into same spinal cord segment as neurons from areas where pain is felt; perception of pain in unaffected areas		Pain is felt in part of body separate from source of pain and may assume any characteristic.	Myocardial infarction, which may cause referred pain to jaw, left arm, and left shoulder; kidney stones, which may refer pain to groin
RADIATING Sensation of pain extending from initial site of injury to another body part		Pain feels as though it travels down or along body part. It may be intermittent or constant.	Low-back pain from ruptured intravertebral disk accompanied by pain radiating down leg from sciatic nerve irritation

Location. To assess pain location the nurse asks the client to point to all areas of discomfort. To localize the pain more specifically, the nurse then has the client trace the area from the most severe point outward. This is difficult to do if pain is diffuse, involves several sites, or involves large segments of the body. Some assessment tools have body diagrams (Fig. 43-6) on which the nurse can draw the location of the pain. This can be useful as a baseline if the pain should change.

When recording pain location, the nurse uses anatomical landmarks and descriptive terminology. The statement, "The pain is localized in the upper right abdominal quadrant," is more specific than "The client states the pain is in the abdomen." Knowing a client's disease or illness can

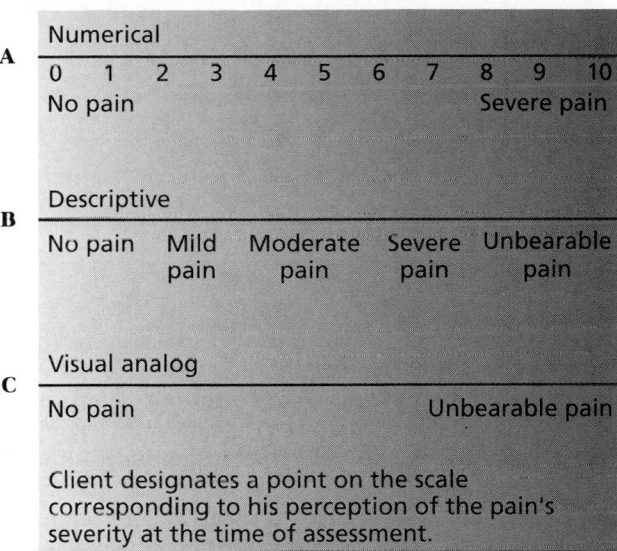

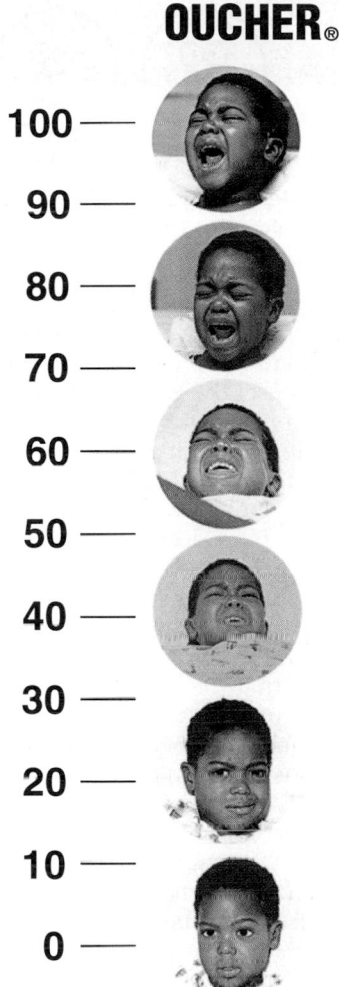

Fig. 43-7 Sample pain scales. **A**, Numerical. **B**, Verbal descriptive. **C**, Visual analog.

Fig. 43-8 African American version of the Oucher Pain Scale. (© *Denyes Villarruel, 1990. Used with permission.*)

help the nurse locate pain more easily. Pain, classified by location, may be superficial or cutaneous, deep or visceral, or referred or radiating (Table 43-5).

Severity. The most subjective characteristic of pain may be its severity, or intensity. Clients are often asked to describe pain as mild, moderate, or severe. However, the meaning of these terms differs for the nurse and client. This type of information is also difficult to verify over time.

Descriptive scales are a more objective means of measuring pain severity (Fig. 43-7). A verbal descriptor scale (VDS) consists of a line with three- to five-word descriptors equally spaced along the line. The descriptors are ranked from "no pain" to "unbearable pain." The nurse shows the client the scale and asks the client to choose the current intensity of pain. The nurse also asks how much the pain hurts at its worst and how much it hurts at its best. The VDS enables a client to choose a category for describing pain. Numerical rating scales (NRS) may be used instead of word descriptors. In this case clients rate pain on a scale of 0 to 10. The scales work best when assessing pain intensity before and after therapeutic interventions. When scales are used to rate pain, a 10-cm baseline is recommended (AHCPR, 1992).

A visual analog scale (VAS) does not have labeled subdivisions. It consists of a straight line, representing a continuum of intensity, and has verbal descriptors at each end. This scale gives the client total freedom in identifying the severity of pain. The VAS may be a more sensitive measure of pain severity because clients can identify any point on the continuum rather than being forced to choose one word or number (McGuire, 1984).

There are some unique tools available to measure pain intensity in children. Beyer et al (1992) have been developing the "Oucher," which consists of two separate scales: a 0 to 100 scale on the left for older children and a six-picture photographic scale on the right for younger children. Photographs of the face of a child (in increasing levels of discomfort) are designed to cue children into understanding

what pain is and its severity. A child merely points to the selection, thus simplifying the task of describing the pain. New ethnic versions of the tool have also been developed (Fig. 43-8). Wong and Baker (1988) developed the Faces Scale to assess pain in children (Fig. 43-9). The scale consists of six cartoon faces ranging from a smiling face ("no pain") to increasingly less happy faces, to a final sad, tearful face ("worst pain"). Children as young as 3 years of age can use the scale. Researchers are beginning to test the Faces Scale with older adults.

A pain scale should be designed so that it is easy to use and is not time consuming for the client to complete. If the client can read and understand the scale, the description of pain should be more accurate. Descriptive scales are useful not only in assessing the severity of pain, but also in evaluating changes in a client's condition. The nurse can use the scales after therapy or when symptoms become aggravated to judge whether the pain has decreased or increased.

The nurse does not use pain scales to compare one client with another. Although the scales lend relative objectivity to measurement, the severity of pain is too subjective to permit comparisons between individuals.

Fig. 43-9 Faces Scale. *(From Wong DL, Baker CM: Pain in children: comparison of assessment scales,* Oklahoma Nurs, *33(1):8, 1988.)*

Quality. Another subjective characteristic of pain is its quality. Because there is no common or specific pain vocabulary in general use, the words a client may choose to describe pain can apply to any number of things. Often, a client describes pain as crushing, throbbing, sharp, or dull. A client's pain is often indescribable.

The nurse should not provide descriptive words for a client. Assessment is more accurate if a client can describe the sensation after open-ended questions. For example, the nurse might say, "Tell me what your pain feels like." The only time that the nurse offers to list descriptive terms is when the client cannot describe the pain. McCaffery and Beebe (1989) report that the qualities of pricking, burning, and aching are useful to describe pain initially. Later the client may choose more descriptive terms.

There is some consistency in the way people describe certain types of pain. The pain associated with a myocardial infarction is often described as *crushing* or *viselike,* whereas the pain of a surgical incision is often described as *sharp* and *stabbing.* When the client's descriptions fit the pattern forming in the nurse's assessment, a clearer analysis can be made of the nature and type of pain.

Pain Pattern. Various factors affect the character of pain. It helps to assess specific events or conditions that precipitate or aggravate pain. The nurse asks the client to describe activities that cause pain, such as physical movement, coffee ingestion, or urination. The nurse may also ask the client to demonstrate actions that cause a painful response, such as coughing or turning a certain way. In the example of a ruptured intravertebral disk, the lower-back pain and radiation down the leg is aggravated by bending over or lifting objects. Swallowing and talking typically aggravate the pain of pharyngitis. After the nurse identifies precipitating or aggravating factors, it is easier to plan interventions to prevent pain from occurring or worsening.

Relief measures. It is useful to know whether a client has an effective way for relieving pain, such as changing position, using ritualistic behavior (pacing, rocking, rubbing), eating, meditation, or applying heat or cold to the painful site. The client's methods often work best for the nurse, too. Clients gain comfort from knowing that the nurse is willing to try their relief measures. Copp (1990) discovered that clients develop methods to reduce the intensity of oncoming pain. They used a range of muscular activities, verbal methods (prayer and cursing), and concentration exercises. In the home, the nurse must be sure that relief measures (such as ice packs) are used safely. Assessment of relieving factors should also include identification of practitioners (e.g., internist, orthopedist, acupuncturist, chiropractor, or dentist) whose services the

client has sought. Clients with chronic pain are more likely to try alternative health care methods.

Concomitant Symptoms. Concomitant symptoms are those that often occur with pain (e.g., nausea, headache, dizziness, urge to urinate, constipation, and restlessness). Certain types of pain have predictable accompanying symptoms. For example, severe rectal pain often results in constipation. The pain of an inflamed gallbladder or a kidney stone frequently causes nausea and vomiting. Concomitant symptoms may be as much a treatment priority as the pain itself.

EFFECTS OF PAIN ON THE CLIENT

Pain is a stressful event that can alter lifestyle and psychological well-being. In the case of cancer pain, it can cause suffering, loss of control, and impaired quality of life throughout the client's course of care, even for the client whose condition is stable and whose life expectancy is long (Jacox et al, 1994). By recognizing the effects pain has on clients, the nurse can better identify the nature and existence of pain.

Physical Signs and Symptoms. The physiological response to pain can reveal the existence and nature of pain and the potential threat to the client's welfare. When a client has pain, the nurse should assess vital signs, conduct a focused physical examination, and observe for autonomic nervous system involvement (see Table 43-2). Physiological signs can reveal pain in a client who tries not to complain or admit discomfort. There is no predictable level or extent of change in a client's condition that indicates pain.

At the onset of acute pain, the heart and respiratory rates and blood pressure increase. The nurse compares vital signs with baseline measurements recorded before onset. A change in vital signs is significant, but the nurse should take into account all signs and symptoms before determining that pain is the cause. The nurse should not confuse signs and symptoms of pain with other pathological changes. For example, a client who is highly anxious also has elevated heart and respiratory rates. The nurse performs a physical and neurological assessment based on the client's pain history. The painful area should be examined to see if palpation or manipulation of the site increases pain (Jacox et al, 1994). During a general overview, the nurse looks for cues indicating pain (e.g., posturing or guarding a painful area).

If pain is unrelieved, the nurse looks for signs of physical exhaustion. Decreasing vital sign values indicate parasympathetic nerve response. The client becomes less responsive to stimuli within the environment. The nurse should measure vital signs more often if the client's condition deteriorates.

Behavioral Indicators of Effects of Pain

VOCALIZATIONS
- Moaning
- Crying
- Gasping
- Grunting

FACIAL EXPRESSIONS
- Grimace
- Clenched teeth
- Wrinkled forehead
- Tightly closed or widely opened eyes or mouth
- Lip biting

BODY MOVEMENT
- Restlessness
- Immobilization
- Muscle tension
- Increased hand and finger movements
- Pacing activities
- Rhythmic or rubbing motions
- Protective movement of body parts

SOCIAL INTERACTION
- Avoidance of conversation
- Focus only on activities for pain relief
- Avoidance of social contacts
- Reduced attention span

▶ RESEARCH HIGHLIGHT

RESEARCH ABSTRACT
Confused, disoriented, or nonverbal older clients frequently suffer from painful conditions. A sample of 26 clients from the Alzheimer's unit of a large Midwestern nursing home was studied for behaviors that indicated pain. Each client's medical record confirmed the presence of a painful disorder such as cancer and degenerative joint disease. A pain assessment was performed on each client by a certified nurse practitioner. Most clients had no pain behaviors despite their diagnosis. Only three clients showed typical pain behaviors. Staff were surveyed and found to be surprised that the identified clients were in pain. Further review resulted in staff being able to describe client's pain behaviors. Clients who normally moaned and rocked became quiet and withdrawn when in pain. Clients who were friendly and outgoing became agitated and combative. Clients who were outgoing and easily involved in activities began to cry easily and withdraw when pain developed. Some clients refrained from eating when in pain.

IMPLICATIONS FOR PRACTICE
▶ There is a lack of objective assessment tools and criteria for assessing pain in the nonverbal elderly.
▶ Nurses must become very familiar with the "normal behavior" of this population in order to detect pain.
▶ Family can be a source to help identify behavioral changes.

REFERENCE
Marzinski LR: The tragedy of dementia: clinically assessing pain in the confused, nonverbal elderly, *J Gerontol Nurs* 17(6):25, 1991.

Behavioral Effects. When a client has pain, the nurse assesses verbalization, vocal response, facial and body movements, and social interaction (see the box above). A verbal report of pain is a vital part of assessment. The nurse must be willing to listen and understand. Many clients cannot verbalize discomfort because of the inability to communicate. An infant or a client who is unconscious, disoriented or confused, aphasic, or who speaks a foreign language is unable to explain the pain experience. In these cases, it is especially important for the nurse to be alert for behaviors that indicate pain (see the box at right).

Groaning, grunting, and crying are examples of vocalizations used to express pain. Certain vocalizations may be involuntary and may occur without warning when acute pain occurs. For some clients, vocalizations are culturally acceptable ways to communicate and do not necessarily indicate a higher severity of pain or reduced tolerance.

Subtle facial expressions or body movements often reveal more about the character of pain than does precise questioning. For example, the client may grimace or begin to toss and turn at regular intervals. The amount of restlessness or protective movement may increase as the assessment progresses. Some nonverbal expressions characterize sources of pain. The client with chest pain often grabs or holds the chest. A child or adult with severe abdominal pain often assumes a fetal position. The nonverbal expression of pain may support or contradict other information about pain. If a woman in labor reports that her labor pains are occurring more frequently and if she begins to massage her abdomen more frequently, her report is confirmed. If a client complains of severe abdominal pain but continues to grasp the chest, a more detailed assessment may be necessary.

The nature of pain causes a person to attend to the discomfort and fight it or to give in to the discomfort and withdraw socially. The extent to which a client interacts with the environment can provide a clue for the nurse about the intensity or nature of pain. Severe pain can seriously hamper a person's lifestyle.

Influence on Activities of Daily Living. Clients who live with daily pain are less able to participate in routine activities. Assessment of these changes reveals the extent of the client's disability and adjustments necessary to help clients participate in self-care.

The nurse asks whether pain interferes with sleep. There may be an initial difficulty falling asleep. Sleeping pills or other medications may be needed to induce sleep. The pain may awaken the client during the night and create difficulty in falling back to sleep (see Chapter 42). If a cancer client is taking opioids for pain control, the drugs frequently cause sleep disturbances.

Depending on the location of the pain, the client may have difficulty performing normal hygiene measures. The nurse determines whether the client can dress independently or shampoo hair. The pain may restrict mobility to the point that the client is no longer able to bathe in a bathtub. The client may have problems performing other activities of daily living. For example, a client with severe arthritis may find it painful to grasp eating utensils. The nurse determines the client's need for assistance with self-care activities. The nurse also considers the need for family members or friends to assist the client with basic hygiene.

Pain can impair the ability to maintain normal sexual relations. Conditions such as arthritis, degenerative diseases of the hip, and chronic back pain make it difficult for a person to assume usual positions during intercourse. Prolonged use of opioids for cancer pain is known to affect sexual function and libido in men and women (Jacox et al, 1994). When assessing the extent to which pain has affected sexual activity, the nurse determines the frequency of sexual relations before and after the onset of pain. It also helps to learn whether a client is physically unable to participate or if the desire for sexual intercourse has been reduced by the pain.

The ability of people to work can be seriously threatened by pain. The more physical activity required in a job, the greater the risk of discomfort when the pain is associated with musculoskeletal and certain visceral alterations. Pain related to emotional stress is probably increased in individuals whose jobs involve tension-laden decision making. The nurse assesses the work that clients do and their abilities to function in regular jobs. The daily chores of homemakers are assessed in the same manner as the duties involved in jobs outside the home. The nurse assesses whether it is necessary for clients to stop activity occasionally because of pain. Often the nurse can help clients select ways of minimizing or controlling the pain so that they can remain productive.

It is also important to include an assessment of the effect of pain on social activities. The pain may be so debilitating that the client becomes too exhausted to socialize. The nurse identifies the client's normal social activities, the extent to which they have been disrupted, and the client's wish to participate.

NEUROLOGICAL STATUS

A client's neurological function can easily influence the pain experience. Any factor that interrupts or influences normal pain reception or perception affects the client's awareness and response to pain. For example, a client who has a spinal cord injury, **peripheral neuropathy**, as in the

Examples of NANDA Nursing Diagnoses for Pain

Anxiety *related to:*
- Unrelieved pain

Pain *related to:*
- Physical injury or trauma
- Reduced blood supply to tissues
- Natural childbirth processes

Chronic pain *related to:*
- Tissue scarring
- Inadequate pain control

Hopelessness *related to:*
- Chronic malignant pain

Ineffective individual coping *related to:*
- Chronic pain

Impaired physical mobility *related to:*
- Musculoskeletal pain
- Incisional pain

Risk for injury *related to:*
- Reduced pain reception

Self-care deficit *related to:*
- Musculoskeletal pain

Sexual dysfunction *related to:*
- Arthritic hip pain

Sleep pattern disturbance *related to:*
- Low-back pain

case of diabetes mellitus, or a neurological disease such as multiple sclerosis, is less likely to sense pain than is a client who has normal neurological function. Some therapies influence pain perception and response. Analgesics, sedatives, and anesthetics depress functions of the central nervous system. It is important for the nurse to conduct a neurological assessment (see Chapter 33) of a client at risk for being insensitive to pain. This client could suffer injury easily and thus requires preventive nursing care.

Sample Nursing Diagnostic Process for Chronic Pain

ASSESSMENT ACTIVITIES	DEFINING CHARACTERISTICS	NURSING DIAGNOSIS
Have client describe character of pain.	Pain is colicky, worse after eating, often associated with nausea. Pain is constant; rated 5 on a scale of 0 to 10.	**Chronic pain** related to tissue invasion by abdominal cancer.
Assess onset and location of pain.	Pain present for 7 months; localized in right lower abdomen, radiates to right shoulder and neck.	
Observe client behaviors.	Moves slowly, stays in bed during much of day, has a blank facial expression.	
Assess influence pain has had on daily activities.	Client's appetite is reduced. Spouse reports client awakens frequently during night, gets little sleep.	
Review medical history.	Client is diagnosed with metastatic cancer of the colon.	

Nursing Diagnosis

The development of an accurate nursing diagnosis for a client in pain results from thorough data collection and analysis (see the diagnostic process box on p. 1170). A nurse must not diagnose pain simply because it is presumed that a client will be uncomfortable. Too often a nurse may choose the diagnosis of pain because a client is about to have surgery or a specific disease condition implies pain.

An accurate diagnosis is made only after a complete assessment of all variables. In the example of the diagnosis of pain, the nurse may assess the client's withdrawal from communication, rigid posturing, moaning, and the client's verbalization of discomfort. In contrast, the diagnosis of anxiety may be made by observing a client's facial tension and appearance, poor eye contact, restlessness, and verbalizations of feeling scared. The two diagnoses have similar defining characteristics. The nurse sorts out patterns of data to identify pain as the correct diagnosis.

The nursing diagnosis should focus on the specific nature of the pain to help the nurse identify the most useful types of interventions for alleviating pain and minimizing its effect on the client's lifestyle and function. Pain related to physical trauma versus pain related to natural childbirth processes require very different nursing interventions. Accurate identification of related factors ensures appropriate nursing therapies will be chosen.

The nurse may make diagnoses other than that of pain. The extent to which pain affects a client's lifestyle and general state of health determines whether other nursing diagnoses are relevant (see the nursing diagnoses box on p. 1170). For example, the nurse's assessment may reveal that a client suffers from pain of the hands and shoulders. As a result, the client is unable to remove or fasten necessary items of clothing. The client has the pain of crippling arthritis. The nursing diagnosis would be that of dressing/grooming self-care deficit related to arthritic pain. The client would have a nursing diagnosis of chronic pain to direct the nurse's interventions toward pain relief. The additional diagnosis of self-care deficit would lead the nurse to assist the client with alternative measures for performing self-care.

Planning

For each nursing diagnosis identified, the nurse develops a care plan for the client's needs (see the care plan below). Together the nurse and client discuss realistic expectations for pain-relief measures, the degree of pain relief to expect, and the anticipated effects on lifestyle and function. It is not inappropriate to reassure clients and families that most pain can be relieved safely and effectively (Jacox et al, 1994). This of course will depend on a comprehensive and well-managed plan of care. Expected outcomes and goals are selected on the basis of the nursing diagnosis and client's condition. Appropriate therapies are chosen on the basis of the related factor contributing to the client's pain or health problem. For example, pain related to acute incisional pain responds to analgesics, whereas pain related to early labor contractions can be reduced with relaxation exercises.

A therapy that works for one client will not work for all. In the home, the nurse uses some of the remedies that the client has adopted. However, the nurse cannot use therapies that are unsafe.

Sample Nursing Care Plan for Chronic Pain

NURSING DIAGNOSIS: **Chronic pain** related to tissue invasion by abdominal cancer.
DEFINITION: Chronic pain is the state in which an individual experiences pain that continues for more than 6 months (Kim, McFarland, and McLane, 1995).

GOALS	EXPECTED OUTCOMES	INTERVENTIONS	RATIONALE
Client and spouse will actively participate in pain management plan within 2 weeks.	Client and spouse initiate pain-control therapies.	Implement drug regimen with transdermal Fentanyl. Explain to client and spouse expected side effects, schedule for patch replacement, method to treat breakthrough acute pain.	Transdermal drug bypasses gastrointestinal absorption (McKenry and Salerno 1994). Indicated for clients with constant pain (Jacox, et al, 1994).
		Have client select therapies that have relieved pain in past (e.g., distraction while playing cards, lying in semi-Fowler's position in bed).	Personal control refers to a person's ability to shape immediate circumstances through own actions (e.g., choosing among options) (Wallston et al, 1987).
	Client maintains daily log of pain-control therapies and responses.	Have client complete a pain log of type of pain, measures used to control pain, and relief obtained.	Recording pain experience and relief measures increases client's perception of control (Kim, McFarland, and McLane, 1995).
		Teach spouse how to perform slow-stroke back massage.	Slow-stroke back massage is easy to do, takes a brief time, and has been shown to induce relaxation (Meek, 1993).

When developing the care plan, the nurse selects priorities based on the client's level of pain and its effect on the client's condition. For acute, severe pain it is important to provide relief as soon as possible. Analgesics can provide relatively rapid relief and lessen the chance of pain worsening. After a client gains some relief from pain, the nurse plans other therapies such as relaxation or the application of heat to enhance the effect of analgesics.

A comprehensive plan includes a variety of resources for pain control. It is important to include the family in the care plan. The family may need to administer care in the home. In an acute care setting the family must understand the nature and extent of the client's pain and the forms of therapy to be used. Family members who show a disinterest or a prejudicial view toward pain can delay recovery. Additional resources available include nurse specialists, physical therapists, and occupational therapists. An oncology nurse specialist is very familiar with therapies most effective for chronic, malignant pain. Physical therapists can plan exercises that strengthen muscle groups and lessen pain in affected areas. Occupational therapists may devise splints to support painful body parts. When the nurse is caring for a client experiencing pain, client-centered goals might include the following:

1. Stating a sense of well-being and comfort
2. Maintaining the ability to perform self-care
3. Maintaining existing physical and psychosocial function
4. Explaining factors contributing to the pain experience
5. Using therapies administered within the home safely.

To establish an effective care plan, the nurse establishes a therapeutic relationship with the client and educates the client about pain.

THERAPEUTIC RELATIONSHIP

People in pain are highly vulnerable and not always convinced that someone is concerned with their welfare. A client in pain needs someone to trust. If the family is unsupportive or if the nurse is unable to establish a therapeutic relationship with the client, any resultant mistrust can heighten the awareness of pain. Unless clients have means to express concerns or fears about pain, their reactions to the pain may become inappropriate. Often, clients become angry or complain when needs for pain relief are ignored.

The nurse can best help by seeing the client as a total person and conveying a sense of caring. Giving careful attention to the client's concerns during assessment is one way of building confidence in the nurse. Promptness in attending to the client's needs further establishes a strong therapeutic relationship. Making judgments about the validity of pain, bartering pain relief in return for "good" client behavior, and controlling sources of pain relief destroy the client's trust in the nurse.

A successful nurse-client relationship depends in part on the nurse's ability to respect the client's response to pain. Many nurses value firm self-control. However, a client may need to cry or moan or even become angry. The client should never feel ashamed or fearful that the nurse will not be accepting.

EDUCATION

Clients are better prepared to handle almost any situation when they understand it. The experience of pain is no exception. Teaching clients about the pain experience reduces anxiety and helps clients achieve a sense of control. For example, clients entering a clinic or hospital for the first time may know tests will be performed but do not understand them. As a result, they might fantasize about the experience. Fears are enhanced if friends have had unpleasant experiences in similar circumstances. Fear increases the perception of painful stimuli.

During the anticipatory phase of the pain experience, the nurse plans to teach clients about the procedures and associated discomfort. For example, prior to an intravenous (IV) insertion, the nurse should explain the sensation caused by the tourniquet application as well as the needle stick itself. Explaining the procedure in a confident tone conveys a sense that the nurse will care for the client correctly. When clients receive instruction about an upcoming painful experience, they often perceive the actual experience as less unpleasant.

For some clients, early warning of pain can be a problem. The highly anxious or fearful client may be irrational and unable to learn from the nurse's explanations. Such clients tend to fantasize horrible events if they receive information too early about painful procedures. If clients seem unlikely to benefit from advance preparation, it is best to explain invasive procedures a short time before they occur. It is not always easy to know whether clients can accept impending unpleasant experiences. If clients are typically anxious or if previous teaching has not relieved anxiety, the nurse must judge when to tell clients about procedures.

Relevant play is a type of teaching that works well with children. Play reduces anxiety that might otherwise be created if the nurse tried to explain complicated procedures. For example, if a child is to have a laceration of the arm sutured, it helps to let the child put sutures into a doll's arm. Almost any procedure or situation can be acted out with dolls or other appropriate toys.

 Implementation

The nature of pain and the extent to which it affects a person's well-being determine the choice of pain-relief therapies. Pain therapy requires an individualized approach, perhaps more so than any other client problem. The nurse and client must be partners in using pain-control measures. Nurses administer and monitor therapies ordered by physicians for pain relief and independently use pain-relief measures that complement those prescribed by a physician. Client remedies are often most successful, especially when the client has already had experience with pain. Generally, the least invasive or safest therapy should be tried first. If there is doubt about a nursing therapy, the nurse should consult a physician.

CARING IN PROMOTING COMFORT

Regardless of the type of therapies used, the nurse's ability to show caring toward clients enhances their comfort. Kolcaba (1992) stresses the importance of recognizing the holistic nature of comfort. Comfort is physical and mental, and a nurse's responsibility does not end with physical care. A nurse's competence in developing interpersonal relationships with clients centers on the ability to establish and maintain a caring relationship that affirms the worth of the client. A skilled nurse quickly communicates respect for a client, enhances the client's sense of worth, and acquires the client's trust. This conveys to the client a sense of comfort and security.

The nurse can convey caring in many ways: careful repositioning of the client; displaying a friendly, reliable, and accessible image; remaining attentive and responsive to requests; and personalizing every aspect of care. Clients are able to perceive a nurse's caring approach. This reinforces the trust that builds as a nurse forms a relationship with a client. Caring involves a sense of dedication to an individual, but it involves more than having concern for another person; it involves integrating behaviors into everyday nursing practice.

Pain can be minimized through caring behaviors. Burnside (1988) suggests that two types of touching—*task-oriented* and *affective*—can be effective with clients. Task-oriented touching occurs when a nurse takes a client's blood pressure or helps the client walk. Affective touching is less routine and is intended to show concern, such as gently stroking the client's back during a conversation. Often one can combine task-oriented and affective touching (e.g., placing a hand on the client's shoulder while giving medication). Simply sitting and holding a client's hand, allowing a client to move at his own speed, speaking in a soft tone of voice, and staying with a client for a time after a procedure are all caring behaviors. When a nurse can successfully convey compassion, maintain the client's dignity, and consistently strive to minimize discomfort or suffering, pain-relieving measures will be more successful.

HOLISTIC HEALTH STRATEGIES

Because comfort affects a person's physical and mental functioning, **holistic health** approaches are becoming important interventions for maintaining a person's wellness. Holistic health is an ongoing state of wellness that involves taking care of the physical self, expressing emotions appropriately and effectively, using the mind constructively, being creatively involved with others, and becoming aware of higher levels of consciousness (Association for Holistic Health, 1981). The use of holistic health approaches assumes a person's own capacity for healing and returns responsibility for health back to the individual (Edelman and Mandle, 1994). The concept of holistic health parallels the values nursing has always had in maintaining the integrity of the whole person.

Holistic health is more than just self-care, (e.g., maintaining proper nutrition, exercise [Fig. 43-10], and coping strategies). It also is a process of personal inquiry. A person learns to look at the emotional meaning of any health problems they might have and the significance of the problem in light of their purpose in life (Edelman and Mandle, 1994). A person becomes consciously aware of the relationship between emotional health and physical health. The role of clients is to participate actively in their own well-being. Common holistic health approaches include wellness education, regular exercise, and management of interpersonal relationships. When a person develops pain or other symptoms of discomfort, there are tools the nurse can offer.

Therapeutic Touch. Developed 23 years ago by Kunz and Krieger, **therapeutic touch** derives in part from the an-

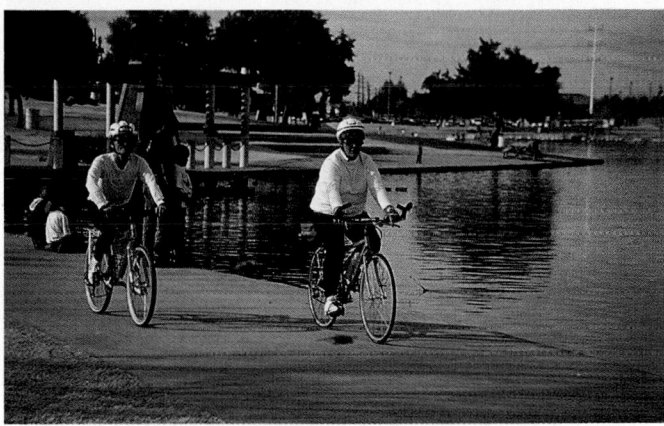

Fig. 43-10 Regular exercise is important for health maintenance.

cient practice of the "laying on of hands" (Mackey, 1995). The approach suggests that, in a healthy person, there is an equilibrium between inward and outward energy flow. Illness represents an imbalance of the energy field. Therapeutic touch involves the use of the hands to consciously direct an energy exchange. Advanced training is required. There are four basic steps to the technique: centering, assessment, treatment, and evaluation. Each step generally flows into the next, with the whole process lasting about 25 minutes.

The technique begins with the nurse *centering* or moving into a meditative state. This part of the technique can take time to master; however, once it occurs, a nurse can become focused after taking only 3 to 4 deep breaths. With an intent to help and with attention focused on the client, the nurse begins the *assessment* process. This involves moving the hands symmetrically around the client 2 to 6 inches from the body, allowing energy fields to interact. The experienced nurse can sense differences in energy flow as the hands move across the client's body (Mackey, 1995). The nurse notes sensations of temperature variations, pressure, tingling, or pulsation.

After finding areas of imbalance, the nurse begins *treatment* to restore balance to the client's energy field. This transfer stage may be done in silence or with a verbal exchange. The nurse warms a cool area, and directs energy toward a deficient or empty area using visualization and movement of the hands. After performing the treatment, the nurse *evaluates* the energy field for balance. Research has shown the analgesic properties of therapeutic touch in creating a generalized relaxation response.

Acupressure. Based on the theory of Asian medicine that a life force, in the form of energy, circulates throughout the body in well-defined cycles, **acupressure** opens congested energy pathways to promote a healthier state. Nurse therapists learn the energy pathways or body meridians and apply pressure over particular points along the pathways. For example, if a client has a headache, pressure over the Hoku point (Fig. 43-11) will relieve the discomfort. As the pressure points are touched, the nurse begins to feel a subtle sensation or pulse under the fingers. At first, the pulses at various points will feel different, but as they con-

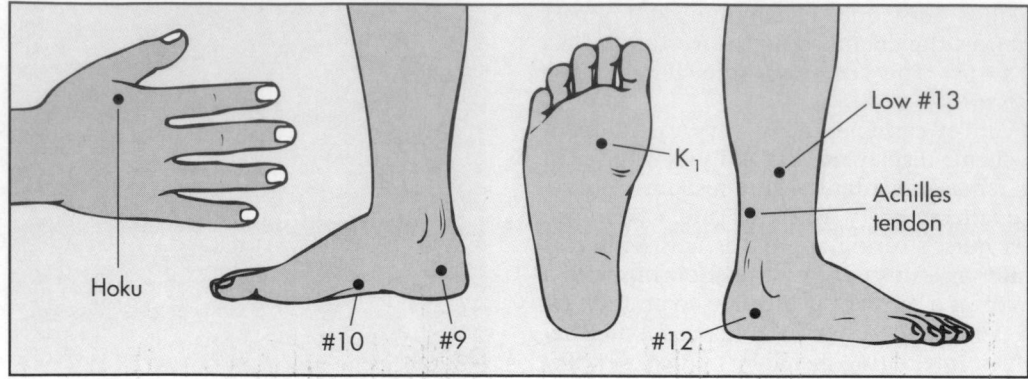

Fig. 43-11 Examples of pressure points used in acupressure *(From Edelman CL, Mandle CL:* Health promotion throughout the lifespan, *ed 3, St Louis, 1994, Mosby.)*

tinue to be held, they come into balance. Once the points are balanced the nurse gently removes the fingers. Many simple, easy acupressure techniques can be taught to clients for primary pain prevention. A complete acupressure session takes about 1 hour.

Relaxation and Guided Imagery. Clients can alter affective-motivational and cognitive pain perception through relaxation and guided imagery. **Relaxation** is mental and physical freedom from tension or stress. Relaxation techniques provide individuals with self-control when discomfort or pain occurs, reversing the physical and emotional stress of pain. Relaxation techniques can be used at any phase of health or illness. They are preventive measures to help the body bounce back and regenerate each day and are alternatives to alcohol, smoking, or overeating (Edelman and Mandle, 1994). Clients who use relaxation techniques successfully experience several physiological and behavioral changes (see the box on p. 1175). Relaxation techniques include meditation, yoga, Zen, guided imagery, and progressive relaxation exercises.

Relaxation with or without guided imagery relieves tension headaches, labor pain, anticipated episodes of acute pain (e.g., a needlestick), and chronic pain disorders. It may take 5 to 10 training sessions before clients can effectively minimize pain (Carney, 1983). Relaxation training can be practiced indefinitely and usually has no side effects. Carney (1983) notes studies showing that 60% to 70% of clients with tension headache can reduce headache activity by at least 50% with relaxation.

For effective relaxation, the individual's participation and cooperation are needed. Relaxation techniques are taught only when the client is not in acute discomfort because the inability to concentrate makes the exercise ineffective. The nurse explains the technique in detail and describes common sensations the client may experience (e.g., a decrease in temperature or numbness of a body part). The client should use these sensations as feedback.

The nurse is a coach, guiding the client slowly through steps of the exercise. The environment should be free of noises or other irritating stimuli. The client may sit in a comfortable chair or lie in bed (see the box on p. 1175). A light sheet or blanket for warmth often helps the client feel more comfortable. The client may use guided imagery and relaxation exercises together or separately.

In **guided imagery** the client creates an image in the mind, concentrates on that image, and gradually becomes less aware of pain. The nurse coaches the client in forming the image and concentrating on the sensory experience. Initially the nurse asks the client to think of a pleasant scene or experience that promotes the use of all senses. The client describes the image and the nurse records it so that it can be used during later exercises. The nurse uses specific information given by the client and does not make changes in the client's image. The following is an example of a portion of a guided imagery exercise:

Imagine yourself lying on a cool bed of grass with the sounds of rushing water from a nearby stream. It's a balmy day. You turn to see a patch of blue wildflowers in bloom and can smell their fragrance.

The nurse sits closely enough to the client to be heard but is not intrusive. The nurse's calm, soft voice helps the client focus more completely on the suggested image. While relaxing, the client focuses on the image, and it becomes unnecessary for the nurse to speak continuously. If the client shows signs of agitation, restlessness, or discomfort, the nurse should stop the exercise and begin later when the client is more at ease.

Progressive relaxation of the entire body takes about 15 minutes. The client pays attention to the body, noting areas of tension. Tense areas are replaced with warmth and relaxation. Some clients relax better with their eyes closed. Soft background music can help.

Progressive relaxation exercise involves a combination of controlled breathing exercises and a series of contractions and relaxation of muscle groups. The client begins by breathing slowly and diaphragmatically, allowing the abdomen to rise slowly and the chest to expand fully. When the client establishes a regular breathing pattern, the nurse coaches the client to locate any area of muscular tension, to think about how it feels, to tense muscles fully, and then completely to relax them. This creates the sensation of removing all discomfort and stress. Gradually the client can relax the muscles without first tensing them. When full relaxation is achieved, pain perception is lowered and anxiety toward the pain experience becomes minimal. The following is an example of how a nurse coaches a client:

Let's begin by finding as comfortable a position as possible. Arms at your side . . . legs uncrossed. . . . Move until you feel at ease. . . .

Effects of Relaxation
▪ Decreased pulse, blood pressure, and respirations
▪ Decreased oxygen consumption
▪ Decreased muscle tension
▪ Decreased metabolic rate
▪ Heightened global awareness
▪ Lack of attention to environmental stimuli
▪ No voluntary change of position
▪ Sense of peace and well-being
▪ Deep, wakeful, restful period of alertness

Body Positions for Relaxation
SITTING
▪ Sit with entire back resting against back of chair.
▪ Place feet flat on floor.
▪ Keep legs separated.
▪ Hang arms at the side or rest on chair arms.
▪ Keep head aligned with spine.
LYING
▪ Keep legs separated with toes pointed slightly outward.
▪ Rest arms at sides without touching sides of body.
▪ Keep head aligned with spine.
▪ Use thin, small pillow under head.

Take a deep breath. Feel your stomach and chest slowly rise. . . . Relax. . . . Now breathe out slowly. . . slowly . . . and relax.

Count to 4, inhaling on 1 and 2, exhaling on 3 and 4. . . . Continue to breathe slowly. . . . Your body is beginning to relax. . . . Think "relax." . . . Feel the parts of your body. . . . Notice any tension in your muscles. . . . Continue to breathe slowly . . . and relax.

Concentrate on your face . . . your jaws . . . your neck. . . . Notice any tightness. . . . Breathe in warmth and relaxation. . . . Concentrate on any tension in your hands. . . . Notice how it feels. . . . Now make a fist—a tight fist! As you begin to exhale, relax your fist. . . . Good! Notice how your hand feels. . . . Think "relax." . . . Your hand feels warm . . . heavy or light. . . . Just relax more . . . and more. Now focus on your forearms. . . . Notice any tension. . . . Relax your arms. . . . Feel your body relaxing. . . . Let the feelings of relaxation spread from your fingers and hands through the muscles of your arms.

If the client becomes agitated or uncomfortable, the nurse stops the exercise. If the client seems to have difficulty relaxing only part of the body, the nurse slows the progression of the exercise and concentrates on the tensed body part. The client must also know from the beginning that the exercise can be stopped at any time. With practice the client can soon perform relaxation exercises independently.

MAINTAINING WELLNESS

Pain can seriously disable and immobilize a person, which can impair the ability to perform self care activities. Pain can also cause social isolation, depression, and changes in self-concept. Change in function can mean a significant loss to a client. The nurse helps the client and family members find ways to cope with pain and maintain a functional lifestyle.

The nurse minimizes potential effects of immobilization (see Chapter 37) from pain by using good positioning techniques. Families can learn a simple routine of range of motion exercises. Passive exercises should not be carried out if they increase pain (Jacox et al, 1994). Painful body parts can be further protected by using elastic bandages, braces, splints, or pillows for support. These devices can be used in the home as well as in any health care facility. If crutches or other assistive devices are needed, the nurse ensures that they are used safely and properly. Otherwise, the client may be at risk for further injury or pain.

Painful disorders of the upper extremities create difficulty in eating, bathing, grooming, and dressing. The nurse may refer a client to an occupational therapist who can devise ways to maintain function, even when finger movement or grasp is impaired. Eating utensils, a comb and brush, and a toothbrush can be attached to extension devices. These devices have enlarged handles or splints that allow clients to pick up the items. Clothing fasteners made from Velcro tape make it easier for clients to remove or apply clothing. Shirts or blouses can be sewn so that garments can simply be pulled on or off over the head.

Measures that promote a sense of well-being in a client with pain include warm baths, thorough personal hygiene measures, and a schedule for adequate rest. The nurse should plan rest periods before exhaustive procedures or visits by friend. Clients with chronic pain should rest before social activities in the home.

A person with pain may avoid sexual activity for fear that it will cause or aggravate discomfort. However, the need for sexual warmth is not negated by pain. Clients can learn to express themselves sexually regardless of pain. A client whose movement is restricted by pain may not be able to assume the positions for intercourse. Alternative positions may be less uncomfortable and strenuous. Nurses should also caution clients about the fact that tranquilizers, muscle relaxants, and narcotics decrease libido and potency.

NONPHARMACOLOGICAL PAIN-RELIEF MEASURES

One of the most basic nursing responsibilities is protecting the client from harm. There are a number of nonpharmacological therapies that lessen the reception and perception of pain and which can be used in acute and tertiary care as well as in the home and restorative care settings. Similarly, these therapies are used in combination with pharmacological measures. Nonpharmacological measures include cognitive-behavioral interventions and physical agents. The goals of cognitive-behavioral interventions are to change clients' perceptions of pain, to alter pain behavior, and to provide clients with a greater sense of control. Relaxation and guided imagery discussed as holistic health approaches are examples. Physical agents have the goal of providing comfort, correcting physical dysfunction, altering physiological responses, and reducing fears associated with pain-related immobility. The AHCPR guidelines for acute pain management (1992) cite nonpharmacological interventions to be appropriate for clients who meet the following criteria:

- Find such interventions appealing
- Express anxiety or fear
- May benefit from avoiding or reducing drug therapy

- Are likely to experience and need to cope with a prolonged interval of postoperative pain
- Have incomplete pain relief after use of pharmacological therapies.

In the case of cancer clients, the nurse's responsibility is to evaluate the effects of nonpharmacological measures to ensure pain relief so that clients are not excluded from the use of pharmacological therapies as needed.

Anticipatory Guidance. Modifying anxiety directly associated with pain relieves pain and adds to the effects of other pain-relief measures. Moderate anxiety may be useful when a client anticipates a painful experience. Clients should receive a detailed description of all medical procedures and expected postoperative discomfort to learn what is to be expected during a painful procedure or event. Knowledge about pain helps a client control anxiety and cognitively gain a level of pain relief. An example of anticipatory guidance is preoperative teaching (see Chapter 48).

The nurse gives clients information that prevents misinterpretation of the painful event and promotes understanding of what to expect. Information given to clients includes explanations of the following:

1. Occurrence, onset, and expected duration of pain
2. Quality, severity, and location of pain
3. Information on how the client's safety is ensured
4. Causes for the pain
5. Methods the nurse and client take for pain relief
6. Expectations of the client during a procedure

The nurse cannot say that the client will experience no pain. Anticipatory guidance gives an honest explanation of the pain experience. The nurse also gives instruction on pain-relief techniques so that the client will be prepared to cope with discomfort. In clients with high levels of anxiety, too much information can worsen pain.

Distraction. The reticular activating system inhibits painful stimuli if a person receives sufficient or excessive sensory input. With meaningful sensory stimuli, a person can ignore or become unaware of pain. Pleasurable stimuli cause the release of endorphins. Persons who are bored or in isolation have only their pain to think about and thus perceive it more acutely. Distraction directs a client's attention to something else and thus can reduce the awareness of pain and even increase tolerance. There is one disadvantage. If it works, health care personnel or family may question the existence or severity of pain. Distraction may work best for short, intense pain lasting a few minutes, such as during an invasive procedure or while waiting for an analgesic to work.

The nurse assesses activities enjoyed by the client that may act as distractions. These might include singing, praying, describing photos or pictures aloud, listening to music, and playing games. Most distractions can be used in a hospital, home, or long-term care facility.

One effective distraction is music, which decreases physiological pain, stress, and anxiety by diverting the person's attention away from pain. Music has been shown to have the effect of lowering the heart rate, decreasing anxiety and depression, relieving pain, reducing blood pressure, and altering time perception (Guzetta, 1989). The nurse can use music creatively in many clinical situations. Clients generally prefer to perform (play an instrument or sing a song) or listen to music. Music that initially matches a person's mood is usually best. For example, a lonely person might initially enjoy playing a solo instrument or listening to a classical orchestral piece. Classical, popular, and nontraditional music (music with no vocals, periods of silence) are used in music therapy. Popular music does not usually produce a deep level of relaxation because it is short with a steady beat and words. Music produces an altered state of consciousness through sound, silence, space, and time. It must be listened to for at least 15 minutes to be therapeutic. In an acute care setting, listening to music can be highly effective in reducing a client's postoperative pain. The box below suggests ways to use music effectively.

Biofeedback. Biofeedback is a behavioral therapy that involves giving individuals information about physiological responses (e.g., blood pressure or tension) and ways to exercise voluntary control over those responses (NIH, 1986). The therapy is used to produce deep relaxation, and is especially effective for muscle tension and migraine headaches. When headaches are treated, electrodes are attached externally over each temple. The electrodes measure skin tension in microvolts. A polygraph machine visibly records the tension level for the client to see. The client learns to achieve optimal relaxation using feedback from the polygraph, while lowering the actual level of tension experienced. The therapy takes several weeks to learn. Biofeedback can stop headaches and lessen the risk of development of future headaches.

Self-Hypnosis. Hypnosis can help alter pain perception through the influence of positive suggestion. A holistic health approach, self-hypnosis uses self-suggestion and images of relaxation and peace. The person enters the relaxation state using a variety of seed thoughts and then conditions a certain response to them (Edelman and Mandel, 1994). Self-hypnosis is like daydreaming. The intense concentration reduces apprehension and stress as a person concentrates on only one thought.

Reducing Pain Perception. One simple way to promote comfort is by removing or preventing painful stimuli (see the box on p. 1177). This is especially important for

---

Using Music to Control Pain

- Match musical selections to a client's taste. Consider age and background.
- Use earphones to avoid annoying other clients or staff and help client to concentrate on music.
- Be sure controls on the radio or tape player are easy to press, manipulate, and distinguish.
- Have family members bring tapes from home.
- If pain is acute, increase the volume of music. As pain decreases, reduce the volume.
- If background music is provided, select general types suited to the client's preferences.
- Have the client concentrate on the music and emphasize rhythm by tapping fingers or patting the thigh.
- Avoid interruptions by dimming lights and closing the drapes or door.
- Instruct client not to analyze the music: "Go wherever it takes you."
- Leave clients alone as they listen to the music.

Controlling Painful Stimuli in the Client's Environment

- Tighten and smooth wrinkled bed linen.
- Position tubing on which client is lying.
- Loosen constricting bandages (unless specifically applied as a pressure dressing).
- Change wet dressings.
- Position client in anatomical alignment.
- Check temperature of hot or cold applications, including bath water.
- Lift client in bed—do not pull.
- Position client correctly on bed pan.
- Avoid exposing skin or mucous membranes to irritants (e.g., diarrheal stool, wound drainage).
- Prevent urinary retention by keeping Foley catheters patent and free flowing.
- Prevent constipation with fluids, diet, and exercise.

---

clients who are immobilized or unable to sense discomfort. Pain can also be prevented by anticipating painful events. For example, a client who is allowed to become constipated may suffer from distention and abdominal cramping. The nurse actively intervenes to ensure that the normal elimination process continues. Before performing procedures, the nurse considers the client's condition, aspects of the procedure that may be uncomfortable, and techniques to avoid causing pain. For example, in a client with severe arthritic knee pain, the nurse knows that any extreme flexion of the knee causes much pain. Before walking the client to the bathroom, the nurse makes sure that an elevated toilet seat is available. The client can then be seated and can rise with minimal discomfort. It takes only simple consideration of the client's comfort and a little extra time to avoid pain-producing situations.

Cutaneous Stimulation. **Cutaneous stimulation** is the stimulation of the skin to relieve pain. A massage, warm bath, ice bag, and transcutaneous electrical nerve stimulation (TENS) are simple ways to reduce pain perception. The specific way in which cutaneous stimulation works is unclear. One suggestion is that it causes release of endorphins, thus blocking the transmission of painful stimuli. The gate-control theory suggests that cutaneous stimulation activates larger, faster transmitting A-beta sensory nerve fibers. This decreases pain transmission through small-diameter A-delta and C fibers. Synaptic gates close to the transmission of pain impulses. Meek (1993) suggests that touch and massage are sensory integration techniques that influence autonomic nervous system activity. When a person perceives touch to be relaxing, the relaxation response is elicited.

An advantage to cutaneous stimulation is that the measures can be used in the home, giving clients and families some control over pain symptoms and treatment. The proper use of cutaneous stimulation can reduce pain perception and help to reduce muscle tension that might otherwise increase pain. When slow-stroke back massage (SSBM) has been used with terminally ill clients, there has been a decrease in systolic and diastolic blood pressure. The

technique for SSBM may involve several approaches, but one method is to slowly and rhythmically stroke the client's skin with the hands at a rate of 60 strokes a minute. The hands cover an area 2 inches wide on both sides of the spinous processes, from the crown of the head to the sacral area; the technique lasts for 3 minutes. Chapter 40 reviews the technique for back massage.

When using cutaneous stimulation methods, the nurse eliminates sources of environmental noise, helps the client to assume a comfortable position, and explains the purpose of the therapy. Cutaneous stimulation should not be used directly on sensitive skin areas (e.g., burns, bruises, skin rashes, inflammation, and underlying bone fractures).

Cold and heat applications (see Chapter 49) relieve pain and promote healing. The selection of heat versus cold therapies varies with clients' conditions. For example, moist heat relieves the early morning stiffness of arthritis, but cold applications reduce the acute pain and inflamed joints of the disease (Ceccio, 1990). When using any form of heat or cold application, the nurse instructs the client to avoid injury to the skin by checking the temperature and avoiding direct application of the cold or hot surface to the skin. Especially at risk are clients with spinal cord or other neurological injury, older adults, and confused clients.

Ice massage and application of cold packs are two types of cold therapy that are particularly effective for pain relief. Ice massage involves the use of a large ice cube or a small paper cup filled with water and frozen (water rises out of the cup as it freezes to create a smooth surface of ice for massage). The massage is simple. A nurse or the client can apply the ice with firm pressure to the skin, followed by a slow, steady, circular massage over the area. Cold may be applied near the pain site, on the opposite side of the body corresponding to the pain site, or on a site located between the brain and pain site. It takes 5 to 10 minutes to apply cold. Each client responds differently to the site of application that is most effective. Application near the actual site of pain tends to work best. A client feels cold, burning, and aching sensations and numbness. When numbness occurs, the ice should be removed. Cold is particularly effective for tooth or mouth pain when ice is placed on the web of the hand between the thumb and index finger. This point on the hand is an acupuncture point that apparently influences nerve pathways to the face and head. Cold applications are also effective before invasive needle punctures.

Another form of cutaneous stimulation, sometimes called counterstimulation, is **transcutaneous electrical nerve stimulation (TENS)**, involving stimulation of the skin with a mild electrical current passed through external electrodes. The therapy requires a physician's order. The TENS unit consists of a battery-powered transmitter, lead wires, and electrodes. The electrodes are placed directly over or near the site of pain. Hair or skin preparations should be removed before attaching the electrodes. When a client feels pain, the transmitter is turned on and a buzzing or tingling sensation is created. The client may adjust the intensity and quality of skin stimulation. The tingling sensation can be applied until pain relief occurs. TENS is effective for postsurgical pain control and reduction of pain caused by postoperative procedures (e.g., removing drains and cleaning and repacking surgical wounds) (Hargreaves and Lander, 1989).

PHARMACOLOGICAL PAIN THERAPY

Several pharmacological agents provide pain management. All require a physician's order. The nurse's judgment in the use of medications and management of clients receiving pharmacological therapies helps ensure the best pain relief possible.

Acute Pain Management. Nurses care for clients who undergo surgery and medical procedures (e.g., endoscopy), and who are victims of trauma. The approach to therapy ranges from having no set strategy to using a comprehensive team approach. The AHCPR (1992) has established a pain-treatment flow chart (Fig. 43-12) for the aggressive treatment of postoperative pain. The guidelines are also applicable to clients recovering from painful medical procedures and trauma. The systematic approach ensures quick response on the part of care givers to client discomfort. The key to success is ongoing evaluation of therapies: Is relief obtained? Are their unacceptable side effects of medications? The health care team collaborates to find the combination of therapy that works best for a client.

Analgesics. **Analgesics** are the most common method of pain relief. Although analgesics can effectively relieve pain, nurses and physicians still tend to undertreat clients because of incorrect drug information, concerns about addiction, anxiety over errors in using **narcotic analgesics**, and administration of less medication than was ordered. Nurses must understand the drugs available for pain relief and their pharmacological effects.

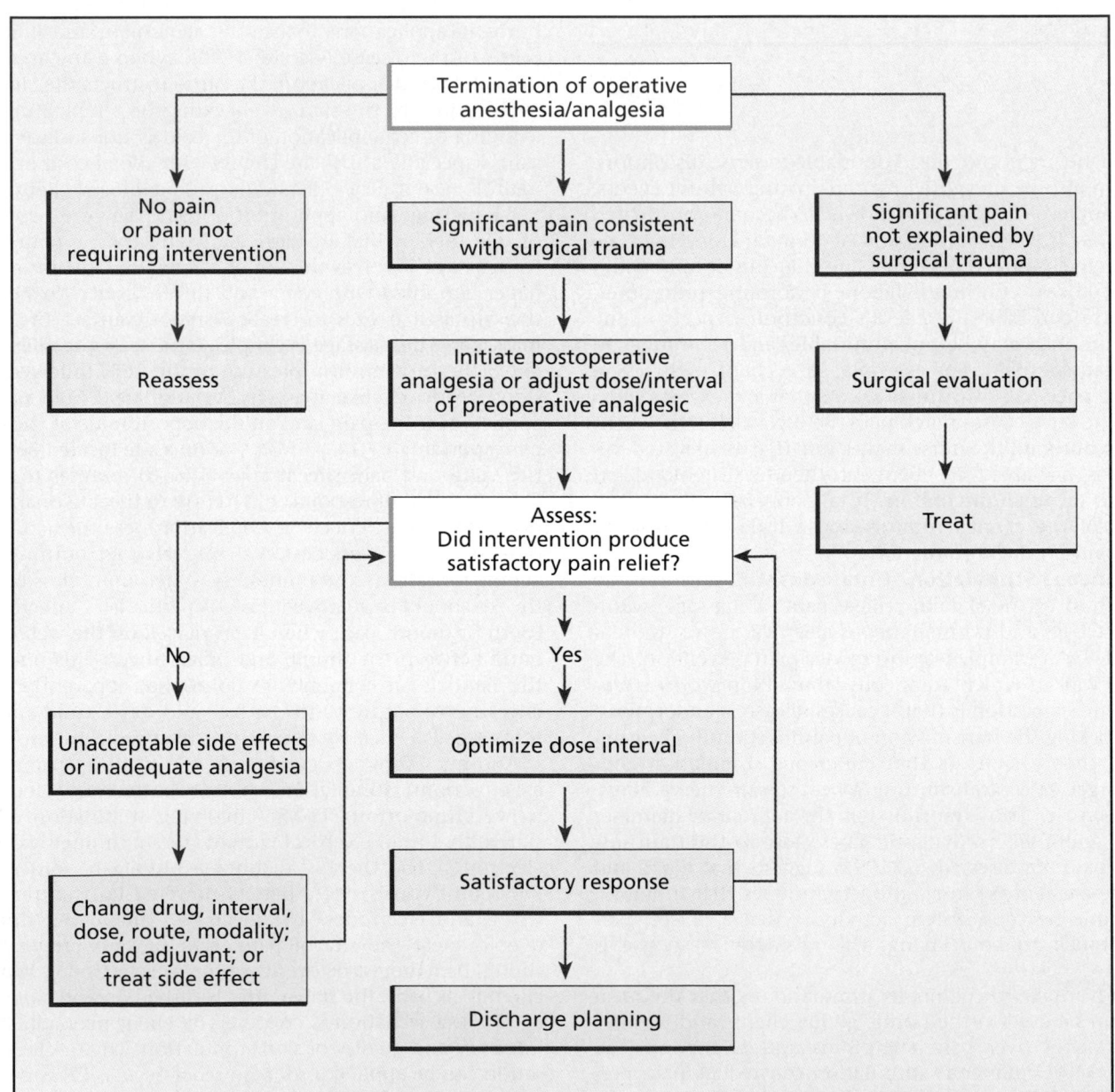

Fig. 43-12 Pain treatment flow chart: postoperative phase. *(From Acute Pain Management Guideline Panel: Acute pain management: operative or medical procedures and trauma, clinical practice guideline, AHCPR Pub No 92-0032. Rockville, MD, 1992, AHCPR, PHS, USDHHS.)*

Table 43-6	Analgesics and Indications for Therapy
DRUG CATEGORY	**INDICATIONS**
NONNARCOTIC ANALGESICS	
Acetaminophen (Tylenol)	Mild postoperative pain
Acetylsalicylic acid (aspirin)	Fever
NSAIDs	
Ibuprofen (Motrin, Nuprin)	Dysmenorrhea
Naproxen (Naprosyn)	Vascular headaches
Indomethacin (Indocin)	Rheumatoid arthritis
Tolmetin (Tolectin)	Soft tissue athletic injury
Piroxicam (Feldene)	Gout
Ketorolac (Toradol)	Postoperative pain
	Severe traumatic pain
NARCOTIC ANALGESICS	
Meperidine (Demerol)	Cancer pain (except meperidine)
Methylmorphine (codeine)	Myocardial infarction
Morphine sulfate	
Fentanyl (Sublimaze)	
Butorphanol (Stadol)	
Hydromorphone HCL (Dilaudid)	
ADJUVANTS	
Amitriptyline (Elavil)	Anxiety
Hydroxyzine (Vistaril)	Depression
Chlorpromazine (Thorazine)	Nausea
Diazepam (Valium)	Vomiting

There are three types of analgesics: (1) nonnarcotic and nonsteroidal antiinflammatory drugs (NSAIDs), (2) narcotic analgesics or opioids, and (3) adjuvants or coanalgesics (Table 43-6). Nonnarcotic NSAIDs generally provide relief for mild to moderate pain, such as the pain associated with rheumatoid arthritis, minor surgical and dental procedures, episiotomy, and low-back problems. One exception, ketorolac (Toradol), is the first injectable analgesic NSAID that is comparable to morphine in efficacy (McKenry and Salerno, 1995). Treatment of mild to moderate postoperative pain should begin, unless contraindicated, with an NSAID (AHCPR, 1992). Although the exact mechanism of action is unknown, NSAIDs are believed to act by inhibiting the synthesis of prostaglandins (McKenry and Salerno, 1995) and by inhibiting the cellular responses during inflammation. Most NSAIDs act on peripheral nerve receptors to reduce transmission and reception of pain stimuli. Unlike opioids, NSAIDs do not cause sedation or respiratory depression, nor do they interfere with bowel or bladder function (AHCPR, 1992).

Opioid or narcotic analgesics are generally prescribed for moderately severe to severe pain, such as postoperative and malignant pain. They act on the central nervous system to produce a combination of depressing and stimulating effects. Adjuvants such as sedatives, antianxiety agents, and muscle relaxants enhance pain control or relieve other symptoms associated with pain, such as depression and nausea. They may be given alone or with analgesics. Sedatives are often prescribed to chronic pain sufferers. These drugs can cause drowsiness and impairment of coordination, judgment, and mental alertness. Misuse of sedatives and antianxiety agents is a serious health problem that can cause disabling illness behaviors.

Narcotic analgesics, when given orally or by injection, act on higher centers of the brain and spinal cord by binding with opiate receptors to modify perception of and reaction to pain. Morphine sulfate is a derivative of opium and has the following characteristic analgesic effects:

1. Raising the pain threshold, thereby reducing pain perception
2. Reducing anxiety and fear, which are components of the reaction to pain
3. Inducing sleep even in the presence of severe pain

The danger of morphine sulfate and other narcotic analgesics is the potential for depression of vital nervous system functions. Opiates cause respiratory depression by depressing the respiratory center within the brainstem. Clients also experience side effects such as nausea, vomiting, constipation, and altered mental processes. Characteristics of an ideal analgesic should include:

1. Rapid onset
2. Prolonged effectiveness
3. Effectiveness in all age groups
4. Oral and parenteral use
5. Lack of severe side effects
6. Nonaddicting nature
7. Inexpensive

The proper use of analgesics requires careful assessment, application of pharmacological principles, and common sense (see the box on p. 1180). A person's response to an analgesic is highly individualized. An NSAID may be as effective as a potent narcotic for some clients, or an orally administered analgesic may bring the same relief as an injectable form. Nurses must stay familiar with comparative doses of different analgesics. In addition, nurses must know the route of administration most effective for a client so that controlled, sustained pain relief is achieved.

The nurse should always know the comparative potencies of analgesics in oral and injectable form. For example, a physician may order meperidine 50 to 100 mg intramuscularly or orally every 3 to 4 hours as necessary. This order leaves much to the judgment of the nurse and requires clarification. Such an order can create confusion. The nurse must select the best dose, route, and interval. A 75-mg dose of meperidine (Demerol) has about the same analgesic strength as 10 mg of morphine intramuscularly (McKenry and Salerno, 1995). The lowest dose, 50 mg, by mouth is equal to the strength of two aspirin. If nurses on succeeding shifts choose different routes for the same doses, the client will not receive the same level of analgesia, and pain control will be poor. Nurses must provide controlled, sustained pain relief. Equianalgesic charts that convert recommended adult doses to children's doses are available. These charts consider age and body size. Older adults also require special considerations (see the box on p. 1180).

Patient-Controlled Analgesia. Clients benefit from having control over pain therapy. When clients depend on nurses for **analgesia**, an erratic cycle of alternating pain and analgesia often occurs. The client feels pain and asks for medication, but the nurse must first assess the client and then prepare the medication. Within an hour analgesia finally occurs, but pain relief may last only 30 minutes, and

Nursing Principles for Administering Analgesics

Know the Client's Previous Response to Analgesics
- Determine whether relief was obtained.
- Ask whether a nonnarcotic was as effective as a narcotic.
- Identify previous doses and routes of administration to avoid undertreatment.
- Determine whether the client has allergies.

Select Proper Medications When More Than One is Ordered
- Use nonnarcotic analgesics or milder narcotics for mild to moderate pain.
- Know that nonnarcotics can be alternated with narcotics.
- In older adults, avoid combinations of narcotics.
- Remember that morphine and hydromorphone are the narcotics of choice for long-term management of severe pain.
- Know that injectable medications act quicker and can relieve severe, acute pain within 1 hour and that oral medication may take as long as 2 hours to relieve pain.

- Use a narcotic with a nonnarcotic analgesic for severe pain because such combinations treat pain peripherally and centrally.
- For chronic pain, give an oral drug for sustained relief.

Know the Accurate Dosage
- Remember that doses at the upper end of normal are generally needed for severe pain.
- Adjust doses, as appropriate, for children and older clients.

Assess the Right Time and Interval for Administration
- Administer analgesics as soon as pain occurs and before it increases in severity.
- Do not give analgesics only by ordered schedules. Remember that an around-the-clock administration schedule is usually best.
- Give analgesics before pain-producing procedures or activities.
- Know the average duration of action for a drug and the time of administration so that the peak effect occurs when pain is most intense.

GERONTOLOGICAL PRINCIPLES for Pain Control

- In older adults there is fear that pain will result in crippling and forced dependency.
- Older adults are at high risk for pain-inducing situations.
- The potential for lowered pain tolerance exists with diminished adaptive capacity.
- Changes in peripheral vascular function, skin, and transmission of pain impulses place the older adult at risk for being unable to sense pain (Ebersole and Hess, 1994).
- It is not uncommon for acuity of symptoms or severity of pain to be less dramatic in older persons than in younger persons.
- Older adults may be susceptible to side effects of narcotics because of changes in serum proteins, liver and renal function, and a reduction in cardiac output.
- The risk for gastric and renal toxicity from NSAIDs is increased among older adults.
- Older adults are more sensitive to the analgesic effects of opioid drugs because they experience a higher peak and longer duration of pain relief.
- Pain is *not* normal with aging. Presence of pain requires aggressive assessment and management.

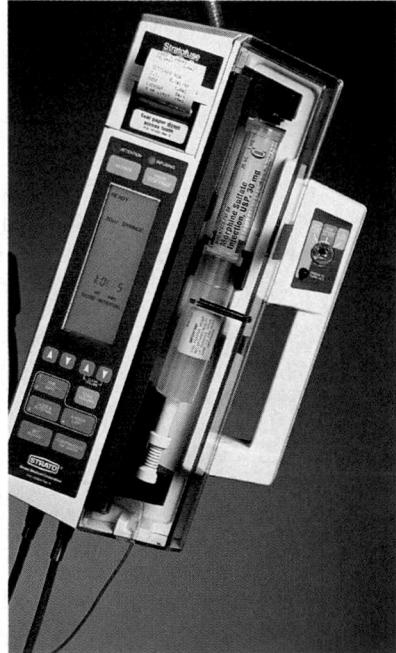

Fig. 43-13 Patient-controlled analgesic device.

the client may be sedated as long as an hour. Then, gradually, the client again feels discomfort, and the cycle begins again.

A drug delivery system called **patient-controlled analgesia (PCA)** is a safe method for postoperative, traumatic, and cancer pain management that most clients prefer to intermittent injections. It is a drug delivery system that allows clients to administer pain medications when they want them without risk of overdose. The goal is to maintain a constant plasma level of analgesic so that the prob-

lems of as-needed (prn) dosing are avoided. Systemic PCA usually involves IV drug administration, but it can also be given subcutaneously. PCAs are portable infusion pumps (usually computerized), containing a chamber for a syringe (Fig. 43-13), or specifically designed devices such as a wristwatch doser that delivers a small, preset dose of medication. The analgesic of choice is morphine. To receive a dose the client pushes a button attached to the PCA device. The system is designed to deliver no more than a specified number of doses either every hour or 4 hours (depending on the

CLIENT TEACHING and Preparation for PCA

OBJECTIVES
Client will be able to explain purpose of PCA in managing pain.
Client will use the PCA device correctly.
Client achieves pain control.

TEACHING STRATEGIES
Teach the use of PCA before any sedative is administered so that clients can understand how to use it after awakening from anesthesia or sedation.
Instruct client on the purpose of PCA, the operating instructions, expected pain relief, precautions, and potential side effects (Intravenous Nurses Society [IVNS], 1990), emphasizing that the client controls medication delivery.
Explain that the pump prevents the risk of overdose.
Tell family members or friends that they should not operate the PCA device for the client.
Have the client demonstrate use of the PCA delivery button.

EVALUATION
Ask client to tell you the purpose of the PCA device.
Observe the client administer a dose.
Evaluate the severity of the client's pain 15 to 20 minutes after use of the PCA.

pump) to avoid overdoses. A typical PCA prescription relies on a series of "loading" doses; for example, 3 to 5 mg of morphine, repeated every 5 minutes until initial postoperative pain diminishes. A low-dose basal infusion (0.5 to 1 mg/hr) at night allows uninterrupted sleep. On-demand doses typically add 1 mg morphine every 6 minutes, with a total hourly limit of 10 mg (AHCPR, 1992). Most pumps have locked safety systems that prevent tampering by clients or their family members. Even though a dose can be released over only a select number of minutes, a small bell alarms in some PCA units each time the client pushes the button.

Benefits of PCA include the control clients gain over their pain, pain relief that does not depend on nurse availability, the tendency for clients to take less medication, and that small doses of narcotics are delivered at short intervals, stabilizing serum drug concentrations for sustained pain relief. Client preparation and teaching is critical to the safe and effective use of PCAs (see the box above). Clients must be able to understand the use of the equipment and be physically able to locate and press the button to deliver the dose. Clients who are confused and unresponsive, those with neurological disease, and those with impaired renal or pulmonary function are not candidates for PCA.

Nurses must check the intravenous line and PCA device regularly to ensure proper functioning. Certain pumps keep track of accumulative dosage and print out the information on demand. Even though clients control administration of analgesics, the nurse must routinely check that the PCA device operates correctly. The nurse also documents drug dosages and tracks any waste of narcotics.

Local and Regional Anesthetics. Local anesthesia is the loss of sensation to a localized body part. Physicians use local anesthesia while suturing a wound, delivering an infant, and performing simple surgery. Local anesthetics have fewer risks than general anesthetics, which cause loss of consciousness and depress vital functions. Local anesthetics can be applied topically on skin and mucous membranes or injected to anesthetize a body part. The drugs produce temporary loss of sensation by inhibiting nerve conduction; they also block motor and autonomic functions when administered as nerve blocks. Local anesthetics block the function of sensory, motor, and autonomic neurons supplying the affected area. Thus when the client temporarily loses sensation in a body part, motor and autonomic function is also lost. Smaller sensory nerve fibers are more sensitive to local anesthetics than are large motor fibers. As a result, the client loses sensation before losing motor function, and conversely, motor activity returns before sensation.

Local anesthetics can cause side effects, depending on their absorption into the circulation. Itching or burning of the skin or a localized rash is common after topical applications. Application to vascular mucous membranes increases the chance of systemic effects such as a change in heart rate. Injection of anesthetics increases the risk of systemic side effects, depending on the amount of drug used and the area injected.

Table 43-7 summarizes the types of local anesthesia by injection. Each produces a different level of anesthesia as a result of the amount of anesthetic used and location of the spinal nerve affected.

The nurse provides emotional support to clients receiving local anesthesia by explaining insertion sites and warning clients that they will temporarily lose sensory function. It is common for clients to fear paralysis because epidural and spinal injections come close to the spinal cord. Autonomic function (bowel and bladder control) may also be temporarily lost. To reassure the client, the nurse explains application of the anesthetic and the sensations experienced. Injection can be painful unless the physician numbs the injection site. The nurse prepares clients for such discomfort. Before a client receives an anesthetic, the nurse checks for allergies. To monitor systemic effects, the nurse assesses blood pressure and pulse. Spinal anesthesia may also cause respiratory changes.

After administration of a local anesthetic, the nurse protects the client from injury until full sensory and motor function return. Pain is a protective mechanism. Until a local anesthetic is absorbed and metabolized, the client must be careful in using an anesthetized body part. Clients can easily injure themselves without knowing it. For example, after an injection into a joint, the nurse warns the client to avoid using the joint until function returns. For clients with topical anesthesia, the nurse avoids applying heat or cold to numb areas. After spinal anesthesia, the client stays in bed until sensory and motor function return. The nurse assists the client during the first attempt at getting out of bed.

Epidural Analgesia. Epidural analgesia is a form of local anesthesia and an effective therapy for the treatment of acute postoperative pain, labor and delivery pain, and chronic pain, especially that associated with cancer (McNair, 1990). It permits control or reduction of severe pain without the more

Table 43-7	Local Anesthesia Techniques		
TYPE	**AREA OF INJECTION**	**AREA ANESTHETIZED**	**INDICATIONS FOR USE**
Infiltration	In superficial area under skin or mucous membranes	Small peripheral nerves to area infiltrated	Small incisions of skin, insertion of sutures to close cuts or wounds, minor dental repairs
Peripheral nerve block	In area surrounding large peripheral nerve at point above bifurcation of nerve	Wider area than with infiltration, numbing entire body part (e.g., hand, upper gums, foot)	Major dental repairs, manipulation or reduction of extremity fractures, minor hand and foot surgery
Epidural or peridural nerve block	In lumbosacral region of spinal cord, around major nerve roots exiting base of spinal cord at site outside dura mater	Lower trunk and extremities	Delivery of newborn, major surgery to lower trunk and extremities (e.g., hemorrhoidectomy, appendectomy, vascular repair)
Spinal nerve block	Around major nerve root within subarachnoid space of spinal cord	Lower trunk and extremities	Major surgery to lower trunk and extremities, clients at risk with general anesthesia

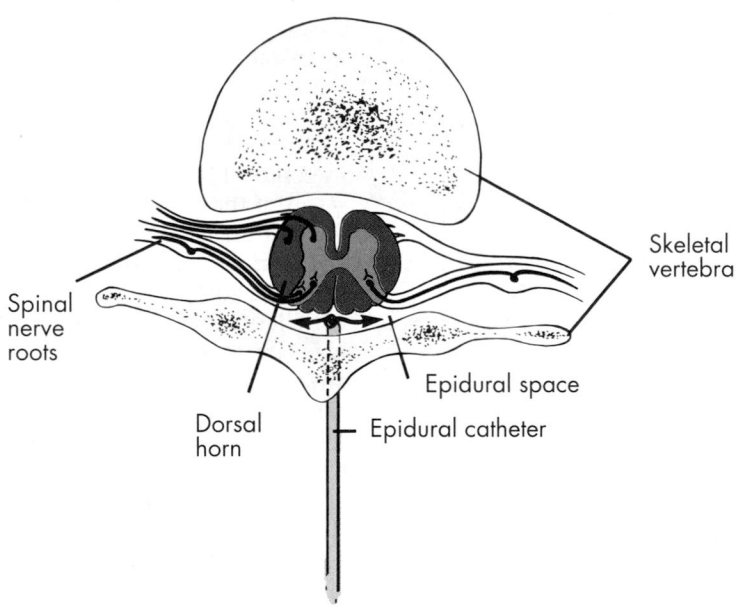

Fig. 43-14 Anatomical drawing of epidural space.

serious sedative effects of parenteral or oral narcotics. (However, intraspinal morphine can produce the same side effects of nausea, mental clouding, and sedation, since it is absorbed into the circulation of the epidural vascular plexus). Epidural analgesia can be short or long term, depending on the client's condition and life expectancy. Short-term therapy is used for pain after intrathoracic, abdominal, and orthopedic surgery. Long-term therapy is used for intractable pain in the lower part of the body, particularly when it is bilateral (DuPen and Williams, 1992). McNair (1990) lists several advantages of epidural analgesia, including:

- Production of excellent analgesia
- Occurrence of minimal sedation
- Action of long duration
- Facilitation of early ambulation

- Avoidance of repeated injections
- No significant effect on sensation
- Little effect on blood pressure or heart rate

Epidural analgesia is administered into the spinal **epidural space.** The physician inserts a blunt-tip needle into the spinous processes of the lumbar vertebra (L3 and L4). Unlike with spinal anesthesia, the needle for epidural anesthesia does not enter the subarachnoid space. When the needle reaches the space, solutions may be freely injected and small catheters may be passed into it. Once a catheter is advanced into the epidural space (Fig. 43-14) and the needle is removed, the remainder of the catheter is secured with occlusive dressing and taped up the back of the client (Fig. 43-15). If the catheter is only temporary, it is connected to tubing positioned along the spine and over the brightly colored intermittent injection cap on the catheter tubing. Labeling the catheter "epidural catheter" also helps. Continuous infusions must be administered through electronic infusion devices for proper control (IVNS, 1990). Because of the catheter location, strict surgical asepsis is needed to prevent a serious and potentially fatal infection. Physicians are notified immediately of any signs or symptoms of infection or pain at the insertion site. Thorough nursing care is needed during hygiene procedures to keep the catheter system clean and dry.

Nurses receive special training for the administration of epidural analgesia. Narcotics used commonly for epidural analgesia include preservative-free morphine sulfate, fentanyl, sufentanil, and hydromorphone. Morphine has a long-lasting effect but also causes more side effects (Sabbe and Yaksh, 1990). The medications act like the neurotransmitter enkephalin, an endorphin, blocking transmission of pain stimuli in the spinal cord (McNair, 1990).

Frequently a local anesthetic such as bupivacaine is also administered. The anesthetic blocks pain conduction through local peripheral nerve fibers around the site of insertion. Bupivacaine also blocks the sympathetic nervous system, causing side effects such as hypotension, reduced intestinal peristalsis, and bladder dysfunction.

The nursing implications for managing epidural analgesia are numerous (Table 43-8). Monitoring of the medication's effects differs, depending on whether infusions are intermittent or continuous. Complications of epidural narcotic use include respiratory depression (rare but most serious), nausea and vomiting, urinary retention, constipation, and pruritus. When clients are started on epidural analgesia, monitoring occurs as often as every 15 minutes, including assessment of respiratory rate, respiratory effort, and skin color. Once stabilized, monitoring can move to every hour (refer to agency policy). The client must receive thorough education about epidural analgesia in terms of the action of the medication and its advantages and disadvantages. Clients should know about the potential for respiratory depression and should be instructed to notify a

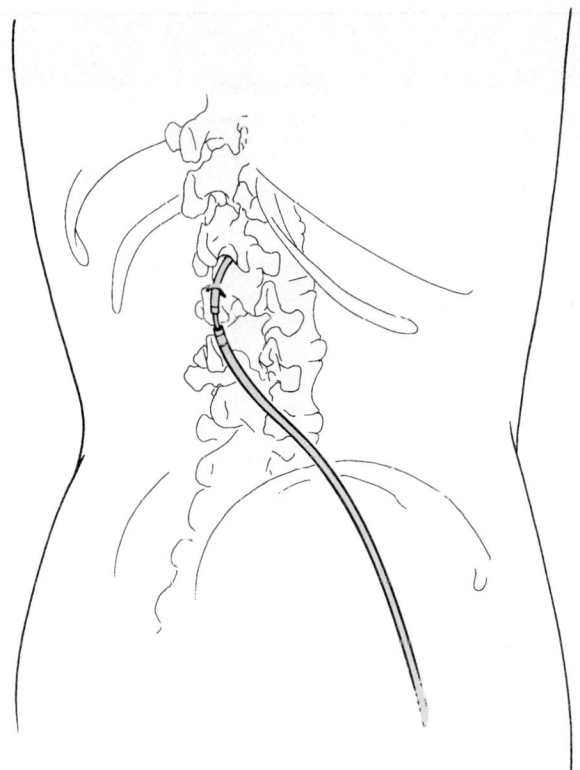

Fig. 43-15 Epidural catheter.

client's shoulder. The end of the catheter can then be placed on the client's chest for the nurse's access. Permanent catheters may be tunneled through the skin and exit at the client's side.

The catheter is connected to a continuous epidural infusion pump, a port or reservoir, or is capped off for bolus injections. To reduce the risk of accidental epidural injection of drugs intended for intravenous use, it helps to place a

Table 43-8	**Nursing Care of Clients with Epidural Infusions**
GOAL	**ACTIONS**
Prevent catheter displacement.	Secure catheter (if not connected to implanted reservoir) carefully to outside skin.
Maintain catheter function.	Check external dressing around catheter site for dampness or discharge. (Leak of cerebrospinal fluid may develop.) Use transparent, adhesive dressing to aid inspection. Inspect catheter for breaks.
Prevent infection.	Use strict aseptic technique when caring for catheter (see Chapter 34). Do not routinely change dressing over site. Change tubing every 24 hours.
Monitor for respiratory depression.	Monitor vital signs, especially respirations, per policy. Pulse oximetry and apnea monitoring may be used.
Prevent undesirable complications.	Assess for pruritis (itching) and nausea and vomiting. Administer antiemetics as ordered.
Maintain urinary and bowel function.	Monitor intake and output. Assess for bladder and bowel distention. Assess for discomfort, frequency, and urgency.

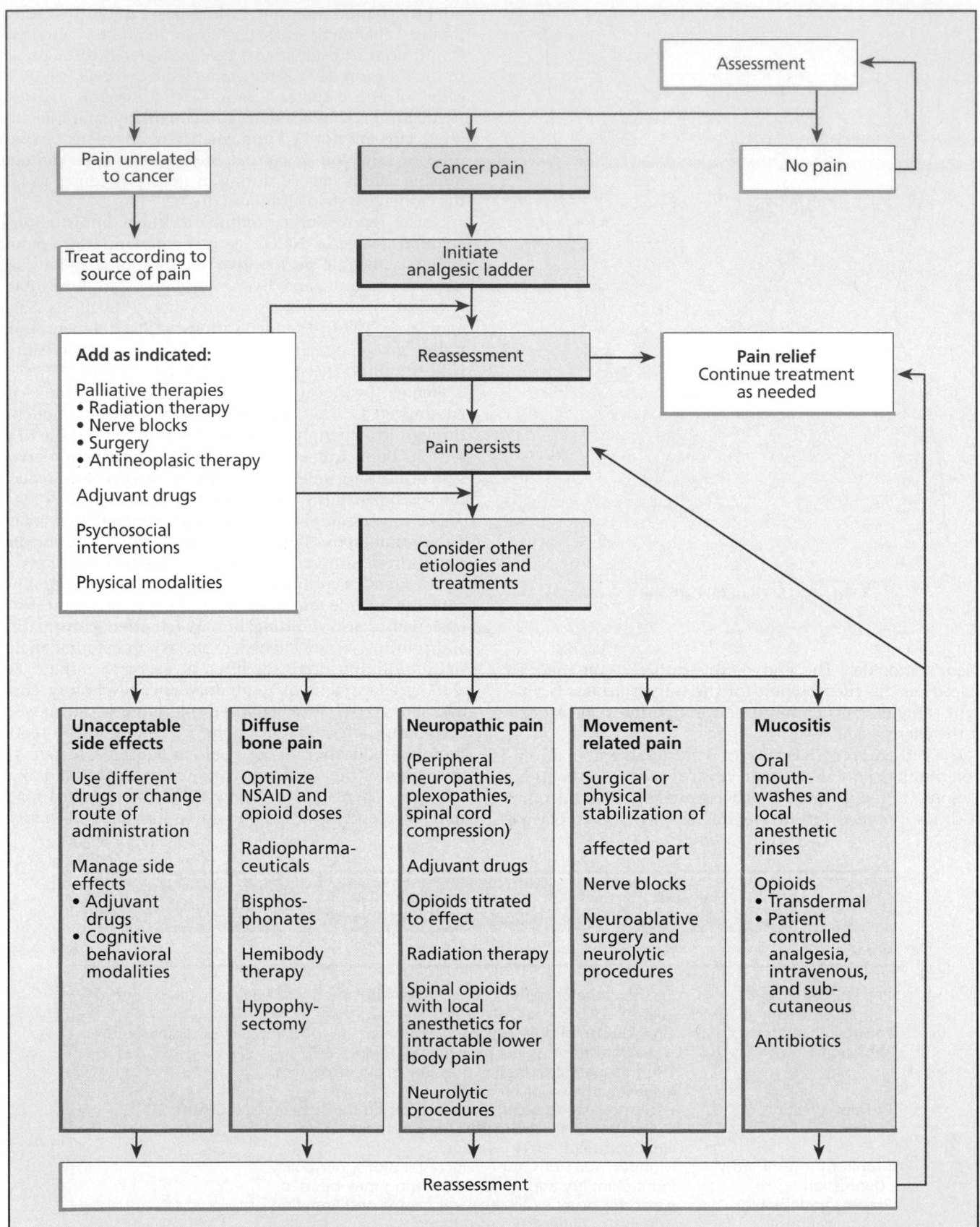

Fig. 43-16 Flow chart: continuing pain management in patients with cancer. *(From Jacox A, Carr DB, Payne R, et al: Management of cancer pain. Clinical practice guideline No. 9 AHCPR Pub. No. 94-0592, Rockville, MD, 1992, Agency for Health Care Policy and Research, USDHHS, PHS.)*

health care provider if breathing difficulty develops. If respiratory depression develops, the infusion is turned off immediately. A client on long-term therapy can be taught to safely administer infusions in the home with minimal ongoing intervention by the nurse.

SURGICAL MEASURES FOR PAIN RELIEF

When a client's pain persists despite medical treatment and it is clear that the pain is physical and not psychological, surgical therapies may give relief. Neurosurgical treatment is appropriate for clients in whom more conservative treatment is neither tolerated nor effective (Jacox et al, 1994). The risks include new pain symptoms from nerve damage or nerve division, recurrence of pain, and postoperative neurological impairment. Surgery involves resection of either peripheral nerve roots or pain pathways in the spinothalamic tract. For example, a **dorsal rhizotomy** involves surgically cutting the dorsal (posterior) nerve roots as they enter the spinal cord. It is effective for relieving localized acute pain in the area supplied by the nerve root and deep visceral pain. The client loses sensation of pain but retains full motor function. A **chordotomy** is more extensive and involves resection of the spinothalamic tract. The procedure is used to treat intractable or unrelieved pain. The risks of the procedure are great because permanent paralysis may result from edema of the spinal cord or accidental resection of motor nerves. After the procedure, the client has a permanent loss of pain and temperature sensation in the affected areas.

When nurses care for these clients, it is important to be aware of the area of resection to assess for paresthesias, change in temperature sensation, and loss of motor function. When performed correctly, these procedures can relieve persistent pain without causing serious neurological deficits.

CLIENTS WITH INTRACTABLE PAIN

Intractable pain cannot be permanently relieved. The pain can become so debilitating that a client will try anything to gain relief. Chronic intractable pain encompasses a client's total existence and can often lead clients to reject active treatment programs and even to consider or commit suicide (Jacox et al, 1994). One of the greatest nursing challenges is to care for the client with intractable pain. The AHCPR released clinical practice guidelines for the management of cancer pain (Jacox et al, 1994). The guidelines are designed to treat cancer pain in a more comprehensive and aggressive manner. Similarly, they provide clients and families more options for pain relief. Fig. 43-16 is a flow chart depicting cancer pain management from assessment to various treatment options. The best choice of treatment often changes as the client's condition and the characteristics of pain change. Nonpharmacological therapies as well as pharmacological therapies can be used together.

Administering analgesics to treat cancer-related pain requires applying principles different from those used to treat acute pain. The World Health Organization (1990) recommends a three-step approach to managing cancer pain (Fig. 43-17). Basically, therapy begins with using NSAIDs and/or adjuvants and progresses to strong opioids if pain persists. When a client with cancer first experiences pain, it is best to begin with a higher dosage than will be needed

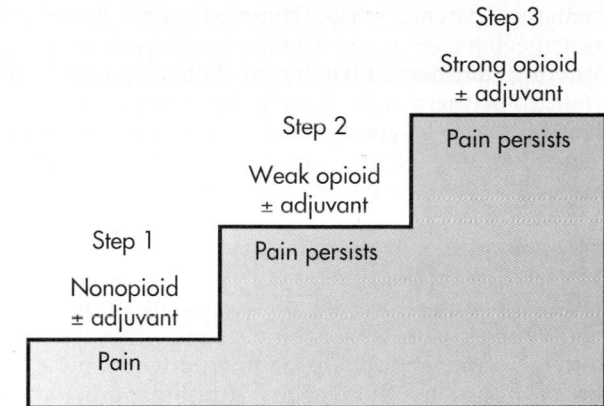

Fig. 43-17 WHO analgesic ladder is a three-step approach to using drugs in cancer pain management. ±*adjuvant,* with or without adjuvant medications. *(From World Health Organization: Cancer pain relief and palliative care: report of a WHO Expert Committee, WHO Tech Rep Series NO 804, Geneva, 1990, The Organization.)*

for relief. The physician can slowly decrease the dosage to the amount needed, thus providing the client with immediate pain relief. In addition, there is aggressive treatment of the side effects of analgesia such as nausea and constipation so that analgesia can be continued.

Studies show that drug dependence is low among clients with cancer-related pain. Giving the right drug and the required dose at the proper interval alleviates the fear of pain, protects the client from drug-seeking behavior, and reduces dependence. It has also been shown that terminally ill clients with prolonged pain develop a tolerance to analgesics. As a result, clients require higher doses of analgesics to attain pain relief. Higher analgesic doses in clients who have become tolerant to narcotics are not lethal because these clients also develop a tolerance to life-threatening side effects.

For clients with cancer, the aim of drug therapy is to anticipate and minimize pain rather than cure it. It is therefore necessary to give required doses on a regular basis. Prescribing analgesics on a prn basis for cancer clients is ineffective and causes more suffering. The cancer client must take an analgesic regularly, even when the pain, nausea, and other symptoms subside. Regular administration maintains blood levels for ongoing pain control.

Various medications and routes of administration can provide some relief for chronic pain sufferers. Some medications can provide pain relief. Epidural analgesia has been highly effective. Intrathecal infusion (administration of opioids via catheters placed within the brain's ventricles) is also helpful in select clients. In addition, there are relatively new analgesics with fewer side effects. Long-acting or controlled-release morphine sulfate has been very successful. Two of these medications are MS Contin and Roxanol SR. Pain relief can be obtained with MS Contin for 8 to 12 hours and with Roxanol SR for up to 6 hours (Wilkie, 1990).

Transdermal drug systems administer drugs such as fentanyl over predetermined rates up to 48 to 72 hours. This route is useful when clients are unable to take drugs orally. Clients find these systems easy to use and they allow for continuous opioid administration without needles or pumps.

Self-adhesive patches release the medication slowly over time, achieving effective analgesia. Caution is needed in administering transdermal patches to clients who are hyperthermic. Hyperthermia causes more rapid drug absorption.

Analgesics may be given rectally when clients have nausea and vomiting or are fasting before or after surgery (Jacox et al, 1994). The route is contraindicated if clients have diarrhea or if cancerous lesions involve the anus or rectum. Morphine, hydromorphone, and oxymorphone are available in suppositories.

Another popular measure for treatment of severe intractable cancer pain is morphine sulfate administered by continuous intravenous drip or intermittently by a PCA pump. Continuous intravenous infusions provide improved, uniform pain control with fewer peaks and valleys in plasma concentration, more effective drug action, and lower drug dosages overall. Thus there are fewer side effects. Although a client receives a continuous infusion of morphine sulfate, the total daily dose may be less than with conventional intramuscular injections. Candidates for continuous infusions include clients with severe pain, for whom oral and injectable narcotics provide minimal relief; clients with severe nausea and vomiting; clients with clotting disorders who bruise from injections; and clients unable to swallow oral medications.

Continuous-drip morphine sulfate is given in acute care settings and in the home. The morphine sulfate is delivered by an infusion control pump to ensure a safe, accurate, and steady rate of infusion. Each agency has guidelines for morphine dose and infusion rates. The drug can cause numerous side effects that initially require the nurse's ongoing assessment. Clients receiving the drug at home are taught how to monitor the drug's effects (see the box below). Adjuvant drugs, such as antiemetics, corticosteroids, anticonvulsants, neuroleptics, biphosphonates, and calcitonin (given for bone pain), or antidepressants may be needed to enhance pain control and prevent side effects (Paice, 1991; Jacox et al, 1994).

When a client is first placed on continuous-drip morphine sulfate, it is essential that an intravenous access is patent and the intravenous site is without complications (see Chapter 45). A central line catheter such as a Hickman, an implanted venous access port, or a peripherally inserted central catheter (PICC) are usually best suited for long-term IV infusion. When infusions begin, the nurse records baseline blood pressure and respiratory rates to begin monitoring for central nervous system depression. After an infusion starts, the nurse monitors vital signs as often as every 15 to 30 minutes for the first few hours until the client gains relief at a constant dosage. If blood pressure or respirations decrease, the infusion rate is reduced according to the physician's order or agency policy. If the client shows signs of severe respiratory depression, the physician orders that the infusion be discontinued. The narcotic antagonist naloxone (Narcan) should be available to reverse respiratory depression.

In the home, clients may use ambulatory infusion pumps. State-of-the-art ambulatory pumps are small devices, often no larger than a deck of cards, that contain a 1- to 30-day supply of medication. The pumps are lightweight and allow free movement. The pump is battery powered and worn in a pouch attached to a belt or harness. The bag of medication and intravenous fluid fits inside the pump.

CLIENT TEACHING
on Ambulatory Infusion Pumps

OBJECTIVES
Client and family will identify and be alert for side effects of excess morphine infusion.
Client and family will take proper action in the case of pump malfunction.
Client and family will identify precautions to take in managing daily pump care.
Family will know when and how to react in an emergency.

TEACHING STRATEGIES
■ Tell client and family to observe for the following side effects: dizziness or fainting, nausea, vomiting, slow and shallow respirations, constipation, mood changes, euphoria, inability to empty bladder fully, dry mouth, weakness, agitation, tremors, strange dreams.
■ Instruct family on how to administer naloxone (Narcan) intramuscularly to reverse respiratory depression.
■ Teach client and family how to keep central venous catheter patent, maintain pump flow rate, and irrigate the catheter routinely with heparin flush.
■ Tell client how to prevent air from entering central venous catheter and to clamp catheter when infusion has stopped.
■ Explain how to prevent infection at catheter site and to keep site clean with soap and water.

■ Have client follow a preventive bowel routine using stool softeners, laxatives, dietary fiber, hydration, and routine exercise.
■ Warn client against wearing pump in shower or submerging in bathtub. Device can be temporarily disconnected during shower or placed in a plastic bag hung outside shower or tub.
■ During sleep, keep the pump on the bed or adjacent nightstand. During lovemaking, the pump can be set to the side so it does not interfere with closeness and intimacy.
■ Instruct the client and family on the purpose of the pump alarms and how to respond when they go off.
■ Keep a 24-hour emergency telephone number nearby.

EVALUATION
Ask client and family to describe the common side effects to expect from morphine overdose.
Give the client and family situations involving pump malfunction and have them explain the action they would take to correct the problem.
Ask client and family to describe routine precautions to take while wearing the pump.
Have family explain what to do should the client develop respiratory depression.

Although the pumps are programmed by physicians, pharmacists, or nurses, clients must be highly motivated to care for the pump properly. The client must show the capacity to learn the procedures and to assume responsibility for proper pump operation (Bernstein et al, 1993). In addition, it is important that the client have the physical capabilities to make adjustments to the pump (e.g., change batteries). The client and family learn to manage the pump, to observe for side effects, and to maintain function of the central venous catheter. Because the client is initially managed on morphine sulfate in the hospital before going home, the risk of side effects is not as great unless the client or family member increases drug doses. A home health care nurse makes routine visits to be sure that the client manages the pump correctly. The intravenous fluid bag and tubing are changed routinely by the nurse. This maintains the sterility of the system.

The nurse uses all available pain-relief measures for the client with cancer. The nurse-client relationship can help the client adapt to chronic pain. The client must feel that those responsible for managing the pain are competent and dependable.

PAIN CLINICS AND HOSPICES

During the last decade, health professionals from the United States and Canada have recognized pain as a significant health problem. With an increased awareness of the multiple problems that pain can cause for clients, programs have been designed for pain management. Pain clinics offer several options. A comprehensive pain center can treat persons on inpatient and outpatient bases. Staff members representing all health care disciplines such as nursing, medicine, physical therapy, and dietetics work with clients to find the most effective pain-relief measures. A comprehensive clinic provides not only diverse therapy but also research into new treatments and training for professionals.

There are also syndrome-oriented and modality-oriented pain centers. A syndrome-oriented center cares for clients with only specific types of pain, such as back pain or arthritis. Modality-oriented centers offer only specific types of treatment, such as biofeedback, acupuncture, or TENS.

Hospices are programs for care of the terminally ill. Hospice comes from the Latin word *hospes*, which means "a place to rest." Often, hospice programs are affiliated with hospitals. The programs help terminally ill clients continue to live at home in comfort and privacy with the help of a hospice health care team. Pain control is a priority for hospices. Clients receive the proper dosage and form of analgesics that provide pain relief. Under the guidance of hospice nurses, families learn to monitor clients' symptoms and become the primary care givers. A hospice client may become hospitalized in the event of a brief acute care crisis or family problem.

 ## Evaluation

The evaluation of pain is one of many nursing responsibilities that requires effective critical thinking. The client's behavioral responses and cues to pain relief therapies are not always so obvious. For example, some clients fear loss of control over the influence of pain medications and thus are not always honest about their effectiveness. The nurse must be an intent observer and know what responses to anticipate on the basis of the type of pain therapy, the timing of the therapy, the physiological nature of any injury or disease, and the client's previous responses.

The client is usually the best resource for evaluating the effectiveness of pain-relief measures. The nurse must continually determine whether the character of the client's pain changes and whether individual therapies are effective. The family often is another valuable resource, particularly in the case of the client with cancer, who may not be able to express discomfort during the latter stages of terminal illness. The nurse is successful in treating pain when the goals of care are met. The nurse uses evaluative criteria in determining the outcome of pain-relief therapies (see the evaluation box below).

If the nurse determines that a client continues to have discomfort after therapy, it may be necessary to try different or additional therapies. For example, if an analgesic provides only partial relief, the nurse may add relaxation exercises or guided-imagery exercises. The nurse may also consult with the physician about trying different analgesics.

The nurse also evaluates the client's perceptions of the effectiveness of therapy. The client may help decide the best times to attempt a treatment. For example, the client is the best judge of whether a therapy works better when anxiety and irritability are absent or when the pain is most severe.

 ## Sample Evaluation of Interventions for Pain

GOALS	EVALUATIVE MEASURES	EXPECTED OUTCOMES
Client and spouse will actively participate in pain-management plan.	Have client and spouse describe schedule for fentanyl patch placement. Ask client to discuss distraction techniques used for pain control. Have client and spouse discuss satisfaction with pain-control measures.	Client and spouse initiate pain-control therapies.
	Ask client during home visit to show you pain control log (review entries).	Client maintains daily log of pain-control therapy and responses.
Client achieves pain control.	Have client rate pain severity on visual analog scale.	Client reports pain severity of less than 4.

The nurse also determines tolerance to therapy and the overall relief obtained. For example, if a nurse administers an analgesic, side effects from the medication and the client's reported pain relief must be assessed. Similarly, after turning a client, the nurse should return to determine whether the client is tolerating the new position and whether pain has subsided. If a therapy aggravates discomfort, the nurse stops it immediately and seeks an alternative.

The nurse and client should not become frustrated if a therapy does not act quickly. Time and patience are necessary to maximize the effectiveness of a therapy. The nurse considers factors that may be influencing the client's perceptions or reactions to pain. For example, a backrub may prove ineffective if the client has just learned the results of diagnostic tests and has had no opportunity to express concerns. The nurse evaluates the entire pain experience to determine therapies that are most effective and times that they should be administered.

■ KEY CONCEPTS ■

▶ Pain is a subjective experience.

▶ A nurse's misconceptions about pain often result in doubt about the degree of the client's suffering and unwillingness to provide relief.

▶ Knowledge of the three components of the pain experience—reception, perception, and reaction—provides the nurse with guidelines for determining pain-relief measures.

▶ An interaction of psychological and cognitive factors affects pain perception.

▶ A person's cultural background influences the meaning of pain and how it is expressed.

▶ It is common for older clients not to report pain.

▶ Clients who are in chronic pain are likely to show more subtle behavioral changes than those in acute pain.

▶ The difference between acute and chronic pain involves duration of discomfort, physical signs and symptoms, and the client's perceptions regarding pain relief.

▶ The nurse does not collect a pain history when the client is experiencing severe discomfort.

▶ Pain scales are used to objectively evaluate the effectiveness of pain therapies.

▶ Pain can cause physical signs and symptoms similar to the signs and symptoms of certain disease processes.

▶ Clients waiting to undergo invasive tests may gain some pain relief by anticipatory guidance.

▶ To provide maximum pain relief the nurse develops a therapeutic caring relationship with the client.

▶ The nurse individualizes pain therapy by collaborating closely with the client, using assessment findings, and trying a variety of therapies.

▶ Eliminating sources of painful stimuli is a basic nursing measure for promoting comfort.

▶ Proper administration of analgesics requires the nurse to know the client's response to the drugs, to select the proper medication, and to administer an accurate dose in a timely manner.

▶ Using a regular schedule for analgesic administration is more effective than an as-needed schedule in controlling pain.

▶ A patient-controlled analgesic device gives clients pain control with low risk of overdose.

▶ While caring for a client who receives local anesthesia, the nurse protects the client from injury.

▶ Nursing implications for administering epidural analgesia include preventing infection and monitoring closely for respiratory depression.

▶ The aim of therapy for cancer clients is to anticipate and prevent pain rather than treat it.

▶ Evaluation of the client's pain therapy requires consideration of the changing character of pain, response to therapy, and the client's perceptions of a therapy's effectiveness.

■ KEY TERMS ■

Acupressure, p. 1173

Analgesics, p. 1178

Analgesia, p. 1179

Association cortex, p. 1156

Biofeedback, p. 1176

Chordotomy, p. 1185

Concomitant symptoms, p. 1168

Cutaneous stimulation, p. 1177

Dorsal rhizotomy, p. 1185

Epidural space, p. 1182

Euphoria, p. 1160

Exacerbations, p. 1160

Guided imagery, p. 1174

Holistic health, p. 1173

Intractable pain, p. 1160

Local anesthesia, p. 1181

Narcotic analgesics, p. 1178

Neuroregulators, p. 1156

Neurotransmitters, p. 1155

Nociceptors, p. 1155

Pain, p. 1154

Patient-controlled analgesia (PCA), p. 1180

Peripheral neuropathy, p. 1170

■ CRITICAL THINKING EXERCISES ■

1. Sarah is 80 years old and has remained independent, living in a small apartment two blocks from her daughter. The nurse at the physician's office has seen Sarah regularly over the last 10 years. She notices that Sarah is less lively, her posture is more stooped, and she regularly holds her hand over her abdomen. During examination, Sarah grimaces during abdominal palpation. When the nurse asks whether she has discomfort, Sarah says, "No, it just tickles." What should the nurse consider in further assessing Sarah for pain?

2. Mr. Rodriguez has come to the ambulatory care center for a same-day endoscopy. He has not had the procedure before. He is asking you appropriate questions as you begin to prepare him for the procedure. He will have an IV inserted prior to the endoscopy. What nonpharmacological methods might you use to provide comfort to this client?

3. Identify the pharmacological therapies best suited for the following situations:

   a. Jeff Newton is a 20-year-old who suffered a sprained ankle during a soccer game. He comes to the urgent care center; x-rays are negative.

   b. Mia Romero was admitted to the hospice program 3 months after being diagnosed with terminal breast cancer. She has bone metastasis with constant back pain.

   c. Linette Simpson underwent an abdominal hysterectomy this morning. She has awakened from anesthesia and is complaining of severe incisional pain.

4. As the nurse, you are making morning rounds and find Mr. Sarti lying on his side, arms wrapped around his knees. He groans while turning over to his back. He has a nasogastric tube in place and an intravenous catheter in his right arm. The progress notes from the night shift reveal that Mr. Sarti was admitted at midnight for acute abdominal pain. What measures might you take to promote Mr. Sarti's comfort?

REFERENCES

AHCPR, Acute Pain Management Guideline Panel: Acute pain management: operative or medical procedures and trauma. Clinical Practice Guideline. AHCPR Pub No. 92-0032. Rockville, MD: Agency for Health Care Policy and Research, Public Health Service, 1992, U.S. Dept of Health and Human Services.

Association for Holistic Health: *Statement on holistic health practitioners,* San Diego, California, 1981, The Association.

Bender JS: Approach to the acute abdomen, *Med Clin North Am* 73:1413, 1989.

Bernstein LH et al: Portable medicine pumps in primary care, *Patient Care* 27:91, 1993.

Beyer JE, Denyes MJ et al: The creation, validation, and continuing development of the Oucher: a measure of pain intensity in children, *J Pediatr Nurs* 7(5):335, 1992.

Burnside I: *Nursing and the aged,* ed 3, St Louis, 1988, Mosby.

Calvillo ER, Flaskerud JH: Review of literature on culture and pain of adults with focus on Mexican-Americans, *J Transcult Nurs* 2(2):16, 1991.

Carney RM: Clinical applications of relaxation training, *Hosp Pract* 18(7):83, 1983.

Ceccio CM: Heat vs cold as treatment for arthritic pain, *RN* 53:83, 1990.

Clancy J, McVicar A: Subjectivity of pain, *Br J Nurs* 1(1):8, 1992.

Copp LA: The spectrum of suffering, *Am J Nurs* 90:35, 1990.

Donahue P: *Nursing: the finest art,* St Louis, 1989, Mosby.

DuPen SL, Williams AR: Management of patients receiving combined epidural morphine and bupivacaine for the treatment of cancer pain, *J Pain Symptom Manage* 7(2):125, 1992.

Ebersole P, Hess P: *Toward healthy aging,* ed 3, St Louis, 1994, Mosby.

Edelman CL, Mandle CL: *Health promotion throughout the lifespan,* ed 3, St Louis, 1994, Mosby.

Flor H et al: Assessment of pain-related cognitions in chronic pain patients, *Behav Res Ther* 31(1):63, 1993.

Fortin F, Kirouac S: A randomized controlled trial of preoperative patient education, *Int J Nurs Stud* 13:11, 1976.

Gil K: Psychologic aspects of acute pain, *Anesthesiol Rep* 2(2):246, 1990.

Guzetta CE: Effects of relaxation and music therapy on patients in a coronary care unit with presumptive acute myocardial infarction, *Heart Lung* 18:609, 1989.

Hargreaves A, Lander J: Use of transcutaneous electrical nerve stimulation for postoperative pain, *Nurs Res* 38(3):159, 1989.

Harrison A: Assessing patients' pain: identifying reasons for error, *J Adv Nurs* 16:1018, 1991.

Herr KA, Mobily PR: Complexities of pain assessment in the elderly, *J Gerontol Nurs* 17(4):12, 1991.

International Association for the Study of Pain, Subcommittee on Taxonomy. Pain terms: a list with definitions and notes on usage, *Pain* 6:249, 1979.

Intravenous Nurses Society: Intravenous nursing standards of practice, *J Intravenous Nurs* S70, 1990.

Jacox A, Carr DB, Payne R, et al: *Management of cancer pain.* Clinical Practice Guideline No. 9. AHCPR Pub. No. 94-0592, Rockville, MD, 1994, Agency for Health Care Policy and Research, U.S. Dept HHS, PHS.

Jones RL, Cory PC: Mechanisms of pain, *J Am Acad Phys Assist* 3(5):378, 1990.

Kim MJ, McFarland GK, McLane AM: *Pocket guide to nursing diagnoses,* ed 6, St Louis, 1995, Mosby.

Kolcaba KY: A taxonomic structure for the concept comfort, *Image J Nurs Sch* 23(4):237, 1991.

Kolcaba KY: Holistic comfort: operationalizing the construct as a nurse-sensitive outcome, *Adv Nurs Sci* 15(1):1, 1992.

Mackey RB: Discover the healing power of therapeutic touch, *Am J Nurs* 95:27, April 1995.

Mahon SM: Concept analysis of pain: implications related to nursing diagnoses, *Nurs Diag* 5(1):14, 1994.

Martinelli AM: Pain and ethnicity: how people of different cultures experience pain, *AORN J* 46(2):273, 1987.

Marzinski LR: The tragedy of dementia: clinically assessing pain in the confused, nonverbal elderly, *J Gerontol Nurs* 17(6):25, 1991.

McCaffery M: *Nursing management of the patient with pain,* ed 2, Philadelphia, 1979, Lippincott.

McCaffery M: *Pain: assessment and intervention in nursing practice course syllabus,* St Louis, 1986, Barnes Hospital.

McCaffery M: Understanding your client's pain, *Nurs '80* 10:26, 1980.

McCaffery M, Beebe A: Pain in the elderly: special considerations. In McCaffery M, Beebe A: *Pain: clinical manual for nursing practice,* St Louis, 1989, Mosby–Year Book.

McGuire DB: The measurement of clinical pain, *Nurs Res* 33(3):152, 1984.

McGuire DB: Comprehensive and multidimensional assessment and measurement of pain, *J Pain Symptom Manage* 7(5):312, 1992.

McKerry LM, Salerno E: *Pharmacology in nursing,* ed 19, St Louis, 1994, Mosby.

McNair ND: Epidural narcotics for postoperative pain: nursing implications, *J Neurosci Nurs* 22(5):275, 1990.

Meek SS: Effects of slow-stroke back massage on relaxation in hospice clients, *Image J Nurs Sch* 25(1):17, 1993.

Meinhart NT, McCaffery M: *Pain: a nursing approach to assessment and analysis,* Norwalk, CT, 1983, Appleton-Century-Crofts.

Melzack R, Wall PD: Pain mechanisms: a new theory, *Science* 150:971, 1965.

National Institutes of Health Consensus Develop Panel: New gains against pain, *Emerg Med* 143, Nov 1986.

Paice JA: Unraveling the mystery of pain, *Oncol Nurs Forum* 18(5):843, 1991.

Puntillo KA: The phenomenon of pain and critical care nursing, *Heart Lung* 17:262, 1988.

Ryan P, Vortherms R, Ward S: Cancer pain: knowledge, attitudes of pharmacologic management, *J Gerontol Nurs* 20(1):7, 1994.

Sabbe MB, Yaksh TL: Pharmacology of spinal opioids, *J Pain Symptom Manage* 5(3):191, 1990.

Schultheis K et al: Preparation for stressful medical procedures and person treatment interactions, *Clin Psych Rev* 7:329, 1987.

Van Aernam B, Lindeman C: Nursing intervention with the presurgical patient: the effects of structured and unstructured preoperative teaching, *Nurs Res* 20:319, 1971.

Walker AC et al: Impact of culture on pain management: an Australian nursing perspective, *Holist Nurs Pract* 9(2):48, 1995.

Wallston BS et al: Choice and predictability in the preparation for barium enema: a person-by-situation approach, *Res Nurs Health* 10(1):13, 1987.

Whaley L, Wong D: *Nursing care of infants and children,* ed 5, St Louis, 1995, Mosby.

Wilkie DJ: Cancer pain management: state-of-the-art nursing care, *Nurs Clin North Am* 25(2):331, 1990.

Wong DL, Baker CM: Pain in children: comparison of assessment scales, *Oklahoma Nurse* 33(1):8, 1988.

World Health Organization: Cancer pain relief and palliative care, report of a WHO expert committee (World Health Organization Technical Report Series, 804) Geneva, Switzerland, 1990, WHO.

ADDITIONAL READINGS

Daake DR, Gueldner SH: Imager instruction and the control of postsurgical pain, *Appl Nurs Res* 2(3):114, 1989.

Holm K et al: Effect of personal pain experience on pain assessment, *Image J Nurs Sch* 21(2):72, 1989.

LaFoy J, Geden EA: Postepisiotomy pain: warm versus cold sitz bath, *JOGNN* 18:399, 1989.

Lubenow TR, Ivankovich AD: Patient-controlled analgesia for postoperative pain, *Crit Care Nurs Clin North Am* 3(1):35, 1991.

Melzack R: The McGill pain questionnaire: major properties and scoring methods, *Pain* 1:277, 1975.

Turnage G et al: Spinal opioids: a nursing perspective, *J Pain Symptom Manage* 5(3):154, 1990.

Villarruel AM, Montellano BO: Culture and pain: a Mesoamerican perspective, *Adv Nurs Sci* 15(1):21, 1992.

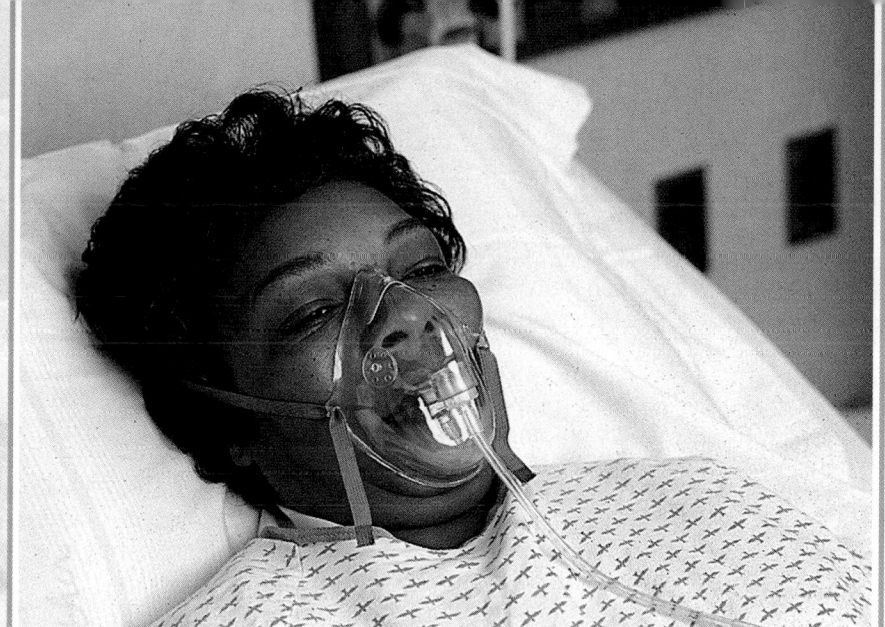

## Chapter 44

Oxygenation

Objectives

Mastery of content in this chapter will enable the student to:

▶ Define the key terms listed.

▶ Describe the structure and function of the cardiopulmonary system.

▶ Identify physiological processes in maintaining cardiac output, myocardial blood flow, and coronary artery circulation.

▶ Describe the electrical conduction system of the heart.

▶ Describe how cardiac output can be altered by preload, afterload, contractility, and heart rate.

▶ Identify physiological processes involved in ventilation, perfusion, and exchange of respiratory gases.

▶ Describe neural and chemical regulation of respiration.

▶ Explain the ways a client's level of health, age, lifestyle, and environment can affect tissue oxygenation.

▶ Identify causes and effects of disturbances in conduction, altered cardiac output, impaired valvular function, myocardial ischemia, and impaired tissue perfusion.

▶ Identify causes and effects of hyperventilation, hypoventilation, and hypoxemia.

▶ Perform a nursing assessment of the cardiopulmonary system.

▶ Develop nursing diagnoses for altered oxygenation.

▶ Describe nursing interventions to increase activity tolerance, maintain or promote lung expansion, promote mobilization of pulmonary secretions, maintain a patent airway, promote oxygenation, and restore cardiopulmonary function.

▶ Develop evaluation criteria for the nursing care plan for the client with altered oxygenation.

xygen is required to sustain life. The nurse often encounters clients who are unable to meet oxygen needs. The cardiac and respiratory systems function to supply the body's oxygen demands.

Cardiac physiology involves the delivery of oxygenated blood from the pulmonary circulation to the left side of the heart and to tissues and delivery of deoxygenated blood to the pulmonary system. Respiratory physiology involves oxygenation of the body through the mechanisms of ventilation, perfusion, and transport of respiratory gases. Neural and chemical regulators control fluctuations in respiratory rate and depth to meet changing tissue oxygen demands.

CARDIOVASCULAR PHYSIOLOGY

The function of the cardiac system is to deliver oxygen, nutrients, and other substances to the tissues and to remove the waste products of cellular metabolism through the cardiac pump, the circulatory vascular system, and the integration of other systems (e.g., respiratory, digestive, and renal) (McCance and Huether, 1994).

Structure and Function

The right ventricle pumps blood through the pulmonary circulation while the left ventricle pumps blood to the systemic circulation supplying oxygen and nutrients to the tissues and removing wastes from the body (Fig. 44-1). The

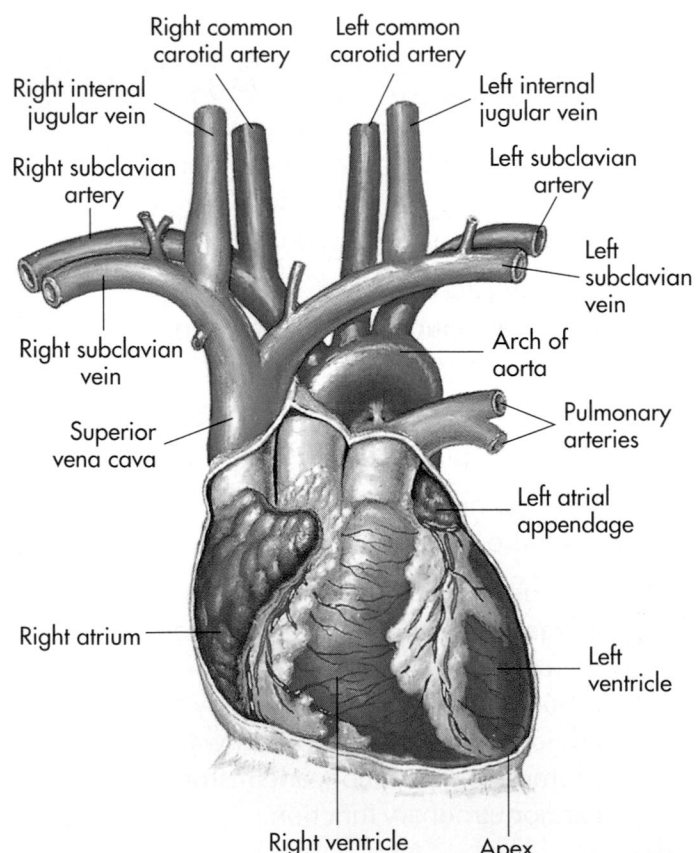

Fig. 44-1 Diagram showing serially connected pulmonary and systemic circulation. Right heart chambers propel unoxygenated blood through the pulmonary circulation; left heart chambers propel oxygenated blood through systemic circulation. *(From Canobbio MM:* Cardiovascular disorders, *St Louis, 1990, Mosby.)*

circulatory system exchanges respiratory gases, nutrients, and waste products between the blood and the tissues.

MYOCARDIAL PUMP

The pumping action of the heart is essential to maintain oxygen delivery. Decreased pump effectiveness, as in coronary artery disease (CAD) and cardiomyopathic conditions, results in a diminished stroke volume, the volume of blood ejected from the ventricles. Hemorrhage and dehydration decrease pump effectiveness by reducing the circulating blood volume, thereby decreasing the amount of blood ejected from the ventricles.

The chambers of the heart fill during diastole and empty during systole. The effectiveness of the diastolic and systolic events of the cardiac cycle can be assessed by monitoring the client's blood pressure (see Chapter 32).

The myocardial fibers have contractile properties that enable them to stretch during filling. In a healthy heart, this stretch is proportionally related to the strength of contraction. As the myocardium stretches, the strength of the subsequent contraction increases; this is known as the *Frank-Starling (Starling's) law* of the heart. In the diseased heart, Starling's law does not apply because the stretch of the myocardium is beyond the heart's physiological limits. The subsequent contractile response results in insufficient ventricular ejection (volume) and blood begins to "back up" in the pulmonary (left heart failure) or systemic circulation (right heart failure).

MYOCARDIAL BLOOD FLOW

To maintain adequate blood flow to the pulmonary and systemic circulations, myocardial blood flow must supply sufficient oxygen and nutrients to the myocardium itself.

The one-way flow of blood through the heart is ensured by the four heart valves (Fig. 44-2). During ventricular diastole the atrioventricular (mitral and tricuspid) valves open and blood flows from the higher pressure atria into the relaxed ventricles. After ventricular filling, the systolic phase begins. As the systolic intraventricular pressure rises, the atrioventricular valves close, preventing the back flow of blood into the atria, and ventricular contraction begins.

During the systolic phase, ventricular pressure rises, causing the semilunar (aortic and pulmonic) valves to open. As the ventricles eject blood the intraventricular pressure falls and the semilunar valves close, thus preventing the back flow into the ventricles. Clients with valvular diseases may have back flow or regurgitation of blood through the incompetent valve, causing a murmur that is heard on auscultation (see Chapter 33).

CORONARY ARTERY CIRCULATION

Blood flow through the atria and ventricles does not supply oxygen and nutrients to the myocardium itself. The coronary circulation is the branch of the systemic circulation that supplies oxygen and nutrients to and removal of waste from the myocardium (see the box on p. 1193). These arteries arise from the aorta just above and behind the aortic valve through openings called the *coronary ostia*. The most abundant blood supply feeds the left ventricular myocardium, which is more muscular and does most of the heart's work. The coronary arteries fill during ventricular diastole (McCance and Huether, 1994).

The figure labels are:
Right common carotid artery, Left common carotid artery, Right internal jugular vein, Left internal jugular vein, Right subclavian artery, Left subclavian artery, Left subclavian vein, Right subclavian vein, Arch of aorta, Superior vena cava, Pulmonary arteries, Left atrial appendage, Right atrium, Left ventricle, Right ventricle, Apex

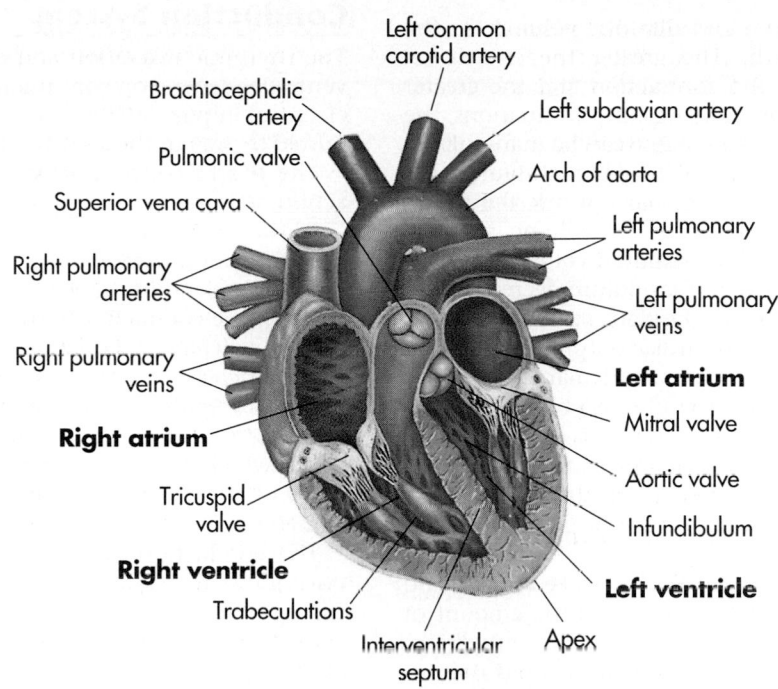

Fig. 44-2 Structures that direct blood flow through the heart. Arrows indicate path of blood through chambers, valves, and major vessels. *(Modified from Canobbio MM:* Cardiovascular disorders, *St Louis, 1990, Mosby.)*

SYSTEMIC CIRCULATION

The arteries and veins of the systemic circulation deliver nutrients and oxygen to and remove waste from the tissues. Oxygenated blood flows from the left ventricle by way of the aorta and into large systemic arteries. These arteries branch into smaller arteries, arterioles, and finally into the smallest vessels, the capillaries. At the capillary level the exchange of respiratory gases, nutrients, and wastes occurs, and the tissues are oxygenated. The waste products exit the capillary network by way of the venules that join to form veins. These veins form larger veins, which carry deoxygenated blood to the right side of the heart where it is returned to pulmonary circulation.

REGULATION OF BLOOD FLOW

The amount of blood ejected from the left ventricle each minute is the **cardiac output.** The normal cardiac output is 4 to 6 L/min in the healthy 150-lb (70-kg) adult at rest. The circulating volume of blood changes according to the oxygen and metabolic needs of the body. For example, during exercise, pregnancy, and fever, the cardiac output increases, but during sleep the cardiac output decreases. Cardiac output is represented by the following formula:

Cardiac output (CO) = Stroke volume (SV) × Heart rate (HR)

Cardiac output in the older adult may be affected by increased arterial wall tension and moderate myocardial hypertrophy due to an increased systolic blood pressure.

Cardiac index (CI) is the adequacy of the cardiac output for an individual. It takes into account the body surface area (BSA) of the client. The CI is determined by dividing the CO by the BSA. The normal range is 2.5 to 4 L/min/m³ (Urban et al, 1995).

Coronary Arteries

RIGHT CORONARY ARTERY
Right Atrium, Anterior Right Ventricle
Supplies:
Posterior aspect of septum (90% of population)
Posterior papillary muscle
Sinus and AV nodes (80%-90% of population)
Inferior aspect of left ventricle

LEFT CORONARY ARTERIES
Left Anterior Descending (LAD)
Supplies:
Anterior left ventricular wall
Anterior interventricular septum (septal branches supply conduction system, bundle of His, and bundle branches)
Anterior papillary muscle
Left ventricular apex

CIRCUMFLEX
Supplies:
Left atrium
Posterior surfaces of left ventricle
Posterior aspects of septum

From Canobbio MM: *Cardiovascular disorders,* St Louis, 1990, Mosby.

Stroke volume is the amount of blood ejected from the left ventricle with each contraction. It can be affected by the amount of blood in the left ventricle at the end of diastole (preload), the resistance to left ventricular ejection (afterload), and myocardial contractility.

Preload is essentially the end diastolic volume. As the ventricles fill, they stretch. The greater the stretch on the ventricle, the greater the contraction and the greater the stroke volume (Starling's law). In clinical situations, the preload and subsequent stroke volume can be manipulated by changing the amount of circulating blood volume. For example, in the client with hemorrhagic shock, fluid therapy and replacement of blood increases volume, thus increasing the preload and cardiac output. If volume is not replaced, preload decreases, the cardiac output decreases, and ultimately the venous return to the right atrium decreases, further decreasing preload and cardiac output.

Afterload is the resistance to left ventricular ejection; the work the heart must overcome to fully eject blood from the left ventricle. The diastolic aortic pressure is a good clinical measure of afterload. In a client with an acute hypertensive crisis, the afterload is increased, increasing the cardiac workload. Afterload in this situation can be manipulated by decreasing systemic blood pressure.

Myocardial contractility also affects stroke volume and cardiac output. Poor contraction decreases the amount of blood ejected by the ventricles during each contraction. Myocardial contractility can be increased by drugs that increase the force of contraction, such as digitalis preparations, epinephrine, and sympathomimetic drugs (drugs that mimic the effects of the sympathetic nervous system). Myocardial contractility can be decreased by injury to the myocardial muscle, such as an acute myocardial infarction. The myocardium of the older adult is more rigid and slower in recovering its contractility (Lueckenotte, 1994).

Heart rate affects blood flow because of the interaction between rate and diastolic filling time. With a sustained heart rate greater than 160 beats/min, diastolic filling time decreases, decreasing stroke volume and cardiac output. The heart rate of the older adult is slow to increase under stress. To compensate for this, the stroke volume may increase to increase the cardiac output and blood pressure (Lueckenotte, 1994).

Conduction System

The rhythmic relaxation and contraction of the atria and ventricles depend on continuous, organized transmission of electrical impulses. These impulses are generated and transmitted by way of the cardiac conduction system (Fig. 44-3).

The heart's conduction system generates the necessary action potentials that conduct the impulses required to initiate the electrical chain of events resulting in the heartbeat. The autonomic nervous system influences the rate of impulse generation as well as the speed of transmission through the conductive pathway and the strength of atrial and ventricular contractions. Sympathetic nerve fibers, which increase the rate of impulse generation and the speed of impulse transmission, innervate all parts of the atria and ventricles. Parasympathetic fibers from the vagus nerve, which decrease this rate, also innervate these parts as well as the sinoatrial and atrioventricular nodes (McCance and Huether, 1994).

The conduction system originates with the **sinoatrial (SA) node**, the "pacemaker" of the heart. The SA node is in the right atrium next to the entrance of the superior vena cava (McCance and Huether, 1994). Impulses are initiated at the SA node at an intrinsic rate of 60 to 100 beats/min. The resting adult rate is approximately 75 beats/min.

The electrical impulses are then transmitted through the atria along intraatrial pathways to the **atrioventricular (AV) node.** The AV node mediates impulses between the atria and the ventricles. It assists atrial emptying by delaying the impulse before transmitting it through the **bundle of His** and the ventricular **Purkinje network.**

The electrical activity of the conduction system is reflected by an **electrocardiogram (ECG).** An ECG monitors the regularity and path of the electrical impulse through the conduction system, however, it does not reflect muscular work of the heart. The normal sequence on the ECG is called **normal sinus rhythm (NSR)** (Fig. 44-4).

NSR indicates the impulse originates at the SA node and follows the normal sequence through the conduction sys-

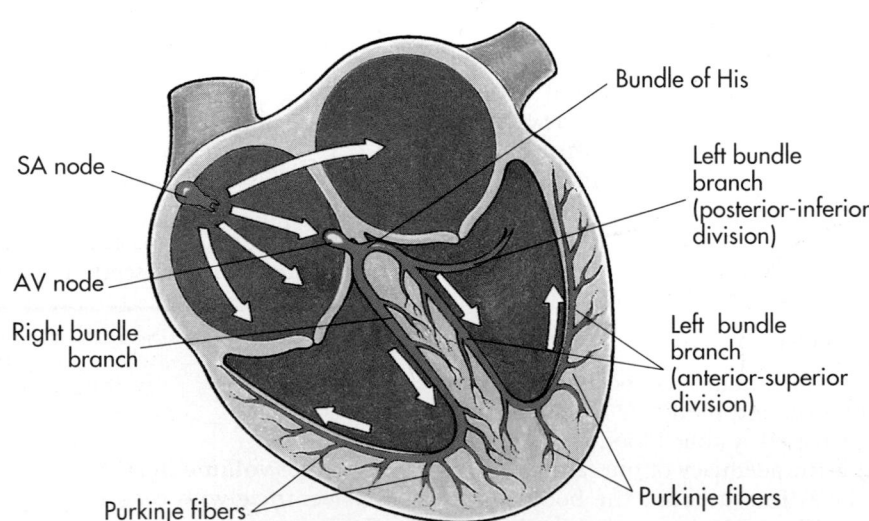

Fig. 44-3 Electrical conduction system. *(From Canobbio MM:* Cardiovascular disorders, *St Louis, 1990, Mosby.)*

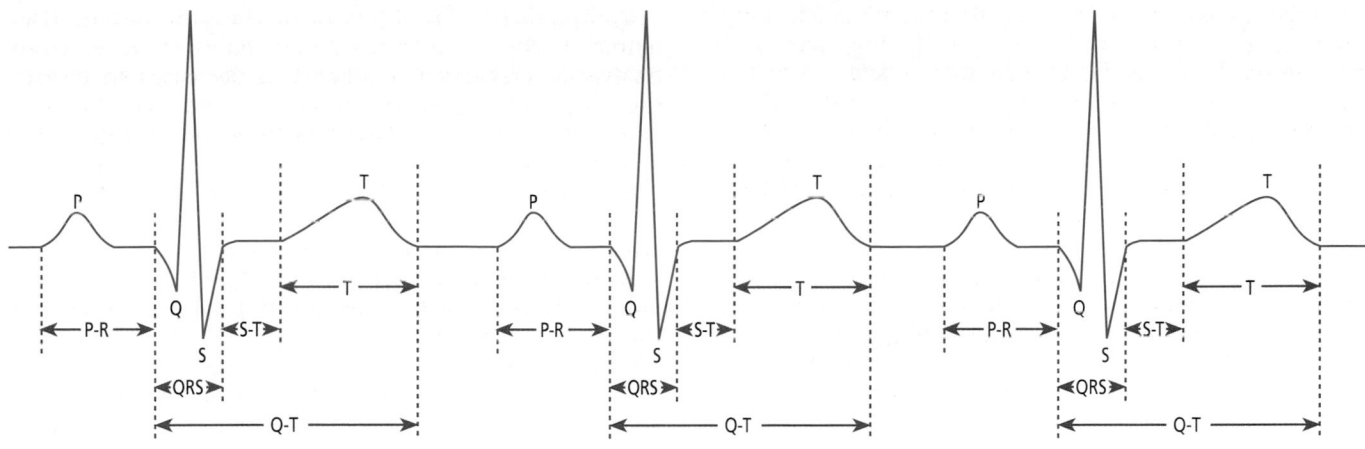

Fig. 44-4 Normal ECG waveform.

tem. The P-wave represents the electrical conduction through the artia. Normally, atrial contraction follows the P-wave. The *PR interval* represents the impulse travel time through the AV node, the bundle of His, and to the Purkinje fibers. The normal length for the PR interval is 0.12 to 0.20 seconds. An increase in the time indicates that there is a block in the impulse transmission though the AV node, whereas a decrease indicates the initiation of the electrical impulse from a source other than the SA node.

The QRS complex indicates the electrical impulse has traveled through the ventricles. Normal *QRS duration* is .06

to 0.12 seconds. Increase in QRS duration indicates a delay in conduction time through the ventricles. Ventricular contraction usually follows the QRS complex.

The *QT interval* represents the time needed for ventricular depolarization and repolarization. The normal QT interval is 0.12 to 0.42 seconds. Changes in electrolyte values, such as hypocalcemia, or therapy with drugs such as quinidine, disopyramide, amiodarone, and theophylline can increase the QT interval. Shortening of the QT interval occurs with digitalis therapy, hyperkalemia, and hypercalcemia (Purcell, 1993).

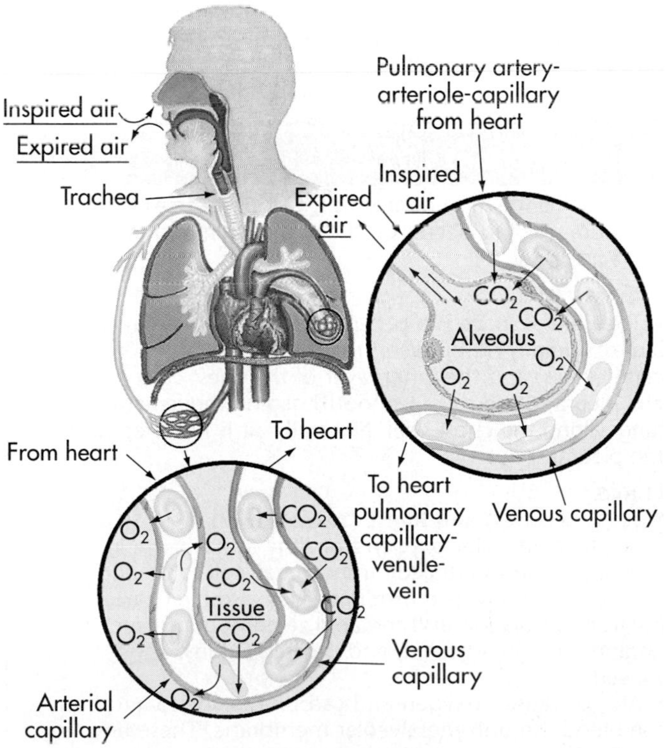

RESPIRATORY PHYSIOLOGY

Most cells in the body obtain their energy from chemical reactions involving oxygen and the elimination of carbon dioxide. The exchange of respiratory gases occurs between environmental air and the blood. There are three steps in the process of oxygenation: ventilation, perfusion, and diffusion (McCance and Huether, 1994). For the exchange of respiratory gases to occur, the organs, nerves, and muscles of respiration must be intact and the central nervous system able to regulate the respiratory cycle (Fig. 44-5).

Structure and Function

Respiration can be altered by conditions or diseases that change the structure and function of the lung. The respiratory muscles, pleural space, lungs, and alveoli (Fig. 44-6) are essential for ventilation, perfusion, and exchange of respiratory gases (see the box on p. 1196).

Ventilation

Ventilation is the process of moving gases into and out of the lungs. Ventilation requires coordination of the muscular and elastic properties of the lung and thorax, and intact innervation. The major inspiratory muscle of respiration is the diaphragm. It is innervated by the phrenic nerve, which exits the spinal cord at the fourth cervical vertebra.

WORK OF BREATHING

Breathing is the effort required to expand and contract the lungs. The work of breathing is determined by the degree of compliance of the lungs, airway resistance, presence of active expiration, and use of accessory muscles of respiration.

Fig. 44-5 Structures of the pulmonary system. The circle denotes the aveoli. *(Modified from Wilson SF, Thompson JM: Mosby's clinical nursing series: respiratory disorders, St Louis, 1990, Mosby.)*

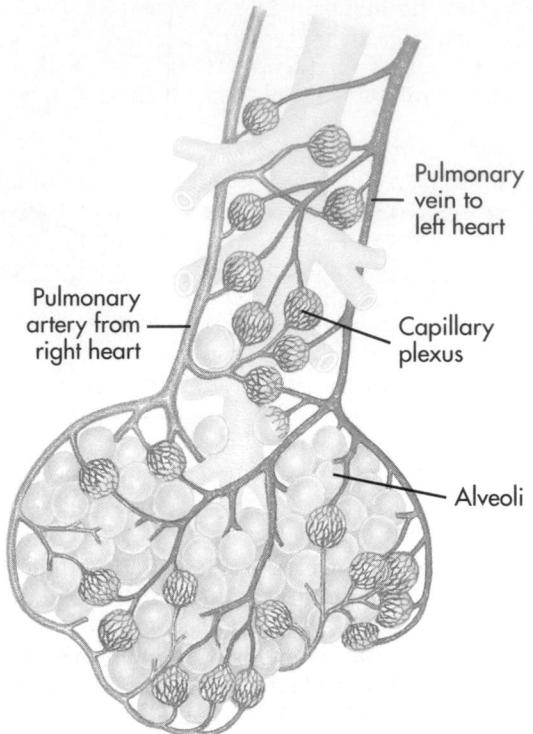

Pulmonary vein to left heart

Pulmonary artery from right heart

Capillary plexus

Alveoli

Fig. 44-6 Alveoli at the terminal end of the lower airway. *(From Thompson J et al: Mosby's manual of clinical nursing, ed 3, St Louis, 1993, Mosby.)*

Compliance is the ability of the lungs to distend (Dettenmeier, 1992) or to expand in response to increased intraalveolar pressure. Compliance is decreased in diseases such as pulmonary edema, interstitial and pleural fibrosis, and congenital or traumatic structural abnormalities, such as kyphosis or fractured ribs.

Surfactant is the chemical produced in the lung by alveolar type 2 cells that maintains the surface tension of the alveoli and keeps them from collapsing.

Airway resistance is the pressure difference between the mouth and the alveoli in relation to the rate of flow of inspired gas. Airway resistance can be increased by an airway obstruction, small airway disease (such as asthma), and tracheal edema. When resistance is increased, the amount of air traveling through the anatomical airways is decreased.

Expiration is normally a passive process that depends on elastic recoil properties and requires little or no muscle work. Elastic recoil is produced by elastic fibers in lung tissue and by surface tension in the fluid film lining the alveoli (Dettenmeier, 1992). Clients with advanced chronic obstructive pulmonary disease lose the elastic recoil of the lung and thorax. As a result the client's work of breathing is increased.

Accessory muscles of respiration can increase lung volume during inspiration. Clients with chronic obstructive pulmonary disease, especially emphysema, frequently use these muscles to increase lung volume. During assessment the nurse may observe elevation of the client's clavicles during inspiration.

Decreased compliance, increased airway resistance, active expiration, or use of accessory muscles increases the work of breathing, resulting in an increased energy expenditure. To meet this expenditure the body increases its metabolic rate and the need for oxygen, as well as the elimination of carbon dioxide. This sequence is a vicious cycle for a client with

---

Major Anatomical Structures of the Thorax and Their Functions

INSPIRATORY MUSCLES

Diaphragm

■ Contraction causes the diaphragm to descend, creating a negative pleural pressure and increasing the vertical dimension of the lungs, which contributes to inflation of the lungs. The increase in vertical dimension and the decrease in intrapulmonary pressure (negative with respect to atmospheric pressure) cause air to enter the lungs.

External Intercostal

■ Contraction elevates the anterior ends of the ribs, causing them to move upward and outward. This increases the anteroposterior dimension of the thorax.

Accessory Muscles

■ Accessory muscles include the scalene, sternocleidomastoid, and trapezius muscles. Contraction elevates the first two ribs and the sternum.

EXPIRATORY MUSCLES

Internal Intercostal

■ Contraction pulls ribs down and in, thereby decreasing the anteroposterior diameter of the thorax.

Abdominal Respiratory

■ Abdominal respiratory muscles include the rectus, transverse abdominis, internal oblique, and external oblique

muscles. Contraction depresses lower ribs, forces the diaphragm up, and decreases the vertical dimension of the thoracic cavity.

PLEURAL SPACE

■ The pleural space is a potential space that is only a thin film of liquid lying between the outer layer of the lung (visceral pleura) and the inner layer of the chest cavity (parietal pleura). It permits a smooth, gliding movement of the lungs along the chest wall. Normally air is not present in the pleural space.

LUNGS

Left (Two Lobes) and Right (Three Lobes)

■ The lungs transfer oxygen from the atmosphere into the alveoli and carbon dioxide from the alveoli to the lungs to be excreted as a waste product. They also filter toxic material from circulation and metabolize compounds such as angiotensin I, bradykinin, and prostaglandins.

Alveoli

■ Alveoli transfer oxygen and carbon dioxide to and from the blood through the alveolar membrane. These tiny air sacs expand during inspiration, greatly increasing the surface area over which exchange of gases occurs.

impaired ventilation, causing further deterioration of respiratory status and ability to oxygenate adequately.

LUNG VOLUMES

Normal lung volumes are measured through pulmonary function testing. Spirometry measures the volume of air entering or leaving the lungs. Variations in lung volumes may be associated with health states such as pregnancy, exercise, obesity, or obstructive and restrictive conditions of the lung. The amount of surfactant, degree of compliance, and strength of respiratory muscles can affect pressures and volumes within the lungs.

PRESSURES

Gases are moved into and out of the lungs through pressure changes (Fig. 44-7). Intrapleural pressure is negative or less than atmospheric pressure, which is 760 mm Hg at sea level. For air to flow into the lungs, intrapleural pressure must become more negative, setting up a pressure gradient between the atmosphere and alveoli.

Perfusion

The primary function of pulmonary circulation is to move blood to and from the alveolar-capillary membrane so gas exchange can occur. Pulmonary circulation is a reservoir for blood so the lung can increase its blood volume without large increases in pulmonary artery or venous pressures. The pulmonary circulation also acts as a filter, removing small thrombi before they can reach vital organs.

PULMONARY CIRCULATION

Pulmonary circulation begins at the pulmonary artery, which receives poorly oxygenated mixed venous blood from the right ventricle. Blood flow through this system depends on the pumping ability of the right ventricle, which has an output of approximately 4 to 6 L/min. The flow continues from the pulmonary artery through the pulmonary arterioles to the pulmonary capillaries where blood comes in contact with the alveolar-capillary membrane and the exchange of respiratory gases occurs. The oxygen-rich blood then circulates through the pulmonary venules and pulmonary veins returning to the left atrium.

DISTRIBUTION

Pressures within the pulmonary circulatory system are low in comparison to those in the systemic circulatory system. The normal pulmonary systolic arterial pressure is between 20 and 30 mm Hg, the diastolic pressure is less than 12 mm Hg, and the mean pressure is less than 20 mm Hg (Daily and Schroeder, 1994). The walls of the pulmonary vessels are

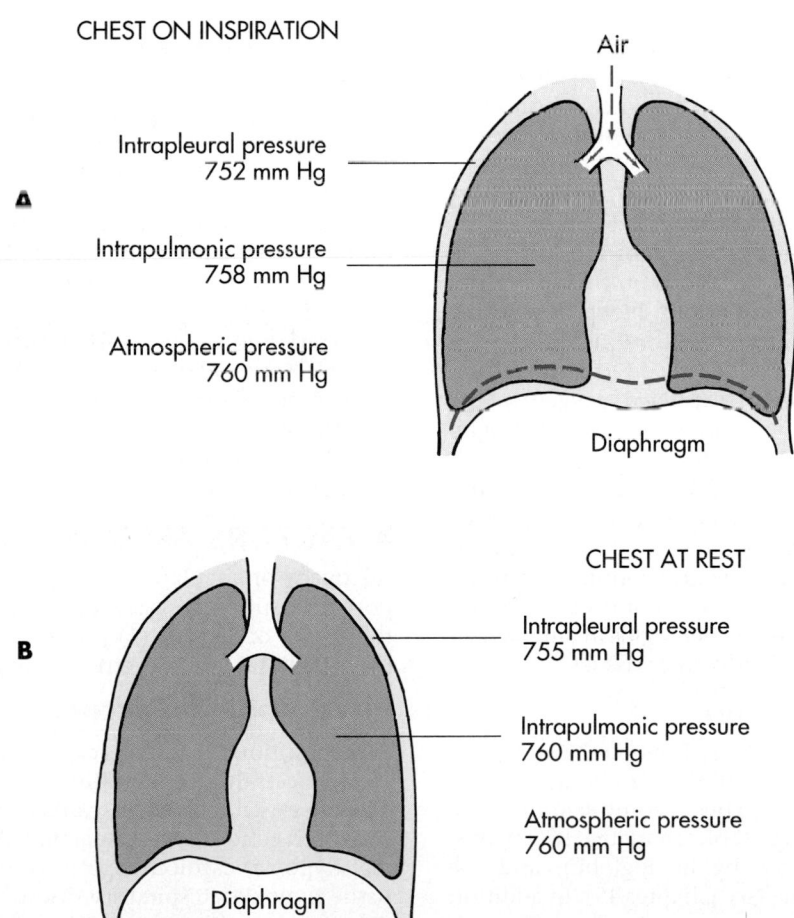

CHEST ON INSPIRATION

Air

A

Intrapleural pressure
752 mm Hg

Intrapulmonic pressure
758 mm Hg

Atmospheric pressure
760 mm Hg

Diaphragm

CHEST AT REST

B

Intrapleural pressure
755 mm Hg

Intrapulmonic pressure
760 mm Hg

Atmospheric pressure
760 mm Hg

Diaphragm

Fig. 44-7 A, Contraction of the diaphragm to increase vertical dimensions of the lungs. **B,** Relaxation of the diaphragm, decreasing vertical dimensions of the lungs. *(Modified from Wade JF: Comprehensive respiratory care, ed 3, St Louis, 1982, Mosby.)*

thinner than those in the systemic circulation and contain less smooth muscle, because of the low pressure and resistance. The lung accepts the total cardiac output from the right ventricle and, except in cases of alveolar hypoxia, does not direct blood flow from one region to another.

Exchange of Respiratory Gases

Respiratory gases are exchanged in the alveoli and the capillaries of the body tissues. Oxygen is transferred from the lungs to the blood, and carbon dioxide is transferred from the blood to the alveoli to be exhaled as a waste product. At the tissue level, oxygen is transferred from the blood to tissues, and carbon dioxide is transferred from tissues to the blood to return to the alveoli and be exhaled. This transfer is dependent on the process of diffusion.

DIFFUSION

Diffusion is the movement of molecules from an area of higher concentration to an area of lower concentration. Diffusion of respiratory gases occurs at the alveolarcapillary membrane, and the rate of diffusion can be affected by the thickness of the membrane.

Increased thickness of the membrane impedes diffusion because gases take longer to transfer across. Clients with pulmonary edema, pulmonary infiltrates, or a pulmonary effusion have an increased thickness of the alveolar-capillary membrane resulting in slowed diffusion, slowed exchange of respiratory gases, and impaired delivery of oxygen to tissues.

The surface area of the membrane can be altered as a result of a chronic disease (i.e., emphysema), an acute disease (i.e., pneumothorax), or a surgical process (i.e., lobectomy). When fewer alveoli are functioning, the surface area is decreased.

OXYGEN TRANSPORT

The oxygen transport system consists of the lungs and cardiovascular system. Delivery depends on the amount of oxygen entering the lungs (ventilation), blood flow to the lungs and tissues (perfusion), rate of diffusion, and oxygen carrying capacity. The capacity of the blood to carry oxygen is influenced by the amount of dissolved oxygen in the plasma, amount of hemoglobin, and tendency of hemoglobin to bind with oxygen (Ahrens, 1990).

Only a relatively small amount of required oxygen, about 3%, is dissolved in the plasma. Most oxygen is transported by hemoglobin, which serves as a carrier for oxygen and carbon dioxide. The hemoglobin molecule combines with oxygen to form oxyhemoglobin. The formation of oxyhemoglobin is easily reversible, allowing hemoglobin and oxygen to dissociate, which frees oxygen to enter tissues.

CARBON DIOXIDE TRANSPORT

Carbon dioxide diffuses into red blood cells and is rapidly hydrated into carbonic acid (H_2CO_3) because of the presence of carbonic anhydrase. The carbonic acid then dissociates into hydrogen ($H+$) and bicarbonate (HCO_3^-) ions. The hydrogen ion is buffered by hemoglobin, and the HCO_3^- diffuses into the plasma (see Chapter 45). In addition some of the carbon dioxide in red blood cells reacts with amino acid groups, forming carbamino compounds. This reaction can occur rapidly without the presence of an enzyme. Reduced hemoglobin (deoxyhemoglobin) can com-

---

> ### Neural and Chemical Regulation of Respiration
>
> **NEURAL REGULATION**
> - Maintains rhythm and depth of respiration and balance between inspiration and expiration.
>
> **Cerebral Cortex**
> - Voluntary control of respiration delivers impulses to the respiratory motor neurons by way of the spinal cord; accommodates speaking, eating, and swimming.
>
> **Medulla Oblongata**
> - Automatic control of respiration occurs continuously.
>
> **CHEMICAL REGULATION**
> - Maintains appropriate rate and depth of respirations based on changes in the blood's carbon dioxide (CO_2), oxygen (O_2), and hydrogen ion (H^+) concentration.
>
> **Chemoreceptors**
> - Located in the medulla, aortic body, and carotid body. Changes in chemical content of O_2, CO_2, and H^+ stimulate chemoreceptors, which in turn stimulate neural regulators to adjust the rate and depth of ventilation to maintain normal arterial blood gas levels. Chemical regulation can occur during physical exercise and in some illnesses. It is a short-term adaptive mechanism.

bine with carbon dioxide more easily than oxyhemoglobin, and therefore venous blood transports the majority of carbon dioxide.

Regulation of Respiration

The main purpose of respiratory regulation is to supply sufficient oxygen to meet the body's demands, such as during exercise, infection, or pregnancy. Respiratory regulation promotes exhalation of metabolically produced carbon dioxide, which is a determinant of acid-base status (see Chapter 45).

Respiration is controlled by neural and chemical regulators. Neural regulation includes the central nervous system control of respiratory rate, depth, and rhythm. Chemical regulation involves the influence of chemicals such as carbon dioxide and hydrogen ions on the rate and depth of respiration (see the box above).

■ FACTORS AFFECTING OXYGENATION

Adequacy of circulation, ventilation, perfusion, and transport of respiratory gases to the tissues are influenced by four types of factors: (1) physiological, (2) developmental, (3) behavioral, and (4) environmental.

Physiological Factors

Any condition that affects cardiopulmonary functioning directly affects the body's ability to meet oxygen demands. The general classifications of cardiac disorders include disturbances in conduction, impaired valvular function, myocardial hypoxia, cardiomyopathic conditions, and peripheral tissue hypoxia. Respiratory disorders include hyperventilation, hypoventilation, and hypoxia.

Other physiological processes affecting a client's oxygenation include alterations that affect the oxygen-carrying capacity of blood, such as the anemias; increases in the

Table 44-1	Physiological Processes Affecting Oxygenation
PROCESS	**EFFECT ON OXYGENATION**
Anemia	Decreases oxygen-carrying capacity of blood
Toxic inhalant	Decreases oxygen-carrying capacity of blood
Airway obstruction	Limits delivery of inspired oxygen to alveoli
High altitude	Decreases inspiratory oxygen concentration because atmospheric oxygen concentration is lower
Fever	Increases metabolic rate and tissue oxygen demand
Decreased chest wall motion (e.g., from musculoskeletal impairments)	Prevents lowering of diaphragm and reduces anteroposterior diameter of thorax on inspiration, reducing volume of air inspired

body's metabolic demands, such as pregnancy or fever and infection; and alterations that affect the client's chest wall movement or the central nervous system (Table 44-1).

DECREASED OXYGEN-CARRYING CAPACITY

Hemoglobin carries 97% of the diffused oxygen to tissues. Any process that decreases or alters hemoglobin, such as anemia and inhalation of toxic substances, decreases the oxygen-carrying capacity of blood.

Anemia is characterized by below-normal levels of hemoglobin. Anemia is the result of decreased hemoglobin production, increased red cell destruction, and/or blood loss. Clinical findings include fatigue, decreased activity tolerance, increased breathlessness, pallor, and increased heart rate.

Carbon monoxide is the most common toxic inhalant that decreases the oxygen-carrying capacity of blood. The affinity for hemoglobin to bind with carbon monoxide is 210 times greater than its affinity to bind with oxygen, creating a functional anemia (Ahrens, 1993). Because of the bond's strength, carbon monoxide is not easily dissociated from hemoglobin, making the hemoglobin unavailable for oxygen transport.

DECREASED INSPIRED OXYGEN CONCENTRATION

When the concentration of inspired oxygen declines, the oxygen-carrying capacity of the blood is decreased. Decreases in the fraction of inspired oxygen concentration (Fio_2) can be caused by an upper or lower airway obstruction limiting delivery of inspired oxygen to alveoli, decreased environmental oxygen (as occurs at high altitudes), or decreased inspiration as the result of an incorrect oxygen concentration setting on respiratory therapy equipment.

HYPOVOLEMIA

Hypovolemia is a reduced circulating blood volume resulting from extracellular fluid losses that occurs in conditions such as shock and severe dehydration. If the fluid loss is significant the body tries to adapt by increasing the heart rate and peripheral vasoconstriction to increase the volume of blood returned to the heart and increase the cardiac output.

INCREASED METABOLIC RATE

Increases in metabolic activity of the body result in an increased oxygen demand. When body systems are unable to meet this increased demand, the level of oxygenation declines. An increased metabolic rate is a normal response of the body to pregnancy, wound healing, and exercise because the body is building tissue. Most people can meet the increased oxygen demand and do not display signs of oxygen deprivation.

Fever increases the tissues' need for oxygen; and, as a result, carbon dioxide production also increases. If the febrile state persists, the metabolic rate remains high and the body begins to break down protein stores resulting in muscle wasting and decreased muscle mass. Respiratory muscles such as the diaphragm and intercostals are also wasted. The body attempts to adapt to the increased carbon dioxide levels by increasing the rate and depth of respiration to eliminate excess carbon dioxide. The client's work of breathing increases and the client will eventually display signs and symptoms of hypoxemia. Those clients with pulmonary diseases are at greater risk for hypoxemia and hypercapnia. Assessment reveals increased rate and depth of respiration, use of the accessory muscles of respiration, use of pursed-lip breathing, and decreased activity tolerance.

CONDITIONS AFFECTING CHEST WALL MOVEMENT

Any condition that reduces chest wall movement can result in decreased ventilation. If the diaphragm cannot fully descend with breathing, the volume of inspired air decreases and less oxygen is delivered to the alveoli and subsequently to tissues.

Pregnancy. As the fetus grows during pregnancy, the greater size of the uterus pushes abdominal contents upward against the diaphragm. In the last trimester of pregnancy the inspiratory capacity declines, resulting in dyspnea on exertion and increased fatigue.

Obesity. Obese clients have reduced lung volumes from the heavy lower thorax and abdomen, particularly when in the recumbent and supine positions. Obese clients have a reduction in compliance as a result of encroachment of the abdomen into the chest, increased work of breathing, decreased lung volumes, and may have fatigue and carbon dioxide retention (Burns et al, 1994).

In some clients an obesity-hypoventilation syndrome develops in which oxygenation is decreased and carbon dioxide is retained, resulting in daytime sleepiness. Obese clients may also develop obstructive sleep apnea. This is characterized by excessive daytime somnolence, and loud snoring and periods of apnea when sleeping. The obese client is also susceptible to pneumonia after an upper respiratory tract infection because the lungs cannot fully expand and pulmonary secretions are not mobilized in the lower lobes.

Musculoskeletal Abnormalities. Musculoskeletal impairments in the thoracic region reduce oxygenation. Such impairments may result from abnormal structural configurations, trauma, muscular diseases, and diseases of the central nervous system.

Abnormal structural configurations. Abnormal structural configurations impairing oxygenation include those that affect the rib cage, such as pectus excavatum, and those that affect the vertebral column, such as kyphosis. Pectus excavatum is a depression of the sternum that interferes with lung expansion. Kyphosis is an abnormal condition of the vertebral column characterized by increased convexity of the thoracic spine, producing a structural barrier to lung expansion. The angle of curvature can progress with time, resulting in severe hypoventilation and hypoxemia.

Trauma. Trauma to the chest wall may also impede inspiration. The person with multiple rib fractures can develop a flail chest, a condition in which fractures cause instability in part of the chest wall and paradoxical breathing. In paradoxical breathing, the lung underlying the injured area contracts on inspiration and bulges on expiration, resulting in hypoxia.

Chest wall or upper abdomen incisions may also decrease chest wall movement. The client may use shallow respirations to minimize chest wall movement to avoid pain. Excessive or high doses of narcotic analgesics may depress the respiratory center, thus decreasing respiratory rate and chest wall expansion.

Muscle diseases. Muscle diseases such as muscular dystrophy affect oxygenation of tissues by decreasing the client's ability to expand and contract the chest. Ventilation is impaired and atelectasis, hypercapnia, and hypoxemia can occur.

Nervous system diseases. Myasthenia gravis, Guillain-Barré syndrome, and poliomyelitis are examples of nervous system diseases that can affect respiratory functioning and result in hypoventilation. Myasthenia gravis interferes with normal transmission of impulses from nerves to muscles, involving the whole body, including muscles of respiration.

Guillain-Barré syndrome and poliomyelitis cause inflammation and paralysis of muscle groups. Guillain-Barré syndrome usually results in an ascending pattern of paralysis. Respiratory muscles become paralyzed as paralysis ascends to the thoracic region. Poliomyelitis may lead to general or local paralysis. Both may reverse, but poliomyelitis usually results in more residual paralysis.

Central nervous system alterations. Diseases or trauma involving the medulla oblongata and spinal cord may result in impaired respiration. When the medulla oblongata is affected, neural regulation of respiration is damaged and abnormal breathing patterns may develop. Damage to the spinal cord can affect respiration in two ways. If the phrenic nerve is damaged, the diaphragm may not descend, thus reducing inspiratory lung volumes and causing hypoxemia. Cervical trauma at C3 to C5 can result in paralysis of the phrenic nerve. Spinal cord trauma below the fifth cervical vertebra usually leaves the phrenic nerve intact but damages nerves that innervate the intercostal muscles, preventing anteroposterior chest expansion.

Influences of Chronic Disease. Oxygenation can be decreased as a direct consequence of chronic disease. It can also be decreased as a secondary effect, as with anemia. The physiological response to chronic hypoxemia is the development of a secondary polycythemia. This adaptive response is the body's attempt to increase the amount of circulating hemoglobin to increase the available oxygen-binding sites.

Developmental Factors

The developmental stage of the client and the normal aging process can affect tissue oxygenation.

PREMATURE INFANTS

Premature infants are at risk for hyaline membrane disease, which is thought to be caused by a surfactant deficiency. The surfactant-synthesizing ability of the lungs develops late in pregnancy, about the seventh month, and may therefore be lacking in preterm infants.

INFANTS AND TODDLERS

Infants and toddlers are at risk for upper respiratory tract infections as a result of frequent exposure to other children and exposure to secondhand smoke (Huebner, 1994; Whatling, 1994). In addition, during the teething process some infants develop nasal congestion, which encourages bacterial growth and increases the potential for respiratory tract infection. Upper respiratory tract infections are usually not dangerous, and infants or toddlers recover with little difficulty. Common airway infections are nasopharyngitis (e.g., rhinoviruses, respiratory syncytial virus, and adenovirus), pharyngitis (e.g., viral and beta-hemolytic streptococci), hemophilus influenza, and tonsillitis. Airway obstruction can also occur with aspirated foreign objects, such as food, buttons, and candy.

SCHOOL-AGE CHILDREN AND ADOLESCENTS

School-age children and adolescents are exposed to respiratory infections and respiratory risk factors such as secondhand smoke and cigarette smoking. A healthy child usually does not have adverse pulmonary effects from respiratory infections. A person who starts smoking in adolescence and continues to smoke into middle age, however, has an increased risk for cardiopulmonary disease and lung cancer.

YOUNG AND MIDDLE-AGE ADULTS

Young and middle-age adults are exposed to multiple cardiopulmonary risk factors: an unhealthy diet, lack of exercise, stress, drugs, and smoking. Reducing these modifiable factors may decrease the client's risk for cardiac or pulmonary diseases.

GERONTOLOGICAL PRINCIPLES for Breathing Patterns

The breathing patterns of older clients are dependent on intra-abdominal pressure changes. The respiratory rate is generally higher in the older client, with a normal rate of 16 to 25 breaths per minute. This rate does not affect carbon dioxide levels because older adults' tidal volume is usually decreased (Pierson, 1992).

Positioning and increased abdominal pressure can greatly affect the older client's breathing pattern. The nurse should position the client to maximize ventilation, such as up in the chair or semi-Fowler's or high Fowler's position. The older client should be encouraged to eat frequent, small meals to reduce pressure on the diaphragm from an overdistended abdomen.

OLDER ADULTS

The cardiac and respiratory systems undergo changes throughout the aging process. In the arterial system atherosclerotic plaques develop and the systemic blood pressure may rise.

Chest wall compliance is decreased in the older client due to osteoporosis and calcification of the costal cartilages. The respiratory muscles weaken and the pulmonary vascular circulation becomes less distensible (see the box on p. 1200). The trachea and large bronchi become enlarged from calcification of the airways, and alveoli enlarge, decreasing the surface area available for gas exchange. In addition, the number of functional cilia are reduced. Decreased ciliary action and effectiveness of cough mechanisms put the older adult at increased risk for respiratory infections (Lueckenotte, 1996).

Ventilation and transfer of respiratory gases decline with age. Osteoporotic changes of the thoracic cage and kyphosis of the vertebrae occur normally with aging. With these changes the lungs are unable to expand fully, leading to lower oxygenation levels (Table 44-2).

Behavioral Factors

Behavior or lifestyle may directly or indirectly affect the body's ability to meet oxygen requirements. Lifestyle factors that influence respiratory functioning include nutrition, exercise, cigarette smoking, substance abuse, and stress (see the boxes on p. 1202).

NUTRITION

Nutrition affects cardiopulmonary function in several ways. Severe obesity decreases lung expansion, and the increased body weight increases oxygen demands to meet metabolic needs. The malnourished client may experience respiratory muscle wasting, resulting in decreased muscle strength and respiratory excursion. Cough efficiency is reduced secondary to respiratory muscle weakness, putting the client at risk for retention of pulmonary secretions. Diets high in fat increase cholesterol and atherogenesis in the coronary arteries. Clients who are obese and/or malnourished are at risk for anemia. Diets high in carbohydrates may play a role in increasing the carbon dioxide load for clients with carbon dioxide retention. As carbohydrates are metabolized, an increased load of carbon dioxide is created and excreted via the lungs (Weilitz, 1993).

EXERCISE

Exercise increases the body's metabolic activity and oxygen demand. The rate and depth of respiration increase, enabling the person to inhale more oxygen and expire excess carbon dioxide.

A physical exercise program has many benefits (see Chapter 37). People who exercise 3 to 4 times per week for 20 to 40 minutes have a lower pulse rate, blood pressure, decreased cholesterol, increased blood flow, and greater oxygen extraction by working muscles (see the box on p. 1202). Fully conditioned people can increase oxygen

Table 44-2	**Changes in the Aging Lung**	
FUNCTION	**PATHOPHYSIOLOGICAL CHANGE**	**KEY CLINICAL FINDINGS**
Breathing Mechanics	Decreased chest wall compliance Loss of elastic recoil Decreased respiratory muscle mass and strength	Decreased vital capacity Increased reserve volume Decreased expiratory flow rates
Oxygenation	Increased ventilation/perfusion mismatch Decreased cardiac output Decreased mixed venous oxygen Increased physiological deadspace Decreased alveolar surface area Decreased carbon dioxide diffusion capacity	Decreased Pao_2 Increased alveolar-arterial oxygen gradient Decreased cardiac output
Ventilation Control and Breathing Pattern	Decreased responsiveness of central and peripheral chemoreceptors to hypoxemia and hypercapnia	Deceased tidal volume Increased respiratory rate Increased minute ventilation
Lung defense mechanisms	Decreased number of cilia and effectiveness of the mucociliary clearance Diminished cough reflex Decreased humoral and cellular immunity Decreased IgA production	Decreased airway clearance Increased risk for infection Increased risk of aspiration
Sleep and breathing	Decreased ventilatory drive Decreased tone of upper airway muscles Decreased arousal	Increased risk of apnea, hypopnea and arterial oxygen desaturation during sleep Increased risk of aspiration Snoring Obstructive sleep apnea
Exercise capacity	Muscle deconditioning and efficiency Decreased muscle mass Decreased reserves	Decreased maximum oxygen consumption Breathlessness at low exercise levels

Modifed from Pierson DJ: Effects of aging on the respiratory system. In Pierson DJ, Kacmarek RM, editors: *Foundations of respiratory care,* New York, 1992, Churchill Livingstone.

Cardiovascular Health Promotion

- Maintain ideal body weight
- Low fat, low salt diet
- Regular exercise program
- Stress reduction
- No smoking
- Monitor cholesterol and triglycerides
- Have blood pressure checked annually

Respiratory Health Promotion

- No smoking
- Avoid secondhand smoke
- Regular exercise program
- Use mask when working in areas such as woodworking, mowing the lawn, painting
- Annual flu vaccine
- Pneumococcal vaccine
- Cover your mouth and nose when coughing or sneezing
- Avoid large crowds during flu season

---

consumption by 10% to 20% because of increased cardiac output and increased efficiency of the myocardial muscle.

CIGARETTE SMOKING

Cigarette smoking is associated with a number of diseases, including heart disease, chronic obstructive lung disease, and lung cancer. Cigarette smoking can worsen peripheral vascular and coronary artery diseases. Inhaled nicotine causes vasoconstriction of peripheral and coronary blood vessels, increasing blood pressure and decreasing blood flow to peripheral vessels. The risk of lung cancer is 10 times greater for a person who smokes than for a non-smoker (Dettenmeier, 1992). Exposure to sidestream smoke increases the risk of lung cancer in the nonsmoker. The number of women smokers has increased substantially over the past 30 years. This has resulted in a tenfold increase in the number of women diagnosed with lung cancer (ACS, 1994). Women who take birth control pills and smoke cigarettes are at increased risk for cardiovascular problems such as thrombophlebitis and pulmonary emboli.

The 5-year survival rate for all lung cancer clients is only 13%, regardless of the diagnosis (ACS, 1994). Frequently lung cancer is diagnosed only when it has reached an advanced stage. Only 16% of lung cancers are diagnosed when the disease is still localized (ACS, 1994).

SUBSTANCE ABUSE

Excessive use of alcohol and other drugs can impair tissue oxygenation in two ways. First, the person who chronically abuses substances often has a poor nutritional intake. With the resultant decrease in intake of iron-rich foods, hemoglobin production declines. Second, excessive use of alcohol and certain other drugs can depress the respiratory center, reducing the rate and depth of respiration and the amount of inhaled oxygen. Substance abuse by either

---

▶ RESEARCH HIGHLIGHT

RESEARCH ABSTRACT

Sixteen subjects aged 60 to 72 years who did not routinely exercise and who had no evidence of cardiopulmonary disease or history of smoking were enrolled in the study. Subjects completed a timed 440 yard (400 meter) walking test, walking as fast as they could while remaining comfortable. Subjects then completed surveys about perceived frustration, tension, and coping ability related to stress. All subjects engaged in a supervised exercise program 3 days a week for 50 to 60 minutes each session, working out at 50% to 60% of their individual predicted maximal heart rate reserves.

All subjects increased their walking capacity. Of the 14 subjects that completed the study, 12 showed a reduction in the incidence of respiratory tract infections and related symptoms. Eleven of the subjects improved their scores on the stress survey, reporting less self-perceived stress.

IMPLICATIONS FOR PRACTICE

▶ Aerobic activity may produce a buffering effect against stress; nurses should encourage clients to exercise within their capacity.

▶ The secondary benefits of exercise include improved cardiovascular function, improved musculoskeletal strength, endurance, improved joint flexibility, and reduced incidence of respiratory infections and related symptoms. Nurses should educate their clients about the benefits of regular exercise and help them develop a plan for health promotion.

REFERENCE

Karper WB, Boshen MB: Effects of exercise on acute respiratory tract infections and related symptoms, *Geriatric Nursing* 14(1):15, 1993.

---

smoking or inhaling, such as crack cocaine or inhaling fumes from paint or glue cans, causes direct injury to lung tissue that can lead to permanent lung damage and impaired oxygenation.

Environmental Factors

The environment can also influence oxygenation. The incidence of pulmonary disease is higher in smoggy, urban areas than in rural areas. In addition, the client's work place may increase the risk for pulmonary disease. Occupational pollutants include asbestos, talcum powder, dust, and airborne fibers. For example, farm workers in dry regions of the southwestern United States are at risk for coccidioidomycosis, a fungal disease caused by inhalation of spores of the airborne bacterium *Coccidioides immitis*.

Asbestosis is an occupational lung disease that develops after exposure to asbestos. The lung in asbestosis is characterized by diffuse interstitial fibrosis, creating a restrictive lung disease. It can also cause pleural mesotheliomas and pleural plaques. Clients at risk to develop asbestosis include those working with textiles, fireproofing, milling, production of paints, plastics, and some prefabricated construction. Clients exposed to asbestos who also smoke are at increased risk of developing lung cancer.

ANXIETY

A continuous state of severe anxiety increases the body's metabolic rate and the oxygen demand. The body responds to anxiety and other stresses by an increased rate and depth of respiration. Most people can adapt, but some, particularly those with chronic illnesses or acute life-threatening illnesses such as a myocardial infarction, cannot tolerate the oxygen demands associated with anxiety.

ALTERATIONS IN CARDIAC FUNCTIONING

Alterations in cardiac functioning are caused by illnesses and conditions that affect cardiac rhythm, strength of contraction, blood flow through the chambers, myocardial blood flow, and peripheral circulation.

Disturbances in Conduction

Some disturbances in conduction are the result of electrical impulses that do not originate from the SA node. These rhythm disturbances are called **dysrhythmias**, meaning a deviation from the normal sinus heart rhythm (Table 44-3). Dysrhythmias may occur as a primary conduction disturbance; as a response to ischemia, valvular abnormality, anxiety, and drug toxicity; as a result of caffeine, alcohol, or tobacco use; or as a complication of acid-base or electrolyte imbalance (see Chapter 45).

Dysrhythmias are classified by cardiac response and site of impulse origin. Cardiac response can be either tachycardiac (greater than 100 beats/min), bradycardiac (less than 60 beats/min), premature (early beat), or blocked (delayed or absent beat).

Tachydysrhythmias and bradydysrhythmias can lower cardiac output and blood pressure. Tachydysrhythmias reduce cardiac output by decreasing diastolic filling time. Bradydysrhythmias lower cardiac output because of the decreased heart rate.

Abnormal impulses originating above the ventricles are referred to as *supraventricular dysrhythmias*. The abnormality on the waveform is the configuration and placement of the P-wave. Ventricular conduction usually remains normal, and a normal QRS complex is observed.

Junctional dysrhythmias represent an abnormal site of impulse conduction above or below the AV node. The P-wave can occur before, during, or after the QRS complexes, and is often inverted if visible. Because the beat originates above the ventricle, ventricular conduction and the QRS complex are usually normal.

Ventricular dysrhythmias represent an ectopic site of impulse formation within the ventricles. The configuration of the QRS complex is usually widened and bizarre. P-waves may or may not be present, often they are buried in the QRS complex. Ventricular tachycardia and ventricular fibrillation are life-threatening rhythms that require immediate intervention.

Altered Cardiac Output

Failure of the myocardium to eject sufficient volume to the systemic and pulmonary circulations can result in heart failure. Failure of the myocardial pump results from primary coronary artery disease, cardiomyopathic conditions, valvular disorders, and pulmonary disease.

Left-sided heart failure is an abnormal condition characterized by impaired functioning of the left ventricle due to elevated pressures and pulmonary congestion. If left ventricle failure is significant, the amount of blood ejected from the left ventricle drops greatly, resulting in decreased cardiac output. Assessment findings may include decreased activity tolerance, breathlessness, dizziness, and confusion as a result of tissue hypoxia from the diminished cardiac output. As the left ventricle continues to fail, blood begins to pool in the pulmonary circulation causing pulmonary congestion. Clinical findings include crackles on auscultation, hypoxia, shortness of breath on exertion and often at rest, cough, and paroxysmal nocturnal dyspnea (Canobbio, 1990).

Right-sided heart failure results from impaired functioning of the right ventricle characterized by venous congestion in the systemic circulation. Right-sided heart failure more commonly results from pulmonary disease or as a sequela to left-sided failure. The primary pathological factor in right-sided failure is elevated pulmonary vascular resistance (PVR). As the PVR continues to rise, the right ventricle must generate more work, and the oxygen demand of the heart increases. As the failure continues, the amount of blood ejected from the right ventricle declines, and blood begins to "back up" in the systemic circulation. Clinically the client has weight gain, distended neck veins, hepatomegaly and splenomegaly, and dependent peripheral edema.

Impaired Valvular Function

Valvular heart disease is an acquired or congenital disorder of a cardiac valve characterized by stenosis and obstructed blood flow or valvular degeneration and regurgitation of blood (Canobbio, 1990).

When stenosis occurs in the semilunar valves (aortic and pulmonic valves), the adjacent ventricles must work harder to move the ventricular volume beyond the stenotic valve. Over time the stenosis can cause the ventricle to hypertrophy (enlarge), and if the condition is untreated, left- or right-sided heart failure can occur. If stenosis occurs in the atrioventricular valves (mitral and tricuspid valves), the atrial pressure rises, causing the atria to hypertrophy.

When regurgitation occurs, there is a back flow of blood into an adjacent chamber. For example, in mitral regurgitation the mitral leaflets do not close completely. When the ventricle contracts, blood escapes back into the atria, causing a murmur, or "whooshing" sound (see Chapter 33).

Myocardial Ischemia

Myocardial ischemia results when the supply of blood to the myocardium from the coronary arteries is insufficient to meet the oxygen demands of the organ. Two common manifestations of this ischemia are angina pectoris and myocardial infarction.

Angina pectoris is usually a transient imbalance between myocardial oxygen supply and demand. The condition results in chest pain that is aching, sharp, tingling, burning, or feels like pressure. The chest pain may be left-sided or substernal and may radiate to the left or both arms, jaw, neck, and back. In some clients anginal pain may not radiate. The pain can last from 1 to 15 minutes. Clients report that pain is often precipitated by activities that increase myocardial oxygen demand (e.g., exercise, anxiety,

Table 44-3	Common Basic Cardiac Dysrhythmias

RHYTHM CHARACTERISTICS	ETIOLOGY	CLINICAL SIGNIFICANCE	MANAGEMENT
SINUS TACHYCARDIA			
Regular rhythm, rate 100-180 beats/min (higher in infants), normal P-wave, normal QRS complex	Rate increase may be normal response to exercise, emotion, or stressors such as pain, fever, pump failure, hyperthyroidism, and certain drugs (e.g., caffeine, nitrates, atropine, epinephrine, isoproterenol, nicotine)	May have hemodynamic consequence in client with damaged heart that is unable to sustain increased workloads (increased myocardial oxygen consumption) brought on by persistent increases in heart rate	Correct underlying factors, remove offending drugs

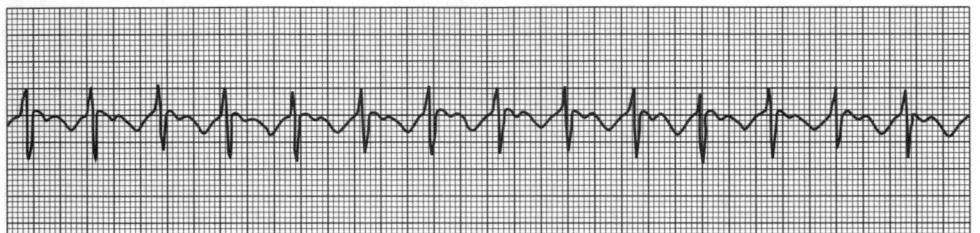

RHYTHM CHARACTERISTICS	ETIOLOGY	CLINICAL SIGNIFICANCE	MANAGEMENT
SINUS BRADYCARDIA			
Regular rhythm, rate less than 60 beats/min, normal P-wave, normal PR interval, normal QRS complex	Rate decrease may be normal response to sleep or in well-conditioned athlete; abnormal drops in rate may be caused by diminished blood flow to SA node, vagal stimulation, hypothyroidism, increased intracranial pressure, or pharmacological agents (e.g., digoxin, propranolol, quidinine, procainamide)	No clinical significance unless associated with signs of impaired symptoms of dizziness, syncope, chest pain	

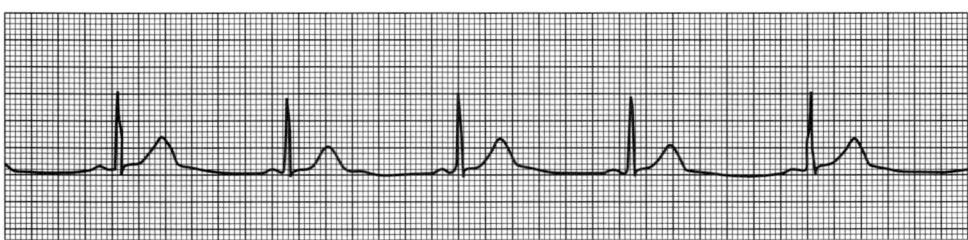

RHYTHM CHARACTERISTICS	ETIOLOGY	CLINICAL SIGNIFICANCE	MANAGEMENT
SINUS DYSRHYTHMIA			
Irregular rhythm; possibly phasic with respiration, slowing during inspiration and increasing with expiration; rate of 60-100 beats/min; normal P-wave; normal PR interval; normal QRS complex	Sinus rhythm with cyclic variation caused by vagal impulses that influence rhythm during respiration; occurs commonly in children, young adults, and older adults; usually disappears as heart rate increases	No clinical significance unless heart rate decreases and symptoms of dizziness occur with decreased rate	None indicated unless heart rate decreases and symptoms occur

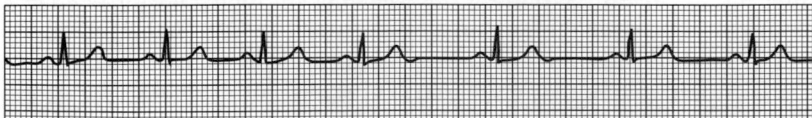

Modified from Canobbio MM: Cardiovascular disorders, St Louis, 1990, Mosby.
PSVT Management: Vagal stimulation such as carotid sinus massage or Valsava maneuver to decrease ventricular response with medication to block AV conduction; adenosine 6 mg IV over 1-3 seconds; adenosine 12 mg IV over 1-3 seconds; assess complex width; narrow-check blood pressure, normal verapamil 2.5-5 mg IV; blood pressure low or unstable proceed to synchronized cardioversion; wide complex, lidocaine 1-1.5 mg/kg IV push, procainamide 20-30 mg/min; synchronized cardioversion is resistant to drug therapy (ECC, 1992).
Sinus Bradycardia Management: Correct underlying causes. If symptomatic, e.g., hypotension, chest pain, decreased level of consciousness, shortness of breath, administer atropine 0.04 mg/kg IV; transcutaneous pacing if available; dopamine 5-20 μg/kg/minute; epinephrine 2-10 μg/min; temporary transvenous pacemaker if resistant to drug therapy (ECC, 1992).

Table 44-3	Common Basic Cardiac Dysrhythmias—cont'd		
RHYTHM CHARACTERISTICS	**ETIOLOGY**	**CLINICAL SIGNIFICANCE**	**MANAGEMENT**

PAROXYSMAL SUPRAVENTRICULAR TACHYCARDIA (PSVT)

| Sudden, rapid onset of tachycardia with stimulus originating above AV node; regular rhythm; rate 150-250 beats/min; P-wave uniform, possibly buried in preceding T-wave; PR interval variable, often difficult to measure; normal QRS complex | May begin and end spontaneously or be precipitated by excitement, fatigue, or caffeine, smoking, or alcohol use | Usually no significant impairment; client complains of palpitations and shortness of breath; if persistent or occurring in client with preexisting organic heart disease, may cause decrease in cardiac ouput and/or blood pressure resulting in pump failure or shock | |

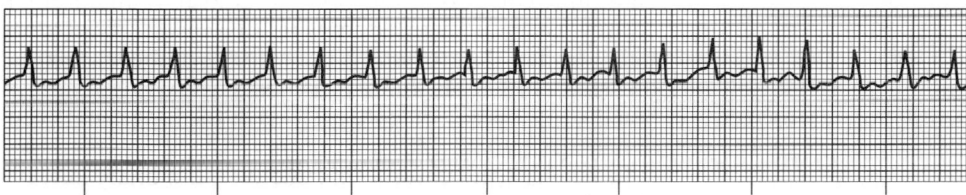

PREMATURE VENTRICULAR CONTRACTIONS (PVCs)

| Irregular rhythm with ectopic beats followed by full compensatory pause; rate normal or increased depending on number of ectopic beats; P-wave absent in ectopic beat; PR interval absent; QRS complex widened and distorted; T-wave in opposition to R-wave | Caused by irritable focus within ventricle, commonly associated with myocardial infarction; other causes include hypoxia, hypocalcemia, acidosis | PVCs occurring frequently (more than 6/min) or in pairs indicating increased ventricular irritability | Suppress PVCs; if PVCs frequent, administer IV bolus of lidocaine 1-1.5 mg/kg IV push followed by continuous IV infusion; administer additional antiarrhythmic agents as needed |

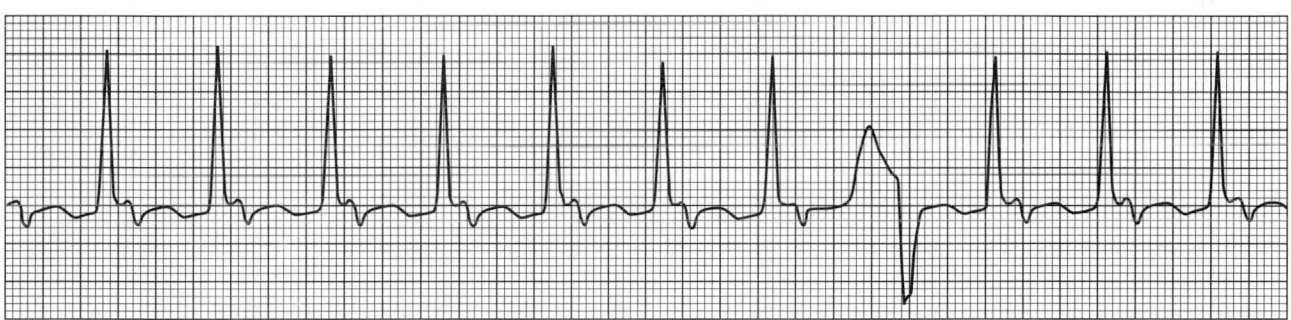

VENTRICULAR TACHYCARDIA

| Rhythm slightly irregular, rate 100-200 beats/min, P-wave absent, PR interval absent, QRS complex wide and bizarre, >0.12 seconds | Caused by irritable ventricular foci firing repetitively, commonly caused by myocardial infarction | Often a forerunner of ventricular fibrillation; if condition persistent and rapid, causes decreased cardiac output because of decreased ventricular filling time | Most episodes terminate abruptly without treatment; administer lidocaine bolus 1-1.5 mg/kg IV followed by continuous intravenous drip; perform defibrillation |

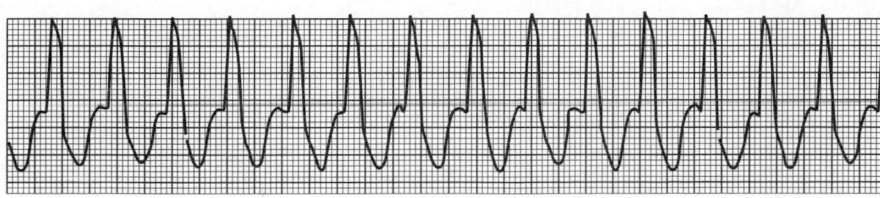

and stress). The pain is usually relieved with rest and coronary vasodilators, the most common being a nitroglycerine preparation.

Myocardial infarction results from sudden decreases in coronary blood flow or an increase in myocardial oxygen demand without adequate coronary perfusion. Infarction occurs because of ischemia (which is reversible) and necrosis (which is not reversible) of myocardial tissue and is not reversible (Canobbio, 1990).

Chest pain associated with myocardial infarction is usually described as crushing, squeezing, or stabbing. The pain may be retrosternal and left precordial and may radiate down the left arm, to the neck, jaws, teeth, epigastric area, and back. The pain occurs at rest or exertion, lasts more than 30 minutes, and is unrelieved by rest, position change, or sublingual nitroglycerin administration.

■ ALTERATIONS IN RESPIRATORY FUNCTIONING

Alterations in respiratory functioning are caused by illnesses and conditions that affect ventilation or oxygen transport. The three primary alterations are hyperventilation, hypoventilation, and hypoxia.

Hyperventilation

The goal of ventilation is to produce a normal arterial carbon dioxide tension (Pa_{CO_2}) and maintain a normal arterial oxygen tension (Pa_{O_2}) (Dettenmeier, 1992). *Hyperventilation* and *hypoventilation* refer to alveolar ventilation and not to the client's respiratory rate.

Hyperventilation is a state of ventilation in excess of that required to eliminate the normal venous carbon dioxide produced by cellular metabolism. Hyperventilation can be induced by anxiety, infections, drugs, an acid-base imbalance, and hypoxia associated with pulmonary embolus or shock. Acute anxiety can lead to hyperventilation and may cause loss of consciousness from excess carbon dioxide exhalation. Fever can cause hyperventilation. For each increase of 1 degree Fahrenheit, there is a 7% increase in the metabolic rate, thereby increasing carbon dioxide production. The clinical response is an increased rate and depth of respiration.

Hyperventilation may also be chemically induced. Salicylate (aspirin) poisoning causes excessive stimulation of the respiratory center as the body's attempt to compensate for excessive carbon dioxide. Amphetamines also increase ventilation by raising carbon dioxide production.

Hyperventilation can also occur as the body tries to compensate for metabolic acidosis by producing a respiratory alkalosis. Ventilation increases to reduce the amount of carbon dioxide available to form carbonic acid (see Chapter 45).

Alveolar hyperventilation produces many signs and symptoms that can be assessed (see the box below, left). Hemoglobin does not release oxygen to tissues as readily, and tissue hypoxia results. As symptoms worsen the client may become more agitated, which further increases the respiratory rate and can result in respiratory alkalosis.

Hypoventilation

Hypoventilation occurs when alveolar ventilation is inadequate to meet the body's oxygen demand or to eliminate sufficient carbon dioxide. As alveolar ventilation decreases, Pa_{CO_2} is elevated. Severe atelectasis can produce hypoventilation. **Atelectasis** is a collapse of the alveoli that prevents normal respiratory exchange of oxygen and carbon dioxide. As alveoli collapse, less of the lung can be ventilated and hypoventilation occurs.

In clients with chronic obstructive pulmonary disease, the inappropriate administration of excessive oxygen can result in hypoventilation. These clients have adapted to a high carbon dioxide level, and their carbon dioxide–sensitive chemoreceptors are essentially not functioning. Their stimulus to breathe is a decreased Pa_{O_2}. If excessive oxygen is administered, the oxygen requirement is satisfied and the stimulus to breathe is negated. High concentrations of oxygen (e.g., greater than 24% to 28% [1 to 3 L/min]) prevent the Pa_{O_2} from falling and obliterate the stimulus to breathe, resulting in hypoventilation. The excessive retention of CO_2 may lead to a respiratory arrest.

Signs and symptoms of hypoventilation are in the box below. If untreated, the client's status can rapidly decline. Convulsions, unconsciousness, and death can result.

Treatment for hyperventilation and hypoventilation begins by treating the underlying cause then improving tissue oxygenation, restoring ventilatory function, and achieving acid-base balance.

Hypoxia

Hypoxia is inadequate tissue oxygenation at the cellular level. This can result from a deficiency in oxygen delivery or oxygen utilization at the cellular level. Hypoxia can be

---

Signs and Symptoms of Alveolar Hyperventilation

- Tachycardia
- Shortness of breath
- Chest pain
- Dizziness
- Lightheadedness
- Disorientation
- Paresthesia
- Numbness (extremities, circumoral)
- Tinnitus
- Blurred vision
- Disorientation
- Tetany (carpopedal spasm)

Signs and Symptoms of Alveolar Hypoventilation

- Dizziness
- Headache (may be occipital only on awakening)
- Lethargy
- Disorientation
- Decreased ability to follow instructions
- Cardiac dysrhythmias
- Electrolyte imbalances
- Convulsions
- Coma
- Cardiac arrest

Signs and Symptoms of Hypoxia

- Restlessness
- Apprehension, anxiety
- Disorientation
- Decreased ability to concentrate
- Decreased level of consciousness
- Increased fatigue
- Dizziness
- Behavioral changes
- Increased pulse rate
- Increased rate and depth of respiration
- Elevated blood pressure
- Cardiac dysrhythmias
- Pallor
- Cyanosis
- Clubbing
- Dyspnea

caused by (1) a decreased hemoglobin level and lowered oxygen-carrying capacity of the blood; (2) a diminished concentration of inspired oxygen, which may occur at high altitudes; (3) the inability of the tissues to extract oxygen from the blood as with cyanide poisoning; (4) decreased diffusion of oxygen from the alveoli to the blood, as in pneumonia; (5) poor tissue perfusion with oxygenated blood as with shock, and (6) impaired ventilation as with multiple rib fractures or chest trauma.

The clinical signs and symptoms of hypoxia include apprehension, restlessness, inability to concentrate, declining level of consciousness, dizziness, and behavioral changes (see the box above). The client with hypoxia is unable to lie down and appears fatigued and agitated. Vital sign changes include an increased pulse rate and increased rate and depth of respiration. During early stages of hypoxia the blood pressure is elevated unless the condition is caused by shock. As the hypoxia worsens, the respiratory rate may decline as a result of respiratory muscle fatigue.

Cyanosis, a blue discoloration of the skin and mucous membranes caused by the presence of desaturated hemoglobin in capillaries, is a late sign of hypoxia. The presence or absence of cyanosis is not a reliable measure of oxygenation status. Central cyanosis, observed in the tongue, soft palate, and conjunctiva of the eye, where blood flow is high, indicates hypoxemia. Peripheral cyanosis, seen in the extremities, nailbeds, and earlobes is often the result of vasoconstriction and stagnant blood flow.

Hypoxia is a life-threatening condition. Untreated, it can produce cardiac dysrhythmias that result in death. Hypoxia is managed by administration of oxygen and treatment of the underlying cause, such as airway obstruction.

■ NURSING PROCESS AND OXYGENATION

 Assessment

The nursing assessment of a client's cardiopulmonary functioning should include data collected from the following areas:

1. Nursing history of the client's normal and present cardiopulmonary function, past impairments in circulatory or respiratory functioning, and measures the client may use to optimize oxygenation
2. Physical examination of the client's cardiopulmonary status, including inspection, palpation, percussion, and auscultation
3. Review of laboratory and diagnostic test results, including complete blood count (CBC), electrocardiogram (ECG), pulmonary function test (PFT), sputum, and oxygenation such as arterial blood gases (ABGs) or pulse oximetry

NURSING HISTORY

The nursing history should focus on the client's ability to meet oxygen needs. The nursing history for cardiac function includes pain and characteristics of pain, dyspnea, fatigue, peripheral circulation, cardiac risk factors, and the presence of past or concurrent cardiac conditions. The nursing history for respiratory function includes presence of a cough, shortness of breath, wheezing, pain, environmental exposures, frequency of respiratory tract infections, pulmonary risk factors, past respiratory problems, current medication use, and smoking history or secondhand smoke exposure.

Fatigue. Fatigue is a subjective sensation in which the client reports a loss of endurance. Fatigue in the client with cardiopulmonary alterations is often an early sign of a worsening of the chronic underlying process. To provide an objective measure of fatigue, the client may be asked to rate the fatigue on a scale of 1 to 10, with 10 being the worst level of fatigue and 1 representing no fatigue.

Dyspnea. Dyspnea is a clinical sign of hypoxia and manifests as breathlessness. It is the subjective sensation of difficult or uncomfortable breathing (Gift, 1990). Physiological dyspnea is shortness of breath associated with exercise or excitement. Pathological dyspnea is the inability to catch a breath without relation to activity or exercise.

Dyspnea can be associated with clinical signs such as exaggerated respiratory effort, use of the accessory muscles of respiration, nasal flaring, and marked increases in the rate and depth of respirations. The use of a visual analog scale can help the client to make an objective assessment of their dyspnea. This allows the nurse and client to determine if specific nursing interventions are having an effect on the client's dyspnea. The visual analog scale is a 100-mm vertical line with 0 equated with no dyspnea, and the 100-mm marker equated with the worst breathlessness the client has experienced. Studies have validated the use of the visual analog scale to evaluate a client's dyspnea in the clinical setting (Gift, 1989).

The nursing history of dyspnea includes the circumstances under which it occurred, such as with exertion, stress, or respiratory tract infection. The nurse also determines whether the client's perception of dyspnea affects the ability to lie flat. **Orthopnea** is an abnormal condition in which the person must use multiple pillows when lying down or must sit to breathe. The presence of orthopnea is usually quantified by the number of pillows required to sleep, such as two- or three-pillow orthopnea.

Cough. Cough is a sudden, audible expulsion of air from the lungs. The person breathes in, the glottis is partially closed, and the accessory muscles of expiration contract to expel the air forcibly. Coughing is a protective reflex to clear the trachea, bronchi, and lungs of irritants and secretions. The carina, the point of bifurcation of the right and left mainstem bronchus, is the most sensitive area for cough production.

A cough is difficult to evaluate and almost everyone has periods of coughing. Clients with a chronic cough tend to deny, underestimate, or minimize their coughing, often because they are so accustomed to it that they are unaware of how frequently it occurs.

Coughing is classified according to the time when the client most frequently coughs. Clients with chronic sinusitis may cough only in the early morning or immediately after rising from sleep. This clears the airway of mucus resulting from sinus drainage. Clients with chronic bronchitis generally produce sputum all day, although greater amounts are produced after rising from a semirecumbent or flat position. This is the result of the dependent accumulation of sputum in the airways and is associated with reduced mobility (see Chapter 37). Once the nurse determines that the client has a cough, it must be identified as productive or nonproductive and its frequency must be assessed. A **productive cough** results in sputum production, material coughed up from the lungs that may be swallowed or expectorated. Sputum contains mucus, cellular debris, and microorganisms, and may contain pus or blood. The nurse must collect data about the type and quantity of sputum (see the box below). The client is instructed to try to produce some sputum, being careful not to simply clear the throat to produce a sample of saliva. The nurse then inspects it for color, consistency, odor, and amount.

If **hemoptysis** (bloody sputum) is reported, the nurse determines if it is associated with coughing and bleeding from the upper respiratory tract, from sinus drainage, or from the gastrointestinal tract (**hematemesis**). In addition, the hemoptysis should be described according to amount, color, and duration and whether it is mixed with sputum. When a client reports bloody or blood-tinged sputum, diagnostic tests, such as examination of sputum specimens, chest x-ray examinations, bronchoscopy, and other x-ray studies, should be performed.

Sputum Characteristics

COLOR
- Clear
- White
- Yellow
- Streaked with blood
- Green
- Brown
- Red

QUALITY
- Same as usual
- Increased
- Decreased

CHANGES IN COLOR
- Same color throughout the day
- Clearing with coughing
- Progressively darker

CONSISTENCY
- Frothy
- Watery
- Tenacious, thick

ODOR
- None
- Foul

PRESENCE OF BLOOD
- Occasional
- Early morning
- Bright or dark red
- Blood-tinged

Wheezing. Wheezing is characterized by a high-pitched musical sound caused by high-velocity movement of air through a narrowed airway. Wheezing may be associated with asthma, acute bronchitis, or pneumonia. Wheezing can occur on inspiration, expiration, or both. The nurse should determine any precipitating factors such as respiratory infection, allergens, exercise, or stress.

Pain. The presence of chest pain needs to be thoroughly evaluated with regard to location, duration, radiation, and frequency. Cardiac pain does not occur with respiratory variations and is most often on the left side of the chest and radiates. Pericardial pain resulting from an inflammation of the pericardial sac is usually nonradiating and may occur with inspiration.

Pleuritic chest pain is peripheral and may radiate to the scapular regions. It is worsened by inspiratory maneuvers, such as coughing, yawning, and sighing. Pleuritic pain is often caused from an inflammation or infection in the pleural space and is described as knifelike lasting from a minute to hours, always associated with inspiration.

Musculoskeletal pain may be present following exercise, rib trauma, and prolonged coughing episodes. This pain is also aggravated by inspiratory movements and may easily be confused with pleuritic chest pain.

Environmental or Geographical Exposures. Environmental exposure to many inhaled substances is closely linked with respiratory disease. The nurse should investigate exposures in the client's home and work place. The most common environmental exposures in the home are cigarette smoke, carbon monoxide, and radon. The nurse should determine whether a client who is a nonsmoker is passively exposed to smoke. Carbon monoxide poisoning can result from a blocked furnace flue or fireplace. The client may have vague complaints of general malaise, flu-like symptoms, and excessive sleepiness. Clients are particularly at risk in the late fall when they turn the heat on or begin to use the fireplace again. Radon gas, a radioactive substance, enters homes through the ground. When homes are underventilated this gas is not able to escape into the atmosphere and becomes trapped in the home.

An employment history is obtained to assess exposure to substances such as asbestos, coal, cotton fibers, fumes, or chemical inhalants. It is particularly important with middle-age and older adults who may have worked in places without regulations to protect workers from carcinogens.

Exposure to substances may occur during travel. Schistosomiasis infection can be acquired in Asia, Africa, the Caribbean, and South America. Coccidioidomycosis (valley fever) can be acquired in southwestern desert regions, at chicken farms, and in the Ohio and Mississippi river valleys.

Respiratory Infections. A nursing history should contain information about the client's frequency and duration of respiratory tract infections. Although everyone occasionally experiences a cold, for some people it can result in bronchitis or pneumonia. Determine if the client has had a pneumovax or flu vaccine in the past. The nurse also asks about any known exposure to tuberculosis and the results of the tuberculin skin test.

Determine the client's risk for human immunodeficiency virus (HIV) infection. Clients with a history of IV drug use, multiple unprotected sexual partners, or a homosexual lifestyle are at risk of developing HIV infection. The client may not display any symptoms of HIV infection until they present with *Pneumocystis carinii* (PCP) or *Mycobacterium pneumonia*. Presentation with PCP or mycobacterium pneumonia indicates a significant depression of the client's immune system and progression to AIDS.

Risk Factors. The nurse must also investigate familial and environmental risk factors such as a family history of lung cancer or cardiovascular disease. Document which blood relatives have had the disease and their present level of health or age at time of death. Other family risk factors include the presence of infectious diseases, particularly tuberculosis. The nurse should determine who in the client's household has been infected and the status of treatment.

Medications. The last component of the nursing history should describe medications the client is using. These include prescribed, over-the-counter, and illicit drugs and substances. Such medications may have adverse effects by themselves or because of interactions with other drugs. A person using a prescribed bronchodilator drug, for example, may decide that using an over-the-counter inhalant as well will be beneficial. This product may react with the prescribed medication by potentiating or decreasing the effect of the prescribed medication.

As with all medication, the nurse assesses clients' knowledge and ability to use the "five rights" of medication administration (see Chapter 35). Of particular importance is the nurse's assessment of clients' understanding of potential side effects of the medications. Clients should be able to recognize adverse reactions and be aware of the dangers in combining prescribed medications with over-the-counter drugs.

When clients are prescribed drugs for which toxic levels can be monitored by blood analyses, the nurse needs to review these laboratory values. Common drugs that can be monitored include theophylline preparations (theophylline levels), digitalis preparation (digitalis levels), and phenobarbital (phenobarbital levels). Toxic effects of these medications can impair cardiopulmonary functioning. Illicit drugs, particularly parenterally administered narcotics, which are often diluted with talcum powder, can cause pulmonary disorders resulting from the irritant effect of talcum powder on lung tissues.

PHYSICAL EXAMINATION

The physical examination performed to assess the client's level of tissue oxygenation includes evaluation of the entire cardiopulmonary system. Inspection, palpation, auscultation, and percussion techniques are used (see Chapter 33).

Inspection. Using inspection techniques, the nurse performs a head-to-toe observation of the client for skin and mucous membrane color, general appearance, level of con-

Table 44-4	Inspection of Cardiopulmonary Status	
ABNORMALITY	**CAUSE**
EYES	
Xanthelasma (yellow lipid lesions on eyelids)	Hyperlipidemia
Corneal arcus (whitish opaque ring around junction of cornea and sclera)	Hyperlipidemia in young to middle adults, normal finding in older adults with arcus senilius
Pale conjunctivae	Anemia
Cyanotic conjunctivae	Hypoxemia
Petechiae on conjunctivae	Fat embolus or bacterial endocarditis
MOUTH AND LIPS	
Cyanotic mucous membranes	Decreased oxygenation (hypoxia)
Pursed-lip breathing	Associated with chronic lung disease
NECK VEINS	
Distention	Associated with right-sided heart failure
NOSE	
Flaring nares	Air hunger, dyspnea
CHEST	
Retractions	Increased work of breathing, dyspnea
Asymmetry	Chest wall injury
SKIN	
Peripheral cyanosis	Vasoconstriction and diminished blood flow
Central cyanosis	Hypoxemia
Decreased skin turgor	Dehydration (normal finding in older adults as a result of decreased skin elasticity)
Dependent edema	Associated with right- and left-sided heart failure
Periorbital edema	Associated with kidney disease
FINGERTIPS AND NAILBEDS	
Cyanosis	Decreased cardiac output or hypoxia
Splinter hemorrhages	Bacterial endocarditis
Clubbing	Chronic hypoxemia

Table 44-5	Respiratory Pattern	
TYPE/ PATTERN	**RATE (BREATHS PER MINUTE)**	**CLINICAL SIGNIFICANCE**
Eupnea	16-20	Normal
Tachypnea	>35	Respiratory failure Response to fever Anxiety Shortness of breath Respiratory infection
Bradypnea	<10	Sleep Respiratory depression Drug overdose Central nervous system (CNS) lesion
Apnea	Periods of no respiration lasting >15 seconds	May be intermittent such as in sleep apnea Respiratory arrest
Hypernea	16-20	Can result from anxiety or response to pain Can cause marked respiratory alkalosis, paresthesia, tetany, confusion
Kussmaul's	Usually >35, may be slow or normal	Tachypnea pattern associated with diabetic ketoacidosis, metabolic acidosis, or renal failure
Cheyne-Stokes	Variable	Increasing and decreasing pattern caused by alterations in acid-base status. Underlying metabolic problem or neurocerebral insult
Biot's	Variable	Periods of apnea and shallow breathing caused by CNS disorder; found in some healthy clients
Apneustic	Increased	Increased inspiratory time with short grunting expiratory time; seen in CNS lesions of the respiratory center

From Weilitz PB: *Pocket guide to respiratory care*, St Louis, 1991, Mosby.

sciousness, adequacy of systemic circulation, breathing patterns, and chest wall movement (Tables 44-4 to 44-6). Any abnormalities should be investigated during palpation, percussion, and auscultation.

Palpation. Palpation of the chest provides assessment data in several areas. It documents the type and amount of thoracic excursion, elicits any areas of tenderness, and can identify tactile fremitus, thrills, heaves, and the cardiac point of maximal impulse. Palpation also allows the nurse to feel for abnormal masses or lumps in the axilla and breast tissue. Palpation of the extremities provides data about the peripheral circulation, the presence and quality of peripheral pulses, skin temperature, color, and capillary refill (see Chapter 33).

Percussion. Percussion is the tapping of an object to determine the presence of air, liquid, or solid in the underlying tissue (Malasanos, Barkauskas, and Stoltenberg-Allen, 1990). Percussion elicits vibrations from the underlying area from 4 to 6 cm deep (Seidel et al, 1995). The five tones of percussion are resonance, hyperresonance, dullness, flatness, and tympany. Percussion allows the nurse to detect the presence of abnormal fluid, air in the lungs, or diaphragmatic excursion (see Chapter 33).

Auscultation. The use of auscultation enables the nurse to identify normal and abnormal heart and lung sounds (see Chapter 33). Auscultation of the cardiovascular system should include assessment for normal S_1 and S_2 sounds, the presence of abnormal S_3 and S_4, and murmurs and rubs. The examiner must identify location, radiation, intensity, pitch, and quality of a murmur. Auscultation is also used to identify a bruit over the carotid arteries, abdominal aorta, and femoral arteries.

Auscultation of lung sounds involves listening for movement of air throughout all lung fields; anterior, posterior, and lateral. Adventitious breath sounds occur with collapse of a lung region, fluid in a lung field, or an airway obstruction. Auscultation also evaluates the response of a client to interventions for improving respiratory status.

DIAGNOSTIC TESTS

Tests to Determine Adequacy of the Cardiac Conduction System. Tests used to determine the cardiac conduction of the heart include electrocardiogram, Holter monitor, exercise stress test, and electrophysiological studies.

Electrocardiogram. The electrocardiogram (ECG) produces a graphic recording of the heart's electrical activity, detecting transmission of impulses and the electrical position of the heart (the axis).

Holter monitor. The **Holter monitor** is a portable device that records the heart's electrical activity and produces a continuous ECG over a specified period, such as 12 hours or longer. The Holter monitor allows clients to continue with their normal activities while recording the heart's electrical activity. Clients keep a diary of activity, noting when they experience rapid heart beats or periods of dizziness. Correlation between activities and abnormal electrical activity can then be determined.

Exercise stress test. **Exercise stress tests** are used to evaluate the cardiac response to physical stress. These provide information on myocardial response to increased oxygen requirements and determine the adequacy of coronary blood flow. Heart rate, electrical activity, and cardiac recovery

Table 44-6	Assessment of Abnormal Chest Wall Movement	
ABNORMALITY		**CAUSE**
Retraction—sinking in soft tissues of chest between and around cartilaginous and bony ribs such as intercostal space, intraclavicular space, trachea, and substernally* worsening with need for increased inspiratory effort		Any condition that causes increased inspiratory effort (e.g., airway obstruction, asthma, tracheobronchitis)
Paradoxical breathing—asynchronous breathing; chest contraction during inspiration and expansion during expiration		Flail chest resulting from rib fractures due to chest trauma or CPR
Increased anteroposterior diameter		Emphysema, chronic obstructive pulmonary disease, advancing age

*Infants can experience sternal and substernal retractions with only slight inspiratory effort because of chest pliability.

time are reflected in the ECG tracing (Canobbio, 1990). In addition, data about the client's blood pressure, presence of chest pain, changes in respiration, color, and rate of muscular fatigue are monitored.

Electrophysiological studies. An electrophysiological study (EPS) is an invasive measure of electrical activity. An electrode catheter is inserted into the right atrium, usually via the femoral vein. Electrical stimulation is then delivered through the catheter while ECG monitors and computers record the heart's electrical response to the stimulus. Specific dysrhythmias can also be induced to determine the pathways through the heart, provide more specific information about difficult to treat dysrhythmias, and assess the adequacy of antidysrhythmic medication.

Tests to Determine Myocardial Contraction and Blood Flow. Echocardiography, scintigraphy, cardiac catheterization, and angiography are used to determine myocardial contraction and blood flow.

Echocardiography. Echocardiography is a noninvasive measure to evaluate the internal structures of the heart and heart wall motion. Sonar (radar) technology is used to measure ultrasonic waves and translate them into formed images. The echocardiogram graphically demonstrates overall cardiac performance.

Scintigraphy. Scintigraphy, or radionuclide angiography, is a noninvasive imaging technique that uses radioisotopes to evaluate cardiac structures, myocardial perfusion, and contractility (Canobbio, 1990).

Cardiac catheterization and angiography. Cardiac catheterization and angiography are invasive procedures used to visualize cardiac chambers, valves, the great vessels, and coronary arteries, and measure pressure and volumes within the four chambers. The procedures require insertion of a catheter into the heart via a percutaneous venous puncture. A contrast material is injected through the catheter, and fluoroscopic pictures are obtained. Both right- and left-sided catheterization can be performed.

Cardiac catheterizations performed for diagnostic purposes are usually done as an outpatient. If there are no complications from the procedure, the client may go home in as few as 6 to 8 hours afterward. Some clients may need to stay overnight for observation. Complications associated with the cardiac catheterization procedure include dysrhythmias, bleeding at the puncture site, hematoma, and stroke.

Tests to Measure Adequacy of Ventilation and Oxygenation. Pulmonary function tests, peak expiratory flow rates, arterial blood gas tests, oximetry, and complete blood counts are used to assess the adequacy of ventilation and oxygenation.

Pulmonary function tests. Pulmonary function tests determine the ability of the lungs to efficiently exchange oxygen and carbon dioxide. Basic ventilation studies are performed with a spirometer and recording device as the client breathes through a mouthpiece into a connecting tube. Measurements include tidal volume (V_T), inspiratory reserve volume (IRV), residual volume (RV), and forced expiratory volume in 1 second (FEV_1) (Table 44-7).

Pulmonary function tests are usually performed in a pulmonary function laboratory. The nurse prepares the client by explaining the procedure. A nose clip prevents air from being inhaled or exhaled through the nose. The client breathes through a mouthpiece attached to a spirometer for measuring lung volume. The client is asked at certain times in the test to inhale or exhale as much air as possible. The client's cooperation is critical to ensure accurate results.

Peak expiratory flow rate. Peak expiratory flow rate (PEFR) is the point of highest flow during maximal expiration, and reflects changes in large airway sizes. The measure is similar to and correlates well with the FEV_1 (Walsh, 1992). The peak expiratory flow meter is a hand-held instrument that allows clients with asthma to follow the degree of airway openness. Information about peak expiratory flow rate is essential assessment data for clients with asthma.

Arterial blood gas tests. Arterial blood gas measurement is performed in conjunction with pulmonary function tests to determine the hydrogen ion concentration, partial pressure of carbon dioxide and oxygen concentration, and oxyhemoglobin saturation. Arterial blood gas tests provide information about diffusion of gas across the alveolar-capillary membrane and adequacy of tissue oxygenation (see Chapter 45).

Oximetry. Continuous measurements of capillary oxygen saturation are available with cutaneous **oximetry** (Procedure 44-1). Oxygen saturation (O_2 sat) is the percentage of hemoglobin saturated with oxygen. Transcutaneous oximeter measurements have the advantages of being easy to use, noninvasive, and readily available (Whitney, 1990). Oximetry is painless when compared to an arterial punc-

Table 44-7	Pulmonary Function Measurements		
DESCRIPTION	**AVERAGE VALUE**	**AVERAGE VALUE**	**CLINICAL SIGNIFICANCE**
TIDAL VOLUME (V_T) Volume of air in (ml) inhaled or exhaled per breath	5-10 ml/kg	Decreased	Decreased in restrictive lung disease and older client
RESIDUAL VOLUME (RV) Volume of air (ml) left in the lungs after maximal exhalation	1200 ml	Increased by as much as 25%	Increased in clients with COPD and older clients due to changes in elastic recoil of the lung, chest wall compliance, and decreased respiratory muscle mass and strength
FUNCTIONAL RESIDUAL CAPACITY (FRC) Volume of air (ml) left in the lung after a normal exhalation	2400 ml	Increased	Increased in clients with obstructive lung disease and older clients due to changes in chest wall compliance, and elastic recoil of the lung, and decreased respiratory muscle mass and strength
VITAL CAPACITY (VC) Volume of air (ml) exhaled after a maximal inhalation	4800 ml	Decreased by as much as 25%	Decreased associated with decreased flow rates found in pulmonary edema, atelectasis, and changes associated with aging such as decreased respiratory muscle strength and chest wall compliance
TOTAL LUNG CAPACITY (TLC) Total volume of air (ml) in the lungs following a maximal inhalation	6000 ml	Unchanged	Decreased in restrictive lung disease; increased in obstructive lung disease

ture. Clients with ventilation/perfusion abnormalities such as pneumonia, emphysema, chronic bronchitis, asthma, pulmonary embolism, or congestive heart failure are ideal candidates for pulse oximetry (Ahrens and Rutherford, 1993).

The most common oximetry is the pulse oximeter. This type of oximeter reports the amplitude of the pulse with the oxygen saturation reading. The nurse usually attaches a noninvasive sensor to the client's finger, toe, or nose that monitors capillary blood oxygen saturation. The nasal probe is recommended for extreme low perfusion states. The blood flow in the nasal septum anterior ethmoid artery remains greater than the flow to the fingers in compromised flow states (Ahrens and Rutherford, 1993). Continuous monitoring of oxygen saturation is useful in assessing sleep disorders, exercise tolerance, weaning from mechanical ventilation, and transient decreases in oxygen saturation.

The accuracy of the pulse oximetry value is directly related to the perfusion of the probe area. Clients with poor tissue perfusion caused by shock, hypothermia, or peripheral vascular diseases may not have reliable oximetry measures. The accuracy of the pulse oximetry is decreased when the systolic blood pressure is less than 90 mm Hg. Spot check oximetry readings have little clinical value. Trends over time provide the best information about the client's oxygenation.

Complete blood count. A complete blood count determines the number and type of red and white blood cells per mm³ of blood. The nurse obtains a venous blood sample by using venipuncture. Normal values for a complete blood count vary with age and gender.

The complete blood count measures the hemoglobin level within the red blood cells (erythrocytes). A deficiency in red blood cells decreases the blood's oxygen-carrying capacity because there are fewer hemoglobin molecules available to carry oxygen to tissues.

When the number of red blood cells is increased, such as polycythemia in chronic lung conditions and cyanotic heart conditions, the oxygen-carrying capacity of the blood is increased. However, increased red blood cells increase blood viscosity and the client's risk for thrombus formation.

Tests to Visualize Structures of the Respiratory System. Chest x-ray examination, bronchoscopy, and lung scan are used to visualize structures of the respiratory system.

Chest x-ray examination. A chest x-ray examination consists of a radiograph of the thorax that allows the physician and nurse to observe the lung fields for fluid (i.e., occurs with pneumonia), masses (i.e., lung cancer), fractures (i.e., rib and clavicular fractures), and other abnormal processes (i.e., tuberculosis). Usually a PA (posterior-anterior) and lateral film are taken to adequately visualize all the lung fields.

Bronchoscopy. Bronchoscopy is visual examination of the tracheobronchial tree through a narrow, flexible fiberoptic bronchoscope. Bronchoscopy is performed to obtain biopsy and fluid or sputum samples and to remove mucus plugs or foreign bodies that have become lodged in the airways.

The client is usually kept NPO before bronchoscopy. The nurse administers medications such as a sedative or atropine to reduce oral secretions. The nurse continues to observe the client after the procedure for signs and symptoms of respiratory distress or hypoxia. Before beginning oral fluids, assess that the client's gag/swallow reflex is intact.

Pulse Oximetry

STEPS	RATIONALE

1. Identify client who will benefit from pulse oximetry.

    a. Assess client's respiratory status: oxygen therapy, hemoglobin level

    b. Review client's medical record for physician's order

    c. Identify clients who may have oxygen desaturation with sleep, activity, suctioning

Allows nurse to monitor trends in client's level of oxygen. Enables nurse to use objective criteria to adjust nursing intervention to optimize oxygen saturation.

Identifies hypoxemia before signs and symptoms develop.

2. Obtain equipment and place at bedside:

    a. Pulse oximeter

    b. Sensor probe

Type of sensor	Client's weight*
(1) Adhesive neonatal	Less than 3 kg (6.6 lb);
(2) Adhesive infant	From 1 kg (2.2 lb) to 20 kg (44 lb)
(3) Adhesive pediatric	From 10 kg (22 lb) to 50 kg (110 lb)
(4) Adhesive adult	More than 30 kg (66 lb)
(5) Adhesive adult nasal	More than 50 kg (110 lb)
(6) Finger clip	More than 40 kg (88 lb)

Ensures error-free data regarding oxygen saturation.

    c. Continuous printout (optional)

3. Explain purpose of procedure to client and family.

Ensures client and family understanding and increases compliance.

4. Wash hands.

Reduces transmission of microorganisms.

5. Select appropriate area to apply sensor based on peripheral circulation and extremity temperature.

Peripheral vasoconstriction alters oxygen saturation.

    a. Determine adequacy of peripheral circulation by assessing capillary refill (toe and finger sites).

    b. Do not use adhesive adult nasal sensor if client has large-bore nasogastric tube or nasoendotracheal tube (nose).

Interferes with oxygen saturation readings because of poor peripheral circulation and excessive equipment or dressings.

    c. Determine use of vasoactive drugs.

    d. Align photoelectron and light-emitting diode.

Permits transmission of light. Alignment ensures accurate oxygen saturation readings.

6. Prepare selected site:

    a. Remove nail polish and artificial nails.

    b. Remove earrings.

    c. Wash selected site, wipe with alcohol, and air dry.

Body oils, nail polish, and artificial nails interfere with transmission of light through nail, tissue, venous and arterial blood, and skin pigmentation (Sonnesso, 1991).

7. Attach sensor probe to appropriate site.

8. Instruct client to breathe normally.

Prevents large fluctuations in minute ventilation and possible changes in oxygen saturation.

9. Attach pulse oximeter sensor to client cable.

    a. Turn machine on.

    b. Listen for audible beep.

Senses with each pulse and indicates how well oximeter monitors pulse.

    c. Observe waveform for bar of light.

Light or waveform fluctuates with each pulsation and reflects pulse strength. Poor light on small waveform usually indicates that signal is too weak to give accurate oxygen saturation reading.

10. Ensure that alarm limits for *both* high and low oxygen saturation and high and low pulse are set according to physician's order and *turned on.*

Manufacturers preset limits, and adjustments can be made according to client's underlying physical condition, therapy, and risks (Sonnesso, 1991).

Provides an audible and visual signal that high or low limits have been exceeded.

*Sonnesso G: *Nurs '91* 21(8):60, 1991.

Continued.

PROCEDURE 44-1

Pulse Oximetry—cont'd

STEPS	RATIONALE
11. Read saturation level as ordered and while performing nursing interventions.	Documents oxygen saturation levels at rest, with activity such as ambulation, during procedure such as suctioning, and with changes in physical condition.
12. Move a finger sensor every 4 hr and a spring-tension sensor every 2 hr (see the illustration below).	Allows nurse to assess for and prevent impaired skin integrity caused by pressure from sensor.
13. Record in nurses' notes client's use of continuous pulse oximetry and record oxygen saturation.	Documents use of equipment for third-party payers, documents oxygen saturation.
14. Correlate oxygen saturation value with arterial blood gas measurements if available.	Documents reliability of oximeter.
15. Report oxygen saturation and response to changes in therapy to oncoming shift.	Provides oncoming nurse with baseline information and response to therapy.

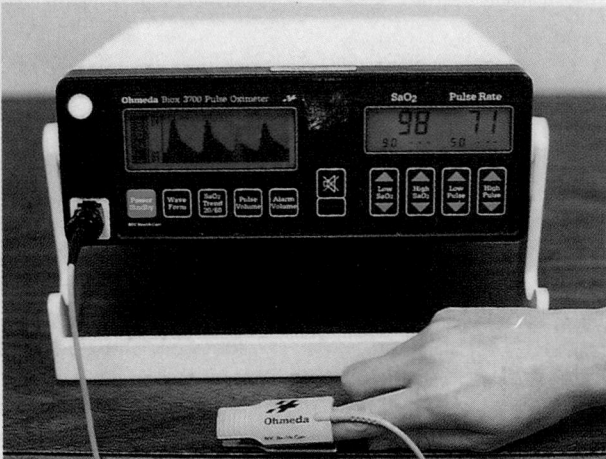

Step 12

Lung scan. The most common lung scan is the computed tomography (CT) scan. CT scanning combines x-ray and computer technology. X-ray beams pass through a section or plane of the thorax from different angles, and the computer calculates tissue absorption and displays a printout and scan picture of the tissues showing densities of various intrathoracic structures. A CT scan can identify abnormal masses by size and location but cannot identify tissue types, which requires a biopsy.

Tests to Determine Abnormal Cells or Infection in the Respiratory Tract. Tests to determine whether there are abnormal cells or infection in the respiratory tract include throat cultures, sputum specimens, skin testing, and thoracentesis.

Throat cultures. A throat culture sample is obtained by swabbing the oropharynx and tonsillar regions with a sterile swab. The throat culture determines the presence of pathogenic microorganisms. If a sensitivity is ordered, the antibiotics to which they are most sensitive can also be determined.

When obtaining a throat culture, the nurse inserts the swab into the pharyngeal region and passes it along reddened areas and areas of exudate. Some clients have an active gag reflex, making it difficult to obtain the specimen. The reflex may be less active if the client is sitting straight and leaning forward slightly. The client may be able to control gagging if informed that the procedure will take only a few seconds.

Sputum specimens. Sputum specimens are obtained to identify the type of organism growing in the sputum. *A sputum culture and sensitivity* (C and S) identifies a specific microorganism and its drug resistance and sensitivities. A sputum specimen may also be obtained to identify the presence of the tubercle bacillus (TB), *sputum for acid-fast bacillus* (AFB). The AFB specimen is obtained 3 consecutive days in the early morning. *Sputum for cytology* is a sputum specimen obtained to identify abnormal lung cancer by cell type. It involves a serial collection of three early morning specimens.

The nurse must ensure the sputum specimen consists of mucus from deep in the bronchus and not saliva. Record the color, consistency, amount, and odor of the sputum and document the date and time the specimen was sent to a specific laboratory for analysis.

Skin testing. Skin testing enables the clinician to determine the presence of bacterial, fungal, or viral pulmonary diseases. The antigen is injected intradermally (see Chapter 35), the injection site is circled, and the client instructed not to wash off the circle (see the box on p. 1215). This procedure enables the clinician to evaluate the response. Tuberculin skin tests are read at 48 hours.

Positive results are based on the size of the induration. An induration is a palpable, elevated, hardened area around the client's injection site. It is caused from edema and inflammation from the antigen/antibody reaction. If induration is present, it is measured in millimeters. Reddened flat areas are not positive reactions and should not be measured. TB testing in older adults is less reliable (see the box below).

Thoracentesis. **Thoracentesis** is surgical perforation of the chest wall and pleural space with a needle to aspirate fluid for diagnostic or therapeutic purposes or to remove a specimen for biopsy. The procedure is performed with aseptic technique using a local anesthetic. The client usually sits upright with the anterior thorax supported by pillows or an over-the-bed table (Fig. 44-8).

Whether this procedure is painful depends on the client's tolerance to pain (see Chapter 43). The nurse can reduce the client's anxiety by explaining the procedure and telling the client what to expect. The client must understand the importance of holding the breath as requested and of not coughing during the procedure. Sudden movements may result in lung puncture by the thoracentesis needle. The client is instructed to notify the physician before coughing or sneezing so the needle can be withdrawn.

After the procedure the nurse monitors the client for signs of pneumothorax; sudden shortness of breath, tracheal deviation, oxygen desaturation, and anxiety. The development of a pneumothorax following a thoracentesis is

GERONTOLOGICAL PRINCIPLES for Tuberculosis

Tuberculin skin testing in the older client is an unreliable indicator of tuberculosis. Due to reduced immune system activity, the older client frequently displays a false negative skin test (Kovach, 1991). It is recommended that the standard 5-TU Mantoux technique test be given and then repeated with the 5-TU or the second strength 250-TU test to create a booster effect. The nurse needs to be aware of the effect of changes associated with aging on TB skin testing to ensure the client's test is valid. Explain to the client that two injections will be necessary. The nurse should also be aware that older clients are at increased risk for reactivation of dormant organisms that have been present for decades. The changes in the older clients immune system increase the risk for developing reactivation TB (Kovach, 1991).

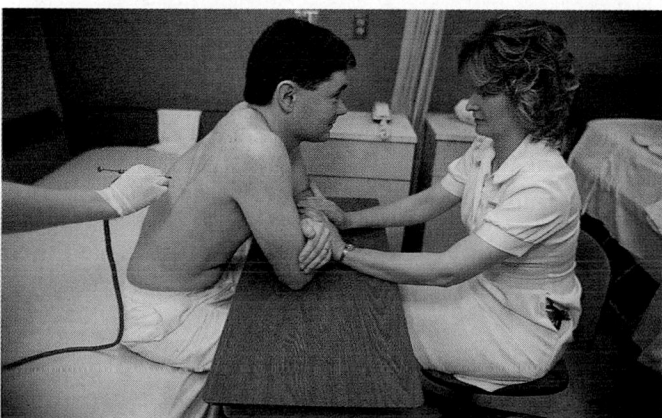

Fig. 44-8 Position for thoracentesis. *(From Wilson SF, Thompson JM: Respiratory disorders, St Louis, 1990, Mosby.)*

an emergency. This type of pneumothorax is known as a *tension pneumothorax* and can result in cardiopulmonary arrest if not treated promptly.

Nursing Diagnosis

Clients with an altered level of oxygenation can have nursing diagnoses that are primarily from a cardiovascular or pulmonary origin (see the nursing diagnoses box below). Each nursing diagnosis should be based on specific defining characteristics and include the related etiology. The diagnostic label is validated by the defining characteristics or signs and symptoms (see the diagnostic process box on p. 1216).

Planning

Clients with impaired oxygenation require a nursing care plan directed toward meeting the actual or potential oxygenation needs of the client (see the care plan on p. 1216). Individual goals are derived from client-centered needs. The nurse identifies specific outcomes of nursing care. The plan includes one or more of the following client-centered goals:

1. Client maintains a patent airway.
2. Client achieves maintenance and promotion of lung expansion.
3. Client mobilizes pulmonary secretions.
4. Client achieves improved activity tolerance.
5. Tissue oxygenation is maintained or improved.
6. Client's cardiopulmonary function is restored and maintained.

The client's level of health, age, lifestyle, and environmental risks affect the level of tissue oxygenation. Clients with severe impairments in oxygenation frequently require

Examples of NANDA Nursing Diagnoses for Cardiopulmonary Dysfunction

Ineffective airway clearance *related to:*
- Impaired cough
- Incisional pain
- Decreased level of consciousness

Impaired gas exchange *related to:*
- Decreased lung expansion
- Presence of pulmonary secretions
- Inadequate oxygen intake

Ineffective breathing pattern *related to:*
- Immobility
- Depressed ventilation from use of narcotics
- Neuromuscular damage
- Airway obstruction

Decreased cardiac output *related to:*
- Irregular cardiac rhythm
- Rapid heart rate

Risk for infection *related to:*
- Stasis of pulmonary secretions

Activity intolerance *related to:*
- Weakness
- Inadequate nutritional intake
- Fatigue

Sample Nursing Diagnostic Process Cardiopulmonary Dysfunction

ASSESSMENT ACTIVITIES	DEFINING CHARACTERISTICS	NURSING DIAGNOSIS
Observe client while breathing.	Dyspnea Tachypnea Use of accessory muscles Nasal flaring Diaphoresis	**Ineffective airway clearance** related to thickened pulmonary secretions
Inspect client's skin and mucous membranes.	Cyanotic nailbeds Circumoral cyanosis Pale mucous membranes	
Auscultate lung fields.	Lower lobe crackles Inspiratory wheezes throughout fields	
Observe cough and inspect sputum.	Poor cough Client tires trying to produce sputum Thick, yellow sputum	

Sample Nursing Care Plan for Ineffective Airway Clearance

NURSING DIAGNOSIS: **Ineffective airway clearance related to thickened pulmonary secretions**
DEFINITION: Ineffective airway clearance is the state in which an individual is unable to clear secretions or obstructions from the respiratory tract to maintain airway patency (Kim, McFarland, McLane, 1995).

GOAL	EXPECTED OUTCOMES	INTERVENTIONS	RATIONALE
Pulmonary secretions will be removed within 3 days.	Adventitious lung sounds will be absent within 48 hr.	Turn, cough, and deep breathe client every 2 hr.	Major complication of reduced mobility is retained secretions, which predisposes client to atelectasis and pneumonia (Dettenmeier, 1992).
		Perform postural drainage with percussion every 3 hr.	Postural drainage moves secretions from smaller to larger airways. Percussion provides additional mechanical force to loosen secretions adhered to walls of airways. Both techniques facilitate secretion removal (Dettenmeier, 1992).
		If client is unable to clear airway, suction for retained secretions.	Main indication for suctioning is when clients are unable to clear airways of mucus and adventitious lung sounds continue (Weilitz, 1991).
	Sputum will be clear, white, and frothy within 48 hr.	Increase fluid intake to 1000 ml within 24 hr, if tolerated. Add high-humidity face mask.	Fluids and humidification help liquify secretions for easy removal (Dettenmeier, 1992). Providing upper airway humidification prevents mucosal drying, keeps secretions moist, and maintains integrity of mucociliary clearance system (Dettenmeier, 1992).

nursing interventions directed toward all six goals. A critical pathway can provide care guidelines for clients who have pulmonary disease and require care from multiple health care disciplines (Fig. 44-9).

Implementation

Nursing interventions for promoting and maintaining adequate oxygenation are included in the domain of nursing: administering and monitoring therapeutic interventions and regimens (Benner 1984). These include independent

nursing actions such as health promotion and prevention behaviors, positioning, coughing techniques, and interdependent or dependent interventions such as oxygen therapy, lung inflation techniques, hydration, medications, chest physiotherapy.

Health Promotion in a Primary Care Setting

Maintaining the client's optimal level of health is important in reducing the number and/or severity of respiratory symptoms. Prevention of respiratory infections is foremost in maintaining optimal health. The nurse practices in the teaching-coaching function domain (Benner, 1984) to provide respiratory-related health information (see the box on p. 1219).

INFLUENZA AND PNEUMOCOCCAL VACCINE

Annual influenza vaccines are recommended for older clients and those with chronic illnesses. The value of vaccination of immunocompromised clients is not completely understood. HIV-positive clients may receive the flu vaccine, however, they may require a second vaccine to gain protection (CDC, 1993). HIV-positive clients can also receive the pneumoccal vaccination. Persons who should not be vaccinated include those with a known hypersensitivity to eggs or other components of the vaccine, and adults with an acute febrile illness (CDC, 1993).

The vaccines are formulated annually based on worldwide surveillance data (Stein, 1993). Pneumococcal vaccine is recommended for clients at increased risk of developing pneumonia, those with chronic illnesses or immunosuppression, those living in special environments such as nursing homes or the American Indian population, and clients over the age of 65 (Butler et al, 1993; Fedson et al, 1994). Studies have shown declining antibody levels to certain antigens 5 to 10 years after vaccination. Revaccination has been recommended for clients vaccinated prior to 1983, due to reformulation of the vaccine from a 14-valent to a 23-valent pneumococcal vaccine in 1983 (Butler et al, 1993).

Admitting Diagnosis: COPD Sub-Acute Stay
DRG# _____
Target LOS _____

Summary of Acute Stay	Hosp. day	SUB-ACUTE DAY 1	SUB-ACUTE DAY 3	SUB-ACUTE DAY 6
		DATE:	DATE:	DATE:
Consults done: _____date._____ _____date:_____	CONSULTS	Interdisciplinary discharge planning team (to include Pulmonary Rehab, PT, OT, Dietary, Social Worker, Case Manager)	Notify dietician via HIS if patient is consuming less than 1/2 meals.	
Most recent results: ABG's _____ date: _____ CXR _____ date: _____ Serum Theo _____ date: _____ Pulse ox _____ date: _____ Other_____ date: _____	TESTS	Daily pulse oximetry to evaluate & determine pt's O2 needs at rest and exertion. Target O2 sat. >/= 90%. ABG's prn, Serum theophylline level after any changes in dosage.	Daily pulse oximetry to evaluate/determine pt's O2 needs at rest and exertion. Target O2 sat. >/= 90%. ABG's prn, Serum theophylline level after any changes in dosage.	ABG's prn Serum theophylline level after any changes in dosage ABG's and theophylline level prior to discharge
Specimen results. Sputum _____ date: _____ Urine _____ date: _____	SPECIMENS			
	TREATMENTS	Oxygen at _____ Titrate oxygen to 90% saturation Nebulized bronchodilator/respiratory tx as ordered, controlled coughing after tx	Oxygen at _____ Titrate oxygen to 90% saturation Nebulized bronchodilator/respiratory tx as ordered, controlled coughing after tx	Oxygen at _____ Titrate oxygen to 90% saturation Nebulized bronchodilator/respiratory tx as ordered, controlled coughing after tx
Treatment Regime: Most current Oxygen: _____ Most current resp tx orders: _____ _____ _____	VITAL SIGNS	Every 8 hours	Every 8 hours	Every 8 hours
	I & O	Every 8 hours if receiving IV fluid Daily weights if on IV fluids, otherwise weights weekly	Every 8 hours if receiving IV fluid Daily weights if on IV fluids, otherwise weights weekly	Weeky weights
Vital sign range: Temp _____ Resp _____ Pulse _____ B/P _____	DIET	DAT specify _____ Small frequent meals if indicated Encourage po fluids unless contraindicated Offer supplements — Pulmocare or milkshakes	DAT specify _____ Small frequent meals if indicated Encourage po fluids unless contraindicated Offer supplements — Pulmocare or milkshakes	DAT specify _____ Small frequent meals if indicated Encourage po fluids unless contraindicated Offer supplements — Pulmocare or milkshakes
	IVs			
Diet tolerance:	MEDS	Bronchodilators, antibiotics, steroids, expectorants, as ordered Avoid narcotics, sedatives, tranquilizers, antiemitcs, antihistamines, & hypnotics	Bronchodilators, antibiotics, steroids, expectorants, as ordered Avoid narcotics, sedatives, tranquilizers, antiemitcs, antihistamines, & hypnotics	Bronchodilators, antibiotics, steroids, expectorants, as ordered Avoid narcotics, sedatives, tranquilizers, antiemitcs, antihistamines, & hypnotics If unresponsibe to relax. techniques, consider selective anxioletics/antidepressant
Activity tolerance.	ACTIVITY	Encourage pursed-lip breathing Ambulate TID with pulse oximeter — gradually increase activity as tolerated Schedule care activities to allow for rest HOB ↑ 45 degrees; may decrease as patient condition allows Provide pillows for propping Keep overbed table in reach	Encourage pursed-lip breathing Ambulate TID with pulse oximeter — gradually increase activity as tolerated Schedule care activities to allow for rest Provide pillows for propping Keep overbed table in reach HOB ↑ 45 degrees; may decrease as patient condition allows When off oxygen, encourage self-reliant activities	Encourage pursed-lip breathing Ambulate TID with pulse oximeter Gradually ↑ activity as tolerated Schedule care activities to allow for rest Provide pillows for propping Keep overbed table in reach When off oxygen, encourage self-reliant activities
Sleep pattern:				
Assessment status: Resp:				
Anxiety level: Mental status:	NURSING ASSESSMENT	Check resp. rate, pattern, breath sounds, color/amt. of sputum, dietary intake, activity tolerance, sleep pattern, anxiety level, comprehension of teaching, mental status, tremor, asterixis & V.S. changes	Check resp. rate, pattern, breath sounds, color/amt. of sputum, dietary intake, activity tolerance, sleep pattern, anxiety level, comprehension of teaching, mental status, tremor, asterixis & V.S. changes	Resp. rate, pattern, breath sounds, color/amt. of sputum, dietary intake, activity tolerance, sleep pattern, anxiety level, comprehension of teaching, mental status, tremor, asterixis, & vital sign changes
Other: Comprehension of teaching:	TEACHING	Assessment/orientation	Begin phase I of teaching; Continue through phases according to patient's understanding	Continue instruction according to patient's understanding
Current D/C plan:	DISCHARGE PLANNING	Notify PT, OT, ST for screening Notify Social Worker of admission if pt is a short stay Assess need for home health care, nsg. home placement, outpatient pulmonary rehab. Discharge plan is to:		If home health care is to follow, call HHC for resp. therapist or other representative to visit prior to D/C Consider and make referrals to community resources as indicated

Nurse signature _____ Shift ____/____   _____ Shift ____/____   _____ Shift ____/____
Nurse signature _____ ____/____   _____ ____/____   _____ ____/____
Nurse signature _____ ____/____   _____ ____/____   _____ ____/____

Fig. 44-9 Portion of CareMap® for COPD, subacute stay. *(Courtesy Baptist Hospital, Pensacola, Fla, and The Center For Case Management, South Natick, Mass.)*

Continued.

TEACHING OUTLINE

Patient Name _____

Room Number _____

Diagnosis _____ COPD — Sub-Acute Stay

	Responsible	Date	Signature
1. <u>Assessment/Orientation:</u> Review CareMap with pt/family. Re-evaluate learning needs: current knowledge, med compliance, level of anxiety, support systems, and understanding of instruction provided in acute care. Provide instruction books, "Rising to the Challenge of Managing Lung Disease" and "Occupational Therapy COPD Program". Explain self report scale, provide relaxation tape, review pt's perception of stressful events.	Respiratory and/or Nsg. Day 1		
2. <u>PHASE I: Disease Process, Treatment/Exercise, and Preventing Infection:</u> Define COPD, review normal anatomy and physiology of the pulmonary system. Review COPD type appropriate to patient (pg. 4-14). Emphasize need to stop smoking if indicated (pg. 15). Inform patient of Health Management Services classes, "Freedom from Smoking" (434-4747). Describe all components of treatment, from pursed lip breathing & diaphramatic/abdominal breathing (pg. 16-18). Review benefits of exercise, precautions, rehab, upper and lower body stretches (pg. 19-21). Emphasize handwashing, annual vaccine, avoidance of people with colds/flu.	Respiratory Therapy/Nsg. Day 2		
Review Section A, OT Booklet, Intro to COPD and Related Effects on your Body and your Surroundings.	Occupational Therapy Day 2		
3. <u>PHASE II: Medications/Oxygen/Aerosol Therapy, Managing Mucus:</u> Review and highlight medications specific to patient, emphasize medication guidelines (pg. 23-29). Review oxygen therapy and guidelines if indicated (pg. 30-31). Review MDI/nebulizer use as instr~~~ regimen. Review guidelines (pg. 32-34). Re~~~ controlled cou~~~	Respiratory Thorapy/Nsg.		

SUMMARY
PATIENT PROBLEMS/OUTCOME CRITERIA

Admitting Diagnosis ____ COPD — Sub-Acute ____   Target LOS _____

Date	Initial	Patient Problem	Outcome Criteria/Goal	Date d/c	Initial
		1. Ineffective airway clearance and impaired gas exchange r/t excessive secretions, ineffective cough & disease process	By discharge the patient will: 1. re-establish usual compensated baseline of PaCO2 and PO2. 2. Demonstrate effective cough 3. Return of baseline breath sounds		
		2. Anxiety r/t dyspnea	By discharge the patient will: 1. Be free of signs/symptoms of anxiety. 2. Demonstrate use of accessory muscles appropriate to activity level.		
		3. Alteration in nutrition: less than body requirements r/t reduced appetite, decreased energy levels, and dyspnea	By discharge the patient will: 1. Be consuming at least 3/4 of meals 2. Verbalize strategies for adequate caloric intake.		
		4. Activity intolerance r/t fatigue and dyspnea	By discharge the patient will: 1. Be able t~~~		

Fig. 44-9, cont'd Portion of CareMap® for COPD, subacute stay.

Both the influenza vaccine and pneumococcal vaccine can be used in pregnant women. There are no contraindications to the pneumococcal vaccine (CDC, 1991), and influenza vaccine can be given after the first trimester (CDC, 1993). However, in all cases it is important to consult the client's obstetrician before administering either vaccine.

ENVIRONMENTAL POLLUTANTS

Avoiding exposure to secondhand smoke is essential to maintaining optimal cardiopulmonary function. Most businesses and restaurants now ban smoking or have separate areas designated as smoking areas. If clients are exposed to secondhand smoke in their home environments,

CLIENT TEACHING
for Cardiopulmonary Health Promotion

OBJECTIVE
- Client will be able to verbalize and demonstrate behaviors that reflect cardiopulmonary health promotion.

TEACHING STRATEGIES
- Educate the client about the importance of regular blood pressure checkups and taking blood pressure medications as prescribed.
- Educate the client about the importance of monitoring the serum cholesterol and triglyceride levels.
- Educate the client about the basic food groups and recommended servings of each.
- Educate client about low fat, low salt, proper caloric diet and provide sample menus.
- Educate client about need for regular aerobic exercise 3 to 4 times per week for 30 to 40 minutes.
- Discuss strategies for minimizing and reducing stress in the client's life, such as setting realistic goals, relaxation and meditation techniques, and getting adequate amounts of rest, relaxation, and sleep.
- Discuss the importance and benefits of pneumococcal vaccine and annual influenza vaccine.
- Discuss the importance of monitoring pollution indexes and limiting exposure on days when the index is high.
- Discuss the need to avoid smoking and secondhand smoke exposure.
- If clients smoke, enroll them in a structured smoking cessation program.
- Discuss strategies to avoid or control secondary infection exposure, such as avoiding prolonged exposure to crowds during the flu season.
- Educate the client about the need to cover the mouth and nose with a scarf when going out into cold air.

EVALUATION
- Have the client verbalize the importance of regular blood pressure checkups.
- Determine the frequency of the client's return visits.
- Obtain client's weight and blood pressure.
- Ask clients to list what they eat in a day.
- Ask clients to describe what they are doing for exercise.
- Ask clients to describe stressful situations in their lives and how they are handling them.
- Ask the client to demonstrate relaxation techniques.
- Determine if the client is smoking.

RESEARCH HIGHLIGHT

RESEARCH ABSTRACT
Clients with dyspnea were studied to determine if the use of a taped relaxation message would reduce their breathlessness. Twenty-six adult COPD clients with dyspnea were randomly assigned to two groups. The treatment group was taught relaxation using a prerecorded tape while the control group was instructed to sit quietly. Skin temperature, heart rate, and respiratory rate were recorded for a total of four weekly sessions. Anxiety, dyspnea, and airway obstruction were measured at the start and end of the study. The relaxation group achieved the study relaxation criteria and reduced their dyspnea, anxiety, and airway obstruction. The control group remained the same or became worse.

IMPLICATIONS FOR PRACTICE
- Alternative methods to relieve dyspnea have been shown to be effective.
- There is a connection between the psychological response and the physiological response of dyspnea.
- Relaxation techniques are appropriate alternative methodologies for controlling breathlessness.
- A nursing care plan for a client experiencing dyspnea should include a component of relaxation.

REFERENCE
Gift AG, Moore T, Soeken K: Relaxation to reduce dyspnea and anxiety in COPD patients, *Nurs Res* 41(4):242, 1992.

counseling and support may be necessary to assist the smoker in successful smoking cessation or alterations in behavior patterns such as smoking outside.

Exposure to chemicals and pollutants in the work environment must also be considered. Clients such as farmers, painters, carpenters, and others benefit from the use of particulate filter masks to reduce inhalation of particles.

Acute and Tertiary Care

Clients with acute pulmonary illnesses require nursing interventions directed toward halting the pathological process, as with a respiratory tract infection; shorten the duration and severity of the illness, such as hospitalization with pneumonia; and prevent complications from the illness or treatments, such as nosocomial infection resulting from invasive procedures.

DYSPNEA MANAGEMENT

Dyspnea is difficult to quantify and to treat. Treatment modalities need to be individualized for each client, and more than one therapy is usually implemented (see the box above). The underlying process that causes or worsens dyspnea must be treated and stabilized initially, then four additional therapies: pharmacological measures, oxygen therapy, physical techniques, and psychosocial techniques, are implemented (Gift, 1990). Pharmacological agents may include bronchodilators, steroids, mucolytics, and antianxiety medications. Oxygen therapy can reduce dyspnea associated with exercise. Physical techniques, such as cardiopulmonary reconditioning, breathing techniques, and cough control, can help to reduce dyspnea (DeVito, 1990). Relaxation techniques, biofeedback, and meditation are physiosocial measures that can lessen the sensation of dyspnea (Gift, 1990; Gift, Moore, and Soeken, 1992; Carrieri-Kohlman et al, 1993).

MAINTENANCE OF A PATENT AIRWAY

The airway is patent when the trachea, bronchi, and large airways are free from obstructions. Three types of interventions are used to maintain a patent airway: coughing techniques, suctioning, and insertion of an artificial airway.

Coughing Techniques. Coughing is effective for maintaining a patent airway. Coughing permits the client to remove secretions from both the upper and lower airways. The normal series of events in the cough mechanism are deep inhalation, closure of the glottis, active contraction of the expiratory muscles, and glottis opening. Deep inhalation increases the lung volume and airway diameter allowing the air to pass partially obstructing mucus plugs or other foreign matter. Contraction of the expiratory muscles against the closed glottis causes a high intrathoracic pressure to develop. When the glottis opens, a large flow of air is expelled at a high speed, providing momentum for mucus to move to the upper airways where it can be expectorated or swallowed.

The effectiveness of coughing is evaluated by sputum expectoration, the client's report of swallowed sputum, or clearing of adventitious sounds by auscultation. Clients with chronic pulmonary diseases, upper respiratory tract infections, and lower respiratory tract infections should be encouraged to deep breathe and cough at least every 2 hours while awake. Clients with a large amount of sputum should be encouraged to cough every hour while awake and every 2 to 3 hours while asleep until the acute phase of mucus production has ended. Cough techniques include deep breathing and coughing for the postoperative client, cascade, huff, and quad coughing.

Cascade cough. With the cascade cough, the client takes a slow, deep breath and holds it for 2 seconds, while contracting expiratory muscles. Then the client opens the mouth and performs a series of coughs throughout exhalation, thereby coughing at progressively lowered lung volumes. This technique promotes airway clearance and a patent airway in clients with large volumes of sputum.

Huff cough. The huff cough stimulates a natural cough reflex and is generally effective only for clearing central airways. While exhaling, the client opens the glottis by saying the word *huff*. With practice the client inhales more air and may be able to progress to the cascade cough.

Quad Cough. The quad cough technique is used for clients without abdominal muscle control, such as those with spinal cord injuries. While the client breathes out with a maximal expiratory effort, the client or nurse pushes inward and upward on the abdominal muscles toward the diaphragm, causing the cough.

Suctioning Techniques. When a client is unable to clear respiratory tract secretions with coughing, the nurse must use suctioning to clear the airways. The three primary suctioning techniques are oropharyngeal and nasopharyngeal suctioning, orotracheal and nasotracheal suctioning, and suctioning an artificial airway.

These techniques are based on common principles. Because the oropharynx and trachea are considered sterile, sterile technique is required for suctioning. The mouth is considered clean, and therefore the suctioning of oral secretions should be performed after suctioning of the oropharynx and trachea. Each type of suctioning requires the use of a rounded-tipped catheter with a number of holes along the sides of the catheter at the distal end. Frequency of suctioning is determined by client assessment. If secretions are identified by inspection or auscultation techniques, suctioning is required. Sputum is not produced continuously or every 1 or 2 hours but occurs as a response to a pathological condition. Therefore there is no rationale for routine suctioning of all clients every 1 to 2 hours.

Oropharyngeal and Nasopharyngeal Suctioning. The oropharynx extends behind the mouth from the soft palate above the level of the hyoid bone and contains the tonsils. The nasopharynx is located behind the nose and extends to the level of the soft palate. Oropharyngeal or nasopharyngeal suctioning is used when the client is able to cough effectively but is unable to clear secretions by expectorating or swallowing. The suction procedure is used after the client has coughed (Procedure 44-2). As the amount of pulmonary secretions is reduced and the client is less fatigued, the client may be able to expectorate or swallow the mucus and suctioning is no longer required.

Orotracheal and Nasotracheal suctioning. Orotracheal or nasotracheal suctioning is necessary when the client with pulmonary secretions is unable to cough and does not have an artificial airway present (see Procedure 44-2). A catheter is passed through the mouth or nose into the trachea. The nose is the preferred route because stimulation of the gag reflex is minimal. The procedure is similar to nasopharyngeal suctioning, but the catheter tip is moved farther into the client to suction the trachea. The entire procedure from catheter passage to its removal cannot take more than 15 seconds because oxygen does not reach the lungs during suctioning. Unless in respiratory distress, the client should be allowed to rest between passes of the catheter. If the client is using supplemental oxygen, the oxygen cannula or mask should be replaced during rest periods. Suctioning causes desaturation and hypoxemia. The client may experience dysrhythmias and hypotension secondary to the suctioning procedure.

Artificial Airways. An artificial airway is indicated for clients with decreased level of consciousness, airway obstruction, mechanical ventilation, and removal of tracheal-bronchial secretions.

Tracheal suctioning. Tracheal suctioning is accomplished through an artificial airway such as an endotracheal tube or tracheostomy tube. The suction catheter should be no greater than one half the size of the internal diameter of the artificial airway. Secretion removal should be as atraumatic as possible. To avoid trauma, suction should never be applied during insertion of the catheter. The catheter is rotated and suction is applied intermittently during withdrawal. It is recommended that the nurse wear a mask and goggles when suctioning to prevent splashes with body fluids.

Two methods of suctioning are currently used. Open suctioning involves using a freshly opened sterile suction catheter that is handled with a sterile glove. Closed suctioning involves a multiple use suction catheter that is encased in a plastic sheath and used for 24 hours. Closed suctioning most often used on clients who require mechanical ventilation to support their respiratory efforts, because it permits continuous delivery of oxygen while suctioning is performed (Fig. 44-10). Although sterile gloves are not used in this procedure, nonsterile gloves are recommended to prevent splashes with body fluids.

Oral airway. The oral airway, the simplest type of artificial airway, prevents obstruction of the trachea by displacement of the tongue into the oropharynx (Fig. 44-11). The oral airway extends from the teeth to the oropharynx, maintaining the tongue in the normal position. The correct size

Text continued on p. 1226.

Suottioning*

STEPS	RATIONALE
1. Assess for signs and symptoms indicating presence of upper airway secretions: gurgling respirations, restlessness, vomitus in mouth, drooling.	Physical signs and symptoms result from decreased oxygen to tissues as well as pooling of secretions in upper airway.
2. Explain to client how procedure will help to clear airway and relieve some breathing problems. Explain that coughing, sneezing, or gagging is normal.	Explanation of procedure relieves client's anxiety.
3. Prepare necessary equipment and supplies:	Ensures that procedure is completed quickly and efficiently.
a. Portable or wall suction unit with connecting tubing with Y connector if needed	
b. Sterile catheter	
c. Yankauer catheter (oropharyngeal)	
d. Sterile water or normal saline, sterile basin	Cleans catheter.
e. Sterile gloves, nonsterile gloves (Yankauer only)	
f. Drape or towel	Protects linen and client's bedclothes.
g. Nasal or oral airway if indicated	Ensures access to airway.
h. Mask/goggles	Provides protection for care giver.
4. Close door or pull curtain.	Ensures privacy.
5. Properly position client:	
a. Place conscious client with functional gag reflex for oral suctioning in semi-Fowler's position with head turned to one side. Place such a client for nasal suctioning in semi-Fowler's position with neck hyperextended.	Gag reflex helps prevent aspiration of gastrointestinal contents. Positioning of head to one side or hyperextending neck promotes smooth insertion of catheter into oropharynx or nasopharynx, respectively.
b. Place unconscious client in side-lying position facing nurse.	Prevents client's tongue from obstructing airway, promotes drainage of pulmonary secretions, and prevents aspiration of gastrointestinal contents.
6. Place towel on pillow or under client's chin.	Prevents soiling of bed linen or bedclothes from secretions. Secretions on towel can be discarded, thus reducing spread of bacteria.
7. Select proper suction pressure for client and type of suction unit. For wall suction units, this is 110-150 mm Hg in adults, 95-110 mm Hg in children, and 50-95 mm Hg in infants.	Provides safe but effective negative pressure according to client's age. Decreases possibility of damage to mucous membranes and hypoxemia.
8. Wash hands.	Reduces transmission of microorganisms.
9. a. Yankauer catheter:	
(1) Apply nonsterile gloves.	Reduces transmission of microorganisms.
(2) Connect one end of connecting tubing to suction machine and other to Yankauer suction catheter. Fill cup with water	Prepares suction apparatus.
(3) Check that equipment is functioning properly by suctioning small amount of water from cup.	Ensures equipment function and lubricates catheter.
(4) Remove oxygen mask, if present.	
(5) Insert catheter into mouth along gum line to pharynx. Move catheter around mouth until secretions are cleared.	Provides continuous suction. Care must be taken not to allow suction tip to invaginate oral mucosal surfaces. Do not use Yankauer that has fallen on floor.
(6) Encourage client to cough. Replace oxygen mask.	Moves secretions from lower airway into mouth and upper airway.
(7) Rinse catheter with water in cup or basin until connecting tubing is cleared of secretions. Turn off suction.	Rinses catheter and reduces probability of transmission of microorganisms. Clean suction tubing enhances delivery of set suction pressure.
(8) Reassess client's respiratory status.	Directs nurse to initiate or cease intervention.
(9) Remove towel, place in laundry. Remove gloves and dispose in receptacle.	Reduces transmission of microorganisms.

*Yankauer catheters, nasopharyngeal or nasotracheal suction, artificial airway.

Continued.

Suctioning—cont'd

STEPS	RATIONALE

9. a. Yankauer catheter—cont'd

(10) Reposition client; Sims' position encourages drainage and should be used if client has decreased level of consciousness.

Facilitates drainage of oral secretions.

(11) Discard remainder of water into appropriate receptacle.

Reduces transmission of microorganisms and maintains medical asepsis.

(12) Place connecting tubing in clean dry area.

(13) Wash hands.

Reduces transmission of miroorganisms to other clients.

b. Nasopharyngeal or nasotracheal suction:

(1) Turn suction device on and set vacuum regulator to appropriate negative pressure.

Excessive negative pressure damages nasal pharyngeal and tracheal mucosa and can reduce greater hypoxia.

(2) If indicated, increase supplemental oxygen to 100% or as ordered by physician.

Reduces suction-induced hypoxemia. (The literature is inconclusive as to the necessity of hyperoxygenation.)

(3) Connect one end of connecting tubing to suction machine and place other end in convenient location.

Prepares for connection of suction catheter to suction apparatus.

(4) If using suction kit:

(i) Open package. If sterile drape is available, place it across client's chest or use towel.

Reduces transmission of microorganisms.

(ii) Open suction catheter package. Do not allow suction catheter to touch any surface other than inside of its package.

Maintains medical asepsis.

(iii) Unwrap or open sterile basin and place on bedside table. Be careful not to touch inside of basin. Fill with about 100 ml sterile normal saline.

Saline is used to clean tubing after each suction pass.

(5) Open lubricant. Squeeze onto open sterile catheter package without touching package.

Prepares lubricant while maintaining sterility. Water-soluble lubricant is used to avoid lipoid aspiration pneumonia.

(6) Apply mask and goggles.

Prevents splashing of secretions into care giver eyes and mouth.

(7) Apply sterile glove to each hand or apply nonsterile glove to nondominant hand and sterile glove to dominant hand.

Reduces transmission of microorganisms and allows nurse to maintain sterility of suction catheter.

(8) Pick up suction catheter with dominant hand without touching nonsterile surfaces. Pick up connecting tubing with nondominant hand. Secure catheter to tubing (see the illustration below).

Maintains catheter sterility. Connects catheter to suction.

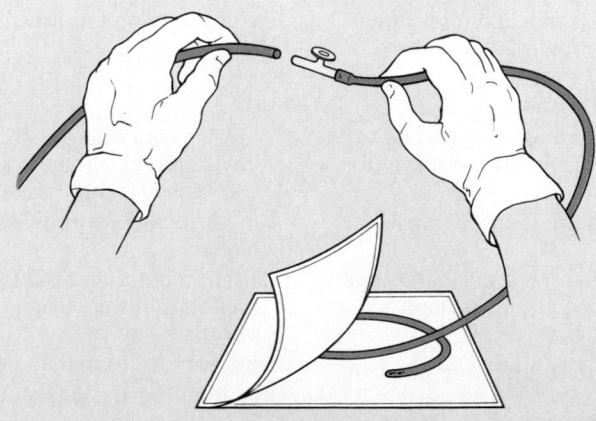

Step 9b(8)

Suctioning—cont'd

STEPS	RATIONALE

9. b. Nasopharyngeal or nasotracheal suction—cont'd

(9) Check that equipment is functioning properly by suctioning small amount of normal saline from basin.

Ensures equipment function. Lubricates internal catheter and tubing.

(10) Coat distal 6-8 cm of catheter with water-soluble lubricant.

Lubricates catheter for easier insertion.

(11) Remove oxygen-delivery device, if applicable, with nondominant hand. Without applying suction, gently but quickly insert catheter with dominant thumb and forefinger into naris using slight downward slant or through mouth when client breathes in. Do not force through naris (see the illustration at right).

Application of suction pressure while introducing catheter into trachea increases risk of damage to mucosa, as well as increases risk of hypoxia due to removal of oxygen present in airways. Epiglottis is open on inspiration and facilitates insertion into trachea. Client should cough. If client gags or becomes nauseated, catheter is most likely in esophagus.

  (i) *Pharyngeal suctioning:* In adults, insert catheter about 16 cm; in older children, 8-12 cm; in infants and young children, 4-8 cm. Rule of thumb is to insert catheter distance from tip of nose to base of ear lobe.

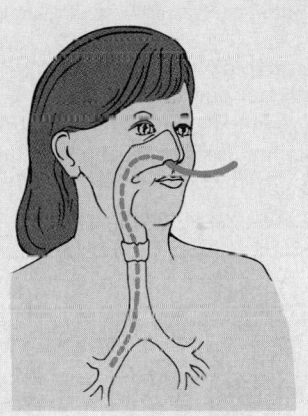

Step 9b(11)

(12) Apply intermittent suction for up to 10 sec by placing and releasing nondominant thumb over vent of catheter and slowly withdraw catheter while rotating it back and forth between dominant thumb and forefinger. Encourage client to cough. Replace oxygen device, if applicable.

Prevents injury to mucosa. If catheter "grabs" mucosa, remove thumb to release suction. Suctioning longer than 10 sec can cause cardiopulmonary compromise.

(13) Rinse catheter and connecting tubing with normal saline until cleared.

Removes secretions from catheter.

c. Artificial airway:

(1) Wash hands.

Reduces transmission of microorganisms.

(2) Turn suction device on and set vacuum regulator to appropriate negative pressure (see Step 7).

Excessive negative pressure damages tracheal mucosa and can induce greater hypoxia.

(3) Connect one end of connecting tubing to suction machine and place other end in convenient location.

Prepares suction apparatus.

(4) If using sterile suction kit:

  (i) Open package. If sterile drape is available, place it across client's chest.

Prevents contamination of clothing.

  (ii) Open suction catheter package. Do not allow suction catheter to touch any nonsterile surface.

Prepares catheter and prevents transmission of microorganisms.

  (iii) Unwrap or open sterile basin and place on bedside table. Be careful not to touch inside basin. Fill with about 100 ml sterile normal saline.

Prepares catheter and prevents transmission of microorganisms.

Continued.

Suctioning—cont'd

STEPS	RATIONALE
9. c. Artificial airway—cont'd	
(5) Apply mask and goggles.	Reduces risk of care giver being splashed.
(6) Apply one sterile glove to each hand or apply nonsterile glove to nondominant hand and sterile glove to dominant hand.	Reduces transmission of microorganisms and allows nurse to maintain sterility of suction catheter.
(7) Pick up suction catheter with dominant hand without touching nonsterile surfaces. Pick up connecting tubing with nondominant hand. Secure catheter to tubing.	Maintains catheter sterility.
(8) Check that equipment is functioning properly by suctioning small amount of saline from basin.	Ensures equipment function; lubricates catheter and tubing Promotes easier catheter insertion. If lubricant is needed, it must be water soluble to prevent petroleum-based aspiration pneumonia. Excessive lubricant can adhere to artificial airway.
(9) Remove oxygen- or humidity-delivery device with nondominant hand.	Exposes artificial airway.
(10) Hyperinflate and/or oxygenate client before suctioning, using manual resuscitation (Ambu) bag or sigh mechanism on mechanical ventilator.	Decreases atelectasis caused by negative pressure. Preoxygenation converts large proportion of resident lung gas to 100% oxygen to offset amount used in metabolic consumption while ventilator or oxygenation is interrupted and offsets volume lost out of suction catheter.
(11) Without applying suction, gently but quickly insert catheter with dominant thumb and forefinger into artificial airway (best to time catheter insertion with inspiration).	Places catheter in tracheobronchial tree. Application of suction pressure while introducing catheter into trachea increases risk of damage to tracheal mucosa, as well as increased hypoxia due to removal of oxygen present in airways.
(i) *Tracheal suctioning:* In adults, insert catheter 20-24 cm; in older children, 14-20; and in young children and infants, 8-14 cm.	
(ii) *Positioning:* In some instances turning client's head to right helps nurse suction left mainstem bronchus; turning head to left helps nurse suction right mainstem bronchus.	
If resistance is felt after insertion of catheter for recommended distance, nurse has probably hit carina. Pull catheter back 1 cm before applying suction.	
(12) Insert catheter until resistance is met, then pull back 1 cm.	Stimulates cough and removes catheter from mucosal wall.
(13) Apply intermittent suction by placing and releasing nondominant thumb over vent of catheter and slowly withdraw catheter while rotating it back and forth between dominant thumb and forefinger. Encourage client to cough.	Prevents injury to tracheal mucosal lining. If catheter "grabs" mucosa, remove thumb to release suction.
(14) Replace oxygen-delivery device. Encourage client to deep breathe.	Reoxygenates and reexpands alveoli. Suctioning can cause hypoxemia and atelectasis.
(15) Rinse catheter and connecting tubing with normal saline until clear. Use continuous suction.	Removes catheter secretions. Secretions left in tubing decrease suction and provide environment for microorganism growth.
(16) Repeat Steps 9c(10-15) as needed to clear secretions. Allow adequate time (at least 1 full min) between suction passes for ventilation and reoxygenation.	Clears airway of excessive secretions and promotes improved oxygenation.
(17) Assess client's cardiopulmonary status between suction passes.	Suctioning can induce arrhythmias, hypoxia, and bronchospasm.

Suctioning—cont'd

STEPS	RATIONALE
9. c. Artificial airway—cont'd	
(18) When artificial airway and tracheobronchial tree are sufficiently cleared of secretions, perform nasal and oral pharyngeal suctioning to clear upper airway of secretions. After this suctioning is performed, catheter is contaminated; do not reinsert into endotracheal or tracheostomy tube.	Removes upper airway secretions. Upper airway is considered clean, whereas lower airway is considered sterile. Therefore same catheter can be used to suction from sterile to clean areas but not from clean to sterile areas.
(19) Disconnect catheter from connecting tubing. Roll catheter around fingers of dominant hand. Pull glove off inside out so that catheter remains in glove. Pull off other glove in same way. Discard into appropriate receptacle. Turn off suction device.	Reduces transmission of microorganisms.
(20) Remove towel and place in laundry, or remove drape and discard in appropriate receptacle.	Reduces transmission of microorganisms.
(21) Reposition client.	Promotes comfort. Sims' position encourages drainage and reduces risk of aspiration.
(22) Discard remainder of normal saline into appropriate receptacle. If basin is disposable, discard into appropriate receptacle. If basin is reusable, place it in soiled utility room.	Reduces transmission of microorganisms.
(23) Remove mask and goggles.	
(24) Wash hands.	Reduces transmission of microorganisms.
10. Prepare equipment for next suctioning.	Provides ready access to suction equipment, especially if client is experiencing respiratory distress.
11. Observe client for absence of airway secretions, restlessness, oral secretions.	Indicates that secretions have been removed from oral and pharyngeal areas.
12. Record the amount, consistency, color, and odor of secretions and client's response to procedure; document client's presuctioning and postsuctioning respiratory status.	Documents that procedure was completed and client's status before and after.

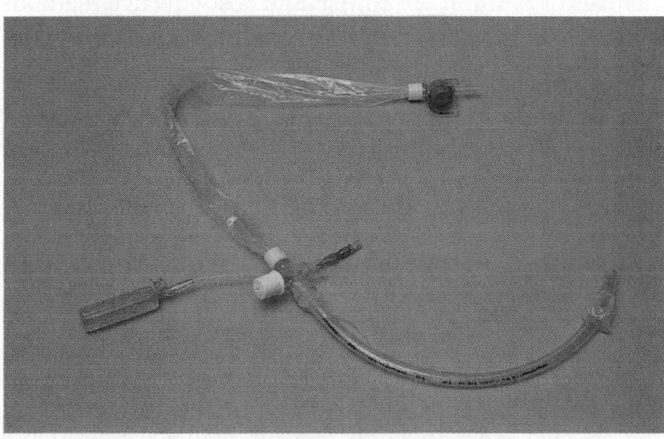

Fig. 44-10 Ballard trach care closed suction.

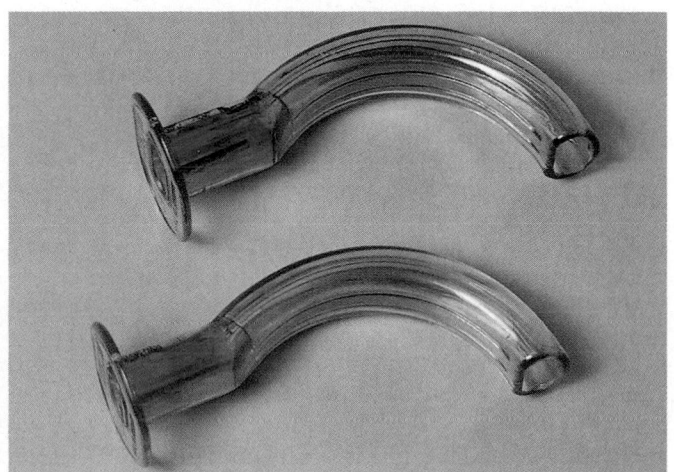

Fig. 44-11 Artificial oral airways.

airway must be used. Proper oral airway size is determined by measuring the distance from the corner of the mouth to the angle of the jaw just below the ear. The length is equal to the distance from the flange of the airway to the tip (Weilitz, 1991). If the airway is too small, the tongue is not held in the anterior portion of the mouth; if too large, it may force the tongue toward the epiglottis and obstruct the airway.

The airway is inserted by turning the curve of the airway toward the cheek and placing it over the tongue. When the airway is in the oropharynx, the nurse turns it so that the opening points downward. Correctly placed, the airway moves the tongue forward away from the oropharynx and the flange, the flat portion of the airway, rests against the client's teeth. Incorrect insertion merely forces the tongue back into the oropharynx.

Tracheal airway. Tracheal airways include endotracheal, nasotracheal, and tracheal tubes. These allow easy access to the client's trachea for deep tracheal suctioning. Because of the presence of the artificial airway, the client no longer has normal humidification of the tracheal mucosa. The nurse should ensure that humidity is being supplied to the airway through nebulization or with the oxygen-delivery system. This humidification is protective and helps reduce the risk of airway plugging.

MOBILIZATION OF PULMONARY SECRETIONS

The ability of a client to mobilize pulmonary secretions may make the difference between a short-term illness and a long recovery involving complications. Nursing interventions that promote mobilization of pulmonary secretions include hydration, humidification, nebulization, and chest physiotherapy.

Hydration. Maintenance of adequate systemic hydration keeps mucociliary clearance normal. In clients with adequate hydration, pulmonary secretions are thin, white, watery, and easily removable with minimal coughing. Excessive coughing to clear thick, tenacious secretions is fatiguing and energy depleting. The best way to maintain thin secretions is to provide a fluid intake of 1500 to 2000 ml per day, unless contraindicated by cardiac status. Adequacy of hydration can be determined by the color, consistency, and ease of secretion expectoration.

Humidification. Humidification is the process of adding water to gas. Temperature is the most important factor affecting the amount of water vapor a gas can hold. The percentage of water in the gas in relation to its capacity for water is the relative humidity. Air or oxygen with a high relative humidity keeps the airways moist and helps loosen and mobilize pulmonary secretions.

Humidification is necessary for clients receiving oxygen therapy. Oxygen delivered to the upper airways, as with a nasal catheter, nasal cannula, or face mask, can be humidified by bubbling it through water. Generally humidification is added when oxygen flow rates exceed 4 L/min.

The humidity tent is used for infants and children with illnesses such as croup and tracheitis to liquefy secretions and help reduce fever. The nebulizer at the top of the humidity tent must remain filled with water to prevent non-humidified air or oxygen from entering the tent. Air in the humidity tent can become cool and fall below 20° C (68° F),

causing the child to become chilled. The nurse monitors the child's body temperature as well as respiratory status. Children in humidity tents require frequent changes of clothing and bed linen to remain warm and dry.

When humidity is used, the nurse needs to ensure sterile saline for inhalation is used for humidification and the solution is changed according to agency procedures. Humidification can be a source for nosocomial infections in clients as the moist environment supports the growth of pathogens.

Nebulization. Nebulization is a process of adding moisture or medications to inspired air by mixing particles of varying sizes with the air. A nebulizer uses the aerosol principle to suspend a maximum number of water drops or particles of the desired size in inspired air. The moisture added to the respiratory system through nebulization improves clearance of pulmonary secretions. Nebulization is often used for administration of bronchodilators and mucolytic agents.

When the thin layer of fluid that supports the mucus layer over the cilia is allowed to dry, the cilia are damaged and cannot adequately clear the airway. Humidification through nebulization enhances mucociliary clearance, the body's natural mechanism for removing mucus and cellular debris from the respiratory tract.

The major types of nebulizers are the jet-aerosol nebulizer and the ultrasonic nebulizer. A jet-aerosol nebulizer uses gas under pressure, and the ultrasonic nebulizer uses high-frequency vibrations to break up the water or medication into fine drops or particles. When inspired with air or administered oxygen, the drops of particles are then deposited throughout the tracheobronchial tree.

MAINTENANCE OR PROMOTION OF LUNG EXPANSION

Nursing interventions to maintain or promote lung expansion include noninvasive techniques. These techniques include positioning and chest physiotherapy, procedures using equipment such as incentive spirometry, and invasive procedures such as management of a chest tube.

Positioning. In the healthy, completely mobile person, adequate ventilation and oxygenation are maintained by frequent position changes during daily activities. However, when a person's illness or injury restricts mobility, there is an increased risk for respiratory impairment. Frequent changes of position are simple and cost-effective methods for reducing the risks of stasis of pulmonary secretions and decreased chest wall expansion.

The most effective position for clients with cardiopulmonary diseases is the 45-degree Semi-Fowler's position (Burns et al, 1994), using gravity to assist in lung expansion and reduce pressure from the abdomen on the diaphragm. When the client uses this position, the nurse needs to ensure that the client does not slide down in bed, which could reduce lung expansion. Unilateral lung disease, such as pneumothorax, atelectasis, pneumonia, thoracotomy, and multiple trauma affecting one lung should be positioned with the "good lung down." This promotes better perfusion of the healthy lung, improving oxygenation. In the presence of pulmonary abscess or hemorrhage, place the affected lung down to prevent drainage toward the healthy lung (Yeaw, 1992).

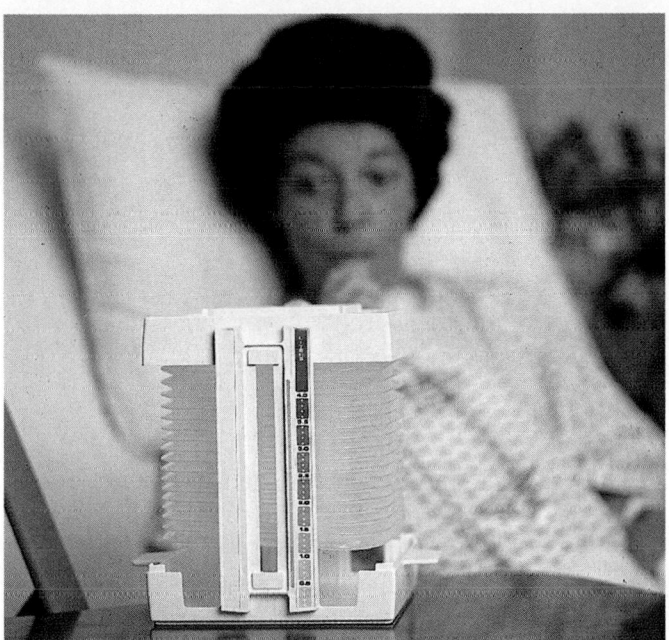

Fig. 44-12 Volume-oriented spirometer.

Incentive Spirometry. Incentive spirometry is a method of encouraging voluntary deep breathing by providing visual feedback to clients about inspiratory volume. Incentive spirometry is used to promote deep breathing to prevent or treat atelectasis in the postoperative client. Studies have shown no respiratory benefit to postoperative incentive spirometry when compared to deep breathing and early ambulation (Bell, 1993).

Flow-oriented incentive spirometers consist of one or more plastic chambers that contain freely moving colored balls. The client inhales slowly and with an even flow to elevate the balls and to keep them floating as long as possible to ensure a maximally sustained inhalation.

Volume-oriented incentive spirometry devices have a bellows that is raised to a predetermined volume by an inhaled breath (Fig. 44-12). An achievement light or counter is used to provide feedback. Some devices are constructed so that the light will not turn on unless the bellows is held at a minimum desired volume for a specified period to enhance lung expansion.

Incentive spirometry encourages clients to breathe to their normal inspiratory capacities. A postoperative inspiratory capacity one half to three fourths of the preoperative volume is acceptable because of postoperative pain. Administration of pain medications prior to incentive spirometry will help the client achieve deep breathing by reducing pain and splinting (see Chapter 48).

Chest Physiotherapy. Chest physiotherapy (CPT) is a group of therapies used in combination to mobilize pulmonary secretions (see the box above). These therapies include postural drainage, chest percussion, and vibration. Chest physiotherapy should be followed by productive coughing and suctioning the client who has a decreased ability to cough. Chest physiotherapy is recommended for clients who produce greater than 30 cc of sputum per day or have evidence of atelectasis by chest x-ray. Eid et al.

(1991) present a practical clinical synopsis of CPT maneuvers for a variety of clinical problems.

Chest percussion involves striking the chest wall over the area being drained. The hand is positioned so that the fingers and thumb touch and the hand is cupped (Fig. 44-13). Percussion on the surface of the chest wall sends waves of varying amplitude and frequency through the chest changing the consistency and location of the sputum. Chest percussion is performed by alternating hand motion against the chest wall (Fig. 44-14). Percussion is performed over a single layer of clothing, not over buttons, snaps, or zippers. The single layer of clothing prevents slapping the client's skin. Thicker or multiple layers of material dampen the vibrations.

Percussion is contraindicated in clients with bleeding disorders, osteoporosis, or fractured ribs. Caution should be taken to percuss the lung fields and not the scapular regions or trauma may occur to the skin and underlying musculoskeletal structures.

Vibration is a fine, shaking pressure applied to the chest wall only during exhalation. This technique is thought to increase the velocity and turbulence of exhaled air, facilitating secretion removal (Dettenmeier, 1992). Vibration increases the exhalation of trapped air and may shake mucus loose and induce a cough. Vibration is not recommended in infants and young children.

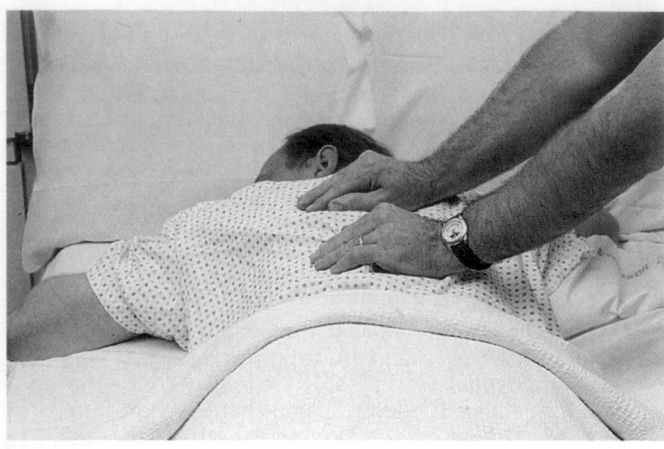

Fig. 44-13 Hand position for chest wall percussion during physiotherapy.

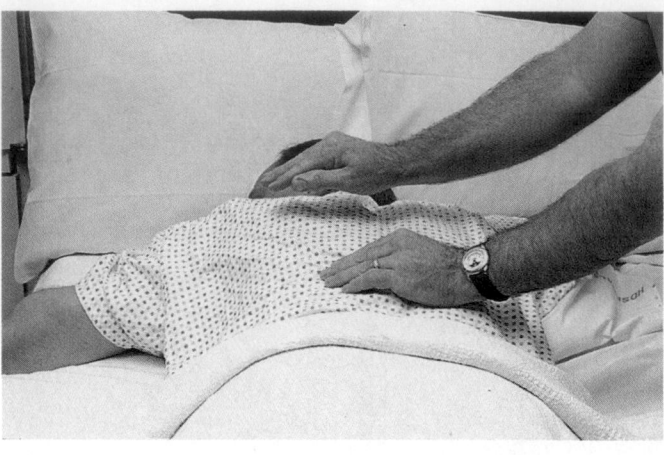

Fig. 44-14 Chest wall percussion, alternating hand motion against the client's chest wall.

Table 44-8	Positions for Postural Drainage		
LUNG SEGMENT	**POSITION OF CLIENT**	**LUNG SEGMENT**	**POSITION OF CLIENT**
ADULT Bilateral	High Fowler's	Right upper lobe— posterior segment	Side lying with right side of chest elevated on pillows
Apical segments Right upper lobe— anterior segment	Sitting on side of bed Supine with head elevated	Left upper lobe— posterior segment	Side lying with left side of chest elevated on pillows
Left upper lobe— anterior segment	Supine with head elevated	Right middle lobe— anterior segment	Three-fourths supine position with dependent lung in Trendelenburg position

Table 44-8	**Positions for Postural Drainage—cont'd**

LUNG SEGMENT	**POSITION OF CLIENT**	**LUNG SEGMENT**	**POSITION OF CLIENT**
Right middle lobe— posterior segment	Prone with thorax and abdomen elevated	Both lower lobes— posterior segment	Prone in Trendelenburg position

Both lower lobes— anterior segments	Supine in Trendelenburg	**CHILD** Bilateral—apical segments	Sitting on nurse's lap, leaning slightly forward flexed over pillow

Left lower lobe—lateral segment

Bilateral—middle anterior segments   Sitting on nurse's lap, leaning against nurse

Right lower lobe—lateral segment

Bilateral lobes— anterior segments   Lying supine on nurse's lap, back supported with pillow

Right lower lobe—posterior segment

Care of the Client With Chest Tubes

STEPS	RATIONALE
1. Assess client for decreased respiratory distress and chest pain, breath sounds over affected lung area, and stable vital signs.	Signs and symptoms reflect improvement in respiratory distress and chest pain after insertion of chest tube.
2. Observe for increased respiratory distress.	Signs and symptoms of increased respiratory distress and/or chest pain, decrease in breath sounds over the affected and nonaffected lungs, marked cyanosis, asymmetric chest movements, presence of subcutaneous emphysema around tube insertion site or neck, hypotension, tachycardia, and/or mediastinal shift are critical and indicate a severe change in client status, such as excessive blood loss or tension pneumothorax. Notify physician immediately.
3. Observe:	
a. Chest tube dressing	Ensures that dressing is patent and notes any drainage.
b. Tubing for kinks, dependent loops, or clots	Maintains a patent, freely draining system, preventing fluid accumulation in chest cavity.
c. Chest drainage system, which should be upright and below level of tube insertion	System must be in this position to function properly.
d. Water seal for fluctuations with client's inspiration and expiration	Fluid should rise in water seal with inspiration and fall with expiration, indicating that system is functioning properly.
e. Bubbling in water-seal bottle or chamber (see Table 44-9)	When system is initially connected to client, bubbles are expected in chamber from air that was present in system and in client's intrapleural space. After a short period, bubbling will stop. Fluid will continue to fluctuate in water seal on inspiration and expiration until lung is reexpanded or system becomes occluded.
f. Type and amount of fluid drainage: Nurse should note color and amount of drainage, client's vital signs, and skin color.	Sudden gush of drainage may be retained blood and not active bleeding. Increase in drainage can be result of client position change.
(1) Less than 50-200 ml/hr immediately postoperative in mediastinal chest tube (Johanson et al, 1988); approximately 500 ml in first 24 hr; dark red drainage is expected early in postoperative period, turning serous with time.	Reexpansion of lungs forces drainage into tube. Coughing can also cause large gushes of drainage.
(2) Between 100-300 ml of fluid may drain in posterior chest tube during first 2 hr after insertion; rate will decrease after 2 hr, 500-1000 ml can be expected in first 24 hr; drainage will be grossly bloody during first several hours after surgery and then change to serous.	Excessive amounts and/or continued presence of frank, bloody drainage after first several hours of surgery should be reported to physician, along with client's vital signs and respiratory status.
g. Bubbling in the suction-control chamber (when suction is being used) (see Table 44-9)	Suction-control chamber has constant, gentle bubbling. Tubing to suction source should be free of obstruction, and suction source should be turned on to appropriate setting.
4. Provide two shodded hemostats for each chest tube, attached to top of client's bed with adhesive tape. Shodded hemostats have a covering to prevent hemostat from penetrating chest tube.	Chest tubes are only clamped under specific circumstances:
	a. To assess air leak (see Table 44-9)
	b. To empty or change collection bottle or chamber; performed by nurse who has received training in procedure
	c. To change disposable systems, have new system ready to be connected before clamping tube so that transfer can be rapid and drainage system reestablished
	d. To change a broken water-seal bottle in event that no sterile solution container is available
	e. To assess if client is ready to have chest tube removed, which is done by physician's order in this situation, nurse must monitor client for re-creation of pneumothorax (see Table 44-9)

Care of the Client With Chest Tubes—cont'd

STEPS	RATIONALE
5. Position the client:	Permits optimal drainage of fluid and/or air.
a. Semi-Fowler's to high Fowler's position to evacuate air (pneumothorax)	Air rises to highest point in chest. Pneumothorax tubes are usually placed on anterior aspect at midclavicular line, second or third intercostal space.
b. High Fowler's position to drain fluid (hemothorax)	Permits optimal drainage of fluid. Posterior tubes are placed on midaxillary line, eighth or ninth intercostal space.
6. Maintain tube connection between chest and drainage tubes intact and taped.	Secures chest tube to drainage system and reduces risk of air leaks causing breaks in airtight system.
a. Water-seal vent must be without occlusion.	Permits displaced air to pass into atmosphere.
b. Suction-control chamber vent must be without occlusion when suction is used.	Provides safety factor of releasing excess negative pressure into atmosphere.
7. Coil excess tubing on mattress next to client. Secure with rubber band and safety pin or system's clamp.	Prevents excess tubing from hanging over edge of mattress in dependent loop. Drainage could collect in loop and occlude drainage system.
8. Adjust tubing to hang in straight line from top of mattress to drainage chamber. If chest tube is draining fluid, indicate time (e.g., 0900) that drainage was begun on drainage bottle's adhesive tape of bottle setup or on write-on surface of disposable commercial system.	Promotes drainage. Provides a baseline for continuous assessment of type and quality of drainage.
9. Strip or milk chest tube only if indicated:	Stripping is controversial and should be performed only if hospital policy permits and there is physician's order. Stripping creates high degree of negative pressure and has potential of pulling lung tissue or pleura into drainage holes of chest tube.
a. Postoperative mediastinal chest tubes are manipulated if nursing assessment indicates obstruction of drainage secondary to clots or debris in tubing.	
b. Postoperative assessment is done every 15 min for the first 2 hr. This assessment interval then changes *based on client's status.*	
10. Wash hands.	Reduces transmission of infection.
11. Record in nurses' notes patency of chest tubes, presence of drainage, presence of fluctuations, client's vital signs, and level of comfort.	Documents accurate functioning of chest tubes and client's physical status.

Postural drainage is the use of positioning techniques that draw secretions from specific segments of the lungs and bronchi into the trachea. Coughing or suctioning normally removes secretions from the trachea. The procedure for postural drainage can include most lung segments (Table 44-8). Because clients may not require postural drainage of all lung segments, the procedure is based on clinical assessment findings. For example, clients with left lower lobe atelectasis may require postural drainage of only the affected region, whereas a child with cystic fibrosis may require postural drainage of all lung segments.

Chest Tubes. Chest tubes are inserted to remove air and fluids from the pleural space, to prevent air or fluid from reentering the pleural space, and to reestablish normal intrapleural and intrapulmonic pressures (Dettenmeier, 1992). A **chest tube** is a catheter inserted through the thorax to remove fluid or air. Chest tubes are used after chest surgery and chest trauma and for pneumothorax or hemothorax to promote lung reexpansion (Procedure 44-3).

A **pneumothorax** is a collection of air or other gas in the pleural space. The gas causes the lung to collapse because it obliterates the negative intrapleural pressure and a counterpressure is exerted against the lung, which is then un-

able to expand. There are a variety of mechanisms for a pneumothorax. It may occur spontaneously or from chest trauma. For example, a pneumothorax is caused by stabbing or trauma from an automobile accident; from the rupture of an emphysematous bleb on the surface of the lung (a large bulla resulting from the destruction caused by emphysema); or from an invasive procedure, such as insertion of a subclavian intravenous line.

A client with a pneumothorax usually feels pain as atmospheric air irritates the parietal pleura. The pain may be sharp and pleuritic. Dyspnea is common and worsens as the size of the pneumothorax increases.

Hemothorax is an accumulation of blood and fluid in the pleural cavity between the parietal and visceral pleurae, usually as the result of trauma. It produces a counterpressure and prevents the lung from full expansion. A hemothorax can also be caused by rupture of small blood vessels from inflammatory processes, such as pneumonia or tuberculosis. In addition to pain and dyspnea, signs and symptoms of shock can develop if blood loss is severe.

The one-bottle system is the simplest closed drainage system because the single bottle serves as a collector and a water seal (Fig. 44-15, *A*). During normal respiration the fluid

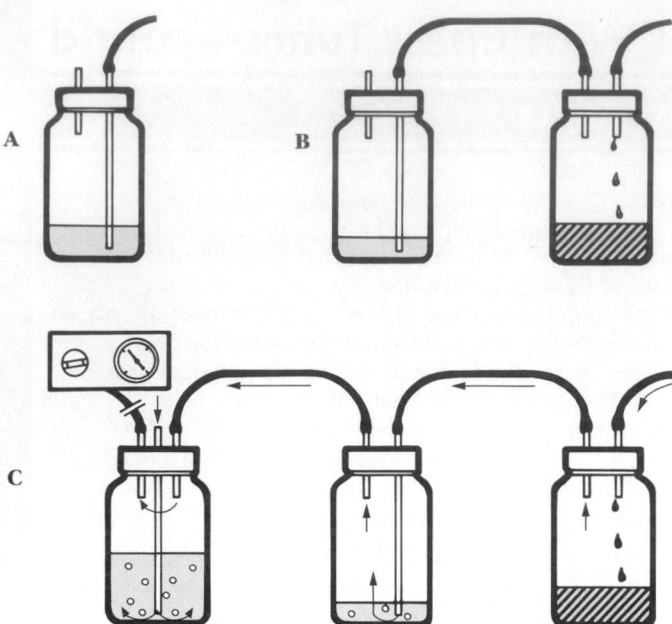

Fig. 44-15 Chest tube drainage. **A**, One-bottle system. **B**, Two-bottle system. **C**, Three-bottle system with suction.

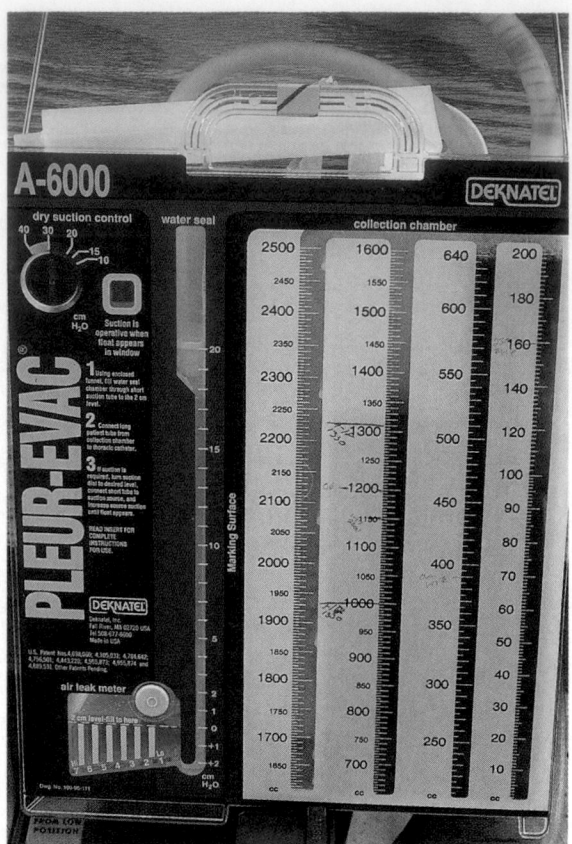

Fig. 44-16 Disposable, commercial chest drainage system.

should ascend with inspiration and descend with expiration. The one-bottle system is used for smaller amounts of drainage, such as an empyema. An empyema is a collection of infected fluid or pus in the pleural space.

A two-bottle system permits the liquid to flow into the collection bottle and air flows into the water-seal bottle (Fig. 44-15, *B*). Fluctuations in the water-seal tube are still anticipated. The two-bottle system allows for more accurate measurement of chest drainage and is used when larger amounts of drainage are expected.

A three-bottle system is used to evacuate any volume of air or fluid with controlled suction (Fig. 44-15, *C*). The suction-control bottle contains a long tube, submerged under water, and vented to the atmosphere. There are two short tubes, one tube connects bottles two and three and the second tube is connected to an external suction source. The suction pressure causes gentle, continuous bubbling in bottle three. Suction pressure is measured in centimeters of water and is equated with length of the long tube submerged in water. Usually −15 to −20 cm water is used for adults. This means the long tube is submerged in 15 to 20 centimeters of water. Children require lesser amounts of pressure.

The disposable systems, such as a Thora-Sene III or Pleur-Evac chest drainage system (Dekental), are a one-piece molded plastic unit that duplicates the three-bottle system (Fig. 44-16). The disposable units appear to be the system of choice because they are cost effective and some facilitate autotransfusion, a common practice in open-heart surgeries. Knowledge of the basics of chest tube management and troubleshooting maneuvers reduces the client's risk of complications (Table 44-9).

Special considerations. Clamping chest tubes is contraindicated when the client is ambulating or being transported. The nurse should handle the chest drainage unit or bottles carefully and maintain the drainage device below the

client's chest. If the tubing disconnects from the bottles, the nurse should instruct the client to exhale as much as possible and to cough. This maneuver rids the pleural space of as much air as possible. The nurse needs to cleanse the tips of the tubing and reconnect them to the bottles quickly. If the chest bottle breaks, quickly submerge the end of the tubing in a container of water to reestablish the seal. Clamping the chest tube may result in a tension pneumothorax, which is a life-threatening event.

Removal of chest tubes requires client preparation. A recent study investigated clients reported sensations during chest tube removal. The most frequent sensations reported included burning, pain, and a pulling sensation (Gift, Bolgiano, and Cunningham, 1991).

MAINTENANCE AND PROMOTION OF OXYGENATION

Promotion of lung expansion, mobilization of secretions, and maintenance of a patent airway assist the client in meeting oxygenation needs. Some clients, however, also require oxygen therapy to keep a healthy level of tissue oxygenation.

Goals of Oxygen Therapy. The goal of oxygen therapy is to prevent or relieve hypoxia. Any client with impaired tissue oxygenation can benefit from controlled oxygen administration. Oxygen is not a substitute for other treatment, however, and should be used only when indicated. Oxygen should be treated as a drug. It is expensive and has dangerous side effects. As with any drug, the dosage or concentration of oxygen should be continuously monitored.

Table 44-9	**Problem Solving with Chest Tubes**	

PROBLEM	**SOLUTION**
Air leak is present. 　Continuous bubbling is seen in water-seal bottle/chamber, indicating that leak is between client and water seal. 　Bubbling continues, indicating that air leak has not been corrected. 　Bubbling continues, indicating that leak is not in the client's chest or at the insertion site. 　Bubbling continues, indicating that leak is not in tubing	Locate leak. 　Tighten loose connections between client and water seal. Loose connections cause air to enter system. Leaks are corrected when constant bubbling stops. 　Cross-clamp chest tube close to client's chest. If bubbling stops, air leak is inside client's thorax or at chest tube insertion site. *Unclamp tube and notify physician immediately.* Reinforce chest dressing. Leaving chest tube clamped causes a tension pneumothorax and mediastinal shift. 　Gradually move clamps down drainage tubing away from client and toward suction-control chamber, moving one clamp at a time. When bubbling stops, leak is in section of tubing or connection distal to the clamp. Replace tubing or secure connection and release clamp. 　Leak is in drainage system. Change drainage system.
Tension pneumothorax is present. 　Severe respiratory distress 　Chest pain 　Absence of breath sounds on affected side 　Hyperresonance on affected side 　Mediastinal shift to unaffected side 　Tracheal shift to unaffected side 　Hypotension 　Tachycardia	Determine that chest tubes are not clamped, kinked, or occluded. Obstructed chest tubes trap air in intrapleural space when air leak originates within client. Notify physician immediately. Prepare immediately for another chest tube insertion; obtain a flutter (Heimlich) valve or large-gauge needle for short-term emergency release of air in intrapleural space; have emergency equipment (e.g., oxygen and code cart) near client.
Dependent loops of drainage tubing have trapped fluid.	Drain tubing contents into drainage bottle. Coil excess tubing on mattress and secure in place.
Water seal is disconnected.	Connect water seal and tape connection.
Water-seal bottle is broken.	Insert distal end of water-seal tube into sterile solution so that tip is 2 cm below surface and set up new water-seal bottle. If no sterile solution is available, double clamp chest tube while preparing new bottle.
Water-seal tube is no longer submerged in sterile fluid.	Add sterile solution to water-seal bottle until distal tip is 2 cm under surface or set water-seal bottle upright so that tip is submerged.

The nurse should routinely check the physician's orders to verify that the client is receiving the prescribed oxygen concentration. The five rights of medication administration also pertain to oxygen (see Chapter 35).

Safety Precautions With Oxygen Therapy. Oxygen is a highly combustible gas. Although it will not spontaneously burn or cause an explosion, it can easily cause a fire to ignite in a client's room if it contacts a spark from a cigarette or electrical equipment. Oxygen in high concentrations has a great combustion potential and fuels fire readily.

With increasing use of home oxygen therapy, clients and health care professionals must be aware of the dangers of combustion. The nurse should promote safety by using the following measures:

1. "No smoking" signs should be placed on the client's room door and over the bed. The client, visitors and roommates, and all personnel should be informed that smoking is not permitted in areas where oxygen is in use.

2. The nurse determines that all electrical equipment in the room is functioning correctly and is properly grounded (see Chapter 36). An electrical spark in the presence of oxygen can result in a serious fire.

3. The nurse should know the fire procedures and the location of the closest fire extinguisher.

4. The nurse should always check the oxygen level of portable tanks before transporting to ensure there is enough oxygen remaining in the tank.

Supply of Oxygen. Oxygen is supplied to the client's bedside either by oxygen tanks or through a permanent wall-piped system. Oxygen tanks are transported on wide-based carriers that allow the tank to be placed upright at the bedside. Regulators are used to control the amount of oxygen delivered. One common type is an upright flow meter with a flow-adjustment valve at the top. A second type is a cylinder indicator with a flow-adjustment handle.

In the hospital or home, oxygen tanks are delivered with the regulator in place. In the hospital, connecting the reg-

Applying a Nasal Cannula

STEPS	RATIONALE
1. Inspect client for signs and symptoms associated with hypoxia and presence of airway secretions.	Left untreated, hypoxia can produce cardiac dysrhythmias and death. Presence of airway secretions decreases effectiveness of oxygen delivery.
2. Explain to client and family what procedure entails and purpose of oxygen therapy.	Decreases client's anxiety, which reduces oxygen consumption and increases client cooperation.
3. Assemble needed supplies and equipment (see the illustration below):	Ensures that procedure is completed quickly and efficiently.
a. Nasal cannula	
b. Oxygen tubing	
c. Humidifier	
d. Sterile distilled water	
e. Oxygen source with flowmeter	
f. "No smoking" signs	
4. Wash hands.	Reduces transmission of infection.
5. Attach nasal cannula to oxygen tubing and attach to humidified oxygen source adjusted to prescribed flow rate.	Prevents drying of nasal and oral mucous membranes and airway secretions.
6. Place tips of cannula into client's nares and (see the illustration below, right) adjust elastic headband or plastic slide until cannula fits snugly and comfortably (see the illustration on p. 1235).	Directs flow of oxygen into client's upper respiratory tract. Client is more likely to keep cannula in place if it fits comfortably.
7. Maintain sufficient slack on oxygen tubing and secure to client's clothes.	Allows client to turn head without dislodging cannula and reduces pressure on tips of nares.
8. Check the cannula every 8 hr and keep humidification jar filled at all times.	Ensures patency of cannula and oxygen flow. Prevents inhalation of dehumidified oxygen.
9. Observe client's nares and superior surface of both ears for skin breakdown.	Oxygen therapy can cause drying of nasal mucosa. Pressure on ears from cannula tubing or elastic can cause skin irritation.

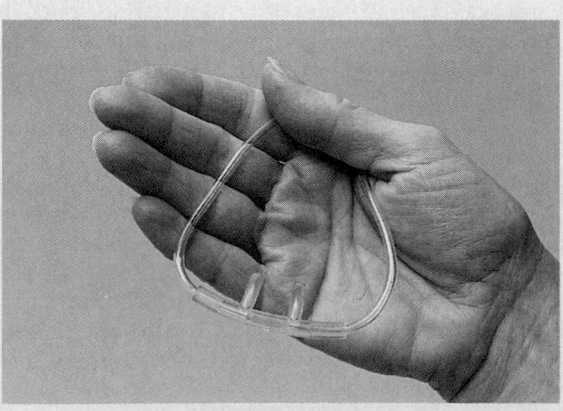

Step 3

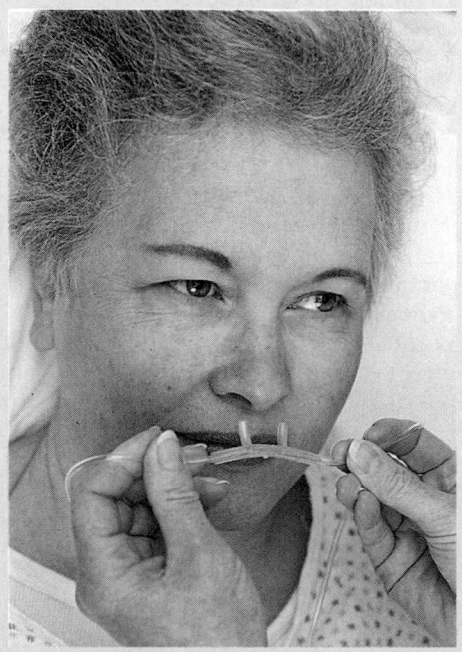

Step 6

Applying a Nasal Cannula—cont'd

STEPS	RATIONALE

10. Check oxygen flow rate and physician's orders every 8 hr (see the illustration below, right).

Ensures delivery of prescribed oxygen flow rate and patency of cannula.

11. Wash hands.

Reduces transmission of microorganisms.

12. Inspect client for relief of symptoms associated with hypoxia.

Indicates that hypoxia is corrected or reduced.

13. Record in nurses' notes method of oxygen delivery, flow rate, patency of oxygen cannula, client response, and respiratory assessment.

Documents correct use of oxygen therapy and client's response.

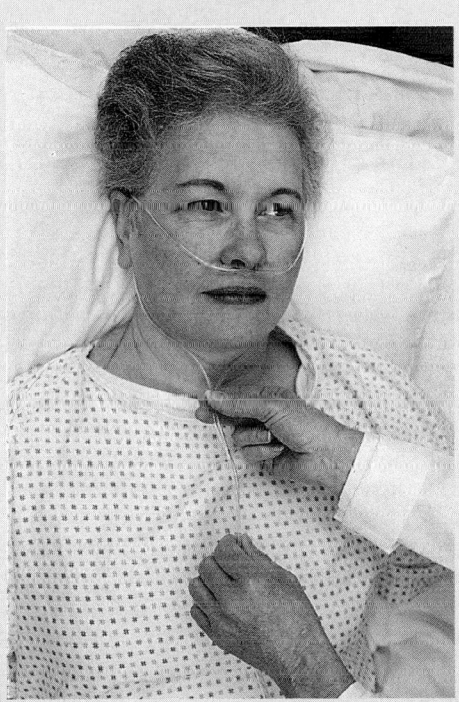

Step 6

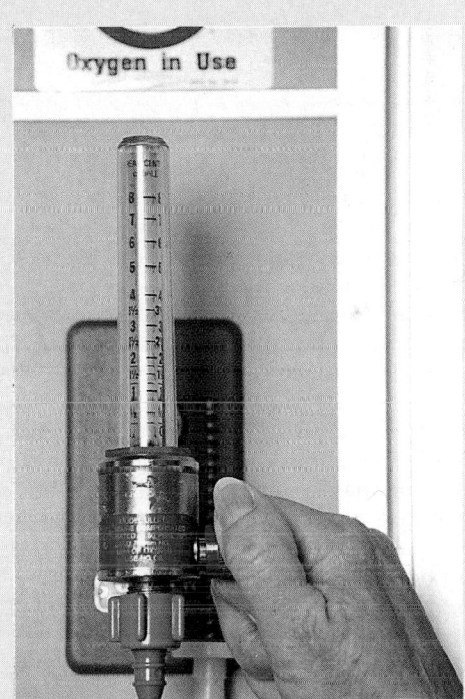

Step 10

ulator is usually done by the respiratory care department. Home care vendors are usually responsible for connecting the oxygen tank to the regulator for home use.

Methods of Oxygen Delivery. Oxygen can be delivered to the client by nasal cannula, nasal catheter, face mask, or mechanical ventilator.

Nasal cannula. A **nasal cannula** is a simple, comfortable device (Procedure 44-4). The two cannulae, about 1.5 cm (½ inch) long, protrude from the center of a disposable tube and are inserted into the nares. Oxygen is delivered via the cannulae with a flow rate of up to 6 L/min. Flow rates greater than 4 L/min are not often used due to the drying effect on the mucosa and the relatively little increase in delivered oxygen. The nurse must know what flow rate produces a given percentage of inspired oxygen concentration (FiO_2) (Table 44-10). The nurse must also be alert for skin

Table 44-10	Approximate FiO_2 with Different Delivery Devices		
NASAL CANNULA		**SIMPLE FACE MASK**	
1 L	24%	5-6 L	40%
2 L	28%	6-7 L	50%
3 L	32%	7-8 L	60%
4 L	36%		
5 L	40%		
6 L	44%		

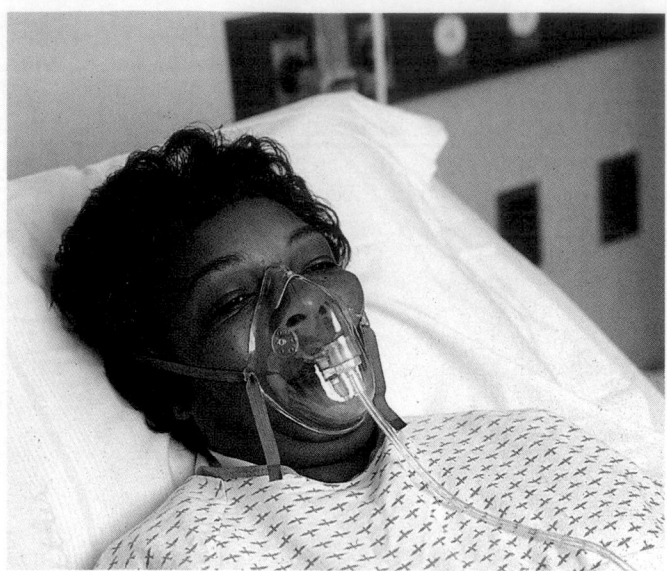

Fig. 44-17 Simple face mask.

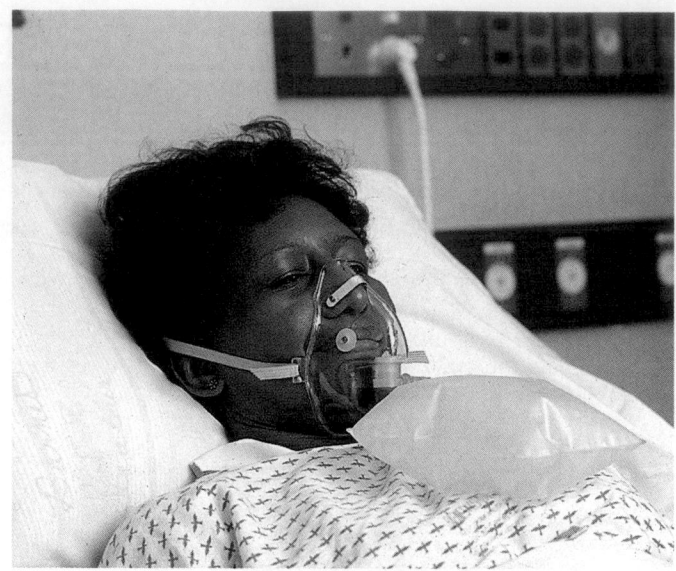

Fig. 44-18 Plastic face mask with reservoir bag.

breakdown over the ears and in the nares from too tight an application of the nasal cannula.

Nasal catheter. Nasal catheters are used less frequently than nasal cannulae, but they are not obsolete. The procedure involves inserting an oxygen catheter into the nose to the nasopharynx. Because securing the catheter can cause pressure on the nostril, the catheter must be changed at least every 8 hours and inserted into the other nostril. For this reason the nasal catheter is often a less desirable method because the client may have pain when the catheter is passed into the nasopharynx and because trauma can occur to the nasal mucosa.

Transtracheal oxygen. Transtracheal oxygen (TTO) is a method of oxygen delivery for clients with chronic lung diseases in which a small, intravenous-size catheter is inserted directly into the trachea through a surgical tract in the lower neck and oxygen is delivered directly into the trachea.

The advantages to TTO are: (1) no oxygen lost to the atmosphere; (2) clients achieve adequate oxygenation at lower flow rates, therefore oxygen delivery is more efficient, less expensive, and produces fewer side effects; and (3) clients are more likely to use oxygen because of the mobility, comfort, and cosmetic improvement.

Once the tracheal stoma is healed, the client is taught to remove and irrigate the catheter with normal saline at least three times a day to maintain catheter patency. The final oxygen flow rate, usually less than 4 L/min, is delivered through an 8 Fr catheter through the mature tract (Reinke, Hoffman, and Wesmiller, 1992).

Oxygen masks. An oxygen mask is a device used to administer oxygen, humidity, or heated humidity. It is shaped to fit snugly over the mouth and nose and is secured in place with a strap. There are two primary types of oxygen masks: low and high concentration.

The simple face mask (Fig. 44-17) is used for short-term oxygen therapy. It fits loosely and delivers oxygen concentrations from 30% to 60%. The mask is contraindicated for clients with carbon dioxide retention because retention can be worsened.

A plastic face mask with a reservoir bag (Fig. 44-18) and a Venturi mask (Fig. 44-19) are capable of delivering higher concentrations of oxygen. When used as a nonrebreather, the plastic face mask with a reservoir bag can deliver from 80% to 90% oxygen (70% when used as a rebreather) with a flow rate of 10 L/min. This oxygen mask maintains a high-concentration oxygen supply in the reservoir bag.

The nurse should frequently inspect the bag to make sure it is inflated. If it is deflated, the client may be breathing large amounts of exhaled carbon dioxide.

The Venturi mask can be used to deliver oxygen concentrations of 24% to 28%, 30%, 35%, 40%, 45%, 55% with oxygen flow rates of 2 to 3, 4, 6, 8, 14 L/min, respectively, depending on which flow control meter is selected (Dettenmeier, 1992).

Home oxygen. Indications for home oxygen therapy include an arterial partial pressure (Pao_2) of 55 mm Hg or less or an arterial oxygen saturation (Sao_2) of 88% or less on room air at rest, on exertion, or with exercise (Dettenmeier, 1992). Clients with a Pao_2 from 56 to 59 mm Hg may also receive oxygen if there is also evidence of cor pulmonale, pulmonary hypertension, erythrocytosis, central nervous system dysfunction, impaired mental status, or increasing hypoxemia with exertion.

When home oxygen is required, it is usually delivered by nasal cannula. When a client has a permanent tracheostomy, however, a T-tube or tracheostomy collar is necessary. Three types of oxygen are used: compressed oxygen, liquid oxygen, and oxygen concentrators. The advantages and disadvantages (Table 44-11) of each type are assessed, along with the client's needs and community resources, before placing a certain delivery system in the home. In the home the major consideration is the oxygen delivery source.

Clients requiring home oxygen need extensive teaching to be able to continue oxygen therapy at home efficiently and safely (Procedure 44-5). This includes oxygen safety, regulation of the amount of oxygen, and how to use the prescribed home oxygen delivery system. The nurse coordi-
Text continued on p. 1243.

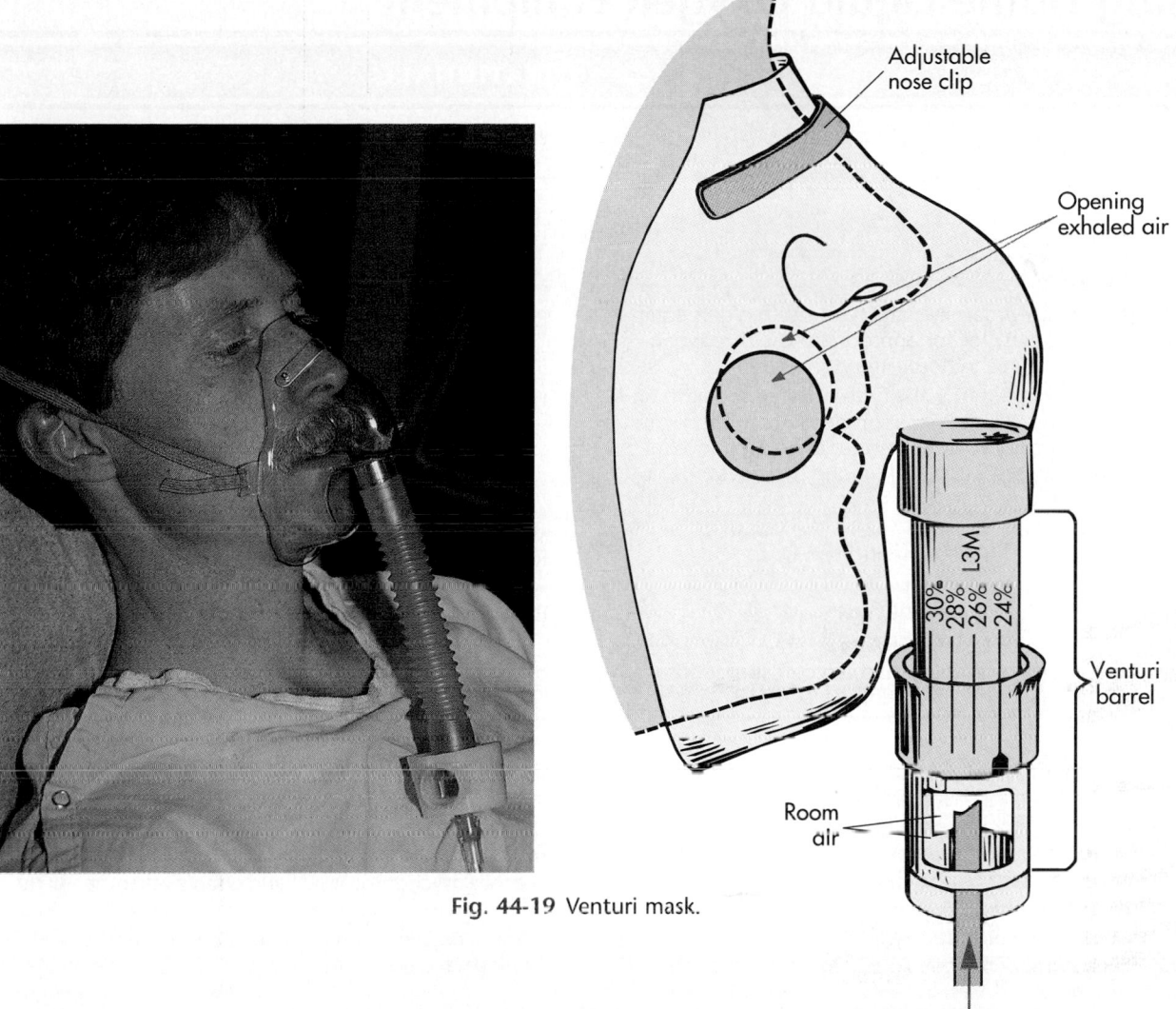

Fig. 44-19 Venturi mask.

Labels in figure: Adjustable nose clip; Opening exhaled air; Venturi barrel; Room air; 30%; 28%; 26%; 24%; L3M

Table 44-11	Home Oxygen Systems		
PRIMARY USE	**ADVANTAGES**	**DISADVANTAGES**	
COMPRESSED GAS CYLINDERS Intermittent therapy, such as for exercise or sleep only	100% oxygen, relatively inexpensive, no loss of gas during storage, relatively portable, delivery of up to 15 L/min	Bulky, possibly unsightly, frequent refilling necessary with continuous use	
LIQUID OXYGEN SYSTEMS High liter flows and active clients	100% oxygen, conveniently portable, portable units refilled at home, delivery of up to 6 L/min	Usually weekly delivery necessary for refill, evaporates if not used, potential for frostbite at connections and if liquid is spilled	
CONCENTRATORS Moderate liter flows and clients with limited mobility inside or outside home	Fixed monthly cost, minimal interruption of household by supplier, no refills of "main tank," most units with delivery of up to 4 or 5 L/min	Oxygen concentration decreases as liter flow increases (usually 85% to 90%), power supply necessary, electric bill increase of $15 to $20 a month, second system for portability necessary (usually gas cylinders)	

Modified from Dettenmeier PA: *Pulmonary nursing care,* St Louis, 1992, Mosby.

Using Home Liquid Oxygen Equipment

STEPS	RATIONALE

1. Assess:
   a. The client for need for home oxygen therapy.

   Candidates for home oxygen have a $PaO_2 \leq 55$ mm Hg or oxygen saturation of 88% on room air or PaO_2 55 to 59 mm Hg or an oxygen saturation of 86% to 89% with evidence of right heart failure, cor pulmonale, or polycythemia.

   b. The client's or family's ability to use oxygen equipment properly, or for appropriate use of oxygen equipment in the home setting.

   Physical or cognitive impairments may require instructing family members or significant others how to operate home oxygen equipment.

   c. Client's and family's ability to observe for signs and symptoms of hypoxia: apprehension, anxiety, decreased ability to concentrate, decreased level of consciousness, increased fatigue, dizziness, behavioral changes, increased pulse, increased respiratory rate, pallor, or cyanosis of the mucous membranes.

   Hypoxia can occur at home, despite the use of oxygen therapy. It can be caused by worsening of the client's physical condition or another underlying condition such as a change in the respiratory status.

2. Explain procedure to client and family.

   Reinforces information given to client and family; allows opportunity to ask questions.

3. Prepare needed equipment:
   a. Nasal cannula (see Procedure 44-4)

   Ensures that procedure is completed quickly and efficiently.

   b. Primary and portable liquid oxygen source for ambulation (see the illustration on p. 1239)
      (1) Nasal cannula
      (2) Oxygen tubing
      (3) Primary liquid oxygen source
      (4) Portable liquid oxygen source

4. Wash hands.

   Reduces transmission of infection.

5. Demonstrate steps for preparation and completion of oxygen therapy.

   Teaches psychomotor skill and enables client to ask questions.

6. Prepare primary and portable oxygen
   a. Place primary oxygen source in clutter-free environment.

   Primary oxygen source replaces compressed oxygen cylinders.

   b. Check oxygen levels of both sources by reading gauge on top (see the illustrations on p. 1239).

   Ensures adequate amount of oxygen available for use and timely refills of primary source.

   c. Refill portable source by placing on top of primary source and pressing down firmly. Check oxygen gauge to determine fullness of portable source (see the illustration on p. 1239).

   Provides secure connection and prevents leakage of oxygen into the room. If not seated securely, the cold liquid oxygen will leak out creating a snowlike precipitate.

   d. Select prescribed rate.

   Ensures delivery of prescribed amount of oxygen.

   e. Connect nasal cannula and oxygen tubing to oxygen source.

   Connects oxygen source to delivery method.

7. Have client and family perform each step with guidance from the nurse.

   Allows nurse to correct for errors in technique and discuss their implications.

8. Discuss signs and symptoms of respiratory tract infection: fever, increased sputum, change in sputum color, foul odor. Instruct client or family to notify physician for signs of hypoxia or infection.

   Respiratory tract infections increase oxygen demand and may affect oxygen transfer from lungs.
   Can prevent severe exacerbation of client's pulmonary disease.

9. Wash hands.

   Reduces transmission of infection.

10. Record teaching plan, information given to client, and validation of understanding.

    Provides written documentation of teaching for client and family; documents client's and family's understanding.

Using Home Liquid Oxygen Equipment—cont'd

STEPS	RATIONALE

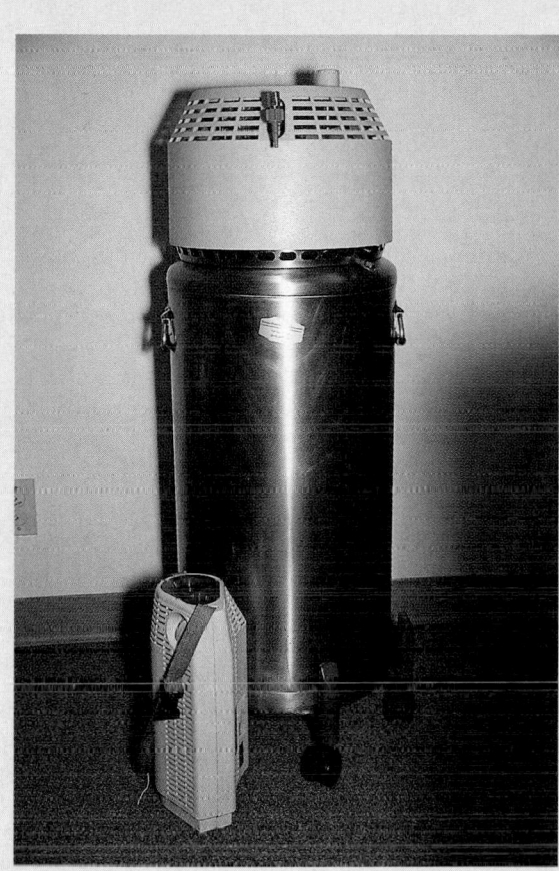

Step 3b

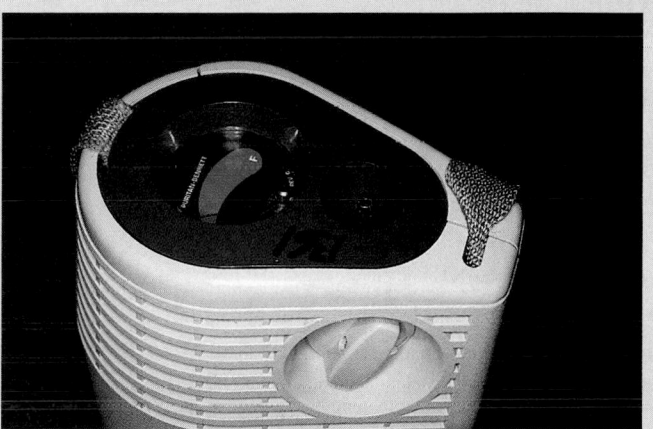

Step 6b

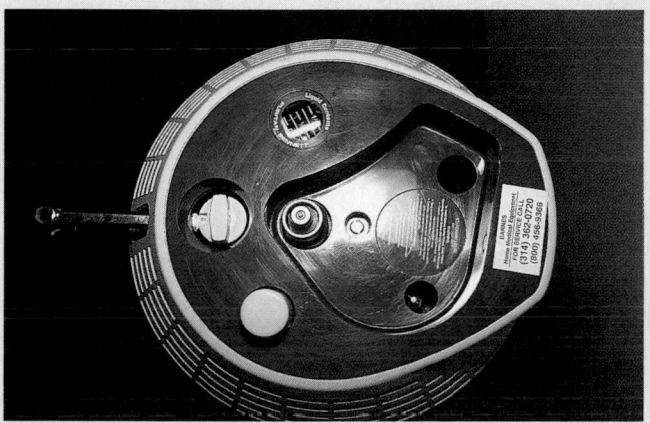

Step 6b

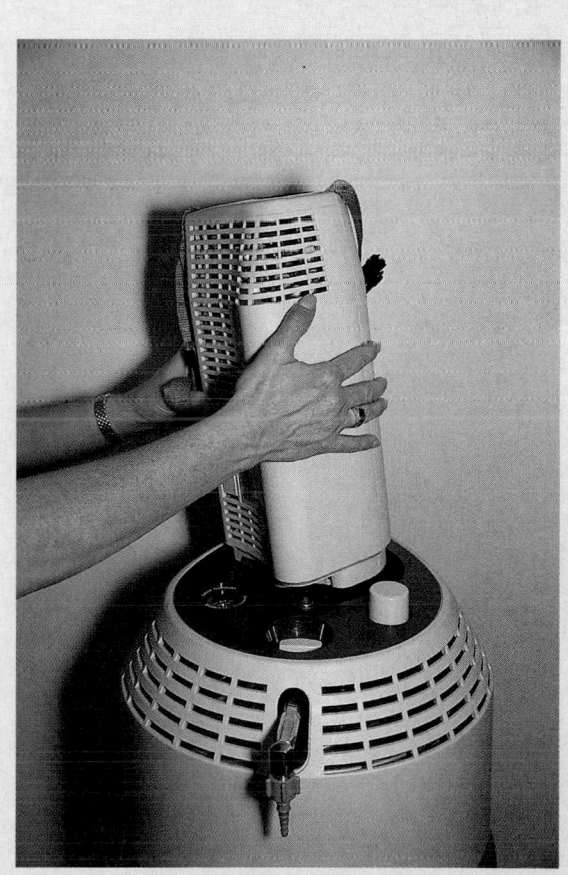

Step 6c

Cardiopulmonary Resuscitation

STEPS	RATIONALE

ONE NURSE

1. Assess for unresponsiveness, observe for spontaneous respirations, palpate carotid pulse; ask victim, "Are you OK?"

2. Call for help: in hospital setting, call a "code"; in community setting, call emergency phone number. For child or infant, complete 1 minute CPR before calling for help.

3. Place victim supine on firm, flat surface or use backboard.

4. Kneel at victim's side.

5. Open victim's airway:

    a. Head-tilt/chin-lift maneuver (adults and children): Place one hand on victim's forehead and apply firm, backward pressure with palm to tilt head back. Place fingers of other hand under bony part of lower jaw near chin and lift to bring chin forward and teeth almost to occlusion, thus supporting jaw and helping to tilt head back (see the illustration at right). The fingers must not press deeply into the soft tissue under the chin. Thumb should not be used to lift chin.

Prevents injury from attempted resuscitation of person who has not suffered a cardiac or respiratory arrest.

Activates mechanism for additional personnel.

Facilitates external compression of heart. Heart is compressed between sternum and hard surface.

Allows performance of rescue breathing and chest compressions without moving knees.

This maneuver is more effective in opening airway than previously recommended head-tilt/neck-lift.

Removes tongue or epiglottis as airway obstruction.

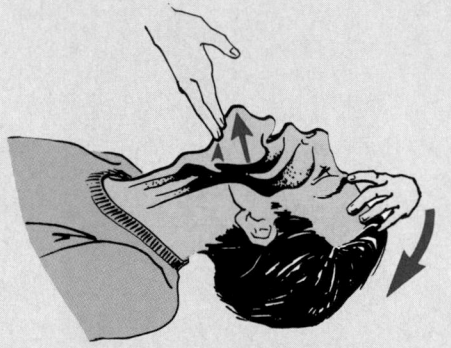

Step 5a

    b. Jaw thrust maneuver (adults and children): Grasp angles of victim's lower jaw and lift with both hands, one on each side, displacing mandible forward while tilting head backward.

6. Prepare for artificial respiration:

    a. For mouth-to-barrier resuscitation of adult, pinch victim's nose and mouth. For infant, place over infant's nose and mouth.

    b. For Ambu bag resuscitation, use proper size face mask and apply it over victim's mouth and nose.

7. Administer artificial respiration:

    a. For mouth-to-barrier resuscitation of adult, take a deep breath and seal lips around victim's mouth, creating air-tight seal. Give two slow breaths, $1^{1}/_{2}$ to 2 seconds each, followed by 10 to 12 breaths per min.

    b. For mouth-to-barrier resuscitation of infant or child, administer two slow breaths, 1-$1^{1}/_{2}$ seconds per breath with pause between for rescuer to take a breath, followed by 20 breaths per min.

This technique without head-tilt is the safest first approach to opening airway of victim with suspected neck injury because it can usually be accomplished without extending neck.

Use of a barrier helps reduce risk of transmission of communicable disease. However, lack of an available barrier should not delay CPR. Forms airtight seal and prevents air from escaping from nose.

Forms airtight seal as bag is compressed and oxygen enters client.

In most adults this volume of air is 800 ml and is sufficient to make chest rise. Adequate ventilation is indicated by observing chest rise and fall and hearing air escape during exhalation. Excess, rapid volume causes pharyngeal pressures to exceed esophageal opening pressures, allowing air to enter stomach.

Since an infant's air passages are smaller with resistance to flow quite high, it is difficult to make recommendations about the force or volume of the rescue breaths. However, three factors should be remembered: (1) rescue breaths are the single most important maneuver in assisting a nonbreathing child, (2) an appropriate volume is one that makes the chest rise and fall, and (3) slow breaths provide an adequate volume at the lowest possible pressure, thereby reducing the risk of gastric distention.

Cardiopulmonary Resusitation—cont'd

STEPS	**RATIONALE**

7. Administer artificial respiration—cont'd

  c. For artificial respiration with an Ambu bag in an adult, compress the bag fully for two breaths.

  d. For Ambu bag resuscitation in a child, use two small compressions of bag.

    Prevents overinflation of child's lungs.

8. Observe for rise and fall of chest wall with each respiration. If lungs do not inflate, reposition head and neck and check for visible airway obstruction, such as vomitus.

    Ensures artificial respirations are entering lungs.

9. Suction any secretions from airway. If suction is unavailable, turn victim's head to one side.

    Prevents airway obstruction. Allows gravity to drain secretions.

10. Assess for presence of carotid pulse; pulse check should take 5 to 10 sec.

    Carotid artery pulse will persist when more peripheral pulses are no longer palpable. Performing external cardiac compressions on a victim who has a pulse may result in serious medical complications.

  a. Carotid pulse is most central and accessible artery in children over 1 yr. However, in an infant the short, stubby neck makes carotid difficult to palpate; brachial artery is recommended instead.

11. If victim is pulseless, begin external cardiac compressions.

    Properly performed external chest compressions can produce systolic blood pressure peaks of more than 100 mm Hg, but diastolic pressure is low, with mean blood pressure in carotid arteries seldom exceeding 40 mm Hg. Blood flow through carotid artery is only one fourth to one third of normal.

Adult

  a. Proper hand position (see the illustration below):

    (1) Rescuer's hand locates lower margin of victim's rib cage on side next to rescuer.

    (2) Fingers are moved up rib cage to notch where ribs meet the lower sternum In center of lower part of chest.

      Results in maximum compression of heart between sternum and vetebrae. If compressions occur over xiphoid process, victim's liver can be lacerated.

    (3) Place heel of hand on lower half of sternum and place other hand on top of hand on sternum so that hands are parallel.

    (4) Fingers may be extended or interlaced but should be kept off chest.

      Reduces risk of rib fracture during compression.

  b. Lock elbows, maintain arms straight and shoulders directly over hands on victim's sternum (see the illustration below, right):

      Thrust for each compression is straight down on sternum.

    (1) Compress chest 3.8 to 5.0 cm (1½-2 in)

    (2) Compress chest 80 to 100 times/min. Perform 15 external compressions with mnemonic "one and, two and, three and. . ." to 15.

      Increases blood flow with increased flow to brain and heart. Allows pause for ventilation in two-rescuer CPR.

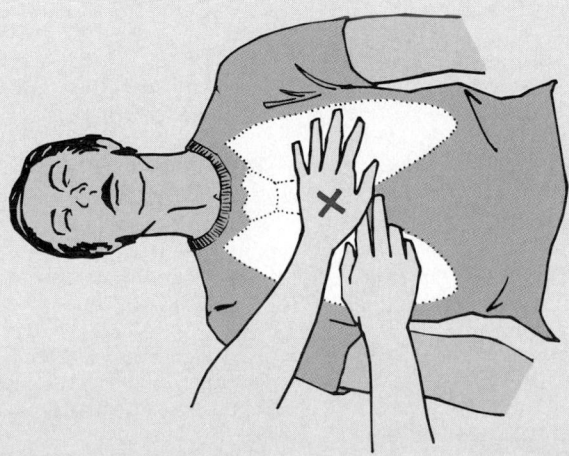

Step 11a

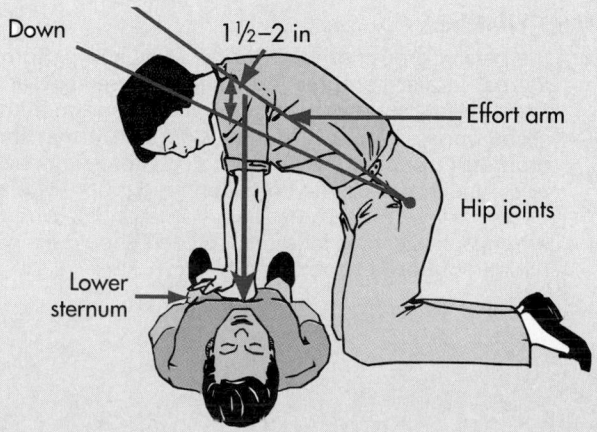

Down   1½–2 in   Effort arm   Hip joints   Lower sternum

Step 11b

From Emergency Cardiac Care Committee and Subcommittee, American Heart Association: Guidelines for cardiopulmonary resuscitation and emergency cardiac care, *JAMA* 268:2171, 1992.

Continued.

Cardiopulmonary Resuscitation—cont'd

STEPS	RATIONALE

Adult—cont'd

(3) Compression should be 50% of the compression-release cycle.

c. Ventilate lungs with two slow rescue breaths as in Step 7a. 1½-2 seconds.

d. Reassess victim after four complete cycles (15 compressions, 2 ventilations each cycle).   Determines return of pulse and respiration and need to continue CPR.

Infant (1-12 mo)

a. Proper hand position: Results in maximum compression.

(1) Draw imaginary line between nipples over breast bone (sternum).

(2) Place index finger of hand farthest from infant's head just under inframammary line where it intersects sternum.   Area of compression is one finger's width below this intersection at the location of middle and ring fingers.

b. Using two or three fingers, compress 1.3 to 2.5 cm (½-1 inch) at least 100 times/min.   Promotes adequate cardiac output.

c. At end of every fifth compression, allow a pause for ventilation (1½ seconds).   Promotes adequate ventilation during CPR.

d. Reassess victim after ten cycles (5 compressions, 1 ventilation each cycle).   Determines return of pulse and respiration and need to continue CPR.

Child (1-7 yr)

a. Proper hand position: Results in maximum compression.

(1) Locate lower margin of victim's rib cage on side next to rescuer with middle and index fingers.

(2) Follow margin of rib cage with middle finger to notch where ribs and sternum meet.

(3) Place index finger next to middle finger.

(4) Place heel of hand next to point where index finger was located, with long axis of heel parallel to sternum.

(5) Rescuer's other hand maintains child's head position.

b. Compress sternum with one hand 2.5 to 3.8 cm (1-1½ inches) at rate of 100 times/min.   Promotes adequate cardiac output.

c. At end of every fifth compression, allow a pause for ventilation (1-1½ seconds).   Promotes adequate ventilation during CPR.

d. Reassess victim after 10 cycles (5 compressions, 1 ventilation each cycle).   Determines return of pulse and respiration and need to continue CPR.

TWO NURSES

1. One person is positioned at victim's side and performs external cardiac compression while other remains at victim's head, maintains an open airway, and monitors carotid pulse. Compression rate is 80 to 100/min and compression should be 50% of the compression-release cycle. The compression-ventilation ratio is 5:1 with a pause for slow rescue breath (1½-2 seconds). When compressor becomes fatigued, rescuers should exchange positions as soon as possible.

nates the efforts of the client and family, home care nurse, home respiratory therapist, and home oxygen equipment vendor. The social worker usually assists with arranging the home care nurse and oxygen vendor. The nurse must assist the client and family in learning about home oxygen and ensure their ability to maintain the oxygen delivery system.

RESTORATION OF CARDIOPULMONARY FUNCTIONING

If a client's hypoxia is severe and prolonged, cardiac arrest may result. A cardiac arrest is a sudden cessation of cardiac output and circulation. When this occurs, oxygen is not delivered to tissues, carbon dioxide is not transported from tissues, tissue metabolism becomes anaerobic, and metabolic and respiratory acidosis occur. Permanent heart, brain, and other tissue damage occurs within 4 to 6 minutes.

Cardiopulmonary Resuscitation. Cardiac arrest is characterized by an absence of pulse and respiration. If the nurse determines that the client has cardiac arrest, **cardiopulmonary resuscitation (CPR)** must be initiated. CPR is a basic emergency procedure of artificial respiration and manual external cardiac massage (Procedure 44-6). The "ABCs" of cardiopulmonary resuscitation are: establish an *a*irway, initiate *b*reathing, and maintain *c*irculation. When an airway cannot be established, the nurse must reassess proper head position and assess for airway obstruction. There is no clinical benefit to cardiac compressions if an airway cannot be established. The purpose of CPR is to circulate oxygenated blood to the brain to prevent permanent tissue damage (ECC, 1992).

Restorative Care

Restorative care may emphasize cardiopulmonary reconditioning as a structured rehabilitation program. **Cardiopulmonary rehabilitation** is actively assisting the client to achieve and maintain an optimal level of health through controlled physical exercise, nutrition counseling, relaxation and stress management techniques, prescribed medications and oxygen, and compliance. As physical reconditioning occurs, the client's complaints of dyspnea, chest pain, fatigue, and activity intolerance should decrease. The client's anxiety, depression, or somatic concerns also often decrease. Goals of rehabilitation are defined by the client and the rehabilitation team.

RESPIRATORY MUSCLE TRAINING

Respiratory muscle training improves muscle strength and endurance, resulting in improved activity tolerance.

Respiratory muscle training may prevent respiratory failure in clients with chronic obstructive pulmonary disease.

One method for respiratory muscle training is the **incentive spirometer resistive breathing device (ISRBD)**. Resistive breathing is achieved by placing a resistive breathing device into a volume-dependent incentive spirometer. Muscle training is achieved when the client uses the ISRBD on a scheduled routine, for example, twice a day for 15 minutes or four times a day for 15 minutes (Celli, 1994). A study by Larson et al. (1988) investigated clients with chronic obstructive pulmonary disease and measured muscle training following use of the ISRBD. Subjects used the ISRBD once daily for 30 minutes for 8 weeks. They were randomized into either 15% PI_{max} or 30% PI_{max}. The PI_{max} represents the effort required to complete each breath. Subjects demonstrated an increase in exercise endurance time and minimal increase in 12-minute walk distance as well as increase in respiratory muscle strength and sputum expectoration.

BREATHING EXERCISES

Breathing exercises include techniques to improve ventilation and oxygenation. The three basic techniques are deep breathing and coughing exercises, pursed-lip breathing, and diaphragmatic breathing (Celli 1994). Deep breathing and coughing exercises are routine interventions for postoperative clients (see Chapter 48).

Pursed-lip breathing involves deep inspiration and prolonged expiration through pursed lips to prevent alveolar collapse. While sitting up, the client is instructed to take a deep breath and to exhale slowly through pursed lips. Clients need to gain control of the exhalation phase so that exhalation is longer than inhalation (Dettenmeier, 1992). The client is usually able to perfect this technique by counting inhalation time and gradually increasing the count during exhalation.

Diaphragmatic breathing is more difficult and requires the client to relax intercostal and accessory respiratory muscles while taking deep inspirations. The client concentrates on expanding the diaphragm during controlled inspiration. The client is taught to place one hand flat below the breastbone above the waist and the other hand 2 to 3 cm below the first hand. The client is asked to inhale while the lower hand moves outward during inspiration. The client observes for inward movement as the diaphragm ascends. These exercises are initially taught with the client in the supine position and then practiced while the client sits and stands. The exercise is often used with the pursed-lip breathing technique.

Sample Evaluation of Interventions for Ineffective Airway Clearance

GOALS	EVALUATIVE MEASURES	EXPECTED OUTCOMES
Pulmonary secretions will be removed.	Auscultate all lung fields after coughing and postural drainage maneuvers.	Adventitious lung sounds will be absent within 48 hr.
	Observe client while coughing for amount of secretions, fatigue, dyspnea.	
	Inspect sputum after cough and/or suctioning.	Sputum will be clear, white, and frothy within 48 hr.

Diaphragmatic breathing is also useful for clients with pulmonary disease, for postoperative clients, and for women in labor to promote relaxation and provide pain control. The exercise improves efficiency of breathing by decreasing air trapping and reducing the work of breathing.

 ## Evaluation

Nursing interventions and therapies are evaluated by comparing the client's progress to the goals and desired outcomes of the nursing care plan. Each goal and category of interventions has objective evaluation criteria (see the evaluation box on p. 1243).

When nursing measures directed to improve oxygenation are unsuccessful, the nurse must immediately modify the nursing care plan. New interventions are then developed. The nurse should not hesitate to notify the physician about a client's deteriorating oxygenation status. Prompt notification can avoid an emergency situation or even the need for cardiopulmonary resuscitation.

■ KEY CONCEPTS ■

► The primary function of the heart is to deliver deoxygenated blood to the lungs for oxygenation and to deliver oxygen and nutrients to the tissues.

► Cardiac output is altered by preload, afterload, contractility, and heart rate.

► Cardiac dysrhythmias are classified by cardiac activity and site of impulse origin.

► The primary function of the lungs is to transfer oxygen from the atmosphere into the alveoli and to transfer carbon dioxide out of the body as a waste product.

► Ventilation is the process of providing adequate oxygenation from the alveoli to the blood.

► Compliance, or the ability of the lungs to expand and contract, depends on the function of musculoskeletal and neurological systems and on other physiological factors.

► The process of inspiration (active process) and expiration (passive process) is achieved with lung changes in pressures and lung volumes.

► Respiration is controlled by the central nervous system and by chemicals within the blood.

► Decreased hemoglobin levels alter the client's ability to transport oxygen.

► Impaired chest wall movement reduces the level of tissue oxygenation.

► Hyperventilation is a respiratory rate greater than that required to maintain normal levels of carbon dioxide.

► Hypoventilation causes carbon dioxide retention.

► Hypoxia occurs if the amount of oxygen delivered to tissues is too low.

► The nursing assessment includes information about the client's cough, dyspnea, fatigue, wheezing, chest pain, environmental exposures, respiratory infection, cardiopulmonary risk factors, use of medications, and physical functioning.

► Diagnostic and laboratory tests may be needed to complete the data base for a client with decreased oxygenation.

► Pursed-lip breathing is an effective intervention to control breathing and increase oxygenation.

► Breathing exercises improve ventilation, oxygenation, and sensations of dyspnea.

► Relaxation techniques and imagery are valuable interventions in controlling dyspnea and anxiety in clients with COPD.

► Nebulization delivers small drops of water or particles of medication to the airways.

► Chest physiotherapy includes postural drainage, percussion, and vibration to mobilize pulmonary secretions.

► Coughing and suctioning techniques are used to maintain a patent airway.

► Oxygen therapy is used to improve levels of tissue oxygenation and is delivered by nasal cannula, nasal catheter, or oxygen mask.

► Cardiac arrest requires the use of cardiopulmonary resuscitation.

■ KEY TERMS ■

Accessory muscles, p. 1196

Afterload, p. 1194

Airway resistance, p. 1196

Angina pectoris, p. 1203

Angiography, p. 1211

Atelectasis, p. 1206

Atrioventricular (AV) node, p. 1194

Bronchoscopy, p. 1212

Bundle of His, p. 1194

Cardiac catheterization, p. 1211

Cardiac index (CI), p. 1193

Cardiac output, p. 1193

Cardiopulmonary rehabilitation, p. 1243

Cardiopulmonary resuscitation (CPR), p. 1243

Chest percussion, p. 1227

Chest physiotherapy (CPT), p. 1227

Chest tube, p. 1231

Compliance, p. 1196

Cough, p. 1207

■ CRITICAL THINKING EXERCISES ■

1. Mr. Havens is a 65-year-old man with a history of congestive heart failure and poor activity tolerance. What data are important in determining the cardiac response to exercise? What criteria are used to determine when the exercise demand has exceeded cardiac workload capacity?

2. Your client experiences chest pain. State how you assess this pain. What are three important interventions for a client with chest pain?

3. You are caring for a client who had abdominal surgery 24 hours ago. This client has a 10-year history of chronic obstructive pulmonary disease. What are the important aspects of assessment and intervention necessary to maintain a patent airway?

4. You receive a physician's order to obtain a pulse oximetry reading on Mr. Aubuchon who was admitted for increasing shortness of breath, history of COPD, and atherosclerosis. What do you need to consider as you prepare to obtain the pulse oximeter reading?

REFERENCES

Ahrens TS: Svo₂ monitoring: is it being used appropriately? *Crit Care Nurs* 10(7):70, 1990.

Ahrens TS, Pulmonary anatomy and physiology. In Kinney MR, Packa DR, Dunbar SB: *AACN's Clinical reference for critical-care nursing,* St Louis, 1993, Mosby.

Ahrens TS, Rutherford K: *Essentials of Oxygenation,* Boston, 1993, Jones and Bartlett Publishers.

American Cancer Society: *Cancer facts and figures 1994,* Atlanta, 1994, American Cancer Society.

Bell DA: Do incentive spirometers reduce the rate of postoperative pulmonary complications?, *Persp Resp Nurs* 4(3):1, 1993.

Benner P: *From novice to expert,* Philadelphia, 1984, Addison Wesley.

Bowers AC, Thompson JM: *Clinical manual of health assessment* ed 4, St Louis, 1992, Mosby.

Burns SM et al: Effect of body position on spontaneous respiratory rate and tidal volume in patients with obesity, abdominal distention and ascites, *Am J of Crit Care* 3(2):102, 1994.

Butler JC et al: Pneumococcal polysaccharide vaccine efficacy: an evaluation of current recommendations, *JAMA* 270(15):1826, 1993.

Canobbio MM: *Cardiovascular disorders,* St Louis, 1990, Mosby.

Carrieri-Kohlman V et al: Desensitization and mastery: treatment approaches for the management of dyspnea, *Heart Lung* 22(3):226, 1993.

Celli BR: Physical reconditioning of patients with respiratory diseases: legs, arms, and breathing retraining, *Resp Care* 39(5):481, 1994.

Centers for Disease Control and Prevention: Update on adult immunization, *MMWR* 40(RR-12), 1991.

Centers for Disease Control and Prevention: Prevention and control of influenza: part I, vaccines, *MMWR* 42(RR-6):1, 1993.

Daily EK, Schroeder JS: *Techniques in bedside hemodynamic monitoring,* ed 6, St Louis, 1994, Mosby.

Dettenmeier PA: *Pulmonary nursing care,* St Louis, 1992, Mosby.

DeVito AJ: Dyspnea during hospitalizations for acute phase of illness as recalled by patients with chronic obstructive pulmonary disease, *Heart Lung* 19(2):186, 1990.

Eid N et al: Chest physiotherapy in review, *Resp Care* 36(4):270, 1991.

Emergency Cardiac Care Committee and Subcommittee, American Heart Association: Guidelines for cardiopulmonary resuscitation and emergency cardiac care, *JAMA* 268:2171, 1992.

Fedson DS et al: Pneumococcal vaccine after 15 years of use, *Arch Intern Med* 154:2531, 1994.

Gift AG: Validation of a vertical visual analog scale as a measure of clinical dyspnea, *Rehab Nurs* 14: 323, 1989.

Gift AG: Dyspnea, *Nurs Clin North Am* 25(4):955, 1990.

Gift AG, Bolgiano CS, Cunningham J: Sensations during chest tube removal, *Heart Lung* 20(2):131, 1991.

Gift AG, Moore T, Soeken K: Relaxation to reduce dyspnea and anxiety in COPD patients, *Nurs Res* 41(4):242, 1992.

Huebner A: Where there's smoke . . tobacco smoke in the air is a hazard to children, *Am Baby for Expectant & New Parents* 56(7):28, 1994.

Johanson BC et al: *Standards for critical care*, ed 3, St Louis, 1988, Mosby–Year Book.

Karper WB, Boshen MB: Effects of exercise on acute respiratory tract infections and related symptoms, *Geriatr Nurs* 14(1):15, 1993.

Kim MJ, McFarland GK, McLane AM: *Pocket guide to nursing diagnoses*, ed 6, St Louis, 1995, Mosby.

Kovach CR: Managing a tuberculosis outbreak, *Geriatr Nurs* 12(1), 29, 1991.

Larson J et al: Inspiratory muscle training with a pressure threshold breathing device in patients with chronic obstructive pulmonary disease. *Am Rev Resp Dis* 138(3):689, 1988.

Lueckenotte AG: *Gerontologic assessment*, ed 2, St Louis, 1994, Mosby.

Lueckenotte AG: *Textbook of gerontologic nursing*, St Louis, 1996, Mosby.

Malasanos L, Barkauskas V, Stoltenberg-Allen: *Health assessment*, ed 4, St Louis, 1990, Mosby.

McCance KL, Huether SE: *Pathophysiology: the biologic basis for disease in adults and children*, ed 2, St Louis, 1994, Mosby.

Pierson DJ: Effects of aging on the respiratory system. In Pierson DJ, Kacmarek RM, editors: *Foundations of respiratory care* , New York, 1992, Churchill Livingstone.

Purcell JA: Cardiac electrical activity. In Kinney MR, Packa DR, Dunbar SB: *AACN's clinical reference for critical-care nursing*, ed 3, St Louis, 1993, Mosby.

Reinke LF, Hoffman LA, Wesmiller SW: Transtracheal oxygen therapy: an alternative delivery approach, *Pers Respir Nurs* 3(3):3, 1992.

Seidel HM et al: *Mosby's guide to physical examination*, ed 3, St Louis, 1995, Mosby.

Sonnesso G: Are you ready to use pulse oximetry? *Nurs 91* 21(8):60, 1991.

Stein BE: adult vaccinations: protecting your patients from avoidable illness, *Geriatrics* 48(9):46, 1993.

Thompson J et al: *Mosby's manual of clinical nursing*, ed 3, St Louis, 1993, Mosby.

Urban NA et al: *Guidelines for critical care nursing*, St Louis, 1995, Mosby.

Walsh M: Peak expiratory flow-rate monitoring, *Perspect Respir Nurs* 3(1):1, 1992.

Weilitz PB: *Pocket guide to respiratory care*, St Louis, 1991, Mosby.

Weilitz PB: Pulmonary embolism and chest trauma. In Ahrens, Prentice D: *Critical care certification preparation & review*, ed 3, Norwalk, Conn, 1993, Appleton & Lange.

Whatling J: Childhood asthma and passive smoking, *Nurs standard* 8(46):25, 1994.

Whitney JD: The measurement of oxygen tension in tissues, *Nurs Res* 39(4):203, 1990.

Wilson SF, Thompson JM: *Respiratory disorders*, St Louis, 1990, Mosby.

Yeaw EMJ: How position affects oxygenation good lung down? *Am J Nurs* 92(3):27, 1992.

ADDITIONAL READINGS

Ahrens TS: Changing perspectives in the assessment of oxygenation, *Crit Care Nurs* 13(4):78, 1993.

American Association of Respiratory Care: AARC clinical practice guideline: postural drainage therapy, *Resp Care* 36(12):1418, 1991.

Breslin EH: Dyspnea-limited response in chronic obstructive pulmonary disease: reduced unsupported arm activities, *Rehab Nurs* 17(1): 12, 1992.

Foyt MM: Impaired gas exchange in the elderly, *Geriatr Nurs* 13(5):262, 1992.

Gift AG: Therapies for dyspnea relief, *Holistic Nurs Pract* 7(2):57, 1993.

Hardy KA: A review of airway clearance: new techniques, indications, and recommendations, *Resp Care* 39(5):440, 1994.

Hess D, Kacmarek RM: Techniques and devices for monitoring oxygenation, *Resp Care* 38(6):646, 1993.

Landis K: Discharge teaching for patients with COPD, *Perspect Resp Nurs* 4(2):1, 1993.

Lewis SM, Collier IC: *Medical-surgical nursing assessment and management of clinical problems*, ed,4, St Louis, 1995, Mosby.

Nelson LD: Assessment of oxygenation: oxygenation indices, *Resp Care* 38(6):631, 1993.

Perry AG, Potter PA: *Clinical nursing skills and techniques: basic, intermediate, and advanced*, ed 3, St Louis, 1994, Mosby.

Pierce JD, Piazza D, Naftel DC: Effects of two chest tube clearance protocols on drainage in patients after myocardial revascularization surgery, *Heart Lung* 20(2):125, 1991.

Thompson JM et al: *Mosby's clinical nursing*, ed 3, St Louis, 1993, Mosby.

Statz E: Reducing COPD patients' dyspnea during activities involving their upper extremities, *Perspect Resp Nurs* 4(4):1, 1993.

Stiesmeyer J: A four-step approach to pulmonary assessment, *Am J Nurs* 8(93):22, 1993.

Thompson JM et al: *Mosby's clinical nursing*, ed 3, St Louis, 1993, Mosby.

Weaver TE, Narsavage GL: Physiological and psychological variables related to functional status in chronic obstructive pulmonary disease, *Nurs Res* 41(5):286,1992.

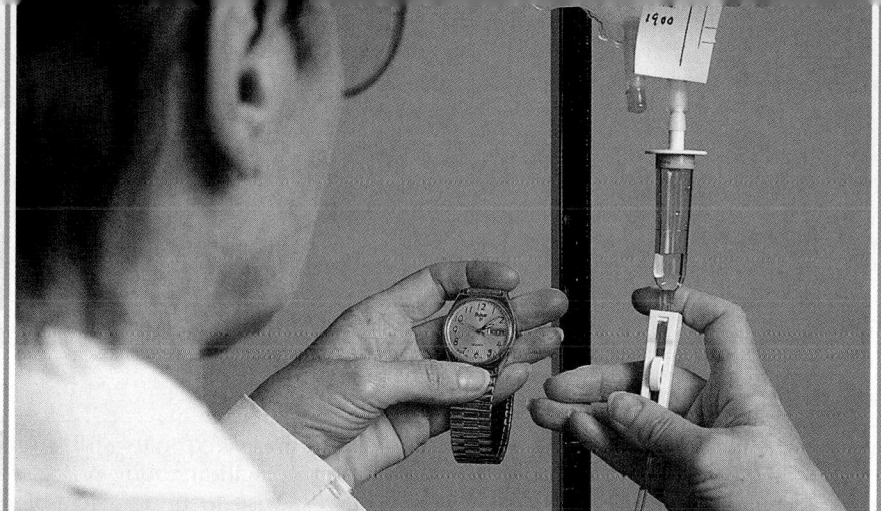
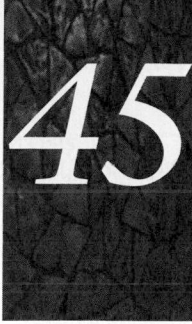

## Chapter 45

Fluid, Electrolyte, and Acid-Base Balances

Objectives

Mastery of content in this chapter will enable the student to:

► Define the key terms listed.

► Describe the distribution, composition, movement, and regulation of body fluids.

► Describe the regulation of sodium, potassium, calcium, magnesium, chloride, bicarbonate, phosphate, and acid-base.

► Describe the isotonic fluid imbalances of fluid volume excess and fluid volume deficit.

► Discuss the alterations in serum osmolality caused by water excess and deficit.

► Discuss the variables affecting normal fluid, electrolyte, and acid-base balances.

► Compile a nursing history and complete a physical examination of a client for fluid, electrolyte, and acid-base balances.

► Describe laboratory studies associated with fluid, electrolyte, and acid-base imbalances.

► Develop a nursing care plan for clients with fluid, electrolyte, and acid-base imbalances.

► Discuss the purpose of intravenous therapy.

► Describe the procedure for initiating and maintaining an intravenous line and calculating intravenous flow rate.

► Demonstrate how to change intravenous solutions, tubing, and dressings and to discontinue an infusion.

► Discuss the complications of intravenous therapy.

► Discuss the procedure for administering a blood transfusion and nursing actions for a transfusion reaction.

Fluid, electrolyte, and acid-base balances within the body are necessary to maintain health. These balances are maintained by the intake, distribution, and output of water and electrolytes, and their regulation by the renal and pulmonary systems. Imbalances may result from many factors including illnesses. Therefore nursing care for many different kinds of clients includes assessment and correction of imbalances or maintenance of balance.

A healthy, mobile, well-oriented adult can usually maintain normal fluid, electrolyte, and acid-base balances because of the body's adaptive mechanisms. However, the infant, the severely ill adult, the disoriented or immobile client, and the older adult are frequently unable to respond independently; and, after time, the body's adaptive capacities can no longer maintain balance without assistance.

■ FLUID AND ELECTROLYTE BALANCES

Distribution of Body Fluids

Body fluids are distributed in two distinct compartments: extracellular fluids (ECF) and intracellular fluids (ICF).

Extracellular fluids include **interstitial fluid** (ISF) and intravascular fluid. Interstitial fluid fills the spaces between most cells of the body and provides a substantial portion of the body's liquid environment. About 15% of body weight consists of interstitial fluids. Intravascular fluid is plasma, the watery, colorless, fluid portion of the lymph and blood in which the leukocytes, erythrocytes, and platelets are suspended. Plasma composes 5% of body weight.

Intracellular fluids (ICF) are liquids within cell membranes containing dissolved substances or solutes essential to fluid and electrolyte balance and metabolism. Intracellular fluids constitute 40% of body weight. Many of the solutes in the intracellular fluid compartment are the same as those located in the extracellular fluid space. However, the proportion of the substances is different. For example, a larger proportion of potassium exists in intracellular fluids than in extracellular fluids.

Composition of Body Fluids

The fluids circulating throughout the body in extracellular and intracellular fluid spaces contain electrolytes, minerals, and cells.

An **electrolyte** is an element or compound that, when melted or dissolved in water or another solvent, dissociates into ions and is able to carry an electric current. Positively charged electrolytes are **cations.** Negatively charged electrolytes are **anions.** The concentration of each electrolyte differs in extracellular and intracellular fluids. However, the total number of anions and cations in each fluid compartment should be the same.

Electrolytes are vital to many body functions including neuromuscular function and acid-base balance. Electrolytes are commonly measured in milliequivalents per liter (mEq/L), which is a measure of chemical activity representing the amount of cation or anion that will react with a given amount of another cation or anion (Weldy, 1992).

Minerals, which are ingested as compounds, are usually referred to by the name of a metal, nonmetal, radical, or phosphate rather than by the name of the compound of which they are a part. They are constituents of all body tissues and fluids and are important in maintaining physio-logical processes. Minerals also act as catalysts in nerve response, muscle contraction, and metabolism of nutrients in foods. In addition, they regulate electrolyte balance and hormone production and strengthen skeletal structures. Examples of minerals include iron and zinc.

Cells are the functional basic units of all living tissue. Examples of cells within body fluids are the red blood cell (RBC) and the white blood cell (WBC).

Movement of Body Fluids

Body fluids are not static. Fluids and electrolytes shift from compartment to compartment to facilitate body processes such as tissue oxygenation, response to illness, acid-base balance, and response to drug therapies. Body fluids and electrolytes move by diffusion, osmosis, active transport, or filtration. Such movement depends on cell membrane permeability or the ability of the membrane to allow fluids and electrolytes to pass through it.

DIFFUSION

Diffusion is a process in which solid, particulate matter, such as sugar in a fluid, moves from an area of higher concentration to an area of lower concentration, resulting in an even distribution of the particles in the fluid or across a cell membrane permeable to that substance (Fig. 45-1). Another way to express this is: substances that are diffusing move down their concentration gradients (Weldy, 1992).

OSMOSIS

Osmosis is the movement of a pure solvent, such as water, through a semipermeable membrane from a solution that has a lower solute concentration to one that has a higher solute concentration (Fig. 45-2). The membrane is permeable to the solvent, but it is impermeable to the solute, the particulate matter. The rate of osmosis depends on the concentration of the solutes in the solutions, the temperature of the solutions, the electrical charges of the solutes, and the differences between the osmotic pressures exerted by the solutions. The concentration of a solution is

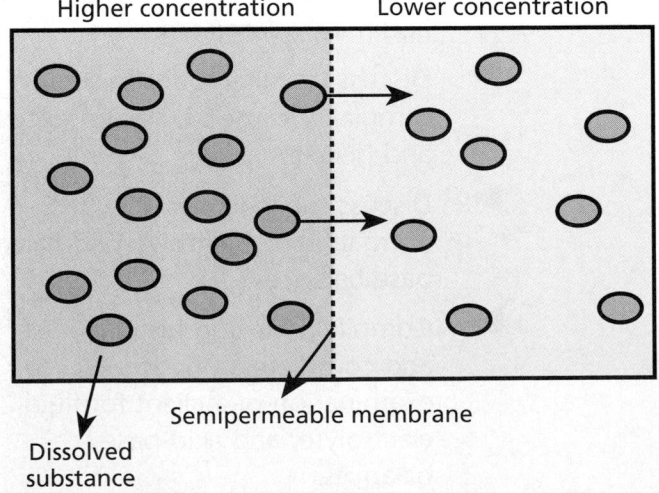

Higher concentration   Lower concentration

Semipermeable membrane

Dissolved substance

Fig. 45-1 Diffusion is the movement of molecules of a substance from an area of higher concentration to an area of lower concentration (along its concentration gradient).

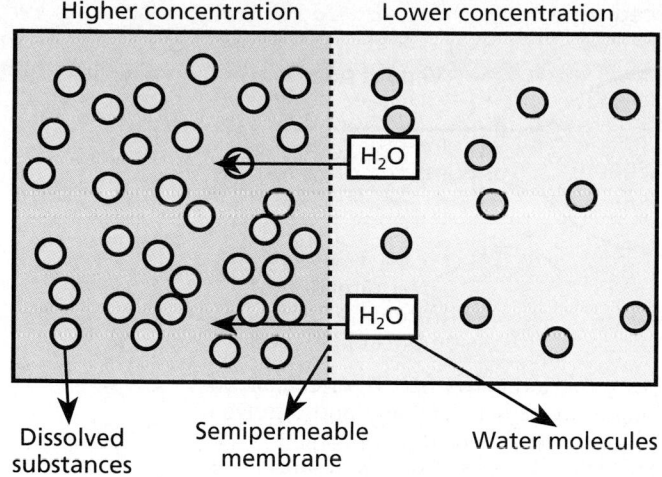

Higher concentration   Lower concentration

H₂O

H₂O

Dissolved substances   Semipermeable membrane   Water molecules

Fig. 45-2 In osmosis, water molecules move from the less concentrated area to the more concentrated area in an effort to equalize the concentration of solutions on two sides of a membrane.

measured in osmols, which reflect the amount of a substance in solution in the form of molecules, ions, or both.

Osmotic pressure is the drawing power for water and depends on the number of molecules in solution. A solution with a high solute concentration has a high osmotic pressure and draws water into itself. Osmotic pressure is exerted through a semipermeable membrane and depends on the activity of the solute separated by the membrane. If the concentration of the solute is greater on one side of the semipermeable membrane, the rate of osmosis is quicker, and a more rapid transfer of solvent across the membrane occurs. This continues until an equilibrium is reached. The osmotic pressure of a solution is also called its **osmolality**, which is expressed in osmols, or milliosmols per kilogram (mOsm/kg), of the solution. The normal serum osmolality is 280 to 295 mOsm/kg.

A solution with the same osmolality as blood plasma is called **isotonic**. The intravenous (IV) administration of an isotonic solution prevents shifting of fluid and electrolytes from intracellular compartments. A **hypotonic** IV solution that has a lesser concentration of solutes than plasma does will move water into the cells. Conversely, administration of a **hypertonic** IV solution with a greater concentration of solutes than plasma will move water out of the cells (Table 45-1).

The osmotic pressure of the blood is affected by plasma proteins, especially albumin, a serum protein naturally produced by the body. Albumin exerts colloid osmotic or **oncotic pressure**, which tends to keep fluid in the intravascular compartment. At the venous end of capillaries, this oncotic pressure and decreased venous hydrostatic pressure draw water and waste products back into the capillaries to be filtered through the kidneys.

FILTRATION

Filtration is the process by which water and diffusible substances move together in response to fluid pressure. This process is active in capillary beds, where hydrostatic pressure differences or gradients determine the movement of water, electrolytes, and other dissolved substances between the capillaries and interstitial fluid.

Hydrostatic pressure is the pressure exerted by a liquid in a column. Arterial blood and fluid enter the capillaries at a pressure greater than interstitial pressure, so fluid and solutes move from the capillaries toward the cells. At the venous end of the capillary bed, because hydrostatic pressure is less than interstitial pressure, fluid and waste products move from the cells back into the capillaries (Fig. 45-3).

ACTIVE TRANSPORT

Unlike diffusion and osmosis, **active transport** requires metabolic activity and expenditure of energy to move materials across cell membranes. This allows cells to admit larger molecules than they would otherwise be able to admit or to move molecules from areas of lesser concentration to areas of greater concentration. Examples of active transport are the sodium and potassium pump (Fig. 45-4). Sodium is pumped out of the cell and potassium is pumped in, against the concentration gradient.

Active transport is enhanced by carrier molecules within a cell that bind themselves to incoming molecules. For example, glucose is able to enter cells after it binds with the transport vehicle insulin. Active transport is the mechanism by which cells absorb glucose and other substances to carry out metabolic activities.

Table 45-1	Differences in Tonicity of Solutions	
SOLUTION TYPES	**DEFINITION**	**EXAMPLES**
Isotonic	Solution with same osmolality as plasma	0.9% normal saline or lactated ringer's
Hypotonic	Solution with lesser solute concentration than plasma	0.45% saline 0.33% saline 2.5% dextrose
Hypertonic	Solution with greater solute concentration than plasma	5% dextrose in 0.45% saline 5% dextrose in normal saline 5% dextrose in lactated ringer's 3% saline

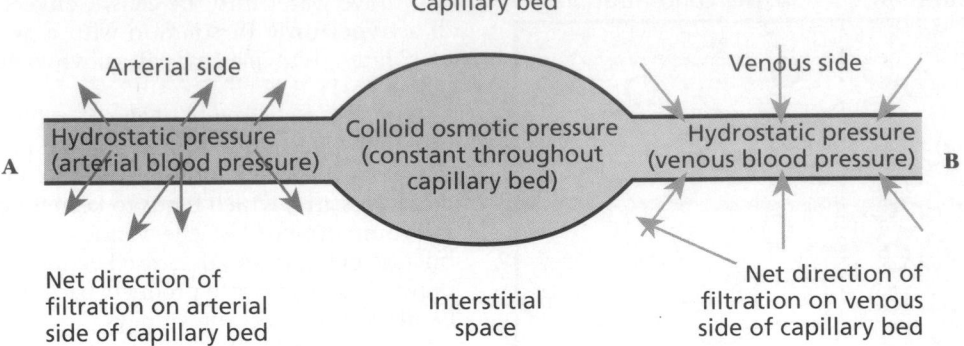

Fig. 45-3 An example of filtration pressure changes within a capillary bed. **A,** Arterial blood pressure exceeds colloid osmotic pressure, resulting in movement of water and dissolved substances out of the capillary into the interstitial space. **B,** Venous blood pressure is less than colloid osmotic pressure, resulting in the movement of water and dissolved substances into the capillary.

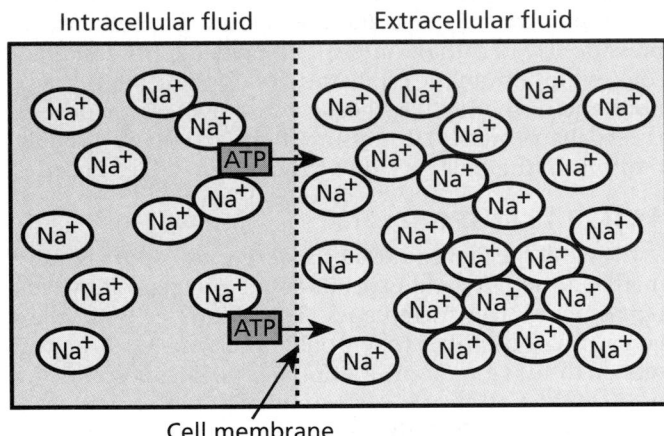

Fig. 45-4 An example of active transport. Energy (ATP) is used to move sodium molecules across a semipermeable membrane against sodium's concentration gradient (i.e., from an area of lesser concentration to an area of greater concentration).

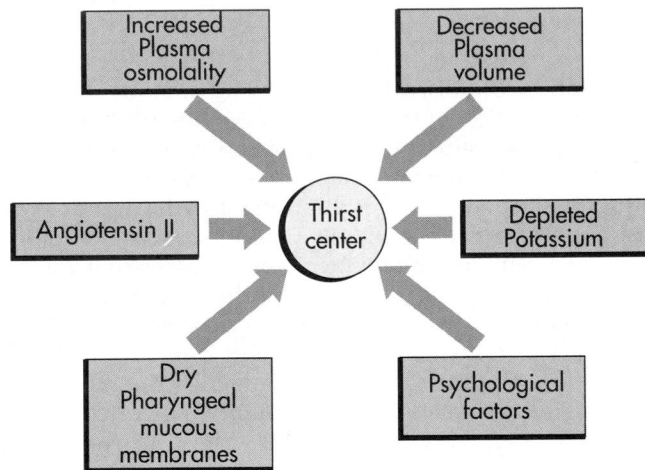

Fig. 45-5 Stimuli affecting the thirst mechanism.

Regulation of Body Fluids

FLUID INTAKE

Fluid intake is regulated primarily through the thirst mechanism. The thirst-control center is located within the hypothalamus in the brain. Major physiological stimuli to the thirst center are increased plasma concentration and decreased blood volume. Receptor cells called **osmoreceptors** continually monitor osmolality. When too much fluid is lost, the osmoreceptors detect the loss and activate the thirst center. As a result the person feels thirsty and seeks water. Other factors affecting the thirst center are dry oral pharyngeal mucous membranes, angiotensin II, potassium depletion, and psychological factors (Potter and Perry 1995) (Fig. 45-5).

Water is also acquired from food intake, such as fruits, vegetables, and meat, and from the oxidation of food substances during digestion. Also, about 220 ml of water is produced every day during the metabolism of carbohydrates,

proteins, and fats (Weldy, 1992). Oral fluid intake requires an alert state. Infants, clients with neurological or psychological impairments, some older adults, and clients who are restrained are unable to perceive or respond to their thirst mechanisms. As a result, they are at risk for dehydration.

FLUID OUTPUT

Fluid output occurs mainly through the kidneys and the gastrointestinal tract. Average daily fluid losses are summarized in Table 45-2.

In the adult, the kidneys receive about 125 ml of plasma to filter each minute and produce about 60 ml (40 to 80 ml) every hour or a total of about 1.5 L of urine a day (Horne et al, 1991). The amount of urine produced by the kidneys is influenced by antidiuretic hormone (ADH) and aldosterone. These hormones affect water and sodium excretion and are stimulated by changes in blood volume.

Water loss from the skin is regulated primarily by the sympathetic nervous system, which activates the sweat glands. Stimulation of the sweat glands can result from muscular exercise, elevated environmental temperature,

Table 45-2	Average Daily Fluid Output in a 70-kg (187-lb) Adult	
ORGAN OR SYSTEM	**AMOUNT (ML)**	
Kidneys	1500	
Skin		
Insensible loss	600-900	
Sensible loss	600	
Lungs	400	
Gastrointestinal tract	100	
Total	3200-3500	

and increased metabolic activity as in a febrile state. Water loss from the skin can be a sensible or insensible loss.

Insensible water loss is continuous and is not perceived by the person. The average insensible water loss from the skin in the adult is about 6 ml/kg/24 hours (Horne et al, 1991). **Sensible water loss** occurs through excessive perspiration and is perceived by the person. The amount of sensible perspiration is directly related to the amount of exercise, environmental temperature, and metabolic activity. As these factors increase, so does the amount of sweat produced and water lost through the skin. Sensible water loss can range up to 1000 ml or more per 24 hours, depending on exercise and external and body temperatures (Horne et al, 1991).

The lungs also expire an insensible water loss of approximately 400 ml of water daily (Horne et al, 1991). This loss may increase in response to changes in respiratory rate and depth as with increased exercise or fever. In addition, devices for oxygen administration can increase insensible water loss from the lungs. This is because the oxygen is drier than the room air.

The average fluid loss from the gastrointestinal tract is approximately 100 ml/day. Vomiting or diarrhea increases fluid loss by preventing the normal absorption of water and electrolytes that have been secreted by the digestive process.

HORMONES

The major hormones affecting fluid and electrolyte balance are ADH and aldosterone. ADH is released by the posterior pituitary gland in response to an increase in blood osmolality, which indicates a state of water deficit. It decreases the production of urine by increasing the reabsorption of water by the kidney tubules. During transient periods of fluid volume deficit such as with vomiting and diarrhea or hemorrhage, the amount of ADH in the blood increases. As a result, the water reabsorbed by the kidney tubules increases and is returned to the circulating blood volume. Thus urinary output declines in response to the hormone's action.

Aldosterone is a mineralocorticoid produced by the adrenal cortex. It regulates sodium and potassium balance by causing the kidney tubules to excrete potassium and reabsorb sodium. As a result, water is also reabsorbed and returned to the blood volume. Fluid volume deficits such as

those produced by hemorrhage or gastrointestinal losses can stimulate the secretion of aldosterone into the blood.

A third class of hormones, glucocorticoids, affects water and electrolyte balance. Normal glucocorticoid hormone secretion does not result in major fluid imbalance; however, excesses of the hormone in the circulation result in Cushing's syndrome, in which the body retains sodium and water. Thus a client receiving steroid medications, such as cortisone or prednisone, retains sodium and water.

Regulation of Electrolytes

CATIONS

The major cations—sodium ($Na+$), potassium ($K+$), calcium (Ca^{2+}), and magnesium (Mg^{2+})—are located in the extracellular and intracellular fluid. Their actions affect neurochemical and neuromuscular transmissions, which influence muscular function, cardiac rhythm and contractility, mood and behavior, and gastrointestinal functioning, as well as other processes. (see Table 45-4 on p. 1255).

Sodium Regulation. Sodium is the most abundant cation in the extracellular fluid. Sodium ions are involved in maintaining water balance, transmitting nerve impulses, and contracting muscles. The normal laboratory value for serum sodium is 135 to 145 mEq/L.

Water follows sodium in fluid and electrolyte balances. For example, if the kidneys retain sodium, water is retained. Conversely, if the kidneys excrete sodium, water is excreted. The reason for administering many drugs (e.g., diuretics) is based on this principle.

Sodium is regulated by salt intake, aldosterone, and urinary output. The major sources of sodium are table salt, processed meats, snacks, and canned foods. In individuals with normal renal function the excretion of urine sodium can be increased to keep the serum sodium level within normal limits.

Potassium Regulation. Potassium is the predominant intracellular cation, which regulates neuromuscular excitability and muscle contraction. Sources include whole grains, meat, legumes, fruits, and vegetables. Potassium is needed for glycogen formation, protein synthesis, and correction of acid-base imbalances. The normal laboratory value for serum potassium is 3.5 to 5.3 mEq/L.

Potassium assists in regulating the acid-base balance because the potassium ion can be exchanged with the hydrogen ion (H^+). Potassium is regulated primarily by the kidneys. Any condition that decreases urine output decreases potassium excretion. With increased aldosterone secretion, more potassium is excreted through the urine and the serum potassium level can fall. Another mechanism of regulation is the exchange with the sodium ion in the kidney tubule. When sodium is retained, potassium is excreted.

Calcium Regulation. There is abundant calcium in the body (Long et al, 1993). The body requires calcium for cell membrane integrity and structure, adequate cardiac conduction, blood coagulation, bone growth and formation, and muscle relaxation. Calcium is in the following forms in body fluids:

1. Ionized (4.5 mg/100 ml)
2. Nondiffusible, which is calcium complexed to protein anions (5 mg/100 ml)
3. Calcium salts such as calcium citrate and calcium phosphate (1 mg/100 ml)

The normal ionized serum calcium laboratory value is 4 to 5 mEq/L. Calcium in body fluid is a small percentage of the total body calcium. The major portion of calcium is in bones and teeth.

Calcium in extracellular fluid is regulated through the actions of the parathyroid and thyroid glands. Parathyroid hormone (PTH) controls the balance among bone calcium, gastrointestinal absorption of calcium, and kidney excretion of calcium. Thyrocalcitonin from the thyroid gland also has a minor role in determining serum calcium levels by inhibiting release of calcium from bones.

Magnesium Regulation. Magnesium is the second most important cation of the intracellular fluids and is essential for enzyme activities, neurochemical activities, and muscular excitability. The normal laboratory value for serum magnesium is 1.5 to 2.5 mEq/L.

Magnesium is primarily excreted through renal mechanisms. Altered magnesium levels are often associated with serious disease and produce symptoms reflecting altered neuromuscular and cardiovascular function (Long et al, 1993).

ANIONS

The major anions are chloride (Cl^-), bicarbonate (HCO_3^-), and phosphate (PO^{3-}). Like cations, they are found in the extracellular and intracellular spaces. Anions affect fluid, electrolyte, and acid-base balances and functions.

Chloride Regulation. Chloride is found in extracellular and intracellular fluid. Chloride balance is maintained through dietary intake and renal excretion and reabsorption. The normal laboratory value for serum chloride is 100 to 106 mEq/L.

Chloride is regulated through the kidneys. The amount excreted is related to dietary intake. A person with normal kidneys who has a high chloride intake will excrete a higher amount of chloride in the urine.

Bicarbonate Regulation. Bicarbonate is the major chemical base buffer within the body. The bicarbonate ion is found in extracellular and intracellular fluid. Normal laboratory arterial bicarbonate levels range between 22 and 26 mEq/L. In venous blood, bicarbonate is measured as carbon dioxide content, and the normal value for adults is 24 to 30 mEq/L.

The kidneys regulate bicarbonate. When the body needs to retain more base, the kidneys reabsorb greater quantities of bicarbonate and return it to the extracellular fluid. The bicarbonate ion is an essential component of the carbonic acid–bicarbonate buffering system essential to acid-base balance.

Phosphate Regulation. Phosphate is a buffer anion in intracellular and extracellular fluid. Phosphate and calcium help develop and maintain bones and teeth. Phosphate also promotes normal neuromuscular action, participates in carbohydrate metabolism, and assists in acid-base regulation. The normal laboratory value for serum phosphate is 2.5 to 4.5 mg/100 ml.

Serum phosphate concentration is regulated by the kidneys, parathyroid hormone, and activated vitamin D (Long et al, 1993). Phosphate is normally absorbed through the gastrointestinal tract. Calcium and phosphate are inversely proportional. If one rises, the other falls.

■ ACID-BASE BALANCE

Acid-base balance exists when the net rate at which the body produces acids or bases equals the rate at which acids or bases are excreted. This balance results in a stable concentration of hydrogen ions in body fluids. The concentration of hydrogen ions in a body fluid is expressed as the pH value. The **pH** is a scale for measuring the acidity or alkalinity of a fluid. A pH value of 7 is neutral. Below 7 is acid, and above 7 is alkaline. An increase in the number of hydrogen ions in the bloodstream increases the acid component, thereby lowering the pH. Normal arterial pH laboratory values range from 7.35 to 7.45.

The human body has regulatory mechanisms for maintaining the acid-base balance and for adapting to short-term changes in hydrogen ion concentration. Such changes occur during physical exercise, moderate anxiety states, and minor gastrointestinal upsets. The body can make adjustments (compensate) for transient changes in pH. However, with severe trauma, uncontrolled diabetes mellitus, or shock, the body's normal compensatory mechanisms are unable to maintain the pH within a physiological range. The types of acid-base regulators within the body are chemical, biological, and physiological buffering systems. A **buffer** is a substance or group of substances that can absorb or release hydrogen ions to correct an acid-base imbalance.

Chemical Regulation

The largest chemical buffer in extracellular fluid is the carbonic acid–bicarbonate buffer system. This system responds within seconds to changes in pH, making it the fastest buffering system. It is an adaptive system, and has a relatively brief effect. This system can be expressed as the following equation:

$$\underset{\substack{\text{carbon} \\ \text{dioxide}}}{CO_2} + \underset{\text{water}}{H_2O} \rightleftarrows \underset{\substack{\text{carbonic} \\ \text{acid}}}{H_2CO_3} \rightleftarrows \underset{\text{hydrogen}}{H^+} + \underset{\text{bicarbonate}}{HCO_3^-}$$

The excretion of carbon dioxide resulting from metabolism is controlled primarily by the lungs. The excretion of hydrogen and bicarbonate ions is controlled by the kidneys. The reaction of these substances buffers a strong acid or base to maintain a relatively constant pH (Fig. 45-6).

A second chemical buffering system involves the plasma proteins (albumin, fibrinogen, and prothrombin) and the gamma globulins, which constitute about 6% to 7% of blood plasma. These proteins can bind with or release hydrogen

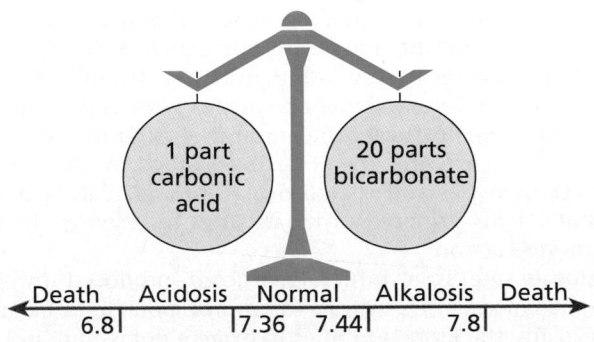

Fig. 45-6 Carbonic acid-bicarbonate ratio and pH.

ions to correct acidosis or alkalosis. However, their capacity to maintain the acid-base balance of extracellular fluid is limited, and they cannot correct long-term imbalances.

Biological Regulation

Biological buffering occurs when hydrogen ions are absorbed or released by body cells. The hydrogen ion has a positive charge and must be exchanged with another positively charged ion, frequently potassium. In conditions with excessive acid, a hydrogen ion enters the cell, and a potassium ion leaves the cell and enters the extracellular fluid. The extracellular fluid is thus less acidic because fewer hydrogen ions are present. As a result of this exchange, however, the serum is high in potassium. After the acidosis is corrected, potassium reenters the cells, and potassium levels return to normal. This biological buffering occurs after short-term chemical buffering and takes 2 to 4 hours.

A second type of biological buffer is the hemoglobin-oxyhemoglobin system. Carbon dioxide diffuses into the RBC and forms carbonic acid. The carbonic acid dissociates into hydrogen and bicarbonate ions. The hydrogen ions attach to the hemoglobin, and the bicarbonate ion becomes available for buffering by exchanging with extracellular chloride (Kokko and Tannen, 1990).

Physiological Regulation

LUNGS

The physiological buffers in the body are the lungs and the kidneys. The lungs can provide a rapid adaptation to an acid-base imbalance. In fact, they can act to return the pH to normal before the biological buffers can.

Ordinarily hydrogen ions and carbon dioxide provide the stimulus for respiration. When the concentration of hydrogen ions is altered, the lungs react to correct the imbalance by altering the rate and depth of respiration. In alkalosis, the rate of respiration is reduced, and the person retains carbon dioxide. The carbon dioxide combines with water in the blood to form carbonic acid, which helps increase the acid component and balance the alkaline excess. If an excess in acid occurs, respiratory rate is increased and the lungs excrete larger amounts of carbon dioxide (Weldy, 1992). Therefore less carbon dioxide is available to combine with water and create carbonic acid.

KIDNEYS

The kidneys can take from a few hours to several days to regulate acid-base abnormalities. They use three mechanisms to regulate hydrogen ion concentration. They can reabsorb bicarbonate during acid excess and excrete it during acid deficit. The kidneys use a phosphate ion (PO_4^{3-}) to carry hydrogen ions by excreting phosphoric acid (H_3PO_4) and forming an acid base. The kidneys also convert ammonia (NH_3) to ammonium (NH_4^+) by attaching a hydrogen ion.

∎ DISTURBANCES IN FLUID, ELECTROLYTE, AND ACID-BASE BALANCES

Disturbances in fluid, electrolyte, and acid-base balances seldom occur alone and can disrupt normal body processes. A client who loses body fluids through burns, illness, or trauma is at risk for electrolyte imbalances. In addition, un-

treated electrolyte imbalances (e.g., potassium loss) result in acid-base disturbances.

Fluid Disturbances

The basic types of fluid imbalances are isotonic and osmolar. Isotonic deficit and excess exist when water and electrolytes are gained or lost in equal proportions. In contrast, osmolar imbalances are losses or excesses of only water so that the concentration (osmolality) of the serum is affected. Another type of imbalance, third-space syndrome, occurs when fluid is trapped in a space from which it is not easily exchanged with the extracellular fluid. Table 45-3 lists the causes and symptoms of common disturbances.

ISOTONIC IMBALANCES

Fluid volume deficit (FVD) results when water and electrolytes are lost in isotonic proportions. Unless other imbalances are present, serum electrolyte levels remain unchanged. Clients at risk include those with gastrointestinal losses of fluid and electrolytes such as from vomiting, gastric suction, diarrhea, or fistulas. The very young and old are quickly affected by these losses (Weldy, 1992) (see the box below). Other causes can include hemorrhage, diuretic administration, profuse sweating, fever, and decreased oral intake.

Fluid volume excess (FVE) results when water and sodium are retained in isotonic proportions, resulting in hypervolemia with unchanged levels of serum electrolytes. Clients at risk include those with congestive heart failure, renal failure, and cirrhosis (Weldy, 1992).

THIRD-SPACE SYNDROME

The client with a severe **third-space syndrome** experiences the effects of an extracellular FVD. This syndrome occurs when there is a shift of extracellular fluid into a body

---

 CLIENT TEACHING on Preventing Dehydration in Infant Diarrhea

OBJECTIVE
Client will be normovolemic despite watery diarrhea after out-patient treatment, avoiding hospitalization.

TEACHING STRATEGIES
∎ Educate parents/family about dangers of diarrhea, especially in children.
∎ Teach parents/family how water or sugar water may actually increase dehydration.
∎ Encourage family to keep a small supply of a rice and water oral rehydration treatment such as Ricelyte (Mead Johnson Nutritionals, Evanston, Ind) in the home. It can be purchased in grocery or drug stores.
∎ Teach family to contact a physician as they continue to administer the treatment.

EVALUATION
∎ Ask family about signs and symptoms of dehydration in children.
∎ Have family describe first-line treatment.

From Cusson R: Rice based oral rehydration fluid in the treatment of infant diarrhea, *J Pediatric Nursing* 7:(6) 414, 1992.

Table 45-3	Fluid Disturbances

CAUSES	SIGNS AND SYMPTOMS

ISOTONIC IMBALANCES

Fluid volume deficit (FVD)

Losses from the gastrointestinal system such as from diarrhea, vomiting, or drainage from fistulas or tubes

Loss of plasma or whole blood, such as with burns or hemorrhage

Excessive perspiration

Fever

Decreased oral intake of fluids

Use of diuretics

Physical exam: weak rapid pulse, collapsed veins, hypotension, rapid respiratory rate, lethargy, oliguria, dry skin and mucous membranes, inelastic skin turgor, rapid weight loss

Laboratory findings: urine specific gravity >1.025, false increased hematocrit >50%, false increased blood urea nitrogen (BUN) >25 mg/100 ml

Fluid volume excess (FVE)

Congestive heart failure

Renal failure

Cirrhosis

Increased serum aldosterone and steroid levels

Excessive sodium intake

Physical exam: bounding pulse, rapid respirations, hypertension, neck vein distention, increased venous pressure, crackles in lungs, rapid weight gain

Laboratory findings: false decreased BUN < 10 mg/100 ml

THIRD-SPACE SYNDROME

Portal hypertension

Small bowel obstruction

Peritonitis

Burns

Physical exam: hypotension, increased abdominal girth (with small bowel obstruction, ascites)

Laboratory findings: decreased serum sodium < 135 mEq/L and decreased albumin < 3.5 g/100 ml (lost in trapped fluids)

OSMOLAR IMBALANCES

Hyperosmolar imbalance

Diabetes insipidus

Interruption of neurologically driven thirst drive

Diabetic ketoacidosis

Administration of hypertonic fluids

Osmotic diuresis

Physical exam: weight loss, dry sticky mucous membranes, thirst, elevated body temperature, irritability, convulsions, coma

Laboratory findings: increased serum sodium >145 mEq/L and increased serum osmolality > 295 mOsm/kg

Hypoosmolar imbalance

SIADH

Excessive water intake

Physical exam: decreased level of consciousness, convulsions, coma

Laboratory findings: decreased serum sodium < 136 mEq/L and decreased serum osmolality < 280 mOsm/kg

---

space, where it becomes trapped. The net result is a deficit in extracellular fluid volume. A small bowel obstruction or burn can result in the shift of up to 5 to 10 L out of the extracellular fluid spaces. The volume of third-space losses cannot be measured precisely (Long et al, 1993).

OSMOLAR IMBALANCES

Hyperosmolar imbalance **(dehydration)** occurs when there is a loss of water without a proportionate loss of electrolytes, especially sodium, or when there is a gain in osmotically active substances. This results in an increased serum sodium level and osmolality (concentration) and intracellular dehydration.

Risk factors for dehydration include conditions that impair sufficient oral intake (e.g., alterations in neurological function). Frail, infirm older clients are at great risk for developing dehydration because there is a marked decrease in intracellular fluid, decrease in renal concentrating ability, decrease in responsiveness to thirst, and increase in proportion of body fat, which limits the older client's reserve in situations of water deficit (Horne et al, 1991).

A decrease in ADH secretion (diabetes insipidus) can lead to profound water losses. A hyperosmolar imbalance can be caused by any condition associated with an osmotic diuresis and administration of hypertonic tube-feeding formulas or IV solutions that increase the number of solutes and the concentration of the blood (see Table 45-3). In these conditions, water moves out of the intracellular fluid to maintain extracellular fluid volume. Eventually cellular function is impaired, and circulatory collapse occurs (Long et al, 1993).

Hypoosmolar imbalance (water excess) occurs when there is an excess intake of water (psychogenic polydipsia) or excess ADH secretion. The overall effect is dilution of the extracellular fluid volume with osmosis of water into the cells (Long et al, 1993). Brain cells are particularly sensitive, and this process can lead to cerebral edema, which can cause decreased level of consciousness, coma, and even death.

Electrolyte Imbalances

SODIUM IMBALANCES

Sodium excess and deficit share many characteristics with osmolar fluid disturbances. Hyponatremia is a less-

| Table 45-4 | Electrolyte Imbalances |

CAUSES	SIGNS AND SYMPTOMS
HYPONATREMIA Kidney disease Adrenal insufficiency Gastrointestinal losses Increased sweating Use of diuretics (especially along with low sodium diet) Interruption of sodium-potassium pump with decreased cell potassium and decreased serum sodium Metabolic acidosis	Physical exam: weak rapid pulse, hypotension, dizziness, apprehension and anxiety, abdominal cramps, nausea and vomiting, diarrhea, coma and convulsions, fingerprints remaining on sternum after palpation, cold clammy skin, personality change Laboratory findings: serum sodium < 135 mEq/L, serum osmolality < 280 mOsm/kg, and urine specific gravity < 1.010
HYPERNATREMIA Ingestion of large amounts of concentrated salt solution Iatrogenic administration of hypertonic saline solution IV Excess aldosterone secretion	Physical exam: low-grade fever, postural hypotension, dry tongue and mucous membranes, agitation, convulsions, restlessness, excitability, oliguria or anuria, thirst, dry and flushed skin Laboratory findings: serum sodium > 145 mEq/L, serum osmolality > 295 mOsm/kg, and urine specific gravity > 1.030 (if water loss not caused by renal dysfunction)
HYPOKALEMIA Use of potassium-wasting diuretics Diarrhea, vomiting, or other gastrointestinal losses Alkalosis Cushing's syndrome or adrenal hormone–producing tumors Polyuria Extreme sweating Excessive use of potassium-free IVs	Physical exam: weak irregular pulse, shallow respirations, hypotension, weakness, decreased bowel sounds, heart block (severe hypokalemia), paresthesia, fatigue, decreased muscle tone, intestinal distention Laboratory findings: serum potassium < 3 mEq/L results in ST depression, flat T wave, taller U wave; levels < 2 mEq/L result in widened QRS, depressed ST, inverted T wave (Raimer, 1994)
HYPERKALEMIA Renal failure Hypertonic dehydration Massive cellular damage such as from burns and trauma Iatrogenic administration of large amounts of potassium IV Adrenal insufficiency Acidosis Rapid infusion of stored blood Use of potassium-retaining diuretics	Physical exam: irregular slow pulse, hypotension, anxiety, irritability, paresthesia, weakness Laboratory findings: serum potassium > 5.3 mEq/L result in faster repolarization (peaked T wave, heart rate 60-110), levels > 7 mEq/L result in impaired interatrial conduction (low, broad P-wave), and levels > 8 mEq/L result in no atrial activity (no P-wave) (Raimer, 1994)
HYPOCALCEMIA Rapid administration of blood containing citrate Hypoalbuminemia Hypoparathyroidism Vitamin D deficiency Neoplastic diseases Pancreatitis	Physical exam: numbness and tingling of fingers and circumoral region, hyperactive reflexes, positive Trousseau's sign (carpopedal spasm with hypoxia), positive Chvostek's sign (contraction of facial muscles when facial nerve tapped), tetany, muscle cramps, pathological fractures with chronic hypocalcemia Laboratory findings: serum calcium < 4.3 mEq/L and ECG changes
HYPERCALCEMIA Hyperparathyroidism Metastatic bone tumors Paget's disease Osteoporosis Prolonged immobilization	Physical exam: decreased muscle tone, anorexia, nausea and vomiting, weakness, lethargy, low back pain from kidney stones, decreased level of consciousness, cardiac arrest Laboratory findings: serum calcium > 5 mEq/L, x-ray showing generalized osteoporosis, widespread bone cavitation, and radiopaque urinary stones, elevated BUN > 25 mg/100 ml, elevated creatinine > 1.5 mg/100 ml caused by FVD or renal damage due to urolithiasis
HYPOMAGNESEMIA Inadequate intake: malnutrition and alcoholism Inadequate absorption: diarrhea, vomiting, nasogastric drainage, fistulas, excessive dietary calcium (competes with magnesium for transport sites) small intestine diseases Hypoparathyroidism Excessive loss resulting from thiazide diuretics Aldosterone excess Polyuria	Physical exam: muscular tremors, hyperactive deep tendon reflexes, confusion, disorientation, tachycardia, positive Chvostek's and Trousseau's signs Laboratory findings: serum magnesium > 1.5 mEq/L (also associated with hypocalcemia and hypokalemia)
HYPERMAGNESEMIA Renal failure Excessive parenteral administration of magnesium	Physical exam: in acute hypermagnesemia: hypoactive deep tendon reflexes, shallow and slow respirations and heart rate, hypotension, flushing Laboratory findings: serum magnesium > 2.5 mEq/L

than-normal concentration of sodium in the blood, which can take place when a net sodium loss or net water excess occurs (Table 45-4). Usually hyponatremia results in a decrease in the osmolality of plasma and extracellular fluid (Long et al, 1993).

When a sodium loss occurs, the body initially adapts by reducing water excretion to maintain serum osmolality at near-normal levels. As sodium loss continues, the body attempts to preserve the blood volume. As a result, the proportion of sodium in the extracellular fluid lessens. However, hyponatremia caused by sodium loss can result in vascular collapse and shock. When a pure sodium deficit occurs, there is a distinct loss of extracellular fluid volume, a condition different from hyponatremia associated with normal or increased extracellular fluid volume. Severe hyponatremia can result in neurological changes at a serum sodium level of 120 mEq/L and in irreversible neurological alterations or death at 110 mEq/L. Any trend of decreasing serum sodium levels should be promptly reported to the client's physician.

Hypernatremia is a greater-than-normal concentration of sodium in the extracellular fluid, which can be caused by extreme water loss or overall sodium excess (see Table 45-4). If the cause of hypernatremia is increased aldosterone secretion, sodium is retained and potassium is excreted. When hypernatremia occurs, the body attempts to conserve as much water as possible through renal reabsorption. Interstitial osmotic pressure increases, and fluid shifts from the cells into the extracellular fluid, causing the cells to shrink and interrupting most of the physiological cellular processes.

POTASSIUM IMBALANCES

Hypokalemia is a condition in which an inadequate amount of potassium circulates in the extracellular fluid. When severe, hypokalemia can affect cardiac conduction by causing dangerous irregularities. Because the normal range of potassium is so narrow, there is little tolerance for fluctuations in serum potassium levels.

Hypokalemia can result from several conditions (see Table 45-4). The most common cause is the use of potassium-wasting diuretics such as thiazide and loop diuretics. This is a particular problem when clients are also receiving digitalis preparations because hypokalemia is the most common cause of digitalis toxicity. Hyperkalemia is a greater-than-normal amount of potassium in the blood. The primary cause of hyperkalemia is renal failure, but other illnesses also result in increased potassium (see Table 45-4). Any decrease in renal function diminishes the amount of potassium the kidney can excrete (Weldy, 1992).

CALCIUM IMBALANCES

Hypocalcemia represents a drop in serum and ionized calcium levels and can result from several illnesses, some of which directly affect the thyroid and parathyroid glands (see Table 45-4). The signs and symptoms of hypocalcemia correlate directly to the physiological role of serum calcium in neuromuscular function.

Hypercalcemia is an increase in the total serum concentration of calcium and ionized calcium. Frequently, hypercalcemia is a symptom of an underlying disease resulting in excess bone resorption with release of calcium (see Table 45-4).

MAGNESIUM IMBALANCES

Hypomagnesemia occurs when the serum concentration level drops below 1.5 mEq/L. The causes of hypomagnesemia (Table 45-4) produce symptoms similar to hypocalcemia. Magnesium acts directly on the neuromuscular junction. Decreases in the serum magnesium concentration increase neuromuscular irritability (Weldy, 1992). Hypermagnesemia occurs when the serum concentration of magnesium rises above 2.5 mEq/L (Table 45-4). Hypermagnesemia diminishes the excitability of muscle cells.

CHLORIDE IMBALANCES

Hypochloremia occurs when the serum chloride level falls below 100 mEq/L. Vomiting or prolonged and excessive nasogastric or fistula drainage can result in hypochloremia. A newborn can quickly develop hypochloremia as a result of diarrhea. Some diuretic medications also result in increased chloride excretion. When serum chloride levels fall, the body adapts by increased reabsorption of the bicarbonate ion, affecting acid-base balance.

Hyperchloremia occurs when the serum chloride level rises above 106 mEq/L, resulting in a decreased serum bicarbonate value. Hypochloremia and hyperchloremia rarely occur as single disease processes but are commonly associated with acid-base imbalance. No single set of symptoms is associated with these alterations.

Acid-Base Imbalances

The primary types of acid-base imbalance are respiratory acidosis, respiratory alkalosis, metabolic acidosis, and metabolic alkalosis (Table 45-5).

RESPIRATORY ACIDOSIS

Respiratory acidosis is marked by an increased arterial carbon dioxide concentration ($Paco_2$), excess carbonic acid, and an increased hydrogen ion concentration (decreased pH). Respiratory acidosis is caused by hypoventilation or any condition that depresses ventilation (see Table 45-5). Decreased ventilation may begin in the respiratory system (respiratory failure) or outside the respiratory system (drug overdose). In clients with respiratory acidosis the cerebrospinal fluid and brain cells become acidic, causing neurological changes. Hypoxemia (decreased oxygen levels) occurs because of respiratory depression, resulting in further neurological impairments (see Chapter 44). Electrolyte changes such as hyperkalemia may accompany acidosis.

RESPIRATORY ALKALOSIS

Respiratory alkalosis is marked by decreased $Paco_2$ and decreased hydrogen ion concentration (increased pH). Respiratory alkalosis results from excessive exhalation of carbon dioxide, or hyperventilation (see Table 45-5). Like respiratory acidosis, respiratory alkalosis can begin outside the respiratory system (anxiety) or within the respiratory system, such as in the initial phases of an asthmatic attack.

METABOLIC ACIDOSIS

Metabolic acidosis results from a rise in hydrogen ion concentration (decreased pH) in the extracellular fluid, caused by an increase in hydrogen ion levels or a decrease in bicarbonate levels (Weldy, 1992). Metabolic acidosis is caused

Table 45-5	Acid-Base Imbalances	
CAUSES	**SIGNS AND SYMPTOMS**	

RESPIRATORY ACIDOSIS
Pneumonia
Respiratory failure
Atelectasis
Drug overdose
Paralysis of respiratory muscles
Traumatic injury
Obesity
Airway obstruction
Head injuries
Stroke
Drowning
Cystic fibrosis

Physical exam: rapid bounding pulse, rapid shallow respirations, hypertension, warm and flushed skin, abdominal cramps, lethargy, convulsions, confusion, dizziness, headache

Laboratory findings: arterial blood gas changes: pH < 7.35, $PaCO_2$ > 45 mm Hg, $PaCO_2$ < 80 mm Hg, SaO_2 normal or < 95%, bicarbonate level normal (if uncompensated) or > 26 mEq/L (if compensated by the kidneys) and potassium > 5.3 mEq/L

RESPIRATORY ALKALOSIS
Anxiety
Fear
Anemia
Hypermetabolic states
Central nervous system injuries, infections
Asthma
Inappropriate mechanical ventilator settings

Physical exam: headache, irritability, dizziness, tachycardia, tachypnea, and tingling of extremities

Laboratory findings: arterial blood gas changes: pH > 7.45, $PaCO_2$ < 35mm Hg, PaO_2 and SaO_2 normal, bicarbonate level normal (if acute or pneumonia uncompensated) or < 22 mEq/L (if compensated), potassium level < 3.5 mEq/L

METABOLIC ACIDOSIS
Starvation
Diabetic ketoacidosis
Renal failure
Shock
Diarrhea
Drug use (methanol, ethanol, formic acid, paraldehyde, aspirin)
Renal tubular acidosis

Physical exam: headache, lethargy, confusion, flushed skin, tachycardia, tachypnea with deep respirations, abdominal cramps

Laboratory findings: arterial blood gas changes: pH < 7.35, $PaCO_2$ normal (if uncompensated) or < 35 mm Hg (if compensated), PaO_2 normal or increased (with rapid deep respirations), SaO_2 normal, bicarbonate < 22 mEq/L, potassium > 5.3 mEq/L

METABOLIC ALKALOSIS
Excessive vomiting
Prolonged gastric suctioning
Hypokalemia
Hypercalcemia
Cushing's syndrome
Drug use (steroids, diuretics, sodium bicarbonate)

Physical exam: headache, lethargy, irritability, tachycardia, slowed respirations, numbness, tingling, tetany, abdominal and muscle cramps

Laboratory findings: arterial blood gas changes: pH > 7.45, $PaCO_2$ normal (if uncompensated) or > 45 mm Hg (if compensated), PaO_2 and SaO_2 normal, bicarbonate > 26 mEq/L, potassium > 3.5 mEq/L

by many conditions (see Table 45-5). The types of metabolic acidosis, normochloremic and hyperchloremic, are classified according to the client's plasma chloride concentration.

METABOLIC ALKALOSIS

Metabolic alkalosis is marked by heavy loss of acid from the body or by increased levels of bicarbonate. The most common cause is vomiting. Metabolic alkalosis may also result when a client with a gastric acid disturbance ingests large amounts of sodium bicarbonate. Other causes are listed in Table 45-5.

VARIABLES AFFECTING NORMAL FLUID, ELECTROLYTE, AND ACID-BASE BALANCES

Fluid, electrolyte, and acid-base status is neither a static nor single physiological entity. Many variables can change the distribution of body fluid and electrolytes. In some instances (e.g., with normal changes during pregnancy and exercise), fluid and electrolyte alterations are normal and expected responses. In other situations, however, fluid, electrolyte, and acid-base imbalances can have severe consequences.

During assessment the nurse identifies altered fluid, electrolyte, and acid-base states. To assess clients effectively, the nurse considers variables influencing fluid, electrolyte, and acid-base status, the way normal balance changes, and whether the change is a normal anticipated change or a consequence of a pathological process. The major factors that can affect normal fluid, electrolyte, and acid-base status include age, body size, environmental temperature, and lifestyle.

Age

Age affects distribution of body fluids and electrolytes. The major differences are observed in infants and older adults. Fluid and electrolyte changes occur normally with developmental changes. However, when an illness is also present, the client may be unable to adapt adequately to these changes. Therefore when assessing clients the nurse needs to account for fluid changes associated with aging and development.

INFANTS

Infants' proportions of total body water are greater than those of school-age children, adolescents, or adults. However, although infants have greater proportions of body water, they are not protected from fluid loss (e.g., from diarrhea) because they ingest and excrete a relatively greater daily water volume than adults (Weldy, 1992). In fact, infants are at greater risk for FVD or hyperosmolar imbalances because their body water losses are proportionately greater per kilogram of body weight.

CHILDREN

In childhood illnesses, the regulatory and compensatory responses to imbalances are less stable and tend to operate within a more narrow range with less tolerance for large changes in balance. Children frequently respond to illness with fevers of higher temperature or longer duration than those of adults. At any age, fever in childhood can increase the rate of insensible water loss.

ADOLESCENTS

In adolescence, major rapid changes occur in anatomical and physiological processes. The increased growth rate increases metabolic processes and, as a result, the amount of water produced as an end product of metabolism. Changes in fluid balance are greater in adolescent girls because of hormonal changes associated with the menstrual cycle.

OLDER ADULTS

The older client's risk of fluid and electrolyte imbalance may be closely associated with decreased renal function and an inability to concentrate urine. The older client may also have chronic illness, such as diabetes mellitus, cardiovascular disorders, or cancer, which can impair fluid balance. In addition, the total amount of body water decreases with age (Horne et al, 1991). Other risk factors that particularly affect the older adult are use of diuretics, often given for hypertension and congestive heart failure; overuse of laxatives and enemas; and colon-cleansing procedures used in preparation for diagnostic tests. Common imbalances associated with aging include hyperosmolar fluid disturbance and hypernatremia (see Tables 45-3 and 45-4). The nurse investi-

gates these imbalances and other treatable causes when older adults suddenly develop changes in mental status.

Obtaining assessment data related to fluid and electrolyte disturbance requires modification when caring for a senior client. For example, skin turgor is best tested over the forehead or sternum because skin elasticity remains most normal in these areas. The normally low baseline temperature must be identified to detect elevations associated with hyperosmolar imbalances or hypernatremia. This client may not become thirsty because of a diminished thirst mechanism (Horne et al, 1991). Last, there is decreased salivation, so mucous membrane moistness is assessed by inspecting the area under the tongue for a pool of saliva. Other elements of fluid balance assessment include using intake and output measurements and daily weight measurements so that trends can be detected despite the normal decreased renal function.

Body Size

Body size and composition have an effect on total body water. Because fat contains no water, the obese client has proportionately less body water. Women have more fat deposits in the breasts and hips than men. As a result, the total body water in women is less than in men of the same age.

Environmental Temperature

The body responds with fluid changes to excessive environmental temperature. It increases peripheral vasodilation, which allows more blood to come to the surface for cooling. Sweating increases body fluid loss, which results in loss of sodium and chloride ions. The body also increases cardiac output and pulse rate. Finally, increased aldosterone secretion occurs, resulting in sodium retention and potassium excretion by the kidneys (Weldy, 1992). Each of these responses can affect overall fluid and electrolyte balance, and the nurse needs to assess the environment to determine actual or potential alterations in fluid and electrolyte balance.

If the surrounding temperature rises above 90° F (32.2° C) or if the body temperature is above 101° F (38.3° C), significant sweating occurs. This cools the peripheral blood to reduce body temperature (Metheny, 1996).

Since sweating varies in volume from 0 to 1000 ml/hour or even more, dehydration can occur without adequate fluid replacement. However, normally the thirst mechanism stimulates such replacement (Metheny, 1996).

Lifestyle

Lifestyle can have an indirect effect on fluid, electrolyte, and acid-base balance. Habits that can affect fluid balance include diet, stress, and exercise.

DIET

Dietary intake of fluids, salt, potassium, calcium, magnesium, and necessary carbohydrates, fats, and proteins helps maintain normal fluid, electrolyte, and acid-base status. When nutritional intake is inadequate, the body tries to preserve its protein stores by breaking down glycogen and fat stores. When excess free fatty acids are released, metabolic acidosis can occur because the liver converts free fatty acids to ketone, a strong acid. However, after those resources are depleted, the body begins to destroy protein stores. When serum protein levels drop below normal, hypoalbuminemia results. In hypoalbuminemia the serum colloid osmotic pressure is decreased, and fluid shifts from the circulating blood volume and enters the interstitial fluid space in the peritoneal cavity.

STRESS

The impact of stress on fluid and electrolyte balance can be understood in terms of the general adaptation syndrome (see Chapter 22). Stress increases aldosterone and glucocorticoid levels, leading to sodium and water retention. In addition, increased ADH secretion decreases urine output. The effect of the stress response is to increase fluid volume. As a result, cardiac output, blood pressure, and perfusion to the major organs are increased.

EXERCISE

Exercise results in increased sensible water loss through sweat. The client who exercises can respond to the thirst mechanism and help maintain fluid and electrolyte balance by increasing fluid intake. Athletes undergoing sustained vigorous exercise must replace fluid loss with a liquid that contains electrolytes. One such substance is Gatorade, which contains glucose, sodium, chloride, and potassium (see Table 45-7, p. 1268).

▶ RESEARCH HIGHLIGHT

RESEARCH ABSTRACT
The diarrhea associated with chemotherapy in the treatment of metastatic colorectal carcinoma can be fatal. Some clients do not respond to the often successful treatment of this diarrhea with Lomotil. This study tested the effect of escalating continuous high dose infusion of octreotide acetate along with bowel rest (nothing by mouth) and intravenous fluid hydration. Eight men and eight women (N=16), aged 41 to 75 years, who were unresponsive to Lomotil treatment were studied. All had received chemotherapy for colorectal cancer. Complete resolution of the diarrhea occurred in 15 of the 16 clients (94%). No toxic reactions occurred. The one remaining client responded to the test regimen with three loose stools instead of fourteen in 24 hrs. Then Lomotil resolved the situation. A study is needed to compare subcutaneous administration of octreotide acetate with the intravenous route.

IMPLICATIONS FOR PRACTICE
▶ Uncontrolled chemotherapy-related diarrhea can be fatal, especially in the older client who carries a smaller percentage of total body fluid than the adult.
▶ Treatment is available for clients with this problem.
▶ Nurses should assess intake and output and electrolyte balance of clients with diarrhea to identify fluid, electrolyte, and acid-base imbalances.

REFERENCE
From Petrelli NJ et al: Bowel rest, intravenous hydration, and continuous high-dose infusion of octreotide acetate for the treatment of chemotherapy-induced diarrhea in patients with colorectal carcinoma, *Cancer* 72:1543, 1993.

■ NURSING PROCESS AND FLUID, ELECTROLYTE, AND ACID-BASE IMBALANCES

 Assessment

The nurse conducts an assessment to identify clients who are at risk or who show signs and symptoms of actual fluid, electrolyte, and acid-base imbalances. Certain conditions such as burns require frequent, indepth assessment. Other cases, such as recovering postoperative clients and clients recovering from gastroenteritis, require routine monitoring.

The nurse also assesses fluid, electrolyte, and acid-base imbalances, which may be associated with treatments of other diseases. For example, if a client is taking some of the anti-cancer chemotherapeutic medications, a fatal fluid volume deficit can result from the diarrhea, an adverse reaction of the treatment (see the box below, left). The implications for nursing assessment are critical.

Fluid, electrolyte, and acid-base assessment helps the nurse anticipate the need for nursing care. For example, a client with edema who is placed on diuretic therapy should have a care plan to anticipate elimination or dietary needs, such as increased use of the bathroom, bedpan, or urinal or instruction about a salt-restricted diet.

One of the most important nursing assessment functions is to identify risk factors for fluid, electrolyte, and acid-base imbalances (see the box below). The nurse compiles a nursing history consisting of information about the client's past or current health problems that cause risk of such imbal

---

Risk Factors for Fluid, Electrolyte, and Acid-Base Imbalances

AGE
- Very young
- Very old

CHRONIC DISEASES
- Cancer
- Cardiovascular disease such as congestive heart failure
- Endocrine disease such as Cushing's disease and diabetes mellitus
- Malnutrition
- Chronic obstructive pulmonary disease
- Renal disease such as progressive renal failure
- Changes in level of consciousness

TRAUMA
- Crush injuries
- Head injuries
- Burns

THERAPIES
- Diuretics
- Steroids
- IV therapy
- Total parenteral nutrition (TPN)

GASTROINTESTINAL LOSSES
- Gastroenteritis
- Nasogastric suctioning
- Fistulas

ances. Following is a discussion of components of a nursing history.

SURGERY

Surgical procedures result in changes in fluid balance during the second to fifth day after surgery because of the body's stress response to surgical trauma. The more extensive the surgery, the greater the body response. For 24 to 48 hours increases in aldosterone and glucocorticoid secretion result in sodium, chloride, and fluid retention while potassium is excreted. An increase in ADH secretion results in decreased urinary output. During this fluid retention phase, these mechanisms and the sympathetic nervous system response help maintain circulating blood volume and pressure after surgery. After the second postoperative day, a diuretic phase begins: hormone levels return to normal causing excess sodium and water to be excreted.

After surgery, clients can exhibit many acid-base changes. The client who is reluctant to breathe deeply and cough may develop respiratory acidosis due to retained $Paco_2$. The client with nasogastric suction may develop metabolic alkalosis due to the loss of gastric acid, fluid, and electrolytes.

BURNS

In clients with severe second- or third-degree burns, body fluids are lost. The greater the body surface burned, the greater the fluid loss. The burned client loses body fluids by one of five routes. First, plasma leaves the intravascular space and becomes trapped edema. This is also called the plasma-to-interstitial fluid shift. It is accompanied by a loss of serum proteins. Second, plasma and interstitial fluids are lost as burn exudate. Third, water vapor and heat are lost in proportion to the amount of skin that is burned away. Fourth, blood leaks from damaged capillaries, adding to the intravascular fluid volume loss. Last, sodium and water shift into the cells, further compromising extracellular fluid volume (Long et al, 1993).

CARDIOVASCULAR DISORDERS

The failing heart has a diminished cardiac output. As a result, perfusion to the kidneys is decreased, and urinary output drops. The client retains sodium and water resulting in circulatory overload, which may lead to pulmonary edema.

Fluid and electrolyte imbalances associated with heart failure can be controlled for a time with medications and with fluid and sodium restrictions. The goal of fluid reduction is to reduce the work of the left ventricle by reducing the excess circulating fluid volume.

RESPIRATORY DISORDERS

Many alterations in respiratory function predispose the client to respiratory acidosis. For example, the changes involved in pneumonia, sedative overdose, and chronic obstructive pulmonary disease interfere with the elimination of carbon dioxide. As the carbon dioxide builds up in the bloodstream, the body's compensatory mechanisms (buffers, renal processes) can no longer adapt. Thus the arterial pH decreases. Any condition that causes hyperventilation (e.g., decreased arterial oxygen level, anxiety, or fever) can result in respiratory alkalosis that is often acute and quickly reversed when the cause is removed.

RENAL DISORDERS

Failing kidneys alter fluid and electrolyte balance. There is an abnormal retention of sodium, chloride, potassium, and water in the extracellular fluid. The plasma levels of metabolic waste products such as BUN and creatinine are elevated because the kidneys are unable to filter and excrete the waste products of cellular metabolism. This elevation is toxic to cellular processes. Metabolic acidosis results when hydrogen ions are retained due to decreased renal function. Because of the renal disorder, the usual renal compensatory mechanisms such as bicarbonate reabsorption are not available, so the body's ability to restore normal acid-base balance is limited.

The severity of fluid and electrolyte imbalance is proportional to the degree of renal failure. Occasionally, acute renal failure induced by shock or a decrease in extracellular fluid may be reversible. Although chronic renal failure is progressive, the client may be treated successfully with dietary control of protein and salt intake, diuretic medications, and fluid restrictions.

CANCER

The types of fluid and electrolyte imbalances that are observed in a client with cancer depend on the type and progression of the cancer. All electrolyte imbalances can occur in the client with cancer and are caused by anatomical distortion and functional impairment from tumor growth and tumor-caused metabolic and endocrine abnormality. For instance, a tumor in the peritoneal cavity produces excess serous fluid resulting in ascites (Long et al, 1993).

HEAD INJURY

Head injury can result in cerebral edema. Occasionally this edema creates pressure on the pituitary gland, and as a result, ADH secretion is changed. Two alterations can occur. Diabetes insipidus occurs when too little ADH is secreted and the client excretes large volumes of dilute urine with a low specific gravity. The second alteration is SIADH, in which there is continued secretion of ADH, which results in a gradual increase of extracellular fluid volume, hyponatremia, and hypoosmolality (Horne et al, 1991). In addition, physical assessment and laboratory findings are consistent with fluid volume overload.

GASTROINTESTINAL DISTURBANCES

Gastroenteritis and nasogastric suctioning result in loss of fluid, potassium, and chloride ions. Hydrogen ions are also lost, causing a disturbance in acid-base balance. Timely education of infant and child caretakers can prevent dehydration resulting from the diarrhea of rotaviral infections (see the box on p. 1253).

Gastrointestinal fistulas can also result in a loss of potassium, resulting in increased risk for hypokalemia. The loss of potassium increases the risk for acid-base disturbances.

PHYSICAL EXAMINATION

Because fluid, electrolyte, and acid-base disturbances can affect all systems, the nurse must systematically identify any abnormalities during the physical assessment (Table 45-6).

DAILY WEIGHTS

Nurses have a responsibility to weigh daily all clients with and who are at risk for fluid and electrolyte distur-

Table 45-6	**Physical and Behavioral Nursing Assessment for Fluid, Electrolyte, and Acid-Base Imbalances**

ASSESSMENT	IMBALANCE
WEIGHT CHANGES	
2%-5% loss	Mild FVD*
5%-10% loss	Moderate FVD*
10%-15% loss	Severe FVD*
15%-20% loss	Death*
2% gain	Mild FVE
5% gain	Moderate FVE
8% gain	Severe FVE
HEAD	
History:	
Headache	FVD*, metabolic or respiratory acidosis, metabolic alkalosis
Dizziness	FVD*, respiratory acidosis or alkalosis, hyponatremia
Observation:	
Irritability	Metabolic or respiratory alkalosis, hyperosmolar imbalance, hypernatremia, hypokalemia
Lethargy	FVD*, metabolic acidosis or alkalosis, respiratory acidosis, hypercalcemia
Confusion, disorientation	FVD*, hypomagnesemia, metabolic acidosis, hypokalemia
Fontanels (infant)	
Inspection:	
Depressed	FVD*
Bulging	FVE*
Eyes	
Inspection:	
Sunken, dry conjunctivae, decreased or absent tearing	FVD
Periorbital edema, papilledema	FVE
History:	
Blurred vision	FVE
Throat and mouth	
Inspection:	
Sticky, dry mucous membranes, dry cracked lips, decreased salivation	FVD, Hypernatremia
Longitudinal tongue furrows	
CARDIOVASCULAR SYSTEM	
Inspection:	
Flat neck veins	FVD
Distended neck veins	FVE
Dependent body parts: legs, sacrum, back	
Slow venous filling	FVD*
Palpation:	
Edema (dependent body parts: back, sacrum, legs)	FVE*
Dysrhythmias (also noted as ECG changes)	Metabolic acidosis, respiratory alkalosis and acidosis, potassium imbalance, hypomagnesemia
Increased pulse rate	Metabolic alkalosis, respiratory acidosis, hyponatremia, FVD, FVE, hypomagnesemia
Decreased pulse rate	Metabolic alkalosis, hypokalemia
Weak pulse	FVD, hypokalemia
Decreased capillary filling	FVD
Bounding pulse	FVE
Auscultation:	
Blood pressure low or without orthostatic changes	FVD, hyponatremia, hyperkalemia, hypermagnesemia
Third heart sound	FVE
Hypertension	FVE
RESPIRATORY SYSTEM	
Inspection:	
Increased rate	FVE, respiratory alkalosis, metabolic acidosis
Dyspnea	FVE
Auscultation: Crackles	FVE

*Data from Horne M et al: *Fluid, electrolyte, and acid-base balance*, St Louis, 1991, Mosby.   *Continued.*

Table 45-6	Physical and Behavioral Nursing Assessment for Fluid, Electrolyte, and Acid-Base Imbalances—cont'd
ASSESSMENT	**IMBALANCE**

GASTROINTESTINAL SYSTEM

History:	
Anorexia	Metabolic acidosis
Abdominal cramps	Metabolic acidosis
Inspection:	
Sunken abdomen	FVD
Distended abdomen	Third-space syndrome
Vomiting	FVD, hypercalcemia, hyponatremia
Diarrhea	Hyponatremia
Auscultation:	
Hyperperistalsis with diarrhea, or hypoperistalsis	FVD, hypokalemia

RENAL SYSTEM

Inspection:	
Oliguria or anuria	FVD, FVE
Diuresis (if kidneys normal)	FVE
Increased urine specific gravity	FVD

NEUROMUSCULAR SYSTEM

Inspection:	
Numbness, tingling	Metabolic alkalosis, hypocalcemia, potassium imbalances
Muscle cramps, tetany	Hypocalcemia, metabolic or respiratory alkalosis
Coma	Hyperosmolar or hypoosmolar imbalances, hyponatremia
Tremors	Respiratory acidosis, hypomagnesemia
Positive Chvostek's sign	Hypocalcemia, hypomagnesemia
Palpation:	
Hypotonicity	Hypokalemia, hypercalcemia*
Hypertonicity	Hypocalcemia, hypomagnesemia, metabolic alkalosis
Percussion:	
Decreased or absent deep tendon reflexes	Hypercalcemia, hypermagnesemia
Increased or hyperactive deep tendon reflexes	Hypocalcemia, hypomagnesemia

SKIN

Body temperature:	
Increased	Hypernatremia, hyperosmolar imbalance, metabolic acidosis
Decreased	FVD
Inspection: Dry, flushed	FVD, hypernatremia, metabolic acidosis
Palpation: Inelastic skin turgor, cold, clammy skin	FVD

bances daily. In this way, fluid retention can be detected early because 5 to 10 pounds of fluid is retained before edema appears. Five pounds of fluid is approximately 2.5 L of fluid volume or about 2400 ml volume. The client is weighed at the same time each day, using the same scale, and wearing the same clothes; if a bed scale is used, the same number of sheets should be on the scale with each weighing.

MEASURING FLUID INTAKE AND OUTPUT

Measuring and recording all liquid intake and output during a 24-hour period helps complete the assessment data base for fluid, electrolyte, and acid-base balances. Intake includes all liquids taken orally, by feeding tube, and parenterally.

Oral intake includes all liquids taken by mouth, such as gelatin, ice cream, soup, juice, and water. Liquid intake also includes fluids given through nasogastric or jejunostomy feeding tubes, liquids given as IV fluids, and blood or its components. Liquid output includes urine, diarrhea, vomitus, gastric suction, and drainage from postsurgical tubes. Frequently the recording of such data is referred to as the *I & O.*

Generally, I & O are routinely measured for clients after surgery and clients whose conditions are unstable, who have fever, whose fluids are restricted, or who are receiving diuretic or IV therapy. The nurse neither needs nor should wait for the physician's order to begin I & O measurements. Clients with chronic cardiopulmonary or renal illnesses and those whose health status has declined also receive such measurements.

Each health care agency has a specific policy regarding when I & O measurements are kept and totalled. Often they are attached to the bedside chart or room door. The records note the type of I & O and are broken down into at least 8-hour segments (Fig. 45-7). At the end of each 8-hour shift, I & O are totalled. The 24-hour totals are then recorded in the client's permanent chart.

Accurate measurement of I & O is a nursing responsibility that may require involvement of the client and family. The nurse explains the reasons that measurements are

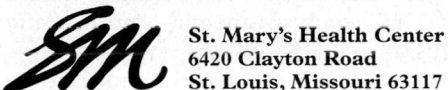

St. Mary's Health Center
6420 Clayton Road
St. Louis, Missouri 63117

PATIENT LABEL

INTAKE AND OUTPUT SUMMARY

	DATE 6-10-xx	2200 – 0600	0600 – 1400	1400 – 2200	24 Hr.		
INTAKE	P.O. Intake	120	800	650	1570	**TOTAL**	**INTAKE**
	Tube Feedings						
	Hyperalimentation						
	I.V. Primary						
	I.V.P.B.	50		50	100		**1670**
	Blood/Blood Products						
OUTPUT	Urine	325	700	500	1525	**TOTAL**	**OUTPUT**
	Emesis						
	G.I. Suction						
	Drainage	50	75	30	155		**1855**
	Chest tube	75	50	50	175		

	DATE	2200 – 0600	0600 – 1400	1400 – 2200	24 Hr.		
INTAKE	P.O. Intake					**TOTAL**	**INTAKE**
	Tube Feedings						
	Hyperalimentation						
	I.V. Primary						
	I.V.P.B.						
	Blood/Blood Products						
OUTPUT	Urine					**TOTAL**	**OUTPUT**
	Emesis						
	G.I. Suction						
	Drainage						

	DATE	2200 – 0600	0600 – 1400	1400 – 2200	24 Hr.		
INTAKE	P.O. Intake					**TOTAL**	**INTAKE**
	Tube Feedings						
	Hyperalimentation						
	I.V. Primary						
	I.V.P.B.						
	Blood/Blood Products						
OUTPUT	Urine					**TOTAL**	**OUTPUT**
	Emesis						
	G.I. Suction						
	Drainage						

	DATE	2200 – 0600	0600 – 1400	1400 – 2200	24 Hr.		
INTAKE	P.O. Intake					**TOTAL**	**INTAKE**
	Tube Feedings						
	Hyperalimentation						
	I.V. Primary						
	I.V.P.B.						
	Blood/Blood Products						
OUTPUT	Urine					**TOTAL**	**OUTPUT**
	Emesis						
	G.I. Suction						
	Drainage						

Fig. 45-7 Twenty-four hour intake and output record. *(Courtesy St. Mary's Health Center, St Louis.)*

needed. A client using a toilet should be instructed to use a calibrated insert, which attaches to the rim of the toilet bowl. The client should be instructed to notify the nurse after each urination. The nurse then measures, records and empties the urine and rinses the insert. Occasionally, clients may also be instructed to measure and record their own output.

The output of a client who has an indwelling Foley catheter, drainage tube, or suction is recorded at the end of each nursing shift or even more frequently (e.g., every hour) as the client's condition requires.

Clients occasionally receive a specific amount of a liquid medication. Over 24 hours, this hourly medication can amount to a significant intake and should always be recorded on the I & O record. For example, antacids are commonly ordered in 30-ml doses every hour or two for clients who have or are at risk for gastrointestinal bleeding.

Recording I & O is essential for obtaining an accurate data base. The nurse looks for trends over 24-, 48-, and 72-hour periods. This information helps maintain an ongoing evaluation of hydration status to prevent severe imbalances.

LABORATORY STUDIES

Laboratory tests are performed to obtain further objective data about fluid, electrolyte, and acid-base balances. These tests include serum electrolyte levels, complete blood count (CBC), BUN levels, blood creatinine levels, urine specific gravity, and arterial blood gas level. The nurse must be familiar with the normal values of common laboratory tests (see the box below).

Serum electrolyte levels are measured to determine the hydration status, the electrolyte concentration of the blood plasma, and the acid-base balance. Electrolytes frequently measured in venous blood include sodium, potassium, chloride, and bicarbonate ions and carbon dioxide combining power. The severity of the illness determines the frequency of the electrolyte measurements. Serum electrolytes are routinely measured when a client is admitted to the hospital, to provide baseline data for electrolyte status.

The CBC is a determination of the number and type of red and white blood cells per cubic millimeter of blood. Changes in the CBC, especially in the hematocrit, occur in

response to dehydration or overhydration. Serious alterations in the CBC, such as anemia, can also affect oxygenation status.

Blood creatinine levels are useful in measuring kidney function. Creatinine is a normal by-product of muscle metabolism and is excreted at fairly constant levels, regardless of factors such as fluid intake, diet, and exercise.

The urine specific gravity test measures the urine's degree of concentration. The specific gravity can be measured at the bedside using a urinometer. Normally the urine specific gravity ranges between 1.003 and 1.030. Because water has a specific gravity of 1.000, urine with a lower specific gravity (1.003) is more dilute than urine with a higher specific gravity (1.030).

Arterial blood gas tests provide information on the status of acid-base balance and on the effectiveness of ventilatory function in providing normal oxygen–carbon dioxide exchange. The arterial pH tests measure the hydrogen ion concentration. A decreased pH is associated with acidosis, whereas an elevated pH is associated with alkalosis.

The $Paco_2$ measures the partial pressure of carbon dioxide in the arterial blood. Alveolar hypoventilation results in an elevated $Paco_2$, whereas hyperventilation is associated with a decreased $Paco_2$. Regulation of carbon dioxide is the pulmonary component of acid-base balance, and changes in the $Paco_2$ may help explain an abnormal pH. $Paco_2$ measures the partial pressure of oxygen in the arteries. This provides information concerning the ventilatory effectiveness of the lungs. $Paco_2$ levels provide no direct information concerning acid-base balance. The oxygen saturation (Sao_2) measures the degree to which hemoglobin is saturated by oxygen.

The serum bicarbonate is another component of arterial blood gases. An elevated bicarbonate level is associated with alkalosis, either primary or as a compensation for respiratory acidosis. A decreased bicarbonate level is usually the result of metabolic acidosis. Bicarbonate levels reflect the renal portion of acid-base regulation. Using these results, the presence and severity of hypoxia and the type and severity of acid-base imbalances can be determined.

 ## Nursing Diagnosis

The three parts of the nursing diagnosis statement are very important in directing the development of the plan of care and evaluation for each individual client (see the nursing diagnoses box on p. 1265).

Assessment reveals clusters of data indicating problems with fluid, electrolyte, acid-base balance, or other related problems (see Tables 45-4, 45-5, 45-6). Nursing diagnoses are derived from supporting defining characteristics and expected causes or related factors that are contained within the data base (see the diagnostic process box on p. 1265).

The identification of the expected causes of the problem or factors related to it leads to the specific plan of care and evaluation for that particular client. This means that the nurse may be caring for two clients, each with a fluid volume deficit but be implementing a different plan of care for each client. For example, one client may have a fluid volume deficit because of an intestinal infection associated with fever and diarrhea. For this client the nurse should

---

Normal Blood Chemistry Values
■ Calcium levels: 4-5 mEq/L
■ Carbon dioxide content (bicarbonate in venous blood): 24-30 mEq/L
■ Chloride level: 100-106 mEq/L
■ Magnesium level: 1.5-2.5 mEq/L
■ Phosphate level: 2.5-4.5 mEq/L
■ Potassium level: 3.5-5.3 mEq/L
■ Sodium level: 135-145 mEq/L
■ Serum osmolality: 280-295 mOsm/kg
■ Urine specific gravity: 1.003-1.030
■ Arterial blood gas levels
pH: 7.35-7.45
$Paco_2$: 35-45 mm Hg
Pao_2: 80-100 mm Hg
Sao_2: 95%-99%
Bicarbonate level: 22-26 mEq/L

Examples of NANDA Nursing Diagnoses for Fluid, Electrolyte, and Acid-Base Disturbances

Risk for or fluid volume deficit *related to:*
- Loss of plasma associated with burns
- Vomiting
- Failure of regulatory mechanisms

Fluid volume deficit *related to:*
- Sodium retention
- Compromised regulatory mechanisms

Impaired tissue integrity *related to:*
- Edema

Impaired gas exchange *related to:*
- Altered oxygen supply
- Alveolar-capillary membrane changes
- Altered blood flow
- Altered oxygen-carrying capacity of blood

Decreased cardiac output *related to:*
- Dysrhythmia associated with electrolyte imbalance

From Kim M et al: *Nursing diagnoses,* ed 6, St Louis, 1995, Mosby.

give ordered antibiotics, antidiarrheals, antipyretics, and administer ordered intravenous fluid replacement in order to treat the specific cause of the problem. This treatment plan is very different from that for another client whose fluid volume deficit is related to a traumatic amputation of the left leg. Antidiarrheal and antipyretic medications would do nothing to treat this client's fluid deficit. The specific plan of care for this client should include ordered intravenous fluids, including blood products, vasopressor medications, and emergency surgery to stop the bleeding.

Another very important portion of the nursing diagnostic statement are the supporting signs and symptoms of the

problem, which becomes the specific yardstick for evaluating the client's progress in response to the actions or therapies that the nurse implements. Continual assessment of these signs and symptoms answers the questions: Are the treatments working? Is the client's health improving or deteriorating? For example, the first client above was experiencing seven watery stools per day. After receiving antibiotics and antidiarrheal medications for an appropriate time, the client should be experiencing less than seven stools per day of a more formed consistency. The reassessment of these specific signs and symptoms would mean that this client's body fluid volume was returning to normal. However, if the client were continuing to have more than seven watery stools per day, the nurse should reassess the client and examine the plan of care for reasons for this poor response to therapy. In this way, the client's plan of care can be revised in order to help achieve the goal of normal fluid levels.

Planning

After identifying a nursing diagnosis, the nurse develops a care plan (see the care plan on p. 1266). The care plan is individualized according to the client's acute or chronic fluid, electrolyte, or acid-base imbalance. The nursing care plan is directed at meeting actual or potential fluid needs. The plan includes one or more of the following goals:

1. Client will have normal fluid, electrolyte, and acid-base balance.
2. Causes of imbalance are identified and corrected.
3. Client will have no complications from therapies needed to restore balance.

It is particularly important to include the client and family in this planning process. Fluid, electrolyte, and acid-base imbalances often result in subtle changes in behavior or status, and only the family may be familiar enough with the client's usual behavior to be able to identify these

Sample Nursing Diagnostic Process for Fluid, Electrolyte, and Acid-Base Disturbances

ASSESSMENT ACTIVITIES	DEFINING CHARACTERISTICS	NURSING DIAGNOSES
Obtain daily weight measurements.	Client experiences sudden weight loss.	**Fluid volume deficit** related to loss of gastrointestinal fluids via vomiting.
Observe volume of urine output related to intake and specific gravity.	Decreased volume of output in comparison to intake; increased urine specific gravity is present.	
Palpate skin turgor.	Inelastic skin turgor noted.	
Ask if client is thirsty or weak.	Client verbalizes thirst and weakness.	
Inspect mucous membranes for degree of moisture.	Dry mucous membranes are noted.	
Observe for abnormal losses of fluids.	Client is vomiting.	
Observe client's orientation to person, place, and time.	Client is confused to place and time.	**Impaired gas exchange** related to alveolar-capillary membrane changes due to large amount of thick creamy lung secretions.
Observe frequency and purposefulness of behavior.	Client is restless.	
Monitor $Paco_2$.	$Paco_2$ is 56 mm Hg.	
Observe amount and character of sputum.	Client has large amount of thick, creamy lung secretions.	

Sample Nursing Care Plan for Fluid Volume Deficit

NURSING DIAGNOSIS: Fluid volume deficit related to active loss of gastrointestinal fluid via vomiting.
DEFINITION: Fluid volume deficit is the state in which an individual experiences vascular, cellular, or intracellular dehydration related to active loss (Kim, McFarland, McLane, 1995).

GOAL	EXPECTED OUTCOMES	INTERVENTIONS	RATIONALE
Client will have normal fluid, electrolyte, and acid-base balance within 48 hrs.	Vital signs will return to normal within 24 hrs.		
	Weight will stabilize by 1/25.	Encourage and measure intake of small amount of fluids containing electrolytes.	Ingesting small volumes may prevent further vomiting. Presence of electrolytes prevents further depletion (Horne et al, 1991).
	Urine output will increase (>70 ml/hr) by 1/24.	Discourage intake of plain water.	Ingestion of plain water causes sodium content in stomach to increase as body attempts to make water isotonic to allow absorption.
	Specific gravity will decrease (<1.030) by 1/24.	Administer parenteral antiemetics as ordered by the physician. Alter environment to lessen stimuli for vomiting (e.g., keep unpleasant odors to minimum).	If vomiting occurs before IV fluid absortion, more fluids and electrolytes are lost.
	Client will have elastic skin turgor by 1/24.	Promote bed rest. Measure amount of vomitus.	This prevents triggering vomiting center in brain. Sudden, quick movements may trigger vomiting.
	Client will verbalize no thirst or weakness by 1/25.	Measure amount of fluid output and any profuse diuresis.	This allows precise replacement of lost fluid and electrolytes.
	Client will have moist mucous membranes by 1/25. Client will exhibit no vomiting by 1/26.	Implement physician orders to provide parenteral fluids containing electrolytes during prolonged periods of vomiting. Measure intake of these fluids.	These fluids will precisely replace losses along with oral fluids.

---

changes in a timely manner. The client and family must know preventive measures, signs and symptoms to report, and measures that can be implemented if the imbalance occurs (see the case study on p. 1267). When medications, special diets, or oral or IV fluids are administered in the home, the client and family need careful teaching so that these interventions are performed safely. In the hospital, the nurse anticipates these needs and initiates teaching before discharge so that the client and family are ready for these procedures. The home health care nurse continues the teaching and evaluates the effectiveness of the home interventions.

Implementation

Prevention of fluid, electrolyte, and acid-base imbalances is important. When imbalances occur, the nurse removes or treats the cause of the imbalance if possible. Other nursing interventions aim to correct fluid and electrolyte imbalances.

When volume is depleted, fluids and electrolytes can be replaced orally, with IV administration of fluids and blood components, or through TPN if the fluid deficit is caused by

malnutrition. For clients with FVE, the nurse implements measures to reduce fluids, such as fluid intake restrictions, reduced sodium intake, and administration of diuretics.

Correcting Fluid and Electrolyte Imbalances

ENTERAL REPLACEMENT OF FLUIDS

Fluids are replaced enterally via the oral route and tube feedings.

Oral. Unless contraindicated, oral replacement of fluids and electrolytes is appropriate as long as the client is not vomiting, is not experiencing a profound fluid loss, or does not have a mechanical obstruction in the gastrointestinal tract. Clients unable to tolerate solid foods may still be able to ingest fluids. Oral fluid replacement is easily implemented in the home and hospital. Mild illnesses such as viral diarrhea and respiratory tract infections, as well as fevers, may cause fluid and electrolyte disturbances. In addition, clients recovering from anesthesia or gastrointestinal surgery usually receive clear liquids first and then advance to a regular diet if they tolerate the liquids. When replacing fluids by mouth in a client with a FVD, the nurse

CASE STUDIES

ISOTONIC EXCESS

Mr. P. is 87 years old and has a history of heart failure. He has been unable to afford the cardiotonic and diuretic medications ordered to treat the heart failure. He is admitted to the hospital because of severe shortness of breath. He recalls that his shoes have been getting tighter and that he has gained 10 pounds over the last 2 weeks. During physical examination, the nurse notes bilateral jugular vein distension and crackles throughout all lung fields.

This example illustrates two important factors: (1) clients need resources (e.g., financial, psychosocial support, information), and (2) clients and significant others should be able to recognize signs and symptoms of worsening conditions. In this situation, if Mr. P. had recognized the significance of dependent edema and weight gain, the development of pulmonary edema might have been prevented.

POSTOPERATIVE FLUID AND ELECTROLYTE SHIFT*

Mr. W. is 72 years old and has just returned to the coronary step down unit following an emergency appendectomy. He has been healthy except for a history of hypertension, a myocardial infarction at age 60, and a history of congestive heart failure.

The nurse checks his chart and notes that on admission to the emergency room he had no peripheral edema and his vital signs were 101-80-24 and 148/70. As she admits him to the division now, his vital signs are 97.6-88-24, 122/62, his buccal mucous membranes are dry, his skin is pale and cool, and he is hypokalemic, hypernatremic, and has 2 plus pedal edema. His IV is running at 100 ml per hour with 40 mEq of KCl/liter and he is NPO.

The nurse knows that due to the coolness of the operating room, Mr. W's resulting vasoconstriction and lowered cardiac output have stimulated his renin-angiotensin system to conserve sodium and water. As sodium is absorbed, potassium is lost. Also the incisional inflammatory response has resulted in a third-space shift of fluid. Thus Mr. W. appears to be hypovolemic intravascularly, yet he actually has excess body fluid as evidenced by the pedal edema. The nurse knows that for the first 24 to 48 hours, this postoperative response is normal.

If the nurse administers the IV at no more than 100 ml/hr, (no more than 1 L / 24 hours more than urinary output for a client with a cardiac history) and replenishes potassium in the

IVs, after 48 hours the fluids and electrolytes will shift again.

On the second postoperative day, Mr. W.'s vital signs are 98.4-98-28 and 154/84. His serum sodium and potassium levels are approaching normal, his pedal edema is 1+ plus. The nurse knows that Mr. W.'s excess fluid is shifting from his third-space to his intravascular space where his normal kidneys are excreting that excess. His heart is working harder to handle that excess fluid, so the doctor orders a diuretic parenterally and lowers the IV rate to 50 ml/ hr when the nurse tells him of Mr. W.'s vital signs. He also decreases the IV potassium to 40 mEq every other liter of IV fluid.

This example demonstrates how fluid, sodium, and potassium shift postoperatively. It also shows how the nurse must protect the cardiac client from postoperative fluid overload during the diuretic stage after 48 hours.

RESPIRATORY ACIDOSIS

Mrs. D. is 68 years old and has smoked more than 1 pack of cigarettes per day for 48 years. She has had chronic obstructive lung disease for 6 years. She developed a productive cough and fever 3 days before. She believed that she could decrease the production of sputum by decreasing her daily intake of fluids. This resulted in a thick sputum that she cannot expectorate. The retained secretions result in a decreased exchange of oxygen and carbon dioxide across the alveolar-capillary membrane.

She is admitted to the hospital and arterial blood gases reveal the following: pH of 7.32, Pao_2 of 49 mm Hg, $Paco_2$ of 56 mm Hg, and bicarbonate level of 26 mEq/L. The decreased pH is associated with an acidotic state, and the elevated Pco_2 is the result of carbon dioxide retention by the lungs, causing acidosis. Decreased diffusion from the alveoli to the capillaries causes the markedly decreased Pao_2, resulting in cellular hypoxia. The bicarbonate level is normal because the renal buffering mechanism has not had time to respond.

In this situation, immediate medical and nursing care for Mrs. D. includes measures to remove the pulmonary secretions (see Chapter 44), provide support for her ventilatory efforts, and treat the respiratory infection. Before discharge, the nurse must teach Mrs. D. the occurrences that place her at risk for respiratory failure, ways to prevent them, and procedures to follow if they recur. ■

*Modified from Bove L: How fluids and electrolytes shift after surgery, *Nursing 94* 24(8):34, 1994.

should choose fluids with adequate calories and electrolyte content (Table 45-7), but if fluids are replaced through a feeding tube, the physician usually prescribes a nutritional supplement (see Chapter 41).

A feeding tube may be appropriate when the client's gastrointestinal tract is healthy but the client cannot ingest fluids (e.g., after oral surgery or with impaired swallowing). All feeding tubes such as nasogastric, gastrostomy, or jejunostomy feeding tubes require a physician's order (see Chapter 41).

RESTRICTION OF FLUID

Clients who have FVE require restricted fluid intake. Such clients may have renal failure, congestive heart failure, cor pulmonale, or SIADH.

Fluid restriction is often difficult for clients, particularly if they are taking medications that dry the oral mucous membranes. The nurse should explain the reason that fluids are restricted, how much fluid is permitted, and that ice chips, gelatin, and ice cream are fluids.

Given this information, the client should help decide how to divide the total amount of fluid with each meal, between meals, before bed, and with medications. Frequently clients on fluid restriction can swallow a number of pills with as little as 1 ounce (30 ml) of liquid.

A good rule of thumb for fluid restrictions is to allow half the allotted total oral fluids between 8 AM and 4 PM, the period when clients usually are more active and receive two meals and most of their oral medications. Then an additional two fifths of the allotted total fluid is permitted between 4 PM and 11 PM, permitting fluids with meals and evening visitors. Between the hours of 11 PM and 8 AM the remainder of the total fluid allotment is permitted. Because the client is usually asleep during this period, fluid needs decrease.

The nurse should also ensure that clients receive their favorite fluids (unless contraindicated). For example, if a client can have only 200 ml of fluid with breakfast and hates cranberry juice but likes apple or grape juice, the nurse should be sure that the diet kitchen has this information.

Table 45-7	Oral Fluids								
SOLUTION	NA mEq/L	CA mEq/L	PO₄ mEq/L	K mEq/L	MG mEq/L	CL mEq/L	BASE BUFFER†	GLUCOSE* G/L	OSMOLALITY mOsm/L
Water‡									
Gastrolyte	50-90			20		52-65	30(C)	20	NA~
Rehydralyte	75			20		65	30(C)	25	310
Lytren	50			25		45	30(C)	20	NA
Pedialyte	45			20		35	30(C)	25	250
Resol	50	4	5	20	4	50	34(C)	20	290
Infalyte	50			20		40	30(B)	20	NA
Apple juice	1-5			24-43				12-32*	870
Cola	1-7			0.1-0.6			7.3-13.4	5-12*	680
Lemon-lime soda	5			1-2				33	520
Gatorade	24			3				50	350
Ginger ale	1-7			0.1-0.4				7-12	510
Grape juice									1170
Orange juice									935
Tea				Trace					NA
Beef broth	55								NA
Jello	6-17			0.1-0.9				8	285-320

Modified from *Drug facts and comparisons,* Philadelphia, 1992, Lippincott; Goepp JG, Katz SA: Oral rehydration therapy, *Am Fam Phys 49*:843, 1993; Groër MW: *Physiology and pathophysiology of the body fluids,* St Louis, 1981, Mosby.
*Carbohydrate source of calories is sucrose
†*B,* bicarbonate; *C,* citrate; *NA,* information not available
‡Contains no calories or electrolytes

Standard Precautions to Prevent Transmission of HIV Through IV Therapy

Gloves must be worn when there is a reasonable expectation that there may be contact with blood (e.g., during venipuncture or while changing IV administration sets).

Gloves should be changed after contact with each client.

Hands and other skin surfaces should be washed immediately and thoroughly if contaminated with blood or other body fluids (see Chapter 34). Hands should be washed immediately after gloves are removed.

To prevent needlestick injuries, needles should not be recapped, purposely bent or broken by hand, removed from disposable syringes, or otherwise manipulated by hand.

Contaminated needles, syringes, and IV fluid equipment should be placed in puncture-resistant containers that are properly labeled as a biohazard for disposal. These containers should be located as close as practical to the use area. When full, they are to be sealed and disposed of properly.

Health care workers who have exudative lesions or weeping dermatitis should refrain from all direct care and from handling invasive equipment until the condition resolves.

Pregnant health care workers are not known to be at greater risk of contracting HIV infections than health care workers who are not pregnant. However, if a health care worker develops HIV infection during pregnancy, the infant is at risk of infection resulting from perinatal transmission. Because of this risk, pregnant health care workers should strictly adhere to precautions to minimize the risk of transmission.

PARENTERAL REPLACEMENT OF FLUID AND ELECTROLYTES

Fluid and electrolytes may be replaced by infusion directly into the blood rather than intake through the digestive system. Parenteral replacement includes total parenteral nutrition (TPN), IV fluid and electrolyte therapy, and blood replacement.

With increasing risk to health care workers for transmission of HIV, AIDS, and other infectious diseases, the principles of standard precautions must be practiced when administering parenteral fluids (see Chapter 34). The Centers for Disease Control and Prevention (CDC) has issued guidelines pertaining to exposure to blood and body fluids (see the box at left).

Vascular Access Devices. Vascular access devices are catheters, cannulas, or infusion ports designed for long-term repeated access to the vascular system (Fig. 45-8). Infusion ports are safer than peripherally placed catheters and have improved mechanisms for delivering long-term IV therapy. Recently, peripherally inserted central catheters (PICC) have begun to be used for clients with poor peripheral venous access who need infusion therapy for only 1 week to 3 months (Silvestri and Masoorli, 1990). Increased use of central venous catheters and implanted infusion ports require nurses to be educated in the care of these devices.

Total Parenteral Nutrition (TPN). TPN is a nutritionally adequate hypertonic solution consisting of glucose and other nutrients and electrolytes given through an indwelling peripheral or central IV catheter. Chapter 41 fully describes TPN administration.

IV Therapy. The goal of IV fluid administration is to correct or prevent fluid and electrolyte disturbances. For example, a client with third-degree burns over 40% of the

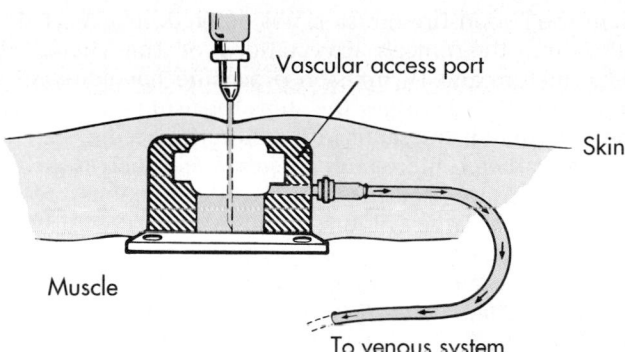

Fig. 45-8 Example of implantable vascular access device.

body is critically ill and needs careful regulation of IV therapy because of continual changes in fluid and electrolyte balance. A client allowed to ingest nothing by mouth for 2 days after an appendectomy receives IV fluid replacement to prevent fluid and electrolyte imbalances. The infusion is discontinued with resumption of normal oral intake.

When IV fluid administration is required and ordered by the physician the nurse must identify the correct solution, equipment needed, and procedures required to initiate, regulate, and maintain the system. The nurse must also identify and correct problems and discontinue the infusion.

Types of solutions. Many prepared electrolyte solutions are available for use. Electrolyte solutions fall into the following categories: isotonic, hypotonic, and hypertonic. A solution is isotonic if its osmolarity approximates that of plasma. A hypotonic solution has an osmolarity less than that of plasma, and a hypertonic solution has an osmolarity greater than that of plasma.

In general, isotonic fluids are used for extracellular volume replacement (e.g., FVD after prolonged vomiting). The decision to use a hypotonic or hypertonic solution is based on the specific electrolyte imbalance.

Certain additives are frequently instilled into IV solutions, most commonly vitamins and potassium chloride (KCl). The physician's order includes required additives, for example:

Bottle #1: 1000 ml—D5W with 20 mEq KCl and 1 ampule of multivitamins

Clients with normal kidneys who are receiving nothing by mouth should have potassium added to IV solutions. If the physician's order for such a client does not include potassium, the nurse should double-check the order. The body has no conservation mechanism for potassium, and even when the serum level falls, the kidneys continue to excrete potassium. If there is no potassium intake orally or parenterally, hypokalemia can quickly develop. The nurse collects and, if necessary, prepares the solution using the five rights of medication administration described in Chapter 35.

Equipment. Correct selection and preparation of equipment make safe and quick placement of an IV line possible. Because fluids are instilled into the bloodstream, sterile technique is necessary. Standard equipment includes IV solution and tubing, needle or catheter (Procedure 45-1), antiseptic, tourniquet, gloves, and dressing. An armboard to restrict hand movement may also be used for some clients.

The arm board is used to reduce movement of the extremity with the IV infusion in place or to maintain the extremity in a flat position.

Other IV equipment includes solution containers, various types of tubing, and volume control devices. Often an injectable antibiotic medication such as ampicillin may be added to a small IV solution bag containing 50 to 100 ml and "piggybacked" into the main line to be administered over 30 to 60 minutes (see Chapter 35).

The type and amount of solution depend on the medication added and the client's physiological status. For example, when ampicillin is administered parenterally, it must be infused within 1 hour after it is prepared. Otherwise the medication loses its potency. Different tubing types are used to administer medications. A drug given rapidly needs to be infused with macrodrip tubing, which delivers large drops so that a rapid rate can be maintained. In addition, clients may require IV extension tubing to increase mobility or facilitate changes in position. **Volume control devices** are used with children, clients with renal or cardiac failure, and critically ill clients to prevent sudden, uncontrolled rapid infusion of large volumes. (Additional information on volume control devices is presented in the section on regulating the infusion flow rate.)

Initiating the intravenous line. After the equipment is collected at the bedside, the nurse assesses the client for the venipuncture site (Procedure 45-1). A **venipuncture** is a technique in which a vein is punctured transcutaneously by a sharp, rigid stylet (e.g., a butterfly needle or a metal needle) partially covered by a plastic catheter (over-the-needle catheter or ONC) or by a needle attached to a syringe. The general purposes of venipuncture are to collect a blood specimen, instill a medication, start an IV infusion, and inject a radiopaque or radioactive tracer for special examinations. Procedure 45-1 describes venipuncture for IV fluid infusion.

The nurse assessing clients for potential venipuncture sites should consider conditions, cautions, and contraindications that exclude certain sites. If possible, nondominant extremities should be used for all clients. In addition, generally the nurse should look for distal sites first and then proximal ones. Because very young and old clients have fragile veins, the nurse should avoid sites that are easily moved or bumped such as the dorsal surface of the hand (see the box on p. 1270). It is often difficult to insert IV lines in clients who have had many venipunctures because their veins may be sclerosed with scar tissue. Obese clients present problems for venipuncture because of the difficulty in locating superficial veins. The veins of thin and emaciated clients are also difficult to puncture. Although they may be visible, the veins are quite fragile, and as a result the nurse may puncture through entire veins instead of placing needles or catheters within them. When clients are severely dehydrated or have decreased extracellular fluid, such as with shock, the veins may collapse due to decreased circulating blood volume. When veins collapse, venipuncture becomes extremely difficult, but it is also a lifesaving measure. For these difficult clients, venipuncture should be performed by someone with expertise. Some agencies have IV therapy teams whose members have special expertise in performing venipunctures and maintaining IV infusions.

Venipuncture is contraindicated in a site that has signs of infection, infiltration, or thrombosis (clotting). An infected

GERONTOLOGICAL PRINCIPLES
for Intravenous Therapy

■ In older clients, use the smallest gauge catheter or needle possible (e.g., 24-26 gauge). This is less traumatizing to the vein and allows better blood flow to provide increased hemodilution of the IV fluids or medications. This gauge can be used for hourly flow rates of 75 to 100 ml/hr.

■ Avoid the back of the older adult's hand or the dominant arm for venipuncture because these sites greatly interfere with the older adult's independence.

• If the older adult has fragile skin and veins, use minimal tourniquet pressure.

■ When the older adult has lost subcutaneous tissue, the veins lose stability and will roll away from the needle. To stabilize the vein, apply traction to the skin below the projected insertion site.

■ Using an angle of 5 to 15 degrees on insertion is helpful because the older adult's veins are more superficial.

■ In the older person with fragile skin, prevent skin tears by minimizing the amount of tape used.

Modified from Coulter K: Intravenous therapy for the elder patient: implications for the intravenous nurse, *J Intraven Nurs* 15(suppl):S18, 1992.

site is red, tender, swollen, and possibly warm to the touch. Exudate may be present. An infected site is not used because of the danger of introducing bacteria from the skin surface into the bloodstream.

Common IV puncture sites include the hand and arm (Fig. 45-9). However, the superficial veins of the foot can be used if the client is not ambulatory and policy allows. The use of the foot for an IV site is more common with pediatric clients but is usually avoided in the adult.

After locating the venipuncture site, the nurse carefully explains the procedure to the client. The nurse should ex-plain the reason the infusion was ordered, its expected results, and the nurse's expectations of the client. The venipuncture and IV infusion procedure has many steps. Procedure 45-1 describes the steps for using an ONC, but the procedure is the same with a butterfly needle.

Large catheters placed into a central vein such as the subclavian vein are used to monitor central venous pressure and to deliver large volumes of fluids and TPN. Although these catheters are inserted by physicians, nurses are responsible for maintaining the catheter and the IV.

Regulating the infusion flow rate. After the IV infusion is secured and the IV line is patent, the nurse must regulate the rate of infusion according to physician's orders (Procedure 45-2). An infusion rate that is too slow can lead to further cardiovascular and circulatory collapse in a client who is dehydrated, in shock, or critically ill. An infusion rate that is too rapid can result in fluid overload, which is particularly dangerous in some cardiovascular, renal, and neurological disorders. The nurse calculates the infusion rate to prevent too-slow or too-rapid administration of fluids.

Infusion pumps regulate the flow of IV fluids. They are designed to deliver a measured amount of fluid over a specified period or to deliver fluids based on the flow rate or drops per minute. Some infusion pumps have an electronic eye that counts the number of drops flowing from an IV administration set. The electronic eye must be placed on the drip chamber below the origin of the drop and above the fluid level in the chamber. In such a pump, if the required number of drops per minute is not achieved, an alarm will sound.

All IV pumps have alarms that sound if the IV bag is empty, the infusion tubing is kinked or contains air, or the vein is clotted. If an alarm sounds, the nurse investigates and corrects the cause of the problem. IV flow rates can be affected by the patency of the IV needle or catheter, infiltration, a knot or kink in the tubing, the height of the solution, and the position of the client's extremity.

Patency of the IV needle or catheter means that the needle and catheter are open, allowing the solution to flow.

Text continued on p. 1275.

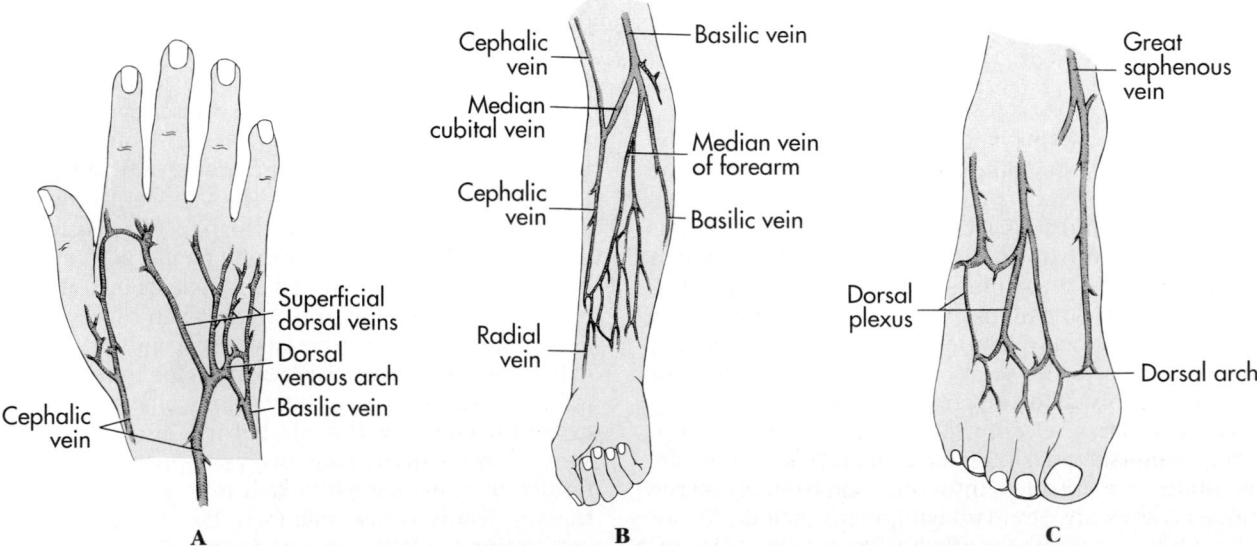

Fig. 45-9 Possible IV sites. **A,** Dorsal surface of the hand. **B,** Inner arm. **C,** Dorsal surface of the foot.

Venipuncture With an Over-the-Needle Plastic Catheter

STEPS	RATIONALE
1. Observe for signs and symptoms indicating fluid or electrolyte imbalances:	Because fluid and electrolyte disturbances can affect every system in the body, nurse must systematically assess client to identify abnormalities related to fluid or electrolyte imbalance. Daily weights document fluid loss or retention. Change in body weight of I kg corresponds to I L (1000 ml) of fluid retention or loss.

1. Observe for signs and symptoms indicating fluid or electrolyte imbalances:
   a. Sunken eyes
   b. Edema
   c. More than 2% increase or decrease in body weight
   d. Dry mucous membranes
   e. Flat or distended neck veins
   f. Hypotension, tachycardia
   g. Regular pulse
   h. Crackles in lungs
   i. Inelastic skin turgor
   j. Increased, decreased bowel sounds
   k. Decreased urine output
   l. Behavioral changes
   m. Confusion

2. Review physician's fluid replacement orders.

3. Assemble necessary equipment for initiating IV line:
   a. Correct solution
   b. Proper needle
   c. Infusion set (infants and children require a microdrip (60 drop/ml) and often a volume control device)
   d. IV tubing
   e. Alcohol and povidone-iodine cleansing swabs
   f. Tourniquet
   g. Arm board, if needed
   h. Gauze or transparent dressing and povidone-iodine solution or ointment
   i. Tape
   j. Towel for under client's hand
   k. IV pole
   l. Disposable gloves
   m. IV gown

Rationale (step 1): Because fluid and electrolyte disturbances can affect every system in the body, nurse must systematically assess client to identify abnormalities related to fluid or electrolyte imbalance. Daily weights document fluid loss or retention. Change in body weight of I kg corresponds to I L (1000 ml) of fluid retention or loss.

Rationale (step 2): Venipuncture is an invasive technique; IV fluids are medications. Both require a physician's order and sterile technique.

Rationale (step 3): Correct solution and preparation of equipment assist in safe and quick placement of IV line.

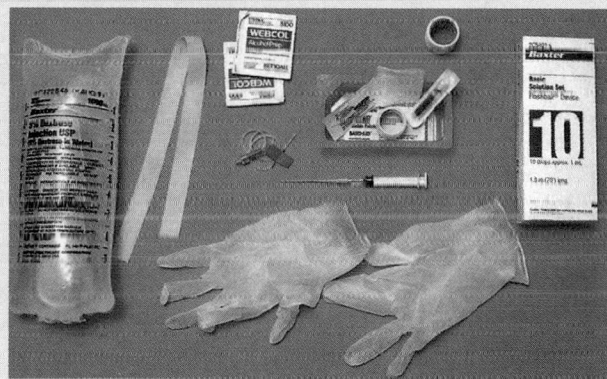

Step 5

4. Identify client and explain procedure. Change client's gown to IV gown.

Reduces anxiety and promotes cooperation. Makes removal of gown easier.

5. Organize equipment on clutter-free bedside stand or overbed table (see the illustration at right).

Reduces risk of contamination and accidents.

6. Identify accessible vein for placement of IV needle or catheter:
   a. Avoid bony prominences.
   b. Use most distal portion of vein first.
   c. Avoid placing IV line over client's wrist, inflamed area, antecubital space, extremity with decreased sensation, or dominant hand.

Promotes ease of placement of IV catheter or needle.

7. Wash hands.

Reduces transmission of microorganisms.

8. Open sterile packages using sterile technique (see Chapter 34).

Maintains sterility of equipment and reduces the spread of microorganisms.

9. Check solution using five rights of drug administration. Make sure prescribed additives such as potassium and vitamins are added, if ordered.
Note: When using bottled IV solution, remove metal cap and metal and rubber discs beneath cap.

IV solutions are medications and should be checked carefully to reduce risk of error.

Permits entry of infusion tubing into solution.

Venipuncture With an Over-the-Needle Plastic Catheter—cont'd

STEPS	RATIONALE
10. Open infusion set, maintaining sterility of both ends.	Prevents bacteria from entering infusion equipment.
11. Place roller clamp just below drip chamber (see the illustration below) and move roller clamp to off position.	Close proximity of roller clamp to drip chamber allows more accurate regulation of flow rate. Prevents accidental spillage of fluid on client, nurse, bed, or floor.
12. Insert infusion set into fluid bag:	Maintains sterility of solution.
a. Remove protective cover from IV bag without touching opening (see the illustration below).	
b. Remove protector cap from tubing insertion spike, not touching spike, and insert spike into opening of IV bag (see the illustration below). Or insert spike into black rubber stopper of IV bottle.	Permits entry of infusion solution into tubing. Prevents contamination of solution from contaminated insertion spike.

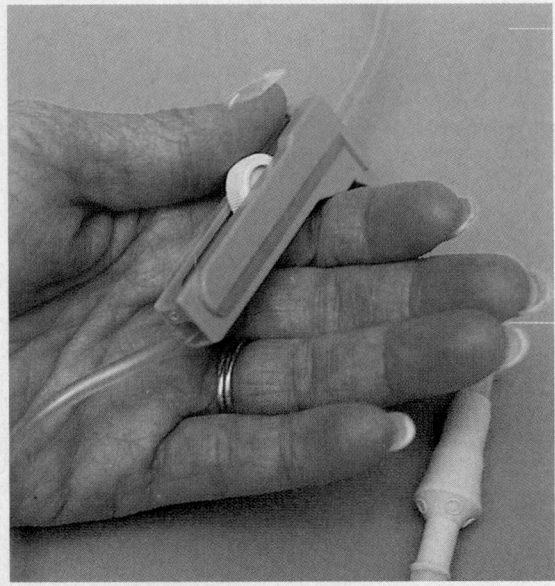

Step 11

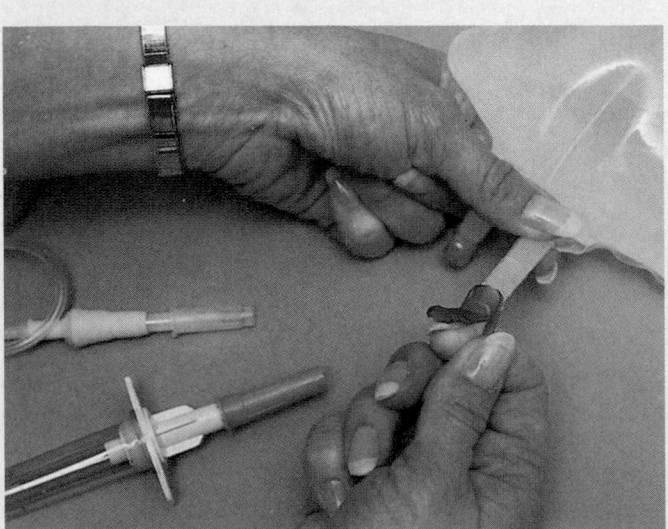

Step 12a

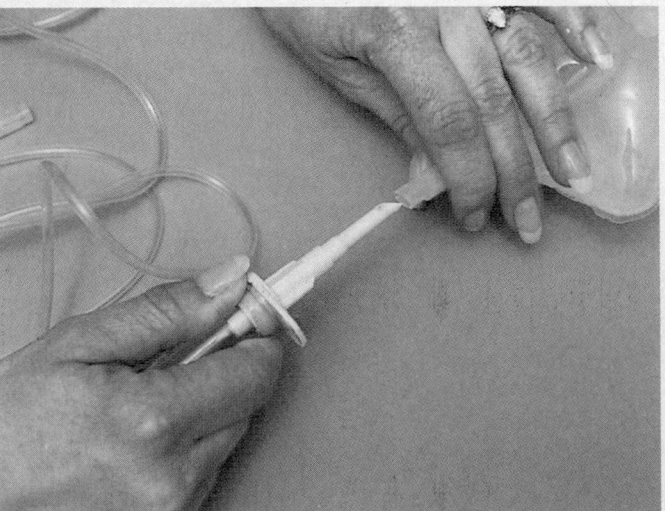

Step 12b

Venipuncture With an Over-the-Needle Plastic Catheter—cont'd

STEPS	RATIONALE

13. Fill infusion tubing:
  a. Compress drip chamber and release. — Creates suction effect. Fluid enters drip chamber.
  b. Remove needle protector and release roller clamp to allow fluid to travel from drip chamber through tubing to needle adapter. Return roller clamp to off position after tube is filled. — Removes air from tubing and permits it to fill with solution.
  c. Be certain tubing is clear of air and air bubbles. — Large bubbles can act as emboli.
  d. Replace needle protector. — Maintains system sterility.
14. Select distal site of vein to be used. — If sclerosing or damage to vein occurs, proximal site of same vein still usable.
15. If large amount of body hair is present at needle insertion site, clip it. — Reduces risk of contamination from bacteria on hair. Also assists in maintaining intactness of IV dressing and makes removal of adhesive tape less painful.

Shaving may cause microabrasions and predisposes to infection (Metheny, 1996).

16. If possible, place extremity in dependent position. — Permits venous dilation and visibility
17. Place tourniquet 10 to 12 cm (4-5 inches) above insertion site. Tourniquet should obstruct venous, not arterial flow (see the illustration below). Check distal pulse. — Diminished arterial flow prevents venous filling.
18. Select well-dilated vein (see the illustration below). Methods to foster vein dilation include stroking extremity from proximal to distal, opening and closing fist, lightly tapping over vein, and applying warmth. Note: Be sure needle adapter end of infusion set is nearby and on sterile gauze or towel. — Increases venous dilation.

Permits smooth, quick connection of infusion to needle after vein is punctured.

19. Apply disposable gloves. — Decreases exposure to HIV, hepatitis, and other blood-borne organisms.
20. Cleanse insertion site with firm, concentric, circular motion outward from insertion site using povidone-iodine solution. Allow to dry (see the illustration below). If client is allergic to iodine, use 70% alcohol for 30 seconds. — Povidone-iodine is topical antiinfective that reduces skin surface bacteria. It must be dry to be effective.

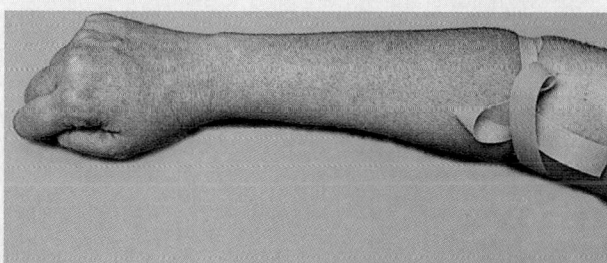

Step 17

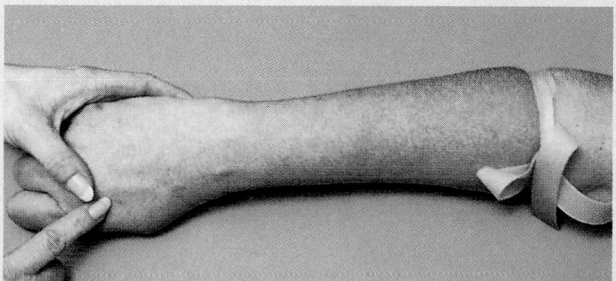

Step 18

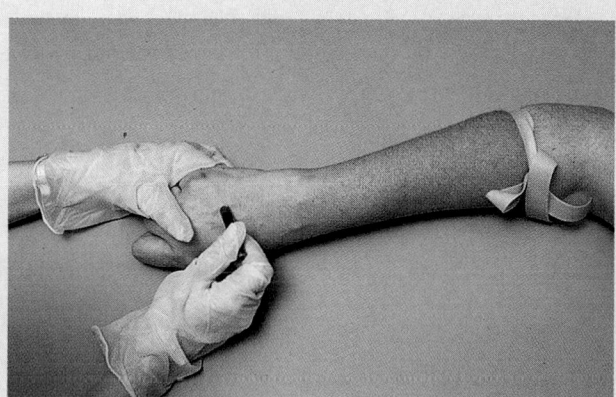

Step 20

Continued.

PROCEDURE 45-1

Venipuncture With an Over-the-Needle Plastic Catheter—cont'd

STEPS	RATIONALE

21. Perform venipuncture. Anchor vein by placing thumb over vein and by stretching skin against direction of insertion 5-7 cm (2 to 3 inches) distal to site:

   a. ONC: insert bevel at 20 to 30 degree angle in direction of venous blood return distal to actual site of venipuncture.

Allows nurse to place needle parallel with vein. Thus when vein is punctured, risk of puncturing both sides is reduced.

   b. Butterfly needle: place needle at 20 to 30 degree angle with bevel up, about 1 cm (half inch) distal to site of venipuncture.

Increased venous pressure from tourniquet increases back flow of blood into catheter or tubing. Stylet helps puncture skin and advance catheter but must be removed to avoid puncture of vein.

22. Look for blood return through tubing of butterfly needle or flashback chamber on ONC, indicating that needle has entered vein. Lower needle until almost flush with skin. Advance catheter about one-quarter inch into vein and then loosen stylet (see the illustration below). Continue advancing flexible catheter or butterfly needle until hub rests at venipuncture site.

23. Stabilizing catheter with one hand, release tourniquet and remove stylet from ONC.

Reduces back flow of blood.

24. Connect needle adapter of infusion to hub of ONC or needle. Do not touch point of entry of needle adapter or inside hub of ONC.

Prompt connection of infusion set maintains patency of vein. Maintains sterility.

25. Release roller clamp to begin infusion at rate to maintain patency of IV line.

Permits venous flow and prevents clotting of vein and obstruction of flow of IV solution.

26. Secure IV catheter or needle:

   a. Place narrow piece (half inch) of tape under hub of catheter with adhesive side up and cross tape over hub.

Prevents accidental removal of catheter from vein.

   b. Place small amount of povidone-iodine solution or ointment at venipuncture site. Allow solution to dry according to agency policy.

Povidone-iodine solution or ointment is topical antiseptic that reduces bacteria on skin and decreases risk of local or systemic infection. When transparent dressing is used, povidone-iodine solution is recommended; ointment interferes with adherence of dressing to skin.

   c. Place second piece of narrow tape directly across catheter's hub.

Prevents accidental disconnection of IV infusion.

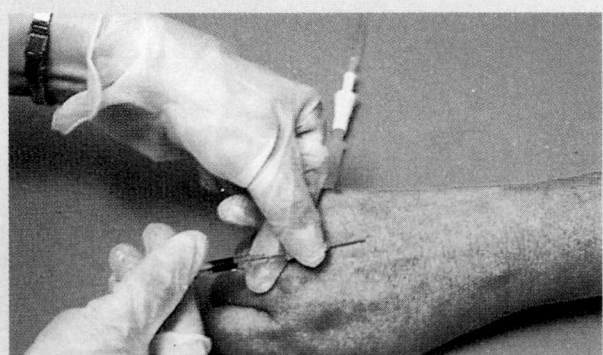

Step 22

Venipuncture With an Over-the-Needle Plastic Catheter—cont'd

STEPS	RATIONALE

26. Secure IV catheter or needle—cont'd

  d. Place transparent dressing over venipuncture site, following manufacturer's directions (see the illustration at right). (Alternate method: place 2 × 2 gauze dressing over venipuncture site and catheter hub. Do not cover connection between IV tubing and catheter hub. Secure it with two 1-inch pieces of tape.) Gloves may be removed to prevent sticking to dressing.

Transparent dressing allows continual observation of venipuncture site. Allows for tubing change without disturbing dressing.

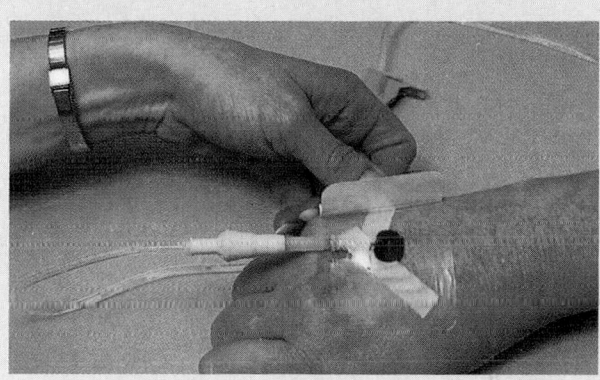

Step 26d

  e. Secure infusion tubing to catheter with piece of 1-inch tape.

Further stabilizes connection of infusion to catheter.

27. Write date, time of placement of IV line, size of needle, and nurse's initial and title on IV dressing.

Provides immediate data as to time of IV insertion and subsequent dressing changes.

28. Adjust flow rate to correct gtts/min.

Maintains correct rate of flow for IV solution.

29. Discard gloves and supplies and wash hands

Reduces transmission of microorganisms.

30. Observe client every hour to determine response to fluid therapy:

  a. Correct amount of solution as prescribed

  b. Proper flow rate (gtts/min)

  c. Patency of IV

  d. Absence of infiltration, phlebitis, or inflammation

Provides continuous evaluation of type and amount of fluid delivered to client. Hourly inspection prevents accidental fluid overload or inadequate hydration.

31. Record in nurses' notes type of fluid, insertion site, flow rate, size and type of IV catheter or needle, and time infusion was begun. Note response to IV fluid, amount infused, and integrity and patency of IV system (whether infusing by gravity or by pump), according to agency policy.

Documents initiation of IV fluid therapy as ordered by physician. Follow-up documentation provides data about response to therapy.

The nurse can assess patency by lowering the IV bag below the level of the insertion site and observing for a blood return. If no blood return occurs and fluid does not flow easily from the drip chamber when the roller clamp is opened, a clot may be present at the catheter tip.

A knot or kink in the tubing can decrease the flow rate. If the tubing is kinked under the IV dressing, the nurse must open the dressing to straighten the tubing. Frequently the flow rate resumes after the tubing is straight. The client may also occlude the tubing by lying or sitting on it. The height of the IV bag can affect flow rates. Raising the bag may increase the rate because of gravity.

The extremity position can decrease flow rates, particularly with IV sites at the wrist or elbow. Occasionally the use of an arm board helps keep the joint extended. Sometimes the best option for the client is an infusion in a new location. However, before discontinuing an infusion hampered by an extremity position, the nurse must be sure that the client has other accessible veins.

These influences on IV flow rates can occur with any client at any time. When caring for a client with an infusion, the nurse should assess the site and the infusion rate at least every hour.

Children, older adults, clients with severe head trauma,

Regulating IV Flow Rates

STEPS	RATIONALE
1. Observe patency of IV line and needle:	For fluid to infuse at proper rate, IV line and needle must be free of kinks, knots, and clots.
a. Open drip regulator and observe for rapid flow of fluid from IV solution into drip chamber, and then close drip regulator to prescribed rate.	Rapid flow of fluid into drip chamber denotes patency of IV line. Closing drip to prescribed rate prevents fluid overload.
b. If fluid does not flow, lower IV fluid bottle or bag below level of infusion site and observe for blood return.	May indicate that needle is patent and in vein. Venous pressure is greater than pressure in IV tubing.
2. Check medical record for correct solution and additives. Usual order includes solution for 24 hours, usually divided into 2 or 3 L. Occasionally, IV order contains only 1 L to keep vein open (KVO). Record also shows time over which each liter is to infuse.	IV fluids are medications. Five rights are followed to decrease chance of medication error.

3. Know drop factor in gtt/ml of infusion set, for example:
Microdrip: 60 gtt/ml
Macrodrip (Perry and Potter, 1994):
   Abbott Lab.   15 gtt/ml
   Travenol Lab. 10gtt/ml
   McGaw Lab.   15 gtt/ml
   Baxter   10 gtt/ml
	Microdroppers, also called *minidrip*, universally deliver 60 gtt/ml. However, commercial parenteral administration sets for macrodrip exist. Nurse should know infusion set drop factor.

4. Select one of the following formulas to calculate flow rate (gtt/min) after calculating ml/hr if necessary (Perry and Potter, 1994):
total volume (ml) ÷ hours of infusion = ml/hr
   a. ml/hr ÷ 60 min = ml/min
   b. ml/hr × drop factor ÷ 60 min = gtt/min
	After hourly rate has been determined, formula will give correct flow rate in gtt/min.

5. If infusion pump or volume control device is used, place it at the bedside.	Increases accuracy of fluid delivery rate.

6. Determine hourly rate by dividing volume by hours, for example:
   1000 ml ÷ 8 hrs = 125 ml/hr
or if 4 L are ordered for 24 hours:
   4000 ml ÷ 24 hrs = 166.7 or 167 ml/hr
	Provides for infusion of fluid at steady rate during prescribed period.

7. Place volume label vertically on IV bottle or bag next to volume markings. Mark adhesive tape base on hourly flow rate. For example: if entire volume of fluid is to be infused over 8, 10, or 12 hr, respective designations will be marked on tape (see the illustration below).	Gives nurse visual cue whether fluids are being administered over correct period.

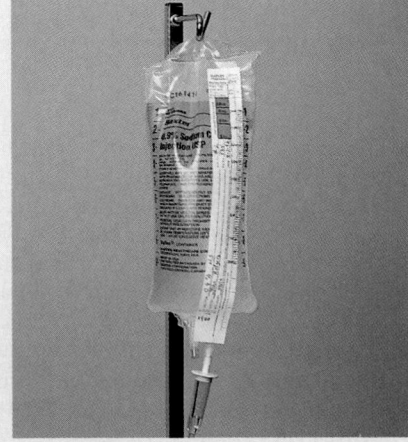

Step 7

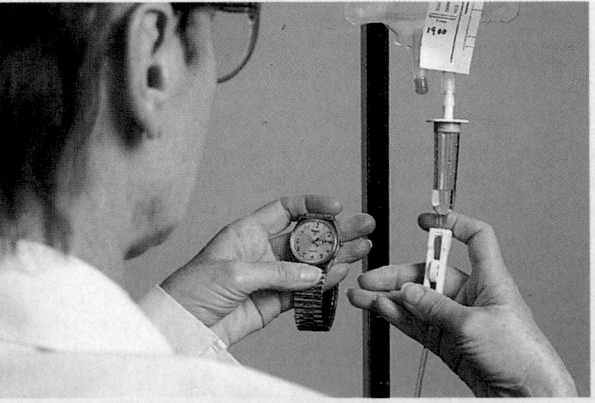

Step 9

Regulating IV Flow Rates—cont'd

STEPS	RATIONALE

8. After hourly rate has been determined, calculate minute rate based on drop factor of infusion set. Minidrip or microdrip infusion set has drop factor of 60 gtt/ml. Regular drip or macrodrip used in this example has drop factor of 15 gtt/ml. Using formula, calculate minute flow rates: Bottle 1: deliver 125 ml/hr.

Allows nurse to calculate minute flow rate based on this formula:

Microdrip:

$$\frac{125 \text{ ml} \times 60 \text{ gtt/min}}{60 \text{ min}} = \frac{7500}{60} = 125 \text{ gtt/min}$$

Total volume × drop factor ÷ Infusion time in minutes = gtt/min

Macrodrip:

$$\frac{125 \text{ ml} \times 15 \text{ gtt/min}}{60 \text{ min}} = 31 \text{ to } 32 \text{ gtt/min}$$

9. Time flow rate by counting drops in drip chamber for 1 minute by watch, and then adjust roller clamp to increase or decrease rate of infusion (see the illustration on p. 1276). Repeat until flow rate is accurate.

Ensures accurate rate of infusion. Determines whether fluids are being administered too slowly or too fast.

10. Follow this procedure for:

  a. Infusion pump:

    (1) Place electronic eye on drip chamber below origin of drop and above fluid level in chamber (see the illustration below).

IV infusion pumps monitor fluids based on flow rate or gtt/min. Infusion pump has electronic eye that counts number of drops flowing from administration set.

    (2) Place IV infusion tubing with ridges of control box in direction of flow (i.e., portion of tubing nearest IV bag at top and portion of tubing nearest client at bottom) (see the illustration below, right). Required gtt/min or volume per hour is selected, door to control chamber is closed, power button is turned on, and start button pressed.

Infusion pumps move fluid by compressing and milking tubing, thus propelling fluid through tubing.

    (3) Ensure that drip rate regulator on tubing is in open position while infusion pump is in use.

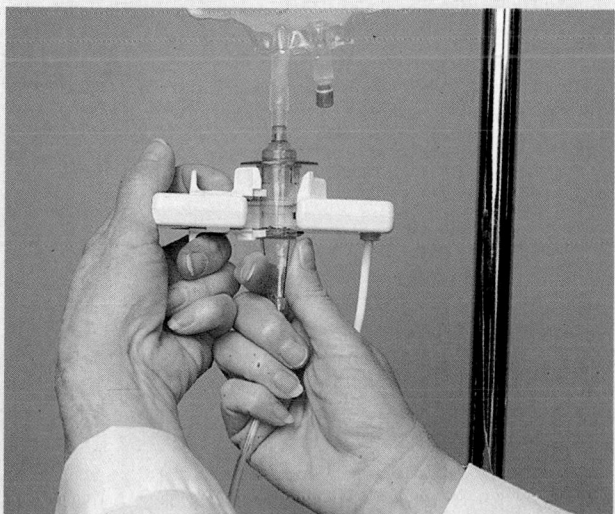

Step 10a(1)

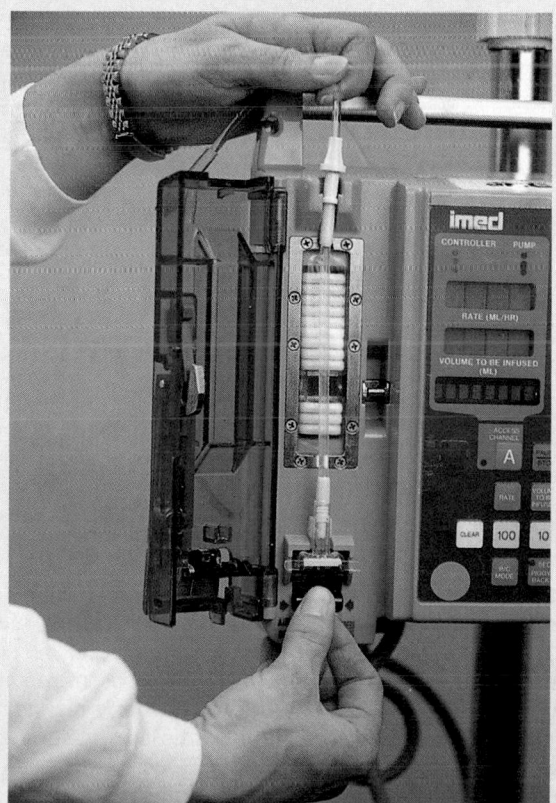

Step 10a(2)

Continued.

Regulating IV Flow Rates—cont'd

STEPS	RATIONALE
10. Follow this procedure for—cont'd	
a. Infusion pump—cont'd	
(4) Monitor infusion rate at least hourly.	Infusion pumps are not infallible and do not replace frequent, accurate assessments.
(5) Assess patency of IV system when alarm sounds.	Alarm indicates that electronic eye has not noted precise number of drips from drip chamber.
b. Volume control device:	
(1) Place volume control device between IV bag and insertion spike of infusion set (see the illustration below).	Reduces risk of sudden increases in fluid volume.
(2) Place 2 hr portion of fluid into device.	Prevents IV line from running dry if nurse does not return it exactly 1 hr. In addition, if accidental increase in flow rate occurs, client receives 2 hr portion of fluid at most.

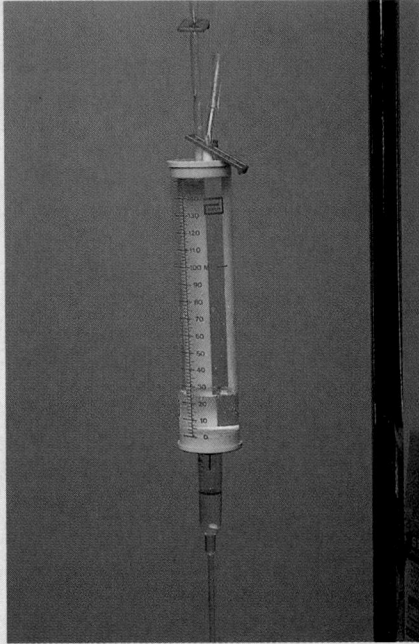

Step 10b(1)

STEPS	RATIONALE
(3) Assess IV system at least hourly and add fluid to device. Regulate flow rate.	Maintains patency of IV system.
11. Observe client hourly to determine response to IV therapy and restoration of fluid and electrolyte balance. Also check IV site for signs of infiltration, inflammation, and phlebitis.	Signs and symptoms of dehydration or overhydration warrant changing rate of fluid infused. Signs of infiltration, inflammation, and phlebitis warrant changing IV site.
12. Record rate of infusion, gtt/min and ml/hr, in client's chart as required by agency policy.	Documents that prescribed IV flow is being delivered to client.

and clients susceptible to volume overload must be protected from sudden increases in infusion volumes. Sudden increases can occur accidentally. For example, a restless client may, with a sudden movement, loosen the roller clamp and increase the flow rate, or the flow rate may be accidentally increased if the client ambulates. A sudden increase in IV volume can result in serious illness or death. Volume control devices, such as a Volutrol or buret, can prevent sudden increases in volume (see Chapter 35).

A volume control device is placed between the IV bag and insertion spike of the infusion set or may be part of the infusion set. Most control devices can hold 150 ml. Nurses usually put 2 hours' worth of fluid in the buret. If the nurse does not return to the client in exactly 1 hour, the IV line does not run dry. In addition, if an accidental increase in flow rate occurs, the client receives at most 2 hours' allotment of fluid instead of 500 or 1000 ml.

Maintaining the system. After the IV line is in place and the flow rate is regulated, the nurse must maintain the system. The nurse provides comfort and assistance with hygiene measures, meals, and ambulation. IV catheters and drugs, especially those with potassium, can cause

Changing IV Solutions and Tubing

STEPS	RATIONALE

CHANGING IV SOLUTION

1. Identify client. Review physician's orders and have next solution prepared at least 1 hr before needed. If solution is prepared in pharmacy, be sure it has been delivered to floor. Check that solution is correct and properly labeled.

Ensures that correct client undergoes procedure.
Prevents finding empty IV bag without having replacement. Checking prevents medication error. If order is written for KVO, change solution every 24 hrs. Sterility of solution cannot be ensured longer than 24 hrs.

2. Prepare to change solution when less than 50 ml remains in bottle or bag.

Prevents air from entering IV tubing and maintains patency of tubing and catheter or needle.

3. Be sure drip chamber is half full.

Provides IV fluid to vein while bag is being changed.

4. Wash hands.

Reduces transmission of microorganisms.

5. Prepare new solution for changing. If using plastic bag, remove protective cover from entry site. If using glass bottle, remove metal cap, metal disc, and rubber disc. Maintain sterility of entry site on bag or bottle.

Permits quick, smooth, and organized change from old to new solution.

6. Move roller clamp to reduce flow rate.

Prevents solution remaining in drip chamber from emptying while changing solutions.

7. Remove old solution from IV pole.

Brings work to nurse's eye level.

8. Quickly remove spike from old IV solution, and without touching tip, spike new solution bottle.

Reduces risk of solution in drip chamber (Step 3) running dry and maintains sterility.

9. Hang new bag or bottle of solution. Discard empty bag or bottle according to agency policy.

Allows gravity to assist with delivery of IV fluid into drip chamber.

10. Check for and remove air in tubing.

Reduces risk of air embolus.

11. Make sure drip chamber contains solution.

Reduces risk of air entering IV tubing.

12. Regulate flow rate to prescribed rate.

Restores fluid balance and delivers fluid as ordered.

13. Observe IV system for patency, absence of infiltration, phlebitis, and inflammation. Observe response to IV therapy.

Provides ongoing evaluation of response to IV therapy.

CHANGING IV TUBING

14. Determine when new infusion set is warranted:
    a. Hanging first solution of day

Changing tubing prevents infection. Procedure is simplified by changing tubing with new solution.

    b. Puncture of infusion tubing

Punctured tubing can allow entry of bacteria into bloodstream.

    c. Contamination of tubing

Contamination of tubing can allow entry of bacteria into bloodstream.

    d. Occlusion of IV tubing (e.g., after infusion of packed RBCs, whole blood, or albumin)

Whole blood or blood component products may occlude or partially occlude IV tubing.

    e. Date on tubing indicates that tubing has been in place 48 hr.

Tubing should be changed every 48 hrs (Gardner, 1996).

15. Assemble the following:
    a. Infusion tubing
    b. Sterile 2 × 2 gauze
    c. If new IV dressing must be applied:
       (1) Sterile 2 × 2 gauze or transparent dressing
       (2) Povidone-iodine ointment or solution
       (3) Adhesive remover
       (4) Alcohol swabs
       (5) Strips of tape or polyurethane film dressing
       (6) Disposable gloves

Enables nurse to efficiently and safely complete the procedure.

16. Explain procedure to client.

Promotes cooperation and prevents sudden movement of extremity, which could dislodge needle or catheter.

17. Wash hands.

Reduces transmission of microorganisms.

18. Open new infusion set, keeping protective coverings over infusion spike and insertion site for butterfly needle or ONC.

Provides nurse with ready access to new infusion set and maintains sterility of infusion set.

Continued.

PROCEDURE 45-3

Changing IV Solutions and Tubing—cont'd

STEPS	RATIONALE

CHANGING IV TUBING—cont'd

19. Apply nonsterile disposable gloves.

Decreases risk of exposure to HIV, hepatitis, and other blood-borne bacteria.

20. Place sterile 2 × 2 gauze on bed near IV puncture site.

Provides sterile field for new sterile needle adapter before connection to IV needle or catheter.

21. If needle or catheter hub is not visible, remove IV dressing. Do not remove tape that secures needle or catheter to skin.

Needle hub must be accessible to provide smooth transition when removing old tubing and inserting new tubing.

22. Move roller clamp of new IV tubing to off position.

Prevents spillage of solution after new bag or bottle is spiked.

23. Slow rate of infusion by regulating drip rate on old tubing.

Prevents complete infusion of solution remaining in tubing.

24. With old tubing in place, compress drip chamber and fill chamber.

Provides surplus in drip chamber so that there is sufficient fluid to maintain patency while changing tubing.

25. Discontinue old tubing from solution and hang drip chamber over IV pole.

Allows fluid to continue to flow through catheter while new tubing is prepared.

26. Place insertion spike of new tubing into old IV solution opening and hang solution on pole.

Permits flow of solution into new infusion tubing.

27. Compress and release drip chamber on new tubing.

Allows drip chamber to fill and promotes rapid, smooth flow of solution through new tubing.

28. Open roller clamp, remove protective cap from needle adapter, and flush tubing with solution.

Removes air from tubing and replaces it with fluid.

29. Place needle adapter of new IV tubing, with protective cap off, between sterile 2 × 2 gauze near IV site.

Will allow smooth, quick insertion of new tubing into needle hub while maintaining sterility of infusion tubing.

30. Turn roller clamp on old tubing to off position.

Prevents spillage of fluid as tubing is removed from needle hub.

31. Stabilize hub of IV catheter or needle, gently pull out old tubing, and quickly insert needle adapter of new tubing into hub.

Prevents accidental displacement of catheter or needle. Prevents clot formation in catheter or needle.

32. Open roller clamp on new tubing.

Permits solution to enter catheter or tubing.

33. Regulate IV drip according to physician's order and monitor rate hourly.

Maintains infusion flow at prescribed rate.

34. If necessary, apply new dressing (Procedure 45-4).

Reduces risk of bacterial infection from skin.

35. Discard old tubing and gloves in container for contaminated materials, and wash hands.

Reduces transmission of microorganisms.

36. Evaluate flow rate and observe connection site for leakage.

Maintains prescribed rate of flow of IV therapy and determines whether fit is secure.

37. Record changing of tubing and solution on client's record and place piece of tape with date and time below level of drip chamber. Record fluid infused on I & O form.

Documents procedure and records that measures to maintain sterility were implemented. Provides visual cue to all care providers about when IV tubing was changed.

---

discomfort and burning sensations. Clients must be reassured that occasional discomfort is expected. However, the nurse should work with the physician to add a neutralizer to the potassium mixture to prevent this discomfort. Occasionally it is necessary to start a new IV line in a larger vein.

Because a client with an infusion in the arm finds it difficult to meet hygiene needs, the nurse should help with bathing and changing gowns. It helps to use a special IV gown specifically made with snaps along the top sleeve seam to facilitate changing the gown without disturbing the venipuncture site. Gowns without such snaps are changed by following six steps for maximal arm mobility and speed:

1. Remove the sleeve of the gown from the uninvolved arm (without IV).
2. Remove the sleeve of the gown from the involved arm (with IV).
3. Remove the IV bottle or bag from its stand and pass it and the tubing through the sleeve.
4. Place the IV bottle or bag and tubing through the sleeve of the clean gown and hang on its stand.
5. Place the involved arm through the gown sleeve.
6. Place the uninvolved arm through the gown sleeve.

Changing an IV Dressing

STEPS	RATIONALE
1. Assess need to change dressing:	
a. Determine when IV dressing was last changed. Many agencies require nurse to write date and time on dressing itself.	Provides information regarding length of time that present dressing has been in place. In addition, nurse is able to plan for dressing change.
b. Observe present dressing for moisture.	Moisture is medium for bacterial growth. Moisture on sterile dressing renders dressing contaminated.
c. Observe present dressing for intactness.	Nonadhering dressing increases risk of bacterial contamination to venipuncture site or displacement of catheter.
d. Observe IV system for proper functioning or complications: kinks in infusion tubing or IV catheter, infiltration, and inflammation.	Unexplained decrease in flow rate or pain and swelling at venipuncture site require nurse to investigate placement and patency of IV catheter.
2. Assemble necessary equipment:	Enables nurse to efficiently and safely complete procedure.
a. Sterile 2 × 2 gauze or transparent dressing	
b. Povidone-iodine ointment or solution	
c. Adhesive remover	
d. Alcohol swabs	
e. Strips of tape or polyurethane film dressing	
f. Disposable gloves	
3. Explain procedure to client.	Assists in obtaining client cooperation and gives time frame around which client can plan personal activities.
4. Wash hands.	Reduces transmission of microorganisms.
5. Apply disposable gloves.	Reduces risk of contact with HIV, hepatitis, and other bloodborne bacteria.
6. Remove transparent dressing in direction of client's hair growth, or remove tape and gauze from old dressing one layer at a time. For both transparent and gauze dressings, leave tape that secures IV needle or catheter in place.	Prevents accidental displacement of catheter or needle, which can occur if catheter tubing becomes tangled between two layers of dressing.
7. If infiltration, phlebitis, or clot occurs or if ordered to do so by physician, discontinue IV infusion:	
a. Turn roller clamp to off position.	Prevents spillage of IV fluid on bed, client, nurse, floor.
b. Place sterile gauze or alcohol pad over venipuncture site and remove catheter or needle by pulling straight away from site.	Prevents damage to vein. Check catheter or needle to be sure it is intact.
c. Apply pressure to site for 1 to 2 minutes.	Controls bleeding and hematoma formation.
8. If IV is infusing properly, remove tape securing needle or catheter. Stabilize needle or catheter with one hand.	Exposes venipuncture site. Prevents accidental displacement of catheter or needle.
9. Use adhesive remover to cleanse skin and remove adhesive residue.	Adhesive residue decreases ability of new tape to adhere tightly to skin.
10. Using circular motion from site outward, cleanse insertion site with povidone-iodine solution. Allow to dry for 30 seconds.	Circular motion prevents cross-contamination from skin bacteria near venipuncture site. Povidone-iodine is topical antiinfective that reduces skin surface bacteria.
11. Replace strip of half-inch adhesive tape under catheter with adhesive side up to anchor catheter or needle.	Prevents accidental displacement of catheter or needle.
12. Place povidone-iodine ointment or solution on venipuncture site. Allow solution to dry. Place second piece of narrow tape directly across catheter.	Povidone-iodine solution or ointment is topical antiseptic germicide that reduces skin bacteria and reduces risk of local or systemic infection. When transparent dressing is used, povidone-iodine solution is recommended; ointment interferes with adherence of dressing to skin.
13. Place 2 × 2 gauze or transparent dressing over venipuncture site. If transparent dressing is selected, apply it in direction of hair growth (see manufacturer's directions).	Provides barrier against bacteria. Reduces discomfort when dressing is removed.
14. Anchor IV tubing with additional pieces of tape. (Do not cover transparent dressing.)	Prevents accidental displacement of needle or catheter or separation of tubing from needle adapter.

Continued.

Changing an IV Dressing—cont'd

STEPS	RATIONALE
15. Place date and time of dressing change directly on dressing (following agency policy).	Documents dressing change.
16. Discard equipment in appropriate container, remove and dispose of gloves, and wash hands.	Reduces transmission of microorganisms.
17. Reassess functioning and patency of IV system in response to dressing change.	Validates that IV is patent and functioning correctly.
18. Record in nurses' notes time dressing was changed, types of dressing used, patency of IV system, and observation of venipuncture site.	Documents that dressing was changed, description of IV system functioning, and venipuncture site free of infection.

The client with an arm or a hand infusion is able to walk, unless contraindicated. A walking IV pole, a standard IV pole with wheels, is needed. The nurse helps the client out of bed and places the pole next to the involved arm. The client is instructed to hold onto the pole with the involved hand and to push it while walking. The nurse assesses the equipment to make sure that the IV bag is at the proper height, that there is no tension on the tubing, and that the flow rate is correct. The nurse should instruct the client to report any blood in the tubing, a stoppage in the flow, or increased discomfort.

Because clients receiving IV therapy to restore a FVD may require frequent changing of solutions, the nurse should allow adequate time for this. Occasionally, clients require an IV infusion to deliver a drug every 4, 6, or 8 hours. An hourly infusion flow of about 10 to 15 ml/hr is used to keep the vein open (KVO) using a microdrip infusion set. A new solution bag or bottle should be hung at least once every 24 hours, even if the old bag is not empty, because the sterility of the solution cannot be guaranteed for longer than a day. When an IV solution container is changed, the nurse uses sterile technique and follows an organized procedure (Procedure 45-3).

Technically, IV tubing can remain sterile for 48 to 72 hours. Each institution will have a policy determining how often dressings, tubing, and sites should be changed. To prevent entry of bacteria into the bloodstream, sterility must be maintained. The procedure for changing tubing is much easier and more efficient if the nurse changes the infusion tubing when preparing to hang a new IV bag or bottle (Procedure 45-3).

The dressing over the IV insertion site is changed according to hospital policy. Usually, gauze or transparent dressings are used (Procedure 45-4). Transparent dressings enable the nurse to continually assess venipuncture sites. The previously recommended practice of daily dressing changes has been reduced to every 48 to 72 hours when IV sites are changed (Gardner, 1996). This practice is more cost effective and does not increase the risk of infection.

Complications of IV therapy. The major complications of IV therapy are infiltration, phlebitis, fluid overload, bleeding, and infection. An **infiltration** occurs when IV fluids enter the subcutaneous space around the venipuncture site. This is manifested as swelling (from increased tissue fluid) and pallor (caused by decreased circulation) around the venipuncture site. Fluid may be flowing through the IV line at a decreased rate or may have stopped. Pain may also occur, usually resulting from edema, and increases in proportion to the amount of infiltration.

When infiltration occurs, infusion must be discontinued, and if necessary, the needle is reinserted at another site. To reduce discomfort caused by infiltration, the nurse raises the extremity, which promotes venous drainage and helps decrease edema, and wraps the extremity in a warm towel for 20 minutes, which increases circulation and reduces pain and edema.

Phlebitis is an inflammation of the vein caused by the catheter or by the chemical irritation of additives and drugs given intravenously. Signs and symptoms include pain, increased skin temperature over the vein, and in some instances redness at the site or progressing along the path of the vein. The IV line must be discontinued and a new line inserted in another vein. Warm, moist heat on the site of phlebitis can offer some relief to the client. Phlebitis is potentially dangerous because blood clots (thrombophlebitis) can occur and in some cases may result in emboli.

Fluid overload occurs when the client has received too-rapid administration of solutions. Assessment findings are dyspnea, crackles in the lungs, and tachycardia. The nurse should slow the rate of infusion, notify the physician, and be prepared to give diuretic medications. Prompt action is necessary to prevent worsening of the condition or even death.

Bleeding can occur around the venipuncture site during infusion. Bleeding is common in clients who have received heparin or who have a clotting disorder. If bleeding occurs around the venipuncture site and the catheter is within the vein, a pressure dressing may be applied over the site to control it. Bleeding from a vein is usually a slow, continuous seepage and is not fatal.

Infusion-related infections are caused by contamination of the IV system, venipuncture site, or the solution itself. Clinical manifestations of these infections include purulent thrombophlebitis, cellulitis, and site infections, as evidenced by erythema, swelling, and pain at the venipuncture site.

Infusion-related infections can be reduced by four interventions. The nurse uses vigorous handwashing techniques to remove gram-negative organisms before applying gloves for the venipuncture procedure. The nurse also changes IV solutions at least every 24 hours. The nurse should also replace all peripheral venous catheters, including heparin locks, at least every 72 hours. In addition, the nurse maintains sterility of the IV system when changing tubing, solutions, and dressings (Potter and Perry, 1995).

Discontinuing IV infusions. Discontinuing an infusion is necessary after the prescribed amount of fluids has been infused, when an infiltration occurs, if phlebitis is present, or if the infusion catheter or needle develops a clot at its tip. The nurse discontinuing an infusion first removes the tape and dressing in the same manner as for the daily infusion dressing changes. The nurse moves the roller clamp to the *off* position to prevent spillage of IV fluid. The nurse applies disposable gloves and places a gauze or alcohol pad over the venipuncture site and, using the other hand, withdraws the catheter needle by pulling straight back from the puncture site. The nurse applies pressure to the site for 1 to 2 minutes to control bleeding and prevent hematoma formation. Clients who have received heparin require longer pressure because of the action of heparin on blood-clotting mechanisms. If needed, the nurse applies a sterile dressing over the venipuncture site. The nurse records the amount of fluid infused and the time of the discontinuation.

Blood Replacement. Blood replacement or transfusion is the IV administration of whole blood or a component such as plasma, packed RBCs, or platelets. The following list includes objectives for blood transfusion:

1. To increase circulating blood volume after surgery, trauma, or hemorrhage
2. To increase the number of RBCs and to maintain hemoglobin levels in clients with severe anemia
3. To provide selected cellular components as replacement therapy (e.g., plasma-clotting factors to help control bleeding in clients with hemophilia)

Blood groups and types. The most important grouping for transfusion is the ABO system, which includes the following groups: A, B, O, and AB. The determination of blood groups is based on the presence or absence of A and B red cell antigens. Individuals with A antigens, B antigens, or no antigens belong to groups A, B, and O, respectively. The person with A and B antigens has AB blood (Long et al, 1993).

Agglutinins, or antibodies that work against the A and B antigens, are called *anti-A* and *anti-B agglutinins*. These agglutinins occur naturally (Long et al, 1993). Individuals with type A blood naturally produce anti-B agglutinins in their plasma. Similarly, type B individuals naturally produce anti-A agglutinins in their plasma. A type O individual naturally produces both agglutinins, which is why a person with type O blood is considered a universal donor. An AB type individual produces neither antibody, which is why type AB individuals can be universal recipients. If blood that is mismatched with the client's blood is transfused, a transfusion reaction occurs. The transfusion reaction is an antigen-antibody reaction and can range from a mild response to severe anaphylactic shock.

Another consideration when matching for blood transfusions is the Rh factor, an antigenic substance in the RBCs of most people. A person with the factor is Rh positive, whereas a person without it is Rh negative. If the blood given to an Rh-positive person is Rh negative, **hemolysis** (RBC destruction) and anemia occur. If an Rh-negative mother gives birth to an Rh-positive baby, the infant may be exposed to antibodies in the mother's Rh-negative blood and destruction of the infant's RBCs can result.

Autotransfusion. **Autotransfusion** is the collection, anticoagulation, filtration, and reinfusion of blood from an active bleeding site. Because the reinfused blood is the client's own, there are many advantages to autotransfusion. The risk of technical errors of blood typing and crossmatching is eliminated. Possible adverse effects associated with homologous blood transfusion are also eliminated. An homologous transfusion occurs when blood is donated by one person and transfused to another. An homologous transfusion occurs within the same species. Autotransfusion reduces reduces risks of homologous transfusion such as possible exposure to serum hepatitis, HIV, and other blood-borne infections.

When an elective surgical procedure is anticipated and transfusions are required, some individuals choose to give one or more units of their own blood in advance. This blood is stored and is available intraoperatively and postoperatively. This, too, is a type of autotransfusion.

Blood transfusions. Transfusing blood or blood components is a nursing procedure. The nurse is responsible for assessment before and during the transfusion and regulation of the transfusion (Procedure 45-5).

If the client has an IV line in place, the nurse should assess the venipuncture site for signs of infection or infiltration. The nurse should also determine whether the IV venipuncture was performed with an 18- or 19-gauge catheter. The large-gauge catheter promotes flow because the molecules of blood and its components are larger than the molecules of IV fluids. A large catheter also prevents hemolysis. The nurse should determine that the catheter is patent and functioning properly. Tubing for blood transfusion has an in-line filter and must be primed with 0.9% normal saline only. Use of any other IV solution results in hemolysis.

Pretransfusion assessment also includes obtaining information from the client. The nurse asks whether the client knows the reason for the blood transfusion and whether the client has ever had a transfusion or a transfusion reaction. A client who has had a transfusion reaction is usually at no greater risk for a reaction with a subsequent transfusion. However, the client may be anxious about the transfusion, necessitating nursing intervention.

Pretransfusion assessment must include a baseline measurement of vital signs. These values must be recorded before the nurse gives any blood products because a change in vital signs can indicate a reaction.

When giving a transfusion, the nurse explains the procedure, asks the client to report any side effects, and makes sure the client has signed an informed consent. The nurse establishes the IV line, primes it with 0.9% normal saline, and hangs a solution container of 0.9% normal saline for use after the transfusion. The nurse then follows established procedures for obtaining blood products. With another registered nurse, the nurse checks the identity of the blood products, the client, and the compatibility of the blood to be infused against the client's blood. The infusion is begun slowly. The infusion is maintained, side effects are monitored, and the transfusion is recorded.

During blood infusion the client is at risk for a reaction,

PROCEDURE 45-5

Administering a Blood Tranfusion

STEPS	RATIONALE
1. Explain procedure to client. Determine if there have been prior transfusions and note reactions, if any.	Clients who have had blood transfusion reactions in the past may have greater fear of transfusion. Past occurrence of certain reactions may increase possibility of recurrence.
2. Ask client to report chills, headache, itching, or rash immediately.	These are signs of transfusion reaction. Prompt reporting and discontinuation can help minimize reaction.
3. Be sure client has signed consent forms.	Some agencies require clients to sign consent forms before receiving transfusions.
4. Wash hands and apply gloves.	Reduces risk for transmission of HIV, hepatitis, and other blood-borne bacteria.
5. Establish IV line with large-gauge (#18 or 19) catheter.	Large-gauge catheters permit infusion of whole blood and prevent hemolysis.
6. Use infusion tubing that has in-line filter. Tubing should also be Y-type administration set (see the illustration below).	Filter removes debris and tiny clots from blood. Y-type set permits administration of additional products or volume expanders easily and immediate infusion of isotonic 0.9% sodium chloride solution after completion of isotonic infusion.
7. Hang solution container of 0.9% normal saline to be administered after blood infusion.	Provides isotonic solution to maintain vein patency. Isotonic solutions prevent hemolysis of RBCs.
8. Follow agency protocol in obtaining blood products from blood bank. Request blood when you are ready to use it.	Whole blood or packed RBCs must remain in cold (1-6 degree C) environment.
9. With another licensed nurse, correctly identify blood product and client:	One nurse reads out loud while other nurse listens and double-checks information. Reduces risk of error.
a. Check compatibility tag attached to blood bag and information on bag itself.	Verifies that ABO group, Rh type, and unit number match.

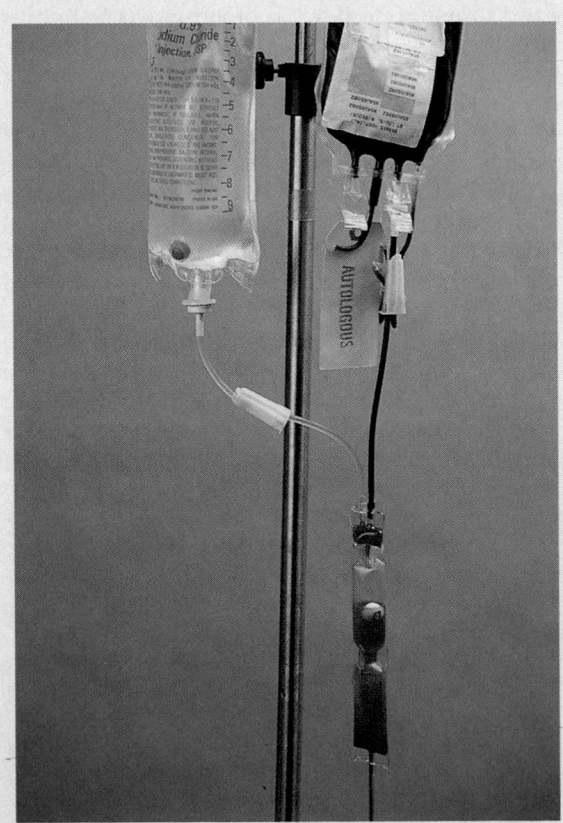

Step 6

Administering a Blood Transfusion—cont'd

STEPS	RATIONALE
9. With another licensed nurse, correctly identify blood product and client—cont'd	
b. For whole blood, check ABO group and Rh type that is on client's chart.	Verifies that information matches that on compatibility tag and blood bag.
c. Double-check blood product with physician's order.	Verifies correct blood component.
d. Check expiration data on bag.	After 21 days, changes in blood structure and chemistry can cause electrolyte and other related problems (Metheny, 1996).
e. Inspect blood for clots.	Anticoagulant citrate-phosphate-dextrose (CPD) is added to blood to preserve it (Metheny, 1996). If clots are present, return blood to blood bank.
f. Ask client's name, and check arm band.	Verifies correct client. Do not administer blood to client without arm band. Identification name and number on wrist band must be identical to those on blood compatibility tag.
10. Obtain baseline vital signs.	Verifies pretransfusion vital signs.
11. Begin transfusion:	
a. Prime infusion line with 0.9% normal saline.	Isotonic saline prevents hemolysis.
b. Begin transfusion slowly by first filling in-line filter.	If filter is not filled, transfusion will not infuse properly.
c. Adjust rate to 2 ml/min for first 15 minutes and remain with client. If you suspect reaction, stop transfusion, flush line with normal saline slowly, and notify blood bank and physician.	Allows detection of reaction while infusing smallest possible volume of blood product. Flushing line prevents further infusion of blood product.
12. Monitor vital signs:	
a. Take vital signs every 5 minutes for first 15 minutes of transfusion and every hour thereafter according to agency policy.	Documents change in vital sign status that could indicate early warning of reaction.
b. Observe client for flushing, itching, dyspnea, hives, rash.	May be early sign of reaction.
13. Maintain prescribed infusion rate using infusion pumps, if necessary.	Infusion pumps maintain prescribed rate.
14. Remove and dispose of gloves. Wash hands.	Reduces transmission of microorganisms.
15. Continually observe for adverse reactions.	Adverse reactions can occur at any point during transfusion (Table 45-8).
16. Record administration of blood or blood product. Record as fluid intake according to agency policy.	Documents administration of blood component.
17. When infusion is completed, return blood bag and tubing to blood bank.	Provides material for analysis if reaction is later discovered.

particularly during the first 15 minutes. Therefore the nurse should remain with the client and assess skin color and vital signs. The nurse continues to monitor the client and obtain vital signs periodically during the transfusion as directed by agency policy (often every 15 minutes). The nurse takes vital signs when a reaction is suspected. The rate of a transfusion is usually specified in the physician's orders. Ideally a unit of whole blood or packed RBCs is transfused in 2 hours. However, a client with a low fluid tolerance can have a transfusion over 4 hours (Potter and Perry, 1995).

Transfusion reactions. A **transfusion reaction** is a systemic response by the body to blood incompatible with that of the recipient. It is caused by RBC incompatibility or allergic sensitivity to the leukocytes, platelets, or plasma protein components of the transfused blood or to the potassium or citrate preservative in the blood. Blood transfusion can also result in disease transmission.

Several types of reactions can result from blood transfu-

sions. General adverse reactions (Table 45-8) range from immediate onset of fever, chills, and skin rash to hypotension, shock, and a delayed reaction that may not occur until several days or weeks after the transfusion.

A second category of reactions includes diseases transmitted by blood donors who have no symptoms or problems. Some diseases transmitted through transfusions are malaria, hepatitis, and HIV infection. Because all units of blood collected must undergo serological testing and HIV screening, the risk of acquiring blood-borne infection from transfusions is reduced.

Correct administration of blood and blood products reduces the risk of transfusion reactions. The nurse, although not actually a participant in the blood labeling process, is responsible for determining that the blood delivered to the nursing unit corresponds to the client's blood type listed in the medical record. Two nurses should check the blood against the client's identification number, blood group, and

Table 45-8	Adverse Reactions to Blood Transfusions				
GENERAL REACTION	**MECHANISM**	**ONSET**	**ASSESSMENT**	**PREVENTION**	**MANAGEMENT**
Acute hemolytic*	ABO-Rh incompatibility; antibodies in recipient's plasma attach to antigens on transfused RBCs, causing those RBCs to break down.	Immediately (or after administration of first 50 ml of blood)	Fever, chills, hypotension, nausea and vomiting, flushing, tachycardia, tachypnea, anxiety, dyspnea, hemoglobinemia and hemoglobinuria (hemoglobin molecules from the donor blood are released into the bloodstream and eliminated by the kidneys), coagulation disorder, renal failure	Careful identification of client when blood samples obtained for blood typing and when blood is released for transfusion. The most common cause is mistaken identification (Lichtor, 1989).	1. Stop transfusion (see pp. 1285). 2. Continue IV normal saline infusion. 3. Notify physician and blood bank. 4. Take vital signs every 15 minutes; monitor for shock: decreased blood pressure, tachycardia, tachypnea. 5. Monitor urine output for oliguria (decreased volume and appearance of dark color secondary to hemoglobin being excreted). 6. Obtain blood and urine samples as directed by agency. 7. Return blood bag and tubing to blood bank. 8. Document reaction as directed by agency.
Delayed hemolytic	Recipient has RBC incompatibility to donor's RBC antigens other than ABO antigens because of previous exposure to blood through transfusion or pregnancy.	2 days or more	Continued anemia; hemoglobinuria, jaundice	Blood bank should do careful cross-matching of donor and recipient blood for subsequent transfusions after first reaction.	1. Since it occurs after the transfusion, it can be missed; monitor blood studies for continued anemia. 2. If detected, notify physician and blood bank.
Febrile, nonhemolytic	Antibodies in recipient react to antigens on donor's white blood cells, platelets, or plasma proteins; it is the most common reaction, especially with multiple transfusions or previous pregnancy.	After first 30 minutes to 6 hours after the transfusion	Fever (>1° C), flushing, chills, headache, anxiety, muscle pain	Use leukocyte-poor blood (filtered).	1. Stop transfusion. 2. Continue IV normal saline infusion. 3. Administer antipyretics as ordered. 4. Monitor temperature every 4 hours.
Circulatory overload	Too rapid infusion expands the vascular volume more than client's heart can tolerate; results in pulmonary edema.	Anytime during or immediately after completion of the transfusion	Dyspnea, cough, anxiety, crackles, tachycardia, tachypnea, orthopnea, increased venous pressure	Administer blood or blood component at a rate based on client's size and health status; administer packed red blood cells rather than whole blood, if ordered; minimize amount of 0.9% normal saline used to maintain patency of IV line before and after each unit of blood; minimize the volume of 0.9% normal saline used to dilute packed red blood cells.	1. Elevate client's head. 2. Notify physician. 3. Slow or stop transfusion as ordered. 4. Administer morphine, diuretics, oxygen as ordered.

Reaction	Cause	Onset	Signs and symptoms	Prevention	Nursing interventions
Sepsis (infection carried through the bloodstream)	Transfusion of blood or blood component contaminated by bacteria or endotoxin.	Within 2 hours of transfusion	Chills, fever, vomiting, diarrhea, markedly decreased blood pressure, shock	Proper care of blood or blood product from time of donation to end of administration (e.g., maintaining proper temperature of blood, beginning transfusion within 30 minutes of blood leaving blood bank, completing transfusion within 4 hours).	1. Stop transfusion. 2. Obtain culture of client's blood. 3. Monitor vital signs every 15 minutes. 4. Administer antibiotics, IV fluids, vasopressors, steroids as ordered.
Urticaria	Recipient allergy to a plasma protein.	During or 1 hour after transfusion	Local flushing, hives, itching	Administer antihistamines before and during transfusion as ordered.	1. Stop transfusion. 2. Notify physician and blood bank. 3. Take vital signs every 15 minutes. 4. Administer antihistamines as ordered.* 5. Transfusion may be restarted if fever or if pulmonary symptoms are not present.
Anaphylactic	Administration of IgA proteins to IgA-deficient recipient who has developed IgA antibody.	Immediately after transfusion begins	Anxiety, urticaria, nausea, vomiting, diarrhea, wheezing, chest pain, hypotension, cardiac arrest	Transfuse washed RBCs with plasma removed; use blood from IgA-deficient donor.	This is life-threatening: 1. Stop transfusion. 2. Continue IV normal saline infusion. 3. Notify physician and blood bank. 4. Take vital signs every 15 minutes. 5. Administer epinephrine if ordered. 6. Initiate cardiopulmonary resuscitation if necessary.
Graft-versus-host disease	Normal donor lymphocytes reproduce in a recipient who is immunocompromised (e.g., clients receiving high-dose chemotherapy); the lymphocytes attack the recipient's tissues as foreign proteins.	Variable, related to rate of lymphocyte reproduction	Fever; skin rash; diarrhea; infection; liver dysfunction manifested by jaundice; bone marrow suppression	Administer irradiated blood if ordered; administer saline-washed blood if ordered.	1. Administer methotrexate, antithymocytic globulin, corticosteroids if ordered.

Modified from La Rocca J, Otto S: *Pocket guide to intravenous therapy*, St Louis, 1993, Mosby; National Blood Resource Education Program's Nursing Education in Working Group: Transfusion nursing: trends and practices for the '90s, *Am J Nurs* 91(6):42, 1991.
*The most serious adverse reaction; can be life threatening if client receives more than 100 ml of incompatible blood.

Arterial Puncture

STEPS	RATIONALE
1. Collect following equipment and bring to bedside:	Permits quick and efficient performance.
a. Heparinized 5-ml syringe	Prevents coagulation of arterial sample.
b. ⅝-inch 20-gauge needle	Promotes atraumatic cannulization of artery.
c. Crushed ice for arterial blood sample	Decreases oxygen metabolism of sample.
d. Local anesthetic	Reduces local pain when more than one attempt is needed and reduces risk of arterial spasm.
e. 2 × 2 gauze	Allows application of pressure after arterial puncture.
f. Disposable gloves	Reduces risk of exposure to HIV, hepatitis, and other blood-borne bacteria.
g. Tape	
2. Check client's identity. Explain procedure and client's responsibility.	Ensures that correct client undergoes procedure. Prevents hyperventilation due to anxiety, resulting in temporary change in blood gases.
3. Palpate radial artery.	Radial artery is selected because it is superficially located, has collateral circulation, and is not adjacent to large vein.
4. Perform Allen's test:	Determines adequate collateral blood flow to hand.
a. Have client make tight fist.	Removes as much blood from hand as possible.
b. Apply direct pressure to radial and ulnar arteries.	Obstructs arterial flow to hand.
c. Have client open hand.	Fingers and hand should be pale and blanched, indicating lack of arterial flow.
d. Release pressure over ulnar artery; observe color of fingers, thumb, and hand. Fingers and hand should flush within 15 seconds. Flushing is positive Allen's test. If test is negative (no flushing), radial artery should be avoided. Check other hand.	If collateral circulation to hand is present through ulnar artery, hand and fingers flush. Ulnar artery can supply blood flow to hand if radial artery is damaged or becomes occluded during procedure.
5. Hyperextend client's wrist over rolled towel.	Maintains radial artery in superficial position.
6. Wash hands. Apply disposable gloves.	Reduces risk of exposure to HIV, hepatitis, and other blood-borne bacteria.
7. Cleanse site with circular motion using povidone-iodine followed by alcohol wipe.	Reduces risk of skin bacteria entering puncture site.
8. Apply local anesthetic. Xylocaine 2% is usually injected subcutaneously.	Anesthetic reduces pain and subsequent hyperventilation in some clients and decreases risk of arterial spasm.
9. Flush 3-ml syringe with small amount of heparin 1000 U/ml and then empty syringe, leaving heparin in needle and hub.	Heparin in needle prevents clotting of blood sample. Excess heparin in syringe affects pH value of blood sample.
10. While palpating artery, insert needle at 45-degree angle while stabilizing client's artery with your free hand (see the illustration below).	Minimizes formation of hematoma at puncture site.

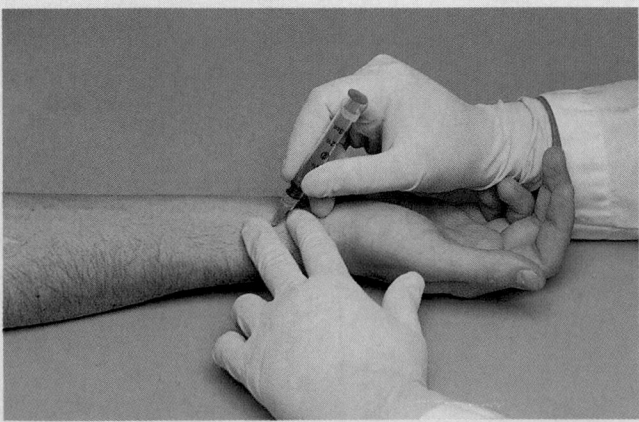

Step 10

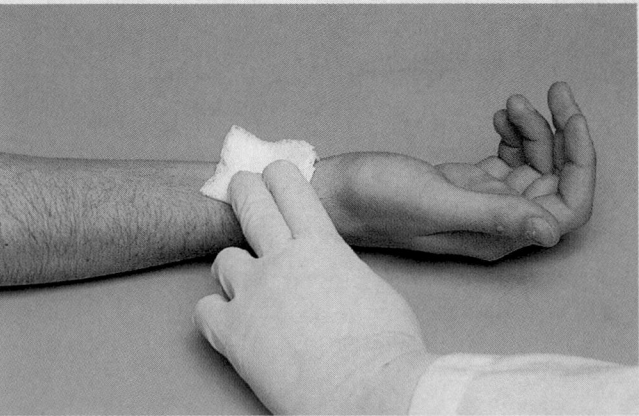

Step 18

Arterial Puncture—cont'd

STEPS	RATIONALE
11. Observe for pulsating flow of blood into syringe.	Indicates puncture of artery.
12. Withdraw 2 ml of blood.	Provides sufficient amount for analysis.
13. Remove needle and syringe from artery. Expel any air in syringe. Cork syringe with air lock.	Prevents entry of air into syringe. If air enters syringe, blood must be discarded to avoid inaccurate blood gas results.
14. Rotate syringe so that blood mixes with heparin.	Prevents clotting of sample.
15. Submerge syringe in crushed ice.	Reduces rate of oxygen metabolism of sampled blood.
16. Label specimen with client's name, body temperature, and (for client on oxygen therapy) inspired oxygen concentration.	Measurement of oxygen concentration is important in evaluating effectiveness of oxygen therapy.
17. Have specimens transported to laboratory immediately.	Prevents alteration of blood gas values by cellular metabolism.
18. Apply pressure to puncture site by applying 2 × 2 gauze over site and holding for 5 minutes. Length of time may be increased for client receiving anticoagulants (see the illustration on p. 1288).	Reduces risk of hematoma formation and damage to artery.
19. Apply tape over gauze if bleeding stops.	Prevents bleeding as extremity is moved.
20. Discard equipment in appropriate container, remove and dispose of gloves, and wash hands.	Reduces transmission of microorganisms.
21. Record in nurses' notes time of arterial blood gas test and extremity from which specimen was drawn.	Documents that arterial blood gas specimen was obtained.

complete name. If even a minor discrepancy exists, the blood should not be given and the blood bank laboratory should be notified immediately.

In addition to allergic reactions and the transmission of illnesses, certain risks (hyperkalemia, hypocalcemia, and circulatory overload) are associated with blood transfusions. Stored blood may cause hyperkalemia. Potassium levels in blood stored 1, 2, and 3 weeks has a potassium content of 12, 18, and 22 mEq/L, respectively (Metheny, 1996). The increase in potassium is related to the destruction of red blood cells. At the end of 21 days, 20% to 30% of cells are destroyed. Because the major intracellular cation is potassium, potassium enters the plasma as cells are destroyed. The potassium level of a client receiving several units of blood should be measured frequently. If the potassium level is elevated, measures to lower the serum level may be used, such as ion exchange resin (e.g., sodium polystyrene sulfonate [Kayexalate]) or hemodialysis.

Clients receiving massive transfusions can develop hypocalcemia because of the action of the citrated blood as it combines with ionized calcium (Metheny, 1996). The preservative often added to blood, CPD contains more citrate than is needed to combine with calcium in the blood collected for the transfusion. Therefore when transfused blood is infused into the bloodstream, the preservative combines with the ionized calcium, and tetany can result. The risk of hypocalcemia increases with the number of blood transfusions the client receives.

Iron overload (**hemosiderosis**) can occur in clients who receive frequent transfusions. Hemosiderosis is an abnormal deposit of iron in a variety of tissues, usually in the form of hemosiderin, an iron-rich pigment that is a product of hemolysis. Clients at risk for hemosiderosis are those with ill-nesses involving chronic, extensive destruction of RBCs, such as anemias, thalassemia major, or splenic dysfunction.

Circulatory overload is a risk when a client receives massive whole blood or packed RBC transfusions for hemorrhagic shock or when a client with normal blood volume receives blood. Clients particularly at risk for circulatory overload are older adults and those with cardiopulmonary and renal failure diseases.

Transfusion reactions are life threatening, but prompt nursing intervention can maintain the client's physiological stability. In the event of a suspected reaction, the nurse should do the following:

1. Stop the transfusion immediately.
2. "Piggyback" 0.9% normal saline into the IV line closest to the access site. The nurse should not turn off the blood and turn on the 0.9% normal saline on the Y- tubing infusion set, which merely infuses the blood in the Y-tubing into the client. Even a small amount of mismatched blood can cause a major reaction.
3. Notify the physician.
4. Remain with the client, observe signs and symptoms, and monitor vital signs every 5 minutes.
5. Prepare to administer emergency drugs, such as antihistamines, vasopressors, fluids, and steroids.
6. Prepare for cardiopulmonary resuscitation.
7. Obtain a urine specimen and send it to the laboratory.
8. Save the blood container and tubing for return to the laboratory.
9. Complete the necessary paperwork, such as reports about transfusion reactions and nurses' notes.

Although anaphylactic transfusion reactions are relatively rare, they can occur with any client. Correct administration of blood and blood products prevents reactions.

When a client has a transfusion reaction, prompt nursing actions can decrease the severity of the response.

Correcting Acid-Based Imbalances

Nursing interventions to promote acid-base balance are performed to support prescribed medical therapies. Physicians often order a variety of drug therapies to correct acid-base imbalances. Because acid-base disturbances can be life threatening and require rapid correction, the nurse must maintain a functional IV line and frequently check the physician's orders for new medications or fluids. Prescribed drugs, such as insulin or sodium bicarbonate, and fluid and electrolyte replacement should be given promptly.

The nurse implements appropriate nursing measures to promote ventilation and oxygenation (see Chapter 44). This is particularly important for the client with respiratory acidosis. Stasis of pulmonary secretions and decreased lung expansion intensify the acidotic condition. Nursing interventions to mobilize pulmonary secretions and promote lung expansion can make the difference between life and death.

For clients with respiratory alkalosis resulting from anxiety, the nurse initiates nursing measures to reduce the anxiety after first correcting respiratory alkalosis. To correct respiratory alkalosis the nurse instructs the client to breathe into a paper bag so that the client rebreathes exhaled carbon dioxide. In this way carbon dioxide combines with water to form carbonic acid, which increases blood acidity. After respiratory alkalosis is corrected, the symptoms disappear. At this point the nurse may be able to assist the client in determining the cause of anxiety and methods to control it. Some clients with repeated anxiety attacks need counseling, and the nurse should make an appropriate and prompt referral.

ARTERIAL BLOOD GASES

Clients with acid-base disturbances usually require repeated arterial blood gas analysis. This procedure requires the removal of blood from an artery to determine acid-base status and adequacy of ventilation and oxygenation. Arterial blood gas samples are drawn from a peripheral artery, such as the radial artery, or from an arterial line. In some agencies nurses are responsible for radial artery punctures. Beginning nursing students do not draw arterial blood gas samples but frequently assist in the sampling process and care for the client after the procedure (Procedure 45-6).

 ## Evaluation

The nurse evaluates the effectiveness of care provided to the client with alterations in fluid, electrolyte, or acid-base imbalances based on expected outcomes. Assessment helps the nurse determine the effectiveness of interventions. For example, if a diuretic is prescribed for a client with congestive heart failure, the nurse assessing the client expects to note a decrease in weight, an increase in 24-hour output, and a decrease in or absence of dependent edema. The nurse uses inspection, palpation, percussion, and auscultation to determine the client's response to nursing interventions. Ongoing assessment enables the nurse to evaluate the response to therapy. Using evaluation data, the nurse determines whether the care goals have been met or whether the care plan requires modification.

Client care goals are developed using objective criteria to measure progress. The criteria in the evaluation box below are examples of expected outcomes based on the specific goals of care.

 ## Sample Evaluation of Interventions for Fluid, Electrolyte, and Acid-Base Disturbances

GOALS	EVALUATIVE MEASURES	EXPECTED OUTCOMES
Client will have normal fluid, electrolyte, and acid-base balance	Inspect the skin for edema or dry, scaly skin. Palpate for inelastic skin turgor, edema, or weak pulse. Inspect oral cavity for dry, sticky mucous membranes, decreased saliva, and longitudinal furrows on tongue.	Elastic skin turgor will return. Clients mucous membranes will be moist. No complaints of thirst.
	Weigh client and be alert for gain or loss.	Weight will be stable at baseline normal.
	Observe for Chvostek's sign, anuria, or oliguria.	Urine output will be ≥ 70 ml/hr. Urine specific gravity ranges 1.010-1.020.
	Auscultate for adventitious lung sounds and third heart sound or dysrhythmias. Obtain vital signs for tachycardia, bradycardia, hypotension, hypertension, and orthostatic hypotension. Obtain laboratory findings and observe for abnormal electrolyte levels.	Vital signs will return to baseline. No vomiting.

■ KEY CONCEPTS ■

► Body fluids are distributed in extracellular and intracellular fluid compartments.

► Body fluids are composed of electrolytes, minerals, cells, and water.

► Body fluids are regulated through fluid intake, output, and hormonal regulation.

► Acid-base balance depends on the hydrogen ion concentration in the blood.

► Biological buffering occurs when hydrogen ions are absorbed or released by the cells to compensate for acid-base imbalances.

► Physiological buffering involves compensatory responses in the lung or kidneys.

► Volume disturbances include isotonic and osmolar fluid volume deficits and excesses.

► Clients who are very young, older adults, or those with chronic and severe acute illnesses are at risk for fluid, electrolyte, and acid-base imbalances.

► Assessment for fluid, electrolyte, and acid-base balances includes the nursing history, physical and behavioral assessment, measurements of intake and output, daily weighing, specific laboratory data such as complete blood count and measurement of serum electrolyte and BUN levels, urine specific gravity, and arterial blood gas levels.

► Fluid volume deficits can be corrected by oral or parenteral administration of fluid.

► Complications of intravenous therapy include infiltration, phlebitis, fluid overload, and bleeding at the infusion site.

► Blood transfusions replace fluid volume loss from hemorrhage, treat anemia, and replace coagulation factors.

► The risks of transfusion include transfusion reactions, hyperkalemia, hypocalcemia, circulatory overload, and blood-borne infections.

► Respiratory acidosis is characterized by increased carbon dioxide concentration, excess carbonic acid, and increased hydrogen ion concentration.

► Respiratory alkalosis is characterized by decreased carbon dioxide and hydrogen ion concentrations.

► Metabolic acidosis is characterized by a rise in hydrogen ion concentration.

► Metabolic alkalosis is characterized by a decrease in hydrogen ion concentration.

► The goals of therapy for acid-base imbalances are treatment of the underlying illness and restoration of the arterial pH to normal.

■ KEY TERMS ■

Active transport, p. 1249
Agglutinins, p. 1283

Anions, p. 1248
Arterial blood gas, p. 1264
Autotransfusion, p. 1283
Buffer, p. 1252
Cations, p. 1248
Dehydration, p. 1254
Diffusion, p. 1248
Electrolyte, p. 1248
Extracellular fluids, p. 1248
Fluid volume deficit (FVD), p. 1253
Fluid volume excess (FVE), p. 1253
Hemolysis, p. 1283
Hemosiderosis, p. 1289
Hydrostatic pressure, p. 1249
Hypertonic, p. 1249
Hypotonic, p. 1249
Infiltration, p. 1282
Infusion pumps, p. 1270
Insensible water loss, p. 1251
Interstitial fluid, p. 1248
Intracellular fluids, p. 1248
Isotonic, p. 1249
Metabolic acidosis, p. 1256
Metabolic alkalosis, p. 1257
Oncotic pressure, p. 1249
Osmolality, p. 1249
Osmoreceptors, p. 1250
Osmosis, p. 1248
Osmotic pressure, p. 1249
Patency, p. 1270
pH, p. 1252
Phlebitis, p. 1282
Respiratory acidosis, p. 1256
Respiratory alkalosis, p. 1256
Sensible water loss, p. 1251
Third-space syndrome, p. 1253
Total parenteral nutrition (TPN) p. 1268
Transfusion reaction, p. 1285
Vascular access devices, p. 1268
Venipuncture, p. 1269
Volume control devices, p. 1269

■ CRITICAL THINKING EXERCISES ■

1. The client has a recorded I & O of 1300 ml and 1500 ml, respectively, for a 24-hour period. This client is eating a regular diet. Discuss the specifics involved in this client's total intake and output in order to determine their equality/ inequality.

2. You are expecting an auto accident victim. You are told that the client has a traumatic below-the-knee amputation of the right leg. Which fluid imbalance would this client be likely to be experiencing? What assessments would you perform in order to confirm your guess? What type of fluid replacement would you expect?

3. Your newly postoperative client who had a general anesthetic has a blood pH of 7.25 and a $Paco_2$ of 50 mm Hg. He is complaining of incisional pain and has not turned or dangled at bedside since his return from the recovery room 1 hour ago. Identify the problem based on this data. What factors are related to the problem? Discuss the physiology of the problem. How would you express this problem in Nursing Diagnosis form? What would your first action be? Identify other actions you would implement.

REFERENCES

Bove L: How fluids and electrolytes shift after surgery, *Nurs 94* 24(8):34, 1994.

Coulter K: Intravenous therapy for the elder patient: implications for the intravenous nurse, *J Intraven Nurs* 15 (suppl): S18, 1992.

Cusson R: Rice based oral rehydration fluid in the treatment of infant diarrhea, *J Pediatr Nurs* 7(6):414, 1992.

Drug facts and comparisons, Philadelphia, 1992, Lippincott.

Gardner JS et al: Guideline for isolation precautions in hospitals, Parts 1 and 2, *Am J Infect Contr* 24(2): 24, 1996.

Goepp JG, Katz SA: Oral rehydration therapy, *Am Family Phys* 49(4):843, 1993.

Groer MW: *Physiology and pathophysiology of the body fluids,* St Louis, 1981, Mosby.

Horne M et al: *Fluid, electrolyte, and acid-base balance,* St Louis, 1991, Mosby.

Kim M et al: *Nursing diagnoses,* ed 6, St Louis, 1995, Mosby.

Kokko J, Tannen R: *Fluids and electrolytes,* ed 2, Philadelphia, 1990, Saunders.

LaRocca J, Otto S: *Pocket guide to intravenous therapy,* St Louis, 1989, Mosby.

Lichtor JL: Transfusion reactions...part 1, *Curr Rev Nurs Anesth* 12(3):18, 1989.

Long B et al: *Medical-surgical nursing,* ed 3, St Louis, 1993, Mosby.

Metheny N: *Fluid and electrolyte imbalance,* ed 3, Philadelphia, 1996, Lippincott.

National Blood Resource Education Program's Nursing Education Working Group: Transfusion nursing: trends and practices for the '90's, *Am J Nurs* 91(6):42, 1991.

Perry A, Potter P: *Pocket guide to basic skills and procedures,* ed 3, St Louis, 1994, Mosby.

Petrelli NJ et al: Bowel rest, intravenous hydration, and continuous high-dose infusion of octreotide acetate for the treatment of chemotherapy-induced diarrhea in patients with colorectal carcinoma, *Cancer* 72:1543, 1993.

Potter P, Perry A: *Basic nursing,* ed 3, St Louis, 1995, Mosby.

Raimer F: How to identify electrolyte imbalances on your patient's E.C.G., *Nurs 94* 24(6):54, 1994.

Silvestri A, Masoorli S: PICC lines: a new dimension in home health care, *J Home Health Care Pract* 2(4):1, 1990.

Weldy N: *Body fluids and electrolytes,* ed 6, St Louis, 1992, Mosby.

ADDITIONAL READINGS

Ankum W et al: The spring balance: a simple monitoring system for fluid overload during steroscopic surgery, *Lancet* 343(8901):836, 1994.

Dennison R et al: Myths and facts...about fluid balance, part 1, *Nurs* 22(1):22, 1992.

Dennison R et al: Myths and facts...about electrolyte imbalance, part 2, *Nurs* 22(2):26, 1992.

Gaskill D et al: The nutritionally vulnerable patient: a pilot study to compare nurses' assessment of intake and actual intake, *J Clin Nurs* 1(2):101, 1992.

Gould S et al: Hypovolemic shock, *Crit Care Clin* 9(2): 239, 1993.

Gulanick M et al: *Nursing care plans,* ed 3, St Louis, 1994, Mosby.

McVicar A et al: Which infusate do I need? Physiological basis of fluid therapy, *Prof Nurs* 7(9):544, 1992.

Ozuna L et al: Development of a vital-sign/ fluid-balance flow sheet, *Oncol Nurs* 20(1):113, 1993.

Porth C: Physiology of thirst and drinking:implications for nursing practice, *Heart and Lung* 21(3):22, 1992.

Price S, Wilson L: *Pathophysiology,* ed 4, St Louis, 1992, Mosby.

Sheehy S: *Emergency nursing,* ed 3, St Louis, 1992, Mosby.

Workman M: Fluid and electrolytes,*Clin Issues Crit Care Nurs, Am Assoc Crit Care Nurs* 3(3):653, 1992.

## Chapter 46

Urinary Elimination

Objectives

Mastery of content in this chapter will enable the student to:

▶ Define the key terms listed.

▶ Describe the process of urination.

▶ Identify factors that commonly influence urinary elimination.

▶ Compare and contrast common alterations in urinary elimination.

▶ Obtain a nursing history for a client with urinary elimination problems.

▶ Identify nursing diagnoses appropriate for clients with alterations in urinary elimination.

▶ Obtain urine specimens.

▶ Describe characteristics of normal and abnormal urine.

▶ Describe the nursing implications of common diagnostic tests of the urinary system.

▶ Discuss nursing measures to promote normal micturition and reduce episodes of incontinence.

▶ Insert a urinary catheter.

▶ Discuss nursing measures to reduce urinary tract infection.

▶ Irrigate a urinary catheter.

▶ Identify two modalities of renal replacement therapy.

Normal elimination of urinary wastes is a basic function most people take for granted. When the urinary system fails to function properly, virtually all organ systems will be eventually affected. Clients with alterations in urinary elimination may also suffer emotionally from body image changes. The nurse provides understanding and a sensitivity to all clients' needs. The nurse must understand the reasons for problems and find acceptable solutions.

■ PHYSIOLOGY OF URINE ELIMINATION

Urinary elimination depends on the function of the kidneys, ureters, bladder, and urethra. Kidneys remove wastes from the blood to form urine. Ureters transport urine from the kidneys to the bladder. The bladder holds urine until the urge to urinate develops. Urine leaves the body through the urethra. All organs of the urinary system must be intact and functional for successful removal of urinary wastes (Fig. 46-1).

Kidneys

Kidneys are paired, reddish-brown, bean-shaped organs that lie on either side of the vertebral column posterior to the peritoneum and against deep muscles of the back. The kidneys extend to the twelfth thoracic and third lumbar vertebrae. Normally the left kidney is 1.5 to 2 cm (⁶/₁₀ to ⁸/₁₀ inch) higher than the right because of the anatomical position of the liver. Each kidney typically measures approximately 12 cm by 7 cm (5 by 3 inches) and weighs 120 to 150 g. An adrenal gland lies on the superior pole of each kidney but is not directly related to urinary elimination. Each kidney is covered by a tough capsule and surrounded by a cushion of fat.

Waste products of metabolism that collect in the blood are filtered in the kidneys. Blood reaches each kidney by a **renal** (kidney) artery that branches from the abdominal aorta. The renal artery enters the kidney at the hilum. Approximately 20% to 25% of the cardiac output circulates daily through the kidneys. Each kidney contains 1 million nephrons. The **nephron**, the functional unit of the kidney, forms the urine. The nephron is composed of the glomerulus, Bowman's capsule, proximal convoluted tubule, loop of Henle, distal tubule, and collecting duct (Fig. 46-2).

Blood reaches nephrons through the afferent arterioles. A cluster of these blood vessels forms the capillary network of the **glomerulus,** which is the initial site of filtration of the blood and the beginning of urine formation. The glomerular capillaries are porous and permit filtration of water and substances such as glucose, amino acids, urea, creatinine, and major electrolytes into Bowman's capsule. Large proteins and blood cells do not normally filter through the glomerulus. The presence of large proteins in the urine **(proteinuria)** is a sign of glomerular injury. The glomerulus filters approximately 125 ml of filtrate per minute. Initially the filtrate closely approximates blood plasma minus the large proteins.

Not all of the glomerular filtrate is excreted as urine. After the filtrate leaves the glomerulus, it passes through a system of tubules and collecting ducts, where water and substances such as glucose, amino acids, uric acid, and sodium and potassium ions are selectively reabsorbed back into the plasma. Other substances such as hydrogen ions, potassium ions (in the presence of aldosterone), and ammonia are secreted back into the tubules where they are lost in the urine. About 99% of the filtrate is reabsorbed into the plasma, with the remaining 1% excreted as urine. Thus the kidneys play a key role in fluid and electrolyte balance (see Chapter 45). Although output does depend on intake, the normal adult 24-hour output of urine is about 1500 to 1600 ml. An output of 60 ml of urine per hour is generally normal. An output of less than 30 ml per hour may indicate renal alterations. The kidneys also produce several hormones vital to production of red blood cells (RBCs), blood pressure regulation, and bone mineralization.

The kidneys are responsible for maintaining a normal

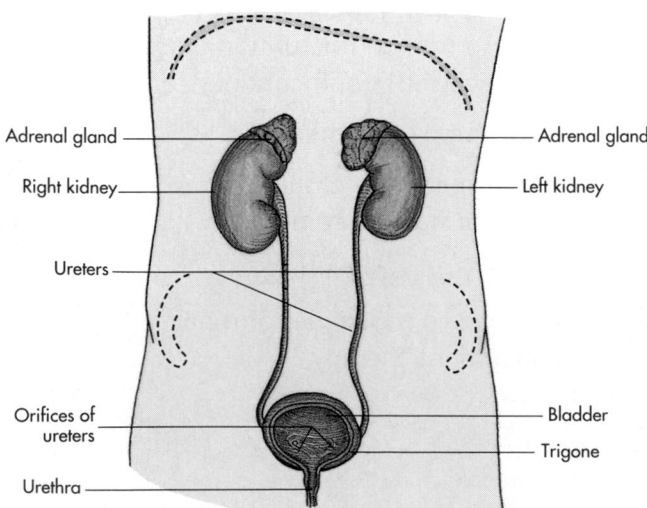

Fig. 46-1 Organs of the urinary system.

Adrenal gland
Right kidney
Ureters
Orifices of ureters
Urethra
Adrenal gland
Left kidney
Bladder
Trigone

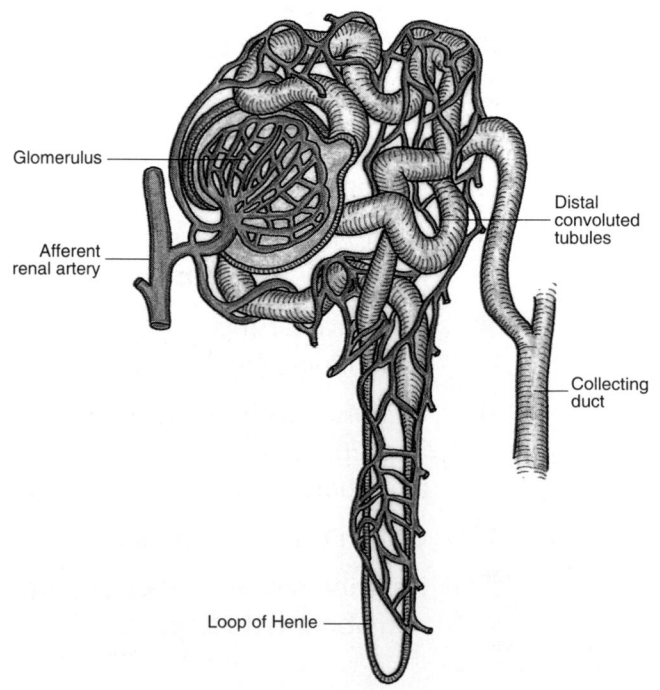

Fig. 46-2 Renal nephron.

Glomerulus
Afferent renal artery
Distal convoluted tubules
Collecting duct
Loop of Henle

RBC volume. They produce **erythropoietin**, a hormone released primarily from specialized glomerular cells that sense decreased RBC oxygenation (local hypoxia). After it is released from the kidney, erythropoietin functions within the bone marrow to stimulate erythropoiesis (production and maturation of RBCs) by converting certain stem cells into erythroblasts (McCance and Huether, 1994). Erythropoietin also prolongs the life of mature RBCs. Clients with chronic alterations in kidney function cannot produce sufficient quantities of this hormone, therefore they are prone to anemia.

Renin is another hormone produced by the kidneys. Its major role is the regulation of blood flow in times of renal ischemia (decreased blood supply). Renin is synthesized and released from juxtaglomerular cells, which are located on the juxtaglomerular apparatus of the nephron (Fig. 46-3).

Renin functions as an enzyme to convert angiotensinogen (a substance synthesized by the liver) into angiotensin I. As angiotensin I circulates through the lungs, it is converted to angiotensin II and angiotensin III. Angiotensin II exerts its effect on vascular smooth muscle to cause vasoconstriction and stimulates aldosterone release from the adrenal cortex. Aldosterone causes retention of water, which increases blood volume. Angiotensin III exerts similar effects but to a lesser degree. The net effect of both of these mechanisms is an increase in arterial blood pressure and renal blood flow (McCance and Huether, 1994).

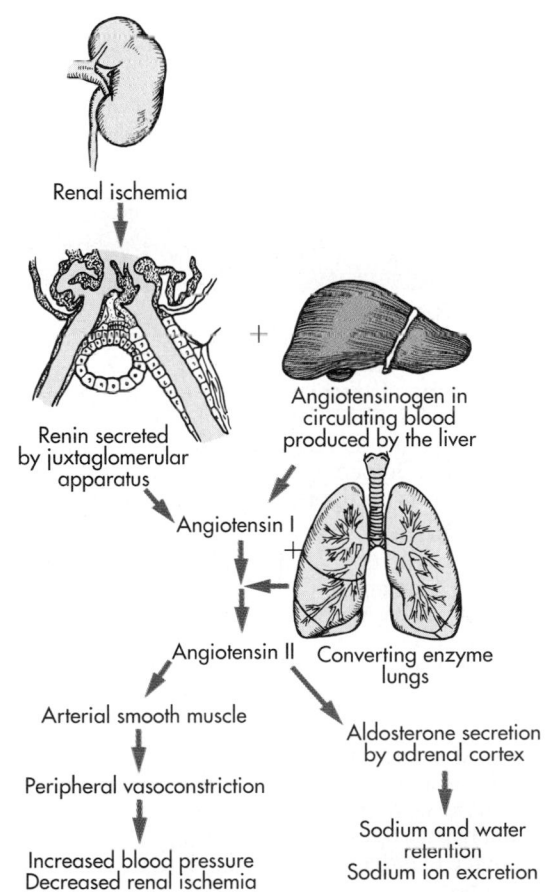

Fig. 46-3 Physiological effects of renin-angiotensin mechanism.

The kidneys also play a role in calcium and phosphate regulation. They are responsible for producing a substance that converts vitamin D into its active form (see Chapter 45). Clients with chronic alterations in kidney function do not make sufficient amounts of the active vitamin D metabolite. Therefore they are prone to develop renal bone disease resulting from the demineralization of bone secondary to impaired intestinal calcium absorption unless the active form of vitamin D is supplied.

Ureters

Urine leaves the tubules and enters collecting ducts that transport it to the renal pelvis. A ureter joins each renal pelvis as the initial exit route for urinary wastes. Ureters are tubular structures measuring 25 to 30 cm (10 to 12 inches) in length and 1.25 cm (½ inch) in diameter in the adult. They extend retroperitoneally to enter the urinary bladder in the pelvic cavity at the ureterovesical junction. Urine draining from the ureters to the bladder is usually sterile.

Three layers of tissue form the wall of the ureter. The inner layer is a mucous membrane continuous with the lining of the renal pelvis and urinary bladder. The middle layer consists of smooth muscle fibers that transport urine through the ureters by peristaltic waves stimulated by distention with urine. An outer layer of fibrous connective tissue supports the ureters.

Peristaltic waves cause the urine to enter the bladder in spurts rather than steadily. The ureters enter obliquely through the posterior bladder wall. This arrangement normally prevents the reflux of urine from the bladder into the ureters during the act of **micturition** by the compression of the ureter at the ureterovesical junction (the juncture of the ureters with the bladder). An obstruction within a ureter, such as a kidney stone (**renal calculus**), results in strong peristaltic waves that attempt to move the obstruction into the bladder. These strong peristaltic waves result in pain often referred to as *renal colic*.

Bladder

The urinary bladder is a hollow, distensible, muscular organ that is a reservoir for urine and the organ of excretion. When empty, the bladder lies in the pelvic cavity behind the symphysis pubis. In men the bladder lies against the rectum posteriorly, and in women it rests against the anterior wall of the uterus and vagina.

The bladder's shape changes as it becomes filled with urine. The walls of the bladder can expand. Pressure within the bladder is usually low, even when partly full, a factor that protects against infection. It can hold approximately 600 ml of urine, although a normal voiding is about 300 ml.

When the bladder is full, it expands and extends above the symphysis pubis. A greatly distended bladder may reach the umbilicus. In a pregnant woman the fetus pushes against the bladder, causing a feeling of fullness and reducing the bladder's capacity. This can occur either in the first or third trimester.

The trigone (a smooth triangular area on the inner surface of the bladder) is at the base of the bladder. An opening exists at each of the trigone's three angles. Two are for the ureters, and one is for the urethra.

The wall of the bladder has four layers: the inner mucous coat, a submucous coat of connective tissue, a muscular coat, and an outer serous coat. The muscular layer has bundles of muscle fibers that form the detrusor muscle. Parasympathetic nerve fibers stimulate the detrusor muscle during urination. The internal urethral sphincter, made of a ringlike band of muscle, is at the base of the bladder where it joins the urethra. The sphincter prevents escape of urine from the bladder and is under voluntary control.

Urethra

Urine travels from the bladder through the urethra and passes outside of the body through the urethral meatus. Normally the turbulent flow of urine through the urethra washes it free of bacteria. Mucous membrane lines the urethra, and urethral glands secrete mucus into the urethral canal. The mucus is believed to be bacteriostatic and forms a mucous plug to prevent entrance of bacteria. Thick layers of smooth muscle surround the urethra.

In women the urethra is approximately 4 to 6.5 cm (1½ to 2½ inches) long. The external urethral sphincter, located about halfway down the urethra, permits voluntary flow of urine. The short length of the urethra predisposes women to infection. Bacteria can easily enter the urethra from the perineal area. In men the urethra, which is a urinary canal and a passageway for cells and secretions from reproductive organs, is 20 cm (8 inches) long. It has three sections: the prostatic urethra, the membranous urethra, and the cavernous or penile urethra.

In a woman the urinary **meatus** (opening) is located between the labia minora, above the vagina and below the clitoris. In a male the meatus is located at the distal end of the penis.

Act of Urination

Several brain structures influence bladder function, including the cerebral cortex, thalamus, hypothalamus, and brainstem. Together they suppress contraction of the bladder's detrusor muscle until a person wishes to urinate or void. Two centers in the pons modulate micturition or voiding; the *M* center triggers the detrusor reflex and the *L* center coordinates pelvic floor tone. Once voiding occurs the response is a contraction of the bladder and coordinated relaxation of pelvic floor muscles.

The bladder normally holds as much as 600 ml of urine. However, the desire to urinate can be sensed when the bladder contains a smaller amount of urine (150 to 200 ml in an adult and 50 to 200 ml in a child). As the volume increases, the bladder walls stretch, sending sensory impulses to the micturition center in the sacral spinal cord. Parasympathetic impulses from the micturition center stimulate the detrusor muscle to contract rhythmically. The internal urethral sphincter also relaxes so that urine may enter the urethra, although voiding does not yet occur. As the bladder contracts, nerve impulses travel up the spinal cord to the pons and cerebral cortex. A person is thus conscious of the need to urinate. Older children and adults can respond to or ignore this urge thus making urination under voluntary control. If the person chooses not to void, the external urinary sphincter remains contracted, and the micturition reflex is inhibited. However, when a person is ready to void, the external sphincter relaxes, the micturition reflex stimulates the detrusor muscle to contract, and efficient emptying of the bladder occurs.

If the urge to void has been ignored repeatedly, the bladder capacity may be reached and the resulting pressure on the sphincter may make continued voluntary control impossible.

Damage to the spinal cord above the sacral region causes loss of voluntary control of urination, but the micturition reflex pathway may remain intact, allowing urination to occur reflexively. This condition is called a **reflex bladder.**

■ FACTORS INFLUENCING URINATION

Many factors influence the volume and quality of urine and the client's ability to urinate. Some alterations may be acute and reversible (urinary tract infection) while others may be chronic and irreversible (slow, progressive development of renal dysfunction). Disease processes that primarily affect renal function (changes in urine volume or quality) are generally categorized as *prerenal, renal,* or *postrenal* in origin (see the box below).

Prerenal alterations in urinary elimination decrease circulating blood flow to and through the kidneys with subsequent decreased perfusion to renal tissue. In other words, the alterations are outside of the urinary system. The decrease in renal perfusion leads to **oliguria** (diminished capacity to form urine) or, less commonly, **anuria** (inability to produce urine). Renal alterations result from factors that cause injury directly to the glomeruli or renal tubule, interfering with their normal filtering, reabsorptive, and secretory functions. Postrenal alterations result from obstruction to the urinary collecting system anywhere from the calyces (drainage structures within the kidney) to the urethral meatus (that is, outside of the kidney but within the urinary system). Urine is formed by the urinary system but cannot be eliminated by normal means.

In addition to disease alterations, other factors should be

Conditions Causing Alterations in Urinary Elimination

PRERENAL CONDITIONS
Decreased intravascular volume: dehydration, hemorrhage, burns, shock
Altered peripheral vascular resistance: sepsis, anaphylactic (allergic) reactions
Cardiac pump failure: congestive heart failure, myocardial infarction, hypertensive heart disease, valvular disease, pericardial tamponade

RENAL CONDITIONS
Nephrotoxic agents (e.g., gentamycin)
Transfusion reactions
Diseases of the glomeruli (e.g., glomerulonephritis)
Renal neoplasms
Systemic diseases (e.g., diabetes mellitus)
Hereditary diseases (e.g., polycystic kidney disease)
Infections

POSTRENAL CONDITIONS
Ureteral, bladder, or urethral obstruction: calculi, blood clots, tumors, stricture
Prostatic hypertrophy
Neurogenic bladder
Pelvic tumors

considered when clients have symptoms related to urinary elimination. Problems related to the act of urination may be the result of cognitive, functional, or physical means resulting in incontinence, retention, or infection.

Growth and Development

Infants and young children cannot effectively concentrate urine. Their urine thus appears light yellow or clear. In relation to their small body size, infants and children excrete large volumes of urine. For example, a 6-month-old child who weighs 6 to 8 kg (10 to 16 pounds) excretes 400 to 500 ml of urine daily. The child weighs about 10% of an adult's weight but excretes 33% as much urine.

A child cannot control micturition voluntarily until age 18 to 24 months. A child must be able to recognize the feeling of bladder fullness, to hold urine for 1 to 2 hours, and to communicate the sense of urgency to an adult. The young child needs parents' understanding, patience, and consistency. A child may not gain full control of micturition until age 4 or 5. Boys are generally slower than girls. Daytime control of micturition is easier to accomplish than nighttime control and occurs earlier in the child's development, usually by 2 years of age.

The adult normally voids 1500 to 1600 ml of urine daily. The kidney concentrates urine, producing a normal, amber-colored urine. A person does not normally wake to void during sleep because of reduction of renal blood flow during rest and the kidney's ability to concentrate urine.

Aging impairs micturition. Problems of mobility sometimes make it difficult for the older adult to reach a toilet in time. An older person may be too weak to rise from a toilet seat without assistance. Chronic neurological disease such as parkinsonism or cerebrovascular accident (stroke) impairs the sense of balance and makes it difficult for a man to stand while voiding or a woman to walk to the toilet. If an older person loses control of thought processes, the ability to control micturition is unpredictable. The person may lose the ability to sense a full bladder or be unable to recall the procedure for voiding.

Changes in kidney and bladder function also occur with aging. The glomerular filtration rate declines but the kidney's ability to concentrate urine also declines. Thus the older adult often experiences **nocturia** (excessive urination at night). The bladder loses its muscle tone and capacity to hold urine, resulting in increased **urinary frequency**. Because the bladder cannot contract as effectively, an older person often retains urine in the bladder after voiding **(residual urine)**. Older men may also suffer from benign prostatic hypertrophy, which makes them prone to urinary retention and incontinence. These changes increase the risk for bacterial growth and development of urinary tract infections (UTIs).

Sociocultural Factors

Cultural norms vary on the privacy of urination (see the box above). North Americans expect toilet facilities to be private, whereas some European cultures accept communal toilet facilities. Social expectations (e.g., school recesses) influence the time of urination. Indoor plumbing for toilet facilities may be rare in many poor rural areas such as Appalachia, the interior of Maine, and other remote mountain communities.

 CULTURAL ASPECTS OF CARE

The bathroom behavior of some clients may be foreign to many health care workers. For example, Mr. Kim, an older Korean client, had been admitted with pneumonia while visiting relatives in the United States. The physician's orders included strict bedrest to assist in decreasing oxygen demand. The nurse explained to Mr. Kim, who understood some English, and to his family that he would need to use the bedpan for defecation and the urinal for voiding. The nurse gave Mr. Kim the urinal, showed him the bedpan, and gave him the call light. A short time later the nurse entered the room to find Mr. Kim out of bed squatting over the bedpan, which was on the floor. He had not used the urinal but rather voided into the bedpan as well. The nurse discovered that in Mr. Kim's native Korea, farmers used a hole in the ground for elimination and only recently have indoor toilets been introduced throughout the country. Elimination is considered unclean and could not be done in the bed. The nurse consulted with the physician and the client was permitted bathroom privileges with assistance (Galanti, 1991).

The nurse's approach to a client's elimination needs must consider cultural and social habits. If a client prefers privacy, the nurse tries to prevent interruptions as the client voids. A client who is less sensitive to the need for privacy should be treated with understanding and acceptance.

Psychological Factors

Anxiety and emotional stress may cause a sense of urgency and increased frequency of urination. An anxious person may have the urge to void even after voiding only a few minutes earlier.

Anxiety may also prevent a person from being able to urinate completely. Emotional tension makes it difficult to relax abdominal and perineal muscles. If the external urethral sphincter is not completely relaxed, voiding may be incomplete, and urine is retained in the bladder. Attempting to void in a public restroom may result in a temporary inability to void.

Personal Habits

Privacy and adequate time to urinate are usually important to most people. Some people need distractions (e.g., reading) to relax.

Muscle Tone

Weak abdominal and pelvic floor muscles impair bladder contraction and control of the external urethral sphincter. Poor control of micturition can result from muscle wasting caused by prolonged immobility, stretching of muscles during childbirth, menopausal muscle atrophy, and damage to muscles from trauma.

Continuous drainage of urine through an indwelling catheter causes loss of bladder tone and/or damage to urethral sphincters. The bladder remains relatively empty when a client has an indwelling catheter in place, and thus it is never stretched to capacity. When a muscle is not stretched regularly, atrophy develops. When a catheter is removed, the client may have difficulty regaining urinary control.

Volume Status

The kidneys maintain a sensitive balance between retention and excretion of fluids (see Chapter 45). If fluids and the concentration of electrolytes and solutes are in equilibrium, an increase in fluid intake causes an increase in urine production. Ingested fluids increase the body's circulating plasma and thus increase the volume of glomerular filtrate and urine excreted.

This amount varies with food and fluid intake. The volume of urine formed at night is about half that formed during the day because both intake and metabolism decline. This results in a decline in renal blood flow. Nocturia can be a sign of renal alteration. In a healthy person, the intake of water in food and fluids balances the output of water in urine, feces, and insensible losses in perspiration and respiration.

Ingestion of certain fluids directly affects urine production and excretion. Alcohol inhibits the release of antidiuretic hormone (ADH) and thus promotes urine formation. Coffee, tea, cocoa, and cola drinks that contain caffeine increase **diuresis** (increased formation and excretion of urine). Foods that contain a high fluid content, such as fruits and vegetables, may also increase urine production.

Febrile conditions affect urine production. The client who becomes diaphoretic loses a large amount of fluids through insensible water loss, which decreases urine production. However, the increased body metabolism associated with fever increases accumulation of body wastes. Although urine volume may be reduced, it is highly concentrated.

Disease Conditions

Several diseases can affect the ability to micturate. Any lesion of peripheral nerves leading to the bladder causes loss of bladder tone, reduced sensation of bladder fullness, and difficulty in controlling urination. For example, diabetes mellitus and multiple sclerosis cause neuropathic conditions that alter bladder function.

Diseases that slow or hinder physical activity interfere with the ability to void. Rheumatoid arthritis, degenerative joint disease, and parkinsonism are examples of conditions that make it difficult to reach and use toilet facilities. A client with rheumatoid arthritis often cannot sit on or rise from a toilet without an elevated seat.

Diseases that cause irreversible damage to the glomerulus or tubules result in permanent alterations in renal function. *Chronic* or *end-stage renal disease (ESRD)* are the terms used to describe the resulting decline in kidney function from these processes. The client with ESRD manifests numerous metabolic disturbances that require treatment for survival. These alterations are caused by the accumulation of nitrogenous waste products and various acid-base and biochemical derangements. The associated symptoms experienced by the client occur as a result of the **uremic syndrome.** This syndrome is characterized by an increase in nitrogenous wastes in the blood, altered regulatory functions (causing marked fluid and electrolyte abnormalities), nausea, vomiting, headache, coma, and convulsions. Treatment options in-

---

Indications for Dialysis

Renal failure that can no longer be controlled by conservative management (i.e., dietary modifications and administration of medications to correct electrolyte abnormalities)

Worsening of uremic syndrome associated with ESRD (i.e., nausea, vomiting, neurological changes, neuropathic conditions, pericarditis)

Severe electrolyte or fluid abnormalities that cannot be controlled by simpler measures (e.g., hyperkalemia, pulmonary edema)

---

clude methods to correct these biochemical derangements. The problem may be managed conservatively, with medications and a regimen of dietary and fluid restrictions. However, as continued deterioration in renal function or worsening of the uremic symptoms becomes evident, more aggressive treatment is indicated. These treatments are known as **renal replacement therapies.** Dialysis and organ transplantation are the two methods of renal replacement. The two methods of dialysis are peritoneal and hemodialysis (see the box above).

Peritoneal dialysis is an indirect method of cleansing the blood of waste products using the processes of osmosis and diffusion. The peritoneum is the serous membrane covering the abdominal organs and lining the peritoneal cavity. It functions as a semipermeable membrane with a capillary bed that delivers the blood. Excess fluid and waste products are readily removed from the bloodstream when a sterile electrolyte solution (dialysate) is instilled into the peritoneal cavity by gravity via a surgically placed catheter. The dialysate is left in the cavity for a prescribed time interval and then is drained out by gravity taking accumulated wastes and excess fluid and electrolytes with it.

Hemodialysis involves using a machine equipped with a semipermeable filtering membrane (artificial kidney) that removes accumulated waste products from the blood. In the dialysis machine, dialysate fluid is pumped through one side of the filter membrane (artificial kidney) while the client's blood passes through the other side. The processes of diffusion, osmosis, and ultrafiltration cleanse the client's blood and it is returned through a specially placed vascular access device (Gore-Tex graft). Both dialysis modalities can be applied for a short or long time, and they require specialized equipment and trained nurses.

Organ transplantation is the replacement of the client's diseased kidneys with a healthy one from a living or cadaveric donor of compatible blood and tissue type. After the client (recipient) is deemed medically and psychosocially suitable, the organ is surgically implanted. Special medications (immunosuppressives) are administered for life to prevent the body from rejecting the transplanted organ. Unlike the other treatments, successful organ transplantation offers the client the potential for restoration of normal kidney function.

Surgical Procedures

The stress of surgery initially triggers the general adaptation syndrome (see Chapter 22). The posterior pituitary gland releases an increased amount of ADH, which increases water reabsorption and reduces urine output. The surgical client is often in an altered state of fluid balance before surgery due to the disease process or preoperative fasting, which aggravates the reduction in urine output. The stress response also elevates the level of aldosterone, resulting in reduction in urine output in an effort to maintain circulatory fluid volume.

Anesthetic and narcotic analgesics may slow the glomerular filtration rate, reducing urine output. These pharmacological agents also impair sensory and motor impulses traveling between the bladder, spinal cord, and brain. Clients recovering from anesthesia and deep analgesia are often unable to sense bladder fullness and are unable to initiate or inhibit micturition. Spinal anesthetics, in particular, create the risk of **urinary retention** because of an inability to sense the need to void and a possible inability of the bladder muscles and sphincters to respond.

Surgery of lower abdominal and pelvic structures can impair urination because of local trauma to surrounding tissues. The edema and inflammation associated with healing may obstruct the flow of urine from the kidneys to the bladder or from the bladder or urethra, interfere with relaxation of pelvic and sphincter muscles, or cause discomfort during voiding. After returning from surgery involving the ureters, bladder, and urethra, clients routinely have urinary catheters.

The surgical formation of a urinary diversion temporarily or permanently bypasses the bladder and urethra as the exit routes for urine. Urinary diversions may be needed in the client with cancer of the bladder. The client with a urinary diversion has a **stoma** (artificial opening) on the abdomen to drain urine.

Medications

Diuretics prevent reabsorption of water and certain electrolytes to increase urine output. Urinary retention may be caused by use of anticholinergics (e.g., atropine), antihistamines (e.g., Sudafed), antihypertensives (e.g., Aldomet), and beta-adrenergic blockers (e.g., Inderal). Some medications change the color of urine (see the box at right). Clients with alterations in kidney function require dosage adjustments in medications excreted by the kidneys.

Diagnostic Examination

Examination of the urinary system can influence micturition. Procedures such as an intravenous pyelogram or urogram require that the client not take fluids orally before the test. A restriction in fluid intake commonly lowers urine output. Diagnostic examinations (e.g., cystoscopy) that involve direct visualization of urinary structures may cause localized edema of the urethral passageway and spasm of the bladder sphincter. The client often has urinary retention after such a procedure and may pass red or pink urine because of bleeding resulting from trauma to the urethral or bladder mucosa.

■ ALTERATIONS IN URINARY ELIMINATION

Clients with urinary problems most commonly have disturbances in the act of micturition. These disturbances result from impaired bladder function, obstruction to urine outflow, or inability to voluntarily control micturition. Some clients may have permanent or temporary changes in the normal pathway of urinary excretion. The client with a urinary diversion has special problems because urine drains to the outside through a stoma.

Urinary Retention

Urinary retention is the marked accumulation of urine in the bladder as a result of the inability of the bladder to empty. Urine continues to collect in the bladder, stretching its walls and causing feelings of pressure, discomfort, tenderness over the symphysis pubis, restlessness, and diaphoresis (sweating).

Normally urine production slowly fills the bladder and prevents activation of stretch receptors until it distends to a certain level of stretch. The micturition reflex occurs and the bladder empties. In urinary retention the bladder becomes unable to respond to the micturition reflex and thus unable to empty.

As retention progresses, retention with overflow may develop. Pressure in the bladder builds to a point where the external urethral sphincter is unable to hold back urine. The sphincter temporarily opens to allow a small volume of urine (25 to 60 ml) to escape. As urine exits, the bladder pressure falls enough to allow the sphincter to regain control and close. With retention overflow the client voids small amounts of urine two or three times an hour with no real relief of distention or discomfort. The nurse should be aware of the volume and frequency of voiding in order to assess this condition in the client. Bladder spasms may occur with voiding.

In acute retention key signs are absence of urine output over several hours and bladder distention. The client under the influence of anesthetics or analgesics may feel only pressure, but the alert client has severe pain as the bladder dis-

Medications that Discolor Urine
YELLOW URINE Vitamin B$_2$ Pyridium (in alkaline urine)
ORANGE TO RUST URINE Azo-Gantrisin Sulfonamides Pyridium Warfarin Sodium (Coumadin)
PINK TO RED URINE Thorazine Ex-Lax Phenytoin (Dilantin) Cascara (in alkaline urine)
GREEN TO BLUE URINE Amitriptyline (Elavil) Methylene Blue Dyrenium
BROWN TO BLACK URINE Injectable iron compounds Levodopa (L-Dopa) Nitrofurantoin Metronidazole (Flagyl)

tends beyond its normal capacity. In severe urinary retention the bladder may hold as much as 2000 to 3000 ml of urine. Retention occurs as a result of urethral obstruction, surgical trauma, alterations in motor and sensory innervation of the bladder, medication side effects, and anxiety.

Lower Urinary Tract Infections

UTIs are the most common hospital-acquired (nosocomial) infections in the United States. They are responsible for more than 5 million physician visits a year (Johnson, 1991). Bacteria in the urine (bacteriuria) may lead to the spread of organisms into the bloodstream and kidneys.

Microorganisms most commonly enter the urinary tract through the ascending urethral route. Bacteria inhabit the distal urethra, external genitalia, and vagina in women. Organisms enter the urethral meatus easily and travel up the inner mucosal lining to the bladder. Women are more susceptible to infection because of the proximity of the anus to the urethral meatus and because of the short urethra. Older adults and clients with progressive underlying disease or decreased immunity are also at increased risk. In men, prostatic secretions that contain an antibacterial substance and the length of the urethra reduce the susceptibility to UTIs. It is estimated that 20% to 30% of hospitalized older adults have significant bacteriuria (Yoshikawa, 1993).

In a healthy person with good bladder function, organisms are flushed out during voiding. However, bladder distention reduces blood flow to the mucosal and submucosal layers, and tissues become more susceptible to bacteria. Residual urine in the bladder becomes more alkaline and is an ideal site for microorganism growth.

The most common cause of infection is the introduction of instruments into the urinary tract. For example, the introduction of a catheter through the urethra provides a direct route for microorganisms. In young adults a single intermittent catheterization carries a 1% chance of infection, while the same procedure has an infection risk of 20% in older adults (Yoshikawa,1993). With an indwelling bladder catheter, bacteria ascend along the outside of the catheter on the urethral wall or travel up the catheter's lumen. The catheter interferes with the normal voiding mechanism that acts as a defense against organisms entering the urethra. Local irritation to the urethra or bladder further predisposes tissues to bacterial invasion. UTIs acquired in health institutions also result from poor handwashing by personnel, contaminated irrigation fluids, and faulty catheterization technique.

Poor perineal hygiene is a common cause of UTIs in women. Inadequate handwashing, failure to wipe from front to back after voiding or defecating, and frequent sexual intercourse predispose women to infection. Any interference with the free flow of urine can cause infection. A kinked, obstructed or clamped catheter and any condition resulting in urinary retention increase the risk of a bladder infection.

Clients with lower UTIs have pain or burning during urination (dysuria) as urine flows past inflamed tissues. Fever,

Table 46-1	Types of Urinary Incontinence		
DESCRIPTION	**CAUSES**	**SYMPTOMS**	
FUNCTIONAL Involuntary, unpredictable passage of urine in a client with intact urinary and nervous systems	Change in environment; sensory, cognitive, or mobility deficits	Urge to void that causes loss of urine before reaching appropriate receptacle The client with cognitive changes may have forgotten what to do	
OVERFLOW (REFLEX) Involuntary loss of urine occurring at somewhat predictable intervals Volume may be large or small	Inhibition of micturition by anesthesia or medications, spinal cord dysfunction (either inhibition of cerebral awareness or impairment of the reflex arc)	Unawareness of bladder filling, lack of urge to void, uninhibited bladder spasm contraction	
STRESS Increased intraabdominal pressure that causes leakage of a small amount of urine	Coughing, laughing, vomiting, or lifting with full bladder; obesity, full uterus in third trimester; incompetent bladder outlet; weak pelvic musculature	Loss of urine with increased intraabdominal pressure; urinary urgency and frequency	
URGE Involuntary passage of urine after a strong sense of urgency to void	Decreased bladder capacity; irritation of bladder stretch receptors; alcohol or caffeine ingestion; increased fluid intake, infection	Urinary urgency, often with frequency (more often than every two hr); bladder spasm or contracture; voiding in either small (less than 100 ml) or large (more than 500 ml) amounts	
TOTAL Total uncontrolled and continuous loss of urine	Neuropathy of sensory nerves; trauma or disease of spinal nerves or urethral sphincter; fistula between bladder and vagina	Constant flow of urine at unpredictable times; nocturia, unawareness of bladder filling or incontinence	

chills, nausea and vomiting, and malaise develop as the infection worsens. An irritated bladder causes a frequent and urgent sensation of the need to void. Irritation to bladder and urethral mucosa results in blood-tinged urine (**hematuria**). The urine appears concentrated and cloudy because of the presence of white blood cells (WBCs) or bacteria. If infection spreads to the upper urinary tract (kidneys— **pyelonephritis**), flank pain, tenderness, fever, and chills are common.

Urinary Incontinence

Urinary incontinence is the loss of control over micturition. It may be temporary or permanent. The client can no longer control the external urethral sphincter. Leakage of urine may be continuous or intermittent. The five types of incontinence are functional, reflex (overflow), stress, urge, and total (Table 46-1).

Incontinence should not be associated only with older adults. It may develop in people of every age, although it is more common in older adults. It is estimated that 37% of women aged 60 or over have some degree of incontinence (Brooks, 1993). Incontinence can impair body image. Clothing may become wet with urine, and the accompanying odor adds to embarrassment. As a result clients with this problem often avoid social activities.

Older adults may have special problems with incontinence because of physical limitations and the environments in which they live. Older persons with restricted mobility have greater chances of being incontinent because of their inability to reach toilet facilities in time. Low-set chairs and beds raised well above the floor may be obstacles for older adults who must get up to reach a toilet. Older clients who have difficulty undoing buttons or manipulating zippers face another obstacle. Older clients often lack the energy to walk very far at one time. The toilet may be too far away for clients with urge incontinence.

Continued episodes of incontinence create the potential for skin breakdown. The acidic character of urine is irritating to skin. The immobilized client who has frequent incontinence is especially at risk for pressure ulcers (see Chapter 38).

Urinary Diversions

A urinary stoma to divert the flow of urine from the kidneys directly to the abdominal surface is done for several reasons (see the box below). Such a **urinary diversion** may be temporary or permanent. Fig. 46-4 illustrates several urinary diversions.

Possible indications for Urinary Diversions
Cancer of the bladder, prostate, urethra, vagina, uterus, cervix
Trauma
Radiation injury to bladder
Vesicovaginal fistula
Urethrovaginal fistula
Neurogenic bladder
Chronic cystitis

The ileal loop or conduit (one of the more common approaches to urinary diversion) involves separating a loop of intestinal ileum with its blood supply intact. The surgeon implants the ureters into the isolated segment of ileum, which is then an outlet for urine drainage. The remaining ileum is reconnected to the rest of the digestive tract. The ileal segment can then be used merely as a conduit and urine will drain continuously or it can be fashioned into a reservoir (Moore et al, 1993). Recent advances in surgical reconstruction of the bowel have led to development of techniques for building a continent reservoir for urine constructed of small or large bowel. A pouch is constructed of ileum, providing urinary flow into a reservoir in a nonrefluxing manner. The portion of the ileum connected to the abdominal wall acts as a continent nipple, requiring intermittent catheterization for emptying. The disadvantage of either an ileal conduit or reservoir is that if urine outflow becomes obstructed, irreversible damage to the kidneys can occur secondary to chronic infections or hydronephrosis.

A **ureterostomy** involves bringing the end of one or both ureters to the abdominal surface. To avoid the need for two collecting devices, a transureteroureterostomy connects the ureters and brings one out through the abdominal wall. In some cases a tube may need to be placed directly into the renal pelvis to provide urinary drainage. This procedure is called a **nephrostomy**.

The client with an incontinent urinary diversion must wear a stomal pouch continuously because there is no sphincter control for regulation of urine flow. Local irritation and skin breakdown occur when urine comes in contact with the skin for long periods.

A urinary diversion poses threats to a client's body image. The client must wear an artificial device to collect urine and must learn to manage it. However, the client can

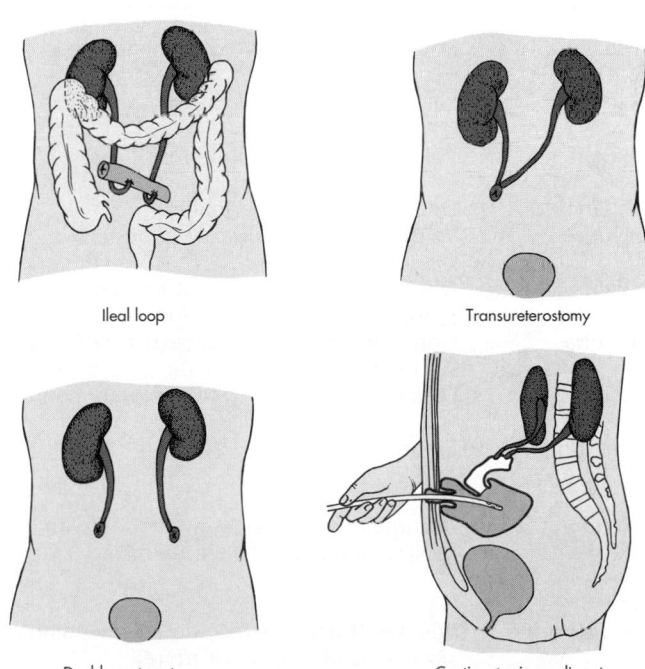

Ileal loop   Transureterostomy

Double ureterostomy   Continent urinary diversion

Fig. 46-4 Types of urinary diversions.

wear normal clothing, engage in physical activity, travel, and have sexual relations.

A client with a urinary diversion should be referred to the enterostomal therapist (a nurse with specialized training in this area). The therapist can be an invaluable resource to assist the client with matters pertaining to all aspects of care. The enterostomal therapist will often meet with the client prior to surgery. The client should also be referred to the United Ostomy Association. This organization may help in providing information regarding support groups to enhance coping and adaptation to lifestyle and body-image changes.

■ NURSING PROCESS FOR URINARY PROBLEMS

Assessment

To identify a urinary elimination problem and gather data for a care plan, the nurse obtains a nursing history, performs a physical assessment, assesses the client's urine, and reviews information from diagnostic tests and examinations.

Nursing History

The nursing history includes a review of the client's elimination patterns and symptoms of urinary alterations, and an assessment of other factors that may be affecting the ability to urinate normally.

PATTERN OF URINATION

The nurse asks the client about daily voiding patterns, including frequency and times of day, normal volume at each voiding, and any recent changes. Frequency varies among individuals and varies with intake and other types of fluid losses. The common times for urination are on awakening, after meals, and before bedtime. Most people void an average of five or more times a day. The client who voids frequently during the night may have renal disease or prostate enlargement. Information about the pattern of urination establishes a baseline for comparison.

SYMPTOMS OF URINARY ALTERATIONS

Certain symptoms specific to urinary alterations may occur in more than one type of disorder. During assessment the nurse asks the client about the symptoms listed in Table 46-2. The nurse also assesses whether the client is aware of conditions or factors that precipitate or aggravate symptoms.

FACTORS AFFECTING URINATION

The nurse summarizes factors in the client's history that normally affect urination such as age, environmental factors, and medication history. Older adults require careful assessment. Normal changes of aging predispose the elderly to certain elimination problems (see the box on p. 1303). The name, amount, and frequency of prescription drugs should be noted. Over-the-counter drugs and exposure to cleaning solvents, pesticides, or other nephrotoxic agents are also important aspects of the history. Environmental barriers at

Table 46-2	Common Symptoms of Urinary Alterations	
SYMPTOMS	**DESCRIPTION**	**CAUSES OR ASSOCIATED FACTORS**
Urgency	Feeling of need to void immediately	Full bladder, bladder irritation or inflammation from infection, incompetent urethral sphincter, psychological stress
Dysuria	Painful or difficult urination	Bladder inflammation, trauma or inflammation of urethral sphincter
Frequency	Voiding at frequent intervals	Increased fluid intake, bladder inflammation, increased pressure on bladder (pregnancy, psychological stress)
Hesitancy	Difficulty initiating urination	Prostate enlargement, anxiety, urethral edema
Polyuria	Voiding large amounts of urine	Excess fluid intake, diabetes mellitus or insipidus, use of diuretics, postobstructive diuresis
Oliguria	Diminished urinary output in relation intake (usually less than 400 ml in 24 hours)	Dehydration, renal failure, UTI, increased ADH secretion, congestive heart failure
Nocturia	Urination, particularly excessive or frequent at night	Excess fluid intake before bed (especially coffee or alcohol), renal disease, aging process
Dribbling	Leakage of urine despite voluntary control of micturition	Stress incontinence, overflow from urinary retention
Hematuria	Blood in the urine	Neoplasms of kidney or bladder, glomerular diseases, infection of kidneys or bladder, trauma to urinary structures, calculi, blood dyscrasias
Retention	Accumulation of urine in bladder, with inability of bladder to empty fully	Urethral obstruction, bladder inflammation, decreased sensory activity, neurogenic bladder, prostate enlargement, after anesthesia, side effects of medications (e.g., anticholinergics, antispasmodics, antidepressants)
Residual urine	Volume of urine remaining after voiding (volumes of 100 ml or more)	Inflammation or irritation of bladder mucosa from infection, neurogenic bladder, prostate enlargement, trauma, or inflammation of urethra

GERONTOLOGICAL PRINCIPLES
for Urinary Problems

- Although the nurse uses the same assessment process for clients of all ages, several factors that are of special concern in the older adult include those changes that occur normally with aging, those changes that are pathological in nature, and the effect that environmental barriers may have on the health of the urinary system.
- Some common physiological changes in renal/urinary function are: decrease in renal blood flow, number of glomeruli, concentration ability, response to ADH, ability to conserve sodium, and an increase in potassium retention.
- Pathological conditions that have an impact on urinary system functioning are: strictures of urethra or ureters, bladder neck obstruction (particularly benign prostatic hypertrophy), and bladder neuropathies related to diabetes mellitus. The normal decrease in immune system function makes the older adult more susceptible to urinary tract infections (Yoshikawa,1993).
- The nurse should note that incontinence is not a normal sign of aging and the older client deserves a thorough assessment to detect reversible causes of incontinence and primary interventions to regain continence.

home or in a health care setting are also evaluated. The client may need an elevated toilet seat, grab bars, or a portable commode. The nurse observes for sensory restrictions such as clients with visual problems who may have trouble reaching toilet facilities. If the client has difficulty with hand coordination, the nurse assesses the type of clothing and ease in using clothing fasteners.

Past illness such as UTI or urinary tract surgery that increases the risk for recurrent problems is important also. Chronic diseases (e.g., multiple sclerosis) that impair bladder function require the nurse to consider preventive care measures such as frequent toileting to keep client's skin dry and free from irritation. The nurse asks the client about the presence of urinary diversion. If the client has a urinary diversion, the nurse determines the rationale for its creation, type of diversion, and usual methods for management (type of appliance or pouch, type of skin barriers or applications, methods used to reduce skin irritation, frequency of appliance changes, and the type of nighttime drainage system). Personal habits also affect urination. If a client is hospitalized the nurse assesses the extent to which personal habits are altered. Privacy is often difficult to accomplish in a health care setting, particularly if a client must use a bedpan.

The nurse assesses for the presence of an indwelling catheter. A client recovering from major surgery or suffering critical illness or disability often has an indwelling catheter to aid urinary drainage and provide a measurement of urine output. The presence of a catheter places a client at risk for infection. A client's physical condition affects the frequency with which the nurse monitors fluid intake (see Chapter 45). Regular intake and output (I & O) measurements help assess a client's overall fluid balance.

Physical Assessment

A physical examination (see Chapter 33) provides the nurse with data to determine the presence and severity of urinary elimination problems. The primary organs reviewed include the skin, kidneys, bladder, and urethra.

SKIN

The nurse assesses skin condition. Problems with urinary elimination are often associated with fluid and electrolyte disturbances. By assessing skin turgor and the oral mucosa the nurse assesses the client's hydration status.

KIDNEYS

If the kidneys become infected or inflamed, flank pain typically develops. The nurse can assess for flank tenderness early in the disease by percussing the costovertebral angle (the angle formed by the spine and twelfth rib). Inflammation of the kidney results in pain during percussion. Auscultation is also performed to detect the presence of a renal artery bruit (sound resulting from turbulent blood flow through a narrowed artery).

Nurses with advanced examination skills learn to palpate the kidneys during abdominal examination. The position, shape, and size of the kidneys can reveal problems such as tumors.

BLADDER

In adults the bladder rests below the symphysis pubis and cannot be examined by the nurse. When distended, the bladder rises above the symphysis pubis at the midline of the abdomen and may extend to just below the umbilicus. On inspection the nurse may note a swelling or convex curvature of the lower abdomen. The nurse lightly palpates the lower abdomen. The bladder normally feels smooth and rounded. As the nurse applies light pressure to the bladder, the client may feel tenderness or even pain. Even when the bladder is not visible palpation may cause the urge to urinate. Percussion of a full bladder yields a dull percussion note.

URETHRAL MEATUS

The nurse assesses the urinary meatus to note the presence of discharge, inflammation, and lesions. This assessment screens for infections and other abnormalities. To examine the female, a dorsal recumbent position provides full exposure of the genitalia. While wearing gloves, the nurse retracts the labial folds to see the urethral meatus. Normally the meatus is pink and appears as a small slitlike opening below the clitoris and above the vaginal orifice. There is normally no discharge from the meatus. If present, specimens of urethral discharge should be obtained before the client voids.

Women with vaginal infections are susceptible to UTIs because vaginal discharge may travel easily to the urethral meatus. Older women commonly have vaginitis as a result of hormonal deficiencies. The nurse inspects the vaginal orifice carefully and describes any drainage. Infection may also be indicated by reddened, inflamed vaginal mucosa.

A man's urethral meatus is normally a small opening at the tip of the penis. The nurse inspects the meatus for discharge, inflammation, and lesions. It may be necessary to retract the foreskin in uncircumcised men to see the meatus.

Assessment of Urine

Assessment of urine involves measuring the client's fluid intake and urine output and observing characteristics of the client's urine.

INTAKE AND OUTPUT

The nurse assesses the client's average daily fluid intake. If an accurate measurement of fluid intake is needed from the client who is at home, the nurse may ask the client to show a commonly used glass or cup on which the intake estimate is based.

In a health care setting the nurse measures a client's fluid intake either when the physician orders I & O measurements (see Chapter 45) or when nursing judgment warrants a more precise measurement. The nurse includes all sources, including oral intake, intravenous fluid infusions, tube feedings, and fluid instilled into nasogastric or gastric tubes.

Because it is often difficult for the client to estimate volumes of urine voided, the nurse must obtain measurements. A change in urine volume is a significant indicator of fluid alterations or kidney disease. While caring for the client, the nurse assesses volume by measuring (with plastic receptacles, bedpans, or urinals) urinary output with each voiding. Special receptacles (urimeters) attach between indwelling catheters and drainage bags and are a convenient means of measuring urine volume regularly. A urimeter holds 100 to 200 ml of urine. After measuring urine from a urimeter, the nurse can drain the cylinder into

the urinary drainage bag or into a receptacle for disposal. Urimeters are indicated when precise hourly measurements of urine are needed.

When urine from a drainage bag is measured, it is best to use a separate plastic graduate receptacle (Fig. 46-5). Scales on the bags offer only an approximate volume. Each client should have a graduated receptacle for their exclusive use to prevent potential cross-contamination.

The nurse reports any extreme increase or decrease in volume. An hourly output of less than 30 ml for more than 2 hours is cause for concern. Similarly, consistently high volumes of urine (**polyuria**), over 2000 to 2500 ml daily, should be reported to a physician.

CHARACTERISTICS OF URINE

The nurse inspects the client's urine for color, clarity, and odor.

Color. Normal urine ranges from a pale, straw color to amber, depending on its concentration. Urine is usually more concentrated in the morning or with fluid volume deficits. As the person drinks more fluids, urine becomes less concentrated.

Bleeding from the kidneys or ureters causes urine to become dark red; bleeding from the bladder or urethra causes a bright red urine. Various medications also change urine color (see the box on p. 1299). Eating beets, rhubarb, or blackberries may cause red urine. Special dyes used in intravenous diagnostic studies eventually discolor urine. Dark amber urine may be the result of high concentrations of bilirubin caused by liver dysfunction. Urine containing bilirubin (**bilirubinuria**) can also be detected by the appearance of yellow foam when a specimen is shaken. The nurse documents and reports any abnormal color or sediment, especially if the cause is unknown.

Clarity. Normal urine appears transparent at voiding. Urine that stands several minutes in a container becomes cloudy. Freshly voided urine in clients with renal disease may appear cloudy or foamy because of high protein concentrations. Urine also appears thick and cloudy as a result of bacteria.

Odor. Urine has a characteristic odor. The more concentrated the urine, the stronger the odor. Stagnant urine has an ammonia odor, which is common in clients who are repeatedly incontinent. A sweet or fruity odor occurs from acetone or acetoacetic acid, by-products of incomplete fat metabolism seen with diabetes mellitus or starvation.

URINE TESTING

The nurse often collects urine specimens for laboratory testing. The type of test determines the method of collection. All specimens are labeled with the client's name, date, and time of collection. Specimens should be transported to the laboratory in a timely fashion to ensure accuracy of test results. Agency infection-control policies require the adherence to standard precautions by all personnel during specimen handling (see Chapter 34).

Specimen Collection. The nurse collects random, clean-voided or midstream, sterile, and timed specimens.

Random specimen. A random routine urine specimen can be collected with a client voiding naturally or from a Foley catheter or urinary diversion collection bag. The specimen should be clean but need not be sterile. Random specimens

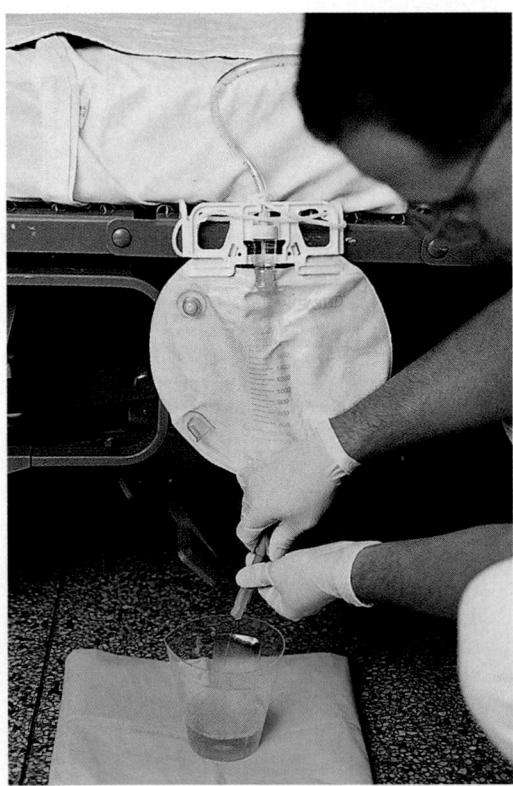

Fig. 46-5 Urimeter drainage bag.

Collecting Midstream (Clean-Voided) Urine Specimen

STEPS	RATIONALE
1. Refer to agency policy for specimen collection.	Agency policies may vary regarding collection method or handling of specimens.
2. Assess status of client	
a. When client last voided	May indicate bladder fullness.
b. Level of awareness or developmental stage	Reveals client's ability to cooperate during procedure.
c. Mobility, balance, and physical limitations	Determines level of assistance.
3. Assess client's understanding of purpose of test and method of collection.	Information allows you to clarify misunderstandings and promotes client cooperation.
4. Prepare following equipment and supplies:	Agency policy may determine type of equipment to use.
a. Soap, washcloth, and towel	Used to clean, rinse, and dry perineum.
b. Commercial kit for clean-voided urine (see the illustration), sterile cotton balls, or 2 × 2 gauze pads	
c. Antiseptic solution (e.g., povidone-iodine) Check for client allergies	

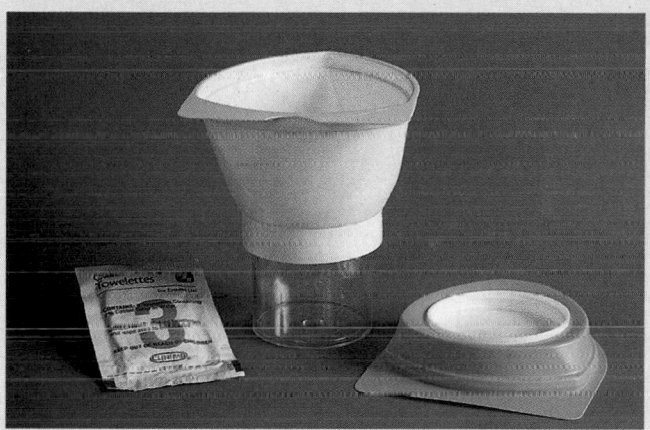

Step 4b

STEPS	RATIONALE
d. Sterile water	Rinses antiseptic solution. Antiseptic solution can alter the results if allowed to enter specimen.
e. Sterile specimen container (may be contained in commercial kit)	
f. Sterile and nonsterile gloves	
g. Bedpan (for non-ambulating clients), specimen hat, bedside commode, or potty chair	Women can void in normal fashion. Children are more likely to use familiar facilities.
h. Completed specimen label	Completion of label and requisition before collecting specimen prevents confusion and allows accurate transport to laboratory.
5. Explain procedure to client:	
a. Reason midstream specimen is needed	Helps client provide specimen independently.
b. Ways client and family can assist	
c. Ways to obtain specimen free of feces	Feces change characteristics of urine and may cause abnormal values.
6. Provide fluids to drink ½ hour before collection unless contraindicated (i.e., fluid restriction) if client does not feel urge to void.	Improves likelihood of client being able to void.
7. Provide privacy for client by closing door or bed curtain.	Privacy allows client to relax and produce specimen more quickly.
8. Give client or family member soap, washcloth, and towel to cleanse perineal area.	Client may prefer to wash own perineal area.
9. Apply nonsterile gloves and assist nonambulatory client with perineal care. Assist female client onto bedpan.	Prevents transmission of microorganisms to nurse. Provides easy access to perineal area to collect specimen.
10. Change gloves if necessary.	Reduces transfer of infection.

Continued.

Collecting Midstream (Clean-Voided) Urine Specimen—cont'd

STEPS	RATIONALE
11. Using surgical asepsis, open sterile kit or prepare sterile supplies. Apply sterile gloves at the appropriate time (see Chapter 34).	Sterile technique is essential to maintain sterility of equipment and specimen. Sterile gloves prevent the transfer of microorganisms to the specimen from the nurse or from the client to the nurse.
12. Pour antiseptic over cotton balls or gauze pads unless kit contains prepared gauze pads in antiseptic solution.	Cotton balls or gauze pads are used to cleanse perineum.
13. Open sterile container and place cap with sterile inside surface up and do not touch inside of container or cap.	Contaminated specimen is most frequent reason for inaccurate reporting of urine cultures and sensitivities.
14. Assist or allow client to independently cleanse perineum and collect specimen: a. Male:	
(1) Hold penis with one hand and using circular motion and antiseptic swab, cleanse end of penis, moving from center to outside (see the illustration below).	Cleanse from area of least contamination to area of greatest contamination to decrease bacteria levels.
(2) If agency procedure indicates, rinse area with sterile water and dry with cotton balls or gauze pad.	Prevents contamination of specimen with antiseptic solution.
(3) After client has initiated urine stream, pass specimen collection container into stream and collect 30 to 60 ml (see the illustration below).	Initial urine flushes out microorganisms that normally accumulate at urinary meatus and prevents their collection in the specimen.

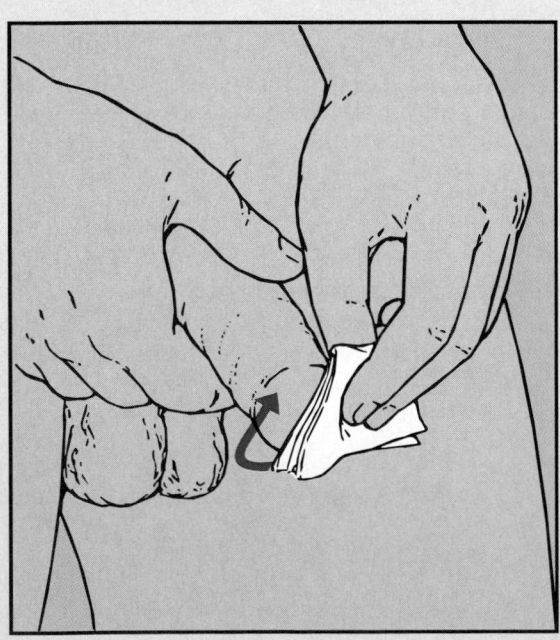

Step 14a(1)

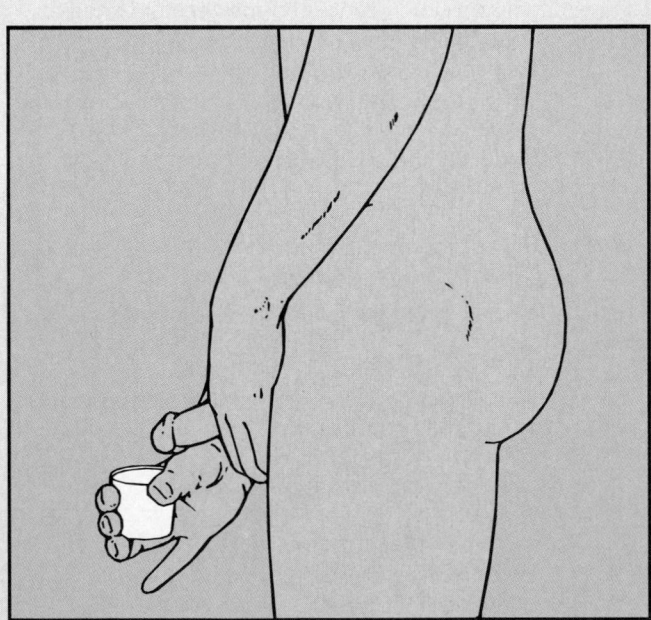

Step 14a(3)

Collecting Midstream (Clean-Voided) Urine Specimen—cont'd

STEPS	RATIONALE

14. Assist or allow client to independently cleanse perineum and collect specimen—cont'd

   b. Female:

     (1) Spread labia with thumb and forefinger of non-dominant hand

         Provides access to urethral meatus.

     (2) Cleanse area with cotton ball or gauze, moving from front (above urethral orifice) to back (toward anus) (see the illustration below).

         Cleanse from area of least contamination to area of greatest contamination to decrease bacteria levels.

     (3) If agency procedure indicates, rinse area with sterile water, and dry with cotton.

         Prevents contamination of specimen with antiseptic solution.

     (4) While continuing to hold labia apart, client should initiate stream and after stream is achieved, pass specimen container into stream and collect 30 to 60 ml (see the illustration below).

         Initial stream flushes out microorganisms that accumulate at urethral meatus.

15. Remove specimen container before flow of urine stops and before releasing labia or penis. Client finishes voiding into bedpan or toilet.

         Prevents contamination of specimen with skin flora.

16. Replace cap securely on specimen container (touch only outside).

         Retains sterility of inside of container and prevents spillage of urine.

17. Cleanse any urine from exterior surface of container, and place in a plastic specimen bag.

         Prevents transfer of microorganisms to others.

18. Remove bedpan (if applicable) and assist client to a comfortable position.

         Promotes relaxing environment.

19. Label specimen and attach laboratory requisition.

         Prevents inaccurate identification that could lead to errors in diagnosis or treatment.

20. Remove gloves, dispose in proper receptacle, and wash hands.

         Reduces transmission of infection.

21. Transport specimen to laboratory within 15 minutes or refrigerate immediately.

         Bacteria grow quickly in urine, and specimen should be analyzed immediately to obtain correct results.

22. Record date and time urine specimen was obtained in nurses' notes.

         Documents implementation of physician's order.

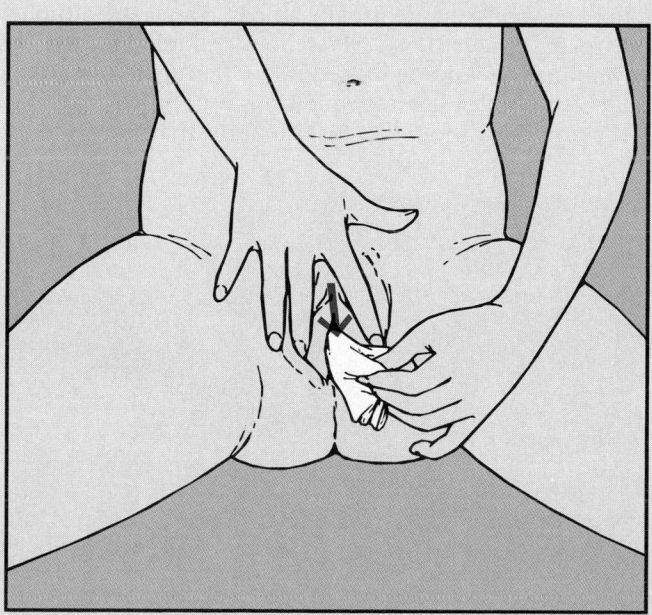

Step 14b(2)

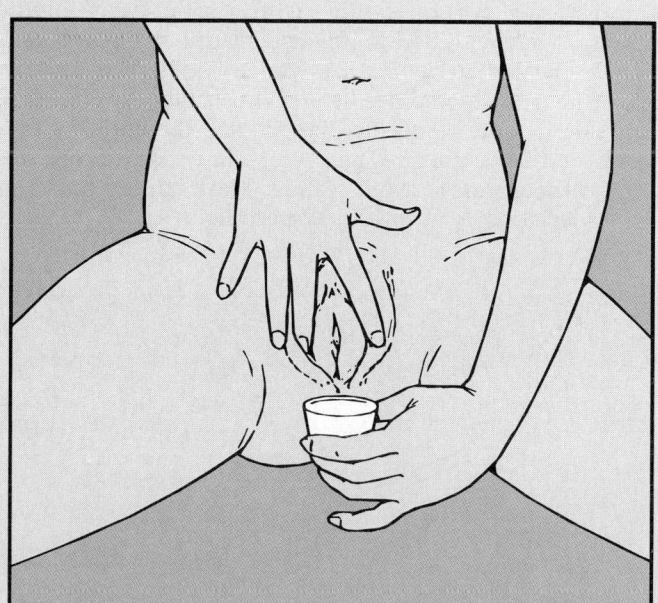

Step 14b(4)

are used for urinalysis testing or measurements of specific gravity, pH, or glucose levels.

The client voids into a clean urine cup, urinal, or bedpan. Many clients are able to do this independently. However, mobility restrictions or poor vision may require the nurse to assist. It is easier to collect a specimen if the client drinks a glass of fluid 30 minutes before the procedure. A client should void before defecating so that feces do not contaminate the specimen. Female clients are also instructed not to place toilet tissue in the bedpan. Only 120 ml (4 oz) of urine is needed for accurate testing. After the specimen is collected the nurse places the lid tightly on the specimen container, washes off any urine that splashed on the outside of the container, places the container in a plastic bag, and sends the labeled specimen promptly to the laboratory.

Clean-voided or midstream specimen. To obtain a specimen relatively free of the microorganisms growing in the lower urethra, the nurse instructs the client on the method for obtaining a clean-voided specimen (Procedure 46-1). This type of specimen is needed to test urine for culture and sensitivity. After appropriate cleansing of the external genitalia, a client begins the urinary stream allowing the initial portion to escape; then during the middle portion of voiding, the client collects the specimen. The initial stream of urine cleans or flushes the urethral orifice and meatus of resident bacteria. It is easiest for a client to obtain clean-voided specimens while using toilet facilities.

Sterile specimen. Another method for collecting a urine specimen for culture is by obtaining it from an indwelling catheter. It is no longer recommended to catheterize a client just to obtain a specimen because the risk of causing an infection is high. A urine specimen is also not collected for culture from a urine drainage bag unless it is the first urine drained into a new sterile bag. Bacteria grow rapidly in the drainage bags and could cause a false measurement.

For an indwelling retention catheter, the nurse uses a sterile syringe to withdraw urine. The nurse washes hands and applies nonsterile gloves to prevent transmission of microorganisms. A 3-ml syringe with a small-gauge needle (23- or 25-gauge) is best to prevent creation of a permanent hole in the catheter port. However, if blood is suspected in the urine, a large-bore needle prevents breakdown of RBCs. It is safe to insert a needle directly into the end of a self-sealing rubber catheter (Fig. 46-6). Silastic, plastic, or silicone catheters are not self-sealing. Most urinary catheters have special ports to withdraw specimens (Fig. 46-7). First,

the nurse clamps the tubing just below the site chosen for withdrawal, allowing fresh, uncontaminated urine to collect in the tube. The nurse then wipes the catheter or port with an antimicrobial swab. Inserting the needle at a 30-degree angle ensures entrance into the catheter lumen. While aspirating 3 to 5 ml of urine the nurse must be careful not to raise the tubing, which would cause urine to flow back into the bladder.

After obtaining the specimen the nurse transfers the urine into a sterile container using sterile aseptic technique (see Chapter 34). The nurse removes the gloves, properly disposes of equipment, and washes hands to reduce the transfer of microorgansims to other clients and health care workers. The laboratory requisition should indicate the method of collection.

Timed urine specimens. Some tests of renal function and urine composition, such as measuring levels of adrenocortical steroids or hormones, creatinine clearance, or protein quantitation tests, require collection of urine over 2-, 12-, or 24-hour intervals.

The timed collection period begins after the client urinates. The nurse discards the sample and indicates the starting time on the collection container and on the laboratory requisition (check agency policy). The client then collects all urine voided in the timed period.

Each voiding is collected in a clean container and immediately emptied into the larger container. Some tests require the client to void at specific times. Each specimen must be free of feces or toilet tissue.

Any missed specimens will make test results inaccurate. The nurse should remind the client to void before defecating so that urine is not contaminated by feces. The collection container may contain a preservative or require refrigeration. The laboratory should be consulted for instructions. The client should void the last specimen at the end of the timed period.

Urine collection in children. Specimen collection from infants and children is often difficult. Adolescents and school-age children are usually able to cooperate, although they may be embarrassed. Preschool children and toddlers have difficulty voiding on request. Offering a young child fluids 30 minutes before requesting a specimen may help. The nurse must use terms for urination that the child can

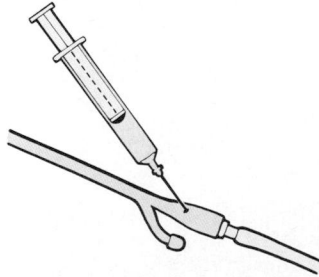

Fig. 46-6 Urine specimen collection; aspiration from a self-sealing rubber catheter. *(Redrawn from McConnell EA:* Care of Patients with Urologic Problems, *Philadelphia, 1983, Lippenworth.)*

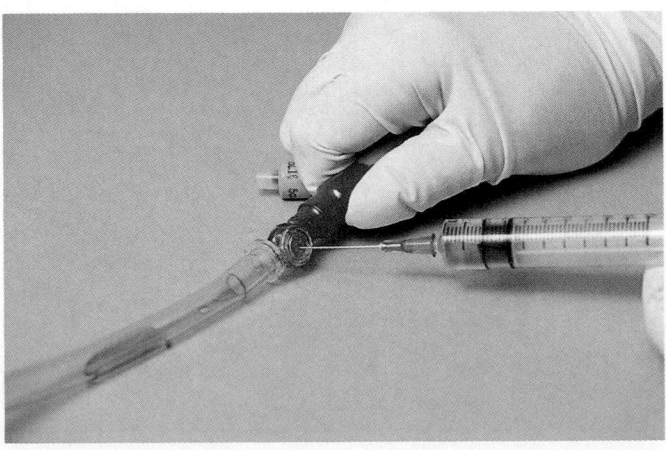

Fig. 46-7 Urine specimen collection; Aspiration from a collection port in drainage tubing of an indwelling catheter.

understand. A young child may be reluctant to void in unfamiliar receptacles. A potty chair or specimen hat placed under the toilet seat is usually effective. The nurse must use special collection devices for infants or toddlers who are not toilet trained. Clear plastic, single-use bags with self-adhering material can be attached over the child's urethral meatus.

The nurse prepares an infant by first washing the genitalia, perineum, and surrounding skin with soap and water or an antiseptic. Thorough drying is necessary because the bag's adhesive does not stick to a moist, powdered, or oily surface. The nurse attaches the bag from back to front, first to the perineum and then toward the symphysis pubis. In girls the perineum should be gently stretched to ensure that the bag has a leak-proof fit. In boys the scrotum and penis fit inside the collection bag. A diaper is placed over the bag. The nurse checks the bag often and removes it as soon as urine is available. An active child can easily loosen the bag and cause a leak. For a clean-voided specimen the nurse uses a sterile collection bag. Specimens should not be obtained by squeezing urine from the diaper material.

Common Urine Tests. Urine tests include urinalysis, specific gravity, and urine culture.

Urinalysis. The laboratory performs a **urinalysis** on a specimen obtained by any of the previously described methods. Table 46-3 lists normal values for a urinalysis. The specimen should be examined as soon as possible, preferably within 2 hours. It should be the first voided specimen in the morning to ensure a uniform concentration of constituents. For a quick screening the nurse can perform certain portions of the urinalysis with special reagent strips.

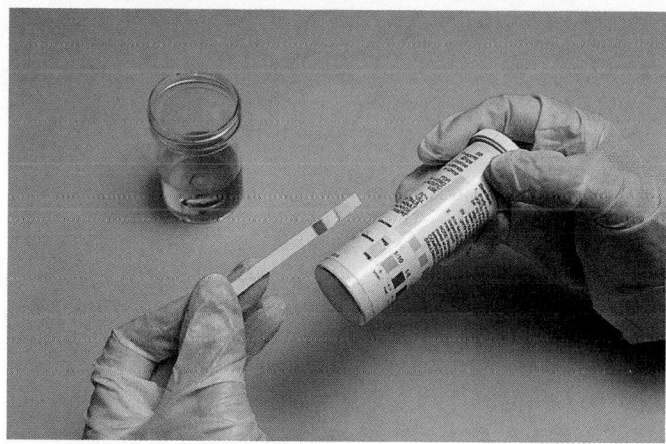

Fig. 46-8 Checking results of a chemical reagent strip dipped in urine.

The nurse dips the strips into the urine and then observes for a color change in the time interval designated on the package (Fig. 46-8).

Specific gravity. The **specific gravity** is the weight or degree of concentration of a substance compared with an equal volume of water. To measure specific gravity a urinometer and cylinder are used. The urinometer has a specific gravity scale at the top and a weighted mercury bulb at the bottom. A urine specimen is poured into a special clean, dry cylinder. The weighted urinometer is suspended and lightly twirled into the cylinder of urine. The concen-

Table 46-3	Routine Urinalysis	
MEASUREMENT AND NORMAL VALUE	**INTERPRETATION**
pH (4.6-8.0)	pH helps indicate acid-base balance. Urine that stands for several hours becomes alkaline. An acid pH helps protect against bacterial growth.
Protein (up to 10 mg/100 ml)	Normally protein is not present in urine. It is seen in renal disease because damage to glomerulus or tubules allows protein to enter urine.
Glucose (not normally present)	Diabetic clients have glucose in urine as a result of inability of tubules to reabsorb high glucose concentrations (over 180 mg/100 ml). Ingestion of high concentrations of glucose may cause some glucose to appear in urine of healthy persons.
Ketone (not normally present)	Clients whose diabetes mellitus is poorly controlled experience breakdown of fatty acids. End product of fat metabolism is ketones. Clients with dehydration, starvation, or excessive aspirin ingestion also have **ketonuria.**
Blood (up to 2 RBCs)	Damage to glomerulus or tubules may cause RBCs to enter urine. Trauma, disease, or surgery of lower urinary tract also may cause blood to be present. In women, blood in a urine specimen may indicate contamination with menstrual fluid.
Specific Gravity (1.010-1.030)	Specific gravity measures concentration of particles in urine. High specific gravity reflects concentrated urine, and low specific gravity reflects diluted urine. Dehydration, reduced renal blood flow, and increase in ADH secretion elevate specific gravity. Overhydration, early renal disease, and inadequate ADH secretion reduce specific gravity.
Microscopic examination WBCs (0 to 8 per high-powered field)	Greater numbers may indicate urinary tract infection.
Bacteria (not normally present)	Bacteria indicate urinary tract infection.
Casts (not normally present)	Casts are cylindrical bodies whose shapes take on likeness of objects within the renal tubule. There are several types, namely hyaline, WBCs, granular cells, and epithelial cells. Their presence in urine is an abnormal finding and indicates renal alterations.

tration of dissolved substances in the urine determines the depth at which the urinometer floats. This measurement is always done as part of a complete urinalysis. The nurse in a critical care unit may be responsible for doing periodic measurement of specific gravity in the assessment of the client.

With the urinometer at eye level the nurse reads the measurement at the base of the meniscus at the level of the urine. The specific gravity of a morning urine specimen voided by a fasting client reflects the kidney's maximum concentrating ability. A specific gravity below 1.010 reflects an inability of the kidneys to concentrate urine or an insufficient secretion of ADH. When the kidneys become diseased, they lose their ability to concentrate urine. Therefore the specific gravity becomes "fixed" at a low value (1.010 or lower). An elevated specific gravity can indicate dehydration. Radiopaque substances or high molecular weight substances in the urine (e.g., protein or glucose) may cause a falsely high specific gravity.

If questions regarding the accuracy of specific gravity measurements arise, a urine osmolality test should be obtained. Although both tests measure urine concentration, the osmolality test is more accurate because it measures the total number of particles in a solution (see Chapter 45).

Urine culture. A urine culture requires a sterile or clean-voided sample of urine. It takes approximately 48 hours before the laboratory can report findings of bacterial growth. While awaiting results, a broad spectrum antibiotic may be ordered as soon as a culture has been obtained. The test for sensitivity determines which specific antibiotics are effective. The results (sensitivities) of a urine culture may indicate a change in choice of medication.

Diagnostic Examinations. The urinary system is one of the few organ systems amenable to accurate diagnostic study by several radiographic techniques. The two approaches for visualization of urinary structures, direct and indirect techniques, can be quite simple or very complex, requiring extensive nursing intervention. These procedures are further subdivided into invasive or noninvasive categories.

Abdominal Roentgenogram. Abdominal roentgenogram, also referred to as *plain film, KUB,* or *flat plate,* of the abdomen is commonly used to assess the gross structures of the urinary tract for abnormalities. It can determine size, symmetry, shape, and location of the kidneys, ureters, and bladder structures. It is also useful in visualizing calculi (if they are calcified) or tumors in these organs. In addition, the ribs or other surrounding support structures can be assessed for fractures or abnormalities. This is important if the client has suffered some type of traumatic injury. Lack of positive findings on the roentgenogram does not rule out the possibility of abnormalities in the urinary tract. Additional diagnostic studies may be needed.

The nursing implications for clients undergoing this procedure include explanation of the procedure and alleviation of client anxiety. No special bowel preparation is needed unless the physician chooses otherwise.

Intravenous pyelogram. To view the entire urinary system, the physician orders the excretory urogram or intravenous pyelogram (IVP). This procedure visualizes the collecting ducts and renal pelvis and outlines the ureters, bladder, and urethra. Although this procedure is noninvasive, it requires the client to receive an intravenous injection of a ra-

diopaque dye. The injected medium takes only a few minutes to circulate and be excreted. The dye is not visible until it is filtered and concentrated by the kidneys. Because the kidneys and ureters lie behind the intestines, it is necessary that the client receive a bowel preparation to empty the intestines before the procedure. Procedures using barium should not be performed 2 to 3 days before an IVP because residual barium in the intestines obscures the view (see Chapter 47).

During the IVP, x-ray studies are taken at specific intervals over 30 to 60 minutes as the dye concentrates. The client may also be asked to void during the procedure to measure bladder emptying. Diseases or disorders of the urinary tract that should be investigated by this means include renal artery occlusion, tumors, cysts or calculi, **vesicoureteral reflux,** and traumatic injuries.

Nursing implications before the test include recognizing clients at risk for alterations in renal function as a result of the intravenous injection of the contrast dye. Any client with renal insufficiency is at risk. Older clients are prone to the nephrotoxic effects of contrast dye because of the fluid loss during bowel preparation. Nursing assessment of volume status and its maintenance before this procedure is of utmost importance (see Chapter 45). Additional nursing implications follow:

1. Signed informed consent (if agency policy)
2. Assess client for history of iodine allergy, which predicts allergies to the IVP dye.
3. Administer cathartic on evening before test.
4. Ensure that client follows the appropriate intake restriction prior to the test. (May be NPO after midnight or clear liquids only after a clear liquid supper.)
5. Explain that facial flushing is normal during dye injection and that client may feel dizzy or warm.
6. Explain that an intravenous infusion for dye injection is started before the test.
7. Explain that the test involves x-ray studies taken at several intervals and that client will void near the end of the test.

Not all agencies employ nurses in the radiology department. If a nurse is not present, the physician or radiology technician assumes these responsibilities. Implications during the test include the following:

1. Assess intravenous site for signs of infiltration of dye into tissues (e.g., swelling, redness, and pain).
2. Observe for signs of allergic reaction to dye (e.g., respiratory distress, fall in blood pressure, and hives).
3. Remind client of normal sensations caused by dye injection.

Nursing implications after the test include the following:

1. Ensure that client receives usual diet afterward.
2. Encourage fluid intake to minimize dehydration caused by bowel prep and to avoid the potential nephrotoxic effects of the contrast material.
3. Monitor I & O and promptly report alterations to physician.
4. Observe for possible delayed allergic reactions.

Renal Scan. Radionuclide tests such as renal scans allow indirect visualization of urinary tract structures after an intravenous injection of radioactive isotopes. Selection of an isotope depends on the physiological process to be studied. The emissions from the radionuclides can be photographed by special cameras. The isotope can be detected without the need of bowel preparation. A very low dosage of radioisotope is used. Therefore no precautions against radioactive exposure are needed except for the use of disposable gloves if the client uses a bedpan or urinal to void. Rinse bedpan or urinal and double flush urine down the toilet to dilute any possible remaining radiation hazard.

After a radionuclide is injected, it circulates through the kidneys and is excreted. The renal scan measures radioactive concentrations. Except for the venipuncture, it is painless. The scanning procedure is completed in about 1 hour. Information pertaining to renal blood flow, anatomical structures, and their excretory function can be obtained from this procedure. The physician can diagnose abnormalities such as renal artery occlusion, urinary obstruction, and many other diseases of the kidney. This procedure is indicated for clients unable to receive IVP dyes. The nurse does not routinely give a sedative before the test unless the physician views the client as highly anxious. Nursing implications before the test include the following:

1. Signed informed consent (if agency policy).
2. Explain that radioisotope is injected intravenously through an existing IV line or needle.
3. Explain that the machine measuring the isotope uptake is similar to a Geiger counter.
4. Explain that client will feel no discomfort but must lie still.
5. Explain that there is no risk of radioactive exposure.

Nursing implications during the test include the following:

1. Assist the client in changing positions during the test. (Technician may do this.)

No specific nursing implications after the test.

Computerized Axial Tomography. Computerized tomography (CT) is a computerized x-ray procedure used to obtain detailed images of structures within a selected plane of the body. The tomographic scanner is a large machine that contains specialized computers and x-ray detector systems that function simultaneously to photograph internal structures in thin, transverse cross-sections (Fig. 46-9). The computer, through a series of complex manipulations, is able to "reconstruct" the cross-sectional image as a recognizable photograph on the television monitor. With this

procedure it is possible to visualize abnormal pathological conditions such as tumors, obstructions, retroperitoneal masses, and lymph node enlargement. The CT scan can detect masses of less than 2 cm in size. Although this procedure is noninvasive, in some examinations oral or intravenous contrast material is used to enhance the areas under study. If intravenous contrast is used, it may be necessary to administer a bowel cleansing solution orally (such as GoLytely) or an enema, especially if additional organs in the abdominal cavity will be examined. The nursing implications before, during, and after this test are the same as those listed under the IVP examination. However, the nurse explains that the client will be placed in a large machine, which may cause feelings of claustrophobia in susceptible individuals.

Renal Ultrasound. Ultrasonography is a valuable noninvasive diagnostic tool in the assessment of urinary disorders. It makes use of high-frequency, inaudible sound waves that reflect off tissue structures. A conductive gel is applied to the skin and functions as a transmitter for sound waves. A transducer passed over the conductive gel emits a sound beam as it is also passed over body tissues of varying density. Some of the sound waves are reflected back to the transducer as echoes. The echoes are converted into electrical impulses that are displayed on an oscilloscope, presenting an image of the tissues being studied. The velocity of the sound waves varies with tissue density. The client is usually prone during the procedure but can be positioned in a sitting position. Ultrasound is frequently used to identify gross renal structures and structural abnormalities of the kidneys or lower urinary tract and to assist with percutaneous biopsy. Abnormalities such as tumors or cysts in the kidney are easily identified. If a Doppler is used with the transducer, examination of blood flow through the kidney can also be performed. This procedure is painless.

Nursing implications before the procedure involve explanation of the test and possibly encouraging the client to ingest oral fluids to cause bladder distention. No specific client care is indicated after the test.

Cystometrogram (CMG) is a test that determines the level of function of the detrusor muscle. This test is used to rule out causes of incontinence. A catheter is inserted, residual volume is measured and discarded and the bladder is filled with either sterile saline or carbon dioxide gas in predetermined increments. Pressure readings are taken at those increments. During the filling time the client's perceptions related to bladder fullness, urge to void, and the ability to inhibit voiding are documented.

Nursing implications before the test involve explanation of the procedure and the need to report sensations as they occur. After the test is completed the client should be instructed to report the following sensations: sweating, pain, nausea, bladder fullness, or a strong urge to void

Invasive Procedures. Invasive procedures include cystoscopy, biopsy, and angiogram.

Cystoscopy. A cystoscopy allows the physician to view the interior of the bladder and urethra. The cystoscope looks much like a urinary catheter, although it is not as flexible and is generally larger. It is inserted through the client's urethra. The instrument has an outer plastic or rubber sheath, an obturator that keeps the scope rigid during insertion, a telescope for viewing the bladder and urethra,

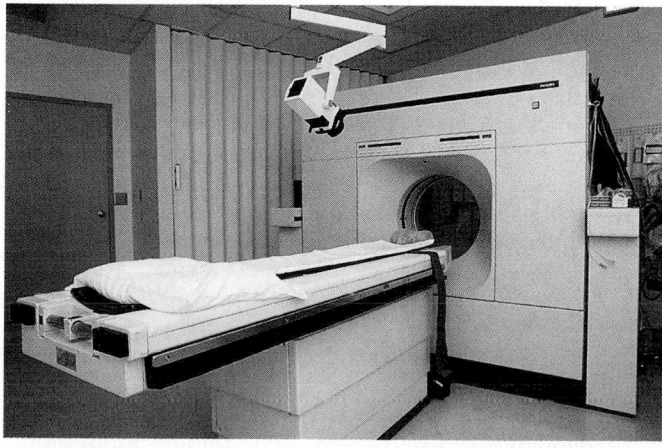

Fig. 46-9 CT equipment. *(From Brundage DJ: Renal disorders, St Louis, 1992, Mosby.)*

and a channel for inserting catheters or special surgical instruments.

The procedure is painful during instrument insertion. There is risk of bladder perforation if the client is not relaxed and cooperative. Local, spinal, or general anesthesia may be given. Because the test requires insertion of a foreign object into a sterile cavity, the client receives large amounts of fluids (intravenously or orally) before and during the procedure to maintain a continuous urine flow and to flush out any bacteria. Antibiotics may also be administered intravenously. During the test, urine and tissue specimens may be collected.

The physician usually performs the cystoscopy in a hospital cystoscopy room. Special cystoscopy tables minimize the stress and fatigue that clients may experience from maintaining one position for a prolonged time. Nursing implications before the test include the following:

1. Signed informed consent.
2. Perform a bowel preparation or enema or administer a cathartic on the evening before the test if ordered.
3. If local anesthetic will be used, encourage intake of oral fluids.
4. If general anesthetic is to be used, instruct client to take nothing by mouth after midnight.
5. Explain that insertion of the cystoscope is similar to insertion of urethral catheter.
6. Explain the importance of lying still during the test.
7. Explain that an intravenous line will be started to give fluids during the test.
8. Administer a sedative and analgesic per the physician's orders.

Nursing implications during the test include the following:

1. Assist client to assume a lithotomy position (see Chapter 33).
2. Prepare perineal area with antiseptic solution.
3. Explain (if client is awake) that insertion of cystoscope causes an urge to void.
4. Remind client to lie still if awake.

Nursing implications after the test include the following:

1. Instruct the client to remain in bed as ordered.
2. Assess for signs of possible urinary retention and time of first voiding.
3. Observe volume and characteristics of urine, including bloody or cloudy urine for each voiding.
4. Encourage increased fluid intake and monitor I & O.
5. Observe for fever, dysuria, or change in blood pressure.
6. Administer medications to alleviate bladder spasms and/or lower back pain.

Renal biopsy. A renal biopsy determines the nature, extent, and prognosis of renal disease. This procedure involves obtaining a piece of renal cortical tissue for examination with sophisticated microscopic techniques. The procedure can be performed by percutaneous (closed) or surgical (open) methods. The use of ultrasound examinations to localize the kidney has revolutionized the percutaneous approach. Tissue diagnosis allows differentiation between disease processes causing alterations in renal function. Therefore more specific treatment interventions can be applied. Nursing implications before this procedure include the following:

1. Signed informed consent
2. Answer any further questions about procedure after physician has initially explained it.

3. Assess hematological studies (e.g., complete blood count, bleeding time, prothrombin time, platelet count, and type and crossmatch for possible blood transfusion) that were ordered as part of preprocedure work-up.
4. Obtain urine specimens for routine analysis, culture, and sensitivity.
5. Instruct client in appropriate positioning (prone) with pillows placed under the abdomen to elevate the kidneys and breathing techniques (client may be asked to hold the breath when biopsy needle is introduced) during the procedure. (Holding the breath during inspiration immobilizes the kidneys as the needle is inserted.)
6. Administer a sedative to relieve anxiety.

Nursing implications during the test include the following:

1. Provide emotional support to the client.
2. Coach client about breathing and positioning.
3. Remind client of expected sensations caused by local administration of analgesics and biopsy instrument.

Nursing implications after the test include the following:

1. Monitor vital signs, noting changes consistent with internal hemorrhage and hemorrhagic shock (see Chapter 48).
2. Observe color, amount, and character of urine, noting bloody urine. The nurse may need to save specimens. (Observe agency policy.)
3. Assess hematological studies (complete blood count) after the biopsy.
4. Encourage client to consume fluids orally.
5. Instruct client to remain in bed for prescribed time (usually 24 hours).
6. Assess biopsy site for signs of bleeding and note complaints of pain.
7. Maintain pressure dressings on biopsy site.
8. Instruct client to refrain from strenuous activity for at least 2 weeks.

Angiography (arteriogram). A renal angiogram is an invasive radiographical procedure that evaluates the renal arterial system. The arteriogram is most often used to examine the main renal artery or its branches to detect any narrowing or occlusion. In addition, this procedure evaluates masses (e.g., neoplasms or cysts) to determine changes in blood flow. The arteriogram is performed by placing a catheter into one of the femoral arteries and advancing it to the level of the renal arteries. Radiopaque contrast material is injected through the catheter while x-ray images are taken in rapid succession.

Pretest nursing implications include the following:

1. Signed informed consent.
2. Assess for iodine allergy, which predicts allergy to the dye used in angiograms.
3. Ensure client takes nothing by mouth after midnight.
4. Explain that facial flushing is normal during dye injection and that client may feel dizzy or warm.
5. Explain that the test involves x-ray studies to be taken at several intervals after the dye is injected.

Nursing implications after either arteriogram or venogram include the following:

1. Monitor vital signs hourly until client is stable and then advance intervals to every 2 hours and 4 hours, respectively.
2. Ensure that the client maintains bed rest for 8 to 12 hours.

3. Check pulse, assess the circulation in the cannulated extremity, and ensure that the extremity is kept in straight alignment.
4. Observe for bleeding, increased tenderness, and hematoma formation at the catheter insertion site for 24 hours.
5. Maintain a pressure dressing over the site for 24 hours (check agency policy).
6. Observe client for possible delayed reactions to the contrast material.
7. Monitor the client's I & O and report abnormalities in urine volume to the physician. Fluids are usually increased either intravenously or by mouth after the test to help flush the dye and minimize the dye's nephrotoxic effects.

 ## Nursing Diagnosis

A thorough assessment of the client's urinary elimination function reveals patterns of data that allow the nurse to make relevant and accurate nursing diagnoses. The nurse thinks critically by reflecting on knowledge of previous clients, reviewing defining characteristics identified, applying knowledge of urinary function, and then making a specific diagnosis. The diagnosis may be an actual problem or a problem that the client is at risk of developing (see the nursing diagnoses box at right).

The diagnosis may focus on a urinary elimination alteration or associated problems such as impaired skin integrity related to urinary incontinence.

Identification of defining characteristics leads the nurse to select an appropriate diagnosis (see the diagnostic process box below). Specifying related factors for each diagnosis allows selection of individualized nursing interventions. For the nursing diagnosis urinary retention with overflow the long-term nursing interventions vary depending on the related cause. For the client with permanent neurological impairment such as multiple sclerosis the nurse needs to plan for alternative methods of bladder emptying such as long-term catheter placement. In contrast the client with urinary retention with overflow related to anesthesia probably has no need of any intervention after a single catheter insertion empties the bladder. Full recovery from the anesthesia eliminates the problem.

 ### Examples of NANDA Nursing Diagnoses for Urinary Elimination

Pain *related to:*
- Urethral inflammation
- Ureteral obstruction

Toileting self-care deficit *related to:*
- Cognitive impairment
- Limited mobility

Impaired skin integrity or risk for impaired skin integrity *related to:*
- Incontinence of urine

Altered urinary elimination *related to:*
- Sensory-motor impairment

Body image disturbance *related to:*
- Feelings about urinary diversion
- Feelings about incontinence

Risk for infection *related to:*
- Poor personal hygiene
- Urethral catheter insertion

Functional incontinence *related to:*
- Diuretic therapy
- Mobility limitations

Reflex incontinence *related to:*
- Neurological impairment
- Anesthesia use for surgery

Stress incontinence *related to:*
- Increased intraabdominal pressure
- Weak pelvic musculature

Urge incontinence *related to:*
- Irritation of bladder mucosa
- Decreased bladder capacity

Total incontinence *related to:*
- Presence of fistula
- Neurological impairment

Urinary retention *related to:*
- Bladder neck obstruction
- Inhibition of reflex arc

 ### Sample Nursing Diagnostic Process for Urinary Elimination

ASSESSMENT ACTIVITIES	DEFINING CHARACTERISTICS	NURSING DIAGNOSIS
Ask client about sensations to void.	Sensation of bladder fullness or urge to void	**Urinary retention** (with overflow) related to weakened detrusor muscle.
	Sensation of pain during and after voiding	
Assess for occurrence of small, frequent voidings or dribbling.	Reports of frequent voiding in small amounts	
Palpate over symphysis pubis for distention	Palpable bladder	
	Increased urge to void with palpation	
	Possible dribbling with palpation	

Sample Nursing Care Plan for Urinary Retention

NURSING DIAGNOSIS: **Urinary retention** related to weakened detrusor muscle
DEFINITION: Urinary retention is the state in which an individual experiences incomplete emptying of the bladder (Kim, McFarland, McLane, 1995).

GOAL	EXPECTED OUTCOMES	INTERVENTIONS	RATIONALE
Client will reestablish usual voiding pattern within 2 days after catheter removal.	Bladder will not be distended after voiding. Client will deny feelings of fullness after voiding. Client will achieve complete bladder emptying within 24 hours of catheter removal.	Have client attempt voiding at regular scheduled times. Instruct client in pelvic floor (Kegel) exercises during nonvoiding times. Have client use exercise with each voiding. Have client use bladder compression (Credé method) during voiding.	Training bladder to empty regularly can reduce incidence of dribbling. Pelvic floor (Kegel) exercises assist in strengthening muscles when pelvic nerves are intact (AHCPR, 1992). Credé method helps stimulate micturition and bladder emptying.

Planning

In developing a plan of care the nurse establishes goals and expected outcomes for each diagnosis. The plan incorporates health promotion activities and therapeutic interventions for clients with urinary elimination problems. Preventive interventions may be required for clients at risk for urinary problems (see the care plan above). The nurse also plans therapies according to the severity of risks to the client. The therapies, if effective, will achieve the outcomes established in the plan.

It is important in the nursing process to consider the client's home environment and normal elimination routines when planning therapies. In planning the care for some clients, consultation with other health professionals may be needed. For example, the physical therapist can design an exercise plan to increase strength and endurance so the client will be able to ambulate to the bathroom. Reinforcement of good health habits that are already followed improves compliance with the care plan.

The alert client with actual or risks for alterations in urinary elimination learns to recognize signs of change and may be able to prevent serious problems. Alterations in urinary elimination pose a high risk to a client's overall state of health.

Planning care also involves an understanding of the client's need to control body function. Alterations in urinary elimination can be embarrassing, uncomfortable, and often frustrating. The nurse and client work together to establish ways of maintaining client involvement in nursing care and to maintain normal urinary elimination. Goals for the client include the following:

1. Understanding normal urinary elimination
2. Promoting normal micturition
3. Achieving complete bladder emptying
4. Preventing infection
5. Maintaining skin integrity
6. Gaining a sense of comfort

Associated problems such as anxiety may require interventions that often have no direct effect on urinary elimination. Unless the nurse intervenes, however, associated problems are likely to continue. Problems involved with urinary elimination alterations are often interrelated and complex. The nurse must also anticipate problems that may develop as a result of therapy. For example, diagnosis of risk for infection is appropriate when a client has an indwelling catheter.

For hospitalized clients, planning should include preparations for discharge (Fig. 46-10). The nurse determines any assistive devices that will be required and the client's educational needs. Teaching throughout the hospital stay is important. Teaching for self-care is continuously reinforced, and return demonstrations of important psychomotor and self-care skills are performed by the client. For example, a client being discharged with an indwelling catheter will need to perform catheter care, understand ways to empty the drainage bag safely, measure urine accurately, and know signs and symptoms of urinary infection. The need for home health services should be explored, and appropriate referrals should be made. The nurse's role in planning these interventions will result in the client's smooth transition through each phase of the nursing process.

Implementation

Implementation is the action phase of the nursing process. The nurse will carry out the independent and collaborative behaviors needed to assist the client in achieving the desired outcomes and goals. The independent activities are those in which nurses use their own judgment. An example of this is teaching self-care activities to the client. Collaborative activities are those prescribed by the physician and carried out by the nurse, such as medication administration.

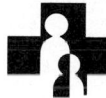

NANTICOKE MEMORIAL HOSPITAL
801 MIDDLEFORD ROAD
SEAFORD, DELAWARE 19973

adapted from CareMap with permission
of The Center for Case Management,
South Natick, MA

UTI WITH SYSTEMIC INVOLVEMENT (PYELONEPHRITIS)

DRG 320   LOS   5 DAYS

Admit Date: _____   Discharge Date: _____

Pathway	Day 1	Day 2	Day 3-4	Day 5
Critical Path Implemented (initial):				
Diagnostic Studies	•CBC •UA, Urine C&S •Chem 7 •CXR •Blood Culture x____ •Consider: KUB/ABD Xray if flank pain present	•Consider: •CBC •Lytes	Consider: •CBC •Lytes •Repeat Blood Culture If pain and fever persist past 72Hrs of therapy Consider: Ultrasound or CT to R/O urological pathology, otherwise D/C	•Repeat urine culture 2 weeks p therapy as O.P.
Treatments	•Strain all urine if flank pain present			
IV/Meds	•IV____@____cc/hr •Antibiotics •Analgesic/Antipyretic •Antiemetic		•Transition to p.o. meds if afebrile X48H•Heplock IV	
Consults	•Social Services if ind			
Nursing	•Physical assessment Q Shift/PRN, esp fluid volume parameters (turgor, lytes, I&O, mucous membranes) •VS Q2HX6H, then Q4HX24H, then Q8H, monitor temp & notify physician of spike >____° •I&O Q4HX24H, then Q shift, notify MD of UO<600cc/24H, adm weight •Skin care, assist with ADL's, daily re-evaluation of skin risk assessment with appropriate interventions, obtain skin care evaluation if indicated •Collaborate with pt on pain management, use 1-5 pain scale •Provide emotional support to pt/family to help reduce anxiety			
Diet	•Clear liquids, advance as tolerated			
Activity & Safety	•OOB as tolerated •Routine safety measures	•OOB as tolerated	•Consider discharge if stable	•Discharge
Teaching Patient & Family	•Teach 1-5 pain scale •Orient to environment •Explain tests/procedures to pt/family •Explain diet, meds, activity	•Explain relationship between disease process, resulting symptoms & therapy prescribed •Implement UTI teaching plan •Implement related procedural teaching plans		
Discharge Planning	•Initial assessment •Advance Directives reviewed •Assess educational needs	•Facilitate phys/RN/family conference for discharge planning & medical follow up		

new 11/94

Fig. 46-10 CareMap® for urinary tract infections. *(Courtesy Nanticoke Memorial Hospital, Seaford, Del, and The Center for Case Management, South Natick, Mass.)*

Health Promotion

The focus of health promotion is to assist the client to understand and participate in self-care practices that will preserve and protect healthy urinary system function. This focus can be achieved using several means.

CLIENT EDUCATION

Success of therapies aimed at eliminating or minimizing urinary elimination problems depends in part on successful client education (see the box below). The nurse instructs clients on their specific elimination problems. For example, clients who practice poor hygiene benefit from learning about normal sterility of the urinary tract and ways to prevent infection. It may also be useful to discuss the basic mechanism for urine production and voiding for clients with elimination alterations. Knowledge of factors that promote normal urine production and voiding can also help. Clients learn the significance of symptoms of urinary alterations so that early preventive health care can be initiated.

The nurse can easily incorporate teaching when giving nursing care. For example, if the nurse is attempting to increase the client's fluid intake, a good time to discuss the benefits is while giving fluids with medications or meals. The nurse may be more successful in teaching about perineal hygiene while giving a bath or performing catheter care.

PROMOTING NORMAL MICTURITION

Maintaining normal urinary elimination will help to prevent many urination problems. Many nursing measures have been designed to promote normal voiding in clients at risk for urination difficulties and in clients with established urination problems. The nurse can initiate many of these measures independently.

Stimulating Micturition Reflex. The client's ability to void depends on feeling the urge to urinate, being able to

control the urethral sphincter, and being able to relax during voiding. The nurse can help a client learn to relax and stimulate the reflex to void by assuming the normal position for voiding. A woman is better able to void in a squatting or sitting position. This position promotes contraction of the pelvic and intraabdominal muscles that assist in sphincter control and bladder contraction. If the client is unable to use toilet facilities, the nurse positions the client in a squatting position on a bedpan (see Chapter 47) or bedside commode. A man voids more easily in the standing position. If the man cannot reach toilet facilities, he may stand at the bedside and void into a urinal, a metal or plastic receptacle for urine (Fig. 46-11). At times it may be necessary for one or more nurses to assist a man to stand.

Other measures that promote relaxation and the ability to void include sensory stimuli. The sound of running water helps many clients void through the power of suggestion. Stroking the inner aspect of the thigh may stimulate sensory nerves and promote the micturition reflex. Placing the client's hand in a pan of warm water often promotes voiding. It is easier for a person to relax and void when sitting on a bedpan that has been warmed. The nurse can also pour warm water over the client's perineum and create the sensation to urinate. If urine output is to be measured, the nurse must first measure the volume of water to be poured over the perineal area. Offering fluids the client will drink may also promote voiding.

Maintaining Elimination Habits. Many clients follow routines to promote normal voiding. In a hospital or long-term care facility the nurse's routines may conflict with those of clients. Integrating clients' habits into the care plan fosters normal voiding and will assist in preventing problems related to urination.

Maintaining Adequate Fluid Intake. A simple method of promoting normal micturition is maintaining good fluid intake. A client with normal renal function who does not have heart disease or alterations requiring fluid restriction should drink 2000 to 2500 ml of fluid daily. However, an average daily intake of 1200 to 1500 ml of fluids is usually adequate.

When fluid intake is increased, the excreted urine flushes out solutes or particles that may collect in the urinary system. Adequate fluid intake may minimize urge incontinence in older adults by diluting the bladder irrita-

CLIENT TEACHING for Urinary Elimination Problems

OBJECTIVE
- Client will adhere to health practices to prevent UTI.

TEACHING STRATEGIES
- Instruct client or care giver about observations to make regarding urinary output.
- Inform clients about pertinent signs and symptoms of infection such as frequency, burning, and urgency of urination. Discuss the importance of contacting the physician.
- Remind client and care givers about recommended levels of fluid intake.
- Reinforce correct perineal hygiene measures.
- Establish client's and family's knowledge about medications and provide instructions on those medications that affect urination, urine color, or volume.

EVALUATION
- Observe client or care giver perform perineal hygiene.
- Observe client correctly measure fluid intake and output.
- Have client give feedback on benefits of adhering to recommended fluid intake.
- If client is determined to be at risk for recurrent UTI provide for follow-up care.

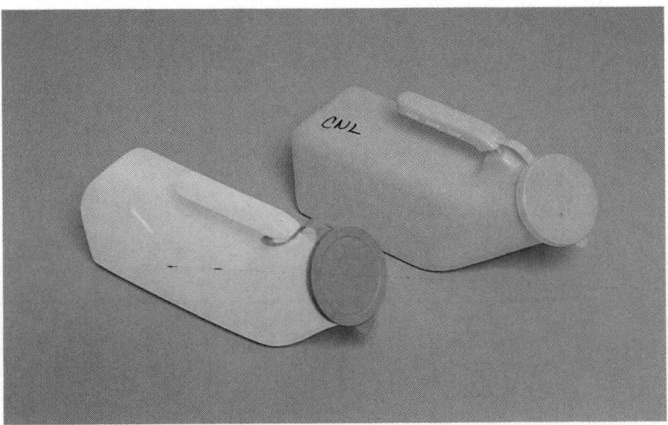

Fig. 46-11 Types of male urinals.

tion caused by concentrated urine (Colling, Owen, and McCready, 1994). Because a client is usually unwilling to drink 2500 ml of water daily, the nurse should encourage fluids that the client prefers. Many vegetables and fruits also have a high fluid content. At home it may help to set a schedule for drinking fluids (e.g., with meals or medications). To minimize nocturia, fluids should be avoided 2 hours before bedtime.

PROMOTING COMPLETE BLADDER EMPTYING

Under normal conditions, a small amount of the client's urine remains in the bladder after voiding because urinary sphincters close. The sphincters provide more pressure than the pressure of urine remaining in the bladder. Thus persons normally remain continent and dry. Urinary incontinence may occur because pressure in the bladder is too great or because the sphincters are too weak. Urinary retention occurs from a strong or contracted sphincter or a weak detrusor muscle that prevents normal bladder emptying.

Measures that promote micturition may help clients with incontinence or retention. Additional measures are used to promote and control bladder emptying so that clients gain a sense of elimination control (Table 46-4). Most urinary elimination problems can be grouped in two major classifications, failure to store or failure to empty (Thayer, 1994).

Table 46-4	Treatment Options for Urinary Incontinence
PRIMARY TREATMENT	**OTHER TREATMENTS/ INTERVENTIONS**
FUNCTIONAL INCONTINENCE	
Habit training	Environmental alterations
	Scheduled toileting
	Skin care
	Protective undergarments
	Condom catheters (for men)
OVERFLOW (REFLEX) INCONTINENCE	
Alpha-Adrenergic blockers	Credé method
Surgery	Indwelling or external
Intermittent catheterization	catheter
STRESS INCONTINENCE	
Pelvic floor conditioning exercises (Kegel)	Estrogen
	Artificial sphincter
Surgery	Biofeedback
URGE INCONTINENCE	
Anti-cholinergic drug therapy	Biofeedback
Bladder retraining	
Treatment of associated UTI or vaginitis	Estrogen
TOTAL INCONTINENCE	
Condom catheter	
Indwelling urinary diversion	

Modified from Thayer D: How to assess and control urinary incontinence, *Amer J Nurs* 94:42, 1994.

PREVENTION OF INFECTION

One of the most important considerations for a client with urinary alterations is the need to prevent infection of the urinary system. Good perineal hygiene that includes cleansing the urethral meatus after each voiding or bowel movement is essential. A daily fluid intake of 2000 to 2500 ml dilutes urine and promotes regular micturition, which flushes the urethra of microorganisms.

Acidifying Urine. Urine is normally acidic and tends to inhibit growth of microorganisms. Meats, eggs, wholegrain breads, cranberries, prunes, and plums increase urine acidity. These foods metabolize into acid end products that eventually enter the urine. Although large quantities of cranberry juice must be ingested to have any effect on urine pH, a study reported out of Harvard did support evidence of significant reduction of bacteriuria in the studied population (NewsWatch, 1994). High doses of ascorbic acid may lower urine pH.

Acute Care

MAINTAINING ELIMINATION HABITS

Clients usually require time to void. Asking clients to void quickly so that they can be transported to x-ray testing or requesting a urine specimen as soon as possible does not contribute to relaxation and normal voiding habits. Clients should be given at least 30 minutes to provide a specimen. The nurse learns the times when clients normally void, such as on awakening or before meals, and offers the opportunity to use toilet facilities then. Also important is the need to respond to clients' urges to urinate. Delay in assisting clients to the bathroom may interfere with normal micturition and contribute to incontinence.

Privacy is essential for normal voiding. If the client cannot reach the bathroom, the nurse makes sure that the bedside area is enclosed by a curtain. In the home the debilitated client may prefer using a bedside commode enclosed behind a partition or room divider. Some clients are embarrassed by the sound of voiding. Running water or flushing the toilet masks the sound. Young children are often unable to void in the presence of persons other than their parents.

If the client typically uses special measures to void, the nurse should encourage their continued use at home and, when possible, in the institution. The client may be able to relax and void more easily while reading or listening to music. Having a cup or glass of fluids may also promote urination.

MEDICATIONS

Drug therapy given alone or with other therapies can help problems of incontinence and retention. There are three types of medications. One relaxes a spastic bladder thereby increasing bladder capacity; one stimulates the bladder to contract thus improving emptying; and the other causes relaxation of the prostatic smooth muscle, reducing obstruction to urethral flow.

The bladder is innervated by the parasympathetic nervous system. When urine is present in the bladder, urge incontinence may result from hyperactivity of the bladder muscle that suddenly increases intravesicular pressure. Uncontrolled bladder contractions may be caused by local bladder irritants such as calculi or infection. Drugs that depress the neurotransmitter acetylcholine, which stimulates the bladder, reduce incontinence caused by bladder irritation. Examples of these anticholinergic drugs include propantheline (Pro-Banthine) and oxybutynin chloride (Ditropan). The anticholinergics can cause cardiac dysrhythmias and should be used with caution in clients with heart disease. Anticholinergics may also cause constipation and a dry mouth.

When the bladder empties, the detrusor muscle contracts in response to parasympathetic stimulation. Incomplete bladder emptying results from impaired innervation or weakness of the detrusor muscle. The client experiences retention and possible overflow incontinence. Cholinergic drugs increase contraction of the bladder and improve emptying. Bethanechol (Urecholine) stimulates parasympathetic nerves to increase bladder wall contraction and relax the sphincter. Bethanechol can be given by subcutaneous or oral routes. Cholinergic drugs may cause diarrhea as a side effect.

The dribbling or overflow incontinence seen in men with prostatic enlargement can be treated with an alpha-1 adrenergic blocker, such as terazosin (Hytin). Terazosin is given orally and relaxes prostatic smooth muscle thus relieving obstructive symptoms. This drug may cause hypotension and it is also used in treatment of hypertension.

CATHETERIZATION

Catheterization of the bladder involves introducing a rubber or plastic tube through the urethra and into the bladder. The catheter provides a continuous flow of urine in clients unable to control micturition or those with obstructions. It also provides a means of assessing hourly urine outputs in hemodynamically unstable clients. Because bladder catheterization carries the risk of UTI and trauma to the urethra, it is preferable to rely on other measures for either specimen collection or management of incontinence.

Types of Catheterization. Intermittent and indwelling retention catheterization are the two forms of catheter insertion. With the intermittent technique a straight single-use catheter (Fig. 46-12, *A*) is introduced long enough to

Text continued on p. 1326.

Guidelines for Appropriate Catheter Selection

The catheter size should be determined by the size of the client's urethral canal. When the French system is used, the larger the gauge number the larger the catheter. Generally, children require an 8 to 10 Fr., women require a 14 to 16 Fr., and men usually require a 16 to 18 Fr.

The length of the catheterization period should dictate the type of material selected.

Plastic catheters are only suitable for intermittent use because they are stiff and inflexible.

Latex or rubber catheters are recommended for medium-term use (up to 3 weeks)

Pure silicone or teflon catheters are recommended for long-term use (2 to 3 months) because the material causes less encrustation at the urethral meatus. Both of these types are fairly expensive initially but last for a longer time. Delamination may be a problem with silicone types.

Polyvinylchloride (PVC) catheters are also very expensive. They are suitable for intervals of 4 to 6 weeks. They soften at body temperature and conform to the urethra.

Determining the appropriate balloon size is also an important aspect of catheterization. Balloon sizes range from 3 ml (pediatric) to large postoperative volumes (75 ml). The 5 ml and 30 ml sizes are most common. The 5 ml volume is appropriate for standard catheterizations. This small volume allows for optimal drainage of the bladder and does not interfere with bladder emptying. The 30 ml balloon catheter is usually reserved for use after prostatectomies as an aid in achieving postoperative hemostasis of the prostatic bed.

Only sterile water should be used to inflate the balloon. Normal saline may crystallize, thus causing incomplete deflation of the balloon at time of intended removal. Additional water should not be instilled into the balloon as a remedy for a leaking catheter as it distorts the catheter tip and leads to bladder irritation and incomplete emptying.

A change in catheter size (or even antispasmodic medication) may be warranted to control leakage.

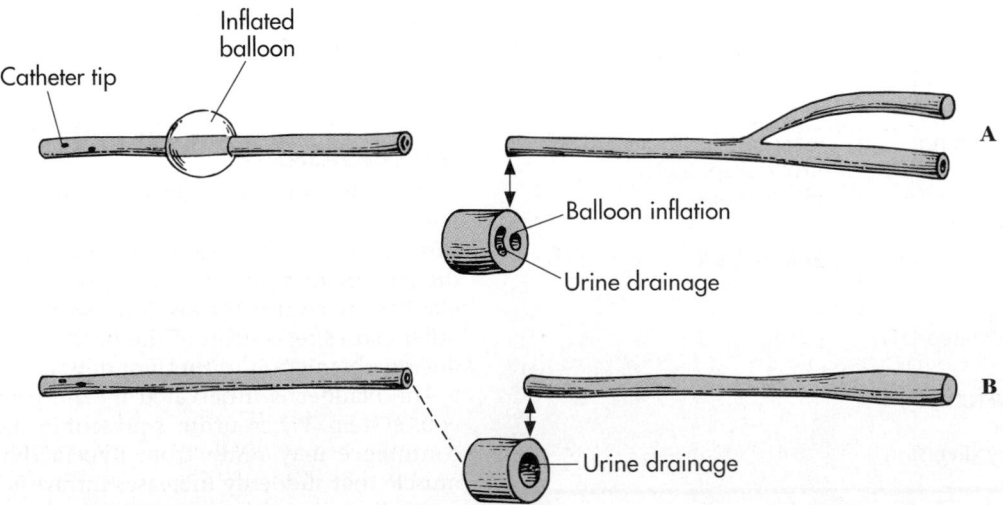

Fig. 46-12 Types of urinary catheters. **A**, Indwelling (Foley) catheter; **B**, straight catheter.

Inserting a Straight or Indwelling Catheter

STEPS	RATIONALE
1. Assess status of client:	
a. When client last voided	May indicate degree of bladder fullness.
b. Level of awareness or developmental stage	Reveals client's ability to cooperate during procedure.
c. Mobility and physical limitations	Affects way that client may be positioned and indicates necessity for assistance.
d. Age	Determines catheter size to use No. 8 to 10 is generally used for children and 14 to 16 for women. No. 12 may be considered for young women. No. 16 to 18 is used for men unless larger size is ordered by physician.
e. Pathological condition that may impair passage of catheter (e.g., enlarged prostate)	Obstruction prevents passage of catheter through urethra into bladder.
f. Allergies	Determines allergies to antiseptic, tape, or rubber (latex).
g. Review of physician's order for catheterization	Catheterization requires physician's order. Physician may order catheterization after surgery or childbirth if the client has not voided for 8 hr. Catheterization may also be ordered for specimen collection or accurate monitoring of critical clients.
2. Prepare necessary equipment and supplies:	
a. Sterile gloves*	Procedure is considered sterile.
b. Sterile drapes, one fenestrated	
c. Sterile lubricant*	Minimizes urethral trauma.
d. Antiseptic cleaning solution*	
e. Cotton balls or gauze squares	
f. Forceps	
g. Prefilled syringe with sterile water	Used to inflate balloon of indwelling catheter.
h. Catheter of correct size and type for procedure (intermittent or indwelling) (see the illustration)	

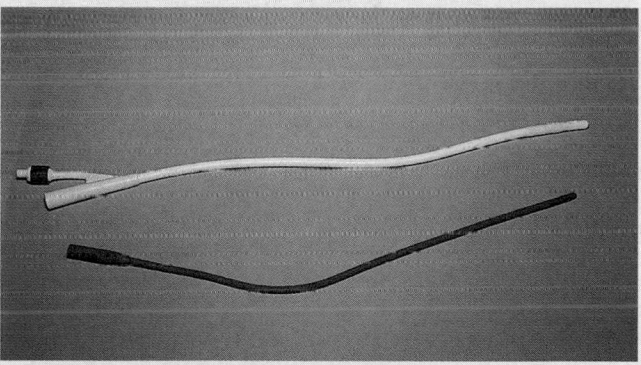

Step 2h

STEPS	RATIONALE
i. Flashlight or gooseneck lamp	Helps in seeing urinary meatus of female client.
j. Bath blanket	Provides client privacy.
k. Waterproof absorbent pad	Prevents soiling of bed linen.
l. Trash receptacle	
m. Disposable gloves, basin with warm water, soap, washcloth, and towel	Providing perineal hygiene before introducing catheter helps reduce risk of UTI. Provides opportunity to examine women's urethral meatus or to retract foreskin of uncircumcised male. Able client can provide own perineal care.
n. Sterile drainage tubing and collection bag (may be preattached to catheter), tape, safety pin, elastic band	If indwelling catheter will be inserted, tape, elastic band, or pin help secure position of catheter, thus preventing trauma to external urethral sphincter.
o. Sterile receptacle or basin (usually bottom of tray)	Provides area for urine to drain when intermittent catheter is used or indwelling catheter is not preattached.
p. Sterile specimen container	For sterile urine specimen collection.

*These items may be contained on catherization tray or may need to be added after sterile field is established. This depends on whether disposable or non-disposable trays are used. Check outer label for contents.

Continued.

PROCEDURE 46-2

Inserting a Straight or Indwelling Catheter—cont'd

STEPS	RATIONALE

3. Explain procedure to client. Describe pressure sensation that will be felt during catheter insertion.

Reduces anxiety and promotes cooperation.

4. Arrange for extra nursing personnel to assist, if necessary.

May be necessary to assist with positioning dependent client. Promotes use of correct body mechanics and safety.

5. Raise bed to appropriate working height.

Promotes use of correct body mechanics.

6. Wash hands.

Reduces transmission of infection.

7. Facing client, stand at left side of bed, if right-handed (on right side if left-handed). Clear bedside table and arrange equipment.

Successful catheter insertion requires nurse to assume comfortable position with all equipment easily accessible.

8. Raise side rail on opposite side of the bed.

Promotes client safety.

9. Close cubicle or room curtains.

Provides privacy and promotes relaxation.

10. Place waterproof pad under client.

Prevents soiling bed linen.

11. Position client:

  a. Female: assist to dorsal recumbent position (supine with knees bent). Ask client to relax thighs so as to externally rotate them (legs may be supported with pillows) (see the illustration below), or position in side-lying (Sims') position with upper leg flexed at knee if unable to be supine (optional).

Provides good view of perineal structures. Alternate position if client cannot abduct leg at hip joint (e.g., arthritic joint). Also this position may be more comfortable for client. Support client with pillows, if necessary, to maintain position.

  b. Male: assist to assume supine position with thighs slightly abducted.

Supine position prevents tensing of abdominal and pelvic muscles.

12. Drape client:

  a. Female: drape with bath blanket. Place blanket diamond fashion over client; one corner at neck, one over each arm and side and last corner over perineum. Raise gown over hips.

Avoids unnecessary exposure of body parts and maintains comfort.

  b. Male: drape upper trunk with bath blanket and cover lower extremities with bed linen, exposing only genitalia (see the illustration p. 1321).

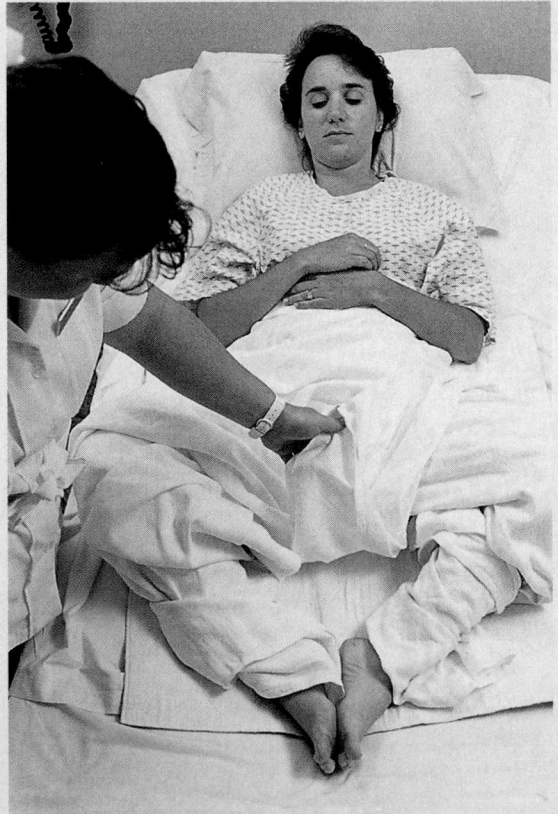

Step 11a

Inserting a Straight or Indwelling Catheter—cont'd

STEPS	RATIONALE
13. Apply disposable gloves. Wash perineal area with soap and water as needed; dry.	Presence of microorganisms is reduced.
14. Remove and dispose of used gloves. Wash hands.	Prevents transmission of microorganisms.
15. Position lamp to illuminate perineal area. (If using a flashlight, have assistant hold it.)	Permits accurate identification and good view of urethral meatus.
16. Open catheterization kit and catheter (if packaged separately) according to directions.	Prevents transfer of microorganisms from work surface to sterile supplies.
17. Apply sterile gloves (see Chapter 34).	Allows handling of sterile supplies without contamination.
18. Organize supplies on sterile field. Open inner sterile package containing catheter. Pour sterile antiseptic solution into compartment containing sterile cotton balls. Open packet containing lubricant. Remove specimen container (cap should be loosely placed on top) and prefilled syringe from collection compartment of tray and set them aside on sterile field.	Maintains surgical asepsis and organizes work area. All activities requiring you to use both hands must be completed before cleansing of urethral meatus.
19. Before inserting indwelling catheter, test balloon by injecting fluid from prefilled syringe into balloon valve (see the illustration below, right). Balloon should inflate fully without leaking. Withdraw fluid and leave syringe on port of catheter, if possible.	Checks integrity of balloon. Balloon that leaks or inflates improperly should not be used.
20. Apply sterile drape:	
a. Female: allow top edge of drape to form a cuff over both hands. Place drape down on bed between client's thighs. Slip cuffed edge just under buttocks, taking care not to touch contaminated surface with gloves. Pick up fenestrated sterile drape and allow it to unfold without touching unsterile objects. Apply drape over perineum, exposing labia and being sure not to touch contaminated surface.	Outer surface of drape covering your hands remains sterile until touched by buttocks. Sterile drape against sterile gloves is sterile. Maintains sterility of work surface.
b. Male: apply drape over thighs just below penis. Pick up fenestrated drape. Allow it to unfold, and drape it over penis with fenestrated slit positioned over penis.	
21. Place sterile kit and its contents on sterile drape between client's thighs, and open urine specimen container (if needed), keeping inside surfaces sterile.	Allows easy access to supplies during catheter insertion.

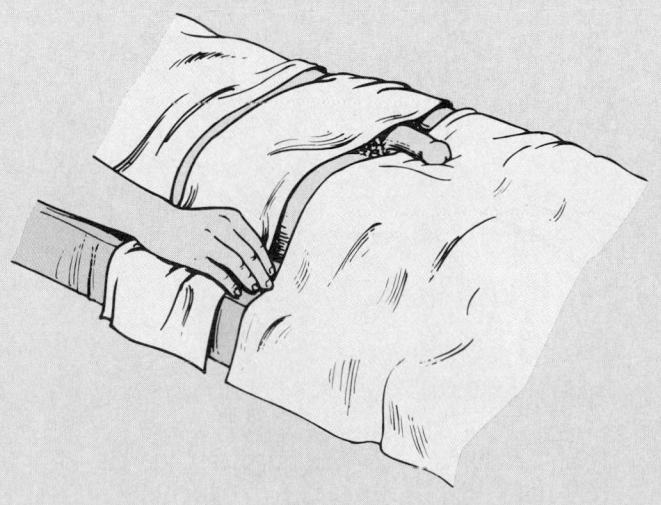

Step 12b

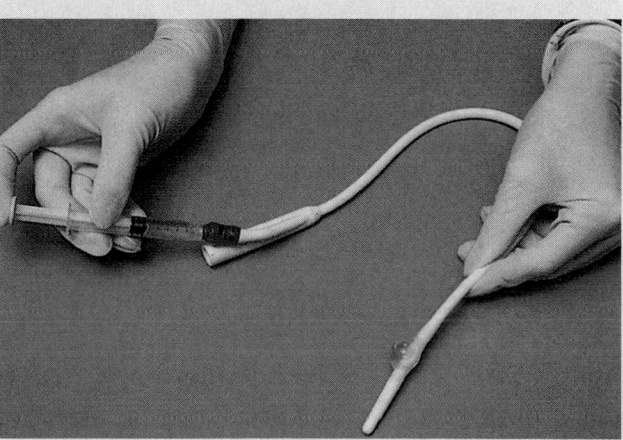

Step 19

Continued.

Inserting a Straight or Indwelling Catheter—cont'd

STEPS	RATIONALE

22. Apply lubricant along sides of catheter tip:
   a. **Female:** 2.5 to 5 cm (1-2 inches)
   b. **Male:** 7.5 to 12.5 cm (3-5 inches)

Allows easy insertion of catheter tip through urethral meatus.

23. Cleanse urethral meatus:
   a. Female:
   (1) With nondominant hand, carefully retract labia to fully expose urethral meatus. Maintain position of nondominant hand throughout procedure.

Provides full visualization of meatus. Full retraction prevents contamination of meatus during cleansing. Closure of labia during cleansing requires that procedure be repeated because area has become contaminated.

   (2) With dominant hand, pick up cotton ball with forceps and clean over perineal area, wiping front to back from clitoris to anus. Use new clean cotton ball for each wipe: along near labial fold, along far labial fold, directly over meatus (see the illustration below).

Cleansing reduces number of microorganisms at urethral meatus. Use of single cotton ball for each wipe prevents the transfer of microorganisms. Preparation moves from area of least contamination to area of most contamination. Dominant hand remains sterile.

   b. Male:
   (1) If client is not circumcised, retract the foreskin with nondominant hand. Grasp penis at shaft just below glans. Retract urethral meatus between thumb and forefinger. Maintain nondominant hand in this position throughout catheter insertion.

Minimizes chance of erection. (If erection develops, discontinue procedure.) Release of foreskin or dropping of penis during cleansing requires process to be repeated because area has become contaminated.

   (2) With dominant hand pick up cotton ball with forceps and clean penis. Begin at meatus. Using a circular motion, advance down toward base (shaft). Repeat this process three times, changing cotton ball each time (see the illustration below).

Reduces number of microorganisms at meatus and moves from area of least contamination to the most contamination. Dominant hand remains sterile.

24. Pick up catheter with gloved dominant hand approximately 5 cm (2 inches) from catheter tip. Hold end of catheter loosely coiled in palm of dominant hand. Place distal end of catheter in urine tray receptacle (if not already attached to drainage tubing and bag).

Collection of urine prevents soiling of bed linen and allows accurate measurement of urine output.

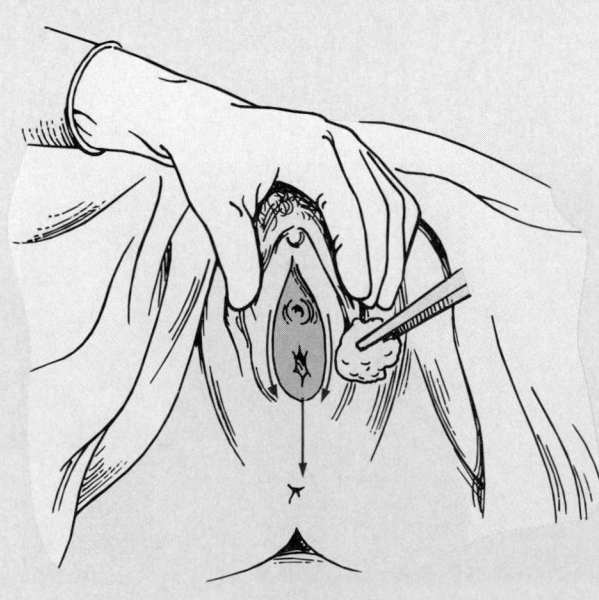

Step 23a(2)

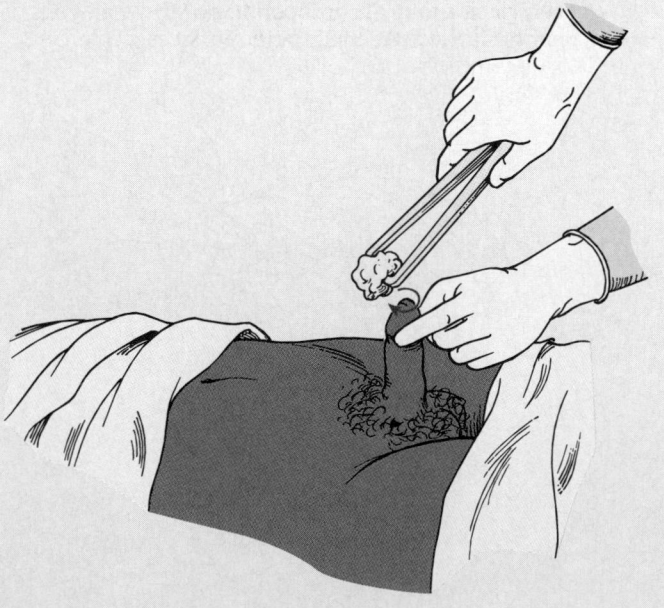

Step 23b(2)

Inserting a Straight or Indwelling Catheter—cont'd

STEPS	RATIONALE

25. Insert catheter:

a. Female: grasp catheter in dominant hand with non-dominant hand continuing to retract labia.

   (1) Ask client to take deep breath, slowly insert catheter through meatus (see the illustration below). (If no urine appears after advancing a few centimeters, catheter may be in vagina. If catheter is in vagina, leave in place; obtain and insert another catheter and remove first catheter.)

                                  Relaxation of external sphincter aids in insertion of catheter. (Catheter in vagina is no longer sterile.) Leaving first catheter in place helps prevent inserting second catheter in vagina.

   (2) Advance catheter approximately 5 to 7.5 cm (3 inches) in adults, 2.5 cm (1 inch) in child, or until urine appears. If inserting indwelling catheter, advance another 5 cm (2 inches) after urine appears. Do not force catheter against resistance.

                Female urethra is short. Appearance of urine indicates that catheter tip is in bladder or lower urethra. Further advancement of catheter ensures bladder placement. Balloon of indwelling catheter must be advanced into bladder. Forceful insertion may traumatize urethra.

   (3) Release labia and hold catheter securely with nondominant hand.

                Bladder or sphincter contraction may cause accidental expulsion of catheter.

b. Male: lifting penis to position perpendicular to client's body and applying light upward traction:

                Straightens urethral canal to ease catheter insertion.

   (1) Ask client to bear down as if voiding, slowly insert catheter through meatus.

                Relaxation of external sphincter aids in catheter insertion.

   (2) Advance catheter 17.5 to 22.5 cm (7-9 inches) in adults, 5 to 7.5 cm (2-3 inches) in young child, or until urine appears. If resistance is felt, withdraw catheter; do not force it through urethra.

                Adult male urethra is long. Appearance of urine indicates that catheter tip is in bladder or urethra. Further advancement of catheter ensures bladder placement. Resistance to catheter passage may be caused by strictures or enlarged prostate.

   If inserting indwelling catheter, advance another 5 cm (2 inches) after urine appears.

                Ensures that balloon is advanced into bladder.

   (3) Release penis and hold catheter securely with nondominant hand.

                Bladder or sphincter contraction may cause accidental expulsion.

26. Collect urine specimen as needed: Fill specimen cup or jar to desired level (20-30 ml) by holding end of catheter in dominant hand over the cup (or collect specimen from sterile drainage bag). With dominant hand pinch catheter to stop urine flow temporarily, and then release catheter to allow remaining urine in bladder to drain into collection tray. Cover specimen cup and set aside for labeling.

                Allows sterile specimen to be obtained for culture analysis.

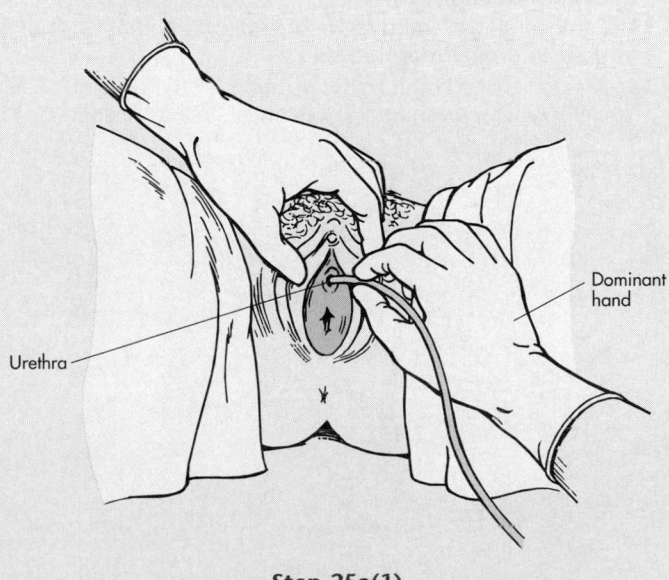

Urethra

Dominant hand

Step 25a(1)

Continued.

Inserting a Straight or Indwelling Catheter—cont'd

STEPS	RATIONALE
27. Allow bladder to empty fully (unless agency policy restricts maximal volume of urine to drain with each catheterization).	Retained urine may serve as a reservoir for growth of microorganisms. (Rapid emptying of large volume may cause engorgement of blood vessels and hypovolemic shock.)
28. Remove single use intermittent catheter. Withdraw catheter slowly and smoothly until removed.	Minimizes client discomfort.
29. Inflate balloon of indwelling catheter:	
a. While holding catheter at urinary meatus with nondominant hand, take end of catheter; place it between first two fingers of nondominant hand.	Catheter should be anchored while syringe is manipulated.
b. Take dominant hand and attach syringe (if not already attached) to injection port at end of catheter.	Port connects to lumen leading to balloon.
c. Slowly inject total amount of solution (see the illustration below). If client complains of sudden pain, aspirate solution and advance catheter farther. Inject no more fluid than balloon size indicates.	Balloon within bladder is inflated. If balloon is malpositioned in urethra, pain occurs during inflation.
d. After inflating balloon fully, release catheter with nondominant hand and pull gently to feel resistance (see the illustration below). Then move catheter slightly back into bladder. Disconnect syringe.	Inflation of balloon anchors catheter tip in place above bladder outlet to prevent removal of catheter. Gentle pulling ensures proper placement and anchoring. Advancing catheter upward minimizes pressure on bladder neck.
30. Attach end of catheter to collecting tube and drainage bag unless preattached. Place bag in dependent position (see the illustration on p. 1325). Do not place bag on side rails of bed.	Closed system for urine drainage is established. Dependent position of drainage bag promotes flow of urine away from bladder. Bags attached to side rails may be raised above level of bladder if rail is raised.
31. Secure catheter:	
a. Female: use elastic strap or tape to secure catheter to inside of thigh. Allow for slack so that movement of thigh does not create tension on catheter (see the illustration on p. 1325).	Anchoring of catheter minimizes trauma to urethra and meatus during movement. Catheter positioned over thigh prevents kinking. Elastic strap or nonallergic tape prevents skin irritation.
b. Male: tape catheter to top of thigh or lower abdomen (with penis directed toward abdomen). Allow some slack in catheter so movement does not cause tension on catheter (see the illustration on p. 1325).	Anchoring catheter to lower abdomen is thought to reduce pressure on urethra at junction of penis and scrotum, thus reducing possibility of tissue necrosis.
32. Be sure there are no obstructions or kinks in tubing. Place excess coil of tubing on bed and fasten it to bottom sheet with clip from drainage set or with rubber band and safety pin.	Patent tubing allows free drainage of urine by gravity and prevents backflow of urine into bladder.
33. Remove gloves and dispose of equipment, drapes, and urine in proper receptacles.	Prevents transmission of microorganisms.
34. Assist client to comfortable position. While wearing clean gloves, wash and dry perineal area as needed.	Client's comfort and security are maintained.

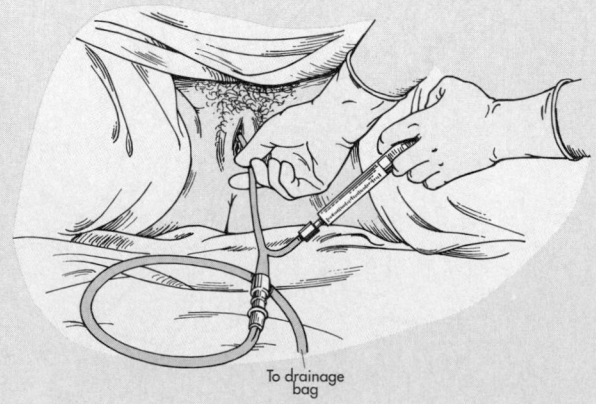

To drainage bag

Step 29c

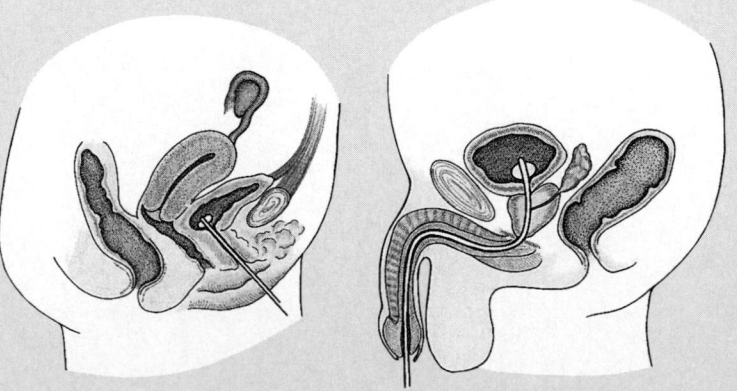

Step 29d

Inserting a Straight or Indwelling Catheter—cont'd

STEPS	RATIONALE
35. Instruct client on ways to lie in bed with catheter: side-lying facing drainage system with catheter and tubing draped over lower thigh or side-lying facing away from system with catheter and tubing between legs.	Urine should drain freely without obstruction. Placing catheter under extremities can result in obstruction from compression of tubing from client's weight. When client is on one side facing away from system, tubing should not be placed over upper thigh; this forces urine to attempt to drain up hill.
36. Caution client against pulling on catheter.	Reduces trauma to urethral meatus.
37. Wash hands.	Reduces spread of infection.
38. Palpate bladder and ask if client is comfortable.	Determines relief of distention.
39. Observe character and amount of urine in drainage system.	Determines if urine is flowing adequately.
40. Report and record type and size of catheter inserted, amount of fluid used to inflate the balloon, and characteristics and amount of urine.	Documents and communicates pertinent information to all members of the health team.

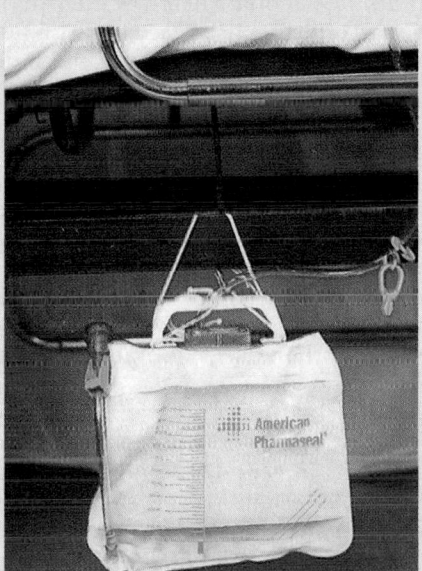

Step 30

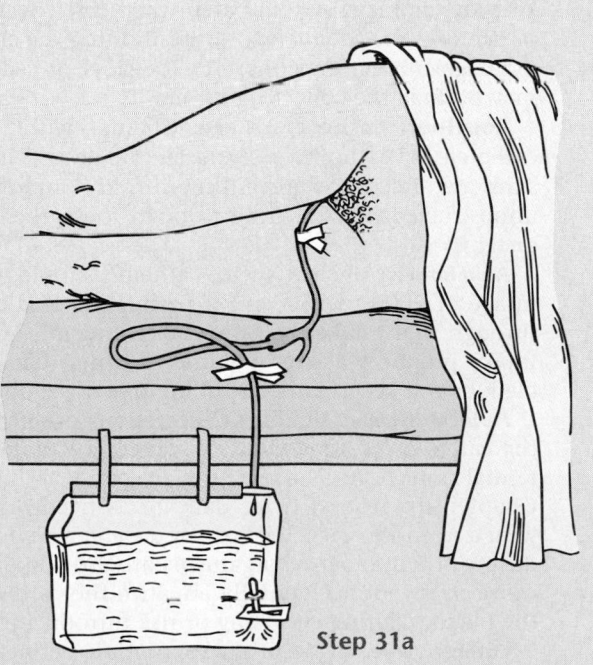

Step 31a

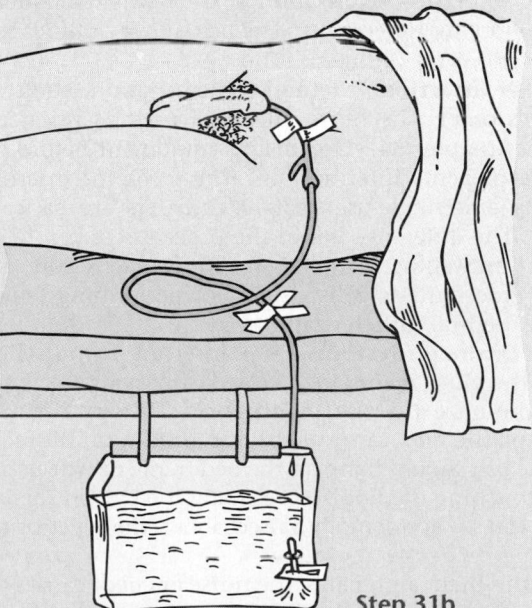

Step 31b

drain the bladder (5 to 10 minutes). When the bladder is empty, the nurse immediately withdraws the catheter. Intermittent catheterization can be repeated as necessary but repeated use increases the risks. An indwelling or Foley catheter remains in place for a longer period until a client is able to void completely and voluntarily or as long as accurate hourly measurements are needed. It may be necessary to change indwelling catheters periodically.

The straight single-use catheter has a single lumen with a small opening about 1.3 cm (½ inch) from the tip. Urine drains from the tip, through the lumen, and to a receptacle. An indwelling Foley catheter has a small inflatable balloon that encircles the catheter just below the tip. When inflated, the balloon rests against the bladder outlet to anchor the catheter in place. The indwelling retention catheter also has two or three lumens within the body of the catheter (Fig. 46-12, B). One lumen drains urine through the catheter to a collecting tube. A second lumen carries sterile water to and from the balloon when it is inflated or deflated. A third (optional) lumen may be used to instill fluids or medications into the bladder. It is easy to determine the number of lumens by the number of drainage and injection ports at the catheter's end.

A third type of catheter has a curved tip. A Coudé catheter is used on male clients who may have enlarged prostates that partly obstruct the urethra. The Coudé catheter is less traumatic during insertion because it is stiffer and easier to control than the straight-tip catheter.

Catheters come in many diameters to fit the size of a client's urethral canal. Suggestions on how to make appropriate decisions regarding catheter selection are provided (see the box on p. 1318).

Indications for Catheterization. Catheterization may be indicated for many reasons. When catheterization time will be short and minimizing infection is a priority, the intermittent method is best. Intermittent catheterization is also preferred for persons with spinal cord injuries who have no bladder control. By intermittently draining the bladder on a routine basis, these clients have fewer infections. Indwelling catheterization is used when long-term bladder emptying is necessary. The box above outlines specific indications for catheterization.

Catheter Insertion. Urethral catheterization requires a physician's order. The nurse must use strict aseptic technique (see Chapter 34). Organizing equipment before the procedure prevents interruptions. The steps for inserting indwelling and single-use straight catheters are basically the same. The difference lies in the procedure taken to inflate the indwelling catheter balloon and secure the catheter. Procedure 46-2 lists steps for performing female and male urethral catheterization.

Closed Drainage Systems. After inserting an indwelling catheter, the nurse maintains a closed urinary drainage system to minimize the risk of infection. Urinary drainage bags are plastic and can hold about 1000 to 1500 ml of urine. The bag should hang on the bed frame or wheelchair without touching the floor. Never hang the bag on the bed rail as it can be accidentally raised above the level of the bladder.

When the client ambulates, the nurse or client carries the bag below the client's waist. The nurse or other health care personnel should never raise a drainage bag and tubing

Indications for Catheterization

INTERMITTENT CATHETERIZATION
- Relief of discomfort of bladder distention, provision of decompression
- Obtaining sterile urine specimens
- Assessment of residual urine after bladder empties
- Long-term management of clients with spinal cord injuries, neuromuscular degeneration, or incompetent bladders

SHORT-TERM INDWELLING CATHETERIZATION
- Obstruction to urine outflow (e.g., prostate enlargement)
- Surgical repair of bladder, urethra, and surrounding structures
- Prevention of urethral obstruction from blood clots
- Measurement of output in critically ill clients
- Continuous or intermittent bladder irrigation

LONG-TERM INDWELLING CATHETERIZATION
- Severe urinary retention with recurrent episodes of UTI
- Skin rashes, ulcers, or wounds irritated by contact with urine
- Terminal illness when bed linen changes are painful for client

above the level of the client's bladder. Urine in the bag and tubing can become a medium for bacteria, and infection is likely to develop if urine flows back into the bladder.

Most drainage bags contain an antireflux valve to prevent urine in the bag from reentering the drainage tubing and contaminating the client's bladder. A spigot at the base of the bag provides a means for emptying the bag. The spigot should always be clamped, except during emptying, and tucked into the protective pouch at the bag's side. To keep the drainage system patent the nurse checks for kinks or bends in the tubing, avoids positioning the client on the drainage tubing, and observes for clots or sediment that may occlude the collecting tubing.

Routine Catheter Care. Clients with indwelling catheters have a number of special care needs. Nursing measures are directed at preventing infection and maintaining unobstructed flow of urine through the catheter drainage system.

Fluid intake. All clients with catheters should have a daily intake of 2000 to 2500 ml if permitted. This can be met through oral intake or intravenous infusion. A high fluid intake produces a large volume of urine that flushes the bladder and keeps catheter tubing free of sediment.

Perineal hygiene. Buildup of secretions or encrustation at the catheter insertion site is a source of irritation and potential infection. Nurses provide perineal hygiene (see Chapter 40) at least twice daily or as needed for a client with a retention catheter. Soap and water are effective in reducing the number of organisms around the urethra. The nurse must not accidentally advance the catheter up into the bladder during cleansing or risk introducing bacteria.

Catheter care. In addition to routine perineal hygiene, many institutions recommend that clients with catheters

Indwelling Catheter Care

STEPS	RATIONALE
1. Assess for episode of bowel incontinence or client's report of discomfort at catheter insertion site. (Frequency may also be by agency policy.)	Accumulation of secretions or feces causes irritation to perineal tissues and acts as source of bacterial growth.

2. Prepare necessary equipment and supplies:
  a. Catheter care kit:
    (1) Gloves
    (2) Cotton balls or application swabs
    (3) Clean washcloth and towel
    (4) Warm water and soap
    (5) Antibiotic ointment (check agency policy)
  b. Bath blanket
  c. Waterproof absorbent pad
	Ensures orderly procedure.
	
	Used to drape client.
	Prevents soiling of bed linen.

3. Explain procedure to client. Offer opportunity to perform self-care to able client.	Reduces anxiety and promotes cooperation. Embarrassment may motivate client to perform own hygiene.
4. Close door or bedside curtain.	Maintains client privacy.
5. Wash hands.	Reduces transmission of infection.

6. Position client:
  a. Female: dorsal recumbent position
  b. Male: supine position
	
	Ensures easy access to perineal tissues.

7. Place waterproof pad under client.	Protects bed linen from soiling.
8. Drape bath blanket on bed clothes so that only perineal area is exposed.	Prevents unnecessary exposure of body parts.
9. Apply gloves.	
10. Remove anchor device to free catheter tubing.	

11. With nondominant hand:
  a. Female: gently retract labia to fully expose urethral meatus and catheter insertion site, maintaining position of hand throughout procedure.
  b. Male: retract foreskin if not circumcised and hold penis at shaft just below glans, maintaining position throughout procedure.
	
	Provides full visualization of urethral meatus. Full retraction prevents contamination of meatus during cleansing.
	
	Accidental closure of labia or dropping of penis during cleansing requires procedure to be repeated.

12. Assess urethral meatus and surrounding tissues for inflammation, swelling, and discharge. Note amount, color, odor, and consistency of discharge. Ask client if burning or discomfort is felt.	Determines presence of local infection and status of hygiene.

13. Cleanse perineal tissue:
  a. Female: use clean cloth, soap, and water. Clean toward anus. Repeat process to clean labia minora, and then cleanse around urethral meatus moving down catheter. Be sure to cleanse each side. Dry area well.
  b. Male: while spreading urethral meatus, cleanse around catheter first, and then wipe in circular motion around meatus and glans.
	
	Reduces the number of microorganisms at urethral meatus. Use of clean cloth prevents transfer of microorganisms.
	
	Cleansing moves from area of least to most contamination.

14. Reassess urethral meatus for discharge.	Determines if cleansing is complete.
15. With towel, soap, and water, wipe in a circular motion along length of catheter for 10 cm (4 inches).	Reduces presence of secretions or drainage on exterior catheter surface.
16. Apply antibiotic ointment at urethral meatus and along 2.5 cm (1 inch) of catheter if ordered by physician or part of agency policy.	Further reduces growth of microorganisms at insertion site.
17. Place client in safe, comfortable position.	Promotes comfort.
18. Dispose of contaminated supplies, remove gloves, and wash hands.	Prevents spread of infection.
19. Record and report condition of perineal tissues, time procedure was performed, client's response, and any abnormalities noted.	Provides data to document procedure and informs staff of client's condition.

receive special care three times a day and after defecation or bowel incontinence to help minimize discomfort and infection (Procedure 46-3).

Ostomy Care. For clients with urinary diversion special nursing care is required to prevent complications related to the collection devices. It is important that the device fit snugly against the skin surface to prevent constant exposure to urine. Urine that remains in contact with the skin causes breakdown and denuding of the skin surface. When this happens the device will not adhere and leakage becomes a major problem. Urine is constantly produced so the pouch may need frequent emptying throughout the day and may need to be hooked to a larger drainage bag for nighttime use.

PREVENTION OF INFECTION

Infection can develop in a catheterized client in many ways. Maintaining a closed urinary drainage system is important in infection control. A break in the system can lead to introduction of microorganisms. Sites at risk are the site of catheter insertion, drainage bag, spigot, tube junction, and the junction of the tube and the bag (Fig. 46-13).

In addition, the nurse monitors the patency of the system to prevent pooling of urine within the tubing. Urine in the drainage bag is an excellent medium for microorganism growth. Bacteria can travel up drainage tubing to grow in pools of urine. If this urine flows back into the client's bladder, an infection will likely develop. Yoshikawa (1993) has demonstrated that almost 100% of clients with indwelling catheters are bacteriuric after 3 to 4 weeks. Suggestions for ways to prevent infections in catheterized clients are provided (see the box at right).

Catheter Irrigations and Instillations. To maintain the patency of indwelling urinary catheters, it sometimes becomes necessary to irrigate or flush a catheter. Blood, pus, or sediment can collect within tubing and result in bladder

distention and the buildup of stagnant urine. Instillation of a sterile solution ordered by the physician clears the tubing of accumulated material. For clients with bladder infections, a physician may order bladder irrigations to include instillation of antiseptic or antibiotic solutions to wash out the bladder or treat local infection. In both irrigations, sterile aseptic technique is followed.

Before performing an irrigation, the nurse assesses the catheter for blockage. If the amount of urine in the drainage bag is less than the client's intake or less than the output during the previous shift, blockage can be expected. If urine does not drain freely, the nurse milks the tubing. Milking is done by gently squeezing then releasing the drainage tube in an alternating fashion. The nurse should always milk from the client to the drainage bag so a clot or sediment will not be forced back into the catheter.

Burgener (1987) recommends that a closed system be maintained during intermittent irrigations or instillations. The nurse uses a sterile 30- to 50-ml syringe with a 19- to 22-gauge, 1-inch needle to inject a prescribed solution into the catheter. This technique is effective for irrigating a partially blocked catheter or for bladder instillations. Steps for using this closed system are in Procedure 46-4.

A single intermittent irrigation is safer and less likely to introduce infections into the urinary tract. There are two additional methods for catheter irrigation. One is a closed bladder irrigation system (Procedure 46-4). This system pro-

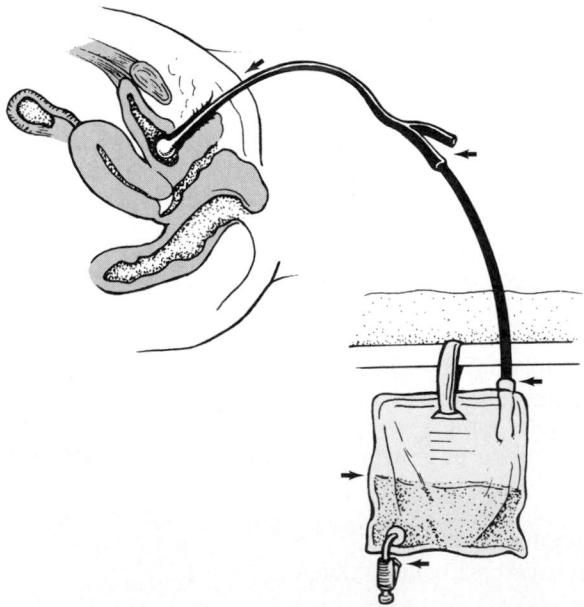

Fig. 46-13 Potential sites for introduction of infectious organism into a urinary drainage system.

Tips for Preventing Infection in Catheterized Clients

- Follow good handwashing techniques (see Chapter 34).
- Do not allow the spigot on the drainage system to touch a contaminated surface.
- Do not open the drainage system at connection points to obtain specimens.
- If the drainage tube becomes disconnected, do not touch the ends of the catheter or tubing. Wipe the end of the tube and catheter with an antimicrobial solution before reconnecting.
- Ensure that each client has a separate receptacle for measuring urine to prevent cross-contamination.
- Prevent pooling of urine in the tubing and reflux of urine into the bladder.
  - Avoid raising the drainage bag above the level of the client's bladder.
  - If it becomes necessary to raise the bag during transfer of the client to a bed or stretcher, clamp the tubing or empty the tubing contents to the drainage bag first.
  - Avoid allowing large loops of tubing to lie on the bed.
  - Provide for drainage of urine from tubing into the bag.
  - Before exercise or ambulation, drain all urine from tubing into drainage bag.
- Avoid prolonged kinking or clamping of the tubing.
- Empty the drainage bag at least every 8 hours. If large outputs are noted, empty it more frequently.
- Remove the catheter as soon as medically warranted.
- Tape or secure the catheter appropriately for client (see Procedure 46-2).
- Perform routine perineal hygiene per agency policy and after defecation or bowel incontinence (see Procedure 46-3).

Closed and Open Catheter Irrigation

STEPS	RATIONALE
1. Assess physician's order for type of irrigation and irrigating solution to use.	Ensures proper selection of equipment.
2. Assess color of urine and presence of mucus or sediment.	Determines if client is bleeding, has infection, or is sloughing tissue.
3. Determine type of catheter in place:	Indicates method for irrigation.
a. Triple lumen (one lumen to inflate balloon, one to instill irrigation solution, one to allow outflow of urine)	
b. Double lumen (one lumen to inflate balloon, one to allow outflow of urine)	
4. Determine patency of drainage tubing.	Ensures that drainage tubing is not kinked, clamped incorrectly, or looped below bladder level.
5. Assess amount of urine in drainage bag.	Volume must be subtracted from volume that drains after irrigation to ensure that all irrigant returns.
6. Collect necessary equipment and supplies:	
a. Closed intermittent method:	
(1) Sterile irrigating solution at room temperature	Cold solution may cause bladder spasm.
(2) Sterile graduated container	
(3) Sterile 30- to 50-ml syringe	Used to instill irrigant into bladder.
(4) Sterile 19- to 22-gauge 1-inch needle	
(5) Antiseptic swab	
(6) Clamp for catheter or tubing	Occludes catheter as irrigant is instilled.
(7) Bath blanket	
b. Closed continuous method:	
(1) Sterile irrigating solution, correct bag of solution at room temperature	Cold solution may cause bladder spasms.
(2) Irrigation tubing and clamp (with or without Y-connector)	Clamp regulates irrigation flow. Y-connector allows two bags to be connected to tubing.
(3) IV pole	
(4) Antiseptic swab	
(5) Y-connector (optional)	Can connect irrigation tubing to double lumen catheter.
(6) Bath blanket	
c. Open method:	Don't use if at all possible as it increases risk of infection.
(1) Sterile irrigation set with tray	
(2) Bulb syringe or 60-ml piston-type syringe	Provides necessary force to dislodge clot.
(3) Sterile collection basin	
(4) Waterproof drape	Prevents soiling of bed linen.
(5) Sterile solution container	
(6) Antiseptic swabs	
(7) Sterile gloves	Keeps system sterile.
(8) Correct irrigation solution at room temperature	Cold solution may cause bladder spasms.
(9) Tape or elastic band to resecure catheter	
(10) Bath blanket	
7. Explain procedure and purpose to client.	Helps client relax and cooperate during procedure.
8. Wash hands and don clean gloves for closed methods.	Prevents transmission of microorganisms.
9. Provide privacy by pulling bed curtains closed. Fold back covers so that catheter is exposed. Cover client's upper torso with bath blanket.	Promotes client comfort.
10. Assess lower abdomen for bladder distention.	Detects whether catheter is malfunctioning or blocking urinary drainage.
11. Position client in dorsal recumbent or supine position.	Promotes client comfort and provides easy access to catheter. Promotes flow of irrigating solution into bladder.

Continued.

Closed and Open Catheter Irrigation—cont'd

STEPS	RATIONALE

12. Closed intermittent irrigation:

   a. Prepare prescribed sterile irrigating solution in sterile graduated cup.

   b. Draw sterile solution into syringe using aseptic technique.   Ensures that irrigating fluid remains sterile.

   c. Clamp indwelling retention catheter below soft injection port.   Occlusion of catheter provides resistance against which irrigant can be forcefully instilled into catheter.

   d. Cleanse catheter injection port with antiseptic swab (same port used for specimen collections).   Reduces transmission of infection.

   e. Insert needle of syringe through port at 30-degree angle.   Ensures that needle tip enters lumen of catheter.

   f. Slowly inject fluid into catheter and bladder.   Slow, continuous pressure dislodges clots and sediment without traumatizing bladder wall.

   g. Withdraw syringe, remove clamp, and allow solution to drain into urinary drainage bag. OPTIONAL: keep tubing clamped and allow solution to remain in bladder for a short time (20-30 min). Don't forget to unclamp catheter.   Allows drainage to flow by gravity.

13. Closed continuous irrigation (see the illustration below):   Prevents entrance of microorganisms.

   a. Using aseptic technique, insert tip of sterile irrigation tubing into bag of irrigation solution.

   b. Close clamp on tubing and hang bag of solution on IV pole.

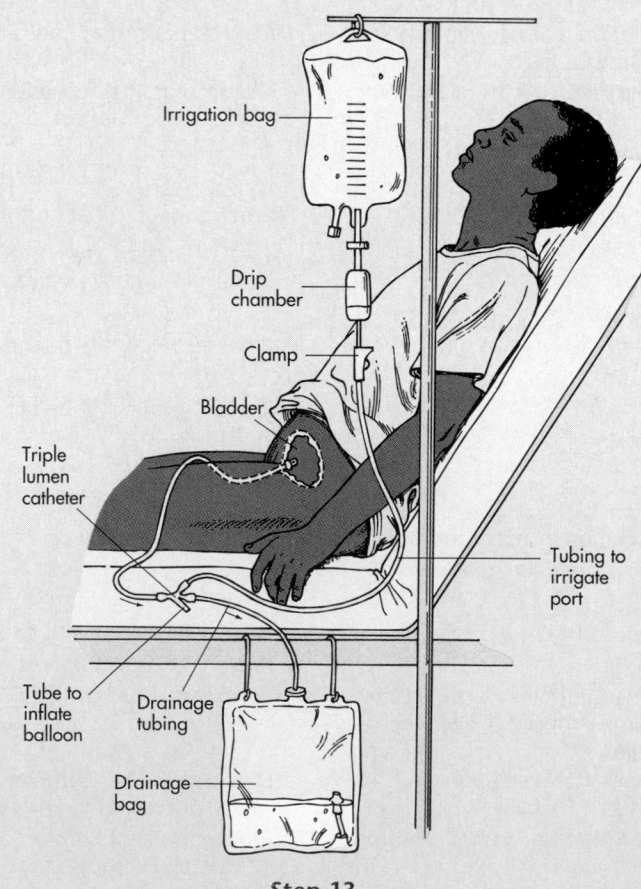

Irrigation bag

Drip chamber

Clamp

Bladder

Triple lumen catheter

Tubing to irrigate port

Tube to inflate balloon

Drainage tubing

Drainage bag

Step 13

Closed and Open Catheter Irrigation—cont'd

STEPS	RATIONALE
13. Closed continuous irrigation—cont'd	
c. Open clamp and allow solution to flow through tubing, keeping end of tubing sterile. Close clamp.	Removes air from tubing.
d. Wipe off irrigation port of triple lumen catheter or attach sterile Y-connector to double lumen catheter, and then attach to irrigation tubing.	Third lumen or Y-connector provides means for irrigating solution to enter bladder. System must remain sterile.
e. Be sure that drainage bag and tubing are securely connected to drainage port of triple lumen catheter or other arm of Y-connector.	Ensures that urine and irrigating solution will drain from bladder.
f. For intermittent flow, clamp tubing on drainage system, open clamp on irrigation tubing, and allow prescribed amount of fluid to enter bladder (100 ml is normal for adults). Close irrigation tubing clamp, and then open drainage tubing clamp.	Fluid instills through catheter into bladder, flushing system. Fluid drains out after irrigation is completed.
g. For continuous irrigation, calculate drip rate and adjust clamp on irrigation tubing accordingly. Be sure that clamp on drainge tubing is open and check volume of drainage in drainage bag. Make sure drainage tubing is patent and avoid kinks.	Ensures continuous, even irrigation of catheter system. Prevents accumulation of solution in bladder, which may cause bladder distention and possible injury.
14. Open irrigation:	
a. Open sterile irrigation tray, establish sterile field, pour required amount of sterile solution into sterile container, and replace cap on large container of solution.	Adheres to principles of surgical asepsis.
b. Apply sterile gloves (see Chapter 34).	Reduces transmission of infection.
c. Position sterile waterproof drape under catheter.	Prevents soiling of bed linen.
d. Aspirate 30 ml of solution into sterile irrigating syringe.	Prepares irrigant for instillation into catheter.
e. Move sterile collection basin close to client's thigh.	Prevents soiling of bed linen and prohibits reaching over sterile field.
f. Disconnect catheter from drainage tubing, allowing urine to flow into sterile collection basin. Cover open end of drainage tubing with sterile protective cap. Position this tubing in a safe place.	Maintains sterility of inner aspect of catheter lumen and drainage tubing and reduces potential of introducing pathogens into bladder.
g. Insert tip of syringe into catheter lumen and gently instill solution.	Gentle instillation reduces incidence of bladder spasm but clears catheter of obstruction.
h. Withdraw syringe, lower catheter, and allow solution to drain into basin. Repeat instilling solution and draining several times until drainage is clear.	Allows drainage to flow by gravity. Provides for adequate flushing of catheter.
i. If solution does not return, have client turn onto side facing you. If changing position does not help, reinsert syringe and gently aspirate solution.	Change of position may move catheter tip in bladder, increasing likelihood that fluid instilled will flow out.
j. After irrigation is complete, remove protector cap from tubing, cleanse end with alcohol swab (or recommended agency solution), and reestablish drainage system.	Reduces entrance of microorganisms into system.
15. Reanchor catheter to client with tape or elastic band.	Prevents trauma to urethral tissue.
16. Assist client to comfortable position.	Promotes relaxation and rest.
17. Lower bed to lowest position.	Promotes client safety.
18. Dispose of contaminated supplies, remove gloves, and wash hands. Put side rails up if appropriate.	Prevents spread of infection.
19. Calculate fluid used to irrigate bladder and catheter and subtract from total volume drained.	Determines accurate urinary output.
20. Assess characteristics of output: viscosity, color, and presence of matter (e.g., sediment, clots).	Evaluates results of irrigation.
21. Record type and amount of solution used as irrigant, amount returned as drainage, and character of drainage.	Documents procedure and client's response.

vides for frequent intermittent or continuous irrigation without disruption of the sterile catheter system. It is used most often in clients who have had genitourinary surgery and are at risk for blood clots and mucus fragments occluding the catheter. The other system involves opening the closed drainage system to instill bladder irrigations (Procedure 46-4). This technique poses greater risk for causing infection. However, it may be needed when catheters become blocked and it is undesirable to change the catheter (e.g., after recent prostate surgery).

Removal of Indwelling Catheter. When removing an indwelling catheter, the nurse promotes normal bladder function and prevents trauma to the urethra.

To remove a catheter the nurse requires a clean, disposable towel; a trash receptacle; and a sterile syringe the same size as the volume of solution within the catheter's inflated balloon. Disposable gloves are also recommended. The end of each catheter contains a label that denotes the volume of solution (5 to 30 ml) within a balloon.

The nurse positions the client in the same position as during catheterization. Some institutions recommend collecting a sterile urine specimen at this time or sending the catheter tip for culture and sensitivity tests. After removing the tape, the nurse places the towel between a female client's thighs or over a male client's thighs. The nurse inserts the syringe into the injection port. Most ports are self-sealing and require that only the tip of the syringe be inserted. The nurse slowly withdraws all of the solution to deflate the balloon totally. If a portion of the solution remains, the partially inflated balloon will traumatize the urethral canal as the catheter is removed. After deflation the nurse explains that the client may feel a burning sensation as the catheter is withdrawn. The nurse then pulls the catheter out smoothly and slowly.

It is normal for the client to experience some dysuria, especially if the catheter has been in place several days or weeks. The catheter causes inflammation of the urethral canal. Until the bladder regains full tone, the client may also experience frequency of urination.

The nurse assesses the client's urinary function by noting the first voiding after catheter removal and documents the time and amount of voiding for the next 24 hours. If amounts are small, frequent assessment of bladder distention is necessary. If over 8 hours elapse without voiding, it may become necessary to reinsert the catheter.

Alternatives to Urethral Catheterization. To avoid the risks associated with catheters inserted through the urethra, there are two alternatives for urinary drainage. Suprapubic catheterization involves surgical placement of a catheter through the abdominal wall above the symphysis pubis and into the urinary bladder. The physician performs the procedure under local or general anesthesia. The catheter is anchored in place with sutures, a commercially prepared body seal, or both. Urine drains into a urinary drainage bag. The suprapubic catheter is relatively painless and reduces the incidence of infection commonly seen with retention catheters. Women who have undergone a vaginal hysterectomy may also benefit temporarily from the insertion of a suprapubic catheter after surgery.

The suprapubic catheter can become blocked by sediment, clots, or the abdominal wall itself. Nurses must monitor the client's I & O carefully, observe for signs of kidney infection (e.g., flank tenderness, chills, and fever), and monitor the appearance of urine. Spread of infection to the kidneys may indicate removal of the catheter. Adequate fluid intake will help to minimize risk of blockage by sediment or infection due to stagnation. The suprapubic catheter must remain patent at all times. The nurse also administers skin care around the insertion site.

The second alternative to catheterization is the condom catheter (Procedure 46-5). It is suitable for incontinent or comatose men who still have complete and spontaneous bladder emptying. The condom is a soft, pliable, rubber sheath that slips over the penis. It may be worn at night only or continuously, depending on the client's needs. There are three general methods of securing the condom catheter. One method uses a strip of elastic tape or rubber that encircles the top of the condom to secure it in place. Another condom uses a self-adhesive inside the sheath. The third method uses an inflatable ring within the condom to secure placement. Care must be taken to ensure that whatever type or size is used, blood supply to the penis is not impaired. Standard adhesive tape should never be used to secure a condom catheter because it does not expand with change in penis size.

The end of the condom fits into a plastic drainage tubing. A drainage bag can be attached to the side of the bed or strapped to the client's leg. The condom catheter itself poses little risk of infection. Infections with condom catheters usually result from buildup of secretions around the urethra, trauma to the urethral meatus, or buildup of pressure in the outflow tubing.

The nurse should change a condom catheter daily to check for skin irritation. With each catheter change the nurse cleans the urethral meatus and penis thoroughly. Twisting of the condom at the drainage tube attachment irritates the skin and obstructs urine outflow. The drainage tubing must be checked often for patency.

For a man with a retracted penis, maintaining of a conventional condom catheter may prove difficult. Special devices are available to help alleviate this problem (Fig. 46-14). Manufacturers' guidelines for product application should be consulted.

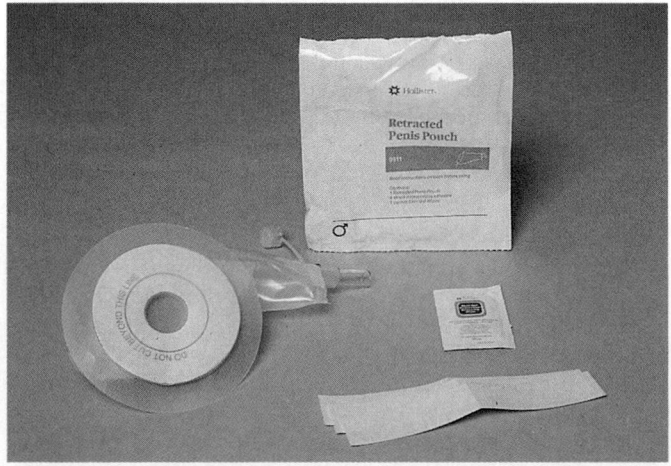

Fig. 46-14 Retracted penis pouch external urinary device.

Applying a Condom Catheter

STEPS	RATIONALE
1. Assess status of client to determine need for condom catheter.	Client continuously incontinent of urine is at high risk for skin breakdown.
2. Prepare equipment and supplies:	
a. Rubber/latex condom sheath (proper size)	
b. Strip of elastic tape (if needed), skin preparation	
c. Urinary collection bag with tubing or leg bag with straps	Leg bag allows mobility.
d. Basin with warm water and soap	
e. Towels and washcloths	
f. Disposable gloves	Protects hands; reduces risk of infection.
g. Bath blanket	
h. Hair clippers or scissors (optional)	
3. Explain procedure to client.	Reduces anxiety and promotes cooperation.
4. Provide privacy by closing door or bed curtains.	Maintains client's self-esteem.
5. Wash hands and don gloves.	Reduces transmission of infection.
6. Assist client into supine position. Place bath blanket over upper torso. Fold bedsheets so that lower extremities are covered; only genitalia should be exposed.	Promotes client comfort and prevents unnecessary exposure of body parts.
7. Assess condition of penis.	Provides a baseline to compare changes in condition of skin after condom application.
8. Provide perineal care (see Chapter 40) and dry thoroughly. Clip hair at base of penis.	Removes irritating secretions. Rubber/latex sheath rolls onto dry skin more easily. Hair adheres to base of condom and pulls during condom removal.
9. Prepare urinary drainage collection or leg bag for connection to condom catheter. Clamp off all drainage exit ports. Secure collection bag to bed frame or leg bag to client leg. Have drainage tubing ready for connection.	Provides easy access to drainage equipment after condom is applied.
10. Apply skin preparation to shaft of penis and allow to dry (30-60 sec).	Prepares penis for easy condom placement and increased adhesion.
11. With nondominant hand, grasp penis along shaft. With dominant hand hold condom sheath at tip of penis and smoothly roll sheath onto penis (see the illustrations below).	
12. Allow 2.5 to 5 cm (1-2 in) of space between end of condom and tip of glans penis.	Allows free passage of urine into collecting tubing when client passes urine. Prevents pressure on glans.
13. Encircle penile shaft with elastic tape (if needed). Strip should only touch condom sheath, not skin. Apply snugly but not too tightly.	Condom must be secured so that it is snug and will stay on but not so tightly as to impair blood flow.

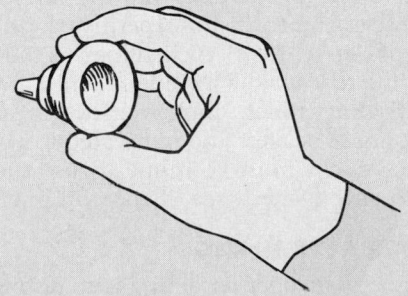 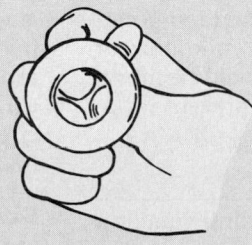 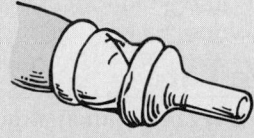

Step 11

Continued.

Applying a Condom Catheter—cont'd

STEPS	RATIONALE
14. Connect drainage tubing to end of condom catheter. A urine drainage bag or leg bag (see the illustration below) attached above or below the knee may be used. Be sure that condom sheath is not twisted (see the illustration below).	Allows urine to be collected and measured. Keeps client dry. Twisted condom obstructs urine flow.
15. Secure so that tubing is not looped and promotes free drainage of urine.	Prevents buildup of urine in sheath.
16. Place client in a safe, comfortable position (lying or sitting but not obstructing urine flow).	Promotes client's comfort.
17. Dispose of contaminated supplies. Remove gloves and wash hands.	Prevents spread of infection.
18. Return in 30 to 60 minutes to observe for urinary drainage.	Determines if normal voiding is occurring.
19. Regularly inspect skin of penile shaft for signs of breakdown or irritation.	Indicates if condom or urine is causing irritation or elastic band is constricting (if used).
20. Record and report time of condom application, condition of skin, and voiding pattern.	Provides data to other members of the health care team.

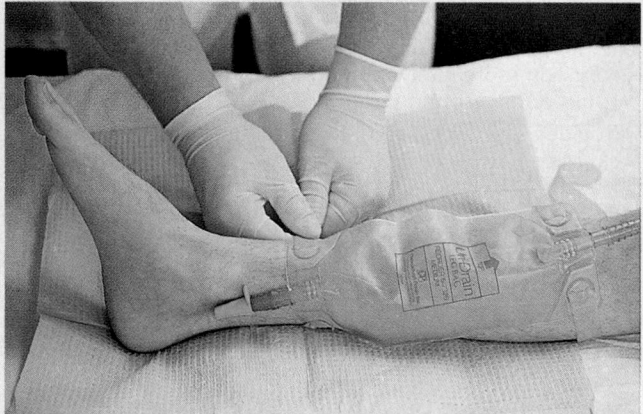

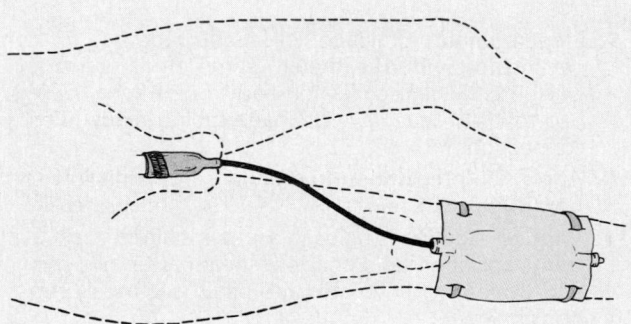

Step 14

There are no collection devices for women as effective as the condom catheter, so frequently the only incontinent devices used are pads and protective clothing. To maintain dignity, pads and protective clothing should not be referred to as adult diapers and should be changed frequently to control odor. These devices should be only used temporarily while treatment methods are being used to minimize or prevent episodes of incontinence. Clients should be monitored frequently and good skin care given to prevent irritation caused by urine.

Restorative Care

The client may regain normal urinary voiding function through special activities such as bladder retraining or habit training. If either of those activities are not possible then self-catheterization may restore a measure of control to the client.

STRENGTHENING PELVIC FLOOR MUSCLES

Clients who have difficulty starting or stopping the urine stream may benefit from pelvic floor (Kegel) exercises (Table 46-5). **Kegel exercises** improve the strength of pelvic floor muscles and consist of repetitive contractions of muscle groups (Burke, 1992). A client begins these exercises during voiding to learn the technique. They are then practiced at nonvoiding times. Improvement is usually gradual. Clients should be alert and motivated to perform the exercises. The client must continue to use these exercises to maintain effectiveness (see the box on p. 1336).

BLADDER RETRAINING

The goal of bladder retraining is to restore a normal pattern of voiding by inhibiting or stimulating voiding (AHCPR, 1992). For bladder retraining to be successful, clients must be alert and physically able to follow a train-

Table 46-5	Pelvic Floor Exercises	
EXERCISE STEPS	**RATIONALE**	

EXERCISE I
Instruct client to concentrate on pelvic muscles.

Have client try to stop flow of urine during urination and then restart it.
Practice with each voiding.

Rationale: Assists client to feel anterior muscles of pelvic floor.
Teaches control technique.

EXERCISE II
Have client assume sitting or standing position.
Instruct client to tighten muscles around anus.

Rationale: Assists client to feel posterior muscles of pelvic floor.

EXERCISE III
Have client tighten posterior muscles and then slowly contract anterior muscles while counting to four.
Then have client relax muscles completely.
Repeat exercise four times per hour while awake, for 3 months.

Rationale: Improves pelvic muscle control, and aids in relaxation of sphincters during voiding.

EXERCISE IV
If feasible, teach client to do modified sit-ups (bent knee).

Rationale: Strengthens abdominal muscles for bladder control.

---

ing program. The program includes education, scheduled voiding, and positive reinforcement. Bladder function may be temporarily disrupted after a period of catheterization (Resnick, 1993).

The nurse first assesses the client's pattern of urination. This information allows the nurse to plan a program that often takes 2 weeks or more to learn. Although the program may be started in the hospital or rehabilitation unit it may need to be continued in an extended-care facility or at home. If the client has an underlying UTI, this should be treated at the same time. The following measures may help the incontinent client gain control over urination and are part of restorative and rehabilitative care:

1. Learning exercises to strengthen the pelvic floor
2. Initiating a toileting schedule on awakening, every 2 hours during the day and evening, before getting into bed, and every 4 hours at night
3. Using methods to initiate voiding (e.g., running water and stroking the inner thigh)
4. Using methods to relax to aid complete bladder emptying (e.g., reading and deep breathing)
5. Never ignoring the urge to void (only if problem involves infrequent voidings that result in retention)
6. Taking fluids approximately 30 minutes before planned voiding times
7. Avoiding tea, coffee, alcohol, and other caffeine drinks
8. Taking prescribed diuretic medication or fluids that increase diuresis (such as tea or coffee) early in the morning
9. Progressively lengthening or shortening periods between voiding
10. Offering protective undergarments to contain urine and reduce the client's embarrassment (not diapers)
11. Following a weight-control program if obesity is a problem
12. Providing positive reinforcement when continence is maintained

These guidelines help the client to establish a routine for voiding and control factors that might increase the number of incontinent episodes.

HABIT TRAINING

A client with functional incontinence may benefit from habit training, which helps clients improve voluntary control over urination. A flexible toileting schedule based on the client's pattern is established.

The nurse helps the client to the bathroom before incontinent episodes occur. Fluids and medications are timed to prevent interference with the toileting schedule. Clients

with moderate or severe mental or physical dysfunction can benefit. When combined with positive reinforcement to reward successful voiding this approach is also called *prompted voiding*.

SELF-CATHETERIZATION

Some clients with chronic disorders such as spinal cord injury learn to perform self-catheterization. The client must be able to physically manipulate equipment and assume a position for successful catheterization. The nurse teaches the client the structures of the urinary tract, clean versus sterile technique, the importance of adequate fluid intake, and the frequency of self-catheterization. Generally, the goal is to have clients perform self-catheterizations every 6 to 8 hours but the schedule should be individualized.

RESEARCH HIGHLIGHT

RESEARCH ABSTRACT

The problem of incontinence is a pervasive and costly one in the United States. Incontinence affects 15% to 39% of elders living in the community and is the second leading cause for nursing home placement. Incontinence is often accompanied by social isolation and depression . Early research had demonstrated the effectiveness of pelvic muscle exercises on the reduction of persistent incontinence, especially stress incontinence. The Visiting Nurse Association of Trenton, New Jersey embarked on a Continence Program to study the effectiveness of pelvic muscle exercises in reducing urge incontinence among community residing elders. Fifty clients were referred for the purpose of restoration of continence. Thirty-seven clients were part of the program as those clients with concurrent urinary tract infection were excluded. The screening involved a thorough assessment of urinary function. The goal was a 70% reduction in urinary incontinence episodes per week. The primary behavioral focus was pelvic muscle exercises but corollary interventions included measures to establish and maintain bowel regularity, adequate diet, and hydration. The results of the intervention program showed a significant 82.39% reduction in incontinent episodes over 12 weeks with most clients showing marked improvement after only 4 to 5 weeks. The pelvic muscle exercise intervention was equally effective in both urge and mixed stress/urge incontinence.

IMPLICATIONS FOR PRACTICE

▶ Nurses are in key positions to identify and treat urinary incontinence in older adults.

▶ Nurses can make a significant impact on the quality of life for many community residing older adults.

▶ Although the economic benefits of reducing incontinent episodes are great, even more important are the return of dignity and feelings of self-esteem.

▶ Pelvic muscle exercises should be included as a primary intervention for urge incontinence (more prevalent in older adults) and not limited to treatment of stress incontinence.

REFERENCE

Flynn L, Cell P, Luisi E: Effectiveness of pelvic muscle exercises in reducing urge incontinence among community residing elders, *J of Gerontological Nurs* 20(5):23, 1994.

MAINTENANCE OF SKIN INTEGRITY

The normal acidity of urine is irritating to skin. Urine allowed to be in contact with the skin becomes alkaline causing encrustations or precipitates to collect on the skin, fostering breakdown. Continuous exposure of the perineal area or skin around an ostomy leads to gradual maceration and excoriation (see Chapter 38). Washing with mild soap and warm water is the best way to remove urine from skin. Body lotion keeps skin moisturized and petroleum-based ointments provide a barrier to the urine. Clients who wet their clothing should receive partial baths and clean sets of clothes after voiding.

When the skin becomes irritated or inflamed, the physician may prescribe a cream or spray containing steroids (e.g., Kenalog) to reduce inflammation. If fungal growth develops, the antifungal drug nystatin (Mycostatin), available in cream or powder, is effective.

The client with an ostomy has a special hygiene problem because urine drains continuously from the ostomy site. Skin barriers provide a layer of protection between the client's skin and ostomy pouch. It is important that the appliance that fits snugly against the skin's surface around the stoma. Urine that remains in contact with the abdominal skin for extended periods of time will breakdown. If breakdown occurs, the pouch system will not adhere to the denuded tissue and leakage becomes a major problem causing additional skin breakdown.

PROMOTION OF COMFORT

Clients with urinary alterations become uncomfortable as a result of the symptoms of urinary problems. Frequent or unpredictable voiding, dysuria, and painful distention are sources of discomfort.

The incontinent client gains comfort from having clean, dry clothing. When stress incontinence is the problem, a protective pad offers protection against soiling. Wet clothing adheres to the skin and can cause rubbing and irritation.

Dysuria may be relieved by giving urinary analgesics that act on the urethral and bladder mucosa. Phenazopyridine (Pyridium) helps relieve dysuria, burning, and itching. It may also be found with sulfonamide antibiotics in preparations such as Azo-Gantanol and Azo-Gantrisin. The sulfonamide provides additional antibacterial action. Clients taking drugs with phenazopyridine should be aware that their urine may appear orange. They must drink large amounts of fluids to prevent toxicity from the sulfonamides and to maintain optimal flow through the urinary system.

If the client has local discomfort from an inflamed urethra, a warm sitz bath may provide pain relief. The warm water soothes inflamed tissues near the urethral meatus by improving blood supply. The client is often relaxed after a sitz bath, so voiding occurs easily. Pain of distention cannot be relieved unless the client is able to empty the bladder. Methods for stimulating micturition may be the only sources of pain relief.

Evaluation

To evaluate outcomes and responses to nursing care the nurse measures the effectiveness of all interventions. The optimal goal is the client's ability to urinate voluntarily without symptoms (e.g., urgency, dysuria, or frequency). The urine should be an amber color, clear, without abnormal constituents, and within the normal range of pH and specific gravity. The client should be able to identify factors that may influence normal voiding. The nurse also evaluates specific interventions designed to promote normal urinary function and prevent complications of urinary alterations (see the evaluation box on p. 1337).

The nurse collects data related to the client's voiding pattern, exposure to risks for urinary tract alteration, and physical condition. Laboratory analysis of urine specimens and diagnostic review of urinary structures provide further information.

Nursing interventions promote normal urination and provide support to clients unable to maintain continence.

Sample Evaluation of Interventions for Urinary Retention

GOALS	EVALUATIVE MEASURES	EXPECTED OUTCOMES
Client will reestablish usual voiding pattern within 2 days after catheter removal.	Palpate bladder for distention after voiding. Ask client about sensations of bladder fullness after voiding. Evaluate volume of urine output.	Bladder will not be distended after voiding. Client will deny feelings of fullness after voiding. Client will achieve complete bladder emptying within 24 hours of catheter removal.
Client will achieve understanding of normal urinary elimination.	Ask client to explain normal voiding. Ask client to describe factors that promote or impair urinary elimination.	Client will verbalize understanding of urinary elimination and follow appropriate health care practices promoting elimination.
Client will be free of infection.	Observe client's toileting self-care habits. If ordered, obtain a midstream sample for culture. Assess client for signs of urgency, frequency, dysuria, burning, or itching at urethral meatus. Observe characteristics of urine.	There will be no bacterial growth. Client will remain free of symtoms. Urine will be clear, amber, and without sediment.

Because of the urinary tract's vulnerability to infection, one of the nurse's primary concerns is infection control. The client with urinary alterations may also suffer embarrassment, social isolation, and depression. Whether the alteration is temporary (e.g., catheterization) or long term (e.g., ileal loop), the nurse must maintain the client's privacy and dignity. The nurse also evaluates the client's need for additional support services (e.g., home health care, physical therapy, counseling) and initiates the referral.

The provision of quality care has become a paramount goal of the profession. To this end, nurses are actively involved in developing methods toystematically evaluate the nursing process. Nursing research is being conducted to validate nursing interventions. Quality improvement is evolving as a tool to evaluate nursing care delivery. The goal is the ensure the delivery of competent, state-of-the-art nursing care with positive outcomes for each client.

■ KEY CONCEPTS ■

▶ The act of micturition or voiding is influenced by voluntary control from higher brain centers and involuntary control from the spinal cord.

▶ Symptoms common to urinary disturbances include urgency, dysuria, polyuria, oliguria, and difficulty in starting the urinary stream.

▶ When collected properly, a clean-voided urine specimen does not contain bacteria from the urethral meatus.

▶ A client can better understand the importance of perineal hygiene by knowing that the urinary tract is normally sterile.

▶ Methods of promoting the micturition reflex assist clients in sensing the urge to urinate and controlling urethral sphincter relaxation.

▶ An increased fluid intake results in increased urine formation that flushes particles and solutes from the urinary system.

▶ An indwelling urinary catheter remains in the bladder for an extended period, making the risk of infection greater than with intermittent catheterization.

▶ Because urine drains almost continuously from a ureterostomy, there is a risk of skin breakdown around a stoma site.

▶ A primary function of the elimination process is fluid balance.

▶ Catheter irrigation becomes necessary when the catheter becomes occluded with sediment or blood clots.

▶ A catheter drainage system should be positioned to allow free drainage of urine by gravity.

▶ Condom catheters are applied snugly but not so tightly as to constrict blood flow.

▶ Incontinence is classifed as functional, overflow, stress, urge, or total. Each type has specific nursing interventions.

▶ Specific guidelines for catheter selection should be followed so that the catheter docs not cause harm during insertion.

▶ Alterations in the urinary system can cause alterations in other organ systems.

■ KEY TERMS ■

■ CRITICAL THINKING EXERCISES ■

1. Mrs. MacGill is a 55-year-old widow who has experienced sudden loss of urine when coughing or sneezing. As a result she no longer visits with her married children because she doesn't want to ride in the car for any distance. She has also given up her Tuesday morning bridge club and only goes to church with an adult incontinent pad in place. The embarrassment of having an "accident" is more than she can bear, and she is terrified of leaving the house.

   a. What are actual and potential nursing diagnoses?

   b. For two of those diagnoses what are the expected outcomes?

   c. For one of those two diagnoses, give two nursing interventions.

2. Mr. Hermann is a 37-year-old man who has been admitted with a possible renal calculus. He has severe renal colic and an intravenous of normal saline has been started to infuse at 150 ml/hour. He is to undergo an IVP in 4 hours.

   a. What is the purpose of the IVP?

   b. Discuss rationale for the rate of IV fluids.

   c. Give at least two nursing responsibilities for the client undergoing an IVP.

3. Miss Josea is a 70-year-old woman who has arthritis in her hips and knees. She is at her family practitioner's office. You are the family nurse practitioner in joint practice with him. As you assess her for her arthritis she tells you that she has noticed that she is unable to get to the bathroom in time and has " wet her pants" more times than she can remember. She asks you to recommend a pad that she can wear that won't let her "smell." What assessments does the nurse need to complete before planning interventions for Miss Josea's care?

REFERENCES

Agency for Health Care Policy and Research (AHCPR), Urinary Incontinence Guideline Panel, *Urinary incontinence in adults: clinical practice guideline,* AHCPR Pub No 92-0038, Rockville, Md, 1992, U.S. Dept of Health and Human Services.

Brooks MJ: Urinary incontinence assessment, treatment and reimbursement, *Home Health Care Nurse* 11(4):41, 1993.

Brundage D: *Mosby's clinical nursing series: renal disorders,* St Louis, 1992, Mosby.

Burgener S: Justification of closed intermittent urinary catheter irrigation/installation: a review of current research and practice, *J Adv Nurs* 12:229, 1987.

Burke MM, Walsh MB: *Gerontological nursing: care of the frail elderly,* St Louis, 1992, Mosby.

Colling JC, Owen TR, McCready MR: Urine volume and voiding patterns among incontinent nursing home residents, *Geriatric Nurs* 15(4):188, 1994.

Flynn L, Cell P, Luisi E : Effectiveness of pelvic muscle exercises in reducing urge incontinence among community residing elders, *J Gerontological Nurs* 20(5):23, 1994.

Galanti GA: *Caring for patients from different cultures,* Philadelphia, 1991, University of Pennsylvania Press.

Johnson CC: Definition, classification, and clinical presentation of urinary tract infections, *Med Clin North Am* 75(2):241, 1991.

Kim MJ, McFarland GK, McLane AM: *Pocket guide to nursing diagnoses,* ed 6, St Louis, 1995, Mosby.

McCance KL, Huether SE: *Pathophysiology: the biological basis for disease in adults and children,* St Louis, 1994, Mosby.

Moore S et al: Treating bladder cancer: new methods new management, *Am J Nurs* 93(5):32, 1993.

NewsWatch: Cranberry juice beneficial, *Geriatric Nursing* 15(4):184, 1994.

Resnick B: Retraining the bladder after catheterization, *Am J Nurs* 93(11):43, 1993.

Thayer D : How to assess and control urinary incontinence, *Am J Nurs* 94(10):42, 1994.

Yoshikawa TT: Chronic urinary tract infections in elderly patients, *Hosp Pract* 28(6):103, 1993.

ADDITIONAL READINGS

Dellasaga C, Clark D, McCreary D: Nursing process: teaching elderly clients, *J Gerontological Nurs* 20(1):31, 1994.

Fiers S, Siebert C: Urinary incontinence: a multidisciplinary appraoch, *Ostomy/Wound Management* 39(7):14, 1993.

Fox B: Recurring urinary tract infections: incidence and risk factors, *Am J Public Health* 80(3):331, 1990.

Fuller N: Clean intermittent catheterization:an intervention for overflow voiding or overflow incontinence, *Ostomy/Wound Management* 38(7):29, 1992.

Gray M: *Mosby's clinical nursing series: genitourinary disorders,* St Louis, 1992, Mosby.

Hesnan K: ET nurses expanding our practice, *Ostomy/Wound Management* 38(7):12, 1992.

Kaltrieder DL et al: Can reminders curb incontinence? *Geriatr Nurs* 11(1):17, 1990.

Pagana KD, Pagana TJ: *Diagnostic testing and nursing implications: a case study approach,* ed 4, St Louis, 1994, Mosby.

Palmer MH et al: Risk factors for urinary incontinence one year after nursing-home admission, *Res Nurs Health* 14:405, 1991.

Powers I, Williams D: Urinary incontinence: helping a patient gain control, *Nursing 92* 22(12):46, 1992.

Toto K: Acute renal failure: a question of location, *Am J of Nurs* 92(11):44, 1992.

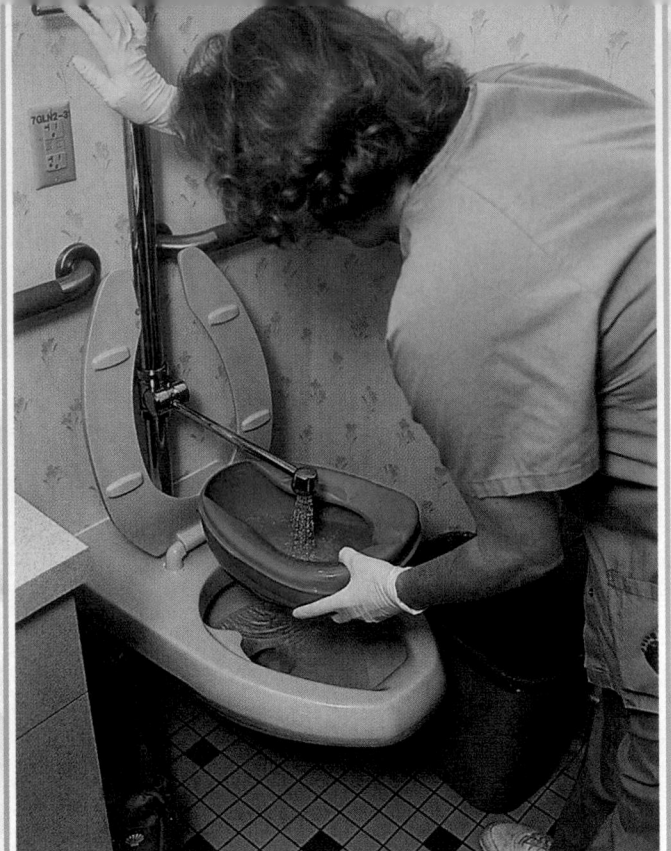

## Chapter 47

Bowel Elimination

Objectives

Mastery of content in this chapter will enable the student to:

▶ Define the key terms listed.

▶ Discuss the role of gastrointestinal organs in digestion and elimination.

▶ Describe four functions of the large intestine.

▶ Explain the physiological aspects of normal defecation.

▶ Discuss psychological and physiological factors that influence the elimination process.

▶ Describe common physiological alterations in elimination.

▶ Assess a client's elimination pattern.

▶ Perform a guaiac test for occult blood.

▶ List nursing diagnoses related to alterations in elimination.

▶ Describe nursing implications for common diagnostic examinations of the gastrointestinal tract.

▶ Administer an enema.

▶ List nursing measures that promote normal elimination.

▶ List nursing measures included in bowel training.

▶ Discuss the relationship between the structure and function of bowel diversions and nursing care required.

Regular elimination of bowel waste products is essential for normal body functioning. Alterations in elimination can cause problems with the gastrointestinal and other body systems. Because bowel function depends on the balance of several factors, elimination patterns and habits vary among individuals. However, there is evidence that frequent, high-volume, normal feces is consistent with a lower incidence of colorectal cancer (Robinson and Weigley, 1989).

To manage clients' elimination problems, the nurse must understand normal elimination and factors that promote or impede elimination. Supportive nursing care respects the client's privacy and emotional needs. Measures designed to promote normal elimination should also minimize discomfort.

▌ NORMAL DIGESTION AND ELIMINATION

The gastrointestinal (GI) tract is a series of hollow mucous membrane–lined muscular organs. The purposes of these organs are to absorb fluid and nutrients, prepare food for absorption and use by the body's cells, and provide for temporary storage of feces (Fig. 47-1). The volume of fluids absorbed by the GI tract is high, making fluid balance a key function of the GI system. In addition to ingested fluids and foods, the GI tract also receives many secretions from organs such as the gallbladder and the pancreas (Table 47-1). Any condition that seriously impairs normal absorption or secretion of GI fluids could cause fluid imbalance.

Mouth

The GI tract mechanically and chemically breaks down nutrients into a suitable size and form. All digestive organs work together to ensure that the mass, or **bolus**, of food reaches the areas of nutrient absorption safely and effectively. Mechanical and chemical digestion begin in the mouth. The teeth **masticate** (chew) food, breaking it down to a suitable size for swallowing. Salivary secretions contain enzymes, such as ptyalin, that initiate digestion of certain food elements. Saliva dilutes and softens the bolus of food in the mouth for easier swallowing.

Esophagus

As food enters the upper esophagus, it passes through the upper esophageal sphincter, which is a circular muscle that prevents air from entering the esophagus and food from **refluxing** (moving backward) into the throat. The bolus of food travels approximately 25 cm (10 inches) down the esophagus. Food is pushed along by slow **peristalsis** produced by alternating involuntary contractions and relaxations of smooth muscle. As a portion of the esophagus contracts above the food bolus, the circular muscle below (or in front) of the bolus relaxes. This alternate contraction-relaxation of smooth muscle propels food toward the next wave (Fig. 47-2).

In 15 seconds the bolus of food moves down the esophagus and reaches the lower esophageal sphincter. The lower esophageal sphincter lies between the esophagus and stomach (Tortora, 1989). Factors influencing lower esophageal sphincter pressure include antacids, which minimize reflux, and fatty foods and nicotine, which increase reflux.

Stomach

In the stomach, food is temporarily stored and mechanically and chemically broken down for digestion and absorption (see Chapter 41). The stomach secretes hydrochloric acid (HCl), mucus, the enzyme pepsin, and intrinsic factor. The concentration of HCl influences stomach acidity and the body's acid-base balance (see Chapter 45). HCl

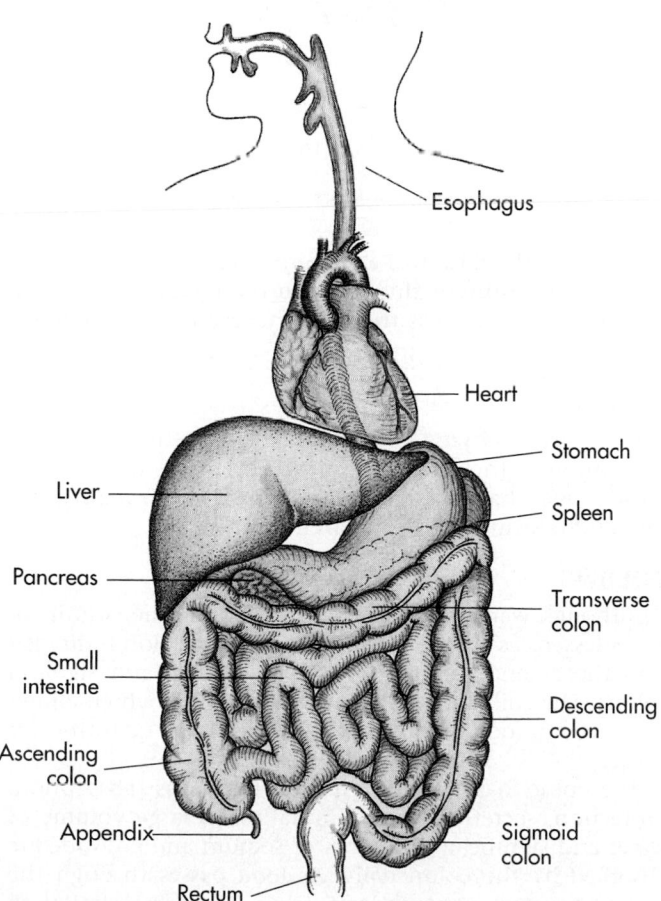

Fig. 47-1 Organs of the gastrointestinal tract (with the heart as a reference point).

Esophagus

Heart

Stomach

Spleen

Transverse colon

Descending colon

Sigmoid colon

Liver

Pancreas

Small intestine

Ascending colon

Appendix

Rectum

Table 47-1	Gastrointestinal Tract Fluid Balance	
Item	**Ingested and Secreted (ml)**	**Absorbed (ml)**
Food and drink	1500	
Saliva	1500	
Gastric juice	3000	
Pancreatic juice	2000	
Bile	500	
Small intestine fluid		5850
Colon		2500
Feces		150
Total	8500	8500

Segmentation

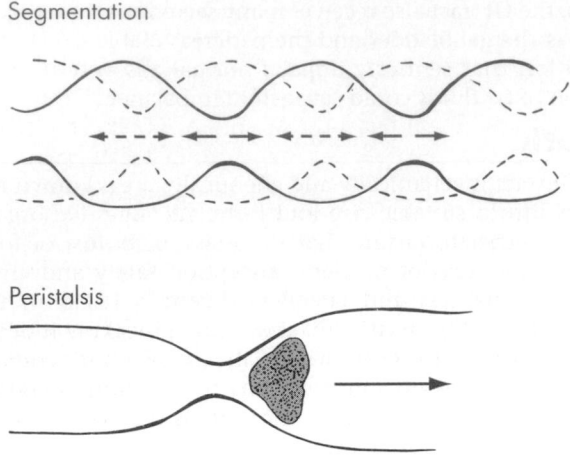

Peristalsis

Fig. 47-2 Segmented and peristaltic waves.

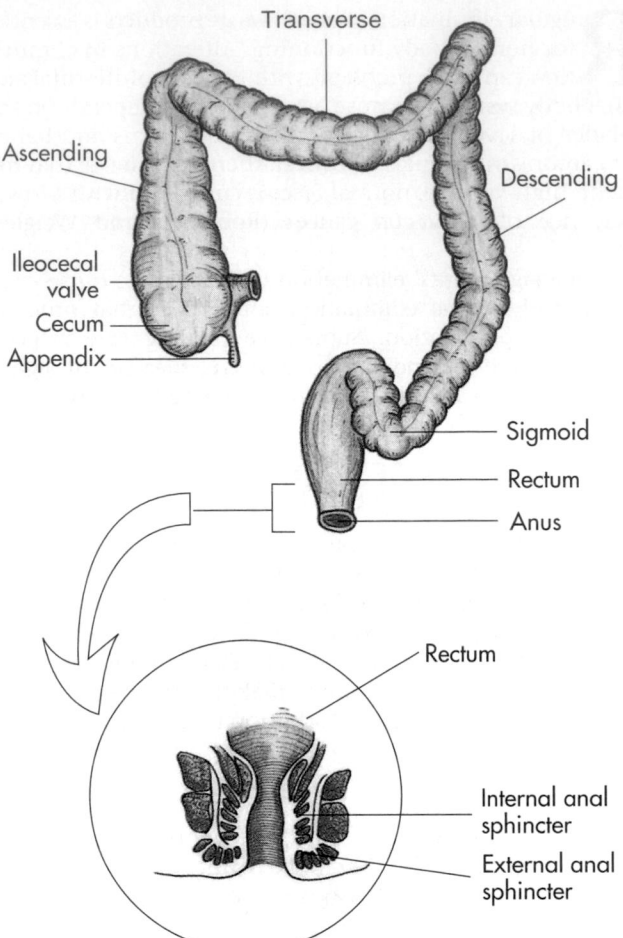

Fig. 47-3 Divisions of the large intestine.

helps mix and break down food in the stomach. Mucus protects the stomach mucosa from acidity and enzyme activity. Pepsin digests proteins, although not much digestion occurs in the stomach. Intrinsic factor is the essential component needed for vitamin B_{12} absorption in the intestine and subsequent normal red blood cell formation. Lack of this intrinsic factor results in pernicious anemia.

Before food leaves the stomach, it is changed into a semi-fluid material called **chyme**. Chyme is more easily digested and absorbed than solid food. Clients who have portions of their stomachs removed or who have rapid stomach emptying (as with gastritis) may have serious digestive problems because food is not broken down into chyme.

Small Intestine

During normal digestion, chyme leaves the stomach and enters the small intestine. The small intestine is a tube about 2.5 cm (1 inch) in diameter and 6 m (20 feet) long. It contains three divisions: duodenum, jejunum, and ileum. Chyme mixes with digestive enzymes (e.g., bile and amylase) while traveling through the small intestine. Segmentation (alternating contraction and relaxation of smooth muscle) churns the chyme, further breaking down food for digestion (see Fig. 47-2). As chyme mixes, forward peristaltic movement temporarily ceases, permitting absorption. Chyme travels slowly through the small intestine to allow absorption.

Most nutrients and electrolytes are absorbed in the small intestine. Enzymes from the pancreas (e.g., amylase) and bile from the gallbladder are released into the duodenum. The enzymes in the small intestine break down fats, proteins, and carbohydrates into basic elements (see Chapter 41). Nutrients are almost entirely absorbed by the duodenum and jejunum. The ileum absorbs certain vitamins, iron, and bile salts. If its function is impaired, the digestive process is greatly altered. For example, inflammation, surgical resection, or obstruction can disrupt peristalsis, reduce the area of absorption, or block passage of chyme.

Large Intestine

The lower GI tract is called the large intestine **(colon)** because it is larger in diameter than the small intestine. How-

ever, its length of 1.5 to 1.8 m (5 to 6 feet) is much shorter. The large intestine is divided into the cecum, colon, and rectum (Fig. 47-3). It is the primary organ of bowel elimination.

CECUM

Unabsorbed chyme enters the large intestine at the cecum through the ileocecal valve. This valve is a circular muscle layer that prevents colon contents from **regurgitating** and returning to the small intestine.

COLON

Although watery chyme enters the colon, the volume of water lessens as chyme moves along it. The colon is divided into the ascending, transverse, descending, and sigmoid colons. The colon is made of muscular tissue, which allows it to accommodate and thus eliminate large quantities of waste.

The colon has four interrelated functions: absorption, protection, secretion, and elimination. A large volume of water and significant amounts of sodium and chloride are absorbed by the colon daily. As food passes through the colon, **haustral contractions** occur. These are similar to segmental contractions of the small intestine but last longer—up to 5 minutes. The contractions produce large sacs in the colon's wall, providing a large surface area for absorption.

As much as 2.5 L of water can be absorbed by the colon in 24 hours. On the average, 55 mEq of sodium and 23 mEq of chloride are absorbed daily. The amount of water absorbed from chyme depends on the speed at which colonic contents move. Chyme is normally a soft, formed mass. If the speed of peristaltic contractions is abnormally fast, there is less time for water to be absorbed and the stool will be watery. If peristaltic contractions slow down, water continues to be absorbed and a hard mass of stool forms, resulting in constipation.

The colon protects itself by releasing a supply of mucus. Mucus is normally clear to opaque with a stringy consistency. Mucus lubricates the colon, preventing trauma to its inner walls. Lubrication is especially important near the distal end of the colon, where contents become drier and harder.

The secretory function of the colon aids in electrolyte balance. Bicarbonate is secreted in exchange for chloride. About 4 to 9 mEq of potassium are released each day by the large intestine. Serious alterations in colon function, such as diarrhea, can cause electrolyte imbalance.

Finally, the colon eliminates waste products and gas (**flatus**). Flatus results from air swallowing, diffusion of gas from the bloodstream into the intestine, and bacterial action on nonabsorbable carbohydrates. Fermentation of carbohydrates (such as in cabbage and onions) produces intestinal gas, which can stimulate peristalsis. An adult normally forms 400 to 700 ml of flatus daily.

Slow peristaltic contractions move contents through the colon. Intestinal content is the main stimulus for contraction. Waste products and gas exert pressure against the walls of the colon. The muscle layer stretches, stimulating the reflex that initiates contraction. Mass peristaltic movements push undigested food toward the rectum. These movements occur only three or four times daily, unlike the frequent peristaltic waves in the small intestine (usually heard during auscultation).

When these mass peristaltic movements occur, large segments of the colon contract as a result of gastrocolic and duodenocolic reflex responses. These occur when the stomach or duodenum is filled with food. Filling initiates nerve impulses that stimulate the colon's muscular walls. Mass peristalsis is strongest during the hour after mealtime.

RECTUM

Waste products that reach the sigmoid portion of the colon are called **feces**. The sigmoid stores feces until just before defecation.

The rectum is the final division of the GI tract. Its length varies according to age:

Infant	2.5 to 3.8 cm (1 to 1.5 inches)
Toddler	5 cm (2 inches)
Preschooler	7.5 cm (3 inches)
School-ager	10 cm (4 inches)
Adult	15 to 20 cm (6 to 8 inches)

Normally the rectum is empty of feces until defecation. It contains vertical and transverse folds of tissue. Each vertical fold contains an artery and veins. If the veins become distended from pressure during the straining, hemorrhoids form. Hemorrhoids can make defecation painful.

When the fecal mass or gas moves into the rectum to distend its walls, **defecation** begins. The process involves involuntary and voluntary control. The internal sphincter is a smooth muscle innervated by the autonomic nervous system. As the rectum distends, sensory nerves are stimulated and carry impulses that cause the internal sphincter to relax, allowing more feces to enter the rectum. At the same time, impulses travel to the brain to create awareness of the need to defecate.

As the internal sphincter relaxes, so does the external sphincter. Adults and toilet-trained children can voluntarily control the external sphincter. If the time for defecation is not right, constriction of the levator ani muscles closes the anus and defecation is delayed. At the time of defecation, the external sphincter relaxes. Pressure can be exerted to expel feces through an increase in intraabdominal pressure or a Valsalva maneuver. A **Valsalva maneuver** is voluntary contraction of abdominal muscles during forced expiration with a closed glottis (holding one's breath while straining).

▌ FACTORS AFFECTING ELIMINATION

Many factors influence the process of bowel elimination (Table 47-2). Knowledge of these factors lets the nurse anticipate measures required to maintain a normal elimination pattern.

Age

Developmental changes that affect elimination occur throughout life. An infant has a small stomach capacity and less secretion of digestive enzymes. Some foods such as complex starches are tolerated poorly. Food passes quickly through an infant's intestinal tract because of rapid peristalsis. The infant is unable to control defecation because of a lack of neuromuscular development. This development usually does not take place until 2 to 3 years of age. During adolescence, there is rapid growth of the large intestine. The secretion of HCl increases, particularly in boys. Adolescents typically eat more.

Older adults often experience changes in the GI system that impair digestion and elimination (Lueckenotte, 1994). Some of the changes in the GI tract that occur with aging are listed in Table 47-3. Some persons may lose their teeth and thus the ability to chew food thoroughly. Food enters the digestive tract only partially chewed and cannot be digested because the amount of digestive enzymes in saliva and the volume of gastric acids decrease with aging. The inability to digest fat-containing foods reflects a loss of the enzyme lipase.

Hospitalized older adults are at particular risk of altered bowel function. One study indicated a 91% incidence of diarrhea or constipation in a population of 33 hospitalized persons with a mean age of 76 years (Ross, 1990).

In addition, peristaltic action declines with age, and esophageal emptying slows. Sluggish emptying of the esophagus can cause discomfort in the epigastric section of the abdomen. Absorptive properties of the intestinal mucosa change, causing protein, vitamin, and mineral deficiencies. Older adults also lose muscle tone in the perineal floor and anal sphincter. Although the integrity of the external sphincter may remain intact, older adults may have difficulty controlling bowel evacuation. Because of slowing

Table 47-2	Factors Affecting Elimination
FACTORS PROMOTING ELIMINATION	**FACTORS IMPAIRING ELIMINATION**
Stress-free environment	Emotional stress (anxiety or depression)
Ability to follow personal bowel habits, privacy	Failure to heed defecation reflex, lack of time or privacy
High-fiber diet	High-carbohydrate, high-fat diet
Normal fluid intake (fruit juices, warm liquids)	Reduced fluid intake
Exercise (walking)	Immobility or inactivity
Ability to assume squatting position	Inability to squat because of immobility, advanced age, musculoskeletal deformities, pain, pain during defecation
Properly administered laxatives and cathartics	Use of narcotic analgesics, antibiotics, and general anesthetics, and overuse of cathartics

Table 47-3	Normal Changes in the GI Tract from Aging	
PORTION OF GI TRACT	**CHANGES**	**CAUSES**
Esophagus	Reduced motility, especially in lower third	Degeneration of neural cells.
Stomach	Decrease in: Acid secretions	Degeneration of gastric mucosa. Alkaline gastric medium contributes to malabsorption of iron. Loss of parietal cells also leads to loss of intrinsic factor, which is needed for vitamin B_{12} absorption. Although digestive enzymes are decreased, enough remain available for digestion.
	Motor activity Mucosal thickness	Delayed gastric emptying and fewer hunger contractions.
Small intestine	Fewer absorbing cells	Absorption not significantly affected.
Large intestine	Weakened musculature	Increase in pouches on the weakened intestinal wall called *diverticulosis*.
	Decreased peristalsis	Constipation.
	Duller nerve sensations	Missed defecation signal.
Liver	Size decreased	Reduced storage capacity and ability to synthesize protein.

Data from Lueckenotte AG: *Pocket guide to gerontologic assessment,* ed 2, St Louis, 1994, Mosby.

of nerve impulses, some are less aware of the need to defecate and are likely to become constipated.

Diet

Regular daily food intake helps maintain a regular pattern of peristalsis in the colon. The food that a person eats influences elimination. **Fiber,** the undigestible residue in the diet, provides the bulk in fecal material. Bulk-forming foods absorb fluids, thereby increasing stool mass. The bowel walls are stretched, creating peristalsis and initiating the defecation reflex. An infant's immature bowel cannot usually tolerate fiber-containing foods until several months of age. By stimulating peristalsis, bulk foods pass quickly through the intestines, keeping the stool soft. The following foods contain a high amount of fiber (bulk):

1. Raw fruits (apples, oranges)
2. Cooked fruits (prunes, apricots)
3. Greens (spinach, kale, cabbage)
4. Raw vegetables (celery, zucchini)
5. Whole grains (cereal, breads)

Ingestion of a high-fiber diet improves the likelihood of a normal elimination pattern if other factors are normal. Gas-producing foods such as onions, cauliflower, and beans also stimulate peristalsis. The gas formed distends intestinal walls, increasing colon motility. Some spicy foods can increase peristalsis but can also cause indigestion and watery stools.

Some foods, such as milk and milk products, are difficult or impossible for some people to digest. This is caused by a **lactose intolerance.** Lactose, a simple form of sugar found in milk, is normally broken down by the enzyme lactase. Intolerance to specific foods may result in diarrhea, gaseous distention, and cramping.

Fluid Intake

An inadequate intake of fluids or disturbances causing loss of fluid (such as vomiting) affect the character of feces. Fluid liquefies intestinal contents, easing its passage through the colon. Reduced fluid intake slows passage of food through the intestine. An adult should drink 6 to 8 glasses (1400 to 2000 ml) of fluid daily. Hot beverages and fruit juices soften stool and increase peristalsis. A large ingestion of milk may slow peristalsis in some persons and cause constipation.

Physical Activity

Physical activity promotes peristalsis, whereas immobilization depresses colonic motility. Early ambulation after illness is encouraged to promote maintenance of normal elimination.

Maintaining tone of skeletal muscles used during defecation is important. Weakened abdominal and pelvic floor muscles impair the ability to increase intraabdominal pressure and to control the external sphincter. Muscle tone may be weakened or lost as a result of long-term illness or neurological disease that impairs nerve transmission.

Psychological Factors

The function of almost all body systems can be impaired by prolonged emotional stress (see Chapter 22). If an individual becomes anxious, afraid, or angry, the stress response is initiated, which allows the body to restore defenses. The digestive process is accelerated, and peristalsis is increased to provide nutrients needed for defense. Side effects of increased peristalsis are diarrhea and gaseous distention. If a person becomes depressed, the autonomic nervous system slows impulses and peristalsis can decrease. A number of diseases of the GI tract may be associated with stress. These include ulcerative **colitis**, gastric ulcers, and **Crohn's disease.** Repeated research endeavors have failed to prove the myth that clients with such diseases have underlying psychopathological conditions. However, anxiety and depression may be a result of such chronic problems (Cooke, 1991).

Personal Habits

Personal elimination habits influence bowel function. Most people benefit from being able to use their own toilet facilities at a time that is most effective and convenient for them. A busy work schedule may disrupt habits and result in alterations such as constipation. A person should learn the best time for elimination. The **gastrocolic reflex** is most easily stimulated to cause defecation after breakfast.

Hospitalized clients can rarely maintain privacy during defecation. Bathroom facilities are often shared with a roommate whose hygienic habits might be quite different. The client's illness often limits physical activity and requires the use of a bedpan or bedside commode. The sights, sounds, and odors associated with sharing toilet facilities or using bedpans are often embarrassing. Embarrassment prompts clients to ignore the urge to defecate, which can begin a vicious cycle of discomfort.

Position During Defecation

Squatting is the normal position during defecation. Modern toilets are designed to facilitate this posture, allowing the person to lean forward, exert intraabdominal pressure, and contract the thigh muscles. However, an older client or one with joint disease such as arthritis may be unable to rise from a low toilet seat. Attachments that raise the seat enable the client to get off the toilet without assistance. Clients who use such attachments, and short people, might require a footstool for proper hip flexion.

For the client immobilized in bed, defecation is often difficult. In a supine position it is impossible to contract the muscles used during defecation. Assisting the client to a more normal sitting position on a bedpan enhances the ability to defecate.

Pain

Normally the act of defecation is painless. However, a number of conditions, including hemorrhoids, rectal surgery, rectal fistulas, abdominal surgery, and childbirth can result in discomfort. In these instances the client often suppresses the urge to defecate to avoid pain. Constipation is a common problem for clients with pain during defecation.

Pregnancy

As pregnancy advances and the size of the fetus increases, pressure is exerted on the rectum. A temporary obstruction created by the fetus impairs passage of feces. Constipation is a common problem during the last trimester. A pregnant woman's frequent straining during defecation can result in formation of permanent hemorrhoids.

Surgery and Anesthesia

General anesthetic agents used during surgery cause temporary cessation of peristalsis (see Chapter 48). Inhaled anesthetic agents block parasympathetic impulses to the intestinal musculature. The anesthetic's action slows or stops peristaltic waves. The client who receives local or regional anesthesia is less at risk for elimination alterations because bowel activity is affected minimally or not at all.

Surgery that involves direct manipulation of the bowel temporarily stops peristalsis. This condition, called **paralytic ileus,** usually lasts about 24 to 48 hours. If the client remains inactive or is unable to eat after surgery, return of normal bowel function may be further delayed.

Medications

Medications are available for promoting defecation. **Laxatives** and **cathartics** soften the stool and promote peristalsis. Although similar, laxatives are milder in action than cathartics. When used correctly, laxatives and cathartics safely maintain normal elimination patterns. However, chronic use of cathartics causes the large intestine to lose muscle tone and become less responsive to stimulation by laxatives. Laxative overuse can also cause serious diarrhea that can lead to dehydration and electrolyte depletion. Mineral oil, a common laxative, decreases fat-soluble vitamin absorption. Laxatives can influence the efficacy of other medications by altering the **transit time** (i.e., the time the medication remains in the GI tract).

Medications such as dicyclomine HCl (Bentyl) suppress peristalsis and treat diarrhea. Several medications have side effects that can impair elimination. Narcotic analgesics depress peristalsis. Opiates commonly cause constipation. Anticholinergic drugs, such as atropine or glycopyrrolate (Robinul), inhibit gastric acid secretion and depress GI motility. Although useful in treating hyperactive bowel disorders, anticholinergics can cause constipation. Many antibiotics produce diarrhea by disrupting the normal bacterial flora in the GI tract. If the diarrhea and associated abdominal cramping become severe, the client might need

Nursing Interventions to Prevent Osmotic Diarrhea Caused by Hyperosmolar Medications

- Dilute medications with 30 to 60 ml water.
- Administer drugs separately.
- Irrigate feeding tube before and after each medication (30 ml each time).
- Report occurrence of diarrhea from either initiation of or continuous consumption of a medication or tube feeding.
- Consult a pharmacist for possible alternative drug preparations.
- Monitor client responses to treatment.
- Consider parenteral route if possible.

Modified from Fruto LV: Current concepts: management of diarrhea in acute care, *Journal of Wound, Ostomy, and Continence Nursing (WOCN)* 21(5):199, 1994.

Common Causes of Constipation

- Irregular bowel habits and ignoring the urge to defecate can cause constipation.
- Clients who have a low-fiber diet high in animal fats (e.g., meats, dairy products, eggs) and refined sugars (rich desserts) often have constipation problems. Also, low fluid intake slows peristalsis.
- Lengthy bed rest or lack of regular exercise causes constipation.
- Heavy laxative use causes loss of normal defecation reflex. In addition, the lower colon is completely emptied, requiring time to refill with bulk.
- Tranquilizers, opiates, anticholinergics, iron, diuretics, antacids with calcium or aluminum, and antiparkinsonism drugs can cause constipation.
- Older adults experience slowed peristalsis, loss of abdominal muscle elasticity, and reduced intestinal mucus secretion. Older adults often eat low-fiber foods.
- Constipation is also caused by GI abnormalities such as bowel obstruction, paralytic ileus, and diverticulitis.
- Neurological conditions that block nerve impulses to the colon (e.g., spinal cord injury, tumor) can cause constipation.
- Organic illnesses such as hypothyroidism, hypocalcemia, or hypokalemia can cause constipation.

to change medications. Nursing interventions that can be used to prevent osmotic diarrhea caused by hyperosmolar medications have been described by Fruto (1994) (see the box above).

Diagnostic Tests

Diagnostic examinations involving visualization of GI structures often require that portions of the bowel be empty of contents. A client is not allowed to eat or drink after midnight of the day preceding examinations such as a barium enema, (LGI) endoscopy of the lower GI tract, or an upper GI (UGI) series. In the case of a barium enema or endoscopy, the client usually receives cathartics and an enema. Such emptying of the bowel can interfere with elimination until normal eating is resumed.

Barium examination procedures pose an additional problem. Barium hardens if allowed to stay in the GI tract. This can lead to constipation or bowel impaction. A client should receive a cathartic to promote elimination of barium after the procedure. Failure to evacuate all barium might require that the client receive a cleansing enema.

■ COMMON BOWEL ELIMINATION PROBLEMS

The nurse might care for clients who have or are at risk for elimination problems because of emotional stress (anxiety or depression), physiological changes in the GI tract, surgical alteration of intestinal structures, other prescribed therapy, or disorders impairing defecation.

Constipation

Constipation is a symptom, not a disease. It is a decrease in frequency of bowel movements, accompanied by prolonged or difficult passage of hard, dry stools. Straining during defecation is an associated sign. When intestinal motility slows, the fecal mass becomes exposed over time to the intestinal walls and most of the fecal water content is absorbed. Little water is left to soften and lubricate stool. Passage of a dry, hard stool may cause rectal pain.

Each person has an individual defecation pattern that the nurse must assess. It is important to remember that not every adult has a daily bowel movement (Ebersole and Hess, 1994). A bowel movement only every 4 or more days is considered abnormal (Lueckenotte, 1994). A usual bowel movement pattern of every 2 to 3 days without any difficulty, pain, or bleeding may be normal for an elderly person (Ebersole and Hess, 1994; Lueckenotte, 1994). If daily records start to suggest a decrease in the frequency of defecation there is cause for concern. The causes of constipation are summarized in the box above.

Constipation is a significant hazard to health. Straining during defecation causes problems to the client with recent abdominal, gynecological, or rectal surgery. The effort to pass a stool can cause sutures to separate, reopening the wound. In addition, clients with histories of cardiovascular disease, diseases causing elevated intraocular pressure (glaucoma), and increased intracranial pressure should prevent constipation and avoid using the Valsalva maneuver (see Chapter 32). Exhaling through the mouth during straining avoids a Valsalva maneuver. Older adults may have constipation from certain medications that they are taking. Some of these medications are aspirin, antihistamines, diuretics, tranquilizers, hypnotics, antacids with aluminum or calcium, and drugs used to control Parkinson's disease (Lueckenotte, 1994).

Impaction

Fecal **impaction** results from unrelieved constipation. It is a collection of hardened feces, wedged in the rectum, which cannot be expelled. In cases of severe impaction, the mass can extend up into the sigmoid colon. Clients who are debilitated, confused, or unconscious are most at risk for impaction. They are too weak or unaware of the need to defecate.

An obvious sign of impaction is the inability to pass a

stool for several days, despite a repeated urge to defecate. When a continuous oozing of diarrheal stool suddenly develops, impaction should be suspected. The liquid portion of feces located higher in the colon seeps around the impacted mass. Loss of appetite (anorexia), abdominal distention and cramping, and rectal pain may accompany the condition. The nurse who suspects an impaction can gently perform a digital examination of the rectum and palpate the impacted mass.

Diarrhea

Diarrhea is an increase in the number of stools and the passage of liquid, unformed feces. It is a symptom of disorders affecting digestion, absorption, and secretion in the GI tract. Intestinal contents pass through the small intestine and colon too quickly to allow the usual absorption of fluid. Irritation within the colon can result in an increased mucus secretion. As a result, feces become watery, so the client may be unable to control the urge to defecate.

It is often difficult to assess diarrhea in infants. An infant who is bottle-fed may have one firm stool every second day, whereas a breast-fed baby may pass five to eight small, soft stools daily. The mother or nurse should note any sudden increase in number of stools, any reduction in fecal consis-

tency with an increase in fluid content, and a tendency for feces to be greenish.

Excess loss of colonic fluid can result in serious fluid and electrolyte or acid-base imbalances. Infants and older adults are particularly susceptible to associated complications (see Chapter 45). Because repeated passage of diarrheal stools also exposes the skin of the perineum and buttocks to irritating intestinal contents, meticulous skin care is needed to prevent skin breakdown (see Chapter 38) and containment of fecal drainage is needed (Bosley, 1994; Fruto, 1994).

Many conditions cause diarrhea (Table 47-4). The aims of treatment are to remove precipitating conditions and to slow peristalsis. The box below lists nursing responsibilities for managing the client with diarrhea.

Incontinence

Fecal **incontinence** is the inability to control passage of feces and gas from the anus. Physical conditions that impair anal sphincter function or control can cause incontinence. Conditions that create frequent, loose, large-volume, watery stools also predispose to incontinence.

Incontinence can harm a client's body image (see Chapter 23). In many situations the client is mentally alert but physically unable to avoid defecation. The embarrassment of soiling clothes can lead to social isolation. The client must depend on the nurse for a basic need.

Flatulence

As gas accumulates in the lumen of the intestines, the bowel wall stretches and distends (**flatulence**). It is a common cause of abdominal fullness, pain, and cramping. Normally, intestinal gas escapes through the mouth (belching) or the anus (passing of flatus). However, if there is a reduction in intestinal motility resulting from opiates, general anesthetics, abdominal surgery, or immobilization, flatulence can become severe enough to cause abdominal distention and severe sharp pain.

Hemorrhoids

Hemorrhoids are dilated, engorged veins in the lining of the rectum. They are either external or internal. External hemorrhoids are clearly visible as protrusions of skin. If the

Table 47-4 Conditions That Cause Diarrhea	
CONDITION	**PHYSIOLOGICAL EFFECTS**
Emotional stress (anxiety)	Increased intestinal motility
Intestinal infection (streptococcal or staphylococcal enteritis)	Inflammation of intestinal mucosa, increased mucus secretion in colon
Food allergies	Reduced digestion of food elements
Food intolerance (greasy foods, coffee, alcohol, spicy foods)	Increased intestinal motility, increased mucus secretion in colon
Tube feedings	Hyperosmolarity of some enteral solutions results in diarrhea, because hyperosmolar fluids draw fluids into the gastrointestinal tract
Medications	
Iron	Irritation of intestinal mucosa
Antibiotics	Suprainfection allowing overgrowth of normal flora, inflammation and irritation of mucosa
Laxatives (short term)	Increased intestinal motility
Colon disease (colitis, Crohn's disease)	Inflammation and ulceration of intestinal walls, reduced absorption of fluids, increased intestinal motility
Surgical alterations	
Gastrectomy	Loss of reservoir function of stomach, improper absorption because food is moved into duodenum too quickly
Colon resection	Reduced size of colon, reduced amount of absorptive surface

---

Summary of Nursing Responsibilities in the Management of Diarrhea

- Provide general supportive measures to maintain fluid status and electrolyte balance.
- Observe systemic manifestations such as fever, leukocytosis, fluid volume deficits, hypokalemia, and metabolic acidosis.
- Identify relationship between onset of diarrhea and initiation of enteral feeding.
- Report symptoms promptly and look for association of occurrence of diarrhea with either initiation or continuous consumption of hyperosmolar medications.
- Consult dietitians and pharmacists regarding drug-nutrient interactions and alternative regimens.
- Maintain perianal skin integrity.

From Fruto LV: Current concepts: management of diarrhea in acute care, *Journal of Wound, Ostomy, and Continence Nursing (WOCN)* 21(5):199, 1994.

underlying vein is hardened, there can be a purplish discoloration. Internal hemorrhoids have an outer mucous membrane. Increased venous pressure from straining at defecation, pregnancy, congestive heart failure, and chronic liver disease can cause hemorrhoids.

■ BOWEL DIVERSIONS

Certain diseases cause conditions that prevent normal passage of feces through the rectum. This creates the need for a temporary or permanent artificial opening **(stoma)** in the abdominal wall. Surgical openings (ostomies) are most commonly formed in the ileum **(ileostomy)** or colon **(colostomy)** (McGarity, 1992) (Fig. 47-4). Ends of the intestines are then brought through an opening in the abdominal wall to create the stoma. Depending upon the type of surgical procedure done, the client will either have no control over when the fecal material exits the stoma (incontinent ostomy) or will have control (continent ostomy). For incontinent ostomies, the stoma is covered with a pouch (appliance) or what clients refer to as "a bag" to collect fecal material.

Incontinent Ostomies

The location of the ostomy determines the consistency of stool. An ileostomy bypasses the entire large intestine. As a result, stools are frequent and liquid. The same is true for a colostomy of the ascending colon. A colostomy of the transverse colon generally results in a more solid, formed

stool. The sigmoid colostomy emits near-normal stool. The location of a colostomy is determined by the client's medical problem and general condition. There are three types of colostomy construction:

1. Loop colostomy
2. End colostomy
3. Double-barrel colostomy

A *loop colostomy* is usually performed in a medical emergency when closure of the colostomy is anticipated. These are usually temporary large stomas constructed in the transverse colon (Fig. 47-5, *A-D*). The surgeon pulls a loop of bowel onto the abdomen (Fig. 47-5, *E*). An external supporting device such as a plastic rod, bridge (Fig. 47-5, *C* and *D*), or rubber catheter (Fig. 47-5, *A*) is temporarily placed under the bowel loop to keep it from slipping back (Fig. 47-5, *A*). The surgeon then opens the bowel and sutures it to the skin of the abdomen (Fig. 47-5, *F*). A communicating wall remains between the proximal and distal bowel. The loop ostomy has two openings through the stoma (Fig. 47-5, *D* and *G*). The proximal end drains stool while the distal portion drains mucus. Within 7 to 10 days the external supporting device is removed.

The *end colostomy* consists of one stoma formed from the proximal end of the bowel with the distal portion of the GI tract either removed or sewn closed (called *Hartmann's pouch*) and left in the abdominal cavity. For many clients, end colostomies are a result of surgical treatment of colorectal cancer. In such cases the rectum might also be re-

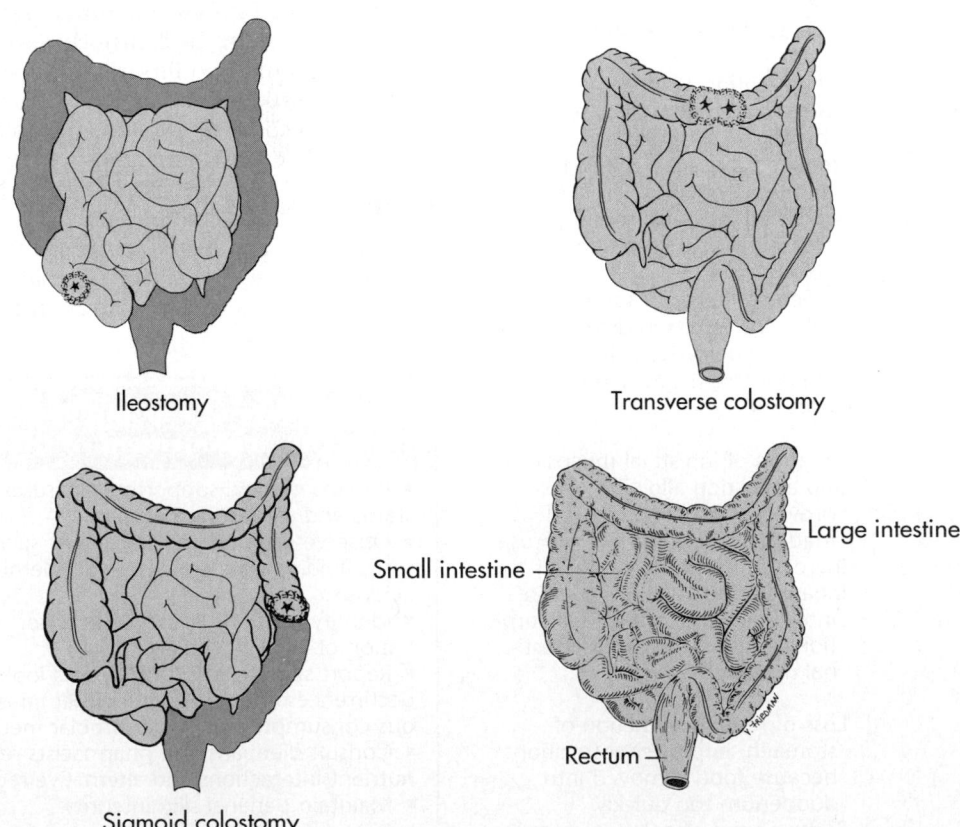

Ileostomy

Transverse colostomy

Sigmoid colostomy

Large intestine

Small intestine

Rectum

Fig. 47-4 Normal intestines *(bottom right)* and three types of ostomies. Shaded areas indicate excised tissue.

Fig. 47-5 A, A transverse loop colostomy supported with a flexible red rubber catheter. *(A Courtesy Hollister, Inc, Libertyville, Ill.)* **B,** Abdominal view of loop colostomy in transverse colon. **C,** Loop colostomy construction is much the same as construction of loop ileostomy. Stoma is created with longitudinal incision through sacculations in colon. **D,** Loop colostomy matured. **E,** Loop ostomy construction, loop of bowel exteriorized. **F,** Support device placed to maintain position of bowel on abdominal surface. Distal bowel of ileum is incised, mesentery. Stitch placed to designate proximal bowel. **G,** Loop ileostomy matured with protruding functional limb. *(B to G From Hampton BG, Bryant RA:* Ostomies and continent diversions: nursing management, *St Louis, 1992, Mosby.)*

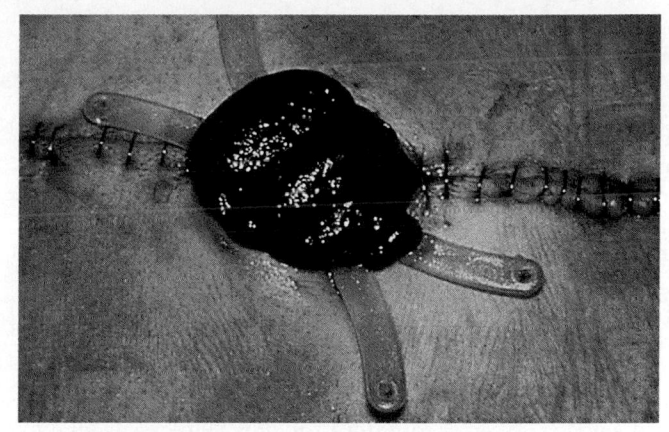

A

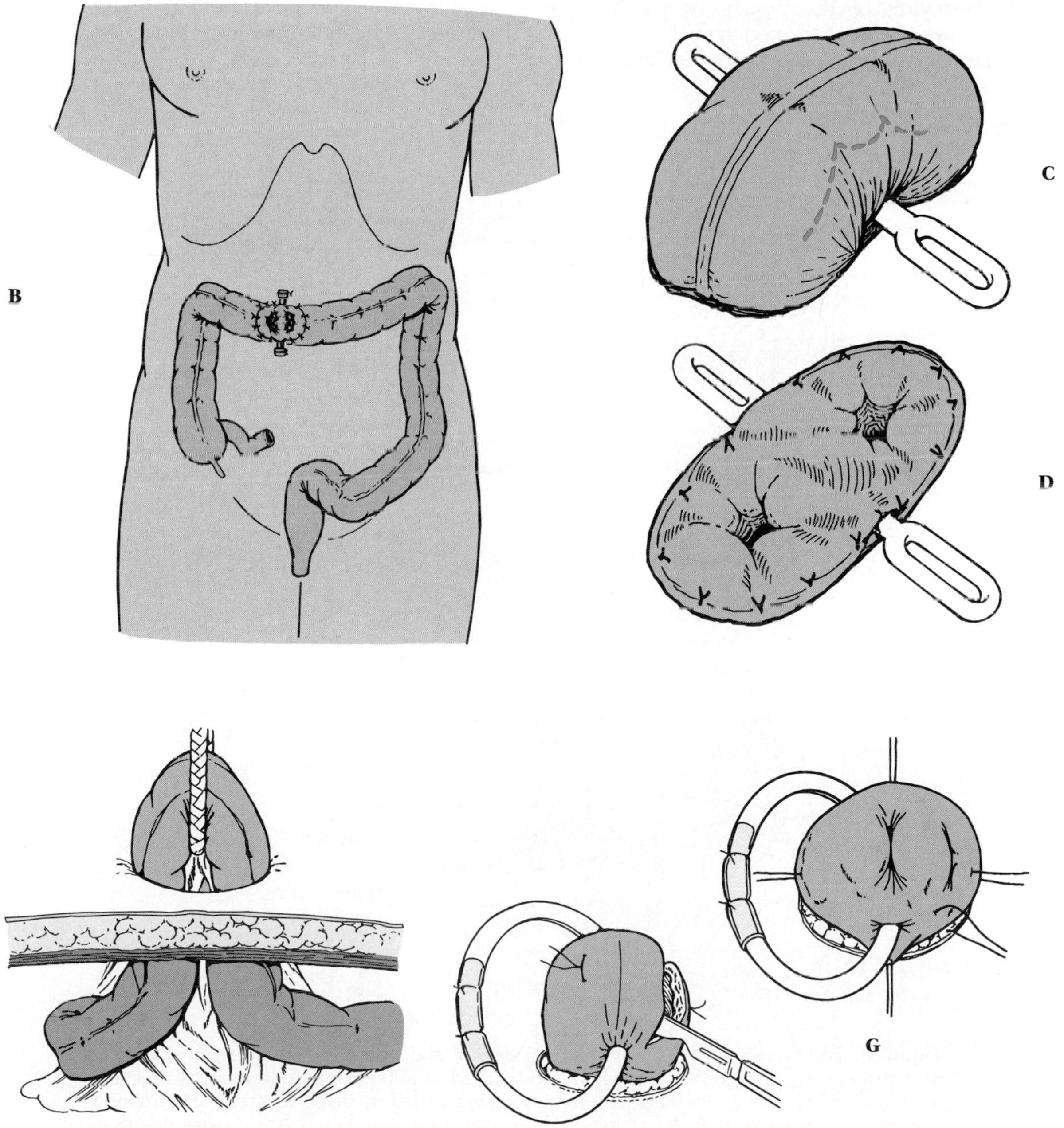

B

C

D

E

F

G

moved. Clients with diverticulitis who are treated surgically often have a temporary end colostomy with a Hartmann's pouch (Fig. 47-6).

Unlike the loop colostomy, the bowel is surgically severed in a *double-barrel colostomy* (Fig. 47-7, *A*) and the two ends are brought out onto the abdomen (Fig. 47-7, *B*). The double-barrel colostomy consists of two distinct stomas: the proximal functioning stoma and the distal nonfunctioning stoma.

Ostomies that emit frequent liquid stools (e.g., ileostomy) create a management challenge. A pouch must always be worn. Control of defecation cannot be achieved because of a continuous oozing of liquid stool. The pouch must be emptied, washed, and if a two-piece ostomy system is being used, even replaced throughout the day. Skin care is vital to prevent exposure to fecal irritants.

A colostomy in the transverse or sigmoid colon needs less frequent emptying of the pouch. Although some clients might choose to not wear a pouch at all times, most clients with sigmoid colostomies wear a pouch at all times even though bowel movements may occur only once or twice daily. Selected foods can be eaten at prescribed intervals so that bowel movements occur at a convenient time.

A physician might order ostomy irrigations similar to an enema for clients with a transverse, descending, or sigmoid colostomy. This allows the person to empty the bowel regularly and regain control as to the time of elimination of feces from the stoma.

Since the late 1980s, some progress has been made toward the development and successful use of a colostomy plug, which can provide continence for up to 28 hours (Bellan, 1990). This two-piece system consists of an adhesive base plate that is put around the stoma and a soft, pliable, carbon-filtered plug that is inserted into the stoma. Usually the client does an irrigation before inserting the plug. This increases the length of time that the client has fecal continence (Clague and Heald , 1990). The plug is not usually used by clients that have frequent, liquid ostomy stools, excessive gas, or abdominal cramping.

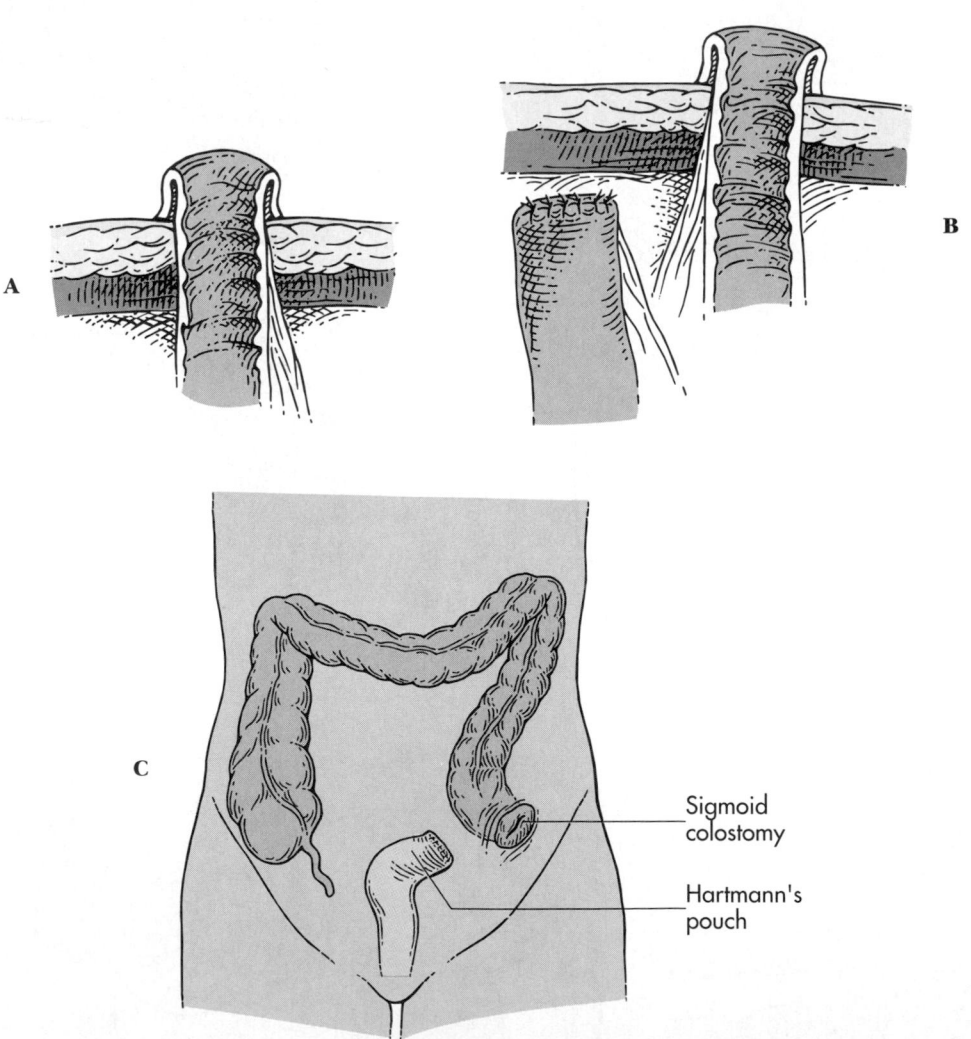

Fig. 47-6 End colostomy. **A,** Cross-sectional view of end stoma. **B,** Cross-sectional view of end stoma with distal bowel oversewn and secured to anterior peritoneum at stoma site. **C,** Sigmoid colostomy. Distal bowel is oversewn and left in place to create Hartmann's pouch. *(From Hampton BG, Bryant RA: Ostomies and continent diversions: nursing management, St Louis, 1992, Mosby.)*

Continent Ostomies

Certain types of surgery may provide continence for select colectomy clients. These continent ostomies are also called *continent diversions* or *continent reservoirs*. In a procedure called an *ileoanal pull-through,* the colon is removed and the ileum is anastomosed or connected to an intact anal sphincter (Corman, 1989; Dalton-Lochner and Connor, 1989). Not every colectomy client is a candidate for this procedure. Selection criteria require close coordination between the client and surgeon.

Some newer surgical procedures based on the ileoanal pull-through are the ileoanal reservoir (IAR) (Rolstad and Hoyman, 1992; Beitz, 1994). The ileoanal reservoir is also called a *restorative proctocolectomy, ileal pouch-anal anastomosis,* or *pelvic pouch*. In this procedure, the client has no permanent external stoma and therefore does not need to wear an ostomy pouch. Clients have an internal pouch created from their ileum. These ileum pouches can be constructed in various configurations such as in a lateral, *S, J,* or *W* shape. The end of the pouch is then sewn or anastomosed to the anus (Fig. 47-8). The surgery is done in several stages and the client may have a temporary ostomy until the surgically created ileum pouch has healed. When healing has occurred and the client has successfully learned Kegel exercises to strengthen the pelvic floor, the temporary ostomy is removed. The client then has bowel movements from only the anal area. Nursing care for clients with an ileoanal reservoir should focus on emotional support, perianal skin care, use of medications, sphincter reeducation, and prompt recognition of complications (Rolstad and Hoyman, 1992; Beitz, 1994).

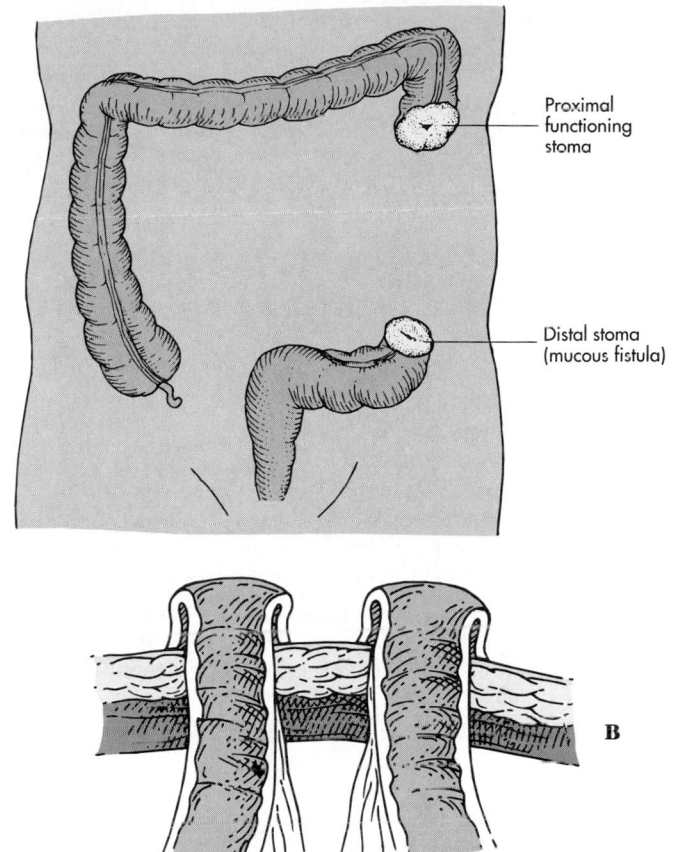

Fig. 47-7 Double-barrel colostomy. **A,** Double-barrel colostomy in the descending colon. **B,** Cross-sectional view of double barrel stoma. *(From Hampton BG, Bryant RA. Ostomies and continent diversions: nursing management, St Louis, 1992, Mosby.)*

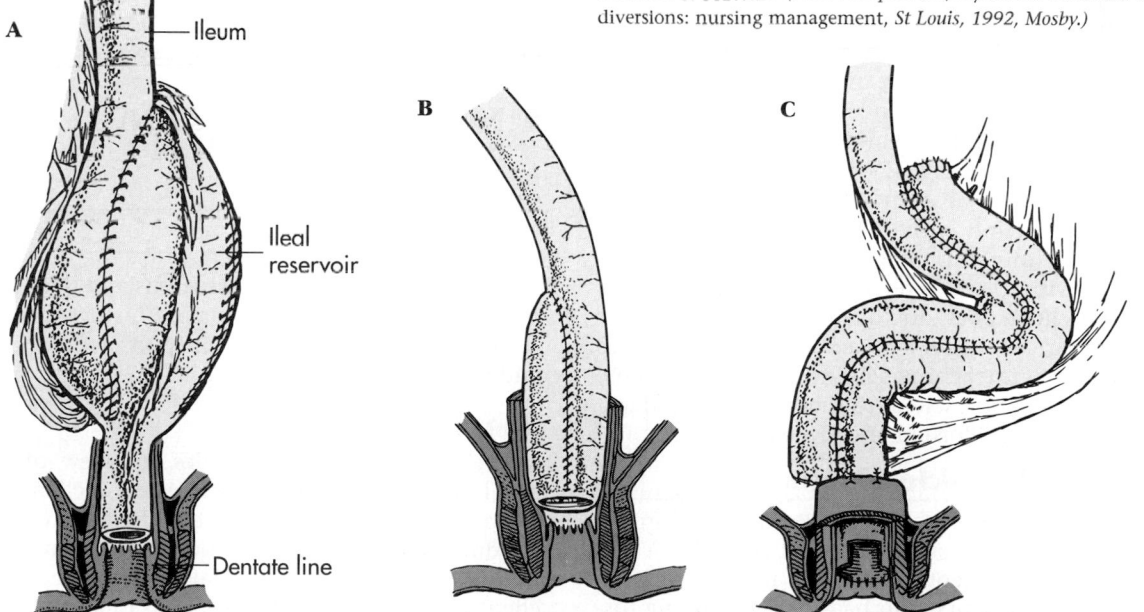

Fig. 47-8 Ileaoanal reservoirs (IAR). **A,** *S*-shaped configuration for IAR. Three 10-cm limbs of ileum are used, antimesenteric surface of each limb opened, and adjacent bowel walls anastomosed. **B,** *J*-shaped configuration for IAR. Distal ileum is aligned in *J*-shape; antimesenteric surface of *J*-shape is opened, and adjacent bowel walls anastomosed. Side-to-end anastomosis of bowel to dentate line is evident. **C,** Lateral or side-by-side ileoanal pouch configuration. *(From Hampton BG, Bryant RA: Ostomies and continent diversions: nursing management, St Louis, 1992, Mosby.)*

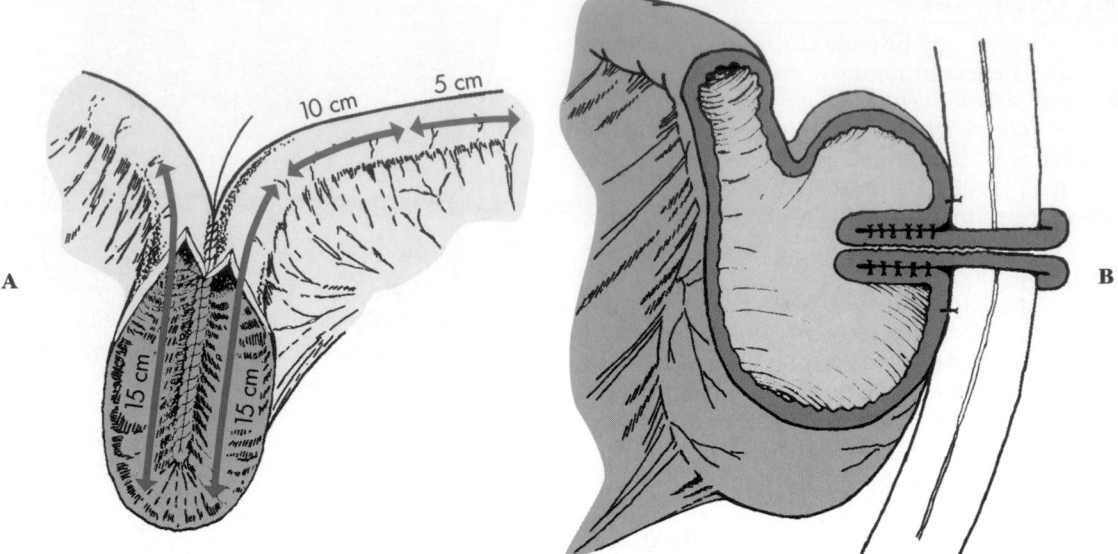

Fig. 47-9 Construction of Kock continent Ileostomy—Kock pouch. **A,** Two 15-cm limbs are used to create pouch, and one 15-cm limb is used to fashion a nipple valve and stoma. **B,** Distal limb is intussuscepted into reservoir to create one-way valve and accomplish continence. Sutures or staples, or both, are placed to stabilize and maintain intussuscepted nipple. Anterior surface of reservoir is anchored to anterior peritoneal wall. *(From Hampton BG, Bryant RA: Ostomies and continent diversions: nursing management, St Louis, 1992, Mosby.)*

The Kock continent ileostomy is yet another new type of continent ostomy (Rolstad and Hoyman, 1992). In this procedure an internal reservoir or pouch is created from a piece of the client's small intestine (Fig. 47-9, *A*). Part of the pouch is brought out onto the client's abdomen as an enteral stoma (Fig. 47-9, *B*). Unlike other ostomy stomas, the external stoma from a Kock continent ileostomy is usually very low on the client's abdomen; usually below the line of the client's underpants. At the end of the internal part of the pouch is a one-way nipple valve, which is how continence is accomplished (see Fig. 47- 9, *B*). This valve only allows fecal contents to drain from the pouch when an external catheter is intermittently placed into the stoma. As fecal contents are only eliminated from the Kock pouch when intubated with the catheter, unlike other people with an ostomy, the client does not have to wear an ostomy pouch. Nursing care of clients with a Kock reservoir focuses on emotional support, teaching self-intubation technique, determining an intubation schedule, diet teaching, and recognizing complications (Rolstad and Hoyman, 1992).

Psychological Considerations

An ostomy can cause serious body image changes, particularly if it is permanent. A study reported by Walsh et al. (1995) measured the perception of body image in clients who had an ostomy. Clients who had a long-standing history of chronic bowel disease such as Crohn's disease or ulcerative colitis had improved quality of life, but a lower body image. Conversely, clients who needed an ostomy because of cancer had a higher body image but a reduced quality of life.

Clients often perceive a stoma as a form of mutilation. Even though clothing conceals the ostomy, the client feels different. Many clients have difficulty maintaining or initiating normal sexual relations (see Chapter 24). An important factor in the client's reactions is the character of fecal secretions and the ability to control them. Foul odors, spillage, or leakage of liquid stools and inability to regulate bowel movements give the client a loss of self-esteem (Mihalopoulos et al, 1994) (see the box on p. 1353).

▌NURSING PROCESS AND BOWEL ELIMINATION

 ### Assessment

To assess bowel elimination patterns and determine abnormalities, the nurse takes a nursing history, does a physical assessment of the abdomen, inspects fecal characteristics, and reviews pertinent test results.

NURSING HISTORY

The nursing history provides a review of the client's usual bowel pattern and habits. What a client describes as "normal" or "abnormal" may be different from factors and conditions that tend to promote normal elimination. Identifying normal and abnormal patterns, habits, and the client's perception of normal and abnormal in regard to bowel elimination allows the nurse to determine the client's problems. Much of the nursing history can be organized around the factors that affect elimination:

1. Determination of the usual elimination pattern. Frequency and time of day are included. Accurate assessment of a client's current bowel elimination pattern can be enhanced by having the client or care

RESEARCH HIGHLIGHT

RESEARCH ABSTRACT
Ninety-seven ostomy clients, at least 50 years old, agreed to participate in this study. The sample consisted of 47 men, 50 women, the mean age of the participants was 68 years, and 68 were married.

The six instruments used in this research were: Surgical Preparedness Inventory, Surgical Adjustment Scale, Social Interaction Inventory, Self-Esteem Inventory, Geriatric Depression Scale, and Life Satisfaction Inventory. Men reported a lower satisfaction with life and twice as many men than women reported symptoms of depression. Older women reported a poorer health status. For both sexes, current health status was associated with positive psychological well-being. Men and women who reported good to excellent current health also reported a positive adjustment to operation, better social interactions, higher self-esteem, fewer symptoms of depression, and more life satisfaction. Clients who did not feel hindered by their ostomies reported high scores of well-being on all outcome measures. The longer the time since the operation, the better the client felt and the less depression.

IMPLICATIONS FOR PRACTICE
▶ Health status affects clients' psychological well-being
▶ Level of health has a direct relationship to postoperative adjustment.
▶ Depression lessens as client moves through the postoperative and restorative care phases.

REFERENCE
Mihalopoulos NG et al: The psychologic impact of ostomy surgery on persons 50 years of age and older, *Journal of Wound, Ostomy, and Continence Nursing* 21(4):149, 1994.

giver complete a bowel elimination or defecation diary (Doughty, 1992). As with any client teaching, the nurse must make sure that the person completing the diary understands what information must be recorded.

2. Identification of routines followed to promote normal elimination. Examples are drinking hot liquids, using laxatives, eating specific foods, or taking time to defecate during a certain part of the day.

3. Description of any recent change in elimination pattern. This information is perhaps the most significant because elimination patterns are variable and the client can best detect change.

4. Client's description of usual characteristics of stool. The nurse determines whether the stool is usually watery or formed or soft or hard, as well as the typical color.

5. Diet history. The nurse determines the client's dietary preferences for a day. The nurse measures servings of fruits, vegetables, cereals, and breads.

6. Description of daily fluid intake. This includes the type and amount of fluid. The client might have to estimate the amount using common household measurements.

7. History of exercise. The nurse asks the client to specifically describe the type and amount of daily exercise.

8. Assessment of the use of artificial aids at home. The nurse assesses whether the client uses enemas, laxatives, or special foods before having a bowel movement.

9. History of surgery or illnesses affecting the GI tract. This information can often help explain symptoms.

10. Presence and status of bowel diversions. If the client has an ostomy, the nurse assesses frequency of fecal drainage, character of feces, appearance and condition of the stoma (color, swelling, and irritation), type of appliance used, and methods used to maintain the ostomy's function.

11. Medication history. The nurse asks whether the client takes medications (such as laxatives, antacids, iron supplements, and analgesics) that might alter defecation or fecal characteristics.

12. Emotional state. The client's emotions can significantly alter frequency of defecation. During assessment, observation of the client's emotions, tone of voice, and mannerisms can reveal significant behaviors that indicate stress.

13. Social history. Clients have many different living arrangements. Where clients live may affect their toileting habits. If the client is sharing living quarters, how many bathrooms are there? Do clients have their own bathroom or do they need to share and thus adjust the time they use the bathroom to accommodate others? If clients lives alone, are they capable of ambulating to the toilet safely? If the client is not independent in bowel management, the nurse determines who assists the client and how.

14. Mobility and dexterity. The client's mobility and dexterity need to be evaluated to determine if the client needs assistive devices or personnel.

PHYSICAL ASSESSMENT

The nurse conducts a physical assessment (see Chapter 33) of body systems and functions likely to be influenced in the presence of elimination problems. Table 47-5 gives a summary of some of the assessments to include when doing a physical examination on a client to evaluate bowel function (Doughty, 1992).

Mouth. An assessment includes inspection of the client's teeth, tongue, and gums. Poor dentition or poorly fitting dentures influence the ability to chew (see Chapter 33).

Abdomen. The nurse inspects all four abdominal quadrants for contour, shape, symmetry, and skin color. Inspection also includes noting masses, peristaltic waves, scars, venous patterns, stomas, and lesions. Normally, peristaltic waves are not visible. However, observable peristalsis can be a sign of intestinal obstruction.

Abdominal distention appears as an overall outward protuberance of the abdomen. Intestinal gas, large tumors, or fluid in the peritoneal cavity may cause distention. A distended abdomen feels tight, and the skin appears taut, as if stretched.

The nurse auscultates the abdomen with the stethoscope to assess bowel sounds in each quadrant (see Chapter 33). Normal bowel sounds occur every 5 to 15 seconds and last ½ second to several seconds. While auscultating, the nurse

Table 47-5	Focused Physical Examination for Bowel Function Evaluation
PARAMETER	**ASSESSMENT STRATEGY**
Mobility	*In ambulatory clients*—Observe gait; determine need for assistive devices or personnel. *In wheelchair-bound clients*—Note degree of needed assistance to transfer from chair to commode or toilet.
Dexterity	Ask client to demonstrate hand motions that would be required to insert suppository or perform digital stimulation (e.g., grasping a pencil, rotation of forefinger).
Anorectal sensation	*In clients with fecal leakage without the urge to defecate*—Insert urinary catheter with 30 cc balloon into rectum; slowly inflate balloon and instruct client to notify you when rectal distension is perceived. Failure to respond to 30 cc is indicative of impaired function.
Anal sphincter function	Inspect anus at rest. Then perform digital exam while asking client to contract and relax sphincter followed by Valsalva's maneuver. The inability to sense rectal distension, to voluntarily contract anus, or to "bear down" is indicative of impaired function.
Abdominal muscle contractility	Instruct client to "bear down" (or to push against the examiner's hand) while lightly palpating the abdominal wall. Check for presence, volume, and consistency of stool in rectum. The presence of large amounts of stool is indicative of decreased sensation and/or impaired emptying.

Modified from Doughty D: A step-by-step approach to bowel training, *Progressions* 4(2):18, 1992.

notes the character and frequency of bowel sounds. An increase in pitch or a "tinkling" sound may be heard with abdominal distention. Absent or hypoactive sounds (less than five sounds per minute) occur with paralytic ileus, such as after abdominal surgery. High-pitched and hyperactive bowel sounds (35 or more sounds per minute) occur with small intestine obstruction and inflammatory disorders.

The nurse palpates the abdomen for masses or areas of tenderness (see Chapter 33). It is important for the client to relax. Tensing abdominal muscles interferes with palpating underlying organs or masses.

Percussion detects lesions, fluid, or gas within the abdomen. Familiarity with the five percussion notes (see Chapter 33) also permits identification of underlying abdominal structures. Gas or flatulence creates a tympanic note. Masses, tumors, and fluid are dull to percussion.

Rectum. The nurse inspects the area around the anus for lesions, discolorations, inflammation, and hemorrhoids. Abnormalities should be carefully recorded (see Chapter 33). To examine the rectum the nurse uses gentle palpation. After applying a clean disposable glove, the nurse applies a lubricant to the index finger. The nurse then asks the client to bear down and as the client does so, the nurse passes the index finger through the relaxed anal sphincter toward the client's umbilicus. The sphincter usually constricts around the nurse's finger. The nurse should methodically palpate all sides of the client's rectal wall for nodules or irregularities in texture. The rectal mucosa is normally smooth and soft. Pushing the index finger forcefully against the rectal wall or extending the finger too far may cause discomfort.

FECAL CHARACTERISTICS

Inspection of fecal characteristics (Table 47-6) reveals information about the nature of elimination alterations. Several factors can influence each characteristic. A key to assessment is knowing whether there have been any recent changes. The client can best provide this information.

LABORATORY AND DIAGNOSTIC TESTS

Laboratory and diagnostic examinations yield useful information concerning elimination problems. Laboratory analysis of fecal contents can detect pathological conditions such as tumors, hemorrhage, and infection.

Fecal Specimens. The nurse is directly responsible for ensuring that specimens are accurately obtained, properly labeled in appropriate containers, and transported to the laboratory on time. Institutions provide special containers for fecal specimens. Some tests require specimens to be placed in chemical preservatives.

Medical aseptic technique should be used during collection of stool specimens (see Chapter 34). Because about 25% of the solid portion of a stool is bacteria from the colon, the nurse should wear disposable gloves when handling specimens.

Handwashing is necessary for anyone who might come in contact with the specimen. Often the client can obtain the specimen if properly instructed. The nurse explains that feces cannot be mixed with urine or water. For this reason the client must defecate into a clean, dry bedpan or special container placed under the toilet seat.

Tests performed by the laboratory for occult (microscopic) blood in the stool (Procedure 47-1) and stool cultures require only a small sample. The nurse collects about an inch of formed stool or 15 to 30 ml of liquid diarrheal stool. Tests for measuring the output of fecal fat require a 3- to 5-day collection of stool. All fecal material must be saved throughout the test period.

After obtaining a specimen, the nurse labels and tightly seals the container and completes laboratory requisition forms. The nurse then records specimen collections in the client's medical record. It is important to avoid delays in sending specimens to the laboratory. Some tests such as measurement for ova and parasites require the stool to be warm. When stool specimens are allowed to stand at room temperature, bacteriological changes that alter test results can occur.

Table 47-6	**Fecal Characteristics**		
CHARACTERISTIC	**NORMAL**	**ABNORMAL**	**ABNORMAL CAUSE**
Color	Infant: yellow; adult: brown	White or clay	Absence of bile
		Black or tarry (melena)	Iron ingestion or upper GI bleeding
		Red	Lower GI bleeding, hemorrhoids
		Pale with fat	Malabsorption of fat
Odor	Pungent; affected by food type	Noxious change	Blood in feces or infection
Consistency	Soft, formed	Liquid	Diarrhea, reduced absorption
		Hard	Constipation
Frequency	Varies: infant 4 to 6 times daily (breast fed) or 1 to 3 times daily (bottle fed); adult daily or 2 to 3 times a week	Infant more than 6 times daily or less than once every 1-2 days; adult more than 3 times a day or less than once a week	Hypomotility or hypermotility
Amount	150 g per day (adult)		
Shape	Resembles diameter of rectum	Narrow, pencil shaped	Obstruction, rapid peristalsis
Constituents	Undigested food, dead bacteria, fat, bile pigment, cells lining intestinal mucosa, water	Blood, pus, foreign bodies, mucus, worms	Internal bleeding, infection, swallowed objects, irritation, inflammation

Guaiac test. A common laboratory test that can be done at home or at the client's bedside is the **guaiac test**, or fecal occult blood testing (FOBT), which measures microscopic amounts of blood in the feces. Small amounts of blood are normally lost daily in the feces from minor abrasions of nasopharyngeal and oral surfaces. Quantities of lost blood greater than 50 ml arising from the upper GI tract can be seen as **melena** (blood in the stool). Guaiac tests help reveal visually undetectable blood. It is a useful diagnostic screening test for colon cancer (see the box at right). There are client characteristics, especially cultural, which must be considered when nurses plan colon cancer screening programs (see the box at right).

Clients who are receiving anticoagulants or who have a bleeding disorder or a GI disorder known to cause bleeding (e.g., intestinal tumors, bowel inflammation, or ulcerations) should be guaiac tested. The most common guaiac test is the hemoccult slide test (Procedure 47-1).

Diagnostic Examinations. A client may have a diagnostic test as an outpatient or inpatient. Visualization of GI structures may be by direct or indirect approach.

Direct visualization. Instruments introduced through the mouth (upper GI viewing or UGI) or the rectum (lower GI viewing) allow the physician to inspect the integrity of mucosa, blood vessels, and organ parts. A **fiberoptic endoscope** is an optical instrument with a lens viewer, a long flexible tube, and a light source at the end. It allows viewing of structures at the tip of the tube and insertion of special instruments for biopsy.

Proctoscopes and sigmoidoscopes are rigid, tube-shaped instruments with attached light sources. The proctoscope looks like a speculum with a light. These instruments are less flexible than fiberoptic scopes and more capable of causing discomfort.

UGI **endoscopy** or **gastroscopy** allows visualization of the esophagus, stomach, and duodenum. The physician inspects for tumors, vascular changes, mucosal inflammation,

---

Screening for Colon Cancer

RISK FACTORS
- Age: over 50
- Family history: colon polyps or colorectal cancer
- History of inflammatory bowel disease (colitis, Crohn's disease)
- Living in urban area
- Diet: high intake of fats, low fiber intake

WARNING SIGNS
- Change in bowel habits
- Rectal bleeding

SCREENING TESTS
- Digital rectal examination every year after age 40
- Guaiac test for occult blood every year after 50
- Proctoscopy every 3-5 years after age 50, after two annual negative examinations

---

CULTURAL ASPECTS OF CARE

Colorectal cancer is one of the most frequently occurring cancers among elderly African Americans. While the use of fecal occult blood testing (FOBT) to detect colorectal cancer early has decreased mortality rates in the general population, the mortality rate in African Americans has increased. This may be because elderly African Americans are least likely to participate in early detection and therefore when they are diagnosed their cancers are at an advanced stage. Increasing the participation in FOBT by elderly African Americans is a national nursing priority and must be part of African American clients' primary prevention screening activities.

Powe BD: Fatalism among elderly African Americans: effects on colorectal cancer screening, *Cancer Nursing* 18(5):385, 1995.

PROCEDURE 47-1

Measuring Occult Blood in Stool

STEPS	RATIONALE

1. Assess client's medical history for bleeding or GI disorder.

Routine screening can be instituted by nurse.

2. Assess type of medications client receives. Note drugs that can cause GI mucosal bleeding.

Anticoagulants increase risk of bleeding in GI tract, even from minor trauma to mucosa. Long-term use of steroids, nonsteroidal antiinflammatory drugs (NSAIDS), and acetylsalicylic acid can irritate mucosa.

3. Refer to physician's order for medication or dietary modifications/restrictions before test. Such restrictions include pretest avoidance of partially cooked red meat, broccoli, turnips, horseradish, and uncooked cantaloupe.

These foods can give false positive results. Iron supplements and supplemental vitamins should be avoided because they can provide false positive results (Eastwood, Avundu, 1988). Rare meats can cause false positive results.

4. Prepare necessary equipment and supplies:
  a. Paper towel
  b. Hemoccult test supplies (see the illustration):
    (1) Cardboard hemoccult slide (read and follow specific directons)
    (2) Wooden applicator
    (3) Hemoccult developing solution
  c. Disposable gloves
  d. Read and follow the directions for the specific brand of cardboard hemoccult slide

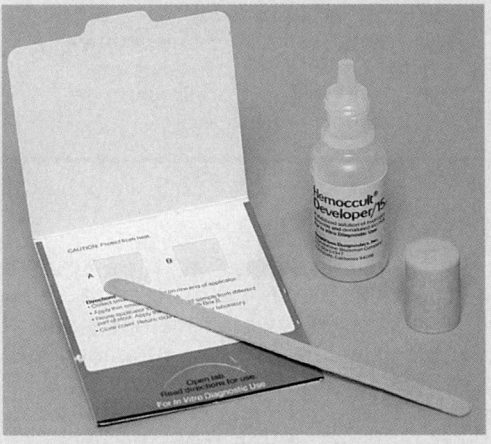

Step 4b

5. Explain purpose of test and ways that client can assist.

Client's understanding of test's purpose provides cooperation and minimizes anxiety.

6. Be sure that dietary or medication restrictions were followed.

Ensures accurate test results.

7. Wash hands.

Reduces transmission of infection.

8. Apply clean disposable gloves.

Reduces transmission of microorganisms from fecal specimen to your hands.

9. Obtain uncontaminated stool specimen.

Specimen is obtained in clean, dry container and not contaminated with urine, water, or toilet tissue.

10. Use tip of wooden applicator to transfer a small portion of feces from the specimen container to the cardboard hemoccult slide.

Small specimen is sufficient for measuring blood content in feces.

11. Perform hemoccult slide test:
  a. Open flap of slide and apply thin smear of stool on paper in first box.

Guaiac paper inside box is sensitive to fecal blood content.

  b. Obtain second fecal specimen from different portion of stool and apply thinly to slide's second box* (see the illustration on p. 1357).

Findings of occult blood are more conclusive for GI bleeding when entire specimen contains blood.

  c. Close slide cover and turn slide over to reverse side. Open cardboard flap and apply 2 drops of hemoccult developing solution on each box of guaiac paper (see the illustration on p. 1357).

Developing solution penetrates underlying fecal specimen. Blood is indicated by change in color of guaiac paper.

Make sure you use hemoccult developing solution not developing solution for other cardboard tests such as gastric pH. The developing solution bottles may look similar, but the solutions aren't the same and can't be used interchangeably.

---

*Some institutions require the slide to be sent to lab for completion of test. Follow institution policy and procedure.

Measuring Occult Blood in Stool—cont'd

STEPS	RATIONALE
11. Perform hemoccult slide test—cont'd	
d. Read results of test after 30-60 sec. Note color changes.	Bluish discoloration indicates occult blood (guaiac positive). No change in color indicates negative results.
e. Dispose of test slide in proper receptacle.	Reduces transfer of microorganisms.
12. Wrap wooden applicator in paper towel, remove gloves, and dispose in proper receptacle.	Feces contain large numbers of microorganisms.
13. Wash hands.	Reduces spread of infection.
14. Record results of test in client's record and note unusual fecal characteristics.	All test results should be documented promptly. Findings may indicate need for further diagnosis and intervention.

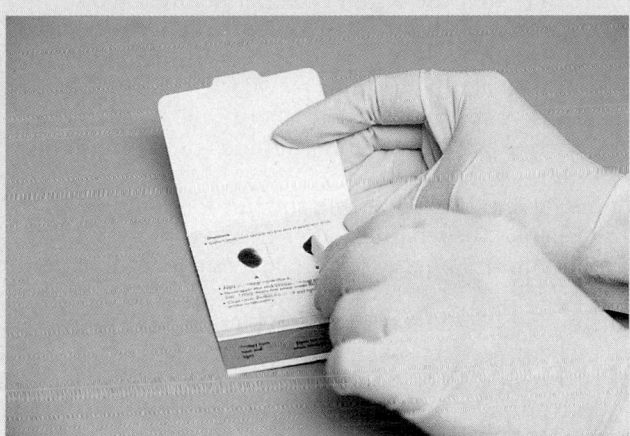

Step 11b

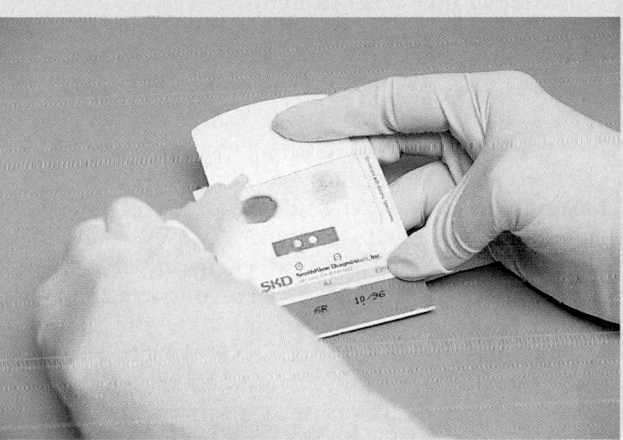

Step 11c

ulcers, hernias, and obstructions. A gastroscope enables the physician to remove tissue specimens (or **biopsy**), remove abnormal tissue growth (**polyps**), and coagulate sources of bleeding. Nursing implications before the test include the following:

1. Client signs informed consent.
2. Client takes nothing by mouth after midnight.
3. Client removes dentures.
4. Nurse explains that the client may feel fullness in the throat and a sense of gagging during the test.
5. Nurse explains that the client will be unable to speak as the endoscope enters the esophagus.
6. Nurse positions the client in the left Sims' or left lateral position.
7. Nurse gives a sedative and an anticholinergic as prescribed.

Nursing implications during the test include the following:

1. Nurse describes steps of the test to the client.
2. Nurse places tissue specimens in a properly labeled container that is sealed tightly.
3. Nurse has emergency equipment available in case of respiratory complications.

Nursing implications afterward include the following:

1. Because the client's throat is anesthetized, the nurse instructs the client to avoid eating or drinking until the gag reflex returns (2 to 4 hours). To check for the gag reflex the nurse places a tongue blade at the back of the client's tongue.
2. Nurse explains that hoarseness and a sore throat are normal for several days; cool fluids and normal saline gargling relieve soreness.
3. Nurse observes for bleeding, fever, abdominal pain, difficulty with swallowing, and difficulty breathing.

Sigmoidoscopy allows visualization of the anus, rectum, and sigmoid colon. Proctoscopy allows visualization of the anus and rectum. Both tests enable the physician to collect tissue specimens and coagulate sources of bleeding. Nursing implications before the test include the following:

1. Client signs an informed consent.
2. Client receives an enema the night before and the morning of the test; laxatives are optional.
3. Client may be allowed a light breakfast.
4. Nurse explains that the client will feel discomfort and the urge to defecate as the instruments are inserted.

5. During the test the physician uses air to distend the bowel for better visualization; the nurse explains that the client will feel "gas pains."
6. Nurse positions the client in a knee-chest position face down; Sims' position on the left side is acceptable. If a proctoscope table is being used, the nurse has the client kneel and lean over the table.
7. Nurse drapes the client to avoid unnecessary exposure and minimize embarrassment.

Nursing implications during the test include the following:

1. Nurse keeps the client draped and observes for respiratory distress (especially in clients with lung disease who cannot tolerate a head-down position).
2. Nurse provides the physician with long cotton swabs for removing mucus.
3. Nurse places tissue specimens in a properly labeled container that is sealed tightly.
4. The nurse comforts the client.

Nursing implications after the test include the following:

1. Nurse observes for rectal bleeding, rectal or abdominal pain, and fever.
2. Nurse cautions the client to observe for blood in stools and to report any bleeding.

Indirect visualization. When direct visualization is impossible (as with deeper GI structures), the physician relies on indirect x-ray examination. The client ingests a **contrast medium** or has the medium given as an enema. One of the most common media is barium, a white, chalky, radiopaque substance that the client drinks like a milkshake. It is used in UGI studies and barium enemas. Contrast media usually contain a flavoring agent for better taste.

Upper GI (UGI) study is an x-ray study of an ingested contrast medium that allows the physician to visualize the lower esophagus, stomach, and duodenum. The physician notes ulcerations, inflammation, tumors, and anatomical malposition of organs. The patency of organs and the pyloric valve are also observed. Nursing implications before the test include the following:

1. Client signs an informed consent.
2. Client takes nothing by mouth after midnight.
3. Nurse explains that the test might take several hours and requires frequent position changes; nurse explains that discomfort is minimal except for lying on a hard examination table.
4. Nurse explains that barium has a chalky taste (some preparations contain artificial flavoring).

A nursing implication during the test follows:

1. The test is done in the radiology department; a technician explains the steps of the test.

Nursing implications after the test include the following:

1. Client can resume eating after the test.
2. Client must expel the barium to avoid bowel impaction; nurse instructs the client to increase fluid intake (at least 2 L after the test). The physician may order a mild laxative or enema. Stools are lightly colored until the barium is expelled.

Small bowel follow-through (continuation of UGI) allows the physician to examine the small intestine. The flow of barium through the intestine may suggest motility problems. A barium enema allows indirect visualization of the lower colon to reveal location of tumors, polyps, and **diverticula.** The physician can also detect positional abnormalities. Nursing implications before the test include the following:

1. Client sometimes is required to sign informed consent.
2. Bowel preparation varies; client may receive any of the following the evening before the test:
   a. Clear liquids for lunch and supper
   b. One glass of water 8 to 10 hours before the test
   c. Stimulant cathartics
   d. Enemas till clear are given
3. On the day of the test the client receives additional cathartic by suppository.
4. Nurse explains the purpose of extensive bowel preparation.
5. Nurse explains that a lengthy procedure might cause fatigue.
6. Nurse observes the results of enemas and cathartics to ensure that the bowel is empty before the test.
7. Nurse explains that the client might feel cramping and fullness after the barium is instilled. Sometimes air may also be instilled.
8. Nurse explains that the client will be instructed to change positions often (supine, prone, and side-lying).

A nursing implication during the test follows:

1. Client expels barium after first set of x-ray films (30 minutes); a repeat film is taken to check for barium retention.

Nursing implications after the test include the following:

1. Client may resume eating after the test.
2. Nurse instructs the client to increase intake of oral fluids to promote barium evacuation and to counteract dehydrating effects of the cathartics.
3. Nurse instructs the client to observe stools for barium; the physician might order a mild cathartic or enema.

 Nursing Diagnosis

The nurse's assessment of the client's bowel function reveals data that may indicate an actual or potential elimination problem or a problem resulting from elimination alterations (see nursing diagnoses box on p. 1359). Associated problems, such as body-image changes or skin breakdown, require interventions unrelated to bowel function impairment. However, in some instances the nurse must direct as much attention to the elimination problem as to the associated problem.

The nurse's ability to identify the correct diagnosis depends not only on the thoroughness of assessment but also on recognition of defining characteristics and factors that can impair elimination (see the diagnostic process box on p. 1359). The nurse determines the client's risk and institutes measures to ensure maintenance of normal bowel function.

 Planning

The care plan should establish goals and outcomes by incorporating the client's elimination habits or routines as much as possible. If the habits caused the elimination problem, the nurse helps the client learn new ones. Defecation patterns vary among individuals. For this reason, the nurse and client must work together closely to plan effective interventions (see the care plan on p. 1361).

When clients are disabled or debilitated by illness, it is necessary to include the family in the plan of care. Often family members have the same ineffective elimination habits as the client. Thus client and family teaching is an important part of the care plan. Other health team members such as dietitians and enterostomal therapists (ET nurses) can be valuable resources. When clients require surgical intervention, a critical pathway may be used to coordinate the activities of the multidisciplinary health care team (Fig. 47-10).

The goals of care for clients with elimination problems include the following:

1. Understanding "normal" elimination
2. Attaining regular defecation habits
3. Understanding and maintaining proper fluid and food intake
4. Achieving a regular exercise program
5. Achieving comfort
6. Maintaining skin integrity
7. Maintaining self-concept

Implementation

Success of the nurse's interventions depends on improving the client's and family members' understanding of bowel elimination. In the home, hospital, or long-term care facility, clients capable of learning can be taught effective bowel habits.

The nurse should teach the client and family about proper diet, adequate fluid intake, and factors that stimulate or slow peristalsis, such as emotional stress. This often can best be done during the client's mealtime. The client should also learn the importance of establishing regular bowel routines and regular exercise and taking appropriate measures when elimination problems develop.

PROMOTION OF REGULAR BOWEL HABITS

One of the most important habits a nurse can teach regarding bowel habits is to take time for defecation. To establish regular bowel habits, a client must know when the

Examples of NANDA Nursing Diagnoses for Bowel Elimination Problems

Constipation *related to:*
- Immobility
- Lack of privacy
- Less than adequate fluid intake

Colonic constipation *related to:*
- Less than adequate fiber intake
- Less than adequate fluid intake
- Chronic use of medication and enemas

Perceived constipation *related to:*
- Cultural/family health beliefs
- Impaired thought processes

Diarrhea *related to:*
- Stress and anxiety
- Dietary intake

Bowel incontinence *related to:*
- Neuromuscular involvement
- Depression, severe anxiety

Pain *related to:*
- Hemorrhoidal inflammation

Toileting self-care deficit *related to:*
- Decreased strength and endurance
- Intolerance to activity

Risk for or impaired skin integrity *related to:*
- Fecal incontinence

Body image disturbance *related to:*
- Presence of ostomy
- Fecal incontinence

Sample Nursing Diagnostic Process for Bowel Elimination Problems

ASSESSMENT ACTIVITIES	DEFINING CHARACTERISTICS	NURSING DIAGNOSIS
Ask client about usual bowel routine, including ease of bowel movement, frequency, time of day, and stool consistency.	Straining at stool Change from daily stool to once every 3 days	**Constipation** related to inadequate dietary intake of fiber and limited fluid intake
Ask client to complete defecation diary.	Describes small, marblelike, hard stools	
Ask client about dietary intake of fiber, fruit, and vegetables.	24-hr dietary review reveals diet of cheese, beef, fried potatoes, no fruits and vegetables	
Palpate lower abdomen.	Abdominal tenderness in left lower quadrant Palpable mass in left lower quadrant	
Obtain daily fluid intake status, including types and amount.	Client drinks 2 cups of coffee, 1 soda/day, rarely drinks water or juice	

					1

BARNES

CARE PATH® 550
MAJOR SMALL & LARGE
BOWEL PROCEDURE

SERVICE		PHYSICIAN		
PRIMARY NURSE		PRIMARY NURSE		
DC DATE	ADM DATE	DATE OF SURGERY	**A-8**	

Problem Number	PATIENT PROBLEMS / NURSING DIAGNOSES
#1	ALTERATION IN COMFORT RELATED TO ABDOMINAL SURGERY
#2	ALTERATION IN BOWEL ELIMINATION RELATED TO ABDOMINAL SURGERY
#3	ALTERATION IN SKIN INTEGRITY RELATED TO ABDOMINAL INCISION AND RECOVERY FROM SURGERY
#4	LACK OF KNOWLEDGE RELATED TO HOSPITALIZATION AND SURGICAL PROCEDURE
#5	ALTERATION IN BODY IMAGE RELATED TO ABDOMINAL SURGERY AND OSTOMY
	* IF APPROPRIATE

#	1, 2, 3	3, 4, 5	4	4	1, 4
	ASSESSMENT / MONITORING	**CONSULTS**	**PROCEDURES / TEST**	**TREATMENT**	**ACTIVITY**
DAY 1 PRE OP	Assessment: Nursing Admission lab results Monitoring: VS routine O₂ saturation x1 I & O	Nurse specialist (if ostomy is a consideration).	CBC, 6, 12, PT, PTT T & C x2 units (admission labs) EKG ≥ 40 years old CXR ≥ 50 years old UA with micro *Mark ostomy site	Antithrombolytic stockings Mechanical bowel preparation	UAL
DAY 2 DOS	Assessment: Wound/dressing q 4 hrs. Bowel function q 4 hrs. Stoma appearance q 4 hrs. Pulmonary status q 2 hrs. Comfort level q 2 hrs. Braden score x1 Patency of tubes and characteristics of drainage q 8 hrs. IV patency & site appearance q 8 hrs. Fall risk factors Monitoring: VS q 1 hr. x 2 q 2 hrs. x2 then q 4 hrs. I & O q 4 hrs. O₂ saturation x1 x2	Respiratory Therapy for O₂		Antithrombolytic stockings O₂ to maintain O₂ saturation ≥ 92% Oral care q 4 hrs. Assist with Incentive Spirometer and TCDB q 2 hrs. Gastric decompression and tube irrigation	Bedrest
DAY 3 POD 1	Assessment: Wound/dressing q 4 hrs. Bowel function q 4 hrs. Stoma appearance q 4 hrs. Pulmonary status q 2 hrs. Comfort level q 2 hrs. Braden score x1 Patency of tubes and characteristics of drainage q 8 hrs. IV patency & site appearance q 8 hrs. Fall risk factors Lab results **O₂ saturation ≥ 92%** Monitoring: VS q 4 hrs. I & O q 8 hrs. Room air O₂ saturation x1 x2	Social Work Respiratory (if O₂ or tx needed) Nurse specialist (if ostomy placed).	CBC, 6	Antithrombolytic stockings Oral care q 4 hrs. Assist with Incentive Spirometer q 2 hrs. Gastric decompression and tube irrigation d/c foley d/c O₂	Up in chair with assist x1 x2 x3 Ambulate in room with assist x1 x2 Bed bath
DAY 4 POD 2	Assessment: Wound/dressing q 4 hrs. Bowel function q 4 hrs. Stoma appearance q 4 hrs. Pulmonary status q 2 hrs. Comfort level q 2 hrs. Braden score x1 Patency of tubes and characteristics of drainage q 8 hrs. IV patency & site appearance q 8 hrs. Fall risk factors Lab results **Voiding without difficulty (UO ≥ 240 cc q 8 hrs.)** Monitoring: VS q 4 hrs. I & O q 8 hrs.	Dietary screening		Antithrombolytic stockings Oral care q 4 hrs. Assist with Incentive Spirometer q 2 hrs. Gastric decompression and tube irrigation *Abdominal wound wet to dry dressing Change TID	Up in chair with assist x1 x2 x3 Ambulate in room with assist x1 x2 Bed bath

SIGNATURE	INIT.	SIGNATURE	INIT.	SIGNATURE	INIT.

Fig. 47-10 Example of a portion of a care path for major small and large bowel procedure.
(Courtesy Barnes-Jewish Hospital, St Louis.)

Sample Nursing Care Plan for Constipation

Nursing Diagnosis: Constipation related to inadequate dietary intake of fiber and limited fluid intake.
Definition: Constipation is the state in which an individual experiences a change in normal bowel habits characterized by a decrease in frequency and/or passage of hard, dry stools (Kim, McFarland, McLane, 1995).

GOALS	EXPECTED OUTCOMES	INTERVENTIONS	RATIONALE
Client will understand and ingest food and fluid intake required to promote soft, formed stools by 2/20.	Client will describe dietary sources high in fiber by 2/18. Client will explain the normal fluid intake to promote defecation by 2/19. Client will prepare 24-hr menu, including high-fiber foods and fluids by 2/20. Client will drink 1400-2000 ml daily.	Instruct client on preferred foods that stimulate peristalsis (wheat, bread, apples, lettuce, celery, apricots).	High-fiber foods increase peristalsis and help propel intestinal content through GI tract by increasing stool mass and fluid content (Brown, Everett, 1990).
Client attains regular defecation schedule by 2/22.	Client will pass soft-formed stools without excess straining.	Administer 8 6-oz glasses of fluids (prefers orange and grape juice) daily. Encourage client to take time to defecate 30-60 min after breakfast. Obtain verbal commitment from client to attempt to defecate within 5 min after sensing urge to defecate.	Adequate fluid intake helps keep fecal material soft (Swartz, 1989). Gastrocolic reflex is most sensitive in morning and after meals (Goldfinger, 1991). Behavioral contracts between client and nurse have demonstrated success for behavioral modification (Gilpatrick, 1989).

urge to defecate normally occurs. The nurse advises the client to begin establishing a routine during a time when defecation is most likely to occur, usually an hour after a meal. If a client is restricted to bed or requires assistance in ambulating, the nurse should offer a bedpan or help the client reach the bathroom.

Many clients have established rituals for defecation. In a hospital or long-term care facility, the nurse should make certain that treatment routines do not interfere with these schedules. It is also important to provide privacy. When clients forced to use a bedpan share rooms with other persons, the nurse should pull the curtain around the area so that clients can relax, knowing that interruptions will not occur. The call light should always be placed within clients' reach. Bathroom doors should be closed, although the nurse may stand close in case clients need assistance.

PROMOTION OF NORMAL DEFECATION

To help clients evacuate bowel contents normally and without discomfort, a number of interventions can stimulate the defecation reflex, affect the character of feces, or increase peristalsis.

Squatting Position. The nurse might need to assist clients who have difficulty squatting because of muscular weakness and mobility problems. Regular toilets are too low for clients unable to lower themselves to a squatting position because of joint- or muscle-wasting diseases. Clients can purchase elevated toilet seats for the home. With such a seat, less effort is needed to sit or stand.

Positioning on Bedpan. Clients restricted to bed must use bedpans for defecation. Women use bedpans to pass both urine and feces, whereas men use bedpans only for defecation. Sitting on a bedpan can be extremely uncomfortable. The nurse should help position clients comfortably.

Two types of bedpans are available (Fig. 47-11). The regular bedpan, made of metal or hard plastic, has a curved smooth upper end and a sharp-edged lower end and is about 5 cm (2 inches) deep. A fracture pan, designed for clients with body or leg casts, has a shallow upper end about 1.3 cm (½ inch) deep. The upper end of the pan fits

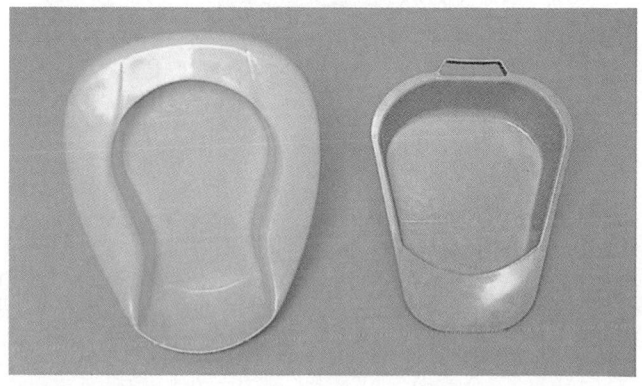

Fig. 47-11 Types of bedpans. *From left,* regular bedpan and fracture bedpan.

under the buttocks toward the sacrum, with the lower end just under the upper thighs. The pan should be high enough so that feces enter the pan. A metal bedpan should be warmed with water first, then dried.

When positioning a client, it is important to prevent muscle strain and discomfort. A client should never be placed on a bedpan and then left with the bed flat unless activity restrictions demand it. If the bed is flat, the hips remain hyperextended. It may be necessary to have the bed flat when placing the client on the bedpan. After the client is on it, the nurse raises the head of the bed 30 degrees. Raising the client to a 90-degree angle makes positioning difficult. In a sitting position, the client must rise straight up while using the strength of the arms as the nurse positions the pan. Most clients are too weak to accomplish this. Clients who have had abdominal surgery are hesitant to exert strain on suture lines. Furthermore, the nurse risks injury in trying to lift the client onto the bedpan.

Fig. 47-12 shows proper and improper positions on bedpans. The best method is to be sure the client is positioned high in bed. The nurse raises the client's head about 30 degrees, to prevent hyperextension of the back and provide support to the upper torso as the client raises the hips by bending the knees and lifting the hips upward. The nurse places a hand palm up under the client's sacrum, resting the elbow on the mattress and using it as a lever to help in lifting, while slipping the pan under the client. Gloves should always be worn by the nurse when handling a bedpan.

If the client is immobile or it is unsafe to allow the client to exert such effort, the client can roll onto the bedpan by using the following steps:

1. Lower the head of the bed flat and assist the client to roll onto one side, backside toward you.
2. Apply powder lightly to back and buttocks to prevent skin from sticking to the pan.
3. Place the bedpan firmly against the buttocks, down into the mattress with the open rim toward the client's feet (Fig. 47-13).
4. Keeping one hand against the bedpan, place the other around the client's far hip. Ask the client to roll back

onto the pan, flat in bed. Do not shove the pan under the client.

5. With the client positioned comfortably, raise the head of the bed 30 degrees.
6. Place a rolled towel or small pillow under the lumbar curve of the client's back for added comfort.
7. Raise the knee gatch or ask the client to bend the knees to assume a squatting position. Do not raise the knee gatch if contraindicated.

The nurse should maintain the privacy of a client using a bedpan. The call light and a supply of toilet paper should be within easy reach. When the client finishes, the nurse responds to the call signal immediately and removes the pan. The client might require assistance with wiping. To remove the pan the nurse asks the client to roll off to the side or raise the hips. The nurse holds the pan steady to avoid spilling. The nurse should avoid pulling or shoving the pan from under the client's hips because this can pull the client's skin and cause tissue injury such as a pressure ulcer (see Chapter 38). After the pan is removed, the nurse, while wearing gloves, cleans the anal and perineal areas.

After assessing the stool, the nurse should immediately empty the bedpan's contents into the toilet or in a special receptacle in the utility room. A spray faucet attached to most toilets allows the nurse to rinse the bedpan thoroughly. The client uses the same bedpan each time. The nurse should chart the characteristics of the feces.

The nurse should offer the bedpan often. Clients may accidentally soil bedclothes if forced to wait. Many clients try to avoid using a bedpan because it is embarrassing and uncomfortable. They may try to get to the bathroom even though their conditions prohibit ambulation. The nurse must warn clients about the risk of falls or accidents.

Cathartics and Laxatives. Often a client is unable to defecate normally because of pain, constipation, or impaction. Cathartics and laxatives have the short-term action of emptying the bowel. They are also used in bowel evacuation for clients undergoing GI tests and abdominal surgery. Although the terms *cathartic* and *laxative* are often used interchangeably, cathartics have a stronger effect on the intestines. Five types of laxatives and cathartics are available (Table 47-7).

Cathartics and laxatives are available in oral, tablet, and powder suppository dosage forms (see Chapter 35). Although the oral route is most commonly used, cathartics that come prepared as suppositories are more effective because of their stimulant effect on the rectal mucosa. Cathar-

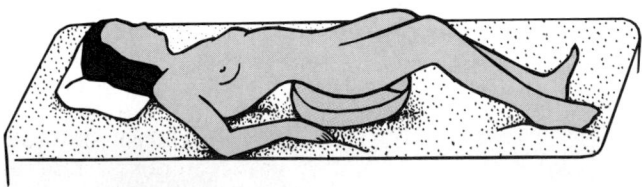

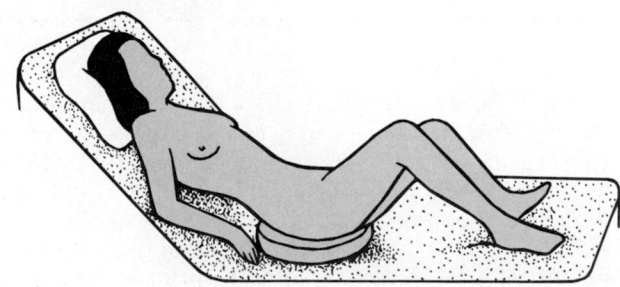

Fig. 47-12 Positions on a bedpan. *Top,* Improper positioning of client. *Bottom,* Proper position reduces client's back strain.

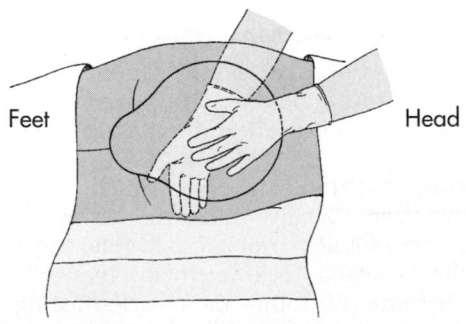

Feet   Head

Fig. 47-13 Positioning an immobilized client on a bedpan.

Table 47-7	Common Types of Laxatives and Cathartics		
AGENT/BRAND NAME	**ACTION**	**INDICATIONS**	**RISKS**
BULK FORMING Methylcellulose (Cologel, Hydrolose) Psyllium (Metamucil, Naturacil)	High-fiber content absorbs water and increases solid intestinal bulk. Agents stretch intestinal wall to stimulate peristalsis.	Agents are least irritating, most natural, and safest cathartics. Agents are drugs of choice for chronic constipation (e.g., pregnancy, low-residue diet). Agents may also be used to relieve mild, watery diarrhea.	Agents can cause obstruction if not mixed with at least 240 ml of water or juice and swallowed quickly. Caution is used with bulk-forming laxatives that also contain stimulants. Agents are not used in clients for whom large fluid intake is contraindicated.
EMOLLIENT OR WETTING Docusate sodium (Colace, Disonate) Docusate calcium (Surfak) Docusate potassium (Dialose)	Stool softeners are detergents that lower surface tension of feces, allowing water and fat to penetrate. They may increase secretion of water by intestine.	Agents are used for short-term therapy to relieve straining on defecation (e.g., hemorrhoids, perianal surgery, pregnancy, recovery from myocardial infarction).	Agents are of little value for treatment of chronic constipation.
SALINE Magnesium citrate or citrate of magnesia (Citroma) Magnesium hydroxide (Milk of Magnesia) Sodium phosphate (Fleet Phospho-Soda, Fleet Enema)	Agents contain salt preparation not absorbed by intestines. Osmotic effect increases pressure in bowel to act as stimulant for peristalsis. Agents may also lubricate feces.	Agents are used only for acute emptying of bowel (e.g., endoscopic examination, suspected poisoning, acute constipation).	Agents are not used in long-term management of constipation. Agents are not used in clients with kidney dysfunction (toxic buildup of magnesium). Phosphate salts are not used for clients on fluid restriction.
STIMULANT CATHARTICS Bisacodyl (Dulcolax) Castor oil (Neoloid, Purge) Casanthranol (Dialose Plus, Peri-Colace) Danthron (Modane Bulk) Phenolphthalein (Doxidan, Correctol, Ex-Lax)	Agents irritate intestinal mucosa to increase motility. Agents decrease absorption in small bowel and colon. Phenolphthalein and danthron may cause pink or red urine.	Agents may be used to prepare bowel for diagnostic procedures.	Agents may cause severe cramping. Agents are not for long-term use. Chronic use may cause fluid and electrolyte imbalances. Agents are avoided during pregnancy and lactation.
LUBRICANTS Mineral oil (Haley's MO, Petrogalar Plain)	Agents coat fecal contents, allowing easier passage of stool. Agents reduce water absorption in colon.	Agents are used to prevent straining on defecation (e.g., hemorrhoids, perianal surgery).	Agents decrease absorption of fat-soluble vitamins (A, D, E, and K). Agents can cause dangerous form of pneumonia if aspirated into lungs. Mineral oil when taken with emollients can increase risk for fat emboli.

tic suppositories such as bisacodyl (Dulcolax) can act within 30 minutes. Older adults often get a strong sudden urge to defecate with Dulcolax.

Antidiarrheal Agents. For clients with diarrhea, frequent passage of liquid stools becomes a problem. The most effective antidiarrheal agents are opiates such as codeine phosphate, opium tincture (Paregoric), and diphenoxylate (Lomotil). Antidiarrheal opiate agents decrease intestinal muscle tone to slow passage of feces. Opiates inhibit peristaltic waves that move feces forward, but they also increase segmental contractions that mix intestinal contents. As a result, more water is absorbed by the intestinal walls. Antidiarrheal agents should be used with caution because opiates are habit forming.

Enemas. An enema is the instillation of a solution into the rectum and sigmoid colon. The primary reason for an enema is to promote defecation by stimulating peristalsis. The volume of fluid instilled breaks up the fecal mass, stretches the rectal wall, and initiates the defecation reflex. Enemas are also given as a vehicle for drugs that exert a local effect on rectal mucosa.

The most common use for an enema is temporary relief of constipation. Other indications include removing impacted feces; emptying the bowel before diagnostic tests, surgery, or childbirth; and beginning a program of bowel training.

Types of enemas. There are several types of enemas. Cleansing enemas promote the complete evacuation of feces from the colon. They act by stimulating peristalsis through the infusion of a large volume of solution or through local irritation of the colon's mucosa. Suggested maximum volumes follow:

Infant	150 to 250 ml
Toddler	250 to 350 ml
School-ager	300 to 500 ml
Adolescent	500 to 750 ml
Adult	750 to 1000 ml

Cleansing enemas include tap water, normal saline, soapsuds solution, and low-volume hypertonic saline. Each solution exerts a different osmotic effect (see Chapter 45), influencing the movement of fluids between the colon and interstitial spaces beyond the intestinal wall. Infants and children should receive only normal saline because they are at risk for fluid imbalance.

Tap water is hypotonic and exerts a lower osmotic pressure than fluid in interstitial spaces. After infusion into the colon, tap water escapes from the bowel lumen into interstitial spaces. The net movement of water is low. The infused volume stimulates defecation before large amounts of water leave the bowel. Tap water enemas should not be repeated because water toxicity or circulatory overload can develop if large amounts of water are absorbed.

Physiologically normal saline is the safest solution to use because it exerts the same osmotic pressure as fluids in interstitial spaces surrounding the bowel. The volume of infused saline stimulates peristalsis. Giving saline enemas does not create the danger of excess fluid absorption. If prepared saline is not available at home, the client may be instructed by the physician or nurse to mix 500 ml (1 pint) of tap water with 1 teaspoon of table salt.

Hypertonic solutions infused into the bowel exert osmotic pressure that pulls fluids out of interstitial spaces. The colon fills with fluid, and the resultant distention promotes defecation. Clients unable to tolerate large volumes of fluid benefit most from this type of enema, which is, by design, low volume. Contraindications for this type of enema are clients who are dehydrated and young infants. A hypertonic solution of 120 to 180 ml (4 to 6 oz) is usually effective. The commercially prepared Fleets Enema™ is the most commonly used.

Soapsuds may be added to tap water or saline to create the effect of intestinal irritation to stimulate peristalsis. Only pure castile soap is safe. Harsh soaps or detergents can cause serious bowel inflammation. The recommended ratio of soap to solution is 5 ml (1 teaspoon) of castile soap to 1000 ml of warm water or saline.

A physician may order a high or low cleansing enema. The terms *high* and *low* refer to the height from which and hence the pressure with which the fluid is delivered. High enemas are given to cleanse the entire colon. Fluid is delivered at a high pressure by raising the enema container to a high level. During administration of a regular enema, the enema can or bag is held 30 cm (12 inches) above the client's hips. With a high enema the bag or can is raised to 30 to 45 cm (12 to 18 inches) or slightly higher above the hips. The client is asked to turn from the left lateral to the dorsal recumbent, over to the right lateral position. The position change ensures that fluid reaches the large intestine. With a low enema the nurse holds the bag 7.5 cm (3 inches) or less above the client's hips. A low enema cleans only the rectum and sigmoid colon.

Oil-retention enemas lubricate the rectum and colon. The feces absorb the oil and become softer and easier to pass. To enhance action of the oil, the client retains the enema for several hours if possible.

Carminative enemas provide relief from gaseous distention. They improve the ability to pass flatus. An example of a carminative enema is MGW solution, which contains 30 ml of magnesium, 60 ml of glycerin, and 90 ml of water.

A return-flow enema, or Harris flush, is a mild colonic irrigation that helps expel flatus. The nurse first administers a small amount (100 to 200 ml) of mild enema solution into the client's rectum and colon. Then the nurse lowers the enema container to allow the solution to flow back through the rectal tube and into the container. Repeating this process several times aids in reducing flatus and promoting peristalsis.

Medicated enemas contain drugs. An example is sodium polystyrene sulfonate (Kayexalate), used to treat clients with dangerously high serum potassium levels. This drug contains a resin that exchanges sodium ions for potassium ions in the large intestine. Another medicated enema is neomycin solution, an antibiotic used to reduce bacteria in the colon before bowel surgery.

Enema administration. The nurse administers enemas in commercially packaged, disposable units or with reusable equipment prepared before use. Sterile technique is unnecessary because the colon normally contains bacteria. However, the nurse wears gloves to prevent the transmission of fecal microorganisms.

The nurse should explain the procedure, including the position to assume, precautions to take to avoid discomfort, and the length of time necessary to retain the solution before defecation. If the client is to receive the enema at home, the nurse explains the procedure to a family member.

Often the physician orders "enemas till clear." This means that the enema is repeated until the client passes fluid that is clear and contains no fecal material. It may be necessary to give as many as three enemas, but the nurse should caution the client against using more than three. Excess enema use seriously depletes fluids and electrolytes. If the enema fails to return a clear solution after three times (check agency policy) or if the client seems to not be tolerating the rigors of repeated enemas, the physician should be notified.

Giving an enema to a client who is unable to contract the external sphincter can pose difficulties. The nurse gives the enema with the client positioned on the bedpan. Giving the enema with the client sitting on the toilet is unsafe because the curved rectal tubing can abrade the rectal wall. Procedure 47-2 outlines the steps for an enema administration.

Administering a Cleansing Enema

STEPS	RATIONALE
1. Assess status of client; last bowel movement, normal bowel patterns, presence of hemorrhoids, mobility, external sphincter control. Assess if any contraindications for giving an enema exist.	Determines presence of factors that indicate need for enema and that influence method of administration.
	Enemas are usually not given to clients with increased intracranial pressure or who have had recent rectal or prostate surgery.
2. Review physician's order for enema.	Determines number of enemas to adminster and type of enema to be given (e.g., oil retention, carminative, medicated).
	Organizes nurse's activities, thereby increasing efficiency.
3. Collect appropriate equipment:	
a. Prepackaged enema:	Contains solution and smooth tip for insertion.
(1) Prepackaged disposable bottle with rectal tip	
(2) Disposable gloves	
(3) Lubricating jelly	
(4) Waterproof pad	
(5) Bath blanket	
(6) Toilet tissue	
(7) Bedpan or commode	
(8) Washcloth, towel, and basin	
b. Enema bag administration:	
(1) Enema solution container	Depends on type of enema to be administered.
(2) Tubing and clamp, if not already attached to container, as in disposable set	
(3) Appropriately sized rectal tube *Adult:* #22 – #30 Fr *Child:* #12 = #18 Fr	Rectal tubing should be small enough to fit diameter of anus and large enough to prevent leakage of solution from around tube.
(4) Ordered correct type and volume of solution warmed to 40.5°-43° C (105°-109° F) for adult and 37° C (98.6° F) for child	You must be aware of the type and how much fluid client can safely tolerate. Hot water can burn intestinal mucosa; cold water can cause abdominal cramping and is difficult to retain.
(5) Bath thermometer	Used to measure temperature of solution.
(6) Lubricating jelly	Reduces friction and irritation to rectal mucosa.
(7) Waterproof pad	
(8) Bath blanket	
(9) Toilet tissue	
(10) Bedpan, plus either commode chair or access to toilet	
(11) Disposable gloves	Protects hands and reduces spread of microorganisms.
(12) Washcloths, towel, and basin	Used to cleanse client after procedure, depending on client's level of mobility.
(13) Intravenous pole	Used to hang solution container.
4. Correctly identify client and explain procedure.	Reduces anxiety and promotes cooperation.
5. Assemble enema bag with appropriate solution and rectal tube.	
6. Wash hands.	Reduces transmission of infection.
7. Provide privacy by closing curtains around bed or closing door to room.	Reduces embarrassment for the client.
8. Raise bed to appropriate working height, and raise side rail on opposite side.	Promotes use of good body mechanics and client safety.
9. Assist client into Sims' position with right knee flexed. Children may also be placed in dorsal recumbent position. Position clients with poor sphincter control on bedpan in comfortable dorsal recumbent position.	Allows enema solution to flow downward by gravity along natural curve of sigmoid colon and rectum, thus improving retention of solution. (Clients with poor sphincter control cannot retain all enema solution.)
10. Place waterproof pad under client's hips and buttocks.	Prevents soiling of linen.

Continued.

Administering a Cleansing Enema—cont'd

STEPS	RATIONALE
11. Cover client with bath blanket, exposing only rectal area.	Provides warmth, reduces exposure of body parts, and allows client to feel more relaxed and comfortable.
12. Place bedpan or commode in easily accessible position. If client will be expelling contents in toilet, ensure that toilet is free.	Ensures access in case client is unable to retain enema solution.
13. Put on disposable gloves.	Prevents transmission of microorganisms from feces.
14. Administer enema:	
a. Using prepackaged disposable container:	
(1) Remove plastic cap from rectal tip. Tip is already lubricated, but more jelly can be applied as needed.	Lubrication provides for smooth insertion of rectal tube without causing rectal irritation or trauma.
(2) Gently separate buttocks and locate rectum. Instruct client to relax by breathing out slowly through mouth.	Breathing out promotes relaxation of external anal sphincter.
(3) Insert tip of bottle gently into rectum. Advance tip 7.5-10 cm (3-4 in) in adult, 5-7.5 cm (2-3 in) in child, or 2.5-3.75 cm (1-1.5 in) in infants.	Prevents trauma to rectal mucosa.
(4) Squeeze bottle until all solution has entered rectum and colon. (Most bottles contain about 250 ml of solution.)	Hypertonic solutions require only small volumes to stimulate defecation.
b. Using enema solution bag:	
(1) Add warmed solution to enema bag. (Warm tap water as it flows from faucet. Place saline container in basin of hot water before adding it to enema bag.) Check temperature of solution with bath thermometer or by pouring small amount of solution over inner wrist.	Hot water can burn intestinal mucosa. Cold water can cause abdominal cramping and is difficult to retain.
(2) Raise container, release clamp, and allow solution to flow long enough to fill tubing.	Removes air from tubing.
(3) Reclamp tubing.	Prevents further loss of solution.
(4) Lubricate 7.5-10 cm (3-4 in) of tip of rectal tube with lubricating jelly.	Allows smooth insertion of rectal tube without risk of irritation or trauma to mucosa.
(5) Gently separate buttocks and locate rectum. Instruct client to relax by breathing out slowly through mouth.	Breathing out promotes relaxation of external anal sphincter.
(6) Insert tip of rectal tube slowly by pointing tip in direction of umbilicus. Length of insertion is 7.5-10 cm (3-4 in) for adult, 5-7.5 cm (2-3 in) for child, and 2.5-3.75 cm (1-1.5 in) for infant.	Prevents trauma to rectal mucosa from accidental lodging of tube against rectal wall. Insertion beyond proper limit can cause bowel perforation.
(7) Hold tubing in rectum constantly until end of fluid instillation.	Bowel contraction can cause expulsion of rectal tube.
(8) Open regulating clamp and allow solution to enter slowly with container at client's hip level.	Rapid infusion can stimulate evacuation of rectal tube.
(9) Raise height of enema container slowly to appropriate level above hips: 30-45 cm (12-18 in) for high enema, 7.5 cm (3 in) for low enema. Infusion time varies with volume of solution administered (e.g., 1 L in 10 min) and with client's ability to withstand given infusion rate.	Allows continuous, slow infusion of solution. Raising container too high causes rapid infusion and possible painful distention of colon. High pressure can cause rupture of bowel in infants.
(10) Lower container or clamp tubing if client complains of cramping or if fluid escapes around rectal tube.	Temporary cessation of infusion prevents cramping. Cramping may prevent client from retaining all fluid, altering effectiveness of enema.
(11) Clamp tubing after all solution is infused.	Prevents entrance of air into rectum.
15. Place layers of toilet tissue around tube at anus and gently withdraw rectal tube.	Provides for client comfort and cleanliness.

Administering a Cleansing Enema—cont'd

STEPS	RATIONALE
16. Explain to client that feeling of distention is normal. Ask client to retain solution for 5-10 min or as long as possible while lying quietly in bed. (For infant or young child, gently hold buttocks together for few minutes.)	Solution distends the bowel. Length of retention varies with type of enema and client's ability to contract anal sphincter. Longer retention promotes more effective stimulation of peristalsis and defecation.
17. Discard enema container and tubing in proper receptacle or rinse out thoroughly with warm soap and water if container is to be reused.	Controls transmission and growth of microorganisms.
18. Remove gloves by pulling them inside out and discarding in trash can.	Prevents transmission of microorganisms.
19. Assist client to bathroom or help position client on bedpan or commode chair.	Normal squatting position promotes defecation.
20. Observe character of feces and solution (caution client against flushing toilet before inspection). Inspect character of stool and fluid passed.	When enemas are ordered "until clear," it is essential to observe contents of solution passed. Determines whether stool is evacuated or fluid is retained.
21. Assist client as needed to wash anal area with warm soap and water.	Fecal content can irritate skin. Hygiene promotes comfort.
22. Wash hands.	Reduces transmission of infection.
23. Observe client (especially elderly) for any signs and symptoms of fluid or electrolyte disturbances and/or changes in pulse rate.	Clients can have depletion of fluid and electrolytes from enemas.
24. Record pertinent information, including type and volume of enema given and color, amount, and consistency of fecal return.	Communicates pertinent information to all members of health care team. Prompt recording improves documentation of treatment results.

Digital Removal of Stool. For clients with an impaction, the fecal mass may be too large to be passed voluntarily. If enemas fail, the nurse must break up the fecal mass with the fingers and remove it in sections. The procedure can be very uncomfortable for the client. Excess rectal manipulation may cause irritation to the mucosa, bleeding, and stimulation of the vagus nerve, which results in a reflex slowing of the heart rate. Because of the procedure's potential complications, a physician's order is necessary for the nurse to remove a fecal impaction.

The steps for removing stool digitally follow:

1. Explain the procedure. Take baseline vitals prior to the procedure. Help the client lie on the side with knees flexed and back toward you.
2. Drape the trunk and lower extremities with a bath blanket and place a waterproof pad under the buttocks. Keep a bedpan next to the client.
3. Apply disposable gloves and lubricate the index finger of your dominant hand with lubricating jelly.
4. Gently insert the gloved index finger into the rectum and advance the finger slowly along the rectal wall toward the umbilicus.
5. Gently loosen the fecal mass by massaging around it. Work the finger into the hardened mass.
6. Work the feces downward toward the end of the rectum. Remove small pieces at a time and discard into bedpan.
7. Reassess the client's heart rate and look for signs of fatigue. Stop the procedure if the heart rate drops significantly or the rhythm changes.

8. Continue to clean feces and allow the client to rest at intervals.
9. Once completed, offer a washcloth and towel to wash and dry the buttocks and anal area. Assist as needed.
10. Remove bedpan and dispose of feces. Remove gloves by turning them inside out, then discard.
11. Assist client to toilet or clean bedpan if urge to defecate develops.
12. Wash hands. Record results of disimpaction by describing fecal characteristics.
13. The procedure may be followed by enemas or cathartics.
14. Reassess client's vital signs.

Bowel Training. The client with incontinence is unable to maintain bowel control. A **bowel training** program can help some clients achieve normal defecation, especially those who still have some neuromuscular control (Doughty, 1992).

The training program involves setting up a daily routine. By attempting to defecate at the same time each day and using measures that promote defecation, the client gains control of bowel reflexes. The program requires time, patience, and consistency. The physician determines the client's physical readiness and ability to benefit from bowel training. A successful program includes the following:

1. Assessing the normal elimination pattern and recording times when the client is incontinent
2. Choosing a time in the client's pattern to initiate defecation-control measures

3. Giving stool softeners orally every day or a cathartic suppository at least half an hour before the selected defecation time (lower colon must be free of stool so that suppository contacts intestinal mucosa)

4. Offering a hot drink (hot tea) or fruit juice (prune juice) (or whatever fluids normally stimulate peristalsis for the client) before the defecation time

5. Assisting the client to the toilet at the designated time

6. Providing privacy and setting a time limit for defecation (15 to 20 minutes)

7. Instructing the client to lean forward at the hips while sitting on the toilet, to apply manual pressure with the hands over the abdomen, and to bear down but not strain to stimulate colon emptying

8. Not criticizing or conveying frustration if the client is unable to defecate

9. Providing regular meals with adequate fluids and fiber

10. Maintaining normal exercise within the client's physical ability

CARE OF OSTOMIES

Clients who have temporary or permanent bowel diversions face unique health care problems. Their patterns of bowel elimination differ from those of clients with intact colons. Persons with incontinent ostomies must wear pouches or appliances to collect stool emitted from the stomas. Some clients learn to irrigate their ostomies to establish regular bowel elimination routines. Clients with ostomies must also follow good health practices such as maintaining proper dietary habits and exercising regularly to maintain normal elimination patterns. Clients with an ostomy have many education needs (Gawron, 1993).

Pouching Ostomies. An incontinent ostomy requires a pouch to collect fecal material. An effective pouching system protects the skin, contains fecal material, remains odor free, and is comfortable and inconspicuous. A person wearing a pouch should feel secure in participating in any activity.

Many pouching systems are available. To ensure that a pouch fits well and meets the client's needs, the nurse considers the location of ostomy, type and size of the stoma, type and amount of ostomy drainage, size and contour of the abdomen, condition of the skin around the stoma, physical activities of the client, client's personal preference, age, and dexterity, and cost of equipment. An **enterostomal therapist (ET)** is a nurse trained to care for ostomy clients. The staff nurse collaborates with the ET to be sure the correct pouching system is used. An example where a referral to an ET nurse would be appropriate is to plan the care of a client that has a high output ostomy that requires a pouch modification (Oetman and Trout, 1994).

A pouching system consists of a pouch and skin barrier. Some pouching systems such as Squibb-Convatec, Hollister, Coloplast, and Smith & Nephew, are attached to the client's skin from the product's adhesive surface, while some pouching systems like VIP are nonadhesive systems. Pouches come in one- and two-piece systems that are disposable or reusable. Some pouches have the opening precut by the manufacturer; others require the stoma opening to be custom cut by someone to the client's specific stoma size.

Skin barriers include wafers, pastes, powders, and liquid film that are applied to the skin around the stoma. Some wafer skin barriers are permanently attached to the ostomy pouch. These are called a one-piece pouch system. In a two-piece system, the pouch can be detached from the skin barrier for emptying or changing. This allows the skin barrier to remain around the client's stoma for several days, thus minimizing the chance of skin damage from too frequent removal of the skin barrier from the peristomal skin. When using a two-piece pouching system, it is important to remember that the skin barrier and pouch must be the same corresponding size and from the same manufacturer. The pouch from one manufacturer will not fit correctly on the skin barrier from another manufacturer. Make sure you use an ostomy pouch made for collecting fecal matter (colostomy or ileostomy) and not one for collecting urine.

It is important to measure the stoma size carefully when selecting and cutting out the opening on the wafer skin barrier. A good skin barrier protects the skin, prevents irritation from repeated removal of the pouch, and is comfortable for the client to wear. Procedure 47-3 describes steps for applying one type of pouch system.

Irrigating a Colostomy. To establish a pattern of regular defecation, clients with descending and sigmoid colostomies often irrigate their ostomy. The muscular quality of the colon allows it to be safely irrigated with a relatively large volume of water or saline. The irrigation acts like an enema, distending the bowel and stimulating peristalsis. Fluid is instilled into the colon via the stoma. Elimination thus occurs at a time chosen by the client. The irrigation also cleans the colon of gas and odor. Only specific equipment for irrigating an ostomy should be used. NEVER use an enema set to irrigate an ostomy. Gentle irrigation using the correct equipment is performed to reduce the risk of bowel perforation.

Surgical creation of a colostomy can seriously change a person's body image. Regaining control of fecal elimination through irrigation helps emotional adjustment. The client can also gain freedom without the need to wear a stomal pouch continuously, although most clients prefer to wear a smaller pouch over the stoma between irrigations in case of any fecal spillage.

The physician recommends when to begin irrigations and their frequency. Eventually clients develop their own schedules. However, it is usually necessary to perform the proce-

---

Contraindications and Cautions to Colostomy Irrigation

CONTRAINDICATIONS
- Ascending colostomies
- Recent surgery—sutures not yet healed
- Disease in remaining colon (diverticulosis, inflammatory disease)
- Infant or child
- Inadequate sanitary facilities
- Stomal abnormalities (prolapse, hernia)

CAUTIONS
- Physical limitations (arthritis, paralysis)
- Mental limitations (confusion, dementia, retardation)

Pouching a Colostomy or Ileostomy

STEPS	RATIONALE
1. Assess condition of existing pouch/skin barrier for leakage and note appearance of underlying stoma and surgical incision. Question client about discomfort at or around stoma. (Gloves may be necessary.)	Determines need to change pouch/skin barrier. Leakage of contents causes skin irritation. Stoma and peristoma sutures should be inspected daily to note early signs of complications.
2. Note amount of drainage from stoma.	Pouches should be emptied before half full to avoid premature leakage. Liquid output, common in postoperative phase, causes skin barrier to melt down and wear out sooner. Copious output also increases deterioration of appliance skin barrier. Ileostomy output is more corrosive to appliance, skin barrier, and skin and requires more durable equipment.
3. Assess skin around stoma, noting scars, folds, or protuberance of skin.	Determines site for pouch placement and size of underlying skin barrier. Allow $1/2$ in of skin barrier on all sides of stoma to ensure secure seal.
4. Determine client's knowledge and understanding of ostomy.	Reveals client's level of acceptance of ostomy and assists in determining extent to which client needs additional teaching to participate in care.
5. Collect appropriate equipment:	
a. Skin barriers (wafers such as Stomahesive, Hollihesive, or paste or powder)	Maintains skin integrity by protecting skin from feces.
b. Ostomy pouch (see the illustration below)	Contains stool, can be emptied from bottom without removal, and is odor proof. Some one-piece pouches can be cut to fit changing stoma sizes. Pouch should be drainable to avoid frequent changes; therefore it needs clamp or closing device.
c. Clamp or closing device	
d. Hypoallergenic tape and/or belt	Reinforces pouch to skin barrier.
e. Washcloth, towel, wash basin with warm water	
f. Skin cleanser (Sween or Bard) or mild soap	Prevents skin irritation.
g. Disposable gloves	Prevents contact with microorganisms in feces.

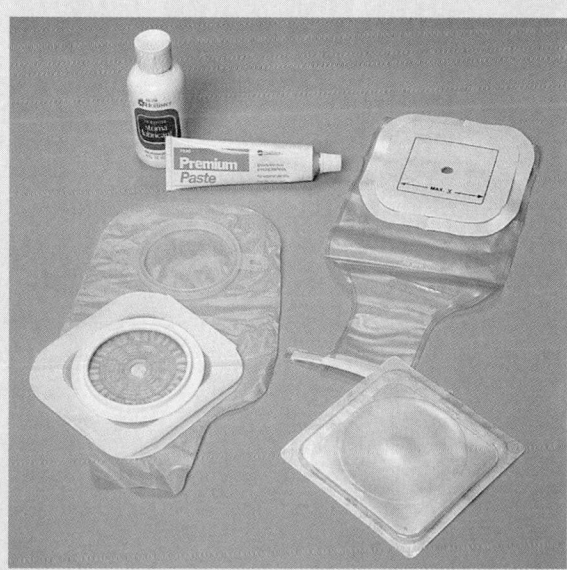

Step 5b

Continued.

Pouching a Colostomy or Ileostomy—cont'd

STEPS	RATIONALE
6. Select optimum time to change pouch/skin barrier (e.g., when client is comfortable, between meals, or before administration of medications that may affect bowel function).	Signs and smells of ostomy may reduce appetite. Changing pouch goes smoother when ostomy is least likely to function.
7. Explain procedure (if client is unfamiliar with technique); otherwise allow client to organize steps for pouch change. Be sure client observes procedure.	Encourages client's participation in care. Ultimately client must assume self-care.
8. Position client supine or sitting for pouch application; if able to stand, help client assume standing position.	When client is lying or standing there are fewer wrinkles in skin and pouch.
9. Wash hands and apply gloves.	Reduces transmission of infection.
10. Close room curtains or door.	Provides privacy.
11. If pouch is full, remove clamp and empty contents through bottom into bedpan.	Prevents spillage on skin.
12. Remove old appliance as one piece.	Reduces trauma; jerking can cause skin tears.
13. Wash skin gently with skin cleanser or with regular soap and water. Remove secretions from skin.	Secretions act as irritant to skin. Bacteria in fecal secretions can enter incisional area (new colostomy) and cause infection.
14. Rinse soap off thoroughly. Blot dry.	Use of any soap could result in film or residue being left behind. These residues can result in chemical reactions or burns and can cause premature leakage because of interference with pouch adhesion. Blot dry gently to avoid trauma to stoma, which normally bleeds easily.
15. If blood appears after washing, reassure client that small amount is normal. Clarify what is abnormal.	Minimizes anxiety. Bowel has rich vascular supply. Client must be able to recognize complications.

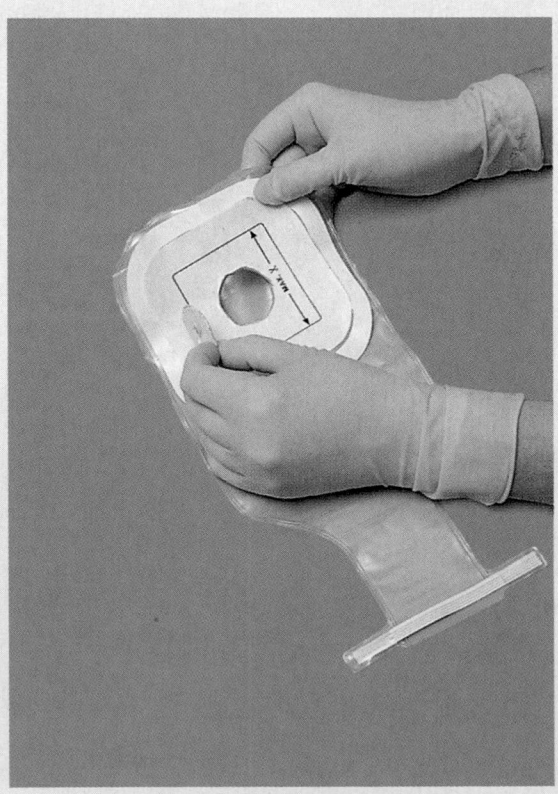

Step 20

Pouching a Colostomy or Ileostomy—cont'd

STEPS	RATIONALE
16. Observe condition of skin and stoma. Encourage client to make these observations daily. Remeasure the stoma size.	Allows for early monitoring of complications. Stoma is at risk for necrosis during first postoperative week. Necrosis is evidenced by dark color, dry appearance, failure to bleed, and sloughing. Client observation aids in acceptance and adjustment; client also develops habit of observing for skin-stomal problems, which are more easily correctable if detected and reported early. Remeasuring the stoma size in the early postoperative period is very important, as the stoma is swollen immediately postoperatively and will normally shrink. The accurate size of the stoma is important in selecting and preparing ostomy pouches and skin barriers.
17. If abdominal crease is present or if contour is irregular, fill in with paste-type barrier.	Provides smooth surface for application of skin barrier and pouch's faceplate.
18. Allow paste to dry for 1-2 min.	Prevents alcohol burns to skin.
19. If abdominal contour is flat or after paste has dried, prepare skin barrier using skin sealant or karaya paste. Cut hole in skin barrier slightly larger than stoma, up to $1/_0$ in. Cut radial slits from center of hole. Cut rounded corners on edges of skin barrier.	Close fit of barrier around stoma prevents contact of skin with effluent. Barrier cut too tight can cut stoma from peristalsis of stoma. Slits allow barrier opening to expand if stoma becomes edematous. Rounded corners adhere better to skin and are more comfortable for client.
20. Prepare ostomy pouch; for non-precut pouches, cut hole in center of faceplate $1/_8$ in larger than hole in barrier (see the illustration on p. 1370).	Avoids risk of paper cut of stoma and ensures better seal with barrier.
21. Remove paper backing from pouch faceplate (see the illustration below) and apply to shiny, noncovered side of barrier.	Reduces risk of wrinkling if wafer is applied to skin before pouch is attached; gives better leakproof seal.
22. Remove backing from barrier and apply it and pouch (see the illustration below) as unit to skin. Smooth out from center. Hold in place for 1-3 min. Apply in position that facilitates emptying.	Creates wrinkle-free secure seal onto skin.

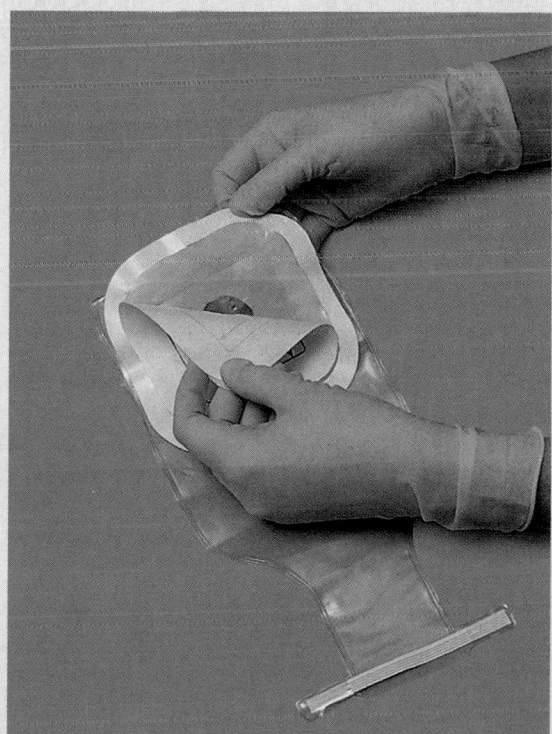

Step 21

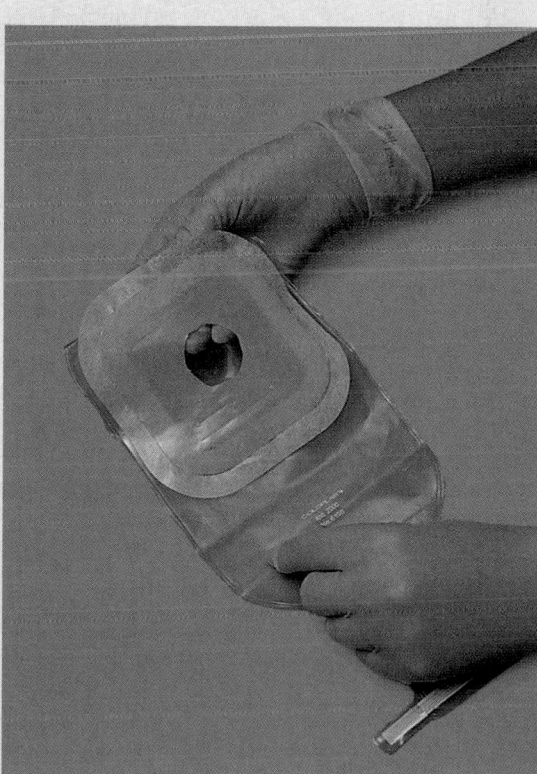

Step 22

Continued.

Pouching a Colostomy or Ileostomy—cont'd

STEPS	RATIONALE
23. Apply hypoallergenic tape and/or belt as needed to edges of faceplate over skin barrier.	Adds extra reinforcement.
24. Fold bottom edges of pouch over to fit clamp or closing device. Secure clamp.	Prevents leakage of pouch contents.
25. Dispose of old appliance in plastic bag and dispose in trash chute. (Be sure this is not reusable appliance because they should be washed and reused several times.)	Avoids odors lingering in room, which is unpleasant to client, family, and staff.
26. Remove soiled gloves and dispose in proper receptacle.	Reduces transmission of infection.
27. Wash hands.	Reduces transmission of infection.
28. Assist client to comfortable position if necessary.	Ensures client comfort.
29. Record pertinent information: type of pouch and skin barrier, amount and appearance of feces, condition of stoma and surrounding skin, client's ability to do ostomy self-care.	Documents care and provides data for later determining change in client's condition.

dure the same way, with the same time of day, and with the same frequency (i.e., every day or every other day, three times a week). Some clients have physical or mental limitations that make colostomy irrigations unwise (see the box on p. 1368). Young children and infants should not receive colostomy irrigations. Infants are at risk for bowel perforation. Young children often cannot sit still for the procedure.

Clients may find irrigation a problem. The procedure is time consuming (45 to 60 minutes), and clients may be unwilling to interrupt their lifestyles. For many, irrigation is unpleasant. The nurse's emotional support can help clients make a choice. Alternate methods of ostomy management are available such as dietary control or laxative use. If a client initially decides against irrigations, the decision can be changed later. Procedure 47-4 outlines the steps for an ostomy irrigation.

MAINTENANCE OF PROPER FLUID AND FOOD INTAKE

In choosing a diet for promoting normal elimination, the nurse should consider the frequency of defecation, characteristics of feces, and types of foods that impair or promote defecation. The client with frequent constipation or impaction requires an increased intake of high-fiber foods and more fluids. However, the client should realize that diet therapy provides only long-term relief of elimination problems and may not give immediate relief from problems such as constipation.

When diarrhea is a problem, the nurse can recommend foods with a low fiber content and discourage foods that typically cause gastric upset or abdominal cramping. Diarrhea caused by illness can be debilitating. If the client cannot tolerate foods or liquids orally, intravenous therapy (with potassium supplements) is necessary. The client returns to a normal diet slowly, often beginning with fluids. Excessively hot or cold fluids stimulate peristalsis, causing abdominal cramps and further diarrhea. As the tolerance to liquids improves, solid foods are ordered.

Diet therapy is important for clients with ostomies. During the first weeks after surgery, many physicians recommend low-fiber diets, particularly for ileostomy clients because the small bowel requires time to adapt to the diversion. Low-fiber foods include bread, noodles, rice, cream cheese, eggs (not fried), strained fruit juices, lean meats, fish, and poultry. As ostomies heal, clients can eat almost any food. High-fiber foods such as fresh fruits and vegetables help ensure a more solid stool needed to achieve success at irrigation. Blockage must be avoided. The stoma's surgical construction can affect the likelihood of blockage. Ileostomy clients should eat slowly and chew food completely. Drinking 10 to 12 glasses of water daily also prevents blockage. High-fiber foods that may cause problems include stringy meats, mushrooms, popcorn, fruits such as cherries, and some seafood such as shrimp and crab. Ostomy clients may benefit from avoiding foods that cause gas and odor, including broccoli, cauliflower, dried beans, and Brussels sprouts.

PROMOTION OF REGULAR EXERCISE

A daily exercise program helps prevent elimination problems. Walking, riding a stationary bicycle, or swimming stimulates peristalsis. Clients who are sedentary at work are most in need of regular exercise.

For a client temporarily immobilized, the nurse should attempt ambulation as soon as possible. If the condition permits, the nurse assists a postoperative client in walking to a chair on the evening of the day of surgery. The client should walk farther each day.

Some clients have difficulty passing stool because of weak abdominal and pelvic floor muscles. Exercises help bedridden clients using a bedpan. The client can practice the exercises as follows:

1. Lie supine; tighten the abdominal muscles as though pushing them to the floor. Hold them tight to the count of three; relax. Repeat five to ten times as tolerated.
2. Flex and contract the thigh muscles by raising one

Irrigating a Colostomy

STEPS	RATIONALE
1. Assess frequency of defecation and character of stool.	Unrelieved constipation characterized by hardened feces can indicate need to irrigate colon.
2. Assess time when client normally irrigates ostomy. With a new ostomy, confer with physician for order.	Maintains established routine for bowel emptying.
3. Assess client's understanding of procedure and ability to perform techniques.	Determines level of client participation.
4. Collect appropriate equipment:	Organizes activities, thereby increasing efficiency.
a. Graduated container	
b. Tubing with regulatory clamp	Provides control of fluid instillation into colon.
c. Cone	Because stoma has no sphincters, there is no way for client to willfully retain solution. Therefore it is given via cone to prevent premature loss of solution.
d. Irrigation sleeve, with or without belt	Directs flow of irrigating fluid from stoma into toilet.
e. Water-soluble lubricant	Makes insertion of cone into stoma easier. Water-soluble lubricants will not harm plastic equipment.
f. Clamps or closure device	May use to close both top and bottom of sleeve, allowing ambulation after solution has returned and while awaiting final results.
g. New appliance/skin barrier	Will need new pouch when irrigation completed.
h. Disposable gloves (clients who do their own irrigation may choose not to wear gloves).	
i. Bedpan, commode, or toilet	
j. Washcloth, towel, wash basin	
k. Intravenous pole	
l. Liquid cleanser	
5. Prepare client by explaining procedure.	Allays client fears by explaining stoma is not painful. Ensures cooperation.
6. Choose proper time for irrigation, about 1 hr after meal.	Coordinates irrigation during normal time of duodenocolic reflex.
7. Assist client with positioning. If ambulatory, have client sit on chair in front of toilet; if confined to bed, have client lie on side.	Allows for directing sleeve into toilet for drainage of fecal contents and irrigant.
8. Wash hands and apply gloves.	Reduces transmission of infection.
9. Close bathroom door or room curtains.	Provides privacy.
10. Remove appliance and cleanse skin as normally done in changing enterostomy pouch.	Allows access to stoma.
11. Apply irrigation sleeve. Roll up so that bottom just touches water in toilet. (For client confined to bed, clip bottom of drain sleeve.)	Directs flow of stool into toilet. Rolling up sleeve prevents it from stopping up plumbing when commode is flushed. Also keeps end of sleeve clean.
12. Fill graduated container with required solution (usually 500-1000 ml tepid water or saline). Hang on intravenous pole so that bottom of container is level with client's shoulder.	Volume of 500-1000 ml is sufficient to distend colon and trigger effective emptying. Cold water results in syncope, and hot water could damage stoma or intestine. Height of bag creates pressure gradient for fluid to enter colon.
13. Attach cone to irrigating tube. Allow enough fluid to run through entire length of tube.	Flushes air out of tube. Air is expelled from tubing because it causes air lock and will not let solution flow.
14. Apply lubricant to cone.	Prevents trauma to stoma.
15. Insert cone through top of irrigation sleeve.	Ensures containment of stool within sleeve.
16. Insert cone gently but firmly into stoma (see the illustration on p. 1374). Stoma should be dilated before first irrigation with gloved, lubricated finger to determine direction of bowel lumen.	Stoma is easily injured. Inserting tube toward direction of bowel facilitates introduction of solution.
17. Begin flow of solution and readjust position of cone as necessary (see the illustration on p. 1374).	To get sufficient distention, solution must not leak around cone. Client or you may need to redirect cone and slowly increase firmness against stoma until solution flows in easily and leakage around cone ceases.

Continued.

Irrigating a Colostomy—cont'd

STEPS	RATIONALE
18. Adjust flow of solution by raising or lowering irrigating container. To aid in this, bottom of irrigator bag should be hung 18 in above stoma.	Too-rapid administration results in cramping and inability to hold sufficient volume for adequate results.
19. Administer 500-1000 ml of solution slowly over 15 min, pausing when client cramps but not removing cone until above amount is given.	Usually 500-1000 ml is required to empty colon. Pauses prevent premature leakage of solution because cone replaces sphincter.
20. When solution runs in, clamp tubing and remove cone, making sure sleeve fits around stoma, close top of irrigation sleeve. Should obtain small gush of fluid, then returns in spurts.	Clamping tubing prevents return of results into irrigator. Sleeve should be placed properly to avoid gush of solution over top of sleeve. If colon was distended sufficiently, contracting of bowel musculature results in return of solution in intermittent spurts.
21. Clamp top of sleeve.	Prevents leakage at top.
22. When most of solution has returned (15-20 min), rinse sleeve with water, fold end up, fasten it to top, and have client ambulate (unless restricted to bed).	Allows ambulation. Prevents leakage. Entire procedure takes about 1 hr, and client may become tired of sitting.
23. When all of feces have returned, rinse sleeve out with water and special liquid cleanser and remove. Then wash sleeve out with soap and water, rinse, and air dry. Do not throw irrigation sleeve away—it is reuseable.	Prevents sleeve from deteriorating, permitting reuse. Controls odor.
24. Apply new pouch according to procedure (see Procedure 47-3).	Avoids leakage and skin problems.
25. Dispose of equipment no longer needed. Remove gloves by turning them inside out and dispose in receptacle.	Reduces transmission of microorganisms.
26. Wash hands.	Prevents cross-contamination.
27. Inspect volume and character of fecal material and fluid that returns after irrigation.	Determines whether irrigant is retained (serious fluid imbalances can occur if retained). Character and amount of stool reveal success of cleaning bowel.
28. Note client's response during irrigant infusion. Ask if client feels cramping or abdominal pain.	Reveals client's tolerance of irrigation.
29. Palpate and auscultate abdomen after return of irrigant.	Evaluates for potential complication of bowel perforation.
30. Assist client to comfortable position.	Ensures client comfort.
31. Record pertinent information, including character of feces and tolerance to procedure. Assess client's ability to do ostomy self-irrigation.	Communicates pertinent information to members of health care team. Evaluation of skill acquisition is a necessary part of teaching a client ostomy self-irrigation technique.
32. If client irrigations are being done to regular evaluations, assess whether there is any fecal drainage or distention between irrigation procedures.	With time, feces will only be eliminated at time of irrigations and not in between irrigations.
33. Record all teaching to client and/or family and further teaching needs in client's record.	Documents care and provides data for later determining change in client's condition.

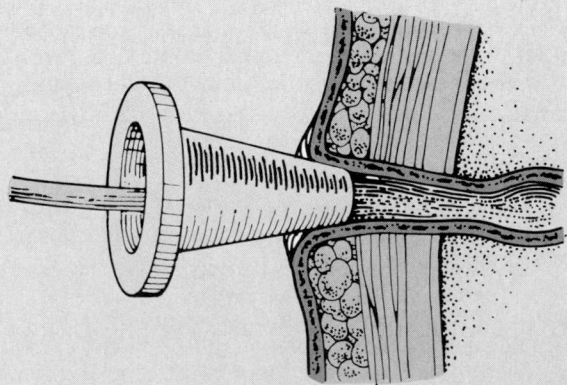

Step 16

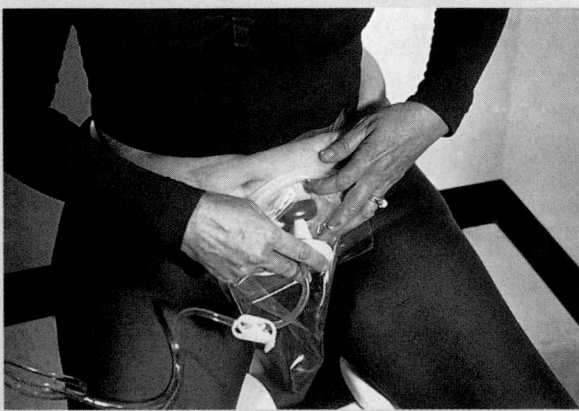

Step 17

knee slowly toward the chest. Repeat for each leg at least five times and increase frequency as tolerated.

PROMOTION OF COMFORT

Many clients have discomfort from alterations in elimination. Pain results when hemorrhoidal tissues are directly irritated. Flatulence can also create discomfort, particularly if distention develops.

The primary goal for the client with hemorrhoids is to have soft-formed, painless stools. Proper diet, fluids, and regular exercise improve the likelihood of stools being soft. If the client becomes constipated, passage of hard stools may cause bleeding and irritation. Local heat provides temporary relief to swollen hemorrhoids. A sitz bath is the most effective means of heat application (see Chapter 49).

To relieve the discomfort of flatulence, the nurse should use measures that reduce flatus or promote its escape. Air swallowing increases flatus. The client can reduce the amount of air swallowed by not drinking carbonated beverages, not using straws for drinking, and not chewing gum or hard candies. When flatulence becomes severe as a result of reduced peristalsis, a nasogastric tube is often used.

When flatulence results in abdominal cramping, ambulation promotes passage of flatus. Having the client walk down the hall may be enough to stimulate peristalsis and relieve gas. When conservative measures fail, flatulence can be relieved by insertion of a rectal tube. The client assumes a side-lying position while the nurse inserts the tube in the same manner as for an enema (Procedure 47-2). Because fluid is not instilled into the bowel, the nurse can advance the tube deeper to reach areas where flatus has accumulated (15 cm or 6 inches in an adult, 5 to 10 cm or 2 to 4 inches in a child).

After inserting the tube the nurse instructs the client to lie quietly in bed. To prevent the tube from being dislodged, the nurse may tape it to one of the buttocks. A gauze dressing or waterproof pad placed around the open end of the rectal tube will catch liquid fecal material.

Continual use of rectal tubes can cause irritation and eventual **excoriation** of the anus and rectal mucosa. A rectal tube should not remain in place longer than 30 minutes. The physician determines the frequency with which the tube can be inserted. If flatulence persists, the nurse should notify the physician.

MAINTENANCE OF SKIN INTEGRITY

The client with diarrhea or fecal incontinence is at risk for skin breakdown when fecal contents remain on the skin. The same problem exists for the client with an ostomy that drains liquid stool (see the box above). Liquid stool is usually acidic and contains digestive enzymes. Irritation from repeated wiping with toilet tissue aggravates skin breakdown. Bathing the skin after soiling helps but may result in more breakdown unless the skin is thoroughly dried.

When caring for a debilitated, incontinent client who is unable to ask for assistance, the nurse should check often for defecation. The anal areas can be protected with petrolatum jelly, zinc oxide, or another ointment that holds moisture in the skin, preventing drying and cracking. Yeast infections of the skin can develop easily. Several powdered antifungal agents are effective against yeast. Baby powder or cornstarch should not be used because they have no

CLIENT TEACHING
for Stomal Care (Incontinent Ostomy)

OBJECTIVE
- Client will demonstrate the correct procedure for stomal care.

TEACHING STRATEGIES
- Instruct client to avoid using alcohol in cleansing around the stoma. Alcohol dilates capillaries and can cause bleeding of the stomal margin.
- Demonstrate how to wash around the stoma with water and a mild soap or with a commercial preparation, such as Peri Wash. Pat the skin dry but do not rub.
- Instruct client not to use cold cream on skin because it prevents the pouch or skin barrier from adhering to the skin.
- Explain to the client that peroxide is an irritant and should not be used.
- Instruct the client that if a yeast infection occurs, thorough cleansing, followed by patting the area dry and applying Kenalog spray or Mycostatin usually resolves the infection.
- Show the client how to inspect the stoma daily and observe a stoma that is moist, shiny, and dark pink to red.
- Teach client to observe for and report excessive bleeding, edema, or abnormal discharge or color to the nurse or physician.
- Teach client how to select and apply correctly sized skin barrier and ostomy pouch
- Teach client how to empty pouch.
- Teach client techniques to reduce odor.

EVALUATION
- Client will correctly state skin care procedures.
- Client will correctly perform stoma skin care procedure.

medical properties and they frequently cake on the skin and become difficult to remove.

PROMOTION OF SELF-CONCEPT

When a client has a bowel elimination problem, a threat to self-concept may be experienced. Frequent incontinence, foul odorous stools, and an ostomy appliance are just a few factors that may cause a client to perceive a change in body image (Mihalopoulos et al, 1994; Walsh et al, 1995). The result could be a client who avoids socializing with others or who is unwilling to assume responsibility for self-care. The nurse can play an important role in restoring a client's self-concept through the following interventions:

1. Give the client an opportunity to discuss concerns or fears about elimination problems.
2. Provide the client and family with information to understand and manage the elimination problem.
3. Give positive feedback when the client attempts self-care measures.
4. Help the client manage the condition but do not expect the client to like it.
5. Provide privacy during care.

Sample Evaluation of Interventions for Constipation

GOALS	EVALUATIVE MEASURES	EXPECTED OUTCOMES
Client will understand and ingest fluid and food required to promote soft-formed stools.	Evaluate meal plan created by client or family member. Measure client's fluid intake.	Client will describe dietary sources high in fiber. Client will prepare 24-hr menu, including high-fiber foods and fluids. Client will explain normal fluid intake to promote defecation. Client will have a minimum fluid intake of 1400-2000 ml daily.
Client will attain regular defecation schedule.	Observe character of stools. Record frequency of defecation. Ask client to describe factors that affect elimination. Ask client to discuss factors in history that may cause elimination problems.	Client will attain a regular schedule of defecation, passing soft-formed stools without excess straining.

6. Show acceptance and understanding. Remember that the client will be watching the nurse during ostomy care and pouch changes for facial expressions and other nonverbal clues that demonstrate acceptance of the ostomy.

Often a client with an elimination problem goes through a process similar to grieving (see Chapter 26). The nurse's support is essential to help the client return to a more normal lifestyle.

Evaluation

The effectiveness of care depends on success in meeting the goals and expected outcomes of care (see the evaluation box above). Optimally the client will be able to regularly defecate soft-formed, painless stools. The client will also gain information needed to establish a normal elimination pattern and to demonstrate ongoing success measured at specific intervals over an extended period. The client will be able to accomplish normal defecation by manipulating natural components of daily living such as diet, fluid intake, and exercise. The client will have minimal reliance on artificial means of defecation such as enemas and laxative use. The client will be comfortable with the ostomy protocol and identify it as one that can be practiced indefinitely.

■ KEY CONCEPTS ■

▶ A primary function of the elimination process is fluid balance.

▶ Mechanical breakdown of food elements, gastrointestinal motility, and selective absorption and secretion of substances by the large intestine influence the character of feces.

▶ Mass peristalsis in the large intestine is strongest an hour after mealtime.

▶ Food high in fiber content and an increased fluid intake keep feces soft.

▶ Regular use of laxatives can lead to constipation.

▶ Vagal stimulation, which slows the heart rate, may occur during straining while defecating, taking rectal temperatures, and enemas.

▶ The greatest danger from diarrhea is development of fluid and electrolyte imbalance.

▶ The location of an ostomy influences consistency of the stool.

▶ Assessment of elimination patterns should focus on bowel habits, factors that normally influence defecation, recent changes in elimination, and a physical examination.

▶ A guaiac test is recommended for clients who take anticoagulants, who have a bleeding disorder or gastrointestinal disorder causing bleeding, or who are at risk for colon cancer.

▶ Indirect and direct visualization of the lower gastrointestinal tract requires cleansing of the bowel before the procedure.

▶ The nurse should consider frequency of defecation, fecal characteristics, and effect of foods on gastrointestinal function when selecting a diet promoting normal elimination.

▶ Proper positioning on a bedpan allows the client to assume a position similar to squatting without experiencing muscle strain.

► Cathartics or laxatives should be administered shortly before the usual time of defecation.

► Proper administration of an enema is the slow instillation of a warm solution in the proper volume.

► Proper selection and use of an ostomy pouching system is necessary to prevent damage to the skin around the stoma. Irrigation of an ostomy follows the same principles as an enema administration except a special irrigating tube is needed and the client cannot control passage of feces.

► Dangers during digital removal of stool include traumatizing the rectal mucosa and promoting vagal stimulation.

► Skin breakdown can occur after repeated exposure to liquid stool.

■ KEY TERMS ■

Biopsy, p. 1357
Bolus, p. 1341
Bowel training, p. 1367
Cathartics, p. 1345
Chyme, p. 1342
Colitis, p. 1345
Colon, p. 1342
Colostomy, p. 1348
Constipation, p. 1346
Contrast medium, p. 1358
Crohn's disease, p. 1345
Defecation, p. 1343
Diarrhea, p. 1347
Diverticula, p. 1358
Endoscopy, p. 1355
Enema, p. 1363
Enterostomal therapist (ET), p. 1368
Excoriation, p. 1375
Feces, p. 1343
Fiber, p. 1344
Fiberoptic endoscope, p. 1355
Flatulence, p. 1347
Flatus, p. 1343
Gastrocolic reflex, p. 1345
Gastroscopy, p. 1355
Guaiac test, p. 1355
Haustral contractions, p. 1342
Hemorrhoids, p. 1347
Ileostomy, p. 1348
Impaction, p. 1346
Incontinence, p. 1347
Lactose intolerance, p. 1344
Laxatives, p. 1345
Masticate, p. 1341
Melena, p. 1355
Paralytic ileus, p. 1345

Peristalsis, p. 1341
Polyps, p. 1357
Refluxing, p. 1341
Regurgitating, p. 1342
Stoma, p. 1348
Transit time, p. 1345
Valsalva maneuver, p. 1343

■ CRITICAL THINKING EXERCISES ■

1. A 24-year-old man with a history of good health is admitted to your unit after a motor vehicle accident. Bed rest has been prescribed for the next 2 weeks. What type of plan would you design to prevent him from becoming constipated during this period of immobility?

2. You are asked to provide an outpatient client with material and instructions for three stool guaiac tests. Identify and explain four important points of information you would want to include in your instructions.

3. An older woman with a new, permanent colostomy is about to be discharged from your unit to her daughter's home. The skin around her stoma has no breakdown. She and her daughter realize the importance of maintaining this skin integrity. How would you advise them?

REFERENCES

Beitz JM: The ileoanal reservoir: an alternative to ileostomy, *J Wound, Ostomy, Continence Nurs (WOCN)*, 21(3):120, 1994.
Bellan A: Coloplast: update on the conseal plug, *Ostomy Internat* 11(2):15, 1990.
Bosley, C: Three methods of stool management for patients with diarrhea, *Ostomy/Wound Management* 40(1):52, 1994.
Brown MK, Everett I: Gentler bowel fitness with fiber, *Geriatr Nurs* 11(1):26, 1990.
Clague MM, Heald RJ: Achievement of stomal continence in one-third of colostomies by use of a disposable plug, *Surg Gynecol Obstet* 170(5):390, 1990.
Cooke DM: Inflammatory bowel disease: primary health care management of ulcerative colitis and Crohn's disease, *Nurs Pract* 16(8):27, 1991.
Corman ML: *Colon and rectal surgery*, ed 2, Philadelphia, 1989, Lippincott.
Dalton-Loehner D, Connor P: Beyond ileostomy: surgery for a normal life, *RN* 52:29, 1989.
Doughty D: A step-by-step approach to bowel training, *Progressions* 4(2):12, 1992.
Eastwood A, Avundu KC: *Manual of gastroenterology: diagnosis and therapy*, Boston, 1988, Little, Brown.
Ebersole P, Hess P: *Toward healthy aging: human needs and nursing response*, St Louis, 1994, Mosby.
Fruto LV: Current concepts: management of diarrhea in acute care, *J Wound, Ostomy, and Continence Nurs (WOCN)* 21(5):199, 1994.
Gawron CL: Unit-based quality assurance: a necessary component of ET nursing practice, *J ET Nurs* 20(2):42, 1993.
Gilpatrick DM: Moving clients towards wellness: behavioral change, *Clin Nurs Spec* 3(1):25, 1989.
Goldfinger SE: Constipation: the hard facts. I. *Harvard Health Letter* 16(4):1, 1991.
Hampton BG, Bryant RA: *Ostomies and continent diversions: Nursing management*, St Louis, 1992, Mosby.
Kim MJ, McFarland GK, McLane AM: *Pocket guide to nursing diagnoses*, ed 6, St Louis, 1995, Mosby.
Lueckenotte AG: *Pocket guide to gerontologic assessment*, ed 2, St Louis, 1994, Mosby.
McGarity WC: Gastrointestinal surgical procedures. In Hampton BG, Bryant RA: *Ostomies and continent diversions: nursing management*, St Louis, 1992, Mosby.

Mihalopoulos NG et al: The psychologic impact of ostomy surgery on persons 50 years of age and older, *J Wound, Ostomy, Continence Nurs (WOCN)* 21(4):149, 1994.

Oetman BK, Trout RJ: Innovative pouch modification for high-output ostomy drainage, *J wound, ostomy, and continence nursing (WOCN)*, 21(1):34, 1994.

Powe BD: Fatalism among elderly African Americans: effects on colorectal cancer screening, *Cancer Nurs* 18(5):385, 1995.

Robinson C, Weigley E: *Basic nutrition and diet therapy*, ed 6, New York, 1989, Macmillan.

Rolstad BS, Hoyman K: Continent diversions and reservoirs. In Hampton BG, Bryant RA: *Ostomies and continent diversions: nursing management*, St Louis, 1992, Mosby.

Ross D: Constipation among hospitalized elders, *Orthop Nurs* 9(3):73, 1990.

Swartz ML: Citrucel (methylcellulose/bulk-forming laxative), *Gastroenterol Nurse* 12(1):50, 1989.

Tortora GJ: *Principles of human anatomy*, ed 5, New York, 1989, Harper & Row.

Walsh BA et al: Psychometric evaluation of body image and quality of life following ostomy surgery. Oral abstract presented at the Wound, Ostomy, Continence Nurses Society (WOCN) 27th Annual Conference, Denver, Colorado, May 18, 1995.

ADDITIONAL READINGS

Allison OC, Porter ME, Briggs GC: Chronic constipation: assessment and management in the elderly, *J Am Acad Nurs Pract* 6(7):311, 1994.

Canty SL: Consitpation as a side effect of opoids, *Onocol Nurs Forum* 21(4):739, 1994.

Fruto LV: Current concepts: management of diarrhea in acute care, *J WOCN* 21(5):199, 1994.

Hall G et al: Managing constipation using a research based protocol, *Medsburg Nurs* 4(1):11, 1995.

Hogstel MO, Nelson M: Anticipation and early detection can reduce bowel elimination complications, *Geriatr Nurs Am J Aging* 13(1):28, 1992.

Kurz JM: Combating antibiotic-induced diarrhea. . .yogurt, *Am J Nurs* 95(6):24K, 1995.

Laim E: Management of constipation in adults, *World Council Enterostomal Ther J* 14(4):11, 1995.

Mahaney-Price AF: Care report. Bacterial overgrowth in a patient with chronic diarreaha, *Nurse Pract Am J Primary Care* 20(9):60, 1995.

Mohle-Boetani JC et al: Communitywide shigellosis: control of an outbreak and risk factors in child day-care centers, *Am J Public Health* 85 (6):812, 1995.

Neal LJ: "Power pudding": natural laxative therapy for the elderly who are homebound, *Home Healthcare Nurs* 13(3):66, 1995.

Ross DG: Altered bowel elimination patterns among hosptialized elderly and middle-aged person: quantatitive results, *Orthop Nurs* 14(1):25 1995.

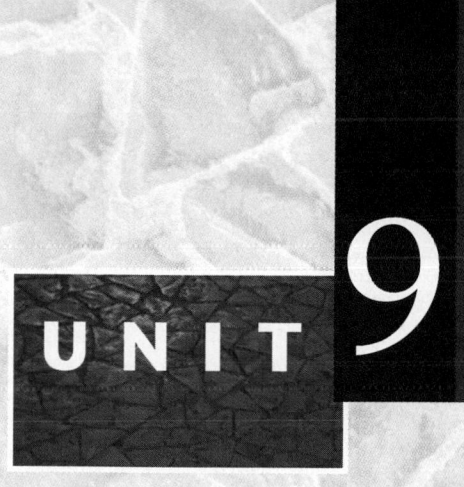

UNIT 9

Caring for the Perioperative Client

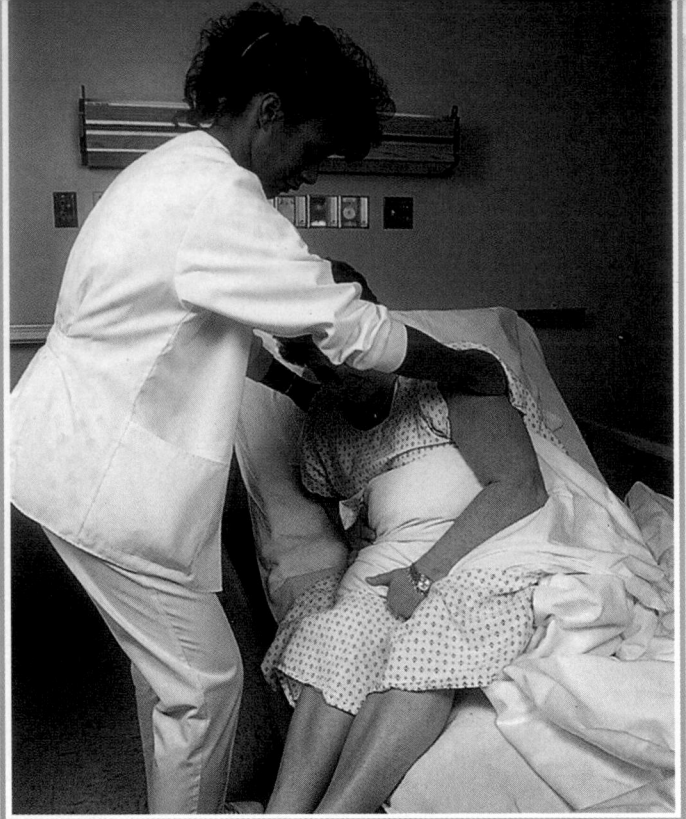

## Chapter 48

Surgical Client

Objectives

Mastery of content in this chapter will enable the student to:

▶ Define the key terms listed.

▶ Explain the concept of perioperative nursing care.

▶ Differentiate between classifications of surgery.

▶ List factors to include in the preoperative assessment of a surgical client.

▶ Describe how to correctly witness a client's informed consent for surgery.

▶ Demonstrate postoperative exercises: diaphragmatic breathing, coughing, turning, and leg exercises.

▶ Provide a client preoperative instruction.

▶ Prepare a client for surgery.

▶ Compare and contrast the actions and side effects of general, regional, and local anesthesia.

▶ Explain the nurse's role in the operating room.

▶ Describe the nurse's role in phase I and II recovery.

▶ Identify factors to include in the postoperative assessment of a client in recovery.

▶ Describe the rationale for nursing interventions designed to prevent postoperative complications.

▶ Explain the difference and similarities in caring for outpatient versus inpatient surgical clients.

Perioperative nursing care includes nursing care given before (preoperative), during (intraoperative), and after surgery (postoperative). It may take place in the hospital, in a free-standing surgical center, in a surgical center attached to a hospital, or in a physician's office. Perioperative nursing is a fast-paced, changing, and challenging field in which to work. It is based on several important characteristics including high quality teamwork; effective and therapeutic communication with the client, client's family, and the surgical team; effective and efficient client assessment in all phases; advocacy for the client and client's family; and understanding of cost containment. The nurse must practice good surgical asepsis; thoroughly document care; and emphasize client safety in all phases. Effective teaching and discharge planning are needed to prevent or minimize complications. **Perioperative nursing** is based on the nursing process and the nurse is called upon to individualize strategies throughout the perioperative period so that the client has a smooth course from admission through convalescence. The continuity of care is stressed in this model.

A client experiences a variety of stressors when facing surgery. Anticipating surgery leads to fear and anxiety for clients who associate surgery with pain, possible disfigurement, dependence, and perhaps even death. The client may be concerned about loss of income or insurance coverage due to hospitalization. Family members often fear a disruption in lifestyle and experience a sense of powerlessness as the surgery approaches. The ability to establish rapport with clients effectively and actively listen to them so that their concerns are addressed is important to the outcome of surgery. The client is better able to cooperate and participate in care if the nurse has provided information about events occurring before and after surgery. This **preoperative teaching** helps to relieve fear of the unknown for the client and family and results in decreased length of hospital stay, decreased use of analgesics postoperatively, and a client who can comply with a postoperative regimen (Dalayon, 1994).

Ambulatory outpatient surgical units are increasingly common. A client enters the unit, undergoes surgery, and returns home the same day. Nurses working in perioperative settings must understand the principles of caring for surgical clients.

HISTORY OF SURGICAL NURSING

Surgery became a medical specialty in the mid–nineteenth century. Surgery gave physicians the means to treat conditions that were difficult or impossible to manage only by pure medicine. However, early surgeons had little knowledge of the principles of asepsis, and anesthesia techniques were primitive and unsafe. Indeed, a surgeon's success was based on speed. However, the discovery of anesthesia in the 1840s made it possible for surgeons to operate on a client who was free of pain. This was a revolution for surgery. Nurses working in the first operating rooms cleaned the rooms and equipment, performed technical tasks such as obtaining supplies, and occasionally accompanied the client to the surgical ward to deliver nursing care.

With the advent of antiseptic and later aseptic practices, surgery became a treatment of choice for many conditions. The development of safer anesthetic gases allowed surgeons to conduct longer operative procedures. All surgery was conducted in hospital settings. Massachusetts General Hospital provided the first operating room education for nurses in 1876. This trend continued into the 1900s as nursing schools included operating room experience in each nurse's clinical instruction.

In 1956 the Association of Operating Room Nurses (AORN) was formed to gain knowledge of surgical principles and explore methods to improve nursing care of surgical clients. The association met many challenges, including overcoming the idea that operating room nurses were only technically skilled practitioners. The organization developed standards of nursing practice to establish the need for registered nurses in the operating room.

During the 1970s a change occurred in nursing education. A focus on the importance of nurses acquiring a broad knowledge base resulted in less emphasis on operating room techniques. Many schools eliminated operating room experience from curriculums. However, today many nursing schools have reinstituted clinical operating room experience.

There has also been a new development in the setting for operative procedures. Ambulatory surgery, sometimes referred to as *outpatient* or *one-day surgery,* is a health care service that is growing rapidly in numbers and types of procedures performed. **Ambulatory surgery** is a scheduled surgical procedure provided for a client who does not remain overnight in a hospital. Biopsies, cosmetic surgery, and cataract extractions are just a few examples of ambulatory procedures. By 1995, more than 60% of all surgery was conducted on an ambulatory basis (Parnass, 1993; Meeker and Rothrock, 1995). The number continues to increase.

There are distinct benefits for the client who has ambulatory surgery. Discovery of anesthetic drugs that metabolize rapidly with few aftereffects allows shorter operative times. Nurses recognize the benefit of early postoperative ambulation and encourage clients to assume an active role in recovery. Ambulatory surgery also offers cost savings by eliminating the need for hospital stays. Frequently, costly diagnostic tests and laboratory data are not required, which also decreases the cost of ambulatory surgery (Meeker and Rothrock, 1995). It also offers a decrease in the possibility of acquiring nosocomial infections as once clients are hospitalized, their normal skin flora changes and they soon become colonized with bacteria found in the hospital (Morales and Andrews, 1993).

In addition to traditional inpatient surgical stays and outpatient ambulatory surgery, most hospitals have same-day surgical programs. In a same-day surgical program a client is admitted early on the morning of surgery, undergoes the surgical procedure and then stays one night during recovery before being discharged.

Procedures such as tumor biopsies and gallbladder removal (**cholecystectomy**) can now be done using laser procedures. For example, a laser or laparoscopic cholecystectomy only involves a few hours to a 24-hour hospital stay and a recovery period of a week. By contrast, a traditional cholecystectomy usually involves a 3 to 5 day hospitalization and at least a 4-week recovery period. Thus many surgeons use laser procedures instead of traditional surgical procedures, thereby decreasing the length of surgery, hospitalization, and the associated costs.

Ambulatory and same-day surgical programs provide challenges for surgical nurses. Before surgery, nurses must find creative ways to educate clients and family members. The preparation time before surgery is shortened, so nurses must perform complete assessments efficiently. Frequently assessments are begun in a preadmission clinic where clients may answer a self-report inventory, a rudimentary physical is completed by a surgical nurse, lab tests may be drawn or completed, teaching is begun, questions are answered, and paperwork is initiated. This streamlines the care required by the client on the day of surgery. The surgical procedures performed in ambulatory surgery also require special considerations by the nurse. Changing trends in care of surgical clients have changed the nurse's role.

CLASSIFICATION OF SURGERY

The types of surgical procedures are classified according to the seriousness, urgency, or purpose of surgery (Table 48-1). A procedure may fall into more than one classification. For example, surgical removal of a disfiguring scar is minor in seriousness, elective in urgency, and reconstructive in purpose. Frequently the classes overlap. An urgent procedure is also considered major in seriousness. The same operation may be performed for different reasons on different clients. For example, a gastrectomy may be performed as an emergency procedure to resect a bleeding ulcer or as an urgent procedure to remove a cancerous growth. The classification indicates to the nurse the level of care a client might require.

PREOPERATIVE SURGICAL PHASE

Surgical clients enter the health care setting in different stages of health. A client may enter the hospital or ambulatory satellite unit on a predetermined day feeling relatively healthy and prepared to face elective surgery. In contrast, a victim of a vehicle accident may face emergency surgery with no time to prepare. The ability to establish rapport and maintain a professional relationship is an essential component of the preoperative phase. Nurses must do this quickly, easily, and effectively (see Chapter 14).

The surgical client may undergo tests and procedures to confirm or rule out alterations requiring surgery. Many tests can be performed in the physician's office or an outpatient laboratory. Usually clients scheduled for ambulatory surgery have tests done several days before surgery. However, the tests can also be done the morning of surgery. Nurses must be familiar with the tests, their purpose and how to monitor results.

NURSING PROCESS AND THE SURGICAL CLIENT

The client meets many health care personnel, including surgeons, nurse anesthetists or anesthesiologists, therapists, and nurses. All play a role in the client's care and recovery. Family members attempt to provide support through their presence but face many of the same stressors as the client. The nurse must effectively communicate with the client and family; the nurse-client relationship is the foundation of care (see Chapter 14). The nurse assesses the client's physical and emotional well-being, recognizes the degree of surgical risk, coordinates diagnostic tests, identifies nursing diagnoses reflecting the client's and family members' needs, prepares the client physically and mentally for surgery, and communicates pertinent information to the surgical team.

 ## Assessment

Assessment of the surgical client involves collecting a nursing history, performing a physical examination, reviewing the client's and family members' emotional health, and analyzing risk factors and diagnostic data. The length of the preoperative period determines the thoroughness of assessment.

For example, if a client is a same-day admission, there may not be enough time to do a comprehensive physical examination. In this case the nurse focuses on key measurements for all body systems to ensure that no obvious problems are overlooked. Even though the physician will screen the client before scheduling surgery, preoperative assessment occasionally reveals an abnormality that delays or cancels surgery. Usually, however, the assessment establishes normal values for the client and alerts the nurse to possible postoperative complications.

Nursing History

The nurse conducts an initial interview to collect a history similar to that described in Chapter 33. In the ambulatory surgical setting the history may be shorter than that collected when the client is hospitalized the evening before surgery because of time constraints. If a client is unable to relate all necessary information the nurse may ask family members.

MEDICAL HISTORY

A review of the client's medical history should include past illnesses and the primary reason for seeking medical care. The client's medical history is an excellent source. Another valuable source of data is medical records from past hospitalizations.

Preexisting illnesses can influence the ability to tolerate surgery and reach full recovery (Table 48-2). Candidates for ambulatory surgery must be carefully screened for medical conditions that may increase the risk for complications during or after surgery.

PREVIOUS SURGERIES

A client's past experience with surgery can influence physical and psychological responses to a procedure. The previous type of surgery, level of discomfort, extent of disability, and overall level of care provided are some factors the client may recall. The nurse assesses any complications that the client experienced. This information helps the nurse anticipate the client's preoperative and postoperative needs.

Previous surgery may also influence the level of physical care required after a surgical procedure. For example, a client who has had a previous thoracotomy for resection of a lung lobe has a greater risk for postoperative pulmonary complications than a client with intact normal lungs.

CLIENTS' AND FAMILY MEMBERS' PERCEPTIONS AND UNDERSTANDING OF SURGERY

The nurse must prepare clients and their families for the surgical experience. Identification of clients' knowledge, expectations, and perceptions allows the nurse to plan teaching and emotional preparation measures. If clients are scheduled for ambulatory surgery, assessment may be per-

Table 48-1	Classification for Surgical Procedures	
TYPE	**DESCRIPTION**	**EXAMPLE**
SERIOUSNESS		
Major	Involves extensive reconstruction or alteration in body parts; poses great risks to well-being	Coronary artery bypass, colon resection, removal of larynx, resection of lung lobe
Minor	Involves minimal alteration in body parts; often designed to correct deformities; involves minimal risks compared with major procedures	Cataract extraction, facial plastic surgery, skin graft, tooth extraction
URGENCY		
Elective	Is performed on basis of client's choice; is not essential and may not be necessary for health	Bunionectomy, facial plastic surgery, hernia repair, breast reconstruction
Urgent	Is necessary for client's health, may prevent additional problems from developing (e.g., tissue destruction or impaired organ function); not necessarily emergency	Excision of cancerous tumor, removal of gallbladder for stones, vascular repair for obstructed artery (e.g., coronary artery bypass)
Emergency	Must be done immediately to save life or preserve function of body part	Repair of perforated appendix, repair of traumatic amputation, control of internal hemorrhaging
PURPOSE		
Diagnostic	Is surgical exploration that allows physician to confirm diagnosis; may involve removal of tissue for further diagnostic testing	Exploratory laparotomy (incision into peritoneal cavity to inspect abdominal organs), breast mass biopsy
Ablative	Is excision or removal of diseased body part	Amputation, removal of appendix, cholecystectomy
Palliative	Relieves or reduces intensity of disease symptoms; will not produce cure	Colostomy, debridement of necrotic tissue, resection of nerve roots
Reconstructive	Restores function or appearance to traumatized or malfunctioning tissues	Internal fixation of fractures, scar revision
Transplant	Is performed to replace malfunctioning organs or structures	Kidney, cornea, or liver transplant; total hip replacement
Constructive	Restores function lost or reduced as result of congenital anomalies	Repair of cleft palate, closure of atrial septal defect in heart

Table 48-2	Medical Conditions That Increase the Risks of Surgery
TYPE OF CONDITION	**REASON FOR RISK**
Bleeding disorders (thrombocytopenia, hemophilia)	Disorders increase risk of hemorrhaging during and after surgery.
Diabetes mellitus	Diabetes increases susceptibility to infection and may impair wound healing from altered glucose metabolism and associated circulatory impairment. Fluctuating blood levels may cause central nervous system (CNS) malfunction during anesthesia. Stress of surgery may cause decreased glucose tolerance.
Heart disease (recent myocardial infarction, dysrhythmias, congestive heart failure)	Stress of surgery causes increased demands on myocardium to maintain cardiac output. General anesthetic agents depress cardiac function.
Upper respiratory infection	Infection increases risk of respiratory complications during anesthesia (e.g., pneumonia and spasm of laryngeal muscles).
Liver disease	Liver disease alters metabolism and elimination of drugs administered during surgery and impairs wound healing and clotting time because of alterations in protein metabolism.
Fever	Fever predisposes client to fluid and electrolyte imbalances and may indicate underlying infection.
Chronic respiratory disease (emphysema, bronchitis, asthma)	Respiratory disease reduces client's means to compensate for acid-base alterations (see Chapter 45). Anesthetic agents reduce respiratory function, increasing risk for severe hypoventilation.
Immunological disorders (leukemia, AIDS, bone marrow depression, and use of chemotherapeutic drugs)	Immunological disorders increase risk of infection and delay wound healing after surgery.
Abuse of street drugs	Persons abusing drugs may have underlying disease (HIV/hepatitis) and altered wellness, which affect healing.

formed in the physician's office or clients' homes.

Each client brings fears to the surgical setting. Some are due to past hospital experiences, warnings from friends and family, or lack of knowledge. The nurse faces an ethical dilemma when a client is misinformed or unaware of the reason for surgery. The nurse asks for a description of the client's understanding of the planned surgery and its implications. The nurse might ask questions such as "Tell me what you think will happen before and after surgery" or "Explain what you know about surgery." The nurse should confer with the physician before revealing specific information about the medical diagnosis. The nurse also determines whether the physician explained routine preoperative and postoperative procedures. When a client is well prepared and knows what to expect, the nurse reinforces the client's knowledge and maintains accuracy and consistency.

MEDICATION HISTORY

If a client regularly uses prescription or over-the-counter drugs, the surgeon or anesthesiologist/anesthetist may temporarily discontinue the drugs before surgery or adjust the dosages (Table 48-3). Certain drugs have special implications for the surgical client. Prescription drugs taken preoperatively are automatically discontinued postoperatively unless a physician reorders them.

ALLERGIES

The nurse is alert for allergies to drugs that may be given during a phase of the surgical experience. If one or more allergies exist, the client receives an allergy identification band to be worn on the wrist before going to surgery. The nurse also makes sure that the front of the client's chart contains a list of allergies.

SMOKING HABITS

The client who smokes is at greater risk for postoperative pulmonary complications than a client who does not. The chronic smoker already has an increased amount and thickness of mucous secretions in the lungs. General anesthetics increase airway irritation and stimulate pulmonary secretions, which are retained as a result of reduction in ciliary activity during anesthesia. After surgery the client who smokes has greater difficulty clearing the airways of mucous secretions (see Chapter 44).

ALCOHOL INGESTION AND SUBSTANCE USE AND ABUSE

Habitual use of alcohol predisposes the client to adverse reactions to anesthetic drugs. The client also experiences a cross-tolerance to anesthetic drugs, necessitating higher-than-normal doses. In addition, the physician may need to increase postoperative dosages of analgesics. Excessive alcohol ingestion can also lead to malnutrition, which may contribute to delayed wound healing. Use of prescription narcotics, barbiturates, and abuse of street drugs may impair the ability of the client to manage pain following surgery as well as affect the level and amount of anesthesia during surgery. IV drug use may impair the vascular system and may make venous access difficult. The client is more likely to be exposed to diseases like HIV and hepatitis.

FAMILY SUPPORT

It is important for the nurse to determine the extent of the client's support from family members or friends. Surgery often results in temporary or permanent disability that requires added assistance during recovery. The client usually cannot immediately assume the same level of physical activity enjoyed before an illness. Often a client returns home with dressings to change or exercises to perform. With ambulatory surgery, clients and families assume responsibility for postoperative care. The family is an important resource for the client with physical limitations and provides the emotional support needed to motivate the client to return to a previous state of health.

Table 48-3	Drugs with Special Implications for the Surgical Client
DRUG CLASS	**EFFECTS DURING SURGERY**
Antibiotics	Antibiotics potentiate action of anesthetic agents. If taken within 2 wk before surgery, aminoglycosides (gentamicin, tobramycin, neomycin) may cause mild respiratory depression from depressed neuromuscular transmission.
Antidysrhythmics	Antidysrhythmics can reduce cardiac contractility and impair cardiac conduction during anesthesia.
Anticoagulants	Anticoagulants alter normal clotting factors and thus increase risk of hemorrhaging. They should be discontinued at least 48 hr before surgery. Aspirin and ibuprofen are commonly used medications that can alter clotting mechanisms.
Anticonvulsants	Long-term use of certain anticonvulsants (e.g., phenytoin [Dilantin] and phenobarbital) can alter metabolism of anesthetic agents.
Antihypertensives	Antihypertensives interact with anesthetic agents to cause bradycardia, hypotension, and impaired circulation. They inhibit synthesis and storage of norepinephrine in sympathetic nerve endings.
Corticosteroids	With prolonged use, corticosteroids cause adrenal atrophy, which reduces body's ability to withstand stress. Before and during surgery, dosages may be temporarily increased.
Insulin	Diabetic client's need for insulin after surgery is reduced because client's nutritional intake is decreased. Stress response and intravenous (IV) administration of glucose solutions can increase dosage requirements after surgery.
Diuretics	Diuretics potentiate electrolyte imbalances (particularly potassium) after surgery.

OCCUPATION

Surgery may result in physical alterations that hinder or prevent a person from returning to work. Ideally the nurse assesses the client's occupational history to anticipate the possible effects of surgery on recovery and eventual work performance. This prepares the nurse to explain any restrictions before a client returns to work. When a client is unable to return to a job, the nurse confers with a social worker and/or occupational therapist to refer the client to job-training programs or to help the client seek economic assistance.

PREOPERATIVE PAIN ASSESSMENT

Surgery, treatments, and positioning may result in postoperative pain for the client. It is very helpful to assess a client preoperatively with regard to previous pain experience, previously used methods of pain control, attitudes about taking pain medication, behavioral responses to pain, client knowledge of, expectations about, and preferences for pain management methods, and family expectations or concerns about pain management (Miaskowski, 1993). Clients believe mistakenly that the nurse will detect their pain and treat it. An objective measurement of pain severity using a visual analog scale (see Chapter 43) provides a baseline for monitoring change in the client's condition. Frequent pain assessments are necessary to alert the nurse to treat the pain. Preoperative explanations by the nurse of anticipated pain sensations and the goals of pain therapy will facilitate the assessment and treatment of postoperative pain (Watt-Watson and Donovan, 1992.)

REVIEW OF EMOTIONAL HEALTH

Surgery is psychologically stressful. The client is anxious about the surgery and its implications. Clients often feel that they have little control over their situation. Family members perceive the client's surgery as a disruption of their lifestyle. Hospitalization and the recovery period at home may be lengthy. The family is usually concerned about the client returning to a normal, productive life. When the client has chronic illness, the family may be fearful that surgery may result in further disability or hopeful that it may improve their lifestyle. To understand the impact of surgery on a client's and family's emotional health, the nurse assesses the client's feelings about surgery, self-concept, body image, and coping resources.

Feelings. The nurse may be able to detect the client's feelings about surgery from mannerisms or behavior. A fearful client often asks many questions, seems uneasy when strangers enter the room, or actively seeks the company of friends and relatives.

It is often difficult to assess feelings thoroughly when ambulatory surgery is scheduled. The nurse usually has less time to establish a relationship with the client. In some outpatient surgical programs the nurse may visit with a client in the home or on the telephone before surgery. In a hospital room the nurse should choose a time for discussion after admitting procedures or diagnostic tests are completed. The nurse should explain that it is normal to have fears and concerns. The client's ability to share feelings depends on the nurse's willingness to listen, be supportive, and clarify misconceptions.

If the client feels powerless, the nurse determines the reason. The medical diagnosis may generate apprehension of increased dependence and loss of physical or mental function. The thought of being "put to sleep" under anesthesia creates concern about loss of control. Many clients feel the need to retain the power to make decisions about treatment. The nurse must assure clients of their right to ask questions and seek information.

A client may be angry about the need for surgery. A young person may feel that it is unfair to have a disorder that typically affects older people. Surgery may occur at a time when it is inconvenient or potentially disruptive. The client may occasionally express anger by verbally attacking the nurse or physician. Being argumentative or overly demanding, refusing to cooperate, and criticizing the nurse's efforts to provide care are manifestations of anger and anxiety.

Self-Concept. Clients with a positive self-concept are more likely to approach surgical experiences appropriately. The nurse assesses self-concept by asking clients to identify personal strengths and weaknesses. Clients who are quick to criticize or scorn personal characteristics may have little self regard or may be testing the nurse's opinion of their characters. Poor self-concept hinders the ability to adapt to the stress of surgery and aggravates feelings of guilt or inadequacy (see Chapter 23).

Body Image. Surgical removal of any diseased body part often leaves permanent disfigurement or alteration in body function. Concern over mutilation or loss of a body part compounds a client's fears.

The nurse assesses for the body image alterations that clients perceive will result from surgery. Individuals will react differently depending on self-concept and degree of self-esteem (see Chapter 23).

Often surgery changes the physical or psychological aspects of clients' sexuality. Excision of breast tissue, colostomies or ureterostomies, or removal of prostate glands may affect clients' perceptions of their sexuality. Surgery such as hernia repair or cataract extraction forces clients to refrain from sexual intercourse until they return to normal physical activity.

The nurse should encourage clients to express concerns about sexuality. The client facing even temporary sexual dysfunction requires understanding and support. Discussions about the client's sexuality should be held with the client's sexual partner so that they can gain a shared understanding of how to cope with limitations in sexual function.

Coping Resources. Assessment of feelings and self-concept helps reveal whether the client can cope with the stress of surgery. The nurse also asks the client about past stress management. If the client has had previous surgery, the nurse determines behaviors that helped resolve any tension or nervousness. The nurse may instruct the client on relaxation exercises that can help control anxiety (see Chapter 22).

The nurse should ask if family members or friends can provide support. The client may want someone else present when the nurse provides instructions or explanations. Often a family member can become the client's coach, offering valuable support during the postoperative period when the client's participation in care is vital.

CULTURE

Clients from different cultures may react to the perioperative experience in different ways. Nursing from a multicultural perspective assists nurses to have a frame of reference in approaching clients with respect and to individually tailor care that promotes recovery.

For example, use of the client's language helps to place an anxious client at ease. The nurse can utilize interpreters, learn foreign languages or some key phrases, and use references like medical dictionaries, which usually have key phrases listed in the appendix. Knowing that eye contact may be disrespectful in Southeast Asian and Native American clients, the nurse limits it. Talking to the male head of the family may be necessary when working with clients from the Middle East and Southeast Asia. Chinese clients may not ask for pain medications and need teaching that helps to explain that being comfortable promotes healing and a quicker recovery (see the box below). These are a few ways to adjust preoperative care for clients who speak a different language than the nurse and come from a different culture.

PHYSICAL EXAMINATION

The nurse conducts a partial or complete physical examination, depending on the amount of time available and the client's preoperative condition. Chapter 33 describes techniques used in physical assessment. Assessment focuses on findings related to the client's medical history and on body systems that will be affected by the surgery.

General Survey. The nurse observes the client's general appearance. Gestures and body movements may reflect weakness caused by illness. The client may appear malnourished to the nurse. Height and body weight are important indicators of nutritional status.

Preoperative assessment of vital signs, including blood pressure while sitting and standing, provides important baseline data with which to compare alterations that occur during and after surgery. Some institutions request that blood pressure be obtained in both arms for comparison. Anxiety and fear commonly cause elevations in heart rate and blood pressure. Anesthetic agents typically depress all vital functions. However, adverse drug reactions may include elevations in heart rate and blood pressure. As the effects of the anesthesia diminish after surgery, the nurse closely monitors vital signs and compares findings with preoperative baseline.

Preoperative assessment of vital signs is also important to rule out fluid and electrolyte abnormalities (see Chapter 45). An elevated heart rate may result from a plasma fluid volume deficit, potassium deficit, or sodium excess. If the pulse is full and bounding, a fluid volume excess may be the cause. Cardiac dysrhythmias are commonly caused by electrolyte imbalances.

An elevated temperature before surgery is a cause for concern. If the client has an underlying infection the surgeon may choose to postpone surgery until the infection has been treated. An elevated body temperature increases the risk of fluid and electrolyte imbalance after surgery.

Head and Neck. The condition of oral mucous membranes reveals the level of hydration. A dehydrated client is at risk for developing serious fluid and electrolyte imbalances during surgery.

Inspection of the soft palate and nasal sinuses can reveal sinus drainage indicative of respiratory or sinus infection. To rule out the possibility of local or systemic infection, the nurse palpates for cervical lymph node enlargement.

The nurse inspects the jugular veins for distention. Excess fluid within the circulatory system or failure of the heart to contract efficiently may lead to jugular vein distention. A client with heart disease is at risk for cardiovascular complications during surgery.

Integument. The nurse carefully inspects the skin overlying all body parts. Particular attention is paid to bony prominences, such as the elbows, sacrum, and scapula. During surgery, a client must lie in a fixed position, often for several hours. Thus a client is susceptible to pressure ulcers (see Chapter 38) if the skin is thin and dry and has poor turgor. The overall condition of the skin also reveals the client's level of hydration. An older adult is at high risk for alteration in skin integrity from positioning and sliding on the OR table causing shear and pressure.

Thorax and Lungs. Assessment of the client's breathing pattern and chest excursion aids in assessing ventilatory capacity. Clients are encouraged to deep breathe and cough postoperatively (see section on preoperative teaching). A decline in ventilatory function may place the client at risk for respiratory complications. For example, a client who has high abdominal surgery will have difficulty breathing deeply because of a painful abdominal incision. Ausculta-

RESEARCH HIGHLIGHT

RESEARCH ABSTRACT

The purpose of this study was to investigate whether nurses provide different amounts of narcotic analgesics to male and female clients, and different amounts to white and ethnic minority clients. A retrospective study was conducted with the medical records of 101 male and 79 female clients who had uncomplicated appendectomies, 40 of whom were ethnic minority members. Narcotic analgesic doses for the entire postoperative period were converted to equianalgesic doses comparable to intramuscular morphine. Male clients received significantly larger initial doses than female clients. There was no gender difference in the total dose received postoperatively. White clients received significantly more total postoperative narcotic analgesics than did ethnic minority clients. The ethnic difference suggests that irrelevant cues may be used in nurses' medication decisions.

IMPLICATIONS FOR PRACTICE

▶ Nurses who respond to clients who make their needs known avoid gender stereotyping.
▶ Undermedication of pain by nurses may be a concern for all clients especially ethnic minority clients. Nurses can improve by accurately assessing pain and evaluating interventions.
▶ Nurses may use irrelevant cues when assessing pain and need to remember that the most reliable indicator is the client's self-report.

REFERENCE

McDonald D: Gender and ethnic stereotyping and narcotic analgesic administration, *Research in Nursing & Health* 17:45, 1994.

tion of breath sounds will indicate whether the client has pulmonary congestion or narrowing of airways. Existing atelectasis or moisture in the airways will be aggravated during surgery. Serious pulmonary congestion may cause postponement of the surgery. Certain anesthetics can cause laryngeal muscle spasm; thus, if the nurse auscultates wheezing in the airways preoperatively, the client is at risk for further airway narrowing during surgery. The nurse should assess for clubbing of the fingers, which may indicate lung disease and possible postanesthetic difficulty (Blackwood, 1986).

Heart and Vascular System. If the client has cardiac disease, the nurse must assess the character of the apical pulse. After surgery the nurse compares the rate and rhythm of the pulse with preoperative baselines. Anesthetic agents, alterations in fluid balance, and stimulation from the surgical stress response can cause cardiac dysrhythmias.

The nurse assesses peripheral pulses, capillary refill time, and the color and temperature of extremities to determine a client's circulatory status. Capillary refill time is assessed by depressing the client's finger or toe nail bed until the skin blanches, releasing the pressure, and then noting the amount of time that it takes for the color to return to the original appearance. Acceptable capillary refill occurs in less than 3 seconds. Sluggish capillary refill is refill time greater than 3 seconds.

Measurement of capillary refill is particularly important for the client having vascular surgery or for a client who may have casts or constricting bandages applied to the extremities after surgery. Postoperative development of a weak or absent pulse in a client who had adequate circulation before surgery indicates impaired circulation.

Abdomen. The nurse assesses the abdomen for size, shape, symmetry, and distention. If the client has abdominal surgery, the nurse makes frequent postoperative assessments of the abdominal incision and compares findings with preoperative data. Distention may indicate postoperative alterations in gastrointestinal function. The nurse should know whether the client has a protuberant abdomen or whether the abdomen has become distended after surgery.

Assessment of preoperative bowel sounds is useful as a baseline. The nurse also determines whether the client has regular bowel movements. If the surgery requires manipulation of the gastrointestinal tract or if a general anesthetic is used, normal peristalsis will not return and bowel sounds will be absent or diminished for several days after surgery.

Neurological Status. During the health history and physical assessment, the nurse observes the client's level of orientation, alertness, and mood, noting whether the client answers questions appropriately and can recall recent and past events. A client who will have surgery for neurological disease (e.g., brain tumor or aneurysm) is likely to demonstrate an impaired level of consciousness or altered behavior. Level of consciousness changes as a result of general anesthesia. However, after the effects of anesthesia disappear, the client should return to the preoperative level of responsiveness.

If the client will have spinal anesthesia, preoperative assessment of gross motor function and strength is important. Spinal anesthesia causes temporary paralysis of the lower extremities. The nurse should be aware of a client entering surgery with weakness or impaired mobility of the lower extremities to avoid becoming alarmed when full motor function does not return as the spinal anesthetic wears off.

RISK FACTORS

Various conditions and factors increase a person's risk in surgery. Knowledge of risk factors enables the nurse to take necessary precautions in planning care.

The American Society of Anesthesiologists (ASA) assigns classification based on a client's physiological condition independent of the proposed surgical procedure (see Table 48-4). Intraoperative difficulties occur more frequently with clients who have a poor physical status classification (Meeker and Rothrock, 1995). Previously, ambulatory surgical experiences were limited to clients ASA classified as 1 and 2. Now, ASA physical status 3 clients are being allowed if the client's medical disease is stable (Parnass, 1993).

Age. Very young and old clients are at risk during surgery because of immature or declining physiological sta-

Table 48-4	Physical Status Classification of the American Society of Anesthesiologists	
CLASS	**DESCRIPTION**	**CHARACTERISTICS**
P1	A normal healthy client	No physiological, biological, organic disturbance
P2	A client with a mild systemic disease	Cardiovascular (CV) disease with minimal restriction on activity Hypertension (HTN), obesity, diabetes mellitus (DM)
P3	A client with a severe systemic disease that limits activity but is not incapacitating	CV or pulmonary disease that limits activity; severe diabetes with systemic complications; history of myocardial infarction (MI), angina pectoris, or poorly controlled HTN
P4	A client with a severe systemic disease that is a constant threat to life	Severe cardiac, pulmonary, renal, hepatic, or endocrine dysfunction
P5	A **moribund** client who is not expected to survive 24 hours with/without the operation	Surgery is done as a last recourse of resuscitative effort; major multisystem or cerebral trauma, ruptured aneurysm, or large pulmonary embolus
P6	A client declared brain dead whose organs are being removed for donor purpose.	

Modified from Meeker M, Rothrock J: *Alexander's care of the patient in surgery,* ed 10, St Louis, 1995, Mosby.

tus. During surgery, nurses and physicians are especially concerned with maintaining an infant's normal body temperature. The infant's shivering reflex is underdeveloped, and often wide temperature variations occur. Anesthesia adds to the risk because anesthetics can cause vasodilation and heat loss.

During surgery an infant has difficulty maintaining a normal circulatory blood volume. The total blood volume of an infant is considerably less than that of an older child or an adult. Even a small amount of blood loss can be serious. A reduced circulatory volume makes it difficult for the infant to respond to the need for increased oxygen during

Table 48-5	Physiological Factors that Place the Older Adult at Risk During Surgery	
ALTERATIONS	**RISKS**	**NURSING IMPLICATIONS**
CARDIOVASCULAR SYSTEM		
Degenerative change in myocardium and valves	Change reduces cardiac reserve.	Assess baseline vital signs.
Rigidity of arterial walls and reduction in sympathetic and parasympathetic innervation to heart	Alterations predispose client to postoperative hemorrhage and rise in systolic and diastolic blood pressure.	
Increase in calcium and cholesterol deposits within small arteries; thickened arterial walls	Problems predispose client to clot formation in lower extremities.	Instruct client on techniques for performing leg exercises and proper turning.
		Apply elastic stockings; SCDs (sequential compression devices).
INTEGUMENTARY SYSTEM		
Decreased subcutaneous tissue and increased fragility of skin	Prone to pressure ulcers and tears.	Assess skin every 4 hours; pad all bony prominences during surgery. Turn or reposition.
PULMONARY SYSTEM		
Rib cage stiffened and reduced in size	Complication reduces vital capacity.	Instruct client on proper technique for coughing, deep-breathing, and use of spirometers.
Reduced range of movement in diaphragm	Greater residual capacity of volume of air is left in lung after normal breath increases, reducing amount of new air brought into lungs with each inspiration.	When possible, have client ambulate and sit in chair frequently.
Stiffened lung tissue and enlarged airspaces	Alteration reduces blood oxygenation.	
RENAL SYSTEM		
Reduced blood flow to kidneys	Reduced flow increases danger of shock when blood loss occurs.	For clients hospitalized before surgery, determine baseline urinary output for 24 hr.
Reduced glomerular filtration rate and excretory times	Problem limits ability to eliminate drugs or toxic substances.	
Reduced bladder capacity	Voiding frequency increases and larger amount of urine stays in bladder after voiding.	Instruct client to notify nurse immediately when sensation of bladder fullness develops.
	Sensation of need to void may not occur until bladder is filled.	Keep call light and bedpan within easy reach.
NEUROLOGICAL SYSTEM		
Sensory losses, including reduced tactile sense and increased pain tolerance	Client is less able to respond to early warning signs of surgical complications.	Orient client to surrounding environment. Observe for nonverbal signs of pain.
Decreased reaction time	Client becomes easily confused after anesthesia.	
METABOLIC SYSTEM		
Lower basal metabolic rate	Lower rate reduces total oxygen consumption.	
Reduced number of red blood cells and hemoglobin levels	Ability to carry adequate oxygen to tissues is reduced.	Administer necessary blood products. Monitor blood test results.
Change in total amounts of body potassium and water volume	Greater risk for fluid or electrolyte imbalance occurs.	Monitor electrolyte levels.

surgery. Thus the infant is highly susceptible to dehydration. However, if blood or fluids are replaced too quickly, overhydration may occur. Other important aspects of a child's surgical care include airway management, fluid maintenance, treatment of seizures, treatment of temperature alterations, identification and treatment of emergence delirium and delayed emergence from anesthesia, treatment of pain and agitation, and availability of appropriate emergency equipment and medication (Bryant and Dierdorf, 1992).

With advancing age a client's physical capacity to adapt to the stress of surgery is hampered because of deterioration in certain body functions. Despite the risk, the majority of clients undergoing surgery are older adults. Table 48-5 summarizes physiological factors that place older clients at risk during surgery.

Nutrition. Normal tissue repair and resistance to infection depend on adequate nutrients. Surgery intensifies this need. After surgery a client requires at least 1500 kcal/day to maintain energy reserves. Increased protein, vitamins A and C, and zinc facilitate wound healing (see Chapters 41 and 49). A malnourished client is prone to improper wound healing, reduced energy stores, and infection after surgery. If a client has elective surgery, nutrient imbalances can be corrected before surgery. However, if a malnourished client must undergo an emergency procedure, efforts to restore nutrients occur after surgery.

Obesity increases surgical risk by reducing ventilatory and cardiac function. The client has difficulty resuming normal physical activity after surgery. The obese client is susceptible to poor wound healing and wound infection because of the structure of fatty tissue, which contains a poor blood supply. This slows delivery of essential nutrients, antibodies, and enzymes needed for wound healing (see Chapter 49). It is often difficult to close the surgical wound of an obese client because of the thick adipose layer. An obese client is also at risk for **dehiscence** (opening of the suture line).

Radiotherapy. For the client with cancer, radiotherapy is often given to reduce the size of the cancerous tumor so that it can be removed surgically. Radiation has some unavoidable effects on normal tissue, such as excess thinning of skin layers, destruction of collagen, and impaired vascularization of tissue. Ideally the surgeon waits to perform surgery 4 to 6 weeks after completion of radiation treatments. Otherwise the client may face serious wound-healing problems.

Fluid and Electrolyte Balance. The body responds to surgery as a form of trauma. As a result of the adrenocortical stress response, hormonal reactions cause sodium and water retention and potassium loss within the first 2 to 5 days after surgery. Severe protein breakdown causes a negative nitrogen balance. The severity of the stress response influences the degree of fluid and electrolyte imbalance. The more extensive the surgery, the more severe the stress. A client who is hypovolemic or who has serious preoperative electrolyte alterations is at significant risk during and after surgery. For example, an excess or depletion of potassium increases the chance of dysrhythmias during or after surgery. If the client has preexisting renal, gastrointestinal, or cardiovascular abnormalities, the risk of fluid and electrolyte alterations is even greater.

DIAGNOSTIC SCREENING

Before a client has surgery, the surgeon may order diagnostic tests to screen for preexisting abnormalities. Many laboratory and diagnostic studies such as ECGs and chest x-rays are no longer done routinely before ambulatory surgery because they have not been cost effective for healthy, asymptomatic individuals (Meeker and Rothrock,

Table 48-6	Diagnostic Screening for Surgical Clients	
TYPE OF TEST	**PURPOSE/SIGNIFICANCE**	**COMMON VALUES**
CBC (Complete Blood Count)	Peripheral venous sample of blood measures red blood cells, white blood cells, hemoglobin, and hematocrit. May reveal infection, low blood volume, and potential for oxygenation problems. Surgeon may order blood replacement.	RBC Men: 4.7-6.l million/mm³ Women: 4.2-5.4 million/mm³ Hgb Men: 14.7-16.1 g/dl Hct Women: 12-16 g/dl Men: 42-52% Women: 37-47% WBC: Adults and children > 2 yrs: 5000-10,000/mm³
Serum Electrolytes	Peripheral venous sample of blood reveals significant fluid and electrolyte imbalances preoperatively. Attention is given to potassium (K⁺) levels. IV fluid replacement may be indicated preoperatively.	Sodium (Na⁺) 135-145 mEq/L Potassium (K⁺) 3.5-5.0 mEq/L Chloride (Cl⁻) 100-106 mEq/L Bicarb (HCO₃⁻) 24-32 mEq/L
Coagulation Studies	PT (prothrombin time), PTT (Partial thromboplastin time), and platelet counts reveal clotting ability of blood. Reveals clients at risk for bleeding tendencies and thrombus formation.	PT Less than 2 sec deviation from control PTT 25-27 sec Platelets 150,000-350,000/mm³
Serum Creatinine	Ability of blood to excrete creatinine, by-product of metabolism, assesses renal function. Elevated level can indicate renal failure.	Creatinine 0.6-1.5 mg/l00 ml
Urinalysis	Analysis of urine screens for urinary infection, renal disease and diabetes.	See Chapter 46 for values

1995). Routine screening tests include a complete blood count (CBC), serum electrolyte analysis, coagulation studies, serum creatinine tests, and urinalysis (see Table 48-6). If diagnostic tests reveal severe problems, the surgeon may cancel surgery until the condition stabilizes.

The nurse is responsible for the preparation of clients for diagnostic studies and for coordinating completion of the tests. The nurse also reviews diagnostic results as they become available to alert physicians to findings and to assist with planning appropriate therapy.

Additional Screening Tests. If a client is over the age of 40 or has heart disease, the physician may order a chest x-ray or an electrocardiogram (ECG). The chest x-ray is an examination of the condition of the heart and lungs. If the physician detects lung abnormalities, a different type and dosage of sedatives or anesthetic agents may be used. Exposure to radiation may cause injury to a fetus so ask the female client if she is pregnant prior to sending her to x-ray. The ECG involves painless application of electrodes to the chest and extremities. An ECG measures the heart's electrical activity to determine whether the heart rate, rhythm, and other factors are normal. The procedure takes less than 5 minutes and requires the client simply to lie flat and relax.

Depending on the type of surgery the client will undergo, there are several diagnostic tests for specific anatomical structures and physiological functions. If the client is likely to lose a large amount of blood during surgery, the physician orders a blood specimen for type and cross-matching. This enables the laboratory to determine the proper blood type and Rh factor. The surgeon usually designates the number of blood units to have available during surgery. Autotransfusion is an option for some clients who choose to donate their own blood before surgery to reduce the risk of transfusion-related infections. The donation usually must be made several weeks before the scheduled surgery. The use of a cell saver in surgery may be possible if physicians are anticipating large blood loss. This unit, while expensive, returns washed red blood cells to the client and decreases the risk of AIDS and hepatitis B by using the client's own blood and has created positive outcomes in terms of length of client stay (Meeker and Rothrock, 1995).

 ## Nursing Diagnosis

The nurse clusters defining characteristics gathered during assessment to identify nursing diagnoses for the surgical client (see the diagnostic process box above). The client with preexisting health problems is likely to have a variety of risk diagnoses. For example, a client with preexisting bronchitis who has abnormal breath sounds and a productive cough will be at risk for ineffective airway clearance. The nature of surgery and the client's health status provide defining characteristics for a number of nursing diagnoses. For example, a client who is to undergo anesthesia for a neurosurgical procedure will be immobilized several hours. A diagnosis of risk for impaired skin integrity will require the nurse's attention during surgery.

The diagnoses establish directions for care that will be provided during one or all surgical phases (see the nursing diagnoses box on p. 1391). Preoperative nursing diagnoses allow the nurse to take precautions and actions so that care

 ## Examples of NANDA Nursing Diagnoses for Preoperative Client

Ineffective airway clearance *related to:*
- Diminished cough
- Increased pulmonary congestion

Anxiety *related to:*
- Knowledge deficit of impending surgery
- Threat of loss of body part

Ineffective family coping: compromised *related to:*
- Temporary role change of client
- Impending severity of surgery

Fear *related to:*
- Impending surgery
- Anticipation of postoperative pain

Knowledge deficit regarding implications of surgery *related to:*
- Lack of experience with surgery
- Information misinterpretation

Altered nutrition: less than body requirements *related to:*
- Preoperative nutrition

Altered nutrition: more than body requirements *related to:*
- Excess intake of food

Powerlessness *related to:*
- Emergency nature of surgery

Risk for impaired skin integrity *related to:*
- Preoperative radiation
- Immobilization during surgery

Sleep pattern disturbance *related to:*
- Fear of surgery
- Schedule of preoperative hospital routines

provided during the intraoperative and postoperative phases is consistent with the client's needs.

Nursing diagnoses made preoperatively may also focus on the potential risks a client may face after surgery. Preventive care is essential so that the surgical client can be managed effectively.

 ## Planning

It is essential to include the surgical client in health care planning. Involving the client early when developing the surgical care plan minimizes surgical risks and postoperative complications. For example, nursing research has shown that structured preoperative teaching can reduce the length of the client's hospital stay (Dalayon, 1994). A client informed about the surgical experience is less likely to be fearful and can prepare to participate in the postoperative recovery phase so that expected outcomes can be met. The family is also an important partner in understanding the outcomes established to achieve recovery. For each diagnosis the nurse establishes the goal of care and the outcomes that must be met to ensure recovery or maintenance of the preoperative state. The care plan on p. 1931 provides a sample relating to a preoperative surgical client.

For the ambulatory surgical client, the preoperative planning phase occurs in the home or in the outpatient surgery unit on the morning of surgery. Ideally it is done in the home by the nurse making phone calls to the client and the

Sample Nursing Diagnostic Process for Clients Facing Surgery

ASSESSMENT ACTIVITIES	DEFINING CHARACTERISTICS	NURSING DIAGNOSES
Ask client about previous surgical experiences.	Client reports no previous surgical experience either personally or involving family Client asks questions about what to expect	**Knowledge deficit** regarding implications of surgery related to first surgical experience.
Ask client about preoperative preparation from physician. Observe client's nonverbal behavior.	Has received minimal preparation by physician Alert and responsive to discussion	
Ask client about previous smoking history. Auscultate client's breath sounds. Assess for presence of a cough, noting, character and productivity. Note client's surgical procedure and type of anesthesia.	History of smoking Abnormal breath sounds Chronic, nonproductive cough present Scheduled for anesthesia Scheduled for abdominal surgery	**Risk for ineffective airway clearance** related to diminished cough and increased pulmonary congestion.

Sample Nursing Care Plan for Knowledge Deficit

NURSING DIAGNOSIS: Knowledge deficit regarding implications of surgery related to first surgical experience
DEFINITION: Knowledge deficit is the state in which specific information is lacking (Kim, McFarland, McLane, 1995).

GOAL	EXPECTED OUTCOMES	INTERVENTIONS	RATIONALE
Client will understand intraoperative and postoperative events prior to scheduled surgery.	Client and family will describe routine procedures that nurses perform after surgery. Client will describe ways to participate in care after surgery. Client and family will describe events that commonly occur in holding area and operating room.	Send teaching booklet and video to client's home. Provide preoperative teaching session to explain common events that occur after surgery (e.g., monitoring, IV care, exercise). Explain events that will occur in holding area (e.g., IV insertion, vital sign check) and in operating room (e.g., positioning, anesthesia).	Structured preoperative teaching has positive influence on recovery. Preparatory Information helps clients form realistic image of surgical experience and be better able to cope and attend to it when it occurs (Lepczyk, 1990).

surgical unit and/or physician's office mailing preoperative information and instructions. This gives the client time to think about the surgical experience, make necessary physical preparations (e.g., altering diet or discontinuing medication use), and ask questions about postoperative procedures. The ambulatory surgical client usually returns home on the day of surgery. Thus well-planned preoperative care ensures that the client is well informed and able to be an active participant during recovery. The family or spouse can also play an active supportive role for the client.

The preoperative care plan is based on individualized nursing diagnoses. However, each client must undergo basic preparations. Goals of care for the surgical client include the following:

1. Understanding physiological and psychological responses to surgery
2. Understanding intraoperative and postoperative events
3. Achieving emotional comfort and relaxation
4. Achieving a return of normal physiological function after surgery (e.g., return of normal vital signs)
5. Maintaining a normal fluid and electrolyte balance
6. Achieving comfort and rest
7. Remaining free of surgical wound infection
8. Remaining safe from harm during the perioperative period

 Implementation

Preoperative nursing interventions provide the client with a complete understanding of the surgery and prepare the client physically for surgical intervention.

**SPECIAL CONSENT TO OPERATION, POST OPERATIVE CARE,
MEDICAL TREATMENT, ANESTHESIA, OR OTHER PROCEDURE**

Patient:_____   Patient No:_____

Washington State law guarantees that you have both the <u>right</u> and <u>obligation</u> to make decisions concerning your health care. Your physician can provide you with the necessary information and advice, but as a member of the health care team, you must enter into the decision making process. This form has been designed to acknowledge your acceptance of treatment recommended by your physician.

IMPORTANT: HAVE PATIENT SIGN FULL OR LIMITED DISCLOSURE BOX AND SIGNATURE LINE AT BOTTOM.

① I hereby authorize Dr._____ and/or such associates or assistants as may be selected by said physician to treat the following condition(s) which has (have) been explained to me: (Explain the nature of the condition(s) in professional and lay language.)

_____

_____

_____

_____

Full Disclosure

I certify that my physician has informed me of the nature and character of the proposed treatment, of the anticipated results of the proposed treatment, of the possible alternative forms of treatment; and the recognized serious possible risks, complications, and the anticipated benefits involved in the proposed treatment and in the alternative forms of treatment, including non-treatment.

_____
PATIENT/OTHER LEGALLY RESPONSIBLE PERSON SIGN
IF APPLICABLE

② The procedures planned for treatment of my condition(s) have been explained to me by my physician. I understand them to be: (Describe procedures to be performed in professional and lay language.)

_____

_____

_____

_____

_____

Limited Disclosure

I certify that my physician has explained to me that I have the right to have clearly described to me the nature and character of the proposed treatment; the anticipated results of the proposed treatment; the alternative forms of treatment; and the recognized serious possible risks, complications, and anticipated benefits involved in the proposed treatment, and in the alternative forms of treatment, including non-treatment.

I do not wish to have these risks and facts explained to me.

_____
PATIENT/OTHER LEGALLY RESPONSIBLE PERSON SIGN
IF APPLICABLE

At:_____
(NAME OF HOSPITAL OR MEDICAL FACILITY)

③ I recognize that, during the course of the operation, post operative care, medical treatment, anesthesia or other procedure, unforeseen conditions may necessitate additional or different procedures than those above set forth. **I therefore authorize my above named physician, and his or her assistants or designees, to perform such surgical or other procedures as are in the exercise of his, her or their professional judgment necessary and desirable.** The authority granted under this paragraph shall extend to the treatment of **all conditions** that require treatment and are not known to my physician at the time the medical or surgical procedure is commenced.

③ **I have been informed that there are significant risks** such as severe loss of blood, infection and cardiac arrest that can lead to death or permanent or partial disability, which may be attendant to the performance of any procedure. **I acknowledge that no warranty or guarantee has been made to me as to the result or cure.**

Any sections below which do not apply to the proposed treatment may be crossed out. All sections crossed out must be initialed by <u>both</u> physician <u>and</u> patient.

⑤ I consent to the administration of anesthesia by my attending physician, by an anesthesiologist, or other qualified party under the direction of a physician as may be deemed necessary. I understand that all anesthetics involve risks of complication and serious possible damage to vital organs such as the brain, heart, lung, liver and kidney and that in some cases may result in paralysis, cardiac arrest and/or brain death from both known and unknown causes.

⑥ I consent to the use of transfusion of blood and blood products as deemed necessary.

⑦ Any tissues or parts surgically removed may be disposed of by the hospital or physician in accordance with accustomed practice.

I certify this form has been fully explained to me, that I have read it or have had it read to me, that the blank spaces have been filled in, and that I understand its contents.

DATE:_____ TIME:_____ A.M. P.M.   _____

DOCTOR'S SIGNATURE:_____   PATIENT/OTHER LEGALLY RESPONSIBLE PERSON SIGN

WITNESS:_____

Fig. 48-1 New special consent to operation, postoperative care, medical treatment, anesthesia, or other procedure.

Informed Consent

Surgery cannot be legally performed until a client understands the need for a procedure, the steps involved, risks, expected results, and alternative treatments. The primary responsibility for informing the client rests with the physician. Consent is not informed if the client is confused, unconscious, mentally incompetent, or under the influence of sedatives. All consent forms must be signed by the client before the nurse administers preoperative medications. Ideally a physician obtains consent before a client is admitted to the hospital or satellite surgical setting. See Fig. 48-1 for an example of a consent form.

The surgeon's explanation should be witnessed by a qualified member of the health care team. The form's structure allows the physician to write information related to the surgery. A client's signature on a consent form implies that the client has been thoroughly informed about the procedure. The nurse frequently witnesses signing of the form and examines the document for the correct date, time, and signature, which must be in ink. A client who is illiterate can sign by making a mark as long as it is properly witnessed. As a witness the nurse is able to attest that the client's signature is on the form but not that the client was properly informed. In many institutions a time limit is placed on consent forms (e.g., 30 days).

In emergencies the client may be unable to sign and family members may be unavailable. The physician is legally permitted to perform surgery without consent in such a case. However, every effort must be made to obtain permission from a responsible family member by telephone, telegram, or in some states by court order. A telephone consent must be witnessed by two persons who hear the family member's oral consent. The two witnesses sign the consent with the name of the family member, noting that an oral consent was obtained. Informed consent is critical to protect not only the client but also health personnel so that the surgical team can practice without fear of legal reprisal.

After the consent form has been completed, the nurse makes sure that the form is placed in the client's medical record. The record goes to the operating room with the client. Chapter 20 discusses in detail the nurse's responsibilities for informed consent.

Preoperative Teaching

Structured preoperative teaching has proven benefits. Preoperative teaching concerning a client's expected postoperative behavior, provided in a systematic and structured format with teaching and learning principles, has a positive influence on the client's recovery. Structured preoperative teaching can influence postoperative factors such as the following:

1. Ventilatory function. Teaching improves the ability to cough and deep breathe effectively.
2. Physical functional capacity. Teaching improves the ability to ambulate and resume activities of daily living early.
3. Sense of well-being. Clients who are prepared for surgery experience less anxiety and report a greater sense of psychological well-being.
4. Length of hospital stay. Structured preoperative teaching can reduce the length of stay.

5. Anxiety about pain and amount of pain medication needed for comfort. Clients who undergo teaching about pain and ways to relieve it are less anxious about pain, ask for what they need, and actually need lesser amounts of pain medication.

The most effective teaching program for surgical clients is planned so that all clients receive the same information. Detailed discussion and demonstration of postoperative exercises are vital. If the client understands why these exercises are important to postoperative recovery and knows how to perform them correctly, the recovery period will be less complicated. Today, because many clients come to the hospital on the day of surgery, preoperative teaching may occur in the home. Printed literature, instructions, and videotapes are made available to clients (Fig. 48-2).

Preadmission nurses may call clients the evening before surgery to clarify questions and reinforce explanations. One study (Lepczyk et al, 1990) demonstrated that it made little difference in knowledge or anxiety measures if clients received perioperative education up to a week before surgery or immediately before. Another study found that clients preferred receiving perioperative information between admission to the hospital and the time of surgery, even if the time span was only a few hours or less (Schoessler, 1989). Therefore it seems ideal to attempt outpatient perioperative education before admission and then to reinforce the information before surgery.

Including family members in perioperative preparation is advised. Often a family member is the coach for postoperative exercises when the client returns from surgery. If anxious relatives do not understand routine postoperative events, it is likely their anxiety will heighten the client's fears or concerns. Perioperative preparation of family members before surgery minimizes anxiety and misunderstanding.

The nurse should provide clients with information about sensations typically experienced after surgery. Preparatory information helps clients anticipate the steps of a procedure and thus helps them form realistic images of the surgical experience. When events occur as predicted, clients are better able to cope and attend to the experiences. For example, in the operating room the anesthesiologist may apply ointment to clients' eyes to prevent corneal damage. Warning clients about sensations of blurred vision will reduce their anxiety on awakening from surgery. Sensations that the nurse may describe include the expected pain at the surgical site, the tightness of dressings, dryness of the mouth, or the sensation of a sore throat resulting from an endotracheal tube.

If the nurse can begin teaching a client 1 or 2 days before surgery, the client may be better able to learn. Anxiety and fear are barriers to learning, and both emotions are heightened as surgery approaches. The nurse assesses the surgical client's readiness and ability to learn. If the client is capable of and receptive to learning, the nurse presents information in a logical sequence, beginning with preoperative events and advancing to intraoperative and postoperative routines. Preoperative teaching checklists give nurses useful guidelines for presenting comprehensive instructions.

The American Nurses Association and the Association of Operating Room Nurses (AORN) (1972) established the following criteria by which the client demonstrates understanding of the surgical experience. Extensive preoperative

Text continued on p. 1398.

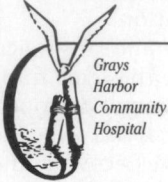

Grays Harbor Community Hospital

YOUR SURGICAL EXPERIENCE
A GENERAL GUIDE TO
WHAT YOU CAN EXPECT

This information packet is designed to help make your scheduled surgery go as smoothly as possible. Please take the time to read all of the information in this packet. If you have any questions about the information presented, please call the pre-admitting nurse or contact your physician/surgeon's office.

Thank you for your cooperation.

DATE OF SURGERY		TIME TO ARRIVE ON DAY OF SURGERY	

PREPARATION FOR YOUR SURGERY

THE DAY BEFORE

1. INFORM your physician if you have a cold, infection, fever, or illness of any kind.
2. If you routinely take any medication for any medical condition, TELL your doctor.
3. Eat a light evening meal.
4. DO NOT smoke or chew gum after 12 midnight the night before your operation.
5. DO NOT EAT OR DRINK ANYTHING AFTER 12 MIDNIGHT THE NIGHT BEFORE YOUR OPERATION, EVEN WATER. This surgical precaution <u>must</u> be strictly observed or your surgery may be cancelled.
6. Do get a good night's rest before your surgery.

POST–OPERATIVELY

1. From the Operating Room, you will be taken to the Recovery Room where you will remain approximately one to four hours, depending on the type of surgery.
2. You will have an IV (intravenous line) to maintain an adequate fluid level until your doctor advances your diet and discontinues the IV.
3. You will be asked to turn, cough, and breathe deeply to help keep your lungs clear and prevent respiratory complications.
4. You may be reminded by your nurse to do leg exercises or other exercises ordered by your physicians.
5. The nursing staff will frequently check your blood pressure, pulse, temperature, and respiration and will help you with your comfort needs, such as positioning and pain medicine as you need it.
6. Your doctor will order specific activity after surgery.

DAY OF SURGERY

1. DO take a complete bath and wash your hair prior to coming to the hospital.
2. DO complete all preparations your doctor has instructed you to do.
*3. Arrive at time given by the Pre-Admission Nurse. Check in at the admitting desk.
4. Wear any kind of comfortable clothing, especially low-heeled shoes.
5. Contact lenses <u>CANNOT</u> be worn in surgery. Bring your container.
6. Do bring a list of medications you are taking.
7. DO NOT wear jewelry or bring valuables with you. (Rings which cannot be removed may be taped over prior to surgery). Please DO NOT wear any makeup.
8. DO NOT bring children with you to the hospital.
9. Young patients may bring favorite toy/blanket.
10. A gown, robe, and slippers will be provided.

AFTER YOUR SURGERY

1. Follow all instructions given by your doctor.
2. Refrain from recreational or work activities. Your body needs and deserves a few hours of quiet rest.
3. DO NOT drive for at least 24 hours after your surgery. You will need a responsible person to drive you home.
4. DO NOT make any important decisions or sign any important papers for 24 hours.
5. DO eat moderately, being aware that food may cause nausea. We recommend you start slowly and increase according to how you feel.
6. DO NOT drink any alcoholic beverages for at least 24 hours.
7. DO NOT SMOKE WHEN ALONE.
8. DO call your doctor's office to arrange for follow-up visit if this is not already done.
9. Do call your doctor if you have any questions or need assistance.

WHEN YOU GET TO THE HOSPITAL

A. Check in at the admitting desk. It is important that you arrive on time.

From the admitting desk, you will be directed to the Day Surgery Department or the Surgical Unit (usually second floor).

B. Upon arrival to the unit, you will be checked in by the nursing staff and shown to your room. Day Surgery patients will be assigned a bed.

You will be given a gown, robe, and slippers to put on. This will be what you will wear to surgery. Usually, you will be asked to remove your undergarments prior to going to surgery.

You will have your temperature, pulse, and blood pressure checked prior to going to surgery.

You may be asked several health/medical questions. Sometimes you will answer the same question asked several times by different people, for example, "When was the last time you had anything to eat or drink?" This helps to insure accuracy of information and it is intended as a safeguard for your care.

Additional tests ordered for you by your doctor may be performed.

An IV (intravenous) catheter will usually be placed so that you will receive adequate fluids. Additional medications may be given through this catheter.

When possible, you will be visited by a physician anesthesiologist or nurse anesthetist.

Your family/friends will be allowed to keep you company while waiting to go to surgery. Due to limited space, please limit your guests to one or two when possible.

C. About one hour before your surgery, you <u>may</u> be given a preoperative medication. This is to help you relax and could make you drowsy. It may make your mouth very dry. After the medication is given, you will be asked to remain in bed and relax. For your safety, the siderails of the bed will be raised and the nurses's call light put within reach. It is <u>very</u> <u>important</u> that you get assistance from the nurse before trying to get out of bed.

D. Depending on the type of surgery you are having, you will be taken to the surgery department between 15 minutes and one hour prior to your surgery time. This is to allow for additional preparation.

IT IS IMPORTANT TO NOTE:

Your surgeon may give you a time estimate of how long the actual surgery will take. This time, however, does not include the additional time required for surgical preparation and anesthetic procedures. This additional time may add a few minutes to an hour. Please keep this in mind when planning for your loved ones while you are in surgery. They may have time to leave and come back.

*PARENTS OF PEDIATRIC PATIENTS SHOULD NOT LEAVE THE HOSPITAL WHILE THE CHILD IS IN SURGERY. IF YOU HAVE QUESTIONS, PLEASE ASK YOUR NURSE.

Fig. 48-2 Surgical instruction sheet. *(Courtesy Grays Harbor Community Hospital, Aberdeen, WA.)*

Demonstrating Postoperative Exercises

STEPS	RATIONALE
1. Assess client's risk for postoperative respiratory complications. Review medical history to identify presence of chronic pulmonary conditions (e.g., emphysema, asthma), any condition that affects chest wall movement, history of smoking, and presence of reduced hemoglobin.	General anesthesia predisposes client to respiratory problems because lungs are not fully inflated during surgery; cough reflex is suppressed, so mucus collects within airway passages. After surgery, client may have reduced lung volume and require greater efforts to cough and deep breathe; inadequate lung expansion can lead to atelectasis and pneumonia. Client is at greater risk to develop respiratory complications if other chronic lung conditions are present. Smoking damages ciliary clearance and increases mucus secretion. Reduced hemoglobin level can lead to inadequate oxygenation.
2. Assess ability to cough and deep breathe by having client take deep breath and observing movement of shoulders and chest wall. Measure chest excursion during deep breath. Ask client to cough after taking deep breath.	Reveals maximum potential for chest expansion and ability to cough forcefully; serves as baseline to measure ability to perform exercises after surgery.
3. Assess risk for postoperative thrombus formation. (Older, immobilized clients are most at risk.) Observe for positive Homan's sign by monitoring calf pain when dorsiflexing client's foot with knee flexed. Observe for calf pain, redness, warmth, swelling, or vein distention.	After general anesthesia, circulation is slowed, and when rate of blood flow is slowed, there is greater tendency for clot formation. Immobilization results in decreased muscular contraction in lower extremities, which promotes venous stasis.
4. Prepare necessary supplies: a. Pillow (optional)	Client may prefer to use pillow to splint incision when coughing to reduce discomfort.
5. Explain postoperative exercises to client, including importance to recovery and physiological benefits.	Information allows client to attend and can motivate learning. Persons tend to learn new skills when benefits can be gained.

DIAPHRAGMATIC BREATHING

6. Assist client to comfortable sitting or standing position. If client chooses to sit, assist to side of bed or to upright position in chair.	Upright position facilitates diaphragmatic excursion.
7. Stand or sit facing client.	Allows client to observe breathing exercise.
8. Instruct client to place palms of hands across from each other, down and along lower borders of anterior rib cage. Place tips of third fingers lightly together (see the illustration below). Demonstrate for client.	Position of hands allows client to feel movement of chest and abdomen as diaphragm descends and lungs expand.
9. Have client take slow, deep breaths, inhaling through nose. Tell client to feel middle fingers separate during inhalation. Demonstrate.	Slow, deep breath prevents panting or hyperventilation. Inhaling through nose warms, humidifies, and filters air.

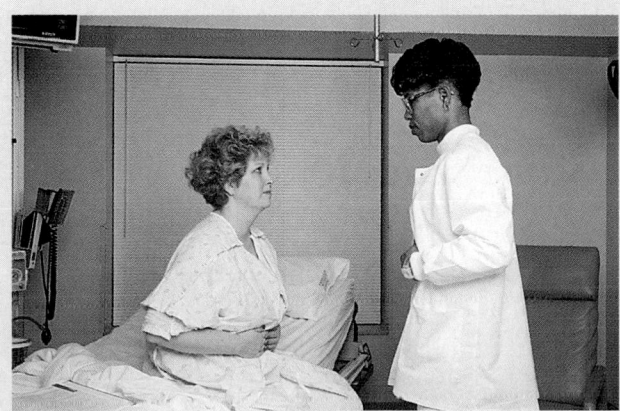

Step 8

Continued.

Demonstrating Postoperative Exercises—cont'd

STEPS	RATIONALE

DIAPHRAGMATIC BREATHING—cont'd

10. Explain that client will feel normal downward movement of diaphragm during inspiration. Explain that abdominal organs descend and chest wall expands.

Explanation and demonstration focus on normal ventilatory movement of chest wall. Client develops understanding of how diaphragmatic breathing feels.

11. Avoid using chest and shoulders while inhaling and instruct client in same manner.

Using auxiliary chest and shoulder muscles increases useless energy expenditure.

12. Have client hold slow, deep breath for count of three and then slowly exhale through mouth. Tell client middle fingertips will touch as chest wall contracts.

Allows for gradual expulsion of all air.

13. Repeat breathing exercise 3 to 5 times.

Allows client to observe slow, rhythmic breathing pattern.

14. Have client practice exercise. Instruct client to take 10 slow, deep breaths every 2 hr while awake during postoperative period until mobile.

Repetition of exercise reinforces learning. Regular deep breathing prevents postoperative complications.

INCENTIVE SPIROMETRY

15. Wash hands.

Reduces transmission of microorganisms.

16. Instruct client to assume semi-Fowler's or high Fowler's position.

Promotes optimal lung expansion during respiratory maneuver.

17. Demonstrate to client how to place mouthpiece so that lips completely cover mouthpiece (see the illustration below).

Demonstration is reliable technique for teaching psychomotor skill and enables client to ask questions.

18. Instruct client to inhale slowly and maintain constant flow through unit. When maximal inspiration is reached, client should hold breath for 2-3 sec and then exhale slowly. Number of breaths should not exceed 10-12 per min (Dettenmeier, 1992).

Maintains maximal inspiration and reduces risk of progressive collapse of individual alveoli. Slow breath prevents or minimizes pain from sudden pressure changes in chest (Dettenmeier, 1992).

19. Instruct client to breathe normally for short period.

Prevents hyperventilation and fatigue.

20. Have client repeat meneuver until goals are achieved.

Ensures correct use of spirometer.

21. Wash hands.

Reduces transmission of microorganisms.

CONTROLLED COUGHING

22. Explain importance of maintaining upright position.

Position facilitates diaphragm excursion and enhances thorax expansion.

23. Demonstrate coughing. Take two slow, deep breaths, inhaling through nose and exhaling through mouth.

Deep breaths expand lungs fully so that air moves behind mucus and facilitates effects of coughing.

24. Inhale deeply third time and hold breath to count of three. Cough fully for two or three consecutive coughs without inhaling between coughs. (Tell client to push all air out of lungs.)

Consecutive coughs help remove mucus more effectively and completely than one forceful cough.

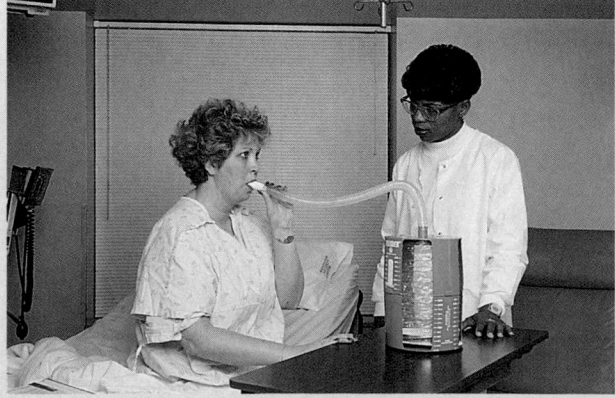

Step 17

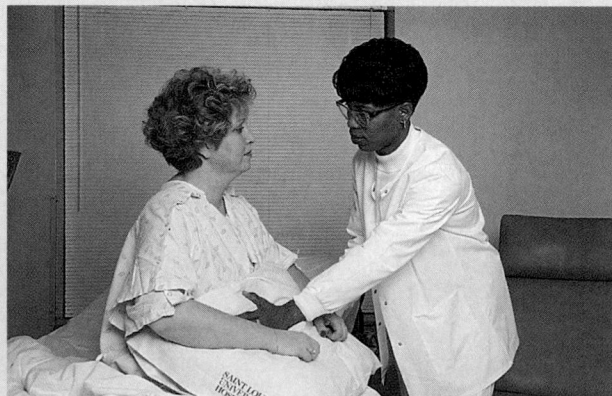

Step 26

Demonstrating Postoperative Exercises—cont'd

STEPS	RATIONALE

CONTROLLED COUGHING—cont'd

25. Caution client against just clearing throat instead of coughing.

Clearing throat does not remove mucus from deep in airways.

26. If surgical incision will be abdominal or thoracic, teach client to place one hand over incisional area and other hand on top of first. During breathing and coughing exercises, client presses gently against incisional area to splint or support it. Pillow over incision is optional (see the illustration on p. 1396, right).

Surgical incision cuts through muscles, tissues, and nerve endings. Deep breathing and coughing exercises place additional stress on suture line and cause discomfort. Splinting incision with hands provides firm support and reduces incisional pulling. (Some clients prefer to have pillow to place over incision.)

27. Client continues to practice coughing exercises, splinting imaginary incision. Instruct client to cough two to three times every 2 hr while awake.

Value of deep coughing with splinting is stressed to effectively expectorate mucus with minimal discomfort.

28. Instruct client to examine sputum for consistency, amount, and color changes.

Sputum consistency, amount, and color changes may indicate presence of pulmonary complication, such as pneumonia.

TURNING

29. Instruct client to assume supine position to right side of bed. Side rails on both sides of bed should be in up position.

Positioning begins on right side of bed so that turning to left side will not cause client to roll toward bed's edge.

30. Instruct client to place left hand over incisional area to splint it.

Supports and minimizes pulling on suture line during turning.

31. Instruct client to keep left leg straight and flex right knee up and over left leg.

Straight leg stabilizes client's position. Flexed right leg shifts weight for easier turning.

32. Have client grab left side rail with right hand, pull toward left, and roll onto left side.

Pulling toward side rail reduces effort needed for turning.

33. Instruct client to turn every 2 hr while awake.

Reduces risk of vascular and pulmonary complications.

LEG EXERCISES

34. Have client assume supine position in bed. Demonstrate leg exercises by performing passive range-of-motion exercises and simultaneously explaining exercise.

Provides normal anatomical position of lower extremities.

35. Rotate each ankle in complete circle. Instruct client to draw imaginary circles with big toe. Repeat five times.

Leg exercises maintain joint mobility and promote venous return to prevent thrombi.

36. Alternate dorsiflexion and plantar flexion of both feet. Direct client to feel calf muscles contract and relax alternately (see the illustration below). Repeat five times.

Stretches and contracts gastrocnemius muscles.

37. Have client continue leg exercises by alternately flexing and extending knees. Repeat five times (see the illustration below).

Contracts muscles of upper legs and maintains knee mobility.

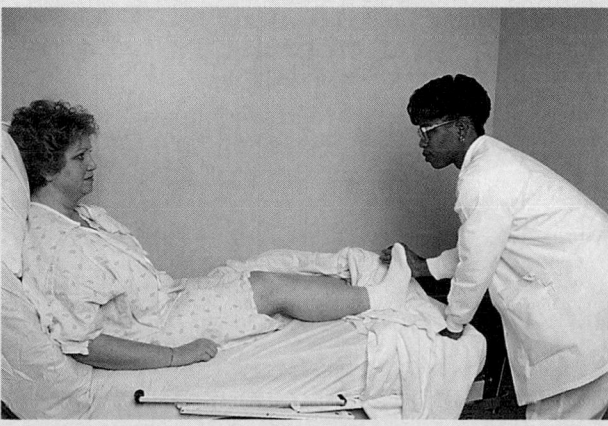

Step 36

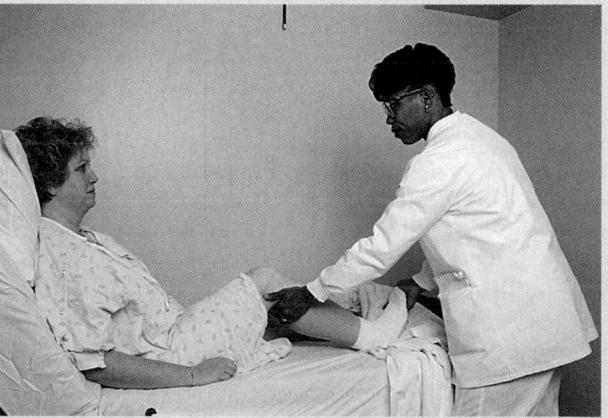

Step 37

Continued.

Demonstrating Postoperative Exercises—cont'd

STEPS	RATIONALE
LEG EXERCISES—cont'd	
38. Have client alternately raise each leg straight up from bed surface, keeping legs straight. Repeat five times.	Promotes contraction and relaxation of quadriceps muscles.
39. Have client practice exercises at least every 2 hr while awake. Instruct client to coordinate turning and leg exercises with diaphragmatic breathing, incentive spirometry, and coughing exercises.	Repetition of sequence reinforces learning. Establishes routine for exercises that develops habit for performance. Sequence of exercises should be leg exercises, turning, breathing, incentive spirometry, and coughing.
40. Observe client's ability to perform all five exercises independently.	Ensures that client has learned correct technique.
41. Record exercises demonstrated and client's ability to perform them independently.	Documents client's education and provides data for instructional follow-up.

teaching not only improves the client's understanding, it also promotes return of normal physiological function.

CLIENT CITES REASONS FOR EACH PREOPERATIVE INSTRUCTION AND EXERCISES

Given a rationale for preoperative and postoperative procedures, the client is better prepared to participate in care. Every preoperative teaching program includes explanation and demonstration of the five postoperative exercises: diaphragmatic breathing, incentive spirometry, coughing, turning, and leg exercises. These exercises are designed to prevent postoperative complications (Procedure 48-1).

When a client is under general anesthesia, the lungs do not ventilate fully. After surgery the client has a reduced lung volume and needs greater effort to breathe. During surgery, venous blood flow to the legs slows. Stasis of circulation may lead to thrombi or clots. A clot can break off and travel to the brain, heart, or lungs to cause potentially fatal complications.

Diaphragmatic breathing improves lung expansion and oxygen delivery without using excess energy. The client learns to use the diaphragm during deep breathing to take slow, deep, and relaxed breaths. Eventually the client's lung volume improves. Deep breathing also helps clear out anesthetic gases remaining in the airways. To facilitate deep breathing the physician may order an incentive spirometer for the client, which encourages effective deep breathing through sustained maximal inspiration (see Chapter 44).

Coughing assists in removing retained mucus in the airways. A deep, productive cough is more beneficial than merely clearing the throat. Postoperative incisional pain makes coughing difficult. The client must anticipate the pain and understand the importance of coughing. The nurse also teaches the client to splint an incision to minimize pain during coughing. Nurses direct clients to cough and deep breathe at least every 2 hours while awake.

Leg exercises and turning improve blood flow to the extremities and thus reduce stasis. Contraction of lower leg muscles promotes venous return, making it difficult for clots to form. The nurse encourages the client to perform exercises at least every 2 hours while awake. If the client is measured for elastic stockings or sequential compression

devices, teaching about the purposes and nursing care that will be required following application is necessary.

After explaining each exercise, the nurse demonstrates it. The nurse acts as a coach, guiding the client through each exercise. For example, the nurse says whether the client is sitting properly and helps the client place the hands in the proper position during breathing. The nurse then allows the client time (at least 15 minutes) for independent practice. The nurse can attend to other duties or ask an assistant to further coach the client before returning to watch each exercise independently. The nurse gives feedback, telling the client what aspect of each exercise is done correctly and what needs improvement.

CLIENT STATES TIME OF SURGERY

The client and family should be told the approximate time that surgery will begin. If the hospital has a busy operating room schedule it is best to let them know how many procedures are scheduled before the client's. It is unwise to tell the client and family the anticipated length of surgery. Unanticipated delays may occur for many reasons. If the client fails to return at the time expected, the family will be highly anxious. Family members should wait in the surgical waiting area for updates from the staff.

CLIENT STATES POSTOPERATIVE UNIT AND LOCATION OF FAMILY DURING SURGERY AND RECOVERY

The unit to which the client is admitted before surgery may be different from the postoperative unit. The family needs to know where the client will be taken after surgery. The nurse also explains where the family can wait and where the surgeon will attempt to find family members after surgery. If the client will be taken to a special unit, it helps to orient the client and family members to the unit's environment before surgery.

CLIENT DISCUSSES ANTICIPATED POSTOPERATIVE MONITORING AND THERAPIES

The client and family want to know about postoperative events. If they understand routine postoperative vital sign monitoring before surgery occurs, they will be less appre-

CNS	DIETARY	RT
HOME HEALTH	OT	OTHER
PT	SW	OTHER

BARNES

CARE PATH® 540
TOTAL MASTECTOMY WITH
MALIGNANCY WITHOUT CC

2

A-8

Problem Number	PATIENT PROBLEMS / NURSING DIAGNOSES

		1	3, 4	2, 3, 4	2, 3	
MEDS / IVS		**NUTRITION**	**PATIENT / FAMILY EDUCATION**	**DISCHARGE PLANNING**	**PSYCHOSOCIAL/ EMOTIONAL/ SPIRITUAL NEEDS**	**INITIALS** (SEE KEY AT BOTTOM)
IVF IM Analgesics Antibiotic if ordered		Clear liquid. Advance as tolerated to diet as prior to admission	Nursing: Pain control Positioning / mobility TCDB Incentive Spirometer Diet IV JP Primary Nursing	**Pt./family** **verbalizes** **understanding** **of Care Path.** **Plan of care** **has been** **mutually set** **with pt./family.**		
DC IVF when tolerating PO well DC IM analgesics Start oral analgesics **Pain controlled with** **oral analgesics**		**Tolerating** **diet as prior** **to admission**	Social Work: Assess resource needs Initiate education re: dx, prosthesis, support groups Nursing: Arm protection S/S infection BSE	Social Work: Complete high risk screening	Social Work: Assess counseling needs Initiate support Nursing: Therapeutic emotional care	
SIGNATURE	**INIT.**	**SIGNATURE**	**INIT.**	**SIGNATURE**	**INIT.**	

Fig. 48-3 Care path for total mastectomy with malignancy. *(Courtesy Barnes-Jewish Hospital, St Louis, Mo.)*

Continued.

				1

BARNES CARE PATH® 540 TOTAL MASTECTOMY WITH MALIGNANCY WITHOUT CC

SERVICE		PHYSICIAN	
PRIMARY NURSE		PRIMARY NURSE	
DC DATE	ADM DATE	DATE OF SURGERY	A-8

Problem Number	PATIENT PROBLEMS / NURSING DIAGNOSES
#1	ALTERATION IN COMFORT
#2	ALTERATION IN COPING
#3	ALTERATION IN SELF-CONCEPT
#4	LACK OF KNOWLEDGE

#	1, 2	2, 3	1	1, 3	1
	ASSESSMENT / MONITORING	CONSULTS	PROCEDURES / TEST	TREATMENT	ACTIVITY
DAY 1 DOS	VS q 4 hrs x1 x2 x3 x4 x5 x6 I & O Pain Control Dressing / JP patency and drainage Ability to void Circulation Emotional response / family coping	Social Work		JP to bulb suction Incentive Spirometer / TCDB Avoid trauma to extremity	Up with assist to bathroom in PM
DAY 2 POD 1	VS q 8 hrs. if stable x1 x2 x3 I & O Pain Control Dressing / JP patency and drainage **Voiding without difficulty** Circulation Emotional response / family coping	Social Work visit Reach to Recovery		JP to bulb suction **Uses Incentive Spirometer independently** Avoid trauma to extremity	Up as tolerated with assist if needed

SIGNATURE	INIT.	SIGNATURE	INIT.	SIGNATURE	INIT.

Fig. 48-3, cont'd Care path for total mastectomy with malignancy.

hensive when nurses make these checks. The nurse can also explain whether the client is likely to have IV lines, dressings, or drainage tubes. The nurse should neither overprepare nor underprepare the client and family. The nurse cannot predict all of the client's postoperative therapies because each surgeon follows different practices for each type of surgery. Although the nurse becomes familiar with each surgeon's preferences, it is easy to misinform a client about a therapy that may not be initiated. Contradictions between the nurse's explanations and postoperative reality can cause great anxiety.

CLIENT DESCRIBES SURGICAL PROCEDURES AND POSTOPERATIVE TREATMENT

After the surgeon has explained the basic purpose of a surgical procedure, the client may ask the nurse additional questions to clarify misunderstandings. The nurse is careful to avoid saying anything that contradicts the surgeon's explanation. Preestablished standards, those integrated in CareMaps® for pre- and postoperative education (Fig. 48-3, beginning on p. 1399) give the nurse an excellent guide for instruction. One way to avoid problems is to first ask what the client has been told. When the client has little or no understanding about the surgery, the physician may need to be notified to reinform the client. The nurse can augment the physician's explanations. Before surgery certain predictable aspects of the client's treatment plan (e.g., dressing changes and respiratory therapy) and level of supportive nursing care are explained. The nurse can also describe plans for postoperative rehabilitation and drug therapy.

CLIENT DESCRIBES POSTOPERATIVE ACTIVITY RESUMPTION

The type of surgery a client undergoes affects the speed with which normal physical activity and regular eating habits can be resumed. The nurse explains that it is normal to progress gradually in activity and eating. If the client tolerates activity and diet well, activity levels will progress more quickly.

CLIENT VERBALIZES PAIN-RELIEF MEASURES

One of the surgical client's greatest fears is pain. The family is also concerned for the client's comfort. Pain after surgery is normal. The nurse informs the client and family of therapies available for pain relief (e.g., analgesics, positioning, splinting, and relaxation exercises) (see Chapter 43). The client needs to know the schedule for analgesic drugs, the route of administration, and their effects.

The client should be encouraged to inform the nurses before the pain becomes a constant discomfort. If a client waits until pain becomes excruciating, an analgesic will not provide relief. Clients who will have patient-controlled analgesia (PCA) after surgery should know how to push the button, to push the button when beginning to feel discomfort, and understand that use of PCA will not cause overmedication. The client should also know the length of time that it takes for a drug to act and that all discomfort is rarely eliminated. The use of a pain scale can be helpful in client evaluation of pain relief. Information from preoperative pain assessment will be helpful to the nurse when teaching about pain-relief measures.

Many surgical clients often avoid taking pain-relief drugs for fear of becoming dependent. But most drug doses and the required intervals between administration are not sufficient to cause dependence. The nurse should encourage the client to use analgesics as needed. Unless the pain is controlled, it will be difficult for the client to participate in postoperative therapy. Hospitalized clients may initially receive intravenous medication depending on the nature of surgery. As they become able to tolerate food, the physician replaces intravenous analgesics with oral forms.

CLIENT EXPRESSES FEELINGS REGARDING SURGERY

The client may feel like part of an assembly line during the preoperative surgical phase. Frequent visits by staff, diagnostic testing, and physical preparation for surgery consume a lot of time, and the client has few opportunities to reflect on the surgical experience. The nurse makes sure that the client feels like an individual. The client and family need time to express feelings about surgery. The client's level of anxiety influences the frequency of discussions. While delivering routine care, the nurse can encourage expression of concerns. The family may wish to discuss concerns without the client so that their fears will not frighten the client. The establishment of a trusting and therapeutic relationship with client and family allows this to happen.

Physical Preparation

The degree of preoperative physical preparation depends on the client's health status, the surgery to be performed, and the surgeon's preferences. A seriously ill client receives more supportive care in the form of medications, IV fluid therapy, and monitoring than the client facing a minor elective procedure. The nurse explains the purpose of all procedures.

MAINTENANCE OF NORMAL FLUID AND ELECTROLYTE BALANCE

The surgical client is vulnerable to fluid and electrolyte imbalances as a result of inadequate preoperative intake or excessive fluid losses during surgery (see Chapter 45). A client takes nothing by mouth (NPO) after midnight on the morning of surgery. The nurse removes fluids and solid foods from the client's bedside and posts a sign over the bed to alert hospital personnel and family members about fasting restrictions. After 6 to 8 hours of fasting, the client's gastrointestinal tract will be relatively empty, so the risks of vomiting or aspirating emesis during surgery are reduced. General anesthetics typically cause slowing of gastrointestinal peristalsis.

A client who is at home the evening before surgery must understand the importance of not taking food or fluids and be willing to follow restrictions. The nurse can allow the client to rinse the mouth with water or mouthwash and brush the teeth as long as the client does not swallow water. The nurse notifies the surgeon if the client eats or drinks during the fasting period.

During surgery, normal mechanisms for controlling fluid and electrolyte balance, including respiration, digestion, circulation, and elimination, are disturbed. The surgical procedure may cause extensive losses of blood and other body fluids. The surgical stress response aggravates any fluid and electrolyte imbalance. The nurse determines whether the client eats and drinks sufficient amounts before fasting to ensure adequate fluid and nutrition intake.

This prevents fluid and electrolyte imbalances and reduces the risk of infection. The client's diet should include foods high in protein, with sufficient carbohydrates, fat, and vitamins. If a client cannot eat because of gastrointestinal alterations or impairments in consciousness, an IV route for fluid replacement is started. The physician relies on serum electrolyte levels to determine the type of IV fluids and electrolyte additives to administer. Clients with severe nutritional imbalances may require supplements with concentrated protein and glucose (see Chapter 41).

REDUCTION OF RISK OF SURGICAL WOUND INFECTION

The risk of developing a surgical wound infection is determined by the amount and type of microorganisms contaminating a wound, susceptibility of the host, and condition of the wound at the end of the operation (largely determined by the surgeon's operative technique). All three factors may interact to cause infection.

The skin is a favorite site for microorganisms to grow and multiply. Without proper skin preparation, the risk of postoperative wound infection is high. Many surgeons have clients bathe or shower the evening before surgery. Some physicians may request clients to bathe or shower more than once, whereas others may have clients give special attention to cleansing the proposed operative site. This attention could include use of antibacterial soaps such as chlorhexidine (Horner, 1993). Depending on the surgical procedure, a client may also shower the morning of surgery.

If the surgical procedure involves the head, neck, or upper chest area, the client may also be required to shampoo the hair. Cleansing and trimming of fingernails and toenails may be necessary.

In the past a surgical client's skin was thoroughly shaved to remove hair around the incision site. The rationale for the procedure was to remove microorganisms residing in body hair. However, studies have shown that shaving the surgical site increases the incidence of postoperative wound infection (Horner, 1993). Shaving with a razor can cause superficial cuts and nicks in the skin that allow microorganisms to grow. The CDC recommends avoiding hair removal or, if necessary, shaving only immediately before the operation (Horner, 1993). **Depilatories** and clipping are preferred over shaving since they do not nick the skin yet both decrease risk of postoperative wound infection. However, there are hospitals and surgical clinics that still require shaving. Frequently this is the job of the surgical orderly. If the nurse is to perform this job, consult an institution's policy and procedure manual.

Another way to reduce the risk of a postoperative wound infection is to keep a client's preoperative hospital stay short. A number of researchers have shown that a short stay is associated with low wound infection rates (Halsey et al, 1981; Morales and Andrews, 1993). Thus clients have less opportunity to acquire pathogens from the hospital.

PREVENTION OF BOWEL AND BLADDER INCONTINENCE

The client may not receive a bowel preparation (e.g., a cathartic or enema) unless surgery involves the gastrointestinal system. Manipulation of portions of the gastrointestinal tract during surgery results in absence of peristalsis for 24 hours and sometimes longer. Enemas and cathartics cleanse the gastrointestinal tract to prevent intraoperative incontinence and postoperative constipation. An empty bowel reduces risk of injury to the intestines and prevents contamination of the operative wound in case a portion of the bowel is incised or opened. The surgeon's order may read "Give enemas until clear." This means that the nurse is to administer enemas until the enema return contains no fecal material (see Chapter 47). Too many enemas given over a short time, however, can cause serious fluid and electrolyte imbalances. Most agencies recommend a limit to the number of enemas (usually three) a nurse may administer successively.

The bladder is not prepared until the morning of surgery. The nurse instructs the client to void just before leaving for the operating room. An empty bladder prevents a client from being incontinent during surgery. This is important during abdominal surgery, when it may become necessary for the surgeon to manipulate the bladder. An empty bladder also makes abdominal organs more accessible during surgery. The nurse in the operating room often inserts a Foley catheter to maintain an empty bladder.

PROMOTION OF REST AND COMFORT

Rest is essential for normal healing. Anxiety about surgery can easily interfere with the ability to relax or sleep. The underlying condition requiring surgery may be painful, further impairing rest.

The nurse should attempt to make the client's environment quiet and comfortable. Frequently the physician orders a sedative-hypnotic or antianxiety agent for the night before surgery. Sedative-hypnotics (e.g., flurazepam [Dalmane]) affect and promote sleep. Antianxiety agents (e.g., alprazolam [Xanax], diazepam [Valium]) act on the cerebral cortex and limbic system to relieve anxiety.

An advantage to ambulatory surgery or same-day surgical admissions is that the client is able to sleep at home the night before surgery. The client is likely to get more rest in a familiar environment.

Day of Surgery

On the morning before surgery the nurse completes a number of routine procedures before releasing the client for surgery.

CHECKING MEDICAL RECORD CONTENTS AND COMPLETING RECORDING

Before the client goes to the operating room, the nurse checks the contents of the medical record to be sure that pertinent laboratory results are present. The nurse checks consent forms for accuracy of information. A preoperative checklist (Fig. 48-4) provides the nurse with guidelines for ensuring completion of nursing interventions. The nurse also checks the nurses' notes to be sure that documentation of care is current. This is especially important if the hospitalized client experienced unpredicted problems the night before surgery.

CHECKING VITAL SIGNS

The nurse makes a final preoperative assessment of vital signs. The anesthesiologist uses these values as a baseline

A-1c PREOPERATIVE/PREPROCEDURAL CHECKLIST

• File with other A-1c's of same date. •

PROCEDURE: _____

DATE OF PROCEDURE: _____

1. Place initials in appropriate box: YES, NO, N/A (not applicable, or was not ordered). Each item must have an entry.
2. Explain any "No." This can be done in the space after the item or in the "Comments" section. Use back of form, if needed.
3. To give more information on any item, use the space after the item. If more space is needed, use the "Comments" section or back of form.

DATE

HOSP. NO.

NAME

BIRTHDATE

ADDRESS

IF NOT IMPRINTED, PLEASE PRINT DATE, HOSP. NO., NAME AND LOCATION.

YES	NO	N/A	
			Special information (e.g., blind, O$_2$, combative)
			Preoperative orders written.
			(If "NO", Dr. _____ notivied at _____ date/time.)
			Consent complete and in medical record.
			Allergies (or NKA) labelled on cover of medical record.
			Specify Allergies:
			Isolation label on cover of medical record. Specify type.
			Ordered lab results in medical record.
			Urinalysis results in medical record.
			Chest x-ray completed. (Report in medical record: Yes____ No____)
			EKG in medical record.
			Type and cross/screen (circle) done. Date drawn:
			History and physical in medical record.
			Forms complete and in medical record:
			1. Nursing documentation with assessment, VS, and wt./ht.
			2. IV Solution Administration Cardex.
			3. Medication Administration Cardex.
			Addressograph plate on cover of medical record. All volumes to procedure, if required.

COMMENTS:

YES	NO	N/A	
			Blood band on patient and legible. Specify location _____ and blood band #_____
			Identification band on patient and legible. Specify location:
			Bathed and in proper attire.
			Nail polish, makeup, and hairpins removed.
			Jewelry removed. Specify item(s) removed and disposition:
			Prosthesis removed: hearing aid, dentures, eye glasses, contact lenses (circle).
			Other: Disposition:
			Anti-embolism stockings on.
			Sequential compression device sleeves on and controller to OR.
			NPO since:
			Teaching completed and documented.
			Preps/tests completed as ordered. Specify:
			Voided/catheterized (circle). Time:
			Medication(s) given.
			Medication(s)/article(s) sent with patient. Specify:

COMMENTS:

Date	Initials	Signature and Title of Individuals Filling Out Form

Date	Initials	Signature of RN Sending Patient to Procedure

41006/4-93/H7528   THE UNIVERSITY OF IOWA HOSPITALS AND CLINICS

Fig. 48-4 Preoperative/procedural checklist. *(Courtesy University of Iowa Hospitals and Clinics.)*

for intraoperative vital signs. If preoperative vital signs are abnormal, surgery may need to be postponed. For example, an elevated temperature may indicate an infection, which may increase the client's surgical risk. The nurse notifies the physician of abnormalities before sending the client to surgery.

PROVIDING HYGIENE

Basic hygiene measures provide additional comfort before surgery. If the hospitalized client is unwilling to take a complete bath, a partial bath is refreshing and removes irritating secretions or drainage from the skin. Because the client cannot wear personal nightwear to the operating room, the nurse provides a clean hospital gown. After being NPO throughout the night, the client usually has a very dry mouth. The nurse may offer mouthwash and toothpaste, again cautioning the client not to swallow water.

CHECKING HAIR AND COSMETICS

During surgery under general anesthesia, the anesthesiologist positions the client's head to introduce an endotracheal tube into the airway (see Chapter 44). This procedure may involve manipulation of the client's hair and scalp. To avoid injury the nurse asks the client to remove hairpins or clips before leaving for surgery. Hairpieces or wigs should also be removed. Long hair can be braided to keep it in place. The client will wear a paper hair net before entering the operating room.

During and after surgery the anesthesiologist and nurses assess skin and mucous membranes to determine the client's level of oxygenation and circulation. Therefore all makeup (lipstick, powder, blush, nail polish) must be removed to expose normal skin and nail coloring.

CHECKING FOR REMOVAL OF PROSTHESES

It is easy for any type of prosthetic device to become lost or damaged during surgery. The client must remove all prostheses, including partial or complete dentures, artificial limbs, artificial eyes, and contact lenses. Hearing aids, false eyelashes, and eyeglasses must also be removed. If a client has a brace or splint, the nurse checks with the physician to determine whether it should remain with the client.

For many clients it is embarrassing to remove dentures or other devices that enhance appearance. Thus privacy should be offered as the dentures are removed. Dentures must be placed in special containers for safekeeping to prevent loss or breakage, and the client is assessed for any loose teeth. A broken tooth can become dislodged during insertion of an endotracheal tube and obstruct the airway.

In many agencies nurses must document an inventory of all prosthetic devices or personal items and have them locked away for safekeeping according to agency policy. It is also common practice for nurses to give prostheses to family members or to keep the devices at the client's bedside. Documentation in the nursing notes or the surgical checklist should reflect these actions.

PREPARING BOWEL AND BLADDER

The client may require an enema or cathartic the morning of surgery. If so, it should be given at least an hour before the client is scheduled to leave, allowing time for the client to defecate without rushing. The client should void before surgery. If the client is unable to void, it should be noted on the preoperative checklist.

APPLYING ANTIEMBOLISM STOCKINGS OR SEQUENTIAL COMPRESSION DEVICES

Many physicians prefer clients to wear **antiembolism stockings** during surgery. These are designed to support the lower extremities and maintain compression of small veins and capillaries. The constant compression forces blood into larger vessels, thus promoting venous return and preventing circulatory stasis. When correctly sized and properly applied, antiembolism stockings can reduce the risk of thrombi. Chapter 37 reviews the procedure for sizing and application. Sequential compression devices may be applied to the lower extremities for the same purpose (Fig. 48-5). These stockings promote circulation by sequentially compressing the legs from ankle upward, promoting venous return. Please check agency policy and procedure manual prior to application. Documentation of application, capillary refill, and client tolerance should be in the nursing notes.

PROMOTING CLIENT DIGNITY

During preoperative preparations, care can become depersonalized unless the nurse maintains the client's privacy and reduces sources of anxiety. Ambulatory and same-day surgical admission clients often must sit in a waiting room before surgery. The nurse provides cover robes and slippers. Hospitalized clients should be ensured privacy by closing room curtains or doors during preoperative preparation. Family may be allowed to stay until it is time for transport to the operating room.

PERFORMING SPECIAL PROCEDURES

A client's condition may warrant special interventions before surgery. The surgeon's orders inform nurses of the need to start IV infusions, insert Foley catheters, or administer medications.

One special procedure involves insertion of a nasogastric (NG) tube, a pliable plastic tube, through the client's nasopharynx into the stomach. The tube has a hollow lumen that allows removal of gastric secretions and introduction of solutions into the stomach. NG intubation has several purposes (Table 48-7). For a surgical client the main pur-

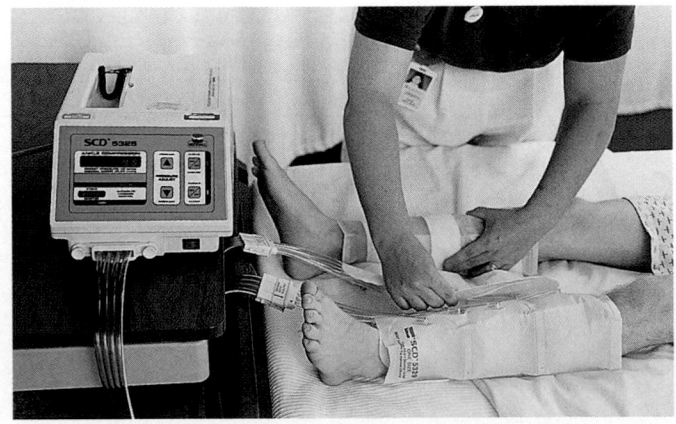

Fig. 48-5 Sequential compression stockings.

Table 48-7	Purposes of NG Intubation	
PURPOSE	**DESCRIPTION**	**TYPE OF TUBE**
Decompression	Removal of secretions and gaseous substances from gastrointestinal tract; prevention or relief of abdominal distention	Salem sump, Levin, Miller-Abbott
Feeding (gavage) (see Chapter 41)	Instillation of liquid nutritional supplements or feedings into stomach for clients unable to swallow fluid	Duo, Dobhoff, Levin
Compression	Internal application of pressure by means of inflated balloon to prevent internal esophageal or gastrointestinal hemorrhage	Sengstaken-Blakemore
Lavage	Irrigation of stomach in cases of active bleeding, poisoning, or gastric dilation	Levin, Ewald, Salem sump

pose is stomach decompression to prevent abdominal distention. The physician often waits to order NG tube insertion until the client is in the operating room.

The Levin and Salem sump tubes are the most common for stomach decompression. The Levin tube is a single-lumen tube with holes near the tip. It may be connected to a drainage bag or an intermittent suction device to drain stomach secretions.

The Salem sump tube is preferable for stomach decompression. The tube has two lumina: one for removal of gastric contents and one to provide an air vent. A blue "pigtail" is the air vent that connects with the second lumen. When the sump tube's main lumen is connected to suction, the air vent permits free, continuous drainage of secretions. The air vent should never be clamped off, connected to suction, or used for irrigation.

Tube insertion (Procedure 48-2) does not require sterile technique. The nurse simply uses clean technique. The procedure is uncomfortable. The client experiences a burning sensation as the tube passes through the sensitive nasal mucosa. When the tube reaches the back of the pharynx, the client may begin to gag. The nurse must help the client relax to make tube insertion easier. Some institutions allow xylocaine jelly to be used when inserting the tube as it increases comfort.

One of the greatest problems in caring for a client with an NG tube is maintaining comfort. The tube is a constant irritation to nasal mucosa. The nurse must assess the condition of the nares and mucosa for inflammation and excoriation. The tape used to anchor the tube becomes soiled. The nurse changes it every day to lessen irritation. Frequent lubrication of the nares also minimizes excoriation. With one naris occluded, the client may breathe through the mouth. Frequent mouth care (at least every 2 hours) helps minimize dehydration. A glass of cool water for rinsing is useful, but the client who is NPO should not swallow the water. The client will frequently complain of a sore throat. An ice bag applied externally to the throat sometimes helps. Gargling with topical xylocaine jelly and/or lozenges may be used if ordered by the physician.

After the tube is introduced, the nurse must maintain its patency. If the tip of the tubing rests against the stomach wall or if the tube becomes blocked with thick secretions, regular irrigation is necessary. Flushing the tube with normal saline by way of a cone-tipped syringe clears blockage within the tube (Procedure 48-2). If an NG tube continues to drain improperly after irrigation, the nurse must reposition it by advancing or withdrawing it slightly. Any change in position requires reassessment of tube placement.

The NG tube can cause distention. The presence of the tube causes many clients to swallow large volumes of air. Channels of gastric secretions also form along the walls of the stomach and bypass the suction holes. Turning the client regularly helps to collapse the channels and promote emptying of stomach contents.

SAFEGUARDING VALUABLES

If a client has any valuables, the nurse should give them to family members or secure them for safekeeping. Many hospitals require clients to sign a release to free the institution of responsibility for lost valuables. Valuables can usually be stored and locked in a designated location. Often clients are reluctant to remove wedding rings or religious medals. A wedding band can be taped in place. However, if there is a risk that the client will experience swelling of the hand or fingers, the band should be removed. Many hospitals allow clients to pin religious medals to their gowns, although the risk of loss increases. Document location of valuables per hospital policy.

ADMINISTERING PREOPERATIVE MEDICATIONS

The use of preoperative medications has been much decreased in the age of ambulatory surgery. However, the anesthesiologist or surgeon may order preanesthetic drugs that reduce the client's anxiety, the amount of general anesthesia required, the risk of nausea and vomiting, and respiratory tract secretions. Tranquilizers, such as chlorpromazine (Thorazine) or diazepam (Valium), reduce anxiety and relax skeletal muscles. Narcotic analgesics, such as morphine or fentanyl (Sublimaze), provide sedation, reduce pain and anxiety, and reduce the amount of anesthetic required during surgery. Drugs such as glycopyrrolate (Robinul) or atropine create anticholinergic effects to inhibit mucous secretions in the oral and respiratory passages

Text continued on p. 1410.

PROCEDURE 48-2

Inserting and Maintaining an NG Tube

STEPS	RATIONALE
1. Apply clean gloves and inspect condition of client's oral cavity.	Baseline condition determines need for special nursing measures for oral hygiene after tube placement.
2. Palpate client's abdomen.	Baseline determination will later serve as comparison after tube is inserted.
3. Check medical record for surgeon's order, type of NG tube to be placed, and whether tube is to be attached to suction or drainage bag.	Procedure requires physician's order. Adequate decompression depends on suction.
4. Prepare equipment and supplies:	
a. 14 or 16 Fr NG tube (smaller lumen for child)	Smaller lumen catheters are not used for decompression because they must be used to remove thick secretions.
b. Water-soluble lubricating jelly	Used to lubricate tube for insertion.
c. pH test strips	Used to measure gastric aspirate acidity.
d. Tongue blade	
e. Flashlight	
f. Asepto bulb or cone-tip syringe	Used to irrigate or instill fluid into tube.
g. 2.5-cm (1-in) wide hypoallergenic tape	Less adhesive than regular tape and reduces loss of skin on nose.
h. Safety pin and rubber band	
i. Clamp, drainage bag, or suction machine	Tube may be open or closed to drainage.
j. Bath towel	
k. Glass of water with straw	
l. Facial tissues	
m. Normal saline	Used for irrigation of tube.
n. Tincture of benzoin (optional)	Increases adhesion of tape to nose.
o. Disposable gloves	
5. Identify client and explain procedure.	Prevents error and gains client's cooperation to facilitate passage of tube and lessen possibility that client will remove tube.

TUBE INSERTION

STEPS	RATIONALE
6. Wash hands and apply gloves.	Reduces transmission of microorganisms.
7. Position client in high Fowler's position with pillows behind head and shoulders. Raise bed to its highest horizontal level.	Promotes client's ability to swallow during procedure. Good body mechanics prevent injury to nurse or client.
8. Assemble all equipment at bedside and place on your side of bed. Pull curtain around bed or close room door.	Procedure should be organized to limit discomfort. Provides privacy.
9. Stand at right side of bed if right-handed and left side if left-handed.	Allows easiest manipulation of tubing.
10. Place bath towel over chest; give tissues to client.	Prevents soiling of gown. Tube insertion through nasal passages may cause tearing.
11. Instruct client to relax and breathe normally while occluding one naris. Then repeat this action for other naris. Select nostril with greater air flow.	Tube passes more easily through naris that is more patent.
12. Measure distance to insert tube:	Tube should extend from nares to stomach; distance varies with each client. Length provides distance from nose to stomach in 98% of clients (Grant, Kennedy-Caldwell, 1988).
a. Traditional method: measure distance from tip of nose to earlobe to xiphoid process to sternum (see the illustration on p. 1407).	
b. Hanson method: first mark 50-cm (20-in) point on tube and then do traditional measurement. Tube insertion should be to midway point between 50 cm and traditional mark.	
13. Mark length of tube to be inserted with piece of tape or note distance from next tube marking.	Marks amount of tube to be inserted from nares to stomach.
14. Cut 10-cm (4-in) long piece of tape. Split one end lengthwise 5 cm (2 in).	Tape will be used after tube insertion to anchor tube securely.

Inserting and Maintaining an NG Tube—cont'd

STEPS	RATIONALE
15. Curve 10-15 cm (4-6 in) of end of tube tightly around index finger; release.	Curving tube tip aids insertion.
16. Lubricate 7.5-10 cm (3-4 in) of end of tube with water-soluble lubricating jelly.	Minimizes friction against nasal mucosa.
17. Initially instruct client to extend neck back against pillow; insert tube slowly through naris with curved end pointing downward (see the illustration below).	Facilitates initial passage of tube through naris and maintains clear airway for open naris.
18. Continue to pass tube along floor of nasal passage, aiming down toward ear. When resistance is felt, apply gentle downward pressure to advance tube (do not force past resistance).	Minimizes discomfort of tube rubbing against upper nasal turbinates. Resistance is caused by posterior nasopharynx. Downward pressure helps tube to curl around corner of nasopharynx.
19. If resistance is met, withdraw tube, allow client to rest, relubricate tube, and insert into other naris.	Forcing against resistance can cause trauma to mucosa. Helps relieve anxiety.
20. Continue insertion of tube until just past nasopharynx by gently rotating tube toward opposite naris:	
a. Stop the advancement, allow client to relax, and provide tissues.	Relieves anxiety; tearing is natural response to mucosal irritation.
b. Explain that next step requires swallowing.	Tube is about to enter esophagus.
21. With tube just above oropharynx, instruct client to flex head forward and dry swallow or suck in air through straw. Advance tube 2.5-5 cm (1-2 in) with each swallow. If client has trouble swallowing and is allowed fluids, offer glass of water. Advance tube with each swallow of water.	Flexed position closes off upper airway to trachea and opens esophagus. Swallowing closes epiglottis over trachea and helps to move tube into esophagus. Swallowing water reduces gagging or choking.
22. If client begins to cough, gag, or choke, stop tube advancement. Instruct client to breathe easily and take sips of water.	Tubing may accidentally enter larynx and initiate cough reflex. Gagging is eased by swallowing water.
23. If client continues to cough, pull tube back slightly.	Tube may enter larynx and obstruct airway.
24. If client continues to gag, check back of pharynx using flashlight and tongue blade.	Tube may coil around itself in back of throat.
25. After client relaxes, continue to advance tube desired distance.	Tip of tube should be within stomach to decompress properly.

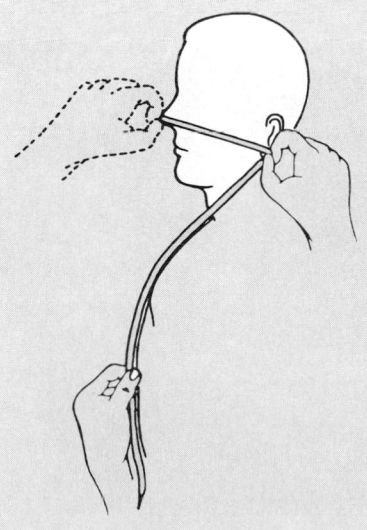

Step 12a

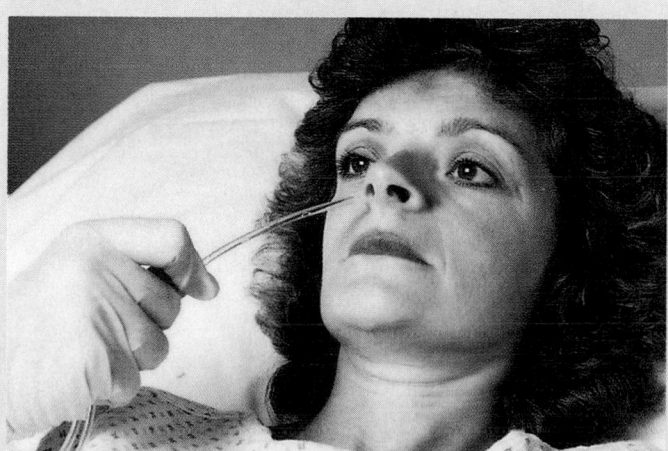

Step 17

Continued.

Inserting and Maintaining an NG Tube—cont'd

STEPS	RATIONALE

CHECKING TUBE PLACEMENT

26. Check posterior pharynx for presence of coiled tube.

Tube is pliable and can coil up in back of pharynx instead of advancing into esophagus.

27. Attach cone-tipped syringe to end of tube. Aspirate gently back on syringe to obtain gastric contents. (Insufflation of air into tube followed by auscultation of sounds is no longer considered most effective in determining tube placement.)

Aspiration of contents provide means to measure fluid pH and thus determine tube tip placement in gastrointestinal tract. (Sounds transmitted by insufflation of air may be transmitted from pleural space to upper abdomen, giving false impression of placement [Metheny, 1988; Metheny et al, 1990].)

28. Measure pH of aspirate with color-coded pH paper with range of whole numbers from 1-11.

Gastric aspirates have decidedly acidic pH values, preferably 4 or less (Metheny et al, 1989).

29. If tube is not in stomach, advance another 2.5-5 cm (1-2 in) and repeat Steps 27 and 28 to check tube position.

Tube must be in stomach to provide decompression.

ANCHORING TUBE

30. After tube is properly inserted, clamp end or connect it to drainage bag or suction machine.

Drainage bag is used for gravity drainage. Intermittent suction is most effective for decompression. Tube is often clamped in client going to operating room.

31. Tape tube to nose; avoid putting pressure on nares.

  a. OPTIONAL: Apply small amount of tincture of benzoin to lower end of nose and allow to dry. Place top end of tape over nose.

  b. Carefully wrap two split ends around tube (see the illustrations below).

Prevents tissue necrosis. Tape anchors tube securely. Benzoin prevents loosening of tape if client perspires.

32. Fasten end of tube to gown by looping rubber band around tube in slip knot. Pin rubber band to gown.

Reduces pressure on nares if tube moves. Pinning provides slack for movement.

33. Unless physician orders otherwise, head of bed should be elevated 30 degrees.

Helps prevent esophageal reflux and minimizes irritation of tube against posterior pharynx.

34. Explain that sensation of tube will decrease somewhat.

Helps adaptation to continued sensory stimulus.

35. Wash hands.

Reduces transmission of microorganisms.

36. Record in nurses' notes time and type of tube inserted, tolerance to procedure, confirmation of placement, character of gastric contents, and whether tube is changed or connected to drainage device.

Documents that procedure was performed correctly. Description of gastric contents provides baseline to determine change.

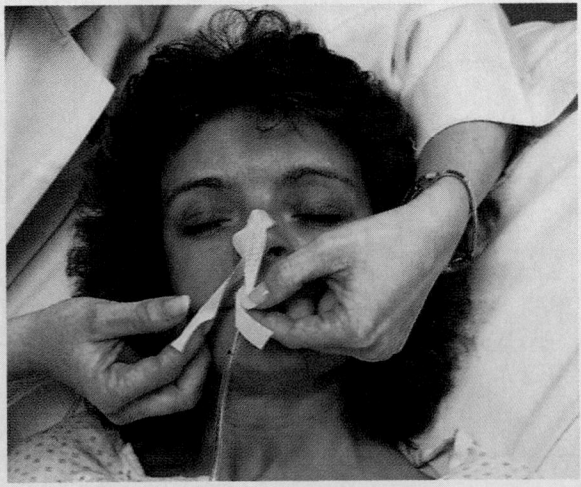 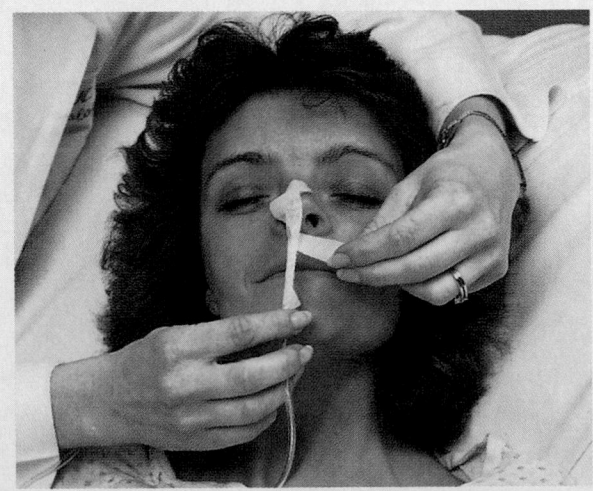

Step 31b

Inserting and Maintaining an NG Tube—cont'd

TUBE IRRIGATION

37. Check tube placement if it remains patent.

Prevents accidental entrance of irrigating solution into lungs.
Minimizes loss of electrolytes from stomach fluids.

38. Draw up 30 ml of normal saline into Asepto or cone-tipped syringe.

39. Clamp connection tubing proximal to connection site for drainage or suction apparatus. Disconnect tubing and lay end on towel.

Reduces backflow of secretions and soiling of gown and bed linen.

40. Insert tip of irrigating syringe into end of tube. Hold syringe with tip pointed at floor and inject saline slowly and evenly. (Do not force solution.)

Position prevents introduction of air into vent tubing, which could cause gastric distention. Solution introduced under pressure can cause trauma.

41. If resistance occurs, check for kinks in tubing. Turn client onto left side. Repeated resistance should be reported to surgeon.

Tip of tube may lie against stomach lining. Buildup of secretions causes distention.

42. After instilling saline, immediately aspirate or pull back slowly on syringe to withdraw fluid. Measure volume returned as output.

Irrigation clears tubing, so stomach should remain empty. Fluid remaining in stomach is measured as intake.

43. Reconnect tube to drainage or suction. (If solution does not return, repeat irrigation.)

Reestablishes drainage collection; may repeat irrigation or repositioning of tube until tube drains properly.

44. Wash hands.

Reduces transmission of microorganisms.

45. Record each irrigation: type and amount of solution used and character and volume of aspirate.

Documents procedure and results.

DISCONTINUATION OF TUBE

46. Apply disposable gloves.

Reduces transmission of microorganisms.

47. Turn off suction and disconnect tube from drainage bag or suction. Remove tape from bridge of nose and unpin tube from gown.

Tube is free of connections before removal.

48. Explain procedure to client and reassure that removal is less distressing than insertion.

Minimizes anxiety and increases cooperation. Tube passes out smoothly.

49. Hand client facial tissue; place clean towel across chest. Instruct client to take and hold deep breath.

Airway will be temporarily obstructed during removal. Client may wish to blow nose after removal.

50. Clamp or kink tubing securely and pull tube out steadily and smoothly while client holds breath.

Clamping prevents tube contents from draining into oropharynx.

51. Measure unit of drainage and note character of content. Dispose of tube and drainage equipment. Remove gloves.

Provides accurate measure of fluid output. Reduces transfer of microorganisms.

52. Clean nares and provide mouth care.

Promotes comfort.

53. Position client comfortably and explain procedure for drinking fluid, if not contraindicated.

Depends on physician's order; usually begins with small amount of ice chips each hour and increases as client is able to tolerate more.

54. Clean equipment and return to proper place. Place soiled linen in "dirty" utility room or proper receptacle.

Proper disposal of equipment prevents spread of microorganisms and ensures proper exchange procedures.

55. Remove gloves, dispose in receptacle, and wash hands.

Reduces transmission of microorganisms.

56. Palpate abdomen periodically, noting distention.

Determines success of abdominal decompression.

57. Inspect condition of nares and nose.

Evaluates onset of skin and tissue irritation.

58. Record removal of NG tube, client's tolerance of procedure, presence of bowel sounds, and abdominal assessment.

Documents procedure and provides baseline information regarding abdominal assessment and bowel sounds.

and prevent spasm of laryngeal muscles. Medications such as droperidol (Inapsine) and metoclopramide (Reglan) may be used to decrease nausea and vomiting.

Typically the physician orders preoperative medications to be administered when the client leaves for the operating room or at an earlier prescribed time. The nurse provides all nursing care measures before giving the client preoperative medications. The consent form needs to be signed prior to the administration of these medications. In addition, the client should be assisted to void. Because the drugs cause sedation, the client should not be allowed to leave the bed or stretcher until surgical personnel arrive to transport the client to the operating room. The client should be warned to expect drowsiness and a dry mouth. The side rails should be raised and the bed or stretcher kept in the low position for client safety.

Evaluation

Often there is limited time to evaluate the outcomes of the preoperative care plan. The client's surgery may be an emergency, or performance of various procedures may make it difficult for the nurse to find time for evaluation. The nurse's interventions may continue during and after surgery so that evaluation does not occur until after surgery. For example, the nurse will not be able to evaluate the success of reducing postoperative wound infection or promoting return of normal physiological function until a few days after surgery.

The nurse evaluates success at preoperative teaching and promoting the client's physiological function, rest, and physical comfort (see the evaluation box below). However, evaluation of these interventions must also continue after surgery.

Transport to the Operating Room

Personnel in the operating room notify the nursing division or ambulatory surgical waiting area when it is time for surgery. In many hospitals a nursing orderly or transporter brings a stretcher for transporting the client. The transporter checks the client's identification bracelet against the client's chart to be sure that the right person is going to surgery. Because the client has already received preoperative drugs, the nurses and transporter assist the client in transferring from bed to stretcher to prevent falls. The family gets one last op-

portunity to visit before the client is transported to the operating room. Nurses then direct the family to a waiting area.

After the client leaves the nursing division the nurse prepares the bed and room for the client's return if the client is returning to the same nursing division. A postoperative bedside unit should include the following:

1. Sphygmomanometer, stethoscope, and thermometer
2. Emesis basin
3. Clean gown
4. Washcloth, towel, and facial tissues
5. IV pole
6. Suction equipment (optional)
7. Oxygen equipment (optional)
8. Extra pillows for positioning the client comfortably
9. Bed pads to protect bed linen from drainage
10. Bed raised to stretcher height with bed linens pulled back

The nurse will be better prepared to care for the client after surgery if the room is readied before the client's return.

■ INTRAOPERATIVE SURGICAL PHASE

Care of the client during surgery requires careful preparation and knowledge of the events that occur during the surgical procedure.

Holding Area

In most hospitals the client enters a holding area outside the operating room. There the nurse explains the steps to be taken in preparing the client for surgery. Nurses in the holding area are usually part of the operating room staff and wear surgical scrub suits, hats, and footwear in accordance with infection-control policies. In some ambulatory surgical settings a perioperative primary nurse admits the client, circulates for the operative procedure, and manages the client's recovery and discharge.

In the holding area the nurse, nurse anesthetist, or anesthesiologist inserts an IV catheter into the arm to establish a route for fluid replacement and IV drugs. A large-bore IV catheter is used for easy infusion of fluids. The nurse also applies a blood pressure cuff. The cuff will remain in place throughout surgery so that the anesthesiologist can assess blood pressure readings.

Because of the preoperative medications, the client begins to feel drowsy. Because the temperature in the holding

Sample Evaluation of Interventions for Knowledge Deficit

GOALS	EVALUATIVE MEASURES	EXPECTED OUTCOMES
Client will understand intraoperative and postoperative events prior to scheduled surgery.	Ask client and family to identify appropriate times of surgery and routine treatment procedures.	Client and family will describe routine procedures that nurses perform after surgery.
	Ask client and family to identify and demonstrate turning, coughing, deep breathing, and spirometry exercises.	Client will describe ways to participate in care after surgery.
	Have client explain postoperative assessments nurses will routinely perform.	Client and family will describe events that commonly occur in holding area and operating room.

area and adjacent operating room suites is usually cool, the client should be offered an extra blanket. The client's stay in the holding area should be brief.

Admission to the Operating Room

Nurses transfer the client to the operating room via stretcher. The client is usually still awake and will notice nurses and physicians wearing complete surgical masks, gowns, and eyewear. The staff carefully transfers the client to the operating table, being sure that the stretcher and table are locked in place. After the client is on the table the nurse fastens a safety strap around the client.

The operating room nurse checks the client's identification and chart; reviews consent forms, medical history, physical assessment findings, and test results; makes sure that prosthetic devices and valuables have been removed; and reviews the preoperative care plan to establish an intraoperative care plan.

The nurse may apply monitoring devices to the client before surgery. Clients receiving general and regional anesthesia undergo continuous ECG monitoring during surgery. Small, plastic electrodes are placed on the chest and extremities to record electrical activity of the heart. A monitor in the operating room displays the heart's electrical activity. Pulse oximetry will be used to monitor oxygen saturation as an index of ventilation quality.

Many ambulatory surgical clients remain awake during the procedure because only local anesthetic is used. The nurse supports the client by explaining procedures and encouraging the client to ask questions. Sights and sounds in the surgical suite can frighten clients.

Introduction of Anesthesia

Clients undergoing surgical procedures receive anesthesia in one of three ways: general, regional, or local.

GENERAL ANESTHESIA

Under **general anesthesia** a client loses all sensation and consciousness. Muscles relax to ease manipulation of body parts. The client also experiences amnesia of all surgical events. Surgery using general anesthesia involves major procedures requiring extensive tissue manipulation.

An anesthesiologist gives general anesthetics by IV and inhalation routes through the four stages of anesthesia. Stage 1 begins with the client awake. The client gradually becomes drowsy and loses consciousness, and a state of analgesia begins. Stage 2 is the stage of excitement. The client's muscles are often tense and almost spasmodic. Swallowing and vomiting reflexes remain intact, and the client may have an irregular breathing pattern. Stage 3 begins with the onset of regular rhythmical breathing. Vital functions are depressed, reflexes are depressed or temporarily lost, and the surgeon begins the operation during this phase. Stage 4 is the stage of complete respiratory depression, which can be fatal. These stages were defined with the use of ether and are sometimes difficult to ascertain with newer anesthetic agents. A more useful designation of stages would likely be induction (stages 1 and 2), maintenance (stage 3), and emergence (stages 2 and 1).

To move the client quickly to maintenance or stage 3 of general anesthesia, the anesthesiologist usually gives an IV dose of a barbiturate pentothal or drug called propofol

(Waugaman and Foster, 1991). To prevent possible aspiration and other respiratory complications, the anesthesiologist puts an endotracheal tube into the client's airway. Succinylcholine, a nerve blocking agent causes temporary paralysis of vocal cords and respiratory muscles while the tube is in place. The anesthesiologist then provides artificial ventilation until succinylcholine's effects wear off and the client again breathes spontaneously. From that point, anesthetic gases or vapors are usually delivered by inhalation through the endotracheal tube. Some commonly used agents are suprane, forane, and halothane. The client also receives a continuous supply of oxygen.

The duration of anesthesia depends on the length of surgery. Surgical risks influence the duration of surgery. The greatest risks from general anesthesia are the side effects of anesthetic agents, including cardiovascular depression or irritability, respiratory depression, and liver and kidney damage.

REGIONAL ANESTHESIA

Induction of **regional anesthesia** results in loss of sensation in an area of the body. The method of induction influences the portion of sensory pathways that is anesthetized. The anesthesiologist gives regional anesthetics by infiltration and local application (see Chapter 43). In major surgery, such as a hernia repair, vaginal hysterectomy, or vascular repair of leg blood vessels, only infiltrative induction is used. Fig. 48-6 provides information as to where medication is introduced to achieve the regional block. Infiltration of anesthetic agents may involve one of the following induction methods:

1. Nerve block. Local anesthetic is injected into a nerve (e.g., brachial plexus in the arm), blocking the nerve supply to the operative site.
2. Spinal anesthesia. The anesthesiologist performs a lumbar puncture and introduces local anesthetic into the cerebrospinal fluid in the spinal subarachnoid space. Anesthesia can extend from the tip of the xiphoid

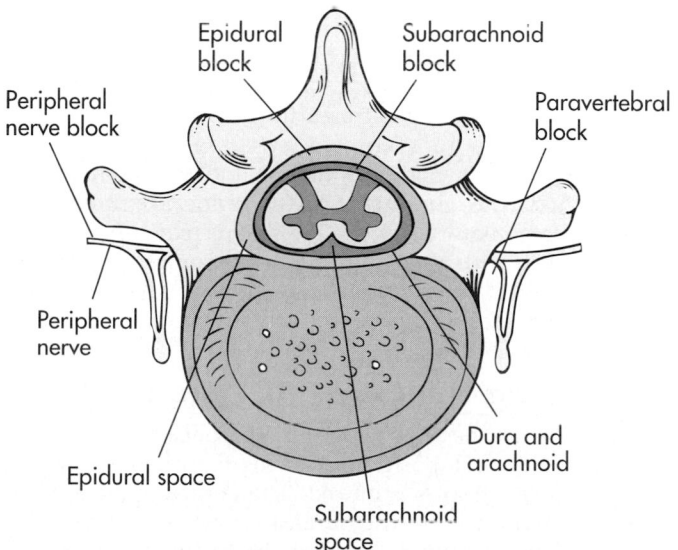

Fig. 48-6 Cross-section of spinal cord placement of needle and medication to achieve regional anesthesia block.

process down to the feet. Positioning of the client influences movement of the anesthetic agent up or down the spinal cord.

3. Epidural anesthesia. This is a safer procedure than spinal anesthesia because the anesthetic agent is injected into the epidural space outside the dura mater and the level of anesthesia is not as great as spinal anesthesia. Because epidural anesthesia provides an effective loss of sensation in the vaginal and perineal areas, it is the best anesthetic for obstetrical procedures. The epidural catheter may be left in so that the client may receive medication via continuous epidural infusion following surgery.

4. Caudal anesthesia. This is a form of epidural anesthesia achieved by giving the local anesthetic at the base of the spine. The anesthesia affects only the pelvic region and legs.

There are risks involved with infiltrative anesthetics, particularly in the case of spinal anesthesia, because the level of anesthesia may rise, which means the anesthetic agent moves upwards in the spinal cord and breathing may be affected. The client may have a sudden fall in blood pressure, which results from extensive vasodilation caused by the anesthetic block to sympathetic vasomotor nerves and pain and motor nerve fibers. If the level of anesthesia rises, respiratory paralysis may develop, requiring resuscitation by the anesthesiologist. The client requires careful monitoring during and immediately after surgery.

The client under regional anesthesia is awake throughout the surgery unless the physician orders a tranquilizer that promotes sleep. Because the client is responsive and capable of breathing voluntarily, it is unnecessary for the anesthesiologist to use an endotracheal tube. Operating room personnel often gain a false sense of security because of the client's relative alertness. Nurses must remember that burns and other trauma can occur on the anesthetized part of the body without the client being aware of the injury. It is therefore necessary to frequently observe the position of extremities and the condition of the skin. It is also important that OR staff use caution in topics discussed in surgery.

LOCAL ANESTHESIA

Local anesthesia involves loss of sensation at the desired site (e.g., a growth on the skin or the cornea of the eye). The anesthetic agent (e.g., lidocaine) inhibits nerve conduction until the drug diffuses into the circulation. The client experiences a loss in pain sensation and touch, motor, and autonomic activities (e.g., bladder emptying). Local anesthesia is commonly used for minor procedures performed in ambulatory surgery. Physicians may infiltrate the operative area with local anesthetics to promote postoperative pain relief. For example, injection of Marcaine may provide relief following herniorrhaphy for 12 hours or more (Rivellini, 1993).

Positioning the Client for Surgery

During general anesthesia, the nursing personnel and surgeon often do not position the client until the stage of complete relaxation is achieved. The choice of position is usually determined by the surgical approach. Ideally the client's position provides good access to the operative site and sustains adequate circulatory and respiratory function. It should not impair neuromuscular structures. The client's

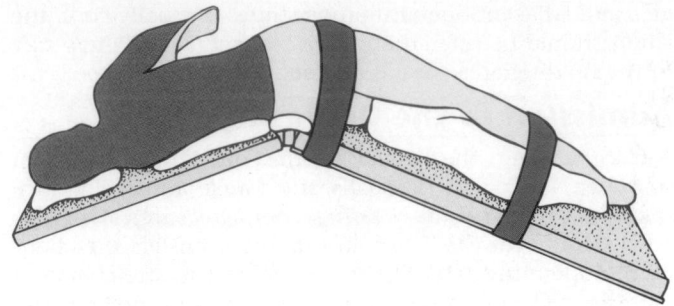

Fig. 48-7 Client's position on operating room table for a nephrectomy.

comfort and safety must be considered. The team must take into account age, weight, height, nutritional status, physical limitations, and preexisting conditions and document them to alert staff who care for the client postoperatively (Walsh, 1993).

It is sometimes difficult for nurses in postoperative divisions to appreciate the discomfort a client may feel after surgery (e.g., discomfort of the left arm or side of a client whose right kidney was removed) (Fig. 48-7). Normal range of joint motion is maintained in an alert person by pain and pressure receptors. If a joint is extended too far, pain stimuli provide a warning that muscle and joint strain are too great. In a client who is anesthetized, normal defense mechanisms cannot guard against joint damage, muscle stretch, and strain. The muscles are so relaxed that it is relatively easy to place the client in a position the individual normally could not assume while awake. The client often remains in a given position for several hours. Although it may be necessary to place a client in an unusual position, the nurse should attempt to maintain correct alignment and protect the client from pressure, abrasion, and other injuries. Attachments to the operating table allow protection and padding of extremities and bony prominences. Positioning should not impede normal movement of the diaphragm or interfere with circulation to body parts. If restraints are necessary, the nurse pads the area to be restrained to prevent skin trauma.

Nurse's Role During Surgery

The nurse assumes one of two roles during the surgical procedure: scrub nurse or circulating nurse. The **scrub nurse** provides the surgeon with instruments and supplies, which requires strict surgical asepsis (see Chapter 34) and familiarity with surgical instruments. Each instrument is designed for a specific purpose during a phase or step in surgery. It takes knowledge and skill to anticipate which instrument the surgeon requires and to pass it quickly and smoothly. The scrub nurse also disposes of soiled gauze sponges and accounts for sponges, needles, and instruments on the surgical field and in body cavities. This role may be assumed by a scrub technician who is not a nurse.

The **circulating nurse** is an assistant to the scrub nurse and surgeon. When the client first enters the operating room the circulator helps position the client and applies necessary equipment and surgical drapes. During surgery the circulator provides the scrub nurse with supplies, disposes of soiled equipment and sponges, and keeps a count of instruments, needles, and sponges used. If there is a need to help reposition the client or move the operating room lights, the circulating nurse is available to assist. Like all members of the surgical team the circulator follows surgical aseptic technique. If a break in asepsis occurs, the circulator assists team members with regowning and regloving.

At the end of each surgical procedure the scrub and circulating nurses count the number of used instruments, needles, and gauze sponges. This procedure prevents the accidental loss of such items within the client's surgical wound. It is not difficult for a sponge saturated with blood to be overlooked within a wound. Careful monitoring of items is essential for the client's safety. The nurse who fails to make accurate counts can be held legally accountable. If a client is injured by a misplaced needle or instrument the nurse may be judged negligent (see Chapter 20).

Documentation of Intraoperative Care

During the intraoperative phase the nursing staff continues the preoperative care plan. For example, strict asepsis must be followed to minimize the risk of surgical wound infection (see Chapter 49). IV fluid infusion and monitoring of urinary and NG output are actions the nurse takes to maintain fluid balance. Throughout the surgical procedure the nurse keeps an accurate record of client care activities and procedures performed by operating room personnel (Fig. 48-8). Documentation of intraoperative care provides useful data for the nurse who cares for the client postoperatively.

■ POSTOPERATIVE SURGICAL PHASE

After surgery a client's care can become complex as a result of physiological changes that may occur. Clients who have undergone general anesthesia are more likely to face complications than those who have only had local anesthesia. The client who requires general anesthesia usually has undergone extensive surgery as well. In contrast an ambulatory surgical client who had local anesthesia with no sedation and has stable vital signs may be immediately discharged. A client who has undergone regional or general anesthesia usually is transferred to the postanesthesia care unit (PACU) to be stabilized prior to discharge while those with local anesthesia may go right to the surgical unit.

To assess a client's postoperative condition the nurse relies on information from the preoperative nursing assessment, knowledge regarding the surgical procedure performed, and events occurring during surgery. This information helps the nurse to detect change. A variation from the client's norm may indicate onset of surgically related complications. The circulating nurse may accompany the client to the PACU and report to the nurse along with the anesthetist or anesthesiologist to provide continuity of care.

A client's postoperative course involves two phases: the immediate recovery period and postoperative convalescence. For an ambulatory surgical client, **recovery** normally lasts only 1 to 2 hours, and **convalescence** takes place at home. For a hospitalized client, recovery may last a few hours, and convalescence takes 1 or more days depending on the extent of surgery and the client's response.

Immediate Postoperative Recovery

Before the arrival of the client in the PACU, the PACU nurse obtains data from the surgical team in the operating room regarding the client's general status and need for special equipment and nursing care. Careful planning allows the nursing staff to consider placement of clients in the PACU. For example, clients who undergo spinal anesthesia are aware of their surroundings and may benefit from being in a quieter part of the PACU, away from clients needing frequent monitoring. The client with a serious infection such as TB should be isolated from other clients. Standard precautions (see Chapter 34) should be used for all clients.

When the client enters the PACU (Fig. 48-9), the nurse and members of the surgical team confer about the client's status. The surgical team's report includes a review of anesthetic agents administered so that the PACU nurse can anticipate the ease with which a client should regain consciousness. A report on IV fluids or blood products administered during surgery alerts the nurse to the fluid and electrolyte balance. The surgeon often reports special concerns (e.g., whether the client is at risk for hemorrhaging or infection). The operating room nurse discusses whether there were complications during surgery, such as excessive blood loss or cardiac irregularities. Frequently this report takes place while PACU staff are admitting the client. The nurse will attach the client to different types of equipment for monitoring such as the noninvasive blood pressure monitor, ECG monitor, and the pulse oximeter. Most clients receive some form of oxygen in this immediate recovery period.

After reviewing events in the operating room the PACU nurse makes a complete assessment of the client's status. The client remains in the PACU until stabilized.

When the client is ready for discharge from the PACU the personnel notify the nursing division of the client's arrival. This allows the nursing staff to inform family members of the client's operative course. The nurse usually advises family members to remain in the designated waiting area so that they can be found when the surgeon arrives to explain the client's condition. The surgeon describes the client's status, the results of surgery, and any complications.

Anxiety can arise if the surgeon has informed the family of the anticipated length of surgery and if the client remains in the operating room past this time. Nurses can help relieve concerns by explaining normal delays, such as room preparation or delay in the previous surgery. If the client's stay in the PACU is extended the nurses can explain to the family that the client is being held longer for observation. If the client has complications it is the surgeon's responsibility to explain what occurred during surgery.

If the surgeon discovered an inoperable condition (e.g., a malignant tumor), the nurse provides support to the family. Directing the family to the location of public telephones, providing a cup of coffee, and encouraging expression of fears in a private location are a few ways to help the family cope with the waiting period. The family's initial shock requires the nurse to be available and serve as a resource for the family.

After the initial assessment on the client's arrival to recovery, the nurse repeats evaluation of vital signs and other key observations at least every 15 minutes, or more frequently depending on client condition and unit policy.

BARNES — OPERATIVE NURSES NOTES AND OR RECORD

| DATE / / | OR RM NO. | SER | ☐ SCHEDULED ☐ EMERGENCY | RECORD NO. |

PREOPERATIVE ASSESSMENT

PATIENT IDENTIFICATION VERIFIED BY: ☐ PATIENT ☐ OTHER _____
☐ ARMBAND ☐ STAMP PLATE ☐ FACE SHEET ☐ CHART REVIEWED
☐ OPERATIVE PERMIT VERIFIED

NPO ☐ YES ☐ NO SINCE _____

☐ ALLERGIES TO: _____
_____ ☐ NKA

VERIFICATION OF PROCEDURE/LOCATION: ☐ VERBAL ☐ CONSENT FORM
☐ SPECIAL PROCEDURE PREMIT (SPECIFY) _____ ☐ NA

MENTAL/EMOTIONAL STATUS: ☐ ALERT/ORIENTED ☐ DROWSY/SEDATED ☐ CONFUSED/DISORIENTED
☐ UNCONSCIOUS/UNRESPONSIVE ☐ INTUBATED/TRACH ☐ NERVOUS/ANXIOUS

PHYSICAL ABNORMALITIES/LIMITATIONS: ☐ NONE ☐ AUDITORY ☐ VISUAL
☐ LANGUAGE ☐ MOBILITY ☐ OTHER _____

PERSONAL ITEMS: ☐ YES ☐ NO LIST: _____
DISPOSITION _____

SKIN CONDITION: ☐ INTACT ☐ OTHER _____

COMFORT MEASURES IMPLEMENTED: ☐ WARM BLANKET ☐ OTHER _____

IV ☐ NA
☐ SITE _____ FLUID _____ ☐ SITE _____ FLUID _____

☐ ARTERIAL LINE ☐ NA LOCATION _____ ☐ O2 ☐ NA ☐ NG TUBE ☐ NA
☐ SWAN GANZ ☐ NA LOCATION _____ ☐ FOLEY CATHETER ☐ NA
☐ CVP LINE ☐ NA LOCATION _____ ☐ OTHER _____ ☐ NA
TIME _____ _____ RN

PATIENT ESCORTED TO OR ROOM BY: ☐ MD ☐ ANESTH ☐ RN
NAME: _____

NURSING DIAGNOSIS: Potential For Anxiety Related To Knowledge Deficit.

PLAN & IMPLEMENTATION-GOAL: Demonstrates Decreased Anxiety.
☐ GIVE CLEAR CONCISE EXPLANATIONS ☐ CONVEY CARING, SUPPORTIVE ATTITUDE
☐ COMMUNICATE PATIENT CONCERNS TO OTHER HEALTHCARE MEMBERS ☐ REMAIN WITH PATIENT DURING INDUCTION ☐ OTHER _____

EVALUATION: Demonstrated Understanding Of EXPLANATIONS. ☐ YES ☐ NO
INITIALS _____ IF NO, EXPLAIN _____

NURSES NOTES: _____

ROOM READY	LC	PT IN OR	LC	INCISION	DRESSING	TIME OUT

PRE-OP DIAGNOSIS

PROCEDURE

☐ X-RAY PROCEDURE ☐ NA ☐ LASER TYPE _____ ☐ NA

POST-OP DIAGNOSIS

| ANESTHETIC ROUTE | ☐ GEN ☐ SPINAL/EPID | ☐ LOCAL ☐ REGIONAL | ☐ MAC ☐ BLOCK TYPE _____ | ☐ NONE | FACTOR |

FIRST PROCEDURE	SECOND PROCEDURE/RELIEF
SURGEON	
1ST ASSISTANT	
2ND ASSISTANT	
3RD ASSISTANT	
OTHER	
ATTENDING ANESTHESIOLOGIST	RELIEF
RESIDENT ANESTHESIOLOGIST	RELIEF
ANESTHETIST	RELIEF

SCRUB NURSES/TITLE/INITIAL/ID# ☐ NA	TIME IN/OUT	TIME IN/OUT	TIME IN/OUT
CIRCULATING NURSES/TITLE/INITIAL/ID#			
CELL SAVER/TITLE/INITIAL/ID# ☐ NA			
PERFUSIONIST/TITLE/INITIAL/ID# ☐ NA			
OBSERVERS ☐ NA			

Fig. 48-8 Operative nurses note. *(Courtesy Barnes-Jewish Hospital, St Louis.)*

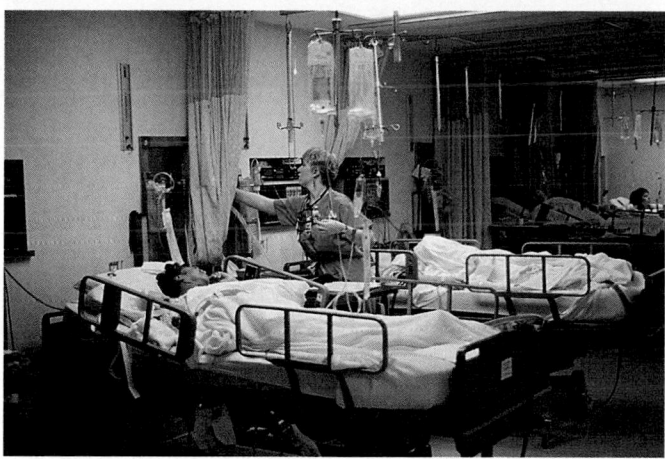

Fig. 48-9 Postanesthesia care unit.

This assessment usually continues until discharge from the PACU.

RESPIRATION

Certain anesthetic agents may cause respiratory depression. Thus the nurse is especially alert for shallow, slow breathing and a weak cough. The nurse assesses respiratory rate, rhythm, depth of ventilation, symmetry of chest wall movement, breath sounds, and color of mucous membranes. If breathing is unusually shallow, placement of the hand over the client's face or mouth allows the nurse to feel exhaled air. Pulse oximetry should reflect 92% to 100% saturation.

The client often has an oral or nasal airway (see Chapter 44) inserted to maintain a patent airway until comfortable breathing at a normal rate resumes. As respiratory function returns, the nurse asks the client to spit out the airway. The ability to do so signifies the return of a normal gag reflex.

One of the nurse's greatest concerns is airway obstruction resulting from aspiration of emesis, accumulation of mucous secretions in the pharynx, or swelling or spasm of the larynx (Odom, 1993). The following measures maintain airway patency:

1. The nurse positions the client on one side with the face down and the neck slightly extended. A small, folded towel supports the head. Neck extension prevents occlusion of the airway at the pharynx. When the face is kept turned downward, the tongue moves forward and mucous secretions flow out of the mouth instead of accumulating in the pharynx. If the nature of the surgery prevents turning the client on one side, the head of the bed is slightly elevated and the client's neck slightly extended, with the head turned to the side. The client should never be positioned with arms over or across the chest because this position reduces maximal chest expansion. The nurse may perform a jaw thrust maneuver and/or chin lift continuously to maintain the airway in some clients.
2. The nurse begins coughing and deep breathing exercises as soon as the client is responsive. This decreases the risk of **atelectasis**, a collapsed or airless portion of the lung due to a mucous plug or fluid.
3. The nurse suctions artificial airways and the oral cavity for mucous secretions (see Chapter 44). Care must be taken to avoid continually eliciting the gag reflex, which might cause vomiting. Before the nurse or client removes an airway, the back of the airway should be suctioned so that mucous plugs and secretions are not retained.
4. The nurse administers oxygen as ordered and monitors oxygen saturation with a pulse oximeter.

CIRCULATION

The client is at risk for cardiovascular complications resulting from actual or potential blood loss from the surgical site, side effects of anesthesia, electrolyte imbalances, and depression of normal circulatory regulating mechanisms. Careful assessment of heart rate and rhythm along with blood pressure reveals the client's cardiovascular status. A rhythm strip is usually obtained, compared with preoperative ECG tracings, and mounted on the PACU record. The values are monitored at least every 15 minutes throughout the recovery phase. The nurse compares preoperative vital signs with postoperative values. The surgeon's postoperative orders may specify when vital sign changes should be reported. For example, a heart rate above 110 beats/min or below 60 beats/min should be reported immediately. However, the nurse must use judgment in reporting vital sign changes. If the client's blood pressure drops progressively after each check or if the heart rate becomes more irregular, the physician should be notified.

The nurse assesses circulatory perfusion by noting the color of nail beds and skin. If the client has had vascular surgery or has casts or constricting devices that may impair circulation, the nurse assesses peripheral pulses distal to the site of surgery. For example, after surgery to the femoral artery, the nurse assesses posterior tibial and dorsalis pedis pulses. The nurse also compares pulses in the affected extremity with those in the nonaffected extremity. Checking for Homans' sign is necessary, particularly for clients undergoing pelvic surgery or clients who were positioned in lithotomy position during surgery as these clients may be predisposed to developing deep vein thromboses.

A common circulatory problem is hemorrhage. Blood loss may occur externally through a drain or incision or internally within the surgical wound. Either type of hemorrhage may result in a fall in blood pressure; elevated heart and respiratory rate; thready pulse; cool, clammy, pale skin; and restlessness. If hemorrhage is external the nurse notes increased bloody drainage on dressings or through drains. If a dressing becomes saturated the blood oozes down the client's sides and collects in a pool under bedclothes. An alert nurse always checks under the client for drainage. When hemorrhage is internal the operative site becomes swollen and tight. For example, if a client bleeds within the abdomen, the abdomen becomes tight and distended. The first signs of suspected hemorrhaging should be reported to the physician immediately. The nurse maintains IV fluid infusion and monitors the client's vital signs every 15 minutes or more frequently until the client's condition stabilizes. Oxygen may be continued and the foot of the bed may be elevated. Medications and volume replacement may be considered.

TEMPERATURE CONTROL

The operating room and recovery room environments are extremely cool. The client's depressed level of body function results in a lowering of metabolism and fall in body temperature. When clients begin to awaken they complain of feeling cold and uncomfortable.

The nurse measures the client's body temperature and provides warmed blankets. If the temperature is 96 or below, an external warming device may be used. Increasing body warmth causes the client's metabolism to rise and circulatory and respiratory functions to improve.

Shivering may not be a sign of hypothermia but rather a side effect of certain anesthetic agents. Demerol may be given in small increments to decrease shivering. Deep breathing and coughing help expel retained anesthetic gases.

In rare instances **malignant hyperthermia**, a life-threatening complication of anesthesia, develops. Malignant hyperthermia causes tachypnea, tachycardia, unstable blood pressure, and muscular rigidity. Despite the name, an elevated temperature is a late sign (Young and Kindred, 1993). Without proper treatment it can be fatal. Immediate administration of dantrolene sodium is the most critical treatment.

NEUROLOGICAL FUNCTIONS

On arrival in the PACU the client may be asleep or reacting to verbal commands in some fashion. However, medications, electrolyte and metabolic changes, pain, and emotional factors can influence the level of consciousness. The nurse rouses the client by calling the name in a moderate tone of voice. The nurse notes whether the client responds appropriately or seems confused and disoriented. If the client remains asleep or unresponsive the nurse attempts arousal through touch or by gently moving a body part. If a painful stimulus is needed to arouse the client the nurse should notify the anesthesiologist.

As the effects of anesthesia wear off, the client's reflexes return, muscle strength is regained, and a normal level of orientation returns. The nurse can easily check for pupillary and gag reflexes (see Chapter 33) and assess grips and movement of extremities. If a client has had surgery involving a portion of the neurological system the nurse conducts a more thorough neurological assessment. For example, if the client had low back surgery the nurse assesses leg movement, sensation, and strength. Clients with regional anesthesia begin to experience a return in motor function before tactile sensation returns. **Dermatome** (a segmental skin area innervated by segments of spinal cord) assessment of the spinal nerves is completed on admission, throughout the PACU period, and on discharge (Fig. 48-10). Typically the nurse assesses dermatome level by touching the client bilaterally and documenting where the client feels touch. The touch can be with hand pressure or a gentle pinch of skin.

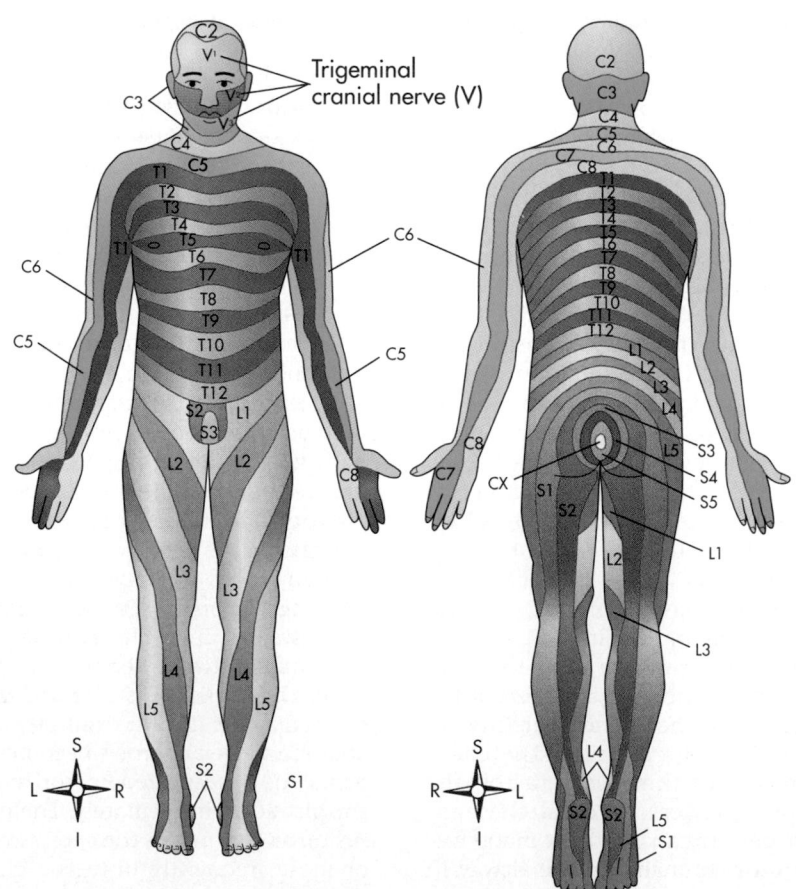

Fig. 48-10 Segmental dermatome distribution of spinal nerves. *C*, Cervical segments; *T*, thoracic segments; *L*, lumbar segments; *S*, sacral segments. *(From Thibodeau G, Patton K: Anthony's textbook of anatomy and physiology, ed 15, St Louis, 1996, Mosby.)*

Orientation to the PACU environment is important in maintaining the client's alertness. The nurse reorients the client, explains that surgery is completed, and describes procedures and nursing measures within the recovery area. The client who was properly prepared before surgery is less likely to be anxious when PACU nurses begin their care.

SKIN INTEGRITY AND CONDITION OF WOUND

In the PACU the nurse assesses the condition of the client's skin, noting rashes, petechiae, abrasions, or burns. A rash may indicate a drug sensitivity or allergy. Abrasions or petechiae may result from inappropriate positioning or restraining that injures skin layers. Burns may indicate that an electrical cautery grounding pad was incorrectly placed on the client's skin. Burns or serious injury to the skin should be documented by an incident report (see Chapter 12).

After surgery most surgical wounds are covered with a dressing that protects the wound site and collects drainage. The nurse observes the amount, color, odor, and consistency of drainage on dressings. The nurse estimates the amount of drainage by noting the number of saturated gauze sponges. If drainage appears on the outer surface of a dressing another way of assessing drainage is by drawing a circle around the outer perimeter of the drainage and dating it with the time noted. This way the nurse can easily note if drainage is increasing (see Chapter 49). However, this is not the most accurate measure of volume of fluid lost.

Many physicians prefer to change dressings the first time so that they can inspect the incisional area. Therefore, the nurse may simply add an extra layer of gauze on top of the original dressing, thereby reinforcing the dressing.

GENITOURINARY FUNCTION

Depending on the surgery a client may not regain voluntary control over urinary function for 6 to 8 hours after anesthesia. An epidural or spinal anesthetic may prevent the client from feeling bladder fullness or distention. The nurse palpates the lower abdomen just above the symphysis pubis for bladder distention. Clients need to be assisted to void if they are unable to void in 8 hours. Because a full bladder can be painful and often causes restlessness in recovery, it may become necessary to insert a catheter. If the client has a Foley catheter there should be a continuous flow of urine of at least 2 ml/kg/hr in adults and 1 ml/kg/hour in children. The nurse observes the color and odor of urine. Surgery involving portions of the urinary tract normally causes bloody urine for at least 12 to 24 hours depending on the type of surgery.

GASTROINTESTINAL FUNCTION

Anesthetics slow gastrointestinal motility and cause nausea. Normally during the immediate recovery phase faint or absent bowel sounds are auscultated in all four quadrants. Inspection of the abdomen rules out distention that may be caused by accumulation of gas. In a client who has had abdominal surgery, distention will develop if internal bleeding occurs. Distention may also occur in the client who develops a **paralytic ileus** from handling of the bowel in surgery. This paralysis of intestines with distention and symptoms of acute obstruction may be also related to the administration of anticholinergic drugs.

To minimize nausea avoid sudden movement of the client. If the client has an NG tube the nurse keeps it patent by regular irrigations. Occlusion of NG tubes results in accumulation of gastric contents within the stomach. Because stomach emptying slows under anesthesia the accumulated contents cannot escape and nausea and vomiting develop. Normally a client does not receive fluids to drink in the PACU because of bowel sluggishness with the risk of nausea and vomiting and because of grogginess from anesthesia.

FLUID AND ELECTROLYTE BALANCE

Because of the surgical client's risk for fluid and electrolyte abnormalities the nurse assesses the hydration status and monitors cardiac and neurological function for signs of electrolyte alterations (see Chapter 45). An important responsibility is maintaining patency of IV infusions. The client's only source of fluid intake immediately after surgery is through IV catheters. The nurse inspects the catheter insertion site to be sure the catheter is properly positioned within a vein so that fluid flows freely. The physician orders a prescribed rate for each infusion. To ensure adequate fluid intake the nurse should not allow infusion of fluids to fall behind. The client may also receive blood products after surgery, depending on blood loss during surgery.

Accurate recording of intake and output helps assess renal and circulatory function. The nurse measures all sources of output, including urine, gastric drainage, and drainage from wounds, and notes any insensible loss from diaphoresis. Mucus suctioned from airways is not included in output measurements.

COMFORT

As clients awaken from general anesthesia the sensation of pain becomes prominent. Pain can be perceived before full consciousness is regained. Acute incisional pain causes clients to become restless and may be responsible for changes in vital signs. It is difficult for clients to begin coughing and deep breathing exercises when they experience pain. The client who had regional or local anesthesia usually does not experience pain initially because the incisional area is still anesthetized.

Assessment of the client's discomfort and evaluation of pain relief therapies are essential nursing functions. Pain scales are an effective method for nurses to assess postoperative pain, evaluate response to analgesics, and to objectively document pain severity (Scott, 1994). Using preoperative pain assessments as a baseline the nurse is able to evaluate the effectiveness of interventions throughout the client's recovery.

It is common to administer narcotic analgesics immediately after surgery for pain relief and to maximize the client's ability to perform respiratory exercises like coughing and deep breathing. Many initial doses are given IV in the PACU and titrated to client comfort. After an anesthetized client is awake and aware, patient-controlled analgesia (PCA) may be utilized. This is given intravenously. Many clients have epidural analgesia that may be continued throughout the recovery period (see Chapter 43).

Recovery in Ambulatory Surgery

The thoroughness and extent of postoperative assessment depends on the ambulatory client's condition, type of surgery, and anesthesia. In many cases the assessment is identical to that conducted for hospitalized clients. However, if the client has undergone minor surgery (e.g., cosmetic removal of a mole), the postoperative recovery phase requires minimal assessment.

If an ambulatory client has received general or regional anesthesia or intensive IV sedation, the client will be transferred to the recovery room. In phase I recovery, clients in need of close monitoring are frequently assessed for vital sign changes, respiratory and circulatory status, level of consciousness, condition of the surgical wound, and pain level.

The time that a client spends in phase I recovery depends on several factors. Outpatient anesthesia is gauged to provide a quick recovery time, few aftereffects, and a speedy return to daily routines. The average time spent in phase I is 1 hour, without complications. Clients are encouraged to gradually sit up on the stretcher or bed and begin to take ice chips or sips of water while regaining full alertness. After clients become stable and no longer require close monitoring the nurse transfers them to phase II recovery. Clients who have undergone minor surgery may be transferred directly to phase II recovery.

Phase II recovery may consist of a room equipped with medical recliner chairs, side tables, and foot rests. Kitchen facilities for preparing light snacks and beverages are usually located in the area, along with bathrooms. The phase II environment is designed to promote the client's and family's comfort and well-being until discharge. The nurse monitors clients but not at the same intensity as phase I. In phase II recovery, nurses initiate postoperative teaching with clients and family members (see the box below).

Postoperative Convalescence

Ambulatory surgical clients are discharged to home when they reach certain criteria such as: can void (if applicable), able to ambulate, alert and oriented, minimal nausea/vomiting, no pain medication for 1 hour, minimal postoperative pain, no excess bleeding or drainage, received written postoperative instructions and prescriptions, verbalize understanding of these instructions, and are being discharged to a responsible adult (Parnass, 1993). In contrast, inpatient clients are kept in the PACU until their condition stabilizes. Then the clients are returned to the postoperative nursing division.

Nursing care focuses on returning the client to a relatively functional level of wellness as soon as possible. The speed of convalescence depends on the type or extent of surgery, risk factors, postoperative complications, and the nurse's care plan.

DISCHARGE FROM PACU

The nurse evaluates readiness for discharge from PACU on the basis of vital sign stability in comparison to the preoperative data. Other outcomes for discharge include body temperature control, good ventilatory function, orientation to surroundings, absence of complications, minimal pain and nausea, controlled wound drainage, adequate urine output, and fluid and electrolyte balance. Many PACU staffs utilize an objective scoring system that helps delineate when clients may be discharged (Levin 1993). If the client's condition is still poor after 2 to 3 hours, the stay lengthens or the surgeon may transfer the client to an intensive care unit (ICU).

When the client is ready to be discharged from the PACU the nurse calls the nursing division to report vital signs, the type of surgery and anesthesia performed, blood loss, level of consciousness, general physical condition, and presence of IV lines or drainage tubes. The nurse's report helps the nurse on the division anticipate special client needs and obtain necessary equipment.

Personnel, which may include nurses, return the client on a stretcher. Staff members assist in safely transferring the client to a bed (see Chapter 37). The PACU nurse, if helping to transport the client, shows the division nurse the recovery room record and reviews the client's condition and course of care. The PACU nurse also points out physician orders that require attention. Before the nurse leaves the division the nurse takes a complete set of vital signs to compare with PACU findings. Minor vital sign variations normally occur after transporting the client.

▌ THE NURSING PROCESS IN POSTOPERATIVE CARE

Once a client returns to a nursing division, postoperative care begins. The nurse must review all relevent preoperative information, assess the client's current status, and then develop and implement an effective plan of care.

 Assessment

Upon return of the client to the nursing division the nurse's assessment includes an initial check of the client's

---

CLIENT TEACHING of Postoperative Instructions for Ambulatory Surgical Client

OBJECTIVE
- The client will verbalize resources to contact for assistance
- The client will describe signs and symptoms of postoperative problems
- The client will list the name and dose of medications
- The client will describe guidelines related to specific surgery.

TEACHING STRATEGIES
- Give instruction sheet with doctor's telephone number, surgery center's number, and follow-up appointment date and time. Allow client and family to ask questions.
- Explain to family member the signs and symptoms of infection for which to observe.
- Explain name, dose, schedule, and purpose of medications. Provide drug information leaflets.
- Explain activity restrictions, diet progression, and any special wound care related to specific surgery. Provide instruction sheet with clear, focused explanations.

EVALUATION
- Client is able to explain when to call doctor with problems
- Client is able to recite date for follow-up appointment
- Client and family member describe signs and symptoms of infection
- Client recites name of drug, dose, and when to take
- Client demonstrates proper activity/movement and wound care

general condition including vital signs, level of consciousness, condition of dressings and drains, IV fluid status, comfort level, and skin integrity.

The same physical measurements and observations performed in the PACU are also carried out on the postoperative division. The nurse routinely assesses the client at least every 15 minutes the first hour, every 30 minutes for 1 to 2 hours, every hour for 4 hours, and then every 4 hours. Frequency of assessment depends on the client's condition. A nurse should not assume that further monitoring is unnecessary if the client appears normal during the initial assessment. A client's postoperative condition can change rapidly. A nurse who fails to follow the assessment schedule is considered neglectful.

The nurse thoroughly documents the initial assessment and makes entries in the nurses' notes. Vital signs, IV fluid intake, and urinary output measurements can be entered on flowsheets. The initial findings are a baseline for comparing postoperative changes.

After the first assessment is completed and immediate needs are attended to, the family is allowed to visit. The nurse can explain the purpose of postoperative procedures or equipment and how the client is doing. The nurse explains whether vital signs are stable and whether the client seems to be awakening without difficulty. The family should know that the client will fall in and out of sleep for most of the rest of the day from the effects of general anesthesia. The family should also be reminded that frequent assessments are to be expected and that loss of sensation and movement in the extremities remains for several hours if the client had spinal anesthesia.

 ## Nursing Diagnosis

The nurse determines the status of problems identified from preoperative nursing diagnoses and clusters new relevant data to identify new diagnoses (see the nursing di-agnoses box below). Previously defined diagnoses, such as impaired skin integrity, may continue as a postoperative problem. The nurse may also identify risk factors leading to identification of new nursing diagnoses (see the diagnostic process box on p. 1420). For example, an older client who has undergone major abdominal surgery and who has a preexisting problem of reduced hip mobility resulting from arthritis will likely have the diagnosis of impaired physical mobility. The surgery itself may add risk factors for the client. The nurse also considers needs of a client's family when making diagnoses. For example, the inability of the family to cope with the client's condition requires the nurse's intervention.

 ## Planning

At the convalescent phase the nurse has much information to plan the client's care. Current physical assessment data and analysis of the preoperative nursing history allow the nurse to plan specific nursing interventions. The surgeon's postoperative orders also offer guidelines. Typical postoperative orders include the following:

1. Frequency of vital sign monitoring and special assessments
2. Types of IV fluids and rates of infusion
3. Postoperative medications (especially those for pain and nausea)
4. Fluids and food allowed by mouth
5. Level of activity that the client is allowed to resume
6. Position that the client is to maintain while in bed
7. Intake and output
8. Laboratory tests and x-ray studies
9. Special directions

The nurse considers the effects of the stress of surgery and limitations it produces when establishing expected outcomes and goals of care for the client. Measurable outcomes help to ensure aggressive but appropriate recovery

---

 ## Examples of NANDA Nursing Diagnoses for Postoperative Client

Ineffective airway clearance *related to:*
- Diminished cough
- Retained secretions
- Prolonged sedation

Ineffective breathing pattern *related to:*
- Incisional pain
- Analgesia effects on ventilation

Pain *related to:*
- Surgical incision
- Nasal irritation from NG tube placement

Ineffective individual coping *related to:*
- Constraints imposed by surgery
- Postoperative therapies

Risk for fluid volume deficit *related to:*
- Wound drainage
- Inadequate fluid intake

Risk for or impaired skin integrity *related to:*
- Wound drainage
- Impaired mobility

Anticipatory grieving *related to:*
- Client's critical condition

Impaired physical mobility *related to:*
- Pain
- Postoperative activity restrictions
- Casts or dressings

Altered oral mucous membrane *related to:*
- Irritation of nasogastric or endotracheal tube
- NPO status

Feeding, bathing/hygiene, dressing/grooming, toileting self-care deficit *related to:*
- Postoperative activity restrictions

Risk for altered body temperature *related to:*
- Lowered metabolism

Risk for infection *related to:*
- Surgical wound incision

Impaired verbal communication *related to:*
- Endotracheal or airway tube placement

Sample Nursing Diagnostic Process for Postoperative Client

ASSESSMENT ACTIVITIES	DEFINING CHARACTERISTICS	NURSING DIAGNOSES
Monitor the rate and depth of client's respirations. Auscultate lungs. Observe client's postoperative coughing technique.	Elevated respiratory rate Shallow respirations Abnormal breath sounds Dyspnea Ineffective cough with splinting	**Ineffective airway clearance** related to incisional pain.
Ask client if discomfort is noted in area of abdominal incision; have client describe nature and character of pain. Observe client's nonverbal behavior while moving and when coughing or deep breathing.	Right upper quadrant incision of 6 in Verbalizes sharp pain present in abdomen, increased with breathing Grimaces when coughs or breathes deeply Attempts to splint abdomen during moving	**Pain** related to trauma of surgical incision.

Sample Nursing Care Plan for Ineffective Airway Clearance

NURSING DIAGOSIS: Ineffective airway clearance related to incisional pain
DEFINITION: Ineffective airway clearance is the state in which an individual is unable to clear secretions or obstructions from the respiratory tract to maintain airway patency (Kim, McFarland, McLane, 1995).

GOAL	EXPECTED OUTCOMES	INTERVENTIONS	RATIONALE
Client will achieve normal ventilatory function with patent airway by second postoperative day (6/4).	Client will be able to breathe deeply by 6/3.	Have client perform diaphragmatic breathing using incentive spirometer every 2 hr while awake.	Adequate lung expansion can prevent atelectasis.
	Cough will be clear and nonproductive by 6/3.	Have client splint abdominal incision while performing coughing exercises.	Splinting incision helps prevent discomfort while performing coughing exercises.
		Offer preferred fluids (iced tea and cranberry juice), 1500 ml/day minimum.	Increased fluid intake helps prevent thickening of mucus.
	Lung sounds will be clear by 6/4.	Turn client side to side every 1-2 hr while awake.	Turning permits lung expansion.

from surgery. For example, the client at risk for impaired mobility should have specific outcomes that outline progressive ambulation, for example, "will walk to end of hall by day 2." After each outcome is met the client will ultimately achieve the goal of independent mobility at a preoperative level or better. The nurse carefully considers all goals of care established during the preoperative surgical phase. Typical goals of care postoperatively include the following:

1. Demonstrating return of normal physiological function
2. Demonstrating absence of postoperative surgical wound infection

3. Achieving rest and comfort
4. Maintaining self-concept
5. Returning to a functional state of health within limitations posed by surgery

See the care plan above for a postoperative surgical client.

Implementation

Regaining Normal Physiological Function

A surgical wound, the effects of prolonged immobilization during surgery and convalescence, and the influence of

Table 48-8	Postoperative Complications	

COMPLICATION	CAUSE

RESPIRATORY SYSTEM

Atelectasis is collapse of alveoli with retained mucous secretions. Signs and symptoms include elevated respiratory rate, dyspnea, fever, crackles auscultated over involved lobes of lungs, and productive cough.

Pneumonia is inflammation of alveoli caused by infectious process. It may involve one or several lobes of lung. Development of pneumonia in lower dependent lobes of lung is common in immobilized surgical client. Signs and symptoms include fever, chills, productive cough, chest pain, purulent mucus, and dyspnea.

Hypoxia is inadequate concentration of oxygen in arterial blood. Signs and symptoms include restlessness, dyspnea, high blood pressure, tachycardia, diaphoresis, and cyanosis.

Pulmonary embolism is embolus blocking pulmonary artery and disrupting blood flow to one or more lobes of lung. Signs and symptoms include dyspnea, sudden chest pain, cyanosis, tachycardia, and drop in blood pressure.

Atelectasis is caused by inadequate lung expansion. Anesthesia, analgesia, and immobilized position prevent full lung expansion. There is greater risk in clients with upper abdominal surgery who have pain during inspiration and repress deep breathing.

Pneumonia is caused by poor lung expansion with retained secretions. Common resident bacterium in respiratory tract is *Diplococcus pneumoniae,* which causes most cases of pneumonia.

Respirations are depressed by anesthetics or analgesics. Increased retention of mucus with impaired ventilation occurs because of pain or poor positioning.

Same factors lead to formation of thrombus or embolus. Immobilized surgical client with preexisting circulatory or coagulation disorders is at risk.

CIRCULATORY SYSTEM

Hemorrhage is loss of large amount of blood externally or internally in short period of time. Signs and symptoms same as hypovolemic shock.

Hypovolemic shock is perfusion of tissues and cells from loss of circulatory fluid volume. Signs and symptoms include hypotension, weak and rapid pulse, cool and clammy skin, rapid breathing, restlessness, and reduced urine output.

Thrombophlebitis is inflammation of vein often accompanied by clot formation. Veins in legs are most commonly affected. Signs and symptoms include swelling and inflammation of involved site and aching or cramping pain. Vein feels hard, cordlike, and sensitive to touch. Pain in calf occurs when client walks or dorsiflexes foot (Homans' sign).

Thrombus is formation of clot attached to interior wall of a vein or artery, which can occlude the vessel lumen.

Embolus is piece of thrombus that has dislodged and circulates in bloodstream until it lodges in another vessel, commonly lungs, heart, or brain.

Hemorrhage is caused by slipping of suture or dislodged clot at incisional site. Clients with coagulation disorders are at greater risk.

In surgical client, hypovolemic shock is usually caused by hemorrhage.

Venous stasis is aggravated by prolonged sitting or immobilization. Trauma to vessel wall and hypercoagulability of blood increase risk of vessel inflammation.

Thrombus is caused by venous stasis (see thrombophlebitis) and vessel trauma. Venous injury is common after surgery of legs, abdomen, pelvis, and major vessels. Thrombi also form from increased coagulability of blood (e.g., polycythemia and use of birth control pills containing estrogen).

GASTROINTESTINAL SYSTEM

Abdominal distention is retention of air within intestines. Signs and symptoms include increased abdominal girth and tympanic percussion over abdominal quadrants. Client complains of fullness and "gas pains."

Constipation is infrequent passage of stools. It should not be immediate concern after surgery, especially if client has preoperative bowel preparation. After client resumes solid diet, failure to pass stool within 48 hr is cause for concern.

Nausea and vomiting are symptoms of improper gastric emptying or chemical stimulation of vomiting center. Client complains of gagging or feeling full or sick to stomach.

Distention is caused by slowed peristalsis from anesthesia, bowel manipulation, or immobilization.

Slowed peristalsis (see causes of distention) and delay in resuming normal diet cause constipation.

Nausea and vomiting are caused by severe pain, abdominal distention, fear, medications, eating or drinking before peristalsis returns, and initiation of gag reflex.

GENITOURINARY SYSTEM

Urinary retention is involuntary accumulation of urine in bladder as result of loss of muscle tone. Signs and symptoms include inability to void, restlessness, and bladder distention. It appears 6-8 hr after surgery.

Retention is caused by effects of anesthesia and narcotic analgesics. Local manipulation of tissues surrounding bladder and edema interfere with bladder tone. Poor positioning of client impairs voiding reflexes.

Continued.

Table 48-8	Postoperative Complications—cont'd
COMPLICATION	**CAUSE**
INTEGUMENTARY SYSTEM *Wound infection* is an invasion of deep or superficial wound tissues by pathogenic microorganisms; signs and symptoms include warm, red, and tender skin around incision. Client may have fever and chills. Purulent material may exit from drains or from separated wound edges. It appears 3-6 days after surgery.	Infection is caused by poor aseptic technique and contaminated wound before surgical exploration.
Wound dehiscence is separation of wound edges at suture line. Signs and symptoms include increased drainage and appearance of underlying tissues. It usually occurs 6-8 days after surgery. *Wound evisceration* is protrusion of internal organs and tissues through incision. It usually occurs 6-8 days after surgery. *Surgical mumps* (parotitis) is swelling of parotid glands due to poor mouth care	Malnutrition, obesity, preoperative radiation to surgical site, old age, poor circulation to tissues, and unusual strain on suture line from coughing cause dehiscence. See dehiscence. Client with dehiscence is at risk for developing evisceration. Obstruction of the parotid gland
NERVOUS SYSTEM Pain that is intractable	Intractable pain may be related to the wound or dressing; anxiety, or positioning.

anesthesia and analgesics are the principal causes for postoperative complications. Nursing interventions are directed at preventing complications so that the client returns to the highest level of functioning possible. Failure of the client to become actively involved in recovery adds to the risk of complications (Table 48-8). Virtually any body system can be affected. The nurse must consider the interrelationship of all systems and therapies provided.

MAINTAINING RESPIRATORY FUNCTION

To prevent respiratory complications the nurse begins aggressive pulmonary hygiene measures early. The benefits of thorough preoperative teaching are realized when clients are able to participate actively. The following measures promote expansion of the lungs:

1. The nurse encourages diaphragmatic breathing exercises at least every 2 hours while clients are awake. Maximal inspirations lasting 3 to 5 seconds open up alveoli.
2. The nurse instructs clients to use incentive spirometers for maximum inspiration (see Chapter 44).
3. The nurse encourages early ambulation. Walking causes clients to assume a position that does not restrict chest wall expansion and stimulates an increased respiratory rate.
4. The nurse assists clients who are restricted to bed to turn on their sides every 1 to 2 hours while awake and to sit when possible. Turning permits expansion of the lungs. Sitting causes lowering of abdominal organs, thus facilitating diaphragmatic movement and lung expansion.
5. Keep the client comfortable. A client who is comfortable will be able to participate in the postoperative regimen. The nurse needs to assess, document, treat, and evaluate clients' pain to be effective.

The following measures promote removal of pulmonary secretions:

1. The nurse encourages coughing exercises every 2 hours while clients are awake and maintains pain control to promote a full productive cough.

2. The nurse provides oral hygiene to expectorate mucus. Oral mucosa become dry when clients are NPO or are placed on limited fluid intake.
3. The nurse initiates orotracheal or nasotracheal suction for clients who are too weak or unable to cough (see Chapter 44).

PREVENTING CIRCULATORY STASIS

Early measures directed at preventing circulatory complications prevent circulatory stasis. The nurse routinely assesses for Homans' (see Chapter 33) sign in the postoperative period and documents findings. Some clients are at greater risk of venous stasis because of the nature of their surgery. The following measures promote normal venous return and circulatory blood flow:

1. The nurse encourages clients to perform leg exercises at least every hour while awake. Exercise may be contraindicated in an affected extremity involving vascular repair or realignment of fractured bones and torn cartilage.
2. The nurse applies elastic antiembolism stockings as ordered by the physician. The stockings should be removed every 8 hours and left off for 1 hour (see Chapter 37).
3. The nurse applies pneumatic **antiembolism stockings.** Each stocking wraps around a client's leg and is kept in place with a velcro attachment. Compressed air inflates the padded plastic stocking systematically from ankle to calf to thigh and then deflates. The alternating inflation and deflation of the stocking reduces venous stasis.
4. The nurse encourages early ambulation. Most clients are expected to ambulate the evening of surgery, depending on the severity of surgery and their condition. The degree of activity allowed progresses as the condition improves. Before ambulation the nurse assesses vital signs. Abnormalities may contraindicate ambulation. If vital signs are normal the nurse first assists the client to sit on the side of the bed. Clients' complaints of dizziness are a sign of postural hypotension. A recheck of blood pressure determines whether ambulation is safe. The nurse

assists with ambulation by standing at the client's side, making sure that the client can walk steadily. In the first few times out of bed, clients may be able to walk only a few feet. This improves each time. The nurse evaluates tolerance to activity by periodically assessing the pulse rate.

5. The nurse avoids positioning clients in a manner that interrupts blood flow to extremities. While in bed, clients should not have pillows or rolled blankets placed under the knees. Compression of the popliteal vessels can cause thrombi. When clients sit in chairs, their legs should be elevated on footstools. A client should never be allowed to sit with one leg crossed over the other.

6. The nurse administers anticoagulant drugs as ordered. Physicians often order small doses of anticoagulants, such as heparin, for clients at greatest risk for thrombus formation. Orthopedic clients often receive aspirin for anticoagulation.

7. The nurse promotes adequate fluid intake orally or intravenously. Adequate hydration prevents concentrated buildup of formed blood elements, such as platelets and red blood cells. When the plasma volume is low, these elements may gather and form small clots within blood vessels.

PROMOTING NORMAL ELIMINATION AND ADEQUATE NUTRITION

Interventions for preventing gastrointestinal complications promote return of normal elimination and faster return of normal nutritional intake. It takes several days for a client who has had surgery on gastrointestinal structures (e.g., a colon resection) to resume a normal diet. Normal peristalsis may not return for 2 to 3 days. In contrast, the client whose gastrointestinal tract is unaffected directly by surgery must recover from the effects of anesthesia before resuming dietary intake. The following measures promote return of normal elimination:

1. The nurse assesses for return of peristalsis every 4 to 8 hours. The nurse routinely auscultates the abdomen to detect return of normal bowel sounds; 5 to 30 loud gurgles per minute over each quadrant indicates that peristalsis has returned. High-pitched tinkling sounds accompanied by abdominal distention suggest the bowel is not functioning properly. The nurse asks if the client is passing gas (flatus). This is an important sign indicating normal bowel function.

2. The nurse maintains a gradual progression in dietary intake. For the first few hours after surgery a client receives only IV fluids. If the physician orders a normal diet the first evening after surgery, the nurse first provides clear liquids, such as water, apple juice, or tea, after nausea subsides. Overloading with large amounts of fluids may lead to distention and vomiting. If the client tolerates liquids without nausea, the diet is advanced as ordered. Clients who have had abdominal surgery are usually NPO the first 24 to 48 hours. As peristalsis returns, the nurse provides clear liquids, followed by full liquids, a light diet of solid foods, and finally a regular diet.

3. The nurse promotes ambulation and exercise. Physical activity stimulates a return of peristalsis. The client who suffers abdominal distention and "gas pain" will obtain relief while walking.

4. The nurse maintains an adequate fluid intake. Fluids keep fecal material soft for easy passage. Fruit juices and warm liquids are especially effective.

5. The nurse administers enemas, rectal suppositories, and rectal tubes as ordered. If constipation or distention develops, the physician attempts to stimulate peristalsis with cathartics or enemas. A rectal tube or return-flow enema promotes passage of flatus (see Chapter 47).

The following measures maintain an adequate dietary intake:

1. The nurse removes sources of noxious odors.

2. The nurse assists the client to a comfortable position during mealtime. The client should sit if possible to minimize pressure on the abdomen.

3. The nurse provides desired servings of food. For example, a client may be more willing to face the first meal when servings are not large.

4. The nurse provides frequent oral hygiene. Adequate hydration and cleansing of the oral cavity eliminate dryness and bad tastes.

5. The nurse provides meals when the client is rested and free from pain. Often a client loses interest in eating if mealtime has been preceded by exhausting activities, such as ambulation, coughing and deep breathing exercises, or extensive dressing changes. When a client has pain, the associated nausea often causes a loss of appetite.

PROMOTING URINARY ELIMINATION

The depressant effects of anesthetics and analgesics impair the sensation of bladder fullness. If bladder tone is reduced, the client has difficulty starting urination. However, clients should void within 8 to 12 hours after surgery. Clients who undergo surgery of the urinary system frequently have Foley catheters inserted to maintain free urinary flow until voluntary control of urination returns. The following measures promote normal urinary elimination (see Chapter 46):

1. The nurse assists the client to assume normal positions during voiding. The male client may need assistance to stand to void. Bedpans make voiding difficult. A female client will have better results if she is able to use a toilet.

2. The nurse checks the client frequently for the need to void. A surgical client restricted to bed needs assistance in handling and using bedpans or urinals. Often the client acquires a sudden feeling of bladder fullness and urgency to void, and the nurse must respond quickly when the client calls for help.

3. The nurse assesses for bladder distention. If a client does not void within 8 hours of surgery, it may be necessary to insert a urinary catheter. A physician's order is needed.

4. The nurse monitors intake and output. An accepted level of urine output is at least 2 ml/kg/hr for adults. If the urine is dark, concentrated, and low in volume, the physician should be notified. A client can easily become dehydrated as a result of fluid loss from the surgical wound. The nurse measures intake and output for several days after surgery until normal fluid intake and urinary output are achieved.

PROMOTING WOUND HEALING

A surgical wound undergoes considerable stress during convalescence. The stress of inadequate nutrition, impaired circulation, and metabolic alterations increase the risk for delayed healing (see Chapter 49). A wound may also undergo considerable physical stress. Strain on sutures from coughing, vomiting, distention, and movement of body parts can disrupt the wound layers. The nurse protects the wound and promotes healing. A critical time for wound healing is 24 to 72 hours after surgery. If a wound becomes infected, it usually occurs 3 to 6 days after surgery. A clean surgical wound usually does not regain strength against normal stress for 15 to 20 days after surgery. The nurse uses aseptic technique during dressing changes and wound care (see Chapters 34 and 49). Surgical drains must remain patent so that accumulated secretions can escape from the wound bed. Ongoing observation of the wound identifies early signs and symptoms of infection. The aging client is at particular risk of developing a postoperative wound infection; the perioperative nurse decreases the risk by providing a safe environment and comprehensive nursing care (Horner, 1993; Saleh, 1993).

ACHIEVING REST AND COMFORT

A surgical client's pain increases as anesthesia wears off. The client becomes more aware of the surroundings and more perceptive of discomfort. The incisional area may be only one source of pain. Irritation from drainage tubes, tight dressings or casts, and the muscular strains caused from positioning on the operating room table can make the client feel miserable.

Pain can significantly slow recovery. The client becomes reluctant to cough, breathe deeply, turn, ambulate, or perform necessary exercises. The nurse assesses the client's pain thoroughly (see Chapter 43). It should not be assumed that the pain is incisional. When the client asks for a pain medication, the nurse determines the nature and character of the pain. The nurse should provide analgesics as often as allowed the first 24 to 48 hours after surgery to improve pain control (AHCPR, 1992). The PCA system allows clients to administer their own IV analgesics from a specially prepared IV pump (see Chapter 43). If clients gain a sense of control over their pain, they usually have fewer postoperative problems. If pain medications are not relieving discomfort, the nurse should notify the physician for additional orders after completing a thorough assessment. The nurse can also utilize other methods of promoting pain relief such as positioning, back rubs, or distraction.

Epidural infusion of narcotics, such as morphine, fentanyl, and meperidine, is also a popular method of postoperative analgesia for many surgical clients (Powell, Bora, 1989; Wild and Coyne, 1992; Gordon et al,1993). Epidural narcotics relieve severe pain, often without the central nervous system depression that can occur with systemic narcotics. Recognizing potential complications and what to do if they occur is an important role for the postoperative nurse (Hambleton, 1994).

MAINTAINING SELF-CONCEPT

The appearance of wounds, bulky dressings, and extruding drains and tubes threatens a client's self-concept. The effects of surgery, such as disfiguring scars, may create permanent changes in the client's body image. If surgery leads to impairment in body function, the client's role within the family can change significantly.

The nurse observes clients for alterations in self-concept. Clients may show a revulsion toward their appearance by refusing to look at incisions, carefully covering dressings with bedclothes, or refusing to get out of bed because of tubes and devices. The fear of not being able to return to a functional role in their families may even cause clients to avoid participating in the care plan.

The family becomes an important part of the efforts to improve the client's self-concept. The nurse explains the client's appearance and ways to avoid nonverbal expressions of revulsion or surprise to the family. The family needs to be accepting of the client's needs and still encourage the client's independence. If the condition is terminal, the family learns to assist the client through the grieving process so that the client can reach a stage of acceptance. The following measures maintain the client's self-concept:

1. The nurse provides privacy during dressing changes or inspection of the wound. Room curtains are kept closed around the bed, and the client is draped so that only the dressing or incisional area is exposed.

2. The nurse maintains the client's hygiene. Wound drainage and antiseptic solutions from the surgical skin preparation dry on the skin's surface and cause irritation. A complete bath the first day after surgery can make the client feel renewed. When the gown becomes soiled by wound drainage, the nurse offers a clean gown and washcloth. The nurse keeps the client's hair neatly combed and offers frequent oral hygiene, especially for the client who is NPO. Room deodorizers may be useful if the odor from drainage seems particularly troublesome to the client and family.

3. The nurse prevents drainage sets from overflowing. Typically the physician orders contents of drainage sets to be measured every 8 hours for output recording. The client sometimes becomes preoccupied with observing the gradual collection of drainage, and some drainage sets can leak contents if they become too full. The nurse should empty the sets periodically to prevent accidental spills and hampering of the client's movement.

4. The nurse maintains a pleasant environment. Self-concept is heightened by being in pleasant, comfortable surroundings. Frequently the room of a surgical client becomes cluttered with extra dressings, rolls of tape, and bottles of antiseptic solution. If the client requires frequent dressing changes, the room may take on the appearance of a supply room. The nurse should store or remove unused supplies and keep the client's bedside orderly and clean.

5. The nurse offers opportunities for the client to discuss feelings about appearance. If the nurse notices that the client avoids looking at an incision, the client may need to discuss any fears or concerns. A client having surgery for the first time is often more anxious than one who has had multiple surgeries. Both male and female clients may worry about permanent scarring. A client is more apt to look at an incision several days after surgery when healing is occurring and energy and well-being are increased. If the client chooses to look at an incision for the first time, the area should be clean. Eventually the client should be able to care for the incision site by applying simple dressings or bathing the affected area.

6. The nurse provides the family with opportunities to dis-

cuss ways to promote the client's self-concept. Encouraging independence can be difficult for a family member who has a strong desire to assist the client in any way. By knowing about the appearance of a wound or incision, family members can be supportive during dressing changes. The topic or tone of a conversation can also help family members distract a client from dwelling on fears and concerns. Family members should not avoid discussing the future. However, the nurse must help them to know when it is appropriate to discuss future plans. Then the client and family can work together to discuss realistic plans for the client's return home.

PROMOTING RETURN TO A FUNCTIONAL STATE OF HEALTH

Throughout the postoperative convalescent period the nurse promotes the client's independence and active participation in care. In those settings where critical pathways are utilized, clients and family members review the anticipated interventions and outcomes in care. The critical pathways is a road map to recovery and gives the client a visible guide that motivates active involvement in care.

When a client is in pain, nauseated, or suffers from complications of surgery, there is less motive for self-care. The nurse must maintain a balance of providing for clients' needs when they are physically dependent and promoting more involvement when their conditions allow.

The goals a nurse sets for a client's involvement in care must be realistic. Surgery may limit the ability to participate effectively. It is unrealistic for the nurse to involve the client if movement is highly restricted or if participation increases discomfort.

The nurse should keep the client and family informed of recovery progress. Many clients become depressed if they think recovery is slow. The nurse explains that it normally takes many days to reach a level of maximal recovery. Surgery may also cause permanent physical limitations that require time for acceptance. The client and family who believe that the stay will be less than 24 hours may be disappointed and upset. Clear, timely communication from the nurse helps them deal effectively with this change.

The nurse plans care daily, keeping in mind the ultimate goals for recovery. From the moment the client enters the hospital, through surgery, and during the postoperative phase, the nurse anticipates the client's return home.

Involvement of family members in the client's care plan can facilitate recovery. If the client requires additional care at home, such as dressing changes, assistance with ambulation, or drug administration, the nurse instructs family members on proper care techniques. If family members are unable to assist the client, the nurse works with the physician and social worker in making plans for home care. The client will be more able to assume a functional state of health when family members understand the limitations a client faces.

 Evaluation

The nurse evaluates the effectiveness of care provided to the surgical client on the basis of expected outcomes following nursing interventions. In all surgical settings the nurse consults with the client and family to gather evaluation data. The nurse can evaluate the ambulatory surgical client's outcomes by making a telephone call to the client's home, asking if complications have developed and if the client understands restrictions or medications. The call is usually placed 24 hours after surgery and reassures the client that the nurse is concerned and allows the nurse to evaluate the progress of recovery.

In an acute care setting the evaluation of a surgical client is ongoing. If a client fails to progress as expected, the nurse revises the care plan based on the priorities of the client's needs. Every effort is made to assist the client to return to as healthy and functional a state as possible.

Part of the nurse's evaluation is determining the extent to which the client and family have learned self-care mea-

---

 Sample Evaluation of Interventions for Postoperative Client

GOALS	EVALUATIVE MEASURES	EXPECTED OUTCOMES
Client will achieve normal ventilatory function with patent airway by second postoperative day.	Measure chest excursion while client deep breathes. Inspect mucus. Auscultate lung sounds after coughing and deep breathing.	Client will be able to breathe deeply. Cough will be clear and nonproductive. Lung sounds will be clear.
Client will remain free of surgical wound infection postoperatively.	Inspect condition of wound edges and character of drainage. Assess body temperature.	Wound edges will be approximated and slightly reddened and drainage will be minimal and clear. Client will remain afebrile postoperatively.
Client will achieve rest and comfort by discharge.	Evaluate client for verbal and non-verbal behaviors indicative of pain.	Client will report less discomfort compared with postoperative baseline.
Client will return to functional state of health by discharge.	Observe client participate in self-care activities. Observe client's level of ambulation.	Client will maintain personal grooming. Client will initiate self-care independently. Client will ambulate 50 yards down hallway by discharge.

sures. A client often has to continue dressing care, follow activity restrictions, continue medication therapy, and observe for signs and symptoms of complications on returning home. A referral to home health care assists clients unable to perform self-care activities. It is useful to have a home health nurse in attendance at discharge to know what a client can effectively perform. The evaluation box on p. 1425 outlines criteria used for postoperative clients.

■ KEY CONCEPTS ■

▶ Perioperative nursing is professional nursing care afforded the surgical client before, during, and after surgery.

▶ Surgery is classified by level of severity, urgency, and purpose.

▶ Previous illnesses, past surgeries, and the nature of nursing care provided influence the client's ability to tolerate surgery.

▶ The preoperative period may be several days or only a few hours long.

▶ All medications taken before surgery are automatically discontinued after surgery unless a physician reorders the drugs.

▶ Family members are important in assisting clients with any physical limitations and in providing emotional support during postoperative recovery.

▶ Preoperative assessment of vital signs and physical findings provides an important baseline with which to compare postoperative assessment data.

▶ A client's feelings about surgery can have a significant impact on relationships with the nursing staff and the client's ability to participate in care.

▶ Surgical removal of a body part may permanently alter a person's body image and sexuality.

▶ Nursing diagnoses of the surgical client may pose implications for nursing care during one or all phases of surgery.

▶ Primary responsibility for informed consent rests with the client's surgeon.

▶ Informed consent cannot be obtained if a client is confused, unconscious, mentally incompetent, or under the influence of sedatives.

▶ Structured preoperative teaching has a positive influence on postoperative recovery.

▶ Basic to preoperative teaching is explanation of all preoperative and postoperative routines and demonstration of postoperative exercises.

▶ Clipping of a surgical site should be done as close as possible to the time of surgery to minimize infection.

▶ In ambulatory surgery, nurses must use the limited time available to educate clients, assess their health status, and prepare them for surgery.

▶ A routine preoperative checklist is a guide for final preparation of the client before surgery.

▶ Many responsibilities of nurses within the operating room focus on protecting the client from potential harm.

▶ Assessment of the postoperative client centers on the body systems most likely to be affected by anesthesia, immobilization, and surgical trauma.

▶ The PACU nurse reports to the nurse on the postoperative division information pertaining to the client's current physical status and risk for postoperative complications.

▶ Accurate pain assessment and intervention are necessary for healing.

■ KEY TERMS ■

Ambulatory surgery, p. 1381
Antiembolism stockings, p. 1422
Atelectasis, p. 1415
Cholecystectomy, p. 1381
Circulating nurse, p. 1412
Convalescence, p. 1413
Dehiscence, p. 1389
Depilatories, p. 1402
Dermatome, p. 1416
General anesthesia, p. 1411
Local anesthesia, p. 1412
Malignant hyperthermia, p. 1416
Moribund, p. 1387
Paralytic ileus, p. 1417
Perioperative nursing, p. 1381
Preoperative teaching, p. 1381
Recovery, p. 1413
Regional anesthesia, p. 1411
Scrub nurse, p. 1412

■ CRITICAL THINKING EXERCISES ■

1. Your 76-year-old client is being admitted for a cataract extraction. Name three of the physiological changes occurring in older adults that place your client at higher risk in surgery.

2. Mrs. B. is a 52-year-old client who will have abdominal surgery in the morning. She has a history of smoking one pack of cigarettes a day for 30 years. What areas would you concentrate on during Mrs. B.'s preoperative teaching?

3. Your client has undergone abdominal surgery to remove a cancerous growth. Describe postoperative measures you would use to promote rest and comfort.

4. Mrs. R. is a 39-year-old client who has undergone a right modified mastectomy. You notice that she refuses to look at her incision and has been remaining in bed even though she has been instructed to increase her activity as tolerated. How can you encourage Mrs. R.'s independence and maintain her self-concept?

5. Mr. H. has been admitted to your unit following a right total knee replacement. He had a lidocaine spinal for anesthesia and currently moans and begs for help. How would you assess his pain, intervene to promote relief, and evaluate the effectiveness of your interventions?

6. Miss C. was admitted through ambulatory surgery for a laparoscopic tubal ligation. What discharge criteria might be used for Miss C.

REFERENCES

Agency for Health Care Policy and Research: *Acute pain management: operative or medical procedures and trauma, Clinical practice guideline*, AHCPR Pub. No. 92-0032, Rockville, Maryland, 1992, Public Health Service, U.S. Department of Health and Human Services.

American Nurses Association, Association of Operating Room Nurses: *Standards of perioperative nursing care*, Kansas City, Mo, 1972, The Associations.

Blackwood S: Back to basics, the preop exam, *Am J Nurs* 86:39, 1986.

Bryant L, Dierdorf S: Postanesthesia recovery, *Seminars in Pediatric Surgery* 1(1):45, 1992.

Dalayon A: Components of preoperative patient teaching in Kuwait, *J Advanced Nursing* 19:537, 1994.

Dettenmeier PA: *Pulmonary nursing care*, St Louis, 1992, Mosby.

Gordon B, Newman S: Factors influencing surgical wound healing and their anesthetic implications, *Semin Periop Nurs* 2(4):221,1993.

Halsey RW et al: Nosocomial infections in U.S. hospitals, 1975-1976: estimated frequency by selected characteristics of patients, *Am J Med* 70:947, 1981.

Horner J: The aging client: a perioperative approach, *Seminars in Perioperative Nursing* 2(4):226, 1993.

Kim MJ, McFarland GK, McLane AM: *Pocket guide to nursing diagnosis*, ed 6, St Louis, 1995, Mosby.

Lepczyk M et al: Timing of preoperative patient teaching, *J Adv Nurs* 15:300, 1990.

Levin D: Assessing and improving quality in the PACU, *Nurs Clin N Am* 28(3):581, 1993.

McDonald D: Gender and ethnic stereotyping and narcotic analgesic administration, *Research in Nursing and Health* 17:45, 1994.

Meeker M, Rothrock J: *Alexander's care of the patient in surgery*, ed 10, St Louis, 1995, Mosby.

Metheny N: Measures to test placement of nasogastric and nasointestinal feeding tubes: a review, *Nurs Res* 37:324, 1988.

Metheny N et al: Effectiveness of the auscultatory method in predicting feeding tube location, *Nurs Res* 39:262, 1990.

Metheny N et al: Effectiveness of pH measurements in predicting feeding tube placement, *Nurs Res* 38:280, 1989.

Miaskowski C: Current concepts in the assessment and management of acute pain, *MedSurg Nursing* 2(1):28, 1993.

Morales C, Andrews J: Postoperative wound care: nursing assessment and management, *Seminars in Perioperative Nursing* 2(4):231, 1993.

Odom J: Airway emergencies in the PACU, *Nurs Clin N Am* 28(3):483, 1993.

Parnass S: Ambulatory surgical patient priorities, *Nurs Clin N Am* 28(3):531, 1993.

Powell AH, Bora MB: How do you give continuous epidural fentanyl? *Am J Nurs* 89(9): 1197, 1989.

Rivellini D: Local and regional anesthesia: nursing implications, *Nurs Clin N Am* 28(3):547, 1993.

Saleh K: The elderly patient in the PACU, *Nurs Clin N Am* 28(3):507, 1993.

Schoessler M: Perceptions of preoperative education in patients admitted the morning of surgery, *Patient Educ Couns* 14:127, 1989.

Scott I: Effectivenesss of documented assessment of perioperative pain, *British J Nurs* 3(10):494, 1994.

Thibodeau G, Patton K: *Anthony's textbook of anatomy and physiology*, ed 15, St. Louis, 1996, Mosby.

Walsh J: Postop effects of OR positioning, *RN* 56(2): 50, 1993.

Watt-Watson J, Donovan M: *Pain management-nursing perspective*, St Louis, 1992, Mosby.

Waugaman W, Foster S: New advances in anesthesia, *Nurs Clin N Am* 26(2):451, 1991.

Wild L, Coyne C: The basics and beyond: epidural analgesia, *AJN* 92(4): 26, 1992.

Young M, Kindred D: Malignant hyperthermia: not just an operating room emergency, *MedSurg Nursing* 2(1):41, 1993.

ADDITIONAL READINGS

Bowman J: Perception of surgical pain by nurses and patients, *Clinical Nursing Research* 3(1):69, 1994.

Curran CR: An interview with Mary Beth Pais, *Nursing economics* 12(1):5, 1994.

Francke A, Theeuwen I: Inhibition in expressing pain, *Cancer Nursing* 17:193, 1994.

Frost E, editor: *Post-anesthesia care unit*, ed 2, St Louis, 1990, Mosby.

Hambleton N: Dealing with complications of epidural analgesia, *Nursing* 94(10):33, 1994.

Litwack K: Post-anesthesia assessment: what medical-surgical nurses need to know, *MedSurg Nursing* 2(4):294, 1993.

Litwack K: *Post anesthesia care nursing*, ed 2, St Louis, 1995, Mosby.

Lorig K: *Patient education: a practical approach*, St Louis, 1992, Mosby.

Metzger RS: The beginning of OR nursing education, *AORN J* 24:73, 1976.

Meyer-Paholuis E et al: The pediatric patient in the PACU, *Nurs Clin N Am* 28(3):519, 1993.

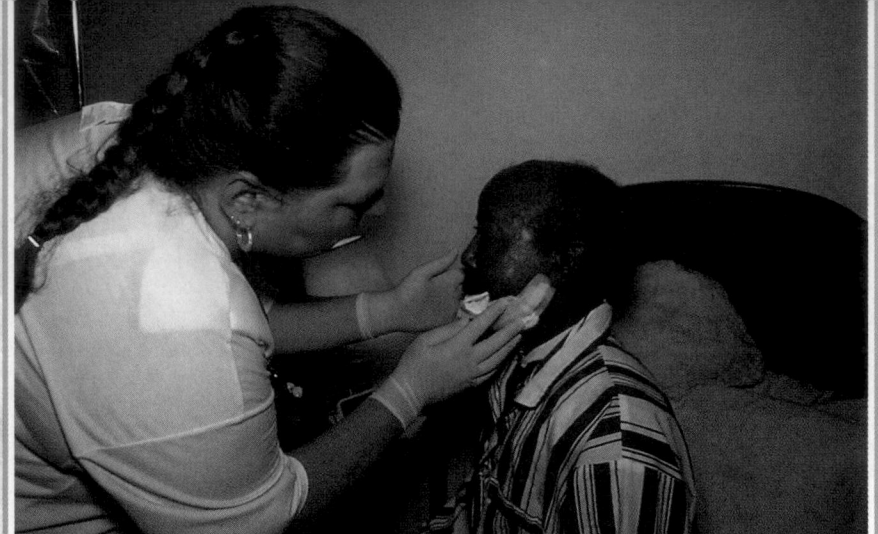
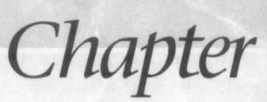
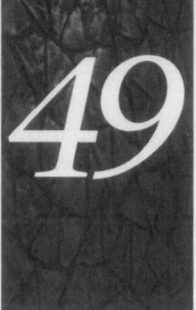

Clients With Wounds

Objectives

Mastery of content in this chapter will enable the student to:

▶ Define the key terms listed.

▶ Discuss normal processes of wound healing.

▶ Describe the differences among wounds healing by primary, secondary, and third intention.

▶ Describe complications of wound healing and their usual time of occurrence.

▶ Explain the factors that impair or promote wound healing.

▶ Describe differences in assessing a wound in a stable versus emergency setting.

▶ Conduct an assessment of a closed and an open wound.

▶ Identify nursing diagnoses related to clients with wounds.

▶ Discuss principles of first aid in wound care.

▶ Explain nursing care implications in the use of dressings.

▶ Apply a sterile dry or wet-to-damp dressing.

▶ Discuss the purpose of bandages and binders.

▶ Describe the effects of heat and cold on wound healing.

▶ Use warm and cold applications safely on an injured body part.

The skin or the integumentary system is the body's largest organ. It composes one sixth of the total body weight (Wysocki, 1995). The integument is a protective barrier against disease-causing organisms; a sensory organ for pain, temperature, and touch; and can synthesize vitamin D. Injury to the integument poses risks to safety and triggers a complex healing response. Knowing the normal healing pattern helps the nurse recognize alterations that require intervention.

NORMAL INTEGUMENT

In relation to wound healing the integument has two principal layers: the epidermis and the dermis (Fig. 49-1). These two layers are separated by a basement membrane, which is often referred to as the *dermal-epidermal junction.* The **epidermis,** or outer layer, has several layers. The stratum corneum is the thin, outermost layer of the epidermis. It consists of flattened, dead, keratinized cells. The cells originate from the epidermal layer, the stratum basale. Cells in the stratum basale divide, proliferate, and migrate toward the epidermal surface. After cells reach the stratum corneum, they flatten and die. This constant movement ensures replacement of surface cells sloughed off during normal **desquamation.** The thin stratum corneum protects underlying cells and tissues from dehydration and prevents entrance of certain chemical agents. However, the stratum corneum does allow evaporation of water from the skin and permits absorption of certain topically applied medications.

The **dermis** is the inner layer of the skin, which provides the tensile strength, mechanical support, and protection to the underlying muscles, bones, and organs. It differs from the epidermis in that it contains mostly connective tissue and few skin cells. **Collagen** (a tough, fibrous protein), blood vessels, and nerves compose it. Fibroblasts, which are responsible for collagen formation, are the only distinctive cell type within the dermis.

Understanding the integument's layers helps the nurse promote wound healing. The epidermis functions to resurface wounds and restore the barrier against invading organisms. The dermis responds to restore the structural integrity (collagen) and the physical properties of the skin. Even though a wound may close in the upper epidermal layer, the client is at risk for infection, circulatory impairment, and tissue breakdown if the underlying dermis fails to heal. A summary of the normal changes in aging skin can be found in the box at right.

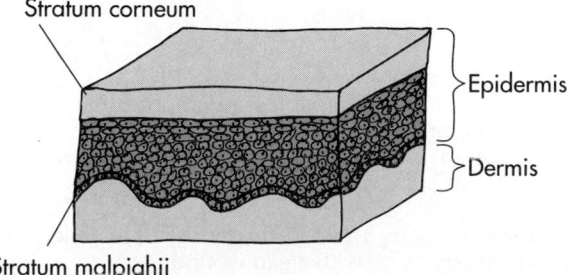

Fig. 49-1 Layers of the integument.

WOUND CLASSIFICATIONS

A **wound** is "a disruption of normal anatomical structure and function that results from pathological processes beginning internally or externally to the involved organ(s)" (Lazarus et al, 1994). There are many ways to classify wounds (Cooper, 1992a). Wound classification systems describe the status of skin integrity, cause of the wound, severity or extent of tissue injury or damage, cleanliness of the wound, or descriptive qualities of the wound such as color (Table 49-1). These classifications overlap. For example, a penetrating knife wound is also an open wound, and a contused wound is a closed wound. Wound classifications enable the nurse to understand the risks associated with a wound and implications for its care. An open wound, for example, presents a greater risk of infection than a closed wound, whereas an abrasion requires less extensive dressings than a deep-penetrating wound.

WOUND HEALING PROCESS

Wound healing involves integrated physiological processes. The nature of healing is the same for all wounds, with vari-

GERONTOLOGICAL PRINCIPLES for Wound Healing

- Diminished epidermal cell activity in elderly skin increases the epidermal cell renewal time by one third. For example, in a young adult, the epithelium renews itself in about 20 days; after the age of 50, epithelium renewal takes 30 or more days.
Clinical significance: Slow replacement of epithelial cells means the elderly have slower wound healing.
- Aging causes atrophy and thinning of both layers of the skin. Clinical significance: The nurse should monitor the elderly client's skin in the buttock area. The sacrum is the most common site of pressure ulcers. With the thinning of the epidermis the skin's barrier function is diminished, so chemicals can easily get into the body. Because the dermis is thinner and flatter, the skin wrinkles.
- There is less surface area in the skin of elderly people as compared with younger skin; there is also a weakening in the epidermis and dermis attachment.
Clinical significance: Because in the elderly the attachment between these two layers of the skin (dermal-epidermal junction) is weakened, the epidermis can "slide," therefore the skin can tear more easily.
- Aging causes impaired immune function of cells located in the skin.
Clinical significance: Altered immune function of elderly skin means the ability to fight infection is decreased in the elderly.
- The hypodermis ("the insulator of the skin") is decreased in size with age.
Clinical significance: Elderly clients have little subcutaneous padding over bony prominences, so are more at risk for skin breakdown and heat stroke.
- Structural changes in collagen occur in elderly skin. Collagen fibers come together as bundles. Also there is a loss in amount of collagen.
Clinical significance: Elderly clients have decreased skin turgor, so they are at greater risk for shearing and tearing injuries.

Table 49-1	Wound Classification		
DESCRIPTION	**CAUSES**	**IMPLICATIONS FOR HEALING**	

STATUS OF SKIN INTEGRITY

Open

Wound involving a break in skin or mucous membranes	Trauma by sharp object or blow (surgical incision, venipuncture, gunshot wound)	Break in skin exposes body to invasion by microorganisms. Loss of blood and body fluids through wound occurs. Function of body part is reduced.

Closed

Wound involving no break in skin	Part of body being struck by blunt object; twisting, straining, or deceleration force against body (bone fracture, tear of visceral organ)	Wound may predispose person to internal hemorrhage. Function of affected body part is reduced.

Acute

Wound that proceeds through an orderly and timely reparative process that results in sustained restoration of anatomical and functional integrity	Trauma from a sharp object	Wounds are usually easily cleaned and repaired. Wound edges are clean and intact.

Chronic

Wound that fails to proceed through an orderly and timely process to produce anatomical and functional integrity	Ulcers, sores exposed to friction, secretions, pressure	Continued exposure to pressure, friction, and secretions impedes wound healing. Wound edges may be necrotic, and drainage may be present.

CAUSE

Intentional

Wound resulting from therapy	Surgical incision; introduction of needle into body part	Incision is usually performed under aseptic technique to minimize chance of infection. Wound edges are usually smooth and clean.

Unintentional

Wound that occurs unexpectedly	Traumatic injury (knife wound, burn)	Wound occurs under unsterile conditions. Wound edges are often jagged.

SEVERITY OF INJURY

Superficial

Wound that involves only epidermal layer of skin	Result of friction applied to skin surface (abrasion, first-degree burn, shearing)	Break creates risk of infection. Wound does not involve underlying injury to tissues or organs. Blood supply to area is intact.

Penetrating

Wound involving break in epidermal skin layer, as well as dermis and deeper tissues or organs	Foreign object or instrument entering deep into body tissues; usually unintentional (gunshot wound, stab wound)	There is high risk of infection because foreign object is contaminated. Wound may cause internal and external hemorrhage; damage to organs causes temporary or permanent loss of function.

Perforating

Penetrating wound in which foreign object enters and exits an internal organ	(See above entry)	There is high risk of infection. Nature of injury depends on organ perforated (lung, compromised oxygenation; major vessel, hemorrhage; intestine, contamination of abdominal cavity by feces).

CLEANLINESS

Clean

Wound containing no pathogenic organisms	Closed surgical wound not entering gastrointestinal, respiratory, genital, or uninfected urinary tract or oropharyngeal cavity	There is low risk of infection.

Clean-contaminated

Wound made under aseptic conditions but involving body cavity that normally harbors microorganisms	Surgical wound entering gastrointestinal, respiratory, genital, or urinary tract or oropharyngeal cavity under controlled conditions	There is greater risk of infection than with clean wound.

Table 49-1	Wound Classification—cont'd	
DESCRIPTION	**CAUSES**	**IMPLICATIONS FOR HEALING**
CLEANLINESS—cont'd **Contaminated** Wound existing under conditions in which presence of microorganisms is likely	Open, traumatic, accidental wounds; surgical wound in which break in asepsis occurred	Tissues are often not healthy and show inflammation. There is high risk of infection.
Infected Bacterial organisms present in wound site, usually above 10^5 organisms per gram of tissue	Any wound that does not properly heal and grows organisms, old traumatic wound, surgical incision into area infected (e.g., ruptured bowel)	Wound presents signs of infection (inflammation, purulent drainage, skin separation).
Colonized Wound containing microorganisms (usually multiple)	Chronic wound (vascular stasis ulcer, pressure ulcer)	Wound healing is slow, and high risk of infection exists.
DESCRIPTIVE QUALITIES **Laceration** Tearing of tissues with irregular wound edges	Severe traumatic injury (knife wound, industrial accident involving machinery, tissues cut by broken glass)	Wound is usually created by contaminated object. Depth of wound determines other complications.
Abrasion Superficial wound involving scraping or rubbing of skin's surface	Wound often resulting from fall (skinned knee or elbow); wound also resulting from dermatological procedure for removing scar tissue	Wound is painful from exposure of superficial nerves; deeper tissues are not involved. There is risk of infection from exposure to contaminated surface.
Contusion Closed wound caused by a blow to body by blunt object; contusion or bruise characterized by swelling, discoloration, and pain	Bleeding in underlying tissues caused by blunt force against body part	Wound is more severe if internal organ is contused. Wound may cause temporary loss of function of body part. Localized bleeding into tissues may form hematoma (collection of blood).

ations depending on the location, severity, and extent of injury. The ability of cells and tissues to regenerate or return to normal structure by cell growth also affects healing. Cells of the liver, renal tubules, and neurons of the central nervous system typically regenerate slowly or not at all.

There are two types of wounds: those with loss of tissue and those without. A clean surgical incision is an example of a wound with little tissue loss. The surgical wound heals by **primary intention.** The skin edges **approximate,** or close together, and the risk of infection is low. Healing occurs quickly. In contrast, a wound involving loss of tissue, such as a burn, pressure ulcer, or severe laceration, heals by **secondary intention.** The wound edges do not approximate. The wound is left open until it becomes filled by scar tissue. It takes longer for a wound to heal by secondary intention, and thus the chance of infection is greater. If scarring from secondary intention is severe, there may be permanent loss of tissue function.

Healing by Primary Intention

An example of the normal healing process is repair of a clean surgical wound. Healing occurs in several stages, described by Doughty (1992) as inflammatory, proliferative, and maturation, or by Krasner (1995) as "the three R's: reaction, regeneration, and remodeling."

INFLAMMATORY PHASE (REACTION)

The inflammation stage is the body's *reaction* to wounding and begins within minutes of injury and lasts about 3 days. Reparative processes control bleeding (**hemostasis**), deliver blood and cells to the injured area (inflammation), and form epithelial cells at the injury site (**epithelialization**). During hemostasis, injured blood vessels constrict and platelets gather to stop bleeding. Clots form a **fibrin** matrix that later provides a framework for cellular repair. Damaged tissue and mast cells secrete histamine, resulting in vasodilation of surrounding capillaries and exudation of serum and white blood cells into damaged tissues. This results in localized redness, edema, warmth, and throbbing. The inflammatory response is beneficial, and there is no value in attempting to cool the area or reduce the swelling unless the swelling occurs within a closed compartment (e.g., ankle or neck).

Leukocytes (white blood cells) reach the wound within a few hours. The primary acting white blood cell is the neutrophil, which begins to ingest bacteria and small debris. The neutrophils die in a few days and leave behind an enzyme **exudate** that attacks bacteria or interferes with tissue repair. In chronic inflammation, the dying neutrophils create pus. The second important leukocyte is the monocyte, which transforms into macrophages. The macrophages are the "garbage cells" that clean a wound of bacteria, dead cells, and debris by phagocytosis. The macrophages also digest and recycle substances, such as amino acids and sugars, that aid in wound repair. Macrophages continue the process of clearing the wound of debris, attracting further macrophages, and stimulating formation of **fibroblasts**, the cells that synthesize collagen. Collagen can be found as early as the second day and is the main component of scar tissue.

After the macrophages clean the wound and make it ready for tissue repair, epithelial cells move from the wound margins under the base of the clot or scab. Epithelial cells continue to gather under the wound space for about 48 hours. Eventually a thin layer of epithelial tissue forms over the wound as a barrier against infectious organisms and toxic materials.

Growth hormones are released by platelets and macrophages. There is increasing evidence that these factors promote wound healing.

The inflammatory phase is prolonged and repair processes are slowed if too little inflammation occurs, as in debilitating disease or after administration of steroids. Too much inflammation also prolongs healing because arriving cells compete for available nutrients.

PROLIFERATIVE PHASE (REGENERATION)

With the appearance of new blood vessels as reconstruction progresses, the proliferative phase begins and lasts from 3 to 24 days. The main activities during this *regeneration phase* are the filling in of the wound with new connective or granulation tissue and the closing of the top of the wound by epithelization. Fibroblasts are the cells that synthesize collagen, which will close the wound defect. Fibroblasts require vitamins B and C, oxygen, and amino acids to function properly. Collagen provides strength and structural integrity to a wound. During this period the wound begins to close with new tissue. As reconstruction progresses, the tensile strength of the wound increases, and the risk of wound separation or rupture is less likely. The degree of stress on a wound influences the amount of scar tissue formed. For example, more scar tissue forms in an extremity wound than in a less mobile area such as the scalp or chest. Impairment of healing during this stage usually results from systemic factors such as age, anemia, hypoproteinemia, and zinc deficiency.

MATURATION (REMODELING)

Maturation, the final stage of healing, may take more than a year, depending on the depth and extent of the wound. The collagen scar continues to reorganize and gain strength for several months. However, a healed wound usually does not have the strength of the tissue it replaces (tensile strength). Collagen fibers undergo *remodeling* or reorganization before assuming their normal appearance. Usually scar tissue contains fewer pigmented cells (melanocytes) and has a lighter color than normal skin.

Healing by Secondary Intention

When tissue loss in a wound is extensive, wound healing takes longer. A large open wound typically drains more fluid than a closed wound. Inflammation is often chronic, and tissue defects become filled with fragile granulation tissue rather than collagen. **Granulation tissue** is a form of connective tissue that has a more abundant blood supply than collagen. Because the wound is larger, the amount of connective tissue scarring is larger.

When epithelial and connective tissue cells are unable to close a wound defect, contraction may occur. **Wound contraction** involves movement of the dermis and epidermis on each side of the wound. The mechanism of contracture is not completely understood. It is known, however, that collagen is not essential and any event that interferes with cell viability at the wound margin inhibits contraction. Wound contraction begins on about the fourth day and occurs simultaneously with epithelization. The cell that provides the motive force is the myofibroblast. Wound contraction results in thinning of surrounding tissues, and the size and shape of the final scar corresponds to tension lines in the damaged area. For example, a square wound in the abdomen assumes the shape of two Ys, end to end. There are areas of the body where contraction gives poor results, such as wounds on the face, sternum, and anterior lower leg. Wound contraction is not the same as a contracture or deformity resulting from muscle shortening and joint fixation.

■ COMPLICATIONS OF WOUND HEALING

Hemorrhage

Hemorrhage, or bleeding from a wound site, is normal during and immediately after the initial trauma. Hemostasis occurs within several minutes unless large blood vessels are involved or the client has poor clotting function. Hemorrhage occurring after hemostasis indicates a slipped surgical suture, a dislodged clot, infection, or erosion of a blood vessel by a foreign object (e.g., a drain). Hemorrhage may occur externally or internally. For example, if a surgical suture slips off a blood vessel, bleeding occurs internally within the tissues, and there are no visible signs of blood unless a surgical drain is present, which is inserted into tissues beneath a wound to remove fluid that collects in underlying tissues. The nurse can detect internal bleeding by looking for distention or swelling of the affected body part, a change in the type and amount of drainage from a surgical drain, or signs of **hypovolemic shock**. A **hematoma** is a localized collection of blood underneath the tissues. It appears as a swelling or mass that often takes on a bluish discoloration. A hematoma near a major artery or vein is dangerous because pressure from the expanding hematoma may obstruct blood flow.

External hemorrhaging is more obvious. The nurse observes dressings covering the wound for bloody drainage. If bleeding is extensive, the dressing soon becomes saturated, and frequently blood escapes along the sides of the dressing and pools beneath the client. The nurse observes all wounds closely, particularly surgical wounds in which the risk of hemorrhage is great during the first 24 to 48 hours after surgery.

Infection

Wound infection is the second most common **nosocomial** (hospital-related) **infection** (see Chapters 34 and 38). According to the Centers for Disease Control (CDC) (Garner, 1985), a wound is infected if purulent material drains from it, even if a culture is not taken or has negative results. A sample of drainage from an infected wound may not reveal bacteria due to poor culture technique or administration of antibiotics. Positive culture findings do not always indicate an infection because many wounds contain colonies of non-infective resident bacteria. In fact, all dermal wounds are considered contaminated with bacteria. What differentiates contaminated wounds from infected wounds is the *amount* of bacteria present. It is generally agreed that wounds with more than 100,000 (10^5) organisms/ml are infected. The *only* exception is when the organism is B-hemolytic strepto-coccus; presence of this organism in colony counts of less than 100,000/ml is considered an infection (Doughty, 1992). The chances of wound infection are greater when the wound contains dead or necrotic tissue, there are foreign bodies in or near the wound, and the blood supply and lo-cal tissue defenses are reduced. Bacterial wound infection in-hibits wound healing.

A contaminated or traumatic wound may show signs of infection early, within 2 to 3 days. A surgical wound infec-tion usually does not develop until the fourth or fifth post-operative day. The client has a fever, tenderness and pain at the wound site, and an elevated white blood cell count. The edges of the wound may appear inflamed. If drainage is pre-sent, it is odorous and **purulent**, which causes a yellow, green, or brown color, depending on the causative organism.

Dehiscence

When a wound fails to heal properly, the layers of skin and tissue may separate. This most commonly occurs before collagen formation (3 to 11 days after injury). **Dehiscence** is the partial or total separation of wound layers. A client with poor wound healing is at risk for dehiscence. However, obese clients have a high risk because of the constant strain placed on their wounds and the poor healing qualities of fatty tissue. Dehiscence often involves abdominal surgical wounds and occurs after a sudden strain, such as coughing, vomiting, or sitting up in bed. Clients often report feeling as though something has given way. When there is an in-crease in serosanguineous drainage from a wound, the nurse should be alert for dehiscence.

Evisceration

With total separation of wound layers, **evisceration** (pro-trusion of visceral organs through a wound opening) may occur. The condition is a medical emergency that requires surgical repair. When evisceration occurs, the nurse places sterile towels soaked in sterile saline over the extruding tis-sues to reduce chances of bacterial invasion and drying. If the organs protrude through the wound, blood supply to the tissues is compromised. The client should be kept NPO, observed for signs and symptoms of shock, and prepared for emergency surgery.

Fistulas

A **fistula** is an abnormal passage between two organs or be-tween an organ and the outside of the body. A surgeon may create a fistula for therapeutic purposes, for example, mak-ing an opening between the stomach and the outer ab-dominal wall to insert a gastrostomy tube for feeding. Most fistulas, however, form as a result of poor wound healing or as a complication of some diseases, such as Crohn's disease or regional enteritis. Trauma, infection, radiation exposure,

---

Risks for Skin Breakdown from Body Fluids

LOW RISK
- Saliva
- Serosanguineous drainage

HIGH RISK
- Gastric drainage
- Pancreatic drainage

MODERATE RISK
- Bile
- Stool
- Urine
- Ascitic fluid
- Purulent exudate

---

and diseases such as cancer prevent tissue layers from clos-ing properly and allow the fistula tract to form. Fistulas in-crease the risk of infection and fluid and electrolyte imbal-ances from fluid loss. Chronic drainage of fluids through a fistula can also predispose a person to skin breakdown (see the box above).

Delayed Wound Closure

Sometimes referred to as *third-intention wound healing*, de-layed wound closure is a deliberate attempt by the surgeon to allow effective drainage of a clean-contaminated or con-taminated wound. The wound is not closed until all evi-dence of edema and wound debris has been removed. An occlusive dressing is used to prevent bacterial contamina-tion of the wound. Then the wound is closed as in primary closure, or first intention. Experimentally, it has been demonstrated that scarring or delayed healing does not sig-nificantly increase when this technique is used (Cooper, 1992).

■ FACTORS INFLUENCING WOUND HEALING

A number of factors influence the rate of wound healing. A client with any factors listed in Table 49-2 is at risk for wound complications. The nurse's knowledge of factors in-fluencing healing helps in providing preventive care and selecting appropriate wound care therapies.

Nutrition

Normal wound healing requires proper nutrition. Physio-logical processes of wound healing depend on the ready availability of protein, vitamins (especially A and C), and the trace minerals zinc and copper. Collagen is a protein formed from amino acids acquired by fibroblasts from pro-tein ingested in food. Vitamin C is needed for synthesis of collagen. Vitamin A reduces the negative effects of steroids on wound healing (see Table 49-2). Trace elements are needed for epithelization (zinc), collagen synthesis (zinc), and collagen fiber linking (copper).

For clients weakened or debilitated by illness, nutritional therapy is especially important. A client who has under-gone surgery (see Chapter 48) and is well nourished still re-quires at least 1500 kcal/day for nutritional maintenance. Alternatives such as enteral feedings (see Chapter 41) and parenteral nutrition (see Chapter 45) are made available for clients unable to maintain normal food intake.

Aging

Although the rates for the stages of healing among older clients may be slowed, the physiological aspects of healing

| Table 49-2 | Factors That Impair Wound Healing |

PHYSIOLOGICAL EFFECTS	NURSING IMPLICATIONS
AGE Aging alters all phases of wound healing. Vascular changes impair circulation to wound site. Reduced liver function alters synthesis of clotting factors. Inflammatory response is slowed. Formation of antibodies and lymphocytes is reduced. Collagen tissue is less pliable. Scar tissue is less elastic.	Instruct client on safety precautions to avoid injuries. Be prepared to provide wound care for longer period. Teach support persons in home wound care techniques.
MALNUTRITION All phases of wound healing are impaired. Stress from burns or severe trauma increases nutritional requirements.	Provide balanced diet rich in protein, carbohydrates, lipids, vitamins A and C, and minerals (e.g., zinc, copper). Provide adequate amounts of calories and fluid.
OBESITY Fatty tissue lacks adequate blood supply to resist bacterial infection and deliver nutrients and cellular elements for healing.	Observe obese client for signs of wound infection and evisceration.
IMPAIRED OXYGENATION Low arterial oxygen tension alters synthesis of collagen and formation of epithelial cells. If local circulating blood flow is poor, tissues fail to receive needed oxygen. Decreased hemoglobin in blood (anemia) reduces arterial oxygen levels in capillaries and interferes with tissue repair.	Provide diet adequate in iron. Vitamin B_{12}, and folic acid. Monitor hematocrit and hemoglobin levels of clients with wounds.
SMOKING Smoking reduces amount of functional hemoglobin in blood, thus decreasing tissue oxygenation. Smoking may increase platelet aggregation and cause hypercoagulability. Smoking interferes with normal cellular mechanisms that promote release of oxygen to tissues.	Discourage client from smoking by explaining its effects on wound healing.
DRUGS Steroids reduce inflammatory response and slow collagen synthesis. Antiinflammatory drugs suppress protein synthesis, wound contraction, epithelization, and inflammation. Prolonged antibiotic use may increase risk of superinfection. Chemotherapeutic drugs can depress bone marrow function, lower number of leukocytes, and impair inflammatory response.	Carefully observe clients receiving these drugs because signs of inflammation may not be obvious. Vitamin A can counter act effects of steroids.
DIABETES Chronic disease causes small blood vessel disease that impairs tissue perfusion. Diabetes causes hemoglobin to have greater affinity for oxygen, so it fails to release oxygen to tissues. Hyperglycemia alters ability of leukocytes to perform phagocytosis and also supports overgrowth of fungal and yeast infection.	Instruct diabetic clients to take preventive measures to avoid cuts or breaks in skin. Provide preventive foot care. Control blood sugar to reduce the physiological changes associated with diabetes.
RADIATION Fibrosis and vascular scarring eventually develop in irradiated skin layers. Tissues become fragile and poorly oxygenated.	Closely observe clients who have surgery after radiation for wound complications.
WOUND STRESS Vomiting, abdominal distention, and respiratory effort may stress suture line and disrupt wound layer. Sudden, unexpected tension on incision inhibits formation of endothelial cell and collagen networks.	Control nausea with ordered antiemetics. Keep nasogastric tubes patent and draining to avoid accumulation of secretions. Instruct and assist client to splint abdominal wound during coughing.

are unchanged from the younger adult. Problems that arise during healing may be difficult to assign to the aging process or to other possible causes, such as poor nutrition, environment, or individual response to stress. Before surgery, the nurse assesses any factors that may influence or alter wound healing in older clients (see Tables 49-1 and 49-2).

PSYCHOSOCIAL IMPACT OF WOUNDS

Although not directly involved in the physiological process of healing, the client's psychological response to any wound is part of the nurse's assessment. Body image changes may impose a great stress on the client's adaptive mechanisms. In addition, body image changes influence self-concept (see Chapter 23) and sexuality (see Chapter 24). The client's personal and social resources for adaptation should also be a part of the assessment. Factors that may affect the client's perception of the wound include the presence of scars, drains (drains may be necessary for weeks or even months after certain procedures), odor from drainage, and temporary or permanent prosthetic devices.

NURSING PROCESS AND WOUND HEALING

 ## Assessment

The nurse often assesses wounds under two conditions: at the time of injury before treatment and after therapy when the wound is relatively stable. Each condition requires the nurse to make different observations and to take different actions.

EMERGENCY SETTING

The nurse may see wounds in any setting, including a clinic, emergency room, rural youth camp, or the nurse's own backyard. The type of wound determines the criteria for inspection. For example, the nurse need not inspect for signs of internal bleeding after an abrasion but should do so in the event of a puncture wound.

When a client's condition is judged to be stable because of the presence of spontaneous breathing, a clear airway, and a strong carotid pulse (see Chapter 44), the nurse inspects the wound for bleeding. An **abrasion** is usually superficial with little bleeding. The wound may appear "weepy" because of plasma leakage from damaged capillaries. A **laceration** may bleed more profusely, depending on the wound's depth and location. For example, minor scalp lacerations tend to bleed profusely because of the rich blood supply to the scalp. Lacerations greater than 5 cm (2 inches) long or 2.5 cm (1 inch) deep can cause serious bleeding. **Puncture** wounds bleed in relation to the depth and size of the wound: for example, a nail puncture does not cause as much bleeding as a knife wound. The primary dangers of puncture wounds are internal bleeding and infection.

The nurse next inspects the wound for foreign bodies or contaminant material. Most traumatic wounds are dirty. Soil, broken glass, shreds of cloth, and foreign substances clinging to penetrating objects can become embedded in the wound.

The size of the wound is the next criterion for inspection.

A deep laceration requires suturing by a physician. A large open wound may expose bone or tissue that should be protected.

When the injury is the result of trauma from a dirty penetrating object, the nurse determines when the client last received a tetanus toxoid injection. Tetanus bacteria reside in soil and in the gut of humans and animals. A tetanus antitoxin injection is necessary if the client has not had one within 5 years.

STABLE SETTING

When the client's condition is stabilized (e.g., after surgery or treatment) the nurse assesses the wound to determine its progress toward healing. If the wound is covered by a dressing and the physician has not ordered it changed, the nurse should not directly inspect the wound unless serious complications are suspected. In such a situation the nurse should inspect only the dressing and any external drains. If the physician prefers to change the dressing, the physician will assess the wound at least daily. When the nurse removes dressings, care is taken to avoid accidental removal or displacement of underlying drains. Because removal of dressings can be painful, it may help to give an analgesic at least 30 minutes before exposing a wound.

Wound Appearance. The nurse notes whether wound edges are closed. A surgical incision should have clean, well-approximated edges. Crusts often form along the wound edges from exudate. A puncture wound is usually a small, circular wound with the edges coming together toward the center. If a wound is open, the wound edges are separated, and the nurse inspects the condition of underlying tissue such as adipose and connective tissue. The nurse also looks for complications such as dehiscence and evisceration. The outer edges of a wound normally appear inflamed for the first 2 to 3 days, but this slowly disappears. Within 7 to 10 days a normally healing wound fills with epithelial cells, and edges close. If infection develops, the wound edges become brightly inflamed and swollen.

Skin discoloration usually results from bruising of interstitial tissues or hematoma formation. Blood collecting beneath the skin first takes on a bluish or purplish appearance. Gradually, as the clotted blood is broken down, shades of brown and yellow appear.

CHARACTER OF WOUND DRAINAGE

The nurse notes the amount, color, odor, and consistency of drainage. The amount of drainage depends on the location and extent of the wound. For example, drainage is minimal after a simple appendectomy. In contrast, wound drainage is moderate for 1 to 2 days after resection of a portion of the small bowel. If the nurse needs an accurate measurement of the amount of drainage within a dressing, the dressing can be weighed and compared with the weight of the same dressing when clean and dry. A rule of thumb is 1 g of drainage equals 1 ml. The color and consistency of drainage vary depending on the components. Types of drainage include the following: **serous, sanguineous, serosanguineous,** and purulent (see Table 49-3).

If the drainage has a pungent or strong odor, an infection should be suspected. The nurse should describe the wound's appearance according to characteristics observed.

Table 49-3	Types of Wound Drainage	
TYPE	**APPEARANCE**	
A. Serous	Clear, watery plasma	
B. Purulent	Thick, yellow, green, tan, or brown	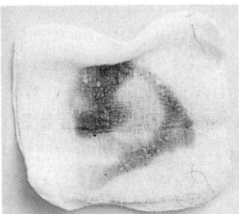
C. Serosanguineous	Pale, red, watery: mixture of serous and sanguineous	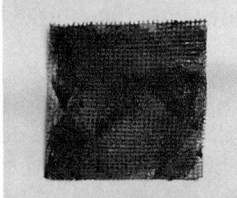
D. Sanguineous	Bright red: indicates active bleeding	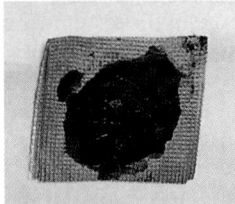

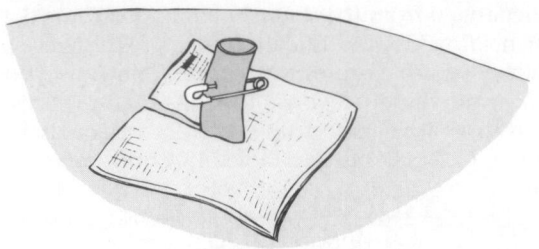

Fig. 49-2 Penrose drain.

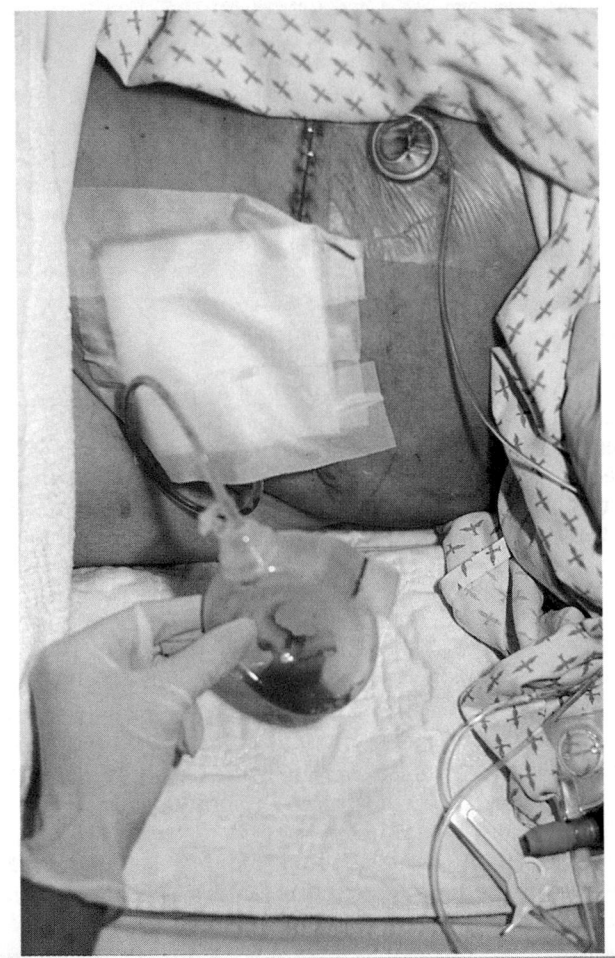

A

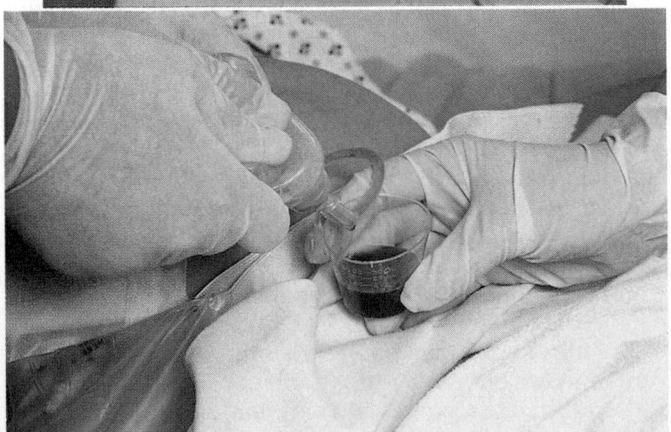

B

Fig. 49-3 Jackson-Pratt drainage device. **A,** Drainage tubes and reservoir. **B,** Emptying drainage reservoir.

An example of accurate recording follows:

Abdominal incision is 5 cm long across RLQ (right lower quadrant); edges well approximated without inflammation or exudate. 1.2-cm diameter circle of serous drainage present on one 4 × 4 gauze.

Drains. The physician inserts a drain into or close to a surgical wound if a large amount of drainage is expected and if keeping wound layers closed is especially important. Some drains are sutured in place. Caution should be exercised when changing the dressing over drains that are not sutured in place to prevent their being accidentally removed. A drain such as a Penrose may lie under a dressing, extend through a dressing, or be connected to a drainage bag or a suction apparatus. The physician often places a pin or clip through the drain to prevent it from slipping farther into a wound (Fig. 49-2). It is usually the physician's responsibility to pull or advance the drain as drainage decreases to permit healing deep within the drain site.

The nurse assesses the number of drains, drain placement, character of drainage, and condition of collecting apparatus. First the nurse observes the security of the drain and its location with respect to the wound. Next the nurse notes the character of drainage. If there is a collecting device, the nurse measures the drainage volume. Because a drainage system must be patent, the nurse looks for drainage flow *through* the tubing as well as *around* the tubing. A sudden decrease in drainage through the tubing may indicate a blocked drain, and the physician should be notified. When a drain is connected to suction, the nurse assesses the system to be sure that the pressure ordered is being exerted. Evacuator units, such as a Hemovac or Jackson-Pratt (JP) (Fig. 49-3), exert a constant low pressure as long as the suction device (bladder or bag) is fully compressed. These type of drainage devices are often referred to as self-suction. When the evacuator device is unable to maintain a vacuum on its own, the nurse notifies the surgeon, who can then order a secondary vacuum system (such as wall suction). If fluid is allowed to accumulate within the tissues, wound healing will not progress at an optimal rate, and the risk of infection is increased.

Wound Closures. Surgical wounds are closed with staples, sutures, or wound closures. A popular skin closure is the stainless-steel staple. The staple provides more strength than nylon or silk sutures and tends to cause less irritation to the skin. The nurse looks for irritation around staple or suture sites and notes whether closures are intact. The nurse may choose to count sutures when the physician has removed a portion of them. Normally for the first 2 to 3 days after surgery the skin around sutures or staples is swollen. Continued swelling may indicate that the closures are too tight. The skin can be cut by overly tight suture material, leading to wound separation. Sutures that are too tight are a common cause of wound dehiscence. Early suture removal reduces formation of defects along the suture line and minimizes chances of unattractive scar formation.

Palpation of Wound. When inspecting a wound, the nurse may observe swelling or separation of wound edges. While wearing gloves the nurse lightly palpates wound edges, detecting localized areas of tenderness or drainage collection. The nurse gently applies the fingertips along the wound edges. If pressure causes fluid to be expressed, the nurse notes the character of the drainage. It may be necessary to collect the drainage for culture. The client is normally sensitive to palpation of wound edges. Extreme tenderness may indicate infection.

Pain. Pain is an important part of wound assessment. If the client experiences serious discomfort while the nurse inspects or palpates the wound, the nurse should look for underlying problems. If the wound is extensive and discomfort seems to be related to dressing removal or application, the nurse plans to administer analgesics before future dressing changes. If discomfort is related to tape removal, use of an adhesive remover may make it painless.

WOUND CULTURES

If the nurse detects purulent or suspicious-looking drainage, collecting a specimen for culture may be necessary (see Chapter 34). The nurse never collects a wound culture sample from old drainage. Resident colonies of bacteria from the skin grow within exudate and may not be the true causative organisms of a wound infection. The nurse cleans a wound first with normal saline to remove skin flora. Aerobic organisms grow in superficial wounds exposed to the air, and anaerobic organisms tend to grow within body cavities. The nurse uses a different method of specimen collection for each type of organism.

To collect an aerobic specimen the nurse uses a sterile swab from a culturette tube (Fig. 49-4). If wound edges are separated, the nurse slowly and gently inserts the tip of the swab into the wound to collect deeper secretions. After collecting the specimen the nurse returns the swab to the culturette tube, caps the tube, and crushes the inner ampule containing the medium for organism growth. The medium must moisten and coat the swab tip. The nurse immediately sends the labeled specimen to the laboratory for quantitative bacterial cultures rather than swab cultures (AHCPR, 1994).

If drainage from a deep body cavity has a foul odor, there is a chance of anaerobic organism growth. The nurse uses a sterile syringe tip to aspirate drainage from the inner wound. Afterward the nurse applies a sterile needle to the syringe, expels air from the syringe and needle, and places a cork over the needle to prevent entrance of air. In some institutions the nurse may inject the specimen into a special vacuum container with a culture medium.

Gram's stains are often performed as well. This test often allows the physician to order appropriate treatment earlier than when only cultures are done. No additional specimens are usually required. The microbiology laboratory needs only to be notified to perform the additional test.

 Nursing Diagnosis

After completing an assessment of the client's wound, the nurse identifies nursing diagnoses that will direct supportive and preventive care (see the nursing diagnoses box on p. 1438). Defining characteristics support existence of a diagnosis for impaired skin integrity. This diagnosis directs the nurse to initiate interventions that promote the wound healing.

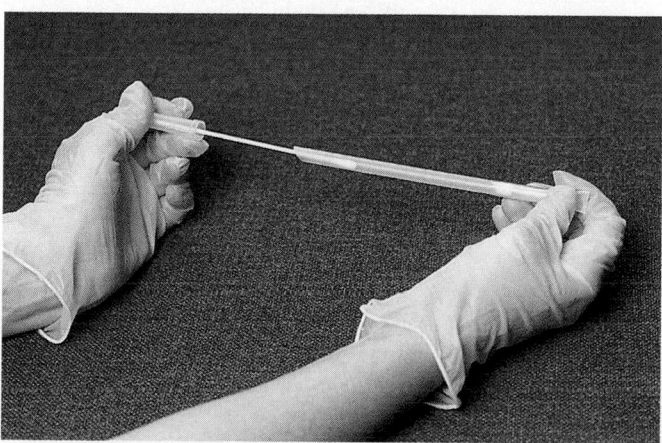

Fig. 49-4 Wound culturette tube.

Examples of NANDA Nursing Diagnoses for Wound Healing

Impaired skin integrity *related to:*
- Surgical incision
- Effects of pressure
- Chemical injury
- Secretions and excretions

Risk for impaired skin integrity *related to:*
- Physical immobilization
- Exposure to secretions

Risk for infection *related to:*
- Malnutrition
- Tissue loss and increased environmental exposure

Pain *related to:*
- Abdominal incision

Impaired physical mobility *related to:*
- Pain of surgical wound

Altered nutrition: less than body requirements *related to:*
- Inability to ingest food

Ineffective breathing pattern *related to:*
- Pain of abdominal incision

Altered tissue perfusion *related to:*
- Interruption of arterial flow
- Interruption of venous flow

Self-esteem disturbance *related to:*
- Perception of scars
- Perception of surgical drains
- Reaction to surgically removed body part

The client may be at risk for poor wound healing because of previously defined factors that impair healing. Thus even though the client's wound may appear normal, the nurse identifies nursing diagnoses such as altered nutrition or altered tissue perfusion that direct nursing care toward support of wound repair.

The nature of a wound can cause problems unrelated to wound healing. Alteration in comfort and impaired mobility are problems that have implications for the client's eventual recovery. For example, a large abdominal incision can cause enough pain to interfere with the client's ability to turn in bed effectively. The nursing diagnostic process box lists nursing diagnoses related to problems of wound healing (see the diagnostic process box below).

Planning

After identifying nursing diagnoses, the nurse develops a care plan for the client needing wound management. The plan is based on the client's identified needs and priorities. Goals and expected outcomes are established, and from the goals the nurse plans therapies according to severity and type of wound and the presence of any complicating conditions (e.g., infection, poor nutrition, immunosuppression, and diabetes) that may affect wound healing.

Because of earlier discharges, it is important to consider the client's home when planning therapies to promote wound healing. Clients and their families may need to continue the objectives of wound management after discharge. The ability of the care giver and the amount of time needed to change a particular dressing need to be considered when selecting a dressing that will be used by the client after discharge. For example, "in the home setting, caregivers may choose more expensive dressing materials to reduce the frequency of dressing changes" (AHCPR, 1994). The nurse and client work together to establish ways of maintaining client involvement in nursing care and to promote wound healing whether the client is in the hospital or home (see Chapter 38).

The nurse's priorities in wound care depend on whether the client's condition is stable or emergent. The type of wound care administered depends on the type of wound, its size and location, and complications. Nursing interventions will be both dependent and independent (see the care plan on p. 1439). Goals of care for clients with wounds include the following:

1. Promoting wound hemostasis
2. Preventing infection
3. Preventing further tissue injury
4. Promoting wound healing
5. Maintaining skin integrity
6. Regaining normal function
7. Gaining comfort

Sample Nursing Diagnostic Process for Wound Healing

ASSESSMENT ACTIVITIES	DEFINING CHARACTERISTICS	NURSING DIAGNOSES
Inspect surface of skin.	Presence of wound Yellow, foul-smelling drainage from wound Edges of wound not approximated Sutures remain in place	**Impaired skin integrity** related to contaminated wound
Inspect wound for signs of healing.	Brown-red drainage 5 days after surgery Edges of wound not approximated	**Risk for infection** related to traumatic, contaminated wound
Obtain client's temperature, heart rate, and white blood cell count.	Client is febrile, heart rate is 125 beats/min, leukocyte (white blood cell) count is 12,000/mm³	

Sample Nursing Care Plan for Impaired Skin Integrity

NURSING: Diagnosis: Impaired skin integrity related to contaminated wound
DEFINITION: Impaired skin integrity is the state in which an individual's skin is adversely altered (Kim, McFarland, McLane, 1995).

GOAL	EXPECTED OUTCOMES	INTERVENTIONS	RATIONALE
Skin integrity will be improved in area of surgical wound (3/20).	Wound will be clean and intact without inflammation, drainage, or maceration (3/18). Wound edges will be approximated.	Keep wound clean and dry. Perform prescribed dressing changes, including debridement and application of treatments. Instruct client or significant other to perform wound assessment and care. Include return demonstration.	Wound healing depends on clean, moist environment for epithelialization and deposition of granulation tissue (Atwater, 1989; Cooper, 1992). Accurate and regular assessment of wound and surrounding skin are critical to nursing care plan for wound management (Cooper, 1992).

Implementation

In an emergency setting the nurse uses first aid measures for wound care. Under more stable conditions the nurse uses a variety of interventions to ensure wound healing.

First Aid for Wounds

When a client suffers a traumatic wound, first aid interventions include stabilizing cardiopulmonary function (see Chapter 44), promoting hemostasis, cleansing the wound, and protecting the wound from further injury.

HEMOSTASIS

After assessing the type and extent of the wound the nurse controls bleeding of a laceration by applying direct pressure on the wound with a sterile or clean dressing, such as a washcloth. After bleeding subsides, an adhesive bandage strip or gauze dressing taped over the laceration allows skin edges to close and a blood clot to form. If a dressing becomes saturated with blood, the nurse adds another layer of dressing, continues to apply pressure, and elevates the affected part. Further disruption of skin layers should be avoided. More serious lacerations should be sutured by a physician. Pressure dressings used the first 24 to 48 hours after trauma help maintain hemostasis.

A puncture wound is allowed to bleed to remove dirt and other contaminants, such as saliva from a dog bite. When a penetrating object, such as a knife blade, is present, it is not removed. Removal could cause massive, uncontrolled bleeding. Except for skull injuries, the nurse may apply pressure around the penetrating object, but not on it; and the client should be transported to an emergency facility.

CLEANSING

The process of cleansing a wound involves selecting both an appropriate wound-cleansing solution and using a mechanical means of delivering that solution without causing injury to the healing wound tissue (AHCPR, 1994). Gentle cleansing of a wound removes contaminants that might serve as sources of infection. However, vigorous cleaning using a method with too much mechanical force can cause bleeding or further injury (see Chapter 38). For abrasions, minor lacerations, and small puncture wounds the nurse first rinses the wound in running water, cleans it with mild soap and water, and may apply an over-the-counter antiseptic. Topical antibiotics applied to wound edges may slow microorganism growth. However, prolonged application of topical antibiotics can foster growth of nonsusceptible organisms. When a laceration is bleeding profusely, the nurse should only brush away surface contaminants and concentrate on hemostasis until the client can be cared for in a clinic or hospital.

Topical Agents for Cleansing Wounds. According to the AHCPR 1994 clinical guidelines, normal saline is the preferred cleansing agent. It is physiological and will not harm tissue. Many topical agents that in the past were used to clean wounds, including povidone-iodine solutions, Dakin's solution (sodium hypochlorite solution), acetic acid solution, and hydrogen peroxide, are toxic to fibroblasts and therefore should not be used to clean wounds.

Saline. Gentle cleansing with normal saline and the application of saline dressings (wet-to-wet, wet-to-damp) are often used in healing wounds and to debride wounds (wet-to-dry). The nurse uses saline to maintain the moist surface needed to promote the development and migration of epithelial tissue. Damp (wet-to-dry) saline dressings should *only* be used to debride wounds (see Chapter 38). They should never be used in a clean granulating wound.

GROWTH FACTORS

Topical and parenteral growth factors have been used to treat nonhealing wounds and fistula formation. The nurse may be responsible for the use of this treatment modality after the physician determines that it may provide a benefit for the client's wound care. Teaching the client or significant other about the use of growth factors is also the nurse's responsibility. The nurse teaches the use of the medication, wound care, and the prevention of wound breakdown and recurrence.

PROTECTION

Regardless of whether bleeding has stopped, the nurse protects the wound from further injury by applying sterile or clean dressings and immobilizing the body part. A light dressing applied over minor wounds prevents entrance of microorganisms. In the case of small abrasions, it is acceptable to leave the wound open to air so that a scab can form.

The more extensive the wound, the larger the dressing required. In the home a clean towel or diaper may be the best dressing. A bulky dressing applied with pressure minimizes movement of underlying tissues and helps immobilize the entire body part. A bandage or cloth wrapped around a penetrating object should immobilize it adequately.

There are alternative dressings that can be used to cover and protect certain types of wounds. Examples are large wounds, wounds with drainage tubes or suction catheters in the wound, wounds that need frequent changing, and fistulas. In these wounds, pouches or special wound collection systems are now used to cover the wound. Some of these newer devices even have a plastic door on the front of the wound pouch so that the nurse can change the wound packing without removing the wound pouch from the skin.

Dressings

The use of dressings requires an understanding of wound healing. A variety of dressing material is commercially available. Unless a dressing is suited to the characteristics of a wound, the dressing can hinder wound repair (Erwin-Toth and Hocevar, 1995; Krasner, 1995; Motta, 1995).

The choice of dressings and the method of dressing a wound influence the progress of wound healing. The proper dressing should not allow a draining wound to become overly dry (desiccated) with extensive scab formation. When this occurs, the dermis dehydrates and crusts. As a result, a barrier forms against normal epidermal cell growth, leaving a depression or defect in the new epidermal surface. Furthermore, dryness of the wound may increase the client's discomfort. Ideally a dressing leaves a wound slightly moist to promote epithelial cell migration. The dressing should also absorb drainage to prevent pooling of exudate that may promote bacterial growth as well as maceration of surrounding skin from wound exudate (Erwin-Toth and Hocevar, 1995; Krasner, 1995; Motta, 1995).

For surgical wounds that heal by primary intention, it is common to remove dressings as soon as drainage stops. In contrast, when the nurse dresses an open wound healing by secondary intention, the dressing material becomes a means for mechanically removing exudate and necrotic tissue.

PURPOSES OF DRESSINGS

A dressing may serve several purposes:
1. Protecting a wound from microorganism contamination
2. Aiding hemostasis
3. Promoting healing by absorbing drainage and debriding a wound
4. Supporting or splinting the wound site
5. Protecting the client from seeing the wound (if perceived as unpleasant)
6. Promoting thermal insulation of the wound surface
7. Providing maintenance of high humidity between the wound and dressing

When the skin becomes broken, a dressing helps reduce exposure to microorganisms. However, when wound drainage is minimal, the healing process forms a natural fibrin seal that can eliminate the need for a dressing. A dressing is always needed for extensive wounds.

Pressure dressings promote hemostasis. Applied with elastic bandages, a pressure dressing exerts localized downward pressure over an actual or potential bleeding site. A pressure dressing eliminates dead space in underlying tissues so that wound healing progresses normally. The nurse checks pressure dressings to be sure that they do not interfere with circulation to a body part. The nurse assesses skin color, pulses in distal extremities, the client's comfort, and changes in sensation. Pressure dressings are not routinely removed.

A primary function of a dressing on a healing wound is to absorb drainage. Most traditional surgical dressings have three layers: a contact or primary layer, an absorbent layer, and an outer protective layer. The contact dressing covers the incision and part of the adjacent skin. Fibrin, blood products, and debris adhere to the contact dressing's surface. A problem occurs if the wound drainage dries, causing the dressing to stick to the suture line. Improper removal of the dressing can cause tearing of the healing epidermal surface. The nurse must either remove the dressing gently and moisten the attached area with sterile normal saline before removal or leave the dressing unchanged for several days.

The dressing technique will vary depending upon the goal of the treatment plan for the wound. For example, if the goal is to maintain a moist environment for a clean granulating wound, it is important for the nurse to prevent the saline-moistened gauze dressing from drying and sticking to the healing wound. This is in direct contrast to the dressing technique that should be used if the goal of care is to mechanically debride the wound using a saline wet-to-dry dressing. When wounds require **debriding**, such as infected or necrotic wounds, the contact dressing debrides necrotic tissue and debris. In this case the contact dressing must be allowed to dry so it sticks to underlying tissue, and debridement occurs during removal.

Dressings applied to a draining wound require frequent changing to prevent microorganism growth and skin breakdown. Bacteria grow readily in the dark, warm, moist environment under a dressing. Skin surfaces become macerated and irritated. Skin breakdown can be minimized by keeping the skin clean and dry and reducing the use of tape.

The absorbent dressing layer serves as a reservoir for additional secretions. The wicking action of woven gauze dressings pulls excess drainage into the dressing and away from the wound.

The final outer layer of a dressing helps prevent bacteria and other external contaminants from reaching the wound surface. Usually the outer dressing is made of a thicker dressing material.

A firmly taped or wrapped dressing supports or immobilizes a body part, minimizing movement of the underlying

- Use a dressing that will keep the ulcer bed continuously moist. Wet-to-dry dressings should be used only for debridement and are not considered continuously moist saline dressings.
- Use clinical judgment to select a type of moist wound dressing suitable for the ulcer. Studies of different types of moist wound dressings showed no differences in pressure ulcer healing outcomes.
- Choose a dressing that keeps the surrounding intact (periulcer) skin dry while keeping the ulcer bed moist.
- Choose a dressing that controls exudate but does not desiccate the ulcer bed.
- Consider care giver time when selecting a dressing.
- Eliminate wound dead space by loosely filling all cavities with dressing material. Avoid overpacking the wound.
- Monitor dressings applied near the anus, since they are difficult to keep intact.

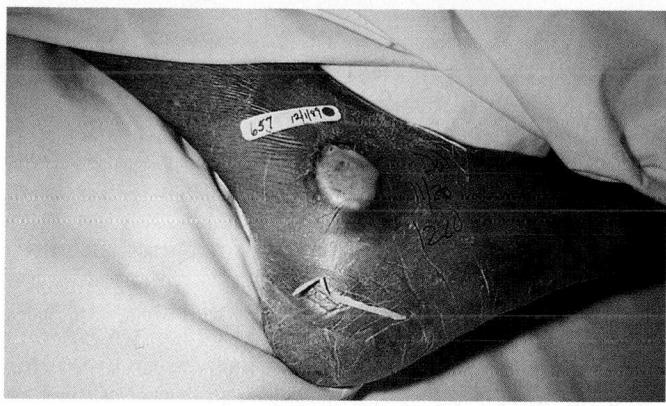

Fig. 49-5 Transparent film dressing.

incision and injured tissues. Finally, a dressing insulates and keeps a wound's surface well hydrated. The humidity between a dressing and the client's skin surface promotes normal epithelial cell growth.

TYPES OF DRESSINGS

Dressings vary by type of material and mode of application (wet or dry) (see Procedure 49-1). They should be easy to apply, comfortable, and made of materials that promote wound healing. The AHCPR (1994) clinical guidelines are helpful when selecting dressings based on the goal of wound treatment (see the box above).

Woven gauze sponges are the oldest and most common dressing. They are absorbent and are especially useful in wounds to wick away the wound exudate (Aronovitch, 1995). They do not interact with wound tissues and thus cause little wound irritation. Gauze is available in different textures and in squares of 10 × 10 cm (4 × 4 inches) or 5 × 5 cm (2 × 2 inches), rectangles of 10 × 20 cm (4 × 8 inches), and rolls of various lengths. These dressings should not be confused with nonwoven sponges. Nonwoven dressings are a blend of synthetic fibers such as rayon and polyester. Because they do not adhere to the skin, they are used to wipe and clean wounds. They are not as useful as woven sponges for packing wounds and wicking away wound exudate (Aronovitch, 1995).

Wet-to-dry dressings are used in treating wounds that require debridement. The nurse moistens the contact dressing layer, increasing the gauze's ability to collect exudate and wound debris, and then applies a dry second layer of absorbent dressing. This wet-to-dry dressing effectively cleanses infected and necrotic wounds.

Nonadherent gauze dressings such as Telfa are used over clean wounds. Telfa gauze has a shiny, nonadherent surface that does not stick to incisions or wound openings but allows drainage to pass through to the softened gauze above.

Another type of dressing is a self-adhesive, transparent film that acts as a temporary second skin (Fig. 49-5). Some examples of these film dressings are Acu-derm, Blisterfilm,

Op-Site, Pro-Crude, Poluskin, Tegaderm, and Uniflex. The transparent dressing is ideal for small, superficial wounds. It can also be used for autolytic debridement of small wounds. It has the following advantages:

1. It adheres to undamaged skin.
2. It serves as a barrier to external fluids and bacteria but still allows the wound surface to "breathe."
3. It promotes a moist environment that speeds epithelial cell growth.
4. It can be removed without damaging underlying tissues.
5. It permits viewing the wound.
6. It does not require a secondary dressing.

Hydrocolloid (HCD) dressings are dressings with complex formulations of colloids, elastomeric, and adhesive components. Some examples are Biofilm, Comfeel, Duo-DERM, Dermiflex, Intact, Intrasite, and Restore. These dressings are occlusive. The wound contact layer of this dressing swells in the presence of exudate and maintains a moist healing environment. Hydrocolloids can be used to heal clean granulating wounds as well as to autolytically debride necrotic wounds. These dressings come in a variety of sizes and shapes. This type of dressing has the following functions:

1. It absorbs drainage through the use of exudate absorbers beneath the dressing.
2. It maintains wound humidity.
3. It slowly liquefies necrotic debris.
4. It provides protective cushioning.
5. It is impermeable to bacteria and other contaminants
6. It is self-adhesive and molds well.
7. It may be left in place for 3 to 5 days, minimizing skin trauma and disruption of healing.

This type of dressing is most useful on shallow to moderately deep dermal ulcers.

Hydrogel dressings are water or glycerin-based amorphous gel impregnated gauze or sheet dressings. They have a high water content and can absorb some but not large amounts of exudate. Hydrogel dressings are used on partial and full thickness wounds, deep wounds with some exudate, necrotic wounds, burns, and radiation-damaged skin. Some examples of these dressings are Aquasorb, Carrasyn Hydrogel wound dressing, ClearSite, Elaso-Gel, IntraSite Gel, Nu-Gel, Transorb, and Vigilon.

Advantages of hydrogel are:
1. It is very soothing and reduces pain in the wound.
2. It provides a moist environment.
3. It can debride the wound.
4. It doesn't stick to the wound and can be removed easily.
5. It can be used in infected wounds.

There are many other types of dressings available. Foam dressings, alginate dressings, and exudate absorbers are used in wounds with exudate and in wounds that need packing. Foam dressings are also used around drainage tubes to absorb drainage. Several manufacturers produce composite dressings. These dressings combine two different dressing types into one dressing. Much research is being done on what type of dressing is best for what type of wound at what point in the wound healing process.

CHANGING DRESSINGS

To prepare for changing a dressing, the nurse must know the type of dressing, the presence of underlying drains or tubing, and the type of supplies needed for wound care. Poor preparation may cause a break in aseptic technique (see Chapter 34) or accidental dislodging of a drain. The nurse's judgment in modifying a dressing change procedure is important during wound care, particularly if the character of a wound changes. Notifying the physician of any change is essential.

The physician's order for changing a dressing should indicate the dressing type, the frequency of changing, and any solutions or ointments to be applied to the wound. An order to "reinforce dressing prn" (add dressings without removing original one) is common right after surgery when the physician does not want accidental disruption of the suture line or bleeding. The medical or operating room record usually tells whether drains are present and from what body cavity they drain. After the first dressing change, the nurse describes the location of drains and the type of dressing materials and solutions to use in the client's care plan. The CDC (Garner, 1985) recommends the following during dressing change procedure:

1. The nurse should perform thorough handwashing before and after wound care.
2. Personnel should not touch an open or fresh wound directly without wearing sterile gloves (see Chapter 34).
3. If a wound is sealed, dressings may be changed without gloves.
4. Dressings over closed wounds should be removed or changed when they become wet or if the client has signs or symptoms of infection.

There is a growing body of literature about sterile versus clean dressings. The AHCPR 1994 clinical practice guidelines recommend that clean dressings and gloves be used on pressure ulcers. For surgical wounds, preliminary research indicates no difference in the healing rate of wounds when clean rather than sterile dressing change technique is used (see the box above).

To prepare a client for a dressing change the nurse:
1. Administers required analgesics so that peak effects occur during the dressing change
2. Describes steps of the procedure to lessen client anxiety
3. Describes normal signs of healing
4. Answers questions about the procedure or the wound

▶ **RESEARCH HIGHLIGHT**

RESEARCH ABSTRACT
The purpose of this research was to determine if there was a difference in the rate of wound healing and cost of supplies when clean or sterile dressing change techniques were used in open surgical wounds in postoperative clients. In this pilot study, the subjects were 15 men and 15 women who had gastrointestinal surgery. The mean age of subjects was 40.6 years (SD 13). The wounds were healing by secondary intention. Subjects were randomized as to either clean or sterile technique. Dressing changes were begun on the first day postoperative. They were repeated three times a day until discharge from the hospital. Subjects were studied for 3 to 9 days. Results showed that there was no difference between the groups in the rate of wound healing. However, the mean cost for the clean dressing technique group was significantly less than for the sterile dressing technique group. The authors caution that the findings of this pilot study need to be confirmed using a large sample size.

IMPLICATIONS FOR PRACTICE
▶ Evaluate which wounds can be managed with a *clean* dressing technique.
▶ Determine which clients must always have sterile dressing changes, for example, clients who are immunosuppressed, and clients receiving radiation.

REFERENCE
Stotts NA et al: Sterile vs clean technique in wound care of patients with open surgical wounds in the post-op period: a pilot study, *Adv in Wound Care* 8(2):13, 1995.

Often the physician orders clients to learn how to change dressings so that they will be prepared for home care. In this situation the nurse must demonstrate dressing change to the client and family and then provide an opportunity for the client or family member to practice (see the box on p. 1446). Usually in this situation wound healing has progressed to the point that risks of complications such as dehiscence or evisceration are minimal. The client should be able to change a dressing independently or with assistance from a family member before discharge. The AHCPR 1994 clinical guidelines state "clean dressing may also be used in the home setting." Disposal of contaminated dressings in the home should be done in a manner consistent with local regulations (See Chapter 34). Procedure 49-1 outlines the steps for changing dry and wet-to-dry dressings.

PACKING A WOUND

The first step in packing a wound is to assess the size, depth, and shape of the wound. These wound characteristics are important in determining the size and type of dressing used to pack a wound. The dressing should be flexible and must be able to be in contact with all of the wound's surface. Make sure that the type of material you are using to pack the wound is appropriate. Nonwoven sponges are usually not used to pack wounds. There are many new dressing materials such as alignates that are also used to

Applying Dry and Wet-to-Dry Dressings

STEPS	RATIONALE
1. Assess size, location, and type of wound to be dressed.	Assists nurse to plan for proper type and amount of supplies needed. Alerts nurse when assistance is needed to hold dressings in place.
2. Assess client's level of comfort.	Removal of dry dressing can be painful; client may require pain medication.
3. Review medical orders for dressing change procedure.	Indicates type of dressing or applications to use.
4. Prepare necessary equipment and supplies:	
a. Gloves: sterile, clean	
b. Dressing set (sterile), scissors, forceps	Used to apply dressing and cut gauze to size.
c. Sterile drape (optional)	
d. Dressings and pads, e.g., fine-mesh gauze (wet-to-dry only)	
e. Sterile basin	
f. Antiseptic ointment (optional for dry dressing)	For antiseptic.
g. Cleansing solution	
h. Solution (wet-to-dry only)	Used to moisten dressing.
i. Tape, ties, or bandage as needed	
j. Waterproof bag	For disposal of old dressing and supplies.
k. Extra gauze dressings, Surgi-Pads, or ABD pads	
l. Bath blanket	
m. Adhesive remover (optional)	
n. Disposable mask (optional) or protective eyewear	Protection from splashes of body fluid from wounds may be needed if vigorous wound cleaning will be done.
5. Explain procedure to client and instruct client not to touch wound area or sterile supplies.	Decreases anxiety. Sudden, unexpected movement by client could result in contamination of wound and supplies.
6. Close room or cubicle curtains; close open windows.	Provides privacy and reduces airborne microorganisms.
7. Position client comfortably and drape with bath blanket to expose only wound site.	Draping provides access to wound and maintains unnecessary exposure.
8. Place disposable bag within reach of work area. Fold top of bag to make cuff.	Ensures easy disposal of soiled dressings. Prevents soiling of bag's outer surface.
9. Apply face mask or protective eyewear (usually required when wound has drainage that may splash into eyes of nurse) and wash hands thoroughly.	Reduces transmission of pathogens to exposed tissues.
10. Put on clean disposable gloves and remove tape, bandage, or ties.	Prevents transmission of infectious organisms from soiled dressings to nurse's hands.
11. Remove tape, pulling parallel to skin and toward dressing. Remove remaining adhesive from skin.	Pulling tape toward dressing reduces stress on suture line or wound edges.
12. With gloved hand, carefully remove gauze dressings, taking care not to dislodge drains or tubes. Keep soiled undersurface away from client's sight. (If dressing sticks on wet-to-dry dressing, do not moisten it; instead warn client of discomfort and gently free dressing.)	Appearance of drainage may be upsetting to client. (Wet-to-dry dressing should debride wound.)
13. Observe character and amount of drainage on dressing and appearance of wound.	Provides estimate of drainage amount and assessment of wound's condition.
14. Dispose of soiled dressings in disposable bag. Discard as per setting policy.	Reduces transmission of microorganisms.
15. Remove gloves by pulling them inside out. Dispose in bag.	Prevents contact of nurse's hands with material on gloves.

Continued.

Applying Dry and Wet-to-Dry Dressings—cont'd

STEPS	RATIONALE

16. Open sterile dressing tray or individually wrapped sterile supplies. Place on bedside table (see the illustration below).

Sterile dressings remain sterile while on or within sterile surface. Preparation of supplies prevents break in technique during dressing change.

   a. **Apply dry dressing:**

      (1) Open bottle of solution and pour into sterile basin.

Keeps supplies sterile.

      (2) Apply sterile gloves.

Allows handling of sterile supplies without contamination.

      (3) Inspect wound for appearance, drainage, and integrity. Avoid contact with contaminated material.

Indicates status of healing.

      (4) Cleanse wound with solution:

         (i) Use separate swab for each cleansing stroke.

Prevents contaminating previously cleaned area.

         (ii) Clean from least contaminated area to most contaminated (see Figs. 49-7 and 49-8).

Prevents introduction of organisms into wound.

      (5) Use dry gauze to swab in same manner as preceding step to dry wound.

Reduces excess moisture, which could eventually harbor microorganisms.

      (6) Apply antiseptic ointment if ordered, using same technique as for cleansing.

Reduces growth of mciroorganisms. Ointment may be applied to dressing if direct application causes discomfort.

      (7) Apply dry sterile dressings to incision or wound site:

         (i)   Apply loose woven gauze as contact layer.

Promotes proper absorption of drainage.

         (ii) Cut 4 × 4 gauze flat to fit around drain, if present. Precut gauze is also available.

Secure drain and promotes drainage absorption at site.

         (iii) Apply second layer of gauze.

Ensures proper coverage and optimal absorption.

         (iv) Apply thicker woven pad (Surgi-Pad).

Protects wound from external environment.

   b. **Apply wet-to-dry dressing:**

      (1) Pour prescribed solution into sterile basin and add fine-mesh gauze.

Contact layer must be totally moistened to increase dressing's absorptive abilities.

      (2) Apply sterile gloves.

Allows handling of sterile supplies without contamination.

      (3) Inspect wound for color, character of drainage, type of sutures, and drains. (see the illustration below, right)

Provides assessment of wound healing.

      (4) Cleanse wound with prescribed normal saline. Clean from least to most contaminated area. (see Figs. 49-7 and 49-8).

Assists in debridement and cleanses wound of debris.

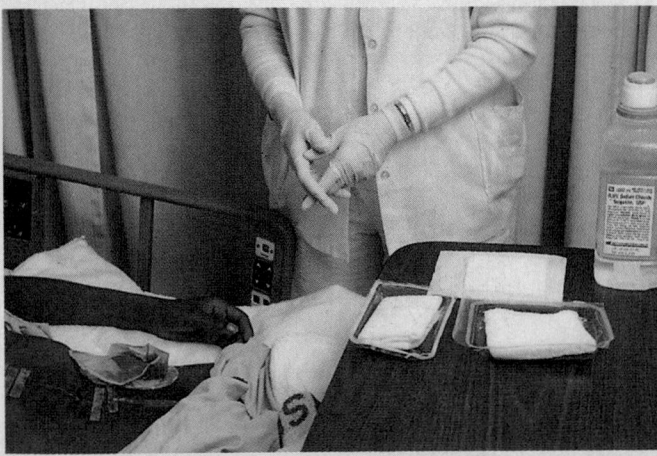

Step 16

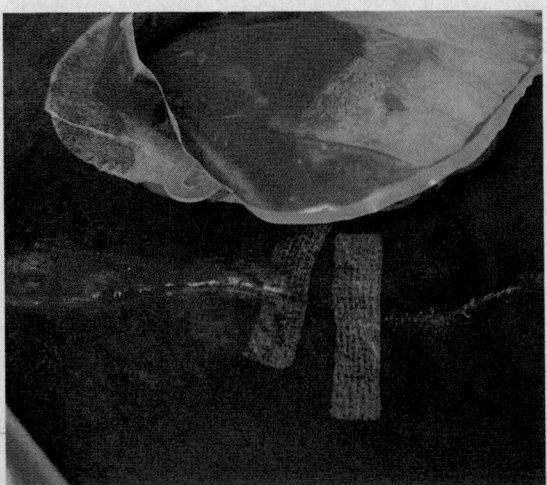

Step 16b(3)

Applying Dry and Wet-to-Dry Dressings—cont'd

STEPS	RATIONALE
16. Open sterile dressing tray or individually wrapped sterile supplies. Place on bedside table—cont'd	
(5) Apply moist, fine-mesh gauze directly onto wound surface. If wound is deep, gently pack gauze into wound with forceps until all wound surfaces are in contact with moist gauze (see the illustrations below).	Moist gauze absorbs drainage and adheres to debris. Wound should be loosely packed to facilitate wicking of drainage into absorbent outer layer of dressing.
(6) Apply dry sterile 4 × 4 gauze over wet gauze.	Pulls moisture from wound.
(7) Cover with ABD pad, Surgi-Pad, or gauze.	Protects wound from entrance of microorganisms.
17. Apply tape over dressing, Kling roll (for circumferential dressings), or Montgomery ties. For application of Montgomery ties:	
a. Expose adhesive surface of tape on end of each tie.	Allows frequent dressing changes without removal of adhesive tape.
b. Place ties on opposite side of dressing (see Fig. 49-6, *A*).	
c. Place adhesive directly on client's skin or use skin barrier.	
d. Secure dressing by lacing ties across it or using safety pins and rubber bands (see Fig. 49-6, *B*).	Ensures dressing remains intact and covers wound.
18. Remove gloves and dispose in bag.	Reduces transmission of infection.
19. Assist client to comfortable position.	Promotes client well-being.
20. Dispose of all supplies and wash hands.	Clean environment enhances comfort. Reduces transmission of infection.
21. Reassess client to determine response to dressing change.	Determines client's comfort level.
22. Monitor status of dressing at least every shift.	Evaluates extent of drainage and integrity of dressing.
23. Record appearance of wound and drainage, client's tolerance, and type of dressing applied in nurses' notes.	Documents progress of wound healing and promotes continuity in dressing change techniques.
24. Record frequency of dressing change and supplies needed on Kardex.	Alerts staff members to dressing change times and supplies needed.

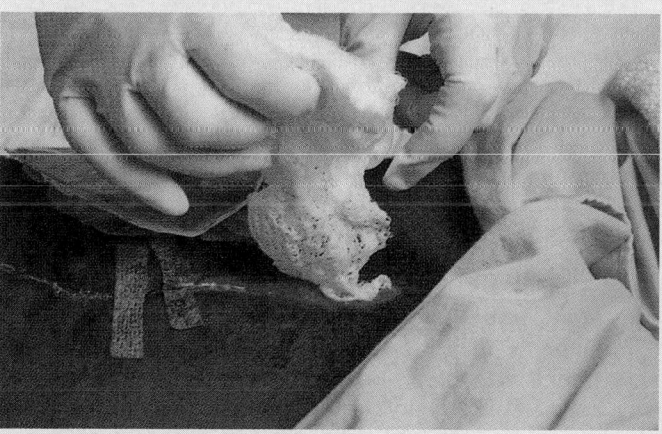

Step 16b(5)

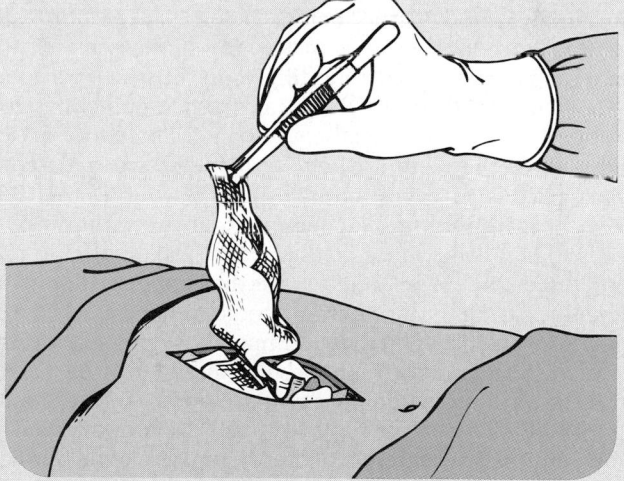

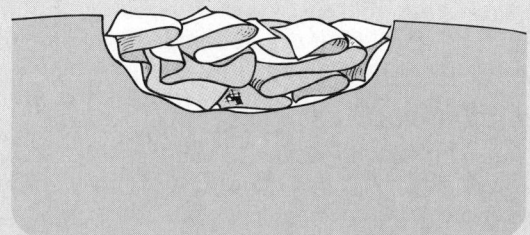

CLIENT TEACHING
for Dressing Application

OBJECTIVE
- Client (or family member) will demonstrate the correct technique for the application of dressing.

TEACHING STRATEGIES
- Discuss with client and significant other the importance of infection control.
- Demonstrate the correct technique for the dressing change for the client and the family member.
- Discuss signs and symptoms of wound infection.

EVALUATION
- Observe family member performing the dressing change.
- Client and family state symptoms of wound infection.

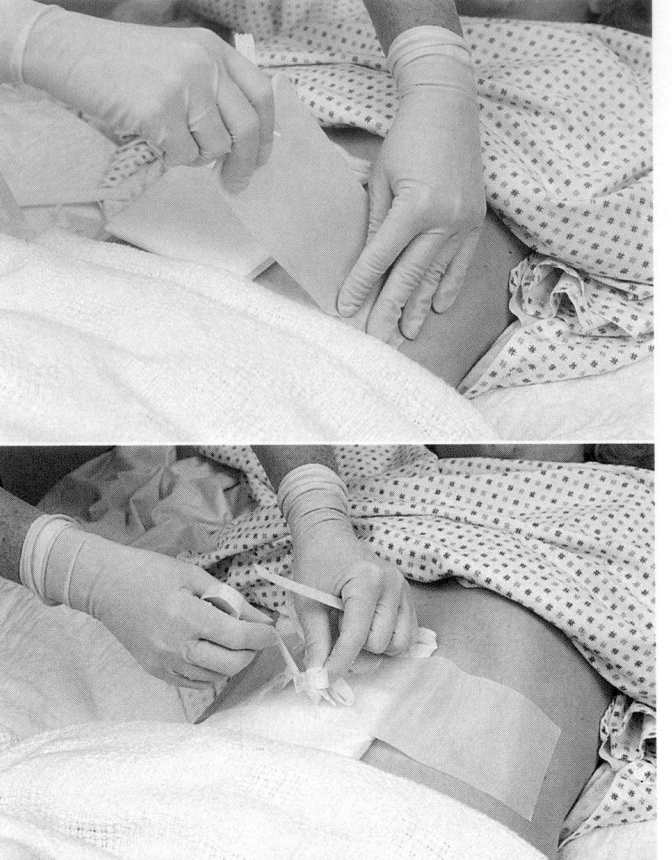

Fig. 49-6 Montgomery ties. **A,** Each tie is placed at side of dressing. **B,** Securing ties encloses dressing.

pack wounds. Because of their ability to absorb wound exudate and conform to the shape of the wound, woven gauze sponges are commonly used to pack wounds that need mechanical debridement (Aronovitch, 1995). After removing the woven gauze from the package, it is essential to fluff the gauze before putting it into the wound (Procedure 49-1). Fluffing (opening up the gauze) increases the amount of surface area of the sponge that can be in contact with the wound surface. The woven gauze sponges should be moistened with normal saline only, as cytotoxic solutions cannot be used in wounds. Using sterile technique, gently fill the wound with the saline-moistened woven gauze. As you are filling the wound, hold the packing material above the wound so that the packing material does not touch the surrounding wound tissue before being packed into the wound (Procedure 49-1). Don't let the sterile packing material drag across the surrounding wound tissue (Procedure 49-1). The AHCPR (1994) clinical practice guidelines recommend that wound dead space be eliminated by *loosely* filling all of the wound cavity with the dressing material. Dead space is "a cavity remaining in a wound" (AHCPR, 1994). It is important to remember that the wound cavity needs to be filled so that areas are not "walled off," to prevent abscesses (AHCPR, 1994). Another important point to remember is that the wound should not be packed too tightly. Overpacking the wound may cause pressure on the tissue in the wound bed. The wound should only be packed until the packing material reaches the surface of the wound (Procedure 49-1); never have so much packing material in the wound that it extends higher than the wound surface. Wound packing that overlaps onto the wound edges can cause maceration of the tissue surrounding the wound (Hess and Miller, 1990). It can also impede the proper healing and closing of the wound.

SECURING DRESSINGS

The nurse may use tape, ties, or bandages, or a secondary dressing and cloth binders to secure a dressing over a wound site. The choice of anchoring depends on the wound size, location, presence of drainage, frequency of dressing changes, and client's level of activity.

The nurse most often uses strips of tape to secure dressings if the client is not allergic to tape. Nonallergenic paper and plastic tapes minimize skin reactions. Common adhesive tape adheres well to the skin's surface, whereas elastic adhesive tape compresses closely around pressure bandages and permits more movement of a body part. Skin sensitive to adhesive tape can become severely inflamed and excoriated and may even slough when the tape is removed.

Tape is available in various widths such as 1.2, 2.5, 5, and 7.5 cm (½, 1, 2, and 3 inches). The nurse chooses the size that sufficiently secures the dressing. For example, a large abdominal wound dressing must remain secure over a large area despite frequent stress from movement, respiratory effort, and possibly abdominal distention. Strips of 7.5-cm (3-inch) adhesive better stabilize such a large dressing so that it does not continually slip off. When applying tape, a nurse ensures that it adheres to several inches of skin on both sides of the dressing and that it is placed across the middle of the dressing. When securing the dressing, the nurse presses the tape gently, exerting pressure away from the wound. This way tension occurs in both directions away from the wound, minimizing skin distortion and irritation. Tape is never applied over irritated or broken skin. Some nurses protect the skin beneath tape with a skin sealant product.

To remove tape safely the nurse loosens the tape ends and gently pulls the outer end parallel with the skin surface toward the wound. The nurse applies light traction to the skin away from the wound as the tape is loosened and removed. The traction minimizes pulling of the skin. If tape covers an area of hair growth, the client experiences less discomfort if the nurse pulls the tape in the direction of hair growth.

To avoid repeated removal of tape from sensitive skin, the nurse can secure dressings with pairs of reusable Montgomery ties (Fig. 49-6). Each tie consists of a long strip; half contains an adhesive backing to apply to the skin and the other half folds back and contains a cloth tie or a safety pin and rubber band combination to be fastened across a dressing and untied at dressing changes. A large, bulky dressing may require two or more sets of Montgomery ties. To provide even support to a wound and immobilize a body part the nurse may apply elastic gauze or cloth bandages and binders over a dressing.

COMFORT MEASURES

A wound can be painful, depending on the extent of tissue injury. The nurse uses several techniques to minimize discomfort during wound care. Careful removal of tape, gentle cleansing of wound edges, and careful manipulation of dressings and drains minimize stress on sensitive tissues. Careful turning and positioning also reduce strain on a wound. Administration of analgesic medications 30 to 60 minutes before dressing changes (depending on a drug's time of peak action) also reduces discomfort.

Cleansing Skin and Drain Sites

Although a moderate amount of wound exudate promotes epithelial cell growth, the physician may order cleansing of a wound or drain site if a dressing does not properly absorb drainage or if an open drain deposits drainage onto the skin. Wound cleansing requires good handwashing and aseptic techniques (see Chapter 34). The nurse may use irrigation to remove debris.

BASIC SKIN CLEANSING

The nurse cleanses surgical or traumatic wounds by applying noncytotoxic solutions with sterile gauze or by irrigation. The following three principles are important when cleaning an incision or the area surrounding a drain:

1. Cleanse in a direction from the least contaminated area, such as from the wound or incision to the surrounding skin (Fig. 49-7) or from an isolated drain site to the surrounding skin (Fig. 49-8).
2. Use gentle friction when applying solutions locally to the skin.
3. When irrigating, allow the solution to flow from the least to most contaminated area.

A wound is thought to be less contaminated than the surrounding skin. After applying a solution to sterile gauze the nurse cleans away from the wound. The nurse never uses the same piece of gauze to cleanse across an incision or wound twice.

A drain site is highly contaminated because the moist drainage harbors microorganisms. If a wound has a dry incisional area and a moist drain site, cleansing moves from the incisional area toward the drain. The nurse uses two separate swabs, one to clean from the top of the incision toward the drain and one to clean from the bottom of the incision toward the drain. To cleanse the area of an isolated drain site the nurse swabs around the drain, moving in circular rotations outward from a point closest to the drain. In this situation the skin near the site is more contaminated than the site itself. To cleanse circular wounds the nurse uses the same technique as cleansing around a drain.

IRRIGATIONS

Irrigations are a special way of cleansing wounds. The nurse uses an irrigating syringe to flush the area with a constant low-pressure flow of solution. The gentle washing action of the irrigation cleans a wound of exudate and debris. Irrigations are particularly useful for open deep wounds involving an inaccessible body part, such as the ear canal, or when cleansing sensitive body parts, such as the conjunctival lining of the eye.

In addition to wound cleansing, irrigations serve to apply heat to an affected area and apply locally acting medications in the form of sterile solutions. The prescribed solution is usually sterile water or saline. Administration of

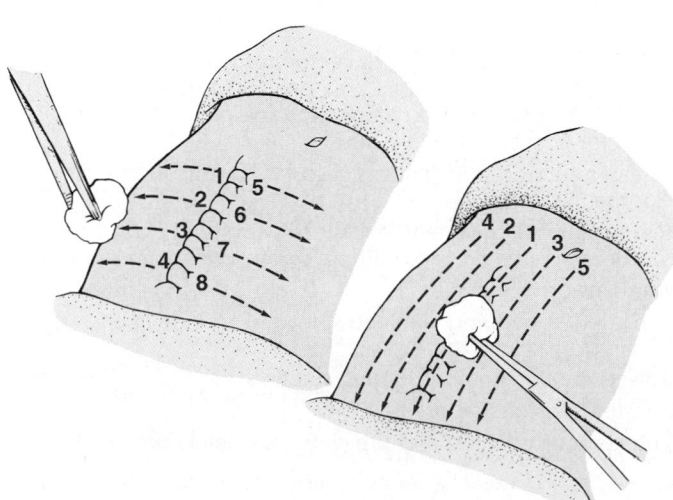

Fig. 49-7 Methods for cleansing a wound site.

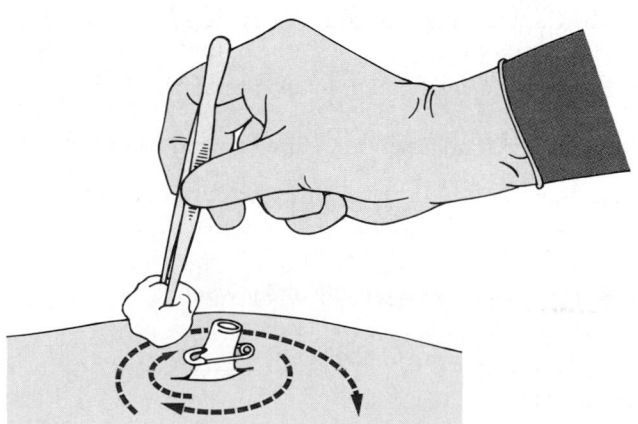

Fig. 49-8 Cleansing a drain site.

Performing Wound Irrigation

STEPS	RATIONALE
1. Assess client's level of pain.	Discomfort may be related directly to wound or indirectly to muscle tension or immobility.
2. Review medical record for physician's prescription for irrigation of open wound and type of solution to be used.	Open wound irrigation requires medical order including type of solutions to use.
3. Identify recent recording of signs and symptoms related to client's open wound:	Data are used as baseline to indicate change in condition of wound.
a. Extent of impairment of skin integrity	
b. Elevation of body temperature	May indicate response to infection.
c. Drainage from wound (amount, color)	Amount will decrease as healing takes place; serous drainage is clear; bright red drainage indicates fresh bleeding; purulent drainage is thick and yellow, pale green, or white.
d. Odor	Strong odor indicates infectious process.
e. Consistency of drainage	Leukocytes produce thick drainage.
f. Size of wounds, including depth, length, and width	Determines stage of healing.
4. Administer prescribed analgesic 30-45 min before starting wound irrigation procedure.	Increased comfort level will permit client to move more easily and be positioned to facilitate infection control during irrigation.
5. Gather equipment at bedside:	Increases efficiency.
a. Sterile basin	Used to hold sterile irrigation solution in preparation for irrigation.
b. 150- to 500-ml prescribed sterile irrigating solution	Warming adds to comfort level.
c. Sterile irrigation syringe, sterile soft catheter, if needed	Used to prevent introduction of additional pathogens during procedure; soft catheter is used to irrigate deep wounds with small openings.
d. Clean basin	Used to collect contaminated irrigating solution.
e. Clean gloves (check policy of institution)	Protect nurse from infection while removing wound dressing.
f. Sterile gloves	Used to maintain asepsis during irrigation and redressing procedures.
g. Waterproof underpad	Prevents soiling of bed linen; is cost and time effective.
h. Sterile dressing tray and supplies for dressing change, including packing, if ordered	Prevents infection and promotes wound healing.
i. Leakproof refuse bag	Used to gather soiled and contaminated dressings and prevent cross-infection.
j. Gown	Gown may or may not be indicated to protect uniform from contamination. Mask and goggles may be indicated if spraying of drainage is possible.
6. Explain procedure.	Reduces anxiety.
7. Position client comfortably to permit gravitational flow of irrigating solution through wound and into collection basin. Position client so that wound is vertical to collection basin.	Directing solution from top to bottom of wound and from clean area to contaminated area prevents further infection. Positioning client during planning stage provides bed surfaces for later preparation.
8. Warm sterile irrigating solution to approximate body temperature.	Increases comfort and reduces vascular constriction response in tissues.
9. Form cuff on leakproof refuse bag and place it near bed.	Helps maintain large opening, thereby permitting placement of contaminated dressing without soiling bag's outer surface.
10. Close room door or bed curtains.	Maintains privacy.
11. Place waterproof underpad on bed surface in front of wound.	Protection of bedding eliminates need to change linens.
12. Place clean basin directly under wound.	Collects contaminated irrigating solution.
13. Wash hands.	Reduces transmission of infection.
14. If gown is needed, apply it now.	Protects your clothing and prevents cross-infection.

Performing Wound Irrigation—cont'd

STEPS	RATIONALE
15. Prepare sterile field using sterile dressing set and supplies.	Reduces risk of introducing microorganisms into wound.
16. Add sterile basin, pour in estimated volume of warm sterile irrigating solution, and set irrigating syringe in basin with solution.	Prepares solution for wound irrigation.
17. Place several strips of adhesive tape within reach and *not* on sterile field.	Provides easy access to tape for securing dressing.
18. Put on clean gloves, remove soiled dressing and discard in leakproof refuse bag.	Reduces transmission of microoganisms.
19. Remove and discard gloves.	
20. Inspect wound and make mental note of healing process, inflammation, drainage, or purulent matter.	Facilitates accurate description later.
21. Apply sterile gloves.	Reduces transmission of microorganisms.
22. Irrigate.	Aids in removal of debris and facilitates healing by secondary intention. This system uses a safe amount of pressure that will not damage the wound tissue.
a. Wound with wide opening:	
(1) Fill syringe with irrigating solution. Put 19-gauge needle on end of syringe.	
(2) Hold syringe tip 2.5 cm (1 in) above upper end of wound.	Prevents trauma to granulation tissue from syringe.
(3) Using slow, continuous pressure, flush wound.	Ensures removal of all debris.
(4) Repeat Steps (1-4) until solution draining into basin is clear.	
b. Deep wound with very small opening:	
(1) Attach soft catheter to filled irrigating syringe.	Permits direct flow of irrigant into wound.
(2) Lubricate tip of catheter with irrigating solution. Gently insert tip of catheter until resistance is felt, and then pull out about 1.2 cm ($^1/_2$ in) to remove tip from fragile inner wall of wound.	
(3) Using slow, continuous pressure, flush wound.	Ensures removal of debris without traumatizing new granulation tissue.
(4) Pinch off catheter just below syringe.	Avoid contamination of sterile solution or basin.
(5) Remove syringe, fill, and reattach to catheter. Repeat until return is clear.	
23. Dry wound edges with sterile gauze.	Prevents maceration of surrounding tissue from excess moisture.
24. Apply sterile dressing.	Maintains sterile protective barrier over wound.
25. Remove and dispose of gloves.	Facilitates placement of adhesive tape.
26. Secure dressing with adhesive tape.	
27. Assist client to comfortable position.	Relieves tension on wound site.
28. Dispose of equipment; retain remaining bottle of sterile solution.	Sterile solution can be used for subsequent irrigations.
29. Wash hands.	Reduces transmission of infection.
30. Inspect dressing periodically.	Determines response to wound irrigation and need to modify care plan.
31. Evaluate skin integrity.	Determines whether extension of wound has occurred.
32. Record wound appearance, irrigation, and client response in nurses' notes.	Fulfills legal responsibility and provides information needed to ensure continuity of care.

irrigating solutions at body temperature enhances comfort and provides the added benefit of local heat application.

Wound Irrigations. Irrigation of an open wound requires sterile technique. The nurse uses a 35-cc syringe with a 19-gauge needle (AHCPR, 1994) to deliver the solution using an irrigation system that has a safe pressure and will not damage healing wound tissue. It is important never to occlude a wound opening with a syringe because this results in the introduction of irrigating fluid into a closed space. The pressure of the fluid could cause tissue damage and discomfort (see Chapter 38). A wound should always be irrigated with the syringe tip over but not in the drainage site. Fluid should flow directly into the wound and not over a contaminated area before entering the wound. Procedure 49-2 lists steps for wound irrigation.

Suture Care

A surgeon closes a wound by bringing the wound edges as close together as possible to reduce scar formation. Proper wound closure involves minimal trauma and tension to tissues with control of bleeding.

Sutures are threads or wire used to sew body tissues together (Fig. 49-9). The client's history of wound healing, site of surgery, tissues involved, and purpose of the sutures determine the suture material to be used. For example, if the client has had repeated surgery for an abdominal hernia, the physician might choose wire sutures to provide greater strength for wound closure. In contrast, a small laceration of the face calls for the use of very fine Dacron (polyester) sutures to minimize scar formation.

Sutures are available in a variety of materials, including silk, steel, cotton, linen, wire, nylon, and Dacron. Sutures come with or without sharp surgical needles attached. Commonly seen are steel staples, a type of outer skin closure that causes less trauma to tissues than sutures, yet provides extra strength. It is also common to see wounds closed with Steri-Strips. A **Steri-Strip** is a sterile butterfly tape applied along both sides of a wound to keep the edges closed.

Sutures are placed within tissue layers in deep wounds and superficially as the final means for wound closure. The deeper sutures are usually an absorbable material that disappears in several days. Sutures are foreign bodies and thus are capable of causing local inflammation. The surgeon can minimize tissue injury by using the finest suture possible and the smallest number necessary.

Policies vary within institutions as to who may remove sutures. If the nurse is allowed to remove them, a physician's order is required. An order for suture removal is not written until the physician believes that the wound has closed (usually 7 to 10 days). Special scissors with curved cutting tips or special staple removers slide under the skin closures for suture removal (Fig. 49-10). The physician usually signifies the number of sutures or staples to remove. If the suture line appears to be healing in certain locations better than in others, the physician may choose to have only some sutures removed (e.g., every other one).

To remove staples, the nurse simply inserts the tips of the staple remover under each wire staple. While slowly closing the ends of the staple remover together, the nurse squeezes the center of the staple with the tips, freeing the staple from the skin.

To remove sutures the nurse first checks the type of suturing used (Fig. 49-11). With intermittent suturing the surgeon ties each individual suture made in the skin. Continuous suturing, as the name implies, is a series of sutures with only two knots, one at the beginning and one at the end of the suture line. Retention sutures are placed more deeply than skin sutures and may or may not be removed by the nurse, depending on agency policy. The manner in

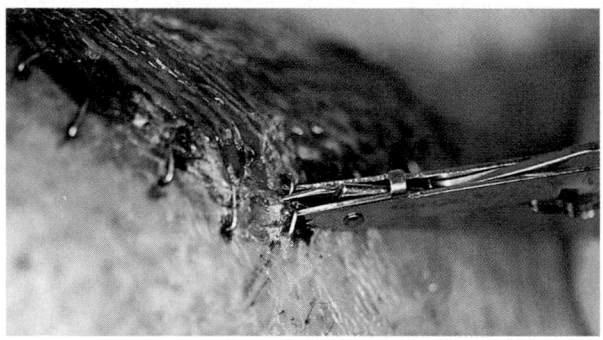

Fig. 49-10 Staple remover.

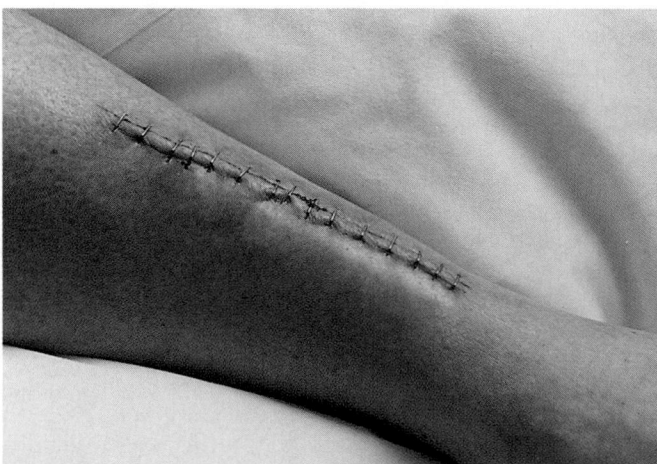

Fig. 49-9 Incision closed with wire staples.

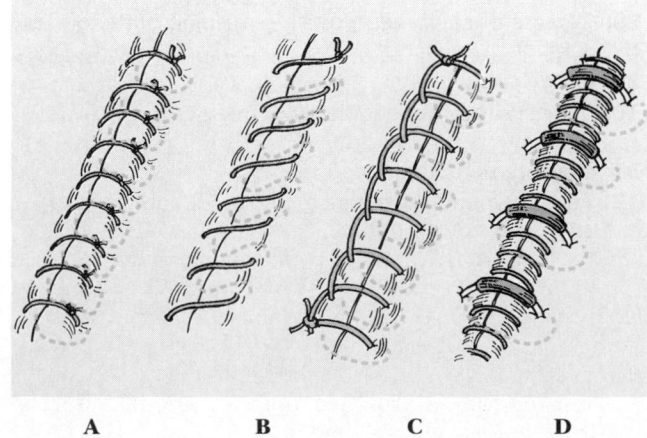

A   B   C   D

Fig. 49-11 Examples of suturing methods. **A,** Intermittent. **B,** Continuous. **C,** Blanket continuous. **D,** Retention.

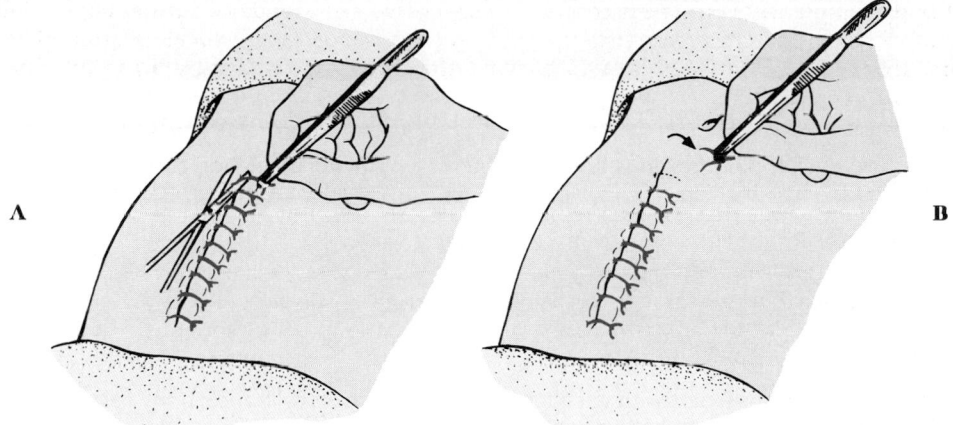

Fig. 49-12 Removal of intermittent suture. **A,** The nurse cuts the suture as close to the skin as possible, away from the knot. **B,** The nurse removes the suture and never pulls the contaminated stitch through tissues.

which the suture crosses and penetrates the skin determines the method for removal. The most important principle in suture removal is to *never* pull the visible portion of a suture through underlying tissue. Sutures on the skin's surface harbor microorganisms and debris. The portion of the suture beneath the skin is sterile. Pulling the contaminated portion of the suture through tissues may lead to infection. The nurse clips suture materials as close to the skin edge on one side as possible and then pulls the suture through from the other side (Fig. 49-12).

Drainage Evacuation

When drainage interferes with healing, drainage evacuation can be achieved by using either a drain alone or a drainage tube with continuous suction. The nurse may apply special skin barriers, similar to those used with ostomies (see Chapter 47), around drain sites. The **skin barriers** are soft, waferlike, plastic materials that are applied to the skin with adhesive. Drainage flows on the barrier but not directly on the skin. **Drainage evacuators** (Fig. 49-13) are convenient, portable units that connect to tubular drains lying within a wound bed and exert a safe, constant, low-pressure vacuum to remove and collect drainage. The nurse ensures that suction is exerted and that connection points between the evacuator and tubing are intact. The evacuator collects drainage that the nurse assesses for volume and character every shift and as needed. When the evacuator fills, the nurse measures output by emptying the contents into a graduated cylinder and immediately resets the evacuator to apply suction.

Bandages and Binders

A simple gauze dressing is often not enough to immobilize or provide support to a wound. **Binders** and bandages applied over or around dressings can provide extra protection and therapeutic benefits by:

1. Creating pressure over a body part (e.g., an elastic pressure bandage applied over an arterial puncture site)
2. Immobilizing a body part (e.g., an elastic bandage applied around a sprained ankle)

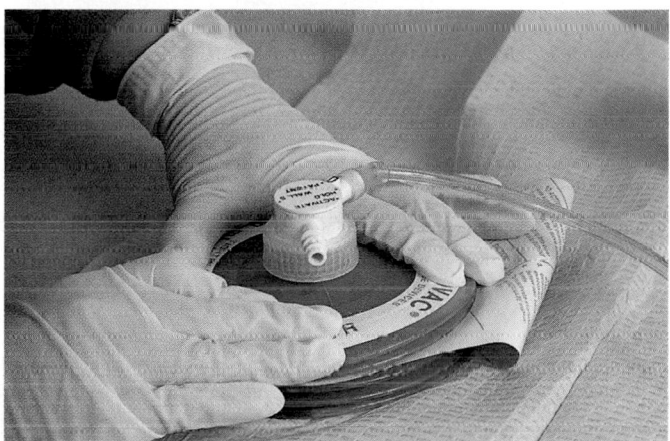

Fig. 49-13 Setting the suction on a drainage evacuator. **1,** With drainage port open, the lever to the vacuum diaphragm is raised. **2,** The nurse pushes straight down on the lever to lower the diaphragm. **3,** Closure of the port prevents escape of air and creates vacuum pressure.

3. Supporting a wound (e.g., an abdominal binder applied over a large abdominal incision and dressing)
4. Reducing or preventing edema (e.g., a well-supporting bra to minimize breast discomfort after delivery of a baby)
5. Securing a splint (e.g., a bandage applied around hand splints for correction of deformities)
6. Securing dressings (e.g., elastic webbing applied around leg dressings after a vein stripping)

Bandages are available in rolls of various widths and materials, including gauze, elasticized knit, elastic webbing, flannel, and muslin. Gauze bandages are lightweight and inexpensive, mold easily around contours of the body, and permit air circulation to prevent skin maceration. Elastic bandages conform well to body parts but can also be used to exert pressure over a body part. Flannel and muslin bandages are thicker than gauze and thus stronger for support-

Table 49-4	Types of Bandage Turns	
TYPE	**DESCRIPTION**	**PURPOSE OR USE**
Circular	Bandage turn overlapping previous turn completely	Anchors bandage at the first and final turn; covers small part (finger, toe)
Spiral	Bandage ascending body part with each turn overlapping previous one by one-half or two-thirds width of bandage	Covers cylindrical body parts such as wrist or upper arm
Spiral—reverse	Turn requiring twist (reversal) of bandage halfway through each turn	Covers cone-shaped body parts such as the forearm, thigh, or calf; useful with nonstretching bandages such as gauze or flannel
Figure eight	Oblique overlapping turns alternately ascending and descending over bandaged part; each turn crossing previous one to form figure eight	Covers joints; snug fit provides excellent immobilization
Recurrent	Bandage first secured with two circular turns around proximal end of body part; half turn made perpendicular up from bandage edge; body of bandage brought over distal end of body part to be covered with each turn folded back over on itself	Covers uneven body parts such as head or stump

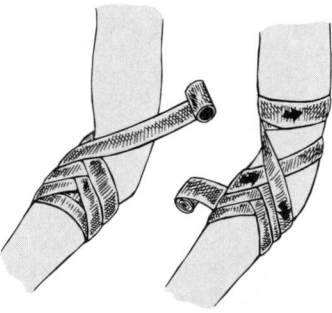

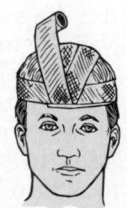
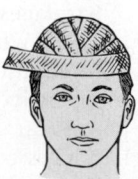

ing or applying pressure. A flannel bandage also insulates to provide warmth.

Binders are bandages that are made of large pieces of material to fit a specific body part. Most binders are made of elastic, cotton, muslin, or flannel. An abdominal binder and a breast binder are examples.

PRINCIPLES FOR APPLYING BANDAGES AND BINDERS

Correctly applied bandages and binders do not cause injury to underlying and nearby body parts or create discomfort for the client. For example, a chest binder must not be so tight as to restrict chest wall expansion. Before a bandage or binder is applied, the nurse's responsibilities include the following:

1. Inspecting the skin for abrasions, edema, discoloration, or exposed wound edges
2. Covering exposed wounds or open abrasions with a sterile dressing
3. Assessing the condition of underlying dressings and changing them if soiled
4. Assessing the skin of underlying body parts and parts that will be distal to the bandage for signs of circulatory impairment (coolness, pallor, or cyanosis, diminished or absent pulses, swelling, numbness, and tingling) to provide a means for comparing changes in circulation after bandage application

Table 49-4 outlines the principles of bandage and binder application. After a bandage is applied, the nurse assesses, documents, and immediately reports changes in circulation, skin integrity, comfort level, and body function such as ventilation or movement. The nurse who applies a bandage can loosen or readjust it as necessary. The nurse should have a physician's order before loosening or removing a bandage applied by a physician. The nurse explains to the client that any bandage or binder feels relatively firm or tight. A bandage should be carefully assessed to be sure that it is properly applied and is providing therapeutic benefit, and soiled bandages should be replaced. Like a damp dressing, a bandage or binder can harbor microorganisms.

BINDER APPLICATION

Binders are especially designed for the body part to be supported. The most common types of binders are the abdominal binder, and T binder (Procedure 49-3). Breast binders, used to provide support after breast surgery, exert pressure to reduce lactation in a woman after childbirth and are now being replaced with well-fitting bras.

Abdominal Binders. An abdominal binder supports large abdominal incisions that are vulnerable to tension or stress as the client moves or coughs (Fig. 49-14). The nurse secures an abdominal binder with safety pins, Velcro strips, or metal stays.

T Binders. As the name implies, the T binder looks like the letter T (Fig. 49-15) and is used to secure rectal or perineal dressings. The single T is for female clients, and the double T fits male clients.

The belt of the binder fits securely around the client's waist with the tail passing between the client's legs from back to front and attaching to the belt's front. The nurse must be sure that the tail fits smoothly and against the dressing. T binders become soiled easily and require frequent changing. Irritation to the urethra or scrotum must be avoided.

SLINGS

Slings support arms with muscular sprains or fractures. A commercially made sling consists of a long sleeve that extends above the elbow, with a strap that fits around the neck. In the home a large triangular piece of cloth can be used. The client may sit or lie supine during sling application (Fig. 49-16). The nurse instructs the client to bend the affected arm, bringing the forearm straight across the chest. The open sling fits under the client's arm and over the chest, with the base of the triangle under the wrist and the triangle's point at the client's elbow. One end of the sling fits around the back of the client's neck. The nurse brings the other end up and over the affected arm while supporting the extremity. The nurse ties the two ends at the side of the neck so that the knot does not press against the cervi-

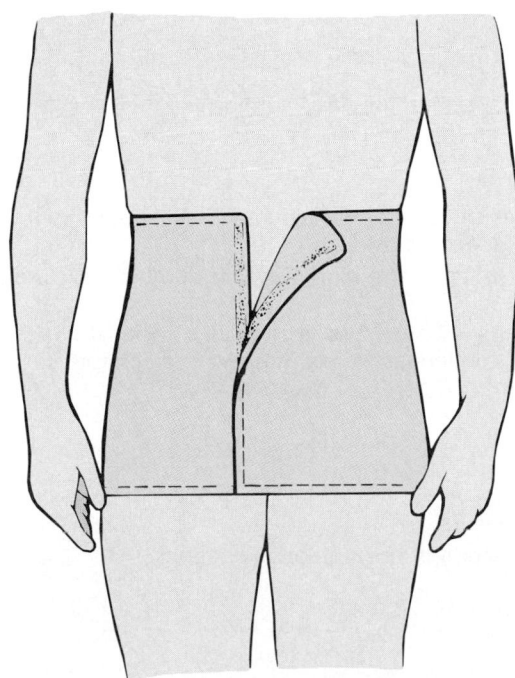

Fig. 49-14 Setting an abdominal binder secures with velcro.

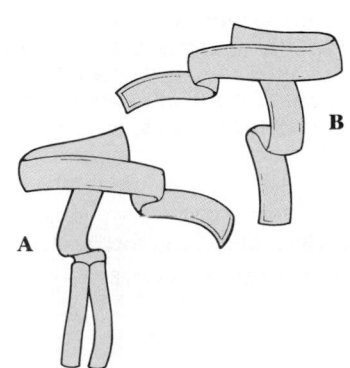

Fig. 49-15 T binders. **A,** Male. **B,** Female.

PROCEDURE 49-3

Applying an Abdominal or T Binder

STEPS	RATIONALE
1. Observe client with need for support of thorax or abdomen. Observe ability to breathe deeply and cough effectively.	Baseline assessment determines client's ability to breathe and cough. Impaired ventilation of lung can lead to alveolar atelectasis and inadequate arterial oxygenation.
2. Inspect skin for actual or potential alterations in integrity. Observe for irritation, abrasions; skin surfaces that rub against each other; allergic response to adhesive tape used to secure dressing.	Impairments in skin integrity can be worsened with application of binder. Binder can cause pressure and excoriation.
3. Review medical record if medical prescription for particular binder is required and reasons for application.	Application of supportive binders may be based on nursing judgment. In some situations, physician input is required.
4. Gather necessary data regarding size of client and appropriate binder.	Ensures proper fit of binder.
5. Prepare necessary equipment and supplies:	
a. Abdominal binder:	
(1) Correct size cloth or elastic straight binder	Binder must be large enough to surround abdomen and overlap to secure closure.
(2) Safety pins (unless Velcro closure is attached)	One pin secures horizontal waistband. Second pin secures each tail, placing pin through all thicknesses at horizontal level.
b. T and double-T binder:	
(1) Correct size binder	
(2) Safety pins: 2 pins for T binder; 3 pins for double-T binder	
6. Explain procedure to client and close curtains or room door.	Promotes understanding. Provides privacy.
7. Wash hands.	Maintains medical asepsis and infection control.
8. Apply abdominal binder:	
a. (1) Position client supine with head slightly elevated and knees slightly flexed.	Minimizes muscular tension on abdominal organs.
(2) Fan-fold far side of binder toward midline of binder.	Reduces time client remains in uncomfortable position.
(3) Instruct and assist client to roll away from you toward raised side rail while firmly supporting abdominal incision and dressing with hands.	Reduces pain and discomfort.
(4) Place fan-folded ends of binder under client.	Permits placement and centering of binder with minimal discomfort.
(5) Instruct and assist client to roll over folded ends.	
(6) Unfold and stretch ends out smoothly on far side of bed. (Binder should extend from just above symphysis pubis to just below costal margin.)	Maintains skin integrity and comfort.
(7) Instruct client to roll back into supine position.	Facilitates chest expansion and adequate wound support when binder is closed.
(8) Adjust binder so that supine client is centered over binder using symphysis pubis and costal margins as lower and upper landmarks.	Centers support from binder over abdominal structures.
(9) Straight binder: Pull distal end of binder over center of client's abdomen. While maintaining tension on that end of binder, pull opposite end of binder over center and secure with Velcro closure tabs or safety pins.	Provides continuous wound support and comfort.
(10) Assess client's ability to breathe deeply and cough effectively.	Determines ventilation and clears airways of pulmonary secretions.
(11) Ask client about comfort level.	Excess discomfort may inhibit expirations.
(12) Adjust binder as necessary.	

Applying an Abdominal or T Binder—cont'd

STEPS	RATIONALE

8. Apply abdominal binder—cont'd

   b. Apply T and double-T binders:

     (1) Assist client to dorsal recumbent position.

     (2) Have client raise hips and place horizontal band around waist (or above iliac crests) with vertical tails extending past buttocks. Overlap waistband in front and secure with safety pins.

       Minimizes muscular tension on perineal organs. Secures binder around client.

     (3) Complete binder application:

       Single-T and double-T binders provide support to perineal muscles and organs.

       (i) *T binder:* Bring remaining vertical strip over perineal dressing and continue up and under center front of horizontal band. Bring end over waistband and secure all thicknesses with safety pin.

       (ii) *Double-T binder:* Bring remaining vertical strips over perineal or suprapubic dressing with each tail supporting one side of scrotum and proceeding upward on either side of penis. Continue upward on either side of penis. Continue drawing ends behind and then downward in front of horizontal band. Secure all thicknesses with one safety pin.

     (4) Assess comfort level with client in lying, sitting, and standing positions. Readjust front pins as necessary. Increase padding if any area rubs against surounding tissues.

       Determines efficacy of binder to maintain dressings and support perineal structures.

     (5) Instruct client regarding removal of binder before defecating or urinating and need to replace binder after these bodily functions.

       Cleanliness of binder reduces infection risk.

9. Wash hands.

   Prevents cross-infections.

10. Observe site for skin integrity, circulation, and characteristics of the wound. Note comfort level of client.

   Determines that binder has not resulted in irritation to skin or underlying organs. Binders should not impede breathing or increase discomfort.

11. Record application of binder, condition of skin and circulation, integrity of dressings, and comfort level.

   Documents procedure. Baseline data ensure continuity of care.

---

cal spine. The loose material at the elbow can be folded evenly around the elbow and pinned. The lower arm and hand should always be supported at a level above the elbow to prevent formation of dependent edema.

BANDAGE APPLICATION

Rolls of bandage can secure or support dressings over irregularly shaped body parts. Each roll has a free outer end and a terminal end at the center of the roll. The rolled portion of the bandage is its body, and its outer surface is placed against the client's skin or dressing. Procedure 49-4 describes the steps for applying an elastic bandage. The nurse may use a variety of bandage turns depending on the body part to be bandaged (see Table 49-4).

Heat and Cold Therapy

Local application of heat and cold to an injured body part can be therapeutic. Before using these therapies, however, the nurse must understand normal body responses to local temperature variations, assess the integrity of the body part, determine the client's ability to sense temperature

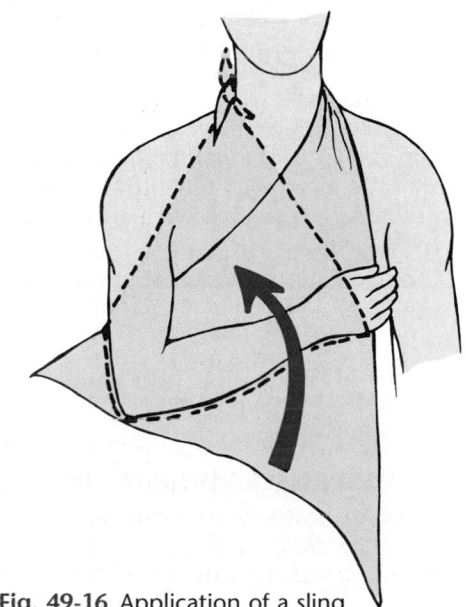

Fig. 49-16 Application of a sling.

Applying an Elastic Bandage

STEPS	RATIONALE
1. Inspect skin for alterations in integrity as indicated by abrasions, discoloration, chafing, or edema. (Look carefully at bony prominences.)	Altered skin integrity contraindicates the use of elastic bandage.
2. Observe adequacy of circulation by noting surface temperature, skin color, and sensation of body parts to be wrapped.	Comparison of area before and after application of bandage is necessary to ensure continued adequate circulation. Impairment of circulation may result in coolness to touch when compared with opposite side of body, cyanosis or pallor of skin, diminished or absent pulses, edema or localized pooling, and numbness or tingling of part.
3. Review medical record for specific orders related to application of elastic bandage. Note area to be covered, type of bandage required, frequency of change, and previous response to treatment.	Specific prescription may direct procedure, including factors such as extent of application (e.g., toe to knee, toe to groin) and duration of treatment.
4. Obtain necessary equipment and supplies (determine if present bandage will be reused or replaced)	
a. Correct widths and number of bandages (Elastic bandages are available in 2, 2$\frac{1}{2}$, 3, 4, 6, and 8 in and 1$\frac{1}{2}$ and 3 yd [5, 6.25, 7.5, 10, 15, and 20 cm and 135 and 270 cm]; 7.5- and 10-cm bandages are most often appropriate.)	Increasingly wider bandages are used as size of body part increases (e.g., 7.5-, 10-, and 15-cm bandages may be used to cover foot, calf, thigh).
b. Safety pins, tape	Secures bandage in place.
5. Explain procedure. Reinforce teaching that smooth, even, light pressure will be applied to improve venous circulation, prevent clot formation, reduce or prevent swelling, immobilize arms, secure surgical dressings, and provide pressure.	Promotes cooperation and reduces anxiety. Improves knowledge level regarding need for elastic bandages.
6. Wash hands.	Reduces transmission of infection.
7. Close room door or curtains. Assist client to assume comfortable, anatomically correct position	Maintains comfort and dignity. Maintains alignment. Prevents musculoskeletal deformity.
8. Hold roll of elastic bandage in dominant hand and use other hand to lightly hold beginning of bandage at distal body part. Continue transferring roll to dominant hand as bandage is wrapped.	Maintains appropriate and consistent bandage tension.
9. Apply bandage from distal point toward proximal boundary using variety of turns to cover various shapes of body parts (Table 49-4).	Bandage is applied in manner that conforms evenly to body part and promotes venous return.
10. Unroll and very slightly stretch bandage. Overlap turns.	Maintains uniform bandage tension. Prevents uneven bandage tension and circulatory impairment.
11. Secure first bandage before applying additional rolls.	Prevents wrinkling or loose ends.
12. Wash hands.	Reduces transmission of microorganisms.
13. Evaluate distal circulation as application is completed and at least twice during 8-hr period (note color, warmth, pulses, and numbness).	Early detection of circulatory difficulties ensures healthy neuromuscular status.
14. Record bandage application and client's response in nurses' notes.	Documents procedures and ensures continuity of care.

variations, and ensure proper operation of equipment. The nurse is legally responsible for safe administration of heat and cold applications.

BODILY RESPONSES TO HEAT AND COLD

Exposure to heat and cold can cause systemic and local responses. Systemic responses occur through heat-loss mechanisms (sweating and vasodilation) or mechanisms promoting heat conservation (vasoconstriction and pilo-erection) and heat production (shivering) (see Chapter 32). Local responses to heat and cold occur through stimulation of temperature-sensitive nerve endings within the skin. This stimulation sends impulses from the periphery to the hypothalamus, which becomes aware of local temperature sensations and triggers adaptive responses for maintenance of normal body temperature. If alterations occur along temperature sensation pathways, the reception and eventual perception of stimuli will be altered.

Table 49-5	Conditions That Increase Risk of Injury from Heat and Cold Application	

CONDITION	RISK FACTORS
Very young clients or older clients	Thinner skin layers in children increase risk of burns. Older clients have reduced sensitivity to pain.
Open wounds, broken skin, stomas	Subcutaneous and visceral tissues are more sensitive to temperature variations. They also contain no temperature and fewer pain receptors.
Areas of edema or scar formation	Reduced sensation to temperature stimuli occurs because of thickening of skin layers from fluid buildup or scar formation.
Peripheral vascular disease (e.g., diabetes, arteriosclerosis)	Body's extremities are less sensitive to temperature and pain stimuli because of circulatory impairment and local tissue injury. Cold application further compromises blood flow.
Confusion or unconsciousness	Perception of sensory or painful stimuli is reduced.
Spinal cord injury	Alterations in nerve pathways prevent reception of sensory or painful stimuli.
Abscessed tooth or appendix	Infection is highly localized. Application of heat may cause rupture with spread of microorganisms systemically.

Table 49-6	Therapeutic Effects of Heat and Cold Applications	

PHYSIOLOGICAL RESPONSE	THERAPEUTIC BENEFIT	EXAMPLES OF CONDITIONS TREATED
HEAT		
Vasodilation	Improves blood flow to injured body part; promotes delivery of nutrients and removal of wastes; lessens venous congestion in injured tissues	Inflamed or edematous body part; new surgical wound; infected wound; arthritis, degenerative joint disease; localized joint pain, muscle strains; low back pain; menstrual cramping, hemorrhoidal, perianal, and vaginal inflammation; local abscesses
Reduced blood viscosity	Improves delivery of leukocytes and antibiotics to wound site	
Reduced muscle tension	Promotes muscle relaxation and reduces pain from spasm or stiffness	
Increased tissue metabolism	Increases blood flow; provides local warmth	
Increased capillary permeability	Promotes movement of waste products and nutrients	
COLD		
Vasoconstriction	Reduces blood flow to injured body part, preventing edema formation; reduces inflammation	Direct trauma (sprains, strains, fractures, muscle spasms); superficial laceration or puncture wound; minor burn; suspected malignancy in area of injury or pain; injections; arthritis and joint trauma
Local anesthesia	Reduces localized pain	
Reduced cell metabolism	Reduces oxygen needs of tissues	
Increased blood viscosity	Promotes blood coagulation at injury site	
Decreased muscle tension	Relieves pain	

The body can tolerate wide variations in temperature. The normal temperature of the skin's surface is 34° C (93.2° F), but temperature receptors usually adapt quickly to local temperatures between 45° and 15° C (113° and 59° F). Pain develops when local temperatures exceed this range. Excessive heat causes a burning sensation. Cold produces a numbing sensation before pain.

The body's adaptive ability creates the major problem in protecting clients from injury resulting from temperature extremes. A person initially feels an extreme change in temperature but within a short time hardly notices it. This can be dangerous because a person insensitive to heat and cold extremes can suffer serious tissue injury. The nurse must recognize clients most at risk for injuries from heat and cold applications (Table 49-5).

LOCAL EFFECTS OF HEAT AND COLD

Heat and cold stimuli create different physiological responses. The choice of heat or cold therapy depends on local responses desired for wound healing.

Effects of Heat Application. Table 49-6 summarizes the benefits of heat application. Heat generally is quite therapeutic, improving blood flow to an injured part. If heat is applied for 1 hour or more, however, blood flow is reduced by a reflex vasoconstriction as the body attempts to control heat loss from the area. Periodic removal and reapplication of local heat restores vasodilation. Continuous exposure to heat damages epithelial cells, causing redness, localized tenderness, and even blistering.

Effects of Cold Application. Table 49-6 also summarizes the benefits of cold application. Prolonged exposure of the skin to cold results in a reflex vasodilation. The cell's inability to receive adequate blood flow and nutrients results in tissue ischemia. The skin initially takes on a reddened appearance, followed by a bluish purple mottling with numbness and a burning type of pain. The skin's tissues can freeze from exposure to extreme cold.

FACTORS INFLUENCING HEAT AND COLD TOLERANCE

The body's response to heat and cold therapies depends on the following factors:

1. Duration of application. A person is better able to tolerate short exposure to temperature extremes.
2. Body part. Certain areas of the skin are more sensitive to temperature variations. These include the neck, inner aspect of the wrist and forearm, and perineal region. The foot and palm of the hand are less sensitive.
3. Damage to body surface. Exposed skin layers are more sensitive to temperature variations.
4. Prior skin temperature. The body responds best to minor temperature adjustments. If a body part is cool and a hot stimulus touches the skin, the response is greater than if the skin were already warm.
5. Body surface area. A person has less tolerance to temperature changes to which a large area of the body is exposed.
6. Age and physical condition. Tolerance to temperature variations changes with age. Clients who are very young and old are most sensitive to heat and cold. If a client's physical condition reduces the reception or perception of sensory stimuli, tolerance to temperature extremes is high, but the risk of injury is also high.

ASSESSMENT FOR TEMPERATURE TOLERANCE

Before applying heat or cold therapies, the nurse assesses the client's physical condition for signs of potential intolerance to heat and cold. The nurse first observes the area to be treated. Alterations in skin integrity, such as abrasions, open wounds, edema, bruising, bleeding, or localized areas of inflammation, increase the client's risk of injury. Because the physician commonly orders heat and cold applications to be placed on traumatized areas, the baseline assessment provides a guide for evaluating skin changes that might occur during therapy.

Assessment includes identification of conditions that contraindicate heat or cold therapy. An active area of bleeding should not be covered by a warm application because bleeding will continue. Warm applications are contraindicated when the client has an acute, localized inflammation such as appendicitis because the heat could cause the appendix to rupture. If a client has cardiovascular problems, it is unwise to apply heat to large portions of the body because the resulting massive vasodilation may disrupt blood supply to vital organs.

Cold is contraindicated if the site of injury is already edematous. Cold further retards circulation to the area and prevents absorption of the interstitial fluid. If the client has impairment in circulation (e.g., arteriosclerosis), cold further reduces blood supply to the affected area. One other contraindication for cold therapy is shivering. Cold applications may intensify shivering and dangerously increase body temperature. The nurse also assesses the client's response to stimuli. Sensation to light touch, pinprick, and mild temperature variations (see Chapter 33) reveals the ability of the client to recognize when heat or cold becomes excessive. If a client has peripheral vascular disease, the nurse pays particular attention to the integrity of extremities. For example, if the physician's order is to apply a cold compress to a lower extremity, the nurse should assess circulation to the leg by observing skin color and palpating skin temperatures, distal pulses, and edematous areas. If signs of circulatory inadequacy are present, the nurse should question the order.

Level of consciousness influences the ability to perceive heat, cold, and pain. If a client is confused or unresponsive, the nurse must make frequent observations of skin integrity after therapy begins.

The nurse must also assess the condition of equipment being used. Electrical equipment should be checked for cracked cords, frayed wires, damaged insulation, and exposed heating components. Equipment containing circulating fluids should not have leaks. The nurse also checks equipment for evenness of temperature distribution. Uneven temperature distribution suggests that the equipment is functioning improperly.

CLIENT EDUCATION AND SAFETY

Before application of heat or cold therapy the client should understand its purpose, the symptoms of temperature exposure, and precautions taken to prevent injury. The box below provides hints for safely applying heat and cold therapy.

APPLYING HEAT AND COLD

A prerequisite to using any heat or cold application is a physician's order, which should include the body site to be

---

Safety Suggestions for Applying Heat or Cold Therapy

- *Do* explain to the client sensations to be felt during the procedure.
- *Do* instruct the client to report changes in sensation or discomfort immediately.
- *Do* provide a timer, clock, or watch so that the client can help the nurse time the application.
- *Do* keep the call light within the client's reach.
- *Do* refer to the institution's policy and procedure manual for safe temperatures.
- *Do not* allow the client to adjust temperature settings.
- *Do not* allow the client to move an application or place hands on the wound site.
- *Do not* place the client in a position that prevents movement away from the temperature source.
- *Do not* leave unattended a client who is unable to sense temperature changes or move from the temperature source.

Table 49-7	Choice of Dry or Moist Applications
ADVANTAGES	**DISADVANTAGES**
MOIST APPLICATIONS Moist application reduces drying of skin and softens wound exudate. Moist compresses conform well to body area being treated. Moist heat penetrates deeply into tissue layers. Warm moist heat does not promote sweating and insensible fluid loss.	Prolonged exposure can cause maceration of skin. Moist heat will cool rapidly because of moisture evaporation. Moist heat creates greater risk for burns to skin because moisture conducts heat.
DRY APPLICATIONS Dry heat has less risk of burns to skin than moist applications. Dry application does not cause skin maceration. Dry heat retains temperature longer because it is not influenced by evaporation.	Dry heat increases body fluid loss through sweating. Dry applications do not penetrate deep into tissues. Dry heat causes increased drying of skin.

treated and the type, frequency, and duration of application. The nurse should consult the agency's procedure manual for correct temperatures to use.

Choice of Moist or Dry. Heat and cold applications can be administered in dry or moist forms. The type of wound or injury, the location of the body part, and the presence of drainage or inflammation are factors considered in selecting dry or moist applications. Table 49-7 summarizes advantages and disadvantages of both.

Hot, Moist Compresses. For open wounds, sterile, hot, moist compresses improve circulation, relieve edema, and promote consolidation of pus and drainage. A **compress** is a piece of gauze dressing moistened in a prescribed warmed solution. A **pack** is a larger cloth or dressing applied to a larger body area.

Heat from hot compresses dissipates quickly. To maintain a constant temperature the nurse must change the compress often or apply a warm aquathermic pad or waterproof heating pad over the compress. Because moisture conducts heat, any device's temperature setting should be lower for a moist compress than for a dry application. A layer of plastic wrap or a dry towel can also be used to insulate the compress and retain heat. Moist heat promotes vasodilation and evaporation of heat from the skin's surface. For this reason a client may feel chilly. The nurse controls drafts within the room and keeps the client covered with a blanket or robe. Procedure 49-5 describes the steps for applying a hot, moist compress.

Warm Soaks. Immersion of a body part in a warmed solution promotes circulation, lessens edema, increases muscle relaxation, and can provide a means to debride wounds and apply medicated solution. A soak can also be accompanied by wrapping the body part in dressings and saturating them with the warmed solution.

The nurse positions the client comfortably, places waterproof pads under the area to be treated, and heats the solution to about 40.5° to 43° C (105° to 110° F). After immersing the body part, the nurse covers the container and extremity with a towel to reduce heat loss. It is usually necessary to remove the cooled solution and add heated solution after about 10 minutes. The problem is to keep the solution at a constant temperature. The nurse never adds a hotter solution while the body part remains immersed. After any soak the nurse dries the body part thoroughly to prevent maceration.

Sitz Baths. The client who has had rectal surgery, an episiotomy during childbirth, painful hemorrhoids, or vaginal inflammation may benefit from a **sitz bath**, a bath in which only the pelvic area is immersed in warm fluid. The client sits in a special tub or chair or in a basin that fits on the toilet seat so that the legs and feet remain out of the water. Immersing the entire body causes widespread vasodilation and nullifies the effect of local heat application to the pelvic area.

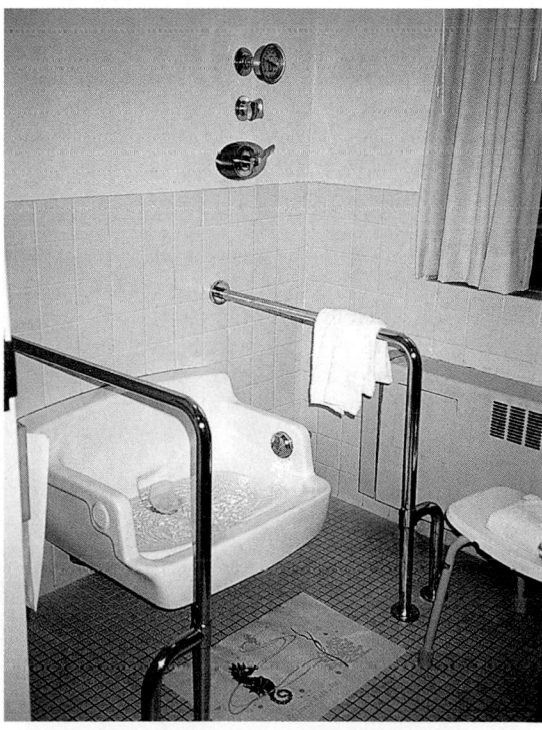

Fig. 49-17 Sitz bath.

Applying a Hot, Moist Compress to an Open Wound

STEPS	RATIONALE
1. Inspect condition of exposed skin and wound on which compress is to be applied (see the illustration below).	Provides baseline to determine changes in skin during heat application. Very thin or damaged skin is more susceptible to injury from heat.
2. Assess client's extremities for sensitivity to temperature and pain using light touch, pinprick, and temperature sensation tests.	Determines whether client is insensitive to heat and cold extremes.
3. Refer to physician's order for type of compress, location and duration of application, and desired temperature.	Ensures likelihood of safe application.
4. Prepare necessary equipment and supplies:	
a. Prescribed solution warmed to proper temperature, approximately 43°-46° C (110°-115° F)	Correct temperature prevents accidental burns.
b. Sterile gauze dressings	
c. Sterile container for solution	
d. Commercially prepared compresses (optional)	Premoistened compress reduces preparation.
e. Sterile gloves	
f. Petrolatum jelly, if desired	Protects untreated skin surface.
g. Sterile cotton swabs	
h. Waterproof pad	Prevents soiling of bed linen.
i. Tape or ties	
j. Dry bath towel	
k. Aquathermic or heating pad (optional)	Provides continuous source of heat.
l. Disposable gloves	
m. Bath thermometer	Measures solution temperature.
n. Bath blanket	
5. Explain steps of procedure and purpose. Describe sensation to be felt (e.g., feeling of warmth and wetness). Explain precautions to prevent burning.	Minimizes anxiety and promotes cooperation.
6. Assist client in assuming comfortable position in proper body alignment.	Compress remains in place for several minutes. Limited mobility in uncomfortable position causes muscular stress.
7. Place waterproof pad under area to be treated.	Prevents soiling of bed linen.
8. Expose body part to be covered with compress and drape client with bath blanket. Close bedside curtains.	Prevents unnecessary cooling and exposure of body part. Provides privacy.
9. Wash hands.	Reduces transmission of infection.

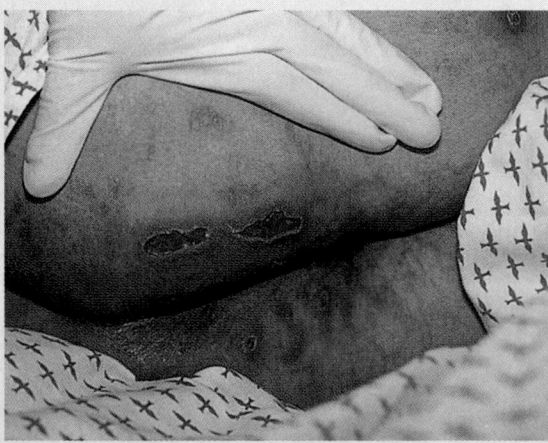

Step 1

Applying a Hot, Moist Compress to an Open Wound—cont'd

STEPS	RATIONALE
10. Assemble equipment. Pour warmed solution into sterile container. (If using portable heating source, keep solution warm. Commercially prepared compresses may remain under infrared lamp until just before use.) Open sterile packages and drop gauze into container to immerse in solution. Turn aquathermic pad (if desired) to correct temperature.	Compresses must retain warmth for therapeutic benefit.
11. Apply disposable gloves. Remove any existing dressing covering wound. Dispose of gloves and dressing in proper receptacle.	Reduces transmission of microorganisms.
12. If wound was covered, assess condition of it and surrounding skin.	Provides baseline to determine skin changes after compress application.
13. Apply sterile gloves.	Allows nurse to manipulate sterile dressing and touch open wound.
14. Apply sterile petrolatum jelly, if desired, with cotton swab to skin surrounding wound. Do not apply jelly on broken areas of skin.	Protects skin from possible burns and maceration.
15. Pick up one layer of immersed gauze and wring out excess water.	Excess moisture macerates skin and increases risk of burns and infection.
16. Apply gauze lightly to open wound. Watch response and ask whether client feels discomfort. In a few seconds, lift edge of gauze to assess for redness.	Skin is sensitive to sudden change in temperature. Redness indicates burn.
17. If client tolerates compress, pack gauze snugly against wound. Be sure all wound surfaces are covered by hot compress.	Prevents rapid cooling from underlying air currents.
18. Wrap or cover moist compress with dry bath towel. If necessary, pin or tie in place.	Insulates compress to prevent heat loss.
19. Change hot compress every 5 min or as ordered.	Prevents cooling and maintains therapeutic benefit of compress.
20. Apply aquathermic or waterproof heating pad over towel (optional). Keep it in place for desired duration of application (about 20-30 min).	Provides constant temperature to compress. Local application of heat for more than 60 min often results in reflex vasoconstriction. Removing hot compress after 30 min and then reapplying in 15 min, if desired, maintains vasodilation and positive therapeutic effects.
21. Ask client periodically whether there is discomfort or burning sensation. Observe area of skin not covered by compress.	Continued exposure to heat can cause burning of skin.
22. Remove pad, towel, and compress in 30 min. Again assess wound and condition of skin.	Continued exposure to moisture will macerate skin.
23. Replace dry sterile dressing as ordered.	Prevents entrance of microorganisms into wound site.
24. Assist client to preferred comfortable position.	Maintains comfort.
25. Dispose of equipment and soiled compress. Remove gloves and wash hands.	Reduces transmission of infection.
26. Inspect affected area covered by compress and heating pad.	Assists in determining effects of application.
27. Ask client whether an unusual burning sensation is noticed that was not felt before.	It may be difficult to assess burn merely by color changes if wound is inflamed or drainage is present.
28. Record type, location, and duration of application. Note temperature used in nurses' notes.	Documents therapy administered.
29. Describe condition of wound, skin, and response.	Documents response to therapy.

The desired temperature for a sitz bath depends on whether the purpose is to promote relaxation or to clean a wound. It may be necessary to add warm water during the procedure, which normally lasts 20 minutes, to maintain a constant temperature. Agency procedure manuals recommend safe water temperatures. A disposable sitz basin contains an attachment resembling an enema bag that allows gradual introduction of warmer water (Fig. 49-17).

The nurse prevents overexposure of the client by draping bath blankets around the client's shoulders and thighs and controlling drafts. The client should be able to sit in the basin or tub with feet flat on the floor and without pressure on the sacrum or thighs. Because exposure of a large portion of the body to heat can cause extensive vasodilation, the nurse should assess the pulse and facial color and ask whether the client feels light-headed or nauseated.

Aquathermia (Water-Flow) Pads. A popular device in health care institutions is the **aquathermia pad** or water-flow pad (Fig. 49-18), used for treating muscle sprains and areas of mild inflammation or edema. The aquathermia unit consists of a waterproof plastic or rubber pad connected by two hoses to an electrical control unit that has a heating element and motor. Distilled water circulates through hollowed channels within the pad to the control unit where water is heated or cooled (depending on temperature setting). Some pads have an absorbent surface to apply moist heat. The units are safer than conventional heating pads. However, the nurse should still check for equipment malfunctions. The temperature setting is fixed by inserting a plastic key into the temperature regulator. In many institutions the central supply room sets the regulators to the recommended temperature (40.5° to 43° C [105° to 110° F]). If the distilled water in the unit runs low, the nurse simply fills the reservoir two-thirds full. Plain tap water is never added because it might leave mineral deposits in the unit.

To avoid burning the client's skin the nurse does not place the pad directly on it. A thin towel or pillow case fits easily over the heating pad. Tape, ties, or a gauze roll holds the pad in place. Pins are never used because they might cause a leak. The nurse checks the client's skin often for signs of burning. An application should last only 20 to 30 minutes. The nurse does not allow a client to lie on a pad. Pressure against a mattress prevents normal heat dissipation. If the pad is to be applied to a region of the back, the client should lie prone or on one side.

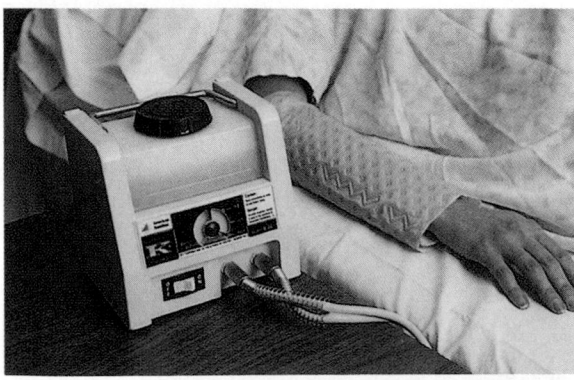

Fig. 49-18 Aquathermia pad.

Warm Air Blower. When wounds require drying (such as the donor site in split-thickness skin grafting), the nurse may use a hair dryer. The hair dryer is set on medium warm setting and held about 8 to 10 inches from the wound. The nurse then gently waves the device over the site for about 5 minutes or the time prescribed by the surgeon. This procedure is repeated 3 or 4 times a day until the wound is completely dry.

Commercial Hot Packs. Commercially prepared, disposable hot packs apply warm, dry heat to an injured area. By striking, kneading, or squeezing the pack, chemicals are mixed and release heat. Package directions recommend the time for heat application.

Electric Heating Pads. Another conventional form of heat therapy is the heating pad, an electric coil enclosed within a waterproof pad covered with cotton or flannel cloth. The pad is connected to an electric cord that has a temperature-regulating unit for a high, medium, or low setting. Nurses should advise clients to avoid using the high setting and never to lie on the pad. Another precaution to note is that a safety pin inserted through a pad can result in an electrical shock.

Cold, Moist, and Dry Compresses. The procedure for applying cold, moist compresses is the same as that for warm compresses. Cold compresses should be applied for 20 minutes at a temperature of 15° C (59° F) to relieve inflammation and swelling. They may be clean or sterile.

There are commercially prepared cold packs similar to the disposable hot packs for dry applications. They come in various shapes and sizes to fit different body parts. When using cold compresses the nurse observes for adverse reactions such as burning or numbness, mottling of the skin, redness, extreme paleness, and a bluish skin discoloration.

Cold Soaks. The procedure for preparing cold soaks and immersing a body part is the same as for warm soaks. The desired temperature for a 20-minute cold soak is 15° C (59° F). The nurse controls drafts and uses outer coverings to protect the client from chilling. It may be necessary to add cold water during the procedure to maintain a constant temperature.

Ice Bags or Collars. For a client who has a muscle sprain, localized hemorrhage, or hematoma or has undergone dental surgery, an ice bag is ideal to prevent edema formation, control bleeding, and anesthetize the body part. Proper use of the bag requires the following steps:

1. Fill the bag with water, secure the cap, invert to check for leaks, and pour out the water.
2. Fill the bag two-thirds full with crushed ice so that the bag can mold easily over a body part.
3. Release any air from the bag by squeezing its sides before securing the cap because excess air interferes with conduction of cold.
4. Wipe off excess moisture.
5. Cover the bag with a flannel cover, towel, or pillow case.
6. Apply the bag to the injury site for 30 minutes; the bag can be reapplied in an hour.

 Evaluation

The nurse evaluates wound healing on an ongoing basis (see the evaluation box on p. 1463). This occurs during

Sample Evaluation of Interventions for Impaired Skin Integrity

GOALS	EVALUATIVE MEASURES	EXPECTED OUTCOMES
Skin integrity will be improved in area of surgical wound.	Inspect skin surfaces next to wound and around drain sites. Observe condition of wound and character of drainage.	Wound will be clean and intact without inflammation, drainage, or maceration. Wound edges will be approximated.

dressing changes, when therapies are administered, and as a client attempts to perform self-care in the presence of a wound. The nurse instructs clients and family members about how to evaluate wound healing after discharge from a health care setting. For example, clients should be warned to notify a physician if signs of infection develop.

The nurse evaluates each intervention designed to promote wound healing and compares the status of the wound with the assessment data. Together the nurse and the client review any teaching plans designed to enable the client and family to care for the wound. The nursing care and teaching plans are modified based on evaluation data. Last, the nurse investigates the client's and family's need for additional support services (e.g., home health care, physical therapy, and counseling) and initiates the referral process.

∎ KEY CONCEPTS ∎

▶ In normal wound healing the epidermal skin layer resurfaces wounds, and the dermis restores the structural integrity and physical properties of the skin.

▶ A clean surgical incision with little tissue loss heals by primary intention.

▶ Healing by primary intention proceeds through three stages: inflammation, proliferation, and maturation.

▶ When there is extensive tissue loss, a wound heals by secondary intention.

▶ The chances of wound infection are greater when the wound contains dead or necrotic tissue, when foreign bodies lie on or near the wound, and when blood supply and tissue defenses are reduced.

▶ Physical stress from vomiting, coughing, or sudden muscular contraction can cause separation of wound edges.

▶ Wound assessment requires a description of the appearance of the wound, palpation of the area, and information regarding character of drainage, drains and wound closures, and pain.

▶ Wound drains remove secretions within tissue layers to promote wound closure.

▶ The nurse never collects a wound culture from old drainage.

▶ Principles of wound first aid include control of bleeding, cleansing, and protection.

▶ The layers of a dry dressing protect the wound edges, absorb drainage, and prevent entrance of bacteria.

▶ The wet-to-dry dressing mechanically removes dead tissue and wound exudate to debride the wound.

▶ When cleaning wounds or drain sites, the nurse cleans from the least to most contaminated area, away from wound edges.

▶ A bandage or binder should be applied in a manner that does not impair circulation or irritate the skin.

▶ The safe use of heat or cold therapy requires an assessment of the client's sensory function, identification of risk factors, and understanding of the physiological effects of heat and cold.

▶ An acute sprain, fracture, or bruise responds best to cold applications.

▶ Warm applications are effective for improving circulation to wound sites and promoting muscle relaxation.

▶ The choice of moist or dry applications depends on the type of wound, location of body part, and presence of drainage or inflammation.

∎ KEY TERMS ∎

Abrasion, p. 1435

Approximate, p. 1431

Aquathermia pad, p. 1462

Binders, p. 1451

Collagen, p. 1429

Compress, p. 1459

Debriding, p. 1440

Dehiscence, p. 1433

Dermis, p. 1429

Desquamation, p. 1429

■ CRITICAL THINKING EXERCISES ■

1. On the second day after surgery, you observe a decreased amount of dark-red drainage in the client's Jackson-Pratt device. What type of action is required?

2. When changing your client's dressing, you note that the Penrose drain is no longer in place. What do you do?

3. While changing your client's dressing, you note a foul odor and observe serous yellow drainage from the suture line. What physician's order would you anticipate?

4. When removing a wet-to-dry dressing, you note that the underlying gauze is wet with saline. The skin surrounding the wound is macerated. What conclusions can you make about the previous dressing? What would you do to avoid recurrence of this type of wet-to-dry application?

REFERENCES

AHCPR, Panel for Treatment of Pressure Ulcers in Adults: *Treatment of pressure ulcers*, (AHCPR Publication No. 95-0653, Clinical Practice Guideline, Number 15), Rockville, Md, 1994, Agency for Health Care Policy and Research, Public Health Service, U.S. Department of Health and Human Services.

Aronovitch S: Selecting the best dressing sponge, *Nurs 95* 25(7):52, 1995.

Atwater EE: Care of the surgically created granulating wound, *Derm Nurs* 1(1):46, 1989.

Cooper DM: Acute surgical wounds. In Bryant RA: *Acute and chronic wounds: nursing management*, St Louis, 1992, Mosby.

Cooper DM: Wound assessment and evaluation of healing. In Bryant RA: *Acute and chronic wounds: nursing management*, St Louis, 1992, Mosby.

Doughty DB: Principles of wound healing and wound management. In Bryant RA: *Acute and chronic wounds: nursing management*, St Louis, 1992, Mosby.

Erwin-Toth P, Hocevar BJ: Wound care: selecting the right dressing, *Am J Nurs* 95(2):46, 1995.

Garner JS: *Guidelines for prevention of surgical wound infections*, Atlanta, 1985, Centers for Disease Control.

Hess CT, Miller P: The management of open wounds: acute and chronic, *Ostom Wound Manage* 31:58, 1990.

Kim MJ, McFarland GK, McLane AM: *Pocket guide to nursing diagnoses*, ed 6, St Louis, 1995, Mosby.

Krasner D: Wound care: how to use the red-yellow-black system, *Am J Nurs*, 5:44, 1995.

Lazarus GS et al: Definitions and guidelines for assessment of wounds and evaluation of healing, *Wound Repair and Regeneration* 2:165, 1994.

Motta GJ: Moistening up for good healing, *Nurs 95* 25:32H, 1995.

Stotts NA et al: Sterile vs clean technique in wound care of patients with open surgical wounds in the post-op period: a pilot study, *Adv Wound Care* 8(2):13, 1995.

Wysocki AB: A review of the skin and its appendages, *Adv Wound Care* 8:53, 1995.

ADDITIONAL READINGS

Bale S, Harding KG: Using modern dressings to effect debridement, *Prof Nurs* 5:244, 1990.

Collier M: Assessing a wound, *Nurs Standard* 8(49):3, 1994.

Cuzzell JZ: The new RYB color code: next time you assess an open wound, remember to protect red, cleanse yellow, and debride black, *Am J Nurs* 88:1342, 1988.

Cuzzell JZ, Stotts NA: Wound care: trial and error yields to knowledge, *Am J Nurs* 90:53, 1990.

Fowler E, Cuzzell JZ, Papen JC: Healing with thin-film dressing, *Am J Nurs* 91:36, 1991.

Hansborough N: Nursing care of donor site wounds, *J Burn Care Rehab* 16(3):337, 1995.

Hill PD: Effects of heat and cold on the perineum after episiotomy/laceration, *JOGNN* 18:124, 1989.

Hudson-Goodman P, Girard N, Jones MB: Wound repair and the potential use of growth factors, *Heart Lung* 19:379, 1990.

Hunt TK: Basic principles of wound healing, *J Trauma* 30:S122, 1990.

Hutchinson JJ, McGuckin M: Occlusive dressing: a microbiologic and clinical review, *Am J Infect Control* 18:257, 1990.

Lange MP et al: Management of multiple enterocutaneous fistulas, *Heart Lung* 18:386, 1989.

LaVan FB, Hunt TK: Oxygen and wound healing, *Clin Plast Surg* 17:463, 1990.

Mash N: Protocols for wound management: standards of care as a systematic approach, *Ostomy/Wound Manage* 22:23, 1989.

Norris SD, Provo B, Stotts NA: Physiology of wound healing and risk factors that impede the healing process, *AACN Clin Iss Crit Care Nurs* 1:545, 1990.

Schmidt JM, Schimpeler SM: Obstetric and gynecologic abdominal wound infections: a comprehensive nurse-managed program, *J Perinat Neonat Nurs* 4:25, 1990.

Sitton E: Early and late radiation-individual skin alterations: nursing care of irradiated skin, Part 2, *Oncol Nurs Forum* 19(6):907, 1992.

Thomas AC, Wysocki AB: The healing wound: a comparison of three clinically useful methods of measurement, *Decubitus* 3:18, 1990.

Ting M: Wound healing and peripheral vascular disease, *Crit Care Nurs Clin North Am* 3(3):515.

Wysocki AB, Bryant RA: Skin. In Bryant RA: *Acute and chronic wounds: nursing management*, St Louis, 1992, Mosby.

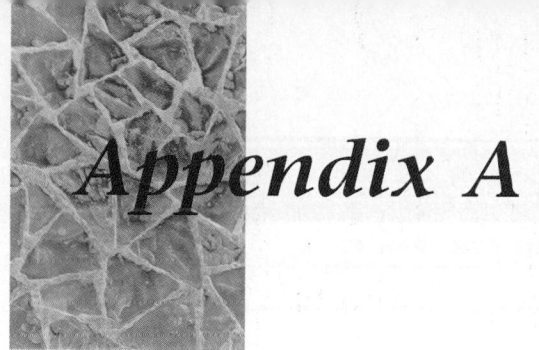

Appendix A

Normal Reference Laboratory Values

	REFERENCE RANGE	
DETERMINATION	CONVENTIONAL	SI
Acetoacetate plus acetone	0.3-2.0 mg/100 ml	3-20 mg/L
Aldolase	1.3-8.2 mU/ml	12-75 nmol · s^{-1}/L
Alpha amino nitrogen	3.0-5.5 mg/100 ml	2.1-3.9 mmol/L
Ammonia	80-110 μg/100 ml	47-65 μmol/L
Ascorbic acid	0.4-1.5 mg/100 ml	23-85 μmol/L
Barbiturate	0; coma level: phenobarbital, approximately 10 mg/100 ml; most other drugs, 1-3 mg/100 ml	0 μmol/L
Bilirubin (van den Bergh test)	1 minute: 0.4 mg/100 ml	Up to 7 μmol/L
	Direct: 0.4 mg/100ml	Up to 17 μmol/L
	Total: 1.0 mg/100 ml	
	Indirect is total minus direct	
Blood volume	8.5%-9.0% of body weight in kg	80-85 ml/kg
Bromide	0; toxic level: 17 mEq/L	0 mmol/L
Bromsulfalein (BSP)	Less than 5% retention 45 min after 5 mg/kg IV	<0.051
Calcium	8.5-10.5 mg/100 ml (slightly higher in children)	2.1-2.6 mmol/L
Carbon dioxide content	24-30 mEq/L; 20-26 mEq/L in infants (as HCO$_3^-$)	24-30 mmol/L
Carbon monoxide	Symptoms with over 20% saturation	0(1)
Carotenoids	0.8-4.0 μg/ml	1.5-7.4 μmol/L
Ceruloplasmin	27-37 mg/100 ml	1.8-2.5 μmol/L
Chloride	100-106 mEq/L	100-106 mmol/L
Cholinesterase (pseudocholinesterase)	0.5 pH U or more/hr; 0.7 pH U or more/hr for packed cells	0.5 or more arb. unit
Copper	Total: 100-200 μg/100 ml	16-31 μmol/L
Creatine phosphokinase (CPK)	Female 5-35 mU/ml	0.08-0.58 μmol · s^{-1}/L
	Male 5-55 mU/ml	
Creatinine	0.6-1.5 mg/100 ml	60-130 μmol/L
Ethanol	0.3%-0.4%, marked intoxication; 0.4%-0.5%, alcoholic stupor; 0.5% or over, alcoholic coma	65-87 mmol/L
		87-109 mmol/L
		>109 mmol/L

Modified from Kaye DA, Rose LF: *Fundamentals of internal medicine,* St Louis, 1983, Mosby Year Book. Adapted from *New Engl J Med* 302:37, 1980.
Abbreviations used: *SI,* Système international d'Unités (The SI for the Heath Professions. World Health Organization, Office of Publications, Geneva, Switzerland, 1977); *d,* 24 hours; P, plasma; *S,* serum; *B,* blood; *U,* urine; *L,* liter; *hr,* hour; and *sec,* second.

Continued.

Blood, Plasma, or Serum Values—cont'd

DETERMINATION	REFERENCE RANGE	
	CONVENTIONAL	SI
Glucose	Fasting: 70-110 mg/100 ml	3.9-5.6 mmol/L
Iron	50-150 μg/100 ml (higher in males)	9.0-26.9 μmol/L
Iron-binding capacity	250-410 μg/100 ml	44.8-73.4 μmol/L
Lactic acid	0.6-1.8 mEq/l	0.6-1.8 mmol/L
Lactic dehydrogenase	60-120 U/ml	1.00-2.00 μmol · $^{-1}$/L
Lead	50 μg/100 ml or less	Up to 2.4 μmol/L
Lipase	2 U/ml or less	Up to 2 arb. unit
Lipids		
Cholesterol	120-220 mg/100 ml	3.10-5.69 mmol/L
Cholesterol esters	60-75% of cholesterol	
Phospholipids	9-16 mg/100 ml as lipid phosphorus	2.9-5.2 mmol/L
Total fatty acids	190-420 mg/100 ml	1.9-4.2 g/L
Total lipids	450-1000 mg/100 ml	4.5-10.0 g/L
Triglycerides	40-150 mg/100 ml	0.4-1.5 g/L
Lithium	Toxic level 2 mEq/L	2 mmol./L
Magnesium	1.5-2.0 mEq/L	0.8-1.3 mmol/L
5'Nucleotidase	0.3-3.2 Bodansky U	30-290 nmol · s^{-1}/L
Osmolality	285-295 mOsm/kg water	285-295 mmol/kg
Oxygen saturation (arterial)	96%-100%	0.96-1.00 L
P$_{CO_2}$	35-43 mm Hg	4.7-6.0 kPa
pH	7.35-7.45	Same
P$_{O_2}$	75-100 mm Hg (dependent on age) while breathing room air; above 500 mm Hg while on 100% O_2 10.0-13.3 kPa	
Phenylalanine	0-2 mg/100 ml	0-120 μmol/L
Phenytoin (Dilantin)	Therapeutic level: 5-20 μg/ml	19.8-79.5 μmol/L
Phosphorus (inorganic)	3.0-4.5 mg/100 ml (infants in 1st yr up to 6.0 mg/100 ml)	1.0-1.5 mmol/L
Potassium	3.5-5.0 mEq/L	3.5-5.0 mmol/L
Primidone (Mysoline)	Therapeutic level: 4-12 μg/ml	18-55 μmol/L
Protein: Total	6.0-8.4 g/100 ml	60-84 g/L
Albumin	3.5-5.0 g/100 ml	35-50 g/L
Globulin	2.3-3.5 g/100 ml	23-35 g/L
Electrophoresis	% of total protein	Of total protein
Albumin	52-68	0.52-0.68
Globulin		
Alpha$_1$	4.2-7.2	0.042-0.072
Alpha$_2$	6.8-12	0.068-0.12
Beta	9.3-15	0.093-0.15
Gamma	13-23	0.13-0.23
Pyruvic acid	0-0.11 mEq/L	0-0.11 mmol/L
Quinidine	Therapeutic: 1.5-3 μg/ml	4.6-9.2 μmol/L
	Toxic: 5-6 μg/ml	15.4-18.5 μmol/L
Salicylate:	0	
Therapeutic	20-25 mg/100 ml; 25-30 mg/100 ml to age 10 yr 3 hr postdose	1.4-1.8 mmol/L 1.8-2.2 mmol/L
Toxic	Over 30 mg/100 ml	>2.2 mmol/L
	Over 20 mg/100 ml after age 60	>1.4 mmol/L
Sodium	135-145 mEq/l	135-145 mmol/L
Sulfate	0.5-1.5 mg/100 ml	0.05-1.2 mmol/L
Sulfonamide	0 mg/100 ml; therapeutic: 5-15 mg/100 ml	0 mmol/L
Transaminase (SGOT) (aspartate amino-transferase)	10-40 U/ml	0.08-0.32 μmol · s^{-1}/L
Urea nitrogen (BUN)	8-25 mg/100 ml	2.9-8.9 mmol/L
Uric acid	3.0-7.0 mg/100ml	0.18-0.42 mmol/L
Vitamin A	0.15-0.6 μg/ml	0.5-2.1 μmol/L
Vitamin A tolerance test	Rise to twice fasting level in 3 to 5 hr	

Urine Values

DETERMINATION	CONVENTIONAL	SI
Acetone plus acetoacetate (quantitative)	0	0 mg/L
Alpha amino nitrogen	64-199 mg/d; not over 1.5% of total nitrogen	4.6-14.2 mmol/d
Amylase	24-76 U/ml	24-76 arb. unit
Calcium	150 mg/d or less	$3.8 \leq$ mmol/d
Catecholamines	Epinephrine: under 20 μg/d	<55 nmol/d
	Norepinephrine: under 100 μmg/d	<590 nmol/d
Copper	0-100 μg/d	0-1.6 μmol/d
Coproporphyrin	50-250 μg/d	80-380 nmol/d
	Children under 80 lb 0-75 μg/d	
Creatine	Under 100 mg/d or less than 6% of creatine. In pregnancy: up to 12%. In children under 1 yr: may equal creatinine. In older children: up to 30% of creatinine	<0.75 mmol/d
Cystine or cysteine	0	0
Follicle-stimulating hormone:		
Follicular phase	5-30 IU/d	Same
Midcycle	15-60 IU/d	
Luteal phase	5-15 IU/d	
Menopausal	50-100 IU/d	
Men	5-25 IU/d	
Hemoglobin and myoglobin	0	
5-Hydroxyindole acetic acid	2-9 mg/d (women lower than men)	10-45 μmol/d
Lead	0.08 μg/ml or 120 μg or less/d	$\leq$0.39 μmol/L
Phenolsulfonphthalein (PSP)	At least 25% excreted by 15 min, 40% by 30 min; 60% by 120 min	0.25 l
Phosphorus (inorganic)	Varies with intake; average 1 g/d	32 mmol/d
Porphobilinogen	0	0
Protein:		
Quantitative	<150 mg/d	<0.15 g/d
Steroids		

17-Ketosteroids (per day)	Age	Male (mg)	Female (mg)	Male (μmol/d)	Female (μmol/d)
	10	1-4	1-4	3-14	3-14
	20	6-21	4-16	21-73	14-56
	30	8-26	4-14	28-90	14-49
	50	5-18	3-9	17-62	10-31
	70	2-10	1-7	7-35	3-24

DETERMINATION	CONVENTIONAL	SI
17-Hydroxysteroids	3-8 mg/d (women lower than men)	8-22 μmol/d as hydrocotrisone
Sugar		
Quantitative glucose	0	0 mmol/L
Identification of reducing substances		
Fructose	0	0 mmol/L
Pentose	0	0 mmol/L
Titratable acidity	24-40 mEq/d	20-40 mmol/L
Urobilinogen	Up to 1.0 Ehrlich U	To 1.0 arb. unit
Uroporphyrin	0	0 nmol/d
Vanillylmandelic acid (VMA)	Up to 9 mg/d	Up to 45 μmol/d

Continued.

Special Endocrine Tests

	REFERENCE RANGE	
DETERMINATION	**CONVENTIONAL**	**SI**
STEROID HORMONES		
Aldosterone	Excretion: 5-19 μg/d	14-53 nmol/d
Fasting, at rest,	Supine: 48 ± 29 pg/ml	180 ± 64 pmol/L
210 mEq sodium diet	Upright: (2 hr) 65 ± 23 pg/ml	
Fasting, at rest,	Supine: 107 ± 45 pg/ml	279 ± 125 pmol/L
110 mEq sodium diet	Upright: (2 hr) 239 ± 123 pg/ml	663 ± 341 pmol/L
Fasting, at rest,	Supine: 175 ± 75 pg/ml	485 ± 208 pmol/L
10 mEq sodium diet	Upright: (2 hr) 532 ± 228 pg/ml	1476 ± 632 pmol/L
Cortisol		
Fasting	8 AM: 5-25 μg/100 ml	0.14-0.69 μmol/L
At rest	8 PM: Below 10 μg/100 ml	0-0.28 μmol/L
20 U ACTH	4 hr ACTH test: 30-45 μg/100 ml	0.83-1.24 μmol/L
Dexamethasone at midnight	Overnight suppression test: Below 5 μg/100 ml	<0.14 nmol/L
	Excretion: 20-70 μg/d	55-193 nmol/d
11-Deoxycortisol	Responsive: over 7.5 μg/100 ml (after metyrapone)	>0.22 μmol/L
Testosterone	Adult male: 300-1100 ng/100 ml	10.4-38.1 nmol/L
	Adolescent male: over 100 ng/100 ml	>3.5 nmol/L
	Female: 25-90 ng/100 ml	0.87-3.12 nmol/L
Unbound testosterone	Adult male: 3.06-24.0 ng/100 ml	106-832 pmol/L
	Adult female: 0.09-1.28 ng/100 ml	3.1-44.4 pmol/L
POLYPEPTIDE HORMONES		
Adrenocorticotropin (ACTH)	15-70 pg/ml	3.3-15.4 pmol/L
Calcitonin	Undetectable in normals	0
	>100 pg/ml in medullary carcinoma	>29.3 pmol/L
Growth hormone		
Fasting, at rest	Below 5 ng/ml	<233 pmol/L
After exercise	Child: Over 10 ng/ml	>465 pmol/L
	Male: Below 5 ng/ml	<233 pmol/L
	Female: Up to 30 ng/ml	0-1395 pmol/L
After glucose	Male: Below 5 ng/ml	<233 pmol/L
	Female: Below 10 ng/ml	0-465 pmol/L
Insulin		
Fasting	6-26 μU/ml	43-187 pmol/L
During hypoglycemia	Below 20 μU/ml	<144 pmol/L
After glucose	Up to 150 μU/ml	0-1078 pmol/L
Leuteinizing hormone	Male: 6-18 mU/ml	6-18 u/L
Pre- or postovulatory	Female: 5-22 mU/ml	5-22 u/L
Midcycle peak	30-250 mU/ml	30-250 u/L
Parathyroid hormone	<10 μl equiv/ml	<10 mEq/L
Prolactin	2-15 ng/ml	0.08-6.0 nmol/L
Renin activity		
Normal diet	Supine: 1.1 ± 0.8 ng/ml/hr	0.9 ± 0.6 (nmol/L)hr
	Upright: 1.9 ± 1.7 ng/ml/hr	1.5 ± 1.3 (nmol/L)hr
Low-sodium diet	Supine: 2.7 ± 1.8 ng/ml/hr	2.1 ± 1.4 (nmol/L)hr
	Upright: 6.6 ± 2.5 ng/ml/hr	5.1 ± 1.9 (nmol/L)hr
Low-sodium diet	Diuretics: 10.0 ± 3.7 ng/ml/hr	7.7 ± 2.9 (nmol/L)hr
THYROID HORMONES		
Thyroid-stimulating hormone (TSH)	0.5-3.5 μU/ml	0.5-3.5 mU/L
Thyroxine-binding globulin capacity	15-25 μg T_4/100 ml	193-322 nmol/L
Total triiodothyronine by radioimmunoassay (T_3)	70-190 ng/100 ml	1.08-2.92 nmol/L
Total thryoxine by RIA (T_4)	4-12 μg/100 ml	52-154 nmol/L
T_3 resin uptake	25%-35%	0.25-0.35
Free thyroxine index (FT_4I)	1-4 ng/100 ml	12.8-51.2 pmol/L

Hematologic Values

DETERMINATION	REFERENCE RANGE	
	CONVENTIONAL	SI
Coagulation factors		
Factor I (fibrinogen)	0.15-0.35 g/100 ml	4.0-10.0 μmol/L
Factor II (prothrombin)	60%-140%	0.60-1.40
Factor V (accelerator globulin)	60%-140%	0.60-1.40
Factor VII-X (proconvertin-Stuart)	70%-130%	0.70-1.30
Factor X (Stuart factor)	70%-130%	0.70-1.30
Factor VIII (antihemophilic globulin)	50%-200%	0.50-2.0
Factor IX (plasma thromboplastic cofactor)	60%-140%	0.60-1.40
Factor XI (plasma thromboplastic antecedent)	60%-140%	0.60-1.40
Factor XII (Hageman factor)	60%-140%	0.60-1.40
Coagulation screening tests		
Bleeding time (Simplate)	3-9 min	180-540 sec
Prothrombin time	Less than 2-sec deviation from control	Less than 2-sec deviation from control
Partial thromboplastin time (activated)	25-37 sec	25-37 sec
Whole-blood clot lysis	No clot lysis in 24 hr	0/d
Fibrinolytic studies		
Euglobin lysis	No lysis in 2 hr	0 (in 2 hr)
Fibrinogen split products	Negative reaction at greater than 1:4 dilution	0 (at > 1:4 dilution)
Thrombin time	Control ± 5 sec	Control ± 5 sec
Complete blood count		
Hematocrit	Male: 45%-52%	Male: 0.42-0.52
	Female: 37%-48%	Female: 0.37-0.48
Hemoglobin	Male: 13-18 g/100 ml	Male: 8.1-11.2 mmol/L
	Female: 12-16 g/100 ml	Female: 7.4-9.9 mmol/L
Leukocyte count	4300-10,800/mm³	4.3-10.8 × 10⁹/L
Erythrocyte count	4.2-5.9 10⁶/mm³	4.2-5.9 × 10¹²/l
Mean corpuscular volume (MCV)	80-94 μm³	80-94 fl
Mean corpuscular hemoglobin (MCH)	27-32 pg	1.7-2.0 fmol
Mean corpuscular hemoglobin concentration (MCHC)	32%-36%	19-22.8 mmol/L
Erythrocyte sedimentation rate (Westergren method)	Male: 1-13 mm/hr	Male: 1-13 mm/hr
	Female: 1-20 mm/hr	Female: 1-20 mm/hr
Erythrocyte enzymes		
Glucose-6-phosphate dehydrogenase	5-15 U/gHb	5-15 U/g
Pyruvate kinase	13-17 U/gHb	13-17 U/g
Ferritin (serum)		
Iron deficiency	0-20 ng/ml	0-20 μg/L
Iron excess	Greater than 400 ng/L	>400 μg/L
Folic acid		
Normal	Greater than 1.9 ng/ml	>4.3 mmol/L
Borderline	1.0-1.9 ng/ml	2.3-4.3 mmol/L
Haptoglobin	100-300 mg/100 ml	1.0-3.0 g/L
Hemoglobin studies		
Electrophoresis for A₂ hemoglobin	1.5%-3.5%	0.015-0.035
Hemoglobin F (fetal hemoglobin)	Less than 2%	<0.02
Hemoglobin, met- and sulf-	0	0
Serum hemoglobin	2-3 mg/100 ml	1.2-1.9 μmol/L
Thermolabile hemoglobin	0	0
LE (lupus erythematosus) preparation		
Heparin as anticoagulant	0	0
Defibrinated blood	0	0
Leukocyte alkaline phosphatase		
Quantitative method	15-40 mg of phosphorus liberated/hr 10¹⁰ cells	15-40 mg/hr
Qualitative method	Males: 33-188 U	33-188 U
	Females: (off contraceptive pill): 30-160 U	30-160 U

Continued.

Hematologic Values—cont'd

DETERMINATION	REFERENCE RANGE	
	CONVENTIONAL	SI
Muramidase	Serum, 3-7 μg/ml	3-7 mg/L
	Urine, 0-2 μg/ml	0-2 mg/L
Osmotic fragility of erythrocytes	Increased if hemolysis occurs in over 0.5% NaCl; decreased if hemolysis is incomplete in 0.3% of NaCl	
Peroxide hemolysis	Less than 10%	<0.10
Platelet count	150,000-350,000/mm³	150-350 $\times$ 10⁹/L
Clot reaction	50%-100%/2 hr	0.50-1.00/2 hr
Platelet aggregation	Full response to ADP, epinephrine, and collagen	1.0
Platelet factor 3	33-57 sec	33-57 sec
Reticulocyte count	0.5%-1.5% red cells	0.005-0.015
Vitamin B₁₂	90-280 pg/ml (borderline: 70-90)	66-207 pmol/L (borderline: 52-66)

Cerebrospinal Fluid Values

DETERMINATION	REFERENCE RANGE		DETERMINATION	REFERENCE RANGE	
	CONVENTIONAL	SI		CONVENTIONAL	SI
Bilirubin	0	0 μmol/L	Glucose	50-75 mg/100 ml (30-50% less than blood)	2.8-4.2 mmol/L
Chloride	120-130 mEq/L (20 mEq/L higher than serum)		Pressure (initial)	70-180 mm of water	70-80 arb. units
Albumin	Mean: 29.5 mg/100 ml	0.295 g/L	Protein		
	$\pm$2 SD: 11-48 mg/100 ml	$\pm$2 SD: 0.11-0.48	Lumbar	15-45 mg/100 ml	0.15-0.45 g/L
			Cisternal	15-25 mg/100 ml	0.15-0.25 g/L
IgG	Mean: 4.3 mg/100 ml	0.043 g/L	Ventricular	5-15 mg/100 ml	0.05-0.15 g/L
	$\pm$2 SD: 0-8.6 mg/100 ml	$\pm$2 SD: 0-0.086			

Miscellaneous Values

	REFERENCE RANGE	
DETERMINATION	**CONVENTIONAL**	**SI**
Autoantibodies in serum		
Thyroid colloid and microsomal antigens	Absent	
Stomach parietal cells	Absent	
Smooth muscle	Absent	
Kidney mitochondria	Absent	
Rabbit renal collecting ducts	Absent	
Cytoplasm of ova, theca cells, testicular interstitial cells	Absent	
Skeletal muscle	Absent	
Adrenal gland	Absent	
Carcinoembryonic antigen (CEA) in blood	0-2.5 ng/ml, 97% healthy nonsmokers	0-2.5 μg/L, 97% healthy nonsmokers
Cryoprecipitable proteins in blood	0	0 arb. unit
Digitoxin in serum	17 $\pm$ 6 ng/ml	22 $\pm$ 7.8 nmol/L
Digoxin in serum		
0.25 mg/d	1.2 $\pm$ 0.4 ng/ml	1.54 $\pm$ 0.5 nmol/L
0.5 mg/d	1.5 $\pm$ 0.4 ng/ml	1.92 $\pm$ 0.5 nmol/L
Duodenal drainage:		
pH	5.5-7.5	5.5-7.5
Amylase	Over 1200 U/total sample	>1.2 arb. unit
Trypsin	Values from 35%-160% "normal"	0.35-1.60
Viscosity	3 min or less	180 sec or less
Gastric analysis	Basal	0.6 $\pm$ 0.5
	Females 2.0 $\pm$ 1.8 mEq/hr	0.8 $\pm$ 0.6 μmol/sec
	Males 3.0 $\pm$ 2.0 mEq/hr	
	Maximal (after histalog or gastrin)	4.4 $\pm$ 1.4 μmol/sec
	Females 16 $\pm$ 5 mEq/hr	6.4 $\pm$ 1.4 μmol/sec
	Males 23 $\pm$ 5 mEq/hr	
Gastrin-1 in blood	0-200 pg/ml	0-95 pmol/L
Immunological tests		
Alpha-feto-globulin	Abnormal if present	
Alpha 1-antitrypsin	200-400 mg/100 ml	2.0-4.0 g/L
Antinuclear antibodies	Positive if detected with serum diluted 1:10	
Anti-DNA antibodies	Less than 15 units/ml	
Complement, total hemolytic	150-250 U/ml	
C3	Range 55-120 mg/100 ml	0.55-1.2 g/L
C4	Range 20-50 mg/100 ml	0.2-0.5 g/L
Immunoglobulins in blood:		
IgG	1140 mg/100 ml	11.4 g/L
	Range 540-1663	5.5-16.6 g/L
IgA	214 mg/100 ml	2.14 g/L
	Range 66-344	0.66-3.44 g/L
IgM	168 mg/100 ml	1.68 g/L
	Range 39-290	0.39-2.9 g/l
Viscosity	1.4-1.8 expressed as relative viscosity of serum compared to water	
Iontophoresis	Children: 0-40 mEq sodium/L	0-40 mmol/L
	Adults: 0-60 mEq sodium/L	0-60 mmol/L
Propranolol (includes bioactive 4-OH metabolite) in serum 4 hr after last does	100-300 ng/ml	386-1158 nmol/L
Stool fat	Less than 5 g in 24 hr or less than 4% of measured fat intake in 3-day period	<5 g/day
Stool nitrogen	Less than 2 g/day or 10% of urinary nitrogen	<2 g/day

Continued.

Miscellaneous Values—cont'd

DETERMINATION	REFERENCE RANGE	
	CONVENTIONAL	SI
Synovial fluid		
Glucose	Not less than 20 mg/100 ml lower than simultaneously drawn blood sugar	See blood glucose mmol/L
Mucin	Type 1 or 2	1-2 arb. unit
	Grades as:	
	Type 1-tight clump	
	Type 2-soft clump	
	Type 3-soft clump that breaks up	
	Type 4-cloudy, no clump	
D-Xylose absorption	5-8 g/5 hr in urine	33-53 mmol
	40 mg/100 ml in blood 2 hr after ingestion of 25 g of D-Xylose	2.7 mmol/L

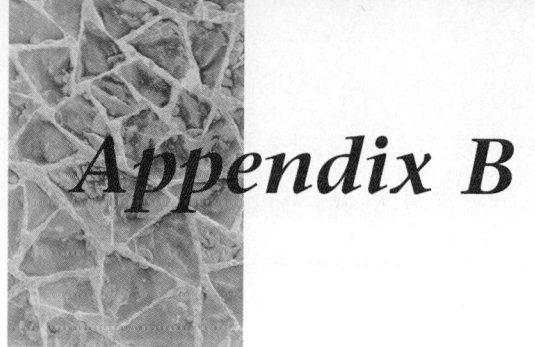

Appendix B

Height and Weight Table: Weights for Persons 29 to 59 Years According to Build*

	Men					Women		
Height[†]		**Small Frame**	**Medium Frame**	**Large Frame**	**Height**[†]		**Small Frame**	**Medium Frame**	**Large Frame**
Feet	**Inches**				**Feet**	**Inches**			
5	2	128-134	131-141	138-150	4	10	102-111	109-121	118-131
5	3	130-136	133-143	140-153	4	11	103-113	111-123	120-134
5	4	132-138	135-145	142-156	5	0	104-115	113-126	122-137
5	5	134-140	137-148	144-160	5	1	106-118	115-129	125-140
5	6	136-142	139-151	146-164	5	2	108-121	118-132	128-143
5	7	138-145	142-154	149-168	5	3	111-124	121-135	131-147
5	8	140-148	145-157	152-172	5	4	114-127	124-138	134-151
5	9	142-151	148-160	155-176	5	5	117-130	124-141	137-155
5	10	144-154	151-163	158-180	5	6	120-133	130-144	140-159
5	11	146-157	154-166	161-184	5	7	123-136	133-147	143-163
6	0	149-160	157-170	164-188	5	8	126-139	133-150	146-167
6	1	152-164	160-174	168-192	5	9	129-142	139-153	149-170
6	2	155-168	164-178	172-197	5	10	132-145	142-156	152-173
6	3	158-172	167-182	176-202	5	11	135-148	145-159	155-176
6	4	162-176	171-187	181-207	6	0	138-151	148-162	158-179

Source of basic data *Build study,* Society of Actuaries and Association of LIfe Insurance Medical Directors of America, 1980. Copyright 1983 Metropolitan Life Insurance Company.
*Indoor clothing weighing 5 pounds for men and 3 pounds for women.
†Shoes with 1-inch heels.

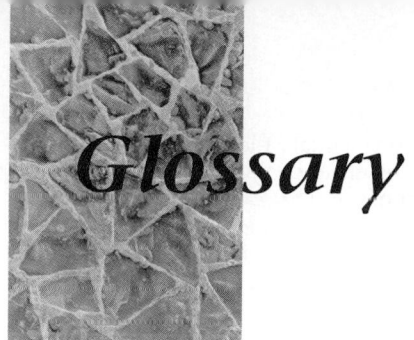

Glossary

ablate (ablation) An amputation, an excision of any body part, or removal of a growth or harmful substance.

abnormal reactive hyperemia Hyperemia over a pressure site lasting longer than 1 hour following removal of pressure; surrounding skin does not blanch.

abrasion Scraping or rubbing away of epidermis; may result in localized bleeding and later weeping of serous fluid.

absorption The passage of substances across and into tissues (e.g., intestinal and parenteral absorption).

abstract A short summary of the purpose of a study, the subjects included in the research, the way the study was conducted, and the results obtained in the investigation.

accessory muscles Muscles in the anterior thorax that increase or decrease chest expansion (e.g., sternocleidomastoid, trapezius).

accountability State of being answerable for one's actions—the professional nurse answers to the self, the client, the profession, the employing institution, and society for the effectiveness of nursing care performed.

accrediting (accreditation) A process whereby a professional association or nongovernmental body grants recognition to a school or institution for demonstrated ability in a special area of practice or training, as the accreditation of hospitals by the Joint Commission of Accreditation for Hospitals or of nursing schools by the National League for Nursing.

acculturation Process of intercultural borrowing between diverse peoples, resulting in new and blended patterns.

acne Inflammatory, papulopustular skin eruption, usually occurring on the face, neck, shoulders, and upper back.

acquired immunodeficiency syndrome A disease involving a defect in cell-mediated immunity that has a long incubation period, follows a protracted and debilitating course, is manifested by recurrent opportunistic infections, and has a poor prognosis.

acromegaly Chronic metabolic condition caused by overproduction of growth hormone and characterized by gradual, marked enlargement and elongation of bones of the face, jaw, and extremities.

active strategies of health promotion Activities that depend on the client being motivated to adopt a specific health program.

active transport Movement of materials across the cell membrane by means of chemical activity that allows the cell to admit larger molecules than would otherwise be possible.

activities of daily living Activities usually performed in the course of a normal day in the client's life, such as eating, dressing, bathing, brushing the teeth, and grooming.

activity tolerance Kind and amount of exercise or work that a person is able to perform.

actual health care problem Health problem currently being perceived or experienced by the client.

acuity charting Mechanism by which entries describing client care activities are made over a 24-hour period. The activities are then translated into a rating score or acuity score that allows for a comparison of clients who vary by severity of illness.

acupressure A therapeutic technique of applying digital pressure in a specified way on designated points on the body to relieve pain, produce anesthesia, or regulate body function.

acute illness Illness characterized by symptoms that are of relatively short duration, are usually severe, and affect the functioning of the client in all dimensions.

adaptation Process by which changes occur in any of a person's dimensions in response to stress.

adolescence The period of development between the onset of puberty and adulthood.

adult day care Services within the community that are directed toward the needs of older adults who require assistance with medications, eating, and supervision.

advance directives A written agreement established between a client and physician to withhold heroic measures or life-sustaining treatment if the patient's condition becomes irreversible. Advance directives are usually written at a time when clients are healthy or able to make conscious decisions regarding their welfare.

advanced practice nurse (APN) A nurse with a master's degree in nursing, advanced education in pharmacology and physical assessment, and certification and expertise in a specialized area of practice. An APN usually works in a critical, acute, restorative, or community health care agency.

adventitious sounds Abnormal lung sounds heard with auscultation.

adverse reaction Harmful or unintended effect of a medication, diagnostic test, or therapeutic intervention.

advocacy Process whereby a nurse objectively provides clients with the information they need to make decisions and supports clients in whatever decisions they make.

aerobic Of or pertaining to the presence of air or oxygen. Requiring oxygen for the maintenance of life.

aerobic metabolism Production of energy and body fuels by the tissues in the presence of oxygen.

afebrile Without fever.

affective learning Acquisition of behaviors involved in expressing feelings in attitudes, appreciations, and values.

afterload The resistance to ventricular ejection.

ageism Attitude that disadvantages, separates, and stigmatizes older adults on the basis of age-related characteristics.

agent Element of the agent-host-environment model of health and illness; any biological, chemical, physical or mechanical, or psychosocial factor whose presence or absence can lead to disease or illness.

agglutinins Antibodies that interact with antigens, resulting in agglutination.

air-lock technique An intramuscular technique, which is less irritating to the SQ tissues. A small volume of air is injected behind a bolus of medication, and the air clears the needle of medication and prevents tracking of the drug through the SQ tissue.

air pollution Contamination of the environmental atmosphere with substances known as pollutants that are not normally found in the air.

airway resistance The pressure difference between the mouth, nose, or other airway opening and the alveoli.

Allen's test A test for the patency of the radial artery. The client's hand is formed into a fist while the nurse compresses the ulnar artery. Compression of the ulnar artery is continued while the fist is opened. If blood perfusion through the radial artery is adequate, the hand should flush and resume normal pinkish coloration.

allergic reaction A hypersensitive response to an allergen to which an organism has previously been exposed and to which the organism has developed antibodies.

alopecia Partial or complete loss of hair; baldness.

Alzheimer's disease A brain disorder that causes gradual and progressive decline in cognitive functioning. The most frequent cause of irreversible dementia; also known as senile dementia of the Alzheimer type, or SDAT.

AMBULARM A safety device that alerts health care personnel that a client is attempting to get up. Provides an alternative to restraints.

ambulatory surgery Scheduled outpatient procedures provided for clients who do not remain overnight in a hospital.

amenorrhea Absence of menstruation.

American Nurses Association (ANA) Organization of professional nurses in the United States that focuses on standards of health care, nurses' professional development, and economic and general welfare of nurses.

amino acid An organic compound composed of one or more basic groups and one or more carboxyl groups. Amino acids are the building blocks that construct proteins and the end products of protein digestion.

anabolism Constructive metabolism characterized by conversion of simple substances into more complex compounds of living matter.

anaerobic The absence of oxygen.

anaerobic metabolism Production of energy and body fuels by the tissues without oxygen.

analgesic Relieving pain; a drug that relieves pain.

analogy Resemblance made between things otherwise unlike.

anemia Disorder characterized by a decrease in hemoglobin in the blood.

aneurysm Localized dilation of the wall of a blood vessel, usually caused by atherosclerosis, hypertension, or a congenital weakness in the vessel wall.

angina pectoris Episodic chest pain caused most often by myocardial anoxia, resulting from atherosclerosis of the coronary arteries. Pain radiates down the inner aspect of the left arm and is often accompanied by feeling of suffocation and impending death.

angiography A radiographic visualization of internal anatomy of the heart and blood vessels after the introduction of a radiopaque contrast medium.

animism The attribution of life to inanimate; objects often results in statements such as "Trees cry when their branches are broken."

anions Negatively charged electrolytes.

anonymity Nondisclosure of a client's or other person's name or identification, such as is used in research to ensure the privacy of research subjects.

anorexia nervosa A disease characterized by a prolonged refusal to eat, resulting in emaciation, amenorrhea, emotional disturbance concerning body image, and an abnormal fear of becoming obese.

antagonistic muscles Group of muscles that work together to bring about movement at the joint.

anthropometry Measurement of various body parts to determine nutritional and caloric status, muscular development, brain growth, and other parameters.

antibody Immunoglobulin, essential to the immune system, that is produced by lymphoid tissue in response to bacteria, viruses, or other antigens.

anticipatory grief Grief response in which the person begins the grieving process before an actual loss.

antiembolic stockings Elasticized stockings that prevent formation of emboli and thrombi, especially after surgery or during bed rest.

antigen Substance, usually a protein, that causes the formation of an antibody and reacts specifically with that antibody.

antigravity muscles Muscles involved with stabilization of joints by opposing the effect of gravity on the body.

antipyretic Of or pertaining to a substance or procedure that reduces fever.

anuria Cessation of urine production.

Apgar score Rating describing a newborn's physiological status at birth and thereafter. Assists in determining the newborn's ability to adjust to extrauterine life.

aphasia Neurological disorder influencing the production and understanding of language.

apical impulse Point at which apex of the heart touches the anterior chest wall. Best site for auscultation of heart sounds. Also called PMI, point of maximal impulse.

apical pulse The heartbeat taken with the bell or diaphragm of a stethoscope placed on the apex, or pointed extremity of the heart.

apnea Cessation of airflow through the nose and mouth.

apocrine gland One of the large, deep exocrine glands located in the axillary, anal, genital, and mammary areas of the body; secretes sweat having a strong odor.

apothecary system A system of graduated liquid volumes based on the minim and on a system of graduated amounts arranged in order of heaviness and based on the grain.

approximate To come close together, as in the edges of a wound.

aquathermia pad A heat application unit that consists of a waterproof plastic or rubber pad connected by two hoses to an electrical control unit that has a heating element and motor.

arthritis An inflammatory condition of the joints, characterized by pain and swelling.

artificialism The belief that all things in the universe have been created by man (Piagetian term).

asepsis Absence of germs or microorganisms.

assault Unlawful threatening or inflicting of harm on another.

assertiveness (training) A technique focusing on the direct, honest statement of feelings and beliefs, both positive and negative, helping individuals become more self-assertive and self-confident.

assessment First step of the nursing process; activities required in the first step are data collection, data validation, data sorting, and data documentation. The purpose is to gather information for health problem identification.

association cortex Part of the cerebral cortex involved in the integration of sensory information, also called the association area.

asymptomatic Without symptoms.

atelectasis Collapse of alveoli, preventing the normal respiratory exchange of oxygen and carbon dioxide.

atherosclerosis Common arterial disorder characterized by yellowish plaques of cholesterol, lipids, and cellular debris in the inner layers of the walls of the large- and medium-sized arteries.

atrioventricular (AV) node A portion or the cardiac conduction system located on the floor of the right atrium; it receives electrical impulses from the atrium and transmits them to the bundle of His.

at risk health problem Alerts the nurse to the need for preventive interventions; the contributing factors for "risk" and "at risk" nursing diagnoses represent those situations that increase the vulnerability of a client or group.

atrophy Wasting or diminution of size or physiological activity of a part of the body caused by disease or other influences.

attachment The deep emotional tie between parent and child that is reciprocal and becomes progressively stronger during the first year.

attitudinal isolation Social isolation that occurs because of the older adult's personal or cultural values.

auditory Related to, or experienced through, hearing.

auscultation Act of listening for sounds within the body to evaluate the condition of body organs; usually performed with a stethoscope.

auscultatory gap Disappearance of sound when obtaining a blood pressure; typically occurs between the first and second Korotkoff's sounds.

autocratic leader A leadership style whereby the leader retains all authority and responsibility and is concerned with tasks and goal accomplishment. Control of employees with little delegation of decision making is characteristic of this style.

automated speech recognition Voice-recognition computer technology that allows an individual to speak and enter data into a computer through voice tones.

autonomy Ability or tendency to function independently.

autopsy Examination performed after a person's death to confirm or determine the cause of death.

autotransfusion The collection, anticoagulation, filtration, and reinfusion of blood from an active bleeding site.

bactericidal Destructive to bacteria.

bacteriostasis A state in which the development or reproduction of bacteria is suspended.

bacteriuria Presence of bacteria in the urine.

basal cell carcinoma A malignant, epithelial cell tumor that begins as a papule and enlarges peripherally, developing a central crater that erodes, crusts, and bleeds. Metastasis is rare. Primary cause is excessive exposure to the sun or to x-rays.

basal energy expenditure (BEE) A measurement of the amount of nutrients needed to meet the body's energy demands while maintaining a stable weight.

basal metabolism rate (BMR) Amount of energy used in a unit of time by a fasting, resting subject to maintain vital functions.

basic human needs Needs for things such as food, water, safety, and love, that people require to maintain vital functions.

battery Legal term for touching of another's body without consent.

bed rest Placement of the client in bed for therapeutic reasons for a prescribed period.

behavioral isolation Social isolation that occurs because of the older adult's socially unacceptable behaviors.

beneficence The doing or active promotion of doing good. One of the four principles of the ethical theory of deontology.

bereavement Response to loss through death; a subjective experience that a person suffers after losing a person with whom there has been a significant relationship.

bilirubinuria The abnormal presence of bilirubin in the urine.

binder Bandage made of a large piece of material to fit a specific body part.

bioavailability The degree of activity or amount of an administered drug or other substance that becomes available for activity in the target tissue.

biofeedback A behavioral therapy that involves giving individuals information about physiological responses (such as blood pressure or tension) and ways to exercise voluntary control over those responses.

biological clock Cyclical nature of body functions; functions controlled from within the body as synchronized with environmental factors; same meaning as biorhythm.

biomedical research Concerned mainly with discovering the causes and treatments of disease.

biopsy Removal of a small piece of living tissue from an organ or other part of the body for microscopic examination.

bisexual Sexual orientation involving erotic preferences for members of either sex.

blanching Whitening of the skin from pressure, vasoconstriction, hypotension.

blastocyst Embryonic form that arises as a cavity within the morula, where cellular differentiation begins.

blended family Family formed when parents bring together unrelated children from previous marriages.

blood pressure (BP) The pressure exerted by the circulating volume of blood on the walls of the arteries, veins, and chambers of the heart. The pressure in the aorta and the large arteries of a healthy young adult is approximately 120 mm Hg during systole and 70 mm Hg during diastole.

body image Mental picture of one's body internally and externally.

body mechanics Coordinated efforts of the musculoskeletal and nervous systems to maintain proper balance, posture, and body alignment.

bolus Round mass of chewed food ready to be swallowed.

bonding Parent's emotional tie to child that usually develops soon after birth as a result of their interaction.

bone resorption Destruction of bone cells and release of calcium into the blood.

borborygmus Audible abdominal sound produced by hyperactive intestinal peristalsis.

bowel training A program of exercises through which the client gains control of bowel reflexes by setting up a daily routine, attempting to defecate at the same time each day, and using measures that promote defecation.

bradycardia Slower than normal heart rate; heart contracts fewer than 60 times per minute.

bradypnea An abnormally slow rate of breathing. Also called oligopnea.

Braxton Hicks contraction Irregular, short uterine contractions.

broad-spectrum antibiotic An antibiotic that is effective against a wide range of infectious microorganisms.

bronchophony An increase in intensity and clarity of the vocal resonance that may result from an increase in the lung tissue density, such as in the consolidation of pneumonia.

bronchoscopy Visual examination of the tracheal and bronchial tree using a flexible fiberoptic bronchoscope.

bruit Abnormal sound or murmur heard while auscultating an organ, gland, or artery.

buccal Of or pertaining to the inside of the cheek or the gum next to the cheek.

buffer Substance or group of substances that can absorb or release hydrogen ions to correct an acid-base imbalance.

bulbar synchronizing region (BSR) Area in the pons and medial forebrain region releasing serotonin from specialized cells believed to aid in sleep.

bulimia nervosa An insatiable craving for food, often resulting in episodes of continuous eating, and often followed by purging, depression, and self-deprivation.

bundle of His A portion of the cardiac conduction system that arises from the distal portion of the AV node and extends across the AV groove to the top of the intraventricular septum, where it divides into right and left bundle branches.

burnout Popular term for the condition of mental or physical energy depletion after a period of chronic, unrelieved job-related stress characterized sometimes by physical illness.

cachexia General ill health and malnutrition marked by weakness and emaciation.

calorie Amount of heat required to raise 1 gram of water 1° centigrade at atmospheric pressure; a kilocalorie or large calorie, used to represent energy values of food, is 1000 times as large as the small calorie, the unit used in physics to describe energy exchange in the body.

Canadian Nurses Association (CNA) Organization of professional nurses in Canada that focuses on standards of health care, nurses' professional development, and economic and general welfare of nurses.

capillary closing pressure The pressure needed to close the capillaries, e.g., when the pressure exceeds the normal capillary pressure range of 16 to 32 mm Hg.

capitation A method of paying a physician, hospital, or managed care system for annual services based on a fee per client.

carbohydrates Dietary classification of foods comprising sugars, starches, cellulose, and gum.

carbon monoxide (CO) Colorless, odorless, poisonous gas produced by the combustion of carbon or organic fuels.

cardiac catheterization A diagnostic procedure in which a catheter is introduced into a large vein, usually of an arm or leg, and threaded through the circulatory system to the heart.

cardiac output The volume of blood expelled by the ventricles of the heart, equal to the amount of blood ejected at each beat (the stroke output), multiplied by the number of beats in the period of time used in the computation.

cardiopulmonary rehabilitation Process of actively assisting the cardiopulmonary client to achieve and maintain an optimal level of health through controlled physical exercise, nutritional counseling, relaxation and stress management techniques, prescribed medication, oxygen therapy, and adherence to the rehabilitation program.

cardiopulmonary resuscitation (CPR) Basic emergency procedures for life support consisting of artificial respiration and manual external cardiac massage.

CareMap® A multidisciplinary collaborative treatment plan that details the series of interventions and anticipated outcomes for specific clients of a selected case type across a course of treatment or hospital stay. A trademark and concept of The Center for Case Management, South Natick, Massachusetts.

caries An abnormal condition of a tooth characterized by decay.

caring The sense of dedication to another person.

carrier Animal or person who harbors and spreads a disease-causing organism but who does not become ill.

cartilage Nonvascular, supporting connective tissue located mainly in the joints and in the thorax, trachea, larynx, nose, and ear.

cartilaginous joint Slightly movable, highly elastic cartilage that unites bony surfaces.

case management Organized system for delivering health care to an individual client or group of clients. Includes assessment and development of a plan of care, coordination of all services, referral, and follow-up; usually assigned to one professional.

catabolism Complex metabolic process in which energy is liberated for use in work, energy, storage, or heat production by oxidation of carbohydrates, lipids, and proteins; carbon dioxide and water, as well as energy, are produced.

cataplexy Condition characterized by sudden muscular weakness and loss of muscle tone.

cathartic Drug that acts to promote bowel evacuation.

catheterization Introduction of a catheter into a body cavity or organ to inject or remove fluid.

cations Positively charged electrolytes.

center of gravity Midpoint or center of the weight of a body or object.

centigrade Denotes a temperature scale in which 0° is the freezing point of water and 100° is the boiling point of water at sea level; also called Celsius.

certified nurse-midwife (CNM) Nurse who is educated in midwifery and possesses certification in accordance with criteria of the American College of Midwives.

cerumen Waxy substance secreted in the ear.

Chadwick's sign A bluish appearance of the cervix is an early sign of pregnancy.

chancre Small open ulcers that drain serous material, found on genitalia and are associated with syphilis.

change Dynamic process by which alterations occur within the behavior and function of a person, family, group, or community.

change-of-shift reports Reports that occur between two scheduled nursing work shifts. Nurses communicate information about their assigned clients to nurses working on the next shift of duty.

change process *See* change.

channel A passageway or groove that conveys fluid, as the central channels that connect the arterioles with the venules.

charting by exception A charting methodology in which data is entered only when there is an exception from what is normal or expected. Reduces time spent documenting.

cheilosis Disorder of the lips and mouth characterized by scales and fissures.

chest percussion Striking the chest wall with a cupped hand to promote mobilization and drainage of pulmonary secretions.

chest physiotherapy Group of therapies used to mobilize pulmonary secretions.

chest tube A catheter inserted through the thorax into the chest cavity for removing air or fluid; used following chest or heart surgery or pneumothorax.

cholecystectomy Surgical removal of the gallbladder.

cholecystitis Inflammation of the gallbladder; may be acute or chronic.

chordotomy Surgical resection of the anterolateral nerve tracts in the spinal cord for pain relief.

chronic illness Illness that persists over a long period of time and affects physical, emotional, intellectual, social, and spiritual functioning.

chronic obstructive pulmonary disease (COPD) A progressive and irreversible condition characterized by diminished inspiratory and expiratory capacity of the lungs.

chyme Viscous, semifluid contents of the stomach present during digestion of a meal, which eventually passes into the intestines.

circadian rhythm Repetition of certain physiological phenomena within a 24-hour cycle.

circulating nurse Assistant to the scrub nurse and surgeon whose role is to provide necessary supplies, dispose of soiled instruments and supplies, and keep an accurate count of instruments, needles, and sponges used.

cirrhosis Chronic degenerative disease of the liver.

citation Reference notation to the source of an idea or quotation.

civil law The law established by a nation or state for its own jurisdiction.

clarification Restating what has been stated or sent to the receiver of a communicated message.

classification A mental process during the school years. The young child can separate objects into groups according to shape or color, but the school-age child understands that the same element can exist in two classes at the same time.

client-centered goal Specific measurable objective designed to reflect the client's highest possible level of wellness and independence in function.

climacteric Physiological, developmental change that occurs in the male reproductive system between the ages of 45 and 60.

clinical nurse specialist (CNS) Nurse with a master's degree in nursing and expertise in a specific area of practice.

clinical nursing problem A difference between the way things are and the way they ought to be in a clinical situation, or between what one knows and what one needs to know to eliminate the clinical problem.

clubbing A bulging of the tissues at the nail base that is due to insufficient oxygenation at the periphery resulting from conditions such as chronic emphysema and congenital heart disease.

cognitive learning Acquisition of intellectual skills that encompass behaviors such as thinking, understanding, and evaluating.

coitus interruptus Withdrawal of the penis from the vagina during intercourse before ejaculation. While ineffective, it is often practiced by adolescents as a method of contraception.

colitis Inflammatory condition of the large intestine.

collaboration The working together of health team members in the delivery of care to a client or group of clients.

collaborative intervention Therapy that requires the knowledge, skill, and expertise of multiple health care professionals.

collagen Substance that combines to form the white, glistening, inelastic fibers of tendons, ligaments, and fasciae.

colon Portion of the large intestine from the cecum to the rectum.

colonized Referring to the establishment of a mass of microorganisms, often nonpathogenic, in or on the body.

colostomy Surgical formation of an opening of the colon onto the surface of the abdomen through which fecal matter is emptied.

common law One source for law that is created by judicial decisions as opposed to those created by legislative bodies (statutory law).

communicable disease Any disease that can be transmitted from one person or animal to another by direct or indirect contact, or by vectors.

communication Ongoing, dynamic series of events that involves the transmission of information or feelings from sender to receiver.

comparison group Group of subjects in a study who are equivalent to the subjects in the experimental group but do not receive the treatment or intervention the study is examining; also known as a control group.

complement An inactive protein compound found in blood serum. It is activated when an antigen and antibody bind together. After a complement is activated, a rapid sequence of catalytic activity changes the shape of antigenic cells.

compliance Person's fulfillment of the prescribed course of treatment.

compress Soft pad of gauze or cloth used to apply heat, cold, or medications to the surface of a body part.

computer-based patient care record (CPCR) A comprehensive computerized system utilized by all health care practitioners to permanently store information pertaining to a client's health status, clinical problems, and functional abilities. The CPCR can store numerous data bases including structured assessment data, clinical decision support systems, and diagnostic artificial intelligence. The CPCR will store information pertaining to a given client from any health care event, providing access to information across a client's lifespan.

concentration (concentrate) A substance, particularly a liquid, that has been strengthened and reduced in volume though evaporation or other means.

conceptual model Global ideas of interest to the individuals, groups, situations, or events that pertain to a specific discipline.

concomitant symptoms Symptoms that accompany a primary symptom.

concrete operation A thought process based on concrete rather than abstract points of reference.

conductive hearing loss A form of hearing loss in which sound is inadequately conducted through the external or middle ear to the sensorineural apparatus of the inner ear.

confabulation Defense mechanism in which the person fabricates experiences or situations and often recounts them in a detailed and plausible way in order to fill in and cover up gaps in memory.

confidentiality Privacy; a nurse must maintain the confidentiality of information related to a client's health care.

Congress for Nursing Practice Unit of the ANA whose activities concern the scope of nursing practice, legal aspects of nursing practice, public recognition of the significance of nursing in health care, and implications of health care trends for nursing practice.

conjunctivitis A highly contagious eye infection. The crusty drainage that collects on eyelid margins can easily spread from one eye to the other.

connotative Tending to suggest meaning by a word apart from the thing it explicitly describes.

conservation The child's ability to recognize that the amount or quantity of a substance remains the same even when its shape or appearance changes.

constipation Condition characterized by difficulty in passing stool or an infrequent passage of hard stool.

consultation Process in which the help of a specialist is sought to identify ways to handle problems in client management or in the planning and implementation of programs.

continuing education Formal educational programs designed to further the knowledge, skills, and professional attitudes of practicing nurses.

contraception Prevention of pregnancy by means of a medication, device, or method that blocks or alters one or more of the processes of reproduction in such a way that sexual union can occur without impregnation.

contrast medium Radiopaque substance injected into the body to improve visualization of internal structures that are otherwise difficult to see on x-ray examination.

controlled substance A drug whose distribution is controlled by federal and/or state government regulation. An example is narcotics.

convalescence Period of recovery after an illness, injury, or surgery.

coping mechanism Any effort directed toward stress management, including task-oriented and ego-defense mechanisms.

core temperature Temperature of deep body tissues and organs.

corpus luteum Ovarian site of ruptured graafian follicle after ovulation. The corpus luteum is maintained through the secretory phase of the menstrual cycle and produces progesterone.

cough Sudden, audible expulsion of air from the lungs.

counseling Implementation method that helps the client use a problem-solving process to recognize and manage stress and that facilitates interpersonal relationships between the client and the family, significant others, or the health care team.

crepitus A crackling sound produced when an examiner palpates gas-filled tissue or when bone fragments rub together.

crime Act that violates a law and that may include criminal intent.

criminal law The law of crimes and their punishment.

crisis Stressful encounter with a change or obstacle to life goals that is perceived as insurmountable.

crisis intervention Use of therapeutic techniques directed toward helping a client resolve a particular and immediate problem.

crisis intervention centers Agencies providing emergency psychiatric and counseling assistance to clients experiencing extreme stress or conflict, often involving attempted suicide, drug or alcohol abuse, or other crisis behaviors.

critical pathway Tool used in managed care. A critical pathway incorporates the treatment interventions of care givers from all disciplines who normally care for a client. Designed for a specific case type, a pathway is used to manage the care of a client throughout a projected length of stay.

critical period The time when development of a specific attribute (physical, cognitive, or psychosocial) is most vulnerable to both advantageous and harmful agents.

critical thinking The examination of data, the gathering of information from the literature, the organization of observations, and drawing upon past experiences.

Crohn's disease Disease involving inflammation of the small intestine.

crutch gait Gait assumed by a person on crutches by alternately bearing weight on one or both legs and on the crutches.

culture Nonphysical traits such as values, beliefs, attitudes, and customs shared by a group and passed from one generation to the next.

cutaneous stimulation Stimulation of a person's skin to prevent or reduce pain perception. A massage, warm bath, application of liniment, hot and cold therapies, and transcutaneous electric nerve stimulation are some ways to reduce pain perception.

cyanosis Bluish discoloration of the skin and mucous membranes caused by deoxygenated hemoglobin in the blood or a structural defect in hemoglobin.

cystitis Inflammation of the urinary bladder, characterized by pain, urgency, and frequency of urination.

cystocele A portion of the vaginal wall and bladder may prolapse or fall into the anterior vaginal orifice.

cytolysis The rupturing of a cell wall, usually occurring after water or ions have entered the cell.

darkly pigmented skin The obvious color of intact dark skin remains unchanged (does not blanch) when pressure is applied over a bony prominence, irrespective of the client's race or ethnicity.

Data, Actions, client Response (DAR) The format used in focus charting for recording client information.

data base Information about a client's level of health, health practices, past illnesses, present illnesses, and physical exam combined to serves as the basis for the plan of care.

debridement Removal of dead tissue from a wound.

decenter A process that enables a child to concentrate on more than one aspect of a situation.

decibel Unit of measure of the intensity of sound.

decision making A process involving critical appraisal of information that results from recognition of a problem and ends with the generation, testing, and evaluation of a conclusion.

defamation of character To harm the reputation of a person by libel or slander.

defecation Passage of feces from the digestive tract through the rectum.

defining characteristics Cluster of signs and symptoms that are observed in the client having a specific nursing diagnosis.

dehiscence Separation of a wound's edges, revealing underlying tissues.

dehydration Excessive loss of water from the body tissues, accompanied by a disturbance of body electrolytes.

delegation The process of assigning another member of the health care team aspects of client care, e.g., assigning nurse assistants to bathe a client.

delirium Syndrome involving impairment of memory and other cognitive abilities and characterized by clouding of consciousness.

dementia Irreversible mental state characterized by decreased impairment of memory, intellectual function, and other cognitive abilities that can have a variety of causes.

democratic style People-centered leadership style in which the group participates openly in decision making for group goals.

demography Focusing on the distribution, density, and vital information about a population.

denotative Denoting or tending to denote.

depersonalization Extreme form of identity confusion in which a person is unable to distinguish between inner and outer realities or between the self and others.

depilatory Substance that removes hair.

dermatitis Inflammation of skin characterized by itching, redness, and skin lesions.

dermatome An area on the surface of a body innervated by afferent fibers from one spinal root.

dermis Layer of skin just below the epidermis, containing blood and lymphatic vessels, nerves and nerve endings, glands, and hair follicles.

desquamation Normal process in which the dead cells of the epidermal skin layer slough off.

development Qualitative or observable aspects of the progressive changes an individual makes in adapting to the environment.

developmental crises Occur when a person is unable to complete the developmental tasks of a psychosocial stage and is therefore unable to continue developing.

diagnostic process Process of determining a client's health status and evaluating the factors influencing that status.

diagnostic reasoning A process that enables an observer to assign meaning and to classify phenomena in clinical situations by integrating observations and critical thinking.

diagnosis related groups (DRGs) Group of patients classified for measuring a hospital's delivery of care; classification is based on the following variables: primary and secondary diagnosis, primary and secondary procedures, age, and length of stay.

diaphoresis Secretion of sweat, especially profuse secretion associated with an elevated body temperature, physical exertion, or emotional stress.

diaphragmatic breathing Respiration in which the abdomen moves out while the diaphragm descends on inspiration.

diarrhea Increase in the number of stools and the passage of liquid, unformed feces.

diastole Period of time between contractions of the atria or the ventricles during which blood enters the relaxed chambers.

diastolic pressure The minimum level of blood pressure measured between contractions of the heart.

diffusion Movement of molecules from an area of higher concentration to an area of lower concentration.

direct-question interview Type of inquiry that requires one- or two-word answers.

disability The loss, absence, or impairment of physical or mental fitness.

discharge planning Set of decisions and activities involved in providing continuity and coordination of nursing care when a client is discharged from a health care agency.

disenfranchised grief Occurs when persons experience a loss that is not or cannot be openly acknowledged, publicly mourned, or socially supported.

disinfection The process of killing pathogenic organisms.

dissociation Defense mechanism by which an idea, thought, emotion, or other mental process is separated from the unconsciousness and thereby loses emotional significance.

distention Swelling of a body cavity; may be caused by fluid, gas, or a mass.

diuresis Increased formation and excretion of urine.

diverticula Pouchlike herniations through the muscular wall of a tubular organ; may be present in the stomach, small intestine, or most commonly the colon.

diverticulitis An inflammatory disease of the diverticulum, which requires a moderate- or low-residue diet until the infection subsides.

documentation Act of authenticating events or activities by keeping written records.

drainage evacuators Convenient portable units that connect to tubular drains lying within a wound bed and exert a safe, constant, low-pressure vacuum to remove and collect drainage.

drug abuse Use of a chemical substance for nontherapeutic purposes that do not comply with cultural or social standards.

drug dependence Psychological or physiological reliance on a chemical agent.

drug interaction A modification of the effect of a drug when administered with food or another drug. The effect may increase or decrease the action of the drug or other substance.

drug rehabilitation centers Agencies providing long-term care for a gradual return to the community of a person with chemical or drug dependency.

durable medical equipment (DME) Equipment leased or sold to clients for use in their homes, e.g., wheelchairs, hospital beds, walkers, and canes.

durable power of attorney for health care A document that designates an agent or proxy to make health care decisions for a client who is unable to do so.

dysarthria Difficulty in articulating speech.

dysfunctional grief Actual or perceived object loss; objects may include people, possessions, a job, status, home, and parts of the body.

dyspareunia Painful intercourse for a woman.

dysphagia Difficulty in swallowing.

dyspnea A shortness of breath or difficulty in breathing that may be caused by certain heart or lung conditions or strenuous exercise.

dysrhythmia Deviation from the normal pattern of the heart beat.

dysuria Painful urination resulting from bacterial infection of the bladder and obstructive conditions of the urethra.

eccrine glands Two types of sweat glands; eccrine glands are present throughout the body and promote cooling by evaporation of their secretions.

echocardiography A diagnostic procedure that uses ultrasonic waves for studying the structure and motion of the heart.

ectropion Eversion of the eyelid, exposing the conjunctival membrane and part of the eyeball.

eczema Superficial dermatitis of unknown cause.

edema Abnormal accumulation of fluid in interstitial spaces of tissues.

ego-defense mechanism Unconscious behavior that protects a person from an emotional stress.

electrocardiogram A graphic record of the electrical activity of the myocardium.

electrolyte Element or compound that, when melted or dissolved in water or other solvent, dissociates into ions and can carry an electrical current.

electrophysiological study (EPS) An invasive measure of electrical activity. An electrode catheter is inserted into the right atrium, usually via the femoral vein. Electrical stimulation is then delivered through the catheter while ECG monitors and computers record the heart's electrical response to the stimulus.

embryo Stage of human development from implantation of the fertilized ovum to the eighth week of intrauterine life.

empirical data Information that has been collected through the human senses and can be verified through research.

endogenous infections Infections produced within a cell or organism.

endoscopy Visualization of the interior of body organs and cavities with an endoscope.

enema Procedure involving introduction of a solution into the rectum for cleansing or therapeutic purposes.

enteral nutrition Provision of nutrients through the gastrointestinal tract when the client cannot ingest, chew, or swallow food but can digest and absorb nutrients.

enterostomal therapist Specially trained nurse for care of clients with ostomies.

entropion A condition in which the eyelid turns inward toward the eye.

enuresis Involuntary passage of urine; incontinence.

environment The physical environment in which a person works or lives can increase the likelihood that certain illnesses will occur (e.g., some kinds of cancer and other diseases are more likely to develop when industrial workers are exposed to certain chemicals or when people live near toxic waste disposal sites).

enzyme Protein produced by living cells that catalyzes chemical reactions in organic matter.

epidemiology Study of the occurrence, distribution, and causes of disease.

epidermis Superficial, avascular layers of the skin, made up of an outer, dead, cornified portion of cells and a deeper, living cellular portion.

epidural Type of nerve block local anesthesia in which an anesthetic is injected in the lumbosacral region of the spinal cord to prevent or eliminate pain in the lower trunk and extremities.

epithelialization Refers to the stage of wound healing that is characterized by growth of epithelial tissue.

erythema Redness or inflammation of the skin or mucous membranes that is a result of dilation and congestion of superficial capillaries; sunburn is an example.

erythropoietin (EPO) A glycoprotein hormone synthesized mainly in the kidneys and released into the bloodstream in response to anoxia.

eschar Scab or dry crust that results from excoriation of the skin.

esteem and self-esteem needs The fourth level in Maslow's hierarchy of needs, which involve self-confidence, usefulness, achievement, and self-worth.

estrogen Hormonal steroid compound that promotes the development of female secondary sex characteristics.

ethic of care The delivery of health care based on ethical principles and standards of care.

ethics Principles or standards that govern proper conduct as they apply to professional issues or problems.

ethnicity Cultural group's sense of identification associated with the group's common social and cultural heritage.

ethnocentrism The strong belief that one's own cultural group is the best and that all that this group believes and teaches is truth.

etiology Identification of the cause of a problem. The cause may be a direct or a contributing factor in the development of a client problem or need.

euphoria An exaggerated sense of physical and emotional well-being.

eupnea Normal respiration that is quiet, effortless, and rhythmical.

euthanasia Deliberately bringing about the death of a person who is suffering from an incurable disease or condition; actively, as by administering a lethal drug, or passively, as by allowing the person to die without medical treatment.

evaluation Category of nursing behavior in which a determination is made and recorded regarding the extent to which the client's goals have been met.

evisceration Protrusion of visceral organs through a surgical wound.

exacerbation Increase in the seriousness of a disease or disorder as marked by greater intensity in signs or symptoms.

excoriation Injury to the skin's surface caused by abrasion.

exercise Performance of any physical activity for the purpose of conditioning the body, improving health, maintaining fitness, or as a therapeutic measure.

exercise stress test An evaluation of the client's cardiopulmonary endurance during physical activity. An ECG and analysis of respiratory function is usually performed during the test.

exogenous infection Infection originating outside an organ or part.

exophthalmos Abnormal protrusion of one or both eyeballs.

exostosis An abnormal benign growth on the surface of a bone.

expected outcome Expected condition of a client at the end of therapy or of a disease process, including the degree of wellness and the need for continuing care, medications, support, counseling, or education.

experiment Research study designed to examine a cause-and-effect relationship.

experimental group The group that receives some form of treatment or intervention in a clinical research project.

expressive aphasia Inability to name common objects or to express simple ideas in words or writing.

extended care facility Institution providing medical, nursing, or custodial care for clients over a prolonged period.

extended family Form of family composed of the nuclear family and all other relatives in both of the couple's families.

external stressor Stressor originating outside a person.

extracellular fluid Portion of the body fluid composed of the interstitial fluid and blood plasma.

exudate Fluid, cells, or other substances that have been slowly discharged from cells or blood vessels through small pores or breaks in cell membranes.

Fahrenheit A scale for measurement of temperature in which the boiling point of water is 212° and the freezing point is 32° at sea level.

faith As more than a set of beliefs but a way of relating to self, others, and God and integrating our past, present, and future with God as center.

family A group of people related by heredity, such as parents, children, and siblings. A group of interacting individuals composing a basic unit of society. Although concepts of what constitutes a family vary, the family usually has some degree of permanence, commitment, and attachment.

family as client Nursing perspective in which the family is viewed as a unit of interacting members having attributes, functions, and goals separate from those of the individual family members; the nurse provides care to the family as a whole.

family as context Nursing perspective in which the primary focus of care is on an individual within a family.

family diversity Recognition that different family forms exist, and that each family is unique in and of itself.

family functioning Focuses on the processes used by the family to achieve its goals. These processes include communication among family members, goal setting, conflict resolution, nurturing, and use of internal and external resources.

family functions Processes by which the family operates as a whole, including communication and manipulation of the environment for problem solving.

family health Phenomenon that is more than the sum of the health of individual family members, including the achievement of satisfying family functioning and the attainment of family goals.

family structure Composition of the family organization of relationships among family members.

fatty acids Nutrients composed of chains of carbon atoms and hydrogen atoms with an acid group on one end of the chain and a methyl group at the other.

febrile Pertaining to or characterized by an elevated body temperature.

feces Waste or excrement from the gastrointestinal tract.

feedback In communication theory, information produced by a receiver and perceived by a sender that informs the sender about the receiver's reaction to the message. Feedback is a cyclical part of the process of communication that regulates and modifies the content of messages.

felony Crime of a serious nature that carries a penalty of imprisonment or death.

fetus Stage of human development from the end of the embryonic period until birth.

fever Elevation in the hypothalamic set-point so that body temperature is regulated at a higher level.

fiber A nutrient that contains cellulose, pectin, hemicellulose, and lignin. Sources are mainly fruits and vegetables.

fiberoptic endoscope An optical instrument with a lens viewer, a long flexible tube, and a light source at the end. It allows viewing of structures at the tip of the tube and insertion of special instruments for biopsy.

fibrin Protein product formed from the action of thrombin on fibrinogen in the clotting process.

fibroblasts Cells that are responsible for collagen formation and are the only distinctive cell type within the dermis.

fibrocystic disease Characterized by lumpy painful breasts and sometimes nipple discharge. Symptoms are more apparent before the menstrual period.

fibrous joint Tough layer of fibrous connective tissue that binds bones firmly together.

fidelity The quality or state of being faithful.

fistula Abnormal passage from an internal organ to the body surface or between two internal organs.

flat bones Bones providing for structural contours of the skeleton.

flatulence Condition characterized by the accumulation of gas within the lumen of the intestines.

flatus Intestinal gas.

"flight-or-fight" response Set of physiological responses to a stressor that prepares a person to attempt to overcome or avoid stress.

flow sheet Document on which frequent observations or specific measurements are recorded.

fluid volume deficit An alteration characterized by the loss of fluids and electrolytes in an isotonic fashion.

fluid volume excess An alteration characterized by the abnormal retention of fluids and electrolytes in an isotonic fashion.

focus charting A charting methodology for structuring progress notes according to the focus of the note, e.g., symptoms and nursing diagnosis. Each note includes data, actions, and client response (DAR).

focusing Centering information on the key elements or concepts of the message that has been sent. Focusing eliminates vagueness in communication by limiting the area of discussion.

FOCUS-PDCA Acronym for a process improvement model that includes nine steps: Find a process to improve, organize a team, clarify knowledge of the process, understand sources of process variation, select the process improvement, and then plan, do, check, and act on the improvement. A multidisciplinary team familiar with a process of care participates in the FOCUS-PDCA activity.

Food and Drug Administration (FDA) Federal agency responsible for the enforcement of federal regulations regarding the manufacture and distribution of food, drugs, and cosmetics to ensure protection against the sale of impure or dangerous substances.

food poisoning Toxic processes resulting from the ingestion of a food contaminated by toxic substances or by bacteria containing toxins.

footboard Board placed perpendicular to the mattress, parallel to and touching the plantar surface of the client's foot, and used to maintain dorsiflexion of the feet.

footdrop An abnormal neuromuscular condition of the lower leg and foot, characterized by an inability to dorsiflex, or evert, the foot.

fracture Breakage of bone caused by violence to the body; disruption of bone tissue continuity.

friction Effect of rubbing or the resistance that a moving body meets from the surface on which it moves; a force that occurs in a direction to oppose movement.

frostbite Traumatic effect of extreme cold on the skin and subcutaneous tissues, first manifested by distinct pallor.

functional capacity The client's baseline level of functioning.

functional health patterns A method for organizing assessment data based on the level of client function in specific areas, e.g., mobility.

functional illiteracy An inability to read or comprehend above a fifth grade level.

fungus Simple parasitic plant dependent on other life forms for food.

gait Manner or style of walking, including rhythm, cadence, and speed.

gastrocolic reflex Mass peristaltic activity in the colon in response to food entering the stomach.

gastroscopy A diagnostic procedure that allows visualization of the esophagus, stomach, and duodenum; also called endoscopy.

gastrostomy tube feeding Long, hollow, flexible tube inserted into the stomach through a stab wound in the upper left abdominal quadrant.

gender dysphoria A feeling of being "trapped" in a specific gender; e.g., a man may think of himself as a woman in a man's body, or a woman may describe herself as a man trapped in a woman's body.

gender identity Awareness of being male or female that develops from infancy.

gender role (sex role) Expression of one's maleness or femaleness to both oneself and others.

general adaptation syndrome (GAS) Generalized defense response of the body to stress, consisting of three stages: alarm, resistance, and exhaustion.

general anesthesia Intravenous or inhaled medications that cause the client to lose all sensation and consciousness.

geographic isolation Social isolation of the older adult resulting from urban crime, institutional barriers, and distance from family.

geriatrics Branch of health care dealing with the physiology and psychology of aging and with the diagnosis and treatment of illnesses affecting the older adult.

germicide A chemical preparation that kills germs and that can be applied on skin and tissues, as well as inanimate objects.

gerontological nursing A nursing specialty that focuses on the health care needs of the older adult. Gerontological nurses have a broad focus, assisting older adults in maximizing their functional capabilities.

gerontology Study of all aspects of the aging processes and their consequences.

gingivitis Inflammatory condition in which the gums are red, swollen, and bleeding.

glomerulonephritis An inflammation of the glomerulus of the kidney.

glomerulus Cluster or collection of capillary vessels within the kidney involved in the initial formation of urine.

glossitis An inflammation of the tongue resulting from infectious disease or injury from a burn, bite, or other injury.

gluconeogenesis Formation of glucose or glycogen from substances that are not carbohydrates, such as protein or lipid.

glycogen Polysaccharide that is the major carbohydrate stored in animal cells.

glycogenesis Anabolism of glucose into glycogen for storage.

glycogenolysis Catabolism of glycogen into glucose, carbon dioxide, and water.

glycosuria Abnormal presence of glucose in the urine.

goals Desired results of nursing actions, set realistically by the nurse and client as part of the planning stage of the nursing process.

goniometer Measures the precise degree of motion in a particular joint and is used mainly in clients who have a suspected reduction in joint movement. The instrument has two flexible arms with a 180-degree protractor in the center.

graafian follicle Ovarian follicle that continues to mature through a given menstrual cycle and ruptures to release an ovum at the time of ovulation.

granulation tissue Soft, pink, fleshy projections of tissue that form during the healing process in a wound that is not healing by primary intention.

graphic user interface Mechanism whereby user accesses computer functions through trackball, touch pads, mouse, and icons.

grief Form of sorrow involving the person's thoughts, feelings, and behaviors, occurring as a response to an actual or perceived loss.

grieving process Sequence of affective, cognitive, and physiological states through which the person responds to and finally accepts an irretrievable loss.

grounded Having a three-prong electrical plug; the rounded, longer prong is the ground prong and carries any stray electrical current back to the ground.

growth Quantitative or measurable aspect of an individual's increase in physical measurements.

guaiac test Test of feces for the presence of occult (hidden) blood.

guided imagery Method of pain control in which the client creates a mental image, concentrates on that image, and gradually becomes less aware of pain.

gustatory Pertaining to the sense of taste.

halitosis Offensive breath resulting from poor oral hygiene, dental or oral infection, ingestion of certain foods, or systemic disease.

handicap A congenital or acquired physical, emotional, cognitive, or intellectual defect that has the potential to interfere with a person's ability to function.

hand rolls A roll of cloth that keeps the thumb slightly adducted and in opposition to the fingers.

handwashing A vigorous, brief rubbing together of all surfaces of hands lathered in soap, followed by rinsing under a stream of water.

hand-wrist splints Splints individually molded for the client to maintain proper alignment of the thumb, slight adduction of the wrist, and slight dorsiflexion.

hardiness A combination of three personality characteristics that are thought to mediate against stress: a sense of control over life events, commitment to meaningful activities, and anticipation of challenge as an opportunity for growth.

haustral contraction Type of peristaltic contraction that occurs in the large intestine; produces a large sac in the colon wall to increase surface area for nutrient absorption.

health Dynamic state in which an individual adapts to internal and external environments so that there is a state of physical, emotional, intellectual, social, and spiritual well-being.

health behavior Activities through which a person maintains, attains, or regains good health and prevents illness.

health belief model Conceptual framework that predicts a person's health behavior as an expression of personal health beliefs.

health education Material provided to clients through video media, demonstration, written material, and classes directed at minimizing the effects of preventable diseases and assisting clients to make intelligent, informed decisions about their health and lifestyle.

health-illness continuum Scale by means of which a person's level of health can be described, ranging from high-level wellness to severe illness. The scale takes into account the presence of risk factors.

health maintenance organization (HMO) Group health care agency that provides basic and supplemental health maintenance and treatment services to voluntary enrollees who prepay a fixed periodic fee that is set without regard to the amount or kind of services received.

health promotion Activities directed toward maintaining or enhancing the health and well-being of clients.

health protecting behaviors Considered a third subcategory of health behavior and may, through assessment, reveal needs for vehicular safety, home safety, domestic violence recognition, recreational safety, and occupational safety and health.

heat exhaustion An abnormal condition characterized by weakness, vertigo, nausea, muscle cramps, and loss of consciousness; caused by depletion of body fluid and electrolytes resulting from exposure to intense heat or the inability to acclimatize to heat.

heatstroke A severe and sometimes fatal condition resulting from the failure of the temperature-regulating capacity of the body, caused by prolonged exposure to the sun or to high temperatures.

hematemesis Vomiting of blood indicating upper gastrointestinal bleeding.

hematocrit Measure of the packed cell volume of red cells, expressed as a percentage of the total blood volume.

hematoma Collection of blood trapped in the tissues of the skin or an organ.

hematuria Abnormal presence of blood in the urine.

hemiparesis Muscular weakness of one half of the body.

hemiplegia Paralysis of one side of the body.

hemolysis Breakdown of red blood cells and release of hemoglobin as may result by administration of hypotonic intravenous solutions that cause progressive swelling and rupture of the erythrocytes.

hemoptysis Coughing of blood from the respiratory tract.

hemorrhage External or internal loss of a large amount of blood in a short period of time.

hemorrhoids Permanent dilation and engorgement of veins within the lining of the rectum.

hemosiderosis Abnormal deposition of iron in a variety of tissues.

hemostasis Termination of bleeding by mechanical or chemical means or by the coagulation process of the body.

hemothorax Accumulation of blood and fluid in the pleural cavity between the parietal and visceral pleurae.

heparin lock An intravenous needle connected to a small "well" that allows for the intermittent injection of medication without the need for repeated venipuncture.

hepatitis An inflammatory condition of the liver.

heritage consistency Theoretical model that assesses a client's acculturation to a new culture on a continuum.

heritage inconsistency The degree to which people move away from the dominant and traditional culture of birth or origin.

heterosexual Sexual orientation involving erotic preference for members of the opposite sex.

hierarchy of basic human needs Categorization of human needs from the most basic to those at a higher level.

hirsutism Excessive body hair in a masculine distribution caused by heredity, hormonal dysfunction, or medication.

holistic health A system of comprehensive or total client care that considers the physical, emotional, social, economic, and spiritual needs of the person; the response to the illness; and the effect of the illness on the person's ability to meet self-care needs.

Holter monitor Portable ECG device, similar to the size of a miniature tape recorder; records a continuous ECG over 24 hours or longer.

home health care Professional and paraprofessional services and equipment provided to clients and families in their place of residence for purposes of health promotion and maintenance, client and family education, illness prevention, diagnosis and treatment of disease, and palliation and rehabilitation.

home health care agencies Organizations providing skilled, intermittent health care services usually in the form of nursing, home care aides, or rehabilitative therapies.

home IV therapies The delivery of intravenous (IV) therapy to the client in the home, usually provided by professional nurses through home care agencies.

homeostasis State of relative constance in the internal environment of the body, maintained naturally by physiological adaptive mechanisms.

homophobia Irrational fears of homosexuality or homosexuals.

homosexual Sexual orientation involving erotic preference for members of one's own sex.

hope Confident, yet uncertain, expectation of achieving a future goal.

hospice and hospice care Philosophy of client care that advocates physical and psychosocial support for palliative care of persons in the last months of an incurable illness so that life can be lived as fully and comfortably as possible.

host Element of the agent-host-environment model of health and illness. A host is a person or group who, because of risk factors, may be susceptible to disease or illness.

human immunodeficiency virus A type of retro virus that causes the acquired immunodeficiency syndrome (AIDS).

human relations movement Leadership theory that emphasizes the role of interpersonal relationships and human needs for improving productivity in the workplace.

humidification The process of adding water to gas.

hydrocephalus An abnormal accumulation of cerebrospinal fluid in the ventricles of the brain.

hydrostatic pressure Pressure exerted by a liquid.

hygiene Science of health.

hypercapnia Greater than normal amounts of carbon dioxide in the blood; also called hypercarbia.

hyperglycemia Elevated serum glucose levels.

hypertension Disorder characterized by an elevated blood pressure persistently exceeding 140/90 mm Hg.

hyperthermia Situation in which body temperature exceeds the set-point.

hypertonic Situation in which one solution has a greater concentration of solute than another solution; therefore the first solution exerts more osmotic pressure.

hyperventilation Respiratory rate in excess of that required to maintain normal carbon dioxide levels in the body tissues.

hypervitaminosis A condition caused by excessive intake of a vitamin; is less likely to occur with water-soluble vitamins.

hypervolemia Increase in the amount of fluid in the circulating blood volume.

hypnotic Class of drug that causes insensibility to pain and induces sleep.

hypoglycemia Reduced serum glucose levels.

hypospadias A congenital defect in which the urinary meatus is on the underside of the penis.

hypotension Abnormal lowering of blood pressure in which pressure is inadequate for normal perfusion and oxygenation of tissues.

hypothalamus Portion of the diencephalon of the brain that activates, controls, and integrates the peripheral autonomic nervous system, endocrine processes, and many bodily functions such as body temperature, sleep, and appetite.

hypothermia Abnormal lowering of body temperature below 93° F or 35° C, usually caused by prolonged exposure to cold.

hypothesis A statement derived from a theory that predicts a relationship among variables representing concepts, constructs, or events.

hypotonic A situation in which one solution has a smaller concentration of solute than another solution; therefore the first solution exerts less osmotic pressure.

hypoventilation Reduction in the volume of air that enters the lung for gas exchange; oxygen exchange is insufficient to meet metabolic demands of the body.

hypovolemia Decreased circulatory blood volume resulting from extracellular fluid losses.

hypovolemic shock State of physical collapse caused by massive blood loss, circulatory dysfunction, and inadequate tissue perfusion.

hypoxemia Abnormal deficiency of oxygen in arterial blood.

hypoxia Inadequate cellular oxygenation that may result from a deficiency in the delivery or use of oxygen at the cellular level.

iatrogenic infection Infection caused by a treatment or diagnostic procedure.

ideal self Consists of the aspirations, goals, values, and standards of behavior that a person considers ideal and strives to attain.

identification Internalizing beliefs, values, and behavior of another through imitation and introjection with a unique individual expression.

identity Component of self-concept; sense of continuity and sameness; one's persisting consciousness of being oneself, separate, unique, and distinct from others.

identity confusion Form of self-concept disturbance in which a person does not maintain a clear consciousness of a consistent and continuous self; sense of fragmentation or distortion.

idiosyncratic reactions An individual sensitivity to effects of a drug caused by inherited or other bodily constitution factors.

ileostomy Surgical formation of an opening of the ileum onto the surface of the abdomen, through which fecal matter is emptied.

illness Abnormal process in which any aspect of a person's functioning is diminished or impaired as compared with the previous condition.

illness behavior Ways in which people monitor their bodies, define and interpret their symptoms, take remedial actions, and use the health care system.

illness prevention Health education programs or activities directed toward protecting clients from threats or potential threats to health and toward minimizing risk factors.

imitation A child acquires knowledge, skills, or behaviors from members of the social or cultural group.

immanent justice The notion that the world is equipped with a built-in code of law and order.

immobility Inability to move about freely, caused by any condition in which movement is impaired or therapeutically restricted.

immune response A defense function of the body that produced antibodies to destroy invading antigens and malignancies.

immunization The process by which resistance to an infectious disease is produced or augmented. Immunity is acquired after the oral administration or injection of an antigen, which causes production of an antibody within the body.

immunocompromised Abnormal condition of the immune system in which cellular or humoral immunity is inadequate.

immunoglobulin Humoral antibody produced by the body and present in serum and external secretions; formed in response to specific antigens.

impaction Presence of large or hard fecal mass in the rectum or colon.

implementation Category of nursing behavior in which the action necessary for achieving the projected outcomes of the health care plan are initiated and completed.

incentive spirometry Method of encouraging voluntary deep breathing by providing visual feedback to clients of the inspiratory volume they have achieved.

incontinence Inability to control urination.

individual practice association Prospective payment plans requiring the client to pay a fixed annual payment; the plan pays the provider when the services are used.

individuation Process whereby an individual looks to gain an understanding of the self as distinct yet also in relationship with others.

indurated Hardened tissue, particularly the skin, due to edema, inflammation, or infiltration by a tumor.

induration Hardening of a tissue, particularly the skin, because of edema or inflammation.

infancy Stage of life from 1 month to 1 year of age.

inference Taking one proposition as a given and guessing that another proposition follows.

infertility Man's, woman's, or couple's involuntary inability to conceive.

infiltration Dislodging an intravenous catheter or needle from a vein into the subcutaneous space.

inflammatory bowel disease Chronic, episodic inflammation of the large intestine and rectum, characterized by profuse watery diarrhea containing blood, mucus, and pus.

inflammatory response A protective vascular and cellular reaction that neutralizes pathogens and repairs body cells.

informed consent Process of obtaining permission from a client to perform a specific test or procedure after describing all risks, side effects, and benefits.

infradian rhythm Repetition of certain physiological phenomena within a cycle exceeding 24 hours.

infusion Introduction of a substance such as a fluid, drug, electrolyte, or nutrient directly into a vein by means of gravity flow.

infusion pump Device that delivers a measured amount of fluid over a period of time.

inhibition Process of socialization in which one learns to refrain from a behavior even when motivated to engage in that behavior.

inpatient Client admitted for treatment within a hospital over the course of more than 1 day.

insensible water loss Loss of fluid from the body by evaporation, as normally occurs during respiration.

in-service education Instruction or training provided by an agency or institution to nurses practicing within the agency or institution.

insomnia Condition characterized by chronic inability to sleep or remain asleep through the night.

inspection Assessment process during which the nurse observes the client.

instillation Procedure in which a fluid is slowly introduced into a cavity or passage of the body (e.g., rectum) and allowed to remain for a specific length of time before being withdrawn or drained.

integument Skin and its appendages: hair, nails, and sweat and sebaceous glands.

interferon A protein that interferes with the ability of viruses to multiply and protects body cells from simultaneous infection with other viruses.

internal stressor Stress-causing stimulus that arises within a person.

International Council of Nurses (ICN) International organization for professional nurses; the ANA and CNA are members.

interpersonal communication Exchange of information between two persons or among persons in a small group.

Interpersonal competence The ability to relate well with others whether the "others" be clients, co-workers, peers, or those who hold positions of authority.

interpersonal conflict Occurs when one or more persons have opposing or incompatible expectations for an individual in a particular role.

interrole conflict Occurs when pressures or expectations associated with one role oppose pressures or expectations associated with another.

interstitial fluid Fluid that fills the spaces between most of the cells of the body and provides a substantial portion of the liquid environment of the body.

interview Type of communication with a client initiated for a specific purpose and focused on a specific content area.

intraarterial Within an artery.

intraarticular Within a joint.

intracardiac Within the myocardium.

intracellular fluid Liquid within the cell membrane.

intractable pain Pain not easily relieved, as may occur with some types of cancer.

intradermal A layer within the tissue of the skin, under the epidermis.

intramuscular Tissue within the interior of a muscle.

intraosseous Tissue within the interior of bone.

Intraperitoneal Within the peritoneal cavity.

intrapersonal communication Communication that occurs within an individual, e.g., a person who "talks with the self" silently or forms an idea in the mind.

intrapleural Pertaining to, or affecting, the potential space between the parietal and visceral pleurae.

intraprofessional and interprofessional competence Refers to a demonstrated ability to relate well with one's own nursing peers and with members of other professions or disciplines.

intrathecal Within the sheath surrounding the spinal cord.

intravenous Pertaining to the inside of a vein.

intravenous (IV) bolus Involves introducing a concentrated dose of a drug directly into systemic circulation by way of venous access.

invasion of privacy Release of personal information (e.g., health records, financial statements, or employment history) without the person's permission.

invasive Referring to procedures that involve puncture, incision, or insertion of a foreign object, such as a needle or catheter, into the body.

irregular bones Bones of the vertebral column and some bones of the skull.

irrigation Process of washing out a body cavity or wounded area with a stream of fluid.

irritable bowel syndrome Abnormally increased motility of the small and large intestines, generally associated with emotional stress.

ischemia Decreased blood supply to a body part such as skin tissue or to an organ such as the heart.

isometric contraction Increased muscle tension without muscle shortening.

isotonic Situation in which two solutions have the same concentration of solute; therefore both solutions exert the same osmotic pressure.

isotonic contraction Increased muscle tension resulting in muscle contraction and muscle shortening.

jaundice Yellow discoloration of the skin, mucous membranes, and sclera, caused by greater than normal amounts of bilirubin in the blood.

jejunal feeding tube A hollow tube inserted into the jejunum through the abdominal wall for administration of liquefied foods.

job stress Condition in which some factor or combination of factors at work disrupts the worker's psychological or physiological balance.

joint contracture Abnormal and usually permanent condition of a joint, characterized by flexion and fixation and caused by disuse, atrophy, and shortening of muscle fibers.

joints Connections between bones; classified according to structure and degree of mobility.

justice Fairness or equity in the manner decisions are made. One of the principles of the ethical theory of deontology.

Kardex Trade name for card-filing system that allows quick reference to the particular need of the client for certain aspects of nursing care.

Kegel exercises Pelvic exercises designed to improve the strength of pelvic floor muscles through repetitive contractions of muscle groups.

ketoacidosis Acidosis accompanied by an accumulation of ketones in the body, resulting from faulty carbohydrate metabolism.

ketonuria Presence in the urine of excessive amounts of ketone bodies (products of fat metabolism), such as occurs in diabetes mellitus.

kinesthesia Perception of position of body parts, weight, and movement.

kinship system A unit comprising members of a family related biologically or by marriage. The system incorporates roles and responsibilities of each member.

Korotkoff sounds Sounds heard during the taking of blood pressure using a sphygmomanometer and stethoscope.

Korsakoff's syndrome Psychosis characterized by disorientation of time, place, and person by amnesia for recent events and by confabulation.

kyphosis An exaggeration of the posterior curvature of the thoracic spine.

laceration Torn, jagged wound.

lactation Process and period in which the mother produces milk for the infant.

lactose intolerance A gastric disorder in which some foods, such as milk and milk products, are difficult or impossible to digest.

laissez-faire Philosophy characterized by an individual freedom of choice and action.

land pollution Contamination of soil by improper disposal of radioactive or bioactive waste products.

lanugo Fine hair that normally covers the fetus after the fifth month of intrauterine life and is mostly shed by birth.

laxative Drug that acts to promote bowel evacuation.

leader Person with the ability to influence the behavior of others toward the accomplishment of common goals; not necessarily a manager.

learning Acquisition of new knowledge and skills as a result of reinforcement, practice, and experience.

learning objectives Written statements that describe the knowledge or skill a teacher expects an individual to gain following a learning activity.

left-sided heart failure or left heart failure An abnormal cardiac condition characterized by the impairment of the left side of the heart and by elevated pressure and congestion in the pulmonary veins and capillaries.

legalism An often strict and literal adherence to law or code.

lesbian Female with homosexual partner preference.

leukocytosis Abnormal increase in the number of circulating white blood cells.

leukoplakia Thick, raised, pearly-white patch of precancerous tissue found on the lips, buccal mucosa, penis, or vulva.

libel Written false statement about a person that may injure reputation.

libido Psychological term for sexual desire.

licensed practical or vocational nurse Person trained in basic nursing techniques and direct client care who practices under the supervision of a registered nurse.

lifesaving measure Independent, dependent, or interdependent nursing intervention that is implemented when a client's physiological or psychological status is threatened.

ligaments White, shiny, flexible bands of fibrous tissues binding joints together and connecting various bones and cartilage.

lipid emulsion A soybean oil or safflower oil–based solution that is isotonic and may be infused with amino acid and dextrose solution through a central or peripheral line.

lipoatrophy A breakdown of subcutaneous fat at the site of an insulin injection.

lipogenesis The process during which fatty acids are synthesized.

listening A nonverbal method to convey interest in the client's needs, concerns, and problems. It requires complete attention and involves an attempt to understand the entire verbal and nonverbal message that a person is communicating.

living will Instrument by which a dying person makes wishes known to care givers; a living will has no legal validity in most states.

local adaptation syndrome (LAS) Localized response of tissue, an organ, or a system that occurs as a direct reaction to stress.

local anesthesia Loss of sensation at the desired site of action.

localized As in infection, in which the infectious process is limited to a particular area, such as a wound infection.

long bones Bones that contribute to height of the person, to the length of an extremity such as the arm, or to the length of a portion of an extremity such as the hand.

lordosis An increased lumbar curvature.

love and belonging needs The third level in Maslow's hierarchy of needs, which includes friendship, social relationships, and sexual love.

lymphokines A product of cell-mediated immunity, these cells attract macrophages and stimulate them to attack antigens.

maceration Softening something solid, such as the skin, by soaking.

magicoreligious folk medicine Represents a human's use of charms, holy words, and holy actions to prevent and cure illnesses.

malabsorption syndrome Set of symptoms resulting from disorders in the intestinal absorption of nutrients, characterized by anorexia, weight loss, bloating of the abdomen, and muscle cramps.

malignant hyperthermia An autosomal dominant trait characterized by often fatal hyperthermia in affected people exposed to certain anesthetic agents.

malnutrition Any nutritional disorder such as unbalanced, insufficient, or excessive diet or impaired absorption, assimilation, or utilization of food.

malpractice Injurious or unprofessional actions that harm another.

managed care A health care system in which there is administrative control over primary health care services. Redundant facilities and services are eliminated and costs are reduced. Preventive care is emphasized along with health education.

management process (as described by Fayol) Involves planning, organizing, directing, and controlling activities so that what is planned actually happens.

manager Person with an official organizational position to guide and direct the work of subordinate employees.

masticate To chew or tear food with the teeth while it becomes mixed with saliva.

mastication Chewing, tearing, or grinding food with the teeth while it becomes mixed with saliva.

maturation Process of becoming fully developed and grown, involving the individual's biological ability and environmental opportunities to alter functions and learning.

maturational loss Loss, usually of an aspect of self, resulting from the normal changes of growth and development.

maturity State of adulthood in which the person has attained independence with a balanced development in physiological, psychosocial, and cognitive dimensions.

meatus Opening through any part of the body, e.g., the urethral meatus.

Medicaid State medical assistance based on Title XIX of the Social Security Act. States receive 50% in matching federal funds to provide medical care and services to people meeting categorical and income requirements. Covers home health services based on Medicare guidelines. Many innovative home health programs can be covered by Medicaid as long as they meet the recipient's needs and cost less than institutionalization.

medical diagnosis Identification of a specific disease or pathological process.

Medicare Federal government insurance coverage for persons over 65 years of age (or disabled and under 65) who have paid into the Social Security or Railroad Retirement system. Covers inpatient hospital charges and some home health services.

medication A substance used in the diagnosis, treatment, cure, relief, or prevention of disease.

medulla oblongata Portion of the brain that controls vital functions necessary for homeostasis and survival.

melanin Black or dark brown pigment that occurs naturally in the skin, hair, and iris.

melanoma A group of malignant neoplasms, primarily of the skin, that are composed of melanocytes. Common in fair-skinned people having light-colored eyes and in persons who have had a sunburn. Any black or brown spot having an irregular border, pigment appearing to radiate beyond that border, a red, black, and blue coloration observable on close examination.

melena Abnormal black, tarry stool containing digested blood; indicative of gastrointestinal bleeding.

melting pot Theory that with subsequent generations, cultural customs and values would be lost, or melted down.

menarche Onset of a girl's first menstruation, usually occurring between 9 and 16 years of age.

menopause Natural cessation of menses by the ovaries; normally occurs in women between ages 45 and 60.

menstrual cycle Recurring cycle of changes in the ovaries, uterus, and hormone levels, involving the development of an egg, ovulation, and implantation of the egg or sloughing of the corpus luteum and lining. The cycle can be divided into proliferative and secretory phases by uterine changes or follicular, ovulation, and luteal phases based on ovarian activity.

message Information sent or expressed by sender in the communication process.

metabolic acidosis Abnormal condition of high hydrogen ion concentration in the extracellular fluid caused by either a primary increase in hydrogen ions or a decrease in bicarbonate.

metabolic alkalosis Abnormal condition characterized by the significant loss of acid from the body or by increased levels of bicarbonate.

metabolism Aggregate of all chemical processes that take place in living organisms, resulting in growth, generation of energy, elimination of wastes, and other functions concerned with the distribution of nutrients in the blood after digestion.

metacommunication Dependent not only on what is said but also on the relationship to the other person involved in the interaction. It is a message that conveys the sender's attitude toward the self and the message and the attitudes, feelings, and intentions toward the listener.

metastasis Process by which tumor cells are spread to the distant parts of the body.

metric system A decimal system of measurement based on the meter (39.37 inches) as the unit of length; on the gram (15.432 grains) as the unit of weight or mass; and as a derived unit, on the liter (0.908 U.S. dry quart or 1.0567 U.S. liquid quart) as the unit of volume.

microorganism Any microscopic entity capable of carrying on living processes, such as bacteria, viruses, and fungi.

micturition Urination; act of passing or expelling urine voluntarily through the urethra.

mild stress situation Type of stress situation that is encountered by most people on a daily or weekly basis.

minerals Inorganic elements essential to the body because of their role as catalysts in biochemical reactions.

misdemeanor Lesser crime; the penalty is usually a fine or imprisonment for less than 1 year.

mobility Person's ability to move about freely.

moderate stress situation Stress situation that lasts from several hours to a number of days.

modern Present-day beliefs and practices of the providers within the American, or western, health care delivery system.

moist wound healing environment An environment for wound healing that affects both the rate of epithelialization and the amount of scar formation. A moist wound environment provides the optimum condition for rapid healing.

molding Overlapping and shaping of the soft skull bones during birth, usually resolved during the first few days of life.

monosaturated fatty acids A fatty acid that has one carbon bond.

moral reasoning Decision making based on moral principles and standards.

morals Personal conviction that something is absolutely right or wrong in all situations.

moribund Near death, or in the process of dying.

morning sickness Pregnant woman's symptoms of nausea and vomiting related to changes in serum hormone levels.

mortician Person trained in the care of the dead.

morula Early stage of human development in which a solid mass of cells forms from the zygote approximately 3 days after fertilization.

motivation Internal impulse that causes a person to take action.

mourning A psychological process of reaction activated by an individual to assist in overcoming a great personal loss. The process is finally resolved when a new object relationship is established.

multicultural competence A cultivated and fine-tuned sensitivity to diverse groups within one's own country and world; an appreciation of the fact that we are members of a global village closely united as a result of travel, communications, and information revolution. An ability to act in a manner that manifests each of the above.

murmur A low-pitched fluttering or humming sound, such as a heart murmur.

muscle tone Normal state of balanced muscle tension.

myocardial contractility Contractile strength of the myocardial muscle fibers, which in turn affects stroke volume and cardiac output.

myocardial infarction Necrosis of a portion of cardiac muscle caused by obstruction in a coronary artery.

myocardial ischemia A cardiac condition that results when the supply of blood to the myocardium from the coronary arteries is insufficient to meet the oxygen demands of the organ.

myotonia A normal sexual response in which the muscles do not relax after contracting.

narcolepsy Syndrome involving sudden sleep attacks that a person cannot inhibit; uncontrollable desire to sleep may occur several times during a day.

narcotic Drug substance, derived from opium or produced synthetically, that alters perception of pain and that with repeated use may result in physical and psychological dependence.

narcotic analgesics Act on higher centers of the brain and spinal cord by binding with opiate receptors to modify perception of and reaction to pain.

nasal cannula A device for delivering oxygen by way of two small tubes that are inserted into the nares.

National League for Nursing (NLN) Organization of nurses and lay people concerned with improving nursing education, nursing service, and the delivery of health care in the United States. The NLN is the official accrediting agency for nursing schools.

natural folk medicine Human's earliest uses of the natural environment; the use of herbs, plants, minerals, and animal substances to prevent and treat illnesses.

natural immunity An inherited resistance to infection (e.g., humans are resistant to the distemper virus that attacks dogs and cats).

near-death experience The subjective observations of people who have either been close to clinical death or who may have recovered after having been declared dead.

nebulization Process of adding moisture to inspired air by the addition of water droplets.

necrotic Of or pertaining to the death of tissue in response to disease or injury.

negative nitrogen balance Condition occurring when the body excretes more nitrogen than it takes in.

negligence Careless act of omission or commission that results in injury to another.

neonate Stage of life from birth to 1 month of age.

nephron Structural and functional unit of the kidney containing a renal glomerulus and tubule.

nephrostomy A surgical procedure in which an incision is made on the flank of the client so that a catheter can be inserted into the kidney pelvis for the purpose of drainage.

nesting A period during the last month of pregnancy when the woman may experience a burst of energy, during which she cleans house and prepares for the baby by shopping for baby supplies.

neuropathy Abnormal condition characterized by inflammation and degeneration of peripheral nerves that alter sensory or motor function.

neuroregulators Substances that affect the transmission of nerve stimuli; are divided into two groups: neurotransmitters and neuromodulators.

neurotransmitter Chemical that transfers the electrical impulse from the nerve fiber to the muscle fiber.

nitrogen balance Relationship between the nitrogen taken into the body, usually as food, and the nitrogen excreted from the body in urine and feces. Most of the body's nitrogen is incorporated into protein.

nociceptors Somatic and visceral free nerve endings of thinly myelinated and unmyelinated fibers. They usually react to tissue injury but may also be excited by endogenous chemical substances.

nocturia Urination at night; can be a symptom of renal disease or may occur in persons who drink excessive amounts of fluids before bedtime.

nocturnal enuresis Incontinence of urine during the night.

noise pollution Noise level in an environment when it becomes uncomfortable to its inhabitants.

nonmaleficence The duty to do no harm to another person. One of the principles of the ethical theory of deontology.

nonREM or NREM sleep Abbreviation for nonrapid eye movement, which occurs during the first four stages of normal sleep.

nonverbal communication Communication using expressions, gestures, body posture, and positioning rather than words.

norm Measure of a phenomenon generally accepted as the ideal standard performance against which other measures of the phenomenon may be measured.

normal reactive hyperemia Hyperemia over a pressure site lasts 1 hour or less following removal of pressure; surrounding skin does blanch.

normal sinus rhythm (NSR) The wave pattern on an electrocardiogram that indicates normal conduction of an electrical impulse through the myocardium.

nosocomial infection Infection acquired during hospitalization or stay in a health care facility.

noxious Painful or harmful to health.

nuclear family Form of family consisting of husband and wife and their children.

nurse administrator Nurse in management position with an agency who focuses on the delivery of nursing services.

nurse anesthetist Nurse with advanced training and accreditation in the speciality of nurse anesthesia; manages the anesthetic care of clients in certain surgical situations.

nurse-client relationship Association between the nurse and the client that has as a mutual concern the well-being of the client.

nurse educator Nurse with a background in clinical nursing who works in a school of nursing as a faculty member, in a staff development department of a health care agency, or in an inpatient education department.

nurse-initiated intervention The response of the nurse to the client's health care needs and nursing diagnoses. This intervention is an independent action based on scientific rationale that is executed to benefit the client.

nurse practice acts Statutes enacted by the legislature of any state delineating the legal scope of the practice of nursing within the geographical boundaries of the jurisdiction.

nurse practitioner Nurse with advanced training or education who provides primary care for nonemergency clients, usually in an outpatient or community setting.

nurse researcher Nurse with graduate nursing education who investigates problems related to nursing practice.

nursing care plan Written guidelines of nursing care, documenting specific nursing diagnoses for the client and goals, interventions, and projected outcomes.

nursing diagnosis A statement that describes the client's actual or potential response to a health problem that the nurse is licensed and competent to treat.

nursing health history Data collected about a client's present level of wellness, changes in the life patterns, sociocultural role, and mental and emotional reactions to illness.

nursing interface Mechanism for nurse to access information on computerized systems.

nursing intervention Any action by a nurse that implements the nursing care plan or any specific objective of the plan.

nursing process Systematic problem-solving method by which nurses individualize care for each client. The five steps of the nursing process are assessment, diagnosis, planning, implementation, and evaluation.

nursing research A detailed process in which a systematic study of a problem in the field of nursing is performed.

nursing theory Organized framework of concepts and purposes designed to guide the practice of nursing.

nutrient density The proportion of essential nutrients to the number of calories.

nutrients Foods that contain elements necessary for body function, including water, carbohydrates, proteins, fats, vitamins, and minerals.

nystagmus Involuntary, rhythmic movements of the eyes. The oscillations may be horizontal, vertical, rotary or mixed.

objective data Data relating to a client's health problem that are obtained through observation or diagnostic measurements.

object permanence The Piagetian term for the understanding that a person or object out of sight still exists.

occlusion A blockage in a canal, vessel, or passage of the body.

occupational therapist Health care professional certified to develop and use adaptive devices that help the chronically ill or handicapped carry out activities of daily living.

olfactory Pertaining to the sense of smell.

oliguria Diminished capacity to form and pass urine.

oncotic pressure The total influence of the protein on the osmotic activity of plasma water.

open-ended question interview Inquiry aimed at obtaining a full client response and discussion between the client and the nurse.

ophthalmologist A medical doctor whose practice is limited to diseases, conditions, and trauma to the eyes. An ophthalmologist also prescribes corrective lenses for clients whose visual acuity is impaired.

ophthalmoscope An instrument used to illuminate the structures of the eye in order to examine the fundus, which includes the retina, choroid, optic nerve disc, macula, fovea centralis, and retinal vessels.

oral hygiene Condition or practice of maintaining the tissues and structures of the mouth.

organogenesis A period of fetal development in which there is rapid organ growth.

orthopnea Abnormal respiratory symptom in which a person must sit or stand to breathe deeply or comfortably.

orthostatic hypotension A drop in systolic blood pressure of 15 mm Hg or more when a person rises from a recumbent position to a sitting or standing position.

osmolality The concentration or osmotic pressure of a solution expressed in osmols or milliosmols per kilogram of water (normal = 280-295 mOsm/kg).

osmoreceptors Receptors that are sensitive to fluid concentration in the blood plasma and regulates the secretion of antidiuretic hormone.

osmosis Movement of a pure solvent through a semipermeable membrane from a solution with a lower solute concentration to one with a higher solute concentration.

osmotic pressure Drawing power for water, which depends on the number of molecules in the solution.

osteoporosis A disorder characterized by abnormal rarefaction of bone, occurring most frequently in postmenopausal women, in sedentary or immobilized individuals, and in clients on long-term steroid therapy.

otolaryngologist A medical doctor whose practice is limited to diseases, conditions, and trauma to the ears.

otoscope An instrument, with a special ear speculum, used to examine the deeper structures of the external and middle ear.

ototoxic Having a harmful effect on the eighth cranial (auditory) nerve or the organs of hearing and balance.

ototoxicity Referring to any drug or substance that has a harmful effect on the eighth cranial nerve or the organs of hearing and balance.

outcome indicators Condition of a client at the end of treatment, including the degree of wellness and the need for continuing care, medication, support, counseling, or education.

outpatient services Health care centers that provide primary, acute, and restorative care services to clients. Activities in outpatient settings can include smoking cessation programs, health screening, and rehabilitation.

over-the-counter drug Drug available to a consumer without a prescription.

ovulation Second phase of the menstrual cycle, in which a mature egg is released from the ovary and moves down the fallopian tubes.

oximeter; oximetry A device used to measure oxyhemoglobin in the blood; measurement of oxyhemoglobin.

oxygen saturation The amount of hemoglobin fully saturated with hemoglobin, given as a percent value.

pack A dressing procedure in which gauze with or without medication is placed into an open wound to promote wound healing.

pain Subjective, unpleasant sensation caused by noxious stimulation of sensory nerve endings.

palliative therapy Treatment designed to relieve or reduce intensity of uncomfortable symptoms but not to produce a cure.

palpation Use of the hands and the sense of touch to gather data.

pancreatitis An inflammation of the pancreas.

Papanicolaou (Pap) smear A painless screening test for cervical cancer. Specimens are taken of squamous and columnar cells of the cervix.

paralytic ileus Usually temporary paralysis of intestinal wall that may occur after abdominal surgery or peritoneal injury and that causes cessation of peristalsis. Leads to abdominal distention and symptoms of obstruction.

paraphrasing Restating a passage or phrase to give the same meaning in another form.

parenteral Not in or through the digestive system; typically refers to administering medications by injection.

parenteral nutrition The administration of nutrition into the vascular system.

partial bed bath Bath in which body parts that might cause the client discomfort if left unbathed (i.e., face, hands, axillary areas, back, and perineum) are washed in bed.

passive immunity A form of acquired immunity resulting from antibodies that are transmitted naturally through the placenta to a fetus or through the colostrum to an infant or artificially by injection or antiserum for treatment or prophylaxis.

passive strategies of health promotion Activities that involve the client as the recipient of actions by health care professionals.

patency A term indicating that there are no clots at the tip of the needle or catheter and that the catheter or needle tip is not against the vein wall.

paternalism Doing what an individual believes is in another person's best interests, at times regardless of the person's own determinations.

pathogen Any microorganism capable of producing disease.

pathogenicity The ability of a pathogenic agent to produce disease.

pathological fractures Fractures resulting from weakened bone tissue; frequently caused by osteoporosis or neoplasms.

patient-controlled analgesia (PCA) Drug delivery system that allows clients to self-administer analgesic medications when they want.

payor mix The proportion of different third-party payors whose enrollees use a health care institution (e.g., payor mix will include Medicare, Medicaid, private insurance, and HMO's).

peak expiratory flow rate (PEFR) The maximal flow rate, measured in liters, that can be generated during a forced expiratory maneuver.

peptic ulcers Sharply circumscribed loss of the mucous membrane of the stomach, duodenum, or any other part of the GI system exposed to gastric juices containing acid and pepsin, also called gastric ulcers.

perception Person's mental image or concept of elements in the environment, including information gained through the senses.

percussion Tapping of various body organs and structures to produce vibration and sound and to detect underlying abnormalities.

perfusion The passage of a fluid, such as blood, through a specific organ or an area of the body.

perineal care Cleansing procedure prescribed for cleansing the genital and anal areas as part of the daily bath or after various obstetrical and gynecological procedures.

periodontal disease (pyorrhea) Disease of the tissues around the tooth, such as inflammation of the periodontal membrane or ligament.

perioperative nursing Refers to the role of the operating room nurse during the preoperative, intraoperative, and postoperative phases of surgery.

peripheral neuropathy A functional or organic disorder of the peripheral nervous system.

peripheral vascular resistance A resistance to the flow of blood through a blood vessel as determined by the tone of the vascular musculature and the diameter of the blood vessels.

peripherally inserted central catheter (PICC) A peripherally inserted catheter that extends to the superior vena cava or right atrium.

peristalsis Coordinated, rhythmical, serial contractions of smooth muscle that force food through the digestive tract.

peritoneal dialysis A dialysis procedure performed to correct an imbalance of fluids or electrolytes in the blood or to remove toxins, drugs, or other wastes normally excreted by the kidney.

peritonitis Inflammation of the peritoneum produced by bacteria or irritating substances introduced into the abdominal cavity by a penetrating wound or perforation of an organ in the GI tract or the reproductive tract.

PERRLA Acronym for "pupils equal, round, reactive to light, accommodative"; the acronym is recorded in the physical examination if eye and pupil assessments are normal.

personal space Area surrounding an individual that is perceived as private by the individual, who may regard a movement into the space by another person as intrusive.

petechiae Tiny purple or red spots that appear on skin as minute hemorrhages within dermal layers.

pH Reflection of the hydrogen ion concentration of a liquid.

phagocytosis Process by which certain cells, such as macrophages, engulf and dispose of microorganisms.

pharmacist Licensed professional who formulates and dispenses medications.

pharmacokinetics Study of how drugs enter the body, reach their site of action, are metabolized, and exit from the body.

phenomena Data that can be observed in reality.

phlebitis Inflammation of a vein.

photophobia Abnormal sensitivity of the eyes to light.

physical examination Scrutinization of all body parts through the use of inspection, palpation, percussion, and auscultation.

physical therapist Health care professional licensed to assist in the management of physically disabled or handicapped clients through techniques such as special exercise, application of heat and cold, and sonar wave methods.

physician Health care professional who has the degree of Doctor of Medicine (MD) or Doctor of Osteopath (DO) and is licensed to provide medical, surgical, and other treatment.

physician assistant Health care professional trained in aspects of the practice of medicine to provide support to physicians.

physician-initiated intervention Based on the physician's response to a medical diagnosis; the nurse responds to the physician's written orders.

physiological adaptation The body's ability to maintain a state of relative balance. This adaptive ability is a dynamic form of equilibrium in the body's internal environment.

physiological anorexia A decrease in appetite that occurs with slower growth rates, decreased caloric need, and smaller food intake during toddlerhood.

physiological needs Needs necessary for human survival, including those for oxygen, fluid, nutrition, temperature, elimination, and shelter.

piggyback infusion Method for administering intravenous medications intermittently, a piggyback IV set is a supplementary set that connects with the primary IV tubing.

pigmentation Organic coloring material, such as melanin, that gives color to the skin.

pituitary gland Small gland attached to the hypothalamus that supplies numerous hormones for the control of vital functions and the maintenance of homeostasis.

placebo Dosage form that contains no pharmacologically active ingredients but may relieve pain through psychological effects.

placenta Organ surrounding the embryo and fetus through which nutrients and other substances from the mother and waste products from the fetus pass.

planning The process of designing interventions to achieve the goals and outcomes of health care delivery.

plaque (dental) A thin film on teeth made up of mucin and colloidal material found in salvia and often secondarily invaded by bacteria.

pneumothorax Collection of air or gas in the pleural space.

podiatrist Practitioner trained to diagnose and treat diseases and other disorders of the feet.

point of maximal impulse (PMI) Anatomical point along the fourth to fifth intercostal space at the midclavicular line where the heart beat can most easily be palpated through the chest wall.

poison Any substance that impairs health or destroys life when ingested, inhaled, or absorbed by the body in relatively small amounts.

poison control center One of a network of facilities that provides information regarding all aspects of poisoning or intoxication, maintains records of their occurrence, and refers clients to treatment centers.

pollutant A harmful chemical or waste material discharged into the water or atmosphere.

polyp A small tumorlike growth that projects from a mucous membrane surface.

polypharmacy The use of a number of different drugs by a patient who may have one or several health problems.

polysomnogram Monitoring device that involves placement of electrodes on the scalp, face, chin, and legs to measure brain waves, eye movements, and muscle activity; used to diagnose sleep disorders.

polyunsaturated fatty acids Fatty acids that have two or more carbon double bonds.

polyuria Excretion of an abnormally large volume of urine.

posterior rhizotomy A procedure that involves surgically cutting the dorsal (posterior) roots of a spinal nerve.

postural drainage Use of positioning along with percussion and vibration to drain secretions from specific segments of the lungs and bronchi into the trachea.

postural hypotension Abnormally low blood pressure occurring when an individual assumes the standing posture; also called orthostatic hypotension.

posture Position of the body in relation to the surrounding space.

preadolescence The transitional period between childhood and adolescence, between the ages of 10 and 12.

precertification Preliminary screening process used by third-party payors to approve use of health care services by enrollees of a health plan.

preconceptual thought Characterized by perceptual-bound thinking, in which children judge persons, objects, and events by their outward appearance or what seems to be.

Preferred Provider Organization (PPO) Group of physicians or hospital that provides company employees and their dependents with comprehensive health services at a discount.

preload The volume of blood in the ventricles at the end of diastole, immediately before ventricular contraction.

premenstrual syndrome (PMS) Complex of physical and psychological symptoms experienced by some women just before menstruation.

prenatal Stage of life from conception to birth.

preoperational thought Children can think about things not physically present by using mental representations but are limited by their inability to use logic.

presbycusis Condition that affects the client's ability to hear high-pitched sounds and sibilant consonants such as "s," "sh," and "ch" because of the aging process.

presbyopia Farsightedness with inability to focus on near objects, resulting from loss of elasticity of the lens; occurs with age.

preschooler Stage of life from 3 to 5 years of age.

presentational isolation Social isolation that occurs because of the older adult's socially unacceptable appearance or presentation of self to others.

pressure reducing A device in skin care that reduces the interface pressure, but not necessarily below 32 mm Hg, the capillary closing pressure.

pressure relieving A skin-care device that reduces the interface pressure, the pressure between the body and the support surface, below 32 mm Hg, the capillary closing pressure.

pressure ulcer Inflammation, sore, or ulcer in the skin over a bony prominence.

preventive nursing action Interventions directed toward preventing illness and promoting health to avoid the need for secondary or tertiary health care.

primary care The first contact in a given episode of illness that leads to a decision regarding a course of action to resolve the health problem.

primary care generalists Have competencies in health promotion and disease prevention, assessment and evaluation of symptoms and physical signs, management of common acute and chronic medical conditions, and identification and appropriate referral for other needed health care services.

primary health care system One in which essential health care services are universally accessible to individuals and families within a specific community, made available to them through their full participation, and provided at a cost that the community and county can afford.

primary intention Primary union of the edges of a wound, progressing to complete scar formation without granulation.

primary prevention Activities directed toward decreasing the probability of specific illnesses or dysfunctions.

primary source Research report written by an investigator in an original study.

private duty agencies Organizations that provide professional and paraprofessional home health care services on a continuous basis.

problem-oriented medical record (POMR or POR) Method of recording data about the health status of a client that fosters a collaborative problem-solving approach by all members of the health care team.

problem-seeking interview Type of inquiry that focuses on gathering data to identify problems the client needs to resolve.

problem solving A methodical, systematic approach to explore conditions and develop solutions, including analysis of data, determination of causative factors, and selection of appropriate actions to reverse or eliminate the problem.

problem-solving interview Type of inquiry that focuses on specific problems that have been identified by the client or nurse.

process indicator Specific measures that evaluate the manner in which care is delivered (e.g., correct procedure for dressing changes).

productive cough A sudden expulsion of air from the lungs that effectively removes sputum from the respiratory tract and helps clear the airways.

Professional nursing competence Because the depth and breadth of nursing practice is expanding rapidly, if one is to remain competent, nurses have a professional obligation to remain current with the literature, continuing education, certification and recertification programs as well as pursue advanced degrees.

professional organization Association of professionals created to deal with issues of concern to the profession as a whole.

professional standards review organization Focuses on evaluation of nursing care provided in a health care setting. The quality, effectiveness, and appropriateness of nursing care for the client is the focus of evaluation.

proprioception Sensation achieved through stimuli from within the body regarding spatial position and muscular activity.

proprioceptors Nerve endings located in muscles, tendons, and joints that respond to stimuli originating from within the body regarding spatial position or movement.

prospective payment Procedure by which the federal government sets rates for hospitals in advance for treatment of specific illnesses; this replaces the previous policy of reimbursing each hospital based on actual cost.

prostaglandins Potent hormonelike substances that act in exceedingly low doses on target organs. They can be used to treat asthma and gastric hyperacidity.

protein Any of a large group of naturally occurring, complex, organic nitrogenous compounds. Each is composed of large combinations of amino acids containing the elements carbon, hydrogen, nitrogen, oxygen, usually sulfur, and occasionally phosphorus, iron, iodine, or other essential constituents of living cells. Protein is the major source of building material for muscles, blood, skin, hair, nails, and the internal organs.

proteinuria Presence in the urine of abnormally large quantities of protein, usually albumin. Persistent proteinuria is usually a sign of renal disease or renal complications of another disease, or hypertension or heart failure.

protocol Written and approved plan specifying the procedures to be followed during an assessment or in providing treatment.

proxemics The study of spatial distances between people and its effect on interpersonal behavior.

psychomotor learning Acquisition of ability to perform motor skills.

psychosocial moratorium The period of adolescence when society allows the physically mature teenager to delay the assumption of adult responsibilities. This is a time for youth to try a variety of ideological and vocational roles before making a commitment.

ptosis Abnormal condition of one or both upper eyelids in which the eyelid droops; caused by weakness of the levator muscle or paralysis of the third cranial nerve.

puberty Developmental period of emotional and physical changes, including the development of secondary sex characteristics and the onset of menstruation and ejaculation.

public communication Interaction between one person and a large group of people.

puerperium Period of approximately 6 weeks after childbirth during which the woman's reproductive system is in transition to the nonpregnant state.

pulmonary function tests Procedures for determining the capacity of the lungs to exchange oxygen and carbon dioxide efficiently.

pulse deficit Condition that exists when the radial pulse is less than the ventricular rate as auscultated at the apex or seen on an electrocardiogram. The conditions indicate a lack of peripheral perfusion for some of the heart contractions.

pulse pressure The difference between the systolic and diastolic pressures, normally 30 to 40 mm Hg.

puncture A type of wound made by piercing the skin.

Purkinje network A complex network of muscle fibers that spread through the right and left ventricles of the heart and carry the impulses that contract those chambers almost simultaneously.

pursed-lip breathing Deep inspiration through the nose and mouth, not using pursed lips, followed by prolonged expiration through pursed lips.

purulent Producing or containing pus.

pyelonephritis Infection spreads in the kidneys, causing flank pain, tenderness, low-grade fever, and chills.

pyorrhea A purulent inflammation of the tissues surrounding the teeth.

pyrexia Abnormal elevation of the temperature of the body above 37° C (98.6° F) because of disease. Same as fever.

pyrogen Any substance that causes a rise in body temperature, as in the case of bacterial toxins.

qualitative research The exploration of little-known phenomena that are not easily quantified or categorized using inductive reasoning to develop generalizations or theories from specific observations or interviews.

quality improvement The monitoring and evaluation of processes and outcomes in health care or any other business to identify opportunities for improvement.

quality indicator A quantitative measure of an important aspect of care that determines whether quality of service conforms to requirements or standards of care.

quantitative research Rigorous, systematic, objective examination of specific concepts and their relationships to test theory by focusing on numerical data, statistical analysis, and controls to eliminate bias.

radial pulse Pulse of the radial artery palpated at the wrist over the radius. The radial pulse is the one most often taken.

radiation A method of temperature regulation used by the body to lower body temperature.

range of motion The range of movement of a joint, from maximum extension to maximum flexion, as measured in degrees of a circle.

reality orientation Therapeutic modality for restoring an individual's sense of the present.

receiver Person to whom message is sent during the communication process.

receptive aphasia Abnormal neurological condition in which language function is defective because of an injury to certain areas of the cerebral cortex; specifically language is not understood.

recommended daily allowances (RDAs) Suggested or recommended amounts of various nutrients used in planning diets.

record Written form of communication that permanently documents information relevant to health care management.

recovery room Area adjoining the operating room to which surgical clients are taken while still under anesthesia.

rectocele A bulging of the posterior vaginal wall, caused by prolapse of the rectum.

referent Factor that motivates a person to communicate with another individual.

reflex bladder A condition usually resulting from spinal cord trauma in which micturition reflex pathway may remain intact, allowing urination to occur reflexively.

reflux Abnormal backward flow or return of fluid, as in the case of gastric contents reentering the esophagus.

refractive error Defect in the ability of the lens of the eye to focus light, such as occurs in nearsightedness and farsightedness.

regional anesthesia Loss of sensation in an area of the body supplied by sensory nerve pathways.

registered nurse Health care professional who has completed a course of study at an accredited school of professional nursing and has passed an examination administered by a state board of nursing or the Canadian Nurses Association Testing Service.

rehabilitation Restoration of an individual to normal or near-normal function following a physical or mental illness, injury, or chemical addiction.

rehabilitation center Facility that provides therapy and training to restore a client to an optimal level of functioning and independence.

reinforcement Provision of a contingent response to a learner's behavior that increases the probability of the behavior recurring.

relative humidity Amount of moisture in the air as compared with the maximum amount that the air could contain at the same temperature.

relaxation Act of being relaxed or less tense.

religion Belief in a divine or superhuman power or powers to be obeyed and worshipped as the creator(s) and ruler(s) of the universe.

reminiscence Recalling the past for the purpose of assigning new meaning to past experiences.

remission Partial or complete disappearance of the clinical and subjective characteristics of a chronic or malignant disease; remission may be spontaneous or the result of therapy.

REM sleep Abbreviation for rapid eye movement, occurring during stage of sleep in which dreaming and rapid eye movements are prominent; important for mental restoration.

renal Of or pertaining to the kidney.

renal calculus Calcium stone in the renal pelvis.

renal failure An inability of the renal system to filter and excrete urinary waste products.

renal replacement therapy Treatments designed to carry out kidney function. Currently two methods of renal replacement exist: dialysis, peritoneal and hemodialysis and organ transplantation.

renin A proteolytic enzyme, produced by and stored in the juxtaglomerular apparatus that surrounds each arteriole as it enters a glomerulus. The enzyme affects the blood pressure by catalyzing the change of angiotensinogen to angiotensin, a strong repressor.

report Transfer of information from the nurses on one shift to the nurses on the following shift. Report may also be given by one of the members of the nursing team to another health care provider (e.g., physician or therapist).

research process Systematic collection and analysis of data to obtain new knowledge, add to existing knowledge, or find solutions to problems.

research utilization Systematic process for determining the scientific worth of a group of conceptually related nursing research studies and whether or not the findings can be used to solve a nursing care problem with a particular group of clients in a setting other than the one in which the studies were conducted.

resident Individual client who resides in a long-term care facility.

residual functional capacity The reduced functional capacity created by one or more health problems.

residual functional deficit The difference in functioning between the original functional capacity, before the health problem occurred, and the residual functional capacity.

residual urine Volume of urine remaining in the bladder after a normal voiding; the bladder normally is almost completely empty after micturition.

resocialization Technique that assists older adults to expand their social networks within their community.

respect for persons An ethical principle that implies that humans should revere their own lives and the lives of others. The principle holds that life is the most basic possession humans have.

respiration A physiological phenomenon that involves two distinctly different processes: external respiration, or the movement of air between the environment and lungs, and internal respiration, or the movement of oxygen between hemoglobin and single cells.

respiratory acidosis Abnormal condition characterized by increased arterial carbon dioxide concentration, excess carbonic acid, and increased hydrogen ion concentration.

respiratory alkalosis Abnormal condition characterized by decreased arterial carbon dioxide concentration and decreased hydrogen ion concentration.

respiratory therapist Health care professional licensed to deliver treatment to improve ventilatory function or oxygenation.

respite care Gives the primary care provider the opportunity to have time away. Respite care services can take place in the client's home, a hospital, or an extended care setting.

responsibility Carrying out duties associated with a particular role.

restorative care Restorative care settings include, but are not limited to, inpatient and outpatient rehabilitation facilities, subacute care facilities, clinics, and home health care agencies. The services provided in the restorative settings are those designed to bring the client to the maximal level of health and function.

restorative health care team Health care providers that support the client's efforts to maximize independence within the constraints of the residual functional capacity and, as soon as possible, to reintegrate the client into the community in the previous or modified role and setting.

restraint Device to aid in the immobilization of a client or client's extremity.

reticular activating system Group of specialized nerve cells located in the brainstem, upper spinal cord, and cerebral cortex.

reticular formation Small cluster of neurons in the brainstem and spinal cord that continuously monitor and control vital functions to maintain homeostasis.

return demonstration Demonstrations after the client has first observed the teacher and then practiced the skill in mock or real situations.

reversibility The child's ability to trace a line of thinking back to where it originated.

review of systems A systematic method for collecting data on all body systems.

right-sided heart failure or right heart failure An abnormal cardiac condition characterized by the impairment of the right side of the heart and by elevated pressure and congestion in the systemic veins and capillaries.

risk adjusted Outcome measures adjusted for groups of clients of different acuities and comorbidities.

risk factor Any internal or external variable that makes a person or group more vulnerable to illness or an unhealthy event.

role A person's pattern of behavior in a particular social group or situation.

role ambiguity State in which a person has unclear role expectations and feels unable to predict the outcomes of behavior.

role conflict State in which a person experiences incongruent or incompatible expectations within one role or between two or more simultaneously held roles.

role strain Generalized state of frustration or anxiety produced by the stress of role conflict and ambiguity.

saccharides Classification of sugars in carbohydrates.

safety and security needs Needs for freedom from threats to one's physical and psychological well-being.

sanguineous Fluid containing red blood cells.

saturated fatty acids Fatty acids in which each carbon in the chain has an attached hydrogen atom.

scientific approach A logical, orderly, and objective means of generating research questions and testable hypotheses.

scientific management theory Leadership theory that emphasizes technology and task analysis, rather than human factors, as a means of improving productivity.

scientific method A codified sequence of steps used in the formulation, testing, evaluation, and reporting of scientific ideas.

scientific rationale Reason, based on supporting literature, for choosing a specific nursing action.

scintigraphy A diagnostic technique that produces a photographic recording showing the distribution and intensity of radioactivity in various tissues and organs after the administration of a radiopharmaceutical.

scoliosis A lateral spinal curvature.

scrub nurse Registered nurse or operating room technician who assists surgeons during operations.

sebum Normal secretion of the sebaceous glands of the skin; when combined with sweat, forms a moist, oily, acidic film that protects the skin from drying.

secondary intention Wound closure in which the edges are separated, granulation tissue develops to fill the gap, and finally epithelium grows in over the granulation, producing a larger scar than results with healing by primary intention.

secondary prevention Activities directed toward early diagnosis and prompt intervention, thereby shortening severity of a condition and enabling the client to return to the highest level of health at the earliest possible point.

secondary sex characteristics Physical characteristics other than genitals that distinguish females from males (e.g., the breasts).

secondary source Report that interprets research data written by someone not involved in the original research.

sedative Medication that produces a calming effect by decreasing functional activity, diminishing irritability, and allaying excitement.

seizure Brief, temporary malfunctions of nerve cells in the brain may result in seizure activity. A generalized tonic-clonic seizure is characterized by loss of consciousness, tonicity (rigidity), and clonicity (jerking).

seizure precautions Measures that protect the client from injury during a seizure.

self-actualization State of being in which one is fully achieving one's potential and is able to cope realistically with problems.

self-concept Complex, dynamic integration of conscious and unconscious feelings, attitudes, and perceptions about one's identity, physical being, worth, and roles. How people perceive and define themselves.

self-esteem Feeling of self-worth characterized by feelings of achievement, adequacy, self-confidence, and usefulness.

sender Person who initiates interpersonal communication by conveying a message.

senile keratosis A slowly developing, localized thickening of the outer layers of the skin as a result of chronic, excessive exposure to the sun. Commonly develops in older adults.

senile lentigo Smooth, brown, irregularly shaped spots that initially appear on the backs of the hands and on forearms.

sensory cortex A portion of the brain that processes and integrates all sensory information.

sensory deficit Defect in the function of one or more of the senses, resulting in visual, auditory, or olfactory impairments.

sensory deprivation State in which stimulation to one or more of the senses is lacking, resulting in impaired sensory perception.

seriation The ability of a child to place objects in order according to their increasing or decreasing size.

serosanguineous Thin red drainage composed of serum and blood.

serous fluid Clear fluid that reduces friction between structures covered by serous membranes, such as the lung.

serum concentration The amount of a medication within the client's blood at a given time.

serum half-life Time needed for excretion processes to lower the serum drug concentration by half.

severe stress situation Chronic stress situation that may last from several weeks to years.

sex Classification of male or female based on many criteria, among them anatomical and chromosomal characteristics. Also refers also to biological aspects of sexuality and genital sexual activity.

sexual dysfunction Inability or difficulty in sexual function caused by physiological or psychological factors or both.

sexual health The integration of the somatic, emotional, intellectual, and social aspects of sexual being, in ways that are positively enriching and that enhance personality, communication, and love.

sexuality Dynamic and diverse facet of the personality involving the biological, psychological, sociological, spiritual, and cultural dimensions, depending in part on the person's sense of sexual identity and affecting the person's values, attitudes, behaviors, and relationships with others.

sexually transmitted diseases (STDs) Infectious diseases transmitted to any part of the body through contact with body fluids during sexual activities.

sexual orientation Clear, persistent desire of a person for one sex rather than the other.

sexual response cycle Four phases of biological sexual response: excitement, plateau, orgasm, and resolution as defined by Masters and Johnson.

shearing force Friction exerted when a person is moved or repositioned in bed by being pulled or allowed to slide down in bed.

shivering A process used by the body to raise body temperature.

short bones Bone clusters that when combined with ligaments and cartilage permit movement of the extremities.

side effects Any reaction or consequence that results from medication or therapy.

single-parent family A form of family composed of single, divorced, or widowed parents and their children.

sinoatrial (SA) node Located in the right atrium next to the entrance of the superior vena cava, normal conduction originates in this node; it is considered the pacemaker of the heart.

situational crisis Crisis occurring suddenly in response to a specific external event or conflict.

situational leadership A leadership theory developed by Hersey and Blanchard that is concerned with the extent of structure and socioemotional support provided by a leader on the basis of subordinates' maturity.

situational loss Loss of a person, thing, or quality resulting from a change in a life situation, including changes related to illness, body image, environment, and death.

sitz bath Bath in which only the hips or buttocks are immersed in fluid.

skilled nursing facility An institution or part of an institution that meets criteria for accreditation established by the sections of the Social Security Act that determine the basis for Medicaid and Medicare reimbursement for skilled nursing care, including rehabilitation and various medical and nursing procedures. Law requires that policies designate which level of care giver is responsible for implementation of each policy, that the care of every client be under the supervision of a physician, that a physician be available on an emergency basis, that records be maintained regarding the condition and care of every client, that nursing service be available 24 hours a day, and that at least one full-time registered nurse be employed.

skin barrier An artificial layer of skin, made of plastic or vinyl-like material, applied to skin before application of tape or ostomy drainage. Protects skin from chronic irritation.

slander Utterance of a false statement about another that harms that person's reputation.

sleep State marked by reduced consciousness, diminished activity of the skeletal muscles, and depressed metabolism.

sleep apnea The cessation of breathing for a time during sleep.

sleep deprivation Condition resulting from a decrease in the amount, quality, and consistency of sleep.

sloughing Shedding off of dead tissue cells.

SOAP Acronym for subjective, objective, assessment, and plan, the four parts of the written account of a client's health problem in a problem-oriented record.

social worker Professional trained to counsel clients and families to help them seek community and financial resources and to assist them in selecting long-term and extended care facilities.

socialization Process that begins in infancy by which a person acquires values, behavior, skills, and roles from social norms and significant others.

solution Mixture of one or more substances dissolved in another substance. The molecules of each of the substances disperse homogeneously and do not change chemically. A solution may be a liquid, gas, or solid.

somnambulism Sleep walking.

source record Method for organizing a client's health care record, placing information in sections organized for each discipline that cares for the client.

specific gravity Measurement of the degree of concentration of a liquid.

sphygmomanometer Device for measuring the arterial blood pressure that consists of an arm or leg cuff with an air bladder connected to a tube, a bulb for pumping air into the bladder, and a gauge for indicating the amount of air pressure being exerted against the artery.

spiritual advisor Offers spiritual support and guidance to clients and families and may be employed by an agency or institution or be provided by a religious affiliation within the community. Spiritual advisors are ministers, priests, nuns, rabbis, or lay members of religious congregations.

spiritual distress State of being out of harmony with a system of beliefs, a supreme being, or God.

spiritual health Awareness and openness to a system of beliefs, a supreme being, or God; a presence with or in each person and in the world.

spirituality Spiritual dimension of a person, including the relationship with humanity, nature, and a system of beliefs, a supreme being, or God.

standard Measure or guide that serves as a basis for comparison when evaluating similar phenomena or substances.

standards of care The minimum level of care accepted to ensure high quality of care to clients. Standards of care define the types of therapies typically administered to clients with defined problems or needs.

standing order Written and approved document containing rules, policies, procedures, regulations, and orders for the conduct of client care in various stipulated clinical settings.

statutory law Of or related to laws enacted by a legislative branch of the government.

stenosis An abnormal condition characterized by the constriction or narrowing of an opening or passageway in a body structure.

stereognosis Ability to recognize objects by the sense of touch.

stereotype A generalization about a form of behavior, an individual, or a group.

sterile field Specified area, such as within a tray or on a sterile towel, that is considered free of microorganisms.

sterilization Rendering a person unable to produce children; accomplished by surgical, chemical, or other means.

Steri-strip Trade name for butterfly tape used as a wound closure.

stethoscope An instrument consisting of two earpieces connected by a flexible tubing to a diaphragm, which is placed against the skin to hear sounds produced by the body.

stoma Artificially created opening between a body cavity and the body's surface (e.g., a colostomy) formed from a portion of the colon pulled through the abdominal wall.

stomatitis Any inflammatory condition of the mouth.

strabismus Abnormal ocular condition in which the eyes are crossed.

stratum corneum The horny, outermost layer of the skin, composed of dead cells converted to keratin that continually flakes away.

stress Physiological or psychological tension that threatens homeostasis or a person's psychological equilibrium.

stressor Any event, situation, or other stimulus encountered in a person's external or internal environment that necessitates change or adaptation by the person.

striae A streak or linear scar that results from rapidly developing tension in the skin, commonly seen on the abdomen after pregnancy.

stroke volume The amount of blood ejected by the ventricle during a ventricular contraction.

subacute care Level of medical specialty care provided to clients who need a greater intensity of care than that provided in a skilled nursing facility but who do not require acute care. Often subacute care is an interim level of treatment before a client is moved to a rehabilitation or long-term care facility.

subcutaneous layer Continuous layer of connective tissue over the entire body between the skin and the deep fascia.

subjective data Data relating to a client's health problem described in the client's own words.

subjects People or events selected for a study in order to examine a particular variable or condition.

sublingual A route of medication administration in which the medication is placed underneath the client's tongue.

substitution A child replaces one behavior with another, which provides the same personal gratification.

summarization A concise review of main ideas that have been discussed. It sets the tone for further interactions between the nurse and client.

sundown syndrome Nocturnal confusion in clients who are usually not confused at other times during the day. Institutional tempo changes, sensory deficit, and environmental change are major contributors to this confusion.

suture Surgical stitch taken to repair an incision or wound.

syncope A brief lapse in consciousness caused by transient cerebral hypoxia.

synergistic effect When two drugs act synergistically, the effect of the two drugs combined is greater than the effect that would be expected if the individual effects of the two drugs acting alone were added together.

synergistic muscles Muscles that contract together to accomplish the same movement.

synostotic joint A joint type that occurs when bones are jointed by bones. No movement is associated with this type of joint, and the bony tissue that forms between the bones provides strength and stability.

synovial joint A true and freely movable joint in which contiguous bony surfaces are covered by articular cartilage and are connected by ligaments lined with a synovial membrane.

syntax Arrangement of words as elements in a phrase, clause, or sentence.

systemic Of or pertaining to the whole body rather than to a localized area.

systole Contraction of the heart, driving blood into the aorta and pulmonary arteries. The occurrence of systole is indicated by the first heart sound heart on auscultation and by the palpable apex beat.

systolic pressure The pressure exerted in the aorta and large arteries of a human during systolic contraction of the left ventricle. Indicated during blood pressure measurement as the point when sound can first be heard during deflation of the pressure cuff.

tachycardia Rapid, regular heart rate ranging between 100 and 150 beats per minute.

tachypnea An abnormally rapid rate of breathing, as seen with hyperpyrexia.

tactile Relating to the sense of touch.

tactile fremitus A tremulous vibration of the chest wall during breathing that is palpable on physical examination.

task-oriented behavior Actions involving a person's cognitive abilities in an attempt to solve problems, resolve conflicts, and gratify the person's needs in order to reduce or avoid stress.

technique Method followed in performing a specific procedure such as administering medication, changing a client's dressing, or inserting a Foley catheter.

temperament The child's characteristic style of approaching and reacting to people and situations.

temperature A measure of sensible heat associated with the metabolism of the human body, normally maintained at a constant level of 98.6° F (37° C).

tendon White, glistening, strong, flexible, and inelastic fibrous bands of tissue that connect muscle to bone.

teratogen Chemical or physiological agent that may produce adverse effects in the embryo or fetus.

territoriality Persistent attachment of a person to a specific area or space.

tertiary prevention Activities directed toward rehabilitation rather than diagnosis and treatment.

testosterone Naturally occurring male sex hormone.

theory X and theory Y Developed by McGregor to differentiate the attitudes about human nature often reflected in managing behavior.

therapeutic effect The desired benefit of a medication, treatment, or procedure.

therapeutic touch The use of the hands to provide comfort to the client. Touch can communicate caring and thus help clients relax.

thermoregulation Internal control of body temperature.

third-party reimbursement A method of payment for health care services received by the client, for which the client's bills are submitted to an insurance company or to Medicare.

third space syndrome A shift of body fluid into a space from which it is not easily exchanged with the extracellular fluid.

thoracentesis Surgical perforation of the chest wall and pleural space with a needle for the aspiration of fluid or to obtain a specimen for diagnostic or therapeutic purposes.

threshold Point at which a person first perceives a painful stimulus as being painful.

thrill A continuous palpable sensation like the purring of a cat.

thrombus Accumulation of platelets, fibrin, clotting factors, and the cellular elements of the blood attached to the interior wall of a vein or artery, sometimes occluding the lumen of the vessel.

tidal volume Amount of air inhaled and exhaled during normal ventilation.

time orientation Value that a client places on promptness, future planning, and keeping appointments, which are important in the planning of long-term care and self-care discharge therapies.

tissue ischemia The point at which tissues receive insufficient oxygen and perfusion.

toddlerhood Stage of life from 1 to 3 years of age.

tolerance The ability to endure hardship, pain, or ordinarily injurious substances, such as drugs, without apparent physiological or psychological injury.

topical Pertaining to a drug or treatment applied to the surface of a part of the body.

tort Act that causes injury for which the injured party can bring civil action.

total parenteral nutrition (TPN) The administration of a nutritionally adequate hypertonic solution consisting of glucose, protein hydrolysates, minerals, and vitamins through an indwelling catheter into the superior vena cava.

toxic effects Resulting from an excess amount of medication in a client's blood, these effects may be caused by excessive use of medication, overdose, impaired excretion, or idiosyncratic reaction to the medication itself.

traditional Ancient ethnocultural-religious beliefs and practices handed down through the generations.

trait development theory Leadership theory that analyzes successful leadership in terms of the leader's personal qualities, including intelligence, energy level, aggressiveness, and friendliness.

transcultural communication Each person attempts to understand the other's point of view from that person's cultural frame of reference. Effective transcultural communication is facilitated by identification of areas of commonalities.

transcultural nursing Represents an effort by nurses from all cultural backgrounds and clinical areas to come together and define concepts that enable them to develop the knowledge and skills needed to provide culturally sensitive care.

transcutaneous electrical nerve stimulation (TENS) Technique in which a battery-powered device blocks pain impulses from reaching the spinal cord by delivering weak electrical pulses directly to the skin's surface.

transfer report A verbal report exchanged between care providers when a client is moved from one nursing unit or health care setting to another. The report includes information necessary to maintain a consistent level of care from one setting to another.

transfusion reaction A systemic response by the body to the administration of blood incompatible with that of the recipient.

transit time Time required to propel a bolus of intestinal contents from one location in the gastrointestinal tract to another.

transsexual Person whose gender identity is opposite the biological sex identity.

transtracheal oxygen Method for delivering oxygen directly into the trachea by way of a catheter placed in a tracheal stoma that was surgically placed between two tracheal rings inferior to the cricothyroid membrane.

transvestism Tendency to achieve psychic and sexual relief by dressing in clothing of the opposite sex.

trapeze bar Metal triangular-shaped bar that can be suspended over a client's bed from an overhanging frame; permits clients to move up and down in bed while in traction or some other encumbrance.

triage A process in which a group of clients is sorted according to their needs for care. The kind of illness or injury, the severity of the problem, and the facilities available govern the process.

trochanter roll Rolled towel support placed against the hips and upper leg to prevent external rotation of the legs.

tumescence To become swollen, as with genital vasocongestion during sexual arousal.

turgor Normal resiliency of the skin caused by the outward pressure of the cells and interstitial fluid.

ultradian rhythm Repetition of certain physiological phenomena within a cycle lasting less than 24 hours.

universal access Ensures that health care is provided to all citizens regardless of their employment or insurance status.

unsaturated fatty acids Fatty acids in which an unequal number of hydrogen atoms are attached and the carbon atoms attach to each other with a double bond.

uremic syndrome Symptoms characterized by the presence of urinary constituents in the blood and altered regulatory functions, causing marked fluid and electrolyte abnormalities, nausea, vomiting, headache, coma, or convulsions.

ureterostomy Diversion of urine away from a diseased or defective bladder through an artificial opening in the skin.

urinalysis Routine laboratory testing on a voided urine specimen.

urinary diversion A surgically created diversion of the ureter to the abdominal wall for the drainage of urine following removal of a diseased bladder.

urinary frequency Symptom involving increased voiding.

urinary incontinence Inability to control urination.

urinary retention Retention of urine in the bladder; condition frequently caused by a temporary loss of muscle function.

urinary stasis A filling of the renal pelvis before urine enters the ureters.

urticaria An allergic response producing a pruritic skin condition characterized by transient erythematous wheals of varying shapes.

user interface Traditional mechanism whereby a user of a computer accesses functions and information via keyboard and monitor.

utilization review (UR) An assessment of the appropriateness and economy of an admission to a health care facility or continued hospitalization.

vaginismus An intense contraction of the perineal and vaginal musculature that closes the vaginal introitus; is only occasionally associated with painful genital conditions. Instead, it is most often a psychological response and frequently associated with rape or childhood sexual abuse.

validation therapy Technique used with severely confused and disoriented older adults to provide a sense of dignity and self-worth and validate their feelings.

Valsalva maneuver Any forced expiratory effort against a closed airway, as when an individual holds the breath and tightens the muscles in a concerted, strenuous effort to move a heavy object or to change positions in bed.

value Personal belief about the worth of a given idea or behavior.

values clarification Technique for clarifying values, developed by Louis Raths; process designed to give an individual the opportunity to find meaning and significance in personal values.

value system Values that are related to one another form a value system (e.g., religious and cultural values can shape health values).

valvular heart disease An acquired or congenital disorder of a cardiac valve characterized by stenosis and obstructed blood flow or valvular degeneration and regurgitation of blood.

variance The unexpected event that occurs during client care and that is different from what is predicted on a CareMap®. Variance or exceptions are interventions or outcomes that are not achieved as anticipated. Variance may be positive or negative.

varicosity Abnormal condition of a vein, characterized by swelling and irregular shape or course.

vascular access devices Catheters, cannulas, or infusion ports designed for long-term, repeated access to the vascular system.

vasocongestion Pooling of blood in the genitals and female breasts during sexual arousal.

vegetarianism The consumption of a diet consisting predominantly of plant foods.

venipuncture Technique in which a vein is punctured transcutaneously by a sharp, rigid stylet or by a needle attached to a syringe.

ventilation Respiratory process by which gases are moved into and out of the lungs.

ventricular gallop An abnormal low-pitched extra heart sound (S_4) heard in early diastole.

veracity The ability to tell the truth.

verbal communication The sending of messages from one individual to another or to a group of individuals through the spoken word.

vernix caseosa A grayish-white cheeselike substance consisting of sebaceous gland secretions, lanugo, and epithelial cells that coats the skin of the fetus and newborn.

vesicoureteral reflex An abnormal backflow of urine from the bladder to ureter, resulting from a congenital defect, obstruction of the outlet of the bladder, or infection in the lower urinary tract.

vibration Fine, shaking pressure applied by hands to the chest wall only during exhalation.

virulent Of or pertaining to a very pathogenic or rapidly progressive condition.

vital capacity The amount of air exhaled after a maximal full inspiration.

vital signs Temperature, pulse, respirations, and blood pressure.

vitamins Organic compounds essential in small quantities for normal physiological and metabolic functioning of the body. With few exceptions, vitamins cannot be synthesized by the body and must be obtained from the diet or dietary supplements.

volume control devices Devices designed to prevent sudden, uncontrolled rapid intravenous infusion of large volume. Commonly used with children, with clients with renal or cardiac failure, and with critically ill clients.

volunteer agencies Not-for-profit health care agencies established within a community to meet specific needs.

walking belt Leather device with handles that enables the nurse to help the client walk.

water pollution Contamination of lakes, rivers, and streams by industrial pollutants.

Wernicke's syndrome Illness occurring with advanced stages of vitamin B_1 depletion and accompanied by nystagmus, papillary abnormalities, ataxia, tremor, and stupor.

wheezes Adventitious lung sound caused by a severely narrowed bronchus.

whispered pectoriloquy The transmission of a whisper through the pulmonary structures so that it is heard as normal audible speech on auscultation.

work redesign Formal process used to analyze the work of a certain work group and to change the actual structure of the jobs performed.

wound A disruption of normal anatomical structure and function that results from pathological processes beginning internally or externally to the involved organ(s).

wound contraction A process that involves movement of the dermis and epidermis on each side of the wound.

Z-track injection A technique for injecting irritating preparations into muscle without tracking residual medication through sensitive tissues.

zygote Fertilized ovum created by the joining of the mother's ovum and father's sperm.

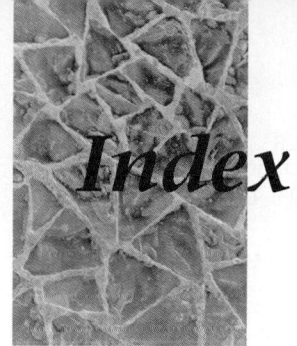

Index

A

A-delta fiber, 1155
AACN; *see* American Association of Colleges of Nursing; American Association of Critical-Care Nurses
Abdellah's theory, 213-214
Abdomen
  aging and, 576
  middle adult, 560
  physical examination, 709-713, 1353-1354
  preoperative assessment, 1387
  vitamin and mineral deficiency, 988
Abdominal binder, 1453, 1454-1455
Abdominal distention, 1421
Abdominal reflexes, 736
Abdominal respiratory muscles, 1196
Abdominal roentgenogram, 1310
Abducens nerve, 732
Abduction, 725, 906
Ablative surgery, 1383
Abnormal reactive hyperemia, 955
Abnormal structural configurations, 1200
ABO system, 1283
Abortion, 343, 424
Abrasion, 1020, 1435
Absorption, 1096-1097
  of drug, 794
  of water, 1342-1343
Absorptive dressing, 984
Abstract, 293
Abstract thinking, 731
Abuse
  child, 427
    nursing research in, 484
    physical examination and, 652-653
  domestic, 652
  drug, 793
    adolescent and, 542
    dietary patterns and, 1108
    older adult and, 577
    oxygenation and, 1202
    physical examination and, 653
    preoperative assessment, 1384
    risks of surgery, 1383
    skin indications, 658
    sleep and, 1137
    young adult and, 555
  older adult, 652
  sexual, 427, 429
Acceptance, 241, 266
Accessory muscles, 1196
Accidents
  adolescent, 543
  prevention of, 882
  school-age child, 536, 537
Accommodation, grieving and, 461

Accountability, 101, 322-323
Accreditation
  documentation and, 180
  licensure and, 217-218
Acculturation, 353
Accuracy of documentation, 183
Acetaminophen, 1179
Acetylsalicylic acid, 1179
Achilles reflex, 736
Achilles tendon, 896
Acid-base balance, 1247-1292
  assessment of, 1259-1264
  blood replacement and, 1283-1290
  body fluids and, 1248-1251
  correction of imbalances, 1290
  disturbances in, 1253-1257
  enteral replacement of fluids, 1266-1267, 1268
  evaluation of, 1290
  intravenous therapy, 1268-1290
    complications of, 1282-1283
    discontinuation of, 1283
    equipment, 1269
    initiating line, 1269-1270
    maintaining system, 1278-1282
    regulating infusion flow rate, 1270-1278
    solutions in, 1269
    vascular access devices, 1268, 1269
  nursing diagnosis in, 1264-1265
  planning in, 1265-1266, 1267
  pressure ulcer and, 957
  regulation of, 1251-1252
  restriction of fluid, 1267
  variables affecting, 1257-1259
Acid-fast bacillus, 1214
Acidifying urine, 1317
Acne, 1020
Acquired immunodeficiency syndrome
  adolescents and, 542
  legal issues, 343-344
  nursing research in, 753
  risks of surgery, 1383
  sexual transmission of, 426
Acromegaly, 665
Acting on values, 314
Active participation, 267, 274
Active sleep, 1133
Active strategies of health promotion, 11-12
Active transport, 1249, 1250
Activities of daily living
  assisting with, 160
  incorporating active exercises into, 943
  pain and, 1169-1170
Activity
  bowel elimination and, 1345
  Healthy People 2000 on, 51

Activity—cont'd
  hospitalized young child and, 524-525
  newborn and, 509
  school-age child and adolescent, 531
Activity theory of aging, 572-573
Activity tolerance, 910-911
Actual health problem, 128
Acuity charting, 193, 194-195
Acupressure, 1173-1174
Acupuncture, 362
Acute care, 61-78
  admission procedures, 65-68
  client in, 63, 64
  continuum of care, 64-65
  delivery of nursing care, 73-77
  discharge planning, 68-70
  in infection, 755
  nursing roles and responsibilities, 71-73
  physician in, 63-64
  in pulmonary disease, 1219-1243
    cardiopulmonary resuscitation, 1240-1242, 1243
    dyspnea management, 1219
    maintenance of lung expansion, 1226-1232, 1233
    maintenance of patent airway, 1219-1226
    mobilization of pulmonary secretions, 1226
    oxygen therapy in, 1232-1239
  regulatory requirements, 65
  services in, 64
  sexual health and, 436
  staff in, 62-63
  urinary elimination, 1317-1334
    catheterization, 1318-1328
    infection control, 1328-1334
    maintaining elimination habits, 1317
    medications and, 1317-1318
Acute hemolytic reaction, 1286
Acute illness
  illness behavior and, 15
  spiritual distress and, 443
Acute pain, 1160-1161, 1178
Adaptation, 370-387
  assessment in, 376-380
  concepts of stress, 371-373
  evaluation of, 385
  health promotion and, 380-385
  in hearing loss, 1007-1008
  learning and, 265
  nursing diagnosis in, 380, 381
  planning in, 380, 381
  response to stress, 374-376, 377
  to stressors, 373-374
Adaptation model, 372
Adaptational model of poverty, 7
Adduction, 725, 906